Principles of Perinatal–Neonatal Metabolism

Second Edition

Springer Science+Business Media, LLC

Richard M. Cowett, MD
Brown University School of Medicine, Department of Pediatrics,
Women and Infants Hospital of Rhode Island, Providence, RI

Editor

Principles of Perinatal–Neonatal Metabolism

Second Edition

With 383 Figures

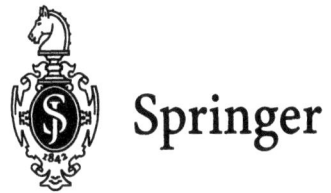
Springer

Richard M. Cowett, MD
Department of Pediatrics
Brown University School of Medicine
Women and Infants Hospital of Rhode Island
101 Dudley Street
Providence, RI 02905-2401, USA

Library of Congress Cataloging-in-Publication Data
Principles of perinatal–neonatal metabolism/[edited by] Richard M.
 Cowett.—2nd ed.
   p. cm.
  Includes bibliographical references and index.
  ISBN 978-1-4612-7227-4   ISBN 978-1-4612-1642-1 (eBook)
  DOI 10.1007/978-1-4612-1642-1
  1. Infants (Newborn)—Metabolism. 2. Fetus—Metabolism.
 3. Maternal-fetal exchange. I. Cowett, Richard M.
  [DNLM: 1. Fetus—metabolism. 2. Infant. Newborn—metabolism.
 3. Maternal-Fetal Exchange—physiology. 4. Pregnancy—metabolism.
 WQ 210.5 P957 1998]
 RJ252.P75 1998
 618.3'2—dc21   97-24816

Printed on acid-free paper.

© 1998 Springer Science+Business Media New York
Originally published by Springer-Verlag New York, Inc. in 1998
All rights reserved. This work may not be translated or copied in whole or in part without the written permission of the publisher Springer Science+Business Media, LLC.
except for brief excerpts in connection with reviews or scholarly analysis. Use in connection with any form of information storage and retrieval, electronic adaptation, computer software, or by similar or dissimilar methodology now known or hereafter developed is forbidden.
The use of general descriptive names, trade names, trademarks, etc., in this publication, even if the former are not especially identified, is not to be taken as a sign that such names, as understood by the Trade Marks and Merchandise Marks Act, may accordingly be used freely by anyone.
While the advice and information in this book are believed to be true and accurate at the date of going to press, neither the authors nor the editors nor the publisher can accept any legal responsibility for any errors or omissions that may be made. The publisher makes no warranty, express or implied, with respect to the material contained herein.

Production coordinated by Chernow Editorial Services, Inc., and managed by Natalie Johnson; manufacturing supervised by Joe Quatela.
Typeset by Best-set Typesetter Ltd., Hong Kong.

9 8 7 6 5 4 3 2 1

ISBN 978-1-4612-7227-4

In Memory of the Past:

*To my Father,
Allen Abraham Cowett;*

and

in Anticipation of the Future:

*To my Children,
Beth Ellen
Allison Ann
Allen Manz
Michael Elliott Drake
Hannah Michelle Kazin*

Preface to the Second Edition

In the Preface to the first edition we suggested that sufficient time had passed in the field of perinatal–neonatal medicine generally to require a cogent analysis of the metabolic principles of the period. At the time of publication of the first edition there was and, continuing today, there is no other comprehensive metabolic research reference text that evaluates this period as a continuum. The first edition focused on the metabolism of the period from physiological and biochemical perspectives with emphasis, of necessity, on the former. In the intervening period, enormous strides have been made in our understanding of the metabolism of the perinatal–neonatal period by investigators in the field. Especially significant are the advances made from cellular and molecular perspectives, which have assisted mechanistically in furthering our understanding of earlier physiological observations. These advances continue to be catalogued and analyzed comprehensively in this edition.

There is no more obvious indication of the trends occurring in science in general and in perinatal–medicine in particular than the websites on the Internet, which allow investigators to collaborate over long distances and update their databases on-line. Certainly one of the most useful and probably most widely used websites is that of the National Library of Medicine: {http://www.nlm.nih.gov}. In particular, this has allowed us to update, complete, and confirm many of the reference citations in this text.

We have carefully followed the suggestions of those individuals who wrote critiques of the first edition in the medical literature. In the medical literature. Meticulous care has been taken in the editing of this textbook to make the writing style and conventions as uniform as possible from chapter to chapter and section to section in spite of its multiauthored nature.

There is a thorough updating of the topics that were discussed in the first edition because of advances in each particular area.

Section I to focuses on the general principles of metabolism and evaluation of metabolic principles of the normal nonpregnant adult as the "gold standard." There are new chapters on: breath testing; analysis of proteins, peptides and small molecules; and glucose transporters from molecular, biochemical and physiological perspectives.

Section II continues to focus on the maternal metabolism in pregnancy. There is a completely revised discussion of glucose metabolism in pregnancy and a new chapter on mineral metabolism in pregnancy.

Section III retains its focus on metabolism in the fetus and placenta. There are new chapters or: growth factors; developmental endocrinology; the sympathoadrenal system; and a thorough revision of the discussion of respiration in the fetus and placenta.

Section IV is an entirely new section that focuses on organ specific metabolism during the perinatal period. The brain, the heart, the lung, the liver, the gastrointestinal tract, and muscle are each evaluated in organ specific discussions of the perinatal period. The kidney is not treated as a separate discussion because of the thorough evaluations of water and electrolyte metabolism in the fetus and placenta and neonatal water and electrolyte metabolism that appear elsewhere in the text.

The last section, Section V, continues its focus on neonatal metabolism. There is an entirely new discussion of inborn errors of carbohydrate metabolism; inborn errors of amino acid and organic acid metabolism; and body composition; and new chapters concerning inborn errors of lipid metabolism (mitochondrial fatty acid oxidation), bilirubin metabolism, nutritional support of the neonate by human milk feeding; and finally an approach to evaluation of the neonate with a potential metabolic defect.

In effect, this reference text has increased from 37 chapters in the first edition to 53 chapters. As a result, the number of text pages has increased by 66% and their size has increased by 33%. A concerted attempt has been made to cross-reference the text between chapters, as well as to provide a detailed index. Clinical correlations are explored wherever germane. One of the major strengths continues to be the exhaustive up-to-date reference list that accompanies each chapter. We trust that this text will continue to provide a comprehensive evaluation of each topic for those individuals interested in metabolism in this continuum known as the perinatal–neonatal period.

As time has marched on, a number of changes have occurred in the lives of individuals mentioned in the Preface to the first edition. Dr. Irwin B. Hanenson passed away after a long illness. I will always remember him with a great deal of fondness. Dr. Robert Schwariz has become an emeritus Professor of Medical Science at Brown. He graciously agreed to update a previously published discussion of his on the subject of inborn errors of carbohydrate metabolism for this edition. I am quite appreciative of his encyclopedic knowledge of carbohydrate metabolism in the perinatal–neonatal period. He has been a major contributor to this area for a number of the decades. Dr. William Oh remains the Chairperson of the Department of Pediatrics at Brown University School of Medicine and Pediatrician-in-Chief of the Hasbro Children's' Hospital. After almost a quarter of a century of providing energy and vision, he reliquinshed the Chair of the Department of Pediatrics at Women & Infants of Rhods Island (i.e., the Division of Neonatology of the Department of Pediatrics of the Brown University School of Medicine). He recruited Dr. James F. Padbury who has assumed the position. Jim is providing welcomed renewed exuberance as the neonatal group continues to move at the cutting edge of this discipline as well as contributing a new chapter on the sympathoadrenal system of the fetus and placenta to this text.

Of course, my father, Allen, remains the ultimate guiding force for me. I think about him daily with affection and respect, as we appreciate the present and anticipate the future.

Many individuals have assisted in completing the many tasks that are critical to the success of a major text such as this book. At Springer-Verlag publishers Laura Gillan has been a motivating and enthusiastic proponent of the effort. I am deeply indebted to her and her associates, including Jeff Sands, as well as to Barbara Chernow, David Kapian, and Kathy Jackson. Likewise, I am quite appreciative of the assistance of Janet Crager and Frank Kellerman of the Sciences Library of Brown University. They have been major contributors to the success we have had in finalizing the references lists that accompany each chapter. The above individuals, probably more than even the individual contributors, will be happy that this second edition is nearing completion.

Finally, I am deeply indebted to all of the individual contributors, all 67 of them, who have been as conscientious as I had originally hoped they would be in evaluating that specific area of perinatal–neonatal metabolism for which they are an "academic household name." I hope the reader continues to be as pleased as I am with the depth of this compendium and finds it as useful.

Providence, Rhode Island   Richard M. Cowett, MD
December, 1997

Preface to the First Edition

Over the fast quarter century or so, specialization within obstetrics and gynecology, and pediatrics has resulted in the development of the disciplines of maternal-fetal medicine and neonatology respectively. A primary focus of maternal-fetal medicine has been to understand the mechanism(s) of premature delivery and develop treatment modalities for improving the length of gestation. A primary focus of neonatology has been to understand the causes of respiratory distress in the neonate. Success has resulted, not only in the lengthening of gestation, but an improved understanding of the causes and treatment of neonatal respiratory disease. With increasing success has come the necessity to understand the metabolic principles of the parturient, the fetal/placenta unit, and the neonate. These principles are clearly very important from multiple aspects. Increased understanding of metabolism of the pregnant woman would explain the aberrations occurring in normal and abnormal pregnancy and improve nutritional support for the parturient. A prime example of altered metabolism is the parturient with diabetes. Understanding metabolism of the fetal/placenta unit is necessary to increase the probability that the fetus will be born appropriate for size irrespective of the gestational age. The various component of neonatal metabolism are important, not only for understanding the changes in physiology and biochemistry occurring in the developing neonate, but the principles by which nutritional support should be provided.

Enough time has lapsed so that cogent analyses are possible for each component of the metabolic principles of the perinatal-neonatal period. A general survey of the literature documents that separate discussions of metabolism exist. There are chapters on maternal metabolism as part of maternal-fetal medicine texts. There are textbooks on altered metabolism such as diabetes mellitus in pregnancy. Texts of principles of fetal physiology have been published, as have various analysis of neonatal metabolism and nutrition as single texts or chapters of general neonatology texts. To my knowledge there is no comprehensive metabolic reference text which has evaluated the perinatal-neonatal period as a continuum. It is obvious that the perinatal-neonatal period is a continuum in which each stage is inexorably intertwined with the other. It is this continuum that we have attempted to capture from a physiological and biochemical perspective metabolically.

In Section I the general principles of metabolism are analyzed. The first half evaluates methodology used to study metabolism. Kinetic techniques have been responsible for major advances that provide information above and beyond that of static measurements. No analysis of metabolism in the 1990s would be complete without a consideration of the evolving techniques of a cellular and molecular basis which are ever increasingly providing an explanation of metabolic parameters. It is also apparent that animal modeling is required to evaluate mechanisms which cannot be analyzed by human investigation.

Within Section I metabolic control of glucose, protein and lipid is evaluated in the normal non-pregnant adult as a "gold standard." Subsequently, biochemical and physiological aspects of insutin, the contrainsulin hormones, and somatomedins are considered in the non pregnant adult.

Section II evaluates maternal metabolism during pregnancy. Metabolism of glucose, protein, lipids, and prostaglandins are analyzed in detail from the perspective of changes occurring during pregnancy. Studies that evaluate energy metabolism in pregnancy are considered. The final chapter is a subject which is emerging as a major topic in the metabolism of pregnancy–the effects of exercise.

Section III considers metabolism in the fetal/placenta unit. Glucose, protein, and lipid are discussed comprehensively. Since metabolism is influenced to a great degree by respiration and circulation within the fetal/placenta unit, these topics are considered as well. Finally, water metabolism, of critical importance to the fetus is explored in detail.

Section IV analyzes the various components of neonatal metabolism. A great deal of research in metabolism of a perinatal-neonatal nature has evaluated the neonate and the various components are considered comprehensively. Glucose metabolism and the inborn errors of carbohydrate metabolism are analyzed as are neonatal protein metabolism and inborn errors of amino acids and organic acids. Extensive research has been performed on lipid and carnitine, on neonatal minerals, trace metals, vitamins, both fat soluble and water soluble, and these topics are explored. Neonatal energy metabolism is discussed in detail as is an offshoot of that subject, neonatal thermal regulation. Extensive research has been performed on water metabolism in the neonate and this is analyzed as are studies of body composition which have been published. Two specific aberrations of the norm are considered from a neonatal perspective; the first, the small for gestational age neonate and the second, the infant of the diabetic mother. Increasing success has occurred over the last quater century relative to neonates undergoing surgery and their metabolic needs are evaluated. Finally, nutritional support of the neonate, specifically alternate fucls and routes of administration, are evaluated.

The text is cross referenced between sections. With some topics there has been enough research to allow for separate discussions (e.g., glucose, protein, lipid and water) in separate sections. With other (e.g., minerals, trace elements, and vitamins) the authors have evaluated the topics in a single chapter. Clinical correlations are provided throughout the text.

We believe that this reference text will privide a comprehensive evaluation for those individuats interested in metabolism in this continuum known as the perinatal-neonatal period.

It is appropriate to acknowledge a few individuals who have been most influential in my carcer. Dr. Irwin B. Hanenson, Professor Emeritus of Medicine at the University of Cincinnati College of Medicine, whom I first met when I was a teenager, introduced me to research and allowed me to work as a technician in his laboratory at the May Institute for Medical Research of the Jewish Hospital in Cincinnati, Ohio. He remains a very close friend to this day. Professor Margaret Shea Gilbert. Professor of Biology Emeritus at Lawrence College (University) in Appleton, Wisconsin, who recently passed away, provided support and enthusiasm for my budding interest in research during an undergraduate honor's thesis. Dr. Robert Schwartz, Professor of Pediatries and Medical Sciences at Brown University, I first met when he was Chairman of the Department of Pediatrics at Cleveland Metropolitan General Hospital, and Professor of Pediatrics at Case Western Reserve University where I was an intern and junior assistant resident in Pediatrics. He probably more than anyone should be given the credit for my interest in carbohydrate metabolism in the perinatal-neonatal period. This interest was enhanced when we both separately came to the Department of Pediatrics at Brown University in the early 1970s. He remains a mentor, colleague and close friend. Dr. Leo Stern, who passed away in 1989 unexpectedly, recruited me to

Brown University as a fellow in neonatology, and, during his lifetime as Chairman of the Department of Pediatrics at Brown University, remained a special influence on me personally and professionally. I first met Dr. William Oh when Dr. Stern recruited him to be Chief of the Division of Neonatology and Professor of Pediatrics and Medical Sciences at Brown University. Dr. Oh, now Chairman of the Department of Pediatrics at Brown University, has been a unique guide for me not only from a personal but from a professional standpoint. He remains a mentor, colleague and close friend. The above individuals and especially my father, Allen, whom I remember with love and affection, should probably be given credit for my success, but none of the blame for my short comings. I remain deeply indebted to all of them.

Many individuals at Springer-Verlag Publishers have been important from the beginning of this book to its completion. I am deeply indebted to all of them and to my former secretary Mrs. Lori D. Krahenbill at Women and Infants' Hospital.

Finally, it goes without saying, that each of the senior authors that have contributed to this text are "academic household names" in the areas about which they have written. I very much appreciate the thoroughness that each of them has evidenced in completing their assignment. I hope the reader is as pleased with the text as I am.

Providence, Rhode Island Richard M. Cowett, MD
March, 1991

Contents

Preface to the Second Edition vii
Preface to the First Edition ix
Contributors xvii

Section I Methodology for the Study of Metabolism and General Principles

1 Methodology for the Study of Metabolism: Kinetic Techniques 3
  Dennis M. Bier

2 Methodology for the Study of Metabolism: Breath Testing 17
  Peter D. Klein and Hans Helge

3 Methodology for the Study of Metabolism: Analyses of
  Proteins, Peptides, and Small Molecules 27
  Jacob A. Canick

4 Methodology for the Study of Metabolism: Cellular
  and Molecular Techniques 41
  Lewis P. Rubin

5 Methodology for the Study of Metabolism: Physiologic
  Modeling in Animals 79
  John B. Susa

6 Control of Metabolism in the Normal Adult 91
  Robert R. Wolfe

7 Glucose Transporters: Molecular, Biochemical, and
  Physiologic Aspects 121
  Rebecca A. Simmons

8 Insulin: Molecular, Biochemical, and Physiologic Aspects 135
  Philip A. Gruppuso

9 Counterregulatory Hormones: Molecular, Biochemical, and
  Physiologic Aspects 155
  John E. Gerich and Philip E. Cryer

Section II Maternal Metabolism During Pregnancy

10 Glucose Metabolism in Pregnancy 183
    Patrick M. Catalano, Tatsua Ishizuka, and Jacob E. Friedman

11 Protein Metabolism in Pregnancy 207
    Satish C. Kalhan

12 Lipid Metabolism in Pregnancy 221
    Robert H. Knopp, Bartolome Bonet, and Xiaodong Zhu

13 Essential Fatty Acids and Prostaglandins in Pregnancy 259
    Paul L. Ogburn, Jr.

14 Mineral Metabolism in Pregnancy 281
    Karen M. Davidson and John T. Repke

15 Energy Metabolism During Pregnancy 309
    John V.G.A. Durnin

16 Exercise in Pregnancy: Effects on Cardiorespiratory
    Physiology and Metabolism 319
    Marshall W. Carpenter

Section III Fetal-Placental Metabolism

17 Glucose Metabolism in the Fetal-Placental Unit 337
    William W. Hay, Jr.

18 Protein Metabolism in the Fetal-Placental Unit 369
    Edward A. Liechty and David W. Boyle

19 Lipid Metabolism in the Fetal-Placental Unit 389
    Robert E. Kimura

20 Growth Factors in the Fetal-Placental Unit 403
    Philip A. Gruppuso

21 Developmental Endocrinology in the Fetal-Placental Unit 425
    Ram K. Menon and Mark A. Sperling

22 The Sympathoadrenal System in the Fetal-Placental Unit 437
    Yi-Tang Tseng and James F. Padbury

23 Respiration in the Fetal-Placental Unit 451
    Robert W. Rothstein and Lawrence D. Longo

24 Circulation in the Fetal-Placental Unit 487
    Abraham M. Rudolph

25 Water and Electrolyte Metabolism in the Fetal-Placental Unit 511
    E. Marelyn Wintour

Section IV Organ-Specific Metabolism During the Perinatal Period

26 Brain Metabolism in the Fetus and Neonate 537
    Susan J. Vannucci and Robert C. Vannucci

27 Cardiac Metabolism in the Fetus and Neonate 551
    G. Wesley Vick, III and David J. Fisher

28 Lung Metabolism in the Fetus and Neonate 567
    Luc J.I. Zimmermann and Lambert M.G. van Golde

29 Liver Metabolism in the Fetus and Neonate 601
    Jean-Paul Pégorier and Jean Girard

30 Gastrointestinal Tract Metabolism in the Fetus and Neonate 627
    Robert E. Kimura

31 Muscle Metabolism in the Fetus and Neonate 641
    Ulrich A. Walker and Armand F. Miranda

Section V Neonatal Metabolism

32 Neonatal Glucose Metabolism 683
    Richard M. Cowett and Hussien M. Farrag

33 Inborn Errors of Carbohydrate Metabolism 723
    Robert Schwartz

34 Neonatal Protein Metabolism 773
    Willi E. Heine

35 Inborn Errors of Amino Acid and Organic Acid Metabolism 799
    Gerard T. Berry

36 Neonatal Lipid Metabolism 821
    Margit Hamosh

37 Inborn Errors of Lipid Metabolism (Mitochondrial
    Fatty Acid Oxidation) 847
    Charles A. Stanley

38 Neonatal Carnitine Metabolism 857
    Charles A. Stanley

39 Neonatal Bilirubin Metabolism 865
    William J. Cashore

40 Neonatal Calcium and Phosphorus Metabolism 879
    Jeffrey L. Loughead and Reginald C. Tsang

41 Neonatal Trace Element Metabolism 909
    Peter J. Aggett

42 Neonatal Vitamin Metabolism: Fat Soluble 943
    Frank R. Greer and Richard D. Zachman

43 Neonatal Vitamin Metabolism: Water Soluble 977
    Richard J. Schanler

44 Neonatal Energy Metabolism 1001
    Pieter J.J. Sauer

45 Neonatal Thermoregulation 1027
    Pieter J.J. Sauer

46 Neonatal Water and Electrolyte Metabolism 1045
    Andrew T. Costarino and Stephen Baumgart

47 Body Composition of the Neonate 1077
    Kenneth J. Ellis

48 The Small-for-Gestational-Age Neonate 1097
    Edward S. Ogata

49 The Infant of the Diabetic Mother 1105
    Richard M. Cowett

50 Metabolism of the Neonate Requiring Surgery 1131
    Arnold G. Coran, Agostino Pierro, and David J. Schmeling

51 Nutritional Support of the Neonate I: Alternate
    Fuels and Routes of Administration 1153
    Jane P. Balint and Robert M. Kliegman

52 Nutritional Support of the Neonate II: The Rationale for
    Human Milk Feeding 1181
    Richard J. Schanler

53 Evaluation of the Neonate with a Potential Metabolic Defect 1201
    Pinar T. Ozand

Index 1243

Contributors

Peter J. Aggett, MSc FRCP
Head, Lancashire Postgraduate School of Medicine and Health, University of Central Lancashire, Preston PR12HE UK

Jane P. Balint, MD
Assistant Professor, Division of Pediatric Gastroenterology and Nutrition, Department of Pediatrics, Medical College of Wisconsin, Milwaukee, WI 53226, USA

Stephen Baumgart, MD
Professor and Vice Chair, Department of Pediatrics, Thomas Jefferson University, Jefferson Medical College, Philadelphia, PA 19107, USA

Gerard T. Berry, MD
Professor, Department of Pediatrics, University of Pennsylvania School of Medicine, Senior Physician, Division of Biochemical Development and Molecular Diseases, Children's Hospital of Philadelphia, Philadelphia, PA 19104, USA

Dennis M. Bier, MD
Professor, Department of Pediatrics, Baylor College of Medicine, Director, Children's Nutritional Research Center, Houston, TX 77030, USA

Bartolome Bonet, MD, PhD
Assistant Professor, Universidad San Paolo, Centre de CC Experimentales y Tecnicas, Urbanización Montprincipe, Head, Division of Pediatrics, Fundacion Hospital de Alcorcon 28668 Madrid, Spain

David W. Boyle, MD
Associate Professor, Division of Neonatal-Perinatal Medicine, Department of Pediatrics, Indiana University School of Medicine, Indianapolis, IN 46223, USA

Jacob A. Canick, PhD
Professor, Department of Pathology and Laboratory Medicine, Brown University School of Medicine, Director, Prenatal AFP and Endocrinology Laboratories, Women and Infants Hospital of Rhode Island, Providence, RI 02905, USA

Marshall W. Carpenter, MD
Associate Professor, Department of Obstetrics and Gynecology, Brown University School of Medicine, Director, Division of Maternal-Fetal Medicine, Women and Infants Hospital of Rhode Island, Providence, RI 02905, USA

William J. Cashore, MD
Professor, Department of Pediatrics, Brown University School of Medicine, Associate Chief, Department of Pediatrics, Women and Infants Hospital of Rhode Island, Providence, Rhode Island 02905, USA

Patrick M. Catalano, MD
Professor, Department of Reproductive Biology, Case Western University School of Medicine, Director, High Risk Pregancy and Diabetes Clinic, MetroHealth Medical Center, Cleveland, OH 44109, USA

Arnold G. Coran, MD
Professor, Department of Surgery, Head, Section of Pediatric Surgery, University of Michigan Medical School, Surgeon-in-Chief, C.S. Mott Children's Hospital, Ann Arbor, MI 48109, USA

Andrew T. Costarino, MD
Associate Professor, Departments of Anesthesia and Pediatrics, University of Pennsylvania School of Medicine, Director, Pediatric Critical Care Medicine Fellowship Program, Children's Hospital of Philadelphia, Philadelphia, PA 19104, USA

Richard M. Cowett, MD
Professor, Department of Pediatrics, Brown University School of Medicine, Neonatologist, Department of Pediatrics, Women and Infants Hospital of Rhode Island, Providence, RI 02905, USA

Philip E. Cryer, MD
Irene E. and Michael M. Karl Professor of Endocrinology and Metabolism, Department of Medicine, Director, Division of Endocrinology, Diabetes and Metabolism, Director, General Clinical Research Center, Washington University School of Medicine, Physician, Barnes-Jewish Hospital, St. Louis, MO, 63110, USA

Karen M. Davidson, MD
Clinical Instructor, Department of Obstetrics, Gynecology and Reproductive Biology, Harvard Medical School, Associate Obstetrician and Gynecologist, Brigham and Women's Hospital, Boston, MA 02115, USA

J.V.G.A. Durnin, MA, MB, ChB, DSc, FRCP, FIBiol, FRSE
Professor, Department of Human Nutrition, University of Glasgow, Yorkhill Hospitals, Glasgow G3 8SJ UK

Kenneth J. Ellis, MD
Professor, Department of Pediatrics, Baylor College of Medicine, Director, Body Composition Laboratory, Children's Nutritional Research Center, Houston, TX 77030, USA

Hussien M. Farrag, MD
Assistant Professor, Department of Pediatrics, Tufts University School of Medicine, Staff Neonatologist, Department of Pediatrics, Bayside Medical Center, Springfield, MA 01109, USA

David J. Fisher, MD
Professor and Vice Chair, Department of Pediatrics, The Ohio State University College of Medicine, Executive Director, Children's Hospital Education Institute, Children's Hospital, Columbus, OH 43205, USA

Jacob E. Friedman, PhD
Assistant Professor, Departments of Nutrition and Biochemistry, Case Western University School of Medicine, Cleveland OH 44106, USA

John E. Gerich, MD
Professor, Departments of Medicine and Physiology, Director, General Clinical Research Center and the Diabetes Research Laboratory, University of Rochester School of Medicine and Dentistry, Strong Memorial Hospital, Rochester, NY 14642, USA

Jean Girard, PhD DSc
Research Director, Centre National de la Recherche Scientifique, Director, Laboratoire de la Endocrinologie, Metabolisme et Developpement, 92190 Meudon, France

Frank R. Greer, MD
Professor, Departments of Pediatrics and Nutritional Sciences, University of Wisconsin, Wisconsin Perinatal Center, Meriter Hospital, Madison, WI 53715, USA

Philip A. Gruppuso, MD
Professor, Department of Pediatrics and Professor (Research), Department of Biochemistry, Brown University School of Medicine, Director, Division of Pediatric Endocrinology and Metabolism, Rhode Island Hospital and Hasbro Children's Hospital, Providence, RI 02903, USA

Margit Hamosh, PhD
Professor, Department of Pediatrics, Chief, Division of Developmental Biology and Nutrition, Georgetown University Medical Center, Washington, DC 20007, USA

William W. Hay, Jr., MD
Professor, Department of Pediatrics, Director, Training Program in Neonatal-Perinatal Medicine, Director, Neonatal Clinical Research Center, University of Colorado School of Medicine, Denver, CO 80262, USA

Willi E. Heine, MD, (Professor Dr. Med)
Professor, Department of Pediatrics, University of Rostock Children's Hospital, 18057 Rostock, Federal Republic of Germany

Hans Helge, MD
Professor and Chairman Emeritus, Department of Pediatrics, Free University of Berlin, D/14059 Berlin, Federal Republic of Germany

Tatsuya Ishizuka, MD, PhD
Postdoctoral Fellow, Departments of Nutrition and Biochemistry, Case Western University School of Medicine, Cleveland, OH 44106, USA

Satish C. Kalhan, MBBS, FRCP, DCH
Professor, Department of Pediatrics, Case Western University School of Medicine, Division of Neonatology, Rainbow Babies and Children's Hospital, Cleveland, OH 44106, USA

Robert E. Kimura, MD
Professor and Vice Chair, Department of Pediatrics, Director, Division of Neonatology, Rush-St. Luke's Presbyterian Medical Center, Chicago, IL 60612, USA

Peter D. Klein, PhD
Professor Emeritus, Departments of Pediatrics and Medicine, Baylor College of Medicine, Vice President, Research and Development, Meretek Diagnostics Inc., Houston, TX 77030, USA

Robert M. Kliegman, MD
Professor and Chair, Department of Pediatrics, Medical College of Wisconsin, Milwaukee, Wisconsin 53226, USA

Robert H. Knopp, MD
Professor, Department of Medicine, University of Washington School of Medicine, Chief, Division of Metabolism, Endocrinology and Nutrition, Director, Northwest Lipid Research Center, Harborview Medical Center, Seattle, WA 98104, USA

Edward A. Liechty, MD
Professor, Division of Neonatal-Perinatal Medicine, Department of Pediatrics, Indiana University School of Medicine, Indianapolis, IN 46223, USA

Lawrence D. Longo, MD
Professor, Departments of Physiology and Obstetrics and Gynecology, Director, Center for Perinatal Biology, School of Medicine, Loma Linda University, Loma Linda, CA 92350, USA

Jeffrey L. Loughead, MD
Assistant Clinical Professor, Department of Pediatrics, Wright State University School of Medicine, Newborn Medicine, The Children's Medical Center, Dayton, OH 45404 USA

Ram K. Menon, MD
Associate Professor, Department of Pediatrics, University of Pittsburgh School of Medicine, Division of Pediatric Endocrinology, Children's Hospital of Pittsburgh, Pittsburgh, PA 15213, USA

Armand F. Miranda, MD
Professor of Clinical Pathology Emeritus, Department of Pathology, Consultant in Neurology, Department of Neurology, MDA H. Houston Merritt Clinical Research Center for Muscular Dystrophy and Related Diseases, College of Physicians and Surgeons of Columbia University, New York, NY 10032, USA

Edward S. Ogata, MD
Raymond and Hazel Speck Berry Professor, Departments of Pediatrics, Obstetrics and Gynecology, Northwestern University School of Medicine, Associate Chief of Staff, Children's Memorial Hospital, Chicago, IL 60614, USA

Paul L. Ogburn, Jr., MD
Associate Professor and Chair, Department of Obstetrics, Mayo Clinic School of Medicine, Rochester, MN 55905, USA

Pinar T. Ozand, MD, PhD
Head, Section of Inborn Errors of Metabolism, Department of Pediatrics, King Faisal Specialist Hospital and Research Centre, Riyadh 11211, Saudi Arabia

James F. Padbury, MD
Professor and Vice Chair, Department of Pediatrics, Brown University School of Medicine, Pediatrician-in-Chief, Department of Pediatrics, Women and Infants Hospital of Rhode Island, Providence, RI 02905, USA

Jean-Paul Pegorier, PhD, DSc
Research Director, Centre National de la Recherche Scientifique, 92190 Meudon, France

Agostino Pierro, MD
Reader, Department of Pediatric Surgery, University College London Medical School, Institute of Child Health and Great Ormond Street Hospital for Children, NHS Trust, London WC1N 1EH, UK

John T. Repke, MD
Chris J. and Marie A. Olson Professor of Obstetrics and Gynecology, University of Nebraska College of Medicine, Obstetrician-in-Chief, Department of Obstetrics and Gynecology, University of Nebraska Medical Center, Omaha, NE 68198, USA

Richard W. Rothstein, MD
Assistant Professor, Department of Pediatrics, Tufts University School of Medicine, Staff Neonatologist, Department of Pediatrics, Bayside Medical Center, Springfield, MA 01109, USA

Lewis P. Rubin, MD
Associate Professor, Department of Pediatrics, Brown University School of Medicine, Neonatologist, Department of Pediatrics, Women and Infants Hospital of Rhode Island, Providence, RI 02905, USA

Abraham M. Rudolph, MD
Professor Emeritus, Department of Pediatrics, University of California School of Medicine, San Francisco, CA 94143, USA

Pieter J.J. Sauer, MD
Professor and Chair, Department of Pediatrics, University of Groningen, Pediatrician-in-Chief, Beatrix Children's Hospital, Groningen University Hospital, 9700 RB Groningen, The Netherlands

Richard J. Schanler, MD
Professor, Department of Pediatrics, Baylor College of Medicine, Children's Nutritional Research Center, Houston, TX 77030, USA

David J. Schmeling, MD
Partner, Pediatric Surgical Associates, Ltd, Attending Physician, Department of Surgery, Minneapolis Children's Hospital, Minneapolis, MN 55404, and Attending Physician, Department of Surgery, St. Paul Children's Hospital, St Paul MN 55102

Robert Schwartz, MD
Professor, Department of Pediatrics, Emeritus Professor of Medical Science, Brown University School of Medicine, Staff Endocrinologist, Division of Pediatric Endocrinology and Metabolism, Rhode Island Hospital and Hasbro Children's Hospital, Providence, RI 02903, USA

Rebecca A. Simmons, MD
Assistant Professor, Department of Pediatrics, University of Pennsylvania School of Medicine, Attending Physician, Division of Neonatology, Children's Hospital of Philadelphia, Philadelphia PA 19104, USA

Mark A. Sperling. MD
Professor and Chair, Department of Pediatrics, University of Pittsburgh School of Medicine, Pediatrician-in-Chief, Children's Hospital of Pittsburgh, Pittsburgh, PA 15213, USA

Charles A. Stanley, MD
Professor, Department of Pediatrics, University of Pennsylvania School of Medicine, Division of Endocrinology/Diabetes, Director, General Clinical Research Center Core Laboratory, Children's Hospital of Philadelphia, Philadelphia, PA 19104, USA

John B. Susa, PhD
Associate Professor(Research), Department of Pediatrics, Brown University School of Medicine, Division of Pediatric Endocrinology and Metabolism, Rhode Island Hospital and Hasbro Children's Hospital, Providence, RI 02903, USA

Reginald C. Tsang, MBBS
Professor, Department of Pediatrics, University of Cincinnati College of Medicine, Children's Hospital Medical Center, Cincinnati, OH 45267, USA

Yi-Tang Tseng, PhD
Assistant Professor(Research), Department of Pediatrics, Brown University School of Medicine, Women and Infants Hospital of Rhode Island, Providence, RI 02905, USA

Lambert M.G. van Golde, PhD
Professor and Chairman, Division of Biochemistry, Department of Basic Sciences, Faculty of Veterinary Medicine, University of Utrecht, 3508TD Utrecht, The Netherlands

Robert C. Vannucci, MD
Professor, Department of Pediatrics, Pennsylvania State University College of Medicine, Division of Pediatric Neurology, Penn State Geisinger Health System, Hershey, PA 17033, USA

Susan J. Vannucci, Ph D
Associate Professor, Departments of Pediatrics and Neuroscience and Anatomy, Pennsylvania State University, Hershey, PA 17033, USA

G. Wesley Vick, III, MD, PhD
Assistant Professor, Department of Pediatrics, Baylor College of Medicine, Associate, Lillie Frank Abercrombie Section of Pediatric Cardiology, Texas Children's Hospital, Houston, TX 77030, USA

Ulrich A. Walker, MD
Postdoctoral Fellow, Department of Neurology, MDA H. Houston Merritt Clinical Research Center for Muscular Dystrophy and Related Diseases, College of Physicians and Surgeons of Columbia University, New York, NY 10032, USA

E. Marelyn Wintour, PhD, DSc
Senior Principal Research Fellow, Howard Florey Institute of Experimental Pathology and Medicine, University of Melbourne, Parkville, Victoria 3052, Australia

Robert R. Wolfe, PhD
Professor (Metabolism), Department of Surgery, University of Texas Medical Branch, Chief, Metabolism Unit, Shriners Burns Institute, Galveston, TX 77550, USA

Richard D. Zachman, PhD, MD
Professor, Departments of Pediatrics and Nutritional Sciences, University of Wisconsin, Wisconsin Perinatal Center, Meriter Hospital, Madison, WI 53715, USA

Xiaodong Zhu, MD
Senior Research Fellow, Division of Metabolism, Endocrinology and Nutrition, Department of Medicine, University of Washington School of Medicine, Seattle, WA 98104, USA

Luc J.I. Zimmermann, MD, PhD
Department of Pediatrics, Erasmus University, Division of Neonatology, Sophia Children's Hospital, 3015GJ Rotterdam, The Netherlands

Section I
Methodology for the Study of Metabolism and General Principles

1
Methodology for the Study of Metabolism: Kinetic Techniques

Dennis M. Bier

Metabolic research in the pregnant woman and human neonate is generally limited by several basic ethical constraints. First, the studies must be noninvasive or minimally so, except in unusual circumstances. Second, if blood or tissue samples are needed, they should be invariably small, particularly those samples obtained from the fetus or very low birth weight neonate whose problems continue to be the focus of intense study. Third, given the limited direct access to most organ systems, the approaches used must allow extrapolation from the sampled data to events occurring in otherwise inaccessible areas. Fourth, the maximal information possible must be obtained from any given individual analysis owing to the difficulty of identifying and recruiting appropriate mothers and neonates for study and the need to study the smallest number of subjects necessary to evaluate adequately the proposed hypotheses.

Additionally, the information obtained should be of a dynamic rather than static nature. Metabolic pathways are, after all, concerned with the movement of materials along them; and, in general, there is constant activity. Classic concepts of the virtual cessation of certain enzymatic reactions while others proceed unabated have been replaced by the realization that competing metabolic events are generally occurring simultaneously, albeit at different rates. This results in the regulation of substrate flow, the amplification of substrate delivery or signaling, and occasionally the regulation of heat production by hydrolysis of adenosine triphosphate (ATP).[1,2] Perhaps the most striking, intensively studied example of this concept is the *glucose paradox*, where the postprandial regulation of glycogen deposition is determined by relative, simultaneously occurring activities of the glycogenolytic and gluconeogenic pathways in addition to the enzymes of glycogen synthesis.[3] It should be readily apparent that static measurements of metabolite concentrations provide only limited insight into the dynamics of such systems.

An extension of this concept applies to studies of interorgan substrate transport. The blood glucose concentration may decrease because peripheral glucose uptake increases or hepatic glucose production declines. Hypoglycemia resulting from insulin administration is due to a combination of the two, with the latter predominating initially. Measurements of substrate or effector concentrations have provided invaluable information and have formed the basis for the prevailing pathophysiologic hypotheses. If it were not for the development of microfluorometric techniques,[4] high performance liquid and gas chromatographic analyses,[5,6] radioimmunoassay procedures, assorted laboratory micromethods,[7] and the ready availability of various automated microanalytical instruments in clinical chemistry laboratories, research studies of pregnancy and the very low birth weight neonate would be limited. Static measurements alone do not permit satisfactory assessment of dynamic mechanisms. This constraint holds equally well for the classic balance approach to nitrogen or mineral homeostasis, where net effects can be measured but insight into the adaptive mechanisms responsible for attaining balance (or not) cannot be deduced unambiguously.

Many of the above constraints on perinatal metabolic investigation have been reduced or eliminated by methodologic advances to be discussed. Depending on the question or application, some of these approaches are still in various stages of development, whereas others are routine and have been proven in human perinatal research. This discussion reviews selected current methods, including mass spectrometry, nuclear magnetic resonance spectroscopy, positron emission tomography, stable isotope tracers, and compartmental modeling. The continued development and enhanced application of these methods allow us to answer pressing questions about perinatal metabolic events and their regulation in health and disease.

Mass Spectrometry

Mass spectrometry is the most sensitive and specific general analytical tool available to the investigator of the perinatal period. The basic principles of mass spectrometry are simple.[5,8-11] The substance of interest is introduced into the source of the instrument. Commonly, the material enters the source through a gas inlet valve, as the effluent of a chromatography column, or by direct introduction using one of several methods. In the source the neutral sample molecules are ionized by one of several methods: electron impact bombardment; protonation in the gas phase (chemical ionization); or bombardment with fast atoms; ions (secondary ion mass spectrometry); radioactive fission fragments (plasma desorption mass spectrometry); laser photons (laser desorption mass spectrometry); or various other means. Depending on the method of ionization, the ionized molecules remain intact or are broken into several constituent fragment ions. The ions are ejected from the source into the analyzer region of the instrument, where they are separated on the basis of their mass-to-charge ratios. Because the ions are usually singly charged, the separation is effectively one of mass and is usually achieved using a magnetic field or electrical means. The ions are recorded at the detector. Depending on the ionization mode and instrument characteristics, one can assess the molecular weight, structural information from the fragment ions, isotopic content, or even exact atomic composition in some cases using instruments of mass resolving power.[11] The existence of naturally occurring isotopes was discovered using mass spectrometry in 1919. As discussed in some detail subsequently, this technique remains unparalleled for precise quantitative analysis of various stable isotopes when they are used as biologic tracers.

Because the signal in mass spectrometry is a function of mass and all substances have mass, the method is a universal one and is potentially applicable to every biochemical compound of interest. In practice, there are limits, which generally have been related to the ability of the substance to enter the vapor phase—the prerequisite for molecular analysis by all mass spectrometers. Biochemical compounds amenable to mass spectrometric analysis were limited to low-molecular-weight compounds, which were volatilized easily in their native state or to materials that could be converted to more volatile derivatives and analyzed subsequently by combined gas chromatography/mass spectrometry. The mass range was limited to compounds with molecular weights of approximately 1000 daltons (d) or less.

This limitation has been largely removed with the development of methods that permit vaporization and ionization of large molecules of biological significance.[12-22] In particular, fast atom or ion bombardment approaches, including plasma desorption and laser ionization methods, have allowed mass spectra analysis of materials at molecular weights previously considered inconceivable.[12-22] Analysis of molecules within the 1000 to 5000 d range is now relatively routine. In specialized laboratories, mass spectral information has been obtained on peptides, proteins, and other biopolymers up to 250,000 d in mass.[19,21,22] Because only a small number of molecules in the sample actually enters the vapor phase for analysis, the above methods require only small amounts of material; the methods are nondestructive with virtually complete recovery of the original sample.

At the low mass range the advent of thermal ionization methods and of inductively coupled plasma mass spectrometry now allows vaporization and analysis of inorganic trace minerals of nutritional interest.[23-26] The commercial availability of mass spectrometers coupled to high performance liquid chromatography systems has further broadened the applications of mass spectrometry to biomedical questions. To improve access to these methods, the National Center for Research Resources at the National Institutes of Health has established several mass spectrometry resource centers throughout the United States.

Few methods can approach mass spectrometry in regard to sensitivity and specificity. Although there are other methods that have high sensitivity, only rarely can they achieve such sensitivity with the virtually certain specificity of mass spectrometry. This specificity is provided by the propagated effects of the selectivity of the derivative used for volatilization, the gas or liquid chromatography stationary phase chosen for separation, the mode of ionization, the choice of molecular or fragment ions used for analysis, and the power of the mass spectrometer to resolve ions of the same nominal mass but different exact masses.[8,11] Furthermore, because molecules fragment in the instrument source according to the nature of their chemical bonds, a mass spectrum can be used to derive the structure of an unknown parent compound. Classically, such interpretation of completely unknown molecules was limited to materials of relatively low molecular weight.[11] However, by applying the newer ionization methods, complete structural and sequence analysis of large biopolymers has been accomplished.[14,17,27-29]

Nuclear Magnetic Resonance

For structural analysis, nuclear magnetic resonance (NMR) is the perfect complement to mass spectrometry.[30-34] Like mass spectrometry, the principle of the method is deceptively simple, given the immense information content of an NMR spectrum. The signal generated is the result of realignment of spinning nuclei in a magnetic field after their orientation is altered by applying an external pulse of radiofrequency energy.[30-34] Theoretically, one might expect all spinning nuclei, or at least all spinning nuclei of the same element, to behave essentially the same and so generate little specific information. However, unique atomic and molecular information is obtained because (1) isotopes with spinning nuclei each have a characteristic rate of precession, known as the Larmor frequency, around the axis of the magnetic field; (2) each nuclide has a characteristic inherent sensitivity, called the magnetogyric ratio, to an applied magnetic field; and (3) the resonance frequency of a nucleus is related directly to the local magnetic field experienced by the nucleus. Because the magnitude of the local magnetic field around a nucleus is related to the electronic environment of the nucleus, which is a function of its neighboring nuclei, different chemical environments (i.e., different chemical structures) produce different resonance frequencies, called chemical shifts.

Additional information is obtained by the rate at which the nuclei return to their undisturbed alignment within the external magnetic field. This rate is determined by interactions with neighboring spinning nuclei (spin-spin relaxation, or T2) and by the exchange of energy with the molecular framework or lattice (spin-lattice relaxation, or T1). The assessment of these relaxation parameters is particularly important in magnetic resonance imaging (MRI), where alterations in relaxation patterns characterize abnormal molecular environments (i.e., pathologic tissue states).

Table 1.1 shows selected nuclides of biologic interest that have a nuclear spin and are candidate nuclei for magnetic resonance experiments. Immediately apparent is the absence of (^{12}C) and (^{16}O), which do not have spinning nuclei. This apparent problem can be an advantage when one employs an appropriate isotope (e.g., ^{13}C) as a tracer because the "background" is reduced to zero. Using appropriate techniques, quantitative carbon magnetic resonance measurements of ^{13}C enrichments in biologic samples are identical to those made by mass spectrometry even at relatively low enrichment levels above natural abundance.[35] As discussed subsequently, the simultaneous measurement of the major (tracee) nuclide (e.g., ^{12}C) and the minor (tracer) nuclide (e.g., ^{13}C) using mass spectrometry has great practical significance for quantitative tracer kinetic measurements.

From Table 1.1 it is readily apparent that, aside from sodium, phosphorus, and fluorine, which are not present to any extent in tissue, the inherent sensitivity of other biologically important nuclides is low compared with that of the body's most abundant nuclide, the proton. The concentrations of these nuclides are considerably less than that of the proton, further compounding the problem. This situation translates to limited sensitivity for studying in vivo metabolic events using magnetic resonance spectroscopy (e.g., low millimolar range for ^{13}C) and limited spatial resolution when imaging is attempted with nuclides other than the proton. The facts of inherently high nuclear sensitivity and relatively high body nuclide concentration account for the predominance of phosphorus magnetic resonance metabolic studies in vivo.

Nevertheless, the real value of magnetic resonance spectroscopy lies in its ability to study biochemical events in situ in a completely noninvasive fashion. The advances in NMR have been impressive in this regard, and the National Center for Research Resources of the National Institutes of Health has established several NMR resources nationwide. There have been numerous animal studies, and progress has been made in areas inaccessible to human investigation.[36-45] Nevertheless, the number of in vivo human investigations, including those in infants and children, now is in the thousands.[46,47] By the late 1980s, forearm muscle studies alone numbered nearly 1000.[46]

The regulation of muscle intracellular pH and the maintenance of normal oxidative metabolism have been studied extensively.[36,46,47] Likewise, alterations in metabolic milieu secondary to various myopathies and inborn errors of metabolism have been described in some detail[48-58] (see Chapter 33). For example, during exercise, subjects with muscle phosphorylase deficiency (McArdle's disease), muscle phosphofructokinase (PFK) deficiency, and glycogen branching enzyme deficiency, exhibit an abnormal increase or diminished decline in muscle pH and abnormal ratio ATP/phosphocreatine.[54-58] During the recovery period after exercise, reestablishment of a normal phosphocreatine level is normal in subjects with McArdle's disease, whereas it is delayed in individuals with muscle PFK deficiency because muscle phosphate has been trapped in sugar phosphate intermediates.[54-58] Studies of muscle metabolism in the very low birth weight neonate using phosphorus magnetic resonance have shown dramatic changes in the ATP/ phosphocreatine and phosphocreatine/inorganic phos-

TABLE 1.1. Magnetic resonance properties of selected biologically significant nuclides.

Nucleus	Natural abundance (%)	Relative sensitivity for equal no. of nuclei	Relative sensitivity at natural abundance
^1H	99.985	1000	1000
^2H	0.015	9.7	0.0015
^{13}C	1.10	16	0.176
^{14}N	99.63	1	0.176
^{15}N	0.37	1	0.0037
^{17}O	0.037	29	0.0107
^{19}F	100	830	830.1
^{23}Na	100	93	93.0
^{31}P	100	66	66.0
^{39}K	93.10	0.5	0.466

phate (Pi) ratios during limited muscle activity, suggesting that skeletal muscle in the neonate has limited functional energy reserve compared to that in the adult.[59]

Carbon magnetic resonance has been used to quantify muscle glycogen synthesis in normal individuals and in subjects with non–insulin-dependent diabetes mellitus to show that the principal pathway of plasma glucose disposal in both groups during a hyperglycemic-hyperinsulinemic clamp is muscle glycogen synthesis.[60,61] Cardiac metabolism has been studied in some detail using phosphorus magnetic resonance[47] including individuals with myocardial infarction[47] and myopathies.[47] There has been limited success with imaging cardiac energy phosphate metabolites in three dimensions.[62] Similarly, informative measurements of the muscle energy state in subjects with genetic mitochondrial myopathies[46,47,49,50] have been conducted, including assessment of the effects of pharmacologic attempts to bypass the enzymatic block.[49,50]

Proton magnetic resonance imaging of the human brain has become an indispensable tool in clinical medicine[63,64] and is contributing importantly to understanding the pathophysiology of brain development and injury in the neonate.[65,66] Although some progress has been made in metabolic studies of the animal brain, magnetic resonance studies of human cerebral metabolism have been more limited.[40–44] Adult studies have focused largely on postischemic events using phosphorus magnetic resonance studies of the intracellular energy state.[46,47] Understandably, neonatal proton magnetic resonance studies have concentrated on the effects of asphyxia where significant changes in the ATP/phosphocreatine and phosphocreatine/Pi ratios have been observed whose magnitude may relate to prognosis.[67–70] Understandable as well have been related studies in neonatal seizures[42,70] and intraventricular hemorrhage, where alterations in cerebral metabolism may persist for weeks after the acute insult.[71] Important findings of the various neonatal investigations have been (1) the observation that the highest proton magnetic resonance peak in neonatal brain is due to the phosphomonoesters (PME), phosphorylethanolamine, and phosphorylcholine; and (2) that the PME/ATP ratio declines as the brain matures, providing an index of neuronal tissue maturation[70] (see Chapter 26).

Positron Emission Tomography

Unlike mass spectrometry and magnetic resonance spectroscopy, positron emission tomography (PET) does not have the capability of providing intramolecular structural information. Moreover, it is dependent on radiotracers rather than on stable isotopes.[72] It is a powerful approach

TABLE 1.2. Characteristics of nuclides used for PET scanning.

Nuclide	Half-life (min)	Stable daughter
^{11}C	20.40	^{11}B
^{13}N	9.96	^{13}C
^{15}O	2.07	^{15}N
^{18}F	109.07	^{18}O

for measuring substrate fuel kinetics within organs in a completely noninvasive fashion. Because only short-lived radioisotopes are used, the effective absorbed dose is comparable to that of current clinical nuclear medicine procedures and computed tomography scanning.[73,74]

Many biologically important elements have isotopes that decay by emitting positively charged electrons (positrons). The most prominent are (^{11}C), (^{13}N), and (^{15}O) (Table 1.2). These isotopes can be produced using a cyclotron and are then incorporated into appropriate substrate tracers. In a case where this process is not possible or is disadvantageous, another positron emitter, (^{18}F), can be used to label the substrate. When the labeled substrate is injected into the subject and the nuclide decays, the emitted positron soon collides with one of the numerous electrons in the immediate environment. This collision destroys both particles and converts them into energy in the form of two 511-keV photons that travel in opposite directions. When a pair of radiation monitors 180° on either side of the event detect coincident photons, a signal is recorded. In practice, a ring detector array is placed around the subject, and a positron radiation "metabolite image" is constructed from coincident photon detection in a manner similar to that used for computed tomography.[72,75]

Cardiac and cerebral metabolism have been studied extensively. In the latter case, regional and whole-brain glucose consumption has been measured using 2-deoxy[U-^{11}C]glucose and 2-deoxy-2[^{18}F]fluoroglucose, which give essentially identical rates of 27.72 ± 1.28 and 31.44 ± 2.06 μmol·100g^{-1}·min^{-1}, respectively, for whole-brain glucose utilization in the adult.[76] These values fit well within the range of 25 to 33 μmol·100g^{-1}·min^{-1} measured by the more classic Kety-Schmidt technique.[76] Similar studies have been carried out in more than 100 children. Chugani et al.[74] selected 29 of these subjects who had had only transient neurologic injury and whose glucose consumption rates might be considered representative of normal rates during childhood. In the neonate, cerebral glucose consumption averaged 84% that of the adult, but there was some overlap in range; given the small number of subjects studied, the difference was not statistically significant. Within the limits of both data sets, these measurements essentially confirmed earlier speculation about neonatal brain glucose consumption based on stable isotope studies of glucose production in the human neonate.[77] By 2 years of age brain glucose consumption was identical to that of the adult, but it continued to increase and peaked at about twice the adult rate from about age 4 to age 8. Thereafter it declined to the adult rate. Given the limited number of children at any age, the precise shape of the age relations cannot be defined with certainty and should be considered preliminary. Chugani et al.[74] were further able to define maturational changes in regional rates of brain glucose consumption that qualitatively resembled the adult rates by 2 years of age but which were quantitatively greater than those of the adult from toddler ages to the second decade of life. Similarly, PET scanning has been used by Volpe et al.[78–80] to study the pathogenesis of intraventricular hemorrhage in the neonate and by several other investigators to assess cerebral blood flow and energy metabolism in pathologic states in the adult.[81,82]

Of real potential interest but as yet not applied to the neonate are PET methods employing ^{11}C- or ^{13}N-labeled amino acids to study local cerebral protein synthesis rates.[83–85] Using [1-^{11}C]leucine tracer, the rate of leucine incorporation into cerebral proteins in the adult is about 50 to 60 nmol·100 g^{-1} min^{-1}. In a single study of three children with phenylketonuria, the rate of [^{11}CH$_3$]methionine incorporation appeared to be reduced,[86] although there are no systematic normal cerebral protein synthesis data spanning the pediatric age range with which to compare these results. Indeed, there are no other cerebral protein synthesis studies in children with pathologic conditions other than this single investigation.[86] This deficit is somewhat glaring, given the importance of the developmental pathophysiology of cerebral protein synthesis and the large amounts of data on whole-body protein synthesis obtained using [^{13}C]leucine tracers in humans. In this regard, the first measurements of whole-body protein synthesis rates in children with phenylketonuria made with [1-^{13}C]leucine tracer and gas chromatography/mass spectrometry analysis have been reported.[87] In another area of amino acid physiology, Berglund et al.[88] reported modeling amino acid transport across the placenta of monkeys using PET scanning with [^{11}CH$_3$]methionine tracer.

Cardiac metabolism has been studied by positron emission tomography in some detail using various short-lived radiotracers.[75] ^{13}NH$_3$ and H$_2$^{15}O have been used extensively for measuring cardiac blood flow, and myocardial oxygen consumption has been assessed with C^{15}O$_2$ and ^{15}O$_2$. Cardiac fuel consumption has been measured using [^{11}C]palmitate to quantify fatty acid metabolism[75,89] and [^{18}F]fluorodeoxyglucose to measure glucose utilization in healthy individuals and subjects with myocardial ischemia.[75] Cardiac β-adrenergic, muscarinic, and benzodiazepine receptors have been imaged with appropriate ^{11}C-labeled antagonists.[75] Although no cardiac PET studies have been carried out in the human neonate, the potential is there for studying cardiac fuel and receptor metabolism during the critical period of developmental physiology.

Stable Isotope Tracers

Although nuclear magnetic resonance has proven reliable as a tool for quantifying selected stable isotope tracers in vivo, it does not generally achieve the speed, sensitivity, or precision possible using mass spectrometry. This technique has been used for most of the human studies that employed stable isotope tracers. Although the history, safety, and advantages of stable isotope studies have been reviewed in detail,[9,90–96] it is important to reemphasize several of the practical advantages of using stable isotope tracers in conjunction with mass spectrometric quantitation for studying metabolic fuel transport in children. First, substrate and isotopic enrichment are measured simultaneously. This method is different from conventional radiotracer approaches where specific activity is calculated as the ratio of radioactivity, measured with one set of preparative procedures, to substrate content, determined generally with a completely different preparative and analytical method. The sample is not only processed twice, but precision is diminished through additional error propagation. Using mass spectrometry where the labeled and unlabeled ions can be measured simultaneously, there is only a single preparative procedure, and both isotopes are determined with the high precision that is routine with this analytical approach. Furthermore, a single preparative/analytical procedure almost invariably reduces the size of the sample required for measurement, which is no trivial advantage in neonatal studies. Some studies are just not practical using nuclear magnetic resonance or using a radiotracer if this option were, theoretically, available.

For example, Frazer et al.[97] and Bougnères et al.[98] quantified gluconeogenesis from alanine and glycerol, respectively, in neonates. The amount of blood required to make these measurements would have been prohibitive using nuclear magnetic resonance, and either the dose of ^{14}C or the amount of blood required for counting precision would have been excessive using this radiotracer.

An additional advantage of mass spectrometry and nuclear magnetic resonance is the ability to determine the intramolecular location of label with relative ease. Although it can be accomplished with a radiotracer, the process is difficult and requires tediously degrading the molecule in question carbon by carbon. Matthews et al.[99,100] were able to study leucine and valine turnover, transamination, reamination, and irreversible oxidation in the fed and fasted human using infusions of branched-chain amino acids labeled with both ^{15}N and ^{13}C. They simultaneously measured the plasma leucine and valine molecules that had both labels, ^{15}N alone, ^{13}C alone, or no tracer at all. These studies would have been theoretically possible but realistically impractical using nuclear magnetic resonance because of its low sensitivity. Similarly, our understanding of glucose carbon's contributions to glycogen synthesis and the earlier discussed glucose paradox[3] have been furthered by mass spectrometrically examining the location and pattern of glucose carbon labeling after administration of [U-^{13}C]glucose.[101]

There is the generally appreciated advantage that these compounds are safe. The extension of this fact is that several tracers can be used simultaneously and repeatedly in the same subject. This ability is no trivial advantage in perinatology or neonatology, where longitudinal observations are highly advantageous. Repeated studies are rarely possible with radiotracers because of exposure limits. PET studies are limited in this regard.

The benefits of using several tracers at once are obvious. First, the information content of any given experiment is maximized, and fewer subjects are needed to answer the same number of questions. Second, simultaneous use of several tracers often allows the investigator to control for, or provide additional information on, various assumptions of the method or study design. Third, studying the same subject repeatedly allows the use of paired statistics and the subject to serve as his or her own control. In summary, these advantages serve to reduce the number of subjects necessary to test a single hypothesis and increase the number of hypotheses that can be evaluated using the same number of subjects.

It is important to point out one significant limitation. If one studies precursor–product relationships using stable isotope tracers, there is often considerable dilution of the administered tracer. For example, if one studies amino acid metabolism with [^{15}N, 1-^{13}C]leucine, as mentioned above, the tracer can be infused at a rate sufficient to enrich the free leucine pool to several percent. Nevertheless, the isotopic enrichment in protein amino acids, excreted urea, and expired $^{13}CO_2$ might be on the order of 0.002% to 0.100% above natural abundance, as depicted in Figure 1.1.[92] There is no single mass spectrometer that has this dynamic analytical range. Gas chromatography/mass spectrometry measurements, which can be made easily on picomole amounts of sample, have an isotope detection limit of about one part minor isotope (i.e., tracer) per 1000 parts major isotope (tracee). Isotope ratio mass spectrometric measurements, on the other hand, can precisely measure several parts of tracer per million parts of tracee, but it is done at the expense of significant sample size (micromoles to millimoles of carbon or nitrogen) and sample purification and preparation.[92]

The number of stable isotope studies of metabolic fuel transport carried out in adults now numbers well into the thousands and those carried out in children certainly well above a thousand. They have been reviewed elsewhere[90–96] and are included in material presented in Chapters 2, 5, 6, 8–11, 16, 32–34, 44, and 47–53. It is fair to say that the use of stable isotope tracers in metabolic investigations is now commonplace enough that no review is either comprehensive or up to date. Given the success investigators have had studying metabolic events during the perinatal period, and given that there are limited alternative means to obtain dynamic metabolic data in the pregnant woman and the neonate, the application of stable isotope tracer approaches to important perinatal issues has been underutilized.

Stable isotope tracers have been used to (1) study glucose production, gluconeogenesis, alanine kinetics, and ureagenesis in healthy and diabetic pregnant women;[102–106] (2) deduce that although alanine de novo synthesis occurs in the term fetus,[107] the fetal liver does not produce glucose just prior to birth;[101] (3) quantify the onset of gluconeogenesis immediately after birth;[97,108] (4) determine the magnitude of neonatal glucose production[77,109] and its regulation;[110–119] (5) assess the sources of new glucose carbon;[97,98] and (6) evaluate insulin sensitivity in the neonate in conjunction with the euglycemic hyperinsulinemic clamp.[120] In the neonate these tracers have been employed to quantify free fatty acids and ketone fuel kinetics,[98,121] amino acid and protein turn-

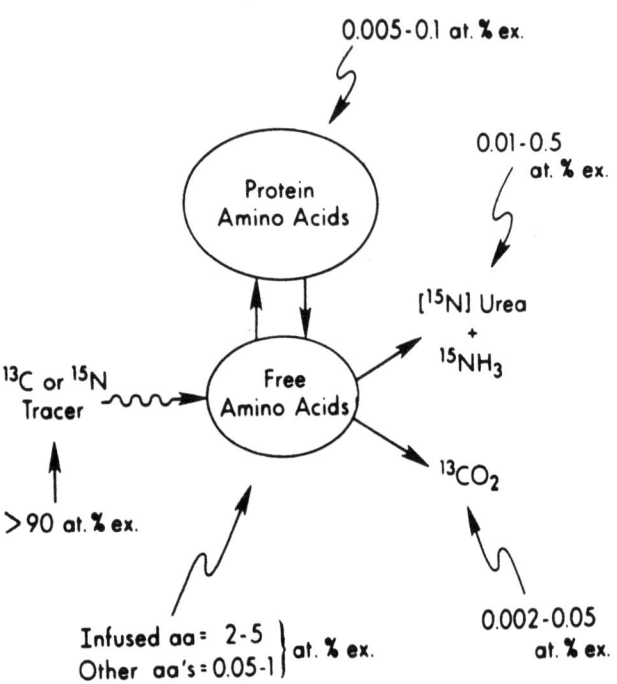

FIGURE 1.1. Approximate dilutions of amino acid stable isotope tracer in vivo. The tracer is infused into the plasma compartment.

TABLE 1.3. Metabolic fuel turnover rates calculated from stable isotope dilution studies in man.

Substrate	Infants ($\mu mol \cdot kg^{-1} min^{-1}$)	Adults ($\mu mol \cdot kg^{-1} min^{-1}$)
Glucose	25–35	12–14
Lactate	30–60	15–20
Alanine	13–17	4–6
Glycine	6–15	4–5
Leucine	2.3–3.3	1.3–2.0
Lysine	2.5–3.0	1.3–2.0
Free fatty acids	13–25	4–8
Glycerol	4–5	1.5–2.0
Ketone bodies	13–25	4–8

over,[121-138] and the fractional synthesis rates of albumin and fibronectin.[122,138] Whole-body protein dynamics have been measured in pregnant[139] and lactating[140] women. Table 1.3 lists the interorgan metabolic fuel transport rates determined in children and adults using stable isotope tracers.[93]

Similar advances have been made in related areas of nutritional significance, particularly in the fields of energy and trace element metabolism. In the former area the use of doubly labeled water ($^2H_2^{18}O$) to measure total daily energy expenditure over the long term in the free-living condition has become an important investigational tool[141-145] that has already been used to quantify energy during early infancy,[146-149] during adolescence,[150,151] and in children recovering from malnutrition.[152,153] In addition, doubly labeled water measurements of energy metabolism in young infants born to lean or overweight mothers has provided evidence that reduced energy expenditure is an important contributor to excessive weight gain during the first year of life.[150] In reference to mineral and trace element metabolism, stable isotopes have been valuable,[92,154] permitting dynamic studies of iron,[155-157] copper,[158-161] zinc,[160-164] selenium,[165] calcium,[26,166-173] and magnesium[174] metabolism (see Chapters 40 and 41).

Mathematical Modeling

Considering the limited access to samples other than plasma, urine, or stool in the neonate, understanding metabolic fuel dynamics in inaccessible areas or tissues requires a model. In fact, positron emission tomography cannot be carried out without a detailed model of the organ under study. The basic theory and practice of modeling has been well described,[175-183] and the adaptations required for the use of stable isotope tracers have been presented.[184]

Building a model is constructing a hypothesis that describes the events under study. The model remains valid so long as it continues to adequately represent the dynamics of subsequently measured events. It is important to discriminate between two models: a model of these data and one of the system.[179] In the former, one refers to a mathematical description of these data. This model does not necessarily define specific biochemical masses, spaces, or events and is frequently called *empirical modeling*.[181] It is often the first step in developing a model of the system that uses all currently available physiologic information to construct a biologically plausible and relevant structure that fits these data.[179] This process is sometimes called *model-based compartmental analysis*.[181]

Understandably, the clinical investigator is interested in system models. In practice, detailed information on the system is often necessary to construct a model that is identifiable (i.e., one in which it is possible to have unique solutions to all of the unknown model parameters). Identifiability is no trivial problem in biologic investigations, where "the principal difficulty attached to the mathematical analysis of physiological and medical systems stems from the mismatch between the complexity of the processes in question and the limited data available from such systems, especially from in vivo studies."[177] This problem may be accentuated when working within the sample size limitations of studies on the neonate, especially one who is low birth weight.

An alternative approach is to simplify the model so it becomes identifiable. The simplifications must be physiologically plausible, or conclusions drawn from the model will have little physiologic meaning. Simplification results in uncertain domains of validity and in loss of the fine details apparent in a more complex model. Complete simplification to the so-called noncompartmental approach poses two problems. First, one cannot solve for structural details of the system. Second, although the noncompartmental approach is often referred to as "model-independent," in fact the opposite is true. With this type of model, kinetic events in the sampled pool reflect those of the system as a whole only when all de novo entries and all irreversible losses occur from the accessible pool. Rarely can these assumptions be satisfied in a biological system, and deductions based on the model may be in error.[185]

Although the limited information available from noncompartmental approaches or simple models is often sufficient to answer useful and practical medical questions, more complex physiologic models are frequently required to understand fully the dynamics of the system and to quantify events taking place outside the accessible compartments, as in plasma. It is precisely this kind of information that is generally sought when tracers are utilized. In pediatrics there is virtually no way to obtain such information other than by compartmental modeling. In addition, once a detailed general model of the system has been developed and validated, the model can be employed in entirely new circumstances. If the model of the system is correct, it does not change as a function of the experiment. The sizes of the various pools and the rate of movement of substrates between these pools may vary; the system, however, if constructed properly in the first place, does not vary. In other words, a properly constructed general model of the system allows one to test how the system responds to various specific conditions.

This concept is perhaps best illustrated by the *minimal model* for assessing insulin sensitivity in vivo.[186-188] Once developed and validated, this model has been used to quantify insulin sensitivity in vivo in children,[189] diabetics,[190] and individuals genetically at risk for developing diabetes.[191] In addition, it has been employed in a variety of experiments to test the effects of islet cell transplantation[192] and growth hormone[193] on insulin sensitivity. Stable isotope modifications of the model have substantially improved its usefulness and extended its potential application in perinatal medicine.[194]

Compartmental modeling has two important but often overlooked advantages. First, fitting these observed data to the model allows the investigator to evaluate if the idea(s) of the system is compatible with these data. In other words, the exercise can help determine which models are not compatible with experimental observations and so lead the investigator to refine his or her description of the system. Second, availability of a detailed compartment model permits the investigator to calculate what information or domains of validity are lost when more simplified models are used to assess the system. This approach provides the clinical investigator with a means to evaluate the "error limits" of data interpretation in clinical studies where sample constraints frequently dictate use of the more simplified models.

Implications

In vivo metabolic studies during the perinatal period are never simple, from either the ethical or the technical point of view. Information on virtually every aspect of intermediary metabolism is absolutely essential and sorely lacking during this critical period of life. Measurements of substrate content can provide a limited and uncertain picture of dynamic physiologic events. Investigative tools are available that can help supply the necessary information. It is imperative that these tools continue to be developed for use during the perinatal period and that clinical investigators begin to apply them in an intensive and imaginative fashion to the myriad unanswered questions.

Acknowledgment. This work was supported with federal funds from the U.S. Department of Agriculture, Agricultural Research Service, under Cooperative Agreement No. 58-6250-6-001.

References

1. Crabtree B, Newsholme EA. A quantitative approach to metabolic control. Curr Top Cell Regul 1985;25:21–76.
2. Crabtree B, Newsholme EA. A systematic approach to describing and analyzing metabolic control systems. Trends Biochem Sci 1987;12:5–12.
3. McGarry JD, Kuwajima M, Newgard CB, et al. From dietary glucose to liver glycogen: the full circle round. Annu Rev Nutr 1987;7:51–73.
4. Lowry OH, Passonneau JV. A flexible system of enzymatic analysis. Orlando: Academic Press, 1972.
5. Goodman SI, Markey SP. Diagnosis of organic acidemias by gas chromatography-mass spectrometry. New York: Alan R. Liss, 1987.
6. Chalmers RA, Lawson AM. Organic acids in man: analytical chemistry, biochemistry and diagnosis of the organic acidurias. London: Chapman & Hall, 1982.
7. Hicks JM, Boecks RL. Pediatric clinical chemistry. Philadelphia: Saunders, 1984.
8. Watson JT. Introduction to mass spectrometry. New York: Raven Press, 1985.
9. Wolfe RR. Tracers in metabolic research. Radioisotope and stable isotope/mass spectrometry methods. New York: Alan R. Liss, 1984.
10. Baillie TA. Stable isotopes. Applications in pharmacology, toxicology and clinical research. Baltimore: University Park Press, 1978.
11. McLafferty FW. Interpretation of mass spectra. 3rd ed. Mill Valley: University Science Books, 1980.
12. Burlingame AL, Millington DS, Norwood DL, et al. Mass spectrometry. Anal Chem 1990;62:268R–303R.
13. Cotter RJ. Plasma desorption mass spectrometry: coming of age. Anal Chem 1988;60:781A–793A.
14. Chowdhury SK, Chait BT. Recent developments in the mass spectrometry of peptides and proteins. Annu Rep Med Chem 1989;24:253–263.
15. Gaskell SJ. Mass spectrometry at high mass: virtues and vices of some new approaches. Trends Physiol Sci 1990;11:99–101.
16. Caprioli RM. Continuous-flow fast atom bombardment mass spectrometry. Anal Chem 1990;62:477A–485A.
17. Stults JT. Peptide sequencing by mass spectrometry. Biomed Appl Mass Spectrom 1989;34:145–201.
18. Cotter RJ. Time-of-flight mass spectrometry: an increasing role in the life sciences. Biomed Environ Mass Spectrom 1989;18:513–532.
19. Spengler B, Cotter RJ. Ultraviolet laser desorption/ionization mass spectrometry of proteins above 100,000 daltons by pulsed ion extraction time-of-flight analysis. Anal Chem 1990;62:793–796.
20. Loo JA, Edmonds CG, Smith RD. Primary sequence information from intact proteins by electrospray ionization tandem mass spectrometry. Science 1990;248:201–204.

21. Hillenkamp F, Karas M. Ultraviolet laser desorption/ionization of biomolecules in the high mass range. In: Proceedings of the American Society of Mass Spectrometry Conference on Mass Spectrometry and Allied Topics. 1989;37:1168–1169.
22. Loo JA, Edmonds CG, Smith RD, et al. Comparison of electrospray ionization and plasma desorption mass spectra of peptides and proteins. Biomed Environ Mass Spectrom 1990;19:286–294.
23. Olivares JA. Inductively coupled plasma-mass spectrometry. Methods Enzymol 1988;158:205–222.
24. Ting BT, Mooers CS, Janghorbani M. Isotopic determination of selenium in biological materials with inductively coupled plasma mass spectrometry. Analyst 1989;114:667–674.
25. Schuette S, Vereault D, Ting BT, et al. Accurate measurement of stable isotopes of magnesium in biological materials with inductively coupled plasma mass spectrometry. Analyst 1988;113:1837–1842.
26. Moore LJ, Machlan LA, Lim MO, et al. Dynamics of calcium metabolism in infancy and childhood. I. Methodology and quantification in the infant. Pediatr Res 1985;19:329–334.
27. Biemann K. Colloquium: some recent applications of mass spectrometry to biochemistry; tandem mass spectrometry applied to protein structure problems. Biochem Soc Trans 1989;17:237–243.
28. Biemann K, Scoble HA. Characterization by tandem mass spectrometry of structural modific proteins. Science 1987;237:992–998.
29. Gibson BW, Biemann K. Strategy for the mass spectrometric verification and correction of structures of proteins deduced from their DNA sequences. Proc Natl Acad Sci USA 1984;81:1956–1960.
30. Gadian DG. Nuclear magnetic resonance and its applications to living systems. Oxford: Clarendon Press, 1982.
31. Shaw D. Fourier transform N.M.R. spectroscopy. 2nd ed. Amsterdam: Elsevier, 1984.
32. Price RR, Stephens WH, Partain CL. NMR physical principles. In: Partain CL, Price RR, Patton JA, et al., eds. Magnetic resonance imaging. Vol. II. Physical principles and instrumentation. 2nd ed. Philadelphia: Saunders, 1988:971–986.
33. Willicott MR. NMR chemical principles. In: Partain CL, Price RR, Patton JA, et al., eds. Magnetic resonance imaging. Vol. II. Physical principles and instrumentation. 2nd ed. Philadelphia: Saunders, 1988:987–1002.
34. Malloy CR. Nuclear magnetic resonance in clinical medicine: an overview. Semin Perinatol 1990;14:193–200.
35. Brainard JR, Downey RS, Bier DM, et al. Use of multiple ^{13}C-labeling strategies and ^{13}C NMR to detect low levels of exogenous metabolites in the presence of large endogenous pools: measurement of glucose turnover in a human subject. Anal Biochem 1989;176:307–312.
36. Chance B, Leigh JS Jr, McLaughlin AC, et al. Phosphorous-31 spectroscopy and imaging. In: Partain CL, Price RR, Patton JA, et al., eds. Magnetic resonance imaging. Vol. II. Physical principles and instrumentation. 2nd ed. Philadelphia: Saunders, 1988:1501–1520.
37. Cohen SM. Carbon-13: NMR spectroscopy. In: Partain CL, Price RR, Patton JA, et al., eds. Magnetic resonance imaging. Vol. II. Physical principles and instrumentation. 2nd ed. Philadelphia: Saunders, 1988:1521–1535.
38. Thomas SR. The biomedical applications of fluorine-19 NMR. In: Partain CL, Price RR, Patton JA, et al., eds. Magnetic resonance imaging. Vol. II. Physical principles and instrumentation. 2nd ed. Philadelphia: Saunders, 1988:1536–1552.
39. Narayana PA, Kulkarni MV, Mehta SD. NMR of ^{23}Na in biological systems. In: Partain CL, Price RR, Patton JA, et al., eds. Magnetic resonance imaging. Vol. II. Physical principles and instrumentation. 2nd ed. Philadelphia: Saunders, 1988:1553–1563.
40. Avison MJ, Herschkowitz EJ, Novotny OAC, et al. Proton NMR observation in phenylalanine and an aromatic metabolite in the rabbit brain in vivo. Pediatr Res 1990;27:566–570.
41. Nioka S, Chance B, Smith DS, et al. Cerebral energy metabolism and oxygen state during hypoxia in neonate and adult dogs. Pediatr Res 1990;28:54–62.
42. Young RSK, Petroff OAC. Neonatal seizure: magnetic resonance spectroscopic findings. Semin Perinatol 1990;14:238–247.
43. Corbett RJT. In vivo multinuclear magnetic resonance spectroscopy investigations of cerebral development and metabolic encephalopathy using neonatal animal models. Semin Perinatol 1990;14:258–271.
44. Petroff OAC, Young RSK, Cowan BE, et al. ^1H nuclear magnetic resonance spectroscopy study of neonatal hypoglycemia. Pediatr Neurol 1988;4:31–34.
45. Shalwitz RA, Becker NN. In vivo ^{13}C nuclear magnetic resonance studies of hepatic glucose and glycogen metabolism. Semin Perinatol 1990;14:224–230.
46. Radda GK, Rajagopalan B, Taylor DJ. Biochemistry in vivo: an appraisal of clinical magnetic resonance spectroscopy. Magn Reson Q 1989;5:122–151.
47. Bottomly PA. Human in vivo NMR spectroscopy in diagnostic medicine: clinical tool or research probe? Radiology 1989;170:1–15.
48. Radda GK, Bore PJ, Gadian DG, et al. ^{13}P NMR examination of two patients with NADH-CoQ reductase deficiency. Nature 1982;295:608–609.
49. Argov Z, Bank WJ, Maris J, et al. Treatment of mitochondrial myopathy due to complex III deficiency with vitamins K_3 and C: a ^{31}P NMR follow-up study. Ann Neurol 1986;19:598–602.
50. Eleff S, Kennaway NG, Buist NMR, et al. ^{31}P NMR study of improvement in oxidative phosphorylation by vitamins K_3 and C in a patient with a defect in electron transport at complex III in skeletal muscle. Proc Natl Acad Sci USA 1984;81:3529–3533.
51. Argov Z, Maris J, Fischbeck K, et al. In vivo studies of human lipid myopathies by ^{31}P magnetic resonance imaging. Ann Neurol 1985;18:119–120.
52. Hayes DJ, Hilton-Jones D, Arnold DL, et al. A mitochondrial encephalomyopathy: a combined ^{31}P magnetic resonance and biochemical investigation. J Neurol Sci 1985;71:105–118.

53. Gadian DG, Radda GK, Ross BD, et al. ^{31}P NMR examination of a myopathy. Lancet 1981;2:774–775.
54. Argov Z, Bank WJ, Maris J, et al. Muscle energy metabolism in human phosphofructokinase deficiency as recorded by ^{31}P nuclear magnetic resonance spectroscopy. Ann Neurol 1987;22:46–51.
55. Chance B, Elleff S, Bank W, et al. ^{31}P NMR studies of control of mitochondrial function in phosphofructokinase-deficient human skeletal muscle. Proc Natl Acad Sci USA 1982;79:7714–7718.
56. Argov Z, Bank WJ, Boden B, et al. Muscle ^{31}P-NMR in partial glycolytic block: in vivo study of phosphoglycerate mutase deficient patient. Arch Neurol 1987;4:614–617.
57. Ross BD, Radda GK, Gadian DG, et al. Examination of a case of suspected McArdle's syndrome by ^{31}P NMR. N Engl J Med 1981;304:1338–1342.
58. Duboc D, Jehenson P, Tran Dinh S, et al. Phosphorous NMR spectroscopy study of muscular enzyme deficiencies involving glycogenolysis and lycolysis. Neurology 1987;37:663–671.
59. Bertocci LA, Mize CE. The use of nuclear magnetic resonance to study muscle metabolism in very low birth weight infants. Semin Perinatol 1990;14:231–237.
60. Jue T, Rothman DL, Shulman GI, et al. Direct observation of glycogen synthesis in human muscle with ^{13}C NMR. Proc Natl Acad Sci USA 1989;86:4489–4491.
61. Schulman GI, Rothman DL, Jue T, et al. Quantitation of muscle glycogen synthesis in normal subjects and subjects with non-insulin-dependent diabetes by ^{13}C nuclear magnetic resonance spectroscopy. N Engl J Med 1990;322:223–228.
62. Bottomley PA, Hardy CJ, Roemer PB. Phosphate metabolite imaging and concentration measurements in human heart by nuclear magnetic resonance. Magn Reson Med 1990;14:425–434.
63. Heiken JP, Glazer HS, Lee JKT. Manual of clinical magnetic resonance imaging: a practical guide to conducting magnetic resonance imaging examinations of the head and body. New York: Raven Press, 1986.
64. Young SW. Magnetic resonance imaging: basic principles. 2nd ed. New York: Raven Press, 1988.
65. Dietrich RB. Magnetic resonance imaging of normal brain maturation. Semin Perinatol 1990;14:201–211.
66. Dubowitz LMS, Bydder GM. Magnetic resonance imaging of the brain in neonates. Semin Perinatol 1990;14:212–223.
67. Cady EB, Dawson MJ, Hope PL, et al. Non-invasive investigation of cerebral metabolism in newborn infants by phosphorous nuclear magnetic resonance spectroscopy. Lancet 1983;1:1059–1062.
68. Hope PL, Cady EB, Tofts PS, et al. Cerebral energy metabolism studied with phosphorus NMR spectroscopy in normal and birth-asphyxiated infants. Lancet 1984;2:366–370.
69. Younkin DP, Delivoria-Papadopoulos M, Wagerle LC, et al. In vivo ^{31}P NMR spectroscopy in neonatal neurologic disorders. In: Plum F, Pulsinelli W, eds. Cerebrovascular disease. New York: Raven Press, 1985:149–159.
70. Delivoria-Papadopoulos M, DiGiacomo JE. ^{31}P nuclear magnetic resonance spectroscopy in the human neonatal brain. Semin Perinatol 1990;14:248–257.
71. Younkin DP, Medoff-Cooper B, Guillet R, et al. In vivo ^{31}P nuclear magnetic resonance measurement of chronic changes in cerebral metabolites following neonatal intraventricular hemorrhage. Pediatrics 1988;82:331–336.
72. Reivich M, Alavi A. Positron emission tomography. New York: Alan R. Liss, 1985.
73. Powers WJ, Stabin M, Howse D, et al. Radiation absorbed dose estimates for oxygen-15 radiopharmaceuticals ($H_2^{15}O$, $C^{15}O$, $O^{15}O$) in newborn infants. J Nucl Med 1988;29:1961–1970.
74. Chugani HT, Phelps ME, Mazziotta JC. Positron emission tomography study of human brain functional development. Ann Neurol 1987;22:487–497.
75. Syrota A. In vivo investigation of myocardial perfusion, metabolism and receptors by positron emission tomography. Int J Microcirc Clin Exp 1989;8:411–422.
76. Reivich M. Cerebral glucose consumption: methodology and validation. In: Reivich M, Alavi A, eds. Positron emission tomography. New York: Alan R. Liss, 1985:131–151.
77. Bier DM, Leake RD, Haymond MW, et al. Measurement of "true" glucose production rates in infancy and childhood with 6,6-dideuteroglucose. Diabetes 1977;26:1016–1023.
78. Volpe JJ, Herscovitch P, Perlman JM, et al. Positron emission tomography in the newborn: extensive impairment of regional cerebral blood flow with intraventricular hemorrhage and hemorrhagic intracerebral involvement. Pediatrics 1983;72:589–601.
79. Altman DI, Powers WJ, Perlman JM, et al. Cerebral blood flow requirement for brain viability in newborn infants is lower than in adults. Ann Neurol 1988;24:218–226.
80. Volpe JJ. Edward B. Neuhauser lecture: current concepts of brain injury in the premature infant. AJR 1989;153:243–251.
81. Baron JC, Frackowiak RSJ, Herholz K. Use of PET methods for measurement of cerebral energy metabolism and hemodynamics in cerebrovascular disease. J Cereb Blood Flow Metab 1989;723–742.
82. Powers WJ. Positron emission tomography in cerebrovascular disease: clinical applications? In: Theodore WH, ed. Clinical neuroimaging. New York: Alan R. Liss, 1988:49–74.
83. Bustany P, Comar D. Protein synthesis evaluation in brain and other organs in human by PET. In: Reivich M, Alavi A, eds. Positron emission tomography. New York: Alan R. Liss, 1985:183–201.
84. Keen RE, Barrio JR, Huang S-C, et al. In vivo cerebral protein synthesis rates with leucyl-transfer RNA used as a precursor pool: determination of biochemical parameters to structure tracer kinetic models for positron emission tomography. J Cereb Blood Flow Metab 1989;9:429–445.
85. Hawkins RA, Huang S-C, Barrio JR, et al. Estimation of local cerebral protein synthesis rates with L-[1-^{11}C] leucine and PET: methods, model, and results in animals and humans. J Cereb Blood Flow Metab 1989;9:446–460.
86. Comar D, Saudubray JM, Duthilleul A, et al. Brain uptake of ^{11}C-methionine in phenylketonuria. Eur J Pediatr 1981;136:13–19.

87. Thompson GN, Pacy PJ, Watts RWE, et al. Protein metabolism in phenylketonuria and Lesch-Nyhan syndrome. Pediatr Res 1990;28:240–246.
88. Berglund L, Andersson J, Lilja A, et al. Amino acid transport across the placenta measured by positron emission tomography and analyzed by compartment modelling. J Perinat Med 1989;18:89–100.
89. Geltman EM, Bergmann SR, Sobel BE. Cardiac positron emission tomography. In: Reivich M, Alavi A, eds. Positron emission tomography. New York: Alan R. Liss, 1985:345–385.
90. Klein PD, Klein ER. Stable isotopes: origins and safety. J Clin Pharmacol 1986;26:378–382.
91. Bier DM, Matthews DE. Stable isotope tracer methods for in vivo investigations. Fed Proc 1982;41:2679–2685.
92. Matthews DE, Bier DM. Stable isotope methods for nutritional investigation. Annu Rev Nutr 1983;3:309–339.
93. Bier DM. The use of stable isotopes in metabolic investigation. Bailliere Clin Endocrinol Metab 1987;1:817–836.
94. Pacy PJ, Cheng KN, Thompson GN, et al. Stable isotopes as tracers in clinical research. Ann Nutr Metab 1989;33:65–78.
95. Halliday D, Rennie MJ. The use of stable isotopes for diagnosis and clinical research. Clin Sci 1982;63:485–496.
96. Hachey DL, Wong WW, Boutton TW, et al. Isotope ratio measurement in nutrition and biomedical research. Mass Spectrom Rev 1987;6:289–327.
97. Frazer TE, Karl IE, Hillman LS, et al. Direct measurement of gluconeogenesis from L-[2,3^{13}C$_2$]alanine in the human neonate during the first eight hours of life. Am J Physiol 1981;240:E615–E621.
98. Bougnères PF, Karl IE, Hillman LS, et al. Lipid transport in the human newborn: palmitate and glycerol turnover and the contribution of glycerol to neonatal hepatic glucose output. J Clin Invest 1982;70:262–270.
99. Matthews DE, Bier DM, Rennie MJ, et al. Regulation of leucine metabolism in man: a stable isotope study. Science 1981;214:1129–1131.
100. Staten MA, Bier DM, Matthews DE. Regulation of valine metabolism in man: a stable isotope study. Am J Clin Nutr 1984;40:1224–1234.
101. Katz J, Lee W-NP, Wals PA, et al. Studies of glycogen synthesis and the Krebs cycle by mass isotopomer analysis with [U-^{31}C]glucose in rats. J Biol Chem 1989;264:12994–13001.
102. Kalhan SC, D'Angelo LJ, Savin SM, et al. Glucose production in pregnant women at term gestation: sources of glucose for human fetus. J Clin Invest 1979;63:388–394.
103. Kalhan SC, Tserng KY, Gilfillan C, et al. Metabolism of urea and glucose in normal and diabetic pregnancy. Metabolism 1982;31:824–833.
104. Cowett RM, Susa JB, Kahn CB, et al. Glucose kinetics in nondiabetic and diabetic women during the third trimester of pregnancy. Am J Obstet Gynecol 1983;146:773–780.
105. Cowett RM. Hepatic responsiveness to a glucose infusion in pregnancy. Am J Obstet Gynecol 1985;153:272–279.
106. Kalhan SC, Gilfillan CA, Tserng KY, et al. Glucose-alanine relationship in normal human pregnancy. Metabolism 1988;37:152–158.
107. Gilfillan CA, Tserng KY, Kalhan SC. Alanine production by the human fetus at term gestation. Biol Neonate 1985;47:141–147.
108. Kalhan SC, Bier DM, Savin SM, et al. Estimation of glucose turnover and ^{13}C recycling in the human newborn by simultaneous [1-^{13}C]glucose and [6,6-^{2}H$_2$] glucose tracers. J Clin Endocrinol Metab 1980;50:456–460.
109. Gilfillan CA, Tserng KY, Kalhan SC. Glucose-lactate relation in the human newborn. Pediatr Res 1985;19:312A.
110. Cowett RM, Wolfe MH, Wolfe RR. Lactate turnover is increased in the neonate relative to the adult. Pediatr Res 1985;19:311A.
111. Kalhan SC, Savin SM, Adam PAJ. Measurement of glucose turnover in the human newborn with [1-^{13}C] glucose. J Clin Endocrinol Metab 1976;43:704–707.
112. Cowett RM, Oh W, Schwartz R. Persistent glucose production during glucose infusion in the neonate. J Clin Invest 1983;71:467–475.
113. Kalhan SC, Olivne A, King KC, et al. Role of glucose in the regulation of endogenous glucose production in the human newborn. Pediatr Res 1986;20:49–52.
114. Cowett RM, Susa JB, Oh W, et al. Glucose kinetics in glucose-infused small for gestational age infants. Pediatr Res 1984;18:74–78.
115. Kalhan SC, Savin SM, Adam PAG. Attenuated glucose production rate in newborn infants of insulin-dependent diabetic mothers. N Engl J Med 1977;296:375–376.
116. King KC, Tserng KY, Kalhan SC. Regulation of glucose production in newborn infants of diabetic mothers. Pediatr Res 1982;16:608–612.
117. Cowett RM, Susa JB, Giletti B, et al. Glucose kinetics in infants of diabetic mothers. Am J Obstet Gynecol 1983;146:781–786.
118. Denne SC, Kalhan SC. Glucose carbon recycling and oxidation in human newborns. Am J Physiol 1986;251:E71–E77.
119. Cowett RM, Andersen GE, Maguire CA, Oh W. Ontogeny of glucose kinetics in low birth weight infants. J Pediatr 1988;112:462–465.
120. Farrag HM, Nawrath LM, Healey JE, et al. Persistent glucose production and greater peripheral sensitivity to insulin in the neonate vs. the adult. Am J Physiol 1997;272:E86–E93.
121. Bougnères PF, Lemmel C, Ferré P, et al. Ketone body transport in the human neonate and infant. J Clin Invest 1986;77:42–48.
122. Yudkoff M, Nissim I, McNellis W, et al. Albumin synthesis in premature infants: determination of turnover with [^{15}N]glycine. Pediatr Res 1987;21:49–53.
123. Denne SC, Kalhan SC. Leucine metabolism in human newborns. Am J Physiol 1987;253:E608–E615.
124. Nicholson JF. Rate of protein synthesis in premature infants. Pediatr Res 1970;4:389–397.
125. De Benoist B, Abdulrazzak Y, Brooke OG, et al. The measurement of whole body protein turnover in the preterm infant with intragastric infusion of L-[l-^{13}C] leucine and sampling of the urinary leucine pool. Clin Sci 1984;66:155–164.

126. Catzeflis C, Schutz Y, Micheli J, et al. Whole body protein synthesis and energy expenditure in very low birth weight infants. Pediatr Res 1985;19:679–687.
127. Pencharz PB, Steffee WP, Cochran W, et al. Protein metabolism in human neonates: nitrogen-balance studies, estimated obligatory losses of nitrogen and whole-body turnover of nitrogen. Clin Sci Mol Med 1977;52:485–498.
128. Pencharz PB, Masson M, Desgranges F, et al. Total-body protein turnover in human premature neonates: effects of birth weight, intra-uterine nutritional status and diet. Clin Sci 1981;61:207–215.
129. Duffy B, Gunn T, Collinge J, et al. The effect of varying protein quality and energy intake on the nitrogen metabolism of parenterally fed very low birthweight (<1600 g) infants. Pediatr Res 1981;15:1040–1044.
130. Pencharz PB, Farri L, Papageorgiou A. The effects of human milk and low-protein turnover and urinary 3-methyl-histidine excretion of preterm infants. Clin Sci 1983;64:611–616.
131. Heine W, Plath C, Richter I, et al. ^{15}N-tracer investigations into the nitrogen metabolism of preterm infants fed mother's milk and a formula diet. J Pediatr Gastroenterol Nutr 1983;2:606–612.
132. Heine W, Richter I, Plath C, et al. Evaluation of different ^{15}N-tracer substances for calculation of whole body protein parameters in infants. J Pediatr Gastroenterol Nutr 1983;2:599–605.
133. Bier DM, Young VR. Assessment of whole body protein-nitrogen kinetics in the human infant. In: Fomon SJ, Heird WD, eds. Energy and protein needs during pregnancy. Orlando: Academic Press, 1986:107–125.
134. Pencharz PB, Protein metabolism in premature infants. Can J Physiol Pharmacol 1988;66:1247–1252.
135. Pencharz PB, Beesley J, Sauer P, et al. Total-body protein turnover in parenterally fed neonates: effects of energy source studied by using [^{15}N]glycine and [l-^{13}C]leucine. Am J Clin Nutr 1989;50:1395–1400.
136. Pencharz PB, Clarke R, Papageorgiou A, et al. A reappraisal of protein turnover values in neonates fed human milk or formula. Can J Physiol Pharmacol 1989;67:282–286.
137. Young VR, Fukagawa NK, Storch KJ, et al. Stable isotope probes: potential for application in studies of amino acid metabolism in neonate. In: Lindblad BS, ed. Perinatal nutrition. Orlando: Academic Press, 1988:221–241.
138. Polin RA, Yoder MC, Douglas SD, et al. Fibronectin turnover in the premature neonate measured with [^{15}N]glycine. Am J Clin Nutr 1989;49:314–319.
139. DeBenoist B, Jackson AA, Hall HStE, et al. Whole-body protein turnover in Jamaican women during pregnancy. Hum Nutr Clin Nutr 1985;339C:167–179.
140. Motil KJ, Montandon CM, Hachey DL, et al. Whole-body metabolism in lactating and nonlactating women. J Appl Physiol 1989;66:370–376.
141. Schoeller DA. Measurement of energy expenditure in free-living humans by using double labeled water. J Nutr 1988;118:1278–1289.
142. Jones PJ, Winthrop AL, Schoeller DA, et al. Validation of doubly labeled water for assessing energy expenditure in infants. Pediatr Res 1987;21:242–246.
143. Prentice AM. Stable isotopic methods for measuring energy expenditure. Proc Nutr Soc 1988;47:259–268.
144. Roberts SB. Use of the doubly labeled water method for measurement of energy expenditure, total body water, water intake, and metabolizable energy intake in humans and small animals. J Physiol Pharmacol 1989;67:1190–1198.
145. Wong WW, Butte NF, Garza C, et al. Comparison of energy expenditure estimated in healthy infants using the doubly labeled water and energy balance methods. Eur J Clin Nutr 1990;44:175–184.
146. Roberts SB, Savage J, Coward WA. Energy expenditure and intake in infants born to lean and overweight mothers. N Engl J Med 1988;318:461–466.
147. Davies PS, Ewing G, Lucas A. Energy expenditure in early infancy. Br J Nutr 1989;62:621–629.
148. Roberts SB, Coward WA, Ewing G, et al. Effect of weaning on accuracy of doubly labeled water method in infants. Am J Physiol 1988;254:R622–R627.
149. Butte NF, Wong WW, Ferlic L, et al. Energy expenditure and deposition of breast-fed and formula-fed infants during early infancy. Pediatr Res 1990;28:631–640.
150. Bandini LG, Schoeller DA, Edwards J, et al. Energy expenditure during carbohydrate overfeeding in obese and nonobese adolescents. Am J Physiol 1989;256:E357–E367.
151. Bandini LG, Schoeller DA, Dietz WH. Energy expenditure in obese and nonobese adolescents. Pediatr Res 1990;27:198–203.
152. Fjeld CR, Schoeller DA. Energy expenditure of malnourished children during catch-up growth. Proc Nutr Soc 1988;47:227–231.
153. Fjeld CR, Schoeller DA, Brown KH. A new model for predicting energy requirements of children during catch-up growth developed using doubly labeled water. Pediatr Res 1989;25:503–508.
154. Turnlund JR. The use of stable isotopes in mineral nutrition research. J Nutr 1989;119:7–14.
155. Turnlund JR, Smith RG, Kretsch MJ, et al. Milk's effect on the bioavailability of iron from cereal-based diets in young women by use of in vitro and in vivo methods. Am J Clin Nutr 1990;52:373–378.
156. Fomon SJ, Janghorbani M, Ting BT, et al. Erythrocyte incorporation of ingested 58-iron by infants. Pediatr Res 1988;24:20–24.
157. Fomon SJ, Ziegler EE, Rogers RR, et al. Iron absorption from infant foods. Pediatr Res 1989;26:250–254.
158. Turnland JR. Stable isotope studies of the effect of dietary copper on copper absorption and excretion. Adv Exp Med Biol 1989;258:21–28.
159. Turnland JR, Keyes WR, Anderson HL, et al. Copper absorption and retention in young men at three levels of dietary copper by use of the stable isotope ^{65}Cu. Am J Clin Nutr 1989;49:870–878.
160. Ehrenkranz RA, Gettner PA, Nelli CM, et al. Zinc and copper nutritional studies in very low birth weight infants: comparison of stable isotopic extrinsic tag and chemical balance methods. Pediatr Res 1989;26:298–307.
161. August D, Janghorbani M, Young VR. Determination of zinc and copper absorption at three dietary Zn-Cu ratios

by using stable isotope methods in young adult and elderly subjects. Am J Clin Nutr 1989;50:14–57.
162. Serfass RE, Ziegler EE, Edwards BB, et al. Intrinsic and extrinsic stable isotopic zinc absorption by infants from formulas. J Nutr 1989;119:1661–1669.
163. Ziegler EE, Serfass RE, Nelson SE, et al. Effect of low zinc intake on absorption and excretion of zinc by infants studied with ^{70}Zn as extrinsic tag. J Nutr 1989;119:1647–1653.
164. Turnland JR, Durkin N, Costa F, et al. Stable isotope studies of zinc absorption and retention in young and elderly men. J Nutr 1986;116:1239–1247.
165. Janghorbani M, Marti RF, Kasper LJ, et al. The selenite-exchangeable metabolic pool in humans: a new concept for the assessment of selenium status. Am J Clin Nutr 1990;51:670–677.
166. Yergey AL, Abrams SA, Vieira NE, et al. Recent studies of human calcium metabolism using stable isotopic tracers. Can J Physiol Pharmacol 1990;68:973–976.
167. Price RI, Kent GN, Rosman KJ, et al. Kinetics of intestinal calcium absorption in humans measured using stable isotopes and high-precision thermal ionization mass spectrometry. Biomed Environ Mass Spectrom 1990;19:353–359.
168. Fairweather-Tait SJ, Johnson A, Eagles J, et al. Studies on calcium absorption from milk using a double-label stable isotope technique. Br J Nutr 1989;62:379–388.
169. Eastell R, Vieira NE, Yergey AL, et al. One-day test using stable isotopes to measure true fractional calcium absorption. J Bone Miner Res 1989;4:463–468.
170. Hillman LS, Tack E, Covell DG, et al. Measurement of true calcium absorption in premature infants using intravenous ^{46}Ca and oral ^{44}Ca. Pediatr Res 1988;23:589–594.
171. Moore LJ, Machlan LA, Lim MO, et al. Dynamics of calcium metabolism in infancy and childhood. I. Methodology and quantification in the infant. Pediatr Res 1985;19:329–334.
172. Smith DL, Atkin C, Westenfelder C. Stable isotopes of calcium as tracers: methodology. Clin Chim Acta 1985;146:97–101.
173. Ehrenkranz RA, Ackerman BA, Nelli CM, et al. Absorption of calcium in premature infants as measured with a stable isotope ^{46}Ca extrinsic tag. Pediatr Res 1985;19:178–184.
174. Schuette SA, Ziegler EE, Nelson SE, et al. Feasibility of using the stable isotope ^{25}Mg to study Mg metabolism in infants. Pediatr Res 1990;27:36–40.
175. Carson ER, Cobelli C, Finkelstein L. The mathematical modeling of metabolic and endocrine systems: model formulation, identification, and validation. New York: Wiley, 1983.
176. Cobelli C. Modeling and identification of endocrine-metabolic systems: theoretical aspects and their importance in practice. Math Biosci 1984;72:263–289.
177. Cobelli C, Carson ER, Finkelstein L, et al. Validation of simple and complex models in physiology and medicine. Am J Physiol 1984;246:R259–R266.
178. Shipley RA, Clark RE. Tracer methods for in vivo kinetics: theory and applications. Orlando: Academic Press, 1982.
179. DiStefano JJ III, Landaw EM. Multiexponential multicompartmental, and noncompartmental modeling. I. Methodological limitations and physiological interpretations. Am J Physiol 1984;246:R651–R664.
180. Landaw EM, DiStefano JJ III. Multiexponential, multicompartmental, and noncompartmental modeling. II. Data analysis and statistical consideration. Am J Physiol 1984;246:R665–R677.
181. Green MH, Green JB. The application of compartmental analysis to research in nutrition. Annu Rev Nutr 1990;10:41–61.
182. Cramp DG. Quantitative approaches to metabolism: the role of tracers and models in clinical medicine. New York: Wiley, 1982.
183. Finkelstein L, Carson ER. Mathematical modelling of dynamic biologial systems. 2nd ed. New York: Wiley, 1985.
184. Cobelli C, Toffolo G, Bier DM, et al. Models to interpret kinetic data in stable isotope tracer studies. Am J Physiol 1987;253:E551–E564.
185. Cobelli C, Toffolo G, Ferrannini E. A model of glucose kinetics and their control by insulin, compartmental and noncompartmental approaches. Math Biosci 1984;72:291–315.
186. Bergman RN, Ider YZ, Bowden CR, et al. Quantitative estimation of insulin sensitivity. Am J Physiol 1979;236:E667–E677.
187. Bergman RN. Toward physiologial understanding of glucose tolerance: minimal-model approach. Diabetes 1989;38:1512–1527.
188. Ader M, Bergman RN. Insulin sensitivity in the intact organism. Bailliere Clin Endocrinol Metab 1987;1:879–910.
189. Cutfield WS, Bergman RN, Menon RK, et al. The modified minimal model: application to measurement of insulin sensitivity in children. J Clin Endocrinol Metab 1990;70:1644–1650.
190. Finegood DT, Hramiak IM, Dupre J. A modified protocol for estimation of insulin sensitivity with the minimal model of glucose kinetics in patients with insulin-dependent diabetes. J Clin Endocrinol Metab 1990;70:1538–1549.
191. Johnston C, Raghu P, McCulloch DK, et al. β-Cell function and insulin sensitivity in nondiabetic HLA-identical siblings of insulin-dependent diabetics. Diabetes 1987;36:829–837.
192. Finegood DT, Warnock GL, Kneteman NM, et al. Insulin sensitivity and glucose effectiveness in long-term islet-autotransplanted dogs. Diabetes 1989;39:189–191.
193. Ader M, Agajanian T, Finegood DT, et al. Recombinant deoxyribonucleic acid-derived 22K- and 20K-human growth hormone generate equivalent diabetogenic effects during chronic infusion in dogs. Endocrinology 1987;120:725–731.
194. Avogaro A, Bristow JD, Bier DM, et al. Stable-label intravenous glucose tolerance test minimal model. Diabetes 1989;38:1048–1055.

2
Methodology for the Study of Metabolism: Breath Testing

Peter D. Klein and Hans Helge

The breath test based on the use of ^{13}C-labeled substrate offers the pediatric gastroenanterologist and other physicians interested in metabolism, an important metabolic and diagnostic tool. Because they are nonradioactive as well as noninvasive, they may be used safely in children in all stages of development, including the preterm neonate. The substrate is administered orally in most applications, and the breath samples required for isotopic determination can be collected from either an awake or sleeping subject. The ^{13}C breath test is characterized by the administration of a substrate in which a small labeled functional group is attached by a target bond. When an appropriate enzyme cleaves this bond, the functional group is released and rapidly metabolized to labeled CO_2, which can be detected in breath samples from the subject. Breath tests are conventionally divided into two categories: the endolytic test, which reflects organ targeted enzyme function, and the xenolytic test, which reflects enzyme activity of gastric or intestinal organisms.

Background and Origins of ^{13}C Breath Tests

Twenty-five years ago, breath tests were exemplified by measurement of fat malabsorption using ^{14}C-palmitic acid,[1] of lactase deficiency by ^{14}C-lactose,[2] detection of ^{14}C-bile salts deconjugation,[3] and metabolism of ^{14}C-pyruvate in various endocrinologic disorders.[4] In 1966, Dr. Bert Tolbert, then director of the Division of Biology and Medicine at the Atomic Energy Commission, undertook a program to reduce the cost of ^{13}C by expanding the market for its use. To implement this program, scientists were drawn from three of the Atomic Energy Commission National Laboratories: Dr. Walton Shreeve, a nuclear medicine specialist from Brookhaven; Dr. Peter Klein, an analytical biochemist from Argonne; Dr. Eugene Robinson, a physical chemist in charge of the isotope distillation facilities at Los Alamos; Dr. Donald Ott, a synthetic organic chemist at Los Alamos; and Dr. Nicholas Matwiyoff, a nuclear magnetic resonance expert from Los Alamos. In early meetings in 1968, Los Alamos was assigned responsibility for isotope production and synthesis of substrates, Brookhaven for the development of clinical applications, and Argonne for the development of the required analytical methodology.

The market strategy originally visualized by Tolbert was to improve the use of ^{13}C through the development of a breath test that required large quantities of labeled substrate. The test best suited to this purpose was deemed to be the oxidation of ^{13}C-glucose to differentiate the normal from the diabetic subject. As convoluted as this logic now seems, it served to establish a program of ^{13}C-labeled organic compound syntheses that supported many academic investigators over the years.

At that time, the measurement of ^{13}C abundance in CO_2 was still the domain of geochemists studying climatic records in tree rings or limestone deposits. Such determinations required the ability to measure the natural abundance of ^{13}C, nominally about 11,350 parts per million to within 0.1 part per million. This process first required the removal of water vapor and other atmospheric gases by cryogenic isolation of the CO_2 sample in liquid nitrogen. The thawed gas was then admitted to one side of a manometer in which its pressure was matched against that of a reference CO_2 sample of known isotopic composition. The sample and standard gases were admitted alternately to a dual-inlet gas-isotope ratio mass spectrometer in which the ratio of the $^{13}CO_2/^{12}CO_2$ ion beam intensities was compared to a reference standard. This process required purification of 2 to 5 ml CO_2 on a vacuum line and a measurement procedure, which permitted about one sample per hour to be analyzed.

Adaptation of this procedure to the analysis of clinical breath samples was undertaken by Dr. Dale Schoeller, then a postdoctoral fellow at Argonne. Schoeller first demonstrated that the natural variability of $^{13}CO_2$ in breath of fasting subjects was ±0.7‰ (parts per thousand $^{13}CO_2$) or approximately 8 ppm in total CO_2.[5] This finding signified that the measurement process could be derated to an accuracy of ±0.1‰ without loss of diagnostic resolution. Second, Schoeller and Klein[6] reported that breath samples could be collected and injected by syringe into evacuated test tubes (Vacutainers®) and stored for up to 6 weeks without change in isotopic composition. The Vacutainers®, which at that time were 50 ml in volume, provided the basis not only for the collection, storage, and transport of clinical samples, but also for automated sample withdrawal and mass spectrometric analysis. In 1979, Schoeller and Klein[7] described the first computer-controlled instrument for the automated cryogenic purification and isotopic analysis of breath CO_2 samples. Although the analysis of the initial sample required 40 minutes, subsequent samples were analyzed at intervals of 20 minutes. This system, which provided the basis of subsequent commercial instruments, had the capacity to analyze up to 80 samples per 24 hours.

In 1986, a British instrument manufacturer, Europa Scientific, introduced a new concept in gas-isotope ratio mass spectrometry with the Automated Breath Carbon Analyzer (ABCA). This concept embodied two advances: first, improved low-drift amplifiers and ion source controllers eliminated the need for within-measurement comparison of sample and standard; and second, a gas chromatographic separation of CO_2 from the other breath gases eliminated the cryogenic separation step. The helium stream carrying the CO_2 peak was introduced into the ion source, and the isotope ratio was measured during its elution. Every tenth sample was a standard gas sample, from which drift corrections could be applied if necessary. Most significantly, the analysis time was reduced to five minutes per sample. A later version of this instrument, the 20/20, further reduced the cycle time to less than 200 seconds. The resultant configuration now enabled a throughput of 130 to 140 samples in an 8-hour shift. As will be seen, these developments proved to be crucial in the establishment of centralized high volume ^{13}C breath test analysis facilities.

Categories of Proposed ^{13}C Breath Tests

Over the years, a variety of substrates has been employed to explore a number of organ functions (Table 2.1). To date, no tests based on these substrates are available outside the research laboratory; none has been approved by the U.S. Food and Drug Administration (FDA) and none is covered under any medical reimbursement sys-

TABLE 2.1. Categories of ^{13}C breath tests.

Organ	Function	Substrate	References
Liver	P_{450} mixed-function oxidase	Aminopyrine	8–21
Liver	P_{445} mixed-function oxidase	Caffeine	22–33
Liver	Mitochondrial	δ-Keto isocaproic acid	34
Liver	Bile salt production, oxidation	Palmitic acid	35–38
Pancreas	Lipase, fat absorption	Triglycerides	39–49
Stomach	Gastric emptying	Acetate, octanoic acid	50–58
Intestine	Bacterial overgrowth	Cholylglycine, xylose	59–61
Intestine	Transit time	Lactosylureide	62
Inborn error	Establish genotype	Phenylalanine, leucine, galactose	63–65

tem. One must conclude, therefore, that these tests make no significant contribution in the day-to-day management of the patient, which leads one to question whether the study of ^{13}C breath testing is a waste of time except as a theoretical tool.

The Emergence of a ^{13}C Breath Test with Commercial Potential

Until the mid-1980s, ^{13}C breath tests were used exclusively in the research setting. This circumstance was dictated by two factors: first, the lack of clinical access to $^{13}CO_2/^{12}CO_2$ isotope ratio measurements, and second, the lack of reimbursement for test use. The introduction of the Europa ABCA instrument greatly simplified and broadened the isotope ratio measurement process, but not until 1986 did breath tests begin to play a significant role in the diagnosis and treatment of patients.

The discovery in 1983 by Warren[66] of a "campylobacter-like organism" in biopsies of gastric and duodenal ulcers, and the championship of an infectious basis of ulcers by Marshall et al.[67] focused interest on the organism now designated *Helicobacter pylori*. This spiral organism, inhabiting the mucosal layer in the crypts of the gastric mucosa, induces an inflammatory response with leukocyte invasion of the mucosal cells. The gastritis, which is always present in *H. pylori* infection, gives rise to vacuolization and in susceptible individuals progresses to ulcer formation. Alternatively, the infection can progress to atrophic gastritis and eventually to gastric carcinoma.

In a 1994 Consensus Statement, the National Institutes of Health declared ulcers to be an infectious process associated with *H. pylori* and the World Health Organization has designated *H. pylori* as a Class I carcinogen.[10]

H. pylori is characterized by a high content of urease, which serves to protect it against the low pH of the stomach. Urea that passes from the bloodstream through the tight junctions in the crypt cell is hydrolyzed to form CO_2 and ammonia, and the ammoniacal plume surrounding the *H. pylori* raises the ambient pH to 5.

The first use of ^{13}C-urea in a breath test to detect the presence of *H. pylori* was described by Graham et al.[69] in 1987 and was widely reproduced by others in subsequent publications.[70-101] In this test, a baseline breath sample is collected before a 240-calorie meal is consumed to inhibit gastric emptying. A solution containing 125 mg of ^{13}C-urea is then consumed, and one or more postdose breath samples are collected. Today, one sample is collected 30 minutes after substrate ingestion. If *H. pylori* is present in the stomach, the organism will hydrolyze the urea and liberate labeled CO_2, which will be detected as an increase over the baseline abundance. A change as small as 2.4‰, or approximately 26 parts per million of $^{13}CO_2$, is evidence of active *H. pylori* infection.

The test is easy to perform, and many laboratories began to experiment with it in various applications. Use of the ^{13}C-urea breath test to reduce endoscopy costs by pharmaceutical companies that were conducting clinical therapy trials soon ballooned the demand for breath analyses. In April 1993, the first company established to produce breath test kits and analyze breath samples was incorporated by Baylor College of Medicine in Houston, Texas. The company, Meretek Diagnostics, obtained approval for the ^{13}C-urea breath test from the FDA on September 17, 1996, and began commercial sales in January 1997.

By the time FDA approval was obtained, a new environment for ^{13}C breath testing in the United States had been developed. Kits with which to administer the test could be shipped to the physician from a central warehouse. The kits included simplified directions for performance of the test in the physician's office, instructions for return of the breath samples by overnight express mail to the analysis facility, and assurance of prompt transmission of the test result by fax within 24 to 48 hours. This ensemble of components eliminated the need for local isotope ratio measurements and gave all physicians access to the test.

Use of the ^{13}C-urea breath test in Europe has relied much more heavily on measurements performed in the physician's office, chiefly because of the added revenue received by the physician. In addition to the Europa-type of gas-isotope ratio mass spectrometer, a variety of infrared devices have been introduced.[102,103] Although these instruments have a lower analytical precision than mass spectrometry, they have the advantages of lower cost in most cases, simpler operation, and the immediacy of results. The role that this technology will play in other breath test applications remains to be demonstrated.

Nevertheless, in Europe as well as the United States, the arrival of the ^{13}C-urea breath test has introduced a new generation of physicians to the concepts and benefits of this noninvasive diagnostic procedure

The Path from Research Probe to Clinical Tool

Given the length of time over which ^{13}C breath tests have been developing and the numbers of applications that have been proposed, it is appropriate to ask whether these tests have had any significant impact on the practice of medicine. At the present time, only the ^{13}C-urea breath test has FDA approval. Currently the FDA has determined that all subsequent breath tests will be classified as diagnostic devices having a drug component. This ruling means that there is a need for intra-agency cooperation to complete the approval process, but the Center for Device Evaluation and Radiological Health (CDERH) will have the primary responsibility.

The development of the ^{13}C-urea breath test provides a paradigm for the progressive transformation of a breath test from a research probe to an established clinical test. Four different steps were required: (1) establish the medical efficacy of the test, (2) obtain regulatory approval of the test, (3) assess financially how test use will affect costs of health care delivery, and (4) provide the economic resources required to market the test.

Establishment of Medical Efficacy

As stated above, ^{13}C breath tests have been classified by the FDA as diagnostic devices. Thus, any breath test proposed for approval must be compared to a predicate device or "gold standard" that represents the best available method of diagnosis of the condition for which the breath test is to be employed. In the case of the ^{13}C-urea breath test, this has been gastroendoscopic examination, biopsy, culture, and histologic examination. Alternative measures such as serology or in vitro urease assays (CLO test®), have been included, but are less effective in their discrimination abilities.

The efficacy of the test versus the predicate device is determined by simultaneous application of both measures in two groups, infected and noninfected subjects. It is preferable that these two groups be of equal size, which may introduce recruitment problems if there are no alternative indications for use of the invasive endoscopy procedure in otherwise asymptomatic subjects. Good statistical design considerations point to a study size of approximately 60 individuals in each category, or a total of 120 to 150 comparisons to the standard.

Four outcomes of this comparison are possible: the breath test may correctly identify patients with the infection (true positive, TP), those in which the infection is absent (true negative, TN), or falsely identify patients with the infection (false negative, FN) or falsely identify as positive patients in which the infection is absent (false positive, FP). From these outcomes it is possible to calculate the following parameters:

$$\text{Sensitivity} = TP/(TP+FN)$$
$$\text{Specificity} = TN/(TN+FP)$$
$$\text{Positive predictive value} = TP/(TP+FP)$$
$$\text{Negative predictive value} = TN/(TN+FN)$$
$$\text{Accuracy} = (TP+TN)/\text{Total}$$

Each of these measures has an uncertainty associated with it that is expressed as a range above and below the calculated value. For example, a study with a small number of uninfected subjects may have a specificity value of 0.95, but a confidence range from 0.50 to 0.99. To date, such measures have been reported almost exclusively on the ^{13}C-urea breath test, but limited reports on other substrates are now beginning to appear.

Another means of assessing the data is to generate what is called a receiver operational characterization (ROC) curve in which the number of true positives or true negatives is plotted against the value of the diagnostic measure used as a cutoff point. In such plots, a rectilinear curve rising steeply to a maximum and maintaining a plateau is indicative of a test with good discriminative ability.

It is at this stage in the development of a breath test that the first and most serious resource hurdle appears. The problem faced by the academic investigator is that organization and execution of such clinical trials is both complex and expensive. To provide meaningful data, the trial must be conducted in accordance with the rules of good clinical practice. These rules govern the manner in which records of patient selection, assignment, testing, and comparisons are maintained. Personnel with such specialized skills are usually available only to pharmaceutical companies that conduct drug evaluation studies. Moreover, experience has shown that without adequate financial support for their execution, it is extremely difficult to conduct clinical trials on a collaborative basis that meet rigorously defined standards. Ultimately, the quality of the trials will be determined and/or limited by the funds available for their execution. One figure of merit is that real costs per subject will seldom be less than $1000 and can easily reach $5000; for even the most efficiently organized trial, the cost is likely to be $500,000 or more. Under certain fortunate circumstances, it may be possible to find a planned or ongoing clinical drug trial in which the predicate device is being employed. Addition of a breath test as a "piggyback" procedure may entail minimal additional costs while deriving the benefits of the investments supporting the main protocol. Under the most sanguine circumstances, the trial sponsor may anticipate enough benefit from the breath test results to subsidize the test costs.

Regulatory Approval of the Test

In the United States, approval of a noninvasive device such as a breath test hinges primarily on its clinical efficacy and safety. In addition, the substrate must be produced in accordance with chemical, manufacturing, and control processes that follow what are called good manufacturing practices (GMPs). This means that the manufacturer must have demonstrated his experience in the synthesis or preparation of the substrate and must have in place the quality control procedures that identify the source and batch number of each ingredient used in substrate production. The manufacturer is required to prepare a certificate of analysis, which documents the chemical and isotopic purity of the product, using previously validated analytical methods, and is required to document the stability of the bulk substance under conventional and accelerated aging conditions.

The bulk substrate product must then undergo confirmatory analysis by an outside reference laboratory before it can be received by the facility in which doses are packaged. When the bulk material has been dispensed into individual units, six-month real time and accelerated stability studies of the packaged dose must be made. The substrate activity is then verified in release testing by the outside reference laboratory. The packaged substrate is then incorporated into the final kit together with the means of breath collection, storage, and sample return. Included in the kit is a sample box, individual Vacutainers®, a patient form with bar-coded identification, and a return shipping label. The kit contains test performance instructions and the label of the kit must include the indications for which its use is intended.

All suppliers and subcontractors in the kit production must be site-visited and must pass GMP inspections before approval is issued by the FDA. The entire approval process is theoretically completed within 60 working days after all required information has been supplied and accepted; recent statistics show a mean approval time of 105 days and the ^{13}C-urea breath test required more than 400 days.

Financial Assessment of the Impact of Test Use on Health Care Delivery Costs

Food and Drug Administration approval of a diagnostic procedure does not assure its adoption by the medical community. It is necessary to construct an algorithm for the disease process, its presentation, and differential diagnosis. In this algorithm, the costs and outcomes of alternatives to the test are compared with those in which the test is employed. The construction of such an algorithm takes into account the course followed by a prudent physician and identifies the cost savings and benefits from use of the test to the patient as well as to the physician. In today's market, both must benefit if the test is to be commercially successful.

Ultimately, reimbursement decisions stem from the deliberations of the technology assessment committees of the Health Care Finance Administration, the Blue Cross/Blue Shield organizations, and other major health care providers and insurers. Gaining access to these committees and presenting justification of the test use requires extensive experience and detailed knowledge of the health care industry.

Once reimbursement codes and costs have been established, development of the marketing plan is undertaken. The components include direct sales to individual physicians, provision to medical supply companies, marketing by clinical laboratory companies, and establishment of long-term contracts with major health care organizations. Alliances with larger corporate partners may also arise in the course of implementing the plan.

Economic Resources Required

From the description thus far, one can see that demonstrating clinical efficacy and obtaining regulatory approval to offer a breath test for use by physicians is neither simple, rapid, nor inexpensive. Although not explicitly stated previously, development of a test to this point soon exceeds the resources of an individual academic investigator. Supporting use of the test after approval, and preparing to market the test, requires an extensive infrastructure that includes capabilities for drug production and packaging, systems for kit manufacture, distribution and analysis, and the means to track and report patient results and, finally, to carry out physician/patient billing. These capabilities must be created without particular advantage for the first test to be successful, but fortunately all subsequent tests face a much lower threshold for their introduction.

After passing initial drug qualification tests for FDA approval, the manufacturer must produce three batches of the labeled compound, all of which meet the same standards, before kit production can take place. This is a further cost and time-consuming process. Kit manufacture is a less complicated process, but requires linkage of kit component records to an inventory by expiration dates, so that all components are of current manufacture. A unique bar code number links each kit to the sample tubes that it contains and to the patient record forms in the kit. This number provides the basis for tracking kit distribution, enables the instrument to recognize analytical samples, and is used to prepare patient reports and, eventually, billing records. All of these functions must also be anticipated in the design and organization of the management information system at the core facility.

The question arises as to where and how breath test samples should be analyzed. Two models exist for this process. The first is made possible by the advent of overnight express delivery and centralized facilities, which make it unnecessary to own a mass spectrometer to carry out breath tests; all that is required is to collect the samples in the designated tubes, drop them in the prepaid express envelope, and receive the results by fax within 48 hours. Preference for this model is reinforced by the emerging economy of scale in gas-isotope ratio mass spectrometer systems. With analysis cycle times approaching 100 seconds and annual outputs of 300,000 analyses per instrument, this process moves from the laboratory into an industrial setting.

The second model exploits the use of several non–mass spectrometric $^{13}CO_2$ isotope analysis instruments based on infrared or laser-assisted isotope ratio spectrometry for prices ranging from \$25,000 to \$100,000. At the present time in the United States, most physicians are disinclined to operate analytical instruments in their offices, given the requirements of the Clinical Laboratories Improvement Act (CLIA). This legislation requires that any diagnostic procedure carried out in a doctor's office must be performed by individuals with documented training and proficiency, who use standardized protocols that are periodically calibrated against reference materials. Given the existing load of regulatory compliance in the practice of medicine, most U.S. physicians may prefer to send their samples out for analysis.

The Future of ^{13}C Breath Tests and Their Application to Perinatology/Neonatology

One may ask whether other breath tests are likely to achieve the same general clinical use now realized in the application of the urea breath test for *H. pylori*. Inspection of the list given in Table 2.1 shows few candidates likely to find the type of widespread use that would justify the investment required for their commercial development.

Consider, for example, the attempt to determine the proportion of dietary fat malabsorbed and excreted from the amount consumed, a value that cannot be calculated from the amount absorbed and oxidized. Furthermore, correlations between results from breath tests using labeled triglycerides and from fecal fat excretion have not shown a stoichiometric equivalence, and most studies have required breath collections over a 12- to 24-hour period. The attendant personnel costs further reduce any perceived advantage over fecal fat measurements.

The time required to administer a breath test figures largely in its ultimate success. Numerous attempts have been made to reduce the duration of the urea breath test from the original 30 minutes to as few as 10 minutes. If a test is to be accepted into clinical practice, an upper limit of 120 minutes for test performance may be tolerated. Within this time interval, there are three candidates that may eventually become available in commercial form: (1) the assessment of liver function with aminopyrine, (2) solid-phase gastric emptying using a prepackaged meal that requires no cooking, and (3) the genotyping of individuals at risk of inborn errors of metabolism.

The aminopyrine breath test has demonstrated the ability to discriminate among at least three levels of liver injury, as documented by liver biopsy. Moreover, its assessment of the active hepatocyte mass of the liver is not provided by any other method or device. This test also has potential application in longitudinal monitoring of liver transplantation candidates to forecast the urgency of the procedure. Despite its recognized efficacy, the aminopyrine breath test has never been the subject of an organized clinical trial with an established protocol that could be translated into an FDA application. Such an application requires substrate production, stability studies, and documentation of the manufacturing process. After submission and approval of the Investigation of New Drug application, clinical trials may begin. This process is under way.

Solid-phase gastric emptying studies using a ^{13}C breath test have two inherent advantages over conventional radionuclide methods. In addition to the absence of radioactive exposure, elimination of reliance on a nuclear medicine imaging facility and the option of test performance in a doctor's office make development of this test particularly attractive. The obstacle remaining in the existing ^{13}C solid-phase gastric emptying tests with octanoic acid is (in addition to the availability of $^{13}CO_2$ breath measurements) the requirement that the meal be cooked on-site before the test can be administered. A standardized meal is needed, a meal that is reproducible, stable, readily accepted by patients, and can be shipped to the physician and stored until required.

All of the foregoing breath tests are oriented to infectious diseases, or to organ function disorders not commonly addressed by perinatologists or neonatologists. *H. pylori* is acquired in early childhood under low socioeconomic conditions, but not encountered in the neonatal nursery. Although feeding disorders are of increasing concern, even during the perinatal period, they usually are associated with liquid-phase emptying, and liver disease is usually linked with anatomic anomalies. At the present time, only assessment of genetic metabolic disorders lends itself to investigation with breath tests. The most promising candidate in this field is the measurement of whole-body galactose oxidation in the neonate found to be galactosemic by newborn heel-stick assays.[65] Through this assay, neonates who are found to have the S135L mutation lack the ability to oxidize galactose in their red blood cells. Such neonates, nevertheless, have essentially normal whole-body galactose oxidation. Functional assessment of enzyme impairment in this disease, as well as in inborn errors, such as maple syrup urine disease,[64] may aid in the management of such patients and in their outcome prediction. Because of the low frequency of instances in which such tests would be used, their commercialization would have to be developed under an orphan drug program.

The next decade will determine whether the ^{13}C urea breath test for *Helicobacter pylori* was a fluke of circumstances or the forerunner of a flood of applications. At this time, a quarter century after its inception, the ^{13}C breath test remains a singularity in medical practice.

References

1. Schwabe AD, Cozzett FJD, Bennett LR. Estimation of fat malabsorption by monitoring of expired radiocarbon dioxide after feeding a radioactive fat. Gastroenterology 1962;42:285–290.
2. Sasaki Y, Iio M, Kameda H, Ueda H, et al. Measurement of ^{14}C-lactose absorption in the diagnosis of lactase deficiency. J Lab Clin Med 1970;6:824–835.
3. Sherr HP, Sasaki Y, Newman A, et al. Detection of bacterial deconjugation of bile salts by a convenient breath-analysis technic. N Engl J Med 1971;285:656–661.
4. Shreeve WW, Cerasi E, Luft R. Metabolism of [2-^{14}C] pyruvate in normal, acromegalic and HGH-treated human subjects. Acta Endocrinol 1970;65:155–169.
5. Schoeller DA, Schneider JF, Solomons N, et al. Clinical diagnosis with the stable isotope ^{13}C in CO_2 breath tests: methodology and fundamental considerations. J Lab Clin Med 1977;90:412–421.
6. Schoeller DA, Klein PD. A simplified technique for collecting breath CO_2 for isotope ratio mass spectrometry. Biomed Mass Spectrom 1978;5:29–31.
7. Schoeller DA, Klein PD. A microprocessor-controlled mass spectrometer for the fully automated purification and isotopic analysis of breath CO_2. Biomed Mass Spectrom 1979;6:350–355.
8. Schneider JF, Schoeller DA, Nemchausky B, et al. Validation of $^{13}CO_2$ breath analysis as a measurement of demethylation of stable isotope-labeled aminopyrine in man. Clin Chim Acta 1978;84:153–162.
9. Goromaru T, Furuta T, Baba S, et al. Metabolic studies of aminopyrine in rat and man by using stable isotope tracer techniques. Chem Pharm Bull 1981;29:1724–1729.
10. Nau H, Rating D, Koch S, et al. Valproic acid and its metabolites: placental transfer, neonatal pharmacokinetics, transfer via mother's milk and clinical status in neo-

nates of epileptic mothers. J Pharmacol Exp Ther 1981; 219:768–777.
11. Irving CS, Schoeller DA, Nakamura KI, et al. The aminopyrine breath test as a measure of liver function. A quantitative description of its metabolic basis in normal subjects. J Lab Clin Med 1982;100:356–373.
12. Jager-Roman E, Rating D, Platzek T, et al. Development of N-demethylase activity measured with the ^{13}C-aminopyrine breath test. Eur J Pediatr 1982;139:129–134.
13. Schoeller DA, Baker AL, Monroe PS, et al. Comparison of different methods expressing results of the aminopyrine breath test. Hepatology 1982;2:455–462.
14. Rating D, Jager-Roman E, Nau H, et al. Enzyme induction in neonates after fetal exposure to antiepileptic drugs. Pediatr Pharmacol 1983;3:209–218.
15. Sakamoto A, Kakui S, Kawamura I, et al. Quantitative assessment of hepatic microsomal function by breath test using ^{13}C-aminopyrine. Jpn J Gastroenterol 1983;80:2603.
16. Shulman RJ, Irving CS, Boutton TW, et al. Effect of infant age on aminopyrine breath test results. Pediatr Res 1985;19:441–445.
17. Goodnight-White SJ, Miller CC, Haber SE, et al. Lactate kinetics in severe COPD. Implications of an abnormal aminopyrine breath test. Chest 1992;01:268S–273S.
18. Meyer-Wyss B, Renner E, Luo H, et al. Assessment of lidocaine metabolite formation in comparison with other quantitative liver function tests. J Hepatol 1993;19:133–139.
19. Guitton J, Souillet G, Riviere JL, et al. Action of methotrexate on cytochrome P-450 monooxygenases in rats. Study performed with [^{13}C]-aminopyrine micro breath test. Eur J Drug Metab Pharmacokinet 1994;19:119–124.
20. Mion F, Geloen A, Rousseau M, et al. Mechanism of carbon tetrachloride autoprotection: an in vivo study based on ^{13}C-aminopyrine and ^{13}C-galactose breath tests. Life Sci 1994;54:2093–2098.
21. Opekun AR, Klein PD, Graham DY. ^{13}C aminopyrine breath test detects altered liver metabolism caused by low-dose oral contraceptives. Dig Dis Sci 1995;40:2417–2422.
22. Arnaud MJ, Thelin-Doerner A, Ravussin E, et al. Study of the demethylation of [1,3,7-Me-^{13}C] caffeine in man using respiratory exchange measurements. Biomed Mass Spectrom 1980;7:521–524.
23. Brazier JL, Ribon B, Desage M, et al. Study of theophylline metabolism in premature human newborns using stable isotope labelling. Biomed Mass Spectrom 1980;7:189–192.
24. Kotake AN, Schoeller DA, Lambert GH, et al. The caffeine CO_2 breath test: dose response and route of N-demethylation in smokers and nonsmokers. Clin Pharmacol Ther 1982;32:261–269.
25. Lambert GH, Schoeller DA, Kotake AN, et al. The effect of age, gender, and sexual maturation on the caffeine breath test. Dev Pharmacol Ther 1986;9:375–388.
26. Pons G, Blais JC, Rey E, et al. Maturation of caffeine N-demethylation in infancy: a study using the $^{13}CO_2$ breath test. Pediatr Res 1988;23:632–636.
27. Levitsky LL, Schoeller DA, Lambert GH, et al. Effect of growth hormone therapy in growth hormone-deficient children on cytochrome P-450-dependent 3-N-demethylation of caffeine as measured by the caffeine $^{13}CO_2$ breath test. Dev Pharmacol Ther 1989;12:90–95.
28. Kruger N, Helge H, Neubert D. The significance of PCDD's/PCDF's (dioxins) in pediatrics. [German]. Monatsschr Kinderheilkd 1991;139:434–441.
29. Kruger N, Helge H, Neubert D. CO_2 breath tests using ^{14}C-caffeine, ^{14}C-methacetin and ^{14}C-phenacetin for assessing postnatal development of monooxygenase activities in rats and marmosets. Dev Pharmacol Ther 1991;16:164–175.
30. Lewis FW, Adair O, Hossack KF, et al. Plasma glucagon concentration in cirrhosis is related to liver function but not to portal-systemic shunting, systemic vascular resistance, or urinary sodium excretion. J Lab Clin Med 1991;117:67–75.
31. Rost KL, Brosicke H, Brockmoller J, et al. Increase of cytochrome P450IA2 activity by omeprazole: evidence by the ^{13}C-[N-3-methyl]-caffeine breath test in poor and extensive metabolizers of S-mephenytoin. Clin Pharmacol Ther 1992;52:170–180.
32. Rost KL, Brosicke H, Heinemeyer G, et al. Specific and dose-dependent enzyme induction by omeprazole in human beings. Hepatology 1994;20:1204–1212.
33. Rost KL, Roots I. Accelerated caffeine metabolism after omeprazole treatment is indicated by urinary metabolite ratios: coincidence with plasma clearance and breath test. Clin Pharmacol Ther 1994;55:402–411.
34. Lauterburg BH, Grattagliano I, Gmur R, et al. Noninvasive assessment of the effect of xenobiotics on mitochondrial function in human beings: studies with acetylsalicylic acid and ethanol with the use of the carbon 13-labeled ketoisocaproate breath test. J Lab Clin Med 1995;125:378–383.
35. Watkins JB, Klein PD, Schoeller DA, et al. Diagnosis and differentiation of fat malabsorption in children using ^{13}C-labeled lipids: trioctanoin, triolein, and palmitic acid breath tests. Gastroenterology 1982;82:911–917.
36. Arimoto K, Sakuragawa N, Suehiro M, et al. Abnormal ^{13}C-palmitate breath test in epileptic patients treated with valproic acid. Brain Dev 1986;18:354–359.
37. Park W, Paust H, Brosicke H, et al. Impaired fat utilization in parenterally fed low-birth-weight infants suffering from sepsis. J Parenter Enteral Nutr 1986;10:627–630.
38. Arimoto K, Sakuragawa N, Suehiro M, et al. Abnormal ^{13}C-fatty acid breath tests in patients treated with valproic acid. J Child Neurol 1988;3:250–257.
39. Watkins JB, Schoeller DA, Klein PD, et al. ^{13}C-trioctanoin: a nonradioactive breath test to detect fat malabsorption. J Lab Clin Med 1977;90:422–430.
40. Suehiro M, Yamada H, Iio M, et al. ^{13}C-trioctanoin breath test for diagnosis of fat malabsorption (author's transl). Jpn J Nucl Med 1981;18:211–214.
41. Paust H, Park W, Schroder H. Current status of parenteral feeding with fat infusions. Clinical experiences with premature and newborn infants. Infusionstherapie Klin Ernahr 1983;10:216–222.
42. Paust H, Park W, Brosicke H, et al. Fat utilization in newborn infants with and without heparin administration. Comparative study with the ^{13}C-triolein breath test. Infusionstherapie Klin Ernahr 1985;12:85–87.

43. Knoblach G, Paust H, Park W, et al. Determination of the oxidation rate of medium-chain triglycerides in newborn infants with the ^{13}C trioctanoin breath test. Monatsschr Kinderheilkd 1988;136:26–30.
44. Yamada T, Nishida H, Sakamoto S, et al. The effect of MCT oil supplement in very low birth weight infants, with evaluation by the ^{13}C-labeled MCT breath test. Acta Paediatr Jpn 1988;30:564–568.
45. Sulkers EJ, Lafeber HN, Sauer PJ. Quantitation of oxidation of medium-chain triglycerides in preterm infants. Pediatr Res 1989;26:294–297.
46. Vantrappen GR, Rutgeerts PJ, Ghoos YF, et al. Mixed triglyceride breath test: a noninvasive test of pancreatic lipase activity in the duodenum. Gastroenterology 1989; 96:1126–1134.
47. Murphy MS, Eastham EJ, Nelson R, et al. Non-invasive assessment of intraluminal lipolysis using a $^{13}CO_2$ breath test. Arch Dis Child 1990;65:574–578.
48. Hoshi J, Nishida H, Yasui M, et al. [^{13}C] breath test of medium-chain triglycerides and oligosaccharides in neonates. Acta Paediatr Jpn 1992;34:674–677.
49. Kato H, Nakao A, Kishimoto W, et al. ^{13}C-labeled trioctanoin breath test for exocrine pancreatic function test in patients after pancreatoduodenectomy. Am J Gastroenterol 1993;88:64–69.
50. Ghoos YF, Maes BD, Geypens BJ, et al. Measurement of gastric emptying rate of solids by means of a carbon-labeled octanoic acid breath test. Gastroenterology 1993;104:1640–1647.
51. Maes BD, Hiele MI, Geypens BJ, et al. Pharmacological modulation of gastric emptying rate of solids as measured by the carbon labelled octanoic acid breath test: influence of erythromycin and propantheline [published erratum appears in Gut 1994;35:866]. Gut 1994;35:333–337.
52. Maes BD, Ghoos YF, Rutgeerts PJ, et al. [*C]octanoic acid breath test to measure gastric emptying rate of solids. Dig Dis Sci 1994;39:104S–106S.
53. Maes BD, Ghoos YF, Geypens BJ, et al. Combined carbon-13-glycine/carbon-14-octanoic acid breath test to monitor gastric emptying rates of liquids and solids. J Nucl Med 1994;35:824–831.
54. Mossi S, Meyer-Wyss B, Beglinger C, et al. Gastric emptying of liquid meals measured noninvasively in humans with [^{13}C]acetate breath test. Dig Dis Sci 1994;39:107S–109S.
55. Braden B, Adams S, Duan LP, et al. The [^{13}C]acetate breath test accurately reflects gastric emptying of liquids in both liquid and semisolid test meals. Gastroenterology 1995;108:1048–1055.
56. Maes BD, Ghoos YF, Geypens BJ, et al. Influence of octreotide on the gastric emptying of solids and liquids in normal healthy subjects. Aliment Pharmacol Ther 1995;9:11–18.
57. Maes BD, Ghoos YF, Geypens BJ, et al. Relation between gastric emptying rate and energy intake in children compared with adults. Gut 1995;36:183–188.
58. Pfaffenbach B, Wegener M, Adamek RJ, et al. Noninvasive ^{13}C octanoic acid breath test for measuring stomach emptying of a solid test meal—correlation with scintigraphy in diabetic patients and reproducibility in healthy probands. Z Gastroenterol 1995;33:141–145.
59. Solomons N, Schoeller DA, Wagonfeld J, et al. Application of a stable isotope (^{13}C)-labeled glycocholate breath test to diagnose bacterial overgrowth and ileal dysfunction. J Lab Clin Med 1977;90:431–439.
60. King CE, Toskes PP. Breath tests in the diagnosis of small intestinal bacterial overgrowth. Crit Rev Clin Lab Sci 1984;21:269–281.
61. Pressman, JH Hofmann AF, Witztum KF, et al. Limitations of indirect methods of estimating small bowel transit in man. Dig Dis Sci 1987;32:689–699.
62. Heine WE, Berthold HK, Klein PD. A novel stable isotope breath test: ^{13}C labeled glycosylureides as noninvasive markers of intestinal transit time. Am J Gastroenterol 1995;90:93–98.
63. Thompson GN, Walter JH, Leonard JV, et al. In vivo enzyme selectivity in inborn errors of metabolism. Metabolism 1990;39:799–807.
64. Elsas LJ, Ellerine NP, Klein PD. Practical methods to estimate whole body leucine oxidation in maple syrup urine disease. Pediatr Res 1993;33:445–451.
65. Berry GT, Nissim I, Mazur AT, et al. In vivo oxidation of [^{13}C] galactose in patients with galactose-phosphate uridyltransferase deficiency. J Biochem Mol Med 1995; 96:158–165
66. Warren JR. Unidentified curved bacilli on epithelium in active chronic gastritis. Lancet 1983;2:1273–1275.
67. Marshall BJ, McGechie DB, Rogers PA, et al. Pyloric campylobacter infection and gastrointestinal disease. Med J Aust 1985;142:439–444.
68. NIH Consensus Conference: *Helicobacter pylori* in peptic ulcer disease. NIH Consensus Development Panel on *Helicobacter pylori* in Peptic Ulcer Disease. JAMA 1994;272:65–69.
69. Graham DY, Klein PD, Evans DJ Jr, et al. *Campylobacter pylori* detected noninvasively by the ^{13}C-urea breath test. Lancet 1987;1:1174–1177.
70. Rauws EA. Detecting *Campylobacter pylori* with the ^{13}C- and ^{14}C-urea breath test. Scand J Gastroenterol Suppl 1989;160:25–26.
71. Cooreman M, Hengels KJ, Krausgrill P, et al. ^{13}C-urea breath test as a non-invasive method for the detection of *Helicobacter (Campylobacter) pylori*. Dtsch Med Wochenschr 1990;115:367–371.
72. Ormand JE, Talley NJ, Carpenter HA, et al. [^{14}C]urea breath test for diagnosis of *Helicobacter pylori*. Dig Dis Sci 1990;35:879–884.
73. Bell GD, Powell K, Weil J, Harrison G, et al. ^{13}C-urea breath test for *Helicobacter pylori* infection [letter; comment]. Gut 1991;32:551–552.
74. Good DJ, Dill S, Mossi S, et al. Sensitivity and specificity of a simplified, standardized ^{13}C-urea breath test for the demonstration of *Helicobacter pylori*. Schweiz Med Wochenschr 1991;121:764–766.
75. Logan RP, Polson RJ, Misiewicz JJ, et al. Simplified single sample ^{13}C urea breath test for *Helicobacter pylori*: comparison with histology, culture, and ELISA serology. Gut 1991;32:1461–1464.

76. Lotterer E, Ramaker J, Ludtke FE, et al. The simplified ^{13}C-urea breath test—one point analysis for detection of *Helicobacter pylori* infection. Z Gastroentero l1991;29:590–594.
77. Hartman NG, Jay M, Hill DB, et al. Noninvasive detection of *Helicobacter pylori* colonization in stomach using [^{11}C]urea. Dig Dis Sci 1992;37:618–621.
78. Vandenplas Y, Blecker U, Devreker T, et al. Contribution of the ^{13}C-urea breath test to the detection of *Helicobacter pylori* gastritis in children. Pediatrics 1992;90:608–611.
79. Drumm B. *Helicobacter pylori* in the pediatric patient. [Review]. Gastroenterol Clin North Am 1993;22:169–182.
80. Ji J, Li XM, Jiang GH. Diagnosis of *Helicobacter pylori* infection by ^{13}C-urea breath test. Chin J Int Med 1993;32:170–172
81. Klein PD, Graham DY. Minimum analysis requirements for the detection of *Helicobacter pylori* infection by the ^{13}C-urea breath test. Am J Gastroenterol 1993;88:1865–1869.
82. Loffeld RJ, Stobberingh E, Arends JW. A review of diagnostic techniques for *Helicobacter pylori* infection. [Review]. Dig Dis 1993;11:173–180.
83. Lotterer E, Ludtke FE, Tegeler R, et al. The ^{13}C-urea breath test—detection of *Helicobacter pylori* infection in patients with partial gastrectomy. Z Gastroenterol 1993;31:115–119.
84. Lotterer E, Ludtke FE, Tegeler R, et al. The ^{13}C-urea breath test, *Helicobacter pylori* infection, and the operated stomach [letter]. J Clin Gastroenterol 1993;16:82–84.
85. Moulton-Barrett R, Triadafilopoulos G, Michener R, et al. Serum ^{13}C-bicarbonate in the assessment of gastric *Helicobacter pylori* urease activity. Am J Gastroenterol 1993;88:369–374.
86. Adamek RJ, Freitag M, Labenz J, et al. The modified ^{13}C-urea breath test in the diagnosis of *Helicobacter pylori* colonization of the gastric mucosa. Dtsch Med Wochenschr 1994;119:1569–1572.
87. Alcalde M, Perez Garcia JI, Sanchez P, et al. Usefulness of the breath test with urea-^{13}C in the diagnosis of *Helicobacter pylori* infection. Med Clin 1994;103:371–373.
88. Blecker U, Lanciers S, Keppens E, et al. Evolution of *Helicobacter pylori* positivity in infants born from positive mothers. J Pediatr Gastroenterol Nutr 1994;19:87–90.
89. Braden B, Duan LP, Caspary WF, et al. More convenient ^{13}C-urea breath test modifications still meet the criteria for valid diagnosis of *Helicobacter pylori* infection. Z Gastroenterol 1994;32:198–202.
90. Braden B, Haisch M, Duan LP, et al. Clinically feasible stable isotope technique at a reasonable price: analysis of ^{13}CO$_2$/^{12}CO$_2$-abundance in breath samples with a new isotope selective-nondispersive infrared spectrometer. Z Gastroenterol 1994;32:675–678.
91. Klein PD, Gilman RH, Leon-Barua R, et al. The epidemiology of *Helicobacter pylori* in Peruvian children between 6 and 30 months of age. Am J Gastroenterol 1994;89:2196–2200.
92. Mion F, Delecluse HJ, Rousseau M, et al. ^{13}C-urea breath test for the diagnosis of *Helicobacter pylori* infection. Comparison with histology. Gastroenterol Clin Biol 1994;18:1106–1111.
93. Reinauer S, Goerz G, Ruzicka T, et al. *Helicobacter pylori* in patients with systemic sclerosis: detection with the ^{13}C-urea breath test and eradication. Acta Dermatol Venereol 1994;74:361–363.
94. Atherton JC, Washington N, Blackshaw PE, et al. Effect of a test meal on the intragastric distribution of urea in the ^{13}C-urea breath test for *Helicobacter pylori*. Gut 1995;36:337–340.
95. Caspary WF. ^{13}C-urea breath test. Patient-friendly gold standard in the diagnosis of *Helicobacter pylori* infection with long term cost control potential. Dtsch Med Wochenschr 1995;120:976–978.
96. Cutler AF, Havstad S, Mac K, et al. Accuracy of invasive and noninvasive tests to diagnose *Helicobacter pylori* infection. Gastroenterology 1995;109:136–141.
97. Koletzko S, Haisch M, Seeboth I, et al. Isotope-selective non-dispersive infrared spectrometry for detection of *Helicobacter pylori* infection with ^{13}C-urea breath test. Lancet 1995;345:961–962.
98. Nakagawa T, Ohara H, Yamamoto M, et al. ^{13}C-urea breath test for the detection of *Helicobacter pylori* infection and the assessment of therapeutic effect. Jpn J Gastroenterol 1995;92:264.
99. Slomianski A, Schubert T, Cutler AF. [^{13}C]urea breath test to confirm eradication of *Helicobacter pylori*. Am J Gastroenterol 1995;90:224–226.
100. Wildgrube HJ. The ^{13}C-urea breath test in *Helicobacter pylori* colonization of the gastric mucosa (letter). Dtsch Med Wochenschr 1995;120:940–942.
101. Yamashiro Y, Oguchi S, Otsuka Y, et al. *Helicobacter pylori* colonization in children with peptic ulcer disease. III. Diagnostic value of the ^{13}C-urea breath test to detect gastric H. pylori colonization. Acta Paediatr Jpn 1995;37:12–16.
102. Braden B, Haisch M, Duan LP, et al. Clinically feasible stable isotope technique at a reasonable price: analysis of ^{13}CO$_2$/^{12}CO$_2$-abundance in breath samples with a new isotope selective-nondispersive infrared spectrometer. Z. Gastroenterol 1994;12:675–678.
103. Koletzko S, Haisch M, Seeboth I, et al. Isotope-selective nondispersive infrared spectrometry for detection of *Helicobacter pylori* infection with the ^{13}C-urea breath test. Lancet 1995;345:961–962.

3
Methodology for the Study of Metabolism: Analyses of Proteins, Peptides, and Small Molecules

Jacob A. Canick

The ability to measure extremely low concentrations of biologically active molecules in fluid and tissue has enhanced the study of perinatal and neonatal metabolism as it has every other area of biology and medicine. Metabolic processes and biologic regulatory mechanisms are intimately connected, making the measurement of hormones and other biologic agents crucial to the study of metabolism. Even a cursory review of this textbook indicates the key role that such measurements have in a discussion of endocrine, paracrine, and/or autocrine effectors. To measure such effector molecules, both large and small, the technique of immunoassay is most commonly utilized, in which an antibody or group of antibodies can recognize and bind the molecule of interest with high specificity and great sensitivity.

The use of antibodies as a tool to measure specific biological molecules was developed by Solomon Berson and Rosalyn Yalow in the late 1950s during the course of their investigation of insulin-dependent diabetes mellitus. They showed that certain patients who were taking porcine insulin to treat their diabetes were requiring increasing doses of the drug because the patients were developing antibodies against the foreign protein, i.e., their immune systems were responding to the injected porcine insulin. Berson and Yalow made a major intellectual leap by extending these findings into a proposal that antibodies produced by immunizing animals to a foreign antigen could be used to develop in vitro systems to measure that antigen. In 1959, they reported on the first immunoassay for the measurement of insulin,[1,2] and during the next few years, they developed various other immunoassays to measure a variety of protein hormones.[3-5] Soon, methods were developed to produce antibodies against small, nonantigenic molecules, such as amines and steroids, so that both large and small ligand molecules could be measured by immunoassay. Rosalyn Yalow was awarded the Nobel Prize in Medicine in 1975 for developing the method of immunoassay. Unfortunately, Solomon Berson died a few years before the prize was awarded.

Initially, immunoassays were designed as competitive binding assays, in which labeled and unlabeled forms of a particular ligand competed for binding to its antibody. Ligand-antibody complexes are separated from free ligand, and the amount of bound label that is measured is inversely proportional to the concentration of the unlabeled ligand. The first method of labeling was radiolabeling, in which a radioisotope was added to or inserted into the ligand molecule, and the first separation techniques involved precipitation and centrifugation. Assay design methods have expanded markedly in the decades since the first immunoassays were introduced, thanks in part to the development of monoclonal antibodies, alternative nonisotopic labeling systems, and the use of solid-phase supports for the immobilization of both ligands and antibodies. The original competitive binding design is still an important and widely used immunoassay format, especially for the measurement of small molecules, and is described in detail below. The newer immunometric design, which in its most common format is known as a sandwich or two-site assay, is now the method of choice for the measurement of large molecules, and is also described below.

This chapter includes a description of the theory and practice of immunoassay although exhaustive discussions have been published elsewhere.[6-13] This chapter provides students and investigators in perinatal and neonatal metabolism with the essentials needed to understand and intelligently implement appropriate assays for future studies. The focus will be on quantitative immunoassay procedures. Qualitative and in situ immunotechniques such as immunoelectrophoresis, Western blotting, and immunohistochemistry are discussed in Chapter 4.

Goals in Immunoassay Development and Design

The goal in the development and design of any assay, whether it is chemically, enzymatically, or immunologically based, is to optimize its sensitivity, specificity, and precision.

Sensitivity is defined as the minimum amount of analyte that can be measured in an assay. Usually, but not always, the goal is to develop an assay with as high a sensitivity as possible. However, the degree of assay sensitivity that needs to be attained can vary, depending on the range of analyte concentrations expected in the study and the relative importance of defining so-called nondetectable analyte concentrations. For example, during pregnancy, maternal serum human chorionic gonadotropin (hCG) concentration increases from less than $2\,mIU\cdot ml^{-1}$ at the time of implantation to between 10,000 and $100,000\,mIU\cdot ml^{-1}$ by the end of the first trimester. If we want to detect pregnancy as early as possible, high sensitivity is the goal. If, instead, we wish to measure second or third trimester hCG concentration for purposes of prenatal genetic screening, clearly we do not need a high-sensitivity hCG assay.[14]

Specificity is defined as the ability of the assay to measure only the targeted analyte, as determined by the degree of cross-reactivity of structurally similar analytes in the assay. Again, the stringency of specificity requirements is governed by the types and concentration of structurally similar molecules or by the number of metabolic forms of the analyte that may be present in test samples. For example, increased antibody specificity has allowed better discrimination between the structurally related anterior pituitary hormone luteinizing hormone (LH), and the placental hormone hCG.[15] In another example, measurement of parathyroid hormone (PTH) will differ depending on the portion of the hormone molecule targeted by the assay (see Chapter 40).

Precision is defined as the degree of variability of the assay result. It is usually expressed as the ratio of the standard deviation of the result to the mean value obtained, the so-called coefficient of variation (CV) of the assay. Both the within-assay (intraassay) CV, which describes the ability of that assay to produce the same result, and the between-assay (interassay) CV, which describes the ability of separate assays to produce the same result, can be calculated. With immunoassay, intra- and interassay CVs of less than 10% are considered acceptable. More and more, CVs of less than 5% are becoming the norm as immunoassay technology improves. For comparison, excellent precision in the measurement of general chemistry analytes like glucose and sodium, with CVs of less than 5%, has been the norm for many years.

Antibody Production

The development of a good immunoassay rests primarily on the ability to produce a good antibody or antiserum. Antibodies used in immunoassays are predominantly of the immunoglobulin G (IgG) type, synthesized by activated B lymphocytes in response to stimulation of the humoral immune system. Structurally, the IgG molecule consists of four protein subunits, two so-called light chains and two so-called heavy chains, forming a mirror image structure as shown in Figure 3.1. The antigen binding region is at the N-terminal, Fab (antigen binding fragment) region.

Antibody preparations used in immunoassays currently are either polyclonal or monoclonal. Polyclonal antibodies are the secretion products of the immune response in a host animal, consisting of a mixture of individual antibodies from many clonal lines of B cells. Serum containing the mix of polyclonal antibodies can be used as is, or can be partially purified to obtain an enriched IgG fraction and affinity purified to reduce the concentrations of less specific antibody species. In contrast, monoclonal antibodies are the discrete products of B cell clonal lines that have been immortalized by fusion with a malignant cell, forming a so-called hybridoma. The

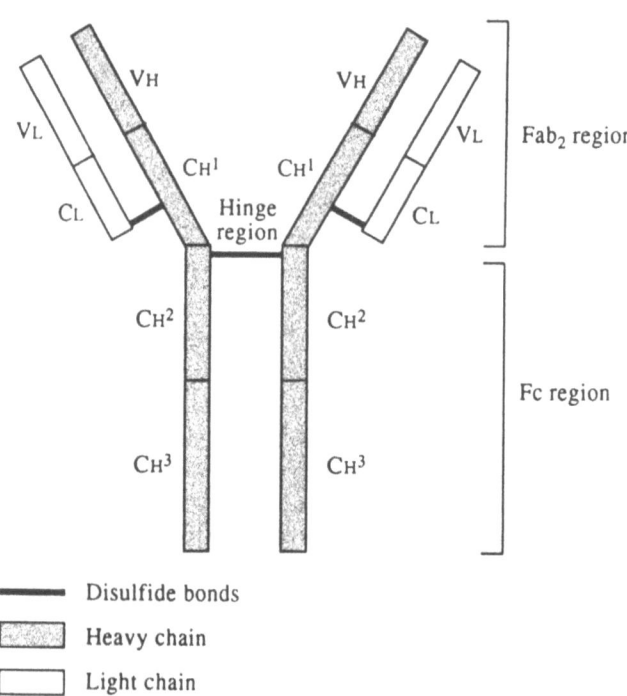

FIGURE 3.1. Immunoglobulin G (IgG) structure: Fab_2 region, antibody-binding site region; Fc region, crystallizable region; V_H, variable domain on the heavy chain; V_L, variable domain on the light chain; C_H^1, C_H^2, C_H^3, constant domains on the heavy chain; C_L, constant domain on the light chain. (From Davies,[64] with permission.)

development of hybridoma technology and the ability to isolate monoclonal antibodies is the result of research by Cesar Milstein and George Kohler,[16,17] for which they were awarded the Nobel Prize in 1984, and has represented the next major step in improving immunoassay methodology.

Antibodies for immunoassay are produced when an immunogen is introduced into a host species. For polyclonal antibody production a rabbit or goat often provides the best results. For monoclonal antibody production, a particular mouse strain is commonly used because the fusion protocol is well characterized and highly efficient. An immunogen, by definition, must be material that can provoke a strong antigenic response. Theoretically, any protein or other large macromolecule taken from one species can elicit a host response when injected into another species. In practice, not all proteins are good immunogens by themselves. In addition, small molecules like peptides, amines, and steroids, are not immunogenic. To provoke an immune response to such nonantigenic or poorly antigenic molecules, the host must be tricked by covalently linking these molecules to a more immunogenic molecule like bovine serum albumin.[18,19] Some large and all small antigens are then mixed with a so-called adjuvant preparation, composed of insoluble, highly inflammatory material designed to boost the immune response, and this preparation is injected into the host, usually subcutaneously, in graded doses over a set time frame.

Antibody Characterization

A good antibody preparation is a valuable commodity. Too often, no matter how precisely immunization procedures are followed, the end results are frustrating, producing antibody preparations that lack one or more of the three required performance characteristics: high titer, high affinity, and high specificity.

Antibody titer describes the concentration of antibody in a particular serum preparation, and is defined in terms of the dilution of the serum preparation required to achieve appropriate assay performance. When antibodies are present in a blood sample taken from the host, they are in limited supply. Therefore, the higher the titer, the more antibody is available for use. A good titer might be in the range of 1:10,000 to 1:100,000, meaning that a few milliliters of antiserum will produce many liters of usable reagent. Lower titers are not necessarily without use, especially if such preparations exhibit high sensitivity and specificity.

Antibody sensitivity or affinity refers to the affinity of the antibody for its antigen and is important in determining whether a particular antibody preparation will be able to measure low concentrations of the antigen. Affinity is expressed quantitatively as the molar dissociation constant (K_d) and is defined as the concentration of antigen at which half maximal binding to the antibody is observed at equilibrium. The K_d is calculated by Scatchard analysis as the plot of the ratio of free over bound antigen versus bound antigen concentration, just as affinity constants are determined for receptor-ligand interactions. Note that the K_d is analogous to the Michaelis constant (K_m) in enzyme kinetics, defined as the concentration of substrate at which there is half maximal velocity. When determining the affinity of a polyclonal antibody preparation made up of a mix of many different specific antibodies, the observed K_d will be an average of the various component affinities, and the Scatchard plot will rarely be a straight line. In the case of a monoclonal antibody, Scatchard analysis should yield a straight line from which the K_d can easily be calculated (see Chapter 4).

Generally, affinity constants should be in the range of 10^{-8} M or less in order to measure the low concentrations of hormones and other effector molecules that are usually found in fluid and tissue. For some hormones, the analogy of measuring a cube of sugar dissolved in a pond indicates the exquisite sensitivity that immunoassay can achieve.

Specificity refers to the differential binding affinity of an antibody for the particular antigen molecule it was intended to measure versus the antibody's ability to recognize molecules of similar but not identical structure. The more specific the antibody, the less concern there is that structurally similar molecules will contribute to the quantitative measurement of the particular analyte under consideration. For example, the anterior pituitary subunit hormones, LH, follicle-stimulating hormone (FSH), and thyroid stimulating hormone (TSH), and the placental subunit hormone, hCG, have almost identical α subunit and similar β subunit peptide sequences. Therefore, to differentially measure each of these hormones, antibodies that recognize unique epitopes on the β subunits of each of these hormones must be selected. In another example, the major estrogen of pregnancy, estriol, is structurally very similar to other important estrogens, estradiol and estrone, which also are increased during pregnancy. Therefore, an antibody used to measure estriol must have high affinity for estriol and comparatively low affinity for estradiol and estrone.

Cross-reactivity is the quantitative expression of specificity, and is experimentally determined through binding studies. It most commonly is calculated by determining the concentration of the intended analyte that produces 50% binding to the antibody, and dividing that by the concentration at which the cross-reacting analyte also produces 50% binding. The final result is expressed as a percentage by multiplying the ratio by 100. If the cross-reacting analyte and the intended analyte both give

50% binding at the same concentration, then the cross-reactivity is 100%. If the concentration of cross-reacting analyte that gives 50% binding is 100 times that of the intended analyte, then the cross-reactivity is 1%. Clearly, measurable cross-reactivity is not acceptable when cross-reacting and intended analytes are present in similar concentrations or especially when the cross-reacting analyte is present in higher concentration than the intended analyte. However, even a high degree of cross-reactivity may be perfectly acceptable if the cross-reacting analyte is always present in very low concentrations relative to the intended analyte.

Components of Immunoassay Design

The major choices in immunoassay design are the type of assay (i.e., competitive binding vs immunometric or noncompetitive), the method of separation of components (i.e., solid vs liquid phase), and the system of signaling (i.e., radioisotopic vs various nonisotopic methods). Decisions on which choices to make are determined by what type and size of analyte is to be measured, what level of sensitivity is needed, whether radioisotope measurement is acceptable, and what type of instrumentation is available in the laboratory.

Type of Assay

There are the two basic types of immunoassay format: competitive, in which labeled and unlabeled antigen compete for binding to a limited amount of antibody; and immunometric, in which antigen is bound to an antibody-coated solid phase and marked for measurement by a second antibody, which has a signal generator attached.

Competitive Immunoassay

Competitive binding immunoassay was originally developed by Berson and Yalow for the determination of insulin concentration and is still commonly used for the measurement of all types of analytes (Figure 3.2).[20] A limited amount of antibody is incubated with a fixed amount of labeled antigen and a sample containing unlabeled antigen, either as a calibration standard, a known control sample, or as a patient sample. The key to competitive assay is that the amount of antibody in the incubation is not enough to bind all the antigen that is added, so that competition between labeled and unlabeled antigen for limited binding sites can occur. After the binding reaction reaches equilibrium, the antigen-antibody complexes, the bound material, are separated from the remaining free antigens and antibody and the bound signal is quantified. The various separation methods are described in the next section. The higher the level of unlabeled antigen that is present in the sample, the less labeled antigen can bind to the antibody. Thus, the amount of labeled antigen-antibody complex is inversely proportional to the amount of unlabeled antigen in the sample.

With competitive immunoassay, a set of calibration standards containing increasing amounts of unlabeled

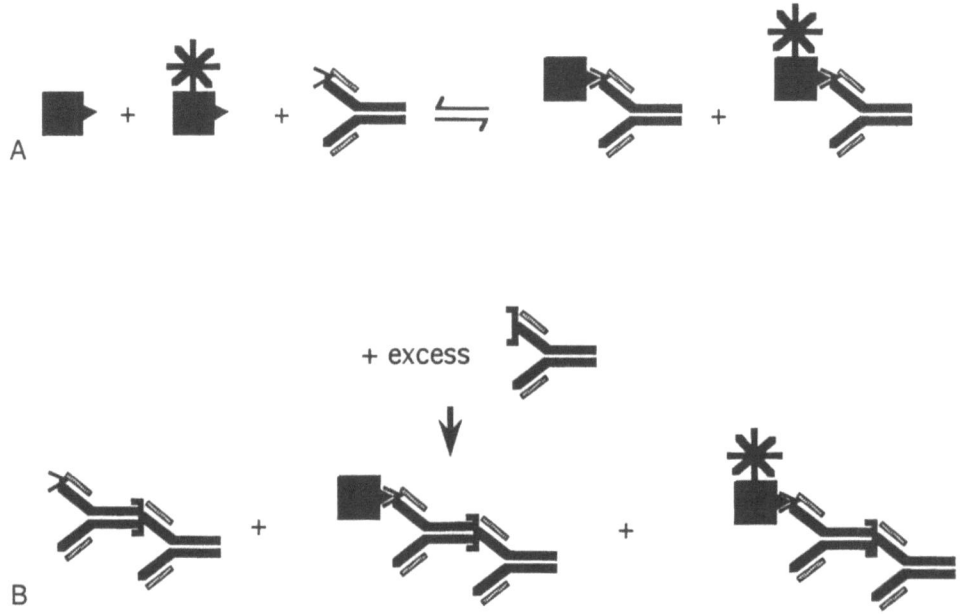

FIGURE 3.2. Competitive immunoassay design. (A) Incubation step: labeled and unlabeled antigen compete for binding to a limited quantity of primary antibody. (B) Separation step: excess second antibody, directed against the primary antibody, causes precipitation of the labeled antigen-primary antibody complex along with all species that have the primary antibody.

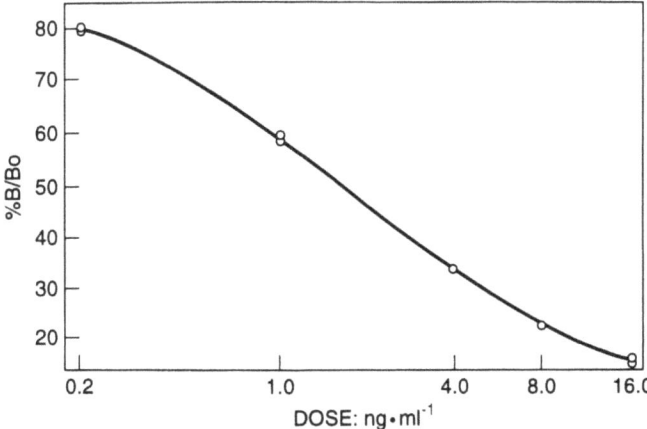

FIGURE 3.3. Example of a standard curve from a competitive radioimmunoassay in which the male sex hormone, testosterone, is measured. In this format, testosterone in the sample competes for binding to a limiting amount of antiserum with a known amount of ^{125}I-labeled testosterone. The more testosterone there is in the sample, the less labeled testosterone can bind to the antiserum, generating a standard curve with a downward slope. The data reduction format for this assay was four parameter logistics.

antigen will generate a standard curve with a downward slope. By convention, the standard curve will be a plot of calibrator concentrations on the x-axis and the percentage of maximum binding of labeled antigen to the antibody on the y-axis. The example shown in Figure 3.3 is a standard curve for the radioimmunoassay of testosterone. Note that the calibrator concentrations are plotted on a logarithmic scale to better show the sigmoid shape of the inverse relationship between increasing amount of calibrator and decreasing amount of radiolabel bound to antibody. Note as well that each calibrator sample is assayed in duplicate to produce better precision. The best fit curve is generated using a data reduction method known as four-parameter logistics.[21,22] This curve-fitting method best accounts for the biologic basis of antibody-antigen interactions in estimating maximum and minimum binding, as well as the steepness of the slope and calculation of curve symmetry. Most assays conform to this type of curve generating method.

Competitive immunoassay is often limited in the range of analyte concentrations it can measure because of the constraints of small amounts of antibody. However, it is the assay of choice for measuring small molecules because size constraints of such analytes will allow only one antibody or one polyclonal antiserum to interact with them at any one time.

Immunometric Assays

The idea of noncompetitive immunoassay or immunometric assay began in the late 1960s with the proposal that labeled antibodies rather than labeled antigen could be used in developing assays with greater sensitivity and precision.[23] Immunometric assay design benefited greatly from the introduction of monoclonal antibody technology. Monoclonal antibodies could be produced in essentially endless supply and allowed unprecedented targeting of specified sites (i.e., epitopes) on high molecular weight analytes. Specific polyclonal antibodies are also used successfully in immunometric assays, often paired with monoclonal antibodies. Immunometric assays differ from competitive binding assays in two basic ways: first, antibody rather than antigen is labeled with signal; and second, antibodies are added in excess rather than in limited supply, allowing antigen-antibody binding to proceed to completion.

Immunometric assays are most commonly developed in a two-site format, in which two antibody preparations are used.[24] One is bound to a solid-phase support and serves to capture the intended analyte, and the other is in solution and has a reporter or signal molecule attached to it. In this way, a highly specific sandwich is formed, with the antigen in the middle and the solid phase and signal antibodies on either side. Such assays can exhibit exceptional specificity because two different antibodies are used, each of which can be selected for its high specificity for the particular antigen.

Sample binding can be accomplished in one or two steps. In the one-step procedure, both sample and signal antibody are added at the same time to the vessel containing the solid-phase antibody (Figure 3.4). After a carefully timed incubation during which all or a portion of the antigen is bound in a sandwich, reagents remaining in solution are washed out. Reporting molecules are either added at this time, or if already present, appropriately quantified. In the two-step procedure, sample alone is first incubated with the solid-phase antibody, reagents

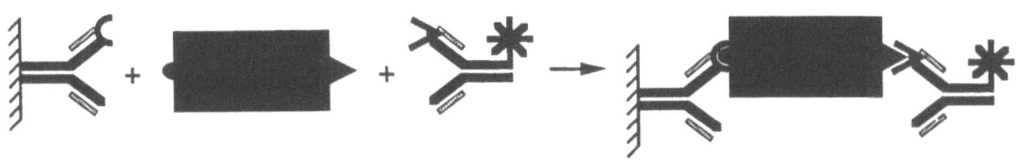

FIGURE 3.4. Immunometric one-step assay design. Excess solid-phase antibody and signal antibody are incubated simultaneously with the antigen-containing sample, after which excess sample and signal antibody are washed out and the bound signal is measured.

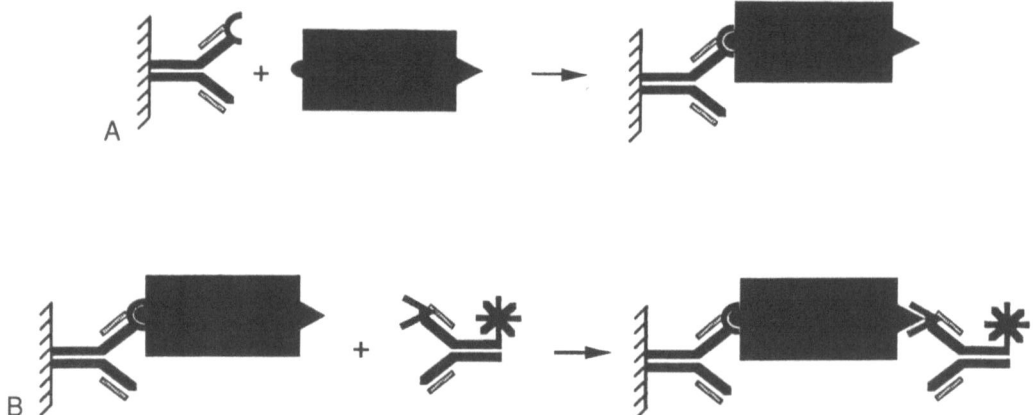

FIGURE 3.5. Immunometric two-step assay design. (A) The antigen-containing sample is incubated with the solid-phase antibody. After incubation, washing steps remove any unbound antigen. (B) The solid-phase antibody-antigen complex is incubated with excess signal antibody to form a sandwich. After incubation, excess unbound signal antibody is washed out and the bound signal is measured.

still in solution are washed out, and then signal antibody is added and will form a sandwich with antigen that was bound in the first step (Figure 3.5). One-step immunometric assays are fast, but by incubating both antibodies simultaneously may display the so-called hook effect.[25] In such a case, a particular sample that contains an unusually high concentration of analyte may display spuriously low apparent binding because, with so much analyte present, separate analyte molecules will bind to the solid-phase antibodies and the signal antibodies, thus preventing a sandwich from being formed. In contrast, while two-step assays require more washing and pipetting steps, they will avoid the possibility of underestimating the analyte concentration because the excess antigen will be washed out before the second antibody is added.

The signal generated in an immunometric assay is directly proportional to the amount of analyte in the sample. Most commonly, the standard curve that is generated will be a plot of calibrator concentration on the x-axis versus the amount of signal bound to the solid phase on the y-axis. In the example shown in Figure 3.6, a two-step immunometric assay in an enzyme-linked immunosorbent assay (ELISA) format was used to measure the gonadal glycoprotein hormone, inhibin A. In

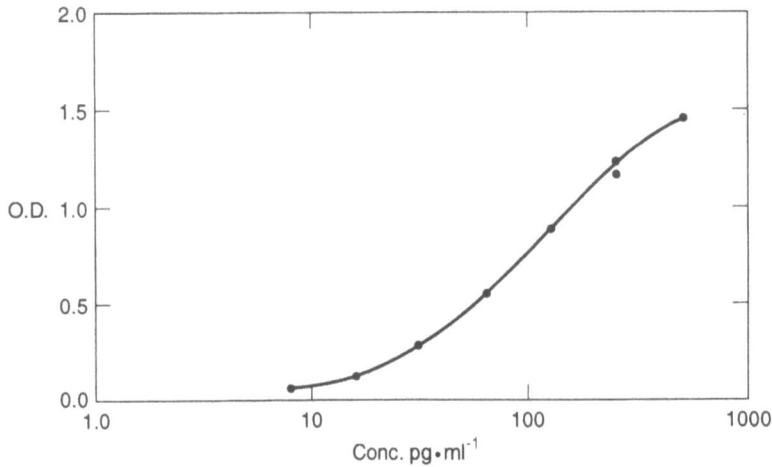

FIGURE 3.6. Example of a standard curve from a two-step immunoenzymetric ELISA format in which the gonadal hormone, inhibin A, is measured. In the first step, inhibin A, an α, β subunit glycoprotein, is captured by a solid-phase antibody that binds to an epitope on the inhibin A β subunit. In the second step, the signal antibody, which has alkaline phosphatase bound covalently linked to it, binds to an epitope on the inhibin A α subunit, forming a sandwich with intact inhibin A. After extensive wash steps, enzyme substrate is added and a blue color is generated. Increasing absorbance is proportional to increasing concentrations of inhibin A. The data reduction format for this assay was four parameter logistics.

contrast to a competitive assay curve, the generation of bound signal increases with addition of increasing amounts of sample. The curve fitting method used in this case was four-parameter logistics, the same method that was used to fit the competitive assay curve (Figure 3.3). Immunometric assays can be designed to be highly sensitive, depending on the activity of the signal reagent and the affinities of the selected antibodies, and often exhibit a wide analytical range limited for the most part by how much solid-phase antibody can be included in the incubation.

Separation Methods

Once the antigen-antibody reaction has taken place, whether in a competitive or immunometric format, the amount of signal in the bound complex must be measured. To do this, the antigen-antibody complex must first be separated from the remaining unbound signal. With the competitive assay format, there is a choice of separation formats, the traditional liquid-phase assay and the newer solid-phase assay. In contrast, immunometric assays are almost always in a solid-phase format. With an almost endless array of solid-phase systems to choose from today, we will focus on a few of the more common types: coated tubes, polystyrene beads, magnetic particles, and the most popular format for in-house solid phase immunoassay, the microtiter plate ELISA.

In a liquid-phase competitive assay, all the initial incubation components, labeled and unlabeled antigen sources, and antibody preparation, are in solution. After equilibrium is attained, the antigen-antibody complex that is still in solution can be precipitated by adding a variety of reagents to the incubation (Figure 3.2). Most typically, a so-called second antibody, also called the precipitating antibody, is added.[26] This antibody has been raised against gamma globulin from the species in which the primary antibody was raised. For example, if the primary antibody in the incubation was raised in rabbit, then the precipitating antibody would be an anti-rabbit gamma globulin antibody preparation raised in another species, typically sheep or goat. The antigen-antibody–second antibody complex tends to be insoluble and can be pelleted by centrifugation. Often, polyethylene glycol, a reagent that by binding to proteins prevents water molecules from interacting with the hydrophilic moieties on the proteins, is added to the second antibody preparation to assist in speeding up the precipitation step and in stabilizing the pellet that is formed by centrifugation.

In a solid-phase immunoassay, whether competitive or noncompetitive, the primary antibody is immobilized, usually by simple adsorption, onto a solid support. Most commonly, the antibody is coated onto the inner surface of the assay tube or microtiter well, and after incubation with the labeled and unlabeled antigen, the incubation mix containing unbound antigens is simply decanted or aspirated away, with bound antigen remaining on the inner surface of the tube or well. Signal associated with the bound antigen is then quantified. Commercially produced solid-phase competitive binding assays often have novel, usually proprietary antibody support systems such as polystyrene beads or stars, or magnetic particles. Such products also have novel methods to separate free from bound material, such as customized bead washers or magnetic bases to complete the separation procedure.

A separation step is necessary in the great majority of immunoassays used today. However, there is a class of competitive immunoassays known as homogeneous assays in which the bound signal generator does not have to be separated from the free signal generator in order to be measured. In this type of assay, the signal changes in some way, depending on whether it is in an antigen-antibody complex or not. For example, the direction of fluorescent emissions will be retarded when bound in the antigen-antibody complex. In this way, the orientation of the fluorescent signal can be measured with no need for separation of the free and bound signal. Likewise, enzyme labels can be oriented such that they function only when in or only when free of the antigen-antibody complex, again obviating the need for the physical separation of free and bound signal. For technical reasons, such homogeneous immunoassays are appropriate only for the measurement of small molecules that are found in high concentration. Therefore, they have been developed mostly for the assay of drugs, steroids, and thyroid hormones. The most well-known homogeneous immunoassays are the so-called fluorescence polarization immunoassay (FPIA)[27] and enzyme multiplied immunoassay (EMIT)[28] methods.

Signaling Methods

The classic signaling method in immunoassay has been the use of radiolabeled antigens and antibodies. Yalow and Berson[1] used the radioisotope iodine-131 (^{131}I) to label or tag insulin in the first immunoassay ever described. ^{131}I, a high-energy gamma emitter that was fairly hazardous to work with and that decayed rapidly, gave way to ^{125}I, a less hazardous gamma emitter with a slower period of decay. For purposes of comparison, the half-life of ^{131}I is 8 days while the half-life of ^{125}I is 60 days. Radioactive iodine is the radiolabel of choice for proteins and peptides if they contain tyrosine residues, because the iodine can be introduced into tyrosine's aromatic ring either chemically or enzymatically. Even if a ligand does not contain a tyrosine residue or other phenol ring structure, as is the case for most steroids, for example, radioactive iodine can be introduced through covalent binding of a phenolic structure to the ligand, being careful to choose a site of attachment of the radiolabel that will not affect the characteristic shape and therefore the recognition of the ligand by its antibody. Alternatively, small molecules can be radiolabeled with radioactive hydrogen (tritium, ^{3}H), which can substitute for hydrogen at multiple locations in the molecular structure. ^{3}H, a beta emitter, was once the dominant label for small molecules. Today, it is not as commonly used as ^{125}I in radioimmunoassay of small molecules because its measurement requires the use of liquid scintillation spectroscopy, a more time-consuming method that generates hazardous chemical waste.

For many years, radioisotopes were the only labels used for immunoassay signal generation. But by the late 1970s, particularly in Europe, nonisotopic alternatives for signal generation were implemented. With today's environmental concerns about the use of radioactivity and the cost and difficulty of radioactive waste management, it would be fair to say that the great majority of assay development today is focused on the use of nonisotopic signaling methods. Today, there is a plentiful supply of alternative, nonradioactive labels from which to choose. For a history of the development of nonisotopic immunoassay, the reader is directed to various interesting review articles.[29-31]

In nonisotopic immunoassay, the signals most commonly generated are color, measured as absorbance of a specific wavelength of light, the emission of fluorescence, and the emission of light or chemiluminescence. Most commonly, in each of these signal generation methods, an enzyme, covalently linked to either the antigen or antibody in the immunoassay, catalyzes the conversion of a substrate to a product that either has a color, emits fluorescence, or emits light. In some fluorescent immunoassays, an enzyme is not required; rather, a molecule that will emit fluorescence after excitation is covalently linked to an antigen or antibody. In enzyme-linked immunoassay, the two enzymes most commonly used are alkaline phosphatase and horseradish peroxidase. Both are excellent choices because of their stability, their high activity (i.e., rapid conversion of substrate to measurable product), and the range of substrates that can be used.

Each nonisotopic signal method has its positive and negative attributes. Color development is the simplest system and therefore is most commonly used, especially when in-house assays must be developed. The generation of fluorescence[32,33] and chemiluminescence,[34] while more technically complex, generally offers the possibility of much greater sensitivity and less background noise, allowing for very low concentrations of ligand to be measured. The signaling methods most commonly in use currently are discussed here. The reader is directed to more detailed reviews for discussion of the most recent innovations in immunoassay design.[6-8]

Practical Considerations in Choosing and Using Immunoassays

With a better understanding of the variety of immunoassay methods available, we can now examine the practical issues in implementing the immunoassay of analytes important in perinatal and neonatal metabolic studies. Clearly, the dominant theme in the transition from prenatal to neonatal life is the development and maturation of biologic systems—systems involving growth, fuel metabolism, mineral and water balance, circulation, nervous function, sexual development, as well as fetal-maternal interactions during pregnancy and at parturition. Integral to each of these are regulatory factors, measured in the circulation and at local sites. These analytes can be grouped in two ways, by similarities in their chemical structure or by their involvement in a particular system. The structural classification of regulatory molecules most often involves the grouping of proteins, peptides, steroids, and thyroid hormones. A functional classification involves the various systems listed above, and these are discussed throughout this text. In addition, certain general issues relating to the implementation of any immunoassay and certain specific issues relating to the various structural classes of regulatory molecules are relevant to the discussion. They are presented as a means to consider the potential problems and issues that can occur when using immunoassay to measure the concentration of specific analytes.

Proteins

Because they are large molecules with complex tertiary structures, proteins and glycoproteins (i.e., proteins with carbohydrate substituents covalently bound) are more and more commonly measured using two-site immunometric assays. However, competitive immunoassay formats are still used. While most proteins are reasonably stable in serum or plasma, it is best to freeze samples for storage if assay is not planned within 24 to 48 hours of sample collection. Certain protein hormones are known to require special handling, including immediate placement on ice, addition of protease inhibitors to the collection tube to prevent enzymatic hydrolysis, and avoidance of repeated freeze-thaw cycles of the sample. It is best to consult published research reports or seek advice from assay kit manufacturers to determine whether any special handling might be necessary before beginning studies on any analyte. Some examples of protein analytes that require more careful handling are adrenocorticotropic hormone (ACTH), parathyroid hormone–related peptide (PTH-RP),[35] calcitonin,[36] osteocalcin, insulin-like growth factor-I (IGF-I), insulin-like growth factor binding protein-1 (IGFBP-1), IGFBP-

2, growth hormone,[37] and the free β subunit of human chorionic gonadotropin.[38]

Peptides

Peptides under about 40 amino acids in length are almost always measured by competitive immunoassay techniques. In contrast, larger peptides can be measured using either two-site immunometric assays or competitive assays. Peptides tend to be less stable than proteins in vitro and in vivo, so that it is more common to consider sample stability when dealing with peptides. Placement of the sample on ice immediately after it is obtained is required. Because of the lack of a complex tertiary structure in most peptides, they are more susceptible to proteolytic digestion than are most proteins. The use of protease inhibitors may be suggested. Again, consult references and the kit manufacturers for information about sample stability.

Peptides commonly circulate while bound noncovalently to larger binding proteins. This is true for the IGFs.[39,40] To measure the total amount of circulating peptide in the sample, it is often necessary to release the bound peptide prior to assay. This is usually accomplished by pretreating the sample with an acid solution, or with a combination of acid and alcohol.[41,42] It may also be important to measure just the free portion of the circulating peptide, because its concentration may be more relevant to its biologic function.[43] In that case, again using the example of the IGFs, it is possible to develop an assay in which the antibody has a low affinity for the bound peptide while being able to recognize and bind the free peptide with high sensitivity and specificity.[44]

Steroids

Because steroids are relatively small molecules (under 500 daltons), they are always measured by competitive immunoassay methods. Steroids are generally stable in serum and plasma. However, it is a good policy not to collect samples for steroid assay in tubes containing gel separation materials. Upon standing in such tubes, progesterone, in particular, and testosterone are adsorbed by the gel, leading to underestimation of their concentrations in the sample.[45,46]

Most steroids circulate noncovalently bound to specific serum-binding proteins, to nonspecific serum proteins, and to a small extent as free or unbound. Estradiol and testosterone are bound with high affinity to circulating sex hormone–binding globulin, while cortisol and progesterone circulate bound predominantly to corticosteroid-binding globulin.[47,48] These steroids bind with lower affinity to albumin and prealbumin. The evidence is strong that only the free or unbound portion of these steroids is available for biologic functions at target tissues.[47] The amount of free steroid in the blood can be measured using either dialysis methods or by direct immunoassay using antibodies with low affinity for the protein-bound steroid.[49,50] To measure the total amount of a particular steroid in a serum or plasma sample, either the sample has to be extracted with an organic solvent such as diethyl ether, which will bring all steroids into the organic phase, or a synthetic steroid analogue must be added in excess to the sample to replace the endogenous protein-bound steroids on the binding proteins. The analogue replacement method is simpler but not always complete. The extraction method is more specific and complete, but it is much more time-consuming and difficult.

An extra factor that makes steroid measurement problematic at times is the great number of structurally similar metabolites that are rapidly formed after a steroid has been secreted into the circulation. For example, there can be more than 20 closely related adrenal steroids found in the circulation at any one time, along with cortisol, the predominant and most active glucocorticoid. These represent intermediates of cortisol biosynthesis, hydroxylated, reduced, and oxidized metabolites of cortisol, and lastly, conjugated forms of cortisol and its metabolites. Conjugates are steroids with sulfates and glucuronates covalently bound by ester linkage and represent the major pathway of steroid excretion into the urine. All these various metabolites present potential specificity problems in the assay of one particular steroid. Generally, an antibody that is selected for use in a particular steroid immunoassay is carefully screened to determine the potential cross-reactivity of relevant steroid metabolites. It is incumbent on an investigator who is studying a particular steroid hormone to determine whether the antibody specificity in the assay is sufficient for the type of sample that will be measured. This point is exemplified by a recent study of testosterone concentration in the neonate with ambiguous genitalia, in which chromatographic purification of the plasma sample was necessary to ensure accurate estimation of testosterone concentration and as a consequence, correct sex assignment.[51]

Thyroid Hormones

The thyroid hormones, thyroxine (T_4) and triiodothyronine (T_3), are iodinated tyrosine derivatives that, because of their relatively small size, are always measured by competitive immunoassay methods. T_4 and T_3 are stable in serum and plasma, and no special precautions in sample handling are required.

The measurement of free versus protein-bound hormone concentration, discussed in the previous section, is as important and perhaps more important in the case of T_3 and T_4. There is no question of the clinical importance of measuring the circulating concentrations of free thyroid hormones in order to differentially diagnose particular forms of thyroid dysfunction.[49,52] Perhaps there are more choices available for the measurement of total and free T_4 and T_3 than for any other analytes measured by immunoassay methods.[53] As is true for the steroid hormones, the thyroid hormones circulate bound primarily to a high-affinity serum-binding protein, thyroid hormone–binding globulin (TBG), and to a lesser extent to albumin. A very small percentage of the total circulating T_3 and T_4 is free and not bound to protein.

Other Small Molecules

Besides steroids and thyroid hormones, other biologic regulatory molecules of low molecular weight that can be measured by competitive immunoassay techniques include prostaglandins (e.g., eicosanoids) and cyclic nucleotides. Prostaglandins and the related arachidonic acid metabolites, prostacyclins, thromboxanes, and leukotrienes are effector molecules involved in a great variety of biologic processes. As discussed in Chapter 13, these analytes tend to be highly unstable and have relatively short half-lives. In addition, prostaglandins are present in a great variety of closely related structures, each of which commonly are in very low concentration. All of these problems make the measurement of prostaglandins by immunoassay relatively unsatisfactory. However, assays to measure the more stable metabolites of the major classes of prostaglandins are available and have been used with reasonable success.[54,55]

The cyclic nucleotides, adenosine 3′,5′-cyclic monophosphate (cAMP) and guanosine 3′,5′-cyclic monophosphate (cGMP), intracellular second messengers involved in receptor-mediated transduction mechanisms, can be measured with good specificity and sensitivity using competitive immunoassay methods.[56] However, the biogenic amines, including the catecholamines and the indolamines and their metabolites are not amenable to measurement by immunoassay because of their poor stability and pH characteristics. These analytes are more commonly measured by high-performance liquid and gas chromatography.

General Issues

Issues that must be addressed in measuring samples by immunoassay are for the most part the same as those encountered when dealing with the measurement of an analyte by any assay method, and excellent in-depth reviews have been published.[57,58] Issues include those of sample collection: Is the analyte concentration affected by the time of day, is it secreted in a noticeably pulsatile fashion, is it influenced by stress, or by dietary intake, or by illness? Does the quality of the sample (i.e., is it hemolyzed or lipemic) affect the measurement? Sample degradation after collection was discussed under the various categories of analytes measured by immunoassay. Finally, have laboratory quality control methods been implemented to assure consistent performance between and within assays?

Most of the answers to questions about sample collection and quality control are available in the literature, in either texts, reviews, or research articles. If they are not, or if they are not directly applicable to samples obtained during the perinatal and neonatal period, then either the question must be tested or, if all else fails, a modicum of caution and common sense should be applied. Store samples on ice as soon as is practical. Spin down the clot or the cells in the shortest acceptable time. If at all practical, to obviate any affect of pulsatile secretion, take two to three small samples over a 40- to 60-minute period, pool the samples, and assay the single pooled sample. Try to obtain samples at the same time of day if possible, and under the same conditions of stress, diet, and wakefulness. If different treatment groups or diagnostic groups are to be compared, try to have the different groups subject to the same degree of control or lack of control.

Implementation of a strict program of quality control is necessary before the assay can be used either clinically or in the research laboratory. The clinical immunoassay laboratory can help by providing pooled or synthetic control samples. It can also provide guidelines for acceptance or rejection of a particular assay run. Some useful steps in quality control should include the use of two or three control samples whose analyte concentrations are targeted to decision points in the reference range for that analyte. Pilot experiments to determine a reference range and whether reference values change with patient age should be carefully planned.

Kits versus In-House Assay

Currently, with the sophistication of immunoassay design and availability of so many different assays, the investigator who intends to measure the concentrations of a particular effector molecule should first determine whether an assay for that analyte already exists. If it does exist, and it is appropriate to the sample type and range of expected concentrations, it is wise to use that assay if possible. The time saved in avoiding the intricacies of assay development will be substantial. An invaluable resource in helping to determine whether kits are available for the measurement of a particular analyte is the British series of books entitled *The Immunoassay Kit Directory*, published by Kluwer Academic Publishers of Lancaster, England. The most recent directory is series A (clinical chemistry), volume 3, edited by John Seth, director of the UK National External Quality Assurance Scheme. Volume 3 is made up of five parts:

Part 1	Peptide hormones	June 1994
Part 2	Steroid and thyroid hormones	December 1994
Part 3	Proteins and tumor markers	May 1995
Part 4	Drugs, eicosanoids, second messengers	November 1995
Part 5	Equipment	December 1995

Ordering information can be obtained at Kluwer Academic Publishers, 101 Philip Drive, Assinippi Park, Norwell, MA 02061, USA, or Kluwer Academic Publishers, PO Box 322, 3300 AH Dordrecht, The Netherlands.

If an assay is not available, or if the assay characteristics are not appropriate to the research at hand, or if the reagent prices are prohibitive, then it may be necessary to develop one's own in-house assay. This is not a minor task. The following outline of the steps required will serve as a brief guide to assay development. The interested reader is referred to various treatises for detailed help.[6,7,9,59] The method of choice in so-called home brew immunoassay is the ELISA format. An ELISA has the advantage of using a robust nonisotopic signaling system, the development of color through enzyme-linked components. If the target analyte is a small molecule, the enzyme can be linked to a purified preparation of the analyte, the labeled antigen, to produce a competitive binding ELISA format. If the target analyte is a large molecule, then the enzyme can be linked to one of two antibodies to produce an immunometric ELISA format. There are a number of steps that must be taken in sequence to ensure an accurate and reproducible assay. Assume that an immunometric-type ELISA is being established. Then the following must be accomplished:

1. Identify a specific capture antibody.
2. Identify and label an appropriate detection antibody or purchase the antibody already labeled.
3. Identify a source of the purified ligand, or be prepared to purify the ligand yourself.
4. Determine the buffer system that will be used.
5. Develop a set of standards covering the targeted range of concentrations.
6. Optimize the kinetics of antibody-antigen binding either by letting the reaction proceed to completion or by precisely timing a partial reaction.
7. Test the linearity of dilution and recovery of patient samples.
8. Establish quality control pools to monitor assay reproducibility.

Summary

Immunoassays can now be considered predictable and robust analytical methods. They enable the investigator to quantify the levels of analytes critical to the patient or to the system being examined. In earlier decades, immunoassay methods were in development at the same time that they were being implemented. For this reason, immunoassay has to this day retained an aura of being difficult and not easily reproducible. Currently this image is not correct. Immunoassay methods have developed to the point that a wide range of analytes can now be routinely measured using automated instrumentation that is almost as predictable and dependable as the chemistry analyzers that routinely measure glucose or uric acid concentrations. While immunoassay automation is still not routinely available in the research setting, easy and fast manual and semiautomated assay methods are currently the rule rather than the exception.

In this chapter, the most common forms of immunoassay have been described both from a theoretical and a practical perspective. Historically, immunoassay began with the development of radioisotope-labeled, competitive binding assays. In the case of small molecules and most peptides, competitive immunoassay, in which labeled and unlabeled antigen compete for binding to a limited amount of antibody, is still the method of choice. For larger peptides and proteins, molecules large enough to allow for unrestricted binding of two separate antibodies, the assay method of choice has become the immunometric or two-site sandwich assay. Whether of competitive or noncompetitive design, the choice of labels or signal generators is vast, as are the varieties of separation techniques now available in immunoassay. Most commonly, if an investigator wants to measure the concentration of a particular analyte, an immunoassay for that analyte will be readily available or the specific assay reagents will be available. Even the task of building an assay has become much easier, with the advent of ELISA technology and kits for nonisotopic signal generation.

What is next for the measurement of analytes by immunoassay? Recombinant technology is affecting assay development and over the next few years genetically engineered antibodies, signal generators, and antigen preparations will become available. The net result will be improvements in the range of analytes that can be measured, the lower limit of detection of these analytes, and the great specificity with which similar molecules will be differentiated from each other. For example, antibody production is being simplified and improved with the use of antibody fragments to more precisely control assay component interactions and antigen-antibody interaction.[60] Antibody-enzyme bioengineered hybrids are also being investigated as a means to improve sensitivity and simplicity in assay design.[61] Improvements in the sensitivity and analyte range of homogeneous immunoassays, in which there is no need to separate free and bound label, will contribute to increased simplicity and acceptance.[62,63]

References

1. Yalow RS, Berson SA. Radiobiology. Assay of plasma insulin in human subjects by immunological methods. Nature 1959;184:1648–1649.
2. Yalow RS, Berson SA. Immunoassay of endogenous plasma insulin in man. J Clin Invest 1960;39:1157–1175.
3. Berson SA, Yalow RS, Auerbach GD, et al. Immunoassay of bovine and human parathyroid hormone. Proc Natl Acad Sci USA 1963;49:613–617.
4. Glick SM, Roth J, Yalow RS, et al. Immunoassay of human growth hormone in plasma. Nature 1963;199:784–787.
5. Yalow RS, Glick SM, Roth J, et al. Radioimmunoassay of human plasma ACTH. J Clin Endocrinol Metab 1964;24:1219–1225.
6. Diamandis EP, Christopoulos TK, eds. Immunoassay. New York: Academic Press, 1996.
7. Wild D, ed. The immunoassay handbook. New York: Stockton Press, 1994.
8. Nakamura RM, Dasahara Y, Rechnitz GA, eds. Immunochemical assays and biosensor technology for the 1990s. Washington, DC: American Association for Microbiology, 1992.
9. Price CP, Newman DJ, eds. Principles and practice of immunoassay. New York: Stockton Press, 1991.
10. Collins WP, ed. Alternative immunoassays. New York: Wiley, 1985.
11. Kricka LJ, ed. Ligand-binder assays. New York: Marcel Dekker, 1985.
12. Albertson BD, Haseltine FP, eds. Non-radiometric assays. Technology and application in polypeptide and steroid hormone detection. New York: Alan R. Liss, 1988.
13. Jaffe BM, Behrman HR, eds. Methods of hormone radioimmunoassay. 2nd ed. New York: Academic Press, 1979.
14. Canick JA. Prenatal screening for Down syndrome using alpha-fetoprotein, unconjugated estriol, and human chorionic gonadotropin. J Clin Immunoassay 1990;13:30–33.
15. Porter P, Coley J, Gani M. Immunochemical criteria for successful matching of monoclonal antibodies to immunoassays of peptide hormones for assessment of pregnancy and ovulation. In: Albertson BD, Haseltine FP, eds. Non-radiometric assays. Technology and application in polypeptide and steroid hormone detection. New York: Alan R. Liss, 1988:181–200.
16. Kohler G, Milstein C. Continuous culture of fused cells secreting antibody of predetermined specificity. Nature 1975;256:495–497.
17. Kohler G, Milstein C. Derivation of specific antibody-producing tissue culture and tumour lines by cell fusion. Eur J Immunol 1976;6:511–519.
18. Lieberman S, Erlanger BF, Beiser SM, et al. Aspects of steroid chemistry and metabolism. Steroid-protein conjugates: their chemical, immunochemical and endocrinological properties. Rec Progr Hormone Res 1959;15:165–200.
19. Erlanger BF. The preparation of antigenic hapten-carrier conjugates: a survey. Meth Enzymol 1980;80:85–104.
20. Yalow RS. Radioimmunoassay of hormones. In: Wilson JD, Foster DW, eds. Williams' textbook of endocrinology. 8th ed. Philadelphia: WB Saunders, 1992:1635–1645.
21. Rodbard D, Lewald JE. Computer analysis of radioligand assay and radioimmunoassay data. Acta Endocrinol (Copenh) 1970;suppl 147:7–103.
22. Healy MJR. Statistical analysis of radioimmunoassay data. Biochem J 1972;130:207–210.
23. Miles LEM, Hales CN. Labelled antibodies and immunological assay systems. Nature 1968;219:186–189.
24. Miles LEM, Lipschitz DA, Bieber CP, et al. Measurement of serum ferritin by a 2-site immunoradiometric assay. Analyt Biochem 1974;61:209–224.
25. Rodbard D, Feldman Y, Jaffe ML, et al. Kinetics of two-site immunoradiometric ("sandwich") assays—II. Studies on the nature of the "high-dose hook effect." Immunochemistry 1978;15:77–82.
26. Schalch D, Parker M. A sensitive double antibody immunoassay for human growth hormone in plasma. Nature 1964;203:1141–1142.
27. Dandliker WB, Feigen GA. Quantification of the antigen-antibody reaction by the polarization of fluorescence. Biochem Biophys Res Commun 1961;5:299–304.
28. Rubenstein KE, Schneider RS, Ullman EF. Homogeneous enzyme immunoassay. New immunochemical technique. Biochem Biophys Res Commun 1972;47:846–851.
29. Schall RF Jr, Tenoso HJ. Alternatives to radioimmunoassay: labels and methods. Clin Chem 1981;27:1157–1164.
30. Howanitz JH. Immunoassay. Innovations in label technology. Arch Pathol Lab Med 1988;112:775–779.
31. Wisdom GB. Recent progress in the development of enzyme immunoassays. Ligand Rev 1981;3:44–49.
32. Hammilä I. Fluoroimmunoassays and immunofluorometric assays. Clin Chem 1985;31:359–370.
33. Diamandis EP. Immunoassays with time-resolved flourescence spectroscopy: principles and applications. Clin Biochem 1988;21:139–150.
34. Weeks I, Woodhead JS. Chemiluminescence immunoassay. J Clin Immunoassay 1984;7:82–89.
35. Pandian MR, Morgan CH, Carlton E, et al. Modified immunoradiometric assay of parathyroid hormone-related peptide. Clinical application in the differential diagnosis of hypercalcemia. Clin Chem 1992;38:282–288.
36. Colton KW, Stevenson JC. Calcium metabolism. In: Wild D, ed. The immunoassay handbook. New York: Stockton Press, 1994:362–365.
37. Jacobs DS, Kasten BL, Demott WR, et al. Laboratory test handbook. 2nd ed. Baltimore: Williams & Wilkins, 1990:215.
38. Stone SJ, Henley R. The stability of blood samples for the measurement of the free beta subunit of chorionic gonadotropin. Prenat Diagn 1995;15:95–96.
39. Baxter RC, Martin JL, Beniac VA. High molecular weight insulin-like growth factor binding protein complex. J Biol Chem 1989;264:11843–11848.
40. Rechler M. Insulin-like growth factor binding proteins. Vitam Horm 1993;47:1–114.
41. Powell DR, Rosenfield RG, Baker BK, et al. Serum somatomedin levels in adults with chronic renal failure: the importance of measuring insulin-like growth factor I (IGF-I) and IGF-II in acid-chromatographed uriemic serum. J Clin Endocrinol Metab 1986;63:1186–1192.

42. Underwood LE, Murphy MG. Radioimmunoassay of the somatomedins. In: Patrono C, ed. Radioimmunoassay in basic and clinical pharmacology (handbook of experimental pharmacology, vol. 82). Heidelberg: Springer-Verlag, 1987:561–574.
43. Lewitt MS, Denyer GS, Cooney GJ, et al. Insulin-like growth factor-binding protein-1 modulates blood glucose levels. Endocrinology 1991;129:2254–2256.
44. Lee PDK, Powell D, Baker B, et al. Characterization of a direct, non-extraction immunoradiometric assay for free IGF-I. Endocrinology 1991;129:462A.
45. Smith RL. Effect of serum-separating gels on progesterone assays. Clin Chem 1985;31:1239.
46. Hilborn S, Krahn J. Effect of time of exposure of serum to gel-barrier tubes on results for progesterone and some other endocrine tests. Clin Chem 1987;33:203–204.
47. Hammond GL. Molecular properties of corticosteroid binding globulin and the sex-steroid binding proteins. Endocr Rev 1990;11:65–79.
48. Cumming DC, Wall SR. Non-sex hormone binding globulin-bound testosterone as a marker for hyperandrogenism. J Clin Endocrinol Metab 1985;61:873–876.
49. Ekins R. Measurement of free hormones in blood. Endocr Rev 1990;11:5–46.
50. Pearce S, Dowsett M, Jeffcoate S. Three methods for estimating the fraction of testosterone and estradiol not bound to sex-hormone-binding globulin. Clin Chem 1989;35:632–635.
51. Fuqua JS, Sher ES, Migeon CJ, et al. Assay of plasma testosterone during the first six months of life: importance of chromatographic purification of steroids. Clin Chem 1995;41:146–1149.
52. Bartalena L. Recent achievements in studies on thyroid hormone-binding proteins. Endocr Rev 1990;11:47–64.
53. Gruhn JG, Barsano CP, Kumar Y. The development of tests of thyroid function. Arch Pathol Lab Med 1987;111:84–100.
54. Dray F, Charbonnel B, Maclouf J. Radioimmunoassays for prostaglandins F_α, E_1 and E_2 in human plasma. Eur J Clin Invest 1975;5:311–318.
55. Kelly RW, Graham BJM, O'Sullivan MJ. Measurement of PGE_2 as the methyl oxime by radioimmunoassay using a novel iodinated label. Prostaglandins Leukot Essent Fatty Acids 1989;27:187–191.
56. Young DS, Bermes EW Jr. Specimen collection and processing; sources of biological variation. In: Burtis CA, Ashwood CR, eds. Tietz textbook of clinical chemistry. 2nd ed. Philadelphia: WB Saunders, 1994:58–101.
57. Westgard JO, Klee GG. Quality management. In: Burtis CA, Ashwood CR, eds. Tietz textbook of clinical chemistry. 2nd ed. Philadelphia: WB Saunders, 1994:548–592.
58. Grammatopoulos D, Stirrat GM, Williams SA, et al. The biological activity of the corticotropin-releasing hormone receptor-adenylate cyclase complex in human myometrium is reduced at the end of pregnancy. J Clin Endocrinol Metab 1996;81:745–751.
59. Crowther JR. ELISA: theory and practice. Methods in molecular biology, vol. 42. Totowa, NJ: Humana, 1995.
60. Ishikawa E. Development and clinical application of sensitive enzyme immunoassay for macromolecular antigens—a review. Clin Biochem 1987;20:375–385.
61. Moore GP. Genetically engineered antibodies. Clin Chem 1989;35:1849–1853.
62. Görög G, Gandolfi A, Paradisi G, et al. Use of bispecific hybrid antibodies for the development of a homogeneous enzyme immunoassay. J Immunol Methods 1989;123:131–140.
63. Ashihara Y, Nishizono I, Suzuki H, et al. Homogeneous enzyme immunoassay for macromolecular antigens using hybrid antibody. J Clin Lab Anal 1987;1:77–79.
64. Davies C. Principles. In: Wild D, ed. The immunoassay handbook. New York: Stockton Press, 1994:3–47.

4
Methodology for the Study of Metabolism: Cellular and Molecular Techniques

Lewis P. Rubin

The history of metabolic investigation is typified by incremental refinements of the understanding of intermediary metabolism. During the late 20th century, successful strategies have included measurement of utilization rates of specific compounds with isotopically labeled substrate and intermediates (stable isotope studies); measurement of intact systems of substrate, product, and enzyme allosteric effector concentrations; use of specific enzyme inhibitors; and kinetic analysis of purified enzymes (see Chapters 1, 2, and 3). However, metabolism is essentially a cellular phenomenon. Small molecules (e.g., sugars, organic acids, fatty acids, amino acids, nucleotides) are the metabolic substrates or products that provide both the components necessary for the biosynthesis of larger molecules as well as the energy needed for cellular function. These larger molecules are the structural constituents of cells and tissues (e.g., polysaccharides, lipids, proteins, nucleic acids). The development of cellular and molecular techniques has greatly expanded the range of questions that can be asked about metabolic physiology.

Genes important for metabolic regulation and the cells that express these genes are the focus of this "new metabolism."[1] Recruitment of particular subsets of genes allows fine-tuning of the cellular response to perturbations of the steady state. Although the genotype is perpetuated as sequences of nucleic acids, genes exert effects by being expressed as intracellular and secreted proteins. Consequently, the ultimate goal of molecular metabolism is an explanation of how certain genes are selectively expressed in response to environmental signals and how their gene products alter cellular function and regulate metabolic pathways. The study of hepatic fuel metabolism has exemplified the potential inherent in this approach. The pathways of glucose metabolism initially were described as a complex, coordinated series of enzymatic reactions. Subsequent investigations delineated how hormones control and integrate these pathways. Currently, there is intense and productive research into the transcriptional and posttranscriptional mechanisms by which hormones and dietary factors exert their effects on the relevant genes and gene products.[2-4]

This chapter explores basic themes and research strategies pertinent to molecular cell biology. The chapter emphasizes experimental methods that are currently used to address specific mechanistic questions, and offers examples relevant for perinatal-neonatal metabolism. The topic is too large for a comprehensive discussion, so this review must be selective. For further background the reader is referred to recent texts[5-9] and to comprehensive technical handbooks available for molecular biology[10-13] and cell biology.[14-16] The first sections of this chapter cover some salient aspects of eukaryotic genomic organization and then review the techniques used for separating and analyzing DNA, RNA, and protein. These methods are covered in the sequence of their development, that is, the blotting of electrophoresed DNA, RNA, and protein, respectively. The essentials of molecular cloning and the polymerase chain reaction (PCR) are then summarized. These two technical innovations have made the development of modern molecular cell biology possible. The subsequent sections review the current understanding of how hormonal and dietary signals interact with cellular receptors and how the resultant ligand-stimulated signaling pathways regulate gene expression. The understanding of receptor action has been advanced by development of new experimental techniques such as radioligand binding, single-channel recording and molecular cloning, and site-directed mutagenesis procedures for modifying receptor structure and function in precise ways. The last sections review features of regulated gene expression important for an understanding of the developmental control of metabolic pathways and relevant methodologies including transgenic organisms. The availability of simplified protocols, relatively inexpensive apparatus, and easily available electronic information ensures that these research strategies will become increasingly important. *BioInformation on the World Wide*

Web 1997 (book and software)[17] is a good introduction to online resources. In 1997, the journal *Current Opinion in Cell Biology* began publishing a selection of World Wide Web sites relevant to reviews of topics published in each issue.[18]

Mammalian Genomic Structure

Each human somatic cell encodes genetic information within a 6μm nucleus that contains 46 chromosomes composed of chromatin, a compact arrangement of proteins and double-stranded deoxyribonucleic acid (dsDNA). Chromatin itself is arranged as individual, repeated units called nucleosomes in which dsDNA is wound around histone proteins. A linear array of human dsDNA is longer than 6×10^6 kilobase (kb) pairs and stretches about 1.8m. The genome directs embryogenesis, development, growth, reproduction, and metabolism, and represents the functional blueprint and evolutionary history of the species. At the time of publication, the Human Genome Project had sampled at least half of the estimated 50,000 to 100,000 human genes.

Native DNA is a double-helical linear polymer containing a two-strand scaffold of phosphodiester bond-linked deoxyribose sugars and nucleotide bases in 5' to 3' linkage. The bases of the two strands are joined by hydrogen bonds in a specific, paired, complementary fashion: adenine (A) only pairs with thymine (T), and guanine (G) only pairs with cytosine (C). During cell division, the two strands unwind so that each strand serves as a template for the DNA polymerase-catalyzed synthesis of a new complementary DNA strand. When genes are expressed, their encoded sequence information (Table 4.1) is first converted into messenger RNA (mRNA) in the process of transcription. RNA is a single-stranded polymer containing a ribose sugar backbone and, instead of thymine, the base uracil (U). RNA sequence information is converted into protein sequences in the process of translation (Figure 4.1). Therefore, gene and protein molecular structure are intimately related.[19-20]

As depicted in Figure 4.1, a structural gene comprises the genomic region lying between the points that correspond to the 5' and 3' terminal bases of the corresponding mRNA. Although transcription commences at the 5' end of the mRNA, it extends beyond the 3' end, which later is generated by cleavage. Since genes essentially are functional units, a broader and more useful definition of a gene also includes regulatory DNA sequences associated with the transcribed DNA segments (i.e., the "coding region"). In other words, a gene is a transcriptional unit that includes one or more promoter sequences, other regulatory regions located upstream (that is, 5' to the coding region), the coding region itself, and sometimes a terminator sequence.

Only about 3% of human genomic DNA is thought to specify the portions of genes that encode proteins; long stretches of noncoding sequence are located between and within genes. An essential feature of eukaryotic gene organization is that the integrity of the coding regions of genes is interrupted by these intervening noncoding DNA sequences. Eukaryotic genes consist of an alternating series of exons, DNA sequences represented in RNA (i.e., exported to the cytoplasm) and introns, or intervening DNA whose sequences remain in the nucleus. Introns are removed by enzymatic splicing (i.e., excision and liga-

TABLE 4.1. Amino acids and their codons.

Amino Acid	Abbreviation	Symbol	Codon
Alanine	ala	A	CGA GCC GCG GCU
Arginine	arg	R	AGA AGG CGA CGC CGC CGU
Asparagine	asn	N	AAC AAU
Aspartic acid	asp	D	GAC GAU
Cysteine	cys	C	UGC UGU
Glutamic acid	glu	E	GAA GAG
Glutamine	gln	Q	CAA CAG
Glycine	gly	G	GGA GGC GGG GGU
Histidine	his	H	CAC CAU
Isoleucine	ile	I	AUA AUC AUU
Leucine	leu	L	UUA UUG CUA CUC CUG CUU
Lysine	lys	K	AAA AAG
Methionine	met	M	AUG
Phenylalanine	phe	F	UUC UUU
Proline	pro	P	CCA CCC CCG CCU
Serine	ser	S	AGC AGU UCA UCC UCG UCU
Threonine	thr	T	ACA ACC ACG ACU
Tryptophan	trp	W	UGG
Tyrosine	tyr	Y	UAC UAU
Valine	va	V	GUA GUC GUG GUU

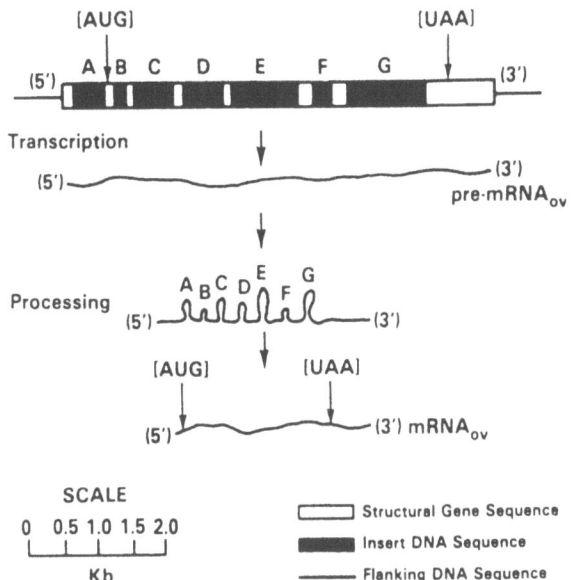

FIGURE 4.1. The flow of genetic information as illustrated by the chicken ovalbumin gene. The structural gene sequences (exons) are interspersed among inserted DNA sequences (introns) labeled A to G. The transcribed intervening sequences are eliminated during processing into a mature mRNA. AUG is the transcription initiation codon and UAA is a polyadenylation site. (From Lewin,[9] with permission.)

tion) of the primary RNA transcript to a mature mRNA. A typical eukaryotic gene comprises several relatively short exons, usually coding for 20 to 80 amino acid residues, sprinkled through a longer length of the genome. This feature explains why, although some genes and their respective mRNAs are similarly sized, most known genes are much longer than would be predicted from mRNA length. Genes can be long indeed; for example, the human dystrophin (Duchenne and Becker muscular dystrophy) gene stretches over 2×10^6 base pairs (bp) and codes for a 500,000 molecular weight (MW) protein.[21]

The apparent minimum exon length roughly corresponds to the information needed to instruct synthesis of the smallest polypeptides that can assume stable folded structures: about 20 to 40 amino acids. Many, but not all, exons also correspond to protein functional domains, supporting the view that proteins have evolved multiple functions by successive genetic incorporation of the information encoded in different exon modules.[22] This evolutionary mechanism permits diversification and increasing complexity of metabolic pathways. By inference, DNA sequences that are shared among genes may represent exons that have migrated among those genes. The human low-density lipoprotein receptor (LDL-R) is a well-known example of a gene in which exons encode distinct functional domains. The 5' portion of the LDL-R coding region contains several exons closely related to DNA sequences that code for complement factor C9. The middle portion of the LDL-R gene contains exons that show sequence homology with certain exons of the epidermal growth factor precursor (preproEGF) gene.[23] Therefore, the LDL-R gene appears to have arisen through an assembly of genetic modules that encoded other proteins. Many large polypeptides, such as extracellular matrix proteins, contain distinct sequence domains for cell adhesion, receptor-like interaction, structural integrity, and growth promotion, and these domains often show significant sequence homologies to other proteins.[24] Sets of genes that are descended by duplication and variation events from some ancestral gene constitute gene families.[25] Gene family members may be clustered together, be dispersed on different chromosomes, or both. When members of a gene family occur at different locations, it may be assumed that one gene was translocated sometime after a duplication event. For example, such an event accounts for the locations of the human parathyroid hormone (PTH) and PTH-related peptide (PTHrP) genes on the short arms of chromosomes 11[26] and 12,[27] respectively.

PTH and PTHrP illustrate the principle that members of a structural gene family usually show related functions, despite expression at different times and in different cell types.[28,29] Repeated genes may exhibit no discernible differences in function. For example, primates have a single insulin gene but rodents have a duplicated insulin gene, one of which lacks a second intron. The rodent insulin genes are coordinately expressed and function identically. Finally, some members of a gene family may be nonfunctional pseudogenes, denoted by the symbol ψ, that are not translated into proteins. Pseudogenes seem to be informational dead ends, descended from once-functioning genetic sequences.

Somatic cells typically express approximately 10,000 to 20,000 genes,[9] a value probably within a factor of 2 to 4 of the total expressed gene number. A subset of ubiquitously expressed genes, numbering perhaps 10,000 in mammals, may be required for functions essential to all cell types. These are the so-called housekeeping or constitutive genes, which do not appear to be subject to regulated expression. Regulated gene expression, which is integral to the regulation of developmental metabolic pathways, is discussed below in the section Analysis of Gene Regulation.

The Manipulation and Analysis of Genomic DNA

The preparation of genomic DNA from nucleated cells, commonly from leukocytes, is a relatively simple procedure. Routinely, 25 to 60 mg of DNA can be isolated per milliliter of whole blood.[30] Other sources of genomic DNA that are relevant for perinatal biology include cultured amniotic fluid cells obtained by amniocentesis, cytotrophoblasts obtained from chorionic villus sampling, and skin fibroblasts cultured from biopsy or necropsy specimens. Once isolated, chromosomal DNA can be stored for years.

The manipulation of DNA in vitro has been made possible by the exploitation of bacterial restriction endonucleases.[31] In prokaryotic dsDNA methylases generate small amounts of 6-methyladenine from adenine and 6-methylcytosine from cytosine. Different bacterial strains have different methylation patterns. Methylation confers host specificity by safeguarding a bacterial strain from contamination with DNA sequences from another strain. This process, called restriction, occurs when the foreign DNA, which lacks methyl groups at the appropriate sites, is attacked by the host strain's restriction endonucleases. The basic feature of this system is that a bacterial strain possesses DNA methylase and restriction endonuclease activity with identical sequence specificity; the methylase adds methyl groups to adenine and cytosine residues in the same target sequence that constitutes the restriction enzyme binding site. Methylation thereby renders the target site resistant to restriction by protecting the DNA sequence from cleavage. In the terminology of molecular biology, all endonucleases that cleave DNA at a specific sequence are considered to be restriction enzymes, even though in most instances there is no direct genetic evidence for the presence of a restriction-methylation system.

Restriction enzymes have become essential tools for in vitro manipulation of DNA sequences studies precisely because they recognize short, specific DNA sequences, often palindromes of 4 to 6 bp (Table 4.2). The enzymes are named in accordance with bacterial strains from which each has been isolated and the order of enzyme isolation from that strain[32] (e.g., *Eco* RI from *Escherichia coli* RY13, *Hin*d III from *Haemophilus influenzae* Rd, *Hpa* I from *Haemophilus parainfluenzae*, or *Pst* I from *Providencia stuartii*. REBASE, a comprehensive, public-domain database of restriction enzymes and their associated methylases (http://www.neb.com/rebase), offers daily updated information about enzyme recognition and cleavage sites and commercial availability.[33] At the time of publication, nearly 3000 restriction enzymes were known.

Often it is useful partially to digest genomic DNA under conditions in which not all restriction endonuclease sites are cut and the DNA fragment distribution approaches a random cleavage of the genome. When the fragments are electrophoresed in an agarose or polyacrylamide gel, they migrate at rates proportional to their molecular weight and produce a smear in which distinct bands usually are not evident.[34,35] DNA within the gel can be detected directly by staining with fluorescent intercalating dyes (e.g., ethidium bromide). When discrete DNA bands are electrophoresed, as little as 1 to 10 ng of DNA can be visualized by direct examination of the gel in ultraviolet light.[36]

TABLE 4.2. Some common restriction enzymes.

Restriction enzyme	Ligation site
Acc I	$5'\ldots GT\,(^A_C)(^G_T)AC\ldots 3'$ $3'\ldots CA(^T_G)(^C_A)TG\ldots 5'$
Bam HI	$5'\ldots GGATCC\ldots 3'$ $3'\ldots CCTAGG\ldots 5'$
Bgl II	$5'\ldots AGATCT\ldots 3'$ $3'\ldots TCTAGA\ldots 5'$
Dde I	$5'\ldots CTNAG\ldots 3'$ $3'\ldots GANTC\ldots 5'$
Eco RI	$5'\ldots GAATTC\ldots 3'$ $3'\ldots CTTAAG\ldots 5'$
*Hin*d III	$5'\ldots AAGCTT\ldots 3'$ $3'\ldots TTCGAA\ldots 5'$
Hpa II	$5'\ldots CCGG\ldots 3'$ $3'\ldots GGCC\ldots 5'$
Pst I	$5'\ldots CTGCAG\ldots 3'$ $3'\ldots GACGTC\ldots 5'$
Sac I	$5'\ldots GAGCTC\ldots 3'$ $3'\ldots CTCGAG\ldots 5'$
Xba I	$5'\ldots TCTAGA\ldots 3'$ $3'\ldots AGATCT\ldots 5'$

It is possible to characterize specific DNA sequences by exploiting the tendency of the complementary base pairs forming dsDNA to be disrupted. Under physiologic conditions, dsDNA separates and reforms at very rapid rates. This property can be mimicked in vitro by denaturation, or melting. The melting temperature (Tm) of dsDNA ranges from 85° to 95°C, depending on a DNA segment's guanine-cytosine (GC) content. Exposure to high salt concentrations or certain reagents (e.g., formamide) facilitates denaturation at lower temperatures. When the denatured (single-stranded) DNA fragments are then allowed to re-anneal, a double helix again forms. This property is a useful measure of the complementarity of a given DNA sample either with other DNA or with RNA, i.e., the capacity to anneal or hybridize and form duplex base paired structures. When the denatured DNA sample is immobilized on a solid support so that it cannot renature (i.e., its two complementary strands cannot reform dsDNA), molecular hybridization becomes a highly specific and sensitive assay.

The most commonly used solid-support DNA hybridization technique is the Southern blot, named for the procedure's originator, E.M. Southern.[37] "Blotting" is a colloquial term used for the transfer of polynucleotides or proteins to a solid support.[38] As depicted in Figure 4.2, in Southern blotting electrophoresed DNA is denatured (e.g., in alkaline solution), neutralized and transferred by capillary action, bulk flow, or electroblotting onto a nitrocellulose filter or nylon screen. Baking or ultraviolet light

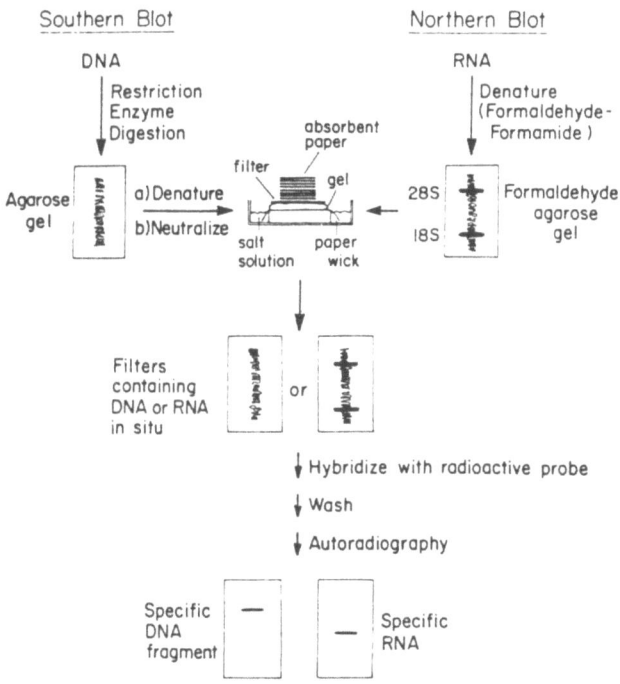

FIGURE 4.2. Southern and northern blotting techniques. (From Goodridge,[242] with permission.)

chemically cross-links the DNA single strands to the solid support.[39] The immobilized DNA can be hybridized in situ with a tagged (i.e., labeled) DNA or RNA probe that contains complementary nucleotide sequence. Tags for probe detection initially were beta emitters (^{32}P), but currently include a range of nonradioactive substances including biotin and digoxigenin. Once hybridized, the blot is washed under conditions that remove non-hybridized probe and the labeled band(s) are visualized by autoradiography, chemiluminescence, etc., in the position(s) determined by the electrophoretic mobility (size) of the hybridized DNA fragment(s).

Variations on traditional DNA gel electrophoresis permit resolution of much larger (megabase, or 10^6 bp) DNA fragments. These analytic techniques include pulsed-field gel electrophoresis (PFGE),[40] field inversion gels (FIG),[41] and contour-clamp homogeneous electric field electrophoresis (CHEF).[42] For purposes of physical mapping of genomic DNA, these techniques can approach the resolution of cytogenetics and, therefore, facilitate large-scale DNA sequencing of the human genome.

Isolated and purified genomic or cloned DNA fragments can be sequenced, analogous to peptide analysis into component amino acid residues. The two most commonly used methods, the dideoxynucleotide chain termination procedure of Sanger et al.[43] and the chemical cleavage procedure of Maxam and Gilbert,[44] permit rapid, accurate, and automated determination of DNA primary structure. Data banks for nucleotide and protein sequence searches and analysis have become indispensable tools for molecular biology. Several single point-of-entry sites that can be routinely accessed through user-friendly Web-browser interfaces are maintained by organizations such as the Baylor College of Medicine Human Genome Center (http://kiwi.imgen.bcm.tmc.edu:8088/search-launcher/launcher.html), Harvard University (http://golgi.harvard.edu/sequences.html), the European Molecular Biology Laboratory (http://www.embl-heidelberg.de/srs/srsc), and the University of Aix-Marseille (http://www-biol.univ-mrs.fr/english/logligne.html).

RNA: Structure and Analysis

Messenger RNAs are synthesized from one DNA strand known as the coding strand during transcription. By convention, the coding DNA strand and the parallel mRNA are written from left to right, from the 5′ to 3′ end. The noncoding strand, or antisense DNA, has the opposite orientation. In eukaryotes, mRNA is synthesized in the nucleus as a large precursor molecule [heterogeneous nuclear RNA or (hnRNA)]. After cleavage and modification steps, the mature mRNAs are exported to the cytoplasm. Most eukaryotic mRNAs, histone mRNAs being a notable exception, contain a polyadenylate sequence at the 3′ end (the "poly(A) tail") that is added in the nucleus to the RNA transcript by poly(A) polymerase. Poly(A) tails distinguish mRNAs, modulate mRNA half-life, and probably perform other, as yet uncharacterized, functions. All eukaryotic mRNAs also are distinguished at the 5′ end by a 7-methylguanylate "cap."

Most mRNAs are substantially longer than is necessary for protein coding. A typical eukaryotic mRNA is 1000 to 2000 bases long, carries 100 to 300 residues of adenylate at the 3′ terminus, a variable length of untranslated 5′ sequence, and a longer 3′ untranslated sequence that is sometimes more than 1000 bases. Ribosomes recognize the mRNA cap, which, in the presence of several initiation factors, facilitates mRNA binding to the ribosomal 40s subunit. An essential attribute of the system is that groups of three consecutive nucleotides in mRNA form codons that comprise the genetic code. Each triplet codon specifies one amino acid (Table 4.1). Triplet combinations of the four ribonucleotides (A,G,C, and U) yield 64 (4^3) possible codons. Since 20 amino acids are represented in proteins, some amino acids are specified by more than one codon. The start (i.e., initiation) and stop (i.e., termination) points of a protein are also specified by codons. Migration along the 40s subunit stops when an AUG (methionine-specifying) initiation codon is encountered, marking the start of the reading frame. During elongation, nascent proteins are assembled from amino acids, amino- to carboxy-terminus, as each mRNA codon recognizes and transiently interacts with the specific, complementary transfer RNA that carries its specified amino acid. This process of protein synthesis from mRNA is known as translation.

Sometimes, more than one mRNA sequence is transcribed from a single gene. The presence of multiple promoter elements (vide infra) may specify different transcription start sites and the use of alternative splicing may generate different 3' ends. Both mechanisms play a role in tissue-specific and developmentally regulated expression of metabolic pathway genes. For example, the mouse amylase gene has two promoters, one used in liver and one used in salivary gland. As a result of the different mRNA 5' ends generated, liver and salivary amylase mRNAs start with different exons[9]; in liver the first 161 bases (b) of the mRNA are coded by exon L, which lies about 4500 bp upstream; in salivary gland, the first 50 b of the mRNA are coded by exon S, which lies about 7300 bp upstream. Since exons L and S encode parts of the 5' untranslated region, both tissues actually synthesize the same amylase protein. In certain other genes, alternative splicing by use of different exons determines whether a tissue synthesizes one or another protein from the same gene, as in the case of calcitonin and calcitonin gene-related protein from their single gene.[45] A third example of the developmental regulation of alternatively spliced transcripts is the expression of structurally and functionally different fetal, neonatal and adult cardiac myosin isoforms.[46]

Since RNA is an inherently unstable molecule, its isolation and subsequent manipulation are more demanding than is the case for dsDNA. RNA is very sensitive to high pH, divalent cations, and omnipresent ribonucleases (RNases). Many investigators treat plasticware, glassware, and solutions with diethyl pyrocarbonate (DEPC) (0.1% in water), which is a strong, but not absolute, inhibitor of RNases,[47] and with baking.[48] The activity of RNases liberated during cell lysis can be inhibited by addition of human placental ribonuclease inhibitor[49] or vanadyl-ribonucleoside complexes.[50] Alternatively, one can disrupt cells and inactivate RNases simultaneously using a combination of potent denaturing agents such as guanidine hydrochloride and guanidinium thiocyanate[51] and reducing agents such as β-mercaptoethanol. These reagents can be used to isolate intact RNA from even RNase-rich tissue such as the pancreas.[52] Numerous straightforward protocols have been developed for the isolation of total RNA from cells and tissues.[52-59] The concentration of the isolated RNA is easily determined by measuring the optical density (OD_{260}) of an aliquot of the final preparation.

A typical mammalian cell contains about 100 pg of RNA, 80% to 85% of which is ribosomal RNA, chiefly 20s, 18s, and 5s. Most of the remaining RNA consists of various low molecular weight species (e.g., transfer RNAs, small nuclear RNAs, etc.). These different RNA subtypes have defined sizes and sequences and can be isolated in virtually pure form by gel electrophoresis, density gradient centrifugation, or anion-exchange or high-performance liquid chromatography.[11] In contrast, mRNAs make up only 1% to 5% of total cellular RNA and they are heterogeneous in size and sequence. The mRNA population collectively encodes virtually all of the polypeptides synthesized by a cell. Since nearly all eukaryotic mRNAs carry 3' terminal poly(A) tails, poly(A)+ RNA can be isolated from the bulk of total cellular RNA by affinity chromatography on oligodeoxythymidine [oligo(dT)]-cellulose columns[60] or by separation using oligo(dT)-linked beads. This step is useful for preparing mRNA templates for the construction of cDNA libraries (vide infra).

Several methods permit quantitation, size determination, and sequence mapping of specific mRNA molecules from preparations of cellular RNA. Specific mRNAs are quantified simply by transferring a known aliquot of the total RNA sample directly onto an immobilized substrate (e.g., nitrocellulose or nylon) using a "dot blot" or "slot blot" vacuum filtration apparatus and hybridizing the RNA with an excess of complementary, labeled probe.[61-63] The amounts of target sequence present in the sample then can be estimated by densitometry.

Total or poly(A)+ RNA also can be denatured in glyoxal or formaldehyde, size fractionated by agarose gel electrophoresis in the presence of denaturants, transferred to nitrocellulose or nylon, and hybridized with a specific probe[62,64-66] (Figure 4.2). This RNA blotting procedure colloquially is called northern blotting, as a takeoff from the eponymous Southern (DNA) blot. Northern blotting is a very sensitive assay of the size (i.e., electrophoretic mobility) and amount (i.e., relative signal intensity) of specific mRNA molecules identified by hybridization. Northern analysis also may suggest regulatory mechanisms for expression of the gene(s) in question by revealing the presence of multiple sizes of mRNAs hybridizing with a specific probe; the multiple transcripts may indicate the existence of several closely related (i.e., cross-hybridizing) genes, or result from use of different transcriptional initiation sites or different polyadenylation sites, alternate splicing of mRNA precursors, or differential transcription of exons. In situations where cell number or absolute RNA concentrations cannot be determined, quantitative Southern analysis using a probe to one of the repetitive genomic DNA sequences (e.g., alu repeat) has been used to enumerate human cells with the intent of establishing absolute transcript levels.[67]

In situ hybridization is a related technique in which RNA hybridization with a probe is assessed directly in prepared tissue sections.[68] This semiquantitative method allows gene expression to be analyzed with single cell resolution.[69,70] Cellular morphology for in situ hybridization is best preserved by limiting exposure to organic solvents and minimizing the stringent posthybridization washes. Asymmetric ^{35}S- or ^{33}P-labeled oligonucleotide probes permit sensitive signal detection and good cellular resolution. The combination of in situ hybridization and immunohistochemistry can be very useful for anatomically mapping metabolic regulatory pathways.[71]

There are more versatile techniques that have much greater sensitivity and specificity than northern hybridization and can yield important quantitative and qualitative data about mRNA structure. In different protection assays, the labeled products of DNA:RNA or RNA:RNA hybridization can be treated under conditions favoring digestion of single-stranded nucleotides only, and the digestion products can be analyzed by polyacrylamide gel electrophoresis (PAGE). In this manner, nuclease S1 mapping can locate the 5′ and 3′ termini of mRNA or DNA templates, locate the 5′ and 3′ splice junctions in restriction endonuclease digested cloned genes, and quantitate the amount of specific classes of mRNA in a sample.[72,73] The assay uses S1 nuclease, an enzyme that has both endonuclease and exonuclease activity and high specificity for single-stranded RNA and DNA, and currently single-stranded probes. S1 nuclease degrades the single-stranded DNA or RNA and the protected fragments (i.e., DNA:RNA or RNA:RNA duplexes) are separated by electrophoresis and detected by autoradiography. A conceptually similar strategy, the RNase protection assay (RPA)[74–78] has become a standard method in many laboratories for quantitating low abundance mRNA molecules, mapping mRNA termini, and determining the position of introns within the corresponding gene. The RPA is based on solution hybridization of a radiolabeled, digoxygenin-labeled or biotinylated antisense cRNA probe ("riboprobe") to target mRNA in a sample. This is followed by RNase digestion of the unhybridized (i.e., single-stranded) RNA and separation of the protected RNA:RNA duplexes by electrophoresis. Primer extension analysis, another related technique, is used primarily to map transcriptional initiation sites.[79]

Reverse transcription (RT) in association with the polymerase chain reaction (PCR) (vide infra) provides a sensitive and rapid alternative method for detection and analysis of RNA, while eliminating the need for large-scale RNA isolation and northern blotting.[80] For RNA detection, the enzyme reverse transcriptase first is used to synthesize a DNA strand complementary to the RNA in question (i.e., cDNA template). This DNA strand is then amplified by PCR. RT-PCR methods are particularly useful for detecting mRNA species present in low abundance[81–83] or in samples containing very few cells.[84] For quantification of RNA, these PCR-based strategies must tackle the considerable problem of how to normalize mRNA expression.[80] This issue may be thought of as analogous to the need to construct a standard curve for interpretation of immunoassay detection of molecules (see Chapter 3). Satisfactory mRNA quantification requires that the RT-PCR product from a gene with variable expression be compared with the RT-PCR product from a reference gene transcript or with an artificial mRNA internal standard. Simultaneous amplification of two different genes (i.e., differential RT-PCR) may yield semiquantitative determination of expression in a series of samples.[85] Competitive quantitative RT-PCR (QC-PCR), controls for tube-to-tube variations in amplification efficiency through addition of a competitive internal standard that is designed to contain primer binding sequences identical to the target gene fragment. Currently, it provides probably the best experimental solution for PCR-based mRNA quantification.[86–89] Since the final ratio of the amplified target to the amplified competitor will exactly reflect the initial ratio of the target to the competitor, the assay should be independent of the number of amplification cycles.[90]

The Analytical Separation of Proteins

Separation of individual proteins from complex mixtures is based on physical properties such as size, charge, and electrophoretic mobility. The choice of an analytic method must strike a balance between power of resolution and preservation of biologic activity.[91] For example, reverse-phase high-performance liquid chromatography (RP-HPLC) is quite useful for separating and analyzing proteins or peptides, but the solvents commonly used as the mobile phase (e.g., acetonitrile with 1% trifluoroacetic acid) denature proteins. Therefore, RP-HPLC may be preferred whenever protein denaturation is acceptable but high resolution is necessary. This situation applies in tryptic digest mapping and amino acid sequencing, where extremely pure protein samples are required and, in fact, denatured proteins are preferred, since tertiary and quaternary structure can interfere with enzymatic cleavage reactions.

Alternatively, if preservation of native protein conformation and function is desirable, ion exchange chromatography usually permits good recovery of activity. The mobile phases are aqueous salt solutions, and separation is based largely on the relative charges of the proteins. Gel filtration and size exclusion chromatography also are useful when high resolution is not needed, for example, during initial steps of protein purification.

Electrophoretic methods separate component proteins in a sample according to mobility or molecular weight. Techniques include zonal electrophoresis in agarose gels or on cellulose acetate membranes, discontinuous PAGE, sodium dodecyl sulfate–PAGE (SDS-PAGE), isoelectric focusing (IEF), and two-dimensional (2-D) PAGE. High-resolution 2-D PAGE separates proteins according to their charges and relative mobilities.[92–94] Conventional one-dimensional SDS-PAGE or IEF can resolve about 100 of the most abundant protein components in a mixture. In contrast, current 2-D PAGE technology allows the resolution of about 3000 to 4000

^{35}S-methionine–labeled polypeptides from any cell line or tissue; of these at least 1000 may correspond to modified variants.[95]

Electrophoresed proteins in a gel, or on a matrix support to which the proteins have been transferred, can be visualized using nonspecific protein stains such as amido black in acetic acid, aniline blue black, Coomassie brilliant blue, India ink, fast green, or colloidal gold or silver stains. Proteins can also be identified in situ by iodination, chlorination, or biotinylation conjugate detection systems.[96]

The critical technical advance in analysis of cellular and secreted proteins has been blotting onto a membrane support so that specific proteins could be identified or probed using antibodies or other ligands. By analogy to DNA (i.e., Southern) blotting, protein transfer from electrophoretic gels to membranes is sometimes called western blotting or, more precisely, either immunoblotting or ligand blotting.[97] Like DNA or RNA, protein solutions also can be directly transferred to a membrane without prior electrophoretic separation (i.e., dot immunoblotting).[98-100] Agarose gels have large pore sizes that do not restrict the movement of protein molecules; they are fragile, and protein transfer must be aided by placing a source of buffer in wet chromatography paper under the gel, as in the original Southern technique (i.e., capillary blotting). As a result, agarose gel electrophoresis rarely is used for protein separation. Polyacrylamide gels, on the other hand, have small pore sizes that hinder free movement of large protein molecules through the sieve-like gel matrix and are better adapted for electrophoretic protein transfer.

Western blot procedures usually separate cellular or serum protein mixtures by SDS-PAGE after reduction by 2-mercaptoethanol or dithiotreitol and denaturing at 100°C. In the initial descriptions of immunoblotting, specific proteins were identified using specific antiserum followed by detection with ^{125}I-labeled protein A[101] or with a second antibody that itself was labeled with ^{125}I, fluorescein, or horseradish peroxidase.[102] Since that time, numerous detection schemes have been adapted for western blot analysis. These techniques generally are not very complex, are sensitive, and can detect single proteins in crude mixtures at positions defined by their size and charge. Monoclonal antibody probes often recognize only a single antigen epitope and so are particularly susceptible to loss of binding activity when electrophoresed proteins (i.e., antigens) are denatured. However, when SDS is omitted from the gel and transfers are performed in alkaline buffer, the proteins retain their native conformation. These "nondenaturing gels" (e.g., PAGE without SDS or isoelectric focusing) make it possible to detect receptors or binding proteins by probing the immobilized native proteins with physiologic ligands.[103]

Protein transfer from polyacrylamide gels is enhanced with vacuum, but electrophoretic transfers are faster and more complete. A commonly used immunoblotting apparatus is illustrated in Figure 4.3. Essentially, a wet membrane is placed in uniform contact with one side of the gel, and gel and membrane are sandwiched between materials (e.g., foam rubber, chromatography paper saturated in transfer buffer) and external plastic grids. The gel sandwich in its plastic cassette is inserted vertically into a buffer tank and a potential gradient is applied across the gel. More recently, horizontal blotting systems have come into wide use. This method dispenses with a buffer tank altogether, the sole source of buffer being buffer-saturated layers of chromatography paper. The wet chromatography paper is placed on the horizontal anode plate, the gel sandwich is positioned over it with the membrane facing the anode (i.e., for SDS gels), and the gel is covered with buffer-soaked paper and the cathode plate. Horizontal protein blotting facilitates blotting several gels simultaneously, uses only small buffer volumes, and does not require cooling.[100]

Like nucleic acids, proteins can be blotted on either nitrocellulose or cationic nylon membranes. In general, these supports must be pretreated with a "blocking agent" (e.g., 3% bovine serum albumin, powdered milk or casein, or serum) to block the unoccupied protein binding sites on the membrane and prevent nonspecific binding of the probe or "background." The primary probes for protein blots may be specific antibodies (e.g., polyclonal or monoclonal, affinity-purified or antiserum), lectins for detection of glycoproteins, DNA or RNA for detection of nucleic acid binding proteins, or ligands (e.g., hormones) for detection of receptors or binding proteins. The primary ligand or specific antibody may be tagged by

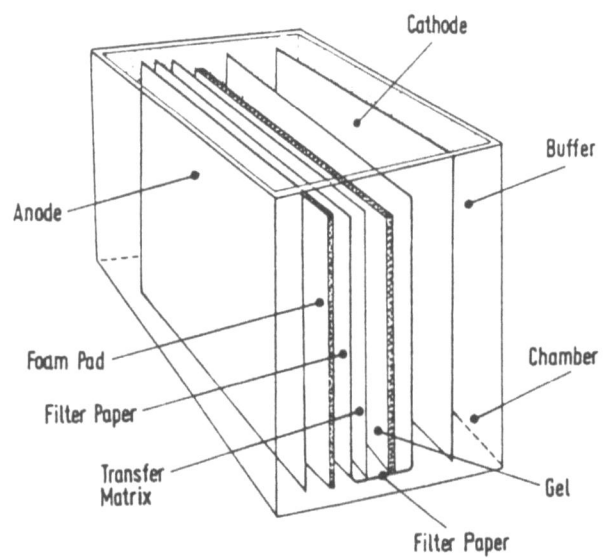

FIGURE 4.3. Vertical protein electroblotting apparatus. (From Stott,[100] with permission.)

radioactivity (^{125}I), fluorescence, or chemiluminescence, but, more commonly, the primary probe is not labeled and, instead, a tagged second or third, indirect, probe is applied. The indirect probe may be antiimmunoglobulin specific for the animal species of primary probe or protein A or protein G, which bind to immunoglobulins and can be themselves detected using a third tagged probe. This "double layer" technique has several advantages: (1) a single labeled second probe can be used for many primary antibodies of different specificities, as well as for suitable negative controls; (2) second antibodies enhance signal detection since several antiimmunoglobulin G (IgG) molecules can bind to the primary probe; and (3) it avoids chemically modifying the primary ligand in ways that might cause nonspecific binding.[104] Western blotting is sometimes combined with high-resolution gel electrophoresis techniques such as isoelectric focusing and 2-D systems to characterize low-abundance proteins of metabolic interest.[99,100] An example of the utility of these techniques has been the detection and identification of putative DNA binding proteins by protein blotting using overlay with labeled DNA, RNA, or histone ligand probes.[105-107]

Generally, however, studies in protein composition and identification have lagged behind the remarkable advances in identification of genes. This lag is partly due to the complexity of the technology required to separate, analyze, and identify the thousands of polypeptides that constitute the "proteome" of a given human cell type. At present, the only available approach to a comprehensive analysis of the human proteome is provided by high-resolution 2D PAGE in combination with methods (vide supra) to identify and quantify the polypeptides present in the individuals spots.[95] Julio E. Celis and colleagues at the Danish Centre for Human Genome Research in Aarhus maintain 2-D PAGE databases for the study of cell regulation and diseases (http://biobase.dk/cgi-bin/celis). When important new cell type-specific protein databases become available they also are published in *Electrophoresis*. All of the known 2-D PAGE database and related servers can be referenced via the Federated 2-D PAGE Database[108] through the ExPASy molecular biology server in Geneva (http://expasy.hcuge.ch/www/expasy-top.html). Recent advances in protein identification techniques (e.g., microsequencing, mass spectrometry, immunoblotting, cDNA expression systems) should make possible further linkage of these gel protein databases to DNA mapping and sequence information with the aim of furnishing an integrated picture of gene and protein expression.

Recombinant DNA Techniques

The methods for amplifying and translating large quantities of individual DNA sequences are collectively known as recombinant DNA technology. Molecular cloning is the process of inserting one DNA molecule of interest into another DNA molecule, usually a bacteriophage or plasmid, that will replicate autonomously as episomes in specially designed host cells, usually bacteria. The gene products of DNA cloning can be synthesized in amounts sufficient for biochemical, structural, and physiologic analysis as well as for medical applications.

Cloning is possible because DNA sequences can be ligated into the genomes of vectors, which are genetically simple carrier elements. Cloning vectors should satisfy several requirements: (1) they must possess suitable restriction enzyme sites so that heterologous (i.e., foreign) DNA can be inserted without disrupting essential vector functions; (2) they must contain an origin for DNA replication and be able to replicate adequately in host cells; and (3) since only a few chimeric plasmids (e.g., foreign plus vector DNA) are generated by the insertion process, cloning vectors must encode suitable selection markers that confer a new bacterial phenotype, usually antibiotic resistance genes.

Relatively small, less than 10kb, DNA fragments usually are cloned into plasmids or phagemids, which are circular dsDNA vector molecules. Phagemids are plasmids into which sequences of the bacteriophage (i.e., bacterial virus) M13 have been engineered. The M13 DNA sequences confer the property to replicate as single-stranded DNA, which is useful for DNA sequencing procedures. Plasmid or phagemid DNA is introduced into host bacteria by transformation, a process in which bacteria, usually *E. coli*, are made permeable (e.g., with divalent cations) to plasmid DNA. In bacterial hosts, plasmid DNA replication is controlled by the enzymes that duplicate the bacterial chromosome. Therefore, mutations engineered in the replicon, the whole genetic unit, can greatly increase plasmid copy number per host cell. Many plasmids are descendants of the cloning vector pBR322.[109] In recent years, plasmid genomes have become progressively more compact; they are designed to be optimally small and to include an expanded capacity for accepting foreign DNA. Plasmid cloning sites, known as polylinkers, contain closely arranged unique synthetic sequences that are targets for restriction endonucleases.

Another common plasmid design feature is specification of resistance to two antibiotics. One gene product identifies (i.e., selects) plasmid-containing bacteria by permitting growth in antibiotic-containing media and the other resistance gene product distinguishes chimeric plasmids; if the insertion site for heterologous DNA lies within this second plasmid gene, insertion of a foreign DNA sequence abolishes that antibiotic resistance. Plasmids propagated in host bacteria routinely are selected by culture in the presence of the appropriate antibiotic(s) and then grown in large quantities. The plasmid DNA is isolated from other bacterial DNA and proteins by chromatography or differential precipitation.[10,11] Plasmid vector systems are especially useful for secondary cloning operations such as the construction of cDNA or cRNA labeled probes, or for large-scale gene expression. As a rule, however, cloning of eukaryotic genomic DNA, where intron-containing genes may span more than 100 kb, requires inserting larger DNA fragments than is possible in plasmids designed for cloning cDNAs. Therefore, bacteriophages, commonly λgt, which are dsDNA viruses, become especially useful for the initial cloning of a gene. Phages can accommodate larger DNA fragments of up to 23 kb. Phage infection of bacteria lyses the host cells, which makes for a convenient plaque assay.

Cosmids are hybrid vector molecules that combine important features of plasmids and bacteriophages. They replicate in *E. coli* like plasmids, but are packaged like bacteriophage particles. Cosmids can accommodate even larger DNA fragments, up to 45 kb, and efficiently infect host cells. Yeast artificial chromosome (YAC) cloning systems can accommodate even larger (i.e., 100–150 kb) DNA fragments[110] and so find application in large-scale genomic sequencing. YACs have been constructed with centromeres and telomeres that allow replication and segregation like normal yeast chromosomes during yeast mitosis. Most recently, various animal virus vectors have been engineered so that animal cells can be infected with cloned genes and gene function can be assayed over time. Delivery of genes to somatic cells in vivo has obvious potential for genetic therapy of metabolic diseases. For example, mutations that disable the cystic fibrosis transmembrane conductance regulator (CFTR) gene cause defects in ion transport across epithelia and the multisystem disease cystic fibrosis. Since adenoviruses show tropism for pulmonary epithelial cells, viral delivery of normal CFTR DNA into the pulmonary epithelium of cystic fibrosis patients may become clinically efficacious.[111]

Several different sources of DNA are suited for molecular cloning, each appropriate for a different purpose. First, if either the gene or its corresponding protein structure is known, DNA can be chemically synthesized. Before the human insulin gene was isolated and sequenced, recombinant human insulin was produced in this fashion working from the protein sequence.[112] A second source is cellular mRNA from which complementary DNA (cDNA) can be synthesized using the enzyme reverse transcriptase and deoxyribonucleotide triphosphates. Finally, chromosomal DNA fragments isolated from nuclei may be cloned into specialized vectors (vide supra).

Particular DNA sequences can be isolated by constructing a set of DNA molecules from a source that contains the sequence of interest. A collection of a sufficient number of clones so that it includes virtually all sequences present in the source cells or tissue is called a library.[113] Libraries are composed of cDNAs of mRNA origin or of digested genomic DNA. The construction of cDNA libraries from various tissues or cells has been a prerequisite for isolating and characterizing numerous eukaryotic genes. Since essentially all mRNAs are represented in the cognate cDNA library, the library really represents that population of genes expressed in that tissue at that time. Plasmids or, more frequently, phage vectors are used to store the large population of cDNAs that form a library.[114] Cloning libraries can be perpetuated indefinitely and be readily retrieved for screening.

A common method for screening of cDNA library is probe hybridization. If a gene has a known product, in principle it is possible to work back from protein sequence to gene. If sufficient peptide can be purified and sequenced, the genetic code will predict the possible DNA sequences.[115] The set of bacterial colonies that compose a cDNA library can be plated on filter paper and hybridized with labeled probes synthesized using the deduced relevant sequences. This recombinant DNA strategy is routinely used in many laboratories for cloning genes that encode specific ligands, receptors, transporters, and metabolic enzymes. Expressing cDNAs of unknown genes in vitro may permit identification of the gene product. A common approach is to express cDNAs in bacteria in the form of fusion proteins linked to some reporter gene (e.g., *E. coli* β-galactosidase). Bacterial colonies are transferred to nitrocellulose and screened with antibody to the enzymatic product using western blot or autoradiography.[116,117] Sometimes a sensitive biologic assay may be available for detection of a specific expressed protein. Transfection into mammalian cells also permits detection of recombinants if the gene in question is expressed on the cell surface or if it alters cell phenotype. Finally, clones of interest can be detected by such methods as hybrid-arrested translation[118] and hybrid-selected translation.[119]

Genomic libraries are important tools for genetic analysis because it is not usually practical to isolate fragments directly from genomic digests. In genomic libraries, in contrast to cDNA libraries, the entire genome (i.e., all genes and DNA sequences) are represented as manageably sized cloned fragments. Furthermore, whereas a cDNA clone represents the amino acid sequence information encoded by its respective mRNA, a genomic clone for that gene contains, in addition to these exon sequences, introns and DNA sequences that flank the transcribed region and may regulate gene expression (vide infra). Clones containing a particular sequence can be selected, usually by colony hybridization. A related strategy, colloquially known as chromosome walking,[120] begins with selecting a genomic clone that contains a known gene or that genetic mapping has shown to lie near a region of interest. DNA fragments subcloned from the ends of this genomic DNA sequence can be used to identify additional clones that contain overlapping sequences. In this manner, genomic regions of several 100 kb can be mapped and subjected to further analysis.

Diagnosis of Metabolic Disease Using Recombinant DNA

Recombinant DNA technology finds wide application in the analysis and diagnosis of metabolic diseases. Increasingly, direct or indirect investigation of DNA is complementing or supplanting biochemical screening for antenatal and neonatal disease identification and carrier detection. In many instances, a genetic defect can be detected without knowing either the primary gene product or even the biochemical derangement causing the disease.

Oftentimes, direct analysis of the genetic disease is possible using allelic probes. For a base-pair change or deletion event responsible for the disease phenotype to be detectable with restriction endonucleases, two conditions must be met: (1) the gene locus must be isolated and cloned so that hybridization probes can be made for examining disease-associated alleles; and (2) gene sequence additions, deletions, or rearrangements that cause the disease must introduce or remove a restriction endonuclease site or must alter the length of DNA between restriction sites.[121]

As a consequence, gene defects that are not gross deletions may remain undetected if a suitable restriction site is not present.[122] In such instances, an alternative approach uses DNA polymorphisms flanking the locus of interest as genetic markers (Figure 4.4). A genetic site is defined as polymorphic when at least 1% of the population encodes a base sequence different from the majority. Specifically, restriction fragment length polymorphisms (RFLPs)[123] are phenotypically neutral base-pair changes that either (1) introduce or remove a restriction site, or (2) introduce sequence insertions, deletions, rearrangements, or variations in the number of short, tandemly repeated DNA sequences, resulting in altered length of DNA between restriction sites. RFLPs are relatively common, consistent with the view that the genome is dynamically heterogeneous. Approximately 1 in 100 to 200 bp in the human genome is polymorphic. For a population, stability of a given RFLP implies that it conveys neither evolutionary advantage nor disadvantage. If a gene contains no detectable polymorphisms, this sort of direct genetic analysis is not possible and the presence of mutations must be inferred from linkage analysis. This latter strategy requires that the genetic markers are located in close proximity (i.e., "linked") to the gene locus

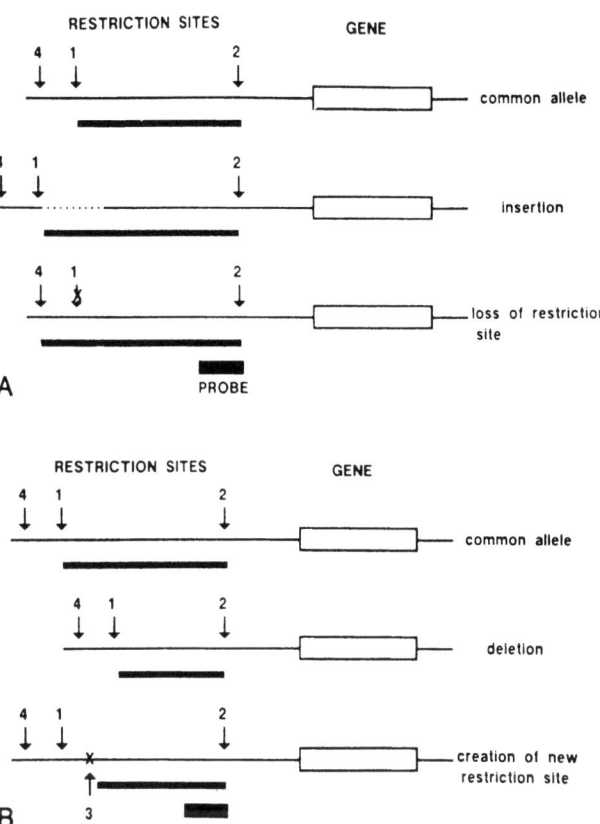

FIGURE 4.4. The molecular basis of RFLPs. (A) A probe (thick bar) is used to determine a restriction fragment (or allele) (thin bar) between sites 1 and 2 near a gene of interest. In the population, larger DNA fragments may arise from insertion of DNA between sites 1 and 2 or from loss of a site (here site 1). (B) Compared with the common allele, smaller fragments also may be generated by deletion of DNA between sites 1 and 2 or by creation of a new restriction site (here site 3). (From Sharp et al,[36] with permission.)

in question (e.g., a disease locus). In the future, "scanning" or "screening" stretches of DNA for the presence of mutations and other sequence differences from the normal sequence may become a reliable, cheap alternative to sequencing.[124]

In principle, any RFLP that distinguishes a disease locus on one chromosome from the normal locus on the allelic diploid chromosome can be used to follow transmission of a mutant allele in a family. When the frequency of an RFLP in a population is high, the likelihood of distinguishing between paired chromosome sets is also high, and the RFLP is said to be "informative."[122] Informative RFLPs are very useful for genetic diagnosis. A compilation of the analysis and diagnosis of human inherited disease using recombinant DNA methods is published annually in *Human Genetics* with quarterly updates (*Gene Diagnosis Newsletter*). The National Center for Biotechnology Information (NCBI) maintains an "Online Mendelian Inheritance in Man" database (http://www.ncbi.nlm.nih.gov/Omim/), a World Wide

Web version of the catalog of human genes and genetic disorders begun by Victor A. McKusick and his colleagues at Johns Hopkins. The database is a compendium of biologic, clinical, and sequence information about human disease-related genes.

The Polymerase Chain Reaction

In recent years, a technical breakthrough by Kary Mullis and other researchers,[124-127] known as the polymerase chain reaction (PCR), has made it possible to bypass molecular cloning and directly amplify short segments of DNA or RNA. Basically, PCR uses repeated cycles of the DNA polymerase-mediated primer extension reaction (Figure 4.5). DNA synthesis of the target sequence requires the presence of two oligonucleotide "primers" that bracket the opposite strands of the DNA target sequence. The use of a thermostable Taq from Thermus aquaticus DNA polymerase and rapid temperature cycling permits repetitive reactions alternating thermal DNA denaturation, primer hybridization, and primer extension reactions in a single test tube without repeated addition of reagents. Typically, a 10^6-fold amplification of the target DNA can be achieved in 2 to 4 hours and 30 cycles. PCR steps are automated and programmable using temperature cycling devices.

Polymerase chain reaction applications have greatly simplified and accelerated analysis of eukaryotic genes.[128-130] As a clinical example, before PCR, rapid, nonisotopic DNA-based genetic diagnosis was practical only for highly abundant target sequences. Detection of rare sequences required long assays, cloning steps, use of hybridization probes, and large tissue samples. In contrast, PCR reaction products are rapidly analyzed using restriction endonuclease digestion and gel electrophoresis[124] (Figure 4.6), followed by sequencing of subclones,[131] direct DNA sequencing,[131-134] transcript sequencing of the amplified DNA,[135] or allele-specific oligonucleotide hybridization.[136] The wide utility of PCR in biologic research and diagnostics has stimulated the development of other in vitro nucleic acid amplification methods that, although in early stages of development, have greater amplification per cycle than PCR.[137,138]

In applied and basic genomics, genes are identified and localized by a process known as transcription mapping. Only a small piece of each cDNA sequence is needed to develop unique gene markers, known as sequence-tagged site (STS) markers, which are detectable in chromosomal DNA by PCR-based assays.[139] To construct a transcript map for the Human Genome Project, cDNA sequences from a master catalog of human genes have been distributed to mapping laboratories in North America, Europe, and Japan. These cDNAs are converted to STSs and their physical locations on chromosomes determined on one of two radiation hybrid panels or YAC libraries containing human genomic DNA. These mapping data have been integrated relative to the human genetic map and then cross-referenced to cytogenetic band maps of the chromosomes. An accurate high-resolution physical map of the human genome is crucial for the localization and positional cloning of genes.

In another PCR application, DNA ligase also can be used to amplify a target sequence by repeated joining of oligonucleotides that hybridize to the target sequence. Basically, two oligonucleotides are hybridized to adjacent sequences on a target strand and joined by DNA ligase to form the product. This synthesized strand is separated from the target sequence by heat denaturation and both the ligation product and target sequence serve as substrates for the next cycle of hybridization and ligation. One important application, ligation-anchored PCR (LA-PCR), is a sensitive and efficient strategy for isolating 5' ends of mRNA transcripts.[140,141] Following first strand cDNA synthesis, the "anchor," lacking an -OH group at the 3' end, is ligated to the 3' end of the first-strand cDNA by T4 RNA ligase. An anchor-specific primer and a primer complementary to a known segment of the cDNA are then used to amplify the 5' end of the transcript.

PCR-based methods are rapidly becoming part of molecular biology procedures in nearly all aspects of gene regulation. In one application, obtaining full-length cDNAs is of critical importance for molecular structure and expression studies. Intact full-length cDNAs, particularly the 5' end of the cDNA, are rarely recovered

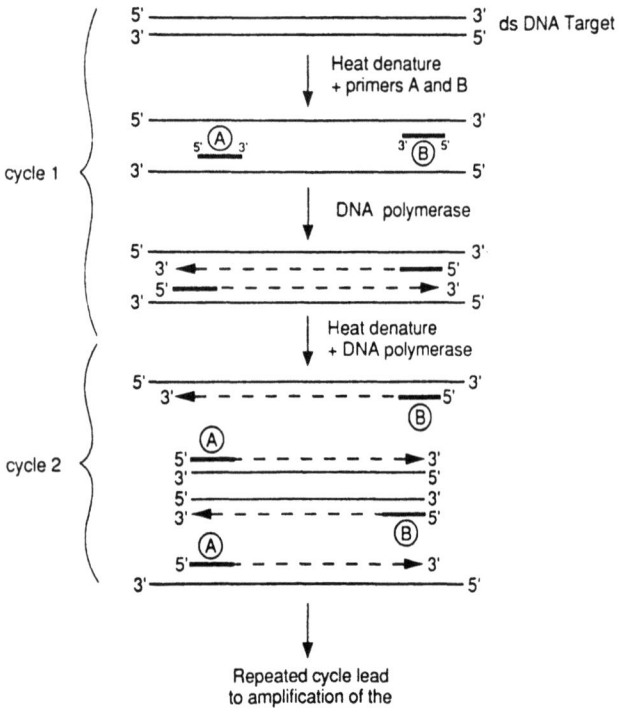

FIGURE 4.5. The polymerase chain reaction. The first two of many repetitive cycles are depicted.

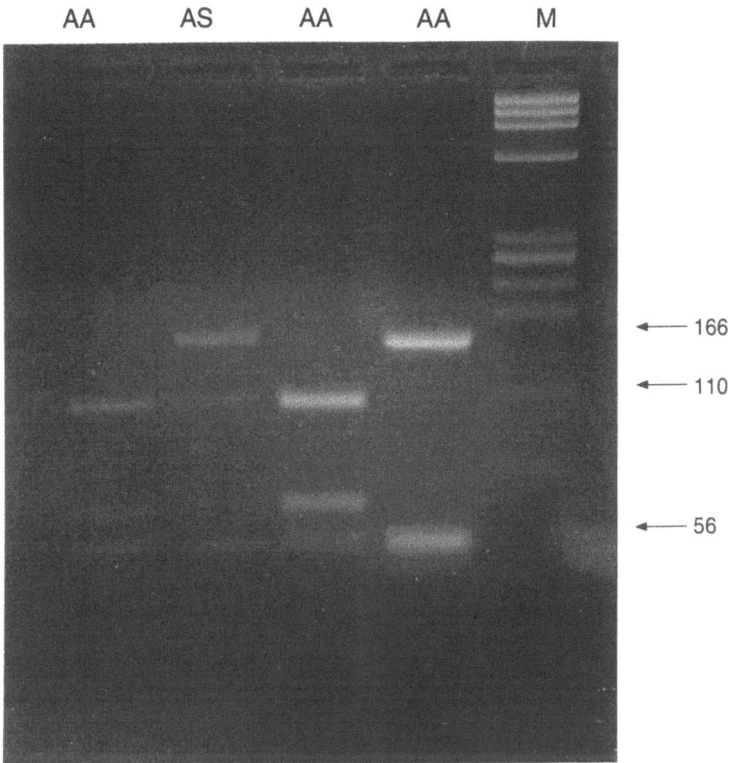

Amplification of beta-globin
gene from umbilical cords

FIGURE 4.6. Detection of sickle cell anemia from umbilical cord samples by PCR and ethidium bromide staining. Lanes labeled AA and AS show β-globin gene amplification products of umbilical cord tissue DNA samples. The amplified product is 166 bp long and includes the single point mutation in the β-globin gene producing hemoglobin S. When control (hemoglobin AA) DNA (4th lane) is digested with Dde I, 110 and 56 bp fragments result (3rd lane). The left (first) lane contains Dde-I– digested amplified DNA from umbilical cord of an infant with genotype AA. The second lane shows amplified product from an umbilical cord of an infant with hemoglobin AS. Dde-I digestion produces the expected 110 and 56 bp bands, as well as an additional uncleaved 166 bp fragment, indicating the presence of a hemoglobin S gene (which contains a point mutation eliminating the Dde I site). (Courtesy of Dr. Beverly Rodgers, Women & Infants' Hospital of Rhode Island.)

from cDNA libraries by screening. Rapid amplification of cDNA ends (RACE)[142,143] is a rapid PCR-based method for amplifying DNA sequences from a mRNA template of a gene of interest between a defined internal site and unknown sequences of either the 5′ or 3′ end of the mRNA. These techniques permit cloning of novel metabolically active genes.[144,145]

Receptor Binding and Initiation of Cell Signaling

An essential principle of endocrinology and cellular metabolism is that messenger molecules, collectively referred to as ligands, exert their metabolic action by their interaction with specific cellular recognition proteins, or receptors. Polypeptide hormones, catecholamines, prostaglandins, neurotransmitters, growth factors, extracellular matrix constituents, certain nutrients, and other small molecules bind to cell surface receptors and alter receptor conformation, triggering intracellular enzymatic signaling systems. On the other hand, "steroid"-type hormones, including glucocorticoids, mineralocorticoids, progestins, and androgens, as well as thyroid hormone, vitamin D metabolites, and retinoic acid (e.g., vitamin A), are relatively apolar, hydrophobic molecules. Free steroids readily diffuse into cells and bind to cytoplasmic or nuclear receptors that are also DNA binding proteins. The characteristic features of both cell surface and steroid receptors are localization in hormone-responsive tissues, high specificity and affinity (i.e., "tight fit") for agonists and antagonist ligands, and the capacity to elicit stereotypical cellular responses once activated by the homologous ligand or an agonist analogue.

Although a particular target cell responds to hundreds or even thousands of different ligands generating a great diversity of specific metabolic responses, these responses

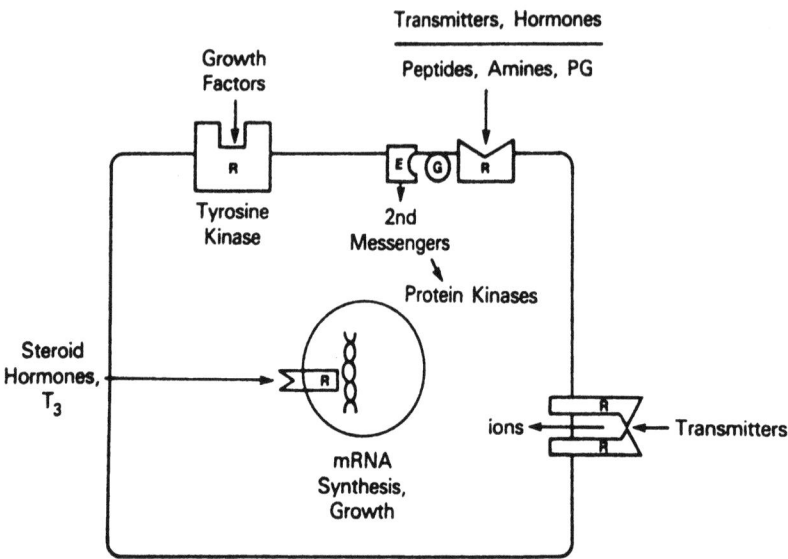

FIGURE 4.7. Cellular mechanisms of action of extracellular ligands. R, receptor; G, receptor-coupled G protein; E, G protein-coupled signal transduction effector (enzyme).

generally are mediated by a relatively few intracellular signaling mechanisms activated by ligand-receptor binding (Figure 4.7). In essence, a multitude of genetically determined target cell responses are generated by a limited set of common enzyme-dependent effector systems.

A comprehensive description of cellular metabolism takes into account the dual functional properties of receptors, namely, recognition (i.e., ligand binding) and activation (i.e., transduction of ligand-receptor binding into specific biologic responses). These essential properties imply that each receptor molecule must contain at least two definable regions or structural domains for, respectively, recognition and transduction of the environmental (e.g., hormonal) stimulus. As a general rule, antagonists bind but generally do not activate their receptors, whereas agonists bind and trigger conformational changes that activate effector systems. Antagonists and agonists, therefore, are important pharmacologic probes in metabolic investigation.

Receptor activation sometimes is triggered in the absence of ligand binding. In particular, lectins or receptor antibodies that cross-link receptor binding sites and alter receptor structure are useful probes of receptor structure and function. Certain receptor antibodies, such as those to receptors for thyroid stimulating hormone,[146] insulin,[147] epidermal growth factor,[148] and prolactin[149] can exert agonist-like effects on their respective target cells. A variation on this theme occurs when receptor-bound gonadotropin-releasing hormone analogues are cross-linked by specific antibody and acquire agonist activity. Luteinizing hormone is then released from the pituitary, presumably as a result of receptor microaggregation and cell activation.[150] Similarly, deglycosylated human chorionic gonadotropin (hCG) derivatives usually act as receptor antagonists, but when cross-linked by anti-hCG antibodies they also can cause target cell activation.

Analysis of Ligand-Receptor Binding

Ligand recognition by its receptor is an example of the broader class of physicochemical phenomena in which a small molecular domain binds stereospecifically to a larger molecule, which generally is a protein. Other examples include the binding of antigen to antibody, substrate to enzyme, and plasma molecule to a specific carrier or binding protein. Some polypeptide ligands display biaxial symmetry (e.g., thyroid-releasing hormone, gonadotropin-releasing hormone, bradykinin, angiotensin II) and bind to complementary, symmetrical subunits in their respective receptors. The symmetries and internal homologies of polypeptides and their subunit receptors may have co-evolved because of the selective advantages conferred by cooperative interactions during receptor binding.[151]

Studies of receptor structure and function aim to comprehend the molecular bases of ligand recognition. Similarly, the investigation of receptor-activated signal transduction pathways aims to understand how ligand-receptor binding generates signals (i.e., so-called postreceptor events) that alter cellular function. The use of radioligand binding studies or, more recently, measurement of ligand concentration by fluorescence, is a mainstay for direct characterization of receptors and measuring specific binding of ligands, usually hormones[152-154] (see Chapter 3). In practice, for binding experiments one incubates a constant receptor concentration with increasing concentrations of labeled ligand, which are known as saturation experiments, or with a fixed concentration of labeled ligand and increasing concentrations of unlabeled, cold ligand that competes with label for receptor binding, which are known as competition experiments. The use of competitive inhibitors that block hormone binding often provides additional, important information about receptor function. In fact, certain receptors, such as those for acetylcholine and catecholamines, have been characterized largely using radioligand-binding experiments with labeled antagonists of high specificity and affinity. This approach is widely used in the pharmaceutical industry as a rapid means of determining the affinity of novel compounds for a particular receptor for which a well-characterized radioligand is available. The presence of high-affinity binding sites, along with the appropriate ligand specificity for agonist and antagonist analogues, is compelling evidence for the presence of a particular receptor.[155]

In general, receptor binding assays ought to satisfy several requirements:

1. *The ligand "tagging" procedure should permit quantification.* Radioactive isotopes (^{125}I, ^{3}H) can be incorporated at high specific activity (high radioactivity per unit ligand) and so frequently are used as ligand tags. It is critical that iodination of polypeptide ligands only minimally alters the peptide's biologic activity; this often is possible with gentle mono-iodination and avoidance of severe oxidizing or reducing conditions. However, tagging with radioiodide atoms can alter biologic activity of natural peptides and tyrosinated peptide analogues. Sometimes the binding characteristics of agonists and antagonists for a specific receptor also may differ.

2. *The receptors must be accessible to the ligand.* Cell surface receptors usually are studied using intact cells or plasma membrane fractions. Intracellular receptors can be assayed in fractionated subcellular preparations of cytosol and/or nuclei. Binding assays derived from these crude receptor preparations often are complicated by problems of ligand degradation, receptor internalization, or nonspecific binding. Preliminary receptor purification steps may minimize these confounders. Additionally, the optimal duration and temperature for ligand-receptor incubation often must be determined empirically. When assays are performed at 37°C, degradation of ligand and receptor complicates in vitro determination of binding constants and thermodynamic properties. For this reason, receptor binding studies are usually performed at lower temperatures (4°–24°C), but at the present there are few experimental data about the kinetic and equilibrium binding properties of peptides and receptors under physiologic conditions.

3. *Bound and unbound (free) ligand must be separable.* Unbound ligand can be separated from particulate or whole cell receptor preparations by centrifugation. Soluble receptor preparations can be subjected to a variety of separation methods, including gel filtration chromatography and polyethylene glycol (PEG) precipitation.

Specificity of the ligand-receptor interaction is measured by comparing binding of labeled ligand in the presence and absence of an excess of unlabeled ligand. For this procedure, one assumes that there is a finite number of receptors and, consequently, that binding capacity is saturable. Total binding is binding obtained in the absence of unlabeled ligand. Any binding of labeled ligand measured in the presence of excess unlabeled ligand is considered to be nonspecific (e.g., biologically irrelevant binding). Specific binding, as a result, is defined as total binding minus nonspecific binding. Knowing the binding characteristics for a receptor preparation and a labeled ligand tracer permits measuring the actual concentrations of ligand present in biologic samples. The principle of this radioreceptor assay is essentially similar to that of radioimmunoassay, except that, instead of binding to an antibody, a ligand binds to its specific receptor (see Chapter 3). Interpretation of binding data must always be tempered by the recognition that many hormone-responsive cells contain so-called spare or excess receptors. Therefore, receptor binding affinity measured by radioligand assays is often lower than the ligand concentration required to elicit half-maximal biologic responses (ED_{50}). In fact, maximal cellular responses may be evoked when only a small proportion of the available receptors are occupied.

It has been suggested that the definition of a hormone receptor should be restricted only to those tissue binding sites that can be associated with defined biochemical or cellular response. However, the demonstration of specific, high-affinity binding sites using radioligand agonists or antagonists also provides a valid index of receptors if appropriate binding conditions are observed. These experimental conditions include the use of labeled biologically active ligands, accurate determination of nonspecific binding, and exclusion of binding due to degradation or other enzymatic activities in sample fractions.[19]

Generally, there are two receptor binding parameters that have practical value: the number of receptor molecules per mass protein or per cell number, known as binding capacity, and the affinity of receptor for the ligand (i.e., "tightness" of binding). It is possible to measure and relate these two terms if ligand-receptor binding equilibrium is established and then ligand is added incrementally to reach binding saturation. As outlined below, it is convenient to deal with affinity as a function of the kinetics of ligand-receptor association and dissociation.

Binding of a ligand, $[L]$, with its specific receptor, $[R]$, may be represented as a simple, bimolecular reversible interaction, assuming that both ligand and receptor are homogeneous and univalent:

$$[L]+[R] \underset{k_d}{\overset{k_a}{\rightleftharpoons}} [LR] \quad (1)$$

where $[LR]$ represents the ligand-receptor complex and k_a and k_d are the association rate constant ($M^{-1}s^{-1}$) and dissociation rate constant (s^{-1}), respectively. Establishment of equilibrium means that the forward and reverse reactions have reached a balance so that for each L and R molecule combining to form LR, an LR complex dissociates into L and R (i.e., the forward and reverse reaction rates are equal). Since the rate constants, as the term implies, remain constant, the change that must occur so that a system to reach equilibrium is a change in the relative concentrations of reactants (L, R) and products (LR). In other words, and as stated in the law of mass action, the rate of a reaction is proportional to the product of the concentrations of the reactants. At equilibrium

$$k_a[L][R] = k_d[LR] \quad (2)$$

so that the product of the reactant concentrations in the forward direction multiplied by the k_a is equal to the product of the reactant concentrations in the reverse direction multiplied by the k_d. Equation 2 can be rearranged to give

$$\frac{k_a}{k_d} = \frac{[LR]}{[L][R]} = K_A \quad (3)$$

The association equilibrium constant (K_A) is defined as the ratio of the association and dissociation rate constants. The dissociation equilibrium constant (K_D), describing the dissociation of LR to form L and R, is then defined as

$$\frac{k_d}{k_a} = \frac{[L][R]}{[LR]} = K_D \quad (4)$$

By convention the equilibrium constants (K) are distinguished from the rate constants (k) by the use of capitalized and lowercase letters, respectively. From Equations 3 and 4 it follows that

$$K_A = 1/K_D \quad (5)$$

K_D has units of moles/liter while K_A has the reciprocal units (i.e., liters/mole). Since the latter are impractical for routine laboratory use, K_D is the equilibrium constant designated as the affinity constant. When the magnitude of K_D is small, the tendency of LR to dissociate to L and R is small.

When increasing amounts of ligand are added to a constant receptor concentration, data like those shown in Figure 4.8A are obtained. Since $[LR]$ indicates bound receptor sites and $[R]$ indicates free receptor sites, the relation between the total receptor concentration ($[R_T]$) and occupied sites is

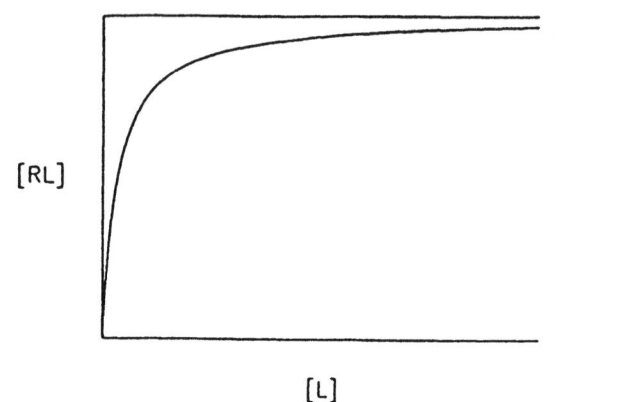

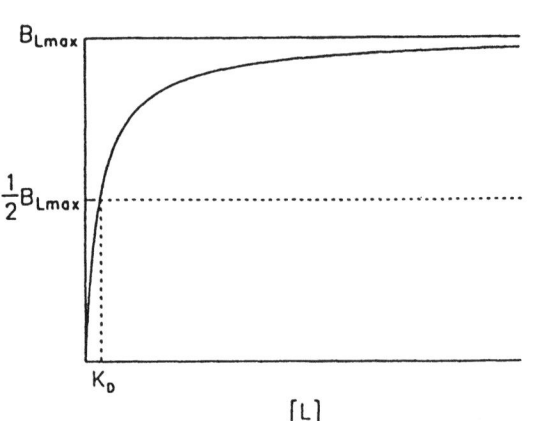

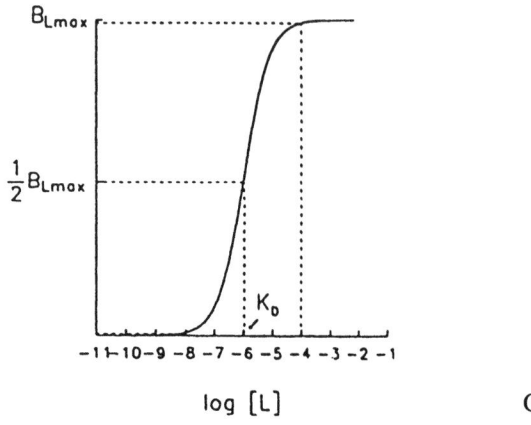

FIGURE 4.8. A plot of data obtained from a radioreceptor assay. As $[L]$ increases (with fixed total $[R]$) the amount of RL increases and approaches horizontal as $[L]$ approaches infinity B. (A) The upper limit of the curve represents the maximal binding, or $B_{L\,max}$. (B) One then locates $\frac{1}{2}B_{L\,max}$ on the ordinate, then moves horizontally to intersect the curve and down to intersect the abscissa, which determines the value of K_D. (C) The data are spread out by plotting B_L vs $\log[L]$.

$$[R_T]=[LR]+[R] \quad (6)$$

$$\text{or} \quad [R]=[R_T]-[LR] \quad (7)$$

The upper limit of the curve in Figure 4.8A, where $[LR]$ equals R_T, represents the condition of maximum ligand binding and is called B_{max}. The amount of ligand bound at any ligand concentration is called B. The equation that describes the relationship shown in Figure 4.8A is obtained by substituting the value $[R]$ from Equation 7 into Equation 4 to give

$$K_D = \frac{([R_T]-[LR])[L]}{[LR]} \quad (8)$$

Expanding terms yields

$$K_D + \frac{[R_T][L]}{[LR]} - \frac{[LR][L]}{[LR]} = \frac{[R_T][L]}{[LR]} - [L] \quad (9)$$

Rearranging gives

$$K_D + [L] = \frac{[R_T][L]}{[LR]} \quad (10)$$

and

$$[LR] = \frac{[R_T][L]}{K_D + [L]} \quad (11)$$

Substituting B_{max} for $[R_T]$ and B for $[LR]$ results in

$$B = \frac{B_{max}[L]}{K_D + [L]} \quad (12)$$

Equation 12 is a representation of the Hill-Langmuir equation,[156,157] which is identical to the Michaelis-Menten equation for enzyme kinetics.[158] $[L]$ is known since it is added for receptor assay. It is now possible to describe ligand-receptor interaction in terms of the two experimental values which must be determined, namely, binding affinity (K_D) and the number of receptors present (B) (Figure 4.8B,C).

Practical considerations apparent for determining K_D and B_{max} are that, for high $[L]$, it may be difficult to measure B_{max} reliably, and that ligands may not be available in large quantities or be expensive. Fortunately, Equation 12 can be rearranged to

$$B = \frac{B_{max}[L]}{K_D + [L]} \quad (13)$$

Further rearrangement of terms gives

$$\frac{B_{max}}{B} = \frac{K_D + [L]}{[L]} \quad (14)$$

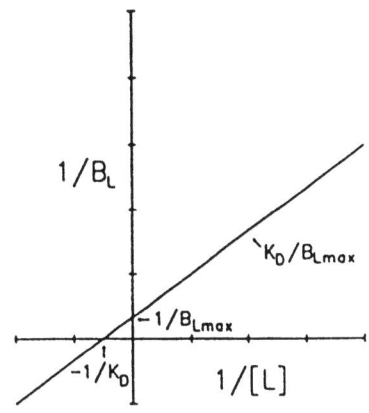

FIGURE 4.9. Plot of $1/B_L$ vs $1/[L]$, the double reciprocal or Lineweaver-Burk equation.

$$\text{or} \quad \frac{B_{max}}{B} = \frac{K_D}{[L]} + 1 \quad (15)$$

$$\text{or} \quad \frac{1}{B} = \frac{1}{[L]}\frac{K_D}{B_{max}} + \frac{1}{B_{max}} \quad (16)$$

which is the double reciprocal of the Langmuir isotherm, known as the Lineweaver-Burk equation.[159] Figure 4.9 shows that plotting $1/B$ vs $1/[L]$ gives a straight line. The $1/B$ axis intercept equals $1/B_{max}$, the $1/[L]$ axis intercept equals $-1/K_D$ and the slope equals K_D/B_{max}. Therefore, it is possible directly to measure B_{max} and K_D. Since the double-reciprocal plot spreads the data poorly, the methods below are the preferred linear transformations for plotting binding data.

Equation 12 also can be transformed by rearranging terms to obtain

$$\frac{B(K_D + [L])}{[L]} = B_{max} \quad (17)$$

and expanding terms to obtain

$$\frac{(B)(K_D)}{[L]} + B = B_{max} \quad (18)$$

and

$$\frac{B}{[L]} = \frac{B}{K_D} + \frac{B_{max}}{K_D} \quad (19)$$

known as the Rosenthal-Scatchard equation.[160-162] Plotting $B/[L]$ vs B yields the graphical representation in Figure 4.10. The $B/[L]$ axis intercept is B_{max}/K_D, the B axis intercept is B_{max}, and the slope is $-1/K_D$. An alternative rearrangement of Equation 18 gives

$$B = -\frac{B}{[L]}(K_D) + B_{max} \quad (20)$$

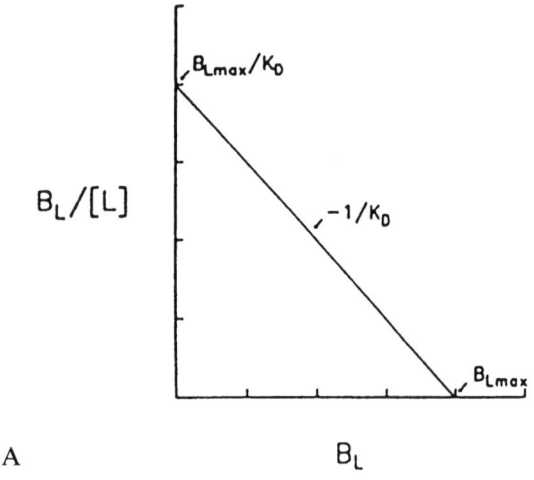

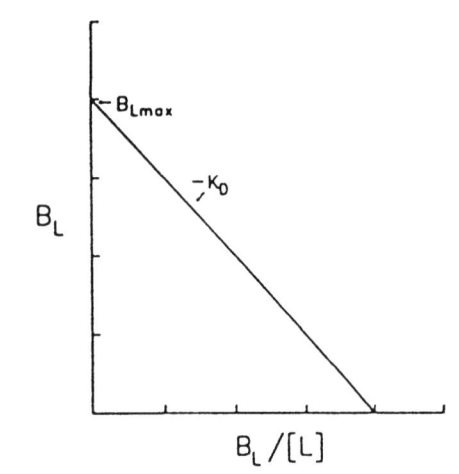

FIGURE 4.10. (A) Plot of $B_L/[L]$ vs B_L, the Rosenthal-Scatchard equation. (B) Plot of B_L vs $B_L/[L]$, the Eadie-Hofstee equation.

which is the Eadie-Hofstee equation.[163,164] Plotting B vs $B/[L]$ yields the graph in Figure 4.10B. The B axis intercept equals B_{max} and the slope equals $-K_D$. All of these calculations assume that one molecule of ligand binds to one receptor site so that the number of binding sites per cell number, or per mass protein, is calculated by multiplying the molar concentration of receptors by Avogadro's number (6.02×10^{23}).

While Scatchard plots are very useful for visualizing data and obtaining estimates of K_D and B_{max}, they are reliable only to the extent that the data are very good and fit a straight line. These qualifications hold because the linear transformation distorts the experimental error. Specifically, the assumptions that the scatter of points around the line follows a Gaussian distribution and that the standard deviation is the same at every experimental value are not true for the transformed data. Simple linear regression overestimates K_D and B_{max}. B, with its associated errors, occurs in both variables, and so it should not be applied to Scatchard or Eadie-Hofstee plots. Because nonlinear Scatchard plots are even more difficult to handle, there is a temptation to fit the data into straight lines. Fortunately, nonlinear least-square methods enhance accuracy for the estimation of binding parameters with their confidence limits.[165] Ligand (Biosoft) and Prism (GraphPad) are commercially available programs designed specifically for the analysis of ligand-binding experiments. In summary, it is inappropriate to analyze data by performing linear regression on a Scatchard plot but it is often helpful to display receptor binding data in this form.

Not all Scatchard or Eadie-Hofstee plots are linear. Nonlinearity may indicate the presence of (1) more than one type of binding site for the ligand at different affinities in the preparation; or (2) allosteric receptor-receptor interactions that, upon initial ligand binding, enhance or decrease further ligand binding (i.e., positive or negative cooperativity). To determine whether there is significant allostery, the data from ligand-receptor binding studies can be further transformed and represented as a Hill plot.[166,167] Allostery is present if the slope of the Hill plot line significantly differs from a value of 1. Other factors producing nonlinear Scatchard plots include artifacts introduced when the analysis is not carried out under equilibrium conditions, inaccurate estimates of nonspecific binding, inaccurate separation of bound and free hormone, and significantly different affinities of labeled and unlabeled ligand for the receptor.[166]

Many peptide hormones and growth factors exhibit the following features: high receptor binding affinity, with K_Ds that typically range from 10^{-11} to $10^{-9} M^{-1}$; high specificity for biologically active hormones and agonist or antagonist derivatives; and saturability at relatively low ligand concentrations. These properties are consistent with the high selectivity and low concentration of receptors, which frequently number only several thousand sites per cell. Quantification of receptor number and affinity for different ligands also permits identification of receptor subtypes. For example, M1 muscarinic cholinergic receptors show high affinity for the drug pirenzipene, while M2 receptors show low affinity for pirenzipene. It is also possible to determine how ions, nucleotides, lipids, and other molecules may modulate ligand-receptor binding.

Receptor Purification and Molecular Analysis

Morphologic techniques, such as receptor autoradiography and immunohistochemistry, and subcellular fractionation can be used to study a receptor's distribution in organs, tissues, or subcellular components, as well as for assay of receptor internalization. The physicochemical characterization of receptors can be a more arduous task because cell surface receptors are relatively insoluble in aqueous solutions. Although occasionally receptors can be dissociated from the cell membrane using limited enzymatic digestion or incubation under hypotonic conditions, receptor solubilization for physicochemical analysis usually requires that receptors be extracted from tissue homogenates or membrane fractions by treatment with mild nonionic detergents (e.g., Triton X-100, Lubrol) or zwitterionic detergents (e.g., Chaps). Detergent-extracted solubilized receptors with their effector systems can be purified and reconstituted into artificial lipid bilayers or into host cell membranes for studies of their activation mechanisms under defined conditions.[168] Alternatively, preformed ligand-receptor complexes, produced by saturation of target cells with labeled ligand, can be extracted with nonionic detergents. These soluble ligand-receptor complexes tend to be more stable and are more amenable to chemical analysis than are free, soluble receptors.

Detergent-solubilized hormone receptors can be purified on a small scale by conventional fractionation procedures, affinity chromatography on gel-ligand complexes, or immunoaffinity techniques. The purified receptors (e.g., those for insulin, EGF, catecholamines, and various glycoproteins) can be quite stable, retaining specificity and high affinity for their ligands. This purification strategy may produce sufficient quantities of receptor protein for partial amino acid sequencing and synthesis of deduced oligonucleotide DNA sequences. Labeled oligonucleotide probes then can be made for hybridization screening of cDNA libraries in order to identify candidate receptor cDNA clones. Antibodies raised to purified receptors also can be used to screen cDNA libraries that are constructed in expression vectors such as λgt 11. These methods have led to discovery of the primary structures and functional organization of numerous receptors important in perinatal metabolism, including the receptors for insulin, EGF, β-adrenergic catecholamines, and low-density lipoprotein. New receptors can also be cloned by nucleotide sequence homology to previously cloned receptors.[169] Once the gene sequence for a receptor is known, it becomes possible to undertake detailed analysis of receptor regulation by expression studies and to explore structure-function relationships by engineering specific alterations in the DNA sequence through site-directed mutagenesis.[170]

Receptors and Target Cell Desensitization

Cell surface receptors exist in a dynamic state in the plasma membrane. Regulation of receptor-mediated events can take place at multiple steps including topologic distribution of receptors in the membrane; interaction with other membrane constituents and intracellular effector systems; and distribution with intracellular sites for recycling, synthesis, and degradation. Many of the metabolic changes associated with pregnancy and fetal and neonatal development are mediated through changes in receptor number and ligand affinity.

Desensitization, also called tachyphylaxis, describes a progressive waning of biologic response despite ongoing stimulation of constant intensity. This phenomenon occurs when a target cell is subjected to prolonged or repeated exposure to an agonist. Desensitization is caused by altered receptor function rather than by agonist degradation and, for many receptors, such as the adrenergic receptor gene family, it involves receptor phosphorylation.[171] Desensitization may be homologous, in which exposure to the specific agonist diminishes the cellular response only to that ligand, or heterologous, in which exposure to one ligand impairs the ability of that effector system [e.g., adenosine 3′,5′-cyclic monophosphate (cAMP) or diacylglycerol accumulation] to respond to other ligands that act on other receptors. Ligand-stimulated adenylate cyclase responses commonly show acute desensitization;[172] the rapid, initial burst of ligand-stimulated cAMP production is followed by a decline to basal levels and a loss of responsiveness to further hormonal stimulation. Since most peptide hormones and neurotransmitters are secreted episodically, these ligand-triggered membrane effector systems may be adapted for optimal target cell activation by an intermittent stimulus.

The other side of desensitization is supersensitivity. In the case of neurotransmitter receptors, prolonged exposure to agonists may induce a state of heightened sensitivity. If, for example, the β-adrenergic antagonist propranolol is abruptly withdrawn after prolonged receptor blockade, deleterious cardiovascular consequences may result because the receptors have a heightened sensitivity to β-adrenergic agonists.

Acute desensitization of an effector system can be distinguished from true ligand-induced receptor loss, or receptor downregulation (i.e., internalization). Ligand-induced receptor downregulation has been demonstrated for receptors for numerous peptide and steroid hormones, growth factors, and neurotransmitters. The phenomenon is similar to the normal entry of essential nutrients and other molecules into a cell (e.g., transferrin or LDL) by receptor-mediated endocytosis. Homologous receptor downregulation, in which increased hormone concentrations decrease the number of specific receptors, and receptor upregulation during reduced hormone exposure have obvious biologic advantages.

The developmental regulation of target cell receptor number and hormone responsiveness are important mechanisms in perinatal-neonatal metabolism. For example, hCG treatment increases luteinizing hormone (LH) receptor number in fetal and neonatal testicular (Leydig) cells but it induces desensitization and receptor loss in the adult testis.[173] An important feature of slower binding and dissociating hormone-receptor systems, such as gonadotropin binding to gonadal target cells, is that the phases of desensitization and receptor loss by internalization may merge, and the initial period of refractoriness due to homologous desensitization may be followed by internalization and degradation of LH-receptor complexes.[174]

Ligand-mediated regulation of receptor number provides a convenient means for differentiating between two general classes of cell surface receptors.[175] Class I receptors are responsible for target cell stimulation and the rapid regulation of metabolic events. Ligand binding (e.g., by a hormone, growth factor, neurotransmitter, chemotactic peptide, etc.) may induce receptor desensitization or downregulation or both, but internalization of the ligand-receptor complex is not essential for receptor activation. In contrast, class II receptors (e.g., so-called nutrient or feeding receptors) govern the cellular uptake of nutrient macromolecules and certain other molecules essential for cell growth and metabolism (e.g., LDL, transferrin, β_2-macroglobulin, EGF). Class II receptors do not, as a rule, undergo downregulation in the sense used above. After receptor-mediated endocytosis they are recycled to the cell surface.

Receptor Types and Signal Transduction Pathways

Several distinct receptor types have been identified, each linked to distinct signal transduction mechanisms. Lipophilic ligands bind to intracellular receptors. Steroids, sterols (e.g., vitamin D metabolites), retinoic acid (e.g., vitamin A), thyroid hormone, and other lipophilic compounds readily pass through the cell membrane, although it is uncertain whether or not this occurs by simple diffusion, and bind to members of a "superfamily" of cytoplasmic and nuclear receptors that are also DNA-binding proteins. Ligand binding activates receptor association with other nuclear transcription factors, binding to specific DNA regulatory sequences and modification of gene expression.

Another broad category of receptors interacts with ligands at the cell surface. Membrane receptors can be classified structurally and functionally into three superfamilies, differing in the number and arrangement of their membrane-spanning segments and signal transduction pathways: (1) two-to-four-transmembrane (2-TM, 3-TM, 4-TM) segment receptors that form ligand-gated ion channels, (2) single-transmembrane segment receptors directly or indirectly coupled to intracellular enzymes, and (3) seven-transmembrane (7-TM) segment receptors coupled to G proteins. Binding of ligand, the "first messenger," initiates an intracellular enzymatic cascade, which ultimately leads to altered cellular function. For many polypeptide hormones, growth factors, and neurotransmitters, the cascades involve the generation of intracellular "second messengers" [e.g., cAMP, guanosine 3',5'-cyclic monophosphate (cGMP), inositol polyphosphates, Ca^{2+}, etc.].

The ligand-gated ion channel receptors are integral transmembrane glycoproteins that contain extracellular ligand binding sites. At least three structurally different channel subfamilies have been defined by molecular cloning combined with pharmacologic and electrophysiologic techniques: 4-TM receptors, including the nicotinic cholinergic receptor, which is a sodium channel, and the γ-aminobutyric acid (GABA) receptor, which is a chloride channel; the excitatory amino acid receptors (3-TM); and the adenosine triphosphate (ATP) (2-TM) receptors. All of the characterized ligand-gated ion channels are multisubunit complexes that exist in one of three functional states: resting (i.e., or closed), open, and desensitized.[176,177] Agonist binding to a resting receptor induces transition to the open state, called gating, and often also a transition to the desensitized state. Because the desensitized state often exhibits higher agonist affinity than does the open one, most ion channels will be in the desensitized state after prolonged exposure to the specific agonist.[178] The physiology of ligand-gated ion channels is amenable to mechanistic investigation because the ligand-stimulated response (i.e., ionic current through open channels measurable with voltage or patch-clamp techniques) is directly proportional to receptor activation. Development of single-channel recording techniques has been an enormous advance for studies of ion channel function. These methods permit direct measurement of the duration of ion channel openings and closings, and so avoid limiting assumptions that are necessary when interpreting macroscopic current records.[179,180] Ligand-operated ion channels have manifold functions in developmental metabolism. Recently, for example, familial persistent hypoglycemia of infancy (i.e., "familial hyperinsulinism" or "nesidioblastosis") has been demonstrated to be caused by several loss-of-function mutations in the high-affinity sulfonylurea receptor, a subunit of the pancreatic islet β-cell ATP-sensitive potassium channel[181,182] (see Chapter 32).

A superfamily of single-transmembrane segment receptors includes receptors with cytoplasmic domain catalytic activity like tyrosine kinase[183] (e.g., mitogenic growth factors, insulin), serine-threonine kinase (e.g., transforming growth factor-β type 1 and 2, activin, inhibin, müllerian inhibiting substance, bone morphogens), guanylate cyclase[184] (e.g., atrial natriuretic peptide type A, B, and C), and phosphotyrosine phosphatase.[185,186] All of the known ligands are polypeptides. Signal transduction is initiated via phosphorylation or dephosphorylation of proteins or by formation of cGMP. Approximately 10% of cellular proteins generally are phosphorylated and the typical cell necessarily contains a great number of protein kinases with different substrate specificity.[187,188] More than 99% of cellular protein kinases phosphorylate serine or threonine residues, whereas fewer than 1% are tyrosine kinases. Ligand binding to tyrosine kinase receptors (i.e., intrinsic enzyme activity) and tyrosine kinase-linked receptors (i.e., associated with cytoplasmic tyrosine kinases) mediates the action of numerous polypeptide hormones, growth factors, cytokines, proto-oncogenes, and oncogenes.[189,190] In general, growth factors constitute a diverse group of polypeptides that modulate cell proliferation. These factors differ somewhat from classical hormones in that neither their site(s) of synthesis nor site(s) of action is restricted to defined tissues. Moreover, many growth factors probably act in paracrine or juxtacrine and, sometimes, autocrine fashion. Oncogenes are genes that, having been altered by mutation, amplification, translocation, or carriage by viruses, can cause malignant transformation. Proto-oncogenes are the respective normal precursors. In transformation, constitutive activation of a positive control element gene or deletion of a normal inhibitory regulator (e.g., negative control element) unregulates some normal developmental growth process.

The basic organizational motifs for protein tyrosine kinase-containing receptors, including receptors for EGF/transforming growth factor-α, insulin, insulin-like growth factor-I (IGF-I), platelet-derived growth factor (PDGF), and nerve growth factor (NGF) are similar. These transmembrane glycoproteins contain a single extracellular ligand-binding domain and a cytoplasmic catalytic (e.g., tyrosine kinase) domain that transduces a hormonal signal and generates a biochemical message. Not surprisingly, the cytoplasmic tyrosine kinase domains of growth factor receptors and many oncogene products are similar. Tyrosine kinase activity is critical for cell proliferation and it underlies the regulation of growth and metabolism by several growth factors and hormones, including insulin (see Chapter 8). Membrane receptors for growth hormone (GH), prolactin, erythropoietin, granulocyte-macrophage colony stimulating factors, interferons, and many interleukins are devoid of intrinsic enzyme activity but associate with cytoplasmic tyrosine kinases like the Janus kinase (JAK) family, and other membrane proteins, to form subunit receptor complexes.[191,192]

Receptors for the majority of polypeptide hormones, all monoamine neurotransmitters, prostaglandins, and extracellular calcium[193] are members of another, related structural superfamily of transmembrane proteins in which a single polypeptide chain is reversibly associated with distinct effector molecules through intermediary guanine-nucleotide binding proteins (G proteins).[194,195] These receptor-coupled G proteins are heterotrimers composed of α, β, and γ subunits.[196] Ligand binding alters receptor conformation, allowing it to associate with a G protein, promoting exchange of guanosine diphosphate (GDP) for guanosine triphosphate (GTP), leading to dissociation of the $\beta\gamma$-subunit from G_α. Essentially, the intracellular signaling is governed by a receptor-dependent GTP (on), GDP (off) switch. The $\beta\gamma$ subunits, which are identical or similar for many receptors, function as a heterodimer.[197] A greater degree of specificity resides in the various α subunits of G proteins (G_a, G_i, G_p, G_{12}, etc.) that activate or inhibit adenylate cyclase, activate phospholipases (PLC and PLA_2) or directly modulate ion channels. The G_α subunits are a multigene family of 39- to 52-kd proteins that share ~45% to 80% amino acid similarity.[198] The most completely described G protein-activated effector system is the accumulation of the second messenger cAMP.[199] A stimulatory G protein, G_s, couples binding of many hormone-activated receptors to allosteric activation of adenylate cyclase, increasing intracellular levels of cAMP (e.g., β-adrenergic receptors). In other instances, an inhibitory G protein, G_i, causes receptor-mediated reduction in adenylate cyclase activity (e.g., α-adrenergic receptors). Cyclic AMP activates cAMP-dependent cytoplasmic protein kinases, which, in turn, phosphorylate key cellular proteins. This is the transduction mechanism that triggers numerous intracellular metabolic pathways, including glycogenolysis and lipolysis.[200]

Specific bacterial toxins such as cholera toxin and pertussis toxin alter specific G protein α-subunit activity by catalyzing the oxidized form of nicotinamide adenine dinucleotide (NAD^+)-dependent adenosine diphosphate (ADP)-ribosylation of critical amino acid residues.[201,202] These reactions are useful experimentally for distinguishing unique G protein α subunits. Specifically, cholera toxin catalyzes the ADP-ribosylation and irreversible activation of G_s and pertussis toxin ADP-ribosylates and irreversibly inactivates G_i. Using the bacterial toxins as pharmacologic probes, G protein-coupled receptors for many metabolically active peptides [e.g., vasopressin, oxytocin, angiotensin, vasoactive intestinal peptide (VIP), cholecystokinin, parathyroid hormone, calcitonin, somatostatin] and small molecules (e.g., α- and β-adrenergic, muscarinic cholinergic, and dopaminergic agonists; prostaglandins; leukotrienes; thromboxanes) have been described.

An important aspect of receptor function is that a single receptor may interact with several different G proteins. Thus, M1 muscarinic adrenergic receptors are coupled to a G protein that stimulates phosphoinositide turnover, while M2 muscarinic receptors are coupled to a

G protein that inhibits adenylate cyclase activity; the pertinent effector coupling and ligand-binding domains of the receptors have been mapped.[203] Additionally, molecular cloning studies of G proteins and biochemical and immunologic analysis have shown that multiple G proteins may have identical bacterial toxin substrate specificity. Thus, a multigene family of "G_i-like" proteins exists, comprising several similar pertussis toxin–sensitive G proteins.[204] Different members of this family regulate a variety of other signaling pathways, including those that involve PLC, PLA_2, and K^+ channels.

Numerous G protein–coupled receptors have been cloned and sequenced. Several cloning strategies have revealed the existence of new receptor subtypes whose existence had not been previously demonstrated pharmacologically.[205,206] Cloning studies also have shown that G protein–coupled receptors share a common structural motif, namely, a pattern of seven conserved hydrophobic membrane-spanning α-helices connected by alternating extracellular and cytoplasmic loops, usually with the peptide amino-terminus exposed to the extracellular face and a cytoplasmic carboxy-terminus. Structure-function relationships for the extracellular ligand-binding and cytoplasmic G protein–coupling domains of many receptors have been examined by site-directed mutagenesis, transient transfection of the altered gene into mammalian cells, and subsequent pharmacologic analysis.[207,208] Numerous G proteins and G protein–coupled receptor mutations have been described that cause syndromes of hormone hyposecretion [e.g., McCune-Albright syndrome, nephrogenic diabetes insipidus, familial adrenocorticotropic hormone (ACTH) resistance, familial GH deficiency, hypergonadotrophic ovarian dysgenesis, male pseudohermaphroditism, familial hypoparathyroidism] or hypersecretion (e.g., familial male precocious puberty, neonatal severe primary hyperparathyroidism).[209] Targeted disruption of a G_α gene has produced knockout mice (vide infra) with growth retardation, thymocyte abnormalities, and a progressive, ultimately lethal form of ulcerative colitis.[210]

General Properties of Second Messengers

Second messengers have several common features: (1) they are small molecules that are derived from abundant precursors or stores, such as ATP, GTP, extra- and/or intracellular Ca^{2+}, and membrane phospholipids;[211] (2) they are generated rapidly, usually within seconds, in response to hormone interaction with the appropriate receptor; (3) under basal conditions they are present in low concentrations, and, although they can increase many-fold during cellular stimulation, these molecules generally remain minor cellular constituents, and (4) they are removed rapidly by metabolism or pumping out of the cytosol (e.g., Ca^{2+}) following the termination of ligand action.[212] These properties allow for the rapid, transient cellular responses characteristic of many metabolic pathways. In other cases, however, second messenger–mediated responses are much longer lasting or are not reversible, such as the activation of cell division or regulation of the transcription of specific genes. These actions may contribute to the trophic effects of certain hormones, such as the actions of ACTH on the adrenal gland or PTH on bone, and mediate the interplay between metabolism and growth.

The role of cAMP, first described in the classic studies of Sutherland et al.,[213] has become a paradigm of second messenger signal transduction. Cyclic AMP is formed by the adenylate cyclase catalyzed cyclization of ATP on the inner face of the plasma membrane. Numerous ligands stimulate adenylate cyclase by activating receptor-coupled G_s [e.g. β-adrenergic agonists, ACTH, thyroid-stimulating hormone (TSH), corticotropin-releasing hormone (CRH), PTH, calcitonin] while others inhibit the enzyme via G_i (e.g., $α_2$-adrenergic, muscarinic, and D_2-agonists; angiotensin II; somatostatin). Cyclic AMP, in turn, binds to its own intracellular receptors, the regulatory subunits of cAMP-dependent protein kinases (PKAs), altering the phosphorylation state of many cellular protein substrates.[200]

Adenylate cyclase and cAMP can be measured by radioimmunoassay. The role of cAMP signal transduction in metabolic pathways is also studied with pharmacologic probes: cholera toxin mimics or potentiates agonist-stimulated adenylate cyclase activity, while pertussis toxin inactivates G_i, preventing the receptor-mediated inhibition of adenylate cyclase; synthetic nonhydrolyzable GTP analogues, such as 5′-guanylyl imidodiphosphate (Gpp(NH)p) and 5′-guanosine γ-thiotriphosphate (GTP-γ-S), activate adenylate cyclase at the GTP binding site; forskolin and cAMP analogues also mimic cAMP-mediated cellular and nuclear effects; fluoride ions inhibit ligand-activated adenylate cyclase and stimulate basal enzyme levels; phosphodiesterase inhibitors (e.g., xanthines) amplify ligand-stimulated cAMP accumulation; and manganese ions constitutively activate adenylate cyclase.

Calcium ions (Ca^{2+}) also play a role in the activation of hormonal secretion (i.e., "stimulus-secretion coupling"),[214] and help to regulate cell metabolism, contraction, growth, differentiation, and death. While indirect studies have long implicated a messenger function for changes in cytosolic Ca^{2+} concentrations ($[Ca^{2+}]_c$), this role has been verified by the development of methods that directly assess Ca^{2+} and Ca^{2+} fluxes in living cells, especially fluorescent dyes (e.g., fura-2), which change their spectral properties upon binding Ca^{2+} in the submicromolar range.[215-217] As a second messenger, Ca^{2+} has numerous intracellular target molecules, including the Ca^{2+}-binding proteins (CaBPs); coordinated activation of different CaBPs, including calmodulin,[218] is essential for integrated cellular function. Upon binding Ca^{2+}, calmodulin undergoes a conformational change that permits it to activate a variety of enzymes and other effector systems, including adenylate cyclases, cyclic nucleotide phosphodiesterase, some protein kinases, and Ca^{2+}-Mg^{2+} adenosine triphosphatase (ATPase).

Under basal conditions, cells pump Ca^{2+} against electrochemical gradients from the cytosol to the extracellular fluid or into sequestered intracellular sites such as endoplasmic reticulum and mitochondria. $[Ca^{2+}]_c$ under resting conditions is about 100 nM, which is four orders of magnitude less than extracellular $[Ca^{2+}]$. Many metabolically relevant ligands can transiently raise $[Ca^{2+}]_c$ by opening voltage sensitive or receptor-operated Ca^{2+} channels, carriers, or pumps located in the plasma membrane or in the membranes of intracellular stores. Agonists can induce steep gradients of $[Ca^{2+}]_c$ because Ca^{2+} is buffered and sequestered efficiently.

The neutral acetoxymethyl esters of fluorescent dyes such as fura-2 are easily loaded into most cells. Ubiquitous intracellular esterases cleave the dyes into nondiffusible, charged forms that fluoresce upon binding Ca^{2+}. Studies of dye-loaded cultured cells have demonstrated that ligand binding induces oscillations in intracellular Ca^{2+} [219,220] that have unique temporal and spatial patterns. The same cell may respond differentially to two different agonists. For example, pancreatic acinar cells display sinusoidal Ca^{2+} oscillations in response to acetylcholine but transient oscillations in response to stimulation with cholecystokinin.[221] Agonist-induced Ca^{2+} signaling in many cell types (e.g., hepatocytes), show both temporal[222,223] and spatial organization.[224-226] An application of these techniques to studying physiologic alterations in pregnancy has demonstrated an exaggerated vasopressin-induced platelet Ca^{2+} response in pregnancies complicated by subsequent preeclampsia.[227]

The regulation of $[Ca^{2+}]_c$ by intracellular Ca^{2+} stores is intimately related to a family of other second messengers, namely the inositol polyphosphates. The complexity of inositol phosphate metabolism is appreciated by HPLC, which separates inositol phosphates with only subtle structural differences.[228] The polyphosphoinositides, phosphatidylinositol-4-monophosphate (PIP) and phosphatidylinositol-4,5-bisphosphate (PIP_2), are minor phospholipid components of the plasma membrane formed by successive phosphorylations of phosphatidylinositol. PIP_2 can be hydrolyzed by the membrane-associated enzyme, phospholipase C, into two second messengers, water-soluble inositol 1,4,5-trisphosphate (IP_3) and diacylglycerol (DG).[229,230] This enzymatic signaling cascade is activated when ligands bind to cell surface receptors coupled to distinct stimulatory or inhibitory G proteins that regulate phospholipase C activity in a fashion akin to the dual regulation of adenylate cyclase.

IP_3 liberates Ca^{2+} from the intracellular pool and contributes to the initial spike in cytosolic Ca^{2+} induced by Ca^{2+}-mobilizing hormones.[228] Further phosphorylation of IP_3 produces inositol-1,3,4,5-tetrakisphosphate (IP_4), which also is a second messenger implicated in uptake of extracellular Ca^{2+}.[231,232] Other, higher order inositol polyphosphates may also be functional.[233] The active inositol polyphosphates rapidly are broken down by phosphatases into inositol, which is recycled into phosphatidylinositol. An important feature of this system is that the second messengers are stored in latent form as inositol lipid, a structural component of the plasma membrane.

Many inositol phosphatases are inhibited by Li^+, providing a convenient means of pharmacologically amplifying hormonally induced changes in this signaling pathway.[234] Inositol phosphates can be measured in ^3H-myo-inositol–labeled cells by HPLC or ion exchange chromatography.[235,236] Pharmacologic probes for IP_3 recognition sites and inositol phosphate analogues resistant to degradation by intracellular phosphatases are also available. The latter may be useful for making high-affinity radioligands for the IP_3 receptor.

The other second messenger generated by PIP_2 hydrolysis, DG, binds and activates isoforms of protein kinase C (PKC),[230] a central regulator of cellular metabolism and proliferation. Tumor-promoting phorbol esters are DG analogues and constitutively activate PKC isoforms. They are widely used pharmacologic probes of PKC activity in different cell types. Increasingly, specific PKC inhibitors have become useful probes for different behaviors of the lipid-dependent domain and of the catalytic domain of PKC isotypes.[237,238] Changes in intracellular Ca^{2+} can directly activate Ca^{2+}-dependent protein kinases such as the Ca^{2+}/calmodulin protein kinases. Increases in intracellular Ca^{2+} levels also stimulate a Ca^{2+}-sensitive PLC, leading to an increase in the level of DG, the endogenous activator of PKC.

The lipid composition of cell membranes is complex and fairly tightly metabolically regulated. In the past several years, it has become evident that tyrosine kinase receptors and G protein–linked receptors can activate several phospholipases [e.g., phospholipase A_2 (PLA_2), inositol lipid-specific PLC, and phosphatidylcholine-specific phospholipase D (PLD)], and give rise to multiple second messengers. Hydrolysis of membrane phospholipids by receptor-activated PLA_2 results in release of arachidonic acid. Further metabolism by cyclooxygenase and lipoxygenase gives rise to multiple bioactive molecules collectively known as eicosanoids (e.g., prostaglandins, thromboxanes, prostacyclin, and leukotrienes), but arachidonic acid itself can act as an intracellular second messenger. Receptor-activated PLD promotes breakdown of phosphatidylcholine as an alternate route of synthesis of DG.[239,240] In a more general sense, the specific lipid composition of the membrane probably modulates the enzymatic activity of many membrane-bound proteins.[241] This heterogeneity in lipid activation, coupled with evidence that PKC isoforms occupy specific subcellular compartments,[211] suggests that specific intracellular signaling mechanisms and their developmental regulation will be deciphered.

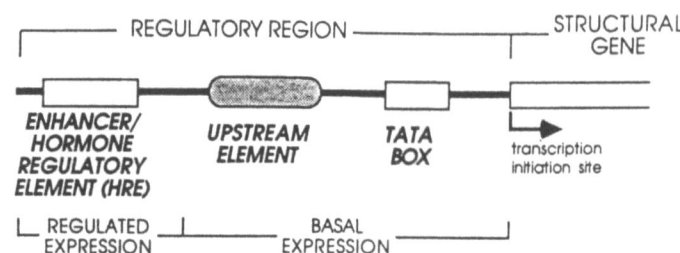

FIGURE 4.11. Stereotypical regulatory regions of a eukaryotic gene. (Modified from Tremp et al.[243])

Analysis of Gene Regulation

Frequently, the major regulatory event in metabolism is the activation of transcription of a specific gene and/or the efficiency of translation in response to some external signal, such as a ligand binding its receptor. For instance, concentrations of enzymes regulating the flow of intermediates through metabolic pathways are regulated by control of the transcriptional activity of the corresponding genes.[4,242,243] Tens of thousands of genes are transcribed in a finely tuned and regulated manner by elaborate sets of enzyme complexes. Gene regulation theoretically can occur at several levels: (1) transcription of a gene into a primary RNA transcript, which is the most common control; (2) processing of the primary transcript into a mature RNA by 3' termination cleavage, 3' end polyadenylation, 5' end capping, or excision of introns; (3) stabilization of the RNA in the nucleus or cytoplasm by several of the above-mentioned modifications or by degradation; (4) translation of mRNA into protein; (5) posttranslational modification of protein; and (6) targeting of the protein either within the cell or for export.[244-247] The regulation of expression of genes important in developmental metabolism commonly occurs at several levels, as might be expected for the tightly regulated and temporally and spatially complex functions of the respective gene products. An excellent example is human insulin-like growth factor-I (IGF-I), a peptide intimately involved with mammalian growth and development, which has a complex tissue-specific and developmental pattern of expression. In different settings, IGF-I may act via endocrine, paracrine, or autocrine pathways. Not surprisingly, both transcriptional and translational mechanisms, including RNA alternative splicing, differential mRNA polyadenylation, and extensive precursor processing, modify IGF-I biosynthesis in different tissues and at different points in the organism's development (see Chapter 20).[248] A second example is the control of cellular iron concentrations, where both mRNA stability and translation of the transferrin receptor and ferritin have effects.[249,250]

The stereochemical terms *cis* and *trans* were introduced into genetics by J.B.S. Haldane[251] to describe markers that are linked on the same chromosome (*cis*), or are unlinked and located on separate chromosomes (*trans*). This terminology persists in molecular genetics, so that regulatory regions are said to contain *cis*-acting elements, which are short, conserved DNA sequences lying within or near a given gene, that function by binding specific nuclear *trans*-acting factors, which are DNA-binding proteins. The *trans*-acting proteins are encoded by other, usually unlinked genes, hence *trans*. Transcription factors, which are grouped in families based on shared DNA-binding motifs, are defined as proteins that are needed to activate or repress transcription rate and interact with, but are not themselves part of, the RNA polymerase complex.[252]

The principal DNA regulatory region of the typical eukaryotic gene is located upstream, that is, 5' to, the coding region (i.e., the structural gene).[9,253] Most regulated genes contain several kinds of these *cis*-acting promoter elements (Figure 4.11). These short, approximately 8 to 20 bp, discrete consensus sequences may be present in tandem repeats and in different combinations. A consensus sequence is defined by aligning all known examples of the sequence so as to maximize their homology. Eukaryotic promoters consist of sometimes distantly separated nucleosome-free hypersensitive DNA sequences that presumably are brought into juxtaposition when they bind to their respective *trans*-acting proteins. Promoter consensus sequences are frequently described as highly conserved "boxes" or motifs and may occur widely in promoters of many different genes.[9,254,255,256]

A "TATA box," which is an AT-rich region containing the sequence TATAAAA, is usually located 25 to 30 bp upstream from the beginning of the transcriptional initiation site (i.e., start point or CAP site) of most genes and is important for accuracy and efficiency of transcription. TATA boxes may be absent in constitutively active or housekeeping genes. This TATA box sequence binds to several proteins (e.g., "general" transcription factors) that are essential for the formation of the RNA polymerase II transcriptional initiation complex.[257] Other protein-binding DNA consensus sequences, often located about 40 to 100 bp upstream from the start point, are collectively known as upstream promoter elements (UPEs). These elements include the so-called CAAT box (GGCCAATCT, ATGCAAAT, CCAAT) and GC box (GGGCGG, GCCACACCC). The TATA box and UPEs act in concert to determine basal gene expression. Choice of the exact start point depends on TATA box location, while the farther upstream CAAT and GC box enhancer sequences, which are the sites for the start of assembly of the enzymatic transcription apparatus, influence the efficiency of transcription.[258,259]

Elements located even farther upstream are recognized by tissue-specific factors (Figure 4.12). These DNA sequences, called response elements or regulatory elements, uniquely identify groups of genes that respond to specific transcription factors. Response elements may be located either in promoters or in sequences called enhancers. Enhancers and silencers (i.e., the inhibitory counterparts of enhancers) are defined as regulatory sequences that can act at great distances in either orientation and may be upstream or downstream from a gene coding region. The distinction between promoters and enhancers becomes blurred, so that enhancers might be viewed as promoter sequences that are grouped closely together and have the capacity to function at large distances (i.e., several kilobases) from the start point.[9] Response elements and enhancers, along with their respective transcription factors, are responsible for the regulated expression of genes by hormones, growth factors, certain nutrients, metals, tissue-specific factors, and stress (e.g., heat shock, mechanodeformation, and shear fluid). Basal transcription factors are required for initiation of transcription in all genes; activator and repressor proteins dictate the rate at which the basal complex initiates transcription. Different genes are controlled by distinct combinations of activators and repressors.[259] External metabolic signals and cell surface acting ligands stimulate effector systems (e.g., cAMP, Ca^{2+}-activated pathways, PKC) that activate these specific transcription factors that bind to consensus response elements. These various response elements may be similar in structure.[256] The hydrophobic ligands such as the steroids, thyroid hormone, and vitamins A and D directly bind to members of a family of ligand-dependent transcription factors. It is becoming increasingly clear that transcriptional repression is at least as important as transcriptional activation for establishing cell-type specific patterns of gene expression during embryogenesis and development.[260]

The glucocorticoid response element (GRE) is a well-studied example of a hormone-responsive sequence; GREs vary in location from several kilobases upstream from the promoter (e.g., the tyrosine aminotransferase gene)[261] to being contained within the first intron of the coding region (e.g., growth hormone gene).[262] Sequences that may serve as negative GREs have been identified for several genes whose transcription is inhibited by glucocorticoids.[263] Additionally, glucocorticoids may inhibit gene transcription by interfering with *trans*-activation of other promoter elements.[264] Genes involved in metabolic pathways often are subject to transcriptional control by a variety of hormones and dietary factors as, for example, the differential regulation of liver pyruvate kinase by insulin, glucagon, thyroid hormone, and glucocorticoids.[265] A common approach to mapping *cis*-acting regulatory elements of a particular gene is to produce

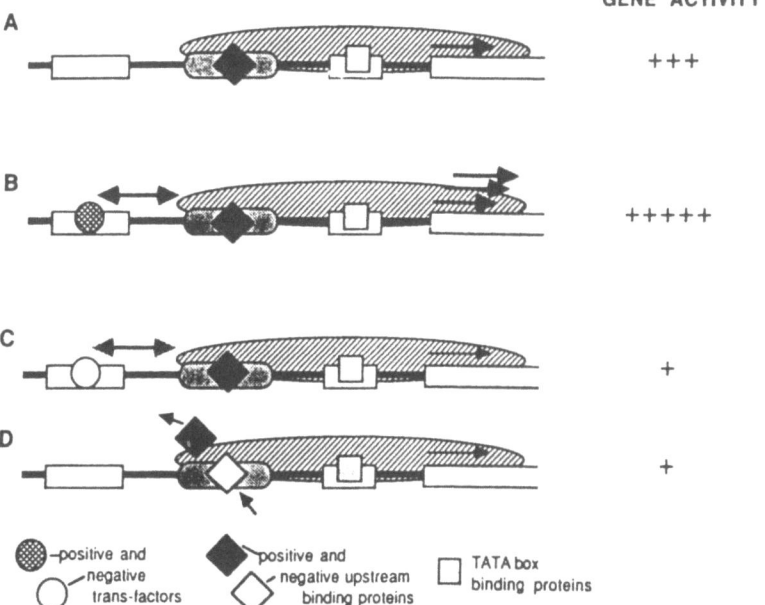

FIGURE 4.12. Some mechanisms of regulation of eukaryotic gene activity. (A) Basal gene activity determined by TATA box and upstream promoter elements. Enhancer/regulatory element-specific *trans*-acting factors increase (B) or decrease (C) basal transcription. (D) Negative gene regulation may also occur by interference of negative regulators with "basal" factors. (Modified from Tremp et al.[243])

deletions of the regulatory region followed by a functional assay of the phenotypic consequences of the deletions (vide infra). Several strategies may be used for generating large deletions, including elimination of internal or terminal sequences by restriction endonuclease digestion, successive removal of DNA with exonucleases,[266] and PCR using two primers abutting the region to be deleted.[267]

Since all somatic cells in an organism contain identical genomic DNA, the combinations of specific transcription factors made by the appropriate cells at appropriate times and in response to specific signals are essential to normal metabolism.[268] For example, the discovery of the four myogenic basic helix-loop-helix transcription factors (e.g., myoD, myogenin, Myt-5, and MRF4), each of which can activate the program for skeletal muscle differentiation, has led to rapid progress toward understanding the molecular mechanisms that regulate muscle gene expression.[269,270] Pit-1, a member of the POU structural family of transcription factors,[271] is synthesized only in pituitary cells, where it regulates pituitary-specific gene expression [e.g., GH, prolactin (PRL)].[272] Mutations in the gene encoding Pit-1 have been identified in patients with panhypopituitarism;[273,274] the mutant Pit-1 still binds to its DNA-binding site in target gene promoters but it does not activate transcription. Several disease-causing mutations also have been characterized in the steroid hormone receptor superfamily.[275]

Steady-state mRNA levels represent the sum of transcriptional and posttranscriptional events, such as processing, degradation, etc.[276] The nuclear run-on transcription assay directly measures an effector's role on transcription.[277] This method allows examination of the role of changes in transcriptional rate synthesis on steady-state mRNA abundance and the effect of stimuli or changed physiologic state on transcriptional rate. Nuclei are isolated from cells or tissue by homogenization and centrifugation. These nuclei are incubated in the presence of labeled ribonucleotides so that elongation of transcription already in progress proceeds. The labeled nascent RNA is hybridized to specific DNA(s) blotted to nitrocellulose of nylon. The detection signals (e.g., autoradiography, chemiluminescence) provides an index of the number of RNA polymerase II molecules engaged in transcription. Since the use of double-stranded probes may give misleading results due to the presence of antisense transcription in some genes, notably in the c-myc gene,[278] it is important to distinguish between sense and antisense transcription in a nuclear run-on assay. Consequently, single-stranded probes are preferred in this procedure.

The molecular analysis of regulatory sequences frequently begins with visual or computer-assisted sequence inspection to identify known motifs. The analysis of protein–DNA interactions is one of the most rapidly advancing areas in molecular biology.[279] DNase footprinting (i.e., hypersensitivity) studies[280] are used to characterize the targets of sequence-specific DNA-binding proteins.[281,282] Eukaryotic chromatin is packaged into nucleosomes and higher-order structures that restrict entry of RNA polymerases and transcription factors. In actively transcribed regions, chromatin is less densely packed, and is accessible for transcription and, experimentally, to nonspecific endonucleases like DNase I. In DNase footprinting a nuclear protein preparation is added to an end-labeled DNA fragment containing a potential binding site. The formed protein-DNA complex is treated with DNase I under conditions that cleave all phosphodiesterase bonds at similar rates. PAGE separation will visualize a "ladder" of end-labeled cleavage products except where tight interaction of a protein with a specific DNA sequence protects it. In those regions the corresponding fragments will be missing from the ladder, giving the appearance of a "footprint."[283] DNase footprinting and subsequent Southern blotting permit analysis of chromatin structures associated with gene activation over long regions of DNA.[281] A caveat is that in vitro binding data may not reflect the in vivo binding patterns of nuclear factors.[284,285] There are numerous variations on this procedure.[279]

The electrophoretic mobility shift assay (EMSA),[285–287] also known as the gel shift or gel retardation assay, uses PAGE to determine whether a labeled DNA fragment binds nuclear proteins and whether the binding is sequence-specific. If the labeled DNA contains a protein-binding site, it migrates more slowly than does the DNA fragment alone; the band is "shifted" upward in the gel relative to the fragment alone. Competition with unlabeled DNA fragments will discriminate nonspecific DNA-protein interaction (Figure 4.13). A variation of EMSA uses binding with antibodies directed against specific nuclear proteins. The "supercomplex" of antibody-nuclear protein-DNA yields a "supershifted" band on PAGE that signals specific interaction between antibody and protein. Binding-site selection assays combine specificity of DNA-protein interactions with PCR amplification to identify a protein's DNA binding site without prior knowledge of the genes it may control. Synthetic potential DNA-binding sequences are incubated with the protein and the protein-bound DNA fragments are separated by EMSA or with an antibody. Protein-DNA interactions are disrupted by heating and the DNA fragments are amplified by PCR using primers complementary to the sequences flanking the random oligonucleotides.[289]

The introduction of reporter genes into mammalian cells for in vitro transcription is another commonly used strategy for the indirect measure of relative rates of transcription and analysis of defined promoter sequences. These techniques have proven invaluable for delineating

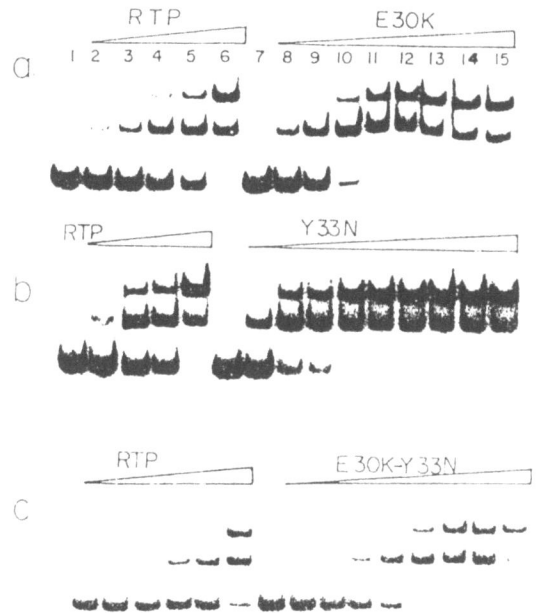

FIGURE 4.13. Autoradiogram of a nondenaturing 8% PAGE showing the binding of the wild type and the mutant forms of a replication terminator protein (RTP) to a 53-bp terminus DNA. The left panels show the gel mobility shifts caused by the binding of increasing amounts of wild-type RTP, and the right panels show the shifts caused by increasing amounts of the indicated mutant form of the protein. In each case, the first shift is due to the filling of the core by a single dimer of RTP, and the second shift is due to the filling of both the core and the auxiliary sites by two dimers involved in cooperative dimer-dimer interaction. The double shift is a diagnostic feature of dimer-dimer interaction, and it is clear that this is retained in each of the mutants. (A and C) Lanes 1–6 correspond to 0 ng, 15 ng, 30 ng, 60 ng, 100 ng, and 300 ng of wild-type RTP, and lanes 7–15 correspond to 0 ng, 15 ng, 30 ng, 60 ng, 100 ng, 200 ng, 300 ng, 400 ng, and 500 ng of the mutant. (B) Lanes 1–5 correspond to 0 ng, 15 ng, 60 ng, 100 ng, and 300 ng of wild-type RTP, and lanes 6–15 correspond to 0 ng, 15 ng, 30 ng, 60 ng, 100 ng, 200 ng, 300 ng, 400 ng, 500 ng, and 600 ng of the mutant. (From Manna et al.,[288] with permission.)

cis-acting elements and performing structure-function analysis of transcription factors including steroid hormone receptors. A change in reporter gene activity implies that the test DNA sequence confers a difference in transcriptional activity. Bacterial chloramphenicol acetyltransferase (CAT) has been a widely used reporter gene for determining strength of promoters and other upstream transcriptional regulatory sequences;[290,291] CAT activity assays combine sensitivity, low background, simplicity, and low expense. These assays are being superseded by the use of firefly luciferase,[292,293] which has much greater sensitivity (i.e., 10–20 RNA molecules), ease of readout, rapid nonradioactive detection by chemiluminescence, and wide dynamic range. Light is produced with high quantum efficiency from the enzymatic reaction of the substrate luciferin with ATP. Transfection of luciferase vectors using viral transcriptional control elements allows scaling down samples to 1/1000th of the size of a standard CAT assay.[294] The numerous CAT and luciferase plasmid vectors offer a variety of cloning sites for delineating basal promoter elements and enhancers, introducing new promoters, performing structure-function analysis of transcription factors, and testing response elements with well-understood promoters of various strengths and properties. Site-directed mutagenesis[170] can be used to determine whether that sequence possesses transcriptional activity.[295]

Since the first demonstration that an antisense RNA transcribed from a transgene could downregulate expression of a eukaryotic gene,[296] various antisense strategies also have been developed for investigating functions of particular genes.[297]

Posttranscriptional control in metabolism and development also occurs, although probably less commonly than transcriptional control.[247,298] Variable RNA processing has been discussed above. Hormones and other factors also may regulate mRNA, and consequently protein, stability. Differential stability is a fundamental property of both mRNAs and proteins that makes biologic regulation possible. The half-lives for eukaryotic mRNAs and proteins may range from a few minutes for highly regulated gene products such as rate-limiting enzymes and oncogenes to greater than 100 hours for very stable species.[276,299,300] An illustration of regulated mRNA stability in perinatal metabolism is the coordinate regulated expression of milk protein genes by insulin, glucocorticoid, and prolactin.[301] In the presence of insulin and glucocorticoid, prolactin stabilizes the casein mRNA by extending the transcript half-life about fourfold.[302,303] The addition of glucocorticoid to mammary explants cultured in the presence of insulin and prolactin also dramatically increases the half-life compared to culture with insulin and prolactin alone. Thus, it appears that initiation of transcription of the casein gene requires insulin and prolactin in the presence of glucocorticoid, while casein transcript stability is dependent on glucocorticoid and prolactin alone. The postulated action of glucocorticoid is inhibition of degradation of the transcript.

Changes in the size of the poly(A) tail of specific mRNAs also affect mRNA stability and translational efficiency.[276,304,305] For example, variation in the length of the poly(A) tail of vasopressin mRNA in the suprachiasmatic nuclei of the brain regulates vasopressin mRNA abundance and is a molecular mechanism for the circadian rhythm of vasopressin peptide levels in the cerebrospinal fluid.[306] The orchestrated extension and shortening of the poly(A) tail length of select mRNAs correlate with their translational activation or inactivation at defined stages of oocyte development.[307,308]

Extensive posttranscriptional control of certain neuroendocrine genes also occurs in "polyproteins," where a single gene is translated into a single protein sequence that then undergoes proteolytic processing to produce distinct, functional polypeptides. Some polyproteins, such as proopiomelanocortin (POMC), have tissue-specific cleavage patterns that determine the products secreted by different cell types.[309] Other polyproteins appear to serve as an amplification mechanism, such as the enkephalin precursor, which is spliced into six copies of met-enkephalin and one copy of leu-enkephalin.

Several experimental approaches are applicable to the analysis of mammalian transcriptional regulation. It is possible to transfect cells with genes having modified signal sequences in their coding regions or modified tissue-specific *cis*-acting elements in their promoters. Specific gene products also can be overexpressed in a measured fashion using heterologous promoters ligated to structural genes. Deletion of specific enzymes and their replacement by genes containing site-specific mutations permits testing of the function of specifically modified enzymes. DNA sequences transfected into mammalian cells greatly facilitate expression studies. Each successfully transfected cell usually takes up many copies of the heterologous DNA. Transfected DNA sequences become incorporated into the nuclear genome and can be transcribed in a regulated fashion. In transient expression assays, the function of the transfected DNA is assayed during the first 24 to 72 hours after transfection, at a time when the heterologous DNA still remains extrachromosomal and, therefore, is not influenced by the site of its integration into the host cell genome.

Transgenic Techniques and Gene Ablation

Since the first successful manipulation of the germ line of mice in 1980,[310] a large number of transgenic animals have been produced worldwide for use in both basic and applied research. Additionally, development of gene targeting protocols involving homologous recombination in mouse embryonic stem cells has resulted in a considerable number of mutant lines with specific phenotypes and well-defined DNA structural changes. Transgenic mice permit the effects of specific genes and gene products upon metabolism, development, and growth to be studied in intact animals, and they expand the range of human disorders that can be studied in mouse models.[311-314] The considerable advantages of these methods must be balanced against expense, complexity, and the fact that function of the integrated transgenes is affected by the site of integration. Transgenic mice are created by injecting plasmids carrying the DNA sequences of interest into the germinal vesicle (i.e., nucleus) of a mouse oocyte or into the pronucleus of a fertilized egg. The egg subsequently is implanted into a pseudopregnant mouse. After birth, the recipient mouse genome is examined (e.g., by Southern blot of tail DNA) to see whether it has integrated the DNA construct, and by northern analysis or RT-PCR to see whether the construct is expressed. Usually, multiple copies of the plasmid become integrated in tandem into a single chromosomal site. The transfected genes are generally expressed in appropriate cells and at the expected time, but copy number and activity may change in the mouse progeny. Using transgenic technology, mutations can be produced to result in (1) aberrant expression of otherwise normal genes, (2) targeted ablations of cell populations, and (3) insertional inactivation of genes by homologous recombination. This "reverse genetics" is a powerful tool for the analysis of development.[312]

Analysis of transgenic mouse lines containing rat liver-type pyruvate kinase gene constructs with varying deletions of the upstream regulatory region have helped define the *cis*-acting sequences involved in the regulation of that gene by diet, glucagon, and tissue type.[315] Similarly, tissue-specific promoters can be used to direct overexpression of potentially rate-limiting reactions in specific organs. This approach is being applied to the study of metabolic pathways and already has been successfully exploited for the study of growth. Several laboratories have created transgenic mice that overexpress human transforming growth factor-α (TGF-α) cDNAs in different mouse tissues. Exposure to abnormally high levels of TGF-α during development had pleiotropic effects in target tissues, shedding light on tissue-specific mechanisms of cell proliferation and differentiation.[316-318]

Similarly, targeted ablation or knockout of a gene can shed light on in vivo functions. The goal of the knockout method is to replace a specific gene of interest with one that is inactive, altered, or irrelevant. To increase the probability that such replacement will occur, both ends of the replacement gene sequence are flanked by long DNA sequences homologous to the sequences flanking the target gene. Such gene constructs permit corresponding stretches of DNA introduced into embryonic stem cells to be exchanged by homologous recombination. Engineering dual selectable markers (e.g., neomycin resistance, gancyclovir sensitivity) allows selection of recombinant cell clones, which are injected into mouse blastocysts. The resultant heterozygous, haplodeficient, mice are bred to each other to produce homozygous (null) mice for the specific gene.[319] As one example, this approach is helping to define more fully the roles of steroid hormones[320,321] and growth factors[322,323] in fetal lung maturation. New methods of inducible inactivation of a target gene in mice may allow tissue- and cell type-specific targeted gene inactivation.[324-326] The Johns

Hopkins University maintains an on-line Transgenic/Targeted Mutation Database (TBASE), which organizes information about transgenic and targeted mutation animals generated and analyzed worldwide (http://www.bis.med.jhml.edu/Dan/tbase/tbase.html). More recently, other model organisms, particularly the zebrafish,[327] have begun to show immense promise for studying the genetic mechanisms underlying vertebrate development.

Implications and Future Directions

Recombinant DNA techniques and recent advances in cellular physiology have dramatically altered the experimental study of metabolism. Cloned complementary or genomic DNA finds manifold uses in the laboratory: the structure of metabolically active proteins can be deduced; base complementarity can be exploited in hybridization strategies, including Southern and northern blots and chromosome mapping using somatic cell hybrids; genes altered by site-directed mutagenesis or in unaltered form can be transferred into heterologous mammalian cells for purposes of analyzing the structure and function of regulatory and coding regions. Transgenic[328] and gene knockout mouse models are opening new avenues for integration of molecular biology and physiology. The application of these genetic methods with total genome sequence and database information on gene expression patterns, morphologic changes during development, and mutant phenotypes should significantly enhance the unraveling of gene expression, differentiation, and metabolic control.[329]

Whenever a gene has a known product, in principle it is possible to work back from the protein to the gene, by synthesizing an oligonucleotide in order to obtain the mRNA that codes for the protein and then using the mRNA directly or indirectly, as a probe to isolate that gene. This strategy has elucidated the gene structure of many classic metabolic regulators (e.g., insulin) as well as novel, developmentally important hormones (e.g., PTHrP). Alternatively, identifying a gene responsible for a metabolic disorder may open the way for identification of the unknown gene product and even the malfunctioning cell type(s). This pathway from RFLP linkage analysis to molecular pathogenesis has proved especially rewarding when applied to many X-linked diseases. At present, it is unraveling the pathobiology of many autosomal disorders, including cystic fibrosis.

Detailed studies of receptor structure and function also suggest etiologies for several metabolic disorders and provide insights into developmental metabolism. For example, receptor mutations have been identified for the LDL-receptor in familial hypercholesterolemia.[330] Organ-specific alterations of receptor coupled G proteins also can have pathologic consequences in acquired and genetic metabolic diseases.[209] In general, it is assumed that each ligand has an intended receptor; EGF/TGF-α and PTH/PTHrP binding to single receptors seem to be intriguing exceptions. Not infrequently, however, elucidation of ligand-receptor interactions reveals that one receptor recognizes several ligands. This theme of receptor "spillover" has important implications for an understanding of normal and disordered metabolism. In some clinical syndromes, pathologic hypersecretion of an agonist may lead to inappropriate stimulation of a receptor with which the ligand has low affinity. Thus, hCG secretion by choriocarcinomas can produce hyperthyroxinemia due to the TSH-like activity of the gonadotropin; IGFs secreted by mesenchymal tumors can induce a physiologic state that mimics hyperinsulinism.

The actions of multiple ligands on a single receptor or receptor class illuminate the interplay between developmental metabolism and growth control. For instance, the existence of an IGF-II/mannose-6-phosphate receptor indicates that two cellular biochemical systems, namely, cell growth (IGF-II) and lysosomal trafficking (e.g., mannose-6-phosphate), may be interrelated.[331] It is well recognized that many hormones also regulate cell proliferation or differentiation or both (e.g., insulin, glucocorticoids, vitamin D, PTH). Description of the molecular mechanisms that underlie these multiple effector functions will enhance the general understanding of perinatal-neonatal metabolism, as well as the particular physiology of the infant and of diabetic mothers, mineral metabolism in pregnant or lactating women and in fetuses, and the mechanisms of intrauterine stresses on fetal growth and maturation.

Finally, the future direction of experimentation in perinatal-neonatal metabolism will be heavily influenced by studies that combine molecular cellular techniques with new methods of cell and tissue culture. Epithelium lining body cavities maintains a high degree of distinct anatomical and functional polarity.[332,333] Traditionally, cell culture restricted in vitro cellular function and differentiation, since epithelial cells attach, grow, and tend to flatten on the impermeable, usually solid polystyrene or glass surface. The development of defined, serumless media and extracellular matrix components for cell culture[334] permits the investigation of the role of cell adhesion molecules, and cell shape in epithelial differentiation, gene expression, and protein secretion.[335–340] Epithelial cells also can be cultured on porous-bottomed dishes that provide independent access to both sides of a cell monolayer and promote differentiation.[341–342] Pertinent applications include biogenesis, sorting, and vectorial transport of macromolecules; hormone secretion and responsiveness; and receptor localization.[332,339–344] Cell biology is being transformed by the development of tools for imaging molecular functions in living cells and tissues and a union of the techniques of microscopy and molecular biology.[345-348]

References

1. Goodridge AG. The new metabolism: molecular genetics in the analysis of metabolic regulation. FASEB J 1990;4: 3099–3110.
2. Granner D, Pilkis S. The genes of hepatic glucose metabolism. J Biol Chem 1990;265:10173–10176.
3. Clarke SD, Abraham S. Gene expression: nutrient control of pre- and posttranscriptional events. FASEB J 1992;6: 3146–3152.
4. Girard J, Perdereau D, Foufelle F, et al. Regulation of lipogenic enzyme gene expression by nutrients and hormones. FASEB J 1994;8:36–42.
5. Bray D, Lewis J, Raff M, et al. Molecular biology of the cell. 3d ed. New York: Garland, 1995.
6. Wolfe SL. An introduction to cell and molecular biology. New York: Wadsworth, 1995.
7. Baltimore D, Berk A, Lodish H. Molecular cell biology. 3d ed. New York: W. H. Freeman, 1995.
8. Berg P, Singer M. Genes and genomes. New York: Univ Sci, 1997.
9. Lewin B. Genes VI. Oxford: Oxford University Press, 1997.
10. Ausubel FM, Brent RB, Kinston RE, et al. Current protocols in molecular biology. New York: Wiley, 1987.
11. Sambrook J, Fritsch EF, Maniatis T. Molecular cloning: a laboratory manual. 2nd ed. Cold Spring Harbor, NY: Cold Spring Harbor Laboratory Press, 1989.
12. Glover D, ed. DNA cloning 3: a practical approach. 2nd ed. New York: IRL Press, 1995.
13. White BA, ed. PCR cloning protocols: from molecular cloning to genetic engineering. Totowa, NJ: Humana Press, 1996.
14. Freshney RI. Culture of animal cells: a manual of basic technique. 3rd ed. New York: Alan R. Liss, 1994.
15. Kaufman PB, Wu W, Kim D, et al. Handbook of molecular and cellular methods in biology and medicine. Boca Raton, FL: CRC Press, 1995.
16. Pollard JW, Walker JM. Animal cell culture. Totowa, NJ: Humana Press, 1990.
17. Smagula CS. BioInformation on the World Wide Web 1997: an annotated directory of molecular biology tools. BIOTA, 1997.
18. Lafont F, Toldo L. The cell biologist and the World Wide Web: World Wide Web sites. Curr Opin Cell Biol 1997;9: 116–117.
19. Catt KJ. Molecular mechanisms of hormone action: control of target cell functions by peptide, steroid, and thyroid hormones. In: Felig P, Baxter JD, Broadus AE, et al. eds. Endocrinology and metabolism. 2nd ed. New York: McGraw-Hill, 1987; pp. 82–165.
20. Blake CC. Exons and the evolution of proteins. Int Rev Cytol 1985;95:149–185.
21. Monaco AP, Kunkel LM. Cloning of the Duchenne/Becker muscular dystrophy locus. Adv Hum Genet 1988;17:61–98.
22. Gilbert W. Genes-in-pieces revisited. Science 1985;228: 823–824.
23. Sudhof TC, Goldstein JL, Brown MS, et al. The LDL-receptor gene: a mosaic of exons shared with different proteins. Science 1985;228:815–822.
24. Engel J. EGF-like domains in extracellular matrix proteins: localized signals for growth and differentiation. FEBS Lett 1989;251:1–7.
25. Maeda N, Smithies O. The evolution of multigene families: human haptoglobin genes. Annu Rev Genet 1986; 20: 81–108.
26. Naylor SL, Sakaguichi AY, Szoka P, et al. Human parathyroid hormone gene (PTH) is on short arm of chromosome 11. Somat Cell Genet 1983;9:609–616.
27. Mangin M, Ikeda K, Dreyer BE, et al. Isolation and characterization of the human parathyroid hormone-like pepetide gene. Proc Natl Acad Sci USA 1989;86:2408–2412.
28. Yasuda T, Banville D, Hendy GN. Characterization of the human parathyroid hormone-like peptide gene: functional and evolutionary aspects. J Biol Chem 1989;264:7720–7725.
29. Stewart AF, Broadus AE. Parathyroid hormone-related proteins: coming of age in the 1990s. J Clin Endocrinol Metab 1990;71:1410–1414.
30. Antonarakis SE, Phillips JA III, Kazazian HH. Genetic diseases: diagnosis by restriction endonuclease analysis. J Pediatr 1982;100:845–856.
31. Roberts RJ. Restriction and modification enzymes and their recognition sequences. Nucleic Acids Res 1983;11: 135–167.
32. Smith HO, Nathans DJ. A suggested nomenclature for bacterial host modification and restriction systems and their enzymes. J Mol Biol 1973;81:419–423.
33. Roberts RJ, Macelis D. REBASE-restriction enzymes and methylases. Nucleic Acids Res 1996;24:223–225.
34. Danna KJ, Sack GH Jr, Nathans D. Studies of simian virus 40 DNA. VII. A cleavage map of the SV40 genome. J Mol Biol 1973;78:363–376.
35. Nathans D, Smith HO. Restriction endonucleases in the analysis and restructuring of DNA molecules. Annu Rev Biochem 1975;44:273–293.
36. Sharp PA, Sugden B, Sambrook J. Detection of two restriction endonuclease activities in *Haemophilus parainfluenzae* using analytical agarose-ethidium bromide electrophoresis. Biochemistry 1973;12:3055–3063.
37. Southern EM. Detection of specific sequences among DNA fragments separated by gel electrophoresis. J Mol Biol 1975;98:503–517.
38. Duman RS, Nestler EJ. Molecular biology III. Tracking DNA: The Southern blot. Am J Psychiat 1997;154:3.
39. Church GM, Gilbert W. Genomic sequencing. Proc Natl Acad Sci USA 1984;81:1991–1995.
40. Schwartz DC, Cantor CR. Separation of yeast chromosome-sized DNAs by pulsed field gradient gel electrophoresis. Cell 1984;37:67–75.
41. Carle GF, Frank F, Olson MV. Electrophoretic separation of large DNA molecules by periodic inversion of the electric field. Science 1986;232:65–68.

42. Chu CG, Vollrath D, Davis RW. Separation of large DNA molecules by contour-clamped homogeneous electric fields. Science 1986;234;1582–2585.
43. Sanger F, Nicklen S, Coulson AR. DNA sequencing with chain-terminating inhibitors. Proc Natl Acad Sci USA 1977;74:5463–5467.
44. Maxam AM, Gilbert W. A new method for sequencing DNA. Proc Natl Acad Sci USA 1977;74:560–564.
45. Jonas V, Lin CR, Kawashima E, et al. Alternative RNA processing events in human calcitonin/calcitonin gene-related peptide gene expression. Proc Natl Acad Sci USA 1985;782:1994–1998.
46. Breitbart RE, Andreadis A, Nadal-Ginard B. Alternative splicing: a ubiquitous mechanism for the generation of multiple protein isoforms from single genes. Annu Rev Biochem 1987;56:467–492.
47. Fedorcsak I, Ehrenberg L. Effects of diethyl pyrocarbonate and methyl methanesulfonate on nucleic acids and nucleases. Acta Chem Scand 1966;20:107–112.
48. Kumar A, Lindberg U. Characterizations of messenger ribonucleoprotein and messenger RNA from KB cells. Proc Natl Acad Sci USA 1972;69:681–685.
49. Blackburn P, Wilson G, Moore S. Ribonuclease inhibitor from human placenta: purification and properties. J Biol Chem 1977;252:5904–5910.
50. Berger SL, Birkenmeier CS. Inhibition of intractable nucleases with ribonucleoside-vanadyl complexes: isolation of messenger ribonucleic acid from resting lymphocytes. Biochemistry 1979;18:5143–5149.
51. Cox RA. The use of guanidium chloride in the isolation of nucleic acids. Methods Enzymol 1968;12B:120–122.
52. Chirgwin JM, Przybyla AK, MacDonald RJ, et al. Isolation of biologically active ribonucleic acid from sources enriched in ribonuclease. Biochemistry 1979;18:5294–5299.
53. Favolaro J, Triesman R, Kamen R. Transcription map of polyoma virus-specific RNA: analysis by two dimensional nuclease S_1 mapping. Methods Enzymol 1981;65:718–749.
54. Cathala G, Savouret JF, Mendez B, et al. A method for isolation of intact, transcriptionally active ribonucleic acid. DNA 1983;2:329–335.
55. Stallcup MR, Washington LD. Region-specific initiation of mouse mammary tumor virus RNA synthesis by endogenous RNA polymerase II in preparations of cell nuclei. J Biol Chem 1983;258:2802–2807.
56. Chomczynski P, Sacchi N. Single-step method of RNA isolation by acid guanidinium thiocyanate-phenol-chloroform extraction. Anal Biochem 1987;162:156–159.
57. MacDonald RJ, Swift GH, Przybyla AK, et al. Isolation of RNA using guanidinium salts. Methods Enzymol 1987;152:219–227.
58. Birnboim HC. Rapid extraction of high molecular weight RNA from cultured cells and granulocytes for Northern analysis. Nucleic Acids Res 1988;16:1487–1497.
59. Chomczynski P. A reagent for the single-step simultaneous isolation of RNA, DNA and proteins from cell and tissue samples. BioTechniques 1993;15:532–537.
60. Aviv H, Leder R. Purification of biologically active globin messenger RNA by chromatography on oligothymidylic acid-cellulose. Proc Natl Acad Sci USA 1972;69:1408–1412.
61. Kafatos FC, Jones CW, Efstratiadis A. Determination of nucleic acid sequence homologies and relative concentrations by a dot hybridization procedure. Nucleic Acids Res 1979;7:1541–1552.
62. Thomas PS. Hybridization of denatured RNA and small DNA fragments transferred to nitrocellulose. Proc Natl Acad Sci USA 1980;77:5201–5205.
63. White BA, Bancroh FC. Cytoplasmic dot hybridization: simple analysis of relative mRNA levels in multiple small cell or tissue samples. J Biol Chem 1982;257:8569–8572.
64. Alwine JC, Kemp DJ, Stark GR. Method for detection of specific RNAs in agarose gels by transfer to diazobenzyloxymethyl-paper and hybridization with DNA probes. Proc Natl Acad Sci USA 1977;74:5350–5354.
65. Goldberg DA. Isolation and partial characterization of the *Drosophila* alcohol dehydrogenase gene. Proc Natl Acad Sci USA 1980;77:5794–5798.
66. Bresser J, Gillespie D. Quantitative binding of covalently closed circular DNA to nitrocellulose in NaI. Anal Biochem 1983;129:357–364.
67. Trapnell BC. Quantitative evaluation of gene expression in freshly isolated human respiratory epithelial cells. Am J Physiol 1993;264:L199–L212.
68. Gee CE, Roberts JL. In situ hybridization histochemistry: a technique for the study of gene expression in single cells. DNA 1983;2:157–163.
69. Angerer RC, Cox KH, Angerer LM. In situ hybridization to cellular RNAs. In: Setlow JK, Hollaender A, eds. Genetic engineering, vol. 7. New York: Plenum Press, 1985:43–65.
70. Singer RH, Lawrence JB, Villnave C. Optimization of in situ hybridization using isotopic and nonisotopic detection methods. Biotechniques 1986;4:230–245.
71. Ronnekliev OK, Naylor BR, Bond CT, et al. Combined immunohistochemistry for gonadotropin releasing hormone (GnRH) and pro-GnRH, and in situ hybridization for GnRH messenger ribonucleic acid in rat brain. Mol Endocrinol 1989;3:363–371.
72. Berk AJ, Sharp PA. Sizing and mapping of early adenovirus mRNAs by gel electrophoresis of S1 endonuclease-digested hybrids. Cell 1977;12:721–732.
73. Sisodia SS, Cleveland DW, Sollner-Webb B. A combination of RNase H and S1 nuclease circumvents an artefact inherent to conventional S1 analysis of RNA splicing. Nucleic Acids Res 1987;15:1995–2011.
74. Zinn K, DiMaio D, Maniatis T. Identification of two distinct regulatory regions adjacent to the human, β-interferon gene. Cell 1983;34:865–879.
75. Melton DA, Krieg PA, Rebagliati MR, et al. Efficient in vitro synthesis of biologically active RNA and RNA hybridization probes from plasmids containing a bacteriophage SP6 promotor. Nucleic Acids Res 1984;12:7035–7056.
76. Krieg PA, Melton DA. In vitro RNA synthesis with SP6 RNA polymerase. Methods Enzymol 1987;155:397–415.
77. Wundrack I, Dooley S. Nonradioactive ribonuclease protection analysis using digoxygenine labeling and chemiluminescent detection. Electrophoresis 1992;13:637–638.

78. Nass SJ, Dickson RB. Detection of cyclin messenger RNAs by nonradioactive ribonuclease protection assay: a comparison of four detection methods. BioTechniques 1995;19:772–778.
79. Agarwal KL, Brunstedt J, Noyes BE. A general method for detection and characterization of an mRNA using an oligonucleotide probe. J Biol Chem 1981;256:1023–1028.
80. Souaze F, Ntodou-Thome A, Tran CY, et al. Quantitative RT-PCR: limits and accuracy. BioTechniques 1996;21:280–285.
81. Fuqua SAW, Fitzgerald SD, McGuire WL. A simple polymerase chain reaction method for detection and cloning of low abundance transcripts. Biotechniques 1990;9:206–211.
82. Rappolee DA, Mark D, Baanda MJ, et al. Wound macrophages express TGF-alpha and other growth factors in vivo: analysis by mRNA phenotyping. Science 1988;241:708–710.
83. Brenner CA, Tam AW, Nelson PA, et al. Message amplification phenotyping (MAPPing): a technique to simultaneously measure multiple mRNAs from small numbers of cells. BioTechniques 1989;7:1096–1103.
84. Alard P, Lantz O, Sebagh M, et al. A versatile ELISA-PCR assay for mRNA quantitation from a few cells. BioTechniques 1993;15:730–737.
85. Frye RA, Benz CC, Liu E. Detection of amplified oncogenes by differential polymerase chain reaction. Oncogene 1989;4:1153–1157.
86. Apostolakos MJ, Schuermann WHT, Frampton MW, et al. Measurement of gene expression by multiplex competitive polymerase chain reaction. Anal Biochem 1993;213:277–284.
87. Siebert PD, Larrick JW. Competitive PCR. Nature 1992;359:557–558.
88. Celi FS, Zenilman ME, Shuldiner AR. A rapid and versatile method to synthesize internal standards for competitive PCR. Nucleic Acids Res 1993;21:1047.
89. Gause WC, Adamovicsz J. The use of the polymerase chain reaction to quantitate gene expression. PCR Methods Appl 1994;3:123–135.
90. Diviacco S, Norio P, Zentilin L, et al. A novel procedure for quantitative polymerase chain reaction by coamplification of competitive templates. Gene 1992;122:313–320.
91. Deutscher MP, ed. Guide to protein purification. Methods Enzymol 1990;182:1–894.
92. O'Farrell PH. High resolution two-dimensional electrophoresis of proteins. J Biol Chem 1975;250:4007–4021.
93. Anderson N, Anderson L. The human protein index. Clin Chem 1982;28:739–748.
94. Garrels J. The Quest system for quantitative analysis of two dimensional gels. J Biol Chem 1989;264:5269–5282.
95. Celis JE, Gromov P, Ostergaard M, et al. Human 2-D PAGE databases for proteome analysis in health and disease. FEBS Lett 1996;398:129–134.
96. Bers G, Garfin D. Protein and nucleic acid blotting and immunohistochemical detection. Biotechniques 1985;3:276–288.
97. Burnette WN. "Western blotting": electrophoretic transfer of proteins from sodium dodecyl sulfate polyacrylamide gels to unmodified nitrocellulose and radiographic detection with antibody and radioiodinated protein A. Anal Biochem 1982;112:195–203.
98. Towbin H, Gordon J. Immunoblotting and dot immunobinding: current status and outlook. J Immunol Methods 1982;72:313–340.
99. Beisiegel U. Protein blotting. Electrophoresis 1986;7:1–18.
100. Stott Dl. Immunoblotting and dot blotting. J Immunol Methods 1989;119:153–187.
101. Renart J, Reiser J, Stark GR. Transfer of proteins from gels to diazobenzyloxymethyl-paper and detection with antisera: method for studying antibody specificity and antigen structure. Proc Natl Acad Sci USA 1979;76:3116–3120.
102. Towbin H, Straehelin T, Gordon J. Electrophoretic transfer of proteins from polyacrylamide gels to nitrocellulose sheets: procedure and some applications. Proc Natl Acad Sci USA 1979;76:4350–4354.
103. Reinhart MP, Malamud D. Protein transfer from isoelectric focusing gels: the native blot. Anal Biochem 1982;123:229–235.
104. Gershoni JM, Palade GE. Electrophoretic transfer of protein S from sodium dodecyl sulfate polyacrylamide gels to a positively charged membrane filter. Anal Biochem 1982;124:396–405.
105. Bowen B, Sternberg I, Laemmli BK, et al. The detection of DNA binding proteins by protein blotting. Nucleic Acids Res 1980;8:1–20.
106. Richter JD, Smith LD. Developmentally regulated RNA binding proteins during oogenesis in *Xenopus laevis*. J Biol Chem 1983;258:4864–4869.
107. Miskimins WK, Robens MP, McClelland A, et al. Use of a protein-blotting procedure and a specific DNA probe to identify nuclear proteins that recognize the promotor region of the transferrin receptor gene. Proc Natl Acad Sci USA 1985;82:6741–6744.
108. Appel RD, Bairoch A, Sanchez JC, et al. Federated 2-DE database: a simple means of publishing 2-DE data. Electrophoresis 1996;17:540–546.
109. Balbas P, Soberon X, Merino E, et al. Plasmid vector pBR322 and its special-purpose derivatives—a review. Gene 1986;50:3–40.
110. Burke DT, Carle GF, Olson MV. Cloning of large segments of exogenous DNA into yeast by means of artificial chromosome vectors. Science 1987;236:806–812.
111. Wilson JM. Adenoviruses as gene-delivery vehicles. N Engl J Med 1996;334:1185–1187.
112. Goeddel DV, Kleid DG, Bolivar F, et al. Expression in *Escherichia coli* of chemically synthesized genes for human insulin. Proc Natl Acad Sci USA 1979;76:106–110.
113. Maniatis T, Hardison RC, Lacy E, et al. The isolation of structural genes from libraries of eucaryotic DNA. Cell 1978;15:687–701.
114. Huynh TV, Young RA, Davis RW. Constructing and screening libraries at ygt 10 and ygt 11. In: Glover D, ed. DNA cloning: a practical approach, vol. 1. Oxford: IRL Press, 1985:49–78.
115. Ullrich A, Berman CH, Dull TJ, et al. Isolation of the human insulinlike growth factor I gene using a single synthetic DNA probe. EMBO J 1984;3:361–364.

116. Young RA, Davis RW. Efficient isolation of genes fusing antibody probes. Proc Natl Acad Sci USA 1983;80:1194–1198.
117. De Wet J, Fukushima H, Dewji NN, et al. Chromogenic immunodetection of human serum albumin and alpha-L-fucosidase clones in a human hepatoma cDNA expression library. DNA 1984;3:437–447.
118. Villa-Komaroff L, Efstratiadis A, Broome S, et al. A bacterial clone synthesizing proinsulin. Proc Natl Acad Sci USA 1978;75:3727–3731.
119. Cleveland DW, Lopata MA, MacDonald RJ, et al. Number and evolutionary conservation of alpha- and beta-tubulin and cytoplasmic beta- and gamma-actin genes using specific cloned cDNA probes. Cell 1981;20:95–105.
120. Bender W, Spierer P, Hogness DA. Chromosomal walking and jumping to isolate DNA from the Ace and rosy loci and the bithorax complex in Drosophila melanogaster. J Mol Biol 1983;168:17–33.
121. Cooper DN, Schmidtke J. Diagnosis of genetic disease using recombinant DNA. Hum Genet 1986;73:1–11.
122. Ostrer H, Hejtmancik JE. Prenatal diagnosis and carrier detection of genetic diseases by analysis of deoxyribonucleic acid. J Pediatr 1988;112:679–687.
123. Kan YW, Dozy AM. Polymorphism of DNA sequence adjacent to human β-globin structural gene: relationship to sickle mutation. Proc Natl Acad Sci USA 1978;75:5631–5635.
124. Saiki RK, Scharf S, Faloona F, et al. Enzymatic amplification of β-globin genomic sequences and restriction site analysis for diagnosis of sickle cell anemia. Science 1985;20:1350–1354.
125. Erlich HA, ed. PCR technology. Principles and applications for DNA applications. New York: Stockton Press, 1989.
126. Mullis KB, Faloona FA. Specific synthesis of DNA in vitro via a polymerase-catalyzed chain reaction. Methods Enzymol 1987;155:335–350.
127. Bloch W. A biochemical perspective on the polymerase chain reaction. Biochemistry 1991;30:2735–2747.
128. Saiki RK, Gelfand DH, Stoffel S, et al. Primer-directed enzymatic amplification of DNA with thermostable DNA polymerase. Science 1988;239:487–491.
129. Eisenstein BI. The polymerase chain reaction: a new method of using molecular genetics for medical diagnosis. N Engl J Med 1990;322:178–183.
130. Reiss J, Cooper DN. Application of the polymerase chain reaction to the diagnosis of human genetic disease. Hum Genet 1990;85:18.
131. Scharf SJ, Horn GT, Erlich HA. Direct cloning and sequence analysis of enzymatically amplified genomic sequences. Science 1986;233:1076–1078.
132. Gyllensten UB, Erlich HA. Generation of single-stranded DNA by the polymerase chain reaction and its application to direct sequencing of the HLA-DQa locus. Proc Natl Acad Sci USA 1988;85:7652–7656.
133. Gyllensten UB. PCR and DNA sequencing. Biotechniques 1989;7:700–708.
134. Tahara T, Kraus JP, Rosenberg LE. Direct sequencing of PCR amplified genomic DNA by the Maxam-Gilbert method. Biotechniques 1990;8:366–368.
135. Stoflet ES, Koerberl DD, Sarkar G, et al. Genomic amplification with transcript sequencing. Science 1988;239:491–494.
136. Saiki RK, Bugavan TL, Horn GT, et al. Analysis of enzymatically amplified, β-globin and HLA-DQ DNA with allele-specific oligonucleotide probes. Nature 1986;324:163–166.
137. Kwoh DY, Davis GR, Whitfield KM, et al. Transcription-based amplification system and detection of amplified human immunodeficiency virus type I with a bead-based sandwich hybridization format. Proc Natl Acad Sci USA 1989;86:1173–1177.
138. Guatelli JC, Whitfield KM, Kwoh DY, et al. Isothermal, in vitro amplification of nucleic acids by a multienzyme reaction modeled after retroviral replication. Proc Natl Acad Sci USA 1990;87:1874–1878.
139. Hudson TJ, Stein LD, Gerety SS, et al. An STS-based map of the human genome. Science 1995;270:1945–1954.
140. Troutt AB, McHeyzer-Williams MG, Pulendran B, et al. Ligation-anchored PCR: a simple amplification technique with single-sided specificity. Proc Natl Acad Sci USA 1992;89:9823–9825.
141. Ansari-Lari MA, Jones SN, Timms KM, et al. Improved ligation-anchored PCR strategy for identification of 5′ ends of transcripts. BioTechniques 1996;21:35–38.
142. Frohman MA, Dush MK, Martin GR. Rapid production of full-length cDNAs from rare transcripts: amplification using a single gene-specific oligonucleotide primer. Proc Natl Acad Sci USA 1988;85:8998–9002.
143. Wang WP, Myers RL, Chiu IM. Single primer-mediated polymerase chain reaction: application in cloning of two different 5′-untranslated sequences of acidic fibroblast growth factor mRNA. DNA Cell Biol 1991;10:771–777.
144. Aksoy IA, Wood TC, Weinshilboum R. Human liver estrogen sulfotransferase: identification by cDNA cloning and expression. Biochem Biophys Res Commun 1994;200:1621–1629.
145. Verhoeven AJ, Carling D, Jansen H. Hepatic lipase gene is transcribed in rat adrenals into a truncated mRNA. J Lipid Res 1994;35:966–975.
146. McKenzie JM, Zakarija M. LATS: new thoughts on an old theme. In: Fisher DA, Burrow GN, eds. Perinatal thyroid physiology and disease. New York: Raven Press, 1975:185–195.
147. Taylor SI, Grunberger G, Marcus-Samuels B, et al. Hypoglycemia associated with antibodies to the insulin receptor. N Engl J Med 1982;307:1422–1426.
148. Schreiber AB, Lax I, Yarden Y, et al. Monoclonal antibodies against receptors for epidermal growth factor induce early and delayed effects of epidermal growth factor. Proc Natl Acad Sci USA 1981;78:7535–7539.
149. Djiane J, Houdebine L-M, Kelly PA. Prolactin-like activity of antiprolactin receptor antibodies on casein and DNA synthesis in the mammary gland. Proc Natl Acad Sci USA 1981;78:7445–7448.
150. Conn PM, Rogers DC, Stewart JM, et al. Conversion of a GnRF agonist to an antagonist: implication for a receptor microaggregate as the functional unit for signal transduction. Nature 1982;296:653–655.

151. Beddell CR, Sheppey GC, Blundell TL, et al. Symmetrical features in polypeptide hormone-receptor interactions. Int J Peptide Protein Res 1977;9:161–165.
152. Lefkowitz RJ, Roth J, Pricer W, et al. ACTH receptors in the adrenal: specific binding of ACTH-125 I and its relation to adenyl cyclase. Proc Natl Acad Sci USA 1970;65:745–752.
153. Haylett DG. Direct measurement of drug binding to receptors. In: Foreman JC, Johansen T, eds. Textbook of receptor pharmacology. Boca Raton, FL: CRC Press, 1996;121–149.
154. Limbird LE. Cell surface receptors: a short course on theory and methods. 2nd ed. Boston: Martins Nijhoff, 1996.
155. Roth J, Lesniak MA, Bar RS, et al. An introduction to receptors and receptor disorders. Proc Soc Exp Biol Med 1979;162:3–12.
156. Langmuir I. The absorption of gases on plane surfaces of glass, mica and platinum. J Am Chem Soc 1918;40:1361–1403.
157. Hill AV. The possible effects of the aggregation of the molecules of haemoglobin on its dissociation curve. J Physiol 1910;40:iv–vii.
158. Michaelis L, Menten ML. Zur kinetik der invertinwirkung. Biochem Z 1913;49:333–369.
159. Lineweaver H, Burk D. The determination of enzyme dissociation constants. J Am Chem Soc 1934;56:658–666.
160. Scatchard G. The attraction of proteins for small molecules and ions. Ann NY Acad Sci 1949;51:660–672.
161. Scatchard G, Coleman JS, Shen AL. Physical chemistry of protein solutions. VII. The binding of some small anions to serum albumin. J Am Chem Soc 1957;79:12–20.
162. Rosenthal HE. A graphic method for the determination and presentation of binding parameters in a complex system. Anal Biochem 1967;20:525–532.
163. Eadie GS. The inhibition of cholinesterase by physostigmine and prostigmine. J Biol Chem 1942;146:85–93.
164. Hofstee BHJ. On the evaluation of the constants Vm and Km in enzyme reactions. Science 1952;116:329–331.
165. Hulme EC (ed.). Receptor-ligand interactions. A practical approach. New York: IRL Press, 1992.
166. Rodbard D. Mathematics of hormone-receptor interaction. 1. Basic principles. In: O'Malley B, Means A, eds. Receptors for reproductive hormones. New York: Plenum, 1973:289–326.
167. Rodbard D, Munson PJ, Thakur AK. Quantitative characterization of hormone receptors. Cancer 1980;46:2907–2918.
168. Levitski A. Reconstitution of membrane receptor systems. Biochim Biophys Acta 1985;833:127–153.
169. Hla T, Maciag T. An abundant transcript induced in differentiating human endothelial cells encodes a polypeptide with structural similarities to G-protein coupled receptors. J Biol Chem 1990;265:9308–9313.
170. Hutchison CA, Phillips S, Edgell M, et al. Mutagenesis at a specific position in a DNA sequence. J Biol Chem 1978;18:6551–6560.
171. Sibley DR, Benovic JL, Caron MG, et al. Regulation of transmembrane signalling by receptor phosphorylation. Cell 1987;48:913–922.
172. Lefkowitz RJ, Wessels MR, Stadel JM. Hormones, receptors, and cyclic AMP: their role in target cell refractoriness. Curr Top Cell Regul 1980;17:205–230.
173. Hubtaniemi IT, Nozu K, Warren DW. Acquisition of regulatory mechanisms for gonadotropin receptors and steroidogenesis in the maturing rat testis. Endocrinology 1982;111:1711–1720.
174. Harwood JP, Conti M, Conn PM, et al. Receptor regulation and target cell responses: studies in the ovarian luteal cell. Mol Cell Endocrinol 1978;11:121–135.
175. Kaplan J. Polypeptide-binding membrane receptors: analysis and classification. Science 1981;212:14–20.
176. Triggle DJ. Desensitization. Trends Pharmacol Sci 1980; 14:395–398.
177. Unwin N. Acetylcholine receptor channel imaged in the open state. Nature 1995;373:37–43.
178. Egeberg J. Molecular structure of ligand-gated ion channels. In: Foreman JC, Johansen T, eds. Textbook of receptor pharmacology. Boca Raton, FL: CRC Press, 1996:85–100.
179. Sakmann B, Neher E, eds. Single channel recording, 2nd ed. New York: Plenum, 1995.
180. Gibb AJ. Receptors linked to ion channels: activation and block. In: Foreman JC, Johansen T, eds. Textbook of receptor pharmacology. Boca Raton, FL: CRC Press, 1996;159–185.
181. Thomas PM, Wohlik N, Huang E, et al. Inactivation of the first nucleotide-binding fold of the sulfonylurea receptor, and familial persistent hyperinsulinemic hypoglycemia of infancy. Am J Hum Genet 1996;59:510–518.
182. Thomas PM, Cote GJ, Wohlik N, et al. Mutations in the sulfonylurea receptor gene in familial persistent hyperinsulinemic hypoglycemia of infancy. Science 1995;268:426–429.
183. Schlessinger J, Ullrich A. Growth factor signaling by receptor tyrosine kinases. Neuron 1992;9:383–391.
184. Garbers DL, Lower DG. Guanylyl cyclase receptors. J Biol Chem 1994;269:30741–30744.
185. Hunter T. Protein kinases and phosphatases: the ying and yang of protein phosphorylation and signaling. Cell 1995;808:225–236.
186. Streauli M. Protein tyrosine phosphatases in signaling. Curr Opin Cell Biol 1996;8:182–188.
187. Hunter T. A thousand and one protein kinases. Cell 1987;50:823–829.
188. Hanks SK, Quinn AM, Hunter T. The protein kinase family. Conserved features and deduced phylogeny of the catalytic domain. Science 1990;241:42–52.
189. Yarden Y, Ullrich A. Growth factor receptor tyrosine kinases. Annu Rev Biochem 1988;57:443–478.
190. Gammeltoft S, Kahn CR. Molecular structure of tyrosine kinase-linked receptors. In: Foreman JC, Johansen T, eds. Textbook of receptor pharmacology. Boca Raton, FL: CRC Press, 1996:101–117.
191. Darnell JE, Kerr IM, Stark GR. Jak-STAT pathways and transcriptional activation in response to IFRNs and other extracellular signaling proteins. Science 1994;264:1415–1421.
192. Inhe JN. Cytosine receptor signaling. Nature 1995;377: 591–594.

193. Brown EM, Hebert SC. Calcium-receptor-regulated parathyroid and renal function. Bone 1997;20:303–309.
194. Emala CW, Schwindinger WF, Wand GS, et al. Signal transducing G proteins: basic and clinical implications. Prog Nucleic Acid Res Mol Biol 1994;47:81–111.
195. Neer EJ. Heterotrimeric G proteins: organizers of transmembrane signals. Cell 1995;80:249–257.
196. Hamm HE, Gilchrist A. Heterotrimeric G proteins. Curr Opin Cell Biol 1996;8:189–196.
197. Clapham DE, Neer EJ. New roles for G-protein βγ-dimers in transmembrane signaling. Nature 1993;365:403–406.
198. Rens-Domiano S, Hamm HE. Structural and functional relationship of heterotrimeric G-proteins. FASEB J 1995;9:1059–1066.
199. Gilman AG. G Proteins and regulation of adenyl cyclase. JAMA 1989;262:1819–1825.
200. Krebs KG. Role of the cyclic AMP-dependent protein kinase in signal transduction. JAMA 1989;262:1815–1818.
201. VanDop C, Tsubokawa M, Bourne HR, et al. Amino acid sequence of retinal transducin at the site ADP ribosylated by cholera toxin. J Biol Chem 1984;259:696–698.
202. West RE Jr, Moss I, Vaughan M, et al. Pertussis toxin catalyzed ADP-ribosylation of transducin. J Biol Chem 1985;260:14428–14430.
203. Kobilka BK, Kobilka TS, Daniel K, et al. Chimeric α_2-β_2-adrenergic receptors: delineation of domains involved in effector coupling and ligand binding specificity. Science 1988;240;1310–1316.
204. Jones DT, Reed RR. Molecular cloning of five GTP-binding protein cDNA species from rat olfactory neuroepithelium. J Biol Chem 1987;262:14241–14249.
205. Peralta KG, Ashkenazi A, Winslow JW, et al. Distinct primary structures, ligand-binding properties and tissue-specific expression of four human muscarinic acetylcholine receptors. EMBO J 1987;6:3923–3929.
206. Regan IW, Kobilka TS, Yang-Feng TL, et al. Cloning and expression of a human kidney cDNA for an α_2-adrenergic receptor subtype. Proc Natl Acad Sci USA 1988;75:6301–6305.
207. Dharmawardhane S, Cubitt AB, Clark AM, et al. Regulatory role of the G 1 subunit in controlling cellular morphogenesis in Dictyostelium. Development 1994;120:3549–3561.
208. Gao P, Watkins DC, Malbon CC. Constitutively active mutant Gs L2 (G203T) induce primitive endoderm from stem cells. Am J Physiol 1995;268:1460–1466.
209. Spiegel AM. Defects in G protein-coupled signal transduction in human disease. Annu Rev Physiol 1996;58:143–170.
210. Rudolf U, Finegold MJ, Rich SS, et al. Ulcerative colitis and adenocarcinoma of the colon in Gi2–deficient mice. Nature Genet 1995;10:141–148.
211. Spiegel S, Foster D, Kolesnich R. Signal transduction through lipid second messengers. Curr Opin Cell Biol 1996;8:159–167.
212. Brown EM. Second messengers and the control of cellular function. In: Posillico JT, ed. Introduction to endocrine investigation 1988: techniques and concepts. Randolph, MA: Serono Symposia, USA Press, 1988:75–88.
213. Sutherland EW, Oye I, Butcher RW. The action of epinephrine and the role of the adenyl cyclase system in hormone action. Recent Prog Horm Res 1965;21:623–646.
214. Douglas WW. Stimulus-secretion coupling: variations on the theme of calcium-activated exocytosis involving cellular and extracellular sources of calcium. Ciba Found Symp 1978;54:61–90.
215. Grynkiewicz G, Peonie M, Tsien RY. A new generation of Ca^{2+} indicators with greatly improved nuorescence properties. J Biol Chem 1985;260:3440–3450.
216. Bright GR, Fisher GW, Rogowska J, et al. Fluorescence ratio imaging microscopy. Methods Cell Biol 1989;30B:157–192.
217. Tsien RY. Fluorescent indicators of ion concentrations. Methods Cell Biol 1989;30B:127–156.
218. Means AR. Calmodulin: properties, intracellular localization, and multiple roles in cell regulation. Recent Prog Horm Res 1981;37:333–367.
219. Berridge MJ. Calcium oscillations. J Biol Chem 1990;265:9583–9586.
220. Berridge MJ, Dupont G. Spatial and temporal signalling by calcium. Curr Opin Cell Biol 1994;6:267–274.
221. Osipchuk YV, Wakui M, Yule Dl, et al. Cytoplasmic Ca^{2+} oscillations evoked by receptor stimulation, G-protein activation, internal application of inositol trisphosphate or Ca^{2+}: simultaneous microfluorimetry and Ca^{2+}: dependent Cl⁻ recording in single pancreatic acinar cells. EMBO J 1990;9:697–704.
222. Woods NM, Cuthbertson KSR, Cobbold PH. Repetitive transient rises in cytoplasmic free calcium in hormone stimulated hepatocytes. Nature 1986;3:600–602.
223. Kawanishi T, Blank LM, Harootunian AT, et al. Ca^{2+} oscillations induced by hormonal stimulation of individual fura-2 loaded hepatocytes. J Biol Chem 1989;264:12859–12866.
224. Saez JC, Connor JA, Spray DC, et al. Hepatocyte gap junctions are permeable to the second messenger, inositol 1,4,5–trisphosphate, and to calcium ions. Proc Natl Acad Sci USA 1989;86:2708–2712.
225. Rooney TA, Sass EJ, Thomas AR. Agonist-induced cytosolic calcium oscillations originate from a specific locus in single hepatocytes. J Biol Chem 1990;265:10792–10796.
226. Lin C, Hajnoczky G, Thomas AP. Propagation of cytosolic calcium waves into the nucleus of hepatocytes. Cell Calcium 1994;16:247–258.
227. Zemel MD, Zemel PC, Berry S, et al. Altered platelet calcium metabolism as an early predictor of increased peripheral vascular resistance and preeclampsia in urban black women. N Engl J Med 1990;323:434–438.
228. Putney JW Jr, Bird GS. The phosphate-calcium signaling system in nonexcitable cells. Endocr Rev 1993;14:610–631.
229. Berridge MJ. Inositol trisphosphate and diacylglycerol: two interacting second messengers. Annu Rev Biochem 1987;56:159–193.
230. Nishizuka Y. Protein kinase C and lipid signaling for sustained cellular responses. FASEB J 1995;9:484–496.
231. Irvine RF, Moor RM. Microinjection of inositol 1,3,4,5–tetrakisphosphate activates sea urchin eggs by a mechanism dependent on external Ca^{++}. Biochem J 1986;240:917–920.

232. Dassouli A, Sulpice J-C, Roux S, et al. Stretch-induced inositol trisphosphate and tetrakisphosphate production in rat cardioimyocytes. J Mol Cell Cardiol 1993;25:973–982.
233. Putney JW Jr, Takemura H, Hughes AR, et al. How do inositol phosphates regulate calcium signaling? FASEB J 1989;3:1899–1905.
234. Sherman WR. Inositol homeostasis, lithium and diabetes. In: Michell RH, Drummond AH, Downes CP, eds. Inositol lipids and cell signaling. Orlando, FL: Academic Press, 1989:39–79.
235. Downes CP, Hawkins PT, Irvine RF. Inositol 1,3,4.5-tetrakisphosphate and not phosphatidylinositol 3,4-bisphosphate is the probable precursor of inositol 1,3,4-trisphosphate in agonist-stimulated parotid gland. Biochem J 1986;238:501–506.
236. Batty IR, Nahorski SR, Irvine RF. Rapid formation of inositol 1,3,4,5-tetrakisphosphate following muscarinic receptor stimulation of rat cerebral conical slices. Biochem J 1985;232:211–215.
237. Nakadate T, Jeng AY, Blumberg PM. Comparison of protein kinase C functional assays to clarify mechanisms of inhibitor action. Biochem Pharmacol 1988;37:1541–1545.
238. Jaken S. Protein kinase C isozymes and substrates. Curr Opin Cell Biol 1996;8:168–173.
239. Foster DA. Intracellular signalling mediated by protein-tyrosine kinases networking through phospholipid metabolism. Cell Signal 1993;5:389–399.
240. Exton JH. Phosphatidylcholine breakdown and signal transduction. Biochim Biophys Acta 1994;12:26–42.
241. Yeagle PL. Lipid regulation of cell membrane structure and function. FASEB J 1989;3:1833–1842.
242. Goodridge AG. Dietary regulation of gene expression: enzymes involved in carbohydrate and lipid metabolism. Annu Rev Nutr 1987;7:157–185.
243. Tremp GL, Boquet D, Ripoche M-A, et al. Expression of the rat L-type pyruvate kinase gene from its dual erythroid- and liver-specific promotor in transgenic mice. J Biol Chem 1989;264:19904–19910.
244. Wiesner RJ, Zak R. Quantitative approaches for studying gene expression. Am J Physiol 1991;260:L179–L188.
245. Latchman DS. Gene regulation: a eukaryotic perspective. 2nd ed. New York: Van Nostrand Reinhold, 1995.
246. Laemmli UK, Tijian R. Nucleus and gene expression. A nuclear traffic jam: unraveling multicompartment machines and compartments. Curr Opin Cell Biol 1996;8:299–302.
247. Hentze MW. Translational regulation versatile mechanisms for metabolic and developmental control. Curr Opin Cell Biol 1995;7:393–398.
248. Rotwein P, DeVol D, Lajara P, et al. Physiological regulation of insulin-like growth factor expression. In: LeRoith D, Raizada MK, eds. Molecular and cellular biology of insulin-like growth factors and their receptors. New York: Plenum Press, 1989:117–124.
249. Klausner RD, Rouault TA, Hartford JB. Regulating the fate of mRNA: the control of cellular iron metabolism. Cell 1993;72:19–28.
250. Harford JB. Iron regulation of transferrin receptor mRNA stability. In: Belasco JG, Brawerman G, eds. Control of messenger RNA stability. San Diego: Academic Press, 1993:239–266.
251. Haldane JBS. The cytological basis of genetical interference. Cytologia 1931;3:54–65.
252. Papavassiliou A, ed. Transcription factors in eukaryotes. New York: Van Nostrand Reinhold, 1996.
253. Maniatis T, Goodbourn S. Fischer JA. Regulation of inducible and tissue-specific gene expression. Science 1987; 236:1227–1244.
254. Chin WW. Hormonal regulation of gene transcription. In: Posillico JT, ed. Introduction to endocrine investigation 1988: techniques and concepts. Randolph, MA: Serono Symposia. USA Press, 1988:27–36.
255. Guarente L. UAEs and enhancers: common mechanism of transcriptional activation in yeast and mammals. Cell 1988;52:303–305.
256. Angel P, Imagawa M, Chiu R, et al. Phorbol ester inducible genes contain a common cis element recognized by a TPA-modulated trans-acting factor. Cell 1987;49:729–739.
257. Pugh BF. Mechanisms of transcription complex assembly. Curr Opin Cell Biol 1996;8:303–311.
258. Buratowski S. The basics of basal transcription by RNA polymerase II. Cell 1994;77:1–3.
259. Tijan R, Maniatis T. Transcriptional activation: a complex puzzle with few easy pieces. Cell 1994;77:5–8.
260. Gray S, Levine M. Transcriptional repression in development. Curr Opin Cell Biol 1996;8:358–364.
261. Becker P, Renkawitz R, Schutz G. Tissue-specific DNase I hypersensitive sites in the 5'-flanking sequences of the tryptophan oxygenase and the tyrosine aminotransferase genes. EMBO J 1984;3:2015–2020.
262. Slater E, Rabenau O, Karin M, et al. Glucocorticoid-receptor binding and activation of a heterologous promotor by dexamethasone by the first intron of the human growth hormone gene. Mol Cell Biol 1985;5:2984–2992.
263. Beato M, Chalepakis G, Schauer M, et al. DNA regulatory elements for steroid hormones. J Steroid Biochem 1989;37:737–747.
264. Akerblom IE, Slater EP, Beato M, et al. Negative regulation by glucocorticoids through interference with a cAMP responsive enhancer. Science 1988;741:350–353.
265. Vaulont S, Munnich A, Decaux J-E, et al. Transcriptional and post-transcriptional regulation of L-type pyruvate kinase gene expression in rat liver. J Biol Chem 1986;261: 7621–7625.
266. Mariana BD, Lingappa JR, Kafatos FC. Temporal regulation in development: negative and positive cis regulators dictate the precise timing of expression of a *Drosophila* chorion gene. Proc Natl Acad Sci USA 1988;85:3029–3033.
267. Imai Y, Matsushima Y, Sugimura T, et al. A simple and rapid method for generating a deletion by PCR. Nucleic Acids Res 1991;19:27–85.
268. Papavassiliou AG. Transcription factors. N Engl J Med 1995;332:45–47.
269. Molkentin JD, Olson EN. Defining the regulatory networks for muscle development. Curr Opin Gen Dev 1996;6:445–453.
270. Rawls A, Olsen EN. MyoD meets its maker. Cell 1997;89: 5–8.

271. Verrijzer CP, Van der Vliet PC. POU domain transcription factors. Biochim Biophys Acta 1993;1173:1–21.
272. Anderson B, Rosenfeld MG. Pit-1 determines cell types during development of the anterior pituitary gland: a gland for transcriptional regulation of cell phenotypes in mammalian organogenesis. J Biol Chem 1994;269:29335–29338.
273. Radovick S, Nations M, Du Y, et al. A mutation in the POU-homeodomain of Pit-1 responsible for combined pituitary hormone deficiency. Science 1992;257:1115–1118.
274. Pfaffle RW, DiMattia GE, Parks JS, et al. Mutation of the POU-specific domain of Pit-1 and hypopituitarism without pituitary hypoplasia. Science 1992;257:1118–1121.
275. Latchman DS. Transcription-factor mutations and disease. N Engl J Med 1996;334:28–33.
276. Belasco JG, Brawerman G, eds. Control of messenger RNA stability. San Diego: Academic Press, 1993.
277. Spindler SR, Mellon SH, Baxter JD. Growth hormone gene transcription is regulated by thyroid and glucocorticoid hormones in cultured rat pituitary tumor cells. J Biol Chem 1982;257:11627–11632.
278. Kindy MS, McCormack J, Buckler A, et al. Independent regulation of the two strands of the c-myc gene. Mol Cell Biol 1987;7:2857–2892.
279. Kneale GG, ed. DNA-protein Interactions: principles and protocols. Totowa, NJ: Humana Press, 1994.
280. Galas D, Schmitz A. DNase footprinting: a simple method for detecting protein-DNA binding specificity. Nucleic Acids Res 1978;5:3157–3170.
281. Elgin SCR. The formation and function of DNase I hypersensitive sites in the process of gene activation. J Biol Chem 1988;263:19259–19262.
282. Leblanc B, Moss T. DNase I footprinting. In: Kneale GG, ed. DNA-protein interactions. Totowa, NJ: Humana Press, 1994:1–10.
283. Sandaltzopoulos R, Becker PB. Solid phase DNase I footprinting: quick and versatile. Nucleic Acids Res 1994;22:1511–1512.
284. Mueller PR, Wold B. In vivo footprinting of a muscle specific enhancer by ligation mediated PCR. Science 1988;246:780–786.
285. Sekhar-Reddy PM, Shen CJ. Protein-DNA interactions in vivo of an erythroid-specific, human β-globin locus enhancer. Proc Natl Acad Sci USA 1991;88:8676–8680.
286. Revzin A. Gel electrophoresis assays for DNA-protein interactions. BioTechniques 1987;7:346–355.
287. Fried M. Measurement of protein-DNA interaction parameters by electrophoresis mobility shift assay. Electrophoresis 1989;10:366–376.
288. Manna AC, Pai KS, Bussiere DE, et al. Helicase-contrahelicase interaction and the mechanism of termination of DNA replication. Cell 1996;87:881–891.
289. Rosenthal N. Recognizing DNA. N Engl J Med 1995;333:925–927.
290. Gorman CM, Moffat LF, Howard BH. Recombinant genomes which express chloramphenicol acetyltransferase in mammalian cells. Mol Cell Biol 1982;2:1044–1051.
291. Nordeen SK, Green PP III, Fowlkes DM. A rapid, sensitive, and inexpensive assay for chloramphenicol acetyltransferase. DNA 1987;6:173–178.
292. DeWet JR, Wood KV, DeLuca M, et al. Firefly luciferase gene: structure and expression in mammalian cells. Mol Cell Biol 1987;7:725–737.
293. Brasier AR, Tate JE, Habener JF. Optimized use of the firefly luciferase assay as a reporter gene in mammalian cell lines. Biotechniques 1989;7:1116–1122.
294. Schwartz O, Virelizier JL, Montagnier L, et al. A microtransfection method using luciferase-encoding reporter gene for the assay of human immunodeficiency virus LTR promotor activity. Gene 1990;88:197–205.
295. Marth JD. Recent advances in gene mutagenesis by site-directed recombination. J Clin Invest 1996;98:S47–50.
296. Izant JG, Weintraub H. Inhibition of thymidine kinase gene expression by anti-sense RNA: a molecular approach to genetic analysis. Cell 1984;36:1007–1015.
297. Dougherty WG, Parks TD. Transgenes and gene suppression: telling us something new? Curr Opin Cell Biol 1995;7:399–405.
298. Williams DL, Sensel M, McTigue M, et al. Hormonal and developmental regulation of mRNA turnover. In: Belasco JG, Brawerman G, eds. Control of messenger RNA stability. San Diego: Academic Press, 1993:161–218.
299. Shapiro DJ, Blume JE, Nielsen DA. Regulation of messenger RNA stability in eukaryotic cells. Bioessays 1987;6:221–226.
300. Hargrove JL, Schmidt FH. The role of mRNA and protein stability in gene expression. FASEB J 1989;3:2360–2370.
301. Vonderhaar BK, Ziska SE. Hormonal regulation of milk protein gene expression. Annu Rev Physiol 1989;51:641–652.
302. Topper YJ, Sankaran L, Chomczynski P, et al. Three stages of responsiveness to hormones in the mammary cell. Ann NY Acad Sci 1986;464:1–10.
303. Chomczynski P, Qasba P, Topper YJ. Transcriptional and posttranscriptional roles of glucocorticoids in the expression of the rat 25,000 molecular weight casein gene. Biochem Biophys Res Commun 1986;134:812–818.
304. Zeevi M, Nevins JR, Darnell JE Jr. Newly formed mRNA lacking polyadenylic acid enters the cytoplasm and the polyribosomes but has a shorter half-life in the absence of polyadenylic acid. Mol Cell Biol 1982;2: 517–525.
305. Palatnik CM, Wilkins C, Jacobson A. Translational control during early Dictyostelium development: possible involvement of poly(A) sequences. Cell 1984;36:1017–1025.
306. Robinson BG, Frim DM, Schwanz WJ, et al. Vasopressin mRNA in the suprachiasmatic nuclei: daily regulation of polyadenylate tail length. Science 1988;241:342–344.
307. Sachs A, Wahle E. Poly(A) tail metabolism and function in eukaryotes. J Biol Chem 1993;268:22955–22958.
308. Jackson RJ, Standart N. Do the poly(A) tail and 3' untranslated region control mRNA translation? Cell 1990;62:15–24.
309. Eberwine JH, Roberts JL. Analysis of pro-opiomelanocortin gene structure and function. DNA 1983;2:1–8.
310. Gordon JW, Scangos GA, Plotkin DJ, et al. Genetic transformation of mouse embryos by microinjection of purified DNA. Proc Natl Acad Sci USA 1980;77:7380–7384.
311. Hanahan D. Transgenic mice as probes into complex systems. Science 1989;246:1265–1275.

312. Landel CP, Chen S, Evans GA. Reverse genetics using transgenic mice. Annu Rev Physiol 1990;52:841–851.
313. Ho Y-S. Transgenic models for the study of lung biology and disease. Am J Physiol 1994;266:L319–L353.
314. Glasser SW, Korfhagen TR, Wert SE, Whitsett JA. Transgenic models for study of pulmonary development and disease. Am J Physiol 1994;267:L489–L497.
315. Vaulont S. Puzenat N, Leviat F, et al. Proteins binding to the liver specific pyruvate kinase gene promotor: a unique combination of known factors. J Mol Biol 1989;209:205–219.
316. Jhappan C, Stahle C, Harkins RN, et al. TGFα over-expression in transgenic mice induces liver neoplasia and abnormal development of the mammary gland and pancreas. Cell 1990;61:1137–1146.
317. Matsui Y, Halter SA, Holt JT, et al. Development of mammary hyperplasia and neoplasia in MMTγ-TGFα transgenic mice. Cell 1990;61:1147–1155.
318. Sandgren EP, Luetteke NC, Palmiter RD, et al. Overexpression of TFGα in transgenic mice: induction of epithelial hyperplasia, pancreatic metaplasia, and carcinoma of the breast. Cell 1990;61:1121–1135.
319. Majzoub JA, Muglia LJ. Knockout mice. N Engl J Med 1996;334:904–907.
320. Cole TJ, Blendy JA, Monaghan AP, et al. Targeted disruption of the glucocorticoid receptor gene blocks adrenergic chromaffin cell development and severely retards lung maturation. Genes Dev 1995;9:P1608–1621.
321. Muglia L, Jacobson L, Dikkes P, et al. Corticotropin-releasing hormone deficiency reveals major fetal but not adult glucocorticoid need. Nature 1995;373:427–432.
322. Stanley E, Lieschke GJ, Grail D, et al. Granulocyte/macrophage colony-stimulating factor-deficient mice show no major pertubation of hematopoiesis but develop a characteristic pulmonary pathology. Proc Natl Acad Sci USA 1994;91:5592–5596.
323. Dranoff G, Crawford AD, Sadelain M, et al. Involvement of granulocyte-macrophage colony-stimulating factor in pulmonary homeostasis. Science 1994;264:713–716.
324. Kuhn R, Schwenk F, Aguet M, et al. Inducible gene targeting in mice. Science 1995;269:1427–1429.
325. Gazit G, Kane SE, Nichols P, et al. Use of the stress-inducible GRP78/BIP promotor in targeting high level gene expression in fibrosarcoma in vivo. Cancer Res 1995;55:1660–1663.
326. Chan CH, Blazar BR, Eide CR, et al. A murine granulocyte-macrophage colony-stimulating factor (GM-CSF) receptor on normal committed bone marrow progenitor cells and GM-CSF-dependent tumor cells. Blood 1995;86:2732–2740.
327. Eisen JS. Zebrafish make a big splash. Cell 1996;87:969–977.
328. Knapp JR, Kopchick JJ. The use of transgenic mice in nutrition research. J Nutr 1994;124:461–468.
329. Miklos GLG, Rubin GM. The role of the Genome Project in determining gene function: insights from model organisms. Cell 1996;87:521–529.
330. Brown MS, Goldstein JL. A receptor-mediated pathway for cholesterol homeostasis. Science 1986;232:34–47.
331. Kiess W, Blickenstaff GD, Sklar MM, et al. Biochemical evidence that the type II insulin-like growth factor receptor is identical to the cation-independent mannose 6–phosphate receptor. J Biol Chem 1988;263:9339–9344.
332. Matlin KS, Valentich JD, eds. Modern cell biology: functional epithelial cells in culture. New York: Alan R. Liss, 1989.
333. Handler JS. Overview of epithelial polarity. Annu Rev Physiol 1989;51:729–740.
334. Kleinman HK, Luckenbill-Edds L, Cannon FW, et al. Use of extracellular matrix components for cell culture. Anal Biochem 1987;166:1–13.
335. Hadley MA, Byers SW. Suarez-Quian CA, et al. Extracellular matrix regulates Sertoli cell differentiation, testicular cord formation, and germ cell development in vitro. J Cell Biol 1985;101:1511–1522.
336. Takeichi M. The cadherins: cell-cell adhesion molecules controlling animal morphogenesis. Development 1988;102:639–655.
337. Panayotou G, End P, Aumailley M, et al. Domains of laminin with growth-factor activity. Cell 1989;56:93–101.
338. Heino J, Massague J. Cell adhesion to collagen and decreased myogenic expression implicated in the control of myogenesis by transforming growth factor a. J Biol Chem 1990;265:10181–10184.
339. Shannon JM, Pitelka DR. The influence of cell shape on the induction of functional differentiation in mouse mammary cells in vitro. In Vitro 1981;17:1016–1028.
340. Mostov KE, Cardone MH. Regulation of protein traffic in polarized epithelial cells. Bioessays 1995;17:129–138.
341. Handler JS, Preston AS, Steele RE. Factors affecting the differentiation of epithelial transport and responsiveness to hormones. Fed Proc 1984;43:2221–2224.
342. Neutra MR, Wilson JM, Weltzin RA, et al. Membrane domains and macromolecular transport in intestinal epithelial cells. Am Rev Respir Dis 1988;138:S10–S16.
343. Amsler K. Sodium-coupled transport processes in cultured epithelial ceils. In: Matlin KS, Valentich JD, eds. Modern cell biology: functional epithelial cells in culture. New York: Alan R. Liss, 1989:193–234.
344. Lisanti MP, Rodriguez-Boulan E. Glycophospholipid membrane anchoring provides clues to the mechanism of protein sorting in polarized epithelial cells. Trends Biochem Sci 1990;15:113–118.
345. Giuliano KA, Taylor DL. Measurement and manipulation of cytoskeletal dynamics in living cells. Curr Opin Cell Biol 1995;7:4–12.
346. Hahn K, Kolega J, Montibeller J, et al. Fluorescent analogues: optical biosensors of the chemical and molecular dynamics of macromolecules in living cells. In: Mason WT, ed. Fluorescent and luminescent probes for biological activity. San Diego: Academic Press, 1993:349–359.
347. Potter SM. Vital imaging: two photons are better than one. Curr Biol 1996;6:1595–1596.
348. Stark H, Orlova EV, Rinke-Appel J, et al. Arrangements of tRNAs in pre- and posttranslocational ribosomes revealed by electron cryomicroscopy. Cell 1997;88:19–28.

5
Methodology for the Study of Metabolism: Physiologic Modeling in Animals

John B. Susa

Overview of Animal Models

Using an animal model to study the metabolic interactions between the mother and her fetus helps the perinatal investigator answer questions that for ethical or practical reasons cannot be dealt with in human clinical investigation. Any investigator who uses animals must determine which animal model is most appropriate for answering the questions that are under investigation.

The diversity, in terms of differences in relative mass of the fetus compared with maternal mass as well as the number of offspring produced by mammals, is striking.[1] In some cases such as in the marsupial, fetal and neonatal weight is similar across the phylum, although the adult weight ranges from 60 g to 60 kg.[2] In other cases fetal and neonatal weight are more closely related to maternal size. One of the smallest mammals, the fruit bat, which weighs 6 g, delivers a neonate that weighs 2 g, while the blue whale, which weighs 1×10^8 g delivers an offspring that may weigh as much as 2×10^6 g.[3] The neonatal fruit bat, which weighs about 33% of its mother's weight, imposes a much higher metabolic demand on its mother than the gigantic blue whale neonate, which represents only 2% of its mother's weight. Consequently, the investigator who is choosing an animal model must be cognizant of the fact that numerous factors must be considered beyond what animal is readily available.

The use of an animal allows the investigator to answer questions that are unanswerable in humans. In other cases, animal studies allow for parallel investigations in both human and animal physiology. This comparative approach is helpful because it allows for more detailed or specific in vivo and/or in vitro studies using animals to answer questions raised during human investigation. In some cases most of what is known about a particular facet of perinatal physiology comes from animal studies that may or may not yet have been confirmed in the human. The need to choose an animal model that will provide information that can be appropriately applied to human clinical problems and practice must be approached with care.

Chemical reactions are similar across all living things. Studies that focus on the chemistry of life, including energy production and utilization, or synthetic and degradative processes, can be studied in a wide variety of animals. In most cases these processes can be studied in vitro as well or better than in vivo. In many instances rodents are used because they have been the animal of choice for so long that the biological chemistry of these animals is well characterized. This extensive study has produced a database of knowledge not available for larger animals. Because of the small size of the mother and the fetus, it is difficult to carry out studies that require fetal manipulation or multiple sampling of the fetal compartment without compromising the pregnancy or causing significant and interfering maternal and fetal stress.

Investigations that require fetal manipulation are better done in the larger animal. The most commonly used large animal for such studies is the sheep. This larger mother and fetus can be studied simultaneously since it is possible to introduce catheters into both the maternal and fetal circulation without compromising either the mother or fetus. If the investigator is willing to wait a few days postsurgery, the effects of the surgical stress dissipate to the point that it is possible to sample both maternal and fetal compartments in an awake, unstressed, and unanesthetized chronic in vivo preparation. Those who choose to use this model must be able to bear the significant costs associated with highly sophisticated research animal facilities with large support staffs and ancillary services that are required to maintain large pregnant animals within the usually urban biomedical research environment.

Although no animal model is identical to the human, those who are formulating research hypotheses that require animals that mimic as closely as possible human physiology or pathophysiology must be cautious in their search. Despite the obvious similarities between human and nonhuman primates, there are major differences in terms of maternal diet and activity levels of captive or free-ranging pregnant animals and pregnant humans. These differences contribute to relative differences in metabolic activity in the mother and her fetus. For example, the human neonate is born with a body fat content of approximately 16%, while nonhuman primates are born with very little body fat, no more than 2%. Therefore, investigation of the control of fetal fat metabolism during gestation would probably be better carried out in an animal whose fetus was equally as fat as the human at birth, if the goal was to understand what is the cause of this relatively large fat production. If the goal is to learn how fetal fat syntheses could be reduced in utero, then fetal nonhuman primate studies may well be appropriate and necessary. As is usually the case in animal research, the question asked often helps to direct the investigator to the appropriate animal model.

Despite major differences between different species it is possible to manipulate experimental conditions in ways that elicit similar metabolic responses. Some experimental manipulations can make the human, sheep, or pig neonate more metabolically similar. For example, to avoid metabolic substrate utilization for heat generation by shivering and nonshivering thermogenesis, the neonatal lamb and piglet can be studied under thermoneutral conditions. Since the human neonate experiences weight loss or no weight gain during the first 24 hours of life and has low intakes of colostrum during this period, food intake by the neonate lamb or piglet must be restricted to mimic the human experience. Care must also be taken to exclude the growth-retarded lamb or piglet since their lipid stores are so limited that they become metabolically dissimilar to the human once these lipid stores are consumed. Manipulating the length of fasting, the gestational and/or postnatal age at study, or the environmental conditions during the study may make a particular animal an appropriate model for human biology in one instance and inappropriate in another.

With the wide diversity of animals that may be utilized, investigators must be cautious to claim that their particular animal model of specific human pathophysiology will allow appropriate conclusions to be drawn that are completely applicable to the human clinical situation. The investigator must acknowledge the differences as well as point out the similarities between any animal model and human biology.

The Ideal Animal Model

According to some animal rights activists, given the diversity in adult and fetal size found in the animal kingdom, finding an animal model that is similar to human perinatal biology is impossible. They argue that the differences in size, diet, behavior and living conditions are too great to allow for the logical and appropriate transfer of knowledge gained from studying the nonhuman mammal to the human. Although there is no appropriate animal model of human biology, our knowledge of the process of fetal growth and development can be greatly enlarged by the study of these events in a variety of different species. It is this appreciation of the diversity and differences found in the animal kingdom that allows us to understand and appreciate the biology all mammals share and the uniqueness of the human animal. Study of fetal physiology in various mammalian species has confirmed that there are common themes that unify mammalian biology. One important similarity is that metabolic rate is a function of weight.[2] The smaller the animal the higher its metabolic fuel consumption and oxygen utilization. This fact means that extrapolation of knowledge about the adult to the neonate in the same species or from one member of an order to another such as from marmosets to gorillas (i.e., the smallest to the largest primates) may lead to invalid conclusions.

If the focus of the studies is on an individual organ system and its metabolism, differences between different mammalian species become less dramatic. At the organ level, most interspecies differences disappear except for the gastrointestinal tract and liver. The gastrointestinal tract and liver place into the circulation the metabolic fuel substrate necessary for sustaining life and growth. Because the food-consuming diversity in mammals ranges from herbivores to insectivores, to carnivores, to omnivores, the metabolic functions of the liver of different mammals must be more variable that any other organ. In contrast the central nervous system of all mammals is metabolically similar since it relies on glucose as its primary metabolic substrate with ketone bodies as secondary substrates becoming increasingly more utilized when the glucose supply is limited. It is much easier to justify the use of an animal as a model of human pathophysiology when studies are focused at the organ, cellular, or subcellular level.

The placenta, common to all mammals, is the great equalizer of fetal metabolic fuel metabolism, because it presents and modulates the fetal fuel supply.[4] All mammalian fetuses share a common diet of glucose, fatty acids, amino acids, organic acids, and ketones made available by the placenta. Thus, the mammalian fetus in general is much more metabolically similar than the adult counterpart.

Once the fetus is born and is separated from the modulating influence of the placenta, it must be prepared to survive in an environment as diverse as the differences found between mammals. The degree to which the neonatal mammal is able to survive in its new extrautero environment varies. At one extreme is the very small marsupial neonate, which is separated from its placental mediator so early in development that it cannot survive, except in its mother's pouch.[5] In that protective environment it must continue to develop for as long as a year before it is able to live outside of the protective environment of the pouch. At the other end of the spectrum is the very large blue whale neonate, which, when it separates from the placenta, is fully developed and is able to survive and function in the same environment as its mother.[3]

Animal Models to Study the Causes of Fetal Macrosomia

Although much is known about the impact of maternal diabetes on her fetus, it is not possible to describe precisely how it is that the infant of a mother with diabetes mellitus (IDM) is often macrosomic. The search for this answer has used many different animal models to study diabetes and related pathophysiology.[6] This body of work has demonstrated that there is no identical animal model to diabetes during pregnancy in the human. However, animal models have been used by investigators to address some important questions.

Animal models of maternal diabetes fall into two categories: those produced experimentally by maternal pancreatic ablation, and cases of spontaneous diabetes. The production of diabetes in the pregnant animal has resulted in mixed results in terms of the production of fetal macrosomia.[7] The increase in fetal body weight appears to be a function of body fat content of the fetus, the severity and duration of the diabetes, and the temporal pattern of maternal hyperglycemia. In sheep or swine, maternal diabetes has little or no effect on fetal size. There are reports that in the rodent the impact of maternal diabetes is variable, ranging from large, to appropriate, to small for gestational-age fetuses.[8,9]

The direct administration of insulin to the fetus has not produced fetal macrosomia in all animals. The pig and sheep fetus appear to be unaffected by direct insulin administration, while the nonhuman primate and rat fetus demonstrate accelerated weight gain. Fetal insulin deficiency, on the other hand, has been shown to cause fetal growth retardation in all animals where it has been produced.[3] Table 5.1 illustrates the effects of spontaneously occurring or experimentally produced diabetes and fetal glucose and insulin manipulations on fetal macrosomia in some common laboratory animals.

Recent studies reveal some important relationships between fetal weight and other factors in the non-obese diabetic mouse (NOD) that are similar to the variable outcomes of human pregnancy complicated by diabetes. The latter depends on the severity and duration of disease based on the commonly used White classification.[10] These animals confirm that maternal hyperglycemia plays an important role in affecting fetal weight when other factors such as maternal age, size, parity, and gestational duration are controlled.

TABLE 5.1. Fetal macrosomia in laboratory animals.

Species	Condition	Birth weight
Nonhuman primate	Experimental diabetes	+
	Spontaneous diabetes	+
	Fetal insulin infusion	+
Sheep	Experimental diabetes	−
	Fetal insulin infusion	−
	Maternal glucose infusion	−
Swine	Experimental diabetes	−
	Fetal insulin infusion	−
Rat	Experimental diabetes	+/−
	Spontaneous diabetes	+/−
	Fetal insulin infusion	+
	Maternal glucose infusion	+
Mouse	Experimental diabetes	+/−
	Spontaneous diabetes	+/−

+, present; −, absent; +/−, variable.

Fetal weight in animals that produce multiple offspring during the pregnancy is also affected by litter size, parity and maternal age. In some respects this is true in the human. The large neonate in the human is associated with an increased parity, hereditary factors, and maternal age.[11] However, the increased weight of the mouse fetus as parity and age increase is associated with a concomitantly decreasing litter size. Since the human normally produces a single offspring per pregnancy and there is an increased incidence of twinning as the mother ages, the reasons for macrosomia in the mouse and the human may not be the result of the same pathophysiology.

Another experimental way to produce diabetes during pregnancy in the rat is to subject the young female, during the third to sixth week of age, to severe protein-energy malnutrition.[12] When the animal becomes pregnant she experiences wide movements of plasma glucose and insulin concentrations. At term the number of offspring per litter is the same as controls, but those fetuses weigh significantly more. The explanation for these data lies in the possibility that during pregnancy the capacity of the maternal pancreas to secrete adequate insulin to maintain maternal substrate concentrations within the normal range is compromised. The increased substrate transfer that occurs during these episodes of elevated glucose concentration results in intermittent periods of hyperinsulinemia that may explain the fetal macrosomia.

Some investigators have utilized the nonhuman primate as the animal model to determine if fetal hyperinsulinemia leads to fetal macrosomia.[13] These investigators have used two different experimental approaches. Some have demonstrated that streptozotocin-produced diabetes in the pregnant rhesus monkey (*Macaca mulatta*) results in the macrosomia and selective organomegaly in the offspring that is similar to that found in the IDM. The presence of hyperglycemia and hyperinsulinemia at delivery and the consequent neonatal hypoglycemia found in the neonate is analogous to that found in the IDM.

Others have taken advantage of the impermeability of the rhesus monkey placenta to insulin in either direction and its permeability to glucose to create fetal euglycemic hyperinsulinemia in the fetus. This experimentally produced fetal hyperinsulinemia accompanied by euglycemia has been used to show that fetal hyperinsulinemia results in the fetal macrosomia and selective organomegaly that is the hallmark of infants born to human and nonhuman primate mothers who have diabetes.[14]

When diabetes during pregnancy in the human was not as well[1] controlled as is standard practice today, selective organomegaly was reported at autopsy in the fetus carried by the mother with diabetes.[15] Besides a 40% increase in expected birth weight, liver, heart, lung, thymus, and adrenal weights were also significantly increased. If fetal insulin concentrations in the rhesus are increased to above $800\mu U \cdot ml^{-1}$, a similar pattern of selective organomegaly is observed.

A more recent postmortem study of fetal weight in a Scandinavian population among infants of mothers whose diabetes was better controlled than in previous generations identified only total fetal weight and heart weight as being significantly increased in a very large population sample.[16] Hyperinsulinemia in the rhesus fetus, with concentrations of approximately $300\mu U \cdot ml^{-1}$, during the latter part of gestation results in a doubling of the rate of fetal weight gain.[17] However, only fetal body weight and heart weight are significantly increased.

Fetal pharmacologic hyperinsulinemia (i.e., plasma insulin concentration greater than $800\mu U \cdot ml^{-1}$) in the nonhuman primate produces changes very similar to those seen in instances of poor diabetes control in the human or when there is an excess of human fetal insulin producing cells. The degree of macrosomia and organomegaly observed during physiologic hyperinsulinemia (i.e., plasma insulin concentration of approximately $300\mu U \cdot ml^{-1}$) is similar to that reported in the human infant born to a mother whose diabetes is better controlled.

Several animal models have been used to show that insulin administration results in increased synthesis of fat.[18] The fetus carried by a mother with diabetes is born with approximately 50% more fat than those carried by women without diabetes. The rhesus monkey fetus that is made chronically hyperinsulinemic is born with visibly greater amounts of fat in the thoracic cavity, the perinephrium, and the pericardium compared with control fetuses of comparable gestational age. Some of the increased weight of these fetuses can be explained by this increased amount of fat. This increased fat is the direct result of the stimulation by insulin of fatty acid synthesis.[19] An increase in the rate of lipogenesis and triglyceride synthesis has been observed in the liver of the fetus carried by the rhesus monkey with streptozotocin-induced diabetes during pregnancy. Even though the rhesus monkey fetus is born lean with no more than 2% of its body weight accounted for by fat, this animal model replicates the increased adiposity of the IDM.

Most of the increased weight of the hyperinsulinemic rhesus fetus is the result of hyperplasia. The liver of this fetus has normal protein to DNA ratios. Microscopic examination reveals parenchymal and hematopoietic cells of normal morphology and size. The protein-to-DNA ratio in heart and skeletal muscle is also normal, and microscopic examination of muscle fibers, including cross-sectional area measurements, confirms the fact that hyperinsulinemia with concurrent normal growth substrate concentrations stimulates cellular hyperplasia.[20] This contrasts with the human IDM where an increased concentration of fetal growth substrates is present and in which both hyperplasia and hypertrophy at the cellular level has been observed.[21]

Use of Bioengineered Rodent Models

Until recently, the appearance of mutations in the mammal that provide opportunities for the study of important scientific questions have been the result of chance occurrence. Occasionally such a chance occurrence in the right gene has produced a mutation that produces an animal strain that has a transmittable genetic defect that is similar to some human pathophysiologic condition. Advances in molecular bioengineering technology allow investigators to create a rodent with planned genetic alterations at specific loci of the genome. This technology has been used to either introduce specific genes from one species into another, to produce an animal that expresses a desired gene product, or to inactivate a specific gene and produce an animal with a specific gene product deficiency.

These processes are the result of the isolation of puripotent embryonic stem cell from the inner mass of the rodent blastocyte.[22] These stem cells can be cultured in vitro without differentiating for sufficiently long periods of time to permit the introduction of specific DNA fragments. DNA introduced into these cultured cells can participate in homologous recombination to alter targeted genes in a predetermined manner. The cultured embryonic stem cell retains its ability to resume normal development in vivo when injected into blastocytes that can then be implanted into the uterus of a "pseudo"-pregnant rodent. The pup delivered by this mother is a mixture of cells originating from the injected embryonic stem cells and the recipient blastocytes. The altered embryonic stem cell genome can be introduced into animals that then transmit that altered genome to future generations. This process allows investigators to introduce genetic material from different species into the rodent to create a transgenic animal model that produces proteins that it previously could not.[23] The other major use of this technology is to produce alterations in the genome that result in the production of an inactive gene product resulting in a "knockout" animal model.

Data from a number of recent clinical studies have been interpreted as demonstrating that other fetal growth factors besides insulin contribute to the overgrowth of the fetus carried by a mother with diabetes.[24,25] These growth factors are the insulin-like growth factors (IGF) I and II, which share structural homology with insulin and exert their effects through receptor-mediated processes. That IGFs play an important role in the control of fetal growth is a hypothesis that is being tested in numerous perinatal research laboratories throughout the world.[23,26,27] It has not yet been possible to experimentally confirm that the overgrowth of the fetus of a mother with diabetes is due to IGFs (see Chapter 20).

These new bioengineered animal models may be used to test this hypothesis much more directly than previously possible, when investigators were dependent on chance for specific point mutations to occur to create a useful animal model. Investigators are now using some of these newer approaches to determine if the overexpression or underexpression of IGFs result in altered fetal growth. One experiment in which data are consistent with the hypothesis that elevated IGFs contribute to fetal overgrowth, is one in which embryos from mice bred for having low and high IGF-I levels were transplanted into a neutral maternal line.[28] Embryos from the high IGF-I line weighed more than those from the low IGF-I line at term. Unfortunately, hormone, growth factor, and metabolic substrate concentration were not measured. It is premature to conclude that the increased fetal weight is due to the elevated IGF-I concentration.

Others have developed a line of transgenic mice that overexpress IGF-I, in most tissue, prenatally and postnatally. These mice produce fetuses that have very elevated plasma and tissue concentrations of IGF-I; however, the pups are normal in size and weight at delivery.[29] Between the first and second month of age the offspring with elevated plasma and tissue concentrations of IGF-I begin to grow at a faster rate so that by 6 months of age they weigh 25% more than controls. These studies show that IGF-I is a potent stimulator of postnatal growth but that it does not stimulate fetal overgrowth.

Studies of growth of mice embryos carrying null mutations of the genes encoding for IGF-I and IGF-II have demonstrated that the absence of either or both of these growth factors results in the deceleration of fetal growth during the last third of gestation.[30,31] At term the IGF-I (–/–) or IGF-II (–/–) fetus weighs approximately 40% less than its wild-type littermate. Postnatal weight gain is also reduced in the IGF-I (–/–) animal such that by 2 months of age it weighs 70% less than its wild type littermate. Thus, studies using transgenic and knockout mice have provide experimental evidence that the absence of IGFs during fetal development leads to fetal growth retardation. In another study the murine embryo that inherited an inactive IGF-II receptor from its father develops normally in utero and postnatally. However, the fetus that inherits that mutation from its mother weighs 25% to 30% more than its wild type littermate and dies at birth.[32]

The elevation of circulating concentrations of these IGFs in fetuses carried by the mother with diabetes needs to be more carefully studied, using both humans and animals. The biologic activity of the IGFs is modulated by protein that binds the growth factors in the plasma. There are as many as six different binding proteins now identified. Each binding protein is unique and may serve a different function, ranging from being a simple carrier of the growth factor to being a stimulatory or inhibitory modulator of its activity.[33] The exact nature of these interactions needs to be clarified. Because the IGFs exert their activities via both autocrine and paracrine processes, the study of these mechanisms needs to be carried out at the cellular and tissue level rather than at the whole-body level.

These early studies with new animal models still provide no support for the hypothesis that the fetal macrosomia observed in the human is attributable to elevated IGF concentrations. The bioengineered rodent model may prove to be the most useful tool for carrying out studies to determine the mechanisms by which IGFs influence fetal growth. Until such studies have been carried out, it is premature to conclude that IGFs play any significant role in producing fetal macrosomia.

Fetal Growth Studies Using Farm Animals

Several studies using insulin-like growth factors have been performed that try to mimic the effect of insulin on fetal growth. That the further one moves philogenetically from humans the less useful the animal model becomes is illustrated by two studies that look at the effect of IGFs on the chicken. The readily available animal model, the chick embryo in ovo, has been used to determine if IGF-I can directly stimulate fetal growth.[34] This model has the benefit of being totally dissociated from maternal factors when such a study is being performed. The administration of IGF-I on days 7 and 14 by direct injection into the allantoic sac failed to have any effect on total body weight, bone length, organ weight, or muscle DNA, RNA, and protein content. IGF-II administration to growing broiler chickens likewise has not been demonstrated to affect weight gain, bone growth, or organ weight.[35] These studies illustrate how the animal model of choice may or may not provide data that clarify or help explain human pathophysiology.

Because it is possible to place catheters into the fetal compartment during swine and ovine pregnancy, dynamic studies can be carried out in these two species that are not possible in other animals. In both cases these animals can endure considerable manipulation of their fetus, including fetal surgery, without experiencing fetal loss. Catheters inserted into the fetus can be maintained in a patent state for weeks, and access to the fetal compartment allows investigators to study fetal metabolic events as gestation progresses. Both the female pig and sheep are tolerant of these manipulations without the requirement of sedation and/or stressful restraint.[36]

Seven days after fetal catheterization, the late gestation fetal pig is insulin sensitive as measured by depressed glucose concentration and elevation in growth hormone and adrenocorticotropic hormone (ACTH) after an intravenous insulin infusion.[37] Delivery of 3 U of insulin per day from days 90 to 104 of gestation, the term being 114 days, had no effect on total body weight and length.[38] These fetuses had significantly elevated somatomedin activity than did controls, again with no apparent biologic effect.[39] These data could be interpreted as providing direct experimental evidence that neither insulin nor insulin-like growth factors directly affect fetal swine growth.

Although spontaneous diabetes has not been reported in swine, alloxan diabetes has been produced in pregnant Yorkshire gilts during the last third of pregnancy.[40] Forty-two days of maternal diabetes with accompanying fetal hyperglycemia failed to raise the fetal insulin concentration above the control concentration. Fetal weight at delivery was unaffected by maternal diabetes, although body composition studies identified a significant increase in fat content in the IDMs. The reason for this increased fat content could not be attributed to hepatic lipogenesis since hepatic lipogenesis was unaffected. The increased fat deposits may be due to increased de novo fatty acid synthesis by the adipose cell or direct incorporation of maternal fatty acids into the fetal adipose cell. Subsequent studies identified an increase in fetal subcutaneous tissue lipogenic enzyme activities, which were increased by as much as 40-fold.[41] Similar data have been reported by investigators who produced alloxan diabetes in a different strain of swine, the Yucatan miniature pig.[42] Therefore, the use of pregnant swine as an animal model for diabetes during pregnancy is a poor choice if one is interested in studying the relationship between fetal hyperinsulinemia and fetal weight.

Administration of alloxan to pregnant sheep results in metabolic and endocrine derangements simulating those found in pregnant women with insulin-dependent diabetes.[43] Despite the fetal hyperglycemia and hyperinsulinemia, these sheep experiments have failed to produce the fetal macrosomia that is the hallmark characteristic of the IDM.[44] A similar conclusion about the effect of insulin on fetal sheep growth has been drawn from two studies in which chronic fetal hyperinsulinemia has been produced with no effect.[45,46]

Investigators, studying the relationship between maternal diabetes and fetal IGF, have used both swine and sheep for their studies. Production of maternal diabetes in pregnant swine results in an increase in IGF-I messenger RNA (mRNA) in fetal skeletal muscle, liver, heart, and kidney as well as in placental tissue. At the same time IGF-I mRNA was reduced in fetal adipose and brain tissue. The elevated tissue mRNA is accompanied by a parallel elevated plasma concentration of IGF-I in the fetuses of pregnant swine with diabetes. This study documents that metabolic and endocrine alterations result in tissue-specific regulation of IGF-I expression during development.[47]

Similar studies have been carried out in the pregnant ewe and its fetus. One study in which ewes were fasted for 72 hours documented that fetal IGF-I concentration drops with fasting and that fetal concentration can be restored to prefasting levels with 4 hours of glucose infusion. Nutrient, in particular glucose, availability seems to be a determinant in control of IGF-I secretion.[48] Since amino acid infusion does not restore the fasting suppressed fetal IGF-I concentration, the hypothesis that the fetal hyperglycemia found in the IDM would lead to elevated IGF-I concentration and to subsequent fetal overgrowth is a conclusion of these studies.[49]

Direct evidence that elevating IGF-I concentration in fetal sheep may result in fetal overgrowth comes from a recent study in which IGF-I was infused into fetal sheep from days 120 to 130 of gestation.[50] Ten days of IGF-I infusion, sufficient to increase fetal plasma IGF-I concentration by 140%, significantly increased the weight of fetal liver, lungs, kidneys, spleen, pituitary, and adrenal glands by 16% to 50%. The selective organomegaly reported in these studies is similar to that found in the chronically hyperinsulinemic fetal rhesus monkey[19] and in the human infant of mothers whose diabetes is poorly controlled.[17] Although not identical, there is an obvious similarity in the pattern and magnitude of selective organomegaly summarized in Figure 5.1. Whether there exists a common mechanistic explanation for these similarities remains to be determined. Although the fetal sheep had elevated IGF-I concentration and the human IDMs probably did, too (it was not measured in 1964), the fetal rhesus monkey did not.[51] Elevated plasma insulin concentration is found in the human IDM and the hyperinsulinemic rhesus. Insulin concentration was suppressed in the IGF-I infused fetal sheep.

Presumably the selective organomegaly is the result of IGF-1 acting through its type 1 receptor. Because of the structural similarity between the type-1 growth factor receptor and the insulin receptor, there is some potential that under conditions of elevated ligand concentration there is cross-reactivity between the ligand and its receptor. The insulin receptor of HepG2 cells, for example, has been found to respond to IGF-1 with increased serine and tyrosine residue phosphorylation at in vitro concentrations of 100 ng of IGF-1·ml^{-1}.[52] This increase in insulin receptor phosphorylation by IGF-1 correlates with the dose-response stimulation of the type 1 receptor by IGF-1. Although the type 1 receptor has a much higher affinity for IGF-1, it does bind insulin if the concentration of insulin is sufficiently high.[53] Although highly specific, IGF-1 receptor binding of IGF-1 can be displaced by insulin in a dose-dependent manner. This displacement results in an increase in receptor tyrosine kinase activity.[54] In addition, insulin and IGF-1 binding by muscle tissue also changes from species to species in both quantity and activity.[55]

The interaction of insulin and insulin-like growth factors in the regulation of energy metabolism, cellular growth and differentiation is not well understood yet. The use of immortalized gonadotropin-releasing hormone (GnRH)-secreting neurons to study these events has revealed that although there are differences in binding of insulin, IGF-I, and IGF-II to specific receptors, both insulin and IGF-I were equally potent mitogens at a dose of only 0.1 ng·ml^{-1}.[56]

The discovery of "atypical" insulin and IGF receptors and receptor hybrids raises the possibility that the control of fetal growth by these peptides may be more complex that previously postulated. The human breast cancer cell has a high binding affinity for insulin, but IGF-1 is five times more potent in inhibiting ^{125}I-insulin binding than insulin itself. Characterization of this binding protein revealed that in addition to the typical insulin and IGF-1 receptors, there is another receptor that binds both insulin and IGF-1 with high affinity.[57] A hybrid IGF-1/insulin receptor has been characterized in human placental tissue that is more effectively stimulated by IGF-1 than by insulin in a dose-dependent manner.[58]

Differences in response of fetal tissue to insulin and IGF-1 may also be a function of differences in the developmental regulation of the expression of their receptors. For example, in the more primitive *Xenopus*, the pattern of developmental expression of the insulin and IGF-1 receptors is different.[59] The differential response of human, nonhuman primate, and sheep fetal tissue to insulin and IGF-1 may be attributable to any number of reasons that require more careful investigation. The lack of increase in fetal weight with IGF-1 infusion into the fetal sheep may be due to the fact that the signal transaction sequence initiated by the type 1 receptor is not fully intact even though the receptor itself is present.[60] Alternatively, the lack of response may mean that IGF-1 plays primarily a permissive role in the stimulation of muscle mass increase. Since the fetal insulin concentration was reduced by IGF-1 infusion, it may be possible that IGF-1 and insulin function synergistically to control muscle growth in the fetus.

The use of fetal sheep to investigate IGF-1 regulation of fetal growth has documented that IGF-1 can promote

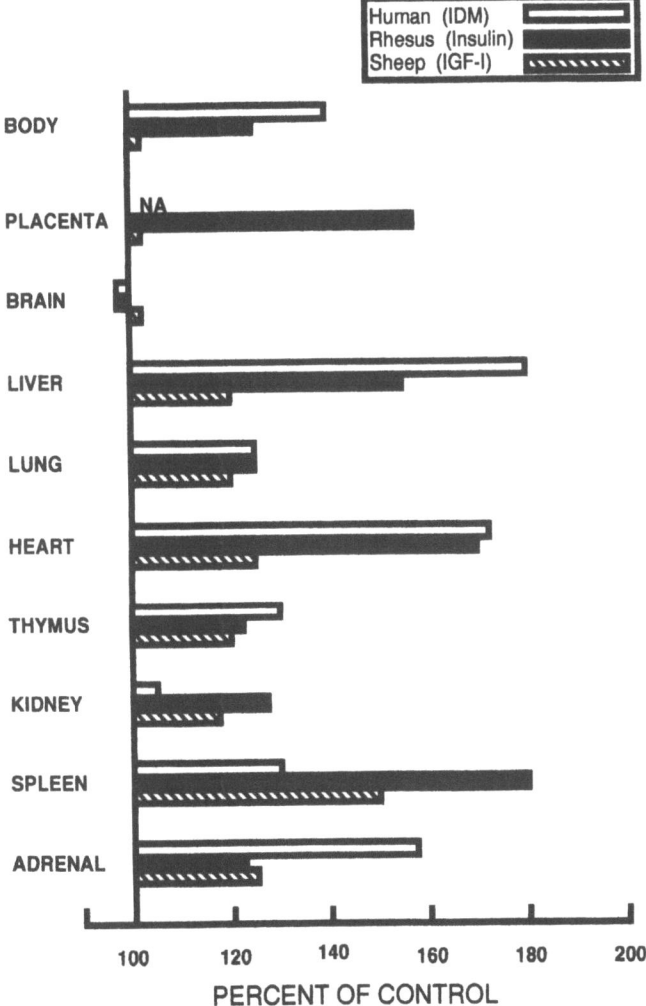

FIGURE 5.1. Selective organomegaly in human infants of mothers with poorly controlled diabetes, insulin-infused rhesus monkey fetuses, and IGF-I–infused sheep fetuses.

the growth (i.e., increased weight) of some fetal tissue. It has provided evidence that IGF-1 has an endocrine role as well as a paracrine role in the fetus. Precisely what that role is and how it is played out remains the subject of future investigation in the sheep and other species.

Metabolic Factors

The mammalian neonate is born at a different developmental stage and with different concentration of the two metabolic fuel reserves—lipids and glycogen.[61] The relative size of lipid stores determines the degree to which the neonate is dependent on the immediate start of nursing from the mother. Those neonates with small lipid reserves must initiate nursing very soon after birth if they are to survive their new and hostile postnatal environment. In anticipation of severance of the relatively constant source of glucose that it receives from its mother, the mammalian fetus has deposited liver and muscle glycogen stores that are two to three times higher than those of its mother.[62] Although distributed throughout the body, the accumulation of glycogen in cardiac muscle and the nervous system serves to protect these vital organs from hypoxic injury in anoxic episodes during labor and vaginal birth.

Table 5.2 illustrates that the amount of readily available metabolic fuel reserves available to the fetus varies greatly in mammals. These differences account for the fact that some neonates such as the rat and pig must have access to mother's milk soon after birth, while others can survive some time before feeding is initiated. Generally, neonates born with large lipid reserves can survive longer than those with very low lipid reserves. When the fetus leaves its protected and metabolically stable in utero environment at birth, major metabolic alterations occur in the neonate. The neonate must make the transition from being an energy storage system to an energy using and replenishing system. The specifics of how this happens is unique to the particular species. In general the investigator must recognize the differences in both neonatal body composition and the neonatal dietary intake reflected in mother's milk composition. The relative composition of maternal milk that the neonate is provided is also variable, as summarized in Table 5.3. Most mammalian milk is relatively rich with 50% to 60% of the caloric content composed of fat (see Chapter 52).[63]

Differences in placental metabolism and function also affect fetal growth and metabolism. In the human the transfer of glucose in a stereospecific manner is very efficient. This efficient system results in glucose being the primary oxidative fuel of the human fetus.[64] The gradient between maternal and fetal plasma glucose concentration varies widely in different species as illustrated in Figure 5.2. These differences are due to the fact that the primate hemochorial placenta is more permeable to glucose than the epitheliochorial placenta of the horse, cow, or sheep. Differences between species exist in the permeability of the placenta to other important metabolic substrates such as amino acids and lipids. To grow normally the fetus must be assured a constant and increasing supply of metabolic substrates. For this to be accomplished, uterine and umbilical blood flow increases in all species as pregnancy progresses. The concentration and relative abundance of these growth substrates is species specific and dependent on maternal diet.

Even though fetal growth rate is species specific, fetal oxidative metabolic rate, corrected for body weight, is relatively constant. This is because the fate of energy derived from this oxidative metabolism is species specific. For example, although human fetal growth rate as expressed as the daily percent increase is only one-third that of the fetal sheep, the two have similar oxidative rates. The human fetus at term has large fat reserves (i.e., 16% of birth weight) but the lamb is very lean (i.e., 2% body fat). Additional energy is required to build up these fat stores in the sheep compared to the human, and that energy is partitioned differently.

TABLE 5.2. Glycogen and fat stores in the neonate of several mammalian species.

Species	Weight at birth (g)	Total lipid stores (g/kg body wt.)	Muscle glycogen stores (g·kg body wt^{-1})	Liver glycogen stores (g·kg body wt^{-1})
Human	3500	160	7.5	3.8
Monkey	500	20	7.5	2.5
Sheep	4500	30	8.8	2.2
Pig	1000	11	20.9	2.1
Guinea pig	100	110	4.5	3.5
Rabbit	50	58	2.3	2.7
Rat	5	11	1.8	5.8

From Jones,[70] with permission.

TABLE 5.3. Milk composition in several mammalian species.

	Percent of total calories		
Species	Fat	Protein	Carbohydrate
Human	53	6	41
Monkey	53	12	35
Cow	50	21	29
Goat	62	20	18
Sheep	62	20	18
Horse	28	22	50
Pig	59	26	15
Dog	63	25	12
Cat	64	28	8
Guinea pig	62	28	10
Rabbit	58	37	5
Rat	69	25	6

From Jones,[70] with permission.

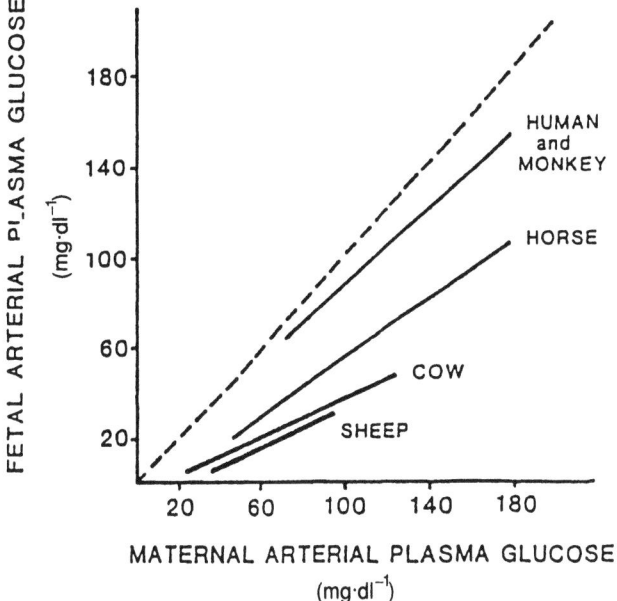

FIGURE 5.2. Relation between fetal and maternal plasma glucose concentration in humans and common large animals used in perinatal research.

Extrauterine life means that the steady supply of metabolic nutrient to the fetus ends when the umbilical cord is severed. Survival in a colder, hostile environment requires that the fetus maintain body temperature and that a new way of accessing nutrients from its mother be established. Because the size and distribution of fetal energy reserves vary in different species, neonatal metabolic responses to birth and survival also differ. Generally, the early response to the stopping of maternoplacental derived nutrients is a decrease in neonatal glucose and amino acid concentrations.[6]

Without feeding, survival depends on the fetus' ability to utilize its own energy reserves for heat production and movement so that it can gain access to maternal colostrum and milk. Fetal glycogen and nonstructural lipid stores are the life-sustaining reserves of the neonate. Based on respiratory quotient data, carbohydrate stores are mobilized first, followed by lipid stores.[65] Although all mammalian fetuses have relatively similar glycogen pool sizes, their lipid pool sizes differ. The human, rabbit, and guinea pig neonates begin to mobilize lipids reserves immediately after birth, while the swine, sheep, and rat, with very small lipid reserves, are very dependent on maternal milk, which in these species has a very high fat content. These differences are illustrated by the fact that the human neonate is able to maintain euglycemia for over 24 hours of fasting at room temperature, while the neonatal pig develops life-threatening hypoglycemia after only 12 hours of fasting at room temperature.

As neonatal glycogen stores are being consumed, neonatal gluconeogenesis increases, reaching a maximal concentration 24 to 48 hours after birth. Critical to the regulation of neonatal plasma glucose concentration is glucagon, which during states of low insulin concentration activates hepatic glycogenolysis, blocks glycogen synthesis, and stimulates gluconeogenesis by promoting the adaptive synthesis of key gluconeogenic enzymes.[66]

The glucose-sparing effect of free fatty acids and ketone bodies that are released into the plasma of the neonate plays an important role in preventing hypoglycemia. Neonatal hypoglycemia occurs sooner in the human intrauterine growth-retarded neonate.[67] Besides the amount of lipid available to the fetus for mobilization, the kind of lipid is also species specific. Brown adipose tissue, which is predominantly utilized for thermal regulation,[68] is found in relatively low abundance in the human and the pig compared with most other mammals.[69] The species to species differences in placental function, fetal metabolism, and energy store deposition during gestation, and then neonatal energy mobilization and access to mother's milk in mammals illustrate the biologic variability and complexity of mammals. This complexity and variability requires familiarity with the biology of mammals for those who seek to use these animals to study human pathobiology.

The ideal animal model mimics human perinatal physiology and metabolism and must include (1) an omnivorous mother; (2) a placenta that readily transfers glucose and amino acids, but transfers lipids more slowly; (3) a fetus that at term weighs about 5% of maternal weight; (4) large fetal lipid stores of about 16% of body weight at birth; (5) mother's milk that is high in lipid and carbohydrate content but low in protein; and (6) a neonate that is developmentally immature.

No single animal model can meet these criteria. Many different mammals have one or more features of their pregnancy that are similar to those of human pregnancy. Therefore, any investigator who is interested in studying a particular aspect of human pathophysiology needs to carefully evaluate the pros and cons of any specific model. That investigator and those who seek to apply the findings of that work in their own studies must be careful when they interpret these studies to explain aspects of human pathophysiology. It is not practical to provide a comparison of all possible animal models of human pathophysiology. Investigators must be thoroughly familiar with the specifics of how maternal metabolic events are altered in a specific species. If those alterations are consistent with similar events in the human, then the animal chosen may prove to be a useful model.

References

1. Battaglia FC. Commonality and diversity in fetal development: bridging the interspecies gap. Pediatr Res 1978;12: 736–745.

2. Dawes GS. Foetal and neonatal physiology. Chicago: Year Book Medical Publishers, 1969; pp. 13–17.
3. Mathews LH. The natural history of the whale. New York: Columbia University Press, 1978.
4. Dancis J. Placental physiology. In: Kretchmer N, Quilligan EJ, Johnson JD, eds. Prenatal and perinatal biology and medicine, vol. 1. New York: Harwood, 1987; pp. 1–33.
5. Tyndale-Biscoe H. Life of marsupials. London: Edward Arnold, 1973.
6. Susa JB, Schwartz R. Model of diabetes: fetal hyperinsulinemia and macrosomia. In: Brans YW, Kuehl TJ, eds. Nonhuman primates in perinatal research. New York: Wiley, 1988:217–230.
7. Fowden AL. The role of insulin in fetal growth. Early Hum Dev 1992;29:177–181.
8. Omori Y, Azuma K, Minei S, Hirata Y. Fetal pancreases in the NOD mouse. In: Taruri S (ed.), Insulitis and type I diabetes: lessons from the NOD mouse. Tokyo: Academic Press, 1986:251–260.
9. Eriksson UJ, Andersson A, Efendic S, et al. Diabetes in pregnancy: effect on fetal and newborn rat with particular regard to body weight, serum insulin concentration and pancreatic contents of insulin, glucagon, and somatostatin. Acta Endocrinol (Copenh) 1980;94:354–364.
10. Bevier WC, Jovanovic-Peterson L, Formby B, Peterson CM. Maternal hyperglycemia is not the only cause of macrosomia: lessons learned from the nonobese diabetic mouse. Am J Perinatol 1994;11:51–56.
11. Kramer MS. Determinates of low birth weight: methodological assessment and meta-analysis. Bull WHO 1987;65:683–737.
12. Eriksson UJ, Swenne I. Diabetes in pregnancy: fetal macrosomia, hyperinsulinism, and islet hyperplasia in the offspring of rats subjected to temporary protein-energy malnutrition early in life. Pediatr Res 1993;34:791–795.
13. Susa JB, Langer O. Diabetes and fetal growth. In: Reece EA, Coustan DR, eds. Diabetes mellitus in pregnancy. 2nd ed. New York: Churchill Livingstone, 1995:79–92.
14. Susa JB, McCormick KI, Widness JA, et al. Chronic hyperinsulinemia in the fetal rhesus monkey: effects on fetal growth and composition. Diabetes 1979;18:1058–1063.
15. Naeye RI. Infants of diabetic mothers: a quantitative morphologic study. Pediatrics 1965;35:980–988.
16. Hulquist GT, Olding LB. Endocrine pathology of infants of diabetic mothers. Acta Endocrinol Suppl (Copenh) 1981;241:1–201.
17. Susa JB, Neave C, Sehgal P, et al. Chronic hyperinsulinemia in the fetal rhesus monkey: effects of physiologic hyperinsulinemia on fetal growth and composition. Diabetes 1984;33:656–660.
18. Persson B. Insulin as a growth factor in the fetus. In: Ritzen M, ed. The biology of normal human growth. New York, Raven Press, 1981; pp. 213–227.
19. Reynolds WA, Chez RA. Observations on the tissue lipids of infants born to diabetic monkeys: lipid composition of tissue. In: Cheek DB, ed. Fetal and postnatal cellular growth. New York: Wiley, 1975; pp. 323–338.
20. Martins EA, Neave C, Susa JB, Singer DB. The effect of insulin on the size of skeletal muscle fibres in fetal rhesus monkeys. Pediatr Pathol 1986;6:377–381.
21. Naeye RL. Infants of diabetic mothers: a quantitative morphologic study. Pediatrics 1965;35:980–986.
22. Koller BH, Smithies O. Altering genes in animals by gene targeting. In: Paul WE, Fathman CG, Metzger H, eds. Annu Rev Immunol 1992;10:705–730.
23. Goodnow CC. Transgenic mice and analysis of B-cell tolerance. In: Paul WE, Fathman CG, Metzger H, eds. Annu Rev Immunol 1992;10:489–518.
24. Bennet A, Wilson DM, Liu F, et al. Levels of insulin-like growth factors I and II in human cord blood. J Clin Endocrinol Metab 1983;57:609–612.
25. Omori Y, Minei S, Shimizu M, et al. Insulin-like growth factor-I and CPR levels in the umbilical cord blood of newborns from diabetic mothers. J Tokyo Wom Med Coll 1985;55:971–978.
26. Reece EA, Wiznitzer A, Le E, Homko C, et al. The relation between human fetal growth and fetal blood levels of insulin-like growth factors I and II, their binding proteins, and receptors. Obstet Gynecol 1994;84:888–895.
27. Verhaeghe J, Van Bree R, Van Herck E, et al. C-Peptide, insulin-like growth factors I and II, and insulin-like growth factor binding protein-I in umbilical cord serum: correlation with birth weight. Am J Obstet Gynecol 1993;169:89–97.
28. Gluckman PD, Morel PCH, Ambler GR, et al. Elevating maternal insulin-like growth factor I in mice and rats alters the pattern of fetal growth by removing maternal constraint. J Endocrinol 1992;134:R1–R3.
29. Mathews LS, Hammer RE, Behringer RR, et al. Growth enhancement of transgenic mice expressing human insulin-like growth factor-I. Endocrinol 1988;123:2827–2833.
30. Baker J, Liu JP, Robertson EJ, Efstratiadis A. Role of insulin-like growth factors in embryonic and postnatal growth. Cell 1993;75:73–82.
31. DeChiara TM, Efstratiadis A, Robertson EJ. A growth deficiency phenotype in heterozygous mice carrying an insulin-like growth factor II gene disrupted by targeting. Nature 1990;345:78–80.
32. Lau MM, Stewart CE, Liu Z, et al. Loss of imprinted IGF2/cation-independent mannose 6-phosphate receptor results in fetal overgrowth and perinatal lethality. Genes Dev 1994;8:2953–2963.
33. Drop SL, Brinkman A, Kortleve DJ, et al. The evolution of insulin-like growth factor binding protein family. In: Spencer EW, ed. Modern concepts of Insulin–like growth factors. New York: Elsevier Science, 1991.
34. Spencer GS, Garssen GJ, Gerrits AR, et al. Lack of effect of exogenous insulin-like growth factor I (IGF-I) on chick embryo growth rate. Reprod Nutr Dev 1990;30:515–521.
35. Spencer GS, Decuypere E, Buyse J, Zeman M. Effect of recombinant human insulin-like growth factor-II on weight gain and body composition of broiler chickens. Poult Sci 1996;75:388–392.
36. Nathanielsz PW. Animal models in fetal medicine, vol. 1. Amsterdam: Elsevier/North Holland Biomedical Press, 1980.
37. Spencer GS, Garssen GJ, Colenbrander B, et al. Glucose, growth hormone, somatomedin, cortisol and ACTH changes in the plasma of unanaesthetised pig foetuses fol-

lowing intravenous insulin administration in utero. Acta Endocrinol (Copenh) 1983;104:240–245.
38. Garssen GJ, Spencer GS, Colenbrander B, et al. Lack of effect of chronic hyperinsulinemia on growth and body composition in the fetal pig. Biol Neonate, 1983;44:234–241.
39. Spencer GS, Hill DJ, Garssen GJ, et al. Somatomedin activity and growth hormone levels in body fluids of the fetal pig: after chronic hyperinsulinemia. J Endocrinol 1983;96:107–114.
40. Ezekwe MO, Martin RJ. The effects of maternal alloxan diabetes on body composition, liver enzymes and metabolism and serum metabolites and hormones of fetal pigs. Horm Metab Res 1980;12:136–139.
41. Kasser TR, Martin RJ, Allen CE. Effect of gestational alloxan diabetes and fasting on fetal lipogenesis and lipid deposition in pigs. Biol Neonate 1981;40:105–112.
42. Phillips RW, Panepinto LM, Will DH, Case GL. The effects of alloxan diabetes on Yucatan miniature swine and their progeny. Metabolism 1980;29:40–45.
43. Miodovnik M, Mimouni F, Berk W, Clark KE. Alloxan-induced diabetes mellitus in the pregnant ewe; metabolic and cardiovascular effects on the mother and her fetus. Am J Obstet Gynecol 1989;160:1239–1244.
44. Lips JP, Jongsama HW, Eskes TK. Alloxan-induced diabetes mellitus in pregnant sheep and chronic fetal catheterization. Lab Anim 1988;22:16–22.
45. Milley JR. The effect of chronic hyperinsulinemia on ovine fetal growth. Growth 1986;50:115–126.
46. Owens JA. Endocrine and substrate control of fetal growth. Reprod Fertil Dev 1991;3:501–517.
47. Ramsay TG, Wolverton CK, Steele NC. Alterations in IGF-I mRNA content in fetal swine tissue in response to maternal diabetes. Am J Physiol 1995;267:R1391–1396.
48. Basset NS, Oliver MH, Breier BH. The effect of maternal starvation on plasma insulin-like growth factor 1 concentrations in late gestation ovine fetuses. Pediatric Res 1990;27:401–404.
49. Oliver MH, Harding JE, Brier BH, et al. Glucose but not mixed amino acid infusion regulates plasma insulin-like growth factor-1 concentrations in fetal sheep. Pediatr Res 1993;34:62–65.
50. Lok F, Owens JA, Mundy L, et al. Insulin-like growth factor-I promotes growth selectively in fetal sheep in late gestation. Am J Physiol 1996;270:R1148–1155.
51. Susa JB, Widness JA, Hintz R, et al. Somatomedins and insulin in diabetic pregnancies: effects on fetal macrosomia in the human and rhesus monkey. J Clin Endocrinol Metab 1984;58:1099–1105.
52. Duronio V. Insulin receptor is phosphorylated in response to treatment of HepG2 cells with insulin-like growth factor 1. Biochem J 1990;270:27–32.
53. Venkatesan N, Davidson MB. Insulin-like growth factor 1 receptor in adult rat liver: characterization and in vivo regulation. Am J Physiol 1990;258:E329–337.
54. Gutierrez J, Parrizas M, Maestro MA, et al. Insulin and IGF-1 binding and tyrosine kinase activity in fish heart. J Endocrinol 1995;146:35–44.
55. Parrzas M, Maestro MA, Banos N, et al. Insulin/IGF-1 binding ratio in skeletal and cardiac muscles of vertebrates: a phylogenetic approach. Am J Physiol 1995;269:R1370–1377.
56. Olson BR, Scott DC, Wetsel WC, et al. Effects of insulin-like growth factors I and II and insulin on the immortalized hypothalamic GTI-7 cell line. Neuroendocrinology 1995;62:155–165.
57. Milazzo G, Yip CC, Maddux BA, et al. High affinity insulin binding to an atypical insulin-like growth factor-1 receptor in human breast cancer cells. J Clin Invest 1992;89:899–908.
58. Kasuya J, Paz IB, Maddux BA, et al. Characterization of human placental insulin-like growth factor receptor-1/insulin hybrid receptors by protein microsequencing and purification. Biochemistry 1993;32:13531–13536.
59. Scavo L, Shuldiner AR, Serrano J, et al. Genes encoding receptors for insulin and insulin-like growth factor 1 are expressed in *Xenopus* oocytes and embryos. Proc Natl Acad Sci USA 1991;88:6214–6218.
60. Jones CT, Clemmons DR. Insulin-like growth factors and their binding proteins: biological actions. Endocr Rev 1995;16:3–34.
61. Girard J, Ferre P. Metabolic and hormonal changes around birth. In: Jones CT, ed. The biochemical development of the fetus and neonate. New York: Elsevier Biochemical Press, 1982:517–551.
62. Shelley HJ. Glycogen reserves and their changes at birth and in anoxia. Br Med Bull 1961;17:137–143.
63. Girard J, Ferre P. Metabolic and hormonal changes around birth. In: Jones CT, ed. The biochemical development of the fetus and neonate. New York: Elsevier Biochemical Press, 1982:517–551.
64. Battaglia FC, Meschia G. An introduction to fetal physiology. Orlando, FL: Academic Press, 1986:49–99.
65. Girard JR, Ferre P, Gilbert M. Fetal metabolic response to maternal fasting in the rat. Am J Physiol 1977;232:E456–463.
66. Park CR, Exton JH. Glucagon and the metabolism of glucose. In: Lefebvre PJ, Unger RH, eds. Glucagon. Oxford: Pergamon Press, 1972:77–108.
67. Cornblath M, Reisner SH. Blood glucose in the neonate. N Engl J Med 1965;273:378–381.
68. Alexander G. Cold thermogenesis. Int Rev Physiol 1979;20:43–155.
69. Heim T. Homeothermy and its metabolic cost. In: Davis JA, Dobbing J, eds. Scientific foundations of paediatrics. London: Heinemann, 1981:91–128.
70. Jones CT. The biochemical development of the fetus and neonate. New York: Elsevier, 1982.
71. Beard RW, Nathanielsz PW. Fetal Physiology and medicine. New York: Marcel Dekker, 1984.

6
Control of Metabolism in the Normal Adult

Robert R. Wolfe

Glucose Metabolism

Glucose Production

Under normal circumstances in the adult many physiologic control mechanisms ensure that there is relatively close matching of the uptake of glucose by tissue and the appearance of glucose in the bloodstream. This matching of uptake and appearance, reflected by a relatively constant blood glucose concentration over a wide range of circumstances, is controlled by regulatory factors governing both uptake and production. Production is considered first (see Chapters 10, 17, and 32).

During periods of fasting the body relies on endogenous glucose production to replace the glucose taken up by glucose-dependent tissue. The primary organs responsible for glucose production are the liver and kidneys. Although other tissue, such as muscle, may be able to synthesize glucose-6-phosphate (G6P), the enzyme glucose-6-phosphatase (G6Pase), which is necessary to convert G6P to glucose, can be found in significant quantities only in the liver and kidney. The liver's relative contribution to total glucose production is far in excess of that of the kidney, but in certain situations (e.g., starvation) the kidney may contribute significantly. Glycogenolysis in the liver and gluconeogenesis in the liver and kidneys are the two primary processes of glucose production.

Glycogenolysis

There are two components of glucose production: glycogenolysis and gluconeogenesis. Following ingestion of a meal or during a glucose infusion, a significant portion of glucose ends up stored as glycogen in the liver by mechanisms to be discussed below. Glycogen exerts a negligible osmotic pressure and can be degraded on demand. In contrast to most tissue in which glycogen can be broken down to provide energy locally via glycolysis, the liver makes little direct use of its stored glycogen.[1] The liver consumes mostly fatty acids for energy.[2] Instead, glycogen is stored in the liver when glucose is abundant (e.g., immediately after a meal) and is released into the circulation during fasting. The exact contribution of glycogen to total glucose production is difficult to quantitate, but estimates range as high as 90% for the contribution of glycogen after an overnight fast.[3] With more prolonged fasting (e.g., 60 hours), hepatic glycogen becomes depleted and gluconeogenesis becomes the entire source of glucose production.

Glycogenolysis is under hormonal control. Hormones released in response to hypoglycemia or stress stimulate net glycogenolysis by both stimulating the rate of glycogen breakdown and inhibiting the rate of glycogen synthesis. Glucagon-stimulated glycogenolysis is one of the most sensitive and reproducible metabolic effects of hormones on any tissue.[4] Other hormones that stimulate glycogenolysis are epinephrine, norepinephrine, vasopressin, and angiotensin II.

The central nervous system (CNS) also plays a role in the regulation of glycogen metabolism. When branches of the splanchnic nerve that innervate the liver are stimulated, the activities of glycogenolytic enzymes are increased more rapidly than after the injection of pharmacological quantities of epinephrine.[5] The locus of control of glucose homeostasis within the CNS has been under investigation ever since Claude Bernard found more than 100 years ago that puncture of the fourth ventricle resulted in glucosuria. The hypothalamus is an important area of control of glucose homeostasis in the CNS. Stimulation of the ventromedial hypothalamus is accompanied by acute increases in glucose, glucagon, and epinephrine and by suppression of insulin secretion; stimulation of the lateral hypothalamus is followed by a decreasing blood glucose concentration.[5]

Gluconeogenesis

Gluconeogenesis refers to the new formation of glucose from noncarbohydrate precursors. Gluconeogenesis is a

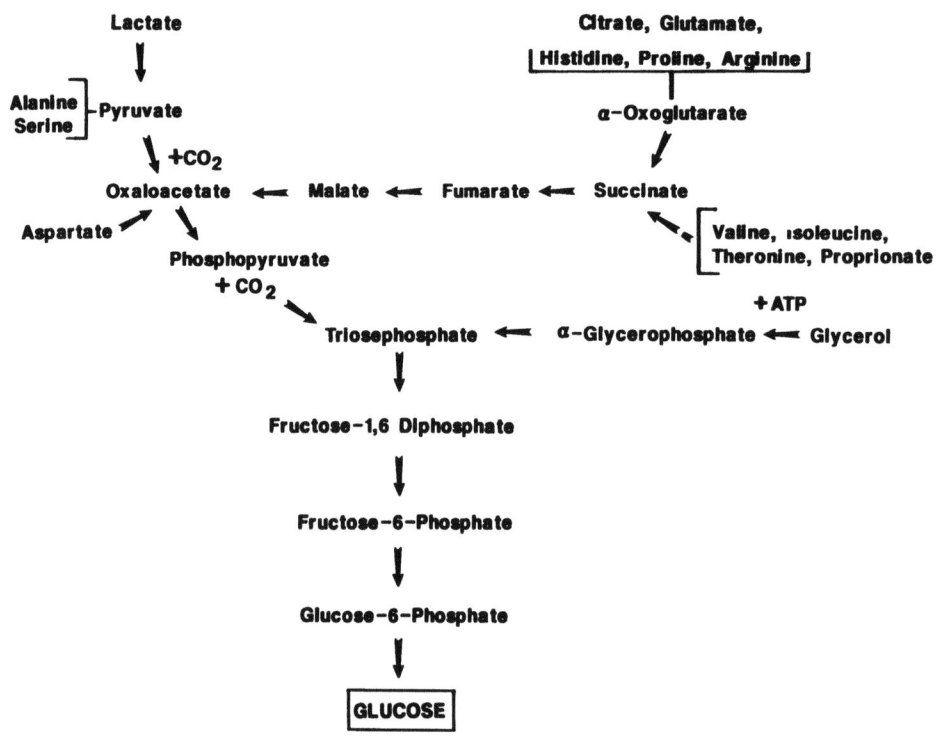

FIGURE 6.1. Pathways of gluconeogenesis from various precursors.

complex reaction sequence comprising many intermediate steps; it involves some reactions of glycolysis in reverse and some additional reactions that overcome the energy barriers, preventing direct reversal of glycolysis. The pathways of gluconeogenesis from various precursors are summarized in Figure 6.1.

Lactate is the single most important gluconeogenic precursor under most conditions. Because much of the lactate is derived from plasma glucose via glycolysis, the resynthesis of glucose from lactate is a cyclic process. This cycle was originally described by Cori[6] and is commonly called the Cori cycle. Resynthesis of glucose from lactate in the liver is the primary route of clearance of lactate produced in other tissue as a consequence of the partial metabolism of glucose. Teleologic advantage of the Cori cycle can be envisioned most easily in a circumstance in which complete oxidation of glucose and fatty acids to carbon dioxide and water is limited because of local tissue hypoxia. Under these circumstances, the Cori cycle maintains a supply of fuel (i.e., glucose) that can provide a certain amount of energy anaerobically. The "net" glucose formation does not increase via the Cori cycle, and in that sense it may be considered a waste of energy, as energy is required to resynthesize the glucose from lactate. However, this energy comes from fat oxidation in the liver, so in situations such as vigorous exercise the Cori cycle results in a transfer of energy from adipose tissue to muscle, with glucose and lactate serving as the "currency."[7] The resting rate of Cori cycle activity in the normal human has been determined to account for approximately 15% of the total glucose production during fasting,[8] but that figure is probably a significant underestimation owing to methodologic limitations.[9]

Alanine and glutamine account for 50% to 60% of the total amino acids released from muscle. In nonacidotic conditions, little glutamine is taken up by the kidney; rather, it is taken up by the mucosal cells of the small intestine and converted to alanine.[10] Alanine is the major amino acid precursor for gluconeogenesis. It is clear that far more alanine is released from muscle than is present in muscle protein. The pyruvate resulting from the glycolytic catabolism of glucose is transaminated, and the resulting alanine is released into the bloodstream and travels to the liver, where the carbons are reincorporated into glucose and the nitrogen is incorporated into urea.[11] Alanine functions in a metabolic cycle analogous to the Cori cycle in that no new "net" glucose is produced. The ammonia group required for the transamination of pyruvate is derived from amino acids that are oxidized by muscle, including the branched-chain amino acids valine, leucine, and isoleucine, as well as aspartate and glutamate. It has been proposed that the role of this process is the transfer of potentially toxic ammonia from muscle to liver in a nontoxic form.

The physiologic role of the glucose-alanine cycle depends on the circumstance. At rest after an overnight fast, alanine-derived gluconeogenesis accounts for a small percentage of the total rate of glucose production. During exercise, the glucose-alanine cycle becomes more active.[12] During starvation, gluconeogenesis from alanine becomes more important for maintaining hepatic glucose output, but in this circumstance most of the carbons in alanine released by muscle are derived from amino acids, rather than from glucose.[13] Much of this gluconeogenesis from alanine represents the "net" synthesis of glucose from non–glucose-derived precursors, rather than a cyclic process.

Glycerol release as a consequence of the peripheral breakdown of stored triglyceride is potentially an excellent gluconeogenic precursor in that it enters the gluconeogenic pathway closer to glucose than any other substrate (Figure 6.1). The extent to which glycerol is converted to glucose is primarily a function of its availability, as the conversion of glycerol to glucose is the major route by which glycerol is cleared from the blood. Glycerol contributes only about 3% of the total glucose produced during a short fast in a normal, lean subject. When there is a stimulus for the mobilization of fat, such as occurs during fasting[14] or with sepsis,[15] the contribution of glycerol can increase to as much as 20% of total glucose production.[16]

Renal Gluconeogenesis

The precise contribution of renal gluconeogenesis to total glucose production is controversial. It is agreed that under most conditions the contribution is not more than 20% of the total, and some investigators have placed the figure much lower. Prolonged starvation is the one circumstance in which the kidney assumes a significant role in gluconeogenesis.[17] Metabolic acidosis is probably the major factor increasing renal gluconeogenesis during starvation. Under acidotic conditions, glutamine uptake by the kidney is increased by an unknown mechanism. First, glutamine is hydrolyzed to glutamate and ammonia in the kidney (i.e., via the enzyme glutaminase); and then glutamate is deaminated to ammonia and α-oxoglutarate, which is converted to glucose. Glutaminase activity is inhibited by glutamate rather than formation of new glutamate from glutamine. The ammonia released in both reactions passes into the renal tubular fluid, enabling the kidney to buffer H^+ ions, and thereby permitting more acid to be secreted.

Control Mechanisms

Rate control of gluconeogenesis is exerted primarily through certain "bottlenecks" of the reaction chain: (1) availability of substrates (i.e., precursors) and the conversion of certain starting materials to the first intermediate step; (2) conversion of pyruvate to phosphoenolpyruvate (PEP); and (3) conversion of fructose-diphosphate to fructose-6-phosphate. All controlling steps occur at points where metabolic alternatives are available. At the initiating step, the alternative to the degradation of the precursor is its nondegradation. Gluconeogenesis is only one of many potential fates of pyruvate, including the tricarboxylic acid (TCA) cycle and its use for synthetic purposes. Finally, at the fructose-diphosphate step, the alternative to gluconeogenesis is the TCA cycle and eventual oxidation.

Substrate Availability

Regulation of the supply of substrates to the liver is a factor in regulating the rate of total gluconeogenesis as well as the relative contribution of a particular precursor to gluconeogenesis.[18] The entry of lactate, pyruvate, and glycerol into the liver does not appear to be under hepatic control. Amino acid uptake by the liver, on the other hand, is influenced by several hormones, but it is not clear if they directly affect transport. Once the precursor is in the liver cell, the rate of gluconeogenesis depends on the rate at which the starting material is degraded. The control mechanism might be via the activity of the initiating enzyme.

Conversion of Pyruvate to PEP

The pathway of the conversion of pyruvate to PEP is shown in Figure 6.2. There are several potential sites of control of this conversion:

1. Entry of pyruvate into the mitochondria is a potential control point that is influenced by glucagon, epinephrine, and cortisol.[19]

2. Pyruvate carboxylase is an enzyme responsible for converting pyruvate to oxaloacetate. Pyruvate carboxylase is activated by a high concentration of acetyl coenzyme A (CoA), directing pyruvate away from oxidation and toward gluconeogenesis. Many other factors may be involved in the regulation of pyruvate carboxylase.[20]

3. The pyruvate dehydrogenase enzyme competes with pyruvate carboxylase for pyruvate; consequently, regulation of pyruvate dehydrogenase is important for determining the eventual fate of pyruvate. The control of pyruvate dehydrogenase is not completely understood, but it involves a phosphorylation-dephosphorylation sequence in which phosphorylation decreases the enzyme activity with a resultant decrease in the amount of pyruvate directed to oxidation.[21]

4. Oxaloacetate in the cytosol is converted to PEP carboxykinase (PEPCK) and then to PEP. There does not appear to be a mechanism for short-term control because the enzyme does not exist in interconvertible forms with differing activities.[19] However, long-term adaptations in gluconeogenesis (e.g., starvation, diabetes) may be mediated through alterations in the rate of synthesis of PEPCK. Cortisol stimulates synthesis, as do hormones acting through the cyclic adenosine mono-

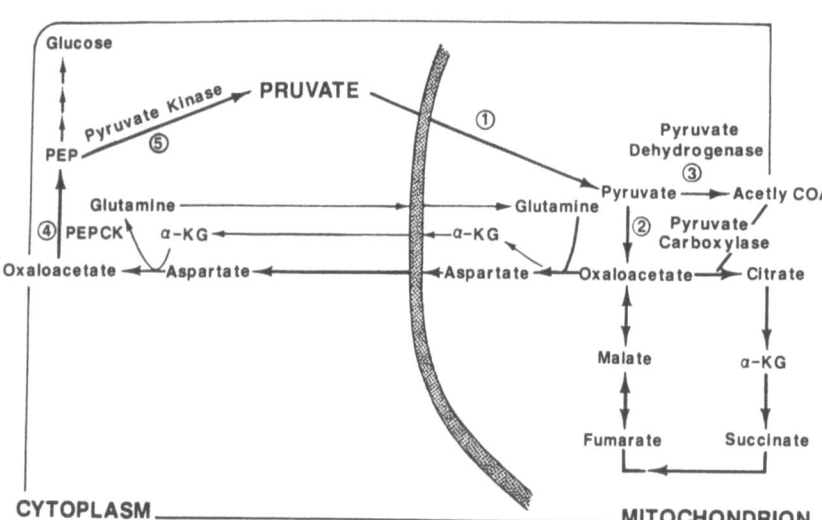

FIGURE 6.2. Potential sites of control of conversion of pyruvate to phosphoenolpyruvate (PEP).

phosphate (cAMP) "second messenger" system (e.g., glucagon, epinephrine). Activity of PEPCK is increased with fasting and experimental diabetes.[7]

5. If the liver is in the gluconeogenic mode, it would be desirable to have pyruvate kinase activity low so that any PEP formed would be directed back toward glucose instead of being reconverted to pyruvate. It is clear that a certain amount of such "futile cycling" does occur during active gluconeogenesis, but there may be some suppression of pyruvate kinase during gluconeogenesis.[22]

Conversion of Fructose Diphosphate to Fructose-6-Phosphate

The direction of the net flux between fructose diphosphate (FDP) and fructose-6-phosphate (F6P) is determined by the relative activities of phosphofructokinase (PFK) and fructose diphosphatase (FDPase). Conditions resulting in the stimulation of one enzyme tend to inhibit the other. For example, in conditions requiring a high rate of glycolysis (e.g., anoxia), PFK is stimulated by adenosine monophosphate (AMP), adenosine diphosphate (ADP), and inorganic phosphorus (Pi). On the other hand, FDPase is inhibited by AMP, and the subsequent accumulation of FDP potentiates the inhibitory action. Total inhibition of one enzyme is unlikely, so there is always a certain amount of "futile cycling."[23]

Futile Cycles

Until the 1970s it was generally thought that "glycolytic" enzymes were completely suppressed during active gluconeogenesis. It has become evident that this proposal is not valid. There are three key steps in glycolysis and gluconeogenesis where potential "futile" cycles exist, meaning that the two opposing reactions are catalyzed by separate enzymes in which adenosine triphosphate (ATP) is hydrolyzed and heat is produced in at least one of the reactions; and two reactions can be active simultaneously. The three potential futile cycles in glucose metabolism are (1) the glucose cycle (glucose → G6P → glucose); (2) the F6P cycle (F6p → FDP → F6P); and (3) the PEP cycle (pyruvate → PEP → pyruvate).[24] The glucose cycle and the F6P cycle are catalyzed by a pair of irreversible enzymes, but the PEP cycle is a complex sequence that differs according to the gluconeogenic precursor. Under normal circumstances in the human, about 25% to 30% of total flux from G6P to glucose is cycled back to G6P.[25] The fructose cycle is less active, although it involves 10% to 15% of total flux in some individuals.[25,26] The PEP cycle is likely the most active of the substrate cycles in glucose metabolism, as 35% of PEP derived from oxaloacetate is recycled to pyruvate/lactate.[27] The rate of the glucose cycle is directly affected by hormones, with glucagon being the predominant stimulator of cycling and insulin its primary antagonist.[28] Glucose cycling is elevated in a number of pathologic conditions (e.g., severe burns,[29] type II diabetes,[30] and acromegaly[31]). In all cases, the rate of glucose cycling increases directly in proportion to the total rate of flux of glucose, which suggests that glucose cycling is not under direct hormonal control but rather is a passive consequence of the total rate of glucose production. The PEP cycle, on the other hand, may serve a physiologic function. For example, in short-term (e.g., 3-day) fasting, the efficiency of the gluconeogenic process is enhanced by a significant decrease from 35% to 15% in the recycling of PEP back to pyruvate/lactate.[27] This decrease in recycling amplifies the extent to which glucose output from the liver is increased when gluconeogenesis is the only source of glucose.

Physiologic Control of Glucose Production

Although all of the specific factors cited above can potentially affect the rate of glucose production, in normal humans the rate of glucose production is primarily under the control of only a few factors. Glucagon is the predominant stimulator of glucose production. For example, in one study in dogs given somatostatin along with intraportal replacement of insulin to create a selective lack of glucagon, and with glucose infused to maintain euglycemia, glucose production fell almost 70%.[32] The same sort of response can be seen in the human,[33] even when glucagon is chronically elevated, as in the case of severe injury.[34] In the dog the basal glucagon effect entirely involves stimulation of glycogenolysis.[35] Glucagon can stimulate gluconeogenesis in vivo,[35] but precise quantitation of this action is made difficult because of problems quantitating gluconeogenesis.

Insulin is the primary inhibitor of glucose production. Selective reduction in the normal basal insulin concentration causes prompt doubling of glucose production.[36] Hyperinsulinemia inhibits both glycogenolysis and gluconeogenesis.[3] The suppressive effect of insulin on glucose production is somewhat difficult to isolate from the direct effect of glucose, as glucose infusion in the absence of a change in insulin concentration inhibits glucose production,[37] provided a basal concentration of insulin is available.[38] In any circumstance in which the insulin concentration is elevated, glucose must be infused to avoid hypoglycemia, thereby complicating interpretation of the effect of insulin.

The rate of delivery of gluconeogenic precursors to the liver seems to play a secondary role in controlling the amount of total glucose production. That is, the amount of precursor available and glucose production are well matched, such that an acute reduction in the delivery of alanine and lactate to the liver causes a decrease in glucose production.[18] On the other hand, infusion of extra gluconeogenic precursors (e.g., alanine and glycerol) fails to stimulate glucose production, even after 3 days of fasting when 100% of glucose production is derived from gluconeogenesis.[18] Thus it seems that, whereas an adequate amount of gluconeogenic precursors is necessary to satisfy the requirements for substrates set by the rate of gluconeogenic reactions as governed by such other factors as glucagon and insulin, total glucose production cannot be "driven" by high rates of delivery of precursors.

Glucose Uptake

Glucose taken up by cells is either stored as glycogen or metabolized. If metabolized, the predominant route is glycolysis. The pyruvate produced by glycolysis can then be converted to lactate and released into the blood, or it can be decarboxylated and then enter the TCA cycle for complete oxidation. The hexose monophosphate shunt is an alternative metabolic pathway of lesser importance.

Glycolysis

Glycolysis involves the anaerobic breakdown of glucose to pyruvate and lactate and occurs in the cytosol of all tissue. With the exception of the end products and the rate at which glycolysis proceeds, the reaction in glycolysis is the same regardless of whether oxygen is present. When oxygen is not available, nicotinamide adenine dinucleotide, reduced (NADH), which is formed during glycolysis, cannot readily be oxidized by the respiratory chain. In this case, the oxidation of NADH proceeds by the lactate dehydrogenase (LDH) reaction, catalyzing the conversion of pyruvate to lactate, thereby allowing glycolysis to proceed.

There are numerous potential control points of glycolysis. The first is the phosphorylation of glucose to form G6P. This reaction is catalyzed by the enzyme hexokinase. Hexokinase has a high affinity for glucose, thereby enabling cells to take up glucose and immediately convert it to G6P even when plasma glucose concentration is low. In addition to hexokinase, the liver possesses a second enzyme, called glucokinase, that catalyzes the conversion of glucose to G6P. The phosphorylation of glucose is important because it is essentially an irreversible reaction, thus trapping the glucose inside the cell unless the specific enzyme G6Pase necessary to convert G6P to glucose is present. G6P is present in significant quantities only in the liver; in other tissues, once the glucose is taken up from plasma it is rapidly converted to G6P and must be either metabolized for energy or stored. Thus, in addition to being the first intermediate in the pathway of glucolysis, G6P is important because it is at a key point in other metabolic pathways as well, including the hexose monophosphate shunt, glycogen synthesis, and gluconeogenesis.

The next potential control point of glycolysis is the conversion of fructose-6-phosphate to fructose-1,6-diphosphate, which is catalyzed by PFK. Phosphofructokinase is an inducible enzyme whose activity is considered to be of prime importance in the regulation of glycolysis. This step is followed by the oxidation reaction, whereby glyceraldehyde 3-(P) forms 1,3-diphosphoglycerate via glyceraldehyde 3-phosphate dehydrogenase. This reaction is nicotinamide adenine dinucleotide (NAD)-dependent, meaning that NAD^+ availability at this step of glycolysis is essential for the reaction to continue.

The last regulated step of glycolysis is the conversion of phosphoenolpyruvate (PEP) plus ADP to pyruvate plus ATP. This step is catalyzed by the enzyme pyruvate kinase. At this point in glycolysis, 2 "net" mol of ATP have been generated for 1 mol of glucose oxidized. As stated above, it is not clear that pyruvate kinase is actively regulated in relation to the rate of the reaction in the opposite direction.

Once pyruvate is formed, the redox state of the tissue determines whether the pyruvate is reduced to lactate by LDH or enters the TCA cycle. Although the state of oxygenation of the tissues is clearly an important issue in determining the fate of pyruvate, other factors may play a role. For example, a high rate of glycolysis, regardless of the state of oxygenation, results in accelerated lactate release owing to a limitation in the activity of pyruvate dehydrogenase, which is responsible for the decarboxylation of pyruvate and formation of acetyl CoA. However, in this case pyruvate release also increases, leaving the lactate/pyruvate ratio relatively constant.

Pyruvate Oxidation

If adequate NAD^+ is available when pyruvate is formed, pyruvate enters the TCA cycle. To enter the TCA cycle, pyruvate must first be transported into the mitochondria and converted to acetyl CoA. This process is catalyzed by several enzymes collectively referred to as the pyruvate dehydrogenase complex. Once acetyl CoA is formed, it can enter the TCA cycle, whereupon it is oxidized. Complete oxidation of 1 mol of glucose yields 38 mol of ATP, which represents about one-half the energy liberated in the process. The remainder of the energy is released as heat. The considerable discrepancy between the amount of energy obtained from the complete aerobic oxidation of glucose and the amount obtained from the anaerobic glycolysis emphasizes the importance of the availability of oxygen.

Hexose Monophosphate Shunt (Pentose Phosphate Pathway)

The hexose monophosphate shunt, an additional pathway for glucose oxidation, occurs in certain tissue. Because a major function of the shunt is the provision of nicotinamide adenine dinucleotide phosphate, reduced (NADPH), which is required for such processes as fatty acid and steroid synthesis, it is not surprising to find the monophosphate shunt occurring in liver and adipose tissue.

Glycogen Deposition

Carbohydrate is stored in the cell in the form of glycogen. It exerts negligible osmotic pressure and can be degraded on demand for energy, or, in the case of the liver, for release of glucose into the bloodstream.

After ingestion of a high-carbohydrate meal or glucose infusion, a significant portion of the absorbed glucose ends up in the liver. However, much of this glycogen is not derived from glucose directly cleared by the liver. Rather, most ingested or infused glucose is taken up peripherally[39] and partially metabolized to lactate[40] or alanine;[41] it is then transported back to the liver, where it is taken up and converted to glycogen.[42] In peripheral tissues, on the other hand, glucose is directly converted to glycogen. It seems likely that the stimulation of glycogen deposition results from activation of the enzyme glycogen synthase, apparently in direct response to the plasma glucose concentration.[1,43]

It is not clear why, when glycogen synthase activity is high in the liver, thereby allowing a high percentage of G6P produced via gluconeogenesis to go to glycogen, there is not a high rate of hepatic glucose uptake and direct glycogen synthesis. Evidence indicates that the gradient of glucose concentration between the portal vein and hepatic artery plays a role in determining the extent of hepatic uptake of glucose, meaning that a greater percentage of ingested carbohydrate is directly deposited in the liver as glycogen than if the same amount of glucose is infused intravenously.[44]

Regulation of Glucose Utilization

After a high-carbohydrate meal, glucose is the major fuel of the body; after several hours of fasting, only about 25% of total CO_2 production is from glucose oxidation.[45] Certain tissues, most notably the brain and erythrocytes, depend on glucose for energy and have a relatively constant rate of glucose uptake under most conditions. An exception is with prolonged starvation, during which the brain adapts to the use of ketone bodies for energy. However, this situation is unusual and is not relevant to the day-to-day regulation of glucose utilization when nutrition is available. Therefore, even though the brain and erythrocytes may account for more than 50% of glucose uptake in the postabsorptive state, they probably do not play a significant role in the fluctuations in the rate of glucose oxidation observed in different physiologic states.

The liver plays an important role in the disposition of a glucose load.[46] Because much of this glucose uptake is converted to glycogen rather than CO_2, however, the liver is not a site where the rate of glucose oxidation varies greatly.

Muscle mass, on the other hand, exerts a profound influence on the overall rate of glucose utilization. Because muscle constitutes approximately 40% of the body mass, any change in the rate of glucose uptake by muscle significantly affects the overall rate of glucose uptake. In the postabsorptive human at rest, it is debatable if the muscle takes up any glucose at all;[47] but with hyperglycemia or during exercise, the rate of glucose utilization by the muscle can increase severalfold.

Muscle Uptake of Glucose

Glucose is rapidly phosphorylated to G6P once inside the cell, so the intracellular concentration of glucose is lower than the extracellular concentration, and movement of glucose into the cell occurs down its concentration gradient. Glucose diffusion is facilitated by a carrier-transport system that, when combined with glucose, renders the glucose, sufficiently lipid-soluble to move through the cell membrane. No energy is expanded in this process, so it is considered a passive, as opposed to active, transport mechanism. The rate of glucose uptake increases in muscle as the blood concentration of glucose increases; for any blood concentration of glucose, insulin increases the ability of the muscle cell to take up glucose. Insulin works on the surface of the cell by binding to specific receptors, which then initiate its action.[48] The maximal metabolic effect of insulin can apparently be elicited when only 2% of the insulin receptors are filled.[49]

Muscle glucose uptake and utilization are increased significantly during exercise,[50] and bed rest causes a decreased ability of muscles to clear glucose.[51] Muscle glucose uptake during exercise is enhanced by an increased insensitivity to the action of insulin, but is not dependent on insulin to occur.[50]

It is generally accepted that insulin regulates muscle glucose utilization by controlling the rate of glucose entry into the cells. It is possible that there is an additional mechanism whereby glucose uptake is controlled in which insulin plays a secondary role. This mechanism was originally described as the glucose–fatty acid cycle[52] and later updated and renamed the glucose-ketone-fatty acid cycle.[53] The cornerstone of the theory is that free fatty acids (FFAs) inhibit glucose utilization. Because insulin inhibits lipolysis and reduces the circulatory levels of FFAs in the plasma, a low concentration of insulin (e.g., during fasting) releases that inhibition and results in a high FFA concentration. The high FFA concentration inhibits glucose utilization, and because the rate of uptake of glucose is reduced, a given blood concentration of glucose can be maintained at a reduced rate of glucose production. The further decrease in glucose production that occurs with prolonged fasting is ascribed to the ketosis that develops. The ketones are proposed to compete with glucose as energy substrates in the brain, further reducing the need for glucose production. This theory focuses on peripheral mechanisms influencing the rate of glucose production secondarily as a consequence of changes in plasma glucose concentration.

In vitro evidence regarding the so-called glucose-FFA cycle is controversial. The net result of many studies suggest that an inhibitory effect of FFAs on glucose oxidation can be demonstrated in certain tissues (e.g., heart and diaphragm),[53] but not in skeletal muscle.[54] In vivo the effect of FFAs on glucose clearance and oxidation has been even more difficult to demonstrate convincingly. During a constant glucose infusion at a high enough rate that the body relies entirely on glucose as an energy substrate [i.e., respiratory quotient (RQ) = 1], the addition of fatty acids, caused by Intralipid plus heparin, has no effect on glucose oxidation.[55] On the other hand, under some circumstances a high FFA concentration may impair the stimulatory action of insulin on glucose uptake.[56] However, even in such a circumstance, the effect of FFAs appears not to involve direct inhibition of glucose oxidation, because the percentage of glucose uptake oxidized remained constant.[56] Rather, an effect of FFAs on glucose transport is likely. This effect can be demonstrated only after FFA concentration has been elevated for several hours.[57] On the other side of the cycle, whereas there is little doubt that insulin inhibits lipolysis, the increase in lipolysis in short-term fasting is not prevented by the continuous infusion of enough glucose to maintain euglycemia.[58] At the least, a drop in insulin concentration is not the sole mechanism whereby lipolysis is stimulated.

Physiologic Response to Infused Glucose

Glucose concentration is maintained by two mechanisms: regulation of production and regulation of uptake. During glucose infusion, glucose production is inhibited by an amount essentially equal to the infusion rate, up to the point at which the rate of glucose infusion exceeds the rate of endogenous production.[45] At this point, the rate of glucose uptake increases, as the total amount of glucose entering the blood increases. Initially, stimulation of glucose uptake is mediated in great part by the insulin response, which results from the increase in plasma glucose concentration. However, as time proceeds, an adaptation occurs whereby the ability of tissues to clear glucose increases.[59] As adaptation becomes evident, the plasma glucose and insulin concentrations decrease.[59] The mechanism responsible for this adaptation is not clear, although it may involve an increased ability to oxidize glucose. Figure 6.3 shows the response to a 6-day glucose infusion in unstressed patients.[59] After 2 days of glucose infusion, the rate of glucose oxidation was higher than after 2 hours, with the result that the plasma glucose concentration was lower. The active role of oxidation in the adaptation of uptake is made less clear, however, when it is considered that subsequent increases in the rate of glucose infusion cause little further increase in glucose oxidation. But the high rate of glucose clearance seen after 2 days at the lower infusion rate was still evident during the higher infusion rate.

The data presented in Figure 6.3 are striking in terms of the amount of infused glucose that is not directly oxidized, despite the fact that the glucose infusion had proceeded long enough to fill the glycogen stores. The fate of

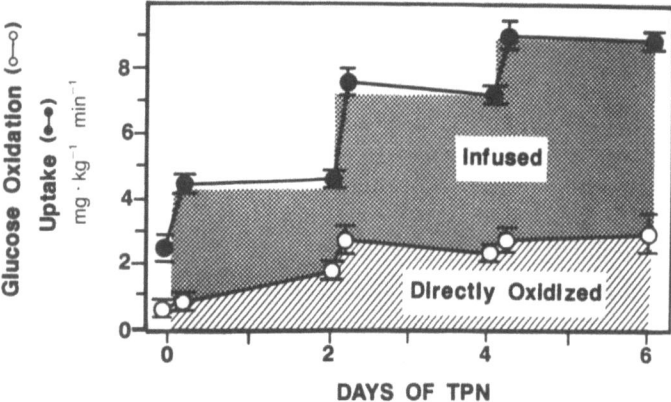

FIGURE 6.3. Glucose oxidation during continuous glucose infusion in moderately stressed patients receiving total parenteral nutrition (TPN). (Adapted from Wolfe et al.[59])

the nonoxidized glucose shown in Figure 6.3 is predominantly hepatic triglyceride synthesis, which is subsequently transported, via very low density lipoproteins (VLDLs) to the periphery for storage. Adding extra insulin during such a constant infusion of glucose lowers the plasma glucose concentration, owing to stimulation of glucose clearance, but does not affect the rate of glucose oxidization.[45]

Lipids in Energy Metabolism

In the normal adult lipids constitute more than 80% of the stored fuel reserve. Furthermore, fat stores, along with small carbohydrate stores, can be almost completely depleted without detriment to the individual. Conversely, the use of protein reserves is limited, as even moderate depletion can adversely affect an organism exposed to stress.[60] Consequently, when an individual must rely on endogenous fuel supplies for the provision of energy, lipids are the physiologically most desirable source of that energy. Most tissues, including heart and skeletal muscle, can readily use fatty acids as substrates for energy metabolism.[61,62] Although the brain cannot directly use fatty acids because of the blood-brain barrier, the use of fatty acids by other tissue preserves the limited carbohydrate stores for use by nervous tissue. Additionally, the brain can use ketone bodies (e.g., β-hydroxybutyrate and acetoacetate) resulting from fatty acid oxidation in the liver. In the postabsorptive state in man, oxidation of fat may supply approximately 50% to 60% of the energy. If food deprivation continues, adaptive mechanisms occur whereby most energy is derived from the metabolism of fat, with body nitrogen being spared as a consequence.[4] The extent to which starvation can be tolerated appears to be related to the ability to rely on fat as an energy source.

The primary lipid fuel reserve is stored in adipose tissue triglyceride, although some fat droplets are present in cells of other tissues (e.g., muscle). Stored triglyceride is derived principally from dietary fat or is synthesized from dietary carbohydrate and, to a lesser extent, dietary protein (see Chapters 12, 19 and 36).[63]

Intestinal Fat Absorption

Ingested fat is hydrolyzed in the gut, with monoglycerides and fatty acids being the main products. These products enter the epithelial cells that line the small intestines, after which most of the fatty acids are synthesized into triglycerides using the monoglycerides as the backbone. The triglycerides are subsequently "packaged" into chylomicrons, which in turn enter the circulation via the intestinal lymphatic system. Approximately 90% of absorbed fat enters the circulation as chylomicrons, with the rest transported as albumin-bound FFAs.

Hepatic Triglyceride Synthesis

In addition to the intestinal origin of triglycerides, the liver synthesizes it from dietary carbohydrates and circulating FFAs. In vitro studies have indicated that fatty acids can be synthesized from certain amino acids, but the in vivo significance of these pathways has yet to be established.[63] Synthesis of triglycerides from carbohydrates appears to be under both "coarse" (i.e., long-term) control and "fine" (i.e., short-term) control.[64] Long-term control involves changes in enzyme activity and is responsible for nutritional adaptations that produce an increased capacity of the liver to synthesize triglycerides when the diet is high in carbohydrates.[65] Fine control is exerted via modulation of enzyme activity by factors such as substrate supply and hormonal regulation. The role of cAMP as an inhibitor of lipogenesis seems particularly important in this regard.[64] Whatever the hepatic triglyceride precursor, these fats are normally packaged into VLDLs and are secreted into the blood for transport to extrahepatic tissues.

Until recently, the rate of hepatic fatty acid synthesis was unknown. However, a new stable isotope methodology called mass isotopomer distribution analysis has made possible the quantitation of the contribution of newly synthesized fatty acids to hepatic VLDL output.[66] Under normal dietary conditions, the rate of hepatic fatty acid synthesis is essentially negligible.[66] Even when 4 days of a hyperenergetic carbohydrate diet (i.e., ≈ 2.5 times energy expenditure) was given to human volunteers, newly synthesized fatty acids contributed only a small fraction of the fatty acids in VLDL.[65] In fact, in that hypercaloric circumstance the adipose tissue is likely to be the main site of de novo lipogenesis.[67]

Triglyceride of intestinal chylomicrons and hepatic VLDLs origin are transported in the blood to extrahepatic tissues. Prior to leaving the vascular system, triglyceride must be hydrolyzed to fatty acids and glycerol.

Clearance of Lipid from Blood by Adipose Tissue

The fate of lipoprotein triglyceride depends primarily on two factors: (1) the presence of lipoprotein lipase (LPL) on the luminal surface of capillary endothelial cells, which is responsible for initiating triglyceride hydrolysis;[68] and (2) blood flow to tissues capable of catabolizing triglyceride. The latter is probably important only in situations in which cardiac output or blood flow to selected tissues is greatly compromised. The major tissue beds responsible for triglyceride fatty acid uptake are adipose tissue, myocardium, and skeletal muscle.[69] During the absorptive state of digestion, most circulating triglyceride fatty acids are taken up by adipocytes; and along with α-glycerophosphate, originating primarily from plasma glucose, they are converted to triglycerides for storage within the fat cell. Insulin plays an important role in this process. Adipose tissue is an insulin-sensitive tissue with regard to glucose transport. Insulin stimulates glucose uptake, thereby promoting the α-glycerophosphate synthesis necessary for fat synthesis. Insulin increases LPL activity in adipose tissue, promoting the catabolism of intravascular triglycerides so its fatty acids can enter fat cells.[70]

Mobilization of Endogenous Fat as an Energy Source

A cell's energy needs from fat are derived primarily from fatty acids. Fatty acids are transported in the blood in two forms: albumin-bound FFAs and triglycerides. Although the quantitative contribution of the albumin-bound FFAs to energy metabolism is more important, once triglyceride fatty acids are released by the action of LPL the two sources become indistinguishable from one another. However, the contribution of fatty acids from circulating triglycerides to energy metabolism constitutes less than 5% of the total from plasma FFAs.[71] Mobilization of endogenous fat as an energy source primarily involves the mechanisms whereby plasma FFAs are made available for tissue oxidation.

When the energy intake of an individual falls below the energy provided by absorbed food, the net storage of fat is reversed and fatty acids are mobilized. The initiating step in the mobilization of FFAs is lipolysis, or the breakdown of stored triglyceride to its component fatty acids and glycerol. This step is catalyzed by hormone-sensitive lipase, which is mediated by cAMP.[72] In this regard, catecholamines are the primary stimulators of lipolysis.[28] Furthermore, the lipolytic effect of epinephrine is elicited at a lower concentration than is the effect of epinephrine on glucose concentration.[73] A number of hormones [e.g., glucagon and adrenocorticotropic hormone (ACTH)], have been shown to stimulate lipolysis in vitro,[64] but their in vivo effect is minimal.[28] In contrast to the tachyphylaxis to chronic hormone stimulation often seen with other processes, chronic adrenergic stimulation seems to enhance responsiveness to further adrenergic stimulation. In response to short-term fasting, for example, increased adrenergic activity plays an important role in stimulating lipolysis.[74] Coincidentally, the lipolytic responsiveness to epinephrine infusion is amplified.[75] Similarly, in severely injured children, lipolysis is stimulated by chronically elevated adrenergic activity, and lipolytic responsiveness to acute epinephrine infusion is amplified.[76]

Countering the stimulatory effect of catecholamines, insulin is probably the most important inhibitor of lipolysis.[28] Lipolysis is regulated to cause fatty acid availability to be inversely related to the plasma glucose concentration, thereby explaining the general reciprocal relation between glucose and fatty acid oxidation. In addition, adenosine is a potent inhibitor of lipolysis, but it does not seem to be a primary regulator in terms of enabling a matching between fatty acid requirements and availability.[77]

Although these various factors cited above can affect the rate of lipolysis, it may be overstating their role to refer to them as "regulators" of lipolysis. This is because, in contrast to the tightly regulated glucose system, the release of FFAs into the plasma is not regulated in relation to substrate requirements. Further, the plasma FFA concentration is unregulated, and may vary over a fivefold range or more, because the factors that control lipolysis are not responsive to changes in FFA availability. Thus, epinephrine is the most important stimulator of lipolysis, but its release is unrelated to FFA concentration. Rather, it is responsive to declines in blood glucose concentration and blood pressure. Similarly, insulin is the most potent inhibitor of lipolysis, but its release is controlled by the blood glucose concentration. Insulin release is not affected by FFA concentration. Adenosine is also a potent inhibitor of lipolysis, yet adenosine concentration is highest when the need for FFA as energy substrates would seemingly be the highest. Thus, adenosine concentration increases during periods of high turnover of ATP, such as during exercise. It is during periods of high ATP utilization that one would anticipate that FFA release would be stimulated to provide more substrate for energy metabolism, yet it is precisely in this circumstance that adenosine inhibits lipolysis.[77]

Whereas it is clear that lipolysis is not regulated in a manner that would likely result in a good matching between the requirement for fatty acids as energy substrates and the availability of plasma FFA, fat oxidation is rarely limited by the availability of plasma FFA. This is because the fatty acids are released as a consequence of lipolysis at a rate well in excess of the rate of fatty acid oxidation.[74] The extra fatty acids released by lipolysis have two fates: they can be recycled directly back into triglycerides within the adipose tissue, or they can be released into the plasma, cleared, and subsequently reesterified within the liver. The extent of either route of recycling of fatty acids back into triglycerides is under hormonal control[28] and varies in a variety of clinical circumstances.[28,76]

Under normal conditions, about 70% of released fatty acids are reesterified, with most recycling occurring via the "extracellular" route involving the FFAs being transported via the plasma to the liver.[78] There are far more plasma fatty acids potentially available than are required for oxidation. When there is an acute stimulus for fatty acid oxidation, in addition to lipolysis increasing, the percent of fatty acids reesterified decreases, thereby making a greater amount of fatty acids available than would be the case if the initial rate of lipolysis had not considerably exceeded the requirement for oxidation. The importance of this mechanism is best illustrated by the response to exercise.[78] At the start of aerobic exercise, the rate of lipolysis responds quickly but incompletely. Fatty acid oxidation nonetheless increases severalfold, because the percentage of released fatty acids that are reesterified falls from the resting value of 70% to about 25%. The extra fatty acids made available for oxidation by this mechanism are about equal to the amount of extra fatty acids resulting from the stimulation of lipolysis.[78] As soon as exercise stops, as much as 90% of released fatty acids are reesterified, thereby resulting in a rapid fall in plasma FFA concentration, despite the maintenance of an accelerated rate of lipolysis for several hours after exercise.[78]

Under most circumstances, almost all fatty acids available for oxidation come from adipose tissue. However, during strenuous exercise there is breakdown of triglycerides stored within the muscle. The fatty acids can be directly metabolized within the muscle, whereas the glycerol will be released into the blood. Thus, the ratio of fatty acids released into the blood/glycerol release can approach 1:1 during exercise,[78] whereas the ratio is close to 3:1 in most circumstances. Because of this direct oxidation of fatty acids released by intramuscular lipolysis that never enter the circulation, the percent of uptake of plasma FFA that is oxidized increases during exercise.

Regulation of FFA Oxidation

With the exception of red blood cells, which lack mitochondria, and the brain, which cannot readily clear FFAs from plasma owing to the blood-brain barrier, all tissue utilizes FFAs as an important energy fuel.[79] FFAs are normally the major source of energy for resting muscle. Plasma FFAs also serve as the predominant energy substrate in the heart.

The first step in the catabolism of fatty acids is the reaction whereby the acetyl CoA of the fatty acid is formed. This reaction is catalyzed by the acetyl CoA synthase for the specific fatty acid. Once the acetyl CoA is formed, it must be transferred to the mitochondria for subsequent oxidation. This process can be accomplished only in the presence of carnitine via an enzyme system called carnitine acyl transferase (CAT).[80] Once inside the mitochondria, fatty acid oxidation occurs by a process of β-oxidation in which 2-carbon units are removed as acetyl CoA from the carboxyl end of the fatty acids. Enzyme activities indicate that β-oxidation can keep pace with the acetyl CoA production.[61] Studies in the rat heart indicate that the availability of flavin adenine dinucleotide (FAD^+) and NAD^+ is important in regulating fatty acetyl CoA oxidation. As a cell becomes more oxidized, flux through the oxidative pathway increases and the acetyl CoA concentration declines.[81] Once the acetyl CoA is produced, oxidation can be completed only by entry into the TCA cycle. Ultimately, then, the rate of fatty acid oxidation is controlled by TCA cycle activity, which is normally regulated by H^+ flux through the electron transport pathway. In general, a decrease in the ATP/(ADP + Pi) ratio in the cytosol stimulates TCA cycle activity because it brings about a decrease in the $NADH/NAD^+$ ratio in the mitochondria. A decrease in the NADH/NAD ratio results in acceleration of TCA cycle activity.[82]

The physiologic regulation of fatty acid oxidation is intertwined with the regulation of glucose oxidation, because under almost all circumstances the sum of glucose and fatty acid oxidation is equal to the total energy derived from nonprotein energy sources. The discussion of the regulation of the rates of appearance in plasma of glucose and fatty acids leads to the conclusion that glucose metabolism is regulated primarily by changes in appearance, whereas fat metabolism is regulated primarily by changes in its rate of oxidation. Expressed differently, availability of glucose largely determines the rate of glucose oxidation, but the availability of FFA does not determine the rate of fat oxidation. The logical extrapolation from this perspective is that fatty acid oxidation is regulated by the rate of intracellular metabolism of glucose. However, this perspective is in contrast to the traditional view of the normal interaction between glucose and fatty acids.

The notion that the intracellular metabolism of glucose controls substrate metabolism is diametrically opposed to certain aspects of the traditional view of glucose–fatty acid interactions was first expressed by Randle et al.[52] in 1963. Randle et al. termed their hypothesis the "glucose–fatty acid cycle." The two essential features of the glucose–fatty acid cycle cited in their seminal paper were (1) the limitation on glucose metabolism imposed by the release of fatty acids from muscle or adipose-tissue glycerides, and (2) the inhibition of release of fatty acids by uptake of glucose. In subsequent years, the cycle was expanded to include hypothesized mechanisms.[83] Thus, the inhibitory effects of FFA on glucose oxidation have been proposed to be mediated by inhibition of pyruvate dehydrogenase (PDH), PFK, and hexokinase (HK). The inhibition of PDH has been proposed to be mediated by an increased ratio of acetyl CoA/CoA, the inhibition of PFK has been proposed to be mediated by an increase in citrate, and HK has been proposed to be mediated by glucose-6-phosphate.[83]

The glucose–fatty acid cycle provides a potential explanation for substrate interactions in a variety of circumstances. For example, a high plasma FFA concentration occurs in many insulin-resistant states, such as obesity, type II diabetes, or severe trauma and sepsis. The glucose–fatty acid cycle potentially provides a link between high FFA concentration and insulin resistance, since the high FFA concentration should inhibit glucose oxidation and thus uptake by virtue of increased FFA oxidation.

The original glucose–fatty acid cycle was based entirely on in vitro results from experiments examining rat heart and diaphragm muscle metabolism.[52] Several in vitro studies have been done since that time, with conflicting results. Whereas some studies have shown an inhibitory effect of FFA on glucose oxidation in rat skeletal muscle,[84] others have found no such effect.[85,86] Maizels et al.[87] proposed that a fatty acid effect on glucose oxidation may only occur in red muscle under some circumstances, such as when the rate of glycolysis is increased. Thus, it appears that under certain circumstances, the glucose–fatty acid cycle functions in specific tissue. However, it is not clear how these in vitro results relate to the situation in vivo.

Direct support for the proposed mechanisms of control of glucose metabolism by FFA in the human subject is lacking. In studies in which FFA concentration has been altered, there has not been a corresponding change observed in either muscle citrate or glucose-6-phosphate concentrations.[85–90] Nonetheless, the glucose–fatty acid cycle has received widespread acceptance as an explanation for substrate interactions in human subjects.[91–93] The reason for this, in part, is the reliance on the euglycemic-hyperinsulinemic clamp procedure to assess the glucose–fatty acid cycle in human subjects. With this procedure, the effect of FFA on glucose oxidation has been assessed in human subjects by acutely elevating the plasma FFA concentration by the infusion of a lipid emulsion plus heparin in the setting of euglycemia-hyperinsulinemia. In this experimental setting, it has generally, but not always, been found that the amount of glucose infusion necessary to maintain euglycemia at any particular insulin concentration is less when FFA concentration is high.[93] Further, in this circumstance glucose oxidation also generally falls,[93] leading to the conclusion that fatty acids inhibit glucose oxidation, i.e., a "validation" of a central component of the glucose–fatty acid cycle.

However, these data can be interpreted differently. There is little doubt that decreased uptake of glucose at any concentration of insulin with an increasing FFA concentration indicates an inhibitory effect of FFA on glucose transport. This is consistent with the observation of an inhibitory effect of FFA on insulin-mediated glucose transport in vitro in soleus muscle.[94] On the other hand, in the same study there was no effect of FFA concentrations on basal glucose transport in either the soleus or epitrochearis muscle, and FFA did not affect insulin-mediated glucose transport in the epitrochearis muscle.[94] Further, FFA actually stimulated glucose uptake in adipose tissue.[94] Regardless of whether or not there is an in vivo effect of FFA on glucose transport at the whole-body level, this is not part of the glucose–fatty acid cycle. The glucose–fatty acid cycle proposes that the inhibitory effect of FFA is exerted intracellularly on oxidation. This distinction is significant, because if the FFA effect is on transport, then a higher concentration of glucose will overcome this limitation and enable a normal rate of glucose oxidation. Thus, there is no evidence that there is any impairment of glucose oxidation by FFA once glucose is in the cell. For example, the data from a representative experiment in which high FFA concentration inhibited glucose uptake during the clamp procedure is summarized in Table 6.1.[93] In this study, glucose uptake and oxidation were both reduced when the FFA concentration was high. However, the percent of glucose uptake oxidized, a parameter not expressed by the investigators, showed no indication of impairment at higher FFA concentrations. To consider this point in simplistic terms, if there isn't any glucose in the cell, it can't be oxidized. If glucose uptake is reduced, glucose oxidation will be reduced simply because there is less glucose available. These results provide no support for an inhibitory effect of FFA on glucose oxidation, and thus do not support the notion that impaired glucose uptake is the result of an intracellular inhibition of glucose oxidation. Nonetheless, this and similar studies, have repeatedly been cited as validating the traditional glucose–fatty acid cycle.[88]

The failure to demonstrate that FFA inhibits glucose uptake by inhibiting glucose oxidation is not surprising when it is considered that there are no studies in the human demonstrating a role of glucose oxidation in con-

TABLE 6.1. Effect of increasing FFA concentration on glucose uptake and oxidation in normal volunteers.

Subjects (N)	Insulin concentration ($\mu U \cdot ml^{-1}$)	FFA concentration ($\mu mol \cdot L^{-1}$)	Glucose uptake ($mg \cdot kg^{-1} min^{-1}$)	Glucose oxidation ($mg \cdot kg^{-1} min^{-1}$)	% Glucose uptake oxidized
9	62 ± 4	161 ± 5	5.9 ± 0.4	2.4 ± 0.1	40
6	62 ± 2	342 ± 13†	4.5 ± 0.2†	1.7 ± 0.1†	38
11	63 ± 4	650 ± 10†	3.5 ± 0.2†	1.6 ± 0.1	46

Data taken from Thiebaud et al.[93]
† Significantly different from low FFA group, $p < .001$.

trolling glucose uptake. This is in part due to the fact that the euglycemic-hyperinsulinemic clamp procedure is not the best means by which to assess the role of changes of FFA concentration on glucose oxidation. With the clamp procedure two potentially important variables are controlled—plasma glucose and insulin concentration. Nonetheless, the most important factor in relation to glucose oxidation (i.e., the rate of glucose uptake) is uncontrolled. Since changes in glucose oxidation during the clamp procedure are normally directly related to the rate of glucose uptake and thus glucose infusion,[95] it is impossible to assess the intracellular regulation of glucose oxidation when the rate of glucose infusion is variable. This can best be appreciated by considering the extreme case of no glucose infusion versus a glucose infusion at $10 mg \cdot kg^{-1} min^{-1}$. Obviously, the rate of glucose oxidation could not be as high in the absence of glucose infusion as during high dose glucose infusion, simply because there is not as much glucose available.

Because of the limitations in interpreting the results of traditional glucose clamp experiments, the effect of an increase in FFA availability on glucose oxidation should be tested in the setting of constant glucose uptake.[96] To maximize the chances of observing an FFA effect on glucose oxidation, a high glucose infusion rate should be used to stimulate glycolysis and ensure that virtually all tissues use glucose as an energy substrate. If some tissues are using fat as an energy substrate already, then it would not be possible for an increase in plasma FFA to cause any further increase in fat oxidation in those tissues. In this circumstance, plasma FFA has minimal effect on either plasma glucose uptake or oxidation.[96]

The conclusion from the study described above, which involved a prolonged glucose infusion and a brief (2-hour) increase in FFA concentration, may have reflected to some extent an adaptation to a prolonged glucose infusion that does not occur over the normal time course of a euglycemic-hyperinsulinemic clamp procedure. Even so, the findings are consistent with some studies using the traditional euglycemic-hyperinsulinemic clamp approach. For example Bevilacqua et al.[97] found no effect of FFA on glucose uptake during the euglycemic clamp in obese subjects.

The effect of changing the plasma FFA concentration on substrate oxidation has also been investigated during exercise. In the absence of any nutrient intake, the utilization of plasma FFA as an energy substrate decreases as a proportion of total energy requirements as the exercise intensity increases.[98] Conversely, the proportionate contribution of energy derived from carbohydrate oxidation increases.[98] In high-intensity exercise, the relationship between lipolysis and the oxidation of fatty acids is different from the situation at rest. Whereas normally at rest the fatty acids are released into plasma at least twice as fast as they are oxidized,[99] during high intensity exercise the rate of fat oxidation actually exceeds the rate of peripheral lipolysis.[98] This is possible because of concurrent intramuscular triglyceride (TG) lipolysis. Therefore, to determine if the availability of fatty acids was limiting for the rate of fatty acid oxidation in high intensity exercise, Intralipid plus heparin was infused to raise FFA concentration during high intensity exercise.[100] In Table 6.2 the relationship between the rate of appearance of plasma FFA (RaFFA) and total fat oxidation from both plasma

TABLE 6.2. Effect of exercise intensity and plasma FFA concentration on fat and carbohydrate metabolism during exercise.

Exercise intensity % of VO₂ max	Peripheral lipolysis ($\mu mol\, glycerol \cdot kg^{-1} min^{-1}$)	Plasma RaFFA ($\mu mol \cdot kg^{-1} min^{-1}$)	Total fat oxidation ($\mu mol\, FA \cdot kg^{-1} min^{-1}$)	Carbohydrate oxidation ($\mu mol\, glucose \cdot kg^{-1} min^{-1}$)
25	9.8 ± 1.6	25.8 ± 2.6	26.8 ± 1.8	15 ± 1.8
65	6.9 ± 0.6	22.8 ± 2.7*	42.8 ± 3.7*	132 ± 7.9*
85	8.5 ± 2.5	17.0 ± 3.4*†	29.6 ± 4.3†	259 ± 8.0
85 + lipid		61.0 ± 10.6*†‡	34.0 ± 4.4‡	230 ± 9.1‡

Data taken from Romijn et al.[98,100]
* Significantly different from 25% VO₂ max, $p < .05$.
† Significantly different from 65% VO₂ max, $p < .05$.
‡ Significantly different from 85% VO₂ max, without lipid ($p < .05$).

and intracellular lipolysis is shown for different exercise intensities, and also the response to increasing RaFFA during exercise at 85% VO$_2$ max is shown. First, at progressively higher intensities of exercise the rate of peripheral lipolysis did not increase, despite the greatly increased demand for energy. This underscores the lack of regulation of lipolysis and RaFFA in relation to substrate requirements. In fact, RaFFA significantly decreased when exercise intensity increased from 65% to 85% VO$_2$ max, which can be explained by a decrease in adipose tissue blood flow.[98] Second, when RaFFA was increased from 17 ± 3.4 to 61.0 ± 10.6 µmol·kg^{-1}·min^{-1} by the infusion of Intralipid plus heparin, the rate of fat oxidation increased less than 5 µmol·kg^{-1}·min^{-1}. Whereas that increase in oxidation was statistically significant, fat provided only 35% of total energy expenditure during the lipid infusion, even though ample FFA were provided to meet most of the energy requirements. Similarly, total carbohydrate oxidation during exercise at 85% VO$_2$ max was significantly reduced by the increase in RaFFA, but the magnitude of change (12%) was of little physiologic significance when compared to the 350% increase in RaFFA (see Chapter 16).

Thus, the in vivo experiments indicate that fatty acids do not directly control the rate of glucose oxidation at a cellular level. Furthermore, evidence indicates that plasma FFA only affects glucose clearance, and thus the plasma glucose concentration, in certain specific circumstances. In particular, FFA may inhibit glucose transport in the insulin-stimulated state, but not in the basal state. Since the inhibitory effect of fatty acids on glucose oxidation is the cornerstone of the glucose–fatty acid cycle,[52] we must reject that traditional explanation of glucose–fatty acid kinetics.

There is no doubt that there is a reciprocal relationship between fatty acid and glucose oxidation. If from the above discussion the conclusion is that this relationship is not controlled by the metabolism of fatty acids, it is logical to propose the reverse of the traditional glucose–fatty acid cycle, i.e., that the intracellular metabolism of glucose controls the rate of fatty acid oxidation. In the following section support for this notion is provided, including evidence for a proposed mechanism whereby this process may be controlled.

The Glucose–Fatty Acid Cycle Reversed

Effect of Glucose on Lipolysis

A glucose effect on fatty acids could be controlled by either regulation of lipolysis and/or control of fatty acid oxidation. Glucose infusion or ingestion inhibits lipolysis and decreases the release of FFA into the blood.[101] The inhibition of lipolysis during glucose infusion is mediated predominantly by insulin. The inhibitory effect of insulin on lipolysis was a key part of the original glucose–fatty acid cycle.[52] The control of lipolysis by insulin was proposed to be the mechanism whereby fatty acid oxidation decreased when carbohydrate availability was high. However, in the preceding sections we have documented that the availability of plasma FFA is not a primary determinant of the rate of fat oxidation. Rather, different rates of fat oxidation for a particular RaFFA are determined by the availability of glucose. As a consequence, "unmetabolized" FFA is cleared from the blood and reesterified into TG. The liver is a major site of fatty acid clearance. Those fatty acids that are taken up by the liver that are not oxidized are reesterified into TG and secreted into the blood as very low density lipoproteins (VLDL-TG). In general, the rate of VLDL-TG secretion is related to the availability of FFA.[102] However, during periods of hyperglycemia-hyperinsulinemia, hepatic oxidation of fatty acids is low, and fatty acids that are taken up by the liver are more efficiently channeled into triglycerides. Thus, in normal volunteers given a continuous high carbohydrate feeding for 4 days, not only was the hepatic secretion of VLDL-TG derived from de novo synthesized FA increased significantly, so too was the rate of secretion of VLDL-TG derived from reesterified fatty acids.[103] Even with the inhibitory effect on lipolysis during prolonged hyperglycemia/hyperinsulinemia, the reesterification of plasma FFA was the predominant pathway for the production of VLDL-TG. This occurred because of an increased fractional reesterification of nonoxidized fatty acids, with the result being sustained hypertriglyceridemia.[103] The channeling of fatty acids in the liver to VLDL-TG production, as opposed to oxidation, can be explained by an inhibition of hepatic FFA acid oxidation by glucose.

Effect of Glucose on Fatty Acid Oxidation

The effect of the acute elevation of glucose availability and oxidation on fatty acid oxidation was tested in the setting of constant FFA concentration.[104] Normal volunteers were studied in the basal state and during a hyperinsulinemic-hyperglycemic clamp (plasma insulin = 1789 ± 119 pmol·L^{-1}, plasma glucose = 7.7 ± 0.2 mm·L^{-1}). In this study it was found that increased availability of glucose inhibited fat oxidation, despite the constant availability of FFA (Table 6.3). This result is precisely contrary to that predicted by the traditional glucose–fatty acid cycle, and leads to the conclusion that the intracellular availability of glucose, rather than FFA, determines the nature of substrate oxidation in the human.

To assess the mechanism by which glucose inhibits fatty acid oxidation, the hypothesis that glucose and/or insulin inhibits entrance of FFA into the mitochondria

TABLE 6.3. Effect of hyperinsulinemia/hyperglycemia on glucose and fatty acid oxidation.

	Basal	Clamp
Glucose concentration (mmol·L^{-1})	4.8 ± 0.1	7.7 ± 0.2*
Glucose oxidation (μmol·kg^{-1}min^{-1})	6.2 ± 0.8	22.3 ± 1.4*
FFA concentration (mmol·L^{-1})	0.38 ± 0.06	0.33 ± 0.07
Fat oxidation (μmol·kg^{-1}min^{-1})	2.6 ± 0.2	0.4 ± 0.3*

Data taken from Sidossis and Wolfe.[104]
*Significantly different from basal value, $p < .01$.

was investigated.[105] Thus, subjects were infused with 1-^{13}C-oleate, a long-chain fatty acid, and 1-^{14}C-octanoate, a medium-chain fatty acid, in the basal state and during a hyperglycemic-hyperinsulinemic state. Plasma oleate enrichment and FFA concentration were kept constant by means of the infusion of Intralipid and heparin. Oleate, but not octanoate, requires the carnitine acyl transferase enzyme in order to gain access to mitochondrial matrix. Thus, if glucose and/or insulin limit long-chain fatty acid entrance into the mitochondria, then long-chain acylcarnitine formation should be decreased during the clamp, causing a decrease in oleate, but not octanoate, oxidation. During the clamp, oleate oxidation decreased from the basal value of 0.9 ± 0.1 to 0.4 ± 0.1 μmol·kg^{-1}min^{-1}. In contrast, octanoate oxidation remained unchanged in the transition from basal to clamp. The conclusion that glucose and/or insulin directly limits fatty acid oxidation by restricting long-chain fatty acid entrance into the mitochondria was supported by a decrease in intramuscular acylcarnitine concentration from 843 ± 390 in the basal state to 296 ± 77 nmol·g^{-1} dry weight during the clamp.[105]

Physiologic Role of Glucose Availability Controlling Metabolism

One of the appealing aspects of the traditional glucose–fatty acid cycle was that it was consistent with certain physiologic and pathologic circumstances. For example, a high plasma FFA concentration is associated with many insulin-resistant states, such as obesity,[106] type II diabetes,[107] or severe trauma and sepsis.[108] The glucose–fatty acid cycle potentially provides a link between high FFA concentration and insulin resistance, since the high FFA concentration should lead to increased FFA oxidation, which in turn should inhibit glucose uptake and oxidation (i.e., cause insulin resistance). However, it has been established in the previous sections that this explanation is not likely. Consequently, it is pertinent to consider physiologic regulation of substrate metabolism with glucose availability as the controlling factor.

Much of the early work describing metabolic regulation from a physiologic perspective came from the study of the response to fasting.[109] With progressive fasting, the FFA concentration increases and the glucose concentration declines, and fat becomes essentially the sole nonprotein energy substrate. According to traditional explanations, the high FFA inhibits glucose uptake, which limits gluconeogenesis and therefore serves to spare protein.[88] In this case, however, the plasma glucose concentration would have to increase to signal the liver, yet this does not happen. Further, there is no evidence either in vitro or in vivo, that a high FFA concentration exerts an inhibitory effect on basal glucose uptake. Thus, enough glucose was infused into normal, fasting volunteers to maintain the normal postabsorptive concentration during fasting.[110] The FFA concentration nonetheless increased, but rather than causing a corresponding decrease in glucose clearance, basal glucose clearance actually increased over the 3-day period.[110] Thus, there are many flaws in the notion that FFA availability controls substrate metabolism in fasting. On the other hand, invoking glucose availability as the controlling factor in modulating changes in substrate metabolism with fasting makes a more consistent explanation possible. The decreased availability of hepatic glycogen with fasting leads to a fall in the availability of plasma glucose, causing a fall in glucose oxidation, thereby releasing the inhibition of fat oxidation.

Contrary to the notion that the increase in FFA concentration stimulates fat oxidation in fasting, it is more likely that the primary physiologic role of the increased rate of lipolysis in fasting is to provide glycerol as a gluconeogenic precursor.[111] After an overnight fast there is already more than enough FFA available to easily satisfy energy requirements, and the stimulation of lipolysis in prolonged fasting is unrelated to any demand for excess energy substrates. The controlling role of the plasma glucose availability in determining the rate of fat oxidation in the liver in fasting is indicated by the marked reduction in plasma ketone concentration, reflecting fat oxidation when the normal postabsorptive plasma glucose concentration is maintained.[110]

Another response that can be better explained by glucose, rather than FFA, controlling substrate metabolism is the fact that excessive carbohydrate intake increases triglyceride concentration,[112,113] yet recent studies indicate a limited capacity for hepatic fatty acid synthesis.[103] In this case, high glucose intake apparently inhibits fatty acid oxidation in the liver, thereby channeling fatty acids into triglyceride formation.

The notion of glucose availability controlling metabolism is also consistent with experimental evidence during exercise. Under normal circumstances, fatty acid oxidation increases as exercise intensity increases from a low 25% VO$_2$ max to a moderate 65% VO$_2$ max, but decreases as intensity exceeds 65%.[98] This can be explained by stimulation of muscle glycogenolysis in high-intensity exercise, which leads to increased glycolytic flux and inhibition of fatty acid oxidation. With endurance training, fat is used to a greater extent than carbohydrate at the same exercise intensity as in the untrained state. This is related to a stimulation of lipolysis in trained individuals, both in the resting state[114] and during exercise.[115] Traditionally, it has been thought that the greater availability of fat with training decreased muscle protein glycogen breakdown by inhibiting glycolysis at the phosphofructokinase step.[88] However, Coggan et al.[116] were unable to confirm this mechanism. In contrast, they reported that muscle glucose-6-phosphate was significantly lower in the trained state, indicating that training-induced reduction in carbohydrate utilization results from attenuation of flux before the phosphofructokinase step in glycolysis.[116] It seems likely that training results in a reduced rate of glycogen breakdown, and FFA oxidation is increased because of decreased availability of pyruvate for oxidation.

Explanation of altered substrate kinetics in diabetes was one of the original reasons for the glucose–fatty acid cycle.[52] In contrast, it is more likely that in insulin-resistant states such as diabetes, an impaired rate of glucose uptake leads to increased fatty acid oxidation, rather than the reverse. A variety of mechanisms may be responsible for the impaired glucose uptake.

Although it is clear that the traditional glucose–fatty acid cycle is flawed, it clearly would not have endured so long if it had absolutely no merit. Indeed, in many circumstances, some FFA effect on glucose can be demonstrated, even if glucose availability predominates in importance. For example, a modest increase in FFA oxidation occurs during exercise when FFA concentration is increased.[100] Thus, whereas glucose availability predominates in determining the mix of substrate oxidation, there is a reciprocal relationship between glucose and FFA in which FFA availability plays a role, albeit a minor one. This is to be expected, considering that the mechanism whereby glucose inhibits fat oxidation is by limiting its entry into mitochondria by inhibiting the carnitine acyl transferase enzyme. For any given enzyme activity, within some range of substrate concentration, a greater concentration of FFA will cause more fatty–acyl CoA to be transferred to the mitochondria. The studies of octanoate metabolism indicate that once inside the mitochondria, there is no inhibitory effect of glucose on β-oxidation of fatty acids. Consequently, the explanation of the normal relationships between glucose and fatty acids presented here places great weight on the predominance of glucose availability as the controlling factor, the mechanism whereby glucose controls metabolism can be overridden to a modest extent in situations in which there are large changes in the FFA concentration. Furthermore, a direct effect of FFA on glucose clearance may also exert some control over substrate oxidation in certain circumstances, provided that the actual rate of glucose uptake is impaired.

Glycerol

The direct oxidation of glycerol is not a major pathway for energy production. However, at high rates of lipolysis, the appearance of glycerol in the plasma increases markedly. Under these circumstances, as much as 30% of glucose production might originate from glycerol.[16] Because glucose is used as an energy substrate, it is evident that glycerol can provide the carbon skeleton for what could quantitatively be an important substrate pool. Additionally, glycerol can effectively spare nitrogen by successfully competing with amino acids as gluconeogenic precursors, making amino acids available for reincorporation into protein and reducing urea production.[18]

Ketones

Ketone bodies, primarily β-hydroxybutyrate and acetoacetic acid, can be used by many tissues, including the brain, as the principal energy source.[117] Ketones are produced in the liver as a consequence of β-oxidation of fatty acids. Normally, in the fed state, ketone production is minimal, but with fasting the rate of ketone production may increase severalfold.[118] The ketogenic response to food deprivation is considered by some to be critical for the adaptive response that normally occurs with starvation.[4] Because ketones can compete with glucose for oxidative pathways in the brain, the demand for glucose production, and consequent depletion of protein, is minimized when ketone concentrations are high. Also, it has been proposed that ketones exert a specific inhibitory effect on protein catabolism.[13] The exact role of the ketones as metabolic regulators has not been established.

Regulation of Protein Synthesis

The net synthesis of protein that is essential for growth and development is the balance between the total rates of synthesis and catabolism. Synthesis and catabolism are constitutive processes of protein turnover. The difference between the absolute rates of synthesis and catabolism is equal to protein balance, with a positive value indicating net protein synthesis and a negative value indicating net protein breakdown. Although the opposing processes of synthesis and catabolism are related, they are apparently independently regulated. Nonetheless, some of the same factors may affect each process. Despite the importance of the regulation of protein catabolism, there is relatively little information regarding its regulation,[119] largely stem-

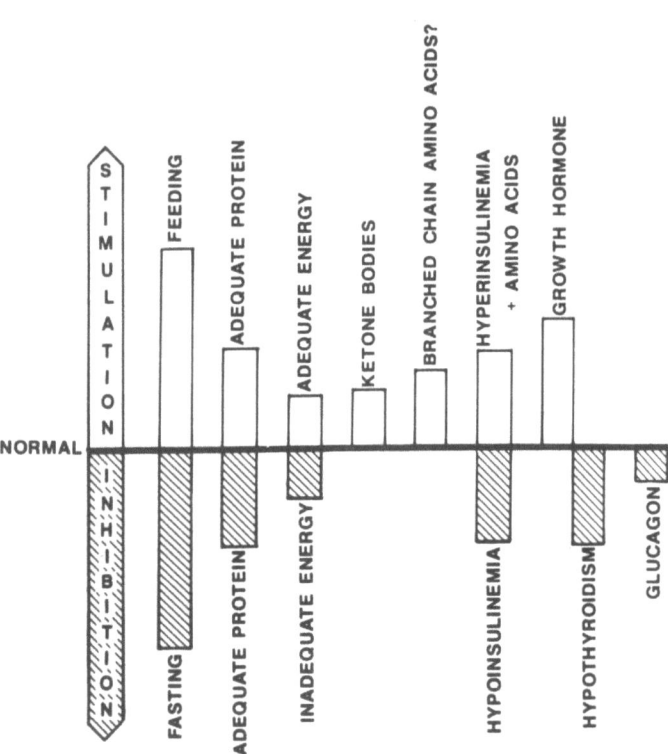

FIGURE 6.4. Possible regulators of protein synthesis rate.

ming from the difficulty of measuring in vivo the rate of breakdown of specific proteins. Consequently, in this section attention is focused on the regulation of protein synthesis. There is an abundance of information available regarding the mechanism and regulation of protein synthesis. There is an abundance of information available regarding the mechanism and regulation of protein synthesis at the molecular level that has been comprehensively described in several excellent overviews of the topic.[120,121] Therefore this discussion focuses on protein synthesis at the tissue, organ, and whole-body level (see Chapters 11, 18, and 34).

Effect of Age on Protein Synthesis

Protein synthesis is highest in the neonate,[122] gradually decreasing with age to reach a constant value to adulthood;[123,124] this rate seems to be maintained into old age[125] (Table 6.4). Even in the neonate the rate is directly related to postconceptional age, being highest (14.3 ± 4.5 g·kg^{-1}day^{-1}) in a group of premature neonates studied at a postconceptional age of 32 weeks and decreasing rapidly to half this rate by term[122] (see Chapter 34). During growth, from infancy to adulthood, there is a further halving of the rate of protein synthesis from about 6.0 to about 3.5 g·kg^{-1} day^{-1}.[123,124] The faster rate of protein synthesis in the young is not due solely to their greater requirement for growth and development, but to the fact that endogenous protein is being degraded at a greatly accelerated rate as well (Figure 6.4). In the rapidly growing infant, about three-fourths of protein synthesis is related to the renewal of endogenous protein to replace that lost by catabolism of preexisting protein, and only one-fourth contributes to protein deposition during growth. For example, the full-term neonate, synthesizing protein at the rate of 8.0 g·kg^{-1}day^{-1}, has a net protein synthesis rate of 1.8 gk·g^{-1}day^{-1} and a renewal rate of 6 g·kg^{-1}day^{-1}.[122] This is twice the absolute rate of protein synthesis in adult man receiving an adequate diet[124] (Table 6.4).

From animal studies it appears that the decrease in whole-body protein synthesis that occurs from infancy to adulthood is mostly due to a marked slowing of the rate of synthesis of skeletal muscle protein, which proportionately is the largest protein store in the body.[126] When the fractional rates of protein synthesis (FSR) of different organs and skeletal muscle are compared in the young and adult rat, there is little change in the FSR of most organs, but skeletal muscle FSR decreases threefold. Despite the net deposition of muscle that occurs during growth, the reduction in FSR is so great with increasing age that the contribution of skeletal muscle protein synthesis to the overall whole-body protein synthesis rate is greatly reduced.[126]

Effect of Feeding and Fasting

The response of protein synthesis to feeding and fasting is uncertain.[127-131] On the one hand, several investigators[127-129] have shown that the switch from continuous feeding of adequate intakes of energy and protein to a 12-

TABLE 6.4. Protein synthesis rates in different age groups in the fed state.

Subjects	Age	Protein synthesis rate (g·kg⁻¹day⁻¹)
Neonates		
Premature	7.4 months[a]	14.3 ± 4.5[b]
	8 months	11.8 ± 2.9
Full term	8.4 months	7.9 ± 2.7
	11 months	7.7 ± 1.4
Infants	1.25 years	6.2 ± 0.6[c]
Adults	32 years	3.5 ± 0.4[d]
Elderly	65 years	3.3 ±[e]

All values are the mean ± SD. They were determined using ^{15}N-glycine.
[a] Postconceptional age for neonates.
[b] Heine et al.[122]
[c] Golden et al.[123]
[d] Jackson et al.[124]
[e] Golden and Waterlow.[125]

to 15-hour fast causes a marked decrease in the absolute rate of protein synthesis, ranging from 40%[127] to 25%.[129] On the other hand, Motil et al.[130] and Melville et al.[131] failed to demonstrate any change in protein synthesis in response to fasting. Although these studies differed in terms of the effect of fasting on the total synthesis rate, these investigators consistently found that protein balance shifted from a positive net protein synthesis to a negative net protein breakdown value as subjects went from the prandial to the postabsorptive state. Equilibrium in protein metabolism during adulthood is maintained by a cycle in which the net postprandial gain in synthesis balances the net postabsorptive loss of protein. Skeletal muscle appears to be the major contributor to this response.[127] Muscle protein synthesis is decreased about 50% by fasting.[127] Because skeletal muscle protein mass could account for as much as 80% of total body protein mass[132] and its synthesis makes up about one-half of the rate of whole-body protein synthesis, it is evident that a major response of muscle synthesis to fasting is reflected at the whole-body level.

In contrast to the response of the absolute synthesis rate, there is a progressive increase in net protein synthesis rate in infants as dietary protein intake increases from marginal level (0.7 g·kg⁻¹day⁻¹) to a surfeit level (5.2 g·kg⁻¹day⁻¹), owing mostly to a progressive reduction in breakdown rate.[125,133,134] This general relation between protein intake and protein synthesis and breakdown rates evident in the fed neonate is consistent with observations from in vitro studies. For example, Fulks et al.[135] found that the addition to a medium in which the diaphragms from fed rats were incubated with amino acids at plasma concentrations caused a 23% increase in protein synthesis and a 19% inhibition of breakdown rate. When the amino acid concentration was increased to five times the plasma concentration, there was no change in synthesis, but the breakdown rate was further decreased by 25%.

Effect of Protein Intake

Several studies have shown that different levels of protein intake have little effect on the absolute rate of protein synthesis in infants.[125,133,134] Golden and Waterlow[125] reported only a modest 6% increase in protein synthesis rate in infants switched from diets supplying an adequate (1.2 g·kg⁻¹day⁻¹) to a surfeit (3.2 g·kg⁻¹day⁻¹) level of protein (Table 6.5). The synthesis rates they reported on 1.2 g·kg⁻¹day⁻¹ confirmed those reported by Picou and Taylor-Roberts.[133] Even lower levels of protein intake appear to be adequate to maintain protein synthesis in infants. Infants given only 0.7 g·kg⁻¹day⁻¹ and 100 kcal·kg⁻¹day⁻¹ maintained a synthesis rate of 6.0 ± 0.7 g·kg⁻¹day⁻¹, which is not different from the rate of synthesis in infants given 1.7 g·kg⁻¹day⁻¹,[103] and is comparable to the data shown in Table 6.5 from other investigators.[125,133] The regulatory mechanisms in response to varying levels of protein intake appear to be different in the adult, in whom there is a progressive increase in protein synthesis rate as dietary intake increases from inadequate to marginal to adequate intake in both the fed and fasted states.[130] Concomitantly, there is a progressive and parallel increase in the catabolism rate as dietary protein intake increases, suggesting that these two processes are closely interdependent.[130] Although a higher protein intake does not necessarily increase net protein synthesis, it does generally cause a higher rate of protein turnover. The potential physiologic significance of protein turnover is discussed below.

TABLE 6.5. Effect of different levels of protein intake on protein kinetics in fed human subjects.

Parameter	Infants[a]			Adults[b]		
	1.2[c]	3.6[c]	5.2[c]	0.1[c]	0.6[c]	1.5[c]
Synthesis	6.2 ± 0.5	6.1 ± 0.6	6.6 ± 0.5	2.4 ± 0.1	3.8 ± 0.3	4.2 ± 0.2
Catabolism	2.5 ± 0.5	4.7 ± 0.4	4.4 ± 0.4	2.4 ± 0.1	3.0 ± 0.2	2.5 ± 0.3
Balance	+0.7	−1.4	+2.2	0	+0.8	+1.7

Values are mean ± SEM.
[a] Data from Golden et al.[123]
[b] Data from Motil et al.[130]
[c] Protein intake (g·kg⁻¹day⁻¹).

TABLE 6.6. Effect of energy intake on protein kinetics in fed and fasted subject.

Parameter	Protein kinetics		
	Energy (44 ± 0.6 kcal·kg^{-1}day^{-1})	Protein (54 ± 0.6 g·kg^{-1}day^{-1})	Δ
Fed			
Synthesis	3.55 ± 0.12	3.71 ± 0.10	0.16
Catabolism	2.67 ± 0.09	2.63 ± 0.12	0.04
Net balance	−0.88 ± 0.12	+1.08 ± 0.12	0.20
Fasted			
Synthesis	3.27 ± 0.13	3.2 ± 0.12	0
Catabolism	3.74 ± 0.09	3.73 ± 0.14	0
Net balance	−0.53 ± 0.08	−0.53 ± 0.08	0

Recalculated from Motil et al.[137]
Values are mean ± SEM.

Effect of Energy Intake

In the adult and the infant receiving a marginal protein intake, it has been shown that even a modest increase in energy intake of 10 kcal·kg^{-1}day^{-1} above the amount required to maintain energy balance leads to an overall improvement of nitrogen balance.[134,136,137] Studies by Motil et al.[137] in normal adults given a marginal protein intake of 0.6 g·kg^{-1}day^{-1} and either an adequate energy intake of 44 kcal·kg^{-1}day^{-1} or excess energy intake of 54 kcal·kg^{-1}day^{-1}, suggested that the overall improvement in nitrogen balance when energy intake is increased is the result of stimulation of protein synthesis in the fed state, as protein breakdown rate does not change. In the fasted state, protein kinetics are not responsive to the preceding level of energy intake (Table 6.6). The data of Jackson et al.[134] suggest that the overall improvement in nitrogen balance with excess energy intake is due to stimulation of protein synthesis. The conclusion that the level of energy intake exerts its effect via changes in the synthesis rate is further supported by results from obese subjects given a marginal protein intake and whose energy intake was decreased from 17 kcal·kg^{-1}day^{-1} to 5 kcal·kg^{-1}day^{-1}.[138] The reduction in energy intake caused a 42% decrease in protein balance owing to the 10% reduction in synthesis rate, whereas the breakdown rate remained constant.

Effect of Various Substrates

Branched-Chain Amino Acids

Not only is the quantity of protein important in the regulation of protein synthesis, but the relative concentrations of specific amino acids may be as well. The most prominent example is leucine, which appears to play a regulatory role beyond that expected on the basis of its function as an essential amino acid for the synthesis of protein.[139–141] Several investigators have shown that the branched-chain amino acids (BCAAs) stimulate protein synthesis and inhibit catabolism in the incubated and perfused rat skeletal and cardiac muscle, an effect not elicited by any other of the plasma amino acids.[135,139,141] Furthermore, the BCAA effect on both synthesis and catabolism can be elicited by leucine alone.[135] When the degradation of leucine is blocked with cycloserine, the leucine effect on synthesis remains intact, but its suppressive effect on protein breakdown is lost.[141] It appears that leucine itself directly stimulates synthesis, but it is one of the degradation products of leucine that inhibits synthesis. Because α-ketoisocaproate (KIC) is capable of inhibiting protein degradation to the same extent as leucine in the rat diaphragm,[141] it is possible that KIC is the mediator of the leucine effect on catabolism. However, KIC is in very low concentration intracellularly when not added exogenously.

The physiologic significance of the leucine effect is not clear. The in vivo situation differs from the in vitro experiments that were the basis for the formulation of the theory that leucine is a regulator of protein metabolism because in vivo there is never a circumstance in which leucine is totally absent. In the human an important regulatory role for leucine has been difficult to demonstrate. When normal volunteers are fed increasing levels of leucine while receiving an otherwise adequate intake of protein, the net protein balance is improved.[142] However, a similar response can be shown for any other essential amino acid deleted from an otherwise complete protein intake.

In starved patients Sherwin[143] reported an improved nitrogen balance in response to an infusion of leucine. Because there was no change in the 3-methylhistidine excretion rate, which is an indicator of muscle protein breakdown, it was deduced that the improved nitrogen balance was due to stimulation of the protein synthesis rate.[112] It was not demonstrated that the leucine effect was unique to that amino acid. Furthermore, in the rat receiving a normal diet or a 2-day starvation diet, there was no change in the rate of protein synthesis in heart, gastrocnemius muscle, or jejunal serosa after administration of leucine.[144] When branched-chained amino acids leucine, valine, and isoleucine were fed to normal volunteers, there was no benefit as compared to the response to the mixture of three other essential amino acids threonine, methionine, and histidine that have never been claimed to play a regulator role.[145]

Because the overall rate of net protein breakdown is greatly accelerated after trauma and infection,[146,147] and the rate of leucine oxidation is dramatically increased in such patients,[147,148] much interest has focused on the clinical utility of leucine in these circumstances to promote net protein synthesis. Initial studies, predominantly in animals, were encouraging.[149–153] However, careful studies in the human have generally failed to document any unique effect of leucine or BCAA on either protein synthesis or catabolism.[154,155] From all of these studies it seems likely that, whereas some amount of leucine does have a unique anabolic effect, that effect is elicited at a concentration of leucine that is generally present under most physiologic circumstances in the human, and extra leucine beyond the requisite amount does not have the same unique effect on protein metabolism.

Glucose

The nitrogen-sparing effect of glucose has been well documented in both fasting normal volunteers and a variety of stressed patients.[156-159] The response of protein metabolism is in part due to the effect of insulin, the release of which is stimulated by glucose. In addition, glucose infusion has a direct inhibitory effect on urea production when the insulin response is blocked by the infusion of somatostatin.[36] There are two potential mechanisms whereby glucose can affect protein kinetics: (1) glucose can directly inhibit protein breakdown;[135,160] and (2) glucose can potentially affect protein balance by inhibiting glucose production,[37] thereby making more amino acids available for reincorporation into protein and decreasing the loss of nitrogen to urea. In the case of this indirect action of glucose, one would expect an increase in the protein synthesis rate due to the increased availability of amino acids. Because whole-body protein synthesis is not stimulated by glucose, it seems likely this mechanism is of minimal importance in net protein balance. This point is particularly true because of the observation that gluconeogenesis persists, at least to some extent, during glucose infusion as a route of glycogen synthesis (vide supra).

Ketones

It has been proposed that ketone bodies have a protein-sparing effect during fasting because the CNS switches from glucose to ketones as its primary metabolic fuel. This adaptation decreases the need for amino acids as fuel for gluconeogenesis, thereby decreasing net protein loss.[161,162] Studies in normal adult volunteers indicate that the anabolic effect of ketones is elicited by stimulation of synthesis.[163,164]

Hormones

Several hormones have regulatory roles in protein metabolism.[104,129,133-149] Of paramount importance is the anabolic hormone insulin, which is known, from studies with diabetic animals, to be important for the maintenance of protein homeostasis and muscle mass.[145,146] Insulin stimulates protein synthesis and inhibits breakdown in a wide variety of cell cultures and in heart, liver, and muscle tissues.[104,128] The low rate of muscle protein synthesis in the diabetic rat is restored to normal by insulin administration,[145] and in the insulin-treated diabetic rat there is a progressive loss of protein, a decrease in the muscle protein synthesis rate, and an increase in the protein breakdown rate following insulin withdrawal.[146]

The overall anabolic effect of insulin at the whole-body level is well established. Early studies have shown that in insulin-deprived type 1 diabetics nitrogen balance is markedly negative, indicating a net catabolism of body protein.[165] More recently, leucine turnover studies suggested that during insulin deficiency the net catabolic state arises from an increase in whole-body protein breakdown.[166-171] Leucine oxidation was found to be increased with insulin deficiency, indicating an increased net loss of an essential amino acid.[166-171] Paradoxically, in the same studies, nonoxidative leucine disposal, an index of whole-body protein synthesis, was found normal or increased in insulin-deprived diabetics.[172-177] The unexpected result of unimpaired protein synthesis during insulin deficiency may represent a methodologic artifact, since the value is not directly measured, but deduced mathematically. However, if insulin deficiency does cause an increase in whole-body protein synthesis, it raises the question of where this increased protein synthesis rate is occurring. Some liver secretory proteins involved in the acute-phase response are increased during insulin deficiency.[177,178] Gut and kidney protein content was also found to be increased in the diabetic rat,[179,180] indicating a stimulation of synthesis with insulin lack. More expectedly, in diabetes muscle protein synthesis was found to be normal[171] or decreased.[181,182]

The apparent discrepancy between whole-body responses to insulin and the prediction, from in vitro studies, that insulin should stimulate synthesis can be partially explained by the apparent potent effect of insulin to whole-protein breakdown in vivo. Using the hyperinsulinemic-euglycemic clamp technique combined with leucine turnover, insulin has been found to reduce whole-body protein breakdown in a dose-dependent manner.[183-185] At physiologic insulin concentration protein breakdown is suppressed up to 20% to 30%.[183-187] Leucine oxidation is also blunted by insulin.[182-187] Thus, by inhibiting protein breakdown, insulin has the effect of reducing the availability of precursor for synthesis of new protein. Infusion of amino acids without insulin stimulates whole-body protein synthesis.[186,187] When amino acids are infused during euglycemic-hyperinsulinemia, insulin does not affect protein synthesis.[186,187] Thus, whereas these data indicate that insulin does not inhibit protein synthesis directly, there are no data at the whole-body level supporting the role of insulin as a stimulator of protein synthesis.

Thus, there is a considerable discrepancy between the in vivo studies, indicating no direct effect of insulin on protein synthesis, and the in vitro experiments showing an important stimulatory effect of insulin on specific proteins. Furthermore, although only certain specific proteins have been shown to be stimulated by insulin in vitro, these include the quantitatively most important contributors to whole-body protein turnover (i.e., muscle protein, collagen, and albumin).[188,189] Thus, if this action were occurring in vivo it would be expected that this would be reflected by the whole-body technique. The best explanation for this discrepancy may be that limitations of the whole-body technique make quantitative assessment of protein synthesis unreliable. In the leucine technique, the rate of protein synthesis is calculated as the difference between protein breakdown and leucine oxidation. Neither breakdown nor oxidation are precisely determined, due to a number of factors.[190]

A number of investigators have used the leg or forearm arteriovenous balance technique to study insulin effects on human skeletal muscle. Taken together, these studies suggest that the in vivo effect of insulin on net muscle protein deposition is dependent on the systemic amino acid concentrations. Thus, systemic physiologic hyperinsulinemia, without amino acid infusion, failed to improve protein balance, and did not modify protein synthesis or degradation, either in the forearm or in the leg.[191,192] Despite the absence of an effect on muscle, in the same studies systemic amino acid concentrations and whole-body protein breakdown were reduced following insulin infusion. Insulin caused these responses by acting primarily at sites other than skeletal muscle. Therefore, it is possible that the lack of a major insulin effect on muscle in these studies was related to the development of hypoaminoacidemia. In other studies, insulin was infused directly into the brachial artery to raise forearm deep venous insulin concentration to high physiologic levels, without affecting systemic amino acid concentration, and therefore not altering amino acid delivery to the forearm. With this experimental model net protein balance markedly increased,[193,194] apparently due to an isolated decrease in breakdown.[193]

Consistent with the interpretation of the importance of amino acid concentrations in influencing the response to insulin, systemic insulin infusion with concomitant amino acid infusion to prevent changes in systemic amino acid concentrations has been shown to improve net muscle protein balance, by means of an isolated decrease in breakdown.[195] Furthermore, hyperaminoacidemia of two or three times the normal postabsorptive concentrations stimulated muscle protein synthesis,[196] and such an effect was enhanced by concomitant insulin infusion.[197] On the other hand, using a new model to quantify muscle protein synthesis that overcomes some of the limitations of previous methods, a small local increase of insulin in the leg significantly stimulated synthesis without affecting breakdown.[172] Thus, insulin at physiologic postprandial concentrations promotes muscle protein anabolism in the presence of either normal or high systemic amino acid concentrations. On the other hand, muscle protein balance was improved despite the fall of amino acid concentrations, at pharmacologically high insulin concentrations.[173]

Physiologic Effects of Insulin on Other Tissues

The effect of insulin on protein metabolism in the liver has been less extensively investigated than the effect of insulin on protein metabolism in muscle. Measurement of protein synthesis in liver is complicated by the simultaneous synthesis of plasma proteins as well as its intracellular liver proteins. Moreover, the arteriovenous balance approach is not possible, because of the difficulty of obtaining portal venous blood, and more importantly, because the liver is able to oxidize all circulating amino acids. Therefore, there is no amino acid that is a suitable representative of liver protein kinetics.

Early studies showed that in diabetes liver protein content was not affected,[174] whereas total serum protein concentrations were reduced, mainly due to a depression of albumin.[171,178] Recently De Feo et al.,[175] using the precursor/product incorporation technique in insulin-deficient diabetic humans, showed that albumin fractional synthetic rate was increased by insulin infusion while fibrinogen synthesis was reduced. With regard to intracellular liver protein, using the constant-infusion technique, Pain and Garlic[181] showed that in the diabetic rat fractional protein synthesis was unaffected in the liver.

The regulation of protein breakdown in liver has been investigated using the organ perfusion technique. The addition of either insulin[176] or amino acids[177] to perfusion of normal liver has an inhibitory effect on protein degradation. Interestingly, the insulin effect was not additive to the effect observed with a maximally effective level of amino acids.[198,199] The role of amino acid availability in regulating liver protein breakdown independently from insulin was also suggested by studies showing that proteolysis in perfused liver from fed normal and diabetic mice was the same.[200] On the other hand, proteolysis was increased to a much greater extent in the fasting diabetic animal than in controls.

It is well known that the gut, the kidney, and skin play a major role in interorgan nitrogen exchange and whole-body protein turnover. The fractional synthetic rates of intestinal mucosa, skin, and kidney protein are several times faster than muscle protein.[201] However, few data are available regarding the effect of insulin on tissue other than muscle and liver. In the diabetic rat gut and kidney, protein content was significantly higher than in controls.[180,194] Therefore, further investigation is required to obtain a comprehensive description of the response of various tissues to insulin.

Protein Breakdown and Insulin

The hydrolysis of intracellular proteins to their constituent amino acids is a highly regulated process that recent studies have revealed to be far more complex than previously believed.[202] Three major pathways have been identified. The most thoroughly characterized is an ATP-independent system of acid proteases (i.e., cathepsins) and hydrolases contained in cellular organelles termed lysosomes.[203] The other two pathways are the Ca^{2+}-dependent proteases,[204] and an ATP-dependent pathway requiring the presence of ubiquitin.[205] Insulin apparently plays an important role only in regulating lysosome protein breakdown.[202,206,207] Under normal physiologic conditions, lysosomes are predominantly involved in the degradation of extracellular and membrane associated proteins in liver.[202,208] Muscle lysosomes normally do not play an important role in myofibrillar protein degradation.[209] However, during insulin withdrawal, lysosomes are involved in muscle protein breakdown.[202] The other proteases are located in the cytosol and show proteolytic activity at neutral pH. The Ca^{2+} dependent proteases are unresponsive to insulin[202] and need unphysiologically elevated Ca^{2+} concentrations, and therefore they may be important primarily in damaged tissues.[208] The most important process in muscle is the ATP-independent system that requires the presence of a specialized protein termed ubiquitin.[205] This system is not sensitive to insulin[202] and is quantitatively the most important degradative system of myofibrillar proteins in muscle under normal conditions.[208] From these in vitro findings, it would be predicted that in vivo insulin lack could result in accelerated breakdown of both liver and muscle protein, and insulin excess would be expected to diminish protein breakdown primarily in the liver.

The protein anabolic effect of growth hormone in the growing young animal is well known.[210] Loss of the pituitary gland causes marked decreases in both protein synthesis and breakdown rates in the growing rat, with the overall decrease in protein synthesis (i.e., 54%) being greater than breakdown (i.e., 30%), which causes cessation of normal growth and muscle development.[210] When the hypophysectomized animal is treated with growth hormone, normal growth is reinitiated and the rate of synthesis of muscle protein increases.[210] In human studies growth hormone has been shown to improve nitrogen balance after severe trauma, in postoperative patients undergoing major surgery[211–213] and in normal volunteers receiving hypocaloric intravenous nutrition. Patients recuperating from major gastrointestinal surgery were treated with growth hormone 0.1 mg·kg^{-1}day^{-1} for 7 days, and both protein synthesis and breakdown rates were two times the rates observed in a control group of patients who received saline instead, resulting in net protein synthesis of 0.3 g·kg^{-1}day^{-1} in the treated group versus a net protein loss of 0.2 g·kg^{-1}day^{-1} in the untreated group.[211] In a similar study of cancer patients who underwent surgery, the net loss of protein in the group treated with growth hormone was 25% less than in the untreated group.[212] Both the animal and human studies suggest that growth hormone stimulates protein synthesis and breakdown rates, but the former to a greater extent than the latter.

Normal concentrations of thyroid hormones have a net protein anabolic effect at the whole-body level and are essential for normal growth and development.[210] Thyroid hormones stimulate the synthesis of liver proteins[214] as well as both synthesis and catabolism in skeletal muscles.[215,216] Although physiologic levels of triiodothyronine (T_3) and thyroxine (T_4) are necessary to induce protein synthesis for normal growth and development in the young hypothyroid rat, high concentrations of thyroid hormones (i.e., hyperthyroidism) cause severe muscle wasting and general loss of body mass. This result is due to the fact that the stimulatory effect on synthesis is maximized at low concentrations of thyroid hormones, but the enhancement of breakdown continues to increase in hyperthyroid conditions.[210]

In vitro and in vivo studies suggest that glucagon acts mainly on the synthesis and breakdown of proteins in the liver,[217] and not in peripheral tissue.[218] Glucagon stimulates the rate of protein breakdown in the perfused rat liver and in liver cell cultures,[217,218–221] and it inhibits liver protein synthesis, especially in the presence of high amino acid concentrations.[217] When normal human subjects were infused with glucagon (i.e., 1 mg·24 hours^{-1}) for 2 days, during an 8-day period of constant dietary intake, there was a significant increase in total nitrogen excretion but no change in the rate of excretion of 3-methylhistidine, suggesting that the net loss of protein was not due to an increased rate of skeletal muscle protein breakdown.[222] Hyperglucagonemia in the presence of hypoinsulinemia and normoinsulinemia has been found to have only a modest inhibitory effect on whole-body protein turnover in the normal human.[223–225] Hyperglucagonemia may have a more pronounced effect on muscle protein breakdown if it occurs with concomitant hypoinsulinemia,[225] but this effect is minimal when normal insulin concentration is maintained, suggesting that insulin deficiency is more important than hyperglucagonemia in terms of causing an increase in protein breakdown.[225] It is possible that the modest increase in net protein loss due to hyperglucagonemia is the result of preferential utilization of intrahepatic amino acids to fuel the increased rate of gluconeogenesis elicited by glucagon; as a consequence, there is an increased rate of ureagenesis and hence an increased net loss of protein.

The anabolic effects of testosterone on skeletal muscle are well established. Although much of the evidence for this statement is anecdotal, arising from the use of testosterone injections by body builders, there is also a scientific basis. Testosterone increases muscle protein synthesis in young men given pharmacologic concentrations of testosterone for 12 weeks.[226] Further, in elderly men in whom the endogenous testosterone concentration had decreased, restoration of the normal young adult concentration increased muscle protein synthesis.[227] Testosterone may function at least in part via the growth hormone (GH) insulin-like growth factor-1 (IGF-I) system.[228]

Significance of Protein Turnover

From the above discussion it is evident that for any given protein balance a variety of rates of protein synthesis and catabolism are possible. Furthermore, many circumstances (e.g., excess protein intake) may alter the absolute rates of synthesis and catabolism without affecting the net balance. Consequently, it is pertinent to consider the physiologic significance of the recycling back of amino acids into protein that results from catabolism. This sort of recycling of amino acids can be called protein turnover; according to this definition, in the fasting state catabolism is always greater than synthesis. Therefore, the amount of protein degraded that is not resynthesized is not a component of the turnover of the protein pool. On the other hand, if synthesis is greater than catabolism in the fed state, it is the rate of catabolism that dictates the rate of turnover. As an example, the fasting situation is considered below.

CASE 1 (NO PROTEIN TURNOVER):
C = 1; S = 0; NB = −1

AMPLIFICATION = 1 − S/NB = 1 − 0/−1 = 1

IF C IS HALVED:

C = 0.5 × 1 = 0.5
S − C = 0.5
NET BALANCE = + 0.5

CASE 2 (PROTEIN TURNOVER = 67% OF TOTAL CATABOLISM)

C = 3; S = 2; NB = −1

AMPLIFICATION = 1 − S/NB = 1 − 2/−1 = 3

IF C IS HALVED:

C = 0.5 × 3 = 1.5
S − C = + 0.5
NET BALANCE = + 1.5 (3 × NB IN CASE 1)

FIGURE 6.5. Theoretical example of amplification of control of the net protein balance as a consequence of protein turnover.

The beneficial effect of a high rate of protein turnover can be argued from the teleologic perspective, as the highest rate of protein turnover under normal conditions is in infants who are rapidly growing. The only time such high rates of turnover are approached during adulthood is in response to injury, a situation that again requires net synthesis of proteins as part of the reparative process. On the other hand, it is self-evident that a high rate of protein turnover per se can have no effect on net protein balance if catabolism is elevated to the same extent as synthesis. This is particularly so as there is an energy cost of protein turnover that has a direct impact on caloric requirements and energy balance. It is necessary to evaluate the physiologic significance of any given rate of protein turnover in relation to the concomitant net protein balance.

One positive benefit of a high rate of protein turnover is that the control of the net production of protein can be amplified, either at the individual protein or whole-body level (Figure 6.5). Thus, if a stimulus doubles the rate of synthesis in the absence of an effect on breakdown, the greater the rate of cycling between synthesis and breakdown before the stimulus the greater the absolute amount of increase caused by a fixed percentage increase of the synthesis. Another possible beneficial effect of protein may be that newer protein functions better than older protein. For example, perhaps muscle concentration is more forceful with newer protein (e.g., crossbridges), thereby explaining the physiologic significance of a higher rate of turnover (i.e., both synthesis and breakdown) in the trained athlete.

Regardless of the physiologic significance of protein turnover, the existence of protein turnover is an important fact. Thus, the regulation of both synthesis and breakdown are crucial in determining net protein balance. As discussed above, the two processes are regulated differently, particularly in vitro. Nonetheless, there is a strong link between the rate of synthesis and breakdown of any protein, raising the possibility that intracellular availability is a determinant of protein synthesis.

Acknowledgment. This work is supported by grant 8490 from the Shriners Hospital and National Institutes of Health Grant DK34817.

References

1. Hers HG. The control of glycogen metabolism in the liver. Annu Rev Biochem 1976;45:167–189.
2. Krebs HA. Some aspects of the regulation of fuel supply in omnivorous animals. Adv Enzyme Regul 1972;1:397–420.
3. Cherrington AD, Stevenson RW, Steiner KE, et al. Insulin, glucagon and glucose as regulators of hepatic glucose uptake and production in vivo. Diabetes Metab Rev 1987;3:307–332.

4. Gahill GF Jr. Starvation in man. N Engl J Med 1970;282: 668–675.
5. Frohman LA. The hypothalamus and metabolic control. In: Ioachim H, ed. Pathobiology annual. New York: Appleton-Century Crofts, 1971: 353–372.
6. Cori CF. Mammalian carbohydrate metabolism. Physiol Rev 1931;11:143–275.
7. Exton JH. Gluconeogenesis. Metabolism 1972;21:945–990.
8. Wolfe RR, Allsop JR, Burke JF. Glucose metabolism in man: responses to intravenous glucose infusion. Metabolism 1979;28:210–220.
9. Hetenyi G Jr. Correction for the metabolic exchange of ^{14}C for ^{12}C atoms in the pathway of gluconeogenesis in vivo. Fed Proc 1982;41:104–109.
10. Windmueller HG, Spaeth AE. Intestinal metabolism of glutamine and glutamate from the lumen as compared to glutamine from blood. Arch Biochem Biophys 1975;171: 662–667.
11. Felig P. The glucose-alanine cycle. Metabolism 1973;22: 179–207
12. Wolfe RR, Wolfe MH, Nadel ER, et al. Isotopic determination of amino acid-urea interactions in exercise in humans. J Appl Physiol 1984;56:221–229.
13. Newsholme EA. Carbohydrate metabolism in vivo: regulation of the blood glucose level. Clin Endocrinol Metab 1976;5:543–578.
14. Wolfe RR, Peters EJ, Klein S, et al. Effect of short-term fasting on the lipolytic responsiveness to epinephrine infusion in normal and obese human subjects. Am J Physiol 1987;252:E189–E196.
15. Wolfe RR, Shaw JHF, Durkot MJ. Effect of sepsis on VLDL kinetics: responses in basal state and during glucose infusion. Am J Physiol 1985;248:E732–E740.
16. Bortz WM, Paul P, Hall AG, et al. Glycerol turnover and oxidation in man. J Clin Invest 1972;51:1537–1546.
17. Owen OE, Felig PF, Morgan AP, et al. Liver and kidney metabolism during prolonged starvation. J Clin Invest 1969;48:574–583.
18. Jahoor F, Peters EJ, Wolfe RR. The relationship between gluconeogenic substrate supply and glucose production in humans. Am J Physiol 1990;258:E288–E296.
19. Exton JH, Mallette LE, Jefferson LS, et al. The hormonal control of hepatic gluconeogenesis. Recent Prog Horm Res 1970;26:411–461.
20. Krebs H. Gluconeogenesis. Proc R Soc Lond [Biol] 1964;159:545–564.
21. Randle PH, Sugdon PH, Kerbey AL, et al. Regulation of pyruvate oxidation and conversation of glucose. Biochem Soc Symp 1981;43:47–67.
22. Cohen SM, Ogawa S, Shulman RG. ^{13}C NMR studies of gluconeogenesis in rat liver cells: utilization of labeled glycerol by cells from euthyroid and hyperthyroid rats. Proc Natl Acad Sci USA 1979;76:1603–1607.
23. Newsholme EA, Gevers W. Control of glycolysis and gluconeogenesis in liver and kidney cortex. Vitam Horm 1967;25:1–87.
24. Katz J, Rognstad R. Futile cycles in the metabolism of glucose. Curr Top Cell Regul 1976;10:237–289.
25. Shulman GI, Ladenson PW, Wolfe MH, et al. Substrate cycling between gluconeogenesis and glycolysis in euthyroid, hypothyroid and hyperthyroid man. J Clin Invest 1985;76:757–764.
26. Karlander S, Roovete A, Vrame M, et al. Glucose and fructose-6 phosphate cycle in humans. Am J Physiol 1986; 251:E530–E536.
27. Wolfe RR, Chinkes DL, Baba H, et al. Response of phosphoenolpyruvate cycle activity to fasting and to hyperinsulinemia in human subjects. Am J Physiol 1996; 271:E159–E176.
28. Miyoshi H, Shulman GI, Peters EJ, et al. Hormonal control of substrate cycling in humans. J Clin Invest 1988; 81:1545–1555.
29. Wolfe RR, Herndon DN, Jahoor F, et al. Effect of severe burn injury on substrate cycling by glucose and fatty acids. N Engl J Med 1987;317:403–408.
30. Efendic S, Wajngot A, Vranic M. Increased activity of the glucose cycle in the liver: early characteristics of type 2 diabetes. Proc Natl Acad Sci USA 1985;82:2965–2969.
31. Karlander S, Vranic M, Efendic S. Increased glucose turnover and glucose cycling in acromegalic patients with normal glucose tolerance. Diabetologia 1986;29:778–783.
32. Cherrington AD, Liljenquist JE, Shulman GI, et al. The importance of hypoglycemia induced glucose production during selective glucagon deficiency. Am J Physiol 1979; 236:E263–E271.
33. Liljenquist JF, Mueller GL, Cherrington AD, et al. Evidence for an important role of glucagon in the regulation of hepatic glucose production in normal man. J Clin Invest 1977;59:369–374.
34. Jahoor F, Herndon DN, Wolfe RR. Role of insulin and glucagon in the response of glucose and alanine kinetics in burn-injured patients. J Clin Invest 1986;78:807–814.
35. Cherrington AD, Williams PE, Shulman GI, et al. Differential time course of glucagon's effect on glycogenolysis and gluconeogenesis in the conscious dog. Diabetes 1981; 30:180–187.
36. Cherrington AD, Lacy WW, Chiasson JL. Effect of glucagon on glucose production during insulin deficiency in the dog. J Clin Invest 1978;62:664–677.
37. Wolfe RR, Shaw JHF, Jahoor F, et al. Response to glucose infusion in humans: role of changes in insulin concentration. Am J Physiol 1986;250:E306–E311.
38. Wahren J, Felig P, Cerasi E, et al. Splanchnic and peripheral glucose and amino acid metabolism in diabetes mellitus. J Clin Invest 1972;51:1870–1878.
39. Katz LD, Glickman MG, Rapoport S, et al. Splanchnic and peripheral disposal of oral glucose in man. Diabetes 1983;32:675–679.
40. Wolfe RR, Burke JF. Effect of glucose infusion on glucose and lactate metabolism in normal and burned guinea pigs. J Trauma 1978;18:800–805.
41. Wolfe RR, Jahoor F, Shaw JHF. Effect of alanine infusion on glucose and urea production in man. JPEN 1987; 11:109–111.
42. Newgard CB, Hirsch LJ, Foster DW, et al. Studies on the mechanism by which exogenous glucose is converted into liver glycogen in the rat. J Biol Chem 1983;258:8046–8052.
43. Hems DA. Short-term hormonal control of hepatic carbohydrate and lipid catabolism. FEBS Lett 1977;80:237–245.

44. Adkins BA, Myers SR, Hendrick GK, et al. Importance of the route of intravenous glucose delivery on hepatic glucose balance in the conscious dog. J Clin Invest 1987;79:557–565.
45. Wolfe RR, Allsop JR, Burke JF. Glucose metabolism in man: response to intravenous glucose infusion. Metabolism 1979;28:210–220.
46. Felig P, Wahren J, Hendler R. Influence of oral glucose ingestion on splanchnic glucose and gluconeogenic substrate metabolism in man. Diabetes 1975;24:468–475.
47. Andres R, Cader G, Zierler KL. The quantitatively minor role of carbohydrate in oxidative metabolism by skeletal muscle in intact man in the basal state: measurements of oxygen and glucose uptake and carbon dioxide and lactate production in the forearm. J Clin Invest 1956;35:671–682.
48. Cuatrecasas P. Insulin-receptor interactions in adipose tissue cells: direct measurement and properties. Proc Natl Acad Sci USA 1971;68:1264–1268.
49. Czech MP. Molecular basis of insulin action. Annu Rev Biochem 1977;46:359–384.
50. Wolfe RR, Nadel ER, Shaw JHF, et al. Role of changes in insulin and glucagon in glucose homeostasis in exercise. J Clin Invest 1986;77:900–907.
51. Stuart CA, Shangraw RE, Prince MJ, et al. Bedrest induced insulin resistance occurs primarily in muscle. Metabolism 1988;37:802–806.
52. Randle P, Garland PB, Hales CN, et al. The glucose-fatty acid cycle: its role in insulin sensitivity and the metabolic disturbances of diabetes mellitus. Lancet 1963;1:785–789.
53. Newsholme EA. Carbohydrate metabolism in vivo: regulation of blood glucose level. Clin Endocrinol Metab 1976;5:543–578.
54. Goodman MN, Berger M, Ruderman NB. Glucose metabolism in rat skeletal muscle at rest: effect of starvation, diabetes, ketone bodies and free fatty acids. Diabetes 1974;23:881–888.
55. Wolfe BM, Peters EJ, Schmidt BF, et al. Effect of elevated FFA on glucose oxidation in normal man. Metabolism 1988;37:323–329.
56. Thiebaud D, DeFronzo RA, Jacot E, et al. Effect of long chain triglyceride infusion on glucose metabolism in man. Metabolism 1982;31:1128–1136.
57. Bonadonna RC, Zych K, Boni C, et al. Time dependence of the interaction between lipid and glucose in humans. Am J Physiol 1989;257:E49–E56.
58. Klein S, Rosenblatt JI, Holland OB, et al. Importance of blood glucose concentration in regulating lipolysis during fasting humans. Am J Physiol 1990;258:E32–E39.
59. Wolfe RR, O'Donnell TF Jr, Stone MD, et al. Investigation of factors determining the optimal glucose infusion rate in total parenteral nutrition. Metabolism 1980;29:892–900.
60. Blackburn GL, Maini BS, Pierce EC. Nutrition in the critically-ill patient. Anesthesiology 1977;47:181–194.
61. Hochachka PW, Neely JR, Driedzic NR. Integration of lipid utilization with Krebs cycle activity in muscle. Fed Proc 1977;36:2009–2014.
62. Neely JR, Rovetto MJ, Oram JF. Myocardial utilization of carbohydrate and lipids. Prog Cardiovasc Res 1972;15:289–329.
63. Feller DD. Conversion of amino acids to fatty acids. In: Renold AE, Cahill GF, eds. Handbook of physiology: sect. 5: adipose tissue. Washington, DC: American Physiological Society, 1965:363.
64. Masoro FJ. Lipids and lipid metabolism. Annu Rev Physiol 1977;39:301–321.
65. Aarsland AA, Chinkes DL, Wolfe RR. Contributions of de novo synthesis of fatty acids and lipolysis to total VLDL-triglyceride secretion during prolonged hyperglycemia/hyperinsulinemia in normal man. J Clin Invest 1996;98:2008–2017.
66. Hellerstein MK, Christiansen M, Kaempfer S, et al. Measurement of de novo hepatic lipogenesis in humans using stable isotopes. J Clin Invest 1991;87:1841–1852.
67. Aarsland A, Chinkes DL, Wolfe RR. Hepatic and whole body fat synthesis in humans during carbohydrate overfeeding. Am J Clin Nutr 1997;65:1774–1782.
68. Linder C, Chernick SS, Fleck TR, et al. Lipoprotein lipase and uptake of chylomicron triglyceride by skeletal muscle of rats. Am J Physiol 1976;231:860–864.
69. Tan MH, Santa T, Havel RJ. The significance of lipoprotein lipase in rat skeletal muscles. J Lipid Res 1977;18:363–370.
70. Garfinkel AS, Nilson-Ehle P, Scholtz MC. Regulation of lipoprotein lipase by induction of insulin. Biochim Biophys Acta 1976;424:264–273.
71. Wolfe RR, Shaw JHF, Durkot MJ. Effect of sepsis on VLDL kinetics: responses in basal state and during glucose infusion. Am J Physiol 1985;248:E732–E740.
72. Storck R, Spitzer JA. Metabolism of isolated fat cells from various tissue sites in the rat: influence of hemorrhagic hypotension. J Lipid Res 1974;15:200–205.
73. Clutter WE, Bier DM, Shah SD, et al. Epinephrine plasma metabolic clearance rates and physiologic thresholds for metabolic and hemodynamic actions in man. J Clin Invest 1980;66:94–101.
74. Klein S, Peters EJ, Holland OB, et al. Effect of short and long-term beta-adrenergic blockade on lipolysis during fasting in humans. Am J Physiol 1989;257:E65–E73.
75. Wolfe RR, Peters EJ, Klein S, et al. Effect of short-term fasting on the lipolytic responsiveness to epinephrine infusion in normal and obese human subjects. Am J Physiol 1987;252:E189–E196.
76. Wolfe RR, Peters EJ, Jahoor F, et al. Regulation of lipolysis in severely burned children. Ann Surg 1987;206:214–221.
77. Peters EJ, Klein S, Wolfe RR. Effect of fasting on the lipolytic response to theophylline. Am J Physiol 1991;26:E500–E504.
78. Wolfe RR, Weber JM, Klein S, et al. The role of the triglyceride-fatty acid cycle in controlling fat metabolism in humans during and after exercise. Am J Physiol 1990;258:E382–E389.
79. Fredrickson DS, Gordon RS Jr. Transport of fatty acids. Physiol Rev 1958;38:585–630.
80. Fritz IB, Yue KTN. Long-chain carnitine acyltransferase and the role of acylcarnitine derivatives in the catalytic increase of fatty acid oxidation induced by carnitine. J Lipid Res 1963;4:279–288.

81. Oram JF, Bennetch SL, Neely JR. Regulation of fatty acid utilization in isolated perfused rat hearts. J Biol Chem 1973;248:5299–5309.
82. Hansford RG, Johnson RN. The steady state concentrations of coenzyme A SH and coenzyme A thioester, citrate, and isocitrate during tricarboxylate cycle oxidations in rabbit heart mitochondria. J Biol Chem 1975;250:8361–8375.
83. Randle PJ, Priestman DA, Mistry SC, Aarsland A. Glucose fatty acid interactions and the regulation of glucose disposal. J Cell Biochem 1994;55S:1–11.
84. Rennie MJ, Winder WW, Holloszy JO. A sparing effect of increased plasma fatty acids on muscle and liver glycogen content in the exercising rat. Biochem J 1976;156:647–655.
85. Berger M, Hagg SA, Goodman MN, et al. Glucose metabolism in perfused skeletal muscle. Biochem J 1976;158:191–202.
86. Goodman MN, Berger M, Ruderman NB. Glucose metabolism in rat skeletal muscle at rest: effect of starvation, diabetes, ketone bodies and free fatty acids. Diabetes 1974;23:881–888.
87. Maizels EZ, Ruderman NB, Goodman MN, et al. Effect of acetoacetate on glucose metabolism in the soleus and extensor digitorum longus muscles of the rat. Biochem J 1977;162:557–568.
88. Boden G, Chen X, Ruiz J, et al. Mechanisms of fatty acid-induced inhibition of glucose uptake. J Clin Invest 1994;93:2438–2446.
89. Boden G, Jadali F, White J, et al. Effects of fat on insulin-stimulated carbohydrate metabolism in normal men. J Clin Invest 1991;88:960–966.
90. Hargreaves M, Kiens B, Richter EA. Effect of increased plasma free fatty acid concentrations on muscle metabolism in exercising men. J Appl Physiol 1991;70:194–201.
91. Balasse EO, Neef MA. Operation of the "glucose-fatty acid cycle" during experimental elevations of plasma free fatty acid levels in man. Eur J Clin Invest 1974;4:247–252.
92. Bonadonna RC, Groop LC, Simonson DC, DeFronzo RA. Free fatty acid and glucose metabolism in human aging: evidence for operation of the Randle cycle. Am J Physiol 1994;266:E501–E509.
93. Thiebaud D, DeFronzo RA, Jacot E, et al. Effect of long chain triglyceride infusion on glucose metabolism in man. Metabolism 1982;31(11):1128–1136.
94. Hardy RW, Ladenson JH, Hendrikson FJ, Holloszy JO. Palmitate stimulates glucose transport in rat adipocytes by a mechanism involving translocation of the insulin sensitive glucose transporter. Biochem Biophys Res Commun 1991;177:343–349.
95. Wolfe RR, Allsop JR, Burke JF. Glucose metabolism in man: responses to intravenous glucose infusion. Metabolism 1979;28(3):210–220.
96. Wolfe BM, Klein S, Peters EJ, et al. Effect of elevated free fatty acids on glucose oxidation in normal humans. Metabolism 1988;37:323–329.
97. Bevilacqua S, Bonadonna R, Buzzigoli G, et al. Acute elevation of free fatty acid levels leads to hepatic insulin resistance in obese subjects. Metabolism 1987;36(5):502–506.
98. Romijn JA, Coyle EF, Sidossis LS, et al. Regulation of endogenous fat and carbohydrate metabolism in relation to exercise intensity and duration. Am J Physiol 1993;265:E380–E391.
99. Wolfe RR. Assessment of substrate cycling in humans using tracer methodology. In: Kinney JM, ed. Energy metabolism: tissue determinants and cellular corollaries [review]. New York: Raven Press, 1991:495–524.
100. Romijn JA, Coyle EF, Zhang X-J, et al. Relationship between fatty acid delivery and fatty acid oxidation during strenuous exercise. J Appl Physiol 1995;79:1939–1945.
101. Wolfe RR, Peters EJ. Lipolytic response to glucose infusion in human subjects. Am J Physiol 1987;252:E218–E223.
102. Hopkins PN, Williams RR. A simplified approach to lipoprotein kinetics and factors affecting serum cholesterol and triglyceride concentrations. Am J Clin Nutr 1981;34:2560–2590.
103. Aarsland A, Chinkes D, Wolfe RR. Contributions of de novo synthesis of fatty acids and lipolysis to VLDL secretion during prolonged hyperglycemia/hyperinsulinemia in normal man. J Clin Invest 1996;98:2008–2017.
104. Sidossis L, Wolfe RR. Hyperglycemia-induced inhibition of fatty acid oxidation: the glucose-fatty acid cycle reversed. Am J Physiol 1996;270:E733–E738.
105. Sidossis L, Stuart CA, Gastaldelli A, et al. Glucose decreases fat oxidation by direct inhibition of fatty acid entry into the mitochondria. Diabetes 1995;44:198A.
106. Wolfe RR, Peters EJ, Klein S, et al. Effect of short-term fasting on lipolytic responsiveness in normal and obese human subjects. Am J Physiol 1987;252:E189–E196.
107. Reaven GM, Hollenbeck C, Jeng CY, et al. Measurement of plasma glucose, free fatty acid, lactate and insulin for 24h in patients in NIDDM. Diabetes 1988;37:1020–1024.
108. Shaw JH, Wolfe RR. An integrated analysis of glucose, fat and protein metabolism in severely traumatized patients. Studies in the basal state and the response to total parenteral nutrition [review]. Ann Surg 1989;209:63–72.
109. Cahill GF, Herrera MG, Morgan AP. Hormone-fuel interrelationships during fasting. J Clin Invest 1966;45:1751–1769.
110. Klein S, Wolfe RR. Carbohydrate restriction regulates the adaptive response to fasting. Am J Physiol 1992;262:E631–E636.
111. Baba H, Zhang X-J, Wolfe RR. Glycerol gluconeogenesis in fasting humans. Nutrition 1995;11(2):149–153.
112. Reaven GM, Lerner RL, Stern MP, Farquhar JW. Role of insulin endogenous hypertriglyceridemia. J Clin Invest 1967;46:1756–1767.
113. Reaven GM, Hill DB, Gross RC, Farquhar JW. Kinetics of triglyceride turnover of very low density lipoproteins of human plasma. J Clin Invest 1965;44:1826–1833.
114. Romijn JA, Klein S, Coyle EF, et al. Strenuous endurance training increases lipolysis and triglyceride-fatty acid cycling at rest. J Appl Physiol 1993;75(1):108–113.
115. Klein S, Weber JM, Coyle EF, Wolfe RR. Effect of endurance training on glycerol kinetics during strenuous exercise in humans. Metabolism 1996;45:357–361.
116. Coggan AR, Spina RJ, Kohert WM, Holloszy JO. Effect of prolonged exercise on muscle citrate concentration be-

fore and after endurance training in men. Am J Physiol 1993;264:E215–E220.
117. Williamson DH, Whitelaw E. Physiological aspects of the regulation of ketogenesis. Biochem Soc Symp 1971; 43:137–161.
118. McGarry JO, Wright PH, Foster DW. Hormonal control of ketogenesis: rapid activation of hepatic ketogenic capacity in fed rats by antiinsulin serum and glucagon. J Clin Invest 1975;55:1201–1209.
119. Jahoor F, Wolfe RR. Regulation of protein catabolism. Kidney Int [Suppl S22] 1987;32:S81–S93.
120. Moldave K. Eukaryotic protein synthesis. Annu Rev Biochem 1985;54:1109–1149.
121. Pain VM. Protein synthesis and its regulation. In: Waterlow JC, Garlick PH, Millward DJ, eds. Protein turnover in mammalian tissues and in the whole body. Amsterdam: Elsevier/North Holland, 1978:16–49.
122. Heine PW, Krienke L, Richter I, et al. ^{15}N tracer kinetic studies on the nitrogen metabolism of very small pre-term infants on a diet of mother's milk. Hum Nutr Clin Nutr 1985;39C:399–409.
123. Golden MHN, Waterlow JC, Picou D. Protein turnover synthesis and breakdown before and after recovery from malnutrition. Clin Sci Mol Med 1977;53:473–477.
124. Jackson AA, Persaud C, Badaloo V, et al. Whole-body protein turnover in man determined in three hours with oral or intravenous ^{15}N-glycine and enrichment in urinary ammonia. Hum Nutr Clin Nutr 1987;41C:263–276.
125. Golden MHN, Waterlow JC. Total protein synthesis in elderly people: a comparison of results with [^{15}N]-glycine and [^{14}C] leucine. Clin Sci Mol Med 1977;53:277–288.
126. Waterlow JC, Garlick PJ, Millward DJ, eds. Protein turnover in mammalian tissues and in the whole body. Amsterdam: Elsevier/North Holland, 1978:531–535.
127. Rennie MJ, Edwards RHT, Halliday D, et al. Muscle protein synthesis measured by stable isotope techniques in man: the effects of feeding and fasting. Clin Sci 1982;63: 519–523.
128. Clugson GA, Garlick PJ. The response of protein and energy metabolism to food intake in lean and obese man. Hum Nutr Clin Nutr 1982;36C:57–70.
129. Hoffer LJ, Yang RD, Matthews DE, et al. Effects of meal consumption on whole-body leucine and alanine kinetics in young adult men. Br J Nutr 1985;53:31–38.
130. Motil KJ, Matthews DE, Bier DM, et al. Whole-body leucine and lysine metabolism: response to dietary protein intake in young men. Am J Physiol 1981;240:E712–E721.
131. Melville S, McNurlan MA, McHardy KC, et al. The role of degradation in the acute control of protein balance in man: failure of feeding to stimulate protein synthesis as assessed by 1-^{13}C-leucine infusion. Metabolism 1989;38:248–255.
132. Millward DJ, Halliday D, Rennie MJ. The extent of protein synthesis in muscle in man. Hum Nutr Clin Nutr 1984; 38C:151–154.
133. Picou D, Taylor-Roberts T. The measurement of total protein synthesis and catabolism and nitrogen turnover in infants in different nutritional states and receiving different amounts of dietary protein. Clin Sci 1969;36: 283–296.
134. Jackson AA, Golden MHN, Byfield R, et al. Whole-body protein turnover and nitrogen balance in young children at intakes of protein and energy in the region of maintenance. Hum Nutr Clin Nutr 1983;37C:433–446.
135. Fulks RM, Li JB, Goldberg AL. Effects of insulin, glucose and amino acids on protein turnover in rat diaphragm. J Biol Chem 1975;250:290–298.
136. Inoue G, Fujita Y, Niiyama Y. Studies on protein requirements of young men fed egg protein and rice protein with excess and maintenance energy intakes. J Nutr 1973;103: 1673–1687.
137. Motil KJ, Bier DM, Matthews DE, et al. Whole-body leucine and lysine metabolism studied with [1-^{13}C]-leucine and [alpha-^{15}N]-lysine: response in healthy young men given excess energy intake. Metabolism 1981;30:783–791.
138. Garlick PJ, Clugston GA, Waterlow JC. Influence of low-energy diets on whole-body protein turnover in obese subjects. Am J Physiol 1980;238:E235–E244.
139. Buse MG, Reid SS. Leucine: a possible regulator of protein turnover in muscle. J Clin Invest 1975;56:1250–1261.
140. Morgan HE, Chua BH, Boyd TA, et al. Branched-chain amino acids and the regulation of protein turnover in heat and skeletal muscle. In: Walser M, Williamson DH, eds. Metabolism and clinical implications of branched chain amino and ketoacids. Amsterdam: Elsevier/North Holland, 1981:217–226.
141. Goldberg AL, Tischler ME. Regulatory effects of leucine on carbohydrate and protein metabolism. In: Walser M, Williamson DH, eds. Metabolism and clinical implications of branched chain amino and ketoacids. Amsterdam: Elsevier/North Holland, 1981:205–216.
142. Cortiella J, Matthews DE, Hoerr RA, et al. Leucine kinetics at graded intakes in young men: quantitative fate of dietary leucine. Am J Clin Nutr 1988;48:998–1009.
143. Sherwin RS. Effect of starvation on the turnover and metabolic response to leucine. J Clin Invest 1978;61: 1471–1481.
144. Garlick PJ, McNurlan MA, Fern EB. Does leucine regulate muscle protein synthesis in vivo? In: Waterlow JC, Stephen JML, eds. Nitrogen metabolism in man. London: Applied Science, 1981:125–131.
145. Ferrando AA, Williams BD, Stuart CA, et al. Oral branched chain amino acids decrease whole-body proteolysis. JPEN 1995;19:47–54.
146. Wolfe RR, Jahoor F, Hartl WH. Protein and amino acid metabolism after injury. Diab Metab Rev 1989;5:149–164.
147. Wolfe RR, Goodenough RD, Burke JF, et al. Response of protein and urea kinetics in burn patients to different levels of protein intake. Ann Surg 1983;197:163–171.
148. Freund H, Hoover HC Jr, Atamian S, et al. Infusion of the branched chain amino acids in postoperative patients. Ann Surg 1979;190:18–23.
149. Blackburn GL, Moldawer LL, Usui S, et al. Branched chain amino acid administration and metabolism during starvation, injury and infection. Surgery 1979;86:307–315.
150. Sakamoto A, Moldawer LL, Usui S, et al. In vivo evidence for the unique nitrogen sparing mechanism of branched-chain amino acid administration. Surg Forum 1979;30:67–69.

151. Sakamoto A, Moldawer LL, Bothe A Jr, et al. Are the nitrogen-sparing mechanisms of branched-chain amino acids administration really unique? Surg Forum 1980;30:99–100.
152. Moldawer LL, Sakamoto A, Blackburn GL, et al. Alterations in protein kinetics produced by branched-chain amino acid administration during infection and inflammation. In: Walser M, Williamson DH, eds. Metabolism and clinical implications of branched chain amino and ketoacids. Amsterdam: Elsevier/North Holland, 1981:533–539.
153. Freund HR, James JH, Fischer JE. Stimulation of protein synthesis in liver and muscle and decrease in protein degradation following branched chain amino aicd infusions in the post-injury rat. In: Walser M, Williamson DH, eds. Metabolism and clinical implications of branched chain amino and ketoacids. Amsterdam: Elsevier/North Holland, 1981:541–546.
154. Yu YM, Wagner DA, Walesreswski JC, et al. A kinetic study of leucine metabolism in severely burned patients. Ann Surg 1988;207:421–429.
155. Millikan WJ Jr, Henderson JM, Galloway JR, et al. In vivo measurement of leucine metabolism with stable isotopes in normal subjects and in those with cirrhosis fed conventional and branched-chain amino acid-enriched diets. Surgery 1985;98:405–413.
156. Robert JJ, Bier DM, Zhao XH, et al. Glucose and insulin effects on de novo amino acid synthesis in young men: studies with stable isotope labeled alanine, glycine, leucine and lysine. Metabolism 1982;31:1210–1218.
157. O'Connell RC, Morgan AP, Aoki TT, et al. Nitrogen conservation in starvation: graded response to intravenous glucose. J Clin Endocrinol Metab 1974;39:555–563.
158. Moldawer LL, O'Keefe SJD, Bothe A Jr, et al. In vivo demonstration of nitrogen-sparing mechanisms for glucose and amino acids in the injured rat. Metabolism 1980;29:173–180.
159. Shaw JHF, Wolfe RR. Whole-body protein kinetics in patients with early and advanced gastrointestinal cancer: the response to glucose infusion and total parenteral nutrition. Surgery 1988;103:148–155.
160. Flaim KE, Kochel PJ, Kira Y, et al. Insulin effects on protein synthesis are independent of glucose and energy metabolism. Am J Physiol 1983;245:C133–C143.
161. Sherwin RS, Hendler RG, Felig P. Effect of ketone infusions on amino acid and nitrogen metabolism in man. J Clin Invest 1975;55:1382–1390.
162. Pawan GLS, Temple SJG. Effect of 3-hydroxybutyrate in obese subjects on very low energy diets and during therapeutic starvation. Lancet 1983;1:15–17.
163. Miles JM, Nissen SL, Rizza RA, et al. Failure of infused beta-hydroxybutyrate to decrease proteolysis in man. Diabetes 1983;32:197–205.
164. Nair KS, Welle SL, Halliday D, et al. Effect of beta-hydroxybutyrate on whole-body leucine kinetics and fractional mixed skeletal muscle protein synthesis in humans. J Clin Invest 1988;82:198–205.
165. Atchley DW, Loeb RF, Richards DW, et al. On diabetic acidosis: a detailed study of electrolyte balances following the withdrawal and reestablishment of insulin therapy. J Clin Invest 1933;12:297–326.
166. Nair KS, Garrow JS, Ford C, et al. Effect of poor diabetic control and obesity on whole-body protein metabolism in man. Diabetologia 1983;25:400–403.
167. Umpleby AM, Boroujerdi MA, Brown PM, et al. The effect of metabolic control on leucine metabolism in type 1 (insulin-dependent) diabetic patients. Diabetologia 1986;29:131–141.
168. Nair KS, Ford GC, Halliday D. Effect of intravenous insulin treatment on in vivo whole-body leucine kinetics and oxygen consumption in insulin-deprived type 1 diabetic patients. Metabolism 1987;36:491–495.
169. Rogert JJ, Beaufrere B, Koziet J, et al. Whole-body de novo amino acid synthesis in type 1 (insulin-dependent) diabetes studied with stable isotope-labelled leucine, alanine and glycine. Diabetes 1985;34:67–73.
170. Tessari P, Nosadini R, Trevisan R, et al. Defective suppression by insulin of leucine-carbon appearance and oxidation in type 1, insulin dependent diabetes mellitus: evidence for insulin resistance involving glucose and amino acid metabolism. J Clin Invest 1986;77:1797–1804.
171. Pacy PJ, Nair KS, Ford C, Halliday D. Failure of insulin infusion to stimulate fractional muscle protein synthesis in type 1 diabetic patients. Anabolic effect of insulin and decreased proteolysis. Diabetes 1989;38:618–624.
172. Darmaun B, Matthews DE, Bier DM. Effect of cortisol on glutamine, alanine, leucine and phenylalanine kinetics in man. Clin Res 1985;33:702.
173. Denne SC, Liechty EA, Liu YM, et al. Proteolysis in skeletal muscle and whole body in response to euglycemic hyperinsulinemia in normal adults. Am J Physiol 1991;261 (Endocrinol Metab 24):E809–E814.
174. Kimbal SR, Flaim KE, Peavy DE, Jefferson LS. Protein metabolism. In: Ellemberg M, Rifkin M, eds. Diabetes mellitus, theory and practice. 4th ed. New York: Elsevier, 1989:41–50.
175. DeFeo P, Gan Gaisano M, Haymond MW. Differential effects of insulin deficiency on albumin and fibrinogen synthesis in humans. J Clin Invest 1991;88:833–840.
176. Mortimore GE, Mondon CE. Inhibition by insulin of valine turnover in liver. Evidence for a general control of proteolysis. J Biol Chem 1970;245:2375–2383.
177. Woodside KH, Mortimore GE. Suppression of protein turnover by amino acids in the perfused rat liver. J Biol Chem 1972;247:6474–6481.
178. McMillan DE. Changes in serum proteins and protein-bound carbohydrates in diabetes mellitus. Diabetologia 1970;6:597–604.
179. Jonsson A, Wales JK. Blood glycoproteins levels in diabetes mellitus. Diabetologia 1976;12:245–250.
180. McNurlan MA, Garlic PJ. Protein synthesis in liver and small intestine in protein deprivation and diabetes. Am J Physiol 1981;241(Endocrinol Metab 4):E238–E245.
181. Pain WM, Garlic PJ. Effect of streptozotocin diabetes and insulin treatment on the rate of protein synthesis in tissues of the rat in vivo. J Biol Chem 1974;249:4510–4514.
182. Pain WM, Albertse EC, Garlick PJ. Protein metabolism in skeletal muscle, diaphragm and heart of diabetic rats. Am J Physiol 1983;245(Endocrinol Metab 6):E604–E610.
183. Fukagawa NK, Minaker KL, Rowe JW, et al. Insulin-mediated reduction of whole-body protein breakdown.

Dose-response effects on leucine metabolism in postabsorptive men. J Clin Invest 1985;76:2306–2311.
184. Tessari P, Trevisan R, Inchiostro S, et al. Dose-response curves of the effects of insulin on leucine kinetics in man. Am J Physiol 1986;251:E334–E343.
185. Shangraw RE, Stuart CA, Prince MJ, et al. Insulin responsiveness of protein metabolism in vivo following bedrest in humans. Am J Physiol 1988;255:E548–E558.
186. Tessari P, Inchiostro S, Biolo G, et al. Differential effects of hyperinsulinemia on leucine-carbon metabolism in vivo. Evidence for distinct mechanisms in regulation of net amino acid deposition. J Clin Invest 1987;79:1062–1069.
187. Castellino P, Luzi L, Simonson DC, et al. Effect of insulin and plasma amino acid concentration on leucine metabolism in man: role of substrate availability on estimates of whole body protein synthesis. J Clin Invest 1987;80:1784–1793.
188. Dillmann WH. Diabetes mellitus-induced changes in the concentrations of specific mRNAs and proteins. Diabetes Metab Rev 1988;4:789–797.
189. Goldstain RH, Poliks CF, Pilch PF, et al. Stimulation of collagen formation by insulin and insulin-like growth factor in cultures of human lung fibroblasts. Endocrinology 1989;124:964–970.
190. Wolfe RR. Radioactive and stable isotope tracers in biomedicine. Principles and practice of kinetic analysis. New York: Wiley-Liss, 1992.
191. Tessari P, Inchiostro S, Biolo G, et al. Effects of acute systemic hyperinsulinemia on forearm muscle proteolysis in healthy man. J Clin Invest 1991;88:27–33.
192. Arfviddsson B, Zachrisson H, Möller-Loswick AC, et al. Effect of systemic hyperinsulinemia on amino acid flux across human legs in postabsorptive state. Am J Physiol 1991;260(Endocrinol Metab 23):E46–E52.
193. Gelfand RA, Barret EJ. Effect of physiologic hyperinsulinemia on skeletal muscle protein synthesis and breakdown in man. J Clin Invest 1987;80:1–6.
194. Pozefsky T, Felig P, Tobbin JD, et al. Amino acid balance across tissues of the forearm in postabsorptive man. Effects of insulin at two dose levels. J Clin Invest 1969;48:2273–2282.
195. Heslin MJ, Newman E, Wolf RF, et al. Effect of hyperinsulinemia on whole body and skeletal muscle leucine carbon kinetics in humans. Am J Physiol 1992;262 (Endocrinol Metab 25):E911–E918.
196. Gelfand RA, Glickman MG, Castellino P, et al. Measurement of L-[1-^{14}C]leucine kinetics in splanchnic and leg tissues in humans. Diabetes 1988;37:1365–1372.
197. Bennett WM, Connacher AA, Scringeour CM, et al. Euglycemic hyperinsulinemia augments amino acid uptake by human leg tissues during hyperaminoacidemia. Am J Physiol 1990;259:E185–E194.
198. Neely AN, Cox JR, Fortney JA, et al. Alterations of lysosomal size and density during rat liver perfusion. Suppression by insulin and amino acids. J Biol Chem 1977;252:6948–6954.
199. Mortimore GE, Poso AR, Kadowaki M, Wert JJ. Multiphasic control of hepatic protein degradation by regulatory amino acids. General features and hormonal modulation. J Biol Chem 1987;262:16322–16327.
200. Hutson NJ, Lloyd CE, Mortimore GE. Regulation of hepatic protein breakdown by food intake in streptozotocin diabetic mice. Fed Proc 1981;40:1692.
201. Waterlow JC, Garlick PJ, Millward DJ. Protein turnover in mammalian tissues and in the whole body. Amsterdam, New York, Oxford: North-Holland, 1978.
202. Kettelhut IC, Wing SS, Goldberg AL. Endocrine regulation of protein breakdown in skeletal muscle. Diabetes Metab Rev 1988;4:751–772.
203. De Duve C. The lysome in retrospect. In: Dingle JT, Fell H, eds. Lysosomes in biology and pathology. Amsterdam: North-Holland:3–42.
204. Mellgren R. Ca^{2+}-dependent proteases: an enzyme system active at cellular membranes. FASEB J 1987;1:110–115.
205. Fagan JM, Waxman L, Goldberg AL. Skeletal muscle and liver contain a soluble ATP + ubiquitin-dependent proteolytic system. Biochem J 1987;243:335–343.
206. Jefferson LS, Rannels ED, Munger BL, Morgan HE. Insulin in the regulation of protein turnover in heart and skeletal muscle. Fed Proc 1974;33:1098–1104.
207. Mortimore GA, Ward WF, Schworer CM. Lysosomal processing of intracellular proteins in rat liver and its general regulation by amino acids and insulin. In: Segal HL, Dole DJ, eds. Protein turnover and lysosome function. New York: Academic Press, 1978:67–87.
208. Furuno K, Goldberg AL. The activation of protein degradation in muscle by Ca^{2+} or muscle injury does not involve a lysosomal mechanism. Biochem J 1986;237:859–864.
209. Lowell BB, Ruderman NB, Goodman MN. Evidence that lysosomes are not involved in the degradation of myofibrillar proteins in rat skeletal muscle. Biochem J 1986;234:237–240.
210. Goldberg AL, Griffin GE. Hormonal control of protein synthesis and degradation in rat skeletal muscle. J Physiol 1977;270:51–52.
211. Ward HC, Halliday D, Lim AJW. Protein and energy metabolism with biosynthetic human growth hormone after gastrointestinal surgery. Ann Surg 1987;206:56–61.
212. Ponting GA, Halliday D, Teale JD, et al. Postoperative positive nitrogen balance with intravenous pyponutrition and growth hormone. Lancet 1988;1:438–440.
213. Wilmore DW, Moylan JA, Bristow BF, et al. Anabolic effects of human growth hormone and high caloric feedings following thermal injury. Surg Gynecol Obstet 1974;138:875–884.
214. Griffin EE, Miller LL. Effects of hypothyroidism, hyperthyroidism and thyroxin on net synthesis of plasma protein by the isolated perfused rat liver. J Biol Chem 1973;248:4716–4723.
215. Flaim KE, Li JB, Jefferson LS. Protein turnover in rat skeletal muscle: effects of hypophysectomy and growth hormone. Am J Physiol 1978;234:E38–E43.
216. Flaim KE, Li JB, Jefferson LS. Effects of thyroxine on protein turnover in rat skeletal muscle. Am J Physiol 1978;235:E231–E236.
217. Woodside KH, Ward WF, Mortimore GE. Effects of glu-

cagon on general protein degradation and synthesis in perfused rat liver. J Biol Chem 1974;249:5458–5463.
218. Pozefsky T, Tancredi RG, Moxley TR, et al. Metabolism of forearm tissues in man: studies with glucagon. Diabetes 1976;25:128–135.
219. Deter RL, Bandhuin P, DeDuve C. Participation of lysosomes in cellular autophagy induced in rat liver by glucagon. J Cell Biol 1967;35:C11–C16.
220. Schworer CM, Mortimore GE. Glucagon-induced autophagy and proteolysis in rat liver: medication by selective deprivation of intracellular amino acids. Proc Natl Acad Sci USA 1979;76:3169–3173.
221. Arstila AU, Trump BF. Studies on cellular autophagocytosis: the formation of autophagic vacuoles in the liver after glucagon administration. Am J Pathol 1968;53:687–733.
222. Fitzpatrick GF, Meguid MM, Gitlitz PH, Brennan MF. Glucagon infusion in normal man: effects on 3-methylhistidine excretion and plasma amino acids. Metabolism 1977;26:477–485.
223. Nair KS, Halliday D, Matthews DE, et al. Hyperglucagonemia during insulin deficiency accelerates protein catabolism. Am J Physiol 1987;253:E208–E213.
224. Pacy PJ, Cheng KN, Ford GC, et al. Influence of glucagon on whole-body and forearm leucine metabolism. Clin Sci 1988;74(suppl 18):50–51.
225. Hartl WH, Miyoshi H, Jahoor F, et al. Bradykinin attenuates glucagon-induced leucine oxidation in human subjects. Am J Physiol 1990;259:E239–E245.
226. Griggs RC, Kingston W, Jozefowicz RF, et al. Effect of testosterone on muscle mass and muscle protein synthesis. J Appl Physiol 1989;66:498–503.
227. Urban RJ, Bodenburg YH, Gilkson C, et al. Testosterone administration to elderly men increases skeletal muscle protein synthesis, strength, and the intramuscular IGF-I system. Am J Physiol 1995;32:E820–E826.
228. Hobbs CJ, Plymate SR, Rosen CJ, Adler RA. Testosterone administration increases insulin-like growth factor-l levels in normal men. J Clin Endocrinol Metab 1993;77:776–779.

7
Glucose Transporters: Molecular, Biochemical, and Physiologic Aspects

Rebecca A. Simmons

Glucose is a vital substrate for the developing fetus. It is required by most cells for oxidative and nonoxidative adenosine triphosphate (ATP) production and serves as a precursor for other carbon-containing compounds. It is the primary fuel used for most specialized cells and is the major fuel used by the brain. Its storage in the liver as glycogen provides a means by which glucose homeostasis can be maintained, particularly during the neonatal period. Glycogen stores also represent the primary source of energy for muscle tissue during exercise in postnatal life. Because of the diverse metabolic roles played by glucose, defects in its uptake or metabolism can alter cellular function and lead to significant morbidity and mortality. This chapter focuses on the molecular biology and regulation of glucose transporters with an emphasis on the fetus and neonate.

The plasma membrane of most mammalian cells, except those of the proximal kidney and small intestine, have a passive mediated transport system for glucose. Facilitative entry of glucose into the cell is controlled by glucose transporters (GLUT), structurally related proteins that are encoded by a gene family[1-7] and expressed in a tissue specific manner (Table 7.1). A different family of proteins, Na^+-coupled transporters (SGLT), actively transport glucose across the apical membranes of polarized intestinal and renal epithelial cells.[8-13] The driving force for active glucose absorption is the electrochemical Na^+ gradient across the membrane.

Most cells contain at least one glucose transporter isoform, and many contain more than one. In most cell types, glucose transporters mediate a net uptake of glucose. Under some circumstances, glucose is transported out of the cell. For example, the Na^+-coupled transporter actively transports glucose into epithelial cells of the small intestine, and a facilitative transporter mediates the efflux of glucose from the cell into the interstitium. In the hepatocyte, the facilitative glucose transporter is responsible for the uptake of glucose from the portal circulation, and the release of glucose generated by glycogenolysis or gluconeogenesis. Thus, glucose transporters ensure efficient tissue uptake and distribution of glucose.

Sodium-Dependent Glucose Transporters

It has long been known that dietary sugars are actively absorbed from the small intestine; however only recently has the molecular mechanism involved been elucidated. Active absorption of glucose across epithelial cells of the small intestine and the kidney proximal tubule is accomplished by Na^+-glucose cotransporters located in the brush border membrane. Transport of each glucose molecule is coupled to either the cotransport of two Na^+ ions (SGLT 1) or one Na^+ ion (SGLT 2). This transport system utilizes the energy from an extracellular to intracellular Na^+-ion electrochemical gradient, generated by Na^+,K^+–adenosine triphosphatase (ATPase), to drive the accumulation of glucose into the cell. To date, three Na^+-glucose cotransporter isoforms have been isolated. These transporters belong to a major class of membrane proteins called cotransporters or symporters. These exist in bacteria, plants, and animal membranes, and actively transport sugars, amino acids, carboxylic acids, and some ions (e.g., Cl, PO_4, SO_4, I) into the cell.

SGLT 1 is a hydrophobic integral membrane protein with approximately 12 membrane-spanning domains (Figure 7.1). The gene encoding the human intestinal SGLT has been localized to the q11.2-qter region of chromosome 22.[14] It is abundantly expressed in the brush border of the small intestine and at a lower concentration in kidney, lung, and liver.

Clinical interest in the intestinal brush border Na^+-glucose cotransporter has focused on diarrhea and malabsorption. Glucose-galactose malabsorption is a rare autosomal recessive disorder characterized by onset of severe, watery diarrhea in the neonatal period. Unless

TABLE 7.1. Glucose transporter isoform distribution

Facilitated-diffusion type (GLUT)	Major site of expression	Chromosomal location
GLUT 1	erythrocytes, blood-tissue barriers (brain, placenta)	1
GLUT 2	Liver, pancreatic β-cell, small intestine	3
GLUT 3	neuron, testis	12
GLUT 4	skeletal and cardiac muscle, adipose tissue	17
GLUT 5	small intestine, sperm	1
GLUT 6	pseudogene	
GLUT 7	liver (endoplasmic reticulum)	N.D.
Na⁺-dependent type (SLGT)		
SGLT 1	small intestine, kidney	22
SGLT 2	kidney	N.D.
SGLT 3 (SAAT/pSGLT2)	kidney	N.D.

glucose and galactose are eliminated from the diet, death rapidly ensues. Wright et al.[15] have demonstrated that a single missense mutation in the gene encoding the intestinal Na⁺-glucose cotransporter is sufficient to cause life-threatening diarrhea.

SGLT 2 cDNA was originally isolated by Hediger et al.[8] from a human cDNA library. The SGLT amino acid sequence is approximately 60% identical to that of SGLT 1, and the proteins have the same predicted secondary structure. The expression of this cotransporter is restricted to the renal cortex and is located in epithelial cells of proximal tubules S1 segments.

Familial renal glycosuria is an autosomal dominant disorder, although an autosomal recessive mode of inheritance has not been excluded in all cases, affecting 0.2% to 0.6% of the general population and is characterized by the excretion of a large amount of glucose in the urine in the presence of a normal blood glucose concentration. The molecular basis for benign renal glycosuria has not been determined. It is possible that mutations in the

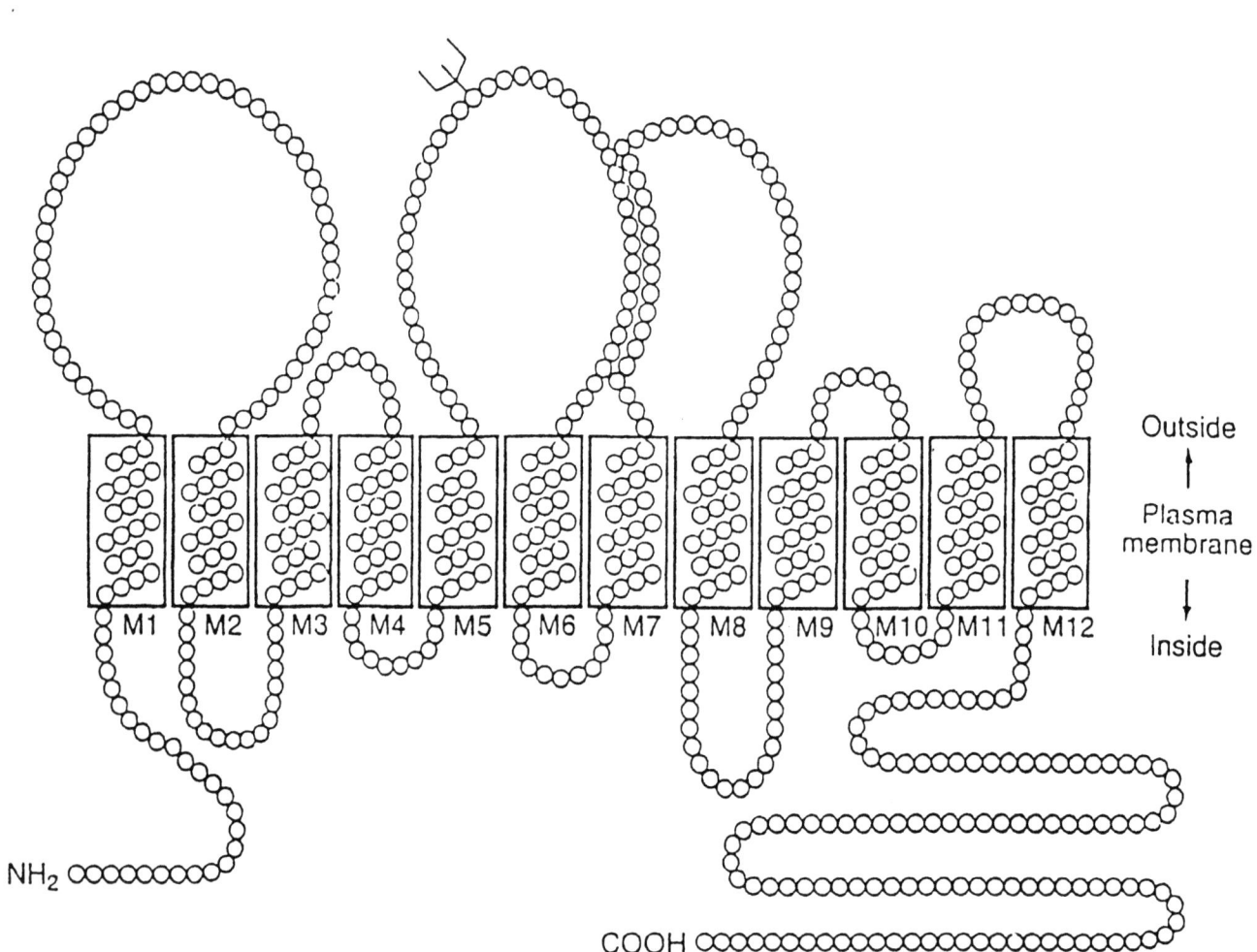

FIGURE 7.1. Schematic of glucose transporter orientation in the plasma membrane.

low affinity Na⁺-glucose cotransporter, SGLT 2, may be responsible for the defect in renal absorption of filtered glucose.

Na⁺-glucose cotransporters appear to be active prenatally, and, as a consequence, the intestine is ready to absorb the first ingested glucose.[16] The cloned cDNAs and specific antibodies for the different Na⁺-glucose cotransporters will be valuable tools for identifying the specific cells in the intestine and kidney that express these proteins, and for studying the regulation of their expression during development and in altered metabolic states such as diabetes mellitus or pregnancy.

Facilitated Glucose Transporters

The energy-independent process of transporting glucose across the cell membrane occurs by facilitative diffusion. Transport of glucose is saturable, stereoselective, and bidirectional. The kinetics of glucose transport inward and outward are not necessarily identical,[17] and, in fact, in the erythrocyte the rate of exchange flux for glucose is faster than net flux. The primary function of the facilitative glucose transporters is to mediate the exchange of glucose between the blood and the cytoplasm of the cell. This may involve a net uptake or output of glucose from the cell, depending on the type of cell in question, its metabolic state, and the metabolic state of the organism. In most cells, cytoplasmic glucose is rapidly phosphorylated by hexokinase or glucokinase, levels of glucose-6-phosphatase are low, and therefore there is little intracellular free glucose. These cells are only involved in net uptake and metabolism of blood glucose. The hepatocyte is a net producer of glucose in the postabsorptive state. Glycogenolysis and gluconeogenesis increase intracellular free glucose above its concentration in the blood, resulting in net efflux of glucose from the cell. In the postprandial state, glucose is transported into the hepatocyte to replenish glycogen stores.

The facilitative glucose transporters are a family of structurally related proteins. Six facilitated glucose transporter isoforms have been identified and are designated as GLUT (i.e., the gene symbol for facilitative glucose transporter). The human genes encoding these proteins are named GLUT 1 to 5 and GLUT 7.[2,3,18–21] GLUT 6 is a pseudogene that is not expressed at the protein level.[22] Isoforms are expressed in a tissue-specific manner, reflecting the unique glucose requirements of various tissues.

These proteins vary in size from 492 to 524 amino acids. They exhibit 39% to 68% sequence identity and 50% to 76% sequence similarity in pair-wise comparisons.[1,3,19,20,23–28] A topology map of the GLUTs has been proposed based on analysis of the primary amino acid sequence of GLUT 1.[20] Each isoform consists of 12 membrane-spanning domains, an intracytoplasmic hydrophilic loop, and an exofacial loop bearing a single N-glycosylation site. Both the NH₂ and COOH terminals are exposed intracellularly (Figure 7.2). Comparisons between the different isoforms have revealed that the sequences of the transmembrane segments and the short cytoplasmic loops connecting these transmembrane regions are highly conserved. These regions most likely are responsible for the transport of glucose. The NH₂ and COOH terminals are quite unique for each of the different isoforms and may contribute to isoform-specific properties, such as kinetics, hormone sensitivity, and subcellular localization.[1,3,18–20,22,24–27]

Structure and Properties of Facilitative Glucose Transporters

GLUT 1

GLUT 1 was the first glucose transporter to be cloned. Antibodies were raised against the purified erythrocyte glucose transporter to screen antigen-expression cDNA libraries from RNA from the human hepatoblastoma cell line (HepG2). The amino acid sequence of GLUT 1 is highly conserved. There is 98% identity between the sequences of human and rat GLUT 1, and 97% identity between the sequences of human and mouse, rabbit, or pig. This high degree of sequence conservation implies that all domains of this 492-residue protein are functionally important.

GLUT 1 is the most ubiquitously distributed of the transporter isoforms. It is found in virtually all tissues of the fetus and in many tissues and cell types of the adult.[29–36]

GLUT 1 has a very high affinity for glucose. These properties make it likely that GLUT 1 is responsible for constitutive glucose uptake. In many organs GLUT 1 is concentrated in endothelial cells of the blood-tissue barrier. Thus, one of the specialized roles of GLUT 1 is to shuttle glucose between blood and the organs that have limited access to small solutes via passive diffusion.

GLUT 1 is the predominant isoform of the fetus. Interestingly, this transporter is also expressed in fetal tissues that fail to express it significantly in the adult. Most fetal cells exhibit rapid growth and differentiation, necessitating an increased supply of energy producing substrate. This may be the reason for the prevalence of GLUT 1 in fetal tissue. After birth, GLUT 1 decreases and other isoforms such as GLUT 2 in the liver and GLUT 4 in the muscle increase.[29,32,35,36] The signals responsible for the decline in GLUT 1 expression during the neonatal period are not known. It is hypothesized that the switch from a carbohydrate to a fat source of fuel may induce this change in some organs.[35]

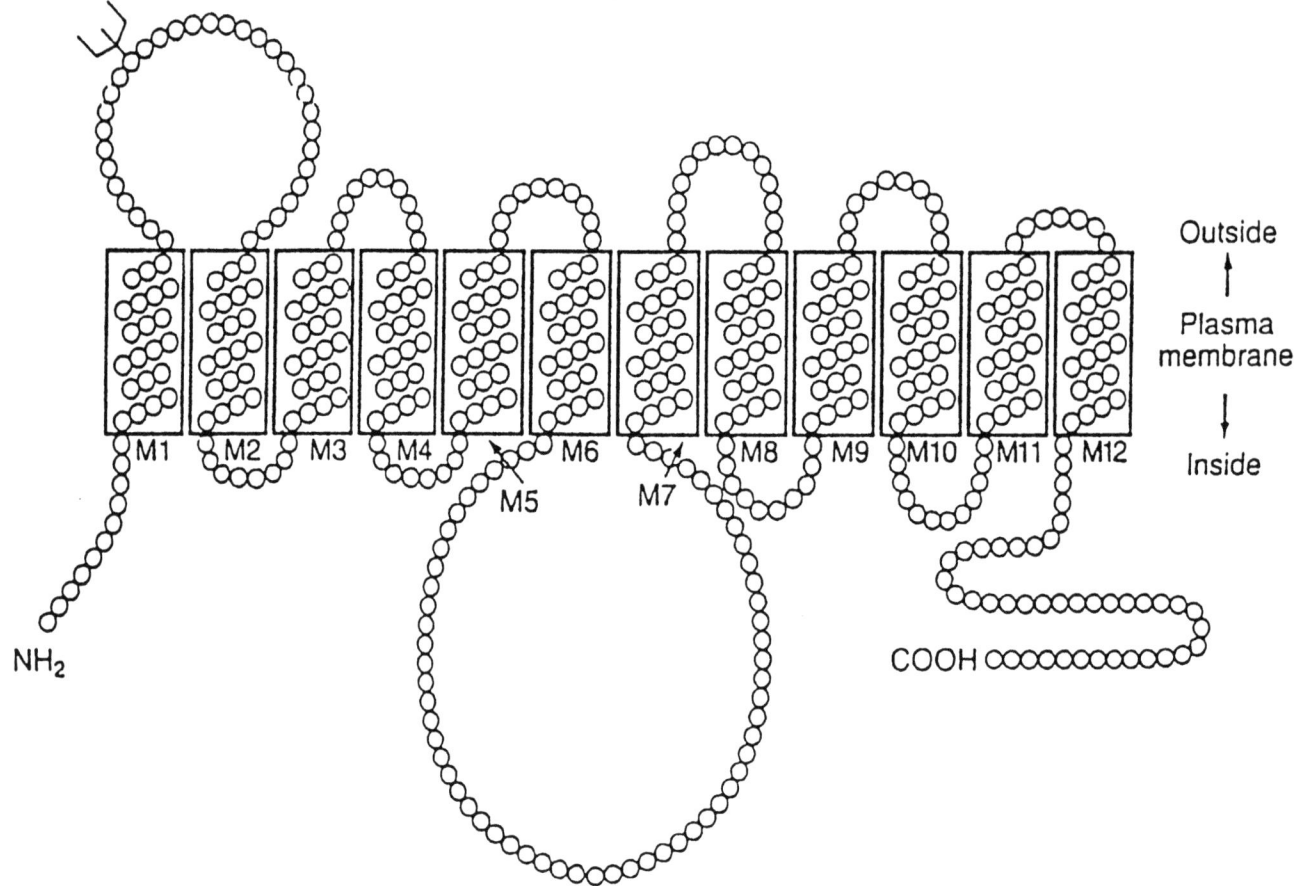

FIGURE 7.2. Schematic of glucose transporter orientation in the plasma membrane.

A majority of the studies concerning the regulation of GLUT 1 have been carried out in cultured cells and cell lines from the human and the rodent. GLUT 1 expression is induced by growth factors and hormones such as insulin, insulin-like growth factor (IGF-I), growth hormone, glucose, estrogen, transforming growth factor-β (TGF-β), thyroid hormone, cyclic adenosine monophosphate (cAMP), fibroblast growth factor, and oncogenes in many different cell types.[37–46] GLUT 1 expression also increases under conditions of cellular stress.[47] There is some evidence that the regulation of GLUT 1 in response to a variety of cellular stresses involves a similar translocation of the transporter to that observed for GLUT 4 in response to insulin.[48]

GLUT 2

GLUT 2 is the major transporter isoform expressed in the adult liver, pancreatic β cells and epithelial cells of the intestinal mucosa and kidney.[24–26] Concentration of this isoform is quite low in the fetus. GLUT 2 has 55% amino acid identity with sequences of GLUT 1, and has a similar structure and orientation in the plasma membrane. In contrast to GLUT 1, whose sequence is highly conserved, there is only 81% identity between the sequences of human and rat GLUT 2. The most characteristic feature of this isoform is its low affinity for glucose. GLUT 2 and glucokinase form a glucose-sensing apparatus in hepatocytes and β cells, which respond to subtle changes in blood glucose concentration by altering the rate of glucose transport into the cell. The transport capacity of GLUT 2 is in excess of the glucokinase-trapping reaction, thus making phosphorylation of glucose the rate-limiting step for glucose uptake in hepatocytes and β cells. In the intestine and kidney, the high-capacity low-affinity system is necessary to be able to transport glucose under conditions of the large transepithelial substrate flux that occurs after meals.

Expression of GLUT 2 appears to be developmentally regulated. β-cell content of GLUT 2 protein in the fetus is approximately half that of the adult rat.[49] Despite the reduction in GLUT 2 content, the poor insulin secretory response seen in fetal islet cells is not due to a limitation of glucose transport. At least a tenfold decrease in transport activity would be required to reduce metabolism of glucose sufficient to perturb glucose-induced insulin secretion.[50,51] Other factors appear to be responsible for the poor insulin secretory response observed in the fetus.

Studies performed in the fetal rat have demonstrated that GLUT 2 concentration is markedly diminished in the fetal hepatocytes compared to the adult.[52-54] Shortly after birth GLUT 2 protein content dramatically increases and subsequently is elevated again, coinciding with the newborn pup's weaning from high fat maternal milk.[53,54] Although an altered hormonal or substrate milieu is often implicated etiologically in the metabolic maturation associated with birth, the mechanism of this change is still unknown.

Studies done in the adult animal have shown that GLUT 2 gene expression is modulated by glucose as GLUT 2 messenger RNA (mRNA) levels increase under a high glucose milieu and decrease with hypoglycemia.[55-58] However, in an experimental model of diabetes, GLUT 2 mRNA and protein expression are decreased in the pancreatic β cells despite ambient in hyperglycemia.[59-61] It has been suggested that the decrease in GLUT 2 expression found in diabetic β cells could further limit glucose-induced insulin secretion.[59] This hypothesis has recently been supported by experiments with transgenic mice expressing GLUT 2 antisense RNA under the control of the rat insulin I promoter. This animal showed an 80% reduction in GLUT 2 in the β cells and an impaired glucose-stimulated insulin secretion, and it developed diabetes.[62]

GLUT 3

GLUT 3 was first isolated from human fetal skeletal muscle.[63] Human GLUT 3 has 64% and 52% identity with human GLUT 1 and GLUT 2, respectively, with an 83% amino acid sequence identity between the sequences of human and mouse GLUT 3. Thus, as with GLUT 2, the sequence of GLUT 3 is not as highly conserved among species as that of GLUT 1. GLUT 3 mRNA is present at variable levels in all human tissue and is most abundant in brain, kidney, and placenta. However, the tissue distribution of GLUT 3 protein is much more restricted. GLUT 3 protein is present predominantly in neuronal processes in all gray matter regions of the brain, but not in peripheral nerve tissue.[64] High levels of GLUT 3 protein are expressed in the testis, with high levels also found in spermatozoa.[64] The monocyte, and to a lesser extent the lymphocyte, also abundantly express GLUT 3.[65] In contrast to the wide distribution of GLUT 3 mRNA in the human, GLUT 3 protein is not detectable in a wide range of other tissue including placenta, lung, liver, kidney, spleen, thyroid, or adipocyte. These data suggest that GLUT 3 may provide a high-affinity glucose transport system in cells that are highly dependent on glucose as a fuel source.

The expression of GLUT 3 in brain indicates that two facilitative glucose transporters are involved in the uptake of glucose. GLUT 1 is primarily responsible for transport of glucose across the blood-brain barrier, and GLUT 3 controls the uptake of glucose into the neuron.

There is relatively little information available about the regulation of GLUT 3. Data derived from fetal rat brain suggest that glucose concentration does not regulate expression of this transporter isoform in the fetus.[66] This is in contrast to GLUT 1, where a high glucose concentration downregulates GLUT 1 protein and mRNA abundance.[39] In the adult, glucose concentration may modulate GLUT 3 expression in some tissue. A high glucose concentration has been shown to decrease GLUT 3 mRNA levels in bovine retinal cells and retinal pericytes.[67] The investigators suggest that a reduction in GLUT 3–mediated glucose transport may be related to the development of diabetic retinopathy.

GLUT 4

GLUT 4 is primarily expressed in adult tissue that exhibits insulin-stimulated glucose transport, such as adipose, skeletal, and cardiac muscle.[39] Several investigators have demonstrated that GLUT 4 is expressed in adult rat brain in the cerebellum, hypothalamus, anterior medulla oblongata, and various brain nuclei.[68,69] This suggests that insulin-sensitive glucose uptake may occur in specific areas of the brain.

Very little GLUT 4 is expressed in fetal tissues,[37] and levels do not increase until well after birth.[33,35] The sequence of human GLUT 4 is highly conserved, and there is 95% and 96% identity between the sequences of human and rat or mouse.

Insulin causes a rapid and reversible increase in glucose uptake in adipocytes and skeletal muscle. This increase results primarily from translocation of a latent pool of glucose transporters from intracellular vesicles to the plasma membrane.[70] Glucose transport in insulin-sensitive tissue has received considerable attention because of the importance of this process in the maintenance of whole-body glucose disposal. The transport step is rate-limiting for glucose uptake into fat and muscle under most conditions.[71,72]

Intense effort has been devoted to studying the role of GLUT 4 in adult-onset diabetes [non–insulin-dependent diabetes mellitus (NIDDM)]. Diabetes mellitus is associated with an insulin-resistant state. The impaired ability of insulin to stimulate glucose utilization occurs in muscle and adipose tissue. Several studies have demonstrated a significant decrease in GLUT 4 content in adipose tissue from patients with NIDDM and gestational diabetes.[73,74] However, there does not appear to be any significant linkage between mutations in GLUT 4 and NIDDM.

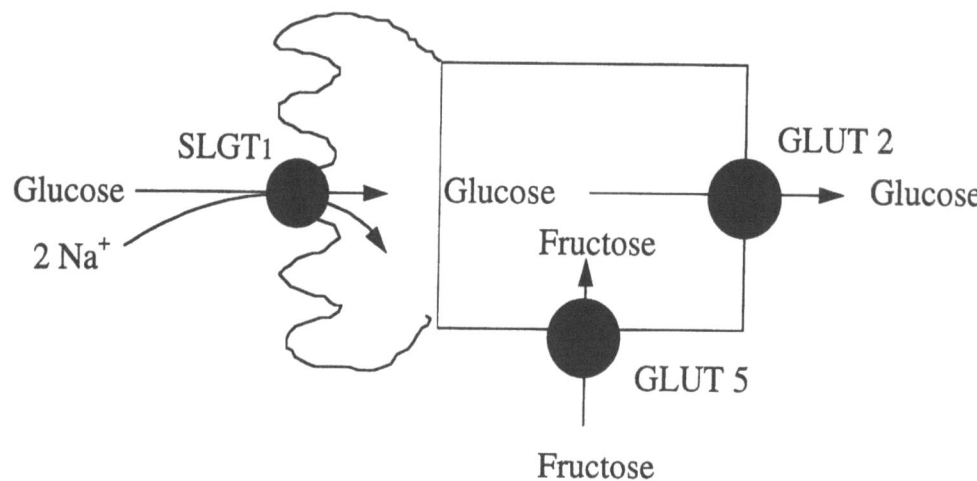

FIGURE 7.3. Glucose transport in the intestinal epithelial cells.

There is little reduction in the GLUT 4 content of skeletal muscle obtained from NIDDM patients despite a marked impairment in insulin-regulated glucose transport in this tissue.[75,76] Thus, it is likely that other defects, possibly in trafficking of GLUT 4 or in the insulin-signaling pathway, result in impaired glucose transport in muscle.

Mice with genetic ablation of GLUT 4 expression are not overtly diabetic, but exhibit only moderate insulin resistance, with postprandial hyperinsulinemia and mild hyperglycemia during an oral glucose-tolerance test.[77] Homozygous GLUT 4 deficiency also results in growth retardation, shortened life span, cardiac hypertrophy, marked reduction in adipose tissue content, and decreased free fatty acids. Interestingly, hyperinsulinemia is even more marked in mice heterozygous for GLUT 4 deficiency.[78] These data suggest that homozygous knockout mice compensate for the lack of GLUT 4 by increased expression or function of another glucose transporter.

Not unexpectedly, overexpression of GLUT 4 in transgenic mice improves glucose uptake. Mice overexpressing GLUT 4 in muscle and adipose tissue demonstrate increased basal and insulin-stimulated glucose transport.[79-83] Overexpression of GLUT 4 in muscle and adipose tissue of db/db diabetic mice results in significant reduction in fasting and fed glucose concentrations and enhanced glucose disposal during a glucose tolerance test.[84]

GLUT 5

GLUT 5 is the most divergent member of the glucose transporter family.[22] Human GLUT 5 shares 42%, 40%, 39%, and 42% identity with human GLUT 1, 2, 3, and 4, respectively.[85] GLUT 5 is expressed at high levels in the apical membrane of intestinal enterocytes and mature spermatocytes in adults. Fructose is transported across intestinal epithelial cells by passive transport (Figure 7.3). There is also a high rate of fructose utilization by testes. In view of these data, it seems likely that GLUT 5 is the major mammalian fructose transporter.

GLUT 5 is also found in smaller quantities in adult human kidney, brain, muscle, and adipose tissue.[86,87] The physiologic significance of GLUT 5 in these tissues is unknown.

GLUT 7

A new isoform, referred to as GLUT 7, has been cloned from rat liver.[88,89] The deduced amino acid sequence shows sequence similarities to GLUT 2. GLUT 7 contains a consensus sequence motif within its COOH-terminal tail for the retention of membrane-spanning proteins in the endoplasmic reticulum.[90,91] It colocalizes with the gluconeogenic enzyme glucose-6-phosphatase. An enzyme complex composed of both glucose-6-phosphatase and GLUT 7 may exist within the endoplasmic reticulum to ensure movement of glucose-6-phosphate in and free glucose out. Its role in human tissue remains to be determined.

Localization and Regulation of Facilitative Glucose Transporters

Embryo

Reverse-transcription polymerase chain reaction (RT-PCR), immunofluorescence, and immunoelectron microscopy techniques have confirmed that GLUT 1 is expressed in all stages of embryonic development of the mouse, rat, rabbit, and cow. Studies, however, have not been performed in the human, including the oocyte and the blastocyst. It is readily detectable in trophectoderm and inner-cell mass cells of the mouse blastocyst, and is associated with the intracellular membrane as well as the plasma membrane of all cell types.[92-95] During organogenesis in the rat embryo, GLUT 1 is localized to the neural tube, as well as the heart tube, gut, and optic vesicle.[96]

GLUT 2 also appears to be an important mediator of glucose uptake in the early embryo. GLUT 2 is expressed as early as the 8-cell blastocyst stage. It is located on trophoectoderm membranes facing the blastocyst cavity.[92,94]

During organogenesis, the embryo is dependent on anaerobic glycolysis, an inefficient pathway for the generation of energy as only 2 mol of ATP are synthesized per mole of glucose. Therefore, high-affinity glucose transporters such as GLUT 1 and GLUT 3 are required for glucose uptake. Expression of GLUT 3 appears by day 10 of gestation in the rat, and is found in the surface ectoderm, yolk sac, and gut.[96] Interestingly, GLUT 3 soon disappears and is found in only very small quantities in fetal brain. This suggests that GLUT 1 can provide for the majority of glucose uptake in the developing fetus.

Placenta

In the human placenta, villi are in direct contact with maternal blood. The surface of the placental villi is covered with a single syncytiotrophoblast layer, formed by the fusion of the underlying cytotrophoblast elements. Fetal capillaries lie directly beneath the syncytiotrophoblast. Transfer of glucose from maternal to fetal blood occurs via the placental villi and is most likely mediated by GLUT 1. GLUT 1 is abundantly expressed in the plasma membranes of both the basal and apical sides of the syncytiotrophoblast. GLUT 1 may facilitate the entry of glucose into the cytoplasm of the syncytiotrophoblast from maternal blood, while GLUT 1 at the basal plasma membrane may aid in the exit of glucose from the cytoplasm of the syncytiotrophoblast to the pericapillary space of the fetus. GLUT 1 on the endothelial cell of the capillary then transfers glucose into the fetal circulation.[94-100] Protein and mRNA levels of GLUT 1 increase in the placenta as the fetus matures underscoring the importance of this transporter in fetal development.[98]

GLUT 3 is found only on amnion epithelial cells and cytotrophoblast.[98,101] While GLUT 3 is much more restricted in its expression in the placenta than is GLUT 1, its function is equally important. GLUT 3 is a high-affinity transporter and is likely to be saturated with maternal-derived glucose under normal physiologic conditions. If maternal glucose availability were to decrease drastically, GLUT 3 would be capable of scavenging maternal glucose for use by the placenta and fetus. Glucose transporter isoforms other than GLUT 1 and 3 have not been detected in human placenta.

Data regarding the regulation of glucose transporter expression in the human placenta are very limited. A few studies have been carried out in the placenta from pregnancy complicated by intrauterine growth retardation (IUGR) and diabetes. The growth-retarded fetus is often hypoglycemic, and impaired placental glucose transport has been implicated as a pathophysiologic mechanism. The growth-retarded fetus has a reduced umbilical venoarterial concentration difference of glucose, and lower fetal weight-specific umbilical volume flow.[102,103] However, placentas from the preterm and term intrauterine growth-retarded neonate have not shown a difference in levels of GLUT 1 protein[104] (see Chapter 48).

Gestational diabetes is associated with placenta overgrowth and an increase in transplacental glucose transfer to the fetus. Despite these changes in the maternal/fetal glucose relationship preliminary data have not found altered GLUT 1 and GLUT 3 expression in the placenta from the diabetic pregnancy.[105,106] These investigations suggest that glucose transporter protein expression is not strongly regulated in the human placenta; however, further studies examining glucose transporter function are needed.

Brain

Brain glucose utilization accounts for approximately 80% of whole-body glucose disposal in the human.[107] Furthermore, there is heterogeneity in glucose utilization among different regions of the brain. Circulating glucose crosses the blood-brain barrier and enters brain parenchyma cells via facilitative glucose transporters. Most studies of GLUT expression in the nervous system of the developing animal have been performed in the rat. Prior to the formation of the blood-brain barrier, GLUT 1 is abundant in the germinal neuroepithelium, which gives rise to both neurons and neuroglia.[108] Just before birth GLUT 1 is abundant in the brain vasculature, meninges, ependyma, and choroid plexus. After birth, GLUT 1 is also found in glial cells.[108] GLUT 1 is developmentally regulated in rat and rabbit brain.[29-31] Its expression is highest in adult brain, followed by fetal and neonatal brain, respectively.

Few localization studies have been done in the human fetus. One report has demonstrated that the localization of GLUT 1 in the mid-to-late-gestation human fetus is similar to the rat (i.e., it is primarily located in the microvascular endothelial cells that constitute the blood-brain barrier).[87] Little GLUT 1 is expressed in the parenchyma. To date, no studies have identified GLUT 3 in the human fetal brain.

After birth, GLUT 3 is found in the cerebellum in neurofilament-positive cellular transverse fibers, cell bodies of Purkinje cells, and other neuronal elements in close proximity to the Purkinje layer.[87] This region-specific pattern of GLUT 3 expression may reflect the differing glucose requirements of anatomically distinct regions of the brain. Localization of GLUT 3 is similar to the distribution of glucose utilization, which during early infancy is mainly infratentorial, and later in development occurs in supratentorial structures as well.[109,110] Regulation of glucose transport in the fetal brain is uniquely different from that in the adult brain. Before birth, low glucose concentrations, both in vivo or in vitro, fail to upregulate glucose transport in the whole fetal rat brain[66] or in isolated glial cells. However, after birth hypoglycemia induces a marked increase in GLUT 1 expression in whole rat brain isolated glial cells.[111] Furthermore, glucose transport in the fetal brain does not respond to insulin or IGF-I,[37] two hormones that increase GLUT 1 expression in glial cells of older animals.[112,113] The mechanisms underlying these differences in regulation of glucose transport that occur with maturation are unknown.

Lung

Glucose is an important metabolic substrate for the lung, providing carbon moieties for energy production and synthesis of surfactant. In adult lung, transport of glucose across the apical membrane of the type II pneumocyte occurs by sodium-coupled transport,[114-116] and across the basolateral membrane by facilitative glucose transport. To date, GLUT 1 is the only isoform found to be expressed in the type II pneumocyte of the fetal rat and humans.[117] It is hypothesized that SGLT 1 is also expressed in the type II pneumocyte; however, no study has thus far been able to localize this transporter in fetal lung.

GLUT 1 is abundantly expressed in the fetal lung when compared to that of the juvenile and adult rat.[36] Glucose utilization and levels of GLUT 1 mRNA and protein dramatically decline as the animal matures.[36,118,119] By day 14 of life, GLUT 1 is undetectable in the rat pup. The factors responsible for this significant decrease in the synthesis of GLUT 1 are unknown.

Insulin and IGF-I are important modulators of glucose transport in the type II pneumocyte of the fetal rat. Physiologic concentrations of insulin and IGF-I stimulate glucose transport,[37] while a higher concentration of insulin inhibits glucose uptake.[120] Several animal studies suggest that hyperinsulinemia, through its inhibitory effects on glucose transport, contributes to the decrease in surfactant synthesis observed in the infant of the diabetic mother. In a model that somewhat mimics human gestational diabetes, diabetes is induced in the pregnant rat by streptozotocin. The fetal rat is hyperglycemic, hyperinsulinemic, and large for gestational age. Type II pneumocytes from these animals exhibit markedly diminished glucose uptake and GLUT 1 expression.[121] It is possible that the decrease in glucose uptake diminishes the supply of glucose available for surfactant synthesis. This could be one factor that increases the risk of respiratory distress syndrome in the infant of the diabetic mother.

Liver

Transport of glucose across the hepatocyte does not appear to be rate limiting for glucose metabolism. However, glucose transport is developmentally regulated in the human and rat, and glucose transport contributes to the changes in glucose metabolic capacity from fetal to extrauterine life. The major glucose transporter in the adult hepatocyte is GLUT 2. GLUT 1 is expressed only in the perivenous hepatocyte.

In contrast, in the fetus, GLUT 1 and GLUT 2 are abundantly expressed in the hepatocyte.[52,54] During the fetal to neonatal transition, there is a shift from abundant GLUT 1 in the hepatocyte to an adult pattern of little GLUT 1 expression.[29,53] Many metabolic and hormonal factors dramatically change during the perinatal period. The factors responsible for the switch in Glut 1 expression remain to be delineated.

Muscle

A majority of the studies regarding glucose transport in muscle have been carried out in the adult. As described earlier, GLUT 4 is the predominant isoform expressed in adult muscle. In response to insulin, this transporter isoform significantly increases the transport of glucose into the myocyte. In contrast to the marked insulin responsiveness observed in the adult, fetal muscle only modestly responds to insulin. Insulin and IGF-I increase GLUT 1 expression 1.5-fold in normal fetal rat muscle explants[37] compared to the 20-fold increase observed in adult muscle.[122,123] Interestingly, insulin does not stimulate GLUT 1 expression in isolated myoblasts from a fetal rat,[35] suggesting that stimulation of glucose transport by insulin requires tissue-specific additional factors.

GLUT 1 is localized to the myoblast and levels are quite high in the fetal and newborn rat pup. GLUT 1 decreases significantly during weaning.[35,124,125] It appears that the switch from GLUT 1 to GLUT 4 expression during this time period is secondary to dietary factors. If rats are weaned to a diet rich in fat, the normal increase in GLUT 4 is prevented.[35,124,125] The molecular mechanisms responsible for this observation are unknown.

Kidney

The kidney, small intestine, and liver can all release glucose during periods of decreased glucose availability. Although the liver is the principal supplier of glucose during a short fast, the kidney also produces glucose during prolonged starvation. The Na$^+$-glucose cotransporter, SGLT 1, transports glucose into the brush-border cell of the proximal tubule of the kidney. GLUT 2, localized on the basolateral membrane of epithelial cells lining the renal tubule, is involved in the net release of glucose into the blood during absorption of renal glucose.

No data are available concerning the regulation of glucose transport in the fetal kidney, and only a few reports have described the ontogeny of renal glucose transport. SGLT 1 is expressed in a lower quantity in the fetal compared to the adult kidney. GLUT 2 is also present in the fetal kidney and its expression increases with maturation.

As described above, a single missense mutation on SGLT 1 has been described in a family affected with the autosomal recessive glucose-galactose malabsorption. It will now be possible to screen families with benign renal glycosuria in hopes of identifying another mutation or defect in SGTL 1.

Implications

Glucose transporters have acquired distinct physiologic and biochemical properties that allow them to serve specific functions in the tissues in which they are expressed. An understanding of the mechanisms underlying tissue-specific expression of these transporters will facilitate an understanding of in vivo glucose utilization and clearance processes that occur in the normal and disease state. Although studies in adults provide insight into the regulation of glucose transport, similar studies are required in the fetus and neonate to fully understand the role of the glucose transporter in fetal and neonatal development.

References

1. James DE, Strube M, Mueckler M. Molecular cloning and characterization of an insulin-regulatable glucose transporter. Nature 1989;333:83–87.
2. Fukumoto H, Serino S, Imura H, et al. Sequence, tissue distribution, and chromosomal localization of mRNA encoding a human glucose transporter-like protein. Proc Natl Acad Sci USA 1988;85:5434–5438.
3. Kayano T, Fukumoto H, Eddy RL, et al. Evidence for a family of human glucose transporter-like proteins: sequence and gene localization of a protein expressed in fetal skeletal muscle and other tissues. J Biol Chem 1988;263:15245–15248.
4. Wheeler TJ, Hinkle PC. The glucose transporter of mammalian cells. Annu Rev Physiol 1985;47:503–517.
5. Lodish HF. Anion-exchange and glucose transport proteins: structure, function, and distribution. Harvey Lect 1988;82:19–46.
6. Gould GW, Bell GI. Facilitative glucose transporters: an expanding family. Trends Biochem Sci 1990;15:18–22.
7. Pilch PF. Glucose transporters: What's in a name? Endocrinology 1990;126:3–5.
8. Hediger MA, Coady MJ, Ikeda TS, Wright EM. Expression, cloning and cDNA sequencing of the Na$^+$/glucose cotransporter. Nature 1987;330:379–381.
9. Meddings JB, DeSouza D, Goel M, Thiesen S. Glucose transport and microvillus membrane physical properties along the crypt-villus axis of the rabbit. J Clin Invest 1990;85:1099–1107.
10. Ikeda TS, Hwang ES, Coady MJ, et al. Characterization of a Na$^+$/glucose cotransporter cloned from rabbit small intestine. J Membr Biol 1989;110:87–95.
11. Malo C, Berteloot A. Proximo-distal gradient of Na$^+$-dependent D-glucose transport activity in the brush border membrane vesicles from the human fetal small intestine. FEBS Lett 1987;220:201–205.
12. Turner DJ, Kempner ES. Radiation inactivation studies of the renal brush-border membrane phlorizin-binding protein. J Biol Chem 1982;257:10794–10797.
13. Takahashi M, Malathi P, Prieser II, Jung CY. Radiation inactivation studies on the rabbit kidney sodium-dependent glucose transporter. J Biol Chem 1985;260:10551–10556.
14. Hediger MA, Budard ML, Emanual BS, et al. Assignment of the human intestinal Na$^+$/glucose gene (SGLT 1) to the q 11.2–q ter region of chromosome 22. Genomics 1989;4:297–300.
15. Wright EM, Turk E, Zakel B, et al. Molecular genetics of intestinal glucose transport. J Clin Invest 1991;88:1435–1440.
16. Buddington RK, Diamond JM. Ontogenetic development of intestinal nutrient transporters. Annu Rev Physiol 1989;51:601–619.
17. Carruthers A. Facilitative diffusion of glucose. Physiol Rev 1990;70:1135–1176.
18. Birnbaum MJ. Identification of a novel gene encoding an insulin-responsive glucose transporter protein. Cell 1989;57:305–315.
19. Birnbaum MJ, Haspel HC, Rosen OM. Cloning and characterization of cDNA encoding the rat brain glucose-transporter protein. Proc Natl Acad Sci USA 1986;83:5784–5788.
20. Mueckler M, Caruso S, Baldwin M, et al. Sequence and structure of a human glucose transporter. Science 1985;229:941–945.
21. Bell GI, Burant CF, Takeda J, Gould GW. Structure and function of mammalian facilitative sugar transporters. J Biol Chem 1993;268:19161–19164.
22. Kayano T, Burant CF, Fukumoto H, et al. Human facilitative glucose transporters: isolation, functional characterization, and gene localization of cDNAs encoding an isoform (Glut 5) expressed in small intestine, kidney,

muscle, and adipose tissue and an unusual glucose transporter pseudo-gene-like sequence (Glut 6). J Biol Chem 1990;265:13276–13282.
23. Shows TB, Eddy RL, Byers MG, et al. Polymorphic human glucose transporter gene (Glut) is on chromosome 1p31.3–p35. Diabetes 1987;36:546–549.
24. Fukumoto H, Seino S, Imura H, et al. Identification of a human liver-type glucose transporter: cDNA sequence, expression and localization of the gene to chromosome 3. Proc Natl Acad Sci USA 1988;85:5434–5438.
25. Thomas B, Sarkar HK, Kaback HR, Lodish HF. Cloning and functional expression in bacteria of a novel glucose transporter present in liver, intestine, kidney, and beta pancreatic islet cells. Cell 1988;55:281–290.
26. Permutt MA, Koranyi L, Keller K, et al. Cloning and functional expression of a human pancreatic islet glucose transporter cDNA. Proc Natl Acad Sci USA 1989;86:8688–8692.
27. Fukumoto H, Kayano T, Buse JB, et al. Cloning and characterization of the major insulin-responsive glucose transporter expressed in human skeletal muscle and other insulin-responsive tissues. J Biol Chem 1989;264:7776–7779.
28. Bell GI, Murray JC, Nakamura Y, et al. Polymorphic human insulin-responsive glucose transporter gene on chromosome 17p13. Diabetes 1989;38:1072–1075.
29. Werner H, Adamo M, Lowe WL, et al. Developmental regulation of rat brain/Hep G2 glucose transporter gene expression. Mol Endocrinol 1989;3:273–279.
30. Sadiq F, Holtzclaw L, Chundu K, et al. The ontogeny of the rabbit brain glucose transporter. Endocrinology 1990;126:2417–2424.
31. Sivitz W, DeSautel S, Walker PS, Pessin JE. Regulation of the glucose transporter in developing rat brain. Endocrinology 1989;124:1875–1880.
32. Devaskar S, Zahm DS, Holtzclaw L, et al. Developmental regulation of the distribution of rat brain insulin-insensitive (Glut 1) glucose transporter. Endocrine 1991;129:1530–1540.
33. Santalucia T, Camps M, Castello A, et al. Developmental regulation of Glut 1 (erythroid/Hep2) and Glut 4 glucose transporter expression in rat heart, skeletal muscle, and brown adipose tissue. Endocrinology 1992;130:837–846.
34. Studelska DR, Campbell C, Pary S, et al. Developmental expression of insulin-regulatable glucose transporter Glut 4. Am J Physiol 1992;263:E102–E106.
35. Leturque A, Postic C, Ferre P, Girard J. Nutritional regulation of glucose transporter and adipose tissue of weaned rats. Am J Physiol 1991;260:E588–E593.
36. Simmons RA, Flozak AS, Ogata ES. Glut 1 gene expression in growth-retarded juvenile rats. Pediatr Res 1994;35:382A.
37. Simmons RA, Flozak AS, Ogata ES. The effect of insulin and IGF-I upon glucose transport in normal and small for gestational age fetal rats. Endocrinology 1993;133:1361–1368.
38. Cartee GD, Bohn EE. Growth hormone reduces glucose transport but not Glut-1 or Glut-4 in adult and old rats. Am J Physiol 1995;268:E902–E909.
39. Simmons RA, Flozak AS, Ogata ES. Glucose regulated Glut 1 function and expression in fetal rat lung and muscle in vitro. Endocrinology 1993;132:2312–2318.
40. Hart CD, Flozak AS, Simmons RA. Modulation of glucose transport in fetal rat lung by estrogen and dihydrotestosterone. Pediatr Res 1995;37:335A.
41. Kitagawa T, Masumi A, Akamatsu Y. Transforming growth factor-B_1 stimulates glucose uptake and the expression of glucose transporter mRNA in quiescent Swiss mouse 3T3 cells. J Biol Chem 1991;266:18066–18071.
42. Weinstein SP, O'Boyle E, Haker RS. Thyroid hormone increases basal and insulin-stimulated glucose transport in skeletal muscle. Diabetes 1994;43:1185–1189.
43. Cornelius P, Marlowe M, Call K, Pekala PH. Regulation of glucose transport as well as glucose transporter and immediate early gene expression in 3T3-L1 preadipocytes by 8-bromo-cAMP. J Cell Physiol 1991;146:298–308.
44. Leuthner SR, Flozak AS, Simmons RA. Regulation of glut 1 gene expression by cAMP in fetal rat brain. Pediatr Res 1994;35:382A.
45. Hiraki Y, Rosen OM, Birnbaum MJ. Growth factors rapidly induce expression of the glucose transporter gene. J Biol Chem 1988;263:13655–13662.
46. Flier JS, Mueckler MM, Usher P, Lodish HF. Elevated levels of glucose transporter and transporter messenger RNA are induced by ras and src oncogenes. Science 1987;235:1492–1495.
47. Pasternak CA, Aiyathurai JEJ, Makinde V, et al. Regulation of glucose uptake by stressed cells. J Cell Physiol 1991;149:324–331.
48. Widnedd C. Control of glucose transport by GLUT 1: regulated secretion in an unexpected environment. Biosci Rep 1995;15:427–443.
49. Hughes SJ. The role of reduced glucose transporter content and glucose metabolism in the immature secretory responses of fetal rat pancreatic islets. Diabetologia 1994;37:134–140.
50. Meglasson MD, Matschinsky FM. Pancreatic islet glucose metabolism and regulation of insulin secretion. Diabetes Metab Rev 1986;2:163–214.
51. Lenzen S. Glucokinase: signal recognition enzyme for glucose-induced insulin secretion. London: Portland Press, 1992:101–125.
52. Lane RH, Flozak AS, Ogata ES, Simmons RA. Hepatic glucose transporter gene expression in altered fetal growth. Pediatr Res 1995;37:312A.
53. Postic C, Leturque A, Printz RL, et al. Development and regulation of glucose transporter and hexokinase expression in rat. Am J Physiol 1994;266:E548–E559.
54. Levitsky LL, Sheng Q, Mink K, Rhoads DB. Glut 1 and Glut 2 mRNA, protein, and glucose transporter activity in cultured fetal and adult hepatocytes. Am J Physiol 1994;267:E88–E94.
55. Asano J, Katagiri H, Tsukuda, et al. Upregulation of Glut 2 mRNA by glucose, mannose, and fructose in isolated rat hepatocytes. Diabetes 1992;41:22–25.
56. Chen L, Alam T, Johnson JH, et al. Regulation of B-cell glucose tranporter gene expression. Proc Natl Acad Sci USA 1990;87:4088–4092.

57. Postic C, Burdelin R, Rencurel F, et al. Evidence for a transient inhibitory effect of insulin on Glut 2 expression in the liver: in vivo and in vitro studies. Biochem J 1993; 293:119–124.
58. Waeber G, Thompson N, Haefliger JA, et al. Characterization of the murin high Km glucose transporter gene and its transcriptional regulation by glucose in a differentiated insulin-secreting cell line. J Biol Chem 1994;269:26912–26919.
59. Johnson JH, Ogawa A, Chen L, et al. Underexpression of B-cell high Km glucose transporters in non-insulin-dependent diabetes. Science 1990;250:546–548.
60. Ohneda M, Johnson JH, Inman LR, et al. Glut 2 expression and function in B-cells of GK rats with NIDDM. Diabetes 1993;42:1065–1072.
61. Orci L, Ravazzola M, Baetens D, et al. Evidence that down-regulation of B-cell glucose transporters in non-insulin-dependent diabetes may be the cause of diabetic hyperglycemia. Proc Natl Acad Sci USA 1990;87:9953–9957.
62. Valera A, Solanes G, Fernandez-Alvarez J, et al. Expression of Glut-2 antisense RNA in B-cells of transgenic mice leads to diabetes. J Biol Chem 1994;269:28543–28546.
63. Yano H, Seino Y, Inagaki N, et al. Tissue distribution and species difference of the brain type glucose transporter (Glut 3). Biochem Biophys Res Commun 1991;174:470–477.
64. Haber RS, Weinstein SP, O'Boyle E, et al. Tissue distribution of the human Glut 3 glucose transporter. Endocrinology 1993;132:2538–2543.
65. Estrad DE, Elliot E, Zinman B, et al. Regulation of glucose transport and expression of Glut 3 transporters in human circulating mononuclear cells: studies in cells from insulin-dependent diabetic and nondiabetic individuals. Metabolism 1994;43:591–598.
66. Simmons RA, Flozak AS, Ogata ES. Glucose regulates Glut 1 function and gene expression in fetal rat brain. Pediatr Res 1993;35:71A.
67. Knott RM, Robertson M, Forrester JV. Regulation of glucose transporter (Glut 3) and aldose reductase mRNA in bovine retinal endothelial cells and retinal pericytes in high glucose and high galactose culture. Diabetologia 1993;36:808–812.
68. Leloup C, Arluison M, Kassis N, et al. Discrete brain areas express the insulin-responsive glucose transporter Glut-4. Mol Brain Res 1996;38:45–53.
69. Raynor DV, Thomas MEA, Trayhurn DA. Glucose transporters (Gluts 1–4) and their mRNAs in regions of the rat brain: insulin-sensitive transporter expression in the cerebellum. Can J Physiol Pharmacol 1994;72:476–479.
70. Slot JW, Gevze HJ, Gigengack S, et al. Immunolocalization of the insulin regulatable glucose transporter in brown adipose tissue of the rat. J Cell Biol 1991;113: 123–135.
71. Koranyi LI, Bouney RE, Vuorinen MH, et al. Levels of skeletal muscle glucose transporter protein correlates with insulin-stimulated whole body glucose disposal in man. Diabetologia 1991;34:763–765.
72. Eriksson J, Koranyi L, Bourey R, et al. Insulin resistance in type 2 (non-insulin-dependent) diabetic patients and their relatives is not associated with a defect in the expression of the insulin-responsive glucose transporter (GLUT-4) gene in human skeletal muscle. Diabetologia 1992;35:143–147.
73. Garvey WT, Maianu L, Huecksteadt TP, et al. Pretranslational suppression of a glucose transporter protein causes insulin resistance in adipocytes from patients with non-insulin-dependent diabetes mellitus and obesity. J Clin Invest 1991;87:1072–1081.
74. Okuno S, Akazawa S, Yasuhi, et al. Decreased expression of the GLUT4 glucose transporter protein in adipose tissue during pregnancy. Horm Metab Res 1995;27:231–234.
75. Pedersen OJ, Bak JF, Andersen PH, et al. Evidence against altered expression of Glut 1 or Glut 4 in skeletal muscle of patients with obesity of NIDDM. Diabetes 1990; 39:865–870.
76. Handberg A, Vaag A, Dansbro H, et al. Expression of insulin regulatable glucose transporters in skeletal muscle from type 2 diabetic patients. Diabetologia 1990;33:625–627.
77. Katz EB, Stenbit AE, Hatton K, et al. Cardiac and adipose tissue abnormalitites but not diabetes in mice deficient in Glut 4. Nature 1995;377:151–155.
78. Rossetti L, Stenbit AE, Katz EB, et al. Disruption of one allele of the murine Glut 4 gene causes marked resistance to the action of insulin. J Invest Med 1996;44:265A.
79. Deems RO, Evans JL, Deacon RW, et al. Expression of human Glut 4 in mice results in increased insulin action. Diabetologia 1994;37:1097–1104.
80. Gulve EA, Ren JM, Marshall BA, et al. Glucose transport activity in skeletal muscles from transgenic mice overexpressing Glut 1: increased basal transport is associated with a defective response to diverse stimuli that activate Glut 4. J Biol Chem 1994;269:18366–18370.
81. Ikemoto S, Thomson KS, Itakura H, et al. Expression of an insulin-responsive glucose transporter (Glut 4) minigene in transgenic mice: effect of exercise and role in glucose homeostasis. Proc Natl Acad Sci USA 1995; 92:865–869.
82. Marshall BA, Mueckler MM. Differential effects of Glut 1 or Glut 4 overexpression on insulin responsiveness in transgenic mice. Am J Physiol 1994;267:E738–E744.
83. Treadway JL, Hargrove DM, Nardone NA, et al. Enhanced peripheral glucose utilization in transgenic mice expressing the human Glut 4 gene. J Biol Chem 1994; 269:956–961.
84. Gibbs EM, Stock JL, McCoid SC, et al. Glycemic improvement in diabetic db/db mice by overexpression of the human insulin-regulatable glucose transporter (Glut 4). J Clin Invest 1995;95:1512–1518.
85. Bell GI, Kayano T, Buse JB, et al. Molecular biology of mammalian glucose transporters. Diabetes Care 1990;13: 198–208.
86. Bell GI, Burant CF, Takeda J, Gould GW. Structure and function of mammalian facilitative sugar transporters. J Biol Chem 1993;268:19161–19164.
87. Mantych GJ, James DE, Chung HD, Devaskar SU. Cellular localization and characterization of Glut 3 glucose transporter isoform in human brain. Endocrinology 1992; 131:1270–1278.

88. Waddell ID, Scott H, Grant A, Burchell A. Identification and characterization of a hepatic microsomal glucose transport protein. Biochem J 1991;275:363–367.
89. Burchell A. Hepatic microsomal glucose transport. Biochem Soc Trans 1994;22:658–663.
90. Jackson MR, Nilsson T, Peterson PA. Identification of a consensus motif for retention of transmembrane proteins in the endoplasmic reticulum. EMBO J 1990;9:3153–3162.
91. Jackson MR, Nilsson T, Peterson PA. Retrieval of transmembrane proteins to the endoplasmic reticulum. J Cell Biol 1993;121:317–333.
92. Aghayan M, Rao LV, Smith RM, et al. Developmental expression and cellular localization of glucose transporter molecules during mouse preimplantation development. Development 1992;115:305–312.
93. Schultz GA, Hojan A, Watson AJ, et al. Insulin, insulin-like growth factors and glucose transporters. Reprod Fertil Dev 1992;4:361–371.
94. Hogan A, Heyner S, Charron MJ, et al. Glucose transporter gene expression in early mouse embryos. Development 1991;113:363–372.
95. Robinson DH, Smith PR, Benos DJ. Hexose transport in preimplantation rabbit blastocysts. J Reprod Fertil 1990;89:1–11.
96. Matsumoto K, Akazawa S, Ishibashi M, et al. Abundant expression of Glut 1 and Glut 3 in rat embryo during the early organogenesis period. Biochem Biophys Res Commun 1995;209:95–102.
97. Takata K, Kasahara T, Kasahara M, et al. Localization of erythrocyte/HepG2-type glucose transporter (Glut 1) in human placental villi. Cell Tissue Res 1992;267:407–412.
98. Arnott G, Coghill G, McArdle HJ, Hundal HS. Immunolocalization of Glut 1 and Glut 3 glucose transporters in human placenta. Biochem Soc Trans 1994;22:272–273.
99. Reid NA, Boyd R. Further evidence for the presence of 2 facilitative glucose isoforms in the brush border membrane of the syncytiotrophoblast of the human full term placenta. Biochem Soc Trans 1994;22:267.
100. Sakata M, Kurachi H, Imai T, et al. Increase in human placental glucose transporter-1 during pregnancy. Eur J Endocrinol 1995;132:206–212.
101. Wolf HJ, Desoye G. Immunohistochemical localization of glucose transporters and insulin receptors in human fetal membranes at term. Histochemistry 1993;100:379–385.
102. Economides DL, Nicolaides KH. Blood glucose and oxygen tension levels in small-for-gestational age fetuses. Am J Obstet Gynecol 1989;160:385–389.
103. Laurin J, Lingman G, Marsal K, Persson PH. Fetal blood flow in pregnancies complicated by intrauterine growth retardation. Obstet Gynecol 1987;69:895–902.
104. Jansson TS, Wennergren M, Illsley NP. Glucose transporter protein expression in human placenta throughout gestation and in intrauterine growth retardation. J Clin Endocrinol Metab 1993;77:1554–1562.
105. Suzuki N, Oka Y, Lir JL. Protein contents of Glut-1 and Glut-3 of human placental tissue at delivery of diabetic mothers do not relate to neonatal birth weight [abstract]. Proceedings of the 1st International Symposium on Diabetes and Pregnancy in the 1990s, 1992:104.
106. Hauguel DE, Mouzon S, Boileau P, Girard J. Structural localization and regulation of glucose transporter expression in placentas of diabetic rats. Diabetes 1994;43:135A.
107. Schienberg P. Observations on cerebral carbohydrate metabolism in man. Ann Intern Med 1963;62:367–371.
108. Bondy CA, Lee WH, Shou J. Ontogeny and cellular distribution of brain glucose transporter gene expression. Mol Cell Neurosci 1992;3:305–314.
109. Chugani HT, Phelps MF, Mazziotta JC. Positron emission tomography study of human brain functional development. Ann Neurol 1987;22:487–497.
110. Chugani HT, Phelps ME. Maturational changes in cerebral function in infants determined by 18 FD6 positron emission tomography. Science 1986;23:840–843.
111. Walker PS, Donovan JA, Van Ness BG, et al. Glucose dependent regulation of glucose transport activity, protein, mRNA in primary cultures of rat brain glial cells. J Biol Chem 1988;263:15594–15601.
112. Clarke DW, Boyd FT, Kappy MS, Raizada MK. Insulin binds to specific receptors and stimulates 2-deoxy-glucose uptake in cultured glial cells from rat brain. J Biol Chem 1984;259:11672–11675.
113. Werner H, Raizada MK, Mudd LM, et al. Regulation of rat brain/HepG2 glucose transporter gene expression by insulin and insulin-like growth factor-I in primary cultures of neuronal and glial cells. Endocrinology 1989;125:314–326.
114. Oelberg DG, Xu F, Shabarek F. Sodium-coupled transport of glucose by plasma membranes of type II pneumocytes. Biochim Biophys Acta 1994;1194:92–98.
115. Basset G, Saumon G, Bouchonnet F, Crone C. Apical sodium-sugar transport in pulmonary epithelium in situ. Biochim Biophys Acta 1988;942:11–18.
116. Clerici C, Soler P, Saumon G. Sodium-dependent phosphate and alanine transports but sodium-independent hexose transport in type II alveolar epithelial cells in primary culture. Biochim Biophys Acta 1991;1063:27–35.
117. Simmons RA, Gounis AS, Bangalore SA, Ogata ES. Intrauterine growth retardation: fetal glucose transport is diminished in lung but spared in brain. Pediatr Res 1992;31:59–63.
118. Simmons RA, Charlton VE. Substrate utilization by the fetal sheep lung during the last trimester. Pediatr Res 1988;23:606–611.
119. Mantych G, Devaskar U, deMello D, Devaskar S. Glut-1 glucose transporter protein in adult and fetal mouse lung. Biochem Biophys Res Commun 1991;180:367–373.
120. Engle MJ, Langan SM, Sanders RL. The effects of insulin and hyperglycemia on surfactant phospholipid synthesis in organotypic cultures of type II pneumocytes. Biochim Biophys Acta 1983;753:6–13.
121. Simmons RA, Atkins VA, Ogata ES. The effect of maternal diabetes on glut 1 function and expression in fetal lung. Pediatr Res 1992;31:182A.

122. Kahn BB, Cushman SW. Mechanisms for markedly hyperresponsive insulin-stimulated glucose transport activity in adipose cells from insulin-treated streptozotocin rats. J Biol Chem 1987;262:5118–5124.
123. Charron MJ, Kahn BB. Divergent molecular mechanisms for insulin-resistent transport in muscle and adipose cells in vivo. J Biol Chem 1990;240:3237–3244.
124. Issad T, Coupe C, Ferre P, Girard J. Insulin resistance during suckling period in rats. Am J Physiol 1987;253:E142–E148.
125. Wallace S, Cambell G, Knott R, et al. Development of insulin sensitivity in rat skeletal muscle. FEBS Lett 1992;301:69–72.

8
Insulin: Molecular, Biochemical, and Physiologic Aspects

Philip A. Gruppuso

For more than half a century insulin has occupied a position as the most intensively studied mammalian hormone. This stems in part from insulin's role as the preeminent anabolic hormone in mammals. The effort put into understanding the physiology and biochemistry of this peptide follows a rich scientific history that has come from its study. The demonstration, by von Mering and Minkowski[1] in 1889, that pancreatectomy in the dog resulted in a syndrome similar to diabetes mellitus eventually led to the discovery of insulin, an accomplishment which is credited to Banting and Best.[2] A number of seminal discoveries that had an impact on all of biochemical physiology followed: quantification of the hormone by radioimmunoassay,[3] sequencing of the peptide,[4] complete synthesis of the hormone,[5,6] and, more recently, cloning of the gene for insulin[7] and synthesis of the recombinant protein for therapeutic use.[8] This progress has paralleled the advances in the understanding of insulin's physiologic role in regulating intermediary metabolism.[9,10] Over the past two decades, intense effort has focused on elucidating the mechanisms by which it exerts its effects at the cellular level. This effort resulted in the cloning of the gene for the insulin receptor.[11] More recently, great strides have been made in defining the cellular mechanisms by which insulin is transduced via activation of the insulin receptor protein tyrosine kinase and subsequent signaling events.

This chapter provides a comprehensive review of our current understanding of insulin biosynthesis, secretion, mechanism of action, and role in the physiologic regulation of metabolism.

Structure and Biosynthesis of Insulin

The insulin molecule consists of two peptides, termed A for acidic and B for basic, with a total molecular weight of approximately 6000. The two chains are joined by two disulfide linkages with a third disulfide bond being internal to the A chain. Once the structure of insulin had been elucidated,[4] speculation began as to the mechanism of insulin biosynthesis. In the early 1960s it was discovered that polypeptides are synthesized stepwise from a messenger RNA (mRNA) template derived from complementary DNA (cDNA). Taken together with the ability to synthesize insulin in vitro via recombination of separate A and B chains, it was widely held that this same mechanism was involved in the in vivo synthesis of insulin. The work of Steiner et al.[12] and Chance et al.[13] subsequently demonstrated that insulin is actually produced by the processing of a precursor protein, proinsulin (Figure 8.1). Proinsulin, in turn, has a precursor, termed preproinsulin, which is cleaved to proinsulin upon synthesis in the endoplasmic reticulum.[14] The N-terminal extension of preproinsulin is involved in binding of the nascent peptide during the early stages of synthesis to a signal recognition particle-ribosome complex. Upon removal of this extension, or leader sequence, proinsulin is released. Folding of this protein results in efficient formation of correct disulfides and the characteristic tertiary structure of insulin.[15]

The biosynthesis of insulin (Figure 8.2) involves the partial proteolytic conversion of proinsulin to insulin. This process, which takes place primarily in newly formed β granules in the pancreatic β cell,[16] involves the action of two recently described endoproteases that act on the carboxylic side of two dibasic amino acid pairs at the insulin/C peptide junctions in the proinsulin molecule (Arg^{31}, Arg^{32} at the B chain/C peptide junction; Lys^{64}, Arg^{65} at the A chain/C peptide junction). The newly exposed COOH-terminal basic amino acids are then rapidly removed by the action of an exopeptidase, carboxypeptidase-H. This processing yields equimolar amounts of mature insulin and C peptide.

The work of Frank et al.[17,18] showed that the structure of the insulin moiety in proinsulin differs little from the structure of insulin. However, the presence of a C peptide that has little discernible order in its tertiary structure is

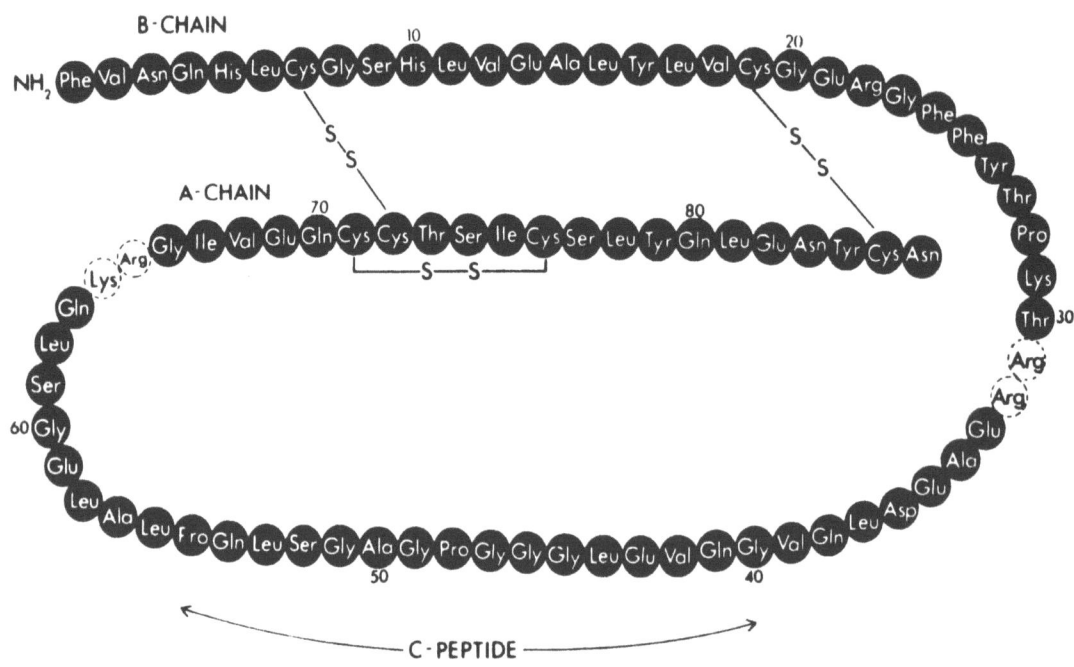

FIGURE 8.1. Amino acid sequence of human proinsulin. The basic residues, indicated in open circles, represent the cleavage sites for conversion of proinsulin to insulin. (From Oyer et al.,[170] with permission.)

sufficient to decrease the ability of proinsulin to interact with the insulin receptor to only 3% to 5% of insulin.[19] Notably, the primary[20] and tertiary[21] structures of proinsulin are closely related to those of insulin-like growth factor I (IGF-I). Proinsulin might therefore be expected to interact potently with IGF receptors. However, studies using recombinant human proinsulin and IGF-I indicate that proinsulin and the partially cleaved proinsulin-insulin conversion intermediates interact minimally with the human IGF-I receptor.[22]

Considerable variation in the amino acid sequence exists among insulins from different species. However, this variation is largely confined to specific areas, with most residues exhibiting a high degree of conservation. Pig and beef insulins vary from human insulin in 1 and 3 residues, respectively. In contrast, cod and human insulins vary in 15 of the 51 amino acids. Nonetheless, all of these insulins have similar biologic potency. C peptide, which is critical to insulin biosynthesis but not action, is poorly conserved. A practical consequence of this is the poor interspecies cross-reactivity of C peptide antisera used for radioimmunoassay. Of interest is the observation that the evolution of the metabolic and growth-promoting functions of insulin may be divergent.[23] That is, the relative potencies of insulins in stimulating glucose oxidation and DNA synthesis vary. This apparent separation of two functional domains is probably a reflection of the evolutionary divergence of insulin and the insulin-like growth factors and the specificities of their respective receptors.

C peptide is present in the circulation[24] and its concentration in plasma and in urine have been used as an indirect measure of insulin secretion in normal adults,[25,26] individuals with diabetes mellitus,[27,28] pregnant women,[29] and neonates.[29-31] The usefulness of C peptide as an indicator of insulin secretion is derived from the fact that while it is secreted with insulin, the two have no structural homology. C peptide is not removed from the circulation by the liver via receptor-mediated endocytosis[32] nor does it bind to insulin antibodies, which are present in the circulation of insulin-treated diabetics[27] and their newborns.[30] However, precise quantification of insulin secretion by C-peptide measurement is problematic, owing largely to the widely disparate half-lives of C peptide (30–45 min) and insulin (2–5 min).[33] The use of plasma C peptide in pregnant women and cord plasma C peptide as a measure of insulin secretion may be further complicated by its extraction and metabolism by the placenta.[34] Nonetheless, measurement of C-peptide immunoreactivity provides an additional means of assessing insulin secretion, especially in the presence of insulin antibodies.

The conversion of proinsulin to insulin in the β cell proceeds to approximately 95% completion. Insulin secretion is accompanied by the release of small amounts of proinsulin and proinsulin-insulin conversion intermediates, which can be detected in the circulation.[35] These conversion intermediates represent partially cleaved forms of proinsulin. This partial proteolysis may occur at the proinsulin-to-insulin conversion sites, or at sites within the C peptide. As might be expected, partial cleavage of proinsulin increases potency, especially if the cleavage results in the uncovering of the N-terminal glycine of the A chain, a region of insulin that is involved in receptor binding.

The presence of proinsulin and the conversion intermediates in serum, first observed by Rubenstein et al.,[36] Roth et al.,[37] was found to be affected by variations in insulin secretion. Since proinsulin contains insulin, it is measured in insulin radioimmunoassays that utilize insulin antibodies cross-reactive with proinsulin. In recent years, specific proinsulin radioimmunoassays have become readily available with the advent of specific proinsulin antibodies that cross-react with neither insulin nor C peptide.[38,39] Studies using these proinsulin radioimmunoassays have largely confirmed the results of older studies that relied on the separation of proinsulin from insulin based on size.

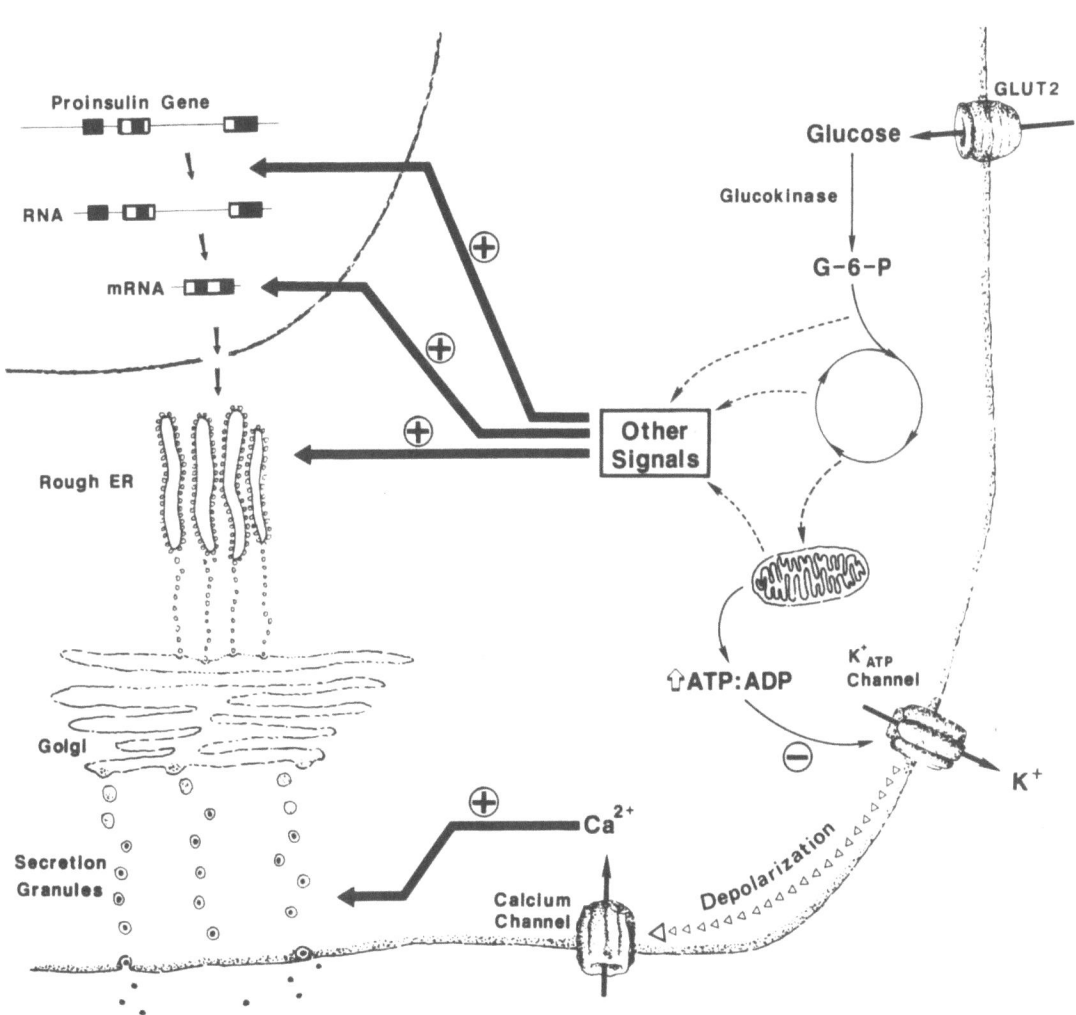

FIGURE 8.2. Scheme depicting the biosynthesis of insulin and its regulation by glucose in the pancreatic β cell. The nucleus, containing the proinsulin gene, translation of proinsulin RNA, and processing to mature proinsulin mRNA, is shown at the upper left. In the rough endoplasmic reticulum (ER), preproinsulin is synthesized and cleaved to proinsulin, which is transferred to the Golgi apparatus where proteolytic conversion to insulin begins. As secretion granules are produced and mature, conversion to insulin continues. This results in a mixture of approximately 95% insulin plus C peptide and 5% proinsulin and conversion intermediates.

Regulation of insulin production and secretion is depicted on the right side of the figure. Glucose undergoes facilitated transport into the β cell via GLUT 2 followed by phosphorylation by glucokinase. Further metabolism of glucose results in the generation of uncharacterized signals, which can activate proinsulin gene transcription, accumulation of proinsulin mRNA largely via increased RNA stability, and translation (heavy arrows). Further metabolism at the level of mitochondria results in an increased ATP/ADP ratio. This causes inhibition of ATP-sensitive potassium channels, leading to membrane depolarization. This, in turn, results in activation of voltage-gated calcium channels and calcium influx, which triggers the fusion of secretion granules with the plasma membrane.

Acute increases in insulin secretion (e.g., in response to an oral glucose load) result in a decrease in the circulating levels of proinsulin and conversion intermediates relative to insulin.[40] Conversely, hypoinsulinemic states are associated with an increase in the percent insulin immunoreactivity due to the proinsulin component.[41,42] Insulinomas,[43] idiopathic hyperinsulinemia in the newborn,[44] and the hyperinsulinism seen in infants of diabetic mothers[45] are all associated with absolute increases in circulating proinsulin and conversion intermediates.

In addition to the pathophysiologic causes of hyperproinsulinemia, several kindreds with familial hyperproinsulinemia have been described.[46-48] In two of these families, substitution of Arg[65] (C-peptide/A-chain junction) results in impaired conversion.[49,50] In the third family, the circulating proinsulin was normal in its in vitro susceptibility to trypsin, indicating normal C-A and C-B junctions.[48] The abnormality in this kindred is due to a point mutation resulting in an aspartic acid for histidine substitution at residue 10 of proinsulin.[51] This apparently results in a distinct conformation of proinsulin that resisted proteolytic conversion to insulin. Most recently, a more generalized defect in prohormone processing was described as resulting in hyperproinsulinemia along with impaired processing of proopiomelanocortin, secondary hypocortisolism, and hypogonadotropic hypogonadism.[52] Interestingly, the abnormality in glucose homeostasis resulting from this putative defect in prohormone convertase-1 (PC1) was a combination of impaired glucose tolerance and reactive hypoglycemia.

The Insulin Gene

The insulin gene, first cloned from the rat by Ulrich et al.,[8] is on the short arm of chromosome 11 in the human.[53] The human insulin gene contains three exons and two introns.[54,55] The exons are organized as follows:

5′ — prepeptide — B chain — C peptide — A chain — 3′.

It was the cloning of the rat insulin genes and their translation in vitro that established preproinsulin as the in vivo translation product.[56]

Structural analysis of the human insulin gene (Figure 8.3) reveals a 5′ flanking region of which approximately 350 base pairs are required to confer both β-cell specific expression and glucose-mediated regulation.[57-59] It is likely that two types of cis-acting elements within the insulin promoter are required for this regulation: E boxes and TAAT boxes. The E-box motifs, of which there are two in the promoter region of the human insulin gene, are thought to serve as binding sites for basic helix-loop-helix transcriptions factors.[60] The TAAT motifs, also known as A boxes, three of which are present in the human insulin gene promoter, have been shown to bind several islet-specific homeodomain-containing transcriptional fac-

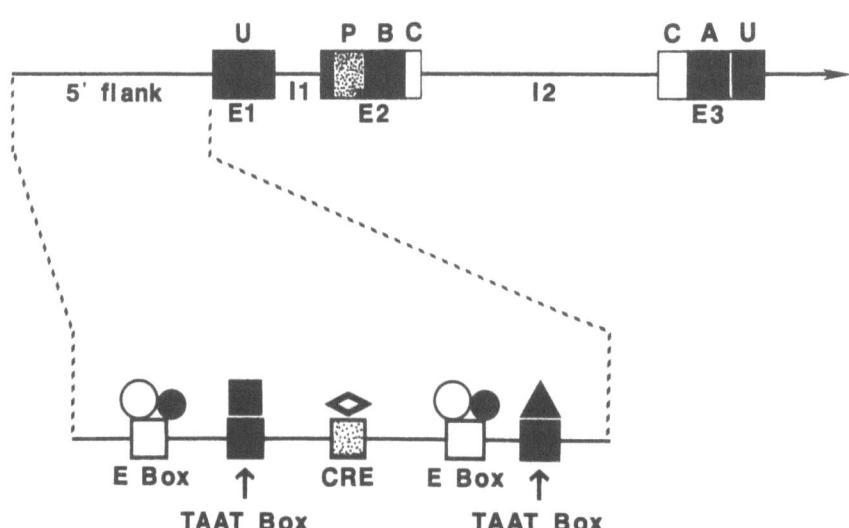

FIGURE 8.3. A diagrammatic representation of the proinsulin gene in vertebrates. The top part of the figure shows the 5′ flanking region, exons (E1, E2, E3) and introns (I1, I2). Within the regions present in mature preproinsulin mRNA, portions that are untranslated (U) regions as well as those that code for the prepeptide coding region (P), B chain (B), C peptide (C), and A chain (A) are shown. The lower part of the figure illustrates the relative positions of key cis-elements within the 5′ flanking region of the gene. These elements interact with numerous binding proteins that have been best characterized for the rat insulin I gene. These include IEF-1 which binds to the E boxes, cAMP response element binding protein (CREB), which binds to the cAMP response element (CRE), and IEF-2, Imx-1, and IUF-1, which bind to the TAAT boxes.

tors.[60] These include isl-1,[61] Imx-1,[62] cdx-3,[62] and IPF-1.[63] These represent candidate factors for the induction of insulin expression during the embryologic development of the pancreas, as well as the aforementioned regulation of expression in the mature β cell. Acute regulation of insulin gene expression, as modulated by nutritional status, for example, involves these factors as well (vide infra).

A number of point mutations in the insulin gene resulting in mutant gene products have been described. These insulinopathies include the three aforementioned kindreds with hyperproinsulinemia expressing two distinct mutations.[48–51] In addition, a variety of point mutations in the insulin molecule itself have been thoroughly characterized. Although such patients represent an exceedingly small proportion of the diabetic population, analysis of these abnormal insulins has contributed to our understanding of the structural requirements for insulin bioactivity. The mutant insulins, first characterized by investigators at the University of Chicago,[64] had substitutions in the 24th or 25th residues of the B chain, identifying this region as contributing to the "active site" of insulin. Subsequently, kindreds have been described in which there are abnormalities in portions of the insulin molecule not considered critical for activity, indicating that even subtle changes in the tertiary structure of insulin can affect its ability to bind to the insulin receptor.

Regulation of Insulin Secretion

In the mature mammal, the secretion of insulin by the pancreatic β cell is regulated primarily by glucose. In general, other factors (e.g., including pancreatic hormones, cytokines, nutrients) may be thought of as modifying the response to glucose. The mechanism by which the β cell translates extracellular glucose concentration into a regulatory signal controlling insulin secretion has not been fully elucidated. However, the overall strategy for this regulatory mechanism and many of its components have been characterized.

The rate of insulin secretion is proportional to the rate of glucose metabolism by the β cell. Nonmetabolizable glucose analogues do not function as insulin secretagogues. The currently held model for control of insulin secretion by glucose is as follows.[65] It is thought that the metabolism of glucose leads to an increase in the β cell adenosine triphosphate (ATP)/adenosine diphosphate (ADP) ratio. This is thought to result in inhibition of an ATP-sensitive K$^+$ channel, which, in turn, causes opening of voltage-gated Ca^{2+} channels. The resulting influx of Ca^{2+} into the β cell is thought to trigger the fusion of insulin-containing vesicles with the plasma membrane (Figure 8.2). Such a mechanism requires a response proportional to extracellular glucose concentration. This requirement led to the concept of a β-cell "glucose sensor." In recent years, two candidate gene products have emerged; the β cell glucose transporter, GLUT 2, and the major hexokinase expressed in β cells, termed glucokinase or hexokinase IV. In both cases, these proteins have a relatively high K_m for glucose (i.e., approximately 17mM for GLUT 2 and 8mM for glucokinase).[66] The entry of glucose into β cells and the initiating step in its metabolism are both proportional to extracellular glucose concentration. Of note, overexpression of the low K_m glucose transporter, GLUT 1, does not alter islet responsiveness to glucose.[67] In contrast, overexpression of glucokinase results in induction of insulin gene expression, supporting glucokinase as the β-cell glucose sensor.[67]

Strong evidence supporting a requirement for glucokinase in the regulation of insulin secretion has come from the recent observations on the nature of maturity-onset diabetes of the young (MODY). This form of non–insulin-dependent diabetes mellitus is inherited in an autosomal dominant manner. Analysis of DNA from family members showed linkage of the disorder with missense or non-sense mutations in the gene for glucokinase.[68] When the mutations were reproduced in glucokinase expressed in bacteria, the abnormal enzymes were found to exhibit a low V_{max} or elevated K_m for glucose.[69] The dominant inheritance of the disorder is presumed to result from interference of normal β-cell glucose metabolism by the abnormal enzyme. No similar linkage between GLUT 2 and any form of diabetes has been identified.

In addition to the acute regulation of insulin release, glucose stimulates proinsulin biosynthesis within approximately 20 minutes. However, this stimulation is insensitive to inhibitors of RNA synthesis, indicating activation of translation.[70] This effect may involve several mechanisms, including activation of translational initiation, augmented transfer of proinsulin mRNA to ribosomes and further redistribution of proinsulin mRNA to membrane-bound ribosomes.[71]

Insulin secretion and proinsulin biosynthesis are regulated in tandem under many conditions. However, their activation can be dissociated, indicating distinct regulatory mechanisms for the two processes.[72] For example, glucose-mediated stimulation of insulin release is a calcium-dependent process, while activation of proinsulin biosynthesis is not. Similarly, increases in β-cell adenosine 3′,5′-cyclic monophosphate (cAMP) stimulate secretion but not biosynthesis.

While the primary acute regulator of insulin secretion and biosynthesis is circulating glucose concentration, numerous other factors function in a regulatory role when basal glucose concentration is held constant.[73] They include amino acids (e.g., particularly arginine and leucine), growth hormone, a number of intestinal peptides, and glucagon, all of which are stimulatory. Somatostatin, epinephrine, norepinephrine, and prostaglandin E are inhibitory. Although the mechanisms for regulation of insulin secretion at the cellular level are becoming well defined, the relative potency of these factors in determining basal insulin secretion in the presence of basal glucose concentrations is unclear.

Longer term nutritional regulation of insulin production by glucose occurs at the level of proinsulin mRNA transcriptional control.[72] This serves to maintain the ability of the β cell to replenish insulin stores by elevating proinsulin mRNA at times of high insulin production. Conversely, prolonged fasting results in diminished proinsulin gene transcription. In vitro studies indicate that these effects of glucose take place in human islets over approximately 4 hours.[74] Other secretagogues, including leucine, seem to increase proinsulin mRNA levels via a similar mechanism. Conversely, somatostatin, a potent inhibitor of insulin secretion, decreases proinsulin mRNA levels by promoting its instability.[75]

In addition to its central role in regulating basal insulin secretion, glucose is a primary physiologic stimulus for insulin secretion in the fed state. In the mature mammal, the insulin response to a persistent glucose stimulus is biphasic. In humans, the acute-phase insulin release peaks at 3 to 5 minutes, while the second phase persists for as long as the stimulus is present. The acute phase represents the secretion of stored insulin. The second phase is a result of de novo synthesis of insulin; inhibitors of protein synthesis suppress second-phase insulin release.[76] It is this phase that is dependent on stimulation of translation.

Studies on the kinetics and regulation of insulin secretion in the fetus have indicated that fetal islets show less of an insulin secretory response to glucose than do adult islets. This has been especially well studied in fetal rat pancreatic islets, as reviewed by Hughs.[77] This presumably relates to an inability of the fetal β cell to generate an increase in cytosolic Ca^{2+} concentration in response to glucose.[78] However, fetal islets and mature islets have indistinguishable cytosolic Ca^{2+} responses to glyceraldehyde, arginine, and leucine. The physiologic significance of these in vitro findings to regulation of basal insulin production in the fetus has not yet been clarified.

A recent advance in understanding the regulation of insulin secretion came from work aimed at defining the receptor for sulfonylureas, a class of insulin secretagogues used to treat non–insulin-dependent diabetes mellitus. Purification and cloning of the sulfonylurea receptor[79] led to the observation that this protein is abnormal in some infants with hyperinsulinemic hypoglycemia.[80] The receptor itself is a member of a new class of ATP binding proteins that appears to associate with the β-cell potassium channel,[81] providing a mechanism for ATP-mediated potassium flux.

Mechanism of Insulin Action: The Insulin Receptor

The fate of insulin following secretion has been demonstrated by Sodoyez et al.[82] using detection of radiolabeled insulin by an external scintillation camera. Within 5 minutes after the intravenous injection of ^{123}I-insulin into humans or experimental animals, insulin is concentrated in the liver. By 30 minutes, most of the insulin has been degraded. Both of these processes and the ability of insulin to exert its metabolic effects depend on the binding of insulin to a specific, high-affinity cell surface receptor. Not surprisingly, the highest insulin receptor concentrations occur in two of insulin's primary target tissues, liver and adipose.[83] Skeletal muscle, the main target for insulin-stimulated glucose uptake, has a lower concentration of insulin receptors. Nonetheless, the receptor abundance in muscle is still in a range which permits insulin signaling at the usual physiologic concentrations of the circulating hormone, 10^{-10} to 10^{-9} M.

The insulin receptor is an integral membrane glycoprotein with an apparent relative molecular mass (M_r) of approximately 350,000. It is composed of two α subunits (M_r = 135,000) and two β subunits (M_r = 95,000) with the four subunits linked by disulfide bonds (Figure 8.4).[84] Prior to the isolation and cloning of the insulin receptor, affinity labeling with ^{125}I-insulin indicated that the insulin binding site is contained within the α-subunit.[85] Both the α and β subunits are glycoproteins. The α subunit is entirely extracellular, while the β subunit contains a membrane spanning domain. The subunit structure of the insulin receptor, originally deduced from protein biochemical analyses, was subsequently confirmed with the determination of the primary structure deduced from the sequence of the human insulin receptor cDNA.[11]

The receptor is synthesized from a polypeptide precursor, which contains both the α and β subunits.[86] Synthesis of the proreceptor is followed by core glycolysis, formation of intra- and intersubunit disulfide bonds, and proteolytic processing. Completion of glycosylation and fatty acid acylation result in the mature receptor.

In 1982, Kasuga et al.[87] demonstrated that the binding of insulin stimulates the phosphorylation of the β subunit of the insulin receptor on tyrosine residues. Subsequent studies showed that the tyrosine kinase activity is intrinsic to the β subunit. Furthermore, β subunit autophosphorylation is dependent on insulin concentration, thereby fulfilling an essential characteristic of an insulin signal transmission mechanism. The precise mechanism by which extracellular insulin binding results in intracellular kinase activation is not known. However, mutational analysis of the β-subunit transmembrane domain is consistent with a subtle change in conformation in this region following insulin binding.[86]

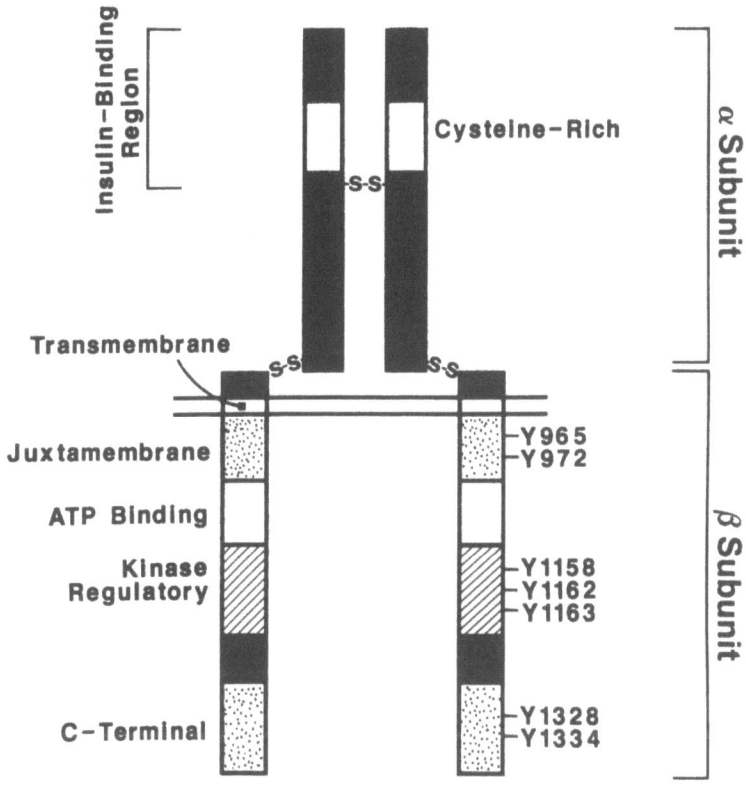

FIGURE 8.4. Schematized drawing of the insulin receptor. As indicated, the two α and two β subunits are joined by disulfide bonds. A cysteine-rich domain within each α subunit composes part of the insulin-binding region. Transmembrane, juxtamembrane, ATP binding, kinase regulatory, and C-terminal domains within the β subunits are shown. The positions of β subunit tyrosine phosphorylated sites, as designated by the single letter amino acid abbreviation Y, are shown for the β subunit at lower right.

Once the receptor is activated, at least six and possibly seven sites in the β subunit undergo tyrosine phosphorylation.[88,89] The tyrosine phosphorylation probably occurs via transphosphorylation.[86] That is, phosphorylation is catalyzed by the paired β subunit rather than occurring as a true autophosphorylation reaction. Three sites, Tyr^{1158}, Tyr^{1162}, and Tyr^{1163}, are within the kinase autoregulatory domain. Mutation of these sites to phenylalanine results in marked impairment of autophosphorylation and kinase activation.[90]

Two additional tyrosine phosphorylation sites in the C-terminal "tail" of the β subunit are not required for kinase activation but may be involved in signaling.[86] A juxtamembrane autophosphorylation site, Tyr^{972}, appears to be involved in both receptor endocytosis and signaling.[86]

In addition to being a substrate for tyrosine phosphorylation, the insulin receptor is phosphorylated on threonine and serine residues. At least three protein kinases are capable of phosphorylating the insulin receptor. Two, cAMP-dependent protein kinase[91] and the calcium/phospholipid-dependent protein kinase, protein kinase-C,[92] phosphorylate distinct sites on the receptor. In both cases phosphorylation inhibits tyrosine kinase activity measured in in vitro assays. It should be pointed out, however, that mutational analysis of Ser/Thr phosphorylation sites has not defined a clear physiologic role for receptor Ser/Thr phosphorylation.

Following the binding of insulin to its receptor at the cell surface, the ligand-receptor complex undergoes internalization.[93] The insulin/receptor complex is first localized to coated pits, regions of the cell surface where the protein clathrin is concentrated. The coated pits form coated vesicles, resulting in internalization via endocytosis. The lumen of the endocytotic vesicle is acidified, which causes the dissociation of insulin from its receptor. The insulin then undergoes lysosomal degradation. The internalized insulin receptor is either recycled to the cell surface or degraded. The process of internalization and insulin/receptor dissociation leads to termination of the insulin signal. Cessation of insulin receptor signaling presumably involves dephosphorylation of the insulin receptor by tyrosine-specific protein phosphatases, a large and diverse family of enzymes.[94] An increase in protein tyrosine phosphatase activity has been shown to occur in experimental insulin resistant states.[95,96] A primary role for these enzymes in insulin resistance has not been established.

The ligand-induced internalization of receptors accounts for the generalized phenomenon termed "downregulation." An inverse relationship between insulin concentration and insulin receptor number has been demonstrated in many cell types. An exception to this relationship has been found in hyperinsulinemic fetuses of diabetic mothers, who have increased binding of insulin to monocytes.[97] However, studies in the fetal rat show that fetal hypoinsulinemia is associated with increased hepatic insulin receptor number.[98] Thus, the aforementioned exception may be specific to regulation of monocyte insulin receptor complement and/or the fetopathy seen with maternal diabetes.

Mechanism of Insulin Action: Postreceptor Events

Based on the discussion in the previous section, the insulin receptor can be viewed as a complex enzyme (i.e., tyrosine kinase) whose activity is regulated by an allosteric activator (i.e., insulin) and covalent modification (i.e., positive regulation via tyrosine phosphorylation; negative regulation via serine/threonine phosphorylation). However, the mechanisms downstream from receptor kinase activation involved in insulin signal transduction defied characterization until recently. The development of antibodies against phosphotyrosine was a critical advance in this area. The use of these antibodies allowed identification of multiple proteins that undergo tyrosine phosphorylation following the exposure of intact cells to insulin. Through this work and parallel studies on growth factor action, it appears that signaling by receptor tyrosine kinases can be explained by two paradigms. One is direct activation of signaling proteins in response to their phosphorylation on tyrosine residues. The second is the formation of signaling complexes in which proteins associate noncovalently via interactions between tyrosine phosphorylated domains and phosphotyrosine binding domains. Both paradigms apply to insulin signaling.

The use of phosphotyrosine antibodies allowed detection of the major soluble substrate for the insulin receptor tyrosine kinase, insulin receptor substrate-1 (IRS-1). This protein with an approximate M_r of 185,000 was found to be rapidly tyrosine phosphorylated following the treatment of intact cells with insulin.[99] It was the use of a mutant insulin receptor in which Tyr^{972} was converted to Phe that suggested that IRS-1 phosphorylation is a required event in insulin signaling. Expression of this mutant receptor in intact cells showed normal insulin binding, receptor kinase activity, and receptor internalization. However, insulin-stimulated glycogen and DNA synthesis did not occur, nor did IRS-1 tyrosine phosphorylation.[100]

Using immunoaffinity purification with phosphotyrosine antibodies, IRS-1 was isolated, eventually leading to sequencing of the rat liver cDNA encoding this protein.[101] These and other studies, summarized elsewhere,[86] defined a protein whose most significant features were the apparent absence of any catalytic activity and the presence of at least 20 tyrosine phosphorylation sites. Cloning of the IRS-1 genes from other species showed a high level of conservation of the amino acids surrounding most of the tyrosine phosphorylation sites.

It now appears that IRS-1 plays an essential role in insulin signal transduction by functioning as a docking protein (Figure 8.5).[86,102] Its tyrosine phosphorylated sites are able to bind a spectrum of signaling proteins including the regulatory (p85) subunit of phosphatidylinositol 3-kinase (PI 3-kinase), the adaptor protein Grb2, which is involved in signaling via Ras (vide infra), and the protein tyrosine phosphatase, Syp. These proteins possess common binding domains, termed *Src*-homology 2 (SH2) domains, which are homologous to a portion of the protein tyrosine kinase, *src*. These regions of the signaling proteins mediate the formation of signaling complexes in which other components with catalytic activity are activated.

PI 3-kinase is a heterodimeric enzyme composed of a regulatory (M_r 85,000; p85) and a catalytic (M_r 110,000) subunit. The enzyme catalyzes the phosphorylation of phosphatidylinositol (PI), PI-4-phosphate, and PI-4,5-diphosphate on the D-3 position of the inositol ring. Insulin stimulation of PI 3-kinase activity was first observed in antiphosphotyrosine immunoprecipitates from insulin treated cells.[103] Subsequently, the ability of tyrosine phosphorylated IRS-1 to bind p85 and activate PI 3-kinase was demonstrated.[101]

The signaling pathway downstream from PI 3-kinase activation has not yet been elucidated. Several lines of evidence indicate that PI 3-kinase activation is involved mediating insulin's effects on glucose transport, protein synthesis, DNA synthesis, and gene expression. Most compelling are studies using several inhibitors of PI 3-kinase–mediated signaling: wortmannin, LY294002, and rapamycin. Overall, these studies have shown a correlation between PI 3-kinase inhibition and loss of some of the biologic effects of insulin. The structurally distinct nature of the three inhibitors decreases the likelihood of a confounding inhibition of another signaling pathway. Especially susceptible to these effects are insulin stimulation of the translocation of GLUT 4, the insulin-sensitive glucose transporter, from microsomal to plasma membranes (Figure 8.5). Nonetheless, establishing a functional link between PI 3-kinase and insulin's biologic effects will require the identification of effectors that are activated by some or all of the D-3 phosphorylated PI species.

In many systems, insulin also activates a pathway involving the small G protein, Ras, and members of the mitogen activated protein (MAP) kinase family of Ser/Thr kinases. MAP kinases are activated by many growth factor receptor tyrosine kinases (see Chapter 20). Initiation of the MAP kinase cascade involves the activation of

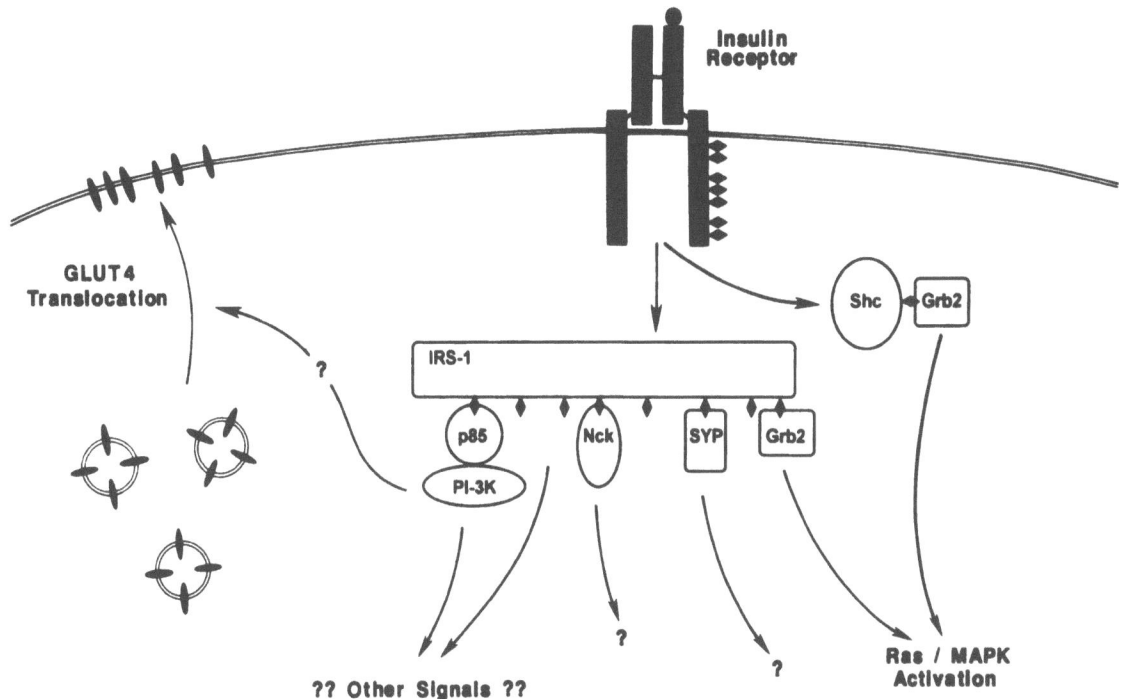

FIGURE 8.5. Current model for insulin signaling via the association of signaling proteins with the primary insulin receptor substrate, IRS-1. In addition to signaling via IRS-1, direct activation of the Ras/MAP kinase pathway via phosphorylation of Shc is shown. The mechanism depicted on the left whereby stimulation of GLUT 4 translocation to the cell surface occurs via PI-3 kinase activation is tentative.

Ras. Activation of this Ras by insulin may involve two potential mechanisms.[102] The first is direct binding of the adapter protein Grb2 to IRS-1. A second mechanism in which the products of the *shc* gene are tyrosine phosphorylated by the insulin receptor kinase leads to association of Shc with Grb2 (Figure 8.5). Both the IRS-1/Grb2 and Shc/Grb2 complexes may associate with the Ras nucleotide exchange factor, *son of sevenless* (SOS). This event targets the complex to the plasma membrane leading to an increase in guanosine triphosphate (GTP)-bound Ras. Ras, activated thusly, binds the initial protein kinase (Raf) in the three-kinase cascade leading to MAP kinase activation. Insulin's effects on gene expression, cell proliferation, protein synthesis, and intermediary metabolism in the hepatocyte may not be mediated by MAP kinases. Insulin does not activate this pathway in either developing fetal rat hepatocytes[103] or mature rat hepatocytes.[104]

Most of the varied actions of insulin can be explained by effects on reversible protein phosphorylation. The first enzyme shown to catalyze the interconversion of another enzyme between two forms was the "PR enzyme" of Cori and Cori.[105] This enzyme converts glycogen phosphorylase *a*, the active form of the enzyme, to phosphorylase *b*. More than a decade passed before Krebs and Fisher[106] demonstrated that phosphorylase was activated by attachment of a phosphoryl group. It was the discovery of phosphorylase kinase that led to the realization that PR enzyme was a protein phosphatase. Subsequently, Robison et al.[107] discovered the second messenger, cAMP, and the mediation of virtually all of its effects via activation of a protein kinase, cAMP-dependent protein kinase (or protein kinase A). The numerous substrates for protein kinase A can explain the effects of cAMP-mediated hormones, including epinephrine and glucagon. However, the pleiotropic effects of insulin cannot be similarly explained based on the action of a single intermediate enzyme. Insulin exerts its acute metabolic effects by promoting the phosphorylation of some proteins and the dephosphorylation of others (Table 8.1).

Among the downstream protein kinases activated by insulin is a particular kinase that phosphorylates ribosomal protein S6, thereby activating protein synthesis. A 90-kd ribosomal S6 kinase (pp90^{rsk}) is activated in response to insulin, probably via MAP kinase activation.[108] A second S6 kinase, pp70^{rsk}, is probably downstream from PI-3 kinase, although it appears that pp70^{rsk} is not required for activation of glucose transport in response to insulin.[109]

The predominant effect of insulin on regulatory enzymes of intermediary metabolism is to promote their dephosphorylation. In general, dephosphorylation of regulatory enzymes generally promotes activity through anabolic pathways, while phosphorylation pro-

TABLE 8.1. Modulation of the net phosphorylation state of various proteins by insulin.

Dephosphorylation	Phosphorylation
Phosphorylase (−)[a]	ATP-citrate lyase (±)
Phosphorylase kinase (−)	Acetyl-CoA carboxylase (±)
Glycogen synthase (+)	Ribosomal protein S6 (+)
Hormone-sensitive lipase (+)	Inhibitor 2 (+)[b]
Pyruvate dehydrogenase (+)	
Acetyl-CoA carboxylase (+)	
Fructose-2,6-bisphosphatase (+)	
6-Phosphofructo, 2 kinase (−)	
eIF-2 (initiation factor for protein synthesis; +)	

[a] Signs in parentheses refer to stimulation (+) or inhibition (−) of activity. In some cases, the effect on enzyme activity is unknown (±).
[b] Denotes stimulation of protein phosphatase activity.

motes catabolic processes. The protein phosphatases that mediate insulin effect have been studied in detail; the deduced amino acid sequence for protein phosphatases types 1 and 2A have recently been obtained.[110,111] However, the mechanism for regulation of these enzymes by insulin has not been fully elucidated. Protein phosphatase type 1 (PP-1) is of particular interest because of its ability to dephosphorylate key regulatory enzymes (vide infra). This enzyme was originally found to be sensitive to two heat-stable inhibitors. Inhibitor 1 was only active when phosphorylated by protein kinase A.[112] Unlike inhibitor 1, inhibitor 2 is actually purified as a component of the PP-1 heterodimer along with a catalytic subunit and appears to be phosphorylated in response to insulin.[113] Furthermore, its phosphorylation results in phosphatase activation.[114] However, inhibitor 2 is not a component of the glycogen particle[115] where PP-1 exerts potent insulin-mediated effects through the dephosphorylation of phosphorylase, glycogen synthase, and phosphorylase kinase. Rather, glycogen-associated PP-1 is bound to a regulatory "G" subunit[116] that can be phosphorylated in response to insulin, thereby mediating phosphatase activation.[117] It appears that this mechanism involving G-subunit phosphorylation, as defined in skeletal muscle, is catalyzed by pp90^{rsk}.

A discussion of insulin signal transduction would be incomplete without mention of the large body of work aimed at discovering an insulin second messenger with a role analogous to that filled by cAMP in β-adrenergic signaling. This search led to the discovery of an inositol-phosphate glycan mediator of insulin action several years ago.[118] While this second messenger, which is derived from the rapid hydrolysis of a membrane glycosyl-phosphatidylinositol, is a purported mediator of protein phosphatase activation,[102] definitive demonstration of its role in insulin action has not been forthcoming. Nonetheless, the generation of small, soluble signaling molecules in response to insulin, in addition to those derived from the activation of PI 3 kinase, should be considered a possible mechanism of insulin signal transduction.

Regulation of Intermediary Metabolism by Insulin

The role of insulin in metabolic regulation is remarkable for the variety of its tissue- and organ-specific effects. Insulin action is mediated via complex mechanisms involving the interaction of allosteric effectors with changes in the phosphorylation state of enzymes. It is ironic that the first enzyme discovered to be regulated by reversible phosphorylation (i.e., phosphorylase) should have a single regulatory site. This has proven to be the exception. Enzymes of intermediary metabolism that are regulated by reversible phosphorylation have been found, in most cases, to have multiple phosphorylation sites that serve as substrates for multiple protein kinases and protein phosphatases. Interaction between these sites occurs with phosphorylation at one site perhaps affecting the phosphorylation or dephosphorylation of a separate site. Finally, as is the case for phosphorylase (vide infra), an allosteric factor can often modify the interaction between the enzyme and its regulatory kinases or phosphatases.

As noted above, many of the key, insulin-regulated enzymes of intermediary metabolism undergo dephosphorylation in response to insulin. The activity of other enzymes, notably, phosphoenolpyruvate carboxykinase and fatty acid synthase complex, is regulated by insulin at the level of enzyme protein content. Figure 8.6 illustrates many of the key regulatory points at which insulin controls carbohydrate metabolism.

Regulation of Glucose Transport

A principal effect of insulin on skeletal muscle and adipose tissue is the stimulation of glucose transport.[119,120] This occurs largely through stimulation of the maximum rate of transport (V_{max}) rather than a change in the affinity of the transport mechanism for glucose.[121] The effect is rapid, with adipocytes exhibiting a 20- to 30-fold stimulation of glucose transport within 10 minutes of insulin treatment.[122] Largely through the work of Cushman and Wardzala,[123] and Kono et al.,[124] the mechanism of insulin-stimulated glucose transport in adipocytes has been shown to involve the translocation of glucose transporters from an intracellular pool to the plasma membrane (Figure 8.5). Furthermore, chronic hyperinsulinemia may lead to an enhanced glucose transport response to insulin by increasing the size of the intracellular pool of transporters.[125]

Recently, the complexity of the regulation of glucose transport has become apparent as transporter proteins

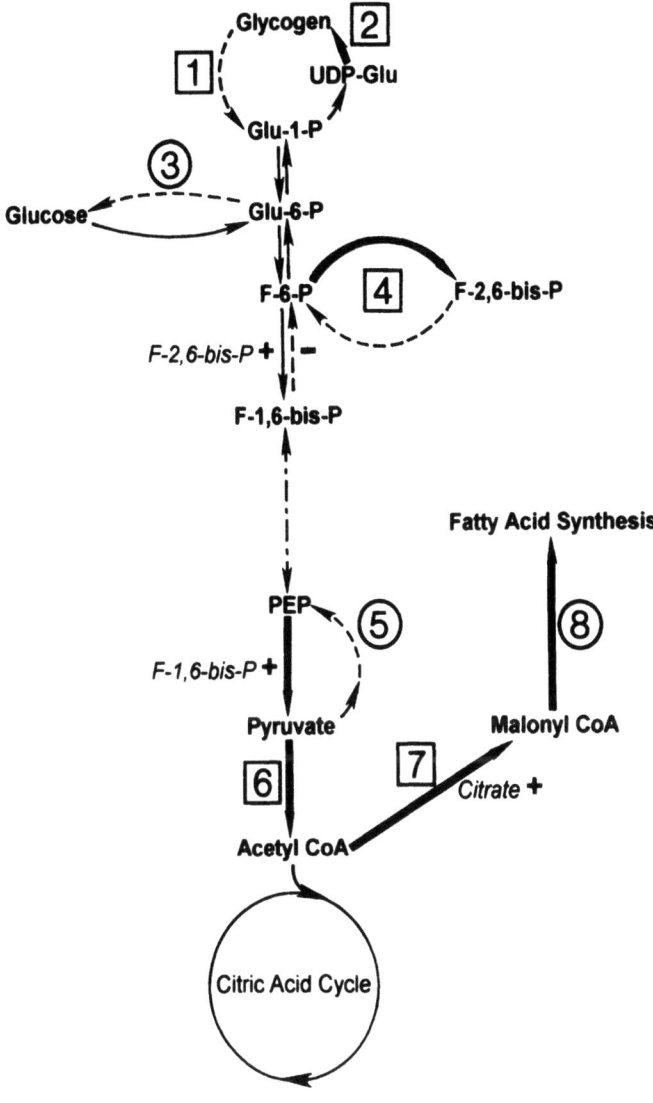

FIGURE 8.6. Key insulin-regulated reactions of intermediary metabolism. Heavy lines represent reactions that show increased activity in the fed state in response to insulin. Dashed lines represent reactions whose activity is decreased in response to insulin. Numbers enclosed in squares denote enzymes that are dephosphorylated in response to insulin. The numbers in circles are enzymes whose content is regulated by insulin. The specific enzymes are 1, phosphorylase; 2, glycogen synthase; 3, glucose-6-phosphatase; 4, bifunctional 6-phosphofructose-2-kinase/fructose-2,6-bisphosphatase; 5, phosphoenolpyruvate carboxykinase; 6, pyruvate dehydrogenase complex; 7, acetyl-CoA carboxylase; 8, fatty acid synthase complex.

have been characterized. Mueckler et al.[126] first reported the sequence and structure of a human glucose transporter (see Chapter 7). These investigators utilized sequencing of a cloned DNA to deduce the structure of a facilitated diffusion glucose carrier from HepG2 cells. This protein, subsequently designated GLUT 1, has 12 membrane-spanning domains that may form a transmembrane pore for the passage of glucose. Despite the human hepatoma origin of the cell line from which the transporter originates, this transporter proved to be identical to the human erythrocyte transporter and distinct from the normal hepatic transporter subsequently sequenced by Lodish.[127] The latter transporter, GLUT 2 is largely confined to liver, kidney, intestine, and pancreatic β cells. Most importantly, neither of these constitutively expressed transporters proved to be the hormone-sensitive transporter that can account for insulin stimulation of adipocyte or skeletal muscle glucose transport. It is the erythroid transporter that represents the predominant placental glucose transport protein.

Pilch's group[128] utilized a novel approach to identify the insulin-responsive glucose transporter. They produced monoclonal antibodies against proteins that were translocated to the surface of rat adipocytes in response to insulin. The lone protein so identified, bound cytochalasin (a characteristic of glucose transporters), was expressed in fat, skeletal muscle, and myocardial muscle, and was distinct from the constitutively expressed transporters. This protein was further characterized as an insulin-regulated transporter, GLUT 4, which is expressed in cardiac muscle, skeletal muscle, and fat.[129]

It should be noted that insulin does not stimulate hepatic uptake of glucose in the presence of euglycemia. In this organ, glucose transport is accomplished by the facilitated diffusion glucose carrier mentioned above. While insulin directly stimulates peripheral uptake of glucose during periods of glucose excess (e.g., in the fed state), it is the level of glycemia that is the main determinant of hepatic glucose uptake in the presence of "permissive" (i.e., basal) portal concentrations of insulin.[130]

The considerable data on the regulation of GLUT 4 translocation and expression has been recently summarized by Stephens and Pilch.[131] As discussed above, the means by which insulin activates the translocation of GLUT 4 from the intracellular to cell surface membrane compartments is unknown. Not all of the components of the membrane vesicles which contain GLUT 4 are similarly translocated.[131] It is possible that regulation of the activity of individual GLUT 4 molecules may also contribute to insulin-sensitive glucose transport. The mechanism for the developmental regulation of GLUT 4, whose expression increases postnatally in insulin sensitive tissues, has not been elucidated.

Hepatic Glycogen Metabolism

The regulation of glycogen metabolism has long been a paradigm for mechanisms of metabolic regulation. The mechanisms by which glucagon activates glycogenolysis have been thoroughly characterized (see Chapter 6). In contrast, the role of insulin in promoting glycogenesis and inhibiting glycogenolysis has been a subject of considerable controversy. This stems, in part, from the fact that much of the basic enzymology of glycogen metabolism has been carried out on enzymes purified from skeletal muscle. The potential for critical differences between muscle and liver enzymes is exemplified by the finding that while muscle glycogen synthase is inhibited upon phosphorylation by cAMP-dependent protein kinase, hepatic synthase lacks the cAMP-dependent phosphorylation site.[132]

The regulation of glycogen metabolism is best viewed as a series of phosphorylation/dephosphorylation cycles with phosphorylation of the rate-limiting enzymes promoting glycogenolysis while their dephosphorylation leads to glycogenesis. Phosphorylase b to a conversion is dependent on phosphorylation at a single site by a single kinase, phosphorylase kinase. Hepatic glycogen synthase, on the other hand, exhibits phosphorylation at multiple sites by multiple protein kinases.[133] Among these, phosphorylase kinase plays a prominent role in the inactivation of hepatic glycogen synthase.[134] Activation of a single regulatory kinase, phosphorylase kinase, can lead to activation of glycogenolysis and simultaneous inactivation of glycogenesis. Similarly, dephosphorylation of both rate-limiting enzymes, as well as the β subunit of phosphorylase kinase, can be carried out by PP-1. The latter is a point of focus for insulin-mediated effects on glycogen metabolism.

The consensus of a number of in vivo animal studies aimed at the effect of insulin on PP-1 is that insulin stimulates its activity.[135-137] Studies by Miller et al.[138] indicate that insulin activates hepatic protein phosphatases directed toward glycogen synthase, resulting in stimulation of glycogenesis. However, the effect of insulin on protein phosphatases is best demonstrated when measured as the ability to counteract phosphatase inhibition by counter-regulatory hormones.[136] In addition, insulin and glucose seem to have synergistic actions on protein phosphatases.[139] Indeed, the physiologic effect of glucose to stimulate glycogenesis probably should place insulin in a secondary role.

Hepatic phosphorylase, but not skeletal muscle phosphorylase, functions as a glucose receptor. The binding of glucose to phosphorylase appears to increase the affinity of phosphorylase for PP-1, leading to phosphorylase a to b conversion via dephosphorylation.[140] Furthermore, the work of Stalmans et al.[141] demonstrated that phosphorylase a is inhibitory for glycogen synthase activation. More recently, this interaction between phosphorylase and glycogen synthase was confirmed by studies showing that phosphorylase a is an allosteric inhibitor of the glycogen-bound form of hepatic PP-1.[142] Glucose can sequentially promote phosphorylase inactivation leading to synthase activation without a requirement for insulin activation of protein phosphatase activity.

The accretion of hepatic glycogen occurs during the second half of the third trimester in most species. Fetal hepatic glycogenesis appears to be best correlated with induction of hepatic glycogen synthase.[143] This process is not impaired by fetal hypoinsulinemia as long as fetal growth is normal. This can be demonstrated using a model of chronic maternal hyperinsulinemia in the pregnant rat.[143] The production of chronic maternal hypoglycemia leads to fetal hypoglycemia and hypoinsulinemia but does not cause significant intrauterine growth retardation. Fetal hepatic glycogen synthase, phosphorylase, protein phosphatase, and, most importantly, glycogen content are unaffected despite an approximately 70% reduction in fetal serum insulin concentrations at term. Taken together with studies showing that epidermal growth factor (EGF)[144] and insulin-like growth factor-I (IGF-I)[145] can promote glycogenesis in fetal rat hepatocytes, it appears that the acquisition of hepatic glycogenesis in the fetus is not solely dependent on insulin.

Hepatic Glycolysis and Gluconeogenesis

The regulation of hepatic glycolysis and gluconeogenesis by hormones that control cAMP levels in liver, most notably, epinephrine and glucagon, occurs at two distinct levels. Activated cAMP-dependent protein kinase phosphorylates a number of regulatory enzymes, thereby controlling their activity acutely. These include pyruvate kinase[146] and the bifunctional enzyme, 6-phosphofructo-2-kinase/fructose-2,6-bisphosphatase.[147] The regulation of pyruvate kinase activity is of particular importance to regulation of gluconeogenesis since most gluconeogenic precursors enter the pathway proximal to this enzyme. Conversely, regulation of fructose 2,6-bisphosphate levels is critical to control of glycolysis, as reviewed by Exton.[148] Fructose 2,6-bisphosphate is a potent allosteric stimulator of 6-phosphofructose-1-kinase and an inhibitor of fructose-1,6-bisphosphatase. Thus, cAMP-dependent phosphorylation of 6-phosphofructo-2-kinase/fructose-2,6-bisphosphatase leads to decreased fructose 2,6-bisphosphate concentrations, resulting in metabolic flux toward gluconeogenesis. Furthermore, fructose 1,6-bisphosphate is an allosteric activator of pyruvate kinase; its accumulation promotes glycolysis. This entire regulatory process can be reversed by protein phosphatases that dephosphorylate cAMP-dependent sites. Although acute effects of insulin on this system have not yet been thoroughly elucidated, it is reasonable to conclude that insulin activates such protein phosphatases.

A long-term effect of cAMP in the liver is to promote the synthesis of phosphoenolpyruvate carboxykinase, a rate-limiting enzyme for gluconeogenesis. This is effected through stimulation of transcription,[149] a process that can be reversed by insulin.[150]

Hepatic Lipid Metabolism and Ketogenesis

Insulin acutely increases the rate of fatty acid synthesis in hepatocytes.[151,152] The key regulatory enzyme for this effect is acetyl-coenzyme A (CoA) carboxylase. This enzyme catalyzes the first committed step of fatty acid synthesis, the conversion of acetyl-CoA to malonyl-CoA by the fixation of bicarbonate. Acetyl-CoA carboxylase is a phosphoenzyme with multiple phosphorylation sites for multiple protein kinases and phosphatases.[153] As is the case for glycogen synthase, interaction between phosphorylation sites may occur. Nonetheless, inactivation of the enzyme in response to elevated intracellular cAMP is probably mediated by phosphorylation at a single site.[154] Inactivation of the enzyme in response to insulin can be accounted for by dephosphorylation at this site. In addition, insulin can activate the carboxylase in the absence of counterregulatory hormones. This effect probably is also dependent on insulin-stimulated dephosphorylation of the enzyme.[153] However, since it has been shown that insulin stimulates an increase in the phosphorylation of specific tryptic peptides distinct from those phosphorylated in response to glucagon or epinephrine,[153] it is possible that insulin exerts its activating effect through stimulation of both protein kinases and phosphatases.

The stimulation of acetyl-CoA carboxylase activity and resulting increase in malonyl-CoA concentrations also accounts for the inhibition of ketogenesis in response to insulin. Malonyl-CoA is a potent inhibitor of carnitine acyltransferase I.[155] This enzyme is located on the outer aspect of the inner mitochondrial membrane. It catalyzes a transesterification between carnitine and fatty acyl-CoA, the initial step in the transport of fatty acids into the mitochondria where they undergo oxidation. Thus, generation of malonyl-CoA for fatty acid synthesis is also inhibitory for fatty acid oxidation.

In addition to the aforementioned acute effects, insulin promotes hepatic lipogenesis by stimulating the synthesis of acetyl-CoA carboxylase, fatty acid synthetase, ATP-citrate lyase, malic enzyme, and glucose-6-phosphate dehydrogenase.[156] Interestingly, insulin stimulates hepatic activity of these enzymes in the chronically hyperinsulinemic fetal rhesus monkey, although no augmented induction of glycogen synthase occurs.[157]

Adipocyte Metabolism

Insulin regulation of adipocyte fatty acid synthesis is regulated, in part, through acute effects on acetyl-CoA carboxylase as it is in liver. In addition, insulin stimulates the phosphorylation of ATP-citrate lyase and the ribosomal protein S6 in isolated rat adipocytes. Insulin may promote dephosphorylation of hormone-sensitive triglyceride lipase, thereby leading to its inactivation. This latter effect directly counteracts the stimulation of lipolysis by cAMP-mediated hormones.[158] Finally, in contrast to liver, insulin potently stimulates adipocyte glucose transport,[131] thereby promoting uptake of substrate for lipogenesis.

Regulation of Protein Synthesis by Insulin

In addition to its ability to regulate the synthesis of specific gene products at the transcriptional level (vide infra), insulin partly fulfills its function as an anabolic hormone by increasing protein synthesis in general. In addition, inhibition of proteolysis is an additional mechanism whereby insulin controls protein accretion, especially in skeletal muscle. Since this tissue is the primary source of gluconeogenic precursors derived from protein, this effect of insulin also results in attenuation of hepatic glucose production.

Insulin promotes protein synthesis in skeletal muscle at several levels. It stimulates amino acid uptake,[159] promotes translation through stimulation of polysome formation and polypeptide initiation,[160] and inhibits lysosomal protein degradation.[161] Similar effects pertain in liver.

The most potent effects of insulin on protein synthesis may be mediated via ribosomal protein S6 phosphorylation, as described above. In addition, insulin can promote initiation of polypeptide synthesis via the dephosphorylation of regulatory phosphoproteins. Among these proteins, eukaryotic initiation factor-2 (eIF-2) is required for translation and is inhibited upon phosphorylation by a cAMP-independent protein kinase. It is a substrate for protein phosphatase type-1.

As discussed above, insulin promotes the accumulation of lipogenic hormones, largely through stimulation of their synthesis. Insulin also stimulates expression of the gene for pyruvate kinase. Conversely, insulin suppresses expression of the gene for phosphoenolpyruvate carboxykinase, thereby opposing the effect of cAMP-mediated hormones. The mechanisms involved in the regulation of gene expression by insulin have not been elucidated. However, several transcription factors whose activity is modulated in response to insulin have been identified. In 3T3-442A adipocytes, multiple DNA binding proteins are rapidly phosphorylated in response to insulin.[162] One of these proteins is nucleolin, a nucleolar constituent that is thought to be involved in the synthesis and transport of preribosomal RNA.

Other transcription factors that may serve as targets for insulin signaling include the cAMP response element binding protein (CREB)[163] and several proteins bearing structural similarity to nuclear lamins.[164] In addition, the AP-1 family of transcription factors, the constituents of which include c-Fos and c-Jun, are phosphorylated in response to insulin in 3T3-442A cells.[165] The regulation of transcription factor activity by insulin via reversible phosphorylation represents an area of intense, ongoing investigation.

Insulin as a Growth Factor

Insulin is a standard constituent of cell culture media and is required for responsiveness of many cell types to agents that promote growth (see chapter 20). However, a direct role for insulin in stimulation of proliferation is less distinct. Many cells will respond to supraphysiologic concentrations of insulin with increased rates of proliferation; however, this probably results from interaction of insulin with type I insulin-like growth factor receptors, which bind insulin with low affinity. Nonetheless, insulin is capable of promoting DNA synthesis in rat hepatocytes.[166] Recent studies indicate that insulin exerts a specific proliferative effect on late gestation fetal rat hepatocytes, which is mediated by a mechanism distinct from that employed by other hepatocyte mitogens such as transforming growth factor-α or hepatocyte growth factor.[167]

Support for an intermediary role for growth factors in mediating insulin effects on growth comes from studies of diabetes mellitus.[168] Experimental diabetes in the rat is associated with decreased IGF-I release from liver; this can be restored by insulin administration. Studies of poorly controlled diabetes in childhood indicate suppressed serum IGF-I concentrations despite elevated growth hormone concentrations. Again, IGF-I serum concentration can be restored by improved metabolic control.

The association between macrosomia and hyperinsulinemia in infants of diabetic mothers has been widely interpreted as supporting a role for insulin as a fetal growth factor. Many aspects of the fetopathy of diabetes in pregnancy can be reproduced by primary hyperinsulinemia in the fetal rhesus monkey.[169] Conversely, experimental intrauterine growth retardation, regardless of cause, is associated with fetal hypoinsulinemia. Pancreatic agenesis with its attendant fetal hypoinsulinemia is a cause of fetal growth retardation. Although a strong association exists between fetal insulinemia and growth, the mechanisms by which insulin can augment growth in specific fetal tissues and organs have not yet been defined.

Conclusion: The Physiologic Integration of Insulin's Biochemical Actions

The physiologic effects of insulin represent the sum of insulin's effects at the cellular level. An understanding of the role of insulin in metabolic physiology requires integration of insulin action and the actions of other peptide hormones, growth factors, steroid hormones, catecholamines, neural mechanisms, etc. Insulin's specialized role may be viewed as promoting fuel storage and acting as a permissive factor in growth. Secretion of insulin in response to increased substrate availability leads to carbohydrate storage as glycogen, lipogenesis in liver and fat cells and protein synthesis in virtually all tissues. The molecular mechanisms involved in these processes allow for an extraordinary multiplicity of control points, accounting for the exquisite fine-tuning of metabolic regulation.

References

1. von Mering J, Minkowski O. Diabetes mellitus nach pankreasextirpation. Arch Exp Pathol Pharmakol 1889;26:371–387.
2. Banting FG, Best CH. The internal secretion of the pancreas. J Lab Clin Med 1922;7:251–266.
3. Yalow RS, Berson SA. Immunoassay of endogenous plasma insulin in man. J Clin Invest 1960;39:1157–1175.
4. Sanger F. Chemistry of insulin. Br Med Bull 1960;16:183–188.
5. Katsoyannis PG, Tometsko A, Fukuda K. Insulin peptides: IX: the synthesis of the A-chain of insulin and its combination with natural B-chain to generate insulin activity. J Am Chem Soc 1963;85:2863–2865.
6. Meienhofer J, Schnabel E, Brinkoff O, et al. Synthese der insulin ketten und ihre kombination zu insulin-aktiven präparaten. Z Naturforsch (C) 1963;18h:1120.
7. Hodgkin DC, Mercola D. The secondary and tertiary structure of insulin. In: Steiner DF, Freinkel N, eds. Endocrine pancreas, vol. 1, sect. 7, endocrinology. Handbook of physiology. Washington, DC: American Physiologic Society, 1972:139–157.
8. Ulrich A, Shine J, Chirgwin J, et al. Rat insulin genes: construction of plasmids containing the coding sequences. Science 1977;196:1313–1319.
9. Goeddel DV. Expression in *Escherichia coli* of chemically synthesized genes for human insulin. Proc Natl Acad Sci USA 1979;76:106–110.
10. Cohen P, Parker PJ, Woodgett JR. The molecular mechanism by which insulin activates glycogen synthase in mammalian skeletal muscle. In: Czech MP, ed. Molecular basis of insulin action. New York: Plenum Press, 1985:213–233.
11. Rosen OM. After insulin binds. Science 1987;237:1452–1458.
12. Steiner DF, Hallund W, Rubenstein AH, et al. Isolation and properties of proinsulin, intermediate forms, and other minor components from crystalline bovine insulin. Diabetes 1968;17:725–736.
13. Chance RE, Ellis RM, Bromer WW. Porcine proinsulin: characterization and amino acid sequence. Science 1968;161:165–167.
14. Chan SJ, Keim P, Steiner DF. Cell-free synthesis of rat preproinsulins: characterization and partial amino acid se-

quence determination. Proc Natl Acad Sci USA 1976; 73:1964–1968.
15. Steiner DF. The biosynthesis of insulin: genetic, evolutionary, and pathophysiologic aspects. Harvey Lect 1984;78: 191–228.
16. Rhodes CJ, Alarcon C. What beta-cell defect could lead to hyperproinsulinemia in NIDDM? Diabetes 1994;43:511–517.
17. Frank BH, Veros AJ. Physical studies on proinsulin—association behavior and conformation in solution. Biochem Biophys Res Commun 1968;32:155–160.
18. Frank BH, Veros AJ, Pekar AH. Physical studies on proinsulin. A comparison of the titration behavior of the tyrosine residues in insulin and proinsulin. Biochemistry 1972;11:4926–4931.
19. Gavin III JR, Kahn CR, Gorden P, et al. Radioreceptor assay of insulin: comparison of plasma and pancreatic insulins and proinsulin. J Clin Endocrinol Metab 1975;41:438–445.
20. Rinderknecht E, Humbel RE. The amino acid sequence of human insulin-like growth factor I and its structural homology with proinsulin. J Biol Chem 1978;253:2769–2776.
21. Blundel TL, Bedarkar S, Rinderknecht E, et al. Insulin-like growth factor: a model for tertiary structure accounting for immunoreactivity and receptor binding. Proc Natl Acad Sci USA 1978;75:180–184.
22. Gruppuso PA, Frank BH, Schwartz R. Binding of proinsulin and proinsulin conversion intermediates to human placental insulin-like growth factor I receptors. J Clin Endocrinol Metab 1988;67:194–197.
23. King JL, Kahn CR. Non-parallel evolution of metabolic and growth-promoting functions of insulin. Nature 1981;292:644–646.
24. Rubenstein AH, Clark JL, Melani F, et al. Secretion of proinsulin C-peptide by pancreatic beta cells and its circulation in blood. Nature 1969;224:697–699.
25. Eaton RP, Allen RC, Schade DS, et al. Prehepatic insulin production in man: kinetic analysis using peripheral connecting peptide behavior. J Clin Endocrinol Metab 1980;51:520–528.
26. Horwitz DL, Rubenstein AH, Katz AI. Quantitation of human pancreatic beta cell function by immunoassay of C-peptide in urine. Diabetes 1977;26:30–35.
27. Kuzuya H, Blix PM, Horwitz DL, et al. Determination of free and total insulin and C-peptide in insulin-treated diabetics. Diabetes 1977;26:22–29.
28. Kuzuya T, Matsuda A, Sakamoto T, et al. C-peptide immunoreactivity (CPR) in urine. Diabetes 1978;27(suppl 1):210–215.
29. Gero L, Baranyi E, Bekefi D, et al. Investigation on serum C-peptide concentrations in pregnant diabetic women and in newborns of diabetic mothers. Horm Metab Res 1981;14:516–520.
30. Block MB, Pildes RS, Mossabhoy NA, et al. C-peptide immunoreactivity: a new method for studying infants of insulin-treated mothers. Pediatrics 1974;53:923–928.
31. Sosenko IR, Kitzmiller JL, Loo SW, et al. The infant of the diabetic mother: correlation of increased cord C-peptide levels with macrosomia and hypoglycemia. N Engl J Med 1979;301:859–862.
32. Polonsky K, Jaspan JB, Pugh W. Metabolism of C-peptide in the dog. In vivo demonstration of the absence of hepatic extraction. J Clin Invest 1983;72:1114–1123.
33. Polonsky KS, Rubenstein AH. C-peptide as a measure of the secretion and hepatic extraction of insulin. Pitfalls and limitations. Diabetes 1984;33:486–494.
34. Gruppuso PA, Susa JB, Sehgal P, et al. Metabolism and placental transfer of ^{125}I-proinsulin and ^{125}I-tyrosylated C-peptide in the pregnant rhesus monkey. J Clin Invest 1987;80:1132–1137.
35. De Haen C, Litle SA, May JM, et al. Characterization of proinsulin-insulin intermediates in human plasma. J Clin Invest 1978;62:727–737.
36. Rubenstein AH, Cho S, Steiner DF. Evidence for proinsulin in human urine and serum. Lancet 1968;1:1353–1355.
37. Roth J, Gorden P, Pastan I. "Big insulin": a new component of plasma insulin detected by immunoassay. Proc Natl Acad Sci USA 1968;61:138–145.
38. Deacon CF, Conlon JM. Measurement of circulating proinsulin concentrations using a proinsulin-specific antiserum. Diabetes 1985;34:491–497.
39. Cohen RM, Nakabayashi T, Blix PM, et al. A radioimmunoassay for circulating human proinsulin. Diabetes 1985;34:84–91.
40. Gorden P, Roth J. Plasma insulin: fluctuations in the "big" insulin component in man after glucose and other stimuli. J Clin Invest 1969;48:2225–2234.
41. Gorden P, Sherman BM, Simopoulos AP. Glucose intolerance with hypokalemia: an increased proportion of circulating proinsulin-like component. J Clin Endocrinol Metab 1972;34:235–240.
42. Gorden P, Hendricks CM, Roth J. Circulating proinsulin-like component in man: increased proportion in hypoinsulinemic states. Diabetologia 1974;10:469–474.
43. Sherman BM, Gorden P, Roth J, et al. Circulating insulin: the proinsulin-like properties of "big" insulin in patients without islet cell tumors. J Clin Invest 1971; 50:849–858.
44. Kuhl C, Hvorslev V, Tygstrup I, et al. Elevated serum proinsulin in beta cell nesidioblastosis. Report of a case in a newborn. Scand J Gastroenterol 1979;14(suppl 53):49–52.
45. Heding LG, Persson B, Stangenberg M. B-cell function in newborn infants of diabetic mothers. Diabetologia 1980;19:427–432.
46. Gabbay KH, DeLuca K, Fisher JN Jr, et al. Familial hyperproinsulinemia: an autosomal dominant defect. N Engl J Med 1976;294:911–915.
47. Kanazawa Y, Hayashi M, Ikeuchi M, et al. Familial proinsulinemia: a rare disorder of insulin biosynthesis. In: Baba S, Kaneko T, Yanihara N, eds. Proinsulin, insulin, C-peptide. Amsterdam: Excerpta Medica, 1979:262–269.
48. Gruppuso PA, Gordon P, Kahn CR, et al. Familial hyperproinsulinemia due to a proposed defect in proinsulin to insulin conversion. N Engl J Med 1984;311:629–634.

49. Robbins DC, Shoelson SE, Rubenstein AH, et al. Familial hyperproinsulinemia. Two cohorts secreting indistinguishable type II intermediates of proinsulin conversion. J Clin Invest 1984;73:714–719.
50. Shibasaki Y, Kawakami T, Kanazawa Y, et al. Posttranslational cleavage of proinsulin is blocked by a point mutation in familial hyperproinsulinemia. J Clin Invest 1985;76:378–380.
51. Chan SJ, Seino S, Gruppuso PA, et al. A mutation in the B chain coding region is associated with impaired proinsulin conversion in a family with hyperproinsulinemia. Proc Natl Acad Sci USA 1987;84:2194–2197.
52. O'Rahilly S, Gray H, Humphreys PJ, et al. Brief report: impaired processing of prohormones associated with abnormalities of glucose homeostasis and adrenal function. N Engl J Med 1995;333:1386–1390
53. Owerbach D, Bell GI, Rutter WJ, et al. The insulin gene is located on the short arm of chromosome 11 in humans. Diabetes 1981;30:267–270.
54. Bell GI, Pictet RL, Rutter WJ, et al. Sequence of the human insulin gene. Nature 1980;284:26–32.
55. Ullrich A, Dull TJ, Gray A, et al. Genetic variation in the human insulin gene. Science 1980;209:612–615.
56. Chan SJ, Noyes BE, Agarwal KL, et al. Construction and selection of recombinant plasmids containing full-length complementary DNAs corresponding to rat insulins I and II. Proc Natl Acad Sci USA 1979;76:5036–5040.
57. Walker MD, Edlund T, Boulet AM, Rutter WJ. Cell-specific expression controlled by the 5'-flanking region of insulin and chymotrypsin genes. Nature 1983;306:557–561.
58. Fromont-Racine M, Bucchini D, Madsen O, et al. Effect of 5'-flanking sequence deletions on expression of the human insulin gene in transgenic mice. Mol Endocrinol 1990;4:669–677.
59. Dandy-Dron F, Itier JM, Monthioux E, et al. Tissue-specific expression of the rat insulin I gene in vivo requires both the enhancer and promoter regions. Differentiation 1995;58:291–295.
60. Clark AR, Petersen HV, Read ML, et al. Human insulin gene enhancer-binding proteins in pancreatic a and b cell lines. FEBS Letts 1993;329:139–143.
61. Karlsson O, Thor S, Norberg T, et al. Insulin gene enhancer binding protein Isl-1 is a member of a novel class of proteins containing both a homeo- and a cys-his domain. Nature 1990;344:879–882.
62. German MS, Wang J, Chadwick RB, Rutter WJ. Synergistic activation of the insulin gene by a LIM-homeodomain protein and basic helix-loop-helix protein: building a functional insulin minienhancer complex. Genes Dev 1992;6:2165–2176.
63. Ohlsson H, Karlsson K, Edlund T. IPF1, a homeodomain-containing transactivator of the insulin gene. EMBO J 1993;12:4251–4259.
64. Tager HW. Abnormal products of the human insulin gene. Diabetes 1984;33:693–699.
65. Matschinsky FM. A lesson in metabolic regulation inspired by the glucokinase glucose sensor paradigm. Diabetes 1996;45:223–241.
66. Meglasson MD, Matschinsky FM. Pancreatic islet glucose metabolism and regulation of insulin secretion. Diabetes Metab Rev 1986;2:163–214.
67. German MS. Glucose sensing in pancreatic islet beta cells: the key role of glucokinase and the glycolytic intermediates. Proc Natl Acad Sci USA 1993;90:1781–1785.
68. Vionnet N, Stoffel M, Takeda J, et al. Nonsense mutation in the glucokinase gene causes early-onset non-insulin-dependent diabetes mellitus. Nature 1992;356:721–722.
69. Gidh-Jain M, Takeda J, Xu LZ, et al. Glucokinase mutations associated with non-insulin-dependent (type 2) diabetes mellitus have decreased enzymatic activity: implications for structure/function relationships. Proc Natl Acad Sci USA 1993;90:1932–1936.
70. Permutt MA, Kipnis DM. Insulin biosynthesis. 1. On the mechanism of glucose stimulation. J Biol Chem 1972;247:1194–1199.
71. Welsh M, Schrerberg N, Gilmore R, Steiner DF. Translational control of insulin biosynthesis. Evidence for regulation of elongation, initiation and signal-recognition-particle-mediated translational arrest by glucose. Biochem J 1986;235:13690–13694.
72. Docherty K, Clark AB. Nutrient regulation of insulin gene expression. FASEB J 1994;8:20–27.
73. Ward WK, Beard JC, Halter JB, et al. Pathophysiology of insulin secretion in non-insulin-dependent diabetes mellitus. Diabetes Care 1984;7:491–502.
74. Hammonds P, Schofield PN, Ashcroft SJH, et al. Regulation and specificity of glucose-stimulated insulin gene expression in human islets of Langerhans. FEBS Letts 1987;223:131–137.
75. Philippe J. Somatostatin inhibits insulin gene expression through a posttranscriptional mechanism in a hamster islet cell line. Diabetes 1993;42:244–249.
76. Curry DL, Bennett LL, Grodsky GM. Dynamics of insulin secretion by the perfused rat pancreas. Endocrinology 1968;83:572–578.
77. Hughs SJ. The role of reduced glucose transporter content and glucose metabolism in the immature secretory responses of fetal rat pancreatic islets. Diabetologia 1994;37:134–140.
78. Weinhaus AJ, Poronnik P, Cook DI, Tuch BE. Insulin secretagogues, but not glucose, stimulate an increase in $[Ca^{2+}]_i$ in the fetal rat beta-cell. Diabetes 1995;44:118–124.
79. Aguilar-Bryan L, Nichols CG, Wechsler SW, et al. Cloning of the beta cell high-affinity sulfonylurea receptor: a regulator of insulin secretion. Science 1995;268:423–426.
80. Thomas PM, Cote GJ, Wohlik N, et al. Mutations in the sulfonylurea receptor gene in familial persistent hyperinsulinemic hypoglycemia of infancy. Science 1995;268:426–429.
81. Inagaki N, Gonoi T, Clement JP, et al. Reconstitution of IKATP: an inward rectifier subunit plus the sulfonylurea receptor. Science 1995;270:1159–1162.
82. Sodoyez JC, Sodoyez-Goffaux F, Guillaume M, et al. [^{123}I] insulin metabolism in normal rats and humans: external

detection by a scintillation camera. Science 1983;219:865–867.
83. Kahn CR, Baird KI, Flier JS, et al. Insulin receptors, receptor antibodies, and the mechanism of insulin action. Recent Prog Horm Res 1981;37:447–538.
84. Pessin JE, Mottola C, Yu K-T, et al. Subunit structure and regulation of the insulin-receptor complex. In: Czech M, ed. Molecular basis of insulin action. New York: Plenum Press, 1985:3–30.
85. Pilch PF, Czech MP. The subunit structure of the high affinity insulin receptor. Evidence for a disulfide-linked receptor complex in fat cell and liver plasma membranes. J Biol Chem 1980;19:70–75.
86. Cheatham B, Kahn CR. Insulin action and the insulin signaling network. Endocr Rev 1995;16:117–142.
87. Kasuga M, Karlsson FA, Kahn CR. Insulin stimulates the phosphorylation of the 95,000–dalton subunit of its own receptor. Science 1982;215:185–187.
88. Goren HJ, White MF, Kahn CR. Separate domains of the insulin receptor contain sites of autophosphorylation and tyrosine kinase activity. Biochemistry 1987;26:2374–2381.
89. Feener EP, Backer JM, King GL, et al. Insulin stimulates serine and tyrosine phosphorylation in the juxtamembrane region of the insulin receptor. J Biol Chem 1993;268:11256–11264.
90. Wilden PA, Kahn CR, Siddle K, White MF. Insulin receptor kinase domain autophosphorylation regulates receptor enzymatic function. J Biol Chem 1992;267:16660–16668.
91. Roth R, Beaudoin J. Phosphorylation of purified insulin receptor by cAMP kinase. Diabetes 1987;36:123–126.
92. Jacobs S, Cuatrecasas P. Phosphorylation of receptors for insulin and insulin-like growth factor I. J Biol Chem 1986;261:934–939.
93. Heidenreich KA, Olefsky JM. The metabolism of insulin receptors: internalization, degradation, and recycling. In: Czech MP, ed. Molecular basis of insulin action. New York: Plenum Press, 1985:45–66.
94. Stone RL, Dixon JE. Protein-tyrosine phosphatases. J Biol Chem 1994;269:31323–31326.
95. Boylan JM, Brautigan DL, Madden J, et al. Differential regulation of multiple hepatic protein tyrosine phosphatases in alloxan diabetic rats. J Clin Invest 1992;90:174–179.
96. Ahmad F, Goldstein BJ. Alterations in specific protein-tyrosine phosphatases accompany insulin resistance of streptozotocin diabetes. Am J Physiol 1995;268:E932–E940.
97. Neufeld ND, Kaplan SA, Lippe BM. Increased monocyte receptor binding of 125I-insulin in infants of gestational diabetic mothers. J Clin Endocrinol Metab 1978;47:590–595.
98. Gruppuso PA. Effects of fetal hypoinsulinemia on fetal hepatic insulin binding in the rat. Biochim Biophys Acta 1989;1010:270–273.
99. White MF, Maron R, Kahn CR. Insulin rapidly stimulates tyrosine phosphorylation of a Mr 185,000 protein in intact cells. Nature 1985;318:183–186.
100. White MF, Livingston JN, Backer JM, et al. Mutation of the insulin receptor at tyrosine 960 inhibits signal transmission but does not affect its tyrosine kinase activity. Cell 1988;54:641–649.
101. Sun XJ, Rothenberg P, Kahn CR, et al. The structure of the insulin receptor substrate IRS-1 defines a unique signal transduction protein. Nature 1991;352:73–77.
102. Saltiel AR. Diverse signaling pathways in the cellular actions of insulin. Am J Physiol 1996;270:E375–E385.
103. Boylan JM, Gruppuso PA. In vitro and in vivo regulation of hepatic mitogen-activated protein kinases in fetal rats. Am J Physiol 1994;267:G1078–G1086.
104. DiGuglielmo GM, Baass PC, Ou W-J, et al. Compartmentalization of SHC, GRB2 and mSOS, and hyperphosphorylation of Raf-1 by EGF but not insulin in liver parenchyma. EMBO J 1994;13:4269–4277.
105. Cori GT, Cori CF. The enzymatic conversion of phosphorylase a to b. J Biol Chem 1945;158:321–332.
106. Krebs EG, Fisher EH. The phosphorylase b to a converting enzyme of rabbit skeletal muscle. Biochim Biophys Acta 1956;20:150–157.
107. Robison GA, Butcher RW, Sutherland EW, eds. Cyclic AMP. New York: Academic Press, 1971:91–144.
108. Sturgill TW, Ray LB, Erikson E, Maller JL. Insulin-stimulated MAP-2 kinase phosphorylates and activates ribosomal protein S6 kinase II. Nature 1988;334:715–718.
109. Fingar DC, Hausdorff SF, Blenis J, Birnbaum MJ. Dissociation of pp70 ribosomal protein S6 kinase from insulin-stimulated glucose transport in 3T3-L1 adipocytes. J Biol Chem 1993;268:3005–3008.
110. Berndt N, Campbell DG, Caudwell FB, et al. Isolation and sequence analysis of a cDNA clone encoding a type-1 protein phosphatase catalytic subunit: homology with protein phosphatase 2A. FEBS Lett 1987;223:340–346.
111. da Cruz e Silva O, Alemany S, Campbell DG, et al. Isolation and sequence analysis of a cDNA clone encoding the entire catalytic subunit of a type-2A protein phosphatase. FEBS Lett 1987;221:415–422.
112. Goris J, Defreyn G, Vandenheede JR, et al. Protein inhibitors of dog-liver phosphorylase phosphatase dependent on and independent of protein kinase. Eur J Biochem 1978;91:457–464.
113. Lawrence JC Jr, Hiken J, Burnette B, et al. Phosphorylation of phosphoprotein phosphatase inhibitor-2 (I-2) in rat fat cells. Biochem Biophys Res Commun 1988;150:197–203.
114. Villa-Moruzzi E, Ballou LM, Fisher EH. Phosphorylase phosphatase. Interconversion of active and inactive forms. J Biol Chem 1984;259:5857–5863.
115. Stralfors P, Hiraga A, Cohen P. The protein phosphatases involved in cellular regulation. Purification and characterization of the glycogen-bound form of protein phosphatase-1 from rabbit skeletal muscle. FEBS Lett 1985;149:295–303.
116. Cohen P. The structure and regulation of protein phosphatases. Annu Rev Biochem 1989;58:453–508.
117. Dent PA, Lavoinne S, Nakielny FB, et al. The molecular mechanism by which insulin stimulates glycogen synthesis in mammalian skeletal muscle. Nature 1990;348:302–308.

118. Saltiel AR, Fox JA, Sherline P, et al. Insulin-stimulated hydrolysis of a novel glycolipid generates modulators of cAMP phosphodiesterase. Science 1986;233:967–972.
119. Levine R, Goldstein M. On the mechanism of action of insulin. Recent Prog Horm Res 1955;11:343–380.
120. Park CR, Reinwein D, Henderson MJ, et al. The action of insulin on the transport of glucose through the cell membrane. Am J Med 1959;26:674–684.
121. Crofford OB, Renold AE. Glucose uptake by incubated rat epididymal adipose tissue: characteristics of the glucose transport system and action of insulin. J Biol Chem 1965;240:3237–3244.
122. Karnieli E, Zarnowski MJ, Hissin PJ, et al. Insulin-stimulated translocation of glucose transport systems in the isolated rat adipose cell: time course, reversal, insulin concentration-dependency and relationship to glucose transport activity. J Biol Chem 1981;256:4772–4777.
123. Cushman SW, Wardzala LJ. Potential mechanism of insulin action on glucose transport in the isolated rat adipose cell. Apparent translocation of intracellular transport systems to the plasma membrane. J Biol Chem 1980;255:4758–4762.
124. Kono T, Robinson FW, Blevins TL, et al. Evidence that translocation of the glucose transport activity is the major mechanism of insulin action on glucose transport in fat cells. J Biol Chem 1982;257:10942–10947.
125. Kahn BB, Horton ES, Cushman SW. Mechanism for enhanced glucose transport response to insulin in adipose cells from chronically hyperinsulinemic rats. Increased translocation of glucose transports from an enlarged intracellular pool. J Clin Invest 1987;79:853–858.
126. Mueckler M, Caruso C, Baldwin SA, et al. Sequence and structure of a human glucose transporter. Science 1985;229:941–945.
127. Lodish HF. Anion-exchange and glucose transport proteins: structure, function and distribution. Harvey Lect 1987;82:19–46.
128. James DE, Brown R, Navarro J, Pilch PF. Insulin regulatable tissues express a unique insulin-sensitive glucose transport protein. Nature 1988;333:183–185.
129. Kasanicki MA, Pilch PF. Regulation of glucose transporter function. Diabetes Care 1990;13:228–243.
130. Cherrington AD, Stevenson RW, Steiner KE, et al. Insulin, glucagon, and glucose as regulators of hepatic glucose uptake and production in vivo. Diabetes Metab Rev 1987;3:307–332.
131. Stephens JM, Pilch PF. The metabolic regulation and vesicular transport of GLUT4, the major insulin-responsive glucose transporter. Endocr Rev 1995;16:529–546.
132. Wang Y, Bell AW, Hermodson MA, et al. Liver isozyme of rabbit glycogen synthase. Amino acid sequences surrounding phosphorylation sites recognized by cyclic AMP-dependent protein kinase. J Biol Chem 1986;261:16909–16915.
133. Imazu M, Strickland WG, Chrisman TD, et al. Phosphorylation and inactivation of liver glycogen synthase by liver protein kinases. J Biol Chem 1984;259:1813–1821.
134. Akatsuka A, Singh TJ, Huang K-P. Phosphorylation of rat liver glycogen synthase by phosphorylase kinase. J Biol Chem 1984;259:7878–7883.
135. Shahed AR, Mehta PP, Chalker D, et al. Stimulation of rat liver phosphorylase phosphatase activity by insulin. Biochem Int 1980;1:486–492.
136. Farkas I, Toth B, Got G, et al. Hormonal regulation of phosphorylase phosphatase activity in rat liver. FEBS Lett 1986;203:253–256.
137. Toth B, Bollen M, Stalmans W. Acute regulation of hepatic protein phosphatases by glucagon, insulin, and glucose. J Biol Chem 1988;263:14061–14066.
138. Miller TB Jr, Garnache A, Cruz J. Insulin regulation of glycogen synthase phosphatase in primary cultures of hepatocytes. J Biol Chem 1984;259:12470–12474.
139. Witters LA, Avruch J. Insulin regulation of hepatic glycogen synthase and phosphorylase. Biochemistry 1978;17:406–410.
140. Stalmans W, De Wulf H, Lederer B, et al. The effect of glucose and of a treatment by glucocorticoids on the inactivation in vitro of liver glycogen phosphorylase. Eur J Biochem 1970;15:9–12.
141. Stalmans W, De Wulf H, Hue L, et al. The sequential inactivation of glycogen phosphorylase and activation of glycogen synthetase in liver after the administration of glucose to mice and rats. The mechanism of the hepatic threshold to glucose. Eur J Biochem 1974;41:127–134.
142. Alemany S, Cohen P. Phosphorylase a is an allosteric inhibitor of the glycogen and microsomal forms of rat hepatic protein phosphatase-1. FEBS Lett 1986;198:194–202.
143. Gruppuso PA, Brautigan DL. Induction of hepatic glycogenesis in the fetal rat. Am J Physiol 1989;256:E49–E54.
144. Freemark M. Epidermal growth factor stimulates glycogen synthesis in fetal rat hepatocytes: comparison with the glycogenic effects of insulin-like growth factor I and insulin. Endocrinology 1986;119:522–526.
145. Freemark M, D'Ercole AJ, Handwerger S. Somatomedin-C stimulates glycogen synthesis in fetal rat hepatocytes. Endocrinology 1985;116:2578–2582.
146. Ekman P, Dahlqvist U, Humble E, et al. Comparative kinetic studies on L-type pyruvate kinase from rat liver and the enzyme phosphorylated by cyclic 3'5'-AMP-stimulated protein kinase. Biochim Biophys Acta 1976;429:374–382.
147. Pilkis SJ, Regen DM, Stewart HB, et al. Evidence for two catalytic sites on 6-phosphofructo-2-kinase/fructose 2,6-bisphosphatase. J Biol Chem 1984;259:949–958.
148. Exton JH. Mechanisms of hormonal regulation of hepatic glucose metabolism. Diabetes Metab Rev 1987;3:163–183.
149. Beale EG, Hartley JL, Granner DK. $N_6,0_2'$-dibutyryl cyclic AMP and glucose regulate the amount of messenger RNA coding for hepatic phosphoenolpyruvate carboxykinase (GTP). J Biol Chem 1982;257:2022–2028.
150. Cimbala MA, Larmers WH, Nelson K, et al. Rapid changes in the concentration of phosphoenolpyruvate carboxykinase mRNA in rat liver and kidney. J Biol Chem 1982;257:7629–7636.
151. Geelen MJH, Beynen AC, Christiansen RZ, et al. Short-term effects of insulin and glucagon on lipid synthesis in isolated rat hepatocytes. FEBS Lett 1978;95:326–330.

152. Beynen AC, Vaartjes WJ, Geelen MJH. Opposite effects of insulin and glucagon in acute hormonal control of hepatic lipogenesis. Diabetes 1979;28:828–835.
153. Witters LA. Regulation of acetyl CoA carboxylase by insulin and other hormones. In: Czech MP, ed. Molecular basis of insulin action. New York: Plenum Press, 1985:315–326.
154. Ha J, Daniel S, Broyles SS, Kim KH. Critical phosphorylation sites for acetyl-CoA carboxylase activity. J Biol Chem 1994;269:22162–22168.
155. McGarry JD, Mannaerts GP, Foster DW. A possible role for malonyl-CoA in the regulation of hepatic fatty acid oxidation and ketogenesis. J Clin Invest 1977;60:265–270.
156. Lakshmanan MR, Nepokroeff CM, Porter JW. Control of the synthesis of fatty-acid synthetase in rat liver by insulin, glucagon, and adenosine 3′:5′ cyclic monophosphate. Proc Natl Acad Sci USA 1972;69:3516–3519.
157. McCormick KL, Susa JB, Widness JA, et al. Chronic hyperinsulinemia in the fetal rhesus monkey. Effects on hepatic enzymes active in lipogenesis and carbohydrate metabolism. Diabetes 1979;28:1064–1068.
158. Fain JN. Hormonal regulation of lipid mobilization from adipose tissue. In: Litwack G, ed. Biochemical actions of hormones, vol. VII. New York: Academic Press, 1980:119–204.
159. Narahara HT, Holloszy JO. The actions of insulin, trypsin, and electrical stimulation on amino acid transport in muscle. J Biol Chem 1974;249:5435–5443.
160. Kimball SR, Jefferson LS. Cellular mechanisms involved in the action of insulin on protein synthesis. Diabetes Metab Rev 1988;4:773–787.
161. Kettelhut IC, Wing SS, Goldberg AL. Endocrine regulation of protein breakdown in skeletal muscle. Diabetes Metab Rev 1988;4:751–772.
162. Csermely P, Schnaider T, Cheatham B, et al. Insulin induces the phosphorylation of nucleolin: a possible mechanism of insulin-induced RNA efflux from nuclei. J Biol Chem 1993;268:9747–9752.
163. Holcomb B, Hsieh P, Hoeffler J, Draznin B. Insulin inhibits nuclear phosphatase PP-2A to promote phosphorylation of the transcription factors ATF-1 and CREB. Clin Res 1993;41:210A.
164. Csermely P, Kahn CR. Insulin induces the phosphorylation of DNA-binding nuclear proteins including lamins in 3T3-F442A. Biochemistry 1992;31:9940–9952.
165. Kim SJ, Kahn CR. Insulin stimulates phosphorylation of c-Jun, c-Fos and Fos-related proteins in cultured adipocytes. J Biol Chem 1994;269:11887–11892.
166. Koch KS, Shapiro S, Skelly H. Rat hepatocyte proliferation is stimulated by insulin-like peptides in defined medium. Biochem Biophys Res Commun 1982;109:1054–1060.
167. Grupposo PA, Boylan JM, Bienieki TC, Curran TC. Evidence for a direct hepatotrophic role for insulin in the fetal rat: implications for the impaired hepatic growth seen in fetal growth retardation. Endocrinology 1994;134:769–775.
168. Hill DJ, Milner RDG. Insulin as a growth factor. Pediatr Res 1985;19:879–886.
169. Susa JB, Schwartz R. Effects of hyperinsulinemia in the primate fetus. Diabetes 1985;34:36–41.
170. Oyer PE, Cho S, Peterson JD, Steiner DF. Studies on human proinsulin. Isolation and amino acid sequence of the human pancreatic C-peptide. J Biol Chem 1971;246:1375–1386.

9
Counterregulatory Hormones: Molecular, Biochemical, and Physiologic Aspects

John E. Gerich and Philip E. Cryer

Normal nutrient homeostasis depends on the balance between the effects of insulin and those of the counterregulatory hormones.[1-4] Classically these hormones have been defined as those that oppose the actions of insulin, and they include glucagon, catecholamines, growth hormone, and cortisol. Of the catecholamines (i.e., epinephrine and norepinephrine), epinephrine is currently considered to act as a circulating hormone, whereas norepinephrine probably acts mainly as a neurotransmitter. Although thyroxine and triiodothyronine affect various aspects of metabolism,[5] circulating thyroid hormone levels are not acutely altered by nutrient signals, and fluctuations in their daily secretion do not influence metabolic processes. For these reasons, thyroxine and triiodothyronine are not generally considered among the classic counterregulatory hormones.

In recent years, evidence has been offered that amylin, a cosecretory product of insulin by the pancreatic β cell,[6] tumor necrosis factor α (TNFα) and leptin,[7] both of which are secretory products of adipocytes, and certain cytokines released from inflammatory tissues[8] may affect insulin sensitivity in various tissues. The physiologic and pathogenetic roles of these factors have not been established. Consequently, only a brief summary of some of them will be provided.

Regulating factors in addition to insulin and the classic counterregulatory hormones also affect metabolic balance. These include various neurotransmitters (e.g., norepinephrine from sympathetic postganglionic and sympathetic postganglionic neurons, and acetylcholine from parasympathetic neurons and neuropeptides) as well as substrates including glucose and fatty acids. Their roles have been reviewed elsewhere.[1-4]

Glucagon

Background

Glucagon, a 29 amino acid polypeptide with a molecular weight of 3485 daltons(d) (Figure 9.1), was discovered as a "contaminant" hyperglycemic factor in pancreatic extracts by Kimball and Murlin[9] in 1923 and finally sequenced by Bromer and Behrens[10] in the late 1950s. Studies of its mechanism in the 1960s by Sutherland et al.[11] led to the discovery of the second messenger cyclic adenosine monophosphate (cAMP). Full appreciation of its importance for normal fuel homeostasis in humans and in patients with diabetes mellitus did not come until the 1970s when the availability of somatostatin, an inhibitor of glucagon secretion, permitted investigation of its lack under various experimental conditions.[12]

Biosynthesis

Glucagon is secreted by A cells of pancreatic islets. Normally, these cells constitute approximately 15% to 20% of the total islet cell mass. In most species, A cells are located at the periphery of islets juxtaposed to both B cells, which secrete insulin, and D cells, which secrete somatostatin. Glucagon is synthesized initially as a large molecule of approximately 12,000 d. This peptide undergoes cleavage to a 9000-d molecule, which in turn is cleaved to a 4900-d molecule, which is finally cleaved to yield the 3485-d molecule.[13,14] The whole process takes about 90 minutes. All of these peptides are immunoreactive, but only the 3485-d molecule is biologically active.

Plasma Glucagon

Plasma glucagon concentration varies considerably from individual to individual. The main factors responsible for this variation are the specificity of the antiserum used in the immunoassay and the relative proportion of the total immunoreactivity accounted for by the 3485-d molecule.[12,15,16] In dogs and humans, the pancreas is not the sole source of glucagon. A cells, similar to those in pancreatic islets, have been found in the stomach and in the small and large intestine.[17,18] These cells contain a peptide that is immunologically and physicochemically similar or identical to pancreatic A-cell glucagon and that

H-His-Ser-Gln-Gly-Thr-Phe-Thr-Ser-Asp-Tyr-Ser-Lys-Tyr-Leu-Asp-
  1   2   3   4   5   6   7   8   9 10 11 12 13 14 15

Ser-Arg-Arg-Ala-Gln-Asp-Phe-Val-Gln-Trp-Leu-Met-Asn-Thr-OH
 16 17 18 19 20 21 22 23 24 25 26 27 28 29

FIGURE 9.1. Amino acid sequence of glucagon.

TABLE 9.1. Composition of plasma glucagon immunoreactivity in normal humans.

Species	40,000 dalton	9000 dalton	3500 dalton	2000 dalton
Mean	48.3%	10.7%	25.6%	15.4%
S.E.	6.8	2.1	3.7	2.1
Range	8–97	1–32	1–51	1–33

Data from refs. 35 and 38 are based on Bio-Gel P-30 chromatography of plasma from 18 overnight-fasted subjects.

has a glucagon-like biologic activity.[19–21] These observations could explain the presence of circulating glucagon immunoreactivity following total pancreatectomy in humans[22–25] and other species.[26–28] The relative contribution of pancreatic and extrapancreatic A cells to plasma glucagon and substrate homeostasis remains to be established.[29–30] Control of extrapancreatic glucagon secretion seems to differ from that of pancreatic glucagon.[21,24,27,31]

Normally, in humans and most other mammalian species, arterial and peripheral venous plasma immunoreactive glucagon concentrations range between 35 and 200 pg·ml^{-1} (1.0–6.0 × 10^{-8} M) after a 12- to 16-hour fast. Portal venous levels can average 1.5 to 3.0 times those present in arterial blood because of extraction of glucagon by the liver.[32–39] As with other peptide hormones, circulating glucagon immunoreactivity is heterogeneous.[16] By using chromatography, four immunoreactive species with apparent molecular weights of >40,000, 9000, 3500, and 2000 have been found (Figure 9.2) (Table 9.1) There is considerable individual and species variation in the proportions of each component found in plasma.[34,35] In humans, the 3500-d species, the only fraction unequivocally demonstrated to be biologically active, usually constitutes only about 25% of total plasma glucagon immunoreactivity. The 9000-d molecule, which has similar immunoreactivity but substantially less bioactivity than the 3500-d molecule, can be converted by trypsin to a smaller immunoreactive peptide of approximately 3500 d[40]; it is thought to represent the biosynthetic precursor of glucagon (i.e., proglucagon?) found in the pancreas, which is also convertible to glucagon by trypsin.[41] Increased amounts of the 9000-d molecule are found in the plasma of patients with the glucagonoma syndrome,[42] with renal failure,[36] and with hepatocellular damage or carcinoma of the pancreas.[15] The 2000-d molecule probably represents an inactive degradation product of glucagon.

The heterogeneity of plasma glucagon can complicate the interpretation of in vivo studies of glucagon secretion and metabolism. Changes in plasma glucagon immunoreactivity during stimulation or suppression of A cell secretion are due almost exclusively to changes in the 3500-d fraction.[40,43,44] Although the overall distribution of plasma glucagon is not altered in diabetes and most other pathologic conditions in which the study of A cell function might be of interest,[16] the relative contribution of the fractions can vary considerably among individuals. Thus, comparisons, based on absolute levels of total plasma glucagon immunoreactivity, may be misleading.

The pancreatic content of glucagon varies considerably among species; the human pancreas contains approximately 700 to 1000 μg of glucagon. Glucagon is stored within A cells in distinctive granules and is secreted by a process called emiocytosis,[45] which involves migration of secretory granules to the periphery of cells, fusion of granules with the plasma membranae, and extrusion of granule contents into the extracellular space. Like insulin secretion, secretion of glucagon probably involves a cAMP-calcium interaction,[46,47] is dependent on the presence of extracellular calcium,[48] and is influenced by the concentration of ions such as potassium, calcium, and magnesium.[49] In vivo secretion of glucagon is the net result of the influence of substrate, neural, ionic, hormonal, and local factors on islet A cell function. The plasma concentration of glucagon depends on the balance between rates of secretion and degradation and also on the sampling site (e.g., peripheral venous versus portal venous). Basal (nonstimulated) secretion rates of gluca-

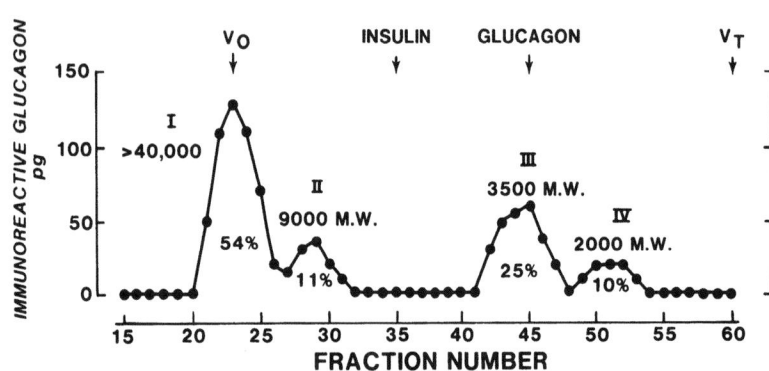

FIGURE 9.2. Immunoheterogeneity of human plasma glucagon.

gon can be estimated from data on portal venous-arterial differences and portal venous plasma flow rates. Secretion rates of glucagon may also be estimated on the basis of the clearance of glucagon under steady-state conditions; such estimation yields a value of approximately 1400 pg·kg^{-1}·min^{-1} in humans.[50] It should be pointed out, however, that these values underestimate secretion of glucagon and merely represent posthepatic delivery of glucagon. From what is known of the pancreatic content of glucagon and secretory rates of glucagon, it can be estimated that at least 25%, and probably more, of the pancreatic content of glucagon is secreted each day.

Glucagon Catabolism

In normal humans, the metabolic clearance rate of glucagon is independent of the prevailing plasma glucagon level. Estimates range between 7 and 14 ml·kg^{-1}·min^{-1}.[50,51] Normal concentrations have been reported in patients with diabetes[51] or liver disease,[52] whereas decreases have been found in renal failure[53] and starvation.[50] The liver and kidney seem to be the major sites of glucagon catabolism, but the relative contribution of each remains controversial.[52,53]

Initial reports suggested that the liver was not a major site of glucagon degradation.[32,36,38] The conflicting results reported may, however, be reconciled if the heterogeneity of circulating glucagon immunoreactivity is taken into account. When portal venous and peripheral venous plasma is subjected to gel filtration, it seems that the liver does not appreciably extract the biologically inactive 9000- and >40,000-d plasma glucagon immunoreactivity.[36] Thus, the portal-peripheral gradient of glucagon immunoreactivity is almost totally accounted for by extraction of the biologically active 3500-d molecule; this averages approximately 60% and results in a portal-peripheral gradient of 2.5 to 3 for the biologically active molecule.

It has long been known that the kidney is capable of degrading exogenous glucagon. Arteriovenous gradients across the kidney in normal animals indicate extraction of 23% to 39% of the presented glucagon.[34,54,55] Because less than 2% of the extracted hormone appears in urine and because nonfiltering kidneys continue to extract appreciable amounts of glucagon,[55] it seems that both tubular reabsorption and postglomerular capillary tubular uptake precede renal parenchymal degradation of glucagon. The hyperglucagonemia found in uremic man is due primarily to decreased clearance of the 9000-d molecule and cannot be accounted for by increased secretion of glucagon (3500-d molecule) or its decreased catabolism.[56] Because bilateral nephrectomy decreases the metabolic clearance rate of 3500-d glucagon approximately 30%,[34] the liver and kidney can account for 80% to 90% of the metabolic clearance of the biologically active glucagon fraction of plasma glucagon immunoreactivity.

Regulation of Glucagon Secretion

Glucose is the most important physiologic regulator of glucagon secretion. Hyperglycemia decreases and hypoglycemia increases glucagon secretion.[46] In vitro studies, such as those using the isolated perfused pancreas in which most variables operative in vivo can be controlled, indicate that the A cell is as exquisitely sensitive to changes in the ambient extracellular glucose concentration as is the B cell[57]; thus, glucose suppresses basal and stimulated glucagon release at concentrations as low as 5 mM glucose (90 mg·dl^{-1}). In vivo, a decrease in plasma glucose of 1 to 2 mM increases plasma glucagon.[58]

Other substrates also influence glucagon secretion. Various amino acids stimulate A cell release of glucagon,[59] while free fatty acids[60] and ketone bodies[61] suppress glucagon secretion. Amino acid stimulation of glucagon release may be important in preventing hypoglycemia, which might otherwise occur because of insulin release accompanying ingestion of a noncarbohydrate meal. Suppression of glucagon secretion by free fatty acids and ketone bodies may be part of a negative feedback system regulating ketogenesis.

The islets of Langerhans are richly innervated.[62] Like insulin release, glucagon secretion is influenced by both sympathetic and parasympathetic nervous systems; epinephrine, norepinephrine, and acetylcholine,[63-67] and electrical stimulation of mixed pancreatic, splanchnic, and vagus nerves augment glucagon release.[68-70] Both A and B cell secretion are influenced in the same direction by parasympathetic (i.e., increase),[58] β-adrenergic (i.e., increase),[63,67] and α-adrenergic (i.e., decrease)[59,70] mechanisms. The observation that glucagon secretion is increased by epinephrine while insulin release is simultaneously decreased[63] can best be explained by postulating that the A cell contains a preponderance of β-adrenergic receptors, while the B cell contains a preponderance of α-adrenergic receptors. Neural input to the A cell is probably important in modulating the increases in plasma glucagon observed during stress and perhaps also after mixed meals.

A variety of hormones have been reported to alter A cell function; epinephrine, gastrin, pancreozymin, vasoactive interspinal peptide, and gastric inhibitory polypeptide increase glucagon release,[71,72] while secretin apparently suppresses glucagon secretion.[73] Whether these represent true physiologic interactions or merely pharmacologic effects is unclear. Hyperglucagonemia, relative or absolute, has been found in states of growth hormone,[74] cortisol,[75] and thyroid hormone excess.[76]

Conceivably, this might play a role in the associated abnormalities of carbohydrate and lipid metabolism.

Alterations in nutrition also influence A cell function. Acute ingestion of pure or high carbohydrate meals suppresses glucagon release, whereas pure or high protein–containing meals stimulate glucagon release. Concomitant changes in plasma glucose and amino acid levels are probably responsible for these changes.[77] Prolonged (i.e., weeks or days) alterations in diet also alter A cell function. During total starvation, there is an acute increase in plasma glucagon lasting 1 to 2 days, probably as a result of increased secretion.[78] Prolonged ingestion of high-carbohydrate or isocaloric high-fat diet decreases basal and meal-stimulated plasma glucagon levels.[79,80] Conversely, low-carbohydrate diets or high-protein diets increase basal and stimulated glucagon secretion.[79,80] In obesity, normal plasma glucagon responses to protein meal ingestion,[81] and either increased[82] or decreased[83] responses to amino acid stimulation have been reported.

Hypoglycemia stimulates glucagon secretion through both intraislet and central nervous system mediated autonomic signals.[84] Within the islets low glucose concentrations increase A-cell glucagon secretion directly and, by reducing B-cell secretion, decrease tonic A-cell inhibition by insulin. Autonomic adrenergic (i.e., norepinephrine), cholinergic, and peptidergic neural and adrenomedullary hormonal (epinephrine) signals, triggered by hypoglycemia, also increase A-cell glucagon secretion.

Role of Glucagon in Carbohydrate Homeostasis

At concentrations that approximate those found in the portal vein in vivo, glucagon is a potent stimulator of hepatic glycogenolysis, gluconeogenesis, and ketogenesis in vitro.[85] These actions of glucagon and the increases in plasma glucagon observed during hypoglycemia,[58] exercise,[86] trauma,[87] infection,[88] and other stress[89] provide evidence that glucagon is important in the maintenance of euglycemia in the postabsorptive state and at times when there are increased demands for fuels and when the organism must rely on mobilization of endogenous substrate. Under these conditions, when β-cell function is normal, the major action of glucagon would be to counteract the actions of insulin on storage of glucose and other fuels. Conversely, when β-cell function is deficient, glucagon could accentuate the metabolic consequences of insulin deficiency and be an important determinant of the magnitude of hyperglycemia and hyperketonemia found in diabetes.

Substantial evidence for the role of glucagon in glucose homeostasis has been provided from studies employing somatostatin; this peptide is a potent inhibitor of glucagon and insulin secretion and does not itself directly affect substrate metabolism at doses used in vivo. Infusion of somatostatin in normal man[90] results in an acute decrease in the glucose production rate, which is accompanied by a decrease in plasma glucose; this occurs despite a concomitant decrease in plasma insulin and can be prevented by replacement infusion of glucagon. These observations suggest that in the postabsorptive state, glucagon action on the liver balances insulin action on the liver to maintain an appropriate output of glucose to match glucose utilization and, therefore, maintain stable euglycemia. With prolongation of the glucagon deficiency during infusion of somatostatin, glucose production does not exceed normal rates. These changes reflect the effects of the concomitant insulin deficiency and the unopposed actions of other counterregulatory factors. When insulin deficiency is avoided by infusion of replacement amounts of insulin along with somatostatin, which results in an isolated deficiency of glucagon, plasma glucose decreases more than that observed during infusion of somatostatin alone, and both it and the glucose production rate remain suppressed below normal.

In addition to a role for glucagon in the maintenance of euglycemia by antagonizing the effects of postabsorptive (i.e., low) plasma insulin concentrations, there is considerable evidence that glucagon acts in the defense against hypoglycemia by antagonizing the effects of excess plasma insulin.[91,92] When hypoglycemia is produced in humans by injection of insulin, the restoration of euglycemia is due to a compensatory increase in hepatic glucose production. Although secretion of catecholamines, growth hormone, and cortisol are stimulated along with that of glucagon, only the increases in plasma glucagon and catecholamines coincide with or precede the compensatory increase in the glucose production rate.[92,93] That glucagon is the major acute glucose counterregulatory hormone is suggested by the fact that inhibition of the plasma glucagon responses by somatostatin markedly attenuates the compensatory increase in the glucose production rate and impairs restoration of euglycemia following insulin administration (Figure 9.3). Prevention of cortisol secretion,[94] adrenergic blockade,[92] adrenalectomy,[91] or acute growth hormone deficiency[92] does not appreciably affect immediate glucose counterregulation. The effects of glucagon during restoration of euglycemia involves both glycogenolysis and gluconeogenesis.[95]

The role of glucagon in disposal of ingested carbohydrate is unclear. The liver is the main organ responsible for clearance of glucose appearing in the portal vein after ingestion of carbohydrate and presumably also that derived from a meal.[96,97] The increases in the portal venous insulin and glucose concentrations act to promote formation of glycogen from the ingested glucose. Suppression of glucagon secretion is probably also important in the

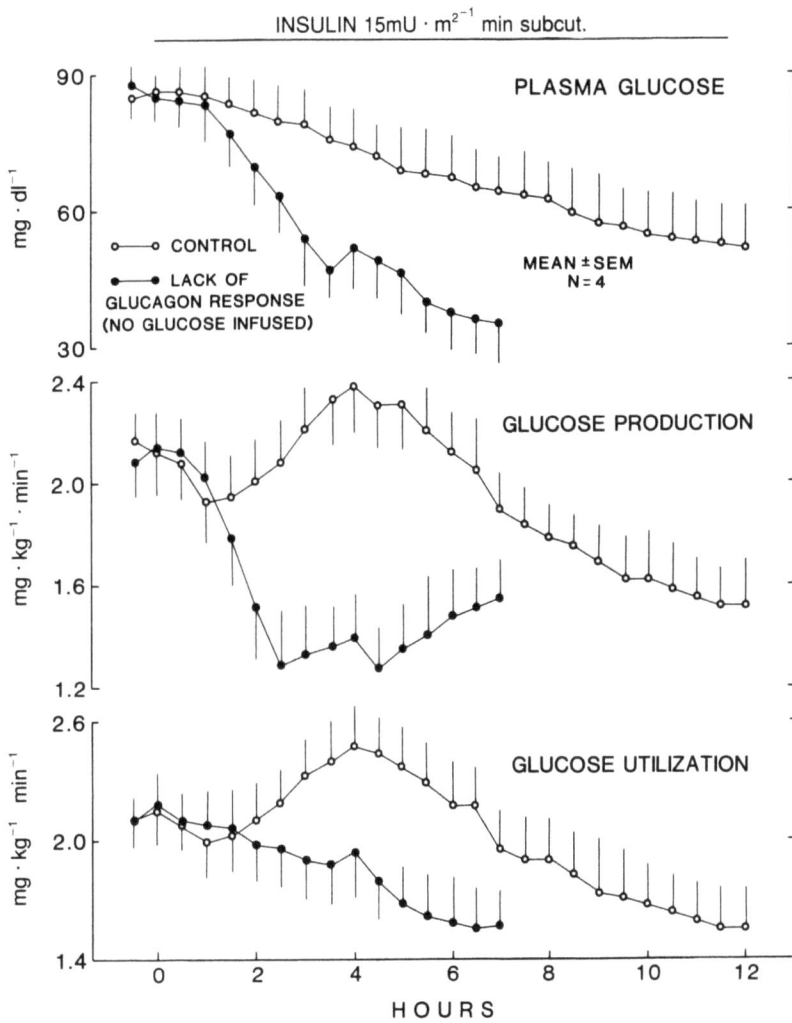

FIGURE 9.3. Effect of isolated glucagon deficiency on hypoglycemic action of insulin in normal human volunteers.

decrease in endogenous glucose output and in the formation of glycogen from the ingested glucose. In insulin-dependent diabetics incapable of insulin secretion, suppression of increases in plasma glucagon following ingestion of a mixed meal or glucose load improves postprandial glucose tolerance.[98] Moreover, the effectiveness of exogenous insulin in preventing postprandial hyperglycemia and improving diabetic control is markedly augmented when glucagon secretion is suppressed by somatostatin.[99]

Role of Glucagon in Ketone Body Homeostasis

Circulating levels of ketone bodies (e.g., acetone, acetoacetic acid, and β-hydroxybutyrate) are determined by the net balance between rates of ketone body production and removal. The plasma ketone body concentration and insulin seem to be the major factors affecting removal of ketone bodies by tissues.[100,101] While there is no evidence to suggest that glucagon influences this process, there are considerable data, mainly from animal studies, that indicate that glucagon may play a key role in the formation of ketone bodies.

Ketone body formation results from β-oxidation of free fatty acids derived from intra- and extrahepatic sources. Two key factors are necessary for ketone body formation: sufficient substrate in the form of free fatty acids and a shift in the hepatic handling of free fatty acids from triglyceride synthesis (i.e., esterification) to oxidation. Several studies have demonstrated that glucagon can directly act on the liver in vitro to augment ketogenesis.[102-104] This is thought to involve the promotion of transport of free fatty acids across the mitochondrial membrane by acylcarnitine transferase, an important rate-limiting step for free fatty acid oxidation.[105] Glucagon apparently does not directly affect this enzyme but indirectly causes its activation by lowering intrahepatic levels of malonylcoenzyme A (CoA), an inhibitor of acylcarnitine transferase.[106] It has been postulated that glucagon is essential for switching the liver to a ketogenic mode (i.e., from an organ primarily esterifying free fatty acids to one oxidizing them) to permit maximal rates of ketogenesis to occur.[105,106]

Few studies have directly examined the effect of glucagon on ketogenesis in vivo. In one study, using the hepatic-venous catheter technique, it was demonstrated that in humans glucagon would directly increase net splanchnic ketone body production and lipolysis.[107] However, plasma glucagon concentration exceeded 5000 pg·ml^{-1}, concentrations probably occurring only in extreme cases of diabetes ketoacidosis and in patients with glucagonsecreting islet cell tumors. In another study in dogs using the same method and infusion of somatostatin,[108] it was reported that deficiency of insulin did not augment splanchnic ketone body release if glucagon was also deficient, but that if basal plasma glucagon concentrations were maintained during insulin deficiency, splanchnic ketone body release increased. It was further demonstrated that during insulin deficiency, a given increase in circulating free fatty acid concentrations results in greater ketone body production if basal plasma glucagon concentrations were maintained than if they were suppressed by somatostatin. By using a combination of the hepatic catheter and isotopic techniques, it has been shown[109] that in dogs with combined glucagon and insulin deficiency, there is little change in plasma free fatty acids and ketone body concentrations and fatty acids are mainly oxidized to CO_2 or esterified.[109] In contrast, when insulin deficiency occurs without glucagon deficiency, ketogenesis is increased, and fatty acids are preferentially converted into ketone bodies rather than esterified. Under these conditions, no effect of glucagon on extrahepatic lipolysis was observed. Since no net increase in fatty acid uptake by the liver was also observed, the above changes could be explained most readily on the basis of increased availability of free fatty acids due to intrahepatic lipolysis and altered hepatic metabolism of free fatty acids derived from both intra- and extrahepatic sources.

Most studies in humans have involved changes in circulating ketone body concentration and not rates of ketone body production. Pharmacologic doses of glucagon given as a bolus have been reported to increase both plasma free fatty acid and ketone body concentrations in normal subjects despite concomitant increases in plasma insulin.[110] Following acute withdrawal from insulin in insulin-dependent diabetics, the expected hyperketonemia can be markedly attenuated by suppression of glucagon secretion with somatostatin.[11] Under such conditions (e.g., insulin withdrawal and somatostatin administration), infusion of physiologic amounts of glucagon, producing circulating glucagon concentrations less than those reported in ketoacidosis, results in a marked degree of hyperketonemia. There are thus two prerequisites for glucagon to stimulate ketogenesis: adequate substrate (e.g., free fatty acids) and insulin deficiency or the inability to increase plasma insulin concentrations.

Mechanism of Action

It is well established that the actions of glucagon on glycogenolysis, gluconeogenesis, and ketogenesis are mediated mainly by cAMP.[112] Binding of glucagon with its receptor activates the catalytic subunit of the membrane-bound enzyme adenylate cyclase, which catalyzes the conversion of adenosine triphosphate (ATP) to cAMP, which in turn leads to activation of intracellular kinases. For glycogenolysis, this results in phosphorylation of phosphorylase, which activates the enzyme. Thus, glycogen formation is inhibited and glycogen breakdown is stimulated.[113]

The actions of glucagon on gluconeogenesis are more complex and involve several steps.[114] Glucagon increases hepatic uptake of amino acids, but its major effect is intrahepatic. Glucagon stimulates gluconeogenesis mainly by increasing the rate of phosphoenolpyruvate production and decreasing the rate of its disposal by pyruvate kinase. It does this by modulating flux through pyruvate carboxylase, pyruvate kinase, phosphoenolpyruvate carboxykinase, fructose-1,6-bisphosphatase, and phosphofructokinase. Glucagon activates pyruvate kinase by altering its phosphorylation state by a cAMP-dependent process. Glucagon also stimulates the phosphorylation of phosphofructokinase and fructose-1,6-bisphosphatase, predominantly by altering the level of fructose 2,6-bisphosphate instead of by phosphorylation. Pyruvate carboxylase and phosphoenolpyruvate carboxykinase activities are altered by changes in the level of substrates and other metabolites that affect the enzymes.

Stimulation of ketogenesis by glucagon is linked to some of the biochemical steps involved in its stimulation of gluconeogenesis,[115] namely, an inhibition of glycolysis. The rate-limiting step of ketogenesis is the transport of fatty acid CoA esters across the mitochondrial membrane where they undergo β-oxidation. The enzyme catalyzing this transfer is fatty acid carnitine acyl transferase II. This enzyme is inhibited by malonyl-CoA. The inhibition of glycolysis by glucagon lowers intracellular levels of malonyl-CoA and results in activation of the fatty acid acyl transferase.

Glucagon Secretion in Diabetes Mellitus

In human diabetics, plasma glucagon concentrations are inappropriate for the prevailing plasma glucose concentration[116] and are markedly increased in diabetic ketoacidosis.[117] In contrast to nondiabetics, carbohydrate ingestion does not suppress plasma glucagon in diabetics,[118] and excessive increases in plasma glucagon are observed with protein meals,[119] mixed meals,[98] and infusion of amino acids.[120] Some of these abnormalities, such as the fasting hyperglucagonemia and excessive responses to infusion of arginine, protein, or mixed-meal ingestion, can be improved or corrected by administration of physiologic quantities of insulin, suggesting that they were, in part, the result of insulin deficiency.

In contrast to the above, in most studies[98,121-125] acute administration of physiologic or even pharmacologic amounts of insulin have not been able to correct abnormal A-cell responses to glucose in human diabetes. These observations suggest that abnormal A-cell responses to glucose may not be solely due to insulin deficiency. Evidence for a selective defect in A-cell glucose recognition independent of insulin deficiency is provided by the findings that plasma glucagon can be suppressed normally in human diabetes by elevation of circulating free fatty acid levels but not by hyperglycemia,[123] and that the diabetic A cell fails to respond appropriately to hypoglycemia or to hyperglycemia.[125]

Metabolic Consequences of A-Cell Dysfunction in Diabetes Mellitus Patients

At the present time, the preponderance of evidence suggests that the full-blown manifestations of diabetes cannot be explained solely on the basis of insulin deficiency, and that abnormal A-cell function is an important determinant of the magnitude of hyperglycemia and hyperketonemia found in diabetes. The evidence for this can be summarized as follows. Fasting hyperglycemia and insulin requirements are lower in pancreatectomized patients lacking glucagon.[29] Moreover, in such individuals[29] and in insulin-dependent diabetics whose glucagon secretion is suppressed with somatostatin,[111] hyperglycemia and hyperketonemia following acute withdrawal of insulin are markedly diminished. In insulin-dependent diabetics, acute suppression of glucagon secretion decreases plasma glucose to concentrations only slightly above normal, and chronic suppression markedly improves diabetic control.[122,126]

Epinephrine

Background

Composed of the sympathetic nervous system and the chromaffin cells, largely those that constitute the adrenal medullae, the sympathochromaffin (sympathoadrenal) system is the prototype neuroendocrine system.[127-130] Although it releases an array of other neurotransmitter or neuromodulators and potential hormones, the principal products of the sympathochromaffin system are catecholamines. Defined as compounds with a dihydroxyphenyl (catechol) nucleus and an amine side chain, the natural catecholamines are dopamine, norepinephrine (noradrenaline), and epinephrine (adrenaline) (Figure 9.4). These are small modified amino acids with molecular weights of 153, 169, and 183 d, respectively. Their chemical structures have been known since the turn of the century.[131] Thus, epinephrine is the oldest of the chemically characterized hormones.

All three natural catecholamines function as neurotransmitters in the central nervous system. In the periphery, norepinephrine functions primarily as a neurotransmitter released from sympathetic postganglionic neurons.[128,129,132] Under some conditions, its plasma concentrations are high enough for it to serve a hormonal function as well. Although extraadrenal epinephrine secretion occurs,[133,134] the adrenal medullae can be considered the exclusive source of biologically active plasma epinephrine concentrations, at least in adults.[133,135-137] Thus, epinephrine is a hormone in the classic sense. The role of dopamine, other than as a biosynthetic precursor of norepinephrine and epinephrine, in the periphery is not well defined.[128,129] The discussion that follows focuses largely on the counterregulatory hormone epinephrine.

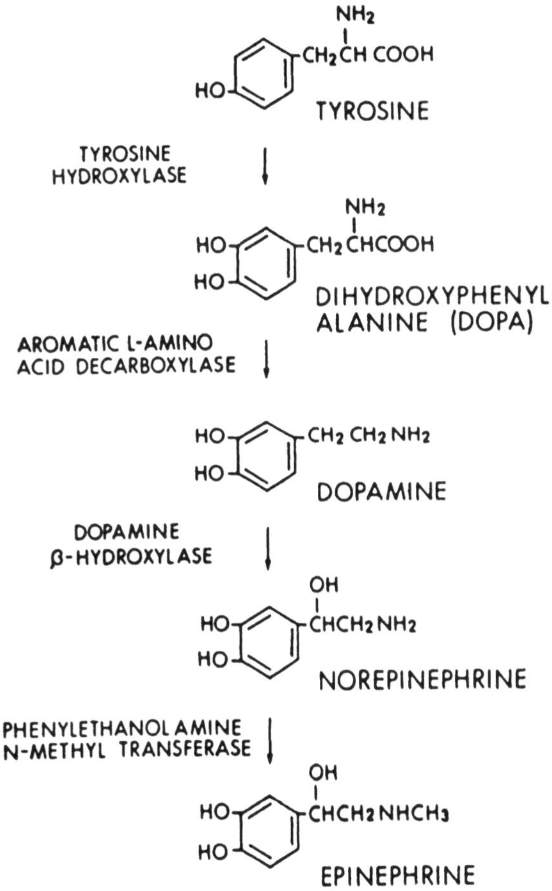

FIGURE 9.4. Biosynthesis and chemical structures of the catecholamines.

Biosynthesis and Release

The catecholamines are synthesized from tyrosine, derived from the diet or formed from phenylalanine, through this sequence: tyrosine → dihydroxyphenylalanine (DOPA) → dopamine → norepinephrine → epinephrine (Figure 9.4).[128–130] Tyrosine hydroxylase, which catalyzes the hydroxylation of tyrosine to form DOPA, is the rate-limiting enzyme. Its activity is product inhibited by catecholamines, and its synthesis is increased by high firing rates of the preganglionic neurons. DOPA is decarboxylated to form dopamine by the nonspecific enzyme aromatic L-amino acid decarboxylase; dopamine is hydroxylated to form norepinephrine by dopamine-β-hydroxylase (DBH), and norepinephrine is o-methylated to form epinephrine by phenylethanolamine N-methyltransferase (PNMT). Whereas sympathetic postganglionic neurons and some adrenomedullary cells lack PNMT, and thus synthesize, store, and release norepinephrine, most adrenomedullary chromaffin cells contain the entire set of biosynthetic enzymes and synthesize, store, and release epinephrine.

Tyrosine hydroxylase and amino acid decarboxylase are cytoplasmic enzymes, but DBH is localized in chromaffin granules, along with chromogranins, ATP, and catecholamines. Thus, norepinephrine formation occurs within these vesicles. Because PNMT is cytoplasmic in location, norepinephrine must leave the granules to be converted to epinephrine, which then reenters granules for storage.

In response to firing of preganglionic acetylcholine releasing neurons and depolarization of the chromaffin cell membrane, catecholamines and the remaining soluble contents of the chromaffin granules are released, by exocytosis, into the extracellular fluid.

Inactivation, Degradation, and Elimination

Catecholamines are degraded by two principal enzyme systems: monoamine oxidase (MAO) and catechol-O-methyl transferase (COMT).[128–130] Conjugation, largely to the sulfate in humans, also occurs. COMT converts the catecholamines to their O-methyl derivatives (e.g., metanephrine from epinephrine), which can be further metabolized to form substrates for MAO resulting in the formation of vanillylmandelic acid (VMA). MAO converts catecholamines to dihydroxymandelic acid, which ultimately forms substrates for COMT, again resulting in the formation of VMA.

The vast majority of the norepinephrine released from axon terminals of sympathetic neurons is dissipated locally through either reuptake into the terminals (uptake 1), where it is either restored in granules or degraded largely by MAO, or uptake (uptake 2) and metabolism, largely by COMT, in cells adjacent to the sympathetic cleft. Thus, only a small fraction, perhaps, about 10%, enters the circulation. Thus, the plasma norepinephrine concentration is only an index of sympathetic neural norepinephrine release. Indeed, under some conditions, such as hypoglycemia, it is only an index of sympathochromaffin activity, since the adrenal medullae contribute substantially to the plasma norepinephrine pool. The extent to which epinephrine released from chromaffin cells is dissipated locally is not well defined, but a substantial fraction enters the circulation.

Catecholamines are cleared, in part into adrenergic axon terminals (uptake 1) throughout the body, although uptake 2 is thought to account for the bulk of clearance of circulating catecholamines. Quantitatively, the liver and the kidneys are the major sites of metabolic clearance of circulating catecholamines. Less than 5% are excreted in the urine unchanged.

Mechanisms of Actions

Like the peptide hormones, and unlike the thyroid and steroid hormones, catecholamines interact with receptors on the plasma membranes of target cells to initiate their actions.[128,129,138] On the basis initially of agonist potency sequences and later the use of specific antagonists and ligand-binding techniques, the adrenergic receptors (adrenoceptors) are divided into two types, α-adrenergic receptors and β-adrenergic receptors. There are subtypes of both of these. The subtypes of α-adrenergic receptor, α_1- and α_2-adrenergic receptors, both of which exhibit the agonist potency sequence epinephrine (E) > norepinephrine (NE) > isoproterenol. The subtypes of β-adrenergic receptors include β_1- and β_2-adrenergic receptors. These exhibit the agonist potency sequences isoproterenol > E ≈ NE and isoproterenol > E > NE, respectively. A β_3-adrenergic receptor that exhibits the potency sequence isoproterenol ≈ NE > E has also been cloned.[139]

β-Adrenergic receptors are linked through a stimulatory guanine and nucleotide protein, G_s, to adenylate cyclase. The cellular actions mediated through these receptors are thought to result from increased intracellular cAMP levels and activation of the corresponding protein kinase. α_2-adrenergic receptors are linked through an inhibitory guanine nucleotide protein, G_i, to adenylate cyclase. The cellular actions mediated through these receptors are the result, at least in part, of decreased intracellular cAMP levels. Agonist occupancy of α_1-adrenergic receptors activates phospholipase C. The cellular actions mediated through these receptors are attributed to increased intracellular inositol phosphate and diacylglycerol levels.

Regulation of Secretion

Physiologic regulation of sympathochromaffin catecholamine release is accomplished via the central nervous system. Although the latter includes sympathetic reflexes mediated at the spinal cord level, adrenomedullary activity is regulated by the brain. For example, hypoglycemia is normally a potent stimulus to adrenomedullary epinephrine secretion. However, there is no epinephrine response to hypoglycemia in individuals who have suffered a spinal cord transection.[140] Sympathochromaffin activity is regulated by a variety of brain regions.[129] Changes can be the result of mechanisms initiated within the brain, or of afferent signals integrated in the brain into a sympathochromaffin response.

Although plasma catecholamine concentrations are elevated in response to a variety of stresses, the sympathochromaffin system can no longer be viewed simply as a stress response system. Biologically active sympathochromaffin activation also occurs in a variety of common physiologic conditions. For example, plasma epinephrine concentrations increase during assumption of the upright posture, during mild physical exercise, during public speaking, and during decrements in plasma glucose to concentrations just below the physiologic range (Figure 9.5).[141,142]

Plasma catecholamine concentrations increase rapidly, and often markedly, during stimulation. For example, plasma epinephrine concentrations can rise by 100-fold or more during hypoglycemia.[127,128,143] They also fall rapidly, with plasma half-times of 1 to 2 minutes, when stimulation stops. Thus, the sympathochromaffin system is a rapid communication system, with its neural signals transmitted in seconds and its hormonal signals transmitted within minutes.

Metabolic Actions

The catecholamines in general, and epinephrine in particular, have long been known to exert potent metabolic,[144] as well as cardiovascular, actions. Epinephrine is known to affect carbohydrate, lipid, and protein metabolism.[128,129,135-137,145] However, the physiologic role of epinephrine in metabolic regulation has only begun to emerge. This is particularly the case with respect to carbohydrate metabolism.

Epinephrine raises the plasma glucose concentration. The mechanisms of the glycemic effect are complex. They involve both direct and indirect (i.e., other hormone-mediated) actions, are the result of both stimulation of the glucose production rate and limitation of glucose utilization, and are mediated through both β- and α-adrenergic receptors in humans.[135-137,145-151] These are shown schematically in Figure 9.6.

Epinephrine stimulates both renal and hepatic glucose production.[152] The renal effect is sustained and most likely due to β-adrenergic stimulation of gluconeogenesis since the kidney normally contains little glycogen. The hepatic effect is transient and is mediated largely through $β_2$-adrenergic receptors in humans, although a small α-adrenergic component has been described.[151] Both glycogenolysis and gluconeogenesis are stimulated, the former by direct actions (e.g., increased phosphorylase and decreased glycogen synthase activities) and the latter largely by mobilization of gluconeogenic precursors (e.g., lactate, alanine, glycerol). Acting through β-adrenergic receptors, epinephrine also limits glucose utilization directly. This is a sustained effect. Thus, in contrast to glucagon, epinephrine produces a sustained increment in the plasma glucose concentration. Finally, the hormone stimulates lipolysis via β-adrenergic receptors and in-

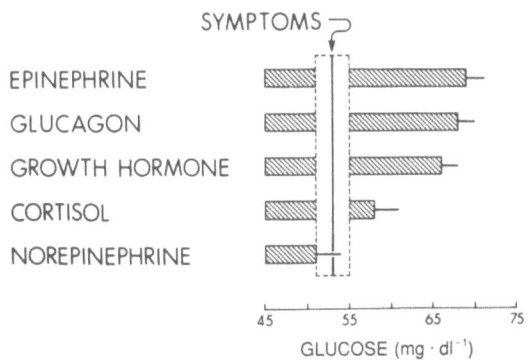

FIGURE 9.5. Venous plasma glucose thresholds of activation of glucose counterregulatory systems (e.g., increments in plasma glucagon, epinephrine, glucagon growth hormone, cortisol, and norepinephrine concentrations) and for symptoms during decrements in the plasma glucose concentration in normal humans. (From Schwartz et al.,[141] with permission.)

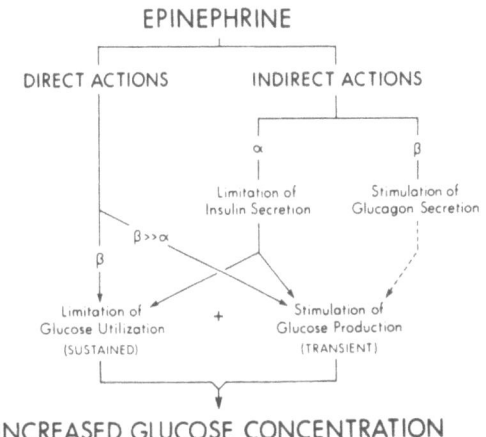

FIGURE 9.6. Mechanisms of the hyperglycemic effect of epinephrine in humans. (From Clutter et al.,[137] with permission.)

creased fatty acid levels drive glucose production and limit glucose utilization.

If these direct actions, mediated through β-adrenergic receptors, were the sole mechanism of the glycemic response to epinephrine, a potent β-adrenergic agonist such as isoproterenol would be expected to produce marked hyperglycemia. In fact, it has little glycemic effect because of β_2-adrenergic stimulation of insulin secretion.[153] This underscores the fundamental importance of the indirect glycemic actions of epinephrine, specifically the role of modulated insulin secretion.

As alluded to earlier, epinephrine is a mixed agonist. It interacts with both α- and β-adrenergic receptors. α_2-adrenergic limitation of insulin secretion is an important indirect glycemic action of epinephrine. It permits the glycemic response, triggered by the β-adrenergic actions, to occur. However, as the plasma glucose concentration rises, some limited insulin secretion occurs. This, too, is a critical event in that it limits the magnitude of the glycemic response.[136,137] Indeed, the glycemic response to comparable epinephrine levels is about fourfold greater in persons who cannot increase insulin secretion, such as those with insulin-dependent diabetes mellitus, than in normal individuals.[136] Among other potential indirect glycemic actions of epinephrine, increments in glucagon do not appear to play a major role.[137,149]

Epinephrine is a potent stimulator of lipolysis,[135,137,148,149] an effect generally attributed to β_1-adrenergic receptor–mediated action.[154] However, it is conceivable that β_3-adrenergic receptors are also involved.[139] α_2-Adrenergic receptor–mediated inhibition of lipolysis has been described, but the stimulatory effect predominates. Increments in circulating nonesterified fatty acid (NEFA) levels resulting from increased lipolysis are the major reason that epinephrine also stimulates ketogenesis. In addition, indirect actions (e.g., limitation of insulin secretion, stimulation of glucagon secretion) might be involved, and evidence of direct stimulation of hepatic ketogenesis has been reported.[155] Interestingly, in contrast to its restraining influence on the glycemic response, insulin secretion does not limit the magnitude of the lipolytic and ketogenic responses to epinephrine.[136] This is best explained by the fact that the increments in insulin secretion are small but in a site, the hepatic portal circulation, critical to limitation of glucose production but not to limitation of lipolysis.

Epinephrine also causes decreased net proteolysis with decreased circulating amino acid (i.e., except alanine) concentrations.[156,157] It stimulates alanine flux from muscle to liver.[157] Finally, epinephrine stimulates thermogenesis.[158–160]

Basal epinephrine concentrations probably have little effect on metabolic processes. However, these processes are sensitive to physiologic plasma epinephrine elevations. Venous plasma epinephrine thresholds for stimulation of lipolysis and thermogenesis have been estimated to be 75 to 125 pg·ml^{-1} (410–600 pmol·L^{-1}),[137] only about two- to fourfold basal levels.[127] The thresholds for the glycemic, ketogenic, and presumed glycolytic effects of the hormone are about 100 to 200 pg·ml^{-1} (550–1100 pmol·L^{-1}).[137] Because arterial epinephrine concentrations are approximately twice venous levels, the biologic thresholds for these metabolic effects are higher than those cited.

Role in Metabolic Regulation

Although likely involved in the physiologic regulation of lipid, ketone, and protein metabolism, a physiologic role for epinephrine is best established with respect to carbohydrate metabolism, specifically defense against hypoglycemia.

As mentioned earlier, in defense against decrements in plasma glucose, dissipation of insulin is important, and glucagon plays a primary counterregulatory role. Epinephrine is not normally critical. However, it compensates largely and becomes critical when glucagon is deficient.[3,91,92,161–166] Thus, hypoglycemia develops or progresses when both glucagon and epinephrine are deficient and insulin is present. This combination occurs all too frequently in patients with insulin-dependent diabetes mellitus, as discussed below.

Metabolic Consequences in Diabetes Mellitus

As discussed earlier, patients with insulin-dependent diabetes mellitus (IDDM) exhibit increased glycemic sensitivity to epinephrine because they cannot release insulin as the plasma glucose concentration rises. Epinephrine also stimulates lipolysis and ketogenesis. Thus, it is reasonable to suggest that epinephrine, among other factors, might contribute to metabolic decompensation (e.g., in diabetic ketoacidosis). It does not appear, however, that increased sympathochromaffin activity plays a major role in the pathophysiology of IDDM.[161] Decreased sympathochromaffin activity, however, does play an important role.[3,161]

As mentioned earlier, deficient glucagon secretory responses to plasma glucose decrements are the rule in IDDM. To the extent that they have deficient glucagon responses, patients with IDDM are dependent on epinephrine to prevent or correct hypoglycemia.[3,167–169] Deficient epinephrine secretory responses to plasma glucose decrements develop in many patients with IDDM.[1–4,161,168,169] These patients have defective counterregulation that is associated with, and best attributed to, combined deficiencies in their glucagon and epinephrine responses to developing hypoglycemia. They have been shown, in prospective studies,[170,171] to have at least a 25-fold increased risk of severe iatrogenic

FIGURE 9.7. Effect of defective glucose counterregulation, associated with and best attributed to combined deficiencies of the glucagon and epinephrine secretory responses to plasma glucose decrements, on the occurrence of severe hypoglycemia during the intensive treatment of insulin-dependent diabetes mellitus. (Data from White et al.,[170] with permission.)

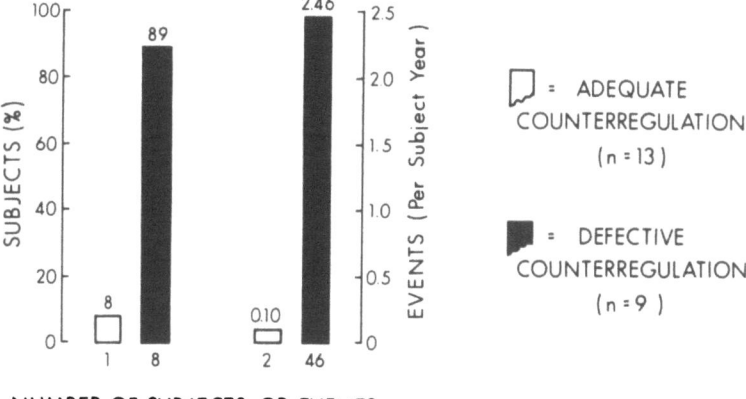

hypoglycemia, at least during intensive therapy (Figure 9.7).

Growth Hormone

Background

Human growth hormone (HGH), a 191 single-chain peptide (molecular weight 22,650 d) having two intramolecular disulfide bonds (Cyc_{53}-Cys_{165} and Cyc_{182}-Cys_{189}),[172] is secreted by the somatotrophs of the anterior pituitary (Figure 9.8). Smaller and larger variants due to alternative messenger RNA (mRNA) processing, interchain disulfide dimers, and nondissociable aggregates occur, but are probably of no physiologic significance.

Growth hormone (GH) is structurally related to human chorionic somatomammotropin (HCS) and prolactin. HCS also has 191 amino acids of which 161 are identical to those of growth hormone; it is, however, only 0.1% as potent as HGH. Prolactin is a 199 amino acid peptide which has 16% homology with HGH; it also is

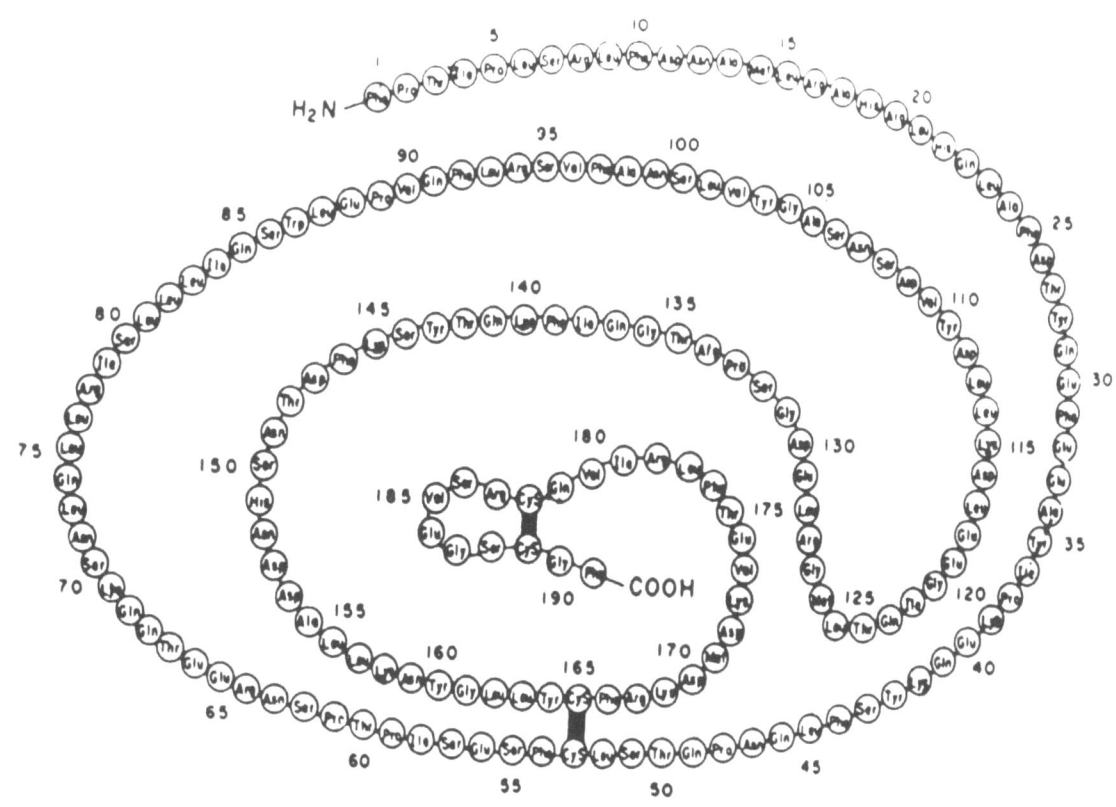

FIGURE 9.8. Amino acid sequence of human growth hormone.

much less potent as a growth promoting hormone than HGH and arises from a different gene (i.e., chromosome 6) than HGH (i.e., chromosome 17).[173]

Biosynthesis

Synthesis of growth hormone is affected by a variety of factors, the most important of which are growth hormone–releasing hormone (GRH), growth hormone release-inhibiting factor, commonly called somatostatin, thyroid hormone, and corticosteroids. GRF is a 44 amino acid peptide synthesized mainly in the arcuate nucleus of the hypothalamus; its release into the hypothalamic hypophysial portal system stimulates not only growth hormone release but also its synthesis.[174] Somatostatin, synthesized in neurons in the anterior periventricular region of the hypothalamus, exists as a 14 and 28 amino acid peptide.[175] The latter may represent more than a biosynthetic precursor, since there is evidence for discrete receptors for the two peptides; they both inhibit secretion and synthesis of growth hormone. Corticosteroids and thyroid hormone also directly stimulate growth hormone synthesis. Pituitary cells grown in tissue culture lacking thyroid hormone and corticosteroids have markedly reduced levels of GH mRNA.[176]

Regulation of Secretion

Growth hormone secretion is subject to a complex system of regulation. Of primary importance is the balance between GRF and somatostatin. GRF stimulates growth hormone secretion via a cAMP mechanism, whereas somatostatin inhibits growth hormone release by reducing pituitary cell potassium/calcium transport. All known stimuli to growth hormone secretion are inhibited by somatostatin.[175] Its secretion is also subject to feedback inhibition by two mechanisms: one involves direct stimulation of somatostatin release by growth hormone[177]; the other involves somatomedins, the growth hormone–dependent growth factors, which can directly act on the somatotrope to inhibit GH release[178] and stimulate release of somatostatin.[179]

There is also evidence that central α-adrenergic, serotonin, and cholinergic pathways augment GH release. Glucose and free fatty acids suppress GH release, whereas hypoglycemia, amino acids, α_2-adrenergic agonists (e.g., clonidine), exercise, short-term fasting, and stress all increase GH secretion. Responses to these stimuli are augmented by β-adrenergic receptor blockade and reduced by α-adrenergic receptor blockade.

Throughout the day, GH is secreted in episodic pulses.[180] The largest of these occur 1 to 2 hours after the onset of sleep coincident with EEG stages 3 and 4. These can be attenuated by cholinergic blockade, but not by glucose or α-adrenergic blockade. Estrogens augment growth hormone secretion; responses to various stimuli are greater in premenopausal women than in men. Growth hormone secretion varies with age, being greater in pubertal children than in prepubertal children and in adults. Both the frequency and magnitude of secretory episodes are greatest in puberty.[181] Basal plasma growth hormone levels are generally less than $3\,ng\cdot ml^{-1}$; peaks during pulsatile episode can be as high as $30\,ng\cdot ml^{-1}$.

In obesity, growth hormone secretion is reduced, whereas in poorly controlled diabetes mellitus GH secretion and responses to various stimuli are increased; this hypersecretion can be corrected with long-term intensive insulin treatment, which restores plasma glucose to near normal.

Degradation

Liver and kidney are the main tissues responsible for growth hormone degradation. Most of the growth hormone filtered by the kidney is reabsorbed so that urinary growth hormone is not a reliable index of its secretion.

Metabolic Effects

Growth hormone exerts effects on growth and metabolism. The effects of growth are largely considered to be indirect, the consequences of somatomedins (particularly somatomedin C, insulin-like growth factor-I), whereas the metabolic effects are largely direct. Administration of growth hormone produces early insulin-like effects lasting 1 to 2 hours followed by sustained anti-insulin effects.[182] When growth hormone is infused into normal volunteers at rates that produce high physiologic or pharmacologic levels ($\sim 30\,ng\cdot ml^{-1}$) under conditions in which plasma insulin and glucagon concentrations are fixed, plasma glucose concentration decreases initially due to both a suppression of hepatic glucose output and an increase in glucose clearance. Human forearm studies have demonstrated an early action of growth hormone to stimulate free fatty acid uptake by muscle.[183,184] Such effects occur too rapidly to be mediated by stimulation of somatomedin production and thus probably represent direct effects of growth hormone, consistent with the presence of its receptors in liver, muscle, and adipose tissue. It had once been thought that these insulin-like effects were due to impurities in growth hormone preparations or variants of the hormone; however, their demonstration with recombinant human growth hormone indicates that they are intrinsic properties of the hormone. The mechanism for these insulin-like effects is unknown.

The anti-insulin effects of growth hormone include increased hepatic glucose production, decreased peripheral glucose uptake, decreased glucose oxidation, increased lipolysis, increased fat oxidation, and increased ketone body production. When growth hormone is infused into normal volunteers at rates that raise circulating levels to ~30 ng·ml^{-1} under conditions in which plasma insulin and glucagon levels remain fixed, by 4 hours impaired suppression of hepatic glucose output and a reduction in peripheral glucose clearance is demonstrable.[182] In studies in which HGH was infused into normal volunteers for 12 hours at a rate that raised circulating levels to 8 ng·ml^{-1}, fasting plasma insulin concentrations increased nearly twofold along with a slight increase in plasma glucose.[178] During subsequent insulin clamp studies, the sensitivity of the liver and peripheral tissues to insulin was impaired without a change in insulin binding to monocytes.[178] In studies in which an oral glucose tolerance test was administered 2 hours after starting an infusion of growth hormone in normal volunteers, which raised plasma HGH to about 9 ng·ml^{-1}, there was greater postglucose hyperglycemia, greater insulin secretion as measured by splanchnic C-peptide release, and impaired suppression of hepatic glucose output and of circulating free fatty acid levels.[185]

Infusion of growth hormone into obese volunteers undergoing a prolonged fast, which raised plasma growth hormone levels to only about 5 mg·ml^{-1}, increased plasma insulin, glucose, free fatty acids, glycerol, and ketone bodies, but did not change urinary nitrogen secretion[186]; the failure of urinary nitrogen excretion to decrease despite the increase in circulating insulin levels suggests an antianabolic effect on protein metabolism. Infusion of growth hormone to patients with insulin-dependent diabetes mellitus who cannot respond with a compensatory increase in insulin secretion produces a marked deterioration in glycemic control.[187]

Mechanism of Action

Growth hormone exerts its effects initially by binding to its cell surface receptor, a member of the cytokine/hemapoietin superfamily.[188] One molecule of growth hormone binds to two of its receptors, leading to dimerization of the receptors and activation of an associated tyrosine kinase (JAK2).[189] Then the growth hormone receptor becomes phosphorylated and other protein kinases become activated, e.g., mitogen-activated protein (MAP) kinase.[190] There is also evidence that activation of phosphatidylinositol-3 kinase, protein kinase C, as well as alterations in intracellular calcium levels and effects on transcription factors that are involved in mediation of growth hormone tissue actions.[190]

However, the exact mechanisms responsible for the anti-insulin effects of growth hormone remain unclear.[191,192] In humans, they do not appear to be mediated by changes in insulin receptor binding.[178] In vitro studies indicate that inhibition of DNA-mediated RNA synthesis is involved,[193] consistent with the lag time observed in studies in vivo.[178,185] Growth hormone has been shown to inhibit insulin activation of phosphatidylinositol phospholipase C in mouse adipose tissue.[194] Moreover, there is evidence that growth hormone may affect other mediators of the intracellular insulin signaling pathway such as MAP kinase, insulin receptor substrate (IRS)-1 and IRS-2.[190] Another possibility is that some of the effects of growth hormone are indirect, being mediated via the increased circulating free fatty acid due to the glucose–fatty acid cycle.[191] In general, the effects of HGH on fat metabolism occur earlier and are more pronounced than those on glucose metabolism.

Role of Endogenous Growth Hormone

Individuals who are growth hormone deficient have reduced plasma glucose and insulin concentrations and reduced hepatic glucose output, are more sensitive to exogenous insulin, and have a tendency to become hypoglycemic during prolonged fasting.[195] These abnormalities are reversed with HGH treatment.[195] Conversely, individuals with acromegaly have increased plasma glucose and insulin concentrations and increased hepatic glucose output, are resistant to insulin, and are generally glucose intolerant.[195] These abnormalities can be reversed with successful treatment.[196] These observations point to a role for growth hormone in setting the organism's sensitivity to insulin on a long-term basis.

Patients with poorly controlled insulin-dependent diabetes mellitus have increased circulating growth hormone concentrations and are insulin resistant.[197,198] Improvement in glycemic control with intensive insulin treatment normalizes plasma growth hormone concentrations and improves tissue insulin sensitivity implying a role for growth hormone.[197,199] Suppression of growth hormone secretion in such patients with somatostatin also improves glycemic control and insulin sensitivity.[122] Finally, suppression of growth hormone secretion in insulin-dependent diabetic patients undergoing withdrawal from insulin markedly reduces the increase in plasma-free fatty acid and ketone bodies,[200] indicating a role for growth hormone in the pathogenesis of diabetic ketoacidosis.

Growth hormone normally plays a significant role as a counterregulatory hormone in defense against hypoglycemia. Its secretion is stimulated when the plasma glucose concentration decreases to about 70 mg·dl^{-1}.[201] Prevention of this increase during infusion of insulin results in greater hypoglycemia because of less of an increase in hepatic glucose output and greater glucose utilization (Figure 9.9).[202] However, growth hormone is primarily important during protracted hypoglycemia since little influence of its lack of increase is observed until after 2 to 4 hours.[202] The plasma growth

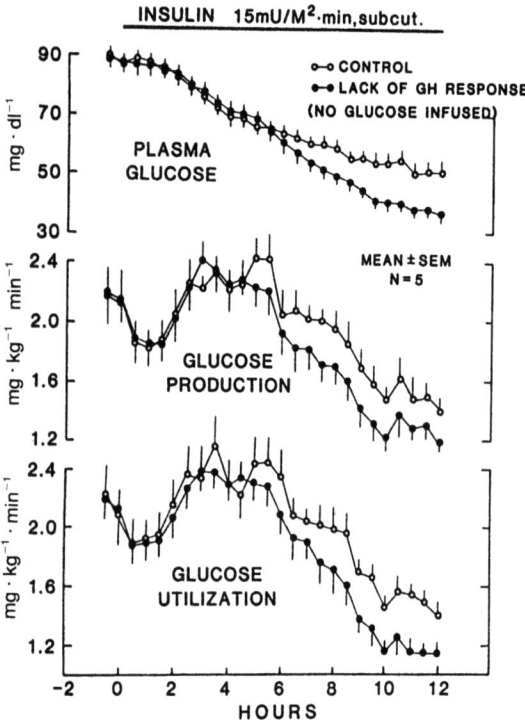

FIGURE 9.9. Effect of isolated growth hormone deficiency on hypoglycemic action of insulin. (From Bolli and Garich,[206] with permission.)

hormone response to hypoglycemia is sometimes deficient in patients with long-standing insulin-dependent diabetes and can predispose them to more severe and prolonged hypoglycemia.[201]

Two other areas where growth hormone plays an important role are the Somogyi phenomenon and the dawn phenomenon. The Somogyi phenomenon refers to the rebound hyperglycemia that can occur in patients with insulin-dependent diabetes following an episode of hypoglycemia.[203] The insulin resistance that usually results can cause increases in fasting and postprandial plasma glucose concentrations.[204] These increases are attenuated when the growth hormone response to hypoglycemia is prevented.[205]

The dawn phenomenon refers to the early morning increase in insulin requirements found in both nondiabetic and diabetic individuals.[206,207] In nondiabetic individuals, an increase in insulin occurs and plasma glucose concentrations remain stable.[208] In diabetic individuals who cannot increase their insulin secretion adequately, plasma glucose concentrations increase as much as 50 mg·dl^{-1}.[208] Studies using somatostatin have demonstrated that the nocturnal surges of growth hormone secretion that occur during sleep are largely responsible for this phenomenon (Figure 9.10).[209] When the nocturnal surges were prevented in patients with insulin-dependent diabetes, no increases in plasma glucose occurred; when the spontaneous surges were simulated with exogenous growth hormone, the early morning increases in plasma glucose were reproduced.

Cortisol

Background

The adrenal cortex produces glucocorticoids, mineralocorticoids, and sex steroids.[210] In humans, the principal glucocorticoid is cortisol. It has prominent effects on carbohydrate, lipid, and protein metabolism.[210,211] Relative to insulin, glucagon, and epinephrine, cortisol, like growth hormone, stands relatively low in the hierarchy of glucoregulatory hormones. Nonetheless, cortisol is appropriately considered a counterregulatory hormone. Its excess produces insulin resistance and often hyperglycemia in susceptible individuals.[211] Its deficiency can sometimes result in postabsorptive hypoglycemia.[211] Recently, like growth hormone, it has been shown to be involved in defense against prolonged hypoglycemia, in contrast to its lack of an important role in the correction of short-term hypoglycemia.[1-4]

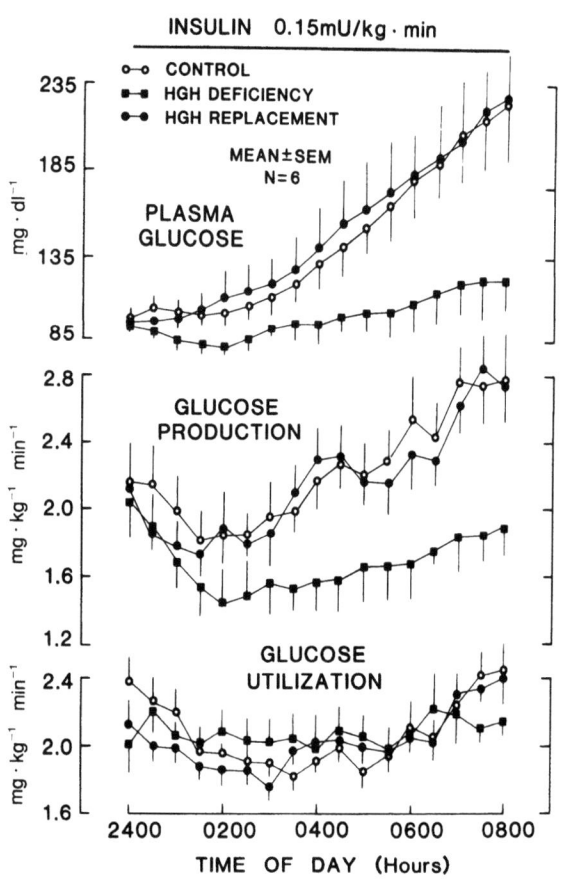

FIGURE 9.10. Role of growth hormone in the dawn phenomenon. (From DeFeo et al.,[202] with permission.)

Biosynthesis, Release, and Transport

Cortisol is synthesized, through a series of enzymatic reactions, from cholesterol (Figure 9.11). Although cholesterol can be synthesized from acetate within the adrenal cortex, the bulk of the cholesterol utilized in steroid biosynthesis is derived from circulating lipoproteins, predominantly low-density lipoproteins (LDL), through LDL (B,E) receptors on adrenocortical cells. The mitochondrial side chain cleavage enzyme system, which converts cholesterol to pregnenolone, includes the rate-limiting step in steroid biosynthesis. In the zona fasciculate and zona reticularis of the adrenal cortex it is stimulated by adrenocorticotropin (ACTH) resulting in increasing formation of cortisol, the mineralocorticoid deoxycorticosterone, and sex steroids. ACTH, through increments in intracellular cAMP, stimulates both the biosynthesis and release of these steroids. Aldosterone, the principal mineralocorticoid, is synthesized in the zona glomerulosa. Its secretion is stimulated transiently by ACTH, but other factors, notably the renin-angiotensin system and the serum potassium concentration, are the primary determinants of aldosterone secretion.

In the circulation, cortisol is largely (90–97%) bound to proteins, particularly corticosteroid binding globulin but also albumin. It is the unbound, or free, cortisol that gains access to target tissues, but cortisol dissociates from its binding proteins rapidly. Thus, the circulating protein-bound cortisol provides a reservoir of cortisol.

Degradation and Elimination

Cortisol has a relatively long plasma half-time, approximately 80 to 120 minutes. It is inactivated, primarily in the liver, through reduction to dihydro- and tetrahydrocortisol and subsequent glucuronidation. Cortisol is also converted to cortisone, which is metabolized in similar fashion. The water-soluble reduced and glucuronidated metabolites are then excreted in the urine. Although cortisol is filtered through the renal glomerulus, it is largely reabsorbed. Less than 1% of circulating cortisol is excreted in the urine unchanged.

Mechanisms of Action

Cortisol diffuses into cells and binds to intracellular receptors. Glucorticoid receptors, in contrast to those for other steroid hormones, are found in most tissues. Therefore, cortisol affects the vast majority of body tissues. The cortisol-receptor interaction is thought to result in a

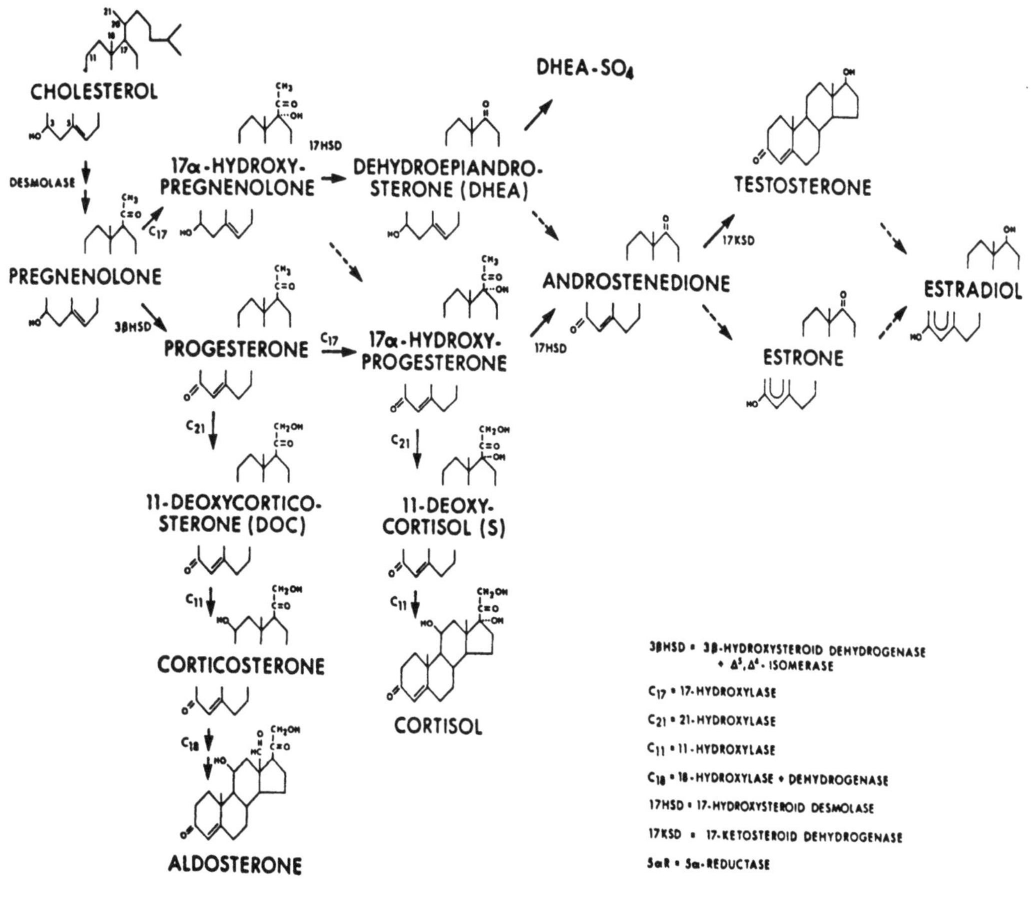

FIGURE 9.11. Adrenocortical steroid biosynthesis.

conformational change in the receptor that permits it to interact with glucocorticoid response elements of relevant genes. This interaction results in altered transcription of mRNA from the gene and can be either stimulatory or inhibitory. For example, cortisol stimulates transcription of mRNAs for several hepatic enzymes but inhibits transcription of proopiomelanocortin mRNA in the pituitary. The general pattern is for cortisol to stimulate RNA and protein synthesis in the liver and to inhibit synthesis and stimulate breakdown in many peripheral tissues including skeletal muscle with a lesser influence on these in brain and cardiac tissue.[210] The possibility that cortisol also exerts nontranscriptional regulatory effects cannot be excluded. For example, rapid negative feedback of cortisol on ACTH secretion is thought to occur too rapidly to be mediated by an effect on transcription.

Regulation of Secretion

Although other factors may well be involved,[210] the dominant regulator of cortisol secretion is ACTH. Pituitary ACTH secretion is controlled by hypothalamic stimulatory factors including corticotropin-releasing hormone and vasopressin among others. The major determinants of ACTH secretion are CNS-mediated diurnal and other rhythms, psychological and physical stress, and negative feedback by cortisol at both the hypothalamic and pituitary levels. Hypoglycemia is a potent stimulus to ACTH and cortisol secretion.

Metabolic Actions

Cortisol stimulates glucose production and limits glucose utilization.[210,211] These effects are normally counteracted by increased insulin secretion such that glucose homeostasis is maintained. Cortisol also stimulates lipolysis and proteolysis.[210,211]

The mechanisms by which cortisol limits glucose utilization, presumably in insulin-sensitive tissues, have not been fully defined. Although a variety of effects on insulin receptors have been described and long-term cortisol excess appears to decrease insulin binding in vivo, downregulation of insulin receptors does not appear to be an important factor.[211] Cortisol is thought to decrease glucose transport into cells, at least in part, by decreasing the activity of glucose transporters in the plasma membranes of relevant target cells.[212]

Studies with the euglycemic clamp technique have clearly documented earlier suggestions that long-term (i.e., hours) cortisol elevations reduce insulin-mediated glucose disposal in humans.[211] Thus, the dose-response curve for stimulation of glucose utilization by insulin is shifted to the right, i.e., sensitivity to insulin is decreased.[213]

The mechanisms by which cortisol stimulates glucose production are multiple. The hormone stimulates hepatic and renal gluconeogenesis[214,215] by increasing the delivery of gluconeogenic precursors (e.g., amino acids including glutamine, alanine, lactate, and glycerol) and by enhancing the activity of key gluconeogenic enzymes such as phosphoenolpyruvate carboxykinase.[210,211] Although glucocorticoids enhance glycogen formation, at least in part the result of enhanced gluconeogenesis, in the liver they also increase the activity of glucose-6-phosphatase and, therefore, the release of glucose derives from either pathway from the liver. Finally, there is considerable evidence that glucocorticoids enhance the glycemic responses to other hormones such as glucagon and epinephrine, i.e., they play a permissive role in the actions of these hormones.[216]

In humans, long-term (i.e., hours) cortisol elevations produce rather small increments in glucose production.[211,213,216] However, the dose-response curve for suppression of glucose production by insulin is clearly shifted to the right,[213] i.e., sensitivity to insulin is decreased with respect to suppression of glucose production, as well as to stimulation of glucose utilization as mentioned earlier. It should be emphasized that these effects require several hours of cortisol elevation in vivo. Indeed, an initial decrease in glucose production has been reported in careful studies employing hepatic venous sampling in dogs.[217] It is also notable that whereas cortisol antagonized the effects of insulin on glucose metabolism, it enhances the glycemic response to glucagon and epinephrine.[216]

Role in Metabolic Regulation

Cortisol, unlike growth hormone, is critical to survival. Demonstrable systemic metabolic abnormalities, such as postabsorptive hypoglycemia, sometimes occur in persons with long-standing cortisol deficiency. However, clinical hypoglycemia is uncommon in untreated patients, and hypoglycemia is not demonstrable after 3 days of glucocorticoid withdrawal in patients with Addison's disease[218] or those with hypopituitarism.[219] Thus, postabsorptive hypoglycemia, when it occurs, might be the indirect result of malnutrition—with hepatic glycogen depletion perhaps in concert with depletion of gluconeogenic substrates—in patients with adrenocortical insufficiency.

Although it produces substantial resistance to insulin actions, glucocorticoid excess, whether the result of endogenous overprotection of therapeutic administration, generally does not result in substantial hyperglycemia in persons with normal insulin secretion. However, it can produce marked metabolic decompensation in patients with diabetes mellitus, even those with rather minimal impairment of insulin secretion.

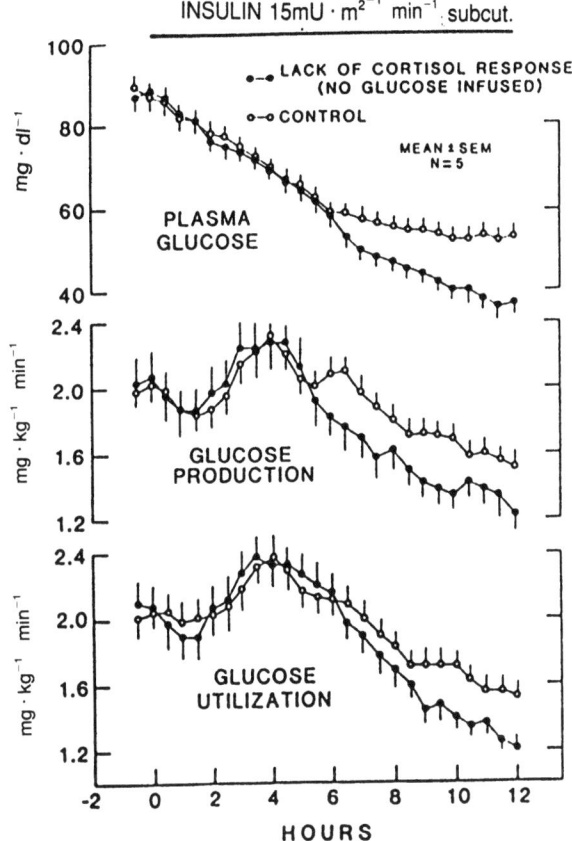

FIGURE 9.12. Effect of isolated cortisol deficiency on the hypoglycemic action of insulin. (From DeFeo et al.,[221] with permission.)

As would be expected from the delayed glycemic actions of the hormone, it is now well established that cortisol does not play an important role in the prevention of hypoglycemia in otherwise normal individuals or in recovery from short-term hypoglycemia.[3,91,92,211,220] As discussed earlier, these are the province of insulin and glucagon, and in the absence of glucagon, epinephrine.[1–4,91,92] However, there is now good evidence that cortisol and growth hormone are involved in recovery from prolonged hypoglycemia. For example, isolated cortisol deficiency, produced pharmacologically in normal individuals (Figure 9.12),[221] or cortisol and growth hormone deficiency resulting from hypopituitarism,[222] results in lower plasma glucose concentrations during relatively low-dose insulin infusions. This is largely the result of reduced limitation of glucose utilization.[221]

Metabolic Consequences in Diabetes

Insulin-treated patients with cortisol deficiency with or without growth hormone deficiency are more sensitive to insulin and, therefore, generally require lower insulin doses. This might be expected to result in more frequent, or more severe, iatrogenic hypoglycemia. Although the latter has not been well documented, the evidence discussed earlier that cortisol is involved in defense against prolonged hypoglycemia is consistent with that expectation. However, glucocorticoid replacement is relatively simple and should reverse this effect.

Cortisol, along with growth hormone, contributes to the late insulin resistance following hypoglycemia in patients with insulin-dependent diabetes mellitus, and thus is a factor in the pathogenesis of the Somogyi phenomenon.[223] It is not involved in the pathogenesis of the dawn phenomenon.[209,223]

Glucocorticoid excess is not an insurmountable obstacle to glycemic control in patients with insulin-requiring diabetes mellitus, although greater insulin doses are required. However, as mentioned earlier, it can be a major problem for those with relatively mild diabetes who are not being managed with insulin. Indeed, glucocorticoid excess can convert a diabetic patient with fasting euglycemia on treatment with diet alone to a patient with symptomatic hyperglycemia requiring treatment with insulin.

Other Potential Counterregulatory Hormones

Amylin

Amylin[6] is a 37 amino acid peptide, structurally similar to calcitonin gene-related peptide, which is cosecreted from pancreatic β cells along with insulin. In humans, plasma amylin levels generally range from 2 to 20 pmol·L^{-1} and parallel changes in those of insulin.[224] The metabolic role of amylin is presently poorly understood. It does not appear to affect insulin and glucagon secretion, at least acutely.[225–227] Although the liver has amylin receptors that activate adenylate cyclase,[228] most in vitro studies have not observed a direct effect on liver glucose metabolism.[229–231] In contrast, in muscle tissue in vitro, amylin has been shown to activate glycogen phosphorylase, inhibit glycogen syntheses, inhibit hexokinase, inhibit glycogen formation, increase glycogen breakdown, and cause insulin resistance.[6,232–235]

In vivo effects have varied among species. In rats, amylin has consistently been shown to cause insulin resistance by inhibiting stimulation of glycogen synthesis[233,234,236–238] and by impairing suppression of glucose production.[236–238] In cats, injection of amylin causes glucose intolerance.[239] In dogs, conflicting results regarding induction of insulin resistance have been reported.[240,241] In humans, no effect has been found on plasma glucose and insulin levels, rates of glucose production and disposal, or insulin sensitivity.[225,242,243] It is possible nevertheless that amylin may have long-term effects on insulin sensitivity since insulin-resistant states are associated with high circulating amylin levels.[6]

Tumor Necrosis Factor-α (TNF-α)

Tumor necrosis factor-α is a cytokine released by adipocytes and macrophages that has actions on carbohydrate, lipid, and protein metabolism.[8,244,245] Formally called cachectin, because of its involvement in the metabolic alterations accompanying cancer, endotoxemia and trauma, this peptide has recently been found to be expressed in adipocytes and has been proposed to be responsible for at least some of the insulin resistance associated with obesity,[244] since its administration causes insulin resistance and since it is overrepresented in genetically obese rodents.

In addition to indirect effects due to its stimulation of cortisol, glucagon, and catecholamine release,[246] TNF-α has been shown to have direct actions on muscle and adipose tissue and possibly the liver. For example, in adipocytes and myocytes it downregulates GLUT 4 mRNA levels,[247,248] reduces catalytic activity of the insulin receptor,[249] and impairs insulin-stimulated glucose transport.[250] In the liver it inhibits autophosphorylation of the insulin receptor and phosphorylation of IRS-1.[251]

Tumor necrosis factor-α binds to widely distributed cell membrane receptors (e.g., TNF-R_1 and -R_2).[252] Several mechanisms of action have been proposed, including activation of phospholipase A_2, multiple protein kinases and phosphoprotein phosphatases, and transcription factors.[244] Since its effects on tissues take several days to become apparent, it is likely that TNF-α acts as a long-term modulator of tissue insulin sensitivity rather than an acute humoral regulator such as glucagon, catecholamines, growth hormone, and cortisol.

Leptin

Leptin is the peptide product of the ob gene. It is exclusively expressed in adipose tissue and released into the circulation, and it acts on the hypothalamus to reduce food intake and regulate energy expenditure in rodents.[253–255] Food intake, obesity, insulin, and glucocorticoids increase its expression (i.e., mRNA levels), whereas caloric restriction has the opposite effects.[256]

In humans, plasma concentrations normally are in the range of 5 to 20 ng·mmol^{-1} and are increased after acute overfeeding,[257] during prolonged insulin infusion,[257] and in both lean and obese insulin-resistant women with polycystic ovary syndrome,[258] as well as in obese individuals with and without diabetes.[259,260] Circulating concentrations are reduced after hypocaloric dieting, exercise training,[261] and in women with anorexia nervosa,[262] but are unaffected by acute infusions of insulin or meals.[263,264] Circulating leptin concentrations are positively correlated with body fat, are lower in men than in women, and are inversely related to age.[265]

Recent studies indicate that leptin may, in addition to being a satiety factor, modulate insulin secretion and sensitivity. It has been reported[7] that the liver possesses leptin receptors and that leptin reduces insulin-induced IRS-1 phosphorylation and insulin inhibition of gluconeogenesis. Leptin receptors have also been found on pancreatic β-TC-3 cells.[266] Because plasma leptin concentrations do not change acutely, it is likely that leptin would be a long-term modulator of insulin sensitivity and secretion. Further studies are needed in this area.

Summary

The key anti-insulin hormones in humans are glucagon, epinephrine, cortisol, and growth hormone. Thyroid hormone, amylin, TNF-α, and leptin are not acutely important regulators of insulin sensitivity. Glucagon and epinephrine are rapidly acting insulin antagonists whose mechanism of action has been well established. The mechanisms by which cortisol and growth hormone antagonize the actions of insulin are less well understood; these hormones are slow-acting, compared with glucagon and epinephrine. Glucagon is most important in the moment-to-moment control of glucose homeostasis by its actions on the rate of hepatic glucose production; it is the key hormone for immediate counterregulation to a decrement in plasma glucose, and abnormalities of its secretion contribute substantially to those due to inadequate insulin secretion in the pathogenesis of diabetes mellitus. Also, increases in epinephrine, cortisol, and growth hormone secretion exacerbate this situation beyond what can be directly explained by insulin deficiency. Next to glucagon, epinephrine is the most important counterregulatory hormone via its actions to increase hepatic glucose output and to limit glucose utilization in insulin-sensitive tissues. It is important in recovery from both acute and prolonged hypoglycemia and its role becomes critical when glucagon secretion is impaired, such as in long-standing, insulin-dependent diabetes mellitus. Cortisol and growth hormone become important as counterregulatory hormones during prolonged hypoglycemia; both also play a role in rebound hyperglycemia (i.e., Somogyi phenomenon), whereas growth hormone is the principal factor responsible for the dawn phenomenon. Chronic excess of any of these hormones can lead to impaired glucose tolerance and, in susceptible individuals, frank diabetes mellitus. On the other hand, deficiencies of any of these hormones can, under certain conditions, cause hypoglycemia.

References

1. Cryer PE. Hypoglycemia and insulin-dependent diabetes mellitus. In: Alberti KGMM, Krall LP, eds. Diabetes annual. 4th ed. Amsterdam: Elsevier Science, 1988: 272–310.

2. Gerich JE. Glucose counterregulation and its impact on diabetes mellitus. Diabetes 1988;37:1608–1617.
3. Cryer PE, Binder C, Bolli GB, et al. Hypoglycemia in IDDM. Diabetes 1989;38:1193–1199.
4. Cryer PE, Gerich JE. Hypoglycemia in insulin-dependent diabetes mellitus: insulin excess and defective glucose counterregulation. In: Rifkin H, Porte D, eds. Ellenberg and Rifkin's diabetes mellitus, theory and practice. New York: Elsevier Science, 1990:526–546.
5. Müller M, Seitz H. Thyroid hormone action on intermediary metabolism. Klin Wochenschr 1984;62:11–18,49–55, 97–102.
6. Cooper G. Amylin compared with calcitonin gene-related peptide: structure, biology, and relevance to metabolic disease. Endocr Rev 1994;15:163–201.
7. Cohen B, Novick D, Rubinstein M. Modulation of insulin activities by leptin. Science 1996;274:1185–1188.
8. Mitch W, Goldberg A. Mechanisms of muscle wasting: the role of the ubiquitin-proteasome pathway. N Engl J Med 1996;335:1897–1905.
9. Kimball C, Murlin J. Aqueous extracts of pancreas III. Some precipitation reactions of insulin. J Biochem 1923; 58:337–348.
10. Bromer W, Winn L, Behrens O. The amino acid sequence of glucagon V. Location of amide groups, acid degradation studies and summary of sequential evidence. J Am Chem Soc 1957;79:2807–2810.
11. Sutherland E, Robison G, Butcher R. Some aspects of the biological role of adenosine 3′,5′-monophosphate (cyclic AMP). Circulation 1968;37:279–306.
12. Gerich J. Physiology of glucagon. Int Rev Physiol 1981; 24:244–275.
13. Patzelt C, Schiltz E. Conversion of proglucagon in pancreatic alpha cells: the major endproducts are glucagon and a single peptide, the major proglucagon fragment, that contains two glucagon-like sequences. Proc Natl Acad Sci USA 1984;81:5007–5011.
14. Conlon J. The glucagon-like polypeptides—order out of chaos? Diabetologia 1980;18:85–88.
15. Weir G. Glucagon in normal physiology and diabetes mellitus. In: Brownlee E, ed. Diabetes mellitus. New York: Garland STPM Press, 1981:207–259.
16. Jaspan J, Rubenstein A. Circulating glucagon: plasma profiles and metabolism in health and disease. Diabetes 1977;26:887–902.
17. Munoz-Barragan L, Rufener C, Srikant C, et al. Immunocytochemical evidence for glucagon-containing cells in the human stomach. Horm Metab Res 1977;9:37–39.
18. Morita S, Doi K, Yip C, Vranic M. Measurement and partial characterization of immunoreactive glucagon in gastrointestinal tissues of dogs. Diabetes 1976;25:1018–1025.
19. Sasaki H, Rubalcava B, Baetens D, et al. Identification of glucagon in the gastrointestinal tract. J Clin Invest 1975; 56:135–145.
20. Srikant C, McCorkle K, Unger R. Properties of immunoreactive glucagon fractions of canine stomach and pancreas. J Biochem 1977;252:1847–1851.
21. Doi K, Prentki M, Yip C, et al. Identical biologic effects of pancreatic glucagon and a purified moiety of canine gastric immunoreactive glucagon. J Clin Invest 1979;63:525–531.
22. Werner P, Palmer J. Immunoreactive glucagon responses to oral glucose, insulin infusion and deprivation, and somatostatin in pancreatectomized man. Diabetes 1978;27:1005–1012.
23. Müller W, Berger M, Sutter P, et al. Glucagon immunoreactivity and amino acid profile in plasma of duodenopancreatectomized patients. J Clin Invest 1979;63:820–827.
24. Meyata M, Yamamoyo T, Yamaguchi M, et al. Plasma glucagon after total resection of the pancreas in man. Proc Soc Exp Biol Med 1976;152:540–543.
25. Botha J, Vinik A. Plasma-glucagon after pancreatectomy. Lancet 1976;1:1290–1291.
26. Vranic M, Pek S, Kawamori R. Increased glucagon immunoreactivity in plasma of totally depancreatized dogs. Diabetes 1974;23:905–912.
27. Mashiter K, Harding P, Chou M, et al. Persistent pancreatic glucagon but not insulin response to arginine in pancreatectomized dogs. Endocrinology 1975;95:678–693.
28. Matsuyama T, Foa P. Plasma glucose, insulin, pancreatic, and enteroglucagon levels in normal and depancreatized dogs. Proc Soc Exp Biol Med 1974; 147:97–102.
29. Barnes A, Bloom S. Pancreatectomized man: a model for diabetes without glucagon. Lancet 1976;1:219–221.
30. Gerich J, Karam J, Lorenzi M. Diabetes without glucagon. Lancet 1976;1:855–856.
31. Müller W, Brennan M, Tan M, Aoki T. Studies of glucagon secretion in pancreatectomized patients. Diabetes 1974;23:512–516.
32. Brockman R, Manns J, Bergman E. Quantitative aspects of secretion and hepatic removal of glucagon in sheep. Can J Physiol Pharmacol 1976;54:666–670.
33. Röjdmark S, Bloom G, Chou M, et al. Hepatic insulin and glucagon extraction after their augmented secretion in dogs. Am J Physiol 1978;235:88–96.
34. Emmanouel D, Jaspan J, Rubenstein A, et al. Glucagon metabolism in the rat: contribution of the kidney to the metabolic clearance rate of the hormone. J Clin Invest 1978;62:6–13.
35. Jaspan J, Huen A, Morely C, et al. The role of the liver in glucagon metabolism. J Clin Invest 1977;60:421–428.
36. Röjdmark S, Bloom G, Chou M, Field J. Hepatic extraction of exogenous insulin and glucagon in the dog. Endocrinology 1978;102:806–813.
37. Blackard W, Nelson N, Andrews S. Portal and peripheral vein immunoreactive glucagon concentrations after arginine or glucose infusions. Diabetes 1974;23:199–202.
38. Felig P, Gusberg R, Hendler R, et al. Concentrations of glucagon and the insulin glucagon ratio in the portal and peripheral circulation. Proc Soc Exp Biol Med 1974; 147:88–90.
39. Dencker M, Hedner P, Holst J, Tranberg K. Pancreatic glucagon response to an ordinary meal. Scand J Gastroenterol 1975;10:471–474.
40. Kuku S, Jaspan J, Emmanouel D, et al. Heterogeneity of plasma glucagon: circulating components in normal subjects and patients with chronic renal failure. J Clin Invest 1976;58:742–750.
41. Noe B, Bauer G, Steffes M, et al. Glucagon biosynthesis in human pancreatic islets: preliminary evidence for a biosynthetic intermediate. Horm Metab Res 1975;7:314–322.

42. Weir G, Horton E, Aoki T, et al. Secretion of glucagonomas of a possible glucagon precursor. J Clin Invest 1977;59:325–330.
43. Valverdi I, Lemon H, Kessinger A, Unger R. Distribution of plasma glucagon immunoreactivity in a patient with suspected glucagonoma. J Clin Endocrinol Metab 1976;42:804–808.
44. Recant L, Perrino P, Bhathena S, et al. Plasma immunoreactive glucagon fractions in four cases of glucagonoma: increased "large glucagon immunoreactivity." Diabetologia 1976;12:319–326.
45. Carpentier J, Malaisse-Lagae F, et al. Glucagon release from rate pancreatic islets: a combined morphological and functional approach. J Clin Invest 1977;60:1174–1182.
46. Gerich J, Charles M, Grodsky G. Regulation of pancreatic insulin and glucagon secretion. Annu Rev Physiol 1976;38:353–388.
47. Toyota T, Sato S, Kudo M, et al. Secretory regulation of endocrine pancreas: cyclic AMP and glucagon secretion. J Clin Endocrinol Metab 1975;41:81–89.
48. Gerich J, Frankel B, Fanska R, et al. Calcium dependency of glucagon secretion from the in vitro perfused rat pancreas. Endocrinology 1974;94:1381–1385.
49. Epstein G, Fanska R, Grodsky G. The effect of potassium and valinomycin on insulin and glucagon secretion in the perfused rat pancreas. Endocrinology 1978;103:2207–2215.
50. Fisher M, Sherwin R, Hendler R, Felig P. Kinetics of glucagon in man: effects of starvation. Proc Natl Acad Sci USA 1976;73:1735–1739.
51. Alford F, Bloom S, Nabarro J. Glucagon metabolism in man: studies on the metabolic clearance rate and the plasma acute disappearance time of glucagon in normal and diabetic subjects. J Clin Endocrinol Metab 1976;42:830–838.
52. Sherwin R, Fisher M, Bessoff J, et al. Hyperglucagonemia in cirrhosis: altered secretion and sensitivity to glucagon. Gastroenterology 1978;74:1224–1228.
53. Sherwin R, Bastl C, Finkelstein F, et al. Influence of uremia and hemodialysis on the turnover and metabolic effects of glucagon. J Clin Invest 1976;57:722–731.
54. Lefebvre P, Luykx A, Nizet A. Renal handling of endogenous glucagon in the dog: comparison with insulin. Metabolism 1974;23:753–760.
55. Bastl C, Finkelstein F, Sherwin R, et al. Renal extraction of glucagon in rats with normal and reduced renal function. Am J Physiol 1977;233:67–71.
56. Emmanouel D, Jaspan J, Kuku S, et al. Pathogenesis and characterization of hyperglucagonemia in the uremic rat. J Clin Invest 1976;58:1266–1271.
57. Gerich J, Charles M, Grodsky G. Characterization of the effects of arginine and glucose on glucagon and insulin release from the perfused rat pancreas. J Clin Invest 1974;54:833–841.
58. Gerich J, Schneider V, Dippe S, et al. Characterization of glucagon response to hypoglycemia in man. J Clin Endocrinol Metab 1974;38:77–82.
59. Rocha D, Faloona G, Unger R. Glucagon-stimulating activity of 20 amino acids in dogs. J Clin Invest 1972;51:2346–2351.
60. Gerich J, Langlois M, Noacco C, et al. Adrenergic modulation of pancreatic glucagon secretion in man. J Clin Invest 1974;53:1441–1446.
61. Goberna R, Tamarit J, Osorio J, et al. Action of β-hydroxybutyrate, acetoacetate, and palmitate on insulin release from the perfused isolated rat pancreas. Horm Metab Res 1974;6:256–260.
62. Gerich J, Lorenzi M. The role of the autonomic nervous system and somatostatin in the control of insulin and glucagon secretion. In: Ganong W, Martini L, eds. Frontiers in neuroendocrinology. 5th ed. New York: Raven Press, 1977;265–288.
63. Gerich J, Langlois M, Schneider V, et al. Effects of alterations of plasma free fatty acid levels on pancreatic glucagon secretion in man. J Clin Invest 1974;53:1284–1289.
64. Gerich J, Karam J, Forsham P. Stimulation of glucagon secretion by epinephrine in man. J Clin Endocrinol Metab 1973;37:479–481.
65. Iversen J. Effect of acetyl choline on the secretion of glucagon and insulin from the isolated, perfused canine pancreas. Diabetes 1973;22:381–387.
66. Leclercq-Meyer V, Brisson G, Malaisse W. Effect of adrenaline and glucose on release of glucagon and insulin in vitro. Nature New Biol 1971;231:248–249.
67. Iversen J. Adrenergic receptors and the secretion of glucagon and insulin from the isolated perfused canine pancreas. J Clin Invest 1973;52:2102–2116.
68. Marliss E, Girardier L, Seydoux J, et al. Glucagon release induced by pancreatic nerve stimulation in the dog. J Clin Invest 1973;52:1246–1259.
69. Porte D, Girardier L, Seydoux J, et al. J. Neural regulation of insulin secretion in the dog. J Clin Invest 1973;52:210–214.
70. Raneto A, Kosaka K, Nakao K. Effects of stimulation of the vagus nerve on insulin secretion. Endocrinology 1967;80:530–536.
71. Unger R, Ketterer H, Dupre J, Eisentraut A. The effects of secretion, pancreozymin, and gastrin upon insulin and glucagon secretion in anesthetized dog. J Clin Invest 1967;46:630–645.
72. Pederson R, Brown J. Interaction of gastric inhibitory polypeptide, glucose, and arginine on insulin and glucagon secretion from the perfused rat pancreas. Endocrinology 1978;103:610–615.
73. Santeusanio F, Faloona G, Unger R. Suppressive effect of secretion upon pancreatic alpha-cell function. J Clin Invest 1972;51:1743–1749.
74. Goldfine I, Kirsteins L, Lawrence A. Excessive glucagon response to arginine in active acromegaly. Horm Metab Res 1972;4:97–100.
75. Wise J, Hendler R, Felig P. Influence of glucocorticoids on glucagon secretion and plasma amino acid concentration in man. J Clin Invest 1973;52:2774–2782.
76. Seino Y, Goto Y, Taminato T, et al. Plasma insulin and glucagon responses to arginine in patients with thyroid dysfunction. J Clin Endocrinol Metab 1974;38:1136–1140.
77. Unger R. Glucagon physiology and pathophysiology. N Engl J Med 1971;285:443–448.

78. Marliss E, Aoki T, Unger R, et al. Glucagon levels and metabolic effects in fasting man. J Clin Invest 1970;49:2256–2270.
79. Müller W, Faloona G, Unger R. The influence of antecedent diet upon glucagon and insulin secretion. N Engl J Med 1971;285:1450–1454.
80. Lewis S, Wallin J, Kane J, Gerich J. Effect of diet composition on metabolic adaptations to hypocaloric nutrition: comparison of high carbohydrate and high fat isocaloric diets. Am J Clin Nutr 1977;30:160–170.
81. Kalkoff R, Gossain V, Maktute M. Plasma glucagon in obesity. N Engl J Med 1973;289:465–467.
82. Gerich J, Langlois M, Noacco C. Glucagon secretion in obesity. Lancet 1973;1:1323.
83. Wise J, Hendler R, Felig P. Evaluation of alpha-cell function by infusion of alanine in normal, diabetic, and obese subjects. N Engl J Med 1973;288:487–490.
84. Cryer P. Glucagon and Glucose counterregulation in Lefèbvre P, ed. Glucagon I. Berlin: Springer-Verlag, 1996: 149–158.
85. Exton J, Park C. Interaction of insulin and glucagon in the control of liver metabolism. In: Steiner D, Freinkel N, eds. Endocrine pancreas, section 7, handbook of physiology. Baltimore: Williams & Wilkins, 1972:437–455.
86. Galbo H, Holst J, Christensen N. Glucagon and plasma catecholamine response to graded and prolonged exercise in man. J Appl Physiol 1975;38:70–76.
87. Wilmore D, Moylan J, Pruitt B, et al. Hyperglucagonemia after burns. Lancet 1974;1:73–75.
88. Rocha D, Santeusanio F, Faloona G, Unger R. Abnormal pancreatic alpha-cell function in bacterial infections. N Engl J Med 1973;288:700–703.
89. Wilderson J, Hutcheson D, Leshin S, et al. Serum glucagon and insulin levels and their relationship to blood glucose values in patients with acute myocardial infarction and acute coronary insufficiency. Am J Med 1974;57:747–753.
90. Liljenquist J, Müeller G, Cherrington A, et al. Evidence for an important role of glucagon in the regulation of hepatic glucose production in normal man. J Clin Invest 1977;59:369–374.
91. Gerich J, Davis J, Lorenzi M, et al. Hormonal mechanisms of recovery from insulin-induced hypoglycemia in man. Am J Physiol 1979;236:E380–E385.
92. Rizza R, Cryer P, Gerich J. Role of glucagon, catecholamines, and growth hormone in human glucose counterregulation. Effects of somatostatin and combined α- and β-adrenergic blockade on plasma glucose recovery and glucose flux rates after insulin-induced hypoglycemia. J Clin Invest 1979;64:62–71.
93. Garber A, Cryer P, Santiago J, et al. The role of adrenergic mechanisms in the substrate and hormonal response to insulin-induced hypoglycemia in man. J Clin Invest 1976;58:7–15.
94. Feldman J, Plonk J, Bivens C. The role of cortisol and growth hormone in the counterregulation of insulin-induced hypoglycemia. Horm Metab Res 1975;7:378–381.
95. Lecavalier L, Bolli G, Cryer P, Gerich J. Contributions of gluconeogenesis and glycogenolysis during glucose counterregulation in normal humans. Am J Physiol 1989; 256:E844–E851.
96. Felig P, Wahren J, Hendler R. Influence of oral glucose ingestion of splanchnic glucose and gluconeogenic substrate mechanism in man. Diabetes 1975;24:468–475.
97. Kelley D, Mitrakou A, Marsh H, et al. Skeletal muscle glycolysis, oxidation, and storage of an oral glucose load. J Clin Invest 1988;81:1563–1571.
98. Unger R, Madison L, Miller W. Abnormal alpha-cell function in diabetes: response to insulin. Diabetes 1972;21:301–309.
99. Gerich J, Lorenzi M, Karam J, et al. Abnormal pancreatic glucagon secretion and postprandial hyperglycemia in diabetes mellitus. JAMA 1975;234:159–165.
100. Balasse E, Havel R. Evidence for an effect of insulin on the peripheral utilization of ketone bodies in dogs. J Clin Invest 1971;50:801–803.
101. Miles J, Rizza R, Haymond M, Gerich J. Effects of acute insulin deficiency and administration on ketone body and glucose turnover in man. Clin Res 1979;27:658.
102. Witters L, Trasko C. Regulation of hepatic free fatty acid metabolism by glucagon and insulin. Am J Physiol 1979; 237:23–29.
103. Heimberg M, Weinstein I, Kohout M. The effects of glucagon dibutyryl cyclic adenosine 3′,5′-monophosphate, and concentrations of free fatty acid on hepatic lipid metabolism. J Biochem 1969;244:5131–5139.
104. Parrilla R, Goodman N, Toews C. Effects of glucagon: insulin ratios on hepatic metabolism. Diabetes 1974;23: 725–731.
105. McGarry J. New perspectives in the regulation of ketogenesis. Diabetes 1979;28:517–523.
106. McGarry J, Takabayashi Y, Foster D. The role of malonyl-CoA in the coordination of fatty acid synthesis and oxidation in isolated rat hepatocytes. J Biochem 1978;253: 8294–8300.
107. Liljenquist J, Bombay J, Lewis S, et al. Effects of glucagon on lipolysis and ketogenesis in normal and diabetic man. J Clin Invest 1974;53:190–197.
108. Keller V, Chiasson J, Liljenquist J, et al. The roles of insulin, glucagon, and free fatty acids in the regulation of ketogenesis in dogs. Diabetes 1977;26:1040–1051.
109. Asplin C, Hartog M, Goldie D. Change of insulin dosage, circulating free and bound insulin and insulin antibodies on transferring diabetics from conventional to highly purified porcine insulin. Diabetologia 1978;14:99–105.
110. Schade D, Eaton R. Modulation of fatty acid metabolism by glucagon in man. I. Effects in normal subjects. Diabetes 1975;24:502–509.
111. Asplin C, Paquettte T, Palmer J. In vivo inhibition of glucagon secretion by paracrine beta-cell activity in man. J Clin Invest 1981;68:314–318.
112. Rodbell M. The actions of glucagon at its receptor. In: Lefebvre P, ed. Glucagon I. Berlin: Springer-Verlag, 1983: 263–290.
113. Stalmans W. Glucagon and liver glycogen metabolism. In: Lefebvre P, ed. Glucagon I. Berlin: Springer-Verlag, 1983: 291–314.
114. Baetens D, Malaisse-Lagae F, Perrelet A, Orci L. Endocrine pancreas: three-dimensional reconstruction show

two types of islets of Langerhans. Science 1979;206:1323–1325.
115. McGarry D, Foster D. Glucagon and ketogenesis. In: Lefebvre P, ed. Glucagon I. Berlin: Springer-Verlag, 1983:383–398.
116. Unger R, Orci L. Physiology and pathophysiology of glucagon. Physiol Rev 1976;56:779–826.
117. Unger R. Role of glucagon in the pathogenesis of diabetes: the status of the controversy. Metabolism 1978;27:1691–1709.
118. Müller W, Faloona G, Aguilar-Parada E, Unger R. Abnormal alpha-cell function in diabetes: response to protein and carbohydrate ingestion. N Engl J Med 1970;283:109–115.
119. Wahren J, Felig P, Hagenfeldt L. Effect of protein ingestion on splanchnic and leg metabolism in normal man and in patients with diabetes mellitus. J Clin Invest 1976;57:987–999.
120. Seino Y, Ikeda M, Kurachi H, et al. Failure to suppress plasma glucagon concentrations by orally administered glucose in diabetic patients after treatment. Diabetes 1978;27:1145–1150.
121. Buchanan K, Carroll A. Abnormalities of glucagon metabolism in untreated diabetes mellitus. Lancet 1971;2:1394–1395.
122. Gerich J, Schultz T, Tsalikian E, et al. Clinical evaluation of somatostatin as a potential adjunct to insulin in the management of diabetes mellitus. Diabetologia 1977;13:537–544.
123. Raskin P, Fujita Y, Unger R. Effect of insulin-glucose infusions on plasma glucagon levels in fasting diabetics and nondiabetics. J Clin Invest 1975;56:1132–1138.
124. Gerich J, Langlois M, Noacco C, et al. Comparison of suppressive effects of hyperglycemia and evaluation of plasma free fatty acid levels on glucagon secretion in normal and insulin-dependent diabetic subjects: evidence for selective alpha-cell insensitivity to glucose in diabetes mellitus. J Clin Invest 1976;58:320–325.
125. Gerich J, Langlois M, Noacco C, et al. Lack of glucagon response to hypoglycemia in diabetes: evidence for an intrinsic pancreatic alpha-cell defect. Science 1973;182:171–173.
126. Raskin P, Unger R. Hyperglucagonemia and its suppression: importance in the metabolic control of diabetes. N Engl J Med 1978;299:433–436.
127. Cryer PE. Physiology and pathophysiology of the human sympathoadrenal neuroendocrine system. N Engl J Med 1980;303:436–444.
128. Cryer PE. Diseases of the sympathochromaffin system. In: Felig P, Baxter J, Broadus A, Frohman L, eds. Endocrinology and metabolism. 2nd ed. New York: McGraw-Hill, 1994:651–692.
129. Landsberg L, Young JB. Catecholamines and the adrenal medulla. In: Wilson JD, Foster DW, eds. Williams' textbook of medicine. 7th ed. Philadelphia: WB Saunders, 1985:891–965.
130. Nagatus T. Biochemistry of the catecholamines. Baltimore: University Park Press, 1973:3–7.
131. Hermansen K. Tolbutamide, glucose, calcium, and somatostatin secretion. Acta Endocrinol 1982;99:86–93.
132. Silverberg AB, Shah SD, Haymond MW, Cryer PE. Norephinephrine: hormone and neurotransmitter in man. Am J Physiol 1978;234;E252–E256.
133. Shah SD, Tse TF, Clutter WE, Cryer PE. The human sympathochromaffin system. Am J Physiol 1984;247:E380–384.
134. Ricordi C, Shah SD, Lacy PE, et al. Delayed extra-adrenal epinephrine secretion following bilateral adrenalectomy in rats. Am J Physiol 1988;254:E52–E53.
135. Clutter W, Bier D, Shah S, Cryer P. Epinephrine plasma metabolic clearance rates and physiologic thresholds for metabolic and hemodynamic actions in man. J Clin Invest 1980;66:94–101.
136. Berk MA, Clutter WE, Sjot DA, et al. Enhanced glycemic responsiveness to epinephrine in insulin-dependent diabetes mellitus is the result of inability to secrete insulin. J Clin Invest 1985;75:1842–1851.
137. Clutter WE, Rizza RA, Gerich JE, Cryer PE. Regulation of glucose metabolism by sympathochromaffin catecholamines. Diabetes Metab Rev 1988;4:1–15.
138. Leftkowitz RJ, Carbon MG. Adrenergic receptors: models for the study of receptors coupled to guanine nucleotide regulatory proteins. J Biochem 1988;263:4993–4996.
139. Emorine LJ, Marullo S, Briend-Sutren M-M, et al. Molecular characterization of the human β_3-adrenergic receptor. Science 1989;245:1118–1121.
140. Palmer JD, Henry DP, Johnson DG, Ensinck JW. Glucagon response to hypoglycemia in sympathectomized man. J Clin Invest 1976;57:522–525.
141. Schwartz NS, Clutter WE, Shah SD, Cryer PE. The glycemic thresholds for activation of glucose counterregulatory systems are higher than the threshold for symptoms. J Clin Invest 1987;79:777–781.
142. Boyle PJ, Schwartz NS, Shah SD, et al. Plasma glucose concentrations at the onset of hypoglycemia symptoms in patients with poorly controlled diabetes and nondiabetics. N Engl J Med 1988;318:1487–1492.
143. Garber AJ, Cryer PE, Santiago JV, et al. The role of adrenergic mechanisms in the substrate and hormonal response to insulin-induced hypoglycemia in man. J Clin Invest 1976;58:7–15.
144. Cori CF, Buchwald KW. Effect of continuous intravenous injection of epinephrine on the carbohydrate metabolism, basal metabolism and vascular system in normal man. Am J Physiol 1930;95:71–78.
145. Rizza RA, Haymond MW, Cryer PE, Gerich JE. Differential effects of physiologic concentrations of epinephrine on glucose production and disposal in man. Am J Physiol 1979;237:E356–E362.
146. Rizza RA, Haymond MW, Miles JM, et al. Effect of α-adrenergic stimulation and its blockade on glucose turnover in man. Am J Physiol 1980;238:E467–E472.
147. Rizza RA, Cryer PE, Haymond MW, Gerich JE. Adrenergic mechanisms for the effect of epinephrine on glucose production and clearance in man. J Clin Invest 1980;65:682–689.
148. Galster A, Clutter W, Cryer P, et al. Epinephrine plasma thresholds for lipolytic effects in man: measurements of fatty acid transport with [1-13C] palmitic acid. J Clin Invest 1981;67:1729–1738.

149. Gray D, Lickley H, Vranci M. Physiologic effects of epinephrine on glucose turnover and plasma free fatty acid concentration mediated independently of glucagon. Diabetes 1980;29:600–608.
150. Deibert D, DeFronzo R. Epinephrine-induced insulin resistance in man. J Clin Invest 1980;65:717–721.
151. Rosen SG, Clutter WE, Shah SD, et al. Direct α-adrenergic stimulation of hepatic glucose production in postabsorptive human subjects. Am J Physiol 1983;245:E616–E626.
152. Stumvoll M, Chintalapudi U, Perriello G, et al. Uptake and release of glucose by the human kidney: postabsorptive rates and responses to epinephrine. J Clin Invest 1995;96:2528–2533.
153. Sacca L, Morrone G, Cicala M, et al. Influence of epinephrine, norepinephrine and isoproterenol on glucose homeostasis in normal man. J Clin Endocrinol Metab 1980;50:680–684.
154. Mauriege P, DePergola G, Berlan M, Lafontan M. Human fat cell beta-adrenergic receptors: beta-agonist-dependent lipolytic responses and characterization of beta-adrenergic binding sites on human fat cell membranes with highly selective beta1-antagonists. J Lipid Res 1988;29:587–601.
155. Weiss M, Keller U, Stauffacher W. Effect of epinephrine and somatostatin induced deficiency on ketone body kinetics and lipolysis in man. Diabetes 1984;33:738–744.
156. Shamoon H, Jacob R, Sherwin RS. Epinephrine-induced hypoaminoacidemia in normal and diabetic human subjects. Effect of beta blockade. Diabetes 1980;29:875–881.
157. Miles JM, Nissen SL, Gerich JE, Haymond MW. Effects of epinephrine infusion on leucine and alanine kinetics in humans. Am J Physiol 1984;247:E166–E172.
158. Sjostrom L, Schutz Y, Gudinchet F, et al. Epinephrine sensitivity with respect to metabolic rate and other variables in women. Am J Physiol 1973;245:E431–E442.
159. Fellows IW, Bennett T, Macdonald IA. The effect of adrenaline upon cardiovascular and metabolic functions in man. Clin Sci 1985;69:215–222.
160. Staten MA, Matthews DE, Cryer PE, Bier DM. Physiologic increments in epinephrine stimulate metabolic rate in humans. Am J Physiol 1987;253:E322–E330.
161. Cryer PE. Decreased sympathochromaffin activity in IDDM. Diabetes 1989;38:405–409.
162. Rosen SG, Clutter WE, Berk MA, et al. Epinephrine supports the postabsorptive plasma glucose concentration, and prevents hypoglycemia, when glucagon secretion is deficient in man. J Clin Invest 1984;73:405–411.
163. Boyle PJ, Shah SD, Cryer PE. Insulin, glucagon and catecholamines in the prevention of hypoglycemia during fasting in humans. Am J Physiol 1989;256:E651–E661.
164. Tse TF, Clutter WE, Shah SD, et al. Neuroendocrine responses to glucose ingestion in man: specificity, temporal relationships and quantitative aspects. J Clin Invest 1983;72:270–277.
165. Tse TF, Clutter WE, Shah SD, et al. The mechanisms of postprandial glucose counterregulation in man: physiologcial roles of glucagon and epinephrine vis-a-vis insulin in the prevention of hypoglycemia late after glucose ingestion. J Clin Invest 1983;72:278–286.
166. Hirsch IB, Marker J, Smith L, et al. Glucoregulation during exercise: a reassessment (abstract). Diabetes 1989;38:21A.
167. Popp DA, Shah SD, Cryer PE. The role of epinephrine mediated B-adrenergic mechanisms in hypoglycemia in insulin-dependent diabetes mellitus. J Clin Invest 1982;69:315–326.
168. Bolli G, DeFeo P, Compagnucci P, et al. Abnormal glucose counterregulation in insulin-dependent diabetes mellitus: interaction of anti-insulin antibodies and impaired glucagon and epinephrine secretion. Diabetes 1983;32:134–141.
169. DeFeo P, Bolli G, Ventura M, et al. Rapid variations in glucose uptake in vivo: evidence for a rhythm in insulin action in man. Diabetologia 1984;27(A):268.
170. White NH, Skor DA, Cryer PE, et al. Identification of type I diabetic patients at increased risk for hypoglycemia during intensive therapy. N Engl J Med 1983;308:485–491.
171. Bolli G, DeFeo P, DeCosmo S, et al. A reliable and reproducible test for adequate glucose counterregulation in type I (insulin-dependent) diabetes mellitus. Diabetes 1984;33:732–737.
172. Chawla R, Parks J, Rudman D. Structural variants of human growth hormone: biochemical, genetic, and clinical aspects. Annu Rev Med 1983;34:519.
173. Miller W, Eberhardt N. Structure and evolution of the growth hormone gene family. Endocr Rev 1983;4:97.
174. Guillemin R, Brazeau P, Bohlen P, et al. Growth hormone-releasing factor from a human pancreatic tumor that caused acromegaly. Science 1982;218:585–587.
175. Reichlin S. Somatostatin. N Engl J Med 1983;309:1495–1501.
176. Wegnez M, Schachter B, Baxter J, Martial J. Hormone regulation of growth hormone mRNA. DNA 1982;1:145–153.
177. Tannenbaum G. Evidence for autoregulation of growth hormone secretion via the central nervous system. Endocrinology 1980;107:2117–2120.
178. Rizza R, Mandarino L, Gerich J. Effects of growth hormone on insulin action in man: mechanisms of insulin resistance, impaired suppression of glucose production and impaired stimulation of glucose utilization. Diabetes 1982;31:663–669.
179. Berelowitz M, Szabo M, Frohman L, et al. Somatomedian-C mediates growth hormone negative feedback by effects on both the hypothalamus and the pituitary. Science 1981;212:1279–1281.
180. Plotnick L, Thompson R, Kowarski A, et al. Circardian variation of integrated concentration of growth hormone in children and adults. J Clin Endocrinol Metab 1975;40:240–247.
181. Abe H, Kato Y, Chiba T, et al. Plasma immunoreactive somatostatin levels in rat hypophysial portal blood: effect of glucagon administration. Life Sci 1978;23:1647–1654.
182. MacGorman L, Rizza R, Gerich J. Physiologic concentrations of growth hormone exert insulin-like and insulin antagonistic effects on both hepatic and extrahepatic tissues in man. J Clin Endocrinol Metab 1981;53:556–559.

183. Rabinowitz D, Klassen G, Zierler K. Effect of human growth hormone on muscle and adipose tissue metabolism in the forearm of man. J Clin Invest 1965;44:51–61.
184. Moeller N, Jorgensen J, Schmitz O, et al. Effects of growth hormone pulse on total and forearm substrate fluxes in humans. Am J Physiol 1990;258:E86–E91.
185. Bratusch-Marrain P, Smith D, DeFronzo R. Effect of growth hormone on glucose metabolism and insulin secretion in man. J Clin Endocrinol Metab 1982;55:973–982.
186. Felig P, Marliss E, Cahill G. Metabolic response to human growth hormone during prolonged starvation. J Clin Invest 1971;50:411–420.
187. Press M, Tamborlane W, Sherwin R. Importance of raised growth hormone levels in mediating the metabolic derangements of diabetes. N Engl J Med 1984;310:810–815.
188. Bazan J. Hemopoietic receptors and helical cytokines. Immunol Today 1990;11:350–354.
189. Argentsinger L, Campbell G, Yang X, et al. Identification of JAK2 as a growth hormone receptor-associated tyrosine kinase. Cell 1993;74:237–244.
190. Carter-Su C, Schwartz J, Smit L. Molecular mechanism of growth hormone action. Annu Rev Physiol 1996;58:187–207.
191. Davidson M. Effect of growth hormone on carbohydrate and lipid metabolism. Endocr Rev 1987;8:115–131.
192. Cameron C, Kostyo J. Adamafio N, Dunbar J. Metabolic basis for the diabetogenic action of growth hormone in the obese (ob/ob) mouse. Endocrinology 1987;120:1568–1573.
193. Goodman H. Effects of growth hormone on glucose utilization in diaphragm muscle in the absence of increased lipolysis. Endocrinology 1967;81:1099–1103.
194. Chou S, Kostyo J, Adamafio N. Growth hormone inhibits activation of phosphatidylinositol phospholipase C by insulin in ob/ob mouse adipose tissue. Endocrinology 1990;126:62–66.
195. Bougneres P, Artavia-Loria E, Gerre P, et al. Effects of hypopituitarism and growth hormone replacement therapy on the production and utilization of glucose in childhood. J Clin Endocrinol Metab 1985;61:1152–1157.
196. Hansen I, Tsalikian E, Beaufrere B, et al. Insulin resistance in acromegaly: defects in both hepatic and extrahepatic insulin action. Am J Physiol 1986;250:E269–E273.
197. Yki-Jarvinen H, Koivisto V. Natural course of insulin resistance in type I diabetes. N Engl J Med 1986;315:224–230.
198. Hansen A, Johansen K. Diurnal patterns of blood glucose, serum free fatty acids, insulin, glucagon, and growth hormone in normal and juvenile diabetes. Diabetologia 1970;6:27–33.
199. Hansen A. Normalization of growth hormone hyperresponse to exercise in juvenile diabetes after normalization of blood sugar. J Clin Invest 1971;50:1806–1811.
200. Gerich J, Lorenzi M, Bier D, et al. Prevention of human diabetic ketoacidosis by somatostatin: evidence for an essential role of glucagon. N Engl J Med 1975;292:985–989.
201. Bolli G, Dimitriadis G, Pehling G, et al. Abnormal glucose counterregulation after subcutaneous insulin in inmsulin-dependent diabetes mellitus. N Engl J Med 1984;310:1706–1711.
202. DeFeo P, Perriello G, Torlone E, et al. Demonstration of a role of growth hormone in glucose counterregulation. Am J Physiol 1989;256:E835–E843.
203. Bolli G, Gottesman I, Campbell P, et al. Glucose counterregulation and waning of insulin in the Somogyi phenomenon (posthypoglycemic hyperglycemia). N Engl J Med 1984;311:1214–1219.
204. Perriello G, DeFeo P, Torlone E, et al. The effect of asymptomatic nocturnal hypoglycemia on glycemic control in diabetes mellitus. N Engl J Med 1988;319:1233–1239.
205. Kollind M, Adamson V, Lins P. Somatostatin reduces posthypoglycemic insulin resistance in insulin-dependent diabetes mellitus. Acta Endocrinol 1988;118:173–178.
206. Bolli G, Gerich J. The dawn phenmenon—a common occurrence in both noninsulin-dependent and insulin-dependent diabetes mellitus. N Engl J Med 1984;310:746–750.
207. Bhathena S, Voyles N, Smith S, Recant L. Decreased glucagon receptors in diabetic rat hepatocytes. J Clin Invest 1978;61:1488–1497.
208. Bolli G, DeFeo P, DeCosmo S, et al. Demonstration of a dawn phenomenon in normal human volunteers. Diabetes 1984;33:1150–1153.
209. Campbell P, Bolli G, Cryer P, Gerich J. Pathogenesis of the dawn phenomenon in insulin-dependent diabetes mellitus accelerated glucose production and impaired glucose utilization due to nocturnal surges in growth hormone secretion. N Engl J Med 1985;312:1473–1479.
210. Baxter JD, Tyrrell JB. The adrenal cortex. In: Felig P, Baxter JD, Broadus AE, Frohman LA, eds. Endocrinology and metabolism. 2nd ed. New York: McGraw-Hill, 1987:511–650.
211. McMahon M, Gerich J, Rizza R. Effects of glucocorticoids on carbohydrate metabolism. Diabetes Metab Rev 1988;4:17–30.
212. Carter-Su C, Okamota K. Effect of insulin and glucocorticoids on glucose transporters in rat adipocytes. Am J Physiol 1987;252:E441–E453.
213. Rizza R, Mandarino L, Gerich J. Cortisol-induced insulin resistance in man: impaired suppression of glucose production and stimulation of glucose utilization due to a postreceptor defect of insulin action. J Clin Endocrinol Metab 1982;54:131–138.
214. Lecavalier L, Bolli G, Gerich J. Glucagon-cortisol interactions on glucose turnover and lactate gluconeogenesis in humans. Am J Physiol 1990;258:E569–575.
215. Schoolwerth A, Smith B, Culpepper R. Renal gluconeogenesis. Miner Electrolyte Metab 1988;14:347–361.
216. Shamoon H, Hendler R, Sherwin R. Synergistic interaction among anti-insulin hormones in the pathogenesis of stress hyperglycemia in humans. J Clin Endocrinol Metab 1981;52:1235–1241.
217. Lecocq F, Mebane D, Madison L. The acute effect of hydrocortinose on hepatic glucose output and peripheral glucose utilization. J Clin Invest 1964;43:237–246.
218. Malerbi D, Liberman B, Giurno-Filho A, et al. Glucocorticoids and glucose metabolism: hepatic glucose production in untreated Addisonian patients and on two different levels of glucocorticoid administration. Clin Endocrinol 1988;28:415–422.

219. Boyle P, Cryer P. Growth hormone, cortisol, or both are involved in defense against, but are not critical to recovery from, hypoglycemia. Am J Physiol 1991;260:E395–E402.
220. Voorhees ML, Jakubowski AF, MacGillivray MH. The adrenomedullary and glucagon responses of hypopituitary children to insulin-induced hypoglycemia. Pediatr Res 1981;15:912–915.
221. DeFeo P, Perriello G, Torlone E, et al. Contribution of cortisol to glucose counterregulation in man. Am J Physiol 1989;257:E35–E42.
222. Boyle PJ, Cryer PE. Roles of chronic growth hormone and cortisol deficiency in prolonged hypoglycemia. Clin Res 1990;38:11A.
223. Cryer PE. Morning hyperglycemia in insulin-dependent diabetes mellitus: insulin lack versus the dawn and Somogyi phenomenon. In: Mazzaferri EL, ed. Advances in endocrinology and metabolism. Chicago: Year Book Medical, 1990:231–243.
224. Butler P, Chou J, Carter W, et al. Effects of meal ingestion on plasma amylin concentration in NIDDM and nondiabetic humans. Diabetes 1990;39:752–756.
225. Bretherton-Walt D, Gilbey S, Ghater M, et al. Failure to establish islet amyloid polypeptide as a circulating beta cell inhibiting hormone. Diabetologia 1990;33:115–117.
226. Pettersson M, Ahren B. Failure of islet amyloid polypeptide to inhibit basal and glucose-stimulated insulin secretion in model experiments in mice and rats. Acta Physiol Scand 1990;138:389–394.
227. Nagamatsu S, Carroll R, Brodsky G, Steiner D. Lack of islet amyloid polypeptide regulation of insulin biosynthesis or secretion in normal rat islets. Diabetes 1990;39:871–874.
228. Morishita T, Yamaguchi A, Fujita T, Ciba T. Activation of adenylate cyclase by islet amyloid polypeptide with COOH-terminal amide via calcitonin gene-related peptide receptors on rat liver plasma membranes. Diabetes 1990;39:875–877.
229. Nishimura S, Sanke T, Machida K, et al. Lack of effect of islet amyloid polypeptide on hepatic glucose output in the in situ-perfused rat liver. Metabolism 1992;41:431–434.
230. Roden M, Liener K, Furnsinn C, et al. Effects of islet amyloid polypeptide on hepatic insulin resistance and glucose production in the isolated perfused rat liver. Diabetologia 1992;35:116–120.
231. Stephens T, Health W, Hermeling R. Presence of liver CGRP/amylin receptors in only nonparenchymal cells and absence of direct regulation of rat liver glucose metabolism by CGRP/mylin. Diabetes 1991;40:395–400.
232. Leighton B, Cooper G. Pancreatic amylin and calcitonin gene-related peptide cause resistance to insulin in skeletal muscle in vitro. Nature 1988;335:632–635.
233. Young D, Deems R, Deacon R, et al. Effects of amylin on glucose metabolism and glycogenolysis in vivo and in vitro. Am J Physiol 1990;259:E457–E461.
234. Leighton B, Foot E. The effects of amylin on carbohydrate metabolism in skeletal muscle in vitro and in vivo. Biochem J 1990;269:19–23.
235. Deems R, Deacon R, Young D. Amylin activates glycogen phosphorylase and inactivates glycogen synthase via a cAMP-independent mechanism. Biochem Biophys Res Commun 1991;174:716–720.
236. Frontoni S, Hoi S, Banduch D, Rossetti L. In vivo insulin resistance induced by amylin primarily through inhibition of insulin-stimulated glycogen synthesis in skeletal muscle. Diabetes 1991;40:568–573.
237. Molina J, Cooper G, Leighton B, Olefsky J. Induction of insulin resistance in vivo by amylin and calcitonin gene-related peptide. Diabetes 1990;39:260–265.
238. Koopmans S, Mansfeld A, Jansz H, et al. Amylin-induced in vivo insulin resistance in conscious rats: the liver is more sensitive to amylin than peripheral tissues. Diabetologia 1991;34:218–224.
239. Johnson K, O'Brien T, Jordon K, et al. The putative homone islet amyloid polypeptide (IAPP) induces impaired glucose tolerance in cat. Biochem Biophys Res Commun 1990;167:507–513.
240. Kassir A, Upadhyoy A, Lim T, et al. Lack of effect of islet amyloid polypeptide in causing insulin resistance in conscious dogs during euglycemic clamp studies. Diabetes 1991;40:998–1004.
241. Sowa R, Sanke T, Tabata H, et al. Islet amyloid polypeptide amide causes peripheral insulin resistance in vivo in dogs. Diabetologia 1190;33:118–120.
242. Wilding J, Khandan-Nia N, Bennet W. Lack of acute effect of amylin (islet associated polypeptide) on insulin sensitivity during hyperinsulinemic euglycemic clamp in humans. Diabetologia 1994;37:166–169.
243. Nyholm B, Moller N, Gravholt C, et al. Acute effects of the human amylin analog AC137 on basal an insulin-stimulated euglycemic and hypoglycemic fuel metabolism in patients with insulin-dependent diabetes mellitus. J Clin Endocrinol Metab 1996;81:1083–1089.
244. Hotamisligil G, Spiegelman B. Tumor necrosis factor α: a key component of the obesity-diabetes link. Diabetes 1994;43:1271–1278.
245. Evans R, Argiles J, Williamson D. Metabolic effects of tumor necrosis factor alpha (cachectin) and interleukin-1. Clin Sci 1989;77:357–364.
246. Lang C, Dobrescu C, Bagby G. Tumor necrosis factor impairs insulin action on peripheral glucose disposal and hepatic glucose output. Endocrinology 1992;130:43–52.
247. Stephens J, Pekala P. Transcriptional repression of the GLUT4 and C/EBP genes in 3T3-Li adipocytes by tumor necrosis factor-alpha. J Bil Chem 1991;266:21839–21845.
248. Cornelius P, Lee M, Marlowe M, Pekala P. Monokine regulation of glucose transporter mRNA in L6 myotubes. Biochem Biophys Res Commun 1989;165:429–436.
249. Hotamisligil G, Budavari A, Murray D, Spiegelman B. Reduced tyrosine kinase activity of the insulin receptor in obesity-diabetes: central role of tumor necrosis factor-α. J Clin Invest 1994;94:1543–1549.
250. Hotomisligil G, Murray D, Choy L, Spiegelman B. TNF-α inhibits signalling from the insulin receptor. Proc Natl Acad Sci USA 1994;91:4854–4858.
251. Feinstein R, Kanety H, Papa M, et al. Tumor necrosis factor-α suppresses insulin-induced tyrosine phosphorylation of insulin receptor and its substrates. J Biol Chem 1993;268:26055–26058.

252. Bazzoni F, Beutler B. The tumor necrosis factor ligand and receptor families. N Engl J Med 1996;334:1717–1725.
253. Pelleymounter N, Cullen M, Baker M, et al. Effects of the obese gene product on body weight regulation in ob/ob mice. Science 1995;269:540–543.
254. Masuzaki H, Ogawa Y, Isse N, et al. Human obese gene expression: adipocyte-specific expression and regional differences in the adipose tissue. Diabetes 1995;44:855–858.
255. Halaas J, Gajiwala K, Mafferi M, et al. Weight-reducing effects of the plasma protein encoded by the obese gene. Science 1995;269:543–546.
256. Rohner-Jeanrenaud F, Jeanrenaud B. Obesity, leptin and the brain. N Engl J Med 1996;334:324–325.
257. Kolaczynski J, Ohannesean J, Considine R, et al. Response of leptin to short-term and prolonged overfeeding in humans. J Clin Endocrinol Metab 1996;81:4162–4165.
258. Brzechffa P, Jakimiuk A, Agarwal S, et al. Serum immunoreactive leptin concentrations in women with polycystic ovary syndrome. J Clin Endocrinol Metab 1996;81:4166–4169.
259. Sinkha M, Ohannesian J, Heiman M, et al. Nocturnal rise in leptin in lean, obese and non-insulin-dependent diabetes mellitus subjects. J Clin Invest 1996;97:1344–1347.
260. Considine R, Sinha M, Heiman M, et al. Serum immunoreactive-leptin concentrations in normal weight and obese humans. N Engl J Med 1996;334:292–295.
261. Kohrt W, Landt M, Birge S. Serum leptin levels are reduced in response to exercise training, but not hormone replacement therapy, in older women. J Clin Endocrinol Metab 1996;81:3980–3985.
262. Grinspoon S, Gulick T, Asari H, et al. Serum leptin levels in women with anorexia nervosa. J Clin Endocrinol Metab 1996;81:3861–3863.
263. Kolaczynski J, Nyce M, Considine R, et al. Acute and chronic effects of insulin on leptin production in humans: studies in vivo and in vitro. Diabetes 1996;45:699–701.
264. Dagogo-Jack S, Fanelli C, Paramore D, et al. Plasma leptin and insulin interrelationships in obese and nonobese individuals. Diabetes 1996;45:695–698.
265. Ostlund R, Yang J, Klein S, Gingerich R. Relation between plasma leptin concentration and body fat, gender, diet, age and metabolic covariates. J Clin Endocrinol Metab 1996;81:3909–3913.
266. Kieffer T, Heller R, Habener J. Leptin receptors expressed on pancreatic beta-cells. Biochem Biophys Res Commun 1996;224:522–527.

Section II
Maternal Metabolism During Pregnancy

10
Glucose Metabolism in Pregnancy

Patrick M. Catalano, Tatsua Ishizuka, and Jacob E. Friedman

The longitudinal changes in glucose homeostasis that occur during normal human pregnancy provide for both maternal and fetoplacental metabolic demands. There are major adaptations in maternal glucose metabolism during pregnancy in nonobese women that result in increased maternal fat stores in early gestation and increased glucose availability for oxidative needs of the fetus and placenta in late gestation. In industrialized countries, problems relating to insufficient glucose availability are fortunately quite rare. In contrast, maternal and fetal problems associated with a surfeit of maternal glucose are becoming ever more common, particularly in various ethnic groups immigrating to industrialized countries.[1]

This chapter reviews the longitudinal changes in maternal glucose metabolism, i.e., endogenous (primarily hepatic) glucose production, peripheral insulin sensitivity (primarily skeletal muscle and adipose tissue), and pancreatic β cell response in women with normal glucose tolerance and contrast these adaptations to women with abnormal glucose tolerance during pregnancy. In addition to the physiologic and biochemical changes that occur during pregnancy, information is incorporated concerning the potential molecular mechanisms underlying these adaptations in glucose metabolism, and in human gestation when available or in nonpregnant human and animal models. Last, the genetic implications, hormonal factors, and cellular changes associated with the alterations in maternal glucose metabolism are reviewed as well as the potential long-term effects of an abnormal maternal metabolic environment on the developing fetus.

Nonpregnant Glucose Metabolism

Postabsorptive Glucose Metabolism

To understand the changes in glucose metabolism in pregnant women, there must be a basic understanding of the various aspects of glucose metabolism in nongravid individuals in the postabsorptive and postprandial state. The basal or postabsorptive condition refers to the 6 to 10 hours after the last meal. Plasma glucose concentration represents the balance between endogenous glucose production, primarily hepatic ($1.8–2.2\,mg \cdot kg^{-1} min^{-1}$), and glucose uptake by various tissues.[2] Glucose uptake in the postabsorptive period is not dependent on insulin-mediated glucose mechanisms, but rather non–insulin-mediated glucose uptake, which occurs primarily in tissues such as the central nervous system and splanchnic bed.[3] Glucose uptake is facilitated by the non–insulin-dependent glucose transporters; primarily GLUT 1.[4] Glucose that is not used for oxidative requirements undergoes glycolysis to lactate. Lactate and other three-carbon precursors are potentially available as substrates for gluconeogenesis in the liver.[5] Although skeletal muscle is the primary insulin sensitive tissue in the postprandial state, under postabsorptive conditions skeletal muscle primarily utilizes free fatty acids for energy needs. Approximately 80% of oxygen consumed by muscle tissue under postabsorptive conditions is used for oxidation of lipid.[6]

Postabsorptive hepatic glucose production primarily represents glycogenolysis and to a lesser extent gluconeogenesis. The potential nutrient sources for gluconeogenesis and relative glucose uptake by various tissues are shown in Table 10.1.[3] The longer the postabsorptive period, the greater is the percent contribution of gluconeogenesis to total hepatic glucose production. Rothman et al.,[7] using tritiated glucose in conjunction with ^{13}C nuclear magnetic resonance spectroscopy, showed that gluconeogenesis accounted for 64% of hepatic glucose production after 22 hours of fasting, and by 42 hours accounted for essentially all basal hepatic glucose production.

The regulation of hepatic glucose production is the result of the balance between insulin and glucagon. In the postabsorptive period when insulin concentration is

TABLE 10.1 Summary of normal glucose homeostasis in the postabsorptive state.

Plasma glucose	Rate ($\mu mol \cdot kg^{-1} min^{-1}$)	Percent of total
Appearance		
Hepatic output	12	100
Glycogenolysis	9	75
Gluconeogenesis	3	25
Lactate	1.8	15
Alanine	0.5	4
Glycerol	0.2	2
Amino acids	0.5	4
Disappearance		
Brain uptake	6	50
Splanchnic uptake	2.4	20
Muscle uptake	1.8	15
Other uptake (red cells, renal medulla)	1.2	10
Adipose tissue uptake	0.6	5

The rate of glucose output and uptake is measured in micromoles per kilogram of body weight per minute. To convert micromoles of glucose to milligrams, divide by 5.55. (From Dinneen et al.,[3] with permission.)

low, there is increased lipolysis, which makes available free fatty acids for oxidative needs in tissues such as skeletal muscle. Free fatty acids may also inhibit glucose metabolism in muscle tissue because of the Hales-Randle effect.[8] Free fatty acids are involved in basal glucose homeostasis by providing a source of energy for hepatic gluconeogenesis. In contrast, glucagon stimulates hepatic glycogenolysis and inhibits hepatic glycolysis in order to provide glucose required by the central nervous system.[9]

Postprandial Glucose Metabolism

After a meal, increased glucose availability plus increased insulin and decreased glucagon concentrations increase glucose uptake in insulin-sensitive tissue and decrease hepatic glucose production. Splanchnic tissues initially take up approximately 25% and eventually 40% of ingested glucose.[3] As plasma glucose and insulin concentrations increase, hepatic glucose production decreases by approximately 50%.[10] Peripheral, as well as portal insulin may be involved in insulin-mediated decreases in hepatic glucose production.[11] Hepatic glycogen stores are replaced in the postabsorptive state by both direct (i.e., glucose → glycogen) and indirect (i.e., lactate → glucose-6-phosphate → glycogen) routes.[12] The direct route of hepatic glycogen resynthesis occurs through phosphorylation of glucose by glucokinase to glucose-6-phosphate, which is then converted to glycogen. The indirect pathway utilizes three-carbon precursors such as lactate, alanine, glutamine, and pyruvate in the process of gluconeogenesis to increase hepatic glycogen concentration.[13] The indirect pathway may contribute as much as 50% to 60% of newly synthesized glycogen depending on time since the last meal.[13]

As noted previously, skeletal muscle is the primary insulin-sensitive tissue relative to postprandial glucose disposal. Hence, in the transition from the postabsorptive to postprandial state, oxidative needs of skeletal muscle revert from free fatty acids to glucose.[3] Studies by Kelley et al.,[14] using dual stable isotope methodology, showed that 5 hours after ingestion of oral glucose, skeletal muscle takes up approximately 25% of the oral glucose with a 50% decrease in lipid oxidation. Of the glucose taken up by skeletal muscle, approximately 50% is oxidized and 35% stored as glycogen in muscle tissue. The remainder is metabolized to lactate and becomes available for gluconeogenesis in the liver. Additionally, a decrease in glucagon concentration enhances hepatic glycogen storage via gluconeogenesis because of decreased glycogenolysis and increased substrate delivery. Figure 10.1, from the review by Dinneen et al.,[3] summarizes the major changes in glucose metabolism in the transition from the postabsorptive to the postprandial state in the nonpregnant individual.

Molecular Biology of Insulin Signaling

The intracellular events that link the stimulation of insulin receptors to the movement of glucose transporters is the subject of ongoing investigation (see Chapter 7). The initial events include binding of insulin to the α subunit of the insulin receptor on the extracellular surface on the cell, activation of the insulin receptor tyrosine kinase on the β subunit (i.e., autophosphorylation), the subsequent phosphorylation of insulin receptor substrates, and the interaction of these substrates with several downstream signaling molecules that stimulate the translocation of GLUT 4–containing vesicles (Figure 10.2).

Insulin initiates its effects on cellular metabolism by binding to one of the α/β dimers of the receptor, causing a conformational change that activates the β-subunit to undergo autophosphorylation on at least six tyrosine residues.[15] The autophosphorylation of the β-subunit enhances the kinase (i.e., enzyme) activity of the receptor up to 10- to 20-fold toward other protein substrates particularly on tyrosine residues.[16,17] In 1991, a major cytosolic protein involved in insulin signaling, termed insulin receptor substrate-1 (IRS-1) was purified and cloned.[18] IRS-1 has a molecular weight of 185kd on sodium dodecyl sulfate-polyacrylamide gel electrophoresis (SDS-PAGE) and has up to 22 potential tyrosine phosphorylation sites. Upon phosphorylation by the insulin

10. Glucose Metabolism in Pregnancy

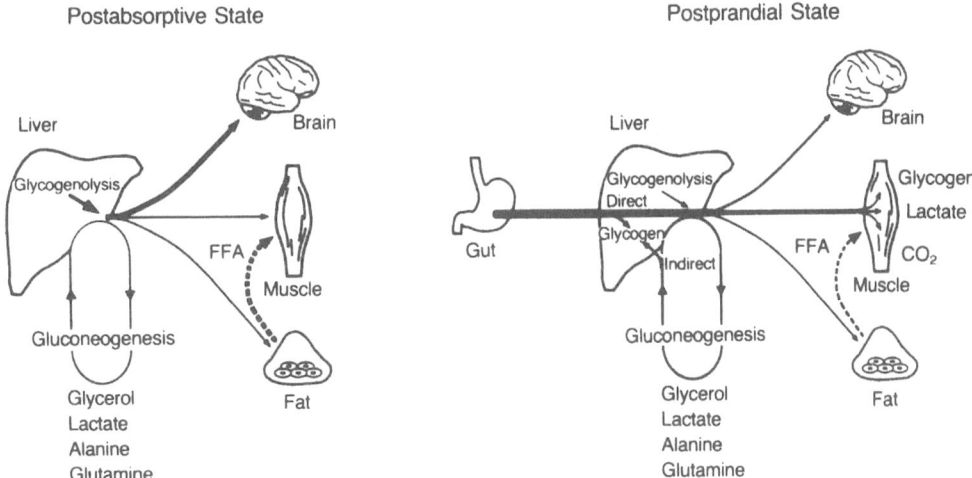

FIGURE 10.1. Major sites of glucose metabolism in the postabsorptive and postprandial states. During the transition from the postabsorptive to the postprandial state, the primary site of glucose uptake shifts from insulin-independent tissues (e.g., the brain) to insulin-dependent tissues (e.g., the liver, muscle, and adipocytes). Substrates for gluconeogenesis are derived predominantly from peripheral tissues, although some (e.g., lactate and pyruvate) may be derived from intrahepatic sources postprandially. The synthesis of hepatic glycogen after glucose is ingested may occur through one or both pathways, direct or indirect (i.e., gluconeogenic). The uptake of free fatty acids (FFA) by muscle decreases after the ingestion of carbohydrate, CO_2, carbon dioxide. (From Dinneen et al.,[3] with permission.)

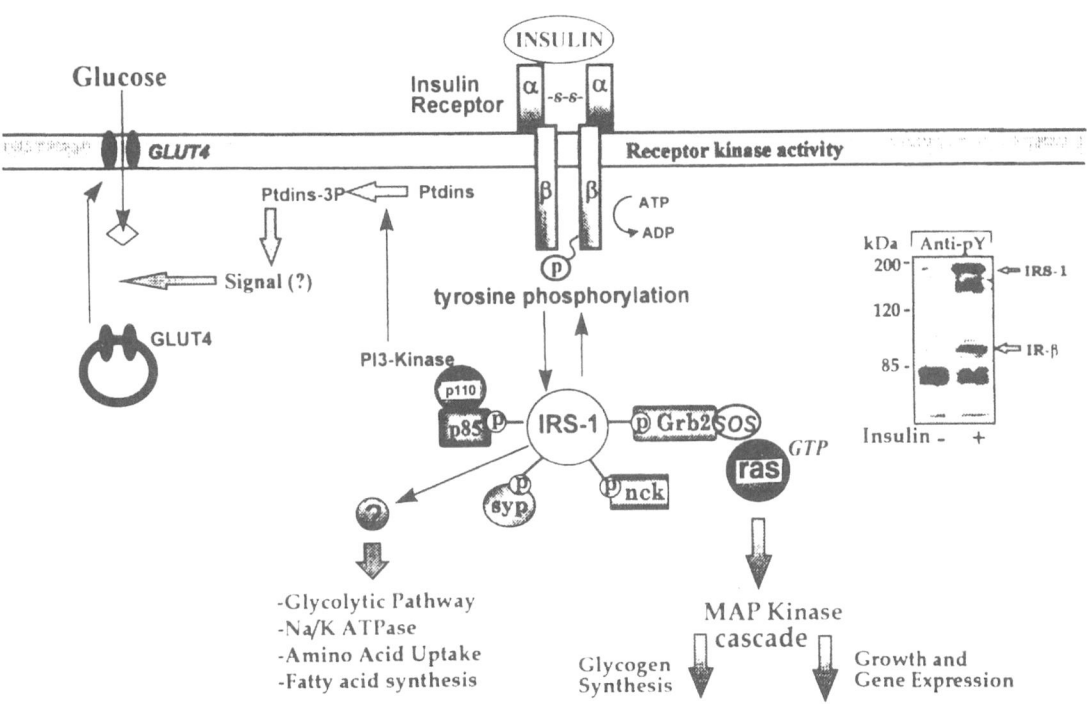

FIGURE 10.2. Components of the proximal insulin signaling network. Insulin binding stimulates intrinsic tyrosine phosphorylation of the insulin receptor and results in phosphorylation of IRS-1, an intracellular substrate protein that binds several proteins. The model depicts several insulin-regulated pathways and some of the components involved. IRS-1 binds several proteins containing Sh2 domains, including the p85 subunit of PI-3-kinase, the protein-tyrosine phosphatase Syp, and two adapter molecules NCK and Grb2. The binding of Grb2 stimulates its association with the guanine nucleotide releasing factor SOS, which complexes with Ras and activates MAP kinase cascade. The association of p85 with phosphorylated IRS-1 activates the catalytic subunit p110 (PI-3-kinase) leading within minutes to accumulation of phosphatidylinositol-3-phosphate and appears necessary for the trafficking of GLUT 4 containing vesicles to the plasma membrane.

receptor, IRS-1 binds to the insulin receptor and both proteins can be detected in their phosphorylated form in skeletal muscle protein extracts separated by SDS-PAGE and immunoblotted using antiphosphotyrosine antibodies (Anti-pY). The phosphorylation of IRS-1 on multiple tyrosine residues within seconds and the binding of several other phosphotyrosine-containing proteins suggest the main function of IRS-1 is as a docking protein for transmitting signals to other targets critical for amplifying the insulin signal cascade.[19,20] In the mouse with a gene knockout of IRS-1, there is growth retardation and a mild form of glucose intolerance, including a 50% reduction in insulin-stimulated glucose transport in skeletal muscle and adipose tissue,[21,22] confirming that the IRS-1 pathway plays an important role in regulation of growth and glucose metabolism. Recently a second IRS protein, IRS-2, has been cloned and purified and found in multiple tissues of normal and IRS-1 knockout mice and mediates IRS-1–like signals (Chapter 8).[22,23]

IRS-1 binds to multiple proteins that contain SH2 (Src-homology-2) domains that are characteristic of signal transduction molecules. Insulin stimulates the binding of an adapter molecule Grb-2 protein (growth receptor binding protein-2)[24,25] to IRS-1. The phosphorylated Grb-2 molecule binds to the son of sevenless (SOS) and activates Ras, a guanine nucleotide exchange protein.[26] The activation of Ras leads to exchange of guanosine triphosphate (GTP) for guanosine diphosphate (GDP) and activates a series of protein kinases known as the mitogen-activated protein (MAP) kinase cascade that links the insulin receptor to identifiable metabolic targets. The activation of the MAP kinase pathway is critical for many of the effects of insulin including DNA synthesis, transcription factor gene expression, and regulation of glycogen synthase activity, the rate-limiting enzyme in glycogen synthesis.[26-28] Insulin stimulates the binding and activation of a lipid kinase enzyme, phosphatidylinositol-3 (PI-3)-kinase, to IRS-1.[29,30] PI-3-kinase is composed of an 85-kd regulatory subunit (p85) that is associated with the phosphorylated IRS-1 and activates the catalytic 110-kd subunit. During insulin stimulation, the 110-kd subunit catalyzes the phosphorylation of a membrane phospholipid phosphatidylinositol at position D3 of the inositol ring.[31] The stimulation of PI-3-kinase activity is directly linked to insulin-stimulated glucose transport in muscle and fat cells by activating the translocation of vesicles containing the GLUT 4 glucose transporter to the plasma membrane.[32,33] It is speculated that the generation of phospholipid products may be involved in targeting vesicles to specific subcellular locations crucial for proper GLUT 4 trafficking in the cell.[34] Phosphorylation of IRS-1 induces binding of NCK, a 47-kd protein involved in cell proliferation,[35] and SYP, a 68-kd tyrosine phosphatase involved in stimulating DNA synthesis in response to insulin.[20]

Glucose Metabolism During Gestation

Early Gestation

In assessing the alterations in maternal glucose metabolism in early gestation, defining baseline or nonpregnant measurements is critical. For example, many investigators have used a cross-sectional study design, where nonpregnant control subjects are matched for significant variables, such as maternal age and weight, with pregnant women. Longitudinal study designs provide an advantage over cross-sectional studies in that each subject acts as her own control, thereby decreasing the intersubject variability. However, longitudinal study designs have their own intrinsic problems when postpartum measurements are used to represent pregravid conditions. Postpartum factors such as breast-feeding,[36] type of contraception,[37] weight gain during pregnancy, and effects of parity[38] are variables that need to be considered in assessing the effect of pregnancy on glucose metabolism in the postpartum period.

Early pregnancy, defined as the first 20 weeks of gestation, can be considered a maternal anabolic state. Fetoplacental demands for glucose are relatively minimal during organogenesis, and, at least in nonobese women, maternal metabolism is geared toward storage of adipose tissue to meet the increased energy demands of late gestation. Estimates of maternal adipose tissue accretion vary according to the population being examined. Longitudinal studies initiated prior to conception in women from various European countries have shown increases in body fat ranging from 0.5 kg at 10 weeks' gestation[39] to 3.5 kg at 18 weeks' gestation.[40] The increases in body fat in early pregnancy represent between 20% and 60% of total fat accretion in pregnancy and approximately 80% of weight gain in the first 12 weeks of gestation.[41] Furthermore the accretion of maternal body fat may be related to the changes in insulin sensitivity in early gestation (vide infra).

Postabsorptive Glucose Metabolism

Based on the early pregnancy studies of Spellacy et al.,[42] there were no significant differences in fasting insulin or glucose concentrations between early gestation and in the same subjects evaluated at 6 weeks postpartum. These results were confirmed in studies showing no significant changes in basal glucose or insulin concentrations after an overnight fast in parturients compared with their own pregravid measurements.[43] In these same subjects when basal hepatic glucose production was estimated using steady-state stable isotope methodology, there were no significant differences between mean pregravid and 12- to 14-week estimates of glucose turnover, even when corrected for fat free mass. Prolonged fasting defined as

12 to 84 hours, however, has been shown by Felig and Lynch[44] to result in decreases of 15 to 20 mg·dl^{-1} in plasma glucose concentration of pregnant women compared with very little change in nongravid control subjects. These data are consistent with the energy requirements of the relatively small amount of fetoplacental tissue in early gestation and the observation that basal hepatic glucose production is primarily used to provide glucose for oxidative needs in non–insulin-dependent tissue.

Postprandial Glucose Metabolism

The available information regarding postprandial glucose metabolism in early pregnancy is controversial. Earlier studies by Spellacy et al.[42] reported that there was no significant difference in insulin response to an intravenous glucose challenge at 13 to 15 weeks' gestation compared with the postpartum response at least 6 weeks after delivery in the same subjects. In contrast, Catalano et al.[45] reported that there was a significant 120% increase in the first-phase insulin response (i.e., 0–6 min) and a 50% increase in second-phase (i.e., 6–60 min) insulin response to an intravenous glucose challenge in early pregnancy (12–14 weeks) as compared with pregravid measurements in the same nonobese subjects prior to conception. Whether significant increases in insulin response persist postpartum and may explain these differences between studies remains unknown.

Tissue sensitivity to infused insulin involves both liver and skeletal muscle. Insulin infusion decreases hepatic glucose production and increases skeletal muscle glucose uptake. Insulin sensitivity, as commonly considered, refers to the quantity of glucose taken up by peripheral tissues (i.e., primarily skeletal muscle) relative to a defined amount of insulin. Decreased insulin sensitivity and increased insulin resistance are common features of a variety of metabolic conditions such as obesity, non–insulin-dependent diabetes, and pregnancy. Estimates of insulin sensitivity during pregnancy have included quantification of the insulin response either to a fixed oral or intravenous glucose challenge or the ratio of insulin to glucose under a variety of experimental circumstances. Although these measures can sometimes give qualitative information regarding changes in maternal insulin sensitivity, because of changes in maternal plasma volume and maternal-fetal glucose transport they may lead to underestimates in early gestation and overestimates in late gestation (see Chapter 17).

In recent years, newer methodologies such as the Bergman minimal model technique[46] and the euglycemic-hyperinsulinemic clamp coupled with the infusion of stable isotopes of glucose have improved our ability to quantify tissue insulin sensitivity. However, these methods have their limitations, particularly during pregnancy. For example, although the euglycemic-hyperinsulinemic clamp, defined as the glucose infusion rate required to maintain euglycemia during a constant insulin infusion, as first described by DeFronzo et al.,[47] is considered the "gold standard," the insulin infusions used to estimate glucose uptake are sometimes elevated and not always physiologic. In contrast, the Bergman minimal model technique relies on mathematical modeling to estimate insulin sensitivity based on the rate of glucose disappearance and insulin kinetics during a frequently sampled intravenous glucose tolerance test. Refinements of the original minimal model methodology have included the addition of intravenous tolbutamide or insulin 20 minutes after the infusion of glucose in order to improve the mathematical fitting.[48] The correlation of the estimates of the insulin sensitivity using the minimal model and the euglycemic-hyperinsulinemic clamp in nongravid women have ranged between $r = 0.62$[49] and $r = 0.89$.[50] The correlation of these two methodologies to estimate insulin sensitivity during pregnancy has yet to be published.

On the basis of enhanced glucose disappearance during an intravenous glucose challenge relative to nongravid control subjects, Kalkhoff et al.[51] first postulated that there was an increase in insulin sensitivity in early gestation. Prospective longitudinal studies in nonobese women with normal glucose tolerance using the euglycemic-hyperinsulinemic clamp by Catalano et al.,[45] however, have reported a 40% decrease in maternal insulin sensitivity by 12 to 14 weeks' gestation. However, when the glucose infusion rate was adjusted for the insulin concentration achieved during the clamp, insulin sensitivity decreased only 7% to 10%. Of interest in these same subjects there was an increase in the rate of glucose disappearance (k-value) during an intravenous glucose tolerance test from the time prior to conception (1.84) to 12 to 14 weeks' gestation (1.94). The 30% to 40% increase in maternal plasma volume and therefore volume of distribution of glucose in early pregnancy may help explain the apparent discrepancy between the improvement in glucose disappearance rates with the intravenous glucose tolerance test and decreases in glucose infusion rates using the euglycemic-hyperinsulinemic clamp as estimates of insulin sensitivity in early gestation.

An noted previously, a second estimate of insulin sensitivity is the ability of infused insulin to decrease hepatic glucose production. By adding a known amount of a stable isotope of glucose to the glucose infusion required to maintain a stable glucose concentration during the euglycemic-hyperinsulinemic clamp, it is possible to estimate suppression of hepatic glucose production.[52] When this technique was used in women with normal glucose tolerance, there was greater than 90% suppression of hepatic glucose production during insulin infusion both prior to conception and in early gestation compared with basal hepatic measurements. The insulin infusion rate used in these studies (40mU·m$^{2-1}$min^{-1}) has previously been shown to almost completely suppress hepatic glucose production in subjects with normal glucose tolerance but is low enough to demonstrate impaired suppression of hepatic glucose production in subjects with non–insulin-dependent diabetes mellitus (NIDDM).[47]

Relationship Between Weight Gain and Insulin Sensitivity

Studies in nonpregnant individuals have reported an association between reduced insulin sensitivity and weight gain over time. Swinburn et al.[53] in studies of Pima Indians reported that subjects with decreased insulin sensitivity gained less weight as compared with insulin-sensitive subjects (3.1 vs. 7.6kg, $p < .0001$) over a period of 4 years. Furthermore, the percent weight change per year was significantly correlated with insulin sensitivity using euglycemic clamps. Preliminary data in pregnant women[41] have supported the findings of Swinburn et al.[53] In nonobese insulin-sensitive women, increases in body fat during early pregnancy were significantly correlated with the decrease in insulin sensitivity. In support of the relationship between weight gain and insulin sensitivity, there was a recent report on the changes in weight gain during gestation in women with gestational diabetes mellitus (GDM) in comparison with women with normal glucose tolerance.[54] Total weight gain during pregnancy was less in women with GDM (decreased insulin sensitivity) as compared with normal glucose tolerance. Even when adjusted for pregravid weight, maternal age, and gestational age at delivery, nonobese women with gestational diabetes had significantly (2.8kg) less weight gain as compared with a matched control group. Although the exact mechanism for the relationship between increased insulin sensitivity and weight gain is unknown, Ravussin and Swinburn[55] speculated that lower rates of glucose oxidation in subjects with decreased insulin sensitivity may be related to a reciprocal increase in fat oxidation, thereby limiting fat storage. Alternatively, insulin resistance associated with increases in percent body fat may induce cellular changes in obesity during pregnancy that limit further adipose tissue expansion.

Late Gestation

It has been assumed that with advancing gestation there is a greater maternal reliance on fatty acids as an energy source as glucose and amino acids are preferentially used by the placenta and transported to the fetus for oxidative needs and growth requirements. Morphologic evidence for these maternal metabolic adaptations is found in the data of Taggart et al.,[56] where skinfold measurements, as an estimate of maternal adipose stores, increase in early and mid-gestation and then decreased starting at 30 weeks' gestation through the postpartum period (Figure 10.3). Additional evidence for these metabolic adaptations is found in the work of Freinkel.[57] In late gestation, increases in glucose and insulin after an oral glucose challenge are accompanied by increases in plasma triglyceride concentration and decreases in plasma glucagon concentration as compared with nongravid subjects. The prolonged hyperglycemia after a glucose challenge in late pregnancy results in increased amounts of glucose available for transport to the fetus and placenta via facilitated transport mechanisms. In contrast free fatty acids and triglycerides cross the placenta poorly, relative to glucose, and become available for maternal metabolic needs, thereby sparing glucose for the fetus. Longitudinal

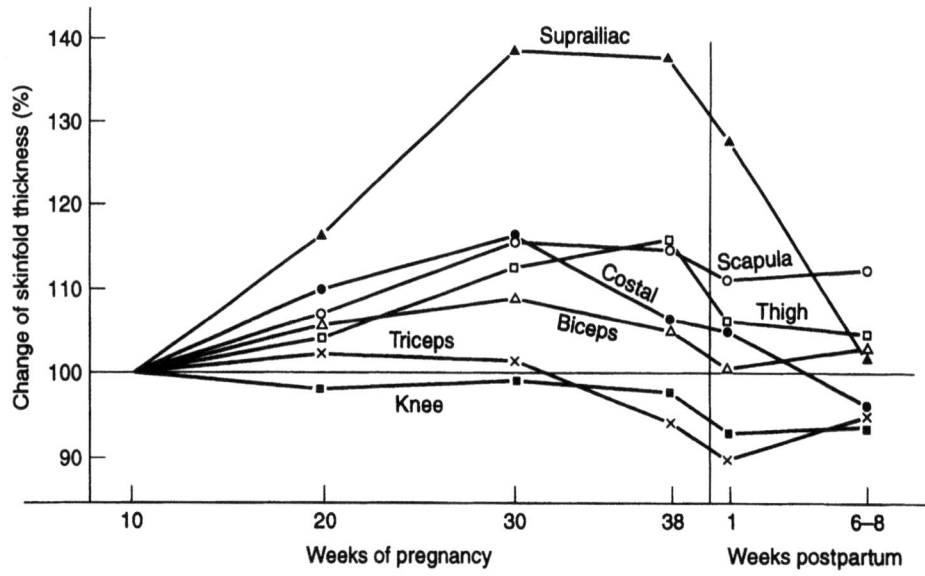

FIGURE 10.3. Proportional skinfold thicknesses during and after pregnancy. (From Taggart et al.,[56] with permission.)

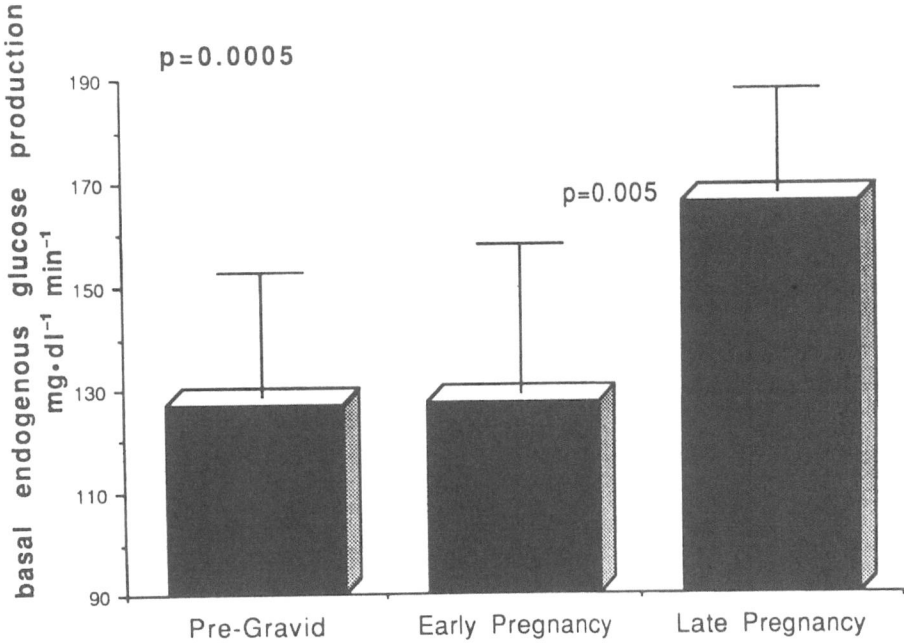

FIGURE 10.4. Changes in total basal endogenous glucose production (primarily hepatic) from pregravid through early and late gestation (mean ± SD). (From Catalano et al.,[43] with permission.)

research using indirect calorimetry to estimate nutrient utilization has shown a progressively lower respiratory quotient (RQ) during euglycemic-hyperinsulinemic clamps with advancing gestation,[41] thereby supporting increasing maternal reliance on postprandial lipid metabolism in late gestation. These alterations in maternal glucose and lipid metabolism have been the basis for the consideration of late pregnancy as a state of decreased insulin sensitivity.

Postabsorptive Glucose Metabolism

Increases in the volume of distribution of glucose and increased fetoplacental utilization with advancing gestational age have been cited as explanations for the decrease in fasting glucose concentrations in late pregnancy. Studies by Kalhan et al.,[58] and by Cowett et al.[59] using stable isotope methodology, have shown that there were no significant differences in basal hepatic glucose production in pregnant women at term as compared with a nonpregnant control group, when the data were expressed per kilogram of body weight. However, when the data were expressed in relationship to pregravid weight, there was an increase in hepatic glucose production in late pregnancy. When estimates of hepatic glucose production were evaluated prior to and during a planned pregnancy in nonobese women using stable isotope methodology,[43] there was a 30% increase in basal hepatic glucose production by late gestation relative to pregravid estimates (Figure 10.4). A significant increase in hepatic glucose production with advancing gestation persisted even when corrected for fat free body mass. The increases in hepatic glucose production occurred despite significant increases in fasting insulin concentration in late pregnancy. These data are consistent with a decrease in basal hepatic insulin sensitivity in late gestation. Furthermore, the increases in basal maternal free fatty acids, glycerol, and ketones in late pregnancy as described by Freinkel,[57] support the possibility of a decreased effect of insulin on other maternal nutrients.

Postprandial Glucose Metabolism

As noted previously, increased insulin response to a glucose challenge with advancing gestation, as reported by Spellacy and Goetz,[60] in comparison with the same subjects postpartum, represents one of the earliest documentation of decreased insulin sensitivity in late pregnancy. Additionally, Burt[61] demonstrated that pregnant women experienced less hypoglycemia in response to exogenous insulin in comparison with nonpregnant subjects. Later research by Fisher et al.[62] using a high-dose glucose infusion test, Buchanan et al.[63] using the Bergman minimal model, and Ryan et al.[64] and Catalano et al.[45] using the euglycemic-hyperinsulinemic clamp all have demonstrated a significant decrease in insulin sensitivity ranging from 33% to 78% in late pregnancy. The longitudinal changes in insulin sensitivity as estimated from euglycemic-hyperinsulinemic clamp studies in nonobese women are shown in Figure 10.5. It should be noted, however, that all these quantitative estimates of maternal insulin sensitivity are probably overestimates of true maternal skeletal muscle insulin sensitivity. Non–insulin-mediated glucose disposal particularly in late gestation by the human fetus and placenta can only be estimated but may represent a significant amount of total glucose

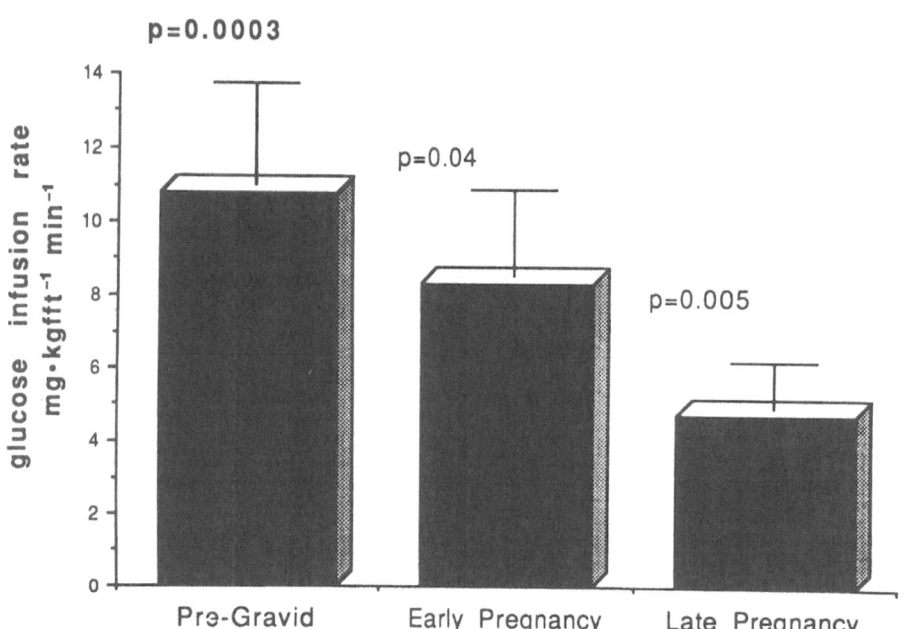

FIGURE 10.5. Changes in glucose infusion rate (i.e., insulin sensitivity) in nonobese pregnant women with normal glucose tolerance during the euglycemic-hyperinsulinemic clamp (mean ± SD). (From Catalano et al.,[45] with permission.)

utilization. Hay et al.[65] reported that in the pregnant ewe model approximately one third of maternal glucose utilization was accounted for by uterine, placental, and fetal tissue. Furthermore, fetal blood sampling studies by Marconi et al.[66] in pregnant women have also shown that fetal glucose concentration was a function of gestational age in addition to maternal glucose concentration.

As noted previously, there is a significant increase in insulin response to a glucose challenge in late pregnancy. However, although β-cell function is usually assessed by measuring insulin concentration in response to such a challenge, ideally information regarding insulin clearance, the impact of changing glucose tolerance, and degree of insulin sensitivity should be noted. Data regarding insulin clearance in pregnancy are scant and contradictory. Previous investigators have described either no change or increases in the metabolic clearance rate of insulin in pregnancy. In separate studies, Bellman and Hartman,[67] Lind et al.,[68] and Burt and Davidson[69] have reported no difference in the insulin disappearance rate when insulin was infused intravenously at various concentrations in pregnant women in late gestation and nonpregnant subjects. In contrast, Goodner and Freinkel,[70] using an ^{131}I insulin infusion, described a 25% increase in insulin turnover in the pregnant as compared with nonpregnant rat model. Preliminary longitudinal studies assessing insulin clearance during the euglycemic clamp in pregnant women support the data of Goodner and Freinkel, showing a significant increase in the metabolic clearance rate of insulin in pregnant women.[71] However, definitive studies, as described by Polonsky,[72] evaluating insulin kinetics in nonpregnant women, have not yet been performed.

There is a progressive and significant increase in first- and second-phase insulin response to intravenous glucose with advancing gestation in normal pregnant women.[45] First-phase insulin response is defined as the insulin response in the first 5 to 10 minutes after an intravenous glucose challenge. First-phase insulin response is considered a sensitive early indicator of β-cell dysfunction, and a decrease in first-phase response has been associated with a deterioration of glucose tolerance.[73] There is evidence for a progressive increase in first- and second-phase insulin response with advancing gestation that mirrors the decrease in insulin sensitivity described previously.[45] The mechanisms that lead to the increases in insulin secretion are not known with certainty. There is evidence from animal studies for both increases in maternal islet cell size and secretion during pregnancy. Hellerman[74] described a significant increase in pancreatic islet cell size in pregnant rats at delivery as compared with nonpregnant controls. However, the 10% to 15% increase in human islets does not account for the two- to threefold increase in insulin response observed during gestation.[75] In a separate report Kalkhoff and Kim[76] reported that pregnant rats secrete significantly more insulin per unit of islet cell mass as compared with virgin rats using an in vitro islet cell preparation. However, the cellular mechanisms responsible for the increased responsiveness of the islet cells during pregnancy have yet to be definitively identified. These in vitro results suggest that there may be a shift in the glucose utilization curve to a lower threshold for insulin secretion. This mechanism could involve a change in GLUT 2 or glucokinase activity, but has yet to be investigated in pregnancy.

It is of interest to note that most insulin assays employed recognize proinsulin as well as insulin. Phelps et al.[77] and Kuhl[78] have reported a normal relationship between insulin and proinsulin in pregnant women, confirming that the increases in insulin concentration during pregnancy are not the result of only increased proinsulin moieties.

In contrast to the well-documented studies of decreased glucose uptake in peripheral tissues, estimates of hepatic insulin sensitivity in late gestation are less definitive. Glucose turnover with insulin infusion during the euglycemic-hyperinsulinemic clamp was almost completely suppressed (>90%) in late pregnancy in nonobese women with normal glucose tolerance.[43] The insulin infusion of $40\,mU \cdot M^{2-1} min^{-1}$ resulted in a plasma insulin concentration of approximately $100\,\mu U \cdot ml^{-1}$. However, estimates of hepatic insulin sensitivity to exogenous insulin in the pregnant rabbit model, by Hauguel et al.,[79] reported that there was decreased insulin sensitivity in late as compared with midpregnancy at a similar basal glucose concentration. Preliminary longitudinal studies in the human, using lower-dose insulin infusions ($\sim 20\,mU \cdot M^{2-1} min^{-1}$), however, have shown decreased suppression of endogenous glucose production in late as compared with midpregnancy.[80]

Hormones Associated with Alterations in Glucose Metabolism

There is a considerable body of information implicating the hormonal milieu of pregnancy contributing to the decrease in insulin sensitivity in pregnancy. For example, in the woman with insulin-dependent diabetes, the significant increase in the insulin requirement during pregnancy rapidly decreases with delivery of the placenta. Additionally, a number of reproductive hormones that increase with advancing gestation have been implicated in the decrease in insulin sensitivity to glucose:

1. In early gestation, increases in estrogen and progesterone have been implicated in the alterations of maternal glucose metabolism. Estrogen treatment of the female rat has been shown to enhance insulin action. After estrogen administration, there was a significant decrease in glucose concentration after an intravenous glucose challenge in comparison with control animals. The improvement was associated with an almost twofold increase in insulin concentration.[81] In studies of women treated with various estrogen preparations for 6 months, there was no significant alteration of either oral glucose tolerance or insulin response, although women with borderline or frankly abnormal glucose response curves tended to show a slight improvement after estrogen therapy.[82] Progesterone, like estrogen, has been associated with a 60% to 70% increase in insulin response to a glucose challenge but does not alter glucose tolerance.[83] Costrini and Kalkhoff[81] concluded that, unlike estrogen, which may primarily enhance insulin response, progesterone may secondarily enhance insulin response because of its action as an insulin antagonist and not as the result of primary pancreatic β-cell stimulation. Nelson et al.,[84] using tracer infusions to estimate endogenous glucose turnover and euglycemic clamps to estimate glucose uptake in the oophorectomized rat model, have shown that chronic progesterone therapy does not alter insulin-mediated glucose uptake in peripheral tissues, but rather reduces the ability of insulin to suppress endogenous glucose production. Furthermore, based on additional studies in the rat model, progesterone has been shown to alter the route of glucose metabolism and result in increases in glucose oxidation in muscle tissue.[85]

2. In late pregnancy, maternal concentrations of cortisol both bound and free, are approximately 2.5-fold higher than in the nonpregnant state.[86] Under experimental conditions of a 24-hour infusion of cortisol, Rizza et al.[87] reported a significant increase in hepatic glucose production rates and decreased insulin sensitivity as estimated by decreased glucose uptake during multidose euglycemic-hyperinsulinemic clamps. Because of a shift to the right with near-maximal glucose utilization during high insulin infusion and normal insulin binding to monocytes and erythrocytes, the investigators proposed that the decreases in insulin action were best explained by a postreceptor defect. These results were consistent with the findings of Ryan et al.,[64] who proposed a potential postreceptor defect to explain the decrease in insulin sensitivity to glucose in pregnancy because of a shift to the right in the dose-response curve to increasing insulin infusions and normal insulin binding to erythrocytes.

3. Human placental lactogen (or human chorionic somatomammotropin) is a polypeptide hormone secreted by the syncytiotrophoblast primarily into the maternal circulation and is believed to be one of the hormones primarily responsible for the decreased insulin sensitivity with advancing gestation. It accounts for approximately 10% of total placental protein production at term and is believed to share many of the biologic properties of human growth hormone.[88] Twelve-hour overnight infusions of human placental lactogen at approximately $300\,\mu g \cdot kg^{-1} hr^{-1}$ result in mean plasma concentrations of $2.3\,\mu g \cdot ml^{-1}$, a concentration similar to that observed in late gestation, have been shown by Beck and Daughaday[89] to result in impaired glucose tolerance as manifested by an increase in insulin and glucose concentration to an oral glucose challenge. Furthermore, Kalkhoff et al.[90] reported that postpartum infusions of human placental lactogen resulted in increases in plasma glucose response to an oral glucose challenge but no change in insulin response in women with normal glucose

tolerance. In contrast, in women with subclinical diabetes mellitus, infusions of human placental lactogen resulted in frankly abnormal glucose tolerance with increases in both glucose and insulin response. The mechanisms by which human placental lactogen results in altered glucose tolerance are undefined.

4. Maternal plasma prolactin concentration increases five- to tenfold during pregnancy and have been implicated in the decrease in insulin sensitivity during pregnancy. Gustafson et al.[91] measured plasma glucose and insulin response to an oral glucose challenge in women with hyperprolactinemia and an age- and weight-matched control group. The basal insulin concentration as well as postchallenge glucose and insulin response were greater in the women with an elevated prolactin concentration. These data were supported by animal research in which short-term prolactin administration in the adult female rat resulted in increased insulin response to intravenous glucose administration.[92] Whether these alterations in insulin response were the result of decreased insulin sensitivity or enhanced β-cell response remains unknown.

Cellular Mechanisms Controlling Carbohydrate Metabolism in Pregnancy

Control of Hepatic Glucose Output

The regulation of hepatic glucose production in pregnancy involves a complex integration of short-term and long-term regulatory processes. Hepatic glucose production consists of both gluconeogenesis and glycogenolysis, and is controlled primarily by substrate delivery and by the hormones glucagon, cortisol, and insulin. Several factors probably contribute to increased hepatic glucose production in late pregnancy. There is an increase in hepatic glucose production, which is driven by an increase in glycerol, lactate, and fatty acid concentrations. The increased substrate delivery increases the intramitochondrial concentrations of acetyl–coenzyme A (CoA) and adenosine triphosphate (ATP), and increases the shuttle of glutamate or malate across the mitochondrial inner membrane, allowing increased nicotinamide adenine dinucleotide, (NADH) formation outside of the mitochondria. In addition to the increased delivery of substrates, hormone-mediated changes in activity of two key gluconeogenic enzymes, fructose-1,6-bisphosphatase and a bifunctional enzyme phosphofructokinase-2/fructose bisphosphatase-2 (PFK-2/FBPase-2) regulate the gluconeogenic pathway. Glucagon inhibits pyruvate kinase and stimulates the gluconeogenic enzyme fructose-1,6-bisphosphatase, which regulates the conversion of fructose 1,6-bisphosphate to fructose-6-phosphate and bypasses the glycolytic enzyme phosphofructokinase (PFK-1). The activity of PFK-2/FBPase-2 is controlled by adenosine 3′,5′-cyclic monophosphate (cAMP), which inactivates PFK-2 and reduces the level of the metabolite fructose 2,6-bisphosphate, effectively removing the allosteric activation of PFK-1, thereby slowing glycolysis and allowing gluconeogenesis to proceed without futile cycling. The final step in hepatic glucose production is controlled by the relative activities of glucose-6-phosphatase and glucokinase. Given the increased hepatic glucose production, lower plasma glucose (below K_m for glucokinase), and hepatic insulin resistance in pregnancy, one would expect the balance of the substrate flux to be shifted toward activation of glucose-6-phosphatase leading to increased transport of free glucose by the liver glucose transporter GLUT 2.

In the long term, from hours to days, an increased concentration of cortisol in pregnancy favors stimulation of gluconeogenesis by increasing the synthesis rate of key gluconeogenic enzymes at the level of gene expression. The expression of phosphoenolpyruvate carboxykinase, fructose-1,6-bisphosphatase, glucose-6-phosphatase, and GLUT 2 are coordinately upregulated in response to cortisol and glucagon and their expression is inhibited by insulin.[93] The fact that there is a resistance to the action of insulin in suppressing hepatic glucose production in late pregnancy suggests there may be impairment in insulin's ability to suppress expression of liver genes involved in gluconeogenesis. While there is insulin resistance with regard to the ability to suppress hepatic glucose production, however, the ability of insulin to stimulate other metabolic processes in the liver such as triglyceride synthesis is increased in pregnancy,[94] suggesting that hepatic insulin resistance may be specific to particular metabolic pathways.

The increased β-oxidation of fatty acids in the liver mitochondria provides energy for driving gluconeogenesis. However, the hypertriglyceridemia in pregnancy suggests increased acetyl-CoA derived from fatty acid oxidation may be partially diverted to form citrate, which is necessary to synthesize hepatic triglycerides. In such a case, replenishing reactions such as transamination of aspartate and another α-keto acid to form oxaloacetate may be needed to allow the oxaloacetate to condense with acetyl-CoA to form citrate. Whether insulin's effectiveness at activating the rate-limiting enzymes of fatty acid synthesis, acetyl-CoA carboxylase, and fatty acid synthetase is increased in pregnancy remains to be studied. However, hepatocytes incubated in the presence of glucocorticoids have been shown to potentiate insulin's ability to stimulate fatty acid synthesis and lipogenesis.[95]

Insulin Secretion

The normal response to the insulin resistance of pregnancy includes a compensation in β-cell function and increased insulin secretion. The exact metabolic signals that trigger the insulin secretory response from the β cell in response to glucose have not been identified, although several candidates have been suggested. Changes in the β-cell ATP to adenosine diphosphate (ADP) ratio brought about by glucose metabolism, the so-called fuel hypothesis,[96,97] suggests that inhibition of the ATP-sensitive K$^+$ channel and stimulation of Ca^{2+} entry into β cells are regulated by glucose and result in depolarization and increased insulin secretion. Recent work has focused on the first two steps of glucose metabolism, namely GLUT 2 and glucokinase, whose activities change throughout the range of blood glucose concentrations. Under normal conditions, the low-affinity (i.e., K_m 17mM) GLUT 2 glucose transporter in liver and islet cells mediates glucose transport activity that greatly exceeds the rate of glucose utilization, and therefore glucokinase has been postulated to be the point at which glucose utilization is controlled.[96,98] Recent support for this hypothesis has come from molecular and genetic studies of families with an autosomal dominant form of non–insulin-dependent diabetes termed maturity-onset diabetes of the young (MODY). These families have been shown to have at least 28 different mutations in the glucokinase gene,[99,100] which in heterozygous individuals appears to result in a much higher threshold for glucose-stimulated insulin secretion, and the total amount of insulin released is less than in normal patients.[101,102]

Skeletal Muscle Glucose Metabolism— Basic Mechanisms

One of the most prominent metabolic adaptations during pregnancy is the reduction in insulin-stimulated whole-body glucose disposal. In the nonpregnant state, despite the high levels of glucose uptake that occur in skeletal muscle, the intracellular concentration of free glucose does not change under euglycemic-hyperinsulinemic conditions.[103] This indicates that glucose is quickly metabolized by muscle, and that glucose transport across the cell membrane is the rate-limiting step in glucose utilization. The regulation of glucose disposal in skeletal muscle occurs in response to changes in availability of ATP, availability of substrates, and in response to hormonal and nervous stimulation. The principal hormonal regulator of glucose disposal in skeletal muscle is insulin, which activates glucose transport and glycogen synthase, and stimulates glucose oxidation by activating pyruvate dehydrogenase complex (PDC) activity. Epinephrine, via cAMP, and Protein Kinase A (PKA) stimulate glycogen phosphorylase and the activity of PFK-1, the rate-limiting step in glycolysis. PFK-1 is allosterically controlled by ATP, AMP, Ca^{2+}, and citrate. Citrate, a potential inhibitor of glycolysis, has been shown to rise in response to fatty acid oxidation and increased acetyl-CoA in skeletal muscle.[104] The rise in citrate inhibits PFK activity, increasingly slowing glycolysis and increasing glucose-6-phosphate. The rise in glucose-6-phosphate may then inhibit hexokinase II and reduce glucose transport, leading to decreased glycogen synthesis.[105] The elevation in acetyl-CoA can allosterically inhibit PDC activity, and increases the NADH/NAD ratio, slowing overall Krebs cycle activity. This reciprocal relationship between increased fatty acid metabolism and reduced glucose oxidation has been termed by Randle et al.[8] the glucose–fatty acid cycle, and has particular relevance for the pregnant state, since the increased utilization of fatty acids in pregnancy may serve to reduce the muscle's metabolism of glucose, for the benefit of the fetus (see Chapter 6).

In the case of euglycemic-hyperinsulinemic clamp studies, the term nonoxidative glucose disposal is frequently used to indicate the pathway of glucose → glucose-6-phosphate → glycogen, primarily in skeletal muscle. Glycogen synthase (GS) is the rate-limiting enzyme controlling glycogen synthesis in skeletal muscle. In muscle, GS exists mainly in an active dephosphorylated form and a less active phosphorylated form. The conversion between the two forms of GS is controlled by insulin and cAMP via a series of kinases and phosphatases that phosphorylate and activate phosphoprotein phosphatase-1 (PP-1), thus activating GS, and by allosteric activation by the presence of increased glucose-6-phosphate concentration. The second messenger system linking the activation of insulin receptor to stimulation of PP-1 is regulated by the MAP kinase pathway. Using nuclear magnetic resonance (NMR) spectroscopy in the human, the rate of glycogen synthesis in skeletal muscle and the concentration of glucose-6-phosphate have been shown to be directly linked to the rate of glucose transport.[106] Thus, any decrease in insulin-mediated glucose disposal in pregnancy could be primarily due to a reduction in skeletal muscle glucose transport.

The metabolism of glucose by skeletal muscle is controlled initially by the transport of glucose across the cell membrane, which takes place by facilitated diffusion. This energy-independent process is mediated by a unique family of facilitative glucose transporters termed GLUT 1 to GLUT 5, which are tissue-specific[107] (see Chapter 7). The GLUT 4 glucose transporter is a 509 amino acid protein and is the major glucose transporter expressed in skeletal muscle, adipose tissue, and cardiac muscle. GLUT 4 has a 65% homology with GLUT 1 and is the only glucose transporter isoform capable of being recruited to the cell surface membrane in response to insulin. Skeletal muscle expresses small amounts of GLUT 1 and GLUT 5 isoform; however, the amount of these proteins is much smaller in muscle, accounting for less than 5% of total transporters in human muscle.[108] GLUT 1 is highly expressed in neurons, red blood cells, and in the capillary endothelial cell, making its exact quantitation in skeletal muscle difficult. In all cells GLUT 1 is primarily located at the cell surface membrane, and is believed to facilitate non–insulin-mediated glucose transport across the muscle membrane in the basal state.[4] GLUT 4, on the other hand, undergoes translocation from unique intracellular vesicles to the cell surface and transverse tubules in response to insulin.[109]

Glucose Metabolism in Women with Diabetes Mellitus

Diabetes mellitus is a chronic metabolic disorder characterized by either absolute or relative insulin deficiency, resulting in increased glucose concentrations. Although glucose intolerance is the common outcome of diabetes mellitus, the pathophysiology remains heterogeneous. To develop uniformity in diagnosis, a classification of diabetes mellitus was published by the National Diabetes Data Group in 1979.[110] The two major classifications of diabetes are type 1, or insulin-dependent diabetes mellitus (IDDM), and type 2 or non–insulin dependent diabetes mellitus (NIDDM). During pregnancy, classification of women with diabetes mellitus has often relied upon the White classification[111] first proposed in the 1940s. This classification is based on factors such as the duration and age of onset of diabetes as well as end organ involvement, primarily retinal and renal. In this chapter, glucose metabolism is reviewed in pregnant women with the two major forms of diabetes mellitus.

Insulin-Dependent Diabetes Mellitus

Insulin-dependent diabetes mellitus (IDDM) is usually characterized by an abrupt appearance at a young age and absolute insulinopenia with lifelong requirements for insulin replacement. These patients may have a genetic predisposition for autoantibodies directed against their islet cells.[112] The degree of concordance for the development of IDDM in monozygotic twins is approximately 33%, suggesting the events subsequent to the development of autoantibodies and appearance of diabetes are related to environmental factors.[113] Because of their insulinopenia and increased dependence on lipid metabolism for energy needs during pregnancy, these women are at increased risk for the development of diabetic ketoacidosis when pregnant. Additionally, because intensive insulin therapy is used in women with IDDM to decrease the risk of spontaneous abortion and congenital anomalies in early pregnancy, these women are at increased risk of hypoglycemic reactions. Studies by Diamond et al.[114] and Rosenn et al.[115] have shown that women with IDDM are at increased risk for hypoglycemic reactions during pregnancy because of diminished counterregulatory epinephrine and growth hormone responses to hypoglycemia. This deficiency in counterregulatory response may also be in part due to an independent effect of pregnancy.

The alterations in carbohydrate metabolism in women with IDDM are not well characterized. Because of maternal insulinopenia, insulin response during gestation can only be estimated relative to pregravid insulin requirements. Estimates of the alteration in insulin requirements are complicated by degree of preconceptual glucose control and frequent presence of insulin antibodies. Weiss and Hofman[116] reported on the change in insulin requirements in IDDM women who had achieved strict glucose control either prior to conception or before 10 weeks' gestation. Their mean blood glucose control was $91 \pm 11\,mg \cdot dl^{-1}$ with a range of 72 to $105\,mg \cdot dl^{-1}$. There was a 12% decrease in insulin requirements from 10 to 17 weeks' gestation and a 50% increase in insulin requirements from 17 weeks' gestation until delivery as compared with pregravid requirements. After 36 weeks' gestation there was a decrease in insulin requirements (Figure 10.6). A 5% decrease in insulin requirements after 36 weeks' gestation was also noted by McManus and Ryan.[117] The decrease in insulin requirements was associated with longer duration of diabetes mellitus but not with adverse perinatal outcome.

Schmitz et al.[118] have evaluated the longitudinal changes in insulin sensitivity using the euglycemic-hyperinsulinemic clamp in women with IDDM in early (i.e., 13 weeks) and late (i.e., 34 weeks) pregnancy and postpartum in comparison with nonpregnant women with IDDM. In the pregnant women there was a significant 50% decrease in insulin sensitivity only in late pregnancy. There was no significant difference in insulin sensitivity in the pregnant women with IDDM as compared with the nonpregnant women with IDDM either in early gestation or within one week of delivery. Of interest there was a significant inverse relationship between the serum concentration human placental lactogen and insulin sensitivity from early to late gestation. Based on the available data, women with IDDM appear to have a similar decrease in magnitude in insulin sensitivity in late pregnancy as compared with women with normal glucose tolerance.

Non–Insulin-Dependent Diabetes Mellitus

The pathophysiology of NIDDM involves abnormalities of both insulin-sensitive tissue as noted by decreased skeletal muscle and hepatic sensitivity to insulin, and β-cell response as noted by inadequate insulin response for a given degree of glycemia. Initially in the course of the development of NIDDM, the insulin response to a glucose challenge may be increased relative to that of indi-

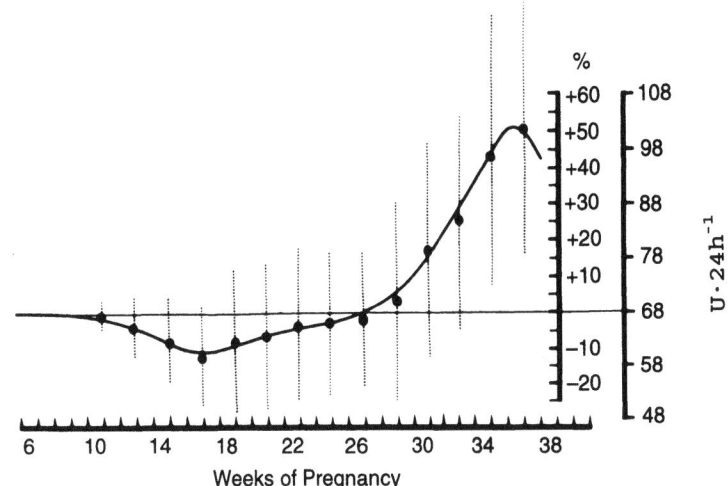

FIGURE 10.6. Insulin requirement in the course of pregnancy of 12 selected patients (White B-R) with particularly strict metabolic control even before the 10th gestational week (mean ± SD). The calculations were carried out for 36 weeks of therapy with 87 dose adjustments. The weeks of gestation are evaluated two by two. 100% = insulin requirement at institution of therapy. (From Weiss and Hofman,[116] with permission.)

viduals with normal glucose tolerance but inadequate to maintain normoglycemia. Whether or not insulin resistance precedes β-cell dysfunction in the development of NIDDM continues to be debated. Arguments and experimental data support both contentions, and as noted by Sims and Calles-Escadon,[119] heterogeneity of metabolic abnormalities exists in any classification of diabetes mellitus.

Despite the limitations of any classification system, certain clinical generalizations can be made regarding individuals with NIDDM or who develop gestational diabetes mellitus (GDM) during pregnancy. These individuals are typically older and most often heavier than IDDM patients, and the onset of the disorder is usually insidious. Individuals with NIDDM may or may not require insulin therapy for maintenance of normoglycemia and usually do not develop ketoacidosis. Data in monozygotic twins have reported a lifetime risk of both twins developing NIDDM that ranges between 58 to almost 100%, suggesting the disorder has a strong genetic component.[120,121]

Women with NIDDM are usually listed as class B according to White's ordering.[111] Recent studies have shown that many women developing GDM (i.e., glucose intolerance recognized for the first time during pregnancy), share many of the metabolic characteristics of individuals with NIDDM. Although earlier studies reported the incidence of islet cell antibodies in women with GDM as measured by immunofluorescence techniques to be between 10%[122] and 35%,[123] more recent data using more specific monoclonal antibodies have found a much lower incidence, on the order of 1% to 2%,[124] suggesting very little evidence for IDDM disorders in women with GDM. Furthermore, metabolic research employing both the minimal model[125] and the euglycemic-hyperinsulinemic clamp[126] techniques have demonstrated defects in insulin secretory response and decreased insulin sensitivity in women with a history of GDM when evaluated postpartum, indicating typical NIDDM abnormalities are present in women with GDM. Thus in these women it is believed that the hormonal events of pregnancy may represent an unmasking of a genetic susceptibility to NIDDM.

Decreased insulin response to a glucose challenge has been demonstrated by several investigators in late gestation in women with GDM, although the degree of insulin sensitivity reported in these women varied considerably. Yen et al.[127] described a decrease in first-phase insulin response and a decrease in glucose disposal using the intravenous glucose tolerance test in women with GDM in late gestation. In contrast, Fisher et al.,[128] in an investigation of nonobese women with GDM using a glucose infusion test, described an increase in insulin sensitivity in late pregnancy. These investigators suggested that the increase in insulin sensitivity was consistent with the low insulin response in their study subjects. Recently, Buchanan et al.,[63] using the minimal model technique in late pregnancy, showed that women with GDM had a significant decrease in first-phase insulin and that insulin sensitivity was similar to that of a pregnant woman with normal glucose tolerance. In a prospective longitudinal study of nonobese women with normal glucose tolerance prior to conception who developed GDM during pregnancy, in comparison with a matched control group, Catalano et al.[129] showed that there was a progressive decrease in first-phase insulin response in late gestation in women developing GDM (Figure 10.7). The decrease in first-phase insulin response, however, developed gradually with advancing gestation along with a progressive decrease in insulin sensitivity.

Decreased insulin sensitivity has been proposed as a potential mechanism in the pathophysiology of GDM. Ryan et al.[64] reported a 40% decrease in insulin sensitivity in women with GDM in comparison with a pregnant control group in late gestation using the euglycemic-hyperinsulinemic clamp. Using similar techniques, Catalano et al.[129] described the longitudinal changes in

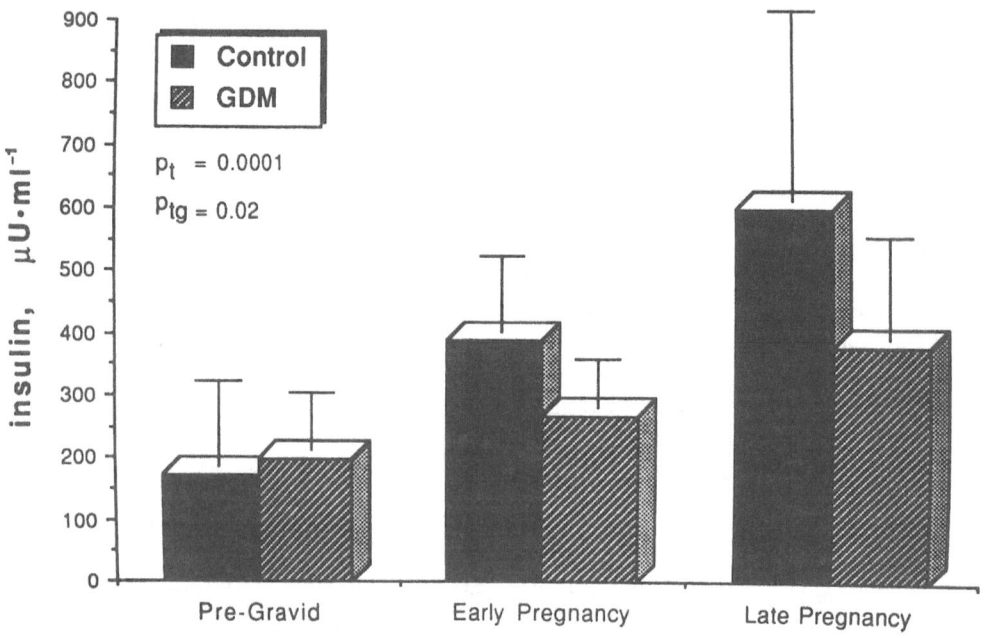

FIGURE 10.7. Longitudinal changes in first-phase insulin response during the intravenous glucose tolerance test in women with normal glucose tolerance and gestational diabetes. Pt, change over time pregravid through late pregnancy; Ptg, group/time interaction (mean ± SD). (From Catalano et al.,[129] with permission.)

insulin sensitivity prior to conception through early and late gestation in a nonobese control group and women developing GDM. Although women developing GDM had decreased insulin sensitivity in comparison with the matched control group, the differences in insulin sensitivity between the two groups were greatest before conception and in early pregnancy and by 34 to 36 weeks' gestation the difference in insulin sensitivity between groups was less pronounced (Figure 10.8).

Garvey et al.[130] reported that the GLUT 4 content was normal in rectus abdominus muscle from pregnant women and those with GDM. By contrast, in adipocytes Ciraldi et al.[131] found that insulin receptor kinase activity was unaltered, yet maximal glucose transport was de-

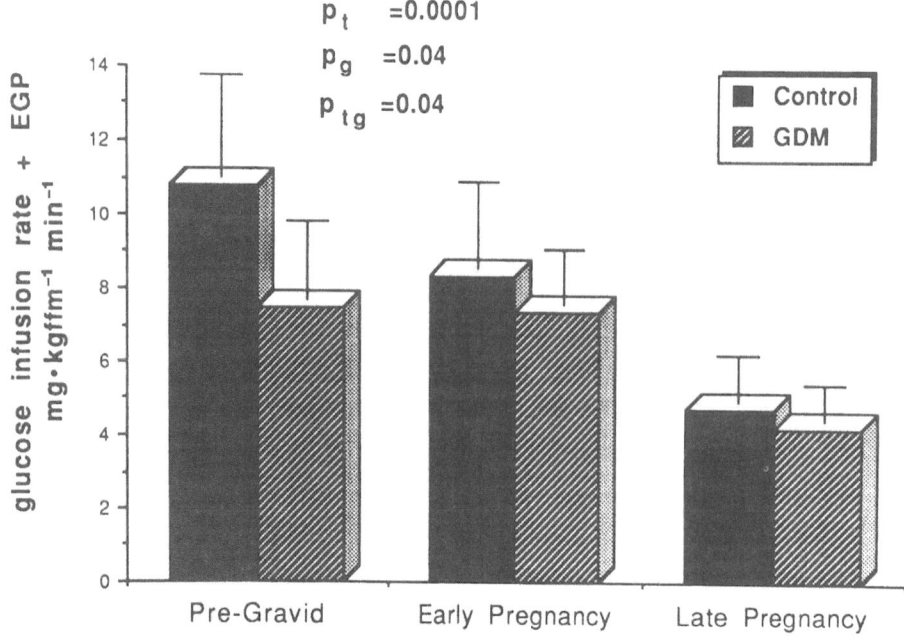

FIGURE 10.8. Longitudinal changes in insulin sensitivity as estimated from glucose infusion rate plus residual endogenous glucose production (EGP) during the euglycemic-hyperinsulinemic clamp in women with normal glucose tolerance and gestational diabetes. Pt, changes over time pregravid through late gestation; Pg, difference between groups; Ptg, group time interaction (mean ± SD). (From Catalano et al.,[129] with permission.)

creased threefold in adipocytes obtained from pregnant subjects matched with a similar level of obesity [body mass index (BMI) >27 kg·m^{-2}], suggesting that insulin resistance in fat cells may be related to postreceptor changes in GLUT 4 trafficking to the cell surface as well as reduced GLUT 4 gene expression as noted by Garvey et al.[132] These data suggest that knowledge gained concerning the nature of insulin resistance in fat cells may not apply to skeletal muscle, and that the most important explanation for the decreased whole-body glucose disposal in pregnancy and GDM remains unknown.

In women with GDM, there was essentially no change in insulin sensitivity from the time prior to conception through early pregnancy compared with the 40% decrease in insulin sensitivity in the control group. Furthermore, in some very insulin-resistant women there was actually a small increase in insulin sensitivity in early gestation relative to pregravid measurements. This paradoxical increase in insulin sensitivity in early gestation in these women may explain the 12% decrease in insulin requirements in early gestation in women with insulin-dependent diabetes,[116] many of whom are known to have decreased insulin sensitivity.[133]

Basal hepatic glucose production has been reported to be similar in women with normal glucose tolerance and GDM. Studies by Kalhan et al.,[58] Cowett et al.,[59] and Catalano et al.,[43] employing various stable isotope methodologies have demonstrated similar increases in basal hepatic glucose production in late gestation in control subjects and women with GDM. Studies employing the euglycemic-hyperinsulinemic clamp to estimate insulin suppression of hepatic glucose production in women with GDM have shown less suppression of hepatic glucose production in late gestation in women with GDM (80%) as compared with women with normal glucose tolerance (95%).[129] Taken together these data illustrate that abnormalities in insulin response, decreased hepatic sensitivity to infused insulin, and decreased peripheral insulin sensitivity over the course of a full-term pregnancy all contribute to the development of glucose intolerance during gestation in women with GDM. Furthermore, the results of these studies in women with GDM may provide a paradigm for the development of NIDDM over a period of years in this high-risk population.

Potential Cellular Mechanisms Contributing to Abnormalities in Glucose Metabolism in Pregnancy and GDM

Changes in the Insulin Receptor in Pregnancy

The cellular mechanisms responsible for insulin resistance in pregnancy are unknown, but probably are related to alterations in the insulin receptor and/or changes in the events that occur after insulin binds to the receptor, the so-called postreceptor processes. The division between receptor and postreceptor defects when discussing insulin resistance refers to the fact that insulin resistance can occur in the presence of normal to increased insulin binding. Since plasma insulin concentration is increased in pregnancy, one would expect the insulin receptor to be downregulated. Several groups have reported lower binding affinity of the insulin receptor in adipocytes from pregnant compared with nonpregnant women.[134–136] However, insulin binding to hepatocytes[137,138] and skeletal muscle,[139,140] quantitatively the most important tissue for insulin-stimulated glucose disposal, have been found to be similar in pregnant and nonpregnant women. These data suggest that insulin resistance in pregnancy is possibly tissue-specific and may be related to postreceptor events that change specific metabolic pathways for glucose disposal. The diversion of ingested nutrients away from skeletal muscle toward storage in maternal adipose tissue and transport to the fetal compartment suggests postreceptor events may figure prominently in the mechanisms underlying the adaptation to pregnancy.

Proximal Post–Insulin Receptor Defect(s)

Although insulin resistance is a universal finding in pregnancy and GDM, very few studies have investigated the mechanism of the insulin resistance in skeletal muscle of pregnant women at the cellular or molecular level. In studies in adipose tissue, approximately 50% of the patients with GDM have a profound cellular depletion of GLUT 4, whereas the other subgroup demonstrated normal total cellular GLUT 4 with an abnormal subcellular distribution. Insulin-stimulated translocation of GLUT 4 was severely decreased in all patients with GDM, and glucose transport activity was reduced by 60%.[141] However, there have been no follow-up studies to see whether these defects are present before gestation or if it persists postpartum. It is entirely possible these defects are acquired as a result of chronic hyperglycemia or hyperinsulinemia during gestation. With regard to skeletal muscle, there is no information on glucose transport or postreceptor alterations in pregnancy or GDM. The levels of GLUT 4 protein are completely normal, suggesting the marked insulin resistance in skeletal muscle during pregnancy and in GDM is accounted for almost entirely by a postreceptor defect in insulin signaling. Recent data in rectus abdominus muscle from pregnant subjects indicate the levels of Insulin Receptor β (IRβ) and IRS-1 protein are significantly decreased compared to nonpregnant subjects matched for a similar percent body fat,[142] suggesting a reduction in signal transduction from the insulin receptor to IRS-1 could be an important adaptation producing whole-body insulin resistance in pregnancy. However, longitudinal studies of the same subjects before and after delivery are needed to confirm these findings. Ciaraldi et al.[136] found no change in insulin-stimulated tyrosine kinase activity in fat cells from pregnant patients. However there are no biochemical data with respect to the postreceptor mechanism of insulin receptor signaling in either adipose or skeletal muscle in pregnancy and GDM.

Altered Protein Tyrosine Phosphatase Activity

Insulin receptor autophosphorylation and IRS-1 tyrosine phosphorylation are balanced by dephosphorylation reactions carried out by cellular and membrane-bound protein tyrosine phosphatases (PTPase). They have been postulated as a pathogenetic factor in the insulin resistance of obesity and NIDDM. Data of skeletal muscle from insulin-sensitive and insulin-resistant nondiabetic Pima Indians demonstrated a 33% increased basal cytosolic PTPase activity in insulin-resistant subjects that failed to suppress in response to insulin. Insulin infusion produced a rapid 25% suppression of PTPase activity in the insulin-sensitive subjects, but not in those who were insulin resistant.[143] Specific type 1B PTPase messenger RNA (mRNA) levels are increased in insulin-resistant subjects after a euglycemic-hyperinsulinemic clamp, whereas they are suppressed by 50% in insulin-sensitive subjects.[144] Another study by Kusari et al.,[145] however, in a different population showed a lowered PTPase activity in obese nondiabetic and NIDDM subjects associated with a 38% decrease in PTPase 1B activity. The conflicting data regarding PTPase activity suggest that multiple factors, both genetic and environmental, as well as variations in specific PTPases and their intracellular targets may be involved in the modulation of PTPase activity. The clinical significance of PTPase activity in humans is suggested by studies using the potent phosphatase inhibitor vanadate. A number of studies have shown that vanadate given orally normalizes hyperglycemia in diabetic humans[146] and animals by enhancing glucose uptake by skeletal muscle[147] possibly via increasing the phosphorylation state of the insulin receptor or receptor substrates.[148,149] However, it is unknown to what extent the regulation of PTPases plays in the insulin resistance of human pregnancy.

Changes in β-Cell Response

The factors involved in the loss of first-phase insulin secretion in the GDM patient are not known. A major stumbling block in understanding the molecular basis for defective glucose-stimulated insulin secretion is the lack of in vitro systems that mimic the secretory abnormality. Multiple candidate defects have been proposed but no single hypothesis can explain all the characteristics of the secretory abnormalities.[150] Although in vitro studies using the isolated perfused pancreas have emphasized the importance of hyperglycemia in mediating the blunted response to glucose, the abnormal first phase of insulin secretion persists in the patient whose diabetic control has been greatly improved, supporting the hypothesis that the patient with NIDDM and perhaps GDM may have an intrinsic defect in the β cell.[151,152]

Tumor Necrosis Factor

The cytokine tumor necrosis factor-α (TNF-α) has recently been proposed to play a role in the insulin resistance of obesity and NIDDM[153] (see Chapter 20). Infusion of TNF-α results in increased insulin resistance in rats and in human skeletal muscle cells incubated in culture.[154,155] TNF-α mRNA expression is elevated in the adipose tissue of obese animals and in humans with obesity and correlates with the extent of obesity and degree of hyperinsulinemia.[156] Although the concentration of circulating TNF-α in plasma of obese patients is extremely low compared with that found in burn patients and patients with cachexia, recent evidence indicates skeletal muscle expresses the mRNA for TNF-α and may be acting in a paracrine fashion.[157] Neutralization of TNF-α in obese and insulin-resistant rats improves insulin sensitivity and insulin receptor autophosphorylation.[158] TNF-α mediates insulin resistance at multiple levels and appears to act primarily by producing an increase in the serine phosphorylation of IRS-1 in a manner that blocks the autophosphorylation of the insulin receptor β subunit.[159] In adipose tissue, exposure to TNF-α downregulates several fat-specific genes and reduces expression of GLUT 4 protein. However, muscle levels of GLUT 4 are not downregulated in animal models of obesity in which TNF-α is expressed, and neutralization of TNF-α has no effect on GLUT 4 mRNA expression despite improvements in insulin sensitivity. These effects are consistent with the effects of TNF-α on downregulating the proximal insulin-signaling pathway. Recently, the levels of TNF-α have been reported to increase in the blood from early to late pregnancy and correlate with the reduction in insulin sensitivity and increase in percent body fat.[160] These data suggest the possibility that a rise in TNF-α could be linked to a change in insulin receptor phosphorylation, and may be involved in the insulin resistance and diminished insulin-stimulated glucose disposal in late pregnancy. The hormonal mediators that trigger the increase in TNF-α in pregnancy and obesity are not known but could be related to insulin, insulin-like growth factor-1 (IGF-1), or glucocorticoids.

Genetic Defects in Insulin Action in GDM

Women with GDM, especially those who are diagnosed early in pregnancy, have an additional component of insulin resistance that is not specifically related to pregnancy.[63,124,125] Furthermore, in women with a history of GDM, there is a significantly increased risk of the subsequent development of NIDDM, estimated to be about 2% to 3% per year of follow-up.[161,162] It seems likely that in most women, GDM represents an unmasking of the genetic predisposition of NIDDM induced by the hormonal milieu of pregnancy. However, in the absence of specific genetic markers for NIDDM, this is difficult to prove.

Examination of insulin action in women with a previous history of GDM indicates that decreased insulin sensitivity and glucose disposal persists in the majority of patients after delivery, suggesting that the genetic components of insulin resistance are present in skeletal muscle of former GDM patients. Most of the molecular abnormalities that lead to tissue insulin resistance in GDM may be similar to those in NIDDM. The chronically elevated basal concentration of insulin that is indicative of insulin resistance may produce downregulation of the insulin receptor and IRS-1, a decrease in insulin receptor kinase activity, and other postreceptor alterations in insulin action that may persist in former GDM after pregnancy.[163–165] Studies of insulin action at the cellular level in subjects with previous GDM are important for several reasons: (1) They tell us about the defects found in diabetes that may be unrelated to hyperglycemia or insulin deficiency. In patients with established diabetes, regardless of the type, it is possible to trace a vicious series of events that is compounded by insulin resistance, insulin deficiency, and hyperglycemia. (2) The studies determine which defects found in GDM are the earliest and which are secondary. This information provides an understanding of disease progression and the basis for prevention. (3) Most importantly, these studies can provide a guide to search for the diabetic gene(s).

There is ample evidence for multiple genetic factors in the pathogenesis of NIDDM; however, unlike NIDDM, it is clear in GDM that the environmental factors involved in diabetes are no longer present after delivery. Studies of women with a prior history of GDM or who exhibit GDM for the first time at delivery represent a unique opportunity to determine whether the defects that occur during GDM are reduced after delivery or represent the genetic factors for developing insulin resistance and subsequent NIDDM.

Potential Long-Term Effects of Abnormal Glucose Metabolism on Postnatal β-Cell Function and Insulin Sensitivity

Abnormal maternal glucose metabolism has a multitude of both short- and long-term effects on the developing fetus. Although there is a genetic component involved in the development of NIDDM, metabolic milieu during pregnancy may affect the long-term risks for development of diabetes mellitus and obesity in the offspring of women with abnormal glucose tolerance during pregnancy. In comparison to the 5% to 6% risk of IDDM in the offspring of fathers with IDDM, the risk to the offspring of women with insulin-dependent diabetes is approximately 1% to 2%.[166] In contrast, the risk of GDM is only 7% in women whose fathers had a history of NIDDM, whereas the risk of GDM was approximately 35% if there was a maternal history of NIDDM.[167] Additional studies in various ethnic groups have reported an additional in utero environmental risk above and beyond that of the genetic risk of developing glucose intolerance in the offspring of women with abnormal glucose tolerance (see Chapter 49).[168,169]

A number of animal models have been developed to study mechanisms underlying dietary-environment triggers and genetic factors involved in glucose intolerance and obesity in the offspring of the diabetic mother. While none of the animal models is a perfect reflection of the human condition, information from these models may give important mechanistic data that provide potential avenues for investigation in human pregnancy. Gauguir et al.,[170] using glucose infusion to render a pregnant rat model hyperglycemic, reported that females born of these rats were both glucose intolerant and had impaired insulin secretion. These defects in glucose metabolism persisted into the third generation in offspring of female hyperglycemic rats. Their offspring were hyperglycemic, hyperinsulinemic, as well as macrosomic, and displayed glucose intolerance as adults. Van Assche et al.[171] have demonstrated abnormalities in β-cell function and insulin sensitivity in the offspring of a streptozocin hyperglycemic pregnant rat model. Islet cell hyperplasia and β-cell degranulation were found in the fetuses of up to the third generation of offspring of diabetic mothers, while pancreatic islets were normal in fetuses from control mothers even if the father was an offspring of a diabetic mother. Holemans et al.[172] used the euglycemic-hyperinsulinemic clamp to study insulin sensitivity in adult offspring of streptozocin diabetic rats. The steady-state glucose infusions were 50% to 60% lower in the offspring of the streptozocin diabetic rats in comparison with age- and weight-matched controls, indicating decreased insulin sensitivity. Patel's group[173] evaluated the metabolic consequences in the progeny of rats fed an isocaloric high carbohydrate formula in their early postnatal life. The rats fed the isocaloric high carbohydrate diet from day 4 through 24 of life were hyperinsulinemic on day 45 and had a significantly greater growth rate from day 60 onward. There was evidence of adipose tissue hypertrophy by day 100 in contrast with a control population. These metabolic changes were found to persist in the next generation of offspring of these artificially reared animals without dietary manipulation. Additionally, when basal insulin release was assessed in these animals and their offspring, the rats fed the isocaloric high carbohydrate diet had a greater basal insulin response but failed to increase insulin response above basal values with a glucose challenge.[174] Again these abnormalities in β-cell response persisted into the second generation.

As predicted by Freinkel,[57] the diabetic intrauterine environment appears to have lasting effects on the anthropometric development and glucose metabolism of the offspring of women with glucose intolerance, i.e., fuel-mediated teratogenesis. Pettitt et al.[175] have followed the long-term effects of diabetes in offspring of Pima Indian women. The offspring of the women with diabetes mellitus during pregnancy were more obese, had greater glucose concentrations after a glucose challenge, and had a nearly 10-fold greater risk of diabetes than the offspring of prediabetic women by the age of 20. Additionally, Silverman et al.[176] in a follow-up study of children born to women with a diagnosis of diabetes mellitus prior to conception or GDM reported an increased risk of impaired glucose tolerance in these children, particularly after the age of 10. Impaired glucose tolerance was not associated with the etiology of the mother's diabetes, i.e., whether or not she had diabetes mellitus prior to conception or GDM. Amniotic fluid insulin concentrations and obesity were independent factors in the development of impaired glucose tolerance in this population.

Impact of GDM on Fetal Growth and Metabolism: Environment vs. Genetics

These data suggest the effects of the intrauterine environment may be of greater importance than genetic factors when considering the effects on glucose metabolism and body composition of the offspring. However, the severity of the early and later metabolic abnormalities appears to vary among offspring, despite a similar exposure to hyperglycemia. Thus, while exposure to hyperglycemia in utero is a risk factor for the development of future diabetes, it is not the sole factor (see Chapter 49).

The original Pederson[177] hypothesis proposed that neonatal macrosomia in offspring of diabetic mothers was caused by fetal hyperinsulinemia, secondary to elevated maternal glucose. Holemans et al.[178] have reported that the adult offspring of streptozocin diabetic mothers are not only insulin resistant but also glucose intolerant, indicating that transmission of hyperglycemia may also occur as a result of exposure to maternal diabetes in utero. It is clear that maternal glucose is not the sole determinant of fetal hyperglycemia and macrosomia, since not all littermates of a given mother exposed to similar maternal glucose develop macrosomia. A similar disparity has also been noted among infants of white, black, and Hispanic mothers with gestational diabetes, despite similar degrees of maternal metabolic dysregulation in the three groups,[179] suggesting genetic factors are an important determinant of the fetal response to hyperglycemia. In addition Gloria-Bottini et al.[180] have shown a relationship between genetic variability around the locus coding for IGF-1 and an increase in fetal body mass in offspring of diabetic mothers, suggesting some component in the expression of fetal macrosomia may be related to genetic variability in the IGF-1 locus.

In addition to hyperglycemia associated with insulin deficiency induced by streptozocin treatment, two other models have been used including hyperglycemia produced by chronic glucose infusion, and diabetes in the C57BL/KsJ-db+/+ mouse. Of these models only the db/+ mouse develops diabetes spontaneously, and can be easily identified by black coat color, whereas the C57BL/KsJ+/+ pregnant mouse has a misty coat color and is normoglycemic during pregnancy.[181] Studies of the C57BL/KsJ-db+/+ mouse indicate the mother is glucose intolerant during pregnancy, and the offspring are significantly heavier than offspring from C57BL/KsJ+/+ controls.[182] This suggests the db gene may interact with the hormones of pregnancy to trigger gestational diabetes and cause macrosomia in the offspring. The db/+ mouse model has a distinct advantage over other streptozocin diabetic models because the diabetes is caused by a mutation in a single gene on the C57BL/KsJ strain. Therefore, it should be possible to predict based on genotyping which offspring are genetically programmed for obesity and the impact of altering the maternal environment on the risk of obesity and diabetes in mature animals. Metabolic interventions that reduce the risk of diabetes and obesity in offspring need to be developed based on an understanding of the disruptions in maternal metabolism during pregnancy.

References

1. Green JR, Pawson IG, Schumacher LB, et al. Glucose tolerance in pregnancy: ethnic variation and influence of body habitus. Am J Obstet Gynecol 1990;163:86–92.
2. DeFronzo RA, Lilly Lecture, 1987. The triumvirate: β cell, muscle, liver: a collusion responsible for NIDDM. Diabetes 1988;37:667–687.
3. Dinneen S, Gerich J, Rizza R. Carbohydrate metabolism in non-insulin dependent diabetes mellitus. N Engl J Med 1992;327:707–713.
4. Burant CF, Sivitz WI, Fukumoto H, et al. Mammalian glucose transporters: structure and molecular regulation. Recent Prog Horm Res 1991;47:349–389.
5. Consoli A, Nurjhan N, Reilly JJ, et al. Contribution of liver and skeletal muscle to alanine and lactate metabolism in humans. Am J Physiol 1990;259:E677–684.

6. Dagenais GR, Tancredi RG, Zierler KL. Free fatty oxidation by forearm muscle at rest, and evidence for an intramuscular lipid pool in the human forearm. J Clin Invest 1976;58:421–431.
7. Rothman DL, Magnusson I, Katz LD, et al. Quantitation of hepatic glycogenolysis and gluconeogenesis in fasting humans with ^{13}C NMR. Science 1991;254:573–576.
8. Randle PJ, Garland PB, Hales CN, et al. The glucose-fatty acid cycle: its role in insulin sensitivity and the metabolic disturbances of diabetes mellitus. Lancet 1963;1:785–789.
9. Exton J, Park C. Interaction of insulin and glucagon in the control of liver metabolism. In: Steiner D, Freinkel N, eds. Handbook of physiology. Baltimore: Williams & Wilkins, 1972:437–455.
10. Ferrannini E, Bjorkman O, Reichard GA, et al. The disposal of an oral glucose load in healthy subjects: a quantitative study. Diabetes 1985;34:580–588.
11. Kryshak EJ, Butler PC, Marsh C, et al. Pattern of postprandial carbohydrate metabolism and effects of portal and peripheral insulin delivery. Diabetes 1990;39:142–148.
12. McGarry JD, Kuwajima M, Newgard CB, et al. From dietary glucose to liver glycogen: the full circle round. Ann Rev Nutr 1987;7:51–73.
13. Radziuk J. Hepatic glycogen in humans. I. Direct formation after oral and intravenous glucose or after a 24 hour fast. Am J Physiol 1989;257:E145–157.
14. Kelley D, Mitrakou A, Marsh H, et al. Skeletal muscle glycolysis, oxidation and storage of an oral glucose load. J Clin Invest 1988;81:1563–1571.
15. White MF, Shoelson SE, Keutmann H, et al. A cascade of tyrosine autophosphorylation in the B-subunit activates the insulin receptor. J Biol Chem 1988;263:1969–2975.
16. Wilden PA, Siddel K, Haring H, et al. The role of insulin receptor kinase domain autophosphorylation in receptor-mediated activities. J Biol Chem 1992;267:13719–13726.
17. White MF, Kahn CR. The insulin signaling system. J Biol Chem 1994;269:1–4.
18. Sun XJ, Rothenberg P, Kahn CR, et al. The structure of the insulin receptor substrate IRS-1 defines a unique signal transduction protein. Nature 1991;352:73–78.
19. Waters SB, Yamauchi K, Pessin JE. Functional expression of insulin receptor substrate-1 (IRS-1) is required for insulin-stimulated mitogenic signaling. J Biol Chem 1993;268:22231–22237.
20. Sun XJ, Crimmins DL, Myers MG, et al. Pleiotropic insulin signals are engaged by multisite phosphorylation of IRS-1. Mol Cell Biol 1993;13:7418–7428.
21. Araki E, Lipes MA, Patti ME, et al. Alternative pathway for insulin signaling in mice with targeted disruption of the IRS-1 gene. Nature 1994;372:186–189.
22. Sun XJ, Wang LM, Zhang Y, et al. The structure and function of IRS-2: a common element in insulin/IGF-1 and IL-4 signaling. Nature 1995;377:173–177.
23. Yamauchi T, Tobe K, Tamemoto H, et al. Insulin signaling and insulin actions in the muscles and livers of insulin-resistant, insulin receptor substrate-1 deficient mice. Mol Cell Biol 1996;16:3074–3084.
24. Skolnik EY, Lee CH, Baltzer AG, et al. The SH2/SH3 domain-containing protein GRB2 interacts with typrosine-phosphorylated IRS-1 and Shc: implications for insulin control of ras signalling. EMBO J 1993;12:1929–1936.
25. Tobe K, Matsuoka K, Tamemoto H, et al. Insulin stimulates association of IRS-1 with the protein abundant Src homology/growth factor receptor-bound protein. J Biol Chem 1993;268:11167–11171.
26. Yonezawa K, Ando A, Kaburagi Y, et al. Signal transduction pathways from insulin receptors to Ras. J Biol Chem 1994;269:4634–4640.
27. Honda RY, Tobe K, Kaburagi K, et al. Upstream mechanisms of glycogen synthase activation by insulin and insulin-like growth factor-1. J Biol Chem 1995;270:2729–2734.
28. Yamauchi K, Pessin JE. Insulin receptor substrate-1 (IRS-1) and Shc compete for a limited pool of Grb2 in mediating insulin downstream signaling. J Biol Chem 1994;269:31107–31114.
29. Russell M, Lange-Carter CA, Johnson GL. Direct interaction between Ras and the kinase domain of mitogen-activated protein kinase (MEKK1). J Biol Chem 1995;270:11757–11783.
30. Cheatham B, Vlahos CJ, Cheatham L, et al. Phosphatidylinositol 3-kinase activation is required for insulin stimulation of pp 70 S6 kinase, DNA synthesis, and glucose transporter translocation. Mol Cell Biol 1994;14:4902–4911.
31. Okada T, Kawano Y, Sakadibara T, et al. Essential role of phosphatidylinositol 3-kinase in insulin-induced glucose transport and antilipolysis in rat adipocytes. J Biol Chem 1994;269:3568–3573.
32. Backer JM, Myers MG, Sun XJ, et al. Association of IRS-1 with the insulin receptor and the phosphatidylinositol 3′ kinase. Formation of binary and ternary signaling complexes in intact cells. J Biol Chem 1993;268:8204–8212.
33. Clarke JF, Young PW, Konezawn K, et al. Inhibition of the translocation of GLUT1 and GLUT4 in 3T3L-1 cells by the phosphatidylinositol 3-kinase inhibitor, wortmannin. Biochem J 1994;300:631–641.
34. Yeh JI, Gulve EA, Rameh L, et al. The effects of wortmannin on rat skeletal muscle. Dissociation of signaling pathways for insulin- and contraction-activated hexose transport. J Biol Chem 1995;270:2107–2113.
35. White MF. The IRS-1 signaling system. Curr Opin Genet Dev 1994;4:47–52.
36. Kjos SL, Henry O, Lee RM, et al. The effect of lactation on glucose and lipid metabolism in women with recent gestational diabetes. Obstet Gynecol 1993;82:451–455.
37. Skouby SO, Anderson O, Saurbrey N, et al. Oral contraception and insulin sensitivity: in vivo assessment in normal women and women with previous gestational diabetes. J Clin Endocrinol Metab 1987;64:519–523.
38. Klitz-Silverstein D, Barrett-Connor E, Wingard OL. The effect of parity on the later development of non-insulin-dependent diabetes mellitus or impaired glucose tolerance. N Engl J Med 1989;321:1214–1219.
39. Durnin JVGA, McKillop FM, Grant S, et al. Energy requirements of pregnancy in Scotland. Lancet 1987;2:897–900.
40. Forsum E, Sadurskis A, Wager J. Resting metabolic rate and body composition of healthy Swedish women during pregnancy. Am J Clin Nutr 1988;47:942–947.

41. Catalano PM, Calles J, Roman NJ, et al. Longitudinal changes in body composition, energy expenditure and route of glucose disposed in pregnant control subjects and women with gestational diabetes. Abstract #S-114, Society for Gynecologic Investigation, Toronto, Canada, March 31–April 3, 1993.
42. Spellacy WN, Goetz FC, Greenberg BZ, et al. Plasma insulin in normal "early" pregnancy. Obstet Gynecol 1965;25:862–865.
43. Catalano PM, Tyzbir ED, Wolfe RR, et al. Longitudinal changes in basal hepatic glucose production and suppression during insulin infusion in normal pregnant women. Am J Obstet Gynecol 1992;167:913–919.
44. Felig P, Lynch U. Starvation in human pregnancy: hypoglycemia, hypoinsulinemia, and hyperketonemia. Science 1970;170:990–992.
45. Catalano PM, Tyzbir ED, Roman NM, et al. Longitudinal changes in insulin release and insulin resistance in nonobese pregnant women. Am J Obstet Gynecol 1991;165:1667–1672.
46. Pacini G, Bergman RN. MINMOD: a computer program to calculate insulin sensitivity and pancreatic responsivitity from the frequently sampled intravenous glucose tolerance test. Comput Methods Programs Biomed 1986;23:113–122.
47. DeFronzo RA, Tobin JD, Andres R. Glucose clamp technique: a method for quantifying insulin secretion and resistance. Am J Physiol 1979;237:E214–223.
48. Bergman RN. Lilly Lecture, 1989. Toward physiological understanding of glucose tolerance, minimal model approach. Diabetes 1989;38:1512–1527.
49. Saad MF, Anderson RL, Laws A, et al. A comparison between the minimal model and the glucose clamp in the assessment of insulin sensitivity across the spectrum of glucose tolerance. Diabetes 1994;43:1114–1121.
50. Bergman RN, Prager R, Volund A, et al. Equivalence of the insulin sensitivity index in man derived by the minimal model method and the euglycemic glucose clamp. J Clin Invest 1987;79:790–800.
51. Kalkhoff RK, Kissebah AH, Kim HJ. Carbohydrate and lipid metabolism during normal pregnancy: relationship to gestational hormone action. In: Merkatz IR, Adam PA, eds. The diabetic pregnancy—a perinatal prospective. New York: Grune & Stratton, 1979:3–21.
52. Black PR, Brooks DR, Bessey PQ, et al. Mechanisms of insulin resistance following injury. Ann Surg 1982;196:420–435.
53. Swinburn BA, Nyomba BC, Saad MF, et al. Insulin resistance associated with lower rates of weight gain in Pima Indians. J Clin Invest 1991;88:168–173.
54. Catalano PM, Roman NM, Tyzbir ED, et al. Weight gain in women with gestational diabetes. Obstet Gynecol 1993;81:523–528.
55. Ravussin E, Swinburn BA. Pathophysiology of obesity. Lancet 1992;340:404–408.
56. Taggart NR, Holliday RM, Billewicz WZ, et al. Changes in skinfolds during pregnancy. Br J Nutr 1967;21:439–451.
57. Freinkel N. Banting lecture 1980: of pregnancy and progeny. Diabetes 1980;29:1023–1035.
58. Kalhan SC, D'Angelo LJ, Savin SM, et al. Glucose production in pregnant women at term gestation: sources of glucose for human fetus. J Clin Invest 1979;63:388–394.
59. Cowett RA, Susa JB, Kahn CB, et al. Glucose kinetics in nondiabetic and diabetic women during the third trimester of pregnancy. Am J Obstet Gynecol 1983;146:773–780.
60. Spellacy WN, Goetz FC. Plasma insulin in normal late pregnancy. N Engl J Med 1963;268:988–991.
61. Burt RL. Peripheral utilization of glucose in pregnancy. III. Insulin intolerance. Obstet Gynecol 1956;2:558–664.
62. Fisher PM, Sutherland HW, Bewsher PD. The insulin response to glucose infusion in normal human pregnancy. Diabetologia 1980;19:15–20.
63. Buchanan TZ, Metzger BE, Freinkel N, et al. Insulin sensitivity and β-cell responsiveness to glucose during late pregnancy in lean and moderately obese women with normal glucose tolerance or mild gestational diabetes. Am J Obstet Gynecol 1990;162:1008–1014.
64. Ryan EA, O'Sullivan MJ, Skyler JS. Insulin action during pregnancy: studies with the euglycemic clamp technique. Diabetes 1985;34:380–389.
65. Hay WW, Sparks JW, Wilkening RB, et al. Partition of maternal glucose production between conceptus and maternal tissues in sheep. Am J Physiol 1983;245:E347–350.
66. Marconi AM, Paolini C, Buscaglia M, et al. The impact of gestational age and fetal growth on the maternal-fetal glucose concentration difference. Obstet Gynecol 1996;87:937–942.
67. Bellman O, Hartman E. Influence of pregnancy on the kinetics of insulin. Am J Obstet Gynecol 1975;122:829–833.
68. Lind T, Bell S, Gilmore E. Insulin disappearance rate in pregnant and non-pregnant women and in non-pregnant women given GHRIH. Eur J Clin Invest 1977;7:47–51.
69. Burt RL, Davidson IWF. Insulin half-life and utilization in normal pregnancy. Obstet Gynecol 1974;43:161–170.
70. Goodner CJ, Freinkel N. Carbohydrate metabolism in pregnancy: the degradation of insulin by extracts of maternal and fetal structures in the pregnant rat. Endocrinology 1959;65:957–967.
71. Catalano PM, Calles J, Mead P, et al. Pancreatic beta cell secretion and metabolic clearance rate of insulin in pregnant control subjects and women with gestational diabetes. Abstract #S-111, Society for Gynecologic Investigation, Toronto, Canada, March 31–April 3, 1993.
72. Polonsky KS. Lilly Lecture 1994. The β cell in diabetes: from molecular genetics to clinical research. Diabetes 1995;44:705–717.
73. Calles-Escadon J, Robbins DC. Loss of early phase of insulin release in humans impairs glucose tolerance and blunts thermic effects of glucose. Diabetes 1987;36:1167–1172.
74. Hellerman B. The islets of Langerhans in the rat during pregnancy and lactation with special reference to the changes in the B/A cell ratio. ACTA Obstet Gynecol Scand 1960;39:331–342.
75. Van Assche FA, Aerts L, De Prins F. A morphological and histoenzymatic study of the endocrine pancreas in non-pregnant and pregnant rats. Am J Obstet Gynecol 1974;118:39–41.

76. Kalkhoff RK, Kim HJ. Effects of pregnancy on insulin and glucose secretion by perfused rat pancreatic islets. Endocrinology 1978;102:623–631.
77. Phelps RL, Bergenstal R, Freinkel N, et al. Carbohydrate metabolism in pregnancy. XIII. Relationships between plasma insulin and proinsulin during late pregnancy in normal and diabetic patients. J Clin Endocrinol 1975;41:1085–1091.
78. Kuhl C. Serum proinsulin in normal and gestational diabetic pregnancy. Diabetologia 1976;12:295–300.
79. Hauguel S, Gilbert M, Girard J. Pregnancy-induced insulin resistance in liver and skeletal muscles of the conscious rabbit. Am J Physiol 1987;252:E165–169.
80. Catalano PM, Drago NM, Highman T. Longitudinal changes in amino acid sensitivity during pregnancy. Abstract for Society for Gynecologic Investigation, Philadelphia, PA, March 20–23, 1996.
81. Costrini NV, Kalkhoff RK. Relative effects of pregnancy, estradiol and progesterone on plasma insulin and pancreatic islet insulin secretion. J Clin Invest 1971;50:992–999.
82. Spellacy WN, Buhi WC, Birk SA. The effect of estrogens on carbohydrate metabolism: glucose, insulin and growth hormone studies on one hundred and seventy-one women ingesting premarin, mestranol, and ethinyl estradiol for six months. Am J Obstet Gynecol 1972;114:378–392.
83. Kalkhoff RK, Jacobson M, Lemper D. Progesterone, pregnancy and the augmented plasma insulin response. J Clin Endocrinol 1970;31:24–28.
84. Nelson T, Schulman G, Grainger D, Diamond MP. Progesterone administration induced impairment of insulin suppression of hepatic glucose production. Fertil Steril 1994;62:491–496.
85. Sutter-Dub MT, Dazey B, Vergnaad MT, et al. Progesterone and insulin resistance in the pregnant rat. Diabetes Metab (Paris) 1981;7:97–104.
86. Gibson M, Tulchinsky D. The maternal adrenal. In: Tulchinsky D, Ryan KJ, eds. Maternal-fetal endocrinology. Philadelphia: Saunders, 1980:129–143.
87. Rizza RA, Mandarino LJ, Gerich JE. Cortisol-induced insulin resistance in man: impaired suppression of glucose production and stimulation of glucose utilization due to a postreceptor defect of insulin action. Clin Endocrinol Metab 1982;54:131–138.
88. Osathanondh R, Tulchinsky D. Placental polypeptide hormones. In: Tulchinsky D, Ryan KJ, eds. Maternal-fetal endocrinology. Philadelphia: Saunders, 1980:17–42.
89. Beck P, Daughaday WH. Human placental lactogen: studies of its acute metabolic effects and disposition in normal man. J Clin Invest 1967;46:103–110.
90. Kalkhoff RK, Richardson BL, Beck P. Relative effects of pregnancy, human placental lactogen and prednisolone on carbohydrate tolerance in normal and subclinical diabetic subjects. Diabetes 1969;18:153–175.
91. Gustafson AB, Banasiak MF, Kalkhoff RK. Correlation of hyperprolactinemia with altered plasma insulin and glucagon: similarity to effects of late human pregnancy. J Clin Endocrinol Metab 1980;51:242–246.
92. Gustafson A, Banasiak M, Kalkhoff R, et al. Prolactin-induced hyperinsulinemia (abstract). Clin Res 1978;26:720A.
93. Pilkis SJ, Granner D. Molecular physiology of the regulation of hepatic gluconeogenesis and glycolysis. Annu Rev Physiol 1992;54:885–909.
94. Phelps RL, Metzger BE, Freinkel N. Diurnal profiles of glucose, insulin, free fatty acids, triglycerides, cholesterol, and individual amino acids in late normal pregnancy. Am J Obstet Gynecol 1981;140:730–736.
95. Amatruda JM, Livingston JN, Lockwood DH. Cellular mechanisms in selected states of insulin resistance: human obesity, glucocorticoid excess, and chronic renal failure. Diabetes Metab Rev 1985;1:293–317.
96. Melasson MD, Matschinsky FM. Pancreatic islet glucose metabolism and regulation of insulin secretion. Diabetes Metab Rev 1986;2:163–175.
97. Landgraf R, Kotler-Brajburg J, Matschinsky FM. Kinetics of insulin from the perfused rat pancreas caused by glucose, glucoseamine and galactose. Proc Natl Acad Sci USA 1971;68:546–549.
98. Hellman B, Lernmark B, Sehlin J, et al. Effects of phlorizin on metabolism and function of pancreatic b-cells. Metabolism 1972;21:60–65.
99. Froguel P, Vaxillaire M, Sun F, et al. Close linkage of glucokinase locus on chromosome 7p to early-onset noninsulin-dependent diabetes mellitus. Nature 1992;356:162–167.
100. Vionnet N, Stoffel M, Taqkeda J, et al. Nonsense mutation in the glucokinase gene causes early-onset noninsulin-dependent diabetes mellitus. Nature 1992;356:721–726.
101. Vehlo G, Froguel P, Clement K, et al. Primary pancreatic beta-cell secretory defect caused by mutations in glucokinase gene in kindreds of maturity onset diabetes of the young. Lancet 1992;340:444–448.
102. Byrne MM, Sturis J, Clemment K, et al. Insulin secretory abnormalities in subjects with hyperglycemia due to glucokinase mutations. J Clin Invest 1994;93:1120–1129.
103. Ziel F, Venkatesan N, Davidson M. Glucose transport is rate limiting for skeletal muscle glucose metabolism in normal and streptozotocin induced diabetic rats. Diabetes 1988;37:885–890.
104. Wolfe BM, Klein S, Peters EJ, et al. Effect of elevated free fatty acids on glucose oxidation in normal humans. Metabolism 1988;37:323–329.
105. Rennie MJ, Holloszy JO. Inhibition of glucose uptake and glycogenolysis by availability of oleate in well-oxygenated perfused skeletal muscle. Biochem J 1977;168:161–170.
106. Rothman DL, Magnusson I, Cline G, et al. Decreased muscle glucose transport/phosphorylation is an early defect in the pathogenesis of non-insulin-dependent diabetes mellitus. Proc Natl Acad Sci USA 1995;92:983–987.
107. Bell GI, Kayano T, Buse JB, et al. Molecular biology of mammalian glucose transporters. Diabetes Care 1990;13:198–216.
108. Shepherd PR, Gibbs EM, Wesslau C, et al. Human small intestine facilitative fructose/glucose transporter GLUT5 is also present in insulin responsive tissues and brain: investigation of biochemical characteristics and translocation. Diabetes 1992;41:1360–1365.
109. Friedman JE, Dudek RW, et al. Immunolocalization of glucose transporter GLUT4 within human skeletal muscle. Diabetes 1991;40:150–154.

110. National Diabetes Data Group. Classification and diagnosis of diabetes mellitus and other categories of glucose intolerance. Diabetes 1979;28:1039–1057.
111. White P. Pregnancy complicating diabetes. Am J Med 1949;7:609–616.
112. Srikanta S, Ganda OP, Rabizadeh A, et al. First-degree relatives of patients with type 1 diabetes mellitus, islet cell antibodies and abnormal insulin secretion. N Engl J Med 1985;313:461–464.
113. Olmos P, A'Hearn R, Heaton DA, et al. The significance of the concordance rate of type 1 (insulin-dependent) diabetes in identical twins. Diabetologia 1988;31:747–750.
114. Diamond MP, Reece EA, Caprios L, et al. Impairment of counterregulatory hormone responses to hypoglycemia in pregnant women with insulin-dependent diabetes mellitus. Am J Obstet Gynecol 1992;166:70–77.
115. Rosenn BM, Middounik M, Khoury JC, et al. Counter-regulatory hormonal responses to hypoglycemia during pregnancy. Obstet Gynecol 1996;87:568–574.
116. Weiss PAM, Hofman H. Intensified conventional insulin therapy for the pregnant diabetic patient. Obstet Gynecol 1984;64:629–637.
117. McManus RM, Ryan EA. Insulin requirements in insulin-dependent and insulin-requiring GDM women during the final month of pregnancy. Diabetes Care 1992;15:1323–1327.
118. Schmitz O, Klebe J, Moller J, et al. In vivo insulin action in type 1 (insulin-dependent) diabetic pregnant women as assessed by the insulin clamp technique. J Clin Endocrinol Metab 1985;61:877–881.
119. Sims EAH, Calles-Escadon J. Classification of diabetes: a fresh look for the 1990's? Diabetes Care 1990;13:1123–1128.
120. Newman B, Selby M-C, Slemenda C, et al. Concordance for type 2 (non-insulin dependent) diabetes mellitus in male twins. Diabetologia 1987;30:763–768.
121. Elbein SC, Bragg KL, Hoffman MD, et al. The genetics of NIDDM. Diabetes Care 1994;17:1523–1533.
122. Steel JM, Irvine WJ, Clark BF. The significance of pancreatic islet cell antibody and abnormal glucose tolerance during pregnancy. J Clin Lab Immunol 1980;4:83–86.
123. Ginsberg-Fellner F, Mark EM, Nechemias C, et al. Autoantibodies to islet cells: comparison of methods (Letter). Lancet 1982;2:1218.
124. Catalano PM, Tyzbir ED, Sims EAH. Incidence and signficance of islet cell antibodies in women with previous gestational diabetes mellitus. Diabetes Care 1990;13:478–482.
125. Ward WK, Johnson CLW, Beard JC, et al. Abnormalities of islet β-cell function, insulin action, and fat distribution in women with histories of gestational diabetes: relationship to obesity. J Clin Endocrinol Metab 1985;61:1039–1045.
126. Catalano PM, Bernstein IM, Wolfe RR, et al. Subclinical abnormalities of glucose metabolism in subjects with previous gestational diabetes. Am J Obstet Gynecol 1986;155:1255–1263.
127. Yen SCC, Tsai CC, Vela P. Gestational diabetogenesis: quantitative analysis of glucose-insulin interrelationship between normal pregnancy and pregnancy with gestational diabetes. Am J Obstet Gynecol 1971;111:792–800.
128. Fisher PM, Sutherland HW, Bewsher PD. The insulin response to glucose infusion in gestational diabetes. Diabetologia 1980;19:10–14.
129. Catalano PM, Tyzbir ED, Wolfe RR, et al. Carbohydrate metabolism during pregnancy in control subjects and women with gestational diabetes. Am J Physiol 1993;264:E60–67.
130. Garvey WT, Maianu L, Hancock JA, et al. Gene expression of GLUT4 in skeletal muscle from insulin-resistant patients with obesity, IGT, GDM, and NIDDM. Diabetes 1992;41:465–475.
131. Ciraldi TP, Kettel M, El-Roeiy A, et al. Mechanisms of cellular insulin resistance in human pregnancy. Am J Obstet Gynecol 1994;170:635–641.
132. Garvey WT, Maianu L, Zhu JH, et al. Multiple defects in the adipocyte glucose transport system cause cellular insulin resistance in gestational diabetes. Diabetes 1993;42:1773–1785.
133. Yri-Jarvinen H, Koivisto VA. Natural course of insulin resistance in type 1 diabetes. N Engl J Med 1986;315:224–230.
134. Pagano G, Cassader M, Massobrio M, et al. Insulin binding to human adipocytes during late pregnancy in healthy, obese and diabetic state. Horm Metab Res 1980;1212:177–181.
135. Hjollund E, Pedersen O, Espersen T, et al. Impaired insulin receptor binding and post-binding defects of adipocytes from normal and diabetic pregnant women. Diabetes 1982;35:598–603.
136. Ciraldi TP, Kettel M, El-Roeiy A, et al. Mechanisms of cellular insulin resistance in human pregnancy. Am J Obstet Gynecol 1994;170:635–641.
137. Davidson MB. Insulin resistance of late pregnancy does not include the liver. Metab Clin Exp 1984;33:532–537.
138. Martinez C, Ruiz P, Andres A, et al. Tyrosine kinase activity of liver insulin receptor is inhibited in rats at term gestation. Biochem J 1989;263:267–272.
139. Damm P, Handber A, Kuhl C, et al. Insulin receptor binding and tyrosine kinase activity in skeletal muscle from normal pregnant women and women with gestational diabetes. Obstet Gynecol 1993;82:251–259.
140. Toyoda N, Deguchi T, Murata K, et al. Postbinding insulin resistance around parturition in the isolated rat epitrochlearis muscle. Am J Obstet Gynecol 1991;165:1475–1480.
141. Garvey WT, Maianu L, Zhu JH, et al. Multiple defects in the adipocyte glucose transport system cause cellular insulin resistance in gestational diabetes. Diabetes 1993;42:1773–1185.
142. Friedman JE, Ishizuka T, Huston L, et al. Altered expression of insulin signaling intermediates in human skeletal muscle during late gestation. Diabetes 1996;45(suppl 2):57A.
143. McGuire MC, Fields RM, Nyomba BL, et al. Abnormal regulation of protein tyrosine phosphatase activities in skeletal muscle of insulin-resistant humans. Diabetes 1991;40:939–942.

144. Thompson DB, Degregorio M, Sommercorn J. Insulin resistance alters immediate early gene expression in human skeletal muscle in vivo. Diabetes 1992;41(suppl 1):89A.
145. Kusari J, Kenner KA, Suh KI, et al. Skeletal muscle protein tyrosine phosphatase activity and tyrosine phosphatase 1B protein content are associated with insulin action and resistance. J Clin Invest 1994;93:1156–1159.
146. Halberstam M, Cohen N, Shlimovich P, et al. Oral vanadyl sulfate improves insulin sensitivity in NIDDM but not obese nondiabetic subjects. Diabetes 1996;45:659–666.
147. Carey JO, Azevedo JL, Morris PG, et al. Oxalaic acid, vanadate, and phenylarsine oxide stimulate 2-deoxyglucose transport in insulin-resistant human skeletal muscle. Diabetes 1995;44(6):682–686.
148. Posner BI, Faure R, Burgess JW, et al. Peroxovandium compounds—a new class of potent phosphotyrosine phosphatase inhibitors which are insulin mimetics. J Biol Chem 1994;269:4596–4602.
149. Elberg G, Li J, Shechter Y. Vanadium activates or inhibits receptor and nonreceptor protein tyrosine kinases in cell-free experiments, depending on its oxidation state. J Biol Chem 1994;269:9521–9526.
150. Leahy JL. Detrimental effects of chronic hyperglycemia on the pancreatic b-cell. In: LeRoith D, Taylor SI, Olefsky JM, ed. Diabetes mellitus, a fundamental and clinical text. Philadelphia: Lippincott-Raven, 1996:103–113.
151. Pfifer MA, Halter JB, Porte D. Insulin secretion in diabetes mellitus. Am J Med 1981;70:579–584.
152. Garvey WT, Olefsky JM, Griffin J, et al. The effect of insulin treatment on insulin secretion and insulin action in type II diabetes mellitus. Diabetes 1985;34:222–227.
153. Hotamisligil GS, Spiegelman BM. TNF alpha: a key component of obesity-diabetes link. Diabetes 1994;43:1271–1283.
154. Lang C, Dobrescu C, Bagby G. Tumor necrosis factor impairs insulin action on peripheral glucose disposal and hepatic glucose output. Endocrinology 1992;130:43–48.
155. Hurel S, Ofei F, Wells A. TNF-alpha and insulin sensitivity in humans: effects in vivo of antibody blockade in obese NIDDM patients and in vitro upon human cultured myotubes. Exp Clin Endocrinol Diabetes 1996;104(suppl 2):59.
156. Hotamisligil GS, Arner P, Caro JF, et al. Increased adipose tissue expression of tumor necrosis factor-alpha in human obesity and insulin resistance. J Clin Invest 1995;95(5):2409–2415.
157. Saghizadeh M, Ong JM, Garvey WT, et al. The expression of TNF alpha by human muscle. Relationship to insulin resistance. J Clin Invest 1996;97(4):1111–1116.
158. Hotamisligil GS, Shargill NS, Spiegelman BM. Adipose expression of tumor necrosis factor alpha: direct role in obesity-linked insulin resistance. Science 1993;259:87–90.
159. Hotamisligil GS, Peraldi P, Budavari A, et al. IRS-1 mediated inhibition of insulin receptor tyrosine kinase activity in TNF-alpha and obesity-induced insulin resistance. Science 1996;271:665–668.
160. Catalano P, Highman T, Huston L, et al. Relationship between reproductive hormones/TNF-alpha and longitudinal changes in insulin sensitivity during gestation. Diabetes 1996;45(suppl 2):175a.
161. Kjos SL, Buchanan TA, Greenspoon JS, et al. Gestational diabetes mellitus: the prevalence of glucose intolerance in diabetes mellitus in the first two months post-partum. Am J Obstet Gynecol 1990;163:93–99.
162. O'Sullivan JB. Diabetes mellitus after GDM. Diabetes 1991;40(suppl 2):131.
163. Kahn CR. Insulin action, diabetogenes, and the cause of type II diabetes (Banting lecture). Diabetes 1994;43:1066–1084.
164. Flier JS. Syndromes of insulin resistance. From patient to gene and back again. Diabetes 1992;41:1207–1219.
165. Bogardus C. Insulin resistance in the pathogenesis of NIDDM in Pima Indians. Diabetes Care 1993;16:228–231.
166. Warram JH, Krolewski AS, Gottleib MS. Differences in risk of insulin dependent diabetes in offspring of diabetic mothers and fathers. N Engl J Med 1984;311:149–152.
167. Martin AO, Simpson JL, Ober C, et al. Frequency of diabetes mellitus in mothers of probands with gestational diabetes: possible maternal influence on the predisposition to gestational diabetes. Am J Obstet Gynecol 1985;151:471–475.
168. Ekoe JM, Thomas F, Balkau B, et al. Effect of maternal diabetes on the pattern of selected insulin resistance syndrome parameters in normal glucose tolerance subjects of two Algonquin Indian communities in Quebec. Diabetes Care 1996;19:822–826.
169. Klein BEK, Klein R, Moss SE, et al. Parental history of diabetes in a population based study. Diabetes Care 1996;19:827–830.
170. Gauguir D, Bihoreau MT, Ktorza A, et al. Inheritance of diabetes mellitus as consequence of gestational hypoglycemia in rats. Diabetes 1990;39:734–739.
171. Van Assche FA, Aerts L. Long-term effect of diabetes and pregnancy in the rat. Diabetes 1985;34(suppl 2):116–118.
172. Holemans K, Aerts L, Van Assche FA. Evidence for an insulin resistance in the adult offspring of pregnant streptozotocin-diabetic rats. Diabetologia 1991;34:81–85.
173. Valdlamuoi S, Kalhan S, Patel MS. Persistence of metabolic consequences in the presence of rats fed a high carbohydrate (HC) formula in their early postnatal life. Am J Physiol 1995;269(Endocrinol Metab 32):E731–738.
174. Laychock SG, Vadlamuoi S, Patel MS. Neonatal rat dietary carbohydrate affects pancreatic insulin secretion in adults and progeny. Am J Physiol 1995;269(Endocrinol Metab 32):E739–744.
175. Pettitt DJ, Nelson RG, Saad MF, et al. Diabetes and obesity in the offspring of Pima Indian women with diabetes during pregnancy. Diabetes Care 1993;16:310–314.
176. Silverman BC, Metzger BE, Cho NH, et al. Impaired glucose intolerance in adolescent offspring of diabetic mothers. Diabetes Care 1995;18:611–617.
177. Pedersen J. Weight and length at birth of infants of diabetic mothers. Acta Endocrinol 1954;16:330–343.
178. Holemans K, Van Bree R, Verhaeghe J, et al. In vivo glucose utilization by individual tissues in virgin and pregnant offspring of severely diabetic rats. Diabetes 1993;42(4):530–536.
179. Dooley SL, Metzger BE, Cho N. Gestational diabetes:

influence of race on disease prevalence and perinatal outcome in a U.S. population. Diabetes 1991;40(suppl 2):25.
180. Gloria-Bottini F, Gerlini G, Lucarini N. Both maternal and foetal genetic factors contribute to macrosomia of diabetic pregnancy. Hum Hered 1994;44:24–30.
181. Kaufman RC, Amankwah KS, Dunaway G, et al. An animal model of gestational diabetes. Am J Obstet Gynecol 1981;141:479–482.
182. Kaufmann RC, Amankwah KS, Colliver JA, et al. Diabetic pregnancy: the effect of genetic susceptibility for diabetes on fetal weight. Am J Perinatol 1987;4:72–74.

11
Protein Metabolism in Pregnancy

Satish C. Kalhan

Gestation in humans and animals is associated with profound anatomic, physiologic, and metabolic adaptation in the mother in order to support the needs of the growing conceptus. Although glucose is the primary source of energy for the fetus, protein accretion is an essential component for fetal growth and the synthesis of new fetal and maternal tissues. Therefore, study of protein and nitrogen metabolism has interested a number of investigators over the past many years. Using contemporary methods, these investigators have attempted to examine alterations in protein metabolism throughout mammalian pregnancy, their efforts often leading to conflicting results. This chapter discusses these data, with particular focus on human pregnancy. These results and methodologic problems, as they relate to quantification of protein metabolism, are emphasized.

The minimum protein costs of pregnancy in humans have been studied in the following ways: (1) chemical analysis of the fetus, other products of conception, and maternal pregnancy-induced tissue growth; (2) nitrogen balance techniques wherein the difference between daily nitrogen intake and nitrogen losses is measured and calculated; (3) calculations of fat-free body nitrogen accumulation based on whole-body accumulation of potassium as measured by ^{40}K counting; and (4) estimates of gain in fat-free body mass by body density and total body water measurements (see Chapter 47).

Direct and indirect chemical analysis of fetal and maternal tissues in humans have suggested that the total protein cost of pregnancy is approximately 925 g, or 148 g nitrogen.[1] Calloway[2] pointed out that a discrepancy (3345 g) existed between the estimated and observed gain in the weight of the pregnancy-related tissues and that if this difference is also included in lean body mass, the actual protein cost of pregnancy in humans will increase to 250 g nitrogen.

Nitrogen balance studies in the human have shown nitrogen retention in excess of the theoretical protein cost throughout pregnancy.[3] This remains true even when careful accounting for the unmeasured nitrogen losses such as in hair, nails, sweat, exhaled ammonia, and vaginal secretions is made.[3] These data support the concept that maternal nitrogen gain in the form of lean body mass represents a significant protein cost over and above that deposited in the fetus and products of conception.[4] Similar conclusions were drawn when the increase in lean body mass was estimated by ^{40}K counts in pregnant teenagers.[4] It should be pointed out that in lean adult tissue potassium (K) and nitrogen (N) are deposited in a constant ratio of 2.7 mEq K per gram N. However, the K/N ratio of fetal and maternal tissue deposited during pregnancy has been found to be lower than that in the normal adult. Whole-carcass analysis of the human infant showed a K/N ratio of 2.15 mEq·g N^{-1} [5], and the ratio in fetal and maternal tissue has been shown to be similar.[6] Recognition of this change in K/N ratio is important when one calculates N retention using ^{40}K counting method.

Using morphometric methods in combination with body density, tracer measurement of total body water and ^{40}K counting, Pipe et al.[1] measured changes in body composition during normal pregnancy and postpartum. Total body potassium incorporation was used to derive the fat-free mass accumulated during pregnancy. Their data showed a net accretion of 0.92 kg lean tissue between 12 and 37 weeks of gestation, which represents 29.4 g of nitrogen or a nitrogen accretion rate of 0.17 g·day^{-1}. These cited studies point to the discrepancies in measurement of nitrogen accretion in the mother and the fetus in the human. These differences may be related to the analytical methods or the subject population studied. In any case, these data point to the need for more accurate estimation of nitrogen/protein metabolism in vivo.

Plasma Amino Acids in Pregnancy

Inasmuch as changes in plasma amino acids may reflect the overall alterations in maternal protein metabolism, a

TABLE 11.1. Plasma amino acid levels in nonpregnant and pregnant women at 16 to 20 weeks' gestation after a 12-hour fast.

	Concentration ($\mu mol \cdot L^{-1}$), mean ± SEM		
Amino acid	Nonpregnant women ($n = 11$)	Pregnant women ($n = 12$)	p
Taurine	51.5 ± 2.5	36.0 ± 2.9	<.001
Threonine	138.0 ± 11.3	150.9 ± 7.0	
Serine	126.3 ± 6.0	107.4 ± 4.6	<.025
Proline	151.3 ± 10.1	93.8 ± 4.9	<.001
Citrulline	27.2 ± 1.2	18.9 ± 0.8	<.001
Glycine	197.4 ± 14.6	120.8 ± 7.6	<.001
Alanine	279.3 ± 15.1	221.6 ± 9.0	<.005
α-Aminobutyrate	22.0 ± 3.1	20.4 ± 1.6	
Valine	201.4 ± 11.7	169.8 ± 3.9	<.025
Cystine	94.8 ± 5.4	69.1 ± 3.0	<.001
Methionine	18.0 ± 1.7	16.7 ± 0.7	
Isoleucine	51.4 ± 2.7	47.0 ± 1.8	
Leucine	99.5 ± 2.0	91.0 ± 2.5	<.025
Tyrosine	40.4 ± 3.3	34.5 ± 1.7	
Phenylalanine	45.8 ± 2.4	42.3 ± 1.1	
Ornithine	71.8 ± 7.6	33.7 ± 5.0	<.001
Lysine	164.1 ± 12.1	175.8 ± 13.9	
Histidine	81.4 ± 5.5	100.7 ± 5.7	<.025
Arginine	55.5 ± 6.6	51.0 ± 7.6	

Data from Felig et al.,[8] with permission.

number of investigators have examined plasma amino acid concentrations through pregnancy in humans and animals. It has been recognized for a long time that pregnancy in humans and in animals is characterized by hypoaminoacidemia. Felig et al.,[8] in a study of normal pregnant women at between 16 and 19 weeks' gestation observed a significant reduction in most amino acids in the postabsorptive state (Table 11.1). Similar decreases in plasma amino acid concentrations have been documented by other investigators.[9-14] As has been described in relation to glucose, adaptive changes in maternal plasma amino acids can be seen early in gestation, prior to significant changes in total body water and expansion in plasma volume.[8,9,11,12] Although, the plasma concentration of total alpha-amino nitrogen tends to decrease further as gestation advances, the change is not statistically significant.[9,12] Between 30 and 40 weeks' gestation, the mean total serum amino acid concentration in nine subjects after a 14 hour fast was $3.21 \pm 0.18 \, mmol \cdot L^{-1}$ (mean ± SEM) as compared with 3.92 ± 0.17 ($p < .05$) during the postpartum period.[9] Postpartum, a rapid increase in the plasma amino acid concentration was demonstrated by Gard and Handley;[15] however, the pattern and time course of these increases differed with different amino acids. A decrease in plasma amino acid concentration during early gestation has been demonstrated in the rhesus monkey and in the rat.[16,17] This decrease has been more marked for glucogenic amino acids. The mechanism and the significance of the pregnancy-induced plasma hypoaminoacidemia is not understood. Because this early gestation hypoaminoacidemia cannot be explained simply due to volume expansion, a role of pregnancy-related hormone progesterone and placental lactogen has been postulated.[18,19] In addition studies by Pastor-Anglada et al.[20] have shown that at least in the rat pregnancy hypoaminoacidemia is not due to any changes in specific tissue amino acid pool.

Effect of Fasting and Feeding

The plasma amino acid response to fasting has been reported in the human in early gestation by Felig et al.[8] and in the pregnant rat by Metzger et al.[21] During 48 hours of fasting in the 20-day pregnant rat, a rapid and profound reduction in gluconeogenic amino acids (e.g., alanine, serine, threonine, glutamine, and glutamate), was observed. These changes occurred coincident with the development of maternal hypoglycemia. The investigators speculated that the low blood glucose concentration in the mother may be related to a limitation in the availability of glucogenic substrates.[21] In contrast, fasting in humans in early gestation resulted in only a small decrease in plasma alanine concentration.[8] The changes in other amino acids were qualitatively similar to those seen in fasting nonpregnant women, except that the changes were observed early in fasting, thus supporting the concept of "accelerated starvation."[22] Because alanine is considered a key glucogenic substrate, a reduction in its circulating concentration was considered to be of primary importance in the limitation of hepatic gluconeogenesis during prolonged starvation in nonpregnant subjects. These investigators speculated that substrate (i.e., alanine) lack contributed to the fasting hypoglycemia characteristic of pregnancy.[8]

Studies in the human during late gestation have demonstrated that the plasma amino acid response to a standardized calorie intake are of lower magnitude as well as of lesser duration.[23,24] These plasma amino acid responses to feeding are in contrast to the exaggerated glucose, triglyceride, and insulin responses seen in these subjects.[23,25] It is possible that the heightened insulin response may result in accelerated uptake of these amino acids. On the other hand, a delay in digestion of ingested protein and absorption of amino acids from the gut cannot be excluded.[24]

As discussed above, the significance of the change in circulating amino acids is not well understood. It could be a mechanism to conserve maternal amino nitrogen and make it available for fetal utilization. The concentrations of circulating amino acids have been related to the fetal outcome, in particular birth weight, by three groups of investigators, both in early and late human gestation.[26-28] Their data show a positive correlation between total amino acid concentrations and certain individual amino acids (e.g., serine, threonine, lysine, proline, ornithine, and arginine), and neonatal birth weight.[26] In addition, the concentration of total amino acids in plasma from gestationally malnourished (i.e., small for gestational age) infants was significantly lower than that from mothers having normal neonates.[27] These studies suggest that the homeostatic changes in maternal amino acids may have important influence both on maternal metabolism and on fetal growth and body weight.

Urea Synthesis During Pregnancy

Urea is the end product of protein catabolism and estimates of the rates of urea excretion have been used to assess protein catabolism and oxidation. The rates of urea synthesis have been measured in the human and in the rat either during fasting or in response to the administration of exogenous amino acids. Studies in the pregnant rat have demonstrated an attenuated rise in blood urea concentration in response to intraperitoneal administration of alanine or casein hydrolysate.[29] Similarly Metzger et al.[30,31] observed a decreased rate of urea synthesis when a supramaximal dose of alanine was administered to an isolated liver preparation from pregnant rats. The later observation was significant because the urea production was decreased in the presence of appropriate increase in glucose production and a marked increase in ammonia production in the pregnant state, suggesting an intrahepatic mechanism for the decreased urea synthesis. Nitzan and Klipper-Orbach[32] observed a lower blood urea concentration in pregnant rats at 6, 12, and 24 hours following bilateral nephrectomies as compared with nonpregnant rats, suggesting a pregnancy-induced decrease in urea synthesis. The above studies are in contrast to the studies of Herrera et al.,[34] who demonstrated an increase in total nitrogen and urea excretion rates in pregnant rats after 24 and 48 hours of fasting. Such a prolonged fast was also associated with an increase in urinary ammonia excretion that correlated with the marked ketosis and ketonuria observed in these animals. These studies in the pregnant rat late in gestation suggest a nitrogen-sparing effect of pregnancy during the immediate postabsorptive state and an increased rate of protein catabolism (i.e., "accelerated starvation") during fasting.[22]

Studies in human pregnancy late in gestation suggest a maternal adaptive response to conserve nitrogen as evidenced by a decrease in urea excretion. However, few investigators have actually quantified the rates of urea synthesis.[13,34] A decreased blood urea response to oral alanine administration in pregnant women was reported by McGarrity et al.[35] In contrast, Felig[36] found no differences in the daily excretory rates of urinary urea, ammonia and total nitrogen between nonpregnant and pregnant women following a 24-hour fast. However, the latter study was performed early in gestation, a time when fetal nitrogen accretion has not as yet significantly increased. Using stable isotope labeled [$^{15}N_2$]urea and steady-state tracer dilution method, Kalhan et al.[13] quantified the rates of urea synthesis during the antepartum and postpartum periods. Their data are displayed in Table 11.2. As shown, pregnancy was associated with a decrease in plasma urea nitrogen concentration as well as a decrease in the rate of urea nitrogen synthesis (S_U). The decrease in urea synthesis and consequent decrease in urinary urea excretion (E_U) accounted for the decrease in urinary nitrogen excretion rate (E_N) observed in pregnant subjects. The mechanism of decrease in urea synthe-

TABLE 11.2. Nitrogen metabolism in human pregnancy.

Time of assay	Plasma urea N (mg·dl^{-1})	S_U (mg·kg^{-1}hr^{-1})	E_U (mg·kg^{-1}hr^{-1})	E_{NH}^3 (mg·kg^{-1}hr^{-1})	E_N (mg·kg^{-1}hr^{-1})
Antepartum	8.22 ± 2.24[a]	4.17 ± 1.28	3.82 ± 0.86	0.24 ± 0.09	5.29 ± 1.42
Postpartum	11.49 ± 3.16[b]	6.84 ± 2.52[+]	5.68 ± 2.96	0.23 ± 0.12	7.47 ± 3.68

S_U, urea N synthesis rate; E_U urea N excretion rate; E_{NH}^3 ammonia N excretion rate; E_N total N excretion rate.
Results are mean ± SD of eight determinations.
[a,b] Significantly different by paired t-test $p < .03^a$ or $p < .002^b$ compared with antepartum.
Data from Kalhan et al.[13]

sis remains unclear. It may be the consequence of the decrease in plasma amino acid concentrations and thus a decrease in the delivery of ureogenic substrate or due to a decrease in the urea cycle activity. The available data suggest that the decreased ureogenesis, at least in man, is probably the result of a decreased hepatic extraction of circulating amino acids. Recently, Forrester et al.[34] have quantified rates of urea production in normal pregnant women in Jamaica using [^{15}N$_2$]urea tracer as intermittent intravenous dose throughout the day, and measuring the dilution of the tracer in urinary urea. Although the dietary protein and calorie intake was higher throughout pregnancy in their subjects as compared with nonpregnant controls, the urea production was not significantly increased. In fact, the urea production rate during the third trimester was significantly less than that in the first trimester. Of interest, urea salvage (i.e., reutilization of urea N) through the metabolic activity of the colonic microflora was higher in pregnancy. The investigators interpreted these data as implying heightened maternal N demands.

Alanine Metabolism in Pregnancy

As alanine is considered quantitatively a major nitrogen carrier from the skeletal muscle to the liver, and is a significant contributor to urea nitrogen in the liver, the metabolism of alanine has been examined to define the mechanism of nitrogen conservation observed during pregnancy.[37–41] Thus far, alanine metabolism has been quantified in the human[42,43] and the rat,[44–48] with conflicting results. Using stable isotope labeled L-[2,3^{13}C]alanine tracer, alanine turnover and its incorporation into glucose were examined by Kalhan et al.[41,42] during isotopic steady state using the tracer dilution method. Studies were preformed in 15 normal pregnant women during the third trimester of pregnancy after an overnight fast of at least 10 hours. Their data showed that pregnancy had no significant effect either on circulating alanine concentration or on the rate of alanine turnover (Table 11.3). However, the fraction of alanine carbon incorporated into glucose was significantly reduced in the pregnant subjects. Because the pregnant subjects had a higher respiratory quotient (0.83 ± 0.04 vs 0.77 ± 0.02, $p < .005$) as compared with nonpregnant subjects, suggesting increased carbohydrate oxidation, the fraction of alanine carbon appearing in CO_2 was slightly increased, although not statistically significant. Similar results (i.e., unchanged alanine kinetics) have been reported in well-controlled diabetic subjects during pregnancy.[42] In contrast to the studies in humans, a significant increase in alanine turnover rate was observed by Pastor-Anglada et al.[43] in pregnant rats studied at 12 days of gestation (Table 11.3). These studies were performed in the fed state using L-[2,3,^{3}H$_2$]alanine tracer. In addition, alanine degradation rate quantified by the appearance of [^{3}H]tracer in body water was also significantly increased. The fractional extraction of alanine by the liver, measured by changes in hepatic afferent and efferent vessels, was also increased by day 12 of gestation.[44] These investigators further demonstrated an increased alanine utilization by isolated hepatocytes from the pregnant rats[45,46] and a greater capacity for Na$^+$-dependent transport in plasma membrane vesicles from livers of pregnant rats at 12 and 21 days gestation.[45] Similarly increased hepatic uptake of alanine during pregnancy in rats has been demonstrated by other investigators.[47] In addition, isolated liver and hepatocyte preparation from pregnant rats show an increased capacity to incorporate alanine C into glucose.[30,47]

It is important to recognize that Pastor-Anglada et al.[43] utilized [^{3}H]alanine to quantify alanine turnover in pregnant rats. As shown by Yang et al.,[48] [^{3}H] labeled alanine, as a result of greater loss of tracer (possibly due to futile cycling), gives rise to higher estimates of alanine turn-

TABLE 11.3. Alanine metabolism in pregnancy of humans and rats.

Subject	Blood alanine ($\mu mol \cdot L^{-1}$)	Alanine turnover ($\mu mol \cdot kg^{-1} min^{-1}$)	Alanine to glucose (%)	Alanine to CO_2 (%)
Humans[a]				
Pregnant, third trimester ($n = 15$)	223.5 ± 37.2	4.43 ± 0.82	23.5 ± 8.3^b	37.8 ± 7.9
Nonpregnant ($n = 8$)	200.4 ± 46.8	4.11 ± 1.08	30.8 ± 8.2	33.0 ± 5.8
			Alanine degradation ($\mu mol \cdot kg^{-1} min^{-1}$)	
Rats[c]				
Pregnant, gestation 12 days ($n = 6$)	214 ± 12	35.5 ± 3.0^d	26.4 ± 2.3^d (74%)	
Virgin ($n = 6$)	250 ± 25	26.6 ± 2.1	17.5 ± 2.2 (66%)	

Values are given as mean ± SD.
[a] Data of Kalhan et al.[41,42] [2,3,^{13}C$_2$]alanine tracer.
[b] $p < .03$ compared with nonpregnant subjects.
[c] Data of Pastor-Anglada et al.[43] [2,3,^{3}H$_2$]alanine tracer.
[d] $p < .05$ compared with controls.

over. Thus, the higher rate of alanine turnover observed by these investigators may be due to a greater rate of futile cycling of alanine to pyruvate. In addition, they performed their measurements during the fed state, only 2 hours after the removal of food. The increase in hepatic uptake and catabolism as documented above are in contrast with other studies in rats, which show a decreased hepatic alanine transaminase activity,[49] or lack of an increase in hepatic gluconeogenesis in response to a load of alanine in fasted rats during late pregnancy.[50] The conflict in data from various studies in rat pregnancy is probably related to the nutritional state of the animal (e.g., duration of fast, etc.) and the in vivo or in vitro nature of the study.

Nonetheless, in contrast to studies in humans, data in the rat suggest an increased alanine turnover and increased hepatic uptake during pregnancy. The observed differences may be related to species differences, differences in the fetal maternal weight ratio in these species, experimental conditions such as duration of fasting and anesthesia, and may be related to the characteristics of the experimental model used (e.g., isolated liver, hepatocytes, etc). In any case, these data suggest a central role of liver in the regulation of urea nitrogen flux and nitrogen-sparing during pregnancy. At least in the case of the rat, this regulation is not related to a decreased uptake of one of the ureogenic amino acid (i.e., alanine) and may be due to an intracellular mechanism.[51,52]

As suggested by Pastor-Anglada,[51] either a low ornithine content or a depletion of N-acetyl-glutamate may be responsible for this change. In addition, a decreased activity of hepatic alanine aminotransferase has been demonstrated late in gestation in the rat.[49]

Protein Turnover in Pregnancy

Very few studies have examined the dynamic aspects of protein metabolism in vivo during pregnancy in humans or other mammalian species. Furthermore, failure to control a number of experimental variables (e.g., time of gestation, calorie and protein intake) and lack of appropriate nonpregnant control groups, make these data difficult to interpret. In addition, as discussed by Kalhan et al.,[41] a major problem in terms of expression of data in the pregnant subjects remains. Should the quantitative data be expressed in relation to unit mass or in relation to prepregnancy weight remains unresolved. This is particularly important when protein kinetic studies are considered. Pregnancy in the human and other mammalian species is associated with increase in body weight, which is a sum of the total fetal mass and changes in maternal body weight. In small mammals with a large fetal to maternal body weight ratio, the body weight changes are influenced by the mass of the conceptus; in larger mammals with a small fetal to maternal body weight ratio, the body weight reflects mostly changes in the maternal body weight. The latter is a composite change in the multiple body compartments including protein and fat. Probably, the dynamic aspects of protein metabolism should best be expressed in relation to the total protein mass of the mother and conceptus. Estimation of the protein mass is difficult during pregnancy, particularly in the human. Thus, the protein kinetics data should be interpreted with caution particularly when comparisons are made between different mammalian species. At best, attempts have been made to express the experimental data based on the estimates of fat free mass.[53]

Protein Turnover and Its Measurement

It has long been recognized that the body proteins are in a constant state of flux or turnover consisting of both breakdown and resynthesis (see Chapter 34). Since this process of breakdown and synthesis requires energy, and since protein turnover in vivo has been shown to be related to energy consumption,[54-57] much attention has been focused at quantifying the dynamic aspects of protein turnover in vivo. In addition, it has also been demonstrated that protein accretion (i.e., growth) is closely related to protein turnover.[56] Rapidly growing organisms such as the fetus and neonate have a higher rate of protein turnover when compared with a mature adult.[58,59] A simplified model for the whole-body protein metabolism in vivo is shown in Figure 11.1. As shown, the breakdown of proteins intracellularly results in the liberation of free amino acids, which are also the precursor pool for the synthesis of new proteins. The intracellular amino acid pool is in equilibrium with the plasma amino acids. The other sources of plasma amino acids are the dietary ingested proteins. The amino acids/proteins are catabolized and excreted either as breath CO_2 or urinary nitrogen. As shown in Figure 11.2, in cases of pregnancy this simple model is made more complex by the fetal amino acid pool and fetal protein metabolism, which further contributes to the maternal plasma amino acid pool. However, the fetal contribution to the overall protein metabolism in the mother remains difficult to quantify in humans.

A number of isotopic tracer methods have been employed for the measurement of whole-body protein turnover. These have been reviewed by Waterlow et al.[60,61] and Williams et al.[62] These methods can be classified into two types: (1) direct, where the incorporation of the tracer amino acid into proteins is measured;[62-64] and (2) indirect, where the turnover of an essential amino acid (i.e., an amino acid that is not synthesized in vivo, such as leucine,[65,66] lycine,[67] or phenylalanine,[68]) is quantified, or the turnover of the total body nitrogen, such as by [^{15}N]glycine tracer, is measured.[69] By knowing the flux of

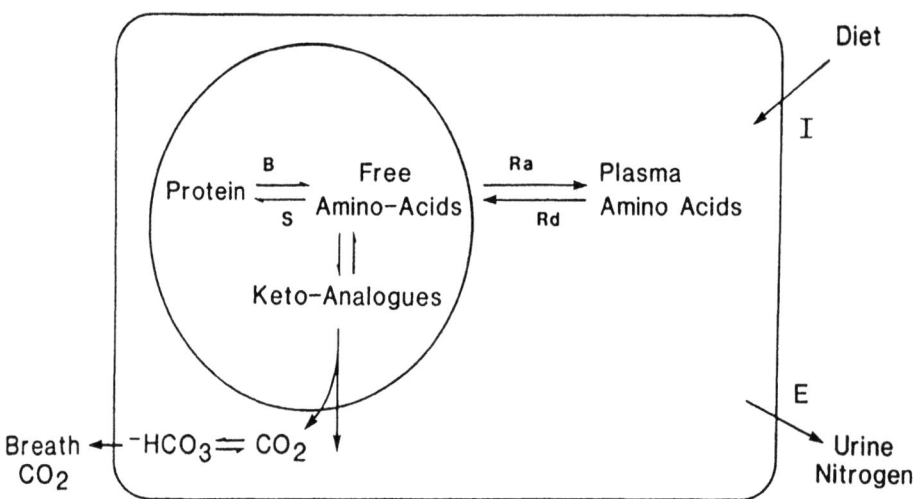

FIGURE 11.1. Simplified model for the whole-body protein metabolism in vivo. As shown, breakdown (B) of proteins results in free amino acids within the cell. This intracellular amino acid pool is the precursor pool for protein synthesis (S). The sources of plasma amino acids include the intracellular amino acid pool and the dietary ingested protein (I). The catabolism of protein is represented by urinary nitrogen (E) and expired carbon dioxide. As discussed in the text, protein breakdown and synthesis can be estimated by measuring the turnover rate and oxidation of essential amino acids in the plasma using tracer dilution techniques.

the essential amino acid and its catabolism, the amount of amino acid available for protein synthesis can be calculated by a simple balance equation. For such measurements, the whole-body protein pool is considered to be a single, well-mixed pool. By knowing the fraction of the specific amino acid in body proteins, the synthesis and breakdown rates of whole-body proteins can be calculated. The advantages and disadvantages, along with the limitations, of these tracer methods have been reviewed.[60,61]

Whole-Body Amino Acid and Nitrogen Kinetics in Pregnancy

As discussed above, whole-body kinetics of essential amino acids have been utilized to estimate the rates of protein breakdown and synthesis. Using [^{15}N]leucine tracer, Krishnamurti and Schaefer[70] quantified the rates of leucine turnover in five pregnant ewes at 111 to 124 days' gestation. The tracer was infused at constant rate for 8 hours. Although they did not report data on non-

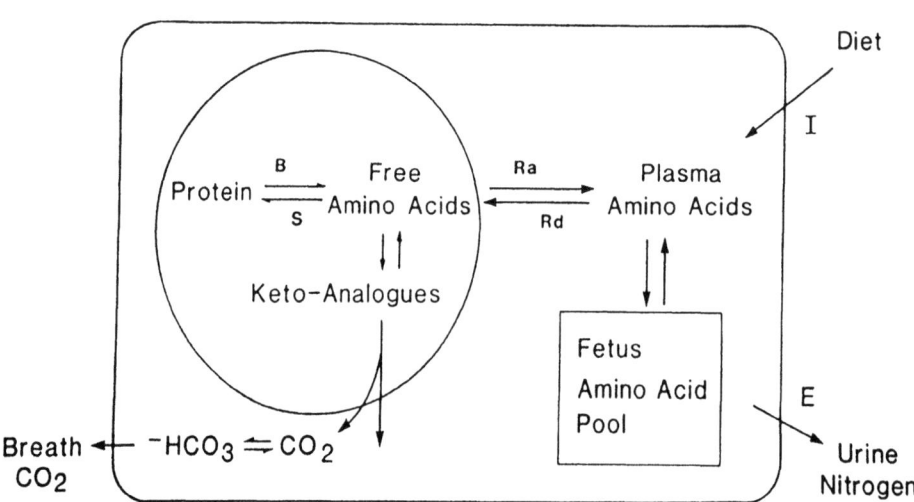

FIGURE 11.2. Model for protein metabolism in pregnancy. The essential components are similar to those in Figure 11.1 except for the addition of the fetal and placental amino acid pools and the fetal-placental protein turnover and protein catabolism. In humans the fetal contribution to the overall maternal-fetal protein metabolism cannot be quantified because of ethical considerations.

pregnant sheep in that study, such data were presented subsequently on nonpregnant ewes that were studied under similar conditions.[71] The rates of leucine turnover quantified by tracer dilution method in pregnant ewes who had free access to feed and water during tracer infusion, was $60.2 \pm 12.1 \,\mu\text{mol}\cdot\text{kg}^{-1}\text{hr}^{-1}$ (mean $\pm$ SD, $n = 5$, range 43.3–$72\,\mu\text{mol}\cdot\text{kg}^{-1}\text{hr}^{-1}$). This rate of leucine flux was almost 50% of that reported by the same investigators in three nonpregnant ewes—mean $135\,\mu\text{mol}\cdot\text{kg}^{-1}\text{hr}^{-1}$ ($n = 3$; $143, 118, 145\,\mu\text{mol}\cdot\text{kg}^{-1}\text{hr}^{-1}$). Because the animals had free access to feed during the isotopic tracer infusion and because the dietary intake during the study could not be that were quantified, the effect of pregnancy on leucine/protein turnover could not be measured. However if one assumes similar dietary intake during the study period, these data would suggest a decreased rate of leucine turnover in pregnant ewes. Inasmuch as leucine turnover is an indirect measure of body protein breakdown rate, these data indicate a lower protein breakdown rate during pregnancy in sheep late in gestation. The effect of pregnancy on the rate of leucine/protein oxidation was not measured in these studies.

The effect of pregnancy on whole-body leucine kinetics in the rat was examined by Ling et al.[72] using [1-^{14}C]leucine tracer. Pregnant rats were studied at day 17 and 20 of gestation. Again, these investigators also did not include nonpregnant animals as controls. Their data are displayed in Table 11.4 along with the data in nonpregnant rat from Vazquez et al.[73] Whole-body leucine flux appears to be higher in pregnant rats at day 17 and 20 of gestation. However, when expressed per 100g body weight, whole-body leucine flux appears to be actually lower than in the nonpregnant animals. In contrast, both the fraction of leucine turnover oxidized and the total amount of leucine oxidized appear to be higher in the pregnant animals. Of significance, the fraction of leucine turnover oxidized decreased from day 17 to day 20. Finally, leucine incorporation into protein appears to remain unchanged in the pregnant rat or, if at all, a small increase was observed in these postabsorptive rats at day 20 of gestation. These data demonstrate a small increase in protein/leucine turnover and a marked increase in leucine oxidation in the pregnant rat. These data are particularly of interest since the rat has a relatively high fetal/maternal mass ratio as compared with, for example, humans, and would be expected to have a high rate of protein turnover. Inasmuch as leucine oxidation is considered a measure of protein oxidation, the study of Ling et al.[72] would suggest increased contribution of protein to oxidative metabolism in rat pregnancy, a conclusion not supported by other available data from animal and human pregnancies.

Mayel-Afshar and Grimble[74] serially quantified the changes in protein metabolism with advancing gestation in the rat using [^{14}C]tyrosine tracer. Their data are displayed in Table 11.5. In contrast to the leucine turnover data, a marked increase in the total tyrosine flux was seen by day 17 of gestation. The increase in tyrosine flux persisted even when the data were normalized per 100g body weight. Although the fraction of tyrosine oxidized was significantly lower on days 17 and 21 of gestation as compared with nonpregnant rats, the total amount of tyrosine oxidized was decreased only on day 21 of gestation. The decreased rate of tyrosine oxidation is consistent with the decreased rate of protein oxidation as measured by rates of urea synthesis.

Taken as a whole, the leucine and tyrosine flux data in the rat indicate an increase in whole-body amino acid and therefore protein turnover in pregnancy. However, certain inconsistencies remain. Since leucine and tyrosine, respectively, constitute 7% and 3% of whole-body protein in the rat, an increase in whole-body protein turn-

TABLE 11.4. Whole-body leucine kinetics in rats.

Leucine kinetics	Nonpregnant rats[a]	Pregnant rats[b]	
		Day 17	Day 20
Concentration ($\mu\text{mol}\cdot\text{ml}^{-1}$)	0.090 ± 0.010	0.110 ± 0.004	0.130 ± 0.010
Flux			
($\mu\text{mol}\cdot\text{hr}^{-1}$)	62.7 ± 5.1	74.3 ± 4.9	78.5 ± 2.9
($\mu\text{mol}\cdot 100\text{g}^{-1}\text{hr}^{-1}$)	43.2 ± 3.5	28.0^c	30.4^c
Oxidation			
$\mu\text{mol}\cdot\text{hr}^{-1}$	11.3 ± 0.8	25.4 ± 2.6	25.0 ± 2.4
% Oxidized	18.0^c	39.2 ± 2.3	31.7 ± 1.9^d
Incorporation into protein ($\mu\text{mol}\cdot\text{hr}^{-1}$)	47.7 ± 5.4	48.8 ± 3.3	53.6 ± 1.5

Results are given as mean $\pm$ SE.
[a] Data of Vasquez et al.[73] $n = 7$; male fed rats.
[b] Data of Ling et al.[72] $n = 7$; studies performed after a 12-hour fast.
[c] Calculated from mean data.
[d] $p < .05$ compared with day 17.

TABLE 11.5. Whole-body tyrosine kinetics in pregnant rats.

Parameter	Day 0	Day 8	Day 12	Day 17	Day 21
Flux					
μmol/hr	77 ± 5	86 ± 9	90 ± 5	125 ± 3	117 ± 16[a]
μmol·100 g^{-1}·hr^{-1}	31	32.5	32.4	42.2	34.9
Oxidation					
μmol·hr[b]	13.1	14.4	14.7	17.9	11.9
μmol·100 g^{-1}·hr[b]	5.3	5 + 5	5 + 3	6.0	3.6
% Oxidized	17.50 ± 0.45	16.69 ± 0.35	16.32 ± 1.08	14.36 ± 0.25[c]	10.2 ± 0.85[c]

Results are given as mean ± SE.
[a] Significantly different from nonpregnant values, $p < .05$.
[b] Calculated from mean data.
[c] Significantly different from nonpregnant values, $p < .001$.
Data from Mayel-Afshar and Grimble.[74]

over should result in proportionally greater increase in leucine turnover as compared with tyrosine turnover. Instead, actual measurements show a greater increase in tyrosine turnover than leucine turnover (Tables 11.4 and 11.5), suggesting that pregnancy-related changes in protein turnover are not necessarily uniformly manifested and that there probably is a more marked increase in turnover of certain proteins containing greater amounts of tyrosine.

Studies in Humans

Whole-body protein turnover was quantified by de Benoist et al.[75] in a cross-sectional study of Jamaican women during normal pregnancy. Six different subjects were studied at 12, 24, and 33 weeks' gestation. After appropriate dietary preparation, [^{15}N]glycine tracer was administered orally by a slight modification of Picou and Taylor-Roberts'[76] method. Six nonpregnant subjects were studied as controls. The nitrogen flux was calculated form the ^{15}N enrichment in both urea and ammonia. The data revealed higher nitrogen flux rate in early gestation. There was greater variation when enrichments in urea were used for calculation of flux rate than when enrichments in ammonia were used. The nitrogen flux calculated from the harmonic average, which assumes equal rates of flux in the two pools, is displayed in Table 11.6. As shown, the nitrogen flux was higher in pregnant subjects as compared with nonpregnant subjects; however, the differences were not statistically significant. Furthermore, the nitrogen flux was higher in early gestation and decreased toward the end of pregnancy. Similarly, the calculated rate of protein synthesis and breakdown was also lower at 33 weeks' gestation as compared with that at 12 weeks. There was also a small decrease in protein oxidation with advancing gestation. Again, the calculated rates of protein synthesis were higher in pregnant women as compared with nonpregnant women, while protein oxidation was slightly, although not significantly, decreased in pregnancy.

In contrast to the study of de Benoist et al.,[75] Fitch and King,[77] in their study of eight pregnant and nine nonpregnant women, did not show any effect of pregnancy on protein turnover, protein synthesis, and catabolism. In this study [^{15}N]glycine tracer was administered orally as a single dose and protein metabolism was quantified from the excretion of ^{15}N in urinary ammonia over the next 10 hours. Interestingly, even though Fitch and King had used ^{15}N ammonia enrichments to calculate protein turnover, their data were similar or slightly higher than that of de Benoist et al. Because [^{15}N]glycine studies are done during normal feeding, these differences in the two studies may be the result of differences in dietary nitrogen intake and because of the differences in the experimental protocol (i.e., single dose versus repeated multiple oral doses of the tracer glycine). Denne et al.[78] quantified

TABLE 11.6. Whole-body protein and nitrogen metabolism in human pregnancy.

		Pregnant women		
Parameter	Nonpregnant women ($n = 6$)	12 Weeks ($n = 6$)	24 Weeks ($n = 6$)	33 Weeks ($n = 6$)
Nitrogen flux (mg N·kg^{-1}·day^{-1})	524.5 ± 43.5	770.2 ± 89.0	664.9 ± 34.6	561.9 ± 29.6
Protein synthesis (g·kg^{-1}·day^{-1})	1.86 ± 0.37	3.79 ± 0.54	2.81 ± 0.34	2.13 ± 0.18
Protein breakdown (g·kg^{-1}·day^{-1})	1.72 ± 0.36	3.26 ± 0.46	2.29 ± 0.39	1.37 ± 0.36
Protein oxidation (g·kg^{-1}·day^{-1})	1.05 ± 0.21	1.03 ± 0.24	0.98 ± 0.39	0.91 ± 0.26

Results are given as mean ± SE.
Data from deBenoist et al.[75]

FIGURE 11.3. Leucine flux and oxidation rates in relation to gestational age in human pregnancy during fasting. Each data point represent one subject. (From Denne et al.,[78] with permission.)

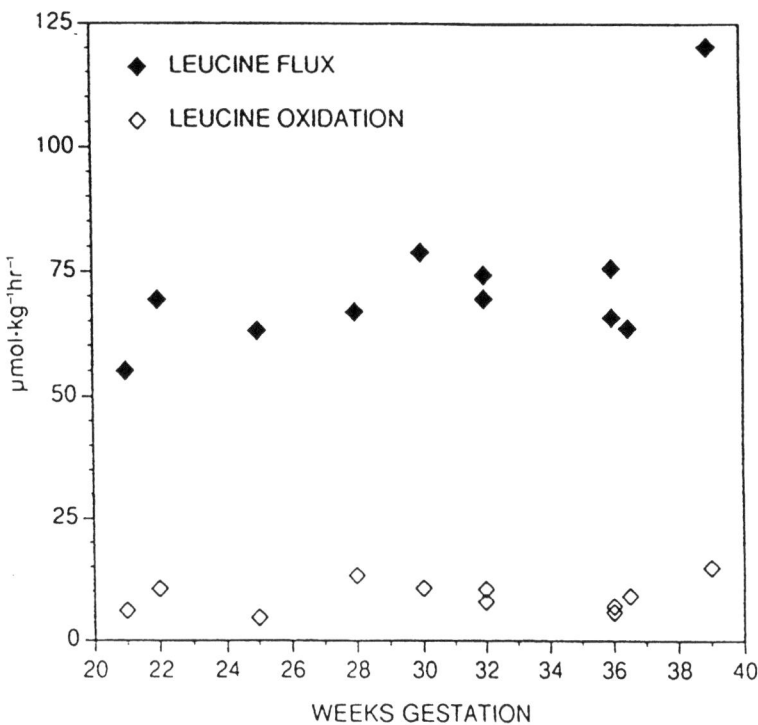

whole-body rates of leucine turnover in 11 women during the third trimester of pregnancy along with quantification of rates of urea nitrogen excretion and respiratory quotient. The data of leucine flux (turnover) and oxidation are displayed in Figure 11.3. In this cross-sectional study, there was no significant change in leucine kinetics between 20 and 40 weeks' gestation. When compared with nonpregnant women, there was a significant decrease in leucine turnover during pregnancy (pregnant $68.2 \pm 7.0\,\mu mol\cdot kg^{-1}hr^{-1}$, mean ± SD; nonpregnant $81.7 \pm 12.5\,\mu mol\cdot kg^{-1}hr^{-1}$, $p < .01$). As before, urea excretion rate was also lower in pregnancy. Similar observations have been reported in well-controlled diabetes in pregnancy.[79] Finally, Thompson and Halliday[53] studied six women serially through pregnancy using [^{13}C]leucine, and expressed the protein turnover data based on their estimation of fat-free mass. Their data suggest, based on fat-free mass, an increase in the rate of protein breakdown and synthesis with advancing gestation. Since leucine turnover is considered to reflect whole-body protein breakdown rate, these data indicate that fasting, in the third trimester of human pregnancy, does not result in increased proteolysis. Thus, the studies of whole-body protein turnover in the human suggest a slight decrease in protein breakdown rate during fasting,[75,78] or an increase if the data are expressed based on fat-free mass,[53] and a small increase in nitrogen turnover throughout the day.[77]

All these data should be considered with caution because (1) the cross-sectional nature of studies may have masked the differences, if any, between pregnant and nonpregnant states; and (2) there may be a change in the kinetics of tracer glycine and its various compartments during pregnancy, which may affect the results of whole-body protein kinetics. The differences in leucine and tyrosine kinetics in the rat[72,74] may be due to differences in metabolism of these two amino acids in pregnancy, or may reflect a greater increase in the turnover of proteins with a greater tyrosine content.

Partitioning of the Whole-Body Protein Metabolism in Pregnancy

The measured whole-body protein kinetics are a sum of the kinetics of a large number of proteins, some turning over at more rapid rates than others. Therefore, measurement of whole-body kinetics may mask significant changes in individual components; for example, an acceleration or increase in one component may be balanced by a deceleration or decrease in another component. Therefore, attempts have been made to quantify the contribution of individual tissues (e.g., liver, skeletal muscle, uterus, and fetus) to whole-body protein kinetics in pregnancy. The protein kinetics in the individual tissue is quantified by measuring the specific activity of an amino acid (e.g., leucine, tyrosine, or valine) free in the plasma or tissue homogenate and covalently bound in protein during the infusion of tracer amino acid or following a flooding dose of tracer amino acids. As summarized by Attaix et al.,[80] the tissue protein fractional synthesis rate (FSR $\%\cdot day^{-1}$) is highest in the liver followed by small

TABLE 11.7. Protein metabolism in skeletal muscle in pregnancy.

Parameter	Day 0	Day 8	Day 12	Day 17	Day 21
Rat (gastrocnemius)[a]					
Weight (g)	5.38	5.88	5.93	6.24	6.13
Protein (F)	0.025	0.026	0.024	0.025	0.025
K_s/day	0.037	0.049	0.048	0.042	0.037
K_d/day		0.023	0.063	0.022	0.04
Prot sy (g·day^{-1})	0.027	0.045	0.041	0.040	0.035
Prot br (g·day^{-1})		0.021	0.054	0.021	0.038
Rat (rectus)[b]					
K_s/day				0.034	0.034
Prot sy (g·day^{-1})				0.65	0.51
Mouse (gastrocnemius)[c]		Virgin	Day 10	Day 18	
K_s/day		0.049	0.049	0.049	
Prot sy/day (mg·day^{-1})		2.23	2.26	2.44	

F, fraction; K_s, fractional protein synthesis; K_d, fractional protein destruction; Prot sy, protein synthesis; Prot br, protein breakdown.
Only mean data are presented.
[a] Data of Mayel-Afshar and Grimble[82] using [^{14}C]tyrosine tracer.
[b] Data of Ling et al.[72] using [^{14}C]leucine tracer.
[c] Data of Millican et al.[83] using [4^{3}H]phenylalanine tracer.

intestine, skin, and muscle, in descending order across several animal species. However, because of its large mass, skeletal muscle contributes the most (~33%) to the whole-body protein synthesis.

Skeletal Muscle

Measurements of protein synthesis and breakdown rates in skeletal muscle of the pregnant rat remain inconsistent.[81] Mayel-Afshar and Grimble,[82] using [^{14}C]tyrosine, quantified the changes in protein metabolism in the gastrocnemius muscle of pregnant rats throughout gestation. Their data (Table 11.7) show that there was very little change in the protein content of the skeletal muscle during pregnancy, and the fractional rate of protein synthesis and the total protein synthesis appeared to increase in early pregnancy (i.e., days 8 and 12) followed by a decrease later in gestation. The decrease was most apparent on day 21 of gestation. These data are in contrast to those of Ling et al.[72] in the rat and of Millican et al.[83] in the mouse, which did not demonstrate any change in the protein metabolism in the gastrocnemius muscle during late gestation. The reasons for these differences are not readily apparent and may be related to the isotopic tracer used and the tracer infusion method utilized.

The changes in the skeletal muscle protein metabolism in humans were examined by quantifying the rate of urinary excretion of 3-methylhistidine (3-MH) during pregnancy.[84] 3-Methylhistidine is a characteristic amino acid of contractile protein actin and the heavy chain of myosin in skeletal muscle. During the intracellular breakdown of these proteins, 3-MH is released and because it is not reutilized, the urinary excretion rate of 3-MH has been used as a measure of the breakdown rate of the skeletal muscle myofibrillar protein both in human subjects and in rats.[85] However, as discussed by Rennie and Millward,[86] a number of problems, particularly the contribution of the rapidly turning over nonskeletal muscle proteins, cast doubt on the validity of this method. In spite of these flaws, 3-MH excretion has been reported in two studies of human pregnancy. Naismith and Emery[84] serially measured 3-MH excretion in eight women throughout pregnancy at 5-week intervals. Their data showed no consistent change in early or midpregnancy, and a marked increase in 3-MH excretion from the 30th to 35th week of gestation. However, they did not correct the dada for the urinary creatinine excretion or for the weight of the subject. Fitch and King[77] studied nine nonpregnant and eight pregnant women at 30–36 weeks' gestation on a standardized diet. It is significant to note that the subjects were not on a meat-free diet so that dietary meat protein may have contributed to the 3-MH excretion. These investigators observed a significantly higher rate of 3-MH excretion during pregnancy (pregnant 0.157 ± 0.015 μmol·mg creatinine^{-1}, nonpregnant 0.121 ± 0.26, mean ± SD), suggesting an increased rate of muscle protein breakdown late in gestation.

In summary, the data regarding changes in skeletal muscle protein metabolism in pregnancy remain controversial. It is likely that alterations in skeletal muscle protein turnover make minimal contribution to the adaptation in protein metabolism in the pregnant mother.

The lack of any significant effect on skeletal muscle protein metabolism is also consistent with the unchanged rates of alanine turnover, observed by Kalhan et al.[41,42] in humans during the third trimester of pregnancy.

Liver

Estimates of rates of hepatic protein synthesis have been performed in studies of the pregnant rat and mouse.[72,82] In this context, it should be recognized that hepatic proteins consist of two distinct components: (1) the fixed proteins, and (2) the soluble liver-produced secretory proteins. As pointed out by Garlick et al.,[64] if the latter are not included in the measurements of protein synthesis, e.g., in the constant rate infusion method in which the liver-produced protein will leave the hepatic tissue by the time steady-state measurements are made, it will result in an underestimation with persistent lower values of the hepatic protein synthesis rate. At least this argument has been used to explain the lower rates observed with constant rate amino acid infusion method as compared with the single-dose flooding methods. The data from three studies quantifying the liver protein metabolism in pregnancy are summarized in Table 11.8. As shown, with the advancing gestation in the pregnant rat, and with the increase in the mother's body weight, there is an increase in the weight of the liver. Although the total protein content also increased with gestation, the fraction of liver weight represented by proteins showed only a small increase from 15% to 18%. However, a significant increase in the fractional rate of protein synthesis was observed irrespective of the tracer amino acid used, whether it was tyrosine or leucine. Furthermore, in the study of Millican et al.,[83] who used the phenylalanine flooding dose method and thus included the liver produced secretory proteins in their measurement, an almost 75% increase in daily fractional rate of protein synthesis was observed. Because the total hepatic protein content also increased during gestation, an increase in the fractional synthesis rate indicated an increase in the absolute rate of protein synthesis. The small decrease in the hepatic protein content between days 17 and 21 would suggest a greater rate of hepatic protein breakdown as compared with synthesis. Similarly an increased 47% incorporation of labeled leucine into protein per unit of RNA—ribosomal activity—or hepatic protein synthesis was demonstrated by Harris and Kretchmer[87] in an in vitro liver ribosomal preparation from the pregnant rat.

Thus, all the studies in the pregnant rat taken together point to a key adaptive role for the liver in relation to amino acid and protein metabolism. At least in rat pregnancy, there is a marked increase in hepatic protein turnover throughout gestation, with a marked increase in the absolute and fractional rate of protein synthesis and breakdown. In the rat, the last part of gestation is characterized by a greater increase in hepatic protein breakdown rate relative to the rate of protein synthesis. Such a change would result in a net increase in amino acid efflux from the liver. These amino acids may become available for fetal protein synthesis.

Uterus

During pregnancy, the uterus undergoes major adaptive growth in order to accommodate the growing conceptus. Studies by Morton and Goldspink[88] have shown that in the rat, this uterine growth involves both cellular hypertrophy and hyperplasia.

Quantitative measurements of the protein turnover in the pregnant uterus using [^{3}H]phenylalanine by the flooding dose method show that although the total rate of protein synthesis increases markedly in the second half of gestation (day 0, 17.2 ± 3.2 g·day^{-1} vs day 20, 245 ± 44 g·day^{-1}), the fractional rate of protein synthesis (K_s) did not change (44 ± 5%·day^{-1}). Thus, the growth and protein accretion by the uterus is the result of a decrease in the rate of protein breakdown. Such a conclusion is also supported from the measured decrease in the specific activity of uterine hydrolase cathepsin D.[88]

Fetus

Although no direct quantitative measurements of fetal protein turnover are available in the human, the data in

TABLE 11.8. Liver protein metabolism in rat pregnancy.

Gestation (days)	Body weight (g)	Liver weight (g)	Protein (g)	Fractional protein synthesis by tracer amino acid (K_s·day^{-1})		
				Tyrosine[a]	Leucine[b]	Phenylalanine[c]
0	246.00	9.62	1.5 (15.6%)	0.544	—	0.643
10					0.656	
17	296.00	12.10	1.82 (15.0%)	0.525	0.573	—
18						1.12
21	335.00	11.00	1.98 (18.0%)	0.636	0.787	—

K_s, fractional protein synthesis.
[a] Data of Mayel-Afshar and Grimble.[82]
[b] Data of Ling et al.[72]
[c] Data of Millican et al.[83]

the human neonate, both premature and term, and studies in sheep fetus indicate a higher rate of protein turnover in the fetus as compared with the adult.[60,89-93] Further, studies in the sheep fetus suggest a decline in the fractional rate of protein synthesis and breakdown with advancing gestation, i.e., as the size of the fetus increases.[91,92] The magnitude of the fetal contribution to the overall protein metabolism in the pregnant subject remains undetermined. At least in large mammals where the fetal maternal body weight ratio is low, the fetal contribution to the overall amino acid/protein flux would be expected to be low. Chien et al.[94] have quantified leucine and phenylalanine accretion by the human fetus at term gestation. Pregnant women undergoing elective cesarean section were infused with [1-^{13}C]leucine and [^{15}N]phenylalanine tracers, and tracer-tracee gradients across the umbilical and uterine circulations were quantified. Their data show a net fetal uptake of leucine ($2.22 \pm 0.29\,\mu mol \cdot kg^{-1} min^{-1}$) and phenylalanine ($0.80 \pm 0.11\,\mu mol \cdot kg^{-1} min^{-1}$) with net outputs of CO_2 ($6.11 \pm 1.12\,ml \cdot kg^{-1} min^{-1}$) and of α-ketoisocaproic acid ($1.04 \pm 0.32\,\mu mol \cdot kg^{-1} min^{-1}$). They estimated fetal whole-body accretion of leucine C to be 69% of the umbilical uptake. Fetal phenylalanine accretion was 78% of the umbilical uptake. These data, although of interest, should be interpreted with caution because of the rapid changes in umbilical circulation at the time of delivery of the fetus.

References

1. Hytten FE, Leitch I. The gross composition of the components of weight gain. In: The physiology of human pregnancy. 2nd ed. London: Blackwell Scientific, 1971:371–387.
2. Calloway DH. Nitrogen balance during pregnancy. In: Winick M, ed. Nutrition and fetal development. New York: Wiley, 1972:79–94.
3. King JC. Protein metabolism during pregnancy. Clin Perinatol 1975;2:243–254.
4. King JC, Calloway DH, Morgen S. Nitrogen retention, total body ^{40}K and weight gain in teenage pregnant girls. J Nutr 1973;103:772–785.
5. Fee BA, Weil WB Jr. Body composition on infants of diabetic mothers by direct analysis. Ann N Y Acad Sci 1963;110(II):869–897.
6. Forbes GB. Pregnancy. In: Anonymous human body composition. New York: Springer-Verlag, 1987:196–208.
7. Pipe NGJ, Smith T, Halliday D, et al. Changes in fat, fat-free mass and body water in human normal pregnancy. Br J Obstet Gynaecol 1979;86:929–940.
8. Felig P, Kim YJ, Lynch V, et al. Amino acid metabolism during starvation in human pregnancy. J Clin Invest 1972;51:1195–1202.
9. Cox BD, Calame DP. Changes in plasma amino acid levels during the human menstrual cycle and in early pregnancy. A preliminary report. Horm Metab Res 1978;10:428–433.
10. Metzger BE, Unger RH, Freinkel N. Carbohydrate metabolism in pregnancy. XIV. Relationships between circulation glucagon, insulin, glucose and amino acids in response to a "mixed meal" in late pregnancy. Metabolism 1977;26:151–156.
11. Christensen PJ, Date JW, Schonheyder F, Volqvartz K. Amino acids in blood plasma and urine during pregnancy. Scand J Clin Lab Invest 1957;9:54–61.
12. Schoengold DM, DeFiore RH, Parlett RC. Free amino acids in plasma throughout pregnancy. Am J Obstet Gynecol 1978;131:490–499.
13. Kalhan SC, Tserng K, Gilfillan C, Dierker LJ. Metabolism of urea and glucose in normal and diabetic pregnancy. Metabolism 1982;31:824–833.
14. Lindblad BS, Baldesten A. The normal venous plasma free amino acid levels of non-pregnant women and of mother and child during delivery. Acta Paediatr Scand 1967;56:37–48.
15. Gard PR, Handley SL. Human plasma amino acid changes at parturition. Horm Metab Res 1985;17:112.
16. Kerr GR. The free amino acids of serum during development of *Macaca mulatta* II. During pregnancy and fetal life. Pediatr Res 1968;2:493–500.
17. Pastor-Anglada M, Remesar X. Development of the gestational plasma hypoaminoacidemia in the rat. Comp Biochem Physiol 1986;85A:735–738.
18. Landau RL, Lugibihl K. The effect of progesterone on the concentration of plasma amino acids in man. Metabolism 1967;16:1114–1122.
19. Handwerker S, Fellows RE, Crenshaw MC, et al. Ovine placental lactogen: acute effects on intermediary metabolism in pregnant and non-pregnant sheep. J Endocr 1976;69:133–137.
20. Pastor-Anglada M, Lopez-Tejero D, Remesar X. Free amino acid pools in some tissues of the pregnant rat. Horm Metab Res 1986;18:590–594.
21. Metzger BE, Hare JW, Freinkel N. Carbohydrate metabolism in pregnancy IX: plasma levels of gluconeogenic fuels during fasting in the rat. J Clin Endocrinol Metab 1971;33:869–872.
22. Freinkel N, Metzger BE, Nitzan M, et al. "Accelerated starvation" and mechanisms for the conservation of maternal nitrogen during pregnancy. Israel J Med Sci 1972;8:426–439.
23. Phelps RL, Metzger BE, Freinkel N. Carbohydrate metabolism in pregnancy. XVII. Diurnal profiles of plasma glucose, insulin, free fatty acids, triglycerides, cholesterol, and individual amino acids in late normal pregnancy. Am J Obstet Gynecol 1981;140:730–736.
24. Fitch WL, King JC. Plasma amino acid, glucose, and insulin responses to moderate-protein and high-protein test meals in pregnant, nonpregnant, and gestational diabetic women. Am J Clin Nutr 1987;46:243–249.
25. Metzger BE, Phelps RL, Freinkel N, Navickas IA. Effects of gestational diabetes on diurnal profiles of plasma glucose, lipids, and individual amino acids. Diabetes Care 1980;3:402–409.
26. Kalkhoff RK, Kandaraki E, Morrow PG, et al. Relationship between neonatal birth weight and maternal plasma amino

acid profiles in lean and obese nondiabetic women and in type I diabetic pregnant women. Metabolism 1988;37:234–239.
27. McClain PE, Metcoff J, Crosby WM, Costiloe JP. Relationship of maternal amino acid profiles at 25 weeks of gestation to fetal growth. Am J Clin Nutr 1978;31:401–407.
28. Moghissi KS, Churchill JA, Kurrie D. Relationship of maternal amino acids and proteins to fetal growth and mental development. Am J Obstet Gynecol 1975;15:398–410.
29. Beaton GH. Urea formation in the pregnant rat. Arch Biochem Biophys 1957;67:1–9.
30. Metzger BE, Agnoli FS, Hare JW, Freinkel N. Carbohydrate metabolism in pregnancy X. Metabolic disposition of alanine by the perfused liver of the fasting pregnant rat. Diabetes 1973;22:601–612.
31. Metzger BE, Agnoli FS, Freinkel N. Effect of sex and pregnancy on formation of urea and ammonia during gluconeogenesis in the perfused rat liver. Horm Metab Res 1970;2:367–368.
32. Nitzan M, Klipper-Orbach J. Effects of pregnancy on the development of acute uremic syndrome in the rat. Israel J Med Sci 1976;12:129–133.
33. Herrera E, Knopp RH, Freinkel N. Carbohydrate metabolism in pregnancy. VI. Plasma fuels, insulin, liver composition, gluconeogenesis, and nitrogen metabolism during late gestation in the fed and fasted rat. J Clin Invest 1969;48:2260–2272.
34. Forrester T, Badaloo AV, Persaud C, Jackson AA. Urea production and salvage during pregnancy in normal Jamaican women. Am J Clin Nutr 1994;60:341–346.
35. McGarrity WJ, McHenry HB, Van Wyck HB, et al. An effect of pyridoxine on blood urea in human subjects. J Biol Chem 1949;178:511–516.
36. Felig P. Maternal and fetal fuel homeostasis in human pregnancy. Am J Clin Nutr 1973;26:998–1005.
37. Galim EB, Hruska K, Bier DM, et al. Branched-chain amino acid nitrogen transfer to alanine in vivo in dogs. Direct isotopic determination with [15N]leucine. J Clin Invest 1980;66:1295–1304.
38. Haymond MW, Miles JM. Branched chain amino acids as a major source of analine nitrogen in man. Diabetes 1982;31:86–89.
39. Felig P, Pozefsky T, Marliss E, Cahill GF Jr. Alanine: key role in gluconeogenesis. Science 1970;167:1003–1004.
40. Felig P. The glucose-analine cycle. Metabolism 1973;22:179–207.
41. Kalhan SC, Gilfillan CA, Tserng K, Savin SM. Glucose-alanine relationship in normal human pregnancy. Metabolism 1988;37:152–158.
42. Kalhan SC, Hertz RH, Rossi KQ, Savin SM. Glucose-alanine relationship in diabetes in human pregnancy. Metabolism 1991;40:629–633.
43. Pastor-Anglada M, Champigny O, Ferre P, et al. Alanine turnover rate and its hepatic metabolism are increased in midpregnant rat. Biol Neonate 1988;54:126–132.
44. Pastor-Anglada M, Remesar X, Bourdel G. Alanine uptake by liver at midpregnancy in rats. Am J Physiol 1987;252:E408–E413.
45. Felipe A, Remesar X, Pastor-Anglada M. Na$^+$-dependent alaine transport in plasma membrane vesicles from late-pregnant rat livers. Pediatr Res 1989;26:448–451.
46. Casado J, Remesar X, Pastor-Anglada M. Hepatic uptake of amino acids in late-pregnant rats. Effect of food deprivation. Biochem J 1987;248:117–122.
47. Cuezva JM, Valcarce C, Chamorro M, et al. Alanine and lactate as gluconeogenic substrates during late gestation. FEBS Lett 1986;194:219–223.
48. Yang RD, Matthews DE, Bier DM, et al. Alanine kinetics in humans: influence of different isotopic tracers. Am J Physiol 1984;247:E634–E638.
49. Palou A, Remesar X, Arola L, Alemany M. Glucose-alanine relationships during rat pregnancy and lactation. Mol Physiol 1981;1:301–309.
50. Zorzano A, Lasuncion MA, Herrera E. Role of the availability of substrates on hepatic and renal gluconeogenesis in the fasted late pregnant rat. Metabolism 1986;35:297–303.
51. Pastor-Anglada M. Letter to the editor. Metabolism 1989;38:290.
52. Kalhan SC. Response to letter to the editor. Metabolism 1989;38:290–291.
53. Thompson GN, Halliday D. Protein turnover in pregnancy. Eur J Clin Nutr 1992;46:411–417.
54. Garlick PJ. Protein turnover in the whole animal and specific tissues. In: Florkin M, Stotz EH, eds. Comprehensive biochemistry—protein metabolism, part I. Amsterdam: Elsevier, 1980:77–152.
55. Reeds PJ, James WPT. Nutrition: the changing scene; protein turnover. Lancet 1983;1:571–574.
56. Young VR, Steffee WP, Pencharz PB, et al. Total human body protein synthesis in relation to protein requirements at various ages. Nature 1975;253:192–194.
57. Garlick PJ, Clugston GA, Swick RW, Waterlow JC. Diurnal pattern of protein and energy metabolism in man. Am J Clin Nutr 1980;33:1983–1986.
58. Millward DJ, Garlick PJ, Stewart RJC, et al. Skeletal-muscle growth and protein turnover. Biochem J 1975;150:235–243.
59. Milley JR. Fetal protein metabolism. Semin Perinatol 1989;13:192–201.
60. Waterlow JC. Protein turnover in the whole animal. Invest Cell Pathol 1980;3:107–119.
61. Waterlow JC, Golden MHN, Garlick PJ. Protein turnover in man measured with ^{15}N: comparison of end products and dose regimes. Am J Physiol 1978;235:E165–E174.
62. Williams IH, Sugden PH, Morgan HE. Use of aromatic amino acids as monitors of protein turnover. Am J Physiol 1981;240:E677–E681.
63. Goldspink DF, Kelly FJ. Protein turnover and growth in the whole body, liver and kidney of the rat from the foetus to senility. Biochem J 1984;217:507–516.
64. Garlick PJ, McNurlan MA, Preedy VR. A rapid and convenient technique for measuring the rate of protein synthesis in tissues by injection of [^{3}H]phenylalanine. Biochem J 1980;192:719–723.
65. Matthews DE, Motil KJ, Rohrbaugh DK, et al. Measurement of leucine metabolism in man from a primed,

continuous infusion of L-[1-^{13}C]leucine. Am J Physiol 1980;238:E473–E479.
66. Irving CS, Thomas MR, Malphus EW, et al. Lysine and protein metabolism in young women. J Clin Invest 1986; 77:1321–1331.
67. Thompson GN, Pacy PJ, Merritt H, et al. Rapid measurement of whole body and forearm protein turnover using a [^{2}H$_5$]phenylalanine model. Am J Physiol 1989;256:E631–E639.
68. Denne SC, Kalhan SC. Leucine metabolism in human newborns. Am J Physiol 1987;253:E608–E615.
69. Stein TP, Leskiw MJ, Buzby GP, et al. Measurement of protein synthesis rates with [^{15}N]glycine. Am J Physiol 1980;239:E294–E300.
70. Krishnamurti CR, Schaefer AL. Measurement of plasma leucine flux and protein synthesis in pregnant ewes using gas chromatography and mass spectrometry. Nutr Rep Int 1987;35:683–692.
71. Krishnamurti CR, Janssens SM. Determination of leucine metabolism and protein turnover in sheep, using gas-liquid chromatography-mass spectrometry. Br J Nutr 1988;59:155–164.
72. Ling PR, Bistrian BR, Blackburn GL, Istfan N. Effect of fetal growth on maternal protein metabolism in postabsorptive rat. Am J Physiol 1987;252:E380–E390.
73. Vazquez JA, Paul HS, Adibi SA. Relation between plasma and tissue parameters of leucine metabolism in fed and starved rats. Am J Physiol 1986;250:E615–E621.
74. Mayel-Afshar S, Grimble RF. Tyrosine oxidation and protein turnover in maternal tissues and the fetus during pregnancy in rats. Biochim Biophys Acta 1982;716:201–207.
75. DeBenoist B, Jackson AA, Hall JSE, Persaud C. Whole-body protein turnover in Jamaican women during normal pregnancy. Hum Nutr Clin Nutr 1985;39C:167–179.
76. Picou D, Taylor-Roberts T. The measurement of total protein synthesis and catabolism and nitrogen turnover in infants in different nutritional states and receiving different amounts of dietary protein. Clin Sci 1969;36:283–296.
77. Fitch WL, King JC. Protein turnover and 3-methylhistidine excretion in non-pregnant, pregnant and gestational diabetic women. Hum Nutr Clin Nutr 1987;41C:327–339.
78. Denne SC, Patel D, Kalhan SC. Leucine kinetics and fuel utilization during a brief fast in human pregnancy. Metabolism 1991;12:1249–1256.
79. Kalhan SC, Denne SC, Patel DM, et al. Leucine kinetics during a brief fast in diabetes in pregnancy. Metabolism 1994;43:378–384.
80. Attaix D, Aurousseau E, Manghebati A, Arnal M. Contribution of liver, skin and skeletal muscle to whole-body protein synthesis in the young lamb. Br J Nutr 1988; 60:77–84.
81. Goldspink DF, Lewis SEM, Kelley FJ. Protein synthesis during the developmental growth of the small and large intestine of the rat. Biochem J 1984;217:527–534.
82. Mayel-Afshar S, Grimble RF. Changes in protein turnover during gestation in the foetuses, placentas, liver, muscle and whole body of rats given a low-protein diet. Biochim Biophys Acta 1983;756:182–190.
83. Millican PE, Vernon RG, Pain VM. Protein metabolism in the mouse during pregnancy and lactation. Biochem J 1987; 248:251–257.
84. Naismith DJ, Emery PW. Excretion of 3-methylhistidine by pregnant women: evidence for a biphasic system of protein metabolism in human pregnancy. Eur J Clin Nutr 1988;42:483–489.
85. Young VR, Munro HN. N^t-Methylhistidine (3-methylhistidine) and muscle protein turnover: an overview. Fed Proc 1978;37:2291–2300.
86. Rennie MJ, Millward DJ. 3-Methylhistidine excretion and the urinary 3-methylhistidine/creatinine ratio are poor indicators of skeletal muscle protein breakdown. Clin Sci 1983;65:217–225.
87. Harris JE, Kretchmer N. Synthesis of hepatic protein during pregnancy in the rat. J Nutr 1988;118:1319–1324.
88. Morton AJ, Goldspink DF. Changes in protein turnover in rat uterus during pregnancy. Am J Physiol 1986;250:E114–E120.
89. Pencharz PB. The 1987 Borden Award Lecture: protein metabolism in premature human infants. Can J Physiol Pharmacol 1988;66:1247–1252.
90. Catzeflis C, Schultz Y, Micheli J, et al. Whole body protein synthesis and energy expenditure in very low birth weight infants. Pediatr Res 1985;19:679–687.
91. Meier PR, Peterson RG, Bonds DR, et al. Rates of protein synthesis and turnover in fetal life. Am J Physiol 1981;240:E320–E324.
92. Van Veen LCP, Teng C, Hay WW Jr, et al. Leucine disposal and oxidation rates in the fetal lamb. Metabolism 1987;36:48–53.
93. Kennaugh JM, Bell AW, Teng C, et al. Ontogenetic changes in the rates of protein synthesis and leucine oxidation during fetal life. Pediatr Res 1987;22:688–692.
94. Chien PFW, Smith K, Watt PW, et al. Protein turnover in the human fetus studied at term using stable isotope tracer amino acids. Am J Physiol 1993;265:E31–E35.

12
Lipid Metabolism in Pregnancy

Robert H. Knopp, Bartolome Bonet, and Xiaodong Zhu

It is not a new idea that lipid metabolism is altered during pregnancy. Virchow[1] and Becquerel and Rodier[2] observed lipemia during pregnancy in the 19th century and concluded that it represented an elevation in plasma lipids. It is also an old observation that certain fatty acids are essential in the diet, and it follows that the mother must supply these fatty acids to the fetus.[3] What is new is the understanding of how maternal lipid metabolism adapts to the needs of fetal growth and development and how derangements in lipid metabolism can impair fetal growth and development. This knowledge has been spurred by the expansion of our understanding of lipoprotein physiology, and the awareness that lipoprotein lipid lowering can prevent arterial wall injury.[4,5] This chapter describes what is known about alterations in lipid and lipoprotein metabolism in pregnancy and the ways in which altered lipid metabolism in pregnancy may affect fetal growth and development.

Basic Principles of Lipid and Lipoprotein Physiology

Essential Fatty Acids

The body's fat store is derived from exogenous or dietary sources as well as endogenous synthesis. Fats with an obligatory dietary requirement are the polyunsaturated essential fatty acids such as linolenic acid, 18:2, or linolenic acid, 18:3 (i.e., carbon chain length:unsaturated bonds). These fatty acids are elongated in the body to become precursors for prostaglandin and leukotriene metabolism. In the case of the 18:2 omega-6 series, arachidonic acid, 20:4, is the elongation product. In the omega-3 fatty acid series, 18:3 is elongated to eicosapentenoic acid, 20:5, and docosahexanoic acid, 22:6. These 20- and 22-carbon fatty acids are converted to prostaglandins, which have competitive or alternative effects on a variety of biologic processes such as vascular reactivity, platelet function, and respiratory physiology. The omega-3 series has been reported to be essential for photoreceptor development in animals studied by Connor's group,[6] which showed that omega-3 fatty acid–deficient subhuman primates give birth to offspring with diminished visual capacity owing to a deficiency of 22:6 fatty acids in the photoreceptor membranes of the retina. Transfer of fatty acids across the placenta is discussed in a later section (see also Chapter 19).

Fat Absorption and Recycling

Apart from the requirement for essential fatty acids from the diet by both fetus and mother, all other fats, including cholesterol and fatty acids of varied lengths and saturation, that are required for normal physiologic functions are synthesized by the body. Approximately 1.0 to 1.2 g of cholesterol enters and leaves the body's metabolism per day in the nonpregnant individual, and the situation seems to be similar during pregnancy.[7] About 300 to 500 mg of cholesterol is ingested per day but only about one half of the cholesterol ingested in the diet is absorbed. Studies by Kesaniemi et al.[8] showed that the fraction of cholesterol absorbed is subject to some autoregulation depending on the low-density lipoprotein (LDL) cholesterol concentration and the apoprotein (apo) E phenotype present at two alleles in combinations of three isoforms: E_2, E_3, and E_4. Even with these effects and possibly others on cholesterol absorption, the percentage of cholesterol absorbed from the diet varies only between 40% and 60%.[8] Nothing is known about the effect of pregnancy on this process. Most cholesterol entry into the body pool in the nonpregnant individual and probably the pregnant woman is derived from endogenous synthesis. This process occurs largely in the liver, to a lesser extent in the intestine, and in certain instances of high metabolic demand in the adrenal, ovary, and testis. In contrast, fatty acid absorption is essentially complete in the human and nearly so in the laboratory rodent.

Cholesterol is made available to body tissue that requires it for new cell growth or cellular renewal largely by the lipoprotein cascade. By this process, dietary cholesterol, hepatic cholesterol, and cholesterol stored in various tissues of the body, either normally or abnormally, are continually recycled so as to deliver cholesterol to sites that are in need. One site that is predominantly in need of cholesterol is the growing placenta during normal pregnancy, which synthesizes approximately 400 to 500 mg of steroid hormones daily, or nearly one half the estimated daily net cholesterol input and output of the body in a nonpregnant individual. Whether this proportionality applies to pregnancy is uncertain, as cholesterol synthesis has never been measured in human pregnancy. Apart from cholesterol losses in the form of steroid hormones, the single metabolic pathway for sterol excretion in the body is via cholesterol and bile acid secretion in the bile. A schema for lipoprotein metabolism that describes the entry of cholesterol and fat via the diet, its cycling to and from the liver, and its excretion in the bile is shown in Figure 12.1.

Similar to the storage and metabolism of cholesterol, fatty acids are stored in the form of triacylglycerol (i.e., triglyceride) largely in adipose tissue, which composes 15% to 25% of female nonpregnant body weight. Although in situ synthesis of fatty acids in adipose tissue has been demonstrated in the nonpregnant and pregnant animal model, little de novo fatty acid synthesis is believed to occur in human adipose tissue; and the circulating lipoprotein cascade is responsible for the delivery of fatty acids derived either from the diet or hepatic synthesis to adipose tissue stores.[9,10] In summary, a recycling transport system delivers cholesterol and fatty acids, the two main fats of the body, to sites where they are required for new cell synthesis, energy provision, and a host of metabolic signaling processes involving phospholipids, inositol, diacyl glycerol, and prostaglandins and their metabolites.

The Lipoprotein Cascade

The normal lipoprotein transport is depicted in Figure 12.1. Cholesterol and fatty acids, esterified to triglyceride, are absorbed from the intestine and incorporated into chylomicrons in the intestinal enterocyte. They are then slowly secreted into the lymphatic circulation, where they enter the general circulation via the lymphatic duct. These chylomicrons are 2000 Å or more in diameter, are opaque to light, and carry as their primary apoprotein apo B-48, a large hydrophobic apoprotein made entirely in the gut. In subhuman species and the young infant, apo B-100 may be formed in the intestine, but this possibility appears not to be the case in the mature human. Smaller apoproteins are associated with chylomicrons during their formation in the gut. They include apo C-I, apo C-II, and apo C-III, which play a catalytic role in chylomicron triglyceride hydrolysis; apo A-I, apo A-II, and apo A-IV, which predominate in high-density lipoprotein (HDL); and apo E, mentioned above, which plays a role in chylomicron clearance by the liver. The enzyme responsible for chylomicron triglyceride clearance is lipoprotein lipase (LPL), which is synthesized in a variety of cells but particularly adipose tissue and muscle. It has a protein structure that allows it to migrate to the capillary endothelial cell, where it is anchored by a hydrophobic tail while its catalytic component extends into the capillary lumen. This catalytic component can penetrate the polar surface coat of the chylomicron particle, consisting of free cholesterol and phospholipids and protein, and it enters the neutral lipid, triglyceride-containing core where it initiates triglyceride hydrolysis. The process requires apo C-II as a cofactor and is inhibited by apo C-III. The C-II/C-III ratio declines during hypertriglyceridemia and in pregnancy, but the significance of these minor changes on triglyceride hydrolysis is not known.[11] The process of LPL-mediated chylomicron triglyceride clearance is rapid, since there is a half-life of minutes, and it provides an efficient mechanism for transporting fat, usually about 35% of daily caloric intake, quickly through the circulation.

Lipoprotein lipase is subject to regulation, increasing in adipose tissue capillary beds during feeding and with insulin exposure, declining with fasting and insulin deficiency. Reciprocally lipoprotein lipase increases in heart and in muscle during caloric deprivation and declining during the fed state. In this manner, dietary fatty acids are delivered to these tissues appropriately based on metabolic demand. With repeated exposures of the neutral lipid core to LPL, the chylomicron particle progressively becomes smaller, and a relatively cholesterol ester-rich remnant particle emerges. This remnant particle contains variable amounts of apo E, a small 299-amino-acid, arginine- and lysine-rich peptide with a midprotein sequence that binds to a chylomicron remnant receptor present primarily on hepatocyte surfaces in the liver.[12,13] The remnant receptor has some features of the LDL receptor and is suited to binding lipoproteins bearing multiple copies of apo E but not apo B-48 or B-100. For this reason it is known as the LDL receptor–

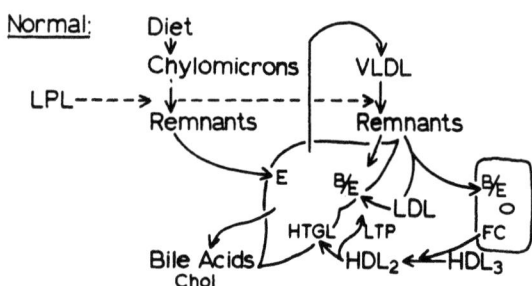

FIGURE 12.1. Lipoprotein metabolism in the normal adult.

related protein (LRP). The receptor has other specificities including α_2-macroglobulin and tissue factor pathway inhibitor.[13] This metabolic arrangement assures that the liver is the main site for the regulation of fatty acid and cholesterol metabolism (Figure 12.1) and largely precludes the direct delivery of dietary cholesterol, which is highly intermittent, to other tissues. The importance of apo E in mediating this removal and uptake process is illustrated by the accumulation of chylomicron remnants in individuals who have deletions or substitutions of amino acids in the receptor-binding region of the apo E molecule, resulting in so-called type III hyperlipidemia or remnant removal disease.[14,15]

Cholesterol delivered to the liver via chylomicron remnants mixes with cholesterol newly synthesized in the liver from acetyl coenzyme A (CoA) under regulation by the enzyme hydroxy-3-methylglutaryl (HMG) CoA-reductase, the last rate-limiting enzyme in the sequence. This cholesterol is incorporated into large triglyceride-rich particles called very low density lipoproteins (VLDL), which are slightly smaller than chylomicrons but are otherwise similar in structure and composition, with apo B-100 being the major structural apoprotein. Apo B-100 has a larger molecular weight than intestinal apo B-48 in the ratio of 100:48. Triglyceride for VLDL synthesis is derived from fatty acids that enter the liver via the chylomicron remnant or from free fatty acids mobilized from peripheral adipose tissue stores. Free fatty acids are removed from the circulation by many tissues; nearly all tissues are capable of oxidizing fatty acids. The disappearance rate of free fatty acids is rapid, on the order of a few minutes, and resembles the speed and efficiency of chylomicron triglyceride removal from the circulation. The importance of the liver in removing free fatty acids from the circulation relates to the limited availability of albumin to bind free fatty acids and the toxicity to mitochondrial respiration that occurs if free fatty acids exceed a certain molar ratio in relation to albumin. Thus, the conversion of circulating free fatty acids to triglycerides in the liver serves as a detoxification mechanism. Hepatic triglyceride homeostasis is maintained by exporting fat from the liver into the circulation in the form of VLDL. Hepatic synthesis of apoprotein B and the rate of its intracellular degradation also influence the rate of VLDL synthesis and secretion. Genetic disorders in this process contribute to various forms of combined hyperlipidemia, that is, combined elevations of cholesterol and triglyeride, which can be seen in pregnancy (vide infra).

The catabolism of VLDL is similar to that of chylomicrons (Figure 12.1). LPL in tissues that utilize fatty acids for storage or energy cleave the triglyceride fatty acids from the neutral lipid VLDL core, again forming VLDL remnants that contain apo E and apo B, which predominate in the intermediate density lipoprotein (IDL) fraction, which has physical properties between VLDL and LDL. Because of the ability of apo E to bind to the LDL (i.e., apo B/apo E) receptor, these remnants can be taken up directly by the liver. It is believed that the putative apo E receptor plays little role in this process. Further removal of triglyceride by hepatic triglyceride lipase (an LPL relative), converts VLDL remnants to LDL, which is then taken up by the liver or peripheral tissue by the classic LDL receptor described by Brown and Goldstein.[15]

Recently, a VLDL receptor has been described that has many properties of the LDL receptor, but its gene resides on a different chromosone. The VLDL receptor also recognizes apo E–rich VLDL remnants. The receptor is highly expressed in triglyceride fatty acid metabolizing tissue, indicating an alternative route for triglyceride fatty acids entering tissues besides via lipolysis.[16] The VLDL receptor has an essential role in egg lipid accumulation.[17]

Low-density lipoprotein transports the majority of cholesterol in the blood. Because of the abundance of cholesterol in the human diet, individuals living in affluent Western society metabolize relatively little LDL cholesterol in peripheral tissues by the LDL receptor. Most cholesterol (i.e., about 70%) recycles back into the liver (Figure 12.1). Thus, LDL concentration is particularly sensitive to LDL receptor regulation in the liver. One of the important influences is dietary fat intake. If dietary cholesterol intake increases, heightened amounts of chylomicron remnants are delivered to the liver, the hepatic cholesterol supply increases, and the LDL receptor is downregulated, causing an accumulation of LDL cholesterol in the circulation.[18,19] Similarly, dietary saturated fatty acids downregulate the LDL receptor and cause LDL levels to increase.

Cholesterol recycling in the process of cell senescence and renewal is accomplished by "reverse cholesterol transport." In this process, HDL serves as a free cholesterol acceptor and delivers cholesterol back to the central processing station (i.e., the liver), as is depicted in Figure 12.1. The most lipid-poor, protein-rich of the HDL species, HDL_3, serves as an acceptor for free cholesterol and binds to cell surfaces in proportion to the amount of cholesterol contained in cells, at least in fibroblast and smooth muscle cell models.[20–22] Free cholesterol absorbed onto the polar surface of HDL_3 is esterified by the enzyme lecithin cholesterol acyl transferase (L-CAT) where fatty acids from lecithin are transferred to cholesterol to form cholesterol ester and lysolecithin. The lipophilic cholesterol ester passes to the neutral lipid core of the HDL particle, where it progressively accumulates. By this mechanism, the HDL particle becomes more lipid-rich and attains the buoyancy of HDL_2.

The conversions between HDL_3 and HDL_2 depend on the HDL apoproteins (i.e., apo A-I and apo A-II). Some

HDL species contain apo A-I and apo A-II. There are several molecular weight forms of HDL that contain only apo A-I, whereas others contain both of these apoproteins.[23] Finally, much of the uptake of cholesterol from cells and changes in HDL structure occur in the lymph and may not be possible to trace in the general circulation.

Once formed, cholesterol ester-rich HDL_2 can deliver its cholesterol to the liver catalyzed by hepatic triglyceride lipase (HTGL) (Figure 12.1), which serves not only as a triglyceride lipase for the more dense lipoproteins, VLDL remnants, LDL, and HDL but as a phospholipase. For this reason it is also known as hepatic lipase. The catabolism of surface phospholipids in HDL_2 appears to alter the chemical gradient for cholesterol between HDL and the liver, thereby promoting the transfer of cholesterol ester to the liver.[24] Additionally, cholesterol can be retained in the circulation by direct transfer of cholesterol ester from HDL_2 to LDL and VLDL (depicted only with LDL in Figure 12.1) by lipid transfer protein (LTP). LTP associates with HDL and transfers cholesterol ester to VLDL and LDL in exchange for the alternative neutral lipid, triglyceride, from VLDL and LDL. Differences in cholesterol ester triglyceride exchange among lipoproteins in various species may relate as much to the balance between lipid transfer protein and lipid transfer protein inhibitor as much as to the absolute level of lipid transfer protein itself.[25,26] In addition, phospholipid transfer between VLDL, IDL, and HDL is facilitated by a phospholipid transfer protein (PLTP), which may prove to have clinical significance and currently is under intense study.[27,28]

Cholesterol is excreted from the body through the bile. The pool of cholesterol in the liver serves as a substrate for 7-α-hydroxylation of cholesterol and its conversion to bile acids apparently regardless of its origin. Bile acids, cholesterol, and phospholipids are secreted into the bile and can be reabsorbed in the gut, constituting the enterohepatic circulation. Even sterols excreted in the bile can be recycled via dietary chylomicrons to further conserve the body's supply of cholesterol.

Effects of Estrogens and Progestins on Lipoprotein Metabolism

Little is known about the hormonal determinants of hyperlipidemia in pregnancy, but mechanistic inferences can be drawn from analogous conditions, such as exposure of women to specific sex steroid regimens. This subject has been reviewed recently.[29–32]

The effects of estrogens and estrogen plus progestin are depicted in Figure 12.2 and Table 12.1. There is no information that estrogen alters the absorption of dietary nutrients from the intestine or that cholesterol absorption (vide supra) is altered by estrogen. The increase in triglyceride concentrations typically seen with estrogen administration is the result of the induction of the formation and secretion of apo B and VLDL particles from the liver.[33,34] LPL activity is usually unchanged.[35,36] The VLDL particles as they are measured in the plasma appear to have normal percentage composition,[37] and cholesterol content of VLDL tends to fall when estrogen is given concurrently.[38] The failure of cholesterol to accumulate disproportionately in VLDL with cholesterol feeding may be related to the ability of estrogen to

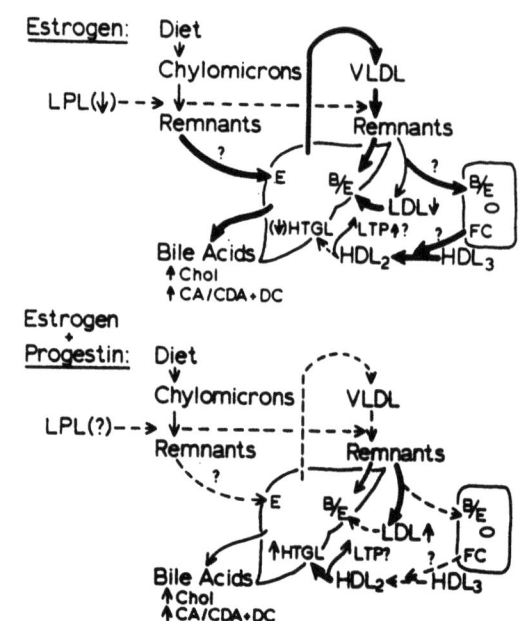

FIGURE 12.2. Effects of estrogen and progestins and lipoprotein metabolism. (From Knopp,[277] with permission.)

TABLE 12.1. Comparison of the effects of estrogens, estrogen plus progestin, and the menstrual cycle on plasma lipoprotein concentrations.

Lipoprotein	Estrogen[a]	Estrogen plus progestin[b]	Menstrual cycle[c]	
			Follicular	Luteal
Triglyceride (TG)	↑	↓	—	—
Cholesterol (C)	—	—	—	↓
VLDL-TG	↑	↓	—	—
LDL-C	↓	(—,↑)	—	↓
HDL-C	↑	↓	—	(—,↑)

[a] Estrogen effects are most clearly described in the postmenopausal women.
[b] Estrogen plus progestin effects are expressed as the change seen versus those seen with estrogen alone. Whether an LDL-C rise is seen may relate to the relative dose and androgenicity of the progestin and is more likely to be seen with oral contraceptive use than with postmenopausal estrogen-progestin use.
[c] Of numerous reports, LDL-C is consistently lower during the second half of the menstrual cycle. Only one report has found a higher HDL-C level during the luteal phase (see ref. 78 for review).

upregulate the LDL receptor[39,40] and to enhance the removal of remnants of triglyceride-rich lipoprotein particle catabolism and LDL particles.[41,42] Individuals who have remnant accumulation due to an abnormal apo E phenotype (i.e., type III hyperlipidemia) usually experience an improvement in their hyperlipidemia when treated with estrogen,[41] and VLDL remnant removal is enhanced, as demonstrated by increased uptake of labeled IDL.[42] Because the extent to which remnants of chylomicron or VLDL origin are removed by the VLDL, LRP, and LDL receptors is not clear, it is not known whether the improvement in type III hyperlipidemia in response to estrogen is due solely to an increase in LDL receptors or to an increase in the other receptor types as well. The situation with LDL is clearer.[43-46]

With respect to cholesterol removal from cells and the process of reverse cholesterol transport, it may be hypothesized that this pathway is upregulated because of the increased concentration of HDL_2 that is seen in the circulation. This effect has not been demonstrated directly. It is uncertain if estrogen has any effect on the transfer of free cholesterol from cell walls to HDL_3 or if HDL_3 binding to its putative receptor is altered. What is known is that apoprotein A-I entry into the circulation is increased by estrogen.[33,46] Another basis for the increase in HDL_2 cholesterol concentration is the reduction in hepatic triglyceride lipase, which was first shown with estrogen exposure by Applebaum-Bowden et al.[38] and recently confirmed by Brinton.[47] It is possible that the recycling of cholesterol from HDL_2 to LDL and VLDL in exchange for triglyceride (TG) may be enhanced based on the fact that HDL and LDL TG concentrations are increased with estrogen exposure, as first shown by Gustafson and Svanborg[48] during the 1970s and confirmed in our studies.[37] An increase in LDL cholesterol as a result of this recycling process usually does not occur presumably because of the estrogen-induced upregulation in the LDL receptor. Whether lipid transfer protein activity or its inhibitor protein activity or levels are altered with estrogen exposure is not well studied, but LTP activity is increased in pregnancy.[49] Finally, it is established that bile acid secretion is increased with estrogen exposure along with an increase in biliary cholesterol secretion (Figure 12.2), which may be related to the increased tendency for women to develop gallstones. With respect to the bile acid composition itself, cholic acid is increased relative to chenodeoxycholic and deoxycholic acids.[50]

The effect of progestins/androgens on lipoprotein metabolism is modeled in Figure 12.2 and is designated as the effect of progestin/androgen. In general, the effects of progestins/androgens oppose the effects of estrogen, but depending on their potency can have their own effect. Under the effect of estrogen plus progestin, there is no known alteration in dietary fat absorption or LPL activity. VLDL entry into the circulation falls as does triglyceride concentration.[51,52] It is possible that remnant removal is impaired owing to its decreased removal by the liver. We have found in the woman treated with a progestin-dominant, androgenic oral contraceptive progestin that VLDL cholesterol concentration is increased relative to triglyceride, suggesting secretion of a more cholesterol-rich VLDL or impaired remnant removal.[37] Opposite evidence in the rat has been reported by Khoka et al.,[53] where *dl*-norgestrel, a potent androgenic progestin, given alone enhances remnant removal but impairs LDL cholesterol removal. The mechanism of enhancement of remnant removal under the influence of this progestin could be due to an upregulation of hepatic lipase,[54] but the increase in LDL cholesterol suggests a downregulation of the LDL receptor. In this respect the effect of a progestin is opposite that of estrogens, where LDL cholesterol concentration typically falls.[43,44] Wolfe and Huff[55] found increased remnant removal in the postmenopausal woman treated with estrogen plus progestin, an observation compatible with an estrogen effect alone.[41,42]

It is known that HDL cholesterol concentrations, particularly HDL_2, are reduced by exposure to androgen or potent androgenic progestin.[37,44,56] This reduction in HDL_2 could reflect diminished reverse cholesterol transport due to diminished apoprotein A-I synthesis. Alternatively, it could be a result of increased HDL_2 cholesterol uptake by the liver by increased hepatic triglyceride lipase activity.[54] Finally, the fall in HDL cholesterol concentrations with progestin therapy can be hypothetically related to the observed reduction in chylomicron and VLDL triglyceride concentrations and transport, which result in diminished transfer of surface remnants from VLDL particles to HDL and reduces HDL mass. When extrapolating these progestin effects to pregnancy, it is important to keep in mind that natural progesterone does not appear to have the same antiestrogenic profile as the C-19 synthetic progestins or cyproterone or medroxyprogesterone acetate. The effects may still be marked, however, because of the high plasma hormone concentrations reached.

Sex Differences in Lipoprotein Metabolism

One way to study the integrated effects of natural estrogen and progesterone on fat metabolism is to consider metabolic differences between men and women (Table 12.2). The male-female difference is important because it is the baseline onto which the metabolic change during pregnancy is engraved and because it serves as a model of the effect of natural sex steroids on metabolism independent of the fetal demand for nutrients. In general, women

TABLE 12.2. Effects of male-female differences on metabolism in the reproductive age range.

Parameter	Men	Women
Adipose fat mass	—	↑
Basal insulin concentration	—	↑
FFA concentrations	—	—,↑
FFA turnover	—	↑
Triglyceride secretion	—	↑
Triglyceride turnover	—	↑
HDL cholesterol concentration	—	↑
FFA rise with fasting	—	↑
Glucose fall, fasting	—	↑

FFA, free fatty acids.

differ from men in that they have accelerated rates of fat and glucose metabolism (Figure 12.3). Compared to men, women have increased adipose tissue stores, increased basal insulin concentration, increased insulin secretion in response to a glucose stimulus, increased plasma–free fatty acid response to starvation in some studies, increased free fatty acid clearance by the liver,[57] and elevated LPL activity.[58] Triglyceride secretion and removal are increased.[59-61] Plasma LDL concentration is lower in the estrogen-exposed reproductive-age woman than in men[62,63] and is higher postmenopausally than in men. Reverse cholesterol transport is hypothesized to be increased based on the higher HDL cholesterol levels in women versus men[62-64] (Figure 12.3). Very recently, we have compared LDL and HDL responses to a National Cholesterol Lowering Program step-II saturated fat restricted diet (i.e., <7% of calories) and found equivalent LDL decreases in men and women after 6 months, but an HDL-C decrease twice as great in women (6.4%) as in men (3%).[65] The mechanism and significance of this difference are unknown.

The origin of the higher insulin concentration in women is probably hormonal,[66] and there is evidence that insulin sensitivity is normal or enhanced in normal women, especially in view of the increased amount of glucose metabolism by muscle in women.[67] When normalized for the amount of muscle tissue, glucose utilization in women is 45% higher than in men.[67] The higher insulin concentration could lead to a greater degree of fat synthesis and storage, with the hyperinsulinemia and insulin sensitivity driven by sex hormones.[66,68]

The male-female difference is especially apparent during fasting, where plasma–free fatty acid concentrations are more markedly elevated[69] and plasma glucose and insulin concentration more sharply decreased than in men for equal periods of fasting.[69] Whether the greater free fatty acid concentration elevation is due to the increased store of fat mass in women compared to that in men or is a direct hormonally mediated effect is uncertain. Because these accelerated adaptations to starvation so closely resemble the changes that occur in human

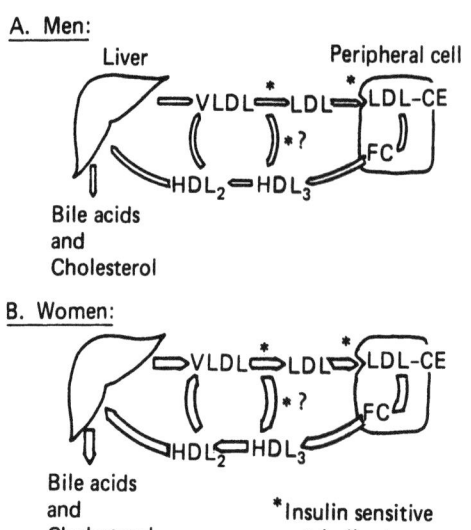

FIGURE 12.3. Male-female differences in lipoprotein metabolism.

pregnancy during fasting (vide infra), this similarity emphasizes the important role of sex steroids themselves in addition to the fetus when explaining the metabolic changes of pregnancy.

The important point to be drawn about interactions between estrogen and natural progesterone as seen during the menstrual cycle is that LDL cholesterol concentration is lower during the luteal phase than during the follicular phase of the menstrual cycle.[70-79] The increase in metabolic rate and basal body temperature in the luteal phase may have some effect on LDL concentration.[80]

During the luteal phase, although progesterone concentration is higher as a result of increased secretion from the corpus luteum, estrogen concentration is higher compared to the first half of the menstrual cycle. It appears that it is the estrogen effect that predominates over the progesterone effect during the normal menstrual cycle, and this observation provides another clue as to what to expect in pregnancy. No consistent effects have been reported for HDL cholesterol, although an increase was reported once;[78] nor have there been consistent effects on total triglycerides during the menstrual cycle (Table 12.1).[64]

Fat Storage, Free Fatty Acid Metabolism, and Appetite Regulation in Pregnancy

It is well known that the weight gain of pregnancy is associated not only with an increase in the mass of the uterus and its contents and the breasts, but also an accumulation of subcutaneous and intraabdominal adipose tissue. Measurement of total body fat accumulation in

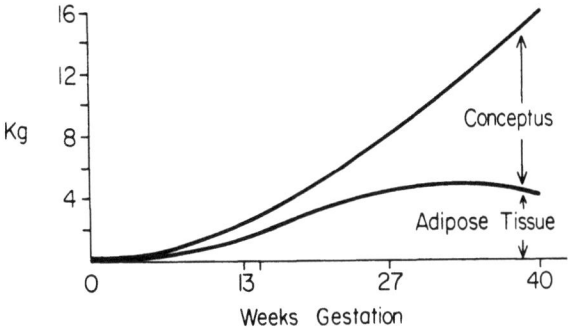

FIGURE 12.4. Body fat accumulation in pregnancy. (From Hytten,[279] with permission.)

pregnancy was first reported in the human by Hytten et al.[81] using deuterium measurements of total body water. By their estimates, body fat accumulation reaches a maximum at midgestation and does not increase further or even declined slightly (Figure 12.4). Similar patterns of weight gain have been seen in most animal models with variation in time course probably related to species, strain of animal, and dietary conditions.[82-84] In the pregnant rat model, the attenuation of fat mass accumulation toward the end of gestation is associated with a de novo reduction of fatty acid synthesis and heightened incorporation of glucose into glycerol, suggesting increased fatty acid reesterification.[10] A similar trend is seen in the hamster.[85] This pattern of redirection of glucose to fatty acid reesterification rather than de novo lipogenesis indicates an increase in insulin resistance and intracellular contrainsulin effects. Studies in the rodent and the human indicate a reduction in insulin sensitivity of about 70%.[86,87] This effect occurs during the third trimester of gestation, in keeping with evolving glucose intolerance during late gestation and a heightened tendency to fatty acid mobilization, especially during fasting.[88,89] Heightened free fatty acid mobilization from adipose tissue has been shown in the fasted pregnant rat and in human pregnancy.[90,91] Sharply increased plasma-free fatty acid and ketone concentrations have been reported with fasting in both animal[92] and human[93] pregnancy.

The realignment in the disposition of circulating fuels during pregnancy is illustrated in Figure 12.5. Maternal metabolic events can be divided into early and late gestation, reflecting an early growth of adipose tissue stores and late attenuation of this storage. Throughout this time the mother's caloric intake is increased consistently to 250 to 300 kilocalories·day^{-1}. What is different is the fate of the extra incoming calories between early and late gestation. During early gestation (Figure 12.5, top) incoming glucose and triglyceride fatty acids are used by muscle and adipose tissue, respectively, with little glucose being utilized by the fetus, which has a minimal metabolic requirement at this time. Later and particularly during the last third of pregnancy (Figure 12.5, bottom) fetal growth is rapid, the fetal glucose requirement for energy is great, and fetal adipose tissue formation is substantial. A large amount of glucose is transferred to the growing fetus. Competition between maternal tissue, particularly muscle, and the growing fetus for glucose is obviated by the development of maternal insulin resistance, which is attributed to at least six hormones that are increased during pregnancy: progesterone, prolactin, cortisol, thyroxine, placental lactogen, and placental growth hormone (GH-V) (variant).[94,95] As an alternative to glucose, muscle can oxidize fat for energy, a phenomenon most dramatically seen in the fasted state, where free fatty acid and ketone body concentrations are greatly elevated.[92,93]

Lipoprotein lipid metabolism follows this general pattern. In the fed state, alimentary chylomicron or VLDL triglyceride fatty acids can be oxidized by muscle, which retains some LPL activity.[96] In addition, the uterus has increased LPL activity[97] and the placenta has LPL activity,[98,99] including human placental trophoblast and macrophages,[100] and can oxidize fatty acids.[101] However, adipose tissue LPL activity decreases throughout gestation, as has been reported by numerous investigators.[96-98,102-104] Most recently, Alvarez et al.[104] reported a reduction in total heparin releasable LPL in the third trimester of human gestation. These data extend an earlier observation by Kinnunen et al.[105] It appears that aggregate releasable LPL activity is reduced in late gestation pregnancy, with the greatest reduction occurring in adipose tissue. This reduction in adipose tissue LPL activity may help explain the attenuation in growth of the fat store during the second half of pregnancy because, as mentioned above, in situ formation of free fatty acids from glucose in adipose tissue does not occur to

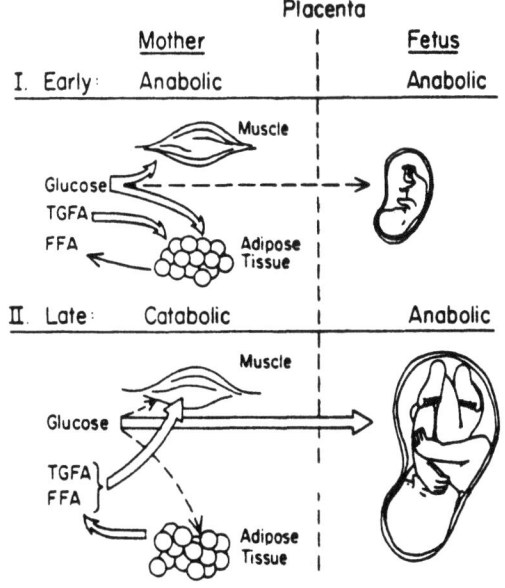

FIGURE 12.5. Reallocation of body fuels in pregnancy after an overnight fast. (From Knopp,[278] with permission.)

an appreciable extent in the human. Lasunción and Herrera[106] found reduced uptake of triglyceride-rich lipoprotein by isolated adipocytes from pregnant rats.[106] An exception to this generalization has been encountered by Argiles and Herrera,[107] who found that in vivo adipose tissue uptake of chylomicron [^{14}C]triglyceride was unimpaired during late rat gestation, albeit at higher plasma triglyceride concentrations, although they found attenuation of carcass fat storage during late gestation.[108] Most evidence indicates that tissue enzymes that participate in the disposition of triglyceride fatty acid calories in pregnancy are regulated by the changes in pregnancy hormones, insulin concentration, and insulin sensitivity, as are the other fuels of pregnancy (i.e., glucose and amino acids).

The elevation in free fatty acid concentrations at any moment in pregnancy are dependent on the dietary status of the mother, which has led to variable degrees of free fatty acid elevation being reported in pregnancy after an overnight fast but with rising concentration toward term.[65,93,109,110] What is unequestioned is that, with progressive caloric restriction, the tendency to fatty acid mobilization is higher;[90-93] in fact, even in the fed state in the pregnant rat model, increased fatty acid mobilization from adipose tissue, along with increased fatty acid reesterification and recycling, is observed.[90,91] A certain amount of caloric wastage due to fatty acid recycling within adipose tissue itself appears to occur during pregnancy, resulting in generation of extra heat energy. The extent to which this "futile cycle" may be greater in nonobese versus obese pregnant women is worthy of further investigation.

Apart from the already-mentioned effects of pregnancy to accelerate adipose tissue fat storage during early gestation and then to slow it during late gestation, marked differences among individuals are observed in the extent to which they enter pregnancy lean or obese and then augment weight gain during the course of pregnancy. In general, it has been observed that the obese woman tends to gain less fat mass during gestation and may undergo an actual loss in body fat storage, in contrast to the lean, primiparous individual, who usually gains a substantial amount of adipose tissue mass during the first pregnancy.[111,112] The mechanism controlling the augmented accumulation of fat in the lean person and the restricted or even negative fat accumulation in an already obese person is uncertain. It has been speculated that the hypothalamus becomes more sensitized to body signals[112] that reflect fat storage accumulation, such as the central nervous system insulin concentration.[113] Alternatively, a more markedly elevated basal and stimulated insulin concentration in an obese versus a lean pregnancy might reach such a level as to inhibit appetite center receptors insensitive to lower levels of insulin feedback. Other feedback signal alterations, such as in adipsin and leptin require investigation.[114,115] It has been recently reported that leptin concentration is increased 67% in late pregnancy, which is attributed to the increase in fat mass, insulin concentration, and possibly pregnancy hormones.[115] Interestingly, leptin administration to infertile ob/ob mice which lack leptin restored fertility.[116] Precedent also exists for sex steroid hormones having an effect on the hypothalamus. For instance, progesterone heightens the respiratory drive and is used therapeutically to treat hypoventilation in the pickwickian syndrome, a condition of severe hypoxemia related to severe obesity.[94] Similarily, Megace, a synthetic progestin, is used to stimulate appetite in wasting conditions.[117]

In conclusion, adipose tissue mass in pregnancy is sensitive to hormonal effects in its intermediary metabolism and to alterations in maternal appetite. The increase in caloric intake expands the adipose tissue store until late gestation, when these forces are opposed by contrainsulin pregnancy hormones as well as leptin, which may function to oppose the increased appetite stimulated by steroid hormones (see Chapter 9).

Lipoprotein Changes in Normal Pregnancy

Fat and Cholesterol Absorption and Synthesis

As mentioned in an earlier section, cholesterol absorption appears to be regulated to permit only 40% to 50% of cholesterol ingested to be absorbed. Whether pregnancy hormones alter this absorption is unknown, but some speculation can be made on the basis of the absorption of other nutrients during pregnancy. For instance, increased amounts of iron are required during pregnancy and in fact are absorbed during the course of gestation.[118] Increased amounts of calcium are absorbed from the gut throughout gestation under the influence of vitamin D, which is present in increased amounts beginning early in gestation.[94] By analogy, it is plausible that an increased amount of cholesterol should be absorbed as well, particularly to meet the increased cholesterol requirements of pregnancy, as 400 to 500mg of steroid hormone is excreted in the urine daily. Using the sterol balance method, Potter and Nestel[7] found a rise in bile acid production but a fall in neutral sterol excretion and concluded there was not a net increase in sterol synthesis in pregnancy.

With respect to triglyceride fatty acid absorption, a study in the pregnant rat model by Argiles and Herrera[107] indicated that triglyceride fatty acid absorption is complete and undelayed, in contrast to the nonpregnant rat where fat absorption is not necessarily complete. The rate of fat absorption could be altered in human pregnancy owing to reduced gastrointestinal mobility,[119] and postprandial chylomicronemia might be more prolonged in pregnancy, because of the underlying hypertriglyceridemia and third trimester reduction in LPL activity,[104] although the matter requires direct observation.

TABLE 12.3. Comparison of lipoprotein lipid and apoprotein concentrations (mg·dl⁻¹; mean ± SD) in 36-week gestation pregnancy compared to nonpregnant control subjects.

	Nonpregnant	36-week gestation
Total	(23)[a]	(23)[a]
Triglyceride	59 ± 19	222 ± 60
Cholesterol	171 ± 26	251 ± 32
VLDL		
Triglyceride	33 ± 14	107 ± 41
Cholesterol	11 ± 6	22 ± 9
Apo B	7 ± 6	20 ± 11
LDL		
Triglyceride	14 ± 10	72 ± 21
Cholesterol	104 ± 23	161 ± 39
Apo B	61 ± 10	84 ± 23
HDL		
Triglyceride	12 ± 6	29 ± 9
Cholesterol	56 ± 12	64 ± 9
Apo A-1	128 ± 23	164 ± 16
HDL$_2$	(19)	(18)
Cholesterol	22 ± 8	38 ± 12
HDL$_3$		
Cholesterol	34 ± 5	31 ± 6

Note: All data taken from Montes et al.[276] except those of HDL$_2$ and HDL$_3$ which are from Fähraeus et al.[127]

[a] Number of subjects denoted in parentheses.

From Knopp et al.,[124] with permission.

TABLE 12.4. Reference values for lipoprotein lipid concentrations at 36 weeks' gestation and 6 weeks postpartum.

	Concentration (mg·dl⁻¹), by percentile				
	5th	10th	50th	90th	95th
36 weeks' gestation					
Total TG	133	146	209	341	387
Total C	185	196	243	299	318
VLDL-TG	48	58	105	200	246
LDL-C	89	106	148	200	218
HDL-C	42	46	64	86	93
6 weeks postpartum					
Total TG	48	54	77	137	157
Total C	152	161	200	254	265
VLDL-TG	16	20	41	95	122
LDL-C	74	92	125	164	177
HDL-C	44	46	58	79	88

From Knopp et al.,[63] with permission.

Serial Changes in Lipoprotein Lipids in Pregnancy

The modern era of lipid measurements in pregnancy began during the 1930s with the report by Boyd,[120] who found that total plasma lipids in pregnancy were increased 50%, cholesterol was increased from 181 to 205 mg·dl⁻¹ and neutral fat was increased from 154 to 353 mg·dl⁻¹. Through 1976, 12 subsequent studies of lipoprotein lipids in the fasting state and seven studies of nonfasting subjects have been reviewed and were confirmatory and added significant details.[121] In general, plasma total triglyceride concentration increases two- to fourfold, and total cholesterol increases 25% to 50%. We have confirmed these increases[122] and have measured LDL cholesterol, which increases 50%, and HDL cholesterol, which increases to a maximum of 30% in midgestation followed by a slight decline.[89,122-124] Typical third trimester elevations are shown in Table 12-3. Reference percentile values for lipoprotein lipid concentration at 36 weeks' gestation have been reported and are presented in Table 12.4.[63] A confirmatory population study of lipoprotein lipid and apoprotein values has appeared.[125]

These changes in total triglyceride and cholesterol, VLDL cholesterol, LDL cholesterol, HDL cholesterol, VLDL triglyceride, LDL triglyceride, and HDL triglyceride are shown in Figures 12.6, 12.7, and 12.8, respectively, as measured in subjects studied serially throughout gestation in our laboratory.[89,122-124] Similar increases have been observed by Potter and Nestel,[126] Fahraeus et al.,[127] Desoye et al.,[128] and others.[129-131]

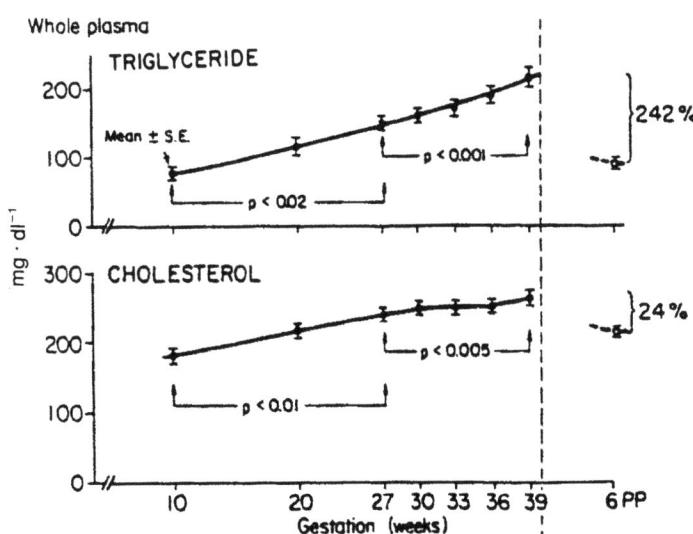

FIGURE 12.6. Serial changes in total triglyceride and cholesterol in pregnancy and postpartum (8–20 subjects). (From Knopp et al.,[124] with permission.)

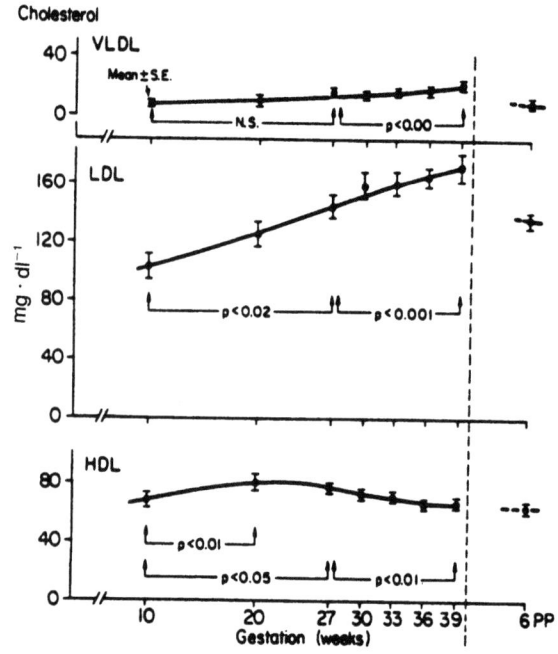

FIGURE 12.7. Serial lipoprotein cholesterol changes in pregnancy and postpartum (8–20 subjects). (From Knopp et al.,[89] with permission.)

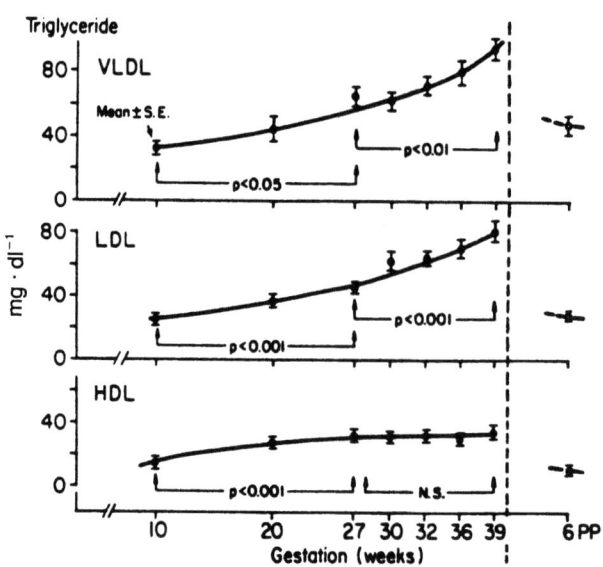

FIGURE 12.8. Serial lipoprotein triglyceride changes in pregnancy and postpartum (8–20 subjects). (From Knopp et al.,[89] with permission.)

The increase in LDL lipids occurs in the density range of 1.006 to 1.019 (IDL or LDL_1) and the true LDL range, or LDL_2 (density 1.019–1.063).[123,132] A linear rise in VLDL and LDL apo B is seen.[128,133] Most recently, Silliman et al.[134] have observed that the form of LDL in late gestation is small and dense and inverse in degree to the extent of the triglyceride elevation, typical of nonpregnancy hypertriglyceridemia.[134] Fahraeus et al.[127] and Desoye et al.[128] have reported the same rise and fall in HDL cholesterol that we saw. Similar trends are seen in the data of Potter and Nestel[126] in subjects studied cross-sectionally. In addition, Fahraeus et al., Desoye et al., and our group[124] have seen that the HDL rise is largely due to an increase in HDL_2 cholesterol concentration. Changes in HDL cholesterol concentration and the HDL subfractions in our own investigations are shown in Figure 12.9, where HDL_2 concentrations peak, like total HDL cholesterol, at about 20 weeks' gestation. Most recently, Alvarez et al.[104] found that the HDL_2 cholesterol increase occurred in the HDL_{2b} fraction, the estrogen-sensitive fraction. In keeping with the increase in HDL_2 is an increase largely in apo A-I, in contrast to apo A-II, which does not increase (Figure 12.10), although apo A-II was reported to be increased by Desoye et al.[128] It is noteworthy that the increase and later slight decline in HDL cholesterol (Figure 12.9) is not matched by a decline in apo A-I concentration (Figure 12.10). These data suggest independent effects on HDL apoprotein mass versus HDL lipid content as a function of time. It is likely that the decrease in HDL cholesterol in the third trimester is driven by the increase in HDL triglyceride content, a result of the lipid transfer reaction. In this process, plasma VLDL triglyceride concentration increases, and an increased amount of triglyceride is available for exchange with HDL cholesterol. HDL triglyceride concentration remains elevated through late gestation, unlike HDL cholesterol (Figure 12.7). The lipid transfer reaction is mediated by cholesterol ester transfer protein (CETP), which is increased 30% to 40% in pregnancy, favoring increased lipid transfer.[49,104]

Some dispute revolves around the pregnancy associated changes in Lp(a), a glycopeptide associated with apo B of lipoproteins in the approximate density range of 1.050 to 1.075. Zechner et al.[135] observed a rise in midgestation and then a fall. Panteghini and Pagani[136] observed an increase especially in the second trimester (Table 12.5). Finally, Lp(a) is reportedly elevated in normal pregnancy but not in the pregnant woman who

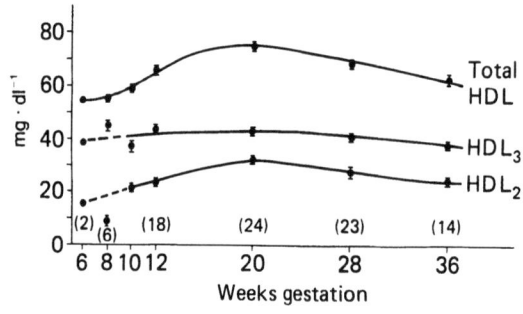

FIGURE 12.9. HDL cholesterol and HDL_2 and HDL_3 changes during pregnancy. ( ) denotes number of subjects.

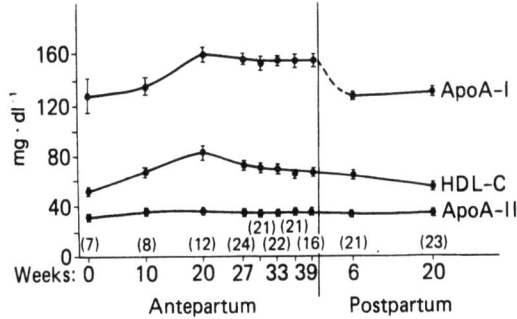

FIGURE 12.10. Apo A-I and apo A-II changes in pregnancy.

Mechanisms of Changes in Lipoprotein Metabolism in Pregnancy

A schema explaining some of the changes in pregnancy is presented in Figure 12.11; the nonpregnant situation is represented at the top, midgestation at the middle, and late gestation on the bottom. The schema, overall, is an exaggeration of the difference between women and men (Figure 12.3). In a normal nonpregnant individual, the liver secretes VLDL, which is converted at least in part to LDL, which is taken up by the LDL receptor in peripheral tissues as well as the liver, although the liver effect is not illustrated (see Figure 12.1 for more detail). Reciprocally, HDL takes up cholesterol from peripheral tissue, and surface coat components (i.e., apo C, apo E, phospholipid, free cholesterol) are acquired from VLDL. Reciprocally, there is net movement of cholesterol ester to VLDL (and LDL, not shown) in exchange for triglyceride moving to HDL via the cholesterol ester transfer protein mechanism (LTP in Figures 12.1 and 12.2).

smokes.[137] The significance and mechanism of this change are unknown. In the nonpregnant woman and in men, Lp(a) is a potent heart disease risk factor, possibly related to its structural homology to plasminogen, which is believed to confer an antithrombolytic effect. In this connection, a family has been reported with history of recurrent thromboembolsim, placental ischemia, and an Lp(a) concentration in excess of the 99th percentile.[138]

With respect to the effect of diet on hyperlipidemia in pregnancy, high carbohydrate feeding has surprisingly little triglyceride-raising effect compared to the normal "carbohydrate induction" seen in the nonpregnant woman or the exaggerated carbohydrate induction seen in the postpartum lactating woman.[139] As for the effect of dietary cholesterol, McMurry et al.[140] have reported that cholesterol restriction from 600–1000 to 0 mg·dl^{-1} results in an approximately 20% decrease in cholesterol. Lipids in pregnancy can be influenced by the cholesterol content of the diet but less by the carbohydrate content. Studies of changes in polyunsaturated fatty acids on lipoproteins are not available.

During midgestation and late gestation (Figure 12.11), the increasing hypertriglyceridemia of pregnancy progressively reflects increased secretion of VLDL from the liver. This adatation has been observed in the perfused liver by Wasfi et al.[141] and has been shown following triton blockade of LPL removal of VLDL in the pregnant rat.[124] Conversely, VLDL triglyceride could accumulate as a result of the reduction in LPL activity reported by many investigations.[96–98,102–104,142] In an attempt to quantify triglyceride-rich lipoprotein flux in an animal model of pregnancy, Humphrey et al.[124,143] radiolabeled rat chylomicrons and injected them into normal and pregnant rats during mid- and late gestation. In this investigation, the triglyceride transport rate was double during late pregnancy compared to the nonpregnant state and 10 days

TABLE 12.5. Median (and range) of serum concentrations of Lp(a) compared with other lipids and lipoproteins.

Week of pregnancy	n	Lp(a) (mg·L^{-1})	Triglycerides	Total chol	LDL chol	HDL chol	Apo A-I	Apo B
				(g·L^{-1})				
0–8	39	71 (2–517)	0.60 (0.29–1.94)	1.67 (1.23–2.34)	0.87 (0.52–1.47)	0.63 (0.47–0.93)	1.52 (1.19–2.01)	0.87 (0.52–1.34)
9–16	29	74 (2–533)	0.66 (0.38–2.00)	1.94 (1.28–2.82)	0.98 (0.58–1.73)	0.73 (0.51–1.13)	1.74 (1.16–2.52)	0.97 (0.63–1.64)
17–24	34	89 (2–491)	1.23 (0.58–3.30)	2.47 (1.98–3.11)	1.29 (0.85–1.99)	0.87 (0.49–1.22)	2.04 (1.44–2.47)	1.31 (0.98–1.85)
25–32	47	138 (2–570)^a	1.60 (0.86–3.77)	2.69 (1.95–4.65)	1.48 (0.80–3.22)	0.84 (0.46–1.17)	2.02 (1.44–2.90)	1.55 (0.86–2.77)
33–40	44	141 (2–788)^b	1.98 (0.82–3.81)	2.75 (1.83–3.65)	1.58 (0.85–2.41)	0.77 (0.43–1.27)	2.02 (1.47–2.66)	1.59 (1.02–2.06)
Postpartum (1 week)	39	84 (2–646)	1.76 (0.34–4.04)	2.25 (1.46–3.37)	1.31 (0.55–2.70)	0.62 (0.33–1.02)	1.62 (0.99–2.44)	1.41 (0.62–2.02)
Nonpregnant controls	100	61 (2–702)	<2	<2	—	—	—	—

Significantly different from nonpregnant controls at $^a p < .01$, $^b p < .001$ (Wilcoxon test).
Chol, cholesterol; LDL, low-density lipoprotein; HDL, high-density lipoprotein; apo, apolipoprotein.
From Panteghini et al.,[136] with permission.

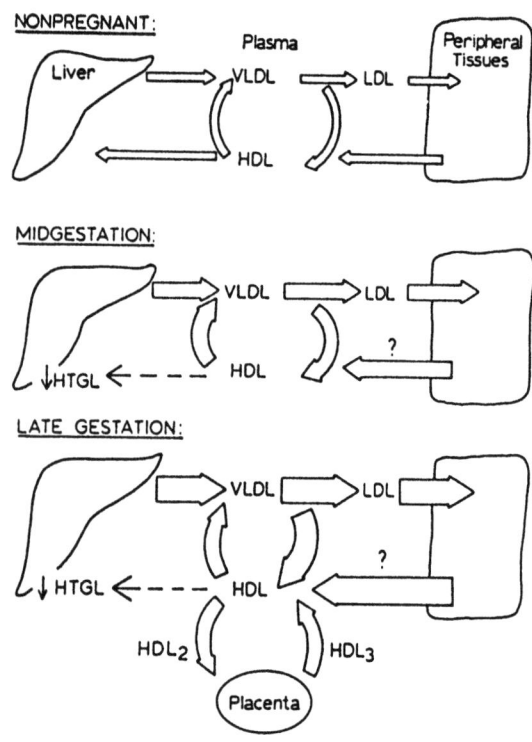

FIGURE 12.11. Changes in lipoprotein flow in pregnancy.

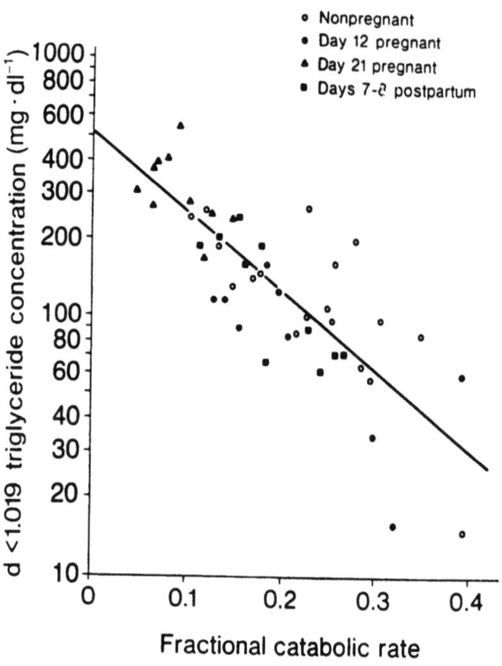

FIGURE 12.12. Clearance of chylomicron triglycerides in rat pregnancy. (From Humphrey et al.,[143] with permission.)

postpartum (Figure 12.12). On the other hand, the fractional catabolic rate was roughly one half of normal at day 21 of rat gestation compared to the nonpregnant, the gestational day 12, or the 10-day postpartum measurements. It could not be directly determined from these investigations whether the reduction in fractional catabolic rate is due to an increase in pool size or to an absolute reduction in the LPL-mediated rate of triglyceride fatty acid removal. In an attempt to resolve this question, the relation between fractional catabolic rate and density <1.019 lipoprotein triglyceride concentrations was plotted, and a logarithmic, continuous inverse relation was seen, suggesting that the relation between concentration and fractional catabolic rate is a continuous function in the pregnant and nonpregnant states. This analysis led to the conclusion that the reduction in fractional catabolic rate is largely due to the increase in plasma triglyceride pool size and an increase in VLDL secretion, rather than a primary reduction in removal, although a VLDL rise is expected from the reduction in LPL activity and could not be ruled out.[96–98,102,103,142]

Another approach to the problem of assessing triglyceride fatty acid removal in the pregnant rat model consisted in comparing plasma triglyceride concentration at known times after the cessation of ad libitum feeding in the rat.[96] In this investigation, triglyceride fatty acid clearance was equivalent after 8 hours in pregnant and nonpregnant rats. More rapid clearance at 4 hours in nonpregnant rats may have been due to the fact that endogenous triglyceride concentration is higher in the pregnant rat than in the nonpregnant rat, resulting in competition for LPL-mediated removal sites, as well as to a higher prior food intake in the pregnant rat compared to nonpregnant rat, resulting in more fat absorption at 4 hours than in the nonpregnant rat. The conclusion was that plasma disposition of a fat load is unimpaired in the pregnant rat, a conclusion also drawn by Argiles and Herrera.[107]

What is one to make of the sharp reductions in LPL in the rat and human model in adipose tissue and in total postheparin lipolytic activity[96–98,102,103,142] and postheparin LPL activity?[104,105] Additional sites of triglyceride fatty acid removal during pregnancy are the uterus[98] and the placenta.[99,124] Bonet et al.[100] have demonstrated high activity levels of the LPL in cultured human trophoblast, confirming whole-placenta measurements.[99,124] LPL activity is substantial, not only in trophoblastic cells but in placental macrophages, which are present in abundance.[100] It is possible that the trophoblasts and macrophages of the placenta oxidize major amounts of triglyceride fatty acid or conceivably transfer them to the placenta.[100,101] Whether heparin-induced release of lipoprotein lipase in vivo in human pregnancy adequately reflects the extent of this process is problematical because of the nature of the placental circulation, which is a low-pressure, large-volume system into which fetal chorionic villi project.[144] Until the relative activities of total-body muscle LPL versus adipose tissue LPL activities are quantified and the extent to which these tissues and the placenta oxidize or store triglyceride fatty acids is known, the question of whether hypertriglyceridemia in pregnancy is due to overproduction or diminished removal, or both, cannot be resolved. What seems likely is that the usual high LPL activity for triglyceride uptake by adipose tissue is diminished during late pregnancy, making triglyceride-rich lipoproteins more available to other tissue (e.g., muscle, heart, breast, uterus, and placenta). Teleologically, the hyperlipidemia of pregnancy could be intensifying that diversion.

Because of the inability to study human pregnancy with anything but stable isotopes, nothing is yet known about the kinetics of lipoprotein metabolism in pregnancy. The increase in VLDL triglyceride concentrations in mid- and late gestation should reflect predominantly increased entry into the circulation (as shown in Figure 12.11) and possibly some element of diminished removal. Because LDL is primarily a catabolic product of VLDL, there should be an increased traffic in LDL cholesterol, similar to that seen in VLDL. Whether LDL receptor-mediated LDL cholesterol clearance is enhanced in pregnancy is a matter of debate. No studies have been done in humans, and studies of two animal models are conflicting. Shiomi et al.[145] found that LDL clearance was increased in the pregnant compared to the nonpregnant homozygous Watanabe heritable hyperlipidemic (WHHL) rabbits. In the nonpregnant state, these rabbits have less than 5% normal functioning LDL receptors, comparable to the human LDL receptor deficiency state.[145] Shiomi et al. found a decrease in LDL cholesterol concentrations from 562 to 114 mg·dl^{-1} without a reduction in VLDL input, as measured by hepatic VLDL secretion using triton inhibition of LPL-mediated VLDL clearance. On the other hand, Belknap and Sharp[146] found a decrease in receptor-mediated LDL clearance by the liver and by the whole animal in rat pregnancy using ^{125}I-labeled rat LDL cholesterol. Nonreceptor-mediated clearance of LDL is reduced late in gestation by day 21 in these studies. This effect occurs in the rat despite an increase in LDL clearance via the placenta.[147] If the putative decrease in pregnant rat LDL clearance reflects hepatic uptake, as in the human,[18] it could be due to a marked increase in maternal hepatic cholesterol synthesis, which has been reported in the rat.[148]

It is uncertain if these studies on LDL metabolism in the rat can be extrapolated to the human. The pregnant rat does show about a twofold increase in LDL cholesterol concentration.[149] However, LDL cholesterol concentration is low in the pregnant rat compared to the human, with the LDL cholesterol concentration rising from an average of 8 to 14 mg·dl^{-1}, comparing the nonpregnant and the term animal. In comparison, plasma triglyceride concentrations increase from approximately 78 to 160–175 mg·dl^{-1} at term in the rat.[150] Some species difference may be important with respect to LDL cholesterol. An additional species difference is seen in the subhuman primate, where plasma triglyceride, LDL cholesterol, and HDL cholesterol concentrations decline markedly during gestation.[150] Extrapolations from one species or animal model to the human may be hazardous. Although certain effects may be consistent, such as enhanced hepatic secretion of VLDL triglyceride, the plasma concentration always reflects the balance between entry and removal. If removal of VLDL triglyceride is greater or less than entry at any given moment, and the same for LDL or HDL lipid, increases or decreases are observed. Only direct kinetic measurements during human pregnancy can answer the questions relating to increased entry versus decreased removal as mechanisms for the differences in lipoprotein concentrations observed among the species.[124,149,150] One bit of physiologic information about LDL in human pregnancy is that the high LDL triglyceride concentration is inversely related to the reductions in hepatic and lipoprotein lipase activities (Table 12.6).

Only inferences can be drawn about whether VLDL remnants are removed more slowly during pregnancy. We attempted to approach this question by examining VLDL cholesterol/total triglyceride ratios in the pregnant woman compared to the oral contraceptive user and the nonpregnant subject. As shown in Figure 12.13, a smooth exponential decline in the VLDL cholesterol/triglyceride ratio is seen as VLDL triglyceride concentrations increase. In contrast, at a low concentration of triglyceride, both the oral contraceptive user and the pregnant woman have a lower VLDL cholesterol/VLDL

TABLE 12.6. Lineal semilogarithmic regressions between the changes in plasma lipoprotein triglyceride content and the changes in lipase activities in women during pregnancy, postpartum, and postlactation.

	Log HL	Log LPL
VLDL-TG		
n	76	65
r	−0.466	−0.351
p	<0.001	0.004
LDL-TG		
n	78	66
r	−0.652	−0.398
p	<0.001	0.001
HDL-TG		
n	74	63
r	−0.757	−0.344
p	<0.001	0.006

Lineal semilogarithmic regression analysis formula, $Y = a + b (\log X)$. The values correspond to the differences between two consecutive periods (2nd minus 1st trimester, 3rd minus 2nd trimester, postpartum minus 3rd trimester, and postlactation minus postpartum).
From Alvarez et al.,[104] with permission.

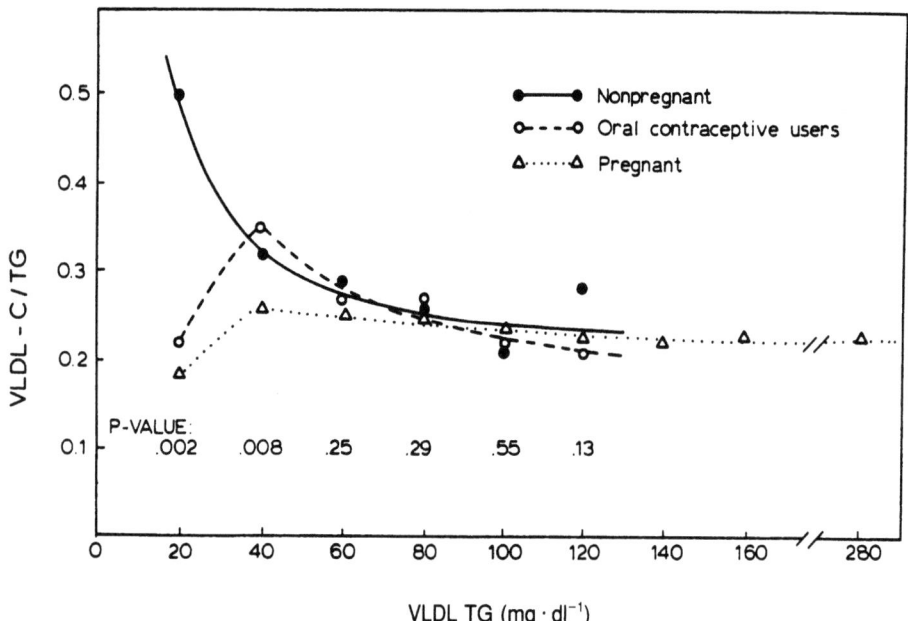

FIGURE 12.13. Lipoprotein cholesterol/triglyceride ratios in normal women, oral contraceptive users, and pregnancy. (From Knopp et al.,[151] with permission.)

triglyceride ratio. That is, triglyceride is more abundant relative to the amount of cholesterol. As VLDL triglyceride concentration increases, the oral contraceptive curve becomes superimposed over the nonpregnant curve, and the pregnant curve remains below the nonpregnant curve until reaching a VLDL triglyceride concentration of 100 to 120 mg/dl. Above that point, the pregnancy curve appears to be an extension of the nonpregnant relation. The interpretation of these curvilinear relationships is that there is no accumulation of cholesterol in VLDL relative to triglyceride during pregnancy compared to that in the normal nonpregnant woman. These data are compatible with normal remnant clearance from the VLDL density range. As for the VLDL triglyceride itself, increases are inversely proportional to decreases in activities of hepatic lipase and lipoprotein lipase (-0.466 and -0.351; $p < .001$ and $.004$, respectively).[104]

We have previously reported a roughly threefold increase in IDL lipoprotein during late gestation.[132] The reduction in hepatic triglyceride lipase (HTGL)[104,105] could retard remnant clearance in pregnancy as it does in the nonpregnant person; however, the increase in IDL is proportional to the VLDL and LDL increases. Therefore, selective reduction in IDL removal seems unlikely on this account. An increased incidence 1.1% of β-migrating VLDL was seen in a survey of normal pregnant women compared to no cases among nonpregnant controls.[63] Perhaps the common E_2/E_2 phenotype might become manifest as β-VLDL under the pressure of an increased rate of VLDL entry into the circulation, diminished HTGL activity, or both. Obviously, direct assessment of remnant removal is required during pregnancy.

The regulation of HDL metabolism has been studied in the pregnant rat model. This model differs from the human in that an increase in HDL cholesterol concentration is not observed. To determine if HDL protein and cholesterol ester plasma transport increased or changed during the course of gestation, Sakuma et al.[152] prepared in vitro doubly labeled ^{125}I HDL protein and tritiated HDL cholesterol ester from nonpregnant rats and reinjected the HDL into recipient late-gestation pregnant rats. The fractional catabolic rate is not altered in the pregnant animal compared to the nonpregnant control. However, because of the two- to threefold increase in plasma volume, calculated total transport through the plasma compartment was increased two- to threefold proportionately. Whether these observations in the rat can be extrapolated to human pregnancy is uncertain.[152] The probability in human pregnancy is that the unusual association of a rising total plasma triglyceride concentration with a rising HDL apoprotein and cholesterol content, at least through the first half of pregnancy, reflects an increasing estrogen effect that could both augment the apo A-I synthesis rate[47] and diminish HDL-C removal[45] owing to a reduction in hepatic triglyceride lipase.[104,105] In fact, Alvarez et al.[104] have found an inverse association between HDL_{2b}, the subfraction with the greatest increase, and a reduction in hepatic lipase activity ($r = -.456$, $p = .001$). The change in HDL_{2b} level was also positively associated with change in lipoprotein lipase activity over the course of gestation.[104]

The slight decline in HDL cholesterol concentration after the peak level is reached at gestational week 20 may have at least three explanations. The first is that transfer of cholesterol ester from HDL to LDL and VLDL may be enhanced in return for triglyceride (Figure 12.2) via lipid transfer protein reaction because of its increased activity and because of the increased concentration of substrate.[49,104] Second, late gestation insulin resistance and increased fat mobilization could have an adverse effect on HDL cholesterol similar to that seen in type II diabetes[153] as well as obesity and endogenous hypertriglyceridemia.[154] A third possible mechanism for the decline in HDL cholesterol concentration is increased uptake of HDL cholesterol containing lipoprotein by the placenta itself (Figure 12.14). We have observed that HDL_2 cholesterol is a donor for progesterone secretion in the cultured trophoblast[155] (vide supra). In contrast, HDL_3 tends to remove cholesterol from trophoblast and reduce progesterone secretion.[155] It is further noteworthy that the decline in HDL during later gestation is associated with a fall in HDL_2 rather than HDL_3. Utilization of HDL_2 could explain the decline in HDL cholesterol concentration. Only further studies can differentiate among these possibilities. However, because the decline in HDL cholesterol is unaccompanied by a decline in apo A-I (Figure 12.10), an alteration in lipid metabolism, rather than apoprotein metabolism in HDL, appears to be responsible. A final point is that HDL appears to be a hormonal secretagogue, stimulating human chorionic gonadotropin (hCG) secretion.[156] In summary, HDL appears to become cholesterol-poor relative to midgestation by several possible mechanisms.

Excretion of cholesterol and bile acids into the bile seems not to be increased during the last two trimesters of pregnancy, although the composition of bile is altered such that cholesterol excretion is increased relative to that of bile acids and phospholipids. Chenodeoxycholic acid declines, and cholic acid excretion increases. The enterohepatic circulation is reduced during pregnancy.[157] These changes resemble those of estrogen (Figure 12.2). Surprisingly, changes in fecal sterol excretion are the opposite of the changes in bile, with a peak in bile acid excretion at midgestation and a decrease in neutral sterol excretion of cholesterol and its degradation products.[7] Possibly this difference reflects increased cholesterol absorption during pregnancy.

Hormonal Basis for the Lipoprotein Changes in Pregnancy

The lipoprotein lipid increases during pregnancy are generally thought to be due to the sex steroids of pregnancy. Two investigations have examined the correlations of hormones and lipoproteins. We have examined the association between lipoprotein lipid concentration at 36 weeks' gestation and insulin, estradiol, estriol, progesterone, and placental lactogen in 290 pregnant women after an overnight fast[124] (Table 12.7). Plasma triglyceride concentration is significantly positively associated with plasma estriol concentration, and VLDL triglyceride concentration correlates positively with insulin. Montelongo et al. has also observed a positive association of plasma VLDL, IDL, and HDL triglyceride in pregnancy with plasma estradiol, progesterone, and prolactin concentrations.[158] LDL cholesterol is negatively associated with progesterone concentration, and HDL cholesterol is positively associated with both estradiol and progesterone concentrations. Although cause and effect are not established by these associations, the observations are consistent with some of the data about the effects of hormones on lipoproteins presented earlier. An increase in plasma insulin concentration is thought to be associated with an increase in triglyceride secretion, particularly in the presence of obesity. Sex steroids such as estradiol and estriol are believed to increase hepatic secretion of triglyceride and VLDL. HDL concentration increase under the influence of estrogen. A negative association between LDL cholesterol and progesterone is more difficult to explain, but could reflect increased utilization of LDL cholesterol by the placenta

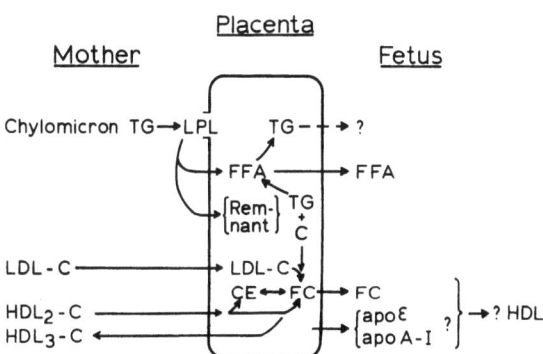

FIGURE 12.14. Hypothetical model of cholesterol transfer to the fetus.

TABLE 12.7. Correlations of hormone and lipoprotein cholesterol and triglyceride concentrations during pregnancy.

Hormone or lipoprotein	Spearman correlation coefficients			
	TG	VLDL-TG	LDL-C	HDL-C
Insulin	0.09	0.14[b]	−0.09	0.00
Estradiol	0.09	0.05	0.01	0.13[a]
Estriol	0.13[a]	0.09	−0.07	0.06
Progesterone	0.04	0.02	−0.15[b]	0.15[c]
hCS	0.07	0.03	−0.03	0.03

hCS, placental lactogen (human chorionic somatomammotropin).
A total of 290 pregnant women were studied after an overnight fast at 36 weeks' gestation. See Knopp et al.[124] for descriptions of the population studied and the results, Sigel for the nonparametric correlation method of Spearman, and Walden et al. for assay methodology.
Statistical significance: [a] $p < .05$; [b] $p < .02$; [c] $p < .01$.
From Knopp et al.,[124] with permission.

in the course of progesterone secretion. That is, if progesterone secretion were greater, LDL cholesterol concentrations would be lower.

Using a different approach, Desoye et al.[128] examined the relation between the increase in various lipoprotein constituents during pregnancy over time and the corresponding increase in chorionic gonadotropin, estradiol, progesterone, placental lactogen, and insulin. In this time course analysis, lipoprotein constituents increased, as did estradiol, progesterone, placental lactogen, and insulin; and, not surprisingly, positive associations were consistently seen. In contrast, the hCG concentration declined as expected between the first and third trimesters of pregnancy, and a negative association with the rising concentrations of lipoprotein constituents was observed. In this approach, associations could be causal or coincidental. Alvarez et al.[104] have performed a similar analysis relating change in hepatic lipase and lipoprotein lipase activities to change in estradiol, progesterone, and prolactin. In all these instances, the associations are negative, and the interpretation about causality is probable in the case of estrogen, unlikely in the case of progesterone, and uncertain for prolactin.[104]

Role of the Placenta in Lipid and Lipoprotein Lipid Removal and Transfer to the Fetus

A teleologic rationale for the rise in lipoprotein lipids in pregnancy is to enhance delivery of lipoprotein lipids to the fetoplacental unit. This scenario includes free fatty acids as well as lipoprotein triglyceride, cholesterol, and phospholipid-associated fatty acids, the last carrying a polyunsaturate as one of their fatty acids. With respect to fatty acid transport, the presence of unusual or essential fatty acids of dietary origin acids in the fatty acid profile of the fetal circulation indicates that essential fatty acids can traverse the placenta.[3,159] For a time it was believed that free fatty acid transfer was limited in the rodent model.[160] Subsequently, Shafrir and Barash[160] modified the interpretation of these early observations to say that free fatty acid transfer was sufficient for the amount of fat assimilation by the rat fetus, which is, unlike most other species, low at the time of delivery. It appears that the fetus does not use fatty acids for oxidation, probably a desirable situation because of the high oxygen requirement for fat oxidation.[161] Subsequent investigations indicate that species specificity imposes high selectivity on the rate of transplacental free fatty acid transport to the fetus. For instance, Hershfield and Nemeth[162] compared several species and found that a much greater proportion of fatty acid comes from the mother in the guinea pig and rabbit than in the rat, sheep, or human. In fact, fatty acid transport in the guinea pig is so great that lipemia develops in the growing fetus.[162] Regardless of species, however, free fatty acid transport is rapid, within minutes in the rhesus and cynomolgus monkey models, as reported by Portman et al.[163] Transport in the reverse direction does occur, but the dominant direction from mother to fetus appears to be a function of the maternal-fetal gradient, which favors flow in the downhill direction from mother to fetus.[124,164] The other reasonably consistent point is that essential fatty acids are transported more than nonessential fatty acids.[162,163,165,166] Ruyle, Connor et al.[165] have shown that docosahexanoic acid is preferentially transferred via the umbilical erythrocytes. This effect supports the retinal and CNS developmental needs for long-chain ω-3 fatty acids.[6,166]

The extent of the human maternal-fetal gradients at birth are presented in Table 12.8, which shows the significant differences in the arteriovenous circulation concentrations of glucose and free fatty acids (FFA). That the FFA gradient from maternal to fetal circulation and the further downhill FFA gradient between umbilical vein and artery reflects the fact that net FFA transport is supported by the positive correlation between maternal and fetal FFA concentrations ($r = .37; p < .05$).[124] This association confirms previous reports.[167-169] Further evi-

TABLE 12.8. Fuel and total protein concentrations at delivery in maternal vein and fetal umbilical vein and artery.

Assay	Maternal venous conc.	Fetal umbilical conc.		$\frac{\text{Vein} - \text{artery}}{\text{vein}} \times 100$
		Venous	Venous-arterial	
Glucose ($mg \cdot dl^{-1}$)	150 ± 51	107 ± 7	12.5 ± 2.0	11.7
FFA ($\mu Eq \cdot L^{-1}$)	672 ± 39	320 ± 23	25.7 ± 9.7	8.0
TG ($mg \cdot dl^{-1}$)	208 ± 14	28.9 ± 2.8	0.21 ± 0.47	0.72
Cholesterol ($mg \cdot dl^{-1}$)	206 ± 5	69.6 ± 2.0	0.52 ± 0.75	0.74
Total protein ($mg \cdot dl^{-1}$)	7.89 ± 0.19	7.00 ± 0.14	0.32 ± 0.15	0.46

Results are given as the means ± SE.
EDTA or Na oxalate F plasma was obtained from blood withdrawn by needle and syringe from the umbilical artery and vein from the umbilical cord clamped at placental and fetal extremes and simultaneously from a maternal antecubital vein. All pregnant women were healthy, had vaginal term deliveries, and were receiving saline intravenously, but not glucose.
From Knopp et al.,[124] with permission.

dence of the significance of FFA transport to the fetus is that the maternal concentrations of FFAs in these studies are associated with neonatal birth weight.[167,169,170]

Free fatty acid transfer across the placenta does appear to be subject to maternal metabolic regulation to the extent that when FFA concentrations increase, a greater amount of fatty acid transport across the placenta is observed, with accumulation of fat in fetal stores, including liver and adipose tissue in rabbits fasted for 48 hours[171] or in animals treated with heparin.[172] The rapidity of fatty acid transfer from mother to fetus within minutes, as demonstrated by Portman et al.,[163] argues against an intermediate metabolic step in FFA metabolism during the course of transplacental transport.

On the other hand, Freinkel[173] and Szabo et al.[174] showed that fatty acids can be taken up by placental tissue to form triglyceride and that glyceride accumulated during rat gestation in increasing amounts in the placenta.[101] Fasting causes a further increase in placental triglyceride concentration, suggesting that the placenta may protect the fetus from excessive FFA transfer.[175] With the increase in triacylglycerol concentrations in the placental tissue in their rat model, Diamant et al.[101] found increased oxidation of carbon dioxide per milligram of DNA oxidized from oleic acid. These observations indicate that increased amounts of fatty acids can be oxidized during late gestation, and the triglyceride accumulation may reflect relative saturation of fatty acid oxidative mechanisms.[101] Coleman and Haynes[176,177] have also shown that placental cells can form fatty acids de novo and esterify and release them and that the enzymes of triglyceride synthesis and breakdown are present in placenta, and in the case of the rat at concentrations comparable to liver.[178]

Phospholipids, as one might expect, do not cross the placenta, as was demonstrated by Popjak and Beeckmans[179] during the late 1940s. However, it was established by these investigators[180] and subsequently by Biezenski and Carrozza[181,182] that phospholipids can be hydrolyzed into their constituent phosphorus-containing moieties and fatty acids transferred into the umbilical vein as such or reformed into phospholipids and then transferred. The fact that the observations of Biezenski and Carrozza indicated that placental phospholipid can reach the circulation suggests that a mechanism for phospholipid assembly into lipoprotein exists in the placenta and for the subsequent transfer to the fetal circulation, possibly as HDL, the most phospholipid-rich lipoprotein (vide infra).

With respect to the question of whether triglyceride fatty acids have access to the placenta or cross it, the argument begins with whether LPL is present in the placenta itself. The first demonstration of LPL activity with typical inhibitory characteristics of sodium chloride and protamine was reported by Mallov and Alousi[99] in 1965 in the rat and human placenta. Subsequently, LPL activity has been described in other species including the guinea pig, rabbit, and sheep,[183–185] and in human cultured trophoblast and macrophages.[100] That triglyceride could cross the placenta unchanged seems to be unlikely considering the size of the triglyceride particle. In other tissues triglyceride fatty acids enter and leave the cell only in the free fatty acid form and are esterified only for the purpose of storage within the cell or for transport in extracellular fluid in the form of lipoproteins.[176,178]

To study VLDL triglyceride fatty acid access to the placenta, Hummel et al.[186] injected radiolabeled chylomicron VLDL lipoprotein triglycerides into the pregnant rat and found that measurable amounts of fatty acids arising from these injections appear in the fetal circulation. We confirmed this observation in our laboratory (E. Herrera, J. Humphrey, and R.H. Knopp, unpublished data). These data indicate that maternal triacylglycerol fatty acids reach the placental circulation but do not indicate in what form. Lasunción et al.[187] have, in unpublished data, attempted to demonstrate direct triglyceride fatty acid transfer across the placenta by infusing triglyceride in the isolated uterine horn model they developed. Infusions lasting 15 minutes have not indicated any significant triglyceride fatty acid transport (personal communication). In the rat, the mechanism of fatty acid transport across the placenta arising from triglycerides involves hydrolysis of triglycerides by the LPL of extraplacental tissues and uptake and transfer by the placenta as fatty acids. However, it is possible that species differences exist, as the rat transfers less free fatty acid than other species.[160,162] Further research is required to explore this point.

The earliest investigation of whether neutral lipids are transferred across the placenta was made by Boyd and Wilson[188] in 1935, who tested for an umbilical vein-artery gradient for neutral lipid in the cord at delivery. They found none. In confirmation, in our studies (Table 12.8) a statistically significant gradient for plasma triglyceride concentrations across the umbilical venous arterial circuit was not observed.[124] It is possible that hemoconcentration may occur on the venous side of the umbilical circulation so that protein concentrations may be slightly higher on the venous than on the arterial side of the fetal umbilical circulation. Such a trend is seen in the data presented in Table 12.8. Some artifact may arise, depending on the technique for sampling umbilical blood.[124] On the other hand, triglyceride secretion by the placenta may occur under specific conditions. For instance, Elphick et al.[189] found a triglyceride gradient only during Intralipid (triglyceride-phospholipid emulsion) infusion. Regarding mechanisms for the secretion of triglyceride from the placental trophoblast to the fetal circulation, it is noteworthy that the placenta did not generate an apo B message in a study where liver and intestine did.[190] On the other hand, rat placenta does contain apo B message.[191] This matter requires more study. Alternatively, triglyceride may be associated with secretion of another type of lipoprotein particle; again, HDL is a possibility, since it seems capable of assembly in a variety of tissues even as a process of repair of injury,[192] and the placenta can secrete phospholipid.[193]

With respect to cholesterol transfer across the placenta, in the pregnant rat fed deuterated cholesterol in classic studies, cholesterol reached the fetal tissue.[194] In the rat, earlier studies indicated that about 20% of fetal cholesterol is derived from maternal circulation and about 80% is synthesized locally.[195] These early studies in the rat have been challenged by Belknap and Dietschy,[147] who injected radiolabeled water into the pregnant rat and found that sterol synthesis rates were several times higher per unit weight in the fetus than in the dam, particularly in the fetal liver. When maternal cholesterol synthesis is suppressed by cholesterol feeding, there is minimal reduction in the rate of appearance of newly synthesized sterol in the fetus, placenta, and fetal membranes at 17 days' gestation. Whereas the placenta does take up LDL at about one half the rate of the maternal liver, none of the apolipoprotein or cholesterol is transferred to the fetus over short observation times. The extent of the dispute with previous data may relate to the differences between the 15% to 20% of transfer reported in a French study in the late gestation rat[195] in contrast to that reported by Belknap and Dietschy,[147] who found almost none. It is noteworthy that Chevalier[195] found that higher amounts (65%) of fetal cholesterol were derived from the mother during early gestation.

The possibility of species differences was again raised by the studies of Pitkin et al.,[196] who calculated that 42.6% of the serum cholesterol in the term fetus originates by transfer from the maternal blood in the rhesus monkey. The transfer of isotope seems to be largely unidirectional, with transfer from mother to fetus reaching equilibrium 10 to 12 days after injection, whereas fetal injection of isotopic cholesterol results in no more than 5% of fetal specific activity being reached in maternal cholesterol. In a similar study in baboons, Khansi et al.[197] found that equilibration of labeled maternal cholesterol with fetal cholesterol occurred after 5 days. With respect to the human, evidence for transplacental cholesterol transfer has been obtained in studies of Lin et al.[198] Another possibility is that mevalonate may be an important maternal precursor for fetal cholesterol synthesis.[199]

In summary, there may be species differences in cholesterol transport, as there is variation in the quantity of fatty acid transfer across the placenta and in placental anatomy. These differences may relate to the substantial variation in fat stores in the animal models of pregnancy, as mentioned above (see Biezenski[200] for review). The early literature on lipid transfer across the placenta has been reviewed by Robertson and Sprecher[201] and Roux and Yoshioka.[202] (See discussion about animal models in metabolic research in Chapter 3.)

With respect to lipoprotein cholesterol uptake by the placenta, uptake and degradation of LDL and small amounts of HDL have been observed.[203–205] Using cultured trophoblast cells from human subjects, we have found that LDL cholesterol is taken up by the placenta, as LDL-cholesterol–^{14}C stimulated placental secretion of ^{14}C-labeled progesterone.[155,206] This process is specific as it is blocked by anti-LDL receptor antibody. The placental syncytiotrophoblast LDL receptor also appears to be specifically regulated and sensitive to estrogen in the placenta[207,208] as it is elsewhere.[39,40] We have found that HDL stimulated progesterone secretion, with HDL sometimes providing more stimulus to progesterone secretion than LDL, depending on the viability of the LDL receptor.[155,206] In any case, HDL_3, which is associated with the reverse cholesterol transport pathway (vide supra), tends to inhibit the secretion of progesterone by the placenta and to reduce placental cholesterol content.[155] These observations have led to the hypothesis that HDL_2 may serve as an alternative cholesterol donor to the placenta, as it does to other endocrine organs (see Gwynne and Strauss[209] for review). In this way, women deficient in LDL (hypobetalipoproteinemia) have only minor reductions in steroid hormone production and can still conceive and bear children.[210]

Although much remains to be learned about transplacental lipid transport, a hypothetical model based on the above discussion is presented in Figure 12.14. In this scenario, chylomicron or VLDL triglycerides can reach the placenta from the maternal circulation and be cleaved into free fatty acids under the influence of placental LPL. It is also possible, although not yet proven, that apo E containing chylomicrons or VLDL, or their remnants, may be taken up by the placenta via detecting LDL receptor–related protein (LRP),[211] the VLDL receptor,[212] the LDL receptor, or all three. Overbergh et al.[213] are of the opinion that the LRP (macroglobulin receptor) is most important. In this case, triglyceride would be taken up as part of the lipoprotein particle by the placental cell and cleaved intracellularly by lysosomal lipases to free fatty acids. Once within the placenta, free fatty acids can be secreted to the fetus unchanged or can be reesterified to triglyceride within the placenta, whereupon they are largely stored or oxidized. LDL cholesterol is taken up by the LDL receptor, whereas HDL_2 is more likely to deliver cholesterol by a nonspecific transfer process, as has been described for the ovary,[214] though a docking protein interaction appears likely.[22] Once within the cell, free cholesterol or cholesterol ester can be cyclically esterified and deesterified and possibly secreted to the fetal circulation via assembly of HDL on the fetal side involving apo E and apo A-I. It is notable that the amount of apo E in cord blood HDL is unusually high (5.8 mg·dl⁻¹) relative to cholesterol (39.7 mg·dl⁻¹) and that the HDL has an unusual size distribution.[215,216] As cord LDL cholesterol concentration is only 25 mg·dl⁻¹, it was speculated that HDL may be a major carrier of cholesterol in the fetus.[215] HDL_3 may serve to withdraw cholesterol from the placenta back into the maternal or fetal circulation.[155,206] Secretion of apo E by the placenta may facilitate this process.[217] An additional determinant of placental cholesterol balance is the extent to which progesterone and its metabolites are formed in this endocrine organ. Based on the discrepancies in the rat model between the report of Belknap and Dietschy[147] and the primate studies of Pitkin et al.[196,198] and others,[194,195,197] there appears to be some uncertainty as to the extent to which cholesterol traverses the placenta completely and reaches the fetus. Placental morphology, species, and extent of fetal maturity in utero may prove to be important predictors of the quantity of cholesterol, free fatty acid, and triglyceride transport, collectively, across the placenta.

Effects of Modified Lipoproteins on the Placenta

The final consideration bearing on access of cholesterol to the placenta is pathophysiologic. It is well known that oxidative stress can modify circulating lipoproteins, especially LDL-C. These modified lipoproteins are taken up by scavenger receptors.[218] This system is relevant to pregnancy and placental function. Recently, Bonet et al.[219] found that cultured placental trophoblast and macrophages from normal healthy elective cesarean-section deliveries contain scavenger receptors. This finding was demonstrated using acetylated LDL, a model of an oxidatively modified lipoprotein such as malonyldialdehyde modified LDL.[218] A most interesting finding was that the uptake and degradation of acetylated LDL by trophoblast was tenfold greater than for normal labeled LDL in trophoblast (Figure 12.15). In contrast, the acetylated LDL uptake in placental macrophages was only three- to fourfold greater than normal LDL, meaning that at least in these primary cell culture conditions, the activity of scavenger receptors/LDL receptors was greater in trophoblast than even macrophages, the classic cell type involved in acquisition and processing of damaged biologic material including modified lipids and lipoproteins. These studies demonstrated acetylated LDL uptake by immunochemically identified trophoblast and macrophages, thereby extending the observations by Alsat et al.[220] and Malassine et al.[221] of acetylated LDL uptake by placental microvillous membranes and syncytiotrophoblast. These observations indicate that the placental villous surface of syncytiotrophoblast is equipped to ingest or assimilate damaged LDL and conceivably other damaged entities at a higher rate than LDL itself. The observation suggests that this mechanism provides a basis for the placenta to protect itself from the damaging effect of modified lipoprotein and the possibility of passing such material to the fetus. By virtue of its very high scavenger receptor activity, the trophoblast barrier appears to be the first line of defense against maternal modified lipoproteins.

To investigate if the uptake of modified LDL had equivalent access as substrate for progesterone synthesis, progesterone manufacture by cultured trophoblast was determined in the presence of acetylated LDL (Figure 12.16) or copper oxidized LDL (Figure 12.17).[219] As shown, progesterone formation was much less stimulated

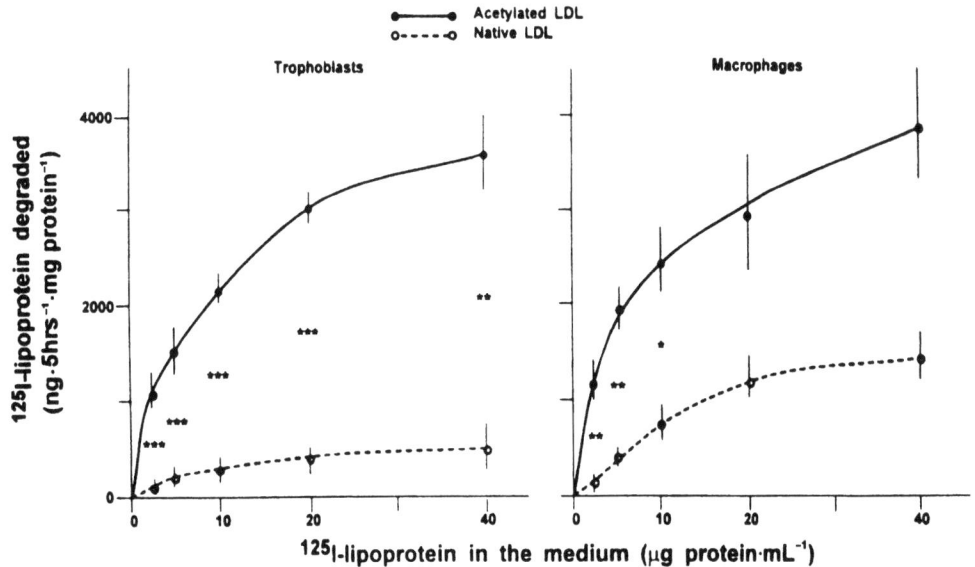

FIGURE 12.15. Uptake and degradation of acetylated LDL by trophoblasts. (From Bonet et al.,[219] with permission.)

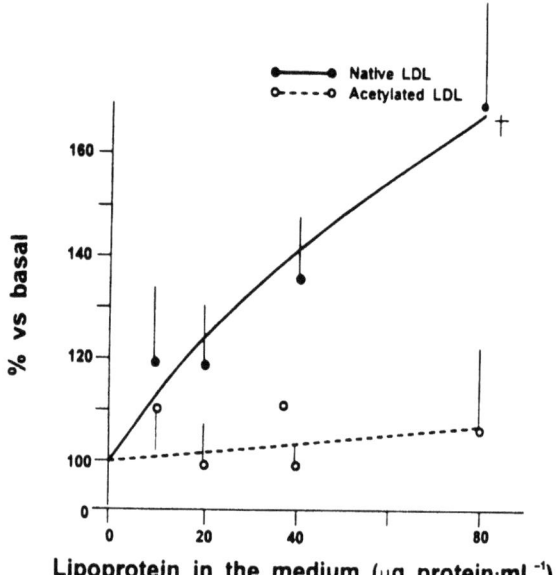

FIGURE 12.16. Progesterone secretion in trophoblasts incubated with increasing concentrations of LDL (•) or ac-LDL (○). Trophoblasts from human placenta were incubated for 48 h in HAM's F-10 medium containing 10% lipoprotein deficient serum with several changes of medium to deplete cells of cholesterol. DbcAMP 0.5 mM was added to stimulate progesterone secretion. After 48 h, the medium was removed and new medium was added to the wells. Increasing concentrations of ac-LDL or LDL were added. The medium was removed after 24 h for determination of progesterone concentration. Mean ± SE of five observations. †Denotes a significant increase above baseline in progesterone secretion stimulated by native LDL ($p < .05$). (From Bonet et al.,[219] with permission.)

placental trophoblast and macrophages was observed as measured by the appearance of ^{51}Cr into prelabeled cells[224] and generation of lipid peroxides. This process was likened to oxidation of the LDL itself, because the cytotoxicity (i.e., Cr leak) was inhibited by addition of divalent metal ion chelator [ethylenediaminetetraacetic acid (EDTA)], culture medium containing metal ions, and antioxidants such as butylated hydroxytoluene (BHT).[224–226] Interestingly, the trophoblast seemed less susceptible to cytotoxic stress than macrophages, conceivably another example of its resiliency as a first line of defense.

Because estrogens are known antioxidants[227–229] and because progestins and androgens might oppose the antioxidant effect of estrogen as these hormones oppose other physiologic effects of estrogen,[94] we studied the effects of estrogen, progestin, and testosterone on the oxidation of LDL by cultured trophoblast and placental macrophages in the presence of copper Cu^{2+} ion and again measured cytotoxicity in the form of ^{51}Cr release.[225,226] The expected result was observed. Estrogen inhibited LDL oxidation and diminished the cytotoxic effect of the incubation on trophoblast and macrophages. Progesterone and testosterone had the opposite effects, being pro-oxidant and procytotoxic. All effects were pro-

by the modified LDLs than by native LDL, even though the scavenger receptor activity was much greater than the LDL receptor activity.[219] These data suggest that modified LDL taken up by the trophoblast scavenger receptors has a different fate that prevents its access to the pathways of normal cholesterol metabolism in the trophoblast. This apparent sequestration may be another way in which the trophoblast presents a line of defense of the placenta against the potential injurious effects of modified LDL. It remains to be seen how the intracellular processing of modified LDL accomplishes this effect and whether the sequestration of damaged LDL extends to preventing its transfer to the fetal circulation.

What might be the deleterious effect of oxidized LDL on placental cell function? It has already been shown that oxidized LDL can be cytotoxic to cells of the arterial wall, thereby constituting a mechanism for the inflammatory response associated with atherosclerosis in hypercholesterolemia or even acute atherosis observed in toxemia of pregnancy.[222,223] For this reason, when placental trophoblast and macrophages were incubated with LDL under conditions that favor LDL oxidation, in the presence of copper, absence of albumen, an increase in damage to

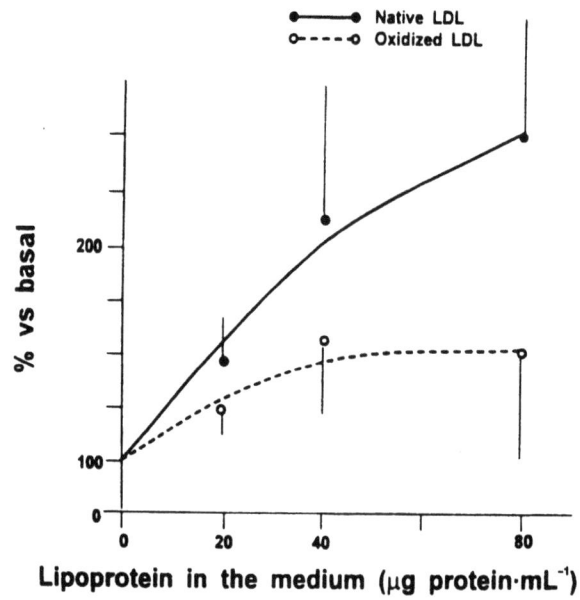

FIGURE 12.17. Progesterone secretion in trophoblasts incubated with increasing concentrations of LDL (•) or ox-LDL (○). Trophoblasts from human placenta were incubated as described in the legend to Figure 12.16. After 48 h, the medium was removed and new medium was added to the wells. Increasing concentrations of ac-LDL or LDL were added with 0.5 mM Dbc AMP. The medium was removed after 24 h for determination of progesterone concentration. Values correspond to the mean ± SE of three observations. (From Bonet et al.,[219] with permission.)

portional to the degree of LDL oxidation.[226] These data confirmed that LDL oxidation can be injurious to placental cells and that sex steroid hormones among other factors could modulate this process. These data would suggest that an estrogen deficiency or a decrease in the estrogen-progestin ratio in pregnancy might favor placental/oxidative injury, or, by extension, arterial wall injury in many different circumstances such as menopause or eclampsia.

In summary, the placental trophoblasts are directly exposed to maternal blood in a slow, low-flow environment where maternal lipoprotein has prolonged exposure to the syncytiotrophoblast surface of the placenta. Such an environment, especially under conditions of placental injury, could favor oxidation of LDL and injury to other cell types.[224,225]

Oxidative Stress in Pregnancy and Relationships to Preeclampsia and Eclampsia

As long ago as 1978, Ishihara[230] observed that plasma lipid peroxide concentration increased with duration of gestation in normal pregnant women. This observation was confirmed by Maseki et al.[231] and both investigators found increased concentration of plasma lipoperoxides in toxemic pregnancy, as noted by Hubel et al.[232] In laboratory studies, Bonet and Knopp[233] found an increase in susceptibility of LDL to oxidation as gestation proceeds in normal pregnancy and a further increased susceptibility in plasma of first-trimester insulin-dependent diabetes mellitus (IDDM) pregnant women. These findings parallel a similar tendency of diabetes in the nonpregnant non-IDDM (NIDDM) and IDDM individual and diabetic animal model.[234-236] Of course, toxemia is more common in the diabetic pregnancy.[237] Taken together, these data point to pregnancy as an oxidative stress that is exaggerated in diabetes and toxemia.

The role of hyperlipidemia in the pathogenesis of toxemia has been explored by a number of investigators. In 1978, Potter and Nestel[126] found that toxemic pregnant women had an elevated plasma triglyceride concentrations. Several investigators have confirmed this observation, including Hubel et al.,[238] Franz and Wendler[239] and Rosing et al.[240] who found plasma triglyceride and free fatty acid concentrations were significantly increased above noneclamptic pregnancy concentrations both antepartum and postpartum. The eclamptic subjects had a 50% increase in plasma total malonyldialdehyde concentration, which decreased postpartum, though not in controls. Elevations in LDL were not observed. These results suggest that hypertriglyceridemia is a risk factor or covariate of toxemia since it persists postpartum and because obesity is still another risk factor for toxemia, as noted by Sattar et al.[241] Hubel et al.[238] hypothesized that the dyslipidemia associated with toxemia might contribute to the endothelial dysfunction of toxemia.

Current theory holds that preeclampsia and eclampsia originate in an abnormal implantation of trophoblast into the muscular layers of the spiral arteries of the uterus, thereby blocking the normal dilatation of spiral arteries and increases in blood flow.[242] The physiologic adrenergic denervation at the base of the spiral artery does not occur, resulting in diminished placental perfusion and production of placental mitogens and cytokines such as tumor necrosis factor-α (TNF-α), which are increased in maternal plasma in preeclampsia.[242] Eicosanoids are produced as are other vasoactive compounds, all of which may contribute to the maternal vasoconstriction, capillary leak, and vasoconstriction.[242] The affected placenta reflects this damage by increasing its production of lipid peroxides and the vasoconstrictor eicosanoid thromboxane relative to prostacycline.[243] A number of previous investigators have found increased amounts of lipid peroxides in placentas of preeclamptic and eclamptic pregnancies.[243,244]

All of these results indicate that amounts of lipid peroxides are increased in toxemic pregnancy plasma and in the placenta itself. Could LDL be involved as a mediator for lipid peroxidation and endothelial and even trophoblast damage even though the concentration is not elevated in eclamptic versus normal pregnancy? The matter has not been examined directly, but Branch et al.[245] have found concentration of antibodies to oxidized LDL in plasma of eclamptic and preeclamptic women just as they have found antibodies to oxidized LDL in the plasma of individuals with hyperlipidemia and atherosclerosis. Whether the immune process is itself pathologic or protective is not known. What is clear is that lipoprotein oxidation is involved in the pathogenesis of preeclampsia and eclampsia. Given our demonstration of placental cell cytotoxicity by oxidized LDL, and possibly apoptosis (Zhu X et al., unpublished data), it is tempting to speculate that the initial process of placental injury can lead to a vicious cycle of lipoprotein oxidation, maternal arterial injury, further LDL oxidation, further placental damage, and so forth. Much further work is necessary to explore and validate this hypothesis. Interestingly, two early studies established the consistency of the oxidative stress, pregnancy, and hypertension association.[246,247]

Effects of Lipid and Lipoprotein Levels on Fetal Growth

Maternal free fatty acids have ready access to the fetus, in proportion to greater chain length and unsaturation, and these free fatty acids can contribute to adipose tissue growth. Therefore, it might be expected that neonatal birth weight might be related to maternal plasma fatty acid concentrations. At least three studies have found associations.[167,169,170] A positive association might not be observed in all instances, since FFA increases most markedly with caloric deprivation, which would have a negative effect on fetal growth. For instance, in preliminary data from the Diabetes in Early Pregnancy Project, first trimester ketone body concentration is inversely associated with birth weight.[248] When positive associations are seen in normal pregnancy between maternal FFA concentration and fetal growth, what may be represented is the success of the conversion of the mother to a fat-based energy economy in late gestation when the fetal glucose requirements are greatest.[94]

Regarding the role of plasma triglyceride fatty acid associations with fetal growth and development, an investigation of 881 normal pregnant women, women with a positive 1-hour 50-g glucose screening test, and gestational diabetic pregnant women showed a positive association between plasma triglyceride concentrations and infant growth up to the 90th percentile of plasma triglyceride concentration (Figure 12.18).[249,250] This triglyceride association with neonatal birth weight corrected for gestational age is stronger than that for glucose using a single measurement of each at the time of glucose screening at 28 weeks' gestation. This observation suggests a direct relationship between maternal triglyceride concentration by means of hydrolysis to FFA by placental LPL and transport to the fetus. Of great interest is the fact that there appears to be a maximum to this effect at a triglyceride concentration at the 85th to 90th percentile, followed by a lower birth weight at an even higher plasma triglyceride level (Figure 12.18). Could a toxic effect ensue as a result of serious hypertriglyceridemia or is triglyceride concentration above the 90th percentile associated with or a consequence of some deleterious process such as eclampsia? As discussed above, at present it is not

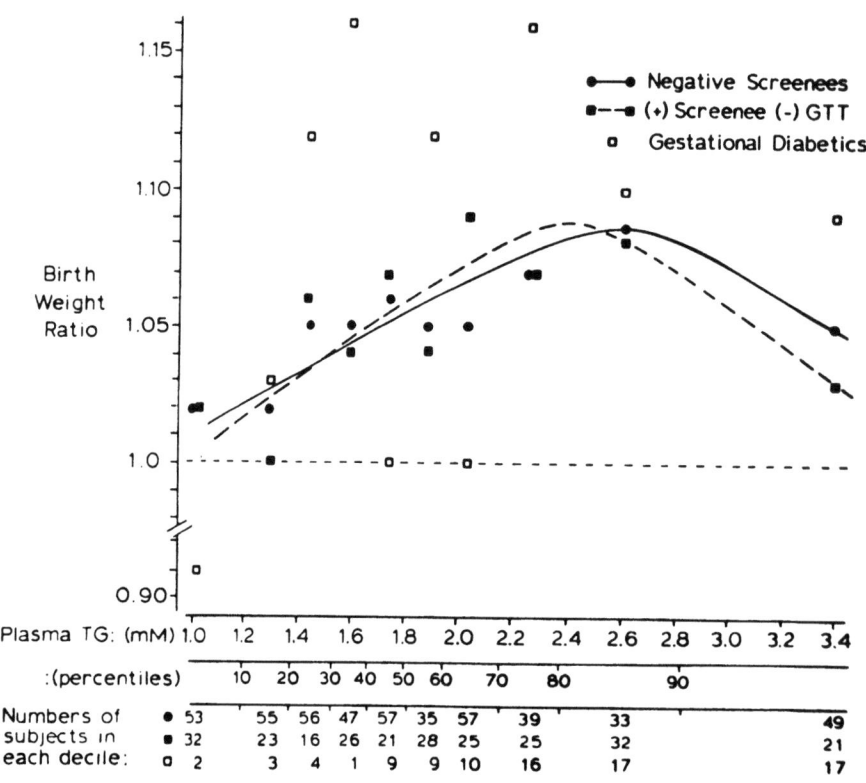

FIGURE 12.18. Relationship between birth weight ratio (infant birth weight adjusted for gestational age) and plasma triglyceride (TG) concentration (on the topmost bottom horizontal axis). A birth weight ratio of 1.00 denotes an infant birth weight at the 50th percentile value for a given gestational age using the Portland sea level tables. A value other than 1.00 is the ratio of the observed birth weight divided by the 50th percentile birth weight for that gestational age. The percentile values of plasma TG (on the middle horizontal axis) are based on the distribution of plasma TG concentrations in nondiabetic pregnant subjects in this study. The percentile scale is more expanded at higher TG levels because of the upward skewness of the plasma TG distribution. The lowest horizontal axis refers to the numbers of subjects studied within each TG decile. Between the 0 and 10th TG percentiles, there are 53 negative screenees, 32 GTT$^-$ subjects, and 2 GDM subjects. The slopes of the negative screenee and GTT$^-$ groups are significantly different from horizontal ($p < .05$ in each instance). The relationship between birth weight ratio and TG in the GDM subjects is more unstable, possibly because of fewer subjects, especially in the lower TG percentiles, and is not statistically significantly different from the horizontal. The GDM data points nonetheless follow the trend of the negative screenees and GTT$^-$ groups. Above the 75–90th percentile of TG, birth weight ratio tends to drop ($p < .05$ when all three groups are combined). (From Knopp et al.,[250] with permission.)

12. Lipid Metabolism in Pregnancy

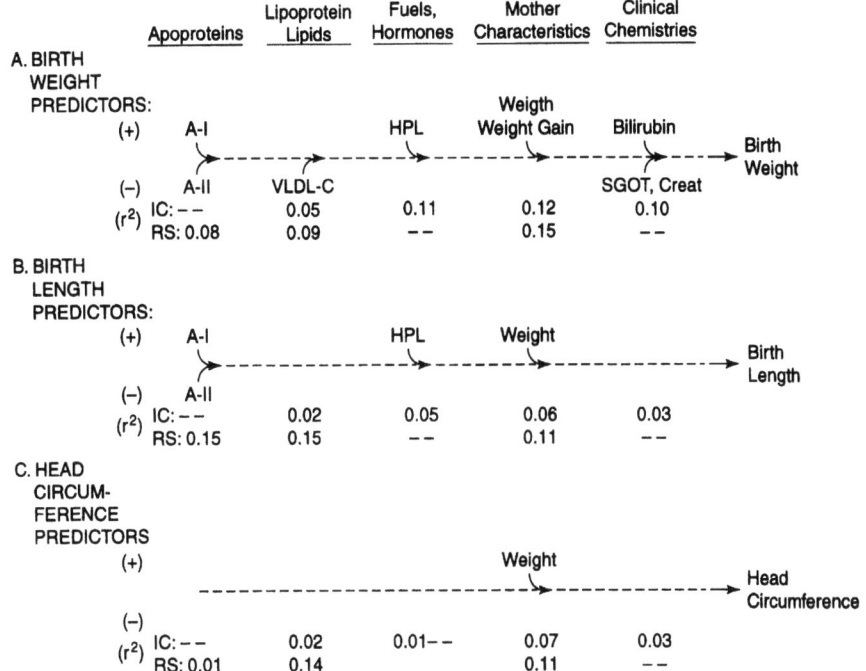

FIGURE 12.19. Parameters significantly associated positively (+) or negatively (−) with birth weight or birth weight ratio, birth length, and head circumference. Values for r^2 for each category are presented below each line for the initial cohort of subjects (IC) where the n approximates 210–273, and the random sample (RS) where the n approximates 75. The value of r^2 denotes the amount of variation in the outcome variable explained by each group of variables rather than the cumulative r^2 values, which are presented in the tables. (From Knopp et al.,[252] with permission.)

known if the hypertriglyceridemia of toxemia is a cause or an effect, but the asymptote between birth weight and triglyceride elevation in these data could be a respresentation of this association. More studies are needed to verify this observation. The triglyceride/birth weight association appears to be a durable one, having been described earlier by Skryten et al.[251]

In another investigation of normal subjects, a positive association has been shown between apo A-I concentration, a major apolipoprotein of HDL_2, and birth weight adjusted for gestational age. In contrast, apo A-II concentration, predominantly associated with HDL_3, is inversely associated with adjusted neonatal birth weight and birth length, but not head circumference.[252] These results are summarized in Figure 12.19, which shows that placental lactogen, maternal weight and weight gain, and bilirubin, which is an endogenous antioxidant, are also positively associated with birth weight and length. Only maternal prepregnancy weight was associated with head circumference at birth. These apoprotein associations provide independent evidence for the idea that availability of cholesterol from the maternal side in the form of lipoproteins can influence fetal growth and development. Possible mechanisms may relate to the effect of HDL_2 to deliver cholesterol to cells, to promote progesterone secretion, and for HDL_3 to inhibit these processes as noted by Lasunción et al.[155] The main conclusion is that apoprotein A-I and A-II rank with other known maternal predictors of birth size, including indices of placental size (HDL) and maternal prepregnancy weight and weight gain. These data indicate that the lipoprotein cascade is as important as any other circulating nutrient in the regulation and prediction of birth weight.

Effects of Diabetes on Lipoprotein Levels in Pregnancy

The lipoprotein changes in diabetic pregnancy have been examined by several investigations and the data are influenced by whether the diabetic population is composed of type I or type II diabetics and the type of statistical analysis. In an early investigation we found that diabetes in NIDDM subjects was associated with hypertriglyceridemia but not IDDM (Table 12.9).[253] These triglyceride elevations and associated reductions in HDL tended to be less marked or to disappear postpartum (Figure 12.20). Similarly, we have seen elevated triglyceride concentrations in gestational diabetics at 24 to 28 weeks' gestation (Table 12.10).[250] Of interest, placental saturated fatty acid content and total lipid content is elevated in gestational diabetic pregnancy.[254] Hollingsworth and Grundy[255] also observed increased total and lipoprotein triglycerides and reduced HDL-C concentrations in NIDDM and gestational diabetic pregnancy. On the other hand, Montelongo et al.[157] found little difference in plasma concentrations of gestational diabetics and overt diabetics versus normal pregnant subjects, but attribute this to lower plasma sex hormone concentrations in these pregnant subjects. Most recently, Koukkou et al.[256] confirmed a total triglyceride increase

TABLE 12.9. Plasma triglyceride and cholesterol in normal and diabetic pregnancy.

	Triglyceride (mg·dl^{-1})	Cholesterol (mg·dl^{-1})	Age (mg·dl^{-1})	Gestation (mg·dl^{-1})
Normal (38)	189 ± 58*	211 ± 28	26 ± 6	35 ± 3
Gestational diabetic subjects (22)	207 ± 110	209 ± 46	30 ± 5†	36 ± 4
Overt diabetic subjects (10)	180 ± 72	221 ± 29	29 ± 4	33 ± 4

Number of subjects in parentheses.
* Mean ± SD.
† Different from normal ($p < .02$).
From Knopp et al.,[253] with permission.

and a lower LDL-C in gestational diabetics. They also found a trend toward a lower total cholesterol level as we had in an earlier study.[257]

In a more extensive study of insulin-dependent diabetic subjects,[258] we found no difference in plasma triglyceride, but a lower total cholesterol level (Figure 12.21) that was due to a selective reduction in HDL and in the HDL$_3$ fraction of HDL (Figure 12.22) and an absence of the usual increment in HDL apoproteins A-I and A-II (Figure 12.23).

In summary, these data indicate that the obese gestational diabetes mellitus (GDM) and NIDDM pregnant subject has the features of the nonpregnancy obese diabetic, though somewhat magnified by the pregnancy. On the other hand, a rather focal defect in HDL metabolism appears to exist in IDDM (type I) diabetic pregnancy, again directing attention to the importance of HDL in progesterone secretion, birth weight prediction, and redox state. Since HDL functions as a plasma antioxidant, it is interesting that HDL-C concentration was low in early gestation in two infants of diabetic mothers with congenital malformations.[258] It is known that oxidative stress is an important cause of congenital malformation (Table 12.11).[259,260] The lower HDL-C is not consistently explained by poorer diabetic control or hypertriglyceridemia in IDDM pregnancy, so the explanation remains to be found.

Lipoprotein Lipid Changes During Lactation

The lactating mother delivers as many as 480 to 830 calories/day to her neonate. Approximately one half of these calories are delivered in the milk in the form of triacylglycerol or triglyceride.[261] This process places a substantial demand on maternal lipoprotein triglyceride homeostasis. Numerous investigators have been interested in the source of triglyceride fatty acids for the lactating breast. Originally, Otway and Robinson[142] in 1968

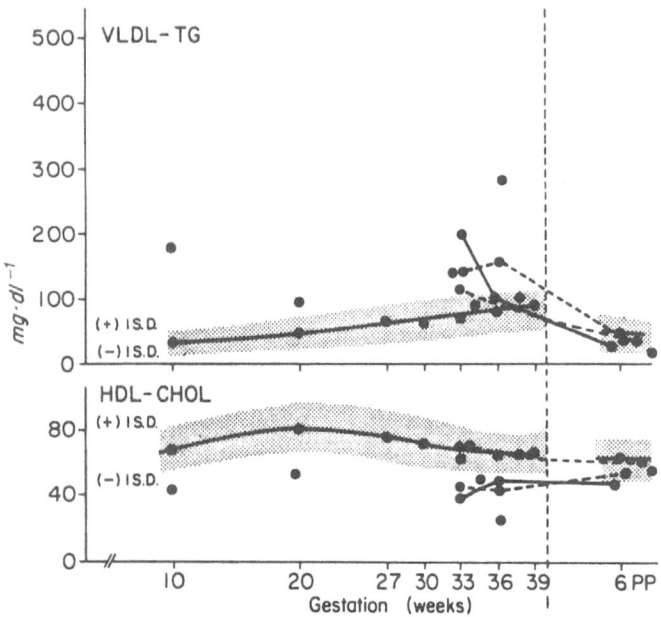

FIGURE 12.20. VLDL triglyceride (TG) and HDL cholesterol (CHOL) concentrations in adult-onset (type II) diabetic subjects studied at various stages in pregnancy and 6 weeks postpartum (PP). These subjects are compared with the mean ± 1 SD (hatched area) for VLDL-TG and HDL-CHOL concentration for 12–22 serially studied normal pregnant subjects. Solid and dotted lines connect serially studied subjects. (From Knopp et al.,[253] with permission.)

TABLE 12.10. Screening test and 3-h glucose tolerance test (GTT) results in the three pregnancy groups.

	Negative screenees (521)	Positive screenees (GTT⁻) (264)	Gestation diabetes mellitus (GDM) (96)
Screening test			
Glucose (mM)	6.27 ± 0.94	8.71 ± 0.72*	9.55 ± 1.11†‡
GHb (%)	4.7 ± 0.6	4.9 ± 0.7*	5.2 ± 0.7†‡
GPro (%)	2.8 ± 1.0	3.0 ± 1.0*	3.1 ± 1.0†
IRI (pM)	410 ± 273	662 ± 453*	791 ± 648†
TG (mM)	1.86 ± 0.68	1.92 ± 0.68	2.29 ± 0.68†‡
3 h GTT			
Glucose (mM)			
0 h	—	4.77 ± 0.44	5.27 ± 0.61‡
1 h	—	8.55 ± 1.28	10.93 ± 1.28‡
2 h	—	7.10 ± 0.99	9.43 ± 1.28‡
3 h	—	5.94 ± 1.33	7.32 ± 1.78‡
Sum of increments	—	21.0 ± 2.2	26.6 ± 2.3‡
Cord plasma (n)	324–325	184–187	70–72
Glucose (mM)	2.72 ± 1.50	2.78 ± 1.78	2.94 ± 1.83
IRI (pM/L)	108 ± 86	108 ± 72	151 ± 144†‡

Values are means ± SD. (n), number of subjects. Glucose, GHb, GPro, IRI, and TG are all measured 1 h post 50-g oral glucose load after overnight fast.
*GTT⁻ differs from negative screenees ($p < .005$).
† GTT⁺ differs from negative screenees ($p < .005$).
‡ GDM differs from GTT⁻ ($p < .005$).
From Knopp et al.,[250] with permission.

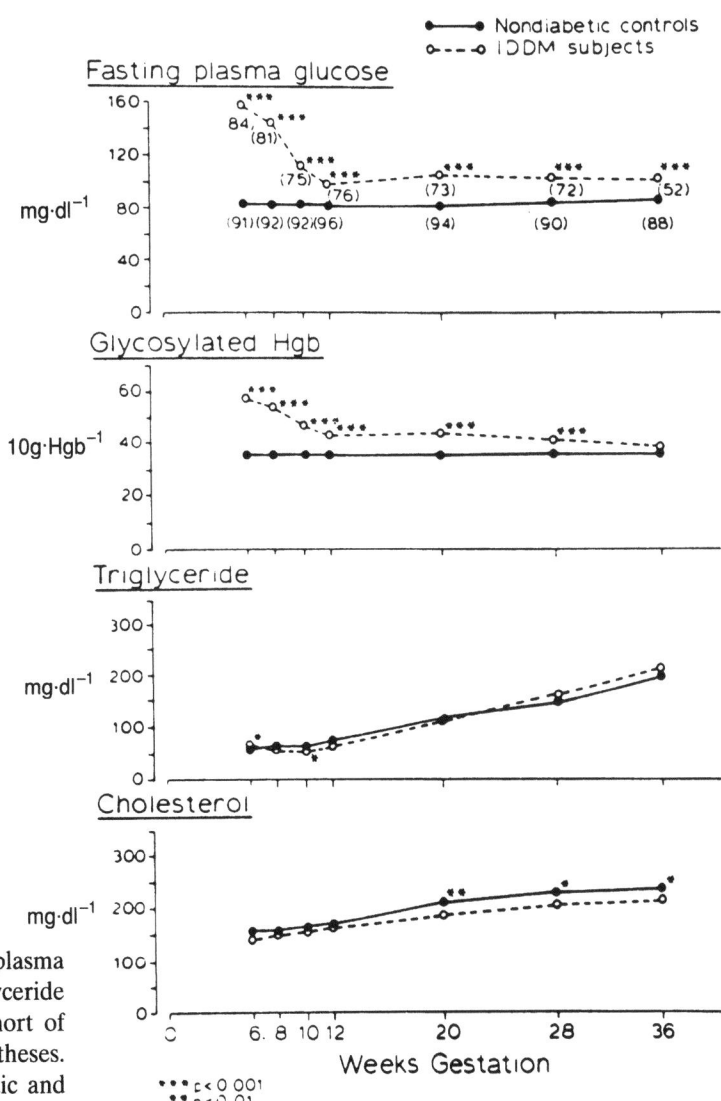

FIGURE 12.21. Median plasma concentrations of fasting plasma glucose, glycosylated hemoglobin, and total plasma triglyceride and cholesterol throughout gestation in the entire cohort of subjects. The numbers of subjects studied are in parentheses. Asterisks denote statistical significance between diabetic and normal subjects. (From Knopp et al.,[258] with permission.)

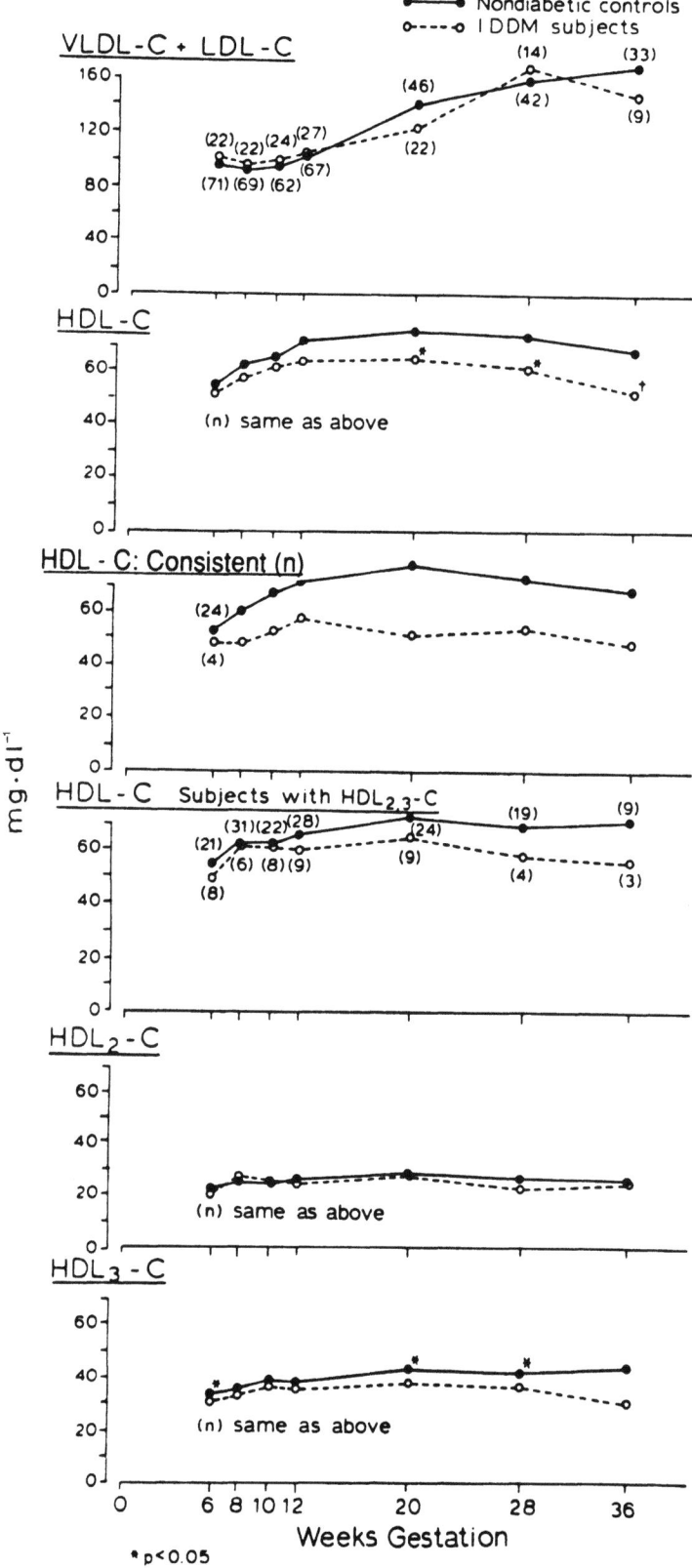

FIGURE 12.22. Median plasma concentrations of VLDL + LDL-C and HDL-C throughout gestation. HDL-C values are also shown for 24 normal and 4 diabetic subjects who had measurements made at each visit and for those who had HDL_2-C and HDL_3-C measurements made. The numbers of subjects studied are in parentheses. Asterisks and dagger denote statistical significance between diabetic and normal subjects. (From Knopp et al.,[258] with permission.)

FIGURE 12.23. Mean ± SE of the percent increase, between 12 and 28 weeks' gestation, in apoprotein A-I and A-II levels in nondiabetic and diabetic subjects. Significant increases in apoprotein A-I and A-II were seen in normal control subjects but not in type I diabetic subjects. (From Knopp et al.,[258] with permission.)

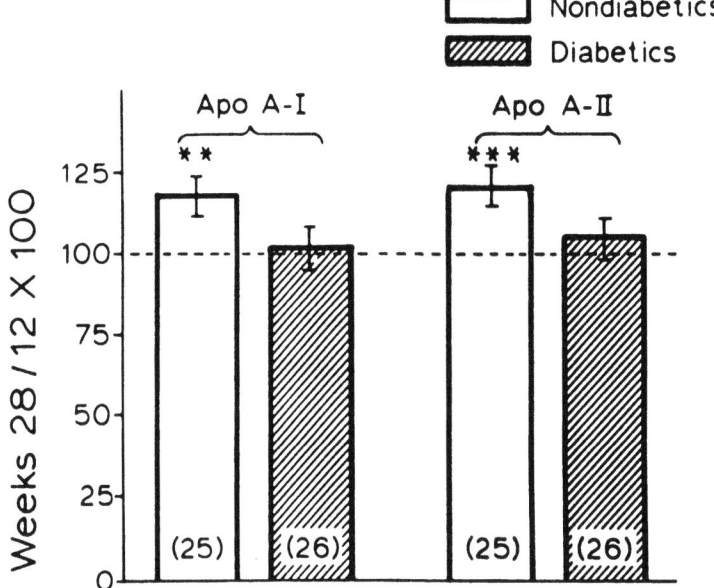

showed that with parturition adipose tissue LPL concentrations fell dramatically, whereas LPL activity in the lactating breast increased markedly. These observations were confirmed by Hamosh et al.,[102] Chajek-Shaul et al.,[262] and Ramirez et al.[98] The role of prolactin in this process was investigated by Zinder et al.,[263] who showed that prolactin given to nonpregnant animals increases the LPL activity in the lactating mammary gland and reduces it in adipose tissue. Blocking the increase in circulating prolactin levels in the late pregnant rat by administering progesterone has also been shown to block the increase in LPL activity in the mammary gland,[98] which further emphasizes the relation between prolactin and mammary gland LPL activity. Zinder et al.[264] showed that chylomicron triacylglycerol and cholesterol could be taken up by the perfused rat mammary tissue and that this process is associated with the level of LPL activity. Finally, Hachey et al.[265] have shown that long-chain fatty acids labeled with stable isotopes and orally administered to the lactating mother can be taken up by the breast and appear in

TABLE 12.11. Glycemic status and lipoprotein lipids in two mothers of congenitally malformed infants.

Status, lipids	Weeks' gestation						
	6	8	10	12	20	28	36
Glucose (mg·dl⁻¹)							
002 McR	184	258	137	58	84	200	136
356 DEN	174	148	135	183	92	83	—
Diabetic means	165	144	150	115	127	124	119
Glycosylated hemoglobin (ng·log⁻¹)							
002 McR	66	58	58	44	56	57	54
356 DEN	42	—	50	41	—	—	—
Diabetic means	62	57	53	48	49	46	42
Triglyceride (mg·dl⁻¹)							
002 McR	92	122	109	—	190	310	239
356 DEN	38	71	71	66	8	163	—
Diabetic means	64	61	70	78	129	226	243
Cholesterol (mg·dl⁻¹)							
002 McR	125	119	122	—	160	178	156
356 DEN	131	145	153	163	187	225	—
Diabetic means	154	162	164	174	194	232	217
HDL-C (mg·dl⁻¹)							
002 McR	49	54	58	—	64	60	60
356 DEN	45	46	48	49	53	56	—
Diabetic means	54	62	71	69	62	58	—

002 McR, microcephaly with developmental delay.
356 DEN, anencephaly.
From Knopp et al.,[258] with permission.

TABLE 12.12. Effects of lactation on lipoproteins.

Lipoproteins	Postpartum concentrations (mg·dl^{-1})			Postpartum difference from antepartum (mg·dl^{-1})		
	Lac	non-Lac	p	Lac	non-Lac	p
Total						
TG	92	112	<0.02	129	116	NS
Chol	207	188	<0.01	39	50	NS
VLDL						
TG	54	78	<0.01	63	57	NS
Chol	14	17	NS	14	12	NS
LDL						
TG	26	24	NS	44	35	NS
Chol	129	121	NS	25	21	NS
PL	70	70	NS	15	15	NS
Apo-B	76	66	NS	29	24	NS
HDL						
TG	12	10	NS	20	22	NS
Chol	65	51	<0.001	−1	17	<0.0001
PL	141	123	<0.005	1	23	<0.01
Apo A-I	142	126	<0.02	31	46	<0.01
Apo A-II	34	31	<0.01	−3	4	<0.001

TG, triglyceride; Chol, cholesterol; PL, phospholipid, Lac, lactating; NS, not significant.
From Knopp et al.,[261] with permission.

breast milk. They also demonstrated in situ fatty acid synthesis in the human mammary gland.[266] Lipoprotein cholesterol is delivered to the lactating breast as chylomicrons and denser lipoproteins.[267] Finally, a reduction occurs in human adipose tissue LPL activity with lactation, as in animals.[268]

The effects of this process on lipoproteins in the postpartum lactating mother have been quantified in our laboratory. The investigation was designed to measure lipoprotein lipid concentrations in 72 women at 36 weeks' gestation and at 6 weeks postpartum, when 56 were lactating and 16 were not.[261] Postpartum data in lactating and nonlactating groups were compared, as were the changes from antepartum measurements at 36 weeks' gestation (Table 12.12). No statistically significant differences were detected in the 36-week gestation measurements in the two groups. However, postpartum nonlactating subjects had slightly higher plasma triglyceride concentrations and slightly lower total cholesterol concentrations than lactating subjects. In VLDL, plasma triglyceride concentrations were significantly higher. LDL cholesterol concentrations were not statistically significantly different. A marked difference in cholesterol was seen in HDL, where the HDL cholesterol concentration was 65 mg·dl^{-1} in lactating subjects and 51 mg·dl^{-1} in nonlactating subjects. Phospholipid, apo A-I, and apo A-II concentrations were similarly higher in the lactating than in the nonlactating groups. These differences in HDL were confirmed by calculating the differences between predelivery and postdelivery lipoprotein measurements in the lactating and nonlactating groups; the differences in total triglyceride cholesterol and VLDL triglyceride did not test significantly different. The increase in apo A-II as well as apo A-I suggests that the HDL cholesterol rise in postpartum lactating women is associated with HDL$_3$ as well as HDL$_2$ cholesterol increases. Because the absolute concentrations of VLDL triglyceride are lower in the lactating than in the nonlactating subject and the antepartum-postpartum differences show similar trends, the possibility exists that the difference in the postpartum measurements reflects increased utilization of maternal triglycerides. Alternatively, less VLDL triglyceride may be entering the circulation because of the lesser secretion of ovarian estrogen in lactating women.

Desoye et al.[128] measured lipoprotein lipids during the first and second halves of the menstrual cycle and 6 to 8 weeks postpartum in 23 women on whom they had performed studies during pregnancy. Nine of these subjects were still lactating, and none was using oral contraceptives. These investigators reported no differences in any lipoprotein lipid or apoprotein as a result of lactation. However, the relative body weight of nonlactating women was greater than that of lactating subjects. In addition, reference was not made in that study to the antepartum lipoprotein concentration, nor was any attempt made to normalize the postpartum results in light of the antepartum differences should they exist.

The observation that postpartum lactating women have higher HDL concentrations, including all constituents of HDL, raises mechanistic questions. The postpartum lactating woman is normally amenorrheic and has low estrogen concentrations in the circulation. Under such a circumstance, one would expect HDL cholesterol concentrations to be low rather than high. However, an alternative explanation for these changes can be offered. If circulating plasma triglycerides, either from the diet as chylomicrons or from the liver as VLDL, are taken up by the lactating breast at an increased rate, triglyceride lipoprotein transport through the circulation may be increased, especially if plasma triglyceride concentrations are not consistently lower with lactation.[261] By some mechanism, VLDL production may be maintained despite the absence of estrogen. Alternatively, the reduction in adipose tissue LPL may offset the increase in mammary gland LPL such that plasma triglyceride flux is not altered. In the former instance, an increase of VLDL flux in the circulation could generate increased quantities of surface remnants that transfer to HDL and augment HDL mass. An increase in dietary fat intake during lactation could have the same effect. Kinetic studies are required to distinguish among these possibilities.

With respect to dietary fat and cholesterol, Mellies et al.[269] have found that milk fatty acid patterns generally parallel dietary fatty acid intake. Similarly, these investigators have found that increased intake of maternal phytosterols, plant sterols such as sitosterol, in the diet lead to an increase in breast milk content and neonatal phytosterol concentrations in plasma. Mellies et al. did not find any effect on breast milk of feeding high cholesterol diet to lactating mothers. In hypobetalipoproteinemic women, a deficiency of chylomicrons, VLDL, and LDL leads to a reduction in lipoprotein triglyceride delivery to the breast and increased endogenous synthesis, resulting in low essential fatty acid content of the expressed milk.[270]

Management of Lipid Disorders in Pregnancy

Severe hypertriglyceridemia during pregnancy with plasma triglyceride concentration exceeding 2000 mg·dl^{-1} has become increasingly recognized as being due to specific mutations in the lipoprotein lipase gene resulting in low LPL levels.[271] This condition of severe hypertriglyceridemia can subject the pregnant woman to severe hemorrhagic pancreatitis. Treatment of such individuals is best accomplished with a low fat diet; in one clinical study in our center, feeding 6 to 8 g daily of omega-3-rich fatty acids, as fish oil, was successful in reducing plasma triglyceride concentration and reversing early symptomatic pancreatitis.[272] This subject has recently been reviewed.[273] Hypercholesterolemia has no known deleterious effect on the fetus and should receive no more than dietary treatment in light of uncertainties about the safety of lipid-lowering drugs for fetal growth and development. As mentioned earlier, cholesterol restriction reduced plasma cholesterol levels during pregnancy.[140] A recent report has also appeared of successful LDL apheresis treatment of homozygous familial hypercholesterolemia in pregnancy.[274] There is no proof that the hyperlipidemia of pregnancy per se is atherogenic.[275] Elevations in triglyceride and cholesterol during pregnancy may predict underlying hyperlipidemia in one third to one half of cases (R.H. Knopp, unpublished data), and a fall in LDL cholesterol with a rise in triglyceride during pregnancy may signify combined hyperlipidemia (Figure 12.24).[276] Further studies are

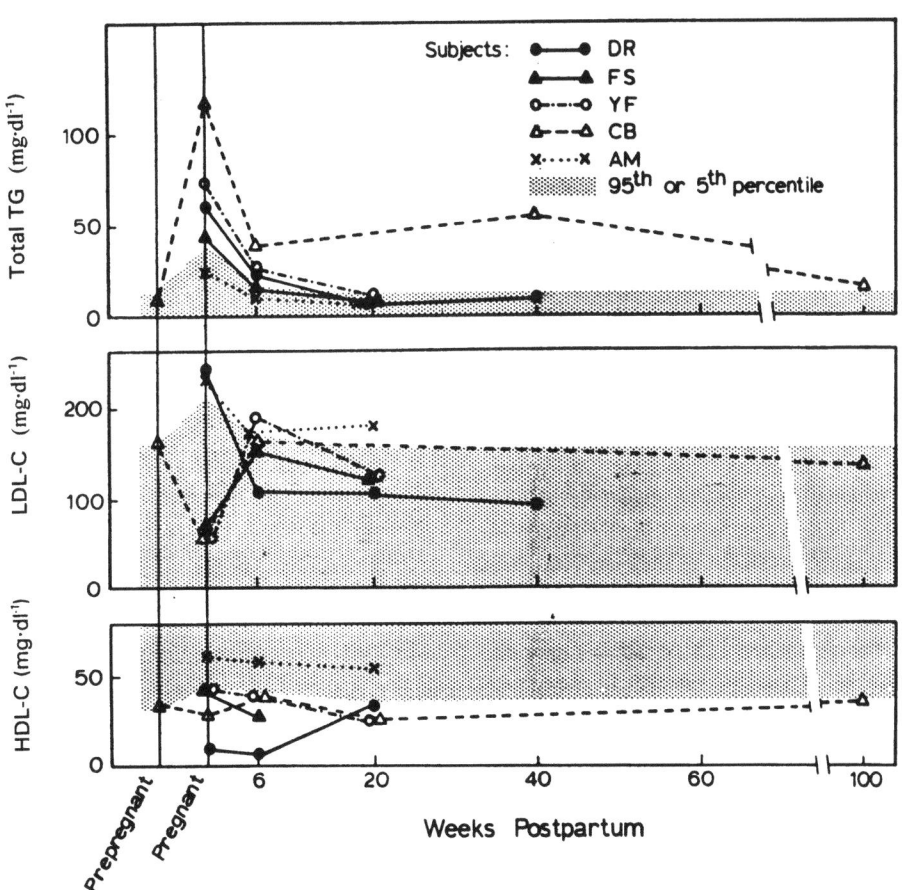

FIGURE 12.24. Plasma total triglyceride and LDL and HDL cholesterol concentrations antepartum, at 36 weeks of gestation, and at various times postpartum in four hypertriglyceridemic subjects in pregnancy compared with the 95th or 5th percentiles of a random population of pregnant women or nonpregnant women aged 20 to 29 years. Total triglyceride for subject YF (aged 33) is above the 95th percentile for women aged 20–29 at 20 weeks postpartum, but below the 95th percentile for women aged 30–39. (From Montes et al.,[276] with permission.)

needed to verify this hypothesis. When considering postpartum lipid screening it is important to keep in mind that LDL cholesterol does not return to baseline for 9 months to 1 year after delivery.[276]

Summary

This review of lipid metabolism during pregnancy spanned investigations of many years and described not only changes in circulating lipids but also underlying changes in whole-body lipid metabolism in the pregnant woman and placenta, the possible transfer to the fetus, the role of lipoproteins in postpartum lactation, and derangements associated with diabetes and toxemia. Future research in this area requires that investigators pass the descriptive stage and begin kinetic studies of lipoprotein metabolism during pregnancy using nonradioactive isotopic methods and that they make parallel studies on the effects of individual sex hormones on lipoproteins. Finally, the effects of oxidized lipids in pregnancy on placental trophoblast and arterial wall function is needed to understand the pathophysiology of eclampsia and its management. Such studies are now beginning and promise to enhance our understanding of the pivotal role of lipid metabolism in reproduction.

Acknowledgments. This work was supported by grant DK-35816 and the USA-Spain Cooperative Research Agreement CCA-8510/06 and the Robert B. McMillen Family Trust.

References

1. Virchow R. Zur Entwicklungsgeschichte des Krebses: Bemerkungen uber Fettbildung im thierischen Korper und pathologische Resorption. Virchow Arch 1847;1:94.
2. Becquerel A, Rodier A. La composition du sang. Gaz Med 1844;20:127.
3. Soderhjelm L. Fat absorption studies. VI. The passage of polyunsaturate fatty acids through the placenta. Acta Soc Med Up 1953;58:239–243.
4. Scandinavian Simvastatin Survival Study Group. Randomised trial of cholesterol lowering in 4444 patients with coronary heart disease: the Scandinavian Simvastatin survival study (4S). Lancet 1994;344:1383–1389.
5. Sheperd J, Cobbe SM. Ford I, et al. Prevention of coronary heart disease with pravastatin in men with hypercholesterolemia. N Engl J Med 1995;333:(20)1301–1307.
6. Neuringer M, Connor WE, VanPetten C. Dietary omega-3 fatty acid deficiency and visual loss in infant rhesus monkeys. J Clin Invest 1984;73:272–276.
7. Potter J, Nestel PJ. Cholesterol balance during pregnancy. Clin Chem Acta 1978;87:57–61.
8. Kesaniemi A, Enholm C, Miettenin TA. Intestinal cholesterol absorption efficiency in man is related to apoprotein E phenotype. J Clin Invest 1987;80:578–581.
9. Herrera E, Knopp RH. Pentose monophosphate shunt dehydrogenases and fatty acid synthesis in late rat pregnancy. Experientia 1972;28:646–647.
10. Knopp RH, Saudek CD, Arky RA, O'Sullivan JB. Two phases of adipose tissue metabolism in pregnancy: maternal adaptations for fetal growth. Endocrinology 1973;92:984–988.
11. Montes A, Knopp RH. Lipid metabolism in pregnancy. IV. C apoprotein changes in very low and intermediate density lipoproteins. J Clin Endocrinol Metab 1977;45:1060–1063.
12. Willnow TE, Sheng Z, Ishibashi S, Herz J. Inhibition of hepatic chylomicron remnant uptake by gene transfer of a receptor antagonist. Science 1994;264:1471–1474.
13. Warchawsky I, Brose GJ Jr, Schwartz AL. The low density lipoprotein receptor-related protein mediates the cellular degradation of tissue factor pathway inhibitor. Proc Soc Exp Biol Med 1994;91:6664–6668.
14. Mahley RW. Apolipoprotein E: cholesterol transport protein with expanding role in cell biology. Science 1988;240:622–630.
15. Brown MS, Goldstein J. Lipoprotein receptors in the liver: control signals for plasma cholesterol traffic. J Clin Invest 1983;72:743–747.
16. Jingami H, Yamamoto T. The VLDL receptor: wayward brother of the LDL receptor. Curr Opin Lipidol 1995;6:104–108.
17. Beisiegel U, St Clair RW. An emerging understanding of the interactions of plasma lipoproteins with the arterial wall that leads to the development of atherosclerosis. Curr Opin Lipidol 1996;7:265–268.
18. Brown MS, Goldstein JL. A receptor-mediated pathway for cholesterol homeostasis. Science 1986;232:34–47.
19. Coetzee GA, van der Westhuyzen DR. Lipoprotein receptors in perspective. Curr Opin Lipidol 1992;3:60–66.
20. Francis GA, Knopp RH, Oram JF. Defective removal of cellular cholesterol and phospholipids by apolipoprotein in A-I in tangier disease. J Clin Invest 1995;96:(1)78–87.
21. Pietersw MN. Schouten D, VanBerkel TJC. In vitro and in vivo evidence for the role of HDL in reverse cholesterol transport. Biochim Biophys Acta 1994;1225:125–134.
22. Steinberg D. A docking receptor for HDL cholesterol esters. Science 1996;271:460–461.
23. Cheung MC, Albers JJ. Characterization of lipoprotein particles isolated by immunoaffinity chromatography. J Biol Chem 1984;259:12201–12209.
24. Johnson WJ, Bamberger ML, Latta RA, et al. The bidirectional flux of cholesterol between cells and lipoproteins: effects of phospholipid depletion on high density lipoprotein. J Biol Chem 1986;261:5766–5776.
25. Ikewaki K, Nishiwaki M, Sakamoto T, et al. Increased catabolic rate of low density lipoproteins in humans with cholesterol ester transfer protein deficiency. J Clin Invest 1995;96:1573–1581.
26. Nishide T, Tollefson JH, Albers JJ. Inhibition of lipid transfer by a unique high density lipoprotein subclass

containing an inhibitor protein. J Lipid Res 1989;30:149–158.
27. Albers JJ, Tu A, Wolbauer G, et al. Molecular biology of phospholipid transfer protein. Curr Opin Lipidol 1996;7:88–93.
28. Cheung MC, Wolfbauer G, Albers JJ. Plasma phospholipid mass transfer rate: relationship to plasma phospholipid and cholesterol ester transfer activities and lipid parameters. Biochim Biophys Acta 1996;1303:101–110.
29. Knopp RH, Zhu X, Lau J, Walden CE. Sex hormones and lipid interactions: implications for cardiovascular disease in women. Endocrinologist 1994;4;286–301.
30. Knopp RH, Zhu X, Bonet B. Effects of estrogens on lipoprotein metabolism and cardiovascular disease in women. Atherosclerosis 1994;110:S83–S91.
31. Knopp RH, Zhu X, Bonet B, Bagatell C. Effects of sex steroids on lipoproteins, clotting and the arterial wall. Semin Reprod Endocrinol 1996;14:(1)15–27.
32. Sacks FM, Gerhard M, Walsh BW. Sex hormones, lipoproteins and vascular reactivity. Curr Opin Lipidol 1995;6:161–166.
33. Schaefer EJ, Foster DM, Zech LA, et al. The effects of estrogen administration on plasma lipoprotein metabolism in premenopausal females. J Clin Endocrinol Metab 1983;57:262–267.
34. Walsh BW, Schiff I, Rosner B, et al. Effects of postmenopausal estrogen replacement on the concentrations and metabolism of plasma lipoproteins. N Engl J Med 1991;325:1196–1204.
35. Applebaum DM, Goldberg AP, Pykalisto OJ, et al. Effect of estrogen on post heparin lipolytic activity: selective decline in hepatic triglyceride lipase. J Clin Invest 1977;59:601–608.
36. Iverius PH, Brunzell JD. Relationship between lipoprotein lipase activity and plasma sex steroid level in obese women. J Clin Invest 1988;82:1106–1112.
37. Knopp RH, Walden CE, Wahl PW, et al. Oral contraceptive and postmenopausal estrogen effects on lipoprotein triglyceride and cholesterol in an adult female population: relationships to estrogen and progestin potency. J Clin Endocrinol Metab 1981;53:1123–1132.
38. Applebaum-Bowden D, McLean P, Steinmetz A, et al. Lipoprotein, apolipoprotein and lipolytic enzyme changes following estrogen administration in postmenopausal women. J Lipid Res 1989;30:1895–1906.
39. Kovanen PT, Brown MS, Goldstein JL. Increased binding of low density lipoproteins to liver membranes from rats treated with 17a-ethinyl estradiol. J Biol Chem 1979;254:11367–11373.
40. Ma PTS, Yamamoto T, Goldstein JL, Brown MS. Increased mRNA for low density lipoprotein receptor in livers of rabbits treated with 17a-ethinyl estradiol. Proc Natl Acad Sci USA 1986;83:792–796.
41. Hazzard WR. Primary type I hyperlipoproteinemia. In: Rifkind BM, Levy RL, eds. Hyperlipidemia—diagnosis and therapy. Orlando, FL: Grune & Stratton, 1977:137–175.
42. Chait A, Brunzell JD, Albers JJ, Hazzard WR. Type III hyperlipoproteinemia ("remnant removal disease"): insight into the pathogenic mechanism. Lancet 1977;1:1176–1178.
43. Tikkanen MJ. Nikkila EA, Vartainen E. Natural estrogen as an effective treatment for type II hyperlipoproteinemia in postmenopausal women. Lancet 1978;2:490–492.
44. Wahl PW, Walden CE, Knopp RH, et al. Effect of estrogen/progestin potency on lipid/lipoprotein cholesterol. N Engl J Med 1983;308:862–867.
45. The Writing Group for the PEPI Trial. Effects of estrogen or estrogen/progestin regimens on heart disease risk factors in postmenopausal women: the postmenopausal estrogen/progestin intervention trial. JAMA 1995;273:199–208.
46. Arbeeny CM, Eder HA. Effects of 17a-ethinyl estradiol on the serum lipoproteins of cholesterol fed diabetic rats. J Biol Chem 1980;255:10547–10550.
47. Brinton A. Oral estrogen replacement therapy in postmenopausal women selectively raises levels and production rates of lipoprotein A-I and lowers hepatic lipase activity without fractional catabolic rate. Arterioscler Thromb Vasc Biol 1996;16:431–440.
48. Gustafson A, Svanborg A. Gonadal steroid effects on plasma lipoproteins and individual phospholipids. J Clin Endocrinol Metab 1972;35:203–207.
49. Silliman K, Tall AR, Kretchmer N, Forte TM. Unusual high-density lipoprotein subclass distribution during late pregnancy. Metabolism 1993;42:(12)1592–1599.
50. Everson GT, Fennessey P, Kern F Jr. Contraceptive steroids alter the steady-state kinetics of bile acids. J Lipid Res 1988;29:68–76.
51. Wolfe BM, Grace DM. Norethindrone acetate inhibition of splanchnic triglyceride secretion in conscious glucose-fed swine. J Lipid Res 1979;20:175–182.
52. Kenagy R, Weinstein L, Heimberg M. The effects of 17b-estradiol and progesterone on the metabolism of free fatty acid by perfused livers from normal female and ovariectomized rats. Endocrinology 1981;108:1613–1621.
53. Khoka R, Huff MW, Wolfe BM. Divergent effects of d-norgestrel on the metabolism of rat very low density and low density apolipoprotein B. J Lipid Res 1986;27:699–705.
54. Tikkanen MJ, Nikkila EA. Regulation of hepatic lipase and serum lipoproteins by sex steroids. Am Heart J 1987;113:562–567.
55. Wolfe BM, Huff MW. Effects of combined estrogen and progestin administration on plasma lipoprotein metabolism in postmenopausal women. J Clin Invest 1989;83:40–45.
56. Olsson AG, Orö L, Rossner S. Effects of oxandrolone on plasma lipoproteins and the intravenous fat tolerance in man. Atherosclerosis 1974;19:337–346.
57. Kushlan MC, Gollan JL, Ma WL. Sex differences in hepatic uptake of long chain fatty acids in single-pass perfused rat liver. J Lipid Res 1981;22:431–436.
58. Huttunen JK, Enholm C, Kekki M, Nikkila EA. Postheparin plasma lipoprotein lipase and hepatic lipase in normal subjects and in patients with hypertriglyceridemia: correlations to sex, age, and various parameters of triglyceride metabolism. Clin Sci Mol Med 1976;50:249–260.

59. Soler-Argilage C, Wilcox HG, Heimberg M. The effect of sex on the quantity and properties of the very low density lipoprotein secreted by the liver in vitro. J Lipid Res 1976;17:139–145.
60. Nikkila EA, Kekki M. Polymorphism of plasma triglyceride kinetics in normal human adult subjects. Acta Med Scand 1971;190:149–59.
61. Tollin C, Ericsson M, Johnson O, Backman C. Clearance of triglycerides from the circulation and its relationship to serum lipoproteins: influence of age and sex. Scand J Clin Lab Invest 1985;45:679–684.
62. Anonymous. The Lipid Research Clinics Population Studies data book, vol. I. 1980; NIH Publication No. 80-1527. Washington, DC: USDHHS.
63. Knopp RH, Bergelin RO, Wahl PW, et al. Population based lipoprotein lipid reference values for women classified by sex hormone usage. Am J Obstet Gynecol 1982;143:626–637.
64. Knopp RH. Cardiovascular effects of endogenous and exogenous sex hormones over a woman's lifetime. Am J Obstet Gynecol 1988;158:1630–1643.
65. Walden CE, Retzlaff BM, Buck BL, et al. Lipoprotein response to the national cholesterol education program step II diet by hypercholesterolemic and combined hyperlipidemic women and men. Arterioscler Thromb Vasc Biol 1997;17:375–382.
66. Costrini NV, Kalkhoff RK. Relative effects of pregnancy, estradiol, and progesterone on plasma insulin and pancreatic islet insulin secretion. J Clin Invest 1971;50:992–999.
67. Yki-Jarvinen H. Sex and insulin sensitivity. Metabolism 1984;33:1011–1015.
68. Guerre-Millo M, Leturque A, Girard J, Lavaw M. Increased insulin sensitivity and responsiveness of glucose metabolism in adipocytes from female versus male rats. J Clin Invest 1985;76:109–116.
69. Merrimee TJ, Fineberg SE. Homeostasis during fasting. II. Hormone substrate difference between men and women. J Clin Endocrinol Metab 1973;37:698–702.
70. Barclay M, Barclay RK, Skipski VP, et al. Fluctuations in human lipoproteins during the normal menstrual cycle. Biochem J 1965;96:205–209.
71. Kim H, Kalkhoff RK. Changes in lipoprotein composition during the menstrual cycle. Metabolism 1979;28:663–668.
72. Basdevant KA, DeLignieres B, Bigorie B, Guy-Grand B. Estradiol, progesterone, and plasma lipids during the menstrual cycle. Diabetes Metab Rev 1981;7:1–4.
73. Mattson L, Silferstolpe G, Samsioe G. Lipid composition of serum lipoproteins in relation to gonadal hormone during the normal menstrual cycle. Eur J Obstet Gynecol Reprod Biol 1984;17:327–335.
74. Ahumada-Hemer H, Valles De Bourges V, Juarez-Ayala J, et al. Variations in serum lipids and lipoproteins throughout the menstrual cycle. Fertil Steril 1985;44:80–84.
75. Tikkanen MJ, Kuusi T, Nikkila EA, Stenman UH. Variation of postheparin plasma hepatic lipase by menstrual cycle. Metabolism 1986;35:99–104.
76. Woods M, Schaefer EJ, Morrill A, et al. Effect of menstrual cycle phase on plasma lipids. J Clin Endocrinol Metab 1987;65:321–323.
77. Webb P. 24-hour energy expenditure and the menstrual cycle. Am J Clin Nutr 1986;44:614–619.
78. Jones DY, Judd JT, Taylor PR, et al. Menstrual cycle effects on plasma lipids. Metabolism 1988;37:1–2.
79. Lussier-Cacan S, Nestruck AC, Arslanian H, et al. Influence of a triphasic oral contraceptive preparation on plasma lipids and lipoproteins. Fertil Steril 1990;53:(1)28–34.
80. Meijer GAL, Westerterp KR, Saris WHM, ten Hoor F. Sleeping metabolic rate in relation to body composition and the menstrual cycle. Am J Clin Nutr 1992;55:637–640.
81. Hytten RE, Thomson AM, Taggart N. Total body water in normal pregnancy. Obstet Gynaecol Br Commonw 1966;73:553–561.
82. Beaton GH, Beare J, Ryu MH, et al. Protein metabolism in the pregnant rat. J Nutr 1954;54:291–304.
83. Knopp RH, Childs MT, Warth MR. Dietary management of the pregnant diabetic. Curr Concepts Nutr 1979;6:119–139.
84. Lopez-Luna P, Munoz T, Herrera E. Body fat in pregnant rats in mid and late gestation. Life Sci 1986;39:1389–1393.
85. Bhatia AJ, Wade GN. Effects of pregnancy and ovarian steroids on fatty acid synthesis and uptake in Syrian hamsters. Am J Physiol 1990;260:R153–R158.
86. Knopp RH, Ruder HJ, Herrera E, Freinkel N. Carbohydrate metabolism in pregnancy. VII. Insulin tolerance during later pregnancy in the fed and fasted pregnant rat. Acta Endocrinol 1970;65:352–360.
87. Buchanan TA, Metzger BE, Freinkel N, Bergman RN. Insulin sensitivity and b-cell responsiveness to glucose during late pregnancy in lean and moderately obese women with normal glucose tolerance or mild gestational diabetes. Am J Obstet Gynecol 1990;162:1008–1014.
88. Freinkel N. Banting lecture 1980: of pregnancy and progeny. Diabetes 1980;29:1023–1035.
89. Knopp RH, Montes A, Childs MT, et al. Metabolic adjustments in normal and diabetic pregnancy. Clin Obstet Gynecol 1981;24:21–49.
90. Knopp RH, Herrera E, Freinkel N. Carbohydrate metabolism in pregnancy. VIII. Metabolism of adipose tissue isolated from fed and fasted rats in late gestation. J Clin Invest 1970;49:1438–1446.
91. Elliott JA. The effect of pregnancy on the control of lipolysis in fat cells isolated from human adipose tissue. Eur J Clin Invest 1975;5:159–163.
92. Herrera E, Knopp RH, Freinkel N. Carbohydrate metabolism in pregnancy. VI. Plasma fuels, insulin, liver composition, gluconeogenesis, and nitrogen metabolism during late gestation in the fed and fasted pregnant rat. J Clin Invest 1969;48:2260–2272.
93. Metzger BE, Ravnikar V, Vileisis RA, Freinkel N. Accelerated starvation: and the skipped breakfast in late normal pregnancy. Lancet 1982;1:588–592.
94. Knopp RH, Magee MS. Physiological changes in pregnancy. In: Patten HD, Fuchs A, Hille B, et al., editors. Textbook of physiology. 21th ed. Philadelphia: WB Saunders, 1989:1386–1407.
95. Knopp RH. Hormone mediated changes in nutrient metabolism in pregnancy: a physiological basis for normal fetal development. In: Jacobsen MS, Rees JM, Golden

NH, Irwin CE, eds. Adolescent nutritional disorders: prevention and treatment. N.Y.: Academy of Sciences, 1997:251–271.
96. Childs MT, Tollefson JH, Knopp RH, Bowden DA. Lipid metabolism in pregnancy. VIII. Effects of dietary fat vs. carbohydrate on lipoprotein and hepatic lipids and tissue triglyceride lipases. Metabolism 1981;30:27–35.
97. Gray JM, Greemwood MRC. Uterine and adipose lipoprotein lipase activity in hormone treated and pregnant rats. Am Physiol Soc 1983;E132–E137.
98. Ramirez I, Llobera M, Herrera E. Circulating triacylglycerols, lipoproteins, and tissue lipoprotein lipase activities in rat mothers and offspring during perinatal period: effect of postmaturity. Metabolism 1983;32:333–341.
99. Mallov S, Alousi AA. Lipoprotein lipase activity of rat and human placenta. Proc Soc Exp Biol Med 1965;119:301–306.
100. Bonet B, Knopp RH, Brunzell JD, Gown A. Metabolism of very low density lipoprotein triglyceride by human placental cells: the role of lipoprotein lipase. Metabolism 1992;41:596–603.
101. Diamant YZ, Diamant S, Freinkel N. Lipid deposition and metabolism in rat placenta during gestation. Placenta 1980;1:319–325.
102. Hamosh M, Clary TR, Chernick SS, Scow RO. Lipoprotein lipase activity of adipose and mammary tissue and plasma triglyceride in pregnant and lactating rats. Biochim Biophys Acta 1970;210:473–482.
103. Knopp RH, Boroush MA, O'Sullivan JB. Lipid metabolism in pregnancy. II. Postheparin lipolytic activity and hypertriglyceridemia in the pregnant rat. Metabolism 1975;24:481–493.
104. Alvarez JJ, Montelongo A, Iglesias A, et al. Longitudinal study on lipoprotein profile, high density lipoprotein subclass and postheparin lipases during gestation in women. J Lipid Res 1996;37:299–308.
105. Kinnunen PKJ. Unnerus H, Ranta T, et al. Activities of postheparin plasma lipoprotein lipase and hepatic lipase during pregnancy and lactation. Eur J Clin Invest 1980;10:469–474.
106. Lasunción MA, Herrera E. Effect of pregnancy on the uptake of lipoprotein triglyceride fatty acids by isolated adipocytes in the rat. Biochem Biophys Res Commun 1981;98:227–233.
107. Argiles J, Herrera E. Appearance of circulating and tissue ^{14}C lipids after oral ^{14}C tripalmitate administration in the late pregnant rat. Metabolism 1989;38:104–108.
108. Herrera E, Lasunción MA, Gomez-Coronado D, et al. Role of lipoprotein lipase activity on lipoprotein metabolism and the fate of circulating triglycerides in pregnancy. Am J Obstet Gynecol 1988;158:1575–1583.
109. McDonald-Gibson RG, Young M, Hytten RE. Changes in plasma nonesterified fatty acids and serum glycerol in pregnancy. Br J Obstet Gynaecol 1975;82:460–466.
110. Burt RL. Plasma nonesterified fatty acids in normal pregnancy and the puerperium. Obstet Gynecol 1960;15:460–464.
111. Subcommittee on Nutritional Status and Weight Gain During Pregnancy, Subcommittee on Dietary Intake and Nutrient Supplements During Pregnancy, Committee on Nutritional Status During Pregnancy and Lactation, Food and Nutrition Board, Institute of Medicine, National Academy of Sciences. Nutrition during pregnancy: part I weight gain, part II: nutrient supplements. Washington, DC: National Academy Press, 1997.
112. Hytten FE, Leitch I. The physiology of human pregnancy. 2nd ed. Oxford: Blackwell Scientific, 1971.
113. Baskin DG, Figlewicz DP, Woods SC, et al. Insulin in the brain. Annu Rev Physiol 1987;49:335–347.
114. Flier JS, Cook KS, Usher P, Spiegelman BM. Severely impaired adipsin expression in genetic and acquired obesity. Science 1987;237:405–408.
115. Butte NF, Hopkinson JM, Nicolson MA. Leptin in human reproduction: serum leptin levels in pregnant and lactating women. J Clin Endocrinol Metab 1997;82:585–589.
116. Chehab FF, Lim ME, Ronghua L. Correction of the sterility defect in homozygous obese female mice by treatment with the human recombinant leptin. Nat Genet 1996;12:318–320.
117. Oster MH. Enders SR, Samuels SJ, et al. Megestrol acetate in patients with AIDS and cachexia. Ann Intern Med 1994;121:400–408.
118. Heinrich HC, Bartels H, Heinisch B, et al. Intestinale 59 Fe-Resorption und Pralatenter Eisenmangel Während der Gravidität des Menschen. Klin Wochenschr 1968;46:199–202.
119. Davison JS, Davison MC, Hay DM. Gastric emptying time in late pregnancy and labour. J Obstet Gynaecol Br Commonw 1970;77:37–41.
120. Boyd ELM. The lipemia of pregnancy. J Clin Invest 1934;13:347–363.
121. Knopp RH, Montes A, Warth MR. Carbohydrate and lipid metabolism in normal pregnancy. In: Food and Nutrition Board, ed. Laboratory indices of nutritional Status in Pregnancy. Washington, DC: National Academy of Sciences, 1978:35–88.
122. Knopp RH, Humphrey J, Irvine S. Biphasic metabolic control of hypertriglyceridemia in pregnancy. Clin Res 1977;25:161A.
123. Knopp RH. Physiological and clinical significance of hyperlipidemia in pregnancy. Perspect Lipid Disord 1984;2:12–16.
124. Knopp RH, Warth MR, Charles D, et al. Lipoprotein metabolism in pregnancy, fat transport to the fetus and the effects of diabetes. Biol Neonate 1986;31:913–921.
125. Piechota W, Staszewski A. Reference ranges of lipids and apolipoproteins in pregnancy. Eur J Obstet Gynecol Reprod Biol 1992;45:27–35.
126. Potter JM, Nestel PJ. The hyperlipidemia of pregnancy in normal and complicated pregnancies. Am J Obstet Gynecol 1979;133:165–170.
127. Fahraeus L, Larsson-Cohn U, Wallentin L. Plasma lipoproteins including high density lipoprotein subfractions during normal pregnancy. Obstet Gynecol 1985;66:468–472.
128. Desoye G, Schweditsch MO, Pfeiffer KP, et al. Correlation of hormones with lipid and lipoprotein levels during pregnancy and postpartum. J Clin Endocrinol Metab 1987;64:704–712.

129. Loke DFM, Viegas OAC, Kek LP, et al. Lipid profiles during and after normal pregnancy. Gynecol Obstet Invest 1991;32:144–147.
130. Mazurkiewicz JC, Watts GF, Warburton FG, et al. Serum lipids, lipoproteins, and apolipoproteins in pregnant non-diabetic patients. J Clin Pathol 1994;47:728–731.
131. Uberos-Fernández J, Muñoz-Hoyos A, Molina-Carballo A, et al. Lipoproteins in pregnant women before and during delivery: Influence on neonatal haemorheology. J Clin Pathol 1996;49:120–123.
132. Warth MR, Arky RA, Knopp RH. Lipid metabolism in pregnancy. III. Altered lipid composition in intermediate, very low, low and high density lipoprotein fractions. J Clin Endocrinol Metab 1975;41:649–655.
133. Steitz HO, Brockerhoff P, Holzer A, et al. Verteilungsmuster von Apolipoprotein A und B in den Lipoproteinfraktionen des Serums bei Schwangeren und Pos Partum. Z Geburtshilfe Perinatol 1987;191:243–249.
134. Silliman K, Shore V, Forte TM. Hypertriglyceridemia during late pregnancy is associated with the formation of small dense low-density lipoproteins and the presence of large buoyant high-density lipoproteins. Metabolism 1994;43:1035–1041.
135. Zechner R, Desoye G, Schweditsch MO, et al. Fluctuations of plasma lipoprotein(a) concentrations during pregnancy and postpartum. Metabolism 1986;35:333–336.
136. Panteghini M, Pagani F. Serum conditions of lipoprotein(a) during normal pregnancy and postpartum. Clin Chem 1991;37:2009.
137. Wersch JWJ, VanMackelenbergh BAHA, Ubachs JMH. Lipoprotein(a) in smoking and non-smoking pregnant women. Scand J Clin Lab Invest 1994;54:361–364.
138. Berg K, Roald B, Sande H. High Lp(a) lipoprotein level in maternal serum may interfere with placental circulation and cause fetal growth retardation. Clin Genet 1994;46:52–56.
139. Warth MR, Knopp RH. Lipid metabolism in pregnancy. V. Interactions of diabetes, body weight, age and high carbohydrate diet. Diabetes 1977;26:1056–1062.
140. McMurry MP, Connor WE, Goplerud CP. The effects of dietary cholesterol upon the hypercholesterolemia of pregnancy. Metabolism 1981;30:869–879.
141. Wasfi I, Weinstein I, Heimberg M. Increased formation of triglyceride from oleate in perfused livers from pregnant rats. Endocrinology 1980;107:584–590.
142. Otway S, Robinson DS. The significance of changes in tissue clearing-factor lipase activity in relation to the lipaemia of pregnancy. Biochem J 1968;106:677–682.
143. Humphrey JL, Childs MT, Montes A, Knopp RH. Lipid metabolism in pregnancy. VII. Kinetics of chylomicron triglyceride removal in fed pregnant rat. Am J Physiol 1980;239:E81–E87.
144. Lee MM, Dempsey EW. Microcirculation of the rat placenta: scanning and transmission electron microscope observations on fetal blood vessels. Am J Obstet Gynecol 1976;126:495–505.
145. Shiomi M, Takashi I, Watanabe Y. Increase in hepatic low-density lipoprotein receptor activity during pregnancy in watanabe heritable lipidemic rabbits: an animal model for familial hypercholesterolemia. Biochim Biophys Acta 1987;917:92–100.
146. Belknap WM, Sharp C. Hepatic low density lipoprotein (LDL) clearance is reduced during pregnancy in the rat. Gastroenterol 1988;94:52A.
147. Belknap WM, Dietschy JM. Sterol synthesis and low density lipoprotein clearance in vivo in pregnant rat, placenta, and fetus: sources for tissue cholesterol during fetal development. J Clin Invest 1988;82:2077–2085.
148. Feingold KR, Wiley T, Moser AH, et al. De novo cholesterogenesis in pregnancy. J Lab Clin Med 1983;101:256–263.
149. Montes A, Humphrey J, Knopp RH. Lipid metabolism in pregnancy. VI. Lipoprotein composition and hepatic lipids in fed pregnant rat. Endocrinology 1978;103:1031–1038.
150. McMahan MR, Clarkson TB, Sackett GP, Rudel LL. Changes in plasma lipids and lipoproteins in *Macaca nemestrina* during pregnancy and the postpartum period. Proc Soc Exp Biol Med 1980;164:199–206.
151. Knopp RH, Bergelin RO, Wahl PW, Walden CE. Effects of pregnancy, postpartury lactation and oral contraceptive use on the lipoprotein cholesterol triglyceride ratio. Metabolism 1985;34:893–899.
152. Sakuma N, Oshima T, Knopp RH. Sex hormone and lipid metabolism: effects of pregnancy on lipoprotein lipids in third trimester Japanese women and HDL apoprotein and cholesterol kinetics in the experimental rat. J Jpn Atheroscl Soc 1982;10:617–624.
153. Walden CE, Knopp RH, Wahl PW, et al. Sex differences in the effect of diabetes mellitus on lipoprotein triglyceride and cholesterol concentrations. N Engl J Med 1984;311:953–959.
154. Walden CE, Knopp RH, Wahl PW, et al. Hyperlipidemia in the Pacific Northwest Bell Telephone Company Health Survey: Lipoprotein lipid interrelationships. Arteriosclerosis 1983;3:125–131.
155. Lasunción MA, Bonet B, Knopp RH. Mechanism of the HDL_2 stimulation of progesterone secretion in cultured placental trophoblast. J Lipid Res 1991;32:1073–1087.
156. Wu YQ, Joprgensen EV, Handwerker S. High density lipoproteins stimulate placental lactogen release and adenosine 3′,5′-monophosphate (cAMP) production in human trophoblast cells: evidence for cAMP as a second messenger in human placental lactogen release. Endocrinology 1988;123:1879.
157. Kern F, Everson GT, DeMark B, et al. Biliary lipids, bile acids, and gallbladder function in the human female: effects of pregnancy and the ovulatory cycle. J Clin Invest 1981;1229–1242.
158. Montelongo A, Lasunción MA, Pallardo LF, Herrera E. Longitudinal study of plasma lipoproteins and hormones during pregnancy in normal and diabetic women. Diabetes 1992;41:1651–1659.
159. McConnell KP, Sinclair RG. Passage of elaidic acid through the placenta and also into the milk of the rat. J Biol Chem 1937;118:123–129.
160. Shafrir E, Barash V. Placental function in maternal-fetal fat transport in diabetes. Biol Neonate 1987;51:102–112.

161. Battaglia FC, Hay WW Jr. Energy and substrate requirements for fetal and placental growth and metabolism. In: Beard RW, Nathanielsz PW, eds. Fetal physiology and medicine. New York: Marcel Dekker, 1984:601–628.
162. Hershfield MS, Nemeth AM. Placental transport of free palmitic and linoleic acids in the guinea pig. J Lipid Res 1968;9:460–468.
163. Portman OW, Behrman RE, Soltys P. Transfer of free fatty acids across the primate placenta. Am J Physiol 1969;216:143–147.
164. Noble RC, Shand JH, Bell AW. Fetal to maternal transfer of palmitic and linoleic acids across the sheep placenta. Biol Neonate 1979;36:113–118.
165. Ruyle M, Connor WE, Anderson GJ, Lowensohn RI. Placental transfer of essential fatty acids in humans: venous-arterial difference for docosahexanoic acid in fetal umbilical erythrocytes. Proc Natl Acad Sci USA 1990;87:7902–7906.
166. Dancis J, Jansen V, Kayden HJ, Bjornson L, Levitz M. Transfer across perfused human placenta: III. Effect of chain length on transfer of free fatty acids. Pediatr Res 1974;8:796–799.
167. Whaley WH, Zuspan FP, Nelson GH. Correlation between maternal and fetal plasma levels of glucose and free fatty acids. Am J Obstet Gynecol 1966;94:419–421.
168. Sabata V, Wolf H, Lausmann S. The role of free fatty acids, glycerol, ketone bodies and glucose in the energy metabolism of the mother and fetus during delivery. Biol Neonate 1968;13:7–17.
169. Sheath J, Grimwade HJ, Waldron K, et al. Arteriovenous nonesterified fatty acids and glycerol differences in the umbilical cord at term and their relationship to fetal metabolism. Am J Obstet Gynecol 1972;113:358–362.
170. Szabo AJ, Oppermann V, Hanover B, et al. Fetal adipose tissue development: relationship to maternal free fatty acid levels. In: Camerini-Davalos RA, Cole HS, eds. Early diabetes in early life. New York: Academic Press, 1975:167–176.
171. Edson JL, Hudson DG, Hull D. Evidence for increased fatty acid transfer across the placenta during a maternal fast in rabbits. Biol Neonate 1975;27:50–55.
172. Muller PS, Soloman F, Brown JR. Free fatty acid concentration in maternal plasma and fetal body fat content. Am J Obstet Gynecol 1964;88:196.
173. Freinkel N. Effects of conceptus on maternal metabolism during pregnancy. In: Leibel BS, ed. On the nature and treatment of diabetes. Amsterdam: Excerpta Medica Foundation, 1965:679–691.
174. Szabo AJ, deLellis R, Grimaldi RD. Triglyceride synthesis by the human placenta. I. Incorporation of labeled palmitate into placental triglycerides. Am J Obstet Gynecol 1973;115:257–266.
175. Herrera E, Freinkel N. Metabolism in the liver, brain and placenta of fed and fasted and fetal rats. Horm Metab Res 1975;7:247–249.
176. Coleman RA. The role of the placenta in lipid metabolism and transport. Semin Perinatol 1989;13:180–191.
177. Coleman RA, Haynes EB. Synthesis and release of fatty acids by human trophoblast cells in culture. J Lipid Res 1987;28:1335–1341.
178. Coleman RA, Haynes EB. Microsomal and lysosomal enzymes of triacylglycerol metabolism in rat placenta. Biochem J 1984;217:391–397.
179. Popjak G, Beeckmans ML. Are phospholipids transmitted through the placenta? Biochem J 1950;46:99–103.
180. Popjak G. The origin of fetal lipids. Cold Spring Harb Symp Quant Biol 1954;19:200–208.
181. Beizenski JJ. Role of placenta in fetal lipid metabolism. Am J Obstet Gynecol 1969;104:1177.
182. Biezenski JJ, Carrozza J, Li JR. Role of placenta in fetal lipid metabolism. III. Formation of rabbit plasma phospholipids. Biochim Biophys Acta 1971;239:92–97.
183. Thomas CR, Lowy C, St Hillaire RJ, et al. Studies on the placental hydrolysis and transfer of lipids to the fetal guinea pig. In: Miller RR, Thiede HA, eds. Fetal nutrition metabolism, and immunology: the role of the placenta. New York: Plenum, 1984:135–146.
184. Elphick MC, Hull D. Rabbit placental clearing factor lipase and transfer to the fetus of fatty acids derived from the triglycerides injected into the mother. J Physiol (Lond) 1977;273:475–487.
185. Clegg R. Placental lipoprotein lipase activity in the rabbitt, rat and sheep. Comp Biochem Physiol 1981;69B:585–591.
186. Hummel L, Schwartze A, Schirrmeister W, Wagner H. Maternal plasma triglycerides as a source of fetal fatty acids. Acta Biol Med Ger 1976;35:1635–1641.
187. Lasunción MA, Testar X, Palacin M, et al. Method for the study of metabolite transfer from rat mother to fetus. Biol Neonate 1983;44:85–92.
188. Boyd ELM, Wilson KM. The exchange of lipids in the umbilical circulation at birth. J Clin Invest 1935;14:7–15.
189. Elphick MC, Filshie GM, Hull D. The passage of fat emulsion across human placenta. Br J Obstet Gynaecol 1978;85:610–618.
190. Deeb SS, Motulsky A, Albers JJ. A partial cDNA clone for human apolipoprotein B. Proc Natl Acad Sci USA 1985;82:4983–4986.
191. Demmer LA, Lavin MS, Elovson J, et al. Tissue-specific expression and developmental regulation of the rat apolipoprotein B gene. Proc Natl Acad Sci USA 1986;83:8102–8106.
192. Rothblat GH, Mahlberg FH, Johnson WJ, Philips MC. Apolipoproteins, membrane cholesterol domains and the regulation of cholesterol efflux. J Lipid Res 1992;33:1091–1097.
193. Stammers JP, Hull D, Silver M, et al. Release of lipid from the equine placenta during in vitro incubation. Placenta 1994;15:857–872.
194. Goldwater WH, Stettin D. Studies in fetal metabolism. J Biol Chem 1947;169:723–738.
195. Chevalier F. Transferts et synthese du cholesterol chez le rat au cours de sa croissance. Biochim Biophys Acta 1964;84:316–339.

196. Pitkin RM, Connor WE, Lin DS. Cholesterol metabolism and placental transfer in the pregnant rhesus monkey. J Clin Invest 1972;51:2584–2592.
197. Khansi F, Merkatz I, Soloman S. The conversion of acetate to cholesterol in the fetus of the baboon and the transfer of cholesterol from mother to fetus. Endocrinology 1971;91:6–12.
198. Lin DS, Pitkin RM, Connor WE. Placental transfer of cholesterol in the human fetus. Am J Obstet Gynecol 1977;128:735–739.
199. Feingold KR, Wilet MH, MacRae G, Siperstein MD. Mevalonate metabolism in pregnant rats. Metabolism 1980;29:285–291.
200. Beizenski JJ. Fetal lipid metabolism. In: Wyann RM, ed. Obstetrics and gynecology annual. New York: Appleton-Century-Crofts, 1975:39–70.
201. Robertson AF, Sprecher H. A review of human placental lipid metabolism and transport. Acta Pediatr 1968;183:1–18.
202. Roux JF, Yoshioka T. Lipid metabolism in the fetus during development. Clin Obstet Gynecol 1970;13:595–620.
203. Winkel GA, Snyder JM, MacDonald PC, Simpson ER. Regulation of cholesterol and progesterone synthesis in human placental cells in culture by serum lipoproteins. Endocrinology 1980;80:1054–1060.
204. Cummings SW, Hatley W, Simpson ER, Ohashi M. The binding of high and low density lipoproteins to human placental membrane fractions. J Clin Endocrinol Metab 1982;54:903–908.
205. Winkel CA, Gilmore J, MacDonald PC, Simpson ER. Uptake and degradation of lipoproteins by human trophoblastic cells in primary culture. Endocrinology 1980;107:1892–1898.
206. Knopp RH, Lawson R, Li JR. Effect of high density lipoprotein on progesterone secretion by cultured placental cells. Circulation 1981;64:271 (abstract).
207. Albrecht ED, Henson MC, Pepe GJ. Regulation of placental low density lipoprotein uptake in baboons by estrogen. Endocrinology 1991;128:450–458.
208. Albrecht ED, Babischkin JS, Koos RD, Pepe GJ. Developmental increase in low density lipoprotein receptor messenger ribonucleic acid levels in placental syncytiotrophoblasts during baboon pregnancy. Endocrinology 1995;136:5540–5546.
209. Gwynne JT, Strauss JF. The role of lipoproteins in steroidogenesis and cholesterol metabolism in steroidogenic glands. Endocr Rev 1982;3:299–329.
210. Parker CR Jr, Illingworth DR, Bissonnette J, Carr BR. Endocrine changes during pregnancy in patient with homozygous familial hyperbetalipoproteinemia. N Engl J Med 1986;314:557–560.
211. Gåfvels ME, Coukos G, Sayegh R, et al. Regulated expression of the trophoblast a$_2$-macroglobulin receptor/low density lipoprotein receptor-related protein. Differentiation and cAMP modulate protein and mRNA levels. J Biol Chem 1992;267:21230–21234.
212. Wittmaack FM, Gåfvels ME, Bronner M, et al. Localization and regulation of the human very low density lipoprotein/apolipoprotein-E receptor: trophoblast expression predicts a role for the receptor in placental lipid transport. Endocrinology 1995;136:340–348.
213. Overbergh L, Lorent K, Torrekens S, et al. Expression of mouse alpha-macroglobulins, lipoprotein receptor-related protein, LDL receptor, apolipoprotein E, and lipoprotein lipase in pregnancy. J Lipid Res 1995;36:1774–1786.
214. Parinaud J, Perret B, Ribbes H, et al. High density lipoprotein utilization by human granulosa cells for progesterone synthesis in serum-free culture: respective contributions of free and esterified cholesterol. J Clin Endocrinol Metab 1987;64:409–417.
215. Blum CB, Davis PA, Forte RM. Elevated levels of apolipoprotein E in the high density lipoproteins of human cord blood plasma. J Lipid Res 1985;26:755–760.
216. Davis PA, Forte TM, Nichols AV, Blum CB. Umbilical cord blood lipoproteins: isolation and characterization of high density lipoproteins. Arteriosclerosis 1983;3:357–365.
217. Rindler MJ, Traber MG, Bersinger NA, Dancis J. Synthesis and secretion of apolipoprotein E by human placenta and choriocarcinoma cell lines. Placenta 1991;12:615–624.
218. Steinberg D, Parthasarathy S, Carew TE, et al. Beyond cholesterol: modifications of low-density lipoprotein that increase its atherogenecity. N Engl J Med 1989;320:915–924.
219. Bonet B, Chait A, Gown A, Knopp RH. Metabolism of modified LDL by cultured human placental cells. Atherosclerosis 1995;112:125–136.
220. Alsat E, Mondon F, Rebourcet R, et al. Identification of specific binding sites for acetylated low density lipoprotein in microvillous membranes from human placenta. Mol Cell Endocrinol 1985;41:229–235.
221. Malassine A, Alsat E, Besse C, et al. Acetylated low density lipoprotein endocytosis by human syncytiotrophoblast in culture. Placenta 1990;11:191.
222. Henriksen T, Evensen SA, Carlander B. Injury to human endothelial cells in culture induced by low density lipoproteins. Scand J Clin Lab Invest 1979;39:361–368.
223. Chisholm GM. Cytotoxicity of oxidized lipoproteins. Curr Opin Lipidol 1991;2:311–316.
224. Hauge-Gillenwater H, Bonet B, Meekins D, Knopp RH. LDL oxidation and human placental trophoblast and macrophage cytotoxicity. Proc Soc Exp Bio Med 1998:217 (in press).
225. Zhu X, Knopp RH. Effect of sex steroid hormones on oxidative modification of low density lipoproteins by placental macrophages and trophoblast and their susceptibility to cytotoxicity. Circulation 1993;88:I-32 (abstract).
226. Zhu X, Bonet B, Knoop RH. 17b-estradiol, progesterone and testosterone inversely modulate LDL oxidation and cytotoxicity in cultured placental trophoblast and macrophages. Am J Obstet Gynecol 1997;177:196–209.
227. Mazière C, Auclair M, Ronveaux MF, et al. Estrogens inhibit copper and cell-mediated modification of low density lipoprotein. Atherosclerosis 1991;89:175–182.
228. Rifci VA, Khachadurian AK. The inhibiton of low density lipoprotein oxidation by 17ß-estradiol. Metabolism 1992;14:1110–1117.

229. Nègre-Salvayre AM, Pieraggi T, Mabile L, Salvayre R. Protective effect of 17b-estradiol against the cytoxicity of minimally oxidized LDL to cultured bovine aortic endothelial cells. Atherosclerosis 1993;99:207–217.
230. Ishihara M. Studies on lipoperoxide of normal pregnant women and of patients with toxemia of pregnancy. Clin Chem Acta 1978;84:1–9.
231. Maseki M, Nishigaki I, Hagihara M, et al. Lipid peroxide levels and lipid content of serum lipoprotein fractions of pregnant subjects with or without preeclampsia. Clin Chem Acta 1981;115:151–161.
232. Hubel CA, Roberts JM, Taylor RN, et al. Lipid peroxidation in pregnancy: new perspectives on preeclampsia. Am J Obstet Gynecol 1989;161:1025–1034.
233. Bonet B, Knopp RH. Accelerated LDL oxidation in diabetic gestation. Program of the 2nd International Graz Symposium on Gestational Diabetes 1992; Abstract.
234. Baynes JW. Role of oxidative stress in development of complications in diabetes. Diabetes 1991;40:405–412.
235. Bowie A, Owens D, Collins P, et al. Glycosylated low density lipoprotein is more sensitive to oxidation: implications for the diabetic patient? Atherosclerosis 1993;102:63–67.
236. Tsai EC, Hirsch IB, Brunzell JD, Chait A. Reduced plasma peroxyl radical trapping capacity and increased susceptibility of LDL to oxidation in poorly controlled IDDM. Diabetes 1994;43:1010–1014.
237. Kitzmiller JL, Brown ER, Phillipe M, et al. Diabetic nephropathy and perinatal outcome. Am J Obstet Gynecol 1981;141:741–751.
238. Hubel CA, McLaughlin MK, Evans RW, et al. Fasting serum triglycerides, free fatty acids, and malondialdehyde are increased in preeclampsia, are positively correlated, and decrease within 48 hours post partum. Am J Obstet Gynecol 1996;174:975–982.
239. Franz H, Wendler D. A controlled study of maternal serum concentrations of lipoproteins in pregnancy-induced hypertension. Arch Gynecol Obstet 1992;252:81–86.
240. Rosing U, Samsioe G, Ölund A, et al. Serum levels of apolipoprotein A-I, A-II and HDL-cholesterol in second half of normal pregnancy and in pregnancy complicated by pre-eclampsia. Horm Metab Res 1989;21:276–382.
241. Sattar N, Gaw A, Packard CJ, Greer IA. Potential pathogenic roles of aberrant lipoprotein and fatty acid metabolism in pre-eclampsia. Br J Obstet Gynaecol 1996;103:614–620.
242. Zuspan FP, Samuels P. Preventing preeclampsia. N Engl J Med 1993;329:1265–1266.
243. Walsh SW, Wang Y. Secretion of lipid peroxides by the human placenta. Am J Obstet Gynecol 1993;169:1462–1466.
244. Walsh SW, Wang Y. Trophoblast and placental villous core production of lipid peroxides, thromboxane, and prostacyclin in preeclampsia. J Clin Endocrinol Metab 1995;80:1888–1893.
245. Branch DW, Mitchell MD, Miller E, et al. Pre-eclampsia and serum antibodies to oxidised low density lipoprotein. Lancet 1994;343:645–646.
246. Stamler FW. Fetal eclamptic disease of pregnant rat fed antivitamin E stress diet. Am J Pathol 1959;35:207–231.
247. McKay DG, Goldenberg V, Kaunitz H, Csavossy I. Experimental toxemia. An electron microscope study and review. Arch Pathol 1967;84:557–597.
248. Jovanovic L, Metzger BE, Knopp RH, et al. Diabetes in Early Pregnancy Study. First trimester β-hydroxybutyrate (β-OH B) in Type I diabetic pregnancy compared to normal pregnancy. 1997, submitted.
249. Knopp RH, Magee MS, Larson MO, et al. Alternative screening tests and birth weight associations in pregnant women with abnormal glucose screening. Diabetes 1988;37:110A (abstract).
250. Knopp RH, Magee MS, Walden CE, et al. Prediction of infant birth weight by GDM screening tests: importance of plasma triglyceride. Diabetes Care 1992;15:1605–1613.
251. Skryten A, Johnson P, Samsioe G, Gustafson A. Studies in diabetic pregnancy. I. Serum lipids. Acta Obstet Gynecol Scand 1976;55:211–215.
252. Knopp RH, Bergelin RO, Wahl PW, Walden CE. Relationships of infant birth size to maternal lipoproteins, apoprotein, fuel, hormones, clinical chemistries and body weight at 36 weeks gestation. Diabetes 1985;34(suppl II):71.
253. Knopp RH, Chapman M, Bergelin RO, et al. Relationship of lipoprotein lipids to mild fasting hyperglycemia and diabetes in pregnancy. Diabetes Care 1980;3:416–420.
254. Delmis J, Ivanisevic M, Bukovic D. Placental lipid contents in gestational diabetic pregnancy. Coll Antropol 1994;18:323–327.
255. Hollingsworth DR, Grundy SM. Pregnancy-associated hypertriglyceridemia in normal and diabetic women. Differences in insulin-dependent, non-insulin-dependent and gestational diabetes. Diabetes 1982;31:1092–1097.
256. Koukkou E, Watts GF, Lowy C. Serum lipid, lipoprotein and apolipoprotein changes in gestational diabetes mellitus: a cross-sectional and prospective study. J Clin Pathol 1996;49:634–637.
257. Knopp RH, Warth MR, Carroll CJ. Lipid metabolism in pregnancy. I. Changes in lipoprotein triglyceride and cholesterol in normal pregnancy and the effects of diabetes mellitus. J Reprod Med 1973;10:95–101.
258. Knopp RH, Van Allen M, McNeeley M, et al. Effects of insulin dependent diabetes mellitus on plasma lipoproteins in diabetic pregnancy. J Reprod Med 1993;38:703–710.
259. Eriksson UJ. The pathogenesis of congenital malformations in diabetic pregnancy. Diabetes Metab Rev 1995;11:63–82.
260. Eriksson UJ, Siman CM. Pregnant diabetic rats fed the antioxidant butylated hydroxytoluene show decreased occurrence of malformations in offspring. Diabetes 1996;45:1497–1502.
261. Knopp RH, Walden CE, Wahl PW, et al. Effect of post-partum lactation on lipoprotein lipids and apoproteins. J Clin Endocrinol Metab 1985;60:542–547.
262. Chajek-Shaul T, Friedman G, Halperin G, et al. Role of lipoprotein lipase in the uptake of cholesterol ester by rat lactating mammary gland in vivo. Biochim Biophys Acta 1981;666:216–222.

263. Zinder O, Hamosh M, Fleck TR, Scow RO. Effect of prolactin on lipoprotein lipase in mammary glands and adipose tissue of rats. Am J Physiol 1974;226:742–748.
264. Zinder O, Mendelson CR, Blanchette-Mackie EF, Scow RO. Lipoprotein lipase and uptake of chylomicron triglycerol and cholesterol perfused by rat mammary tissue. Biochim Biophys Acta 1976;431:526–537.
265. Hachey DL, Thomse MR, Emken EA, et al. Human lactation: maternal transfer of dietary triglycerides labelled with stable isotopes. J Lipid Res 1987;28:1185–1192.
266. Hachey DL, Silber GH, Wong WW, Garza C. Human lactation. 2. Endogenous fatty acid synthesis by the mammary gland. Pediatr Res 1989;25:63–68.
267. Kris-Etherton PM, Frantz ID Jr. The contribution of chylomicron cholesterol to milk cholesterol in the rat. Proc Soc Exp Biol Med 1980;165:502–507.
268. Rebuffe-Scrive M, Enk L, Crona N, et al. Fat cell metabolism in different regions in women: effect of menstrual cycle, pregnancy and lactation. J Clin Invest 1985;75:1973–1976.
269. Mellies MJ, Ishikawa T, Gartside P, et al. Effects of varying maternal dietary cholesterol and phytosterol in lactating women and their infants. Am J Clin Nutr 1978;31:1347–1354.
270. Wang CS, Illingworth DR. Lipid composition and lipolytic activities in milk from a patient with homozygous familial hypobetalipoproteinemia. Am J Clin Nutr 1987;45:730–736.
271. Ma Y, Ooi TC, Liu M, et al. High frequency of mutations in the human lipoprotein lipase gene in pregnancy-induced chylomicronemia: possible association with E2 isoform. J Lipid Res 1994;35:1066–1075.
272. Knopp RH, The Staff of the NW Lipid Research Clinic. What's new in the nutritional management of hyperlipidemia? In: Program of the American Dietetic Association Annual Meeting, San Francisco: 1988:14.
273. Hsia SH, Connelly PW, Hegele RA. Successful outcome in severe pregnancy-associated hyperlipemia: a case report and literature review. Am J Med Sci 1995;309:213–218.
274. Kroon AA, Swinkels DW, van Dongen PWJ, Stalenhoef AFH. Pregnancy in a patient with homozygous familial hypercholesterolemia treated with long-term low-density lipoprotein apheresis. Metabolism 1994;43:1164–1170.
275. Bengtsson C. Ischaemic heart disease in women. Acta Med Scand 1973;549:11–28.
276. Montes A, Walden CE, Knopp RH, et al. Physiologic and supraphysiologic increases in lipoprotein lipids and apoproteins in late pregnancy and postpartum: possible markers for the diagnosis of "prelipidemia." Arteriosclerosis 1984;4:407–417.
277. Knopp RH. Oral contraception into the 1990s. New York: Parthenon, 1989.
278. Knopp RH. Fuel metabolism in pregnancy. Contemp Obstet Gynec 1978;12:83–90.

13
Essential Fatty Acids and Prostaglandins in Pregnancy

Paul L. Ogburn, Jr.

Essential fatty acids (EFAs) are a subgroup of polyunsaturated fatty acids (PUFA) that are required constituents of the diet; otherwise, illness and eventually death will occur. All living cells contain these lipids, especially in the phospholipids of membranes. EFAs serve as more than building blocks for tissue; they are also the obligate precursors for prostaglandins and related eicosanoids, which are essential for human and other animal metabolism.

The prostaglandins and related compounds are potent substances that occur naturally in the body. Because they usually are produced in exceedingly small quantities and have a short half-life, they are considered to have effects near the site of their production. Prostaglandins are important mediators of smooth muscle activity, vascular tone, coagulation, inflammation, immune responses, lipid and glucose metabolism, renal function, and reproductive physiology and pathology.

A large and growing number of oxygenated polyunsaturated fatty acid compounds have been described. This family of compounds, which includes the prostaglandins and leukotrienes, has been called eicosanoids[1] (Figure 13.1). This chapter considers the prostaglandins, the essential fatty acids, and other oxygenated products from these fatty acids, because of their roles in normal and abnormal fetal and maternal metabolism.

Essential Fatty Acids

That certain fatty acids are required in the diet was first reported by Burr and Burr,[2,3] who studied rats maintained on a diet without lipids. These animals lost weight, developed scaly skin and hair loss, and had reproductive failure and hematuria. Atrophy of the adrenal glands and hemorrhagic renal necrosis were associated with death. Capillary damage and leakage were common findings in these fat-deprived animals. These changes could be prevented by adding adequate amounts of linoleic acid or arachidonic acid to the diet. Although mammalian systems can produce monounsaturated fatty acids (e.g., oleic acid) and polyunsaturates from the oleic acid family, they cannot produce linoleic or arachidonic acids de novo. This family of essential fatty acids is called omega-6 because the first double bond is six carbons from the noncarboxyl end of the fatty acid. Omega-6 fatty acids include linoleic acid (18:2ω6) and dihomolinolenic acid (20:3ω6), both of which are found in plant sources. Arachidonic acid (20-4ω6) is produced from these substances by mammals.[2-4]

The essential fatty acids are used by the body to produce phospholipids for cell membranes, endoplasmic reticulum, and mitochondria. From the maternal circulation the fetus and placenta receive a relatively high proportion of the essential fatty acids necessary for rapid growth and development. The brain is especially dependent on arachidonic acid, linoleic acid, linolenic acid (18:3ω3), and their respective chain elongation products for adequate growth (Figure 13.2). Lipids make up more than 50% of the solid matter of the brain. For the human fetus, adequate sources of essential fatty acids must be available for somatic and especially neurologic tissue growth[5,6] (Figure 13.3).

Biosynthesis of Prostaglandins

During the early 1900s it was discovered that semen causes smooth muscle contraction and vasodilation in vitro. The term prostaglandins was used to describe these active substances contained in seminal plasma.[7-12] The prostaglandins have great biologic activity, are found in small quantities in most normal conditions, and have short half-lives. For these reasons, early investigators had difficulty determining these chemical structures. Eventually, pure compounds were derived from the seminal vesicles of sheep,[13-15] and even greater quantities were found to be available in a gorgonian coral (*Plexaura*

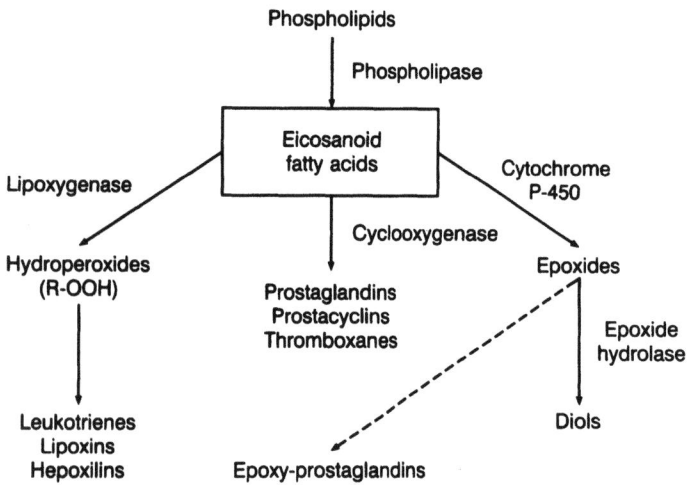

FIGURE 13.1. Family of oxygenated, polyunsaturated fatty acids called eicosanoids includes the prostaglandins and other cyclooxygenase products, which play key roles in normal and pathological pregnancies. (Redrawn from Pace-Asciak,[1] with permission.)

homomalla).[16] Corey[17] achieved total synthesis of prostaglandins in 1971. Much of the early work with prostaglandins focused on prostaglandins $F_{2\alpha}$ ($PGF_{2\alpha}$) and E_2 (PGE_2) for termination of pregnancy.[18–22]

Quantitation of prostaglandins in physiologic conditions has continued to be a difficult problem because of the low concentrations normally present and the short half-life of these compounds[18] (Figure 13.4). Gas chromatography mass spectrometry was initially used to identify and quantitate the prostaglandins.[23,24] A more sensitive, but less accurate, means of measuring prostaglandins includes radioimmunoassay methods.[25–27] The initial investigators studying prostaglandins tried to measure these substances directly. Generally it is more common to measure the prostaglandin metabolites that have longer half-lives and are found in greater quantities in urine, plasma, and various tissues. This method avoids the possibility that the measured prostaglandin concentration is altered significantly during sample collection. However, because different clearances of these metabolites may occur in different situations, and because of cross-reactivity that may occur in radioimmunoassays, one must be cautious when interpreting results that report specific effects or specific concentration of any individual prostaglandin or its metabolite.

Prostaglandins are classically derived from 20-carbon fatty acids with three, four, or five double bonds in the carbon chains.[28–34] Carbon atoms 8 and 12, as counted from the carboxyl group, are bound to each other to form a five-membered carbon ring in the middle of this chain. The position of double bonds, hydroxy groups, and ketone groups define the name of the particular prostaglandin. The subscript 1, 2, or 3 designates the number of double bonds in the aliphatic side chains of the compounds (Figure 13.5). The immediate stable precursors of the prostaglandins are polyunsaturated fatty acids.[28–33] Nonesterified arachidonic acid is the obligate precursor of $PGF_{2\alpha}$ and PGE_2.[28–31] The first step in the production of prostaglandins may be the release of the precursor polyunsaturated fatty acid from its esterified state to its nonesterified free state. Phospholipids contain relatively high quantities of polyunsaturated fatty acids and may serve as the storage depot for substrate used in prostaglandin production. Phospholipase A_2 has been shown to be an important enzyme for releasing arachidonic acid for prostaglandin production.[31–35] Other lipolytic enzymes, including other phospholipases, may play a part in releasing arachidonic acid and other polyunsaturated fatty acids for prostaglandin production. Once arachidonic acid is released, it may be converted to prostaglan-

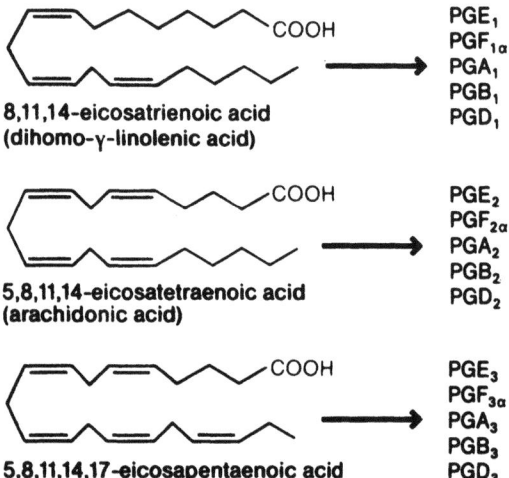

FIGURE 13.2. Three essential fatty acids that serve as precursors for prostaglandins also are necessary building blocks for phospholipids to construct somatic and neural tissues. Dihomo-γ-linolenic acid and arachidonic acid are ω-6 fatty acids, whereas eicosapentaenoic acid is a ω-3 fatty acid. (Redrawn from Ogburn and Brenner,[18] with permission.)

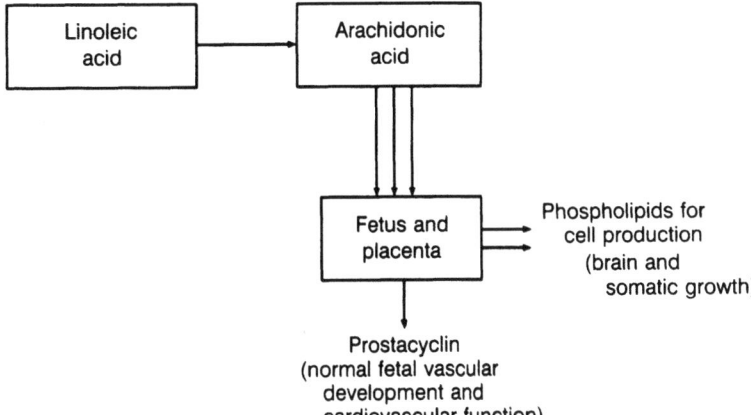

FIGURE 13.3. Fetus depends on adequate transfer of the essential fatty acids from the maternal blood to support adequate growth and prostacyclin production.

dins and related compounds by the cyclooxygenase pathway or to other eicosanoids (Figure 13.6).

Prostaglandin synthetase, a complex of enzymes that converts polyunsaturated fatty acids to prostaglandin is associated with the microsomal fraction.[35-38] The prostaglandin synthetase complex is made up of two membrane-bound enzymes, cyclooxygenase and endoperoxide isomerase, and the soluble enzyme peroxidase.[38-40] After polyunsaturated fatty acid is released from its esterified state, molecular oxygen is added to the free polyunsaturated fatty acid molecule by cyclooxygenase. The two atoms of the first oxygen molecule attach to carbons 9 and 11, and a single atom of the second oxygen molecule attaches to carbon 15 to form PGG_2. Peroxidase converts PGG_2 to $PGH_{2\alpha}$, which is converted to $PGF_{2\alpha}$ or PGE_2. An alternative pathway in which PGG_2 is converted to PGE_2 through 15-hydroxyperoxy-PGE_2 has been described.[37-49] Prostaglandins of the A and B series are produced from the corresponding PGE by dehydration with or without isomerization.[42]

Prostaglandins are produced quickly from their corresponding polyunsaturated fatty acids. Small quantities of these compounds produce great changes and are metabolized quickly to substances that are much less active or that may even inhibit prostaglandin production or action.[46-52] When PGE_2 or $PGF_{2\alpha}$ is injected into the bloodstream, the half-life is less than 1 minute, whereas the half-life of each primary metabolite is about 8 minutes.[50-52] These metabolites are the 15-keto-13,14-dihydroprostaglandins, which are produced by the successive action of two enzyme systems: prostaglandin-15-hydroxy-dehydrogenase and prostaglandin-13-ketoreductase. The 15-keto-13,14-dihydroprostaglandins are further metabolized by beta and omega oxidation to produce two primary urinary metabolites, 7α-hydroxy-5,11-diketotetranorprostane-1,16-dioic acid (from PGE_2) and $5_\alpha,7_\alpha$-dihydroxy-5,11-ketotetranorprostane-1,16-dioic

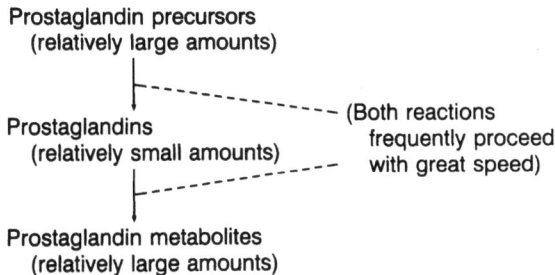

FIGURE 13.4. Quantities of the active prostaglandins are small compared to their respective precursors and metabolites. (Redrawn from Ogburn and Brenner,[18] with permission.)

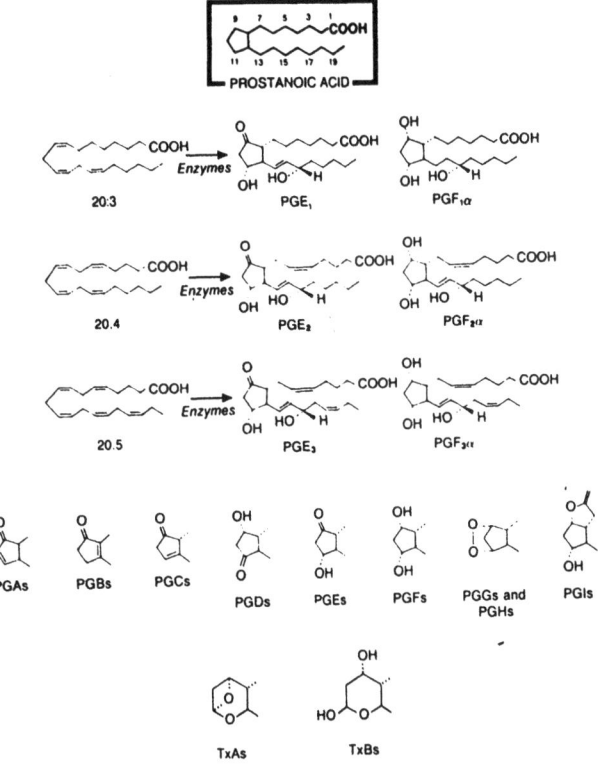

FIGURE 13.5. Structures and nomenclature for the major prostaglandins. PGI, the prostacyclins; TXAs, the thromboxane As. (From Pace-Asciak,[1] with permission.)

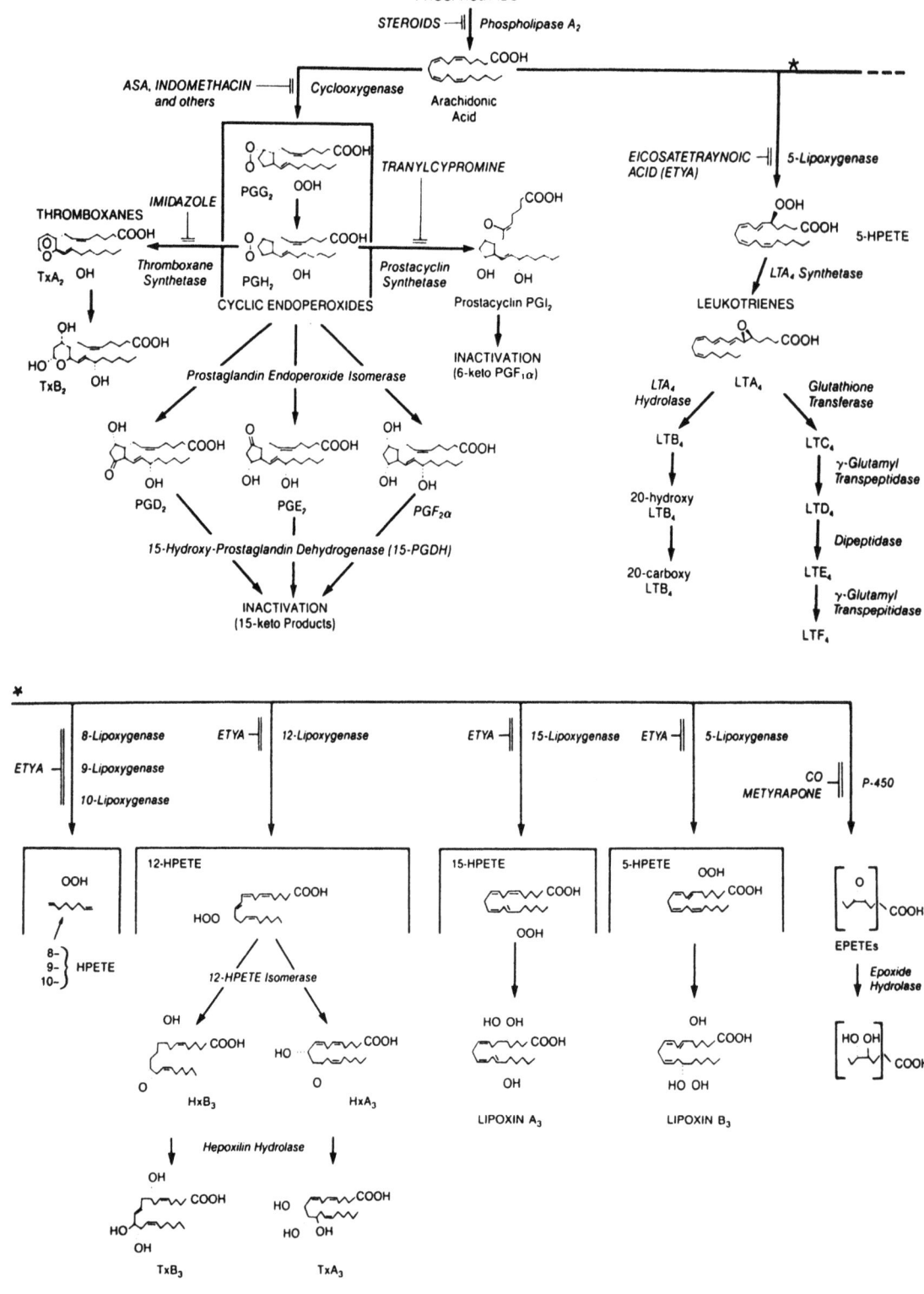

FIGURE 13.6. A & B: This outline of the arachidonic acid cascade shows indomethacin and aspirin (ASA) to inhibit cyclooxygenase, eicosatetraenoic acid to inhibit the various lipoxygenases, and carbon monoxide and metyrapone to inhibit cytochrome P-450. (From Pace-Asciak,[1] with permission.)

acid from $PGF_{2\alpha}$.[50,51] Total prostaglandin production in the adult human over a 24-hour period has been estimated to be 1 to 2 mg.[52]

Prostaglandin synthetase is inhibited by aspirin, indomethacin, and many other nonsteroidal anti-inflammatory agents.[53,54] These agents seem to work by inhibiting cyclooxygenase and by competing with polyunsaturated fatty acid substrate to bind the enzymatic active site.[55] The effects of these agents on inflammation, pain, platelet activation, and other prostaglandin-mediated responses may be the result of their antiprostaglandin-synthetase activity. These agents may inhibit term and preterm labor by the same mechanism.

Metabolic pathways that produce other eicosanoids from arachidonic acid were first discovered in the human platelet.[41,56,57] Platelet aggregation is associated with conversion of arachidonic acid to PGH_2 through the cyclooxygenase pathway. Subsequently, PGH_2 is converted to two principal products: hydroxyheptadecatrienoic acid and thromboxane A_2. Thromboxane A_2 and its more stable, much less active metabolite thromboxane B_2 induce platelet aggregation and arterial constriction.[58] A different compound, which inhibits platelet aggregation and relaxes smooth muscle, is produced from PGH_2 in blood vessel walls and is called prostacyclin (PGI_2).[59,60]

Prostaglandins interact with individual cells at specific receptor sites and activate adenyl cyclase or guanyl cyclase, or both. The prostaglandins of the E series are thought to stimulate the production of cyclic adenosine monophosphate (cAMP) by adenyl cyclase, and those of the F series the production of cyclic guanosine monophosphate (cGMP) by guanyl cyclase in some tissues. These nucleotides, cAMP and cGMP, may account for some of the different effects that prostaglandins E and F may have on the same tissue. The cyclic nucleotides are eventually metabolized by phosphodiesterase, and the effects of the prostaglandins cease. In certain circumstances, the prostaglandins in both E and F series elicit the same cellular response. This situation may be due to (1) cross-reactivity of these two prostaglandin types for the same receptor site, (2) their activation of the same nucleotide cyclase through different receptors, or (3) activation of the same enzymes by both adenyl cyclase and guanyl cyclase intracellularly.[61-68]

Lipoxygenase Products

An alternative pathway for the metabolism of arachidonic acid in the platelet and other tissues is favored when cyclooxygenase is inhibited by aspirin or a similar compound. In this reaction, one of several lipoxygenase compounds convert arachidonic acid to a respective hydroperoxy fatty acid (Figure 13.6). One of these fatty acids is 12-hydroperoxy-5,8,10,14-eicosatetraenoic acid (12-HPETE), which is subsequently converted to 12-hydroxy-5,8,10,14-eicosatetraenoic acid (12-HETE).[52,54] The production of PGI_2 is inhibited by 12-HPETE.[69]

A group of compounds called leukotrienes has been described that arise from arachidonic acid through the 5-lipoxygenase pathway. The addition of the tripeptide glutathione to the unstable leukotriene A produces leukotriene C. Leukotriene C and its metabolic product leukotriene D are probably primary mediators of immediate-type hypersensitivity reactions[1,70-77] (Figure 13.7). Indeed, leukotriene D_4 has been identified as slow-reacting substance of anaphylaxis (SRS-A).[68] Leukotriene A_4 may be converted to the 5,12-dihydroxyeicosatetraenoic acid (leukotriene B_4).[73]

Physiologic Actions and Effects of Prostaglandins

Vascular System

The prostaglandins and related eicosanoids play critical roles in maintaining normal vascular patency and hemostasis. Vascular endothelium produces prostacyclin (PGI_2) and PGE_2, which promote normal vasodilation and inhibit platelet aggregation. Platelets produce pri-

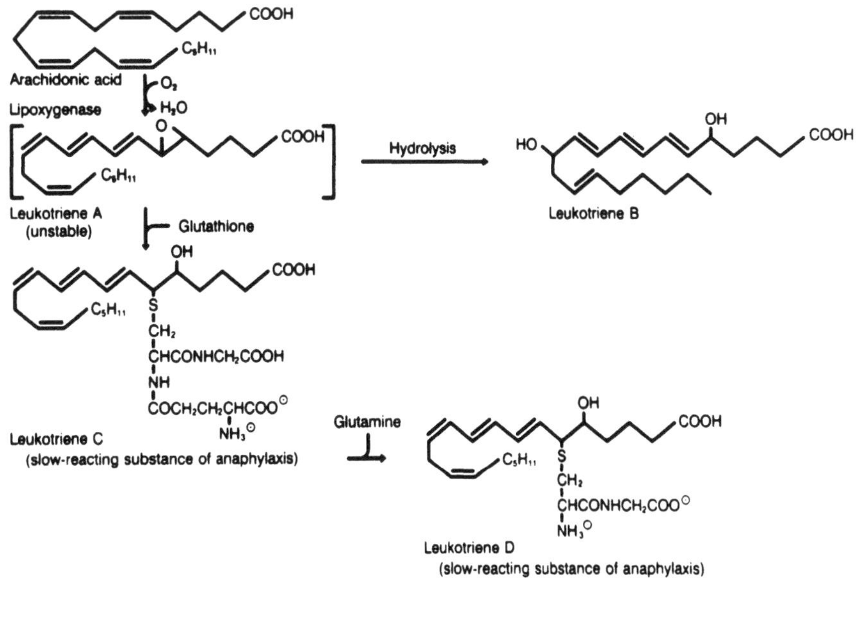

FIGURE 13.7. Slow-reacting substance of anaphylaxis (SRS-A) has been determined to be derived from arachidonic acid through a lipoxygenase pathway. (Redrawn from Ogburn and Brenner,[18] with permission.)

marily thromboxane and 12-HETE, which promote thrombosis and vasospasm. In this way injury to the endothelium promotes vasospasm and thrombosis. This reaction is necessary for normal hemostasis, such as is seen in laceration injuries, and it may explain why atherosclerotic coronary artery injuries lead to sudden occlusion and myocardial infarction.[4,18] The vasospasm, capillary injury, and occasional platelet consumption reaction seen with severe preeclampsia may be similarly associated with thromboxane production (vide infra).[18]

Respiratory System

Prostaglandin E_2 promotes bronchodilation, but $PGF_{2\alpha}$ and thromboxane A_2 are both strong bronchoconstrictors. The lipoxygenase products of arachidonic acid, including the leukotrienes, cause bronchospasm and mucus production and may be partially responsible for such pathologic states as asthma and adult respiratory distress syndrome.[18,74]

Renal System

Through vasodilation, PGE_2 and prostacyclin increase glomerular filtration. They produce an increase in water and sodium excretion, as well as an increase in renin production. These changes are part of the physiology of normal pregnancy.[18,74] The dilation of the renal collecting system seen during normal pregnancy may reflect the smooth muscle relaxing effects of prostacyclin. Thromboxane production associated with inflammation or other pathologic conditions can cause intrarenal vasoconstriction with a decrease in renal function, which may explain the oliguria seen in severe preeclampsia.[72]

Gastrointestinal System

The delayed stomach emptying and decreased motility of the intestines and gallbladder may reflect the smooth muscle relaxing effects of prostacyclin during pregnancy. The uterine-stimulating prostaglandins (e.g., $PGF_{2\alpha}$ and PGE_2) cause the increased gastrointestinal motility with diarrhea, nausea, and vomiting that is seen with exogenous administration or endogenous production of these substances.[18,74] The nausea and vomiting of the active stage of labor may be due to high circulating concentrations of the prostaglandins.

Immune System

Prostacyclin and PGE_2 seem to work in a number of ways to inhibit T cell proliferation and macrophage activation. These substances have been associated with reversing the cell-mediated immune response associated with organ transplant rejection. Thromboxane A_2 and leukotrienes have been associated with progression of the rejection process.[74] The increased production of prostacyclin and PGE_2 in the fetal placental unit may play a part in preventing the premature rejection of the conceptus by the maternal immune system.

Reproduction

Prostaglandins play important roles in the reproductive system of both sexes (Table 13.1).[75-77] Prostaglandins are produced from the seminal vesicles and are normally found in human seminal fluid in extremely high concentrations.[78,79] The stimulation of smooth muscle and vascular activity of prostaglandins suggest that they may be active in the physiology of erection and ejaculation.[76] They may play a role in male fertility and in the transport of sperm to the ovum. A decreased concentration of PGE_2 was found in the semen of men who were infertile.[80,81] Prostaglandins secreted in the seminal fluid may facilitate sperm penetration through the cervical mucus, or they may help propel spermatozoa toward their rendezvous with the ovum by stimulating contractions of the smooth muscle of the uterus and the fallopian tubes.[82,83]

Prostaglandins may play an important part in fertilization by affecting tubal motility under the influence of a proper balance of estrogen and progesterone. Prostaglandins of the F series usually cause contraction of the tube, and prostaglandins of the E series usually cause relaxation of the tube except for the interstitial segment, in which they cause contractions. The E prostaglandins in

TABLE 13.1. Possible roles of prostaglandins in reproduction.

Male partner
   Erection
   Ejaculation
   Facilitation of sperm transport
Female partner
   Sperm transport
   Tubal peristalsis
   Ovulation
   Luteolysis
   Implantation
   Menstruation
   Endometriosis
Uterine activity
   Myometrial relaxation in pregnancy
   Dysmenorrhea
   Term and preterm labor
   Abortion
   Postpartum involution
Fetus
   Vascular development
   Fetal malformations
   Vascular dynamics
Preeclampsia
Diabetes (effects on the fetus and the pregnancy)

seminal plasma may be associated with uterine contractions and relaxation of the ampullary portion of the tube to allow ovum transport to the midtubal portion so that fertilization can take place. Contraction of the interstitial end of the tube would prevent premature dumping of the fertilized ovum into the endometrial cavity.

Progesterone increases the response of the tubes to the E prostaglandins and decreases their response to prostaglandin $F_{2\alpha}$, which is produced in the tubal tissue. If estrogen concentrations are increased during the secretory phase or because of exogenous pharmacologic intervention, the increase may stimulate $PGF_{2\alpha}$ and lead to increased tubal motility and loss of the zygote. Progesterone dominance and subsequent PGE effects may inhibit transport of the fertilized ovum to the endometrium until sufficient blastocyst development has occurred.[76,84,89]

Normal ovulation involves prostaglandins in the following ways: (1) $PGF_{2\alpha}$ increases intraovarian pressure; (2) prostaglandins in the E series stimulate ovulation; (3) prostaglandins may stimulate the synthesis and release of luteinizing hormone, whereas prostaglandin synthetase inhibitors can inhibit its release; (4) preovulatory graafian follicles show progressively increasing amounts of $PGF_{2\alpha}$ as ovulation approaches, but aspirin and other nonsteroidal, anti-inflammatory agents block production of prostaglandins in these follicles and inhibit ovulation in animals; (5) luteinizing hormone and human chorionic gonadotropin increase $PGF_{2\alpha}$ content in the graafian follicle. This increased $PGF_{2\alpha}$ concentration may bring about follicular rupture by causing contraction of smooth muscle in the ovary, including the muscles of the follicular wall.[87-93] Prostaglandins have been shown to participate in luteolysis in animals. Although this situation can stimulate labor in animals, the progesterone needed to maintain pregnancy in humans comes from the placenta after 9 weeks' gestation. Labor produced in the human is thought to be due to direct uterine stimulation by prostaglandin rather than by luteolysis.[94-101]

Clinical and experimental studies suggest that prostaglandins are probably important participants in menstruation. Prostaglandins E_2 and $F_{2\alpha}$ are present in menstrual blood, and their concentrations in blood are elevated during menstruation. Concentrations of prostaglandins in the endometrium increase before menstruation and may be augmented by additional estrogen. Some studies have suggested that dysmenorrhea was associated with an elevated concentration of $PGF_{2\alpha}$ in the endometrium and an increase in the $PGF_{2\alpha}/PGE_2$ ratio during menstruation. Treatment with agents that inhibit prostaglandin production may significantly relieve dysmenorrhea.[102-108]

Prostaglandins may play an important role in the pathophysiology of endometriosis. $PGF_{2\alpha}$ and PGE_2 concentrations have been found to be higher in samples of endometrial tissue from patients with endometriosis.[107] Elevated prostaglandin concentrations may contribute to the infertility that is often seen with this condition in addition to stimulating an inflammatory response and causing pain.[108] Other possible effects of increased prostaglandins in endometriosis include luteolysis and toxic effects on the blastocyst.[103,104,109] Inflammation and adhesions may develop secondary to either prostaglandins or lipoxygenase products of arachidonic acid.

Prostaglandins and Pregnancy

It has been known for some time that prostaglandins E and F stimulate uterine contractility in the pregnant woman. Prostaglandins that are oxytocic differ in potency in the following order from maximum to minimum: PGE_1 and $PGE_2 > PGF_{2\alpha} > PGF_{1\alpha}$.[107] There is evidence that prostaglandins may be the agents responsible for spontaneous labor. During spontaneous labor $PGF_{2\alpha}$ concentrations are elevated in the blood and amniotic fluid as well as in the myometrium and placenta.[110-116] Prostaglandin synthetase inhibitors have been used to stop preterm labor. Plasma concentration of $PGF_{2\alpha}$ has been shown to change cyclically, with higher concentrations being seen immediately after uterine contractions.[115]

Prostaglandins and Arachidonic Acid During Labor

Normal and preterm labor seem to be associated with the production of prostaglandins. At the onset of labor, arachidonic acid is liberated, and prostaglandins are produced (Figure 13.8). The presumed sequence of events is as follows: Lysosomes of the fetal membranes are disrupted, releasing the enzyme phospholipase A_2, which acts on the phospholipids of the fetal membranes to release arachidonic acid. Progesterone protects the lysosomes from rupture, thereby maintaining pregnancy. Free arachidonic acid is converted to prostaglandins, possibly in the decidua, where high concentrations of prostaglandin synthetase have been detected. The prostaglandins produced from arachidonic acid cause uterine contractions. This theory is supported by the finding of significantly elevated concentrations of arachidonic acid and $PGF_{2\alpha}$ in amniotic fluid during labor,[113,114,116-123] and by the fact that labor has been initiated by injection of arachidonic acid into the amniotic cavity in human subjects.[123]

Pregnancy and Lipid Metabolism

Arachidonic acid is a polyunsaturated fatty acid that, in addition to being the precursor to the prostaglandins and other eicosanoids, is essential to phospholipid production and cell growth. Other lipids are utilized for fetal struc-

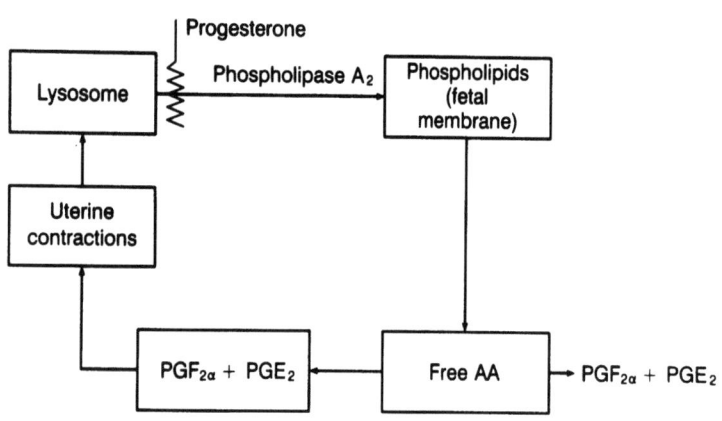

FIGURE 13.8. Normal and preterm labor perpetuate themselves through the cycle of arachidonic acid (AA) release, prostaglandin formation (PGE_2 and PGF_α), and uterine contractions. (Redrawn from Ogburn and Brenner,[18] with permission.)

tural growth and energy metabolism as pregnancy progresses. During the first two trimesters of pregnancy, the mother stores fat as adipose tissue. During the third trimester the rate of maternal fat synthesis is reduced and mobilization of fatty acids from the fat stores is increased. The third trimester is the time for the greatest fetal growth. This growth coincides with the development of relative insulin resistance in the pregnant woman, which would favor transfer of glucose and fatty acids to the fetus and require that the woman use more fatty acids as metabolic fuel. Human placental lactogen and progesterone have been implicated in the insulin resistance that results in higher concentrations of free fatty acids in maternal plasma during the third trimester of pregnancy[124–126] (see Chapter 10).

Prostaglandins may have a role in the release and metabolism of free fatty acids, particularly free arachidonic acid.[127] Oxytocin has been shown to increase circulating free fatty acids and could account for some of their elevated levels during labor.[128] During normal pregnancy, serum concentrations of free fatty acids increase with each trimester, and they increase to an even greater concentration during labor. The serum concentration of arachidonic acid in free form is elevated at the time of labor. However, the percentage of total free fatty acids consisting of arachidonic acid is uniformly decreased during labor[18,129] (Figures 13.9 and 13.10). It should be noted that the percentage of free fatty acids consisting of arachidonic acid is much higher in cord blood than in maternal blood (Figure 13.10). This difference is consistent with the concept that essential fatty acids, including arachidonic acid, are preferentially transported across the placenta to the fetus for growth and prostaglandin production.

Progressive decreases in circulating essential fatty acids have been documented in normal human pregnancy.[130] The patterns of diminished essential fatty acids in pregnancy are extreme enough to resemble nutritional deprivation and disease states in the nonpregnant individual.[131] This pattern of essential fatty acid scarcity that occurs in the plasma during pregnancy is maintained during lactation in the postpartum woman.[131] The possibility that EFAs move from the plasma to maternal tissues (e.g., RBCs) has been suggested.[132]

Preeclampsia

Preeclampsia, a condition of pregnancy characterized by hypertension, proteinuria, edema, and vasospasm, remains a significant cause of maternal, fetal, and neona-

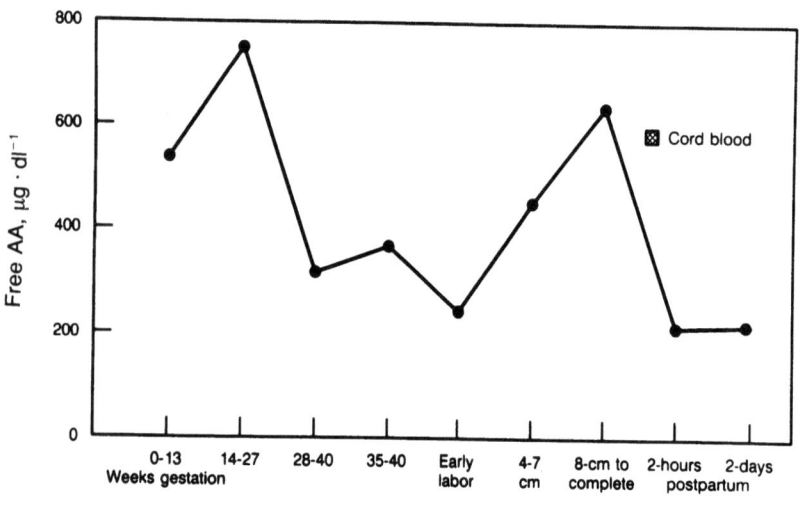

FIGURE 13.9. Concentrations of nonesterified arachidonic acid (free AA) are increased in the maternal plasma during active labor. Concentrations in cord blood are similar to those in maternal blood. (From Ogburn and Brenner[18] and Ogburn et al.,[129] with permission.)

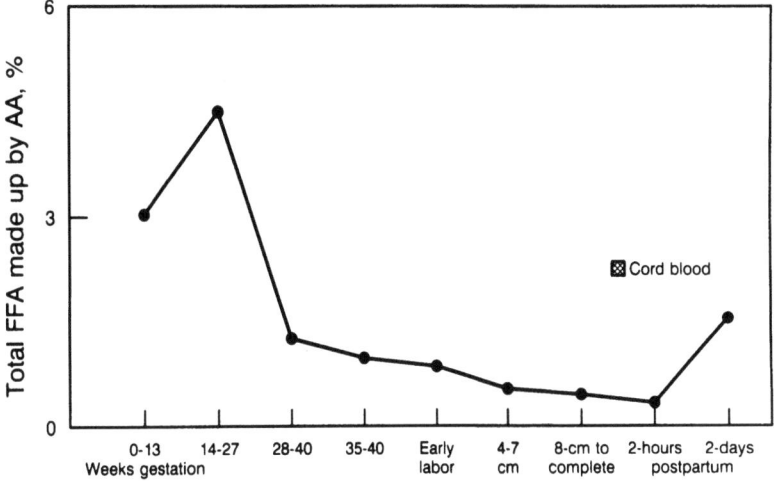

FIGURE 13.10. Percentage of nonesterified fatty acids (FFA) made up by arachidonic acid (AA) is highest in maternal blood during the first and second trimesters. Cord blood contains a much higher proportion of nonesterified AA than does maternal blood near the time of delivery. (From Ogburn and Brenner,[18] with permission.)

tal death.[133] The etiology of the condition is unknown, but it may be associated with a relative increase in the thromboxane A_2/PGI_2 ratio above that of normal pregnancy.[134-136] PGI_2 production may be increased in normal pregnancy compared to that in the nonpregnant state.[136-138]

Prostacyclin (PGI_2) is produced from arachidonic acid and is a potent vasodilator and inhibitor of platelet aggregation.[139] It is produced by the endothelium of all studied blood vessels, the myometrium, the placenta, and the fetus.[139-142] It has a half-life of approximately 3 minutes but produces a stable metabolite, 6-keto-$PGF_{1\alpha}$, which may be quantitated.[143] Prostacyclin seems to be responsible for the vasodilation, decreased blood pressure, and smooth muscle relaxation seen with normal pregnancy.[144-146] Gant et al.[147] showed that pregnant women are normally resistant to the pressor effects of angiotensin II. Normal pregnant women needed more exogenous angiotensin II to develop a rise in diastolic blood pressure than do nonpregnant women and preeclamptic patients.[147,148] Other studies using cyclooxygenase inhibitors suggest that prostacyclin may cause this resistance to angiotensin II in normal pregnancies.[149] Failure to produce increased prostacyclin in response to angiotensin II may predict preeclampsia months before clinical symptoms occur.

As outlined earlier, thromboxane A_2 is another metabolite of arachidonic acid and is a potent vasoconstrictor and platelet aggregator. It is produced primarily by the platelets, and it has a half-life of approximately 30 seconds. The measurable stable metabolite of this substance is thromboxane B_2.[150] The thromboxane effect would explain the following clinical conditions seen in preeclampsia-eclampsia: (1) elevated blood pressure; (2) vasospasm, resulting in tissue ischemia and dysfunction of the kidneys, liver, and brain; and (3) platelet activation, resulting in thrombocytopenia and capillary plugging.[133]

Several investigators have found preeclampsia to be associated with increases in the thromboxane A_2/prostacyclin ratio, measured as the thromboxane B_2/6-keto-$PGF_{1\alpha}$ ratio.[151-153] Work by Walsh[154] has shown that the altered thromboxane A_2/prostacyclin metabolism of preeclampsia is maintained in tissue culture of placentas incubated for 48 hours. The thromboxane B_2/prostacyclin theory of preeclampsia has gained enough support to engender the use of low-dose aspirin to promote a decrease in this ratio as an experimental therapy.[155,156] Magnesium sulfate, the conventional therapy for preeclampsia, seems to promote production of prostacyclin by human umbilical endothelial cells in vitro.[157] Magnesium sulfate improved uterine and probably other organ perfusion in vivo, suggesting that it works by promoting prostacyclin production in vivo as well.[155] Recent evidence that prenatal exposure to magnesium sulfate prevents cerebral palsy and mental retardation in very low birth weight neonates may be related to improved uterine, placental, and/or fetal perfusion due to the prostacyclin induced by magnesium sulfate.[158]

If the clinical manifestations of preeclampsia are caused by a relative increase in the thromboxane A_2/prostacyclin ratio, the etiology of preeclampsia can be defined by finding the cause of the altered thromboxane A_2/prostacyclin ratio. The two major theoretical mechanisms for this reasoning are (1) endothelial injury–platelet activation, and (2) essential fatty acid deficiency (EFAD)–lipoxygenase product production. These two theories are not mutually exclusive. Endothelial injury, platelet activation, and lipooxygenase production have been described as part of the pathophysiology of preeclampsia.[133,144,159] EFAD has been described in preeclampsia and may be explained by inadequate transfer of essential fatty acids to the fetus through the placenta.[160-162] This inadequacy may result from preexisting maternal vascular disease or, classically, in primigravid pregnancies that have inadequate invasion of the

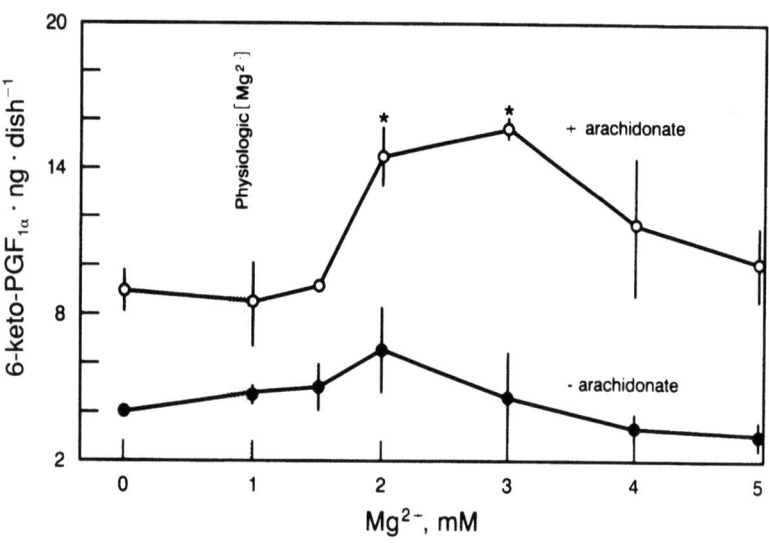

FIGURE 13.11. Stimulation of 6-keto-PGF$_{1\alpha}$ (i.e., stable metabolite of prostacyclin) production by umbilical vessel endothelial cell cultures exposed to various concentrations of magnesium sulfate. *$p < .005$; $n = 14$. (From Watson et al.,[157] with permission.)

myometrial spiral arteries by the trophoblasts. Neonates born to mothers with preeclampsia are frequently growth-retarded and have placental insufficiency. Their skin may be peeling, and subcutaneous tissue may be without fat.[133,159] This clinical picture is classic for essential fatty acid deficiency as described in humans and animals[2,3,163].

Relevant preliminary studies have suggested the following:

1. Magnesium sulfate promoted increased prostacyclin production by cultured umbilical vessel endothelial cells exposed to preeclampsia serum[157] (Figure 13.11), which may explain its usefulness in the clinical treatment of preeclampsia.
2. EFAD patterns were present in cord blood of preeclamptic pregnancies;[160] Lewis et al.[144] have suggested that EFAD patterns inhibited normal prostacyclin production. The specific EFAD pattern seen in preeclamptic cord blood is a relative elevation of the oleic acid/arachidonic acid ratio (OA/AA) (Figure 13.12).

There is evidence that EFAD may inhibit prostacyclin production by means of lipoxygenase products of the nonessential fatty acids. This could potentially explain the relative increase in the thromboxane B_2/6-keto-PGF$_{1\alpha}$ ratio of preeclampsia. A theoretical model of preeclampsia is shown in Figures 13.3, 13.13, 13.14, and 13.15.[41,160]

Blood concentrations of free fatty acids and arachidonic acid may be elevated in preeclampsia.[18,129] Because albumin binds free fatty acids, the decrease in plasma albumin concentration that occurs in preeclampsia may result in the cascade of pathologic events associated with the disorder. The increased blood concentration of non–albumin-bound arachidonic acid would stimulate platelet activation and possibly aggregation. Platelet activation and aggregation would release thromboxane A_2, a potent vasoconstrictor that could cause the hypertension seen in preeclampsia. With increased platelet coagulation, thrombocytopenia or diffuse intravascular coagulation, or both, could occur. Based on the fact that omega-3 PUFA, which are concentrated in fish oil, can serve as precursors for prostacyclin I_3, but not thromboxanes, there is a good possibility that dietary fish oil may decrease preterm labor and preeclampsia.[164]

Elevated serum concentrations of fatty acids are hepatotoxic; hepatic dysfunction increased concentra-

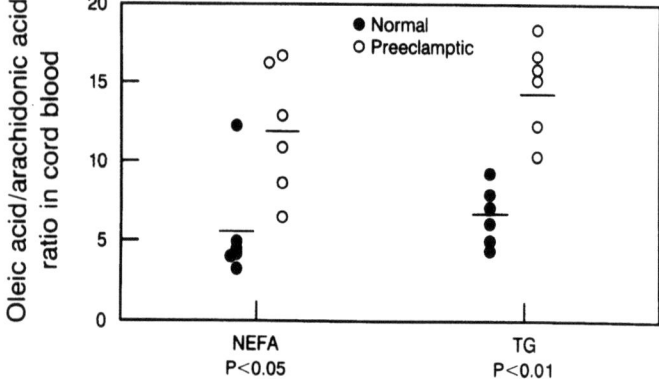

FIGURE 13.12. Elevated samples oleic acid/arachidonic acid ratios were seen in a group of cord blood samples from preeclamptic patients in the nonesterified (NEFA) and triglyceride (TG) fractions. (From Ogburn et al.,[161] with permission.)

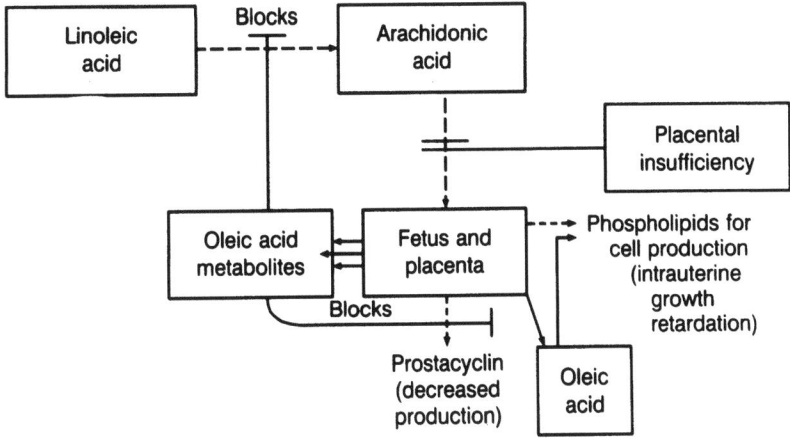

FIGURE 13.13. With classic preeclampsia, maternal vascular or placental insufficiency leads to relative essential fatty acid deficiency in the fetus. The fetus responds by making oleic acid to supply some of the fatty acid substrate for phospholipids to support fetal growth. Oleic acid and its metabolites decrease arachidonate availability and prostacyclin production.

tions of free fatty acids.[165,166] The relative increase in serum concentrations of free fatty acid and arachidonic acid may be responsible for the hypertension, vasospasm, thrombocytopenia, coagulopathy, and hepatic dysfunction that can occur with preeclampsia (Figure 13.16). This theory may be further supported by studies that suggested that the placenta made its own arachidonic acid and may even have transferred it to maternal blood.[129,162,167]

Low-Dose Aspirin Therapy

Low-dose aspirin has been documented to increase the prostacyclin/thromboxane ratio in pregnant women and nonpregnant individuals by inhibiting the cyclooxygenase in platelets, thereby inhibiting thromboxane production while not affecting the prostacyclin production of endothelial cells. For this reason, low-dose aspirin has been proposed as a treatment to prevent severe preeclampsia by starting it during the second trimester or treating preeclampsia during the third trimester.[168-178] Some investigators have suggested that low-dose aspirin does not reach the fetus in amounts high enough to be detected, to cause inhibition of fetal platelets, or to close the ductus arteriosus prematurely.[172] As early as 1978, Goodlin et al.,[173] demonstrated the possible use of low-dose aspirin to prevent recurrent preeclampsia. Sanchez-Ramos et al.[174] have presented data that suggest that low-dose aspirin may promote angiotensin II resistance, probably through increasing the $PGI_2:TXA_2$ ratio as a means of decreasing the frequency of preeclampsia. Sibai et al.[175] have found low-dose aspirin to decrease preeclampsia by 25% in a large prospective study involving otherwise normal primigravidas. In other studies, low-dose aspirin was more associated with delaying the onset of preeclampsia and preventing preterm birth.[176]

Phospholipid antibodies, including anticardiolipin antibody and lupus anticoagulant, have been described as associated with severe preeclampsia, abruptio placentae, intrauterine growth retardation, and recurrent fetal death in utero and spontaneous abortion. There is some evidence that much of the recurrent severe preeclampsia may be related to one or more of these circulating antibodies. Lupus anticoagulant, especially, has been associated with recurrent deep venous thrombosis in some patients, both pregnant and nonpregnant. A fair amount of clinical experience has been reported in the literature, which suggests that the combination of prednisone 40 mg and 1 infant aspirin a day (i.e., 60–80 mg) may be effective treatment for these phospholipid antibodies.[177] Some investigators have suggested that low-dose aspirin may be just as effective by itself as in combination with prednisone.[178] Others have shown the addition of heparin to be beneficial in the treatment of this condition.[179,180]

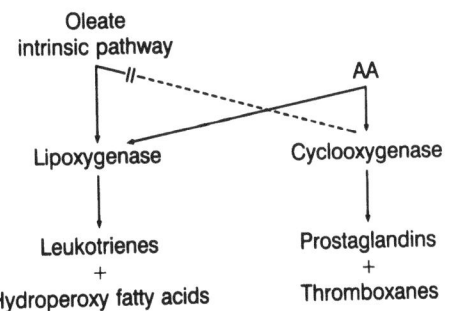

FIGURE 13.14. Oleic acid and its metabolites can be hydroxylated by the lipoxygenase pathways but cannot serve as a substrate for prostaglandin production. (From Lewis et al.[141] and Ogburn et al.,[160] with permission.)

Fetal Circulation

Prostacyclin is preferentially produced by fetal vascular tissue. It may play an important role in maintaining fetal

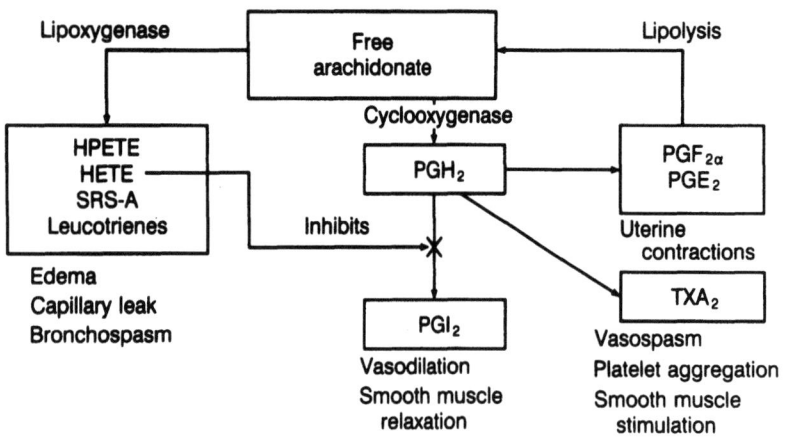

FIGURE 13.15. With preeclampsia, the lipoxygenase products of oleic acid metabolites as well as arachidonic acid may inhibit the prostaglandin production needed to maintain normal vasodilation. This reaction would shift the balance toward thromboxane production. (From Ogburn et al.,[161] with permission.)

and umbilical cord circulation. The prostacyclin released from the uterus during pregnancy may cause the decrease in maternal blood pressure that frequently occurs during the first and second trimesters of pregnancy.[181,182]

Prostaglandins may maintain the patency of the fetal ductus arteriosus before birth. In the normal neonate elevation in the partial pressure of oxygen causes the ductus arteriosus to close, which allows normal neonatal circulation to occur (see Chapter 24). Products of arachidonic acid (e.g., PGE_2 and prostacyclin) are associated with relaxation of the ductus arteriosus in vitro. In the premature neonate, the ductus arteriosus tissue is less likely to respond to oxygen by contracting. On occasion this lack of response results in persistent patent ductus arteriosus in the neonate. Inhibitors of prostaglandins and prostacyclin production (e.g., nonsteroidal anti-inflammatory agents) have promoted contraction of the ductus arteriosus tissue in vitro and closure of the ductus arteriosus in premature neonates.[183,184] The use of indomethacin to inhibit preterm labor has been associated with transient constriction of the ductus arteriosus. This effect disappears if the duration of indomethacin is limited to 48 hours.

Glucose Metabolism

Glucose metabolism may be significantly altered by prostaglandins, which may participate with insulin in favoring the uptake of glucose into skeletal muscle.[185] In contrast, insulin secretion is inhibited by certain prostaglandins in the human.[186] The condition of diabetes mellitus may be affected by the quantity and types of prostaglandin present. Indeed, the insulin response to glucose in diabetes mellitus is improved by the administration of salicylates, which are inhibitors of prostaglandin production.[186]

Insulin-dependent diabetes is associated with a number of major problems, not only in the mother but

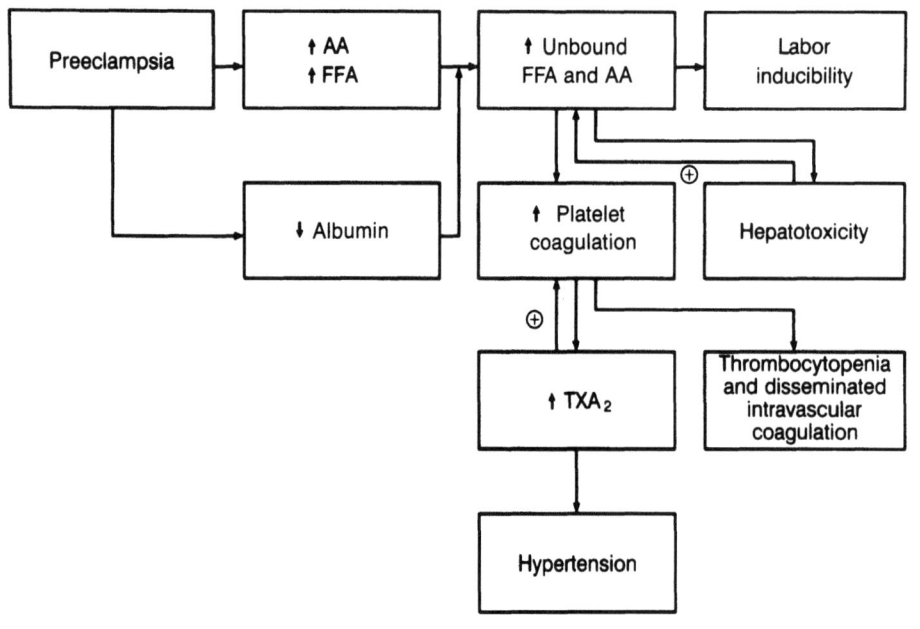

FIGURE 13.16. Decreased albumin in maternal circulation in preeclampsia may increase nonesterified fatty acids (FFA) and arachidonic acid (AA), which are not bound to albumin. These lipids may serve to activate platelets and cause hepatic dysfunction, which frequently accompanies severe preeclampsia. (From Ogburn and Brenner,[18] with permission.)

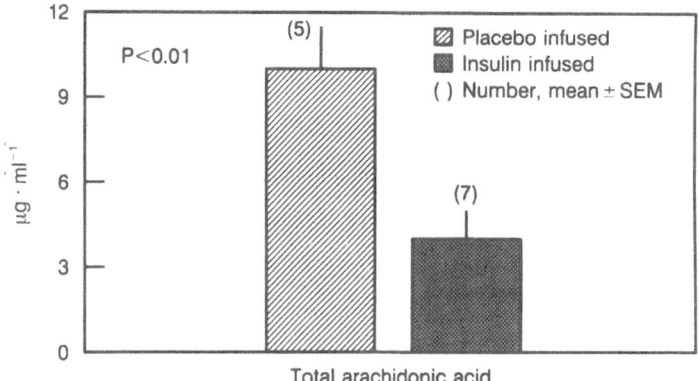

FIGURE 13.17. Chronic infusion of insulin to fetal lambs decreased circulating arachidonic acid. (From Stonestreet et al.,[190] with permission.)

also in the neonate, as documented elsewhere in this text (see Chapters 10 and 49). These problems include but are not limited to the following: (1) fetal macrosomia; (2) fetal malformation associated with hyperglycemia; (3) fetal vascular thrombosis; (4) fetal death in utero near term associated with poor diabetic control; and (5) maternal preeclampsia associated with preexisting vascular disease, poor diabetic control, or both.

Fetal macrosomia is associated with maternal hyperglycemia and increased transfer of glucose to the fetus with subsequent increased fetal insulin production. This condition leads to conversion and deposition of glucose into triglycerides and extra body fat. There is a significantly increased rate of growth of the nonlipid tissues of the fetus. It is fairly well documented that fetal hyperinsulinemia seems to result in fatty acids, including the essential fatty acids, moving out of the circulating bloodstream and into the lipid and nonlipid tissues of the fetus.[187-191] Hyperinsulinemia in the fetal sheep model has been associated with decreasing quantities of circulating arachidonic acid[192] (Figure 13.17). This essential fatty

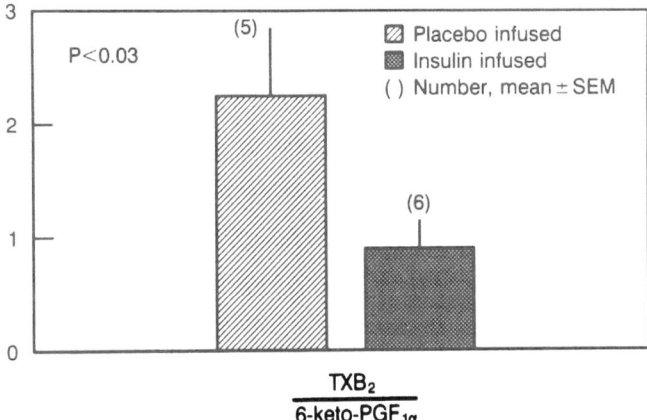

FIGURE 13.18. Chronic infusion of insulin into fetal lambs decreased the circulating thromboxane (TXB$_2$)/prostacyclin (measured as the 6-keto-PGF$_{1\alpha}$ metabolite) ratio. (From Stonestreet et al.,[190] with permission.)

acid is required not only for adipose tissue production, but for normal growth of nonadipose tissues including the brain.

Poorly controlled diabetes mellitus is thought to be associated with changes in the thromboxane/prostacyclin ratio. A number of investigators have shown that elevated glucose concentration and low insulin concentration are associated with an increased thromboxane/prostacyclin ratio possibly due to the vascular injury, platelet activation, and increased blood pressure associated with diabetes.[193-198] Similar changes in the arachidonic acid–thromboxane-prostacyclin system have been seen in the infants of diabetic women.[199,200] Some investigations have shown that fetal hyperinsulinemia with resultant hypoglycemia not only diminishes arachidonic acid availability in the circulating bloodstream, but decreases the thromboxane/prostacyclin ratio overall[190] (Figure 13.18).

Hyperglycemia in the adult is associated with a relative increase in serum oleic acid and a relative decrease in arachidonic acid, a condition analogous to the essential fatty acid deficiency pattern[201] (vide supra) (Figure 13.19). Elevated maternal free oleic acid plasma levels have been documented in human diabetic pregnancies.[202] This relative increase in oleic acid and decrease in arachidonic acid was ameliorated by improving glycemia control.[201] In the same way, the fetal rat conceptus model has shown malformations in the fetal rat and yolk sacs in vivo and in vitro when an elevated glucose concentration was present[203] (Figures 13.20 to 13.23). Striking diminutions in these fetal malformations are produced by adding a high concentration of free arachidonic acid to the incubation under in vitro conditions of these fetal rats. Oleic acid was found to be increased in the embryonic phospholipids and nonesterified fatty acids of these conceptuses exposed to excess glucose, suggesting increased production of this nonessential monounsaturated fatty acid and an essential fatty acid deficiency pattern.[203,204]

The production of oleic acid in the poorly controlled diabetic pregnant woman may decrease the normal

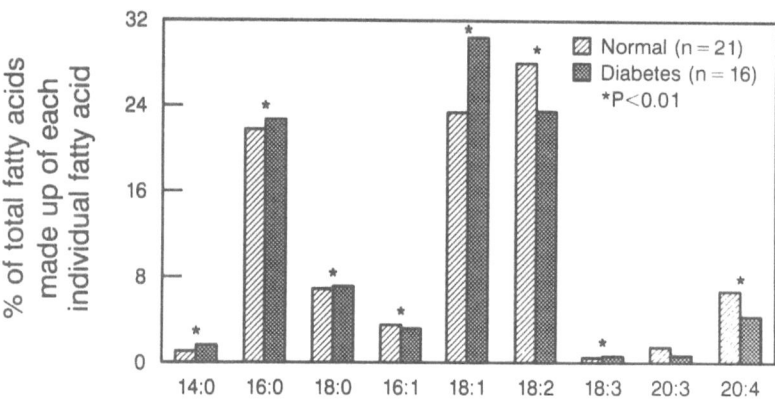

FIGURE 13.19. With poorly controlled diabetes mellitus, an essential fatty acid deficiency pattern is seen, with significantly elevated total oleic acid (18:1) and significantly depressed arachidonic acid (20:4). (From Tuna et al.,[199] with permission.)

amounts of arachidonic acid and prostacyclin available to the fetus. Rosenthal and Whitehurst,[205] have shown the oleic acid added to human endothelial cell cultures from umbilical veins inhibit the usual conversion of linoleic acid to arachidonic acid. Ongari et al.[206] have shown that relative decreases in arachidonic acid decrease the production of prostacyclin by human umbilical artery rings in vitro. In addition, the increase oleic acid and its polyunsaturated chain elongation products, including Mead's acid may be converted to perhydroxides and hydroxides, which promote vascular injury, platelet activation, and thromboxane production[144] (Figures 13.15 and 13.24). The theoretical explanation for the problems of the fetus in poorly controlled diabetes mellitus is as follows:

1. Fetal malformations associated with poor glycemic control during the first trimester may be associated with transient vasospasm in conjunction with an increased thromboxane/prostacyclin ratio. The latter may be secondary to hyperglycemia or to the essential fatty acid

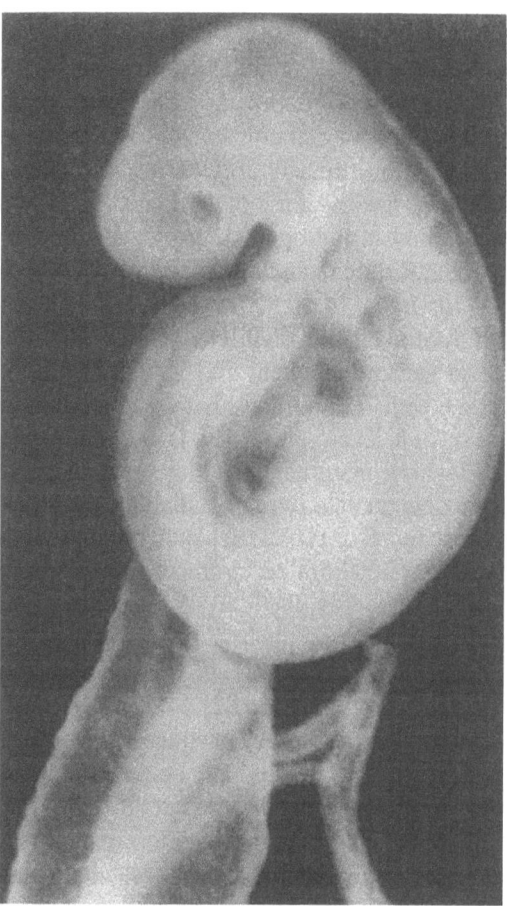

FIGURE 13.20. Normal day 12 rat embryo grown in normal glucose concentration. No abnormalities are seen. (From Pinter and Reece,[203] with permission.)

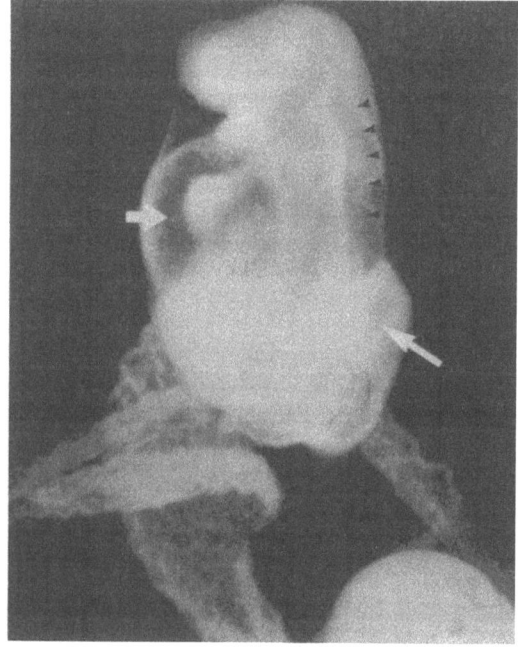

FIGURE 13.21. Day 12 rat embryo grown in high glucose concentration. Abnormalities of the spine and tail are evident (arrows).

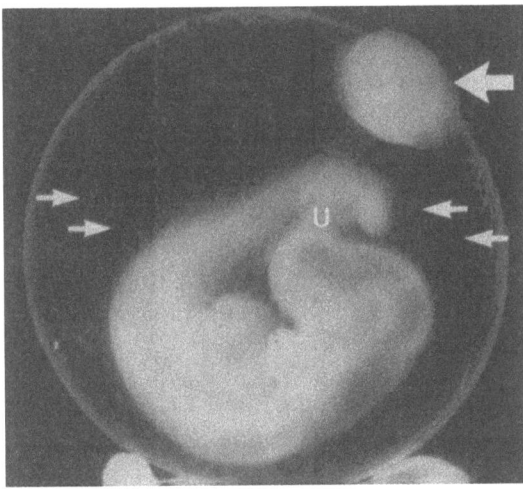

FIGURE 13.22. Normal day 12 rat embryo and yolk sac (large arrow). The membranes are smooth and transparent (small arrows). The umbilical vessels (u) may be seen connecting the yolk sac to the fetus. (From Pinter and Reece,[203] with permission.)

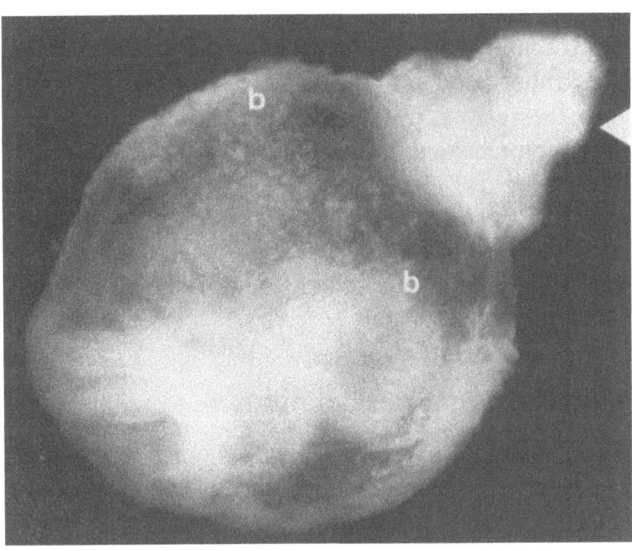

FIGURE 13.23. Day 12 rat embryo, yolk sac, and membranes grown in high glucose concentration. The yolk sac is enlarged and malformed (arrow). The fetal membranes are clouded by numerous vascular malformations. (From Pinter and Reece,[203] with permission.)

deficiency pattern, with increased oleic acid promoting the imbalance in the thromboxane/prostacyclin ratio.

2. Vascular spasm and platelet activation may occur secondary to the same thromboxane/prostacyclin ratio imbalance later in pregnancy, which could result in the vascular thrombosis sometimes described in fetuses of poorly controlled diabetic mothers. Vasospasm of the umbilical cord could result in fetal demise or fetal hypoxia, which is another complication of poor diabetic control in pregnancy. Recurrent episodes of chronic fetal hypoxia secondary to hyperglycemia could result indirectly in other abnormalities including increased erythropoietin, polycythemia, and hyperviscosity, which may be seen in these fetuses. This situation would further compromise normal blood flow and may increase the transient vascular insufficiency or thrombosis previously described.

3. Fetal hyperinsulinemia results in increased deposition of essential and nonessential fatty acids into adipose and nonadipose tissues, resulting in fetal macrosomia.

4. Maternal hyperglycemia exacerbates the essential fatty acids deficiency pattern described previously and

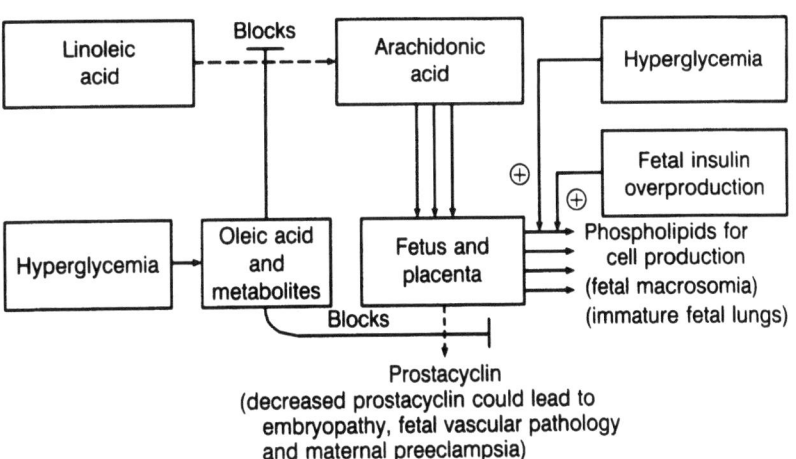

FIGURE 13.24. Pregnancy complicated by poorly controlled diabetes mellitus is associated with increased utilization of arachidonic acid for phospholipid production resulting in an increased risk of macrosomia. Hyperglycemia is associated with an increase in oleic acid, which, with its metabolites, may inhibit the prostacyclin needed to ensure normal fetal vascular development. This mechanism may also explain fetal vascular pathology and maternal preeclampsia seen in poorly controlled diabetes mellitus.

promotes preeclampsia in poorly controlled diabetics. It would occur by virtue of the lipoxygenase products of the nonessential fatty acid (e.g., oleic acid products) diminishing the relative production of prostacyclin and promoting thromboxane production.

This theory seems to explain many of the findings associated with poorly controlled diabetes mellitus and pregnancy. There are suppositions and assumptions that remain to be investigated.

Pharmacologic Considerations

Prostaglandins E_2 and $F_{2\alpha}$ can be given orally, per rectum or vagina, or parenterally to induce abortion, produce cervical softening, or induce labor. Because the natural products are quickly metabolized, a number of active synthetic analogues have been developed that have greater potency and length of action. The uterine contracting properties of prostaglandins E_2, and $F_{2\alpha}$ and certain synthetic analogues have made them useful for treating postpartum hemorrhage. PGE_1 has been used in neonates with ductus-dependent congenital heart disease to maintain patency of the ductus arteriosus until corrective surgery can be done. Other prostaglandins of the E series (e.g., the analogue 16,16-dimethyl-PGE_1) have been used as antiulcer treatment because they inhibit gastric acid secretion.[74] The vasodilatory effects of the prostaglandins of the E series and the A series, as well as that of prostacyclin, have made these prostaglandins useful in experiments to treat Raynaud's disease, peripheral atherosclerosis, pulmonary hypertension, and even the rejection of renal allografts in humans.[74]

Preterm Labor

Preterm delivery occurs in about 7% of all pregnancies but is associated with about 75% of the perinatal morbidity and mortality seen in the United States.[207,208] Preterm labor is associated with production of prostaglandins from arachidonic acid secondary to tissue inflammation or necrosis especially with infection, blood clotting especially with abruptio placentae, or transient hypoxia as with uterine contractions. Prostaglandins may cause preterm labor in the following ways:

1. Myometrial cells increase receptors for oxytocin and increase the number of gap junctions when exposed to prostaglandins. This situation increases irritability and coordination in the myometrium.
2. Intracellular calcium increases to concentrations that stimulate myometrial contractions.
3. Cervical tissue softens.

Effective treatment for preterm labor includes bed rest and hydration with glucose-containing solutions. This treatment increases the blood flow and oxygen to the uterus and eliminates ischemia as a cause of prostaglandin production. Preterm labor has been treated by decreasing myometrial intracellular calcium using β-mimetic agents, magnesium sulfate, or calcium channel blockers. Some of these agents have been reported to cause maternal respiratory distress, especially the combination of β-mimetics and magnesium sulfate.[209,210] Treating infections, especially of the urinary tract, with antibiotics decreases tissue inflammation as a source of prostaglandin production.[205]

The treatment of preterm labor with a short course of indomethacin (i.e., 48 hours) has been effective in prolonging pregnancy safely. The use of indomethacin for longer periods with the fetus in utero have caused permanent constriction of the ductus arteriosus with resultant fetal death.[207,211,212] Indomethacin has increasingly been used to treat persistent ductus arteriosus in the neonatal unit when it is clinically apparent.[74]

Implications

Pregnancy depends on essential fatty acids and their products, including the prostaglandins, prostacyclin, and thromboxane. These substances participate in the following physiologic situations:

1. Normal sexual function in men and women
2. Normal ovulation, fertilization, and implantation
3. Fetal growth, both somatic and neurologic
4. Normal vascular function, including fetal vascular formation and normal maternal and fetal vascular dilation
5. Uterine relaxation and growth, allowing the pregnancy to expand
6. Uterine contractions at term to promote normal parturition.

Abnormalities or disruptions of the normal pregnancy may be related to abnormalities in essential fatty acid metabolism and prostaglandins in the following clinical conditions:

1. Premature delivery or miscarriage
2. Intrauterine growth retardation secondary to insufficient fatty acid available for adequate fetal cell production
3. Preeclampsia
4. Abnormal fetal development secondary to diabetes
5. Fetal macrosomia
6. Abnormalities associated with an infant of a diabetic mother.

Acknowledgment. This work was supported by a grant from the Mayo Foundation.

References

1. Pace-Asciak CR. The eicosanoids. In: Kalant H, Roschlau WHE, eds. Principles of medical pharmacology. 5th ed. Philadelphia: B.C. Decker, 1989:302–310.
2. Burr GO, Burr MM. A new deficiency disease produced by the rigid exclusion of fat from the diet. J Biol Chem 1929;82:345–367.
3. Burr GO, Burr MM. On the nature and role of the fatty acids essential in nutrition. J Biol Chem 1930;86:587–621.
4. Gorman RR, Marcus AJ. Prostaglandins and cardiovascular disease. Current Concepts Series. Kalamazoo: Upjohn, 1981.
5. Raux JF, Yoshioka T. Lipid metabolism in the fetus during development. Clin Obstet Gynecol 1970;13:595–620.
6. Crawford MA, Hassam AG, Stevens PA. Essential fatty acid requirements in pregnancy and lactation with special reference to brain development. Prog Lipid Res 1981;20:31–40.
7. Kurzrok R, Leib CC. Biochemical studies of human semen; action of semen on human uterus. Proc Soc Exp Biol Med 1930;28:268–272.
8. Battez G, Boulet L. Action de l'extrait de prostate humaine sur la vessie et sur la pression arterielle. C R Soc Biol Paris 1913;74:8–9.
9. Von Euler US. Zur Kenntnis der pharmakologischen Wirkungren von Nativsekreten und Extrakten mannlicher accessoricher Geschlectlichsdrusen. Arch Exp Pathol Pharmacol 1934;175:78–84.
10. Von Euler US. On specific vasodilating and plain muscle stimulating substances from accessory genital glands in man and certain animals (prostaglandin and vesiglandin). J Physiol (Lond) 1936;88:213–234.
11. Goldblatt MW. A depressor substance in seminal fluid. J Soc Chem Ind (Lond) 1993;52:1056–1057.
12. Goldblatt MW. Properties of human seminal plasma. J Physiol (Lond) 1935;84:208–218.
13. Bergstrom S, Sjovall J. The isolation of prostaglandin F from sheep prostate glands. Acta Chem Scand 1960;14:1693–1700.
14. Bergstrom S, Sjovall J. The isolation of prostaglandin E from sheep prostate glands. Acta Chem Scand 1960;14:1701–1705.
15. Bergstrom S, Ryhage R, Samuelsson B, et al. Prostaglandins and related factors. 15. The structures of prostaglandin E, $F_{1\alpha}$, $F_{1\beta}$. J Biol Chem 1963;238:3555–3564.
16. Weinheimier AJ, Spraggins RL. The occurrence of two new prostaglandin derivatives (15-epi-PGA_2) in the gorgonian *Plexaura homomalla*. Tet Lett 1969;10:5185–5188.
17. Corey EJ. Studies on the total synthesis of prostaglandins. Ann NY Acad Sci 1971;180:24–37.
18. Ogburn PL Jr, Brenner WE. The physiologic actions and effects of prostaglandins. Kalamazoo: Upjohn, 1981.
19. Karim SMM, Filshie GM. Therapeutic abortion using prostaglandin $F_{1\alpha}$. Lancet 1970;1:157–159.
20. Roth-Brandel U, Bygdeman M, Wiqvist N, et al. Prostaglandins for induction of therapeutic abortion. Lancet 1970;1:190–191.
21. Karim S. Action of prostaglandin in the pregnant woman. Ann NY Acad Sci 1971;180:483–498.
22. Wiqvist N, Beguin F, Bygdeman M, et al. Recent aspects on systemic administration of prostaglandin. In: Southern EM, ed. The prostaglandins: clinical applications in human reproduction. Mount Kisco, NY: Futura, 1972:295–306.
23. Samuelsson B, Hamberg M, Sweeley CC. Quantitative gas chromatography of prostaglandin E_1 at the nanogram level: use of deuterated carrier and multiple ion analyzer. Anat Biochem 1970;38:301–304.
24. Thompson CJ, Los M, Horton EW. The separation, identification, and estimation of prostaglandins in nanogram quantities by combined gas chromatography-mass spectrometry. Life Sci 1970;9:983–988.
25. Granstrom E. Radioimmunoassay of prostaglandins. Prostaglandins 1978;15:3–17.
26. Granstrom E, Kindahl H. Radioimmunoassay for prostaglandin metabolites. Adv Prostaglandin Thromboxane Res 1976;1:81–92.
27. Dray F, Chorbonnel B, Maclouf J. Primary prostaglandins in human peripheral plasma by radioimmunoassay. Adv Prostaglandin Thromboxane Res 1976;1:93–97.
28. Van Dorp DA, Beerthuis RK, Nugteren DH, et al. The biosynthesis of prostaglandins. Biochem Biophys Acta 1964;90:204–297.
29. Van Dorp DA, Beerthuis RK, Nugteren DH, et al. Enzymatic conversion of all-*cis*-polyunsaturated fatty acids into prostaglandins. Nature 1964;203:839–841.
30. Bergstrom S, Danielsson H, Samuelsson B. The enzymatic formation of prostaglandin E_1 from arachidonic acid. 32. Prostaglandins and related factors. Biochem Biophys Acta 1964;90:207–210.
31. Anggard E, Samuelsson B. Biosynthesis of prostaglandins from arachidonic acid in guinea-pig lung. 38. Prostaglandins and related factors. J Biol Chem 1965;240:3518–3521.
32. Kupiecki FP. Conversion of homo-gamma-linolenic acid to prostaglandin $F_{1\alpha}$ by ovine and bovine seminal vesicle extracts. Life Sci 1965;4:1811–1815.
33. Bergstrom S. Prostaglandins from bedside observation to a family of drugs. Prog Lipid Res 1981;20:7–12.
34. Struijk CB, Beerthuis RK, Pabon HJJ, et al. Specificity in the enzymic conversion of polyunsaturated fatty acids into prostaglandin. Recl Trav Chim Pays Bas Belg 1966;85:1233–1250.
35. Flower RJ, Blackwell GJ. The importance of phospholipase-A_2 in prostaglandin biosynthesis. Biochem Pharmacol 1976;25:285–291.
36. Wallach DP. The enzymatic conversion of arachidonic acid to prostaglandin E_2 with acetone powder preparations of bovine seminal vesicles. Life Sci 1965;4:361–364.
37. Wallach DP, Daniels EG. Properties of a novel preparation of prostaglandin synthetase from sheep seminal vesicles. Biochim Biophys Acta 1971;231:445–457.
38. Van Dorp DA. Aspects of the biosynthesis of prostaglandins. Prog Biochem Pharmacol 1967;3:71–82.
39. Samuelsson B, Hambert M. Role of endoperoxides in the biosynthesis and action of prostaglandins. In: Robinson HJ, Vane JR, eds. Prostaglandin synthetase inhibitors. New York: Raven Press, 1974:107–119.

40. Nugteren DH, Hazelhof E. Isolation and properties of intermediates in prostaglandin biosynthesis. Biochim Biophys Acta 1973;326:448–461.
41. Hamberg M, Samuelsson B. Prostaglandin endoperoxides: novel transformations of arachidonic acid in human platelets. Proc Natl Acad Sci USA 1974;71:3400–3404.
42. Van Dorp DA. The biosynthesis of prostaglandins. Mem Soc Endocr 1966;14:39–47.
43. Hamberg M, Samuelsson B. On the mechanism of the biosynthesis of prostaglandins E_1 and $F_{1\alpha}$. J Biol Chem 1967;242:5336–5443.
44. Nugteren DH, Van Dorp DA. The participation of molecular oxygen in the biosynthesis of prostaglandins. Biochim Biophys Acta 1965;98:654–656.
45. Nugteren DH, Beerthuis RK, Van Dorp DA. The enzymic conversion of all-*cis*-8,11,14-eicosatrienoic acid into prostaglandin E_1. Recl Trav Chim Pays Bas Belg 1966;85:405–419.
46. Ryhage R, Samuelsson B. The origin of oxygen incorporated during the biosynthesis of prostaglandin E_1. Biochem Biophys Res Commun 1965;19:279–282.
47. Samuelsson B. On the incorporation of oxygen in the conversion of 8,11,14-eicosatrienoic acid to prostaglandin E_1. J Am Chem Soc 1965;87:3011–3013.
48. Klenberg D, Samuelsson B. The biosynthesis of prostaglandin E_1 studied with specifically ^{3}H-labelled 8,11,14-eicosatrienoic acids. Acta Chem Scand 1965;19:534–535.
49. Hamberg M, Samuelsson B. Detection and isolation of an endoperoxide intermediate in prostaglandin biosynthesis. Proc Natl Acad Sci USA 1973;70:899–903.
50. Hamberg M, Samuelsson B. On the metabolism of prostaglandin E_1 and E_2 in man. J Biol Chem 1971;246:6713–6721.
51. Granstrom E. On the metabolism of prostaglandin $F_{1\alpha}$ in female subjects: structures of two metabolites in blood. Eur J Biochem 1972;27:462–469.
52. Nugteren DH. The determination of prostaglandin metabolites in human urine. J Biol Chem 1975;250:2808–2812.
53. Smith JB, Willis AL. Aspirin selectively inhibits prostaglandin production in human platelets. Nature 1971;231:235–237.
54. Vane JR. Inhibition of prostaglandin synthesis as a mechanism of action for aspirin-like drugs. Nature 1971;231:232–235.
55. Rome LH, Lands WEM. Structural requirements for time-dependent inhibition of prostaglandin biosynthesis by anti-inflammatory drugs. Proc Natl Acad Sci USA 1975;72:4863–4865.
56. Hamberg M, Svensson J, Samuelsson B. Prostaglandin endoperoxides: new concept concerning the mode of action and release of prostaglandins. Proc Natl Acad Sci USA 1975;71:3824–3828.
57. Hinman JW, Weeks JR. The prostaglandins: biology and biochemistry. In: Southern EM, ed. Prostaglandins: clinical applications in human reproduction (Brook Lodge Symposium on the Prostaglandins, Augusta, MI, 1972). Mount Kisco, NY: Futura, 1972:31–36.
58. Hamberg M, Svensson J, Samuelsson B. Thromboxanes: a new group of biologically active compounds derived from prostaglandin endoperoxides. Proc Natl Acad Sci USA 1975;72:2994–2998.
59. Gryglewski RJ, Bunting S, Moncada S, et al. Arterial walls are protected against deposition of platelet thrombi by a substance (prostaglandins X) which they make from prostaglandin endoperoxides. Prostaglandins 1976;12:685–713.
60. Moncada S, Gryglewski RJ, Bunting S, et al. An enzyme isolated from arteries transforms prostaglandins endoperoxides to an unstable substance that inhibits platelet aggregation. Nature 1976;263:663–665.
61. Kuehl FA, Humes JL. Direct evidence for a prostaglandin receptor and its application to prostaglandin measurements (rat-adipocytes-antagonists-analogues-mouse ovary assay). Proc Natl Acad Sci USA 1972;69:480–484.
62. Wakeling AE, Kirton KT. Prostaglandin receptors in the hamster uterus during the estrous cycle. Prostaglandins 1973;4:1–8.
63. Powell WS, Hammarstrom S, Samuelsson B. Prostaglandin $F_{2\alpha}$ receptor in ovine corpora lutea. Eur J Biochem 1974;41:103–107.
64. Powell WS, Hammarstrom S, Samuelsson B. Occurrence and properties of a prostaglandin $F_{2\alpha}$ receptor in bovine corpora lutea. Eur J Biochem 1975;56:73–77.
65. Powell WS, Hammarstrom S, Samuelsson B, et al. Prostaglandin $F_{2\alpha}$ receptor in human corpora lutea. Lancet 1974;1:1120 (letter).
66. Kuehl FA Jr. Prostaglandins, cyclic nucleotides and cell function. Prostaglandins 1974;5:325–340.
67. Dunham EW, Haddox MK, Goldberg ND. Alteration of vein cyclic 3′,5′ nucleotide concentrations during changes in contractility. Proc Natl Acad Sci USA 1974;71:815–819.
68. Elattar TMA. Prostaglandins: physiology, biochemistry, pharmacology, and clinical applications. J Oral Pathol 1978;7:175–207, 239–282.
69. Bunting S, Gryglewski RJ, Moncada S, et al. Arterial walls generate from prostaglandin endoperoxides a substance (prostaglandin X) which relaxes strips of mesenteric and coeliac arteries and inhibits platelet aggregation. Prostaglandins 1976;12:897–913.
70. Hammarstrom S, Murphy RC, Samuelsson B, et al. Structure of leukotriene C: identification of the amino acid part. Biochem Biophys Res Commun 1979;28:1266–1272.
71. Samuelsson B. Leukotrienes: a new group of biologically active compounds. Presented at the Golden Jubilee International Congress on Essential Fatty Acids and Prostaglandins. Minneapolis, 1980.
72. Morris HR, Taylor GW, Piper PJ, et al. Slow-reacting substance of anaphylaxis: studies on purification and characterization. Agents Actions 1979;6(suppl):27–36.
73. Borgeat P, Samuelsson B. Transformation of arachidonic acid by rabbit polymorphonuclear leukocytes: formation of a novel dihydroxyeicosatetraenoic acid. J Biol Chem 1979;245:2643–2646.
74. Hecker M, Foegh ML, Ramwell PW. The eicosanoids: prostaglandins, thromboxanes, leukotrienes, and related

compounds. In: Katzung BG, ed. Basic and clinical pharmacology, Norwalk, CT: Appleton & Lange, 1989:229–241.
75. Embrey MP. The prostaglandins in human reproduction: clinical applications. Edinburgh: Churchill Livingstone, 1975.
76. Karim SMM, ed. Advances in prostaglandin research: prostaglandins and reproduction. Baltimore: University Park Press, 1975.
77. Arrata WS, Tsai AY. Prostaglandins in reproduction. J Reprod Med 1978;20:84–89.
78. Bygdeman M, Samuelsson B. Analyses of prostaglandins in human semen: prostaglandins and related factors. Clin Chim Acta 1966;13:465–474.
79. Eliasson R. Studies on prostaglandin: occurrence, formation, and biological actions. Acta Physiol Scand 1959;46(suppl 158):1–73.
80. Hawkins DF. Relevance of prostaglandin to problems of human subfertility. In: Ramwell PW, Shaw JE, eds. Prostaglandins symposium of Worchester Foundation for Experimental Biology. New York: Interscience, 1968.
81. Bygdeman M, Fredricsson B, Svanborg K, et al. The relation between fertility and prostaglandin content of seminal fluid in man. Fertil Steril 1970;21:622–629.
82. Eskin BA, Azarbal S. Effect of $PGF_{2\alpha}$ upon periovular cervical mucus. Adv Biosci 1973;9:731–735.
83. Labhsetwar AP. Prostaglandins and studies in laboratory animals. In: Karim SMM, ed. Advances in prostaglandin research: prostaglandins and reproduction. Baltimore: University Park Press, 1975:255–256.
84. Sandberg F, Ingleman-Sundberg A, Ryden G. The effect of prostaglandin E_1 on the human uterus and the fallopian tubes in vitro. Acta Obstet Gynecol Scand 1963;42:269–278.
85. Sandberg F, Ingleman-Sundberg A, Ryden G. The effect of prostaglandins E_2 and E_3 on the human uterus and fallopian tubes in vitro. Acta Obstet Gynecol Scand 1964;43:95–102.
86. Sandberg F, Ingleman-Sundberg A, Ryden F. The effect of prostaglandin $F_{1\alpha}$, $F_{1\beta}$, $F_{2\alpha}$, and $F_{2\beta}$ on the human uterus and the fallopian tubes in vitro. Acta Obstet Gynecol Scand 1966;44:585–594.
87. Coutinho EM. Tubal and uterine motility. In: Diczfalusy E, Borell U, eds. Control of human fertility. Nobel Symposium 15. Stockholm: Almqvist & Wiksell; New York: Wiley, 1971:97–115.
88. Spilman CH, Harper MJ. Effects of prostaglandins on oviduct motility and egg transport. Gynecol Invest 1975;6:186–205.
89. Horton EW. Hypothesis on physiological roles of prostaglandins. Physiol Rev 1969;49:122–161.
90. Pharriss BB, Behrman HR. Gonadal function. In: Ramwell PW, ed. The prostaglandins. New York: Plenum Press, 1973:347–363.
91. Armstrong DT, Grinwish DL. Blockade of spontaneous and LH-induced ovulation in rats by indomethacin, an inhibitor of prostaglandin biosynthesis. Prostaglandins 1972;1:21–28.
92. Coutinho EM. Ovarian contractility and ovulation. In: Edwards RG, ed. Research in reproduction, vol. 6. London: International Planned Parenthood Federation, 1974:3–4.
93. Coutinho EM, Maia HS. The contractile response of the human uterus, fallopian tubes, and ovary to prostaglandins in vivo. Fertil Steril 1971;22:539–543.
94. Sato T, Taya K, Jyujyo T, et al. The stimulatory effect of prostaglandins on luteinizing hormone release. Am J Obstet Gynecol 1974;118:875–876.
95. LeMaire WJ, Leidner R, Marsh SM. Pre- and postovulatory changes in the concentration of prostaglandins in rat graafian follicles. Prostaglandins 1975;9:221–229.
96. Sato T, Jyujo T, Hirono M, et al. Effects of indomethacin, an inhibitor of prostaglandin synthesis, on the hypothalamic pituitary system in rats. J Endocrinol 1975;64:395–396.
97. Pharriss B. Prostaglandin induction of luteolysis. Ann NY Acad Sci 1971;180:436–444.
98. Kirton KT, Pharriss BB, Forbes AD. Luteolytic effects of prostaglandin $F_{2\alpha}$ in primates. Proc Soc Exp Biol Med 1970;133:314–316.
99. McCracken JA, Baird DT, Goding JR. Factors affecting the secretion of steroids from the transplantal ovary in the sheep. Recent Prog Horm Res 1971;27:537–582.
100. Arrata WSM, Chatterton RT. Effect of prostaglandin $F_{2\alpha}$ on the luteal phase of the cycle in nonpregnant women. Am J Obstet Gynecol 1974;120:954–959.
101. Kirton KT. Prostaglandins and reproduction of subhuman primates. In: Karim SMM, ed. The prostaglandins: progress in research. New York: Wiley-Interscience, 1972:47–70.
102. Downie J, Poyser NL, Wunderlich M. Levels of prostaglandins in human endometrium during the normal menstrual cycle. J Physiol (Lond) 1974;236:465–472.
103. Sakaena SK, Lau IF. Effect of exogenous estradiol and progesterone on the uterine tissue levels of prostaglandin $F_{2\alpha}$ in ovariectomized mice. Prostaglandins 1973;3:317–322.
104. Lundstrom V, Bygdeman M. Prostaglandin $F_{2\alpha}$ and E_2 in primary dysmenorrhea. Presented at the Fourth International Prostaglandin Conference, Washington, DC, 1979.
105. Lundstrom V, Green K, Wiqvist N. Prostaglandins, indomethacin and dysmenorrhea. Prostaglandins 1976;11:893–907.
106. Rickles VR. The prostaglandins. Biol Rev 1967;42:614–652.
107. Willman EA, Collins WP, Clayton SG. Studies in the involvement of prostaglandins in uterine symptomatology and pathology. Br J Obstet Gynaecol 1976;83:337–341.
108. Halbert DR, Demers LM, Jones DE. Dysmenorrhea and prostaglandins. Obstet Gynecol Surv 1976;31:77–81.
109. McNatty KP, Henderson KM, Sawers RS. Effects of prostaglandin $F_{2\alpha}$ and E_2 on the production of progesterone by human granulosa cells in tissue culture. J Endocrinol 1975;67:231–240.
110. Karim SM. Appearance of prostaglandin $F_{2\alpha}$ in human blood during labor. Br Med J 1968;4:618–621.

111. Karim SM. Identification of prostaglandins in human amniotic fluid. Br J Obstet Gynaecol 1966;73:903–908.
112. Liggins GC, Grieves S. Possible role for prostaglandin $F_{2\alpha}$ in parturition in sheep. Nature 1971;232:626–631.
113. Hillier K, Calder AA, Embrey MP. Concentrations of prostaglandin $F_{2\alpha}$ in amniotic fluid and plasma in spontaneous and induced labours. Br J Obstet Gynaecol 1974;81:257–263.
114. Keirse MJNC, Flint APC, Turbull AC. F prostaglandins in amniotic fluid during pregnancy and labour. Br J Obstet Gynaecol 1974;81:131–135.
115. Sharma SC, Hibbard BM, Hamlett JD, et al. Prostaglandin $F_{2\alpha}$ concentrations in peripheral blood during the first stage of normal labor. Br Med J 1973;1:709–711.
116. Pritchard JA, MacDonald PC. Williams' obstetrics. 15th ed. Norwalk, CT: Appleton-Century-Crofts, 1976:294–297.
117. Schwarz BE, Schultz FM, MacDonald PC, et al. Initiation of human parturition. IV. Demonstration of phospholipase A_2 in the lysosomes of human fetal membranes. Am J Obstet Gynecol 1976;125:1089–1092.
118. Schwarz BE, Schultz FM, MacDonald PC, et al. Initiation of human parturition. III. Fetal membranes content of prostaglandin E_2 and $F_{2\alpha}$ precursor. Obstet Gynecol 1975;46:564–568.
119. MacDonald PC, Porter JC, Schwarz GE, et al. Initiation of parturition in the human female. Semin Perinatol 1978;2:273–286.
120. Schultz FM, Schwarz BE, MacDonald PC, et al. Initiation of human parturition. II. Identification of phospholipase A_2 in fetal chorioamnion and uterine decidua. Am J Obstet Gynecol 1975;123:650–653.
121. Okazaki T, Okita JR, MacDonald PC, et al. Initiation of human parturition. X. Substrate specificity of phospholipase A_2 in human fetal membranes. Am J Obstet Gynecol 1978;130:432–438.
122. Kerise MJNC, Hicks BR, Mitchell MD, et al. Increase of the prostaglandin precursor, arachidonic acid, in amniotic fluid during spontaneous labor. Br J Obstet Gynaecol 1977;84:937–940.
123. MacDonald PC, Schultz M, Duenhoelter JH, et al. Initiation of human parturition. I. Mechanisms of action of arachidonic acid. Obstet Gynecol 1974;44:629–636.
124. Knopp PH. Fuel metabolism in pregnancy. Contemp Obstet Gynecol 1978;12:83–90.
125. Hytten FE, Leitch I. The physiology of human pregnancy. 2nd ed. Oxford: Blackwell Scientific, 1971:333–369.
126. Knopp RH, Saudek CD, Arky RA, et al. Two phases of adipose tissue metabolism in pregnancy: maternal adaptations for fetal growth. Endocrinology 1973;92:984–988.
127. Ogburn PL, Brenner WE, Reitz RC, et al. Arachidonic acid and other free fatty acid changes during abortion by prostaglandin $F_{2\alpha}$. Am J Obstet Gynecol 1978;130:188–193.
128. Gudson JP, Burt RL. Effects of oxytocin on non-esterified fatty acids. Obstet Gynecol 1971;38:444–447.
129. Ogburn PL, Williams PP, Johnson SB, et al. Serum arachidonic acid levels in normal and preeclamptic pregnancies. Am J Obstet Gynecol 1984;148:5–9.
130. Schwartz K. Personal communication.
131. Holman RT, Johnson SB, Ogburn PL. Deficiency of essential fatty acids and membrane fluidity during pregnancy and lactation. Proc Natl Acad Sci USA 1991;88:4835–4839.
132. Kay H. Personal communication.
133. Pritchard JA, MacDonald PC, Gant NF. Williams' obstetrics. Norwalk, CT: Appleton-Century-Crofts, 1985;525–560.
134. Bussolino F, Bernadetto G, Massorbrio M, Camussi G. Maternal vascular prostacyclin activity in preeclampsia. Lancet 1980;2:702.
135. Remuzzi G, Marchesi D, Zoja C, et al. Reduced umbilical and placental vascular prostacyclin in severe pre-eclampsia. Prostaglandins 1980;20:105–110.
136. Ylikorkala O, Viinikkal L. Maternal plasma levels of 6-keto-$PGF1_{\alpha}$ during pregnancy and the puerperium. Prostaglands Med 1981;7:95–99.
137. Lewis PJ, Boylan P, Friedman LA, et al. Prostacyclin in pregnancy. Br Med J 1980;280:1581–1582.
138. Remuzzi G, Zosa G, Marchesi D, et al. Plasmatic regulation of vascular prostacyclin in pregnancy. Br Med J 1981;282:512–514.
139. Dusting GJ, Moncada S, Vane JR. Prostacyclin: its biosynthesis, actions and clinical potential. Adv Prostaglandin Thromboxane Leukotriene Res 1982;10:59–106.
140. Omini C, Folco GC, Pasargiklian, et al. Prostacyclin (PGI_2) in pregnant human uterus. Prostaglandins 1979;17:113–120.
141. Mitchell MD, Hibby JG, Hicks BR, et al. Possible role for prostacyclin in human parturition. Prostaglandins 1978;16:931–937.
142. Kawano M, Mori N. Prostacyclin producing activity of human umbilical, placenta and uterine vessels. Prostaglandins 1983;26:645–662.
143. Greer IA, Walker JJ, et al. Immunoreactive prostacyclin and thromboxane metabolites in normal pregnancy and the puerperium. Br J Obstet Gynaecol 1985;92:581–585.
144. Lewis PJ, Moncada S, O'Grady J, eds. Prostacyclin in pregnancy. New York: Raven Press, 1983:1–230.
145. McGiff JC, Itskoritz HD. Prostaglandins and the kidney. Circ Res 1973;33:479–488.
146. Terragno NA, Terragno DA, Pacholczyk D, et al. Prostaglandins and the regulation of uterine blood flow in pregnancy. Nature 1974;249:57–58.
147. Gant NF, Daley GL, Chand S, et al. A study of angiotensin II pressor response throughout primigravid pregnancy. J Clin Invest 1973;52:2682–2689.
148. Talledo OE, Chesley LC, Zuspan FP. Renin-angiotensin system in normal and toxemic pregnancies. III. Differential sensitivity to angiotensin II and norepinephrine in toxemia of pregnancy. Am J Obstet Gynecol 1968;100:218–221.
149. Worley RJ, Gant NF Jr, Everett RM, et al. Vascular responsiveness to pressor agents during human pregnancy. J Reprod Med 1979;23:115–128.
150. Hamberg M, Svensson J, Samuelsson B. Proc Natl Acad Sci USA 1975;72:2994–2998.

151. Koullapis EN, Micolaides KH, Collins WP, et al. Plasma prostanoids in pregnancy-induced hypertension. Br J Obstet Gynaecol 1982;89:617–621.
152. Martensson L, Wallenburg HCS. Uterine venous concentrations of 6-keto-PGF$_{1\alpha}$ (6-K) in normal pregnancy (NP) and pregnancy-induced hypertensive (PIH) women. Presented at the Society for Gynecologic Investigation, 31st Annual Meeting, San Francisco, 1984: 243.
153. Yamaguchi M, Mori N. 6-Keto-PGF$_{1\alpha}$, thromboxane B$_2$, and 13, 14-dihydro-15-keto prostaglandin F concentration of normotensive and preeclampsic patients during pregnancy, delivery, and the postpartum period. Am J Obstet Gynecol 1985;151:121–127.
154. Walsh SW. Preeclampsia: an imbalance in placenta prostacyclin and thromboxane production. Am J Obstet Gynecol 1985;151:110–115.
155. Louden KA, Heptinstall S, Broughton Pipkin F, et al. The effect of low-dose aspirin on platelet reactivity in pregnancy, PIH and neonates. Presented at the Sixth International Congress, International Society for the Study of Hypertension in Pregnancy, Montreal, 1988, abstract 131.
156. Railton A, Davey DA. Aspirin and dipyridamole in the prevention of preeclampsia: effect on plasma prostanoids 6-keto-PGF$_{1\alpha}$ and TXB$_2$ and clinical outcome of pregnancy. Presented at the Sixth International Congress, International Society for the Study of Hypertension in Pregnancy, Montreal, 1988, abstract 36.
157. Watson KV, Moldow CF, Ogburn PL Jr, et al. Magnesium sulfate: rationale for its use in preeclampsia. Proc Natl Acad Sci USA 1986;83:1075–1078.
158. Schendel DE, Berg CJ, Yeargin-Allsopp M, et al. Prenatal magnesium sulfate exposure and the risk for cerebral palsy or mental retardation among very low-birth weight children aged three to five years. JAMA 1996;276:1805–1810.
159. Chesley LC. Hypertensive disorders of pregnancy. Norwalk, CT: Appleton-Century-Crofts, 1978.
160. Ogburn PL Jr, Turner SI, Williams PP, et al. Preeclampsia and essential fatty acid patterns. Prog Lipid Res 1986;28:417–419.
161. Ogburn PL Jr, Williams PP, Johnson SB, et al. Serum arachidonic acid levels in normal and preeclamptic pregnancies. Am J Obstet Gynecol 1984;148:5–9.
162. Ogburn PL Jr, Turner SI, Williams PP, et al. Essential fatty acid patterns in preeclampsia. Zenrtalbl Gynakol 1986;108:983–939.
163. Holman RT. Essential fatty acids in nutrition and metabolism. Arch Intern Med 1960;105:33–38.
164. Olsen SF, Secher NJ. A possible prevention effect of low-dose fish oil on early delivery and preeclampsia: indications from a 50-year-old controlled trial. Br J Nutr 1990;64:599–609.
165. Nieschlag E, Kremer GJ, Mussgnug U. Insulin, Glucosetoleranz und freie Fettsauren wahrend und nach Akuter Hepatitis. Klin Wochenschr 1970;48:381–385.
166. Brown RE, Madge GE, Schiller HM. Observations on the pathogenesis of Reye's syndrome. South Med J 1971;64: 942–946.
167. Zimmerman T, Winkler L, Moller U, et al. Synthesis of arachidonic acid in the human placenta invitro. Biol Neonate 1979;35:209–121.
168. Wallenburg HC, Dekker GA, Makovitz JW, et al. Low-dose aspirin prevents pregnancy-induced hypertension and preeclampsia in angiotensin-sensitive primigravidae. Lancet 1986;1:1–3.
169. Schiff E, Peleg E, Goldenberg M, et al. The use of aspirin to prevent pregnancy-induced hypertension and lower the ratio of thromboxane A$_2$ to prostacyclin in relatively high risk pregnancies. N Engl J Med 1989; 321:351–356.
170. Benigi A, Gregorini G, Frusca T, et al. Effect of low-dose aspirin on fetal and maternal generation of thromboxane by platelets in women at risk for pregnancy-induced hypertension. N Engl J Med 1989;21:357–362.
171. Heyborne KD, Burke MS, Porreco RP. Prolongation of premature gestation in women with hemolysis, elevated liver enzymes and low platelets: a report of five cases. J Reprod Med 1990;35:53–57.
172. Sibai BM, Mirro R, Chesney CM, et al. Low-dose aspirin in pregnancy. Obstet Gynecol 1989;74:551–557.
173. Goodlin RC, Haesslein HO, Fleming J. Aspirin for the treatment of recurrent toxaemia [letter]. Lancet 1978; 2:51.
174. Sanchez-Ramos L, O'Sullivan MJ, Garrido-Calderon J. Effect of low-dose aspirin on angiotensin II pressor response in human pregnancy. Am J Obstet Gynecol 1987; 156:193–194.
175. Sibai BM, Curitis SN, Thom E, et al. Prevention of preeclampsia with low-dose aspirin in healthy, nulliparous pregnant women. N Engl J Med 1993;329:1213–1218.
176. CLASP Collaborative Group. CLASP: a randomized trial of low-dose aspirin for the prevention and treatment of preeclampsia among 9364 pregnant women. Lancet 1994; 343:619–629.
177. Lubbe WF, Butler WS, Palmer SJ, et al. Lupus anti-coagulant in pregnancy. Br J Obstet Gynaecol 1984;91: 357–363.
178. Lockshin MD, Druzin ML, Qamar T. Prednisone does not prevent recurrent fetal death in women with antiphospholipid antibody. Am J Obstet Gynecol 1989;160: 439–443.
179. Kutteh WH. Antiphospholipid antibody-associated recurrent pregnancy loss: Treatment with heparin and low-dose aspirin is superior to low-dose aspirin alone. Am J Obstet Gynecol 1996;174:1584–1589.
180. Rai R, Cohen M, Dave M, Regan L. Randomised controlled trial of aspirin and aspirin plus heparin in pregnant women with recurrent miscarriage associated with phospholipid antibodies (or antiphospolipid antibodies) BMJ 1997;314:253–257.
181. Terragno NA, Terragno A. Prostaglandin metabolism in the fetal and maternal vasculature. Fed Proc 1979;38:75–77.
182. Terragno NA, Terragno A. McGiff JC, et al. Synthesis of prostaglandins by the ductus arteriosus of the bovine fetus. Prostaglandins 1977;14:721–727.
183. Clyman RI. Developmental responses to oxygen, arachidonic acid, and indomethacin in the fetal lamb

ductus arteriosus in vitro. Prostaglandins Med 1978;1:167–174.
184. Albert BS, Lewins MJ, Rowland DW, et al. Plasma indomethacin (indo) levels in newborns with patent ductus (PDA). Presented at the Fourth International Prostaglandin Conference, Washington, DC, 1979.
185. Dietze G, Matthias W, Bottger I, et al. Possible involvement of kinins and prostaglandins in the translation of insulin action on glucose uptake into skeletal muscle. Adv Exp Med Biol 1979;120A:511–520.
186. Robertson RP, Metz SA. Sounding board: prostaglandins, the glucoreceptor, and diabetes. N Engl J Med 1979;301:1446–1447.
187. Pederson J. The pregnant diabetic and her newborn. 2nd ed. Baltimore: Williams & Wilkins, 1977.
188. Whitelaw A. Subcutaneous fat in newborn infants of diabetic mothers: an indication of quality of diabetic control. Lancet 1977;1:15–18.
189. Susa JB, McCormick KL, Widness JA, et al. Chronic hyperinsulinemia in the fetal rhesus monkey. Diabetes 1979;28:1058–1063.
190. Vileisis RA, Oh W. Enhanced fatty acid synthesis in hyperinsulinemic rat fetuses. J Nutr 1983;113:246–252.
191. Ogburn PL Jr, Goldstein M, Walker J, et al. Prolonged hyperinsulinemia reduces plasma fatty acid levels in major lipid groups in fetal sheep. Am J Obstet Gynecol 1989;161:728–732.
192. Stonestreet BS, Ogburn PL Jr, Goldstein M, et al. Effects of chronic fetal hyperinsulinemia on plasma arachidonic acid and prostaglandin concentrations. Am J Obstet Gynecol 1989;161:894–899.
193. Gerrard JM, Stuart MJ, Rao GHR, et al. Alteration in the balance of prostaglandin and thromboxane synthesis in diabetic rats. J Lab Clin Med 1980;95:950–958.
194. Halushka PV, Roger RC, Loadholt CB, et al. Increased platelet thromboxane synthesis in diabetes mellitus. J Lab Clin Med 1981;97:87–96.
195. Butkus A, Shirey EK, Schumacher OF. Thromboxane biosynthesis in platelets of diabetes and coronary artery disease patients. Artery 1982;11:238–251.
196. Halushka PV, Mayfield R, Colwell JA. Insulin and arachidonic acid metabolism in diabetes mellitus. Metabolism 1985;34(suppl 1):32–36.
197. McDonald JWD, Dupre J, Roger NW, et al. Comparison of platelet thromboxane synthesis in diabetic patients on conventional insulin therapy and continuous insulin infusion. Thromb Res 1982;28:705–712.
198. Axelrod L, Levine L. Plasma prostaglandin levels in rats with diabetes mellitus and diabetic ketoacidosis. Diabetes 1982;31:994–1001.
199. Stuart MJ, Elrad H, Graeber JE, et al. Increased synthesis of prostaglandin endoperoxides and platelet hyperfunction in infants of mothers with diabetes mellitus. J Lab Clin Med 1979;94:12–17.
200. Stuart MJ, Sunderji SG, Walenga RW, et al. Abnormalities in vascular arachidonic acid metabolism in the infant of the diabetic mother. Br Med J 1985;290:1700–1702.
201. Tuna N, Frankhauser S, Goetz FC. Total serum fatty acids in diabetes: relative and absolute concentrations of individual fatty acids. Am J Med Sci 1968;255:120–131.
202. Chen C, Adam P, Laskowski D, et al. The plasma-free fatty acid composition and blood glucose of normal and diabetic pregnant women and of their newborns. Pediatrics 1965;36:843–855.
203. Pinter E, Reece EA. Diabetes-associated congenital malformations: epidemiology, pathogenesis, and experimental methods of induction and prevention. In: Reece EA, Coustan DR, eds. Diabetes mellitus in pregnancy: principles and practice. New York: Churchill Livingstone, 1988:205–245.
204. Pinter E, Reece EA, Ogburn PL Jr, et al. Fatty acid content of yolk sac and embryo in hyperglycemia-induced embryopathy and effect of arachidonic acid supplementation. Am J Obstet Gynecol 1988;159:1484–1490.
205. Rosenthal M, Whitehurst M. Fatty acyl delta 6 desaturation activity of cultured human endothelial cells: modulation by fetal bovine serum. Biochim Biophys Acta 1983;750:490–496.
206. Ongari M, Ritter J, Orchard M, et al. Correlation of prostacyclin synthesis by human umbilical artery with status of essential fatty acid. Am J Obstet Gynecol 1984;149:455–460.
207. Obgurn PL Jr. The treatment of preterm labor. Postgrad Obstet Gynecol 1990;10:1–5.
208. Iams JD, Johansen FF, Creasy RK. Prevention of preterm birth. Clin Obstet Gynecol 1988;31:599–615.
209. Ferguson JE, Hensleigh PA, Kredentser D. Adjunctive use of magnesium sulfate with ritodrine for preterm labor tocolysis. Am J Obstet Gynecol 1984;148:166–171.
210. Ogburn PL Jr, Hansen CA, Williams PP, et al. Magnesium sulfate and betamimetic dual agent tocolysis in preterm labor with single agent failure. J Reprod Med 1985;30:583–587.
211. Niebyl JR, Blake DA, White RB, et al. The inhibition of premature labor with indomethacin. Am J Obstet Gynecol 1980;136:1014–1019.
212. Morales WJ, Smith SG, Angel JL, et al. Efficiency and safety of indomethacin versus ritodrine in the management of preterm labor: a randomized study. Obstet Gynecol 1989;74:567–572.

14
Mineral Metabolism in Pregnancy

Karen M. Davidson and John T. Repke

Nutrition has long been recognized as an important component of good health for the parturient and her fetus. Recently attention has been focused on individual nutrients, vitamins, minerals, and trace elements. Certain minerals have always been recognized as important in the human diet. Sodium, iron, and iodine are known to be essential components of a healthful diet. Lately, recognition of other minerals and trace elements has led to our understanding of their contribution to pregnancy and fetal development. Minerals such as calcium, magnesium, zinc, lead, copper, fluoride, and selenium all make their own unique contribution to maternal and fetal health. All of the above possess unique characteristics of transport across the fetal placental unit. This discussion focuses on the role of these nutrients in the human with specific focus on their role in pregnancy and normal fetal development.

Sodium

Sodium, the principal action of extracellular fluid, acts as the primary regulator of extracellular fluid volume. In addition, sodium regulates osmolarity, acid-base balance, and membrane potentials of the cell. Sodium is actively transported across the cell membrane in exchange for potassium. Its homeostasis is maintained over a wide range of circumstances through a balance achieved between the filtered load and the amount of tubular reabsorption by the kidney.

Bioavailability and Metabolism

The major source of sodium in the diet is sodium chloride. Sodium bicarbonate and monosodiumgluconate make up less than 10% of the usual intake.[1] Drinking water provides less than 10% of the daily sodium intake.[2] Over 75% of dietary salt is added during processing and manufacturing.[3] The usual intake of sodium ranges from $1.8\,g\cdot day^{-1}$ to $5.0\,g\cdot day^{-1}$.[4,5] This variability is due to individual differences in the amount of table salt added to food.

Obligatory losses of sodium in adults are approximately 300 mg of sodium chloride or 115 mg of elemental sodium per day.[3] The recommended dietary allowance of 500 mg of sodium chloride per day is generous enough to allow for replacement of obligatory losses, as well as to cover for excess sweating in warmer climates.[3] The usual dietary intake of sodium chloride easily covers these daily requirements. Sodium deficiency does not occur even with very low sodium diets[6,7] or excessive sweating because of the tight homeostatic control of sodium excretion. Sodium depletion has been found in cases of trauma, chronic diarrhea, or renal disease where sodium retention is impossible.[8]

Sodium balance is maintained under the opposing actions of the renin-angiotensin-aldosterone system and atrial natriuretic peptide (ANP) (Figure 14.1). The renin-angiotensin-aldosterone system is activated by low blood volume and extracellular volume. The result of activation is vasoconstriction and increased sodium retention through decreased renal excretion of sodium. Atrial natriuretic peptide is the major hormone involved in the regulation of extracellular fluid volume.[9] It decreases plasma volume by promoting natriuresis and shifting plasma fluid into the interstitium.[10] In addition, it inhibits the secretion of renin and aldosterone[11] and decreases the vasoconstricting effects of angiotensin.[10,12]

Sodium Metabolism in Pregnancy

There is an increased need for sodium in pregnancy because of the increased extracellular volume of the mother, the requirements of the fetus, and the increases in the amniotic fluid volume. The average total body sodium increases by 60 g (900 mEq NaCl) over the course of pregnancy, with an additional daily requirement of 200 mg (3–4 mEq NaCl).[13,14] The average daily intake of

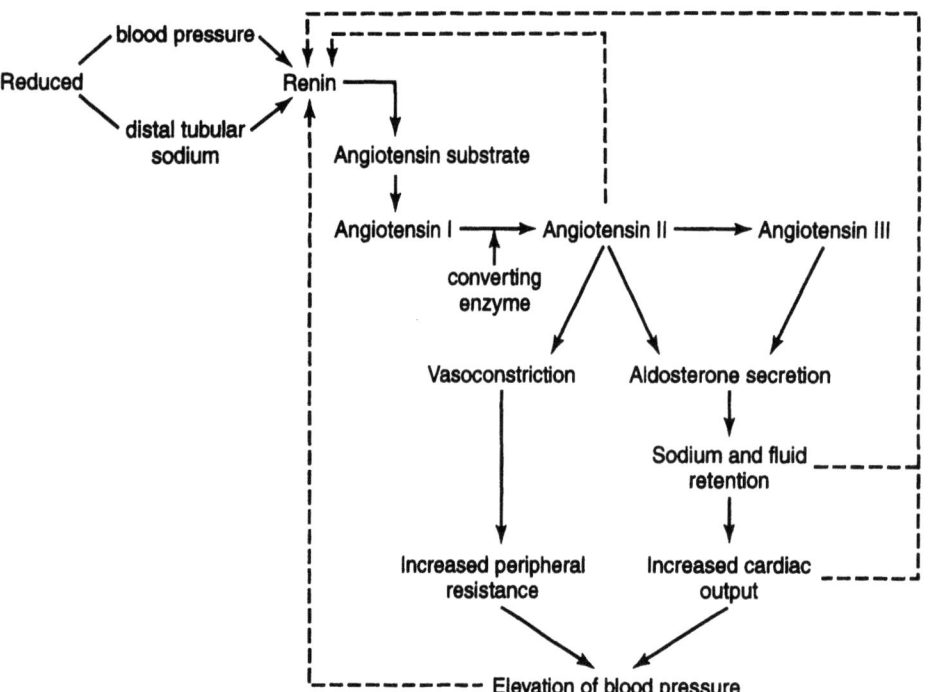

FIGURE 14.1. Role of renin-angiotensin system in the regulation of blood pressure. Solid lines represent positive interactions; broken lines show negative interactions or feedback inhibition.

NaCl easily exceeds this level, making supplementation during pregnancy unnecessary. Sixty percent of the expanded sodium content is distributed in the maternal extracellular fluid compartment.[15] Serum sodium concentration decreases from an average of 140 mEq/L to 137 mEq/L by 12 weeks of gestation and is maintained at this lower concentration for the remainder of the pregnancy.[16] Resetting of this serum concentration by the kidney is the most important adjustment of pregnancy.[17]

Complex alterations in volume homeostasis occur in pregnancy. The glomerular filtration rate (GFR) doubles in the first 2 weeks of pregnancy, paralleling increases in renal blood flow.[18] This increased GFR leads to a 50% increase in the filtered load of sodium and a resultant increased rate of tubular reabsorption of filtered sodium. The mechanism by which changes in the rate of sodium resorption occurs is not clear, but may be related to the effects of progesterone, arginine vasopressin, or ANP. Progesterone concentration increases in pregnancy and produces smooth muscle relaxation and vasodilation. Renal artery vasodilation by progesterone may be responsible for increases in sodium excretion, or progesterone may act independently to inhibit sodium resorption at the level of the nephron.[19,20] In addition, progesterone counteracts the sodium retaining effects of aldosterone. Arginine vasopressin can further inhibit sodium resorption, by unknown mechanisms. Atrial natriuretic peptide concentrations do not change in pregnancy,[11,12] but there may be an increased sensitivity to it with increasing gestational age.[11]

In pregnancy, aldosterone secretion rates increase, with a resultant third-trimester concentration that is 10 to 20 times greater than in the nonpregnant patient.[15] Aldosterone acts to fine-tune the increased reabsorption of sodium seen in pregnancy. As the GFR and filtered load of sodium increases, aldosterone acts to increase sodium delivery to the distal tubule.[22] The renin-angiotensin system is paradoxically stimulated in pregnancy and is thought to be responsible for the increase rate of aldosterone secretion. Despite an increased blood and extracellular fluid volume in pregnancy, renin and angiotensin concentrations rise, possibly due to a compensatory response to the normal fall in systemic vascular resistance[23] or due to a new set point of fluid volume homeostasis associated with pregnancy.[24] Normal pregnancy is characterized by refractoriness to the vasoconstricting actions of angiotensin II starting at the end of the first trimester.[25] The mechanism for this change is thought to be threefold: through a downregulation of angiotensin receptors, through increased vascular synthesis of the vasodilator prostaglandin, and through the presence of an endothelial-derived relaxing factor.[26]

Sodium Metabolism in Preeclamptic Pregnancies

In the preeclamptic pregnancy, there are decreases in renal blood flow, GFR, plasma volume, and prominent sodium retention, and an increased sensitivity to angiotensin II.

Plasma volume reductions can be noted as early as the second trimester, prior to the development of hypertension.[27,28] Extracellular fluid volume is normal in preeclampsia, but there is a redistribution of fluid into the extravascular space due to enhanced capillary permeability and reduced colloid oncotic pressure.[27,29] General endothelial damage is thought to underlie the capillary permeability, independent of proteinuria.[30]

Sodium retention in preeclampsia starts at the onset of the clinical signs of hypertension, proteinuria, and edema.[31] Impaired vasodilatory capacity of damaged renal vascular endothelial cells acts to reduce GFR and renal blood flow. Furthermore, enhanced sensitivity to angiotensin II adds to vasoconstriction in renal vessels and a tendency toward sodium retention.[10,31] Despite sodium retention in preeclampsia, ANP concentration is paradoxically increased.[32-35] This may be a compensatory mechanism to prevent further increases in blood pressure.[35]

The role of sodium in the diet on the development and clinical course of preeclampsia has been debated. The older literature suggested that a low sodium diet may ameliorate the hypertension, edema, and proteinuria in preeclampsia.[36,37] Other research found no effect of dietary sodium on preeclampsia[38] or a lower incidence with high sodium intake.[39] More recent research has noted exacerbations of preeclampsia with sodium restriction.[40,41] It is hypothesized that sodium restriction stimulates the renin-angiotensin system through excessive renal sodium loss.[40]

Calcium

The adult body contains approximately 1200 g of calcium, 99% of which is stored in the skeleton.[42] The remainder is found in the extracellular fluid, intracellular structures, and in the cell membrane. Calcium is essential for nerve conduction, muscle contraction, blood clotting, and membrane permeability. Calcium homeostasis is maintained under tight control, regulated by hormonal factors and membrane transport as discussed in detail in Chapter 40. Alterations in calcium homeostasis occur in pregnancy and have been implicated as a possible factor in the development of hypertensive disorders in pregnant and nonpregnant patients.

Bioavailability and Metabolism

Calcium absorption in the intestine occurs at an average rate of 30% to 40% in normal adults in calcium balance.[43] This rate increases during periods of high requirements, such as childhood and pregnancy, and during periods of low dietary intake. Additional promoters of calcium absorption include vitamin D, parathyroid hormone (PTH), lactose, intestinal acidity, growth hormone, phosphate, and dietary protein.[44] Phytates, oxalates, cortisol, fatty acids, alcohol, and cellulose bind to calcium, making them insoluble and decreasing intestinal absorption.[45] The average dietary intake of calcium in the United States is 500 to 600 mg, well below the recommended daily allowance (RDA) of 800 mg in the adult.[46] In one large study, the overwhelming majority of women in the childbearing years consumed less than 800 mg.[47] Dairy products make up 55% of the dietary intake of calcium, followed by green leafy vegetables, bones in fish, and calcium fortified food.[48]

Throughout life, skeletal bone is constantly turning over with resorption and formation. From birth to approximately age 30, bone formation exceeds resorption. Later in life, bone resorption predominates, with bone mass declining slowly until age 50 with great subsequent acceleration after menopause. This results in a gradual decrease in bone strength and an increase in the risk of fractures. Bone resorption is stimulated by PTH, thyroxine, vitamin D, and growth hormone.[44] Resorption is inhibited by calcitonin, estrogen, and glucocorticoids.[44] Calcium is excreted primarily in urine, but also in feces and sweat. Renal calcium reabsorption is stimulated by PTH, thiazide diuretics, and hypocalcemia.[44] Renal calcium excretion is favored during periods of acidosis, hypercalcemia, hypophosphatemia, and hyperthyroidism.[44] Fine-tuning of intestinal absorption, renal excretion, and bone resorption, under the influence of these multiple factors, maintain the serum calcium concentration in a narrow range under many physiologic circumstances.

Calcium Metabolism in Pregnancy

Calcium requirements increase by 33% during pregnancy, primarily due to fetal needs for skeletal calcification, especially in the third trimester.[49] A net transfer of 25 to 30 g calcium crosses the placenta in an active process, with fetal calcium concentration exceeding that in the maternal blood.[50] Total serum calcium concentration declines progressively during normal pregnancy, primarily because of hemodilution and a fall in albumin concentration.[51-53] Ionized calcium concentration remains constant throughout pregnancy, under the regulation of PTH, vitamin D, and calcitonin.[51-60] Despite increased calcium requirements during pregnancy, the normal pregnant woman is relatively hypercalciuric, with renal excretion of 350 to 600 mg calcium per day, as compared with 100 to 250 mg·day^{-1} in the nonpregnant woman.[61]

Calcium balance is maintained through a 50% increase in intestinal absorption, as well as through alterations in the hormonal control of calcium.[49] Early investigations, measuring breakdown products of PTH, concluded that pregnancy represented a period of physiologic hyperparathyroidism.[52,53,62] An elevated PTH concentration was felt to be responsible for the more efficient intestinal absorption of calcium that has been documented in pregnancy.[63,64] More recent research, using assays capable of directly measuring the hormone, instead of its breakdown products, have revealed no such elevations during pregnancy.[49,65] Instead, increased intestinal absorption of calcium in pregnancy is thought to be secondary to elevated concentration of 1,25-dihydroxyvitamin D, which acts directly on the intestinal tract to increase absorption.[49,61,66]

Vitamin D is a fat-soluble vitamin obtained from dietary sources or through the skin's exposure to ultraviolet light. Vitamin D undergoes activation by a 25-hydroxylation in the liver followed by a 1-hydroxylation in the kidney. The placenta is capable of 1-hydroxylation of vitamin D, probably resulting in the increased concentration of 1,25-dihydroxyvitamin D in pregnancy.[61] It is not clear if renal vitamin D activation is increased in pregnancy. Calcitonin appears to be independently regulated in the fetus and mother, with no consistent changes seen in the maternal serum concentration in pregnancy.[63,66] Estrogen concentrations are elevated early in pregnancy and act to further enhance the efficiency of calcium intestinal absorption during pregnancy.[42] Parathyroid-related peptide (PTHrp) has been found in pregnant ewes to be involved in increasing calcium intestinal absorption, mobilizing calcium from bone, and transporting calcium across the placenta.[67] Further investigation of PTHrp in human pregnancy is necessary.

Calcium in Hypertensive Disorders of Pregnancy

Vascular smooth muscle tone and peripheral vascular resistance are determined by the concentration of free intracellular calcium.[68] Alterations in calcium metabolism have been prosposed as a factor in the development of hypertension in the pregnant and nonpregnant patient. Epidemiologic studies have revealed an inverse relationship between the rate of hypertensive disorders of pregnancy and calcium intake.[69-72] Animal models reveal an association between calcium deprivation and elevated systolic blood pressure.[73-75] Replacement of calcium reversed the blood pressure alterations.

Ionized calcium concentrations have been noted to be decreased in patients with pregnancy-induced hypertension (PIH) and in preeclampsia.[76,77] Other investigations have not shown any changes in ionized calcium, possibly due to nonuniform criteria for the definitions of PIH and preeclampsia.[78-82] Several investigations have noted a decrease in 1,25-dihydroxyvitamin D concentration[83-85] and an increase in PTH concentration in preeclampsia,[83,84] although preeclampsia definitions differ between investigations. Preeclampsia has been associated with a lower mean 24-hour urine calcium when compared to normotensive pregnancy.[80] A 24-hour urine calcium of less than 195 mg prior to 24 weeks reliably predicted those patients destined to develop preeclampsia in one series.[86]

A possible mechanism for the hormonal changes in preeclampsia has been proposed.[61] Reduced placental function in preeclampsia may lead to a reduction in 1-hydroxylation of vitamin D by the placenta reducing the concentration of bioactive vitamin D, 1,25-dihydroxyvitamin D. A lower concentration of 1,25-dihydroxyvitamin D leads to decreased calcium absorption from the intestine, which in turn results in a decline in serum ionized calcium concentration. Lower ionized calcium stimulates a elevation in PTH and a resultant increase in renal conservation of calcium and decrease in urinary calcium concentration. Lower calcium absorption may predispose to the development of preeclampsia by interfering with the production of the vasodilator, endothelial nitric oxide (NO).[87] Release of NO is dependent on transmembrane ionized calcium flux[88] and NO synthase (NOS) is a calcium-dependent enzyme.[89] Decreases in NO and NOS result in vasoconstriction and a lack of the normal resistance to pressor agents such as angiotensin II. Further investigations are required to evaluate the validity of these hypotheses.

Clinical trials have been performed to evaluate the efficacy of calcium supplementation for the prevention of preeclampsia in high-risk groups. A recent meta-analysis of the available randomized controlled trials found an overall substantial reduction in the systolic and diastolic blood pressure in patients supplemented with 1200 to 2000 mg elemental calcium each day.[90] Calcium had a reproducibly preventative effect on the incidence of PIH across series. A larger effect was noted with investigations limited to primiparous patients. A strong correlation was noted between calcium supplementation and a reduced rate of preeclampsia. No significant reduction was noted on the incidence of preterm delivery, cesarean section, intrauterine growth restriction, or perinatal death in patients with calcium supplementation. It was hypothesized that calcium supplementation may prevent the clinical manifestations of preeclampsia and other hypertensive disorders of pregnancy, without necessarily having an impact on the underlying pathologic process leading to preeclampsia. The meta-analysis concluded that calcium may spare up to two thirds of women from mild preeclampsia. The investigators recommended a policy of offering calcium supplementation to all pregnant women in high-risk groups. An ongoing investigation sponsored by the National Institutes of Health (NIH) is further reviewing the possible preventative effects of calcium on hypertensive disorders in pregnancy.

Magnesium

In the adult body, there exists 20 to 28 mg of magnesium. Greater than 50% of magnesium is stored in bones, 40% in muscles and soft tissue, and less than 1% in extracellular fluid, including plasma.[91] Plasma magnesium concentration is kept very constant in the healthy, nonpregnant adult by homeostatic mechanisms, which are poorly understood. As a complex with adenosine triphosphate (ATP), magnesium is required for all biosynthetic processes, including glycolysis, formation of adenosine 3',5'-cyclic monophosphate (cAMP), membrane transport via sodium-potassium and calcium pumps, and transmission of the genetic code.[92] Intracellularly, it is involved in the control of cellular metabolism by modulating the activity of rate-limiting enzymes.[93] Extracellularly, magnesium maintains electrical potentials of nerve and muscle membranes and is involved in the transmission of impulses across the neuromuscular junction.[91] Depletion of magnesium can increase neuronal excitability, enhance neuromuscular transmission[94] and increase the responsiveness to vasopressor substances[95] (see Chapter 40).

Bioavailability and Metabolism

Dietary magnesium is found in the highest concentration in nuts, legumes, unmilled grains, and green vegetables. It is absorbed primarily in the distal intestine by intracellular diffusion and solvent drag mechanisms. Net gut absorption is approximately 50%, but can be stimulated by PTH and vitamin D_3.[96] Phytates and fiber mildly decrease the absorption of magnesium.[97]

Homeostasis of magnesium occurs primarily at the level of the kidney. Its major reabsorption occurs in the loop of Henle under the stimulatory influence of PTH.[98] Bone magnesium stores are in equilibrium with plasma, acting as a buffer against fluctuations in its cellular concentration. Bone resorption is also under the influence of PTH and vitamin D_3.[96]

Magnesium Metabolism in Pregnancy

The net maternal magnesium accumulation during pregnancy is 11.1 g, with the term fetus containing approximately 0.8 g.[99] Its intake must increase during pregnancy to meet the increased demand from growth of both the mother and the fetus. The recommended dietary allowance during pregnancy of 320 mg·day^{-1} should be adequate for healthy women, assuming a 50% dietary absorption.[100] Unfortunately, dietary investigations during pregnancy report that most women consume only two thirds of this amount, especially when eating diets low in fresh vegetables and whole grains.[101]

Total plasma and serum magnesium concentrations decrease progressively during pregnancy, reaching a nadir in the late third trimester, followed by a rise in the postpartum period.[102] The overall extracellular concentration is thought to fall in pregnancy because of hemodilution, reduced concentrations of protein bound cations, and an elevation in the GFR. Extracellular ionized (i.e., free) magnesium concentration decline during pregnancy, despite lack of protein binding.[103]

Because the intracellular compartment comprises up to 40% of the overall magnesium stores, its intracellular concentrations more accurately reflect its overall status. The intracellular concentration has been estimated using muscle, lymphocytes, and erythrocytes. Intracellular estimations performed in this manner have yielded mixed data, with most investigations showing unchanged or slightly decreased concentrations during pregnancy.[104-106] More recently, it has been possible to directly measure intracellular cytosolic magnesium thereby avoiding any confounding factors such as changes in plasma volume and protein binding. Direct intracellular concentrations were noted to be significantly lower in pregnant women compared to nonpregnant controls.[103]

Intracellular and extracellular magnesium decreases in pregnancy are thought to be mediated by the kidney. The combination of the physiologic increase in the GFR with no change in the tubular reabsorption of magnesium is thought to account for its overall decline.[107] In addition, the renal response to decreases in plasma magnesium concentration results in no significant decrease in urine magnesium excretion.

Fetal Magnesium Metabolism and Placental Transport

Fetal magnesium accretion increases throughout the third trimester.[108] Fetal homeostatic mechanisms are poorly defined. By late gestation, fetal plasma concentration is greater than that seen in maternal plasma, implying an active placental mechanism for transporting magnesium against the maternofetal concentration gradient.[109] The placental transfer rate increases with increasing gestational age, with a direct correlation to increasing fetal weight.[109] It has been shown that large fluctuations in maternal serum magnesium concentrations leads to similar changes in the fetus and neonate.[110] These changes may be secondary to a separate passive transport mechanism.

Transport through the placenta to the fetus involves simple diffusion across the fetal capillary endothelium followed by movement across the syncytiotrophoblast. The syncytiotrophoblast acts as a major barrier to maternofetal ion exchange. No specific channels or facilitative transport protein mediating this influx has been identified. Magnesium efflux into the fetal plasma compartment is against an eletrochemical gradient and is an energy requiring process.

Investigations of the perfused rat placenta in sodium-free media have reported a reduction in magnesium efflux.[111] In addition, the rat placenta, treated with amiloride, reduced magnesium clearance.[112] These data suggest the presence of a Na^{2+}/Mg^{2+} exchange mechanism.

The control(s) of placental transport governing the dramatic increases in fetal magnesium concentration late in pregnancy is (are) not clearly defined. Removal of the parathyroid glomic in sheep leads to a reversal of the placental gradient between mother and fetus.[113] The gradient can be reestablished in the sheep model through infusion of the midportion of parathyroid hormone–related peptide (PTHrp), which is thought to stimulate the placental pump responsible for magnesium transport.[113] PTHrp was not found to affect placental transfer in the rat, however, and has not been studied in the human.[114]

Magnesium in Tocolysis and Seizure Prophylaxis

The primary use of magnesium in pregnancy is for tocolysis in patients with preterm labor and for prophylaxis against seizures in patients with preeclampsia.[115] In vitro and in vivo studies have demonstrated a reduction in gravid uterine muscle contractility in the presence of magnesium in supraphysiologic concentrations.[116] Although the etiology of eclampsia is not clear, parenteral magnesium treatment in preeclamptic patients is felt to lead to cerebral vasodilation, with resultant improvement in blood flow and prevention of ischemic damage from causing seizures.[117,118] Long-term use of magnesium can inhibit calcium absorption and produce muscle weakness, cardiac arrhythmias, and sedation. Fetal effects seen with chronic high doses of magnesium include fetal parathyroid gland suppression, transient hypocalcemia, and other abnormalities resembling rickets.[119]

Magnesium Status and Pregnancy Outcome

Magnesium depletion in vitro and in vivo affects vascular tone, blood pressure, capillary lumen size, susceptibility of cells to oxidative stress, and viability of cells in ischemic environments.[117] In particular, isolated human umbilical vessels, incubated in a hypomagnesium extracellular medium, exhibit marked vasoconstriction.[120] Decreased magnesium concentration has also been associated with impaired insulin metabolism, hyperlipidemia, and accelerated atherosclerosis in animal models.[121] In addition, pregnant diabetic animals show a reduced maternofetal placental flux of magnesium and reduced fetal accretion.[122] These abnormalities can be reversed with insulin treatment. From these investigations, it has been theorized that maternal magnesium status can affect susceptibility to the presumably vascularly mediated conditions of preeclampsia, eclampsia, and fetal growth restriction. In addition, diabetic embryotoxicity is felt to be related to alterations in the availability of magnesium to the fetus.[123]

In human dietary recall evaluations, no relationship was found between magnesium intake and the development of pregnancy-induced hypertension (PIH), preeclampsia (PET), preterm labor (PTL), or intrauterine growth restriction (IUGR).[124] In the same population, renal excretion was not different between normal pregnancies and those affected by PIH, PET, PTL, or growth, implying no change in magnesium steady state. In a separate investigation, plasma and erythrocyte magnesium concentrations were not correlated to blood pressure or the development of PET.[125] In a recent prospective, cross-sectional analyses, ionized serum magnesium (the active portion) was decreased in all pregnant patients when compared to nonpregnant controls.[125] There were, however, no differences between normal pregnant patients and those with PET or eclampsia.

A retrospective investigation in 1984 showed that the frequency of IUGR and PET was reduced in association with magnesium supplementation.[126] In contrast, a prospective investigation of magnesium supplementation in a Danish population showed no protective effect.[127] There were fewer preterm deliveries, and accordingly, fewer admissions to the neonatal intensive care unit and a decreased frequency of low birth weight neonates. Two prospective randomized controlled trials have produced conflicting data. Kovács et al.[128] in 1988 studied 985 patients, half of whom were randomized to daily magnesium supplementation. The treatment group was found to have fewer premature births, fewer cases of IUGR, and a reduced incidence of PET. In an investigation of 400 patients with a high incidence of poor nutrition and at high risk for PET, Sibai et al.[129] found that daily magnesium supplementation produced no difference in systolic or diastolic blood pressure, no difference in rates of PET, PTL, delivery at less than 36 weeks, and postterm pregnancy. There were also no differences in birth weight, incidence of IUGR, Apgar scores, or neonatal ICU admissions.

In human studies of nonpregnant diabetics, there was increased renal magnesium excretion, possibly due to a specific tubular magnesium transport defect.[130] Human maternal serum[131] and amniotic fluid[132] magnesium concentrations were also found to be lower in the poorly controlled diabetic pregnancy. Well-controlled diabetics were not found to share these serum abnormalities. Intracellular free magnesium, thought to be the best predictor of magnesium status, was found to be lower in a group of gestational diabetics compared to nondiabetic pregnant controls.[121] In addition, a significant relationship was noted between serum magnesium concentration at

9 weeks and fetal malformations or abortion in insulin-dependent diabetics.[131] There was no correlation between hemoglobin A_1 concentration and magnesium concentration in these patients. This effect was noted experimentally in the rat where induced maternal magnesium deficiency resulted in an increased rate of fetal absorption, reduced fetal ossification, low birth rate, and fetal malformations.[123] The degree of magnesium deficiency in these animal models was, however, far greater than that likely to occur even in poorly controlled human diabetics.

Zinc

Zinc is a trace element and an essential component of more than 400 enzyme systems and 70 metalloenzymes, including DNA and RNA polymerases, alkaline phosphatase, carbonic anhydrase, and alcohol dehydrogenase.[133] The functions of zinc in metalloenzymes are catalytic, structural, and regulatory. Metalloenzymes are required for cellular proliferation and differentiation, nucleic acid metabolism, gene expression, stabilization of membranes, and cellular immunity.[134,135] Zinc has recently been shown to play an important role in forming DNA-binding domains known as zinc fingers.[136] Zinc fingers are highly conserved throughout evolution and furnish one of the fundamental mechanisms for regulating gene expression and cellular differentiation during development. Because of its central role in gene expression and cellular proliferation, normal zinc balance is felt to be essential to human reproduction and to fetal growth and development (see Chapter 41).

Bioavailability and Metabolism

Approximately 70% of dietary zinc is obtained from animal products, with meat, liver, and oysters having high amounts of available zinc.[137] The bioavailability of zinc is variable and influenced greatly by many factors: the dietary content of calcium, iron, copper, and tin, heavy metals such as cadmium, mercury, and lead; fiber; phytates; soy proteins; drugs such as antacids, quinolones, phenytoin, tetracycline, diazepam, captopril, and metronidazole; and the gastrointestinal tract.[138,139] Cigarette smoking decreases the bioavailability of zinc by increasing concentrations of phytates and cadmium.[140] Large dietary intake of milk products[141] and supplementation with iron may limit the bioavailability of zinc.[142]

Zinc uptake is an active process that occurs in the proximal gastrointestinal tract as a complex with metallothionein. Metallothionein is a low molecular weight cytosolic protein that binds divalent metals and has a high affinity for zinc.[143] The complexes are taken up by mucosal cells and expelled into the lumen of the intestinal tract. Functional absorption of zinc from the intestinal lumen is inefficient, varying from 14% to 41%.[144] Damage to the proximal intestine and/or villous atrophy, as seen in Crohn's disease, celiac disease, and intestinal bypass operations, further reduces zinc absorption.[145]

The total zinc concentration in plasma and serum varies greatly based on its distribution. After absorption, approximately 60% to 65% of zinc is albumin bound and transferred via complexes with metallothionein to be sequestered in the liver.[146] Corticosteroids, infection, and acute-phase reactants increase the production of metallothionein complexes, thereby decreasing the serum zinc concentration. It is decreased under conditions of low concentrations of albumin and beta-globulins. In catabolic states and in hemolysis, plasma and serum zinc concentrations increase.

Zinc is stored primarily in the liver, but can be found in almost all tissues. Elimination of zinc occurs primarily via the enteral route, with increased losses found in patients with acute or chronic diarrhea, steatorrhea, and inflammatory bowel disease.[147] Although zinc is excreted in relatively small amounts via the kidney, clinically important losses can be seen with chronic diuretic use.[147] Cutaneous losses of zinc can occur in patients with extensive sweating or burns.

Zinc Metabolism in Pregnancy

The recommended daily allowance of zinc during pregnancy is $15\,\text{mg·day}^{-1}$, which is approximately $3\,\text{mg·day}^{-1}$ more than in the nonpregnant adult.[148] This recommendation assumes a dietary intake of approximately $30\,\text{mg·day}^{-1}$ with mean intestinal absorption of 25% and additional mean daily losses of $3.6\,\text{mg·day}^{-1}$, with the goal to maintain a total body zinc of 2 to $3\,\text{g}$.[148] Dietary bioavailability and absorption of zinc is lower in pregnant patients who smoke, consume a strictly vegetarian diet or large quantities of dairy products, or have large iron supplementation.

Zinc requirements increase during periods of rapid growth or cellular repair. Accordingly, fetal zinc requirements increase by 50-fold during the second and third trimester.[149] During this same period, serum zinc concentration decreases slightly, probably accounted for by maternal volume expansion, reduced circulating albumin, and redistribution of zinc from the maternal to fetal compartment. Few patients increase their dietary zinc intake adequately during pregnancy to compensate for the increased fetal needs. Investigations in animals have revealed possible adaptive mechanisms that alter zinc utilization during pregnancy, thereby meeting this increased demand without increasing dietary intake.[150] It has been speculated that there may be increased fractional zinc absorption and/or decreased endogenous zinc excretion during the latter half of pregnancy. Human investigations have not yet demonstrated such an adaptive change, possibly due to limitations in the sensitivity of measurement of zinc concentration.

Indirect measurements of zinc nutriture in pregnancy have been performed in an attempt to avoid the inaccuracies of serum and plasma measurements. Zinc concentrations in hair, toenails, and erythrocytes have been found to remain unchanged with increasing gestation.[151] No consistent change has been found in amniotic fluid concentration of zinc with advancing gestation and no correlation has been found between maternal serum and amniotic fluid zinc concentration.[151] Amniotic fluid zinc concentrations have been noted to be reduced in patients with chorioamnionitis, possibly due to increased concentrations of metallothionein. A prospective trial, however, has failed to demonstrate any predictive value of the amniotic fluid zinc concentration with regard to pregnancy outcome.[152]

Zinc and Pregnancy Outcome

Because of zinc's central role in normal growth in development on a molecular level, attempts have been made to correlate poor zinc nutriture with adverse pregnancy outcome and abnormal fetal growth. Severe zinc deficiency in animals has been associated with reduced fertility, congenital malformations, labor abnormalities, and growth restriction.[153]

The study of zinc's effect on pregnancy outcome in humans has yielded less clear data. The most severe form of zinc deficiency is found in patients with acrodermatitis enteropathica (AE). These patients have impaired zinc absorption secondary to a defective or absent ligand for zinc absorption in the gut. In the neonatal period, affected patients exhibit failure to thrive, impaired immune function, and gastrointestinal disorders.[154] In one small series of patients who became pregnant while not on zinc supplementation, there was a high incidence of major obstetric complications and congenital malformations in the offspring.[155] With zinc supplementation, there was no difference in rates of malformations compared to the normal population.

Studies of the effect of zinc deficiency on pregnancy outcome in humans without AE have yielded variable conclusions. Mild zinc deficiency has been associated with an increased incidence of pregnancy induced hypertension, prolonged labor, postpartum hemorrhage, and prematurity.[156,157] In addition, supplementation of zinc has been shown to decrease the rate of preterm delivery and need for respiratory assistance in a group of neonates born to teenage mothers.[158] More recent studies have failed to substantiate these data. In a study of 285 pregnant women, serum zinc concentrations at 18 and 30 weeks were not correlated with Apgar scores, rate of maternal infection, or rate of prematurity.[159] In two recent randomized controlled trials of zinc supplementation, there were no differences in blood loss, hypertension, Apgar scores, neonatal abnormalities, or gestational age at birth between the treated and the control groups.[160,161] A third large randomized trial revealed a tendency toward fewer preterm deliveries and fewer neo-

TABLE 14.1. Selected pregnancy outcomes and neonatal measurements in the zinc supplement and placebo subgroups by body mass index (BMI) categories.

	BMI ≥26			BMI <26		
	Zinc supplement ($n = 155$)	Placebo ($n = 145$)	p	Zinc Supplement ($n = 134$)	Placebo ($n = 134$)	p
Maternal characteristics						
Age, y	24.8	24.2	0.32	22.9	21.2	0.01
BMI, kg/m^2	33.4	33.0	0.64	22.3	22.2	0.57
Current smoker, %	7.7	5.5	0.44	3.0	3.0	0.98
Pregnancy outcome						
Birth weight, g	3240	3241	0.99	3190	2942	0.005
Gestational age, wk	39.0	38.7	0.47	38.6	37.9	0.08
Preterm birth <32 wk, %	3.2	5.5	0.33	3.0	6.8	0.15
Birth weight <1500 g, %	3.9	3.5	0.84	2.3	6.0	0.12
Anthropometric measurements						
Crown-heel length, cm	50.2	49.8	0.41	50.3	49.7	0.20
Head circumference, cm	34.3	34.0	0.50	34.1	33.4	0.005
Abdominal circumference, cm	33.3	33.1	0.64	32.8	32.6	0.58
Arm length, cm	9.9	9.7	0.27	9.9	9.6	0.03
Subscapular skinfold, mm	4.2	3.9	0.05	3.9	3.6	0.06
Neonatal outcome						
Neonatal hospital stay, d	3.9	4.5	0.47	3.1	4.9	0.10
Neonatal sepsis, %	0.7	1.4	0.52	0	2.2	0.08

From Goldenberg,[162] with permission.

nates weighing less than 1500 g with zinc supplementation (Table 14.1).[162] These differences were not significant, even after subgroup analyses of women with the lowest body mass indices.

The inconsistencies in the conclusions of these investigations are likely due to several factors. First, there exist great inaccuracies in clinical and serologic assessment of zinc nutriture, especially in pregnancy. In addition, the degree of zinc deprivation imposed on laboratory animals and seen in AE is far greater than that seen in otherwise normal patients. Many of the studies involving zinc supplementation have been small, with initiation after the completion of embryogenesis and using inconsistent doses. Finally, the precise amount of zinc each patient is receiving is difficult to measure because the bioavailability of zinc is influenced greatly by factors such as medications, alcohol, smoking, and dietary differences.

Zinc and Neural Tube Defects

A prominent feature in many experimental models of severe zinc deficiency has been the appearance of an increased rate of neural tube defects. Neural tube defects are seen in unsupplemented patients with AE and patients taking zinc chelators such as valproic acid and phenytoin.[155] Serum zinc concentrations were noted to be significantly lower in mothers delivering anencepalic neonates versus controls.[163] In another study, however, serum and hair zinc concentrations were not noted to be different from normal in mothers delivering anencephalic neonates.[164] In a recent study, high toenail zinc concentration was associated with an odds ratio of 5.0 for delivering a neonate with a neural tube defect when compared to a control population matched for folic acid supplementation, age of mother, and previous history of neural tube defect.[165] The abnormally elevated zinc concentration in the toenails were thought to be secondary to zinc sequestration in the hair, nails, and liver, with relative zinc deficiency at the site of neural tube closure.

Zinc and Birth Weight

Because of its importance in cell growth and differentiation, zinc supplementation has been studied as a means of improving birth weight. Several small, nonrandomized trials of zinc nutriture and supplementation produced mixed results in regards to birth weight. A recent randomized control trial of zinc supplementation in 589 women with low serum zinc concentrations revealed significant increases in birth weight in the supplemented population.[162] This increase was most pronounced in the subgroup with the lowest body mass index. Similarly, a regression analysis of a large group of Egyptian women found that low maternal weight at 3 months of gestation and low second trimester plasma zinc concentration were the best predictors of birth weight.[166] Several other large series, however, have failed to find any association between birth weight and maternal hair, serum, or urinary zinc concentration.[159,167,168]

Iron

Iron is a major constituent of hemoglobin, myoglobin, and several essential enzyme systems. It is necessary for delivering oxygen from the lungs to the tissues of the body and for the function of enzymes required for oxidation reactions and energy release from cells. Iron deficiency is the most prevalent nutrient deficiency in the world, producing anemia in 1.2 billion people worldwide.[169] It represents the most common form of anemia in reproductive age women and is seen in 15.6% to 55% of pregnant women in late pregnancy in the United States[170,171] (see Chapter 41).

Bioavailability and Metabolism

Iron balance is constantly and precisely regulated through changes in its bioavailability and absorption.[172] The major dietary sources of iron are meat, fish, poultry, vegetables, and fortified cereals. Food supplements account for 25% of the daily iron intake in the average U.S. diet.[173] Iron absorption takes place in the duodenum of the small intestine. The amount of iron absorbed is determined by the iron content of the meal, the chemical form of iron ingested, and the iron status of the individual.[174] Heme iron, present in meat, fish, and poultry, is highly bioavailable because it is absorbed intact within a prophyrin ring and is not susceptible to inhibition by ligands in the diet.[175] The percent of heme absorbed from the diet remains constant regardless of the amount ingested. Non-heme iron absorption, in contrast, is profoundly affected by the interaction with promotive and inhibitory substances in the diet that make iron more or less soluble. Absorption is inhibited by phytates, bran, antacids, calcium phosphate, and tannins in tea.[176–178] Promoters of absorption include ascorbic acid and meat proteins.[179] The percent of non-heme iron absorbed varies depending on the overall amount of iron present in the meal. The actual amount of iron absorbed is usually fairly constant. Absorption of non-heme iron varies with the iron status of the individual. An increased percent of iron is absorbed in individuals with low body iron stores.[180] The response to low iron stores may not be sufficient, however, if iron intake is marginal.

The adult female has approximately 2.2 g of iron, the majority of which is incorporated into iron porphyrin complexes such as hemoglobin, myoglobin, and enzyme systems.[180] The remaining iron is present in the storage proteins, ferritin and hemosiderin located in the spleen, liver, and bone marrow, with a small amount in the blood transport protein, transferrin.[181] The average storage reserve in adult females in the United States is 300 mg.[182] The average daily iron loss is variable in women depending on the volume of menstrual blood flow,[182] but can range from 1.0 to 1.5 mg·day^{-1}. A daily intake of 15 mg of elemental iron is sufficient to maintain adequate iron stores in all but 5% of menstruating women.[183] The usual dietary intake of iron in the United States is sufficient to cover this requirement without supplementation.

Iron Deficiency Anemia

When the iron requirements increase or the iron intake decreases, there is a point when the intestine can no longer increase absorption to meet the body's demands. At this point, iron stores get depleted and serum ferritin concentration decreases. As the iron stores become completely empty, transferrin saturation decreases with a resultant fall in erythroid precursors and erythrocyte indices.[184] A microcytic, hypochromic anemia results, with low hemoglobin and, low ferritin concentrations, and decreased erythrocyte indices. Serum ferritin concentration is thought to closely reflect iron stores. A concentration of less than 12 μg·L^{-1}, coupled with a hemoglobin less than 11 g·dl^{-1} indicates iron deficiency anemia.[185] Once depleted, however, serum ferritin no longer reflects the severity of deficiency. Transferrin receptors on cell membranes can now be measured to assess the severity of iron deficiency.[186] With worsening deficiency the concentration of receptors in the circulation increases.

Populations at high risk for iron deficiency anemia include poor, undereducated women with a history of menorrhagia, a diet low in meat and ascorbic acid, a history of donating blood more than three times per year, or chronic aspirin use.[187] Iron deficiency is more common during periods of rapid growth, such as from 6 months to 4 years of age, and during early adolescence. The female reproductive years predispose patients to iron deficiency from menstrual losses and pregnancy. Iron deficiency has been associated with a decreased work capacity,[188] decreased immune function,[189] and possibly impaired school performance in children.[190]

Iron Metabolism in Pregnancy

Iron requirements in pregnancy increase because of the need to replace the usual basal losses, allow for the expansion of red cell mass, provide iron to the fetus and placenta, and replace blood loss at delivery. These increased demands begin at approximately 16 weeks and continue until term. The estimated total pregnancy iron needs are 1000 mg or an additional 1.5 mg each day.[191] This allows for a replacement of approximately 800 mg of lost iron and a retention of 200 mg to maintain iron stores.

To cover the doubling in the iron requirement in pregnancy, there must be an abundant dietary intake of iron that is highly absorbable with large quantities of heme iron, animal protein, and ascorbic acid. In addition, prepregnancy stores must be adequate to buffer the needs of pregnancy. Intestinal absorption increases in pregnancy in response to the increased demands.[192] In the iron-sufficient nonpregnant state, 10% of elemental iron is absorbed. In pregnancy, absorption increases to 20% with adequate iron stores, and up to 40% with iron deficiency.

The fetus obtains its required iron, regardless of the maternal iron status, through a process of active placental transport.[193] Maternal iron, complexed with transferrin, enters the apical trophoblast and is released into the cell.[194] The maternal transferrin is recycled and released back through the cell membrane to the maternal side. The intracellular iron is transported by ferritin to fetal transferrin on the fetal side of the cell and exits to the fetal circulation via the basolateral surface.[195] Fetal iron concentration regulates the amount of iron crossing the placenta by altering the concentration of transferrin membrane receptors on the apical trophoblast.[196] In addition, placental ferritin in cytotrophoblasts and fetal endothelial cells regulate inward flux of iron into the fetal circulation.[197] Two thirds of fetal iron is incorporated into fetal hemoglobin.[194] The remaining one third enters the fetal liver and is used in the first year after birth. Infants born to mothers with severe iron deficiency are at higher risk of iron deficiency in the first few months of life, presumably due to inadequate accumulation of stored iron in the fetal liver.[198,199]

Iron Deficiency in Pregnancy

Hemoglobin concentration falls normally in pregnancy due to an expansion in plasma volume. Typically, hemoglobin falls approximately 2 mg·L^{-1} by the second trimester, and rises again slightly by term.[187] If the additional iron demands of pregnancy are not met by increased dietary intake and absorption, women can develop iron deficiency anemia where the supply of iron in the bone marrow limits the synthesis of hemoglobin. The Centers for Disease Control (CDC) defines anemia as a hemoglobin less than 11.0 g·dl^{-1} in the first and third trimester or less than 10.5 g·dl^{-1} in the second trimester.[200] When accompanied by a low serum ferritin concentration (i.e., less than 12.0 μg·L^{-1}), iron deficiency is presumed to be the cause of anemia.[187] Ferritin concentration, however, normally declines in late gestation due to hemodilution and can be falsely decreased.[201] Transferrin receptor concentration does not change in pregnancy and may give a more accurate diagnosis of iron deficiency anemia when an elevated concentration is found.[202]

Iron deficny has been associated with adverse effects in the mother, the fetus, and the neonate. The pregnant woman with iron deficiency can experience fatigue, a decrease in work performance, and cardiovascular stress from low oxygen saturation.[203] Maternal cell-mediated immunity and leukocyte bactericidal enzyme function have been shown to be impaired with severe iron deficiency.[189,202] Maternal tolerance of blood loss and surgery at the time of delivery may also be theoretically impaired.[203]

Many reports support an increased frequency of adverse pregnancy outcome with iron deficiency anemia theoretically because of impaired hemoglobin oxygen transport to the uterus, placenta, and developing fetus. Investigations from developing countries have found significantly higher rates of low birth weight,[204–207] preterm delivery,[206] intrauterine fetal death,[204] and neonatal death[204,208] in women with severe anemia. Most of these studies, however, did not analyze their results by the cause of anemia, with malaria being the most common cause of anemia in most reports. In addition, these investigation did not control for other factors that may have contributed to poor obstetric outcome.

Studies from industrialized countries report an association with severe anemia and low birth weight,[170,209,210] intrauterine fetal demise,[209,210] and preterm delivery.[209–212] Other studies found no association between low hemoglobin and low birth weight and preterm delivery.[213–215] Most of these studies considered anemia in general and did not control for social class, maternal age, and smoking history. Klebanoff et al.[216] studied over 26,000 women and found an odds ratio (OR) of 1.9 for preterm labor in women with a hematocrit less than the tenth percentile. Although there was no indication as to the type of anemia, nonwhites were found to have an OR of 1.2 to 2.0 for preterm delivery compared to whites (Table 14.2). Lu et al.[214] studied 17,000 women in the first 20 weeks of pregnancy and found an association between early anemia and increased rates of preterm delivery and intrauterine growth restriction. No such association was noted when anemia developed in late pregnancy. Klebanoff et al.[215] found anemia associated with preterm delivery in a population of 35,000 pregnant women. Analysis of the subgroup of African-American women revealed no such association. A prospective cohort study of almost 800 inner city women revealed a rate of anemia of 27.9% with iron deficiency as an etiology in only 12.5%.[211] The subgroup with iron deficiency in the first half of pregnancy was associated with increased rates of preterm delivery, low birth weight, and poor maternal weight gain. Iron deficiency anemia developing in the third trimester was not associated with increased rates of preterm delivery and low birth weight. All other forms of anemia were not associated with adverse pregnancy outcomes, regardless of onset of anemia. In essence, iron deficiency anemia may be associated with preterm delivery and low birth weight if present in the first half of pregnancy. The mechanism by which this occurs is unclear and whether this outcome may be related to other confounding factors, such as poor maternal weight gain and smoking.

From the data on iron deficiency and pregnancy outcome, it appears that the best way to avoid adverse outcome may be to identify and correct the iron deficient state prior to pregnancy. It has been recommended that all patients should receive iron supplementation during pregnancy, since the recommended dietary intake in pregnancy is approximately twice that found in the average diet in the United States.[190] Observational studies in industrialized countries of iron supplementation and pregnancy outcome have reported mixed data. No difference in pregnancy outcome with iron supplementation was noted in several observational investigations,[213,217] while one did note lower rates of preterm delivery and low birth weight with iron supplementation.[218] These investigations were all relatively small with poor statistical

TABLE 14.2. Odds ratios for preterm birth and anemia during pregnancy.

	Black women		White women	
Week of pregnancy	No. of women	Odds ratio (95% confidence interval)	No. of women	Odds ratio (95% confidence interval)
25	1422	1.6 (1.2–2.2)	1110	1.1 (0.7–1.8)
26	1429	1.5 (1.1–2.1)	977	1.2 (0.8–1.9)
27	1524	1.1 (0.8–1.5)	997	2.1 (1.3–3.3)
28	1555	0.8 (0.6–1.1)	1062	1.6 (1.1–2.4)
29	1826	1.2 (0.9–1.5)	1391	1.1 (0.7–1.6)
30	2069	1.1 (0.9–1.5)	2236	0.8 (0.6–1.2)
31	1968	1.0 (0.8–1.3)	2848	1.9 (1.3–2.7)
32	2520	0.8 (0.6–1.0)	2934	1.0 (0.7–1.4)
33	1939	0.9 (0.7–1.2)	2343	1.0 (0.7–1.4)
34	2229	0.7 (0.5–0.9)	2139	1.3 (0.9–1.8)
35	2546	0.6 (0.5–0.8)	2031	0.7 (0.5–1.2)
36	2687	0.6 (0.5–0.8)	2094	1.1 (0.7–1.7)

From Lu,[214] with permission.

power and had no controls for confounding factors such as use of other prenatal supplementation.

Clinical trials of iron supplementation in pregnancy have provided mixed data. Some show no increases in hemoglobin with iron supplementation,[198,211,219] while others have found an improvement in iron status parameters, depending on the dose and formulation of the supplementation.[220,221] Randomized controlled trials of the effect of iron supplementation on clinical outcomes have shown no significant change in rates of low birth weight, preterm delivery, or intrauterine fetal death.[222-226] In a study by Milman et al.[199] iron supplementation did not change maternal hemoglobin concentration but was associated with significant decrease in iron deficiency anemia at term and fewer cases of low ferritin concentration, indicating higher iron stores. Neonates of women with supplementation had significantly higher umbilical cord ferritin concentration, signifying higher iron reserves. Based on these data, it is hypothesized that iron supplementation may decrease iron deficiency in infants in the first several months of life.

Several investigations have suggested the use of selective supplementation of women with low hemoglobin, low serum ferritin, and/or high serum transferrin concentrations.[227,228] It has been suggested that iron supplementation twice each week may be as effective as daily dosing, with fewer side effects.[229] Further research is necessary to determine the optimal dose and frequency of iron supplementation, as well as the appropriate hematologic indices for selective supplementation. In addition, future investigation should focus on methods to improve compliance with supplementation and decrease the overall expenditure per case of iron deficiency anemia.

Lead

Lead is a mineral for which nutritional requirements, if they do exist, are very low and easily met by levels naturally occurring in food, water, and air. The primary concern regarding lead is not in terms of deficiency, but in regard to its excess. High-level lead exposure has been recognized for centuries as being detrimental to human health. Acute, high exposure causes nausea, vomiting, abdominal pain, diarrhea, constipation, and a metallic taste. In addition, central nervous system disorders such as paresthesias, pain, and muscle weakness are frequently noted. Finally, lead inhibits heme synthesis and can result in anemia, hemoglobinuria, and renal damage. A blood lead concentration of greater than $25\,\mu g \cdot dl^{-1}$ has historically been considered high enough by the CDC to warrant medical referral.[230] Recent data indicate that concentration considerably lower than this cutoff may be associated with adverse effects.[231-234]

Bioavailability and Metabolism

Lead exposure occurs primarily from industrial sources, such as mining and smelting plants and coal-fired power plants; manufacturing of batteries, cables, and pipes; as well as household exposures to lead paint and leaded gasoline. Lead enters the body either through inhalation of dust into the upper respiratory tract or through ingestion of contaminated food or beverage. Respiratory secretions are swallowed and absorbed into the intestinal tract or absorbed via aerosols into the lung.[235] The rate of gastrointestinal absorption is approximately 40% in children, as compared to 10% to 15% in adults.[236] This rate is increased with cigarette smoking, alcohol ingestion, and deficiencies in iron and/or calcium.[237] After absorption, lead enters the bloodstream and 99% becomes bound to erythrocytes.[238] It is initially distributed to soft tissues, especially hepatocytes and tubular epithelium of the kidney. This is followed by redistribution to bone, teeth, and hair. Eventually, 95% of total lead stores are found in bone, where the half-life is 20 to 30 years.[239] Lead is eliminated via urine and bile. Blood lead concentration commonly is the most assessed of the recent and active fraction of lead circulating in soft tissues.[240]

Lead Metabolism in Pregnancy

During pregnancy, lead transfers readily from mother to fetus, with cord blood concentration 90% to 100% as high as maternal concentration.[241] The mechanism for transfer of lead across the placenta has not been clearly defined, but probably involves simple diffusion related to the fetal blood flow rate.[242] Fetal uptake across the placenta is constant throughout gestation and cumulative until birth.[243] Lead accumulates mainly in the fetal bone, erythrocytes, and hepatocytes.[244] Maternal blood concentration of lead decreases during pregnancy, to a greater extent than expected from hemodilution alone.[245] An increased efflux of bone lead stores during pregnancy can serve as a reservoir to pass to the fetus without any concurrent environmental source.[246] As such, if maternal lead poisoning has occurred at any time in the past, elevated bone stores can pass to the fetus.

Treatment of high maternal lead concentration consists primarily of removal of the source of lead exposure. Absorption in the gut can be decreased with limiting smoking and alcohol use, as well as with increasing calcium and iron intake. Chelating agents are not useful in prevention of fetal exposure as they do not cross the placenta and have been shown to have no effect on fetal blood lead concentration.[247]

Lead and Fetal Neurotoxicity

The perinatal period appears to be a particularly vulnerable one for neurotoxicity.[248,249] Mature, but not immature, organs can form lead-protein complexes that help to sequester lead away from mitochondria.[249] Immature fetal neuroendothelial cells are more easily damaged by lead, altering the blood-brain barrier and allowing lead to reach newly formed components of the brain. Once in the fetal brain, lead impairs early structuring and modification of neuronal circuits in the rat.[250] Lead disrupts cell acquisition, fiber outgrowth, and synapse formation.[251] In addition, lead disrupts neurotransmission by forming complexes with calmodulin[252] and produces neurotoxins through the inhibition of heme synthesis.[252] In studies of the monkey[253] and the rodent,[254] low-level prenatal lead exposure was shown to alter the developing structures of the central nervous system and produce long-term effects, even with no further postnatal exposures.

Multiple studies have noted early deficits in human neonates with low-level antenatal lead exposure.[255–259] These early deficits, however, were not detectable by school age. Only one study, with very high blood lead concentrations in the neonates, was noted to have deficits that lasted through to school age.[260] In another study, neonatal blood lead concentration correlated with poor test scores at age 4 only in those children with the lowest socioeconomic status.[261] These deficits were not found on testing in any subsets 1 year later at the age of 5.[262] A meta-analysis by the World Health Organization of all studies of antenatal lead neurotoxicity concluded that each increase of $10\mu g \cdot dl^{-1}$ mean blood lead concentration was associated with a 1- to 3-point decline in IQ within blood lead levels of $0-25\mu g \cdot dl^{-1}$.[263] No threshold concentration of lead exposure has been found for this effect.[264]

Although the major site of damage with lead exposure appears to be associated with the central nervous system there exist several reports of other teratogenic effects, as well. In 1984, Needleman et al.[265] retrospectively studied 4354 infants and found an odds ratio of 2.4 for minor anomalies if lead concentrations were greater than $15\mu g \cdot dl^{-1}$. There were no syndromes or patterns to the anomalies and no information in the study on the possible timing of prenatal lead exposure. In two smaller subsequent evaluations, no association was found with minor or major anomalies.[266,267] A case report in 1991 revealed a case of VACTERL syndrome, which entails *v*ertebral, *a*nal, *c*ardiac, *t*racheal, *e*sophageal, *r*enal, and *l*imb anomalies, in a patient with high lead exposure up until the eight week of gestation.[268] A case control study in 1993 evaluated drinking water lead concentration in over 1000 women delivering fetuses with congenital anomalies, fetal demise, or neonatal demise.[269] Lead concentrations greater than the 95th percentile were associated with a relative risk of fetal demise of 2.1. Mildly elevated lead concentrations were associated with ear, face, neck, and cardiovascular anomalies. No association was found with CNS, genitalia, or musculoskeletal anomalies. This study was limited by lack of information on individual drinking water consumption or maternal blood lead concentrations, which might have been quite variable in the population.

Lead and Pregnancy Outcome

Lead toxicity has been long associated with poor pregnancy outcome. Investigations of the impact of lower lead concentration on pregnancy outcome have yielded less clear data. A strong association was initially noted between premature rupture of membranes (PROM) and elevated maternal and fetal lead concentrations in 1976.[270] Three subsequent reports showed either a slightly decreased incidence[265] or no difference in the rate of PROM with elevated blood lead concentrations.[271,272] Cord tissue lead concentration was found to be significantly elevated in PROM in a more recent report.[257] There was no correlation with placental tissue or antenatal blood lead concentrations and PROM. There does not appear to be strong evidence to support an association between lead and PROM.

The association of preterm delivery (PTD) with lead exposure has been studied extensively. Several reports have been published of an increased risk of PTD with elevated lead concentration, but failed to control for other risk factors associated with PTD.[270,273] Others used lead exposure defined as community proximity to a lead smelter.[257,274] These reports are difficult to assess because individual exposure can be quite variable within a community. Three studies used individual exposure status and controlled for confounding risk factors.[258,273,274] Bellinger et al.[258] showed a 2% decreased risk of PTD, with each increase of $1\mu g \cdot dl^{-1}$ maternal blood lead concentration, whereas McMichael et al.[272] found an 11% increase in the rate of PTD with the same increase in lead concentration. The third report failed to find any correlation between maternal lead concentration and rates of PTD.[274]

Investigations of mean gestational age at delivery have shown variable effects of maternal lead status. Using multivariate analysis to control for potential confounders, three studies found maternal blood lead concentration to be unrelated to gestational age at delivery.[255,256,275] Dietrich et al.[276] found a decrease in gestational age by 4 days with each increase of $10\mu g \cdot dl^{-1}$ in antenatal blood lead. Conversely, both Bellinger et al.[258] and Factor-Litvak et al.[274] noted increases in gestational age with increased blood lead concentration. These large, well designed investigations failed to clarify the association, if any, between lead and gestational age.

The incidence of low birth weight, defined as <2500g, was found to be correlated with rising lead concentrations in several case control series.[258,277,278] One using community risks for defining populations, did not find such an association.[272] Mean birth weight was found to be significantly lower with an increasing blood lead concentration. This effect was noted after adjustment for socioeconomic factors, gestational age, and other known risk factors using multivariate regression analysis. The majority of studies clearly support the hypothesis that prenatal lead exposure can adversely affect mean birth weight. One study found that birth weight appeared to be constant until reaching a lead concentration greater than 6.2 µg·dl^{-1}, implying a possible threshold effect.[274]

Copper

Copper is the third most abundant trace element in the body, after iron and zinc. It is essential for the activity of multiple enzyme systems in the body, including cytochrome oxidase in the electron transport chain, superoxide dismutase for free radical detoxification, dopamine β-hydroxylase for production of catecholamines, and lysl oxidase for cross-linking collagen and elastin.[279] Copper is necessary for erythropoiesis, leukopoiesis, thermal regulation, immune and cardiac function, and glucose metabolic regulation (see Chapter 41).

Bioavailability and Metabolism

The adult body has 80 to 150 mg of copper.[280] The major food sources of copper are liver, seafood, and dried beans, peas, and nuts. Copper is primarily absorbed via the proximal intestine, through passive absorption and facilitated mechanisms by the uptake of amino acids.[281] Natural food copper is absorbed at a rate of approximately 36%.[282] Bioavailability is decreased by high vitamin C intake, which reduces and chelates copper in the intestine.[283] In addition, zinc intake above the RDA can decrease copper retention.[284]

After transport across the intestine, albumin carries copper to the liver, where the majority of copper is stored. Once in the liver, more than 95% of copper complexes to ceruloplasmin, a major copper-carrying protein in plasma responsible for the efficient delivery of copper to peripheral tissue.[285] Ceruloplasmin, synthesized in the liver, has ferrous oxidase activity and plays a role in tissue angiogenesis, coagulation, and acute-phase reactions.[279] Ceruloplasmin concentration increases in inflammation, infection, and injury, as well as in response to estrogen and malignancy.[286] Transport of copper across the plasma membrane into the intracellular space is controlled in yeast systems by the gene DTR1.[287] The mammalian gene homologous to CTR1 has not yet been identified. Once inside the cell, excess copper is bound to metallothionein.[281] Excretion of copper is primarily via bile, with small amounts excreted in urine, skin, hair, and sweat.[288] Cholestasis can impair copper excretion and lead to hepatic accumulation of copper.

Copper homeostasis is tightly controlled in the normal adult by mechanisms that have not been clearly defined. Even though the usual dietary intake of most adults is far below the RDA of 1.6 mg·day^{-1}, purely nutritional copper deficiency is extremely rare.[289] Parenterally fed premature infants appear to be at most risk for copper deficiency, probably due to the immaturity of the liver.[290] Clinically, these infants display anemia, neutropenia, skeletal abnormalities, and osteoporosis, as well as neurologic and cardiac problems.

Two inborn diseases, Menkes' kinky hair syndrome and Wilson's disease, result in severely altered copper metabolism. Menkes' disease is a rare X-linked recessive disorder characterized by severe copper deficiency. It is fatal in early childhood and involves severe psychomotor retardation, seizures, hypertonia, temperature instability, skeletal abnormalities, and a characteristic gray steel wool appearance of hair.[291] Wilson's disease is an autosomal recessive disorder characterized by the accumulation of copper in tissues, especially the liver, brain, and kidneys, with resultant severe structural and functional damage.[292] Patients typically present at 10 to 15 years of age with severe hepatic damage and neurologic dysfunction.

The gene defect has recently been localized for both of these diseases: Menkes' at Xq13.3[293] and Wilson's at 13q14.[294] Overall homology between these two genes is 54%, with greater than 78% homology in specific domains.[279] The genes responsible for these diseases encode similar copper transporting P-type adenosine triphosphatases (ATPases).[279] Further description of the function and regulation of these genes may yield information regarding regulation of copper metabolism under normal conditions.

Copper Metabolism in Pregnancy

Maternal serum copper concentration doubles by the end of pregnancy, probably in response to estrogen stimulation of ceruloplasmin production.[286] Animal studies have shown that copper absorption is increased in pregnancy, but this finding has not been replicated in human investigations.[295] The mechanism and control of placental copper transport is not understood. It is known that ceruloplasmin does not cross the placenta because of its high molecular weight.[296] A high concentration of copper is found in the placenta of the fetus with Menkes' disease.[297] Further elucidation of the defect in intracellular transport in Menkes' disease may help to clarify the mechanism of placental transport in normal pregnancy.

The fetus accumulates 15 to 17 mg of copper during pregnancy, 80% during the third trimester.[298] Although maternal serum concentration of copper is 5 to 10 times higher than that of the fetus, fetal liver concentration is ten times higher than in the mother.[296] Fetal hepatic reserves are thought to protect the full-term infant against copper defiency in the first few months of life.

Copper and Pregnancy Outcome

In animal studies, severe copper deficiency has been associated with poor pregnancy outcome. Rats fed severely copper deficient diets had a high incidence of fetal resorption and stillbirths.[299] Sheep fed low copper diets for several generations developed neonatal ataxia in offspring.[296] In the human, copper deficiency is rarely as severe as that induced in animal models. In a study of women in Wales, low serum copper levels were associated with a decrease in neonatal head circumference and an increase in the incidence of neural tube defects.[300] In addition, hair copper content correlated directly to birth weight. These data were not confirmed by subsequent analyses in India, where there was no correlation between low serum copper concentration and neonatal birth weight, length, or head circumference.[301] Because of the changes in serum ceruloplasmin concentration in pregnancy, measures of functional copper nutriture may be more accurate than the serum and tissue concentrations. By more accurately identifying those patients with overall poor copper nutriture, it may be possible to assess the true risk for poor pregnancy outcome.

Fluoride

Fluoride is present in small amounts in all soil, water, plants, and animals.[302] It does not appear to be essential, although this issue is still not clearly settled. Animal research found that fluoride supplementation stimulated growth in rats[303] and protected mice against impaired reproduction and anemia.[304] No such effect was found in several other studies in animals.[305,306] The primary importance of fluoride is in the reduction of dental caries.[307]

Bioavailability and Metabolism

The average daily intake of fluoride is $0.9\,mg \cdot day^{-1}$ without fluorinated water and $1.7\,mg \cdot day^{-1}$ with fluorinated water.[308] The recommended concentration of fluoride in drinking water is 0.7 to 1.2 ppm, depending on the average regional temperature.[309] Residents of warmer climates tend to consume more water and require less fluorination per liter. The major dietary sources of fluoride are tea and marine fish consumed with bones. Food prepared with fluorinated water has a substantially greater content. Cooking in Teflon-coated pans can also increase dietary fluoride content, whereas aluminum decreases content.[310]

Absorption of fluoride occurs primarily via the stomach and proximal small intestine. Absorption is 100% for ionized fluoride found in drinking water, whereas protein bound fluoride found in food is absorbed at a 60% to 70% rate.[309,311] Increased gastric acidity can increase absorption.[312] Plasma fluoride is not protein bound and its concentration is directly proportional to levels of absorbed fluoride, without evidence of any homeostatic mechanisms.[313] Intracellular fluoride concentration change in proportion to plasma concentration, with alkalinization of plasma promoting a net flux out of the cell.[314] In the first 24 hours after ingestion, 50% of absorbed fluoride is incorporated into calcified tissues, with the majority of the remainder excreted in the urine.[315] Alkalinization of the urine can increase renal excretion of fluoride,[313] although bones and tooth enamel hold 99% of the body's stores.[315]

Fluoride and Caries Protection

It is universally accepted that postnatal fluoride imparts a benefit to caries protection, with multiple studies supporting fluoride reduction in dental caries.[307] It protects teeth by replacing hydroxyl ions in developing enamel prior to tooth eruption, forming apatite crystal that are 6 to 10 times more resistant to acid dissolution.[316] The tight crystalline structure prevents pits and fissure formation that allow for decay. This protective effect appears to be greatest during the period of maximal tooth formation, during the first 8 years of life.[316] Posteruptive teeth can benefit, as well, because fluoride facilitates remineralization of carious lesions, inhibits acid production of plaque bacteria, and improves tooth morphology.[317]

Fluoride Metabolism in Pregnancy

Fluoride is metabolized in a very similar manner in the pregnant and the nonpregnant women. Blood concentrations appear to decline toward the end of pregnancy, potentially due to increased urinary excretion, related to increases in the GFR.[318] The mechanism by which fluoride passes through the placenta is not clearly defined. Several investigations of its transplacental flow in both sheep and humans reveal lower concentration in fetal compared to maternal blood,[319,320] with a ratio of 0.86 in one study.[321] Other research has found equal concentrations in maternal and fetal blood, implying passive diffusion as the mechanism of transport.[322-324] Placental tissue has been found to contain a higher content compared to other tissue or circulating blood.[321,325,326] In addition, mixed umbilical cord samples were found not to reflect neonatal fluoride status.[323] These data have led some to hypothesize that the placenta may sequester the cation from both maternal and fetal sources.[323]

Amniotic fluid fluoride concentration has been found to be lower than umbilical cord blood and maternal plasma.[327] No correlation was found between maternal blood concentration and amniotic fluid.[328] Amniotic fluid fluoride concentration was found to increase toward term as compared to midgestation, possibly due to an increasing GFR with fetal growth.[327]

Prenatal Fluoride in Caries Prevention

The development of primary dentition begins at 10 to 12 weeks of gestation. Fluoride is incorporated into the inner enamel during an early, short secretory stage, while surface enamel is enhanced with fluoride during the longer maturation stage.[329] Maturing enamel appears at 8 to 9 months of gestation. The entire maturation stage lasts 1 to 2 years.

Animal research with fetal fluoride treatment reveals an improvement in caries resistance, morphologic characteristics, and color of developing teeth.[330] In addition, surface enamel fluoride concentration of decidual teeth increases with increasing prenatal and postnatal administration. Glenn[331] noted 350% to 400% more fluoride in teeth treated with fluoride prenatally.

Controversy exists regarding the benefits of prenatal fluoride in the prevention of dental caries in the human. Several investigations have shown that infants exposed to fluorinated water both pre- and postnatally were found to have significantly lower rates of caries than infants exposed only postnatally.[332,333] Other research found no association between caries rates and prenatal ingestion of fluorinated water.[334–336] When fluorinated water was combined with prenatal fluoride supplementation, it was found to decrease caries rates in decidual teeth in children.[337–339] At a symposium on prenatal fluoride in the early 1980s, there was a general consensus that some benefit of caries prevention accrues to the primary teeth when the fetus is exposed.[340] Permanent teeth do not clearly benefit from this exposure. Further carefully controlled clinical studies need to be undertaken prior to recommending fluoride supplementation universally to all pregnant patients.

Prenatal exposure to fluorinated water or supplements have not been found to produce any harmful effects on pregnancy outcome. Erickson[341] studied a population of more than 1 million pregnancies exposed to fluorinated water supplies and noted no increase in congenital malformations. In a study of rats, no mutagenic effect of sodium fluoride supplements was noted at high concentration.[342] No infants in a study of approximately 400 were noted to have evidence of fluoride toxicity (fluorosis) following prenatal supplementation to the mother.[339]

Iodine

Iodine is an essential mineral for animals and humans because it is an integral part of the thyroid hormones thyroxine and triiodothyronine. These hormones are necessary for cell proliferation, synapse formation, dendritic proliferation, and microtubular assembly in brain development.[343] Iodine deficiency is a major public health problem, affecting an estimated 800 million people worldwide.[344] It represents the most widespread nutritional cause of impaired brain development and one of the most common preventable causes of mental retardation and cerebral palsy[345] (see Chapter 41).

Bioavailability and Metabolism

Iodine is unevenly distributed in the environment with mountainous areas and areas with frequent flooding having the lowest iodine soil content. The iodine content of food is variable depending on the soil content, fertilizing, and food processing. Iodized table salt provides 76 µg of iodine per gram of salt.[346] Iodates are used in bread making in the United States and dairy products contain iodine from disinfectants used in processing procedures. The usual dietary intake of iodine in the United States is 170 µg·day^{-1}.[347] The recommended dietary allowance is set at 150 µg·day^{-1} to maintain a positive iodine balance.[348] Many areas of Africa, Asia, and South America and parts of Europe have no programs for iodine food supplementation and have widespread iodine deficiency.

Iodine is rapidly and completely absorbed from the intestine and transported to the thyroid gland for synthesis into thyroid hormones, to the salivary and gastric glands, and to the kidneys for excretion into the gastrointestinal tract and urine.[346] All iodine excreted into the gastrointestinal tract is reabsorbed and excreted in the urine. Urinary excretion of iodine in a 24-hour sample is the most reliable indicator of its status. Iodine deficiency has been defined by the World Health Organization as mild with urinary excretion of 50 to 100 µg·day^{-1}, moderate with 25 to 49 µg·day^{-1}, and severe with less than 25 µg·day^{-1}.[348]

Iodine Metabolism in Pregnancy

Pregnancy causes profound changes in iodine and thyroid hormone metabolism.[349–352] Elevated estrogen concentration in pregnancy increases the circulating concentrations of thyroid-binding globulin and increase total serum thyroxine concentration. In addition, chorionic gonadotropin acts as a thyrotropic hormone that stimulates thyroxine secretion. The peripheral conversion of thyroxine to triiodothyronine is enhanced by placental deiodinating activity. Pregnancy increases the urinary loss of iodine through an increased GER and increased renal clearance.[353] There is a reduction of available iodine to the maternal thyroid gland due to shunting of the maternal iodine pool to the fetal-placental complex. The net effect of pregnancy is to increase thyroid hormone requirements while decreasing iodine availability. With borderline deficiency, pregnancy can unmask more clinically significant iodine deficiency.

Iodine Deficiency and Pregnancy Outcome

Severe iodine deficiency during pregnancy has been associated with spontaneous abortions, intrauterine fetal demise, congenital anomalies, maternal and fetal goiter, hypothyroidism, impaired brain function, and endemic cretinism.[354] Endemic cretinism is characterized by two forms: neurologic and myxedematous. Neurologic cretinism is more common in Asia and involves mental deficiency, deaf-mutism, and a spastic-rigid motor disorder.[355] Myxedematous cretinism, a rarer disorder, is seen more commonly in parts of Africa and usually involves fewer difficulties with brain and hearing dysfunction and more severe and persistent hypothyroidism and growth restriction.[356] In addition to frank cretinism, an estimated six times more infants may have lesser degrees of mental and psychomotor retardation and learning disabilities in iodine-deficient regions.[357]

There are few histopathologic studies examining human fetal neurologic tissue affected by iodine deficiency. Animal data of iodine deficiency in the sheep[358,359] and the monkey[360] reveal a decreased weight of offspring, delayed bone maturation, decreased brain weight and brain DNA content, delayed maturation and migration of cells in the hippocampus, decreased dendrite density, and retarded myelination in the cerebral hemispheres and brain stem. Data of these animals with thyroid hormone analogues suggest that restoration of both maternal and fetal thyroid function is necessary for normalization of fetal development.[361] The effects of iodine deficiency appear to be mediated by a combination of maternal and fetal hypothyroidism, with the most vulnerable embryologic time period corresponding to 10 to 18 weeks in human fetuses.[345]

Studies in human abortuses reveal that the fetal thyroid can begin concentrating iodine and synthesizing thyroid hormone by 10 to 11 weeks of gestation.[362] Prior to 10 weeks' gestation maternal thyroid hormone can cross the placenta and influence fetal neurologic development. Neurologic cretinism is felt to be related to a lack of maternal passage of adequate concentration of thyroxine early in gestation prior to the onset of fetal thyroid gland function.[363] This results in abnormalities in the early development of cerebral cortex association areas and basal ganglia. Myxedematous cretinism probably involves adequate early transfer of maternal thyroid hormone followed by a failure of the developing fetal thyroid gland.[363] At birth, severe fetal hypothyroidism results.

Treatment of iodine deficiency prior to pregnancy has been shown to prevent cretinism in population studies in Papua, New Guinea.[364] Treatment after the second trimester had no effect on rates of neurologic impairment, implying an early onset of damage. In Zaire, iodine treatment late in pregnancy was able to decrease the perinatal mortality rate from myxedematous cretinism.[365] It appears that optimum reduction in all forms of iodine-deficiency disorder occurs with correction of iodine deficiency prior to pregnancy. First and early second trimester iodine supplementation in iodine deficient regions is probably helpful in decreasing perinatal morbidity and mortality.[366]

Selenium

Selenium is a trace element that functions as an integral component of the active site of the enzyme glutathione peroxidase.[367] This enzyme catalyzes the reduction of hydrogen peroxide to water and protects against free radical formation and oxidative damage to plasma membrane lipids. Selenium is a part of the active site of iodothyronine deiodinase, an enzyme that facilitates the conversion of thyroxine to triiodothyronine in peripheral tissues.[368]

Bioavailability and Metabolism

The adult human contains 10 to 20 mg of selenium, all of which is derived from dietary sources.[369] Seafood and organ meats contain the largest amounts of selenium, whereas the selenium content of grains and seeds varies with the soil content.[370] Approximately 80% of dietary selenium is absorbed, with organically bound forms retained to a greater degree.[371] The usual adult selenium intake is 70 to 100 $\mu g \cdot day^{-1}$.[371]

Selenium status can be determined by measurements of selenium concentration in whole blood, plasma, erythrocytes, and tissues or through the measurement of glutathione peroxidase activity. Erythrocyte selenium concentration provides a better index of long-term selenium status than plasma concentration, and is easier to perform than the measurement of peroxidase activity. In addition, peroxidase activity is only useful in populations with low selenium intake, as the enzyme activity plateaus at higher intake.[372]

Selenium deficiency in normal adults is rare, as selenium balance can be maintained over a wide range of dietary intakes. Selenium deficiency has been described in inhabitants of a large area in China where the soil content is severely lacking in selenium, as well as in patients receiving total parenteral nutrition (TPN).[373] Clinical signs and symptoms of selenium deficiency include muscle weakness and discomfort. Young children and women in selenium deficient regions of China are prone to a specific form of cardiomyopathy, known as Keshan disease.[374] Several patients receiving TPN with a low selenium concentration have been shown to develop cardiomyopathies.[375]

Selenium Metabolism in Pregnancy

The usual adult dietary intake of approximately $100 \mu g \cdot day^{-1}$ is sufficient to meet the excess selenium needs during pregnancy.[370] Supplementation of selenium during pregnancy is discouraged in healthy women because the amount of selenium to cause toxicity has not been clearly defined. Supplementation of as little as $1 mg \cdot day^{-1}$ caused signs of toxicity in one analysis.[376]

Plasma selenium concentration has been shown to decrease during pregnancy, probably due to an increasing plasma volume.[377] Erythrocyte and whole blood concentrations decrease starting at 16 weeks' gestation.[377] Erythrocyte glutathione concentrations show no change during pregnancy in women without selenium deficiency.[377] Placental transfer of selenium occurs via a saturable transport channel shared with sulfate.[378] Organically bound forms of selenium cross the placenta more readily.[379]

Selenium and Pregnancy Outcome

Because selenium helps to prevent free radical formation, it is theorized that its deficiency may lead to mutagenesis through free radical damage of DNA. Studies of animals with severe deficiency reveal a high rate of embryonic mortality at implantation and idiopathic miscarriage.[380] A recent article by Barrington et al.[369] noted that patients with spontaneous first trimester abortions had significantly lower serum selenium concentration than patients with normal pregnancies and nonpregnant controls, after correction for serum albumin and total protein concentrations. Serum selenium concentration were noted to be significantly lower in mothers of infants with neural tube defects, as well as in the neonatal themselves.[381] More studies are necessary to determine the possible role of maternal selenium status in early embryonic development.

Vascular endothelial damage initiated by free radicals may play a role in the etiology of preeclampsia. It has been hypothesized that deficient selenium concentration may predispose parturients to preeclampsia through free radical formation. This theory has been studied with limited data and conflicting results. Amniotic fluid selenium concentration was found to have no correlation with the development of preeclampsia in forty patients.[382] Lu et al.[389] noted that serum selenium concentration was significantly lower in the patient with preeclampsia compared to nonpregnant controls. Supplementation with selenium was then used in a high-risk group for the prevention of preeclampsia.[384] The treatment group was found to have an 8% incidence of preeclampsia, compared to a 23% incidence in the control group. Unfortunately, this study failed to define their high-risk groups or their criteria for preeclampsia, and only included 100 patients. They did not indicate the baseline selenium status of the patients in the two study groups. Further studies clearly are needed prior to recommending selenium supplementation for the prevention of preeclampsia.

References

1. Sanchez-Castillo CP, Warrender TP, Whitehead TP, et al. An assessment of the sources of dietary salt in a British population. Clin Sci 1987;72:95–102.
2. National Research Council. Drinking water and health. Report of the Safe Drinking Water Committee, Advisory Center on Toxicology, Assembly of Life Sciences. Washington, DC: National Academy Press, 1977.
3. National Research Council. Recommended dietary allowances. 10th ed. Washington, DC: National Academy Press, 1989:250–260.
4. Abraham S, Carroll MD. Fats, cholesterol, and sodium intake in the diet of persons 1–74 years: United States. Advance Data No. 54. U.S. Department of Health, Education, and Welfare, Washington, DC, 1981.
5. Pennington JAT, Wilson DB, Newell RF, et al. Selected minerals in food surveys, 1974 to 1981/82. J Am Diet Assoc 1984;84:771–780.
6. Page LB. Epidemiologic evidence on the etiology of human hypertension and its possible prevention. Am Heart J 1976;91:527–534.
7. Page LB. Hypertension and atherosclerosis in primitive and acculturating societies. In: Hunt JC, ed. Hypertension update, vol. 1. Lyndhurst, NJ: Health Learning Systems, 1979:1–12.
8. Gothberg G, Lundin S, Aurell M, et al. Responses to slow graded bleeding in salt-depleted rats. J Hypertens Suppl 1983;2:24–26.
9. Theunissen IM, Parer JT. Fluid and electrolytes in pregnancy. Clin Obstet Gynecol 1994;37:3–15.
10. Fievet P, Fournier A, deBold A, et al. Atrial natriuretic factor in pregnancy-induced hypertension and preeclampsia: increased plasma concentrations possibly explaining these hypovolemic states with paradoxical hyporeninism. Am J Hypertens 1988;1:16–21.
11. Lowe SQ, Macdonald GJ, Brown MA. Acute and chronic regulation of atrial natriuretic peptide in human pregnancy: a longitudinal study. J Hypertens 1992;10:821–829.
12. Olsson K, Hossaini-Hilali J, Eriksson L. Atrial natriuretic responses to angiotensin II in pregnant conscious goats. Acta Physiol Scand 1992;145:385–394.

13. Durr JA. Maternal fluid adaptation to pregnancy. In: Brace RA, Ross MG, Robillard JE, eds. Reproductive and perinatal medicine, vol. XI: Fetal and neonatal body fluids. Ithaca: Perinatology Press, 1989.
14. Davison JM. Renal disease. In: deSwiet M, ed. Medical disorders in obstetric practice. Oxford: Blackwell Scientific, 1989:306–308.
15. Hytten FE, Leitch I. The physiology of human pregnancy. 2nd ed. Oxford: Blackwell Scientific, 1971.
16. Lind T. Maternal physiology. Washington DC: Council on Resident Education in Obstetrics and Gynecology, 1985.
17. Pitkin RM, Kaminetzky HA, Newton M, et al. Maternal nutrition: a selective review of clinical topics. Obstet Gynecol 1972;40:773–785.
18. Sullivan CA, Martin JN. Sodium and pregnancy. Clin Obstet Gynecol 1994;37:558–573.
19. Ehrlich EN, Nolten WE, Oparil S, et al. Mineralocorticoids in normal pregnancy. In: Lindheimer MD, Katz AI, Zuspan FP, eds. Hypertension in pregnancy. New York: Wiley, 1976:189–191.
20. Lindheimer MD, Katz AI. Renal changes during pregnancy: their relevance to volume homeostasis. Clin Obstet Gynecol 1975;2:345–364.
21. Hatjis CG, Kofinas AD, Greelish JP, et al. Atrial natriuretic factor concentrations during pregnancy and in the postpartum period. Am J Perinatol 1992;9:275–278.
22. Schrier RW. Pathogenesis of sodium and water retention in high-output cardiac failure, nephrotic syndrome, cirrhosis, and pregnancy, II. N Engl J Med 1988;319:1127–1134.
23. Schrier RW, Briner VA. Peripheral arterial vasodilation hypothesis of sodium and water retention in pregnancy: implications for pathogenesis of preeclampsia-eclampsia. Obstet Gynecol 1991;77:632–639.
24. Davison JM, Lindheimer MD. Volume homeostasis and osmoregulation in human pregnancy. Baillieres Clin Endocrinol Metab 1989;3:451–472.
25. Gant NF, Daley GL, Chand S, et al. A study of angiotensin II pressor response throughout primigravid pregnancy. J Clin Invest 1973;52:2682–2689.
26. Brown MA, Gallery EDM. Sodium excretion in human pregnancy: a role for arginine vasopressin. Am J Obstet Gynecol 1986;154:914–919.
27. Fadnes HO, Øian P. Transcapillary fluid balance and plasma volume regulation: a review. Obstet Gynecol Surv 1989;44:769–773.
28. Huisman A, Aarnoudse JG. Increased second trimester hemoglobin concentration in pregnancies later complicated by hypertension and growth retardation. Acta Obstet Gynecol Scand 1986;65:605–608.
29. Pearson JF. Fluid balance in severe preeclampsia. Br J Hosp Med 1992;48:47–51.
30. Brown MA, Zammit VC, Lowe SA. Capillary permeability and extracellular fluid volumes in pregnancy-induced hypertension. Clin Sci 1989;77:599–604.
31. Brown MA, Whitworth JA. The kidney in hypertensive pregnancies: victim and villain. Am J Kidney Dis 1992;20:427–442.
32. Thomsen JK, Storm TL, Thamsborg G, et al. Atrial natriuretic peptide concentrations in preeclampsia. BMJ 1987;294;1508–1510.
33. Kristensen CG, Nakagawa Y, Coe FL, et al. Effect of natriuretic factor in rat pregnancy. Am J Physiol 1986; 250:R589–594.
34. Hirai N, Yanaihara T, Nakayama T, et al. Plasma levels of atrial natriuretic peptide during normal pregnancy complicated by hypertension. Am J Obstet Gynecol 1988; 159:27–31.
35. Fievet P, Fournier A, deBold A, et al. Atrial natriuretic factor in pregnancy-induced hypertension and preeclampsia: increased plasma concentrations possibly explaining these hypovolemic states with paradoxical hyporeninism. Am J Hypertens 1988;1:16–20.
36. Steegers EAP, Eskes TKAB, Jongsma HW, et al. Dietary sodium restriction during pregnancy: a historical review. Eur J Obstet Gynecol Reprod Biol 1991;40:83–90.
37. Chesley LC, Annitto JE, City J. A study of salt restriction and of fluid intake in prophylaxis against preeclampsia in patients with water retention. Am J Obstet Gynecol 1943;45:961–971.
38. Gray MJ, Munro AB, Sims EAH, et al. Regulation of sodium and total body water metabolism in pregnancy. Am J Obstet Gynecol 1964;89:760–765.
39. Robinson M. Salt in pregnancy. Lancet 1958;1:178–181.
40. Millar JA. Salt and pregnancy-induced hypertension. Lancet 1988;2:514.
41. Palomaki JF, Lindheimer MD. Sodium depletion simulating deterioration in a toxemic pregnancy. N Engl J Med 1970;282:88–89.
42. Repke JT. Calcium homeostasis in pregnancy. Clin Obstet Gynecol 1994;37:59–65.
43. National Research Council. Recommended dietary allowances. 10th ed. Washington, DC: National Academy Press, 1989:174–83.
44. Villar J, Belizán JM. Calcium during pregnancy. Clin Nutr 1986;5:55–62.
45. Chu JY, Margen S, Costa FM. Studies on calcium metabolism. II. Effects of low calcium and variable protein intake on human calcium metabolism. Am J Clin Nutr 1975;28:1028–1035.
46. United States Department of Agriculture. Nationwide food consumption survey. Nutrient intakes: Individuals in 48 states. Year 1977-78. Report No. I-2. Consumer Nutrition Division. Human Nutrition Information Service. U.S. Department of Agriculture. Hyattsville, MD: 1984
47. United States Department of Agriculture. Nationwide food consumption survey: Continuing survey of food intakes by individuals. Women 19–50 years and children 1–5 years, 4 days, 1985. Report 85-4. Nutrition Monitoring Division, Human Nutrition Information Service. U.S. Department of Agriculture. Hyattsville, MD: 1987.
48. Block G, Dresser CM, Hartman AM, et al. Nutrient sources in the American diet: quantitative data from the NHANES II survey. I. Vitamins and minerals. Am J Epidemiol 1985;122:13–26.
49. Heaney RP, Skillman TG. Calcium metabolism in normal human pregnancy. J Clin Endocrinol 1971;33:661–670.

50. Care AD. The placental transfer of calcium. J Dev Physiol 1991;15:253–257.
51. Tan CM, Raman A, Sinnathray TA. Serum ionic calcium levels during pregnancy. J Obstet Gynaecol Br Commonw 1972;79:694–697.
52. Pitkin RM, Reynolds WA, Williams GA, et al. Calcium metabolism in normal pregnancy: a longitudinal study. Am J Obstet Gynecol 1979;133:781–790.
53. Drake TS, Kaplan RA, Lewis TA. The physiologic hyperparathyroidism of pregnancy: Is it primary or secondary? Obstet Gynecol 1979;53:746–749.
54. Pitkin RM, Gebhardt MP. Serum calcium concentrations in human pregnancy. Am J Obstet Gynecol 1977;127:775–778.
55. Lund B, Selnes A. Plasma 1,25-dihydroxyvitamin D levels in pregnancy and lactation. Acta Endocrinol Copenh 1979;53:746–749.
56. Richards SR, Nelson DM, Zuspan P. Calcium levels in normal and hypertension and lactation. Am J Obstet Gynecol 1984;149:168–171.
57. Gertner JM, Coustan DR, Kliger AS, et al. Pregnancy as a state of physiologic absorptive hypercalciuria. Am J Med 1986;81:451–456.
58. Davis OK, Hawkins DS, Rubin LP, et al. Serum parathyroid hormone (PTH) in pregnant women determined by an immunoradiometric assay for intact PTH. J Clin Endocrinol Metab 1988;67:850–852.
59. Frolich A, Rudnicki M, Fischer-Rasmussen W, et al. Serum concentrations of intact parathyroid hormone during late human pregnancy: a longitudinal study. Eur J Obstet Gynaecol Reprod Biol 1991;42:85–87.
60. Seki K, Makimura N, Mitsui C, et al. Calcium-regulating hormones and osteocalcin levels during pregnancy: a longitudinal study. Am J Obstet Gynecol 1991;164:1248–1252.
61. Seely EW, Graves SW. Calcium homeostasis in normotensive and hypertensive pregnancy. Compr Ther 1993; 19:124–128.
62. Cushard WG, Creditor MA, Canterbury JM, et al. Physiologic hyperparathyroidism in pregnancy. J Clin Endocrinol 1972;34:767–771.
63. Van den Elzen HJ, Wladimiroff JW, Cohen Overbeek TE, et al. Calcium metabolism, calcium supplementation and hypertensive disorders of pregnancy. Eur J Obstet Gynaecol Reprod Biol 1995;59:5–16.
64. Pitkin RM. Calcium metabolism in pregnancy and the perinatal period: a review. Am J Obstet Gynecol 1985;151: 99–106.
65. Breslau NA, Zerwekh JE. Relationship of estrogen and pregnancy to calcium homeostasis in pseudohypoparathyroidism. J Clin Endocrinol Metab 1986;62:45–51.
66. Cruikshank DP, Pitkin R, Reynolds WA, et al. Calcium regulating hormones and ions in amniotic fluid. Am J Obstet Gynecol 1980;136:621–625.
67. Barlet JP, Davicco MJ. Parathyroid hormone related peptide. Reprod Nutr Dev 1990;30:639–651.
68. Frank GB. The current view of the source of trigger calcium in the excitation concentration coupling in the vertebrate skeletal muscle. Biochem Pharmacol 1980;29: 2399–2406.
69. Belizán JM, Villar J. The relationship between calcium intake and edema—proteinuria and hypertension gestosis: an hypothesis. Am J Clin Nutr 1980;33:2202–2210.
70. Neri LC, Mandel JS, Hewitt D. Relationship between mortality and water hardness in Canada. Lancet 1972;1: 931–934.
71. Marironi R, Koirtyohann SR, Pierce JO, et al. Calcium content of river water, trace element concentration in toenails, and blood pressure in village populations in New Guinea. Sci Total Environ 1976;6:41–53.
72. Langford HG, Watson RL. Electrolytes, environment, and blood pressure. Clin Sci Mol Med 1973;45:111S–113S.
73. Kobayashi J. On the influence of NaCL, KCL, Na_2SO_4, and $CaCO_3$ on the life and blood pressure of rats with calcium and magnesium deficiencies. Jpn J Hygiene 1968;23:106–110.
74. Itokawa Y, Tanaka C, Fujiwara M. Changes in body temperature and blood pressure in rats with calcium and magnesium deficiencies. J Appl Physiol 1974;37:835–839.
75. Belizán JM, Pineda O, Sainz E, et al. Rise of blood pressure in calcium-deprived pregnant rats. Am J Obstet Gynecol 1981;141:163–169.
76. Varner MW, Cruikshank DP, Pitkin RM. Calcium metabolism in the hypertensive mother, fetus, and newborn. Am J Obstet Gynecol 1983;143:762–765.
77. Van Overloop B, Treisser A, Coumaros G, et al. Decreased ionized calcium and increased parathyroid hormone in the serum of mild gestational hypertensive patients at the third trimester: a link between calcium metabolism and hypertension in pregnancy. Clin Exp Hypertens (B) 1992;B11:233–247.
78. Sowers JR, Zemel MB, Bronsteen RE, et al. Erythrocyte cation metabolism in preeclampsia. Am J Obstet Gynecol 1989;161:441–445.
79. Roelofsen JTM, Berkel GM, Uttendorfsky OT, et al. Urinary excretion of calcium and magnesium in normal and complicated pregnancies. Eur J Obstet Gynaecol Reprod Biol 1988;27:227–236.
80. Taufield PA, Ales KL, Resnick LM, et al. Hypocalciuria in preeclampsia. N Engl J Med 1987;316:715–718.
81. Frenkel Y, Barkai G, Maschiach S, et al. Hypocalciuria of preeclampsia is independent of parathyroid hormone level. Obstet Gynecol 1991;77:689–691.
82. August P, Marcaccio B, Gertner JM, et al. Abnormal 1,25-dihydroxyvitamin D metabolism in preeclampsia. Am J Obstet Gynecol 1992;166:1295–1299.
83. Seely EW, Wood RJ, Brown EM, et al. Lower serum ionized calcium and abnormal calciotropic hormone levels in preeclampsia. J Clin Endocrinol Metab 1992;74:1436–1440.
84. Ohara N, Yamasaki M, Morikawa H, et al. Dynamics on the calcium metabolism and calcium-regulating hormones in pregnancy-induced hypertension. Folia Endocrinol Jap 1986;62:882–896.
85. August P, Marcaccio B, Gertner JM, et al. Abnormal 1,25-dihydroxyvitamin D metabolism in preeclampsia. Am J Obstet Gynecol 1992;166:1295–1299.
86. Sanchez-Ramos L, Jones DC, Cullen MT. Urinary calcium as an early marker for preeclampsia. Obstet Gynecol 1991;77:685–688.

87. López-Jaramillo P, Terán E, Moncada S. Calcium supplementation prevents pregnancy-induced hypertension by increasing the production of vascular nitric oxide. Med Hypoth 1995;45:68–72.
88. Luckhoff A, Pohl U, Mulsch A, et al. Differential role of extra- and intracellular calcium in the release of EDRF and prostacyclin from culture endothelial cells. Br J Pharmacol 1988;95:189–196.
89. Palmer RMJ, Moncada S. A novel citrulline forming enzyme implicated in the formation of nitric oxide by vascular endothelial cells. Biochem Biophys Res Commun 1989;158:348–352.
90. Bucher HC, Guyatt GH, Cook RJ, et al. Effect of calcium supplementation on pregnancy-induced hypertension and preeclampsia: a meta-analysis of randomized controlled trials. JAMA 1996;275:1113–1117.
91. Aikawa JK. Magnesium: its biologic significance. Boca Raton, FL: CRC Press, 1981.
92. Wester PO. Magnesium. Am J Clin Nutr 1987;45:1305–1312.
93. Garfinkel L, Garfinkel D. Magnesium regulation of the glycolic pathway and the enzymes involved. Magnesium 1985;4:60–72.
94. Wacker WEC. Magnesium metabolism. N Engl J Med 1968;278:658–660.
95. Lee MI, Todd HM, Bowe A. The effect of magnesium sulphate infusion on blood pressure and vascular responsiveness during pregnancy. Am J Obstet Gynecol 1984;149:705–708.
96. Zofkova I, Kancheva RL. The relationship between magnesium and calciotropic hormones. Magnes Res 1995;8:77–84.
97. Schwartz R, Apgar BJ, Wien EM. Apparent absorption and retention of Ca, Cu, Mg, Mn, and Zn from a diet containing bran. Am J Clin Nutr 1986;43:444–455.
98. Hardwick LL, Jones MR, Brautbar N, et al. Magnesium absorption: mechanism and the influence of vitamin D, calcium, and phosphate. J Nutr 1991;121:13–23.
99. Macy IG, Hunscher HA. An evaluation of maternal nitrogen and mineral needs during embryonic and infant development. Am J Obstet Gynec 1934;27:878–880.
100. National Research Council. Recommended dietary allowances. 10th ed. Washington, DC: National Academy Press, 1989:187–194.
101. Morgan KJ, Stampley GL, Zabik ME, et al. Magnesium and calcium dietary intakes of the US population. J Am Coll Nutr 1985;4:546–550.
102. Lukacsi L, Littner F, Grimes E, et al. Magnesium content of human myometrium and placenta during various stages of gestation, and of different body fluids at term. Magnes Res 1993;6:47–52.
103. Bardicef B, Bardicef O, Sorokin Y, et al. Extracellular and intracellular magnesium depletion in pregnancy and gestational diabetes. Am J Obstet Gynecol 1995;172:1009–1013.
104. Lim P, Jacob E, Dong S, et al. Values for tissue magnesium as a guide in detecting magnesium deficiency. J Clin Pathol 1969;22:417–421.
105. Boston JL, Beauchene RE, Cruikshank DP. Erythrocyte and plasma magnesium during teenage pregnancy: relationship with blood pressure and pregnancy-induced hypertension. Obstet Gynecol 1989;73:169–174.
106. Rosner F, Gorfien PC. Erythrocyte and plasma zinc and magnesium levels in health and disease. J Lab Clin Med 1968;72:213–219.
107. Colussi G, Surian M, DeFerrari ME, et al. The changes in plasma diffusible levels and renal tubular handling of magnesium during pregnancy: a longitudinal study. Bone Miner 1987;2:311–319.
108. Widdowson EM. Changes in body composition during growth. In: Davis JA, Dobbing J, eds. Scientific foundation of pediatrics. London: Heinemann Medical, 1981:330–342.
109. Greer FR. Calcium, phosphorous, magnesium, and the placenta. Acta Paediatr Suppl 1994;405:20–24.
110. Hallak M, Berry SM, Madincea F, et al. Fetal serum and amniotic fluid magnesium concentrations with maternal treatment. Obstet Gynecol 1993;81:185–188.
111. Shaw AJ, Mughal MZ, Maresh MJA, et al. Sodium-dependent magnesium transport across in situ perfused rat placenta. Am J Physiol 1991;261:R369–372.
112. Günther T, Vormann J, Höllriegl V. Effects of amiloride and furosemide on ^{28}Mg transport into fetuses and maternal tissues of rats. Magnes Bull 1988;10:34–37.
113. Barri M, Abbas SK, Pickard DW, et al. Fetal magnesium homeostasis in the sheep. Exp Physiol 1990;75:681–688.
114. Shaw AJ, Mughal MZ, Maresh MJA, et al. Effects of two synthetic parathyroid hormone-related protein fragments on maternofetal transfer of calcium and magnesium and release of cyclic AMP by the in-situ perfused rat placenta. J Endocrinol 1991;129:399–404.
115. Petrie RH. Tocolysis using magnesium sulfate. Semin Perinatol 1981;5:266–273.
116. Altura BM, Altura BT. Magnesium ions and the contraction of vascular smooth muscle; relationship to some vascular diseases. Fed Proc 1981;40:2672–2679.
117. Altura BT, Altura BM. Interactions of Mg and K on cerebral vessels—aspects in view of stroke. Review of present status and new findings. Magnes 1984;3:195–211.
118. Smith LH. Disorders of magnesium metabolism. In: Wyngaarden LH, Smith JB, eds. Cecil textbook of medicine. Philadelphia, PA: WB Saunders, 1982.
119. Lamm CI, Norton KI, Murphy RJ, et al. Congenital rickets associated with magnesium sulphate infusion for tocolysis. J Pediatr 1988;113:1078–1082.
120. Altura BM, Altura BT, Carella D. Magnesium deficiency induced spasm of umbilical vessels: relation to preeclampsia, hypertension, growth retardation. Science 1983;221:376–378.
121. Altura BT, Bruit M, Bloom S, et al. Magnesium dietary intake modulates blood lipid levels and atherogenesis. Proc Natl Acad Sci USA 1990;87:1840–1844.
122. Husain S, Birdsey T, Mughal Z, et al. Effect of diabetes mellitus on magnesium transport in rat placenta. Placenta 1992;13:A24–28.
123. Giavini E, Broccia ML, Prati M. Congenital malformations in offspring of diabetic rats: experimental study on the influence of the diet composition and magnesium intake. Biol Neonate 1990;57:207–217.

124. Skajaa K, Dørup I, Sandstrom B. Magnesium intake and status and pregnancy outcome in a Danish population. Br J Obstet Gynaecol 1991;98:919–928.
125. Handwerker SM, Altura MT, Altura AM. Ionized serum magnesium and potassium levels in pregnant women with preeclampsia and eclampsia. J Reprod Med 1995;40:201–208.
126. Conradt A, Weidinger H, Algayer H. On the role of magnesium in fetal hypertrophy, pregnancy-induced hypertension and pre-eclampsia. Magnes Bull 1984;2:68–72.
127. Spätling L, Spätling G. Magnesium supplementation in pregnancy. A double-blind study. Br J Obstet Gynaecol 1988;95:120–125.
128. Kovács L, Molnár BG, Huhn E, et al. Magnesium substitution in pregnancy: a prospective, randomized double-blind study. Geburtshilfe Frauenheilkd 1988;48:595–600.
129. Sibai BM, Villar MA, Bray E. Magnesium supplementation during pregnancy: a double-blind randomized controlled clinical trial. Am J Obstet Gynecol 1989;161:115–119.
130. Garland HO. New experimental data on the relationship between diabetes mellitus and magnesium. Magnes Res 1992;5:193–202.
131. Minoumi F, Miodovnik M, Tsang RC, et al. Decreased maternal serum magnesium concentration and adverse fetal outcome in insulin-dependent diabetic women. Obstet Gynecol 1987;70:85–88.
132. Minoumi F, Miodovnik M, Tsang RC, et al. Decreased amniotic fluid magnesium concentration in diabetic pregnancy. Obstet Gynecol 1987;69:12–14.
133. Sandstead HH. The role of zinc in human health. In: Hemphill HH, ed. Trace substances in environmental health. Columbia, MO: University of Missouri Press, 1978:37–59.
134. Bettiger WJ, O'Dell BL. A critical physiological role of zinc in the structure and function of biomembranes. Life Sci 1981;28:1425–1429.
135. Keusch G, Wilson C, Waksal S. Nutrition, host defense, and the lymphoid system. In: Gallin JI, Fauci AS, eds. Advances in host defense mechanisms. New York: Plenum, 1983:275–359.
136. Rhodes D, Klug A. Zinc fingers. Sci Am 1993;268(2):56–59.
137. Welsh SO, Marston RM. Zinc levels of the U.S. food supply. Food Technol 1980;36:70–76.
138. Solomons NW. Biologic availability of zinc in humans. Am J Clin Nutr 1982;35:1048–1075.
139. Weismann K. Chelating drugs and zinc. Dan Med Bull 1986;33:208–211.
140. Kuhnert BR, Kuhnert PM, Zarlingo TJ. Associations between placental cadmium and zinc and age and parity in pregnant women who smoke. Obstet Gynecol 1988;71:67–71.
141. Wood RJ, Hanssen DA. Effect of milk and lactose on zinc absorption in lactose-intolerant postmenopausal women. J Nutr 1988;118:982–986.
142. Solomons NW, Jacob RA. Studies on the bioavailability of zinc in humans. IV. Effect of heme and nonheme iron on absorption of inorganic zinc. Am J Clin Nutr 1981;34:475–481.
143. Cousins RJ. Absorption, transport, and hepatic metabolism of copper and zinc: special reference to metallothionein and ceruloplasmin. Physiol Rev 1985;65:238–309.
144. Solomons NW, Cousins RJ. Zinc. In: Solomons NW, Rosenberg IH, eds. Absorption and malabsorption of mineral nutrients. New York: Alan R. Liss, 1984;125–197.
145. Solomons NW. Biologic availability of zinc in humans. Am J Clin Nutr 1982;35:1048–1075.
146. Kilereich S, Christiansen C. Distribution of serum zinc between albumin and α2-macroglobulin in patients with different zinc metabolic disorders. Clin Chem Acta 1986;154:1–6.
147. Wester PO. Tissue zinc at autopsy—relation to medication with diuretics. Acta Med Scand 1980;208:269–271.
148. National Research Council. Recommended dietary allowances. 10th ed. Washington, DC: National Academy Press, 1989;205–213.
149. Chaube S, Nishimura H, Swinyard CA. Zinc and calcium in normal human embryos and fetuses. Arch Environ Health 1973;26:237–240.
150. Swanson CA, King JC. Zinc utilization in pregnant and non-pregnant women fed controlled diets providing the zinc RDA. J Nutr 1982;122:697–707.
151. Solomons NW, Helitzer-Allen DL, Villar J. Zinc needs during pregnancy. Clin Nutr 1986;5:63–71.
152. Rösick U, Rösick E, Brätter P, et al. Determination of zinc in amniotic fluid in normal and high risk pregnancies. J Clin Chem Clin Biochem 1983;21:363–372.
153. Apgar J. Zinc and reproduction. Annu Rev Nutr 1985;5:43–68.
154. Lockitch G, Halstead AC. Pediatric nutrition. In: Soldin SJ, Rifai N, Hicks JMB, eds. Biochemical basis of pediatric disease. Washington, DC: American Association for Clinical Chemistry Press, 1995:30–31.
155. Hambidge KM, Neldner KH, Walraven PA. Zinc, acrodermatitis enteropathica and congenital malformation. Lancet 1975;1:577–578.
156. Scholl TO, Hediger ML, Schall JI, et al. Low zinc intake during pregnancy: its association with preterm and very preterm delivery. Am J Epidemiol 1993;137:1115–1124.
157. McMichael AJ, Dreosti IE, Gibson GT. Maternal zinc status and pregnancy outcome: A prospective study. In: Prasad AS, Dreosti IE, Hetzel BS, eds. Clinical applications of recent advances in zinc metabolism. New York: Alan R. Liss, 1982:53–66.
158. Cherry FF, Sandstead HH, Rojas P, et al. Adolescent pregnancy: associations among body weight, zinc nutriture, and pregnancy outcome. Am J Clin Nutr 1989;50:945–954.
159. Tamura T, Goldenberg RL, Freeberg LE, et al. Maternal serum folate and zinc concentrations and their relationships to pregnancy outcome. Am J Clin Nutr 1992;56:365–370.
160. Mahomed K, James DK, Golding J, et al. Zinc supplementation during pregnancy: a double blind

randomised controlled trial. Br Med J 1989;299(6703): 826–830.
161. Garg HK, Singhal KC, Archad Z. A study of the effect of oral zinc supplementation during pregnancy on pregnancy outcome. Indian J Physiol Pharmacol 1993;37:276–284.
162. Goldenberg RL, Tamura T, Neggers Y, et al. The effect of zinc supplementation on pregnancy outcome. JAMA 1995;274:463–468.
163. Buamah PK, Russell M, Bates M, et al. Maternal zinc status: a determination of central nervous system malformation. Br J Obstet Gynaecol 1984;91:788–790.
164. Ghosh A, Fong LYY, Wan CW, et al. Zinc deficiency is not a cause for abortion, congenital abnormality, and small-for-gestational age infant in Chinese women. Br J Obstet Gynaecol 1985;92:892–898.
165. Milunsky A, Morris JS, Jick H, et al. Maternal zinc and fetal neural tube defects. Teratology 1992;46:341–348.
166. Kirksey A, Wachs TD, Yunis F, et al. Relation of maternal zinc nutriture to pregnancy outcome and infant development in an Egyptian village. Am J Clin Nutr 1994;60:782–792.
167. Bro S, Berendsten H, Norgaard J, et al. Serum zinc and copper concentrations in maternal and umbilical cord blood. Relation to course and outcome of pregnancy. Scand J Clin Lab Invest 1988;48:805–811.
168. Campbell-Brown M, Ward RJ, Haines AP, et al. Zinc and copper in Asian pregnancies—Is there evidence for a nutritional deficiency? Br J Obstet Gynaecol 1985;92:875–885.
169. Vitieri FE. Iron deficiency: ending hidden hunger. Proceedings of a Policy Conference on Micronutrient Malnutrition. WHO, UNICEF, World Bank, CIDA-Canada, USAID, FAO, UNDP, The Task force for Child Survival and Development. Atlanta, GA, 1991.
170. Scholl TO, Hediger ML, Fischer RL, et al. Anemia vs iron deficiency: increased risk of preterm delivery in a prospective study. Am J Clin Nutr 1992;55:985–988.
171. Beard J. Iron deficiency: assessment during pregnancy and its importance in pregnant adolescents. Am J Clin Nutr 1994;59(suppl):502S–510S.
172. Finch CA, Cook JC. Iron deficiency. Am J Clin Nutr 1984;39:471–477.
173. Murphy SP, Calloway DH. Nutrient intakes of women in NHANES II emphasizing trace minerals, fiber, and phytate. J Am Diet Assoc 1986;86:1366–1372.
174. Craig WJ. Iron status in vegetarians. Am J Clin Nutr 1994;59:12335–12375.
175. Bothwell TH. Overview and mechanisms of iron regulation. Nutr Rev 1995;53:237–245.
176. Cook JD, Dassenko SA, Lynch SR. Assessment of the role of nonheme-iron availability in iron balance. Am J Clin Nutr 1991;54:717–722.
177. Hallberg L, Brune M, Erlandsson M, et al. Calcium effect of different amounts on nonheme and heme-iron absorption in humans. Am J Clin Nutr 1991;53:112–119.
178. Cook JD, Dassenko SA, Whittaker P. Calcium supplementation: effect on iron absorption. Am J Clin Nutr 1991;53:106–111.
179. Gillooly M, Bothwell TH, Torrance JD, et al. The effects of organic acids, phytates, and polyphenols on the absorption of iron from vegetables. Br J Nutr 1983;49:331–342.
180. Bothwell TH, Charlton RW, Cook JD, et al. Iron metabolism in man. Oxford: Blackwell Scientific, 1979.
181. National Research Council. Recommended dietary allowances. 10th ed. Washington, DC: National Academy Press, 1989:443–453.
182. Hallberg L, Hogdahl AM, Nilsson L, et al. Menstrual blood loss—a population study. Variation at different ages and attempts to define normality. Acta Obstet Gynecol Scand 1966;45:320–351.
183. National Research Council. Nutrient adequacy: assessment using food consumption surveys. Report of the Subcommittee on Criteria for Dietary Evaluation, Coordinating Committee on Evaluation of Food Consumption Surveys, Food and Nutrition Board, Commission on Life Sciences. Washington, DC: National Academy Press, 1986.
184. Expert Scientific Working Group. Summary of a report on assessment of the iron nutritional status of the United States population. Am J Clin Nutr 1994;60:117–121.
185. Institute of Medicine, Food and Nutrition Board, Committee on Nutritional Status during Pregnancy and Lactation. Nutrition during pregnancy, Part II: Nutrient supplements. Washington, DC: National Academy Press, 1990.
186. Carriaga MR, Skikne BS, Finley B, et al. Serum transferrin receptor for the detection of iron deficiency in pregnancy. Am J Clin Nutr 1991;54:1077–1081.
187. Wada L, King JC. Trace element nutrition during pregnancy. Clin Obstet Gynecol 1994;37:574–586.
188. Vitieri FE, Torun B. Anaemia and physical work capacity. Clin Haematol 1974;3:609–626.
189. Dallman PR. Iron deficiency and the immune response. Am J Clin Nutr 1987;46:329–334.
190. Lozoff B, Brittenham GM. Behavioral aspects of iron deficiency. Prog Haematol 1986;14:23–53.
191. Hallberg L. Iron balance in pregnancy. In: Berger H, ed. Vitamins and mineral in pregnancy and lactation. New York: Raven Press, 1988:115–126.
192. Schwartz WJ, Thurnau GR. Iron deficiency anemia in pregnancy. Clin Obstet Gynecol 1995;38:443–454.
193. Harris ED. New insights into placental iron transport. Nutr Rev 1992;50:329–337.
194. Vanderpuye OA, Kelley LK, Smith CH. Transferrin receptors in the basal plasma membrane of the human placental syncytiotrophoblast. Placenta 1986;7:391–403.
195. Contractor SF, Eaton BM. Role of transferrin in iron transport between maternal and fetal circulation of perfused lobule of human placenta. Cell Biochem Funct 1986;4:69–74.
196. van Dijk JP. Regulatory aspects of placental iron transfer: a comparative study. Placenta 1988;9:215–226.
197. Dumartin B, Canivenc R. Placental iron transfer regulation in the haemophagous region of the badger placenta: ultrastructural localization of ferritin in

trophoblast and endothelial cells. Anat Embryol 1992;185:175–179.
198. Puolakka J. Serum ferritin as a measure of iron stores during pregnancy. Clin Haematol 1985;14:613–628.
199. Milman N, Agger AO, Nielson OJ. Iron status markers and serum erythropoietin in 120 mothers and newborn infants: effect of iron supplementation in normal pregnancy. Acta Obstet Gynecol Scand 1994;73:200–204.
200. Centers for Disease Control. CDC criteria for anemia in children and childbearing aged women. MMWR 1989;38:400–404.
201. Puolakka J, Janne O, Pakarinen A, et al. Serum ferritin as a measure of iron stores during and after normal pregnancy with and without iron supplements. Acta Obstet Gynecol Scand 1980;95:53–56.
202. Farthing MJG. Iron and immunity. Acta Paediatr Scand Suppl 1989;361:44–52.
203. United States Preventive Services Task Force. Routine iron supplementation during pregnancy. JAMA 1993;270:2848–2854.
204. Macgregor MW. Maternal anemia as a factor in prematurity and perinatal mortality. Scot Med J 1963;8:134–140.
205. Reinhardt MC. Maternal anemia in Abidjan: its influence on placenta and newborns. Helv Pediatr Acta 1978;33(suppl):43–63.
206. Bhargava M, Kumar R, Iyer PU, et al. Effect of maternal anemia and iron depletion on foetal stores, birthweight, and gestation. Acta Paediatr Scand 1989;78:321–322.
207. Brabin BJ, Ginny M, Sapau J, et al. Consequences of maternal anemia on outcome of pregnancy in a malaria endemic area in Papua New Guinea. Ann Trop Med Parasitol 1990;84:11–24.
208. Lister UG, Rossiter CE, Chong H. Perinatal mortality. Br J Obstet Gynaecol 1985;92(suppl):86–99.
209. Klein L. Premature birth and maternal prenatal anemia. Am J Obstet Gynecol 1966;83:588–590.
210. Murphy JF, O'Riordan J, Newcombe RG, et al. Relation of haemoglobin levels in first and second trimesters to outcome of pregnancy. Lancet 1986;1:992–994.
211. Garn SM, Ridela SA, Petzoid AS, et al. Maternal hematologic levels and pregnancy outcomes. Semin Perinatol 1981;5:155–162.
212. Lieberman E, Ryan KJ, Monson RR, et al. Association of maternal hematocrit with premature labor. Am J Obstet Gynecol 1988;159:107–114.
213. Knotterus JA, Delgado LR, Knipschild PG, et al. Haematologic parameters and pregnancy outcome: a prospective cohort study in the third trimester. J Clin Epidemiol 1990;43:461–466.
214. Lu ZM, Goldenberg RL, Cliver SP, et al. The relationship between maternal hematocrit and pregnancy outcome. Obstet Gynecol 1991;77:190–194.
215. Klebanoff MA, Shiouo PH, Berendes HW, et al. Facts and artifacts about anemia and preterm delivery. JAMA 1989;262:511–515.
216. Klebanoff MA, Shiouo PH, Selby JV, et al. Anemia and spontaneous preterm birth. Am J Obstet Gynecol 1991;164:59–63.
217. Taylor DJ, Lind T. Haematologic changes during normal pregnancy: iron induced macrocytosis. Br J Obstet Gynaecol 1976;83:760–767.
218. Kullander S, Kallen B. A prospective study of drugs and pregnancy. Acta Obstet Gynecol Scand 1976;55:287–295.
219. Romslo I, Haram K, Sagen N, et al. Iron requirement in normal pregnancy as assessed by serum ferritin, serum transferrin saturation, and erythrocyte protoporphyrin determinations. Br J Obstet Gynaecol 1983;90:101–107.
220. Simmons WK, Cook JD, Bingham KC, et al. Evaluation of a gastric delivery system for iron supplementation in pregnancy. Am J Clin Nutr 1993;58:622–626.
221. Thomson JK, Prien-Larsen JC, Devantier A, et al. Low-dose iron supplementation does not cover the need for iron during pregnancy. Acta Obstet Gynecol Scand 1993;72:93–98.
222. Paintin DB, Thomson AM, Hytten FE. Iron and the haemoglobin level in pregnancy. Br J Obstet Gynaecol 1966;73:181–190.
223. Willoughby MLN. An investigation of folic acid requirements in pregnancy. Br J Haematol 1967;13:503–509.
224. Primbs K. Iron treatment during pregnancy—a comparative study. Geburtshilfe Frauenheilkd 1973;33:552–559.
225. Fleming AF, Martin JD, Hahnel R, et al. Effects of iron and folic acid antenatal supplements on maternal hematology and fetal well-being. Med J Aust 1974;2:429–436.
226. Hemminki E, Rimpela U. A randomized comparison of routine versus selective iron supplementation during pregnancy. J Am Coll Nutr 1991;10:3–10.
227. Institute of Medicine. Iron deficiency anemia: Recommended guidelines for prevention, detection, and management among U.S. children and women of childbearing age. Washington, DC: National Academy Press, 1993.
228. Scholl TO, Hediger ML. Anemia and iron-deficiency anemia: compilation of data on pregnancy outcome. Am J Clin Nutr 1994;59(suppl):492S–501S.
229. Schultink W, Gross R, Gliwitzki M, et al. Effect of daily vs. twice weekly iron supplementation in Indonesian preschool children with low iron status. Am J Clin Nutr 1991;53:112–119.
230. Centers for Disease Control. Preventing lead poisoning in young children: a statement by the Centers for Disease Control. U.S. Dept. of Health and Human Services, 99-2230, 1985:252–255.
231. Needleman HL. Lead at low dose and the behavior of children. Neurotoxicology 1983;4:121–123.
232. Schwartz J, Otto D. Blood lead, hearing thresholds, and neurobehavioral development in children and youth. Arch Environ Health 1987;42:153–160.
233. Yule W, Rutter M. Effect of lead on children's behavior and cognitive performance: a critical review. In: Mahaffey KN, ed. Dietary and environmental lead: human health effects. Amsterdam: Elsevier Science, 1985.
234. Winneke G, Collet W, Lilienthal H. The effects of lead in laboratory animals and environmentally-exposed children. Toxicology 1988;49:219–298.

235. Morrow PE, Beiter H, Amato F, et al. Pulmonary retention of lead: an experimental study in man. Environ Res 1980;21:373–384.
236. Gross SD. Human oral and inhalation exposures to lead: summary of Kehoe balance experiments. J Toxicol Environ Health 1981;8:333–377.
237. Baghurst PA, McMichael A, Vimpani GV, et al. Determinants of blood lead concentration of pregnant women living in Port Pirie and surrounding areas. Med J Aust 1987;146:69–73.
238. DeSilva PE. Determination of lead in plasma and studies on its relationship to lead in erythrocytes. Br J Int Med 1981;38:209–217.
239. Klassen CD. Heavy metal and heavy metal antagonists. In: Gilman AG, Rall TW, Nies AS, eds. The pharmacological basis of therapeutics. New York: Pergamon Press, 1990: 1592–1598.
240. Mushak P. Biologic monitoring of lead exposure in children: Overview of selective biokinetics and toxicology issues. In: Smith MA, Grant LD, Sors AZ, eds. Lead exposure in child development. Boston: Kluwer Academic, 1989:72–74.
241. Cavalleri A, Minoia C, Pozzoli L. Lead in red blood cells and in plasma of pregnant women and their offspring. Environ Res 1978;17:403–408.
242. Goyer RA. Transplacental transport of lead. Environ Health Perspect 1990;89:101–105.
243. Rabinowitz MB, Needleman HL. Temporal trends in the lead concentrations of umbilical cord blood. Science 1982; 216:1429–1431.
244. Mayer-Poken O, Denkhaus W, Konietzko H. Lead content of fetal tissues after maternal intoxication. Arch Toxicol 1986;58:203–204.
245. Alexander FW, Delves HT. Blood lead levels during pregnancy. Int Arch Occup Environ Health 1981;48:35–39.
246. Thompson GN, Robertson EF, Fitzgerald S. Lead mobilization during pregnancy. Med J Aust 1985;143:131–139.
247. Tenenkim M. Poisoning in pregnancy. In: Koren G, ed. Maternal fetal toxicology: a clinician's guide. New York: Marcel Dekker, 1990:80–83.
248. Krigman MR, Mushak P, Bouldin TW. An appraisal of rodent models of lead encephalopathy. In: Roizin L, Sheraki H, Grcevic N, eds. Neurotoxicology. New York: Raven Press, 1997:299–302.
249. Holtzman D, DeVries C, Nguyan H, et al. Maturation of resistance to lead encephalopathy: cellular and subcellular mechanisms. Neurotoxicology 1984;5:167–182.
250. McCauley PT, Bull RT, Tonti AP, et al. The effects of prenatal and postnatal lead exposure on neonatal synaptogenesis in rat cerebral cortex. J Toxicol Environ Health 1982;10:639–651.
251. Regan CM, Cookman GR, Keane GT. The effects of chronic low-level lead exposure on the early structuring of the central nervous system. In: Smith MA, Grant LD, Sors A, eds. Lead exposure and child development: an international assessment. Boston: Kluwer Academic, 1989:100–103.
252. Thomas JH, Gillham B. Wills' biochemical basis of medicine. 2nd ed. London: Wright, 1989.
253. Gilbert SG, Rice DC. Low-level lifetime lead exposure produces behavioral toxicity (spatial discrimination reversal) in adult monkeys. Toxicol Appl Pharmacol 1987; 91:484–490.
254. Cookman GR, Hemmens SE, Keane F, et al. Chronic low level lead exposure precociously induces rat glial development in vitro and in vivo. Neurosci Lett 1988;86: 33–37.
255. Ernhart C, Morrow-Tlucak M, Wolf A, et al. Low level lead exposure in the prenatal and early preschool periods: intelligence prior to school entry. Neurotoxicol Teratol 1989;11:161–170.
256. Cooney G, Bell A, McBride W, et al. Neurobehavioral consequences of prenatal low level exposures to lead. Dev Med Child Neurol 1989;11:95–104.
257. Baghurst P, McMichael A, Wigg N, et al. Environmental exposure to lead and children's intelligence at age of seven years. The Port Pirie cohort study. N Engl J Med 1992; 327:1279–1284.
258. Bellinger D, Stiles K, Needleman H. Low-level lead exposure, intelligence, and academic achievement: a long-term follow-up study. Pediatrics 1992;90:855–861.
259. Dietrich K, Berger O, Succop P, et al. The developmental consequences of low to moderate prenatal and postnatal lead exposure: intellectual attainment in the Cincinnati Lead Study cohort following school entry. Neurotoxicol Teratol 1993;15:37–44.
260. Wasserman G, Graziano J, Factor-Litvak P, et al. Consequences of lead exposure and iron supplementation on childhood development at age 4 years. Neurotoxicol Teratol 1994;16:233–240.
261. Dietrich K, Succop P, Berger O, et al. Lead exposure and the cognitive development of urban preschool children: the Cincinnati Lead Study cohort at age 4 years. Neurotoxicol Teratol 1991;13:203–211.
262. Dietrich K, Succop P, Berger O, et al. Lead exposure and the central auditory processing abilities and cognitive development of urban children: the Cincinnati Lead Study cohort at age 5 years. Neurotoxicol Teratol 1992;14:51–56.
263. World Health Organization. Environmental health criteria on inorganic lead. Geneva: WHO, 1995.
264. Schwartz J. Low-level lead exposure and children's IQ: a meta-analysis and search for a threshold. Environ Res 1994;65:42–55.
265. Needleman H, Rabinowitz M, Leviton A, et al. The relationship between prenatal exposure to lead and congenital anomalies. JAMA 1984;251:2956–2959.
266. Ernhart C, Wolf A, Kennard M, et al. Intrauterine exposure to low levels of lead: the status of the neonate. Arch Environ Health 1986;41:287–291.
267. McMichael A, Vimpani G, Robertson E, et al. The Port Pirie cohort study: maternal blood lead and pregnancy outcome. J Epidemiol Commun Health 1986;40:18–25.
268. Levine F, Muenke M. VACTERL association with high prenatal lead exposure: similarities to animal models of lead teratogenicity. Pediatrics 1991;87:390–392.
269. Aschengrau A, Zierler S, Cohen A. Quality of community drinking water and the occurrence of late adverse pregnancy outcomes. Arch Environ Health 1993;48: 105–113.

270. Fahim MS, Fahim Z, Hall OG. Effects of subtoxic lead levels on pregnant women in the State of Missouri. Res Commun Chem Pathol Pharmacol 1976;13:309–331.
271. Angell NF, Lavery JP. The relationship of blood lead levels to obstetric outcome. Am J Obstet Gynecol 1982; 142:40–46.
272. McMichael AJ, Vimpani GV, Robertson EF, et al. The Port Pirie cohort study: maternal blood lead and pregnancy outcome. J Epidemiol Community Health 1986;40:18–25.
273. Moore MR, Goldberg A, Pocock SJ, et al. Some studies of maternal and infant lead exposure in Glasgow. Scott Med J 1982;27:113–122.
274. Factor-Litvak P, Graziano JH, Kline JK, et al. A prospective study of birthweight and length of gestation in a population surrounding a lead smelter in Kosovo, Yugoslavia. Int J Epidemiol 1991;3:722–728.
275. Ward NI, Watson R, Bryce-Smith D. Placental element levels in relation to fetal development for obstetrically 'normal' births: a study of 37 elements. Evidence for effects of cadmium, lead, and zinc on fetal growth, and for smoking as a source of cadmium. Int J Biosoc Res 1987; 9:63–81.
276. Dietrich KN, Krafft KM, Bornschein RL, et al. Low-level fetal lead exposure effect on neurobehavioral development in early infancy. Pediatrics 1987;80:721–730.
277. Bogden JD, Thind IS, Louria DB, et al. Maternal and cord blood metal concentrations and low birth weight—a case control study. Am J Clin Nutr 1978;31:1181–1187.
278. Bornschein RL, Grote J, Mitchell T, et al. Effects of prenatal lead exposure on infant size at birth. In: Smith MA, Grante LD, Sors AI, eds. Lead exposure and child development: an international development. Lancaster, UK: Kluwer, 1988:307–319.
279. Monaco AP, Chelly J. Menkes and Wilson diseases. Adv Genet 1995;33:233–253.
280. Solomons NW. Biochemical, metabolic, and clinical role of copper in human nutrition. J Am Coll Nutr 1985;4:83–105.
281. Evans GW. Copper homeostasis in the mammalian system. Physiol Rev 1973;53:535–570.
282. Turnlund JR, Keyes WR, Anderson HL, et al. Copper absorption and retention in young men at three levels of dietary copper using stable ^{65}Cu. Am J Clin Nutr 1989;49: 870–878.
283. Jacob RA, Skala JH, Omaye ST, et al. Effect of varying ascorbic acid intakes on copper absorption and ceruloplasmin levels of young men. J Nutr 1987;117:2109–2115.
284. Festa MD, Anderson HL, Dowdy RP, et al. Effect of zinc intake on copper excretion and retention in men. Am J Clin Nutr 1985;41:285–292.
285. Delves HT. The microdetermination of copper in plasma protein fraction. Clin Chem Acta 1976;71:495–500.
286. Johnson NC. Study of copper and zinc metabolism during pregnancy. Proc Soc Exp Biol Med 1961;108:518–519.
287. Dancis A, Yuan DS, Haile D, et al. Molecular characterization of a copper transport protein in S. cerevisiae: an unexpected role for copper in iron transport. Cell 1994;76:393–402.
288. Lewis KO. The nature of the copper complexed in the bile and their relationship to the absorption and excretion of copper in normal subjects and Wilson's disease. Gut 1973; 14:221–232.
289. Klevay LM, Reck RA, Jacob GM, et al. The human requirement for copper. I. Healthy men fed conventional American diets. Am J Clin Nutr 1980;33:45–50.
290. Shaw JCL. Copper deficiency and non-accidental injury. Arch Dis Child 1988;63:448–455.
291. Menkes JH. Kinky hair disease: twenty-five years later. Brain Dev 1988;10:77–79.
292. Brewer GJ, Yuzbasiyan-Gurkan V. Wilson disease: an update, with emphasis on new approaches to treatment. Dig Dis 1989;7:178–193.
293. Beck J, Enders J, Schliephacke M, et al. X; 1 translocation in a female Menkes patient: characterization by fluorescence in situ hybridization. Clin Genet 1994;46:295–298.
294. Bowcock AM, Tomfohrede J, Weissenbach J, et al. Refining the position of Wilson disease by linkage disequilibrium with polymorphic microsatellites. Am J Hum Genet 1994;54:79–87.
295. Davies NT, Williams RB. The effect of pregnancy on the uptake and distribution of copper in the rat. Proc Nutr Soc 1976;35:4A–5A.
296. Allen LH. Trace minerals and outcome of human pregnancy. Clin Nutr 1986;5:72–77.
297. Damsgaard E, Horn N, Heydorn K. Trace elements in the placentas of normal foetuses and male foetuses with Menkes disease determined by neutron activation analysis. In: Bratter P, Schramel P, eds. Trace element-analytical chemistry in medicine and biology, vol. 2. New York: Walter de Gruyter, 1983:499–506.
298. Shaw JCL. Trace elements in the fetus and young infant. II. Copper, manganese, selenium, and chromium. Am J Dis Child 1980;134:74–81.
299. Hall GA, Howell J. The effect of copper deficiency on reproduction in the female rat. Br J Nutr 1969;23:41–47.
300. Morton MS, Elwood PC, Abernathy M. Trace elements in water and congenital malformation of the central nervous system in South Wales. Br J Prev Soc Med 1976;30:36–39.
301. Vir SC, Love AHG, Thompson W. Serum and hair concentrations of copper during pregnancy. Am J Clin Nutr 1981;34:2382–2388.
302. Hodge HC, Smith FA. Minerals: fluorine and dental caries. In: Gould RF, ed. Dietary chemicals vs. dental caries. Advances in Chemistry Series No. 94. Washington, DC: American Chemical Society, 1970:93–115.
303. Milne DB, Schwartz K. Effect of different fluorine compounds on growth and bone fluoride levels in rats. In: Hoekstra WG, Suttie JW, Ganther HE, et al., eds. Trace element metabolism in animals. Baltimore: University Park Press, 1974;710–714.
304. Messer HH, Armstrong WD, Singer L. Influence of fluoride intake on reproduction in mice. J Nutr 1973;103: 1319–1326.
305. Weber CW, Reid BL. Effect of low-fluoride diets fed to mice for six generations. In: Hoekstra WG, Suttie JW, Ganther HE, et al., eds. Trace element metabolism in

animals. Baltimore: University Park Press, 1974:707–709.
306. Tao S, Suttie JW. Evidence for a lack of an effect of dietary fluoride level on reproduction in mice. J Nutr 1976;106:1115–1122.
307. Burt BA. The epidemiologic basis for water fluoridation in the prevention of dental caries. J Public Health Policy 1982;3:391–407.
308. Singer L, Ophaug RH, Harland BF. Fluoride intake of young male adults in the United States. Am J Clin Nutr 1980;33:328–332.
309. National Research Council. Recommended dietary allowances. 10th ed. Washington, DC: National Academy Press, 1989:235–240.
310. Full CA, Parkins FM. Effect of cooking vessel composition on fluoride. J Dent Res 1975;54:192–195.
311. Cremer H-D, Büttner W. Absorption of fluorides. In: Fluoride and human health. Geneva: World Health Organization, 1970:75–89.
312. Whitford GM, Pashley DH. Fluoride absorption: the influence of gastric acidity. Calcif Tissue Int 1984;58:2058–2065.
313. Whitford GM. The metabolism and toxicity of fluoride. Monographs in oral science 13. Basel: Karger, 1989.
314. Whitford GM, Reynolds KE, Pashley DH. Acute fluoride toxicity: influence of metabolic alkalosis. Toxicol Appl Pharmacol 1979;50:31–39.
315. Whitford GM. Intake and metabolism of fluoride. Adv Dent Res 1994;8:5–14.
316. Council on Dental Therapeutics. Fluoride compounds. In: Accepted dental therapeutics, 39th ed. Chicago: American Dental Association, 1982:344–368.
317. Fassman DK. Prenatal fluoridation. NY State Dent J 1993;59:47–51.
318. Gedalia I, Brzezinski A, Bercovici B, et al. Placental transfer of fluorine in the human fetus. Proc Soc Exp Biol Med 1961;106:147–149.
319. Bawden JW, Wolkoff AS, Flowers CE. Placental transfer of F-18 in sheep. J Dent Res 1964;43:678–680.
320. Ericsson SY, Malmans CL. Placental transfer of fluoride investigated with F-18 in man and rabbit. Acta Obstet Gynecol Scand 1962;41:144–150.
321. Shen YW, Taves DR. Fluoride concentration in the human placenta and maternal and cord blood. Am J Obstet Gynecol 1974;119:205–207.
322. Caldera R, Chavinie J, Laurent AM, et al. Preliminary study on transplacental transfer of fluoride. J Gynecol Obstet Biol Reprod (Paris) 1986;15:731–735.
323. Shimonovitz S, Patz D, Ever-Hadani P, et al. Umbilical cord fluoride serum levels may not reflect fetal fluoride status. J Perinat Med 1995;23:279–282.
324. Maduska AL, Ahokas RA, Anderson GD, et al. Placental transfer of intravenous fluoride in the pregnant ewe. Am J Obstet Gynecol 1980;136:84–86.
325. Ericsson SY, Ullberg S. Autoradiographic investigation of distribution of F-18 in mice and rats. Acta Odont Scand 1958;16:363–370.
326. Gedalia I, Brzezinski A, Zukerman H, et al. Placental transfer of fluoride in the human fetus at low and high fluoride intake. J Dent Res 1964;43:669–680.
327. Ron M, Singer L, Menczel J, et al. Fluoride concentration in amniotic fluid and fetal cord and maternal plasma. Eur J Obstet Gynecol Reprod Biol 1986;21:213–218.
328. Brambilla E, Belluomo G, Malerba A, et al. Oral administration of fluoride in pregnant women, and the relation between concentration in maternal plasma and in amniotic fluid. Archs Oral Biol 1994;39:991–994.
329. Speirs RL. The value of prenatally administered fluoride. Dent Update 1983;3:43–51.
330. Gray HS. A morphological study of the influence of fluoride on rat molar teeth. Arch Oral Biol 1973;18:1451–1455.
331. Glenn F. Immunity conveyed by a sodium fluoride supplement during pregnancy. Part II. J Dent Child 1979;46:17–19.
332. Blayney JR, Hill IN. Evanston dental caries study. XXIV Prenatal fluorides—value of waterborne fluorides during pregnancy. J Am Dent Assoc 1964;69:291–294.
333. Tank G, Storvick CA. Caries experience of children one to six years old in two Oregon communities (Corvallis and Albany) I. Effect of fluoride on caries experience and eruption of teeth. J Am Dent Assoc 1964;69:749–757.
334. Carlos JP, Gittlesohn AM, Haddon W. Caries in deciduous teeth in relation to maternal ingestion of fluoride. Public Health Rep 1962;77:658–660.
335. Horowitz H, Heifetz S. Effects of prenatal exposure to fluoridation on dental caries. Public Health Rep 1967;82:297–303.
336. Katz S, Muhler J. Prenatal and postnatal fluoride and dental caries experience in deciduous teeth. J Am Dent Assoc 1968;76:305–311.
337. Kailis DG, Taylor SR, Davis GB, et al. Fluoride and caries observations on the effects of prenatal and postnatal fluoride on some Perth pre-school children. Med J Aust 1968;2:1037–1040.
338. Prichard JL. The prenatal and postnatal effects of fluoride supplements on West Australian school children aged 6, 7, and 8, Perth, 1967. Aust Dent J 1969;14:335–338.
339. Glenn FB, Glenn WD, Duncan RC. Fluoride tablet supplementation during pregnancy for caries immunity: a study of the offspring produced. Am J Obstet Gynecol 1982;143:560–564.
340. Teuscher GW. Editorial. J Dent Child 1981;48:2.
341. Erickson D. Water fluorination and congenital malformations: no association. J Am Dent Assoc 1976;93:981–986.
342. Martin C. Effect of fluoride on murine chromosomes. J Dent Res 1978;57:212–215.
343. Wada L, King JC. Trace element nutrition during pregnancy. Clin Obstet Gynecol 1994;37:574–586.
344. Hetzel BS. An overview of the prevention and control of iodine deficiency disorders. In: Hetzel BS, Dunn JT, Stanbury JB, eds. The prevention and control of iodine deficiency disorders. Amsterdam: Elsevier, 1987:7–34.
345. DeLong GR. Effects of nutrition on brain development in humans. Am J Clin Nutr Suppl 1993;57:286S–290S.
346. National Research Council. Recommended dietary allowances. 10th ed. Washington, DC: National Academy Press, 1989:213–217.

347. Pennington JAT, Young BE, Wilson DB. Nutritional elements in U.S. diets: results from the Total Diet Study, 1982 to 1986. J Am Diet Assoc 1989;89:659–664.
348. Dunn JT. Iodine supplementation and the prevention of cretinism. Ann NY Acad Sci 1993;678:158–168.
349. Hall R, Richards CJ, Lazarus JH. The thyroid and pregnancy. Br J Obstet Gynaecol 1993;100:512–515.
350. Burrow GN. The thyroid gland and reproduction. In: Yen Sc, Jaffee RB, eds. Reproductive endocrinology. Philadelphia: Saunders, 1986:424–440.
351. Burrow GN. Thyroid function and hyperfunction during gestation. Endocr Rev 1993;14:194–202.
352. Glinoer D. Maternal thyroid function in pregnancy. J Endocrinol Invest 1993;16:374–378.
353. Beckers C. Reinwein D. The thyroid and pregnancy. Stuttgart: Schattauer, 1991.
354. Hetzel BS. Iodine deficiency disorders (IDD) and their eradication. Lancet 1983;2:1126–1129.
355. DeLong GR, Stanbury JB, Fierro-Benitez R. Neurologic signs in congenital iodine-deficiency disorder (endemic cretinism). Dev Med Child Neurol 1985;27:317–324.
356. Pharoah POD. Geographical variation in the clinical manifestations of endemic cretinism. Trop Geograph Med 1976;28:259–267.
357. Ma T, Wang YY, Wang D, et al. Neuropsychological studies in iodine deficiency areas in China. In: DeLong GR, Robbins J, Condliffe PG, eds. Iodine and the brain. New York: Plenum, 1989;259–268.
358. Potter BJ, Mano MT, Belling GB, et al. Retarded fetal brain development resulting from severe dietary iodine deficiency in sheep. Neuropath Appl Neurobiol 1982; 8:303–313.
359. MeIntosh GH, Potter BJ, Mano M, et al. The effect of maternal and fetal thyroidectomy on fetal brain development in the sheep. Neuropathol Appl Neurobiol 1983;9:215–223.
360. Mano MT, Potter BJ, Belling GB, et al. Fetal brain development in response to iodine deficiency in a primate model. J Neurol Sci 1987;79:287–300.
361. Comite F, Burrow GN, Jorgensen EC. Thyroid hormone analogs and fetal goiter. Endocrinology 1978;102:1670–1674.
362. Shepard TH. Onset of function in the human fetal thyroid: biochemical and radioautographic studies from organ culture. J Clin Endocrinol Metab 1967;27:945–958.
363. Pharoah POD, Connolly KJ. Iodine and brain development. Dev Med Child Neurol 1995;38:464–469.
364. Pharoah POD, Buttfield IH, Hetzel BS. Neurologic damage to the fetus resulting from severe iodine deficiency during pregnancy. Lancet 1971;1:308–310.
365. Thilly CH. Psychomotor development in regions with endemic goiter. In: Hetzel BS, Smith RM, eds. Fetal brain disorders: recent approaches to the problem of mental deficiency. Amsterdam: Elsevier, 1981:265–282.
366. Hetzel BS. Progress in the prevention and control of iodine deficiency disorders. Lancet 1987;2:266–269.
367. Rotruck JT, Pope AL, Ganther HE, et al. Selenium: biochemical role as a component of glutathione peroxidase. Science 1973;179:588–590.
368. Levander OA, Burk RF. Selenium. In: Shils ME, Olson JA, Shike M, eds. Modern nutrition in health and disease. 8th ed. Philadelphia: Lea & Febiger, 1994:242–251.
369. Barrington JW, Lindsay P, James D, et al. Selenium deficiency and miscarriage: A possible link? Br J Obstet Gynaecol 1996;103:130–132.
370. National Research Council. Recommended dietary allowances. 10th ed. Washington, DC: National Academy Press, 1989:217–222.
371. Pennington JAT, Young BE, Wilson DB. Nutritional elements in U.S. diets: results from the Total Diet Study, 1982 to 1986. J Am Diet Assoc 1989;89:659–664.
372. Levander OA. Considerations on the assessment of selenium status. Fed Proc 1985;44:2579–2583.
373. Levander OA, Burk RF. Report of the 1986 ASPEN Research Workshop on Selenium in Clinical Nutrition. J Parenter Enter Nutr 1986;10:545–549.
374. Keshan Disease Research Group. Epidemiologic studies on the etiologic relationship of selenium and Keshan disease. Chin Med J 1979;92:477–482.
375. Fleming CR, Lie JT, McCall JT, et al. Selenium deficiency and fatal cardiomyopathy in a patient on home parenteral nutrition. Gastroenterology 1982;83:689–693.
376. Institute of Medicine, Food, and Nutrition Board. Committee on Nutritional Status during Pregnancy and Lactation. Nutrition during Pregnancy. Part II: Nutritional Supplements. Washington, DC: National Academy Press, 1990.
377. Zachara BA, Wardak C, Didkowski W, et al. Changes in blood selenium and glutathione concentrations and glutathione peroxidase activity in human pregnancy. Gynecol Obstet Invest 1993;35:12–17.
378. Shennan DB, Boyd CAR. Review article: placental handling of trace elements. Placenta 1988;9:333–343.
379. Levander OA. Selenium. In: Mertz W, ed. Trace elements in human and animal nutrition. 5th ed. Orlando: Academic Press, 1986;2:209–279.
380. Stuart LD, Oehme FW. Environmental factors in bovine and porcine abortion. Vet Hum Toxicol 1982;24:435–441.
381. Güvenç H, Karatas F, Güvenç M, et al. Low levels of selenium in mothers and their newborns with a neural tube defect. Pediatrics 1995;95:879–882.
382. Roy AC, Ratnam SS, Karunanithy R. Amniotic fluid selenium status in pre-eclampsia. Amniotic fluid selenium status in pre-eclampsia. Gynecol Obstet Invest 1989;28:161–162.
383. Lu BY, Zhang SW, Liu WF, et al. Changes of selenium in patients with pregnancy induced hypertension. Clin J Obstet Gynecol 1990;25:325–327.
384. Han L, Zhou SM. Selenium supplement in the prevention of pregnancy induced hypertension. Clin Med J 1994;107:870–871.

15
Energy Metabolism During Pregnancy

John V.G.A. Durnin

It would appear self-evident that when a woman becomes pregnant she will need extra amounts of energy, protein, and other nutrients to meet the increasing demands of the fetal and maternal tissues. Although the amount of the extra energy can be calculated on a theoretical basis with a considerable degree of precision, the actual increase in the energy content of the diet of a pregnant woman seldom seems to match this theoretical quantity. Controversy has existed for many years about whether it would be expected that a woman should eat the amount of extra food energy apparently required, or whether some degree of compensation might occur, for example in a reduction of physical activity or a diminution in basal metabolic rate (BMR), which would lessen the requirement. There is a remarkable scarcity of extensive well-controlled longitudinal studies of this important problem, but most published work suggests that the actual extra energy intake in the diet during pregnancy seldom seems to approach these theoretical requirements. The extra energy and nutrients required by pregnancy can be subdivided into what Hytten and Chamberlain[1] describe as "capital gains" and "running costs."

Energy Cost of Pregnancy—"Capital Gains"

The capital gains comprise the many kinds of additions that are being made to the mother's body during pregnancy: the fetus is growing; the uterus increases in size; the placenta has to be formed; there is a considerable increase in body fluids, including the blood; the breasts grow larger; and a variable amount of fat is deposited, primarily as an energy store for lactation and possibly for late pregnancy. All of these changes involve an energy cost, and this has been quantified for the various components by Hytten and Leitch[2] and subsequently by Hytten and Chamberlain[1] with more or less general acceptance of their calculations (Table 15.1).

Increased Fat Stores in Mother and Their Energy Cost

A large and highly variable constituent in this array is the amount of adipose tissue added to the mother's body. One of the main sources of error in assessing the energy requirements of pregnancy lies in estimating the energy cost of depositing the extra fat that is normally laid down during pregnancy. This is difficult to measure quantitatively, and estimates vary about the amount of energy needed to deposit the extra fat. When fat is added to the body it is deposited not just as fat, or chemical lipid within the fat cell; the enlargement of the fat cells results in an increase in the mass of the cell membranes and there is also an increase in the supportive tissue, so that there is a greater amount of connective tissue and of extracellular fluid. The total mass of these tissues, other than fat, accounts for 10% to 30% of the total mass of additional adipose tissue. If an attempt is made to measure this alteration in the energy stores, most methods assess only the lipid fraction and not the total adipose tissue, because measurements of "fatness" done by densitometry, total body water, total body potassium, impedance, skinfold thickness, etc., depend on basic assumptions about the composition of the fat-free mass (FFM), e.g., that the density of the FFM is 1100 kg L3, the water content of the FFM is 72% of the mass, the K content is $60 mmol \cdot kg^{-1} FFM^{-1}$. The fat mass is simply the difference between the total body mass and the FFM; for example, a 50-kg woman whose FFM was 40 kg might have 10 kg of fat. If she added 10 kg of weight to her body and her FFM was measured at 47 kg, her fat mass would then be 60 minus 47 kg, i.e., 13 kg, showing an increase in fat content of 3 kg. The actual energy cost of depositing fat or lipid within the fat cell is about $10,000 kcal \cdot kg^{-1}$ [41.8 megajoule (MJ)], which includes the actual energy content of the lipid [$7000 kcal \cdot kg^{-1}$ (29.3 MJ)] together with the physiologic cost involved in the transformation. Since the measurement of this increase is a measurement

TABLE 15.1. Mean weight gain and energy costs at two levels of maternal fat gain.

	Weight (kg)	Energy costs (kcal)	(MJ)
Fetus	3.5	8300	34.9
Placenta	0.6	700	3.0
Uterus, fluids, and breasts	5.0	3000	12.6
Fat gain	2.0	22,000	92.4
	5.0	55,000	231.0
Total for tissue costs where fat gain was:	2.0 kg	34,000	142
Total for tissue costs where fat gain was:	5.0 kg	67,000	281
BMR		31,000	130
Grand total	2 kg gain	65,000	273
	5 kg gain	98,000	412

of maternal body fat and not of adipose tissue, the energy cost of this fat deposition is taken as 10,000 to 11,000 kcal·kg^{-1} (41.8 to 46.0 MJ). (see Chapter 47)

Importance of Extra Fat Stores

The quantity of fat laid down in pregnancy and its energy equivalent have importance from two viewpoints. First, if it is accepted that there is a physiologic need for a pregnant woman to increase her fat reserves—as a safety factor related to successful lactation—the amount of energy involved in the deposition of 2 to 3 kg of fat constitutes a considerable proportion of the total energy cost of the capital gains of pregnancy, i.e., the energy needed for the growth of the fetal and maternal tissues. This energy is approximately 11 kcal·day^{-1} (46 kJ) or roughly 20,000 to 30,000 kcal (84–126 MJ) for the 2 to 3 kg, which seems to be the average gain for a population of normally nourished young women. It therefore accounts for more than 50% of the total "capital costs." Second, in any group of pregnant women in a developed industrialized society there is much variability in the amount of added fat, and some women blame a large accumulation of fat during pregnancy for their subsequent development of obesity. They find that with each pregnancy the extra weight acquired is not completely lost following delivery, and there is a gradual insidious retention of some of the extra fat.

For women who intend to breast-feed their neonates, the increase in the amount of body fat presumably represents a useful reserve of energy. However, there is no need for this reserve if the mother has no intention of breast-feeding or if she intends to lactate for only 2 or 3 weeks.

Measurement of Fat Deposition

If there is some concern about the amount of the increase in a mother's weight during the period of gestation, it would be useful to measure the actual amount of fat deposition. This can be done using equations that depend on the relationship of skinfold thickness to density and therefore fatness.[3] However, because of the uncertainty attached to the validity of these equations in pregnant women, when alterations may have occurred in the proportions of body fluids and body density, it is easier and more accurate to use a different approach. An assumption has to be made that by 2 to 4 weeks postpartum, the alterations in the composition of the maternal tissues that have taken place as a result of pregnancy will have regressed so that, with the exception of some increase in breast tissue, which will be mainly a reflection of fluctuating amounts of breast milk, and of some adipose tissue, the maternal body composition will have returned to its prepregnant state. Therefore, the difference in the prepregnant mother's weight and her weight 2 to 4 weeks postpartum will represent the change in maternal adipose tissue.

Weight and Fat Gain

Since the total weight gain by the mother may have an influence on weight retention in the postpartum period, it may be useful to examine some comparative data from a longitudinal study on 135 women.[4] When the women were classified into three equal groups according to total weight and fat gain (Table 15.2 and Figure 15.1), those gaining most weight were more likely to retain significant amounts of fat, even after 6 months of lactation. Similar findings have been reported in studies in Scandinavia[5] and the United States.[6] However, neither the woman's initial body weight (Table 15.2) nor the initial fatness (Table 15.3) appear to have much influence on either the total weight or the total fat gain by the mother.

There are social, cultural, and other influences on what is regarded as a desirable amount of fat to gain during pregnancy. Clearly, large differences in the amount of fat added to the body during pregnancy will result in very different requirements of energy. In an industrialized society with ample food availability, Hytten and Chamberlain[1] have suggested 3.5 kg of additional fat as a reasonable average. At the present time, much obstetric advice recommends indirectly a fat gain of about 2 to 2.5 kg.[5] On the other hand, in the United States a total weight gain of up to 16 kg is advised for normal-weight women[7] in order, supposedly, to reduce the likelihood of low birth-weight babies. This would almost certainly involve an addition of 5 kg or more of the fat to the

15. Energy Metabolism During Pregnancy

TABLE 15.2. Mean weight gains, fat gains, and birth weights, including confidence intervals (C.I.) of 135 women divided into tertiles according to initial body weight.

	Group 1	Group 2	Group 3
Number of subjects	45	45	45
Initial weight (kg)	50.1	56.7	65.8
Weight gain (kg)	11.1[a]	13.0	13.4
(C.I.)	(10.1–12.0)	(11.7–14.2)	(12.0–14.8)
% Increase in body weight	22	23	20
Fat gain (kg)	1.9	2.2	2.6
(C.I.)	(1.3–2.5)	(1.5–3.0)	(1.7–3.4)
Birth weight (kg)	3.37	3.41	3.67[b]
(C.I.)	(3.23–3.51)	(3.27–3.56)	(3.51–3.84)

[a] Weight gain of group 1 significantly less than groups 2 and 3, $p < .05$.
[b] Birth weight of group 3 significantly greater from groups 1 and 2, $p < .05$.

prepregnant body stores, with an energy cost of perhaps more than 55,000 kcal (230 MJ). The energy needed for all these increases in fetal and maternal tissues thus involves a quantity varying from about 34,000 to 67,000 kcal (142–280 MJ). Although these estimates of the energy costs required by pregnancy have been derived partly on theoretical grounds, a longitudinal field study on four population groups provides data that fit reasonably well with the theory. This study measured the energy cost of the different components of pregnancy in groups of Scottish,[4] Dutch,[8] Thai,[9] and Filipino[10] women and part of the data is shown in Table 15.5 (vide infra). A brief description of some aspects of these results is given later.

"Running Costs" Including BMR

What has been considered so far has been the energy required to produce the capital gains of pregnancy, i.e., the increase in the mass or volume of all the differing tissues of the maternal body compared to the prepregnant state. There is also another influence on the energy needs, which may be termed the "running costs." The increase in the mass of the maternal body results in a higher BMR and in a greater expenditure of energy in moving the larger body mass around. Figure 15.2 shows data on the BMR of 96 women originally measured in triplicate on three different occasions chosen to represent different stages of the menstrual cycle in the prepregnant women. Measurements were continued at monthly intervals throughout pregnancy and for 6 months postpartum. There was a small nonsignificant increase in BMR during the first 4 to 5 months and a much steeper rise until the end of pregnancy, resulting in a total augmentation of energy expenditure of about 30,000 kcal (126 MJ).

The equivalent value in the Dutch study[8] was just under 35,000 kcal (146 MJ), which, considering the slightly heavier body mass of the Dutch women, was similar to the Scottish data. There was a suggestion in both studies

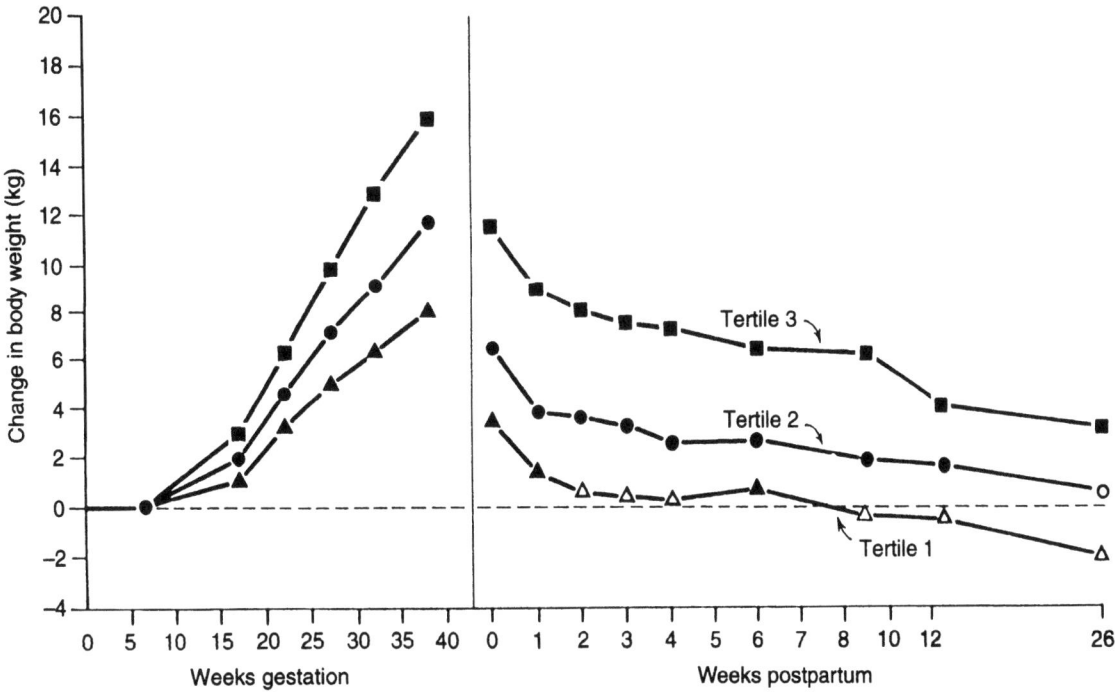

FIGURE 15.1. Change in body weight during pregnancy and up to 6 months postpartum. Filled symbols indicate value is significantly different from initial measurement ($p < .05$).

TABLE 15.3. Mean weight gains, fat gains, and birth weights, including confidence intervals (C.I.) of 135 women divided into tertiles according to initial % body fat.

	Group 1	Group 2	Group 3
n	45	45	45
Initial % fat	21	25	30
Initial weight (kg)	53.7	55.3	63.5
(C.I.)	(51.9–55.4)	(53.8–56.7)	(61.0–66.0)
Weight gain (kg)	11.9	12.5	13.0
(C.I.)	(10.9–12.9)	(11.3–13.8)	(11.6–14.4)
Initial fat mass (kg)	11.3	13.8	19.1
(C.I.)	(10.8–11.9)	(13.4–14.2)	(17.9–20.0)
Gain in fat mass (kg)	2.3	2.5	2.0
(C.I.)	(1.7–2.9)	(1.8–3.1)	(1.4–3.7)
Birth weight (kg)	3.4	3.49	3.56
(C.I.)	(3.25–3.55)	(3.32–3.66)	(3.41–3.70)

that there might have been a slight decrease in the BMR expressed as energy per kilogram of body mass, but this decrease did not obscure the absolute increase in BMR due to the greater body mass as pregnancy progressed. No overall energy saving thus occurred. The physiologic significance of the slight fall in BMR per kilogram of body mass might have no relevance to any improvement of metabolic efficiency, indicating some special adaptation stimulated by pregnancy, but could simply represent the differing metabolic rates of the various tissues being formed in the woman's body (e.g., fluid, fat). These increases in BMR were much lower than the 46,500 kcal (195 MJ) reported in a similar type of study on 19 Swedish women.[11]

Prentice et al.[12] postulated the existence of energy-sparing adaptations in human pregnancy in that thin women demonstrated effects on metabolism that might have been stimulated by low prepregnant fatness. The data on BMR in the Scottish study[4] did not support this hypothesis. A comparison of the influence of the initial body fatness was done by subdividing the 135 women into three groups, with mean initial fat of 21%, 26%, and 31%. The pattern of change in BMR was almost identical in the three groups and none showed any significant fall or rise in BMR until about 21 weeks' gestation, when it increased up to term in a parallel fashion in all three groups. There was much individual variation, with as many fat women showing a fall in BMR during the first 20 weeks as did the thin women.

Total Energy Cost of Pregnancy

Overall, then, the total energy cost of pregnancy, comprising the energy needed to lay down the increased tissue mass, together with the extra energy for the greater BMR, and the large amount of energy for activity, will be from 65,000 kcal (273 MJ) to 98,000 kcal (412 MJ), varying with the amount of the mother's fat gain; the amounts of 2 or 5 kg of fat gain (Table 15.1) are used as examples since they represent amounts that are commonly found in an average population. If these increased energy costs are to be offset in full, then the energy intake in the diet would have to rise by 240 to 360 kcal (1.0 to 1.5 MJ) per day throughout the whole of pregnancy.

Tables 15.4 and 15.5 show equivalent data for weight and fat gain and total energy cost in the four-country study.[4,8–10] It can be seen that the data from Scotland and for the Netherlands are very similar, but they differ from those for Thailand and the Philippines. Table 15.4 illustrates the effect of the initial body mass of these populations on the proportion of weight and of fat

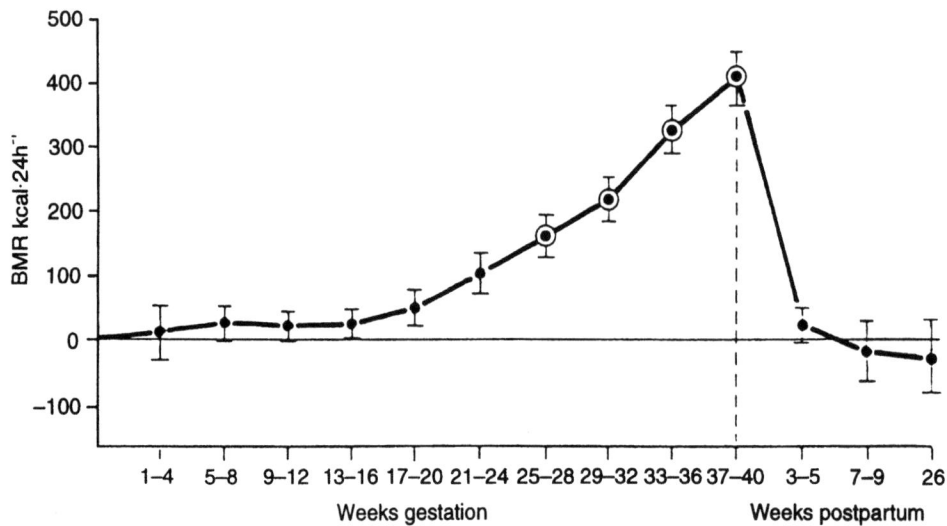

FIGURE 15.2. Increase in BMR throughout pregnancy and during the first 6 months postpartum for 96 women (mean + C.I.).

TABLE 15.4. Weight and fat gain during pregnancy in four-country study.

Country (reference)	Mean (S.E.M.) total weight gain (kg)	Weight gain as % of initial weight	Mean (S.E.M.) fat gain (kg)	Fat gain as % of initial weight
Scotland[4]	11.7 (0.4)	20	2.3 (0.3)	4.0
Netherlands[8]	10.5 (0.5)	17	2.0 (0.3)	3.2
Thailand[9]	8.9 (0.4)	19	1.4 (1.1)	2.9
Philippines[10]	8.5 (0.4)	19	1.3 (0.3)	2.9

gained during pregnancy. In absolute terms the Scottish and Dutch mothers gained more weight and fat than the other groups, but relative to the initial weights of these groups the differences are quite small. If all of the data in Tables 15.4 and 15.5 are standardized for body weight, there are no significant differences in the total energy cost of pregnancy.

A logical conclusion from these data might well be that pregnancy in a normal healthy population necessitates an increased intake of dietary energy of the order of at least 200 to 300 kcal·day^{-1} (approximately 0.8–1.2 MJ).

Any recommendation with an implication that these theoretical values might perhaps be an overestimation of the real requirements is often greeted with horror as potentially jeopardizing the health of this nutritionally very vulnerable group, as we might expect of expert committees concerned with making recommendations. The energy needs of pregnant women recommended for either national or international adoption would almost invariably err on the safe side. Thus, the total energy intake required to replace energy costs, as calculated on the basis given here, should be the amount of energy equivalent to these costs.

Energy Intakes and Requirements

These mainly theoretical recommendations have persisted for so long because of the difficulty of achieving, and the comparative scarcity of, properly controlled scientific observations of the alterations in energy intake occasioned by pregnancy. Until recently, almost all such studies have been largely cross-sectional, so that the same women have not been followed at different stages of pregnancy, the methodology has often not been of satisfactory precision, the sample size has been statistically inadequate to demonstrate reliable findings, and the first set of measurements of food intake has been done late in the first trimester instead of, ideally, in the prepregnant state.

Prepregnant measurements are necessary to provide an absolutely reliable baseline since food intake often falls in the period between gestation weeks 6 to 8 and 12 to 14, presumably due to nausea and morning sickness.

An interesting illustration of the necessity of good baseline data is provided by the study on the energy intakes of pregnant Thai women. In the original investigation[9] the first measurements of energy intakes were done at 10 to 16 weeks' gestation. From this initial level, there was then a gradual increase in energy intake, so that between about 22 and 30 weeks' gestation there was an increment of 300 to 400 kcal·day^{-1} (1.3–1.7 MJ) over the initial measurement, rising to about 500 kcal·day^{-1} (2.1 MJ) at 37 weeks. This result was so out of keeping with other comparable data that a repeat study was undertaken on a slightly larger number of mothers (63 in the second study compared to 44 in the first), and the initial measurements were made before the women became pregnant. It was found that the prepregnant energy intake was 2170 kcal·day^{-1} (9.1 MJ), but by 8 to 12 weeks' gestation the intake had fallen to 1890 kcal·day^{-1} (7.9 MJ). It then gradually increased until by 20 weeks' gestation it was about 150 kcal·day^{-1} (0.63 MJ) higher than in prepregnancy, and it remained approximately at that level until term. However, the extent of this reduction in energy intake during the first few weeks of pregnancy, presumably due to morning sickness, negated the subsequent rise during the second and third trimester, so that the overall increase in energy intake throughout

TABLE 15.5. Energy cost of pregnancy in the four-country study: kcal (MJ).

	Scotland[4]	Netherlands[8]	Thailand[9]	Philippines[10]
Fetus	8100 (34.0)	8190 (34.4)	7100 (29.9)	6880 (28.9)
Placenta	730 (3.05)	740 (3.10)	600 (2.51)	600 (2.51)
Uterus, fluids, and breasts, etc.	2880 (12.1)	2940 (12.3)	2480 (10.4)	2400 (10.1)
Maternal fat	25,200 (106)	21,900 (92.0)	15,330 (64.4)	14,240 (59.8)
BMR	30,000 (126)	34,290 (144)	23,810 (100)	18,810 (79)
Total	66,910 (291)	68,060 (286)	49,320 (208)	42,930 (181)

pregnancy became almost zero. Taking the baseline at 10 to 14 weeks in the first study was producing a quite distorted picture of the real state.

Energy Savings

The conclusion to be reached from the comparatively few published reports where energy intake has been measured at different stages of pregnancy, and particularly from the results obtained by the collaborative project in Scotland, the Netherlands, the Philippines, and Thailand, where the methodology was both comprehensive and carefully standardized,[13,14] would be that, in both industrialized and developing countries, pregnancy appears to necessitate a rather small increase in energy intake, of the order of only 100 to 200 kcal·day^{-1} (420–840 kJ) and even then only in the last 6 to 8 weeks of pregnancy.

There is an enigma here! On the assumption that at least some of the dietary data are valid, and that there has been no increase in energy intake in spite of an increased requirement, this situation could have arisen only if the pregnant mother had been able to reduce her need for the supposed amount of extra energy. She must have been saving energy by some means and presumably this must have excluded using up some of the energy stores of maternal fat, since the assumption has been made that at least 2 kg of fat will have been added to the maternal body. There is no evidence of any reduction in BMR (Figure 15.2) nor in dietary-induced thermogenesis. The only other source of energy saving seems to be via a diminished level of physical activity. While this suggestion might be superficially plausible, there might be some reservations about accepting it unreservedly. In an industrialized society most people—men and women—already lead a relatively sedentary existence and there might be little scope for further reductions in energy expenditure that would be necessary to offset the extra demands of pregnancy.

In developing countries with a predominantly rural economy, most women might be supposed to continue, of necessity, their work in the fields and in tending their households, with little possibility of reducing activity.

Measurement of Energy Intake

The finding that indirectly indicated that some important energy saving must occur during pregnancy—or at least appeared to have been present in the Scottish and Dutch studies—was that the increase in food energy intake was much less than the calculated 240 kcal·day^{-1} (1.0 MJ). However, the validity of the discrepancy between this calculated value and the actual intake depends on how well the field surveys of the food intake of pregnant women were done. For the information from these surveys to be reliable and acceptable, several conditions must be met: (1) The methodology of food intake assessment should be scientifically acceptable. Many reports of food intake have used methods, such as the 24-hour recall, that may suit the convenience of the participant and the investigator, but are too imprecise to allow proper analysis. (2) An appropriate sample size of women is needed, and ideally the measurements should be done before the women become pregnant and should be repeated at suitable intervals throughout the course of pregnancy. (3) Allowance must be made for the normal variability in energy intake that exists within the individual mother, and the investigation must be able to detect differences in energy intake of, at most, about 150 kcal·day^{-1} (0.6 MJ). (4) To obtain data on which we can rely, with a statistical order to the power of 0.9, which might be taken as a desirable biologic level, energy intakes should be assessed during 5 days on about 50 women if we are carrying out a longitudinal survey, or on at least 200 women if it is a cross-sectional survey.

If we accept these statistical requirements, there are almost no studies in the published literature that do not necessitate considerable reservations in the deductions which can be made from their data. This should not necessarily be regarded as a criticism of these investigations. Often they were not specifically designed to examine the energy requirements of pregnancy, although many published reports contain data that might have been expected to provide at least some partial answers to this question. Unfortunately, many studies that report energy intakes of pregnant women 15–21 (Table 15.6) are limited by various deficiencies (e.g., inadequate sample size, and measurements made on only one or two occasions). Only a few studies, such as those on Asian women in Birmingham, England,[22,23] on 71 women from a low socioeconomic group living in Cambridge,[24] on 54 white American women,[25] and the four-country study,[4,8–10] provide data that are relevant to energy needs in pregnancy and are statistically acceptable.

Perhaps it is not surprising that there is such a scarcity of relevant and reliable data. As well as the necessity of repeating the dietary data at several intervals throughout pregnancy, there are also other data that pertain to energy balance, and therefore may indirectly affect the energy intake. These are changes in weight, in body fat stores, BMR, metabolic rate during standardized activity, and activity patterns and energy expenditures.

Possible Influence of Methodology

It has frequently been argued, and it is certainly a possibility, that the mere measurement of energy intake in the diet of an individual may cause an alteration of normal

TABLE 15.6. Reported energy intakes during pregnancy.

Source	n	Gestation stage	Energy intake (kcal/day)
van der Rijst (1962)[27]	499	1st trimester	2620
		2nd trimester	2720
		3rd trimester	2620
English and Hitchcock (1968)[16]	26	2nd trimester	2150
		3rd trimester	2030
Lunnell, Persson, and Sterky (1983)[28]	58	1st trimester	2035
		2nd trimester	2185
		3rd trimester	2137
Blackburn and Calloway (1976)[18]	21	24 weeks	2065
		33 weeks	1801
		39 weeks	2000
Whitehead et al. (1981)[29]	25	2nd trimester	1950
		3rd trimester	2005
Doyle et al. (1982)[30]	68	1st trimester	1613
		2nd trimester	1723
		3rd trimester	1772
Grafe (1983)[31]	89	22 weeks	2753
		34 weeks	2755
Durnin et al. (1987)[4]	162	Prepregnant	2010
		16 weeks	2020
		24 weeks	2030
		32 weeks	2090
		37 weeks	2120
van Raaji et al. (1987)[8]	54	Prepregnant	2160
		16 weeks	2140
		24 weeks	2120
		36 weeks	2200
Schofield, Wheeler, and Stewart (1987)[32]	85	1st trimester	2028
	38	2nd trimester	2059
	107	3rd trimester	1913
Haste et al. (1990)[33]	161	28 weeks	2017
		36 weeks	1924

eating pattern. To investigate further the extent of the discrepancies caused by the variable methodology, the dietary data on the 162 Scottish women were analyzed in subgroups.

Figure 15.3 shows the increase in energy intakes in the Scottish women at various stages of pregnancy. Three groups are illustrated. The first is the entire group of 162 pregnant women. The second group omits 31 women who had energy intakes that were so low as to be unrepresentative of the norm. The third group includes only the women on whom the initial measurements were obtained in the prepregnant state, but here also those with unrepresentative low intakes were excluded; there were 81 women in this group. The three groups show similar patterns, although the total increase in energy intake of the whole group of the 162 women is about 6000 to 7000 kcal (25–29 MJ) less than those of the other groups. This difference is equivalent to about 30 kcal (126 kJ) per day, which is a relatively unimportant quantity. The mean overall increase in energy intake was only about 75 kcal (0.3 MJ) per day, and it was distributed differently during the three trimesters. During the first trimester there was a decrease in intake, presumably due to morning sickness. There was then a gradual increase in energy intake until term, the overall amount of about 75 kcal (0.3 MJ) being considerably less than the theoretical requirement of 240 kcal (1.0 MJ) per day.

Influence of Reduced Physical Activity

It has already been argued that energy savings to offset this difference between actual intakes and the extra requirements must be connected with reduced physical activity. For example, it might be supposed, perhaps on anecdotal evidence, that an increased time in bed, especially in the later stages of pregnancy, would result in a decreased total daily energy expenditure. A reduction in the total duration of physical activity and perhaps a slowing down of such activity as occurs may also be influences. This possibility has been examined with the use of activity diaries, and an attempt was made to record, during

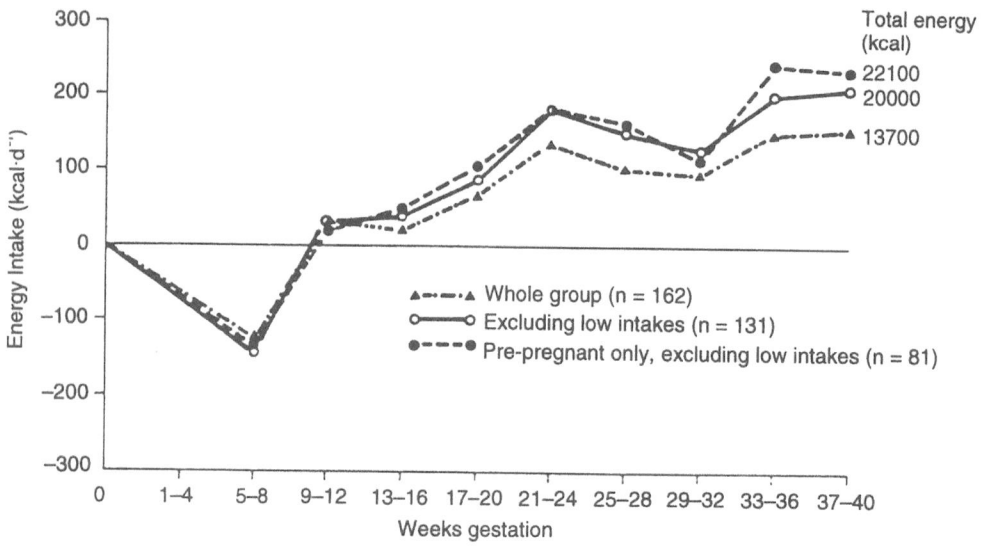

FIGURE 15.3. Energy increments (kcal) throughout pregnancy.

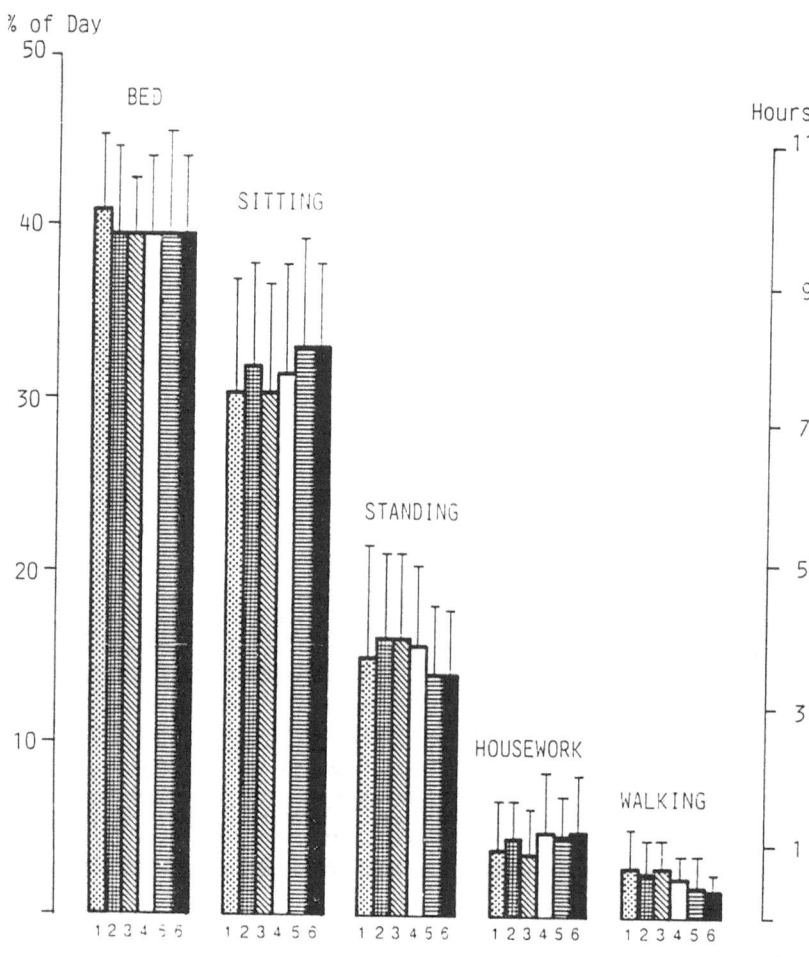

FIGURE 15.4. Average time per day of activities.

TABLE 15.7. Possible energy savings during pregnancy related to changed activity pattern.

	Energy saving	
	kcal·day^{-1}	(kJ·day^{-1})
1 h "standing" replaced by "sitting"	42	(176)
0.5 h "housework" replaced by "sitting"	45	(189)
1 h "sitting" replaced by "lying down"	30	(126)
0.5 h "walking" replaced by "sitting"	48	(202)
Total	165	(693)

several consecutive days and at six different stages of pregnancy, the complete pattern of activity throughout the 24 hours of the day. But as Figure 15.4 shows, the evidence to support this idea is not very persuasive. However, although there was only limited evidence to suggest reduced activity, Table 15.7 shows that reductions could be effective in causing the requisite energy saving and yet be small enough to make detection virtually impossible using any equipment currently available.

It is interesting to note that an earlier study in Papua New Guinea,[26] also demonstrated reductions in physical activity that almost fully compensated for the extra energy cost of both pregnancy and lactation. Although the evidence is not totally convincing, and it is possible that specific population groups of mothers might show different results, the data described here strongly suggest that for an average woman living in a developed country, a very small addition to the prepregnant energy intake could be adequate for the extra energy needs of pregnancy.

The comparatively large number of women who took part in the four-country longitudinal investigation were normal and healthy and behaved normally throughout pregnancy. Their weight gain, fat gain, and the birth weights of their babies were normal. The study was carefully done and did not appear to interfere in any important way with the usual behavior of the mother. The field work was done by postgraduate and postdoctoral research workers trained in nutrition. Almost all of the pregnant woman were highly motivated and diligently supervised. Explanations related to pregnancy in anything other than general terms were avoided in case they might introduce a bias, such as answers to questions about diet in pregnancy. The considerable intraindividual variability in the energy intake from day to day and from one 3- or 5-day period to another makes it highly improbable that there was any consistent bias. Another favorable factor was that this study was an intraindividual comparison in which changes in energy intakes of each individual woman were more important than the absolute values.

Conclusion

A normal pregnant woman living in an industrialized country does not require extra intake of food equivalent to the theoretical energy cost of pregnancy. An allowance of no more than an extra 100 to 150 kcal·day^{-1} (0.4–0.6 MJ) during the second and third trimesters would appear to be at least adequate to cover the energy requirements of pregnancy. Data obtained in the studies in developing countries seem to point to similar conclusions.

References

1. Hytten FE, Chamberlain G. Clinical physiology in obstetrics. Oxford: Blackwell Scientific, 1980.
2. Hytten FE, Leitch I. The physiology of human pregnancy, 2nd ed. Oxford: Blackwell Scientific, 1971.
3. Durnin JVGA, Wormersley J. Body fat assessed from total body density and its estimation from skinfold thickness measurements on 481 men and women aged from 16–72 years. Br J Nutr 1974;32:77–97.
4. Durnin JVGA, McKillop FM, Grant S, et al. Energy requirements of pregnancy in Scotland. Lancet 1987;2:897–900.
5. Rossner S, Ohlin AL. Pregnancy as a risk factor for obesity: lessons from the Stockholm Pregnancy and Weight Development Study. Obes Res 1995;3:1071–1073.
6. Scholl TO, Hediger ML, Schall JI, et al. Gestational weight gain, pregnancy outcome, and post-partum weight retention. Obstet Gynecol 1995;86:423–427.
7. Krasovec K, Anderson MA. Maternal nutrition and pregnancy outcomes: anthropometric assessment. Scientific Publication No. 529. Washington DC: Pan American Health Organization and World Health Organization, 1991.
8. Van Raaji JMA, Vernatt-Miedema SII, Schonk CM, et al. Energy requirements of pregnancy in The Netherlands. Lancet 1987;2:953–955.
9. Thongprasert K, Tamphaichitre V, Valyasevi A, et al. Energy requirements of pregnancy in rural Thailand. Lancet 1987;2:1010–1012.
10. Tuazon MAG, Van Raaji JMA, Hautvast JGAJ, et al. Energy requirements of pregnancy in the Philippines. Lancet 1987;2:1129–1131.
11. Forsum E, Sadurskis A, Wager J. Energy maintenance costs during pregnancy in healthy Swedish women. Lancet 1985;1:107–108.
12. Prentice AM, Goldberg GR, Davies HL, et al. Energy-sparing adaptions in human pregnancy assessed by whole-body calorimetry. Br J Nutr 1989;62:5–22.
13. Durnin JVGA. Energy requirements of pregnancy: an integration of the longitudinal data from the five-country study: Lancet 1987;2:1131–1133.
14. Durnin JVGA. Energy requirements of pregnancy. An integrated study in five countries: background and methods. Lancet 1987;895–896.

15. Thomson AM. Diet in pregnancy. I Dietary survey technique and the nutritive value of diets taken by primigravidae. Br J Nutr 1958;12:446–461.
16. English RM, Hitchcock NE. Nutrient intakes during pregnancy, lactation and after the cessation of lactation in a group of Australian women. Br J Nutr 1968;22:615–624.
17. Emerson K, Saxena BN, Poindexter EL. Caloric cost of normal pregnancy. Obstet Gynecol 1972;40:786–794.
18. Blackburn MW, Calloway DH. Energy expenditure and consumption of mature, pregnant and lactating women. J Am Diet Assoc 1976;69:29–37.
19. Smithells RW, Ankers C, Lennon D, et al. Maternal nutrition in early pregnancy. Br J Nutr 1977;38:497–506.
20. Darke SJ, Disselduff MM, Try GP. Frequency distributions of mean daily intakes of food energy and selected nutrients obtained during nutrition surveys of different groups of people in Great Britain between 1968 and 1971. Br J Nutr 1980;44:243–252.
21. Anderson AS, Whichelow MS. Constipation during pregnancy: dietary fibre intake and the effect of fibre supplementation. Hum Nutr Appl Nutr 1985;39A:202–207.
22. Abraham R, Campbell-Brown M, Haines AP, et al. Diet during pregnancy in an Asian community in Britain—energy, protein, zinc, copper, fibre and calcium. Hum Nutr Appl Nutr 1985;39A:23–25.
23. Eaton PM, Wharton PA, Wharton BA. Nutrient intake of pregnant Asian women at Sorrento Maternity Hospital Birmingham. Br J Nutr 1984;52:457–468.
24. Black AE, Wiles SJ, Paul AA. The nutrient intakes of pregnant and lactating mothers of good socio-economic status in Cambridge, UK: some implications for recommended daily allowances of minor nutrients. Br J Nutr 1986;56:59–72.
25. Beal VA. Nutritional studies during pregnancy. II. Dietary intake, maternal weight gain, and size of infant. J Am Diet Assoc 1971;58:321–326.
26. Greenfield H, Clark J. Energy compensation in childbearing in young Lufa women. Papua New Guinea Med J 1975.
27. van der Rijst, MPJ. Nutrient intake relative to recommended daily allowances. In: van den Berg H, Bruinse HW, eds. On the role of nutrition in normal human pregnancy. Utrecht, Netherlands: University of Utrecht Press 1983:181–185.
28. Lunnell NO, Persson B, Sterky G. Energy and nutrient intake according to parity, smoking behaviour, season and pregnancy outcome. In: van den Berg H, Bruinse HW, eds. On the role of nutrition in normal human pregnancy. Utrech, Netherlands: University of Utrecht Press, 1983: 179–180.
29. Whitehead RG, Paul AA, Black AE, et al. Recommended dietary amounts of energy for pregnancy and lactation in the United Kingdom. Food Nutr Bull 1981;suppl 5:259–265.
30. Doyle W, Crawford MA, Laurance M, et al. Dietary survey during pregnancy in a low socio-economic group. Hum Nutr Appl Nutr 1982;36A:95–106.
31. Grafe HK. Dietary intake during pregnancy. In: van den Berg H, Bruinse HW, eds. On the role of nutrition in normal human pregnancy. Utrech, Netherlands: University of Utrecht Press, 1983:175–178.
32. Schofield C, Wheeler E, Stewart J. The diets of pregnant and post-pregnant women in different social groups in London and Edinburgh: energy, protein, fat and fibre. Br J Nutr 1987;58:369–381.
33. Haste FM. Brooke OG, Anderson HR, et al. Nutrient intakes during pregnancy: observations on the influence of smoking and social class. Am J Clin Nutr 1990;51:29–36.

16
Exercise in Pregnancy: Effects on Cardiorespiratory Physiology and Metabolism

Marshall W. Carpenter

Pregnancy and exercise both demonstrate the profound adaptive response of which the mammalian body is capable. This chapter examines cardiorespiratory physiology as it is affected by pregnancy at rest and under conditions of acute exertion, and the metabolic and endocrine responses to acute exertion in the nonpregnant and pregnant states.

Cardiovascular Physiology During Pregnancy

The cardiovascular changes in early pregnancy anticipate later needs of the conceptus and are largely accomplished in the human by midgestation. Plasma volume increases by 6 to 8 weeks, reaching its maximum (i.e., 45%, 1200 to 1300 cc) at 30 to 34 weeks.[1,2] Red cell volume increases 20% to 30% (i.e., 250 to 450 cc) but peaks later, creating a dilutional anemia.[2]

The relationship between increased intravascular volume and the coincident rise in cardiac output (Q) remains speculative.[3] Compared to prepregnancy values, Q has been noted to increase 23% and stroke volume (SV) to rise 20% by the gestational age of 8 weeks using echocardiography.[4] Earlier data that used postpartum values for comparison found increased Q in the first trimester using several techniques including dye dilution methods[5] and echocardiographic studies.[6,7] A sequential study of Doppler-derived hemodynamic and endocrine measures was performed in 10 women with normal pregnancy outcomes at 5 to 8 weeks of amenorrhea. Only cardiac output increased consistently between the 5th and 8th weeks, which correlated with a rise in left atrial diameter and a fall in total peripheral vascular resistance. A rising 17β-estradiol was detected throughout the 4 weeks of observation. These data suggest that the maternal hemodynamic changes found in the first trimester result from a primary fall in systemic vascular tone.[8] At its maximum, resting cardiac output, estimated from sonographic measurements has been observed to increase 34% from prepregnancy values.[4] This is proportionately greater than the 13% increase in body mass during pregnancy.

Cardiac output later in pregnancy is dependent on body position; it is reduced in the supine position probably because of uterine compression of the vena cava. Resting cardiac output in the lateral decubitus or sitting position appears to continue to increase up to 28 to 32 weeks' gestation and is observed to remain stable or decrease thereafter.[6,9–12] Many published observations of the incremental rise in cardiac output in pregnancy may underestimate the effect of pregnancy because of unstable methods and conditions of measurement and the use of early pregnancy observations as "baseline" values for later comparisons. A small study ($n = 8$) of oxygen extraction (Fick) estimated cardiac output in pregnancy and noted that thoracic electrical bioimpedance estimates of cardiac output were position dependent and inappropriate for pregnancy studies.[13] The limitations of thoracic electrical bioimpedance and two-dimensional and Doppler cardiography are discussed more fully elsewhere.[14] Maternal heart rate increases by 20 beats per minute by 32 weeks with variable increases thereafter.[11,12,15]

Cardiac architecture, imaged by M-mode echocardiography, changes in several ways during pregnancy. Ventricular wall thickness and end-diastolic ventricular volume increase proportionately in each ventricle by the end of the second trimester.[6,7,16] There appears to be no change in end systolic M-mode dimensions at rest. Mitral velocimetry suggests that there may be decreased left ventricular compliance or an increase in preload in pregnancy.[16] Pulsed and continuous-wave Doppler estimates of cardiac output and stroke volume indicated that these values increase from initial 8- to 11-week values through 36 weeks of pregnancy.[16] However, Fick-derived stroke volume appears to decrease from 24 weeks to term such that the pregnancy-related increased cardiac output appears to be maintained during the third trimester by increases in heart rate.[11]

Systemic vascular resistance changes directly with mean arterial pressure (MAP) and inversely with cardiac output. Systemic vascular resistance was measured during recumbency in groups of pregnant women of differing gestational ages.[8] The low first trimester recordings (986 ± 183 dyne·sec^{-1}cm^{-1}) rose linearly through pregnancy to nonpregnant values (1244 ± 152 dyne·sec^{-1}cm^{-1}).[5]

Pregnancy alters regional blood flow at rest. Compared to nonpregnant dimensions, uterine artery diameter doubles by 21 weeks' gestation, increasing 2.4-fold by term. Doppler estimates of volumetric flow suggested a 60% increase in common iliac flow, a 50% reduction in external iliac flow with a term unilateral uterine artery flow of 312 ml·min^{-1}.[17] Compared to postabortal measurements, xenon 133 washout estimates of cerebral blood flow at 7 to 19 weeks showed increased flow to the cerebellum, basal ganglia and all areas of the cerebrum, in the range of 8% to 12%, except the occipital lobes,[18] despite the hypocapnea of pregnancy.

The autonomic response to baroreceptor stimulation may be attenuated by midpregnancy.[19] Some investigators have found no change in tests of autonomic integrity, such as heart rate variation, expiratory/inspiratory pulse ratio, and pulse alterations with standing, performed on 10 normal gravidas who had shown no change from pregnancy to the postpartum period.[20] However, the Valsalva maneuver produces an attenuated tachycardic reaction to blowing in pregnant subjects. Also, in the same study, standing was found to produce a reduced biphasic heart rate response during pregnanncy.[21]

Venous compliance increases by the second trimester and is thought to be mediated by progesterone.[22] Lower extremity increase in venous compliance is greater than that of the upper extremity.[23]

Respiratory Physiology During Pregnancy

The relationship between ventilation and perfusion in the lung appears to be unchanged by pregnancy. Blood volume, cardiac output, and minute volume respiration ($\dot{V}E$) all increase from 34% to 50% during pregnancy.[24] Increased $\dot{V}E$ is a direct result of increased total lung volume and not due to increased breathing frequency.[24–26] Tidal volume measured at 563 ml in the nonpregnant state at several months postpartum increases 12% in early and 27% by late pregnancy.[12] The ratio of ventilation to $\dot{V}O_2$ (the ventilatory equivalent) is increased in pregnancy by 17%. This results in a decrease in arterial P_{CO_2} from 39 to 31 torr[27] and a mild respiratory alkalosis, resulting in an increase in pH of 7.40 to 7.44.

Resting oxygen uptake increases 13% to 30% during pregnancy.[24,25,28] Forty-seven percent of the pregnancy increase occurs by 8 weeks' and 73% of the increase by 15 weeks' gestation.[29] However, data from later in pregnancy have observed that the resting $\dot{V}O_2$ corrected for body mass is not significantly different ante- and postpartum.[30,31]

Acute Cardiovascular Response to Exertion in the Nonpregnant State

The cardiorespiratory system responds to exertion by ensuring an adequate increase in tissue oxygen delivery to exercising muscle. Oxygen consumption ($\dot{V}O_2$) is the product of oxygen delivery in the blood (i.e., cardiac output) and oxygen extraction in the periphery [i.e., arterial-venous oxygen difference ($avDo_2$)] expressed by the rearranged Fick equation[32] $\dot{V}O_2 = Q \cdot avDo_2$. Since cardiac output is determined by heart rate (HR) and stroke volume (SV), this equation can be expanded to $\dot{V}O_2 = HR \cdot SV \cdot avDo_2$. $\dot{V}O_2$ typically increases 10 to 20 times from rest to maximal exercise. $\dot{V}O_2$ increases linearly with increasing exercise intensity, expressed as power output, until maximal oxygen consumption ($\dot{V}O_2$ max) is reached, where a "plateau" may occur (Figure 16.1). $\dot{V}O_2$ max is the most important indicator of cardiorespiratory fitness. Consequently, % $\dot{V}O_2$ max is used to describe relative exercise intensity when the comparison of physiologic responses to exertion between individuals or conditions is made. $\dot{V}O_2$ max is normally limited by the circulatory response to exertion, particularly the increment in cardiac output.

Cardiac output is coupled to $\dot{V}O_2$ during exercise so that each liter increment in $\dot{V}O_2$ is accompanied by a 5- to 6-L increase in Q.[33,34] Both higher brain centers and skeletal muscle afferents are probably involved in maintaining this constant relationship.[35] Cardiac output typically increases four to five times from rest to maximal exercise (Figure 16.2).

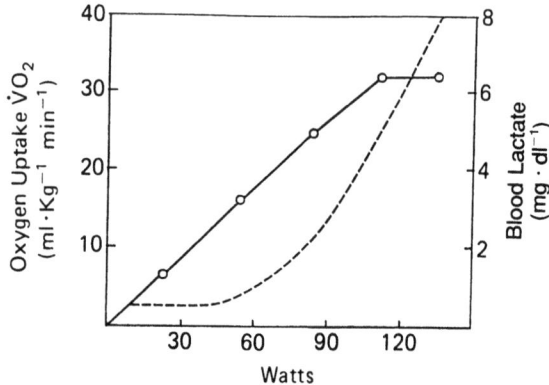

FIGURE 16.1. Characteristic oxygen uptake and blood lactate response to incremental power output (i.e., work load). (Unpublished $\dot{V}O_2$ data from pregnant subjects in our laboratory. Lactate curve adapted from Astrand.[41])

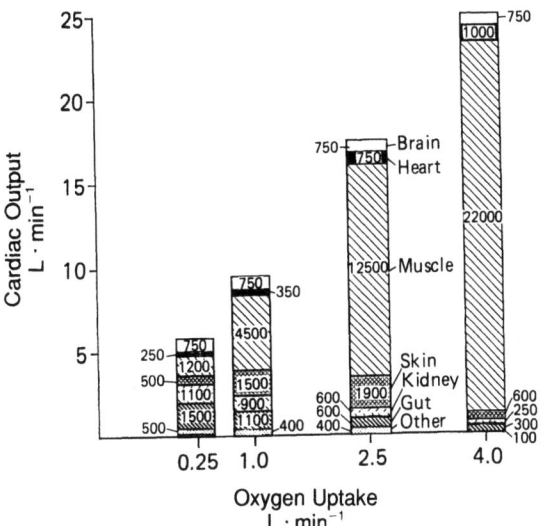

FIGURE 16.2. Changes in distribution of cardiac output to organ systems at four levels of oxygen uptake. (From Horvath,[121] with permission.)

mated by plasma norepinephrine concentration, increases in many tissues including nonactive muscle, the splanchnic region, and kidneys, causing local vasoconstriction. This increase in sympathetic nervous activity is probably due to increased release rather than reduced tissue uptake of catecholamines and is likely uniform throughout the body, except during heavy work where most of the circulating norepinephrine is derived from working muscles.[39] Sympathetic nervous activity in bone, connective tissue, and adipose tissue is unquantified.

The increased plasma norepinephrine concentration is closely related to the intensity of exercise (Figure 16.3) and to elevated exercise heart rate above 100 bpm.[32] The

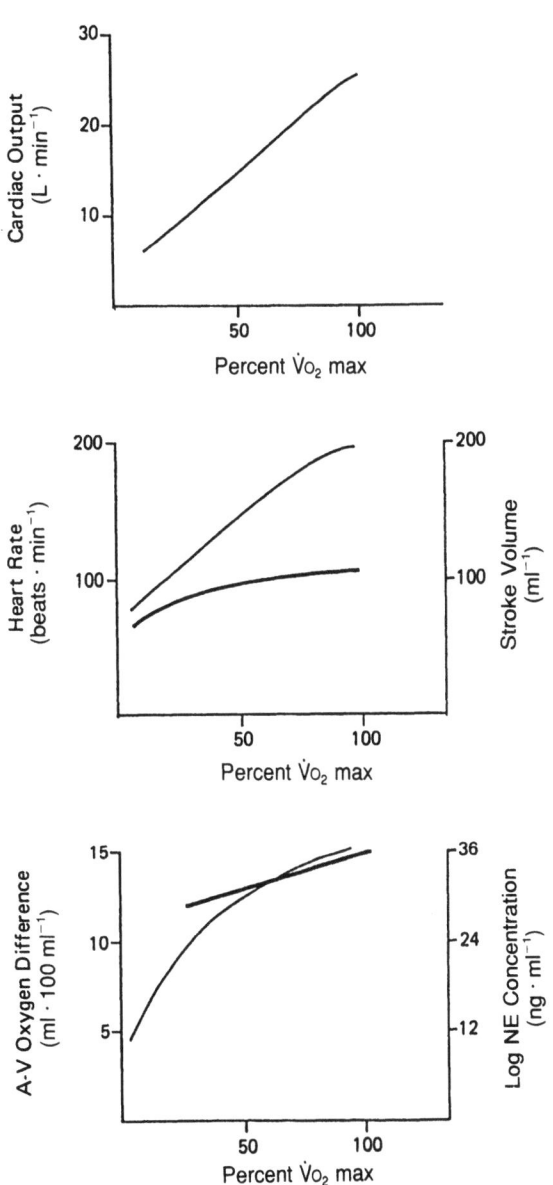

FIGURE 16.3. Characteristic changes in cardiac output, heart rate, stroke volume, atrioventricular (AV) oxygen difference, and norepinephrine concentration as a function of exercise intensity represented as % $\dot{V}O_2$ max. (Adapted from Rowell,[32] with permission.)

Heart rate is linearly related to $\dot{V}O_2$ throughout exercise (Figure 16.3). The initial increment in HR during dynamic exercise is caused by abatement of vagal stimulus to the heart. After the HR reaches approximately 100 bpm during exercise, increased sympathetic nervous activity is responsible for the further rise to maximal levels. Heart rate typically increases two to three times from rest to maximal exercise.

The initiation of the muscle pumping action during exercise in the nonpregnant state increases stroke volume 1.5 to 2.0 times above resting values at exercise intensity less than 40% $\dot{V}O_2$ max (Figure 16.3). Only small additional increases in SV (10%) are seen at higher exercise intensities.[32,36–38] There has been considerable debate over the importance of the Frank-Starling mechanism during exercise. This length-tension relationship indicates that SV is determined by ventricular filling pressure or preload. The Frank-Starling mechanism is operative during low-intensity upright incremental exercise but does not influence SV later at higher exercise intensity.[38] Initially during exercise both end-diastolic volume and SV increase. Above 40% $\dot{V}O_2$ max, end-diastolic volume remains unchanged and the increased SV is accounted for by a decreased end-systolic volume. As exercise intensity rises toward maximal levels, SV remains unchanged as end-systolic volume decreases slightly. These results suggest that during the later stages of vigorous dynamic exercise the elevated SV is due predominantly to increased sympathetic stimulation rather than the Frank-Starling mechanism.

Blood flow is redistributed during exercise to provide working skeletal muscle with adequate oxygen and nutrients[32] (Figure 16.2). Sympathetic nervous activity, esti-

close relationship between relative exercise intensity and regional vasoconstriction is independent of level of exercise training or aerobic capacity. The proportion of total cardiac output available to the exercising muscle, however, varies directly with the level of maximal cardiac output. Endurance athletes with their high maximal cardiac output may deliver 90% of the total cardiac output to working muscle while sedentary individuals may deliver only 70% to 80%, thus maintaining the same low absolute perfusion to nonexercising regions. The stimulus for the rise in sympathetic nervous activity during exercise is under investigation.[35]

The arterial-venous oxygen difference ($avDo_2$) widens with increasing exercise intensity to values at maximal exertion three- to fourfold above those found at rest (Figure 16.3). In some highly trained athletes arterial O_2 saturation may actually decline during maximal exercise, thereby reducing $avDo_2$.[32,40]

Acute Respiratory Response to Exertion in the Nonpregnant State

Ventilation increases linearly with $\dot{V}o_2$, averaging 20 to 25 L of air for each liter of oxygen uptake ($\dot{V}o_2$) during light and moderate exercise. However, the relative increase in ventilation with increasing $\dot{V}o_2$ during exercise intensity exceeding 50% $\dot{V}o_2$ max is greater than at lower intensity and can reach values as high as 35 to 40 L of air per liter $\dot{V}o_2$ during maximal exercise.[36,37,41] Greater tidal volume and breathing frequency contribute to the elevated minute ventilation ($\dot{V}E$) at lower exercise intensities while higher breathing rates primarily increase $\dot{V}E$ at high exercise intensities.[42]

The exercise intensity at which the $\dot{V}E/\dot{V}o_2$ slope rises has been termed the "ventilatory threshold" or "ventilatory inflection point."[36,43] During moderate-intensity exercise, lactic acid accumulates in the blood and is buffered by bicarbonate. The resulting increased production of CO_2 is associated with increased $\dot{V}E$ and clearance of CO_2 ($\dot{V}co_2$). Beyond the ventilatory threshold, the slope of $\dot{V}E/\dot{V}o_2$ increases but that of $\dot{V}E/\dot{V}co_2$ is unchanged.

There has been active debate about the meaning of the ventilatory threshold and whether it really reflects the onset of anaerobic metabolism or lactate accumulation in the blood. Nevertheless, it is a reliable index of exercise performance and may vary independently of $\dot{V}o_2$ max. Training results in a greater increase in ventilatory threshold $\dot{V}o_2$ than in maximal $\dot{V}o_2$. Ventilation does not normally limit $\dot{V}o_2$ max since pulmonary ventilation during maximal exercise is still 60% to 85% of maximal voluntary ventilation.[37]

The partial pressures of oxygen in the alveoli (PAo_2) and arteries (Pao_2) are maintained close to resting levels even during maximal aerobic exercise.[41] The PAo_2 increases slightly and Pao_2 decreases somewhat at very high exercise intensities. This is due to the sigmoid shape of the oxyhemoglobin dissociation curve, which shifts down and to the right during exercise as the temperature increases and pH decreases with exercise (i.e., Bohr effect). During strenuous exercise in highly trained endurance athletes Pao_2 may decrease further because of O_2 diffusion limitation secondary to very short pulmonary capillary transit times.[40]

Effects of Pregnancy on Acute Cardiovascular and Respiratory Exercise Response

Pregnancy is not associated with alteration in the coupling of $\dot{V}o_2$ to cardiac output[28] (Table 16.1), suggesting that the neurogenic control of cardiac output is unaffected by this condition. Pregnancy appears to change (1) the relative contribution of stroke volume to cardiac output, (2) the oxygen uptake at rest and during weight-bearing exercise, (3) the peripheral vascular response to exercise and during the recovery phase, and (4) peak $\dot{V}co_2$ with maximal effort.

Increases in HR and SV contribute to the higher Q in pregnant women at low and moderate exercise intensity. At high-intensity exertion increased SV is primarily responsible for the 15% increase in Q during midpregnancy compared to the postpartum state.[28] The increased contribution of stroke volume to incremental cardiac output at high-intensity exertion in pregnancy is reflected in a lower slope of HR/% $\dot{V}o_2$ max.[28,44] Others have noted the same increase in stroke volume at peak exertion in late pregnancy but have found that the increased stroke volume at 15 weeks is due to increased fractional shortening in contrast to the increase at 34 weeks, which is due to increased end-diastolic left ventricular dimensions.[45]

Electrocardiographic response to exertion may be influenced by pregnancy. In one study of 15 gravidas, treadmill exercise to 85% of age-specific maximal heart rate at 37 weeks produced a higher incidence of ST segment depression (6/15) than found with similar exercise stress

TABLE 16.1. Linear regressions of Q vs. $\dot{V}o_2$ and HR vs. $\dot{V}o_2$.

Relation	Antepartum		Postpartum	
	Slope	y-Intercept	Slope	y-Intercept
$\dot{Q}$ vs. $\dot{V}o_2$	6.15 ± 1.32	5.81 ± 1.23[a]	6.18 ± 1.34	3.59 ± 1.17
HR vs. $\dot{V}o_2$	76.3 ± 19.1[a]	57.8 ± 15.6[a]	94.7 ± 32.7	36.0 ± 19.5

Values are means ± SD; $n = 39$.
[a] $p < .01$ antepartum vs. postpartum.
From Sady et al.,[28] with permission.

at 29 weeks (2/15) and postpartum (1/15). There were no differences among tests of the QRS complex, axis, conduction, P-Q, and Q-T intervals or arrhythmias.[46] Another investigation noted a 12% incidence of ST segment depression in women exercised to a peak heart rate of 174 ± 2 bpm in each trimester and postpartum. Findings were consistent at each testing period.[47]

Maternal blood pH in response to submaximal exertion for 10 minutes does not appear to differ during pregnancy compared to 12 weeks postpartum. Cycle (50 and 75 W) and treadmill exertion (67 m/min at 2.5% and 12% grade) at 37 weeks' gestation produced higher minute ventilation, tidal volume, and ventilatory equivalent for CO_2 compared to postpartum. However, the pH decrease (0.04 units) was comparable between conditions. The decrease in P_{CO_2} and $[HCO_3^-]$ during exertion was less in pregnancy than in the postpartum period.[48]

Maximal oxygen uptake, measured under conditions of incremental power output during cycle ergometry, appears to be unchanged in pregnancy compared to the postpartum periods (Table 16.2).[28,44] Likewise, maximum heart rate appears to be unchanged by pregnancy,[28,49] though the age-specified formula for estimating maximal heart rate (i.e., 220 – age in years) may overestimate this value.[44] The greater stroke volume found during pregnancy may be due to a decrease in end-systolic volume or a continued increase in end-diastolic dimensions secondary to increased venous return. The interaction of gestational age and intensity of exertion on end-systolic and end-diastolic dimensions has not been examined. Change in altitude from sea level to 6000 feet in the third trimester, appears to have no effect on submaximal exertional response in gravidas, but reduces peak $\dot{V}O_2$.[50]

Absolute oxygen consumption ($L \cdot min^{-1}$) is 14% higher at rest, 9% higher during weight-supported exertion (cycle ergometer), and 12% higher during weight-bearing (treadmill) exertion at identical submaximal work loads (approximately 60% $\dot{V}O_2$ max) during pregnancy compared to the postpregnant state.[31] Oxygen uptake during cycle ergometry exercise has not been found to be consistently elevated during pregnancy compared with the postpartum state.[24,25,28,51–53] Weight-bearing exertion under identical work loads, however, results in a consistent increased oxygen uptake during pregnancy.[24,31] When oxygen consumption is expressed as a function of body mass ($ml \cdot kg^{-1} \cdot min^{-1}$), however, differences in oxygen uptake in pregnancy and the postpartum state disappear.

Approximately 75% of the increased absolute oxygen uptake during submaximal weight-bearing exercise in pregnancy is accounted for by maternal weight gain. Differences in $\dot{V}O_2$ at rest amount to 25% of the increase and may be attributed to the increased mass of metabolically active tissue of the conceptus since $\dot{V}O_2$ per unit weight is unchanged. The remaining 50% increase results from the increased caloric cost of movement of the larger body mass during pregnancy. This is demonstrated when weight gain is controlled for experimentally by comparing non–weight-bearing to weight-bearing exercise during pregnancy or by using weight belts postpartum during weight-bearing exertion to mimic pregnancy weight.[31] Provided that $\dot{V}O_2$ max during weight-bearing exertion does not change during pregnancy, these data suggest that pregnant women have a higher resting and exertional percent $\dot{V}O_2$ max. This is probably due to the increased metabolic demands of the conceptus and the increase in "internal" work of exercise due to body changes associated with maternal weight gain. There are no data to suggest that pregnancy causes changes in muscle metabolism at the cellular level resulting in increased $\dot{V}O_2$ at a given work load.

The peripheral vascular response to exercise during pregnancy is similar to that in the nonpregnant state. During cycle ergometric exertion at 75% $\dot{V}O_2$ max the rise in systolic blood pressure and MAP is comparable during pregnancy with that noted 7 weeks postdelivery and shows the same linear increase with exercise intensity.[47]

Likewise, incremental, stepwise, isometric, extensor leg exercise to maximal effort at 29 and 35 weeks and in the postpartum period showed no difference in the relationship between force generation over a period of 45 seconds and rise in MAP compared to that in the postpartum period.[54] Although the pressor response was unaffected by pregnancy, the force generated against a footboard was reduced 13% at 35 weeks.

Others found an increase in MAP during leg extension isometric exercise to exhaustion (4 minutes) during 25 to 36 weeks' gestation, but noted only 19 torr increase in MAP measured somewhat later (3 minutes) after cessation of effort. They found no increase in Doppler esti-

TABLE 16.2. Maximal values for $\dot{V}O_2$, $\dot{V}E$, RER, HR, $\dot{Q}$, SV, and avO_2 difference antepartum and postpartum.

Variable	Antepartum	Postpartum
$\dot{V}O_2$		
$L \cdot min^{-1}$	1.91 ± 0.32	1.83 ± 0.31
$ml \cdot kg^{-1} \cdot min^{-1}$	27.3 ± 4.76	28.0 ± 5.13
$\dot{V}E$ ($L \cdot min^{-1}$)	90.5 ± 13.91	82.1 ± 14.32[a]
RER	1.17 ± 0.054	1.22 ± 0.097[a]
HR (beats/min)	182 ± 7.8	184 ± 7.1
$\dot{Q}$ ($L \cdot min^{-1}$)[b]	16.00 ± 2.46	13.93 ± 2.08[a]
SV ($ml \cdot beat^{-1}$)[c]	88 ± 14.4	76 ± 11.5[a]
$avDo_2$ ($ml \cdot dl^{-1}$)[c]	11.99 ± 1.69	13.19 ± 1.49[a]

Values are means ± SD; $n = 36$.
[a] $p < .01$ antepartum vs. postpartum.
[b] Maximal values estimated by multiplying the average of submaximal exercise stroke volume by the maximal HR.
[c] Maximal values calculated from the Fick relationship.
From Sady et al.,[28] with permission.

mated cardiac output associated with isometric exertion compared to that measured at rest.[55] These observations suggest that the sympathetic response to baroreceptor stimuli during exertion is not altered by pregnancy.

Labor induces changes in oxygen uptake and minute ventilation consistent with mild exertional intensity. Average $\dot{V}O_2$ throughout labor was increased 23% (from 3.6 ± 0.8 to 4.3 ± 0.9 ml·kg^{-1}min^{-1}) compared to resting values in the third trimester. Peak 10-minute averaged $\dot{V}O_2$ during labor was 87% greater (6.8 ± 2.2 ml·kg^{-1}min^{-1}) than that at rest in the third trimester. Likewise, 10-minute averaged peak $\dot{V}E$ was 58% higher.[56]

The pregnant woman differs from the nonpregnant woman during the recovery phase after exercise. In the third trimester, stroke volume after 3 minutes of recovery fell 26% from preceding submaximal exercise values. This contrasts with the 11% decline observed in the same individuals during the postpartum period.[57] Cardiac output changes did not differ between pregnancy and postpartum periods. These differences may be due to increased venous capacitance with resulting venous pooling and may occur despite continued leg movement if the recovery-phase work load is minimal.

Pregnancy does not appear to change the peak $\dot{V}O_2$ of exertion but does result in higher $\dot{V}E$ at rest and throughout all intensities of exertion and a lower peak $\dot{V}CO_2$ during rapidly incremental cycle ergometer exercise. This was associated with a lower $\dot{V}CO_2/\dot{V}O_2$ slope above the anaerobic threshold. This may reflect either decreased exercise-induced lactate production or increased metabolism by the maternal liver or by the fetoplacental unit.[44]

Acute Effects of Maternal Exercise on the Fetus

Exercise causes increased cardiac output and redistribution of aortic blood flow such that an inverse linear relationship exists between % $\dot{V}O_2$ max and splanchnic blood flow.[39] In the pregnant sheep,[58–60] the goat,[61] and probably the human[62–64] uterine blood flow declines in response to moderate and vigorous maternal exercise. The pregnant ewe, exercised for 40 minutes at 70% $\dot{V}O_2$ max, demonstrated an 11% fall in fetal arterial Po_2.[65] In the pregnant ewe exercised to exhaustion, uterine blood flow fell 28% and fetal arterial Po_2 was reduced 30%. Despite these changes and marked lactacidemia in the maternal circulation, neither uterine nor umbilical oxygen uptake was reduced by maternal exhaustive exertion.[40]

These data raised concerns about fetal safety during maternal exercise in humans. In fact, Doppler monitoring of fetal heart rate during maternal treadmill and cycle exercise seemed to indicate that fetal bradycardia might occur even at modest maternal exertional intensity.[66–68] Subsequent studies of 4 gravidas during submaximal maternal exercise using two-dimensional ultrasound did not identify significant change in baseline fetal heart rate.[69] In another study, 45 gravidas were monitored with two-dimensional sonography during 85 submaximal and 79 maximal voluntary exertion tests on a cycle ergometer.[49] Only one fetal bradycardia occurred during exertion and that at mild intensity during a maternal vagal episode. Fifteen bradycardic episodes occurred following maximal exertion (16%), all within 4 minutes of exertional cessation and all followed by physiologic heart rate recordings within 30 minutes of exercise cessation. Postexertional fetal bradycardia was not related to duration of maximal exercise, maternal blood pressures during or after exertion, or peak maternal heart rate. Women achieving higher peak $\dot{V}O_2$ had an increased incidence of postexertional fetal bradycardia (Table 16.3) suggesting that exercise training may predispose toward rather than prevent fetal bradycardia.

Reduction in ambient maternal Po_2 with increased altitude does not appear to affect fetal well-being in the human during maternal exertion. Continuous incremental cycle ergometry to a volitional maximum intensity was performed at sea level and at 6000 feet altitude 2 to 4 days later in sedentary gravidas at 34 weeks who lived at sea level. Fetal heart rate response immediately before and after maternal exertion did not differ between the sea level and increased altitude exertion.[50]

Fetal heart rate (FHR) has been observed to increase following maternal exertion.[70] This response is more pronounced in the mature fetus and greater with prolongation of maternal exertion beyond 20 minutes,[71] but does not appear to be affected by maternal fitness or recent exercise frequency.[72] Fetal heart rate response has been found to have a positive correlation with exercise intensity and duration as well as to gestational age.[73] Others have observed FHR patterns before, during, and

TABLE 16.3. Exercise variables in sessions where fetal bradycardia was present or absent after maximal exercise.

Variable	Fetal bradycardia mean ± SD	
	Present ($n = 15$)	Absent ($n = 64$)
Peak maternal heart rate (bpm)	180.0 ± 9.7	180.0 ± 8.4
Peak maternal oxygen uptake (ml·kg^{-1}min^{-1})	29.0 ± 5.3[a]	25.1 ± 3.6
Duration of maximal exercise period (min)	7.4 ± 2.5	6.9 ± 1.8
Systolic pressure (mmHg)	39.0 ± 18.7	36.0 ± 15.6
Diastolic pressure (mmHg)	18.0 ± 21.8	10.0 ± 12.0
Mean arterial pressure (mmHg)[b]	21.0 ± 14.4	17.0 ± 10.5

[a] $p < .01$, unpaired t-test.
[b] Refers to blood pressure at maximal exertion minus lowest pressure during recovery and includes 12 sessions with and 58 without fetal bradycardia.
From Carpenter et al.,[71] with permission.

after exercise in patients in whom membranes were ruptured for induction of labor.[74] Blinded review of heart rate recordings were unable to detect qualitive changes in FHR patterns related to maternal exercise. The type of maternal exercise may affect FHR response. Compared to 40 minutes of treadmill walking, low-impact aerobic dance of the same duration resulted in a greater rise of FHR. This occurred despite a higher measured relative $\dot{V}o_2$ and minute ventilation achieved in the treadmill group.[75] The study was not of a crossover design.

The systolic/diastolic velocimetry ratio (S/D ratio) has been observed to rise in the uterine artery during incremental maternal cycle ergometer exercise performed at 37 weeks to a peak of 170 bpm and to correlate with maternal exercise heart rate.[76] A similar rise in pulsatility index has also been observed in myometrial vessels in exercising women under similar conditions.[77] Others did not find a change in uterine artery pulsatility index following dancing at 65% $\dot{V}o_2$ max.[78] However, the umbilical S:D ratio does not appear to change with maternal exertion.[76,78]

The frequency of fetal breathing periods >30 seconds, fetal gross body movement frequency and duration were observed for 20 minutes before and immediately after a continuous incremental treadmill exercise protocol extended to 75% age-specific maximum heart rate.[79] Fetal breathing episode frequency fell from 2.3 per 20 minute observation to 0.3 per 20 minute observation. Likewise, fetal gross body movement frequency fell from 1.9 to 0.8. Duration of fetal breathing during the 20-minute observation period fell from 159 to 61 seconds and fetal gross body movement duration fell from 157 to 97 seconds. However, no maternal controls for maternal movement without increased $\dot{V}o_2$ were used.

Acute Metabolic Response to Exercise in the Nonpregnant State

The energy for muscular contraction constitutes the greatest single increase in energy transfer in the body. The energy output measured as oxygen uptake under steady-state conditions may increase more than 10-fold over resting values during very intense exertion.[36,37,41]

Energy expenditure during exercise is usually estimated using indirect calorimetry by measuring oxygen consumption ($\dot{V}o_2$). Exercise intensity can be expressed relative to $\dot{V}o_2$ max as % $\dot{V}o_2$ max or, alternatively, in relation to multiples of resting metabolic rate, METs in which 1 MET = resting $\dot{V}o_2$ = $3.5\,ml\cdot kg^{-1}\cdot min^{-1}$, or in relation to measured or estimated HR max (220 − age).[80] In these terms, light exercise may be considered <40% $\dot{V}o_2$ max, <4 METs, or <60% HR max; moderate exercise may reflect 40% to 70% $\dot{V}o_2$ max, 4 to 6 METs, or 60% to 80% HR max; and heavy exercise may be associated with >70% $\dot{V}o_2$ max or >6 METs or 80% HR max.

Fat stores provide vastly greater potential energy (15 kg, 6×10^5 kJ) than muscle glycogen (300–400 g, 5×10^3 kJ), hepatic glycogen (80–90 g, 1.5×10^3 kJ), and blood glucose (20 g, 3×10^1 kJ). Though protein is present in much larger quantities than carbohydrate, submaximal exertion preferentially uses lipid sources after the first minutes of exercise.

Fat, in the form of free fatty acids (FFA), is the primary fuel for muscle in the postabsorptive state. The ratio of carbon dioxide production to oxygen uptake ($\dot{V}co_2/\dot{V}o_2$), measured at the mouth, is the respiratory exchange ratio (RER) and, under steady-state conditions, may be used to approximate the respiratory quotient (RQ = CO_2 produced/O_2 consumed) as an indirect measure of relative oxidation of fats and carbohydrates. The differing RQ values for carbohydrate (1.0) and fat (0.7) allow estimation of the relative mix of fuel being oxidized under given conditions. Ignoring the small amount of protein oxidized during brief exercise introduces only slight error in the calculation of the RQ.[37] The proportionate oxidation of fat and carbohydrate during exertion depends on several factors including exercise intensity, duration, and type as well as training and nutritional status.

Exercise Intensity

As exercise intensity increases from 60% to 100% $\dot{V}o_2$ max, the contribution of carbohydrates to the total energy supplied increases.[36,37,41,81] Adenosine triphosphate (ATP) is produced in increasing proportions by anaerobic glycolysis at these exercise intensities. It is not surprising that glucose provides an increasing share of energy with higher intensity exercise, from 50% at moderate exercise to nearly 100% at $\dot{V}o_2$ max, becoming the predominant fuel at ≥70% $\dot{V}o_2$ max. The increased plasma lactate concentration under these conditions may directly or indirectly suppress lipolysis, further increasing demands for carbohydrate as an energy source.[82] Thus, the greater the intensity of exercise (% $\dot{V}o_2$ max), the shorter is the duration of exertion that can be sustained.

Protein ordinarily supplies only a small portion of energy at any exercise intensity (<10%) and fat constitutes the remainder.[36,37,41,81,83,84] Though protein may not play a direct role in exercise metabolism, it may provide precursors for glucose and metabolites required for oxidation of carbohydrates and fat.[84,85]

Lactate Threshold

Concentrations of blood lactate remain at or near resting levels during exercise of increasing intensity until 60% to 70% $\dot{V}o_2$ max, at which time lactate begins to rise nonlinearly (Figure 16.1). The lactate or anaerobic threshold is that point at which lactate entry into the blood exceeds its removal. The anaerobic threshold has been defined as "the level of work or O_2 consumption just below that at which metabolic acidosis and the associated changes in gas exchange occur."[86] This model proposes linkages between inadequate muscle oxygen, lactate production, and the increase in pulmonary ventilation as respiratory compensation for metabolic acidosis. This concept has been the subject of long debate.[36,86,87]

Lactate concentration, however, does not always correlate with tissue hypoxia but may reflect an imbalance between pyruvate production and oxidation.[36,43] Lactic acid is produced even at rest, but the relative rates of entry into and clearance from the blood maintain its plasma concentration at low values. The elevated lactate concentration during exercise exceeding 60% to 70% $\dot{V}o_2$ max reflects a greater entry than removal from the blood. Factors assumed to be responsible for this imbalance include hormonally mediated increases in glycogenolysis and glycolysis, recruitment of fast twitch glycolytic fibers, and a redistribution of blood flow from lactate-removing tissues to lactate-producing tissues.[36]

The exercise intensity at which lactate concentration increases in blood is reproducible within individuals but highly variable among people. Many factors influence lactate concentration including exercise duration, alteration in muscle glycogen concentration, and prior endurance training.[87] Lactic acid contributes to the lowering of pH in skeletal muscle, which may impede continuing muscle contraction. However, fatigue occurs despite the wide fluctuation in pH and lactate concentration in muscle and, therefore, is not explained by these changes.

Exercise Duration

Utilization of the three basic systems for energy transfer in the body [Adenosine triphosphate-phosphocreatine (ATP-PC), nonoxidative, and oxidative] depends on the duration of exercise.[36,37,41,88] Initially, ATP and PC which are immediate sources in the muscle provide enough energy for 6 to 8 seconds of maximal muscular activity such as sprinting, 20 to 30 seconds of cross-country racing, or 1 minute of brisk walking. Nonoxidative energy is provided from glycogenolysis and glycolysis for more sustained exercise. Lactic acid is formed in the muscle and diffuses into the blood. This system can provide enough energy to sustain maximal exercise for 1 to 3 minutes. As exercise extends beyond 5 to 10 minutes, blood glucose and FFA become increasingly important as suppliers of fuel. Blood glucose concentration becomes progressively dependent on gluconeogenesis with increasing duration of exercise. Moderate intensity exercise for 40 minutes results in a fourfold rise in splanchnic glucose production. This response can be reduced by both glucose (15–60%) and glucose plus insulin infusion (67%) during exertion.[89]

Prolonged exercise greater than 2 hours relies increasingly on utilization of FFA and less on blood glucose. Under this condition, muscle and hepatic glycogen stores fall, blood glucose concentration decreases, and increased lipolysis occurs. Glycogen typically contributes only a small portion to the overall calories of exercise but depletion of muscle glycogen is related to the onset of fatigue at intensities greater than 70% of $\dot{V}o_2$ max.[36,37,41,81]

Nutritional Status

The timing and type of food ingested is an important determinant of fuel utilization during exercise. A high carbohydrate diet increases muscle glycogen content and enhances endurance performance.[36,37,41] Glycogen-depleting exercise over a few days followed by elevated dietary carbohydrate intake over several days leads to a "supercompensation" of muscle glycogen stores in endurance athletes. In contrast, carbohydrate-restricted diets decrease muscle and liver glycogen. Eating carbohydrates during prolonged exercise increases endurance.[36,37,41]

Acute Metabolic Response to Exercise During Pregnancy

Fasting insulin concentration increases throughout pregnancy,[90] beginning as early as 12 weeks' gestation[91] despite reduced fasting glucose concentration. Twenty-four-hour glucose sampling in pregnant women ingesting their usual mixed-nutrient meals has demonstrated variable degrees of postprandial hyperglycemia, but consistently elevated insulin concentration compared to the nonpregnant state.[92] Insulin sensitivity, quantified as insulin-mediated glucose uptake during a euglycemic hyperinsulinemic clamp, has been found to decrease significantly from prepregnancy values by 12 postconceptional weeks.[93] The insulin resistance that characterizes pregnancy results in an accelerated "starvation ketosis." The exaggerated glycemic responses following meals rapidly change over a period of 4 to 5 hours to elevated FFAs and ketonemia and reduced plasma glucose concentrations.[94]

The relative postabsorptive hypoglycemia may be due in part to the increasing glucose uptake by the enlarging conceptus. However, no data are available that suggest that hepatic capacity for glucose production is limited in pregnancy. The fasting pregnant woman at rest has a higher oxygen uptake and a higher absolute rate of fatty acid oxidation. This results in sparing of glucose for use by the maternal brain and the conceptus. However, the RER at rest has been found to be unchanged[28] or increased during pregnancy (0.83 ± 0.01) compared to postpartum (0.76 ± 0.02, $p < .01$).[24] This increased RER characteristic of the postabsorptive state at rest in pregnancy indicates an increased proportion of carbohydrate oxidation relative to fat oxidation under these conditions.

Submaximal treadmill exercise during pregnancy results in an increased respiratory exchange ratio compared to exercise under identical conditions postpartum.[24] This is consistent with the increased energy costs of weight-bearing exercise during pregnancy.

In one study nonpregnant women and gravidas in the second and third trimester of pregnancy exercised for 30 minutes at a pulse of 140 bpm. Lactate and nonesterified fatty acid levels rose similarly with exercise among all three groups, except that preexertional lactate levels were higher in the third trimester group.[95]

Others have measured higher lactate 2concentrations during exercise in pregnancy. At 80% $\dot{V}O_2$ max exertion, lactate concentration was observed to be 26% higher during pregnancy than during the nonpregnant state.[52] Percent oxidation of lactate to CO_2 during and after exercise appears to be unaltered by pregnancy, suggesting that differences in lactate threshold due to pregnancy may be related to differences in lactate production.[94] The source of lactate production under these conditions, however, has not been documented, and it remains unclear whether this is due wholly to muscle production or, additionally, to lactate production by the conceptus.

Glucose homeostasis during labor in normal pregnancy has been examined using stable isotope label techniques.[97] Compared to controls at 6 months postpartum, glucose turnover was measured in latent labor, active labor, and with fetal and placental expulsion. Plasma insulin concentration did not decrease during labor, as might be expected, and was actually higher during placental expulsion. Despite this, plasma glucose increased throughout labor and was greater than that noted in controls, and plasma FFA concentrations were increased in labor compared to postpartum controls. Glucose production and uptake were greater during labor as was glucose clearance. There were no prelabor control observations in this study, however.

Acute Catecholamine Response to Exertion in the Nonpregnant and Pregnant States

Norepinephrine, released from sympathetic nerve endings, plays a primary role in preventing exercise-related hypoglycemia. It acts directly by stimulating hepatic glycogenolysis and peripheral lipolysis. Indirectly, norepinephrine inhibits insulin release through activation of α-adrenergic receptors and causes glucagon release by stimulation of β-adrenergic receptors.[98]

Norepinephrine secretion increases with moderate degrees of exertion.[99] Norepinephrine and epinephrine increase in parallel with percent $\dot{V}O_2$ max and correlate with pulmonary arterial oxygen saturation. Plasma epinephrine concentration is also associated with norepinephrine and glucose concentration.[73,99] Epinephrine release is associated with more intense exertion than norepinephrine response. During rest, the hepatosplanchnic vascular bed is the major contributor of norepinephrine but becomes the bed of greatest fractional extraction during exertion in dogs. Exercising muscle contributes the most norepinephrine during exertion. In contrast, epinephrine is produced almost entirely by the adrenal medulla, being unmeasurable following adrenal medulla ablation or beta-blockade in the exercising rat.[100] The heart produces minor amounts of norepinephrine at rest, but has a net uptake of epinephrine during exertion.

Plasma epinephrine and norepinephrine concentrations are unchanged during late human pregnancy in the lateral decubitus and supine position. Movement from recumbency to standing results in a 100% increase in plasma norepinephrine during pregnancy in contrast to a significantly greater increase of 190% during the postpartum period.[101]

When subjects arise from recumbency and perform treadmill exercise at 2.3 METs, a 45% rise in norepinephrine but no significant rise in epinephrine is measured.[67] Comparison with the nonpregnant state was not performed in this study. These data are confirmed by ovine experiments showing a 39% increase in norepinephrine with moderate exertion and a threefold rise with severe exertion.[102]

In another study, 30-minute cycle ergometric exertion at 140 bpm produced a 2.5-fold rise in norepinephrine, which peaked at 30 minutes, and a similar increment in epinephrine at 15 minutes of exertion in nonpregnant women. Third-trimester women, however, demonstrated only 30% of the rise in these hormones that occurred in the nonpregnant control group and a delay in peak epinephrine concentrations to 30 minutes.[95] However, since the pregnant subjects exercised at the same pulse as nonpregnant controls in this study, the increment in $\dot{V}O_2$ in pregnant subjects was less in the pregnant group, and may have accounted for their reduced catecholamine response.

Other Acute Endocrine and Metabolic Responses to Exertion in the Pregnant and Nonpregnant State

Glucose Homeostasis During Exercise in Pregnancy

Whole-body glucose uptake increases from rest to exercise 7 to 40 times depending on exertional intensity and duration.[89] Stable glucose concentration and provision

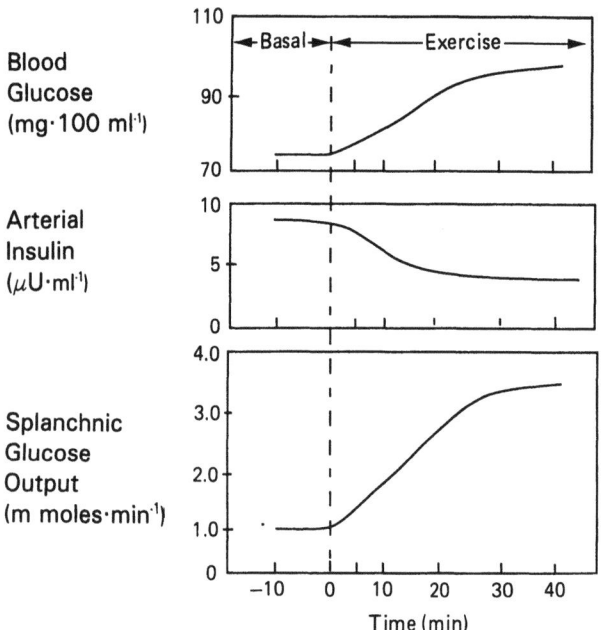

FIGURE 16.4. Influence of exercise on arterial blood glucose, arterial insulin, and splanchnic glucose output in control subjects receiving the saline infusion. (Adapted from Felig and Wahren,[89] with permission.)

of this substrate to both exercising muscle and nonexercising tissue is maintained by increased glucose production, which is stimulated during exercise by hormonal changes that promote glycogenolysis and gluconeogenesis.[32,36,37,41,81,85,103,104]

Moderate intensity exertion for 40 minutes results in a fourfold increase in endogenous glucose production (Figure 16.4), which is reduced 15% to 60% by glucose infusion before and during exercise.[89] Exercise causes a fall in plasma insulin concentration and an elevation in plasma glucagon concentration. Both effects are augmented by increased exercise intensity or duration, and are probably mediated by increased catecholamine release.

Hypoinsulinemia occurs during exercise despite the usual acute 15% to 20% rise in plasma glucose concentration. This results from the inhibition of insulin release by α-adrenergic stimulation of β cells.[104] However, a low insulin concentration ($12 \mu U \cdot ml^{-1}$) is required for uptake of glucose by peripheral tissues during exercise. This is demonstrated by removal of insulin infusion from pancreatectomized dogs, which results in marked reduction in peripheral uptake and increased hepatic production.[105] Beyond this permissive role of insulin, the marked rise in glucose uptake by exercising muscle appears not to be modulated by insulin.[106] Lowered insulin concentration during exertion, therefore, reduces the insulin-dependent uptake of glucose, increases glucose availability by allowing glycogenolysis, and increases the availability of FFAs via lipolysis.

The proportion of endogenous glucose production attributable to gluconeogenesis increases from 25% at rest to 45% with prolonged mild exercise. Whereas mild prolonged exertion results in a twofold rise in splanchnic glucose production, 40 minutes of heavy exercise increases total splanchnic glucose production fivefold. This results in a reduction in the proportion of endogenous glucose production due to gluconeogenesis from 25% to 5%.[107] The small contribution of gluconeogenesis under conditions of prolonged, intense exertion may account for the slow fall in plasma glucose concentration seen in this condition.

Exercise not only inhibits insulin release but also alters its subsequent metabolic effects. Single bouts of exercise appear to increase insulin sensitivity as measured by glucose uptake up to 48 hours postexertion.[108] Isolated exertion augments maximal glucose uptake under conditions of maximal effective insulin concentration (i.e., insulin responsivity).[108] Insulin responsivity does not appear to be augmented by chronic exercise training independent of acute exercise effect; although this postreceptor response to exercise has not been adequately addressed.[109]

Changes in insulin secretion, action, and postreceptor changes characteristic of non–insulin-dependent diabetes have been identified in pregnancy. Compared to normal, nonpregnant women and pregnant women with glucose intolerance, normal pregnant women generally demonstrated higher insulin/glucose ratios during oral glucose tolerance tests. Also, normal pregnant women demonstrated glucose uptake during a euglycemic hyperinsulinemic clamp that is intermediate between the other groups at insulin concentrations of both 40 and $240 mU \cdot M^{2-1} min^{-1}$, suggesting that pregnancy induces changes in both receptor and postreceptor events.[110] Insulin binding sites on red blood cells are reported to be unchanged by pregnancy,[110] but adipocyte insulin binding is reduced during late pregnancy and accompanied by reduced insulin sensitivity and reduced maximal insulin responsiveness.[111] Another study compared nonpregnant controls matched for insulin sensitivity [intravenous glucose tolerance test (IVGTT)] with nonobese pregnant patients at term.[112] The number of high-affinity insulin receptors on adipocytes was lower in pregnant subjects but kinase activity was unaltered. Adipocytes from nonpregnant subjects had a threefold sensitivity and increased insulin responsivity compared to pregnant subjects.

In nondiabetic pregnancy, postprandial walking does not alter mean 24-hour glucose concentration or glucose excretion.[113] Mild exertion for 15 minutes during pregnancy does not alter insulin concentration.[114] Another study had nonpregnant and second- and third-trimester pregnant women perform cycle ergometric exertion for 30 minutes at a pulse of 140 bpm.[95] Compared to nonpregnant women who experienced a 16% fall in glucose during exertion, gravidas in the second and third trimester of pregnancy demonstrated a 25% and 32% drop in glucose. These subjects had eaten 2 hours prior to exertion. This was associated with a 50% higher pre-exertion plasma insulin concentration ($32\mu U \cdot ml^{-1}$) in third-trimester subjects than in second-trimester or nonpregnant subjects, which may have produced the exercise-related fall in glycemia due to inhibition of glucose production.

Pregnancy may alter glucose kinetics during exercise. Third-trimester nondiabetic pregnant subjects exercised at 60% $\dot{V}O_2$ max for 30 minutes demonstrated no significant increase in glucose production measured by $[6,6^{-2}H_2]$ glucose tracer methods. Lactate kinetics were examined by $[U^{-13}C]$ lactate tracer and demonstrated a rise in lactate flux to CO_2 that correlated with rise in $\dot{V}O_2$ during exertion. Plasma concentrations of glucose and lactate were unchanged by exertion in this study.[96] These data imply that under the conditions of this protocol most energy for exercising muscle was derived from local glycogen stores and fatty acids.

Prior exertion may affect maternal glucose disposal during pregnancy. Thirty minutes following a 30-minute bout of cycle exertion, no change in the glucose response to a 75-g oral glucose load was noted, but a significant 23% reduction in the area under the insulin curve could be demonstrated.[115] Others found no significant change in either the insulin or glucose curve after a 600-kcal mixed-nutrient meal consumed 14 hours after a 30-minute bout of exertion.[116]

Glucagon concentration increases only during intense exertion in the dog and the human.[104,117] Glucagon release is mediated by epinephrine stimulation of α cell β-adrenergic receptors. In humans, brief exertion at 100% $\dot{V}O_2$ max raises glucagon 35%, and under this condition the plasma concentration of glucagon rises in parallel with that of norepinephrine. Prolonged exertion at 75% $\dot{V}O_2$ max for a mean duration of 81 minutes increases glucagon concentration to three times resting values despite norepinephrine concentrations similar to those found in brief acute intense exertion.[104] These data suggest that glucagon release may be mediated by factors in addition to α-adrenergic stimulation.

The interplay among insulin, catecholamines, and glucagon in maintaining muscle glucose uptake and euglycemia during exertion is complex. Suppression of insulin release is required to allow a prolonged glycemic response to infused glucagon.[100] However, maintenance of preexertional plasma insulin concentration during exercise alone does not result in hypoglycemia. When insulin is infused during moderate exertion in normal subjects, glucose concentration stabilizes at a lower level but exercise-induced increases in glucose production and uptake are not altered compared to saline infused controls. Glucagon concentration is likewise unaltered under the two conditions and is not increased compared to the preexercise control period.[89]

Glucagon appears to maintain glucose homeostasis during moderate exertion under conditions of pharmacologic sympathectomy. When insulin-dependent diabetic subjects with a constant infusion of insulin exercise at 55% $\dot{V}O_2$ max for 1 hour, treatment with propranolol does not result in hypoglycemia. Compared to those not treated with beta-blockers, those treated with propranolol had increased postexertional glucagon release and increased growth hormone and cortisol release during and after exertion.[118] In contrast, when catecholamine actions are blocked and changes in both insulin and glucagon are prevented, hypoglycemia can be induced by moderate exertion.[98]

These observations suggest that glucagon is not required for glucose homeostasis during exertion except under conditions of extreme exertional intensity and duration, in which glucagon provides amplification of hepatic gluconeogenesis and glycogenolysis. Physiologic glucagon concentration probably does not significantly increase the rate of lipolysis during prolonged exertion. However, glucagon augments ketogenesis and hepatic output of β-hydroxybutyrate in the exercising dog.[119]

Pregnancy-associated insulin resistance is not mediated solely by the increased glucagon concentration that characterizes pregnancy.[90] Glucagon release may respond to even light exercise during pregnancy (mean maternal pulse of 104 bpm), having been observed to rise twofold after 15 minutes of exertion while glucose concentration remained constant.[114] However, this finding was not confirmed in later studies.[67]

Growth Hormone and Cortisol

A rise in growth hormone concentration results in lipolysis but its effect is delayed somewhat after exercise begins and becomes greater with longer durations of exertion.[120] The magnitude of growth hormone release is related to rate of rise of both $\dot{V}O_2$ and lactate. Cortisol stimulates amino acid release from muscle and helps mobilize FFA from adipose tissue. Cortisol is released during prolonged, high-intensity exertion. The hormonal changes observed during exercise are rapidly reversed during the first minutes of recovery, although increments in cortisol and growth hormone may be sustained longer. Secretory response of these hormones to exercise during pregnancy has not been examined.

References

1. Hytten FE, Paintin DB. Increase in plasma volume during normal pregnancy. J Obstet Gynaecol Br Comm 1963; 70:402–407.
2. Lund CJ, Donovan JC. Blood volume during pregnancy. Am J Obstet Gynecol 1967;98:393–403.

3. Longo LD. Maternal blood volume and cardiac output during pregnancy: a hypothesis of endocrinologic control. Am J Physiol 1983;245:R720–R729.
4. Capeless EL, Clapp JF. Cardiovascular changes in early phase of pregnancy. Am J Obstet Gynecol 1989;161:1449–1453.
5. Lees MM, Taylor SH, Scott DB, et al. A study of cardiac output at rest throughout pregnancy. J Obstet Gynaecol Br Comm 1967;74:319–328.
6. Laird-Meeter K, van de Ley G, Bom TH, et al. Cardiocirculatory adjustments during pregnancy—an echocardio-graphic study. Clin Cardiol 1979;2:328–332.
7. Rubler S, Damani PM, Pinto ER. Cardiac size and performance during pregnancy estimated with echocardiography. Am J Cardiol 1977;40:534–540.
8. Duvekot JJ, Cheriex EC, Pieters FAA, et al. Early pregnancy changes in hemodynamics and volume homeostasis are consecutive adjustments triggered by a primary fall in systemic vascular tone. Am J Obstet Gynecol 1993;169:1382–1392.
9. Rose DJ, Bader ME, Bader RA, et al. Catheterization studies of cardiac hemodynamics in normal pregnant women with reference to left ventricular work. Am J Obstet Gynecol 1956;72:233–246.
10. Walters WAW, MacGregor WG, Hills M. Cardiac output at rest during pregnancy and the puerperium. Clin Sci 1966;30:1–11.
11. Ueland K, Novy MJ, Peterson EN, et al. Maternal cardiovascular dynamics. Am J Obstet Gynecol 1969;104:856–864.
12. Spatling L, Falenstein F, Huch A, et al. The variability of cardiopulmonary adaptation to pregnancy at rest and during exercise. Br J Obstet Gynaecol 1992;99:1–40.
13. Clark SL, Southwick J, Pivarnik JM, et al. A comparison of cardiac index in normal term pregnancy using thoracic electrical bio-impedance and oxygen extraction (Fick) techniques. Obstet Gynecol 1994;83:669–672.
14. Van Oppen AC, Stigter RH, Bruinse HW. Cardiac output in normal pregnancy: a critical review. Obstet Gynecol 1996;87:310–318.
15. Wilson M, Morganti A, Zervoudakis J, et al. Blood pressure, the renin-aldosterone system and sex steroids throughout normal pregnancy. Am J Med 1980;68:97–104.
16. Mabie WC, DiSessa TG, Crocker LG, et al. A longitudinal study of cardiac output in normal human pregnancy. Am J Obstet Gynecol 1994;170:849–856.
17. Palmer SK, Zamudio S, Coffin C, et al. Quantitative estimation of human uterine artery blood flow and pelvic blood flow redistribution in pregnancy. Obstet Gynecol 1992;9:1000–1006.
18. Ikeda T, Ikenoue T, Mori N, et al. Effect of early pregnancy on maternal regional cerebral blood flow. Am J Obstet Gynecol 1993;168:1303–1308.
19. Ekholm EMK, Erkkola RU. Autonomic cardiovascular control in pregnancy. Eur J Obstet Gynecol Reprod Biol 1996;64:29–36.
20. Airaksinen KEJ, Salmela PI, Ikaheimo MJ, et al. Effect of pregnancy on autonomic nervous function and heart rate in diabetic and nondiabetic women. Diabetes Care 1987;10:748–751.
21. Ekholm EMK, Piha SJ, Antina KJ, et al. Cardiovascular autonomic reflexes in mid-pregnancy. Br J Obstet Gynaecol 1993;100:177–182.
22. Fawer R, Dettling A, Weihs D, et al. Effect of the menstrual cycle, oral contraception and pregnancy on forearm blood flow, venous distensibility and clotting factors. Eur J Clin Pharmacol 1978;13:251–257.
23. Barwin BN, Roddie IC. Venous distensibility during pregnancy determined by graded venous congestion. Am J Obstet Gynecol 1976;125:921–923.
24. Knuttgen HG, Emerson K. Physiological response to pregnancy at rest and during exercise. J Appl Physiol 1974;36:549–553.
25. Pernoll ML, Metcalfe J, Schlenker TT, et al. Oxygen consumption at rest and during exercise in pregnancy. Respir Physiol 1975;25:285–293.
26. Wolfe LA, Ohtake PJ, Mottola MF, et al. Physiological interactions between pregnancy and aerobic exercise. Exerc Sports Sci Rev 1989;17:295–356.
27. Boutourline-Young H, Boutourline-Young E. Alveolar carbon dioxide levels in pregnant parturient and lactating subjects. J Obstet Gynaecol Br Comm 1956;63:509–528.
28. Sady SA, Carpenter MW, Thompson PD, et al. Cardiovascular response to cycle exercise during and after pregnancy. J Appl Physiol 1989;65:336–341.
29. Clapp JF. Metabolic adaptations during pregnancy. Presented at the New England Perinatal Society Annual Meeting, 1989.
30. Clapp JF. Cardiac output and uterine blood flow in the pregnant ewe. Am J Obstet Gynecol 1978;130:419–423.
31. Carpenter MW, Sady SP, Sady M, et al. Effect of maternal weight gain during pregnancy on exercise performance. J Appl Physiol 1990;68:1173–1176.
32. Rowell LB. Human circulation. Regulation during physical stress. New York: Oxford University Press, 1986.
33. Faulkner JA, Heigenhauser GF, Schork MA. The cardiac output-oxygen uptake relationship of men during graded bicycle ergometry. Med Sci Sports Exerc 1977;9:148–154.
34. Lewis SF, Taylor WF, Graham RM, et al. Cardiovascular responses to exercise as functions of absolute and relative work load. J Appl Physiol 1983;54:1314–1323.
35. Mitchell JH, Schmidt RF. Cardiovascular reflex control by afferent fibers from skeletal muscle receptors. In: Shepherd JT, Abboud FM, eds. Handbook of physiology. Section 2: The cardiovascular system volume III. Peripheral circulation and organ blood flow, part 2. Bethesda, MD: American Physiological Society, 1983:623–660.
36. Brooks GA, Fahey TD. Exercise physiology: human bioenergetics and its applications. New York: John Wiley, 1985.
37. McArdle WD, Katch FI, Katch VL. Exercise physiology, energy, nutrition, and human performance. Philadelphia: Lea & Febiger, 1986.
38. Plotnick GD, Becker LC, Fisher ML, et al. Use of the Frank-Starling mechanism during submaximal versus maximal upright exercise. Am J Physiol (Heart Circ Physiol) 1986;251:H1101–H1105.

39. Christensen NJ, Galbo H. Sympathetic nervous activity during exercise. Annu Rev Physiol 1985;45:139–153.
40. Dempsey JA. Is the lung built for exercise? Med Sci Sports Exerc 1986;143–173.
41. Astrand PO, Rodahl K. Textbook of work physiology. Physiological bases of exercise. New York: McGraw-Hill, 1986.
42. Deuster PA, Chrousos GP, Luger A, et al. Hormonal and metabolic responses of untrained, moderately trained, and highly trained men to three exercise intensities. Metabolism 1989;38:141–148.
43. Jones NL, Ehrsam RE. The anaerobic threshold. Exerc Sport Sci 1982;Rev 10:49–83.
44. Lotgering FK, Struijmk PC, Van Doorn MB, et al. Anaerobic threshold and respiratory compensation in pregnant women. J Appl Physiol 1995;78:1772–1777.
45. Veille JC, Hellerstein HK, Cherry B, Bacevice AE. Effects of advancing pregnancy on left ventricular function during bicycle exercise. Am J Cardiol 1994;73:609–610.
46. Asher UA, Ben-Shlomo I, Said M, Nabil H. The effects of exercise induced tachycardia on the maternal electrocardiogram. Br J Obstet Gynaecol 1993;100:41–45.
47. Van Doorn MB, Lotgering FK, Struijk PC, et al. Maternal and fetal cardiovascular responses to strenuous bicycle exercise. Am J Obstet Gynecol 1992;166:854–859.
48. Pivarnik JM, Lee W, Spillman T, et al. Maternal respiration and blood gases during aerobic exercise performed at moderate altitude. Med Sci Sports Exerc 1992;24:868–872.
49. Carpenter MW, Sady SP, Hoegsberg B, et al. Fetal heart rate response to maternal exertion. JAMA 1988;259:3006–3009.
50. Artal B, Fortunato V, Welton A, et al. A comparison of cardiopulmonary adaptations to exercise in pregnancy at sea level and altitude. Am J Obstet Gynecol 1995;172:1170–1180.
51. Ueland K, Novy MJ, Metcalfe J. Cardiorespiratory responses to pregnancy and exercise in normal women and patients with heart disease. Am J Obstet Gynecol 1973;115:4–10.
52. Lehmann V, Regnat K. Untersuchung sur korperlichen Belastungsfahigkeit schwangeren Frauen. Der Einfluss standardisierter Arbeit auf Herzkreislaufsystem, Ventilation, Gasaustausch, Kohlenhydratstoffwechsel und Saure-Basen-Haushalt. Z Geburtshilfe Perinatol 1976;180:279–289.
53. Blackburn MW, Calloway DH. Heart rate and energy expenditure of pregnancy and lactating women. Am J Clin Nutr 1985;42:1161–1169.
54. Lotgering FK, van den Berg A, Struijk PC, Wallenburg HCS. Arterial pressure response to maximal isometric exercise in pregnant women. Am J Obstet Gynecol 1992;166:538–542.
55. Van Hook JW, Gill P, Eastaerling TR, et al. The hemodynamic effects of isometric exercise during late normal pregnancy. Am J Obstet Gynecol 1993;169:870–873.
56. Eliasson AH, Phllips YY, Stajduhar KC, et al. Oxygen consumption and ventilation during normal labor. Chest 1992;102:467–471.
57. Morton MJ, Paul MS, Campos GR, et al. Exercise dynamics in late gestation: effects of physical training. Am J Obstet Gynecol 1985;152:91–97.
58. Clapp JF. Acute exercise stress in the pregnant ewe. Am J Obstet Gynecol 1986;136:489–493.
59. Lotgering FK, Gilbert RD, Longo LD. Exercise responses in pregnant sheep oxygen consumption, uterine blood flow, and blood volume. J Appl Physiol 1983;55:834–841.
60. Chandler KD, Bell AW. Effects of maternal exercise on fetal and maternal respiration and nutrient metabolism in the pregnant ewe. J Dev Physiol 1981;3:161–176.
61. Hohimer AR, McKean TA, Bissonnette JM, et al. Effect of exercise on uterine blood flow in the pregnant Pygmy goat. Am J Physiol 1984;246:207–212.
62. Morris N, Osborn SB, Payling Wright H. Effect uterine blood-flow during exercise in normal and pre-eclamptic pregnancies. Lancet 1956;2:481–484.
63. Morrow RJ, Knox Ritchie JW, Bull SB. Fetal and maternal hemodynamic responses to exercise in pregnancy assessed by Doppler ultrasonography. Am J Obstet Gynecol 1989;160:138–140.
64. Rauramo I, Forss M. Effect of exercise on placental blood flow in pregnancies complicated by hypertension, diabetes or intrahepatic cholestasis. Acta Obstet Gynecol Scand 1988;67:15–20.
65. Lotgering FK, Gilbert RD, Longo LD. Exercise responses in pregnant sheep: blood gases, temperatures and fetal cardiovascular system. J Appl Physiol 1983;55:842–850.
66. Artal R, Paul RH, Romeo Y, Wiswell R. Fetal bradycardia induced by maternal exercise. Lancet 1984;2(8397):258–260.
67. Artal R, Wiswell R, Romeo Y. Hormonal responses to exercise in diabetic and nondiabetic pregnant patients. Diabetes 1985;34(suppl 2):78–80.
68. Jovanovic L, Kessler A, Peterson CM. Human maternal and fetal response to graded exercise. J Appl Physiol 1985;58(5):1719–1722.
69. Paolone AM, Shangold M, Paul D, et al. Fetal heart rate measurement during maternal exercise—avoidance of artifact. Med Sci Sports Exerc 1987;19:605–609.
70. Collings C, Curet LB. Fetal heart rate response to maternal exercise. Am J Obstet Gynecol 1985;151:498–501.
71. Carpenter MW, Sady SP, Haydon B, et al. Maternal exercise duration and intensity affect fetal heart rate. American College of Sports Medicine Annual Meeting, 1989.
72. Webb KA, Wolfe LA, McGrath MJ. Effects of acute and chronic maternal exercise on fetal heart rate. J Appl Physiol 1994;77:2207–2213.
73. Clapp JF, Little KD, Capeless EL. Fetal heart rate response to sustained recreational exercise. Am J Obstet Gynecol 1993;168:198–206.
74. Spinnewijn WEM, Lotgering FKK, Struijk PC, Wallenburg HCS. Fetal heart rate and uterine contractility during maternal exercise at term. Am J Obstet Gynecol 1996;174:43–48.
75. McMurray RG, Katz VL, Poe MP, Hackney AC. Maternal and fetal responses to low-impact aerobic dance. Am J Perinatol 1995;12:282–285.

76. Erkkola RU, Pirhonen JP, Kivijarvi AK. Flow velocity waveforms in uterine and umbilical arteries during submaximal bicycle exercise in normal pregnancy. Obstet Gynecol 1992;79:611–615.
77. Hackett GA, Cohen-Overbeek T, Campbell S. The effect of exercise on uteroplacental Doppler waveforms in normal and complicated pregnancies. Obstet Gynecol 1992;79:919–923.
78. Asakura H, Makai A, Yamaguchi M, et al. Ultrasonographic blood flow velocimetry in maternal and umbilical arteries during maternal exercise. Acta Obstet Gynecol Jpn 1994;46:308–314.
79. Winn HN, Hess O, Goldstein I, et al. Fetal responses to maternal exercise: effect on fetal breathing and body movement. Am J Perinatol 1994;11:263–266.
80. American College of Sports Medicine. Guidelines for exercise testing and prescription. Philadelphia: Lea & Febiger, 1986.
81. Felig P, Wahren J. Fuel homeostasis in exercise. N Engl J Med 1975;21:1078–1084.
82. Hjemdahl P and Fidholm BB. Direct antilipolytic effect of acedosis in isolated rat adipocytes. Acta Physiol Scand 1977;101:294–301.
83. Brooks GA. Amino acid and protein metabolism during exercise and recovery. Med Sci Sports Exerc 1987;19:S150–S156.
84. Dohm GL. Protein as a fuel for endurance exercise. Exerc Sport Sci 1986;Rev 14:143–173.
85. Horton ES. Exercise and diabetes mellitus. Med Clin North Am 1988;72:1301–1321.
86. Wasserman K, Whipp BJ, Koyal SN, Beaver WL. Anaerobic threshold and respiratory gas exchange during exercise. J Appl Physiol 1973;35:236–243.
87. Gollnick PD, Bayly WM, Hadgson DR. Exercise intensity, training, diet, and lactate concentration in muscle and blood. Med Sci Sports Exerc 1986;18:334–340.
88. Keul J. The relationship between circulation and metabolism during exercise. Med Sci Sports 1973;5:209–219.
89. Felig P, Wahren J. Role of insulin and glucagon in the regulation of hepatic glucose production during exercise. Diabetes 1979;28(suppl 1):71–75.
90. Kuhl C, Holst JJ. Plasma glucagon and insulin:glucagon ratio in gestational diabetes. Diabetes 1976;25(1):16–23.
91. Fischer PM, Hamilton PM, Sutherland HW, et al. The effect of gestation on intravenous glucose tolerance in women. J Obstet Gynaecol Br Cwlth 1974;81:285–290.
92. Lewis SB, Wallin JD, Kuzuya H, et al. Circadian variation of serum glucose, C-peptide immunoreactivity and free insulin in normal and insulin-treated diabetic pregnant subjects. Diabetologia 1976;12:343–350.
93. Catalano PM, Tyzbir ED, McAuliffe T, Sims EAH. Increase in insulin response and insulin resistance in normal pregnant women. Society for Gynecologic Investigation, 36th Annual Meeting. In: Scientific Program and Abstracts. 1989:275.
94. Felig P, Lynch V. Starvation in human pregnancy: hypoglycemia, hypoinsulinemia, and hyperketonemia. Science 1970;170:990–992.
95. Bonen A, Campagna P, Gilchrist L, et al. Substrate and endocrine responses during exercise at selected stages of pregnancy. Exerc Pregnancy 1992.
96. Cowett RM, Carpenter MW, Carr S, et al. Glucose and lactate kinetics during a short exercise bout in pregnancy. Metabolism 1996;2:753–758.
97. Maheux PC, Bonin B, Dizaso A, et al. Glucose homeostasis during spontaneous labor in normal human pregnancy. J Clin Endocrinol Metab 1986;81:209–215.
98. Hoelzer DR, Dalsky GP, Clutter WE, et al. Glucoregulation during exercise: hypoglycemia is prevented by redundant glucoregulatory systems, sympatho-chromaffin activation and changes in islet hormone secretion. J Clin Invest 1986;77:212–221.
99. Christensen NJ, Galbo H, Hansen JF, et al. Catecholamines and exercise. Diabetes 1979;28(suppl 1):58–62.
100. Scheurink AJW, Steffens AB, Bouritius H, et al. Adrenal and sympathetic catecholamines in exercising rats. J Appl Physiol 1989;256:R155–R160.
101. Barron WM, Mujais SK, Zinaman M, et al. Plasma catecholamine responses to physiologic stimuli in normal human pregnancy. Am J Obstet Gynecol 1986;154:80–84.
102. Palmer SM, Oakes GK, Champion JA, et al. Catecholamine physiology in the ovine fetus. Am J Obstet Gynecol 1984;149:426.
103. Calles-Escandon J, Felig P. Fuel-hormone metabolism during exercise and after physical training. Clin Chest Med 1984;5:3–11.
104. Galbo H. Hormonal and metabolic adaptation to exercise. New York: G.T. Verlag, 1983.
105. Vranic M, Kawamori R. Essential roles of insulin and glucagon in regulating glucose fluxes during exercise in dogs. Mechanism of hypoglycemia. Diabetes 1979;28:45–52.
106. Pruett EDR. Plasma insulin during prolonged work at near maximal oxygen uptake. J Appl Physiol 1970;29:155–158.
107. Wahren J. Glucose turnover during exercise in healthy men and in patients with diabetes mellitus. Diabetes 1979;28:82–88.
108. Mikines KJ, Sonne B, Farrell PA. Effect of physical exercise on sensitivity and responsiveness to insulin in humans. Am J Physiol 1988;254(Endocrinol Metab 17):E248–E259.
109. King DS, Dalsky GP, Clutter WE, et al. Effects of exercise and lack of exercise on insulin sensitivity and responsiveness. J Appl Physiol 1988;64:1942–1946.
110. Ryan ED, O'Sullivan MJ, Skyler JS. Insulin action during pregnancy: studies with the euglycemic clamp technique. Diabetes 1985;34:380–389.
111. Hjøllund E, Pedersen O, Espersen T, Klebe JG. Impaired insulin receptor binding and postbinding defects of adipocytes from normal and diabetic pregnant women. Diabetes 1986;35:598–603.
112. Ciaraldi TP, Kettel M, El-Roeiy A, et al. Mechanisms of cellular insulin resistance in human pregnancy. Am J Obstet Gynecol 1994;170:365–341.
113. Hollingsworth DR, Moore TR. Postprandial walking exercise in pregnant insulin dependent (type 1) diabetic

women: reduction of plasma lipid levels but absence of a significant effect on glycemic control. Am J Obstet Gynecol 1987;157:1359–1363.
114. Artal R, Platt LD, Sperling M, et al. Exercise in pregnancy I. Maternal cardiovascular and metabolic responses in normal pregnancy. Am J Obstet Gynecol 1981;140:123–127.
115. Young JC, Treadway JL. The effect of prior exercise on oral glucose tolerance in late gestational women. Eur J Appl Physiol Occup Physiol 1992;64:430–433.
116. Lesser KB, Gruppuso PA, Terry RB, Carpenter MW. Exercise fails to improve postprandial glycemic excursion in women with gestational diabetes. J Matern Fet Med 1996;5:211–217.
117. Böttger I, Schlein EM, Faloona GR, et al. The effect of exercise on glucagon secretion. J Clin Endocrinol Metab 1972;35:117–125.
118. Tuttle KR, Marker JC, Dalsky GP, et al. Glucagon, not insulin, may play a secondary role in defense against hypoglycemia during exercise. Am J Physiol 1988;254 (Endocrinol Metab 17):E713–719.
119. Wasserman DH, Spalding JA, Bracy D, et al. Exercise-induced rise in glucagon and ketogenesis during prolonged muscular work. Diabetes 1989;38:799–807.
120. VanHelder WP, Casey K, Radomski MW. Regulation of growth hormone during exercise by oxygen demand and availability. Eur J Appl Physiol 1987;56:628–632.

Section III
Fetal-Placental Metabolism

17
Glucose Metabolism in the Fetal-Placental Unit

William W. Hay, Jr.

All glucose supplied to the placenta and fetus comes from the maternal glucose pool, produced by maternal glucogenesis or ingested in the mother's diet. The principal control of this glucose supply is the maternal arterial glucose concentration. Regulation of maternal glucose concentration is considered elsewhere (see Chapter 10). Regulation of glucose supply to the placenta and fetus, which is far more complex than a simple direct relation with maternal glucose concentration, has been the subject of considerable research for several decades. This interest is appropriate because glucose appears to be the major substrate for placental and fetal energy metabolism. For example, in the sheep model, glucose accounts directly for a major portion of placental oxygen consumption and indirectly, as glucose plus lactate, for at least 50% of fetal oxygen consumption. Glucose contributes to the production of placental and fetal glycogen and lipid and can exchange its carbon with other carbon-containing compounds such as amino acids.

Although maternal glucose concentration is the driving force for glucose supply to the placenta, glucose transfer to the fetus is driven by the maternal-fetal arterial glucose concentration gradient. This gradient is produced by net glucose consumption in both placenta and fetus.

Despite net transfer of glucose from the pregnant mother to the fetus, tracer experiments have demonstrated bidirectional exchange of glucose molecules at both fetal and maternal surfaces of the placenta. Fetal glucose can enter the placenta from the fetal plasma glucose pool where it can contribute to placental glucose metabolism or transfer into the maternal circulation. These observations indicate that placental and fetal glucose supply and exchange are intimately related. Furthermore, to the extent that fetal glucose metabolism is independent of supply (e.g., by fetal glucogenesis), it can regulate placental-fetal glucose exchange.

Methods for Determining and Quantifying Placental-Fetal Glucose Exchange

Net Flux Measurements: Fick Principle

Early studies of placental-fetal glucose exchange relied on measurement of plasma glucose concentration in the maternal (i.e., uterine) and fetal (i.e., umbilical) circulations. Based on variations in the fetal versus maternal concentration, early investigators such as Widdas[1] proposed placental glucose transport schemes. More recently, measurement of transplacental glucose transport has been accomplished by application of the Fick principle (i.e., computing the product of blood flow times the whole-blood glucose concentration difference across the uterine circulation, to quantify net uterine glucose uptake, and the umbilical circulation to quantify net umbilical glucose uptake).[2] Net umbilical glucose uptake represents the net transfer of glucose to the fetus by the placenta. The difference between uterine and umbilical net uptake rates represents the net rate of glucose consumption by the uteroplacental tissues. Equations are presented in Appendix 17.1 and Figure 17.1, which illustrate these principles and provide numerical examples. Such tissues include the maternal and fetal vasculature, uterine tissues (e.g., myometrium and endometrium), and the trophoblast itself, as well as other intervening cell layers that are unique to each species.[3] Although the portion of net uteroplacental glucose uptake that is strictly placental (i.e., trophoblast) has not been determined, blood flow,[4] the Fick principle,[5] and tracer[6] estimates indicate that in the pregnant sheep at least 70% to 80% of net uteroplacental glucose uptake is placental.

The Fick principle method requires much more accurate measurements of glucose concentration (i.e., at least $0.1 \, mg \cdot dl^{-1}$, preferably $0.01 \, mg \cdot dl^{-1}$), sampling catheters in

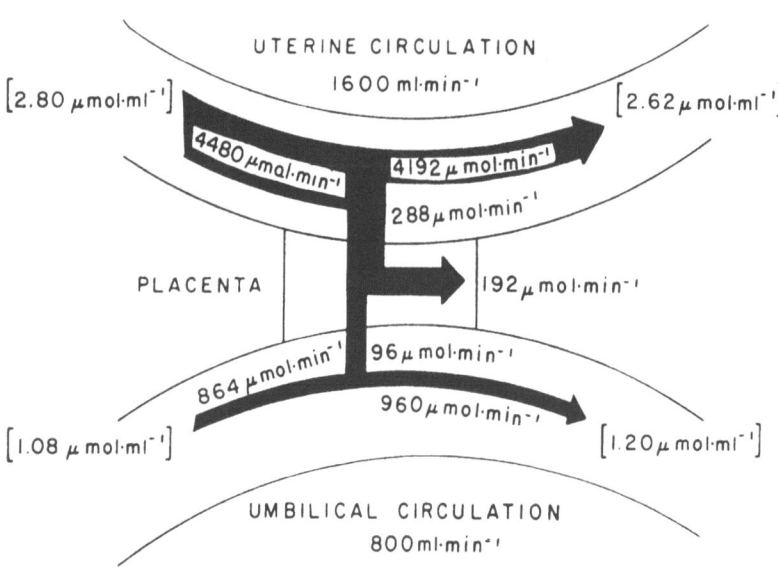

FIGURE 17.1. Numerical example of Fick principle measurements of glucose flux in the uterine and umbilical circulations and the transfer of glucose between these circulations by the uteroplacental tissues.

the uterine artery (or other maternal artery) and vein and the umbilical vein and umbilical artery (or the fetal aorta, iliac, or femoral artery) and an accurate simultaneous measurement of uterine and umbilical blood flow.

Application of the Fick principle to quantify placental-fetal glucose exchange provides estimates of flux that represent net rates; that is, they are rates of consumption and indicative of metabolism. Under certain natural conditions (e.g., fetal glucogenesis producing net hepatic glucose release into the fetal circulation) or under certain experimental situations (e.g., infusion of glucose into the fetal circulation), Fick principle measurements of placental or fetal glucose metabolism are inadequate to measure total glucose utilization. Under these circumstances, tracer methodology has been applied to quantify glucose utilization rates and turnover rates in the various pools of the maternal-placental-fetal system.

Tracer Methodology

Application of tracer methodology to the measurement of maternal-placental-fetal glucose exchange is a complex area of investigation because of the multiple pathways for parallel and divergent fluxes of glucose and tracer glucose and because of different methods of tracer administration, sampling, chemical analysis, and modeling. Such issues have been dealt with in extensive reviews[6,7] (see Chapter 1). The following discussion is designed to present general principles. Symbols and equations are presented in Appendix 17.2.[6,8]

Net Utilization Versus Turnover

The term glucose turnover has been equated with glucose utilization or glucose consumption, terms that imply metabolism when a whole animal under study functions as one compartment.[9] In such a simple, one-compartment system, glucose turnover rate is the steady-state entry rate or exit rate of glucose into or out of the sampled pool, usually the plasma, within the "compartment" studied. It is calculated as:

Glucose turnover rate (GTR) = r^*/SA for radiolabeled glucose tracers or $(r/E_{net}) - r$ for stable isotopic glucose tracers

where r^* = the rate of radiolabeled isotope tracer glucose infusion (e.g., dpm·min^{-1}), r is the rate of stable isotope tracer glucose infusion rate (e.g., μmol·min^{-1}), SA = the measured glucose specific activity (e.g., dpm·mg^{-1}), and E_{net} is the net fractional increase in stable isotopic enrichment (the "$-r$" corrects the calculated turnover rate for the stable isotope tracer glucose infusion rate, which, for stable isotopes, is small but not negligible, as it is for radiolabeled isotope tracers). These equations are derived from the following relations that occur at steady state:

Glucose turnover rate = glucose entry rate
= glucose disappearance (utilization) rate

$$\frac{\text{Glucose entry rate}}{\text{Tracer entry rate}} = \frac{\text{pool glucose concentration}}{\text{pool tracer glucose concentration}}$$
$$= \frac{\text{glucose disappearance rate}}{\text{tracer disappearance rate}}$$

Application of this technique and these equations to the study of fetal metabolism is complicated by the anatomy of the fetal circulation and the permeability of the placenta to tracee glucose and tracer glucose (Figure 17.2).

17. Glucose Metabolism in the Fetal-Placental Unit

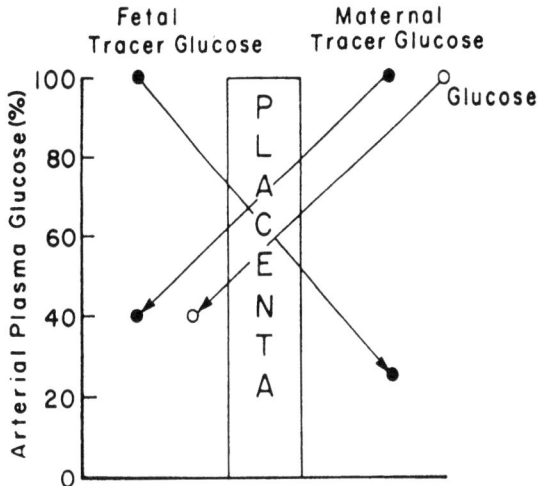

FIGURE 17.2. Concentration differences across the sheep placenta for unlabeled glucose and tracer glucose infused into the fetal inferior vena cava or the maternal femoral vein. The normal glucose gradient is from maternal to fetal circulation, which determines a net glucose flux from mother to fetus. This flux is paralleled by tracer glucose infused into the maternal circulation. For the tracer infused into the fetus, its concentration gradient is from fetal to maternal circulation, and the net tracer flux is from fetus to mother. These relationships define bidirectional transport of glucose across the uteroplacenta in sheep. (From Battaglia and Meschia,[3] with permission.)

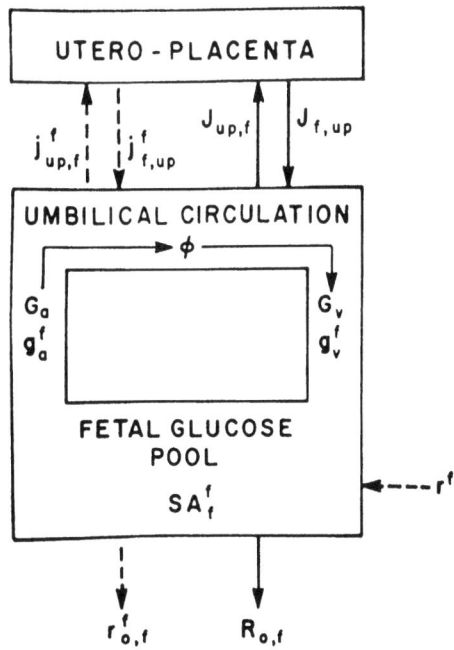

FIGURE 17.3. Steady-state fluxes and glucose (J, unidirectional; R, net) and tracer glucoses (j, unidirectional; r, net) for the fetus and uteroplacenta during a constant infusion of tracer glucose into the fetus (see Appendix 17.2 for symbols and equations). (From Hay and Sparks,[6] with permission.)

As shown in Figure 17.3, in steady state the infusion rate of tracer glucose into the fetus (r^f) is equal to the irreversible disposal (utilization) rate by the fetal organism ($r_{o,f}^f$) plus the net flux of the tracer into the placenta ($j_{up,f}^f - j_{f,up}^f$) which appears to vary according to fetal and maternal glucose concentrations and utilization rates. Glucose turnover rate in the fetus is calculated by dividing each term by SA_f^f (the specific radioactivity of glucose in the fetus using a tracer infusion into the fetus):

$$\left(r^f/SA_f^f\right) = \left[\left(r_{o,f}^f/SA_f^f\right) + \left(j_{up,f}^f/SA_f^f\right) - \left(j_{f,up}^f/SA_f^f\right)\right].$$

Thus the apparent glucose turnover in the fetus, which is the ratio of the rate of tracer infusion divided by the specific activity, is equivalent to:

$$\text{"GTR}_f\text{"} = \left(R_{o,f}\right) + \left(J_{up,f} - J_{f,up}\right)$$

where "GTR$_f$" = the fetal glucose "turnover rate," $R_{o,f}$ = the net tracee flux to the fetal tissues from the fetal glucose pool, and $J_{up,f}$ and $J_{f,up}$ = the unidirectional fluxes of tracee between the fetus and placenta. Thus, fetal glucose turnover rate is the sum of net fetal glucose utilization plus the net rate of exchange of glucose molecules between the fetus and the placenta. The turnover rate calculation defines a physicochemical property of the sampled pool, i.e., for steady state, the rate at which glucose molecules exit the pool to be replaced at the same rate by glucose molecules "new" to the pool.[3] GTR$_f$ overestimates fetal tissue glucose metabolism because of diffusional exchange of tracer and tracee glucose in the uteroplacental unit and cannot be used to calculate or estimate fetal metabolic parameters such as net glucose utilization, clearance, or "endogenous" production by gluconeogenesis or glycogenolysis.[6,10] An example of this problem is presented in Table 17.1.

Fetal Glucose Metabolism Using Tracer Methodology: Rationale and Calculations

The tracer methods described require the use of large experimental animals surgically prepared with chronically indwelling catheters for the sampling of maternal arterial, uterine venous, umbilical arterial, and umbilical venous blood, and the simultaneous measurements of uterine and umbilical blood flows. This relatively complex approach is important; specifically, net glucose flux rates into and out of the fetal and maternal glucose pools can be measured by both tracer and Fick principle methods, allowing direct comparison of utilization and net uptake rates and estimation of endogenous production rates (i.e., utilization greater than exogenous entry) in both fetus and the uteroplacental unit.

The fetus and mother may be represented as two pools of glucose, each representing an anatomical compartment separated by a third pool called the uteroplacenta.

TABLE 17.1. Fetal insulin effect on fetal glucose utilization, umbilical glucose uptake, tracer glucose distribution, and "glucose turnover" (fetal tracer infusion).

Parameter	Control	Insulin infusion
Umbilical blood flow (ml·min^{-1})	800	800
Tracer glucose infusion (dpm·min^{-1})	2,100,000	2,100,000
Tracer glucose (dpm·ml^{-1})		
Umbilical vein	10,750	8675
Umbilical artery	12,141	9691
Glucose (mg·ml^{-1})		
Umbilical vein	0.246	0.207
Umbilical artery	0.223	0.178
Calculations		
Net tracer flux to placenta from fetus (dpm·min^{-1})	800 (12,141 − 10,750) = 1,112,800	800 (9691 − 8675) = 83,083
Net tracer flux into fetal metabolism (dpm·min^{-1})	2,100,000 − 1,112,800 = 987,000	2,100,000 − 813,083 = 1,286,917
Fetal glucose specific activity (dpm·mg^{-1})	54,444	54,530
Fetal glucose utilization (mg·min^{-1})	18.1	23.6
Umbilical glucose uptake (mg·min^{-1})	800 (0.246 − 0.223) = 18.4	800 (0.207 − 0.178) = 23.2
"Glucose turnover" (mg·min^{-1})	38.6	38.5

Note: Insulin enhances fetal glucose and tracer glucose metabolism, lowering their concentrations in fetal blood and leading to equally increased GUR and UGU and to decreased net tracer flux to the placenta from the fetus. Because specific activity does not change, GTR does not change, owing to decreased fetal-placental tracer exchange that balances the increase in fetal glucose utilization. Thus, GTR does not indicate the marked insulin-induced changes in GUR and UGU.

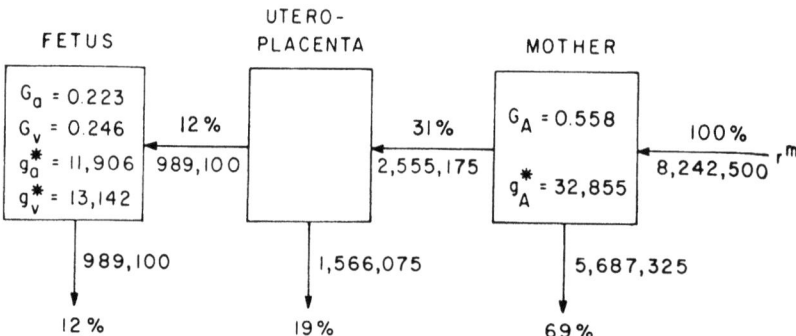

FIGURE 17.4. Example of calculation of maternal, uteroplacental, and fetal glucose utilization with a maternal tracer glucose infusion.

Experimental data
Umbilical blood flow: 800 ml·min^{-1}
Uterine blood flow: 1600 ml·min^{-1}
Tracer glucose infusion rate: 8,242,500 dpm·min^{-1}
Tracer concentrations in blood samples (dpm·ml^{-1}): 32,855 uterine artery, 31,258 uterine vein, 13,142 umbilical vein, 11,906 umbilical artery
Glucose concentrations in blood samples (mg·ml^{-1}): 0.558 uterine artery, 0.532 uterine vein, 0.246 umbilical vein, 0.223 umbilical artery

Calculations
Net tracer flux into uterus: 1600 (32,855 − 31,258) = 2,555,200 dpm·min^{-1}
Net tracer flux into maternal metabolism: 8,242,500 − 2,555,175 = 5,687,325
Maternal glucose specific activity (dpm·mg^{-1}): 32,855/0.558 = 58,880
Maternal (nonuterine) glucose utilization rate: 5,687,325/58,880 = 96.6 mg·min^{-1}
Umbilical (net fetal) glucose uptake: 800 (0.246 − 0.223) = 18.4 mg·min^{-1}
Uterine glucose uptake: 1600 (0.558 − 0.532) = 41.6 mg·min^{-1}
Uteroplacental glucose uptake: 41.6 − 18.4 = 23.2 mg·min^{-1}
Net tracer flux to fetus (and into fetal metabolism) from uteroplacenta: 800 (13,142 − 11,906) = 988,800 dpm·min^{-1}
Fetal glucose specific activity: 11,906/0.223 = 53,390 dpm·mg^{-1}
Fetal glucose utilization rate: 988,800/53,390 = 18.6 mg·min^{-1}
Estimated fetal glucose production rate: 18.5 − 18.4 = 0.1 mg·min^{-1}

17. Glucose Metabolism in the Fetal-Placental Unit

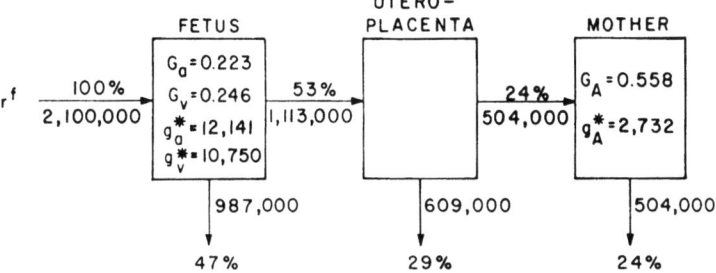

FIGURE 17.5. Example of calculation of fetal glucose utilization with a fetal tracer glucose infusion.

Experimental Data
Umbilical blood flow: 800 ml·min^{-1}
Tracer glucose infusion rate: 2,100,000 dpm·min^{-1}
Tracer glucose concentrations in blood (dpm·ml^{-1}): 10,750 umbilical vein, 12,141 umbilical artery
Glucose concentrations in blood (mg·min^{-1}): 0.246 umbilical vein, 0.223 umbilical artery

Calculations
Net tracer flux to placenta from fetus: 800 (12,141 − 10,750) = 1,112,800 dpm·min^{-1}
Net tracer flux into fetal metabolism: 2,100,000 − 1,112,800 = 987,200 dpm·min^{-1}
Fetal glucose specific activity: 54,444 dpm·mg^{-1}
Fetal glucose utilization rate: 18.1 mg·min^{-1}
Umbilical glucose uptake rate: 800 (0.246 − 0.223) = 18.4 mg·min^{-1}
Estimated fetal glucose production rate: 18.1 − 18.4 = −0.3 mg·min^{-1}

Without any tracer glucose in the system, net glucose flux to the pregnant uterus from the mother ($R_{up,m}$), net glucose flux to the fetus from the placenta ($R_{f,up}$), and net uptake of glucose by the uteroplacenta ($R_{o,up} = R_{up,m} - R_{f,up}$) can be calculated by the Fick principle.

The infusion of tracer glucose at constant rate into either the mother, the fetus, or both creates tracer fluxes within and among the three anatomical spaces. During a maternal tracer infusion (Figure 17.4) a portion of the tracer taken up by the uterine circulation is utilized (i.e., irreversibly disappears) within the uteroplacenta ($r^m_{f,up}$) and some is utilized by the fetus ($r^m_{o,f}$). The rate at which the fetus takes up the maternally infused tracer ($r^m_{f,up}$) is calculated by applying the Fick principle to tracer uptake by the umbilical circulation. Uteroplacental tracer uptake is calculated as the difference between uterine and umbilical tracer uptakes.

Similarly, the infusion rate of tracer into the fetus (r^f) (Figure 17.5) is equal to two exit rates [i.e., fetal net utilization (irreversible disposal) of tracer ($r^f_{o,f}$) and the net flux of tracer into the placenta ($r^f_{up,f}$)]. Of the tracer that enters the placenta, some is utilized (irreversibly disappears) within the uteroplacental mass ($r^f_{up,f}$) and some enters the mother via the uterine circulation ($r^f_{m,up}$) to be utilized (irreversibly disposed of) from the maternal pool ($r^f_{o,m}$).

Fetal Glucose Utilization Kinetics: Models Based on Number of Glucose Pools

The experimental design described above is relatively complex; some investigators have devised a simpler approach that involves one tracer of glucose infused into the mother and another into the fetus combined with measurement of glucose-specific activities in maternal and fetal arterial blood.[11,12] This method assumes that the maternal-placental-fetal glucose system can be represented by a two-pool model even though the intervening tissues of the uteroplacental mass metabolize glucose at a rapid rate.

Two-Pool Model of Glucose Utilization

The steady-state two-pool model of maternal-fetal glucose exchange is shown in Figure 17.6 (top).

In such two-pool models, the equations for calculating glucose utilization by the fetal tissue ($R_{o,f}$) and glucose utilization by the nonuterine maternal tissues ($R_{o,m}$) are as follows:[6]

$$R_{o,f:II} = \left\{ \left[(r^f)(SA^m_m) - (r^m)(SA^f_m) \right] / \left[(SA^m_m)(SA^f_f) - (SA^m_f)(SA^f_m) \right] \right\}$$

$$R_{o,m:II} = \left\{ \left[(r^m)(SA^f_f) - (r^f)(SA^m_f) \right] / \left[(SA^m_m)(SA^f_f) - (SA^m_f)(SA^f_m) \right] \right\}$$

Three-Pool Model of Glucose Utilization

A more complex representation of maternal-fetal glucose exchange is the three-pool model depicted in Figure 17.6 (bottom), which includes the uteroplacental tissues interposed between the maternal and fetal glucose pools.[6] According to reasonable but arbitrary choices, the uteroplacenta is assumed to metabolize tracer and tracee glucose derived from both the maternal and fetal pools but it does not produce glucose new to the system. Additionally, because glucose is transferred across the pla-

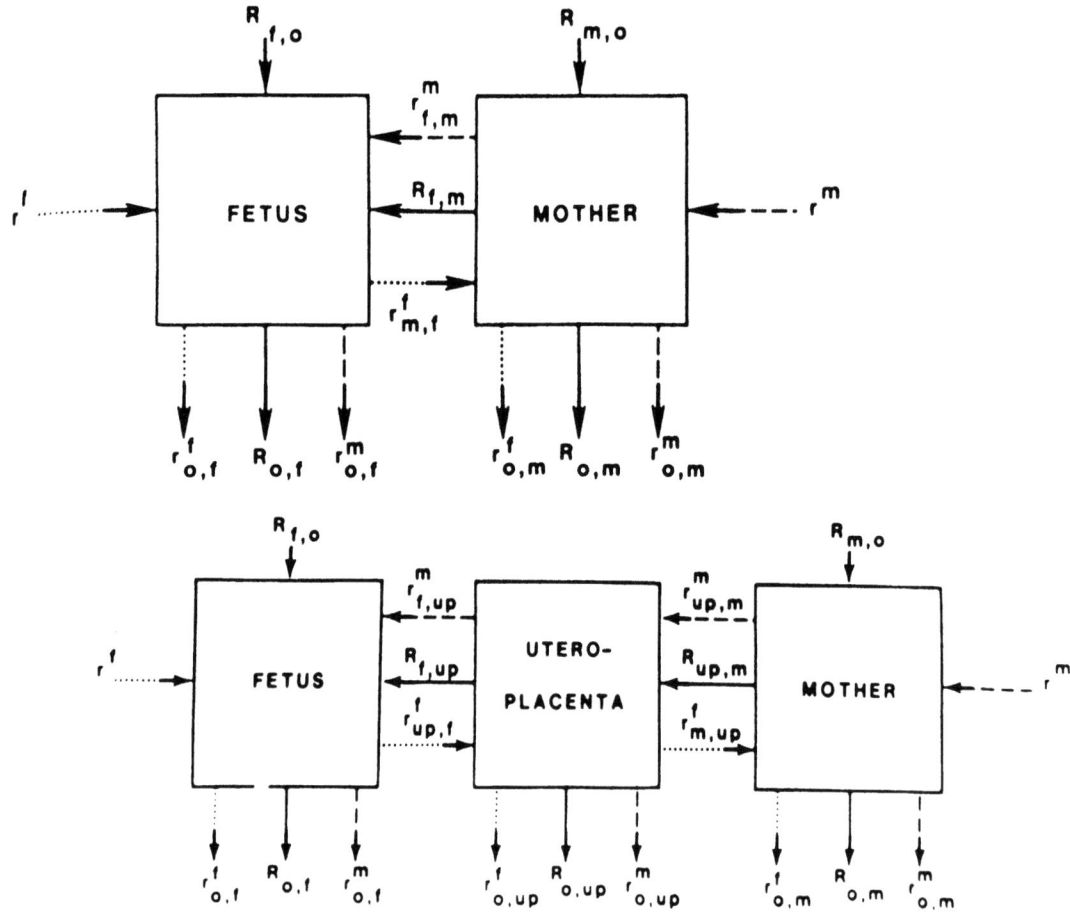

FIGURE 17.6. Top: Two-pool glucose model showing net tracer (r) and tracee (R) fluxes. Bottom: Three-pool glucose model showing net tracer (r) and tracee (R) fluxes. (From Hay et al.,[8] with permission.)

centa in both directions by facilitated diffusion,[1,13] each of the net tracer and tracee fluxes between the fetal, uteroplacental, and maternal pools results from the bidirectional exchange of glucose molecules.

The net rate of fetal glucose utilization ($R_{o,f}$) is calculated by dividing the net rate of fetal tracer utilization ($r_{o,f}^f$ or $r_{o,f}^m$) by the specific activity of the tracer in fetal arterial blood (i.e., SA_f^f or SA_f^m, respectively). The simultaneous infusion of two tracers, one into the fetus and one into the mother, permits two independent estimates of fetal glucose utilization. In several experiments in pregnant sheep, these two rates are not different.[14–16] Although intracardiac shunts produce slightly different mixtures of venous, arterial, and umbilical venous blood, which in turn produce slightly different specific activities among different arteries (e.g., aorta, cerebral arteries), the impact of such differences on whole-body fetal glucose utilization have not been determined; estimates indicate, however, that variations would be less than about 6%.

The equations for the rates of glucose utilization by fetal ($R_{o,f}$) and maternal (i.e., nonuterine) tissues ($R_{o,m}$) are:

$$R_{o,f} = \left\{\left[\left(r^f\right)\left(SA_m^m\right) - \left(r^m\right)\left(SA_m^f\right)\right] - \left(r_{o,up}^f\right)\left(SA_m^m\right) - \left(r_{o,up}^m\right)\left(SA_m^f\right)\right\} / \left[\left(SA_m^m\right)\left(SA_f^f\right) - \left(SA_f^m\right)\left(SA_m^f\right)\right]$$

Similarly,

$$R_{o,m} = \left\{\left[\left(r^m\right)\left(SA_f^f\right) - \left(r^f\right)\left(SA_f^m\right)\right] - \left(r_{o,up}^m\right)\left(SA_f^f\right) - \left(r_{o,up}^f\right)\left(SA_f^m\right)\right\} / \left[\left(SA_m^m\right)\left(SA_f^f\right) - \left(SA_f^m\right)\left(SA_m^f\right)\right]$$

$R_{o,f:III\ pool}$ and $R_{o,m:III\ pool}$ are less than $R_{o,f:II\ pool}$ and $R_{o,m:II\ pool}$ by the expressions:

$$R_{o,f:III} = R_{o,m:II} - \left\{\left[\left(r_{o,up}^f\right)\left(SA_m^m\right) - \left(r_{o,up}^m\right)\left(SA_m^f\right)\right] / \left[\left(SA_m^m\right)\left(SA_f^f\right) - \left(SA_f^m\right)\left(SA_m^f\right)\right]\right\}$$

and

$$R_{o,m:III} = R_{o,m:II} - \left\{\left[\left(r_{o,up}^m\right)\left(SA_f^f\right) - \left(r_{o,up}^f\right)\left(SA_f^m\right)\right] / \left[\left(SA_m^m\right)\left(SA_f^f\right) - \left(SA_f^m\right)\left(SA_m^f\right)\right]\right\}$$

17. Glucose Metabolism in the Fetal-Placental Unit

Both mathematically and experimentally, the differences between II-pool and III-pool values for $R_{o,f}$ and $R_{o,m}$ are equivalent to the net utilization of glucose by the uteroplacenta ($R_{o,up}$), which clearly is derived from both fetal and maternal pools.

The main significance of the three-pool model is that it demonstrates the necessity of considering uteroplacental glucose utilization in the modeling of maternal-fetal glucose exchange. If this exchange is represented by a two-pool model, the glucose utilization by the whole system (i.e., mother, uteroplacenta, and fetus) is partitioned so that a fraction of uteroplacental glucose utilization is assigned to the fetus and a fraction to the mother (Figure 17.7). Unfortunately, the portion assigned to the fetus does not necessarily represent only placental tissues, nor does the portion assigned to the mother necessarily represent only uterine tissues. Because the uteroplacenta can have a higher rate of glucose utilization than the fetus, the large contribution of the fetal glucose pool to uteroplacental glucose consumption cannot be ignored in tracer experiments designed to measure the rate of fetal glucose metabolism.

Fetal Glucose Oxidation and CO_2 Production

The rate of CO_2 produced by the oxidation of glucose in fetal tissues can be calculated as the rate of CO_2 produced from the fetal oxidation of glucose carbon using the equation:[17-19]

$$R_{ox} = r_{ox}/SA_f^f$$

where r_{ox} units are disintegrations per minute (dpm) of $^{14}CO_2$ excreted per minute from the fetus (i.e., calculated as the product of the umbilical arteriovenous $^{14}CO_2$ concentration difference in dpm·ml^{-1} times the umbilical blood flow in ml·min^{-1}), SA_f^f units are dpm·millimole^{-1} of glucose carbon, and R_{ox} units are millimoles CO_2·minute^{-1}. This calculation does not assume that all of the $^{14}CO_2$ produced from the infused ^{14}C-glucose comes from direct fetal oxidation of the labeled glucose carbon. In reality, some of the ^{14}C-glucose infused into a fetus diffuses into the uteroplacenta and is converted to other compounds (e.g., ^{14}C-lactate and, in fetal sheep, ^{14}C-fructose), which are taken up by the fetus and metabolized to $^{14}CO_2$. To the extent that umbilical excretion of $^{14}CO_2$ includes ^{14}C-glucose that is infused into and oxidized directly by fetal tissues and some from the fetal oxidation of ^{14}C compounds produced in the placenta from ^{14}C-glucose not taken up by the fetus, the fetal production of CO_2 from glucose oxidation would be overestimated. Experimental evidence demonstrates that in fetal sheep this overestimate is about 3% from lactate and 16% from fructose.[19] Compounds other than lactate and fructose may be involved as well (e.g., amino acids, keto acids, fatty acids) but their contribution has not been measured.

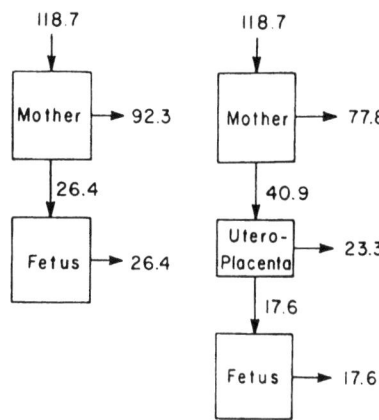

FIGURE 17.7. Comparison of two-pool, three-pool, and Fick principle calculations of fetal, maternal, and uteroplacental glucose fluxes (refer to Figures 17.4 and 17.5 and Appendix 17.2).

Experimental data
$r^f = 2,100,000$ dpm·min^{-1} $SA_f^f = 54,444$
$r^m = 8,242,500$ dpm·min^{-1} $SA_m^f = 7,200$
$R_{o,m}II - R_{o,m}III$
$SA_m^m = 74,126$ $r_{o,up}^f = 609,000$
$SA_f^m = 53,177$ $r_{o,up}^m = 1,566,075$

Calculations
$R_{o,f}II = \{[(2,100,000 \times 74,126) - (8,242,500 \times 7,200)]/[(74,126 \times 54,444) - (53,177 \times 7,200)]\} = 26.4$ mg·min^{-1}

$R_{o,f}III = \{[(2,100,000 \times 74,126) - (8,242,500 \times 7,200)] - [(609,000 \times 74,126) - (1,566,075 \times 7,200)]/[(74,126 \times 54,444) - 53,177 \times 7,200)]\} = 17.1$ mg·min^{-1}

$R_{f,up} = 17.6$ mg·min^{-1}

$R_{o,f}II - R_{o,f}III = 9.3$ mg·min^{-1}

$R_{o,m}II = \{[(8,242,500 \times 54,444) - (2,100,000 \times 53,177)]/[(74,126 \times 54,444) - (53,177 \times 7,200)]\} = 92.3$ mg·min^{-1}

$R_{o,m}III = \{[(8,242,500 \times 54,444) - (2,100,000 \times 53,177)] - [(1,566,075 \times 54,444) - (609,000 \times 53,177)]/[(74,126 \times 54,444) - (53,177 \times 7,200)]\} = 77.8$ mg·min^{-1}

$R_{o,m}II - R_{o,m}III = 14.5$ mg·min^{-1}

$(R_{o,m}II - R_{o,m}III) + (R_{o,m}II - R_{o,m}III) = 23.8$ mg·min^{-1}

$R_{o,up} = 23.3$ mg·min^{-1}

The production of ^{14}C labeled compounds from the tracer, which are oxidized secondarily in the fetus, can occur in the maternal tissues as well as in the placenta, but this contribution to fetal $^{14}CO_2$ excretion also has not been determined.

Fetal Glucose Oxidation Rate

One can estimate the oxidation rate of glucose. To do this, ^{14}C-glucose is infused into the fetus and the net uptake of the tracer by the fetus and the net excretion of

$^{14}CO_2$ from the fetus via the umbilical circulation is calculated by applying the Fick principle. By this method one can estimate the fraction of glucose oxidized by the fetus as the ratio of umbilical $^{14}CO_2$ excretion ($dpm \cdot min^{-1}$) divided by the net ^{14}C-glucose utilized by the fetus ($dpm \cdot min^{-1}$); the glucose oxidation rate is the product of the oxidation fraction and the glucose utilization rate: R_{ox} = (fraction of glucose oxidized) × (fetal glucose utilization rate).[17]

$$R_{ox} = \left[\left(net\ ^{14}CO_2\ excretion\right)/\left(net\ fetal\ ^{14}C\text{-}glucose\ utilization\right)\right] \times \left[\left(net\ fetal\ ^{14}C\text{-}glucose\ uptake\right)/\left(SA_f^f\right)\right]$$

where the rate of $^{14}CO_2$ excretion = (umbilical blood flow × umbilical arteriovenous blood $^{14}CO_2$ concentration difference), [(net fetal ^{14}C-glucose uptake) / (net fetal ^{14}C-glucose utilization rate)] is equal to fetal glucose utilization rate, and SA_f^f = the glucose-specific activity ($dpm \cdot mg^{-1}$) in fetal arterial blood. These calculations assume that all of the $^{14}CO_2$ that is excreted from the fetus is the result of direct fetal glucose oxidation, and that there is proportionality between $^{14}CO_2$ production and glucose oxidation. The latter assumption would be true, for example, if the tracer were 1-^{14}C-glucose and one molecule of $^{14}CO_2$ excreted represented one molecule of glucose completely oxidized. Alternatively, U-^{14}C-glucose could be used, in which case, six molecules of $^{14}CO_2$ excreted would represent one molecule of glucose oxidized. Problems generated from this latter assumption are avoided by expressing the specific activity as $dpm \cdot unit^{-1}$ glucose carbon, as in the equation for calculating the rate of fetal CO_2 production from glucose carbon oxidation.

Validation of Oxidation Methodology

In separate experiments in pregnant sheep, van Veen et al.[20] validated the method for measuring fetal $^{14}CO_2$ production using a constant infusion of ^{14}C-bicarbonate into the fetus to simulate a constant rate of fetal $^{14}CO_2$ production. In these experiments $^{14}CO_2$ excretion from the fetus via the umbilical circulation equaled the rate of ^{14}C entry via the $NaH^{14}CO_2$ infusion. $^{14}CO_2$ excretion from the fetus via the umbilical circulation can be considered equal to fetal $^{14}CO_2$ production from fetal oxidation of a ^{14}C-labeled substrate.

It is important to understand that these calculations of fetal glucose oxidation reflect only the oxidation of glucose leaving the plasma and entering fetal tissues. In situations of intracellular glucose production (e.g., glycogenolysis or gluconeogenesis), the intracellular glucose-6-phosphate specific activity, which is the precursor for glycolysis and glucose oxidation, is diluted relative to plasma, so the total fetal oxidation of glucose carbon is higher. Measurements of this process have not been undertaken.

The rate of uteroplacental $^{14}CO_2$ production from a specific ^{14}C-labeled substrate tracer infused into the fetus or the mother can be measured as the difference between the net rate of $^{14}CO_2$ entry into the uterine circulation (uterine blood flow × uterine venoarterial blood $^{14}CO_2$ concentration difference) and the net uptake of $^{14}CO_2$ by the uteroplacenta from the fetus via the umbilical circulation (umbilical blood flow × umbilical arteriovenous $^{14}CO_2$ concentration difference). This calculation requires highly accurate measurement of blood $^{14}CO_2$ concentration given the magnitude of uterine blood flow.

Fetal Glucose Production

Tracer glucose can be used to quantify fetal "endogenous" glucose production rates. These rates must be distinguished semantically from "production" rates, which are net "entry" rates into the fetal pool and include glucose molecules produced de novo (i.e., "endogenously") in the fetus ($J_{f,o}$) as well as glucose molecules produced in the pregnant woman and transported for the first time into the fetal glucose pool. The latter rate is the portion of the maternal glucose production rate ($J_{m,o}$) that, when reaching the fetus, is new to the fetus. It is calculated as:

$$\left(J_{m,o}\right)\left[\left(J_{f,m}\right)/\left(J_{f,m} + J_{o,m}\right)\right]$$

where $J_{f,m}$ = the unidirectional flux of tracer glucose to the fetus from the mother and $J_{o,m}$ = nonuterine maternal tracer uptake rate. "Endogenous" glucose production rates must be distinguished from the glucose "turnover" rate, which is the total entry or exit of glucose molecules into or out of the fetal glucose pool [i.e., for entry, the sum of glucose produced in the fetus de novo ($J_{f,o}$) + glucose produced in the mother and transported to the fetus ($J_{f,m}$) + glucose entering the fetus from the placenta by exchange or recycling (J_{recyc})]. These entry rates are intimately related. In fact, studies in which insulin was infused at a constant rate into the fetus produced an increased net fetal glucose utilization rate. Glucose turnover rate did not change, implying logically an increase in $J_{f,m}$ but a concomitant decrease in J_{recyc}.[21,22] It is important to appreciate that the transport ($J_{f,m} - J_{recyc}$) is not equal to the Fick principle calculation of net umbilical uptake, which is ($J_{f,up} - J_{up,f}$). Measurement of endogenous glucose production rate in the fetus with tracers requires two isotopes of glucose: one infused into the fetus and one into the mother. The isotope of glucose infused into the fetus (r^f) produces two specific activities: one in the fetus (SA_f^f) and one in the mother (SA_m^f). SA_f^f represents, at steady state, flux for tracer and tracee glucose and, at tracer equilibrium, dilution of r^f by fetal glucose production ($J_{f,o}$) and maternal glucose transferred to the fetus (J_m). Similarly, the isotope of glucose infused into the mother (r^m) produces two specific activities: one in the mother (SA_m^m) and one in the fetus (SA_f^m). SA_m^m represents dilution of r^m by $J_{m,o}$, whereas SA_f^m represents dilution of r^m by $J_{o,f}$ and by $J_{f,m}$. Equations relating the dilution of each isotope in the fetal pool have been developed and have been combined to solve for $J_{f,o}$ or the rate of fetal "endogenous" glucose production:[6]

$$J_{f,o} = \left\{ \left[(r^f)(SA_m^m - SA_f^m) \right] / \left[(SA_m^m)(SA_f^f) - (SA_m^f - SA_f^m) \right] \right\}$$

Fetal "endogenous" glucose production can be estimated as the difference between the rates of fetal glucose utilization measured by tracer techniques and umbilical glucose uptake measured by the Fick principle.

Placental Glucose Flux and Metabolism

Placental Glucose Uptake and Transfer

Glucose Transporters

Placental glucose uptake and transfer occur by facilitated diffusion, based on experimental evidence showing that rates of glucose uptake and transfer reach plateaus at increasing concentrations of maternal glucose.[1,5] In human placentas studied by perfusion techniques in vitro, the transport system for D-glucose is only saturable at maternal plasma glucose concentrations >20 mmol·L^{-1}, which is well above the normal physiologic range.[23] In sheep studied in vivo, saturation of net maternal-to-fetal glucose flux occurs at over twofold above normal maternal glucose concentrations. Placental glucose uptake and transfer are mediated by sodium-dependent, temperature-sensitive transport systems on both the microvillous and basal plasma membranes of the human syncytiotrophoblast that have specificity for hexoses and differential specificity among hexoses favoring D-glucose molecules.[24-26] The specific glucose transporters are protein molecules that are formed intracellularly and move to active sites in the membrane. The regulation of this movement in the trophoblast cell is not known, although there is some evidence that the process does occur in response to changes in the concentration of glucose molecules in the extracellular space.[24] (see Chapter 7)

The predominant molecular isoforms of glucose transporters found in the placenta are GLUT 1 and GLUT 3.[27] GLUT 1 is predominant in humans, localized to both microvillous and basal plasma membranes of syncytiotrophoblast and endothelial cells,[28-32] as well as to all cells of the amnion.[33] Expression of the high-affinity ($K_m \cong 1–1.5$ mmol/L) GLUT 3 isoform in the human placenta is controversial; its messenger RNA (mRNA) has been demonstrated in high levels, but GLUT 3 protein has been found only in rather low abundance. It is not known if this low abundance of GLUT 3 protein in the human placenta is real or due to limited antibody specificity.[27] GLUT 3 expression in the rat and the sheep becomes more prominent in later gestation. Its actual participation in glucose uptake and transport has not been confirmed, although Ehrhardt et al.[34] have shown in preliminary studies in sheep placenta using cytochalasian B competitive binding assays that GLUT 3 could account for as much as 40% of glucose uptake by the end of gestation up from only 8% at mid-gestation. GLUT 3 may be more prominent on the fetal side of the placenta, at least in the rat.[35] More recently, Clarson et al.[36] have shown expression of GLUT 3 mRNA and protein in rapidly dividing cells in the trophoblast, a phenomenon uncharacteristic of GLUT 1, which appears to be unaffected by either growth or differentiation; these investigators attributed a role for GLUT 3, therefore, in maintaining metabolic requirements of dividing trophoblast cells rather than in the transport of glucose into the placenta or into the fetus.

It is not known if the placental glucose transporters function as carriers of glucose across thin portions of the trophoblast, if they transfer glucose molecules to other transporter proteins within the trophoblast intracellular matrix, or if they release glucose molecules to the free intracellular glucose pool for immediate phosphorylation or diffusion to the basolateral surface for transport into the fetus. The number of glucose transporters appears to increase with gestation in sheep, most likely as a result of an increase in placental surface area.[34,37] Similar evidence for a gestational increase in GLUT 1 in the rat and human is less compelling.[27,30] It has not been determined if an increase in glucose transporter concentration occurs as well. The increase in glucose transporter number over gestation probably accounts in part for the gestational increase in placental-fetal glucose transport capacity.

In general, changes in placental glucose transporter mRNA levels have not always been linked to similar changes in protein concentration. Furthermore, time and glucose concentration–dependency have been observed, as well as species differences. For example, in preliminary studies in sheep, acute hyperglycemia, following maternal glucose infusion, increased GLUT 1 protein but this declined to normal levels with chronic hyperglycemia. In contrast, acute and chronic hypoglycemia, produced by a maternal insulin infusion, led to a decrease in GLUT 1 protein.[38] The hypoglycemic effect has been observed in vivo in the rat, whereas in vitro, hypoxia is the principal regulator of GLUT 1 protein, initially increasing its expression but eventually decreasing its expression, even though GLUT 1 mRNA may remain increased.[39] In human and rat trophoblast,

GLUT 1 protein and mRNA are decreased by hyperglycemia in vitro in the human, although only at very high glucose concentrations in the incubation medium,[40] but there is no change in vivo in the rat. Rat GLUT 3 protein has not been found to change in response to glycemia, either in vitro or in vivo.[30,39] Others have reported a relatively acute increase in GLUT 1 protein in the growth restricted rat fetus produced by uterine artery ligation in late gestation, in spite of no change in GLUT 1 mRNA.[41] GLUT 1 mRNA in rat placenta has been found to decrease with maternal insulin-like growth factor-I (IGF-I) treatment; such treatment increased placental and fetal weight, with the placental weight increase disproportionately greater than that of the fetus.[42] Only one study in vitro in human trophoblast cells and one study in vivo in sheep, which showed changes in either GLUT 1 protein or mRNA or both, have compared GLUT 1 expression with transport function; neither study found a change in glucose transport capacity.[43,44] These two studies speculated that transport capacity may have been maintained either by translocation of GLUT 1 to the cell surface or that transport capacity reflected an overall abundance of GLUT 1 protein that was great enough such that even 20% to 50% changes in protein concentration were insufficient to affect transport capacity. Such speculation needs further study, as does the entire field of placental glucose transporter expression, function, and regulation by glucose supply. Clearly there are marked differences in these aspects of glucose transport in the placenta that differ by study design, species, time of gestation, and duration and degree of change in glycemia.[30]

Insulin Receptors

In all species studied to date, the maternal and fetal surfaces of the placenta contain large numbers of insulin receptors, and receptor number increases with gestation. In the human placental trophoblast, receptor number on the maternal surface predominates in early gestation,[45] while in later gestation receptor number predominates on the fetal side where the receptors are confined more to endothelial cells.[46,47] Desoye and Shafrir[48] have hypothesized that this "spatiotemporal" pattern of insulin receptor expression might confer increasing regulation of insulin sensitive functions in the placenta to the developing fetus as its own insulin concentration and insulin secretion capacity increase with gestation, although this has not been tested to date. The physiologic role of insulin receptors on the placental surfaces remains unclear, despite considerable efforts to identify insulin-dependent metabolic processes.[48-50] Insulin binding to these receptors has been observed, but none of the classical effects of insulin, such as acute regulation of placental glucose uptake and transfer,[51-56] glycogen synthesis,[57,58] and inhibition of lipolysis[59] by plasma insulin, has been found on either the maternal or the fetal surface. These observations are true in the rodent and sheep placentas as well.[48] Furthermore, neither GLUT 1 nor GLUT 3, the only glucose transporter proteins identified in the placenta in any species to date, are insulin sensitive.[60] GLUT 4, which is insulin sensitive, has not been found in placental tissue from any species at any stage of gestation.[48] All of these studies have demonstrated that fetal glucose concentration, but not insulin concentration, determines placental glucose transfer to the fetus. The role of placental insulin receptors and the potential for insulin action on the placenta remain obscure despite attempts to link such receptors to insulin-like growth factor function.[61] IGF-I actually decreases GLUT 1 mRNA,[42] amino acid uptake,[62] or the regulation of placental synthesis of peptide and steroid hormones.[48] (see Chapters 8 and 20)

Placental Glucose Transport Kinetics and Placental Glucose Consumption

The description of placental-to-fetal glucose transfer was first quantified according to carrier-mediated, facilitated diffusion by Widdas.[1] Widdas theorized that placental glucose transfer would approach a maximum as maternal and fetal glucose concentrations increased beyond physiologic limits, according to the equation

$$Q_f = V_{max}\left\{\left[G_A/(G_A + K_m)\right] - \left[G_a/(G_a + K_m)\right]\right\}$$

where V_{max} = the maximal flux of glucose, and K_m = the concentration of glucose in the maternal (G_A) or fetal (G_a) plasma at which the transport mechanisms are half-saturated. This model assumes that the placenta acts simply as a diffusion membrane and does not consume glucose. According to the data by Meschia et al.,[2] placental glucose consumption in the late gestation pregnant sheep can account for up to two thirds of uterine glucose uptake. Similar large estimates of placental glucose consumption have been obtained in the guinea pig and human using in situ[63,64] and in vitro[65,66] perfusion models. To test the effect of placental glucose consumption on placental glucose transfer, Simmons et al.[5] infused glucose into the fetus or mother in chronically catheterized pregnant sheep and demonstrated that the relation between placental glucose transfer and the maternal-fetal plasma glucose concentration gradient has a negative intercept. The magnitude of this negative intercept is equal to net fetal to placental glucose transfer (i.e., net placental glucose consumption) when the maternal and fetal glucose concentrations are equal and experimentally accounts for about 75% of uteroplacental glucose uptake. This observation is supported by additional tracer studies showing that as much as 40% of placental glucose consumption could come from the fetal plasma glucose pool. Under normal glycemic conditions,[6] the equation for placental glucose transfer according to Widdas was modified by Simmons et al. to include a negative intercept accounting for net placental glucose consumption[5]:

$$Q_f = V_{max}\{[G_A/(G_A + K_m)] - [G_a/(G_a + K_m)]\} - \dot{q}p$$

where $\dot{q}p$ = the net placental glucose consumption from fetal-to-placental glucose transfer at $G_A = G_a$. At experimentally determined values of $K_m = 70\,mg \cdot dl^{-1}$, $G_A = 70\,mg \cdot dl^{-1}$, $\dot{q}p = 30\,mg \cdot min^{-1}$, $V_{max} = 209$, and $Q_f = 20\,mg \cdot min^{-1}$, G_a would equal $24.5\,mg \cdot dl^{-1}$. If $\dot{q}p$ were zero, G_a would equal about $47.5\,mg \cdot dl^{-1}$.[6] Clearly, net placental glucose consumption contributes significantly to the physiologic hypoglycemia of the fetus and helps to establish the glucose concentration gradient by which the placenta and fetus compete for glucose molecules.

The equation for transplacental glucose transfer by Simmons et al.[5] indicates that changes in maternal or fetal glucose concentration affect transport and should affect uterine glucose uptake and placental glucose consumption. Experiments in near-term pregnant sheep have shown that net glucose uptake from the uterine circulation, placental-to-fetal glucose transfer, and net uteroplacental glucose consumption are directly related to maternal glucose concentration.[66] These experiments involved tightly controlled maternal glucose clamp experiments in which glucose flux across the placenta was quantified by the Fick principle at several steady-state maternal glucose concentrations. The results demonstrate saturation kinetics for all three flux rates (Figure 17.8). The V_{max} for uterine glucose uptake is about $73\,mg \cdot min^{-1}$ reached at a K_s of about $145\,mg \cdot dl^{-1}$, which is approximately twice the normal G_A. The K_m for uterine glucose uptake is about $50\,mg \cdot dl^{-1}$, close to the normal blood glucose concentration in pregnant sheep at this gestation, implying significant regulatory capacity of placental glucose flux by maternal glucose concentration.

Uptake and net consumption of glucose by the placenta demonstrate saturation kinetics with V_{max} of $41\,mg \cdot min^{-1}$; K_m (maternal arterial glucose concentration at $V_{max}/2$) and K_s (maternal arterial glucose concentration at which V_{max} is reached) are $19\,mg \cdot dl^{-1}$ and $145\,mg \cdot dl^{-1}$, respectively—not significantly different from the same parameters for uterine uptake. Interestingly, placental oxygen consumption does not change significantly over these wide ranges of glucose consumption, while lactate production does, and fetal lactate uptake from the placenta and fetal plasma lactate concentration are directly related to fetal glucose concentration.[67] Given the constancy of placental oxygen consumption over this range of placental glucose consumption, these studies raise the possibility that a reciprocal relationship exists between placental glucose oxidation and placental oxidation of

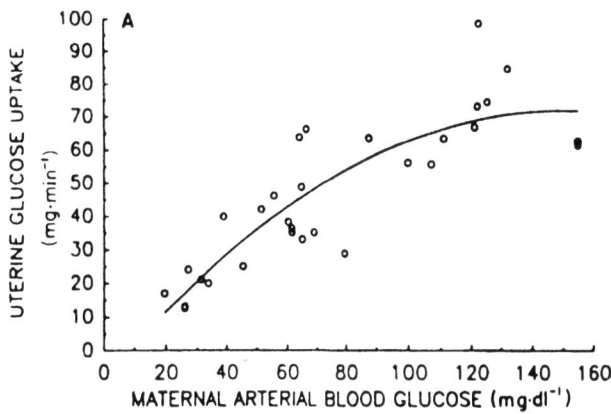

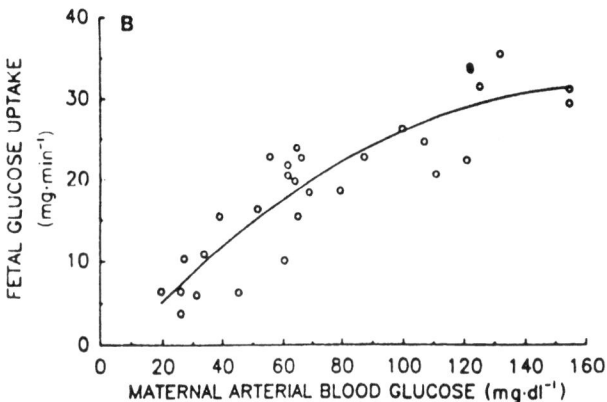

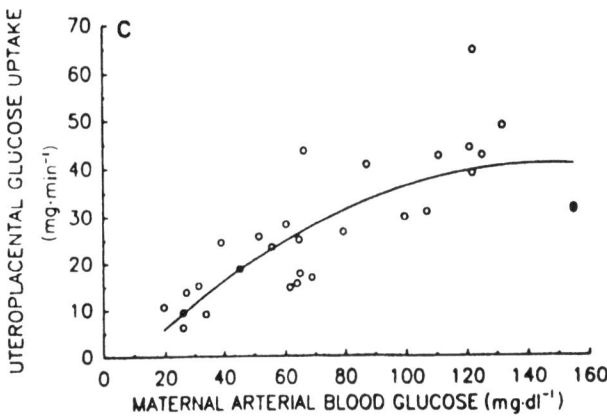

FIGURE 17.8. Experimental data from glucose clamp experiments in pregnant sheep demonstrating saturation kinetics for net uterine glucose uptake (A), net fetal glucose uptake (B), and net uteroplacental glucose uptake (C) versus maternal arterial blood glucose concentration. (From Hay and Meznarich,[66] with permission.)

other substrates. The nature of such substrates (e.g., trophoblast glycogen, lactate, amino acids, ketones) and their quantitative role in placental oxidative metabolism remain to be determined.

The effect of maternal glucose concentration on net placental-to-fetal glucose transfer demonstrates saturation kinetics.[66,68] This relation does not necessarily define the quantitative characteristics of placental-to-fetal glucose transport capacity, because as maternal glucose concentration and placental glucose transport are increased, fetal glucose concentration and utilization rate increase. Other studies in which glucose was infused into the fetus directly have shown a saturation of fetal glucose utilization rate at about the same V_{max} and K_s values as determined by maternal glucose infusions.[69] The maternal glucose infusion technique may reflect fetal glucose consumption kinetics as well as those of placental-to-fetal glucose transfer. To address this experimental problem, other studies have used glucose clamp procedures in maternal and fetal circulations simultaneously, regulating the maternal-to-fetal glucose concentration gradients at different maternal and fetal glucose concentrations.[70] As shown in Figure 17.9, placental-to-fetal glucose transfer, quantified as the change in the umbilical venoarterial glucose concentration difference, is sensitive to a change in fetal glucose concentration gradient, regardless of the maternal glucose level.[71] This study design is important for demonstrating that at a constant maternal glucose concentration uteroplacental glucose consumption is directly related to fetal glucose concentration.

As discussed above, when the transplacental glucose concentration is abolished, approximately three fourths of the glucose consumed by the uteroplacenta is supplied by the fetal circulation.[5] This observation implies that the fetal side of the uteroplacenta is markedly more permeable to glucose than the maternal side, and it indicates that changes in fetal glucose concentration have a strong influence on placental glucose flux and metabolism (Figure 17.10).

The importance of this regulation of placental-to-fetal glucose transfer and net uteroplacental glucose consumption by fetal glucose concentration is shown by observations in chronically hypoglycemic pregnant sheep in which fetal glucogenesis developed.[10,74] This rate of fetal glucose production contributes glucose molecules to the fetal glucose pool and sustains fetal glucose utilization at near-normal rates. As a result, the fetal-to-placental glucose concentration gradient and the placental-to-fetal glucose transfer rate are relatively reduced; under these circumstances, uteroplacental glucose consumption is maintained at near-normal rates for the level of maternal glycemia. Fetal glucose production can compensate for a reduced maternal glucose supply and sustain not only fetal glucose utilization requirements but those of the fetal vital supply organ, the placenta. This phenomenon is a striking example of how fetal metabolic autonomy acts to protect fetal survival without further demand on a limited maternal nutritional supply. Several other placental factors may affect placental glucose transport, includ-

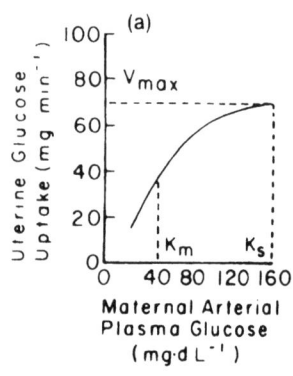
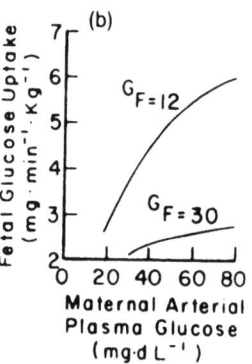
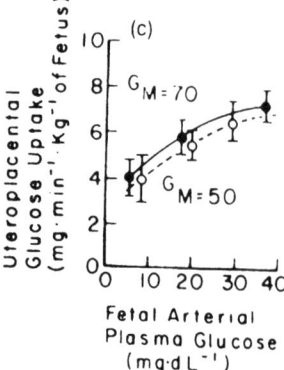

FIGURE 17.9. (a) Schematic representation of effect of maternal glucose concentration on uterine glucose uptake, based on experiments in which glucose was infused into pregnant sheep after an overnight fast to produce a large variety of maternal arterial blood glucose concentrations. Fick principle measurements were then made of net uterine glucose uptake rates versus the maternal arterial blood glucose concentration, which shows saturation kinetics with an approximate K_m value in the physiologic range of maternal glucose concentration (about 50–60 mg·dl^{-1}). (Adapted from data in Hay and Meznarich,[66] with permission.) (b) Fetal glucose uptake (net transfer of glucose from placenta to fetal circulation) plotted against maternal arterial glucose concentration showing a saturable dependence of fetal glucose uptake on maternal glucose concentration. In addition, this relationship is left-shifted as fetal glucose concentration is decreased, showing that as fetal glucose concentration is decreased relative to that of the mother, which increases the maternal-fetal glucose concentration gradient, placental-to-fetal glucose transfer increases. (Adapted from data in Hay et al.,[72] with permission.) (c) Net rate of uteroplacental glucose consumption in sheep, expressed per kilogram of fetus, plotted against fetal arterial plasma glucose. Solid line: values measured while maternal arterial plasma glucose was clamped at about 70 mg/dl. Dotted line: values measured while maternal arterial plasma glucose was clamped at about 50 mg·dl^{-1}. These data show that although maternal glucose concentration determines glucose entry into the uteroplacenta and fetus, actual uteroplacental glucose consumption is regulated largely by the fetal glucose concentration. (Adapted from data in Hay et al.,[71] with permission. Figure 17.9 from Gluckman and Heymann, with permission.)

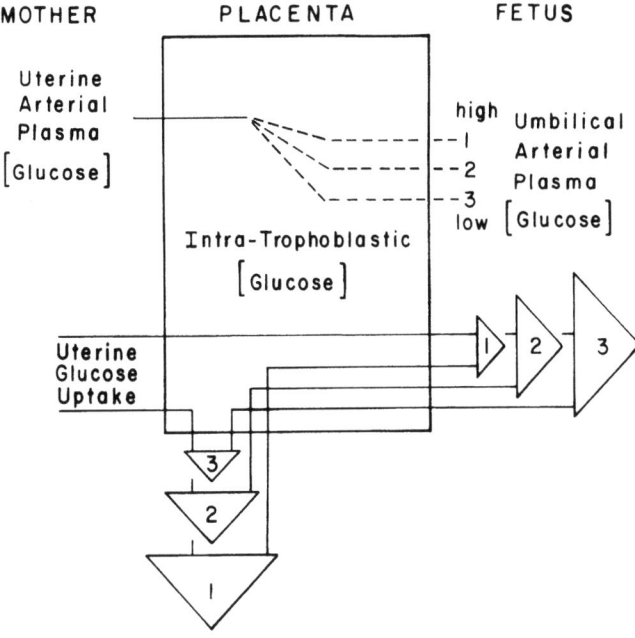

FIGURE 17.10. Schema of effects of fetal glucose concentration on placental glucose transfer to the fetus and uteroplacental glucose consumption, adapted from data in sheep. A decrease in fetal glucose concentration relative to maternal glucose concentration promotes maternal-to-fetal glucose transfer at the expense of uteroplacental glucose consumption. These findings demonstrate a reciprocal relationship between placental glucose transfer and uteroplacental glucose consumption that is determined by the fetal glucose concentration gradient, in contrast to total uterine glucose uptake, which is primarily under the control of the maternal arterial plasma glucose concentration and the maternal-fetal arterial plasma glucose concentration gradient. (From Hay,[73] with permission.)

ing placental surface area, thickness, uterine and umbilical blood flow, and glucose consumption. The effect of changes of placental thickness on glucose transport has not been studied, but there appears to be a direct relation between the maternal-to-fetal arterial glucose gradient and the amount of intervening placental and vascular tissue layers (Figure 17.11).[75] Whether such tissue layers increase the gradient by glucose consumption or by imposing a barrier to transport is unknown.

The effect of placental surface area has been determined by Owens et al.,[76] who performed uterine carunculectomies in nonpregnant sheep. This model, as developed by Alexander,[77] limits the myometrial implantation area, effectively reducing the number of placental cotyledons and the surface area of the placenta. In these studies, fetal weight and fetal glucose consumption were reduced approximately proportional to the reduction in placental weight (Table 17.2). Placental glucose consumption and transport to the fetus were similarly reduced. The fetal/placental weight ratio was greater in the carunculectomy group (12.6 ± 3.9) than in the control group (7.8 ± 1.3), indicating that the placenta may have developed compensatory mechanisms that allow increased nutrient transport in response to the restricted placental size. The maternal-to-fetal glucose concentration gradient increased from the control group level owing to the development of fetal hypoglycemia that, combined with the reduced transport of glucose, indicated that placental glucose transport capacity was reduced. Systematic studies have not been done to determine whether the glucose transport capacity might have been maintained, or amino acid transport capacity actually increased, sufficient to accomplish at least some of the increased nutrient transfer in these growth-restricted but partially growth-compensated fetuses.

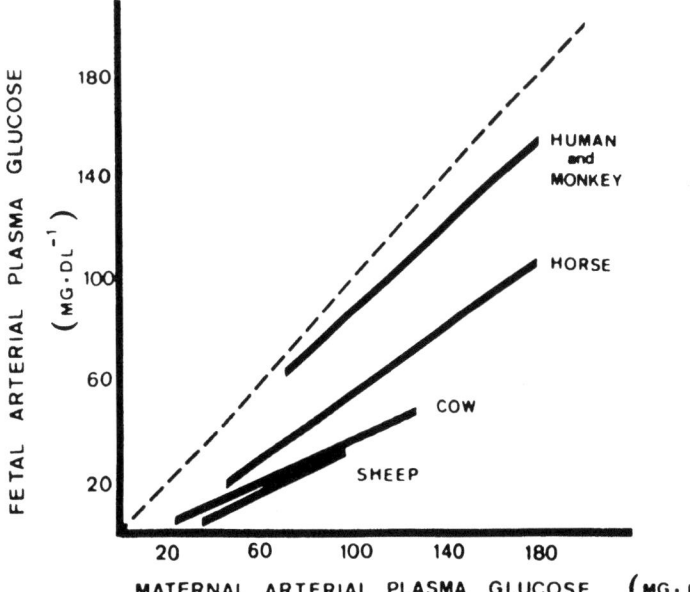

FIGURE 17.11. Relation of fetal arterial plasma glucose concentration to maternal arterial plasma glucose concentration for the human, monkey, horse, cow, and sheep. (From Battaglia and Hay,[75] with permission.)

TABLE 17.2. Placental and fetal metabolic results of uterine carunculectomy in sheep (mean ± SD).

Parameter	Control	Carunculectomy (growth restricted)
Placental weight (g)	485 ± 105	197 ± 91
Fetal weight (g)	3720 ± 807	2198 ± 653
Maternal arterial blood glucose (mM)	1.84 ± 0.46	2.41 ± 0.45
Fetal arterial blood glucose (mM)	0.84 ± 0.24	0.57 ± 0.11
Fetal oxygen consumption		
mmol·min^{-1}	1.208 ± 0.488	0.748 ± 0.215
mmol·min^{-1} total fetal weight	0.325 ± 0.131	0.340 ± 0.100
Fetal glucose consumption		
mg·min^{-1}	18.4 ± 2.7	11.1 ± 4.3
mg·min^{-1}·kg^{-1} total fetal weight	4.9 ± 0.7	5.1 ± 2.0
Estimated placental glucose transfer capacity (fetal glucose consumption/maternal-fetal glucose concentration difference)	0.036	0.018

Gestational Changes in Placental Glucose Transfer

Over the second half of gestation, the functional capacity of the placenta to transfer substances between maternal and fetal circulations increases markedly, as shown previously for placental urea diffusing capacity.[78] A dramatic increase in placental glucose transport capacity has been shown. This increase in transport capacity far exceeds the transport one would expect for the simultaneous increase in maternal-fetal glucose concentration gradient. As shown in Figure 17.12, approximately 60% of the increased placental glucose transport is accounted for by the increase in transport capacity, the remaining 40% being accounted for by the change in gradient.[79,80]

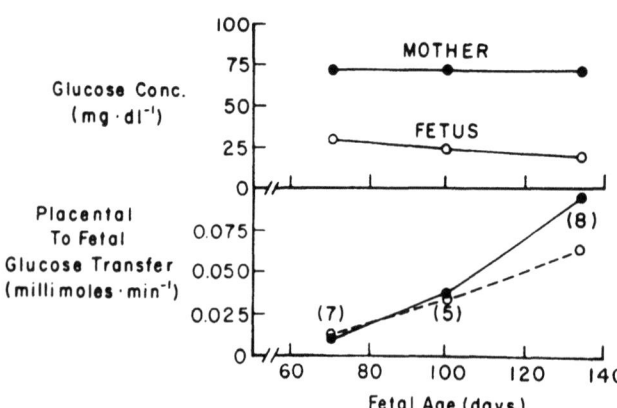

FIGURE 17.12. Placental to fetal glucose transfer in pregnant sheep. The increase in placental glucose transfer (PGT) that occurs over the second half of gestation in sheep is largely accounted for by an increase in placental glucose transfer capacity shown by the comparison of PGT at a fixed transplacental glucose concentration gradient of 45 mg·dl^{-1} with total PGT. (From Hay,[79] with permission.)

This increased transport capacity most likely reflects an increase in surface area and the number of glucose transporters. The regulation of this developmental increase in glucose transporter abundance, other than by remodeling of the trophoblast membrane surface area, is not known. Figure 17.13 presents a schema of how the increase in placental glucose transfer capacity over the second half of gestation in sheep interacts with fetal metabolism to guarantee an increase in placental transfer of glucose to meet the increasing glucose needs of the growing fetus.[81] The fetal metabolic adjustments include increased insulin production and plasma insulin concentration, and increased insulin action that is accounted for largely by and increase in the fraction of fetal body weight accounted for by insulin-sensitive tissues (e.g., primarily skeletal muscle). All of these factors combine to produce increased fetal glucose utilization; increased fetal plasma glucose clearance, defined as the ratio of plasma glucose disposal rate (measured as fetal glucose utilization rate) divided by the plasma glucose concentration rate; a relatively lower fetal plasma glucose concentration; and ultimately an increase in the maternal-fetal plasma glucose concentration gradient leading to increased glucose transfer across the placenta to the fetus.[82] The increasing transplacental glucose concentration gradient could result from a gestational-dependent increase in placental glucose consumption. This does occur in sheep and might be expected to do so in other species.[81] In the human placenta, however, in vitro perfusion experiments by Malek et al.[83] have shown a 40% reduction in glucose consumption between 28 to 33 weeks and term, coupled with a decrease in placental lactate production of 36% over the same period. Whether this represents the results of in vivo conditions or of the in vitro placenta in late gestation has not been determined. The human placenta has not been studied in

17. Glucose Metabolism in the Fetal-Placental Unit

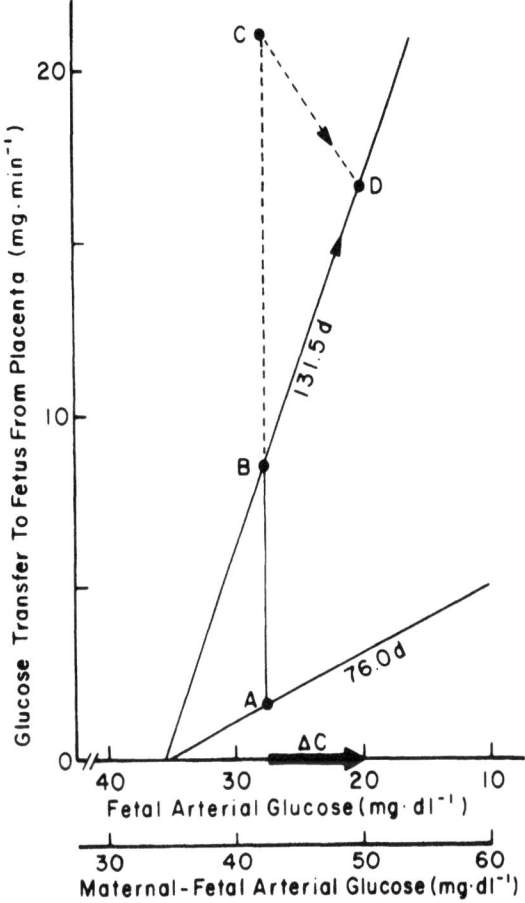

FIGURE 17.13. Graphic illustration of interrelationships among developmental changes in placental glucose transport capacity, fetal glucose demand, and fetal glucose concentration from mid- to late gestation in the sheep model. Placental glucose transfer capacity increases over gestation, shown by the increased slope of the 131.5-day gestational age line versus the slope of the mid-gestation, 76-day line, supplying more glucose to the fetus (A → B). Fetal growth demands more glucose, however, represented by point C. Additional glucose is provided by the simultaneous decrease in fetal plasma glucose concentration relative to that in the maternal plasma, which increases the transplacental glucose concentration gradient (x-axis segment ΔC), producing the actual glucose supply to the fetus at point D (which is less than point C because the lower fetal glucose concentration also decreases the mass action transfer of glucose from the fetal plasma into fetal cells). (From Molina et al.,[81] with permission.)

vivo with respect to the rate of glucose metabolism or transfer to the fetus.[84]

Placental Glucose Metabolism

Glucose carbon consumed by the placenta produces CO_2 and water by oxidation.[6] Based on data in pregnant sheep, such glucose carbon consumption in the placenta could account for about 45% of placental oxygen consumption, assuming all of the glucose that is available for oxidation is oxidized, and that placental lactate and fructose production are derived solely from net placental glucose consumption.[2] Preliminary studies in pregnant sheep in which tracer glucose was infused into the mother indicate that glucose oxidation might account for as little as 15% to 20% of net placental glucose consumption, with lactate production accounting for about 30% to 40%, fructose for about 9% to 10%, and amino acids for about 2% to 3%. This would leave as much as 50% of uteroplacental glucose consumption unaccounted for. This amount of glucose oxidation could account for only about 20% to 30% of placental oxygen consumption. Further experiments are necessary to determine the validity of these observations.

Glucose produces placental glycogen, but rates of production and regulation of this process are not known.[85] Lactate is produced by the placenta of all species in relatively large amounts, averaging 0.1 mmol·min^{-1} in or 30% to 40% of net uteroplacental glucose consumption sheep. Estimates in humans are much smaller. Lactate enters into the maternal and fetal circulations at approximately equal rates, based on data in sheep under normoglycemic conditions.[86] Placental lactate production is a normal aerobic process unaffected by small to moderate changes in maternal or fetal blood PO_2, blood oxygen content, or uterine or umbilical blood flow.[87] In sheep the amount of lactate taken up by the fetus is about half of the net fetal glucose uptake at normal glucose concentrations and about one third of fetal lactate utilization. Most fetal lactate is produced by the fetus, although it is clear that lactate produced in the placenta is a net source of carbon for fetal carbon utilization. Lactate production by the human placenta in vivo has been more difficult to demonstrate; in vitro, human placental lactate production is quite large.[84,88]

Placental production of fructose is unique to ruminants[89] and does not occur to any appreciable extent in humans, although fructose has been found in relative abundance in the urine of neonates over the first hours of life.[90] In the sheep quantitative aspects of placental fructose production and fetal fructose metabolism have been investigated using the Fick principle and tracer methodology.[91] In well-fed, normoglycemic sheep, net placental fructose production averages 1.27 ± 0.7 (SEM) mg·min^{-1}·kg^{-1} fetal weight and enters the umbilical vein exclusively. Tracer studies show placental oxidation of fructose but at a low rate. Fructose does produce a small amount of lactate in the placenta, but there is no net conversion to glucose with release into the uterine or umbilical circulation. The simultaneous tracer-derived fetal fructose utilization rate, 0.97 ± 0.08 (SEM) mg·min^{-1}·kg^{-1} fetal weight, is no different from the net umbilical fructose uptake, demonstrating no evidence for fetal fructose production. Fructose is transported only into the fetus from the placenta. Its transport is dependent on GLUT 5, which is specific to this hexose.[60] GLUT 5 presence or function in the ruminant placenta has not been studied.

Fetal Glucose Metabolism

Fetal Glucose Uptake and Utilization

As discussed (Figure 17.11), early studies of fetal glucose metabolism established that fetal glucose concentration is directly related to maternal glucose concentration. These observations suggest that maternal glucose concentration determines the rate of glucose supply to the fetus. This hypothesis was tested by applying the Fick principle, and data from a number of laboratories have established a direct relation between fetal glucose uptake via the umbilical circulation and maternal glucose concentration.[52] As presented earlier, this relationship is defined by saturation kinetics.[66] More recently, studies using radioactively labeled tracers of glucose have demonstrated a similar relationship for maternal glucose concentration and fetal glucose utilization rate[69] (Figure 17.14).

The near identity of the two correlations, umbilical glucose uptake (UGU) versus glucose concentration in maternal arterial circulation (G_A) and glucose utilization rate in the fetus (GUR_F) versus G_A, has two important implications. First, UGU versus G_A most likely represents the kinetics of GUR_F much more than the kinetics, or at least the capacity, for placental-to-fetal glucose transfer. Second, there is little if any fetal glucogenesis under the conditions of short-term (i.e., 1–4 hour) perturbations in G_A, UGU, G_a, and GUR_F, in which case GUR_F would be expected to be greater than UGU. In human fetuses, stable isotopic tracer infusions into the mother have shown no dilution in fetal plasma sampled by cordocentesis over the second half of gestation and in response to mild hypoglycemia induced by overnight maternal fasting.[92] These data indicate the absence of fetal glucogenesis in the human fetus under normal and acutely mild hypoglycemic conditions, which are similar to results in sheep.

Fetal Insulin Secretion

It is clear from many studies that fetal glucose concentration (G_a) and fetal insulin concentration (I_a) change together. Insulin secretion in response to changes in G_a has been observed over a large portion of late gestation, and several studies have documented that this relation can occur acutely[93] and chronically.[94] In a recent study in sheep it was observed that while basal fetal plasma glucose concentration tended to decrease over the second half of gestation by about 30%, fetal plasma insulin concentration did not change. At the same time, however, fetal plasma volume and extracellular volume increased even more, demonstrating that basal insulin secretion had increased.[95] Furthermore, there was a fivefold increase in glucose- and arginine-stimulated insulin secretion over the same gestational period, demonstrating the development of both insulin secretion capacity and the responsiveness of the fetal pancreatic β cell to normal insulin secretagogues.

Other studies in the fetal sheep have demonstrated that sustained, marked hyperglycemia in the fetus has the unique effect of decreasing fetal insulin concentration

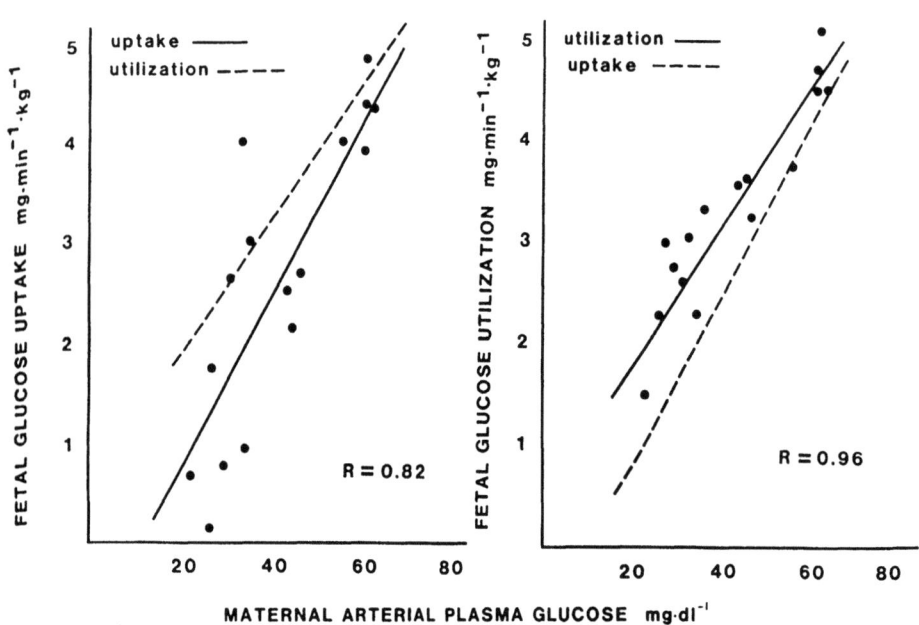

FIGURE 17.14. Comparison of fetal glucose uptake and fetal glucose utilization (determined with [U-^{14}C] glucose tracer infused into the fetal inferior vena cava) with maternal arterial plasma glucose concentration. (Adapted from data presented by Hay et al.[22])

from an initial elevated value, enhanced by glucose stimulation, back to basal concentration. Additional glucose stimulation of insulin secretion also is reduced under these conditions, and eventually this suppression of insulin secretion is extended to other secretagogues such as arginine. These data indicate that chronically high glucose concentrations in the fetus can limit insulin secretion, perhaps as a means of limiting fetal glucose storage and oxidation, which are processes that consume excessive amounts of oxygen and produce excessive amounts of lactate.[96]

Mechanisms that might account for such hyperglycemic suppression of fetal insulin secretion are not known. Preliminary studies indicate that fetal pancreatic GLUT 2, the glucose transporter on the β-cell membrane that is coupled with glucokinase and forms the β-cell glucose sensing mechanism is not altered under conditions of chronic hyperglycemia.[97]

Similar hyperglycemic suppression of fetal insulin secretion has been observed in the fetal rat.[98,99] Such results are in contrast to conventional understanding about the human fetus of a diabetic mother in whom hyperglycemia is presumed to stimulate fetal insulin secretion. Indeed, a variety of observations in human diabetic pregnancies have shown greater amniotic fluid insulin concentrations and greater cord blood concentrations of C-peptide, a marker of insulin secretion, at term delivery.[100] Variability in human maternal glucose concentration has not been shown to be a principal reason for this enhanced fetal insulin secretion, even though this is a reasonable hypothesis given the propensity in late gestation among normal pregnant women and women with gestational diabetes to develop increasingly exaggerated meal-associated hyperglycemia.[101] Pulsatile spikes of hyperglycemia in fetal sheep clearly have been shown to enhance glucose- and arginine-stimulated fetal insulin secretion, a process that is augmented over time.[102] The role of other secretagogues under such conditions has not been studied extensively. Fatty acids are known insulin secretagogues and they tend to be enhanced in concentration in pregnant diabetics and their fetuses, perhaps contributing to the augmented insulin secretion in human fetuses of diabetics.[103] In sheep and other experimental animals, fetal plasma concentrations of fatty acids are quite low and likely do not contribute very much to fetal insulin secretion.[3] Other studies indicated that amino acids might play a significant role in fetal insulin secretion, but most of the studies that led to this conclusion were performed by injecting large doses of amino acids (e.g., arginine) into the fetus, producing pharmacologic concentrations in the fetus.[104] More recently, bolus arginine infusions into fetal sheep in late gestation, at basal and hyperglycemic glucose levels, demonstrated that physiologic concentrations of arginine had little effect on fetal insulin secretion. The change in insulin secretion was not great enough to produce any measurable effect on fetal glucose metabolism until the rapidly increased arginine concentration exceeded the normal plasma arginine concentration by over twofold, which is into the pharmacologic range.[104]

It is much better appreciated that acute and chronic hypoglycemia limit fetal pancreatic insulin secretion, under basal conditions and in response to acute glucose stimulation.[74] The mechanisms that produce these effects of hypoglycemia are not known, although it is presumed that glucose is necessary for stimulation of the insulin gene response elements as well as the mechanisms for insulin secretion from the β cell. The molecular mechanisms involved in fetal insulin production, storage, and secretion have not been elucidated.

Effect of Insulin and Glucose on Glucose Utilization

The simultaneous change of I_a with G_a and earlier observations that bolus infusions of insulin into the fetus could lower G_a indicated that GUR_F could be controlled directly by G_a and I_a separately as well as in combination.[105] Several studies have quantified the separate and combined effects of G_a and I_a on fetal glucose metabolism. Using glucose clamp techniques, Hay and Meznarich[106] showed that insulin alone could enhance fetal glucose utilization to a maximal rate about twice normal. These studies were conducted under euglycemic conditions by infusing glucose into the fetus in response to changes in G_a. Umbilical uptake did not change because the G_{A-a} gradient was held constant and because insulin had no independent effect on umbilical glucose uptake from the placenta. The maximal effect of insulin approximately doubled the glucose oxidation rate, but increased fetal oxygen consumption only by about 15%. These data indicated that a major portion of the increased glucose oxidation substituted for the oxidation of other substrates, allowing fetal oxygen consumption and total substrate oxidation rates to remain relatively constant. These studies were extended to include insulin clamps at a large variety of fetal insulin and glucose concentrations. The results, presented as three-dimensional glucose utilization[43] (Figure 17.15) or oxidation[19] (Figure 17.16) rate response surfaces, emphasize the combined effects of glucose and insulin on fetal glucose metabolism.

Several features of this response are important. First, the separate effects of glucose and insulin are parallel over their maximal effect ranges; that is, their effects are independent and additive, indicating that glucose transport to cells in fetal sheep represents the rate-limiting process by which glucose and insulin both promote glucose metabolism. Second, the V_{max} for GUR_F is about 10.6 mg·min^{-1}·kg^{-1} (at K_s = 45 mg·dl^{-1} for G_a, and K_s = 80 μU·ml^{-1} for I_a), about the same as predicted by the UGU/GUR_F versus G_A relation, again emphasizing that

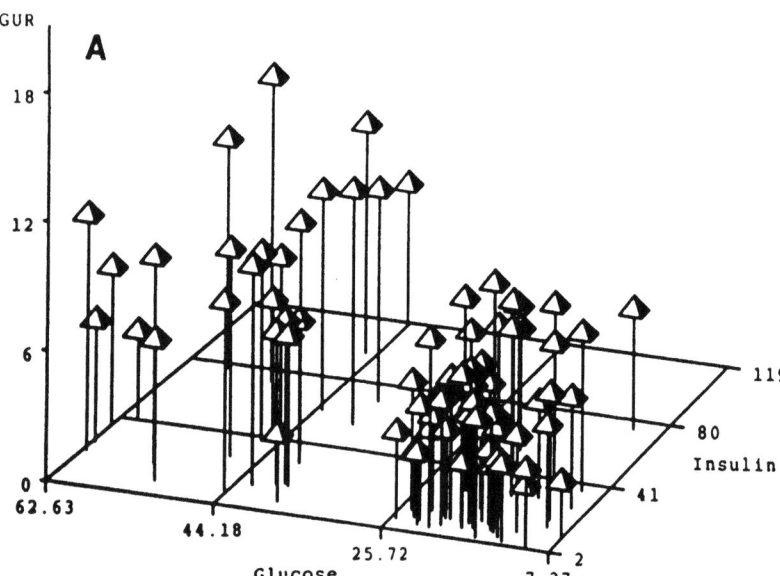

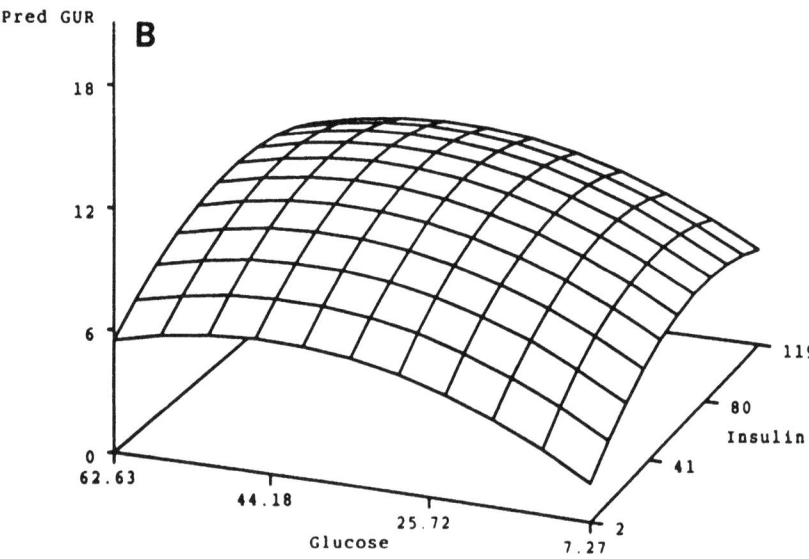

FIGURE 17.15. A: Three-dimensional plot of individual values of glucose utilization rate at different concentrations of insulin and glucose. B: Predicted three-dimensional glucose by insulin surface. Data obtained in near-term fetal sheep. (From Hay et al.,[69] with permission.)

the latter relation is more a reflection of fetal glucose metabolism than the kinetics of placental-to-fetal glucose transfer. Third, bearing in mind that in fetal sheep I_a (in $\mu U \cdot ml^{-1}$) $\cong 0.5$ G_a (in $mg \cdot dl^{-1}$), K_m values can be selected for the combined $G \times I$ surface of $20.6 mg \cdot dl^{-1}$ G_a and $10.0 \mu U \cdot ml^{-1}$ I_a, remarkably similar to normal values for G_a and I_a in normal fetal sheep. Comparability of normal concentrations with K_m values for a substrate-driven reaction is a commonly observed situation in biologic reactions, demonstrating maximum sensitivity in the control of the reaction by a change in substrate concentration. Fourth, the GUR intercept for insulin-dependent GUR is near zero, whereas the GUR intercept for glucose-dependent GUR ranges from about 2 to $6 mg \cdot min^{-1} kg^{-1}$. Additionally, based on an expected unit ($\mu U \cdot ml^{-1}$) change in plasma insulin concentration of about 0.95 times a unit ($mg \cdot dl^{-1}$) change in blood glucose concentration, the GUR_F versus G_a sensitivity is about twice the GUR_F versus I_a sensitivity.[93] These observations indicate that, whereas fetal GUR_F is regulated by physiologic concentrations of glucose and insulin, most glucose utilization in fetal sheep depends primarily on the supply of glucose to the fetus and on physiologic concentrations of glucose secondarily augmented by changes in insulin concentration. Finally, the saturation kinetics of the independent GUR versus glucose concentration relation demonstrate that GUR does not change proportionate to glucose concentration. Fetal glucose clearance decreases with increasing glucose concentration. Insulin acts to increase glucose clearance to approximately the same extent at any glucose concentration but does not change the GUR versus glucose concentration (Table 17.3).

Effect of Other Hormones on Fetal Glucose Metabolism

Fetal glucose utilization is affected by fetal thyroid hormone action, although this appears to occur indirectly by

FIGURE 17.16. (A) Three-dimensional plot of individual values of CO_2 production from glucose carbon oxidation at different concentrations of insulin and glucose. (B) Predicted three-dimensional glucose by insulin surface. Data obtained in near-term fetal sheep. (From Hay et al.,[18] with permission.)

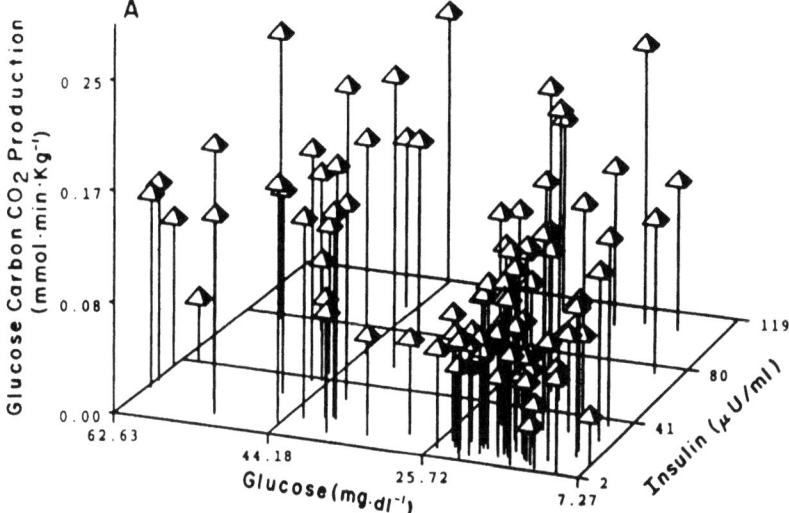

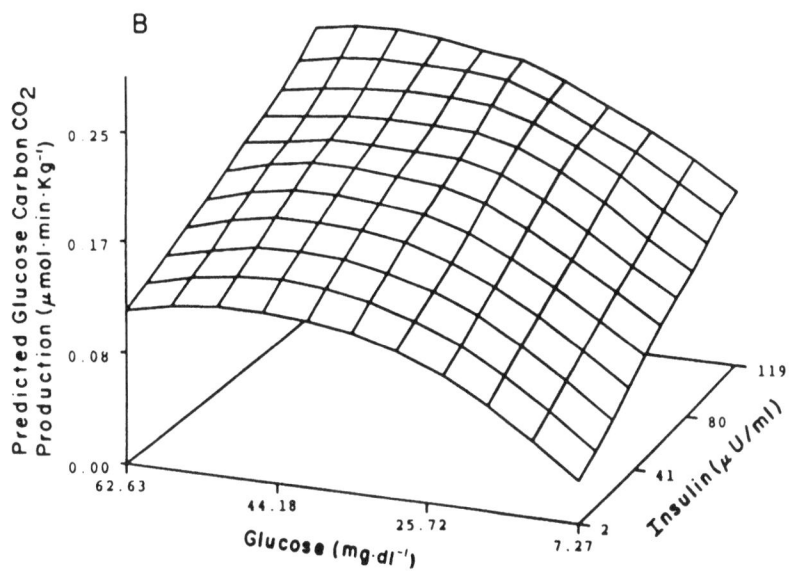

the regulation of fetal metabolic rate (i.e., oxygen consumption) by thyroid hormone.[108] Changes in fetal plasma cortisol concentration during late gestation appear to have little effect on fetal glucose concentrations or on the rates of glucose utilization.[109] Cortisol increases in concentration in the fetal plasma in very late gestation, however, at which time the cortisol dependent increases in fetal hepatic glycogen and gluconeogenic enzyme activities enhance the glucogenic capacity of the fetus and may contribute to the endogenous glucose production observed in normal fetuses just before term and at the time of delivery.[110] Cortisol infusions into the fetus just prior to the cortisol surge divert fetal plasma glutamine into fetal glucose and glycogen production and away from glutamate production.[111] High concentrations of glucagon[112] and physiological concentrations of circulating catecholamines[113] such as adrenal epinephrine and spillover norepinephrine from peripheral nerve endings are normally present in modest concentrations in the fetal plasma, but they do stimulate fetal glucogenesis when infused exogenously into the fetus. IGF-I has little or no effect on fetal glucose kinetics, but glucose concentration itself is a direct regulator of IGF-I production and circulating concentration.[114] In part, these changes in IGF-I concentrations may be due to the simultaneous changes in fetal plasma insulin as insulin can alter IGF-I concentration independently of fetal glucose concentration.[115] These observations suggest that it is the intracellular concentrations of glucose, which is controlled by insulin, that regulates fetal IGF-I production. In turn, IGF-I can inhibit protein breakdown,[116] as does insulin,[117] which is increased in concentration with higher glucose

TABLE 17.3. Effect of hypo- and hyperinsulinemia in the fetus on fetal metabolism.

Metabolite	Hypoinsulinemia	Hyperinsulinemia
Glucose		
Concentration	Increase	Decrease
Umbilical uptake	Decrease	Increase
Utilization	Decrease	Increase
Oxidation	Decrease	Increase
Lactate		
Concentration	Increase	?
Umbilical uptake	No change	?
Fructose		
Concentration	Increase	?
Amino acids		
Concentration	Increase	Decrease
Protein catabolism	?	Decrease
Fat		
FFA concentrations	Increase	?
Deposition	Decrease	Increase
Oxygen		
Arterial content	Increase	Decrease
Consumption	?	Small increase

From Fowden,[107] with permission.

concetrations, thereby enhancing indirectly the capacity for glucose to promote fetal nitrogen balance and growth. This conclusion is supported by evidence collected in chronic fetal sheep studies that show that decreased fetal glucose supply for several weeks leads to decreased placental transfer of leucine to the fetus, produces fetal hypoinsulinemia as well, and results in increased protein breakdown, initially including increased leucine oxidation.[118] As leucine concentration decreases chronically, leucine oxidation decreases, so that over longer periods only protein breakdown is involved. Glucose supply to the fetus, therefore, indirectly affects fetal amino acid metabolism and protein accretion, via insulin, IGF-I, and placental amino acid supply mechanisms.

Fetal Glucose Transporters

Cellular and molecular mechanisms that account for tissue glucose uptake in the fetus have not received much attention experimentally. GLUT 1 is found throughout the fetal tissues and on all endothelial cells and probably accounts for the majority of basal tissue glucose uptake from the fetal plasma.[60] Studies in rat and sheep fetuses show that GLUT 1 expression is upregulated by hypoglycemia and hypoinsulinemia in skeletal muscle and adipose tissue in contrast to no change in the brain, whereas skeletal muscle and adipose tissue GLUT 4, which is insulin-responsive, initially is upregulated but then downregulated toward normal levels of expression.[119,120] In contrast, sustained hyperglycemia, initially with hyperinsulinemia but with subsequent normalization of insulin concentration, produces transient increases in insulin-independent brain GLUT 1 and liver GLUT 2 expression, and increased fat and skeletal muscle GLUT 1, but a reciprocal reduction in fat and skeletal muscle GLUT 4.[121,122] Sustained hyperglycemia and hypoglycemia failed to alter myocardial GLUT 1 expression in these same studies in fetal sheep, and hyperglycemia, initially with hyperinsulinemia but later with normoinsulinemia, had no effect on myocardial GLUT 4 expression.[123] In contrast, sustained hypoglycemia with hypoinsulinemia decreased myocardial GLUT 4 expression. The separate effects of glucose and insulin on such changes in GLUT 1 and 4 expression are not yet known, although glucose-specific and insulin-specific GLUT gene response elements have not yet been identified in any cells.[124] GLUT 1 appears to be responsive by translocation from intracellular storage pools to glucose concentration only in insulin-sensitive cells. This aspect of GLUT 1 function has not been studied very much in the fetus, although Simmons et al.[125] found that insulin and IGF-I increased lung and skeletal muscle cellular GLUT 1 protein and mRNA in cells derived from normal fetuses, but not in growth restricted fetuses. Cell culture of lung and skeletal muscle cells in vitro showed different effects, with low glucose enhancing and high glucose suppressing GLUT 1 protein and mRNA.[126] Obviously, cell, tissue, in vitro, in vivo, and species differences in study design currently limit our ability to make firm conclusions about the regulation of glucose transporter expression in the fetus.

Fetal Glucose Oxidation

Insulin and glucose act independently and additively to promote glucose oxidation as well as glucose utilization. Furthermore, the fraction of glucose oxidized remains constant over the entire GUR versus glucose concentration × insulin concentration surface. Fetal oxygen consumption is enhanced to a minor degree (i.e., <15% maximal increase).

These results emphasize two important aspects of fetal glucose oxidative metabolism. First, glucose oxidation rate, as well as other metabolic pathways for glucose, depends primarily on cellular glucose uptake and not on intracellular regulation of glucose distribution among metabolic pathways. Of course, this conclusion holds for the summation of all tissues in the fetus that consume glucose. Individual tissues may behave differently, as may intracellular glucose pathways in selected cells or tissues. Second, given the near constancy of fetal oxygen consumption over wide ranges of fetal glucose utilization, there must be a reciprocal relation between the oxidation of glucose and that of other substrates. Whether a similar reciprocal relation exists between glucose and substrates for nonoxidative fates of glucose or such fates are specific to glucose and rate-dependent on glucose supply is not known. There are two such pathways: (1) glycogen formation through which glucose can form glycogen directly as well as indirectly through prior formation of 3-carbon glycolytic intermediates and secondary gluconeogenesis, and (2) fat deposition through which glucose can contribute directly or in combination with lactate and acetate.

Fetal Glucose Carbon Contribution to Glycogen Formation

Many tissues in the conceptus, including placenta, brain, liver, lung, heart, and skeletal muscle produce glycogen over the second half of gestation.[127] Liver glycogen content, which increases with gestation (Figure 17.17), is the most important store of glycogen for systemic glucose requirements. Only the liver contains sufficient glucose-6-phosphatase for release of glucose into the circulation.[128] Skeletal muscle glycogen content increases during late gestation, whereas lung glycogen content decreases with change in cell type, leading to loss of glycogen-containing alveolar epithelium, development of type II pneumocytes, and onset of surfactant production.[129] Cardiac glycogen concentration decreases with gestation owing to cellular hypertrophy, but cardiac glycogen appears essential for postnatal cardiac energy supply and cellular function.[130]

At term, liver glycogen concentration in most species is at least twice the adult concentration of 40 to $60 mg \cdot g^{-1}$. Glycogen synthetic rates vary from low, steady rates of accumulation in long-gestation fetuses of about $2 mg \cdot day^{-1} g^{-1}$ (e.g., human and fetal lambs) to exceptionally high rates of about 40 to $100 mg \cdot day^{-1} g^{-1}$ in term fetal rats with short gestations. The latter, remarkably high glycogen synthetic rate amounts to a glucose requirement of about 0.7 to $1.0 mg \cdot min^{-1} kg^{-1}$, representing less than 20% of estimated glucose utilization in the fetal rate. In large, more slowly growing fetuses (e.g., lamb, monkey, and human), glycogen synthesis by the liver accounts for an even smaller portion of fetal glucose utilization.[131]

In the fetus, net synthesis or degradation of glycogen is controlled by the functional balance between two enzymes: glycogen synthase, which promotes glycogen formation, and glycogen phosphorylase, which promotes glycogen degradation. Total content of these two en-

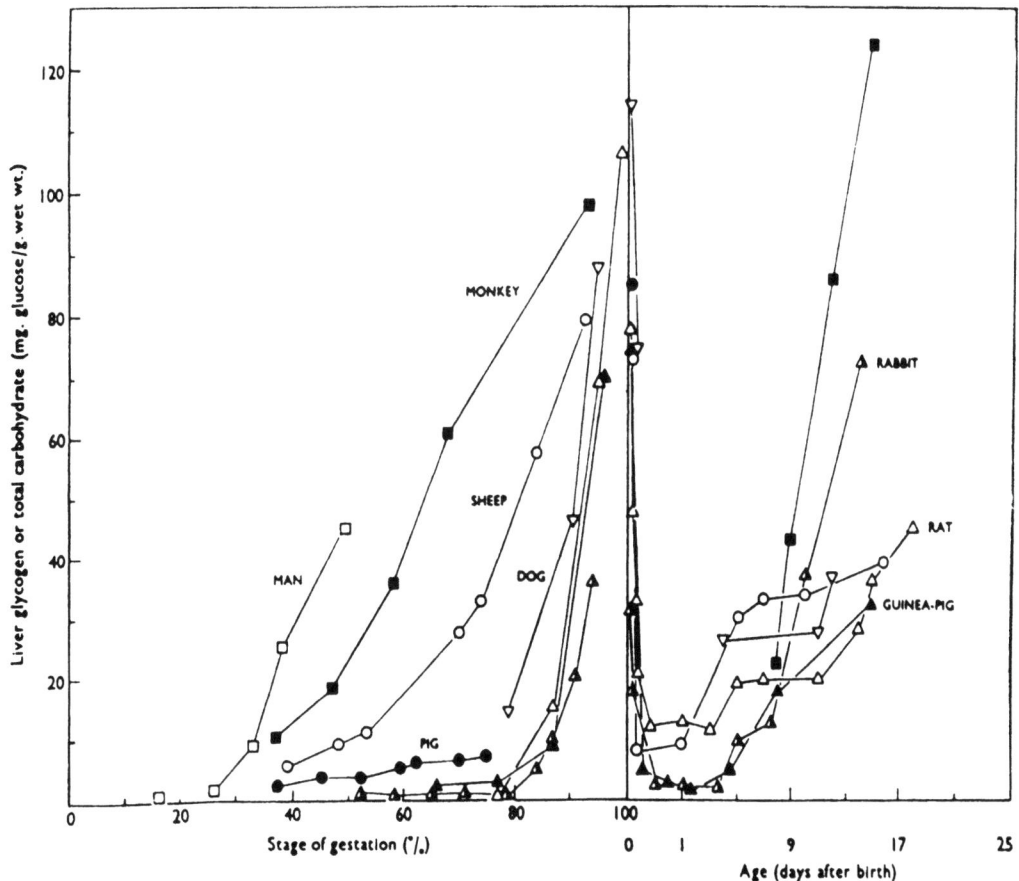

FIGURE 17.17. Liver glycogen in various species before and after birth. Hepatic glycogen content in several species is shown to increase with gestational age, decrease precipitously during the immediate postnatal period, and increase again with a normal neonatal diet. (From Shelly,[127] with permission.)

zymes is relatively constant over gestation. Their functional states are regulated by hormone and substrate concentrations, principally cortisol and glucose, respectively. Experimentally, cortisol depletion by fetal decapitation, hypophysectomy, or adrenalectomy reduces while cortisol infusion enhances fetal glycogen deposition.[109,110] Glucose infusion into mother or fetus, both producing fetal hyperglycemia, increases fetal glycogen deposition by activating glycogen synthase, perhaps via insulin, and experimental hypoglycemia in the fetus reduces glycogen deposition. Glucose acts independently to activate phosphorylase, thereby helping to keep glycogen content constant at higher glucose concentrations.[132] Insulin acts synergistically with glucose to produce hepatic glycogen, and may even act alone in this regard in that pancreatectomized fetal sheep that are hypoinsulinemic but hyperglycemic have less glycogen, and insulin infused, hypoglycemic but hyperinsulinemic fetal sheep have increased hepatic glycogen.[133,134] In the adult liver, glucose enhances synthase by increasing glucose-6-phosphate and inhibiting glucose-6-phosphatase, and gluconeogenic substrates such as fructose enhance glycogen synthesis by inhibiting phosphorylase.[135] As discussed by Sparks et al.,[136] synthase activity in the rat is directly related to fetal adrenal activity. Fetal decapitation in vivo and absence of glucocorticoid activity in vitro prevent an increase of synthase activity. Glucocorticoids given to the decapitated fetus or added to the in vitro system allow synthase activity to increase. Glucocorticoid administration to the pregnant animal (e.g., rat or monkey) hyperstimulates glycogen synthase and glycogen concentration.[136]

Hypoglycemia, glucagon, and cyclic-adenosine monophosphate (cAMP) can induce the fetal liver to release glucose from glycogen by activation of phosphorylase.[137,138] Increased glucose-6-phosphatase activity has been found in the fetus following administration of cortisol, glucagon, cAMP, and fetal hypoglycemia that is secondary to maternal fasting-induced hypoglycemia.[139] Such responses have been measured in vitro in human fetal hepatic tissue.[140] In the human the enzymatic capacity for both hepatic glycogen formation and degradation are present during late fetal life. The nonoxidized rate of net glucose carbon utilization in fetal lambs is probably greater than can be accounted for by net fetal glycogen and fatty acid synthesis. Furthermore, the fetal sheep liver, as early as mid-gestation, contains the enzymes 3-phosphoserine aminotransferase, phosphoserine phosphatase, serine-pyruvate amino-transferase, and 2-phosphoglycerate phosphatase, which catalyze the net conversion of the glycolytic intermediates 3-phosphoglycerate and D-glycerate to serine. These reactions require glutamine and alanine as nitrogen donors, both of which are abundant in the fetal plasma.[141] Net serine release by the fetal liver has been observed.[142] Similar interconversions between glucose carbon and alanine[143] and glycine[144] have been documented. There likely is a significant contribution of fetal glucose carbon to fetal amino acid and protein synthesis, although this process has not been documented or quantified.

Fetuses of hyperglycemic, diabetic mothers have high concentrations and contents of hepatic glycogen, whereas intrauterine growth-restricted fetuses have diminished hepatic glycogen.[145] Based on these observations, glucose has been considered the primary substrate for hepatic glycogen. In fetal baboons, Levitsky et al.[146,147] have demonstrated active glycogen synthesis from lactate and fructose using radioactively labeled tracers. DiGiacomo et al.[148] infused [1-^{13}C]-glucose into fetal sheep at two thirds of gestation to minimize tracer dilution in hepatic glycogen and reported by nuclear magnetic resonance spectroscopy that rearrangement of the labeled first carbon of the tracer may have occurred in newly synthesized glucose molecules of hepatic glycogen.[148] Glucose conversion to glycogen is mostly direct, however, as preliminary studies in fetal sheep hepatocytes, for example, show that about 92% to 94% of glycogen formation is from glucose molecules directly. Only the balance occurs indirectly via prior formation of lactate, fructose, and other glycolytic intermediates with subsequent gluconeogenesis. Together these observations indicate that glucose is the major carbon source for fetal hepatic glycogen synthesis.

In fetal life, there is a large uptake of glutamine from the placenta which is converted to glutamate in the fetal liver, as there is little gluconeogenesis under usual conditions in the fetus. The glutamate in turn is taken up by the placenta where most of it is oxidized to CO_2 and water. Recent studies by Meschia and Battaglia[149] in the fetal sheep have shown that as term approaches, cortisol concentration increases, and parturition begins, fetal hepatic gluconeogenesis increases, particularly from glutamine, as hepatic glutamate production from glutamine and subsequent placental glutamate uptake decreases. Fowden et al.[150] have shown under the same circumstances that increased fetal cortisol acts to increase gluconeogenic enzyme capacities, particularly including glucose-6-phosphatase, which is necessary to release newly formed glucose into the fetal plasma. These coordinated changes demonstrate an important regulation of fetal glucose metabolism that is coupled with amino acid metabolism, placental, and fetal hepatic developmental metabolism, and the requirements for glutamate oxidation in the placenta for other developmentally necessary processes (e.g., perhaps steroidogenesis).

Fetal Glucose Carbon Contributions to Fat Synthesis

The contribution of glucose carbon to fatty acid synthesis has not been quantified in most species including the human, who has the largest proportion of body weight as fat at term—about 16% to 18%. In the fetal sheep, Robertson et al.[151] studied carbon sources for fat synthesis in vitro. Acetate, glucose, and L-lactate provide 50%, 17%, and 33%, respectively, of the C_2 units for fatty acid synthesis in adipose tissue slices, about 30 days prior to birth, or about 80% of gestation. The contributions of acetate and lactate depend directly on their concentrations. Glucose concentration dependence was not studied, but increased glucose in the fetus leads to increased lactate as well. These data indicate a positive contribution of glucose carbon, directly and indirectly, to fat synthesis during hyperglycemia.

Fetal Gluconeogenesis

The ability of the fetus to make new glucose molecules from nonglucose substrates (e.g., lactate, amino acids, glycerol) is highly variable among species. Gluconeogenesis from alanine and lactate has been demonstrated in early calf liver slices.[152] In rats, gluconeogenesis appears limited, not increasing until after birth, coincident with increases in gluconeogenic enzyme levels, particularly phosphoenolpyruvate carboxykinase (PEPCK), and ingestion of fatty acids and triglycerides from maternal milk.[153] In the fetal guinea pig, gluconeogenesis from several substrates has been demonstrated prenatally, although these rates of gluconeogenesis correlate poorly with gluconeogenic enzyme levels.[154,155] In human fetal tissues studies, variable levels of gluconeogenic enzymes are present, but rate-defining activities have not been determined.[156] It is not clear whether postnatal gluconeogenesis in preterm neonates occurs according to developmental stage or is affected by postnatal enzyme induction.

In the fetal lamb near term, all of the enzymes necessary for gluconeogenesis are present.[157] Sparks et al.[136] could not show more than about 3% of fetal lactate utilization entering glucose molecules; a similar low rate of alanine-to-glucose was shown by Prior and Scott.[152] In fetal lambs that had a sustained fasting-induced hypoglycemia for 7 to 10 days, Sparks et al.[158] found that fetal hepatic vein glucose concentration gradually rose above the umbilical vein glucose concentration, indicating net hepatic glucose release, but the source of the hepatic glucose production (i.e., glycogen degradation of gluconeogenesis) was not determined. Given the duration of the marked degree of glucose deprivation with concomitant decreased lactate and fructose supply, it is reasonable to assume that most of this net hepatic glucose release is produced by gluconeogenesis.

In similar studies of fasting-induced hypoglycemia, Hay et al.[15] demonstrated an increasing discrepancy between umbilical glucose uptake and fetal glucose utilization rate at umbilical glucose uptake rates of less than 2.5 mg·min^{-1}·kg^{-1}, indicating the development of net fetal glucose production (Figure 17.18).

This net glucose production rate probably is derived from net glycogen degradation initially. In relation to the indirect conversion of glucose to glycogen and the net contribution of lactate and fructose to glycogen discussed above, it is most likely that ongoing net fetal glucose production is derived from gluconeogenesis, even if it includes intrahepatic cycling via glycogen turnover. Narkewicz et al.[159] showed in chronically hypoglycemic fetal sheep an increase in the cytosolic PEPCK concentration and activity, indicating that the lower glucose and insulin concentrations in these animals acted to stimulate the key regulatory enzyme for gluconeogenesis. This action is regulated primarily by the increase in the fetal plasma glucagon-to-insulin concentration ratio, as hypoinsulinemia coupled with hyperglucagonemia produced by fetal streptozocin injection does result in increased fetal glucose production.[160] However, hypoinsulinemia by itself, as produced by fetal pancreatectomy,[161] results in very little gluconeogenesis.

The rate of gluconeogenesis estimated in these studies is large, approaching 2 mg·min^{-1}·kg^{-1}, or nearly 50% of normal rates of glucose utilization. These flux rates have been confirmed in studies in which sustained maternal

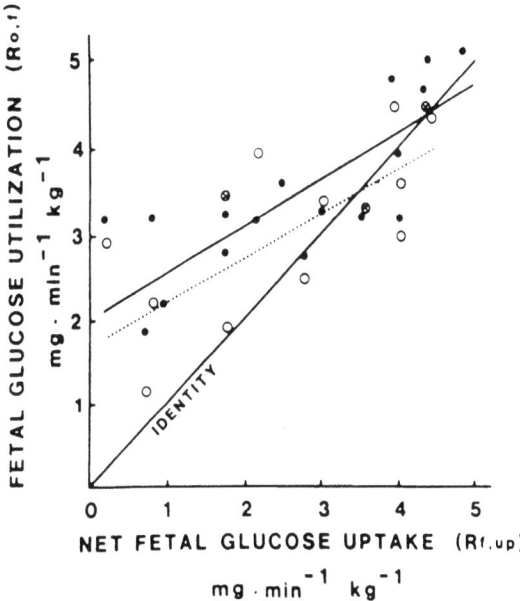

FIGURE 17.18. Fetal glucose utilization rate is compared with net fetal (umbilical) glucose uptake in near-term fetal sheep in which umbilical glucose uptake was varied by fasting-induced hypoglycemia. At fetal (umbilical) glucose uptake rate of less than 2.5 mg·min^{-1}/kg, the fetal glucose utilization rate is significantly greater, indicating the development of net fetal glucose production. ● = [U-^{14}C] glucose infused into the fetal inferior vena cava; O = [6-^{3}H] glucose infused into the maternal femoral vein; ⊕ = [6-^{3}H] glucose infused into the fetal inferior vena cava. (From Hay et al.,[15] with permission.)

and fetal hypoglycemia were produced by prolonged (2 to 3 weeks) insulin infusion in the mother.[10] Umbilical glucose uptake rates fell to approximately $1.2\,\text{mg·min}^{-1}\,\text{kg}^{-1}$, which is 25% of normal, whereas fetal glucose utilization rates decreased only to about $4.0\,\text{mg·min}^{-1}\,\text{kg}^{-1}$, demonstrating, by difference, net fetal glucose production rates of $2.8\,\text{mg·min}^{-1}\,\text{kg}^{-1}$, nearly 60% of normal utilization rates.

The regulation of this fetal glucose production is not well defined. In the above studies an insulin infusion to about $80\,\mu\text{U·ml}^{-1}$ combined with a variable rate glucose infusion that maintained the control-period hypoglycemic concentration of glucose completely abolished the fetal glucose production.[10] At least one regulator of fetal glucose production is the insulin concentration, and its decrease during hypoglycemia may allow glucose production to develop or increase. This same conclusion was reached in different studies in which streptozocin was infused into fetal sheep inducing fetal pancreatic β cell destruction, loss of pancreatic insulin, and a 50% or more reduction in plasma insulin concentrations.[56,160] In these fetuses, glucose concentration increased about 50%, suppressing umbilical glucose uptake and sustaining fetal glucose utilization. A subsequent infusion of insulin reduced the fetal glucose concentration to normal, restoring normal umbilical glucose uptake, but fetal glucose production was not totally inhibited. These studies suggest that insulin deprivation alone could not account for fetal glucose production. Part of the reason for this lack of effect of insulin could be the suppression of insulin action; insulin sensitivity was suppressed peripherally as shown by the normalization of fetal glucose concentration and glucose utilization rate only by pharmacologic concentrations of insulin. In addition, glucagon concentrations doubled following streptozocin injection, which likely acted to promote glucose production by activating PEPCK. In contrast, glucagon concentrations did not change after pancreatectomy in fetal sheep that had marked hypoinsulinemia.[161] In these fetuses, hyperglycemia and glucose production rates were not as marked as in the streptozocin-treated fetuses. These studies implicate glucagon in promoting fetal glucose production. This conclusion is tentative and not supported by convincing studies by Philipps et al.[162] and Devaskar et al.,[163] who reported limited increase in fetal glucose concentration with physiologic increases in glucagon concentration. Unlike the streptozocin and pancreatectomy investigations, these studies were conducted over short-term, several-hour periods in the presence of normal glucose and insulin concentrations. The glucagon effect on fetal glucose production may develop under select conditions. It is also possible that other hormones are involved. For example, Townsend et al.[164] have demonstrated that gluconeogenesis develops in response to fetal cortisol secretion. This same process can be duplicated in utero in the fetus by cortisol infusion.

Fetal Glucose Production and Utilization

Regardless of the regulatory mechanisms and substrate sources, it is clear that the fetus can regulate its own blood glucose concentration. There are several important consequences of this independent regulation of fetal blood glucose concentration. As discussed earlier (Figure 17.9), fetal GUR depends on the fetal arterial glucose concentration. This GUR includes essential oxidative substrate for the brain, red blood cells, myocardium, lung, adrenal gland, and skeletal muscle. Quantification of these essential pathways of fetal glucose metabolism is limited to the brain (about 20% of GUR_F, or 0.8–$1.0\,\text{mg·min}^{-1}\,\text{kg}^{-1}$), the heart (about 5–10% of GUR_F, or about $0.2\,\text{mg·min}^{-1}\,\text{kg}^{-1}$), the hindlimb (about 50–60% of GUR_F, or about $2.0\,\text{mg·min}^{-1}\,\text{kg}^{-1}$), and red blood cells (about 1.0% of GUR_F).[165] The normal rate of fetal glucose oxidation is about $2.5\,\text{mg·min}^{-1}\,\text{kg}^{-1}$; GUR_F during sustained fetal glucose deprivation and hypoglycemia can be as high as 3.5 to $4.0\,\text{mg·min}^{-1}\,\text{kg}^{-1}$, sufficient to sustain essential rates of glucose oxidation. Thus, fetal glucogenesis and maintenance of G_a helps to maintain normal glucose oxidative metabolism.

Fetal Glucose Production and Placental Glucose Flux

Maintenance of G_a limits placental-to-fetal glucose transfer. This limitation diverts placental glucose into placental glucose utilization.[70] It can occur even in the presence of marked reduction of uteroplacental glucose uptake. By maintaining G_a, the fetus can sustain placental and fetal glucose utilization without promoting further drain on the maternal glucose pool, particularly during the periods of maternal glucose deficiency. In this way, the fetus maintains the metabolic integrity of the conceptus with an important degree of autonomy that teleologically can aid survival of both mother and conceptus.

Fetal Glucose Production, Protein Metabolism, and Growth

Fetal oxygen consumption does not vary more than 10% despite a more than 50% reduction or 100% increase in fetal glucose supply.[19] Part of the oxygen consumption is sustained by glucose metabolism provided by gluconeogenesis, presumably in large measure from amino acids. The balance of oxygen consumption is provided by acute increased rates of amino acid oxidation. Van Veen et al.[166] showed a doubling of the leucine oxidation/disposal rate ratio after sustained fasting-induced hypoglycemia

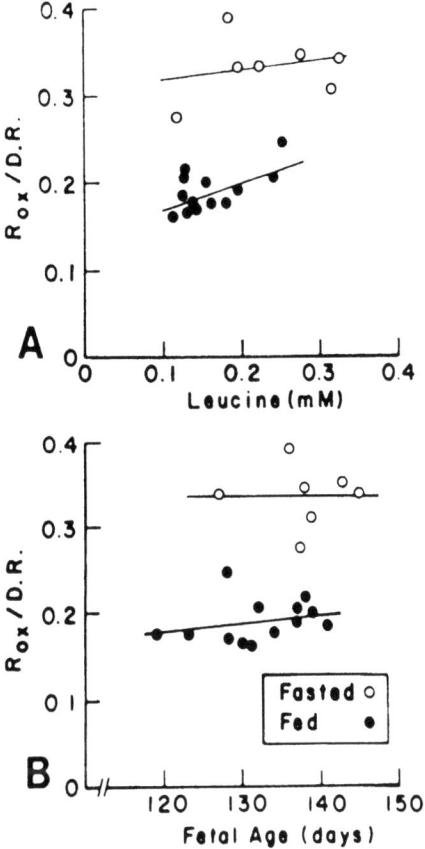

FIGURE 17.19. Leucine oxidation/disposal rate ratio (R_{ox}/D.R.) is compared with the leucine concentration (A) and fetal age (B) in near-term fetal sheep under conditions of fasting-induced hypoglycemia (O) and the normal glycemic fed state (•). These data demonstrate the capacity for fetal oxidation of amino acids—in this case the essential amino acid leucine—to substitute for glucose oxidation when glucose supply is limited. (From van Veen et al.,[166] with permission.)

and diminished umbilical glucose supply (Figure 17.19). Under these conditions, fetal growth is diminished, as the increased supply of amino acids to glucose production and direct oxidation results in reduced availability of nitrogen and carbon for growth. In this reciprocal manner, glucose supply and amino acid metabolism are intimately related such that growth is a variable that appears subservient to fetal oxidative metabolism. A key regulator of this relation is the supply of glucose to the fetus. Supporting this conclusion is evidence from several investigators that hyperinsulinemia by itself acts to decrease fetal protein breakdown, while hyperglycemia does not affect this process, or that of protein synthesis, independently. The strongest determinant of protein synthesis, however, is the plasma concentration amino acids.[167,168]

Acknowledgment. This work was supported by National Institutes of Health grants HD20761 and HD28794.

References

1. Widdas WF. Inability of diffusion to account for placental glucose transfer in the sheep and consideration of the kinetics of a possible carrier transfer. J Physiol (Lond) 1952;118:23–39.
2. Meschia G, Battaglia FC, Hay WW Jr, et al. Utilization of substrates by the ovine placenta in vivo. Fed Proc 1980;39:245–249.
3. Battaglia FC, Meschia G. An introduction to fetal physiology. Orlando: Academic Press, 1986.
4. Makowski EL, Meschia G, Droegemueller W, et al. Measurement of umbilical arterial blood flow to the sheep placenta and fetus in utero. Circ Res 1968;23:623–631.
5. Simmons MA, Battaglia FC, Meschia G. Placental transfer of glucose. J Dev Physiol 1979;1:227–243.
6. Hay WW Jr, Sparks JW. Tracer methods for studying fetal metabolism in vivo. In: Nathanielsz PW, ed. Animal models in fetal medicine, vol. 6. Metabolism. Ithaca, NY: Perinatology Press, 1988:133–177.
7. Hodgson JC. Practical aspects of quantifying metabolic processes in the pregnant dam, conceptus and newborn using radioisotopes. In: Nathanielsz PW, ed. Animal models in fetal medicine, vol. 6. Metabolism. Ithaca, NY: Perinatology Press, 1988:93–132.
8. Hay WW Jr, Sparks JW, Battaglia FC, et al. Maternal-fetal glucose exchange: necessity of a three-pool model. Am J Physiol 1984;246:E528–E534.
9. Shipley RA, Clark RE. Tracer methods for in vivo kinetics. Orlando: Academic Press, 1972.
10. DiGiacomo JE, Hay WW Jr. Regulation of placental glucose transfer and consumption by fetal glucose production. Pediatr Res 1989;25:429–434.
11. Anand RS, Sperling MA, Ganguli S, et al. Bi-directional placental transfer glucose and its turnover in fetal and maternal sheep. Pediatr Res 1979;13:783–787.
12. Hodgson JC, Mellor DJ, Field AC. Rates of glucose production and utilization by the foetus in chronically catheterized sheep. Biochem J 1980;186:739–747.
13. Yudilevich DL, Eaton BM, Short AH, et al. Glucose carriers at maternal and fetal sides of the trophoblast in guinea pig placenta. Am J Physiol 1979;237:C205–C212.
14. Hay WW Jr, Sparks JW, Quissel B, et al. Simultaneous measurements of umbilical uptake, fetal utilization rate, and fetal turnover rate of glucose. Am J Physiol 1981;240:E662–E668.
15. Hay WW Jr, Sparks JW, Wilkening RB, et al. Fetal glucose uptake and utilization as functions of maternal glucose concentration. Am J Physiol 1984;246:E237–E242.
16. Battaglia FC. Placental transport and utilization of amino acids and carbohydrates. Fed Proc 1986;45:2508–2512.
17. Hay WW Jr, Myers SA, Sparks JW, et al. Glucose and lactate oxidation rates in the fetal lamb. Proc Soc Exp Biol Med 1984;173:553–563.
18. Hay WW Jr, DiGiacomo JE, Meznarich HK, et al. Effects of glucose and insulin on fetal glucose oxidation and oxygen consumption. Am J Physiol 1989;206:E704–E713.
19. McGowen JE, Aldoretta PW, Hay WW Jr. Contribution of fructose and lactate produced in the placenta to the

calculation of fetal glucose oxidation rate. Am J Physiol 1995;269:834–839.
20. Van Veen LCP, Hay WW Jr, Battaglia FC, et al. Fetal CO_2 kinetics. J Dev Physiol 1984;6:359–365.
21. Bloch CA, Banach W, Landt K, et al. Effects of fetal insulin infusion on glucose kinetics in pregnant sheep. A compartmental analysis. Am J Physiol 1986;251:E448–E456.
22. Hay WW Jr, Sparks JW, Wilkening RB, et al. Factors affecting tracer glucose distribution among the fetus, placenta and mother in pregnant sheep. Fed Proc 1983;42:467.
23. Haugel S, Desmaizieres V, Challier JC. Glucose uptake, utilization, and transfer by the human placenta as functions of maternal glucose concentration. Pediatr Res 1986;20:269–273.
24. Ingermann RL, Bissonette JM, Koch PL. Glucose-sensitive and -insensitive cytochalasin-B binding proteins from microvillous plasma membranes of human placenta: identification of the D-glucose transporter. Biochim Biophys Acta 1983;730:57–63.
25. Johnson JW, Smith CH. Glucose transport across the basal plasma membrane of human placental syncytiotrophoblast. Biochim Biophys Acta 1985;815:44–50.
26. Stacy TE, Weedon P, Haworth C, et al. Fetomaternal transfer of glucose analogues by sheep placenta. Am J Physiol 1978;234:E32–E37.
27. Hahn T, Desoye G. Ontogeny of glucose transport systems in the placenta and its progenitor tissues. Early Pregnancy Biol Med 1966;2:168–182.
28. Johnson LW, Smith CH. Monosaccharide transport across microvillous membrane of human placenta. Am J Physiol 1980;238:C160–C168.
29. Eaton BM, Mann GE, Yudilevich DL. Kinetics and specificity of glucose transport on the fetal side of the guinea-pig placenta. J Physiol (Lond) 1979;301:87–88P.
30. Jansson T, Wennergren M, Illsley MP. Glucose transporter protein expression in human placenta throughout gestation and in intrauterine growth retardation. J Clin Endocrinol Metab 1993;77:1554–1562.
31. Takata K, Kasahara T, Kasahara M, et al. Localization of erythrocyte/HepG2-type glucose transporter (GLUT 1) in human placental villi. Cell Tissue Res 1992;267:407–412.
32. Hahn T, Hartmann M, Blaschitz A, et al. Localisation of the high affinity glucose transporter protein GLUT 1 in the placenta of human, marmoset monkey (*Callithrix jacchus*) and rat at different developmental stages. Cell Tissue Res 1995;280;49–57.
33. Wolf HG, Desoye G. Immunohistochemical localization of glucose transporters and insulin receptors in human fetal membranes at term. Histochemistry 1993;100:379–385.
34. Ehrhardt RA, McNeill DM, Bell AW. Identification of and developmental increase in glucose transport protein in the sheep placenta. Am J Physiol, in press, 1997.
35. Zhou J, Bondy CA. Placental glucose transporter gene expression and metabolism in the rat. J Clin Invest 1992;91:845–852.
36. Clarson LH, Glazier JD, Sides MK, et al. Expression of the facilitative glucose transporters (GLUT1 and GLUT3) by a choriocarcinoma cell line (JAr) and cytotrophoblast cells in culture. Placenta 1997;18:333–339.
37. Currie MF, Bassett NS, Gluckman PD, Glucose transporter-1 gene expression in ovine placenta. Placenta 1995;15:A11.
38. Das UG, Hay WW Jr, Devaskar SU. Placental glucose transporter (GLUT-1) in fetal sheep is regulated by time-dependent changes in glucose and insulin concentrations. Pediatr Res 1996;39:#1828,307A.
39. Sadiq HF, Morgenthaler TA, Schroeder RE, et al. Effects of hypoxia and glucose on placental glucose transporters. Pediatr Res 1994;35:#1224,206A.
40. Illsley NP. Expression of the human placental glucose transporter (GLUT1) is not subject to significant regulation by glucose concentration. J Soc Gynecol Invest 1995;2#P137,285.
41. Reid GJ, Flozak AS, Simmons RA. Increased expression of glucose transporter protein-1 (GLUT-1) in the growth retarded placenta. J Soc Gynecol Invest 1995;2:#O114,193.
42. Bassett NS, Currie MJ, Woodall SM, et al. The effect of maternal IGF-I treatment on placental GLUT gene expression. Proceedings of the Thorburn Symposium, Hamilton Island, Queensland, Australia, 1994.
43. Barth S, Hahn T, Zechner R, et al. Prolonged hyperglycemia in vitro affects glucose transporter protein GLUT1 and glucose uptake in cultured term trophoblast cells. Placenta 1994;15:A4.
44. Hay WW Jr, Carver TD, Aldoretta PW. Effect of acute and chronic hypo- and hyperglycemia on placental glucose transport capacity in pregnant sheep. Proceedings of the First International Meeting of World Placental Associations, Sydney, Australia, 1994.
45. Posner BI. Insulin receptors in human and animal placental tissue. Diabetes 1974;23:209–217.
46. Desoye G, Hartmann M, Blaschitz A, et al. Insulin receptors in syncytiotrophoblast and fetal endothelium of human placenta: immunohistochemical evidence for developmental changes in distribution pattern. Histochemistry 1994;101:277–285.
47. Jones CJP, Hartmann M, Blaschitz, et al. Ultrastructural localization of insulin receptors in human placenta. Am J Reprod Immunol 1993;30:136–145.
48. Desoye G, Shafrir E. The human placenta in diabetic pregnancy. Diabetes Rev 1996;4:70–89.
49. Desoye G, Shafrir E. Placental metabolism and its regulation in health and diabetes. Mol Aspects Med 1994;15:505–682.
50. Desoye G. Insulin receptors and insulin effects in the human placenta. Curr Trends Exp Endocrinol 1993;1:77–89.
51. Simmons MA, Jones MD Jr, Battaglia FC, et al. Insulin effect on fetal glucose utilization. Pediatr Res 1987;12:90–92.
52. Hay WW Jr, Sparks JW, Gilbert M, et al. Effect of insulin on glucose uptake by the maternal hindlimb and uterus, and by the fetus in conscious pregnant sheep. J Endocrinol 1984;100:119–124.
53. Hay WW Jr, Meznarich HK, Sparks JW, et al. Effect of insulin on glucose uptake in near-term fetal lambs. Proc Soc Exp Biol Med 1985;178:557–564.

54. Jodarski GD, Shanahan MF, Rankin JHG. Fetal insulin and placental 3-O-methyl glucose clearance in near term sheep. J Dev Physiol 1985;7:251–258.
55. Rankin JHG, Jodarski G, Shanahan MF. Maternal insulin and placental 3-O-methyl glucose transport. J Dev Physiol 1986;8:247–253.
56. Hay WW Jr, Meznarich HK. Use of streptozotocin injection to determine the role of normal levels of fetal insulin in regulating uteroplacental and umbilical glucose exchange. Pediatr Res 1988;24:312–317.
57. Shafrir E, Barash V. Placental glycogen metabolism in diabetic pregnancy. Isr J Med Sci 1991;27:449–461.
58. Challier JC, Hauguel S, Desmaizieres V. Effect of insulin on glucose uptake and metabolism in the human placenta. J Clin Endocrinol Metab 1986;62:803–807.
59. Knopp RH, Bonet B, Lasuncion MA, et al. Lipoprotein metabolism in pregnancy. In: Herrera E, Knopp RH, eds. Perinatal biochemistry. Boca Raton, FL: CRC Press, 1992:19–51.
60. Devaskar SU, Mueckler MM. The mammalian glucose transporter. Pediatr Res 1992;31:1–13.
61. Collins JW Jr, Finley SL, Merrick D, et al. Human placental lactogen administration in the pregnant rat: acceleration of fetal growth. Pediatr Res 1988;24:657–662.
62. Greenberg RE, Wogenrich FJ, Garcia P, et al. Fetal insulin increases placental amino acid transport. Clin Res 1989;37:178A.
63. Bissonette JM, Hohimer AR, Cronan JZ, et al. Glucose transfer across the intact guinea-pig placenta. J Dev Physiol 1979;1:415–426.
64. Krauer F, Joyce J, Young M. The influence of high maternal plasma glucose levels, and maternal blood flow on the placental transfer of glucose in the guinea pig. Diabetologia 1973;9:453–456.
65. Challier JC, Hauguel S, Desmaizieres V. Effect of insulin on glucose uptake and metabolism in the human placenta. J Clin Endocrinol Metab 1986;62:803–807.
66. Hay WW Jr, Meznarich HK. Effect of maternal glucose concentration on uteroplacental glucose consumption and transfer in pregnant sheep. Proc Soc Exp Biol Med 1989;190;63–69.
67. Aldoretta PW, Gresores A, Hay WW Jr. Effect of glucose supply on ovine uteroplacental glucose utilization, oxidation, and lactate production. Soc Gynecol Invest Prog 1994;#O104,138.
68. Crandell SS, Palma PA, Morriss FH. Effect of maternal serum insulin on umbilical extraction of glucose and lactate in fed and fasted sheep. Am J Obstet Gynecol 1982;142:219–224.
69. Hay WW Jr, Meznarich HK, DiGiacomo JE, et al. Effects of insulin and glucose concentrations on glucose utilization in fetal sheep. Pediatr Res 1988;23:281–287.
70. Hay WW Jr. Regulation of ovine placental glucose consumption (PGU). Physiologist 1987;30:174A.
71. Hay WW Jr. Placental function. In: Gluckman PD, Heymann MA, eds. Scientific basis of pediatric and perinatal medicine. 2nd ed. London: Edward Arnold, 1996:213–227.
72. Hay WW Jr, Molina RD, DiGiacomo JE, et al. Model of placental glucose consumption and glucose transfer. Am J Physiol 1990;258:R569–R577.
73. Hay WW Jr. Energy and substrate requirements of the placenta and fetus. Proc Nutr Soc 1991;50:321–336.
74. DiGiacomo JE, Hay WW Jr. Fetal glucose metabolism and oxygen consumption during sustained maternal and fetal hypoglycemia. Metabolism 1980;39:193–202.
75. Battaglia FC, Hay WW Jr. Energy and substrate requirements for fetal and placental growth and metabolism. In: Beard R, Nathanielsz P, eds. Fetal physiology and medicine. New York: Marcel Dekker, 1984:601–628.
76. Owens JA, Falconer J, Robinson JS. Effect of restriction of placental growth on fetal and utero-placental metabolism. J Dev Physiol 1987;9:225–238.
77. Alexander G. Studies on the placenta of the sheep (*Ovis arias* L.): effect of surgical reduction in the number of caruncles. J Reprod Fertil 1964;7:307–322.
78. Kulhanek JF, Meschia G, Makowski EL, et al. Changes in DNA content and urea permeability of the sheep placenta. Am J Physiol 1974;226:1257–1263.
79. Hay WW Jr. Placental metabolism of glucose in relation to fetal nutrition. In: Nathanielsz PW, ed. Fetal and neonatal development. Research in perinatal medicine, vol. 7. Ithaca, NY: Perinatology Press, 1988:58–67.
80. Molina RD, Meschia G, Battaglia FC, et al. Maturation of placental glucose transfer (PGT) capacity in the ovine pregnancy. Pediatr Res 1988;23:248A.
81. Molina RD, Meschia G, Battaglia FC, et al. Gestational maturation of placental glucose transfer capacity in sheep. Am J Physiol 1991;261:R697–R704.
82. Molina RD, Carver TD, Hay WW Jr. Ontogeny of insulin effect in fetal sheep. Pediatr Res 1993;34:654–660.
83. Malek A, Sager R, Sakher A, et al. Utilization of glucose by human placental tissue as a function of gestational age. J Soc Gynecol Invest 1995;2:#O150,211.
84. Schneider H. Ontogenic changes in the nutritive function of the placenta. Placenta 1996;17:15–26.
85. Villee CA. The metabolism of human placenta in vitro. J Biol Chem 1953;205:113–123.
86. Sparks JW, Hay WW Jr, Bonds D, et al. Simultaneous measurements of lactate turnover rate and umbilical lactate uptake in the fetal lamb. J Clin Invest 1982;70:179–192.
87. Bloxam DL, Bobinski PM. Energy metabolism and glycolysis in the human placenta during ischaemia and in normal labour. Placenta 1984;5:381–394.
88. Marconi AM, Ferrazzi E, Cetin I, et al. Lactate metabolism in normal and growth retarded human fetuses. Pediatr Res 1990;28:652–656.
89. Setchell BP, Bassett JM, Hinks NT, et al. The importance of glucose in the oxidative metabolism of the pregnant uterus and its contents in conscious sheep with some preliminary observations on the oxidation of fructose and glucose by fetal sheep. Q J Exp Physiol 1972;57:257–266.
90. Good RFW. Fetal fructose in various mammals. Nature 1952;170:750.
91. Meznarich HK, Hay WW Jr, Sparks JW, et al. Fructose disposal and oxidation rates in the ovine fetus. Q J Exp Physiol 1987;72:617–625
92. Marconi A, Cetin E, Davoli A, et al. An evaluation of fetal glucogenesis in intrauterine growth retarded pregnancies:

steady state fetal and maternal enrichments of plasma glucose at cordocentesis. Metabolism 1993;42:860–864.
93. Philipps AF, Carson BS, Meschia G, et al. Insulin secretion in fetal and newborn sheep. Am J Physiol 1978;235:E467-E474.
94. Carson BS, Philipps AF, Simmons MA, et al. Effects of a sustained fetal insulin infusion upon glucose uptake and oxygenation. Pediatr Res 1980;14:147–152.
95. Aldoretta PW, Anderson S, Hay WW Jr. Maturation of glucose-stimulated insulin secretion in fetal sheep. Pediatr Res 1994;35:#1188,200A.
96. Carver TD, Anderson SM, Aldoretta PW, et al. Glucose suppression of insulin secretion in chronically hyperglycemic fetal sheep. Pediatr Res 1995;38:754–762.
97. Lane RH, Xian Y, Hay WW Jr, et al. The role of pancreatic GLUT 2 in the abnormal secretory response of chronically hyperglycemic fetal lambs. Program of the International Congress of Endocrinology 1996;#P3-419,859.
98. Kervran A, Randon J. Development of insulin release by fetal rat pancreas in vitro. Diabetes 1980;29:673–678.
99. Kervran A, Guillaume M, Jost A. The endocrine pancreas of the fetus of diabetic pregnant rat. Diabetologia 1978;15:387–393.
100. Cowett RM. Hypoglycemia and hyperglycemia in the newborn. In: Polin RA, Fox WW, eds. Fetal and neonatal physiology. Philadelphia: WB Saunders, 1992:406–418.
101. Freinkel N, Phelps NL, Metzger BE. Intermediary metabolism during normal pregnancy. In: Sutherland HW, Stowers JM, eds. Carbohydrate metabolism in pregnancy and the newborn. New York: Springer-Verlag, 1978:1–31.
102. Carver TD, Anderson SM, Aldoretta PW, et al. Effect of low-level plus marked "pulsatile" hyperglycemia on insulin secretion in fetal sheep. Am J Physiol 1996;271:E865–E871.
103. Heinze E, Steinke J. Insulin secretion during development: response of isolated pancreatic islets of fetal, newborn and adult rats to theophylline and arginine. Horm Metab Res 1972;4:234–236.
104. Gresores A, Anderson S, Hood, et al. Separate and joint effects of arginine and glucose on ovine fetal insulin secretion. Am J Physiol, 1997;272:E68–E73.
105. Colwill JR, Davis JR, Meschia G, et al. Insulin induced hypoglycemia in the ovine fetus in utero. Endocrinology 1970;87:710–715.
106. Hay WW Jr, Meznarich HK. The effect of hyperinsulinemia on glucose utilization and oxidation and on oxygen consumption in the fetal lamb. Q J Exp Physiol 1986;71:689–698.
107. Fowden AL. The endocrine regulation of fetal metabolism and growth. In: Gluckman PD, Johnston BM, Nathanielsz PW, eds. Advances in fetal physiology: reviews in honor of G.C. Liggins. Ithaca: Perinatology Press, 1989:229–243.
108. Fowden AL, Silver MA. The effects of thyroid hormones on oxygen and glucose metabolism in the sheep fetus during late gestation. J Physiol 1995;482:203–213.
109. Barnes RJ, Comline RS, Silver M. Effect of cortisol on liver glycogen concentrations in hypophysectomized, adrenalectomized and normal foetal lambs during late or prolonged gestation. J Physiol 1978;275:567–579.
110. Fowden AL, Comline RS, Silver M. The effects of cortisol on the concentration of glycogen in different tissues in the chronically catheterized fetal pig. Q J Exp Physiol 1985;70:23–32.
111. Battaglia FC, Meschia G. Personal communication.
112. Padbury JF, Ludlow JK, Ervin MG, et al. Thresholds for physiological effects of plasma catecholamines in fetal sheep. Am J Physiol 1992;252:E530–E537.
113. Devaskar SU, Ganguli S, Styer D, et al. Glucagon and glucose dynamics in sheep: evidence for glucagon resistance in fetus. Am J Physiol 1984;246:E256–E265.
114. Oliver MH, Harding JE, Breier BH, et al. Glucose but not mixed amino acid infusion regulates plasma insulin-like growth factor-I concentrations in fetal sheep. Pediatr Res 1993;34:62–65.
115. Han VKM, Fowden Al. Paracrine regulation of fetal growth. In: Ward RHT, Smith SK, Donnai D, eds. Early fetal growth and development. London: RCOG Press, 1994:275–291.
116. Liechty EA, Boyle DW, Moorehead H, et al. Effects of circulating IGF-I on glucose and amino acid kinetics in the ovine fetus. Am J Physiol 1996;271:E177–E185.
117. Liechty EA, Boyle DA, Moorehead H, et al. Effect of hyperinsulinemia on ovine fetal leucine kinetics during prolonged maternal fasting. Am J Physiol 1992;263:E696–E702.
118. Carver TD, Quick AN, Jr, Teng C, et al. Leucine metabolism in chronically hypoglycemic, hypoinsulinemic growth restricted fetal sheep. Am J Physiol 1997;272:E107–E117.
119. Schroeder RE, Doria-Medina CL, Das UG, et al. Effect of maternal diabetes upon fetal rat myocardial and skeletal muscle glucose transporters. Pediatr Res 1997;41:11–19.
120. Das UG, Schroeder RE, Hay WW Jr, et al. Chronic hypoglycemia causes time-dependent changes in ovine fetal GLUT 1 & GLUT 4 protein expression. Pediatr Res 1995;37:#347,60A.
121. Schroeder RE, Devaskar UP, Trail SE, et al. Effect of maternal diabetes on the expression of genes regulating fetal brain glucose uptake. Diabetes 1993;42:1487–1496.
122. Das UG, Schroeder RE, Hay WW Jr, et al. Chronic hyperglycemia causes time-dependent changes in ovine fetal GLUT 1 & GLUT 4 protein expression. Pediatr Res 1995;37:#1817,305A.
123. Das UG, Hay WW Jr, Devaskar SU. Myocardial glucose transporters in fetal sheep are regulated by time-dependent changes in glucose and insulin concentrations. Pediatr Res 1996;39:#141,26A.
124. Klip A, Tsakiridis T, Marette A, et al. Regulation of expression of glucose transporters by glucose: a review of studies in vivo and in cell cultures. FASEB J 1994;8:43–53.
125. Simmons RA, Gounis AS, Shrikar AB, et al. Intrauterine growth retardation: fetal glucose transport is diminished in lung but spared in brain. Pediatr Res 1992;31:59–63.
126. Simmons RA, Flozak AS, Ogata ES. Glucose regulates GLUT 1 function and expression in fetal rat lung and muscle in vitro. Endocrinology 1993;132:2312–2318.

127. Shelley HJ. Glycogen reserves and their changes at birth and in anoxia. Br Med Bull 1961;17:137–143.
128. Dawkins MJR. Biochemical aspects of developing function in newborn mammalian liver. Br Med Bull 1961;22:28–33.
129. Shellhase E, Kuroki Y, Emrie PA, et al. Expression of pulmonary surfactant apoproteins in the developing rat lung. Clin Res 1989;37:208A.
130. Mott JC. The ability of young mammals to withstand total oxygen lack. Br Med Bull 1961;17:144–148.
131. Sparks JW. Augmentation of glucose supply. Semin Perinatol 1979;3:141–155.
132. Zheng Q, Levitsky LL, Fan J, et al. Glycogenesis in the cultured fetal and adult rat hepatocyte is differently regulated by medium glucose. Pediatr Res 1992;32:714–718.
133. Fowden AI, Comline RS. The effects of pancreatectomy on tissue glycogen concentrations in the fetal sheep. In: Jones CT, ed. Fetal and neonatal development. Ithaca, NY: Perinatology Press, 1988:505–508.
134. Susa JB, McCormick KL, Widness JD, et al. Chronic hyperinsulinemia in the fetal rhesus monkey: effects on fetal growth and composition. Diabetes 1979;28:1058–1063.
135. Youn JH, Youn MS, Bergman RN. Synergism of glucose and fructose in net glycogen synthesis in perfused rat livers. J Biol Chem 1986;261:15960–15969.
136. Sparks JW, Lynch A, Glinsmann WH. Regulation of rat liver glycogen synthesis and activities of glycogen cycle enzymes by glucose, and galactose. Metabolism 1976;25:47–55.
137. Goodner CJ, Thompson DJ. Glucose metabolism in the fetus in utero: the effect of maternal fasting and glucose loading in the rat. Pediatr Res 1967;1:443–451.
138. Bossi E, Greenberg RE. Sources of blood glucose in the rat fetus. Pediatr Res 1972;6:765–772.
139. Glinsmann WH, Eisen HJ, Lynch A, et al. Glucose regulation by isolated near-term monkey liver. Pediatr Res 1975;9:600–604.
140. Raiha NCR, Lindroos K. Development of some enzymes involved in gluconeogenesis in human liver. Ann Med Exp Biol Fenn 1969;47:146–150.
141. Lemons JA, Adcock EW III, Jones MD Jr, et al. Umbilical uptake of amino acids in the unstressed fetal lamb. J Clin Invest 1976;58:1428–1434.
142. Marconi AM, Sparks JW, Battaglia FC, et al. A comparison of amino acid arteriovenous differences across the liver, hindlimb and placenta in the fetal lamb. Am J Physiol 1989;258:E508–E512.
143. Prior RL, Christenson RK. Gluconeogenesis from alanine in vivo by the ovine fetus and lamb. Am J Physiol 1977;233:E462–E468.
144. Cetin I, Marconi AM, Bozzetti P, et al. Umbilical amino acid concentrations in appropriate and small for gestational age infants: a biochemical difference present in utero. Am J Obstet Gynecol 1988;158:120–126.
145. Naeye RL. Infants of diabetic mothers: a quantitative morphologic study. Pediatrics 1965;35:980–988.
146. Levitsky LL, Paton JB, Fisher DE. Gluconeogenesis from lactate in the chronically catheterized baboon fetus. Biol Neonate 1986;50:97–106.
147. Levitsky LL, Paton JB, Fisher DE. Lactate and fructose are glycogenic precursors in the chronically catheterized baboon fetus. Pediatr Res 1987;21:217A.
148. DiGiacomo JE, Hay WW Jr, Chan L, et al. Determination of pathways of fetal glycogen synthesis by NMR spectroscopy. Clin Res 1980;37:177A.
149. Battaglia FC, Meschia G. Personal communication.
150. Fowden AL, Coulson RL, Silver M. Endocrine regulation of tissue glucose-6-phosphatase activity in the fetal sheep during late gestation. Endocrinology 1990:2823–2830.
151. Robertson JP, Faulkner A, Vernon RG. L-Lactate as a source of carbon for fatty acid synthesis in adult and foetal sheep. Biochim Biophys Acta 1981;665:511–518.
152. Prior RL, Scott RA. Ontogeny of gluconeogenesis in the bovine fetus: influence of maternal dietary energy. Dev Biol 1977;58:384–393.
153. Girard JR, Caquet D, Guillet I, Control of rat liver phosphorylase, glucose-6-phosphatase and phosphoenolpyruvate carboxykinase activities by insulin and glucagon in the perinatal period. Enzyme 1973;15:272–285.
154. Robinson RH. Development of gluconeogenic enzymes in the newborn guinea pig. Biol Neonate 1976;29:48–55.
155. Jones CT, Ashton L. The appearance, properties, and functions of gluconeogenic enzymes in the liver and kidneys of the guinea pig during fetal and early neonatal development. Arch Biochem Biophys 1976;174:506–522.
156. Schwartz AL, Rall TW. Hormonal regulation of incorporation of alanine-U-^{14}C into glucose in human fetal liver explants. Diabetes 1975;24:650–657.
157. Warnes DM, Seamark RF, Ballard FJ. The appearance of gluconeogenesis at birth in sheep. Biochem J 1977;162:627–634.
158. Sparks JW, Hay WW Jr, Meschia G, et al. Fetal liver metabolism in the unstressed fetal lamb: experience with a chronic indwelling hepatic venous catheter. Pediatr Res 1982;15:265A.
159. Narkewicz MR, Carver TD, Hay WW Jr. Induction of cytosolic phosphoenolpyruvate carboxykinase in the ovine fetal liver by chronic fetal hypoglycemia and hypoinsulinemia. Pediatr Res 1993;33:493–496.
160. Hay WW Jr, Meznarich HK, Fowden A. Effect of streptozotocin on rates of ovine fetal glucose utilization, oxidation and production in the sheep fetus. Metabolism 1989;38:30–37.
161. Fowden AL, Hay WW Jr. The effects of pancreatectomy on the rates of glucose utilization, oxidation and production in the sheep fetus. Q J Exp Physiol 1988;73:973–984.
162. Philipps AF, Dubin JW, Matty PJ, et al. Influence of exogenous glucagon on fetal glucose metabolism and ketone production. Pediatr Res 1983;17:51–56.
163. Devaskar SV, Ganguli S, Styer D, et al. Glucagon and glucose dynamics in sheep: evidence for glucagon resistance in the fetus. Am J Physiol 1984;246:E256–E265.
164. Townsend SF, Rudolph CD, Rudolph AM. Cortisol induces perinatal hepatic gluconeogenesis. Clin Res 1989;27:209A.

165. Hay WW Jr. Fetal glucose metabolism. Seminars in Perinatol 1979;3:157–176.
166. Van Veen LCP, Teng C, Hay WW Jr, et al. Leucine disposal and oxidation rates in the fetal lamb. Metabolism 1987;36:48–53.
167. Tsalikian EH, Hamilton W. Differential effect of hyperinsulinemia on fetal and neonatal amino acid kinetics. Pediatr Res 1991;29:54A.
168. Milley JR. Effects of insulin on ovine fetal leucine kinetics and protein metabolism. J Clin Invest 1994;93:1616–1624.

Appendix 17.1. Equations for Application of the Fick Principle to Net Glucose Flux Across the Uteroplacental Unit

1. Net uterine glucose uptake (mg·min^{-1}) = uterine blood flow (ml·min^{-1}) × uterine arteriovenous blood glucose concentration difference (mg·ml^{-1})

$$R_{up,m} = \Phi_m (G_A - G_V)$$

2. Net umbilical (fetal) glucose uptake (mg·min^{-1}) = umbilical blood flow (ml·min^{-1}) × umbilical venoarterial blood glucose concentration difference (mg·ml^{-1})

$$R_{f,up} = \Phi_f (G_V - G_a)$$

3. Net uteroplacental glucose uptake (mg·min^{-1}) = net uterine glucose uptake − net umbilical glucose uptake

$$R_{o,up} = R_{up,m} - R_{f,up}$$

Appendix 17.2. Tracer Methodology: Glossary, Nomenclature, Equations

Pool and Compartment Designations

Superscripts

m, f site of tracer infusion into the mother (m) or fetus (f)

Subscripts

o, m, f, up outside, maternal, fetal, and uteroplacenta, respectively

A, V, a, v maternal arterial, uterine venous, umbilical arterial, umbilical venous blood, respectively

The order of subscripts indicates transfer to a sampling site from a sampling site; e.g., $r^m_{f,m}$ = rate of transfer of a tracer infused into the mother, to the fetus, from the mother.

Concentrations and Specific Activities

G_A, G_V, G_a, G_v glucose concentration in A, V, a, and v

$g^f_A, g^f_V, g^f_a, g^f_v$ concentration of tracer infused into the fetus, measured in A, V, a, and v, respectively

$g^m_A, g^m_V, g^m_a, g^m_v$ concentration of tracer infused into mother, measured in A, V, a, and v, respectively

$SA^f_f = g^f_a/G_a$ specific activity of tracer infused into fetus, measured in a

$SA^f_m = g^f_A/G_A$ specific activity of tracer infused into fetus, measured in A

$SA^m_m = g^m_A/G_A$ specific activity of tracer infused into mother, measured in A

$SA^m_f = g^m_a/G_a$ specific activity of tracer infused into mother, measured in a

Flux Rates

Φ_m, Φ_f uterine and umbilical blood flow, respectively

$R_{o,f}$ rate of fetal glucose utilization

$R_{f,o}$ rate of fetal glucose production

$R_{o,m}$ rate of glucose utilization by maternal organs other than gravid uterus

$R_{m,o}$ rate of entry of glucose into maternal pool

$(R_{o,f})_{II}$ rate of fetal glucose utilization, calculated with two-pool model

$(R_{o,m})_{II}$ rate of maternal glucose utilization, calculated with two-pool model

$R_{f,m}$ net glucose flux to fetus from mother, calculated with two-pool model

$J_{f,m}$ unidirectional flux of glucose to mother from fetus in two-pool model

r^f rate of tracer glucose infusion into fetus (fetal tracer)

r^m rate of tracer glucose infusion into mother (maternal tracer)

$r^f_{m,f}$ net flux of tracer infused into fetus, to mother from fetus, in two-pool model

$r^f_{up,f} = \Phi_m(g^f_v - g^f_a)$ net flux of tracer infused into fetus, to uteroplacenta from fetus

$r^f_{m,up} = \Phi_m(g^f_v - g^f_A)$ net flux of tracer infused into fetus, to mother from uteroplacenta

$r^f_{o,f} = r^f - r^f_{up,f}$ irreversible disposal rate by fetal organs of tracer infused into fetus

$r^f_{o,m} = r^f_{m,up}$ irreversible disposal rate of fetal tracer by maternal organs other than gravid uterus

$r^f_{o,up} = r^f_{up,f} - r^f_{m,up}$ irreversible disposal rate of fetal tracer by uteroplacenta

17. Glucose Metabolism in the Fetal-Placental Unit

$r^m_{f,m}$	net flux of tracer infused into mother, to fetus from mother, in two-pool model	$r^m_{o,m} = r^m - r^m_{up,m}$	irreversible disposal rate of tracer infused into mother, by maternal organs other than gravid uterus
$r^m_{up,m} = \Phi_m(g^m_A - g^m_V)$	net flux of tracer infused into mother, to uteroplacenta from mother	$r^m_{o,f} = r^m_{f,up}$	irreversible disposal rate of tracer infused into mother, by fetus
$r^m_{f,up} = \Phi_f(g^m_v - g^m_a)$	net flux of tracer infused into mother, to fetus from uteroplacenta	$r^m_{o,up} = r^m_{up,m} - r^m_{f,up}$	irreversible disposal rate of maternal tracer by uteroplacenta

18
Protein Metabolism in the Fetal-Placental Unit

Edward A. Liechty and David W. Boyle

Protein synthesis and accretion are the cornerstones of growth that provide the structural framework and enzymatic machinery necessary for fetal development. The components the fetus utilizes for protein accretion must be supplied by the maternal uterine circulation. All are derived from the maternal diet or maternal tissue stores. It is important to explore the regulatory processes within the maternal, placental, and fetal compartments that determine fetal amino acid retention. It addition to tissue synthesis, use of free amino acids as oxidative fuel is extensive in the well-nourished fetus and increases significantly during periods of maternal food deprivation. The changes in fetal amino acid utilization represent a significant mechanism by which the fetus adapts to energy deprivation.

Experimental Methodology

Before examining the available data, it is necessary to understand the models and methodology by which the data are derived. In general, four methods have been applied to fetal nitrogen metabolism: (1) carcass analysis, (2) net arteriovenous balance determinations, (3) measurement of the rate of incorporation of a tracer amino acid into fetal protein, and (4) studies of the kinetics of amino acids in the fetal arterial free amino acid pool. Many studies have combined aspects of two or more of the above methods. The following section briefly outlines the assumptions and possible sources of error in these methods (see Chapters 1, 11, 34, and 47).

Carcass Analysis

Many studies describing fetal growth and protein accretion have used the technique of carcass analysis. Fetuses are sacrificed at several points during gestation, and chemical analysis is performed on the carcass. The results obtained are generally expressed as a concentration: mass unit per mass unit. Examples include grams of protein per kilogram wet weight or micromoles of leucine per gram of protein. From these data the total mass of the component at that point in gestation can be calculated.

The slope of a plot of mass against gestational age gives the accretion rate of the component. The growth in mass of an organism is not linear but logarithmic. By analyzing the data in the form of the logistic growth equation,

$$Mass_t = Mass_o \cdot e^{kt}$$

specific growth rates or accretion rates are obtained. The differential form of this equation is

$$dMass/dt = kMass_t$$

This equation states that the change in mass of the component is equal to a constant (k) times the previous mass. In other words, the fetus grows by increasing its mass by a fixed percent per unit time. When applied to total body mass, this constant is called the specific growth rate and contains units of time.[1] Calculation of the specific growth rate facilitates comparison of growth rates or protein accretion rates across species of vastly differing total mass or comparison of growth rates at different points in gestation.

In addition to the growth or accretion rate, it is important to consider changes in body composition that occur as the fetus grows. If body composition is changing, it implies that the rates of accretion differ for two or more body components. When comparing the accretion of one component to that of another throughout gestation, it is often useful to use the allometric (i.e., comparison of two body proportions, Y and X) equation.

$$Y = aX^k$$

A straight line plot results if the log of each component is plotted.

$$\log Y = \log a + k \times \log X$$

The exponent (k) now defines the ratio of the two accretion rates. For instance, if nitrogen content is plotted against mass, and k is more than 1, the organism is becoming progressively enriched with nitrogen (Figure 18.1). On the other hand, if k is less than 1, the overall growth in mass is proceeding faster than the growth in nitrogen, implying that nitrogen, as a percentage of weight, is decreasing, whereas some other component is increasing in percent of weight. The latter situation is characteristic of human gestation, as fat accretion increases much more rapidly than protein accretion during the third trimester.

Carcass analysis and calculation of specific growth rates can give information that is not obtainable by alternative techniques. Generally, the chemical analyses performed in these studies is that each animal represents a single point on the resulting growth curve. The underlying assumption that the dynamic growth curve of a single fetus can be evaluated by static measurements made on multiple fetuses seems reasonable but cannot be tested. Biologic variability and inaccurate estimation of gestational age introduce error into these studies.

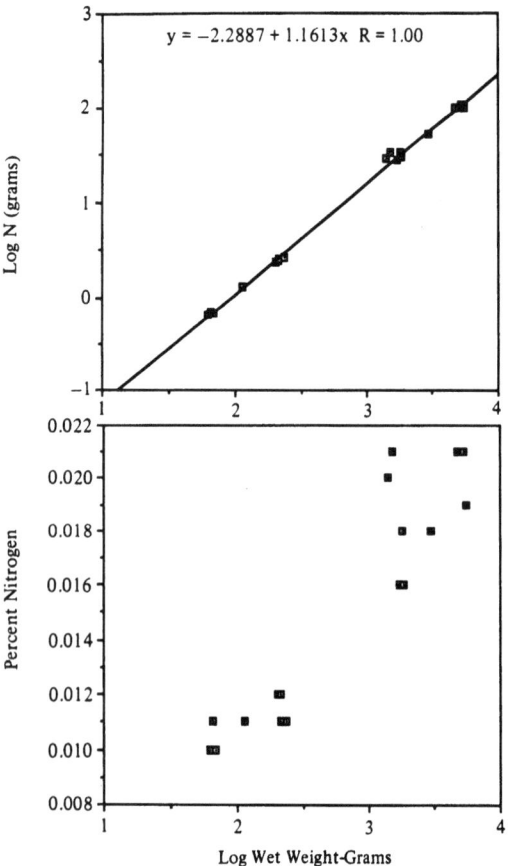

FIGURE 18.1. Nitrogen accretion versus wet weight in the ovine fetus.

Net Arteriovenous Balance Determination

A second important methodology in the study of mammalian amino acid metabolism has been the determination of net rates of amino acid uptake across the umbilical circulation. This methodology relies on the ability to accurately determine umbilical blood flow and amino acid concentration. It has been practical only in large ruminant animals. By the Fick principle, net uptake is equal to the umbilical blood flow multiplied by the whole-blood arteriovenous concentration difference for the amino acid. The error inherent in the determination is equal to the error in the blood flow determination multiplied by the error in the amino acid concentration difference. Precise technology should result in an overall inherent error of less than 10%. If the inherent methodologic error is similar for each amino acid and total amino acid uptake is determined by summation, the potential error rate becomes large. A related problem is the difficulty in detecting real arteriovenous differences for amino acids with an extraction coefficient near the inherent measurement error. It should be emphasized that the Fick principle requires determination of the concentration of the amino acid in whole blood. For certain amino acids, compartmentation between plasma and red blood cells results in considerable error if plasma concentrations rather than whole blood are used.

Measurement of the Rate of Incorporation of Tracer Amino Acid into Fetal Protein

Protein synthesis proceeds at a greater rate than net protein accretion and is counterbalanced by continuing protein breakdown. These processes occur even in a nongrowing animal and allow for the continuing remodeling of body protein. Contraction of body protein stores occurs when breakdown exceeds synthesis; conversely, growth occurs when synthesis exceeds breakdown. Each process may be independently regulated, prompting studies of the control of protein kinetics.

The major tool for studying protein-amino acid kinetics is mathematical modeling based on data derived from tracer dilution experiments. An isotopically labeled tracer molecule is introduced into the fetal plasma, and the rate of loss of label from the plasma or the rate of incorporation of label into tissue protein is determined. To use this model it is necessary to determine the amount of labeled amino acid in the pool that provides precursors for protein synthesis. Generally, this precursor is taken to be the specific activity of the free intracellular tracer amino acid. Although the transfer RNA (tRNA) tracer concentration is more correctly the immediate precursor to protein synthesis, analyzing for specific activity of this pool is difficult. There is evidence that the precursor pool to tRNA may differ from one tissue to another or may exhibit a diurnal variability even within the same tissue.[2] Most studies use the specific activity of either the plasma or the free intracellular pool. It should be remembered that because these specific activities nearly always are lesser or greater than the corresponding tRNA specific activity respectively, rates of protein synthesis are correspondingly over- or underestimated.

The fractional synthetic rate (K_s) of protein refers to the percentage of the total protein mass synthesized per unit time. In the nongrowing animal the fractional degradation rate (K_d) is equal to K_s and equals the fractional rate of protein turnover. In the growing fetus, K_s exceeds K_d, the difference resulting in net protein accretion. Fractional synthetic rates are determined by measuring the rate of incorporation of a tracer amino acid into protein relative to the precursor tracer concentration. Fractional synthetic rates can be determined only at necropsy or by biopsy of the tissues, as determination of the protein-bound label is required. These studies do not allow the investigator to observe dynamic changes in the same organism but do allow calculation of synthetic rates for individual tissues.

Kinetics of Amino Acids in the Fetal Arterial Free Amino Acid Pool

A second concept related to that above is the fetal plasma amino acid turnover rate, or flux. Plasma amino acid flux refers to the flow of an amino acid from the free pool to the protein-bound pool and vice versa. Essential amino acids enter the free pool only from exogenous sources (e.g., transplacental uptake in the case of the fetus) and from protein breakdown. Upon entering the free plasma amino acid pool, the entering substrate molecule dilutes the tracer substrate. In the case of an essential amino acid, both of the above exit the free pool by protein synthesis or by catabolism (i.e., oxidation).

Rate of appearance (Ra) = uptake + breakdown
Rate of disappearance (Rd) = oxidation + synthesis

Rate of appearance is equal to the sum of protein breakdown and exogenous uptake. In addition, if the substrate is a nonessential amino acid, any endogenous synthesis is part of its rate of appearance. The rate of disappearance is equal to the rate of protein synthesis plus the rate of irreversible loss of the amino acid through oxidation. At steady state the rate of appearance is equal to the rate of disappearance (i.e., the sum of protein synthesis and oxidation).

Flux rates determined by this methodology represent integrated summations of the rates of protein synthesis and breakdown from each tissue within the organism. Factors that determine the influence any individual tissue has on the overall flux rate include the rate at which protein is synthesized in the tissue, the percent of total body mass accounted for by that tissue, and the relative percentage of the amino acid within the protein of the tissue. A tissue with a fast turnover rate may influence flux rates out of proportion to its mass. A protein with a slow rate of turnover but a large mass may greatly influence total body flux. The latter is the case with skeletal muscle, which turns over slowly relative to hepatic or gastrointestinal proteins but because of its greater mass still greatly influences total body amino acid flux.

It has become clear that the placenta cannot be accurately modeled solely as a barrier with unidirectional transport between material and fetal blood. The placenta is a metabolically active organ; substrates are metabolized within as well as transported through the placenta. In addition, many substrates undergo bidirectional transfer at the fetal and maternal plasma/trophoblast interface.

This has added complexity to the interpretation of fetal amino acid kinetic experiments, as dilution of a tracer infused into the fetal plasma occurs by flux of unlabeled tracee from the placenta as well as by appearance from endogenous fetal stores. The flux from the placenta exceeds the net umbilical uptake to the degree that flux from the fetal plasma into the placenta occurs. In addition to mediating bidirectional fluxes, the placenta also actively metabolizes some amino acids. This appears to be especially true for the branched-chain amino acids serine and glutamine.

Two methods facilitate the determination of bidirectional placental fluxes. The Fick principle may be used to determine the loss of a fetal tracer to the placenta. The tracer lost via this route, as a percentage of the total fetal tracer infusion, is proportional to the percentage of total fetal tracee disappearance to the placenta. By subtracting this "tracer loss" from the fetal tracer infusion, one effectively removes the fetal to placental flux from the overall rate of disappearance. At steady state, Ra = Rd, and thus the Ra will also be "corrected" by the degree to which the unidirectional placental to fetal flux rate exceeds the net umbilical uptake of tracee. This method has the advantage of requiring only a single tracer, and is done most precisely with radiolabeled tracers. Technical difficulties include the relatively small coefficient of extraction of some amino acids, and the inherent experimental error in determining umbilical blood flow, which is needed for the calculation of tracer loss.

A second method uses a dual-tracer technique, with one tracer infused in the maternal compartment and a differently labeled tracer but same tracee infused into the fetal compartment. By measuring the dilution of the maternal tracer in the fetal compartment, one can estimate the unidirectional maternal to fetal flux rate. Likewise, by measuring the dilution of the fetal tracer in the maternal compartment, one can estimate the unidirectional fetal to maternal flux rate. However, this flux rate is very small relative to overall maternal tracee Ra, and therefore not estimable with precision. The dual tracer method has the advantage of not requiring umbilical blood flow measurement, and is best performed using stable isotopes. The general model of fetal amino acid kinetics in its varying degrees of complexity is depicted in Figure 18.2.

Many older studies in the literature failed to account for the bidirectional fluxes of amino acids at the placental interface, but included them in the overall fetal tracee Ra and/or Rd. Both net umbilical uptake and tracee oxidation were determined independently and subtracted from Ra to determine appearance from protein breakdown or from Rd to determine use for protein synthesis. Therefore, in many of these older studies, both appearance from protein breakdown and use for protein synthesis were overestimated, each to an equal extent. While the quantitative aspects of these older studies should be questioned, conclusions based on the qualitative aspects of the flux rates are likely to be valid.

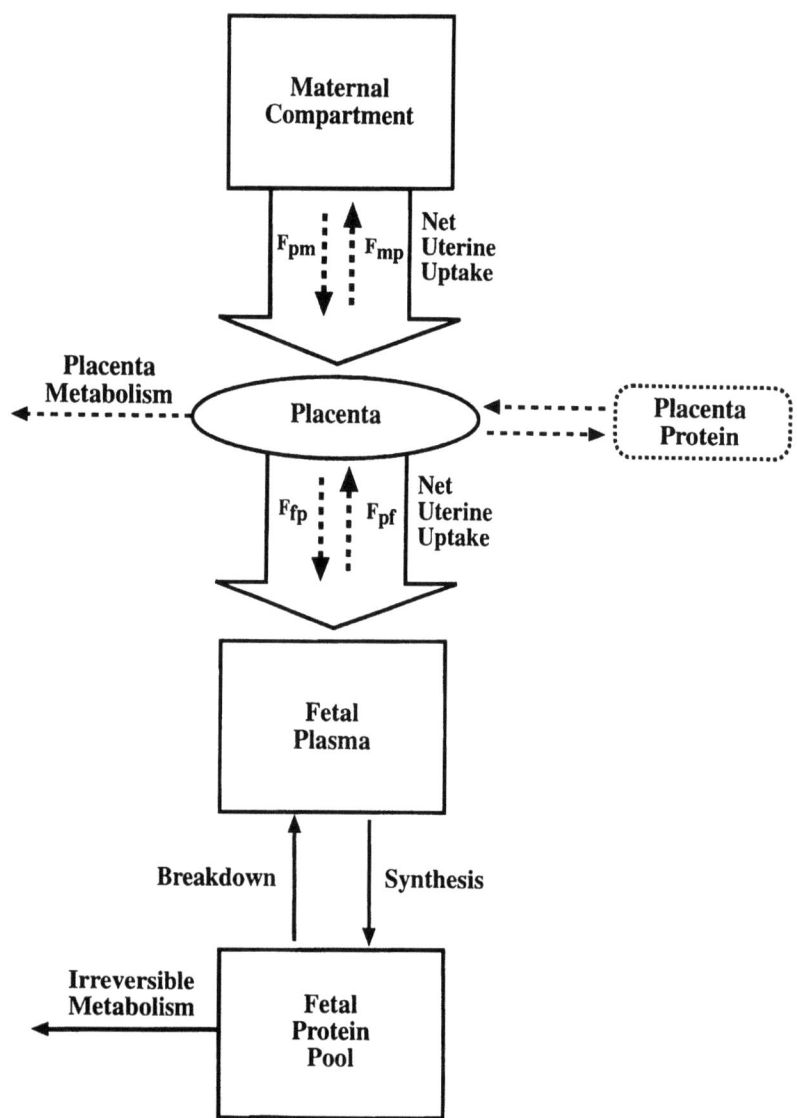

FIGURE 18.2. Steady-state, continuous tracer infusion model for determining fetal amino acid kinetics. The model assumes an essential amino acid as the tracer molecule. Amino acids are transferred from the maternal plasma compartment to the placenta as net uterine uptake. This is the sum of the unidirectional flux rate from the maternal compartment to the placenta (F_{pm}) and the unidirectional flux rate from the placenta to the maternal plasma (F_{mp}). Likewise, amino acids are transferred from the placenta to the fetal plasma as net umbilical uptake, which is the sum of the unidirectional flux rate from placenta to fetal plasma (F_{fp}) and the unidirectional flux rate from fetal plasma to the placenta (F_{pf}). The net uptakes can be determined by the application of the Fick principle. The unidirectional flux rates, however, can only be estimated by means of labeled tracers. Fetal plasma amino acid rate of appearance is equal to the sum of F_{fp} and amino acid appearance from protein breakdown; rate of disappearance is equal to the sum of F_{pf} + rate of irreversible metabolism + rate of use for protein synthesis.

It is important to realize that the first tracer method described, determination of the fractional synthetic rate, directly measures the rate of incorporation of a labeled amino acid from the free pool to the protein-bound pool. The second method, determination of amino acid flux rates, measures the rate of tracer label dilution in the plasma amino acid pool. Protein synthesis is estimated by dividing the flux, calculated from the tracer dilution minus any exogenous intake, by the amount of substrate in total body protein.

The choice of the correct conversion factor relating flux to protein synthesis affects the estimated protein synthetic rate. Although it might seem that simply using the percentage of the tracer in total body protein would give the best estimate, it must be remembered that neither the turnover rate nor the amino acid composition is equal in all tissues or proteins. If the factor chosen heavily weights the estimate to tissues with slower turnovers (e.g., collagen), protein synthetic rates are underestimated. For instance, although leucine makes up 6.6% of total amino acids, the usual factor converting leucine flux rates to protein synthetic rates is 8%, in part because collagen, which makes up 20% of body protein, is relatively scarce in leucine content and turns over slowly.

Fetal Nitrogen Accretion

Carcass analysis data throughout gestation are available for several species, providing daily rate of accretion, increments of total nitrogen,[3] and increments of individual amino acids.[4] These data are given in Tables 18.1 and 18.2. They indicate that despite a widely ranging rate of fetal growth the total growth rate/nitrogen retention rate ratio is similar across species, with the rate of nitrogen retention slightly greater than that of total growth. This finding implies that the fetus has progressively more nitrogen throughout gestation.

It should be noted that for most species the fractional growth rate is not constant throughout gestation. In most species there is a gradual deceleration of growth rate that is most pronounced during the later stages of pregnancy.

TABLE 18.1. Comparison of the fractional rates of growth in wet weight and nitrogen accretion per day (per fraction of gestation).

Species	Fractional growth rate	Fractional N accretion
Rat	0.3 (0.11)	0.53 (0.12)[5]*
Guinea pig	0.07 (0.05)	0.09 (0.07)[6]
Sheep	0.03 (0.08)	0.065 (0.09)[4]
Human	0.015 (0.04)	0.016 (0.04)[1-9]

*Reference number.

TABLE 18.2. Fractional accretion rates for amino acids in ovine fetuses.

Amino acid	K_s
Glu	0.0618
Gly	0.0669
Val	0.0611
Ala	0.0632
Ile	0.0609
Arg	0.0658
Thr	0.0622
Ser	0.0637
Asn	0.0623
Leu	0.0614
Tyr	0.0621
Phe	0.0616
Lys	0.0618
His	0.0633

In the human, cross-sectional studies have shown a marked deceleration after 36 weeks, and in some studies there is a suggestion of negative growth postterm. Sophisticated imaging techniques that allow longitudinal study of an individual fetus have led to doubt as to whether such slowing of growth is a usual phenomenon. In any case, the human fetal fractional growth rate appears to be relatively stable at 1.5% per day from 24 to 34 weeks' gestation.

In the fetal lamb amino acid nitrogen accounts for 82% of total carcass nitrogen. The concentrations of most amino acids decrease slightly over the second half of gestation. Only arginine, glycine, cysteine/cystine, and hydroxyproline evidence increased concentrations.

When the fractional growth and nitrogen accretion rates are analyzed as rates per fraction of gestation, similarities are seen between the rat and sheep and the guinea pig and human. This point is of interest, as the human and guinea pig at term contain much larger amounts of body fat than do the rat and sheep. It may be speculated that such fatty species require a slower rate of growth in lean body mass to accommodate fat accretion, which imposes larger caloric demands on the mother than does accretion of lean body mass.[5] The interrelations between nitrogen accretion, fat accretion, and length of gestation remain to be understood.

Fractional synthetic rates of protein have been shown to be inversely proportional to gestation. Fractional rates of protein or nitrogen accretion are inversely proportional to gestational age, but the slope is less than for the relation between protein synthesis and gestational age.[6] Early in gestation there is a large difference between the two, which progressively narrows as gestation proceeds. The precise mechanism of this finding is unclear. Possible explanations include the increase in the slow-turnover proteins, which constitute the carcass late in gestation, or a decreased requirement for protein remodeling as gestation progresses. Whatever the mechanism, it is clear that alterations in either the fractional synthetic rate or fractional breakdown rate may be important in the regulation of protein accretion.

It has been shown that the increase in absolute protein synthesis is less than the increase in dry weight of the ovine fetus as gestation progresses.[7] This difference is the result of the increase in nonnitrogenous tissue, especially fat and mineralized tissue, which occurs late in gestation.

Umbilical uptake studies have been reliably performed only in the fetal lamb model. These studies uniformly demonstrate that amino acid concentrations are higher in fetal than maternal blood, with the exception of glutamine. The initial studies of Lemons et al.[8] demonstrated that the net uptake of amino acid carbon and nitrogen is significantly greater than would be required based on carcass analysis. The net balance, as demonstrated in Figure 18.3, varies for each amino acid. The neutral amino acids are taken up at a rate double their requirement for carcass accretion. The uptake of acidic and basic amino acids is nearly equal to the carcass accretion requirement; net uptake of glutamate is negative, implying active fetal glutamate synthesis to supply fetal protein synthetic needs. It is possible that the net balance of several other amino acids is less than carcass accretion requirements. Further studies have indicated that, within the limitations of the methodology, no differences are detected when the ewe is fasted despite marked changes in maternal plasma amino acid concentrations.

Determinations of umbilical artery–umbilical vein (UA–UV) concentration differences of amino acids in the rat, measured acutely under anesthesia, are qualitatively similar to those seen in chronically studied sheep, although the actual concentrations are significantly greater.[9] Although it is not possible to accurately determine net umbilical uptake of amino acids in the human, simultaneous determinations of plasma aminograms from umbilical artery and vein in the human have demonstrated differences similar to those seen in the sheep at term[10] and at mid-gestation.[11] It is interesting that the magnitude of the UA–UV concentration difference is greater in the premature human neonate than in mature human neonate.[10] This fact is true not only for those with a positive umbilical balance (UV > UA) but for those amino acids with a negative umbilical balance (e.g., glutamate). Without blood flow data, it is not possible to directly infer that umbilical uptake of amino acids decreased as gestation progressed. However, this observation is consistent with data in fetal sheep demonstrating decreased fractional synthetic rates during late gestation.

Uterine uptake of most amino acids nearly matches simultaneously determined umbilical uptake, implying that the amino acid passes through the placenta unaltered, at least in net quantity (Figure 18.4).[12] The guinea pig placenta has been shown to exhibit active amino acid transport sites on the maternal and fetal sides of the trophoblast. Net transport of amino acids from the mother to the fetus results from different transport rates at the two sites.[13] Contrary to this implication is the evidence that the placenta is rich in amino acid transaminases,[14] especially branched-chain amino acid transaminase,[15,16] and evidence that free ammonia is produced within the placenta.[17] It has been demonstrated that the uterine uptake of the branched-chain amino acids is greater than simultaneous umbilical uptake.[18] Available data suggest that a portion of the glutamate taken from the fetus by the placenta may be converted to glutamine and re-released into the fetus.[12] The purpose of such metabolic interconversions by the placenta remain to be elucidated. The use by the placenta of

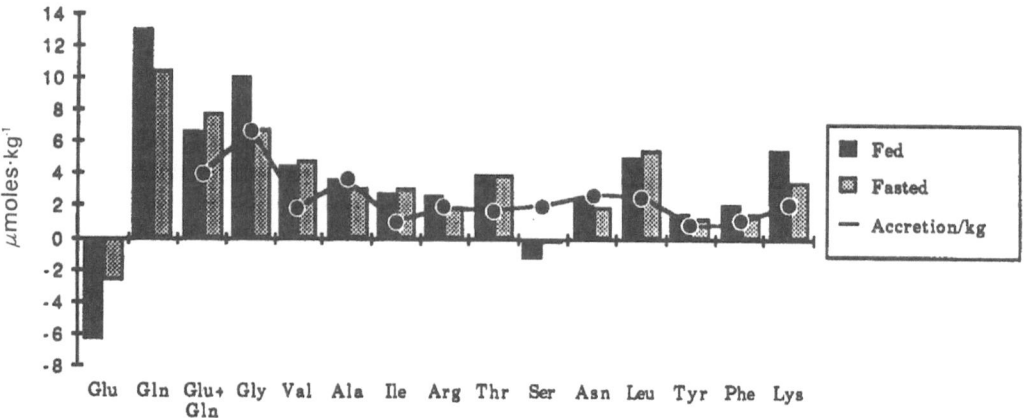

FIGURE 18.3. Comparison of umbilical amino acid uptake versus carcass accretion requirements for the 120-day ovine fetus. Uptake data are from Lemons et al.[8] Fed = those fed 5 to 7 days after operation; the ewe was fed ad libitum. Fasted = ewe was fasted 5 days prior to the study. Accretion data was calculated from Meier et al.[4]

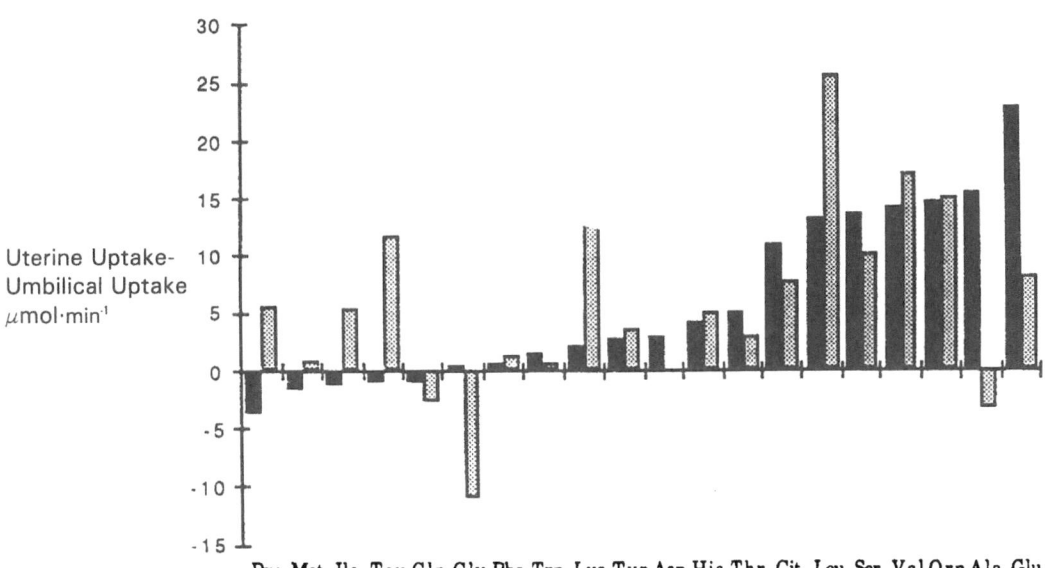

FIGURE 18.4. Differences between the uterine and umbilical uptake of the physiologic amino acids, and the effect on these differences of fasting the ewe. (From Lemons and Schreiner,[18] with permission.)

amino acid carbon skeleton as an oxidative fuel remains to be determined.

Net uterine, but not umbilical, UA–UV differences of amino acids have been determined in several small species, in particular the pig.[19] These differences are consistent with little uptake of acidic amino acids and large uptake of several of the neutral amino acids. A study of the balance of fetal nitrogen must include ammonia. As stated previously, ammonia is produced within the placenta, presumably as the result of transamination of amino acids within trophoblastic tissue.[17] It has not been conclusively shown that α-amino nitrogen is the source of this ammonia. In exercising skeletal muscle, which produces significant amounts of ammonia, the major source appears to be degradation of nucleotides, particularly adenosine.[20,21] As the placenta is metabolically an active organ, with a high rate of oxygen consumption, it is possible that adenosine triphosphate (ATP) degradation could be a significant source of placental ammonia production. Alternatively, the high activities of numerous transaminases make amino acids likely candidates.

The ammonia produced within the placenta effluxes bidirectionally into the maternal and fetal circulations. This efflux of ammonia may account for as much as 14% of total uteroplacental α-amino nitrogen uptake in the pregnant ewe.[22] Absolute uterine ammonia production is relatively constant during the second half of gestation, at approximately 500 mg nitrogen per day. When expressed as a fraction of the total uteroplacental nitrogen requirement, it is inversely proportional to gestational age. At 70 days' gestation, ammonia production may account for 44% of total nitrogen requirements, but by term it accounts for only 12%.

The fetus excretes waste nitrogen through urea synthesized in the fetal liver; the fetal urea is disposed of across the placenta. Initial studies of fetal urea production used ^{14}C-labeled urea to determine fetal urea production and placental urea clearance. Clearance was found to average $20\,ml \cdot kg^{-1} min^{-1}$ and did not change with fasting of the ewe.[23,24] In a primate model, placental urea clearance was found to be $15\,ml \cdot kg^{-1} min^{-1}$.[25] Subsequent studies have primarily relied on the use of this value for clearance rate to calculate fetal urea production rates. On a weight-specific basis, ovine fetal urea synthetic rates are high, averaging $365\,mg \cdot kg^{-1} day^{-1}$ in the fetus of a well-fed ewe. Humans have a significant urea concentration gradient from maternal arterial blood to fetal arterial fetal blood, indicating substantial fetal urea production, although the clearance value for humans is not known.[24] Urea production increases by 100% during fasting of the ewe, with the activities of the five urea cycle enzymes increasing simultaneously.[26]

Protein Metabolism in Specific Fetal Tissues

Rates of protein synthesis and degradation have been determined in a number of fetal tissues. Using ^{14}C-labeled tyrosine in the ovine fetus, Schaeffer and Krishnamurti[27] have shown that fractional synthetic rates tend to be greater for gastrointestinal tissues, with a fractional synthetic rate of more than 75%. Gastrointestinal tissues contribute 20% of total fetal whole-body protein synthesis. Skeletal muscle contributes 20% of total fetal whole-body protein turnover despite a much smaller fractional synthetic rate of only 12%, reflecting the much larger muscle mass in the fetal body.[28] Other fetal tissues, including brain, liver, heart, lung, and kidney, have fractional synthetic rates similar to those of muscle but because of the smaller mass contributed less to whole-body protein turnover.

In the rat, fetal whole-body fractional synthetic rates decline during the gestation, from 73% per day on day 14 to 38% per day on day 20, with term gestation being 21 days. Likewise, the K_s of individual tissues declines; K_s for the kidney declines from 94% on day 18 to 63% on day 20. K_s for liver declines from 112% on day 16 to 98% on day 20.[29] These rates, expressed per day, are much greater than those found in the sheep. However, expressed as a fraction of gestational length, they are comparable.

A number of studies have been performed in fetal sheep using tracer quantities of labeled amino acids. These studies have employed tyrosine, leucine, or lysine labeled with either ^{3}H or ^{14}C. The rates of protein synthesis and amino acid oxidation have been determined from these experiments. Absolute rates of protein synthesis are variable among studies, ranging from 63^{27} to 38.6^{30} to $15 \, g \cdot kg \times kg^{-1} day^{-1}$.[6] All studies have shown much higher rates of protein synthesis in the fetal lamb compartment than are seen simultaneously in the ewe. A more than 50% decrease in protein synthesis rates is seen in fetuses of 48-hour–fasted ewes.[31] This study, which used tyrosine as the tracer, demonstrated a rate of irreversible loss of tyrosine greater than the net utilization. Net placental uptake was negative, and the largest fraction of tyrosine rate of appearance was from endogenous fetal production. A relatively high rate of amino acid oxidation has been observed, as might be predicted from the high rates of fetal urea excretion that are known to occur.[22] Fasting of the ewe has been shown to increase the oxidation rate of both tyrosine and leucine.[32]

Leucine balance and utilization have been extensively documented, and a reasonable net balance of leucine transport and utilization for the fed state ovine fetus can be constructed.[33] Uteroplacental uptake of leucine exceeds umbilical uptake by a considerable degree.[6] Although it has not been shown that placental ammonia production arises from leucine α-amino nitrogen, it can be seen that leucine nitrogen could account for nearly one third of placental ammonia production. The fate of the leucine carbon skeleton is not yet known. A portion is returned to the fetal and maternal circulation as the deamination product α-ketoisocaproate.[33] It is possible that a portion is oxidized within the placenta.

Umbilical leucine uptake accounts for 25% of the total leucine rate of appearance into fetal plasma. The rate of appearance of leucine is the sum of umbilical uptake plus the endogenous leucine produced by protein breakdown. Endogenous leucine appearance accounts for 75% of total leucine flux. Because leucine is an essential amino acid, the endogenous appearance can result only from protein breakdown. It should be noted that in all reported studies the tracer dilution, from which flux is calculated, is determined in arterial plasma, a posthepatic site, but umbilical uptake is estimated from prehepatic sources. Any leucine taken up by the umbilical circulation and the fetal liver is accounted for in the umbilical uptake but does not participate in tracer dilution, resulting in an underestimation of flux due to uptake and overestimation of protein breakdown. Studies in adult sheep have shown that failure to include hepatic uptake of leucine results in a slight (i.e., 5%) underestimation of total flux. It is not known to what extent leucine is taken up by the fetal liver. The activity of branched-chain aminotransferase is low in fetal liver, so it seems reasonable to assume that the error in leucine flux measurements is small.

Leucine oxidation accounts for approximately 20% of total leucine flux and 50% of leucine uptake.[32] This finding is not unexpected, as the rate of leucine accretion into the fetal carcass accounts for only 50% to 60% of leucine umbilical uptake.

By knowing the percentage leucine in the average fetal protein, one can extrapolate the leucine data to ovine fetal protein turnover in general. It is likely that the other branched-chain amino acids, isoleucine and valine, behave in a similar fashion. Most other neutral amino acids, which are taken up in excess to their tissue accretion, are metabolized in a similar fashion. Using 490 μmol leucine per gram of protein, one estimates that the ovine fetal protein turnover rate equals 40 g of protein per day, which compares to a protein accretion rate of 10 to 12 g per day for a 4000-g fetus.[4]

The data of Meier et al.,[6] obtained using lysine as a tracer, give similar estimates of protein turnover (32–53 g·day^{-1}), for late-gestation ovine fetuses. In addition, in this study, the K_s was determined, allowing a second estimate of protein synthesis. The two estimates were close, with the estimate that was determined by the fractional synthetic rate being somewhat greater. Schaeffer and Krishnamurti,[34] using tyrosine as a tracer, have suggested higher estimates of ovine fetal protein turnover than are derived from the leucine and lysine methods. The reasons for this discrepancy are not clear.

Relation Between Protein Synthesis and Energy Consumption

Numerous investigators have noted a correlation between energy consumption and rates of protein synthesis determined from amino acid flux rates. As described above, the allometric equation is used to relate physiologic processes to the dimensions of the organism. Metabolic rate in postnatal animals is generally proportional to body mass and is thought to be a consequence of the necessary equality between heat production and heat dissipation.[35] Heat loss, which occurs at the body surface, must be proportional to body surface area, which should result in the metabolic rate being proportional to the two-thirds power of mass.

It has been found that during prenatal and postnatal life protein synthetic rates scale to an exponent similar to that of energy consumption.[7] Energy requirements for growth may be calculated in several ways. In postnatal life subjects can be studied over long periods. Presumably they are growing at different rates, and a plot of energy intake versus weight gain can be constructed. The slope of this line is an estimate of the calories per gram weight gain needed for growth. In human neonates it has led to an estimate of $0.7\,kcal \cdot g^{-1}$ weight gain.[36] This figure includes the total cost of growth, not simply protein synthesis.

In the fetus, estimates must be made from the known heat of formation of the peptide bonds, which are needed to synthesize protein. Each peptide bond requires 4 ATP = 1 GTP (guanosine triphosphate), leading to an estimate of 0.86 kcal (3.6 kJ) per gram of protein synthesized.[37] If the protein synthetic rate for a hypothetical 3.5-kg fetus is 35 g/day, it can be estimated that approximately 30 kcal ($8.6\,kcal \cdot kg^{-1} day^{-1}$) are devoted to protein synthesis. The oxygen consumption of the late-gestation, 3- to 4-kg fetus is 6 to $7\,ml\,O_2 \cdot kg^{-1} min^{-1}$, equivalent to an energy consumption of about $50\,kcal \cdot kg^{-1} day^{-1}$. Protein synthesis would account for approximately 17% ($8.6\,kcal \cdot 50\,kcal^{-1}$) of the total fetal oxidative metabolism. This figure seems to be a reasonable approximation and is close to that estimated for protein synthesis in other species.

It should not be surprising that these two processes are correlated, as each occurs exclusively in the lean body mass. Whether there is any deeper significance to this relation remains to be determined. Although 17% of energy consumption is a significant amount, much of it is obligatory replacement of protein that has broken down, which is necessary for survival.

Interorgan Metabolism of Amino Acids and Effects of Maternal Fasting

It is accepted that in the postnatal animal active interorgan transport of amino acids takes place, leading to storage of excess amino acids as protein, especially in muscle, during the postabsorptive period.[38] During fasting, release of amino acids for gluconeogenesis takes place. In the postabsorptive state, liver plays a crucial role in maintaining plasma amino acid concentrations; most amino acids, with the exception of the branched-chains amino acids, are removed from portal blood during the first pass through the liver.

In postnatal nonruminant species, branched-chain amino acids are taken up by skeletal muscle. During fasting, transamination of the branched-chain amino acids occurs, and the nitrogen effluxes from skeletal muscle as alanine or glutamine. There is evidence to suggest that the carbon skeleton may efflux as glutamine.[39] Alanine and glutamine are released from skeletal muscle in the largest quantities and together account for more than 50% of total amino acid efflux. Alanine is taken up by the liver, is transaminated to lactate, and then undergoes gluconeogenesis. Glutamine is taken up preferentially by the gut, which then releases alanine, and by the kidney.[40,41] The kidney uses glutamine for secretion of ammonia, important in acid-base balance,[42,43] and for gluconeogenesis. These interrelationships are depicted in Figure 18.5.

During fasting of the pregnant ewe it appears that the fetus undergoes changes in metabolism so that amino acids substitute as oxidative substrate for glucose. This change is necessary, as the supply of glucose to the fetus falls by 50% in response to fasting-induced maternal hypoglycemia. During normoglycemia, glucose accounts for 50% to 75% of oxidative substrate, and amino acids account for 25%. Fasting causes amino acids to substitute as substrate for glucose, resulting in an increase in fetal urea production, which doubles by the fifth day of a prolonged fast. Umbilical uptake of amino acids does not appear to change quantitatively or qualitatively.

Postnatal ruminant species have low activities of branched-chain transaminase in skeletal muscle.[44] Skeletal muscle in these species does not participate as actively in the transformation of waste nitrogen as does skeletal muscle in nonruminants.[45] Studies in the ovine fetus support a scheme similar to that seen in the postnatal ruminant, especially during fasting of the ewe.[46] Figure 18.6 shows the net balance across the ovine fetal hindlimb in the fed and fasted states. Clearly alanine and glutamine are synthesized de novo within fetal skeletal muscle, as the release of these amino acids relative to tyrosine exceeds that which could be derived from protein breakdown. There is a large uptake of the branched-chain amino acids, which increases during fasting. It is interesting to note that the nitrogen exiting the hindlimb is nearly equal to that entering as the branched-chain amino acids. The ketoacids resulting from branched-chain amino acid transamination exit skeletal muscle, indicating active transamination within fetal muscle.

Figure 18.7 shows the difference in fetal and maternal branched-chain amino acid metabolism. The fetus, much like nonruminants, has an increased arteriovenous difference for the branched-chain amino acids as well as an

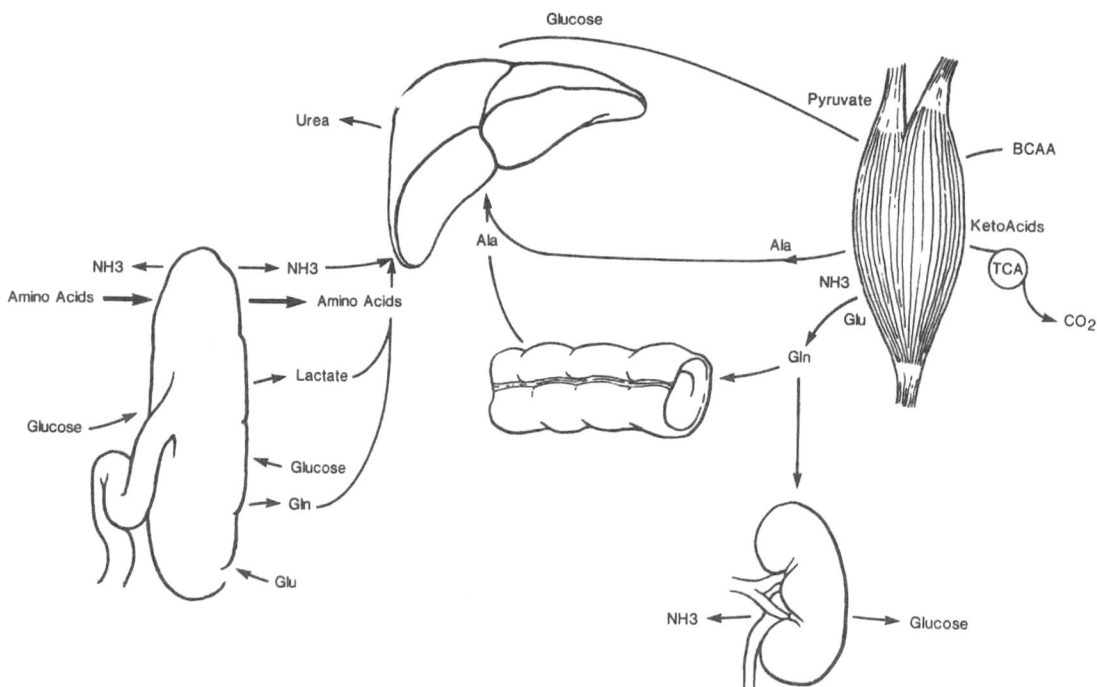

FIGURE 18.5. Relationships between the branched-chain amino acids (BCAA) alanine and glutamine in a postnatal nonruminant species. BCAAs, which may be oxidized or, in the case of ketoisovalerate and ketomethylvalerate, may enter the tricarboxylic acid (TCA) cycle, potentially contributing net carbon, which may exit the TCA as oxaloacetate, subsequently forming glutamate and glutamine. Glutamine nitrogen is derived from the BCAA. Alanine transports nitrogen to the liver for ureagenesis; glutamine is preferentially extracted and partially oxidized by intestine, resulting in alanine formation. Glutamine is an important source of ammonia nitrogen in the kidney.

increase in the activity of transaminase during fasting. The ewe shows little change in either arteriovenous difference or enzyme activity.

The placenta appears to perform several of the metabolic functions that skeletal muscle performs postnatally. The placenta produces both lactate and ammonia, deaminates the branched-chain amino acids, and synthesizes glutamine for umbilical uptake. It concentrates most amino acids, with intracellular concentrations much greater than those in either fetal or maternal plasma, potentially functioning as a buffering reserve if uterine delivery of amino acids falls to a level no longer able to maintain fetal concentrations.[47] The significance of these placental functions remains to be determined.

The ovine fetus responds to maternal fasting in similar ways to that in which a postnatal nonruminant animal responds to fasting, although certain aspects are not yet clear. The only organ bed across which amino acid bal-

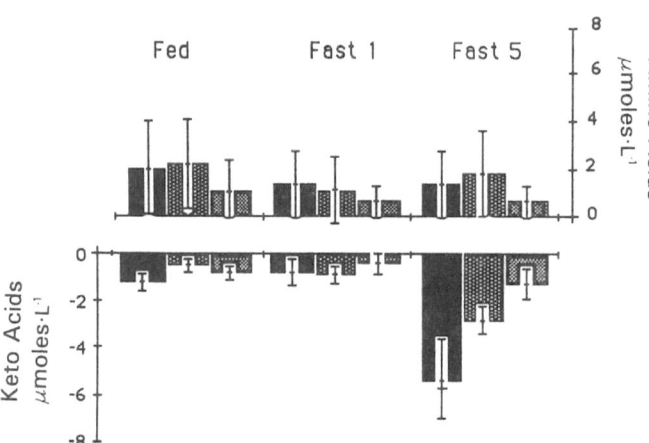

FIGURE 18.6. Effect of maternal fasting on the arteriovenous concentration differences across the ovine fetal hindlimb for the branched-chain amino acids (BCAAs) and their respective α-ketoacids. The data suggest that there is active interorgan transport of the carbon skeleton of the BCAAs that becomes more prominent during fasting. (From Liechty et al.,[46] with permission.)

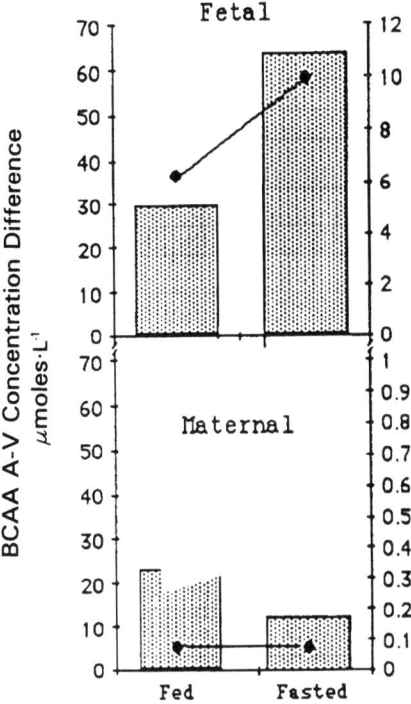

FIGURE 18.7. Fasting the ewe results in differing effects on branched-chain amino acid (BCAA) metabolism in the skeletal muscle of the ewe compared to her fetus. Fetal BCAA transaminase (BCAAT) activity is increased during fasting, whereas that of the ewe is depressed. Note the order of magnitude difference in scale for fetal compared to maternal BCAAT activity. The arteriovenous concentration differences for the BCAAs follow a similar pattern. (From Liechty et al.,[15] with permission.)

ance has been determined is hindlimb skeletal muscle. Although it can be surmised that alanine and glutamine carry nitrogen and possibly carbon from muscle protein stores to the fetal liver and kidney, it has not been demonstrated in the fetus. It has not been conclusively demonstrated that gluconeogenesis from amino acid carbon can be accomplished by the ovine fetus, although there is strong circumstantial evidence that it can occur, at least to a small extent. This evidence includes alanine carbon incorporation into glucose,[48] and the observation that nearly 25% of fetal lactate is derived from noncarbohydrate precursors.[49] Gilfillan et al.[50] demonstrated that alanine is produced by the late-term human fetus. Lemons et al.[51] demonstrated that the enzymes responsible for gluconeogenesis are induced in the ovine fetus in response to maternal fasting. Taken together, these data are suggestive of gluconeogenesis in the ovine fetus. A large body of evidence from the rat fetus and neonate suggests that rodent fetuses are not capable of gluconeogenesis until enzyme induction, which takes place after parturition (see Chapter 17).

Finally, the origin of the excess amino acids for oxidative substrate during maternal fasting is not clear. It has been shown that net umbilical uptake of amino acids does not increase during fasting. One possibility is a diminished growth rate during fasting, freeing the nitrogen that would be used for tissue synthesis for oxidation with no decrease in total body nitrogen. Alternatively, there may be a net catabolism of fetal tissue amino acid stores.

Adaptation and Regulation of Fetal Nitrogen Metabolism

Hormonal Regulation

Insulin

Clinical evidence suggests that insulin is an important regulator of growth in the human fetus. Macrosomia accompanies the fetal hyperinsulinemic syndromes (e.g., maternal diabetes, Beckwith-Wiedemann syndrome, and nesidioblastosis)[52] (see Chapter 32). Conversely, growth retardation is found in the rare infant born with pancreatic aplasia. Chronic hyperinsulinemia in the fetal rhesus monkey induces macrosomia and cardiomegaly.[53] Hyperinsulinemia has profound effects on fetal body composition in the human, with a large increase in the amount and percent of total body fat mass. Lean body mass is greatly increased, although as a percentage of body mass it may be decreased, reflective of a disproportionate increase in body fat mass. Lean body mass is greatly increased, although as a percentage of body mass it may be decreased, reflective of a disproportionate increase in body fat mass.

Milley et al.[54] demonstrated decreased arterial concentration and increased fetal uptake of α-amino nitrogen when the late gestation ovine fetus was infused with exogenous insulin. The increased fetal amino acid uptake resulted in increased tissue synthesis, expansion of intracellular amino acid pools, and increased catabolism, but the partitioning between these fates remains to be determined. It is interesting to note that Milley[55] was not able to document increased birth weight in fetal lambs infused chronically with insulin. Likewise, neither Stagenberg et al.[56] nor Angervall et al.[57] were able to show any increase in body or protein mass in rat fetuses injected with insulin during late gestation. Fetal pigs fail to show any significant effect of insulin on growth.[58] In contrast, Picon[59] has shown a 10% increase in total body nitrogen in insulin-injected rat fetuses. Susa et al.[60] found that chronic insulin infusion in the fetal rhesus monkey resulted in significant 33% increases in body mass. Although chemical analysis of the carcasses was not performed, it can be presumed that the total body nitrogen was increased, although not likely to the same degree as body mass. The protein/DNA ratio was not changed, implying that any increase in lean body mass is mainly the result of tissue hyperplasia rather than hypertrophy.

Investigators have shown that fetal size was substantially less in a diabetic rat model than in controls. Fetal total protein content is decreased in concert with the diminished body size. Fetal fractional synthetic rates are diminished in the rat fetuses of diabetic mothers, whereas fractional breakdown rates are markedly elevated.[61] The placentas of these pups have diminished rates of protein breakdown but normal synthetic rates, the net result being placentomegaly in these fetuses of diabetic mothers.[62] These findings are intriguing because it is generally held that fetal tissue responds to hyperinsulinemia by hypertrophy or hyperplasia or both, whereas the placenta is generally thought not to be an insulin-sensitive organ. Further investigation is warranted to determine if these effects found in the rat can be demonstrated in other species.

Little is known about the effect of insulin on fetal protein kinetics. Generally, in postnatal animals an increasing plasma insulin concentration causes a movement of plasma amino acids into muscle cells, thereby decreasing arterial plasma concentrations. Insulin promotes protein deposition. It is controversial as to whether it occurs primarily because of increased protein synthesis, or decreased protein breakdown.[63] However, evidence using tracer kinetic modeling supports the latter as the major insulin effect.[35,64] In adult human studies, kinetics of the branched-chain amino acids are affected by alterations in the glucose and insulin supply to a greater extent than are those of other amino acids.[65]

Several recent studies have attempted to address the role of insulin's effect on in vivo amino acid kinetics. It has been difficult to differentiate the effects of insulin and glucose, as generally the concentrations are highly correlated. In a series of three studies, Liechty et al.[66–68] have attempted to differentiate these effects. In the first two experiments, glucose was infused into fetal sheep, allowing insulin concentration to rise in response, or not allowing such a rise by means of a somatostatin "insulin clamp." In the final study, hyperinsulinemia was induced by fetal insulin infusion, with glucose concentration held constant by the glucose clamp technique. The results of these experiments are summarized in Table 18.3.

However, the consistent finding among all three experiments was that despite large changes in insulin concentration, no significant changes in leucine rate of appearance were noted in any study. Neither were any consistent changes observed in leucine net umbilical uptake. As the rate of appearance of an essential amino acid is considered reflective of appearance from protein breakdown, these studies have been interpreted as failing to demonstrate a role of insulin in suppressing fetal proteolysis. These studies were analyzed with the simplified model structure, which used only net umbilical uptake, rather than the unidirectional flux of leucine from placenta to fetus (F_{fp}, Figure 18.2), and thus overestimated the quantitative value for protein breakdown. However, unless insulin causes large changes in the flux rates of leucine to and from the placenta, without resulting in a change in the net leucine umbilical uptake, the interpretations should remain qualitatively correct.

Neither does insulin appear to have a direct role in stimulation of fetal protein synthesis. Rather its effect appears to be mediated through increases in glucose utilization, thereby sparing leucine from oxidation. It is then more available for use for protein synthesis. The relationships between glucose, insulin, and leucine oxidation are depicted in Figure 18.8. The overall conclusion from these studies is that insulin has no effect on fetal proteolysis. However, through stimulation of fetal glucose utilization, insulin does have a role in the partitioning of glucose and amino acids to oxidation or tissue accretion, thus increasing protein synthesis.

There is one study that has demonstrated an effect of insulin to suppress fetal proteolysis.[69] In this study of fetal hyperinsulinemia, an amino acid infusion was used to diminish the insulin-induced fall in leucine concentration. The kinetic model employed accounted for disposal of leucine tracer from the fetus to the placenta, which was

TABLE 18.3. Directional changes in ovine fetal leucine, glucose and insulin parameters during four different experimental protocols.

	Glucose		Insulin		Glucose utilization		Leucine Ra		Leucine oxidation	
	Fed	Fasted	Fed	Fasted	Fed	Fasted	Fed	Fasted	Fed	Fasted
Fetal glucose infusion	↑	↑	↑	↑	↔	↔	↔	↔	↔	↓
Hyperinsulinemic glucose clamp	↔	↔	↑	↑	↑	↑	↔	↔	↔	↓
Hyperglycemic insulin clamp	↑	↑	↔	↔	↔	↔	↔	↔	↓	↓
rhIGF-I infusion	↔	↔	↓	↓	↔	↔	↓	↓	↔	↓

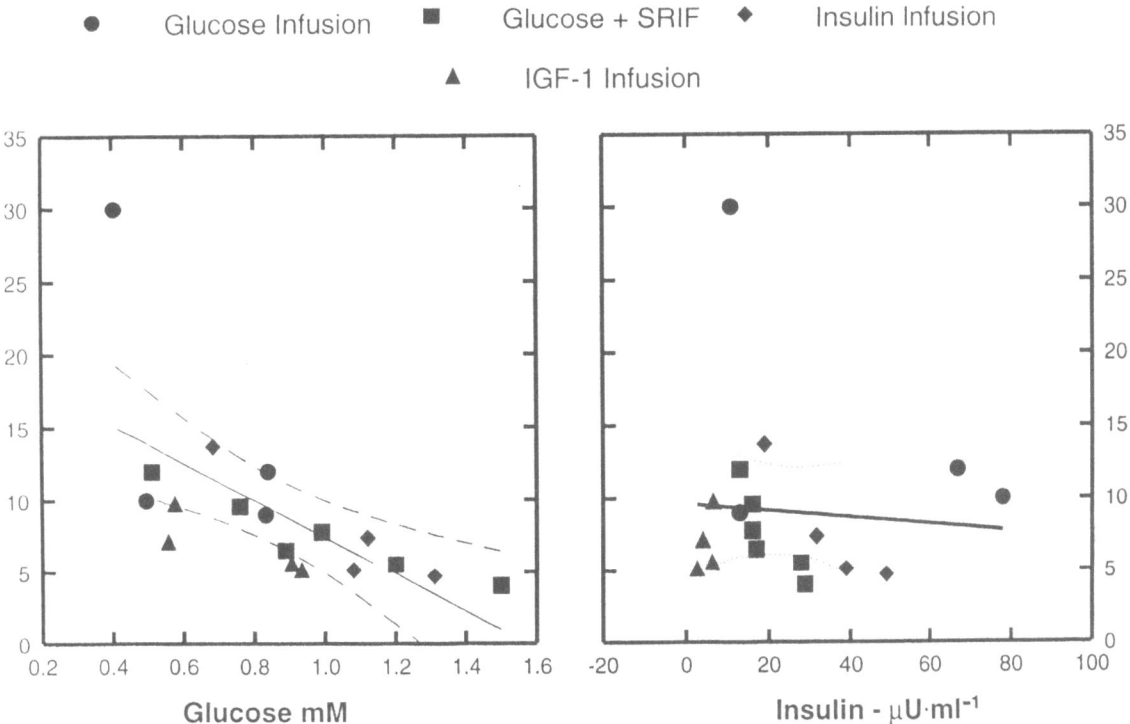

FIGURE 18.8. Relative effects of insulin concentration or glucose concentration on ovine fetal leucine oxidation. There is no correlation between insulin and leucine oxidation, while a significant correlation exists between glucose concentration and leucine oxidation. Data are aggregated from a series of four studies.[66-68,81]

not done in the previously mentioned experiments. Milley[69] was able to demonstrate a small decrease in leucine appearance from protein breakdown, in spite of no statistically significant change in total plasma leucine Ra. It is unclear whether the differences in the findings between these investigations are the result of the model for analysis or differences in experimental protocols. However, it is clear that any effect insulin may have to decrease fetal proteolysis is not of the magnitude of that seen in postnatal subjects, where suppression of proteolysis by 50% is commonly demonstrated.

Other indirect evidence regarding the effect of insulin on amino acid kinetics in the fetus comes from observations during fasting, when the fetal insulin concentration falls to an undetectable concentration. During maternal fasting, use of amino acids as oxidative substrate increases substantially, whereas total umbilical uptake does not change. This situation occurs despite maternal hypoaminoacidemia. Fetal amino acid concentrations in general remain constant or increase during maternal fasting or with other experimental conditions that lower maternal amino acid concentrations.[70]

Postnatally, the lambs' response to fasting is similar to that of the adult, with decreased amino acid concentration and a reduction in protein synthesis coupled with increased protein breakdown.[35] Insulin infusion has no effect on leucine kinetics in fed lambs and causes a decrease in both protein synthesis and protein breakdown in fasted lambs. The relevance of these finding to the fetus is unclear.

Insulin-like Growth Factor-I (IGF-I)

There is evidence that the insulin-like growth factor system may be involved in the regulation of fetal protein metabolism. Although studies of the IGF-I system in the ovine fetus are limited, several investigations in sheep and other mammalian species suggest that IGF-I may be involved in the regulation of fetal growth. Plasma concentrations of IGF-I have been shown to correlate directly with birth weight in humans[71-73] as well as other species.[74,75] In addition, lowered concentrations of IGF-I have been found in association with experimentally induced fetal growth retardation. Such observations have been made in rats and sheep in which fetal growth retardation has been induced by restricting maternal nutrient intake.[76-78] Jones et al.[79] found IGF-I concentration to be reduced by 50% in fetus carried by a ewe with a previous carunclectomy, associated with a 30% decrease in fetal body mass.

It is also clear that the fetal IGF-I system is responsive to nutritional regulation. In the fasted fetal sheep model, provision of intravenous glucose supplementation to the ewe resulted in a rapid (i.e., within 4 hours) return of fetal IGF-I concentrations to normal.[78]

Several studies have documented an effect of IGF-I on ovine fetal amino acid kinetics. Harding et al.[80] demonstrated a 30% decrease in fetal urea production, reflective of a decrease in overall amino acid oxidation, when recombinant human IGF-I was infused into the fetus. Liechty et al.,[81] using a similar rhIGF-I infusion protocol, demonstrated a 10% to 15% decrease in leucine rate of appearance, and a lesser decrease in leucine oxidation. In toto, these data support a role of IGF-I in the fetus to decrease protein breakdown and catabolism, with a net effect of increased tissue accretion. These conclusions are supported by results from an experiment where IGF-I was infused into the fetus from 120 to 130 days of gestation. Infused fetuses had significantly greater liver, lung, kidney, and heart masses than did saline infused controls[82] (see Chapter 20).

Glucagon

Virtually nothing is known about the in vivo effect of other metabolic hormones. Schreiner et al.[83] demonstrated that glucagon concentration rises with prolonged maternal fasting. No obvious correlation exists between glucagon concentration and metabolic parameters, implying that the effect of glucagon on ovine fetal metabolic regulation is minimal. Further studies are necessary to confirm this conclusion.

Intrauterine Growth Retardation

In the preceding sections the importance of amino acids as an oxidative substrate for fetal energy production as well as their role in normal fetal growth has been reviewed. Studies in human pregnancies complicated by intrauterine growth retardation (IUGR) and in animal models of IUGR have demonstrated alterations in amino acid metabolism. The effects on amino acid metabolism under these conditions may be related primarily to a reduction of fetal amino acid availability due to a decrease in transplacental amino acid transport. Alternatively, changes in fetal amino acid utilization may represent an adaptive mechanism to permit survival of the fetus under less than optimal conditions.

Human Studies

Human studies of fetal amino acid metabolism in IUGR have been accomplished by measuring amino acid concentrations in the umbilical artery and/or vein at the time of delivery using the doubly clamped umbilical cord technique, or by transabdominal umbilical cord sampling under ultrasound guidance (i.e., cordocentesis).[84–86] These studies have demonstrated that at term small for gestational age (SGA) infants have decreased plasma concentrations of total α-amino nitrogen compared to normally grown, appropriate for gestational age (AGA) infants.[84,86] This decrease was demonstrated in both the umbilical artery and vein. Most of the difference was accounted for by a decrease in the branched-chain amino acids valine, leucine, and isoleucine. However, lower concentrations of other essential amino acids (e.g., threonine, lysine, and histidine) and nonessential amino acids (e.g., glutamine, glycine, serine, and taurine) were also observed in umbilical venous plasma. The greater differences in amino acid concentrations in the vein as compared with the artery in SGA fetuses may reflect differences in the regulation of amino acid transport by the placenta or altered fetal utilization of amino acids for energy production and protein synthesis. Cetin et al.[84] demonstrated that at term AGA fetuses had significantly positive venoarterial concentration differences for most of the essential amino acids as well as for total α-amino nitrogen. In contrast, SGA fetuses had significantly positive venoarterial concentration differences only for methionine, lysine, histidine, and arginine, but not for total α-amino nitrogen. This latter finding suggests a decrease in umbilical uptake of amino acids (see Chapter 48).

Economides et al.[85] measured plasma concentrations of amino acids in umbilical venous blood samples obtained by cordocentesis in preterm AGA and SGA fetuses from 16 to 36 weeks' gestation. Although there was no difference in total α-amino nitrogen between AGA and SGA fetuses, SGA fetuses were found to have lower concentrations of essential, basic, and branched-chain amino acids. In both preterm and term fetuses positive correlations were found between maternal arterial and umbilical venous amino acid concentrations. Higher concentrations of amino acids were present in the fetal circulation consistent with active placental amino acid transport. Compared to AGA fetuses, SGA fetuses have lower fetomaternal ratios for most amino acids, but in particular for essential and branched chain amino acids.[84–86] This latter finding is consistent with decreased transplacental amino acid transport in SGA fetuses. Of interest is the finding that in preterm SGA fetuses there is a significant correlation between the decrease in plasma concentration and fetomaternal ratio of the essential amino acids and the degree of fetal hypoxemia. This correlation indicates that hypoxemia may be an important etiologic factor for the decrease in amino acid uptake and utilization in IUGR.[85]

Animal Studies

Animal models of IUGR have also demonstrated alterations in fetal amino acid metabolism. In rats, chronic maternal hyperinsulinemia produced by continuous subcutaneous infusion of insulin results in maternal hypoglycemia and lower total plasma amino acid concentration.[87,88] The fetuses from these pregnancies are hypoglycemic, hypoinsulinemic, and growth retarded. In addition, Ogata[88] found the fetuses to have a lower concentration of total plasma amino acids, but did not detect differences in specific amino acids. No difference was found in placental gas exchange in this model. In contrast, bilateral uterine artery ligation in rats results in fetal hypoglycemia, hypoinsulinemia, and IUGR, and in addition results in profound alterations in placental gas exchange with fetal hypoxia and hypercarbia.[89] Similar to the findings in human studies, the SGA rat fetuses had reduced concentrations of valine, leucine, and isoleucine compared to control pups and significantly lower fetomaternal ratios of the branched-chain amino acids. These studies demonstrate that limited maternal fuel availability, specifically glucose and branched-chain amino acids, and fetal hypoxia, hypercarbia, and acidosis are contributing factors in intrauterine growth retardation.

Mechanisms

The specific alterations in fetal and placental amino acid metabolism in IUGR are areas of active investigation. Decreased fetal plasma amino acid concentrations may be the result of reduced umbilical uptake of amino acids, which in turn may be due to decreased placental perfusion, altered transplacental transport, or both. Alternatively, decreased amino acid concentrations may be due to increased fetoplacental amino acid utilization for energy production under conditions of limited glucose availability, as previously described for acute maternal starvation. Depending on the etiology of the fetal growth retardation any one or a combination of several of these factors may contribute to altered amino acid metabolism.

Amino Acid Kinetics

Amino acid kinetics have been studied in IUGR in the ovine fetus using stable and radioactive isotopes of leucine.[90] Leucine is of particular interest in these models of IUGR because leucine is extensively oxidized in the fetus under normal circumstances. In addition, as previously noted, most of the decrease in amino acid concentration observed in SGA fetuses is accounted for by a decrease in the branched-chain amino acids. Furthermore, the rate of leucine oxidation has been shown to increase in response to acute maternal starvation.[68,91]

In the sheep, prolonged uterine blood flow reduction results in hypoxemia and restricted fetal growth as demonstrated by a 20% reduction in daily weight gain and a 38% decrease in linear growth rate.[92] Positive correlations were found between growth rate and arterial oxygen content, once again suggesting a role of oxygen in the regulation of fetal growth. In this model, as in the human SGA fetus, significant reductions were found in the whole-blood concentrations of the branched-chain amino acids. Alanine, tyrosine, and phenylalanine concentrations were increased. The decrease in branched-chain amino acid concentration was associated with a decrease in the net umbilical uptake of isoleucine and leucine as well as the sum of the branched-chain amino acids. In addition, fetoplacental leucine turnover rate was reduced by 20% from 35 µmol/min to 28 µmol/min. In contrast to acute maternal starvation, fetal leucine oxidation decreased by 25% from 8 µmol·min^{-1} to 6 µmol·min^{-1}.[92] The decrease in leucine turnover in this model of IUGR may provide a substantial savings in fetal energy expenditure in the face of reduced oxygen delivery.

Milley[93,94] examined the affect of acute fetal hypoxia on amino acid uptake and protein metabolism. Three hours of fetal hypoxia resulted in decreased umbilical uptake of glucose, lactate, and α-amino nitrogen such that endogenous rather than exogenous substrates were used to support fetal oxidative metabolism.[93] Furthermore, α-amino nitrogen uptake was less than normal nitrogen accretion rates, suggesting that fetal growth must be compromised as a result of hypoxia. In a similar experiment Milley[93] demonstrated that fetal protein synthetic rate declined by 60% during acute hypoxia. It is unclear if similar decreases in protein breakdown took place; but to sustain fetal growth at normal rates, protein breakdown would have to be negligible, a condition that is unlikely. In addition, 3 hours of hypoxia resulted in a significant decrease in fetal oxygen consumption. Milley[94] demonstrated that the decrease in protein synthetic rate accounted for 70% of the decrease in oxygen consumption during fetal hypoxia. It is unclear whether this diminution in protein synthesis is simply a consequence of the decreased tissue pO$_2$, or hormonal regulation; however, it appears that by decreasing protein synthetic rates the fetus is able to diminish its oxygen requirements, albeit at the expense of diminished growth.

Ross et al.[90] have further examined amino acid kinetics in IUGR in fetal sheep. Pregnant sheep were exposed to chronic heat stress beginning early in gestation. This model has been shown to result in fetal growth retardation and hypoglycemia with impaired transplacental glucose transport. By simultaneously infusing distinct leucine tracers into the maternal and fetal circulations, these investigators were able to measure not only leucine flux rates within the fetal compartment, but also the direct flux of maternal leucine across the placenta, and the leucine flux rates between placenta and fetus. Fetal arterial plasma leucine concentration was reduced, and net uterine and uteroplacental uptake were significantly less in IUGR fetuses compared with controls. Net umbilical uptake was also lower in IUGR fetuses; however, this difference did not persist when normalized to fetal weight. As with prolonged uterine blood flow reduction, heat-stressed IUGR fetuses had a 28% decrease in fetal plasma leucine disposal, or turnover rate. Leucine flux from placenta to fetus was nearly 30% lower in IUGR fetuses, primarily as a result of a decrease in the direct flux of leucine from the maternal to fetal circulation. The decrease in maternal leucine transfer was balanced by a 50% reduction in the back-flux of leucine from the fetus to the placenta. Both fetal leucine oxidation and fetal leucine back-flux into the placenta were correlated with leucine concentration. From these data it appears that the decreased plasma leucine concentration in IUGR fetuses is the result of the decrease in leucine flux from the maternal to fetal circulation. The lower fetal plasma concentration in turn determines the back-flux of leucine from the fetus to placenta as well as fetal leucine oxidation.

Amino Acid Transporters

In the heat-stressed model of IUGR net flux of leucine into the uterus and the direct flux of leucine from the maternal to fetal circulation were significantly lower as a function of both fetal and placental weight.[90] These findings are highly suggestive of a reduction in transplacental amino acid transporter activity. The suspicion that a defect in amino acid transport is an important factor in IUGR is supported by the observation that in both human and animal models of IUGR, the branched-chain amino acids, which share the L-transport system, appear to be affected in similar ways. Further support for a primary impairment of amino acid transporter activity in IUGR comes from studies in animal models as well as studies of microvillous membrane vesicles from SGA human pregnancies using artificial analogues of amino acids. In guinea pigs, growth retardation induced by unilateral uterine artery ligation is associated with a significant reduction in the placental transfer of aminoisobutyric acid (AIB), a nonmetabolizable amino acid transported by the system A Na^+-dependent transporter.[95] Similar findings of a defect in the system A transporter have been identified in microvillous membrane vesicles from the placentas of SGA infants using AIB.[96,97] The decrease in AIB uptake by vesicles from placentas of SGA babies was due to a significantly lower V_{max} compared with vesicles from placentas of AGA babies without a difference in the K_m.[96] A reduction in amino acid transport therefore would lead to decreased fetal amino acid availability, decreased protein accretion, and ultimately intrauterine growth retardation.

Effect of Fetal Growth on Maternal Metabolism

The growth of the mammalian fetus represents a large drain on maternal protein and energy stores, especially during the late stages of pregnancy, when absolute growth rates are the greatest. Dietary ingestion of amino acids is episodic, whereas fetal amino acid uptake is continuous. To overcome these problems, alterations in maternal metabolism occur that allow continuous uptake of nutrients by the fetus without it becoming an excessive drain on the mother (see Chapter 10).

The early period of gestation is characterized by maternal storage of fuels. It is most obvious for adipose tissue, but maternal protein stores are also expanded. During a normal pregnancy, a human adult gains 12.5 kg, of which 3.8 kg is fatty tissue and 0.925 kg is protein.[98] Protein gain during early gestation is much greater than the fetal requirement.[99] It is hypothesized that this "storage" protein provides a buffer for the large fetal and neonatal protein requirements of late gestation and lactation.

The latter portion of pregnancy is characterized by metabolic alterations that result in a more rapid switchover from postabsorptive to fasting metabolism than is seen in the nongravid state. The changes in the mother have been termed facilitated anabolism and accelerated starvation.[100] In a postprandial gravida there is an elevated maternal immunoreactive insulin concentration but attenuation of insulin's normal physiologic actions. Exaggerated increments and decrements occur in the maternal concentration of glucose and other substrates, facilitating transfer of these substances, especially glucose, across the placenta.[101] During the postabsorptive period, rapid mobilization of free fatty acids and enhanced ketonemia occurs, potentially sparing glucose and amino acid stores for fetal uptake. Pregnancy is characterized by generalized hypoaminoacidemia compared to the nonpregnant state.[102] Prolonged fasting in pregnant women results in an exaggerated decline in the serum concentrations of most amino acids, most markedly alanine. The relative contributions of alterations in protein synthesis, breakdown, and transplacental clearance that lead to maternal hypoaminoacidemia are not well delineated. Data from rats show increased maternal protein degradation rates in skeletal muscle during late gestation, again emphasizing the importance of maternal storage nitrogen in maintaining late fetal growth rates.[103] Maternal urea synthesis are diminished, suggesting that the increased amino acid flux is crossing the placenta to the fetus, rather than being oxidized by the mother.[104]

Acknowledgment. This work was supported by the James Whitcomb Riley Memorial Association and PHS grant HD 19089.

References

1. Forbes GB. Fetal body composition. In: Forbes GB ed. Human body composition: Growth, aging, nutrition and activity.
2. Zak R, Martin AF, Blough R. Assessment of protein turnover by use of radioisotopic tracers. Physiol Rev 1979;59:407–447.
3. Rattray PV, Garrett WN, East NE, et al. Growth development and composition of the ovine conceptus and mammary gland during pregnancy. J Anim Sci 1974;38:613–626.
4. Meier P, Teng C, Battaglia FC, et al. The rate of amino acid nitrogen and total nitrogen accumulation in the fetal lamb. Proc Soc Exp Biol Med 1981;167:463–468.
5. Sparks JW, Girard JR, Battaglia FC. An estimate of the caloric requirements of the human fetus. Biol Neonate 1980;38:113–119.
6. Meier PR, Peterson RG, Bonds DR. Rates of protein synthesis and turnover in fetal life. Am J Physiol 1981;240:E320–E324.
7. Kennaugh JM, Bell AW, Teng C. Ontogenetic changes in the rates of protein synthesis and leucine oxidation during fetal life. Pediatr Res 1987;22:688–692.
8. Lemons JA, Adcock EW, Jones M, et al. Umbilical uptake of amino acids in the unstressed fetal lamb. J Clin Invest 1976;58:1428–1434.
9. McEvoy-Bowe E, Hislop JH, Wiggens D, et al. Amino acid profiles during development of the fetal rat. Biol Neonate 1987;52:135–140.
10. Hayashi S, Sanada K, Sagawa N, et al. Umbilical vein-artery differences of plasma amino acids in the last trimester of human pregnancy. Biol Neonate 1978;34:11–18.
11. Soltesz G, Harris D, MacKenzie IZ, et al. The metabolic and endocrine milieu of the human fetus at 18–24 weeks of gestation. I. Plasma amino acid concentrations. Pediatr Res 1985;19:91–93.
12. Holzman IR, Lemons JA, Meschia G, et al. Uterine uptake of amino acids and placental glutamine-glutamate balance in the pregnant ewe. J Dev Physiol 1979;1:137–149.
13. Eaton B, Yudilevich DL. Uptake and asymmetric efflux of amino acids at maternal and fetal sides of placenta. Am J Physiol Cell Physiol 1981;241:C106–C112.
14. Jaroszewicz L, Jozwik M, Jaroszewic, K. The activity of aminotransferases in human placenta in early pregnancy. Biochem Med Metab Biol 1971;5:436–439.
15. Liechty EA, Barone S, Nutt M. Effect of maternal fasting on ovine fetal and maternal branched chain amino acid transaminase activities. Biol Neonate 1987;52:166–173.
16. Goodwin G, Gibboney W, Paxton R, et al. Activities of branched-chain amino acid aminotransferase and branched-chain 2-oxoacid dehydrogenase complex in tissues of maternal and fetal sheep. Biochem J 1987;242:305–308.
17. Holzman IR, Lemons JA, Meschia G, et al. Ammonia production by the pregnant uterus. Proc Soc Exp Biol Med 1977;156:27–30.
18. Lemons JA, Schreiner RL. Metabolic balance of the ovine fetus during the fed and fasted states. Ann Nutr Metab 1984;28:268–280.
19. Duee P, Simoes Nunes C, Pégoriez J-P, et al. Uterine metabolism of the conscious gilt during pregnancy. Pediatr Res 1987;22:587–590.
20. Mullen K, Denne SC, McCullough A, et al. Leucine metabolism in stable cirrhosis. Hepatology 1986;6:622–630.
21. Katz A, Salhin K, Heriksson J. Muscle ammonia metabolism during isometric contraction in humans. Am J Physiol Cell Physiol 1986;250:C834–C840.
22. Meschia G, Battaglia FC, Hay WW Jr, et al. Utilization of substrates by the ovine placenta in vivo. Fed Proc 1980;39:245–249.
23. Gresham E, James E, Raye JR, et al. Production and excretion of urea by the fetal lamb. Pediatrics 1972;50:372–379.
24. Simmons MR, Meschia G, Makowski E, et al. Fetal metabolic response to maternal starvation. Pediatr Res 1974;8:830–860.
25. Battaglia FC, Behrman RE, Meschia G. Clearance of inert molecules. Na and Cl ions across the primate placenta. Am J Obstet Gynecol 1968;102:1135–1143.
26. Lemons JA, Snodgrass PJ. Effect of a maternal fast on the urea cycle enzymes of the ovine fetus. J Pediatr Gastroenterol Nutr 1986;5:138–142.
27. Schaefer AL, Krishnamurti CR. Protein synthesis in the gastrointestinal tissues of the ovine fetus. Growth 1984;48:309–320.
28. Schaefer A, Krishnamurti C. Whole body and tissue fractional protein synthesis in the ovine fetus in utero. Br J Nutr 1984;52:359–369.
29. Goldspink D, Kelly F. Protein turnover and growth in the whole body liver and kidney of the rat from the fetus to senility. Biochem J 1984;217:507–516.
30. Noakes D, Young M. Measurement of fetal tissue protein synthetic rat in the lamb in utero. Res Vet Sci 1981;31:336–341.
31. Krishnamurti CR, Schaefer AL. Effect of acute maternal starvation on tyrosine metabolism and protein synthesis in fetal sheep. Growth 1984;48:391–403.
32. Van Veen LCP, Teng C, Hay WW Jr, et al. Leucine disposal and oxidation rates in the fetal lamb. Metab Clin Exp 1987;36:48–53.
33. Liechty EA, Lemons JA, Kien CL. Maternal fasting does not diminish fetal ovine leucine flux. Pediatr Res 1989;25:55A (abstract).
34. Schaefer AL, Krishnamurti CR. Tyrosine turnover and oxidation in the ovine fetus in utero. Can J Anim Sci 1982;62:787–797.
35. Castellino P, Luzi L, Simonson DC. Effect of insulin and plasma amino acid concentrations on leucine metabolism in man—role of substrate availability on estimates of whole body protein synthesis. J Clin Invest 1987;80:1784–1793.
36. Chessex P, Reichman BL, Verellen GJE, et al. Influence of postnatal age, energy intake, and weight gain on energy metabolism in the very low birth weight infant. J Pediatr 1981;99:761–766.
37. Waterlow JC. Protein turnover with special reference to man. Q J Exp Physiol 1984;69:409–438.
38. Cahill GF, Owen OE, Morgan AP. The consumption of fuels during prolonged starvation. Adv Enzyme Reg 1968;6:143–150.

39. Snell K, Duff DAB. Branched chain amino acid metabolism and alanine formation in rat diaphragm muscle in vitro. Biochem J 1984;223:831–835.
40. Kimura R. Glutamine oxidation by the developing rat small intestine. Pediatr Res 1987;21:214–217.
41. Lowenstein JM. Ammonia production in muscle and other tissues: the purine nucleotide cycle. Physiol Rev 1972;52:382–414.
42. Nissim I, Yudkoll M, Segal S. Nitrogen sources for renal ammoniagenesis: study with 15N nitrogen. Am J Physiol Renal Fluid Electrolyte Physiol 1986;251:F995–F1002.
43. Atkinson DE, Bourke E. Metabolic aspects of the regulation of systemic pH. Am J Physiol Renal Fluid Electrolyte Physiol 1987;252:F947–F956.
44. Busboom JA, Merkel EM, Bergen EN. The effect of age on tissue leucine transaminase and alpha ketoisocaproate dehydrogenase in rams. Fed Proc 1983;42:533 (abstract).
45. Pell JM, Calderone EM, Bergman EN. Leucine and alpha ketoisocaproate metabolism and interconversions in fed and fasted sheep. Metab Clin Experiment 1986;35:1005–1016.
46. Liechty EA, Polak MJ, Lemons JA. Branched chain amino acid carbon and nitrogen arteriovenous concentration differences across the ovine fetal hindlimb. Pediatr Res 1987;21:44–48.
47. Velasquez A, Rosado A, Bernal A. Amino acid pools in the fetal-maternal system. Biol Neonate 1976;29:28–40.
48. Prior RL, Christenson RK. Gluconeogenesis from alanine in vivo by the ovine fetus and lamb. Am J Physiol 1977;233:E462–E468.
49. Sparks JW, Hay WW, Bonds D. Simultaneous measurements of lactate turnover rate and umbilical lactate uptake in the fetal lamb. J Clin Invest 1982;70:179–192.
50. Gilfillan CA, Tserng KY, Kalhan SC. Alanine production by the human fetus at term gestation. Biol Neonate 1985;45:141–147.
51. Lemons JA, Moorehead HC, Hage GP. Effects of fasting on gluconeogenic enzymes in the ovine fetus. Pediatr Res 1986;20:676–679.
52. Hill DE. Fetal effects of insulin. Obstet Gynecol Ann 1982;11:133–149.
53. Wigmore PMC, Strickland NC. DNA, RNA, and protein in skeletal muscle of large and small pig fetuses. Growth 1983;47:67–76.
54. Milley JR, Papacostas JS, Tabata BK. Effect of insulin on uptake of metabolic substrates by the sheep fetus. Am J Physiol 1986;251:E349–E356.
55. Milley JR. The effect of chronic hyperinsulinemia on ovine fetal growth. Growth 1986;50:390–401.
56. Stagenberg M, Ekloff AC, Dahlquist G, et al. Lack of effect on body weight and content of nitrogen and fat after insulin administration to fetal rats. Biol Neonate 1981;40:240–245.
57. Angervall L, Karlsson K, Martinson A. Effects on rat fetuses of intrauterine injections of insulin. Diabetologia 1981;20:558–562.
58. Spencer GSG, Hill DJ, Garssen GJ. Somatomedin activity and growth hormone levels in body fluids of the fetal pig. Effect of chronic hyperinsulinemia. J Endocrinol 1983;96:107–114.
59. Picon L. Effect of insulin on growth and biochemical composition of the rat fetus. Endocrinology 1967;81:1419–1421.
60. Susa JB, McCormick KL, Widness JA, et al. Chronic hyperinsulinemia in the fetal rhesus monkey—effects on fetal growth and composition. Diabetes 1979;28:1058–1063.
61. Canavan JP, Goldspink DF. Maternal diabetes in rats. II. Effects on fetal growth and protein turnover. Diabetes 1988;37:1671–1677.
62. Robinson J, Canavan JP, Haj AJE. Maternal diabetes in rats. I. Effects on placental growth and protein turnover. Diabetes 1988;37:1665–1670.
63. Oddy VH, Lindsay DB, Barker PJ, et al. Effect of insulin on hind-limb and whole body leucine and protein metabolism in fed and fasted lambs. Br J Nutr 1987;58:437–452.
64. Tessari P, Trevisan R, Inchiostro S. Dose-response curves of effects of insulin on leucine kinetics in humans. Am J Physiol 1986;251:E334–E342.
65. Vasquez JA, Morse EL, Adibi SA. Effect of dietary fat, carbohydrate, and protein on branched chain amino acid catabolism during caloric restriction. J Clin Invest 1985;76:737–743.
66. Liechty EA, Boyle DW, Moorehead H, et al. Increased fetal glucose concentration decreases ovine fetal leucine oxidation independent of insulin. Am J Physiol Endocrinol Metab 1993;265:E617–E623.
67. Liechty EA, Boyle DW, Moorehead H, et al. Effect of hyperinsulinemia on ovine fetal leucine kinetics during prolonged maternal fasting. Am J Physiol Endocrinol Metab 1992;263:E696–E702.
68. Liechty EA, Denne SC, Lemons JA, et al. Effects of glucose infusion on leucine transamination and oxidation in the ovine fetus. Pediatr Res 1991;30:423–429.
69. Milley JR. Effects of insulin on ovine fetal leucine kinetics and protein metabolism. J Clin Invest 1994;93:1616–1624.
70. Domenich M, Gruppuso PA, Nishino VT, et al. Preserved fetal amino acid concentrations in the presence of maternal hypoaminoacidemia. Pediatr Res 1986;20:1071–1076.
71. Ashton IK, Zapf J, Einschenk I, et al. Insulin-like growth factors (IGF) 1 and 2 in human foetal plasma and relationship to gestational age and foetal size during midpregnancy. Acta Endocrinol 1985;110:558–563.
72. Wang HS, Lim J, English J, et al. The concentration of insulin-like growth factor-I and insulin-like growth factor-binding protein-1 in human umbilical cord serum at delivery: relation to fetal weight. J Endocrinol 1991;129:459–464.
73. Lassarre C, Hardouin S, Daffos F, et al. Serum insulin-like growth factors and insulin-like growth factor binding proteins in the human fetus: relationships with growth in normal subjects and in subjects with intrauterine growth retardation. Pediatr Res 1991;29:219–225.
74. Vileisis RA, D'Ercole AJ. Tissue and serum concentrations of somatomedin-C/insulin-like growth factor I in fetal rats made growth retarded by uterine artery ligation. Pediatr Res 1986;20:126–130.
75. Daughaday WH, Yanow CE, Kapadia M. Insulin-like growth factors I and II in maternal and fetal guinea pig serum. Endocrinology 1986;119:490–494.

76. Bernstein IM, DeSouza MM, Copeland KC. Insulin-like growth factor I in substrate-deprived growth-retarded fetal rats. Pediatr Res 1991;30:154–157.
77. Davenport ML, D'Ercole AJ, Underwood LE. Effect of maternal fasting on fetal growth, serum insulin-like growth factors (IGFs), and tissue IGF messenger ribonucleic acids. Endocrinology 1990;126:2062–2067.
78. Bassett NS, Oliver MH, Breier BH, et al. The effect of maternal starvation on plasma insulin-like growth factor I concentrations in the late gestation ovine fetus. Pediatr Res 1990;27:401–404.
79. Jones CT, Gu W, Harding JE, et al. Studies on the growth of the fetal sheep. Effects of surgical reduction in placental size, or experimental manipulation of uterine blood flow on plasma sulphation promoting activity and on the concentration of insulin-like growth factors I and II. J Dev Physiol 1988;10:179–189.
80. Harding JE, Liu L, Evans PC, et al. Insulin-like growth factor 1 alters feto-placental protein and carbohydrate metabolism in fetal sheep. Endocrinology 1994;134:1509–1514.
81. Liechty EA, Boyle DW, Lee W-H, et al. Effects of circulating IGF-I on glucose and amino acid kinetics in the ovine fetus. Am J Physiol Endocrinol Metab 1996;271:E177–E185.
82. Lok F, Owens JA, Mundy L, et al. Insulin-like growth factor I promotes growth selectively in fetal sheep in late gestation. Am J Physiol Regul Integr Comp Physiol 1996;270:R1148–R1155.
83. Schreiner RL, Nolen PA, Bonderman PW, et al. Fetal and maternal hormonal response to starvation in the ewe. Pediatr Res 1980;14:103–108.
84. Cetin I, Marconi AM, Bozzetti P, et al. Umbilical amino acid concentrations in appropriate and small for gestational age infants: a biochemical difference present in utero. Am J Obstet Gynecol 1988;158:120–126.
85. Economides DL, Nicolaides KH, Gahl WA, et al. Plasma amino acids in appropriate- and small-for-gestational-age fetuses. Am J Obstet Gynecol 1989;161:1219–1227.
86. Cetin I. Umbilical amino acid concentrations in normal and growth retarded fetuses sampled in utero by cordocentesis. Am J Obstet Gynecol 1990;162:253–261.
87. Gruppuso PA, Migliori R, Susa JB, et al. Chronic maternal hyperinsulinemia and hypoglycemia. Biol Neonate 1981;40:113–120.
88. Ogata ES, Paul RI, Finley SL. Limited maternal fuel availability due to hyperinsulinemia retards fetal growth and development in the rat. Pediatr Res 1987;22:432–437.
89. Ogata ES, Bussey ME, Finley S. Altered gas exchange limited glucose and branched chain amino acids and hypoinsulinism retard fetal growth in the rat. Metab Clin Exp 1986;35:970–977.
90. Ross JC, Fennessey PV, Wilkening RB, et al. Placental transport and fetal utilization of leucine in a model of fetal growth retardation. Am J Physiol Endocrinol Metab 1996;270:E491–E503.
91. Loy GL, Quick A, Hay WW Jr, et al. Fetoplacental deamination and decarboxylation of leucine. Am J Physiol Endocrinol Metab 1990;259:E492–E497.
92. Boyle DW, Liechty EA, Denne SC. Effect of prolonged uterine blood flow reduction on feto-placental protein turnover in sheep. Pediatr Res 1996;39:57A (abstract).
93. Milley JR. Protein synthesis during hypoxia in fetal lambs. Am J Physiol 1987;252:E519–E524.
94. Milley JR. Uptake of exogenous substrates during hypoxia in fetal lambs. Am J Physiol Endocrinol Metab 1988;254:E572–E578.
95. Jansson T, Persson E. Placental transfer of glucose and amino acids in intrauterine growth retardation: studies with substrate analogs in the awake guinea pig. Pediatr Res 1990;28:203–208.
96. Mahendran D, Donnai P, Glazier JD, et al. Amino acid (system A) transporter activity in microvillous membrane vesicles from the placentas of appropriate and small for gestational age babies. Pediatr Res 1993;34:661–665.
97. Dicke JM, Henderson GI. Placental amino acid uptake in normal and complicated pregnancies. Am J Med Sci 1988;295:223–227.
98. Van Raaij JMA, Peek MEM, Vernaat-Miedema SH. New equations for estimating body fat mass in pregnancy from body density or total body water. Am J Clin Nutr 1988;48:24–29.
99. King J. Protein metabolism in pregnancy. Clin Perinatol 1975;2:243–254.
100. Freinkel N. Of pregnancy and progeny. Diabetes 1980;29:1023–1035.
101. Phelps RL, Metzger BE, Freinkel N. Carbohydrate metabolism during pregnancy. XVII. Diurnal profiles of plasma glucose, insulin, free fatty acids, triglycerides, cholesterol and individual amino acids in late normal pregnancy. Am J Obstet Gynecol 1981;140:730–736.
102. Felig P, Kim YJ, Lynch V, et al. Amino acid metabolism during starvation in human pregnancy. J Clin Invest 1972;51:1195–1202.
103. Ling PR, Bistrian BR, Blackburn GL, et al. Effect of fetal growth on maternal protein metabolism in the postabsorptive rat. Am J Physiol 1987;252:E380–E390.
104. Kalhan SC, Tserng KY, Gilifan C. Metabolism of urea and glucose in normal and diabetic pregnancy. Metabolism 1982;31:824–833.

19
Lipid Metabolism in the Fetal-Placental Unit

Robert E. Kimura

In utero the fetus is constantly infused with substrates from the placenta. At birth this transfer of substrates is abruptly stopped and the neonate must utilize endogenous substrates to maintain glucose homeostasis. To prepare for this change from exogenous to endogenous sources of substrate, the fetus late in gestation increases fuel storage in the form of glycogen and lipids. During the immediate postnatal period, glycogen is used to maintain glucose homeostasis. Following the depletion of glycogen in the immediate postnatal period, the activation of gluconeogenesis occurs to maintain glucose homeostasis. Equally important, the initiation of oxidation of substrates other than glucose is necessary to decrease the neonate's dependence on glucose as the primary energy source. The activation of lipolysis of fat stores and the initiation of fatty acid and ketone body oxidation provides the neonate with such an alternative energy source. This changing pattern of substrate oxidation is reflected by a fall in the respiratory quotient from 1.0 to 0.7 in the first 3 days of life when fatty acids become preferred substrates in a number of different tissues with high energy demands.[1,2] Specifically, Denne and Kalhan[3] determined that the rate of glucose oxidation could not account for the total cerebral metabolic requirements in the fasted human neonate. These data suggest that alternative metabolic fuels must be utilized in cerebral metabolism.

This chapter discusses developmental changes in fetal lipid metabolism that prepare the fetus for the abrupt changes in substrate availability occurring at birth. Emphasis is placed on the changes in mechanisms that control the relative state of lipid synthesis and storage in the fetus to the activation of lipid utilization in the neonate. By evaluating the control of lipid metabolism during birth, mechanisms of lipid metabolism are delineated.

This chapter also reviews animal studies involved in fetal lipid metabolism. It is important to consider that the rate of fetal growth and timing of maturational events varies greatly from species to species.[4] In addition, significant species differences exist in the body composition of fetuses. For example, human and guinea pig neonates have 16% and 10% of their weight as fat, respectively, whereas only 1% of the rat and the pig's weight is fat. These data indicate that during the later part of gestation in the human and the guinea pig fetus, a greater proportion of substrate is utilized for fat synthesis.[5]

The relative maturity of the fetus at the time of birth and feeding behavior are important when interpreting animal data. For example, compared with the neonatal rat and rabbit, the neonatal guinea pig is mature at birth. The immature rat pup nurses continually while guinea pig and rabbit pups nurse only periodically. Because of the great species variability relative to maturity and feeding patterns, caution should be taken when interpreting metabolic studies and extrapolating from animal models to the human.

Defining Fetal Lipid Metabolism

Fetal lipid metabolism involves processes that result in the production and utilization of lipid. The rate of production of fetal fatty acids and lipids is controlled by both endogenous (i.e., fetal) and exogenous (i.e., placental and maternal) mechanisms. For example, the transfer of maternal lipids to the fetus can have a significant impact on the availability of fatty acids and precursors for fetal fatty acid and lipid synthesis. Similarly, the rate of fetal utilization of fatty acids can be affected by the availability of glucose from the placenta. This chapter considers both fetal and maternal-placental mechanisms that control fetal lipid metabolism. Emphasis is placed on changes in the control mechanisms of lipid metabolism that occur at birth, a period in which the fetus changes from a net accumulator of lipid to a net utilizer of lipid.

Developmental Changes in Fetal Body Composition

Studies of human fetal body composition[6-9] indicate that the number of grams of fat per 100 grams of body weight increases from 0.7 to 3.1 in 23.6- to 25-week gestation fetuses and 10.2 to 16.1 in term neonates. Ziegler et al.[9] estimated that per 100 g of weight gain, 24- to 25-week gestation fetuses gained 4.7 g of lipid while 39- to 40-week gestation fetuses gained 28.9 g. These data clearly demonstrate that the human fetus during the third trimester accumulates significant amounts of lipid.

There is great species variation of the accumulation of adipose tissue prior to birth. For example, in the full-term human neonate fat accounts for 16% of the total body weight, while in the rabbit, rat, and pig only 1% to 2% of the body weight is in the form of fat.[5] Thus, the net requirements for fetal fatty acids vary from species to species.

Changes in Maternal Blood Lipid Concentrations

Mobilization of maternal fat stores occurs late in pregnancy when fetal accumulation of fat is the greatest. Plasma triglyceride concentration increases 100% from 30 to 40 weeks' gestation.[10] Rat plasma free fatty acid concentration increases late in gestation.[11] In studies of maternal rat[11,12] and human[13] adipose tissue, evidence of increased lipolysis with increased triglyceride and fatty acid turnover has been reported. Knopp et al.[14] proposed that the maternal mobilization of lipids late in gestation results in an increase in maternal utilization of lipid as an oxidative substrate and a decrease in the maternal demand of glucose. In this manner, glucose transfer to the fetus late in gestation is maintained. However, as will be discussed in the next section, placental transfer of fatty acids to the fetus may account for a significant proportion of fetal lipid accumulation. Since the rate of placental transfer of fatty acids is in part controlled by the maternal-fetal gradient, the increase in maternal lipolysis that occurs late in gestation may represent a mechanism to increase fetal lipid accumulation.

Factors that Control Placental Fatty Acid Transfer

Fatty acids are transported to the fetus from the maternal circulation in the rat and rabbit. [^{14}C]radioactivity was found in fetal plasma and fetal tissue within 5 minutes after (1-^{14}C) palmitic acid was injected into the pregnant rat[15] and rabbit.[16,17] Factors that have been studied that control the transfer of lipid from the maternal circulation to the fetus include the triglyceride and free fatty acid transplacental gradient, fetal albumin concentration, placental metabolism of maternal lipids, and the utilization of lipid by the fetus.

The Transplacental Fatty Acid Gradient

Studies indicate that there is a causal relationship between increases in maternal plasma triglyceride and fatty acid concentrations seen in late gestation and the increase in the fetal accretion rate of fat during this period. In a streptozocin diabetic rat model in which maternal plasma concentrations of triglycerides and free fatty acids are increased, the fetal carcass and liver have approximately a twofold increase in triglyceride content.[18] In the rabbit an increase in the maternal diet of oil for only 3 days resulted in increased newborn adipose stores.[19] These data indicate that the circulated maternal lipid concentration can alter the amount of lipid stored in the fetus.

Studies suggest that the placental transfer of fatty acids is regulated, in part, by the transplacental fatty acid gradient. Hendrickse et al.[20] measured maternal venous and umbilical cord vein and artery plasma concentrations of free fatty acids of term neonates delivered by cesarean section. They reported a correlation between the maternal venous blood concentration of fatty acid and the umbilical vein-artery concentration difference in free fatty acids. These data suggest that in the human, placental transport of free fatty acids is controlled by maternal free fatty acid concentrations.

Studies on the effect of maternal fetal free fatty acid concentration gradient indicate conflicting results. Using a rabbit placental model Elphick and Hull[21] found that increases in the concentration gradient of fatty acids between maternal and fetal plasma correlates with an increase in net flux of fatty acids across the placenta into the fetal circulation. Thomas and Lowy,[22] using an in situ perfusion preparation of the guinea pig placenta, determined that increases in the transplacental gradient correlates directly with the transfer of fatty acid. However, they reported that this correlation occurred only when the maternal free fatty acid concentration was within normal range. With elevated concentrations of free fatty acids, the correlation did not exist. Thomas and Lowy also reported that an increase in fetal perfusion of the placenta causes an increase in fatty acid placental transfer. An increase in fetal perfusion of the placenta causes an increase in the fatty acid transplacental gradient by lowering the concentration of fatty acids in the perfusate. These data suggest that a decrease in fetal plasma concentration of fatty acids can increase the transplacental transfer of maternal lipids.

In a rabbit model Stephenson et al.[23] artificially increased the maternal fetal gradient and caused an increase in transfer of free fatty acids to the fetus. However, increasing umbilical blood flow had no effect on free fatty acid placental transport to the fetus even though an increase in umbilical blood flow was associated with a decrease in fetal blood free fatty acid concentration and a greater maternal fetal gradient. In addition, net transfer of free fatty acids occurred even with no maternal fetal gradient, suggesting that at physiologic free fatty acid concentrations the maternal fetal gradient may not affect the transfer of lipids to the fetus.

Fetal Albumin and Fetuin Concentrations

Investigations indicate that fetal albumin concentration controls the placental transfer of fatty acids. Dancis et al.,[24] using a human placental preparation, determined that the rate of transfer of fatty acids is inversely proportional to the concentration of albumin present in the perfusate. Thomas and Lowy,[22] using an in situ guinea pig placental preparation in which the fetal vessels were perfused, determined that an elevation in albumin concentration increases palmitic acid transfer. Hershfield and Nemeth[25] concluded that serum albumin concentration and binding affinity for unesterified fatty acids appear to be important for placental transfer of fatty acids in the guinea pig. Stephenson et al.[26] determined that increasing albumin in the rabbit fetus caused an increase in the transfer of free fatty acid to the fetus, while blood pH had no effect on fatty acid transport.

The mechanism by which fetal albumin concentration controls placental transfer of fatty acids has not been delineated. However, Schenker et al.[27] reported that [^{131}I]-labeled albumin is not transferred from the maternal circulation to the fetal circulation, indicating that unesterified fatty acids are transferred across the placenta in an unbound form. It is possible that unesterified fatty acids in the unbound form cannot be released into the fetal circulation. Thus, the release of the fatty acids would be dependent on the albumin concentrations in the fetal blood.

Another newly recognized protein, fetuin, may also control the transfer of fatty acids to the fetus. Fetuin, which binds fatty acids, is 50-fold more efficient than albumin at incorporating fatty acids into cultured aortic smooth muscle cells and ninefold more efficient in human fetal skin fibroblasts.[28] Since fetuin exists in high concentration in the fetus,[29] it may play a role in the transport of lipid in the fetus.[30] The significance of fetuin in lipid transport in the fetus has not been delineated.

Placental Metabolism of Maternal Lipids

Placental metabolism of maternal lipids has been suggested as a control mechanism of the transfer of maternal lipids to the fetus. Utilizing an in situ perfusion guinea pig placental model Thomas et al.[31] determined that maternal lipids are partially oxidized by the placenta prior to transfer to the fetus. They speculated that the partial oxidation occurred in placental peroxisomes. In contrast, Noble et al.[32] determined that incubation of sheep placental homogenates with [1-^{14}C] oleic, linoleic, and linolenic acids results in the incorporation of the [^{14}C] into C20 and C22 polyunsaturated fatty acids products. Knopp et al.[33] reported that fatty acids released from maternal triglycerides by placental lipoprotein lipase are transferred to the fetal compartment.

Fatty Acid Chain Length

Another factor that appears to control placental transfer is fatty acid chain length. In the human placenta, Dancis et al.[24] determined that the transfer of medium- or short-chain fatty acids are transferred more readily than long-chain fatty acids. In contrast, Elphick and Hull[21] in rabbit found no relationship between fatty acid chain length and the rate of transfer across the placenta.

The syncytiotrophoblast plays an important role in the transfer of maternal lipids to the fetus. Lipoprotein lipase on the maternal surface of the syncytiotrophoblast hydrolyzes maternal triacylglycerol.[34] Syncytiotrophoblast lipoprotein lipase activity increases late in gestation when there is a high accretion rate of lipids in the fetus.[34] Fatty acid–binding proteins are responsible for the uptake of free fatty acids. Fatty acid–binding proteins are located on the microvillous membranes of syncytiotrophoblasts facing the maternal circulation.[35,36] This location favors unidirectional flow of maternal fatty acid to the fetus. The very low density lipoprotein/apolipoprotein-E receptor (VLDLR) is expressed in human placental trophoblast cells in a pattern consistent with a role in placental lipid transport.[37] VLDLR expression is high at term relative to that in the first trimester.

Fetal erythrocytes appear to perform a significant role in the placental transfer of docosahexaenoic acid [22:6(n − 3); 22:6(4,−7,10,13,16,19) (DHA)]. DHA, which is required in quantity by the developing nervous system of the fetus, is synthesized from linolenic acid. The umbilical venous-arterial difference for DHA was much greater than the difference of total lipids, suggesting that erythrocytes may play a role in the transport of DHA from the placenta to the fetus.[38]

In summary, many mechanisms involved in the transfer of maternal lipids to the fetus have been proposed. As exemplified by data of the effect of the maternal fetal fatty acid gradient on the flux of lipid across the placenta, conflicting results occur.[22,23] The differences could reflect species differences or differences in experimental conditions. Future studies of the maternal, placental, and fetal factors that control transplacental transfer of lipids under physiologic conditions are needed.

The Significance of Placental Transfer of Maternal Lipids

A question remains as to what extent does the placental transfer of maternal lipids account for the fetal accumulation of lipid as compared to endogenous fetal synthesis of lipids. From various studies there appears to be significant variability in estimates of the significance of placental transfer of maternal lipids. Using umbilical venous arterial differences, Elphick et al.[39] and Persson and Tunell[40] calculated that the net flux of unesterified fatty acids into the fetus from the maternal circulation can account for the fetal requirement of fatty acid during the end of pregnancy. In contrast to these estimates, Dancis et al.,[41] using the perfused human placenta, reported that the rate of transfer of fatty acids from the maternal to fetal circulation could account for approximately 20% of that required for the accumulation of fetal adipose tissue deposited in the last trimester of pregnancy. Coleman[42] estimated that as much as 50% of fetal fatty acid requirements are placentally transferred from mother to fetus. Using the incorporation of ^3H from ^3H_2O into fatty acids as a means of evaluating fetal fatty acid synthesis in the rat, Hummel et al.[43] concluded that fatty acids are obtained equally from the mother and from fetal fatty acid synthesis. In other species such as the rabbit[16] and the monkey,[44] placental transfer of maternal unesterified fatty acid account for total fetal fatty acid requirements.

In summary, placental transfer of lipid is important for the accumulation of fetal lipid late in pregnancy. There appears to be significant species variability. This is not surprising since there is significant species variability in the body composition of the neonate. The maternal fatty acids that are transferred to the fetus can cause an increase in fetal lipid accumulation by two mechanisms: (1) directly providing precursors for adipocytes and (2) providing alternative oxidative substrates. The significance of oxidation of fatty acids is discussed below. It does appear that endogenous synthesis of fatty acids by the fetus accounts for some of the lipid accumulation. The developmental aspects of fetal lipogenesis are reviewed below.

The Effect of Gestational Age on Placental Transport of Lipids

It is clear from the analysis of either fetal blood or neonatal cord blood that the blood concentrations of cholesterol, triglycerides, and apoproteins are low in the preterm fetus or neonate compared to term neonates and are lower than concentrations in the adult.[45–47] Similarly, comparison of cord blood concentrations of essential fatty acids and markers of essential fatty acid deficiency indicate that essential fatty acids are lower in preterm fetus compared to term.[48] Since the accretion of lipids during the third trimester accounts for a significant proportion of growth, the lower preterm essential fatty acid status may reflect a lower demand for lipid. Long-chain polyunsaturated fatty acids in fetal triglycerides increased with gestational age, suggesting that it is caused partially by delta 6- and delta 5-desaturase maturation in the liver.[49] In the human fetus,[50] binding of low-density lipoprotein to fetal liver low-density lipoprotein receptor increased with an increase in gestational age while total cholesterol and low-density protein-cholesterol concentrations decreased. Cai et al.[50] hypothesized that this inverse relation suggests that low-density lipoprotein receptors in human fetal liver may control serum cholesterol concentration.

Analysis of human fetal tissue for lipids indicate that total lipid content increases with gestational age. All fatty acids with the exception of linoleic acid increase with gestational age.[51] There was a significant positive correlation between fetal tissue and maternal RBC linoleic acid content. The correlation between maternal and fetal essential fatty acids (EFA) in phospholipids was more significant after 10 weeks of gestation, suggesting an increase in placental transfer of fatty acids.

Lipogenesis

Pathways of Fatty Acid Synthesis

The three principal pathways of fatty acid synthesis are (1) de novo synthesis in the cytosol of the cell, (2) fatty acid chain elongation by microsomes, and (3) fatty acid chain elongation by mitochondria. De novo synthesis of long-chain fatty acids from acetyl-coenzyme A (CoA) is the primary synthetic pathway in most cells (Figure 19.1). The net reaction involved in de novo synthesis of fatty acids, using palmityl-CoA as an example, is

$$8\ acetyl\text{-}CoA + 14\ NADPH + 14\ H^+ + 7\ ATP + H_2O \leftrightarrow$$
$$palmitic\ acid + 8\ CoA + 14\ NADP + 7\ ADP + 7\ Pi$$

De novo synthesis of fatty acids requires a series of enzyme controlled reactions. The initial reaction of de novo synthesis, the carboxylation of acetyl-CoA to form malonyl-CoA, is catalyzed by the enzyme acetyl-CoA carboxylase (Figure 19.2). This enzyme is thought to be the rate-limiting enzyme for fatty acid synthesis. In the subsequent series of reactions, the fatty acid synthetase complex catalyzes the synthesis of 1 mol of palmitic acid from 7 mol of malonyl-CoA and 1 mol of acetyl-CoA.[52] Adenosine triphosphate (ATP) and nicotinamide adenine dinucleotide phosphate, reduced (NADPH) pro-

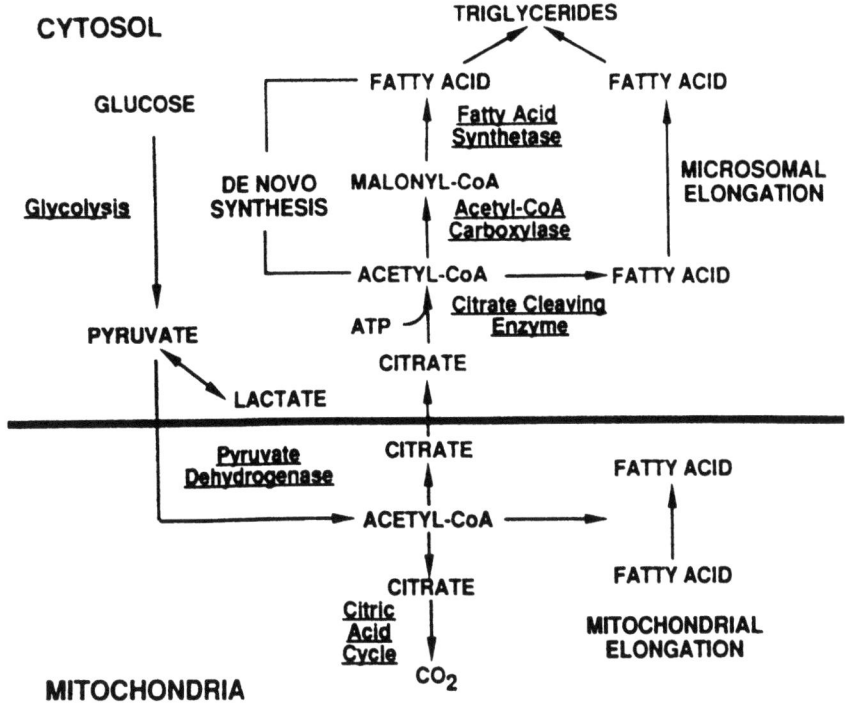

FIGURE 19.1. Biochemical pathways involved in lipogenesis. Names of enzymes are underlined.

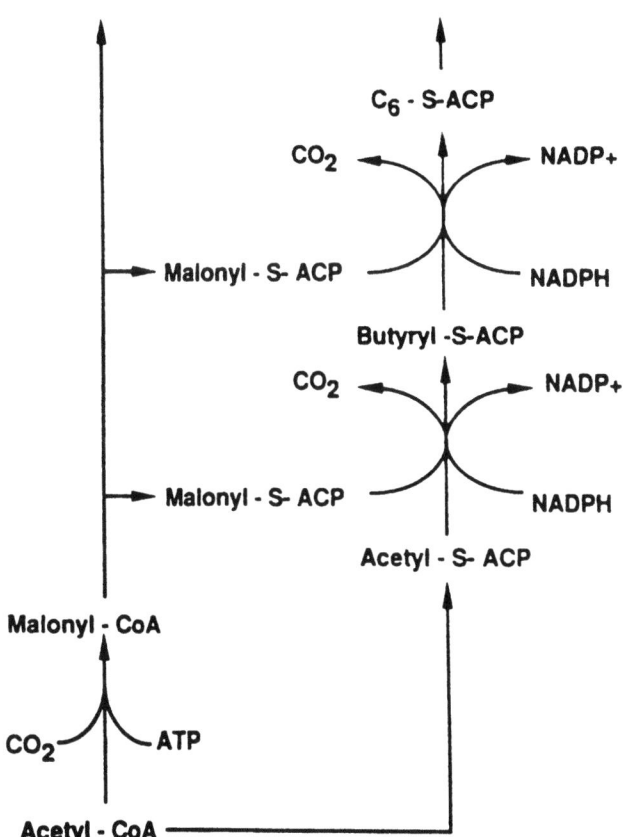

FIGURE 19.2. Biochemical pathways involved in de novo synthesis of fatty acids. Acyl carrier protein (ACP) is a protein involved with the fatty acid synthetase-protein complex.

vide the energy required for these complex series of reactions.

Long-chain fatty acids are also synthesized by the chain elongation of preexisting fatty acids. In mitochondria, the reversal of β-oxidation with the resulting incorporation of acetyl-CoA into preexisting fatty acids results in fatty acid chain elongation by the sequential addition of two carbon subunits. The microsomal and mitochondrial elongation pathways play a relatively minor role in fatty acid synthesis compared to de novo synthesis. One possible exception is the heart, where mitochondrial chain elongation is the only pathway for long-chain fatty acid synthesis.[53]

Evidence of Developmental Changes of Fatty Acid Synthesis

Studies indicate that in the rat, fetal hepatic lipogenesis is most active late in gestation, at the time of rapid adipose tissue accumulation.[54,55] Other studies indicate that the rate of hepatic fatty acids synthesis is high in the late gestation fetus when compared to the adult. Villee and Hagerman[56] reported that the rates of incorporation of acetate, pyruvate, and citrate into lipids by fetal rat liver slices are greater than in the adult. Similarly, Roux[57] determined that the rate of incorporation of acetate into lipid by 20-day-old fetal rabbit liver is 30-fold greater than rates seen in the adult rabbit liver.

The control mechanisms of de novo synthesis of fatty acids involve (1) substrate availability of precursors of acetyl-CoA and (2) the activity of the acetyl-CoA carboxylase and the fatty acid synthetase complex. The in vitro studies comparing the rate of hepatic de novo synthesis of fatty acids in the fetus and the adult suggest an increase in the activity of the enzymes involved in de novo synthesis of fatty acids. In the following sections the effect of these control mechanisms on fetal lipogenesis are examined, specifically changes in hormonal environment on these mechanisms.

Precursors for Fetal Lipogenesis

Carbohydrates in the form of glycogen, glucose, and lactate have been reported to be the major precursors for de novo synthesis of fatty acids in the fetus and the neonate. De novo synthesis of fatty acids in fetal lung has been extensively studied because the synthesis of surfactant is necessary for normal pulmonary function at birth. To investigate the role of glycogen in fetal lung lipid synthesis, Farrell and Bourbon[58] infused [U-^{14}C]glucose into 18.5-day fetuses and measured the fate of the [^{14}C] in lung organ cultures. They determined that as the amount of [^{14}C] decreases in the glycogen pool, it increases in the phospholipid pool, suggesting that glycogen acts as a carbon source for lung lipid synthesis. Other data indicate that lactate, which is present in high concentration in the fetus, may be the preferred lipogenic precursor in fetal lung. In the developing rat lung type II pneumocyte, lactate is the preferred lipogenic precursor for surfactant phospholipid synthesis.[59] Similarly, in fetal rabbit lung explants, glucose and lactate were found to be competitive substrates for surfactant phospholipid fatty acid synthesis.[60] Since serum lactate concentration is elevated in the fetus, these data suggest that lactate may be a major precursor for fetal lung lipogenesis. Lactate has been shown to be a precursor for fatty acid synthesis in fetal lamb adipose tissue[61] and the early neonatal rat brain.[62]

Nearly 40% of all maternal glucose that is perfused into the placenta is metabolized to lactate by the placenta. In vitro studies indicate that lactate may be a major precursor for fetal lipogenesis. One possible reason for the preference of lactate to glucose as a precursor for lipogenesis is that lactate exists in a high redox state. Conversion of lactate to pyruvate results in the conversion of nicotinamide adenine dinucleotide (NAD) to nicotinamide adenine dinucleotide, reduced (NADH). It has been speculated that the major source of NADPH is through hexosemonophosphate shunt activity. However, through transhydrogenases NADP$^+$ can be converted to NADPH while NADH is converted to NAD.

$$NADH + NADP^+ \leftrightarrow NAD^+ + NADPH$$

Lactate may indirectly provide the NADPH required for de novo synthesis of fatty acids. Determination of the presence of transhydrogenases in fetal tissue in which de novo synthesis of fatty acids occurs such as lung, liver, and adipocytes would support this theory. Lactate is an important catabolic and anabolic substrate in the fetus. The placenta is a significant source of lactate to the fetus. Lactate is an important precursor for both glycogen and lipid synthesis. Lactate, because of its oxidative state, produces NADH when it is converted to pyruvate, the direct precursor for amino acid, glycogen, and lipid synthesis. The NADH is an important fuel used in glycogen synthesis and fatty acid synthesis. In fetal lamb 11% to 17% of infused L-[U-^{14}C]lactate was recovered in lipid extracts, indicating that lactate is a significant precursor for fetal lipid.[63] Bolanos and Medina[64] determined that lactate is an important substrate for fetal brain. Late in gestation brain utilization of lactate for oxidation and lipogenesis is maintained while glucose and 3-hydroxybutyrate is decreased.

Other substrates have been investigated as precursors for lipid synthesis. Amino acids were found to be a minor precursor for fetal adipose tissue lipogenesis.[65] Ketone bodies, which are elevated in late fetal and neonatal serum have been examined as possible lipogenic precursors. Seccombe et al.[66] have reported that maternally derived ketone bodies are actively incorporated into lipid of fetal rat liver and brain. Edmond[67] found that ketone bodies are utilized for synthesis of steroids and fatty acids in the developing neonatal rat brain.

To determine in vivo if substrate availability of glucose controls fetal lipogenesis, Ktorza et al.[68] induced a mild hyperglycemia in unrestrained pregnant rats from 20.5 to 23.5 days of pregnancy with the infusion of glucose. They found that total carcass fat is increased over control concentrations and that the rate of lipogenesis is significantly greater in the hyperglycemic fetuses, suggesting that substrate availability does control fetal lipogenesis.

Hormone Regulation of Lipogenesis During Perinatal Development

Short-term hormonal control of the activity of enzymes involved with lipogenesis during the fetal and postnatal period alters the rate of lipogenesis. The plasma insulin-to-glucagon ratio, which is high in the fetus, decreases immediately after birth.[69,70] Insulin and glucagon have antagonistic effects on regulating lipogenesis. Insulin stimulates fatty acid synthesis in isolated adult hepatocytes,[71,72] while glucagon decreases fatty acid synthesis.[73-75] The effect of insulin and glucagon on the regulation of fatty acid synthesis is mediated by acetyl-CoA carboxylase activity. Acetyl-CoA carboxylase activity is increased by insulin and decreased by glucagon or adenosine 3′, 5′-cyclic monophosphate (cAMP).[71,72]

The regulatory effect of insulin during fetal development depends on end-organ response. Picon[76] showed that insulin injected directly into fetal rats increases total body lipids only after 18.5 days' gestation. Similar experiments by Clark et al.[77] showed that insulin administration stimulates the incorporation of precursors into fatty acids only after 18.5 days' gestation in rat. The fetal response to insulin probably relates to the appearance of insulin receptors and the development of postreceptor modulation in the fetus. It has been reported that tissue responsiveness to insulin occurs when surface receptors of insulin increase.[78,79]

The combined effects of substrate availability and insulin effect on lipogenesis by fetal hepatocytes has been studied by Miller et al.[80] The effect of insulin on lipid synthesis from [^{14}C]acetate was measured in fetal and adult hepatocytes. At low concentrations of acetate (<5 mM) insulin induces lipid synthesis in adult hepatocytes but not in fetal hepatocytes. In contrast, at higher acetate concentrations (15–30 mM) lipid synthesis in fetal hepatocytes with and without insulin are greater than adult rates. These experiments suggest that the control of fetal hepatic lipogenesis involves both hormonal and substrate availability.

Other hormones, calcitonin[81] and epidermal growth factor (EGF),[82] have been reported to stimulate synthesis of free fatty acids in the adult rat. Holand and Hardie[82] determined that EGF stimulated fatty acid synthesis in hepatocytes of adult rats that had been starved and then re-fed a low fat diet. When compared to insulin, EGF caused similar stimulation of fatty acid synthesis. Since serum EGF is elevated late in gestation, it may control lipogenesis late in gestation. Further studies on the effect of EGF on the rate of lipogenesis in fetal tissue is required.

Central neural mechanisms may also play a role in controlling fetal lipogenesis and lipid accumulation. Decapitated fetal pigs have been reported to have increased lipid accumulation.[83,84] Martin et al.[83] found that serum insulin, glucagon, and triglyceride concentrations are elevated in decapitated fetuses and that glucose utilization by these fetus are higher than in intact controls. Ramsey et al.[84] determined that fatty acid synthesis from lactate by subcutaneous tissue of decapitated fetal pigs is greater than intact fetuses. These investigators speculated that there are inhibitory factors regulated by a central neural mechanism that control fetal fatty acid synthesis. However, in a recent study, Hausman et al.[85] measured a 2.6-fold increase in lipogenesis activity in adipose tissue in hypophysectomized pigs. In contrast, lipolytic activity in response to norepinephrine in the same adipose tissue was decreased. These data indicate that in the fetus, the presence of enzymes involved with lipolysis and lipogenesis is controlled in part by the pituitary. What are the possible control hormones? Fetal hepatic enzymes involved with gluconeogenesis and lipogenesis are increased with the administration of triiodothyronine to pregnant rats.[86] Since the incorporation of precursors into lipids are increased in the fetuses with maternal triiodothyronine treatment, the increase in enzyme activity appears to have physiologic significance.

Future Studies

With the development of new methods in molecular biology, investigation of the control mechanisms of lipogenesis during late gestation is possible. For example, acetyl-CoA carboxylase is thought to be the rate-controlling enzyme in de novo synthesis of fatty acids. The activation of de novo synthesis of fatty acids by the changes in the insulin-to-glucagon ratio is mediated through acetyl-CoA carboxylase. Do changes in the ratio alter the activity of existing enzyme, or is there a change in the amount of enzyme present? With new techniques in molecular biology, these questions may now be answerable. Towle and Mariash[87] have reported an increase in a species of messenger RNA (mRNA), spot 14, which is associated with stimulation of lipogenesis by feeding rats a high carbohydrate and fat-free diet or with treatment with thyroid hormone. They have yet to relate this change in mRNA to changes in control enzymes associated with lipogenesis. Katsurada et al.[88] measured changes in hepatic antigen, mRNA, and enzyme activity of malic enzyme and glucose-6-phosphate dehydrogenase, enzymes involved in the production of NADPH (Figure 19.3), in the fasted rat re-fed either high carbohydrate, protein, or fat diets. They also measured changes in antigen and enzyme activity of acetyl-CoA carboxylase and fatty acid synthetase complex. By comparing changes in mRNA and enzyme activity, the investigators were able to speculate if changes in enzyme activity were secondary to changes in antigen production of mRNA and/or translation of the mRNA to the enzyme. For example, hepatic malic enzyme activity and antigen was 31% lower in the rat fed only a carbohydrate diet compared to a combined carbohydrate-protein diet. However, mRNA concentration for malic enzyme was equal in the rat fed either a carbohydrate diet alone or a carbohydrate-protein diet. These data suggest that a high-protein diet is required for the translation of the mRNA. Changes in acetyl-CoA carboxylase and fatty acid synthetase activity paralleled changes in antigen in all groups, suggesting that change in enzyme concentration accounted for induction of lipogenesis. Feeding a high-fat diet reduced both the concentration of mRNA and the activity of malic enzyme and glucose-6-phosphate dehydrogenase, suggesting inhibition before translation of mRNA.

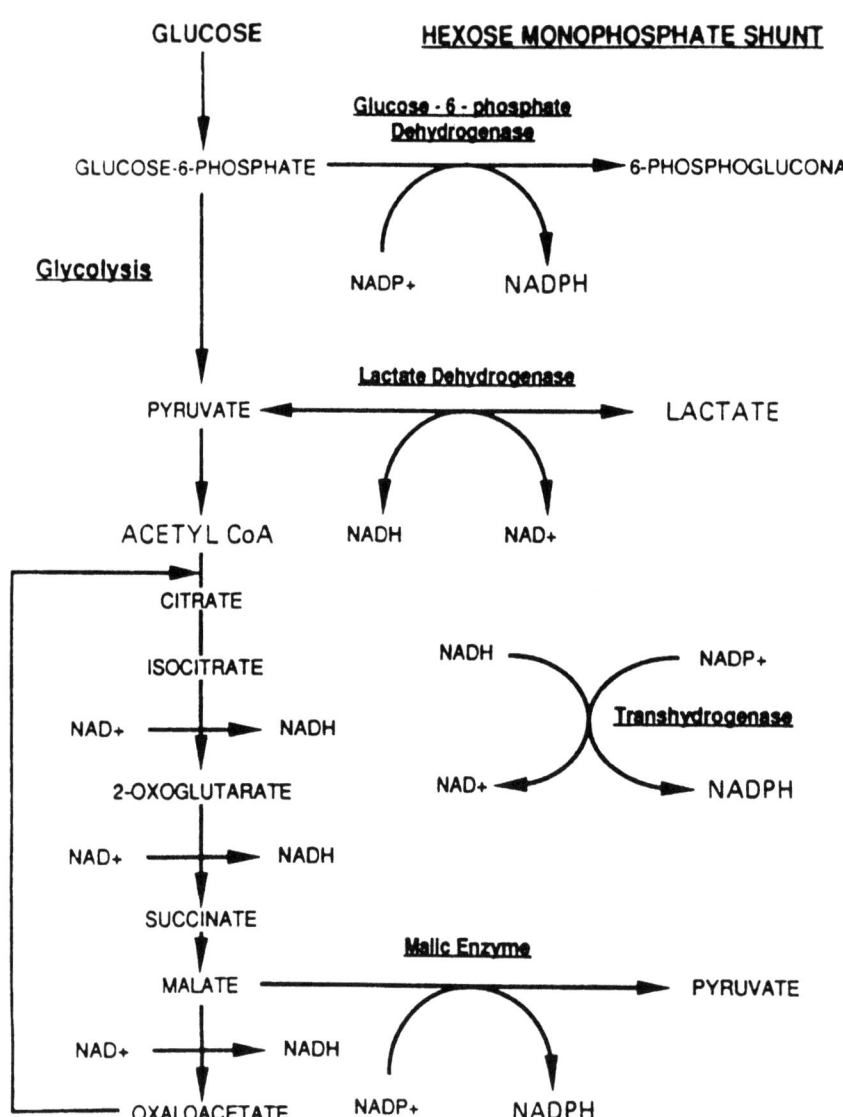

FIGURE 19.3. Biochemical pathways involved in the production of energy for fatty acid synthesis. Names of enzymes are underlined.

The effect of hormones—insulin, glucagon, and epidermal growth factor—and substrates—glucose and lactate—on changes in enzyme activity, in the antigen of the enzyme, and in mRNA in the developing fetus delineates if changes in the control enzymes are secondary to induction of translation of mRNA, translation of mRNA to enzyme, or activation of enzyme that is present.

In summary, lipid accumulation in the fetus late in gestation is important for maintaining energy requirements during the postnatal period. The lipid accumulation is the result of both placental transfer of maternal lipids and the endogenous production of fatty acids by the fetus primarily through de novo synthesis. Glucose and lactate appear to be the major precursors of fetal de novo synthesis. The rate of fetal lipogenesis appears to be controlled by substrate availability, a favorable hormonal environment, a high insulin-to-glucagon ratio, and fetal tissues that can respond to this favorable hormonal environment.

Fatty Acid Oxidation

Late in gestation, the human fetus stores more calories in the form of fat than any other storage fuel.[5] In the postnatal period, oxidation of fatty acids becomes a preferred source of energy for heart and other tissues with high energy demands. The activation of fatty acid oxidation in rabbit hepatocytes within 6 hours after birth[89] indicates that the enzymatic mechanisms involved with fatty acid oxidation must be developed in the fetus and then activated after birth. In this section fatty acid oxidation in the fetus and during the immediate postnatal period is reviewed.

Pathways of Fatty Acid Oxidation

Albumin-bound fatty acids are transported by the bloodstream to sites of oxidation. In the liver, cellular uptake and intracellular transport of fatty acids are thought to

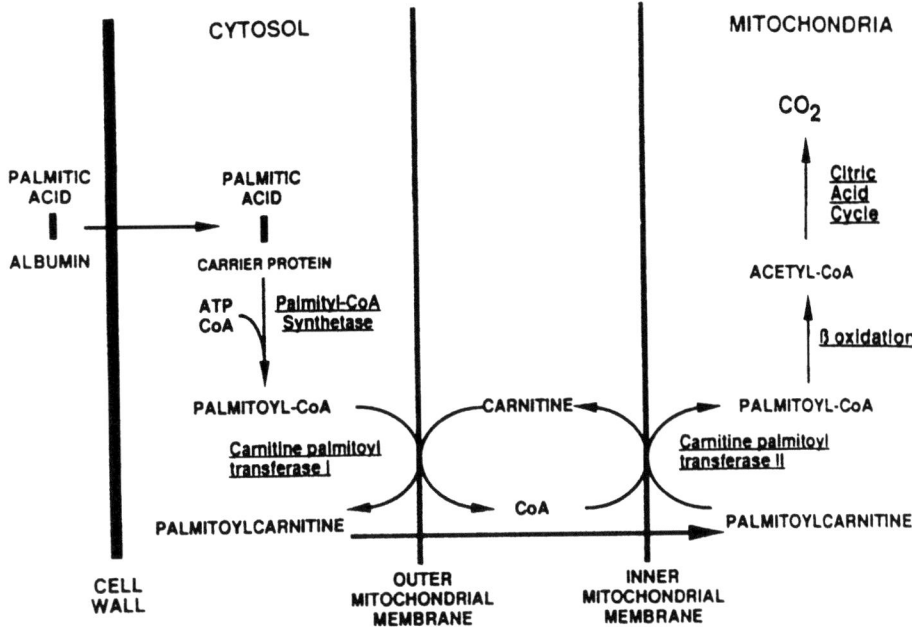

FIGURE 19.4. Biochemical pathways involved in fatty acid oxidation. Names of enzymes are underlined.

involve specialized carrier-binding proteins. Fatty acids are esterified to acyl-CoA esters in the cytosol by acyl-CoA synthetase (Figure 19.4). β-oxidation of fatty acids to acetyl-CoA occurs in the mitochondria. Since the inner mitochondrial membrane is impermeable to acyl-CoA esters, a mitochondrial transport system of the acyl-CoA esters must be present for active fatty acid oxidation. The conversion of acyl-CoA esters to acyl-carnitine esters that readily cross the inner mitochondrial membrane provides a transport mechanism of fatty acids into mitochondria. In the case of palmitic acid, palmitoyl-CoA is converted to palmitoylcarnitine by carnitine palmitoyl transferase I, an enzyme located on the outer surface of the inner mitochondrial membrane. After crossing the mitochondrial membrane palmitoyl carnitine is reconverted to palmitoyl-CoA by carnitine palmitoyl transferase II, which is located on the inner mitochondrial membrane. The palmitoyl-CoA can then undergo β-oxidation, producing acetyl-CoA that can be either further oxidized to CO_2 through the citric acid cycle or converted to ketone bodies.

Fatty Acid Oxidation in the Fetus and the Neonate

Fetal tissues can oxidize fatty acids and ketone bodies.[90] However, the capacity of fetal tissue to oxidize fatty acids is low.[91-93] Zimmermann et al.[94] reported that hepatic oxidation of palmitic acid to CO_2 can account for 25% of the rate of fatty acid oxidation by the whole rat fetus. Hepatic fatty acid oxidation in the 2-day-old rat is more active than in the adult.[92] Ketogenesis from β-oxidation of fatty acids by isolated hepatocytes from fetal rabbits is low and increases eightfold in hepatocytes of 6- and 24-hour-old rabbits.[89] Fatty acids become the preferred fuel in other neonatal rat tissue with high energy demands such as the heart.[95]

Control Mechanisms Involved with Fatty Acid Oxidation in the Fetus and Neonate

An increase in substrate availability, hormone and substrate control of existing enzyme systems, and an increased supply of carnitine and CoA to the neonate may control the postnatal increase in fatty acid oxidation. Since studies indicate that the availability of the substrates significantly controls the rate of β-oxidation of fatty acids in vivo,[96,97] the increase in serum free fatty acid concentration[98-100] may regulate the postnatal increase in fatty acid oxidation.

The increase in postnatal carnitine palmitoyltransferase activity is associated with an increase in fatty acid oxidation, suggesting a regulatory role in the postnatal change in fatty acid oxidation. Carnitine palmitoyltransferase activity in fetal rat heart[91] and liver[101] is low but, increases postnatally and reaches adult values by 30 days of age. Warshaw[91] has demonstrated that the oxidation of palmitoyl-CoA plus carnitine in fetal heart is very limited. However, the rate of oxidation of palmitoylcarnitine is similar in fetal and calf mitochondria.[95] These data suggest that carnitine palmitoyltransferase external to the mitochondrial membrane barrier to palmitoyl-CoA, carnitine palmitoyltransferase I, is rate limiting for fatty acid oxidation in the bovine fetus. Pegorier et al.,[102] using isolated hepatocytes, determined the fate of octanoate in term fetal, 24-hour-old, and adult rabbits. In hepatocytes from 24-hour-old and adult rabbits octanoate is 92% oxidized, while in hepatocytes from term fetal rabbits 43% of the metabolized octanoate is esterified. This difference in the metabolic fate of octanoate reflects the low activity of carnitine acyltransferase, which is required for the transport of the fatty acid into the mitochondria prior to β-oxidation.

The postnatal increase in serum long-chain acyl-CoA esters may increase fatty acid oxidation by inhibiting acetyl-CoA carboxylase.[103] Since malonyl-CoA is a potent inhibitor of carnitine acyltransferase,[74,104] an acute decrease in tissue malonyl-CoA concentration, caused by inhibition of acetyl-CoA carboxylase by acyl-CoA esters, results in an increase in carnitine acyltransferase activity. Studies indicate that an increase in carnitine acyltransferase activity, the rate-limiting step in fatty acid oxidation, causes an increase in fatty acid oxidation.[105] This association between increased availability of fatty acids and the activation of carnitine acyltransferase activity has been reported in rat fetuses of mothers who were either starved or fed a high-fat diet[101] (see Chapter 38).

The association between hepatic fatty acid oxidation, malonyl-CoA concentration, and carnitine acyltransferase activity at the time of birth has been studied extensively by Prip-Buus et al.[106] using the fetal and neonatal rabbit. These investigators determined that oleate oxidation and carnitine palmitoyltransferase-I (CPT-I) activity in isolated hapatocytes increased after birth from 0 to 24 hours. During this same period, malonyl-CoA concentration and the rate of lipogenesis decreased. In addition to the obvious correlation between CPT-I activity and malonyl-CoA concentration, these investigators determined that the inhibitory effect of malonyl-CoA on CPT-I also decreased with time after birth. The concentration of malonyl-CoA needed to inhibit CPT-I was greater in hepatocytes isolated from 24-hour-old rabbits compared to 0- to 6-hour-old rabbits. These data indicate that the increase in fatty acid oxidation at birth is controlled by both the decrease in malonyl-CoA concentration and the sensitivity of the CPT-I to inhibition by malonyl-CoA.

Changes in the sensitivity of CPT-I to malonyl-CoA as a control of fatty acid oxidation has been suggested by Decaux et al.[107] These investigators determined that the capacity of the liver to oxidize fatty acids was decreased from rats weaned on a high-carbohydrate diet. However, no change in intracellular malonyl-CoA concentrations in liver was found even though carnitine palmitoyltransferase I activity was lower. They speculated that the carnitine palmitoyltransferase enzyme was more sensitive to malonyl-CoA. If the sensitivity of an enzyme to an inhibitor can change through different developmental periods, then the modulation of controlling enzymes can be greatly affected. Common to the studies of Decaux et al.[107] and Prip-Buus et al.[106] is the potential effect of lipids and fatty acids on the sensitivity of CPT-I to malonyl-CoA. Twenty-four hours after birth and during the suckling period there is an increase in serum lipids. During these periods of high lipids, CPT-I inhibition by malonyl-CoA is less sensitive compared to the period 0 to 6 hours after birth and after weaning to a high carbohydrate diet when the serum lipid concentrations decrease.

Other possible mechanisms for reduced β-oxidation of fatty acids in the fetal liver are the low tissue concentrations of CoA and carnitine, substrates involved with the activation and transfer of fatty acids into the mitochondria. Escriva et al.[108] reported an increase in hepatic tissue CoA concentration in 16-hour-old pups, which was associated with an increase in hepatic fatty acid oxidation, suggesting a possible control mechanism. Changes in carnitine availability may serve a regulatory role in the development of fatty acid oxidation in the postnatal period. Robles-Valdes et al.[109] has determined that the increase in neonatal rat liver carnitine concentration during the first 24 hours of life parallels a 10-fold increase in plasma ketone concentration. The addition of exogenous carnitine to liver perfusate increases the rate of hepatic fatty acid oxidation.[110] These data suggest that the postnatal increase in hepatic fatty acid oxidation is controlled by increased liver carnitine concentration.

The postnatal increase in plasma glucagon concentration may stimulate fatty acid oxidation. McGarry et al.[110] have reported that glucagon increases the carnitine content in rat liver, suggesting a possible hormonal control mechanism. Glucagon has also been demonstrated to lower the intracellular concentration of malonyl-CoA in the isolated liver cell.[73,106,111] Since malonyl-CoA is an inhibitor of carnitine palmitoyltransferase, a regulatory enzyme of β-oxidation, a decrease in intracellular malonyl-CoA concentration would result in an increase in fatty acid oxidation. In postmature fetal rabbits, the rate of ketone body production is fivefold greater than normal control.[112] In these fetuses the insulin to glucagon ratio decreases threefold because of a 45% decrease in insulin and a 50% increase in glucagon, suggesting a possible role of glucagon for the increase in postnatal fatty acid oxidation. In the isolated hepatocyte from the fetal rabbit, Prip-Buus et al.[106] determined that treatment with glucagon caused not only a decrease in malonyl-CoA concentration but also a decrease in the inhibitory effect of malonyl-CoA on CPT-I. They speculated that the increase in fatty acid oxidation in association with an increase in CPT-I activity was caused in part by the effect of glucagon on decreasing malonyl-CoA concentration and decreasing the sensitivity of CPT-I to malonyl-CoA. In contrast, in the fetal lamb, infusion of glucagon does not induce ketogenesis.[113] It is possible that the difference between these two studies is the maturation age of the fetus and the presence of glucagon receptors and end-organ responses to the glucagon.

Another possible control mechanism of fetal fatty acid oxidation is the presence of high lactate concentration. In addition to serving as a precursor for lipogenesis, studies in cardiac muscle indicate that lactate may regulate the fate of fatty acids, either the incorporation of fatty acids into triglycerides or the oxidation of fatty acids. Bielefeld et al.[114] reported that 5 mM lactate caused a 38% reduction in cardiac muscle fatty acid oxidation. Concomitantly, fatty acid conversion to triglycerides increased 100%. They measured a decrease in the tissue concentration of long-chain acy-carnitine in the presence of lactate. The investigations speculated that lactate inhibited carnitine acyltransferase and, therefore, inhibited fatty acid oxidation. Further studies of the effect of lactate on fatty acid oxidation and carnitine acyltransferase activity in fetal tissue are necessary.

Ketone Oxidation During Development

During the last trimester of human pregnancy the concentration of ketone bodies increases in the maternal blood.[115] In the rat, maternal starvation results in a 50% decrease in fetal glucose concentration and a 36-fold increase in ketone concentrations.[116] Shambaugh et al.[117] have provided evidence in the rat that CO_2 production from ketones is directly proportional to substrate availability. Since there is a good correlation between maternal and fetal blood ketone concentrations in the human[115] and in the rat,[118] these data suggest that fetal ketone oxidation may become significant late in gestation and during periods of maternal starvation when maternal serum lipid concentrations are elevated. Dierkes-Vesting[119] induced fetal liver and kidney acetoacetyl-CoA thiolase and 3-oxoacid CoA transferase, enzymes involved in ketone oxidation, by placing pregnant rats on a high-fat diet, suggesting a significant effect of maternally derived lipids and ketones on fetal ketone oxidation.

In summary, fatty acid oxidation in the fetus is low during a period of time when there is a constant infusion of glucose and lactate from the fetus. Studies suggest that lactate may inhibit fatty acid oxidation by inhibiting carnitine acyltransferase. However, in the immediate postnatal period activation of fatty acids is important for maintenance of energy requirements. Evidence exists that substrate availability of fatty acids, CoA, and carnitine, and the increase in glucagon concentrations in the postnatal period, activate preexisting enzymes involved with β-oxidation of fatty acids.

References

1. Cross KW, Tizard JP, Trythall DA. The gaseous metabolism of the newborn infant. Acta Pediatr Scand 1957;46:265–285.
2. Senterre J, Karlberg P. Respiratory quotient and metabolic rate in normal full-term and small for date newborn infants. Acta Paediatr Scand 1970;59:653–658.
3. Denne SC, Kalhan SM. Glucose carbon recycling and oxidation in human newborns. Am J Physiol 1986;251(Endocrinol Metab 13):E71–E77.
4. Gewolb IH, Warshaw JB. Influences on fetal growth. In: Warshaw JB, ed. The biological basis of reproductive and developmental medicine. Elsevier: New York, 1983:365–389.
5. Widdowson E. Chemical composition of newly born animals. Nature 1950;116:626–628.
6. Camerer W. Die chemische Zusammensetzung des neugeborenen Menschen. Z Biol 1902;43:1–12.
7. Iob V, Swanson WW. Mineral growth of the human fetus. Am J Dis Child 1934;47:302–306.
8. Fee BA, Weil WB. Body composition of infants of diabetic mothers by direct analysis. Ann NY Acad Sci 1963;110:869–897.
9. Ziegler EE, O'Donnell AM, Nelson SE, et al. Body composition of the reference fetus. Growth 1976;40:329–341.
10. Knopp RH. Fuel metabolism in pregnancy. Contemp Obstet Gynecol 1978;12:83–90.
11. Knopp RH, Saudek CD, Arky RA, et al. Two phases of adipose tissue metabolism in pregnancy: maternal adaptations for fetal growth. Endocrinology 1973;92:984–988.
12. Fain JN, Scow RO. Fatty acid synthesis in vivo in maternal and fetal tissues in the rat. Am J Physiol 1966;210:19–25.
13. Elliot JA. The effect of pregnancy on the control of lipolysis in fat cells isolated from human adipose tissue. Eur J Clin Invest 1975;5:159–163.
14. Knopp RH, Montes A, Childs M, et al. Metabolic adjustments in normal and diabetic pregnancy. In: Seeds AE, ed. Clinical obstetrics and gynecology. Hagerstown, MD: Harper & Row, 1981:21–49.
15. Hummel L, Schirrmeister W, Zimmerman T. Transfer of maternal plasma free fatty acids into the rat fetus. Acta Biol Med Germ 1975;34:603–605.
16. Elphick MC, Hudson DG, Hull D. Transfer of free fatty acids across the rabbit placenta. J Physiol (Lond) 1975;252:29–42.
17. Van Duyne CM, Havel RJ, Felts JM. Placental transfer of palmitic acid-1-14C in rabbits. Am J Obstet Gynecol 1962;84:1069–1074.
18. Goldstein R, Levy E, Shafrir E. Increased maternal-fetal transport of fat in diabetes assessed by polyunsaturated fatty acid content in fetal lipids. Biol Neonate 1985;47(6):343–349.
19. Stammers JP, Elphick MC, Hull D. Effect of maternal diet during late pregnancy on fetal lipid stores in rabbits. J Dev Physiol 1983;5:395–404.
20. Hendrickse W, Stammers JP, Hull D. The transfer of free fatty acids across the human placenta. Br J Obstet Gynaecol 1985;92:945–952.

21. Elphick MC, Hull D. The transfer of free fatty acids across the rabbit placenta. J Physiol 1977;264:751–766.
22. Thomas CR, Lowy C. Placental transfer of free fatty acids: factors affecting transfer across the guinea pig placenta. J Dev Physiol 1983;5:323–332.
23. Stephenson TJ, Stammers JP, Hull D. Effects of altering umbilical flow and umbilical free fatty acid concentration on transfer of free fatty acids across the rabbit placenta. J Dev Physiol 1991;15:221–227.
24. Dancis J, Jansen V, Kayden JH, et al. Transfer across perfused human placenta. III. Effect of chain length on transfer of free fatty acids. Pediatr Res 1974;8:796–799.
25. Hershfield MS, Nemeth AM. Placental transport of free palmitic and linoleic acids in the guinea pig. J Lipid Res 1968;9:460–468.
26. Stephenson T, Stammers J, Hull D. Placental transfer of free fatty acids: importance of fetal albumin concentration and acid-base status. Biol Neonate 1993;63:273–280.
27. Schenker S, Dawber NH, Schmid R. Bilirubin metabolism in the fetus. J Clin Invest 1964;43:32–39.
28. Cayatte AJ, Kumbla L, Subbiah MT. Marked acceleration of exogenous fatty acid incorporation into cellular triglycerides by fetuin. J Biol Chem 1990;265:5883–5888.
29. Subbiah MT. Newly recognized lipid carrier proteins in fetal life. Proc Soc Exp Biol Med 1991;198:495–499.
30. Kumbla L, Bhadra S, Subbiah MT. Multifunctional role for fetuin (fetal protein) in lipid transport. FASEB J 1991;5:2971–2975.
31. Thomas CR, Evans JL, Buttriss C, et al. Lipid chain length alterations during placental transfer in the guinea pig. J Dev Physiol 1985;7:305–311.
32. Noble RC, Shand JH, Christie WW. Synthesis of C20 and C22 polyunsaturated fatty acids by the placenta of the sheep. Biol Neonate 1985;47:333–338.
33. Knopp RH, Warth MR, Charles D, et al. Lipoprotein metabolism in pregnancy, fat transport to the fetus, and the effects of diabetes. Biol Neonate 1986;50:297–317.
34. Thomas CR, Lowy C, St. Hillaire RJ, et al. Studies on the placental hydrolysis and transfer of lipids to the fetal guinea pig. In: Miller RK, Tiede HA, eds. Fetal nutrition, metabolism and Immunology: the role of the placenta. New York: Plenum, 1984:135–146.
35. Campbell FM, Taffesse S, Gordon MJ, et al. Plasma membrane fatty-acid-binding protein in human placenta: identification and characterization. Biochem Biophys Res Commun 1995;209:1011–1017.
36. Campbell FM, Dutta Roy AK. Plasma membrane fatty acid-binding protein (FABPpm) is exclusively located in the maternal facing membranes of the human placenta. FEBS Lett 1995;375:227–230.
37. Wittmaack FM, Gafvels ME, Bronner M, et al. Localization and regulation of the human very low density lipoprotein/apolipoprotein-E receptor: trophoblast expression predicts a role for the receptor in placental lipid transport. Endocrinology 1995;136:340–348.
38. Ruyle M, Connor WE, Anderson GJ, et al. Placental transfer of essential fatty acids in humans: venous-arterial difference for docosahexaenoic acid in fetal umbilical erythrocytes. Proc Natl Acad Sci USA 1990;87:7902–7906.
39. Elphick MC, Hull D, Sanders RR. Concentrations of free fatty acids in maternal and umbilical cord blood during elective caesarian section. Br J Obstet Gynaecol 1976;83:539–544.
40. Persson B, Tunell R. Influence of environmental temperature and acidosis on lipid mobilization in the human infant during the first two hours after birth. Acta Paediatr Scand 1971;60:385–398.
41. Dancis J, Jansen V, Kayden JH, et al. Transfer across perfused human placenta II. Free fatty acids. Pediatr Res 1973;7:192–197.
42. Coleman RA. Placental metabolism and transport of lipid. Fed Proc 1986;45:2519–2523.
43. Hummel L, Zimmermann, Wagner H. Quantitative evaluation of the fetal fatty acid synthesis in the rat. Acta Biol Med Germ 1978;37:229–232.
44. Portman OW, Behrman RE, and Soltys P. Transfer of free fatty acids across the primate placenta. Am J Physiol 1969;216:143–147.
45. Legras B, Clerc C, Ruelland A, et al. Blood chemistry of human fetuses in the second and third trimesters. Prenat Diagn 1990;10:801–807.
46. Averna MR, Barbagallo CM, Di Paola G, et al. Lipids, lipoproteins and apolipoproteins AI, AII, B, CII, CIII and E in newborns. Biol Neonate 1991;60:187–192.
47. Kherkeulidze P, Johansson J, Carlson LA. High density lipoprotein particle size distribution in cord blood. Acta Paediatr Scand 1991;80:770–779.
48. Foreman van Drongelen MM, al MD, van Houwelingen AC, et al. Comparison between the essential fatty acid status of preterm and full-term infants, measured in umbilical vessel walls. Early Hum Dev 1995;42:241–251.
49. Hoving EB, van Beusekom CM, Nijeboer HJ, et al. Gestational age dependency of essential fatty acids in cord plasma cholesterol esters and triglycerides. Pediatr Res 1994;35:461–469.
50. Cai HJ, Xie CL, Chen Q, et al. The relationship between hepatic low-density lipoprotein receptor activity and serum cholesterol level in the human fetus. Hepatology 1991;13:852–857.
51. van Houwelingen AC, Puls J, Hornstra G. Essential fatty acid status during early human development. Early Hum Dev 1992;31:97–111.
52. Bressler R, Wakil S. Studies on the mechanism of fatty acid synthesis. I. The conversion of malonyl coenzyme A to long chain fatty acids. J Biol Chem 1961;236:1643–1651.
53. Warshaw JB, Kimura RE. Cellular energy metabolism during fetal development. V. Fatty acid synthesis by the developing heart. Dev Biol 1973;33:224–228.
54. Taylor CV, Bailey E, Bartley W. Changes in hepatic lipogenesis during development of rat. Biochem J 1967;105:717–722.
55. Ballard FJ, Hanson RW. Changes in lipid synthesis in rat liver during development. Biochem J 1967;102:952–958.
56. Villee CA, Hagerman DD. Effect of oxygen deprivation on the metabolism of fetal and adult tissues. Am J Physiol 1958;194:457–464.
57. Roux JF. Lipid metabolism in the fetal and neonatal rabbit. Metabolism 1966;15:856–864.

58. Farrell PM, Bourbon JR. Fetal lung surfactant lipid synthesis from glycogen during organ culture. Biochim Biophys Acta 1986;878:159–167.
59. Maniscalco W, Finkelstein JN, Parkhurst AB. De novo fatty acid synthesis in developing rat lung. Biochim Biophys Acta 1982;711:49–58.
60. Engle MJ, Brown DJ, Dehring AF, et al. Effect of lactate on glucose incorporation into fetal lung phospholipids. Exp Lung Res 1988;14:121–129.
61. Robertson JP, Faulkner A, Vernon RG. L-lactate as a source of carbon for fatty acid synthesis in adult and foetal sheep. Biochem Biophys Acta 1981;665:511–518.
62. Medina JM. The role of lactate as an energy substrate for the brain during the early neonatal period. Biol Neonate 1985;48:237–244.
63. Carter BS, Moores RR Jr, Teng C, et al. Main routes of plasma lactate carbon disposal in the midgestation fetal lamb. Biol Neonate 1995;67:295–300.
64. Bolanos JP, Medina JM. Lipogenesis from lactate in fetal rat brain during late gestation. Pediatr Res 1993;33:66–71.
65. Vernon RG, Finley E, Taylor E. Fatty acid synthesis from amino acids in sheep adipose tissue. Comp Biochem Physiol [B] 1985;82:133–136.
66. Seccombe DW, Harding PGR, Possmayer F. Fetal utilization of maternally derived ketone bodies for lipogenesis in the rat. Biochem Biophys Acta 1977;488:402–416.
67. Edmond J. Ketone bodies as precursors of sterols and fatty acids in the developing rat. J Biol Chem 1974;249:72–78.
68. Ktorza A, Nurjhan N, Girard JR, et al. Hyperglycaemia induced by glucose infusion in the unrestrained pregnant rat: effect on body weight and lipid synthesis in postmature fetuses. Diabetologia 1983;24:128–130.
69. Ktorza A, Bihoreau M, Nurjhan Nea. Insulin and glucagon during the perinatal period: secretion and metabolic effects on the liver. Biol Neonate 1985;48:204–220.
70. Girard JR, Cuendet GS, Marliss EB, et al. Fuels, hormones and liver metabolism at term and during the early postnatal period in the rat. J Clin Invest 1973;52:3190–3200.
71. Witters LZ, Moriarity D, Martin DB. Regulation of hepatic acetyl-CoA carboxylase by insulin and glucagon. J Biol Chem 1979;254:6644–6649.
72. Geelen MJH, Beynen AC, Christiansen RZ, et al. Short-term effect of insulin and glucagon on lipid synthesis in isolated rat hepatocytes. Covariance of acetyl-CoA carboxylase activity and the rat of ^3H_2O incorporation into fatty acids. FEBS Lett 1978;95:326–330.
73. McGarry JD, Takabayashi Y, Foster DW. The role of malonyl-CoA in the coordination of fatty acid synthesis and oxidation in isolated rat hepatocytes. J Biol Chem 1978;253:8294–8300.
74. McGarry JD, Leatherman GF, Foster DW. The site of inhibition of hepatic fatty acid oxidation by malonyl-CoA. J Biol Chem 1978;253:4128–4136.
75. Harris R. Studies on the inhibition of hepatic lipogenesis by N_6, O_2- dibutyryl adenosine 3′, 5′-monophosphate. Arch Biochem Biophys 1975;169:168–180.
76. Picon L. Effect of insulin on growth and biochemical composition of the rat fetus. Endocrinology 1967;81:1491–1421.
77. Clark CM, Cahill GF, Soeldner J. Effects of exogenous insulin on the rate of fatty acid synthesis and glucose C-14 utilization in the twenty-day rat fetus. Diabetes 1968;17:362–368.
78. Blazquez E, Rubalcaua B, Montesano R. Development of insulin and glucagon binding and the adenylate cyclase response in liver membranes of the prenatal, postnatal and adult rat: evidence of glucagon resistance. Endocrinology 1976;98:1014–1023.
79. Maniscalco W, Loo S, Warshaw JB. Ontogeny of insulin action on developing liver. Pediatr Res 1976;10:324.
80. Miller JD, Sinha MK, Sperling MA, et al. Insulin stimulates amino acid and lipid metabolism in isolated fetal rat hepatocytes. Pediatr Res 1986;20:609–612.
81. Yamaguchi M, Momose K, Takahashi K. Stimulatory effect of calcitonin on fatty acid synthesis in the liver of fed rats. Horm Metab Res 1985;17:346–360.
82. Holand R, Haidie DG. Both insulin and epidermal growth factor stimulate fatty acid synthesis and increased phosphorylatin of acetyl-CoA carboxylase and ATP-citrate lyase in isolated hepatocytes. FEBS Left 1985;181:308–312.
83. Martin RJ, Campion DR, Hausman GJ, et al. Serum hormones and metabolites in fetally decapitated pigs. Growth 1984;48(2):158–165.
84. Ramsey TG, Hausman GJ, Martin RJ. Metabolic development of porcine fetal adipose tissue. A role for central regulation. Biol Neonate 1988;53:171–180.
85. Hausman DB, Hausman GJ, Martin RJ. Influence of the pituitary on lipolysis and lipogenesis in fetal pig adipose tissue. Horm Metab Res 1993;25:17–20.
86. Shafrir E, Barash V, Zederman R, et al. Modulation of fetal and placental metabolic pathways in response to maternal thyroid and glucocorticoid hormone excess. 1st J Med Sci 1994;30:32–41.
87. Towle HC, Mariash CN. Regulation of hepatic gene expression by lipogenic diet and thyroid hormone. Fed Proc 1986;45:2406–2411.
88. Katsurada A, Iritani N, Fukuda H, et al. Effects of dietary nutrients on lipogenic enzyme and mRNA activities in rat liver during induction. Biochim. Biophys Acta 1986;877:350–358.
89. Duee PH, Pegorier JP, Mancubl L, et al. Hepatic triglyceride hydrolysis and development of ketogenesis in rabbits. Am J Physiol 1985;249:E478–E484.
90. Roux JB, Myers RE. In vitro metabolism of palmitic acid and glucose in the developing tissue of the rhesus monkey. Am J Obstet Gynecol 1974;118:385–392.
91. Warshaw JB. Cellular energy metabolism during fetal development. IV. Fatty acid activation, acetyl transfer and fatty acid oxidation during development of the chick and rat. Dev Biol 1972;28:537–544.
92. Bailey E, Lockwood E. Some aspects of fatty acid oxidation and ketone body formation and utilization during development of the rat. Enzyme 1973;15:239–253.
93. Augenfeld J, Fritz I. Carnitine palmityltransferase activity in fatty acid oxidation by livers from fetal and neonatal rats. Can J Biochem 1970;48:228–294.
94. Zimmermann T, Hummer L, Wagner H. Quantitative studies on the fetal lipid metabolism in rats: liver fatty acid

esterification and conversion into carbon dioxide, and hepatic output of triglycerides and phospholipids into serum. Biol Neonate 1986;49:43–50.
95. Warshaw JB, Cellular energy metabolism. III. Deficient acetyl-CoA synthetase, acetylcarnitine transferase and oxidation of acetate in fetal bovine heart. Biochem Biophys Acta 1970;223:409–415.
96. Lindsay DB. Fatty acids as energy sources. Proc Nutr Soc 1975;34:241–248.
97. Fritz IB. Factors influencing the rate of long chain fatty acid oxidation and synthesis in mammalian systems. Physiol Rev 1961;41:52–129.
98. Blazquez E, Sagase T, Blazquez M, et al. Neonatal changes in the concentration of rat liver cyclic AMP and serum glucose, FFA, insulin pancreatic glucagon and total glucagon in man and the rat. J Lab Clin Med 1974;83:957–967.
99. Novak M, Melichar V, Hahn P, et al. Release of free fatty acids from adipose tissue obtained from newborn infants. J Lipid Res 1965;6:91–95.
100. Novak M, Monkus E. Metabolism of subcutaneous adipose tissue in the immediate postnatal period of human newborns. I. Developmental changes in lipolysis and glycogen content. Pediatr Res 1972;6:73–80.
101. Chalk PA, Higham FC, Caswell AM, et al. Hepatic mitochondrial fatty acid oxidation during the perinatal period in the rat. Int J Biochem 1983;15:531–538.
102. Pegorier JP, Duee PH, Clouet P, et al. Octanoate metabolism in isolated hepatocytes and mitochondria from fetal, newborn and adult rabbit. Evidence for a high capacity for octanoate esterification in term fetal liver. Eur J Biochem 1989;184:681–686.
103. Ogiwara H, Tanabe T, Nikawa J, et al. Inhibition of rat liver acetyl-coenzyme-A carboxylase by palmitoyl-coenzyme. A. Formation of equimolar enzyme inhibitor complex. Eur J Biochem 1978;89:33–41.
104. McGarry JD, Robles-Valdes C, Foster DW. Role of carnitine in hepatic ketogenesis. Proc Natl Acad Sci USA 1975;72:4385–4388.
105. Bewsher PD, Tarrant ME, Ashmore J. Effects of fat mobilization on liver metabolism. Diabetes 1966;15:346–350.
106. Prip Buus C, Pegorier JP, Duee PH, et al. Evidence that the sensitivity of carnitine palmitoyltransferase I to inhibition by malonyl-CoA is an important site of regulation of hepatic fatty acid oxidation in the fetal and newborn rabbit. Perinatal development and effects of pancreatic hormones in cultured rabbit hepatocytes. Biochem J 1990:269:409–415.
107. Decaux JF, Ferre P, Robin D, et al. Decreased hepatic fatty acid oxidation at weaning in the rat is not linked to a variation of malonyl-CoA concentration. J Biol Chem 1988;263:3284–3289.
108. Escriva F, Ferre P, Robin D, et al. Evidence that the development of hepatic fatty acid oxidation at birth in the rat is concomitant with an increased intramitochondrial CoA concentration. Eur J Biochem 1986;156:603–607.
109. Robles-Valdes C, McGarry JD, Foster DW. Maternal-fetal carnitine relationships and neonatal ketosis in the rat. J Biol Chem 1976;251:6007–6012.
110. McGarry JD, Mannaerts GP, Foster DW. A possible role for malonyl-CoA in the regulation of hepatic fatty acid oxidation and ketogenesis. J Clin Invest 1977;60:265–270.
111. Cook GA, King MT, Veech RL. Ketogenesis and malonyl coenzyme A content of isolated rat hepatocytes. J Biol Chem 1978;253:2529–2531.
112. Herbin C, Duee PH, Pegorier JP, et al. Premature appearance of gluconeogenesis and fatty acid oxidation in the liver of the postterm rabbit fetus. Pediatr Res 1988;23:224–228.
113. Philipps AF, Dubin JW, Matty PJ, et al. Influence of exogenous glucagon on fetal glucose metabolism and ketone production. Pediatr Res 1983;17:51–56.
114. Bielefeld DR, Vary TC, Neely JR. Inhibition of carnitine palmitoylCoA transferase activity and fatty acid oxidation by lactate and oxfenicine in cardiac muscle. J Mol Cell Cardiol 1985;17:619–625.
115. Paterson P, Sheath J, Taft P, et al. Maternal and foetal ketone concentration in plasma and urine. Lancet 1967;1:862–865.
116. Shambaugh GEJ, Mrozak SC, Freinkel N. Fetal fuels. I. Utilization of ketones by isolated tissues at various stages of maturation and maternal nutrition during late gestation. Metabolism 1977;26:263–265.
117. Shambaugh GEJ, Koehler RR, Yokoo H. Fetal fuels. III: Ketone utilization by fetal hepatocyte. Am J Physiol 1978;235:E330–E337.
118. Scow RO, Chernick SS, Smith BB. Ketosis in the rat fetus. Proc Soc Exp Biol Med 1958;98:833–835.
119. Dierkes-Vesting C. Prenatal induction of ketone-body enzymes in the rat. Biol Neonate 1971;19:426–433.

20
Growth Factors in the Fetal-Placental Unit

Philip A. Gruppuso

The term growth factor is generally used to describe small polypeptides that act locally to modulate cell growth and differentiation. Broadening of the use of this term is dictated by recent advances in understanding the means by which cells signal one another at the cell–cell, tissue, and physiologic levels. Growth factors should be considered as one class of extracellular signaling factors. The latter, more encompassing term includes, in addition to growth factors, the classic endocrine hormones, hematopoietic and immune system cytokines, cell–cell adhesion molecules, and matrix proteins. Members of all of these groups are involved in the control of cell growth and differentiation, and all are capable of initiating the sort of signal transduction usually associated with growth factors (see also Chapter 3).

Distinctions between growth factors and other extracellular signaling factors are further blurred by the biologic geography of their actions. While endocrine hormones are thought of as acting at considerable distance from their site of production, all have some local effects. Similarly, some growth factors are secreted in order to have growth regulatory effects on distant organs. It has been shown more recently that growth factors can be synthesized as intrinsic membrane proteins that may function at the level of cell–cell interactions, similar to cell–cell adhesion molecules.

Recent developments in the areas of growth factor synthesis, action, and the basic biology of cancer also make the definition of a growth factor less clear. Indeed, many oncogenes and their normal cellular counterparts (proto-oncogenes) function as growth factors, growth factor receptors, or mediators of growth factor signal transduction. This is particularly relevant to fetal physiology, given that many oncogenes code for "onco-fetal" proteins, that is, proteins whose normal function during fetal life results in aberrant growth regulation when expressed after the completion of development.

This chapter focuses on principles of growth factor production and action. A discussion of general aspects of growth factor biology and physiology is followed by a description of the major classes of polypeptide growth factors.

General Considerations

The Relationship Between Site of Secretion and Action

The classic endocrine mode of action (Figure 20.1) is generally used to describe action on distant tissues, which requires transport of a factor via the bloodstream. Some growth factors clearly function in this mode. Most notable is insulin-like growth factor-I (IGF-I), the hepatic production of which is regulated by growth hormone. Its distant actions, especially at the growing epiphysis, earned its original designation as a somatomedin.[1]

The word paracrine was originally proposed as a description of epithelial cells postulated to have a "peripheral" endocrine function.[2] It was further hypothesized that the products of these cells could have local, "paracrine" actions. Subsequently, the observations linking gut hormones and neurotransmitters established the ubiquitous nature of locally produced factors that could regulate cellular function in a manner similar to endocrine hormones.

When Sporn and Todaro[3] introduced the hypothesis defining autocrine secretion in 1980, they were seeking to describe a mechanism whereby malignant cells could obviate the need for exogenous growth factors. The autocrine hypothesis suggested that the production of growth factors could result in the sustained growth exhibited by tumor cells in culture. The subsequent 10 years demonstrated that autocrine growth factor production pertains to many human tumors as well as the behavior of many normal cells.[4] Furthermore, the definition and characterization of numerous oncogenes has indicated that unrestrained cell growth can bypass the need for

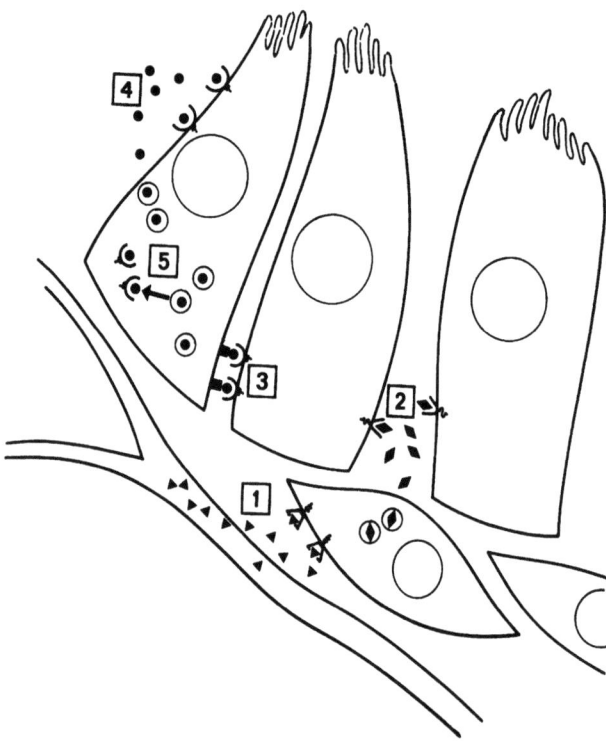

FIGURE 20.1. Local modes of growth factor action. When acting in the classic mode of endocrine action (1), growth factors are released by secreting cells and transported to their targets via the circulation. The local mode of action first described was paracrine (2) in which one cell type secretes a factor that acts on a different, adjacent cell. A variation on paracrine action is juxtacrine (3) action in which a form of the growth factor that remains tethered to the membrane of the secreting cell acts on an adjacent cell. In the autocrine mode of action, as originally described (4), a secreted factor acts on the same cell or cell type responsible for the secretion. In a modification of this mode, internal autocrine action (5), the factor need not be secreted to bind to receptors present in the secreting cell.

autocrine growth factor stimulation. Once oncogene products were shown to be related to growth factors and components of their signal transduction pathways, it became apparent that the autocrine hypothesis should include oncogene-mediated processes.[4]

Other modifications of the autocrine hyopothesis are relevant to the understanding of the role of growth factors in normal physiology. One was that autocrine factors can be growth inhibitors.[5] A second modification was that binding of an autocrine factor to its receptor might occur without secretion into the extracellular space. This was demonstrated by expressing modified growth factors that could not be secreted and showing that they could still exert an autocrine effect.[6,7] Another modification was the inclusion of paracrine involvement in autocrine growth factor function. An example is the requirement for activation of latent transforming growth factor-β (TGF-β) by adjoining smooth muscle cells in the autocrine control of endothelial cell proliferation and migration.[8] Perhaps the most significant modification of the original autocrine hypothesis is its application to normal cellular physiology. Fetal development is one area in which the above principles are most applicable. Local modes of action have obvious and profound implications for studies on the role of growth factors in perinatal biology. Concentrations of growth factors in physiologic fluids may be misleading or, at best, difficult to interpret. Low levels of growth factor expression may not necessarily indicate low biologic activity since growth factors acting at the local level need not be present in high concentrations. Finally, local growth factor action may require a network of cells difficult to reconstruct in an in vitro system.

Cellular Responses to Growth Factors

Proliferation

The cellular response most often associated with growth factor action is the stimulation of cell proliferation. The past decade has seen remarkable progress in defining the basic mechanisms governing cell division and the signaling mechanisms whereby growth factors promote cell growth. Mitogenic signaling involves numerous signal transduction pathways extending from the cell membrane, where receptors activate a signal, to the nucleus, where events required for entry into and progression through mitosis occur. Similarly, progress has been made in delineating the proximal (i.e., membrane) and distal (i.e., nuclear) events that mediate the inhibition of cell proliferation. The mechanisms whereby growth factors control cell proliferation converge at a complex regulatory scheme referred to as the cell cycle.

The mammalian cell cycle may be viewed as a series of four phases. The two gap phases, G1 and G2, allow the cell to prepare for replicative DNA synthesis during S-phases and cell division during M-phases. Progression through the cell cycle (Figure 20.2) is a choreographed series of events, culminating in cell division, which involves the expression of and interactions between cell cycle–dependent protein kinases (CDKs), kinase regulators (cyclins), and recently described CDK inhibitors (CKIs).[9-11] Sequential activation of the CDKs, mediated by binding to their specific cyclins and other regulatory proteins, promotes progression through G1, S, G2, and M. In each case, CDK activation enables the next step. Progression involves complex protein/protein interactions and is regulated by other CDKs, protein phosphatases, and transcription factors. Growth factors promote entry into the cell cycle by mechanisms that are not yet entirely clear. It appears that induction of G1 phase D-type cyclins is critical. Growth factor–dependent accumulation of D-type cyclins brings cells to a restriction (R) point, beyond which cells are committed to pro-

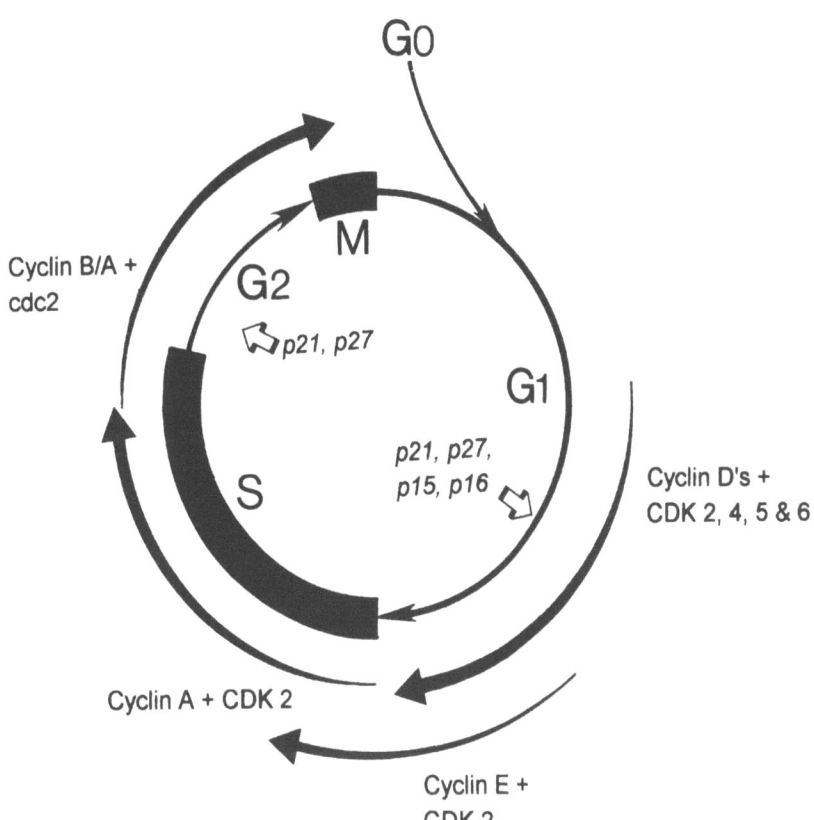

FIGURE 20.2. Interactions between cyclins, cyclin-dependent protein kinases (CDKs), and inhibitors. The loci of action of the inhibitors within the cell cycle are shown by the open arrows.

gression through S-phase and the remainder of the cell cycle.

A key substrate for cyclin D-associated CDKs (i.e., CDK4 and CDK6) is Rb, the product of the retinoblastoma gene. Rb is an inhibitor of the action of a family of transcription factors collectively termed E2F.[12,13] Upon CDK-mediated phosphorylation, Rb and related proteins dissociate from E2F, thereby allowing E2F to stimulate transcription of genes required for S-phase.[12,13]

Mechanisms for negative cell cycle control have been elucidated more recently.[11] This work developed from studies on the tumor suppressor p53. It now appears that the p53 gene product exerts its antigrowth activity by promoting the expression of a 21-kd protein (termed $p21^{Cip1}$, $p21^{Waf1}$, or p21) which binds to CDK/cyclin complexes, thereby inhibiting their activity.[11] Moreover, p21 can also be induced by a p53-independent pathway.[14] This may be particularly relevant to the cessation of cell growth associated with differentiation during development. Recent work on the induction of myogenic differentiation induced by MyoD shows correlation between cell cycle arrest and p21 induction.[15,16] Furthermore, this induction is p53-independent and its effect can be overcome by increasing expression of an active cyclin D1/CDK complex. In this system, a high level of p21 expression is associated not only with cell cycle arrest in G1, but also with quiescence associated with terminal differentiation (G0).

Since the discovery of p21, a variety of cell cycle inhibitors have been characterized. They can be categorized into two families. The first includes p21 plus p27 (Kip1) and p57 (Kip2); p27 appears to be constitutively expressed at nearly constant levels through the cell cycle.[17,18] It may provide for a "threshold" such that increasing CDK activation must overcome the level of p27 in order to result in cell cycle progression.[11] The second family of inhibitors includes $p16^{INK4}$ and its relative, p15. Interestingly, p15 is induced in response to a growth factor that often functions as a growth inhibitor, TGF-β; p15 may well mediate TGF-β–induced growth arrest.[19] While p15 and p16 are inhibitors of G1-phase CDKs, p21 and p27 can inhibit G1/S and G2/M CDKs.

One principle emerging from recent work on cell cycle regulation is that there is a very high level of complexity regarding the function of and interrelations between the multiple cyclins, CDKs and CKIs. Thus, a specific cyclin, CDK or CKI, cannot necessarily be assigned a specific role in a particular cell type. This is also true for the transcriptional regulators, which, in response to cyclins, induce expression of proteins required for cell cycle progression.

Among the cell cycle–regulated transcription factors is the E2F family.[12,13] It is composed of four members (E2F1 through 4). They are involved in the transcriptional regulation of a number of genes critical to G1/S transition, including proliferating cell nuclear antigen (PCNA), cyclin A, cdc2, cyclin E, and enzymes required for DNA synthesis including dihydrofolate reductase. Regulation of transcription by E2Fs involves interactions with Rb (the retinoblastoma protein) and related gene products. When Rb is phosphorylated by G1 CDKs, it dissociates from E2F. Free E2F then interacts with other DNA binding proteins in promoting transcription. Individual E2F family members display a temporal pattern of expression during the cell cycle, which can be used to advantage in studying cell cycle kinetics.

A generally held paradigm for growth factor regulation of the cell cycle states that competence factors [e.g., platelet-derived growth factor (PDGF), epidermal growth factor (EGF), and others] promote entry into G1 while so-called progression factors (the IGFs, insulin) support progression through G1 and entry into S. Progression may be a manifestation of augmented expression of cyclin Ds, suppression of CKIs, or both.

Differentiation

Although it may be counterintuitive to associate growth factors with promotion of cell differentiation, this is in fact a highly prevalent cellular response to these agents. Promotion of differentiation may proceed directly through the activation of gene expression in response to a growth factor signal. In addition, growth inhibition resulting from the action of a growth factor may prime cells for progression to a differentiated phenotype.

One example of the divergent effects of a single growth factor on the growth and differentiation of a single cell type is the action of IGF-I on 3T3-L1 preadipocytes.[20] These fibroblast-like cells are stimulated to proliferate in their undifferentiated state by IGF-I. However, upon growth arrest, IGF-I becomes a potent factor in the induction of differentiation to an adipocyte phenotype. Thus process involves the expression of numerous genes required for lipid storage and synthesis.

Growth factor induction of differentiation is also illustrated by the action of nerve growth factor (NGF) on PC12 cells, a rat pheochromocytoma cell line. PC12 cells, cultured under conditions that support proliferation, undergo a striking transition from an undifferentiated phenotype to one that includes the extension of dendritic processes, the capacity for electrical excitability, and the synthesis of neurotransmitters.[21] Interestingly, there is considerable evidence that the differentiating effect of NGF is mediated by pathways similar to those involved in stimulation of proliferation of these same cells by EGF.[22] However, the amplitude and duration of the signal may be critical to determination of the cellular response.

The examples cited above are representative of the numerous in vitro model systems that have contributed heavily to our understanding of the role of growth factors in promoting cell differentiation. While these model systems may involve established and, therefore, nonphysiologic cell lines, they nonetheless provide tools for studying the normal processes that occur in the developing mammalian fetus.

Apoptosis

Multicellular organisms all possess mechanisms for killing their own cells. Apoptosis is a morphologically recognizable form of physiologic cell death that is characterized by nuclear disassembly, membrane deformation (visible as "blebbing"), DNA fragmentation, and, ultimately, condensation into apoptotic bodies that are easily phagocytosed by macrophages.[23] This sequence of events allows for removal of cells without the release of cellular material, which leads to the inflammatory response associated with necrosis.

Some of the components required for the signaling events that lead to apoptosis have been identified.[24,25] Initiation of the apoptosis signal has been best characterized for Fas,[26] a receptor related to the tumor necrosis factor-α (TNF-α) receptor, and for TNF-α itself.[27] Growth factors that function in a growth inhibitor role may promote apoptosis directly. For example, members of the TGF-β family induce apoptosis in hepatocytes.[28] Whether or not this is dependent on the ability of TGF-β to inhibit cell cycle progression in these cells is unclear.

The most prevalent means by which growth factors regulate apoptosis relates to the fact that for most cells viability is dependent on the presence of growth factors and/or insulin. Hematopoietic cells are particularly susceptible to apoptosis when deprived of growth-promoting cytokines. Growth factors may function as apoptosis inhibitors during development. The IGFs would be especially suited to this role, given that the growth-maintaining effect of the IGFs is so prevalent among various cell types. It appears that many of growth stimulatory effects of the IGFs may relate to their antiapoptosis actions.[29]

During fetal development, apoptosis is clearly an essential component of normal organogenesis and morphogenesis. Its role has been well defined in several distinct areas: determination of cell populations in the developing fetal cerebral cortex,[30] the intrahepatic remodeling that results in bile duct formation,[31] and the formation of limb digits via the apoptotic loss of interdigital tissue.[32]

Cell Migration, Motility, and Morphogenesis

Developmental processes such as angiogenesis and branching morphogenesis require the control of cell migration, which, in turn, is often accompanied by changes in cell morphology. One means by which a cell's migration can be directed is for that cell to respond to a growth factor and for the growth factor, via diffusion, to be present in a concentration gradient within a tissue. In some cases, growth factors may promote cell motility. Such is the case for hepatocyte growth factor (HGF), which, when originally isolated, was also identified as scatter factor.[33] HGF can disrupt the cell–cell adhesion of multiple epithelial cell types in culture. This effect is associated with a transition from an epithelial to mesenchymal cell phenotype. HGF can promote tubular morphogenesis in culture, a process that requires a combination of cell migration, changes in cell–cell adhesion, and proliferation.

Numerous other examples illustrate the direct role growth factors play in morphogenesis. Keratinocyte growth factor (KGF) is probably required for normal development of skin, as indicated by studies in transgenic mice expressing a dominant-negative form of the KGF receptor.[34] Basic fibroblast growth factors (bFGF) is a potent mitogen for capillary endothelial cells in vitro and stimulates angiogenesis in vivo.[35] Acidic FGF (aFGF) can mediate morphologic changes in bladder epithelial cells of the kind described above for HGF.[36] Similar effects can be seen in the same cells in response to TGF-α.[37] This effect is mediated via the EGF receptor.

Normal morphogenesis also requires inhibitory signals so that growth ceases at the appropriate point. Elegant experiments using implantation of slow-release pellets containing TGF-β demonstrated a potent inhibitory effect on the growth of mammary gland ductules in the mouse.[38]

A paradigm for organogenesis in the mammalian fetus is the developing lung. As in all other cases of organogenesis, lung morphogenesis depends on epithelial-mesenchymal interactions, which are required for normal control of cell proliferation and differentiation. Important mechanisms for this interaction involve extracellular matrix proteins, their receptors, and cell–cell adhesion molecules. These mechanisms are complemented by the secretion and action of growth factors.[39] EGF, probably produced by mesenchymal cells and acting on epithelial cells, accelerates lung development. In the early phases of lung development, EGF promotes formation of tracheal and bronchial buds[40] as well as branching morphogenesis.[41] Later in gestation, EGF, functioning as an autocrine factor, promotes surfactant protein expression.[42,43] Various members of the TGF-β family may play distinct roles in lung development, including extracellular matrix protein synthesis.[39] By controlling the composition of the extracellular matrix, TGF-βs may indirectly regulate morphogenesis. TGF-β, produced by immature lung fibroblasts and acting in a paracrine manner, may impede the development of differentiated functions in alveolar epithelial cells.[44] Based on studies delineating the expression of growth factors and their receptors, it is likely that the IGFs, FGFs, and multiple cytokines also contribute to lung morphogenesis.[39] Via regulation of the expression of matrix proteins and cell–cell adhesion molecules, and by their actions on cell proliferation and acquisition of differentiated functions, these multiple factors form a web of regulatory elements that choreograph the complex process of morphogenesis.

A contrasting paradigm for morphogenesis is limb development in the vertebrate fetus. This process is initiated by development of an apical ectodermal ridge. Formation of the ridge involves the cessation of growth in surrounding cells. The maintenance of cell proliferation in the ridge has been attributed to the actions of growth factors, most notably members of the FGF family.[45] As limb development progresses, members of the TGF-β family termed bone morphogenic proteins (BMPs) induce bone formation.[45] It should be noted that the aspect of limb formation that has been best characterized thus far is the expression of genes that determine spatial relationships (e.g., polarization, dorsoventral orientation, etc.). The intercellular signaling factors that control transcription factors involved in this process is an area of intense investigation.

Growth Factor Receptors

Over the past 15 years, remarkable progress has been made in understanding the mechanisms by which growth-promoting signals are initiated at the cell surface and propagated to the nucleus where gene expression is regulated and to the ribosome where protein synthesis, necessary for cell growth is controlled. These signals involve multiple, distinct pathways that allow for signal amplication, divergence of the signal initiated by a particular growth factor, and convergence of signals initiated by multiple growth factors.

Growth factor signal initiation at the cell surface involves specific, high-affinity receptors. The seminal discovery that the oncogene src codes for a tyrosine-specific protein kinase[46] led to the observation by Carpenter and Cohen[47] that the receptor for EGF is a complex allosteric enzyme, also a tyrosine kinase, for which its primary allosteric regulator is its ligand, EGF. While multiple mechanisms for growth factor signal initiation via receptors have been identified, activation of a receptor tyrosine kinase is the most prevalent. The EGF receptor represents a prototype for this receptor subgroup (Figure 20.3). This monomeric receptor with a molecular mass of 170,000 consists of an extracellular ligand-binding domain, a transmembrane domain, and an intracellular tyrosine kinase domain. Binding of the ligand triggers receptor dimerization, tyrosine kinase activation, autophosphorylation of the tyrosine kinase domain of the receptor, and activation of the kinase toward exogenous substrates.[48] Mutation of Lys^{721}, critical to adenosine triphosphate (ATP) binding within the kinase domain, abrogates virtually all cellular responses to EGF.[49,50]

The observation that EGF signaling involved activation of a receptor tyrosine kinase led rapidly to assign-

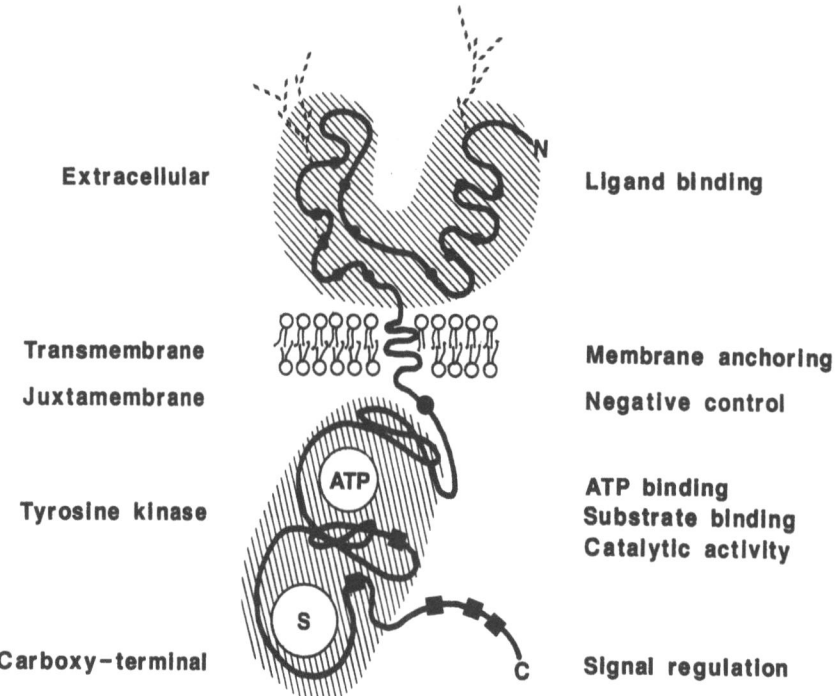

FIGURE 20.3. A schematic representation of the EGF receptor. Major structural domains are shown on the left with corresponding functions on the right. Negative control within the juxtamembrane region refers to kinase inhibition in response to phosphorylation at Thr^{654}. Signal regulation in the carboxy-terminal domain refers to sites of tyrosine autophosphorylation. Tyrosine autophosphorylation sites are shown as squares. S, substrate binding domain; N, amino-terminus; C, carboxy-terminus; ATP, adenosine triphosphate.

ment of a similar mechanism of signaling for the insulin receptor,[51] the type 1 IGF receptor,[52] the receptor for PDGF,[53] and others.[54,55] Receptor tyrosine kinases can be grouped into families based on their structural characteristics (Figure 20.4).[55] All have amino-terminal domains that are responsible for ligand binding. Structural motifs in these domains represent the most distinctive characteristics defining receptor subtypes. Other structural aspects shared by receptor tyrosine kinases include closely related tyrosine kinase domains and carboxy-terminal tails, which are involved in regulation of signal transduction.

Nonreceptor tyrosine kinases also play a role in growth factor signal transduction. Some receptors that do not contain intrinsic tyrosine kinases can signal via tyrosine phosphorylation by utilizing nonreceptor kinases, which are closely associated with the receptors themselves. Most notable are the family of Janus kinases (termed JAKS).[56] Signaling via JAKS, which is most common among cytokines, involves direct tyrosine phosphorylation of so-called STAT proteins (i.e., signal transducers and activation of transcription). Upon tyrosine phosphorylation, these proteins translocate from the cell surface to the nucleus where they act as transcriptional regulators.[56] Growth factor receptor tyrosine kinases such as the EGF receptor can signal via STAT proteins, although this may represent a direct mechanism not involving JAKS activation.[57]

Signaling via Receptor Tyrosine Kinases

Over the past 15 years, a broad range of tyrosine kinase substrates falling into three major categories have been identified: signaling enzymes, adaptor proteins, and structural proteins.[55] In all cases, substrate phosphorylation and/or activation requires binding to the receptor kinases and, in many cases, to other signaling proteins.

Upon receptor activation, binding sites for signaling proteins are generated via receptor autophosphorylation and receptor substrate phosphorylation. The resulting binding interactions depend on tyrosine phosphorylation within specific amino acid sequences and the presence of domains on the adaptor proteins. These binding domains, which have sequence homology to portions of the Src proto-oncogene product, are termed *src* homology, or SH, domains.[58] Within the *src* proto-oncogene product, the SH1 domain is the tyrosine kinase catalytic domain. SH2 and SH3 domains are noncatalytic. They interact with the phosphotyrosine contained in a specific sequence. Via SH domains, tyrosine phosphorylation induces protein–protein binding, which results in the formation of signaling complexes.

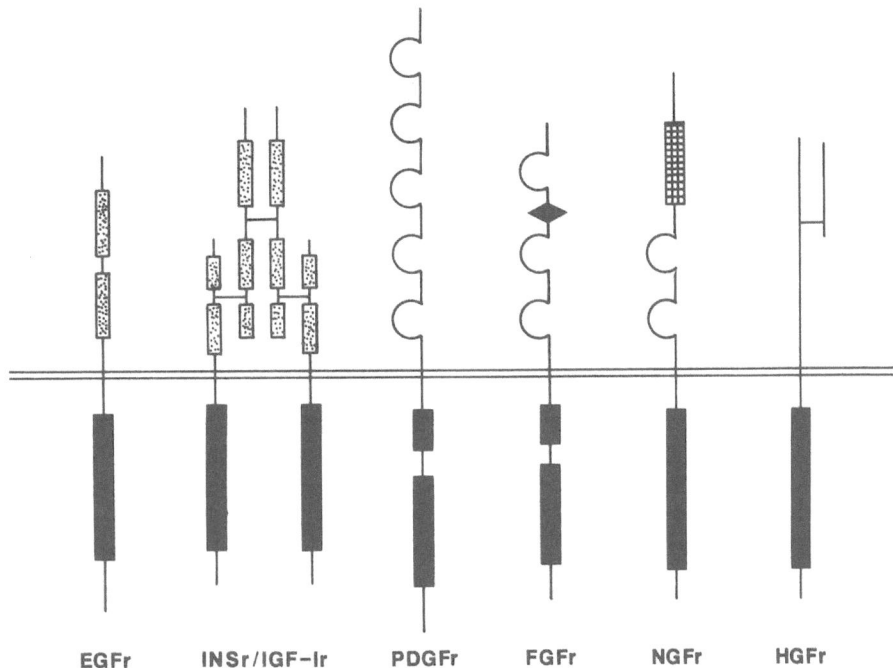

FIGURE 20.4. A schematic representation of several major classes of growth factor receptor tyrosine kinases. The double line indicates the cell membrane with the extracellular space at the top of the figure. Stippled regions represent cysteine-rich domains. Circular motifs represent immunoglobulin (Ig)-like domains. Other symbols in the extracellular region represent other distinguishing structural motifs. In the intracellular portions of the receptors, tyrosine kinase domains are represented by solid bars.

Signaling enzymes represented the first tyrosine kinase substrate category that was identified. An example is phospholipase C-$_{\gamma 1}$ (PLC$_{\gamma 1}$), which, when phosphorylated on a single tyrosine residue, is activated.[59] This enzyme catalyzes the hydrolysis of phosphatidylinositol 4,5-bisphosphate, resulting in the generation of two second messengers: diacylglycerol, an activator of members of the protein kinase C family, and inositol 1,4,5-trisphosphate, which causes release of calcium from intracellular stores. PLC$_{\gamma 1}$ contains SH2 and SH3 domains, which are required for their ability to function as tyrosine kinase substrates.

Another signaling enzyme activated in response to growth factor receptors is phosphatidylinositol 3-kinase (PI 3-kinase). This enzyme is a heterodimer consisting of a 110-kd catalytic subunit and an 85-kd regulatory subunit.[60] The regulatory subunit contains SH2 and SH3 domains.[61-63] Its tyrosine phosphorylation results in activation of the catalytic subunit. While it is established that PI 3-kinase activation results in phosphorylation of multiple phosphorylated phosphoinositides on the D-3 position, the resulting signal transduction mechanism has not yet been elucidated.

A third signaling enzyme is termed *ras*GAP. It activates the guanosine triphosphatase (GTPase) activity of the small G-protein, Ras. This mechanism is involved in the normal inactivation of Ras.[64] The activation of Ras, a critical step in growth factor stimulation of mitogenesis, involves the tyrosine phosphorylation of noncatalytic adaptor proteins.[65]

So-called adaptor proteins represent the second class of receptor tyrosine kinase substrates. Their tyrosine phosphorylation leads to formation of large, multiprotein complexes that have been referred to as signaling particles. Adaptor proteins involved in Ras activation include Shc, Grb2, and SOS. Grb2 and SOS are bound to one another under basal conditions. Grb2, which contains SH2 and SH3 domains, is recruited to the plasma membrane via its direct interaction with growth factor receptors or its interaction with the adaptor protein, Shc.[55] Once translocated to the plasma membrane, SOS can trigger Ras guanosine triphosphate (GTP)-for-guanosine diphosphate (GDP) exchange, resulting in Ras activation. This leads to recruitment of a protein kinase to the plasma membrane that becomes activated. In this manner activation of the mitogen-activated protein (MAP) kinase signaling cascade is triggered (Figure 20.5).[66]

The remainder of the MAP kinase system has been largely characterized in the past several years.[67,68] Raf phosphorylates an intermediary kinase termed MAP or Erk kinase (MEK), which, when phosphorylated, is a

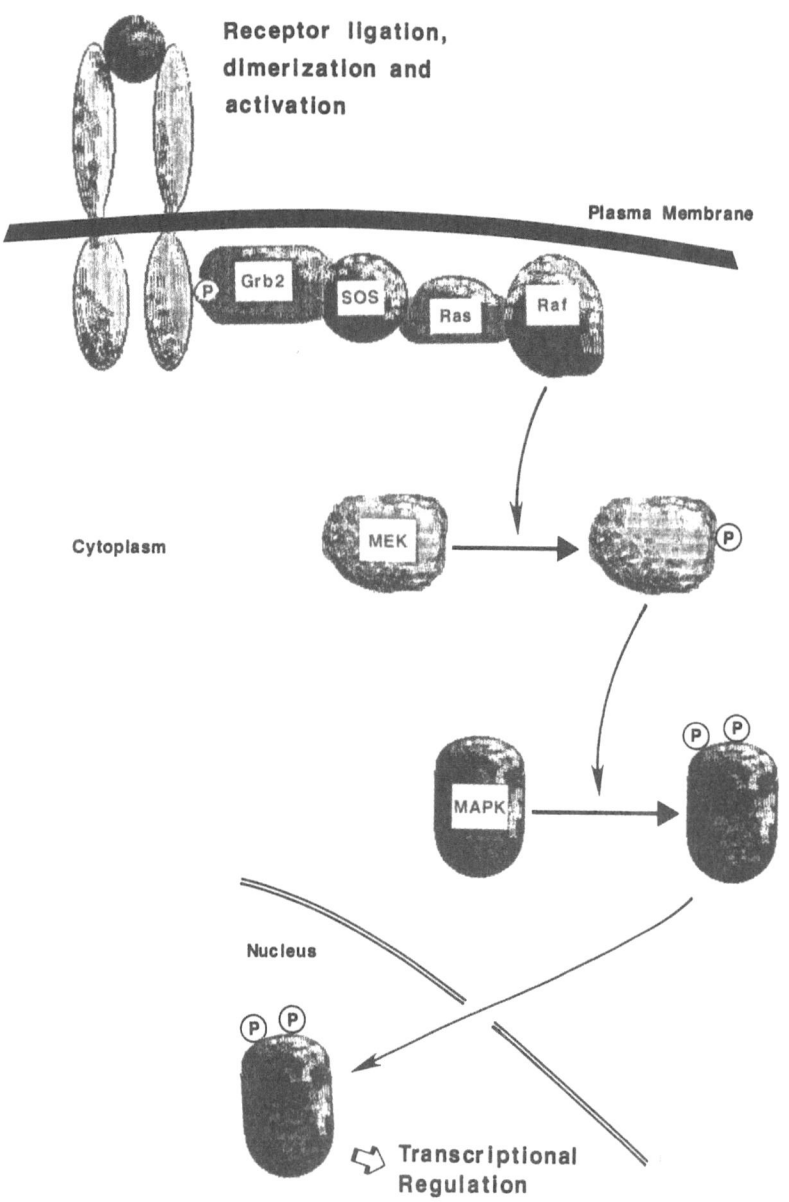

FIGURE 20.5. A model for receptor tyrosine kinase signaling via the Ras/MAP kinase pathway. Receptor ligand binding (top) promotes receptor dimerization and autophosphorylation. Shown here is direct binding of the adaptor protein, Grb2, to the tyrosine phosphorylated receptor. Alternatively, another adaptor protein, Shc, may be tyrosine phosphorylated, resulting in formation of a signaling complex that includes Shc, Grb2, Sos, and Ras. Ras activation, resulting from a GTP-for-GDP exchange, results in translocation of Raf to the plasma membrane. Activation of Raf, a serine/threonine kinase, triggers phosphorylation and activation of MEK. This, in turn, leads to phosphorylation and activation of MAP kinase. Upon translocation to the nucleus, activated MAP kinase can effect transcriptional regulation via phosphorylation of multiple transcription factors.

bifunctional kinase that can phosphorylate MAP kinases on both threonine and tyrosine. This dual phosphorylation results in MAP kinase activation.

The Jun N-terminal kinase (JNK) system is in many ways analogous to the MAP kinase (MAPK) system.[68] JNK was originally identified in parallel by two laboratories as a cyclohexamide-induced or ultraviolet (UV)-induced kinase with specificity for the N-terminal region of c-Jun. Subsequently, JNK was identified as activated in response to TNF-α and interleukin-1 (IL-1). More recent data indicate that TNF-α–mediated activation of JNK may be a required immediate event in liver regeneration following partial hepatectomy in the rat, thus indicating an assigned role in cell cycle entry by normal cells.[69] Unlike the MAP kinase system, multiple JNKs are active in late gestation, developing fetal rat liver.[70]

The actions of the MAPK and JNK signaling pathways are pleiotropic, involving effects at the cell membrane, ribosome, and nucleus, and in the cytoplasm. Substrates for these protein kinase cascades include a variety of effector molecules including other protein kinases, protein phosphatases, enzymes, cytoskeletal elements, ribosomal proteins, and transcription factors. Perhaps the most important downstream mitogenic signaling mechanism is regulation of gene expression by phosphorylation of DNA-binding proteins. One of these downstream ef-factors is the activator protein-1 (AP-1) transcription factor, originally shown to mediate induction of a program of genes in response to a wide variety of stimulants including mitogens, oncogenes, protein kinase C agonists, and cellular stress treatments such as UV light and TNF-α.[71] Subsequent to the discovery of AP-1 activity, it was found that AP-1 was composed of products of the *jun* and *fos* gene families.[72] DNA binding of Fos requires Jun. Also, Jun homodimers and heterodimers (e.g., cJun:JunD) can form Ap-1 complexes in the absence of Fos. Multisite phosphorylation of Jun is the mechanism whereby transcriptional activity of AP-1 is rapidly regulated.[73] It is the N-terminal transcriptional activation sites on Jun that are substrates for JNK.[74] In contrast, the multiple kinases that phosphorylate the Jun C-terminal region are Jun transcriptional inactivators.

The physiologic modulation of mitogenic signaling occurs at multiple levels. Receptor tyrosine kinases can be regulated by a number of distinct and separate mechanisms. Ligand binding to these receptors promotes their internalization. Once internalized, receptors can be degraded or recycled to the cell surface. Thus, cell surface receptor number is a function of receptor synthesis, degradation and recycling.[75] Once receptor-to-ligand binding occurs, the intracellular receptor tyrosine kinase is activated. It has been known for some time that receptor kinase activity can be modified by receptor serine/threonine phosphorylation.[76] The best characterized systems demonstrating this mechanism for receptor kinase modulation are the insulin and EGF receptor systems. In both cases, activation of protein kinase C (PK-C) can lead to receptor phosphorylation with kinase inactivation. Cytokines, such as TNF-α, can induce insulin resistance by decreasing insulin receptor tyrosine kinase activity.[77] Other serine/threonine kinases, including the MAP kinases, can phosphorylate the intracellular domains of these receptors.

Signal transduction by an activated receptor tyrosine kinase can be modified by altered expression or function of downstream effectors, including insulin receptor species-1 (IRS-1) in the case of insulin or Ras. An example of the latter is the disassembly of the Ras nucleotide exchange factor, SOS, from Grb2 during desensitization of Ras signaling by insulin.[78] More recently, it has been demonstrated that the MAPK signaling pathway is subject to negative feedback inhibition.[79] One mechanism accounting for this appears to be phosphorylation SOS by MAPK which leads to inhibition of Ras activation.[80] A novel mechanism for downstream modulation of the MAP kinase pathway has been observed in the fetal rat.[70] While hepatic EGF signaling can be initiated in vivo in the late gestation fetal rat following intraperitoneal injection of EGF, MAP kinase is not activated. This uncoupling of the MAP kinase pathway may represent feedback inhibition resulting from the growth factor–rich environment in the fetus.

In summary, the multiple and diverse signaling pathways utilized by growth factors are regulated in a complex manner. This regulation allows for interaction between the effects of multiple factors. Modulation of growth factor signaling represents a mechanism beyond growth factor expression and receptor expression for modifying growth factor effects during development.

Specific Growth Factors and Growth Factor Families

Epidermal Growth Factor (EGF)/Transforming Growth Factor-α (TGF-α)

Epidermal growth factor was originally identified by Cohen[81] as a fraction purified from mouse submaxillary glands that accelerated eyelid opening and tooth eruption when injected into newborn mice. Its subsequent purification showed it to be a 53 amino acid peptide with a conserved 40 amino acid region containing three disulphide bonds.[82] This region forms a characteristic "active site" required for interaction with the EGF receptor. The human analogue of mouse EGF (hEGF) was originally isolated from human urine as a factor, termed urogastrone, which could inhibit gastric acid secretion.[83] Thirty-seven of its 53 amino acids are identical to those in mouse EGF.

EGF is synthesized as a 1217 amino acid precursor that is encoded by a 4.9-kb mRNA. The 110-kb gene from which this is derived is located on chromosome 4q.[84] The EGF precursor contains a hydrophobic region that allows it to be anchored in cell membranes. Given the great variability in EGF precursor processing between tissues, it is likely that the precursor sometimes functions as a "juxtacrine" factor.

The work that led Todaro and DeLarco[85] to identify TGF-α was based on the observation that cellular transformation is associated with a decreased requirement for serum and exogenous growth factors. They identified a transforming activity that could be derived from the culture medium of murine sarcoma virus-transformed rat kidney cells. Roberts et al.[86] went on to separate this transforming activity into two components, subsequently termed TGF-α and TGF-β. The purification and molecular cloning of TGF-α identified a peptide that has 44% homology to human EGF and that signals via the EGF receptor.[87,88] Like EGF, TGF-α is synthesized as a precursor that is cleaved to generate mature TGF-α after it reaches the cell membrane.[89] This cleavage is highly regulated,[90] and there is considerable evidence that membrane-associated TGF-α precursor acts in a juxtacrine role as both a signaling protein and a mediator of cell–cell adhesion.[91]

Other members of the EGF/TGF-α family include amphiregulan,[92] heparin-binding EGF,[93] cripto,[94] and betacellulin.[95] All were isolated from tumor cells and are able to signal via the EGF receptor. Their varied tissue distributions and potent growth-stimulating activities make it very likely that they play a critical role in normal fetal development.

As members of the EGF/TGF-α family, these peptides are potent mitogens for mesenchymal and epithelial cells. They share a probable role in cell–cell adhesion based on the ability of EGF-like repeats to mediate the formation of stable protein–protein complexes. Since they share the EGF receptor as a mediator for their mitogenic activity, the development of mice containing a null allele at the EGF receptor locus was of particular interest.

Threadgill et al.[96] used gene targeting to develop such "EGF receptor knockout" mice. The resulting phenotype was found to be dependent on the strain of mice used. This was fortuitous in that the variety of lethal mutants that resulted permitted broad insight into the developmental roles of the EGF/TGF-α family members. EGF receptor deficiency in CF-1 mice resulted in peri-implantation death. However, mutant 129/Sv mice survived until mid-gestation. Death in these fetuses resulted from placental defects. Placentas were small with specific and marked reduction in the size of the spongiotrophoblast layer. Most interestingly, CD-1 embryos homozygous for the EGF receptor null mutation survived for up to 3 weeks after birth. Birth weight was normal. However, severe postnatal wasting was observed. Abnormalities in skin and tooth development, predicted by Cohen's original studies identifying EGF, were observed. The gastrointestinal tract showed minor alterations. Liver size was normal, although architectural abnormalities were observed. Analysis of kidney structure indicated that induction of the metanephric blastema was normal, while differentiation of structures derived from the ureteric bud was markedly impaired. Central nervous system development was abnormal in that cortical regions showed decreased cellularity. Of note, lungs of these mice were grossly normal. Lung surfactant protein expression and production were also normal. These results should be interpreted against a background of high redundancy in growth factor function during development. On the other hand, they imply a significant role for EGF/TGF-α family members in the development of multiple organ systems.

Insulin-Like Growth Factors (IGFs), IGF-I and IGF-II

The "somatomedin" hypothesis proposed by Salmon and Daughaday[97] in 1957 stated that the growth-promoting action of growth hormone is mediated by a growth factor. The parallel isolation and characterization of IGF-I and the main growth hormone mediator, somatomedin-C, revealed that they are identical.[98,99] Subsequent isolation of IGF-II showed approximately 70% sequence homology with IGF-I.[100] In addition, both IGF-I and IGF-II were found to have high homology with proinsulin. Like proinsulin, IGF-I and IGF-II contain A and B domains. Unlike mature insulin, a C domain is retained. In addition, an 8 amino acid D domain is present at the carboxy-terminus.

The human IGF-I gene, located on chromosome 12, is composed of 5 exons. Via alternative splicing, two messenger RNAs (mRNAs) are generated, IGF-Ia and IGF-Ib.[101] The differences in the resulting peptides are within a carboxy-terminal E-domain (i.e., 35 amino acids for IGF-Ia and 77 amino acids for IGF-Ib). In the rat, a species used for a great deal of the research on IGFs, considerable heterogeneity in the size of IGF-I transcripts has been observed. While this is developmentally regulated and tissue specific, the physiologic significance of the various transcripts is unclear.[102]

The human IGF-II gene, located on chromosome 11, is paternally imprinted.[103] That is, only the paternal IGF-II gene is active in the offspring with the maternal allele being inactivated. The IGF-II gene codes for a 67 amino acid peptide which, like IGF-I, contains B, C, A, D, and E domains.

While circulating IGF-I is mostly of hepatic origin in the postnatal mammal, as reviewed by Froesch et al.,[104] the IGF-I gene is ubiquitously expressed. The growth hormone dependency of hepatic IGF-I production accounts for the central role of growth hormone in regulating postnatal circulating IGF-I concentrations. In addition, circulating levels of IGF-I are highly influenced by nutritional status and insulin sufficiency.[105-107] The postnatal regulation of IGF-I expression in extrahepatic tissues is, in contrast, multifactorial and highly variable. Tissue-specific examples of IGF-I regulation include the stimulation of its expression in adrenal tissue by adrenocorticotropic hormone (ACTH),[108] and gonadotropins in the gonads.[109]

In the fetus, IGF-II expression exceeds that of IGF-I in most tissues.[110] In contrast, IGF-II expression in the postnatal rat is negligible. In addition, the expression of IGF-II is not growth hormone dependent nor can it be clearly related to nutritional status. From a developmental standpoint, IGF-I may be viewed as a hormonally and nutritionally regulated mediator of growth in the postnatal mammal while IGF-II may be considered an oncofetal, autocrine/paracrine growth factor. This generalization belies the complex nature of the regulation of IGF expression and action. Furthermore, the tissue-specific regulation of IGF-I expression and the co-localization of its production and action requires a broader view of IGF physiology.

The primary cellular action of the IGFs is their mitogenic effect as mediated by the IGF-I, or type I IGF, receptor.[29] While the affinity of the IGF-I receptor for IGF-I is higher than for IGF-II, considerable data indicate that the mitogenic effects of the latter are mediated via this receptor. The IGF-I receptor, originally isolated from human placenta, was found to have structural similarity to the insulin receptor, while having relatively low affinity for insulin.[111] Once cloned, it was confirmed that the IGF-I receptor shares considerable stuctural homology with the insulin receptor, especially in the intracellular, β subunit tyrosine kinase domain, which has 80% sequence homology with the insulin receptor.[112]

The promoter region for the IGF-I receptor gene contains sequences similar to those found both in "housekeeping" genes (i.e., those generally required for normal cellular function) and highly regulated promoters.[113] Expression of the gene occurs in nearly all tissues and in all cell types in culture. The mature receptor, once translated, exhibits considerable heterogeneity. Those forms resulting from altered β-subunit splicing display differential expression during development.[114] The alternative structure that predominates during fetal and early postnatal life (i.e., a 105-, rather than 95-kd β subunit) may have a reduced rate of receptor internalization, thereby augmenting IGF mitogenic signaling.[115] The basis for many other forms of IGF-I receptor heterogeneity have been identified.[116] One form of receptor heterogeneity of particular interest is a hybrid IGF-I/insulin receptor chimera that was identified as IGF-I–binding activity, which could interact with insulin receptor antibodies.[117] The existence of such a receptor may have important physiologic implications for the mitogenic action of insulin and/or the metabolic actions of the IGFs.

The physiologic action of the IGF-I receptor differs from that of the insulin receptor in that the former shows much greater mitogenic potency.[29,116] While signaling pathways that mediate the effects of both receptors have been identified,[116] the molecular basis for the greater mitogenic activity of the IGF-I receptor is still not clear. Like the insulin receptor, the IGF-I receptor interacts with IRS-1.[118] It is probable that the mitogenic activity of the IGFs requires IGF-I receptor-mediated activation of the Ras/MAP kinase pathway, perhaps between a direct interaction between the receptor and Shc.[119] Other signaling pathways that may be required for or involved in mitogenic signaling are activated in response to activation of the IGF-I receptor.[29,116]

As will be discussed below, targeted disruption of the IGF-I receptor gene results in intrauterine growth retardation.[120,121] Interestingly, fibroblasts from these mice showed retarded rates of progression through the cell cycle.[29] Overexpression of the receptors for EGF or PDGF could not substitute for the lack of IGF-I receptor expression.[29] It may be that the IGFs, via the IGF-I receptor, can modulate the rate of cell cycle progression, thus controlling overall rates of cell proliferation. This action could account for the central role that the IGFs seem to play in governing the growth of an organism. This may also account for the interdependence of growth, in general, on other growth factors since expression of the IGF-I receptor is regulated by growth factors including PDGF and basic fibroblast growth factor (bFGF).

The IGF system is made profoundly complex by the panoply of proteins other than the IGF-I receptor that can bind IGF-I and IGF-II. In addition to a family of IGF binding proteins vide infra, there exists the so-called type II IGF receptor (or the IGF-II receptor). It binds IGF-II preferentially while binding IGF-I with a relatively low affinity compared to the IGF-I receptor.[122,123] It does not bind insulin. Unlike the IGF-I receptor, the IGF-II receptor is composed of a single subunit. The assignment of a biologic role in IGF action to the IGF-II receptor was an area of considerable controversy for several years. One difficulty was an inability to determine a potential signaling mechanism, since the IGF-II receptor seemed to possess no intrinsic tyrosine kinase activity. The controversy took an unanticipated turn when molecular cloning showed the cation-independent mannose-6-phosphate (M6P) receptor and the IGF-II receptor to be identical.[124] Thus, the IGF-II/M6P receptor can be considered to have lysosomal-targeting properties. A potential signaling mechanism mediated via stimulation of the influx of calcium into the cell may provide for IGF signaling via the IGF-II receptor.[125] However, no conclusive evidence has been found that provides for a direct mitogenic signaling mechanism via the IGF-II receptor.

In addition to the IGF-I and IGF-II receptors, cells may possess, as noted above, a hybrid IGF-I/insulin receptor. Since these two receptors share considerable structure, the possibility of receptors consisting of an IGF-I receptor αβ dimer plus an insulin receptor αβ dimer was proposed. Several strategies were used to demonstrate that such hybrids could be synthesized in cultured cells.[116] In addition, they were isolated from human placental membranes.[126] While their existence in normal cells is plausible, the role of these receptors in determining the growth versus metabolic actions of the IGFs is uncertain.

Insulin-like growth factors in the circulation and extracellular space are present in a bound form. To date, six IGF-binding proteins (IGFBPs) have been identified, cloned, and characterized. All share structural features, especially in cysteine-rich regions, that account for the capacity to bind IGFs but not insulin.[127] They serve several potential functions including roles as IGF transport proteins, involvement in the control of IGF efflux from the vascular space, the regulation of metabolic clearance of the IGFs, and modulation of the interaction between the IGFs and their receptors.[127] While IGFBPs have been observed most often to inhibit interaction between IGFs and IGF receptors,[128] IGFBP-1 and -3 can augment IGF action in culture.[129] In addition, recent evidence indicates that some of the IGFBPs may have their own role as signaling molecules.

The IGFBPs are synthesized in virtually all cells and tissues that synthesize IGFs. Their expression varies among tissues and under different physiologic conditions, which contributes to the complexity of the IGF system. IGFBP-1, originally purified from amniotic fluid, is produced in liver, kidney, and other tissues in a non–growth hormone–dependent manner.[128] Production of this 25-kd protein is, in general, inversely related to insulin concentration or effect. It may both inhibit and augment IGF action.[127] IGFBP-2, expression of which is particularly high in the fetal rat, is the most abundant IGFBP in cerebrospinal fluid.[130] Its actions have been less well studied than those of IGFBP-1. IGFBP-3, a 46- to 53-kd glycoprotein, accounts for the bound form in which IGFs circulate. Its levels in serum are highly regulated by growth hormone. In addition to its ability to either inhibit or augment IGF action, depending on the system studied,[127] IGFBP-3 may have direct cell signaling properties.[131,132] IGFBP-4, classified as a "low molecular weight IGFBP" along with IGFBP-1 and -2,[127] appears to function as an inhibitor of IGF action. IGFBP-5 is unusual in its ability to adhere to fibroblast extracellular matrix. When localized in this manner, it may augment IGF action.[127] Studies on the actions of IGFBP-6, which has 10-fold higher affinity for IGF-II than for IGF-I, are still quite limited.

The important developmental role of the IGFs in the postimplantation mammalian embryo is suggested by the ubiquitous expression of the IGF-1 receptor. Levels are especially high in the developing nervous system and muscle.[133] However, the developmental role of the IGFs has been best demonstrated through a series of elegant experiments conducted by Efstratiadis and colleagues.[120,121,134,135] By using targeted gene disruption and intercrossing the resulting "knockout" strains, phenotypes suggesting the overall growth regulatory role of the IGF system in fetal development were obtained. The results of these studies, summarized in Table 20.1, have been thoroughly reviewed by several investigators.[29,127,136] It can be concluded that IGF-I and IGF-II, acting via the IGF-I receptor, are required for normal growth of the developing mouse. Their actions are most pronounced during the latter half of gestation. The growth inhibition observed with disruption of this system is generalized, indicating that the IGFs may govern the overall rate of growth of the developing conceptus. Such a role would be consistent with the observation that human fetal serum IGF-1 concentrations correlate with mid-gestation fetal size.[137]

Platelet-Derived Growth Factor (PDGF)

The observation that supplementation of culture medium with serum supported cell proliferation more effectively than plasma supplementation first suggested the existence of platelet-derived mitogens.[138,139] Platelets are a rich source of mitogenic factors, including TGF-β and EGF. The primary mitogen isolated from human platelets was originally termed platelet-derived growth factor (PDGF).[140] Biochemical characterization of PDGF quickly demonstrated multiple forms.[141,142] Unreduced, these proteins exist as dimeric peptides. Further characterization of human PDGF showed that the three possible dimers consisting of A (12kd) and B (18kd) chains (AA, AB, and BB) occur naturally.[143] It appears that the dimeric association of the two chains is random. However, the differing structures of the A and B chains determine a fundamental difference between the resulting PDGF molecules; while PDGF-AA is a secreted protein, PDGF-BB remains associated with intracellular membranes.[144]

Platelet-derived growth factor receptors are present in a wide range of mesenchymal cells.[145] There are two types, α and β, which are encoded on separate genes.

TABLE 20.1. The phenotype of mice with IGF and IGF receptor gene deletions accomplished by targeted disruption through homologous recombination.

Deleted gene	Percent of normal birth weight	Phenotype
IGF-I	60	Small, otherwise normal
IGF-II	60	Small with placental hypoplasia
IGF-I + IGF-II	30	Postnatal respiratory death, placental hypoplasia
IGF-Ir	45	Postnatal respiratory death
IGF-I + IGF-Ir	45	Postnatal respiratory death
IGF-IIr	—	In utero death
IGF-II + IGF-IIr	60	Survival to birth

IGF-Ir, IGF-I receptor; IGF-IIr, IGF-II receptor.
Adapted from Rubin and Baserga[29] and Jones and Clemmons.[127]

While structurally similar, they display distinct ligand affinities.[146,147] The α-receptor binds PDGF A and B chains, while the β-receptor binds only the B chain. The receptor binding of dimeric PDGF promotes receptor dimerization, an initiating step in signal transduction.[148] The divergent structures of the PDGF α- and β-receptors appears to account for distinct biologic effects. Both α- and β-receptors can stimulate cell proliferation, but only β-receptors mediate chemotaxis and membrane ruffling.[149] Since the two receptor forms have different ligand affinities, the difference in receptor signaling confers different biologic actions on the various forms of PDGF.

The primary biologic role of PDGF is to promote cell proliferation. Elegant studies by Olashaw et al.[150] demonstrate that brief exposure of immortalized fibroblasts to PDGF induced a state of competence characterized by entry into G1. Transition through the remainder of the cell cycle then requires the action of so-called progression factors, including EGF and the IGFs. The proliferation of trophoblasts in the first trimester human placenta may represent an example of PDGF-mediated autocrine growth stimulation.[151]

In addition to its mitogenic actions, PDGF acts as a chemoattractant for fibroblasts and smooth muscle cells. It promotes the synthesis of connective tissue matrix proteins. These actions are of obvious importance in the process of wound healing. It is certain that the action of PDGF is central to promoting these processes during embryogenesis and organogenesis. Based on the phenotype displayed by a naturally occurring mutation in the PDGF α-receptor, PDGF is probably required for development of visceral endoderm and mesoderm early in gestation.[152,153] As development proceeds, a role in nervous system development is likely.

The Transforming Growth Factor-β (TGF-β) Family

As noted above for TGF-α, TGF-β was first isolated as a growth promoting, autocrine factor in virus-transformed cells.[85,86] Subsequent purification and molecular cloning identified three closely related mammalian isoforms of TGF-β, designated TGF-$β_1$, -$β_2$, and -$β_3$.[154] TGF-$β_4$ and -$β_5$ were subsequently identified in chickens and frog oocytes, respectively. All of the TGF-βs share common structural features. They are synthesized and secreted in an inactive precursor form that is proteolytically processed to active, disulfide-linked homodimers of about 25 kd. All seem to possess similar biologic activities.

The development of an in vitro model for gonadotropin secretion led to the purification of a long-postulated, gonad-derived inhibitor of this pituitary function. The factor purified from ovarian follicular fluid, inhibin, has structural homology with TGF-β.[155] The active form is an αβ heterodimer, the β subunit of which exists in two forms, A and B. Additional fractions isolated during the purification of inhibin were found to contain related factors, termed "activin."[156] Surprisingly, activin was found to be a dimer of inhibin β subunits (AA, AB, or BB). In the pituitary gland and gonads, inhibin and activin have contrary actions. While inhibin blocks pituitary follicle-stimulating hormone (FSH) secretion and stimulated gonadal steroidogenesis, activin stimulates the former and inhibits the latter.[157,158]

The classic studies of Jost et al.[159] showed that müllerian duct regression in the female was mediated by a nonsteroidal factor produced by the fetal testis. This "antimüllerian hormone" was later purified, cloned and sequenced, thus demonstrating that müllerian inhibitory substance (MIS) is a member of the TGF-β family.[160] MIS, like the TGF-βs, is synthesized as a large dimer that undergoes proteolytic processing, resulting in an active 25-kd homodimer that probably represents the mature, active form.

It is likely that the proteolytic activation of TGF-β family members is a highly regulated process. Latent TGF-β can bind to the IGF-II receptor. This may be required for lysosomal processing of TGF-β precursor.[161] Regulation of TGF-β processing is made all the more important by the ubiquitous distribution of these factors and their receptors.

Members of the TGF-β family are unusual for their ability to stimulate or inhibit cell proliferation, depending on the phenotype of the target cell. In general, mesenchymal cells respond to TGF-β by displaying anchorage-independent growth (i.e., a primary characteristic of cellular transformation). However, this effect may depend on the induction of autocrine growth factors, rather than resulting from direct TGF-β signaling.[162] In contrast, it appears that the growth inhibitory effect of TGF-β on numerous epithelial cell types is direct. However, elucidation of the mechanism for TGF-β growth inhibitory signaling has been difficult.

Three TGF-β receptors were initially described, based on affinity labeling of cell membranes with ^{125}I-TGF-β.[163] The largest of these, the type III TGF-β receptor, is a 280- to 330-kd proteoglycan that has no intracellular signaling domain.[164] The type II receptor may modulate TGF-β biologic availability. Signaling appears to depend on a heterodimeric complex of the 65-kd type I and 85- to 95-kd type II receptors.[165] Both receptor types possess serine/threonine kinase activity.[166,167] It appears that signaling involves intramolecular self-phosphorylation of the type I/II heterodimer followed by phosphorylation of as-yet undefined receptor substrates.

While downstream signaling by TGF-β has not been definitively characterized, multiple signaling pathways have been implicated. A recent development likely to be of great significance is the observation that TGF-β–induced growth inhibition may be mediated by activation of the expression of the cell cycle inhibitor, p15^{INK4B}.[168] Such a mechanism could account for the timing of TGF-β–induced growth arrest (late G1) as well as numerous observations characterizing the phosphorylation of cell cycle proteins induced by TGF-β. Recent evidence suggests the existence of a specific TGF-β response element in the promoter for the cell cycle inhibitor, p21.[169] It is possible that TGF-β may induce growth arrest via regulation of the expression of multiple cyclin-dependent kinase inhibitors.[170] It is likely that growth inhibition in response to TGF-β will depend on direct downregulation of the expression of other proliferative genes, including c-myc and cyclins.[170]

From a developmental standpoint, the regulation of disparate cellular processes other than cell proliferation by TGF-β family members may be key. A survey of TGF-β–mediated biologic actions that could profoundly affect development includes induction of fibronectin and collagen synthesis,[171] regulation of cell migration via chemotaxis,[172] control of osteoblast function and cartilage formation,[173,174] regulation of cell adhesion,[175] induction of apoptosis,[28] and stimulation of angiogenesis.[176]

The Fibroblast Growth Factor (FGF) Family

The FGFs were first discovered by Gospodarowicz et al.,[177,178] who found mitogenic activity toward fibroblasts in extracts of brain and pituitary. The functional specificity of activities within the extracts resulted in isolation of the two primary growth factors in this family, acidic and basic FGF (aFGF, bFGF). Subsequently, five other members were identified based on structural homology with aFGF and bFGF (Table 20.2).[179] Members of the family are produced in a broad spectrum of tissues, including embryonic tissues. While they are mitogenic for fibroblasts, they have a broad spectrum of target cell types as well as actions beyond stimulation of cell proliferation.[180,181]

Among the nine known FGFs, there is considerable structural variability.[182] The family members range in size from 17 to 38 kd. They share only 14% sequence homology. Nonetheless, the human FGFs show considerable cross-species activity as well as cross-reactivity with the four members of the FGF receptor family.

Keratinocyte growth factor (KGF) is unusual among the FGF family members in that it is a mitogen only for epithelial cells.[183] It binds only to the FGF receptor termed FGF-R2, a receptor whose expression is limited to epithelial cells.

The isolation of high-affinity FGF receptors was made difficult by the ability of FGFs to bind heparin, heparan sulfate, and other cationic mucopolysaccharides with high affinity. This led to the alternative designation of FGF family members as heparin-binding growth factors.[180] While the physiologic significance of binding to heparin itself is questionable, it is generally accepted that cationic mucopolysaccharides in the extracellular matrix are involved in FGF ligand-receptor interactions under normal physiologic conditions. The liberation of FGFs from extracellular matrix by heparinase or plasmin may account for a regulatory mechanism controlling the bioavailability of previously synthesized FGFs.[180] Indeed, heparan sulfate binding appears to be required for FGF biologic activity.[184,185]

There are at least 16 FGF family receptors derived as splice variants from four FGF receptor genes.[186] The receptors have intrinsic tyrosine kinase activity. In some cases, cell surface binding of FGF to FGF receptors leads to nuclear translocation of the ligand-receptor complex.[187] Nuclear translocation appears, in these cases, to correlate with mitogenic activity. The complexity of FGF receptor expression is associated with modulation of

TABLE 20.2. Members of the fibroblast growth factor (FGF) family.

FGF	Alternative name	Sites of production
1	Acidic FGF	Neurons, hepatocytes, fibroblasts, keratinocytes, smooth muscle, endothelium
2	Basic FGF	Fibroblasts, macrophages, neurons, keratinocytes, embryonic meso- and ectoderm, others
3	int-2	Embryonic tissues, breast carcinoma
4	hst-1	Embryonic tissues, breast carcinoma
5	Kaposi's growth factor	Embryonic tissues, Kaposi's sarcoma-derived cells
6	hst-2	Embryonic and postnatal skeletal muscle
7	Keratinocyte growth factor	Fibroblasts, uterine smooth muscle, embryonic mesenchymal cells
8	Androgen-induced	Embryonic mesoderm (mouse only)
9	Glia activating factor	Glial cell line

From Baird and Bohlen.[181]

FGF effect. Cells can express more than one receptor isoforms, and some of these isoforms may act as FGF antagonists.[179]

Members of the FGF family have a broad spectrum of biologic activities, all of which relate to fetal development. FGF-6 can induce myoblast proliferation while inhibiting differentiation.[188,189] Branching morphogenesis and alveoli formation in the developing lung appear to involve FGF-7.[190] FGF-4 may be the principal stimulus for mesenchymal differentiation in limb development.[191] Finally, the critical developmental process of angiogenesis may be dependent on FGF action, with these growth factors largely accounting for the "angiogenesis factor" activity described by Folkman.[192]

Nerve Growth Factor (NGF)

Bueker[193] first demonstrated the presence of a diffusible factor in mouse sarcoma tissue, which could stimulate the outgrowth of sensory ganglia. Interestingly, Cohen[194] discovered EGF based on studies of the biologic effects of mouse submaxillary gland extracts, a tissue he found to be a rich source of NGF. As purified from this source, NGF is present in an inactive, 130- to 140-kd (7S) complex. The entire 7S complex consists of two α, two β, and two γ subunits. The active 2.5S NGF preparation from mouse submaxillary glands is a homodimer of the 13-kd β subunits.[195]

The rat pheochromocytoma PC12 cell line has provided an excellent tool for studying NGF action. These cells differentiate into a sympathetic neuronal phenotype upon treatment with NGF. It was from these cells that the two proteins of 75 and 140kd that form the high-affinity NGF receptor were isolated.[196] One of these (p140) was subsequently shown to be a product of the *trk* proto-oncogene and to have tyrosine kinase activity.[197,198] Downstream signaling by NGF in PC12 cells involves Ras and MAP kinase activation, as is usually associated with mitogenic factors.[199] As noted above, NGF is a differentiating factor, not a mitogen, for these cells. The differences in action may be a reflection of differences in the kinetics of activation of mitogenic signaling. In addition, the divergent signaling pathways activated by the NGF receptor may differ from those activated by mitogenic receptor tyrosine kinases.

As indicated by the original studies that led to the identification of NGF, this polypeptide is a diffusible, neurotrophic factor. It exerts its effects on sympathetic and sensory neurons, promoting survival, differentiation, and axonal outgrowth. It is unlikely that NGF exerts a physiologic, mitogenic effect. Injection of antibodies directed at NGF into fetal rats leads to regression of sympathetic and dorsal root ganglia.[200] No such effect is seen postnatally. Conversely, injection of similar neutralizing antibodies in the chick embryo attenuates normal neuronal loss via apoptosis in spinal ganglia.[201] Additional evidence indicates that NGF functions as a diffusible, chemoattractant for developing neurons.[202] This may indicate that peripheral tissues can produce NGF, thereby promoting the neuronal outgrowth required for sensory and sympathetic innervation.

Hepatocyte Growth Factor (HGF)

Hepatocyte growth factor was originally identified as a growth factor for rat hepatocytes derived from rat platelets,[203] one of the sources from which it was originally purified.[204] Two other sources for this activity, sera obtained from rats following partial hepatectomy[205] and from humans with fulminant hepatic failure,[206] supported its identification as a hepatotrophic factor. Subsequent studies showed that HGF was identical to scatter factor, a substance that could induce cell migration and morphologic spreading.[207]

Purified from serum, HGF is a disulfide-linked heterodimer consisting of a 55- to 60-kd α chain and a 32- to 34-kd β chain.[204] It is synthesized as an 85-kd precursor that undergoes cleavage to yield the circulating factor.[208] The role of proteolytic processing of the HGF precursor, a function that may be carried out by tissue plasminogen activator (TPA), could represent an important physiologic activation mechanism.[33]

The HGF receptor is a product of the *c-met* proto-oncogene.[33] Human osteosarcoma cells treated with a chemical carcinogen were the first source in which the activated *met* oncogene was identified. In these cells, gene rearrangement resulting in a truncated form of Met results in a constitutively active tyrosine kinase. Molecular cloning of the *c-met* proto-oncogene revealed that it encoded a receptor-like protein for an undetermined ligand. The observation that HGF stimulates the tyrosine phosphorylation of a 145-kd protein eventually led to identification of the *c-met* product as the HGF receptor.[209,210]

Notwithstanding its designation as hepatocyte growth factor, HGF is a potent mitogen for numerous cell types, including hepatocytes, biliary epithelial cells, keratinocytes, melanocytes, renal tubular epithelial cells, and endothelial cells.[33] HGF's "scattering" activity is observed in many of these same cells. In addition, HGF can act as an in vitro morphogen, promoting the formation of tubular structures when canine kidney epithelial cells are grown in collagen gels.[211]

Hepatocyte growth factor is indeed the most potent proliferative factor for mature hepatocytes. It has a probable role in hepatic carcinogenesis, and may be the primary hepatotrophic factor active in liver regeneration following partial hepatectomy.[212] Given the diversity of its cellular effects, it undoubtedly plays an important role in fetal development.

Conclusion

In addition to the above growth factor families, other broad classes of extracellular signaling molecules (e.g., cytokines, matrix proteins, cell surface adhesion molecules, neurotransmitters, etc.) function in growth-regulating roles. Furthermore, the observation that cancer-causing oncogenes have normal cellular counterparts, proto-oncogenes, provided a mechanism whereby functions assigned to growth factors could be regulated by gene products that can "substitute" for growth factors.[213–215] The first such example was the simian sarcoma virus gene v-*sis*, which was found to encode a protein almost identical to a portion of PDGF.[212] The veritable explosion of research resulting in the discovery of new oncogenes and proto-oncogenes has identified proteins that can function at all levels of the growth factor signaling pathways. Examples include *erb-B*, which codes for a truncated EGF receptor, *src* and *abl*, which code for nonreceptor tyrosine kinases, *raf*, the proximal protein kinase in the MAP kinase cascade, and growth-promoting nuclear transcription factors such as *myc*, *fos*, and *jun*, whose expression may be regulated independent of mitogenic signaling. The further identification of many of these gene products as "onco-fetal proteins" indicates their co-involvement with classic growth factors in the developing conceptus.

References

1. Daughaday WH, Hall K, Raben MS, et al. Somatomedin: proposed designation of sulphation factor. Nature 1972;235:107.
2. Feyrter F. Ueber die These von den peripheren endokrinen Druesen. Wien Z Inn Med 1946;27:9–38.
3. Sporn MB, Todaro GJ. Autocrine secretion and malignant transformation of cells. N Engl J Med 1980;303:878–880.
4. Sporn MB, Roberts AB. Autocrine secretion—10 years later. Ann Intern Med 1992;117:408–414.
5. Tucker RF, Shipley GD, Moses HL, et al. Growth inhibitor from BSC-1 cells closely related to platelet type beta transforming growth factor. Science 1984;226:705–707.
6. Keating MT, Williams LT. Autocrine stimulation of intracellular PDGF receptors in v-sis-transformed cells. Science 1988;239:914–916.
7. Dunbar CE, Browder TM, Abrams JS, et al. COOH-terminal-modified interleukin-3 is retained intracellularly and stimulates autocrine growth. Science 1989;245:1496–1498.
8. Dennis PA, Rifkin DB. Cellular activation of latent transforming growth factor B requires binding to the cation-independent mannose 6-phosphate/insulin-like growth factor type II receptor. Proc Natl Acad Sci USA 1991;88:580–584.
9. Sherr CJ. Mammalian G1 cyclins. Cell 1993;73:1059–1065.
10. Peters G. Stifled by inhibitions. Nature 1994;371:204–205.
11. Sherr CJ, Roberts JM. Inhibitors of mammalian G1 cyclin-dependent kinases. Genes Dev 1995;9:1149–1163.
12. Farnham PJ, Stansky JE, Kollmar R. The role of E2F in the mammalian cell cycle. Biochim Biophys Acta 1993;1155:125–131.
13. Weinberg RA. The retinoblastoma protein and cell cycle control. Cell 1995;81:323–330.
14. Wagner AJ, Kokontis JM, Nissim H. Myc-mediated apoptosis requires wild-type p53 in a manner independent of cell cycle arrest and the ability of p53 to induce $p21^{waf1/cip1}$. Genes Dev 1994;8:2817–2830.
15. Halevy O, Novitch BG, Spicer DB, et al. Correlation of terminal cell cycle arrest of skeletal muscle with induction of p21 by MyoD. Science 1995;267:1018–1021.
16. Parker SB, Eichele G, Zhang P, et al. p53-independent expression of $p21^{Cip1}$ in muscle and other terminally differentiating cells. Science 1995;267:1024–1027.
17. Polyak K, Lee M-H, Erdjument-Bromage H, et al. Cloning of $p27^{Kip1}$, a cyclin-dependent kinase inhibitor and a potential mediator of extracellular antimitogenic signals. Cell 1994;78:59–66.
18. Toyoshima H, Hunter T. p27, a novel inhibitor of G1 cyclin-Cdk protein kinase activity, is related to p21. Cell 1994;78:67–74.
19. Hannon GJ, Beach B. $p15^{INK4B}$ is a potential effector of TGF-beta-induced cell cycle arrest. Nature 1994;371:257–261.
20. Smas CM, Sul HS. Control of adipocyte differentiation. Biochem J 1995;309:697–710.
21. Greene LA, Tischler AS. PC12 pheochromocytoma cultures in neurobiological research. Adv Cell Neurobiol 1982;3:373–414.
22. Qui M-S, Green SH. NGF and EGF rapidly activate $p21^{ras}$ in PC12 cells by distinct, convergent pathways involving tyrosine phosphorylation. Neuron 1991;7:937–946.
23. Martin SJ, Green DR, Cotter TG. Dicing with death: dissecting the components of the apoptosis machinery. TIBS 1994;19:26–30.
24. Steller H. Mechanisms and genes of cellular suicide. Science 1995;267:1445–1449.
25. Vaux DL, Strasser A. The molecular biology of apoptosis. Proc Natl Acad Sci USA 1996;93:2239–2244.
26. Nagata S, Golstein P. The Fas death factor. Science 1995;267:1449–1456.
27. Hannun YA, Obeid LM. Ceramide: an intracellular signal for apoptosis. TIBS 1995;20:73–77.
28. Oberhammer FA, Pavelka M, Sharma S, et al. Induction of apoptosis in cultured hepatocytes and in regressing liver by transforming growth factor beta 1. Proc Natl Acad Sci USA 1992;89:5408–5412.
29. Rubin R, Baserga R. Insulin-like growth factor-I receptor: its role in cell proliferation, apoptosis and tumorigenicity. Lab Invest 1995;73:311–331.
30. Blaschke AJ, Staley K, Chun J. Widespread programmed cell death in proliferative and postmitotic regions of the fetal cerebral cortex. Development 1996;122:1165–1174.
31. Terada T, Nakanuma Y. Detection of apoptosis and expression of apoptosis-related proteins during human

intrahepatic bile duct development. Am J Pathol 1995;146:67–74.
32. Mori C, Nakamura N, Kimura S, et al. Programmed cell death in the interdigital tissue of the fetal mouse limb is apoptosis with DNA fragmentation. Anat Rec 1995;242:103–110.
33. Rubin JS, Bottaro DP, Aaronson SA. Hepatocyte growth factor/scatter factor and its receptor, the c-met proto-oncogene product. Biochim Biophys Acta 1993;1155:357–371.
34. Werner S, Smola H, Liao X, et al. The function of KGF in morphogenesis of epithelium and reepithelialization of wounds. Science 1994;266:819–822.
35. Abraham JA, Mergia A, Whang JL, et al. Nucleotide sequence of a bovine clone encoding the angiogenic protein, basic fibroblast growth factor. Science 1986;233:545–548.
36. Boyer B, Dufour S, Thiery JP. E-cadherin expression during the acidic FGF-induced dispersion of a rat bladder carcinoma cell line. Exp Cell Res 1992;201:347–357.
37. Gavrilovic J, Moens G, Thiery JP, Jouanneau J. Expression of transfected transforming growth factor alpha induces a motile fibroblast-like phenotype with extracellular matrix-degrading potential in a rat bladder carcinoma cell line. Cell Regul 1990;1:1003–1014.
38. Silberstein GB, Daniel CW. Reversible inhibition of mammary gland growth by transforming growth factor-beta. Science 1987;237:291–293.
39. Minoo P, King RJ. Epithelial-mesenchymal interactions in lung development. Annu Rev Physiol 1994;56:13–45.
40. Goldin GV, Opperman LA. Induction of supernumerary tracheal buds and the stimulation of DNA synthesis in the embryonic chick lung and trachea by epidermal growth factor. J Embryol Exp Morphol 1980;60:235–243.
41. Seth R, Shum L, Wu F, et al. Role of epidermal growth factor expression in early mouse embryo lung branching morphogenesis in culture: antisense oligo-deoxynucleotide inhibitory strategy. Dev Biol 1993;158:555–559.
42. Whitsett JA, Weaver TE, Lieberman MA, et al. Differential effects of epidermal growth factor and tranformation growth factor-beta on synthesis of M_r 35,000 surfactant-associated protein in fetal lung. J Biol Chem 1987;262:7908–7913.
43. Raaberg L, Nexo E, Buckley S, et al. Epidermal growth factor transcription, translation and signal transduction by rat type II pneumocytes in culture. Am J Resp Cell Mol Biol 1991;6:44–49.
44. Torday JS, Kourembanas S. Fetal rat lung fibroblasts produce a TGF-beta homolog that blocks alveolar type II cell maturation. Dev Biol 1990;139:35–41.
45. Tickle C, Eichele G. Vertebrate limb development. Annu Rev Cell Biol 1994;10:121–152.
46. Hunter T, Sefton BW. Tranforming gene product of Rous sarcoma virus phosphorylates tyrosine. Proc Natl Acad Sci USA 1980;77:1311–1315.
47. Carpenter G, Cohen S. Epidermal growth factor. J Biol Chem 1990;265:7709–7712.
48. Schlessinger J, Ullrich A, Honegger AM, Moolenaar WH. Signal transduction by epidermal growth factor receptor. Cold Spring Harb Symp Quant Biol 1988;53:515–519.
49. Chen WS, Lazar CS, Poenie M, et al. Requirement for intrinsic protein-tyrosine kinase in the immediate and late actions of the EGF receptor. Nature 1987;328:820–823.
50. Honegger AM, Szapary D, Schmidt A, et al. A mutant epidermal growth factor receptor with defective protein tyrosine kinase is unable to stimulate proto-oncogene expression and DNA synthesis. Mol Cell Biol 1987;7:4568–4571.
51. Kasuga M, Karlsson FA, Kahn CR. Insulin stimulates the phosphorylation of the 95,000-dalton subunit of its own receptor. Science 1982;215:185–187.
52. Ullrich A, Gray A, Tam AW, et al. Insulin-like growth factor 1 receptor primary structure: comparison with insulin receptor suggests structural determinants that define functional specificity. EMBO J 1986;5:2503–2512.
53. Claesson-Welsh L. Platelet-derived growth factor receptor signals. J Biol Chem 1994;269:32023–32026.
54. Van der Geer P, Hunter T, Lindberg RA. Receptor protein-tyrosine kinases and their signal transduction pathways. Annu Rev Cell Biol 1994;10:251–337.
55. Hunter T. Tyrosine phosphorylation: past, present and future. Biochem Soc Trans 1996;24:307–327.
56. Darnell JE, Kerr IM, Stark GR. Jak-STAT pathways and transcriptional activation in response to IFNs and other extracellular signaling proteins. Science 1994;264:1415–1421.
57. Ruff-Jamison S, Chen K, Cohen S. Induction by EGF and interferon-gamma of tyrosine phosphorylated DNA binding proteins in mouse liver nuclei. Science 1993;261:1733–1736.
58. Koch CA, Anderson D, Moran MF, et al. SH2 and SH3 domains: elements that control interactions of cytoplasmic signaling proteins. Science 1991;252:668–674.
59. Nishibe S, Wahl MI, Hernandez-Sotomayor SMT, et al. Increase of the catalytic activity of phospholipase C-gamma 1 by tyrosine phosphorylation. Science 1990;250:1253–1256.
60. Carpenter CL, Duckworth BC, Auger KR, et al. Purification and characterization of phosphoinositide 3-kinase from rat liver. J Biol Chem 1990;265:19704–19711.
61. Escobedo JA, Novankasattusas S, Kavanaugh WM, et al. cDNA cloning of a novel 85 kd protein that has SH2 domains and regulates binding of PI3-kinase to the PDGF beta-receptor. Cell 1991;65:75–82.
62. Skolnik EY, Margolis B, Mohammadi M, et al. Cloning of PI3-kinase-associated p85 utilizing a novel method for expression/cloning of target proteins for receptor tyrosine kinases. Cell 1991;65:83–90.
63. Otsu M, Hiles I, Gout I, et al. Characterization of two 85 kd proteins that associate with receptor tyrosine kinases, middle T/pp60 c-*src* complexes and P13-kinase. Cell 1991;65:91–104.
64. Gibbs JB, Marshall MS, Scolnick EM, et al. Modulation of guanine nucleotides bound to ras in NIH 3T3 cells by oncogenes, growth factors, and the GTPase activating protein (GAP). J Biol Chem 1990;265:20437–20442.
65. Mulcahy LS, Smith MR, Stacey DW. Requirement for *ras* proto-oncogene function during serum-stimulated growth of NIH 3T3 cells. Nature 1985;313:241–248.

66. Stokoe D, Macdonald SG, Cadwallader K, et al. Activation of Raf as a result of recruitment to the plasma membrane. Science 1994;264:1463–1467.
67. Cobb MH, Goldsmith EJ. How MAP kinases are regulated. J Biol Chem 1995;270:14843–14846.
68. Davis RJ. MAPKs: new JNK expands the group. TIBS 1994;19:470–473.
69. Westwick JK, Weitzel C, Leffert HL, Brenner DA. Activation of Jun kinase is an early event in hepatic regeneration. J Clin Invest 1995;95:803–810.
70. Boylan JM, Gruppuso PA. A comparative study of the hepatic mitogen-activated protein kinase and Jun-NH_2-terminal kinase pathways in the late-gestation fetal rat. Cell Growth Diff 1996;7:1261–1269.
71. Dai T, Rubie E, Franklin CC, et al. Stress-activated protein kinases bind directly to the d domain of c-Jun in resting cells: implications for repression of c-Jun function. Oncogene 1995;10:849–855.
72. Angel P, Karin M. The role of Jun, Fos and the AP-1 complex in cell-proliferation and transformation. Biochem Biophys Acta 1991;1072:129–157.
73. Karin M. Signal transduction from the cell surface to the nucleus through the phosphorylation of transcription factors. Curr Opin Cell Biol 1994;6:415–424.
74. Woodgett JR, Pulverer BJ, Plyte S, et al. Nuclear oncoprotein targets of signal transduction pathways. Pigment Cell Res 1994;7:96–100.
75. Schwartz AL. Receptor cell biology: receptor-mediated endocytosis. Pediatr Res 1995;38:835–843.
76. Sibley DR, Benovic JL, Caron MG, Lefkowitz RJ. Regulation of transmembrane signaling by receptor phosphorylation. Cell 1987;48:913–922.
77. Feinstein R, Kanety H, Papa MZ, et al. Tumor necrosis factor-alpha suppresses insulin-induced tyrosine phosphorylation of insulin receptor and its substrates. J Biol Chem 1993;268:26055–26058.
78. Cherniack AD, Klarlund JK, Conway BR, Czech MP. Disassembly of son-of-sevenless proteins from Grb2 during p21ras desensitization by insulin. J Biol Chem 1995;270:1485–1488.
79. Langlois WJ, Sasaoka T, Saltiel AR, Olefsky JM. Negative feedback regulation and desensitization of insulin- and epidermal growth factor-stimulated p21ras activation. J Biol Chem 1995;270:25320–25326.
80. Buday L, Warne PH, Downward J. Downregulation of the ras activation pathway by MAP kinase phosphorylation of Sos. Oncogene 1995;11:1327–1334.
81. Cohen S. Isolation of a mouse submaxillary gland protein accelerating incisor eruption and eyelid opening in the newborn animal. J Biol Chem 1962;237:1555–1562.
82. Cohen S, Taylor JM. Epidermal growth factor: chemical and biological characterization. Recent Prog Horm Res 1974;30:533–550.
83. Gregory H. Isolation and structure of urogastrone and its relationship to epidermal growth factor. Nature 1975;257:325–327.
84. Carpenter G, Wahl MI. The epidermal growth factor family. In: Sporn MB, Roberts AB, eds. Handbook of experimental pharmacology, peptide growth factors and their receptors. I. Berlin: Springer-Verlag, 1990:69–171.
85. Todaro GJ, DeLarco JE. Growth factors produced by sarcoma virus-transformed cells. Cancer Res 1978;38:4147–4154.
86. Roberts AB, Frolik CA, Anzano MA, et al. Transforming growth factors from neoplastic and nonneoplastic tissues. Fed Proc 1983;42:2621–2626.
87. Marquardt H, Hunkapiller MW, Hood LE, et al. Transforming growth factors produced by retrovirus-transformed rodent fibroblasts and human melanoma cells: amino acid sequence homology with epidermal growth factor. Proc Natl Acad Sci USA 1983;80:4684–4688.
88. Marquardt H, Hunkapiller MEW, Hood LE, et al. Rat transforming growth factor type I: structure and relation to epidermal growth factor. Science 1984;223:1079–1082.
89. Derynck R. The physiology of transforming growth factor-alpha. Adv Cancer Res 1992;58:27–52.
90. Pandiella A, Massague J. Cleavage of the membrane precursor for transforming growth factor alpha is a regulated process. Proc Natl Acad Sci USA 1991;88:1726–1730.
91. Massague J. Transforming growth factor-alpha: a model for membrane-anchored growth factors. J Biol Chem 1990;265:21393–21396.
92. Shoyab M, Plowman GD. Purification of amphiregulin from serum-free conditioned medium of 12-O-tetradecanoylphorbol-13-acetate-treated cell lines. Methods Enzymol 1991;198:213–221.
93. Higashiyama S, Abraham JA, Miller J, et al. A heparin-binding growth factor secreted by macrophage-like cells that is related to EGF. Science 1991;251:936–939.
94. Dono R, Montuori N, Rocchi M, et al. Isolation and characterization of the CRIPTO autosomal gene and its X-linked related sequence. Am J Hum Genet 1991;49:555–565.
95. Shing Y, Christofori G, Hanahan D, et al. Betacellulin: a novel mitogen from pancreatic B tumor cells. Science 1993;259:1604–1607.
96. Threadgill DW, Dlugosz AA, Hansen LA, et al. Targeted disruption of mouse EGF receptor: effect of genetic background on mutant phenotype. Science 1995;269:230–238.
97. Salmon WD Jr, Daughaday WH. A hormonally controlled serum factor which stimulates sulfate incorporation by cartilage in vitro. J Lab Clin Med 1957;49:825–836.
98. Rinderknecht E, Humbel RE. The amino acid sequence of human insulin-like growth factor I and its structural homology with proinsulin. J Biol Chem 1978;253:2769–2776.
99. Klapper DG, Svoboda ME, Van Wyk JJ. Sequence analysis of somatomedin-C: confirmation of identity with insulin-like growth factor I. Endocrinology 1983;112:2215–2217.
100. Rinderknecht E, Humbel RE. Primary structure of human insulin-like growth factor II. FEBS Lett 1978;89:283–286.
101. Rotwein P, Pollock KM, Didier DK, et al. Organization and sequence of the human insulin-like growth factor I gene. J Biol Chem 1986;261:4828–4832.
102. Hoyt EC, Van Wyk JJ, Lund PK. Tissue and development specific regulation of a complex family of rat insulin-like

growth factor I messenger ribonucleic acids. Mol Endocrinol 1988;2:1077–1086.
103. DeChiara TM, Robertson EJ, Efstratiadis A. Parental imprinting of the mouse insulin-like growth factor II gene. Cell 1991;64:849–859.
104. Froesch ER, Schmid C, Schwander J, Zapf J. Actions of insulin-like growth factors. Annu Rev Physiol 1985;47: 443–467.
105. Merimee TJ, Zapf J, Froesch ER. Insulin-like growth factors in the fed and fasted states. J Clin Endocrinol Metab 1982;55:99–102.
106. Clemmons DR, Klibanski A, Underwood LE, et al. Reduction of immunoreactive somatomedin-C during fasting in humans. J Clin Endocrinol Metab 1981;53:1247–1250.
107. Boni-Schnetzler M, Binz K, Mary J-L, et al. Regulation of hepatic expression of IGF I and fetal IGF binding protein mRNA in streptozotocin-diabetic rats. FEBS Lett 1989; 251:253–256.
108. Penhoat A, Naville D, Jaillard C, et al. Hormonal regulation of insulin-like growth factor I secretion by bovine adrenal cells. J Biol Chem 1989;264:6858–6862.
109. Oliver JE, Aitman TJ, Powell JF, et al. Insulin-like growth factor I gene expression in the rat ovary is confined to the granulosa cells of developing follicles. Endocrinology 1989;124:2671–2679.
110. Han VK, D'Ercole AJ, Lund PK. Cellular localization of somatomedin (insulin-like growth factor) messenger RNA in the human fetus. Science 1987;236:193–197.
111. Bhaumick B, Bala RM, Hollenberg MD. Somatomedin receptor of human placenta: solubilization, photolabeling, partial purification, and comparison with insulin receptor. Proc Natl Acad Sci USA 1981;78:4279–4283.
112. Ullrich A, Gray A, Tam AW, et al. Insulin-like growth factor 1 receptor primary structure: comparison with insulin receptor suggests structural determinants that define functional specificity. EMBO J 1986;5:2503–2512.
113. Mamula PW, Goldfine ID. Cloning and characterization of the human insulin-like growth factor-I receptor gene 5'-flanking region. DNA Cell Biol 1992;11:43–50.
114. Alexandrides TK, Chen J-H, Bueno R. Evidence for two insulin-like growth factor I receptors with distinct primary structure that are differentially expressed during development. Reg Peptides 1993;48:279–290.
115. Condorelli G, Bueno R, Smith RJ. Two alternatively spliced forms of the human insulin-like growth factor I receptor have distinct biological activities and internalization kinetics. J Biol Chem 1994;269:8510–8516.
116. LeRoith D, Werner H, Beitner-Johnson D, Roberts CT. Molecular and cellular aspects of the insulin-like growth factor I receptor. Endocr Rev 1995;16:143–163.
117. Moxham CP, Duronio V, Jacobs S. Insulin-like growth factor I receptor beta subunit heterogeneity. Evidence for hybrid tetramers composed of insulin-like growth factor I and insulin receptor heterodimers. J Biol Chem 1989;264: 13238–13244.
118. Myers MG, Sun XJ, Cheatham B, et al. IRS-1 is a common element in insulin and insulin-like growth factor-I signaling to the phosphatidylinositol 3'-kinase. Endocrinology 1993;132:1421–1430.
119. Giorgetti S, Pelicci PG, Pelicci G, et al. Involvement of Src-homology/collagen (SHC) proteins in signaling through the insulin receptor and the insulin-like-growth-factor-I-receptor. Eur J Biochem 1994;223:195–202.
120. Liu J-P, Baker J, Perkins AS, et al. Mice carrying null mutations of the genes encoding insulin-like growth factor I (IGF-I) and type I IGF receptor (IGF-IR). Cell 1993; 75:59–72.
121. Baker J, Liu J-P, Robertson EJ, et al. Role of insulin-like growth factors in embryonic and postnatal growth. Cell 1993;75:73–82.
122. Kasuga M, Van Obberghen E, Nissley SP, et al. Demonstration of two subtypes of insulin-like growth factor receptors by affinity cross-linking. J Biol Chem 1981;256:5305–5308.
123. Massague J, Czech MP. The subunit structures of two distinct receptors for insulin-like growth factors I and II and their relationship to the insulin receptor. J Biol Chem 1982;257:5038–5045.
124. Oshima A, Nolan CM, Kyle JW, et al. The human cation-independent mannose 6-phosphate receptor: cloning and sequence of the full-length cDNA and expression of functional receptor in cos cells. J Biol Chem 1988;263: 2553–2567.
125. Okamoto T, Nishimoto I, Murayama Y, et al. Insulin-like growth factor II/mannose 6-phosphate receptor is incapable of activating GTP-binding proteins in response to mannose 6-phosphate, but capable in response to insulin-like growth factor II. Biochem Biophys Res Commun 1990;168:1201–1210.
126. Soos MA, Siddle K. Immunological relationships between receptors for insulin and insulin-like growth factor I. Evidence for structural heterogeneity of insulin-like growth factor I receptors involving hybrids with insulin receptors. Biochem J 1989;263:553–563.
127. Jones JI, Clemmons DR. Insulin-like growth factors and their binding proteins: biological actions. Endocr Rev 1995;16:3–34.
128. Drop SLS, Valiquette G, Guyda HJ, et al. Partial purification and characterization of a binding protein for insulin-like activity (ILas) in human amniotic fluid: a possible inhibitor of insulin-like activity. Acta Endocrinol (Copenh) 1979;90:505–518.
129. Elgin RC, Busby WH, Clemmons DR. An insulin-like growth factor binding protein enhances the biological response to IGF-I. Proc Natl Acad Sci USA 1987;84:3254–3258.
130. Brown AL, Chariotti L, Orlowski CC, et al. Nucleotide sequences and expression of a cDNA clone encoding a fetal rat binding protein for insulin-like growth factors. J Biol Chem 1989;264:5148–5154.
131. Imbenotte J, Liu L, Desauty G, et al. Stimulation by TGF beta of chick embryo fibroblasts-inhibition by an IGFBP-3. Exp Cell Res 1992;199:229–233.
132. Oh Y, Muller HL, Lamson G, et al. Insulin-like growth factor (IGF)-independent action of IGF-binding protein-3 in Hs578T human breast cancer cells. J Biol Chem 1993;268:14964–14971.
133. Bondy CA, Werner H, Roberts CT Jr, et al. Cellular pattern of insulin-like growth factor I (IGF-I) and type I

133. IGF receptor gene expression in early organogenesis: comparison with IGF-II gene expression. Mol Endocrinol 1990;4:1386–1398.
134. DeChiara TM, Robertson EJ, Efstratiadis A. Parental imprinting of the mouse insulin-like growth factor II gene. Cell 1991;643:849–859.
135. DeChiara TM, Efstratiadis A, Robertson EJ. A growth-deficiency phenotype in heterozygous mice carrying an insulin-like growth factor II gene disrupted by targeting. Nature 1990;34:78–80.
136. Heyner S, Garside WT. Biological actions of IGFs in mammalian development. Bioessays 1994;16:55–57.
137. D'Ercole AJ. Somatomedins/insulin-like growth factors and fetal development. J Dev Physiol 1987;9:481–495.
138. Balk SD. Calcium as a regulator of the proliferation of normal, but not transformed, chicken fibroblasts in plasma-containing medium. Proc Natl Acad Sci USA 1971;68:271–275.
139. Ross R, Glomset J, Kariya B, Harker L. Platelet-dependent serum factor that stimulates the proliferation of arterial smooth muscle cells in vitro. Proc Natl Acad Sci USA 1974;71:1207–1210.
140. Heldin C-H, Westermark B, Wasteson A. Platelet-derived growth factor: purification and partial characterization. Proc Natl Acad Sci USA 1979;76:3722–3726.
141. Antoniades HN. Human platelet-derived growth factor (PDGF): purification of PDGF-I and PDGF-II and separation of their reduced subunits. Proc Natl Acad Sci USA 1981;78:7314–7317.
142. Deuel TF, Huang JS, Proffitt RT, et al. Human platelet-derived growth factor—purification and resolution into two active protein fractions. J Biol Chem 1981;256:8896–8899.
143. Hart CE, Bailey M, Curtis DA, et al. Purification of PDGF-AB and PDGF-BB from human platelet extracts and identification of all three PDGF dimers in human platelets. Biochemistry 1990;29:166–172.
144. Thyberg J, Ostman A, Backstrom G, et al. Localization of platelet-derived growth factor (PDGF) in CHO cells transfected with A- or B-chain cDNA: retention of PDGF-BB in the endoplasmic reticulum and Golgi complex. J Cell Sci 1990;97:219–229.
145. Heldin C-H, Westermark B, Wasteson A. Specific receptors for platelet-derived growth factor on cells derived from connective tissue and glia. Proc Natl Acad Sci USA 1981;78:3664–3668.
146. Hart CE, Forstrom JW, Kelly JD. Two classes of PDGF receptor recognize different isoforms of PDGF. Science 1988;240:1529–1534.
147. Heldin C-H, Backstrom G, Ostman A, et al. Binding of different dimeric forms of PDGF to human fibroblasts: evidence for two separate receptor types. EMBO J 1988;7:1387–1393.
148. Heldin C-H, Ernlund A, Rorsman C, et al. Dimerization of B-type platelet-derived growth factor receptor occurs after ligand binding and is closely associated with receptor kinase activation. J Biol Chem 1989;264:8905–8912.
149. Nister M, Hammacher A, Mellstrom K, et al. A glioma-derived PDGF A chain homodimer has different functional activities from a PDGF AB heterodimer purified from human platelets. Cell 1988;52:791–799.
150. Olashaw NE, Olson JE, Drozdoff V, et al. Growth factors: their role in the control of cell proliferation. In: Stein GS, Lian JB eds. Molecular and cellular approaches to the control of proliferation and differentiation. New York: Academic Press, 1992:3–27.
151. Goustin AS, Betsholtz C, Pfeifer-Ohlsson S, et al. Coexpression of the sis and myc proto-oncogenes in developing human placenta suggests autocrine control of trophoblast growth. Cell 1985;41:301–312.
152. Schatteman GC, Morrison-Graham K, Van Koppen A, et al. Regulation and role of PDGF receptor alpha-subunit expression during embryogenesis. Development 1992;115:123–131.
153. Morrison-Graham K, Schatteman GC, Bork T, et al. A PDGF receptor mutation in the mouse (Patch) perturbs the development of a non-neuronal subset of neural crest-derived cells. Development 1992;115:133–142.
154. Roberts AB, Sporn MB. The transforming growth factor-betas. In: Sporn MB, Roberts AB, eds. Peptide growth factors and their receptors. Handbook of experimental pharmacology, vol. 95. Heidelberg: Springer-Verlag, 1990:419–472.
155. Mason AJ, Hayflick JS, Ling N, et al. Complementary DNA sequences of ovarian follicular fluid inhibin show precursor structure and homology with transforming growth factor-beta. Nature 1985;318:659–663.
156. Vale W, Rivier J, Caughan J, et al. Purification and characterization of an FSH releasing protein from porcine ovarian follicular fluid. Nature 1986;321:776–779.
157. Lin T, Calkins JH, Morris PL, et al. Regulation of Leydig cell function in primary culture by inhibin and activin. Endocrinology 1989;125:2134–2140.
158. Gonzalez-Manchon C, Vale W. Activin-A, inhibin and transforming growth factor-beta modulate growth of two gonadal cell lines. Endocrinology 1989;125:1666–1672.
159. Jost A, Vigier B, Prepin J, et al. Studies on sex differentiation in mammals. Recent Prog Horm Res 1973;29:1–41.
160. Cate RL, Mattaliano RJ, Hession C, et al. Isolation of the bovine and the human genes for mullerian inhibiting substance and expression of the human gene in animal cells. Cell 1986;45:685–698.
161. Dennis PA, Rifkin DB. Cellular activation of latent transforming growth factor B requires binding to the cation-independent mannose 6-phosphate/insulin-like growth factor type II receptor. Proc Natl Acad Sci USA 1991;88:580–584.
162. Leof EB, Proper JA, Goustin AS, et al. Induction of c-sis mRNA and activity similar to platelet-derived growth factor by transforming growth factor beta: a proposed model for indirect mitogenesis involving autocrine activity. Proc Natl Acad Sci USA 1986;83:2453–2457.
163. Cheifetz S, Weatherbee JA, Tsang ML, et al. The transforming growth factor-beta system, a complex pattern of cross-reactive ligands and receptors. Cell 1987;48:409–415.
164. Wang XF, Lin HY, Ng-Eaton E, et al. Expression cloning and characterization of the TGF-beta type III receptor. Cell 1991;67:797–805.

165. Wrana JL, Attisano L, Carcamo J, et al. TGF beta signals through a heteromeric protein kinase receptor complex. Cell 1992;71:1003–1014.
166. Bassing CH, Yingling JM, Howe DJ, et al. A transforming growth factor beta type I receptor that signals to activate gene expression. Science 1994;263:87–92.
167. Lin HY, Wang X-F, Ng-Eaton E, et al. Expression cloning of the TGF-beta type II receptor, a functional transmembrane serine/threonine kinase. Cell 1992;68:775–785.
168. Li J-M, Nichols MA, Chandrasekharan S, et al. Transforming growth factor beta activates the promoter of cyclin-dependent kinase inhibitor p15^{INK4B} through an Sp1 consensus site. J Biol Chem 1995;270:26750–26753.
169. Datto MB, Yu Y, Wang X-F. Functional analysis of the transforming growth factor beta responsive elements in the WAF1/Cip1/p21 promoter. J Biol Chem 1995;270:28623–28628.
170. Alexandrow MG, Moses HL. Transforming growth factor beta and cell cycle regulation. Cancer Res 1995;55:1452–1457.
171. Ignotz RA, Massague J. Transforming growth factor-beta stimulates the expression of fibronectin and collagen and their incorporation into the extracellular matrix. J Biol Chem 1986;48:409–415.
172. Wahl SM, Hunt DA, Wakefield LM, et al. Transforming growth-factor beta (TGF-beta) induces monocyte chemotaxis and growth factor production. Proc Natl Acad Sci USA 1987;84:5788–5792.
173. Robey PG, Young MF, Flanders KC, et al. Osteoblasts synthesize and respond to TGF-beta in vitro. J Cell Biol 1987;105:457–463.
174. Seyedin PR, Segarini PR, Rosen DM, et al. Cartilage-inducing factor-beta is a unique protein structurally and functionally related to transforming growth factor-beta. J Biol Chem 1987;262:1946–1949.
175. Ignotz RA, Heino J, Massague J. Regulation of cell adhesion receptors by transforming growth factor-beta: regulation of citronectin receptor and LFA-1. J Biol Chem 1989;264:389–392.
176. Roberts AB, Sporn MB, Assoian RK, et al. Transforming growth factor type-beta: rapid induction of fibrosis and angiogenesis in vivo and stimulation of collagen formation in vitro. Proc Natl Acad Sci USA 1986;83:4167–4171.
177. Gospodarowicz D, Bialecki H, Greenburg G. Purification of the fibroblast growth factor activity from bovine brain. J Biol Chem 1978;253:3736–3743.
178. Gospodarowicz D. Purification of a fibroblast growth factor from bovine pituitary. J Biol Chem 1975;250:2515–2520.
179. Fernig DG, Gallagher JT. Fibroblast growth factors and their receptors: an information network controlling tissue growth, morphogenesis and repair. Prog Growth Factor Res 1994;5:353–377.
180. Burgess WH, Maciag T. The heparin-binding (fibroblast) growth factor family of proteins. Annu Rev Biochem 1989;58:575–606.
181. Baird A, Bohlen P. Fibroblast growth factors. In: Sporn MB, Roberts AB, eds. Peptide growth factors and their receptors. Handbook of experimental pharmacology, vol. 95. New York: Springer-Verlag, 1990:369–411.
182. Miyamoto M, Naruao KI, Seko C, et al. Molecular cloning of a novel cytokine cDNA encoding the ninth member of the fibroblast growth factor family which has a unique secretion property. Mol Cell Biol 1993;13:4251–4259.
183. Rubin JS, Osada H, Finch PW, et al. Purification and characterization of a newly identified growth factor specific for epithelial cells. Proc Natl Acad Sci USA 1989;86:802–806.
184. Rapraeger AC, Krufka A, Olwin BB. Requirement of heparan sulfate for bFGF-mediated fibroblast growth and myoblast differentiation. Science 1991;252:1705–1708.
185. Yayon A, Klagsbrun M, Esko JD, et al. Cell surface, heparin-like molecules are required for binding of basic fibroblast growth factor to its high affinity receptor. Cell 1991;64:841–848.
186. Xu J, Nakahara M, Crabb JW, et al. Expression and immunochemical analysis of rat and human fibroblast growth factor receptor (flg) isoforms. J Biol Chem 1992;267:17792–17803.
187. Imamura T, Enaleka K, Zhan K, et al. Recovery of mitogenic activity of a growth factor mutant with a nuclear translocation sequence. Science 1990;249:1567–1570.
188. de Lapeyriere O, Ollendorf V, Planche J, et al. Expression of the Fgf6 gene is restricted to developing skeletal muscle in the mouse embryo. Development 1993;118:601–611.
189. Coulier F, Pizette S, Ollendorff V, et al. The human and mouse fibroblast growth factor 6 (FGF6) genes and their products: possible implication in muscle development. Prog Growth Factor Res 1994;5:1–14.
190. Peters K, Werner S, Liao X, et al. Targeted expression of a dominant negative FGF receptor blocks branching morphogenesis and epithelial differentiation of the mouse lung. EMBO J 1994;13:3296–3301.
191. Niswander L, Martin GR. FGF-4 and BMP-2 have opposite effects on limb growth. Nature 1993;361:68–71.
192. Folkman J. Tumor angiogenesis. Adv Cancer Res 1985;43:175–203.
193. Buecker ED. Implantation of tumors in the hind limb of the embryonic chick and developmental response of the lumbosacral nervous system. Anat Rec 1948;102:369–390.
194. Cohen S. Purification of a nerve growth promoting protein from the mouse salivary gland and its neurocytotoxic antiserum. Proc Natl Acad Sci USA 1960;46:302–311.
195. Bradshaw RA. Nerve growth factor. Annu Rev Biochem 1978;47:191–216.
196. Hempstead BL, Martin-Zanca D, Kaplan D, et al. High-affinity NGF binding requires coexpression of the *trk* proto-oncogene and the low-affinity NGF receptor. Nature 1991;350:678–683.
197. Kaplan DR, Hempstead B, Martin-Zanca D, et al. The *trk* proto-oncogene product: a signal transducing receptor for nerve growth factor. Science 1991;252:554–558.
198. Klein R, Jing S, Nanduri V, et al. The *trk* proto-oncogene encodes a receptor for nerve growth factor. Cell 1991;65:189–197.
199. Thomas AM, DeMarco M, D'Arcangelo G, et al. Ras is essential for nerve growth factor- and phorbol ester-induced tyrosine phosphorylation of MAP kinases. Cell 1992;68:1031–1040.

200. Aloe L, Cozzari C, Calissano P, et al. Somatic and behavioural postnatal effects of fetal injections of nerve growth factor antibodies in the rat. Nature 1981;291:412–415.
201. Hamburger V, Bruno-Bechtold JK, Yip JW. Neuronal death in the spinal ganglia of the chick embryo and its reduction by nerve growth factor. J Neurosci Res 1981;1:60–71.
202. Korsching S, Thoenen H. Quantitative demonstration of the retrograde axonal transport of endogenous nerve growth factor. Neurosci Lett 1983;39:1–4.
203. Russell WE, McGowan JA, Bucher NLR. Partial characterization of a hepatocyte growth factor from rat platelets. J Cell Physiol 1984;119:183–192.
204. Nakamura T, Nawa K, Ichihara A, et al. Purification and subunit structure of hepatocyte growth factor from rat platelets. FEBS Lett 1987;224:311–316.
205. Nakamura T, Kitazawa T, Ichihara A. Partial purification and characterization of masking protein for beta-type transforming growth factor from rat platelets. Biochem Biophys Res Commun 1986;141:176–184.
206. Ghoda E, Tsubouchi H, Nakayama H, et al. Purification and partial characterization of hepatocyte growth factor from plasma of a patient with fulminant hepatic failure. J Clin Invest 1988;81:414–419.
207. Weidner KMN, Arakaki N, Hartmann J, et al. Evidence for the identity of human scatter factor and human hepatocyte growth factor. Proc Natl Acad Sci USA 1991;88:7001–7005.
208. Nakamura T, Nishizawa T, Hagiya M, et al. Molecular cloning and expression of human hepatocyte growth factor. Nature 1989;342:440–443.
209. Bottaro DP, Rubin JS, Faletto DL, et al. Identification of the hepatocyte growth factor receptor as the c-met proto-oncogene product. Science 1991;251:802–804.
210. Naldini L, Vigna E, Narsimhan RP, et al. Hepatocyte growth factor (HGF) stimulates the tyrosine kinase activity of the receptor encoded by the proto-oncogene c-met. Oncogene 1991;6:501–504.
211. Montasano R, Schaller G, Orci L. Induction of epithelial tubular morphogenesis in vitro by fibroblast-derived soluble factors. Cell 1991;66:697–711.
212. Michalopoulos GK, Zarnegar R. Hepatocyte growth factor. Hepatology 1992;15:149–156.
213. Cooper GM. Cellular transforming genes. Science 1982;218:801–806.
214. Bishop JM. Molecular themes in oncogenesis. Cell 1991;64:235–248.
215. Krontiris TG. Oncogenes. N Engl J Med 1995;333:303–306.

21
Developmental Endocrinology in the Fetal-Placental Unit

Ram K. Menon and Mark A. Sperling

The placenta is a tissue of fetal origin embedded in the maternal uterine wall that permits exchange of vital nutrients and other elements essential for fetal growth, development, and survival. In addition, the placenta is a tissue capable of steroid and polypeptide synthesis. Hormonal products and interconversions resulting from these synthetic pathways appear to be critically important for ordered fetal growth and development. In some instances, notably estradiol (E_2) and estriol (E_3) synthesis, the placenta converts steroid precursors synthesized in the fetal adrenal. Thus, in this instance, the placenta completes a task initiated in the fetal adrenal so that the fetus and placenta act as a unit, the fetoplacental unit. This chapter discusses endocrine aspects of the fetal-placental unit during gestation and their relevance to the physiology of normal intrauterine development as well as selected examples of pathologic disorders.

Steroid Hormones

During pregnancy the placenta synthesizes large amounts of steroids of which the most important are progesterone and estrogen. There is no evidence that the human placenta synthesizes or secretes any other class of steroids such as glucocorticoids or mineralocorticoids. The cholesterol molecule serves as the precursor for all steroids. Plasma low-density lipoprotein (LDL) cholesterol is the principal source of cholesterol in the placenta, fetal adrenal, and corpus luteum, each of which possesses membrane-bound receptors for LDL.[1] Apolipoprotein apo B-100, located on the surface of the LDL particle, binds to these specific membrane-bound receptors, enabling the internalization of the LDL particle by the process of endocytosis. Following entry into the intracellular environment, the LDL-C particle fuses with acid-lipase containing lysosomes, resulting in the release of cholesterol esters via the process of hydrolysis.[2] The number of low-capacity, high-affinity receptors for LDL is regulated by the cellular requirement for cholesterol.

In the normal human pregnancy, after the first 3 to 4 weeks of gestation nearly all the estrogen produced is synthesized in the trophoblast. The unique fact about this process is the mechanism by which the placenta synthesizes this estrogen. The human placenta is devoid of 17α-hydroxylase/17-lyase activity.[3] There is very little conversion of C_{21} steroids to C_{19} steroids; progesterone is not metabolized within the placenta to any significant extent. However, the placenta has a remarkable capacity for aromatization of C_{19} steroids.[4] It is now well established that the human placenta depends on circulating C_{19} precursors for estrogen biosynthesis (Figure 21.1). The principal precursor of placental estradiol is circulating dehydroepiandrosterone sulfate.[5] The principal precursor of placental estriol is plasma 16α-hydroxydehydroepiandrosterone sulfate.[6] Near term the source of the estradiol synthesized by the placenta is equally divided between precursors in the maternal and the fetal circulations. On the other hand estriol produced by the placenta comes mostly from the 16α-dehydroepiandrosterone sulfate originating in the fetal compartment. Placental sulfatase deficiency is an X-linked syndrome associated with ichthyosis. In this condition there is absence of hydrolysis of dehydroepiandrosterone sulfate or 16α-dehydroepiandrosterone sulfate, which results in a deficiency of placental estrogen. The hallmark of this syndrome, extremely low concentrations of estriol in the plasma and urine during pregnancy, may mistakenly lead to a diagnosis of fetal compromise or death.

Although the adrenal glands of the human fetus at term are as large as the adult gland, the morphology of the gland undergoes significant changes during development. Hence, in the fetus the adrenal gland is composed principally of an inner fetal zone that forms 85% of the volume of the gland, whereas the outer cortex (i.e., neo-

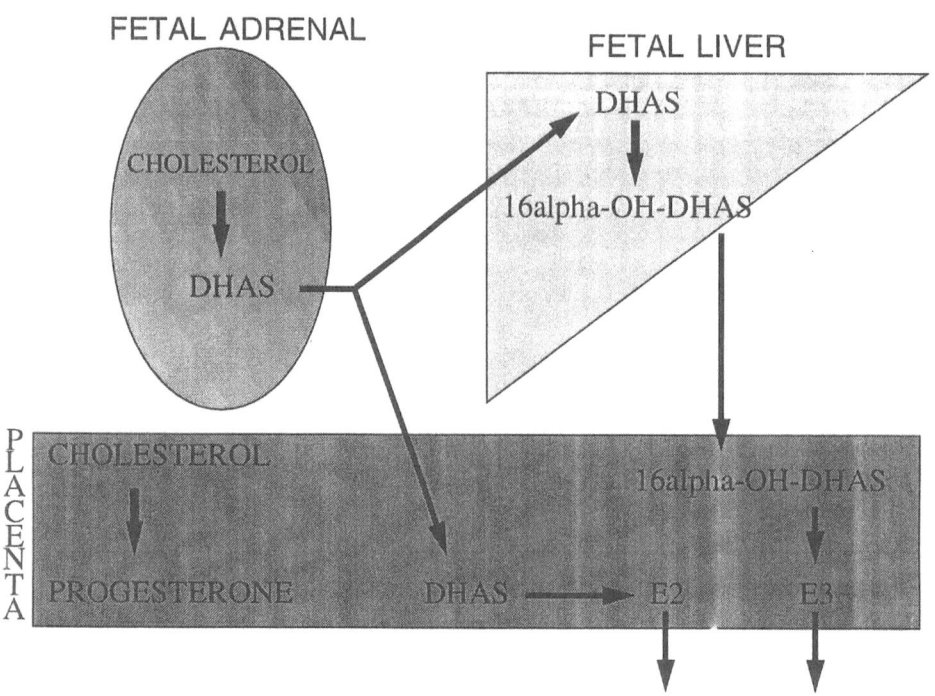

FIGURE 21.1. Steroid biosynthesis in the fetoplacental unit. Schematic representation of the major pathways of steroid hormone synthesis in the fetoplacental unit. DHAS, dehydroepiandrosterone sulfate; E2, estrodiol; E3, estriol. (Adapted from Casey et al.[71])

cortex) that ultimately develops into the cortex in the adult gland accounts for less than 15% of the gland.

The human fetal adrenal gland has a remarkable capacity to synthesize and secrete steroids. At near term the fetal gland secretes 100 to 200 mg of steroid per day, with the principal secretory products being dehydroepiandrosterone sulfate and pregnenolone sulfate. The principal precursor for fetal adrenal gland steroid synthesis is cholesterol; it is estimated that 50% to 70% of the steroids secreted by the fetal adrenal gland are derived from LDL cholesterol and the remainder are derived from cholesterol synthesized de novo in the adrenal gland. High-density lipoprotein (HDL) cholesterol is less of a source, and very low density lipoprotein (VLDL) is not utilized by the fetal adrenal.[7] Because there is a paucity of adipose tissue in the human fetus prior to the 36th week of gestation, the major source of the LDL in the fetus is believed to be the hydrolysis of VLDL in the fetal lungs by lipoprotein lipase, the activity of which is stimulated by prolactin. Hence, it is conceivable that prolactin may be an indirect trophic agent for the fetal adrenal, acting via the regulation of the availability of precursors for fetal adrenal steroid biosynthesis. The major portion of the steroids synthesized by the trophoblast enters the maternal circulation with only a minor fraction entering the fetal compartment. Thus, more than 85% to 90% of the estradiol, estriol, and progesterone synthesized by the trophoblasts enters the maternal compartment.[8]

Patients with congenital lipoid adrenal hyperplasia have a severe defect in the first step in adrenal and go-nadal steroidogenesis, i.e., conversion of cholesterol to pregnenolone. By contrast, the synthesis of pregnenolone in the placenta is unaffected. Initial studies excluded abnormalities in the cholesterol-side-chain cleavage system including the cytochrome P-450 scc gene,[9-12] adrenodoxin reductase, adrenodoxin, and several factors implicated in the transport of cholesterol to mitochondria. Recently, a mitochondrial protein, named the steroidogenic acute regulatory protein (StAR),[13-15] was shown to be mutated in patients with congenital adrenal lipoid hyperplasia.[16-18] The steroidogenic acute regulatory protein stimulates steroidogenesis by forming contact sites between the outer and inner mitochondrial membranes.[19] The messenger RNA (mRNA) for the steroidogenic acute regulatory protein is expressed in the adrenal glands and gonads but not in the placenta. This distribution of expression is consonant with the observation that in contrast to adrenal and gonadal steroidogenesis, placental steroidogenesis is normal in patients with congenital lipoid adrenal hyperplasia.

At term the placenta secretes about 250 mg of progesterone per day. In contrast to the situation with estrogen, the fetus does not contribute to progesterone formation by the placenta. The rate of incorporation of radiolabeled acetate into cholesterol is low, as is the activity of the enzyme hepatic hydroxymethylglutaryl coenzyme A (HMG CoA) reductase, indicating that the rate of de novo synthesis of cholesterol in the placenta is low. In cultured human trophoblasts and choriocarcinoma cells, LDL is the principal source of cholesterol. A finding unique to the trophoblast is the absence of cholesterol esters in trophoblastic tissue. In general, the uptake of LDL by a tissue is associated with increase in the formation of cholesterol esters because of stimulation of acyl-CoA: cholesterol acyltransferase (ACAT) activity by LDL. However, ACAT activity is almost completely inhibited by progesterone in concentrations similar to those present in trophoblastic cells.[20] Thus, in the human placenta ACAT activity is inhibited, thereby preventing the sequestration of cholesterol in the storage form (i.e., cholesterol esters). This mechanism allows for a continuous supply of cholesterol for progesterone biosynthesis; the amino acids derived from the hydrolysis of the protein component of the LDL molecule subserve as the source of essential amino acids for the fetus.

Very little steroid in the maternal circulation enters the fetal compartment. This is partly because of the rapidity of clearance of steroids from the maternal plasma compared to the placental plasma flow rate. In addition, the trophoblasts have an extremely large capacity for aromatization that converts C_{19} steroids to estrogens (Figure 21.1). Hence, circulating C_{19} steroids in the maternal circulation, such as dehydroepiandrosterone sulfate, dehydroepiandrosterone, androstenedione, and testosterone, are converted by the aromatase system to estrogen, resulting in very little or no transfer of these C_{19} steroids from the maternal to the fetal circulation.[21] A clinical correlate of this phenomenon is the relative protection of the fetus from virilizing effects of maternal hormones. In most women with androgen-secreting tumors the fetus does not show signs of virilization. The interdependence of fetal adrenal steroid precursor synthesis, its conversion to potent estrogen by the trophoblasts, and the protective effect of placental aromatase against potentially harmful consequences of maternal androgens form the basis for recognizing the fetus and placenta as a unit, the fetoplacental unit.

Protein Hormones

The human placenta produces many protein hormones. The physiology of the placental production of some of these hormones, such as human chorionic gonadotropin (hCG), human placental lactogen (hPL), luteinizing hormone–releasing hormone (LHRH), thyrotropin-releasing hormone (TRH), and inhibin, is well characterized, while for others, such as adrenocorticotropic hormone (ACTH) and corticotropin-releasing hormone (CRH), the role of the placenta has been less well studied.

Human Chorionic Gonadotropin

Human chorionic gonadotropin is a glycoprotein of molecular weight 39,000 daltons (d), composed of noncovalently linked dissimilar α and β subunits.[22] The gene coding hCG is located on chromosome 6. The α subunit (molecular weight 16,000 d) is virtually identical to the α subunits of human luteinizing hormone (hLH) and human follicle-stimulating hormone (hFSH).[23] Ninety-seven of the 145 amino acids of the β subunit (molecular weight 23,000 d) are identical to the β subunit of hLH. Because of the similarity between the α subunit of hCG and LH, it was difficult in the past to reliably distinguish between these two hormones in routine assays. However, because of the dissimilarity between their β subunits, assays are now available that reliably distinguish between these two hormones, allowing for the gathering of accurate data relating to LH and hCG. Glycosylation plays a role in modulating the biologic actions of hCG by increasing the half-life of the hormone in circulation.

Human chorionic gonadotropin is secreted by the syncytiotrophoblast. Since the cytotrophoblast is the site for production of LHRH it is believed that this organization allows for a paracrine mechanism to exist whereby LHRH of cytotrophoblastic origin stimulates production of hCG by the trophoblasts.[24] Adenosine 3′,5′-cyclic monophosphate (cAMP) and trophoblast-derived interleukin (IL)-6,[25] tumor necrosis factor-α (TNF-α),[26] activin, and inhibin[27] are some of the other regulators of hCG production by the syncytiotrophoblast.

The physiologic role of hCG has not been completely elucidated. One of the purported roles is in the maintenance and conversion of the corpus luteum of menstruation to the corpus luteum of pregnancy.[28] Only a small fraction (i.e., less than 1%) of the hCG produced by the placenta enters the fetal circulation. However, placental hCG likely plays a role in the sexual differentiation of the male fetus by stimulating testosterone production by the fetal testes prior to the onset of secretion of LH by the fetal pituitary.[29]

Placental Lactogen

There is a lack of uniformity regarding the nomenclature of this hormone, with various terms including human chorionic somatomammotropin (hCS), chorionic growth hormone–prolactin (CGP), and human placental lactogen (hPL) used synonymously in the literature for this hormone of molecular weight 22,308 d.[30] In the human, hPL is the product of genes located within the GH/CS gene cluster on the long arm of chromosome 17 at bands q22 to 24. This cluster consists of two human growth hormone (hGH) genes (GH-1 and GH-2) and three placental lactogen genes (CS-P, CS-1, and CS-2). GH-1 (also termed GH-N) is expressed in the pituitary and is the source of circulating growth hormone, whereas GH-2 (hGH-V) is expressed only in the placenta and specifies a gene product that differs from the GH-1 gene product at 13 of the 191 amino acids. hPL is produced by two genes CS-1 and CS-2; the CS-P gene is considered to be a pseudogene because it contains a nucleotide substitution (G to A at the donor splice site of intron 2) that predicts the absence of normal splicing and thus absence of a gene product.

Primate hPL genes evolved from the GH gene and like GH have only a 30% homology to prolactin (PRL).[31] At the amino acid level, hPL has over 80% and 60% homology, respectively, with hGH and human prolactin (hPRL).[32] The secretion of hPL by the syncytiotrophoblast begins with nidation and increases during pregnancy in proportion to the placental mass. The maximum daily production of hPL, estimated to be 1 g or more, is the greatest for any protein hormone in the human. hPL has both lactogenic and somatotropic actions. However, the somatotropic action is much weaker than that of pituitary GH, being only about 1% as potent.[32] hPL does not cross into the fetal compartment. The precise physiologic role of hPL is unclear.

Inhibin

Inhibin is a glycoprotein composed of an α and β subunit and is produced by the ovary, testes, and placenta. Inhibin suppresses the secretion of FSH by the ovary. It is believed that the inhibin produced by the placenta, via its action of inhibition of FSH secretion, prevents ovulation during pregnancy. A paracrine role for inhibin by which it modulates the production of hCG by the syncytiotrophoblast has been suggested.[27,33]

Hypothalamic Peptides

The placenta synthesizes a number of hormonally active peptides that are similar or identical to those produced by the hypothalamus. Thus, the placenta is the site of synthesis of gonadotropin-releasing hormone (GnRH), corticotropin-releasing factor (CRF), TRH, and somatostatin. While the fact that the placenta produces these peptides is not in dispute, their physiologic role is still debatable.

Placental GnRH is chemically and immunologically identical to hypothalamic GnRH.[34] Placental GnRH, acting via GnRH receptors present on trophoblasts, stimulates hCG production and release by the placenta. Inhibin, activin, progesterone, estrogen, vasoactive intestinal peptide (VIP), insulin, prostaglandins, and epinephrine modulate the release of hCG by regulating placental GnRH production or action.[33]

Placental CRH, synthesized in the syncytiotrophoblast and intermediate cells, has identical bioactivity and immunoactivity to the hypothalamic CRH.[35] CRH concentrations in maternal circulation and amniotic fluid are low during most of gestation, but rise significantly during the last 5 weeks of pregnancy.[36] Despite this increase in circulating CRH during the later stages of pregnancy, there is not a corresponding increase in ACTH levels in maternal circulation. This relative resistance of the maternal pituitary gland to the stimulatory effects of CRH is probably due to the presence in the maternal circulation of CRH-binding proteins, which dampen the ACTH-releasing effect of CRH.[37] In contrast, it is believed that the fetal pituitary responds to the increase in placental CRH and produces more ACTH, which in turn stimulates the fetal adrenal to synthesize glucocorticoids. There is experimental evidence to suggest that glucocorticoids have a positive feedback effect on expression of CRH, mRNA, and CRH release by the placenta.[38] This regulatory mechanism may have implications for the role of the fetus in parturition. In some experimental models such as the sheep there is evidence pointing to a relationship between fetal adrenal glucocorticoid activity and the onset of parturition. In the sheep it has been demonstrated that there is an increase in fetal adrenal size and steroid secretory activity late in gestation. In this model the presence of a positive feedback between glucocorticoids and CRH production by the placenta would serve to magnify the surge in cortisol production by the fetal adrenal gland and hence play a role in initiation of labor. However, the role of the fetal adrenal gland in the initiation of labor in the primate has not been elucidated. For example, adrenalectomy in the rhesus monkey fetus does not significantly affect the duration of gestation. In addition, the duration of gestation in the anencephalic neonate and the neonates with X-linked adrenal hypoplasia is not significantly different from that in the control population.[39] As a result of these data, the present consensus is that in the human, fetal adrenal cortisol metabolism does not play an essential role in determining the duration of gestation or the onset of parturition.

Embryology of the Fetal Hypothalamus and Pituitary Gland

The hypothalamus develops from the caudal portion of the neural tube termed the prosencephalon (forebrain). By approximately 34 days postgestation, on the basis of morphologic parameters, the prosencephalon can be separated into the cerebral hemispheres and the diencephalon; the hypothalamus develops from the diencephalon.[40] The primitive neurohypophysis is distinguishable by 37 days, followed by the appearance of the supraoptic-hypophysial tract by 60 days postconception. The hypothalamic-hypophysial portal system is fully organized by the 80th day postconception, and the hypothalamic nuclei are differentiated by the 100th day postconception. All of the classic hypothalamic peptides (e.g., GHRH, TRH, and CRH) are synthesized by neurons that originate in the prosencepahlon. The exception to this pattern is the neurons that secrete GnRH; GnRH neurons develop from the epithelium of the medial olfactory pit.[41-43] These neurons then migrate along the pathway of the olfactory nerve–nervus terminalis complex to reach the developing hypothalamus in the forebrain. GnRH prohormone–containing neurons are detectable in the medial basal fetal hypothalamus by 9 weeks postconception and a functional pulse generator that directs pulsatile secretion of GnRH by these neurons is active by mid-gestation. The clinical significance of the embryologic origin of the GnRH neurons is in the symptomatology of Kallmann's syndrome,[44] which is characterized by the association of hypogonadotropic hypogonadism and anosmia. The X-linked variety of this genotypically heterogeneous disorder is due to the loss of function of a gene, termed the KAL gene, located on the Xp22.3 region. This gene encodes for a 680 amino acid glycoprotein whose structure predicts a role as an extracellular adhesion molecule.[45] The current hypothesis is that loss of function of this gene results in the arrest of the migration of GnRH neurons and aplasia/hypoplasia of the olfactory bulbs and tracts; hence, anosmia with hypogonadotrophic hypogonadism.

Adenohypophysis

Rathke's pouch, the precursor of the adenohypophysis in the human, is ectodermal in origin and develops as a diverticulum of the primitive stomodeum. In the human the craniopharyngeal invagination that forms the Rathke's pouch is apparent by 22 days postconception.[46] By the 35th day the pouch is separated from the stomodeum and the posterior wall comes into contact with the structures destined to become the neurohypophysis (i.e., the primitive infundibular process of the embryonic diencephalon). The anterior wall of the Rathke's pouch forms the adenohypophysis, and the posterior wall forms the intermediate lobe and pars tuberalis of the pituitary gland.[47]

The cellular differentiation of the adenohypophysis takes place after the 40th day postconception with the formation of cell cords that populate the anterior lobe of the primitive pituitary gland. Further differentiation of the cells is apparent by the 8th to 9th week postconception with the appearance of ACTH-containing basophils. The acidophils appear soon thereafter, and by the 14th to 15th week postconception the pituitary gland has achieved the adult organization.

Molecular Events Regulating the Development of the Adenohypophysis

The fully developed pituitary gland contains five distinct cell types: gonadotrophs (producing LH and FSH), thryotrophs [producing thyroid-stimulating hormone (TSH)], somatotrophs (producing GH), lactotrophs (producing prolactin), and corticotrophs [producing proopiomelanocortin (POMC), the precursor of ACTH]. These five cell types develop from a common progenitor cell. The differentiation of this primordial cell into the different hormone specific cell types is an orderly process and has been extensively studied in the rodent.[48,49] In the mouse the first transcript to be detected in the embryonic anterior pituitary is that of the α subunit (common to FSH, LH, and TSH) at postconception day 11. On day 14, transcripts can be detected for POMC and the β subunit of TSH. However, these cells that produce the β subunit of the TSH undergo apoptosis, and the major source of the TSH in the developed pituitary gland are thryotrophs whose differentiation is under the control of the transcription factor Pit-1. At days 16 and 17 expression of the β subunit for LH and FSH can be detected. Transcripts for GH and prolactin appear at embryonic day 17. It is not clear whether the cells that produce prolactin pass through a phase of differentiation where they express both GH and prolactin (i.e., mammosomatotroph). It is of interest to note that not only is there a cell-type specificity but also that each cell type maintains a spatial specificity within the pituitary gland such that each cell type develops within a specific area of the gland.

Pit-1 (also termed growth hormone factor-1, GHF-1) is a member of the POU family of transcription factors. This family of proteins derives its acronym from its principal members Pit-1, Oct-1 and Oct-2, and Unc-86. Oct-1 is a widely expressed transcription factor, Oct-2 is expressed in the brain and lymphocytes, and Unc-86 plays a role in neuronal development in *Caenorhaleditis elegans*. The POU family of transcription factors belong to the helix-loop-helix superfamily of transcription factors. Pit-1 is a pituitary-specific protein that plays an essential role in the transcriptional activation of the GH and prolactin and TSH-β genes in mammals.[50] Via two distinct domains, termed POU-specific (POU-S) and POU-homeo (POU-HD), Pit-1 binds to upstream regulatory elements in the GH, PRL, and TSH genes and increases transcription of these genes. The POU-S is a 75 amino acid region that confers high-affinity site-specific binding to Pit-1 response elements in the regulatory regions of the GH, PRL, and TSH genes.[51] Downstream, i.e., 3′ to the POU-S domain, and separated from it by a nonconserved region of 15 amino acids is the 60 amino acid POU-HD domain that is required for low-affinity binding with relaxed specificity.[52] The POU-HD derives its name from having homology to a conserved sequence motif called homeobox. The amino acid sequence of POU-HD predicts the formation of a helix-loop-helix motif. Genes containing this homeobox motif are known to play essential roles in the regulation of development in *Drosophila* and yeast. Whereas Pit-1 is monomeric in solution, in vivo, in the majority of instances, it binds as dimers to DNA response elements.

In certain cases Pit-1 response elements are able to bind only Pit-1 homodimers, whereas in other examples heterodomers of Pit-1 and other transcription factors such as Oct-1 or retinoic acid receptor interact with Pit-1 response elements.ABnormalities in Pit-1 structure and/or function result in phenotypic alterations by the following mechanisms: (1) the mutant Pit-1 protein may not be able to bind to the cognate DNA response element; (2) in the presence of both wild type and mutant Pit-1, the mutant Pit-1 molecule may form homodimers that compete with the wild-type molecule for binding to the DNA response element or may form heterodimers with the wild-type molecule and thus interfere with the actions of the wild-type molecule; (3) the mutant Pit-1 molecule may interact with and alter the action of other DNA-binding proteins such as Oct-1 or retinoic acid receptor.

Alteration in the characteristics of binding of Pit-1 to DNA response elements results in deficiency of GH, PRL, and TSH. The essential role of Pit-1 in the development of the anterior pituitary gland and in the expression of GH, PRL, and TSH in mammals has been established by studying the Snell and Jackson strains of dwarf mice and by investigating the mechanisms resulting in sporadic and familial combined pituitary hormone deficiency in man. Both the Snell and Jackson strains of mice have hypoplastic anterior pituitary glands and exhibit deficiency of GH, PRL, and TSH.[53] The Snell mouse is homozygous for a missense point mutation in the POU-HD domain (codon 261) that alters a tryptophan to a cysteine residue, resulting in altered ability of the mutant Pit-1 protein to bind to and activate the target genes. In the Jackson mice a gross abnormality (i.e., either a deletion or an insertion) in the Pit-1 gene, completely disrupts the expression of the gene resulting in an absence of Pit-1 protein. In humans several cases of anterior pituitary hormone deficiency have been described that result from mutations in the Pit-1 gene.[54] Although the original publications concerned familial cases of this syndrome, several cases of sporadic mutations in this gene have since been reported. The majority of described cases involve mutations within either the POU-S or POU-HD domains. There is variability in the phenotypic presentation of the various mutations, with the pituitary gland being either normal or decreased in size, and the deficiency in PRL and TSH expression extending from total to partial deficiency.

Ontogeny of Adenohypophysial Hormones

Due to obvious ethical considerations, data on the ontogeny of pituitary hormones in the healthy human fetus are limited; the majority of the data have been obtained from samples from aborted fetuses or at delivery.

Growth Hormone

Growth hormone (GH) can be detected in fetal plasma by the 70th day of gestation, with the concentration rising to a peak of 150 ng·ml^{-1} at 20 to 24 weeks of gestation.[55] Subsequently, the concentration of circulating GH in the fetus decreases to 30 to 50 ng·ml^{-1} in cord blood at term. Available data indicate that alteration in the metabolic clearance of GH is not the major mechanism resulting in high levels of GH in the fetus. On the contrary, direct measurements of the characteristics of GH secretory pattern from the anterior pituitary and estimates of total GH content of the pituitary indicate that increased secretion of GH is the major mechanism for the elevated concentration of GH during fetal life.[56] The secretion of GH is primarily under the stimulatory control of GHRH and the inhibitory control of somatostatin. There is a significant body of evidence that suggests that the increased secretion of GH by the fetal pituitary is due to decreased activity of the somatostatin inhibitory control.[57] Early in gestation the fetal pituitary is relatively resistant to the effects of exogenous somatostatin, providing the basis for the hypothesis that the somatostatin receptor is not fully functional in the fetus. As gestation progresses, there is gradual maturation of the responsiveness of the fetal pituitary to somatostatin. At birth somatostatin is able to effectively block the stimulatory influence of GHRH. In contrast, as early as the 9th week of gestation, experiments using explant cultures of human fetal pituitary gland have corroborated data obtained in the ovine model that GHRH can stimulate GH secretion in a dose-dependent manner.[58] These data support the model that during the early fetal life unrestrained action of GHRH results in an elevated concentration of GH with progressive decline in GH concentration with the maturation of the somatostatin–somatostatin receptor axis.

Luteinizing Hormone and Follicle-Stimulating Hormone

Luteinizing hormone (LH) and follicle-stimulating hormone (FSH) are glycoproteins composed of noncovalently linked α and β subunits. The α subunit has an identical amino acid sequence in LH, FSH, TSH, and hCG, whereas the β subunit confers immunologic and biologic specificity. The cross-reactivity between these hormones as a result of the shared α subunit confounds the interpretation of data generated using the earlier generation immunoassays; the more current generation of assays avoids this problem by the use of anti-β-LH subunit-specific antibodies and strategies such as double-antibody assays.

In the human fetus, gonadotrophin activity is contributed to by hCG (produced by the syncytiotrophoblast) and fetal pituitary LH and FSH. In the fetal circulation hCG reaches its maximum concentration at approximately 12 weeks of gestation and then decreases to a nadir at 18 to 20 weeks. Early in gestation placental hCG, acting via functional hCG/LH receptors present in the fetal testis, plays the major role in stimulating production of testosterone by the fetal testis during the critical period of differentiation of the wolffian ducts and the urogenital sinus and masculinization of the external genitalia. Hence, sexual differentiation is for the most part completed by the time LH and FSH secretion by the fetal pituitary reaches a physiologically significant plateau. This dependence on hCG with independence from fetal pituitary gonadotropins for the early sexual differentiation explains the observation that deficiency of fetal gonadotropins, in conditions such as anencephaly or congenital hypopituitarism, is characterized by the presence of micropenis and undescended testes but not by sexual ambiguity in the male. Using a variety of techniques, both LH and FSH can be detected in the fetal pituitary gland by 10 weeks of gestation.[59-61] The LH content of the pituitary gland increases between 10 and 27 weeks and remains essentially unchanged thereafter. Similarly, the FSH content of the pituitary gland reaches a maximum between 10 and 25 weeks. The pituitary content of both LH and FSH exhibits sexual dimorphism with the concentrations being higher in the female than the male. In general the concentrations of circulating LH and FSH follow a pattern that is similar to the profile of the pituitary content. Hence, pituitary gonadotropins can be first detected in circulation at around 100 days of gestation. These concentrations are highest in mid-gestation, then decrease to reach a nadir at birth.

The principal regulator of fetal gonadotropin secretion is GnRH secreted from the hypothalamus into the hypophysial portal system. The effect of GnRH on the pituitary gonadotrophs is dependent on both the amount of GnRH and more significantly on the pulsatile nature of GnRH secretion. GnRH is detectable in fetal hypothalamic extracts by the 10th week of gestation.[62] The pulsatile nature of GnRH secretion has been demonstrated in the hypothalamus of the mid-gestation human fetus.[63] Plasma concentrations of FSH and LH are high in mid-gestation and decline thereafter. This profile of circulating gonadotropins is attributed to the maturation of negative feedback mechanisms such that the initial unrestrained pulsatile release of GnRH in mid-gestation progressively matures into inhibition of GnRH release from the hypothalamus (Figure 21.2). The negative feedback loop involves the inhibitory effect of the sex steroids, especially progesterone and estrogens, mediated via functional cognate steroid receptors in the fetal hypothalamus and pituitary gland, on fetal hypothalamic GnRH secretion. Given the crucial role of the placenta in fetal steroid metabolism, the modulation of fetal pituitary

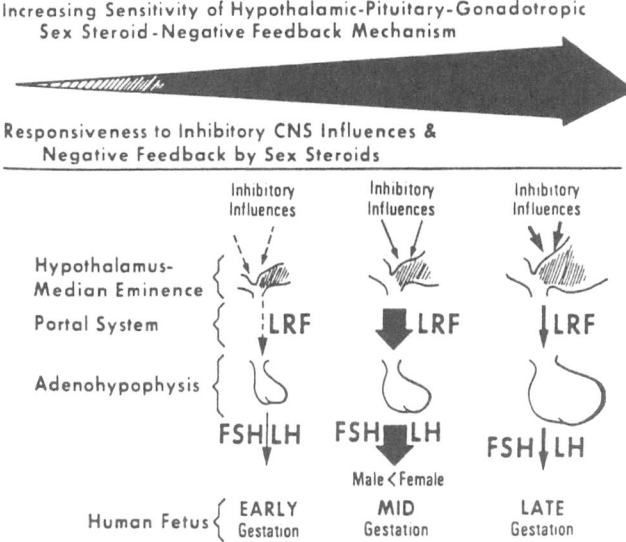

FIGURE 21.2. Ontogeny of regulatory mechanisms for gonadotropin secretion in the human fetus. (See text for details.) (Adapted from Grumbach and Kaplan.[72])

gonadotropins and hypothalamic GnRH by these steroids represents another example of the concept of the fetoplacental unit.

Thyroid Hormones

Role of Placenta in the Regulation of Fetal Thyroid Hormone Status

The placenta acts both as a source of molecules that influence fetal thyroidal function and as a barrier protecting the fetus from the influence of maternal thyroidal hormones (Figure 21.3). In general the fetal thyroidal unit develops independently of maternal influence.

Thyroid-Releasing Hormone

Since thyroid-releasing hormone (TRH), a tripeptide, readily crosses the placenta maternal TRH can gain access to the fetal compartment.[64] However, the low concentration of TRH in the maternal circulation limits the significance of this transport under physiologic conditions. Of more significance is the fact that TRH synthesized by the placenta contributes to the circulating fetal TRH concentration. The role of placentally derived TRH in the regulation of fetal thyroid function remains to be elucidated.

Since the TSH molecule does not cross the placenta, there is no significant effect of maternal TSH on the fetal thyroid. Significantly, hCG, which is produced by the placenta in large amounts during the early period of ges-

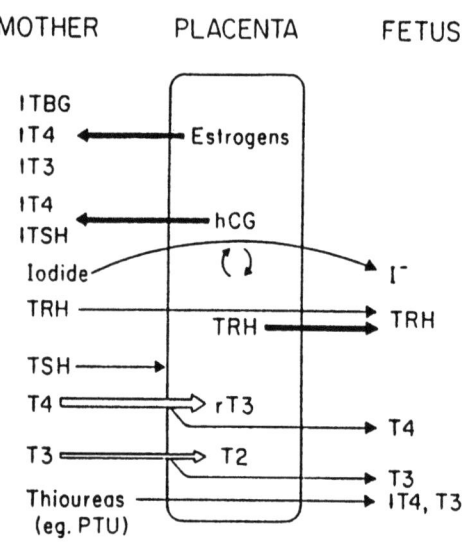

FIGURE 21.3. Permeability of the placenta to maternal and fetal thyroid hormones. Thickness of the arrows indicates the relative amounts of the transfer. Heavy arrows indicate placental production of estrogens, hCG and TRH. (See text for details of the placental role in maternal and fetal thyroid function.) (Adapted from Fisher.[73])

tation and enters fetal circulation, has TSH-like activity. This action of hCG results from the identity of the α subunits of hCG and TSH and the partial homology between the β subunits. However, since hCG is only 0.01% as potent as TSH in stimulating the thyroid gland, the biologic effect of this cross-specificity in action is minimal.[65] One prominent exception to this rule is a hydatiform mole, where the extraordinarily high concentration of hCG can result in some manifestations of hyperthyroidism due to the TSH-like actions of hCG.

There is general consensus that the human placenta is relatively impermeable to maternally derived iodothyronines, in part due to the activity of placental monoiodinase. This inner ring monoiodinase converts the biologically active T_4 and T_3 to the inactive rT_3 and T_2, respectively. Some degree of placental transfer of maternal iodothyronines occurs in the hypothyroid human fetus. It has been postulated that this transferred iodothyronine may play a role in ameliorating some of the potentially deleterious effects of hypothyroidism on fetal organs whose development is particularly sensitive to the thyroidal status.[66]

The human placenta is permeable to iodide. The fetal thyroid gland, much more so than the adult gland, is sensitive to the inhibitory effects of iodine. The effect of exogenous iodide on fetal thyroid function is usually evident after only 70 to 75 days of gestation when the iodide uptake machinery of the gland achieves functional maturity. In the adult thyroid autoregulation of iodide transport into the follicular cells partially compensates for iodide excess or deficiency. This mechanism does not

mature in the fetal gland until near term.[67] The placenta is permeable to a commonly used class of antithyroid drugs, the thiourea group, which includes propylthiouracil. Hence, administration of these drugs to the mother for management of hyperthyroidism can result in alterations in fetal thyroid function. Immunoglobulins of the IgG class, present in the maternal circulation, cross the placenta into fetal circulation. Hence, the function of the fetal thyroid gland can be modulated by the transfer of maternal IgG, most commonly directed against the TSH receptor. The precise clinical effect of these phenomena depends on whether these antibodies are stimulatory or blocking in nature.[68]

Embryology of Thyroid Gland Development

In the human the thyroid gland, a derivative of the primitive buccopharyngeal cavity, is derived from the fusion of two endodermal anlages, the median and the lateral anlagen.[69] The median anlagen is represented by a thickening of the pharyngeal floor, while the lateral anlage originate as paired ultimobranchial bodies derived from the fourth pharyngobranchial pouch. The median and the lateral anlage are first definable at about the 17th day of gestation and fuse together by the 24th day. Subsequent development culminates in the migration of the thyroid gland caudally to its final location in the neck.

Thyroid Hormone Production and Metabolism

The major steps in the synthesis of thyroid hormone by the thyroid gland are the following: (1) active transport of iodide from the plasma into the thyroid cell; (2) synthesis of thyroglobulin by the thyroid follicular cells; (3) organification of the iodide to mono- (MIT) and diiodotyrosines (DIT) bound to the thyroglobulin; (4) formation of triiodothyronine (T_3) and tetraiodothyronine (T_4) by coupling of MIT and DIT; (5) release of T_4, T_3, MIT, and DIT from the thyroglobulin; and (6) recycling of iodine by deiodination of iodotyrosines released within the gland.

Although each of the above-mentioned steps in thyroid hormone synthesis is capable of being modulated in the fetus, and various defects in these processes have been described that result in alteration in the thyroidal status of the fetus, the step that seems to play a major role in the ontogeny of thyroid hormone function in the human is the process of deiodination. Three types of the monodeiodinase (MDI) enzyme catalyze the process of deiodination of the iodotyrosines formed in the thyroid

21. Developmental Endocrinology in the Fetal-Placental Unit

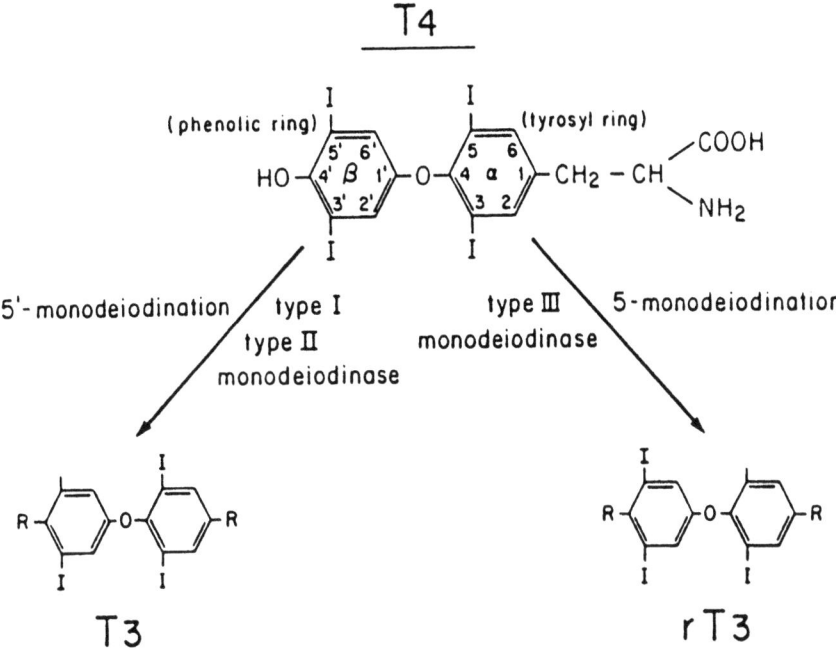

FIGURE 21.4. Pathways of thyroid hormone synthesis. T_4, thyroxine; T_3 triiodothyronine; and rT_3, reverse triiodothyronine. (See text for details.) (Adapted from Fisher.[73])

gland. Two of these enzymes act on the outer ring and the third enzyme acts on the inner ring of the iodothyronine molecule (Figure 21.4). Removal of the iodine molecule on the outer ring of the iodothyronine molecule converts T_4 to T_3, which is the active form of the hormone. In contrast removal of the inner ring converts T_4 and T_3 to rT_3 and DIT, respectively, both inactive metabolites. The inner ring MDI (type III MDI) is widely distributed in fetal tissue including the placenta. This enzyme is very active during fetal life and is the main reason why levels of rT_3 are elevated during fetal life.

The precise profile of the ontogeny of TRH secretion and function in the fetus is undefined at this time. TRH can be detected in the fetal hypothalamus by midgestation. The concentration of immunoreactive TRH increases significantly during the third trimester. The biologic role of TRH from nonhypothalamic sources, such as placenta and pancreas, is undefined. In contrast to TRH, much more is known about the ontogeny of TSH production and secretion by the fetal pituitary gland. Prior to 18 weeks of gestation, the fetal TSH concentration is low; thereafter, the circulating concentration of this hormone increases progressively to peak at term. These data suggest that during the second and third trimester, the fetal thyroid develops under the influence of an elevated concentration of TSH. Parturition is associated with a dramatic transient surge in TSH secretion brought about by the relative cooling of the neonate in the extrauterine environment. Peak concentration of TSH in the perinatal period is reached within 30 minutes of birth and then declines in an exponential manner to reach adult concentration by the first month after birth.

Despite the fact that the iodide transport and thyroglobulin synthesis pathways are operational in the fetal thyroid by 70 to 80 days of gestation, the human fetal thyroid makes very little thyroid hormone until about 125 to 130 days of gestation. From this time onward, the concentration of T_4 (both free and bound) progressively increases until the final weeks of pregnancy (Figure 21.5).

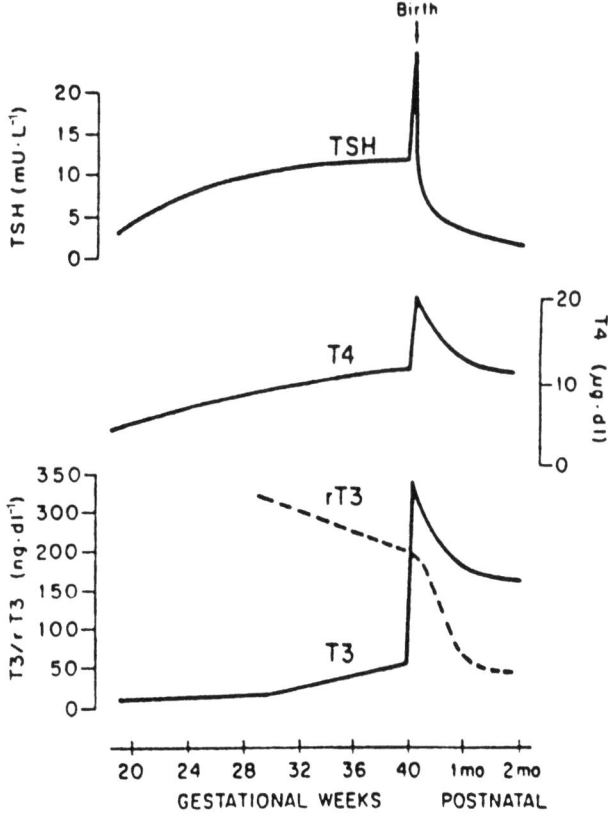

FIGURE 21.5. Profile of thyroid axis in fetal-perinatal period. (See text for details.) (Adapted from Fisher and Polk.[74])

The concentration of T_3 is low (<15–20 ng·dl^{-1}) until 28 to 30 weeks of gestation, after which there is a gradual increase to a concentration of 50 ng·dl^{-1} at term. In contrast the concentration of rT_3 is relatively high in the fetus (300–350 ng·dl^{-1} at 28–30 weeks gestation) and progressively decline until term. This profile of T_3 and rT_3 concentrations is primarily the result of the balance between the activities of two types of monodeiodinase. Hence, fetal life is characterized by high levels of activity of the inner ring (type III) monodeiodinase enzyme that catalyzes conversion of T_3 to rT_3. The increase of T_3 with gestation is the result of maturation of the hepatic type I monodeiodinase that converts T_4 to T_3. Parturition is associated with dramatic changes in the profile of these thyroid hormones.[70] These changes are initiated by a surge in the concentration of TSH, which peaks within 30 minutes of birth. Serum T_3 and T_4 concentrations subsequently increase in response to this TSH surge to peak by 36 to 48 hours of life and then gradually decrease into the adult range by 4 to 6 weeks of life.

References

1. Cummings SW, Hatley W, Simpson ER, Ohashi M. The binding of high and low density lipoproteins to human placental membrane fractions. J Clin Endocrinol Metab 1982;54:903–908.
2. Brown MS, Goldstein JL. A receptor-mediated pathway for cholesterol homoestasis. Science 1986;232:34–37.
3. Little B, Shaw A. The conversion of progesterone to 17α-hydroxy-progesterone by human placenta in vitro. Acta Endocrinol 1961;36:455–461.
4. Ryan KJ. Aromatization of steroids. J Biol Chem 1959;234: 268–272.
5. Siiteri PK, MacDonald PC. The utilization of circulating dehydroepiandrosterone sulfate for estrogen synthesis during human pregnancy. Steroids 1963;2:713–730.
6. Siiteri PK, MacDonald PC. Placental estrogen biosynthesis during human pregnancy. J Clin Endocrinol Metab 1966; 26:751–761.
7. Carr BR, Parker CR, Milewich L, et al. The role of low density, high density, and very low density lipoprotein in steroidogenesis by the human fetal adrenal gland. Endocrinology 1980;106:1854–1860.
8. Gurpide E, Schwers J, Welch MT, et al. Fetal and maternal metabolism of estradiol during pregnancy. J Clin Endocrinol Metab 1966;26:1355–1365.
9. Lin D, Gitelman SE, Saenger P, Miller WL. Normal genes for the cholesterol side chain cleavage enzyme, P450scc, in congenital lipoid adrenal hyperplasia. J Clin Invest 1991;88: 1955–1962.
10. Matteson KJ, Chung BC, Urdea MS, Miller WL. Study of cholesterol side-chain cleavage (20, 22 desmolase) deficiency causing congenital lipoid adrenal hyperplasia using bovine-sequence P450scc oligodeoxyribonucleotide probes. Endocrinology 1986;118:1296–1305.
11. Sakai Y, Yanase T, Okabe Y, et al. No mutation in cytochrome P450 side chain cleavage in a patient with congenital lipoid adrenal hyperplasia. J Clin Endocrinol Metab 1994;79:1198–1201.
12. Fukami M, Sato S, Ogata T, Matsuo N. Lack of mutations in P450scc gene (CYP11A) in six Japanese patients with congenital lipoid adrenal hyperplasia. Clin Pediatr Endocrinol 1995;4:39–46.
13. Epstein LF, Orme-Johnson NR. Regulation of steroid hormone biosynthesis: identification of precursors of a phosphoprotein targeted to the mitochondrion in stimulated rat adrenal cortex cells. J Biol Chem 1991;266: 19739–19745.
14. Stocco DM, Sodeman TC. The 30-kDa mitochondrial proteins induced by hormone stimulation in MA-10 mouse Leydig tumor cells are processed from larger precursors. J Biol Chem 1991;266:19731–19738.
15. Clark BJ, Wells J, King SR, Stocco DM. The purification, cloning, and expression of a novel luteinizing hormone-induced mitochondrial protein in MA-10 mouse Leydig tumor cells: characterization of the steroidogenic acute regulatory protein (StAR). J Biol Chem 1994;269:28314–28322.
16. Bose HS, Sugawara T, Jerome III FS, Miller WL. The pathophysiology and genetics of congenital lipoid adrenal hyperplasia. N Engl J Med 1996;335:1870–1878.
17. Lin D, Sugawara T, Strauss III JF, et al. Role of steroidogenic acute regulatory protein in adrenal and gonadal steroidogenesis. Science 1995;267:1828–1831.
18. Tee MK, Lin D, Sugawara T, et al. T-A transversion 11 bp from a splice acceptor site in the gene for steroidogenic acute regulatory protein causes congenital lipoid adrenal hyperplasia. Hum Mol Genet 1995;4:2299–2305.
19. Stocco DM, Clark BJ. Regulation of the acute production of steroids in steroidogenic cells. Endocr Rev 1996;17:221–244.
20. Simpson ER, Burkhart MF. AcylCoA: cholesterol acyltransferase activity in human placental microsomes: inhibition by progesterone. Arch Biochim Biophys 1980; 200:79–85.
21. MacDonald PC, Siiteri PK. Origin of estrogen in women pregnant with anencephalic fetus. J Clin Invest 1965; 44:465–474.
22. Got R, Bourrillon R. Nouvelle methode de purification de la gonadotropine choriale humaine. Biochim Biophys Acta 1960;42:241–247.
23. Bellisario R, Carlsen RB, Bahl OP. Human chorionic gonadotropin; linear amino acid sequence of the alpha subunit. J Biol Chem 1973;248:6796–6807.
24. Khodr GS, Siler-Khodr TM. The effect of luteinizing hormone-releasing factor on human chorionic gonadotropin secretion. Fertil Steril 1978;30:301–304.
25. Nishino E, Matsuzaki N, Masuhiro K, et al. Trophoblast derived interleukin 6 (IL-6) regulates human chorionic gonadotropin release through IL-6 receptor on human trophoblasts. J Clin Endocrinol Metab 1990;71: 436.
26. Li Y, Matsuzaki N, Masuhiro K, et al. Trophoblast derived tumor necrosis factor-alpha induces release of human chorionic gonadotropin using IL-1 and IL-6 receptor dependent system in the normal human trophoblast. J Clin Endocrinol Metab 1992;74:184–191.

27. Mersol-Barry MS, Miller KF, Choi CM, et al. Inhibin suppresses human chorionic gonadotropin secretion in term, but not first trimester placenta. J Clin Endocrinol Metab 1968;71:1294–1298.
28. Tulsky AJ, Koff AK. Some observations on the role of the corpus luteum in early human pregnancy. Fertil Steril 1957;8:118–130.
29. Serron-Ferre M, Lawrence CC, Jaffe RB. Role of hCG in the regulation of the fetal zone of the human fetal adrenal gland. J Clin Endocrinol Metab 1978;46:834–837.
30. Talamantes F, Ogren L, Markoff E, et al. Phylogenetic distribution, regulation of secretion, and prolactin-like effects of placental lactogens. Fed Proc 1980;39:2582–2587.
31. Bewley TA, Li CH. Structural similarities between human pituitary growth hormone, human chorionic somato-mammotropin and ovine pituitary growth hormone and lactogenic hormones. In: Josmovich JB, Reynolds M, Cobo E, eds. Lactogenic hormones, fetal nutrition and lactation. New York: Wiley, 1975:19–32.
32. Handwerker S, Sherwood LM. Comparison of the structure and lactogenic activity of human placental lactogen and human growth hormone. In: Josmovich JB, Reynolds M, Cobo E, eds. Lactogenic hormones, fetal nutrition and lactation. New York: Wiley, 1975:33–47.
33. Petraglia F, Volpe AO, Genazzani AR, et al. Neuroendocrinology of the human placenta. Front Neuroendocrinol 1990;11:6–37.
34. Khodr GS, Siler-Khodr TM. Placental luteinizing hormone-releasing factor and its synthesis. Science 1980;207:315–317.
35. Shibasaki T, Odagiri E, Shizume K, Ling N. Corticotropin-releasing factor-like activity in human placental extracts. J Clin Endocrinol Metab 1982;55:384–386.
36. Campbell EA, Linton EA, Wolfe CD, et al. Plasma corticotropin-releasing hormone concentrations during pregnancy and parturition. J Clin Endocrinol Metab 1987; 63:1054–1059.
37. Linton EA, Behan DP, Saphier PN, Loury PJ. Corticotropin releasing hormone (CRH)-binding protein. Reduction in the adrenocorticotropin releasing activity of placental but not hypothalamic CRH. J Clin Endocrinol Metab 1990;70:1574–1580.
38. Jones SA, Brooks AN, Challis JRG. Steroids modulate corticotropin-releasing hormone production in human fetal membranes and placenta. J Clin Endocrinol Metab 1989; 68:825–830.
39. Milic AB, Adamsons K. The relationship between anencephaly and prolonged pregnancy. Br J Obstet Gynaecol 1987;76:102–111.
40. Bartelmez GW, Dekaban AS. The early development of the human brain. Contrib Embryol Carnegie Inst 1962;37: 13–32.
41. Schwanzel-Fukuda M, Pfaff DW. Origin of luteinizing hormone-releasing hormone neurons. Nature (Lond) 1989; 338:161–164.
42. Wray S, Grant P, Gainer H. Evidence that cells expressing luteinizing hormone-releasing hormone mRNA in the mouse are derived from progenitor cells in the olfactory placode. Proc Natl Acad Sci USA 1989;86:8132–8136.
43. Wray S, Nieburgs A, Elkabes S. Spatiotemporal cell expression of luteinizing hormone-releasing hormone in the prenatal mouse: evidence for an embryonic origin in the olfactory placode. Dev Brain Res 1989;46:309–318.
44. Prager D, Braunstein GD, Editorial: X-chromosome-linked Kallmann's syndrome: pathology at the molecular level. J Clin Endocrinol Metab 1993;76:824–826.
45. Franco B, Guioli S, Pragliola A, et al. A gene deleted in Kallmann syndrome shares homology with neural cell adhesion and axonal pathfinding molecules. Nature 1991; 353:529–536.
46. O'Rahilly R. The timing and sequence of events in the development of the human endocrine system during the embryonic period proper. Anat Embryol 1983;166:439–451.
47. Ikeda H, Suzuki J, Sasano N, Nizuma H. The development and morphogenesis of the human pituitary gland. Anat Embryol 1988;178:327–336.
48. Schaufele F. Regulation of expression of the growth hormones and prolactin genes. In: Imura H, ed. The pituitary gland. New York: Raven Press, 1994:91–113.
49. Simmons DM, Voss JW, Ingraham HA, et al. Pituitary cell phenotypes involve cell-specific Pit-1 mRNA translation and synergistic interactions with other classes of transcription factors. Genes Dev 1990;4:695–711.
50. Mangalam HJ, Albert VR, Ingraham HA, et al. A pituitary POU domain protein, Pit-1, activates both growth hormone and prolactin promoters transcriptionally. Genes Dev 1989; 3:946–958.
51. Ingraham HA, Flynn SE, Voss JW, et al. The POU-specific domain of Pit-1 is essential for sequence-specific, high-affinity DNA binding and DNA-dependent Pit-1-Pit-1 interactions. Cell 1990;61:1021–1033.
52. Theill LE, Castrillo JL, Wu D, et al. Dissection of functional domains of the pituitary transcription factor GHF-1. Nature 1989;342:945–948.
53. Li S, Crenshaw III EB, Rawson EJ, et al. Dwarf locus mutants lacking three pituitary cell types result from mutations in the POU-domain gene Pit-1. Nature 1990;347: 528–533.
54. Cohen LE, Wondisford FE, Radovick S. Role of Pit-1 in the gene expression of growth hormone, prolactin, and thyrotropin. In: Rosenfield RL, ed. Endocrinology and metabolism clinics of North America. Philadelphia: WB Saunders, 1996;523–540.
55. Kaplan SL, Grumbach MM, Shepard TH. The ontogenesis of human fetal hormones. J Clin Invest 1972;51:3080–3093.
56. Albers N, Bettendorf M, Herrmann H, et al. Hormone ontogeny in the ovine fetus. XXVII. Pulsatile and copulsatile secretion of luteinizing hormone, follicle stimulating hormone, growth hormone, and prolactin in late gestation: A new method for the analysis of copulsatility. Endocrinology 1993;132:701–709.
57. Gluckman PD, Grumbach MM, Kaplan SL. The neuroendocrine regulation and function of growth hormone and prolactin in the mammalian fetus. Endocr Rev 1981;2:363–395.
58. Goodyer CG, Branchaud CL, Lefebvre Y. Effects of growth hormone (GH)-releasing factor and somatostatin on GH secretion from early to midgestation human fetal pituitaries. J Clin Endocrinol Metab 1993;76:1259–1964.
59. Pasteels JL, Sheridan R, Gaspar S, Franchimont P. Synthesis and release of gonadotropins and their subunits

by long-term organ cultures of human fetal hypophyses. Mol Cell Endocrinol 1977;9:1–19.
60. Grumbach MM, Kaplan SL. Ontogenesis of growth hormone, insulin, prolactin and gonadotropin secretion in the human foetus. In: Cross KW, Nathanielsz P, eds. Foetal and neonatal physiology. Proceedings of Sir Joseph Barcroft Centenary Symposium. Cambridge: Cambridge University Press, 1973:462–487.
61. Grumbach MM. Fetal pituitary hormones and the maturation of central nervous system regulation of anterior pituitary function. In: Gluck L, ed. Modern perinatal medicine. Chicago: Year Book Medical, 1974:247–271.
62. Siler-Khodr TM, Khodr GS. Studies in human fetal endocrinology. I. Luteinizing hormone-releasing factor content of the hypothalamus. Am J Obstet Gynecol 1978; 130:795–800.
63. Rasmussen DD, Gambacciani M, Swartz WH, et al. Pulsatile GnRH release from the human mediobasal hypothalamus in vitro: opiate receptor mediated suppression. Neuroendocrinology 1989;49:150–156.
64. Moya F, Mena P, Hensser F, et al. Response of the maternal, fetal and neonatal pituitary thyroid axis to thyrotropin-releasing hormone. Pediatr Res 1986;20:982–986.
65. Harada A, Hershman JM, Reed AW, et al. Comparison of thyroid stimulators and thyroid hormone concentrations in the sera of pregnant women. J Clin Endocrinol Metab 1979;48:793–797.
66. Vulsma T, Gons MH, DeVijlder JJM. Maternal-fetal transfer of thyroxine in congenital hypothyroidism due to a total organification defect or thyroid agenesis. N Engl J Med 1989;321;13–16.
67. Castaign H, Fournet JP, Leger FA, et al. Thyroid of the newborn and postnatal iodine overload. Arch Fr Pediatr 1979;36:356–368.
68. Zakarija M, McKenzie JM. Pregnancy-associated changes in the thyroid stimulating antibody of Graves' disease and the relationship to neonatal hyperthyroidism. J Clin Endocrinol Metab 1983;57:1036–1040.
69. Erickson LE, Fredriksson G. Phylogeny and ontogeny of the thyroid gland. In: Greer ME, ed. The thyroid gland (comprehensive endocrinology). New York: Raven Press, 1990:1–35.
70. Fisher DA, Dussault JH, Sack J, Chopra IJ. Ontogenesis of hypothalamic-pituitary-thyroid function and metabolism in man, sheep and rat. Recent Prog Horm Res 1977;33: 59–116.
71. Casey ML, MacDonald PC, Simpson ER. Endocrinological changes in pregnancy. In: Wilson JD, Foster DW, eds. Williams' textbook of endocrinology. Philadelphia: WB Saunders, 1992:977–991.
72. Grumbach MM, Kaplan SL. Fetal pituitary hormones and the maturation of the contral nervous system regulation of anterior pituitary function. In: Gluck L, ed. Modern perinatal medicine. Chicago: Year Book Medical Publishers, 1974:247–273.
73. Fisher DA. Disorders of the thyroid in the newborn and infant. In: Sperling MA, ed. Pediatric endocrinology. Philadelphia: WB Saunders, 1996:51–70.
74. Fisher DA, Polk DH. The ontogenesis of thyroid hormone function and actions. In: Tulchinsky D, Little AB, eds. Maternal-fetal endocrinology. Philadelphia: WB Saunders, 1994:321–334.

22
The Sympathoadrenal System in the Fetal-Placental Unit

Yi-Tang Tseng and James F. Padbury

Functional development of the sympathoadrenal system is critical to successful fetal and neonatal survival and maturation. During intrauterine life a high degree of sympathetic tone is critical to maintenance of cardiovascular, endocrine, and metabolic homeostasis. At birth, the neonate must successfully initiate air breathing, convert to circulation in series, and sustain energy autonomy and temperature regulation. This chapter reviews relevant concepts in the maturation of the sympathoadrenal system. Because the newest data pertain to novel aspects of catecholamine (CA) metabolism in utero, unique mechanisms for regulation of adrenergic receptors, and developmental aspects of receptor coupling to second messenger systems, these areas are emphasized. Whenever possible, data available for the human are presented. Data from animal studies are used to provide insight not available from human data. The data on neuroanatomic organization and regulation of phenotypic expression in the sympathoadrenal system has been reviewed elsewhere.[1-5] The reader is also referred to past reviews on functional aspects of sympathoadrenal system activity during the transition from fetal to newborn life.

Perinatal Catecholamine Metabolism

Circulating plasma CA concentrations in either the fetus or the adult represent a net expression of the rate of secretion and the rate of clearance from the plasma compartment. Catecholamine clearance represents an integrated summation of reuptake, conjugation, enzymatic degradation, and excretion. In the central nervous system reuptake is the most important mechanism for regulation of extracellular neurotransmitter concentration.[6] Across regional circulations of systemic organ systems, reuptake may account for as much as 80% of CA clearance, as in the heart, versus 10% in the forearm.[7] In vivo methods using radioisotope tracers have been developed and validated to sensitively measure these mechanisms.[8,9] These methods are dependent on the infusion of trace amounts of radiolabeled norepinephrine (^{3}H-NE) and serial measurement of its concentration in circulation to quantitate the rate of norepinephrine production and removal. These approaches are analogous to the now classic methods developed to study glucose production and disposition (see Chapter 33). Pharmacologic agents with specific effects can be administered simultaneously to determine the relative contribution of reuptake and/or enzymatic degradation to norepinephrine turnover.[9]

Circulating CA concentrations are low in the fetus despite a high degree of sympathetic tone, which is important for the maintenance of cardiovascular homeostasis.[1] At birth there are exponential increases in norepinephrine and epinephrine concentrations.[10,11] It was initially unclear whether the low fetal concentrations represented low CA production rates or rapid metabolic clearance. It has been demonstrated, using isotope tracer methods in chronically catheterized fetal sheep, that the fetal sympathoadrenal system is characterized by high CA production and clearance rates.[12-14] These techniques were adapted to examine placental glucose and amino acid transport to the contribution of high placental clearance rates observed in utero. These investigations demonstrated that the placenta is responsible for the high intrauterine clearance rate of CA, contributing to over 50% of the total clearance of norepinephrine in the fetus.[13,15] The high placental clearance was reduced by more than 60% following administration of uptake inhibitors like cocaine or desipramine. Similarly, treatment with these agents results in a threefold increase in circulating plasma CA concentrations.

The mechanism(s) for the placental contribution of intrauterine CA metabolism has been the subject of recent active investigation. The placenta has been shown to express the neuronal reuptake transporters for CA.[15,16] Placental expression is of interest because the placenta is the only noninnervated tissue that expresses these neuronal transporters.[16] To confirm the molecular basis for these observations, an ovine placental cDNA library was evaluated for expression of members of the biogenic amine transporter family expressed in placenta. Both norepinephrine and serotonin transporters from this library were isolated, cloned, and characterized.[17] Both placental transporters had a high degree of homology to the neuronal genes isolated from rat and human neuronal libraries. The factors that determine the placenta as a site of expression and the factors that regulate expression in the placenta were not known. In previous investigations umbilical cord CA concentrations and fetal acid base status were utilized as quantitative measures of fetal distress.[18] More recently human placental norepinephrine transporter (NET) messenger RNA (mRNA) concentration was correlated with quantitative measures of fetal distress at birth and with perinatal clinical complications including fetal growth retardation, fetal distress, and fetal exposure to substances abuse. The human cDNA for the norepinephrine transporter (NET) was used to measure RNA extracted from the placenta following complicated and uncomplicated pregnancies.[19] To compare transporter expression and its relation to fetal condition at birth, plasma CA concentrations, umbilical arterial blood gases, and placental transporter mRNA concentrations were compared by linear regression analysis. Uncomplicated pregnancies had a higher concentration of placental NET mRNA than complicated pregnancies. An inverse relationship between umbilical cord norepinephrine concentration and transporter expression was demonstrated. In patients whose NET mRNA was high, umbilical plasma norepinephrine concentration was low. It was concluded that placental clearance is critical for protection of the fetus from the detrimental effects of high concentrations of circulating plasma CA on the fetal placental vascular bed and derangements in fetal blood flow distribution. This mechanism is dependent on placental expression of plasma membrane neurotransmitter transporters. This further suggests that the high CA production and clearance rates in utero render the fetus particularly susceptible to the adverse consequences of uptake blockers like cocaine.

Perinatal Catecholamine Secretion

Fetal Studies

Understanding of the stimuli and mechanisms for fetal CA release is based largely on studies in fetal sheep. The pioneering studies of Comline and Silver[20-24] demonstrated that prior to complete splanchnic nerve innervation of the adrenal medulla there were marked developmental differences in CA secretion. Immature fetuses, without splanchnic innervation, cannot activate CA release by the usual neural, cholinergic mechanisms. They are still able to release CA in response to stressful stimuli like hypoxia. This direct, nonneuronal response results largely in norepinephrine secretion. Later, when splanchnic innervation has been established and epinephrine is the predominant adrenal amine, the response to hypoxia is greater and there is an increase in the proportion of epinephrine released. Similar findings have been described in the neonatal rat where loss of the direct, nonneurogenic response and development of neural control of CA release occurs after the first postnatal week.[4] In the calf and the foal development of neural control of CA release and secretion of epinephrine as the predominant amine also occurs postnatally.[23,24] The human and the rabbit are presumed to resemble the calf more than the fetal sheep, with development of splanchnic innervation occurring at or near term gestation. However, direct studies in the human are unavailable.

The majority of mammalian species have extramedullary chromaffin tissue as a source of circulating CA. Extramedullary tissue, known as paraaortic tissue or organs of Zuckerkandl, is well developed in rat, rabbit, guinea pig, and the human during fetal and neonatal life and undergoes involution in older animals.[25] Although this tissue arises from the same neural crest origins as the adrenal medullary cell, it is sparsely innervated and is not contiguous with adrenal cortical tissue and locally high circulating concentrations of glucocorticoids.[25] Paraaortic tissue contains greater than 90% norepinephrine and only small amounts of epinephrine.[26,27] This is explained by lack of the terminal enzyme in epinephrine biosynthesis, phenylethanolamine N-methyltransferase (PNMT). Induction of adrenal medullary PNMT activity occurs during development in response to locally elevated glucocorticoid concentrations and results in increased adrenal epinephrine content in most species with advancing gestation.[28] Neonatal hypoglycemia and hypoxia both result in depletion of paraaortic norepinephrine content.[29] Thus, this uniquely fetal/neonatal tissue is viewed as a source of CA at a developmental time when dependence on circulating concentrations may be greatest and assures the availability of high circulating concentrations of CA during fetal and/or neonatal stress.

The chronically catheterized animal provides a useful assessment of the stimuli capable of evoking CA secretion. Fetal sheep release CA in response to hypoxia,[30] hypothermia,[31] hypoglycemia,[32] exercise,[33] hemorrhage,[34] and labor and delivery.[18,35-38] While each of these stimuli is capable of evoking fetal sympathoadrenal responses, the physiologic consequences during fetal life are significantly different compared to the postnatal period. The unique relationship between the fetal sympathoadrenal system and other major organ systems is illustrated by the

22. The Sympathoadrenal System in the Fetal-Placental Unit

TABLE 22.1. Physiologic thresholds for hemodynamic, metabolic, and endocrine responses to circulating plasma catecholamines in adult humans and fetal sheep.

	Epinephrine threshold (pg·ml^{-1})[a]	Norepinephrine threshold (pg·ml^{-1})
Fetal sheep		
Heart rate	N.M.	N.M.
Blood pressure	400–700[b]	600–800
Cardiac contractility	500–600	1000–2500
Glucose	100	2000–3000
Free fatty acids	70–400	3000
Glucagon	700–800	2500–5000
Arteriovenous pressure	1000	6000–8000
Adult humans		
Heart rate	50–100	>1800
Blood pressure	75–125	>1800
Glucose	150–200	>1800
Glycerol	75–125	>1800
Insulin	>400	>1800

[a] Thresholds are as defined in the text.
[b] Values are ranges.
N.M., not measurable.
Data from Padbury et al.,[42] Clutter et al.,[43] and Silverberg et al.[44]

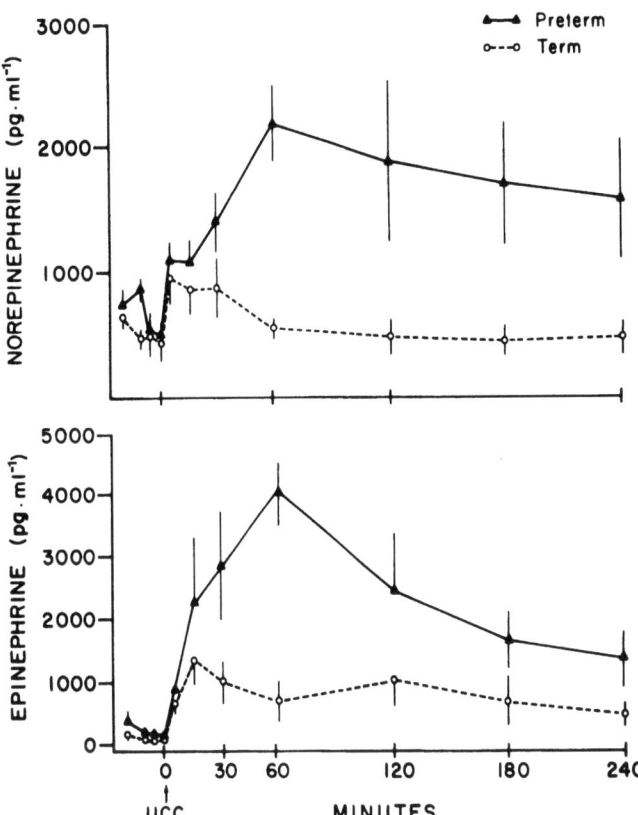

FIGURE 22.1. Plasma catecholamine levels in preterm (▲, 130 days) and term (○, 142 days) sheep following umbilical cord cutting (UCC). Top: norepinephrine (pg·ml^{-1}); bottom: epinephrine (pg·ml^{-1}). (From Padbury et al.,[38] with permission.)

fetal cardiovascular responsiveness to circulating CA. Resting plasma CA concentrations generally are lower in the fetal animal than in the adult animal or the human. Plasma norepinephrine concentrations between 250 and 500 pg·ml^{-1} and epinephrine concentrations less than 50 to 75 pg·ml^{-1} probably represent "well" unstressed animals.[39] These concentrations are below the limits of detection of many assays, but well within the range of enzymatic isotope derivative methods[40] and some high-performance liquid chromatography (HPLC) assays.[41] To quantify fetal responsiveness to changes in circulating CA concentrations, graded infusions of either norepinephrine or epinephrine were administered to the fetal lamb.[42] A variety of cardiovascular, metabolic, and endocrine responses were monitored simultaneously. Dose-response curves were constructed and analyzed to determine the threshold for each CA versus response, that is, the minimum concentration necessary for discernible physiologic effects. The data are summarized in Table 22.1 along with data derived from similar experiments in the adult human. The data demonstrate that for increases in heart rate, blood pressure, and myocardial contractility, the fetal plasma threshold is far greater than in the adult animal or human.[42–45] There are several explanations for this observation including immaturity in receptor development or the mechanisms for coupling receptors to cellular responses.

Catecholamine Release at Birth

Plasma CA concentrations begin to increase during the last 2 to 3 hours of spontaneous labor.[35] Following delivery and umbilical cord cutting, there is a further marked increase in circulating CA (Figure 22.1).[37,38,46] This "surge" in CA at birth has been most carefully investigated in the animal model. The precise stimulus for CA release is not clear, but probably represents an integrated response to compression, mild asphyxia, vestibular and tactile stimulation, hypothermia,[38] and a sudden increase in baroreceptor afferent impulse activity after cord cutting.[47] This increase in CA is vital to the cardiovascular, pulmonary, metabolic, and endocrine adaptations in early postnatal life.[10,11]

Human fetal CA secretion has been documented as early as 21 weeks of gestation by percutaneous umbilical cord sampling[48] from fetal scalp samples obtained during labor and delivery[49–51] and from umbilical cord samples. Elevated concentrations are generally associated with accepted measures of fetal distress. The large umbilical artery to vein concentration gradient noted by the majority of studies of umbilical cord samples implies a fetal origin for the elevated plasma CA.[36,52] The reported values for umbilical plasma CA vary widely depending on the condition of the neonate at birth. Representative data from a number of published studies are shown in Table 22.2. Umbilical arterial CA is clearly elevated in response to fetal distress[36,53] and in association with fetal

TABLE 22.2. Umbilical plasma catecholamine values in the human infant at birth.[a]

Source	Route of delivery[b]	Norepinephrine (pg·ml^{-1}) Mean ± SEM	Range	Epinephrine (pg·ml^{-1}) Mean ± SEM	Range
Lagercrantz and Bistoletti[36]	V	8815 ± 1320		1818 ± 271	
	CS	10,291 ± 1502			
Nakai and Yamada[53]	NS	20,200 ± 8600	3700–36,200	11,200 ± 6300	0–26,000
Eliot et al.[52]	V	3667 ± 393		568 ± 100	
	CS	4248 ± 926		560 ± 123	
Irestedt et al.[54]	V	5374 ± 981		933 ± 139	
	CS/GA	5408 ± 102		183 ± 57	
	CS/EA	1606 ± 242		732 ± 184	
Padbury et al.[18]	V	3354	156–72,210	631	29–13,784
Jones and Greiss[61]	V	4163 ± 510		1984 ± 267	
	CS	2329 ± 301		771 ± 97	
Puolakka et al.[65]	NS	3640 ± 100			
Newnham et al.[63] (prematures)	V	4408 ± 1354		613 ± 153	
	CS/L	10,869 ± 10,369		1211 ± 981	
	CS/NL	5389 ± 1753		350 ± 44	
Falconer and Lake[58]	V	3698 ± 85		1052 ± 49	
	CS/NL	886 ± 120		470 ± 141	
Broberger et al.[66] (infants of diabetic mothers)	V			500	<10–8418
	CS			146	<10–910
Jones et al.[62]	V	2653 ± 457		157 ± 28	
	CS/EA	858 ± 341		161 ± 48	
Paulick et al.[64]	V	10,200	1500–74,100	1120	140–4030
Hertel[60] (infants of diabetic mothers)	V	6270 ± 193		730 ± 49	
	CS	1180 ± 224		230 ± 53	
Greenough et al.[59] (prematures)	NS/L	3414	203–20,027	970	37–3459
	NS/NL	3397	541–12,861	421	<10–2141

[a] The majority are umbilical arterial values.
[b] Route of delivery: V, vaginal delivery; CS, cesarean section; L, labor; NL, no labor; NS, not specified; GA, general anesthesia; EA, epidural anethesia.

heart rate patterns indicative of fetal distress.[18] The fetus demonstrates a "graded" response with log plasma norepinephrine and epinephrine both showing an inverse correlation with scalp pH and pO$_2$.[18] While the duration of labor shows no direct correlation with umbilical arterial plasma CA concentrations,[18] lower cord plasma CA concentrations are observed in neonates delivered by cesarean section without labor than those delivered vaginally.[54] Interestingly, cesarean section with epidural anesthesia is associated with higher cord plasma CA concentrations than cesarean section following general anesthesia.[54]

Fetal sympathoadrenal system activity has been assessed by measurements of CA and CA metabolites in amniotic fluid. Conclusions are generally similar to those reached following measurement of scalp samples. Fetal distress, evidenced by intrauterine growth retardation, is associated with higher amniotic fluid CA[55,56] and metabolite concentrations.[57] However, there is a great deal of variability in concentration ranges and in amniotic fluid composition and volume. Thus, while serving as an index of fetal sympathoadrenal system maturation and general fetal well-being, measurement of amniotic fluid CA or CA metabolites remains adjunctive to other assessments of fetal well-being.

Development and Regulation of Adrenergic Receptors

Multiple Adrenergic Receptors

The adrenergic receptors are members of the guanine nucleotide regulatory protein (G protein)–coupled receptor family, which includes the receptors for a variety of neurotransmitters and hormones.[67] As the site of action of the CA, norepinephrine and epinephrine, adrenergic receptors were first classified into α and β responses based on pharmacologic studies.[68] The α-adrenergic receptors (αAR) were subsequently divided into α_1 and α_2 subtypes.[69] Based on the affinity toward prazocin, α_1AR was further divided into four prazocin-sensitive (α_1A, α_1B, α_1C, α_1D) and one prazocin-insensitive subtypes (α_1L).[70] Subsequently, ligand binding studies and molecular cloning have identified four subtypes of the α_2AR (α_2A, α_2B, α_2C, α_2D).[70] The β-adrenergic receptors

TABLE 22.3. Cloned multiple adrenergic receptors.

Subtype	Tissue distribution	Major G protein	Effector system
$\alpha_1 A$	Vas deferens		
$\alpha_1 B$	Liver, brain	Gq	↑ Phospholipase A_2, C, D; ↑ Ca^{2+} channel
$\alpha_1 C$	Olfactory bulb		
$\alpha_1 D$	Vas deferens, brain		
$\alpha_1 L$	Aorta	?	?
$\alpha_2 A$	Aorta, brain		
$\alpha_2 B$	Liver, kidney	Gi	↓ AC, ↑ Phospholipase C, A_2
$\alpha_2 C$	Brain		↑ K^+, ↓ Ca^{2+} channel, ↑ MAP kinase pathway
$\alpha_2 D$	Brain		
β_1	Heart, pineal gland		
β_2	Lung, prostate	Gs	↑ AC, ↑ Ca^{2+} channel
β_3	Adipose tissue		
β-atypical	Adipose tissue		
β_t	Blood		
β_{4c}	Lung, blood, GI		↑ AC

Data from Berthelsen and Pettinger,[69] Milligan et al.,[70] Lands et al.,[71] Arch and Kaumann,[72] Minneman et al.,[73] and Chen et al.[74]

(βAR) were first divided into two subtypes (β_1, β_2).[71] Later a third cDNA, β_3, was isolated.[72] Other βAR subtypes are being identified, such as the β-atypical[72] and two subtypes expressed on turkey erythrocyte (βtAR, β_{4c}AR),[73,74] which have pharmacologic characteristics distinct from other subtypes. These receptors subtypes are expressed in a tissue-specific manner, are associated with different subtypes of G protein, and hence activate different effector systems (Table 22.3). This allows for multiple functions in different tissue. For example, although β_1 AR is the major subtype in the heart, other subtypes, such as β_2, β_3, α_1, and α_2, have been identified at various parts of the heart. Multiple adrenergic receptor subtypes in the heart have been suggested to serve as backup systems especially during pathologic conditions.[70] These subtypes in the heart contribute to the overall cardiac response not only by their receptor density in the heart but also with their own sensitivity to ligands and effectiveness to couple the different signal transduction pathways.

Hormonal Regulation of the βAR: A Developmental Switch

In light of their critical roles in physiologic homeostasis, such as myocardial contractility and bronchodilation, βAR responsiveness is tightly controlled. It is well established that the βARs are regulated by corticosteroids and thyroid hormones. Corticosteroids have been shown to induce time- and dose-dependent increases in βAR receptor number[75–78] and mRNA levels.[76,77,79] Similarly, thyroid hormones have been shown to increase βAR binding sites.[80] Thyroidectomy decreases βAR mRNA levels in the heart, an effect that can be reversed by thyroxine (T_4) replacement.[81] Most of these studies, however, were done in tissue culture or in an adult animal model. Few studies have been performed in developing animals where corticosteroids and thyroid hormones exert important maturational effects.[82] The regulatory mechanism of βAR found in the adult may not be present during particular stages of development. We showed that while both glucocorticoids and thyroid hormones increased the myocardial βAR number in the neonate, there is no effect in the fetal sheep.[83,84] Recently it has been demonstrated that glucocorticoids alone or in combination with T_4 do not change βAR binding characteristics in the fetal sheep (Table 22.4). The technique of RNase protection assay was adapted to measure β_1AR mRNA levels in these same animals following the various hormone treatments.[85] The steady-state levels of mRNA coding for β_1AR are not changed by these treatments (Figure 22.2). Therefore, these most critical

TABLE 22.4. Effects of betamethasone alone or betamethasone in combination with thyroid hormone (T_4) on fetal sheep myocardial β-adrenergic receptor binding characteristics, as assessed by [^{3}H]dihydroalprenolol binding in membranes from left ventricle of the heart.[a]

Treatment	N	K_d (nM)	B_{max} (fmol·mg protein^{-1})
Control	8	3.51 ± 0.95	164 ± 26
Betamethasone[b]	7	3.52 ± 0.35	176 ± 15
Betamethasone + T_4	4	3.48 ± 0.35	209 ± 27

[a] Data are presented as mean ± SEM.
[b] Fetuses were injected (IM) with either saline, betamethasone (0.5 mg·kg^{-1}), or betamethasone plus T_4 (50 μg·kg^{-1}) under ultrasound guiding 2 days before delivery by cesarean section.
N, Number of sheep heart sample used, each performed in duplicate.

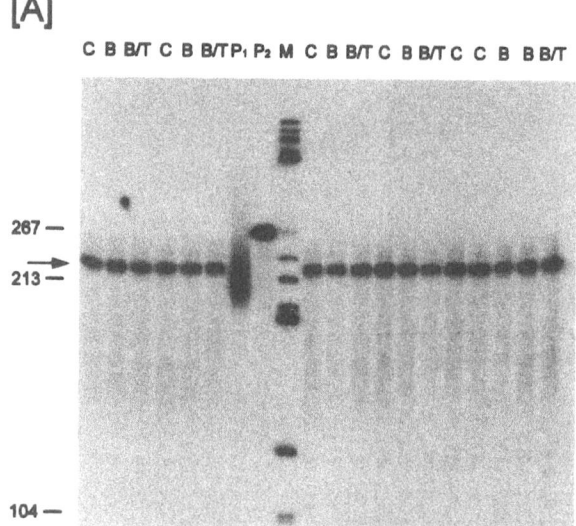

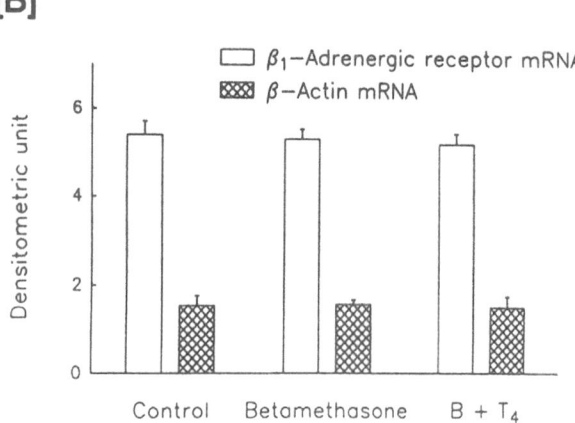

FIGURE 22.2. A: Representative autoradiogram from RNase protection assay of β_1-adrenergic receptor and β-actin mRNAs in fetal sheep treated either with saline (C), betamethasone alone (B), or betamethasone in combination with T_4 (B/T). Numbers on the left side indicate sizes of molecular weight marker in base pair. β-actin levels were used as the internal control. P_1, β-actin cDNA probe. P_2, β_1-adrenergic receptor cDNA probe. Arrow and arrowhead indicate β_1-adrenergic receptor and β-actin transcript, respectively. B: Densitometric measurement of results from RNase protection assay listed in A. Each RNA sample was prepared from a single sheep. Data are presented as mean ± SEM. (From Tseng et al.,[85] with permission.)

regulatory hormones do not induce β_1AR gene expression during this stage of fetal development. Since both glucocorticoid and thyroid hormone receptors are present in fetal sheep at this gestation age[86,87] and there are clearly other genes that are steroid responsive at this gestation stage in fetal sheep,[88] the switch in β_1AR responsiveness to steroid and thyroid hormones may represent a unique form of developmentally regulated transcription.

Steroid hormones mediate their biologic responses by binding to intracellular receptors.[89] These hormone-receptor complexes are translocated to the nucleus where they bind to specific DNA sequences. Several putative core sequence motifs have been identified to which corticosteroid or thyroid hormone receptor complex bind specifically.[90] Such sequence elements, termed glucocorticoid response elements (GRE) and thyroid response elements (TRE), have been identified in the 3'- and 5'-untranslated and open-reading frame domains of the β_2AR gene.[91,92] Binding of corticosteroid and thyroid hormone receptors to these elements results in stimulation of gene transcription. Further, "composite" GREs have been identified that carry binding sites both for receptor and for accessory, nonreceptor factors, which are essential for receptor activity.[93] The interaction between receptor and accessory factors at the "composite" response element determines the activity and specificity of receptor-mediated responsiveness.[94] Our data showing comparable βAR number and β_1AR mRNA levels between the control and hormone-treated animals suggest that the regulation of β_1AR by transcription factors during fetal development is distinct from that of the adult. This could be due to altered expression of distinct transcription factors, such as AP-1, that modulate the transcription mechanism at a "composite" response element, due to the presence of DNA-binding proteins that repress hormone-mediated increase in β_1AR gene expression. Another possibility is that glucocorticoids and thyroid hormones may not act directly on the β_1AR gene but may act indirectly on another transcription factor that is not yet expressed at this stage in the fetus.

To study the detailed transcriptional mechanisms in the developing fetus, the β_1AR gene and 5' flanking sequence from sheep have been cloned.[95,96] The promoter region is shown in Figure 22.3. The entire 2.3 kb of 5' flanking sequence was searched for nucleotide sequences of identified regulatory elements using Genetics Computer Group (GCG) programs and the Transcription Factor Database.[97] Several potential GREs and TREs were identified. The standard procedure is to generate a series of mutant reporter constructs with progressive deletion of the 5' sequence and test its activity in vitro. A series of β_1AR deletion constructs was created and inserted in a luciferase reporter vector (Figure 22.4). The transcription activities were tested in three different cell lines.[98] First, C6 glioma cells were studied because these have been a standard model for studying βAR regulation. Second, the neuronal cell line, SK-N-MC cells, which expresses only β_1AR was evaluated. Last, β_1AR regulation in a new human fetal cardiomyocyte cell line, known

22. The Sympathoadrenal System in the Fetal-Placental Unit

```
   1  CGGTATCGAT AAGCTTGATA TCGAATTCCT GCAGCCCGGG GGATCTCCAG CCCCCTCTTT CTAGCCCTCT
  71  CCTTCCCTCA TTTCCCCTTC TCAGGCTCCC CAACTGGCAG AACTAAGCTG ACAATCCTAA GCCAGGGATG
 141  CAGAAACAAG TAATTCACCC ACATCCACCC ACTGATCATC AAGTTTGGGC CTAAAGCAAA TTTACATGTT
 211  TGGATAAAGA AAAGTTGGGC TTCCCTAGTA GCTGAGACCC ATCTTCAGTC CTTGGATGGG GGAAGATCCC
 281  CTAGAGAAGG AGATGGCAAC CCACTCTAGT ATTCTTGCCT GGAAAATCCC ATAGGCAGAG GAGCCTGGTG
 351  GCTACAGCCC ATGGGGTTGC AAGAGTCAGA CACAACTTAG CTACTAAAAC CACCACCCAT GGCTTATGAA
                                                            TRE rGH
 421  TACACATTGC TGTTAGCTCT CGACTTAGGG AGCTCTCTCC AAGGTAAGAA TATGAGTTTG TTCCTTTCAG
                                              MTV GRE
 491  AAACTATTCT TTTTATTCCA ATGCTAGAAG GATGTGTGAG CATTATGTAA CATTTTCATG CACCCTTAAG
 561  TGGGTAATTA GAAGCTCTTT ATTTCTCAGG ATTCAATTAA AAGCTTTTTA TTTTCAAGGC TGAGTTGAGG
                                                                       TRE rSPOT 14
 631  ACCAGTACTG TGGTGGAATT AGACAAGGGG CTTGCACACC TTTGGCTACA TTGTGTGTTG ATGGGCCACC
                                                                           rCRE
 701  TTCCTGTAGG TACCTCCCCA CATATAGTCA CACCACTGCA GAGCTAACGA CTCACTAATT TTAAACCCAT
 771  TCAGTTGCCA ACCCAACAGC CTTTGATATA ACTTTACATG CTATGGATT TTAATCTTTT TGAGTATTTA
 841  TATATGTTTT CTTCTCTCAT CCCTCCAAAA TTAATCCTAG AGTTTTGAGA ATCTGGGAAC TTGGGCAAAG
 911  GAGAAGGCAA CGCAGCAGAC CAAGAAATTT GAAATCTCAG TTCACTACTG TGTCACCCAA AGTCAATGTA
 981  CCTTTTTTGT TTGGACCGGC CCAGCTCAAG TCATACAATC ACGTGAGTAA CAGACCACAA AATCCAGGTG
                                                         GRE UTEROGLOB
1051  TTATTACTGA ACATGACAAG TCTGAAAAGT AATTACACGT GTTCTAGCTT CCGTGGCGGT GTCATTTACT
1121  CTAACATGCC TGTCCTTAAG CCTCTCTCTC TCTTTACATT ACCGGCACAC ACCGGTGCAC CATACTCACA
1191  CATCCATCAG CTGGGACCTG GGAGTGTGTA TTATTCCAAC TGGTCCTCAG CATTAGCTGT CAGATGTCAC
1261  AACCCCCYGC CGTTTTCTGC ATCTGCTGCC CCGGGAAGCG AGAAGAAGCT TGCAAGAATA GCTCCCGGGA
1331  ACGTTCCTGA AAGATTGGCG CTCTGCTTTA GCAAGGCGCT CGCTGGAAAG TTTCTTCTAA CCGCTCACAC
      SP1
1401  CCGCCTCCGA TCCGATCCCC GAGCTGGCAG GACGCGAGCT GGCTGGGACT CCTCTTGACA GAGGAAGGGC
1471  TTTACACACC ACCCTCCTAG GCTGCCCAAT ACAAGAAACA GTCTTGCAGC CAGACTCCTC CACACCCAGC
       nGRE   rPOMC                              GRE UTEROGLOB (rs)
1541  GAACAGACCG TCCAAGGCGC TCCGGTGTTT CGAGAACACC GAAGTCCCCT CCCTGCTAAA GGGCGCGTGA
                                                                SP1         ➡
1611  GCTCTGCTCT GCAGGAAACC TGGGCACTGG AGGTAGATGG GATGGGTGGC GGCGGGTAGA GCCGGGGCGC
                                                                SP1        TRE rSPOT 14
1681  AGCGGAAAGC AAACGCCGGA GGCAAACGGG GCGCAGGAGA GGGGAGATTG GGTGCCGCCG TAGGGGCCAG
                                                                            TRE rGH
1751  GGTGAAAGCC GGGCGCGGAC GGGAACCGAG GGAACTGGG CACTGGAGCC AAGCGGGCTC TGGAAGGGAC
1821  GCGCGGGCAG GAACCCGCGA GCGCTGGGGA GGGGCTTGCT TGGCGATCTG CCCCGGACTC CCTAGAGCCG
                           SP1                    SP1
1891  CAGAACCGCC GGTGGAGGCG GGGTGCTAGG AGTTGGCGGG GCCGGGTGGG GGTGGGGGGG AACCAGAGAG
1961  GGGCGTGCCT TCGCCAGGAT TGGCTGCAGG AGCCTGACGC GAGNNNCCGG GGGTTGGCTC GGGGGAGTGG
2031  GAGCCGGGTG GGGTGGGTGC TGGGTGCCGG GGCTGCGGGC TCCGCGAGCT CAGAAACATG CTGAGGTCCC
2101  GGCAGCTGTT CCAGCAGCGA CACCACTCCA GCAGCAGCCG CGGCGGCTGC GGCGGCGACA GGCACCGGCT
      SP1
2171  CCGGCGGGGA AGGCGCCCGG CGCCATGCCT CCGGCCCCGC GCCGCGCTGC GCTGACCTGG CCGCGACCTC
                                                           RAREβ
2241  CCTCCGCGCG CCCCGCCGTT CGGGCCTCTG GGGGGTTCCC CAACCGCGGC CCAACTCCGC CACACCCCTC
2311  TCCCCCGGCC TCCGCAGCTC GGC
```

FIGURE 22.3. Ovine β_1-adrenergic receptor gene 5' flanking sequence. Putative regulatory elements in either orientation are indicated. Palindromic sequences of 8 or more bp are in italics and underlined. Two sets of repeats are in bold. The predominant transcription initiation site is indicated by an overlying bold arrow. The large box indicates the location of the 98 bp element common to both the ovine and human β_1-adrenergic receptor genes. (From Padbury et al.,[96] with permission.)

as W1 cells, which has just recently been shown to express many phenotypic characteristics typical for human fetal cardiac myocytes, was evaluated.[99] As shown in Figure 22.4, progressive deletion of the 5' flanking sequence resulted in moderate increases in activity in all three cell lines. The most dramatic increase in transcription activity was seen when sequence −1530 ~ −953 (relative to the translation start site) were deleted. This region contains an AP-1 site and the sequence $5'TGTTCT3'$, which is the most conserved portion of the well-characterized GRE.[100] These data suggest that there may be a "repressor" element within this region that accounts for the negative

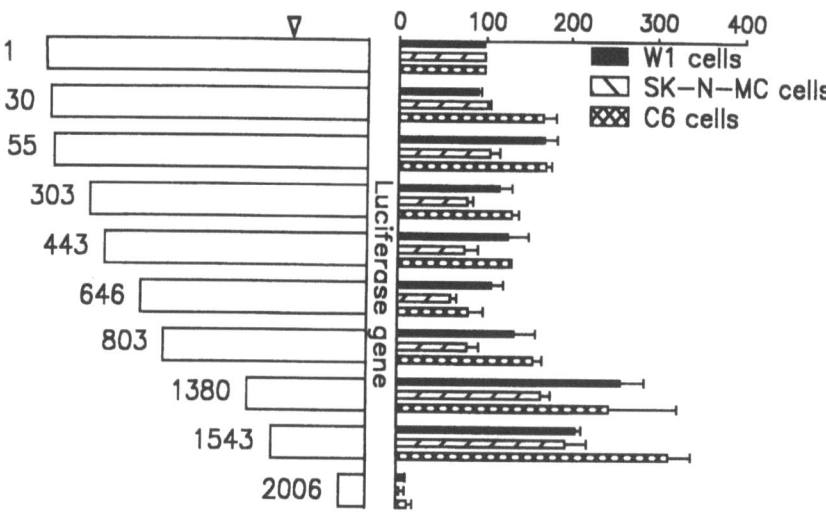

FIGURE 22.4. Schematic of mutant β₁-adrenergic receptor gene promoter constructs (left panel). Each construct was cut at 151 bp upstream from the initiator methionine and ligated directly upstream to the luciferase gene. Results of the basal transcription activities of these constructs in three cell lines are shown on the right panel. Data are mean ± SEM from three separate experiments and are normalized to cotransfected CAT (chloramphenicol acetyltransferase) activity. All activities are expressed as relative to activity of the full-length promoter on top. (From Tseng et al.,[98] with permission.)

regulation of the β₁AR gene. This region needs to be studied further to explain the developmental switch in β₁AR gene regulation.

Desensitization of the βAR

Agonist binding to βAR induces association of guanosine triphosphate (GTP) with the regulatory subunits of the heterotrimeric complex of Gs. This in turn activates adenylyl cyclase (AC) and results in an increase in intracellular adenosine 3′,5′-cyclic monophosphate (cAMP) level.[101] Secondary effects of increased intracellular cAMP can be mediated via cAMP-dependent kinase [protein kinase A (PKA)]. Additionally, cAMP has diverse metabolic and regulatory effects including regulation of gene expression.[102] It is well documented that prolonged agonist occupancy attenuates responsiveness, a phenomenon called desensitization. Desensitization may be mediated by alteration in receptor density,[103] uncoupling of AC to the receptors,[104,105] receptor sequestration or internalization from the cell plasma membrane,[104] or phosphorylation of the receptors by βAR kinases (βARK)[106,107] and PKA.[108] These effects have been observed in numerous studies in vitro[104,109,110] and in vivo.[105,111] Desensitization of the receptors by βARK also requires another protein—β-arrestin.[112] Alteration of adrenergic receptor density and/or sensitivity is important in the pathophysiology of a variety of conditions. It has long been recognized that myocardial adrenergic receptor density is reduced in congestive heart failure due to a variety of causes.[113] This leads to reduced myocardial contractility and an exacerbation of the functional impairment. The receptor downregulation has been attributed to sympathetic nervous system overactivity.[113] There are other conditions associated with sympathetic overactivity and marked alterations in receptor density/sensitivity, including pressure overload–induced hypertrophy,[114] cardiothoracic surgery,[115] hypertension,[116] and cyanotic heart disease.[117] By contrast, there is an increase in receptor density following chronic antagonist treatment.[118]

A unique feature of βAR desensitization is its strict developmental regulation. Receptor downregulation/desensitization is seen in the mature animal following alterations in endogenous CA induced by stimuli as modest as a change in posture only.[119] In contrast, Habib et al.[120] have shown that in the immediate neonatal period when CA concentrations change by several orders of magnitude, there is no change in receptor density or coupling to adenyl cyclase. Prolonged infusion of exogenous agonist also does not change receptor density or sensitivity.[121] In the developing rat, where cardiac sympathetic innervation is not established until after the 2nd week of life, exposure to the same treatment does not alter receptor density and coupling until the 3rd to 4th week.[122] From fetuses to the 1-week-old neonate, a developmental decrease in the sensitivity of AC to βAR agonist stimulation in rat myocardial membrane is accompanied by a decrease in the chronotropic and inotropic sensitivity to βAR agonists.[123] By contrast, there are data demonstrating sensitization in newborn rats chronically treated with βAR agonist.[124] The transition from sensitization to de-

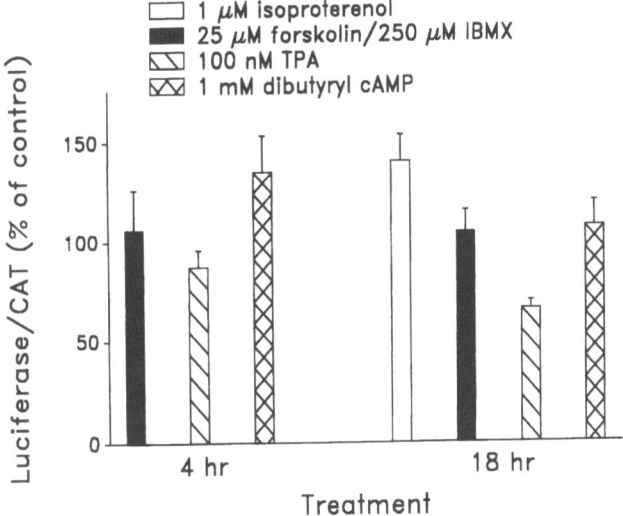

FIGURE 22.5. Effects of β_1-adrenergic receptor agonists on the transcription activity of the ovine β_1-adrenergic receptor full-length promoter transfected into SK-N-MC cells. After 20-hour recovery from transfection, cells were treated with agonists for 4 or 18 hours before harvest for luciferase and CAT activity measurements.

sensitization seems to correlate with sympathetic nerve development.[125] However, other factors may be more relevant such as developmental differences in transcriptional regulation, in the ontogeny of βARK, or in the regulation of G protein expression.[126] These have not been examined.

A series of preliminary studies to begin exploring the mechanism(s) of agonist regulation of the βAR gene has recently been completed. The question asked was whether treatment of SK-N-MC cells with agonist or reagents that increase cAMP content after transfection increases transcription activity. Figure 22.5 shows that isoproterenol and dibutyryl cAMP increased βAR expression. Interestingly, forskolin decreased β_1AR transcription in the dose chosen. These studies were done in cells transfected with the full-length promoter. This suggests the full-length promoter contains sequences that confer responsiveness to cAMP by either direct and/or indirect mechanisms and that the mechanisms of regulation is complex and may involve co-regulation by other genes, e.g., c-fos or c-jun. There is a putative AP-1 site in the proximal promoter (Figure 22.3). A consensus c-AMP response element (CRE) identified in the β_2AR promoter was not found.[127] However, there is a putative reversed CRE at −1600 to −1591 ($^{5'}CACTGCA^{3'}$) found among human β_2AR[127] and other gene promoters such as the rat somatostatin gene,[128] the proenkephalin gene,[129] and the human glycoprotein hormone α unit gene.[130] Further investigations are needed to map precisely the sequences that confer agonist and cAMP-mediated regulation of β_1AR transcription and serve as the basis for future studies to examine the developmental regulation of DNA-binding proteins that regulate βAR expression in vivo.

Implications

This chapter has described several unique aspects of CA physiology and metabolism. Fetal life is characterized by very high CA production and clearance rates and high thresholds for responsiveness to CA. The placenta provides a unique adaptive protection to the fetus through expression of the neuronal reuptake transporters. The high intrauterine production rates may condition the developing animal to sustain the high CA secretion rates vital to successful physiologic adaptation during the early postnatal period. However, the high CA production and clearance rates in utero may render the fetus particularly susceptible to the adverse consequences of uptake blockers like cocaine. This may explain the fetus's unique vulnerability to these agents and some of the severe pathologic effects of fetal cocaine exposure.

The βAR are important, highly regulated plasma membrane receptors that mediate the major intracellular signaling pathways of CA. Their regulation in the adult animal and human by hormones and/or agonists is strictly controlled. By contrast, during development adrenergic receptor expression appears to be constitutively regulated and not responsive to the hormone and agonist dependent alterations in receptor density and responsiveness seen during later life. This may represent a unique form of transcriptional regulation facilitation of development during critical maturational stages. Understanding this mechanism of transcriptional regulation will be important to our understanding of maturation and control of gene expression.

Acknowledgment. This work is supported by United States Public Health Service grants DA 07753 and HD 11343.

References

1. Assali NS, Brinkman CR II, Woods JR Jr, et al. Development of neurohumoral control of fetal, neonatal and adult cardiovascular functions. Am J Obstet Gynecol 1977;129:748–759.
2. Mirkin BL. Ontogenesis of the adrenergic nervous system: functional and pharmacologic implications. Fed Proc 1972;31:65–73.
3. Parvez H, Parvez S. Biogenic amines in development. Amsterdam: Elsevier/North-Holland Biomedical Press, 1980.
4. Slotkin TA, Seidler FJ. Adrenomedullary catecholamine release in the fetus and newborn: secretory mechanisms

and their role in stress and survival. J Dev Physiol 1988; 10:1–16.
5. Whitsett JA, Noguchi A, Moore JJ. Developmental aspects of α- and β-adrenergic receptors. Semin Perinatol 1982;6:125–141.
6. Cass WA, Zahniser NR, Flach KA, Gerhardt GA. Clearance of exogenous dopamine in rat dorsal striatum and nucleus accumbens. J Neurochem 1993;61:2269–2278.
7. Brush JE Jr, Eisenhofer G, Garty M, et al. Cardiac norepinephrine kinetics in hypertrophic cariomyopathy. Circulation 1989;79:836–844.
8. Esler M, Jackman G, Bobik A, et al. Norepinephrine kinetics in essential hypertension. Defective neuronal uptake of norepinephrine in some patients. Hypertention 1981;3:149–156.
9. Esler M, Jennings G, Lambert G, et al. Overflow of catecholamine neurotransmitter to the circulation: source, fate and functions. Pharmacol Rev 1990;70:963–985.
10. Padbury JF. Functional maturation of the adrenal medulla and peripheral sympathetic nervous system. In: Jones CT, ed. Baillière's clinical endocrinology and metabolism, international practice and research. London: Baillière Tindall, 1989;3(3):689–705.
11. Padbury JF, Agata Y, Ludlow JK, et al. Effect of fetal adrenalectomy on catecholamine release and physiologic adaptation at birth in sheep. J Clin Invest 1987;80:1096–1103.
12. Stein H, Oyama K, Martinez A, et al. Plasma epinephrine appearance and clearance rates in fetal and newborn sheep. Am J Physiology 1993;265:R756–R760.
13. Bzoskie L, Blount L, Kashiwai K, et al. Placental norepinephrine clearance: in vivo measurement and physiological role. Am J Physiol 1995;269:E145–E149.
14. Padbury JF, Ludlow JK, Humme JA, Agata Y. Metabolic clearance and plasma appearance rates of catecholamines in preterm and term fetal sheep. Pediatr Res 1986;20:992–995.
15. Bzoskie L, Blount L, Kashiwai K, et al. Placental norepinephrine transporter development in the ovine fetus. Placenta 1997;18:65–70.
16. Ganapathy G, Ramamoorthy S, Leibach F. Transport and metabolism of monoamines in the human placenta. Trophoblast Res 1993;7:35–51.
17. Padbury JF, Tseng YT, McGonnigal B, et al. Placental biogenic amine transporter: cloning and expression. Brain Res (Mol Brain Res) 1997;45:163–168.
18. Padbury JF, Roberman B, Oddie TH, et al. Fetal catecholamine release in response to labor and delivery. Obstet Gynecol 1982;60:607–611.
19. Bzoskie L, Yen J, Tseng YT, et al. Human placental norepinephrine transporter mRNA: expression and correlation with fetal condition at birth. Placenta 1997;18:205–210.
20. Comline RS, Silver M. The release of adrenaline and noradrenaline from the adrenal glands of the foetal sheep. J Physiol 1961;156:424–444.
21. Comline RS, Silver IA, Silver M. Factors responsible for the stimulation of the adrenal medulla during asphyxia in the foetal lamb. Physiology 1965;178:211–238.
22. Comline RS, Silver M. Development of activity in the adrenal medulla of the foetus and newborn animal. Br Med Bull 1966;22:16–20.
23. Comline Rs, Silver M. The development of the adrenal medulla of the foetal and newborn calf. J Physiol 1966;183:305–340.
24. Comline RS, Silver M. Catecholamine secretion by the adrenal medulla of the foetal and newborn foal. J Physiol 1971;216:659–682.
25. Coupland RE. The development and fact of catecholamine secreting endocrine cells. In: Parvez H, Parvez S, eds. Biogenic amines in development. Amsterdam: Elsevier/North-Holland Biomedical Press, 1980:3–28.
26. Coupland RE, Kent C, Kent SE. Normal function of extra-adrenal chromaffin tissues in the young rabbit and guinea-pig. J Endocrinol 1982;92:433–442.
27. Padbury JF, Diakomanolis ES, Lam RW, et al. Ontogenesis of tissue catecholamines in fetal and neonatal rabbits. J Dev Physiol 1981;3:297–303.
28. Bohn MC, Goldstein M, Black IB. Role of glucocorticoids in expression of the adrenergic phenotype in rat embryonic adrenal gland. Dev Biol 1981;82:1–10.
29. Brundin T. Studies on the preaortal paraganglia of newborn rabbits. Acta Physiol Scand Suppl 1966;70:290.
30. Lewis AB, Sischo W. Cardiovascular and catecholamine responses to hypoxemia in chemically sympathetectomized fetal lambs. Dev Pharmacol Ther 1985;8:129–140.
31. Gunn TR, Johnston BM, Iwamoto HS, et al. Haemodynamic and catecholamine responses to hypothermia in the fetal sheep in utero. J Dev Physiol 1985;7:241–249.
32. Harwell CM, Anand RS, Padbury JF, et al. Fetal glucose (G) and catecholamine (CA) response to maternal hypoglycemia. FASEB J 1988;2A:1484.
33. Palmer SM, Oakes GK, Champion JA, et al. Catecholamine physiology in the ovine fetus. III. Maternal and fetal response to acute maternal exercise. Am J Obstet Gynecol 1984;149:426–434.
34. Brace RA, Cheung CY. Fetal cardiovascular and endocrine responses to prolonged fetal hemorrhage. Am J Physiol 1986;251:R417–R242.
35. Eliot RJ, Klein AH, Glatz TH, et al. Plasma norepinephrine, epinephrine, and dopamine concentrations in maternal and fetal sheep during spontaneous parturition and in premature sheep during cortisol-induced parturition. Endocrinology 1981;108:1678–1682.
36. Lagercrantz H, Bistoletti P. Catecholamine release in the newborn infant at birth. Pediatr Res 1973;11:889–893.
37. Padbury JF, Martinez AM. Sympathoadrenal system activity at birth: integration of postnatal adaptation. Semin Perinatol 1988;12:163–172.
38. Padbury JF, Polk DH, Newnham J, Lam RW. Neonatal adaptation: greater sympathoadrenal response in preterm than full-term fetal sheep at birth. Am J Physiol 1985;248:E443–E449.
39. Buhler HU, da Prada M, Haefely W, Picotti GB. Plasma adrenaline, noradrenaline and dopamine in man and different animal spacies. J Physiol 1978;276:311–320.

40. Peuler JD, Johnson GA. Simultaneous single isotope radioenzymatic assay of plasma norepinephrine, epinephrine and dopamine. Life Sci 1977;21:625–636.
41. Hjemdahl P. Catecholamine measurements by high-performance liquid chromatography. Am J Physiol 1984; 247:E13–E20.
42. Padbury JF, Ludlow JK, Ervin MG, et al. Thresholds for physiological effects of plasma catecholamines in fetal sheep. Am J Physiol 1987;252:E530–E537.
43. Clutter WE, Bier DM, Shah SD, Cryer PE. Epinephrine plasma metabolic clearance rates and physiologic thresholds for metabolic and hemodynamic actions in man. J Clin Invest 1980;66:94–101.
44. Silverberg AB, Shah SD, Haymond MW, Cryer PE. Norepinephrine: hormone and neurotransmitter in man. Am J Physiol 1978;234:E252–E256.
45. Stratton JR, Pfeifer MA, Ritchie JL, Halter JB. Hemodynamic effects of epinephrine concentration—effect study in humans. J Appl Physiol 1985;58:1199–1206.
46. Agata Y, Padbury JF, Ludlow JK, et al. The effect of chemical sympathectomy on catecholamine release at birth. Pediatr Res 1986;20:1338–1344.
47. Purves MJ, Biscoe TJ. Development of chemoreceptor activity. Br Med Bull 1967;22:56–60.
48. Weiner CP, Robillard JE, Nakamura KT. Human fetal response to stress—plasma catecholamines, and renin in continuing pregnancies. Pediatr Res 1987;21:381 Am(abstr).
49. Bistoletti P, Nylund L, Lagercrantz H, et al. Fetal scalp catecholamines during labor. Am J Obstet Gynecol 1983; 147:785–788.
50. Bistoletti P, Lagercrantz H, Lunell NO. Fetal plasma catecholamine concentrations and fetal heart-rate variability during first stage of labour. Br J Obstet Gynaecol 1983;90:11–15.
51. Nylund L, Lagercrantz H, Lunell NO. Catecholamines in fetal blood during birth in man. J Dev Physiol 1979;1:427–430.
52. Eliot RJ, Lam RW, Leake RD, et al. Plasma catecholamine concentrations in infants at birth and during the first 48 hours of life. J Pediatr 1980;96:311–315.
53. Nakai T, Yamada R. The secretion of catecholamines in newborn babies with special reference to fetal distress. J Perinat Med 1978;6:39–45.
54. Irestedt L, Lagercrantz H, Hjemdahl P, et al. Fetal and maternal plasma catecholamines levels at elective caesarean section under general or epidural anesthesia versus vaginal delivery. Am J Obstet Gynecol 1982;142:1004–1010.
55. Peleg D, Munsick RA, Diker D, et al. Distribution of catecholamines between fetal and maternal compartments during human pregnancy with emphasis on L-dopa and dopamine. J Clin Endocrinol Metab 1986;62:911–914.
56. Puolakka J, Kauppila A, Vuori J. Amniotic fluid norepinephrine concentration as an indicator of fetal sympathetic nervous activity. Gynecol Obstet Invest 1984;17:265–268.
57. Artal R, Hobel CJ, Lam R, et al. Free metanephrine in human amniotic fluid as an index of fetal sympathetic nervous system maturation. Am J Obstet Gynecol 1979;133:452–454.
58. Falconer AD, Lake DM. Circumstances influencing umbilical-cord plasma catecholamines at delivery. Br J Obstet Gynaecol 1982;9:44–49.
59. Greenough A, Lagercrantz H, Pool J, Dahlin I. Plasma catecholamine levels in preterm infants. Acta Paediatr Scand 1987;76:54–59.
60. Hertel J, Kuhl C, Christensen NJ, Pedersen SA. Plasma noradrenaline and adrenaline in newborn infants of diabetic mothers: relation to plasma lipids. Acta Paediatr Scand 1985;74:521–524.
61. Jones CM III, Greiss FC Jr. The effect of labor on maternal and fetal circulating catecholamines. Am J Obstet Gynecol 1982;144:149–153.
62. Jones CR, McCullouch J, Butters L. et al. Plasma catecholamines and modes of delivery: the relation between catecholamine levels and in vitro platelet aggregation and adrenoceptor radioligand binding characteristics. Br J Obstet Gynaecol 1985;92:593–599.
63. Newnham JP, Marshall CL. Padbury JF, et al. Fetal catecholamine release with preterm delivery. Am J Obstet Gynecol 1984;149:888–893.
64. Paulick R, Kastendieck E, Wentze H. Catecholamine in arterial and venous umbilical blood: placental extraction, correlation with fetal hypoxia, and transcutaneous partial oxygen tension. J Perinatal Med 1985;13:31–42.
65. Puolakka J, Kauppila A, Tuimala R, et al. The effect of parturition on umbilical blood plasma levels of norepinephrine. Obstet Gynecol 1983;61:19–21.
66. Broberger U, Hannson H, Lagercrantz H, Persson B. Sympato-adrenal activity and metabolic adjustment during the first 12 hours after birth in infants of diabetic mothers. Paediatr Scand 1984;73:620–625.
67. Caron MG, Lefkowitz RJ. Catecholamine receptors: structure, function, and regulation In: Bardin CW, ed. Recent progress in hormone research. San Diego: Academic Press, 1993;48:277–290.
68. Ahlquist RP. A study of the adrenotropic receptors. Am J Physiol 1948;153:586–600.
69. Berthelsen S, Pettinger WA. A functional basis for classification of α-adrenergic receptors. Life Sci 1977;21:595–606.
70. Milligan G, Svoboda P, Brown CM. Why are there so many adrenoceptor subtypes? Biochem Pharmacol 1994; 48:1059–1071.
71. Lands AM, Arnold A, McAauliff JP, et al. Differentiation of receptor systems activated by sympathomimetic amines. Nature 1967;214:597–598.
72. Arch JRS, Kaumann AJ. $β_3$-adrenoceptors and atypical β-adrenoceptors. Med Res Rev 1993;13:663–729.
73. Minneman KP, Weiland GA, Molinoff PB. A comparison of the β-adrenergic receptor of the turkey erythrocyte with mammalian β1 and β2 receptors. Mol Pharmacol 1980; 17:1–7.
74. Chen X-H, Harden TK, Nicholas RA. Molecular cloning and characterization of a novel β-adrenergic receptor. J Biol Chem 1994;269:24810–24819.

75. Foster SJ, Harden TK. Dexamethasone increases β-adrenoceptor density in human astrocytoma cells. Biochem Pharmacol 1980;29:2151–2153.
76. Malbon CC, Hadcock JR. Evidence that corticosteroid response elements in the 5'-noncoding region of the hamster β$_2$-adrenergic receptor gene are obligate for corticosteroid regulation of receptor mRNA levels. Biochem Biophys Res Commun 1988;154:676–681.
77. Hadcock JR, Malbon CC. Regulation of β-adrenergic receptors by "permissive" hormones: corticosteroids increase steady-state levels of receptor mRNA. Proc Natl Acad Sci USA 1988;85:8415–8419.
78. Lai E, Rosen OM, Rubin CS. Dexamethasone regulates the β-adrenergic receptor subtype expressed by 3T3-L1 preadipocytes and adipocytes. J Biol Chem 1982;257:6691–6696.
79. Hadcock JR, Wang H, Malbon CC. Agonist-induced destabilization of β-adrenergic receptor mRNA: attenuation of glucocorticoid-induced up-regulation of β-adrenergic receptors. J Biol Chem 1989;264:19928–19933.
80. Williams LT, Lefkowitz RJ. Thyroid hormone regulation of β-adrenergic receptor number. J Biol Chem 1977;252:2787–2789.
81. Lazar-Wesley E, Hadcock JR, Malbon CC, et al. Tissue-specific regulation of α$_{1B}$, β$_1$, and β$_2$-adrenergic receptor mRNAs by thyroid state in the rat. Endocrinology 1991;129:1116–1118.
82. Liggins GC. The role of cortisol in preparing the fetus for birth. Reprod Fertil Dev 1994;6:141–150.
83. Padbury JF, Klein AH, Polk DH, et al. Effect of thyroid status on lung and heart β-adrenergic receptors in fetal and newborn sheep. Dev Pharmacol Ther 1986;9:44–53.
84. Stein HM, Oyama K, Martinez A, et al. Effects of corticosteroids in preterm sheep on adaptation and sympathoadrenal mechanisms at birth. Am J Physiol 1993;264:E763–E769.
85. Tseng YT, Tucker MA, Kashiwa KT, et al. Regulation of β1-adrenoceptors by glucocorticoids and thyroid hormones in fetal sheep. Eur J Pharmacol (Mol Pharmacol Sec) 1995;289:353–359.
86. Polk D, Cheromcha D, Reviczky A, Fisher DA. Nuclear thyroid hormone receptors: ontogeny and thyroid hormone effects in sheep. Am J Physiol 1989;256:E543–E549.
87. McDonald TJ, Myers DA, Nathanielsz PW. Localization of type II glucocorticoid receptor (GR) in the fetal sheep brain at 120 days of gestation (dGA). J Physiol 1993;459:331P.
88. Austin S, Polk DH, Jobe AH, Ikegami M. Hormonal regulation of surfactant protein mRNA expression in preterm fetal lambs. Pediatr Res 1993;33:43A.
89. Gorski J, Gannon F. Current models of steroid hormone action: a critique. Annu Rev Physiol 1976;38:425–450.
90. Evans RM. The steroid and thyroid hormone receptor superfamily. Science 1988;240:889–895.
91. Emorine LJ, Marullo S, Delavier-Klutchko C, et al. Structure of the gene for human β$_2$-adrenergic receptor: expression and promoter characterization. Proc Natl Acad Sci USA 1987;84:6995–6999.
92. Kobilka BK, Frielle T, Dohlman HG, et al. Delineation of the intronless nature of the genes for the human and hamster β$_2$-adrenergic receptor and their putative promoter regions. J Biol Chem 1987;262:7321–7327.
93. Zhang X-K, Dong J-M, Chiu J-F. Regulation of α-fetoprotein gene expression by antagonism between AP-1 and the glucocorticoid receptor at their overlapping bind-ing site. J Biol Chem 1991;266:8248–8254.
94. Pearce D, Yamamoto KR. Mineralocorticoid and glucocorticoid receptor activities distinguished by non-receptor factors at a composite response element. Science 1993;259:1161–1165.
95. Padbury JF, Tseng YT, Waschek JA. A cloning strategy for G-protein-coupled hormone receptors: the ovine β$_1$-adrenergic receptor. Reprod Fertil Dev 1995;7:521–525.
96. Padbury JF, Tseng YT, Waschek JA. Transcription initiation is localized to a TATAless region in the ovine β$_1$-adrenergic receptor gene. Biochem Biophys Res Commun 1995;211:254–261.
97. Ghosh D. Status of the transcription factors database (TFD). Nucleic Acids Res 1993;21:3117–3118.
98. Tseng YT, Waschek JA, Padbury JF. Functional analysis of the 5' flanking sequence in the ovine β$_1$-adrenergic receptor gene. Biochem Biophys Res Commun 1995;215:606–612.
99. Wang Y-C, Neckelmann N, Mayne A, et al. Establishment of a human fetal cardiac myocyte cell line. In Vitro Cell Dev Biol 1991;27A:63–74.
100. Yamamoto KR. Steroid receptor regulated transcription of specific genes and gene network. Annu Rev Genet 1985;19:209–252.
101. Levitzki A. From epinephrine to cyclic AMP. Science 1988;241:800–806.
102. Riabowol KT, Fink JS, Gilman MZ, et al. The catalytic subunit of cAMP-dependent protein kinase induces expression of genes containing cAMP-responsive enhancer elements. Nature 1988;336:83–86.
103. Collins S, Bouvier M, Bolanowski MA, et al. cAMP stimulates transcription of the β2-adrenergic receptor gene in response to short-term agonist exposure. Proc Natl Acad Sci USA 1989;86:4853–4857.
104. Stadel JM, Strulovici B, Nambi P, et al. Desensitization of the β-adrenergic receptor of frog erythrocytes. Recovery and characterization of the down-regulated receptors in sequestered vesicles. J Biol Chem 1983;258:3032–3038.
105. Vatner DE, Vatner SF, Nejima J, et al. Chronic norepinephrine elicits desensitization by uncoupling the β-receptor. J Clin Invest 1989;84:1741–1748.
106. Benovic JL, Strasser RH, Caron MG, Lefkowitz RJ. β-Adrenergic receptor kinase: identification of a novel protein kinase that phosphorylates the agonist-occupied form of the receptor. Proc Natl Acad Sci USA 1986;83:2797–2801.
107. Benovice JL, Onorato JJ, Arriza JL, et al. Cloning, expression, and chromosomal localization of β-adrenergic receptor kinase 2. A new member of the receptor kinase family. J Biol Chem 1991;266:14939–14946.
108. Sibley DR, Peters JR, Caron MG, Lefkowitz RJ. Desensitization of turkey erythrocyte adenylate cyclase.

β-Adrenergic receptor phosphorylation is correlated with attenuation of adenylate cyclase activity. J Biol Chem 1984;259:9742–9749.
109. Motulsky HJ, Cunningham EMS, Deblasi A, Insel PA. Desensitization and redistribution of β-adrenergic receptors on human mononuclear leukocytes. Am J Physiol 1986;250:E583–590.
110. Svartengren J, Svoboda P, Cannon B. Desensitization of β-adrenergic responsiveness in vivo. Decreased coupling between receptors and adenylate cyclase in isolated brown-fat cells. Eur J Biochem 1982;128:481–488.
111. Roscher AA, Wiesmann UN, Honegger UE. Changes in beta adrenergic receptors in submaxillary glands of chronically reserpine- or isoproterenol-treated rats. J Pharmacol Exp Ther 1981;216:419–424.
112. Lohse MJ, Benovic JL, Codina J, et al. β-Arrestin: a protein that regulates β-adrenergic receptor function. Science 1990;248:1547–1550.
113. Bristow MR, Ginsburg R, Minobe W, et al. Decreased catecholamine sensitivity and β-adrenergic-receptor density in failing human heart. N Engl J Med 1982;307:205–211.
114. Galinier M, Senard J-M, Valet P, et al. Changes in beta-adrenergic receptivity during human left ventricular hypertrophy due to pressure overload. J Hypertens 1993;11(suppl 5):S184–185.
115. Smiley RM, Pantuck CB, Chadburn A, Knowles DM. Down-regulation and desensitization of the β-adrenergic-receptor system of human lymphocytes after cardiac surgery. Anesth Analg 1993;77:653–661.
116. Castellano M, Paul Beschi M, et al. Gene regulation of beta-1-adrenergic receptor in genetically hypertensive rats. J Hypertens 1993;11(suppl 5):S64–65.
117. Bernstein D, Voss E, Huang S, et al. Differential regulation of right and left ventricular β-adrenergic receptors in newborn lambs with experimental cyanotic heart disease. J Clin Invest 1990;85:68–74.
118. Bjornerheim R, Golf S, Hansson V. Effects of chronic pindolol treatment on human myocardial β1- and β2-adrenoceptor function. Naunyn Schmiedebergs Arch Pharmacol 1990;342:429–435.
119. Feldman RD, Limbird LE, Nadeau J, et al. Alterations in leukocyte β-receptor affinity with aging. A potential explanation for altered β-adrenergic sensitivity in the elderly. N Engl J Med 1984;310:815–819.
120. Habib DM, Padbury JF, Martinez AM, et al. Neonatal adaptation: cardiac adrenergic effector mechanisms after birth in newborn sheep. Pediatr Res 1991;29:98–103.
121. Stein HM, Oyama K, Saoien R, et al. Prolonged β-agonist infusion does not induce desensitization or downregulation of β-adrenergic receptors in newborn sheep. Pediatr Res 1992;31:462–467.
122. Lau C, Burke SP, Slotkin TA. Maturation of sympathetic neurotransmission in the rat heart. IX. Development of transsynaptic regulation of cardiac adrenergic sensitivity. J Pharmacol Exp Ther 1982;223:675–680.
123. Tanaka H, Shigenobu K. Role of β-adrenergic receptor–adenylate cyclase system in the developmental decrease in sensitivity to isoprenaline in foetal and neonatal rat heart. Br J Pharmacol 1990;100:138–142.
124. Giannuzzi CE, Seidler FJ, Slotkin TA. β-Adrenoceptor control of cardiac adenylyl cyclase during development: agonist pretreatment in the neonate uniquely causes heterologous sensitization, not desensitization. Brain Res 1995;694:271–278.
125. Slotkin TA. Endocrine control of synaptic development in the sympathetic nervous system: the cardiac-sympathetic axis. In: Gootman PM, ed. Developmental neurobiology of the autonomic nervous system. Clifton, NJ: Humana Press, 1986:97–133.
126. Karnik NS, Newman S, Kopf GS, Gerton GL. Developmental expression of G protein alpha subunits in mouse spermatogenic cells: evidence that G alpha I is associated with the developing acrosome. Dev Biol 1992;152:393–402.
127. Collins, S, Altschmied J, Herbsman O, et al. A cAMP response element in the β2-adrenergic receptor gene confers transcriptional autoregulation by cAMP. J Biol Chem 1990;265:19330–19335.
128. Montminy MR, Savarino KA, Wagner JA, et al. Identification of a cyclic-AMP-responsive element within the rat somatostatin gene. Proc Natl Acad Sci USA 1986;83:6682–6686.
129. Comb M, Birnberg NC, Seasholtz A, et al. A cyclic AMP- and phorbol ester-inducible DNA element. Nature 1986;323:353–356.
130. Silver BJ, Bokar JA, Virgin JB, et al. Cyclic AMP regulation of the human glycoprotein hormone alpha-unit gene is mediated by an 18-base-pair element. Proc Natl Acad Sci USA 1987;84:2198–2202.

23
Respiration in the Fetal-Placental Unit

Robert W. Rothstein and Lawrence D. Longo

Development of the embryo, fetus, and neonate requires appropriate respiratory exchange of oxygen and carbon dioxide. During intrauterine life, the placenta serves as the lung for the fetus, permitting respiratory gas exchange and regulating acid-base balance. In this and many other ways, the placenta fulfills the functions of a variety of organs essential to extrauterine existence. With birth, physiologically one of the most tumultuous events of life, the responsibility for respiratory function shifts from the placenta to the neonatal lung, which must change within a matter of seconds from a relatively passive structure with fluid-filled airways to an active member with relatively full functional capacity.

Respiratory Gas Exchange in the Placenta

The placenta serves to couple substrate delivery to the fetus by the mother, in parallel with other vascular beds, as illustrated in Figure 23.1.[1] Under normal physiologic conditions, the oxygen delivery rate exceeds the minimum needed to meet fetal tissue oxygen requirements. In sheep, the oxygen delivery rate is approximately twofold that is necessary to maintain fetal oxidative metabolism and normal fetal acid-base balance.[2] The placenta supplies about $8\,ml\,O_2 \cdot min^{-1}\,kg^{-1}$ fetal mass, about twice that of an adult per weight basis (e.g., $24\,ml \cdot min^{-1}$ for a 3-kg term fetus), and because fetal blood O_2 stores are sufficient only for 1 to 2 minutes, it must be continuous on a moment-to-moment basis. Table 23.1 gives normal values of blood gases and pH in maternal and fetal placental exchange vessels.

Placental Anatomic and Physiologic Classification

The placenta, as illustrated in Figure 23.2, can be separated into two components, a maternal portion consisting of the decidua, and a fetal portion consisting of the chorionic plate and villi.[3] Maternal blood rich in oxygen and low in carbon dioxide is carried to the placenta by terminal branches of the uterine arteries. Blood from the spiral arteries, in the decidual plate, spurts into the intervillous space. Concurrently, fetal blood, oxygen depleted and rich in carbon dioxide, is carried to the placenta by umbilical arteries. Fetal chorionic villi, containing fetal capillaries, project into the pool of maternal blood in the intervillous space, permitting maternal-fetal gas exchange to occur by simple diffusion. Anatomically, the human placenta can be classified as hemochorial, with gas, released from free maternal red blood cells in the intervillous space, traversing the chorionic membrane and fetal endothelial cell wall to reach fetal red blood cells.[4]

As illustrated in Figure 23.3, physiologically the placenta can be classified into a variety of types based on the geometric relationship of the fetal to maternal bloodstream.[5,6] In concurrent exchange maternal and fetal blood in the placental capillary flows in the same direction so that recipient and donor blood equilibrate. Concurrent exchange allows the umbilical venous oxygen tension to be equal to, but not higher than, the oxygen tension in the maternal placental venous blood. In contrast, in countercurrent exchange, maternal and fetal blood flows in the opposite direction, and by providing a large maternal-to-fetal gas gradient throughout the length of the capillary, it provides for very efficient gas exchange. Countercurrent exchange allows the umbilical venous blood oxygen tension to exceed the oxygen tension in the maternal placental venous blood. It must be stressed that the clearance of any exchanger is a function of permeability and flow.[7] If permeability is much less than flow, clearance is virtually equal to permeability and independent of flow, so that the clearance of concurrent and countercurrent exchange becomes equal. If permeability is much greater than flow, clearance is virtually determined by flow. If the two streams are of unequal flow, in countercurrent exchange, the flow-limited clearance is equal to that of the lesser flow.

In addition to concurrent and countercurrent exchange models, a multivillous stream system exists in which fetal

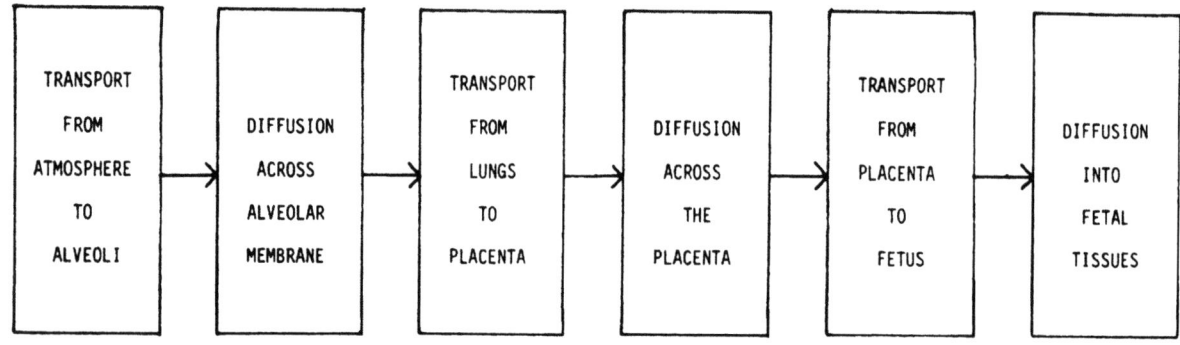

FIGURE 23.1. The transport of oxygen from the atmosphere to the fetal tissues in a sequence of steps that alternate bulk and diffusional transport. (From Meschia,[1] with permission.)

TABLE 23.1. Normal values of O_2, CO_2, and pH in human maternal and fetal blood.

Measurement	Maternal uterine blood		Fetal umbilical blood	
	Artery	Vein	Vein	Artery
P_{O_2} (torr)	95	38	30	22
HbO_2 (% saturation)	98	72	75	50
O_2 content (ml·dl^{-1})	16.4	11.8	16.2	10.9
O_2 content (mM)	7.3	5.3	7.2	4.5
Hb (g·dl^{-1})	12.0	12.0	16.0	16.0
O_2 capacity (ml·dl^{-1})	16.4	16.4	21.9	21.9
O_2 capacity (mM)	7.3	7.3	9.8	9.8
P_{CO_2} (torr)	32	40	43	48
CO_2 content (mM)	19.6	21.8	25.2	26.3
HCO_3	18.8	20.7	24.0	25.0
pH	7.42	7.35	7.38	7.34

P_{O_2} and P_{CO_2}, partial pressures of O_2 and CO_2, respectively; Hb, hemoglobin. From Longo.[12]

blood in different villous capillaries is opposed to maternal blood with varying gaseous concentrations, ranging between that of maternal arterial and venous blood. Alternatively, in the pool system, maternal blood is homogeneously mixed in the intervillous space, eliminating any concentration differences in varying areas of the intervillous space. As shown in Figure 23.4, it is apparent that these exchange models vary in their efficiency of gas transfer, with countercurrent exchange providing the most, and pool exchange the least, efficiency of gas transfer.[5]

Species utilizing countercurrent exchange include the guinea pig, rabbit, domestic cat, and horse, whereas sheep utilize concurrent exchange.[8] Experimental evidence suggests that the near-term human placenta utilizes concurrent exchange, although there is not enough data to exclude, with certainty, other models of exchange.[8] One of the major difficulties encountered in

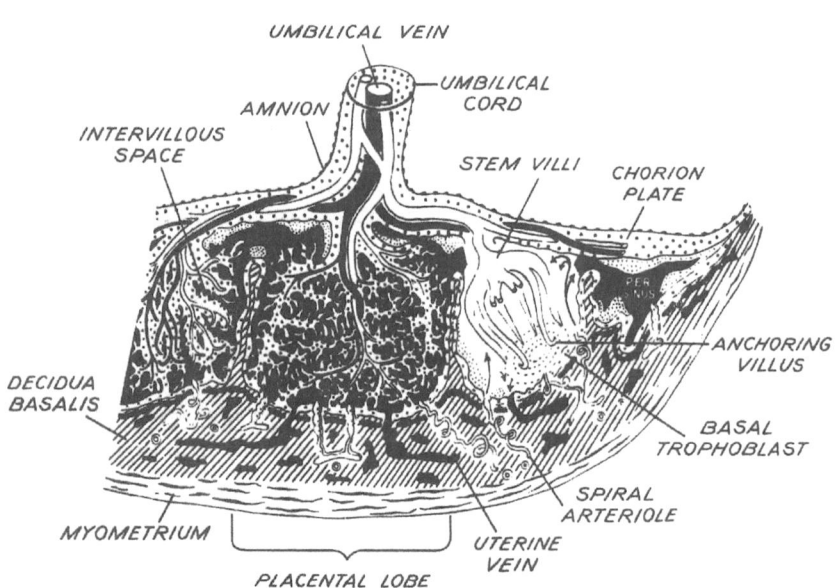

FIGURE 23.2. The architectural plan of the human placenta. (From Dawes,[3] and after Strauss, LQ,[3a] with permission.)

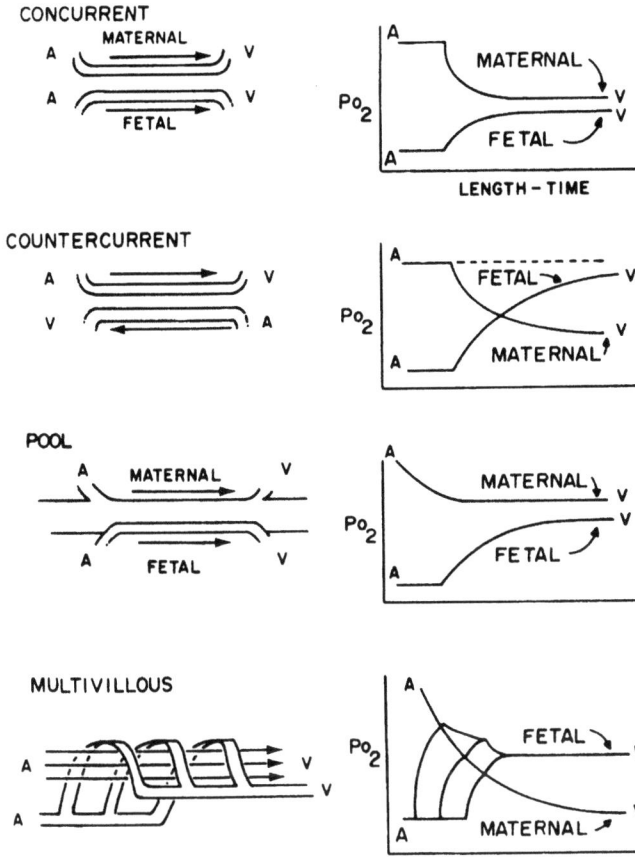

FIGURE 23.3. Physiologic classification of placental types. (From Nelson,[6] after Bartels and Moll,[5] with permission.)

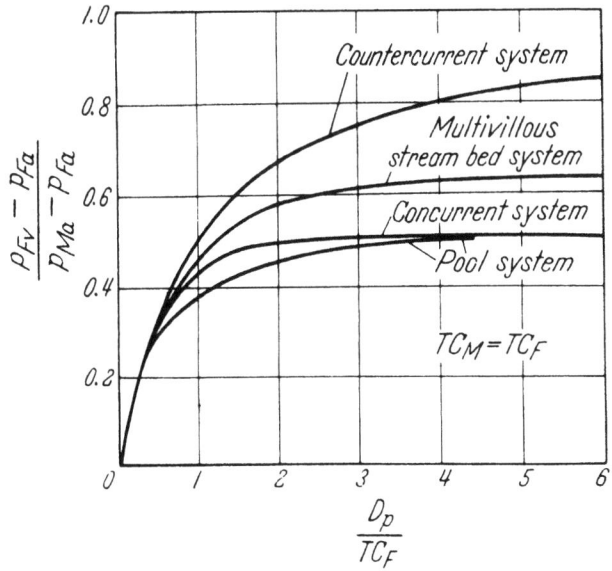

FIGURE 23.4. A comparison of efficiency for oxygen transfer in countercurrent, multivillous, concurrent, and pool placental systems. $(P_{Fv} - P_{Fa})$, increase in partial pressure (O_2) of fetal blood leaving the placenta; $(P_{Ma} - P_{Fa})$, partial pressure (O_2) difference of maternal and fetal blood entering the placenta; D_p, diffusion capacity of the placental membrane; TC_F, fetal transport capacity. If the diffusion capacity is low or the fetal transport capacity is high, the efficiencies of all systems are about equal. (From Bartels and Moll,[5] with permission.)

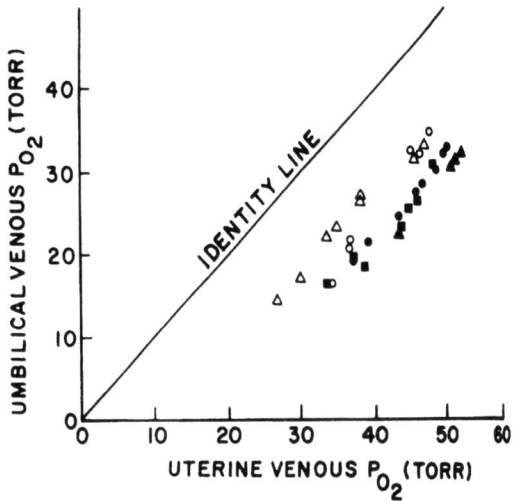

FIGURE 23.5. Relationship of umbilical venous O_2 tension (Po_2) to uterine venous O_2 tension (Po_2). Symbols represent individual measurements on five pregnant sheep, while varying uterine blood flows with a partial aortic occluder. (From Wilkening and Meschia,[2] with permission.)

categorizing the human placenta has resulted from variability in placental venous drainage. This variability is best illustrated by experiments in the rhesus monkey, where tritiated water infused in the fetus drained via the left, right, or both ovarian veins, with drainage shifting during the course of the study.[9] This variability in placental drainage through the ovarian veins invalidates conclusions based on random blood samples, and illustrates the importance of multiple venous sampling on the maternal side, in order to accurately describe placental gas exchange. Recognizing this, Pardi et al.[10] sampled respiratory gases concurrently in both uterine veins and the umbilical vein in human pregnancy, and found that, like the rhesus monkey, there were differences in measured gases depending on which uterine vein was sampled. As in the sheep (Figure 23.5), human umbilical venous Po_2 was always less than the least oxygenated uterine vein, supporting the finding that the human placenta utilizes concurrent exchange.

Factors Affecting Placental Oxygen Transfer

Placental O_2 exchange is altered by varying the properties of maternal or fetal blood (e.g., O_2 capacity or affinity), or by variations in maternal or fetal placental blood flow. As noted above, respiratory gas transfer is dependent on the spatial configuration of the blood vessels, and on the diffusion characteristics of the placental membranes.[11,12] Table 23.2 lists some of these factors and their components. Many of the variables that affect placental gas exchange are interdependent, complicating the de-

TABLE 23.2. Principal factors affecting placental oxygen transfer.

Variable	Associated components
Placental diffusing capacity	Membrane diffusing capacity (area, thickness, O_2 solubility, diffusivity of tissues); capillary blood volume; diffusing capacity of blood (O_2 capacity, hemoglobin reaction rates, concentration of reduced hemoglobin)
Maternal arterial Po_2	Inspired Po_2; alveolar ventilation; mixed venous Po_2; pulmonary blood flow; pulmonary diffusing capacity
Fetal arterial Po_2	Umbilical venous Po_2; fetal O_2 consumption; peripheral blood flow; maternal arterial Po_2; maternal-placental hemoglobin flow; placental diffusing capacity
Maternal placental hemoglobin flow rate	Arterial pressure; placental resistance to blood flow; venous pressure; O_2 capacity of blood
Fetal placental hemoglobin flow rate	Umbilical arterial blood pressure; umbilical venous blood pressure (or maternal vascular pressure under conditions of sluice flow); placental resistance of blood flow; blood O_2 capacity
Spatial relation of maternal to fetal flow	—
Amount of CO_2 exchange	—

From Longo,[12] with permission.

sign and interpretation of experiments. To further complicate matters, the fetus itself can alter its own oxygenation, showing a reduction in Po_2 and oxygen hemoglobin saturation by simply altering its muscular activity.[13] Although the exchange process would ideally be studied by sampling inflowing and end-capillary blood within a single exchange unit, this is experimentally impossible. Uterine and umbilical venous outflow, rather than representing blood from a single exchange unit, consists of blood from numerous compartments with differing O_2 and CO_2 tension and content. This situation probably results from a combination of nonuniform distribution of maternal and fetal placental blood flow, nonuniform distribution of diffusing capacity to blood flow, vascular shunts, and so on. An additional problem for one investigating placental exchange dynamics is that experimental change of a given variable, to stress the system, results in physiologic compensation that masks the effect of a given change. Details of the relative roles of the various factors must be inferred from manipulation of the maternal and fetal arterial input and mixed venous output.

Placental Diffusing Capacity

As in the lung, the quantity of O_2 crossing the placenta is a function of the diffusing capacity and the partial pressure gradient. The diffusing capacity is an index of efficiency of respiratory gas exchange, and expresses the rate of oxygen transfer across the placenta for a given partial pressure difference between maternal and fetal red blood cells. The diffusion characteristics of the placental membrane may be schematically represented as in Figure 23.6, and described by Fick's first law:

$$\frac{dQ}{dt} = \frac{AD\Delta C}{\Delta X} \qquad (1)$$

where dQ/dt = quantity of a given substance (e.g., O_2) crossing the placental membrane per unit time; A = exchange area; D = diffusion constant (cm^2/sec); ΔC = concentration difference (by volume) across the membrane; and ΔX = diffusion distance.[4]

In Fick's first law, the exchange area of the placenta is represented by the villous surface area (VSA), although it is the surface area of the fetal capillaries, rather than the villi itself, that is critical for gas diffusion. The fetal capillary surface area corresponds closely to that of the VSA.[14] The mean VSA in normal pregnancy at 40 weeks' gestation is approximately $11\,m^2$,[14] and ranges between 11

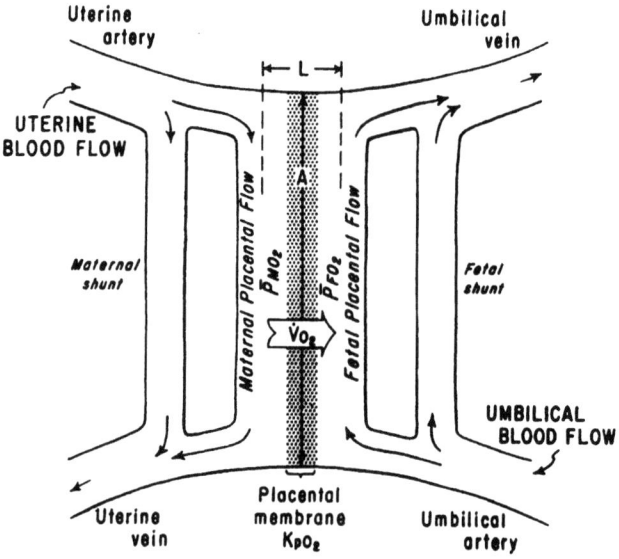

FIGURE 23.6. Schematic representation of placenta and its circulation from the standpoint of gas exchange. Maternal and fetal circulations both contain "shunts" through which blood flows without participating in gas exchange. Gas transfer occurs between the placental streams according to the laws of diffusion (oxygen is used as an example). (From Metcalfe et al.,[4] with permission.)

and 14 m².[15] It is positively and linearly correlated with birth weight[16] at all gestational ages.[14] It is not surprising, that there is a threefold increase in VSA between 28 weeks' gestation and term, which correlates well with the threefold increase in fetal weight during this time period.[14] In addition, in twin pregnancy, VSA does not increase in direct relation to gestational age, but rather in proportion to the combined weight of the two fetuses.[15] Some have speculated that VSA, as a compensatory mechanism, increases in response to conditions resulting in decreased maternal arterial blood oxygen tension, such as severe maternal cardiac failure.[15] This is supported in an animal model where a compensatory adaptation is seen in the placenta of the pregnant guinea pig placed in an isobaric, hypoxic ($F_iO_2 = 12\%$) environment from day 15 through day 60 of gestation. The placental changes included increased branching, increased number of fetal capillaries, as well as decreased trophoblastic thickness, all consistent with adaptation aimed at improving placental diffusing capacity and oxygen transfer.[17]

Since placental diffusion is directly related to the VSA, variations in VSA, as seen in disease states, directly affect gas exchange. It follows that a critical minimal VSA exists, below which fetal life cannot be maintained. This is supported by a small series in which all five fetuses whose VSA was less than 5 m² in the last trimester were stillborn.[14] In mothers who smoke during pregnancy, obliterative endarteritis and small infarcts in the villi may decrease VSA.[18] In preterm preeclampsia, there is an increase in the percent of avascular villi,[19] reducing VSA.[15] A decreased VSA is also seen in pregnancy complicated by eclampsia, hypertension, post-dates, syphilis, erythroblastosis, asphyxia,[15] increased maternal chronological age at conception,[20] and maternal marijuana smoking.[20] Interestingly, there is a 25% increase in VSA in pregnancies complicated by diabetes, secondary to increased branching of peripheral villi.[21] This increase has been directly related to day-to-day variations in maternal blood glucose concentration in some studies,[21] whereas others have found no difference in VSA when comparing the worst metabolically controlled diabetics to the best controlled, based on hemoglobin-A_1C values throughout pregnancy.[22] The values for VSA in gestational diabetics lie almost midway between those of nondiabetics and those with diabetes mellitus.[23] Despite the increase in VSA in pregnancies complicated by diabetes, the placenta behaves as if there is a 25% reduction in VSA, since there is an increase in the number of avascular villi,[15] accompanying the disrupted organization of the cotyledon.[21] Increased prepregnancy weight, in addition to increased rate of weight gain, has also been associated with increased fetal capillary surface area.[20]

In Fick's first law, the diffusion distance varies within a single full-term human placenta, with the minimal distance from the trophoblastic surface to the capillary lumen estimated to be 3.5 µm.[14] During the course of gestation, the diffusion distance across the trophoblast decreases, mostly because vasculosyncytial membranes, which reduce the diffusion distance, develop late in the second trimester.[24] This is one of the many reasons why the preterm placenta is less efficient and less able to tolerate stress than the mature placenta. In pregnancy complicated by diabetes mellitus, the diffusion distance is increased, mostly as a result of thickening of the epithelial and capillary basement membrane, as well as villous edema.[25,26] Despite these detriments to diffusion, the total diffusing capacity in diabetes mellitus is increased, despite the duration and severity of diabetes, as noted by White's classification.[27] This is the result of compensatory adaptations not only in the placenta, but also in the mother and fetus.

The placental membrane is a complex structure, its thickness and permeability varying with location. At a given locus the permeability, diffusibility, and thickness may be treated as constants and combined into a single term that expresses the membrane diffusion characteristics:

$$\frac{dQ}{dt} = \frac{1}{P_z} = D_p \quad (2)$$

where D_p = the placental diffusing capacity in milliliters per minute per torr pressure difference for gas z. For respiratory gases, the Bunsen solubility coefficient (α) and the partial pressure difference (P) are used rather than the concentration difference (C) in derivation from Fick's law. Placental diffusing capacity is commonly expressed as

$$D_p = \frac{V}{P_m - P_f} \quad (3)$$

where V = the quantity of respiratory gas exchanging across the placental membrane per unit time: and $P_m - P_f$ = the mean partial pressure difference between maternal and fetal placental exchange vessels.[28]

Mayhew et al.,[29,30] adapting a morphometric model developed by Longo et al.,[31] described placental diffusing capacity. In this model, there are a series of five histologic compartments arranged in series, with each tissue compartment representing a partial diffusing capacity. These compartments represent the five tissue compartments that oxygen must traverse in moving from the mother to the fetus, and include the maternal erythrocyte, maternal plasma, villous membrane, fetal plasma, and fetal erythrocyte. Since each tissue compartment provides its own resistance to oxygen diffusion, total resistance should be the sum of these five partial resistances, and total oxygen diffusion capacity is represented by the reciprocal of this total resistance. Of the five compartments, the major contributor to oxygen diffusion resistance is the villous membrane, which accounts for 89% of total resistance.[30] Furthermore, within the villous membrane, the harmonic mean thickness is the single most influential variable with an impact on D_p, with alterations in the surface area of the villi and fetal capillaries having a moderate impact on D_p. The harmonic mean thickness normally decreases with advancing gestation[30] and is increased early in gestation in pregnancy complicated by maternal smoking.[32] This model has been applied to understand changes in D_p accompanying advancing gestation,[30] changes in altitude,[33,34] maternal smoking,[32] increased prepregnancy weight and rate of weight gain,[20] and diabetes mellitus.[27]

One must keep in mind that morphometric D_p provides an expression of potential diffusion of oxygen, based solely on physical measurements of the placenta. It follows that values of D_p, morphometrically determined, exceed those determined physiologically, such as by carbon monoxide diffusing capacity determination. This discrepancy results from the morphometric model not taking into consideration vascular shunts, uneven diffusion to perfusion ratios, and placental oxygen consumption.

Ideally, one would study O_2 or CO_2 exchange using these gases, but it is not practical for several reasons. First, significant amounts of the total O_2 exchanging is consumed by the placenta, probably close to one third at term.[35] In addition, uterine and umbilical mixed venous blood samples must be used for the calculations, which represent a mixture of blood from compartments with differing maternal/fetal blood flow ratios[36,37] and probably differing diffusing capacity/blood flow ratios.[38] Under almost all circumstances O_2 exchange is limited by blood flow rather than by diffusion, and, as in the lung, a metabolically inert gas whose exchange is limited by diffusion and that combines with hemoglobin is used.

Carbon monoxide (CO) in low concentration has been shown to be the most practical gas for studies of transplacental diffusion. The placental diffusion capacity for carbon monoxide (D_{PCO}) can be calculated by use of the Haldane relation:

$$\frac{[HbCO]}{[HbO_2]} = \frac{P_{CO} \cdot M}{P_{O_2}} \quad (4)$$

where $[HbCO]$ = carboxyhemoglobin concentration; $[HbO_2]$ = oxyhemoglobin saturation; P_{CO} = CO partial pressure (torr); and M = the relative affinity of hemoglobin for CO and O_2.

Placental CO diffusing capacity equals about $0.5 \, \text{ml} \cdot \text{min}^{-1} \, \text{torr}^{-1} \, \text{kg}^{-1}$ fetal weight in several species (e.g., sheep, dog, macaque monkey);[28,39] in the rabbit and guinea pig, it is severalfold greater.[40,41] Such studies suggest that the mean maternal-fetal partial pressure difference for O_2 is only about 6 torr, a value similar to that of the pulmonary alveolar-capillary P_{O_2} difference.[28] It suggests that the placenta does not constitute a significant barrier to respiratory gas diffusion, and that placental O_2 exchange is limited by blood flow rather than by diffusion.[28]

During the course of gestation, the placental mass and exchange area increase to meet the demands of the developing conceptus. Nonetheless, whereas the fetal mass increases severalfold from 1000 to 3500 g during the last trimester and placental mass doubles, so the placental/fetal mass ratio is halved from 0.22 to 0.14. D_{PCO} calculated in terms of fetal weight remains constant.[39,42] During prolonged antenatal hypoxia in the guinea pig with the mother breathing 12% O_2 from day 15 to 62 of gestation (term is 64 days), D_{PCO} increases about 63%.[41] These changes are associated with an increase in placental vascular volume and a decrease in diffusion distance, which suggests the dependence of D_{PCO} on placental structure.[43] In contrast to the increased D_{PCO} of long-term hypoxia, in the pregnant guinea pig that exercised 15 to 60 minutes/day throughout gestation D_{PCO} decreased about 34%, with the decrease being proportional to exercise duration.[41,44] Again, under these circumstances there was an inverse relation between exercise duration and both D_{PCO} and the maternal and fetal placental exchange area.[45]

Unfortunately, no reliable measurement of D_{PCO} in the human is available. The value would be predicted to decrease in conditions in which the placental membranes are thickened (e.g., syphilis and edema), in association with intrauterine growth retardation, and in association with decreased blood volume or hemoglobin concentration in the placental exchange vessels. None of these clinical associations has been established.

Maternal and Fetal Oxygen Partial Pressures

Theoretical and experimental studies have suggested that placental O_2 exchange is particularly sensitive to changes in maternal or fetal arterial O_2 tensions. Decreases in maternal arterial P_{O_2} to about 70 torr appear to have little effect on placental O_2 exchange and fetal oxygenation, as it would decrease $[HbO_2]$ only about 5%. Above 70 torr the oxyhemoglobin saturation curve is relatively flat, and oxyhemoglobin remains saturated. A decrease in maternal arterial P_{O_2} below this value results in a decreased amount of O_2 crossing to the fetus.[46] In contrast, raising maternal arterial P_{O_2} to about 600 torr by breathing 100% O_2 increases the amount of O_2 in maternal blood slightly and increases fetal umbilical venous O_2 tension 3 to 5 torr. Although of little value under normal circumstances, such an increase in fetal blood O_2 tension may be of greater benefit in instances of fetal hypoxemia.

Fetal arterial O_2 tension influences placental O_2 exchange, the amount of such exchange varying inversely with the umbilical arterial Po_2 value.[11] Fetal arterial Po_2, in turn, is a function of transplacental O_2 exchange, umbilical venous Po_2, and the rate of fetal O_2 consumption. Furthermore, these factors are not independent, but rather produce an impact on each other in order to maintain equilibrium. This is illustrated in fetal sheep, whereby administration of norepinephrine increases fetal oxygen consumption by 25%, without significant change in umbilical arterial or venous Po_2 or oxygen content. Fetal O_2 tension was maintained as a result of a 27% increase in umbilical blood flow.[47] In contrast, administration of a pharmacologic neuromuscular blocker to fetal sheep, with resultant inhibition of fetal movement, decreased fetal oxygen consumption and was accompanied by a significant increase in fetal Po_2 and oxygen saturation. The investigators suggest that umbilical blood flow, which was increased by 6%, is unable to adjust hemodynamically to the increases in fetal Po_2.[48]

Umbilical venous O_2 tension normally is 10 to 15 torr less than that of the uterine venous blood (Table 23.1).[12] The blood gas values shown in Table 23.1 are based on studies in the chronically catheterized sheep and monkey, as well as human data obtained by puncturing the umbilical cord under ultrasonic guidance during cordocentesis. Much of the data presented and discussed are derived from studies in experimental laboratory animals. Concerns are expressed as to whether measurement of fetal oxygen uptake in the experimental animal can be used to estimate that of the human fetus. Despite these differences in body size, composition, and rate of growth, fetal oxygen uptake per gram of wet weight varies ±20% in different species, supporting the theory that fetal animal oxygen uptake data may approximate that in the human.[49]

A number of factors could theoretically affect placental O_2 exchange and account for the O_2 tension difference between uterine and umbilical venous blood. Such factors include the geometric relation of fetal vessels to maternal blood in the exchange area, placental shunts in which uterine or umbilical arterial blood enters the venous circulation without traversing the exchange areas, and nonuniform or uneven distribution of maternal and fetal blood flow in localized regions of the placenta. Such maternal-fetal perfusion inequalities could act as an effective shunt and account for the uterine-umbilical O_2 tension difference.[37,50]

Maternal and Fetal Blood Oxygen Affinity and Capacity

Hemoglobin in maternal blood contributes considerably to placental O_2 transfer. The reduced form of hemoglobin binds with O_2 to form oxyhemoglobin. Because this binding is reversible, hemoglobin can unload O_2 to diffuse across the placenta as the O_2 partial pressure decreases. The ability of hemoglobin to bind oxygen depends not only on the Po_2 but on the hemoglobin-O_2 affinity, as indicated by the sigmoid-shaped oxyhemoglobin saturation curve.

Hemoglobin A (HbA) and hemoglobin F (HbF) have identical oxygen affinities when these molecules are in solution, rather than in the red blood cell, suggesting that differences in affinity are not directly related to structural differences in the hemoglobin molecule.[51] The increased oxygen affinity in HbF is the result of its reduced interaction with 2,3-diphosphoglycerate (2,3-DPG).[52] Studies in fetal sheep receiving isovolemic exchange transfusion with adult blood, having a lower O_2 affinity, reveal that although a high hemoglobin affinity may not be essential to the healthy fetus, it is critical for maintaining normal metabolism in the fetus exposed to hypoxic stress.[53] The in utero transition from predominantly HbF to HbA synthesis occurs at 30 weeks' gestation.[54] This time frame is followed in extrauterine life as well, so that at full-term postconceptual age there is no difference in the relative amount of HbA and HbF synthesis in the neonate born prematurely or at term.[55] At term, roughly 47% to 60% of total hemoglobin being synthesized is HbF,[54,55] which declines, following a sigmoidal curve, to negligible amounts at 4 to 5 months of age.[54]

During placental insufficiency, the fetus compensates for decreased oxygen delivery by increasing HbF synthesis. It is not surprising that HbF concentration is correlated with placental weight, with a smaller placenta being associated with significantly higher fetal umbilical venous HbF concentration.[56] This is illustrated in the term pregnancy complicated by toxemia, where HbF synthesis is significantly higher in the small for gestational age (SGA) neonate when compared to an appropriate for gestational age (AGA) nontoxemic control. One month follow-up of these patients revealed no difference in HbF synthesis between groups.[57] Additionally, in pregnancy complicated by Rh-isoimmunization, the fetus, as early as 20 weeks' gestation, compensates for hemolytic anemia with increased fetal erythropoietin and accompanying extramedullary hematopoiesis.[58] This compensation, in conjunction with increased umbilical blood flow,[59] permits the fetus to maintain normal acid-base balance with decreases in fetal hematocrit of up to 50%.[60] The anemic fetus can increase umbilical blood flow to rates that exceed $120\,ml\cdot min^{-1}\cdot kg^{-1}$ of fetus.[59] Investigators have speculated that in isoimmunization, the increase in umbilical vein blood flow accompanying severe anemia is secondary to compensatory vasodilation of the umbilical vessels.[59] Increased flow may be related to a decrease in resistance associated with a lower blood viscosity resulting from the decreasing red blood cell mass. This relationship is described by Poiseuille's law:

$$R = \frac{8(\eta)L}{\pi r^4} \tag{5}$$

where R = resistance, η = viscosity of fluid, L = length of vessel, and r = radius of vessel.[6] These compensatory increases in umbilical blood flow, associated with a decreased fetal hematocrit, are complemented by an increased placental fractional extraction of oxygen,[61] in addition to a redistribution of fetal blood flow to vital organs.[62]

Compensatory increases in umbilical blood flow, associated with fetal anemia or decreases in fetal hemoglobin affinity, are not immediate. Acute fetal hemorrhage, resulting in a 40% blood loss, is associated with an immediate 52% decrease in umbilical blood flow, with restoration of blood flow by 1 to 2 days, despite a reduced blood volume.[61] Similarly, acute reduction in fetal blood oxygen affinity results in decreased umbilical-placental blood flow 1 hour after fetal blood is isovolumetrically replaced with maternal blood.[63]

The expression P_{50} describes the O_2 partial pressure required to half-saturate hemoglobin. Under standard conditions (i.e., pH 7.40, P_{CO_2} 40 torr, 37°C) the P_{50} for normal adult human blood, including that of the pregnant mother, is 26.5 torr (Figure 23.7). The curve is shifted to the right (i.e., lowered O_2 affinity) in association with increased concentrations of CO_2, hydrogen ion (H^+), 2,3-DPG, adenosine triphosphate (ATP), or chloride ion. In a number of species, the fetal oxyhemoglobin saturation curve is shifted to the left compared to that of maternal blood. The P_{50} for fetal blood near term is about 20 torr (Figure 23.7). Under physiologic conditions in vivo, the maternal curve is shifted to the left (i.e., pH 7.42, P_{CO_2} 34 torr), whereas that of the fetus is shifted to the right (i.e., pH 7.35, P_{CO_2} 45 torr, 37.5°C) so they are almost superimposed (Figure 23.7).

In the erythrocyte, the highly negatively charged 2,3-DPG is a metabolic intermediate of anaerobic glycolysis. By interacting with the two β chains of the hemoglobin tetramere,[64] stabilizing the quaternary structure of deoxyhemoglobin, and by lowering erythrocyte intracellular pH,[65] an increase in erythrocyte 2,3-DPG concentration increases P_{50}. Of the organic phosphates in the human erythrocyte, 2,3-DPG is qualitatively and quantitatively the most effective in lowering oxygen affinity, followed by ATP, adenosine diphosphate (ADP), adenosine monophosphate (AMP), and pyrophosphate. Since erythrocyte glycolysis is sensitive to intracellular pH, which is approximately 0.2 unit lower than plasma pH,[52] it follows that a decrease in plasma pH, as seen in diabetic ketoacidosis, decreases the concentration of erythrocyte 2,3-DPG,[66] and increases oxygen affinity. This increase in oxygen affinity, as illustrated in Figure 23.8, is offset by acidosis decreasing oxygen affinity through the Bohr effect.

In the fetus, due to structural differences in hemoglobin F and A, the effect of 2,3-DPG on the oxyhemoglobin saturation curve is less than half of that for the adult.[52] Additionally, the fetus has a lower concentration of 2,3-DPG when compared to the pregnant woman, where, in the latter, concentration increases significantly from the first to the third trimester.[67] Despite this increase in maternal 2,3-DPG with advancing pregnancy, maternal oxygen affinity (P_{50}) remains unchanged, secondary to the effects of a decreasing CO_2 and increasing pH, as gestation advances.[67]

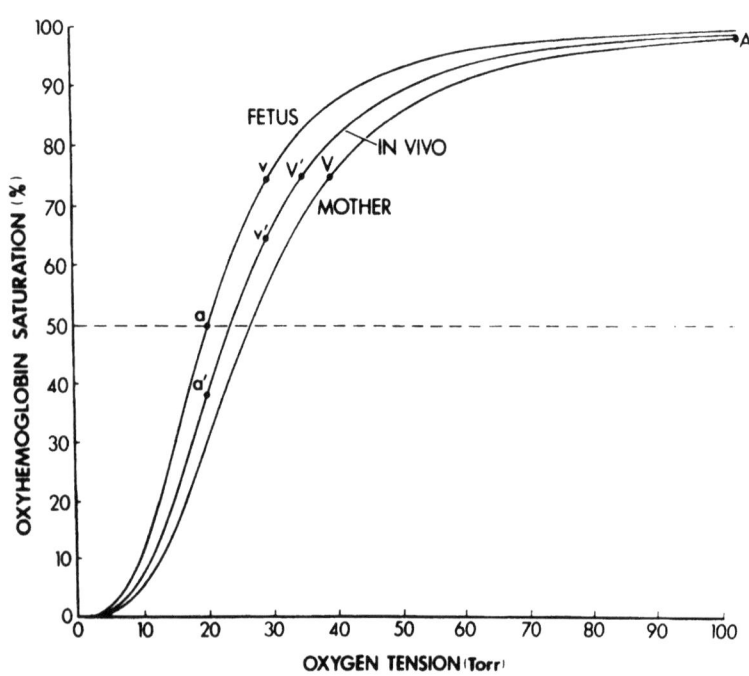

FIGURE 23.7. HbO_2 saturation curves for human maternal and near-term fetal blood. Maternal and fetal HbO_2 affinities (P_{50}) are 26.5 and 20.0 torr, respectively. A, V, maternal arterial and venous values, respectively, under standard conditions; a, v, umbilical arterial and venous values, respectively; V', a', v', probable in vivo maternal venous, umbilical arterial, and umbilical venous values, respectively.

FIGURE 23.8. Diagrammatic representation of the effect of pH changes on hemoglobin affinity of oxygen. (From Bellingham et al.,[66] with permission.)

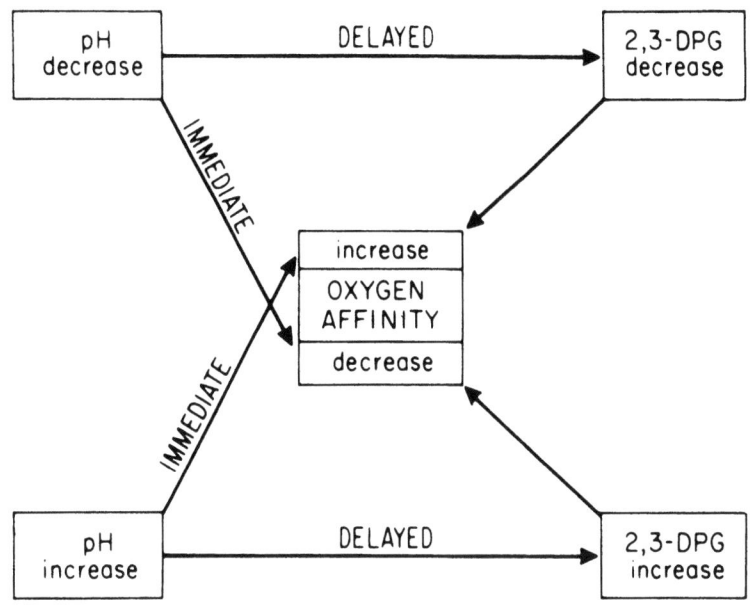

Blood oxygen capacity is the maximum amount of O_2 that can reversibly bind with hemoglobin. With a hemoglobin concentration of $14 \text{ g} \cdot \text{dl}^{-1}$ the nonpregnant woman has a blood O_2 capacity of about $19 \text{ g} \cdot \text{dl}^{-1}$ ([Hb] × 1.36). During the course of gestation physiologic hemodilution occurs as plasma volume increases about 50% and the erythrocyte mass increases about 25%.[68] Near-term maternal hemoglobin concentration decreases to about $11.5 \text{ g} \cdot \text{dl}^{-1}$ with an O_2 capacity of $15.6 \text{ g} \cdot \text{dl}^{-1}$.[69] In the human, fetal hemoglobin concentration increases from $8.5 \text{ g} \cdot \text{dl}^{-1}$ at 10 weeks' gestation, to a mean value of $16.5 \text{ g} \cdot \text{dl}^{-1}$ at term.[70] During the last third of gestation, the fetal blood O_2 capacity exceeds that of the mother.

The placenta is sensitive to changes in maternal hemoglobin concentration. In general, placental hypertrophy accompanies maternal anemia, a compensatory response aimed at increasing placental diffusing capacity with resultant increases in fetal oxygen extraction. If, however, the maternal anemia is severe enough, compensatory placental hypertrophy is hindered, resulting in a significantly smaller placental size.[71] Similar compensatory mechanisms occur with increases in maternal hemoglobin affinity, relative to fetal hemoglobin affinity, in an effort to maintain normal fetal development and growth.[72] This is illustrated in the pregnant ewe, which is homozygous for high oxygen affinity hemoglobin. There is not only a compensatory increase in placental size, but also an increase in uterine blood flow with hemoglobin highly saturated with oxygen.[73] In the pregnant rat transfused with homologous blood, resulting in a lower P_{50} in the maternal versus the fetal blood, similar adaptive placental changes occur.[74]

As noted above, in vivo the maternal and fetal O_2 saturation curves are probably superimposed. Figure 23.9 shows maternal and fetal blood O_2 content as a function of O_2 partial pressure, illustrating that a normal fetal umbilical venous P_{O_2} of only about 28 torr is associated with an O_2 content of $15.5 \text{ ml} \cdot \text{dl}^{-1}$, a concentration as great as the maternal O_2 content of $15.4 \text{ ml} \cdot \text{dl}^{-1}$. Despite the fetal hemoglobin being only about 75% saturated, compared to about 98% in the adult, its greater hemoglobin concentration allows for a higher O_2 content. The maternal and fetal blood oxyhemoglobin saturations have important implications for placental O_2 transfer. An increase of either maternal or fetal O_2 capacity promotes placental O_2 exchange.[11,75] Other factors remaining constant, the larger the sum of maternal and fetal blood O_2 capacity, the more O_2 is exchanged before equilibration of P_{O_2} values is reached in these bloodstreams.

Bohr and Haldane Effects

As maternal and fetal blood course through placental exchange vessels, H^+ and CO_2 diffuse from fetal blood across the placenta, so maternal blood becomes more acidotic and hypercarbic, shifting the oxyhemoglobin saturation curve to the right and increasing the O_2 available for transfer. At the same time, the fetal curve is shifted to the left, promoting O_2 uptake by the fetal erythrocytes. Theoretical studies suggest that this mechanism, the Bohr effect, accounts for about 8% of placental O_2 exchange.[76]

As a consequence of this exchange process, deoxyhemoglobin concentration increases in the maternal-placental blood and decreases in the fetus. Because deoxyhemoglobin binds CO_2 to a greater extent than oxyhemoglobin, CO_2 exchange from fetal to maternal blood is augmented. This Haldane effect is calculated to account for about 46% of placental CO_2 exchange.[76]

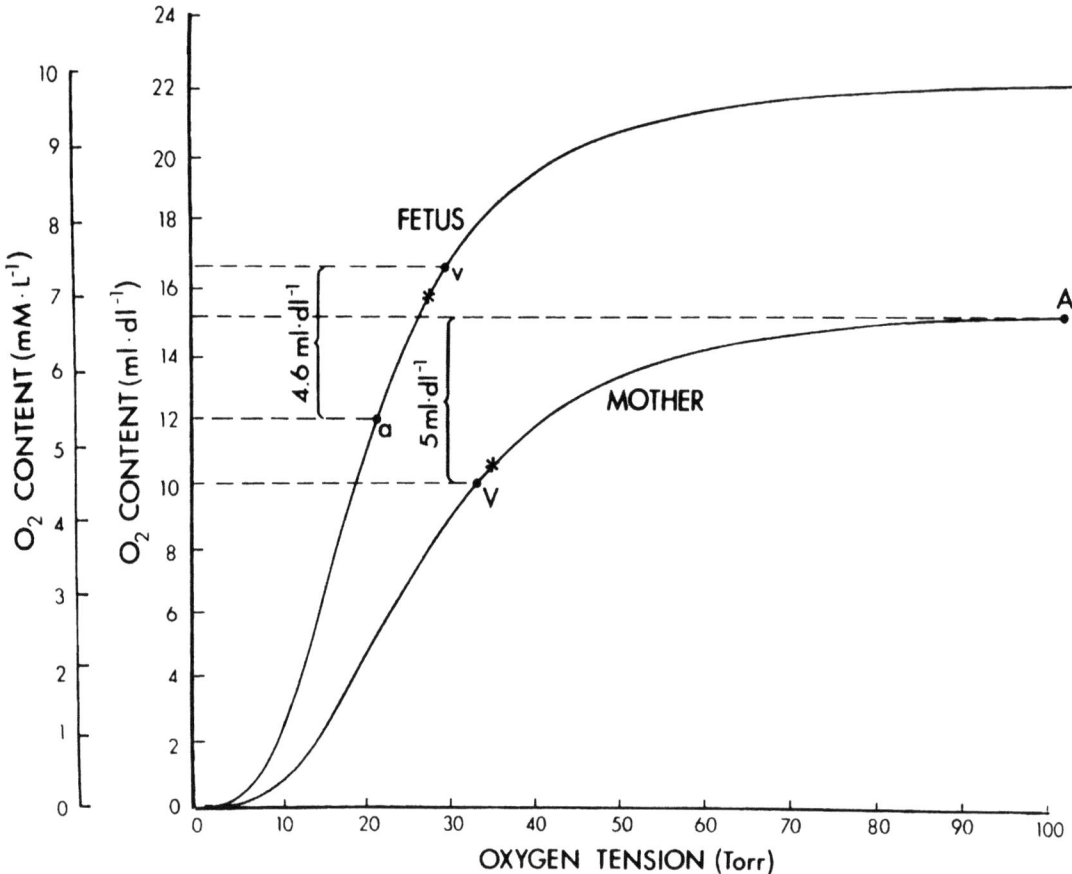

FIGURE 23.9. Blood O_2 content as a function of Po_2 for maternal hemoglobin = $12\,g\cdot dl^{-1}$ and P_{50} = 26.5 torr, and for near-term fetal hemoglobin = $16.5\,g\cdot dl^{-1}$ and P_{50} = 20 torr. *, mean maternal and fetal Po_2; A, V, maternal arterial and venous values; a, v, umbilical arterial and venous values.

Maternal and Fetal-Placental Blood Flow

To a great extent, placental O_2 and CO_2 exchange depend on the rates of uterine and umbilical blood flows. In the human fetus, at term gestation and of normal intrauterine growth, both measured and calculated umbilical venous oxygen content is linearly related to the lowest observable maternal mean arterial blood pressure. This suggests that fetal oxygen availability is a function of maternal uterine blood flow.[56] However, increasing uteroplacental blood flow beyond normal physiologic rates, in nonstressed sheep, does not increase fetal oxygen tension.[77] During the course of gestation uteroplacental blood flow increases from very little to $700-1000\,ml\cdot min^{-1}$ at term.[78,79] About 80% to 90% of this flow supplies the placenta and is available for O_2 and nutrient transfer to the fetus. Data in the monkey,[80] sheep,[81] and other species indicate that placental O_2 exchange varies as a function of uterine blood flow.

Investigators have been unable to demonstrate a significant decrease in fetal blood oxygen tension in association with decreases in uterine blood flow to approximately one half of control. In the near-term sheep, infusion of the adrenergic agonist ritodrine decreases uterine artery blood flow in a dose-dependent fashion. Uterine blood flow decreased as great as 50% of control for 2 hours without deviation in fetal pH, Po_2, and Pco_2 from normal physiologic values.[82] In the near-term sheep, maternal hypotension lasting 20 minutes, accompanying spinal anesthesia, decreased uterine blood flow by 65% with no significant alteration in fetal Po_2.[83] Similar findings, in a chronic sheep preparation, result when uterine blood flow is diminished by inflating an aortic occluder[2] or partially clamping the internal iliac artery.[84] These findings support the conclusion that under normal physiologic conditions, the oxygen delivery rate to the fetus is appreciably greater than the minimum needed to satisfy fetal tissue oxygen requirements.[2] Mathematical models[11] suggest that with a 65% decrease in maternal placenta blood flow, normal oxygen exchange cannot be maintained, unless other compensatory actions occur to maintain normal fetal oxygenation. Such compensatory actions, maintaining fetal and uteroplacental oxygen consumption, include increases in oxygen extraction by both the uterus and the fetal side of the placenta as high as 84% and 50%, respectively.[84]

The role of uterine blood flow in placental O_2 exchange and fetal oxygenation has obvious clinical implications. Uteroplacental blood flow is reduced during the uterine contractions of labor, which is associated with transient decreases in O_2 transfer to the fetus.[12] In the sheep the decrease in uteroplacental oxygen uptake during spontaneous and oxytocin-induced uterine contraction is 3.8% and 10%, respectively.[85] In the sheep, nonlabor uterine contraction is associated with a 2- to 3-torr decrease in fetal arterial Po_2.[13] In addition, blood flow may be decreased in women with vascular disease or hypertensive disorders of pregnancy. Fetal O_2 transfer is highly dependent on the rate of uterine blood flow.[11,56,86,87]

Similar to uteroplacental blood flow, the rate of umbilicalplacental blood flow may partially decrease without affecting fetal oxygen tension. In the near-term fetal sheep, balloon occlusion of the fetal descending aorta resulted in normal fetal oxygen uptake, as long as umbilical oxygen delivery did not decline below 52% of control. Furthermore, decreased umbilical blood flow did not significantly change uterine blood flow.[88] This suggests that, like uteroplacental blood flow, normal umbilical oxygen delivery rate exceeds, by approximately twofold, the minimum oxygen necessary to sustain fetal oxidative metabolism.

As with uteroplacental blood flow, the importance of umbilical flow on placental O_2 exchange is difficult to assess because of compensatory changes in other factors that affect such flow. In an effort to minimize this problem, Power and Jenkins[46] perfused in situ an isolated cotyledon of the sheep placenta with blood of known O_2 tension, content, and flow rate. They demonstrated the dependence of venous outflow O_2 tension and the rate of O_2 transfer on fetal cotyledonary blood flow. Outflow O_2 tension varied inversely with the cotyledonary flow rate, whereas the O_2 exchange rate increased with increased blood flow.[46]

In most vascular beds blood flow is proportional to the hydrostatic pressure difference between arterial and venous vessels. In the placenta, because of the close association of the maternal and fetal circulations, evidence suggests that increases in maternal-placental blood volume may impinge on fetal vessels in placental villi, increasing the resistance of umbilical flow.[89] Under such conditions fetal-placental blood flow would be proportional to the fetal inflow pressure minus that of surrounding maternal-placental blood pressure. Such a "sluice" or "waterfall" relation, in which surrounding pressure affects vascular resistance, has been described in the lung. In addition, evidence suggests that such a mechanism may operate so that increases in fetal-placental blood volume affect maternal placental flow.[90,91] In the near-term pregnant woman lying in the supine position, the gravid uterus may compress the inferior vena cava, impeding uterine venous outflow and causing intervillous space pressure to rise. Fetal-placental vessels would be compressed, increasing vascular resistance and decreasing umbilical flow. Fetal-placental flow would be restored once fetal arterial pressure increased sufficiently.

Regulation of Maternal and Fetal-Placental Blood Flow

As pregnancy advances, there are marked changes in maternal cardiac output and uterine blood flow. The cardiac output doubles in the term sheep, which is the result of a 140% increase in stroke volume and a 20% increase in heart rate at term, when compared to the nonpregnant state.[92] In addition, the percent of cardiac output distributed to the uterus increases from less than 1% prepregnancy to 16% or greater at term.[93] The sevenfold increase in placental blood flow per gram of placental cotyledon, occurring at 90 days' gestation through term, coincides with the time of greatest fetal growth, with 80% of growth occurring in the last 2 months of gestation.[94] Whereas increases in maternal-placental blood flow in the last third of ovine pregnancy is the result of vasodilation,[93,94] increases in fetal-placental blood flow is mostly secondary to increases in the total number of placental vessels.[93] In addition, the distribution of uterine blood flow changes as pregnancy advances, while in the nonpregnant uterus the caruncles, endometrium, and myometrium each receive one third of uterine blood flow, at term 90% of uterine blood flow is distributed to the placental cotyledons.[93]

When discussing the regulation of placental blood flow, one must consider blood flow on both sides of the placenta, namely uterine and umbilical flow. Optimal placental perfusion would be that flow rate below which transplacental exchange would be inadequate, and above which increased perfusion would minimally improve transplacental exchange. In the sheep, a flow ratio of 1,[6,36,95,96] whereby uterine blood flow equals umbilical blood flow, is optimal for exchange of inert molecules, as illustrated in Figure 23.10. This flow ratio is consistent with mathematical models, where the ratio for optimal exchange is 0.9.[11] However, in chronic catheterized sheep models there is a higher uterine to umbilical flow ratio than predicted, measured to be between 1.8 and 3.6.[95] This increased flow ratio may, among other things, reflect increased uterine blood flow required to meet metabolic needs of the placenta, exceeding that flow required to permit transplacental exchange.

As demonstrated in the fetal lamb, a relatively high basal rate of uterine and umbilical blood flow provides a margin of safety for the fetus, enabling the fetus to maintain an almost constant oxygen uptake over a broad range of uterine and umbilical flows.[2] However, despite this protective buffer zone, abnormalities in utero-

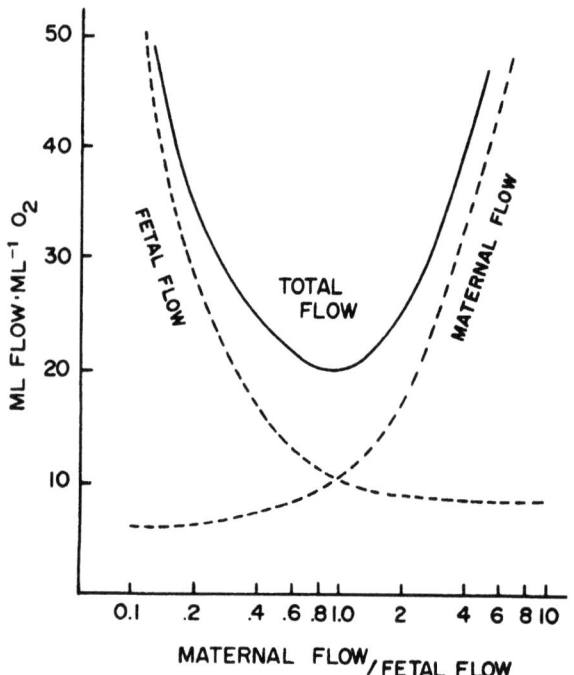

FIGURE 23.10. Efficiency of placental gas transfer. If maternal and fetal blood flow are not well matched, extra maternal or fetal flow work are required with no increase in O_2 transfer. (From Nelson,[6] after Power and Longo,[96] with permission.)

placental blood flow can compromise the fetus by impairing normal implantation, placental growth, and oxygen delivery, if occurring during early, middle, and late pregnancy, respectively.[93] It is of interest to examine how uterine and umbilical blood flow is regulated under normal physiologic conditions and during perturbations, such as pregnancy complicated by maternal diabetes,[97,98] metabolic acidosis,[99] preeclampsia,[98,100] and cigarette smoking,[101] where there is decreased placental intervillous blood flow.

Chemical Mediation of Maternal and Fetal-Placental Blood Flow

Since neurohistochemical techniques applied to the human placenta reveal an absence of adrenergic and cholinergic innervation of umbilical and placental vessels,[102,103] it is apparent that vascular tone is regulated by local mediators. To add to the confusion created by the large number of local mediators of placental blood flow, these mediators may affect uterine vascular tone differently from umbilical vasculature, as illustrated in Table 23.3. A general caveat concerning investigations of these mediators is that plasma concentrations reveal very little information about local physiologic responses, as these mediators are quite labile and are usually found in lower concentration in the peripheral circulation when compared to local concentration where biologic activity occurs. Additionally, physiologic actions of these mediators may work through secondary pathways, rather than direct biologic effects, making observations more difficult to interpret.

Cyclooxygenase metabolites, under normal physiologic conditions and in disease states, regulate placental blood flow. As normal gestation ensues, there is increased maternal production of prostacyclin[104,105] and thromboxane.[106] In human placental in vitro studies,

TABLE 23.3. Regulators of fetoplacental and uteroplacental blood flow.

Variable	Fetoplacental	Uteroplacental	References
Prostacyclin	↓	↓	104, 107, 108, 110, 116
Prostaglandin D_2	↓		108
Prostaglandin E_1	↑		125
	↓		108
Prostaglandin E_2	↑	↑	107, 108, 110, 125
		↓	131
Prostaglandin $F_{2\alpha}$	↑		107, 108, 110, 125
Thromboxane	↑	↑	108, 109, 114
Angiotensin II	↑	↑	93, 119, 122, 124, 125
			107, 109
Bradykinin	↑		107, 125
Leukotrienes	↑	↑	114
Serotonin	↑	↑	107, 110, 125
Norepinephrine/phenylephrine	↑	↑	110, 121, 126
Estrogen		↓	127, 128
Progesterone	↓	↓	129, 132
		↑	131
Relaxin	—	↑	129, 133, 134
Atrial natriuretic factor	↓	↓	141, 174
Nitric oxide	↓	↓	156, 158, 159, 165, 181

↑, increases blood flow; ↓ decreases blood flow; —, no affects on blood flow.

prostacyclin (PGI$_2$) is a potent vasodilator.[107,108] Conversely, thromboxane (Tx) is a potent vasoconstrictor of the human placental vasculature, estimated to be 10- to 100-fold more potent than other placental vasoconstrictors, including prostaglandin E$_2$ (PGE$_2$), prostaglandin F$_{2\alpha}$ (PGF$_{2\alpha}$), angiotensin II (Ang II), 5-hydroxytryptamine (5-HT), noradrenaline (NE), and bradykinin (BK).[107,109,110] Although the circulating concentrations of PGI$_2$ exceed Tx, the human placenta produces equal amounts of both prostacyclin and thromboxane, so that the biologic actions of them on vascular tone should be balanced.[111] Under conditions of hypoxia, however, the human placenta produces increasing amounts of vasodilating prostanoids relative to vasoconstricting prostanoids, suggesting that placental production of prostanoids may participate in the fetoplacental redistribution of blood flow accompanying hypoxia.[112]

The increased uteroplacental production of prostacyclin, as determined by measurements of PGI$_2$ metabolites in sheep, results in a 14-fold increase in PGI$_2$ during pregnancy.[104] Recent evidence, obtained by administration of the cyclooxygenase inhibitor indomethacin to the chronically instrumented sheep in late pregnancy, resulted in questioning the role that prostaglandins play in maintaining basal uteroplacental blood flow in an unstressed pregnancy.[113] Despite a rapid 100% increase in uteroplacental vascular resistance and accompanying 30% decrease in uteroplacental flow, following indomethacin administration the vascular response was transient. By 3 hours, the uteroplacental blood flow had returned to baseline, despite persistent decreases in PGE$_2$ and PGF$_{2\alpha}$ concentrations. Although the investigators concluded that basal uteroplacental blood flow is not maintained by prostaglandins, one must acknowledge the initial increase in vascular resistance observed during prostaglandin inhibition. Additionally, it is possible that other prostaglandins, not measured by the assay, were not significantly inhibited by indomethacin, and were available to regulate basal uteroplacental blood flow.

Prostanoids play an equally important role in the fetoplacental vasculature. Like maternal effects, prostacyclin is a potent vasodilator[107] and Tx a potent vasoconstrictor[109,114] of umbilical vessels. Prostacyclin production by the umbilical artery and vein exceeds production by both uterine and placental vasculature.[105] Furthermore, there is a gradient of prostacyclin production within the umbilical vessels, with increased production in that portion of the vessels closest to the fetus.[115] A similar gradient is seen with Tx production in the umbilical vein but not the umbilical artery.[115] In addition to varying production of vasoactive autocoids along the length of umbilical vessels, there is also varying vasoactive responsiveness, with prostanoids being most potent in juxtafetal segments.[109] Human umbilical artery prostacyclin and Tx production are modulated by fetal oxygen tension, with low oxygen tension preferentially increasing prostacyclin production and high oxygen tension preferentially increasing Tx production.[116] In these studies, the threshold for umbilical artery contraction to oxygen was 36 mm Hg, with maximum contraction at 282 mm Hg, far exceeding the normal in utero human umbilical artery oxygen tension of 15 mm Hg. Similar vasoconstrictive responses to increases in oxygen tension, within physiologic ranges, are not found in the umbilical vein.[117] In contrast, the fetal lamb umbilical vein constricts along the entire length of the vein in response to hypoxemia with little effect on vascular resistance of the umbilical arteries or the placenta. This increase in placental outflow resistance, during hypoxemia, results in pooling of fetal blood in the placenta, and, by increasing surface area for exchange, may permit incresed placental gas transfer.[118]

Like Tx, Ang II is a potent vasoconstrictor, with maternal concentration increasing as normal pregnancy advances.[119] Despite this increase, normal pregnancy results in an attenuated pressor response to systemic infusion of Ang II, when compared to the nonpregnant state.[120] Similar attenuated pressor responses during pregnancy are seen with α-adrenergic agonists as observed with infused phenylephrine and norepinephrine.[121] In the pregnant sheep, physiologic concentrations of infused Ang II increase uteroplacental blood flow, secondary to an increase in maternal mean arterial pressure resulting in improvement of perfusion pressure. At higher doses, however, uteroplacental blood flow decreases, secondary to increases in systemic and uterine vascular resistence.[93] Furthermore, infusion of Ang II increases systemic vascular resistance to a greater extent than uterine and placental vascular resistance, the placental vasculature being relatively refractory to the effects of Ang II.[119] Placental vascular refractoriness during pregnancy is not a universal property, as uteroplacental vascular reactivity to infused phenylephrine or norepinephrine exceeds systemic reactivity.[121] This refractoriness to Ang II during pregnancy may be the result of local increases in vasodilating prostacyclin production stimulated by Ang II.[122] Taken together, investigators speculate that uterine refractoriness to Ang II protects the fetus, maintaining uteroplacental perfusion despite the normal increases in Ang II concentration seen during pregnancy. The exaggerated uterine vasoconstrictive response to α-adrenergic agonists, on the other hand, protects the mother in the fight-or-flight response, decreasing blood flow to the placenta during maternal hypotension, in efforts to ensure survival of the mother.[121]

In the fetus, the renin-angiotensin-aldosterone system contributes to the maintenance of basal vascular tone.[123] In contrast to the blunted uterine-placental vasoconstrictive responses to Ang II, the fetus displays potent umbilical-placental vasoconstriction when Ang II is infused.[124] With respect to α-adrenergic agonists, Ang II causes a

35- to 60-fold increase in umbilical vascular resistance when compared to phenylephrine, the latter having minimal effects except at very high, nonphysiologic concentrations.[125,126] This relative refractoriness of fetoplacental vasculature to α-adrenergic agonists may be a protective mechanism aimed at maintaining umbilical blood flow despite increases in fetal plasma catecholamine concentration. Like prostacyclin, there is a gradient in Ang II production along the length of the umbilical vessels, with production greatest at the juxtaplacental regions.[109]

During pregnancy, there are marked changes in maternal steroid hormone homeostasis, particularly estrogen and progesterone. In general, estrogen dilates placental vasculature.[127] In the sheep, injection of estradiol-17β increased uterine and placental blood flow, with increases significantly greater in early versus late pregnancy.[128] In human pregnancy, Doppler investigation of the uteroplacental circulation reveals that increases in endogenous estradiol-17β concentration contributes to the decrease in uterine vascular resistance observed with advancing gestation.[129] Similarly, high levels of progesterone are maintained in the placental circulation during pregnancy.[130] Although it is generally considered that progesterone opposes estrogen vasodilatory effects in the placenta and that the two hormones working synchronously to control uteroplacental blood flow,[131] the data have been inconsistent. In precontracted human placental artery and vein, administration of exogenous progesterone has been found to cause dose-dependent relaxation, this relaxation being mediated by a receptor-activated adenosine 3′,5′-cyclic monophosphate (cAMP) mechanism.[132] These findings are supported by uteroplacental Doppler studies in which endogenous progesterone, measured in the maternal blood, was found to contribute to the decrease in uterine vascular resistance observed as pregnancy advances.[129] The investigators speculated that inconsistencies in progesterone studies may relate to the fact that synthetic hormones used in a variety of studies may have different vascular effects from endogenous maternal progesterone. Additionally, relaxin, an ovarian peptide synthesized by the corpus luteum that inhibits myometrial contraction induced by vasopressin, may also decrease uterine blood flow during early pregnancy.[129] In contrast, other investigations suggest that relaxin has minor importance in the regulation of uteroplacental circulation,[133] and does not have relaxant effects in the human umbilical artery.[134]

Atrial natriuretic factor (ANF) is a 28 amino acid peptide that is released from atrial myocytes, secondary to atrial distention, and has many renal and cardiovascular functions.[135,136] Included in ANF's function is endothelial-independent vasodilation,[137] resulting from activation of vascular smooth muscle guanylate cyclase and subsequent increase in cellular guanosine 3′,5′-cyclic monophosphate (cGMP).[138] In the human placenta, a small population of cytotrophoblast-like cells is capable of producing ANF.[139] In addition to placentally produced ANF, the fetus produces ANF, with increased release stimulated by elevations in fetal intracardiac pressure. Ventricular messenger RNA (mRNA) for ANF is extremely high in the neonate and decreases rapidly over the first 2 weeks of life.[140] The combination of placentally produced ANF, which is secreted into the fetal-placental circulation, with the ANF produced directly by the fetus, results in a fetal ANF concentration that is three times higher than the maternal concentration.[139] In addition, the placenta is permeable to ANF, as infusion of exogenous atriopeptin into the mother increases atriopeptin in both the mother and the fetus.[140] This placental permeability may further contribute to the increased ANF concentration as noted in the fetus versus the mother.[140] In the human perfused placenta model, infused ANF attenuates ANG II–induced vasoconstriction.[141,142] Some feel that this attenuation occurs only at supraphysiologic doses of ANF.[142] The human fetoplacental vasculature has membrane receptors for ANF.[141] In addition, examination of plasma membranes from placental tissue exposed to either maternal or fetal blood reveals that these receptors are present primarily in placental tissue in closest proximity to the fetal circulation. In placental tissue exposed to maternal blood, such receptors are not found.[143]

Recent investigation suggests that nitric oxide (NO) plays an important role in the regulation of fetoplacental blood flow. The realization that NO modulates vasoreactivity began in 1980, when Furchgott and Zawadzki[144] showed that acetylcholine-induced relaxation of an isolated preparation of rabbit thoracic aorta was dependent on intact endothelium. Later, it was found that this endothelium-derived relaxing factor (EDRF) had identical properties to NO.[145] It is now known that endogenous NO is produced from L-arginine[146] by nitric oxide synthase (NOS) in the endothelial cell.[147] Endogenous NO then diffuses into subjacent smooth muscle, activates guanylate cyclase,[148] with resultant increases in cGMP[149] and subsequent smooth muscle relaxation.[150] Once in the intravascular space, NO has tremendous affinity for the iron of reduced hemoglobin, forming nitrosyl-hemoglobin,[151] and is subsequently metabolized to methemoglobin.[152,153] It is this rapid conversion and inactivation of NO by intravascular hemoglobin that allows it to act locally on vascular smooth muscle.

During pregnancy, there are decreases in placental vascular resistance secondary to dilatation of uteroplacental arteries. The end result of this dilatation is enhanced maternal-fetal blood flow necessary to meet increasing fetal requirements. Although this decrease in vascular resistance was originally thought to result from the trophoblast invading and restructuring the vessel wall, recent evidence in the guinea pig suggests uteroplacental vasodilation is related to increased NOS expression, speculatively constitutive NOS (eNOS), in the periarterial trophoblast cell, followed by local release of NO and resultant dilation.[154] Furthermore, investigations in the rat reveal increased biosynthesis of NO during pregnancy.[155]

The impact of NO in pregnancy has been recently reviewed as it relates to uterine and vascular smooth muscle of the uteroplacental circulation.[156] Pharmacologic agents that generate NO intracellularly[157] result in dose-dependent vasodilation of precontracted fetoplacental vasculature.[158] In the vascular bed of the human placental villus, methylene blue–induced inhibition of guanylate cyclase increases perfusion pressure of the fetoplacental circulation,[158] suggesting that the basal release of NO modulates placental resting vascular tone. Furthermore, villous arteries from uncomplicated pregnancies constrict when NO synthesis is competitively inhibited by L-N-nitro-L-arginine methyl ester (L-NAME), supporting the concept that placental vascular endothelium synthesizes NO, which, in turn, modulates baseline vascular tone.[159] Additionally, basal release of NO in placental cotyledons is sensitive to shear stress, such that increases in flow rate or viscosity increase NO synthesis and release.[160]

Recent investigations aimed at localizing possible sites of placental NO production compared nitric oxide synthase activity in the placental tissue with the placental vascular bed. The data suggest that there is higher inducible NOS activity in the placental tissue when compared to the vascular endothelium.[161] The investigators suggest that regulation of uteroplacental blood flow is, additionally, controlled by the release of placental tissue NO. Furthermore, placental tissue may play a greater role than the uterine vascular endothelium in the production of NO. Similarly, other investigators have found an increase in calcium- and calmodulin-sensitive form of NO synthase in the syncytiotrophoblast of human placental villi.[162] They speculate that NO is released from this cell layer lining the intervillous blood space, and vasodilates the fetal arteriole in the villous core. Physiologically, such an arrangement would be adaptive, since during maternal hypoxia, decreased NO release by the syncytiotrophoblast would cause vasoconstriction of the underlying fetal arteriole. The end result would be improved matching of maternal and fetal perfusion.

Early data with perfused umbilical artery reveals varying responses to a variety of doses of acetylcholine, such that a dose-dependent dilation was not demonstrated.[163] These studies were limited, since at the time they were performed there was no knowledge of the role that endothelium played in modulating vascular responses, and accordingly, there was no mention of endothelial status or efforts to preserve it. It was later found that the endothelium of human umbilical artery and vein was capable of releasing EDRF, although EDRF-stimulated relaxation of precontracted umbilical preparations was not observed.[164] However, in later studies of the human umbilical artery, NO releasing compounds did cause dilation, but vascular relaxation was attenuated when compared to the chorionic plate artery.[165] Vascular relaxation is also attenuated with increasing gestation, as the sensitivity of human umbilical artery smooth muscle to NO decreases as gestation advances.[166] Investigators suggest that the basal release of NO maintains low vascular tone in the fetoplacental vasculature, and may contribute, to a greater extent, than vasodilatory prostanoids in this cause.[167,168] Basal and stimulated release of NO from human umbilical artery is five times and three times, respectively, greater than that of PGI_2. Furthermore, NO relaxes endothelial denuded umbilical vessels significantly more than PGI_2.[168]

Preeclampsia and Placental Blood Flow

In pregnancy complicated by preeclampsia, uteroplacental blood flow is reduced; the more severe the preeclampsia, the more reduced the flow.[100] Although preeclampsia is a disease in the mother, the fetus is also affected. In contrast to normal pregnancy, where Doppler flow velocity waveforms indicate decreases in fetoplacental flow resistance, in pregnancies complicated by hypertension there is increased fetal-placental flow resistance.[169] These alterations in hemodynamics are the result, in part, of an imbalance in prostacyclin and Tx production. The placenta from the preeclamptic human produces more than threefold as much Tx and less than half as much prostacyclin as the normal non-preeclamptic placenta, resulting in sevenfold more Tx produced than prostacyclin.[111] In addition to decreased prostacyclin production in maternal subcutaneous, uterine, and placental vessels,[170] the fetal umbilical artery also demonstrates decreased prostacyclin activity in pregnancy complicated by preeclampsia.[171]

Additionally, the placenta from pregnancy complicated by preeclampsia produces more progesterone than normal, without similar increases in estradiol production.[172] Increases in progesterone concentration, similar to an elevation seen in preeclampsia, were found to inhibit prostacyclin synthesis, without increasing Tx.[173] Additionally, in preeclampsia, low-dose infusion of ANF increases cGMP and causes uteroplacental vasodilation, with resultant increases in the uteroplacental blood flow index by 28%.[174] Similar increases in uteroplacental flow are seen when ANF is infused in a physiologic concentration into maternal guinea pigs, after experimentally induced fetal intrauterine growth retardation (IUGR). Furthermore, this increased placental blood flow was exaggerated in the IUGR versus non-IUGR pregnancy, suggesting upregulation of ANF receptors in vessels supplying these small placentas.[175]

Impairment of NO synthesis or action may be of functional significance in preeclampsia. In isolated-perfused human placental cotyledons from preeclamptic women, inhibition of NO did not significantly change resting perfusion pressure, as observed in normal pregnancy, suggesting decreased basal NO release in preeclampsia.[167] However, measurements of the amount of maternal venous nitrite and nitrate, oxidation products of NO used as an indicator of its production, reveal no significant difference in preeclamptic versus uncomplicated pregnancy. The fetoplacental circulation, however, had a higher concentration of nitrite in preeclampsia, which, the investigators speculate, may be a compensatory response aimed at improving placental blood flow.[176] One must recall that the use of NO oxidation products (e.g., nitrate and nitrite) to estimate NO production has many inaccuracies, as plasma concentrations are affected by diet, intravascular volume, and renal clearance.

Measurements of NOS expression in the placenta and umbilical vessels reveal differences in its expression in terminal villous vessels and the syncytiotrophoblast in pregnancies complicated by preeclampsia.[177] Other investigators have confirmed a lower NOS activity in placental villous homogenates from preeclamptics.[178] Whether this represents a primary vascular alteration of preeclampsia or secondary vascular damage from increases in blood pressure is not clear. Recently, investigators have observed extensive ultrastructural endothelial injury in both placental and nonplacental tissues of preeclamptic patients. This injury was to cytoplasmic organelles and possibly mitochondria, and was not correlated with the degree of hypertension.[179] Others have proposed that a circulating factor of placental origin is shed into the plasma and suppresses maternal endothelial cell proliferation.[180]

Since NO plays such an important role in both uteroplacental and fetoplacental blood flow, much recent research has been directed toward modulating NO release, in efforts to alter placental blood flow. Decreases in both uterine and umbilical artery resistance index is observed following sublingual administration of glyceryl trinitrate (GTN), a pharmacologic agent that generates intracellular NO,[157] to women at 30 weeks' gestation of an uncomplicated pregnancy.[181] Furthermore, in women whose pregnancy was complicated by preeclampsia or IUGR, and having abnormal umbilical artery velocity ratios, sublingual administration of GTN significantly decreased umbilical artery resistance.[182] Similar improvements in uterine artery blood flow are seen following intravenous administration of GTN in normal pregnancies, and in those at increased risk for developing preeclampsia.[183] In these studies, there was no alteration in maternal systemic blood pressure or heart rate associated with GTN administration. Along similar lines, in pregnancies complicated by increased uteroplacental resistance and resultant IUGR, decreases in uterine artery resistance are seen following infusion of L-arginine,[156] a substrate for the synthesis of endogenous NO.[146]

Maternal and Fetal-Placental Oxygen Flow

Fetal oxidative metabolism is unaffected by reductions in oxygen delivery as long as a critical minimum of oxygen delivery to the fetus is exceeded. In the chronic fetal sheep preparation, alterations in oxygen affinity of hemoglobin or decreases in hematocrit do not affect fetal aerobic metabolism as long as fetal oxygen delivery exceeds roughly $12\,ml\cdot min^{-1}\,kg^{-1}$; at lower values there is a decrease in aerobic metabolism resulting in an increasing metabolic acidosis.[53] Oxygen delivery to an organ equals the product of blood flow and blood O_2 content. In many respects a given decrease in hemoglobin concentration has an effect similar to that of decreasing blood flow on O_2 delivery and exchange. In the maternal circulation, decreases in hemoglobin concentration may be compensated for by increases in uteroplacental blood flow. Figure 23.11 depicts how changes in uteroplacental blood flow and O_2 flow affect placental O_2 exchange.

For the fetus, similar principles apply (Figure 23.12). The fetus has a limited ability to increase its already relatively high cardiac output and its uteroplacental blood flow. Despite a low oxygen tension under normal physiologic conditions, the fetus transports large amounts of oxygen to fetal organs. This allows the fetus to meet its metabolic needs and, at the same time, permits ductal arteriosus patency and pulmonary vascular constriction. Adaptive mechanisms facilitating fetal oxygen transport include a high cardiac output relative to body size and metabolic rate, an increased fetal hemoglobin affinity, and a balanced distribution of cardiac output between the placenta and fetus.[49] Under some conditions of fetal hypoxia[184] or asphyxia[185] hemoglobin concentration increases, presumably as a result of water movement from the vascular to the extravascular compartment.

Acid-Base Regulation in the Fetal-Placental Unit

A discussion of respiration in the fetal-placental unit would be incomplete without attention to the impact respiration has on acid-base balance. Fetomaternal acid-base regulation has been recently reviewed.[186] In general, oxidative metabolism in the mother and fetus produces carbon dioxide, which is rapidly hydrated in the presence

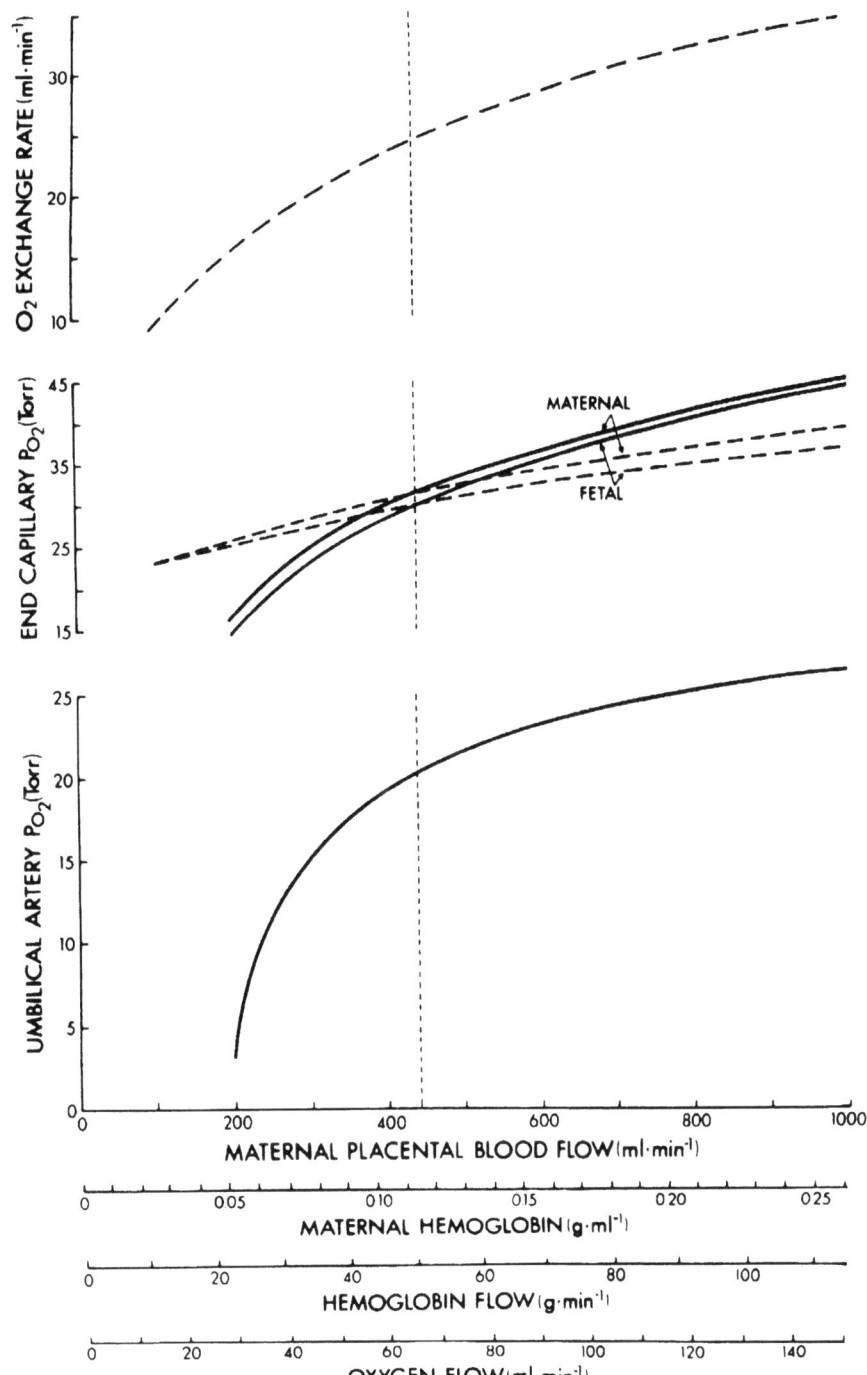

FIGURE 23.11. Calculated effects of changes in maternal-placental blood flow, hemoglobin flow, and O_2 flow on transient maternal and fetal-placental end-capillary Po_2 values and Vo_2 (dashed lines) and on steady-state end-capillary Po_2 values and fetal arterial Po_2 (solid lines).

of carbonic anhydrase to carbonic acid. The carbonic acid then dissociates to form hydrogen and bicarbonate ions, such that

$$CO_2 + H_2O \leftrightarrow H_2CO_3 \leftrightarrow H^+ + HCO_3^- \quad (6)$$

The Henderson-Hasselbach equation shows that the pH of plasma is dependent on the ratio of the concentrations of bicarbonate and carbon dioxide such that

$$pH = 6.1 + \log\left(\left[HCO_3^-/S \times P_{CO_2}\right]\right) \quad (7)$$

where S is the solubility coefficient for CO_2. Under normal physiologic conditions, the serum bicarbonate concentration exceeds that of carbon dioxide by 20-fold. Because of the concentration gradient required to transfer CO_2 across the placenta, the fetal pH is normally 0.1 unit lower than that of the mother. If unstressed, the average pH of human maternal arterial and fetal umbilical arterial blood in the second trimester is 7.373 ± 0.035 and 7.339 ± 0.03, respectively.[187] In the human fetus, pH decreases with increasing gestation.[188]

When placental transfer of oxygen is compromised, there is impaired oxidative metabolism of carbohydrate to carbon dioxide and water, resulting in the accumulation of lactic acid. Incomplete oxidation of fatty acids and

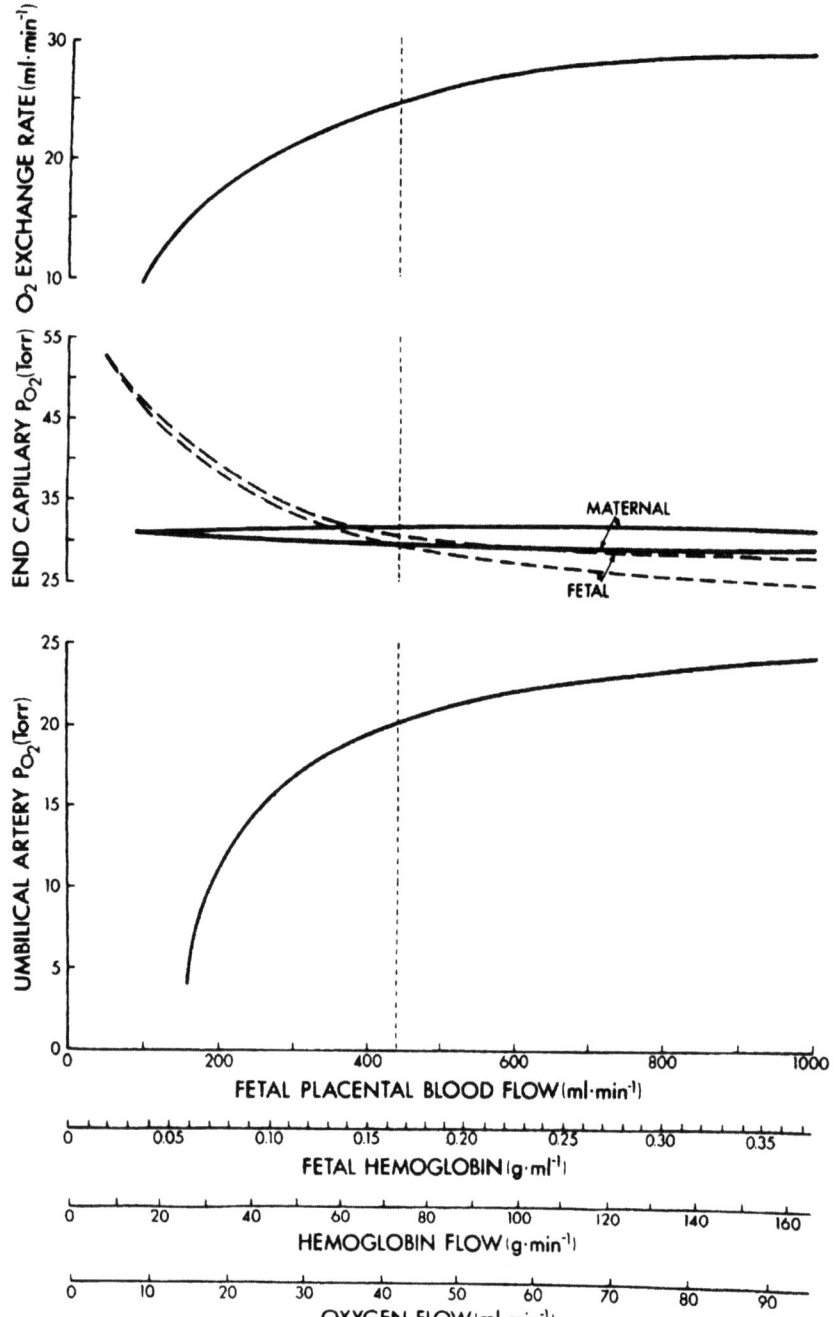

FIGURE 23.12. Calculated effects of changes in fetal-placental blood flow, hemoglobin flow, and O_2 flow on transient maternal and fetal-placental end-capillary P_{O_2} values and V_{O_2} (dashed lines) and on steady-state end-capillary P_{O_2} values and fetal arterial P_{O_2} (solid lines).

altered amino acid metabolism result in excess formation of ketoacid and uric acid, respectively. These nonvolatile acids traverse the placenta very slowly in comparison to the rapid transit of CO_2. Carbon dioxide is carried in the blood in three forms: 62% is carried in the erythrocyte as bicarbonate, 30% is carried by hemoglobin as carbamate, and the remaining 8% is dissolved.[189] The major species of CO_2 crossing the placenta is dissolved CO_2 rather than bicarbonate.[190] Furthermore, fetal bicarbonate transported to the placenta is converted by carbonic anhydrase, located outside the trophoblast, to CO_2.[191] The diffusion constant for CO_2 is approximately 20 times that of oxygen, and since it is so diffusible, its transport is mostly affected by uteroplacental and umbilicoplacental circulation,[189] in addition to anatomic and physiologic vascular shunts.[192]

The placental barriers are poorly permeable to electrically charged bicarbonate. In the sheep there is no appreciable transfer of bicarbonate across the placenta.[190] Administration of sodium bicarbonate to the pregnant sheep does not transfer to the fetus, although it does result in a reduction in uterine blood flow, fetal oxygen tension and saturation, and fetal pH.[193] During human pregnancy, induction of metabolic acidosis by ammonium chloride significantly decreased maternal plasma pH and bicarbonate, without affecting fetal plasma pH or bicarbonate.[194] This suggests that fetal plasma bicarbonate concentration can be independent of that of the mother's. However, other investigators have claimed that the conditions under which Bleacher et al.'s[194] study were performed, such as under general anesthesia during cesarean section, may alter uterine blood flow and placental function, confounding the study results. These investigators, under more physiologic conditions, suggest that bicarbonate does equilibrate across the placenta and is not solely the effects of rapid equilibration of CO_2.[195] The above conflicting conclusions regarding placental bicarbonate transfer may result from the problems encountered when studying the interrelationship between maternal and fetal acid-base balance using in vivo models.[196] These problems include difficulty in separating out placental regulation while changes in fetomaternal metabolism and umbilicouterine blood flow are occurring concurrently, in addition to ongoing equilibration steps in fetomaternal erythrocytes and plasma. To address these confounding variables, isolated placental perfusion models have been employed. Investigations using these models suggest that although an anion exchange system exists for the transport of bicarbonate,[191] it is unlikely that bicarbonate plays a major role in the transfer of CO_2 across the placenta.[190,191,196]

The first line of defense in maintaining both maternal and fetal acid-base homeostasis are buffers. Hydrogen ions are buffered intracellularly and extracellularly. Carbon dioxide produced metabolically diffuses into the erythrocyte, is hydrated by carbonic anhydrase, and the hydrogen ion produced is buffered by erythrocyte hemoglobin, bicarbonate, and inorganic phosphate. Additional buffering is provided by the extracellular carbonic acid-bicarbonate buffer system, forming volatile CO_2, which is rapidly eliminated by the placenta and eventually the maternal lung, provided adequate uterine and umbilical blood flow exists. The placenta itself may even provide a bicarbonate pool that may protect the fetus against changes in maternal pH.[196] Electrically charged nonvolatile acids move slowly across the placenta, and are excreted equally as slowly by the maternal kidney. The fetal kidney has little, if any, function in regulating acid-base balance.

Maternal respiratory changes occur in the first few weeks of pregnancy, with continuous increases in tidal volume. This results in a 60% to 70% increase in alveolar ventilation and a decrease in arterial CO_2 tension to the range of 26.4 to 33.6 torr.[197] The fetal CO_2 tension is maintained in the 35- to 40-torr range. Despite decreases in maternal CO_2, maternal pH remains normal secondary to compensatory increases in renal excretion of bicarbonate.[198] It has been postulated that the lower erythrocyte intracellular pH seen during pregnancy[199] provides continuous stimulus to the central nervous system respiratory centers and evokes hyperventilation.[199] Evidence suggests that increases in maternal progesterone during pregnancy facilitates this hyperventilation, as there is an inverse relationship between plasma progesterone and arterial CO_2 tension.[200] Additionally, in the vagotomized cat, progesterone injected directly into the respiratory area of the medulla, or given intravenously, resulted in dose-dependent stimulation of respiration. Other steroid hormones, including estradiol-17β, testosterone, and cortisol, did not elicit these respiratory effects, and, furthermore, inhibition of progesterone receptors blocked these respiratory effects.[201] This relative hyperventilation is exaggerated at increased altitude[202] and during labor, the latter being affected by such factors as pain, fear, emotional excitement, and misinterpretation of the Lamaze breathing technique, to name a few.

Since CO_2 is so diffusible across the placenta, changes in maternal CO_2 tension are rapidly mirrored in the fetus, with fetal CO_2 exceeding maternal arterial and uterine venous P_{CO_2} (Figure 23.13). In the chronically instru-

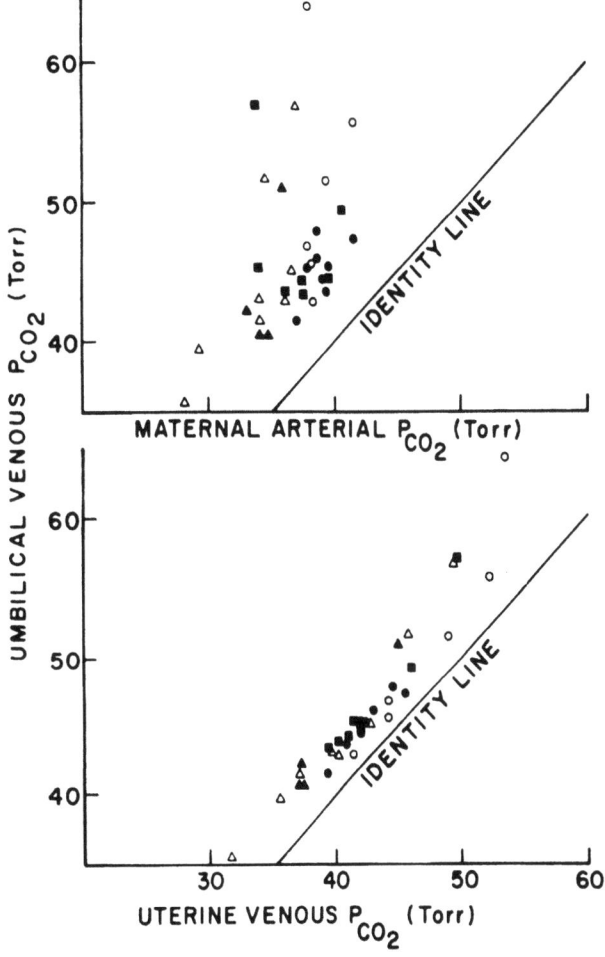

FIGURE 23.13. Plot of umbilical venous CO_2 tension (P_{CO_2}) vs maternal P_{CO_2} (upper panel) and vs uterine venous P_{CO_2} (lower panel). Note that umbilical venous P_{CO_2} is more closely related to uterine venous P_{CO_2}. Symbols represent individual measurements on five pregnant sheep, while varying uterine blood flow with a partial aortic occluder. (From Wilkening and Meschia,[2] with permission.)

mented pregnant sheep, severe maternal and fetal hypercapnia increases uterine vascular resistance, with resultant decreases in uterine blood flow. Additionally, fetal umbilical blood flow increased despite no change in umbilical vascular resistance.[203] Other investigators, however, have not found an accompanying increase in uterine or umbilical artery blood flow with increasing arterial CO_2 tension.[192]

Acute hyperventilation, although enhancing fetal CO_2 exchange by increasing the transplacental CO_2 gradient,[199] may endanger the fetus if extreme. Under normal physiologic conditions, erythrocytes from pregnant women have significantly lower intracellular pH than nonpregnant controls, which, by potentiating oxygen-hemoglobin dissociation, facilitates fetal oxygen delivery.[199] Maternal hyperventilation and associated erythrocyte intracellular alkalosis enhance maternal oxygen affinity secondary to the Bohr effect, and decreases oxygen transfer to the fetus. Additionally, hyperventilation decreases uterine blood flow, which further decreases oxygen transfer to the fetus.[204] The reduction in uterine blood flow may be related to mechanical factors surrounding hyperventilation, rather than direct effects of maternal CO_2 tension and pH on uterine blood flow.[204] The extremely hyperventilated healthy mother, having a CO_2 tension less than 17 torr, delivers a neonate with marked acidosis and delayed onset of respiration.[205] In contrast, voluntary maternal hyperventilation is not associated with marked acidosis;[205,206] however, there is mild, but statistically significant, decrease in fetal oxygen tension.[206] It must be stressed, however, that under normal physiologic conditions, carbon dioxide plays little, if any, role in the regulation of uteroplacental circulation.[203]

Although neonatal acidemia is classically defined as an umbilical artery pH of less than 7.2, pathologic acidemia, defined as that pH capable of causing neonatal morbidity and mortality, is less clearly defined and of poor predictive value.[207,208] Fetal acidosis can be categorized as respiratory and/or metabolic. Respiratory acidosis results from accumulation of fetal CO_2, and is most commonly seen in conditions associated with umbilical cord compression.[189] Metabolic acidosis results from accumulation of acid metabolites and is most commonly seen in conditions associated with fetal hypoxemia.[189] Lactate, although only one of the fixed acids accumulating during metabolic acidosis, is the major end product of anaerobic metabolism. In the full-term fetus, the most common mechanism of increased fetal lactate is decreased perfusion of the intervillous space, resulting in inadequate oxygen delivery.[209] Thus, in a depressed neonate the major source of lactate is the fetus itself.[210] Elevated fetal lactate concentrations are seen in the pregnancy complicated by a prolonged second stage of labor[211] and intrauterine growth retardation.[188] However, even under normal physiologic conditions the fetus has an elevated lactate concentration, which is secondary to increased placental production,[212] and decreased fetal gluconeogenic utilization, of the lactate substrate.[188,213] The end result, under normoxemic conditions, is a gradient of the lactate concentration, with a higher concentration in the umbilical artery and a lower concentration in the maternal arterial circulation.[187,188,210] Increases in fetal CO_2 tension[192] and metabolic decreases in fetal pH[214] do not appear to alter umbilical or uterine blood flow. Infusion of hydrochloric acid directly into fetal sheep shifted the oxygen-hemoglobin dissociation curve to the right of the maternal curve, and although increasing umbilical vein oxygen tension, there was no effect on uterine or umbilical blood flow.[214]

Maternal acidosis is categorized as respiratory and/or metabolic. Since the placenta is so permeable to CO_2, any elevations in maternal CO_2 that exceed that of the fetus result in rapid transfer of CO_2 to the fetus.[190] The fetus is better protected against maternal metabolic acidosis, such that accompanying fetal acidosis does not always occur.[194] Table 23.4 outlines some common maternal, placental, and fetal clinical conditions thought to alter fetal acid-base balance. Also included are conditions that, surprisingly, do not affect fetal acid-base balance. It must be stressed that these different conditions may work through both common and overlapping mechanisms.

Comparison of Gas Exchange in the Placenta and Lung

Sir Joseph Barcroft[240] first explored the question of how respiratory gas exchange in the placenta compares with that of the lung, estimating that the lung is "perhaps twenty times as efficient or more." Of course, the outcome of such a comparison varies depending on the function being compared. Table 23.5 and Figure 23.14 present comparative values for several measures of placental and neonatal pulmonary respiratory gas exchange and blood flow.

Despite the similar weights of these organs, 10- to 20-fold more O_2 is exchanged per minute in the lung than in the term placenta, in rough accord with the mass of the organism supplied. Although in the lung O_2 consumption by parenchymal tissue is an insignificant fraction of the total quantity exchanged, at term 20% to 50% or more of the O_2 derived from maternal blood is consumed by placental tissue before it reaches the fetus.[35] In both organs O_2 and CO_2 exchange mutually enhance one another. The placenta shows double Bohr and Haldane effects because these reactions occur in both maternal and fetal blood.

Both organs receive a generous blood supply. In the placenta 20% to 36% of flow functionally bypasses gas-exchange sites, a fraction much larger than that in the lung except in the neonate, who has a markedly uneven

TABLE 23.4. Maternal, placental, and fetal conditions and effects on fetal acid-base balance.

Variable	Fetal acid-base imbalance	References	Variable	Fetal acid-base imbalance	References
Maternal conditions			Placental conditions		
Decreased O₂ supply to fetus (cyanotic heart disease, anemia, infection, pulmonary disease, hypoventilation, increased altitude)	(+)	186, 202	Placental hypoperfusion	(+)	186
			Placental infarction/separation	(+)	186
			Labor	(+)	232
			Umbilical cord compression	(+)	186, 233
Decreased placental perfusion (hypo- and hypertension, uterine tetany, dehydration)	(+)	186	Fetal conditions		
			Prematurity	(−)	234, 215
			Birth weight	(−)	234, 215
Diabetes mellitus	(+)	186	Twins	(−)	233
Chronic renal failure	(+)	186	Breech	(+)	233
Fever	(−)	215, 216	Intrauterine growth retardation	(+)	10, 188, 235
Chorioamnionitis	(−)	215, 216	Anemia	(+)	186, 213
Glucose infusion/hyperglycemia	(−)	217	Hyperglycemia	(+)	236, 237, 238
	(+)	218, 219	Meconium		
Narcotic analgesia (uncomplicated)	(−)	220, 221	Stained amniotic fluid	(−)	233
Regional anesthesia			Below level of vocal cords	(+)	233
Uncomplicated	(−)	222, 223	Regional anesthesia (complicated by toxic serum levels)	(+)	223
Complicated by					
Maternal hypotension	(+)	223, 224	Delivery route (for same indications)	(−)	239
Prolonged labor	(+)	222	Cocaine	(−)	230
	(−)	223			
Toxic serum levels	(+)	223			
General anesthesia with prolonged induction to delivery interval	(+)	225			
Ethanol	(+)	226, 227			
	(−)	228			
Cigarette smoking	(−)	229			
Cocaine	(−)	230, 231			

(+), associated with fetal acid-base imbalance; (−) not associated with fetal acid-base imbalance.

ventilation/perfusion ratio. Although some of the placental shunt may be anatomical, probably most is physiologic, analogous to nonuniform distribution of ventilation to perfusion in the lung. Both organs have flow characterized by a sluice or waterfall phenomenon. Although the pulmonary circulation displays active and precise regulation, the regulation of maternal and fetal-placental blood flow remains poorly understood.

TABLE 23.5. Comparisons of blood flow and gas exchange in placenta and lung.

Measurement	Placenta	Lungs
CO diffusing capacity (ml·min⁻¹ torr⁻¹)	1.81	25.00
CO diffusing capacity (ml·min⁻¹ torr⁻¹ kg⁻¹ body wt)	0.60	0.42
CO diffusing capacity (ml·min⁻¹ torr⁻¹ kg⁻¹ organ wt)	3.6	42.0
O₂ diffusing capacity (L·min⁻¹torr⁻¹)	2.3	30.0
Mean alveolar-pulmonary capillary Po₂ difference (torr)		8
Mean maternal-fetal placental Po₂ difference (torr)	8	
O₂ transfer rate (ml·min⁻¹)	24	300
O₂ transfer per unit blood flow (ml·min⁻¹)	6	54
Tissue O₂ consumption and CO₂ production	Significant	Insignificant
Interaction of O₂ and CO₂	Double Bohr and double Haldane effects	Bohr and Haldane effects
Fixed acid transfer	Significant	Insignificant
Blood flow (% of cardiac output)	45	100
Distribution	Uneven maternal/fetal flow	Uneven ventilation/blood flow
Shunt (%)	20	2
Type of flow	Sluice (maternal vascular pressure surrounding fetal capillaries)	Sluice (alveolar pressure surrounding pulmonary capillaries)
Regulation	Unknown	Active and precise

From Longo,[12] adapted from Longo,[11] with permission.

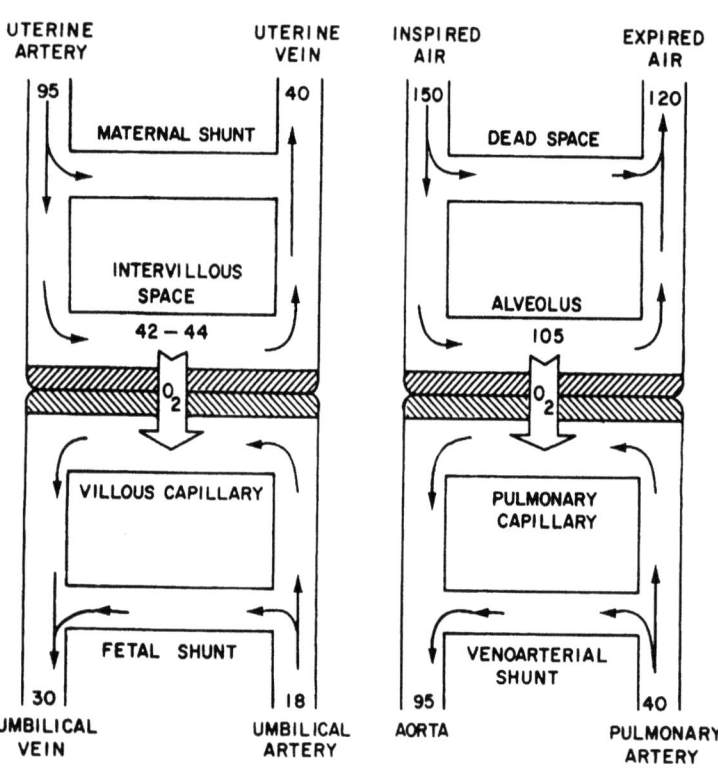

FIGURE 23.14. Analogy of placenta to lung. Oxygen pressures are shown in mm Hg. (From Nelson,[6] with permission.)

Both organs are capable of making vascular adjustment in order to optimize ventilation-perfusion matching. Analogous to hypoxic pulmonary vasoconstriction, perfused placental cotyledons respond to acute decreases in oxygen tension with fetoplacental vasoconstriction. This vasoconstriction is reversed with restoration of oxygen tension and is independent of pH and CO_2 tension.[241] Additionally, there are differences in the acute responses of the lung and placenta to vascular occlusion. In the human, complete occlusion of one pulmonary artery is accompanied by an increase in total ventilation, with, however, a decrease in ventilation of the occluded lung. This ventilatory response, coupled with an increase in perfusion of the unoccluded lung, restores oxygen uptake and arterial oxygen saturation to baseline values.[242,243] Similarly, complete occlusion of one umbilical artery in the pregnant sheep increases perfusion through the unoccluded umbilical artery with increased flux of oxygen across the unoccluded placenta. Despite these compensatory responses, baseline values are not restored, resulting in significant decreases in umbilical venous oxygen tension and saturation.[244] This illustrates a fundamental difference between the lung and the placenta, which is present not only during the duress induced by vascular occlusion, but also during conditions of rest. The lung, which does equilibrate alveolar and pulmonary end capillary oxygen tension, is designed to meet the wide fluctuations in oxygen demands set forth by the mature body, whether it be at rest or during exertion. The placenta, however, does not equilibrate maternal and fetal oxygen tension, and is more designed to accommodate only very small fluctuations in fetal oxygen demand, as fetal oxidative metabolism varies within very small boundaries.[8]

Another question concerns the relative efficiency of placenta O_2 exchange. A large exchange surface with a small barrier, as expressed by the diffusion partial pressure, is advantageous for substrate exchange. The pulmonary surface area per kilogram in an adult is $1.28 m^2$, whereas in the mature fetus the placental surface area per kilogram is 3.98 to $4.33 m^2$.[15] Despite the larger surface area for substrate exchange in the placenta, there also is a larger diffusion distance of $3.5 \mu m$ between the intervillous space and fetal capillary.[14] This exceeds the 0.5 to $0.1 \mu m$ diffusion distance separating the alveolus and pulmonary capillary.[3] In addition, uniform distribution of maternal to fetal-placental flow and a countercurrent flow pattern optimize exchange. Placental efficiency has been considered from several points of view (e.g., the magnitude of the degree of arterialization of umbilical venous blood, the maternal-fetal venous Po_2 or Pco_2 differences, the umbilical arterial-venous Po_2 difference, and the percentage of O_2 extracted from the maternal arterial blood). Until relatively recently, the placenta was believed to be optimally designed to facilitate respiratory gas exchange. We now appreciate that the vascular architecture is not arranged most efficiently, the O_2 consumption and CO_2 production occur in the regions of gas transfer, and that lack of homogeneity of several types introduce further inefficiency. Although it was previously thought that the membranes separating maternal and fetal blood were a significant barrier to diffusion, we now realize that, as in the lung, this tissue constitutes only a minor resistance to exchange.

Altitude and Placental Respiratory Gas Exchange

Despite the hypoxia associated with high altitude, many individuals live at elevations higher than 3000 m, and in the Andes permanent residents live at higher than 4600 m. Because fetal arterial oxygen tension at sea level approximates that of an adult at approximately 5000 m, one would anticipate that the Po_2 of the fetus at high altitude would be much lower than normal. Surprisingly, this is not the case, as not only does the mother and fetus adapt to this hypobaric hypoxic environment, but also there are compensatory mechanisms adapted by the placenta to ensure adequate fetal oxygen delivery. Maternal adaptations observed in pregnant women at 3100 m include hyperventilation[245] and increased hemoglobin concentration.[246] Fetal adaptations to high altitude include increases in fetal hemoglobin[247] and redistribution of blood flow to critical organs.[248] Despite a fetal cardiac output that is significantly lower than that reported at low altitude, the fetal blood flow to the heart and brain are the same in high- versus low-altitude pregnancies.[248] This redistribution of fetal blood flow maintains oxygen delivery to the fetal brain and heart, at the expense of the kidney, gastrointestinal tract, and carcass, where oxygen delivery decreased 31%, 51%, and 58%, respectively.[248] With respect to fetoplacental blood flow, umbilical artery resistance, as measured by Doppler, does not change significantly at altitudes up to 4500 feet above sea level.[249]

Examination of human placenta from both term and preterm pregnancies at high altitude reveal histologic features suggestive of placental hypoxia, including increased incidence of chorioangioma[250] and excessive formation of syncytial knots and cytotrophoblastic cells at terminal villi.[251] Morphologic changes, as classified by Vatnick et al.,[252] observed in high-altitude pregnancies include a shift from type A to predominantly type B placentomes, with additional increases in the percentage of types C and D placentomes.[253] Exposure of the materno-placento-fetal unit to high altitude results in placental adaptations to maintain fetal oxygenation during this hypobaric, hypoxic stress. These placental adaptations to high altitude are aimed at increasing morphometric diffusing capacity of the villous membranes for oxygen. Such changes observed in placentas from pregnancies at high altitude include increased[254,255] and decreased[256] volume of the fetal capillaries, dilation of the fetal capillary sinusoids,[255] increased fetal arteriole and venule branching and capillary coiling,[257] increased fetal and maternal luminal size per vessel,[257] shorter and more tightly clustered peripheral villi,[256,258] decreased total villous surface area and volume with increased intervillous space volume,[34,256,259,260] thinning of the villous membrane,[34,261,262] decreased volume of stromal tissue,[254] and arithmetic and harmonic mean thickness[254] and ratio,[263] which are decreased and increased, respectively. Placental adaptations relate to the nature of the hypoxic stress, as stereologic changes differ in the villi and intervillous space accompanying a variety of settings of hypoxic stress, as is observed in pregnancies complicated by high altitude, diabetes, preeclampsia, anemia, and cigarette smoke.[255,264]

The end result of these maternal, fetal, and placental adaptations to high altitude is best illustrated by blood gas values and intrauterine growth statistics. At altitudes of 3100 m, the neonate, before the onset of respiration, had umbilical arterial oxyhemoglobin saturations averaging 50%, as compared with 58% at 1525 m.[265] Human fetal blood gas values at elevations of 4200 m, obtained during labor by fetal scalp sampling, averaged a Po_2 of 19 torr, which is only slightly less than the sea level value of 22 torr.[266] The fetus is born with a mixed acid-base disturbance, represented by a metabolic acidosis and respiratory alkalosis. The latter correlates with the decreased maternal Pco_2 observed with maternal hyperventilation accompanying acclimatization to high altitude. There is no significant fetal pH difference observed at altitude 4200 m when compared to sea level.

In contrast to chronic exposure to high altitude, acute fetal exposure to high altitudes is not well compensated for, despite attempts to maintain uterine blood flow, redistribute fetal blood flow to vital organs, decrease fetal oxygen consumption, and utilize anaerobic metabolism.[267] This is well illustrated by animal data; sheep and goats acutely exposed to simulated altitude of 3050 m had fetal umbilical venous and arterial oxygen tensions of 15 and 11 torr, respectively.[268] Additionally, in pregnant ewes transported from approximately 1525 to 4300 m, initial umbilical venous and arterial oxyhemoglobin saturation fell from normal values of 74% and 61%, respectively, to 45% and 28%, respectively, during the first few days at the new elevation. Then, over a period of 6 to 18 days, oxyhemoglobin saturation increased to values similar to those at lower altitude.[269] Similarly, clinical concerns surrounding acute altitude affects may occur during accidental decompression of the pressurized aircraft, in an already-stressed fetus necessitating maternal air transport.[267]

The structural adaptations of the placenta to high altitude are more successful on the maternal versus the fetal side of the placenta,[33,34] although compensatory placental morphologic changes occur predominantly in the fetal tissue.[270] Despite attempts to increase total placental diffusive conductance for oxygen, the neonate shows retardation of intrauterine growth[271] and decreased birth weight[34,271,272] at high altitude. Additionally, there is an increased infant mortality rate observed at high altitude, although this occurred in the primarily preterm infant.[271]

Cocaine and Placental Respiratory Gas Exchange

There is increasing abuse of cocaine by women of childbearing age, as 15% of the total number of regular cocaine users are women 18 to 34 years old. Furthermore, in pregnancy the prevalence of cocaine use in mixed populations is between 6.3% and 17%, with increased rates in single, unemployed, low socioeconomic status blacks.[272-274] Cocaine is an alkaloid, derived from the coca plant, which blocks presynaptic reuptake of norepinephrine and dopamine. The resulting excess neurotransmitter at the postsynaptic receptor site produces vasoconstriction.[274] Although there are no characteristic placental histologic or gross structural changes induced by cocaine,[275] it alters placental permeability, with resultant reduction in placental transfer of substrate.[276] Cocaine's lipophilic composition enables its placental transfer, resulting in recently reviewed adverse fetal effects.[274,277]

In the placental circulation, cocaine is a potent vasoconstrictor. In the pregnant sheep, injected cocaine, in doses similar to those used recreationally, causes dramatic, dose-dependent vasoconstriction of uterine arteries, resulting in decreased uterine blood flow and fetal oxygen tension.[230] Residual uterine artery vasoconstriction occurred during α_1-receptor inhibition, suggesting that cocaine vasoconstricts by mechanisms in addition to α_1-adrenergic receptor stimulation.[278] Other suggested mechanisms include increased production of vasoconstricting prostaglandins $PGF_{2\alpha}$ and PGE_2[279] and placental thromboxane.[280] This increase in vasoconstrictors induced by cocaine is further compounded by a significant reduction in placental[280] and umbilical artery[281] vasodilating prostacyclin production.

Cigarette Smoke and Placental Respiratory Gas Exchange

In mothers with a smoking history during pregnancy averaging 18.6 cigarettes per day and who smoked in the range of 1 to 20 cigarettes during labor, fetal carboxyhemoglobin levels in cord blood averaged 9.2%, and are significantly correlated with the number of cigarettes smoked.[282] Furthermore, the affinity of fetal blood for carbon monoxide exceeds that for maternal blood, resulting in a transplacental concentration gradient of carboxyhemoglobin and a higher concentration in the fetal versus the maternal compartment.[282-284] This gradient is further exaggerated by the increased fetal half-life of carboxyhemoglobin, which is three times longer in fetal versus maternal blood.[282]

By displacing oxygen from hemoglobin in arterial blood, carbon monoxide decreases blood oxygen transport capacity.[284] Also, carbon monoxide shifts the oxygen dissociation curve to the left and alters its shape to a more hyperbolic form.[284,285] Furthermore, at the level of the maternal-placental exchange vessels, carbon monoxide lowers maternal oxygen tension, which results in a decreased maternal-fetal oxygen gradient, and diminished oxygen transfer to the fetus.[284] The fetus, secondary to both increased hemoglobin levels and hemoglobin F concentrations, tries to accommodate chronic elevations in carboxyhemoglobin concentration.[285] Despite these compensatory mechanisms, the fetal rhesus monkey exposed to both nicotine-containing and nicotine-free cigarette smoke displayed significant decreases in fetal oxygen tension, with the largest decreases occurring 30 minutes after discontinuation of the cigarette smoking. The investigators speculated that carboxyhemoglobin formation is responsible for the fetal hypoxia.[229] This is supported by investigations in the sheep, where there is a linear decrease in fetal oxygen tension with increases in carboxyhemoglobin concentration.[286] The pregnant woman who smokes one or two packs of cigarettes per day has an associated decrease in fetal blood oxygen tension by 2 to 4 torr for one pack and 4 to 7 torr for two.[283] With respect to oxygenation, it has been calculated that a carboxyhemoglobin level of 9% is equivalent to a 41% decrease in fetal hemoglobin concentration.[287]

Using radioisotope techniques, investigators have shown that cigarette smoke decreases placental intervillous blood flow, with reported decreases of 21% after 5 minutes of smoking. Blood flow was restored to baseline by 15 minutes after smoking ceased. The investigators suggest that sympathomimetic effects of nicotine vasoconstrict uteroplacental vasculature, and, if repeated, may compromise the fetus.[288] Others have shown acute elevations of maternal epinephrine and norepinephrine seen within 3 minutes after initiation of cigarette smoking is responsible for decreased uterine perfusion.[289] Fetal cardiovascular findings accompanying maternal cigarette smoking include transient increases in umbilical blood flow, resulting, in part, from increases in fetal heart rate and umbilical vasodilation.[290] Similarly, increased umbilical venous blood flow is observed when the pregnant, chronic smoker chews high-dose nicotine-containing gum.[291]

Histologically, structural changes are observed in the placenta of the cigarette-smoking woman. These changes in the placental villi include broadening of the basement membrane, edema, increased collagen content and stromal fibrosis, increased calcification and infarction, and decreased vascularization.[18,292,293] Furthermore, as

Fetal Surgery and Placental Respiratory Gas Exchange

In utero surgical therapy addresses life-threatening congenital fetal defects, including congenital diaphragmatic hernia, congenital cystic lung disease, obstructive uropathy, and sacrococcygeal teratoma.[294] In addition to fetal surgery, in utero surgical therapy may be performed directly on the placenta, as seen in fetoscopic laser occlusion of placental vascular communications in monozygotic monochorionic twins.[295] Postoperative preterm labor, relating to the hysterotomy necessary for fetal exposure, remains a limiting factor in human fetal surgery.[296] Recently, endoscopic surgical techniques, termed fetal endohysteroscopic intervention, have been developed to minimize the need for hysterotomy.[297]

In fetal surgery, maintaining placental integrity has been met with many challenges. First of all, fetal anesthesia necessary to produce intraoperative uterine relaxation can affect placental perfusion. In acutely instrumented fetal sheep, inhalational halothane administered during fetal surgery increased placental vascular resistance and, by shunting blood away from the placenta, significantly depressed respiratory gas exchange. Similar placental respiratory gas exchange disturbances, however, were not seen with ketamine.[298] In contrast, other investigators have found that uteroplacental and fetoplacental blood flow are not significantly affected by halothane. This study, however, was performed in the chronically instrumented fetal lamb, which did not experience surgically induced stress, which may explain conflicting data.[299] Additionally, saline volume expansion of the amniotic space, to create the "working space" required to perform fetal endohysteroscopic intervention, may reduce umbilicoplacental and uteroplacental blood flow, impairing placental gas exchange.[300,301] Expansion of the amniotic space, using gas insufflation rather than saline, may provide less alteration of placental gas exchange.[297]

For cardiac conditions in which abnormal fetal flow patterns and pressures result in neonatal anatomic hypoplasia, fetal surgical intervention may be beneficial.[302] Additionally, cardiac surgical intervention may be indicated in fetal conditions having a high rate of intrauterine demise. Human fetal conditions in which cardiac surgical intervention have been applied include critical aortic stenosis and complete heart block.[303,304] One of the many obstacles encountered in fetal cardiac surgery surrounds maintaining the fetal circulation with cardiopulmonary bypass, while accessing the intracardiac defect. In the fetal lamb, bypass circuits,[305] as illustrated in Figure 23.15,

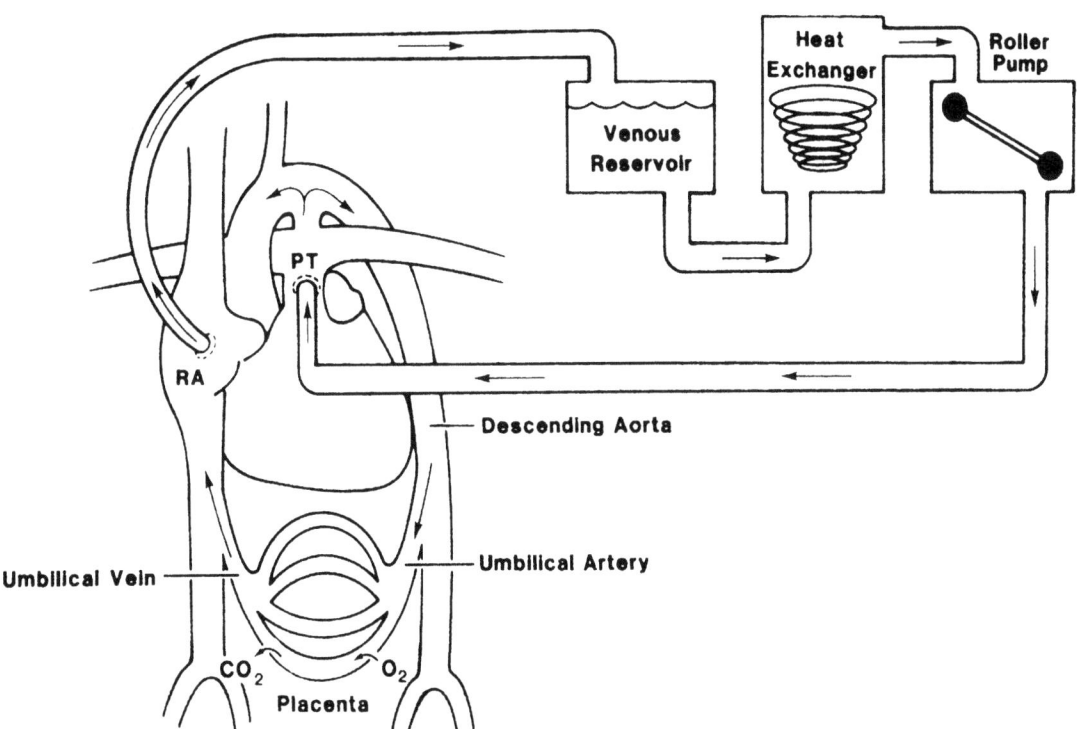

FIGURE 23.15. Extracorporeal circuit used to perform fetal cardiopulmonary bypass. The right atrium (RA) is used for venous uptake and consists of both oxygenated blood returning from the fetus mixing with oxygenated blood returning from the placenta. The blood is then returned from the pump to the fetus via the pulmonary trunk (PT), crosses the ductus arteriosus and supplies the upper body and coronary arteries by retrograde aortic arch flow, and supplies the lower body and placenta by antegrade descending aortic flow. (From Hawkins et al.,[305] with permission.)

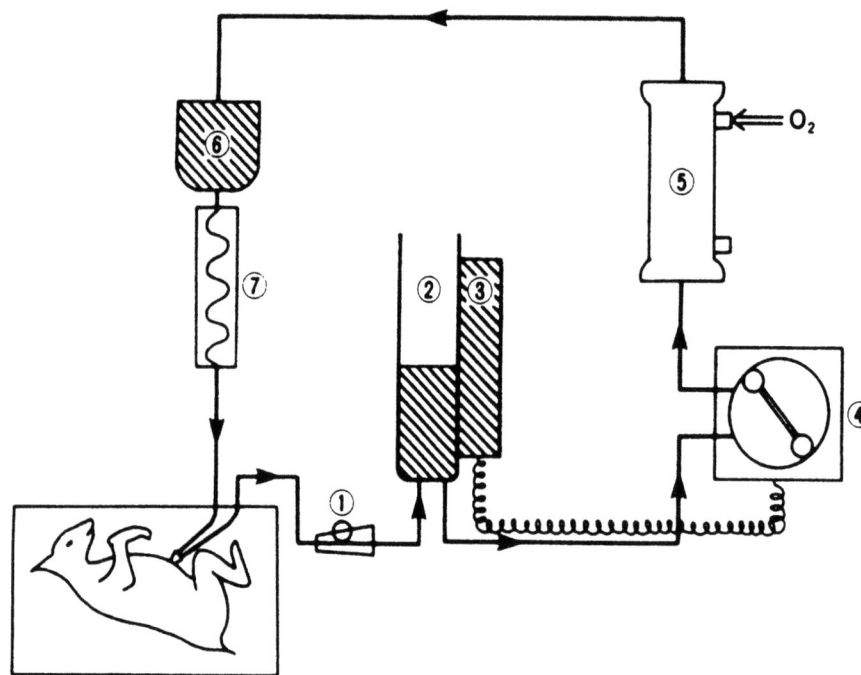

FIGURE 23.16. The extracorporeal blood circuit of the extrauterine fetal incubation system. (1) tube occluder, (2) arterial open-top reservoir, (3) flow detector-controller, (4) blood pump, (5) silicone hollow-fiber membrane oxygenator, (6) closed reservoir, (7) heat exchanger. The oxygenator had a functional surface area for gas exchange of $0.5\,m^2$. The priming volume of the circuit was approximately 230 ml, consisting of anticoagulated, whole blood from donor goats. (From Unno et al.,[314] with permission.)

in which the placenta was used as an in vivo oxygenator, result in disturbances in both placental gas exchange and acid-base balance. Although increasing flow rates of the bypass circuit, coupled with alleviating adverse effects of hypothermia on placental function, improved placental function during the surgical procedure, placental dysfunction again worsened when the fetus was weaned off bypass.[305,306] It has been estimated, using a sheep model, that following bypass, placental blood flow is decreased by 70%.[307] Recent investigations suggest that indomethacin or high-dose steroid administration during fetal cardiac bypass prevents associated increased placental vascular resistance and preserves placental blood flow during and after bypass.[308] Additionally, nitroprusside administration after bypass can partially prevent the observed redistribution of blood flow away from the placenta following bypass, but restoration of placental blood flow is transient.[307] Exclusion of the placenta from the bypass circuit, by using an intact membrane oxygenator to maintain fetal gas exchange, may also improve placental perfusion and function following bypass.[309]

Development of an Artificial Placenta

As our knowledge base of respiration in the fetal-placental unit grows, with concurrent sweeping changes in modern technology, the concept of long-term extrauterine maintenance of fetal life seems more realistic. This is not, however, a new concept since Callaghan et al.[310] in 1963 artificially oxygenated and perfused fetal lambs submerged in artificial amniotic fluid. In 1969, Zapol et al.[311] maintained a fetal lamb at 125 days gestation (term is 147 days), using a silicon membrane oxygenator, nutritional support, and a thermoregulated bath of synthetic amniotic fluid. Four of the eight fetuses survived for periods greater than 20 hours, with two long-term lambs surviving after receiving 4 to 10 hours of extrauterine support. In the exteriorized goat fetus, improved mechanics of fetal catheterization, adding a dialyzing system to the extracorporeal membrane oxygenation (ECMO) circuit to prevent fetal water retention, better control of activated clotting time, and improved regulation of circuit blood flow all contributed to longer survival. The investigators reported survival of exteriorized goat fetuses for up to 10 days, with fetal conditions maintained in the normal physiologic range for most of the course.[312] Recent studies in the exteriorized goat fetus, as illustrated in Figure 23.16, have reported blood gas exchange, oxygen utilization, and cardiovascular function to be within the normal fetal range throughout most of the maintenance of extrauterine fetal life, and have supported fetuses for up to 542 hours.[313,314]

The concept of an artificial placenta has direct applicability to the premature neonate, as incubation in a fluid environment is more physiologic than incubation in air.[314] Similar techniques have been used to maintain exteriorized human previable fetuses, with smaller (300 g) and larger (980 g) fetuses surviving up to 90 minutes and just over 5 hours, respectively.[315,316] There needs to be resolution of problems related to water and nutritional balance, as well as organ maturation before use in the human can be considered.

References

1. Meschia G. Supply the oxygen to the fetus. J Reprod Med 1979;23:160–165.
2. Wilkening RB, Meschia G. Fetal oxygen uptake, oxygenation, and acid-base balance as a function of uterine blood flow. Am J Physiol 1983;244:749–755.
3. Dawes GS. Foetal and neonatal physiology. A comparative study of the changes at birth. Chicago: Year Book, 1968:185.
3a. Strauss L, Goldenberg N, Hirota K, et al. Structure of the human placenta: with observations on ultrastructure of the terminal chorionic villus. Birth Defects Original Article Series 1965;1:13–26.
4. Metcalfe J, Bartels H, Moll W. Gas exchange in pregnant uterus. Physiol Rev 1967;47:782–838.
5. Bartels H, Moll W. Passage of inert substances and oxygen in the human placenta. Pflugers Arch 1964;280:165–177.
6. Nelson NM. Respiration and circulation before birth. In: Smith CA, Nelson NM, eds. The physiology of the newborn infant. Springfield, IL: Charles C. Thomas, 1976:15–116.
7. Meschia G. Physiology of transplacental diffusion. Obstet Gynecol Ann 1976;5:21–38.
8. Wilkening RB, Meschia G. Comparative physiology of placental oxygen transport. Placenta 1992;13:1–15.
9. Wallenburg HCS, van Kreel BK. Placental and nonplacental drainage of the uterus in the pregnant rhesus monkey. Eur J Obstet Gynecol Reprod Biol 1977;7:79–84.
10. Pardi G, Cetin I, Marconi AM, et al. Venous drainage of the human uterus: respiratory gas studies in normal and fetal growth retarded pregnancies. Am J Obstet Gynecol 1992;166:699–706.
11. Longo LD, Hill EP, Power GG. Theoretical analysis of factors effecting placental O_2 transfer. Am J Physiol 1972;222:730–739.
12. Longo LD. Respiratory gas exchange in the placenta. In: Fishman AP, Farhi LE, Tenney SM, eds. Handbook of physiology, sec. 3. The respiratory system, vol. IV. Gas exchange. Washington, DC: American Physiological Society, 1987:351–401.
13. Harding R, Sigger JN, Wickham PJD. Fetal and maternal influences on arterial oxygen levels in sheep fetus. J Dev Physiol 1983;5:267–276.
14. Aherne W, Dunnill MS. Quantitative aspects of placental structure. J Pathol Bacteriol 1966;91:123–139.
15. Clavero JA, Botella Llusia J. Measurement of the villus surface in normal and pathologic placentas. Am J Obstet Gynecol 1963;86:234–240.
16. Blickstein I, Ron A. Can placental surface area and neonatal weight be predicted from placental surface measurements? Gynecol Obstet Invest 1995;40:253–256.
17. Scheffen I, Kaufmann P, Phillippens L, et al. Alterations of the fetal capillary bed in the guinea pig placenta following long-term hypoxia. In: Piiper J, ed. Oxygen transport to tissue, vol. 12. New York: Plenum Press, 1990:779–790.
18. Naeye RL. Effects of maternal cigarette smoking on the fetus and placenta. Br J Obstet Gynaecol 1978;85:732–737.
19. Salafia CM, Pezzullo JC, Lopez-Zeno JA, et al. Placental pathologic features of preterm preeclampsia. Am J Obstet Gynecol 1995;173:1097–1105.
20. Stevens-Simon C, Metlay LA, McAnarney ER. Maternal prepregnant weight and weight gain: relationship to placental microstructure and morphometric oxygen diffusion capacity. Am J Perinatol 1995;12:407–412.
21. Bjork O, Persson B. Villous structure in different parts of the cotyledon in placentas of insulin-dependent diabetic women: a morphometric study. Acta Obstet Gynecol Scand 1984;63:37–43.
22. Stoz F, Schuhmann RA, Schultz R. Morphohistometric investigations of placentas of diabetic patients in correlation to the metabolic adjustment of the disease. J Perinat Med 1988;16:211–216.
23. Stoz F, Schuhmann RA, Haas B. Morphohistometric investigations in placentas of gestational diabetes. J Perinat Med 1988;16:205–209.
24. Salafia CM, Minior VK, Lopez-Zeno JA, et al. Relationship between placental histologic features and umbilical cord blood gases in preterm gestations. Am J Obstet Gynecol 1995;173:1058–1064.
25. Fox J. Pathology of the placenta in maternal diabetes mellitus. Obstet Gynecol 1969;34:792–798.
26. Okudaira Y, Hirota K, Cohen S, et al. Ultrastructure of the human placenta in maternal diabetes mellitus. Lab Invest 1966;15:910–926.
27. Mayhew TM, Sorensen FB, Klebe JG, et al. Oxygen diffusive conductance in placentae from control and diabetic women. Diabetologia 1993;36:955–960.
28. Longo LD, Power GG, Forster RE II. Respiratory function of the placenta as determined with carbon monoxide in sheep and dogs. J Clin Invest 1967;46:812–828.
29. Mayhew TM, Joy CF, Haas JD. Structure-function correlation in the human placenta: the morphometric diffusing capacity for oxygen at full term. J Anat 1984;139:691–708.
30. Mayhew TM, Jackson MR, Haas JD. Microscopical morphology of the human placenta and its effects on oxygen diffusion: a morphometric model. Placenta 1986;7:121–131.
31. Longo LD, Power GG, Forster RE II. Placental diffusing capacity for carbon monoxide at varying partial pressures of oxygen. J Appl Physiol 1969;26:360–370.
32. Jauniaux E, Burton GJ. The effect of smoking in pregnancy on early placental morphology. Obstet Gynecol 1992;79:645–648.
33. Mayhew TM. Scaling placental oxygen diffusion to birth weight: studies on placentae from low- and high-altitude pregnancies. J Anat 1991;175:187–194.
34. Mayhew TM, Jackson MR, Haas JD. Oxygen diffusive conductances of human placentae from term pregnancies at low and high altitudes. Placenta 1990;11:493–503.
35. Meschia G, Battaglia FC, Hay WW Jr, et al. Utilization of substrates by the bovine placenta in vivo. Fed Proc 1980;39:245–249.

36. Longo LD, Power GG. Analysis of PO_2 and PCO_2 differences between maternal and fetal blood in the placenta. J Appl Physiol 1969;26:48–55.
37. Power GG, Longo LD, Wagner HN Jr, et al. Uneven distribution of maternal and fetal placental blood flow, as demonstrated using macroaggregates, and its response to hypoxia. J Clin Invest 1967;46:2053–2063.
38. Power GG, Hill EP, Longo LD. Analysis of uneven distribution of diffusing capacity and blood flow in the placenta. Am J Physiol 1972;222:740–746.
39. Bissonnette JM, Longo LD, Novy MJ, et al. Placental diffusing capacity and its relation to fetal growth. J Dev Physiol 1979;1:351–359.
40. Bissonnette JM, Wickham WK. Placental diffusing capacity for carbon monoxide in unanesthetized guinea pigs. Respir Physiol 1977;31:161–168.
41. Gilbert RD, Cummings LA, Jachau MR, et al. Placental diffusing capacity and fetal development in exercising or hypoxic guinea pigs. J Appl Physiol 1979;46:828–834.
42. Longo LD, Ching K. Placental diffusing capacity for carbon monoxide and oxygen in unanesthetized sheep. J Appl Physiol 1977;43:885–893.
43. Bacon BJ, Gilbert RD, Kaufmann P, et al. Placental anatomy and diffusing capacity in guinea pigs following long-term maternal hypoxia. Placenta 1984;5:465–488.
44. Nelson PS, Gilbert RD, Longo LD. Fetal growth and placental diffusing capacity in guinea pigs following long-term maternal exercise. J Dev Physiol 1983;5:1–10.
45. Smith AD, Gilbert RD, Lammers RJ, et al. Placental exchange area in pigs following long-term maternal exercise: a stereological analysis. J Dev Physiol 1983;5:11–21.
46. Power GG, Jenkins F. Factors affecting O_2 transfer in the sheep and rabbit placenta perfused in situ. Am J Physiol 1975;229:1147–1153.
47. Lorijn RHW, Longo LD. Norepinephrine elevation in the fetal lamb: oxygen consumption and cardiac output. Am J Physiol 1980;239:R115–R122.
48. Wilkening RB, Boyle DW, Meschia G. Fetal neuromuscular blockade: effect on oxygen demand and placenta transport. Am J Physiol 1989;257:H734–H738.
49. Battaglia FC, Meschia G. An introduction to fetal physiology. New York: Academic Press, 1986.
50. Power GG, Dale PS, Nelson PS. Distribution of maternal and fetal blood flow within cotyledons of the sheep placenta. Am J Physiol 1981;241:H486–H496.
51. Allen DW, Wyman J Jr, Smith CH. The oxygen equilibrium of fetal and adult hemoglobin. J Biol Chem 1953;203:81–87.
52. Wimberley PD. Fetal hemoglobin, 2,3-diphosphoglycerate and oxygen transport in newborn premature infants (thesis). Scand J Cin Lab Invest 1982;suppl 160:1–149.
53. Edelstone DI, Darby MJ, Bass K, et al. Effects of reductions in hemoglobin-oxygen affinity and hematocrit level on oxygen consumption and acid-base state in fetal lambs. Am J Obstet Gynecol 1989;160:820–828.
54. Bard H. Postnatal decline of hemoglobin F synthesis in normal infants. J Clin Invest 1975;55:395–398.
55. Bard H. Postnatal fetal and adult hemoglobin synthesis in early preterm newborn infants. J Clin Invest 1973;52:1789–1795.
56. Bonds Dr, Cheek TG, Crosby LO, et al. Term human fetal umbilical vein oxygen content, placental weight and maternal blood pressure. J Perinatol 1987;7:114–117.
57. Bard H. The effect of placental insufficiency on fetal and adult hemoglobin synthesis. Am J Obstet Gynecol 1974;120:67–72.
58. Thilaganathan B, Salvesen DR, Abbas A, et al. Fetal plasma erythropoietin concentration in red blood cell: isoimmunized pregnancies. Am J Obstet Gynecol 1992;167:1292–1297.
59. Jouppila P, Kirkinen P. Umbilical vein blood flow in the human fetus in cases of maternal and fetal anemia and uterine bleeding. Ultrasound Med Biol 1984;10:365–370.
60. Gollin YG, Copel JA. Management of the Rh-sensitized mother. Clin Perinatol 1995;22:545–559.
61. Kwan E, Rurak DW, Taylor SM. Oxygen consumption, acid-base status and behavior during and after acute, severe hemorrhage in fetal lambs. Am J Physiol 1995;269:R758–R766.
62. Fumia FD, Edelstone DI, Holzman IR. Blood flow and oxygen delivery to fetal organs as functions of fetal hematocrit. Am J Obstet Gynecol 1984;150:274–282.
63. Itskovitz J, Goetzman BW, Roman C, et al. Effects of fetal-maternal exchange transfusion and fetal oxygenation and blood flow distribution. Am J Physiol 1984;247:H655–H660.
64. Arnone A. X-ray diffraction study of binding of 2,3-diphosphoglycerate to human deoxyhaemoglobin. Nature 1972;237:146–149.
65. Duhm J. Effects of 2-3-diphosphoglycerate and other organic phosphate compounds on oxygen affinity and intracellular pH of human erythrocytes. Pflugers Arch 1971;326:341–356.
66. Bellingham AJ, Detter JC, Lenfant C. The role of hemoglobin affinity for oxygen and red cell 2,3-diphosphoglycerate in the management of diabetic ketoacidosis. Trans Assoc Am Physicians 1970;83:113–120.
67. Madsen H, Ditzel J. Red cell 2,3-diphosphoglycerate and hemoglobin oxygen affinity during normal pregnancy. Acta Obstet Gynecol Scand 1984;63:399–402.
68. Longo LD, Hardesty JS. Maternal blood volume: measurement, hypothesis of control, and clinical considerations. Rev Perinatol Med 1984;5:35–59.
69. Pritchard JA, Hunt CF. A comparison of the hematologic responses following the routine prenatal administration of intramuscular and oral iron. Surg Gynecol Obstet 1958;106:516–518.
70. Oski FA. Hematological problems. In Avery GB, ed. Neonatology, pathophysiology and management of the newborn. Philadelphia: Lippincott, 1975:379–422.
71. Crowe C, Dandekar P, Fox M, et al. The effects of anaemia on heart, placenta and body weight, and blood pressure in fetal and neonatal rats. J Physiol 1995;515–519.
72. Moore WMO, Battaglia FC, Hellegers AE. Whole blood oxygen affinities of women with various hemoglobinopathies. Am J Obstet Gynecol 1967;97:63–66.

73. Wilkening RB, Molina RD, Meschia G. Placental oxygen transport in sheep with different hemoglobin types. Am J Physiol 1988;254:R585–R589.
74. Hebbel RP, Berger EM, Eaton JW. Effect of increased maternal hemoglobin oxygen affinity on fetal growth in the rat. Blood 1980;55:969–974.
75. Bartels H. Prenatal respiration. Amsterdam: North Holland, 1970.
76. Hill EP, Power GG, Longo LD. A mathematical model of carbon dioxide transfer in the placenta and its interaction with oxygen. Am J Physiol 1973;224:283–299.
77. Crino JP, Harris AP, Parisi VM, et al. Effect of rapid intravenous crystalloid infusion on uteroplacental blood flow and placental implantation-site oxygen delivery in the pregnant ewe. Am J Obstet Gynecol 1993;168:1603–1609.
78. Assali NS, Douglas RA Jr, Baird WW, et al. Measurements of uterine blood flow and uterine metabolism. IV. Results in normal pregnancy. Am J Obstet Gynecol 1953;66:248–253.
79. Metcalfe J, Romney SL, Ramsey LH, et al. Estimation of uterine blood flow in normal human pregnancy at term. J Clin Invest 1955;34:1632–1638.
80. Parer JT, de Lannoy CW, Hoversland AS, et al. Effect of decreased uterine blood flow on uterine oxygen consumption in pregnant macaques. Am J Obstet Gynecol 1968;100:813–820.
81. Fuller EO, Manning MW, Nutter DO, et al. A perfused uterine preparation for the study of uterine and fetal physiology. In: Longo LD, Reneau DD, eds. Fetal and newborn cardiovascular physiology, vol. 2, Fetal and newborn circulation. New York: Garland, 1978:421–435.
82. Ehrenkranz RA, Walker AM, Oakes GK, et al. Effect of ritodrine infusion on uterine and umbilical blood flow. Am J Obstet Gynecol 1976;126:343–349.
83. Lucas WT, Kirschbaum T, Assali NS. Spinal shock and fetal oxygenation. Am J Obstet Gynecol 1965;93:583–587.
84. Hooper SB, Walker DW, Harding R. Oxygen, glucose, and lactate uptake by fetus and placenta during prolonged hypoxemia. Am J Physiol 1995;268:R303–R309.
85. Longo LD, Dale PS, Gilbert RD. Uteroplacental O_2 uptake: continuous measurements during uterine quiescence and contractions. Am J Physiol 1986;250:R1099–R1107.
86. Clapp JF III. The relationship between blood flow and oxygen uptake in the uterine and umbilical circulations. Am J Obstet Gynecol 1978;132:410–413.
87. Dawes GS, Mott JC. Changes in O_2 distribution and consumption in foetal lambs with variations in umbilical blood flow. J Physiol (Lond) 1964;170:524–540.
88. Wilkening RB, Meschia G. Effect of umbilical blood flow on transplacental diffusion of ethanol and oxygen. Am J Physiol 1989;256:H813–H820.
89. Power GG, Longo LD. Sluice flow in placenta: maternal vascular pressure effects on fetal circulation. Am J Physiol 1973;225:1490–1496.
90. Cottle MKW, Van Petten GR, Van Muyden P. Depression of uterine blood flow in response to cord compression in sheep. Can J Physiol Pharmacol 1982;60:825–829.
91. Hasaart THM, De Haan J. Depression of uterine blood flow during total umbilical cord occlusion in sheep. Eur J Obstet Gynecol Reprod Biol 1985;19:125–131.
92. Rosenfeld CR. Distribution of cardiac output in ovine pregnancy. Am J Physiol 1977;232:H231–H235.
93. Rosenfeld CR. Consideration of the uteroplacental circulation in intrauterine growth. Semin Perinatol 1984;8:42–51.
94. Rosenfeld CR, Morriss FH Jr, Makowski EL. Circulatory changes in the reproductive tissue of ewes during pregnancy. Gynecol Invest 1974;5:252–268.
95. Wilkening RB, Anderson S, Martensson L. Placental transfer as a function of uterine blood flow. Am J Physiol 1982;242:H429–H436.
96. Power GG, Longo LD. Graphical analysis of maternal and fetal exchange of O_2 and CO_2. J Appl Physiol 1969;26:38–47.
97. Nylund L, Lunell N-O, Lewander R, et al. Uteroplacental blood flow in a diabetic pregnancy: measurements with indium 113m and a computer-linked gamma camera. Am J Obstet Gynecol 1982;144:298–302.
98. Kaar K, Jouppilka P, Kuikka J, et al. Intervillous blood flow in normal and complicated late pregnancy measured by means of an intravenous ^{133}Xe method. Acta Obstet Gynecol Scand 1980;59:7–10.
99. Blechner JN, Stenger VG, Prystowsky H. Blood flow to the human uterus during maternal metabolic acidosis. Am J Obstet Gynecol 1975;121:789–794.
100. Lunell NO, Nylund LE, Lewander R, et al. Uteroplacental blood flow in preeclampsia. Measurements with indium-113m and a computer-linked gamma camera. J Exp Clin Hypertens 1982;B1:105–117.
101. Rauramo I, Forss M, Kariniemi V, et al. Antepartum fetal heart rate variability and intervillous placental blood flow in association with smoking. Am J Obstet Gynecol 1983;147:967–969.
102. Reilly FD, Russe PT. Neurohistochemical evidence supporting an absence of adrenergic and cholinergic innervation in the human placenta and umbilical cord. Anat Rec 1977;188:277–286.
103. Spivak M. The anatomic peculiarities of the human umbilical cord and their clinical significance. Am J Obstet 1946;52:387–401.
104. Magness RR, Mitchell MD, Rosenfeld CR. Uteroplacental production of eicosanoids in ovine pregnancy. Prostaglandins 1990;39:75–88.
105. Kawano M, Mori N. Prostacyclin producing activity of human umbilical, placental and uterine vessels. Prostaglandins 1983;26:645–662.
106. Ylikorkala O, Viinikka L. Thromboxane A_2 in pregnancy and puerperium. Br Med J 1980;281:1601–1602.
107. Mak KK-W, Gude NM, Walters WAW, Boura ALA. Effects of vasoactive autocoids in the human umbilical-fetal placental vasculature. Br J Obstet Gynaecol 1984;91:99–106.
108. Glance DG, Elder MG, Myatt L. The actions of prostaglandins and their interactions with angiotensin II in the isolated perfused human placental cotyledon. Br J Obstet Gynaecol 1986;93:488–494.

109. Bjoro K, Stray-Pedersen S. Effects of vasoactive autocoids on different segments of human umbilicoplacental vessels. Gynecol Obstet Invest 1986;22:1–6.
110. Maigaard S, Forman A, Anderson KE. Relaxant and contractile effects of some amines and prostanoids in myometrial and vascular smooth muscle within the human uteroplacental unit. Acta Physiol Scand 1986;128:33–40.
111. Walsh SW. Preeclampsia: an imbalance in placental prostacyclin and thromboxane production. Am J Obstet Gynecol 1985;152:335–340.
112. Ekblad U, Erkkola R, Uotila P. Effect of hypoxia on the release of prostaglandin, prostacyclin and thromboxane in perfused human placenta. Contrib Gynec Obstet 1985;13:173.
113. Naden RP, Iliya CA, Arant BS Jr, et al. Hemodynamic effects of indomethacin in chronically instrumented pregnant sheep. Am J Obstet Gynecol 1985;151:484–493.
114. Thorp JA, Walsh SW, Brath PC. Comparison of the vasoactive effects of leukotrienes with thromboxane mimic in the perfused human placenta. Am J Obstet Gynecol 1988;159:1376–1380.
115. Benedetto C, Barbero M, Rey L, et al. Production of prostacyclin, 6-keto PGF_1, alpha and thromboxane B_2 by human umbilical vessels increases from the placenta towards the fetus. Br J Obstet Gynaecol 1987;94:1165–1169.
116. Bjoro K, Haugen G, Stray-Pedersen S. Altered prostanoid formation in human umbilical vasculature in response to variations in oxygen tension. Prostaglandins 1987;34:377–384.
117. McGrath JC, MacLennan SJ, Cameron-Mann A, et al. Contraction of human umbilical artery, but not vein, by oxygen. J Physiol 1986;380:513–519.
118. Paulick RP, Meyers RL, Rudolph CD, et al. Venous responses to hypoxemia in the fetal lamb. J Dev Physiol 1990;14:81–88.
119. Rosenfeld CR, Naden RP. Responses of uterine and nonuterine tissues to angiotensin II in ovine pregnancy. Am J Physiol 1989;257:H17–H24.
120. Chesley LC, Talledo E, Bohler CS, et al. Vascular reactivity to angiotensin II and norepinephrine in pregnant and nonpregnant women. Am J Obstet Gynecol 1965;91:837–842.
121. Magness RR, Rosenfeld CR. Systemic and uterine responses to alpha adrenergic stimulation in pregnant and nonpregnant ewes. Am J Obstet Gynecol 1986;155:897–904.
122. Magness RR, Osei-Boaten K, Mitchell MD, Rosenfeld CR. In vitro prostacyclin production by ovine uterine and systemic arteries: effects of angiotensin II. J Clin Invest 1985;76:2206–2212.
123. Taylor GM, Peart WS, Porter KA, et al. Concentration and molecular forms of active and inactive renin in human fetal kidney, amniotic fluid and adrenal gland: evidence for renin-angiotensin system hyperactivity in 2nd trimester of pregnancy. J Hypertens 1986;4:121–129.
124. Iwamoto HS, Rudolph AM. Effects of angiotensin II on the blood flow and its distribution in fetal lambs. Circ Res 1981;48:183–189.
125. Berman W Jr, Goodlin RC, Heyman MA, et al. Effects of pharmacologic agents on umbilical blood flow in fetal lambs in utero. Biol Neonate 1978;33:225–235.
126. Yoshimura T, Magness RR, Rosenfeld CR. Angiotensin II and alpha agonist. I. Responses of ovine fetoplacental vasculature. Am J Physiol 1990;259:H464–H472.
127. Magness RR, Rosenfeld CR. Local and systemic estradiol-12β: effects on uterine and systemic vasodilation. Am J Physiol 1989;256:E536–E542.
128. Rosenfeld CR, Morriss FH Jr, Battaglia FC, et al. Effect of estradiol-17 beta on blood flow to reproductive and non-reproductive tissues in pregnant ewes. Am J Obstet Gynecol 1976;124:618–629.
129. Jauniaux E, Johnson MR, Jurkovic D, et al. The role of relaxin in the development of the uteroplacental circulation in early pregnancy. Obstet Gynecol 1994;84:338–342.
130. Scommegna A, Baard L, Bienarz J. Progesterone and pregnenolone sulfate in pregnancy plasma. Am J Obstet Gynecol 1972;113:60–65.
131. Rosenfeld CR. Regulation of the placental circulation. In: Polin RA, Fox WW, eds. Fetal and neonatal physiology. Philadelphia: WB Saunders, 1992:56–62.
132. Omar HA, Ramirez R, Gibson M. Properties of a progesterone-induced relaxation in human placental arteries and veins. J Clin Endocrinol Metab 1995;80:370–373.
133. Petersen LK, Svane D, Uldbjerg N, et al. Effects of human relaxin on isolated rat and human myometrium and uteroplacental arteries. Obstet Gynecol 1991;78:757–762.
134. Dombrowski MP, Savoy-Moore RT, Schwartz K, et al. Effect of porcine relaxin on the human umbilical artery. J Reprod Med 1986;31:467–472.
135. Goetz KL. Physiology and pathophysiology of atrial peptides. Am J Physiol 1988;254:E1–E15.
136. Cogan MG. Renal effects of atrial natriuretic factor. Annu Rev Physiol 1990;52:699–708.
137. Garcia R, Thibault G, Nutt RF, et al. Comparative vasoactive effects of inactive and synthetic atrial natriuretic factor. Biochem Biophys Res Commun 1984;119:685–688.
138. Winquist RJ, Faison EP, Waldman SA. Atrial natriuretic factor elicits endothelium-independent relaxation and activates particulate guanylate cyclase in vascular smooth muscle. Proc Natl Acad Sci USA 1984;81:7661–7664.
139. Lim AT, Gude NM. Atrial natriuretic factor production by the human placenta. J Clin Endocrinol Metab 1995;80:3091–3093.
140. Wei Y, Rodi CP, Day ML, et al. Developmental changes in the rat atriopeptin hormone system. J Clin Invest 1987;79:1325–1329.
141. McQueen J, Jardine A, Kingdom J, et al. Interaction of angiotensin II and atrial natriuretic peptide in the human fetoplacental unit. Am J Hypertens 1990;3:641–644.
142. Markenson GR, Foley K, Maslow AS, et al. The effects of atrial natriuretic factor and angiotensin II on fetal-placental perfusion pressure in the ex vivo cotyledon model. Am J Obstet Gynecol 1995;173:1143–1147.
143. Hatjis CG, Grogan BA. Atrial natriuretic peptide receptors in normal human placentas. Am J Obstet Gynecol 1988;159:587–591.

144. Furchgott RF, Zawadzki JV. The obligatory role of endothelial cells in the relaxation of arterial smooth muscle by acetylcholine. Nature 1980;288:373–376.
145. Palmer RMJ, Ferrige AG, Moncada S. Nitric oxide release accounts for the biological activity of endothelium-derived relaxing factor. Nature 1987;327:524–526.
146. Palmer RM, Ashton DS, Moncada S. Vascular endothelial cells synthesize nitric oxide from L-arginine. Nature 1988;333:664–666.
147. Pollock JS, Forstermann U, Mitchell JA, et al. Purification and characterization of particulate endothelium-derived relaxing factor synthase from cultured and native bovine aortic endothelial cells. Proc Nat Acad Sci USA 1991;88:10480–10484.
148. Ignarro LJ, Harbinson GR, Wood KS, et al. Activation of purified soluble guanylate cyclase by endothelium-derived relaxing factor from intrapulmonary artery and vein: stimulation by acetylcholine, bradykinin, and arachidonic acid. J Pharmacol Exp Ther 1986;237:893–900.
149. Ignarro LJ, Burke TM, Wood KS, et al. Association between cyclic GMP accumulation and acetylcholine-elicited relaxation of bovine intrapulmonary artery. J Pharmacol Exp Ther 1983;228:682–690.
150. Murad FD. Cyclic guanosine monophosphate as a mediator of vasodilation. J Clin Invest 1986;78:1–5.
151. Oda H, Kusumoto S, Nakajima T. Nitrosyl-hemoglobin formation in the blood of animals exposed to nitric oxide. Arch Environ Health 1975;30:453–456.
152. Yoshida K, Kasama K. Biotransformation of nitric oxide. Environ Health Perspect 1987;73:201–206.
153. Chiodi H, Mohler JG. Effects of exposure of blood hemoglobin to nitric oxide. Environ Res 1985;37:355–363.
154. Nanaev A, Chwalisz K, Frank H-G, et al. Physiological dilation of uteroplacental arteries in the guinea pig depends on nitric oxide synthase activity of extravillous trophoblast. Cell Tissue Res 1995;282:407–421.
155. Conrad KP, Joffe GM, Kruszyna H, et al. Identification of increased nitric oxide biosynthesis during pregnancy in rats. FASEB J 1993;7:566–571.
156. Neri I, Renzo GCD, Caserta G, et al. Impact of the L-arginine/nitric oxide system in pregnancy. Obstet Gynecol Surv 1995;50:851–858.
157. Ignarro LJ, Lippton H, Edwards JC, et al. Mechanisms of vascular smooth muscle relaxation by organic nitrates, nitrites, nitroprusside and nitric oxide: evidence for the involvement of S-nitrosothiols as active intermediates. J Pharmacol Exp Ther 1981;218:739–749.
158. Myatt L, Brewer A, Brockman DE. The actions of nitric oxide in the perfused fetal-placental circulation. Am J Obstet Gynecol 1991;164:687–692.
159. McCarthy AL, Woolfson RG, Evans BJ, et al. Functional characteristics of small placental arteries. Am J Obstet Gynecol 1994;170:945–951.
160. Wieczorek KM, Brewer AS, Myatt L. Shear stress may stimulate release and action of nitric oxide in the human fetal-placental vasculature. Am J Obstet Gynecol 1995;173:708–713.
161. Morris HN, Eaton BM, Sooranna SR, et al. NO synthase activity in placental bed and tissues from normotensive pregnant women. Lancet 1993;342:679–680.
162. Conrad KP, Vill M, McGuire PG, et al. Expression of nitric oxide synthase by syncytiotrophoblast in human placental villi. FASEB J 1993;7:1269–1276.
163. Gokhale SD, Gulati OD, Kelkar LV, et al. Effect of some drugs on human umbilical artery in vitro. Br J Pharmacol Chemother 1966;27:332–346.
164. Van de Voorde J, Vanderstichele H, Leusen I. Release of endothelium derived relaxing factor from human umbilical vessels. Circ Res 1987;60:517–522.
165. Chaudhuri G, Furuya K. Endothelium-derived vasoactive substances in fetal placental vessels. Semin Perinatol 1991;15:63–67.
166. Izumi H, Garfield RE, Makino Y, et al. Gestational changes in endothelium-dependent vasorelaxation in human umbilical artery. Am J Obstet Gynecol 1994;170:236–245.
167. Gonzalez C, Cruz MA, Gallardo V, et al. Nitric oxide and prostaglandin systems inhibition on the isolated perfused human placenta from normal and pre-eclamptic pregnancies. Gynecol Obstet Invest 1995;40:244–248.
168. Chaudhuri G, Cuevas J, Buga GM, et al. NO is more important than prostacyclin in maintaining low vascular tone in feto-placental vessels. Am J Physiol 1993;265:H2036–H2043.
169. Trudinger BJ, Giles WB, Cook CM, et al. Fetal umbilical artery velocity wave forms and placental resistance: clinical significance. Br J Obstet Gynaecol 1985;92:23–30.
170. Bussolino E, Benedetto C, Massobrio M, et al. Maternal vascular prostacyclin activity in pre-eclampsia. Lancet 1980;2:702.
171. Remuzzi G, Marchesi D, Zoja C, et al. Reduced umbilical and placental vascular prostacyclin production in severe preeclampsia. Prostaglandins 1980;20:105–113.
172. Walsh SW. Progesterone and estradiol production by normal and preeclamptic placentas. Obstet Gynecol 1988;71:222–226.
173. Walsh SW, Coulter S. Increased placental progesterone may cause decreased placental prostacyclin production in preeclampsia. Am J Obstet Gynecol 1989;161:1586–1592.
174. Grunewald C, Nisell H, Jansson T, et al. Possible improvement in uteroplacental blood flow during atrial natriuretic peptide infusion in preeclampsia. Obstet Gynecol 1994;84:235–239.
175. Jannson TB. Low-dose infusion of atrial natriuretic peptide in the conscious guinea pig increases blood flow to the placenta of growth-retarded fetuses. Am J Obstet Gynecol 1992;166:213–218.
176. Lyall F, Young A, Greer IA. Nitric oxide concentrations are increased in the fetoplacental circulation in preeclampsia. Am J Obstet Gynecol 1995;173:714–718.
177. Ghabour MS, Eis ALW, Brockman DE, et al. Immunohistochemical characterization of placental nitric oxide synthase expression in preeclampsia. Am J Obstet Gynecol 1995;173:687–694.
178. Morris NH, Sooranna SR, Learmont JG, et al. Nitric oxide synthase activities in placental tissue from normotensive, pre-eclamptic and growth retarded pregnancies. Br J Obstet Gynaecol 1995;102:711–714.
179. Shanklin DR, Sibai BM. Ultrastructural aspects of preeclampsia. Placental bed and uterine boundary vessels. Am J Obstet Gynecol 1989;161:735–741.

180. Smarason AK, Sargent IL, Redman CWG. Endothelial cell proliferation is suppressed by plasma but not serum from women with preeclampsia. Am J Obstet Gynecol 1996;174:787–793.
181. Luzi G, Abubakari MM, Clerici G, et al. Fetomaternal hemodynamics during maternal glyceryl-trinitrate sublingual administration. Soc Gynecol Invest J 1995;2:177.
182. Giles W, O'Callaghan S, Boura A, et al. Reduction in human fetal umbilical-placental vascular resistance by glyceryl-trinitrate. Lancet 1992;340:856.
183. Ramsay B, De Belder A, Campbell S, et al. A nitric oxide donor improves uterine artery diastolic blood flow in normal early pregnancy and in women at risk of preeclampsia. Eur J Clin Invest 1994;24:76–78.
184. Born GVR, Dawes GS, Mott JC. Oxygen lack and autonomic nervous control of the foetal circulation in the lamb. J Physiol (Lond) 1956;134:149–166.
185. Adamsons K, Beard RW, Myers RE. Comparison of the composition of arterial, venous and capillary blood of the fetal monkey during labor. Am J Obstet Gynecol 1970;107:435–440.
186. Blechner JN. Maternal-fetal acid-base physiology. Clin Obstet Gynecol 1993;36:3–12.
187. Soothill PW, Nicolaides KH, Rodeck CH, et al. Blood gases and acid-base status of human second-trimester fetus. Obstet Gynecol 1986;68:173–176.
188. Nicolaides KH, Economides DL, Soothill PW. Blood gases, pH and lactate in appropriate and small-for-gestational-age fetuses. Am J Obstet Gynecol 1989;161:996–1001.
189. Young BK. Placental regulation of fetal oxygenation and acid-base balance. In: Eden RD, Boehm FH, eds. Assessment and care of the fetus: physiological, clinical and medicolegal principles. Norwalk, CT: Appleton & Lange, 1990:171–177.
190. Longo LD, Delivoria-Papadopoulos M, Forster RE. Placental CO_2 transfer after fetal carbonic anhydrase inhibition. Am J Physiol 1974;226:703–710.
191. Hatano H, Leichtweib HP, Schroder H. Uptake of bicarbonate/CO_2 in the isolated guinea pig placenta. Placenta 1989;10:213–221.
192. Simkovich JW, Cefalo RC, Hellegers AE, et al. Effect of fetal hypercapnia on maternal and fetal cardiovascular and respiratory function. Eur J Obstet Gynecol Reprod Biol 1983;14:311–315.
193. Ralston DH, Shnider SM, deLorimier AA. Uterine blood flow and fetal acid-base changes after bicarbonate administration to the pregnant ewe. Anesthesiology 1974;40:348–353.
194. Blechner JN, Stenger VG, Eitzman DV, et al. Effects of maternal acidosis on the human fetus and newborn infant. Am J Obstet Gynecol 1967;99:46–54.
195. Chang A, Wood C. Fetal acid-base balance. Interdependence of maternal and fetal PCO_2 and bicarbonate concentration. Am J Obstet Gynecol 1976;125:61–63.
196. Aarnoudse JG, Illsley NP, Penfold P, et al. Permeability of the human placenta to bicarbonate: in-vitro perfusion studies. Br J Obstet Gynaecol 1984;91:1096–1102.
197. Huch R. Maternal hyperventilation and the fetus. J Perinat Med 1986;14:3–17.
198. Cruikshank DP, Hays PA. Maternal physiology in pregnancy. In: Gabbe SG, ed. Obstetrics: normal and problem pregnancies. New York: Churchill-Livingstone, 1991:125–146.
199. Bardicef O, Bardicef M, Sorokin Y, et al. "Physiologic" intracellular acidosis in pregnancy. Am J Obstet Gynecol 1995;173:879–880.
200. Machida H. Influence of progesterone on arterial blood and CSF acid-base balance in women. J Appl Physiol 1981;51:1433–1436.
201. Bayliss DA, Millhorn DE, Gallman EA, et al. Progesterone stimulates respiration through a central nervous system steroid receptor-mediated mechanism in cat. Proc Natl Acad Sci USA 1987;84:7788–7792.
202. Yancey MK, Moore J, Brady K, et al. The effect of altitude on umbilical cord blood gases. Obstet Gynecol 1992;79:571–574.
203. Walker AM, Oakes GK, Ehrenkranz R, et al. Effects of hypercapnia on uterine and umbilical circulations in conscious pregnant sheep. J Appl Physiol 1976;41:727–733.
204. Levinson G, Shnider SM, deLorimier AA, et al. Effects of maternal hyperventilation on uterine blood flow and fetal oxygenation and acid-base status. Anesthesiology 1974;40:340–347.
205. Moya F, Morishima HO, Shnider SM, et al. Influence of maternal hyperventilation on the newborn infant. Am J Obstet Gynecol 1965;91:76–84.
206. Miller FC, Petrie RH, Arce JJ, et al. Hyperventilation during labor. Am J Obstet Gynecol 1974;120:489–495.
207. Goldaber KG, Gilstrap LC III, Leveno KJ, et al. Pathologic fetal acidemia. Obstet Gynecol 1991;78:1103–1106.
208. Fee SC, Malee K, Deddish R, et al. Severe acidosis and subsequent neurologic status. Am J Obstet Gynecol 1990;162:802–806.
209. Antoine C, Young BK. Fetal lactic acidosis with epidural anesthesia. Am J Obstet Gynecol 1982;142;55–59.
210. Suidan JS, Antoine C, Silverman F, et al. Human maternal-fetal lactate relationships. J Perinat Med 1984;12:211–217.
211. Katz M, Lunenfeld E, Meizner I, et al. The effect of the duration of the second stage of labour on the acid-base state of the fetus. Br J Obstet Gynaecol 1987;94:425–430.
212. Burd LJ, Jones MD, Simmonds MA, et al. Placental production and foetal utilization of lactate and pyruvate. Nature 1975;254:710–711.
213. Westgren M, Lingman G, Stangenberg M. Oxygenation of the human fetus as a function of hemoglobin concentration. Am J Perinatol 1994;11:9–13.
214. Hellegers AE, Armsted EE, Thomas CE, et al. Effect of fetal metabolic acidosis upon oxygen environment. Am J Obstet Gynecol 1969;105:786–796.
215. Hankins GDV, Snyder RR, Yoemans ER. Umbilical arterial and venous acid-base and blood gas values and the effect of chorioamnionitis on those values in a cohort of preterm infants. Am J Obstet Gynecol 1991;164:1261–1264.

216. Maberry MC, Ramin SM, Gilstrap LC III, et al. Intrapartum asphyxia in pregnancies complicated by intraamniotic infection. Obstet Gynecol 1990;76:351–354.
217. Piquard F, Hsiung R, Schaefer A, et al. Does fetal acidosis develop with maternal glucose infusion during normal labor? Obstet Gynecol 1989;74:909–914.
218. Philipson EH, Kalhan SC, Riha MM, et al. Effects of maternal glucose infusion on fetal acid-base status in human pregnancy. Am J Obstet Gynecol 1987;157:866–873.
219. Kenepp NB, Shelley WC, Gabbe SG, et al. Fetal and neonatal hazards of maternal hydration with 5% dextrose before caesarean section. Lancet 1982;1:1150–1152.
220. Jenkins VR II, Dilts PV Jr. Some effects of meperidine hydrochloride on maternal and fetal sheep. Am J Obstet Gynecol 1971;109:1005–1010.
221. Clark RB, Cooper JO, Stephens SR, et al. Neonatic acid-base studies: effect of heavy medication-narcotic antagonist regimen for labor and delivery. Obstet Gynecol 1969;33:30–34.
222. Shyken JM, Smeltzer JS, Baxi LV, et al. A comparison of the effect of epidural, general, and no anesthesia on funic acid-base values by stage of labor and type of delivery. Am J Obstet Gynecol 1990;163:802–807.
223. Ralston DH, Shnider SM. The fetal and neonatal effects of regional anesthesia in obstetrics. Anesthesiology 1978;48:34–64.
224. Datta S, Alper MH, Ostheimer GW, et al. Method of ephedrine administration and nausea and hypotension during spinal anesthesia for cesarean section. Anesthesiology 1982;56:68–70.
225. Datta S, Ostheimer GW, Weiss JB, et al. Neonatal effect of prolonged anesthetic induction for cesarean section. Obstet Gynecol 1981;58:331–335.
226. Mann LI, Bhakthavathsalan A, Liu M, et al. Placental transport of alcohol and its effect on maternal and fetal acid-base balance. Am J Obstet Gynecol 1975;122:837–844.
227. Horiguchi T, Suzuki K, Comas-Urrutia AC, et al. Effect of ethanol upon uterine activity and fetal acid-base state of the rhesus monkey. Am J Obstet Gynecol 1971;109:910–917.
228. Ayromlooi J, Tobias M, Berg PD, et al. Effects of ethanol on the circulation and acid-base balance of pregnant sheep. Obstet Gynecol 1979;54:624–630.
229. Socol ML, Manning FA, Murata Y, et al. Maternal smoking causes fetal hypoxia: experimental evidence. Am J Obstet Gynecol 1982;142:214–218.
230. Woods JR Jr, Plessinger MA, Clark KE. Effect of cocaine on uterine blood flow and fetal oxygenation. JAMA 1987;257:957–961.
231. MacGregor SN, Keith LG, Chasnoff IJ, et al. Cocaine use during pregnancy: adverse perinatal outcome. Am J Obstet Gynecol 1987;157:686–690.
232. Bowen F. Management issues for the neonatal patient. Clin Perinatol 1996;23:1–30.
233. Goldaber KG, Gilstrap LC III. Correlations between obstetric clinical events and umbilical cord blood acid-base and blood gas values. Clin Obstet Gynecol 1993;36:47–59.
234. Ramin SM, Gilstrap LC III, Leveno KH, et al. Umbilical artery acid-base status in the preterm infant. Obstet Gynecol 1989;74:256–258.
235. Cox WL, Daffos F, Forestier F, et al. Physiology and management of intrauterine growth retardation: a biologic approach with fetal blood sampling. Am J Obstet Gynecol 1988;159:36–41.
236. Robillard JE, Sessions C, Kennedy RL, et al. Metabolic effects of constant hypertonic glucose infusion in well-oxygenated fetuses. Am J Obstet Gynecol 1978;130:199–203.
237. Crandell SS, Fisher DJ, Morriss FH Jr. Effects of ovine maternal hyperglycemia on fetal regional blood flows and metabolism. Am J Physiol 1985;249:E454–E460.
238. Phillips AF, Porte PJ, Stabinsky S, et al. Effects of chronic fetal hyperglycemia upon oxygen consumption in the ovine uterus and conceptus. J Clin Invest 1984;74:279–286.
239. Gilstrap LC III, Hauth JC, Schiano S, et al. Neonatal acidosis and method of delivery. Obstet Gynecol 1984;63:681–685.
240. Barcroft J. The respiratory function of the blood. Part II. Haemoglobin. Cambridge: Cambridge University Press, 1928:1–200.
241. Howard RB, Hosokawa T, Maguire MH. Hypoxia-induced fetoplacental vasoconstriction in perfused human placental cotyledons. Am J Obstet Gynecol 1987;157:1261–1266.
242. Soderholm B. The hemodynamics of the lesser circulation in pulmonary tuberculosis. Effect of exercise, temporal unilateral pulmonary artery occlusion and operation. Scand J Clin Lab Invest 1957;9(suppl 26):1–111.
243. Swenson EW, Finley TN, Gusman SV. Unilateral hypoventilation in man during temporary occlusion of one pulmonary artery. J Clin Invest 1961;40:828–835.
244. Wilkening RB, Meschia G. Effect of occluding one umbilical artery on placental oxygen transport. Am J Physiol 1991;260:H1319–H1325.
245. Moore LG, Jahnigen D, Rounds SS, et al. Maternal hyperventilation helps preserve arterial oxygenation during high-altitude pregnancy. J Appl Physiol 1982;52:690–694.
246. Moore LG, Rounds SS, Jahnigen D, et al. Infant birth weight is related to maternal arterial oxygenation at high altitude. J Appl Physiol 1982;52:695–699.
247. Kaiser IH, Cummings JN, Reynolds SRM, et al. Acclimatization response of the pregnant ewe and fetal lamb to diminished ambient pressure. J Appl Physiol 1958;13:171–178.
248. Kamitomo M, Alonso JG, Okai T, et al. Effects of long-term high-altitude hypoxemia on ovine fetal cardiac output and blood flow distribution. Am J Obstet Gynecol 1993;169:701–707.
249. DeVore GR, Medearis AL, Platt LD. The effect of altitude on the umbilical artery Doppler resistance. J Ultrasound Med 1992;11:317–320.
250. Reshetnikova OS, Burton GJ, Milovanov AP, et al. Increased incidence of placental chorioangioma in high-altitude pregnancies: Hypobaric hypoxia as a possible etiologic factor. Am J Obstet Gynecol 1996;174:557–561.

251. Ali KZM, Ali ME, Khalid MEM. High altitude and spontaneous preterm birth. Int J Gynaecol Obstet 1996;54: 11–5.
252. Vatnick I, Schoknecht PA, Darrigrand R, et al. Growth and metabolism of the placenta after unilateral fetectomy in twin pregnant ewes. J Dev Physiol 1991;15: 351–356.
253. Penninga L, Longo LD. Unpublished data.
254. Reshetnikova OS, Burton GJ, Milovanov AP. Effects of hypobaric hypoxia on the fetoplacental unit: the morphometric diffusing capacity of the villous membrane at high altitude. Am J Obstet Gynecol 1994;171:1560–1565.
255. Burton GJ, Reshetnikova OS, Milovanov AP, et al. Stereological evaluation of vascular adaptations in human placental villi to differing forms of hypoxic stress. Placenta 1996;17:49–55.
256. Jackson MR, Mayhew TM, Haas JD. Morphometric studies on villi in human term placentae and the effects of altitude, ethnic grouping and sex of newborn. Placenta 1987;8:487–495.
257. Krebs C, Longo LD, Leiser R. Term ovine placental vasculature: comparison of sea level and high altitude conditions by corrosion cast and histomorphometry. Placenta 1997;18:43–51.
258. Ali KZ, Burton GJ, Morad N, et al. Does hypercapillarization influence the branching pattern of terminal villi in the human placenta at high altitude? Placenta 1996;17:677–682.
259. Lee R, Mayhew TM. Star volumes of villi and intervillous pores in placentae from low and high altitude pregnancies. J Anat 1995;186:349–355.
260. Jackson MR, Mayhew TM, Haas JD. The volumetric composition of human term placentae: altitudinal, ethnic and sex differences in Bolivia. J Anat 1987;152:173–187.
261. Jackson MR, Mayhew TM, Haas JD. On the factors which contribute to thinning of the villous membrane in human placentae at high altitude. II. An increase in the degree of peripheralization of fetal capillaries. Placenta 1988;9:9–18.
262. Jackson MR, Mayhew TM, Haas JD. On the factors which contribute to thinning of the villous membrane in human placentae at high altitude. I. Thinning and regional variation in thickness of trophoblast. Placenta 1988;9:1–8.
263. Jackson MR, Joy CF, Mayhew TM, et al. Stereological studies on the true thickness of the villous membrane in human term placentae: a study of placentae from high-altitude pregnancies. Placenta 1985;6:249–258.
264. Mayhew TM. Patterns of villous and intervillous space growth in human placentas from normal and abnormal pregnancies. Eur J Obstet Gynecol Reprod Biol 1996; 68:75–82.
265. Howard RC, Bruns PD, Lichty JA. Studies on babies born at high altitudes. III. Arterial oxygen saturation and hematocrit values at birth. Am J Dis Child 1957;93:674–678.
266. Sobrevilla LA, Cassinelli MT, Carcelen A, et al. Human fetal and maternal oxygen tension and acid base status during delivery at high altitude. Am J Obstet Gynecol 1971;111:1111–1118.
267. Parer JT. Effects of hypoxia on the mother and fetus with emphasis on maternal air transport. Am J Obstet Gynecol 1982;142:957–961.
268. Blechner JN, Cotter JR, Hinkley CM, et al. Observations on pregnancy at high altitude. II. Transplacental pressure differences of oxygen and carbon dioxide. Am J Obstet Gynecol 1968;102:794–801.
269. Makowski EL, Battaglia FC, Meschia G, et al. Effect of maternal exposure to high altitude upon fetal oxygenation. Am J Obstet Gynecol 1968;100:852–861.
270. Penninga L, Longo LD. Unpublished data.
271. McCullough RE, Reeves JT. Fetal growth retardation and increased infant mortality at high altitude. Arch Environ Health 1977;32:36–39.
272. Little BB, Snell LM, Palmore MK, et al. Cocaine use in pregnant women in a large public hospital. Am J Perinatol 1988;4:206–207.
273. Neerhof MG, MacGregor SN, Retzky SS, et al. Cocaine abuse during pregnancy: peripartum prevalence and perinatal outcome. Am J Obstet Gynecol 1989;161:633–638.
274. Glantz JC, Woods JR Jr. Cocaine, heroine, and phencyclidine: obstetric perspectives. Clin Obstet Gynecol 1993;36:279–301.
275. Gilbert WM, Lafferty CM, Benirschke K, et al. Lack of specific placental abnormality associated with cocaine use. Am J Obstet Gynecol 1990;163:998–999.
276. Malek A, Ivy D, Blann E, Mattison DR. Impact of cocaine on human placental function using in vitro perfusion system. J Pharmacol Toxicol Methods 1995;33:213–219.
277. Plessinger MA, Woods JR Jr. Maternal, placental and fetal pathophysiology of cocaine exposure during pregnancy. Clin Obstet Gynecol 1993;36:267–278.
278. Dolkart LA, Plessinger MA, Woods JR Jr. Effect of alpha-1 receptor blockade upon maternal and fetal cardiovascular responses to cocaine. Obstet Gynecol 1990;75: 745–751.
279. Ahluwalia BS, Clark JFJ, Westney LS, et al. Amniotic fluid and umbilical artery levels of sex hormones and prostaglandins in human cocaine users. Reprod Toxicol 1992;6:57–62.
280. Monga M, Chmielowiec S, Andres RL, et al. Cocaine alters placental production of thromboxane and prostacyclin. Am J Obstet Gynecol 1994;171:965–969.
281. Cejtin HE, Parsons MT, Wilson L Jr. Cocaine use and its effect upon umbilical artery prostacyclin production. Prostaglandins 1990;40:249–257.
282. Bureau MA, Monette J, Shapcott D, et al. Carboxyhemoglobin concentration in fetal cord blood and in blood of mothers who smoked during labor. Pediatrics 1982;69:371–373.
283. Longo LD, Hill EP. Carbon monoxide uptake and elimination in fetal and maternal sheep. Am J Physiol 1977;232:H324–H330.
284. Longo LD. The biological effects of carbon monoxide on the pregnant woman, fetus and newborn infant. Am J Obstet Gynecol 1977;129:69–103.
285. Bureau MA, Shapcott D, Berthiaume Y, et al. Maternal cigarette smoking and fetal oxygen transport: a study of P50, 2,3-diphosphoglycerate, total hemoglobin, hemat-

285. ocrit and type F hemoglobin in fetal blood. Pediatrics 1983;72:22–26.
286. Longo LD. Carbon monoxide: effects on oxygenation of the fetus in utero. Science 1977;194:523–525.
287. Longo LD. Carbon monoxide in the pregnant mother and fetus and its exchange across the placenta. Ann NY Acad Sci 1970;174:313–341.
288. Lehtovirta P, Forss M. Acute effects of smoking on intervillous blood flow of the placenta. Br J Obstet Gynaecol 1978;85:729–731.
289. Quigley ME, Sheehan KL, Wilkes MM, et al. Effects of maternal smoking on circulating catecholamine levels and fetal heart rates. Am J Obstet Gynecol 1979;133:685–690.
290. Sindberg Eriksen P, Marsal K. Acute effects of maternal smoking on fetal blood flow. Acta Obstet Gynecol Scand 1984;63:391–397.
291. Lindblad A, Marsal K. Influence of nicotine chewing gum on fetal blood flow. J Perinat Med 1987;15:13–19.
292. Brown HL, Miller JM, Khawli O, et al. Premature placental calcification in maternal cigarette smokers. Obstet Gynecol 1988;71:914–917.
293. Asmussen I. Ultrastructure of the human placenta at term. Observations on placentas from newborn children of smoking and non-smoking mothers. Acta Obstet Gynecol Scand 1977;56:119–126.
294. Harrison MR. Fetal surgery. Am J Obstet Gynecol 1996;174:1255–1264.
295. De Lia JE, Cruikshank DP, Keye WR Jr. Fetoscopic neodymium: Yag laser occlusion of placental vessels in severe twin-twin transfusion syndrome. Obstet Gynecol 1990;75:1046–1053.
296. Longaker MT, Golbus MS, Filly RA, et al. Maternal outcome after open fetal surgery. A review of the first 17 human cases. JAMA 1991;265:737–741.
297. Estes JM, MacGillivray TE, Hedrick MH, et al. Fetoscopic surgery for the treatment of congenital anomalies. J Pediatr Surg 1992;27:950–954.
298. Sabik JF, Assad RS, Hanley FL. Halothane as an anesthetic for fetal surgery. J Pediatr Surg 1993;28:542–547.
299. Cheek DBC, Hughes SC, Dailey PA, et al. Effect of halothane on regional cerebral blood flow and cerebral metabolic oxygen consumption in the fetal lamb in utero. Anesthesiology 1987;67:361–366.
300. Skarsgard ED, Bealer JF, Meuli M, et al. Fetal endoscopic ("fetendo") surgery: the relationship between insufflating pressure and the fetoplacental circulation. J Pediatr Surg 1995;30:1165–1168.
301. Tabor BL, Maier JA. Polyhydramnios and elevated intrauternine pressure during amnioinfusion. Am J Obstet Gynecol 1987l;156:130–131.
302. Turley K, Vlahakes GJ, Harrison MR, et al. Intrauterine cardiothoracic surgery: the fetal lamb model. Ann Thorac Surg 1982;34:422–426.
303. Carpenter RJ Jr, Strasburger JF, Garson A Jr, et al. Fetal ventricular pacing for hydrops secondary to complete atrioventricular block. J Am Coll Cardiol 1986;8:1434–1436.
304. Maxwell D, Allan L, Tynan MJ. Balloon dilatation of the aortic valve in the fetus: a report of two cases. Br Heart J 1991;65:256–258.
305. Hawkins JA, Paape KL, Adkins TP, et al. Extracorporeal circulation in the fetal lamb. Effects of hypothermia and perfusion rate. J Cardiovasc Surg 1991;32:295–300.
306. Hawkins JA, Clark SM, Shaddy RE, et al. Fetal cardiac bypass: improved placental function with moderately high flow rates. Ann Thorac Surg 1994;57:293–297.
307. Bradley SM, Hanley FL, Duncan BW, et al. Fetal cardiac bypass alters regional blood flows, arterial blood gases and hemodynamics in sheep. Am J Physiol 1992;263:H919–H928.
308. Sabik JF, Heinemann MK, Assad RS, et al. High-dose steroids prevent placental dysfunction after fetal cardiac bypass. J Thorac Cardiovasc Surg 1994;107:116–125.
309. Fenton KN, Heinemann MK, Hanley FI. Exclusion of the placenta during fetal cardiac bypass augments systemic flow and provides important information about the mechanism of placental injury. J Thorac Cardiovasc Surg 1993;105:502–512.
310. Callaghan JC, Angeles JD, Boracchia B, et al. Studies in the development of an artificial placenta. The possible use of long-term extracorporeal circulation for respiratory distress of the newborn. Circulation 1963;27:686–690.
311. Zapol WM, Kolobow T, Pierce JE, et al. Artificial placenta: two days of total extrauterine support of the isolated premature lamb fetus. Science 1969;166:617–618.
312. Kuwabara Y, Okai T, Kozuma S, et al. Artificial placenta: long-term extrauterine incubation of isolated goat fetuses. Artif Organs 1989;13:527–531.
313. Unno N, Kuwabara Y, Shinozuka N, et al. Development of artificial placenta: oxygen metabolism of isolated goat fetuses with umbilical arteriovenous extracorporeal membrane oxygenation. Fetal Diagn Ther 1990;5:189–195.
314. Unno N, Kuwabara Y, Okai T, et al. Development of an artificial placenta: survival of isolated goat fetuses for three weeks with umbilical arteriovenous extracorporeal membrane oxygenation. Artif Organs 1993;17:996–1003.
315. Chamberlain G. An artificial placenta: the development of an extracorporeal system for maintenance of immature infants with respiratory problems. Am J Obstet Gynecol 1968;100:615–626.
316. Westin B, Nyberg R, Enhorning G. Technique for perfusion of the previable human fetus. Acta Paediatr 1958;47:339–349.

24
Circulation in the Fetal-Placental Unit

Abraham M. Rudolph

Circulation of blood has evolved to transport oxygen and energy substrates to the tissues of the body and to remove carbon dioxide and other metabolites. The circulation carries regulatory hormones to the tissues. Postnatally, respiratory gases enter and leave the body through the lungs, and energy sources are provided from the gastrointestinal tract, entering the portal venous system to be distributed to the liver. In the fetus respiratory gas exchange, substrate supply, and removal of metabolites occur in the placenta. The circulation has been adapted to perform these functions effectively in the fetus. Postnatally, a series of circulatory adjustments are required at the time of birth, particularly in relation to the transfer of gas exchange from the placenta to the lungs.

Course of Blood Flow

Postnatal Circulation

The adult circulation is characterized by serial flow of venous blood into the right atrium (Figure 24.1). It is ejected by the right ventricle into the pulmonary circulation to be oxygenated in the lungs and returns to the left atrium and ventricle to be ejected into the aorta for distribution to body organs. Carbon dioxide is removed and oxygen taken up in the lungs. A variable proportion of oxygen is extracted, and carbon dioxide and metabolites are added to blood by the tissues. Apart from minor amounts of bronchial venous blood that may enter the pulmonary vein and coronary venous blood that may drain directly into the left ventricular cavity, there is essentially no mixing of well-oxygenated pulmonary venous and systemic arterial blood with poorly oxygenated systemic venous and pulmonary arterial blood. Postnatally, metabolic substrates, absorbed from the gastrointestinal tract into the portal venous system, are first delivered to the liver and then enter the systemic venous system and lungs before being delivered to tissues.

Fetal Circulation

Course of Blood Flow in Fetal Liver

Carbon dioxide is removed from, and oxygen is taken up by, fetal blood in the placenta. The oxygenated blood is returned to the fetal body through the umbilical vein in the umbilical cord. The umbilical vein passes from the umbilical ring to the hilum of the liver. It provides branches to the left lobe of the liver and then divides into the ductus venosus and a large arcuate branch, which courses in the hilum to the right, to be joined by the portal vein (Figure 24.2). Branches to the right lobe of the liver are then given off. The ductus venosus passes dorsally and cephalad through the liver parenchyma to join the inferior vena cava immediately underneath the diaphragm. The left hepatic vein joins the ductus venosus at its entry into the inferior vena cava, so there is a common entry orifice. In the sheep fetus this orifice is partly covered by a thin, valve-like membrane on its caudad edge. The right hepatic vein enters the inferior vena cava separately, and the orifice is partly covered by a valve-like structure caudally. The function of these "valves" is not known, but we have conjectured that they may facilitate directional flow of the various venous streams entering the inferior vena cava at this site. It had generally been believed that umbilical and portal venous blood mixed in the porta hepatis and was then distributed to the left and right liver lobes and through the ductus venosus. Lind[1] obtained umbilical venous angiograms in human fetuses immediately after delivery and suggested that umbilical venous blood preferentially passes to the left liver lobe and through the ductus venosus.

Using radionuclide-labeled microspheres, it has been possible to define not only the patterns of blood flow in the fetal liver but the quantities of blood flowing through various channels. From these studies it is evident that umbilical venous blood is distributed to the left lobe of the liver, through the ductus venosus, and to the right liver lobe. Portal venous blood is distributed to the right liver lobe, with only a small proportion passing through the ductus venosus; none is delivered to the left lobe. The flow patterns of the various streams entering the inferior vena cava have been defined by the use of labeled microspheres.

When a right thoracotomy is performed in the fetal lamb, observation of the thoracic portion of the inferior vena cava reveals partial separation of well-oxygenated and poorly oxygenated bloodstreams. The anterior and right portion of the vessel is seen to have a poorly oxygenated stream, but blood flowing in the posterior and left portion is clearly well oxygenated. Studies with microspheres injected simultaneously into abdominal vena caval and umbilical venous tributaries show that umbilical venous and abdominal inferior vena cava blood passes through the inferior vena cava and enters the right and left atria through the foramen ovale. However, umbilical venous blood passing through the ductus venosus is preferentially directed across the foramen ovale into the left atrium and left ventricle. Abdominal inferior vena caval blood, in contrast, preferentially streams across the tricuspid valve into the right atrium and right ventricle. We have conducted similar studies with microspheres injected into the left or right hepatic veins (J. Bristow and A.M. Rudolph, personal observation). Blood from the left hepatic vein tends to follow the course of the ductus venosus stream, being preferentially distributed across the foramen ovale, whereas right hepatic venous blood preferentially streams across the tricuspid valve, following the course of abdominal inferior vena caval blood (Figure 24.3). The streaming patterns in the inferior vena cava have been documented in fetal lambs by ultrasound techniques. Color Doppler studies show that the ductus venosus stream has a high velocity and is directed largely through the foramen ovale, whereas distal inferior vena cava blood has a considerably lower velocity and streams across the tricuspid vale. Ultrasound examinations of human fetuses have also shown similar differences in ductus venosus and distal inferior vena caval velocities, and similar preferential streaming patterns.[4]

Course of Blood Flow in Fetal Heart and Great Vessels

The radionuclide-labeled microsphere technique has proved to be most effective not only for defining patterns of blood flow in the fetal central circulation but for quantitating blood flow through various channels.[5] These studies have confirmed that essentially all superior vena caval blood is distributed through the tricuspid valve into the right ventricle. Right ventricular blood is ejected into the pulmonary trunk, and the larger proportion passes through the ductus arteriosus to the descending aorta, with the remainder entering the pulmonary circulation (Figure 24.4). Blood that passes from the pulmonary trunk through the ductus arteriosus is directed to the descending aorta; none passes retrograde across the aortic isthmus to the ascending aorta and its branches. The left atrium receives blood from the foramen ovale and pulmonary veins, and then empties into the left ventricle, which ejects into the ascending aorta. Most ascending aortic blood is distributed to the coronary circulation, head and cerebral circulation, and upper extremities; only a small proportion passes across the aortic isthmus into the descending aorta.

Admixture of Oxygenated and Systemic Venous Blood

As mentioned above, there is essentially no mixing of oxygenated pulmonary venous and systemic venous blood in the adult circulation. In the fetus, there are several sites of mixing. The first is in the portal veins, where portal and umbilical venous bloods mix. Another mixing site is the inferior vena cava, where ductus veno-

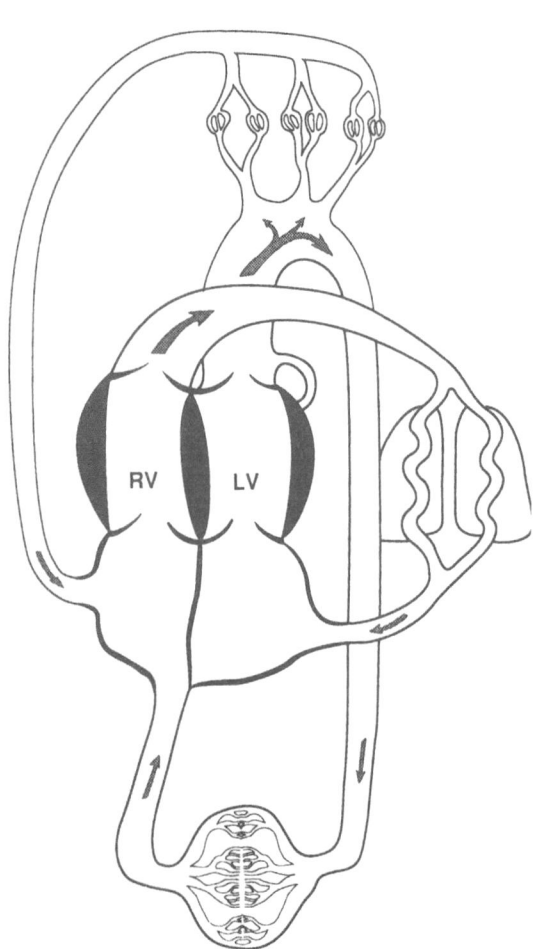

FIGURE 24.1. Course of the adult circulation. Blood flows serially through the pulmonary and systemic circulations.

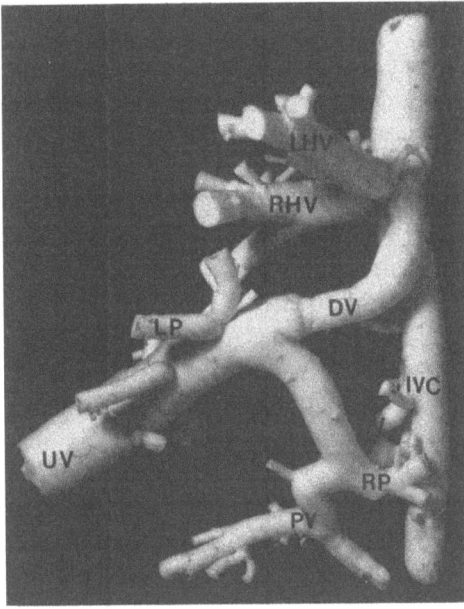
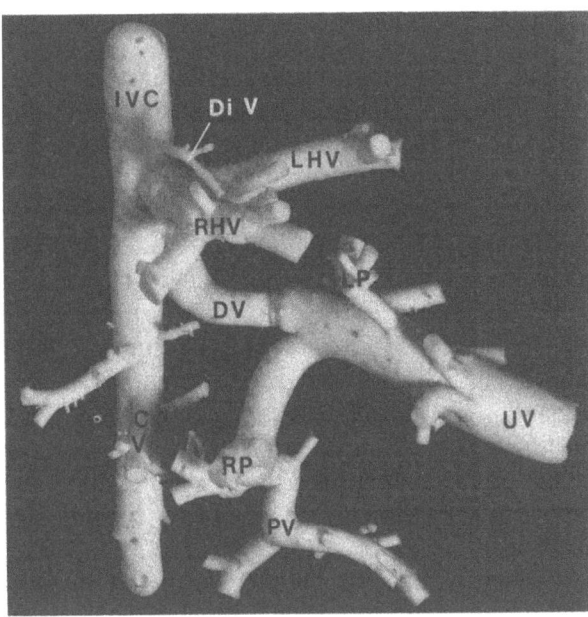

FIGURE 24.2. Silicone rubber cast of veins in the fetal portal sinus and liver seen from the left and right sides. The umbilical vein provides branches to the left liver lobe (LP) and then divides into the ductus venosus (DV) and a large branch, which arches to the right to join the portal vein (Pv). After this junction, portal branches are provided to the right liver lobe (PR). The left hepatic vein (LHV) and ductus venosus join the inferior vena cava (IVC) through a common orifice, and the right hepatic vein (RHV) enters the inferior vena cava through a separate orifice, just underneath the diaphragm. Di V, diaphragmatic vein. (From Bristow et al.,[135] with permission.)

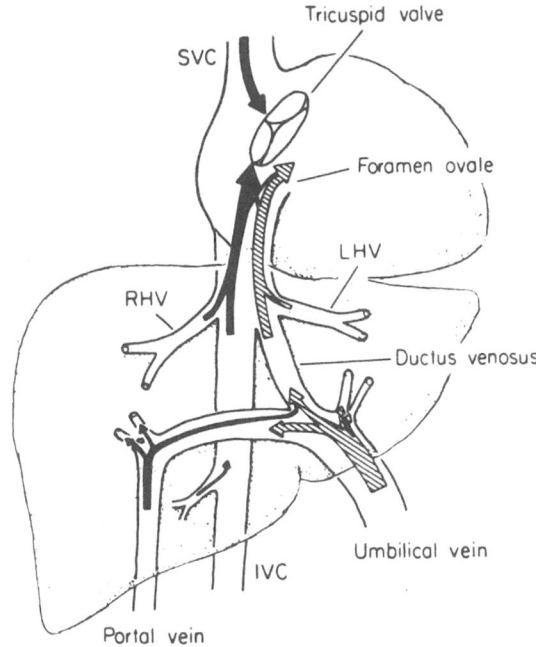
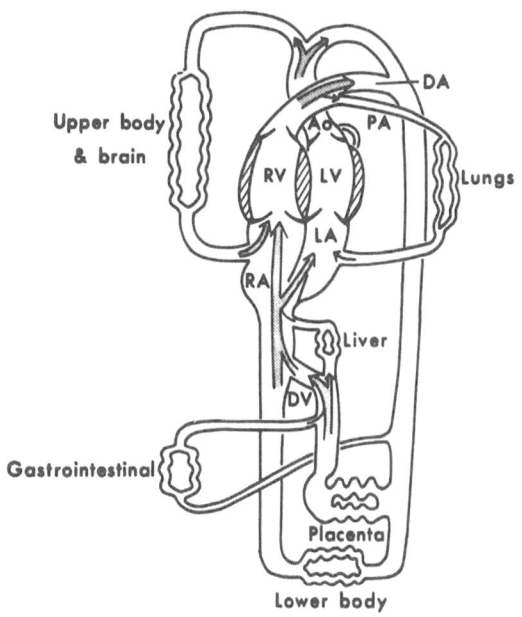

FIGURE 24.3. Course of venous blood flow in the liver and heart of the fetal lamb. Umbilical venous blood supplies the left liver lobe and passes to the ductus venosus and right liver lobe. Portal venous blood is distributed with umbilical venous blood to the right lobe. Only a small amount of portal venous blood passes through the ductus venosus. Ductus venosus and left hepatic venous blood is preferentially distributed through the foramen ovale, whereas abdominal inferior vena caval and right hepatic venous blood preferentially streams through the tricuspid valve. Almost all superior vena caval blood also passes through the tricuspid valve. SVC, superior vena cava. See Figure 24.2 for other abbreviations. (From Rudolph,[136] with permission.)

FIGURE 24.4. Course of blood flow in the fetal circulation of the lamb. Note that right ventricular (RV) blood is largely ejected into the pulmonary trunk and then through the ductus arteriosus (DA) to the descending aorta. Left ventricular (LV) blood supplies the upper body and the cerebral and coronary circulations; only a small proportion crosses the aortic isthmus to the descending aorta (Ao). PA, pulmonary artery; RA, right atrium; DV, ductus venosus: LA, left atrium. (From Rudolph,[137] with permission.)

sus, left and right hepatic venous, and abdominal inferior vena caval blood enters the thoracic portion of the inferior vena cava. Admixture occurs in the left atrium, where blood entering the foramen ovale from the inferior vena cava is joined by pulmonary venous blood. the preferential streaming of blood from several veins to some extent separates the well-oxygenated and poorly oxygenated blood, favoring distribution of oxygenated blood into the left ventricle and ascending aorta and providing blood with a higher oxygen content to the heart, brain, and other upper body tissues. Systemic venous blood is preferentially directed into the right ventricle, pulmonary trunk, and ductus arteriosus to the descending aorta and its branches to the lower body, as well as to the placenta.

Because oxygenated and systemic venous blood is mixed, the blood delivered to the fetal body and the placenta represents a mixture of blood. Hence, some umbilical venous blood is returned to the placenta after passing through the ductus venosus and foramen ovale or ductus arteriosus shunts without first being delivered to fetal tissues to permit oxygen uptake. This situation is equivalent to what occurs postnatally with some congenital heart lesions (e.g., atrial or ventricular septal defect), in which oxygenated blood passes from the left atrium or left ventricle into the right side of the heart to be recirculated to the lung. This condition is known as a left-to-right shunt, and it imposes an additional work load on the heart. Similarly, with congenital heart lesions in which systemic venous blood is shunted through an abnormal communication into the left side of the heart to be distributed back to the body tissues without passing through the lung, a right-to-left shunt is said to occur. Some degree of effective right-to-left shunting is usually present in the fetal circulation because some superior and inferior vena caval blood passes through the foramen ovale and ductus arteriosus and recirculates through fetal body tissues and is not distributed to the placenta for oxygenation. This effective right-to-left shunt contributes to inefficiency of the fetal circulation.

In the sheep fetus under normal conditions, left-to-right shunt represents about 22% of umbilical venous blood, and right-to-left shunt represents about 45% of superior vena caval and 53% of inferior vena caval blood. The combined left-to-right and right-to-left shunts constitute about 33% of the combined ventricular output of the fetal heart.

Fetal Blood Gases and Oxygen Saturation

Maternal arterial blood in the pregnant ewe has a Po_2 of 90 to 100 torr. There is a large Po_2 gradient across the placenta, with a Po_2 of 32 to 35 torr in umbilical venous blood. Umbilical venous blood Pco_2 is 40 torr and pH 7.40. Because the P_{50} (the Po_2 at which hemoglobin is 50% saturated with oxygen) for fetal blood in the sheep is considerably lower (about 27 torr) than that of adult blood (about 38 torr), umbilical venous blood has an oxygen saturation of 85% to 90%. The Po_2 of carotid arterial blood is slightly higher (23 torr) than that of descending aortic blood (21 torr). Fetal arterial blood has a Pco_2 of 43 to 45 torr and a pH of 7.39. Oxygen saturation in carotid arterial blood is about 65%, and in descending aortic blood it is 55%. Pulmonary arterial blood has a Po_2 of 18 to 20 torr and a saturation of about 50%. Superior and inferior vena caval blood has a Po_2 of 12 to 15 torr and an oxygen saturation of about 30% to 40%.

Increasing maternal arterial blood Po_2 by administering 100% oxygen to the ewe increases oxygen saturation to 100% and the Po_2 to more than 400 torr; fetal arterial Po_2 increases to only 30 to 35 torr with an oxygen saturation of about 80%. Umbilical venous blood Po_2 increases to 40 to 60 torr, and oxygen saturation reaches 95% to 100% (see Chapter 23).

Fetal Vascular Pressures

Postnatally, it has become customary to consider atmospheric pressure as the zero reference. When considering effective filling pressures of the cardiac ventricles, it is more appropriate to measure transmural pressure, or intraluminal minus pericardial pressure. Pericardial pressure is generally similar to intrapleural pressure, which is negative (i.e., lower than atmospheric pressure) postnatally. The fetus is surrounded by fluid in the uterus and is subjected to the positive intraabdominal pressure when the uterus is relaxed and to an even higher pressure when the uterus contracts. Fetal vascular pressures are referenced to amniotic cavity pressure as zero.

The ductus arteriosus, a large-diameter vessel connecting the pulmonary trunk with the aorta, tends to equalize pressures in the pulmonary artery and aorta. The similarity of the systolic and diastolic pressures in the aorta and pulmonary artery has been observed in chronically instrumented fetal lambs at gestational age 115 to 145 days (i.e., term). However, there is a tendency for pulmonary trunk pressure to exceed that in the aorta during the last 5 to 7 days of gestation, presumably as a result of mild ductus arteriosus constriction.

Arterial pressure increases with gestational age in the lamb fetus, from a mean of 39 mm Hg at about 80 days' gestation to 55 mm Hg close to term. Figure 24.5 shows the pressures measured in various cardiac chambers in the fetal lamb in utero.

24. Circulation in the Fetal-Placental Unit

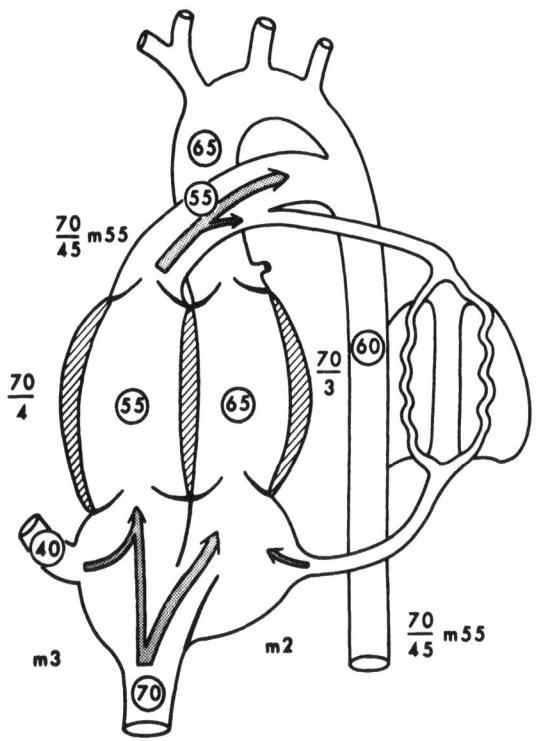

FIGURE 24.5. Pressures (mm Hg) in various chambers and great vessels of the fetal heart. Numbers in circles are percent oxygen saturations in chambers and vessels. (From Rudolph,[137] with permission.)

Methods for Studying the Fetal Circulation

Several methods have been developed for measuring cardiac output in the adult human or animal. They include the Fick method and indicator-dilation methods (e.g., dye dilution, thermodilution, and radioisotope dilution), application of electromagnetic or ultrasonic flow transducers around the aorta or pulmonary artery, and, more recently, application of the Doppler principle using external transducers. Because blood flows serially, measurement of blood flow at any site provides an estimate of cardiac output. Cardiac output represents the volume of blood flowing per unit time through the series circulation. Because both ventricles eject essentially similar stroke volumes, cardiac output is represented as the output of either ventricle.

In the fetus, although similar techniques may be applied, they have to be modified because of the presence of shunts and the exchange of oxygen at the placental site. If it were possible to measure the total amount of oxygen taken up across the placenta, it still would not be possible to measure cardiac output by the Fick method because umbilical-placental blood flow is only a proportion of total output. Because there is mixing of oxygenated blood and systemic venous blood returning to the heart, and because both ventricles contribute blood to the body as well as to the placenta, the concept of cardiac output that is used postnatally cannot apply to the fetus. To indicate the volume of blood ejected by the fetal heart, it is convenient to calculate the total amount of blood ejected by the heart, and the term combined ventricular output has been applied.[5-7]

Early studies of fetal cardiac output were performed in exteriorized lamb fetuses. Barcroft and Torrens[8] reported outputs of 165 to 345 ml/kg fetal body weight per minute in anesthetized fetuses. Mahon et al.[9] used the dye-dilution method, injecting dye into the right and left ventricles and sampling from the pulmonary artery and ascending aorta, respectively. Questions may be raised about the adequacy of mixing of dye because of the short distance between the injection site and the site of sampling. Assali et al.[10] applied electromagnetic flow transducers around the ascending aorta and pulmonary trunk to measure left and right ventricular output separately in exteriorized lamb fetuses.

Rudolph and Heymann[5] developed the radionuclide-labeled microsphere method for measuring blood flow and cardiac output in fetal lambs in utero. They demonstrated that plastic microspheres, labeled with gamma-emitting isotopes, were distributed in relation to blood flow. In early studies 50-µm spheres were used, but 15-µm spheres were used subsequently. When injected into the circulation, these spheres are distributed to tissues in relation to flow to the tissue and are trapped in small vessels. It has been shown that few spheres pass through the capillary bed and are recirculated. By counting the total radioactivity injected and the radioactivity in each organ or tissue, the proportion of total blood flow distributed to the organ can be determined. If the blood flow to any specific organ is determined by some other procedure, blood flow to any other organ can be calculated. In the first application of this technique, umbilical-placental blood flow was calculated using a Fick method, which involves continuous infusion of antipyrine into the fetus and measuring umbilical arterial and venous concentrations when a steady state is reached. The technique has been greatly improved by withdrawing a reference sample from the arterial supply during the injection and circulation of microspheres. A blood sample is withdrawn at constant rate from an arterial catheter in the distribution to the organs of interest, starting immediately before the injection and continuing for a period encompassing that during which the microspheres are circulating. Using the equation.

Organ blood flow $\left(\text{ml}\cdot\text{min}^{-1}\right)$

= Reference sample withdrawal rate $\left(\text{ml}\cdot\text{min}^{-1}\right)$

$\times \dfrac{R_{\text{organ}}}{R_{\text{reference}}}$

where R is the quantity of radioactivity, the blood flow to every organ receiving its blood supply from the artery from which the reference sample is withdrawn can be calculated.[12,13]

In the adult animal, if spheres are injected into the left ventricle, a reference sample can be withdrawn from any branch of the aorta, and blood flow to every organ of the body can be calculated. Cardiac output can be derived from the sum of all the organ blood flows. In the fetus, the patterns of flow preclude the use of a single reference sample to calculate flow to all organs. If spheres were injected into the left ventricle, the concentration of spheres in the ascending aorta and its branches would be higher than that in the descending aorta and its branches because blood passing from the pulmonary artery through the ductus arteriosus would reduce the sphere concentration in descending aortic blood. It is necessary to withdraw a reference sample from arterial branches of both the ascending and the descending aortas during injection of microspheres.

It is possible to take advantage of the presence of venous shunts in the fetus to avoid placing catheters in the cardiac chambers in order to inject microspheres. If microspheres are injected into a tributary of the inferior vena cava, some pass through the foramen ovale into the left atrium and then to the left ventricle and ascending aorta. Some spheres enter the right ventricle and pass to the pulmonary artery through the ductus arteriosus to the descending aorta. If microspheres are injected into a tributary of the fetal inferior vena cava and reference samples are withdrawn simultaneously from branches of the ascending and descending aorta, blood flow to all fetal organs except the lungs can be calculated. To calculate pulmonary blood flow, it is necessary to inject microspheres simultaneously into a superior and an inferior caval tributary.[14] Combined ventricular output and blood flow to each fetal organ and to the placenta can be measured with the microsphere technique if catheters are placed in a hind-limb artery and vein and a forelimb artery and vein, or the carotid artery and jugular vein. The microspheres injected into the superior and inferior caval veins are labeled with different gamma-emitting isotopes. By selecting gamma-emitting radionuclides with appropriate energy spectra, it is possible to quantitate the amount of each isotope in the tissue, enabling repeated studies of combined ventricular output and organ blood flow. The principles of measuring blood flow by the radionuclide-labeled microsphere technique and its application to study in the fetus and adult have been reviewed extensively.[12,13,15] Because of difficulties and expense of disposal of tissues containing radioactive material, the use of the radionuclide-labeled microsphere technique has come into disfavor. Recently, fluorescent microspheres have become available; spheres that fluoresce at different wavelengths may be injected during various experimental conditions. The expenses for equipment and microspheres are comparable to those for the radioactive sphere technique, but disposal is not a problem.[16-19]

The disadvantages of the microsphere method are that a limited number of observations can be made in a single animal and the measurements are not available immediately because tissues must be processed to determine radioactivity. Because flow measurements are obtained only at selected points, it is not possible to observe rapid changes.

Fetal blood flows have been measured continuously by electromagnetic or ultrasonic flowmeters. Assali et al.[10] measured aortic, pulmonary trunk, and ductus arteriosus flows acutely in exteriorized fetal lambs using electromagnetic flowmeters. Rudolph and Heymann[20] and Thornburg and Morton[21,22] have measured ascending aortic flow (i.e., left ventricular output minus coronary blood flow) and pulmonary trunk flow (i.e., right ventricular output) with electromagnetic flowmeters in chronically instrumented fetal lambs. Electromagnetic flow transducers have been used to measure pulmonary,[23] renal,[24] and umbilical blood flow[25] chronically. Using the Doppler principle, ultrasonic flow transducers have been applied around fetal vessels such as the umbilical and iliac arteries. These techniques offer many advantages: continuous measurement of phasic and mean blood flows, ability to assess instantaneous flow changes, and unlimited number of observations. The disadvantages are that they usually require extensive and often complex surgery on the fetus. With electromagnetic flow transducers, growth of the fetus and vessel could be associated with the development of relative narrowing of the vessels because the flow transducer diameter is fixed.

None of the methods mentioned is applicable to measuring flow in human fetuses. The Doppler principle has been applied to measuring blood flows in the descending aorta[26] and umbilical vessels[27] and to assess left and right ventricular output by measuring flow across the mitral and tricuspid valves.[28] An external transducer is applied to the maternal abdomen or, in animal studies, to the surface of the uterus. Attempts have been made to estimate ascending aortic or pulmonary trunk flows in the fetus with external transducers, but depending on fetal position, it may be difficult to maneuver the transducer to achieve an appropriate angle of isonation with the vessel. Another method that could be used for measuring cardiac output is to estimate ventricular volume at end-systole and end-diastole using two-dimensional echocardiography. This method provides a measure of stroke volume that, when multiplied by heart rate, represents cardiac output. The reliability of these measurements has not been tested adequately by confirmation with results obtained by other methods, but one study showed a good relationship between Doppler ultrasound and microsphere measurement of right ventricular output in fetal sheep.[29]

Cardiac Output and Its Distribution

In the adult, cardiac output represents the volume of blood flowing serially through the pulmonary and systemic circulations per unit time. It represents the volume of blood distributed to all body organs, as well as to the lungs. Left and right ventricular outputs are identical apart from intermittent, small variations. Oxygen delivery to the body is the product of arterial oxygen content and cardiac output. Cardiac work is largely determined by the pressure developed by the ventricles and the volume ejected (i.e., cardiac output). In the fetus it is not possible to apply the term cardiac output in the same context. Because blood ejected by both the left and right ventricles is distributed to the organ of gas exchange, the placenta, and because systemic and oxygenated venous bloods mix, different concepts must be considered. The outputs of the two ventricles are usually different. It is convenient in the fetus to consider the total output of the heart, or combined ventricular output. Because the pressures developed by the two ventricles are similar (vide

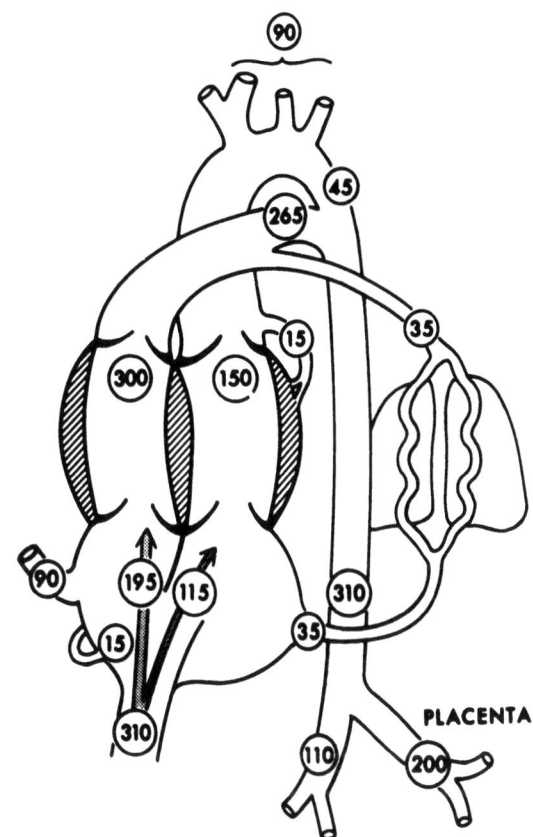

FIGURE 24.7. Quantities of blood (per kilogram of fetal body weight) passing through various cardiac chambers and great vessels of the fetal lamb heart and the placenta. Combined ventricular output is $450\,ml\cdot kg^{-1}\,min^{-1}$. (From Rudolph,[137] with permission.)

infra), cardiac work would be determined by arterial pressure and the output of both ventricles (i.e., combined ventricular output). The combined ventricular output would determine the blood flows to the fetal body and placenta. Umbilical-placental blood flow represents the volume of blood being presented to the site of oxygenation, whereas combined ventricular output minus umbilical-placental blood flow is the volume of blood delivered to the whole fetal body. Umbilical-placental blood flow determines oxygen uptake, and fetal body blood flow determines oxygen delivery to the fetus.

Few measurements of fetal combined ventricular output have been made in humans, and most available information is from studies in the sheep. In chronically instrumented fetal lambs during the latter months of gestation (term is about 145 days), the combined ventricular output is about $450\,ml\cdot min^{-1}kg^{-1}$ fetal body weight,[5,30] umbilical-placental blood flow is about $200\,ml\cdot min^{-1}kg^{-1}$ body weight, and body blood flow is about $250\,ml\cdot min^{-1}kg^{-1}$. The right ventricle ejects about two thirds and the left ventricle about one third of combined ventricular output in the fetal lamb. Figure 24.6 shows the percentages of the combined ventricular output ejected by each ventricle and the proportions passing through various vascular channels. Figure 24.7 indicates the vol-

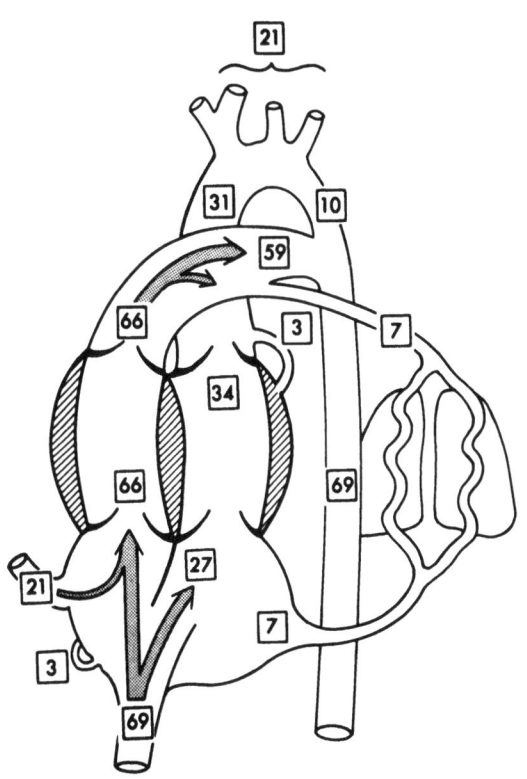

FIGURE 24.6. Percentages of combined ventricular output (CVO) ejected by each ventricle and flowing through chambers and vessels of the fetal lamb heart. The left ventricle ejects only 34%, whereas the right ventricle ejects 66% of CVO. More than half of the CVO passes through the ductus arteriosus (59%) to the descending aorta, and only 10% of the CVO traverses the aortic isthmus. (From Rudolph,[137] with permission.)

TABLE 24.1. Organ blood flow and proportionate distribution of combined ventricular output for organs in the late-gestation fetal lamb under normal in utero conditions.

Organ	Blood flow (ml·100g^{-1}·min^{-1})	% Combined ventricular output
Brain	83 ± 20	2.6 ± 0.6
Myocardium	173 ± 41	2.3 ± 0.5
Gut	57 ± 8	5.8 ± 0.3
Kidney	146 ± 23	1.8 ± 0.2
Lung	87 ± 18	5.4 ± 1.2
Peripheral circulation	30 ± 5	38.6 ± 1.7

Values are means ± SE.
Data are from Rudolph and Heymann.[30]

umes of blood ejected and passing through vessels and shunts.

In the fetus, pressures in the aortic and pulmonary arteries are almost identical. Blood flow to various fetal organs and to the umbilical-placental circulation is determined by local vascular resistance. This parameter is influenced by the size, or cross-sectional area, of the vascular bed and by the degree of vascular constriction or dilatation. The proportions of combined ventricular output and blood flows to organs under normal in utero conditions in the sheep fetus are shown in Table 24.1.

Differences Between Sheep and Humans

Few measurements of cardiac output have been made in the human fetus. Doppler blood flow measurements of left and right ventricular output have been reported, but they are variable.[28,32] A major difference between the human and sheep fetus is the size of the head and brain. Because blood flow to the brain is large in relation to tissue mass, the difference in brain weight could have a marked influence on blood flow patterns. In the sheep fetus the brain represents about 2% of body weight, compared with about 10% in the human fetus. Near term, both human and sheep fetal body weights are about 3.5 kg, and brain weights are about 65 g in the sheep and 350 g in the human. If it is assumed that blood flows to the brain are similar in relation to tissue weight at 120 ml·100g^{-1}·min^{-1}, total brain flows would be 80 ml/min in the sheep and 420 ml/min in the human, or 22 and 120 ml·min^{-1}kg^{-1}, respectively. Because the brain receives its blood supply from the left ventricle, the output of the left ventricle would be at least 250 ml·min^{-1}kg^{-1} body weight. If it is assumed that blood flow to the other body organs and to the placenta are similar in the human and sheep fetuses, the right/left ventricular output ratio would be 1.2:1.0 in the human compared with 2:1 in the sheep.

Regulation of Cardiac Output in the Fetus

The factors that determine ventricular output are heart rate and stroke volume. Stroke volume is influenced by preload, afterload, and myocardial contractility. Extensive studies in isolated myocardial strips and intact hearts have confirmed the importance of the initial length of the myocyte, which influences sarcomere length, in determining the force of muscle contraction. In the intact heart, ventricular volume at end-diastole determines sarcomere length and the force of contraction, and it is the basis of the Frank-Starling mechanism. An increase in initial length or increase in end-diastolic ventricular volume increases the force of contraction of the muscle and, in the intact heart, increases stroke volume if other factors are unchanged. Afterload, or load on the muscle during development of active force, determines the degree of shortening. In the intact circulation, afterload is influenced by several factors (e.g., arterial pressure, compliance of the arterial system, and peripheral vascular resistance). The greater the afterload, the less the degree of muscle shortening and, in the intact heart, the smaller the stroke volume. Contractility is the intrinsic force of contraction of the muscle; with isolated muscle, increased contractility increases the force developed and, in the intact heart, increases stroke volume, or developed pressure. In the cardiovascular system, changing one of the parameters that influence ventricular output may have considerable effect on other factors; it is important to consider possible changes in other parameters when assessing the effects of alteration of one regulatory factor.

Effects of Heart Rate

In the adult circulation, cardiac output remains relatively stable over a wide range of heart rates. With resting rates of about 70 beats per minute (bpm), increasing the rate to 150 bpm or decreasing it to 50 bpm does not alter output. Further increases in heart rate may be associated with a decrease in cardiac output because diastolic filling time is shortened so markedly the ventricles do not receive adequate input to maintain stroke volume. With very slow heart rates, stroke volume is increased to maintain cardiac output, but when maximal diastolic filling has been achieved, further slowing results in a reduction of output.

In studies on the sheep fetus an electromagnetic flow transducer was applied around the ascending aorta or pulmonary trunk to measure left or right ventricular output.[20] It was found that spontaneous increases in heart rate above the resting level of about 160 bpm are associated with ventricular output increases of up to 15% to 20%, and that spontaneous decreases in heart rate results in a fall in output. Because the cause of the spontaneous heart rate change was not known, it is difficult to account for the changes in output on the basis of heart rate change alone. Attempts to examine effects of induced changes in heart rate were made by pacing the right or left atrium to increase the rate and stimulating the cervical vagus nerve to decrease the rate. Pacing the right atrium to increase rates to 240 to 300 bpm results in an increase of up to 15% in left ventricular output and a somewhat lesser increase in right ventricular output. At rates above 300 to 320 bpm, ventricular output falls progressively with increasing rate, presumably because diastolic filling time is too short. When the left atrium is paced, right ventricular output increases, but left ventricular output falls, often dramatically, by 50% or more. These alterations result from a change in phasic pressure relations between the right and left atria. Normally the pressure pulses of the right and left atria are similar in the fetus, with a dominant *a* wave in both chambers, and the right atrial pressure minimally higher than the left in all phases of the cardiac cycle. During pacing the left atrial pressure pulse is altered so the left atrial pressure exceeds that in the right atrium during some phases of the cycle and interferes with flow through the foramen ovale into the left atrium, reducing the left ventricular filling and output.

When heart rate is reduced by stimulating the vagus nerve in the neck, right and left ventricular output falls. Reducing the heart rate to 120 to 140 bpm results in 15% to 20% decrease in cardiac output. Stroke volume increases initially but does not rise with further reductions in rate, so the output falls considerably. Although initial interpretations ascribed this fall to an inability of the fetal myocardium to generate adequate force to increase the stroke output, complex changes in aortic and intrapleural pressures are associated with the vagal stimulation. Aortic pressure initially rises and then increases progressively over 20 to 50 seconds, and intrapleural pressure likewise increases progressively. These concurrent changes could be responsible for the decrease in ventricular output: the increase in aortic pressure could increase afterload, and the increase in intrapleural pressure could effectively decrease venous return and atrial filling. Both these events could contribute to or account for the fall in ventricular output.

Effect of Preload and Afterload

The factors regulating cardiac ventricular output (i.e., preload and afterload) are discussed together because in the intact cardiovascular system there is usually an interaction between them. If afterload is increased, the volume ejected by the ventricle during systole would be reduced and residual ventricular volume would be greater. If volume flowing into the ventricle is maintained, preload would be greater with the next beat. In utero studies of fetal lambs have been performed to assess the role of preload on cardiac output. Because the current methods of measuring ventricular volume in intact animals are not optimal, ventricular end-diastolic or atrial pressures have usually been used as an index of preload. Pressure measurements should be used with caution because at any pressure level the volume is related to ventricular compliance. Studies in isolated myocardium[33] and intact hearts[34] have shown that fetal myocardium is less compliant than that of the adult. In addition, measurement of intracavity pressure alone could further complicate interpretation because the transmural pressure would determine ventricular volume; pericardial pressure could importantly influence the volume of the ventricle.

Studies of fetal lambs in utero have been reported in which preload has been reduced by bleeding the fetus to reduce blood volume and ventricular filling pressure and has been increased by rapid infusion of volume.[21,35,36] Gilbert[35] measured combined ventricular output, whereas Thornburg and Morton[21] and Heymann and Rudolph[36] measured left or right ventricular output with electromagnetic flowmeters. Reducing atrial filling pressure or ventricular end-diastolic pressure results in a marked decrease in ventricular output. Increasing filling pressure by volume infusion is associated with a small increase in output with pressure increases of 2 to 3 mm Hg above resting levels, but further increases in pressure do not cause additional increases in ventricular output, even when filling pressures of 15 to 20 mm Hg are achieved (Figure 24.8). Although heart rate was not regulated in Gilbert's studies, to compensate for changes in rate he examined the relation of filling pressure to calculated stroke volume. Thornburg and Morton maintained a relatively constant heart rate by pretreatment with propranolol, a β-adrenergic blocker, and atropine, a parasympathetic blocker.

Based on these studies, the concept was generated that although the fetal heart exhibits the expected Frank-Starling response at pressures below or slightly above filling pressures, it is limited in its ability to further increase the output with greater filling, which is indicative of restricted myocardial performance or contractility. Several possible explanations for poor myocardial contractility in the fetus have been considered (vide infra). However, Kirkpatrick et al.[37] and Anderson et al.,[38] using different methods for assessing the fetal ventricular response to filling pressures, concluded that left ventricular end-diastolic volume does modulate stroke volume over a "physiological range of filling pressures."

In the studies of Gilbert[35] and of Thornburg and Morton[21,22] the effects of afterload changes on the shape of the ventricular function curves were described by examining the effects of increasing peripheral vascular resistance using methoxamine or phenylephrine or reducing vascular resistance with nitroprusside or

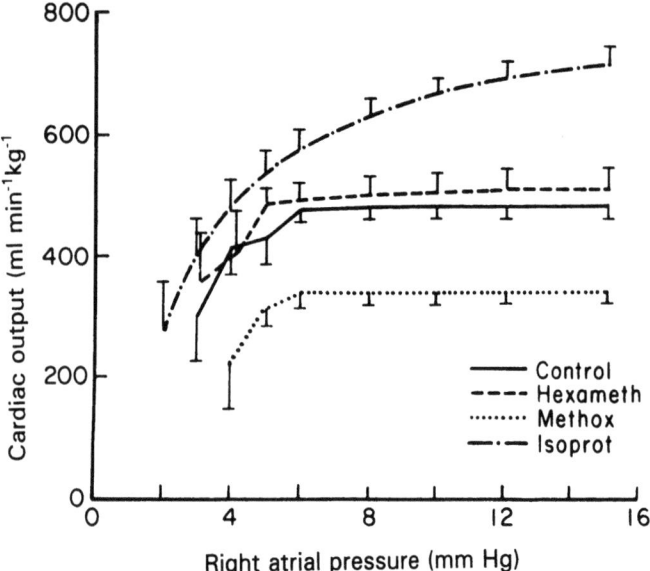

FIGURE 24.8. Response of cardiac output of fetal lambs to changes in right atrial mean pressure decreased by reducing the blood volume by hemorrhage and increased by rapid intravenous infusion. Note that in the control state the cardiac output falls with a decrease of right atrial pressure, but it does not increase when right atrial pressure is raised above 6 mm Hg. Methoxamine, a peripheral vasoconstrictor, reduces cardiac output at the same filling pressure, whereas isoproterenol, a β-adrenoreceptor stimulant, increases cardiac output at similar atrial pressures. (From Gilbert,[138] with permission.)

hexamethonium. In these studies it was observed that reducing afterload raises the whole function curve above the resting curve, but increasing afterload lowers the curve below the resting curve (Figure 24.8). The shape of the curves did not change substantially, and they still showed flattening at atrial filling pressures above the resting values. In all these studies the atrial pressures were increased by rapid fluid infusion, and systemic and pulmonary arterial pressures increased considerably. The effects of this increase in pressure, which probably increased afterload, on the shape of the ventricular function curves was not considered.

In a study in chronically instrumented fetal lambs in which heart rate was controlled, the relations between left ventricular output, left atrial pressure, and aortic pressure were examined by Hawkins et al.[39] This study showed that, at constant left atrial pressure, increasing aortic pressure results in a linear fall of left ventricular output. At any specific level of aortic mean pressure, increasing left atrial pressures are associated with a progressive increase of left ventricular output, even to mean pressures of 10 mm Hg or more. It is apparent that the fetal heart does increase its output above resting atrial filling pressure in response to increased pressure, but that it is sensitive to an increase in afterload.

Myocardial Contractility

Studies of isolated myocardium from fetal and adult sheep have demonstrated that fetal myocardium develops less active tension than adult myocardium at similar muscle lengths. The maximal force that can be generated is considerably lower for fetal than for adult myocardium.[40–42] Several differences in morphologic and biochemical parameters of myocardium have been described that could account for the lesser contractility of fetal myocardium. Friedman[33] has suggested that fetal myocardium contains fewer sarcomeres, or contractile units, in each myocyte, and that a large volume of fetal myocytes is taken up by nuclei and mitochondria, compared with adult myocytes. The earlier in gestation, the less organized is the arrangement of the myofibrils; in the adult heart there is a uniform parallel orientation, whereas in the fetus, particularly during early gestation, there is disorganization of the myofibrillar pattern.[43]

The sarcoplasmic reticulum is important in providing calcium ions, which are essential for myocardial contraction. The fetal myocardial sarcoplasmic reticulum is less well developed than that in the adult,[41,44] but the T-tubular system, representing the extension of the sarcoplasmic reticulum to provide closer relations with the contractile elements, is either poorly developed or absent in immature myocardium.[44–47] Not only are there structural differences in sarcoplasmic reticulum, but in studies with isolated sarcoplasmic reticulum vesicles Mahony[48] has shown that calcium uptake is impaired in fetal myocardium.

Local release of norepinephrine at sympathetic nerve endings is an important mechanism for increasing myocardial contractility. Morphologic studies of fetal hearts using monoamine oxidase fluorescence have demonstrated absent or poor innervation of the immature myocardium. The abundance of sympathetic nerve endings varies greatly at different periods of gestational and postnatal development among species. In the guinea pig, myocardial sympathetic innervation is almost fully developed at birth,[49] whereas in the rabbit[41] and the rat there is almost no innervation at birth; it develops within 14 to 21 postnatal days. The sheep fetus has no detectable sympathetic innervation at 75 days (i.e., mid-gestation), but innervation begins to appear at 90 to 100 days and is abundant but not yet fully developed just before birth.[50]

In addition to the difference in sympathetic innervation, possible differences in β-adrenoreceptor concentration in fetal and adult myocardium have been postulated.[51] Although Cheng et al.[51] could not demonstrate β-adrenoreceptor concentration differences between fetal and adult myocardium in sheep, Chen et al.[52] showed that β-receptors were markedly reduced in fetal mouse myocardium compared with those in the adult. Although these differences in sympathetic innervation and β-adrenoreceptor concentration may not be important in the resting fetal heart, they could influence the ability to respond to stress.

Circulatory Regulation in the Fetus

In the adult circulation the systemic and pulmonary circulations are separate. Each ventricle is subjected to potentially different preload and afterload, and the stroke volume of each ventricle could vary greatly. The Frank-Starling mechanism is useful for adjusting the outputs of the two ventricles so that over a short period the ventricles eject similar volumes. A reduction in venous return to the right atrium would reduce filling pressure and end-diastolic volume of the right ventricle, which would decrease stroke volume. This situation would alter pulmonary blood flow and venous return to the left atrium and ventricle, which in turn would reduce its stroke volume. An increase in systemic arterial pressure would restrict left ventricular stroke volume; end-diastolic volume would increase so that, with the next beat, greater force would be generated to increase stroke volume.

In the fetus the presence of the foramen ovale tends to make right and left atrial pressures equal throughout the cardiac cycle. The ductus arteriosus provides a large communication between the aorta and pulmonary artery, which causes the pressures to be almost identical. During late gestation in fetal lambs, pulmonary trunk pressure may be higher by a few torr than the aortic pressure, probably as a result of increasing constriction of the ductus arteriosus, although it could be related to slower growth of the vessel compared with that of the aorta or pulmonary artery. In view of the similar atrial pressures and similar aortic and pulmonary arterial pressures, the differences in stroke volumes of the left and right ventricles in the fetal lamb are difficult to explain. A possible reason could be that the afterloads of the two ventricles are different, even though pressures are the same. The aortic isthmus, which in the fetus is narrower than the ascending the descending aorta, might functionally separate the upper and lower body circulations. The left ventricle ejects into the ascending aorta and the vessels of the head and neck, a circulation that would be poorly compliant and have a relatively high vascular resistance. The right ventricle ejects into the pulmonary trunk and directly through the large ductus arteriosus into the descending aorta and its branches. This circulation would have a higher compliance and a lower resistance because it includes the umbilical-placental vasculature. Another possible explanation relates to flow patterns in the region of the aortic isthmus and ductus arteriosus, resulting from the velocity of flow from the left and right ventricles. The distance from the pulmonary valve to the ductus arteriosus and descending aorta is short, whereas that from the aortic valve to this region is much longer. The time it takes for blood to reach the junction of the ductus with the descending aorta following ejection of the two ventricles could affect flow patterns during late systole.

Baroreflex Regulation

In the adult the arterial baroreflex modulates arterial pressure over a fairly narrow range. When arterial pressure is increased, the aortic and carotid baroreceptors respond to result in reflex bradycardia, depression of myocardial contractility, and peripheral vasodilatation, all of which tend to decrease arterial pressure. When the aortic and carotid baroreflexes are abolished by bilateral section of the aortic and carotid afferent nerves, there is initially an increase in resting heart rate and arterial pressure, but within 1 to 2 days these parameters return to average levels during the predenervation period. Wide swings of arterial pressure and heart rate occur around the average pressure and rate, in association with stimuli that produce small changes in the normal animal.[53] The function of the arterial baroreceptors in the fetus has been controversial. In fetal lambs the baroreflex sensitivity has been shown to increase with gestational age from about 80 days' gestation, but near term it is as sensitive as in the neonate and adult in terms of the bradycardia induced by arterial pressure increase.[54] It has been suggested that the fetal lamb responds only to large increases in arterial pressure, and that under normal in utero conditions these large alterations of pressure do not occur because the arterial pressure is buffered by the highly compliant umbilical-placental circulation.

To assess the importance of the baroreflex in normal regulation of fetal arterial pressure and heart rate, Itskovitz et al.[55] studied chronically instrumented fetal lambs several days after bilateral section of the aortic and carotid sinus nerves. These lambs show the same wide variation in heart rate and blood pressure that develops in adult animals with sinoaortic denervation. The index of variability described by Guyton et al.[53,56] is similar in fetal lambs and adult sheep, indicating that the baroreflex is fully operative in regulating arterial pressure in the late-gestation fetal lamb.

Chemoreflex Regulation

Based on studies in acutely exteriorized lambs, it had been proposed that the aortic and carotid chemoreceptors are relatively inactive in the fetus.[57-60] Blanco et al.[61] showed that the chemoreceptors do respond to hypoxemia in fetal lambs, predominantly with a cardiorespiratory response manifested by bradycardia. In contrast to the studies by Dawes et al.[58] and Jansen and Chernick,[59,60] Goodlin and Rudolph[62] found that injection of cyanide or nicotine in small amounts results in chemoreceptor stimulation. They attempted to distinguish the carotid and aortic chemoreflex responses. Stimulation of aortic chemoreceptors consistently results in bradycardia and a fall in arterial pressure during the bradycardia, with a subsequent increase in pressure. Carotid chemoreceptor stimulation produces variable responses: tachycardia with hypertension usually results after cyanide stimulation, although bradycardia with hypotension sometimes occurs; and there are variable respiratory responses of single or short bursts of respiratory effort. In studies in chronically instrumented fetal lambs, Itskovitz and Rudolph[63] showed that the chemoreceptors could be stimulated by small quantities of sodium cyanide, indicating that the chemoreceptors are sensitive. The cardiovascular response dominates, with bradycardia and immediate hypotension, but respiratory gasps or, rarely, sequences of respiratory effort are noted. The bradycardia can be abolished if the lambs are pretreated with atropine, indicating that the bradycardia is induced by vagus nerve stimulation. Confirmation of the fact that the cyanide response is the result of chemoreceptor stimulation was obtained by demonstrating the loss of the cardiovascular and respiratory responses in fetal lambs in which sinoaortic denervation had been accomplished.

Recent studies in fetal lambs have shown that the fall in heart rate during acute fetal hypoxemia or cyanide injection is induced by carotid sinus nerve stimulation, and that the aortic nerve is not involved in the responses.[64]

In the adult, chemoreceptor stimulation may be associated with reflex peripheral vasoconstriction. This response has not been studied adequately in the fetus, but it can be inferred that the marked vasoconstriction induced in the peripheral circulation during hypoxia in fetal lambs (vide infra) is partly the result of chemoreceptor stimulation. It is apparent from studies in the fetal lamb that chemoreflex responses are different from those in the adult. The respiratory response in the adult animal dominates, whereas only minor and unsustained respiratory response results in the fetus. Whether it is due to a difference in chemoreceptor response or a difference in central response has not been resolved.

Fetal Circulatory Response to Reduced Oxygen Delivery

The most important stresses placed on the fetus are those related to reduced delivery of oxygen. Oxygen delivery may be decreased by several mechanisms. Maternal arterial oxygen content may be reduced by lung disease in the mother; uterine blood flow may be decreased by either a fall in maternal cardiac output or local factors affecting uterine flow; inadequate placental mass or a placental diffusion disturbance may impede oxygen transport to the fetus; and reduced umbilical blood flow resulting from umbilical cord compression may obstruct umbilical venous return or umbilical arterial supply to the placenta, or both. Much of our knowledge of the effects of reduced oxygen supply on the fetus has been derived from studies in sheep, in which the effect of either complete occlusion of the umbilical cord or decreased maternal arterial oxygen content by administering low-oxygen gas mixtures to the ewe has been examined.

Effects on Oxygen Consumption and Extraction

When fetal oxygen delivery is reduced by maternal hypoxemia or by reducing uterine blood flow, umbilical venous oxygen content falls, but umbilical-placental blood flow is maintained (vide infra). Because total oxygen delivery to the fetus is the product of umbilical blood flow and umbilical venous oxygen content, oxygen delivery is reduced in proportion to the fall in umbilical venous oxygen content.[65,66] When umbilical blood flow is reduced by cord compression, umbilical venous oxygen content does not change significantly, so oxygen delivery is decreased in proportion to the fall in umbilical blood flow.[67]

Reducing oxygen delivery to the fetus by about 50%, by either uterine blood flow restriction or deceasing umbilical venous return, has little effect on fetal oxygen consumption because oxygen extraction increases. The increased extraction is not able to compensate for reductions in oxygen delivery of more than 50%, and oxygen consumption falls precipitously with further decreases in delivery.[67] Normally the fetal lamb extracts about 30% of delivered oxygen, an amount similar to that extracted in the adult. With progressive reduction in oxygen delivery, the fetal lamb has a remarkable ability to extract oxygen, despite the low Po_2 of the blood; with a 75% reduction in oxygen delivery, oxygen extraction is increased to an average of 66%, but in some fetuses extraction reaches 75% to 80%.

Heart Rate and Blood Pressure

In fetal lambs beyond about 110 days' gestation (term is about 145 days), acute hypoxemia produced by administering a low-oxygen gas mixture to the ewe[65] or by reducing uterine blood flow by either arterial occlusion[66] or decreasing the umbilical blood flow[68] results in bradycardia and arterial hypertension. In one study a change of 4 to 5 torr in carotid arterial blood was necessary to produce bradycardia.[68] Recently it has been shown that the magnitude of the bradycardia is directly related to the degree of fall in oxygen saturation of carotid arterial blood.[69] The bradycardia induced by hypoxemia can be abolished by atropine administration, indicating that it is induced reflexly through vagal stimulation. With extreme changes in Po_2, to levels below about 12 torr, the bradycardia cannot be completely prevented by atropine. It has been suggested that with severe hypoxemia the heart is affected directly, producing bradycardia.[68] In the studies with maternal hypoxemia, the changes in fetal heart rate and blood pressure develop after several minutes, and the time relations between their onset are difficult to define. It was first conjectured that the hypertension might be the primary change, related to catecholamine-induced vasoconstriction, and that the bradycardia is a baroreflex response. In studies in which either acute compression of the umbilical cord or acute reduction of uterine blood flow is induced, it is clear that the bradycardia consistently precedes an increase in arterial pressure, suggesting that chemoreflexes are primarily responsible for hypoxemic bradycardia.[67,68] When hypertension occurs, it may contribute to the bradycardia. When severe umbilical cord compression is induced, arterial compression produces an immediate rise in arterial pressure with marked bradycardia, and in this circumstance the baroreflex is involved early.[67] In chronic sinoaortic-denervated fetal lambs, bradycardia does not occur during hypoxemia, adding further support to the role of the aortic and carotid chemoreceptors in this response.[66,70]

When hypoxemia is maintained in the fetus during maternal hypoxemia, within 15 to 30 minutes the heart rate recovers somewhat and blood pressure begins to fall. By about 1 hour after onset of hypoxemia, blood pressure frequently returns to control values and the heart rate might have recovered completely but is usually somewhat decreased compared with the control rate. The mechanism for this recovery is not defined, but it could be due to resetting of chemoreceptor sensitivity.

Studies of the responses to hypoxemia in young fetuses at a gestational age of 85 to 100 days show no decrease of heart rate or increase in arterial pressure bradycardia. The lack of bradycardia in these young fetuses has not been explained, but it could be due to the lack of a chemoreceptor response.[71]

Hepatic and Ductus Venosus Blood Flows

Normally in the fetal lamb about 45% of umbilical venous blood passes through the liver, and 55% enters the ductus venosus. With maternal hypoxemia and with reduced uterine blood flow, a somewhat greater proportion (about 65%) of umbilical venous blood passes through the ductus venosus.[66,72] However, when umbilical blood flow as reduced by 50% there is a dramatic fall in hepatic blood flow, and the proportion of umbilical venous blood that passes through the ductus venosus increases bradycardia.[73] Hepatic blood flow falls by only a modest amount during maternal hypoxemia or uterine blood flow reduction but decreases markedly when umbilical blood flow is reduced (Figure 24.9).

Combined Ventricular Output and Blood Flow Distribution

Hypoxemia induced by reducing maternal arterial oxygen content, decreasing uterine blood flow, or umbilical cord compression is associated with the rapid onset of a 15% to 20% fall in combined ventricular output.[65,66,73] Left and right ventricular outputs fall, and the decrease is associated with bradycardia and a variable, small decrease in stroke volume. The cardiac output gradually begins to recover within 15 to 20 minutes, and by 60 minutes after onset of hypoxemia it has returned to control values. The mechanisms responsible for this reduction in cardiac output have not been defined. It could be related to the increase in afterload associated with peripheral vasoconstriction, to the bradycardia, to a direct vagal myocardial depressant effect, or to a local hypoxic myocardial depression. With mild hypoxemia, atropine administration abolishes both the bradycardia and the decreased cardiac output, indicating that vagal stimulation is involved. With more severe hypoxemia, atropine does not abolish the fall in output completely.

During maternal hypoxemia and uterine blood flow reduction, umbilical-placental blood flow is maintained so the decrease in combined ventricular output is related entirely to a reduction in fetal body flow. Whereas cardiac output falls by 15% to 20%, body flow is reduced by 35% to 40%.[65,66]

With acute umbilical cord compression, which results in a 50% fall in umbilical venous return and umbilical-placental blood flow, combined ventricular output does not change significantly, and fetal body blood flow is not altered.[73]

The distribution of cardiac output is modified to maintain blood flow to vital organs, but flows to most other fetal body organs are reduced. The proportion of cardiac output and the blood flows to the brain, myocardium, and adrenal gland, are increased considerably, and oxygen delivery is maintained to these organs.[6,66,73] With milder degrees of maternal hypoxemia or reduced uterine blood flow, the proportion of cardiac output distributed to the peripheral circulation (e.g., skin, muscle, bone) is reduced somewhat, but blood flow to the other body organs is maintained. With more severe maternal hypoxemia or reduced uterine blood flow sufficient to reduce oxygen delivery to the fetus by 50%, the proportion of cardiac output and actual blood flows to the kidney, gastrointestinal tract, lung, and peripheral circulation are greatly reduced (Figure. 24.10). In contrast, when umbilical

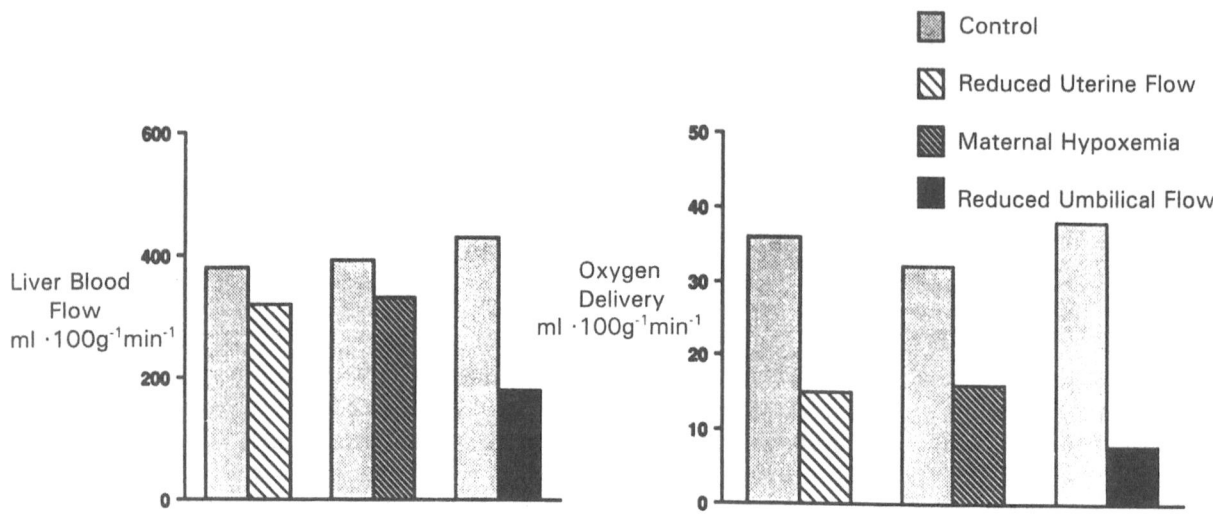

FIGURE 24.9. Effects of various mechanisms of reducing oxygen supply to the fetal lamb to 50% of control level: blood flow and oxygen delivery to the liver. See text for detailed description.

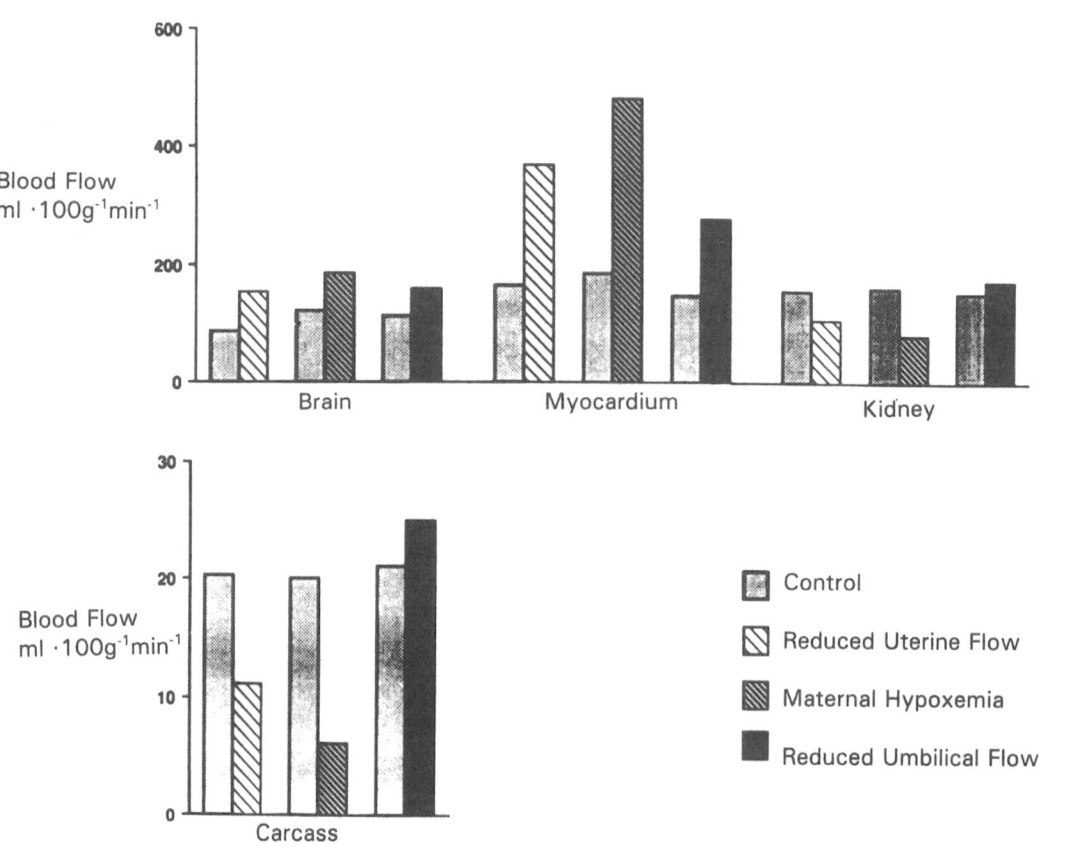

FIGURE 24.10. Effects of various mechanisms of reducing oxygen supply to the fetal lamb to 50% of control levels: blood flow to the brain, myocardium, kidney, and peripheral circulation (carcass).

blood flow is reduced acutely by 50%, which results in a 50% reduction in oxygen delivery to the fetus, pulmonary blood flow is reduced, but there is no significant change in the blood flow to the kidneys, gastrointestinal tract, or peripheral circulation.

The differences in circulatory responses to reducing oxygen supply to the fetus by umbilical cord compression, compared with decreasing maternal arterial oxygen content or uterine blood flow, are of considerable interest because not only is oxygen delivery to tissues maintained but substrate supplies may be different. Although the mechanisms for these differences have not been delineated, it is possible that different degrees of stimulation of the chemoreflexes may be responsible. With maternal hypoxemia and reduced uterine blood flow, umbilical venous Po_2 and oxygen content are reduced. Because umbilical venous blood passes through the ductus venosus and is preferentially distributed through the foramen ovale, the decreased umbilical venous oxygen saturation leads to a marked decrease in carotid arterial oxygen saturation. When umbilical-placental blood flow is reduced, umbilical venous oxygen saturation is maintained. Because a large proportion of umbilical venous blood is shunted through the ductus venosus and then through the foramen ovale preferentially, the fall in carotid arterial oxygen saturation is considerably smaller than with maternal hypoxemia or reduced uterine blood flow. In a series of animals in which uterine blood flow was reduced, causing a 50% decrease in oxygen delivery to the fetus, carotid arterial oxygen saturation fell from 67% to 29%, a decrease of 38%.[66] When oxygen delivery was reduced by 50% by decreasing umbilical blood flow, the carotid arterial oxygen saturation fell from 62% to 40%, a fall of only 22%.[73] Chemoreflex stimulation would be greater with uterine blood flow reduction and with arterial hypoxemia, and it would result in intense peripheral vasoconstriction.

Circulatory Changes After Birth

After birth, the process of gas exchange is transferred from the placenta to the lungs. The umbilical-placental circulation is abolished, and adequate blood flow must be directed to the lungs to permit oxygen uptake and carbon dioxide removal. In addition, to achieve separation of the systemic and pulmonary circulation, the ductus arteriosus and foramen ovale must close. During fetal life, body temperature is maintained by the pregnant female, but after birth the neonate must increase metabolism to maintain temperature. Measurements in fetal and neonatal lambs have demonstrated that fetal oxygen consumption is 6 to $8 ml \cdot min^{-1} kg^{-1}$ body weight. After birth it increases to 15 to $20 ml \cdot min^{-1} kg^{-1}$, the value depending on environmental temperature. Cardiac output tends to be closely related to metabolism, reflected by oxygen consumption, and in the lamb there is a considerable increase in cardiac output after birth (vide infra).

Fetal and Neonatal Pulmonary Circulation

The fetal lungs of the late-gestation lamb receive only 8% to 10% of the combined ventricular output, which represents a flow to the lungs of 35 to $45 ml \cdot min^{-1} kg^{-1}$ fetal body weight. When the series circulation of the adult has been established, the total cardiac output passes through the lung. In neonatal lambs during the first postnatal week, cardiac outputs of 300 to $420 ml \cdot min^{-1} kg^{-1}$ have been reported; thus, pulmonary blood flow increases about 10-fold after birth.[74-76] The exact mechanisms responsible for maintaining the high pulmonary vascular resistance in the fetus and for the dramatic decrease in resistance at birth have not been fully defined. Morphologically, the precapillary vessels of the fetal lung are characterized by a thick medial muscular layer in arterioles of 25 to $50 \mu m$ diameter.[77-80] It had been thought that the medial muscle layer increases in thickness during the latter portion of gestation,[81] but subsequent studies of lamb[78] and human[80] fetal lungs during the second half of gestation fail to show major changes in the thickness of the muscle layer in the arterioles.

Measurements of pulmonary blood flow and pressures have been made acutely in chronically instrumented fetal lamb preparations. Pulmonary arterial pressure is similar to aortic pressure, and both increase during gestation from a mean level of about 39 mm Hg at 80 days' gestation to about 55 mm Hg near term.[30,82] Pulmonary blood flow not only increases progressively with fetal growth, but the blood flow per unit of lung mass increases greatly, from about 40 to about $125 ml \cdot min^{-1} \cdot 100 g^{-1}$ lung weight over the gestational period of 60 days to term. Calculated pulmonary vascular resistance falls dramatically over this period, from 6.0 to $0.3 mm Hg \cdot ml^{-1} min^{-1} \cdot 100 g^{-1}$ lung.[82] The change in pulmonary vascular resistance, representing an increase in total cross-sectional area of the pulmonary vascular bed, is not related to lung growth alone but to a marked increase in the number of vascular units in the same lung volume. In the lamb, Levin et al.[78] found that the number of fifth- to sixth-generation vessels increases from 7.2×10^3 to 61.8×10^3 per milliliter of lung tissue from 85 to 140 days' gestation.[78]

Fetal pulmonary vessels are exposed to Po_2 and Pco_2 of pulmonary arterial blood. In the lamb, pulmonary arterial Po_2 is about 18 torr during the latter third of gestation. It had been conjectured that the relatively low Po_2 is responsible for maintaining fetal pulmonary vasoconstriction, and then at birth ventilation with air increases the Po_2, resulting in vasodilatation. The fact that alveolar ventilation can influence precapillary vessels has been explained by the observation that blood is oxygenated in small precapillary arterioles by diffusion through the wall from surrounding alveoli in adult lungs.[74] Several investigators have examined the role of expansion of the lungs with air. In late-gestation lambs, rhythmic expansion of the lungs with gas that does not change fetal arterial blood gases (3% O_2/5% CO_2 in nitrogen), produces a small increase in pulmonary vascular conductance, but ventilation with air causes pulmonary vascular resistance to increase dramatically.[83,84] It is estimated that physical expasion of the lung with gas could account for only about 30% of the decrease in pulmonary vascular resistance, with oxygen being the dominant factor. Studies were conducted in late-gestation lambs in which pulmonary ventilation was performed in chronically instrumented fetal lambs in utero.[85] Rhythmic ventilation with a gas with about 3% O_2 and 5% CO_2 in nitrogen, which does not significantly alter fetal pulmonary arterial blood gases, results in a marked decrease in mean pulmonary vascular resistance. Ventilation with oxygen increases Po_2 dramatically without altering Pco_2 and causes a further decrease in vascular resistance. Examination of the responses of individual animals is of great interest; in about half of the studies the effects of rhythmic ventilation alone are almost as great or as great as those achieved with ventilation with oxygen to increase Po_2.

These findings clearly demonstrate that postnatal pulmonary vasodilatation may result from two distinct mechanisms; whether the final mediators released by physical expansion with gas and by oxygen are the same has yet to be resolved (vide infra). Lung expansion with air may reduce pulmonary vascular resistance through a mechanical effect. When the alveoli are distended with gas, a gas-fluid interface develops on the alveolar surface, and surface tension forces tend to collapse the alveoli. This situation could exert a force, pulling the alveoli walls inward and distending vessels surrounded by alveoli.

Several vasoactive mechanisms have been proposed for producing postnatal pulmonary vasodilatation, involving either release of a vasodilator or removal of a vasoconstrictor. Bradykinin has been shown to be a potent pulmonary vasodilator in the fetus.[86,87] After birth, plasma bradykinin concentration increases. Heymann et al.[87] showed that increasing fetal blood Po_2 concentration by placing the ewe in a hyperbaric chamber results in a decrease in kininogen, a precursor of bradykinin across the lungs, and is associated with a fall in pulmonary vascular resistance. Leffler et al.[88] suggested that prostaglandins are released from the lung in response to gaseous expansion. Prostacyclin (prostaglandin I_2; PGI_2) is a potent pulmonary vasodilator, and an increase in plasma concentrations across the lung is detected in association with ventilation.[89] It is apparent that PGI_2 alone is not responsible for postnatal pulmonary vasodilation because indomethacin, a prostaglandin synthesis inhibitor, does not abolish the decrease in pulmonary vascular resistance associated with ventilation. It does affect the initial immediate decrease that occurs in 30 to 60 seconds but does not influence the subsequent drop in resistance.[90]

Leukotrienes (LT), particularly LTD_4, are potent pulmonary vasoconstrictors.[91,92] The concept has been presented that leukotrienes are responsible for maintaining pulmonary vasoconstriction in utero, and that either inhibition of leukotriene production or interference with its action results in the decreased pulmonary vascular resistance at birth. Inhibitors of leukotriene synthesis or putative leukotriene blockers have been shown to reduce pulmonary vascular resistance in the normal fetal lamb in utero, with a resultant increase in pulmonary blood flow almost equal to that produced by ventilation in utero.[93] Although these vasoactive agents could be implicated in regulating the pulmonary circulation during the perinatal period, their role has not been conclusively demonstrated.

A vasoactive dilator substance released by endothelial cells, endothelial relaxing factor (EDRF), which has been identified as nitric oxide, has an important role in regulating the pulmonary circulation during the fetal and neonatal periods. Blockade of the release of nitric oxide from arginine by the inhibitor nitro-N-arginine causes pulmonary vasoconstriction in the sheep fetus. It also appears that the vasodilator effect of oxygen on the fetal pulmonary circulation can be related, at least in part, to nitric oxide influence, because the inhibitor nitro-N-arginine markedly attenuates the drop in pulmonary vascular resistance that occurs when the fetal lamb is ventilated with air or oxygen in utero.[94] The decrease in pulmonary vascular resistance resulting from ventilation with 3% O_2 is not significantly affected by nitric oxide inhalation, but is attenuated by the prostaglandin synthesis inhibitor, indomethacin.[95] Currently it is felt that pulmonary vasodilation after birth is associated with at least two mechanisms: physical expansion of the lungs, which releases a prostaglandin, probably PGI_2, and oxygenation, which releases nitric oxide. Possibly other mechanisms may also be involved.

Ductus Arteriosus

During fetal life blood flows through the ductus arteriosus from the pulmonary artery to the descending aorta. The ductus is exposed to blood with a Po_2 of about 18 torr in the pulmonary artery. After birth, if the ductus arteriosus remains patent, blood flows from the aorta to the pulmonary artery shortly after ventilation has occurred. A murmur characteristic of that associated with aortic-to-pulmonary arterial flow (i.e., a continuous murmur), has been heard in animals[96] and humans[97] soon after birth. Initial closure of the ductus is by constriction; subsequently, the vessel is replaced by fibrous tissue, forming the ligamentum arteriosum. Anatomical closure of the ductus arteriosus in the human is usually complete within 14 days after birth.[98] It had generally been believed that ductus arteriosus patency is maintained in the fetus by the low Po_2 of the blood passing through it, and that it constricts in response to the increase in Po_2 after birth.

Perfusion of the isolated lamb ductus arteriosus with electrolyte solution at varying Po_2 levels shows a progressive increase in resistance with increasing Po_2.[99] The responsiveness to O_2 increases with advancing gestational age: the younger the fetus, the higher the Po_2 required to initiate constriction. The older the fetus, the greater the degree of constriction that could be achieved. In isolated rings of ductus arteriosus derived from fetal lambs, the ductus is most relaxed at a Po_2 of about 20 torr. With increasing Po_2, constriction is first noted at about 35 torr and increases progressively to about 100 torr.[100] Reducing Po_2 in the tissue bath results in constriction, with levels below 15 torr. The mechanism responsible for the constrictor effect of oxygen has not yet been resolved. It was proposed by Fay[101] that oxygen may have a direct effect on cytochrome enzymes, but the possibility that oxygen influences some mediator has not been excluded.

Because bradykinin causes constriction of the umbilical vessels, which respond to oxygen similarly to the ductus arteriosus, the possibility that bradykinin may contribute to ductus closure after birth has been proposed.[102] Vagal stimulation has been invoked as a cause of ductus constriction because the vessel is constricted by acetylcholine.[103]

Prostaglandins of the E series were shown to relax isolated ductus rings.[104] The demonstration that salicylates or other nonsteroidal anti-inflammatory agents could cause constriction of the ductus arteriosus in fetal rodents raised the interesting possibility that prostaglandins are involved in normal regulation of the ductus.[105] These agents inhibit the cyclooxygenase enzyme, which generates the production of endoperoxides from arachidonic acid, so that all prostaglandin production is affected. In the chronically instrumented fetal lamb, acetylsalicylic acid results in ductus arteriosus constriction, as evidenced by a reduction of flow and an elevation of pulmonary arterial above aortic pressure.[106] The fact that the constriction results from inhibition of prostaglandin production is confirmed by the demonstration that the ductus is relaxed by infusion of PGE_1.

The prostaglandins that could be generated by isolated ductus tissue are predominantly PGI_2 (prostacyclin) and smaller amounts of PGE_2.[107] PGI_2 is produced by the endothelium of all arteries and is most likely derived from ductus endothelium. The isolated lamb ductus arteriosus, when maximally constricted by oxygen and indomethacin, is relaxed by both PGI_2 and PGE_2. However, the concentrations of PGI_2 required to produce relaxation are much higher than those of PGE_2.[108] Although the possibility that local production of PGE_2 or PGI_2 may be involved in maintaining patency of the ductus is the fetus in utero has not been completely ruled out, the prevailing opinion is that circulating PGE_2 is responsible. Blood PGE_2 concentration is considerably higher in the fetal lamb than in the adult sheep.[109] There is a rapid fall of PGE_2 concentration during the first 3 hours after birth.[110] The origin of the circulating PGE_2 has not been determined, but because the placenta can produce prostaglandins it appears to be the most likely site. Another factor that could contribute to the fall in PGE_2 concentration is metabolism in the lungs. In the adult, almost all PGE_2 is cleared with one passage of blood through the lungs. Although clearance is not as efficient in the fetus and neonate,[111] establishment of ventilation greatly increases pulmonary blood flow in the neonate so that more prostaglandin is presented to the neonatal lung than to the fetal lung (see Chapter 23).

Constriction of the ductus arteriosus resulting from oxygen and from prostaglandin synthesis inhibition is not due to the same mechanism because their effects are additive. The maximum tension that can be developed by ductus rings isolated from 90- to 100-day fetuses and near-term gestation fetuses is comparable.[112] However, the relative contributions of oxygen and indomethacin are different; in young fetal ductus tissue, oxygen constrictor effect is less than in the older fetus, so that a considerably larger proportion of the constrictor effect is related to indomethacin. This finding has led to the proposal that the ductus is much more sensitive to the relaxant effect of PGE_2 in the young fetus than in the older fetus. It has been hypothesized that this greater sensitivity of the ductus arteriosus of the immature fetus to prostaglandin could be responsible for the high incidence of persistent patency of the ductus arteriosus after birth in prematurely born neonates.[113]

The change in the responsiveness of the ductus with advancing gestation has been ascribed to the influence of cortisol. Studies by Clyman et al.[114] on isolated ductus rings from fetal lambs showed that when the lambs at 120 days' gestation had received a cortisol infusion for 48 hours in utero before preparing the rings, the ductus' response to indomethacin is similar to that in term lambs. In two groups of lambs delivered prematurely at about 120 days' gestation, those that had been treated with cortisol infusion for about 2 days before delivery developed a higher vascular resistance across the ductus, indicating more effective constriction than in the control group.[115] Plasma PGE_2 concentration was similar in the two groups over the first 3 hours postnatally. In fetal lambs, plasma cortisol concentration increases slowly during the latter weeks of gestation[116] and increases markedly 2 to 3 days before delivery.[117] The important role of cortisol in effecting postnatal ductus arteriosus closure is evident in preterm neonates in whom the pregnant woman has been given betamethasone to attempt to reduce the incidence of respiratory distress syndrome. The neonates of these treated women have a lower incidence of difficulties relating to persistent patency of the ductus arteriosus.

The relation between prostaglandin concentrations and ductus arteriosus constriction has been applied clinically. In neonates with cyanotic heart disease and reduced pulmonary blood flow, intravenous infusion of PGE_1 has been effective in maintaining patency of the ductus arteriosus after birth, thereby providing adequate pulmonary blood flow, until such time as surgery can be accomplished.[118] Similarly, it has been effective in neonates with aortic coarctation or aortic arch interruption, where patency of the ductus after birth is important for maintaining blood flow to the lower body.[119] In preterm neonates with persistent patency of the ductus arteriosus, indomethacin has been effective in either closing or constricting the ductus to relieve symptoms relating to its patency in a large proportion of these neonates.[120,121]

Although oxygen and prostaglandins appear to be the main factors regulating ductus arteriosus behavior during fetal and postnatal life, it is possible that other mechanisms are important. The role of adenosine has been considered.[122] Adenosine is though to maintain ductus patency in the fetus; after birth plasma adenosine concentration falls following increased oxygenation.

Cardiac Output

As mentioned above, the combined ventricular output in fetal lambs in utero is about $450 ml \cdot kg^{-1} min^{-1}$, with about $300 ml \cdot kg^{-1}$ ejected by the right ventricle and $150 ml \cdot kg^{-1}$ by the left ventricle. Measurements in awake, resting neonatal lambs have yielded values for cardiac output of 300 to $425 ml \cdot kg^{-1} min^{-1}$. The values have depended to a large extent on environmental temperature: the cooler the environment, the higher the output.[123] Because cardiac output represents the volume of blood flowing through the pulmonary and systemic circulations in series postnatally, the output of the two ventricles is 600 to $850 ml \cdot kg^{-1} min^{-1}$, a considerable increase compared with that of the fetus. The basis for this increase and the mechanisms responsible have not yet been fully defined.

Measurements of cardiac output in lambs over the first 6 to 8 weeks after birth have shown a dramatic fall about 425 to about $160 ml \cdot kg^{-1} min^{-1}$. This change parallels the changes in oxygen consumption.[75] Oxygen consumption during fetal life is 7 to $8 ml \cdot kg^{-1} min^{-1}$, increasing to 16 to $20 ml \cdot kg^{-1} min^{-1}$ after birth and falling to about 6 to $8 ml \cdot kg^{-1} min^{-1}$ over the next 6 to 8 weeks. Few measurements of cardiac output changes in association with the birth process have been made. Breall et al.[124] found that left ventricular output increases from the level of about $170 ml \cdot kg^{-1} min^{-1}$ in the fetus to about $340 ml \cdot kg^{-1} min^{-1}$ within 60 minutes after birth and remains constant over the 6 hours of measurement.[124] They note that oxygen consumption increases to $23 ml \cdot kg^{-1} min^{-1}$ and is stable over the next 6 hours.

In an attempt to examine the role of individual birth events on cardiac output, Teitel et al.[125] simulated birth events in fetal lambs in utero.[125] Catheters were placed in various fetal vessels and cardiac chambers in lambs at about 132 to 134 days' gestation; a tracheal tube was inserted and a balloon-cuff occluder placed around the umbilical cord. All catheters were brought to the exterior of the ewe's flank, and the lamb was studied 2 to 3 days after recovery from surgery. Ventilation with 3% O_2/5% CO_2 does not alter fetal blood gases but results in a marked increase in pulmonary blood flow. It is associated with an increase in left ventricular output but a decrease in right ventricular output, so that combined output does not change (Figure 24.11). Ventilation with 100% O_2 markedly increases fetal arterial Po_2 and further increases pulmonary blood flow and left ventricular output, but because right ventricular output decreases again the combined ventricular output does not change. Subsequent occlusion of the umbilical cord does not alter the combined ventricular output. It is apparent that positive-pressure ventilation, oxygenation, or abolition of the umbilical-placental circulation are not responsible for the increase in cardiac output after birth. In association with the marked increase in pulmonary blood flow, left ventricular output increases from 135 to $210 ml \cdot kg^{-1} min^{-1}$ compared with $300-425 ml \cdot kg^{-1} min^{-1}$ noted after birth.

To assess whether the marked change in environmental temperature from that in utero to that in air could account for the changes in cardiac output, measurements were made in fetuses exteriorized into a warm bath at 39°C. Left and right ventricular outputs are identical to those measured in utero. Changing the bath temperature to 25°C has no significant effect on fetal combined ventricular output.[126]

In all the studies performed by Teitel et al.[125] and van Bel et al.,[126] the late-gestation fetuses had not been exposed to the increase in circulating cortisol concentrations and triiodothyronine (T_3) concentrations that occur within 24 to 48 hours before birth. The possible role of thyroid hormone in the postnatal increase in cardiac output was examined in sheep by Breall et al.[124] It has been shown that plasma T_3 concentrations increase rapidly after birth, and because in adults T_3 administration increases cardiac output, it was hypothesized that the two may be related. Breall et al. studied three groups of lambs. All had surgery at about 130 days' gestation, but a second surgical procedure was done at the time of deliv-

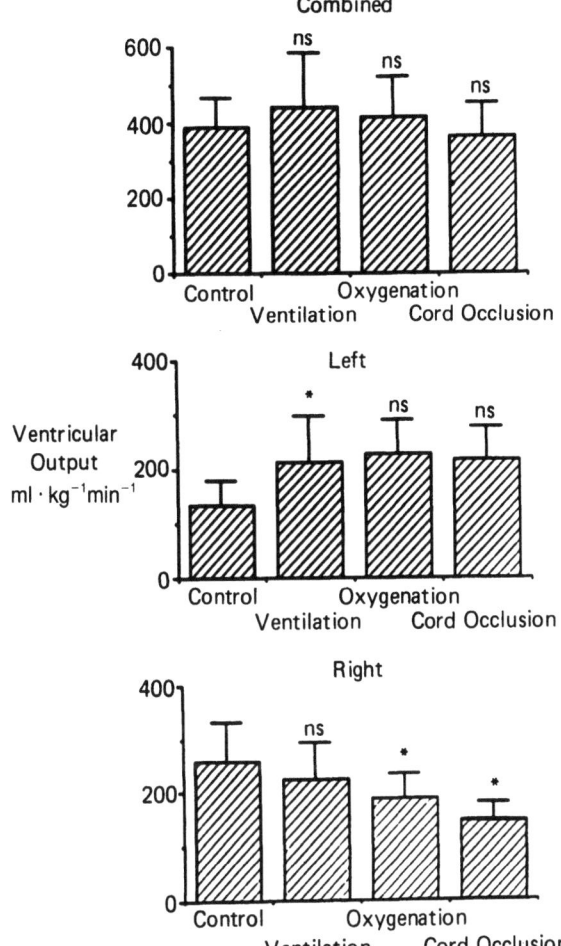

FIGURE 24.11. Effect of simulated birth events on combined ventricular output and on left and right ventricular output in fetal lambs in utero. The period shown as Ventilation represents rhythmic expansion of lungs with no changes in fetal blood gases. The Oxygenation period is during rhythmic ventilation with oxygen. Cord occlusion is the period during which the umbilical cord is completely occluded while the lamb is being ventilated with oxygen. Combined ventricular output does not change significantly, but left ventricular output increases with ventilation and undergoes no further significant changes. Right ventricular output falls somewhat with each event. (From Teitel, et al.,[125] with permission.)

ery for thyroidectomy. In the control group, T_3 concentration was about $1\,ng\cdot ml^{-1}$ at the time of delivery and increased rapidly to 3 to $4\,ng\cdot ml^{-1}$; cardiac output and oxygen consumption increased as expected. In the group that had thyroidectomy at 130 days' gestation, T_3 concentration was in the undetectable range, and there was no change with delivery; in this group, neither cardiac output nor oxygen consumption increased after delivery. In the group of lambs in which the thyroid gland was removed immediately before delivery, plasma T_3 concentration was about $1\,mg\cdot ml^{-1}$ but did not increase after delivery. The cardiac output and oxygen consumption increased to the same levels as in the control group. These studies demonstrate that the postnatal increase in T_3 concentration is not responsible for the increase in cardiac output, but prenatal thyroid action is necessary for cardiac output and oxygen consumption to increase after birth. There are several mechanisms by which thyroidectomy could influence cardiac function. Thyroid hormone is known to increase Na^+,K^+- adenosine triphosphatase (ATPase) activity,[127] to modify cardiac heavy-chain myosin,[128] and to influence β-adrenoreceptor numbers in adult hearts[129] as well as during the perinatal period.[130] Birk et al.[131] showed that at birth the hearts of lambs in which thyroidectomy had been removed at about 130 days' gestation have about half the normal number of β-adrenoreceptors and show a greatly reduced adenylate cyclase response to isoproterenol.

Although it is apparent that thyroid hormone action prenatally is necessary for the postnatal increase in cardiac output, it does not explain the mechanisms responsible. The possibility has been raised that the increase in catecholamine concentration that normally occurs after birth may increase output. Catecholamines increase myocardial contractility and could improve cardiac performance postnatally. Thyroidectomy, by reducing β-adrenoreceptor numbers, could limit the response to catecholamines.

Teitel et al.[132] used a modification of the method of Sunagawa and Sagawa[133] to assess myocardial contractility in lambs at various periods after birth. They found that myocardial contractility falls from the first to the fourth week after birth. In these same animals, isoproterenol infusion has significantly less effect in increasing contractility during the first week and has a progressively greater effect with increasing postnatal age. This finding led to the conclusion that immediately after birth the myocardium is being subjected to a high resting inotropic stimulation by catecholamines and that as the resting inotropic stimulation recedes myocardial contractility is reduced but the response to β-adrenergic receptor stimulation increases. The concept of a high resting myocardial performance during the immediate postnatal period was considered by Klopfenstein and Rudolph,[74] who found that cardiac output is high in relation to body weight early postnatally, but that the response to volume loading is limited. With increasing postnatal age, resting output decreases in relation to body weight, and the percentage increase in response to volume loading is progressively higher with age to about 6 weeks after birth.

If the concept that the increase in cardiac output after birth is due to sympatheticoadrenal stimulation is correct, it might be expected that β-adrenoreceptor blockade would reduce cardiac output to the fetal level. It was not the experience of Klopfenstein and Rudolph,[74] who found that propranolol administration to lambs at varying periods after birth results in only a small decrease (about 10%) in output from resting levels, and there is no significant difference in response from the first to the sixth weeks after birth.

Van Hare et al.[134] used a preparation in the neonate lamb similar to that described in the fetal lamb to examine cardiac output responses at fixed heart rate, with controlled left atrial and aortic pressures.[40] They found that, as with the fetus, left ventricular stroke volume increases progressively with left atrial pressures to a mean level of 10 to 12 mm Hg if aortic mean pressure is kept constant. With increasing aortic pressure, stroke volume falls markedly at constant left atrial pressure. At any left atrial pressure, the same left ventricular stroke volume could be maintained at a much higher aortic pressure in the neonate than in the fetal lamb. It could be related to an increase in myocardial contractility after birth, but this conclusion should not be reached without considering possible differences in loading conditions. The same aortic mean pressure in the fetus and neonate may not reflect the same afterload because of other alterations in the circulation after birth. Similar left atrial pressures may not indicate the same preload because, with ventilation, transmural pressures could be changed dramatically. These factors require further study. The mechanisms involved in the regulation of cardiac output and myocardial performance in the fetus and in the changes after birth are not yet defined.

References

1. Lind J. Changes in the liver circulation at birth. Ann NY Acad Sci 1963;111:110–120.
2. Edelstone DI, Rudolph AM, Heymann MA. Liver and ductus venosus blood flows in fetal lambs in utero. Circ Res 1978;42:426–433.
3. Schmidt KG, Silverman NH, Rudolph AM. Assessment of flow events at the ductus venosus-inferior vena cava junction and at the foramen ovale in fetal sheep by use of multimodal ultrasound. Circulation 1996;93:826–833.
4. Kiserud T, Eik-Nes SH, Hellevik LR, Blaas HG. Ductus venosus—a longitudinal Doppler velocimetric study of the human fetus. J Matern Fetal Invest 1992;2:5–11.
5. Rudolph AM, Heymann MA. The circulation of the fetus in utero. Methods for studying distribution of blood flow, cardiac output and organ blood flow. Circ Res 1967; 21:163–184.
6. Reuss ML, Rudolph AM. Distribution and recirculation of umbilical and systemic venous blood flow in fetal lambs during hypoxia. J Dev Physiol 1980;2:71–84.
7. Rudolph AM, Heymann MA. Control of the foetal circulation. In: Comline KS, Cross KW, Dawes GS, Nathanielsz PW, eds. Proceedings of the Sir Joseph Barcroft Centenary Symposium: foetal and neonatal physiology. Cambridge: Cambridge University Press, 1973:89–111.
8. Barcroft J, Torrens DS. The output of the heart of the foetal sheep. J Physiol 1946:105:22P.
9. Mahon WA, Goodwin JW, Paul WM. Measurement of individual ventricular outputs in the fetal lamb by an indicator dilution technique. Circ Res 1966;19:191–198.
10. Assali NS, Morris JA, Beck R. Cardiovascular haemodynamics in the fetal lamb before and after lung expansion. Am J Physiol 1965;208:122–129.
11. Meschia G, Cotter JR, Makowski EL, Barron DH. Simultaneous measurement of uterine and umbilical blood flows and oxygen uptakes. Q J Exp Physiol 1967;52:1–18.
12. Heymann MA, Payne BD, Hoffman JIE, Rudolph AM. Blood flow measurements with radionuclide-labeled particles. Prog Cardiovasc Dis 1977;20:55–79.
13. Hoffman JIE, Heymann MA, Rudolph AM, Payne BD. Uses and abuses of the radioactive microsphere method of measuring regional blood flow. Bibl Anat 1977;15:20–23.
14. Heymann MA, Creasy RK, Rudolph AM. Quantitation of blood flow pattern in the foetal lamb in utero. In: Comline KS, Cross KW, Dawes GS, Nathanielsz PW, eds. Proceedings of the Sir Joseph Barcroft Centenary Symposium: foetal and neonatal physiology. Cambridge: Cambridge University Press, 1973:129–135.
15. Hoffman JIE, Payne BD, Heymann MA, Rudolph AM. The use of microspheres to measure blood flow. In: Linden RJ, ed. Cardiovascular physiology, techniques in the life sciences. New York: Elsevier Scientific, 1983:P304/1–36.
16. Chien GL, Anselone CG, Davis RF, Van Winkle DM. Fluorescent vs. radioactive microsphere measurement of regional myocardial blood flow. Cardiovasc Res 1995; 30:405–412.
17. Glenny RW, Bernard S, Brinkley M. Validation of fluorescent-labeled microspheres for measurement of regional organ perfusion. J Appl Physiol 1993;74:2585–2597.
18. Austin GE, Tuvlin MB, Martino-Salzman D, et al. Determination of regional myocardial blood flow using fluorescent microspheres. Am J Cardiovasc Pathol 1993;4:352–357.
19. Mori H, Haruyama S, Shinozaki Y, et al. New nonradioactive microspheres and more sensitive X-ray fluorescence to measure regional blood flow. Am J Physiol 1992;263:H1946–H1957.
20. Rudolph AM, Heymann MA. Cardiac output in the fetal lamb: the effects of spontaneous and induced changes of heart rate on right and left ventricular output. Am J Obstet Gynecol 1976;124:183–192.
21. Thornburg KL, Morton MJ. Filling and arterial pressures as determinants of RV stroke volume in the sheep fetus. Am J Physiol 1983;244:H656–H663.
22. Thornburg KL, Morton MJ. Filling and arterial pressures as determinants of left ventricular stroke volume in the fetal lambs. Am J Physiol 1986;251:H961–H968.
23. Lewis AB, Heymann MA, Rudolph AM. Gestational changes in pulmonary vascular responses in fetal lambs in utero. Circ Res 1976;39:536–541.
24. Millard RW, Baig H, Vatner SF. Prostaglandin control of the renal circulation in response to hypoxemia in the fetal lamb in utero. Circ Res 1979;45:172–179.

25. Berman W Jr, Goodlin RC, Heymann MA, Rudolph AM. The measurement of umbilical blood flow in fetal lambs in utero. J Appl Physiol 1975;39:1056–1059.
26. Eldridge MW, Berman W, Greene ER. Serial echo-Doppler measurements of human fetal abdominal aortic blood flow. J Ultrasound Med 1985;114:1023–1028.
27. Eik-Ness SH, Brubakk AO, Ulstein MK. Measurement of human fetal blood flow. Br Med J 1980;280:283–284.
28. De Smedt MCH, Visser GHA, Meijboom EJ. Fetal cardiac output estimated by Doppler echocardiography during mid-late gestation. Am J Cardiol 1987;71:338–342.
29. Shiraishi H, Silverman NH, Rudolph AM. Accuracy of right ventricular output estimated by Doppler echocardiography in the sheep fetus. Am J Obstet Gynecol 1993;168:947–953.
30. Rudolph AM, Heymann MA. Circulatory changes during growth in the fetal lamb. Circ Res 1970;26:289–299.
31. Saxena KK, Jose JV, Chacko J, et al. Intracardiac blood flow velocities and cardiac output in normal fetuses: a prospective pulsed Doppler echocardiographic study. Indian Heart J 1992;44:399–402.
32. Allan LD, Chita SK, Al-Ghazali W, et al. Doppler echocardiographic evaluation of the normal human fetal heart. Br Heart J 1987;57:528–533.
33. Friedman WF. The intrinsic properties of the developing heart. In: Friedman WF, Lesch M, Sonnenblick EH, eds. Neonatal heart disease. Orlando: Grune & Stratton, 1973: 21–49.
34. Romero TE, Covell J, Friedman WF. A comparison of pressure-volume relations of the fetal, newborn, and adult heart. Am J Physiol 1972;222:1285–1290.
35. Gilbert RD. Control of fetal cardiac output during changes in blood volume. Am J Physiol 1980;238:H80–H86.
36. Heymann MA, Rudolph AM. Effects of increasing preload on right ventricular output in fetal lambs in utero. Circulation 1973;48(Suppl IV):37.
37. Kirkpatrick SE, Pitlick PT, Naliboff J, Friedman WF. Frank-Starling relationship as an important determinant of fetal cardiac outpur. Am J Physiol 1976;231:495–500.
38. Anderson PAW, Manring A, Glick KL, Crenshaw CC Jr. Biophysics of the developing heart. III. A comparison of the left ventricular dynamics of the fetal and neonatal lamb heart. Am J Obstet Gynecol 1982;143:195–203.
39. Hawkins J, Van Hare GF, Schmidt KG, Rudolph AM. Effects of increasing afterload on left ventricular output in fetal lambs. Circ Res 1989;65:127–134.
40. Davies P, Dewar J, Tynan M, Ward R. Post-natal developmental changes in the length-tension relationship of cat papillary muscles. J Physiol 1975;253:95–102.
41. Friedman WF, Pool PE, Jacobowitz D, Seagren SS. Sympathetic innervation of the developing rabbit heart. Biochemical and histochemical comparisons of fetal, neonatal and adult myocardium. Circ Res 1968;23:25–32.
42. Nakanishi T, Jarmakani JM. Developmental changes in myocardial mechanical function and subcellular organelles. Am J Physiol 1984;246:H615–H625.
43. Smolich JJ. Ultrastructural and functional features of the developing mammalian heart: a brief overview. Reprod Fertil Dev 1995;7:451–461.
44. Maylie JG. Excitation-contraction coupling in neonatal and adult myocardium of cat. Am J Physiol 1982; 242:H834–H843.
45. Maylie JG, Thornburg KL, Faber JJ. Force-frequency relations of the neonatal cat heart. In: Long LD, Reneau DD, eds. Circulation in the fetus and newborn. New York: Garland, 1978:391–398.
46. Nassar R, Reedy MC, Anderson PAW. Developmental changes in the ultrastructure and sarcomere shortening of the isolated rabbit ventricular myocyte. Circ Res 1987;61:465–483.
47. Page E, Buecker JL. Development of dyadic junctional complexes between sarcoplasmic reticulum and plasmalemma in rabbit left ventricular myocardial cells. Circ Res 1981;48:519–522.
48. Mahony L. Maturation of calcium transport function in cardiac sarcoplasmic reticulum in sheep. Pediatr Res 1986;20:172A.
49. Lipp JM, Rudolph AM. Sympathetic nerve development in the rat and guinea pig heart. Biol Neonate 1972;21:76–82.
50. Lebowitz EA, Novick JS, Rudolph AM. Development of myocardial sympathetic innervation in the fetal lamb. Pediatr Res 1972;6:887–893.
51. Cheng JB, Goldfien A, Cornett LE, Roberts JM. Identification of β-adrenergic receptors using [^{3}H]dihydroalprenolol in fetal sheep heart: direct evidence of qualitative similarity to the receptors in adult sheep heart. Pediatr Res 1981;15:1083–1087.
52. Chen HM, Yamamura HI, Roeski WR. Ontogeny of mammalian myocardial β-adrenergic receptors. Eur J Pharmacol 1979;58:255–264.
53. Cowley WW Jr, Liard JF, Guyton AC. Role of the baroreceptor reflex in daily control of arterial blood pressure and other variables in dogs. Circ Res 1973;32:564–576.
54. Shinebourne EA, Vapaavouri EK, Williams RL, et al. Development of baroreflex activity in unanesthetized fetal and neonatal lambs. Circ Res 1972;31:710–718.
55. Itskovitz J, LaGamma EF, Rudolph AM. Baroreflex control of the circulation in chronically instrumented fetal lambs. Circ Res 1983;52:589–596.
56. Guyton AC. Essential cardiovascular regulation in the control linkages between bodily needs and circulatory function. In: Dickinson CJ, Marks J, eds. Developments in cardiovascular medicine. Baltimore: University Park Press, 1978:265–302.
57. Biscoe TJ, Purves MJ, Sampson SR, Types of nervous activity which may be recorded from the carotid sinus nerve of the sheep foetus. J Physiol (Lond) 1969;202: 1–24.
58. Dawes GS, Duncan SB, Lewis BV, et al. Cyanide stimulation of the systemic arterial chemoreceptors in foetal lambs. J Physiol (Lond) 1969;201:117–128.
59. Jansen AH, Chernick V. Respiratory response to cyanide in fetal sheep after peripheral chemodenervation. J Appl Physiol 1974;36:1–5.

60. Jansen AH, Chernick V. Cardiorespiratory response to central cyanide in fetal sheep. J Appl Physiol 1974;37:18–21.
61. Blanco CE, Dawes GS, Hanson MA, McCooke HB. The response to hypoxia of arterial chemoreceptors in fetal sheep and new-born lambs. J Physiol (Lond) 1984;351:25–37.
62. Goodlin RC, Rudolph AM. Factors associated with initiation of breathing. In: Hodari AA, Mariona FG, eds. Proceedings of the International Symposium: physiological biochemistry of the fetus. Springfield, IL: Charles C. Thomas, 1972:294–318.
63. Itskovitz J, Rudolph AM. Cardiorespiratory response to cyanide of arterial chemoreceptors in fetal lambs. Am J Physiol 1987;252:H916–H922.
64. Bartelds B, van Bel F, Teitel DF, Rudolph AM. Carotid, not aortic, chemoreceptors mediate the fetal cardiovascular response to acute hypoxemia in lambs. Pediatr Res 1993;34:51–55.
65. Cohn HE, Sacks EJ, Heymann MA, Rudolph AM. Cardiovascular responses to hypoxemia and acidemia in fetal lambs. Am J Obstet Gynecol 1974;120:817–824.
66. Jensen A, Roman C, Rudolph AM. Effects of reducing uterine blood flow on fetal blood flow distribution and oxygen delivery. J Dev Physiol 1991;15:309–323.
67. Itskovitz J, LaGamma EF, Rudolph AM. The effect of reducing umbilical blood flow on fetal oxygenation. Am J Obstet Gynecol 1983;145:813–818.
68. Itskovitz J, Goetzman BW, Rudolph AM. The mechanism of late deceleration of the heart rate and its relationship to oxygenation in normoxemic and chronically hypoxemic fetal lambs. Am J Obstet Gynecol 1982;142:66–73.
69. Boekkooi PF, Baan J Jr., Teitel D, Rudolph AM. Chemoreceptor responsiveness in fetal sheep. Am J Physiol 1992;263:H162–H167.
70. Itskovitz J, LaGamma EF, Bristow J, Rudolph AM. Cardiovascular responses to hypoxemia in sinoaortic-denervated fetal sheep. Pediatr Res 1991;30:381–385.
71. Iwamoto HS, Kaufman T, Keil LC, Rudolph AM. Responses to acute hypoxemia in fetal sheep at 0.6–0.7 gestation. Am J Physiol 1989;256:H613–H620.
72. Bristow J, Rudolph AM, Itskovitz J, Barnes RJ. Hepatic oxygen and glucose metabolism in the fetal lamb: response to hypoxia. J Clin Invest 1983;71:1047–1061.
73. Itskovitz J, LaGamma EF, Rudolph AM. Effects of cord compression on fetal blood flow distribution and O_2 delivery. Am J Physiol 1987;252:H100–H109.
74. Klopfenstein HS, Rudolph AM. Postnatal changes in the circulation, and responses to volume loading in sheep. Circ Res 1978;42:839–845.
75. Lister G, Walter TK, Versmold HT, et al. Oxygen delivery in lambs: cardiovascular and hematologic development. Am J Physiol 1979;237:H668–H675.
76. Kuipers JRG, Sidi D, Heymann MA, Rudolph AM. Comparison of methods of measuring cardiac output in newborn lambs. Pediatr Res 1982;16:594–598.
77. Hislop A, Reid L. Intrapulmonary arterial development during fetal life—branching pattern and structure. J Anat 1972;113:35–48.
78. Levin DL, Rudolph AM, Heymann MA, Phibbs RH. Morphological development of the pulmonary vascular bed in fetal lambs. Circulation 1976;53:144–151.
79. Wagenvoort CA, Neufeld HN, DuShane JW, Edwards JE. The pulmonary arterial tree in atrial septal defect. A quantitative study of anatomic features in fetuses, infants and children. Circulation 1961;23:733–739.
80. Reid L. The lung: its growth and remodeling during health and disease. Am J Roentgenol 1977;129:777–788.
81. Naeye RL. Arterial changes during the perinatal period. Arch Pathol 1961;71:121–128.
82. Rudolph AM. Fetal and neonatal pulmonary circulation. Am Rev Respir Dis 1977;115:11–18.
83. Cook CD, Drinker PA, Jacobson HN, et al. Control of pulmonary blood flow in the foetal and newly born lamb. J Physiol 1963;169:10–29.
84. Cassin S, Dawes GS, Mott JC, et al. The vascular resistance of the foetal and newly ventilated lung of the lamb. J Physiol 1964;171:61–79.
85. Teitel DF, Iwamoto HS, Rudolph AM. Changes in the pulmonary circulation during birth-related events. Pediatr Res 1990;27:372–378.
86. Campbell AGM, Dawes GS, Fishman AP, Hyman AI. Bradykinin and pulmonary blood flow in the foetal lung. J Physiol 1966;184:80P.
87. Heymann M, Rudolph A, Nies A, Melmon K. Bradykinin production association with oxygenation of the fetal lamb. Circ Res 1969;25:521–534.
88. Leffler CW, Hessler JR, Terragno NA. Ventilation-induced release of prostaglandin-like material from fetal lungs. Am J Physiol 1980;238:H282–H286.
89. Leffler CW, Hessler JR, Green RS. The onset of breathing at birth stimulates pulmonary vascular prostacyclin synthesis. Pediatr Res 1984;18:938–942.
90. Leffler CW, Tyler TL, Cassin S. Effect of indomethacin on pulmonary vascular response to ventilation of fetal goats. Am J Physiol 1978;234:H346–H351.
91. Leffler CW, Mitchell JA, Green RS. Cardiovascular effects of leukotrienes in neonatal piglets. Circ Res 1984;55:780–787.
92. Schreiber MD, Heymann MA, Soifer SJ. The differential effects of leukotriene C_4 and D_4 on the pulmonary and systemic circulations in newborn lambs. Pediatr Res 1987;21:176–182.
93. LeBidois J, Soifer SJ, Clyman RI, Heymann MA. Piriprost: a putative leukotriene synthesis inhibitor increases pulmonary blood flow in fetal lambs. Pediatr Res 1987;22:350–354.
94. Moore P, Velvis H, Fineman JR, et al. EDRF inhibition attenuates the increase in pulmonary blood flow due to oxygen ventilation in fetal lambs. J Appl Physiol 1992;73:2151–2157.
95. Velvis H, Moore P, Heymann MA. Prostaglandin inhibition prevents the fall in pulmonary vascular resistance as a result of rhythmic distension of the lungs in fetal lambs. Pediatr Res 1991;30:62–68.
96. Dawes GS, Mott JC, Widdicombe JG. The cardiac murmur from the patent ductus arteriosus in newborn lambs. J Physiol 1955;128:344–360.

97. Burnard ED. A murmur from the ductus arteriosus in the newborn baby. Br Med J 1958;1:806–810.
98. Mitchell SC. The ductus arteriosus in the neonatal period. J Pediatr 1957;57:12–17.
99. McMurphy DM, Heymann MA, Rudolph AM, Melmon KL. Developmental changes in constriction of the ductus arteriosus: responses to oxygen and vasoactive substances in the isolated ductus arteriosus of the fetal lamb. Pediatr Res 1972;6:231–238.
100. Oberhansli-Weiss I, Heymann MA, Rudolph AM, Melmon KL. The pattern and mechanisms of response of the ductus arteriosus and umbilical artery to oxygen. Pediatr Res 1972;6:693–700.
101. Fay FS. Guinea pig ductus arteriosus. I. Cellular and metabolic basis for oxygen sensitivity. Am J Physiol 1971;221:470–479.
102. Melmon KL, Cline MJ, Hughes T, Nies AS. Kinins: possible mediators of neonatal circulatory changes in man. J Clin Invest 1968;47:1295–1302.
103. Heymann MA, Rudolph AM. Control of the ductus arteriosus. Physiol Rev 1975;55:62–78.
104. Coceani F, Olley PM. The response of the ductus arteriosus to prostaglandins. Can J Physiol Pharmacol 1973;51:220–225.
105. Sharpe GL, Thalme B, Larsson KS. Studies on closure of the ductus arteriosus: XI. Ductal closure in utero by a prostaglandin synthetase inhibitor. Prostaglandins 1974;8:363–368.
106. Heymann MA, Rudolph AM. Effects of acetylsalicylic acid on the ductus arteriosus and circulation of fetal lambs in utero. Circ Res 1976;38:418–422.
107. Pace-Asciak CR, Rangaraj G. Prostaglandin biosynthesis and catabolism in the lamb ductus arteriosus, aorta and pulmonary artery. Biochim Biophys Acta 1978;529:13–20.
108. Clyman RI, Mauray F, Roman C, Rudolph AM. PGE_2 is a more potent vasodilator of the lamb ductus arteriosus than either PGI_2 or 6 keto $PGF_{1\alpha}$. Prostaglandins 1978;16:259–264.
109. Challis JRG, Dilley SR, Robinson JS, Thorburn GD. Prostaglandins in the circulation of the fetal lamb. Prostaglandins 1976;11:1041–1052.
110. Clyman RI, Mauray F, Roman C, et al. Circulating prostaglandin E_2 concentrations and patent ductus arteriosus in fetal and neonatal lambs. J Pediatr 1980;97:455–461.
111. Clyman RI, Mauray F, Heymann MA, Roman C. Effect of gestational age on pulmonary metabolism of prostaglandin E_1 and E_2. Prostaglandins 1981;21:505–513.
112. Clyman RI, Mauray F, Heymann MA, Rudolph AM. Developmental response to oxygen and indomethacin. Prostaglandins 1978;15:993–998.
113. Clyman RI, Mauray F, Roman C, et al. Effect of gestational age on ductus arteriosus response to circulating prostaglandin E_2. J Pediatr 1983;102:907–911.
114. Clyman RI, Mauray F, Roman C, et al. Effects of antenatal glucocorticoid administration on the ductus arteriosus of preterm lambs. Am J Physiol 1981;241:H415–H420.
115. Clyman RI. Ontogeny of the ductus arteriosus response to prostaglandins and inhibitors of their synthesis. Semin Perinatol 1980;4:115–124.
116. Rose JC, Macdonald AA, Heymann MA, Rudolph AM. Developmental aspects of the pituitary-adrenal axis response to hemorrhagic stress in lamb fetuses in utero. J Clin Invest 1978;61:424–432.
117. Nathanielsz PW. Fetal endocrinology—an experimental approach. New York: North-Holland, 1976.
118. Heymann MA, Rudolph AM. Ductus arteriosus patency maintained by prostaglandin E_1 infusion. Prostaglandins Ther 1977;2:2.
119. Heymann MA, Berman W Jr, Rudolph AM, Whitman V. Dilatation of the ductus arteriosus by prostaglandin E_1 in aortic arch abnormalities. Circulation 1979;59:169–173.
120. Heymann MA, Rudolph AM, Silverman NH. Closure of the ductus arteriosus in premature infants by inhibition of prostaglandin synthesis. N Engl J Med 1976;295:530–533.
121. Friedman WF, Hirschklau MJ, Printz MP, et al. Pharmacological closure of patent ductus arteriosus in the premature infant. N Engl J Med 1976;295:526–529.
122. Mentzer RM, Ely SW, Lasley RD, et al. Hormonal role of adenosine in maintaining patency of the ductus arteriosus in fetal lambs. Ann Surg 1985;202:223–230.
123. Sidi D, Kuipers JR, Heymann MA, Rudolph AM. Effects of ambient temperature on oxygen consumption and the circulation in newborn lambs at rest and during hypoxemia. Pediatr Res 1983;17:254–258.
124. Breall JA, Rudolph AM, Heymann MA. Role of thyroid hormone in postnatal circulatory and metabolic adjustments. J Clin Invest 1984;73:1418–1424.
125. Teitel D, Iwamoto HS, Rudolph AM. Effects of birth-related events on central blood flow patterns. Pediatr Res 1987;22:557–566.
126. van Bel F, Roman C, Iwamotot HS, Rudolph AM. Sympathoadrenal, metabolic, and regional blood flow responses to cold in fetal sheep. Pediatr Res 1993;34:47–50.
127. Philipson KD, Edelman IS. Thyroid hormone control of Na^+, K^+-ATPase and K^+-dependent phosphatase in rat heart. Am J Physiol 1977;232:C196–C206.
128. Fink IL, Morkin E. Evidence for a new cardiac myosin species in thyrotoxic rabbits. FEBS Lett 1977;81:391–394.
129. Williams LT, Lefkowitz RJ, Watanabe SM, et al. Thyroid hormone regulation of β-adrenergic receptor number. J Biol Chem 1977;252:2787–2789.
130. Whitsett JA, Noguchi A, Moore JJ. Developmental aspects of α- and β-adrenergic receptors. Semin Perinatol 1982;6:125–141.
131. Birk E, Rudolph AM, Roberts JM. Fetal thyroidectomy reduces postnatal myocardial β-adrenergic receptor responses in newborn lambs. Pediatr Res 1988;23:431A.
132. Teitel DF, Sidi D, Chin T, et al. Developmental changes in myocardial contractile reserve in the lamb. Pediatr Res 1985;19:948–955.
133. Sunagawa K, Sagawa K. Models of ventricular contration based on time-varying elastance. CRC Crit Rev Biomed Eng 1982;7:193–228.

134. Van Hare GF, Hawkins JA, Schmidt KG, Rudolph AM. The effects of increasing mean arterial pressure on left ventricular output in newborn lambs. Circ Res 1990;67:78–83.
135. Bristow J, Rudolph AM, Itskovitz J. A preparation for studying liver blood flow, oxygen consumption and metabolism in the fetal lamb in utero. J Dev Physiol 1981;3:255–266.
136. Rudolph AM. Hepatic and ductus venosus blood flows during fetal life. Hepatology 1983;3:254–258.
137. Rudolph AM. Congenital diseases of the heart: clinical-physiologic considerations in diagnosis and management. Chicago: Year Book, 1974.
138. Gilbert RD. J Dev Physiol Effects of after load and baroreceptors on cardiac function in fetal sheep. 1982;4:299–309.

25
Water and Electrolyte Metabolism in the Fetal-Placental Unit

E. Marelyn Wintour

The first edition of this book emphasized the fact that the water and electrolyte balances of the fetus were primarily dependent on the water and electrolyte balances of the mother.[1] Thus, when the mother was given fluid intravenously, the treatment would affect the fetus. In addition to being a passive recipient of fluid and electrolyte, however, the fetus did develop some measure of control over fluid and electrolyte loss from its body, predominantly by regulation of fetal renal function. In general, new findings relevant to the possible role of the fetal kidney in the genesis of abnormalities of fetal fluid balance are discussed. In addition, some very recent findings of this investigator, relevant to very early kidney development are discussed.

At the time of writing of the first edition virtually nothing was known of specific water channels, by which water could diffuse rapidly into and out of various cell populations. There has been an explosion of knowledge in the area recently. Although very little has yet been done on the expression of any normal or abnormal water channel gene in pregnancy in mother, fetus, or fetal membranes, a section has been included on the basic properties of the six water channel genes thus far cloned, and suggestions made as to potentially fertile areas of investigation.

Since the first edition there have been many advances in knowledge concerning factors that may regulate blood flow to the placenta, and the ability of the placenta to grow normally and function adequately in the maternal-fetal exchanges of solutes and water. With the discovery of many new substances potentially able to alter the state of constriction or dilation of maternal blood vessels and their permeability, a greater understanding of the regulation of maternal blood volume in both normal and pathologic states has been possible. These are discussed, in particular with relevance to states such as preeclampsia, although the cause(s) and cure(s) are still under intense investigation.

Alterations in Maternal Fluid and Electrolyte Balance During Pregnancy

Previously the changes in total fluid and electrolyte balance during pregnancy were summarized, and the possible hormonal basis of these changes was discussed.[1] There is normally an expansion of maternal plasma volume, but either no change or a decrease in maternal arterial blood pressure, as summarized in Table 25.1. The changes, induced by pregnancy, by a variety of hormones that might cause sodium retention are variable in different species. Two aspects that will be addressed further are (1) changes in hormones promoting sodium loss and/or decrease in blood pressure, and (2) the question of how blood volume changes in pregnancy are sensed in an overall integrative fashion.

Natriuretic Peptides

There are at least three genes coding for prohormones of peptides with natriuretic activity: one encodes the 126 amino acid atrial natriuretic peptide (ANP) prohormone, another the 106 amino acid brain natriuretic peptide (BNP) prohormone, and the third the 126 amino acid C-natriuretic peptide (CNP) prohormone.[2] The ANF prohormone, synthesized predominantly but not exclusively in the atrial myocytes of adult hearts, can be processed to four different biologically active peptides in the heart (ANP_{1-30}–long-acting sodium stimulator; ANP_{31-67}–vessel dilation, ANP_{79-98}–kaliuretic stimulation; ANP_{99-126}–ANF), and a fifth (urodilatin) in the kidney. The four atrial-derived peptides circulate and interact with one or more receptors. BNP, though so named because it was originally isolated from the porcine brain, is actually mainly secreted from the ventricle of the heart,[3] and, in the pregnant woman, is made by the amnion.[4]

TABLE 25.1. Physiologic changes in pregnancy—comparative studies.

	Human	Baboon	Rat	Sheep
Plasma volume	↑	↑	↑	↑
Plasma osmolality	↓	?	↓	→
Systolic B.P.	↓	↓	↓	→
Cardiac output	↑	↑	↑	↑
Heart rate	↑	↑	↑	↑
AII-BP response	↓	↓	↓	↓
Aldosterone	↑↑	↑↑	↑	→
Progesterone	↑↑↑	↑↑↑	↑↑	↑
Estrogens	↑↑↑	↑↑↑	↑	→
Renin-AII	↑	↑	↑	↑

AII, angiotensin II; ↑, small increase; ↓, small decrease; →, no change; ↑↑, moderate increase; ↑↑↑, large increase.

CNP was originally found in the brain,[5] but a more substantial site of production is the atrium.[6] However, CNP is probably not a systemic hormone and it is important to note that CNP messenger RNA (mRNA) has been found in the rat, mouse, and human kidney.[7] There are at least three receptors for natriuretic peptides, encoded by separate genes.[8] These are named, confusingly, GC-A, GC-B, and C. C-receptor is possibly a misnomer, as it binds to the peptide ligand, but does not have any clear second message system linked to natriuresis, and it is called the "clearance" receptor.[9] Both the GC-A and GC-B receptors have intrinsic guanylate cyclase activity, and can be activated by ANP_{99-126}, BNP, CNP, and urodilatin, although the most potent ligand for the GC-B receptor is CNP.[2,10,11] An extensive amount of work has been done on ANP_{99-126}, with less on natriuretic peptide receptors during pregnancy, in both mother and fetus. Much less is known of the secretion of the other natriuretic peptides in the mother and fetus.

In the nonpregnant adult human, ANP_{99-126} has potent diuretic and natriuretic effects by both increasing glomerular filtration rate (GFR) and decreasing proximal tubular sodium reabsorption.[12] Similar findings have been made in the anesthetized rat,[13] dog,[14,15] and conscious sheep.[16] A most interesting facet of the action of ANP_{99-126} is that the natriuretic and diuretic actions are amplified by sodium loading or volume expansion,[17–21] an effect not easily explained by changes in receptor mRNA with sodium loading.[22] BNP has similar actions to ANP_{99-126},[23] is co-released with ANP_{99-126} in hypervolemic states,[3,24] and when both peptides are infused into healthy male subjects, their effects are additive.[25] When BNP was infused, the metabolic clearance rate (MCR) of ANP_{99-126} is decreased, leading to an increase in the plasma concentration of ANP_{99-126}. BNP concentration is not increased in normal pregnancy,[26] although there is a very high concentration of BNP in human amniotic fluid,[4] but an undetectable concentration of ANP_{99-126}.

There is debate about whether plasma ANP_{99-126} concentration changes in human pregnancy. Some cross-sectional data show an increase;[26,27] however, it seems that in all studies there is a wide range found at any particular stage of pregnancy. In one longitudinal study, ANP_{99-126} was temporarily increased only at midpregnancy.[28] Some studies suggest that if posture and sodium intake are controlled strictly, and longitudinal studies performed, there is no effect of pregnancy on the plasma ANP_{99-126} concentration.[29] However, during the pregnancy, volume expansion produces a bigger increment in plasma ANP_{99-126} concentration than occurs in nonpregnant women.[29] Thus, it is probably possible to explain the data of different investigators on the basis of variations in the conditions under which the sampling occurred.

In the experimental animal, a small but significant increase in plasma ANP_{99-126} has been recorded sometimes,[30] whereas others have not seen this difference in cross-sectional studies,[31–32] so possibly the same qualifications apply.

The other peptides, $Pro-ANP_{1-30}$, $Pro-ANP_{31-67}$, and $Pro-ANP_{79-98}$, affect fluid and electrolyte metabolism,[2,33] but may not act on the guanylate-cyclase–linked receptors.[34,35] No systemic study of the secretion or function of these other pro-ANP peptides in pregnancy or in the fetus has been reported.

Why Does Plasma Volume Increase During Pregnancy?

The question as to the mechanism(s) of increased plasma volume during pregnancy can be resolved into two primary ones: (1) Is pregnancy a situation in which the capacity of vasculature is increased, and so is underutilized, that it results in homeostatic mechanisms to fill? (2) Is fluid (i.e., salt and water) primarily retained and adaptations occur so that this overutilized situation does not stimulate responses to return the volume to the normal (i.e., nonpregnant) level? There is some evidence supporting both propositions. There is widespread vasodilation, as well as the arteriovenous shunt of the maternal placental circulation. In addition, a decreased vascular responsiveness to angiotensin II is well established.[36] There is increased production and excretion of guanosine 3′, 5′-cyclic monophosphate (cGMP), a well-established mediator of intracellular vasodilation,[37] and, in the rat, of nitric oxide (NO) synthesis. However, the musculature of the pregnant rat arteries are less sensitive to constriction by α-adrenoreceptor agonists than is that of nonpregnant rats, independent of the production of NO by the endothelium.[37] These would support the underutilized hypothesis, by means of an unidentified agonist.

Altered Sensing of Vascular Volume

In the nonpregnant and early pregnant rat, atrial stretch causes increased ANP secretion, and increased urine output, but this does not occur in the late pregnant rat.[38,39] Furthermore, in the nonpregnant rat atrial distention resulted in a significant increase in c-*fos* expression in the paraventricular nucleus, the medial preoptic area, and the lateral septum, responses markedly attenuated in pregnant rats.[40] These data support the hypothesis that in pregnancy in the rat some factor(s) alter the sensing of an increased volume, so that an expanded plasma volume may be sensed as normal.

Water Channels

A long-held tenet of mammalian physiology was that all cells within the body, with a few special exceptions, were freely permeable to water and water moved passively between compartments in response to osmotic gradients. The most notable exceptions were cells in the thin and thick ascending limb of the loop of Henle in the metanephric kidney, and cells in the collecting ducts, in the inner medulla, in the absence of antidiuretic hormone or arginine vasopressin (AVP). Thus, the osmolality of the extracellular fluid was also the osmolality of the intracellular fluid, and rapid changes in osmolality, especially a decrease, were potentially fatal because of the inabililty of cells, particularly in the brain, to regulate cell volume rapidly. On the other hand, slowly evolving hyponatremia could be tolerated reasonably well because compensatory mechanisms occur, including the intracellular accumulation of organic osmolytes.[41,42] In the first edition of this book there was substantial discussion of the problem of iatrogenic hyponatremia in pregnant women and their fetuses.[1]

It has long been known that the increased water permeability of principal cells of the collecting duct of the kidney, under the influence of increased AVP concentration, resulted from the insertion of vesicles into the apical membranes of these cells. These vesicles were assumed to contain a water channel.[43,44] What has been found, in the past 5 years, is that the rate at which water crosses the cell membrane in many organs and tissues is dependent on the presence of specific water channels, and the structure of the proteins and the genes encoding them has been elucidated.[45-51] The major characteristics of water channel proteins are that in cells containing them (1) water movement is rapid; (2) the Arrhenius activation energy calculated as the slope of ln Pf versus I/RT (ln-log to base e, Pf-water permeability, co-efficient [cm. sec^{-1}], 1, R-gas constant [1·987 cal·deg^{-1}·mole^{-1}], T-absolute temperature) for water movement is low (<5 kcal·mol^{-1}); (3) organic mercurial agents such as p-(chloromercuric) benzenesulfonate (pCMBS) and mercuric chloride ($HgCl_2$) inhibit water movement though the cell membrane, which is true for five sixths of the water channels; and (4) with one exception, the channels are specific for water and do not allow the rapid passage of ions and urea.

The rapid movement of water across the cell membrane is indicated by a ratio of osmotic permeability (Pf) to diffusional permeability (P_{dw}) greater than 1. A Pf > 0.01 cm·sec^{-1} is indicative of a water channel. In membranes without water channels the activation energy for water movement is high, often much greater than 10 kcal·mol^{-1}. Tissues in which a water channel has been found include red blood cells, which must pass continuously through a hypertonic medulla in the postnatal kidney, the proximal tubule and descending thin limb of the loop of Henle, in which a very large volume of the glomerular filtrate is rapidly reabsorbed daily, as well as cells in a wide variety of tissues—heart, spleen, liver, gallbladder, pancreas, stomach, colon, salivary gland, lung, eye, male reproductive tract, brain, and placenta—as detailed in Table 25.2. The most common water channel is aquaporin 1, which was originally called $CHIP_{28}$ (*c*hannel-forming *i*ntegral membrane *p*rotein of 28kd); the human protein was first isolated in 1988,[52] the cDNA sequence published in 1991,[53] and confirmation that it was indeed a water channel was published in 1992.[54] The protein exists in both a nonglycosylated form (28kd) and a larger MR form (40–60kd) believed to be due to N-linked glycosylation on asparagine 42. The tissues in which AQP_1 is located are generally epithelia in which ion transporters generate osmotic gradients to provide a driving force for water movement; for example, in the brain AQP_1 is specifically located in the apical membranes of the epithelial cells of the choroid plexus, which secretes ≈500ml cerebrospinal fluid (CSF) per day in the adult human. It is also strongly expressed in the efferent ducts connecting rete testis to the epididymus in the male rat,[55] in which seminiferous fluid is reabsorbed and sperm concentrated. One of the most interesting locations of AQP_1 is the syncytial trophoblast cells of the human placenta. It would be interesting to know if there is any abnormality of gene expression of AQP_1 in preeclampsia. It would also be of great interest to know if this gene is expressed in decidua, chorion, or amnion.

The rat AQP_1 cDNA sequence was obtained in 1992.[56] When the ontogeny of AQP_1 was studied in the rat it was found that the choroid plexus expressed the gene strongly in late gestation, but red blood cells and kidney did not express the gene until soon after birth.[57] In the human fetal kidney, however AQP_1 was detectable by 14 weeks, strongly expressed in the proximal tubule by 17 weeks and in the thin descending limb of the loop of Henle by 24 weeks.[58] Because the gene for human AQP_1 is located on

TABLE 25.2. Sites of expression of water channel (aquaporin) genes.

Water channel	Organ/tissue	Cell localization
AQP$_1$	Brain	Epithelial cell of chorid plexus—apical microvilli
	Kidney	Proximal tubule—apical cell membrane
		Descending limb of loop of Henle
	Lung	Submucosa of trachea, peribronchial capillary endothelia
	Liver	Bile duct—interlobular and terminal bile ductules cholangiocytes
	Inner ear	
	Eye	Anterior ciliary body epithelium
		Iris epithelium
		Corneal epithelium (fetus only); endothelium (adult)
		Lens epithelium
	Skin	Sweat glands
	Cardiovascular system	Red blood cell membrane
		Nonfenestrated capillaries
	Lacrimal gland	
	Salivary gland	
	Pancreas	
	Skeletal	
	Cardiac smooth muscle	
	Efferent ducts of testis	Apical and basolateral membranes of nonciliated epithelial cells
	Ampulla of vas deferens	Seminal vesicle
AQP$_2$	Kidney	Principal cells of inner medullary collecting ducts
		Apical cell membrane and subapical cytoplasmic vesicles
AQP$_3$	Kidney	Principal cells of inner medullary collecting duct
		Basolateral membranes
	Lung	Tracheal epithelium—basolateral membranes
	Stomach	Gastric parietal cells—basolateral membranes
	Distal colon	Basolateral membrane of villous epithelium
AQP$_4$	Kidney	Principal cells of inner medullary collecting ducts
		Basolateral membranes
	Brain	Astrocytes foot processes surrounding nonfenestrated capillaries
		Cerebellum—Purkinje layer
		Ependymal cells of ventricular lining
		Supraoptic and paraventricular nuclei
	Lung	Tracheal, bronchial epithelium—basolateral membranes
	Stomach	Chief and parietal cells of glandular portion of fundic mucosa
	Eye	Multiple layers of retina, pigmented cells of iris
AQP$_5$	Salivary glands	Parotid, submandibular, sublingual—epithelia
	Lacrimal glands	Epithelium
	Eye	Corneal epithelium
	Lung	Alveolar type I cells

chromosome 7p14,[59] which is coincident with the location of the Colton blood group locus, a search for subjects lacking AQP$_1$ concentrated on those rare individuals who lack Colton antigens.[60] When mutations in the AQP$_1$ gene, which resulted in the absence of functional AQP$_1$ water channels, were found in three people lacking the Colton antigen, water permeability of their red blood cells was decreased, but no obvious pathologic consequences resulted.[60] Whether other compensations occurred could not be determined readily.

As soon as the structure of AQP$_1$ was defined, it was noted that it bore distinct homology to a previously cloned protein—the major intrinsic protein (MIP) of the lens fiber cell of the eye.[61] This 26-kd protein composes over 60% of the membrane protein, but was not believed to be a water channel.[62] However, it has been found, recently, that *Xenopus* oocytes, injected with bovine MIP cRNA, increased their osmotic water permeability.[63] The MIP water channel is less effective than that of AQP_1 since there is a four- to fivefold increase in osmotic water permeability, versus >30-fold for AQP_1, but the MIP protein does now qualify to be called an aquaporin, and, because it is an "ancestral" member of this family it has now been labeled AQP_0. The importance of this protein to normal vision was highlighted by the discovery that natural mutations in this gene underlie cataract formation in the mouse.[64]

Aquaporin 2 (AQP_2) is the AVP-regulated *water channel* of the *collecting duct*, originally called WCH-CD.[65,66] It is located specifically in principal cells of inner medullary collecting ducts, and not in intercalated cells, which are the sites of carbonic anhydrase II (CAII) expression. In mice in which the CAII gene has been knocked out, only AQP_2 expressing principal cells appear. The protein product ($\approx$39kd) in the water-loaded subject is found predominantly in intracellular vesicles, and transferred to the apical membrane under the influence of AVP,[67] by a process involving synaptobrevin and an adenosine triphosphate (ATP)-dependent process.[68,69] Insertion of the protein in the apical membrane increases water permeability quite markedly, and endocytosis of clathrin-coated pits[46,70,71] removes the channels from the membrane when AVP concentration drops.

That the same protein molecules can be recycled more than once was proven recently, when a tagged AQP_2 protein was followed through three rounds of exocytosis and endocytosis, in a kidney cell line in the complete absence of de novo protein synthesis.[72] The human gene is located at chromosome 12q13, and the promoter region contains two GATA consensus sequences, an AP-1 site, an AP-2 site, three E-boxes, and an adenosine 3', 5'-cyclic monophosphate (cAMP) responsive element, suggesting where regulation of expression might occur.[73] Patients have been found with a mutation in the hAQP_2 gene, who suffer from hereditary nephrogenic diabetes insipidus[50,74] (Figure 25.1). More recently it has been shown that treatment of the rat with lithium or induction of hypokalemia also downregulates AQP_2 messenger RNA (mRNA) quite severely.[75,76] There is increased expression of AQP_2 mRNA in dehydration and with AVP treatment,[77] and an increase in the rat made cirrhotic experimentally. The only known ontogeny study is one in the rat, which shows the gene for AQP_2 being expressed by embryonic day 18.[78] While there is convincing and extensive literature

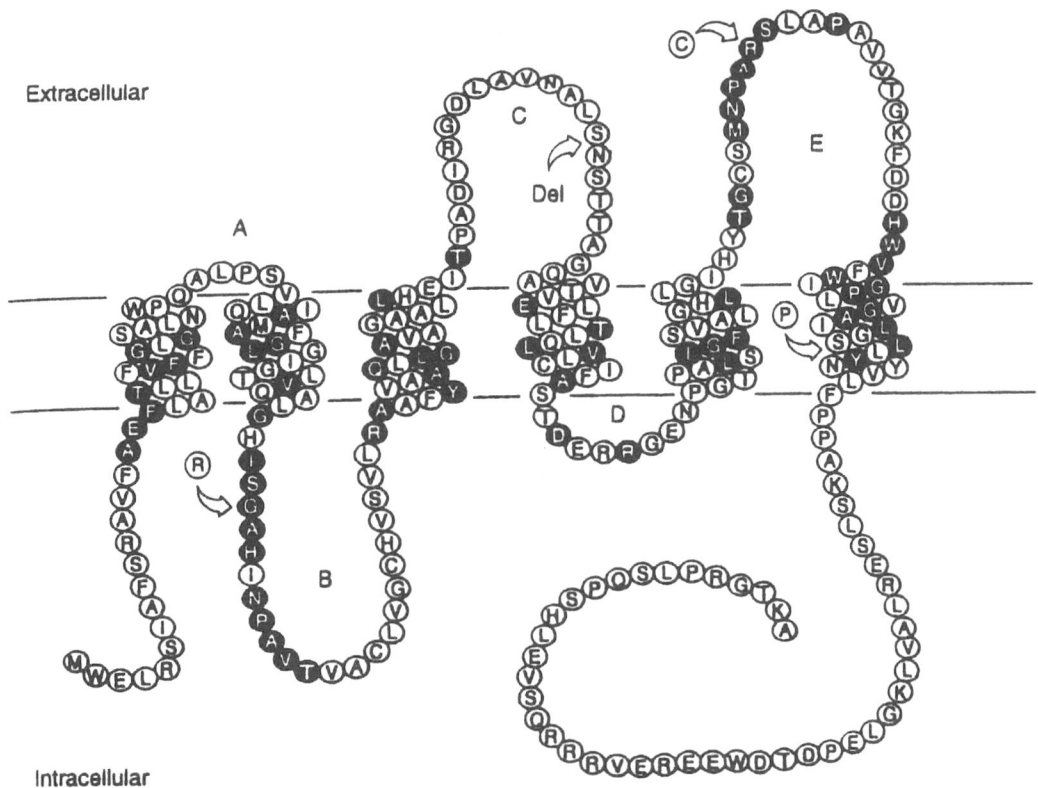

FIGURE 25.1. Proposed transmembrane model of the AQP_2 protein. Filled symbols represent amino acids conserved within the membrane integral protein family.[62] Amino acid substitutions (G64R, R187C, S216P) and the single nucleotide deletion (del) of the four nephrogenic diabetes insipidus patients are indicated by arrows. (From van Lieburg et al.,[49] with permission.)

showing that the ovine fetal kidney can produce a hypertonic urine in response to endogenous or exogenous AVP,[79,80] the sensitivity of the fetal kidney is not as great as that of the adult kidney.[81,82] The concentration and affinity of the AVP-V$_2$ receptor are similar in the ovine fetal and adult kidney, so the requirement for a larger concentration of hormone to produce a negative free water clearance in the fetal kidney may be due to a relatively low level of expression of AQP$_2$. Whether the distribution of AQP$_2$ is the same in development as in adult life is also unknown.

Another aquaporin, AQP$_5$, has been found, which has the closest homology with AQP$_2$.[83] This has the same characteristics as AQP$_1$, but its distribution differs. It is found in the corneal epithelium of the eye, the salivary glands (i.e., secretory lobules), the trachea, and lung, but not in the kidney, intestine, or brain. No record of examination of the reproductive tracts could be found.

Other membranes of the aquaporin family include one that is not exclusively a water channel, but also transports small nonionic molecules such as urea and glycerol and is still inhibited by mercurials (AQP$_3$), and one that is an exclusive water channel, but is not inhibited by mercurial compounds (AQP$_4$). Aquaporin 3 has been called the basolateral integral membrane protein (BLIP) because it is located in the basolateral membrane of principal cell of the collecting duct, as well as in gastric parietal cell.[84-86] It is constitutively located in the membrane, and does not recycle, although the absolute amount of protein can be increased by dehydration.[86] It is thought that entry of water is regulated by the number of AVP-induced apical channels, and then the water exit to the interstitial fluid and blood is facilitated by the presence of the basolateral water channel. The ontogeny of AQP$_3$ is unknown.

Aquaporin 4, the mercurial-insensitive water channel (MIWC) is widely distributed in the brain, being found in ependymal cells lining the aqueduct system at the midline and over the paraventricular and supraoptic nuclei, Purkinje cells of the cerebellum, and glial cells forming the edge of the cerebral cortex and brain stem.[87] It is expressed weakly in other tissues such as eye, kidney, and lung. Of particular interest is that it also localizes in the basolateral membrane of the principal cells of the collecting duct.[88] AQP$_4$ is not expressed in the fetal rat brain, and the ontogeny has not been studied in other species. It is not found in the choroid plexus, so it is not involved in the formation of CSF but may allow fast exit of CSF. The presence of this water channel in ependymal cells lining the third ventricle, and in the vasopressin-secreting cells of the supraoptic and paraventricular nuclei, makes one wonder if it is necessary for osmoreceptor activity, as rapid changes in the cell volume could occur in cells with this water channel. No studies have yet been done on the state of this water channel in the pregnant rat or woman, when the plasma osmolality/plasma arginine vasopressin (Posmol/PAVP) relationship is reset. However, when transgenic mice lacking the AQP$_4$ gene were produced, there was no apparent effect on the growth or development of the young.[88a]

Fluid Balance Across the Lung

The adult lung secretes and reabsorbs fluid; expired air is saturated with water vapor, and some animals use respiratory water loss as a major thermoregulatory mechanism. Excess accumulation of fluid in the adult lung poses a serious threat to life. In the developing fetus, however, lungs are filled with fluid that is essential for the normal growth and development of the lung.[89,90] This fluid must be substantially reabsorbed at birth. There is no doubt that β-adrenergic agents, cortisol, and thyroid hormones are important for adequate fluid reabsorption. Cortisol may also play a part in regulating the secretion rate before birth.[91] The rate of fetal lung liquid secretion is not increased when the fetus is volume loaded,[92] but its secretion rate may be reduced by physiologic increases in arginine vasopressin (AVP) such as occur just prior to parturition[93] or during hypoxic stress in utero.[90] With the advent of the cloning of a number of water channels, or aquaporins, it has been found that AQPs 1, 3, 4, and 5 were expressed in some pulmonary tissue.[94] AQP$_1$ is localized extensively in the vasculature (peribronchial capillaries) but not the epithelium of the alveoli;[51] AQP$_3$ has been found in the basolateral membrane of the trachea; AQP$_4$ localizes to basolateral membranes of airways and trachea; AQP$_5$ mRNA has been found in lung and tracheal extract by Northern blotting.

However, the period during which fluid formation is greatest in the ovine fetus (3–4 ml·h^{-1}kg^{-1}) is during fetal life, and only limited data are available, and then only for the rat. The mRNAs for AQPs 1, 4, and 5 were detected, by RNA protection assay, in the lung before birth; after birth AQP$_1$ mRNA increased greatly, and stayed strongly expressed, whereas the mRNA for AQP$_5$ increased slowly over the first week.[95] The pattern of expression of mRNA for AQP$_5$ differed, in that it increased slowly after birth. AQP$_1$, however, is not expressed in airway epithelium, but occurs predominantly in peribronchial capillaries and visceral pleura.[51] The mRNA level for AQP$_1$ can be increased substantially by glucocorticoid treatment.[51] No mention was made of AQP$_2$, which is the AVP-dependent water channel of the kidney. Given the fact that AVP can alter fluid secretion, on might have expected to find some AQP$_2$ mRNA. On the other hand, if the effect of AVP is via an alteration in the circulation and the volume of blood perfusing the immature alveoli, then one would not expect to find AQP$_2$ mRNA.

The role of water channels in the developing lung and their potential regulation by hormones are exciting areas of investigation for the future.

In summary, there are now known to be at least six genes encoding water channel proteins, and more members of this family may well yet be found. So far the distribution of gene expression of these water channel genes, in adult tissue of the rat, previously, has been described. There has been no systematic study published for the ontogeny of expression during development of the majority of water channel genes, and certainly none outside the rat, and a very limited amount of work in the human fetal kidney. It has not been demonstrated that the level of expression of any these genes, except for AQP_1, AQP_2, and AQP_3, can be up- or downregulated. AQP_1 was found in the term human placenta but the levels of expression of most water channel genes in tissues from pregnant animals have not been reported. It is unknown whether pregnancy can alter the expression of any water channel genes. Consequently it is unknown as to whether any disorders of fluid balance in pregnancy, such as preeclampsia, hydrops fetalis, and oligo- or polyhydramnios, are associated with abnormalities of expression of one or more water channels. Is there a change in the level of expression of AQP_4 in brain osmoreceptor regions in pregnancy?

These recent advances in the understanding of pathways by which water may cross cell membranes have opened new areas of investigation into the water balance of the pregnant mother and the developing fetus.

Water Balance in Pregnancy—Role of Relaxin

As summarized previously, and reviewed extensively elsewhere,[1,96,97] human pregnancy is characterized by a decrease in plasma osmolality (P_{osm}) of approximately $10\,mOsm \cdot kg^{-1}$ water. This decrease in plasma osmolality reflects the retention, within the entire maternal body, of water in excess of solute, and is thought to occur because osmotic thresholds for drinking and for regulation of secretion of AVP have been reset. The decrease in P_{osm} in the pregnant woman begins by week 5 and reaches its fullest extent by week 10, after which time the new concentration remains unaltered until after parturition. The same phenomenon occurs in the pregnant rat, starting between days 10 and 14 of pregnancy. In other species, such as the sheep and the goat, no such change in P_{osm} occurs during pregnancy.[98,99] A summary report of extensive studies by Lindheimer, Davidson, Barron, Durr et al. suggested that the resetting of the thresholds for water drinking and AVP secretion was most likely due to an ovarian hormone, but was not due to the classic steroid hormones, estrogen and progesterone.[97] The effect could be mimicked by treatment of the nonpregnant woman with human chorionic gonadotropin (hCG).[100]

A nonsteroid hormone, produced by the ovary of the pregnant woman and the rat, but not sheep, is the peptide hormone relaxin.[101-104] Relaxin belongs to the family of insulin/insulin-like growth factors, and is better known for its action on tissues of the reproductive tract, such as relaxation of uterine muscle and ripening of the cervix.[105] However, it has become apparent in recent years that relaxin has more extensive biologic activities, one of which is a very potent chronotropic and inotropic agent on the heart.[106]

Specific, displaceable binding sites, with characteristics of receptors, were also found in the brain,[107] and it was of interest that some of these binding sites—the subfornical organ, the organum vasculosum of the lamina terminalis, and the magnocellular portions of the supraoptic and paraventricular nuclei of the hypothalamus—were areas known to be involved in the regulation of water balance, and to be outside the blood-brain barrier. The increase in plasma relaxin concentration in women and rats begins at the same stages of pregnancy, respectively, as the osmolality drop begins.[101,104] There is no functional relaxin gene in the sheep,[102] a species in which P_{osm} does not change in pregnancy.[98] Human chorionic gonadotropin stimulates the ovary to produce relaxin.[108,109] It therefore seemed a very reasonable hypothesis that relaxin would be the ovarian hormone that acts to reset drinking and P_{AVP} osmotic thresholds. There are now a number of experimental studies that support this hypothesis. Relaxin was administered (human recombinant gene-2, $10\mu g \cdot h^{-1}$ i.v.) to groups of ovariectomized rats for 7 days, and compared results with those receiving either no treatment, or intravenous saline ($10\mu \cdot h^{-1}$) for 7 days.[110] Each of these three groups of rats were then subdivided into three groups, which received no osmotic treatment, 24 hours of dehydration, or hypertonic saline 30 minutes prior to being killed. When the rats were killed rapidly, by decapitation, blood was collected for the measurement of plasma osmolality, AVP, and relaxin. The relaxin treatment was able to mimic the fluid changes in pregnancy (Figure 25.2). Osmolality dropped by $10\,mOsm \cdot kg^{-1}$ water, without change in plasma AVP concentration. The relaxin-treated rats drank the same volumes of water as the controls, despite the lowest P_{osm}. Thus, thresholds for both drinking and AVP secretion were altered, by concentrations of relaxin that were equivalent to those seen during normal pregnancy in the rat.

More recently, Thornton and Fitzsimons[111] showed that when porcine relaxin (5ng) was injected into the anterior third ventricle of the rat, there was an immediate stimulation to the drinking of water but not of isotonic or hypertonic saline. The role of endogenous relaxin was

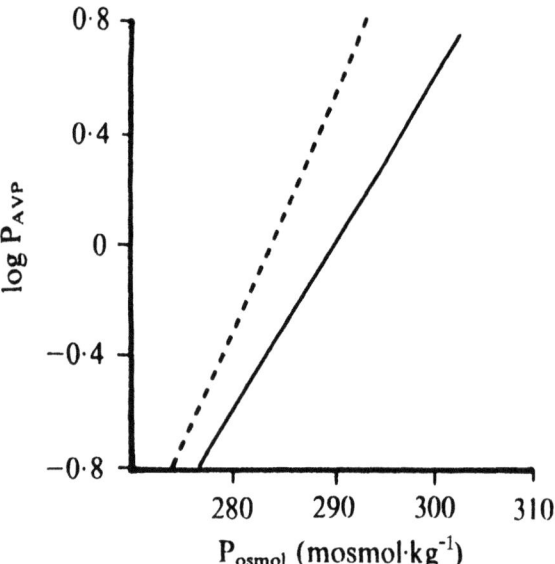

FIGURE 25.2. Calculated regression lines for log plasma arginine vasopressin/plasma osmolality (P_{AVP}/P_{osmol}) in relaxin-treated (broken line) and control (solid line) rats. For relaxin treatment, $y = 0.09x - 25.5$ ($r = .78, n = 15, p > .001$). For control, $y = 0.06x, n = 30, p < .001$. P_{AVP}, pmol·L^{-1}. (From Weisinger et al.,[111] with permission.)

tested by the daily administration of 5 mg (i.v.) of a highly purified monoclonal antibody to relaxin to rats from days 12 to 22 of pregnancy.[112] The mean daily water consumption was decreased by the relaxin-antibody treatment. Unfortunately, no measurements of plasma osmolality were reported for these animals.

Thus, the evidence is accumulating that relaxin is a very important hormone regulating water balance in pregnancy. This is supported by the "natural gene knockout" animal, the sheep, which produces no relaxin, and does not decrease plasma osmolality. It would be of great interest to know if P_{osm} changes in those cases of donor embryo pregnancies, in women without functional ovaries. Although the pregnant ovary is the major source of circulating relaxin in the pregnant woman and rat, the relaxin gene is expressed at low levels in other tissue, including the brain.[105,113] It would be of great interest if overproduction of relaxin, at one of these sites, could be linked to idiopathic hyponatremia.

It is quite possible that in the case of ovarian hyperstimulation syndrome reported recently, in which plasma [Na$^+$] dropped to 117 mmol·L^{-1}, excess relaxin secretion, from multiple corpora lutea, was responsible.[114]

Can relaxin alter the number of water channels in the osmoreceptors, and thus reset the P_{osmol}/P_{AVP} and drinking thresholds? This question remains to be answered.

Mineral Acquisition by the Fetus

For minerals, such as calcium (Ca), that are always in higher concentration in fetal than maternal plasma, there must be active transport by some component of the placenta.[115,116] Although the placenta contains plasma membrane calcium pumps, active transport may involve more of the calcium-binding proteins calbindin D_{9K} and calbindin D_{28}.[117,118] It is highly likely that there is species variation in the exact mechanisms of placental calcium transport, and regulation thereof. While there is good evidence that calbindin D_{9K} is important for placental Ca transport in the normal and diabetic rat,[118,119] it may not be so critical in the human placenta.[120] Fetal parathyroid hormone related peptide (PTHrP) is very important in calcium acquisition by the ovine fetus,[116,121] but may not be so for the rat fetus.[122]

For minerals, such as sodium (Na), for which the maternal plasma concentration is greater than that of fetal plasma, three mechanisms may be involved in placental transport: (1) Na$^+$-H$^+$ exchange, by an amiloride-inhibitible transporter, the NHE-1 (Na$^+$/H$^+$ exchange one) form being predominant in the placenta;[115,123] (2) cotransport with inorganic ions and organic solutes; and (3) Na$^+$ conductance. The Na$^+$-H$^+$ exchanger is thought to be the main transporter on the human placental brush border membrane, and was not affected by hormones such as insulin, angiotensin II, or parathyroid hormone.[123] Mechanisms may differ across species, as there is great variation in placental structure.[124] In the sheep the reflection coefficients for Na$^+$ and Cl$^-$ were found to be significantly less than 1, consistent with a pore size for Na$^+$ of greater than 0.35 but less than 0.4 nm.[125] As there is a greater difference between maternal and fetal plasma [Na$^+$] in the sheep than in the human, due to a much lower permeability of sheep than human placenta to Na$^+$,[126] fructose is synthesized by the placenta and secreted into fetal, but not maternal plasma, to help maintain fetal plasma osmolality.[126] It is not known whether Na$^+$ transport across the ovine placenta can be regulated hormonally.

Maintenance of Placental Blood Flow

Much attention has been focused, recently, on the association of growth during intrauterine life and the susceptibility to diseases of the cardiovascular system and non–insulin-dependent diabetes in adult life.[127–129] This is an additional risk to the well-recognized increase in perinatal morbidity and mortality that is associated with intrauterine growth retardation.[130] The delivery of water, oxygen, and nutrients to the fetus depends on a well-functioning placenta. It is not easy to explain, however, exactly what forces exist to deliver substances such as water and electrolytes to the fetus, particularly in species in which it has been well documented that maternal plasma is always hypertonic to fetal plasma.[1] One thing is certain, however—blood flow to the placenta, on both the maternal and fetal side, must be maintained and balanced.[131] In a prospective combined study across five countries, it was shown that there was a statistically highly significant positive correlation between maternal anemia and placental weight.[132] This finding was confirmed in an even larger study, in which placental weight rose as hemoglobin concentration fell, and this resulted in a large placental to body weight ratio, a known predictor of hypertension in adulthood.[128,133] Inadequate placental function leads to intrauterine growth retardation, and then to an increase in stress and catabolic hormones in the fetus, which may have other effects on fetal fluid balance.[129] Exposure of the immature fetus to higher than normal concentration of glucocorticoid can induce diuresis and natriuresis.[134]

For the above reasons the regulation of placental blood flow, on both the maternal and fetal side, has been the subject of intense study.[135] Some of the factors that have been studied include endothelin,[136-141] endothelin-derived nitric oxide,[136,142-144] eicosanoids,[145] and atrial natriuretic peptide.[146] Endothelin I (Et-1) and its precursor, big Et-1, as well as Et-3, are potent vasoconstrictors in the fetal-placental circulation,[136] acting on both Et-A and Et-B receptors, which are in highest concentration in early pregnancy.[137,139] In growth-retarded fetuses with increased fetoplacental vascular resistance, the fetal plasma concentrations of Et-1 were three to five times that of controls.[138]

The effects of vasoconstrictor endothelins may be antagonized by vasodilator prostaglandins, nitric oxide (NO), and ANP. Local output of NO seemed to make a greater contribution to the low vascular resistance of the fetal vasculature of the human placenta than did the prostaglandins in one study.[145]

ANP_{99-126} receptors are also present in the reproductive tract and placenta of human,[147] sheep,[148] and other species,[149] and appear to be regulated by estrogen and progesterone. It has been shown, experimentally, that low doses of ANP can increase maternal blood flow to the placenta of growth-retarded, but not of normal, guinea pig fetuses.[150]

In addition, the placenta is known to be capable of synthesizing a wide variety of neurohormones, growth factors, cytokines, and steroids,[151] many of which are also capable of affecting placental blood flow.[152]

Preeclampsia

One of the most serious complications of pregnancy is preeclampsia. This is a multisystem disorder, involving primarily placental malfunction, which leads to abnormalities of platelet and clotting functions, vasoconstriction, and, in particular, abnormalities of volume homeostasis.[153-155] It occurs almost always after 20 weeks of gestation, although it may develop before mid-gestation in women with hydatiform mole, or when the fetus has nonimmune fetal hydrops.[155] The volume abnormality involves a redistribution of extracellular fluid such that the plasma volume component is decreased, and the interstitial fluid volume increased.[156] There is a significant correlation between the extent of plasma volume expansion and fetal growth intrauterine growth retardation, which is a serious fetal complication of preeclampsia.[157] The cause of the inequity in plasma and interstitial volume is not known absolutely, but some dysfunction of vascular endothelium is suspected. The primary abnormality is in the placenta, which shows structural changes such as a lack of normal trophoblast invasion of spiral arterioles, as well as the production of various eicosanoids, such as NO, endothelin, and tumor necrosis factor-2, in abnormal amounts.[158-160] In addition, it is proposed that some product secreted, probably by the placenta, into the maternal circulation, acts on the endothelia of systemic blood vessels to alter their normal function, particularly with respect to eicosanoid production.[160,161] The most recent report suggests that this substance is a heat-, acid-, and protease-labile substance that will decrease prostacylin (PGI_2) production of cultured endothelial cells after 72-hour but not 24-hour exposure.[162] The effect is specific for PGI_2 and does not occur with PGE_2. As discussed above, most studies have found that plasma concentrations of some natriuretic peptides, particularly ANP and BNP, are increased in maternal plasma in preeclamptic women.[26,29,162] As ANP enhances transcapillary migration of fluid, this may play a role in the unusual distribution of extracellular fluid in preeclampsia.

Some investigators have long recommended that all pregnant women should be put on a low-salt diet as a prophylactic measure against the development of preeclampsia.[163] However, there is a lack of evidence that a low-salt diet during pregnancy is of any significant advantage,[158] and it has been shown that dietary sodium restriction also reduces the intake of protein, fat, and calcium.[164]

In addition the same group has shown that salt restriction leads to lower stroke volume and cardiac output and higher systemic vascular resistance, which is not ideal for those with genetic susceptibility to developing preeclampsia.[163] In fact, the supposition that preeclampsia is a state of excess salt and water retention is not true for the majority of pregnancy, although total body sodium, relative to body weight, may be higher than normal at one point in gestation.[157,165] Plasma osmolality decreases normally in preeclampsia,[156] and the relaxin concentration is normal.[166] The classic salt-retaining hormonal renin-angiotensin-aldosterone system is actually depressed in preeclampsia, from the increased activity seen in normal human pregnancy.[167] In fact, a number of reports have linked the predisposition to develop preeclampsia to a molecular variant on the angiotensinogen gene.[168,169]

Women with preeclampsia have also been shown to have decreased numbers of mineralocorticoid receptors on peripheral leukocytes.[170,171] They have normal levels of both plasma and urinary cortisol/cortisone ratio, indicating no deficiency of 11β-hydroxysteroid dehydrogenase activity, and no tendency for cortisol to act as mineralocorticoid receptor agonist.[172] Sodium deficiency in pregnancy stimulates increases in the renin-angiotensin-aldosterone system[1] and where the normal pregnant woman shows a decreased pressor responsiveness to exogenous angiotensin II (Ang II) this does not occur in women developing preeclampsia.[36] There is evidence that angiotensin II receptors, at least in platelets, are increased in the preeclamptic woman,[173,174] but not the pregnant woman with gestational hypertension.[175] However, it remains to be proven that vascular Ang II receptors behave in the same way. There is, for example, evidence from rat studies that uterine and glomerular Ang II re-

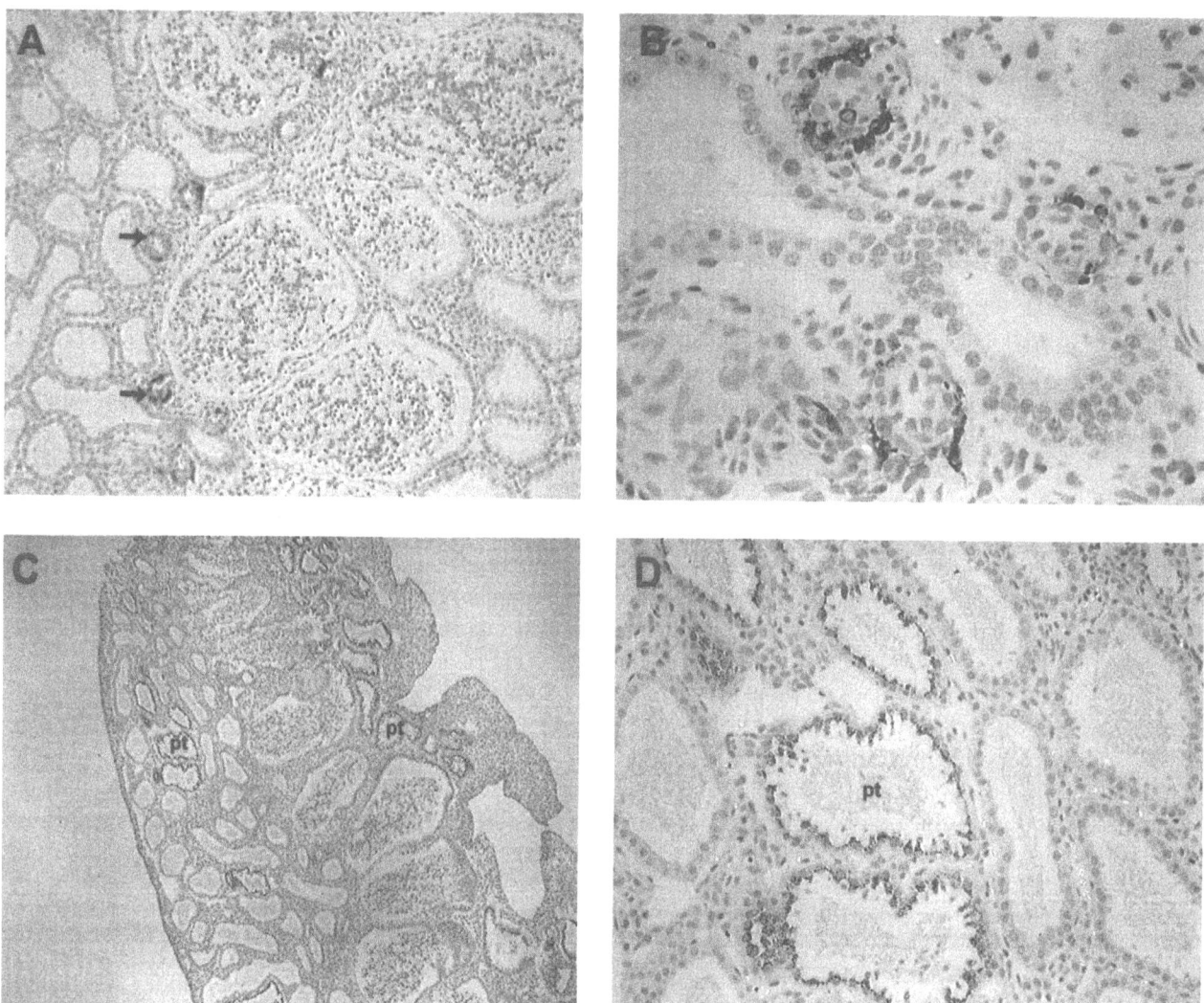

FIGURE 25.3. The renin-angiotensin system in the ovine fetal mesonephric kidney, at 41 days of gestation (term is 145 to 150 days). A, B: Renin immunoreactive cells (arrow, brown staining) are seen in the walls of small and large blood vessels. Magnification A ×100, B ×400. Counterstain—hematoxylin. C, D. Angiotensinogen immunoreactive cells in proximal tubules (pt) of ovine mesonephros. Counterstained with hematoxylin. Magnification C ×40, D ×200. E, F. By hybridization histochemistry the mRNA for angiotensin II receptor, type I, AT_1, is seen in cells in the glomeruli (g) of the ovine fetal mesonephros. E, light field; F, dark field. Magnification E, F ×100. G, H. The mRNA for the angiotensin II receptor, type 2e, AT_2, occurs in the interstitial tissue (it) surrounding the ovine fetal mesonephros. G, light field; H, dark field. Magnification G, H ×100.

ceptors do not alter in pregnancy in parallel, and there are differences in Wistar-Kyoto and spontaneously hypertensive rats.[176] The capacity and affinity of Ang II receptors in human placental blood vessels are lower in the placenta from preeclamptic than from normal pregnant women.[177] For these reasons (i.e., high concentration of natriuretic hormones, lower than normal concentration of antinatriuretic hormones and mineralocorticoid receptors) it seems that there is no valid reason to severely restrict the normal salt intake of pregnant women.

Effect of Inhibition of Angiotensin-Converting Enzyme on the Fetus

For the treatment of many forms of hypertension, angiotensin-converting enzyme (ACE) inhibitors such as captopril or enalapril have been used widely. However, when these drugs were used in the pregnant woman, there were reports of fetal morbidity, which led to warnings about their use by the U.S. Food and Drug Administration.[179,180] This subject has been reviewed by several groups.[180,181] The major adverse effects of the use of ACE inhibitors in pregnancy were fetal hypotension, renal failure, renal tubular dysplasia, pulmonary hypoplasia, growth restriction, hypocalvaria, and increased fetal and neonatal mortality or morbidity.[178,180,182–184] The effects on the fetal kidney are particularly pertinent and are discussed below.

All the components of the renin-angiotensin system (RAS)—renin, angiotensin, ACE, Ang II receptors—are not only present in the developing fetus, but also are found in the fetal kidney itself.[185–201] The components of the RAS are even expressed in the mesonephros—the transient kidney, which functions before the metanephros—as shown in Figure 25.3. In the ovine fetus

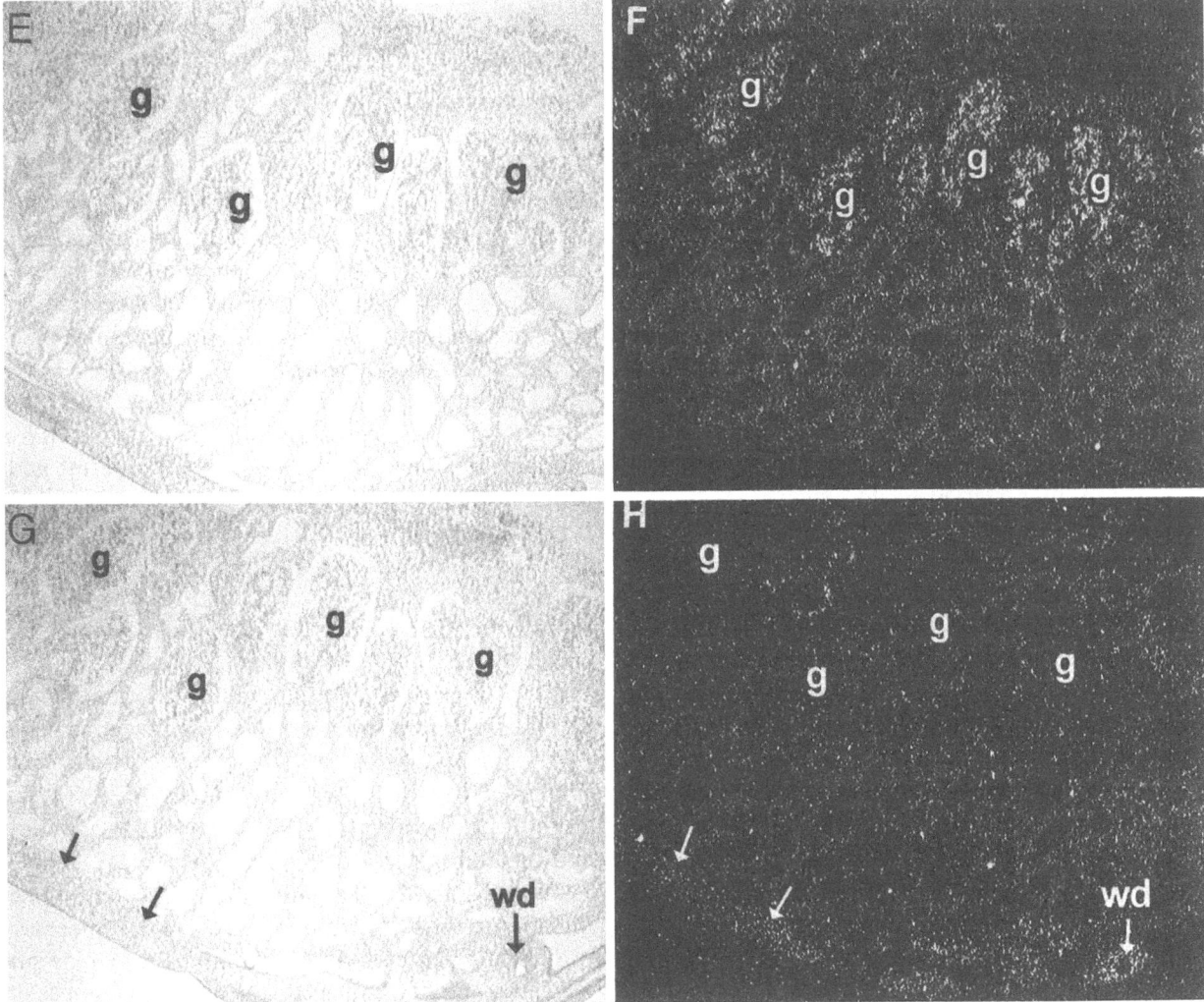

FIGURE 25.3. *Continued*

the mesonephros starts to develop at day 16, reaches maximal size at day 30, and is completely regressed by day 57.[202] The expression of renin, angiotensinogen, and the Ang II receptors AT_1 and AT_2 are very similar in the sheep mesonephros to that found by Schutz et al.[201] in the human mesonephros, which begins at about 3 weeks, reaches maximal size at 8 weeks, and is completely regressed by 16 weeks.[202] In both human and sheep there is a certain period when both mesonephroi and metanephroi coexist, and components of the RAS are expressed simultaneously in both the transient and permanent kidneys.[200,200a,201]

It has been suggested that local, intrarenal production of angiotensin II may be more important in the developing kidney than systemically produced Ang II.[194] This has led to the investigation of the specific role of angiotensin II on renal function in fetal and neonatal life. The argument has been put that, whereas in the adult the major effect of the renin-angiotensin system is salt and water conservation,[203] the major importance of this system in the fetus is the maintenance of normal renal glomerular filtration and urine production, or salt and water excretion into the amniotic compartment.[204] Thus, inhibition of ACE would lead to the previously observed fetal renal failure, and consequent oligohydramnios. Some of the other adverse effects reported with the use of ACE inhibitors, such as pulmonary hypoplasia, would be secondary to oligohydramnios.[205] When studies were done in chronically cannulated ovine fetuses, the short-term (hours) inhibition of the formation of Ang II with ACE inhibitors or the action of Ang II with losartan brought contradictory results, mostly finding only small, if any, effects on fetal blood pressure and renal function in the normal, unstressed fetus.[206–208] The fetal RAS seemed to be more important when the fetus was subjected to some stress, such as hypoxia or hemorrhage, relatively late in gestation.[207,209,210]

Investigators then started to do longer-term studies, more relevant to the situation that might be encountered in the use of ACE inhibitors in the pregnant woman. With long-term treatment, inhibition of Ang II production by ACE inhibitors was shown to cause a severe drop in glomerular filtration rate, even to the point of producing anuria in some fetuses.[211] In the neonatal rat, the administration of an Ang II inhibitor[212] or an ACE inhibitor[213–215] inhibited normal renal growth, impaired renal function, and was associated with increased mortality rates in the neonatal period. The effect of long-term Ang II action could have been due to the fact that Ang II normally induces the formation of a larger proportion of AT_1 receptors than AT_2 receptors. In fetal life, there is a higher proportion of the AT_2 receptor type,[199,216–219] while the functional effects of Ang II on blood pressure and glomerular filtration rate are mediated via the AT_1 receptor.[220] However, in the neonatal rat there was no evidence that the mRNA for the AT_1 receptor was regulated by Ang II binding.[212] A note of caution, nevertheless, must be inserted here. It has been shown that AT_2 receptor mRNA can be present when the actual receptor, as detected by ligand-binding, has not yet appeared.[221]

Another explanation for the greater deleterious effects of long-term rather than short-term ACE inhibition could lie with the actual growth effects of Ang II in the developing kidney. At the time when active nephrogenesis is occurring, before birth in man and sheep, but continuing after birth in the neonate in the rat, ACE inhibition will prevent the normal development of glomeruli.[213,214] However, this cannot be the only explanation of complete anuria, and some importance must be placed on the necessity for Ang II to maintain normal GFR in an underperfused developing kidney.[211] The potential complications of using the standard ACE inhibitors has led to the search for angiotensin II receptor antagonists that may be of less toxicity to the fetus and so can be used safely in hypertension during pregnancy.[222]

The Role of Amniotic Fluid

Amniotic fluid (AF) has been considered, traditionally, as having a major function of providing an aqueous environment in which symmetrical development of the fetus can occur. In the absence of adequate amounts of AF, severe abnormalities of morphologic development occur.[79] In addition, AF has been thought to buffer the fetus from sudden severe changes in temperature or pressure. More recently it has been realized that the AF may perform at least two additional roles: (1) serving as a reservoir of fluid and electrolyte for the fetus; and (2) containing a number of protein, peptide, and steroid factors that may affect growth and development of the fetus after the AF is swallowed, or the hormone/metabolite is absorbed into the fetal circulation. For these reasons there is continued investigation into the regulation of composition and volume of AF.

In species in which a substantial allantoic compartment exists for most of gestation (e.g., sheep, pig, horse, cow, etc.) some of these additional functions may be subserved by the water and solutes of the allantoic fluid (ALLF); however, ALLF cannot be swallowed, and any substance stored in the ALLF for future use must be absorbed via the circulation. Thus, the role of the membranes in secreting such factors is of interest. The presence of receptors in the membranes or placenta allows for paracrine and autocrine effects, as well as endocrine effects of locally produced hormone/growth factors/cytokines.

Amniotic Fluid—Reserve Function, Volume Changes

The volume of amniotic fluid, at any one point in time, can be quite variable, in contrast to the composition, which is much more constant.[79,223] One reason for this may be that fluid is recruited from the AF when the mother becomes dehydrated[221] and dehydration of the mother leads to increased plasma osmolality of mother and fetus, which leads to increased secretion of arginine vasopressin (AVP) by the fetus,[80] which decreases urine flow[81] and lung liquid flow[90]—the prime inputs to the amniotic fluid.

Normal urine flow in the human fetus is of the order of $10\,ml\cdot kg^{-1}hr^{-1}$, which is of the same order as that of the most popular animal model, the ovine fetus. Increased urine flow rates occur if excess hypotonic fluid is delivered to the fetus[225] or if the fetus is exposed to an increased concentration of glucocorticoid at certain periods, generally less than 0.8 of gestation,[134,226,227] or to atrial natriuretic factor.[228] Oligohydramnios results when there is deficient fetal urine input, due either to intrinsic renal defects or to increased AVP output, secondary to fetal hypoxia, hypovolemia, hemorrhage, or maternal indomethacin treatment.[80,202,229] Polyhydramnios may result when there is prolonged, excess urine production, such as is hypothesized to result from high fetal plasma concentrations of atrial natriuretic peptide in the hypertransfused twin of the "stuck twin" syndrome.[230-232] This syndrome is thought to occur when in monozygotic twins sharing a placenta, unbalanced shunting of blood occurs from one twin to the other via a vascular anastomosis.[233,234] The donor twin fails to grow, becomes anemic, and suffers oligohydramnios, the amniotic membrane becomes "stuck" to the fetus. The recipient twin suffers polyhydramnios, which is often quite severe, with up to 20 L of fluid accumulating.[235] As the chronic form often becomes apparent early in gestation, during the second trimester, the mortality rate is very high, probably greater than 70%, due to spontaneous abortion or the very premature delivery of growth-retarded and immature fetuses.

In species with substantial allantoic compartment (e.g., sheep, horse, and cow) abnormalities of allantoic fluid volume are more common than those of amniotic fluid volume.[236,237] When excess urine production is stimulated by exogenous glucocorticoid treatment over days, hydrallantois is the result around mid-gestation.[134,226] However, when urine production rate is increased by hormonal treatment, or by infusion of fluids into the fetus, in the last third of gestation,[223,227] excess fluid does not accumulate for any prolonged period, in either the amniotic or allantoic compartment. This may be due to the fact that there is a substantial blood flow to the fetal membranes of sheep, in the last third of gestation, of some 40 to $50\,ml\cdot min^{-1}$,[208,238] and fluid can cross both amniotic and allantoic membranes relatively rapidly.[239,240]

Protein/Peptide Factors Made by Fetal Membranes

As shown in Table 25.3, human amniotic fluid contains very large quantities of parathyroid-hormone related peptide (PTHrP), vastly in excess of concentrations in maternal and/or fetal plasma. The major source is the amnion, which contains both mRNA and immunoreactive peptide.[241-247] When amniotic cells were cultured, PTHrP secretion was increased, modestly, by human placental lactogen, or growth hormone, as well as by insulin, insulin-like growth factors-I and -II, and epidermal growth factor. Calcitriol and dexamethasone decreased secretion.[247] The receptor mRNA was abundant in the chorio-decidua.[24] 'The roles for PTHrP are unknown, but may involve stimulation of calcium transport to the fetus, vasodilation of placental vessels, and relaxation of the uterus.

Prolactin

Prolactin has long been known to occur in human amniotic fluid in quite high concentrations (Table 25.3). The source of the prolactin is the decidua.[248] There have been many experimental studies to test the hypothesis that prolactin may play a role in the regulation of amniotic fluid volume.[79] Eventually there did appear to be reasonable evidence that this was so. However, the validity of these experiments now comes into question with the finding that the mRNA for the prolactin receptor is found exclusively in the decidua, which could not explain the results on water transfer across the amnion.[249] It is always possible, of course, that the effect is indirect, or that another receptor, not encoded by the prolactin receptor cDNA used in this study, is responsible for the observed effects.[49]

Endothelins

There are three endothelin genes in the human genomic library and they encode three distinct peptides endothelins (ET) 1, 2, and 3, which may act on either or both of two receptors, ET-A and ET-B.[250] The particular peptide found in AF is ET-1 in several molecular weights, which can act on both forms of receptor. The source of AF ET-1 is the nonvascular amnion, which contains the mRNA for prepro-ET-1.[251,252] The level of synthesis and release of ET-1 can be altered by substances normally found in AF: epidermal growth factor

TABLE 25.3. Concentration of certain hormones/peptides found in human amniotic fluid.

Hormone (unit)	Gestation	Amniotic fluid	Maternal plasma	Fetal plasma	Reference
PTHrP ($pmol \cdot l^{-1}$)	16 weeks	21 ± 6	—	—	242,295
	38 weeks	41 ± 9	—	—	
	17 weeks	21.2 ± 3.7	1.4 ± 0.3	1.6 ± 0.1	248
	Term	19 ± 2.7			
Prolactin ($ng \cdot ml^{-1}$)	10–20 weeks	1200–7000	24.8 ± 2.4	—	296
	Term	350	207 ± 47	—	
ET-1	16–17 weeks	203 ± 16	1/10–1/100 AF level		253
	37–40 weeks	70 ± 8			
	in labor	130 ± 13			
BNP ($pmol \cdot l^{-1}$)	First trimester	119 ± 58			4
	Second trimester	108 ± 9			
	Third trimester	28 ± 5	2–3	2–3	
HGF ($ng \cdot ml^{-1}$)	14–16 weeks	12.4 ± 4.5	—	—	261
	38.8 ± 1.2 weeks	10.5 ± 6.6	—	~1	262
Renin ($U \cdot ml^{-1}$)	0–13 weeks	—	162 ± 91	—	297
	36–40 weeks	1470 ± 860	43 ± 17	—	

PTHrP, parathyroid hormone-related peptide; ET-1, endothelin 1; BNP, brain natriuretic peptide; HGF, hepatocyte growth factor.

(EGF), transforming growth factor-β (TGF-β), and cytokines, which could be produced by macrophages or bacteria in situations such as chorioamnonitis.[251] Receptors, both ET-A and ET-B, are present in the amnion, chorion, decidua, as well as the placenta.[253] With respect to AF volume regulation, no effect on water transfer by fetal membranes could be detected in short-term in vitro experiments.[254] However, ET-1 was shown to inhibit basal and stimulated release of prolactin by human decidual cells and thus might indirectly affect AF volume in vivo.[255]

Brain Natriuretic Peptide (BNP)

As discussed above, BNP, a peptide with natriuretic, diuretic, and vasodilator properties, occurs in human AF at values some 50-fold higher than in maternal or fetal plasma, particularly in the first two trimesters.[4] The source is the amnion and secretion is stimulated by TGF-β, and inhibited by cortisol, EGF, at concentrations known to exist in human AF.[256] The role of AF BNP remains to be elucidated.

Hepatocyte Growth Factor (HGF)

Hepatocyte growth factor is another example of a peptide named for one biologic effect but now known to exhibit a wide variety of growth and differential effects.[257]

Originally named because of its potent mitogen effects on hepatocytes, and thought to be important only for liver regeneration,[258] HGF was then recognized as a morphogen for kidney development,[259] and has subsequently been shown to have effects on a wide variety of developmental tissues, including hemopoietic tissue.[257] The highest concentration ever measured in a biologic fluid occurs in human amniotic fluid.[260] This is at least 10 times the concentration found in cord serum at term.[261] The source is both placenta and probably amnion. It acts on the receptor c-*met*, which is expressed widely.[263] The role of HGF in the AF is not yet determined, but when the HGF gene is "knocked out" in mice the embryos die by day 16.[264]

Renin

The renin found in human amniotic fluid is largely inactive or prorenin, and is synthesized in the chorion and decidua.[167] More recently, questions have been raised as to whether most of the renin mRNA, protein, or activity found in fetal membranes is actually there within infiltrating macrophage-like cells.[265] All the Ang II receptor types in the human placenta and fetal membranes appear to be of the AT_1 type, and the fetal membranes, amnion and chorion, contain very few receptors.[266] However, renin appears to be able to cause some effects, e.g., stimulating human amnion prostaglandin E_2 biosynthesis, by a mechanism not involving the production of Ang II and therefore not using, presumably, Ang II receptors.[267] Although infusions of a high dose of angiotensin I into ovine fetuses can increase fetal fluid volumes/hydrops fetalis,[268] these effects are most likely secondary to the cardiovascular and renal effects of the increased Ang II, and not due to any effect on water transfer by the placenta or fetal membranes.[269,270]

Summary of Factors in Amniotic Fluid

Some examples of substances found in human amniotic fluid in high concentrations have been given, but this is by no means an exhaustive list. It does serve to show that AF should be considered as more than just a fluid surrounding the developing fetus. Of interest, one would never guess by looking at the ultrastructure of the amnion that it has such a large protein biosynthetic capacity, as typical granules do not form a prominent part of the epithelial cell ultrastructure.

Human amniotic fluid also contains other hormones, at concentrations significantly lower than those of maternal plasma. Such hormones include relaxin,[271] which occurs at one tenth or less of maternal plasma concentration, and may originate from the maternally derived decidua,[272] and corticotropin-releasing hormone (CRH), which is synthesized in the amnion as well as the placenta and decidua.[273] CRH is present in AF at 16 weeks at a low concentration, which increases only threefold by term, whereas once it appears in maternal plasma (≈18 weeks) the concentration increases, until at term plasma concentration is 100 times that in AF.

Hydrops Fetalis

Hydrops fetalis occurs when fluid accumulates excessively in the tissues and body cavities of the fetus. It is associated with a very high perinatal mortality rate.[274] It is divided, broadly, into two categories—immune and nonimmune.[275] While immune hydrops occurs when there is a fetal hemolytic anemia most commonly secondary to maternal isoimmunization with Rh antigen, nonimmune hydrops can be associated with a wide variety of pathologic mechanisms related to fetal, placental, or maternal disease.[276]

Mechanisms by which hydrops can develop in the fetus have been the subject of intense investigation. One of the more interesting facets of these studies has been the question of how both anemia and hypertransfusion can cause hydrops.

What causes fetal hydrops? Why do some fetuses develop hydrops only, others polyhydramnios, others polyhydramnios and hydrops, others hydrops and oligohydramnios?

Hydrops fetalis has been found in human fetuses that had supraventricular tachycardia,[277] and has been shown to occur with atrial pacing in ovine fetuses,[278,280] probably due to increased central venous pressure, and/or increased plasma ANP. Lymphatic excision but not ligation caused experimental hydrops, although the mechanism was not elucidated.[281]

As it is well known that fetuses with anemia secondary to red cell isoimmunization are very likely to develop hydrops,[275] although only when the blood hemoglobin concentration is 7 to 10 g·dl^{-1} lower than the normal mean,[282] an animal model using the rabbit has been developed to study this phenomenon experimentally.[283] Rapid induction of anemia in ovine fetuses led to hydrops in six fetuses in which central venous pressure (CVP) was increased, and not in another six fetuses in which CVP did not change.[284] Chronic anemia in the ovine fetus leads to increased plasma ANP concentration, increased extracellular fluid volume, as well as increased urine flow, which can be lowered by the administration of a specific blocker of ANP receptors.[285] ANP can decrease plasma volume[286] and increase vascular permeability[287] in the ovine fetus in the last third of gestation. In 15 hydropic human fetuses there was a statistically significant lower plasma colloid osmotic pressure than in the 15 nonhydropic fetuses,[288] which may have been due to decreased production rate of protein, or increased extravasation of protein.[289]

Treatment of ovine fetuses with large doses of angiotensin I over a week or more led to excess fetal fluid accumulation in intact fetuses[268] and to hydrops fetalis in the nephrectomized lamb,[290] which had substantial increases in central venous pressure.

The most recent surveys suggest, as expected, that there are more cases of hydrops fetalis that result from nonimmune causes than otherwise,[275,276] and in such nonimmune cases about 50% show some evidence of right cardiovascular failure.[277] In the twin-to-twin transfusion syndrome both twins may develop hydrops fetalis, from different causes—the donor twin being anemic, while the recipient twin has congestive cardiac failure.[234] Variations in the incidence of hydrops fetalis and polyhydramnios may depend on the hormonal response of the fetus to perturbations of central venous pressure and atrial pressure. In some acute studies in the ovine fetus a 30-minute increase in atrial pressure, induced by pulmonary artery constriction, increased not only ANP, but AVP and renin concentrations in fetal blood.[291] Increases in AVP would tend to decrease urine flow, while increased renin and ANP would tend to increase urine flow.[200] While the causes of hydrops fetalis remain unknown, advanced technology now allows earlier and more reliable diagnosis, and the possibility of treatment.[292,293]

Implications

Since the first edition of this book was published in 1991, there has been an exponential increase in the amount of knowledge of factors and mechanisms regulating salt and water balance in the nonpregnant mammal. To a large extent, these recent discoveries have not been applied yet to the maternal or fetal organism. However, exciting new prospects for discovery are now in sight. With advancing technology, disorders of fluid balance of the fetus can be diagnosed earlier and more accurately. The understanding of the genetic basis for some disorders of water balance, the knowledge of more extensive classes of natriuretic peptides and their receptors, the increasing list of vasoactive compounds that may regulate maternal and fetal cardiovascular functions, and placental transfer of fluid and electrolyte, should all lead to a greater ability to discover the causes of and some cures for disorders of fluid and electrolyte balance in the pregnant woman and fetus.

Acknowledgments. This work is supported by a block grant to the Howard Florey Institute from the National Health and Medical Research Council of Australia. The author wishes to thank Mrs. Helen Mansour for a remarkable effort in typing the manuscript.

References

1. Wintour EM. Water metabolism in the fetal-placental unit. In: Cowett RM, ed. Principles of perinatal-neonatal metabolism. New York: Springer-Verlag, 1991:340–355.
2. Vesely DL. Atrial natriuretic hormones originating from the N-terminus of the atrial natriuretic factor prohormone. Clin Exp Pharmacol Physiol 1995;22:108–114.
3. Mukoyama M, Nakao K, Hosoda K. Brain natriuretic peptide as a novel cardiac hormone in humans. J Clin Invest 1991;87:1402–1412.
4. Itoh H, Sagawa N, Hasegawa M, et al. Brain natriuretic peptide is present in the human amniotic fluid and is secreted from amnion cells. J Clin Endocrinol Metab 1993;76:907–911.
5. Sudoh T, Kanagawa K, Minamino N, et al. C-type natriuretic peptide in porcine brain. Nature 1988;332:78–81.
6. Saito Y, Nakao K, Itoh H, et al. Brain natriuretic peptide is a novel cardiac hormone. Biochem Biophys Res Commun 1989;158:360–368.
7. Dean AD, Vehaskari VM, Greenwald JE. Synthesis and localization of C-type natriuretic peptide in mammalian kidney. Am J Physiol 1994;266:F491–F496.
8. Drewett JG, Garbers DL. The family of guanylyl cyclase receptors and their ligands. Endocr Rev 1994;15:135–162.
9. Maack T, Suzuki M, Almeida FA, et al. Physiological role of silent receptors of atrial natriuretic factor. Science 1987;238:675–678.
10. Nakao K, Ogawa Y, Suga S, et al. Molecular biology and biochemistry of the natriuretic peptide system. II: natriuretic peptide receptors. J Hypertens 1992;10:1111–1114.
11. Jamison RL, Canaan-Kuhl S, Pratt R. The natriuretic peptides and their receptors. Am J Kidney Dis 1992;20:519–530.
12. Brown J, Corr L. Renal mechanisms of human α-atrial natriuretic peptide in man. J Physiol 1987;387:31–46.
13. Harris PJ, Skinner SL, Zhuo J. The effects of atrial natriuretic peptide and glucagon on proximal glomerulotubular balance in anaesthetized rats. J Physiol 1988;402:29–42.
14. Burnett JC, Granger JP, Opgenorth TJ. Effects of synthetic atrial natriuretic factor on renal function and renin release. Am J Physiol 1984;247:F863–F866.
15. Burnett JC, Opgenorth TJ, Granger JP. The renal action of atrial natriuretic peptide during control of glomerular filtration. Kidney Int 1986;30:16–19.
16. Yates NA, McDougall JG, Coghlan JP, et al. Renal effects of atrial natriuretic factor (99–126) in conscious sodium replete sheep. Clin Exp Pharmacol Physiol 1988;15:551–562.
17. Weidmann P, Hellmueller B, Uehlinger DE, et al. Plasma levels and cardiovascular, endocrine and excretory effects of atrial natriuretic peptide receptors in rat tissues. J Clin Endocrinol Metab 1986;62:1027–1036.
18. Metzler CH, Ramsay DJ. Atrial peptide potentiates renal responses to volume expansion in conscious dogs. Am J Physiol 1989;256:R284–R289.
19. Cuneo RC, Espiner EA, Micholls MG, et al. Renal, hemodynamic, and hormonal responses to atrial natriuretic peptide infusions in normal man, and effects of sodium intake. J Clin Endocrinol Metab 1986;63:946–953.
20. Yates NA, Coghlan JP, Murphy GJ, et al. Renal actions of atrial natriuretic factor: modulation of effect by changes in sodium status and aldosterone. Am J Physiol 1990;258:F684–F689.
21. Burgess WJ, Balment RJ. The involvement of vasopressin in the renal actions of atrial natriuretic peptide in conscious fluid-balanced rats. J Endocrinol 1993;138:413–420.
22. Fraenkel MB, Aldred GP, McDougall JG. Sodium status affects GC-B natriuretic peptide receptors mRNA levels, but not GC-A or C receptor mRNA levels, in the sheep kidney. Clin Sci 1994;86:517–522.
23. Holmes SJ, Espiner EA, Richards AM, et al. Renal, endocrine, and hemodynamic effects of brain natriuretic peptide in normal man. J Clin Endocrinol Metab 1993;76:91–96.
24. Yandle T, Richards A, Gilbert A, et al. Assay of brain natriuretic peptide (BNP) in human plasma: evidence for high molecular weight BNP as a major plasma component in heart failure. J Clin Endocrinol Metab 1993;76:832–838.
25. Florkowski CM, Richards AM, Espiner EA, et al. Renal, endocrine, and hemodynamic interactions of atrial and brain natriuretic peptides in normal men. Am J Physiol 1994;266:R1244–R1250.
26. Itoh H, Sagawa N, Mori T, et al. Plasma brain natriuretic peptide level in pregnant women with pregnancy-induced hypertension. Obstet Gynecol 1993;82:71–77.
27. Cusson JR, Gutkowska J, Rey E, et al. Plasma concentration of atrial natriuretic factor in normal pregnancy. N Engl J Med 1985;313:1230–1231.

28. Steegers EAP, van Lakwijk HPJM, Benraad TJ, et al. Atrial natriuretic peptide (ANP) in normal pregnancy: a longitudinal study. Clin Exp Hypertens 1990;B9:273–292.
29. Lowe SA, Macdonald GJ, Brown MA. Acute and chronic regulation of atrial natriuretic peptide in human pregnancy: a longitudinal study. J Hypertens 1992;10:821–829.
30. Mukaddam-Daher S, Gutkowska J, Nuwayhid BS, et al. Atrial natriuretic factor in ovine pregnancy: plasma levels, molecular forms and biological activity. Regul Pept 1994;51:131–139.
31. Robillard JE, Nakamura KT, Varille VA, et al. Plasma and urinary clearance rates of atrial natriuretic factor during ontogeny in sheep. J Dev Physiol 1988;10:335–346.
32. Castro LC, Lam RW, Ross MG, et al. Atrial natriuretic peptide in the sheep. J Dev Physiol 1988;10:235–246.
33. Benjamin BA. Effects of ANF prohormone peptides in conscious monkeys. Clin Exp Pharmacol Physiol 1995; 22:125–129.
34. Dietz JR, Vesely DL, Gower WR, et al. Secretion and renal effects of ANF prohormone peptides. Clin Exp Pharmacol Physiol 1995;22:115–120.
35. Zeidel ML. Regulation of collecting duct Na^+ reabsorption by ANP 31–67. Clin Exp Pharmacol Physiol 1995;22:121–124.
36. Gant NF, Worley RJ, Everett RB, et al. Control of vascular responsiveness during human pregnancy. Kidney Int 1980;18:253–258.
37. McLaughlin MK, Conrad KP. Nitric oxide biosynthesis during pregnancy: implications for circulatory changes. Clin Exp Pharmacol Physiol 1995;22:164–171.
38. Zhang Y, Novak K, Kaufman S. Atrial natriuretic factor release during pregnancy in rats. J Physiol 1995;488:509–514.
39. Kaufman S. Control of intravascular volume during pregnancy. Clin Exp Pharmacol Physiol 1995;22:157–163.
40. Deng Y, Kaufman S. Effect of pregnancy on activation of central pathways following atrial distension. Am J Physiol 1995;269:R552–R556.
41. Kovacs L, Robertson GL. Disorders of water balance—hyponatraemia and hypernatraemia. Baillieres Clin Endocrinol Metab 1992;6:107–127.
42. Trachtman H. Cell volume regulation: a review of cerebral adaptive mechanisms and implications for clinical treatment of osmolal disturbances: II. Pediatr Nephrol 1992;6:104–112.
43. Verkman AS. Water channels in cell membranes. Annu Rev Physiol 1992;54:97–108.
44. Hays RM, Franki N, Simon H, et al. Antidiuretic hormone and exocytosis: lessons from neurosecretion. Am J Physiol 1994;267:C1507–C1524.
45. Sabolic I, Brown D. Water channels in renal and nonrenal tissues. News in Physiol Sci 1995;10:12–17.
46. Brown D, Katsura T, Kawashima M, et al. Cellular distribution of the aquaporins: a family of water channel proteins. Histochem Cell Biol 1995;104:1–9.
47. Verkman AS, Van Hoek AN, Ma T, et al. Water transport across mammalian cell membranes. Am J Physiol 1996; 270:C12–C30.
48. Knepper MA, Wade JB, Terris J, et al. Renal aquaporins. Kidney Int 1996;49:1712–1717.
49. Van Lieburg AF, Knoers NVAM, Deen PMT. Discovery of aquaporins: a breakthrough in research on renal water transport. Pediatr Nephrol 1995;9:228–234.
50. Nielsen S, Marples D, Froklaer J, et al. The aquaporin family of water channels in kidney: an update on physiology and pathophysiology of aquaporin-2. Kidney Int 1996;49:1718–1723.
51. King LS, Nielsen S, Agre P. Aquaporin-1 water channel protein in lung. J Clin Invest 1996;97:2183–2191.
52. Denker BM, Smith BL, Kuhajda FP, et al. Identification, purification, and characterization of a novel M_r 28,000 integral membrane protein from erythrocytes and renal tubules. J Biol Chem 1988;263:15634–15642.
53. Preston GM, Agre P. Isolation of the cDNA for erythrocyte integral membrane protein of 28 kilodaltons: member of an ancient channel family. Proc Natl Acad Sci USA 1991;88:11110–11114.
54. Preston GM, Carroll TP, Guggino WB, et al. Appearance of water channels in *Xenopus* oocytes expressing red cell CHIP28 protein. Science 1992;256:385–387.
55. Brown D, Verbavatz J-M, Valenti G, et al. Localization of the $CHIP_{28}$ water channel in reabsortive segments of the rat male reproductive tract. Eur J Cell Biol 1993;61:264–273.
56. Deen PMT, Dempster JA, Wieringa B, et al. Isolation of a cDNA for rat $CHIP_{28}$ water channel: high mRNA expression in kidney cortex and inner medulla. Biochem Biophys Res Commun 1992;188(3):1267–1273.
57. Bondy C, Chin E, Smith BL, et al. Developmental gene expression and tissue distribution of the $CHIP_{28}$ water channel protein. Proc Natl Acad Sci USA 1993;90:4500–4504.
58. Agre P, Baumgarten R, Preston GM, et al. Human red cell aquaporin CHIP: II. Expression during normal fetal development and in a novel form of congenital dyserythropoietic anemia. J Clin Invest 1994;94:1050–1058.
59. Moon C, Preston GM, Griffin CA, et al. The human aquaporin-CHIP gene. J Biol Chem 1993;268(21):15772–15778.
60. Preston GM, Smith BL, Zeidel ML, et al. Mutation in aquaporin-1 in phenotypically normal humans without functional CHIP water channels. Science 1994;265:1585–1587.
61. Gorin NB, Yancey SB, Cline J, et al. The major intrinsic protein (MIP) of the bovine lens fiber membrane. Cell 1984;39:49–59.
62. Reizer J, Reizer A, Saier MH. The MIP family of integral membrane channel proteins: sequence comparisons, evolutionary relationships, reconstructed pathway of evolution, and proposed functional differentiation of the two repeated halves of the proteins. Crit Rev Biochem Mol Biol 1993;28(3):235–257.
63. Mulders SM, Preston GM, Deen PMT, et al. Water channel properties of major intrinsic protein of lens. J Biol Chem 1995;270:9010–9016.
64. Shiels A, Bassnetts. Mutations in the founder of the *MIP* gene family underlie cataract development in the mouse. Nature Genet 1996;12:212–215.

65. Fushimi K, Uchida S, Hara Y, et al. Cloning and expression of apical membrane water channel of rat kidney collecting tubule. Nature 1993;361:549–552.
66. Ma T, Hasegawa H, Skach WR, et al. Expression, functional analysis, and in situ hybridization of a cloned rat kidney collecting duct water channel. Am J Physiol 1994;266:C189–C197.
67. Nielsen S, Digiovanni SR, Christensen EI, et al. Cellular and subcellular immunolocalization of vasopressin-regulated water channel in rat kidney. Proc Natl Acad Sci USA 1993;90:11663–11667.
68. Jo I, Harris HW, Amendt-Raduege AM, et al. Rat kidney papilla contains abundant synaptobrevin protein that participates in the fusion of antidiuretic hormone-regulated water channel-containing endosomes in vitro. Proc Natl Acad Sci USA 1995;92:1876–1880.
69. Nielsen S, Marples D, Birn H, et al. Expression of VAMP2-like protein in kidney collecting duct intracellular vesicles colocalization with aquaporin-2 water channels. J Clin Invest 1995;96:1834–1844.
70. Yamamoto T, Sasaki S, Fushimi K, et al. Vasopressin increases AQP-CD water channel in apical membrane of collecting duct cells in Brattleboro rats. Am J Pathol 1995;268:C1546–C1551.
71. Brown D, Stow JL, Protein trafficking and polarity in kidney epithelium: from cell biology to physiology. Am Physiol Soc 1996;76:245–297.
72. Katsura T, Ausiello DA, Brown D. Direct demonstration of aquaporin-2 water channel recycling in stably transfected LLC-PK$_1$ epithelial cells. Am J Physiol 1996;270:F548–F553.
73. Uchida S, Sasaki S, Fushimi K, et al. Isolation of human aquaporin-CD gene. J Biol Chem 1994;269:23451–23455.
74. van Lieburg AF, Knoers VVAM, Mallmann R, et al. Normal fibrinolytic responses to 1-desamino-8-D-arginine vasopressin in patients with nephrogenic diabetes insipidus caused by mutations in the aquaporin 2 gene. Nephron 1996;72:544–546.
75. Marples D, Frokiaer J, Dorup J, et al. Hypokalemia-induced downregulation of aquaporin-2 water channel expression in rat kidney medulla and cortex. J Clin Invest 1996;97:1960–1968.
76. Marples D, Christensen S, Christensen EI, et al. Lithium-induced downregulation of aquaporin-2 water channel expression in rat kidney medulla. J Clin Invest 1995; 95:1838–1845.
77. Fujita N, Ishikawa SE, Sasaki S, et al. Role of water channel AQP-CD in water retention in SIADH and cirrhotic rats. Am J Physiol 1995;269:F926–F931.
78. Yamamoto T, Sasaki S, Fushimi K et al. Expression of AQP family in rat kidneys during development and maturation. Am J Physiol 1997;272:F1988–F2004.
79. Wintour EM, Shandley L, Effects of fetal fluid balance on amniotic fluid volume. Semin Perinatol 1993;17:158–172.
80. Ervin MG, Kullama LK, Ross MG, et al. Vasopressin receptors and effects during fetal development. Regul Pept 1993;45:203–208.
81. Wintour EM, Congiu M, Hardy KJ, et al. Regulation of urine osmolality in fetal sheep. Q J Exp Physiol 1982;67:427–435.
82. Horne RSC, MacIsaac RJ, Moritz KM, et al. Effect of arginine vasopressin and parathyroid hormone-related protein on renal function in the ovine foetus. Clin Exp Pharmacol Physiol 1993;20:569–577.
83. Raina S, Preston GM, Guggino WB, et al. Molecular cloning and characterization of an aquaporin cDNA from salivary, acrimal, and respiratory tissues. J Biol Chem 1995;270:1908–1912.
84. Ishibashi K, Sasaki S, Fushima K, et al. Molecular cloning and expression of a member of the aquaporin family with permeability to glycerol and urea in addition to water expressed at the basolateral membrane of kidney collecting duct cells. Proc Natl Acad Sci USA 1994;91:6269–6273.
85. Valenti G, Verbavatz J, Sabolic I, et al. A basolateral CHIP$_{28}$/MIP$_{26}$-related protein (BLIP) in kidney principal cells and gastric parietal cells. Am J Physiol 1994; 267:C812–C820.
86. Ecelbarger CA, Terris J, Frindt G, et al. Aquaporin-3 water channel localization and regulation in rat kidney. Am J Physiol 1995;269:F663–F672.
87. Jung FF, Tang S, Sabolic I, et al. Angiotensin II (ANGII) upregulates CHIP28 expression in immortalized, transformed rat proximal tubule cells (IRPTC). J Am Soc Nephrol 1994;5:274a.
88. Terris J, Ecelbarger CA, Marples D, et al. Distribution of aquaporin-4 water channel expression within the rat kidney. Am J Physiol 1995;269:F775–F785.
88a. Ma T, Young B, Gillespie A et al. Generation and phenotype of a transgenic knock out mouse lacking the mercurial insensitive water channel aquaporin 4. J Clin Invest 1997;100:957–962.
89. Strang LB, Fetal lung liquid: secretion and reabsorption. Physiol Rev 1991;71:991–1016.
90. Hooper SB, Harding R. Fetal lung liquid: a major determinant of the growth and functional development of the fetal lung. Clin Exp Pharmacol Physiol 1995;22:235–247.
91. Wallace MJ, Hooper SB, Harding R. Effects of elevated fetal cortisol concentrations on the volume, secretion and reabsorption of lung liquid. Am J Physiol 1995;269:R881–R887.
92. Davis TA, Gause G, Perks AM, et al. Effects of intravenous saline infusion on fetal ovine lung liquid secretion. Am J Physiol 1992;262:R1117–R1120.
93. Cummings JV, Carlton DP, Poulain FR, et al. Vasopressin effects on lung liquid volume in fetal sheep. Pediatr Res 1995;38:30–35.
94. Matthay MA, Folkesson HG, Verkman AS, Salt and water transport across alveolar and distal airway epithelia in the adult lung. Am J Physiol 1996;270:L487–L503.
95. Umenishi F, Matthay MA, Carter EP, et al. Developmental expression of rat lung water channels in the perinatal period. FASEB 1996;10:144(A25).
96. Monson JF, Williams DJ, Osmoregulatory adaption in pregnancy and its disorders. J Endocr 1992;132:7–9.
97. Lindheimer MD, Barron WM. Water metabolism and vasopressin secretion during pregnancy. Baillieres Clin Obstet Gynaecol 1994;8:311–331.
98. Bell RJ, Laurence BM, Meehan PJ, et al. Regulation and function of arginine vasopressin in pregnant sheep. Am J Physiol 1986;250:F777–F780.

99. Olsson K, Pregnancy—a challenge to water balance. News Physiol Sci 1986;1:131–134.
100. Davison JM, Shiells EA, Philips PR, et al. Serial evaluation of vasopressin release and thirst in human pregnancy. Role of human chorionic gonadotrophin in the osmoregulatory changes of gestation. J Clin Invest 1988;81:798–806.
101. Bell RJ, Eddie LW, Lester AR, et al. Relaxin in human pregnancy serum measured with an homologous radioimmunoassay. Obstet Gynecol 1987;69:585–589.
102. Roche PJ, Crawford RJ, Tregear GW. A single copy relaxin-like gene sequence is present in the sheep. Mol Cell Endocrinol 1993;91:21–28.
103. Eddie LW, Bell RJ, Lester A, et al. Radioimmunoassay of relaxin in pregnancy with an analogue of human relaxin. Lancet 1986;1:1344–1346.
104. Sherwood OD, Crnekovic VE, Gordon WL, et al. Radioimmunoassay of relaxin throughout pregnancy and during parturition in the rat. Endocrinology 1980;107:691–698.
105. Bryant-Greenwood GD, Schwabe C. Human relaxins: chemistry and biology. Endocr Rev 1994;15:5–26.
106. Kakouris H, Eddie LW, Summers RJ. Cardiac effects of relaxin in rats. Lancet 1992;339:1076–1078.
107. Osheroff PL, Phillips HS. Autographic localization of relaxin binding sites in rat brain. Proc Natl Acad Sci USA 1991;88:6413–6417.
108. Gagliardi CL. Goldsmith LT, Saketos M, et al. Human chorionic gonadotropin stimulation of relaxin secretion by luteinized human granulosa cells. Fertil Steril 1992;58:314–320.
109. Johnson MR, Okokon E, Collins WP, et al. The effect of human chorionic gonadotropin and pregnancy on the circulating level of relaxin. J Clin Endocrinol Metab 1991;72:1042–1047.
110. Weisinger RS, Burns P, Eddie LW, et al. Relaxin alters the plasma osmolality/arginine vasopressin relationship in the rat. J Endocrinol 1993;137:505–510.
111. Thornton SN, Fitzsimons JT. The effects of centrally administered porcine relaxin on drinking behaviour in male and female rats. J Neuroendocrinol 1995;7:165–169.
112. Zhao S, Malmgren CH, Shanks RD, et al. Monoclonal antibodies specific for rat relaxin VIII passive immunization with monoclonal antibodies throughout the second half of pregnancy reduces water consumption in rats. Endocrinology 1995;136:1892–1897.
113. Gunnersen JM, Crawford RJ, Tregear GW. Expression of the relaxin gene in rat tissues. Mol Cell Endocrinol 1995;110:55–64.
114. Cremisi HD, Mitch WE. Profound hypotension and sodium retention with the ovarian hyperstimulation syndrome. Am J Kidney Dis 1994;24:854–857.
115. Smith CH, Moe AJ, Ganapathy V. Nutrient transport pathways across the epithelium of the placenta. Annu Rev Nutr 1992;12:183–206.
116. MacIsaac RJ, Heath JA, Rodda CP, et al. Role of the fetal parathyroid glands and parathyroid hormone-related protein in the regulation of placental transport of calcium, magnesium and inorganic phosphate. Reprod Fertil Dev 1991;3:447–457.
117. Strehler E. Recent advances in the molecular characterization of plasma membrane Ca^{2+} pumps. J Membr Biol 1991;120:1–15.
118. Glazier JD, Atkinson DE, Thornburg KL, et al. Gestational changes in Ca^{2+} transport across rat placenta and mRNA for $calbindin_{9k}$ and Ca^{2+}-ATPase. Am J Physiol 1992;263:R930–R935.
119. Husain SM, Birdsey TJ, Glazier JD, et al. Effect of diabetes mellitus on maternofetal flux of calcium and magnesium and $calbindin_{9K}$ mRNA expression in rat placenta. Pediatr Res 1994;35:376–381.
120. Brun P, Durpet JM, Perret C, et al. Vitamin D-dependent calcium-binding proteins (CaPBs) in human fetuses: comparative distribution of 9K CaBP mRNA and 28K CaBP during development. Pediatr Res 1987;21:362–367.
121. Colignon H, Davicco M-J, Barlet J-P. Calcitonin mRNA expression and plasma calciotropic hormones in fetal lambs. Dom Animal Endocrinol 1996;13:269–276.
122. Wintour EM. Water channels and urea transporters. Clin Exp Pharmacol Physiol 1996;24:1–9.
123. Brunette MG, Leclerc M, Claveau D. Na^+ transport by human placental brush border membranes: are there several mechanisms? J Cell Physiol 1996;167:72–80.
124. Leiser R, Kauffman P. Placental structure: in a comparative aspect. Exp Clin Endocrinol 1994;102:122–134.
125. Faber JJ, Anderson DF. Concentration of Na^+ and Cl^- in transplacental ultrafiltrate in sheep. J Physiol 1995;487:159–167.
126. Faber JJ, Thornburg KL. Permeability of the placental membrane for hydrophilic substances. In: Faber JJ, Thornburg KL eds. Placental physiology. New York: Raven Press, 1983:79–89.
127. Law CM, Barker DJP, Bull AR, et al. Maternal and fetal influences on blood pressure. Arch Dis Child 1991;66:1291–1295.
128. Barker DJP, Gluckman PD, Godfrey KM, et al. Fetal nutrition and cardiovascular disease in adult life. Lancet 1993;341:938–941.
129. Robinson JS, Seamark RF, Owens JA. Placental function. Aust N Z J Obstet Gynaecol 1994;34:240–246.
130. Villar JV, de Onis M, Kestler E, et al. The differential neonatal morbidity of the intrauterine growth retardation syndrome. Am J Obstet Gynecol 1990;163:151–157.
131. Silver M, Barnes RJ, Comline RS, et al. Placental blood flow: some fetal and maternal cardiovascular adjustments during gestation. J Reprod Fertil Suppl 1982;31:139–160.
132. Beischer NA, Sivasamboo R, Vohra S, et al. Placental hypertrophy in severe pregnancy anemia. J Obstet Gynaecol Br Commonw 1970;77:398–409.
133. Godfrey KM, Redman WG, Barker DJP. The effect of maternal anaemia and iron deficiency on the ratio of fetal weight to placental weight. Br J Obstet Gynaecol 1991;98:886–891.
134. Wintour EM, Alcorn D, McFarlane A, et al. Effect of maternal glucocorticoid treatment on fetal fluids in sheep at 0.4 gestation. Am J Physiol 1994;266:R1174–R1181.
135. Boura ALA, Walters WAW, Read MA, et al. Autacoids and control of human placental blood flow. Clin Exp Pharmacol Physiol 1994;21:737–748.

136. Myatt L, Brewer AS, Brockman DE. The comparative effects of big endothelin-1, endothelin-1, and endothelin-3 in the human fetal-placental circulation. Am J Obstet Gynecol 1992;167:1651–1656.
137. Robaut C, Mondon F, Bandet J, et al. Regional distribution and pharmacological characterization of [125I] endothelin-1 binding sites in human fetal placental vessels. Placenta 1991;12:55–67.
138. McQueen J, Kingdom JCP, Connell JMC. Fetal endothelin levels and placental vascular endothelin receptors in intrauterine growth retardation. Obstet Gynecol 1993;82:992–998.
139. Kilpatrick SJ, Roberts JM, Lykins DL, et al. Characterization and ontogeny of endothelin receptors in human placenta. Am J Physiol 1993;264:E367–E372.
140. Gude NM, King RG, Brennecke SP. Endothelin: release by and potent constrictor effect on the fetal vessels of human perfused placental lobules. Reprod Fertil Dev 1991;3:495–500.
141. Handwerker S. Endothelins and the placenta. J Lab Clin Med 1995;125:679–681.
142. Gude NM, King RG, Brennecke SP. Role of endothelium-derived nitric oxide in maintenance of low fetal vascular resistance in placenta. Lancet 1990;2:1589–1590.
143. Gude NM. Endothelium-derived relaxing factor (nitric oxide) and the placenta. In: Rice GE, Brennecke SP, eds. Molecular aspects of placental and fetal membrane autacoids. Boca Raton, FL: CRC Press, 1993:263–276.
144. Gude NM, DiIulio J, Brennecke SP, et al. Human placental villous nitric oxide synthase activity. Pharmacol Comm 1994;4:163–171.
145. Gude NM, Xie CY, King RG, et al. Effects of eicosanoid and endothelial cells derived relaxing factor inhibition on fetal vascular tone and responsiveness in the human perfused placenta. Troph Res 1993;7:133–145.
146. Graham CH, Watson JD, Blumenfeld AJ, et al. Expression of atrial natriuretic peptide by third-trimester placental cytotrophoblasts in women. Biol Reprod 1996;54:834–840.
147. Hatjis CG, Greelish JP, Kofinas AD, et al. Atrial natriuretic factor maternal and fetal concentrations in severe preeclampsia. Am J Obstet Gynecol 1989;161:1015–1019.
148. Fujino Y, Ross MG, Ervin MG, et al. Ovine maternal and fetal glomerular atrial natriuretic factor receptors: response to dehydration. Biol Neonate 1992;62:120–126.
149. Potvin W, Varma DR. Down-regulation of myometrial atrial natriuretic factor receptors by progesterone and pregnancy and up-regulation by oestrogen in rats. J Endocrinol 1991;131:259–266.
150. Jansson TB. Low-dose infusion of atrial natriuretic peptide in the conscious guinea pig increases blood flow to the placenta of growth-retarded fetuses. Am J Obstet Gynecol 1992;166:213–218.
151. Petraglia F, Florio P, Nappi C, et al. Peptide signalling in human and membranes: autocrine, paracrine and endocrine mechanisms. Endocr Rev 1996;17:156–186.
152. Clifton VL, Read MA, Boura ALA, et al. Adrenocorticotropin causes vasolidation in the human fetal-placental circulation. J Clin Endocrinol Metab 1996;81:1406–1410.
153. Brown MA. The physiology of pre-eclampsia. Clin Exp Pharmacol Physiol 1995;22:781–791.
154. Easterling TR, Benedetti TJ. Preeclampsia: a hyperdynamic disease model. Am J Obstet Gynecol 1989;160:1447–1453.
155. Cunningham FG, Lindheimer MD. Hypertension in pregnancy. N Engl J Med 1992;326:927–932.
156. Brown MA, Zammit VC, Mitar DM. Extracellular fluid volumes in pregnancy-induced hypertension. J Hypertens 1992;10:61–68.
157. Brown MA, Gallery ED. Volume homeostasis in normal pregnancy and pre-eclampsia: physiology and clinical implications. Bailliers Clin Obstet Gynaecol 1994;8:287–310.
158. Pinto A, Sorrentino R, Sorrentino P, et al. Endothelial-derived relaxin factor released by endothelial cells of human umbilical vessels and its impairment in pregnancy-induced hypertension. Am J Obstet Gynecol 1991;164:507–513.
159. Schiff E, Friedman SA, Baumann P, et al. Tumor necrosis factor-α in pregnancies associated with preeclampsia or small-for-gestational-age newborns. Am J Obstet Gynecol 1994;170:1224–1229.
160. Brown MA. Pre-eclampsia: recognition, prevention and management. Nephrol 1995;1:163–173.
161. Baker PN, Davidge ST, Barankiewicz J, et al. Plasma of preeclamptic women stimulates and then inhibits endothelial prostacyclin. Hypertension 1996;27:56–61.
162. Fievet P, Fournier A, de Bold A, et al. Atrial natriuretic factor in pregnancy-induced hypertension and preeclampsia: increased plasma concentrations possibly explaining these hypovolemic states with paradoxical hyporeninism. Am J Hypertens 1988;1:16–21.
163. Steegers EAP, Eskes TKAB, Hein PR. Dietary sodium restriction during pregnancy; a historical review. Eur J Obstet Gynecol Reprod Biol 1991;40:83–90.
164. van Buul EJA, Steegers EAP, Jongsma HW, et al. Haematological and biochemical profile of uncomplicated pregnancy in nulliparous women; a longitudinal study. Neth J Med 1995;46:73–85.
165. Davey DA, O'Sullivan WJ, McClure Brown JC. Total exhangeable sodium in normal pregnancy and in pre-eclampsia. Lancet 1961;1:519–523.
166. Szlachter BN, Quagliarello J, Jewelewicz R, et al. Relaxin in normal and pathogenic pregnancies. Obstet Gynecol 1982;59:167–170.
167. Hagemann A, Nielsen AH, Poulsen K. The uteroplacental renin-angiotensin system: a review. Exp Clin Endocrinol 1994;102:252–261.
168. Arngrimsson R, Purandare S, Connor M, et al. Angiotensinogen: a candidate gene involved in preeclampsia. Nature Genet 1993;4:114–115.
169. Ward RM. Drug therapy of the fetus. J Clin Pharmacol 1993;33:780–789.
170. Wacker J, E-Mistry N, Bauer H, et al. Mineralocorticoids and mineralocorticoid receptors in mononuclear leukocytes in patients with pregnancy-induced hypertension. J Clin Endocrinol Metab 1992;74:910–913.

171. Armanini D, Zennaro CM, Martella L, et al. Mineralocorticoid effector mechanisms in preeclampsia. J Clin Endocrinol Metab 1992;74:946–949.
172. Walker BR, Williamson PM, Brown MA, et al. 11β-hydroxysteroid dehydrogenase and its inhibitors in hypertensive pregnancy. Hypertension 1995;25:626–630.
173. Baker PN, Broughton Pipkin F, Symonds EM. Platelet angiotensin II binding sites in normotensive and hypertensive women. Br J Obstet Gynaecol 1991;98:436–440.
174. Pawlak MA, Macdonald GJ, Altered number of platelet angiotensin II receptors in relation to plasma agonist concentrations in normal and hypertensive pregnancy. J Hypertens 1992;10:813–819.
175. Baker PN, Broughton Pipkin F. Platelet angiotensin II binding in pregnant women with chronic hypertension. Am J Obstet Gynecol 1994;170:1301–1302.
176. Yang Y, Macdonald GJ, Duggan KA. Differential regulation of uterine and glomerular angiotensin II receptors in normal and hypertensive pregnancy in the rat. Clin Exp Pharmacol Physiol 1994;21:253–256.
177. Knock GA, Sullivan MHF, McCarthy A, et al. Angiotensin II (AT_1) vascular binding sites in human placentae from normal-term, preeclamptic and growth retarded pregnancies. J Pharmacol Exp Ther 1996;271:1007–1015.
178. Rosa FW, Bosco LA, Fossum-Graham C, et al. Neonatal anuria with maternal angiotensin-converting enzyme inhibition. Obstet Gynecol 1989;74:371–374.
179. Piper JM, Ray WA, Rosa FW. Pregnancy outcome following exposure to angiotensin-converting enzyme inhibitors. Obstet Gynecol 1992;80:429–432.
180. Hanssens M, Keirse MJNC, Vankelecom F, et al. Fetal and neonatal effects of treatment with angiotensin-converting enzyme inhibitors in pregnancy. Obstet Gynecol 1991;78:128–135.
181. Brent RL, Beckman DA. Angiotensin-coverting enzyme inhibitors, an embryopathic class of drugs with unique properties: information for clinical teratology counselors. Teratology 1991;43:543–546.
182. Cuniff C, Jones KL, Phillipson K, et al. Oligohydramnios and renal tubular malformation associated with maternal enalapril use. Am J Obstet Gynecol 1990;162:187–189.
183. Pryde PG, Sedman AB, Nugent CE, et al. Angiotensin-converting enzyme inhibitor fetopathy. J Am Soc Nephrol 1993;3:1575–1582.
184. Barr M Jr, Cohen MM Jr. ACE inhibitor fetopathy and hypocalciuria: the kidney-skull connection. Teratology 1991;44:485–495.
185. Mounier F, Hinglais N, Sich M, et al. Ontogenesis of angiotensin-I converting enzyme in human kidney. Kidney Int 1987;32:684–690.
186. Darby IA, Congiu M, Fernley RT, et al. Cellular and ultrastructural location of angiotensinogen in rat and sheep kidney. Kidney Int 1994;46:1557–1560.
187. Olson AL, Perlman S, Robillard JE, Developmental regulation of angiotensinogen gene expression in sheep. Pediatr Res 1990;28:183–185.
188. Olson AL, Robillard JE, Kisker CT. et al. Negative regulation of angiotensinogen gene expression by glucocorticoids in fetal sheep liver. Pediatr Res 1991;30:256–260.
189. Celio MR, Groscurth P, Inagami T. Ontogeny of renin immunoreactive cells in the human kidney. Anat Embryol 1985;173:149–155.
190. Phat VN, Camilleri JP, Bariety J, et al. Immunohistochemical characterization of renin-containing cells in the human juxtaglomerular apparatus during embryonal and fetal development. Lab Invest 1981;45:387–390.
191. Egerer G, Taugner R, Tiedemann K. Renin immunohistochemistry in the mesonephros and metanephros of the pig embryo. Histochemistry 1984;81:385–390.
192. Taylor GM, Peart WS, Porter KA, et al. Concentration and molecular forms of active and inactive renin in human fetal kidney, amniotic fluid and adrenal gland: evidence for renin-angiotensin system hyperactivity in 2nd trimester of pregnancy. J Hypertens 1986;4:121–129.
193. Kon Y, Hashimoto Y, Kitagawa H, et al. An immunohistochemical study on the embyonic development of renin-containing cells in the mouse and pig. Anat Histol Embryol 1989;18;14–26.
194. Gomez AR, Cassis L, Lynch K, et al. Fetal expression of the angiotensinogen gene. Endocrinology 1988;123:2298–2302.
195. Gomez RA, Lynch KR, Sturgill BC, et al. Distribution of renin mRNA and its protein in the developing kidney. Am J Physiol 1989;257:F850–F858.
196. Gomez RA, Pupilli C, Everett AD. Molecular and cellular aspects of renin during kidney ontogeny. Pediatr Nephrol 1991;5:80–87.
197. Yosipiv IV, Dipp S, El-Dahr SS. Ontogeny of somatic angiotensin-converting enzyme. Hypertension 1994;23:369–374.
198. Richoux JP, Amsaguine S, Grignon G, et al. Earliest renin containing cell differentiation during ontogenesis in the rat: an immunocytochemical study. Histochemistry 1987;88:41–46.
199. Gröne H, Simon M, Fuchs E. Autoradiographic characterization of angiotensin receptor subtypes in fetal and adult human kidney. Am J Physiol 1992;262:F326–F331.
200. Wintour EM, Alcorn D, Butkus A, et al. Ontogeny of hormonal and excretory function of the meso- and metanephros in the ovine fetus. Kidney Int 1996;50:1624–1633.
200a. Butkus A, Albiston A, Alcorn D et al. Ontogeny of angiotensin II receptors types 1 and 2 in ovine mesonephros and metanephras. Kidney Int 1997;51:628–636.
201. Schutz S, Le Moullec J-M, Corvol P, et al. Early expression of all the components of the renin-angiotensin-system in human development. Am J Pathol 1996;149:2067–2079.
202. Wintour EM, Alcorn D, Rockell MD, Development and function of the fetal kidney. In: Brace RA, Hanson MA, Rodeck C, ed. Fetus and neonate, vol. 4. Cambridge University Press, 1997:3–5.
203. Rahman ARA, Motwani JG, Lang CC, et al. Circulating angiotensin II and renal sodium handling in man: a dose-response study. Clin Sci 1993;85:147–156.
204. Lumbers ER. Functions of the renin-angiotensin system during development. Clin Exp Pharmacol Physiol 1995;22:499–505.
205. Harding R, Hooper SB, Dickson KA. A mechanism leading to reduced lung expansion and lung hypoplasia in fetal sheep during oligohydramnios. Am J Obstet Gynecol 1990;163:1904–1913.

206. Robillard JE, Gomez RA, Meernik JG, et al. Role of angiotensin II on the adrenal and vascular responses to hemorrhage during development in fetal lambs. Circ Res 1982;50:645–650.
207. Lumbers ER, Stevens AD. The effect of frusemide, saralasin and hypotension on fetal plasma renin activity and on fetal renal function. J Physiol 1987;393:479–490.
208. Lumbers ER, Kingsford NM, Menzies RI, et al. Acute effects of captopril, an angiotensin-converting enzyme inhibitor, on the pregnant ewe and fetus. Am J Physiol 1992;262:R754–R760.
209. Robillard JE, Smith FG, Segar JL, et al. Mechanisms regulating renal sodium excretion during development. Pediatr Nephrol 1992;6:205–213.
210. Gomez AR, Robillard JE. Developmental aspects of the renal responses to hemorrhage during converting-enzyme inhibition in fetal lambs. Circ Res 1984;54:301–312.
211. Lumbers ER, Burrell JH, Menzies RI, et al. The effects of a converting enzyme inhibitor (captopril) and angiotensin II on fetal renal function. Br J Pharmacol 1993;110:821–827.
212. Tufro-McReddie A, Johns DW, Geary KM, et al. Angiotensin II type 1 receptor: role in renal growth and gene expression during normal development. Am J Physiol 1994;266:F911–F918.
213. Fogo A, Yoshida Y, Yared A, et al. Importance of angiogenic action of angiotensin II in the glomerular growth of maturing kidneys. Kidney Int 1990;38:1068–1074.
214. Lane PH. Furosemide treatment, angiotensin II, and renal growth and development in the rat. Pediatr Res 1995;37:747–754.
215. Charbit M, Dechaux M, Blazy I, et al. Deleterious effects of inhibition of the renin-angiotensin system in neonatal rats. Pediatr Nephrol 1995;9:303–308.
216. Zemel S, Millan MA, Feuillan P, et al. Characterization and distribution of angiotensin-II receptors in the primate fetus. J Clin Endocrinol Metab 1990;71(4):1003–1007.
217. Grady EF, Sechi LA, Griffin CA, et al. Expression of AT2 receptors in the developing rat fetus. J Clin Invest 1991;88:921–933.
218. Tsutsumi K, Stromberg C, Viswanathan M, et al. Angiotensin-II receptor subtypes in fetal tissues of the rat: autoradiography, guanine nucleotide sensitivity and association with phosphoinositide hydrolysis. Endocrinology 1991;129:1075–1082.
219. Ciurfo GM, Viswanathan M, Seltzer AM, et al. Glomerular angiotensin II receptor subtypes during development of rat kidney. Am J Physiol 1993;265:F265–F271.
220. de Gasparo M, Levens NR. Pharmacology of angiotensin II receptors in the kidney. Kidney Int 1994;46:1486–1491.
221. Aguilera G, Kapur S, Feuillan P, et al. Developmental changes in angiotensin II receptor subtypes and AT1 receptor mRNA in rat kidney. Kidney Int 1994;46:973–979.
222. Forhead AJ, Fowden AL, Silver M, et al. Haemodynamic responses to an angiotensin II receptor antagonist (GR117289) in maternal and fetal sheep. Exp Physiol 1995;80:285–298.
223. Brace RA. Current topic: progress toward understanding the regulation of amniotic fluid volume: water and solute fluxes in and through the fetal membranes. Placenta 1995;16:1–18.
224. Dickson KA, Harding R. Role of fetal sac fluids during maternal water deprivation in sheep. Exp Physiol 1994;79:147–160.
225. Nijland MJM, Ross MG, Kullama LK, et al. DDAVP-induced maternal hyposmolality increases ovine fetal urine flow. Am J Physiol 1995;268:R358–R365.
226. Tangalakis K, Moritz K, Shandley L, et al. Effect of maternal glucocorticoid treatment on ovine fetal fluids at 0.6 gestation. Reprod Fertil Dev 1995;7:1595–1598.
227. Dodic M, Wintour EM. Effects of prolonged (48 H) infusion of cortisol on blood pressure, renal function and fetal fluids in the immature ovine foetus. Clin Exp Pharmacol Physiol 1994;21:971–980.
228. Fraenkel MB, Potocnik SJ, Wintour EM. Atrial natriuretic peptide receptors are present and functional by midgestation in fetal sheep. Am J Physiol 1994;267:F825–F830.
229. Walker MPR, Moore TR, Cheung CY, et al. Indomethacin-induced urinary flow rate reduction in the ovine fetus is associated with reduced free water clearance and elevated plasma arginine vasopressin levels. Am J Obstet Gynecol 1992;167:1723–1731.
230. Rosen DJD, Rabinowitz R, Beyth Y, et al. Fetal urine production in normal twins and in twins with acute polyhydramnios. Fetal Diagn Ther 1990;5:57–60.
231. Wieacker P, Wilhelm C, Prompeler H, et al. Pathophysiology of polyhydramnios in twin transfusion syndrome. Fetal Diagn Ther 1992;7:87–92.
232. Nageotte MP, Hurwitz SR, Kaupke CJ, et al. Atriopeptin in the twin transfusion syndrome. Obstet Gynecol 1989;73:867–870.
233. Rehan VK, Menticoglou SM, Seshia MMK, et al. Feto-fetal transfusion in twins. Arch Dis Child 1995;73:f41–f43.
234. Lopriore E, Vandenbussche FPHA, Tiersma ESM, et al. Twin-to-twin transfusion syndrome: new perspectives. J Pediatr 1995;127:675–680.
235. Saunders NJ, Snijders RJM, Nicolaides KH. Therapeutic amniocentesis in twin-twin transfusion syndrome appearing in the second trimester of pregnancy. Am J Obstet Gynecol 1992;166:820–824.
236. Wintour EM, Laurence BM, Lingwood BE. Anatomy, physiology and pathology of the amniotic and allantoic compartments in the sheep and cow. Aust Vet J 1986;63:216–221.
237. Henry MM, Morris DD, Pugh DG. Hydrallantois associated with twin pregnancy in a mare. Equine Pract 1991;13:20–23.
238. Hedriana HL, Brace RA, Gilbert WM. Changes in blood flow to the ovine chorion and amnion across gestation. J Soc Gynecol Invest 1995;2:727–734.
239. Gilbert WM, Brace RA. The missing link in amniotic fluid volume regulation: intramembranous absorption. Obstet Gynecol 1989;74:748–754.
240. Gilbert WM, Brace RA. Novel determination of filtration coefficient of ovine placenta and intramembranous pathway. Am J Physiol 1990;259:R1281–R1288.

241. Ferguson JE II, Gorman JV, Bruns DE, et al. Abundant expression of parathyroid hormone-related protein in human amnion and its association with labor. Proc Natl Acad Sci USA 1992;89:8384–8388.
242. Germain AM, Attaroglu H, MacDonald PC, et al. Parathyroid hormone-related protein mRNA in avascular human amnion. J Clin Endocrinol Metab 1992;75:1173–1175.
243. Emly JF, Gregory J, Bowden SJ, et al. Immunohistochemical localization of parathyroid hormone-related peptide (PTHrP) in human term placenta and membranes. Placenta 1994;15:653–660.
244. Dunne FP, Ratcliffe WA, Mansour P, et al. Parathyroid hormone related protein (PTHrP) gene expression in fetal and extra-embryonic tissues of early pregnancy. Hum Reprod 1994;9:149–156.
245. Mitchell MD, Hunter C, Dudley DJ, et al. Significant decrease in parathyroid hormone-related protein concentrations in amniotic fluid with labour at term but not preterm. Reprod Fertil Dev 1996;8:231–234.
246. Bruns ME, Ferguson JE, Bruns DE, et al. Expression of parathyroid hormone-related peptide and its receptor messenger ribonucleic acid in human amnion and choriondecidua: implications for secretion and function. Am J Obstet Gynecol 1995;173:739–746.
247. Dvir R, Golander A, Jaccard N, et al. Amniotic fluid and plasma levels of parathyroid hormone-related protein and hormonal modulation of its secretion by amniotic fluid cells. Eur J Endocrinol 1995;133:277–282.
248. Wu WX, Brooks J, Millar MR, et al. Localization of the sites of synthesis and action of prolactin by immunocytochemistry and in-situ hybridization within the human utero-placental unit. J Mol Endocrinol 1991;7:241–247.
249. Tadokoro N, Koibuchi N, Ohtake H, et al. Localization of prolactin and its receptor messenger RNA in the human decidua. Experientia 1995;51:1216–1219.
250. Sagawa N, Hasegawa M, Itoh H, et al. The role of amniotic endothelin in human pregnancy. Placenta 1994;15:565–575.
251. Sunnergen KP, Word RA, Sambrook JF, et al. Expression and regulation of endothelin precursor mRNA in avascular human amnion. Mol Cell Endocrinol 1990;68:R7–R14.
252. Casey ML, Word RA, MacDonald PC. Endothelin-1 gene expression and regulation of endothelin mRNA and protein biosynthesis in avascular human amnion. J Biol Chem 1991;266:5762–5768.
253. Hasegawa M, Sagawa N, Itoh H, et al. Endothelin receptors in the human amnion, chorion laeve, decidua vera and placenta. Reprod Fertil Dev 1995;7:1585–1589.
254. Eis AW, Mitchell MD, Myatt L. Endothelin transfer and endothelin effects on water transfer in human fetal membranes. Obstet Gynecol 1992;79:411–415.
255. Chao H-S, Myers SE, Handwerker S. Endothelin inhibits basal and stimulated release of prolactin by human decidual cells. Endocrinology 1993;133:505–510.
256. Itoh H, Sagawa N, Hasegawa M, et al. Transforming growth factor-beta stimulates, and glucocorticoids and epidermal growth factor inhibit, brain natriuretic peptide secretion from cultured human amnion cells. J Clin Endocrinol Metab 1994;79:176–182.
257. Matsumoto K, Nakamura T. Emerging multipotent aspects of hepatocyte growth factor. J Biochem 1996;119:591–600.
258. Nakamura T, Nishizawa T, Hagiya M, et al. Molecular cloning and expression of human hepatocyte growth factor. Nature 1989;342:440–443.
259. Woolf AS, Kolatsi-Joannou M, Hardman P, et al. Roles of hepatocyte growth factor/scatter factor and the *met* receptor in the early development of the metanephros. J Cell Biol 1995;128:171–184.
260. Kurauchi O, Itakura A, Ando H, et al. The concentration of hepatocyte growth factor (HGF) in human amniotic fluid at second trimester: relation to fetal birth weight. Horm Metab Res 1995;27:335–338.
261. Khan N, Couper J, Goldsworthy W, et al. Relationship of hepatocyte growth factor in human umbilical vein serum to gestational age in normal pregnancies. Pediatr Res 1996;39:386–389.
262. Saito S, Sakakura S, Enomoto M, et al. Hepatocyte growth factor promotes the growth of cytotrophoblasts by the paracrine mechanism. J Biochem 1995;117:671–676.
263. Bottaro DP, Rubin JS, Faletto DL, et al. Identification of the hepatocyte growth factor receptor as the c-*met* proto-oncogene product. Science 1991;251:802–804.
264. Uehara Y, Minowa O, Mori C, et al. Placental defect and embryonic lethality in mice lacking hepatocyte growth factor/scatter factor. Nature 1995;373:702–705.
265. Hanssens M, Vercruysse L, Verbist L, et al. Renin-like immunoreactivity in human placenta and fetal membranes. Histochem Cell Biol 1995;104:435–442.
266. Kalenga MK, De-Hertogh R, Whitebread S, et al. Distribution of the concentrations of angiotensin II (A II), A II receptors, hPL, prolactin, and steroids in human fetal membranes. Rev Fr Gynecol Obstet 1991;86:585–591.
267. Lundin-Schiller S, Mitchell MD. Renin increases human amnion cell prostaglandin E_2 biosynthesis. J Clin Endocrinol Metab 1991;73:436–440.
268. Anderson DF, Faber JJ. Animal model for polyhydramnios. Am J Obstet Gynecol 1989;160:389–390.
269. Stevenson KM, Lumbers ER. Effects of angiotensin II in fetal sheep and modification of its actions by indomethacin. J Physiol 1995;487:147–158.
270. Moritz KM, Tangalakis K, Wintour EM. Renal, hormonal and cardiovascular responses to chronic angiotensin I infusion in the ovine fetus. Am J Physiol 1997;272:R1912–R1917.
271. Johnson MR, Abbas A, Nicolaides KH, et al. Distribution of relaxin between human maternal and fetal circulation and amniotic fluid. J Endocrinol 1992;134:313–317.
272. Bogic LJ, Mandel M, Bryant-Greenwood GD. Relaxin gene expression in human reproductive tissues by in situ hybridization. J Clin Endocrinol Metab 1995;80:130–137.
273. Warren WB, Silverman AJ, Cellular localization of corticotrophin releasing hormone in the human placenta, fetal membranes and decidua. Placenta 1995;16:147–156.
274. Hansen TN, Gest AL. Hydrops fetalis. In: Brace RA, Ross MG, Robillard JE, eds. Fetal and neonatal body fluids:

the scientific basis for clinical practice. Ithaca, NY: Perinatology Press, 1989:86–116.
275. Santolaya J, Alley D, Jaffe R, et al. Antenatal classification of hydrops fetalis. Obstet Gynecol 1992;79:256–259.
276. Villaespesa AR, Mier SMP, Ferrer PL, et al. Nonimmunologic hydrops fetalis: an etiopathogenetic approach through the postmortem study of 59 patients. Am J Med Genet 1990;35:274–279.
277. Chelliah BP, Cabatu E, Chitkara U, et al. Polyhydramnios and elevated amniotic fluid alpha-fetoprotein caused by fetal supraventricular tachycardia. J Reprod Med 1981;26:45–47.
278. Stevens DC, Hilliard JK, Schreiner RL, et al. Supraventricular tachycardia with edema, ascites and hydrops in fetal sheep. Am J Obstet Gynecol 1982;142:316–322.
279. Nimrod C, Keane P, Harder J, et al. Atrial natriuretic peptide production in association with nonimmune fetal hydrops. Am J Obstet Gynecol 1988;159:625–628.
280. Gest AL, Hansen TN, Moise AA, et al. Atrial tachycardia causes hydrops in fetal lambs. Am J Physiol 1990;258:H1159–H1163.
281. Andres RL, Brace RA. The development of hydrops fetalis in the ovine fetus after lymphatic ligation or lymphatic excision. Am J Obstet Gynecol 1990;162:1331–1334.
282. Nicolaides KH, Clewell WH, Mishaban RS, et al. Fetal haemoglobin measurement in the assessment of red cell isoimmunisation. Lancet 1988;1:1073–1075.
283. Moise JKJ, Rodkey LS, Saade GR, et al. An animal model for hemolytic disease of the fetus and newborn. Am J Obstet Gynecol 1995;173:747–753.
284. Blair DK, Vander Straten MC, Gest AL. Hydrops in fetal sheep from rapid induction of anemia. Pediatr Res 1994;35:560–564.
285. Silberbach M, Woods LL, Hohimer AR, et al. Role of endogenous atrial natriuretic peptide in chronic anemia in the ovine fetus: effects of a non-peptide antagonist for atrial natriuretic peptide receptor. Pediatr Res 1995;38:722–728.
286. Bayer LA, Cheung CY, Brace RA. Autonomic modulation of ovine fetal responses to atrial natriuretic factor infusion. Am J Physiol 1993;265:R596–R601.
287. Silberbach M, Anderson DF, Reller MD, et al. Effect of atrial natriuretic peptide on vascular permeation in the ovine fetus. Pediatr Res 1994;35:555–559.
288. Moise JR, Carpenter RJ, Hesketh DE. Do abnormal starling forces cause fetal hydrops in red blood cell alloimmunization? Am J Obstet Gynecol 1992;167:907–912.
289. Nicolaides KH, Warenski JC, Rodeck CH. The relationship of fetal plasma protein concentration and hemoglobin level to the development of hydrops in rhesus isoimmunization. Am J Obstet Gynecol 1985;341–344.
290. Faber JJ, Anderson DF. Model study of placental water transfer and causes of fetal water disease in sheep. Am J Physiol 1990;258;152:R1257–R1270.
291. Jaekle RK, Sheikh AU, Berry DD, et al. Hemodynamic and hormonal responses to atrial distension in the ovine fetus. Am J Obstet Gynecol 1995;173:694–701.
292. Treadwell MC, Sherer DM, Sacks AJ, et al. Successful treatment of recurrent non-immune hydrops secondary to fetal hyperthyroidism. Obstet Gynecol 1996;87:838–840.
293. Anandakumar C, Biswas A, Chew SSL, et al. Direct fetal therapy for hydrops secondary to congenital atrioventricular heart block. Obstet Gynecol 1996;87:835–837.
294. Ferguson JE, Gorman JV, Bruns DE, et al. Abundant expression of parathyroid hormone-related protein in human amnion and its association with labor. Proc Natl Acad Sci USA 1992;89:8384–8388.
295. Tyson JE, Hwang P, Guyda H, et al. Studies of prolactin secretion in human pregnancy. Am J Obster Gynecol 1972;113:14–20.
296. Skinner SL, Cran EJ, Gibson R, et al. Angiotensins I and II, active and inactive renin, renin substrate, renin activity, and angiotensinase in human liquor amnii and plasma. Am J Obstet Gynecol 1975;121:626–630.

If you have any concerns about our products,
you can contact us on
ProductSafety@springernature.com

In case Publisher is established outside the EU,
the EU authorized representative is:
**Springer Nature Customer Service Center GmbH
Europaplatz 3, 69115 Heidelberg, Germany**

Printed by Libri Plureos GmbH
in Hamburg, Germany

Principles of
Perinatal–Neonatal Metabolism

Second Edition

Springer Science+Business Media, LLC

Richard M. Cowett, MD
Brown University School of Medicine, Department of Pediatrics,
Women and Infants Hospital of Rhode Island, Providence, RI

Editor

Principles of Perinatal–Neonatal Metabolism

Second Edition

With 383 Figures

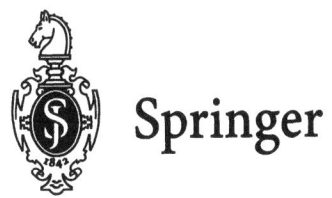

Richard M. Cowett, MD
Department of Pediatrics
Brown University School of Medicine
Women and Infants Hospital of Rhode Island
101 Dudley Street
Providence, RI 02905-2401, USA

Library of Congress Cataloging-in-Publication Data
Principles of perinatal–neonatal metabolism/[edited by] Richard M.
　Cowett.—2nd ed.
　　　p. cm.
　　Includes bibliographical references and index.
　　ISBN 978-1-4612-7227-4　　ISBN 978-1-4612-1642-1 (eBook)
　　DOI 10.1007/978-1-4612-1642-1
　　1. Infants (Newborn)—Metabolism. 2. Fetus—Metabolism.
　3. Maternal-fetal exchange. I. Cowett, Richard M.
　　[DNLM: 1. Fetus—metabolism. 2. Infant. Newborn—metabolism.
　3. Maternal-Fetal Exchange—physiology. 4. Pregnancy—metabolism.
　WQ 210.5 P957 1998]
　RJ252.P75 1998
　618.3′2—dc21　　　　　　　　　　　　　　　　　　　　　　　　　　　　　　97-24816

Printed on acid-free paper.

© 1998 Springer Science+Business Media New York
Originally published by Springer-Verlag New York, Inc. in 1998
All rights reserved. This work may not be translated or copied in whole or in part without the written
permission of the publisher Springer Science+Business Media, LLC,
except for brief excerpts in connection with reviews or scholarly analysis. Use in connection with any
form of information storage and retrieval, electronic adaptation, computer software, or by similar or
dissimilar methodology now known or hereafter developed is forbidden.
The use of general descriptive names, trade names, trademarks, etc., in this publication, even if the former
are not especially identified, is not to be taken as a sign that such names, as understood by the Trade Marks
and Merchandise Marks Act, may accordingly be used freely by anyone.
While the advice and information in this book are believed to be true and accurate at the date of going to
press, neither the authors nor the editors nor the publisher can accept any legal responsibility for any errors
or omissions that may be made. The publisher makes no warranty, express or implied, with respect to the
material contained herein.

Production coordinated by Chernow Editorial Services, Inc., and managed by Natalie Johnson; manufacturing supervised by Joe Quatela.
Typeset by Best-set Typesetter Ltd., Hong Kong.

9 8 7 6 5 4 3 2 1

ISBN 978-1-4612-7227-4

In Memory of the Past:

*To my Father,
Allen Abraham Cowett;*

and

in Anticipation of the Future:

*To my Children,
Beth Ellen
Allison Ann
Allen Manz
Michael Elliott Drake
Hannah Michelle Kazin*

Preface to the Second Edition

In the Preface to the first edition we suggested that sufficient time had passed in the field of perinatal–neonatal medicine generally to require a cogent analysis of the metabolic principles of the period. At the time of publication of the first edition there was and, continuing today, there is no other comprehensive metabolic research reference text that evaluates this period as a continuum. The first edition focused on the metabolism of the period from physiological and biochemical perspectives with emphasis, of necessity, on the former. In the intervening period, enormous strides have been made in our understanding of the metabolism of the perinatal–neonatal period by investigators in the field. Especially significant are the advances made from cellular and melecular perspectives, which have assisted mechanistically in furthering our understanding of earlier physiological observations. These advances continue to be catalogued and analyzed comprehensively in this edition.

There is no more obvious indication of the trends occurring in science in general and in perinatal–medicine in particular than the websites on the Internet, which allow investigators to collaborate over long distances and update their databases on-line. Certainly one of the most useful and probably most widely used websites is that of the National Library of Medicine: {http://www.nlm.nih.gov}. In particular, this has allowed us to update, complete, and confirm many of the reference citations in this text.

We have carefully followed the suggestions of those individuals who wrote critiques of the first edition in the medical literature. In the medical literature. Meticulous care has been taken in the editing of this textbook to make the writing style and conventions as uniform as possible from chapter to chapter and section to section in spite of its multiauthored nature.

There is a thorough updating of the topics that were discussed in the first edition because of advances in each particular area.

Section I to focuses on the general principles of metabolism and evaluation of metabolic principles of the normal nonpregnant adult as the "gold standard." There are new chapters on: breath testing; analysis of proteins, peptides and small molecules; and glucose transporters from molecular, biochemical and physiological perspectives.

Section II continues to focus on the maternal metabolism in pregnancy. There is a completely revised discussion of glucose metabolism in pregnancy and a new chapter on mineral metabolism in pregnancy.

Section III retains its focus on metabolism in the fetus and placenta. There are new chapters or: growth factors; developmental endocrinology; the sympathoadrenal system; and a thorough revision of the discussion of respiration in the fetus and placenta.

Section IV is an entirely new section that focuses on organ specific metabolism during the perinatal period. The brain, the heart, the lung, the liver, the gastrointestinal tract, and muscle are each evaluated in organ specific discussions of the perinatal period. The kidney is not treated as a separate discussion because of the thorough evaluations of water and electrolyte metabolism in the fetus and placenta and neonatal water and electrolyte metabolism that appear elsewhere in the text.

The last section, Section V, continues its focus on neonatal metabolism. There is an entirely new discussion of inborn errors of carbohydrate metabolism; inborn errors of amino acid and organic acid metabolism; and body composition; and new chapters concerning inborn errors of lipid metabolism (mitochondrial fatty acid oxidation), bilirubin metabolism, nutritional support of the neonate by human milk feeding; and finally an approach to evaluation of the neonate with a potential metabolic defect.

In effect, this reference text has increased from 37 chapters in the first edition to 53 chapters. As a result, the number of text pages has increased by 66% and their size has increased by 33%. A concerted attempt has been made to cross-reference the text between chapters, as well as to provide a detailed index. Clinical correlations are explored wherever germane. One of the major strengths continues to be the exhaustive up-to-date reference list that accompanies each chapter. We trust that this text will continue to provide a comprehensive evaluation of each topic for those individuals interested in metabolism in this continuum known as the perinatal–neonatal period.

As time has marched on, a number of changes have occurred in the lives of individuals mentioned in the Preface to the first edition. Dr. Irwin B. Hanenson passed away after a long illness. I will always remember him with a great deal of fondness. Dr. Robert Schwariz has become an emeritus Professor of Medical Science at Brown. He graciously agreed to update a previously published discussion of his on the subject of inborn errors of carbohydrate metabolism for this edition. I am quite appreciative of his encyclopedic knowledge of carbohydrate metabolism in the perinatal–neonatal period. He has been a major contributor to this area for a number of the decades. Dr. William Oh remains the Chairperson of the Department of Pediatrics at Brown University School of Medicine and Pediatrician-in-Chief of the Hasbro Children's' Hospital. After almost a quarter of a century of providing energy and vision, he reliquinshed the Chair of the Department of Pediatrics at Women & Infants of Rhods Island (i.e., the Division of Neonatology of the Department of Pediatrics of the Brown University School of Medicine). He recruited Dr. James F. Padbury who has assumed the position. Jim is providing welcomed renewed exuberance as the neonatal group continues to move at the cutting edge of this discipline as well as contributing a new chapter on the sympathoadrenal system of the fetus and placenta to this text.

Of course, my father, Allen, remains the ultimate guiding force for me. I think about him daily with affection and respect, as we appreciate the present and anticipate the future.

Many individuals have assisted in completing the many tasks that are critical to the success of a major text such as this book. At Springer-Verlag publishers Laura Gillan has been a motivating and enthusiastic proponent of the effort. I am deeply indebted to her and her associates, including Jeff Sands, as well as to Barbara Chernow, David Kapian, and Kathy Jackson. Likewise, I am quite appreciative of the assistance of Janet Crager and Frank Kellerman of the Sciences Library of Brown University. They have been major contributors to the success we have had in finalizing the references lists that accompany each chapter. The above individuals, probably more than even the individual contributors, will be happy that this second edition is nearing completion.

Finally, I am deeply indebted to all of the individual contributors, all 67 of them, who have been as conscientious as I had originally hoped they would be in evaluating that specific area of perinatal–neonatal metabolism for which they are an "academic household name." I hope the reader continues to be as pleased as I am with the depth of this compendium and finds it as useful.

Providence, Rhode Island   Richard M. Cowett, MD
December, 1997

Preface to the First Edition

Over the fast quarter century or so, specialization within obstetrics and gynecology, and pediatrics has resulted in the development of the disciplines of maternal-fetal medicine and neonatology respectively. A primary focus of maternal-fetal medicine has been to understand the mechanism(s) of premature delivery and develop treatment modalities for improving the length of gestation. A primary focus of neonatology has been to understand the causes of respiratory distress in the neonate. Success has resulted, not only in the lengthening of gestation, but an improved understanding of the causes and treatment of neonatal respiratory disease. With increasing success has come the necessity to understand the metabolic principles of the parturient, the fetal/placenta unit, and the neonate. These principles are clearly very important from multiple aspects. Increased understanding of metabolism of the pregnant woman would explain the aberrations occurring in normal and abnormal pregnancy and improve nutritional support for the parturient. A prime example of altered metabolism is the parturient with diabetes. Understanding metabolism of the fetal/placenta unit is necessary to increase the probability that the fetus will be born appropriate for size irrespective of the gestational age. The various component of neonatal metabolism are important, not only for understanding the changes in physiology and biochemistry occurring in the developing neonate, but the principles by which nutritional support should be provided.

Enough time has lapsed so that cogent analyses are possible for each component of the metabolic principles of the perinatal-neonatal period. A general survey of the literature documents that separate discussions of metabolism exist. There are chapters on maternal metabolism as part of maternal-fetal medicine texts. There are textbooks on altered metabolism such as diabetes mellitus in pregnancy. Texts of principles of fetal physiology have been published, as have various analysis of neonatal metabolism and nutrition as single texts or chapters of general neonatology texts. To my knowledge there is no comprehensive metabolic reference text which has evaluated the perinatal-neonatal period as a continuum. It is obvious that the perinatal-neonatal period is a continuum in which each stage is inexorably intertwined with the other. It is this continuum that we have attempted to capture from a physiological and biochemical perspective metabolically.

In Section I the general principles of metabolism are analyzed. The first half evaluates methodology used to study metabolism. Kinetic techniques have been responsible for major advances that provide information above and beyond that of static measurements. No analysis of metabolism in the 1990s would be complete without a consideration of the evolving techniques of a cellular and molecular basis which are ever increasingly providing an explanation of metabolic parameters. It is also apparent that animal modeling is required to evaluate mechanisms which cannot be analyzed by human investigation.

Within Section I metabolic control of glucose, protein and lipid is evaluated in the normal non-pregnant adult as a "gold standard." Subsequently, biochemical and physiological aspects of insutin, the contrainsulin hormones, and somatomedins are considered in the non pregnant adult.

Section II evaluates maternal metabolism during pregnancy. Metabolism of glucose, protein, lipids, and prostaglandins are analyzed in detail from the perspective of changes occurring during pregnancy. Studies that evaluate energy metabolism in pregnancy are considered. The final chapter is a subject which is emerging as a major topic in the metabolism of pregnancy–the effects of exercise.

Section III considers metabolism in the fetal/placenta unit. Glucose, protein, and lipid are discussed comprehensively. Since metabolism is influenced to a great degree by respiration and circulation within the fetal/placenta unit, these topics are considered as well. Finally, water metabolism, of critical importance to the fetus is explored in detail.

Section IV analyzes the various components of neonatal metabolism. A great deal of research in metabolism of a perinatal-neonatal nature has evaluated the neonate and the various components are considered comprehensively. Glucose metabolism and the inborn errors of carbohydrate metabolism are analyzed as are neonatal protein metabolism and inborn errors of amino acids and organic acids. Extensive research has been performed on lipid and carnitine, on neonatal minerals, trace metals, vitamins, both fat soluble and water soluble, and these topics are explored. Neonatal energy metabolism is discussed in detail as is an offshoot of that subject, neonatal thermal regulation. Extensive research has been performed on water metabolism in the neonate and this is analyzed as are studies of body composition which have been published. Two specific aberrations of the norm are considered from a neonatal perspective; the first, the small for gestational age neonate and the second, the infant of the diabetic mother. Increasing success has occurred over the last quater century relative to neonates undergoing surgery and their metabolic needs are evaluated. Finally, nutritional support of the neonate, specifically alternate fucls and routes of administration, are evaluated.

The text is cross referenced between sections. With some topics there has been enough research to allow for separate discussions (e.g., glucose, protein, lipid and water) in separate sections. With other (e.g., minerals, trace elements, and vitamins) the authors have evaluated the topics in a single chapter. Clinical correlations are provided throughout the text.

We believe that this reference text will privide a comprehensive evaluation for those individuats interested in metabolism in this continuum known as the perinatal-neonatal period.

It is appropriate to acknowledge a few individuals who have been most influential in my carcer. Dr. Irwin B. Hanenson, Professor Emeritus of Medicine at the University of Cincinnati College of Medicine, whom I first met when I was a teenager, introduced me to research and allowed me to work as a technician in his laboratory at the May Institute for Medical Research of the Jewish Hospital in Cincinnati, Ohio. He remains a very close friend to this day. Professor Margaret Shea Gilbert. Professor of Biology Emeritus at Lawrence College (University) in Appleton, Wisconsin, who recently passed away, provided support and enthusiasm for my budding interest in research during an undergraduate honor's thesis. Dr. Robert Schwartz, Professor of Pediatries and Medical Sciences at Brown University, I first met when he was Chairman of the Department of Pediatrics at Cleveland Metropolitan General Hospital, and Professor of Pediatrics at Case Western Reserve University where I was an intern and junior assistant resident in Pediatrics. He probably more than anyone should be given the credit for my interest in carbohydrate metabolism in the perinatal-neonatal period. This interest was enhanced when we both separately came to the Department of Pediatrics at Brown University in the early 1970s. He remains a mentor, colleague and close friend. Dr. Leo Stern, who passed away in 1989 unexpectedly, recruited me to

Preface to the First Edition

Brown University as a fellow in neonatology, and, during his lifetime as Chairman of the Department of Pediatrics at Brown University, remained a special influence on me personally and professionally. I first met Dr. William Oh when Dr. Stern recruited him to be Chief of the Division of Neonatology and Professor of Pediatrics and Medical Sciences at Brown University. Dr. Oh, now Chairman of the Department of Pediatrics at Brown University, has been a unique guide for me not only from a personal but from a professional standpoint. He remains a mentor, colleague and close friend. The above individuals and especially my father, Allen, whom I remember with love and affection, should probably be given credit for my success, but none of the blame for my short comings. I remain deeply indebted to all of them.

Many individuals at Springer-Verlag Publishers have been important from the beginning of this book to its completion. I am deeply indebted to all of them and to my former secretary Mrs. Lori D. Krahenbill at Women and Infants' Hospital.

Finally, it goes without saying, that each of the senior authors that have contributed to this text are "academic household names" in the areas about which they have written. I very much appreciate the thoroughness that each of them has evidenced in completing their assignment. I hope the reader is as pleased with the text as I am.

Providence, Rhode Island
March, 1991

Richard M. Cowett, MD

Contents

Preface to the Second Edition vii
Preface to the First Edition ix
Contributors xvii

Section I Methodology for the Study of Metabolism and General Principles

1 Methodology for the Study of Metabolism: Kinetic Techniques 3
   Dennis M. Bier

2 Methodology for the Study of Metabolism: Breath Testing 17
   Peter D. Klein and Hans Helge

3 Methodology for the Study of Metabolism: Analyses of
   Proteins, Peptides, and Small Molecules 27
   Jacob A. Canick

4 Methodology for the Study of Metabolism: Cellular
   and Molecular Techniques 41
   Lewis P. Rubin

5 Methodology for the Study of Metabolism: Physiologic
   Modeling in Animals 79
   John B. Susa

6 Control of Metabolism in the Normal Adult 91
   Robert R. Wolfe

7 Glucose Transporters: Molecular, Biochemical, and
   Physiologic Aspects 121
   Rebecca A. Simmons

8 Insulin: Molecular, Biochemical, and Physiologic Aspects 135
   Philip A. Gruppuso

9 Counterregulatory Hormones: Molecular, Biochemical, and
   Physiologic Aspects 155
   John E. Gerich and Philip E. Cryer

Section II Maternal Metabolism During Pregnancy

10 Glucose Metabolism in Pregnancy 183
    Patrick M. Catalano, Tatsua Ishizuka, and Jacob E. Friedman

11 Protein Metabolism in Pregnancy 207
    Satish C. Kalhan

12 Lipid Metabolism in Pregnancy.. 221
    Robert H. Knopp, Bartolome Bonet, and Xiaodong Zhu

13 Essential Fatty Acids and Prostaglandins in Pregnancy 259
    Paul L. Ogburn, Jr.

14 Mineral Metabolism in Pregnancy...................................... 281
    Karen M. Davidson and John T. Repke

15 Energy Metabolism During Pregnancy................................... 309
    John V.G.A. Durnin

16 Exercise in Pregnancy: Effects on Cardiorespiratory
    Physiology and Metabolism 319
    Marshall W. Carpenter

Section III Fetal-Placental Metabolism

17 Glucose Metabolism in the Fetal-Placental Unit 337
    William W. Hay, Jr.

18 Protein Metabolism in the Fetal-Placental Unit 369
    Edward A. Liechty and David W. Boyle

19 Lipid Metabolism in the Fetal-Placental Unit......................... 389
    Robert E. Kimura

20 Growth Factors in the Fetal-Placental Unit........................... 403
    Philip A. Gruppuso

21 Developmental Endocrinology in the Fetal-Placental Unit 425
    Ram K. Menon and Mark A. Sperling

22 The Sympathoadrenal System in the Fetal-Placental Unit 437
    Yi-Tang Tseng and James F. Padbury

23 Respiration in the Fetal-Placental Unit 451
    Robert W. Rothstein and Lawrence D. Longo

24 Circulation in the Fetal-Placental Unit.............................. 487
    Abraham M. Rudolph

25 Water and Electrolyte Metabolism in the Fetal-Placental Unit 511
    E. Marelyn Wintour

Section IV Organ-Specific Metabolism During the Perinatal Period

26 Brain Metabolism in the Fetus and Neonate 537
    Susan J. Vannucci and Robert C. Vannucci

27 Cardiac Metabolism in the Fetus and Neonate 551
    G. Wesley Vick, III and David J. Fisher

28 Lung Metabolism in the Fetus and Neonate 567
    Luc J.I. Zimmermann and Lambert M.G. van Golde

29 Liver Metabolism in the Fetus and Neonate 601
    Jean-Paul Pégorier and Jean Girard

30 Gastrointestinal Tract Metabolism in the Fetus and Neonate 627
    Robert E. Kimura

31 Muscle Metabolism in the Fetus and Neonate 641
    Ulrich A. Walker and Armand F. Miranda

Section V Neonatal Metabolism

32 Neonatal Glucose Metabolism 683
    Richard M. Cowett and Hussien M. Farrag

33 Inborn Errors of Carbohydrate Metabolism 723
    Robert Schwartz

34 Neonatal Protein Metabolism 773
    Willi E. Heine

35 Inborn Errors of Amino Acid and Organic Acid Metabolism 799
    Gerard T. Berry

36 Neonatal Lipid Metabolism 821
    Margit Hamosh

37 Inborn Errors of Lipid Metabolism (Mitochondrial
    Fatty Acid Oxidation) 847
    Charles A. Stanley

38 Neonatal Carnitine Metabolism 857
    Charles A. Stanley

39 Neonatal Bilirubin Metabolism 865
    William J. Cashore

40 Neonatal Calcium and Phosphorus Metabolism 879
    Jeffrey L. Loughead and Reginald C. Tsang

41 Neonatal Trace Element Metabolism 909
    Peter J. Aggett

42 Neonatal Vitamin Metabolism: Fat Soluble 943
    Frank R. Greer and Richard D. Zachman

43 Neonatal Vitamin Metabolism: Water Soluble 977
    Richard J. Schanler

44 Neonatal Energy Metabolism 1001
    Pieter J.J. Sauer

45 Neonatal Thermoregulation 1027
    Pieter J.J. Sauer

46 Neonatal Water and Electrolyte Metabolism 1045
    Andrew T. Costarino and Stephen Baumgart

47 Body Composition of the Neonate 1077
    Kenneth J. Ellis

48 The Small-for-Gestational-Age Neonate 1097
    Edward S. Ogata

49 The Infant of the Diabetic Mother 1105
    Richard M. Cowett

50 Metabolism of the Neonate Requiring Surgery 1131
    Arnold G. Coran, Agostino Pierro, and David J. Schmeling

51 Nutritional Support of the Neonate I: Alternate
    Fuels and Routes of Administration 1153
    Jane P. Balint and Robert M. Kliegman

52 Nutritional Support of the Neonate II: The Rationale for
    Human Milk Feeding 1181
    Richard J. Schanler

53 Evaluation of the Neonate with a Potential Metabolic Defect 1201
    Pinar T. Ozand

Index 1243

Contributors

Peter J. Aggett, MSc FRCP
Head, Lancashire Postgraduate School of Medicine and Health, University of Central Lancashire, Preston PR12HE UK

Jane P. Balint, MD
Assistant Professor, Division of Pediatric Gastroenterology and Nutrition, Department of Pediatrics, Medical College of Wisconsin, Milwaukee, WI 53226, USA

Stephen Baumgart, MD
Professor and Vice Chair, Department of Pediatrics, Thomas Jefferson University, Jefferson Medical College, Philadelphia, PA 19107, USA

Gerard T. Berry, MD
Professor, Department of Pediatrics, University of Pennsylvania School of Medicine, Senior Physician, Division of Biochemical Development and Molecular Diseases, Children's Hospital of Philadelphia, Philadelphia, PA 19104, USA

Dennis M. Bier, MD
Professor, Department of Pediatrics, Baylor College of Medicine, Director, Children's Nutritional Research Center, Houston, TX 77030, USA

Bartolome Bonet, MD, PhD
Assistant Professor, Universidad San Paolo, Centre de CC Experimentales y Tecnicas, Urbanización Montprincipe, Head, Division of Pediatrics, Fundacion Hospital de Alcorcon 28668 Madrid, Spain

David W. Boyle, MD
Associate Professor, Division of Neonatal-Perinatal Medicine, Department of Pediatrics, Indiana University School of Medicine, Indianapolis, IN 46223, USA

Jacob A. Canick, PhD
Professor, Department of Pathology and Laboratory Medicine, Brown University School of Medicine, Director, Prenatal AFP and Endocrinology Laboratories, Women and Infants Hospital of Rhode Island, Providence, RI 02905, USA

Marshall W. Carpenter, MD
Associate Professor, Department of Obstetrics and Gynecology, Brown University School of Medicine, Director, Division of Maternal-Fetal Medicine, Women and Infants Hospital of Rhode Island, Providence, RI 02905, USA

William J. Cashore, MD
Professor, Department of Pediatrics, Brown University School of Medicine, Associate Chief, Department of Pediatrics, Women and Infants Hospital of Rhode Island, Providence, Rhode Island 02905, USA

Patrick M. Catalano, MD
Professor, Department of Reproductive Biology, Case Western University School of Medicine, Director, High Risk Pregancy and Diabetes Clinic, MetroHealth Medical Center, Cleveland, OH 44109, USA

Arnold G. Coran, MD
Professor, Department of Surgery, Head, Section of Pediatric Surgery, University of Michigan Medical School, Surgeon-in-Chief, C.S. Mott Children's Hospital, Ann Arbor, MI 48109, USA

Andrew T. Costarino, MD
Associate Professor, Departments of Anesthesia and Pediatrics, University of Pennsylvania School of Medicine, Director, Pediatric Critical Care Medicine Fellowship Program, Children's Hospital of Philadelphia, Philadelphia, PA 19104, USA

Richard M. Cowett, MD
Professor, Department of Pediatrics, Brown University School of Medicine, Neonatologist, Department of Pediatrics, Women and Infants Hospital of Rhode Island, Providence, RI 02905, USA

Philip E. Cryer, MD
Irene E. and Michael M. Karl Professor of Endocrinology and Metabolism, Department of Medicine, Director, Division of Endocrinology, Diabetes and Metabolism, Director, General Clinical Research Center, Washington University School of Medicine, Physician, Barnes-Jewish Hospital, St. Louis, MO, 63110, USA

Karen M. Davidson, MD
Clinical Instructor, Department of Obstetrics, Gynecology and Reproductive Biology, Harvard Medical School, Associate Obstetrician and Gynecologist, Brigham and Women's Hospital, Boston, MA 02115, USA

J.V.G.A. Durnin, MA, MB, ChB, DSc, FRCP, FIBiol, FRSE
Professor, Department of Human Nutrition, University of Glasgow, Yorkhill Hospitals, Glasgow G3 8SJ UK

Kenneth J. Ellis, MD
Professor, Department of Pediatrics, Baylor College of Medicine, Director, Body Composition Laboratory, Children's Nutritional Research Center, Houston, TX 77030, USA

Hussien M. Farrag, MD
Assistant Professor, Department of Pediatrics, Tufts University School of Medicine, Staff Neonatologist, Department of Pediatrics, Bayside Medical Center, Springfield, MA 01109, USA

David J. Fisher, MD
Professor and Vice Chair, Department of Pediatrics, The Ohio State University College of Medicine, Executive Director, Children's Hospital Education Institute, Children's Hospital, Columbus, OH 43205, USA

Contributors

Jacob E. Friedman, PhD
Assistant Professor, Departments of Nutrition and Biochemistry, Case Western University School of Medicine, Cleveland OH 44106, USA

John E. Gerich, MD
Professor, Departments of Medicine and Physiology, Director, General Clinical Research Center and the Diabetes Research Laboratory, University of Rochester School of Medicine and Dentistry, Strong Memorial Hospital, Rochester, NY 14642, USA

Jean Girard, PhD DSc
Research Director, Centre National de la Recherche Scientifique, Director, Laboratoire de la Endocrinologie, Metabolisme et Developpement, 92190 Meudon, France

Frank R. Greer, MD
Professor, Departments of Pediatrics and Nutritional Sciences, University of Wisconsin, Wisconsin Perinatal Center, Meriter Hospital, Madison, WI 53715, USA

Philip A. Gruppuso, MD
Professor, Department of Pediatrics and Professor (Research), Department of Biochemistry, Brown University School of Medicine, Director, Division of Pediatric Endocrinology and Metabolism, Rhode Island Hospital and Hasbro Children's Hospital, Providence, RI 02903, USA

Margit Hamosh, PhD
Professor, Department of Pediatrics, Chief, Division of Developmental Biology and Nutrition, Georgetown University Medical Center, Washington, DC 20007, USA

William W. Hay, Jr., MD
Professor, Department of Pediatrics, Director, Training Program in Neonatal-Perinatal Medicine, Director, Neonatal Clinical Research Center, University of Colorado School of Medicine, Denver, CO 80262, USA

Willi E. Heine, MD, (Professor Dr. Med)
Professor, Department of Pediatrics, University of Rostock Children's Hospital, 18057 Rostock, Federal Republic of Germany

Hans Helge, MD
Professor and Chairman Emeritus, Department of Pediatrics, Free University of Berlin, D/14059 Berlin, Federal Republic of Germany

Tatsuya Ishizuka, MD, PhD
Postdoctoral Fellow, Departments of Nutrition and Biochemistry, Case Western University School of Medicine, Cleveland, OH 44106, USA

Satish C. Kalhan, MBBS, FRCP, DCH
Professor, Department of Pediatrics, Case Western University School of Medicine, Division of Neonatology, Rainbow Babies and Children's Hospital, Cleveland, OH 44106, USA

Robert E. Kimura, MD
Professor and Vice Chair, Department of Pediatrics, Director, Division of Neonatology, Rush-St. Luke's Presbyterian Medical Center, Chicago, IL 60612, USA

Peter D. Klein, PhD
Professor Emeritus, Departments of Pediatrics and Medicine, Baylor College of Medicine, Vice President, Research and Development, Meretek Diagnostics Inc., Houston, TX 77030, USA

Robert M. Kliegman, MD
Professor and Chair, Department of Pediatrics, Medical College of Wisconsin, Milwaukee, Wisconsin 53226, USA

Robert H. Knopp, MD
Professor, Department of Medicine, University of Washington School of Medicine, Chief, Division of Metabolism, Endocrinology and Nutrition, Director, Northwest Lipid Research Center, Harborview Medical Center, Seattle, WA 98104, USA

Edward A. Liechty, MD
Professor, Division of Neonatal-Perinatal Medicine, Department of Pediatrics, Indiana University School of Medicine, Indianapolis, IN 46223, USA

Lawrence D. Longo, MD
Professor, Departments of Physiology and Obstetrics and Gynecology, Director, Center for Perinatal Biology, School of Medicine, Loma Linda University, Loma Linda, CA 92350, USA

Jeffrey L. Loughead, MD
Assistant Clinical Professor, Department of Pediatrics, Wright State University School of Medicine, Newborn Medicine, The Children's Medical Center, Dayton, OH 45404 USA

Ram K. Menon, MD
Associate Professor, Department of Pediatrics, University of Pittsburgh School of Medicine, Division of Pediatric Endocrinology, Children's Hospital of Pittsburgh, Pittsburgh, PA 15213, USA

Armand F. Miranda, MD
Professor of Clinical Pathology Emeritus, Department of Pathology, Consultant in Neurology, Department of Neurology, MDA H. Houston Merritt Clinical Research Center for Muscular Dystrophy and Related Diseases, College of Physicians and Surgeons of Columbia University, New York, NY 10032, USA

Edward S. Ogata, MD
Raymond and Hazel Speck Berry Professor, Departments of Pediatrics, Obstetrics and Gynecology, Northwestern University School of Medicine, Associate Chief of Staff, Children's Memorial Hospital, Chicago, IL 60614, USA

Paul L. Ogburn, Jr., MD
Associate Professor and Chair, Department of Obstetrics, Mayo Clinic School of Medicine, Rochester, MN 55905, USA

Pinar T. Ozand, MD, PhD
Head, Section of Inborn Errors of Metabolism, Department of Pediatrics, King Faisal Specialist Hospital and Research Centre, Riyadh 11211, Saudi Arabia

Contributors

James F. Padbury, MD
Professor and Vice Chair, Department of Pediatrics, Brown University School of Medicine, Pediatrician-in-Chief, Department of Pediatrics, Women and Infants Hospital of Rhode Island, Providence, RI 02905, USA

Jean-Paul Pegorier, PhD, DSc
Research Director, Centre National de la Recherche Scientifique, 92190 Meudon, France

Agostino Pierro, MD
Reader, Department of Pediatric Surgery, University College London Medical School, Institute of Child Health and Great Ormond Street Hospital for Children, NHS Trust, London WC1N 1EH, UK

John T. Repke, MD
Chris J. and Marie A. Olson Professor of Obstetrics and Gynecology, University of Nebraska College of Medicine, Obstetrician-in-Chief, Department of Obstetrics and Gynecology, University of Nebraska Medical Center, Omaha, NE 68198, USA

Richard W. Rothstein, MD
Assistant Professor, Department of Pediatrics, Tufts University School of Medicine, Staff Neonatologist, Department of Pediatrics, Bayside Medical Center, Springfield, MA 01109, USA

Lewis P. Rubin, MD
Associate Professor, Department of Pediatrics, Brown University School of Medicine, Neonatologist, Department of Pediatrics, Women and Infants Hospital of Rhode Island, Providence, RI 02905, USA

Abraham M. Rudolph, MD
Professor Emeritus, Department of Pediatrics, University of California School of Medicine, San Francisco, CA 94143, USA

Pieter J.J. Sauer, MD
Professor and Chair, Department of Pediatrics, University of Groningen, Pediatrician-in-Chief, Beatrix Children's Hospital, Groningen University Hospital, 9700 RB Groningen, The Netherlands

Richard J. Schanler, MD
Professor, Department of Pediatrics, Baylor College of Medicine, Children's Nutritional Research Center, Houston, TX 77030, USA

David J. Schmeling, MD
Partner, Pediatric Surgical Associates, Ltd, Attending Physician, Department of Surgery, Minneapolis Children's Hospital, Minneapolis, MN 55404, and Attending Physician, Department of Surgery, St. Paul Children's Hospital, St Paul MN 55102

Robert Schwartz, MD
Professor, Department of Pediatrics, Emeritus Professor of Medical Science, Brown University School of Medicine, Staff Endocrinologist, Division of Pediatric Endocrinology and Metabolism, Rhode Island Hospital and Hasbro Children's Hospital, Providence, RI 02903, USA

Rebecca A. Simmons, MD
Assistant Professor, Department of Pediatrics, University of Pennsylvania School of Medicine, Attending Physician, Division of Neonatology, Children's Hospital of Philadelphia, Philadelphia PA 19104, USA

Mark A. Sperling, MD
Professor and Chair, Department of Pediatrics, University of Pittsburgh School of Medicine, Pediatrician-in-Chief, Children's Hospital of Pittsburgh, Pittsburgh, PA 15213, USA

Charles A. Stanley, MD
Professor, Department of Pediatrics, University of Pennsylvania School of Medicine, Division of Endocrinology/Diabetes, Director, General Clinical Research Center Core Laboratory, Children's Hospital of Philadelphia, Philadelphia, PA 19104, USA

John B. Susa, PhD
Associate Professor(Research), Department of Pediatrics, Brown University School of Medicine, Division of Pediatric Endocrinology and Metabolism, Rhode Island Hospital and Hasbro Children's Hospital, Providence, RI 02903, USA

Reginald C. Tsang, MBBS
Professor, Department of Pediatrics, University of Cincinnati College of Medicine, Children's Hospital Medical Center, Cincinnati, OH 45267, USA

Yi-Tang Tseng, PhD
Assistant Professor(Research), Department of Pediatrics, Brown University School of Medicine, Women and Infants Hospital of Rhode Island, Providence, RI 02905, USA

Lambert M.G. van Golde, PhD
Professor and Chairman, Division of Biochemistry, Department of Basic Sciences, Faculty of Veterinary Medicine, University of Utrecht, 3508TD Utrecht, The Netherlands

Robert C. Vannucci, MD
Professor, Department of Pediatrics, Pennsylvania State University College of Medicine, Division of Pediatric Neurology, Penn State Geisinger Health System, Hershey, PA 17033, USA

Susan J. Vannucci, Ph D
Associate Professor, Departments of Pediatrics and Neuroscience and Anatomy, Pennsylvania State University, Hershey, PA 17033, USA

G. Wesley Vick, III, MD, PhD
Assistant Professor, Department of Pediatrics, Baylor College of Medicine, Associate, Lillie Frank Abercrombie Section of Pediatric Cardiology, Texas Children's Hospital, Houston, TX 77030, USA

Ulrich A. Walker, MD
Postdoctoral Fellow, Department of Neurology, MDA H. Houston Merritt Clinical Research Center for Muscular Dystrophy and Related Diseases, College of Physicians and Surgeons of Columbia University, New York, NY 10032, USA

E. Marelyn Wintour, PhD, DSc
Senior Principal Research Fellow, Howard Florey Institute of Experimental Pathology and Medicine, University of Melbourne, Parkville, Victoria 3052, Australia

Robert R. Wolfe, PhD
Professor (Metabolism), Department of Surgery, University of Texas Medical Branch, Chief, Metabolism Unit, Shriners Burns Institute, Galveston, TX 77550, USA

Richard D. Zachman, PhD, MD
Professor, Departments of Pediatrics and Nutritional Sciences, University of Wisconsin, Wisconsin Perinatal Center, Meriter Hospital, Madison, WI 53715, USA

Xiaodong Zhu, MD
Senior Research Fellow, Division of Metabolism, Endocrinology and Nutrition, Department of Medicine, University of Washington School of Medicine, Seattle, WA 98104, USA

Luc J.I. Zimmermann, MD, PhD
Department of Pediatrics, Erasmus University, Division of Neonatology, Sophia Children's Hospital, 3015GJ Rotterdam, The Netherlands

Section IV
Organ-Specific Metabolism During the Perinatal Period

26
Brain Metabolism in the Fetus and Neonate

Susan J. Vannucci and Robert C. Vannucci

This chapter provides an comprehensive overview of perinatal cerebral metabolism in developing animals and human infants. Substrate and energy transformations in the perinatal brain under physiologic conditions are emphasized. These transformations are perturbed by several acute insults, including hypoxia-ischemia, hypoglycemia, and seizures. Knowledge of specific mechanisms underlying perinatal cerebral oxidative metabolism is fundamental to our understanding how the human brain grows and matures under physiologic conditions.[1]

Cerebral Energy Metabolism

The maintenance of normal cerebral development and function requires a continual supply of energy to the brain in the form of metabolizable substrate, primarily glucose, to fuel the metabolic demands of growth and neuronal activity. Under normal circumstances there exists a delicate balance between the energy-producing and the energy-consuming processes, reflected in the concentration of the primary energy modulator, adenosine triphosphate (ATP). ATP has two ~P bonds, which exist at an energy level capable of providing the necessary driving force for innumerable biochemical reactions and physiologic processes. ATP not only promotes energy-consuming reactions, but also drives physiologic processes, such as ion pumping, by acid hydrolysis. As such, the compound provides the cellular free acid necessary to maintain neuronal viability with its specialized function.

Under physiologic conditions, cellular ATP concentrations are maintained remarkably stable, as the rate of energy consumption by endergonic reactions is exactly balanced by the rate of ATP production. The cell's ability to maintain ATP constant, even under situations of increased energy expenditure, is dependent on those biochemical processes that generate ATP. These processes include substrate and oxidative phosphorylation as well as the energy transformations resulting from the equilibria among the cell's high-energy phosphate reserves, that is, ATP, adenosine diphosphate (ADP), and phosphocreatine.

The most quantitatively important pathway for the generation of ATP is oxidative phosphorylation, which occurs in the mitochondria of all cells (Figure 26.1). Mitochondrial oxidation is a highly efficient process that couples molecular oxidation to the hydrogen atom of nicotinamide adenine dinucleotide, reduced (NADH) or flavin adenine dinucleotide, reduced (FADH) to form water coincident with the phosphorylation of ADP to ATP. In addition, some ATP is formed during substrate-level phosphorylation, which occurs both in the mitochondria and the cytoplasm.

In addition to substrate and oxidative phosphorylation, which are net energy-producing processes, two other mechanisms maintain cellular ATP concentrations constant. These reactions are the creatine phosphokinase and adenylate kinase equilibria, biochemical reactions that simply transfer energy (~P) from one high-energy compound to another. In brain, the primary metabolites that store and transfer energy include ATP, ADP, and phosphocreatine.[2-4] Of the three, ATP plays the critical role in the coupling of energy supply to energy demand via substrate and oxidative phosphorylation (vide supra). Phosphocreatine acts as the predominant energy storage metabolite. Creatine phosphokinase catalyzes a reversible transfer of ~P between phosphocreatine (PCr) and ATP:

$$PCr + ADP + H+ \rightarrow ATP + Cr$$

The adenylate kinase reaction catalyzes the conversion of ADP to ATP:

$$2\ ADP \rightarrow ATP + AMP$$

Owing to their equilibrium constants, both reactions serve to maintain an optimal intracellular concentration of ATP even under situations of reduced ATP synthesis by oxidative phosphorylation.

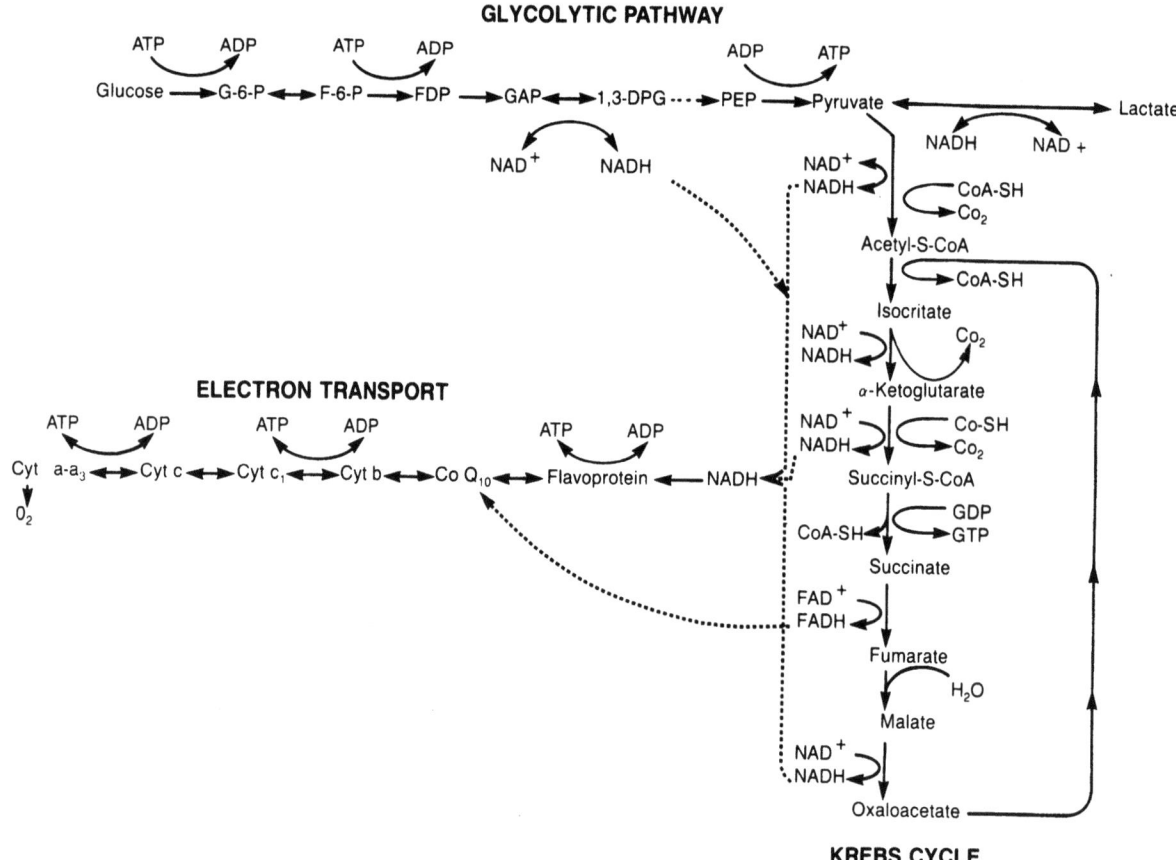

FIGURE 26.1. Schematic diagram of the oxidative pathway. G-6-P, glucose-6-phosphate; F-6-P, fructose-6-phosphate; FDP, fructose diphosphate; GAP, glyceraldehyde phosphate; 1,3-DPG, diphosphoglycerate; PEP, phosphoenopyruvate; ATP, adenosine triphosphate; ADP, adenosine diphosphate; NAD^+, nicotinamide adenine dinucleotide (oxidized form); NADH, nicotinamide adenine dinucleotide (reduced form). (From Vannucci,[1] with permission.)

Cerebral high-energy metabolites have undergone extensive investigation in both perinatal and adult animals. These metabolites can be measured by enzymatic, chromatographic, and magnetic spectroscopic techniques.[5–8] Of the nucleotides, ATP is the predominant form and this is maintained from fetal life through adulthood (Table 26.1). Lower concentrations of ATP have been found in embryonic chick brain tissue.[11] Phosphocreatine is lower in the brains of fetal and newborn animals than in adults, as is total creatine (phosphocreatine + creatine), but the phosphocreatine/creatine ratio changes little with postnatal development. The lower phosphocreatine/creatine ratio in the fetus presumably is the result of a lower brain pH, owing to increased tissue lactate concentrations and mild hypercapnia; the creatine phosphokinase equilibrium reaction is pH dependent.[9]

Magnetic resonance (MR) spectroscopy is a technique whereby the concentration of an organic compound in tissue can be determined by the realignment of selected molecules with a superconducting magnet[12] (see Chapter 1). Either proton (^1H)- or phosphorus (^{31}P)-containing compounds can be analyzed according to the strength, duration, and other characteristics of the magnetic field.[13]

The most frequently examined metabolites in brain are the phosphorus-containing compounds: phosphocreatine; ATP; mono- and diphosphate esters [i.e., includes adenosine monophosphate (AMP) and ADP, respectively]; and inorganic phosphate (Pi).[14–16] Accordingly, MR spectroscopy is capable of ascertaining the energy status of brain tissue in vivo under either physiologic or pathophysiologic conditions, although at present the

TABLE 26.1. Cerebral high-energy reserves in immature and adult rats.

Metabolite	Fetus	Newborn	1 WK	Adult
ATP	2.66	2.63	2.64	2.76
ATP + ADP + AMP	3.11	2.89	3.21	3.17
Phosphocreatine	1.74	3.16*	3.33	4.90*
Creatine	5.35	3.83*	4.65*	5.63*
PCr + creatine	7.10	6.99	7.97*	10.53*
PCr/creatine	0.33	0.83*	0.72	0.87

Values, expressed in mmol/kg wet weight, represent means of four to seven animals in each age group. Fetal, newborn, and 1-week values are from forebrain,[9] whereas adult values are from cerebral cortex.[10] PCr, phosphocreatine.
*$p < .05$ compared with previous age group.

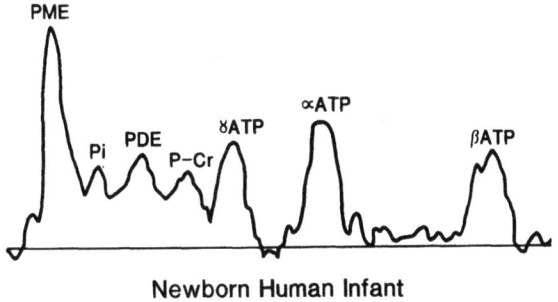
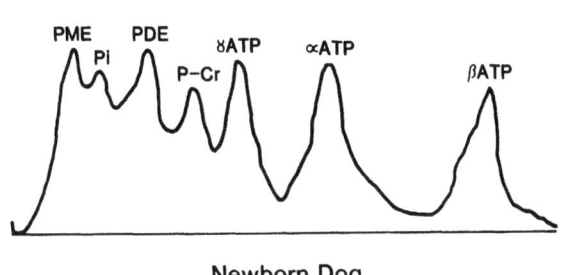

FIGURE 26.2. Representative phosphorus nuclear magnetic spectra of the brains of newborn human infant and a newborn dog. PME, phosphorus monoesters; P_i, inorganic phosphate; PDE, phosphorus diesters; PCr, phosphocreatine; δATP, αATP, and βATP, δ, α, and β adenosine trisphosphate, respectively. (Data for infant derived from Younkin et al.,[15] and data for dog derived from Young.[8] From Vannucci,[1] with permission.)

measurements are semiquantitative in nature (Figure 26.2).

In humans, MR spectroscopy has shown that ATP concentrations remain relatively stable throughout early maturation,[15] although the metabolite almost doubles between birth and adulthood.[17] Concentrations of phosphocreatine, Pi, and the phosphodiesters are low at birth and increase with advancing age. Calculated intracellular pH, measured from the chemical shift of the Pi peak relative to the phosphocreatine peak, is 7.1 in healthy neonates. The phosphocreatine/Pi and the phosphocreatine/ATP ratios are lower in neonates compared with adults. Regional differences in these ratios exist in the newborn brain, with a tendency to lower values in deeper structures (i.e., mostly white matter) compared to superficial structures (i.e., mostly cerebral cortex).[18] It is anticipated that the continued use and greater sophistication of MR spectroscopy will contribute substantially to our understanding of the bioenergetics of the perinatal human brain.

Cerebral Oxidative Metabolism

The oxidative events that operate in the perinatal brain are similar to those of adult animals and humans, although quantitative differences exist. Cellular respiration is that process whereby an organic substrate is consumed to produce energy, primarily in the form of ATP, with carbon dioxide and water as the metabolic byproducts. Respiration is a highly efficient process with minimal energy waste. Under physiologic conditions, 1 mol of glucose, the primary energy fuel, is catalyzed in the presence of oxygen to yield 36 mol of ATP. Other substrates yield proportionately greater or lesser energy depending on their molecular carbon structure and their entry point into the oxidative pathway.

The biochemical machinery that makes up the oxidative pathway is divided into three components: (1) glycolysis, a cytoplasmic process; and (2) the tricarboxylic acid (Krebs) cycle and (3) the cytochrome system, both cycles operate within mitochondria (Figure 26.1). Glycolysis proceeds under both aerobic and anaerobic conditions. In the presence of oxygen, glucose is converted to pyruvic acid, which, in turn, enters the Krebs cycle with little or no conversion to lactic acid. When oxygen is not available, metabolites of the Krebs cycle are depleted, and glycolysis is accelerated with the formation of lactic acid in an attempt to maintain cerebral energy stores. Because anaerobic glycolysis is an inefficient means to generate energy (i.e., only 2 mol of ATP per mol of glucose), brain function cannot be maintained by this process alone.

Glycolytic control points include those reactions in which the activities of specific enzymes govern the rate of metabolism. These enzymes include hexokinase, phosphofructokinase (PFK), and possibly pyruvate kinase. Of these enzymes, PFK is predominantly rate-limiting for glycolysis in both adult and immature brain.[19-21] Metabolites known to inhibit PFK activity and hence glycolysis include ATP, citrate, and hydrogen ions, whereas ADP, AMP, and Pi stimulate PFK activity.[3] These glycolytic regulatory mechanisms are important in the cell's response to hypoxia, acid-base imbalance, and other metabolic disturbances.

Quantitative Aspects of Oxidative Metabolism

Measurements of cerebral oxygen consumption provide a quantitative estimation of energy production by the brain, since oxygen is required for the oxidative phosphorylation of ADP to ATP. Oxygen consumption measurements usually are referred to as the cerebral metabolic rate for oxygen ($CMRO_2$), expressed in terms of ml·100g^{-1}min^{-1}. Oxygen consumption can be calculated in vivo from the Fick principle by measuring cerebral blood flow (CBF) and the arteriovenous difference for oxygen across the brain:

$$CMRO_2 = CBF(A - Vo_2).$$

TABLE 26.2. Cerebral metabolic rates for oxygen ($CMRO_2$) in developing animals and humans.

Species (references)	Fetal	Newborn	Adult
Sheep[22-25]	2.0–3.7	3.9–4.8	4.2
Dog[26,27]	–	1.1	2.8
Monkey[28,29]	–	1.1	3.2
Humans[30-32]	–	1.5	3.2–3.3

Values are expressed in $ml \cdot 100\,g^{-1} min^{-1}$.

$CMRO_2$ has been determined in immature animals of several species, including humans (Table 26.2). Notable species differences exist for the rates of oxygen consumption by brain, which reflect the age and functional immaturity of the animal at the time of the measurement as well as species variations in the brain's intrinsic metabolic requirements. In general, $CMRO_2$ is lower in perinatal animals compared to adults of the same species, and the more functionally immature the animal at birth, the lower the oxygen consumption. This assumption is supported by measurements in newborn dogs, a functionally immature animal at birth, in which both CBF and $CMRO_2$ are 40% of their respective values in adult dogs. In contrast, the newborn lamb is relatively mature at birth and already exhibits a $CMRO_2$ that approximates that of adult sheep (Table 26.2).

Oxygen consumption of the brain has been determined in humans, including newborn infants. The $CMRO_2$ in young, healthy adults is $3.3\,ml \cdot 100\,g^{-1} \cdot min^{-1}$. Settergren et al.[32] measured $CMRO_2$ in infants and children age 11 days to 15 years who were anesthetized with nitrous oxide. The mean value for $CMRO_2$ was $3.2\,ml \cdot 100\,g^{-1} min^{-1}$ for the entire group, and no age-related differences could be ascertained. Garfunkel et al.[31] found $CMRO_2$ values of 1.1 to $2.1\,ml \cdot 100\,g^{-1} min^{-1}$ in three neonates anesthetized with a barbiturate. However, these low values might not apply to healthy, awake infants, since barbiturates are known to depress the $CMRO_2$, and all the infants had severe central nervous system anomalies.

$CMRO_2$ can be determined using positron emission tomography (PET), which is based on computed tomography (CT) except that the source of radiation for external detection is transmitted from within the brain outward rather than passed through the brain as x-rays. In PET, a positron-emitting, rapid decay isotope, prepared by a cyclotron, is administered to the subject. The substance circulates to the brain in which it is metabolized, during which its positrons combine with electrons to form γ-rays. The γ-rays penetrate the brain, skull, and scalp, and are recorded externally on a linear array of scintillation detectors. A computer mathematically reconstructs the spatial distribution of the radioactivity within the brain, which is either quantified or displayed visually (see Chapter 1).

Using PET with ^{15}O-labeled water as the positron-emitting isotope, Altman et al.[33] measured $CMRO_2$ in 11 neonates of gestational ages ranging from 26 to 40 weeks. $CMRO_2$ was low in all of the infants, and values were actually beyond the range of detection in two. In those infants in whom radioactivity was detectable, $CMRO_2$ ranged from $0.2–1.3 \cdot 100\,g^{-1} min^{-1}$, well below the measured value of $3.3 \cdot 100\,g^{-1} min^{-1}$ in human adults. The finding indicates that as in perinatal animals cerebral oxidative metabolism, especially in small premature infants, is low, reflecting the functional immaturity of the brain. A less likely proposal, offered by Altman et al.,[33] is that the energy requirements of the fetal and premature newborn brain are met by nonoxidative metabolism, i.e., anaerobic glycolysis.

Glycolysis

As described above, rates of glycolysis or the glycolytic flux is controlled by specific, rate-limiting enzymes that are either inhibited or activated by changes in the biochemical milieu of the cytoplasm. Aerobic glycolysis is stimulated under those conditions that increase the energy demand of the tissue, such as stimulant drugs and hormones, hyperthermia, and seizures. Anaerobic glycolysis is activated by hypoxia or cerebral ischemia in an attempt to maintain optimal cellular energy balance despite an oxygen debt. Glycolysis is inhibited by sedative and anesthetic agents, hypothermia, and acidosis; these conditions reduce the energy needs of the tissue. Glycolysis can never cease completely, as at least some energy is always required to maintain ion gradients across membranes, without which cellular integrity is compromised.

The extent to which glycolysis and oxidative metabolism can be decreased or increased is not entirely known. In adult animals, barbiturate anesthesia sufficient to produce an isoelectric electroencephalogram reduces oxidative metabolism by no more than 50%.[34] This suggests that up to 50% of cellular energy production is required for maintenance of biochemical and morphologic integrity, while the remaining energy production under physiologic conditions is devoted to the generation of action potentials and to biosynthetic processes. The extent to which glycolysis can be stimulated (i.e., glycolytic capacity) also is conjectural, although studies in experimental animals suggest that glycolytic flux can be accelerated up to 8- to 10-fold during extreme metabolic stress, such as seizures or hypoxia-ischemia.[3]

Both basal glycolytic flux and glycolytic capacity are lower in immature animals than in their adult counterparts, which is in keeping with intrinsically lower rates of oxygen consumption and metabolic demands. For example, the calculated rate of cerebral glycolysis of the perinatal rat is approximately 10 mmol glucose·100 g^{-1}·min^{-1},[35] one tenth the rate calculated for adult rat brain.[36] During total cerebral ischemia, glycolytic flux in newborn rat brain increases fivefold compared with an eightfold increase in adult rat brain.[35,36] The age-specific difference in glycolytic capacity suggests that the ability of perinatal animals to survive longer in hypoxia or anoxia than adults[37] is not related to a heightened capacity of the immature rat to generate energy equivalents via anaerobic glycolysis. Rather, lower cerebral energy demands and hence metabolic requirements underscore the perinatal animal's resistance to cerebral hypoxia-ischemia.[35,36]

Mitochondrial Development

Because the mitochondria produce the vast bulk of energy utilized for cellular needs, these "powerhouses" have been investigated during maturation of the brain. Studies have shown that neither the number nor size of mitochondria per wet weight of tissue changes during postnatal growth of rat brain, although the number of mitochondria per brain cell doubles between birth and adulthood.[38] Oxygen consumption related to mitochondrial protein remains constant throughout maturation, whereas the rate of high-energy phosphate formation actually decreases slightly.[39] Samson et al.[40] have suggested that since oxygen consumption and energy output/mitochondrion are not altered by age, each mitochondrial unit has a phosphorylating capacity that remains relatively constant throughout maturation.

In contrast to the conclusions of Samson et al.,[40] other investigators have shown a relative deficiency in the oxidative phosphorylating capacity of mitochondria that characterizes the immature brain.[41,42] Specifically, the immature brain appears less capable of synthesizing the ATP/molecule of oxygen consumed. This coupling of ATP to oxygen, expressed in terms of the ATP/O or P/O ratio, is 3 for the oxidized form of nicotinamide-adenine dinucleotide (NAD^+)-linked cytochrome components in adult rat brain.[43] Holtzman and Moore[44] have measured P/O ratios in several regions of rat brain during maturation. Ratios of 1.5 for NAD^+-linked substrates were found in animals at postnatal age 1 to 11 days. Thereafter, ratios increased to 2.4 in pons-medulla and 2.8 in cerebral cortex. The data indicate that the brain cell's increasing efficiency for oxidative phosphorylation (i.e., improved coupling) reflects both an increase in the number of mitochondria and an inherent change in their function.

The functional advantage of these mitochondrial changes appears to lie in the pattern of growth of the brain. A striking increase in mitochondrial cell number accompanies neuronal hypertrophy secondary to axonal and dendritic expansion.[45] As individual cells enlarge, the cell surface/volume ratio increases, a circumstance that raises the energy required to maintain ionic gradients across cellular membranes and to propagate action potentials.[40]

Cerebral Energy Utilization

Energy utilization by the brain can be inferred from measurements of oxygen or substrate consumption, since under steady-state conditions energy demand and supply are equivalent. Cerebral energy utilization also can be measured directly in the experimental animal by the Lowry decapitation technique.[19] Lowry et al.[19] devised a novel technique to determine the rate of energy use in brain during the total cerebral ischemia that follows decapitation. The investigators assumed that since the isolated head is a closed metabolic compartment (i.e., no inflow or outflow), rates of depletion of potential (i.e., glucose + glycogen), and endogenous (ATP + ADP + phosphocreatine) high-energy metabolites would be a direct measure of cerebral energy utilization occurring prior to decapitation. Using this method, investigators have shown that the calculated rate of cerebral energy use in perinatal animals, like the $CMRO_2$, is substantially less than in adults.[7,19,35] The energy use rate of 1-day postnatal rat brain is 1.3 mmol~P·kg^{-1}·min^{-1},[35] 20 times less than the calculated rate of 27 mmol~P·kg^{-1}·min^{-1} for adult rat brain.[36] The $CMRO_2$ can be calculated from the rate of cerebral energy use if the ADP/O or P/O ratio is known. P/O ratios for immature rat brain are 1.5 for NAD^+-linked substrates, and they are 1.2 for the oxidized form of flavin-adenine dinucleotide (FAD^+)-linked substrates.[44] A source of ATP other than that derived from oxidative phosphorylation of ADP is substrate phosphorylation, which occurs twice in glycolysis and once in the Krebs cycle. Substrate phosphorylation yields 6 mol of ATP for every mole of glucose consumed; 2 mol are required for the initial phosphorylation of glucose and fructose-6-phosphate in glycolysis. For every mole of glucose consumed, 4 mol of ATP are ultimately generated by a source other than oxidative phosphorylation; this amounts to 20% of the total energy production. Assuming a yield of 3 mol of ~P/mol of oxygen reduced (P/O ratio = 1.5), and taking into account the ATP formed by both oxidative and substrate phosphorylation, the rate of cerebral energy utilization for newborn rat brain translates to a $CMRO_2$ of $[1.3 - (1.3 \times 0.2)]/3 = 0.35$ mmol·kg^{-1}·min^{-1} or 0.78 ml·100 g^{-1}·min^{-1}. This value can be compared with a measured $CMRO_2$ of 5.4 ml·100 g^{-1}·min^{-1} for adult rat brain.[46] The fetal rat at term exhibits a rate of cerebral energy utilization comparable to that of the newborn rat.[35]

The low cerebral energy requirements of most animals at birth reflect an immaturity of the brain at this stage of

TABLE 26.3. Cerebral energy use rates and maximal glycolytic capacities of chick embryos and newly hatched peeps.

Age (D)	Δ~P	ΔLactate	ΔLactate/Δ~P
9	2.84	0.79	0.29
14	3.25	1.51*	0.54*
16	2.76	2.04*	0.78*
19	5.76*	3.22*	0.56*
Peeps	8.98*	5.09*	0.56

Values, expressed in mmol/kg wet weight, represent means of four to six animals in each group. The ratio Δlactate/Δ~P is an indication of the maximal contribution of anaerobic metabolism to the cerebral metabolic rate.
*$p < .05$ compared with the previous age group.
Data derived from Gonya-Magee and Vannucci.[11]

development. It has been suggested that cerebral energy demands in the fetal brain are even less well developed than in the newborn brain,[47] and that energetic demands in embryonic life are met predominantly, if not entirely, by anaerobic glycolysis, with only a small contribution from oxidative metabolism.[45,48] Using the Lowry technique to measure cerebral energy utilization, Gonya-Magee and Vannucci[11] measured rates of cerebral metabolism in chick embryos at 9, 14, 16, and 19 days of incubation and in newly hatched peeps (Table 26.3). Calculated cerebral metabolic rates were not different in the 9-, 14-, and 16-day-old embryos but doubled between 16 and 19 days and doubled again between 19 days and hatching. The extent to which total energy utilization could be derived from anaerobic glycolysis (Δ lactate/ Δ~P) increased from a low at day 9 (0.29) to a maximum at day 16 (0.78). These data suggest that cerebral oxidative metabolism becomes regressively lower with decreasing embryonic age, but a nadir is reached below which metabolism can no longer support cerebral function and growth. Despite the low metabolic activity of the embyronic brain, at no time during development is anaerobic glycolysis capable of entirely supporting the energy needs of the tissue.

The Flow-Metabolism Couple

With the availability of methods to measure cerebral blood flow (CBF) and oxidative metabolism in both animals and humans, a quantitative relationship between these two important biologic processes in brain was quickly ascertained. Further investigation revealed that under physiologic conditions, CBF was predominantly controlled by intrinsic mechanisms that reflect local rate of metabolism, i.e., the extent of tissue carbon dioxide and hydrogen ion accumulation. Accordingly, CBF and oxidative metabolism are tightly linked or coupled. Specifically, when the rate of oxidative metabolism in brain is high, so is CBF, and vice versa. Metabolic diseases are capable of altering this critical relationship, leading to neurologic dysfunction that, if severe enough, produces permanent brain damage.

The brain flow-metabolism couple appears to be a universal phenomenon that encompasses all animal species of all ages and under all physiologic conditions (Figure 26.3). In those animals in which CBF and $CMRO_2$ have been measured simultaneously, the relationship has been apparent regardless of age, despite differences in the intrinsic rates of metabolism among the various species. A regional coupling of CBF to metabolism exists in both adult and immature animals[49-52] when regional CBF (rCBF), determined with an inert, radioactive tracer, is compared with regional cerebral glucose utilization (rCGU) (Figure 26.4). A visual comparison of published

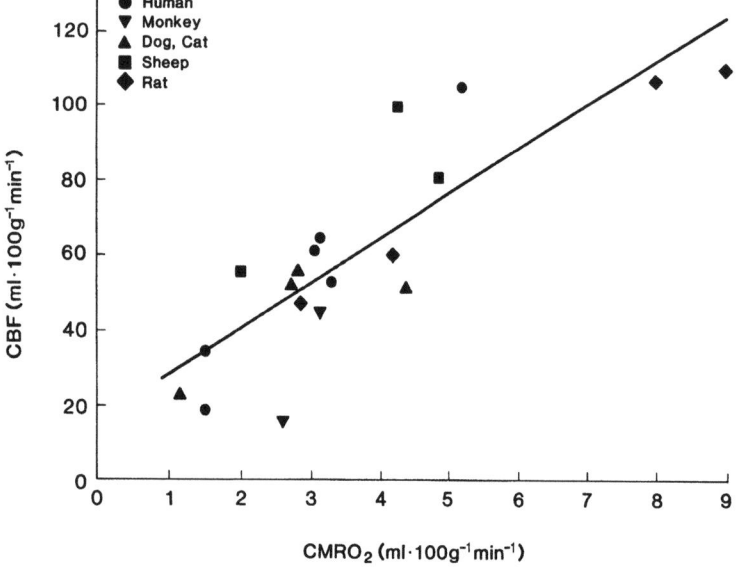

FIGURE 26.3. Relationship between cerebral blood flow (CBF) and the cerebral metabolic rate for oxygen ($CMRO_2$) in several species of animals. Symbols represent values from animals of varying ages. The line denotes the slope of a linear regression analysis with Y = 12.1X + 16.7; $r = 0.85$; $p < .001$. (From Vannucci,[1] with permission.)

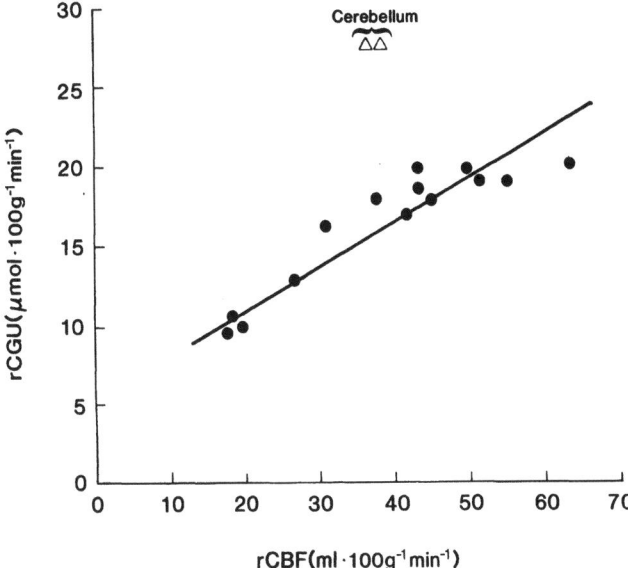

FIGURE 26.4. Relationship between regional cerebral glucose utilization (rCGU) and regional cerebral blood flow (rCBF) in newborn dogs. Symbols represent values from specific regions of brain. The line denotes the slope of a linear regression analysis (excluding cerebellum) with Y = 0.24X + 7.0; r = 0.93; p < .001. (Data from Mujsce et al.[52] From Vannucci,[1] with permission.)

figures depicting rCBF and rCGU, using PET, suggests the existence of a regional CBF-metabolism couple in the human neonate.[53-55] Some exceptions to the rule occur among individual structures, which might reflect local differences in the contribution of glucose versus alternate substrates to overall metabolism or to the use of glucose in biosynthetic processes (vide infra).

Cerebral Glucose Utilization

Glucose is the predominant or exclusive organic fuel for cerebral metabolism under physiologic conditions in all animal species, including humans. Glucose appears to be the predominant substrate for the brain of the fetus and developing postnatal animal. Like $CMRO_2$, glucose consumption in brain can be measured if CBF and the arteriovenous difference for glucose across the brain is known:

$$CMRglucose = CBF\left(A - Vglucose\right)$$

When CMRglucose (or other organic substrate) and $CMRO_2$ are measured simultaneously, the substrate-oxygen quotient can be ascertained, which expresses the relative contribution of the substrate to overall oxidative metabolism:

$$Substrate/O_2 = \frac{CMRsubstrate\left(No.\ C\ atoms\right)}{CMRO_2} \times 100$$

Using these measurements, cerebral glucose utilization has been determined in several perinatal animal species, including fetuses, as well as in human neonates (Table 26.4).[29,32,56-59] As in adult humans,[60,61] glucose serves as the major organic substrate to support cerebral metabolism in all species studied. Furthermore, the vast bulk of glucose consumed is aerobically degraded to carbon dioxide and water or is used in biosynthetic processes with little or no production of lactic acid (i.e., anaerobic glycolysis). Under physiologic conditions glucose is efficiently utilized to produce the maximal amount of chemical energy possible.

In the past only global estimates of cerebral glucose consumption could be ascertained using the method described above. However, the pioneering work of Sokoloff et al.[49,62] now allows for regional measurements of glucose utilization (rCGU) in both experimental animals and humans. Sokoloff et al.[49] used radioactive 2-[^{14}C]-deoxyglucose (2-DG) to measure CGU in 30 or more component structures of adult rat brain. The rationale for the use of 2-DG rather than [^{14}C]-glucose relates to the fact that the radioactive analogue of native glucose is lost from the brain as carbon dioxide and water during the course of an experiment. Accordingly, calculated CGU would underestimate the true CGU value. Deoxyglucose, like glucose, is taken up by brain and phosphorylated by hexokinase but, unlike glucose, is unable to be metabolized further along the glycolytic pathway. The theory and application of the 2-DG technique to the experimental animal now forms the basis of measuring rCGU in humans using PET. Since glucose is the predominant cerebral energy fuel, and glucose utilization is stoichiometrically related to oxygen consumption, the measurement of rCGU under physiologic conditions reflects local rates of cerebral energy utilization and intrinsic functional activity.[62] Using the 2-DG technique, rCGU has been investigated in fetal sheep and guinea pigs as well as in newborn and developing rats, lambs, dogs, and monkeys.[50-52,59,63,64] These studies confirm early in vitro studies that CGU in the perinatal animal is high in brain stem gray matter structures, declining in a caudal to rostral progression through the neuraxis to the cerebral cortex

TABLE 26.4. Substrate equivalents as percent of total cerebral substrate utilization and extent of anaerobic metabolism in newborn animals and humans.

Substrate	Sheep[56]*	Dog[58]	Monkey[29]	Human[32]
Glucose	99.5	93.5	70.4	91.1
β-Hydroxybutyrate	0.5	0.5	14.6	5.5
Acetoacetate	0.0	2.0	4.9	3.4
Lactate	0.0	4.0	10.0	0.0
	100%	100%	100%	100%
% Glucose→lactate	2.6%	0.0%	0.0%	5.2%

*Reference number.

TABLE 26.5. Regional cerebral glucose utilization (rCGU) in developing monkeys.

Structure	Newborn	Pubescent	% Difference
Frontal cortex	28	50	+44*
Parietal cortex	29	47	+38*
Occipital cortex	32	59	+46*
Hippocampus	25	39	+38*
Corpus callosum	15	11	−36
Caudate nucleus	23	52	+56
Thalamus	35	54	+35*
Substantia nigra	28	29	+3
Inferior colliculus	180	103	−75
Cerebellar hemisphere	22	31	+29

Values expressed in $\mu mol \cdot 100 g^{-1} min^{-1}$ represent means of six to seven animals in each group.
*$p < .01$.
Data derived from Kennedy.[50]

(Table 26.5; Figure 26.5). As in adults, CGU is lowest in subcortical and other white matter structures. Duffy et al.[51] equate the hierarchy of rates of glucose consumption to the functional immaturity of the animal with its limited sensory and motor capabilities but with little or no memory or learning abilities in the late fetal or early newborn period.

Using PET with ^{18}fluoro-2-deoxyglucose as the positron-emitting isotope, Chugani and Phelps et al.[52,54] measured rCGU in humans from birth through adulthood (Figure 26.6). In infants 5 weeks of age and younger, glucose utilization was highest in the sensorimotor cerebral cortex, thalamus, midbrain–brain stem, and the cerebellar vermis. This distribution of glucose consumption is similar to that described in term fetal sheep and in newborn dogs and monkeys[50,51,63] (Figure 26.5). By 3 months of age, glucose metabolic activity in the infants had increased in the parietal, temporal, and occipital cortices and in the basal ganglia, with subsequent increases in frontal and various association regions of cerebral cortex occurring by 8 months.[65] Little further change in rCGU was observed between 8 and 18 months of postnatal age. The investigators emphasized that the maturational increases in rCGU measured with PET are in agreement with the behavioral, neurophysiologic, and anatomical changes that occurred during early infant development.

Glucose Transporter Proteins

Although the vital nature of glucose delivery to the brain has been appreciated for some time, the exact mechanism by which glucose, a hydrophilic molecule, traverses the lipid membranes of the microvascular endothelium of the blood-brain barrier (BBB) as well as neurons and glia has been clarified only recently (see Chapter 7). Following

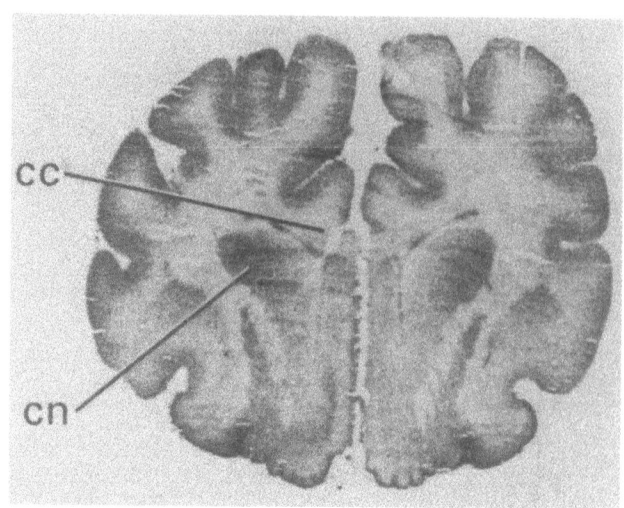
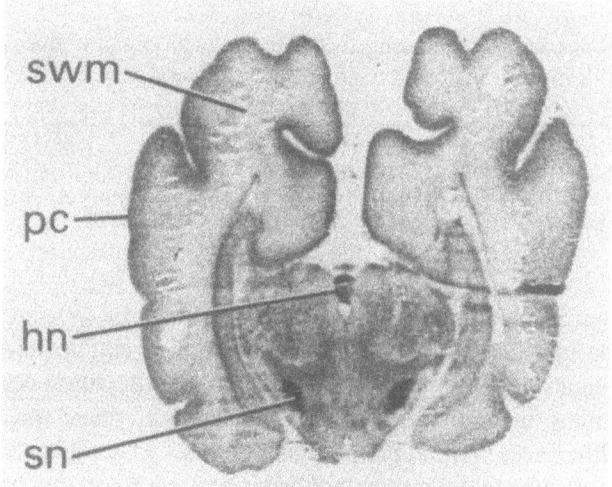
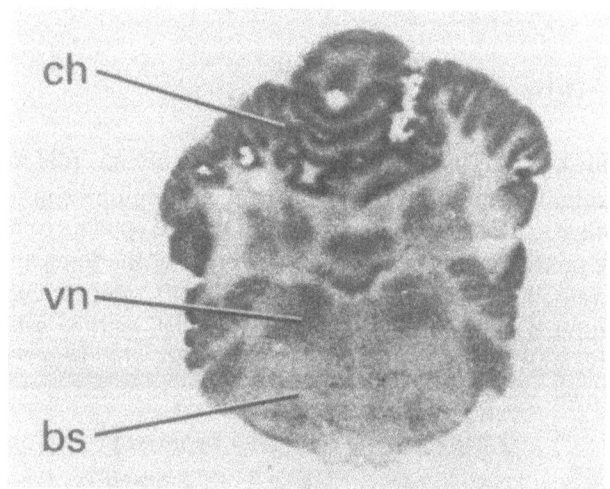

FIGURE 26.5. Representative ^{124}C-deoxyglucose autoradiograms of coronal brain sections from a newborn dog. Darker areas denote regions with higher cerebral glucose utilization. Note the high rates of glucose consumption in selected brain stem structures relative to the cerebral hemispheres. ch, cerebellar vermis; vn, vestibular nucleus; bs, brain stem; swm, subcortical white matter; pc, parietal cerebral cortex; hn, habenular nucleus; sn, subthalamic nucleus; cc, corpus callosum; cn, caudate nucleus. (From Duffy et al.,[51] with permission.)

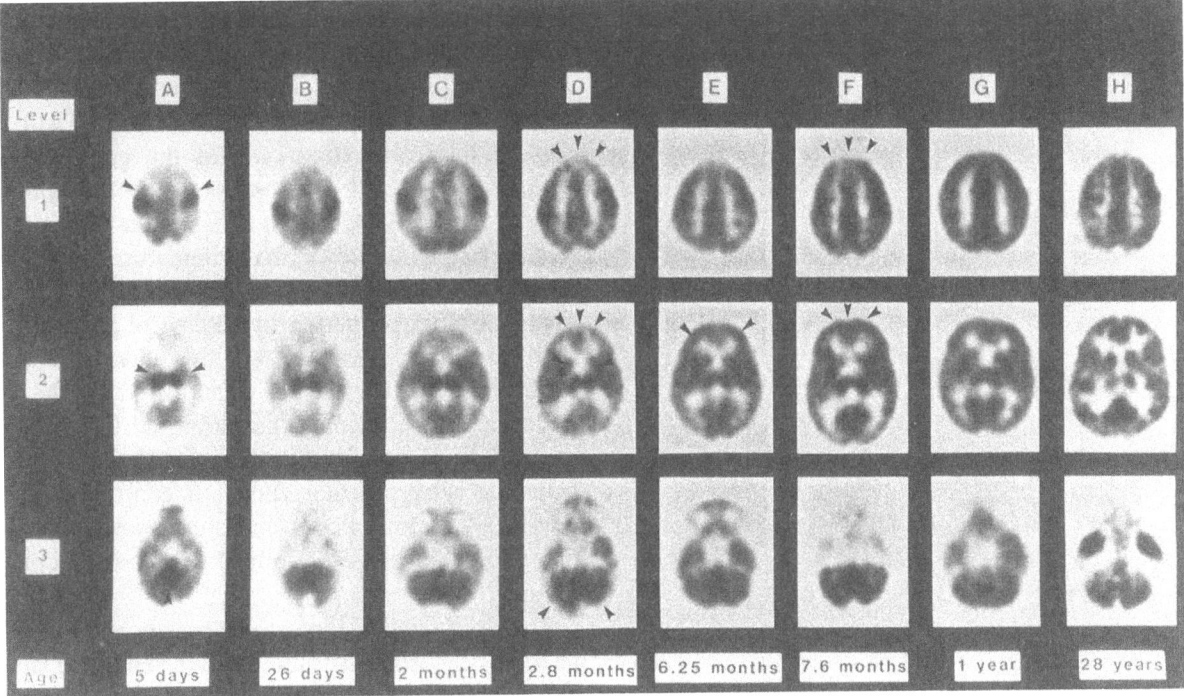

FIGURE 26.6. Representative [18]fluoro-2-deoxyglucose positron emission tomograms during human maturation. Shown are three horizontal levels of brain at ages ranging from 5 postnatal days through 1 year and adulthood. (From Chugani et al.,[54] with permission.)

the pioneering work of Fishman[66] and Crone,[67] it was clear that glucose transport from the blood into the brain occurs by a saturable, stereospecific form of facilitated diffusion which is energy-independent. Twenty years later the first glucose transporter protein was purified from human erythrocytes and provided a tool for the isolation of glucose transporter cDNA clones from both HepG2 cells and rat brain.[68,69] Presently, the mammalian facilitative glucose transporter proteins comprise a 7-gene, 6-protein family of highly homologous, integral membrane proteins, named GLUTs 1 to 7 for the order in which they were cloned.[70,71] All of these proteins are characterized by 12 membrane spanning regions with intracellular NH_2^- and $COOH^-$ termini, and a single site for glycosylation on the extracellular loop between M1 and M2. The amino acid sequences at the COOH terminus are the most divergent among the transporter isoforms and have facilitated the generation of antipeptide antisera as specific probes for the immunologic detection of the proteins.

Although there have been reports of variable levels of expression of all of the family members in brain, GLUTs 1 and 3 are the predominant cerebral glucose transporters[72] (Figure 26.7). GLUT 1, in addition to being a major membrane protein of human erythrocytes, is highly expressed in all blood-tissue barriers, including the BBB and the blood-cerebrospinal barrier, i.e., the choroid plexus. In preparations of isolated cerebral microvessels, i.e., BBB vessels, GLUT 1 is detected as a variably glycosylated protein with an average molecular mass of 55 kd, whereas in vascular-free brain preparations as well as an isolated choroid plexus, GLUT 1 is detected as a less heavily glycosylated protein of 45 kd. The 45-kd GLUT 1 is the predominant transporter of glial cells as well. The function of the differential glycosylation is not known. GLUT 3 is the predominant glucose transporter isoform in neurons, both in vivo and in vitro.[72,73] Although the K_m of GLUT 3 is similar to that of GLUT 1, it is characterized by a higher rate of glucose transport,[74] making it the appropriate transporter isoform for the neural cell with the highest demand for glucose, specifically, the neuron. A third isoform, GLUT 5, has been detected in both ramified and activated microglia in human and rat brain.[75] GLUT 5, originally cloned from a human small intestine cDNA library,[76] normally functions as a fructose transporter and its role in microglia, resident macrophage of the brain, is unclear.

Both the developing and the adult brain display heterogeneous patterns of metabolism and rCGU, and this is also true of the distribution of the glucose transporters. The most reliable information regarding the cell- and region-specific detection of the glucose transporters derives from in situ hybridization analysis of brain sections (Figure 26.8), which can be combined with autoradio-

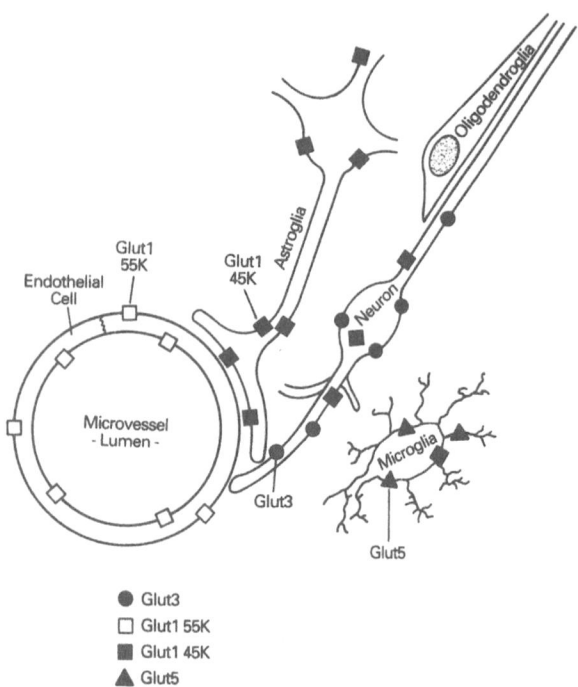

FIGURE 26.7. Schematic representation of the cellular localization of glucose transporter isoforms in the brain. (From Maher et al.[72])

graphic 2-DG analysis. GLUT 1 messenger RNA (mRNA) is routinely detected at high concentrations in cerebral microvessels, choroid plexus, and the ependymal lining of the ventricles. In addition, GLUT 1 mRNA in the mature brain is detected primarily in small nonneuronal cells. GLUT 3 mRNA is detected exclusively in neurons. The regional patterns usually coincide with autoradiographic detection of 2-DG uptake. GLUT 5 is expressed only at very low concentrations in the normal mature brain but is substantially increased in response to injury, such as hypoxia-ischemia, consistent with the microglial response to brain injury.

Although Figure 26.8 depicts the pattern of distribution of the glucose transporters in the mature rat brain, the situation during embryonic and early postnatal life is quite different. GLUT 1 is the predominant glucose transporter isoform of the embryo and is widely expressed in proliferating cells of the germinal neuroepithelium.[77] GLUT 1 is expressed by the endothelial cells of the BBB. Although it has often been suggested that the barrier is "leaky" in the immature brain, it is now fairly well accepted that rat brain endothelial cells start to express barrier properties by 16 days of gestation, while they are still proliferating,[78] and that endothelial cell fenestrations have completely disappeared by the end of gestation.[79] By the end of gestation, GLUT 3 mRNA is expressed in postmitotic neurons, as they migrate away from the subventricular zone.[77] It continues to be expressed by postmitotic neurons during postnatal development to achieve the pattern of expression depicted in Figure 26.8.

The expression of the glucose transporter proteins appears to be closely associated with the energetic demands of the brain, and this relationship is clearly seen in the developing brain. As discussed above, in the newborn rat cerebral glucose uptake and utilization are about 20% of adult rates but increase rapidly to attain adult levels by 21 to 30 days of age. Measurements of GLUT 1 and GLUT 3 proteins in the immature brain during this period reflect these developmental changes[80] (Figure 26.9). Immunoblot analysis of isolated cerebral cortical microvessels as well as total cortical membranes prepared from rats between 1 and 30 days of postnatal age, compared with samples from adult brain, demonstrate that all of the GLUT proteins are at low concentrations during the first postnatal week. These concentrations are in keeping with measured low rates of cerebral glucose utilization. Microvascular GLUT 1 remains somewhat low during the early postnatal period but increases during the next 2 weeks, coincident with increases in BBB glucose uptake. Immunogold electron microscopic analy-

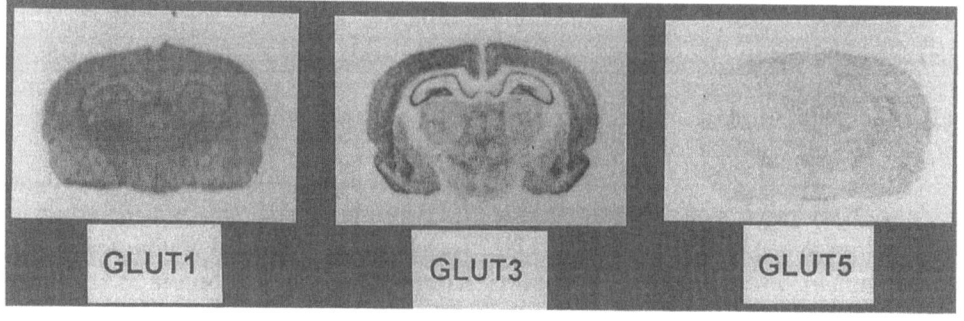

FIGURE 26.8. GLUT 1, 3, and 5 gene expression in 21-day-old rat brain. Autoradiographs of adjacent coronal brain sections following in situ hybridization with [^{35}S]cRNA probes to GLUT 1, mouse GLUT 3, and rat GLUT 5, according to the methodology of Bondy et al.[77]

Alternate Substrates for Cerebral Metabolism

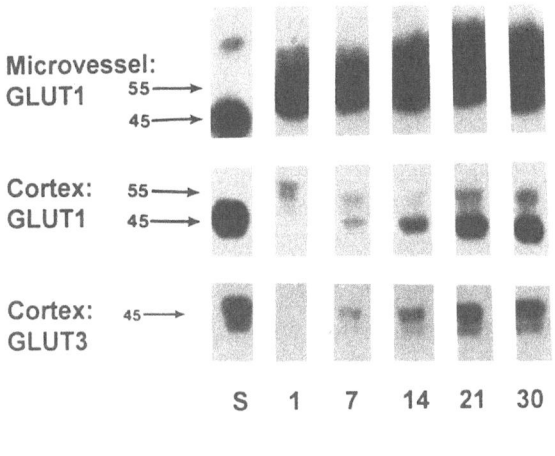

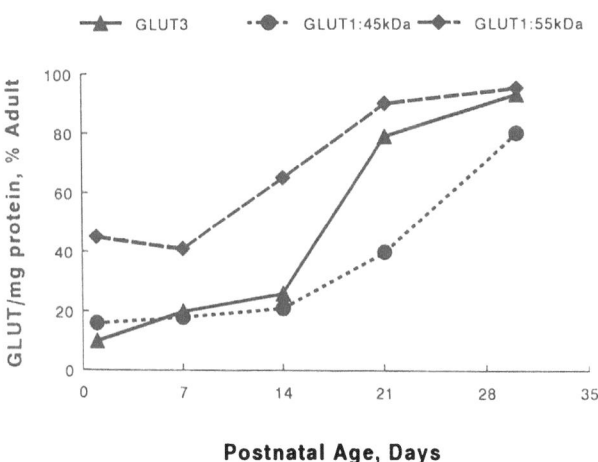

FIGURE 26.9. Developmental expression of GLUT 1 and GLUT 3 proteins in rat brain. Representative Western blot analyses (top panel) of isolated microvessels and total cortical membranes prepared from postnatal rats at 1, 7, 14, 21, and 30 days of age for GLUT 1 and GLUT 3 content, relative to S, a microsomal membrane brain "standard." Densitometric quantitation of five samples at each age, expressed as a percent of the adult value (lower panel) for 55-kd GLUT 1 (microvessel), 45-kd GLUT 1, and GLUT 3 (neuronal/glial membranes). (Derived from data of Vannucci.[80])

sis reveals a similar pattern of BBB GLUT 1 expression in developing rabbit brain.[81] Increases in 45-kd GLUT 1 is more gradual during this period and most probably reflects overall brain growth and increasing reliance on glucose as a fuel during this period. GLUT 3, the neuronal glucose transporter, demonstrates the most marked increase during the second and third postnatal weeks in the rat, which is commensurate with the period of rapid neuronal maturation and synaptogenesis.

As discussed above, glucose is the predominant or exclusive cerebral energy fuel at all ages under physiologic conditions. However, situations occur in which glucose availability to brain is limited by hypoglycemia (i.e., reduced substrate) or by insufficient levels of glucose transporter proteins (i.e., reduced capacity). Under these and other circumstances, the perinatal brain is capable of incorporating and metabolizing substitute organic substrates, especially lactic acid and the ketone bodies, β-hydroxybutyrate, and acetoacetate (vide infra). The immature brain appears capable of consuming a large number of organic metabolites, including free fatty acids and amino acids, as long as these metabolites are available in reasonable concentrations in blood, and the appropriate enzymes for their degradation are present in brain.

The substitute fuels for metabolism in perinatal brain that have received the greatest attention have been the ketone bodies and lactic acid. The transport of these compounds across the BBB and into cells appears to be mediated by the same membrane transporter, the monocarboxylate transporter (MCT), which has now been cloned.[82] Ketone bodies are readily transported from blood to brain in proportion to their concentrations in the circulation.[83] Since all developing mammals are nourished with milk with a high-fat content, these immature animals readily generate ketone bodies in the liver, which appear in substantial concentrations in blood. During suckling, circulating concentrations of ketone bodies can exceed 1 mM and can partially substitute for glucose to sustain cerebral metabolism, accounting for up to 20% of total energy production.[83-86] At the time of weaning, the availability of circulating ketone bodies decreases and measured rates of cerebral glucose utilization increase in the postnatal rat brain with an increased reliance on glucose as the energy substrate.[87] Likewise in adults, nutrient fasting induces endogenous ketone body formation, which contributes significantly to overall cerebral metabolism during starvation-induced hypoglycemia.[88]

Hypoglycemia frequently is encountered in the immediate newborn period prior to the initiation of sustained oral or parenteral feeding. During this time, as well as during fetal life, ketone bodies exist in very low concentrations in blood and, contribute little to cerebral metabolism.[89-91] In contrast, lactic acid is elevated in late fetal and early postnatal life to the extent that its concentration can exceed that of glucose.[92-95] Studies in newborn dogs have shown that during hypoglycemia, lactic acid not only is incorporated into the perinatal brain but is consumed to the extent that the metabolite can support up to 60% of total cerebral oxidative metabolism.[58,96] The versatility of the immature brain to utilize substitute fuels, sparing glucose, contributes to the tolerance of the newborn central nervous system to the known deleterious effects of hypoglycemia.

Acknowledgments. Dr. S.J. Vannucci's research has been supported by grant HD-31521 from the National Institutes of Health. Dr. R.C. Vannucci's research has been supported by grants HD-09109, HD-15738, HD-19913, HD-30704, and HL-19190 from the National Institutes of Health.

References

1. Vannucci RC. Perinatal brain metabolism. In: Polin RA, Fox WW, eds. Fetal and neonatal physiology. Philadelphia: WB Saunders, 1992:1510–1518.
2. McIlwain H, Bachelard HS. Biochemistry and the central nervous system. Baltimore: Williams & Wilkins, 1971.
3. Siesjö BK. Brain energy metabolism. Chichester, England: Wiley, 1978.
4. Erecinska M, Silver I. ATP and brain function. J Cereb Blood Flow Metab 1989;9:2–19.
5. Cohen MM, Lim S. Acid soluble phosphates in the developing rat brain. J Neurochem 1962;9:345–352.
6. Mandel P, Edel-Harth S. Free nucleotides in the rat brain during postnatal development. J Neurochem 1966;13:591–595.
7. Thurston JH, McDougal DB. Effect of ischemia on metabolism of the brain of the newborn mouse. Am J Physiol 1969;216:348–352.
8. Young RSK, Osbakken MD, Briggs RW, et al. ^{31}P NMR study of cerebral metabolism during prolonged seizures in the neonatal dog. Ann Neurol 1985;18:14–20.
9. Vannucci RC, Duffy TE. The influence of birth on carbohydrate and energy metabolism in rat brain. Am J Physiol 1974;226:933–940.
10. Duffy TE, Vannucci RC. Perinatal brain metabolism: effects of anoxia and ischemia. In: Whisnaut JP, Sandok BA, eds. Cerebral vascular disease. New York: Grune and Stratton, 1975:231–235.
11. Gonya-Magee T, Vannucci RC. Ontogeny of cerebral oxidative metabolism in the chick embryo. J Neurochem 1982;38:1387–1392.
12. Leonard JC, Younkin DP, Chance B, et al. Nuclear magnetic resonance: an overview of its spectroscopic and imaging applications in pediatric patients. J Pediatr 1985;106:757–761.
13. Corbett RJT, Laptook AR, Garcia B, Ruley JI. Energy reserves and utilization rates in developing brain measured in vivo by ^{31}P and ^{1}H nuclear magnetic resonance spectroscopy. J Cereb Blood Flow Metab 1993;13:235–246.
14. Cady EB, Dawson MJ, Hope PL, et al. Non-invasive investigation of cerebral metabolism in newborn infants by phosphorus nuclear magnetic resonance spectroscopy. Lancet 1983;1:1059–1062.
15. Younkin DP, Delivoria-Papadolopoulos M, Leonard JC, et al. Unique aspects of human cerebral metabolism evaluated with phosphorus nuclear magnetic resonance spectroscopy. Ann Neurol 1984;16:581–586.
16. Hamilton PA, Cady EB, Wyatt JS, et al. Impaired energy metabolism in brains of newborn infants with increased cerebral echodensities. Lancet 1986;1:1242–1246.
17. Buchli R, Boesiger P, Rumpel H. Developmental changes of phosphorus metabolite concentrations in the human brain: a ^{31}P magnetic resonance spectroscopy study. Pediatr Res 1994;35:431–435.
18. Moorcraft J, Bolas NM, Ives NK, et al. Spatially localized magnetic resonance spectroscopy of the brains of normal and asphyxiated newborns. Pediatrics 1991;87:273–282.
19. Lowry OH, Passonneau JV, Hasselberger FX, Schulz DW. Effect of ischemia on known substrates and cofactors of the glycolytic pathway in brain. J Biol Chem 1964;239:18–30.
20. Lehrer GM, Bornstein MB, Weiss C, Silides DJ. Enzymatic maturation of mouse cerebral neocortex in vitro and in situ. Exp Neurol 1970;26:595–606.
21. Wilson JE. The relationship between glycolytic and mitochondrial enzymes in the developing rat brain. J Biol Chem 1972;239:223–227.
22. Kjellmer I, Karlsson K, Olsson T, Rosén KG. Cerebral reactions during intrauterine asphyxia in the sheep I. Circulation and oxygen consumption in the fetal brain. Pediatr Res 1974;8:50–57.
23. Rosenberg AA, Jones MD, Traystman RJ, et al. Response of cerebral blood flow to changes in PCO_2 in fetal, newborn and adult sheep. Am J Physiol 1982;242:H862–866.
24. Rosenberg A. Cerebral blood flow and O_2 metabolism after asphyxia in neonatal lambs. Pediatr Res 1986;20:778–782.
25. Rosenberg AA, Harris AP, Koehler RC, et al. Role of O_2-hemoglobin affinity in the regulation of cerebral blood flow in fetal sheep. Am J Physiol 1986;251:H56–H62.
26. Brennan RW, Patterson RH, Kessler J. Cerebral blood flow and metabolism during cardiopulmonary bypass: evidence of microembolic encephalopathy. Neurology 1971;21:665–672.
27. Hernandez MJ, Brennan RW, Vannucci RC, Bowman GS. Cerebral blood flow and oxygen consumption in the newborn dog. Am J Physiol 1978;234:R209–R215.
28. Grubb RL, Raichle ME, Phelps ME, Ratcheson RA. Effects of increased intracranial pressure on cerebral blood volume, blood flow and oxygen utilization in monkeys. J Neurosurg 1975;43:385–398.
29. Levitsky LL, Fisher DE, Paton JB, Delannoy CW. Fasting plasma levels of glucose, acetoacetate, D-β-hydroxybutyrate, glycerol and lactate in the baboon infant: correlation with cerebral uptake of substrates and oxygen. Pediatr Res 1977;11:298–302.
30. Kety SS, Schmidt CF. The nitrous oxide method for the quantitative determination of cerebral blood flow in man: theory, procedure and normal values. J Clin Invest 1948;27:476–483.
31. Garfunkel JM, Baird HW, Ziegler J. The relationship of oxygen consumption to cerebral functional activity. J Pediatr 1954;44:64–72.
32. Settergren G, Lindblad BS, Persson B. Cerebral blood flow and exchange of oxygen, glucose, ketone bodies, lactate,

pyruvate and amino acids in anesthetized children. Acta Pediatr Scand 1980;69:457–465.
33. Altman DI, Perlman JM, Volpe JJ, Powers WJ. Cerebral oxygen metabolism in newborns. Pediatrics 1993;93:99–104.
34. Astrup J, Sørensen PM, Sørensen HR. Inhibition of cerebral oxygen and glucose consumption in the dog by hypothermia, pentobarbital and lidocaine. Anesthesiology 1981;55:263–268.
35. Duffy TE, Kohle SJ, Vannucci RC. Carbohydrate and energy metabolism in perinatal rat brain: relation to survival in anoxia. J Neurochem 1975;24:271–276.
36. Swabb DF, Boer K. The presence of biologically labile compounds during ischemia and their relationship to the EEG in rat cerebral cortex and hypothalamus. J Neurochem 1972;19:2843–2853.
37. Vannucci RC, Plum F. Pathophysiology of perinatal cerebral hypoxia-ischemia. In: Gaul E, ed. Biology of brain dysfunction. New York: Plenum Press, 1975:1–45.
38. Gregson NS, Wiliams PL. A comparative study of brain and liver mitochondria from newborn and adult rats. J Neurochem 1969;16:617–626.
39. Dahl DR, Samson FE. Metabolism of rat brain mitochondria during postnatal development. Am J Physiol 1959;196:470–472.
40. Samson FE, Balfour WM, Jacobs RJ. Mitochondrial changes in developing rat brain. Am J Physiol 1960;199:693–696.
41. Milstein JM, White JG, Savaiman KF. Oxidative phosphorylation in mitochondria of developing rat brain. J Neurochem 1968;15:411–415.
42. Murphy MRV, Rappoport DA. Biochemistry of the developing rat brain. II. Neonatal mitochondria oxidations. Biochim Biophys Acta 1963;74:51–59.
43. Moore CL, Strasberg PM. Mitochondrial oxidative metabolism. In: Lajtha A, ed. Handbook of neurochemistry, vol. 3. New York: Plenum Press, 1970:53–85.
44. Holtzman D, Moore CL. Oxidative phosphorylation in immature rat mitochondria. Biol Neonate 1973;22:230–242.
45. Davison A, Dobbing J. The developing brain. In: Davison A, Dobbing J, eds. Applied neurochemistry. Oxford: Blackwell, 1968:253–286.
46. Gjedde A, de La Monte SM, Caronna JJ. Cerebral blood flow and oxygen consumption in rat, measured with microspheres of xenon. Acta Physiol Scand 1977;100:273–281.
47. Mayman CI, Tijerina ML. The effect of hypoglycemia on energy reserves of adult and newborn brain. In: Brierley JB, Meldrum BS, eds. Brain hypoxia. Philadelphia: Lippincott, 1971:242–249.
48. Himwich HE, Bernstein AO, Herrlich H, et al. Mechansims for the maintenance of life in the newborn during anoxia. Am J Physiol 1942;135:387–391.
49. Sokoloff L, Reivich M, Kennedy C, et al. The [^{14}C] deoxyglucose method for the measurement of local cerebral glucose utilization. Theory, procedure, and normal values in the conscious and anesthetized albino rat. J Neurochem 1977;28:897–916.
50. Kennedy C. Energy metabolism in the brain. In: Sinclair JC, Warshaw JB, Bloom RS, eds. Perinatal brain insult. Evansville, IN: Mead Johnson, 1981:30–42.
51. Duffy TE, Cavazzuti M, Cruz NF, Sokoloff L. Local cerebral glucose metabolism in newborn dogs: effects of hypoxia and halothane anesthesia. Ann Neurol 1982;11:233–246.
52. Mujsce DJ, Christensen MA, Vannucci RC. Regional cerebral blood flow and glucose utilization during hypoglycemia in newborn dogs. Am J Physiol 1989;256:H1659–H1666.
53. Chugani HT, Phelps ME. Maturational changes in cerebral function in infants determined by ^{18}FDG positron emission tomography. Science 1986;231:840–843.
54. Chugani HT, Phelps ME, Mazziotta JC. Positron emission tomography study of human brain functional development. Ann Neurol 1987;22:487–497.
55. Volpe JJ, Herscovitch P, Perlman JM, et al. Positron emission tomography in the asphyxiated newborn: parasagittal impairment of blood flow. Ann Neurol 1985;17:287–296.
56. Jones MD, Burd LI, Makowski EI, et al. Cerebral metabolism in sheep: a comparative study of the adult, the lamb, and the fetus. Am J Physiol 1975;229:235–239.
57. Gregoire NM, Gjedde A, Plum F, Duffy TE. Cerebral blood flow and cerebral metabolic rates for oxygen, glucose, and ketone bodies in newborn dogs. J Neurochem 1978;30:63–69.
58. Hernandez MJ, Vannucci RC, Salcedo A, Brennan RW. Cerebral blood flow and metabolism during hypoglycemia in newborn dogs. J Neurochem 1980;35:622–628.
59. Berger R, Gjedde A, Heck J, et al. Extension of the 2-deoxyglucose method to the fetus in utero: theory and normal values for the cerebral glucose consumption in fetal guinea pigs. J Neurochem 1994;63:271–279.
60. Kety SS. Circulation and metabolism of the human brain in health and disease. Am J Med 1950;8:205–210.
61. Alexander SC, Smith TC, Strobel G, et al. Cerebral carbohydrate metabolism of man during respiratory and metabolic alkalosis. J Appl Physiol 1968;24:66–71.
62. Sokoloff L. Localization of functional activity in the central nervous system by measurement of glucose utilization with radioactive deoxyglucose. J Cereb Blood Flow Metab 1981;1:7–36.
63. Abrams RM, Ito R, Frisinger JE, Patlak CS, et al. Local cerebral glucose utilization in fetal and neonatal sheep. Am J Physiol 1984;246:R608–R618.
64. Vannucci RC, Christensen MA, Stein DT. Regional cerebral glucose utilization in the immature rat: effect on hypoxia-ischemia. Pediatr Res 1989;26:208–214.
65. Kinnala A, Suhonen-Polvi H, Äärimaa T, et al. Cerebral metabolic rate for glucose during the first six months of life. An FDG positron emission tomography study. Arch Dis Child 1996;74:F153–F157.
66. Fishman RA. Carrier transport of glucose between blood and cerebrospinal fluid. Am J Physiol 1964;206(4):836–844.
67. Crone C. Facilitated transfer of glucose from blood into brain tissue. J Physiol 1965;181:103–113.

68. Mueckler M, Caruso C, Balwin SA, et al. Sequence and structure of a human glucose transporter. Science 1985; 299:941.
69. Birnbaum MJ, Haspel HC, Rosen OM. Cloning and characterization of a cDNA encoding the rat brain glucose transporter protein. Proc Natl Acad Sci USA 1986;83:5784–5788.
70. Bell GI, Burant CF, Takeda J, Gould GW. Structure and function of mammalian facilitative sugar transporter. J Biol Chem 1993;268:19161–19164.
71. Gould GW, Holman GD. The glucose transporter family; structure, function and tissue-specific expression. Biochem J 1993;295:329–341.
72. Maher F, Vannucci SJ, Simpson IA. Glucose transporter proteins in brain. FASEB J 1994;8:1003–1011.
73. Maher F, Simpson IA. The GLUT3 glucose transporter is the predominant isoform in primary cultured neurons: assessment by biosynthetic and photoaffinity labelling. Biochem J 1994;301:379–384.
74. Maher F, Davies-Hill, TM, Simpson, IA. Substrate specificity and kinetic parameters of GLUT3 in cerebellar granule neurons. Biochem J 1996;315:827–831.
75. Payne J, Mattiaci LA, Maher F, et al. Expression of GLUT5 on microglia in normal and AD brain. Soc Neurosci Abstr 1993;19:1042.
76. Burant CF, Takeda J, Brot-Laroche E, et al. Fructose transporter in human spermatozoa and small intestine in GLUT5. J Biol Chem 1992;267:14523–14526.
77. Bondy CA, Lee W-H, Zhou J. Ontogeny and cellular distribution of brain glucose gene expression. Mol Cell Neurosci 1992;3:305–314.
78. Robertson PL, Dubois M, Bowman PD, Goldstein GW. Angiogenesis in developing rat brain: an in vivo and in vitro study. Dev Brain Res 1985;23:219–223.
79. Yoshida Y, Yamada M, Wakabayashi K, Ikuta F. Endothelial fenestrae in the rat fetal cerebrum. Dev Brain Res 1988;44:211–219.
80. Vannucci SJ. Developmental expression of GLUT1 and GLUT3 glucose transporters in brain. J Neurochem 1994; 62:240–246.
81. Cornford EM, Hyman S, Pardridge WM. An electron microscope immunogold analysis of developmental upregulation of the blood-brain barrier GLUT1 glucose transporter. J Cereb Blood Flow Metab 1993;13:841–854.
82. Garcia CK, Goldstein JL, Pathak RK, et al. Molecular characterization of a membrane transporter for lactate, pyruvate and other monocarboxylates: implications for the Cori cycle. Cell 1994;76:865–873.
83. Hawkins RA, Williamson DH, Krebs HA. Ketone-body utilization by adult and suckling rat brain in vivo. Biochem J 1971;122:13–18.
84. Spitzer JJ, Weng JT. Removal and utilization of ketone bodies by the brain of newborn puppies. J Neurochem 1972;19:2169–2173.
85. Cremer JE, Heath DF. The estimation of rates of utilization of glucose and ketone bodies in the brain of the suckling rat using compartmental analysis of isotopic data. Biochem J 1974;142:527–544.
86. Dombrowski GJ, Swiatek KR, Chao K-L. Lactate, 3-hydroxybutyrate, and glucose as substrates for the early postnatal rat brain. Neurochem Res 1989;14:667–675.
87. Nehlig A, Boyet S, Pereira De Vasconcelos, A. Autoradiographic measurement of local cerebral B-hydroxybutyrate uptake in the rat during postnatal development. Neuroscience 1991;40:871–878.
88. Owen OE, Morgan AP, Kemp KG, et al. Brain metabolism during fasting. J Clin Invest 1967;46:1585–1589.
89. Persson B, Gentz J, Lunnell NO. Diabetes in pregnancy. In: Scarpelli EM, Cosmi EV, eds. Reviews in perinatal medicine, vol. 2. New York: Raven Press, 1978:1–55.
90. Sann L, Ruitton A, Mathieu M, et al. Effect of intravenous L-alanine administration on plasma glucose, insulin and glucagon, blood pyruvate, lactate and beta-hydroxybutyrate concentrations in newborn infants. Acta Pediatr Scand 1978;67:297–302.
91. de Boissieu D, Rocchiccioli F, Kalach N, Bougneres PF. Ketone body turnover at term and in premature newborns in the first two weeks after birth. Biol Neonate 1995;67: 84–93.
92. Stemberg ZK, Hodr J. The relationship between the blood levels of glucose, lactic acid and pyruvic acid in the mother and in both umbilical vessels of the healthy fetus. Biol Neonate 1966;10:227–238.
93. Stanley CA, Anday EK, Baker L, et al. Metabolic fuel and hormone responses to fasting in newborn infants. Pediatrics 1979;64:613–619.
94. Goodwin LS, Hellmann J, Vannucci RC, Maisels MJ. Relationship between cerebrospinal fluid and blood lactate in low birthweight infants. Pediatr Res 1980;14:632A.
95. Nielsen J, Ytrebø LM, Borud O. Lactate and pyruvate concentrations in capillary blood from newborns. Acta Pediatr 1994;83:920–922.
96. Hellmann J, Vannucci RC, Nardis EE. Blood-brain barrier permeability to lactic acid in the newborn dog: lactate as a cerebral metabolic fuel. Pediatr Res 1982;16:40–44.

27
Cardiac Metabolism in the Fetus and Neonate

G. Wesley Vick, III and David J. Fisher

The heart requires a great deal of energy relative to other organs. The recurring nature of cardiac force development demands a reliable source of energy production. The extensive cardiac growth that takes place during the perinatal period places an additional burden on cardiac energy generation. In general, the energy for cardiac contraction and growth comes from metabolism of circulating substrates within the heart. This intracardiac energy metabolism provides the high-energy phosphate bonds that are required for the large amount of chemical, contractile, and mechanical work that is performed by the heart.[1] These are the same high-energy phosphate bonds that couple the processes that yield and require energy in virtually all living organisms.[2]

Cardiac contraction requires both a large amount and a high rate of adenosine triphosphate (ATP) production. The rapid production is necessary to ensure the constancy of the energy source, as there is only a limited capacity within the heart for energy storage relative to demand.[3,4] An additional unique requirement of the heart is a nearly constant ATP concentration, even though cardiac ATP utilization varies greatly in accordance with variations in somatic activity. As the total amount of ATP in a normal mammalian heart is adequate to sustain cardiac contraction for only a few dozen beats, the heart normally avoids an ATP deficit by matching ATP production with utilization. For these reasons, complex mechanisms have evolved in cardiac muscle that facilitate the constant generation of large quantities of ATP.

While the myocardium has a remarkable ability to metabolize and generate energy from a wide variety of circulating substrates, including but not limited to long-chain free fatty acids and carbohydrates, the patterns of substrate utilization are different in the fetus, neonate, and adult. As the type of energy substrate metabolized by the heart can have a significant effect on the capacity of the heart to withstand stresses such as hypoxia or ischemia, investigations of perinatal changes in myocardial metabolism are of central importance to our understanding of normal perinatal physiology as well as the nature and capacity of the cardiac stress response.[5-7]

This chapter describes the perinatal changes in myocardial metabolism. To fully understand the developmental changes, this chapter also provides a comparative discussion of myocardial metabolism in the mature normal adult, including the acquisition of metabolic substrates from the circulation, as well as the normal cardiac substrate metabolism and energy production that results in the generation of ATP and other high-energy phosphate compounds. A description of the processes that govern the use of ATP during normal and abnormal contraction is beyond the scope of this chapter. This information can be found in other sources that describe the transduction of the electrical signal into mechanical contraction.[8]

Substrate Acquisition in the Mature Heart

Substrate availability to the myocardium is determined mainly by the substrate concentration in the blood that perfuses the heart, by the processes that enable substrate entry into the myocardial cell, and by the processes that facilitate the utilization of intracellularly stored substrate. Substrate entry can occur by simple passive diffusion, by facilitated diffusion via a carrier molecule, or by active transport that requires ATP.

Glucose is insoluble in the lipid bilayer that surrounds each cell. Consequently, glucose must be transported across the lipid bilayer of the cell membrane. Glucose is thought to be transported across the cell membrane by a carrier molecule that serves to facilitate diffusion. The transport does not require energy, because glucose concentration in the extracellular fluid is substantially higher than it is intracellularly. The rate of transport is increased by insulin, by increases in cardiac work, and under conditions of tissue hypoxia.[9,10] Glucose transport is inhibited by fatty acid oxidation, and is the rate-limiting step for overall myocardial glucose oxidation at low work loads in the absence of hypoxia and insulin. When there is a high cardiac work load or when high blood insulin levels are present, transport does not limit cardiac glucose utilization.[11]

The main source of energy in the adult heart in the resting postabsorptive state is free fatty acids. These long-chain fatty acids are poorly soluble in water, and are transported in blood bound to albumin, which has several binding sites for fatty acids. Fatty acid uptake by the heart is dependent on the molar ratio of fatty acid to albumin in the circulation.[12] The physiologic range for this ratio is 0.15 to 4.0.[13] As the protein concentration of plasma normally changes relatively little, this ratio is effectively controlled by the fatty acid concentration of plasma, which can range from 0.1 to 2mM. Consequently, as long as albumin concentration is in the physiologic range, fatty acid uptake varies almost linearly with plasma fatty acid concentration and generally does not show saturation kinetics.[14] In contrast to glucose transport, which is sensitive to insulin and accelerated by hypoxia, transport of fatty acid into the cardiac cell seems to be primarily dependent on mass action.

Albumin-bound fatty acids are not directly transported into the myocardial cell. Rather, unbound fatty acids are transported. These free fatty acids, which are present in small quantities in plasma in equilibrium with the bound acids, absorb to the cell membrane and are then transferred to intracellular fatty acid–binding proteins.[15] The equilibrium-transport process is rapid, reversible, and does not require energy expenditure by the cardiomyocyte.

Substrate Catabolic Pathways Utilized in the Mature Heart

Similar to other tissue, there are specific and highly developed catabolic pathways in the myocardium that facilitate the controlled processing of each of the major metabolic substrates and result in the production of ATP. Flux through these pathways is regulated by modulation of substrate availability as outlined above, as well as through changes in activities of key regulatory enzymes.

The three major mechanisms of enzymatic regulation include the alteration of the absolute enzyme concentration, allosteric or noncovalently regulated control, and covalent modification of an enzyme through conversion between active and inactive forms.[16] A further degree of metabolic control is provided by compartmentalization of the different pathways within various internal domains of the cell.[17] The concentration of an enzyme can be altered by changing the rate of enzyme synthesis, the rate of enzyme degradation, or both. Many nutritional, hormonal, and genetic factors are known to affect the rate of enzyme synthesis and degradation. Enzyme molecules subject to allosteric control have at least two distinct binding sites. One of these sites is the region of the molecule that affects enzymatic catalysis, and is known as the catalytic site. The other site is termed the regulatory site. Regulatory molecules can bind to this site and alter the steric configuration of the enzyme in such a manner that its activity is altered. There are many different regulatory molecules, often of small molecular weight. Frequently, they are products of the metabolic pathway in which the enzyme participates and they serve to provide feedback regulation.[18] Covalent modification of enzymes is mediated by other enzymes that add or remove specific chemical groups. Phosphorylation and dephosphorylation are the best-known types of covalent modification, although adenylation, acetylation, and methylation are also used as methods of covalent enzymatic regulation.

Myocardial ATP synthesis can proceed to a limited extent in the absence of oxygen but typically takes place under aerobic conditions.[19] Oxidation of free fatty acids and carbohydrates is the primary mechanism for ATP generation in cardiac muscle. Under certain conditions, lactate, pyruvate, and amino acids can be utilized as an energy substrate. This chapter focuses on the oxidative metabolism of carbohydrates and free fatty acids.

Carbohydrate Metabolism in the Mature Heart

There are four important pathways for myocardial carbohydrate metabolism:[1] glycogen synthesis and degradation, glycolysis, pyruvate metabolism, and the citrate cycle. As the citrate cycle is the final common pathway for both carbohydrate and free fatty acid metabolism, it will be discussed after fat metabolism. Gluconeogenesis does not take place in cardiac muscle (see Chapter 6).

Once transported inside the cell, glucose is phosphorylated by the enzyme hexokinase to form glucose-6-phosphate (Figure 27.1), which cannot easily leave the cell. At high glucose transport rates caused by high cardiac work load, insulin, or hypoxia, the hexokinase reaction becomes the rate-limiting step in glucose metabolism. This reaction is inhibited by high concentrations of glucose-6-phosphate.[20,21] The glucose-6-phosphate that is generated by hexokinase from glucose can be utilized for storage of its potential energy by glycogen synthesis, or for ATP production in the citrate acid cycle after metabolism to pyruvate through glycolysis (Figure 27.1).

Glycogen Synthesis and Glycogenolysis

Glycogen is a large, insoluble carbohydrate polymer that enables the cardiac cell to store relatively large quantities of glucose without osmotic swelling. The cardiac glycogen content is the result of a balance between glycogen synthesis and glycogenolysis; both processes are under hormonal regulation.[22,23] Normal heart muscle contains a fairly constant quantity of glycogen.

Glycogen synthesis begins with the conversion of glucose-6-phosphate to glucose-1-phosphate by phosphoglucomutase. The glucose-1-phosphate is activated, which involves the removal of two terminal phosphate groups from uridine triphosphate, while the remainder of the molecule, uridine monophosphate, is joined to glucose-1-phosphate by a pyrophosphate bridge to form uridine diphosphate glucose. In the reaction catalyzed by glycogen synthetase, uridine diphosphate glucose is transferred to the 4-glucosyl linkage of the glycogen chain. This reaction is thought to be the rate-limiting step in glycogen synthesis and it is necessary for a preexisting glycogen molecule or "primer" to be present for it to proceed.

The glycogen synthetase enzyme is regulated by phosporylation at multiple sites. Several protein kinases phosphorylate glycogen synthetase, which decreases the activity of the enzyme.[24] Glycogen synthetase activity is stimulated by insulin and elevated free fatty acid concentrations. A branching enzyme inserts branching points on the molecule as glycogen is synthesized by transfer of a terminal oligosaccharide fragment of six or seven glucosyl residues from the end of the glycogen chain to the 6-hydroxyl group. Since glycogen synthesis requires high-energy phosphate in the form of uridine triphosphate (UTP), it cannot proceed when high-energy phosphate stores are depleted. This favors the availability of glucose for the generation of ATP when it is required, rather than for storage as glycogen.

Glycogen is broken down by the concerted action of two enzymes, phosphorylase and a specific debranching enzyme, amylo-1,6-glucosidase.[25] Phosphorylase removes glucosyl residues from the outermost chains of the glycogen molecule, thereby forming glucose-1-phosphate molecules during the process. This reaction is the rate-limiting step in glycogen degradation. Phosphorylase can only break down the linear portions of the glycogen molecule. Branches contain only about four residues, which are removed by the debranching enzyme. The glucose-1-phosphate molecules formed by glycogen degradation are then transformed to glucose-6-phosphate by phosphoglucomutase.

Phosphorylase exists in an active "a" form and an inactive "b" form. Phosphorylase is converted from the inactive to the active form in response to epinephrine, norepinephrine, and glucagon.[26,27] This activation does not occur directly. Rather, it occurs indirectly by a second

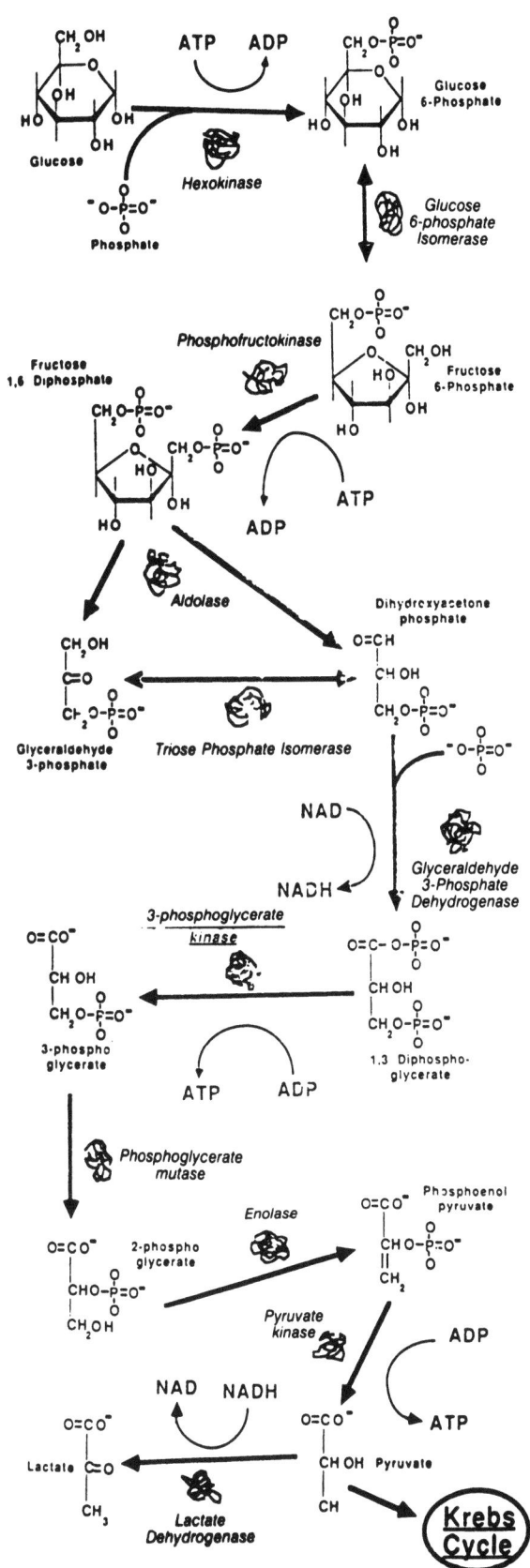

FIGURE 27.1. Glycolysis is the set of enzymatically catalyzed reactions through which glucose is converted into pyruvate with the production of a small amount of ATP.

messenger system mediated by adenosine 3′,5′-cyclic monophosphate (cAMP), which is produced by the enzyme adenylate cyclase. Adenylate cyclase is directly activated by epinephrine, norepinephrine, and glucagon. Thyroid hormone apparently accentuates the effect of epinephrine, norepinephrine, and glucagon by increasing the synthesis of adenylate cyclase. Phosphorylase activity is also stimulated by hypoxia. The mechanism of stimulation in this case is not conversion of phosphorylase b to phosphorylase a, but an increase in activity of phosphorylase b caused by decreased levels of ATP.

Glycolysis

Glycolysis is the primary mode of glucose metabolism (Figure 27.1). This series of reactions is the centerpiece of carbohydrate metabolism, because nearly all sugars can be converted to glucose and used for energy generation. When metabolism is oxidative, glycolysis produces pyruvate, which is further metabolized in the Krebs cycle (Figure 27.2) to provide a total yield of 38 mol of high-energy phosphate bonds per mole of glucose. Under anaerobic conditions, pyruvate cannot be utilized by the Krebs cycle. Although some energy can still be produced by anaerobic glycolysis, anaerobic carbohydrate metabolism produces only 2 mol of high-energy phosphate bonds per mole of glucose. In contrast, the oxidative metabolism of glucose through the glycolytic and Krebs pathways produces a great deal more energy for the myocardium than the anaerobic metabolism of glucose.

Glycolysis takes place in the cytosol. Under aerobic conditions, pyruvate is transferred into the mitochondria where it is metabolized through the Krebs cycle to produce ATP. Under anaerobic conditions, pyruvate is

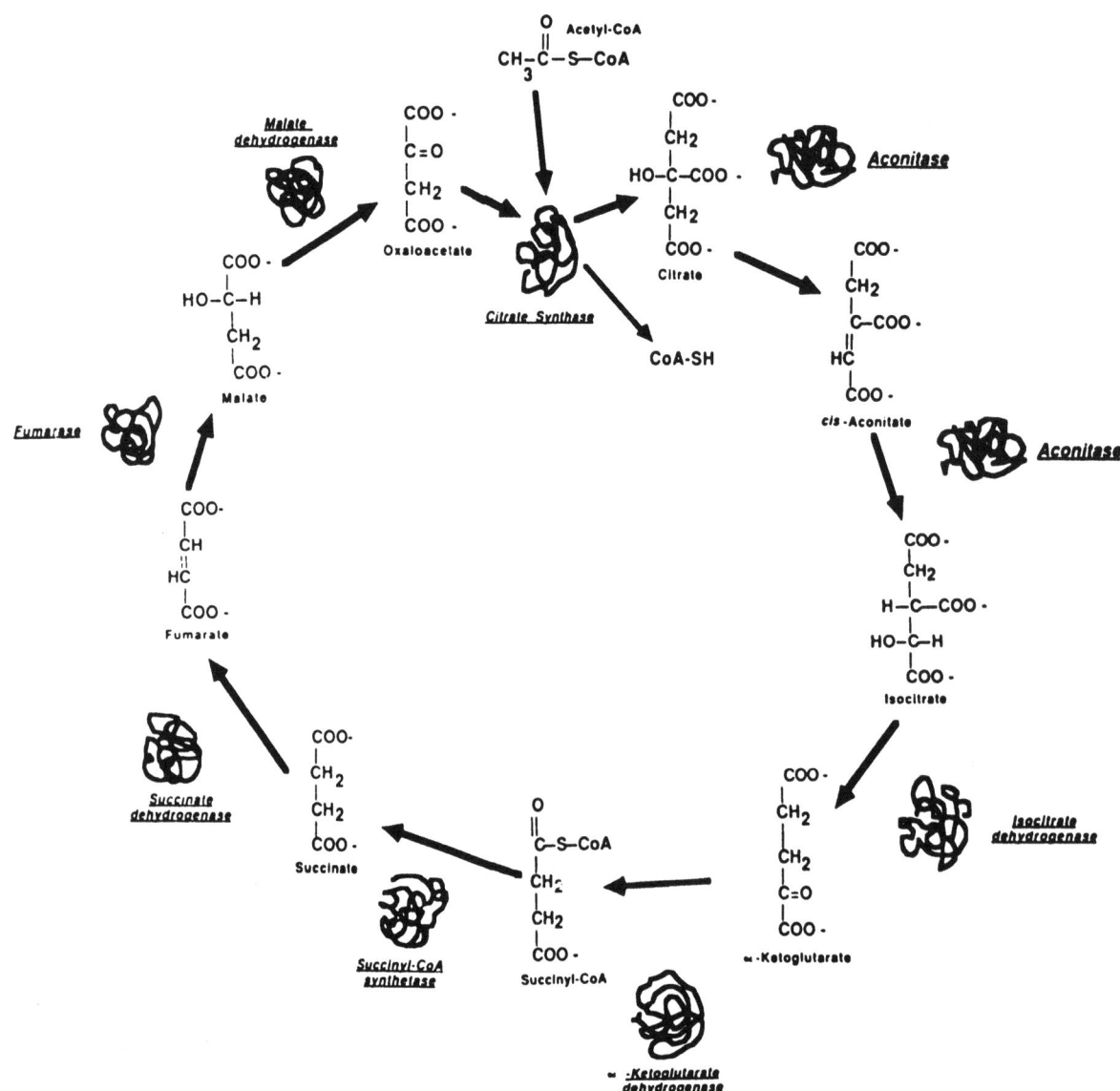

FIGURE 27.2. The citric acid or tricarboxylic acid cycle, also known as the Krebs cycle, is the final common pathway for the oxidative breakdown of carbohydrates, lipids, and protein. This cycle provides the majority of ATP required for cardiac work and growth.

reduced to lactate by the reduced form of nicotinamide adenine dinucleotide (NADH) in a reaction catalyzed by lactate dehydrogenase. This results in limited ATP generation. When there is tissue hypoxia but adequate blood flow, lactate is removed from the cell. When anaerobic conditions occur because of limited blood flow, the lactate remains in the cell. This results in a reduced pH as well as limited ATP generation.

When the supply of glucose is not limiting, and when lactate accumulation is not a problem, the rate of glycolysis is determined primarily by the flux through phosphofructokinase (Figure 27.1). Phosphofructokinase is a large allosterically regulated enzyme that phosphorylates fructose-6-phosphate, converting it to fructose 1,6-diphosphate.[28,29] Phosphofructokinase activity is stimulated by adenosine diphosphate (ADP), adenosine monophosphate (AMP), cAMP, and inorganic phosphate, and inhibited by ATP, citrate, and low pH. During mild ischemia, the rate of glycolysis is stimulated,[30,31] most likely through an increase in activity of phosphofructokinase, which is stimulated by a decrease in intracellular ATP and citrate concentrations and an increase in intracellular AMP, ADP, and inorganic phosphate.[32,33] Lactate production substantially increases when oxygen availability is limited during ischemia. This increase in lactate production is often called the Pasteur effect, because Pasteur had noted that lactate production in yeast was greatly increased during anaerobic conditions.

During severe ischemia, glycolysis is inhibited. One mechanism of this inhibition is thought to be an inhibition of phosphofructokinase by low pH. It is also thought that glyceraldehyde-3-phosphate dehydrogenase is inhibited by the increased lactate and reduced pH in severe ischemia. Glyceraldehyde-3-phosphate dehydrogenase converts glyceraldehyde-3-phosphate to 1,3-diphosphoglycerate, thereby reducing the oxidized form of NAD [NAD^+] to NADH.

Pyruvate Metabolism

Pyruvate can be metabolized in three different ways within the myocardium.[34] It may be reduced to lactate, converted into acetyl coenzyme A (acetyl-CoA) through oxidative decarboxylation by pyruvate dehydrogenase, or it may be converted anaerobically to alanine by transamination. Under normal anaerobic conditions, pyruvate is mainly converted into acetyl-CoA through oxidative decarboxylation by pyruvate dehydrogenase. In liver and kidney, pyruvate can be carboxylated to oxaloacetate by pyruvate carboxylase. There is no pyruvate carboxylase in skeletal or cardiac muscle.

Pyruvate dehydrogenase is a large enzyme complex located on the inner surface of the mitochondria.[35,36] As the pyruvate is generated by the glycolytic pathway in the cytoplasm, pyruvate must be transported into the mitochondria before it can be metabolized. When pyruvate is converted to acetyl-CoA by pyruvate dehydrogenase in the mitochondria, the acetyl-CoA is further metabolized in the Krebs cycle, thereby generating a large amount of ATP.

The pyruvate dehydrogenase step is an important control point of carbohydrate metabolism. Consequently, pyruvate dehydrogenase is a highly regulated enzyme, which can exist in either an active or an inactive form. The active form is converted to the inactive form by phosphorylation and may be restored to its former active status when it is dephosphorylated by pyruvate dehydrogenase kinase. This kinase is inhibited by ADP, NAD^+, CoA, and pyruvate, and activated by acetyl-CoA and NADH. Dephosphorylation of pyruvate dehydrogenase is catalyzed by pyruvate dehydrogenase phosphatase. Pyruvate dehydrogenase is regulated by end-product inhibition from acetyl-CoA and NADH. An increase in cardiac work activates pyruvate dehydrogenase by increasing levels of ADP, NAD^+, and CoA. The active pyruvate dehydrogenase is stimulated by the reduction in NADH levels that occur with increased work load.

In the mature mammalian heart, carbohydrate metabolism is inhibited by fatty acid oxidation mainly through inhibition of pyruvate dehydrogenase. When the adult myocardium receives adequate quantities of the preferred long-chain free fatty acids such as palmitate, the increased quantities of acetyl CoA, NADH, and ATP produced by fatty acid oxidation diminish pyruvate dehydrogenase phosphatase activity and increase pyruvate dehydrogenase kinase activity. Less pyruvate dehydrogenase is then in the active form, and carbohydrate-based oxidation is limited by reduced flux of pyruvate into the tricarboxylic cycle.

A small amount of pyruvate may be converted anaerobically to alanine in a transamination reaction catalyzed by alanine aminotransferase.[37,38] This reaction operates essentially at equilibrium in cardiac muscle. Its rate is dependent on the levels of NAD, NADH, glutamate, and α-ketoglutarate in the cytosol. The relative levels of these reactants are such that the reaction proceeds at a low rate, much below that of the corresponding reaction converting pyruvate to lactate. However, this shunting of pyruvate to alanine might serve to diminish lactate levels in ischemic tissues and thus lessen the inhibition of glycolysis by elevated lactate concentrations. For this reason, it has been suggested that glutamate supplementation of myocardial perfusate is beneficial during cardiopulmonary bypass.[39,40]

Lactate Metabolism

Under anaerobic conditions, the primary metabolic fate of pyruvate is conversion to lactate by lactate dehydrogenase.[41-43] The reaction is reversible, and the direction depends on the relative intracellular concentrations of pyruvate and lactate, and on the ratio of $NADH/NAD^+$ in the cell. Under anaerobic conditions the ratio of NADH to NAD$^+$ and the relative concentration of pyruvate increases, driving the reaction in the direction of lactate production. Under aerobic conditions, the concentration of pyruvate and the ratio of NADH to NAD$^+$ decreases, driving the reaction in the opposite direction. Thus, lactate can be converted to pyruvate and used to produce ATP in the appropriate setting.

Increased in myocardial lactate creation often is an indicator of the presence of anaerobic glycolysis. However, the heart produces lactate even during aerobic metabolism when the rate of glycolysis exceeds the rate of pyruvate oxidation. A more rapid rate of glycolysis than pyruvate oxidation can occur under catecholamine stimulation and in the absence of ischemia or anoxia.[44]

When the blood concentration of lactate is high, as is the case during and immediately after strenuous exercise, lactate is taken up by the myocardium and converted to pyruvate by pyruvate dehydrogenase. Under these circumstances, lactate can be a significant source of energy.

Control of Carbohydrate Metabolism

Cardiac carbohydrate metabolism responds in a coordinated manner to changes in cardiac work load, substrate availability, and hormonal status.[30,45] For instance, increased cardiac work leads to relatively decreased cellular ATP, NADH, and acetyl-CoA, which stimulate phosphofructokinase, pyruvate dehydrogenase, and glycogen phosphorylase activity. As a consequence, glycolysis is accelerated, flux into the citric acid cycle is increased, and glycogenolysis occurs. Increased cardiac work also accelerates glucose transfer across the cell membrane and provides additional substrate for the cardiac cell. These changes result in increased ATP production in support of the increased work load.

In the normal heart at basal conditions, fatty acids are preferentially used as energy substrates. The major determinant of glucose utilization in this situation is glucose transport, which is dependent on the amount of insulin bound to tissue receptors and on fatty acid availability. Glycogenolysis is inhibited since most glycogen phosphorylase is in the inactive form. This occurs when intracellular ATP and glucose-6-phosphate levels are adequate. High levels of ATP and citrate inhibit phosphofructokinase and increase levels of acetyl-CoA and NADH inhibit pyruvate dehydrogenase. Because of the inhibition of glycolysis, glucose is directed to glycogen synthesis.

Hypoxia increases glucose uptake, accelerates glycogen breakdown, and stimulates glycolysis. These changes occur because hexokinase, phosphorylase and phosphofructokinase activities increase secondary to increased levels of ADP, AMP, inorganic phosphate (Pi), and decreased ATP and glucose-6-phosphate. Although hypoxia causes a sustained increase in glycolytic flux, ischemia is associated with a transient elevation in glycolytic flux followed by inhibition of the process. This inhibition is thought to be secondary to inhibition of glyceraldehyde-3-phosphate dehydrogenase by high levels of NADH, lactate, and H$^+$ (i.e., reduced pH).

Lipid Metabolism

Free Fatty Acids

After intracellular uptake, long-chain fatty acids are converted to acyl-CoA by fatty acyl-CoA synthetase.[46–48] For long-chain fatty acids of nine carbons or greater, this reaction takes place in the cytoplasm and requires ATP, reduced CoA, and Mg^{2+}. The rate of the reaction is diminished by AMP and acyl-CoA, which increase during hypoxia. Short-chain fatty acids may be converted to their CoA derivatives inside the mitochondria.

Once acyl-CoA has been formed, it may be transported into the mitochondria or used to form triglyceride or other fatty acid esters. As the mitochondrial membrane is impermeable to CoA and its derivatives, transport of acyl-CoA into the mitochondria for ATP generation takes place by a specific transport mechanism.[49,50] The acyl-CoA derivatives initially are converted to acyl carnitine derivatives by carnitine acyltransferase I, an enzyme located on the inner side of the outer mitochondrial membrane.[51] A carrier protein then transports the acyl carnitine across the membrane and into the mitochondria, where the complex is converted back to acyl-CoA by carnitine acyltransferase II, an enzyme that is located on the inner portion of the mitochondrial membrane. Carnitine acyltransferase I is inhibited by malonyl-CoA, which is synthesized by acetyl-CoA carboxylase from acetyl-CoA. Elevated intracellular acetyl-CoA levels result in an increase in malonyl-CoA. The resulting inhibition of carnitine acyltransferase I reduces transport of acyl-CoA into the mitochondria. Conversely, depressed intracellular acetyl-CoA levels result in depressed malonyl-CoA levels and an increase in acyl-CoA transport into the mitochondria.[52]

Inside the mitochondria, acyl-CoA derivatives are converted to acetyl-CoA by a series of reactions known as β-oxidation. β-oxidation is a four-step cyclical process in which the fatty acyl chain is shortened by two carbons with each turn of the cycle. The first reaction of the cycle is oxidation of acyl-CoA. This is catalyzed by acyl-CoA dehydrogenase, in a reaction that forms enoyl-CoA and reduces FAD to FADH$_2$. The second reaction is the hydration of the enoyl-CoA, catalyzed by enoyl-CoA hydratase, a reaction that requires a molecule of water and results in the formation of hydroxyacyl-CoA. The third reaction in the cycle is the formation of ketoacyl-CoA from hydroxyacyl-CoA, which is catalyzed by hydroxyacyl-CoA dehydrogenase, NAD^+ is reduced to NADH by this reaction. The final reaction is thiolytic cleavage of ketoacyl-CoA by the enzyme thiolase. This reaction produces acetyl-CoA, which can then be further metabolized in the tricarboxylic acid cycle. Thiolase incorporates a new CoA into the remnant of the original acyl chain to create a new acyl-CoA whose chain length is two carbons shorter than the original acyl-CoA chain. The new acyl-CoA then becomes substrate for another cycle of the β-oxidation process.

The final step in β-oxidation of fatty acids with odd numbers of carbons is the creation of a three-carbon fatty acyl compound, propionyl-CoA, which is converted to the tricarboxylic acid cycle compound succinyl-CoA. Besides acetyl-CoA, β-oxidation produces NADH and the reduced form of flavin adenine dinucleotide ($FADH_2$), which are oxidized to produce ATP by the electron transport chain. The acetyl-CoA generated is metabolized in the Krebs cycle to produce additional ATP.

Other Lipid Substrates

In addition to fatty acids, the heart is able to use exogenous triglyceride as a substrate. Heart muscle contains lipoprotein lipase, which can hydrolyze the circulating triglycerides in circulating lipoproteins, principally chylomicrons and very low density lipoproteins, thereby releasing free fatty acids that can be taken up by heart muscle.[51,53]

The ketone bodies, acetoacetate and β-hydroxybutyric acid, may be oxidized by the heart to produce ATP under certain circumstances. Ketone bodies are not usually important sources of energy for the heart, but may be utilized substantially when their circulating concentrations are elevated during starvation or diabetic ketoacidosis.[7,54] Myocardial ketone body metabolism is most likely to occur when circulating long-chain free fatty acid concentration is low and ketone body concentration is elevated.

Control of Lipid Metabolism

The supply of fatty acid substrate is a major controlling factor in myocardial lipid metabolism. Another mechanism of regulation seems to be the limited supply of coenzyme A in the mitochondria. When ATP levels are high, there is a buildup in mitochondrial acetyl-CoA because of reduced flux through the citric acid cycle. Consequently, the level of free CoA decreases, making less available for β-oxidation. A third mechanism of regulation may be through hydroxyacyl-CoA dehydrogenase regulation by the $NADH/NAD^+$ ratio. High levels of ATP in the mitochondria are associated with a high $NADH/NAD^+$ ratio, which inhibits hydroxyacyl-CoA dehydrogenase. Low levels of ATP are generally associated with a low $NADH/NAD^+$ ratio, which increases the activity of this enzyme.

Cardiac usage of fatty acids as a substrate varies in response to external conditions and to the load placed on the heart.[55,56] When extracellular fatty acids are readily available at low levels of cardiac work, free fatty acid oxidation rate is limited by the rate of acetyl-CoA–dependent β-oxidation. Acetyl-CoA produced in excess is transferred to the cytosol and stored there as CoA and carnitine derivatives. Free CoA and carnitine are thereby used, reducing their concentrations and reducing the rate at which free fatty acids can be used as an energy substrate. When cardiac work increases, there is a concomitant increase in the rate of β-oxidation. Concentrations of long-chain acyl-CoA decrease and the concentrations of carnitine and free CoA increase. The rate of activation of free fatty acid increases and free fatty acid uptake increases.

When hypoxia is present, β-oxidation is inhibited by elevated levels of $FADH_2$ and NADH. Concentrations of long-chain acyl-CoA and acyl carnitine increase, which tends to inhibit β-oxidation. Furthermore, at high concentrations the fatty acyl-CoA and fatty acyl carnitine have nonspecific detergent effects, inhibiting many important enzymes, including sodium-potassium adenosine triphosphatase (ATPase).[57]

When lactate content is elevated, such as at peak exercise, fatty acid oxidation is reduced because carnitine acyl-CoA transferase I is inhibited.[58,59] Lactate then becomes an important energy source for the heart. Fatty acid oxidation inhibits glucose utilization, but in most circumstances extracellular glucose does not inhibit or stimulate fatty acid oxidation. The lack of effect of glucose on fatty acid oxidation is probably because fatty acid inhibition of phosphofructokinase and glucose transport prevents the buildup of lactate or pyruvate, which normally inhibits fatty acid oxidation.

Amino Acid Metabolism

Under normal conditions, amino acids do not contribute substantially to energy production by the myocardium.[60] Instead, amino acids apparently serve an important role in providing Krebs cycle intermediates. Two transaminases, glutamic-oxaloacetic transaminase (GOT) and glutamic-pyruvic transaminase (GPT), are present in large quantities in myocardium and enable amino acids to be deaminated and enter the Krebs cycle either as oxaloacetic acid, α-ketoglutaric acid, or as acetyl coenzyme A.[61]

The Tricarboxylic Cycle

The tricarboxylic or citric acid cycle, also termed the Krebs cycle, is the final common pathway for oxidation of acetyl-CoA produced from pyruvate, β-oxidation of fatty acids, or from acetoacetate (Figure 27.2). This cycle is a set of reactions that results in oxidation of acetyl-CoA to carbon dioxide and water, producing the majority of the reducing equivalents for the respiratory chain. This is the major source of ATP production in the heart. In addition to its function in energy production, the citric acid cycle plays a major role in regulation of glycolysis. Citrate, one of the cycle intermediates, is an important inhibitor of phosphofructokinase, which is the rate-limiting enzyme in glycolysis.

Control of the activity of the citric acid cycle is essential for the adaptation of the heart to varying work loads.[62,63] The citric acid cycle enzymes, citrate synthase, isocitrate dehydrogenase, and α-ketoglutarate dehydrogenase, are the primary sites of regulation of the citric acid cycle activity. The regulating factors fall into two major classes. One class of regulatory substances are the carbon substrates and intermediates of the cycle. The second class of regulatory substances is the adenine nucleotides that serve as end products and coenzymes. The cycle intermediates must be present in adequate concentrations for the reactions of the cycle to proceed. If flux through the citric acid cycle begins to increase and the availability of cycle intermediates becomes rate-limiting, amino acids can be converted into cycle intermediates by transamination, as described earlier.

The activity of the citric acid cycle is ultimately regulated by the availability of ADP. When energy consumption in the cardiac cell increases, ATP is broken down to ADP and inorganic phosphate. The resultant increase in ADP augments the rate of those reactions that use ADP to generate ATP, the principal one being oxidative phosphorylation. Thus, the production of ATP increases until it equals the rate of ATP consumption. On the other hand, when energy consumption in the cardiac cell decreases, the ADP and inorganic phosphate (Pi) concentrations tend to decrease. As a consequence, the formation of ATP from oxidative phosphorylation decreases because of lack of phosphate-acceptor, Pi. The rate of ATP formation is inversely proportional to ATP concentration and directly proportional to ADP concentration.

The rate of oxidation of NADH and $FADH_2$ by the respiratory chain is diminished if the relative concentration of ADP falls. As NADH and $FADH_2$ accumulate, the concentration of NAD^+ and FAD drops, causing a diminished rate of oxidation of acetyl-CoA by the citric acid cycle due to lack of these oxidized cofactors.

Oxidative Phosphorylation and the Electron Transport Chain

The breakdown of carbohydrate, fat, and protein produces reducing equivalents in the form of mobile hydrogens. These ultimately combine with oxygen to form water, releasing a great deal of energy, just as burning hydrogen in air releases energy. Part of this energy is lost as heat, but much of it is conserved through the coupled production of ATP, which takes place in the mitochondria. Normally, the coupling between oxidation and phosphorylation is so close that one does not occur without the other. Hence, the process is known as oxidative phosphorylation to distinguish it from other types of phosphorylation not coupled to oxidation. The major portion of the metabolic energy derived from catabolism of energy substrates comes from oxidative phosphorylation, which is the major power source for cardiac contraction, growth, and cellular maintenance.[64-67] For example, in each tricarboxylic acid cycle revolution, there are four steps that result in dehydrogenation. Three of these steps produce an oxidized substrate and NADH and one produces oxidized substrate plus $FADH_2$. These reduced cofactors each donate a pair of electrons to a set of electron carriers known collectively as the electron transport chain. The electrons are passed down this chain from one member to the next, and ultimately combine with oxygen and protons to form water. The electron carrier molecules in the electron transport chain are embedded in the inner membrane of the mitochondrion. With each step of the transfer, the electrons fall to a lower energy level, until they are finally transferred to oxygen molecules that have diffused into the mitochondrion. The energy that is released as the electrons fall to each successively lower energy state is used to pump protons from the inner mitochondrial compartment to the outside. An electrochemical proton gradient is created across the inner mitochondrial membrane. The backflow of protons down this gradient is used to drive a membrane-bound enzyme, ATP synthetase, that catalyzes the conversion of ADP + Pi to ATP, completing the process of oxidative phosphorylation.

One atom of molecular oxygen is reduced to water for each molecule of NADH or $FADH_2$ that is oxidized. The efficiency of oxidative phosphorylation can be expressed as the ratio of phosphorus to oxygen (P/O ratio), that is, the number of ATP molecules produced per oxygen molecule used. The maximum P/O ratios possible for NADH and $FADH_2$ oxidation are 3 and 2, respectively. These maximum P/O ratios are not achieved in practice, because there is some proton leakage across the mitochondrial membrane and because some of the energy derived from the proton gradient is used to transport ADP into or ATP out of the mitochondrion.[68] Thus, experimental measurements on isolated mitochondria indicate that two to three molecules of ATP are synthesized from ADP for each NADH oxidized to NAD^+. For each molecule of $FADH_2$ oxidized to FAD, between one and a half and two molecules of ATP are generated.

When intact, isolated mitochondria are placed in an environment containing oxygen and NADH but not ADP, reduction of NADH stops when the endogenous mitochondrial ADP is depleted. Addition of ADP quickly causes NADH oxidation to resume. Under normal circumstances, mitochondria oxidize NADH and $FADH_2$ only when ADP and Pi are present for ATP generation. This phenomenon is known as respiratory control and is an important characteristic of cardiac metabolism. Cardiac cells oxidize only enough substrate to produce the ATP required for their metabolic activity. When metabolic activity of the heart increases, as it does with exercise or during pressure or volume overload, ADP is produced. The increased level of ADP causes an increased rate of substrate oxidation in the mitochondrion.

Respiratory control occurs because oxidation of NADH, $FADH_2$, and succinate are obligatorily coupled to proton transport across the inner mitochondrial membrane. If the resulting electrochemical gradient created by the proton transport is not reduced by using the protons for ATP synthesis, the gradient increases to very high levels. Eventually, oxidation of NADH stops because the energy requirements to continue increasing the proton gradient become excessive. Uncouplers of oxidative phosphorylation such as 2,4-dinitrophenol act as membrane transporters for H^+, and in the process dissociate ATP production from H^+ movement.

Phosphocreatine and Its Role as an ATP Buffer and in Energy Transport

There is a relatively high concentration of phosphocreatine in the heart, which is approximately twice the concentration of ATP. Phosphocreatine is believed to play an important role in transport of ATP from the mitochondria to the sites of ATP utilization in the myocardial cell.[69] Phosphocreatine acts as an additional reservoir for high-energy phosphate bonds, in that phosphocreatine reacts with ADP to form creatine and ATP (i.e., phosphocreatine + ADP + H^+ ↔ ATP + creatine). This reaction is catalyzed by the enzyme creatine kinase, which is widely distributed in the myocardial cell, within both the mitochondria and the cytosol. It is thought that ATP is converted to phosphocreatine in the mitochondrial inner membrane.[70] Phosphocreatine diffuses into the cytosol and combines with ADP to regenerate ATP and creatine near the sarcoplasmic reticulum and contractile proteins, which require a great deal of energy in the form of ATP.

Cellular Compartmentalization

Three anatomically distinct intracellular compartments play an important role in myocardial energy metabolism. These compartments are the cytosolic space, the outer mitochondrial compartment, and the inner mitochondrial compartment. Furthermore, functional subcompartments exist within these anatomic compartments when enzyme or substrate distribution is not uniform.[71]

The myocardial cell derives considerable advantage from internal compartmentalization, just as the organism as a whole derives advantage by having specialized organs to perform specific functions. Compartmentalization enhances the flexibility of control of pathways that share common intermediates, making possible an additional level of regulation. Compartmentalization can increase the efficiency of catalysis, since higher concentrations of enzymes and substrates are more feasible in a localized compartment than in the entire cell volume, and because diffusion time limitations are minimized by compartmentalization. Compartmentalization makes possible the creation of locally favorable ionic environments, and facilitates intracellular vectorial pumping, such as that employed in oxidative phosphorylation, which must, in principle, take place between two closed compartments separated by a membrane. Compartmentalization does complicate investigation, however, and its possible effects should always be considered in the design of metabolic experiments and interpretation of their results.

The cytoplasmic space is not accessible to many mitochondrial enzymes, cofactors, and substrates, and vice versa. An example is cytoplasmic NAD^+, which, even though it is of relatively low molecular weight, is unable to penetrate the mitochondrial membrane. Other molecules such as sucrose can penetrate the outer but not the inner mitochondrial membrane. The inner mitochondrial membrane is selectively permeable, controlling the entry of important metabolic substrates into the mitochondria. Several carrier systems and membrane-bound translocases make this possible. There are translocases for adenine nucleotides, phosphate, calcium, and carnitine, as well as many other substances.

Thus, multiple mechanisms exist for the transport of substrates between different intracellular compartments. The malate-aspartate shuttle is a good example of a metabolic pathway made necessary by compartmentalization.[72] Substantial quantities of NADH may be produced in the cytoplasm by the glyceraldehyde-3-phosphate dehydrogenase step in glycolysis and may be created when lactate taken up from the circulation is converted to pyruvate before oxidation. If this NADH is not transported into the mitochondria, it inhibits glycolysis by decreasing the activity of glyceraldehyde-3-phosphate dehydrogenase and by decreasing lactate uptake. This transport is mediated through a shuttle mechanism. Oxaloacetate is converted to malate in the cytosol by the enzyme malate dehydrogenase and NADH is converted back to NAD^+ in the process. Malate is transported into the mitochondria in exchange for α-ketoglutarate and is converted back to oxaloacetate, with the generation of intramitochondrial NADH, by mitochondrial malate dehydrogenase. In this manner, the NADH is effectively transferred into the mitochondria. The newly formed mitochondrial oxaloacetate is converted to aspartate and α-ketoglutarate, which are transported out of the mitochondria in exchange for malate and glutamate, respectively. In the cytosol, the newly transported aspartate and α-ketoglutarate are converted to oxaloacetate and glutamate by glutamate-oxaloacetate transaminase. The oxaloacetate can then be used as substrate for malate dehydrogenase, and the glutamate is available for transport back into the mitochondria. The malate-aspartate shuttle is the primary route of disposal of cytosolic NADH in the cardiac cell. Inhibition of this shuttle is followed by intracellular cardiac acidosis and contractile failure. The glycerophosphate shuttle, another shuttle mechanism for transport of cytoplasmic NADH to the mitochondria, has substantial functional importance in brain and skeletal muscle, but not in cardiac muscle.

Regulation of Protein Synthesis and Degradation

Although amino acids do not contribution significantly to energy production in the heart, they are the essential building blocks for the wide variety of intracellular proteins of the heart. Intracellular concentrations of amino acids are determined by several regulated factors, including the rate of entry from extracellular fluid, the rate of exit from the cell, the rate of intracellular amino acid and protein formation, and the rate of intracellular amino acid and protein degradation. As several factors are operative, it is possible for the intracellular concentration of amino acid to fall while the rate of protein synthesis increases. Under normal conditions, the intracellular amino acid supply is not thought to limit protein biosynthesis.

Amino acids enter cardiac cells from the extracellular fluid. There are several transport systems with differing specificities that enable amino acids to enter the cytoplasm. Unfortunately, few studies on amino acid transport have been performed in the cardiac cell, and most of our experimental information comes from studies on other cells, such as Ehrlich ascites tumor cells.[73,74] These studies have demonstrated an A (alanine-preferring) carrier system that facilitates the uptake of amino acids with uncharged, short side chains. This carrier system transports the amino acids into the cell with coupling to Na^+. The high concentration gradient of Na^+ between the extracellular and intracellular space drives the reaction. Of course, the Na^+ must be exported by the Na^+-K^+ pump, and the overall process is an active, or energy-requiring transport mechanism. A second transport system, the L (leucine-preferring) system, preferentially transports aromatic amino acids with large or branched side chains. This transport system is mediated by a permease that is a cell membrane component, and is independent of Na^+. It is a passive system and cannot concentrate amino acids within the cell. Other transport systems for amino acids include a lysine system for transport of the basic amino acids lysine, arginine, and histidine; a transport system for amino acids having a net negative charge, primarily aspartate and glutamate; an iminoglycine system that transports glycine, sarcosine, and proline; and a β-amino transport system for taurine and β-alanine. The β-amino transport system is active in the cardiac cell and where it creates a relatively high taurine concentration.

Cardiac proteins undergo relatively rapid synthesis and degradation, even in the steady state. The average half-time for turnover is 4 to 6 days.[75] Thus, cardiac protein synthesis and degradation is a dynamic process that is ready to respond to external stimuli such as hypoxia, pressure or volume overload, or hormonal and other factors regulating normal and abnormal cardiac growth. Several factors regulate protein synthesis in myocardial cells, including the rate of formation of amino acyl transfer RNA, the availability of genes for transcription, the rate of formation of messenger RNA (mRNA) from genes, the rate at which newly formed mRNA is presented to ribosomes, the rate at which new peptide chains are initiated, and the polymerizing activity of the ribosomes.

There is no evidence suggesting that selective duplication of genes coding for important cardiac proteins occurs during the differentiation of myocardial cells. However, allelic copies of cardiac protein genes are present in the chromosome pairs within cardiac cell nuclei. Many of these genes have been duplicated and are present in multiple copies on the same chromosome. In addition, there is a high incidence of polyploidy (i.e., multiple copies of the chromosomal complement) within the nuclei of mature cardiac cells. Finally, many cardiac muscle cells have multiple separate nuclei. Thus, cardiac cells possess a greater gene-coding transcription potential than most other types of cells, although the functional significance of this observation is unknown.

Since the initiation of peptide chains in the cardiac cell is rapid enough to convert most ribosomal subunits into polysomes under normal circumstances, it follows that cardiac protein synthesis is limited by peptide-chain elongation. Peptide-chain elongation depends on the supply of guanosine triphosphate, ribosomes, amino acyl transfer RNA, and elongation factors. It is uncertain which of these substances is the primary limiting element.

A number of physiologic factors have been demonstrated to affect either protein synthesis or degradation,[76,77] including the relative supplies of carbohydrate and fatty acid, oxygen delivery, hormonal concentrations, availability of amino acids, and the rate of ventricular pressure development and wall stress. Since protein synthesis and degradation require energy, and because cardiac stores of triglyceride and glycogen are limited, the heart requires an external supply of oxidizable substrates. Glucose can support ATP production and cardiac contraction, but will not support linear rates of protein synthesis in the absence of fatty acids. Fatty acids and branched-chain amino acids, particularly leucine, stimulate protein synthesis. The cause is not certain but may be related in part to relatively increased ATP levels in hearts provided with fatty acids as opposed to those provided only with glucose.

Insulin has a substantial effect on myocardial protein balance because it accelerates protein synthesis while inhibiting protein degradation. The primary effect of insulin on protein synthesis appears to be enhancement of peptide-chain initiation which serves to increase the proportion of ribosomes that are in the polysomal form and actively synthesizing protein. Glucagon and catecholamines inhibit protein degradation. Glucocorticoids decrease protein degradation in the presence of insulin and increase protein degradation in the absence of insulin. Somatotropin generally stimulates protein biosynthesis by promoting peptide-chain initiation and ribosome production. Thyroid hormone selectively activates the biosynthesis of cardiac sodium-potassium ATPase and β-receptors. A high concentration of thyroid hormone stimulates the production of the V1 or α isozyme of cardiac myosin. Diabetes is associated with a reduced rate of cardiac protein synthesis and increased cardiac protein degradation.

Both protein synthesis and degradation are energy-requiring processes. Cardiac ischemia reduces myocardial energy stores and slows both protein synthesis and degradation, so that the net effect on myocardial protein balance is small.

Cardiac Metabolism During Development

As the organism develops from fetus to neonate to adult, many changes are occurring within and external to the heart. Many of these perinatal changes exert important effects on myocardial metabolism. External to the heart, the organism changes from a low to a high oxygen content environment. Internally, the heart undergoes many changes in the enzymatic and structural components of the cardiomyocyte. The heart increases in mass through increases in cell number and size during fetal development, and cell size continues to increase postnatally. The interior structure of the cardiac cell and its subcellular components continue to be modified during growth. Of particular note from the standpoint of cardiac metabolism is the increase in mitochondrial complexity and volume relative to cardiac cell size that occurs postnatally. In the embryonic rat heart, mitochondrial volume increases from 22% of cellular volume at day 6 to 34% at day 10. In addition, the cristae, which are the inner mitochondrial membranes where its metabolic enzymes reside, become longer and more densely packed. Similar structural changes occur in the rabbit, hamster, and dog.

Perinatal Arterial Hypoxemia and Oxygen Availability

Experiments with fetal lambs have demonstrated that oxygen consumption per gram of tissue is similar in unanesthetized fetuses and adults.[78] As the fetal lamb is naturally hypoxemic compared with the adult sheep, the fetus achieves this similar degree of oxygen consumption by a greater percentage extraction of oxygen and by a 60% greater resting myocardial blood flow. After birth, the left ventricular myocardial blood flow and oxygen consumption declines compared to the fetus and adult.[79] This information suggests that under normal conditions, myocardial oxygen consumption and metabolism are not limited by arterial oxygen tension or content.[80] Although these observations have not been repeated in fetuses and neonates of other species, the data are in agreement with studies of adults of several species where the in vivo circulating blood oxygen concentration does not appear to be a determinant or limiting factor regarding myocardial oxygen consumption or metabolism.

Perinatal Utilization of Long-Chain Free Fatty Acids

The adult heart can potentially utilize a wide variety of substrates including lipids, carbohydrates, and amino acids. Long-chain free fatty acids are the preferred energy substrate under normal conditions for the mature heart of the human and other species. As described earlier, the long-chain free fatty acids are activated, bound to carnitine at the mitochondrial membrane, transported into the mitochondria, and metabolized mainly by β-oxidation. Carbohydrates and amino acids can become the primary energy substrates for the mature heart when their circulating concentrations are increased or when the circulating free fatty acids concentrations are reduced.[81,82]

In contrast, long-chain free fatty acids do not appear to be an important energy substrate for the fetal mammalian heart. Studies have demonstrated that the cultured fetal mouse myocyte and isolated myocardial mitochondria from most species do not take up free fatty acids.[83-88] Although there are no data on the in vivo uptake of free fatty acids in unanesthetized fetuses, the available in vitro data indicate that much of the lack of utilization of free fatty acids by the fetal heart results from the delayed perinatal maturation of carnitine palmitoyl-CoA transferase.[83,85-88] This enzyme links activated long-chain free fatty acids with the carnitine carrier, a step that is required to transport the activated free fatty acids inside the inner mitochondrial membrane where they are metabolized by β-oxidation. Fetal rat and calf have an additional limitation of diminished content of the carnitine carrier as well as a delay in the maturation of palmitoyl-CoA synthetase, the enzyme that activates long-chain free fatty acids.[83,84]

There appears to be considerable interspecies variability regarding the timing of the postnatal initiation of myocardial free fatty acids utilization. The perfused neonatal pig heart is capable of extracting and metabolizing enough free fatty acids to supply more than 90% of its metabolic requirements,[89] whereas free fatty acids uptake is quite limited in the open chest puppy heart, rat heart homogenates, and in isolated calf, rat, and rabbit mitochondria.[83,84,86,90,91] A great deal of this interspecies variability has been related to the normal postnatal increase in the activity of mitochondrial palmitoyl-CoA transferase.[83,84,90,91] The neonatal rat heart maintains a relative postnatal deficiency in carnitine content longer than most other species.[89,90] Although there is considerable interspecies variability in the perinatal maturation of many of the enzymes and carriers that are required, the entire process of myocardial free fatty acid metabolism appears to be rather fully developed by the end of the first month after birth in the wide variety of species in which this has been studied.[83,84,91,92] Nonetheless, the timing of the perinatal onset of free fatty acid utilization in the human heart is not known.

It may be noteworthy that the concentration of free fatty acids in the fetal circulation is approximately 0.05 M, which is very low compared with the 0.5 M circulating free fatty acid concentration in the adult. The blood free fatty acid concentration increases rapidly after birth. It is possible that the postnatal increase in the enzymatic activities and carriers that are required for free fatty acids oxidation occurs as a function of the postnatal rise in circulating free fatty acids concentration. This hypothesis has not been tested, but it is particularly intriguing if one considers the relationship between the type of substrate and ventricular function.[5-7]

Perinatal Carbohydrate Utilization

Glycogen content of the fetal rat heart decreases by half from the 20th day of gestation to birth (term = 21 days). This trend continues postnatally, as the rat heart at 30 days after birth contains only 10% of the earlier embryonic glycogen content. Coincident with these changes in glycogen content are increases in the myocardial activities of cAMP, phosphorylase, and phosphorylase kinase. The changes in glycogen content and its regulatory enzymes are consistent with decreased reliance of the heart on glucose as an energy source as the perinatal period progresses toward the production of the mature heart.

As free fatty acid concentration is very low in utero, well below the myocardial threshold for fatty acid consumption in the mature heart,[93] it is not surprising that the fetal myocardium utilizes carbohydrates as the predominant alternate to free fatty acids. Activities of the glycolytic enzymes are increased in the hearts of fetal and neonatal guinea pigs and rabbits in comparison with adults of the same species,[94,95] and myocardial carbohydrate uptake rates are higher in the fetal lamb than in adult sheep.[80] However, not all of the fetal consumption of carbohydrates is accounted for by glucose. While glucose is utilized to a relatively greater extent in the fetus compared to the neonate and adult, total glucose uptake accounts for no more than one third of total energy utilization in unanesthetized fetal, neonatal, or adult sheep.[79] The concept that glucose is not the dominant fetal myocardial energy source has been validated from several sources of in vitro data in the monkey, the rat and the mouse.[87,96,97]

Under physiologic conditions, myocardial lactate uptake is sufficient to supply two thirds of the substrate required to meet basal myocardial energy demands in the fetal lamb.[80] In the lamb, the only species for which there is in vivo data, lactate appears to be the dominant fetal myocardial energy substrate. Postnatally, there is a large decrease in myocardial lactate uptake even though there in no change in circulating lactate concentration.[79] This decrease in myocardial lactate uptake is occurring during the period when the enzymes and carriers required for myocardial free fatty acid oxidation are maturing to adult concentrations and activities.

The primary myocardial energy substrate during the perinatal period probably depends on the species and its readiness to utilize long-chain free fatty acids. Prenatally and immediately postnatally, the primary myocardial energy source appears to be carbohydrates.[79,98] Although the myocardium of the older newborn is able to maintain adequate energy availability and function while utilizing glucose, lactate, or pyruvate, the limited available data indicate that long-chain free fatty acids assume a role as the primary myocardial energy source in most species within a few days or weeks after birth.[79,92,98] The in vivo studies have not been repeated in species other than the lamb, and their applicability to the human remains to be determined. However, these in vivo data are at least partially validated by in vitro data. The apparent nondominant role of glucose in fetal myocardial energy metabolism remains a bit of an enigma when considered in light of several reports of a relationship between low blood glucose concentration and cardiomyopathy in the human neonate.[99,100]

Acknowledgment. This work is supported by a grant from the American Heart Association (93-008150).

References

1. Randle PI. Carbohydrate and fatty acid metabolism. In: Berne RM, ed. Handbook of physiology, the cardiovascular system. Bethesda, MD: American Physiological Society, 1979:805–844.
2. Morgan HE, McKee DE. Protein metabolism of the heart. In: Berne RM, ed. Handbook of physiology, the cardiovascular system. Bethesda, MD: American Physiological Society, 1979:845–871.
3. Kammermeier H. Meaning of energetic parameters. Basic Res Cardiol 1993;88:380–384.
4. Jacobus WE. Respiratory control and the integration of heart high-energy phosphate metabolism by mitochondrial creatine kinase. Annu Rev Physiol 1985;47:707–725.
5. Neely JR. Relationship between carbohydrate and lipid metabolism and the energy balance of heart muscle. Annu Rev Physiol 1974:413–459.
6. Lopaschuk GD, Olley SR. Etomoxir, a carnitine palmitoyltransferase I inhibitor, protects hearts from fatty acid-induced ischemic injury independent of changes in long chain acylcarnitine. Circ Res 1988;63:1036–1043.
7. Opie LH. Metabolism of the heart in health and disease. Am Heart J 1968;76:685–698.
8. Taegtmeyer H. Myocardial metabolism. In: Willerson JT, ed. Cardiovascular medicine. New York: Churchill Livingstone, 1995:752–770.
9. Fisher RB. The mechanism of the uptake of sugar by the rat heart and the action of insulin on this mechanism. J Physiol (Lond) 1961;158:73–85.
10. Neely JR, Morgan RH. Effects of ventricular pressure development and palmitate on glucose transport. Am J Physiol 1969;216:804–811.
11. Neely JR, Mochizuki KM. Effects of mechanical activity and hormones on myocardial glucose and fatty acid utilization. Circ Res 1976;38:22–29.
12. Spector AA. Metabolism of free fatty acids. Prog Biochem Pharmacol 1971;6:130–176.
13. Spector AA. Fatty acid binding to plasma albumin. J Lipid Res 1975;16:165–179.
14. Schtacher GE. Uptake and distribution of fatty acids in rat diaphragm and heart muscles in vitro. Arch Biochem Biophys 1963;100:205–213.
15. Mishkin S, Gatmaitan L. The binding of fatty acids to cytoplasmic proteins; binding to Z protein in liver and other tissues of the rat. Biochem Biophys Res Commun 1972;47:997–1003.
16. Dixon M. In: Enzymes. 2nd ed. New York: Academic Press, 1964:301–333.
17. Blum JJ. Metabolic compartmentation. In: Schwartz LM, Azar MM, eds. Advanced cell biology. New York: Van Nostrand Reinhold, 1981:510–526.
18. Rognstad R. Rate-limiting steps in metabolic pathways. J Biol Chem 1979;254:1845–1878.
19. Neely JR, Morgan HE. Relationship between carbohydrate and lipid metabolism and energy balance of heart muscle. Annu Rev Physiol 1964;26:413–459.
20. England PJ. Effectors of rat heart hexokinases and control of rates of glucose phosphorylation in the perfused heart. Biochem J 1967;105:907–920.
21. Purich DL, Rudolph HJ. The hexokinases: kinetic, physical, and regulatory properties. Adv Enzymol 1973;39:250–326.
22. Roach PJ. Glycogen synthetase and glycogen synthase kinases. Curr Top Cell Regul 1981;20:45–105.
23. Krisman CR. A precursor of glycogen biosynthesis: alpha-1-4 glucanprotein. Eur J Biochem 1975;52:117–123.
24. Cohen PD, Krebs EG. Muscle glycogen synthetase. In: The enzymes orlando 1986;17(A):462–497.
25. Cornblath M, Parmeggiani PJ. Regulation of glycogenolysis in muscle. J Biol Chem 1963;238:1592–1597.
26. Carlson GM, Graves PJ. Chemical and regulatory properties of phosphorylase kinase and cyclic AMP-dependent protein kinase. Adv Enzymol 1979;50:41–115.
27. Morgan HE. Regulation of glycogenolysis in muscle. III: Control of muscle glycogen phosphorylase activity. J Biol Chem 1964;239:2440–2445.
28. Hofmann E. The significance of phosphofructokinase in regulation of carbohydrate metabolism. Rev Physiol Biochem Pharmacol 1976;75:2–68.
29. Uyeda K. Phosphofructokinase. Adv Enzymol 1979;48:194–244.
30. Kubler W. Regulation of glycolysis in the ischemic and anoxic myocardium. J Mol Cell Cardiol 1970;1:351–377.
31. Becker WM. Anaerobic production of ATP. In: Zubay G, ed. Biochemistry. Reading: Addison-Wesley, 1983:283–321.
32. Opie LH. Substrate and energy metabolism of the heart. In: Sperelakis N, ed. Physiology and pathophysiology of the heart. Boston: Martinus Nijhoff, 1984:301–336.
33. Garland PB, Newsholme PJ. Citrate as an intermediary in the inhibition of phosphofructokinase in rat heart muscle by fatty acids, ketone bodies, pyruvate, diabetes and starvation. Nature (Lond) 1963;200:169–170.
34. Denton RM. Regulation of pyruvate metabolism in mammalian tissues. Essays Biochem 1979;15:37–77.
35. Garland PB. Control of pyruvate dehydrogenase in the perfused rat heart by the intracellular concentration of acetyl coenzyme A. Biochem J 1964;90:6C–7C.

36. Cooper RH, Denton PJ. Regulation of heart muscle pyruvate dehydrogenase kinase. Biochem J 1974;143:625–641.
37. Taegtmeyer H. De novo alanine synthesis in isolated oxygen deprived rabbit myocardium. J Biol Chem 1977;252:5010–5018.
38. Garber AH, Kipnis IE. Alanine and glutamine synthesis and release from skeletal muscle. I: glyolysis and amino acid release. J Biol Chem 1976;251:826–835.
39. Bittl JA. Protection of ischemic rabbit myocardium by glutamic acid. Am J Physiol 1983;245:H406–H412.
40. Lazar HL. Reversal of ischemic damage with amino acid substrate enhancement during reperfusion. Surgery 1980;88:702–708.
41. Everse J. Lactate dehydrogenases: structure and function. Adv Enzymol 1973;37:61–134.
42. Opie LH. Effects of regional ischemia on metabolism of glucose and fatty acids. Circ Res 1975;36:52–74.
43. Taegtmeyer H. Myocardial metabolism. In: Phelps M, Schelbert HR, Mazziotta JM, eds. Positron emission tomography and autoradiography: principles and applications for the brain and heart. New York: Raven Press, 1986:149–195.
44. Opie LH. Lipid metabolism of the heart and great arteries in relation to ischaemic heart disease. Lancet 1973;1:192–195.
45. Vary TC, Neely DK. Control of energy metabolism of heart muscle. Annu Rev Physiol 1981;43:419–430.
46. Evans JR. Cellular transport of long chain fatty acids. Can J Biochem 1964;42:955–969.
47. Groot PHE, Hulsmann HR. Fatty acid activation: specificity, localization, and function. Adv Lipid Res 1976;14:75–126.
48. Londesborough JC. Fatty acyl CoA synthetases. In: Boyer PD, ed. The enzymes. New York: Academic Press, 1974:469–488.
49. Opie LH. Metabolism of the heart in health and disease. Am Heart J 1968;77:100–122.
50. Oram JF, Neely JI. Regulation of long-chain fatty acid activation in heart muscle. J Biol Chem 1975;250:73–78.
51. Murthy MS. Some differences in the properties of carnitine palmitoyltransferase activities of the mitochondrial outer and inner membranes. Biochem J 1987;248:727–733.
52. Saggerson ED. Carnitine acyltransferase activities in rat liver and heart measured with palmitoyl-CoA and octanoyl-CoA. Biochem J 1982;202:397–405.
53. Ehnholm C. Purification and characterization of lipoprotein lipase from pig myocardium. Biochem J 1975;149:649–655.
54. Ungar I. Studies on myocardial metabolism. IV: Myocardial metabolism in diabetes. Am J Med 1955;18:385–396.
55. Hansford RG. The steady-state concentrations of coenzyme A and coenzyme A thioester, citrate and isocitrate during tricarboxylate cycle oxidations in rabbit heart mitochondria. J Biol Chem 1975;250:8361–8375.
56. Neely JR, Oram MJ. Myocardial utilization of carbohydrates and lipids. Prog Cardiovasc Dis 1972;15:289–329.
57. Katz AM. Lipid-membrane interactions and the pathogenesis of ischemic damage in the myocardium. Circ Res 1981;48:1–16.
58. Bielefeld DR, Neely TC. Site of inhibition of fatty acid oxidation by lactate and oxfenicine in cardiac muscle. Fed Proc 1983;42:1258.
59. Carlsten A, Jagenburg B. Myocardial metabolism of glucose, lactic acid, amino and fatty acids in healthy human individuals at rest and at different work loads. Scand J Clin Invest 1961;13:418–427.
60. Drake AJ, Noble JR. Preferential uptake of lactate by the normal myocardium in dogs. Cardiovasc Res 1980;14:65–72.
61. Krebs HA. Some aspects of the regulation of the fuel supply in omnivorous animals. Adv Enzyme Regul 1972;10:397–420.
62. Williamson JR, Illingworth C. Coordination of citric acid cycle activity with electron transport flux. Circ Res 1976;38 (Suppl 1):39–48.
63. Smith CM. Inhibition of citrate synthase by succinyl-CoA and other metabolites. FEBS Lett 1971;11:35–38.
64. Becker WM. Aerobic production of ATP: electron transport. In: Zubay G, ed. Biochemistry. Reading: Addison-Wesley, 1983.
65. Brunori M. Cytochrome oxidase. Trends Biochem Sci 1982;7:295–299.
66. Thayer W. Synthesis of adenosine triphosphate by an artificially imposed electrochemical proton gradient in bovine heart submitochondrial particles. J Biol Chem 1975;250:5330–5335.
67. Energy conversion: the formation of ATP in chloroplasts, mitochondria, and bacteria. In: Darnell J, Lodish H, Baltimore DH, ed. Molecular cell biology. New York: Scientific American Books, 1986:583–616.
68. Hansford RG. Control of mitochondrial substrate oxidation. Curr Top Bioenerget 1980;10:217–278.
69. Lewandowski ED. The physiological chemistry of energy production in the heart. In: Schlant RC, Alexander RW, eds. The heart arteries & veins. New York: McGraw-Hill, 1994:154–164.
70. Jacobus WE. Creatine kinase of rat heart mitochondria. J Biol Chem 1973;248:4803–4810.
71. Schoolwerth AC. The role of microcompartmentation in regulation of glutamate metabolism by rat kidney mitochondria. J Biol Chem 1980;255:3403–3411.
72. Digerness SB. The malate-aspartate shuttle in heart mitochondria. J Mol Cell Cardiol 1979;8:779–785.
73. Christensen HN. A transport system serving for mono and diamino acids. Proc Natl Acad Sci USA 1964;51:337–344.
74. Christensen HN, Archer M. A distinct Na^+ requiring transport system for alanine, serine, cysteine, and similar amino acids. J Biol Chem 1965;240:3601–3608.
75. Zak R. Comparison of turnover of several myofibrillar proteins and critical evaluation of the double isotope method. J Biol Chem 1977;252:3340–3435.
76. Kira Y, Gordon PJ. Aortic perfusion pressure as a determinant of cardiac protein synthesis. Am J Physiol 1984;246:C247–C58.
77. Everett AW. Regulation of myosin synthesis by thyroid hormone: relative change in the a and b myosin heavy chain mRNA levels in rabbit heart. Biochemistry 1984:1596–1599.

78. Fisher DJ, Heyman MA, Rudolph AM. Regional myocardial blood flow and oxygen delivery in fetal, newborn, and adult sheep. Am J Physiol 1982;243:H729–H731.
79. Fisher DJ, Heyman MA, Rudolph AM. Myocardial consumption of oxygen and carbohydrates in newborn sheep. Pediatr Res 1981;15:843–846.
80. Fisher DJ, Heyman MA, Rudolph AM. Myocardial oxygen and carbohydrate consumption in fetal lambs in utero and in adult sheep. Am J Physiol 1980;238:H399–H405.
81. Shipp JC. Interrelationship between carbohydrate and free fatty acid metabolism of isolated perfused rat heart. Metabolism 1964;13:852–866.
82. Goodale WT. Myocardial carbohydrate metabolism in normal dogs, with effects of hyperglycemia and starvation. Circ Res 1953;1:509–517.
83. Warshaw JB. Cellular energy metabolism during fetal development. II. Fatty acid oxidation by the developing heart. J Cell Biol 1970;44:354–360.
84. Warshaw JB. Cellular energy metabolism during fetal development. IV. Fatty acid activation, acyl transfer and fatty acid oxidation during development of the chick and rat. J Cell Biol 1972;288:537–544.
85. Warshaw JB. Cellular energy metabolism during fetal development. III. Deficient acetyl-CoA synthetase, acetyl carnitine transferase and oxidation of acetate in the fetal bovine heart. Biochem Biophys Acta 1970;223:409–415.
86. Werner JC, Musselman V. Perinatal changes in mitochondrial respiration of the rabbit heart. Biol Neonate 1982;42:208–216.
87. Wildenthal K. Fetal maturation of cardiac metabolism. In: Comline RE, Dawes KW, eds. Fetal and neonatal physiology. Cambridge: Cambridge University Press, 1973:181–185.
88. Barrie SE. Myocardial enzyme activities in guinea pigs during development. Am J Physiol 1977;233:H707–H710.
89. Werner JC, Vary V. Fatty acid and glucose utilization in isolated, working newborn pig hearts. Am J Physiol 1983;245:E19–E23.
90. Wittels B. Lipid metabolism in the newborn heart. J Clin Invest 1965;44:1639–1646.
91. McMillin-Wood J. Carnitine palmityltransferase in neonatal and adult heart and liver mitochondria. J Biol Chem 1975;250:3062–3066.
92. Breuer E, Zlatas E. Developmental changes of myocardial metabolism. II. Myocardial metabolism of fatty acids in the early postnatal period in dogs. Biol Neonate 1968;12:54–65.
93. Zierler KL. Free fatty acids as substrates for heart and skeletal muscle. Circ Res 1976;38:459–463.
94. Wildenthal K. Studies of foetal mouse hearts in organ culture: metabolic requirements for prolonged function in vitro and the influence of cardiac maturation on substrate utilization. J Mol Cell Cardiol 1973;5:87–99.
95. Lopaschuk GD, Marsh MA. Glycolysis is predominant source of myocardial ATP production immediately after birth. Am J Physiol 1991;261:H1698–H1705.
96. Beatty CH, Dwyer MK. Glucose utilization of cardiac and skeletal muscle homogenates from fetal and adult rhesus monkeys. Pediatr Res 1972;6:813–821.
97. Clark CM Jr. Carbohydrate metabolism in the isolated fetal heart. Am J Physiol 1971;220:583–587.
98. Breuer E, Pappova E. Developmental changes of myocardial metabolism: I. Peculiarities of cardiac carbohydrate metabolism in the early postnatal period in dogs. Biol Neonate 1967;9:367–377.
99. Reid MM, Murdock BJ. Cardiomegaly in association with neonatal hypoglycemia. Acta Paediatr Scand 1971;60:295–298.
100. Emmanouilides GC. Neonatal cardiopulmonary distress without congenital heart disease. Curr Probl Pediatr 1979;9:1–39.

28
Lung Metabolism in the Fetus and Neonate

Luc J.I. Zimmermann and Lambert M.G. van Golde

Developmental studies on the metabolism of the perinatal lung have largely been focused on the pulmonary surfactant system, as the fetal lung must produce adequate amounts of this precious lipid-protein complex to ensure the ability of the neonate to initiate regular air breathing at birth. It has been well established for a number of mammalian species, including humans, that there is a spurt in surfactant production in the prenatal lung during the terminal period of gestation.[1-3] Starting with the first breath, this surface-active material has to spread over the alveolar surfaces to protect the alveoli against collapsing at low lung volumes. Pulmonary surfactant also precludes the occurrence of alveolar edema and it reduces the work required to breathe.[4-6] As discussed recently by Enhorning,[7] it might also be of vital importance for maintenance of small airway patency. In addition, there is increasing evidence that surfactant components are involved in several innate defense mechanisms of the lungs against infiltrating pathogens.[8-10]

As the major physiologic function of pulmonary surfactant is undoubtedly to confer mechanical stability to the alveoli, the alveolar gas-exchange processes in the neonate will be severely jeopardized if the surfactant system does not function at birth. This becomes manifest in respiratory distress syndrome (RDS) of the premature neonate, an important clinical condition that is essentially caused by a shortage of surfactant due to immaturity of the lungs.[11,12] The fact that exogenous surfactants are now widely and successfully used for prophylaxis and therapy of RDS supports this notion.[13,14]

In view of the above, this chapter focuses on the pulmonary surfactant system. A general overview of the intra- and extracellular metabolism of lung surfactant is followed by a section on the lipid components of surfactant and their functions. Subsequently, the structure of the surfactant proteins is discussed as well as the crucial roles of these proteins in controlling the dynamics, the metabolism, and the functioning of the overall surfactant system. The next section emphasizes the dramatic developmental changes that take place in the biogenesis of surfactant lipids and proteins as term approaches and the hormonal regulation of these processes. The review concludes with a brief discourse on the influence of surfactant metabolism in therapeutic interventions to prevent or to treat surfactant immaturity at birth.

The Life Cycle of Pulmonary Surfactant

Synthesis of Surfactant in Alveolar Type II Cells

Pulmonary surfactant consists of about 90% lipids. It also contains four unique proteins. According to the now widely accepted nomenclature proposed by Possmayer,[15] these surfactant-associated proteins (SP) are called SP-A, SP-B, SP-C, and SP-D. Figure 28.1 presents a schematic illustration of the overall metabolism and dynamics of the surfactant system. The surfactant lipids and proteins are synthesized at the endoplasmic reticulum of the alveolar epithelial type II cells. There is reasonable evidence from early autoradiography studies[16] as well as from recent immunoelectron microscopy studies[17-19] that the surfactant proteins SP-A, SP-B, and SP-C are routed from the Golgi complex to growing lamellar bodies via multivesicular bodies. The experiments of Chevalier and Collet[16] suggest that the surfactant lipids were not transferred to the lamellar bodies by multivesicular bodies but rather via direct vesicular transport. Although this is a likely scenario, it should be noted that this suggestion requires verification using techniques with a higher resolution power than that of autoradiography. Furthermore, it cannot be excluded that phospholipid transfer proteins are also involved in the transport of the surfactant lipids to lamellar bodies.[20] The mechanism by which the surfactant proteins and lipids are ultimately assembled into the lamellar bodies remains an enigma. This issue is further complicated by the fact that the molecular composition of the surfactant phospholipids, ending up in the lamellar bodies for intracellular storage, differs from that at the site of their synthesis, the endoplasmic reticulum.[21] For example, the lamellar body is enriched in dipalmitoylphosphatidylcholine (DPPC), the major lipid component of surfactant, which implies that there has to be a degree of selectivity, either in the selection of the various lipid molecules for routing to the lamellar bodies or in the assembly of surfactant lipids and proteins into these organelles.[20]

Secretion of Surfactant from Type II Cells

It is generally accepted that surfactant lipids are secreted by exocytosis together with lamellar bodies.[22–25] This view is endorsed by the fact that the lipid patterns of lamellar bodies and extracellular surfactant are strikingly similar.[3] Lamellar bodies from adult and neonatal lung are highly enriched in the hydrophobic proteins SP-B and SP-C.[26,27] They also contain small amounts of SP-A.[26–29] It is very likely that these proteins are co-secreted with the surfactant lipids. This concept has been corroborated by a recent in vivo study in newborn rabbits, which provided evidence for coordinated secretion of SP-B and DPPC of lamellar bodies into the alveolus.[30] However, there is increasing evidence that at least part of the SP-A is secreted by type II cells independently of the lamellar bodies.[31,32]

The secretion of surfactant lipids appears to be under tight regulatory control.[22–25] This process is stimulated in vivo by factors such as labor and ventilation. In addition, it is enhanced by agonists for β-adrenergic, purinergic, and vasopressin receptors. The stimulated secretion of surfactant lipids appears to be associated with a variety of signal-transduction systems involving adenosine 3′,5′-cyclic monophosphate (cAMP)-dependent protein kinase, protein kinase C and intracellular calcium mobilization.[22–25] Factors inhibiting surfactant secretion have been reported. For example, several groups have shown that SP-A effectively inhibits the secretion of surfactant phospholipids by isolated type II cells in culture.[33,34] It remains to be established whether this inhibitory mechanism operates in vivo.

Extracellular Surfactant Metabolism

Low-temperature scanning electron microscopy of rat lung has shown that the alveolar surfaces are lined with a continuous liquid layer with an average thickness of 0.24 μm, with a variation of 25 nm to some micrometers.[35] Upon secretion of the lamellar contents into this liquid layer, at least part of the lamellae transform into a lattice-like structure, called tubular myelin (Figure 28.1). It is

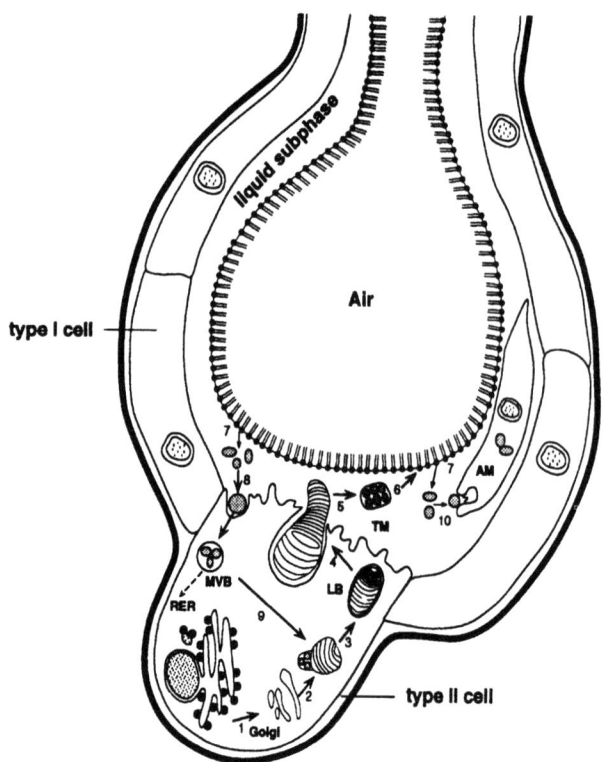

FIGURE 28.1. Schematic representation of the life cycle of pulmonary surfactant. The surfactant lipids and proteins are synthesized at the endoplasmic reticulum (RER) of the type II pneumocyte and thence transported, via the Golgi apparatus, to the lamellar bodies (LB) (processes 1, 2, and 3). The lamellar bodies leave the type II cells by exocytosis (4); in the liquid layer overlying the alveolar epithelium, the secreted lamellae transform into tubular myelin (5), from where the surfactant lipids can be inserted into the surface film (6). This process is highly catalyzed by the hydrophobic surfactant proteins SP-B and SP-C. Surfactant components can be efficiently recycled by the alveolar type II cells (7, 8, 9). Some surfactant can be taken up by the alveolar macrophages (AM) (10) or exit to the larger airways.

generally accepted that this tubular myelin functions as the reservoir from which the surfactant lipids are inserted into the surface film at the air-liquid interface.[36,37] However, it cannot be excluded that other structures in the alveolar lining layer, for example, freshly extruded lamellar body contents, provide lipids to the surface layer directly, i.e., without prior transforming into tubular myelin. In this respect, it is interesting that exogenous surfactants, used for therapy, apparently do not require transformation into tubular myelin for proper spreading.[38]

In a steady state the secretion of surfactant by the type II cells and its clearance from the alveolar spaces should be in equilibrium. It has been estimated from turnover studies that per hour 10% to 30% of the surfactant is cleared from the alveolar spaces.[36] A small part of surfactant exits via the airways and circulation.[37] According to current thinking, reentry of surfactant lipids into the type II cells represents the predominant mechanism for their continuous clearance from the alveolar spaces. The lipids that reenter the type II cells are probably largely recycled directly to lamellar bodies for resecretion. Some of the lipids are catabolized and their degradation products can be reutilized for synthesis of new surfactant components. Evidence has been provided that the surfactant proteins SP-A, SP-B, and SP-C can reenter the type II cells[27,39–41] and that they can recycle with the surfactant phospholipids. The important study of Baritussio et al.[27] has clearly demonstrated that the proteins SP-A, SP-B, and SP-C in newborn rabbits are all cleared more rapidly from the alveolar spaces than the major surfactant phospholipid. Likewise, the clearance of SP-A and SP-B appeared to be faster than that of DPPC in adult rabbit lung.[42,43] This difference in clearance kinetics is most likely due to more efficient recycling of DPPC than of SP-A or SP-B. Although earlier studies in vivo have suggested that the quantity of surfactant lipids cleared by macrophages is relatively small, a recent study by Wright and Youmans[44] demonstrated that isolated alveolar macrophages internalized and degraded both surfactant lipids and SP-A in a time-, temperature-, and concentration-dependent manner. The calculated rates of degradation were consistent with the possibility that the macrophages do contribute significantly to surfactant clearance.[44]

Thus, the extracellular surfactant system is very complex. It comprises freshly secreted lamellar body contents, tubular myelin, the actual surface film at the air-water interface, and vesicles with worn-out surfactant components destined to be cleared from the alveolar spaces. Although it has not been possible to isolate each of these individual fractions, pulmonary surfactant from bronchoalveolar lavage can be routinely separated into two major subfractions: the large and the small surfactant aggregates.[45,46] These subfractions differ in morphologic appearance, buoyant density, surfactant protein composition, and surface activity.[45–49] The large aggregates, which contain multilamellar structures and tubular myelin, represent the surface-active form of alveolar surfactant. The small aggregate fraction, which consists of small vesicles and contains lower amounts of the surfactant proteins, is not capable of reducing surface tension. Pulse-chase experiments have shown that the larger subfractions are the metabolic precursors of the smaller and lighter subtypes.[27,48] The conversion of large into small aggregates in vivo can be reproduced and studied in vitro using a technique known as surface-area cycling.[49] This is a very active field of research as studies with several animal models of acute lung injury have shown that the ratio of small to large aggregates is increased in injured lungs compared with normal lungs.[50] In addition, evidence has been presented that the large surfactant aggregates of preterm animals are more rapidly converted into small aggregates than those of mature neonatal or adult animals.[51]

The Surfactant Lipids: Composition and Functional Aspects

When total surfactants purified from bronchoalveolar lavages of several mammalian species are compared, a highly consistent lipid composition is seen. Phospholipids make up 80% to 90% of the lipids in surfactant. As illustrated in Figure 28.2 phosphatidylcholine (PC) is the major phospholipid class in surfactant and about 60% of these PC molecules contain two saturated acyl residues. Most of this disaturated PC is DPPC. This particular molecular species composes almost half of the surfactant phospholipids. A recent study showed that the proportion of DPPC in calf lung surfactant is lower than that in surfactants of other species (i.e., about one third of surfactant phospholipid).[52] A similar finding has been reported for the proportion of DPPC in total bovine lung tissue, which was substantially lower than that in lung tissue of other mammalian species.[53] Monoenoic PC molecules represent the bulk of the unsaturated PC species in surfactant.

The surfactant phospholipids represent a fluid mixture of saturated and unsaturated molecules that adsorb to the air-liquid interface, generating a surface film with an equilibrium surface tension of about 25 mN·m^{-1}. As will be discussed below, the insertion of the surfactant lipids into the surface film is highly catalyzed by the hydrophobic surfactant proteins SP-B and SP-C. The main component of the surface film is DPPC. In contrast to the unsaturated phospholipids, DPPC is solid at normal body temperature and resists surface compression. After the

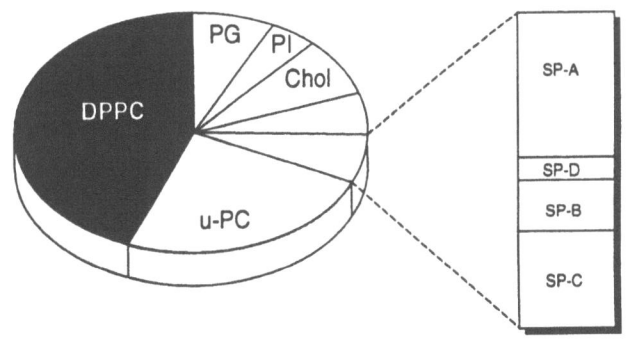

FIGURE 28.2. The lipid and protein composition of pulmonary surfactant. DPPC, dipalmitoylphosphatidylcholine; u-PC, phosphatidylcholines containing at least one unsaturated fatty-acyl chain; PG, phosphatidylglycerol; PI, phosphatidylinositol; chol, cholesterol. SP-A, SP-B, SP-C, and SP-D, surfactant protein A, B, C, and D, respectively.

unsaturated (i.e., more fluid) molecules have been squeezed out of the film at end-expiration, the contractile force at the air-liquid interface decreases to very low values and stabilization of terminal air spaces becomes independent of alveolar size.[4-6] Experimental evidence for this refinement of the surface film by squeeze-out processes, which results in the formation of different types of remnants, has been provided.[54,55] DPPC is the principal surface-active component of pulmonary surfactant that is responsible for the low values of surface tensions that are reached at end-expiration. Although this very low value is often cited as being "near zero," it is theoretically impossible to eliminate surface tension completely.[56] Recruitment of mixed film components occurs when, during inspiration, surface tension transiently increases above its equilibrium value.

It is generally assumed that negatively charged phospholipids contribute to optimal functioning of pulmonary surfactant.[2,20,57] Surfactants of most adult mammalian species, including humans, contain an atypically high proportion of phosphatidylglycerol (PG) that accounts for up to 10% of the phospholipids.[2,3] This is surprising because in mammalian tissues PG serves primarily as a precursor in mitochondrial cardiolipin synthesis and usually does not accumulate. Although this would suggest a specific function for PG in pulmonary surfactant, there is evidence from a number of studies that phosphatidylinositol (PI) can replace PG without affecting the most important physiologic properties of surfactant.[2,20] It may be important that PI and PG substitute for each other, not only because of charge requirements, but also because hydroxyl groups in their head groups might be required in intermolecular interactions in surfactant.[57]

Recent studies using ^{31}P nuclear magnetic resonance (NMR) spectroscopy have provided evidence that a significant proportion of calf surfactant PC (4%) occurs as choline plasmalogen or plasmenylcholine.[58] The plasmalogen analogue of PC contains an alkenylether residue rather than an acyl group at position 1 of the glycerol backbone. Rana et al.[58] suggested that the presence of significant amounts of plasmalogens in surfactant may affect the spreading of surfactant lipids at the air-liquid interface. On the other hand, evidence has been provided that plasmalogens can function as scavengers of radicals and reactive-oxygen species.[59] As the alveolar surfactant is a prime target of air oxidants,[60] it is attractive to speculate that the choline plasmalogen in pulmonary surfactant could perhaps function as a lipophilic antioxidant to protect surfactant constituents against peroxidations. In this context the alveolar type II cells also secrete vitamin E together with surfactant lipids.[61] Kahn et al.[52] recently reported a high-performance liquid chromatography (HPLC) analysis of calf surfactant PC. Although they did find about 2.5% ether-linked PC species in calf surfac-

tant, these ether lipids were largely of the 1-alkyl-2-acyl type and did not contain significant amounts of plasmalogen as reported by Rana et al.[58] The reason for this discrepancy is not clear.

Cholesterol is the most abundant neutral lipid in surfactant, which composes about 7 to 8 weight % or 15 mol % of total surfactant lipid.[57] Its specific function in mammalian pulmonary surfactant remains to be established,[62] although there is evidence to suggest that cholesterol is an important factor in increasing surfactant fluidity and in respreading of the surface film after compression.[57]

The composition of surfactant lipids can be influenced by diet[63,64] and physical effort.[62,65] Age is another factor. It is well known from studies in monkeys and rabbits that bronchoalveolar lavage fluid of newborn animals contains 5 to 10 times more surfactant than lavage from adult animals.[66,67] Experiments with neonatal rats demonstrated that the higher surfactant lipid content in the neonates decreased to the adult concentration during the first 50 days of life.[68] A recent investigation reported that a similar decrease in the total phospholipid content of bronchoalveolar lavage takes place in children between 3 and 8 years of age. The phospholipid composition of surfactant, however, did not change in this period.[69] The changes in surfactant composition in the perinatal period are discussed below.

The Surfactant Proteins: Structure and Functions

In 1972 King and Clements[70] reported that canine surfactant lipids were able to form stable surface films with low surface tension, but that this process was much faster when complete canine surfactant with the proteins included was used. This important early investigation indicated that the presence of the surfactant-associated proteins was essential for an optimal functioning of the lung. In the past decade there has been an enormous increase in our understanding of the structure, function, metabolism, and molecular genetics of the hydrophobic and hydrophilic surfactant proteins. This section presents a general overview of these proteins and their putative functions (Table 28.1).[25,71-77]

The Hydrophobic Surfactant Proteins SP-B and SP-C

Phizackerley et al.[78] were the first to demonstrate the presence of several hydrophobic proteins in organic solvent extracts of lamellar bodies and extracellular surfactant isolated from bronchoalveolar lavage. Initially these proteins did not receive much attention, until it was realized that they play an essential role in determining

TABLE 28.1. Putative functions of the hydrophobic and hydrophilic surfactant proteins.

Hydrophobic proteins function		Hydrophilic proteins function	
SP-B	Promotion of phospholipid insertion into the surface film [71,73,74,79,97,98,128]*	SP-A	Formation of tubular myelin [28,92–94]
	Formation of tubular myelin [92–94]		Regulation of phospholipid insertion into the surface film [54,128,160,161]
	Protection of surfactant against inactivation by plasma proteins [105,106]		Modulation of secretion and uptake of surfactant lipids by type II cells [23,75; but see ref. 169]
SP-C	Promotion of phospholipid insertion into the surface film [73,74,79,97,98,128,129]		Protection of surfactant against inactivation by plasma proteins [163,173]
	Protection of surfactant against inactivation by plasma proteins [105,106]		Role in innate lung defense [8–10,191]
			Activation of alveolar macrophages [192,193]
			Binding and clearance of bacteria [192,196–198] and viruses [201,204]
			Binding to LPS [202]
		SP-D	Role in innate lung defense
			Activation of alveolar macrophages [194]
			Agglutination of bacteria [200]
			Protection against viruses [205]
			Binding to *Pneumocystis carinii* [203]

*Numbers in brackets refer to key references.

the efficacy of surfactants used for replacement therapy. Without these proteins the adsorption of phospholipids to the air-liquid interface, resulting in the generation of a surface film, would be extremely slow.[74] SP-B and SP-C together constitute 1% to 2% of the surfactant weight and the molar ratio of SP-C is about a factor of 2 higher than that of SP-B.[79] Both proteins are secreted by the alveolar type II cells and, in view of their hydrophobic nature, they require specialized intracellular processing events to produce their mature forms.[71,73]

Structure and Biogenesis of SP-B

SP-B is a cysteine-rich positively charged 79-residue polypeptide with a molecular mass of 8.7 kd.[80] Under nonreducing conditions it occurs as a dimer. In the species for which the amino acid sequence has been reported, the primary structure is highly conserved, particularly with respect to the positions of the cysteine residues.[81,82] Although there is an overall excess of aliphatic residues in SP-B that contributes to its hydrophobic properties, the protein does not contain an extremely hydrophobic segment. The seven cysteine residues form a unique disulfide pattern. Three intramolecular disulfide bridges connect distant parts of the peptide chain, leading to tight folding of the SP-B monomer. The remaining cysteine 48 forms an intermolecular disulfide linking two monomeric SP-Bs to dimeric SP-B. Fourier transform infrared spectroscopy studies have shown that almost 50% of SP-B is in an α-helical conformation.[83] It has been predicted that these α-helical regions include at least two amphipathic helices.[71,73,77] These α-helices interact preferentially with superficial parts of lipid bilayers, whereas the charged residues are believed to be important for interactions with negatively charged phospholipids.[71,73,77,83]

Human SP-B is encoded by a single gene on chromosome 2.[71,84] The gene consists of 11 exons and 10 introns. Studies at the cDNA level established that SP-B must be derived from larger precursor forms.[85–89] The primary translation product of the SP-B messenger RNA (mRNA) is a preprotein form with an NH_2-terminally located signal peptide of 23 amino acids. During translocation of the preprotein into the endoplasmic reticulum of the type II cells, the signal peptide is cleaved, yielding the SP-B proprotein. The mature SP-B is processed from the proprotein by subsequent removal of 176 amino acids at the N-terminal and 102 amino acids at the C-terminal end.[71,77,90] The cleavage at the N-terminal side is probably mediated by cathepsin D.[91] Immunoelectron microscopy studies have provided evidence that the processing of SP-B proprotein to the mature SP-B proceeds in multilamellar bodies that are en route to lamellar bodies.[17,18] Dimerization of SP-B monomers probably occurs late in the secretory pathway.[77]

Functional Aspects of SP-B

Suzuki et al.[92] were the first to provide convincing evidence that SP-B is essential for the formation of tubular myelin (Table 28.1). Their elegant experiments showed that it was possible to reconstitute tubular myelin in vitro using Ca^{2+}, surfactant lipids, SP-A, and SP-B. These experiments were confirmed and extended by other investigators.[93,94] SP-B is probably required for this process because it is able to induce calcium-dependent fusion of membranes.[93,95] Interestingly, no tubular myelin was found in neonates with congenital SP-B deficiency, although there was an abundance of alveolar concentric multilamellar structures.[96]

The most important function of SP-B is to enhance the biophysical properties of surfactant lipids (Table 28.1). Experiments with a variety of in vitro systems showed that SP-B greatly promotes the formation of a stable surface film by inducing the insertion of surfactant phospholipids into the surface film.[71,73,74,79,85,97,98] In addition, SP-B combined with lipid mixtures reconstitutes most of the surface activity of natural surfactant in vitro and increases lung compliance in vivo.[79,99] The positively charged residues of SP-B, which are spread over almost the entire peptide chain, are essential for its activity.[74,77,100] They enable SP-B to interact strongly with the negatively charged PG, enhancing phospholipid adsorption and spreading of the phospholipid film.[83,101] SP-B might participate in the refinement of the monolayer by removing PG.[102] During expiration, the surface tension at the air-water interface is reduced and the surface pressure in the monolayer is increased. At a surface pressure higher than 40 to 45 mN·m^{-1}, SP-B is squeezed out of the monolayer, together with two to three phospholipid molecules per SP-B dimer.[103] During subsequent expansion, a new cycle is started by SP-B–catalyzed insertion of phospholipids into the monolayer.[57,98,104]

There is also evidence that the hydrophobic proteins protect against inactivation of surfactant activity due to plasma proteins leaking into the airspaces, and in this respect SP-B appears to be more potent than SP-C[105,106] (Table 28.1).

Instillation of monoclonal antibodies directed against SP-B into the airways of newborn rabbits induced respiratory distress, whereas nonspecific immune sera did not exert this effect.[107] More recently, Nogee et al.[108,109] reported that neonates, unable to produce SP-B due to a genetic defect, develop lethal respiratory distress. The lack of SP-B in these neonates appeared to be due to a frame shift mutation in exon 4.[110] Ablation of the SP-B gene in transgenic mice also led to neonatal respiratory distress.[111] Collectively, these findings provide strong evidence for the critical role of SP-B in pulmonary function.

Structure and Biogenesis of SP-C

SP-C is one of the most hydrophobic peptides that occur in nature. It is only soluble in organic solvents such as chloroform or 80% acetonitrile in water.[112] Depending on the mammalian species, it contains 33 to 35 amino acid residues.[71,73,74,113–116] In its N-terminal part (i.e., amino acids 5 and 6 of human SP-C) it contains two cysteines that are each linked to a palmitoyl group via a thioester-bond. This palmitoylation adds to the hydrophobicity of SP-C.[117] The two cysteines are each flanked by a proline residue, which could be important because these prolines may prevent rotation of the polypeptide backbone.[74] The canine SP-C has only one palmitoyl-cysteine; in that species cysteine 6 is replaced by a phenylalanine.[115] The N-terminal part of the molecule comprises two or three positively charged residues. In human SP-C, for example, lysine and arginine are found at positions 11 and 12. Between positions 13 and 28 SP-C contains only amino acids residues with aliphatic branched chains, including a stretch of up to seven consecutive valines. In the mammalian species that have been analyzed so far, this extremely hydrophobic part of SP-C appears to be highly conserved. The secondary structure of this part of the protein is a regular α-helix[118–120] that is able to span a DPPC bilayer.[120,121] It has been shown that the long axis of the α-helix is oriented parallel to the lipid-acyl chains.[120] Dimeric forms of SP-C have also been reported,[122,123] but their function remains to be clarified.

The human SP-C gene has been located on the short arm of chromosome 8.[124] The gene is organized into six exons.[71] Like SP-B, mature SP-C is contained within the sequence of a much larger proprotein.[124–126] The size of the proprotein is 197 amino acids in the human,[124,125] 194 amino acids in the rat,[126] and 190 amino acids in the dog.[126] In contrast to the proprotein of SP-B, it does not contain a signal sequence. The details of the processing of proprotein SP-C have not yet been fully established. However, recent studies by Beers and Lomax[127] have shown that the processing of the SP-C proprotein involves initial cleavage of C-terminal regions followed by removal of vestigial N-terminal fragments. This processing proceeds in subcellular compartments distal to the trans-Golgi network, probably in multivesicular bodies.[18,19] Palmitoylation probably proceeds prior to cleavage of the proprotein of SP-C.[73] The biochemical aspects of this process in the type II cells are still not understood.

Functional Aspects of SP-C

In contrast to SP-B, SP-C is not required for the biogenesis of tubular myelin[92–94] (Table 28.1). It shares with SP-B the property of accelerating the adsorption of phospholipids to an air-liquid interface.[73,74,79,97,98,116,128,129] Reconstitution experiments with surfactant lipids have shown that the combination of SP-B and SP-C is even more effective in restoring the surface activity of natural surfactant than either of these proteins alone.[128,129] In view of the considerable structural differences between SP-B and SP-C discussed above, it seems justified to speculate that each of these proteins fulfills separate functions in the generation of the surface film in vivo.

The SP-C catalyzed insertion of phospholipids from a subphase into the air-liquid interface is Ca^{2+}-dependent and is preceded by the SP-C–dependent binding of phospholipids to the monolayer.[97,98] The positively charged lysine and arginine at positions 11 and 12 of SP-C are important in this process as they allow binding of the protein to negatively charged phospholipids.[130] It is likely that SP-C is present in the monolayer. When SP-C is squeezed out at high surface pressures, 8 to 10 PC molecules per mole of SP-C accompany the protein, which raises the possibility for SP-C to modify the composition of the monolayer.[131] The function of the palmitoylation of SP-C is not clear, although the in vitro experiments of Creuwels et al.[132] have shown that the palmitoyl groups are probably not necessary for the Ca^{2+}-dependent insertion of phospholipids into the monolayer.

The Hydrophilic Surfactant Proteins SP-A and SP-D

In addition to the two hydrophobic proteins described above, pulmonary surfactant also contains two hydrophilic proteins, SP-A and SP-D. SP-A is the most abundant protein associated with extracellular surfactant. It was the first surfactant protein to be purified and analyzed for its primary structure.[133] There is some doubt as to whether the most recently discovered hydrophilic surfactant protein D[134] should be designated as a true surfactant protein. The majority of this protein is not associated with the surfactant pellet, but is recovered from the supernatant fraction of bronchoalveolar lavage.[135]

Structure and Biogenesis of SP-A

In its monomeric form SP-A has a molecular mass of 28 to 36 kd, depending on the degree of glycosylation. The primary structure of SP-A has been established for a variety of species (e.g., human,[133] dog,[136] rabbit,[137] rat,[138] and mouse[139]). It appears to be highly conserved. The monomeric SP-A consists of four distinct segments: a short amino-terminal segment, a collagenous domain that is amino-terminal to a short stretch of amino acids called the neck region, and a carboxyl-terminal carbohydrate-recognition domain. The amino-terminal segment of mature SP-A comprises only 7 to 10 amino acids, including a cysteine residue at position 6 that forms an interchain disulfide bond, which is important in aligning the SP-A monomers for oligomerization. The amino-terminal part is flanked by a collagen-like domain containing 23 to 24 Gly-X-Y repeats, where X is any amino acid and Y is frequently hydroxyproline. This sequence of repeating triplets is only interrupted between the 13th and 14th repeat by the sequence pro-cys-pro-pro. This structural motif suggests that this region of the molecule is folded into a triple helix. Six of these triple helices are assembled into a bundle of 18 monomers of SP-A. Electron microscopic images of SP-A obtained after rotary shadowing indicated that this region of SP-A is organized into a rod-like structure of approximately 20 nm. The above-mentioned interruption in the collagen-like repeating sequence induces a flexible kink in the collagen rod, causing the individual trimers to bend outward from the central axis into six directions.[140] The collagen-like region is linked to the globular C-terminal region by a short neck region. The C-terminal region comprising 130 amino acids is a carbohydrate-recognition domain (CRD) that has remarkable structural similarities with other C-type (calcium-dependent) lectins or collectins.[141,142] The CRD contains a Ca^{2+}-dependent specific carbohydrate binding site[143,144] and comprises two disulfide bridges between residues 135 and 226 and residues 204 and 218.[145] The positions of the four cysteine residues in the CRD are conserved in all members of the class of calcium-dependent lectins. A complex sialated oligosaccharide is attached to the CRD at asparagine-187.[71,72] The bouquet-like form of the SP-A molecule is very similar to that of the collectin mannose-binding protein.[142,146] As will be described later, two other members of the collectins, conglutinin and SP-D, share a cruciform shape.

The human SP-A locus has been localized to the middle of the long arm of chromosome 10.[147] As it is currently understood, the SP-A locus consists of two functional genes and one pseudogene, and it exhibits extensive variability within the 5' untranslated, coding, and 3' untranslated regions.[76] Interestingly, there is evidence that the two functional genes are differentially regulated during development.[148] In other species that have been investigated there appears to be only one SP-A gene.[71] The primary translation product, which contains a 20 amino acid signal peptide, undergoes extensive modifications, including cleavage of the signal peptide, inter- and intrachain disulfide bridge formation, hydroxylation of specific proline residues, and addition of Asn-linked carbohydrate.[71] It has been proposed that the neck region of SP-A is involved in phospholipid binding.[71] However, more recent studies with chimeras of surfactant proteins A and D have clearly shown that this domain cannot account for all the lipid binding activity of SP-A and that the CRD is also essential for this property of SP-A.[149] This conclusion was substantiated by epitope mapping of SP-A for several monoclonal antibodies against this protein.[150] The latter study provided evidence that the CRD also plays a role in the inhibitory effect of SP-A on secretion of lipids by type II cells[33,34] and on the stimulatory effect of this protein on lipid uptake by type II cells.[37] The region from Glu-202 to Met-207 in the CRD of SP-A may be of particular importance for the expression of these activities of SP-A.[151]

Immunoelectron microscopy studies have demonstrated that SP-A is not only synthesized and secreted by the type II pneumocytes, but also by the Clara cells in the respiratory bronchioli.[152] In addition, immunolocalization and in situ hybridization studies in lungs of human fetuses and neonates have demonstrated abundance of SP-A in tracheal and bronchial glands and epithelium, which underscores the potential importance of nonsurfactant associated functions for SP-A.[153] In fact, a recent study suggested that SP-A is also expressed by epithelial cells of small and large intestine.[154]

The next section discusses the putative functions of SP-A in the dynamics and metabolism of the surfactant system. The potential roles of SP-A and SP-D in lung defense are discussed in a separate section.

Functional Aspects of SP-A in the Surfactant System

As already mentioned, reconstitution experiments in vitro have shown that SP-A is required for the biogenesis of tubular myelin[92-94] (Table 28.1). A role of SP-A in this process was further supported by immunoelectron microscopy studies showing that SP-A is localized at the corners of the tubular myelin network.[28] The latter observation was confirmed more recently by deMello et al.[155] These investigators reported that lungs of neonates dying from RDS appeared to lack tubular myelin and had strongly decreased levels of SP-A, further corroborating a role of SP-A in tubular myelin formation. Recent surface-area cycling investigations have provided evidence that SP-A may also be important in maintaining the integrity of tubular myelin.[156] The molecular mechanisms involved in the biogenesis of tubular myelin are unknown. It has been suggested that the ability of SP-A to simultaneously self-associate through lectin-carbohydrate interactions and to bind to lipid could be responsible for the SP-A–induced formation of tubular myelin.[157] However, more recent studies showing that the carbohydrate moieties of SP-A are not involved in lipid aggregation induced by SP-A do not support this suggestion.[158,159]

Although the presence of SP-A in surfactant preparations has little effect on surface activity on its own, studies in vitro showed that SP-A did enhance the adsorption of surfactant lipids in conjunction with SP-B.[128,160] SP-A also significantly improved lung function in rabbit pups treated with natural surfactant extracts containing SP-B and SP-C.[161] Recent work using the captive bubble technique has suggested that SP-A enhances phospholipid adsorption during dynamic cycling and may promote squeeze-out of non-DPPC lipids during cycling.[54] It is possible that the presence of SP-A is essential when surfactant concentrations are limiting, such as in severe neonatal RDS or when the surfactant is compromised by the presence of inhibitory serum proteins (Table 28.1).[54,162,163]

SP-A may also play a role in regulating surfactant homeostasis.[23,37,71,75] It has been shown that this protein binds specifically to alveolar type II cells[164,165] and that it inhibits the secretion of phospholipids from these cells.[33,34,71,75] A number of studies have demonstrated that SP-A increases the uptake of radioactively labeled phospholipids by alveolar type II cells,[23,166-168] which suggests a potential role for SP-A in the clearance of surfactant lipids from the alveolar spaces (Table 28.1). Very recently, however, Horowitz et al.[169] studied the effect of SP-A on the uptake of fluorescently labeled lipid vesicles by type II cells. By using fluorescence microscopy they were able to follow endocytosis of lipids. The results showed that SP-A did not increase endocytosis of lipids by the type II cells, but rather caused formation of lipid aggregates at the external surface of the type II cells. Another uncertainty concerns the fact that a functional SP-A receptor in the type II cell membrane has not yet been firmly established and characterized. However, several type II cell molecules have been described that bind SP-A, one with a molecular mass of 30 kd[170] and another with a mass of 50 to 55 kd.[171] A very recent investigation provides evidence that the latter binding protein does play a role in SP-A stimulated endocytosis of surfactant lipids.[172]

Studies in vitro have shown that SP-A appears to be quite effective in protecting surfactants containing SP-B and SP-C from inhibition by plasma proteins.[163] Recent experiments with prematurely delivered rabbit pups that intratracheally received surfactants with or without SP-A and increasing amounts of plasma proteins showed that SP-A exerts such a protective effect in vivo (Table 28.1).[173]

Structure and Synthesis of SP-D

The mature human SP-D polypeptide contains 335 amino acid residues, and the molecular mass of this protein is 43 kd under reducing conditions.[174] The amino acid sequence of SP-D has been established for several species (e.g., human,[174,175] rat,[176] and bovine[177]). These investigations have shown that the structural organization of SP-D is similar to that of other collections in that it comprises a short amino-terminal region, a collagen-like domain, a short neck region, and the C-terminal CRD. The collagen-like domain of SP-D is much longer than that of SP-A and contains 59 instead of 23 to 24 Gly-X-Y repeats. In addition, the Gly-X-Y triplets of SP-D are not interrupted. The CRD of SP-D contains all of the invariant residues, including the four conserved cysteine residues, characteristic of the C-type lectins. Interestingly, the nucleotide and deduced amino acid sequences of SP-D revealed a very high similarity (i.e., 87% and 78% identity) with the sequences of conglutinin.[178]

In its functional form SP-D is assembled as multimers of disulfide-bonded trimers composed of 12 apparently identical 43-kd proteins. Electron microscopy studies revealed a highly homogeneous quaternary structure of SP-D in the form of a cross.[179] From the central point, four identical rod-arms of 46 nm emanate and end in a globular terminal expansion comprising the CRD of three SP-D molecules. This cruciform shape of SP-D, which is similar to that reported earlier for conglutinin,[180] seems ideal for agglutination reactions.

The gene encoding human SP-D has been localized to 10q22-q23, close to the SP-A cluster and the locus for the mannose-binding protein gene.[175,181] The primary translation product of SP-D mRNA undergoes several posttranslational modifications, including cleavage of the signal peptide, hydroxylation of lysine and proline, glycoside attachment to hydroxylysine, and attachment of N-linked oligosaccharide within the collagen region.[179] Immunoelectron microscopy studies have demonstrated that SP-D, like SP-A, is synthesized not only by the type II pneumocytes, but also by the Clara cells.[152,182] It has been shown recently that SP-D is also expressed in rat gastric mucosa.[183]

Functional Aspects of SP-D in the Surfactant System

There is no evidence for a role of SP-D in the classic physiologic functions of the surfactant system, although such a role cannot be firmly excluded. For example, the fact that SP-D specifically binds to PI and to glucosylceramide is intriguing, but the physiological significance of this finding is unclear.[184–186] Also, there is one investigation showing that SP-D may counteract the inhibitory effect of SP-A on surfactant lipid secretion by type II cells.[187] However, most investigators believe that the major physiologic functions of SP-D reside in innate lung defense mechanisms (Table 28.1).

Role of the Hydrophilic Surfactant Proteins in Lung Defense

Although animals are equipped with a very efficient and precise mechanism to neutralize and eliminate invading pathogens through highly specific antibody and cell-mediated immune responses, this mechanism cannot provide immediate protection as it takes several days to elicit these responses. The first line of defense against infection is an innate, or nonclonal, immunity that can be activated within minutes. The collectins in the circulation, such as mannose-binding protein and conglutinin, may play an important role in this innate immune defense system. They can selectively recognize configurations of carbohydrates that are present on the surfaces of pathogens and mark these invaders for neutralization by opsonization and complement activation.[141,142,188–190] As described, SP-A and SP-D are also collectins with quaternary structures that are very similar to those of mannose-binding protein and conglutinin, respectively. These observations suggested that SP-A and SP-D could possibly play a similar innate defense role in the airways. In the past few years considerable evidence has been provided to support such a role for the hydrophilic surfactant proteins (Table 28.1). This evidence has been reviewed in depth recently.[8–10,191]

It is highly likely that alveolar macrophages possess specific receptors for both SP-A and SP-D.[8] SP-A[192,193] and SP-D[194] specifically augment the production of oxygen radicals by alveolar macrophages, which can contribute to local killing of microorganisms. SP-A potentiates the antibacterial functions of alveolar macrophages by stimulating the production of inflammatory cytokines and immunoglobulin.[10,195] Several groups have demonstrated that SP-A enhances both serum-dependent[192,196] and serum-independent[197,198] phagocytosis of bacteria by alveolar macrophages.[8] A recent study indicated that SP-A activates a phosphoinositide/calcium signaling pathway in alveolar macrophages leading to this enhanced serum-independent phagocytosis of bacteria.[199] SP-D did not act as an opsonin in the phagocytosis of gram-negative bacteria.[198] However, this protein exerts a very strong agglutinating effect on gram-negative bacteria, which may facilitate their clearance via mucociliary transport.[200] It has also been shown that SP-A can act as opsonin in the phagocytosis of some viruses.[201] Evidence has been provided that SP-A[8,202] and SP-D[200] can bind to lipopolysaccharides (LPS) of a variety of gram-negative bacteria, inhibiting binding of LPS to their regular target cells. SP-D binds to the core region,[200] and SP-A to the lipid A moiety of LPS.[202] A recent study reported that SP-D can interact with gpA, the major surface antigen of *Pneumocystis carinii*, augmenting the binding of this microorganism to alveolar macrophages.[203] Interestingly, both SP-A and SP-D can, at least in vitro, lower the infectivity of some viruses, such as influenza virus A.[204,205]

In some of these effects (e.g., in the activation of alveolar macrophages) the major surfactant lipids exert an effect that is opposite to that of SP-A. It is quite feasible that the local ratio between surfactant lipids and hydrophilic proteins may determine the net effect on the target cell. Disturbances in these ratios, which occur in various lung diseases, could lead to dysregulation of the defense function of pulmonary surfactant.[10]

The Surfactant System in the Developing Lung

Fetal Lung Morphogenesis

It is generally recognized that lung development can be subdivided into five stages:[206] (1) In the embryonic period (i.e., 3 to 6 weeks in the human) the lung originates from a diverticulum of the ventral wall of the primitive gut and soon divides into two bronchial buds. This endodermally derived epithelium later differentiates into both the respiratory epithelium lining the airways and the specialized epithelium that lines the alveoli. The lung bud grows into a mass of mesodermal cells from which blood vessels, smooth muscle, cartilage, and other connective tissues differentiate. Ectoderm contributes to the innervation of the lung. The two lung buds develop lobar buds that subsequently undergo progressive dichotomous branching. As in other organs, mutual interactions between epithelium and mesenchyme are essential for the sequential events of organogenesis. Mesenchyme has been demonstrated to play a determining role in the formation of the characteristic branching morphology. (2) In the pseudoglandular period (i.e., 6 to 16 weeks in the human) 16 to 25 generations of presumptive airways result from the repeated dichotomous branching. These ducts are surrounded by abundant mesenchyme, and in cross section the tissue resembles glandular tissue. The ducts end in terminal sacs, the presumptive alveolar ducts, which are lined by a columnar epithelium. (3) In the canalicular period (i.e., 16 to 24–28 weeks in the human) the functionally important respiratory or gas-exchanging portion of the lung becomes delineated. This period is characterized by the differentiation of the alveolar epithelium, a decrease in the relative amount of connective tissue in the lung, and an increase in the number of blood vessels, with capillaries coming into closer contact with the primitive alveoli. Also, the first appearance of differentiated type II pneumocytes, the producers of surfactant, is noted. All these changes ensure that neonates, born toward the end of this period are potentially viable. However, the relatively small surface area for gas exchange, the still thick intersaccular septa and the high cuboidal epithelium may pose significant problems for gas exchange, especially if surfactant production is deficient and alveolar collapse occurs. (4) In the terminal saccular period of lung development (i.e., 24–28 to 36 weeks in the human) the lungs are further prepared for air breathing after birth. The respiratory portion of the lung further differentiates. Respiratory bronchioles rapidly subdivide into an array of thin-walled primitive alveolar ducts and primitive alveoli, which are lined by type II and flat type I pneumocytes in close contact with a rapidly proliferating capillary network. (5) In the alveolar period (in the human starting before term birth and continuing after birth) true alveoli are formed by indentations of the septal wall. The thinning of the walls continues and the amount of connective tissue decreases further. The number of alveoli increases up to 8 years of life.

It is evident that fetal lung morphogenesis, as described in the five phases, involves major structural changes that are associated with both cell proliferation and cell differentiation. Lung growth is regulated by physical factors and hormones. The effect of these factors may be mediated by intercellular interactions, extracellular matrix components, and growth factors. The cytodifferentiation of the different lung cells is essential for adequate lung function. The regulation of the differentiation of the type II pneumocyte is especially important as it is the producer of pulmonary surfactant.

It can be concluded that, although the lung has no major functions before birth, its almost complete morphologic and biochemical development and maturation before birth is crucial for survival immediately after birth. From the sequence of normal lung development, it is also easy to understand that very premature neonates (i.e., <28 weeks and especially <26 weeks) with lungs in the canalicular stage of development frequently have suboptimal gas exchange, even in the absence of the typical respiratory distress syndrome.

Appearance of Alveolar Type II Cells

During embryonic lung morphogenesis the walls of the lung primordium are lined with undifferentiated columnar epithelial cells, which later differentiate into prospective bronchial epithelium and prospective alveolar epithelium. The acinar tubules during the late pseudoglandular and early canalicular stages of lung development are lined with cuboidal epithelium. At this stage of development, these cells do not contain lamellar bodies, characteristic of mature type II cells. Nevertheless, they do express phenotypic features and possess antigenic determinants of mature type II cells.[207–210] They are frequently called protodifferentiated type II cells or pre-type II cells. During the canalicular period of lung development, the rapid proliferation slows down and the pre-type II cells start to mature. The most striking morphologic feature is the decrease in glycogen content and the increase in number and size of lamellar bodies.[211] In the human fetus, lamellar bodies can be detected within the alveolar epithelium at 20 weeks' gestation, but are not regularly observed until about 24 weeks.[3]

Glycogen Metabolism in the Developing Lung

Fetal lung glycogen content increases during gestation, then decreases rapidly during the period of maximal surfactant synthesis.[211–213] That these processes take place in pre-type II and type II cells has been demonstrated by electron-microscopic studies[214,215] and in an investigation using isolated rat type II cells.[211] This temporal correlation between glycogen depletion and surfactant formation, which has been observed in several species, suggests that glycogen could act as a source of precursor substrates for phospholipid synthesis. In addition, glycogen breakdown may provide the necessary energy and reducing equivalents in the form of nicotinamide adenine dinucleotide phosphate, reduced (NADPH) via the hexose monophosphate pathway.[213] Several studies by Bourbon et al.[216,217] provide evidence for this precursor-product relationship between glycogen and surfactant phospholipids. Radioactive glucose was injected to label fetal rat glycogen in vivo, and explant lung cultures were established one day later. During culture a correlation was demonstrated between the decrease in glycogen content and radioactivity and the increase in pool sizes and radioactivity of disaturated PC (DSPC) and PG.[216] In this study, glucose from the culture medium was used four to five times less than glycogen for DSPC synthesis. Interestingly, Farrell and Bourbon[217] demonstrated that the radioactivity of prelabeled glycogen entered preferentially into surfactant phospholipids instead of membrane phospholipids. The control of glycogen metabolism during lung development is complex and not completely elucidated. During the period of glycogen deposition, increased activities of glycogen synthase have been found.[212,213,218] Increased activities of glycogen phosphorylase have been found to correlate with prenatal glycogen depletion in fetal rabbit and rat lung.[212,213,218] The role of lysosomal acid α-glucosidase in the use of glycogen for surfactant synthesis, as suggested by a study of Bourbon et al.,[219] is not completely clear.[3]

Developmental Changes in Surfactant Lipids

Increasing amounts of surfactant phospholipids are produced by the fetal lung toward the end of gestation.[1,3,220] The main component responsible for this increase is PC. The total amount of PC increases, and the proportion of PC rises in several animal species from 40% to 50–60% of the total phospholipids during lung maturation. The degree of saturation of lung PC also increases significantly during fetal development and rises further after birth. Overall the amount of DSPC almost doubles from the beginning of the canalicular period of lung development to term gestation in rabbits and rats.[3] The changes in phospholipid content and composition at the end of gestation are even more pronounced in lung lavage material and lamellar bodies than in total lung, as might be expected because lavage fluid and lamellar bodies reflect the composition of surfactant more closely than lung tissue.[1,3,220] The increase in the amount of PC in these fractions may be as dramatic as 20- to 30-fold. The proportion of PC in lung lavage phospholipids increases to approximately 70% to 80% at the end of gestation, while there is a compensatory decrease in other lipids, especially sphingomyelin, resulting in a marked increase in lecithin (~PC) to sphingomyelin (L/S) ratio.

In the human fetal lung an accumulation of surfactant PC is found from about 28 weeks, which is much earlier than in experimental animals.[3] This early surge of surfactant PC production may explain why the human neonate can survive a more premature delivery than other species. However, the marked increase of DPPC in the alveolus occurs close to term, which is similar to other species. A continuity exists between fetal lung liquid and amniotic fluid, and in the human fetus large quantities of surfactant enter the amniotic fluid.[221,222] It is possible to assess fetal lung maturation from the analysis of phospholipids in the amniotic fluid.[221] The rapid increase in surfactant concentration is found around weeks 33 to 37. On average, the female matures about 1.5 to 2 weeks earlier than the male.[3] Several conditions are associated with accelerated lung maturity (e.g., such as prolonged rupture of fetal membranes, prolonged labor, and hyperthyroidism) and others with a delay in maturity. It is well known that an increased incidence of RDS is found among infants of diabetic mothers.[223] There is a clear effect of labor on the secretion of PC into the alveolar compartment, as was shown in experiments with rabbits.[224,225] It has also been shown that the L/S ratio in human amniotic fluid increases during labor.[226] These findings may, at least partly, explain that the incidence of RDS at the same gestational age is lower among neonates delivered either vaginally or by cesarean section after some labor than among those delivered without labor.[226]

Besides the marked increase in surfactant PC toward the end of gestation, an important change takes place in the composition of acidic phospholipids in the lung.[1-3,220] In most mammalian species, the relative amount of PG increases, whereas that of PI decreases.[3,227] The functional significance of this switch is not yet completely understood. As discussed earlier, both anionic phospholipids can replace each other without affecting the most important physiologic properties of surfactant. In some species, such as the rhesus monkey, PI remains the dominant anionic phospholipid in the adult.[228] In the human, the proportion of PI increases from about 28 weeks and then decreases at approximately 36 weeks at the same time as the increase occurs in the proportion of PG.[229,230] The decreased availability of inositol may be an important mediator of the switch from PI to PG as the main anionic surfactant phospholipid. This seems to be a plausible explanation as PI and PG have the same precursor, CDP-diacylglycerol, and inositol and glycerol-3-phosphate may compete for this precursor (Figure 28.3).[231] It has been demonstrated in the fetal rat that the concentration of serum inositol is high during gestation but decreases toward birth.[227] Moreover, the uptake of inositol into lung cells via specific transport systems decreases during lung maturation.[232] Also in the human it has been demonstrated that the fetal serum concentration of inositol is much higher than the maternal concentration, and it decreases toward term.[233]

Developmental Changes in Surfactant Phospholipid Synthesis

It is evident that the large changes in the concentrations of surfactant-associated phospholipids during development must be a reflection of increased biosynthesis and secretion of phospholipids by the alveolar type II cells. The pathways of synthesis of the most important surfactant-associated phospholipids are depicted in Figure 28.3. Abundant evidence is available that the synthesis of surfactant PC increases during late gestation.[1-3,220-222] Most of this evidence has come from the many investigations that have demonstrated increased incorporation rates of radioactive precursors into phospholipids and especially into PC toward the end of gestation. Earlier studies were performed in whole-lung slices of several animal species with choline, glycerol, glucose, and palmitate as radioactive precursors for PC. The disadvantage of these whole-lung studies is that cell types other than type II cells contribute to the measured incorporation into PC. Recently, the increased incorporation of glycerol, palmitate, acetate, and choline into PC with advancing gestation was demonstrated in isolated rat fetal type II cells.[234] Carlson et al.[211] showed that this augmented biosynthesis of PC correlated with elevated concentrations of PC in type II cells.

The increased synthesis of PC indicates that alterations must occur in the activities of the enzymes responsible for PC synthesis and/or the availability of their substrates during late gestation. The CDP-choline pathway is the primary pathway for de novo PC synthesis in the developing lung (Figure 28.3).[1-3,20,25,220] Choline is brought into the cell by a facilitated transport system, and is phosphorylated by choline kinase. The synthesis of the activated intermediate, CDP-choline, is catalyzed by CTP: phosphocholine cytidylyltransferase (CT) (EC 2.7.7.15). Finally, the phosphocholine moiety is transferred to diacylglycerol by the CDP-choline: 1,2-diacylglycerol phosphocholinetransferase (Figure 28.3).

Regulation of CTP: Phosphocholine Cytidylyltransferase

Studies with whole lung have shown an increased activity of the CDP-choline pathway during late gestation.[235] Pool size studies have demonstrated that the reaction catalyzed by CT is a rate-limiting step in the CDP-choline pathway in fetal lung and in isolated fetal type II cells.[236,237] In addition, many studies indicate that CT is an important target for developmental[234,238-240] as well as hormonal[241-247] regulation in alveolar type II cells of the developing lung. Although under most circumstances CT has indeed been shown to be the regulatory step, an entire pathway is never regulated by the activity of one single enzyme under all circumstances. Recently, important progress has been made in the understanding of the regulation of CT activity. This was made possible mainly by the purification of the enzyme,[248,249] followed by the availability of antibodies against the enzyme[250-252] and the cloning of its cDNA from rat liver[253] and lung.[254] These recent advancements have important implications for the understanding of the regulation of CT in developing fetal lung.[255]

Cytidylyltransferase is essentially inactive without lipids.[239,256] The amphipathic α-helical domain of the enzyme is involved in its binding to lipid membranes.[257-259] In the type II cell, the most important binding sites involved in the activation of CT are the microsomal membranes[234,240,254,260-264] and the lipids of the cytosolic H-form.[265-269] The currently available data are most compatible with an activation of both cytosolic and microsomal CT activity during fetal lung development and after corticosteroid administration. Cytosolic CT is regulated by phospholipids. The activation of cytosolic CT is accompanied by a conversion of a low molecular weight L-form to a high molecular weight H-form,[265,267,268,270-274] which is a lipoprotein complex consisting of aggregated CT complexed with (phospho) lipids. The H-form is the predominant form in the adult lung.[265-268,270] Fatty acids, either in free form or possibly after incorporation into (phospho) lipids, induce the conversion from the L-form to the H-form.[270-274] They appear to be a very important regulator of CT activity after corticosteroid administration and, most likely, during normal lung development.[275]

Translocation of CT from cytosol to the membranes of the endoplasmic reticulum activates the enzyme.[260] This mechanism is also regulated by fatty acids[276] and plays an important role during lung development.[234,238,240,254,276,277] The cytosolic interconversion from the L-form to the H-form and the translocation of CT from cytosol to endoplasmic reticulum are probably closely related.[270,276]

Taken together, recent studies support the following sequence in the fetal lung after exogenous corticosteroid administration: corticosteroids induce the production of fibroblast-pneumocyte factor (FPF) in lung fibroblasts adjacent to the type II cells[210] at a pretranslational level.[278] This FPF induces fatty acid synthase and other enzymes involved in fatty acid synthesis in fetal type II cells at a pretranslational level,[279] which leads to an increase in fatty acid biosynthesis. Fatty acids, their metabolites, or lipids, into which they become incorporated, ultimately activate CT[25] by increasing the cytosolic H-form and translocation of CT from cytosol to microsomes. A similar sequence could take place during normal type II cell maturation at late gestation or around birth, caused by endogenous corticosteroid production.

Cytidylyltransferase contains several potential sites for phosphorylation by protein kinases.[253,254,280] There is now convincing evidence that CT is phosphorylated and

28. Lung Metabolism in the Fetus and Neonate

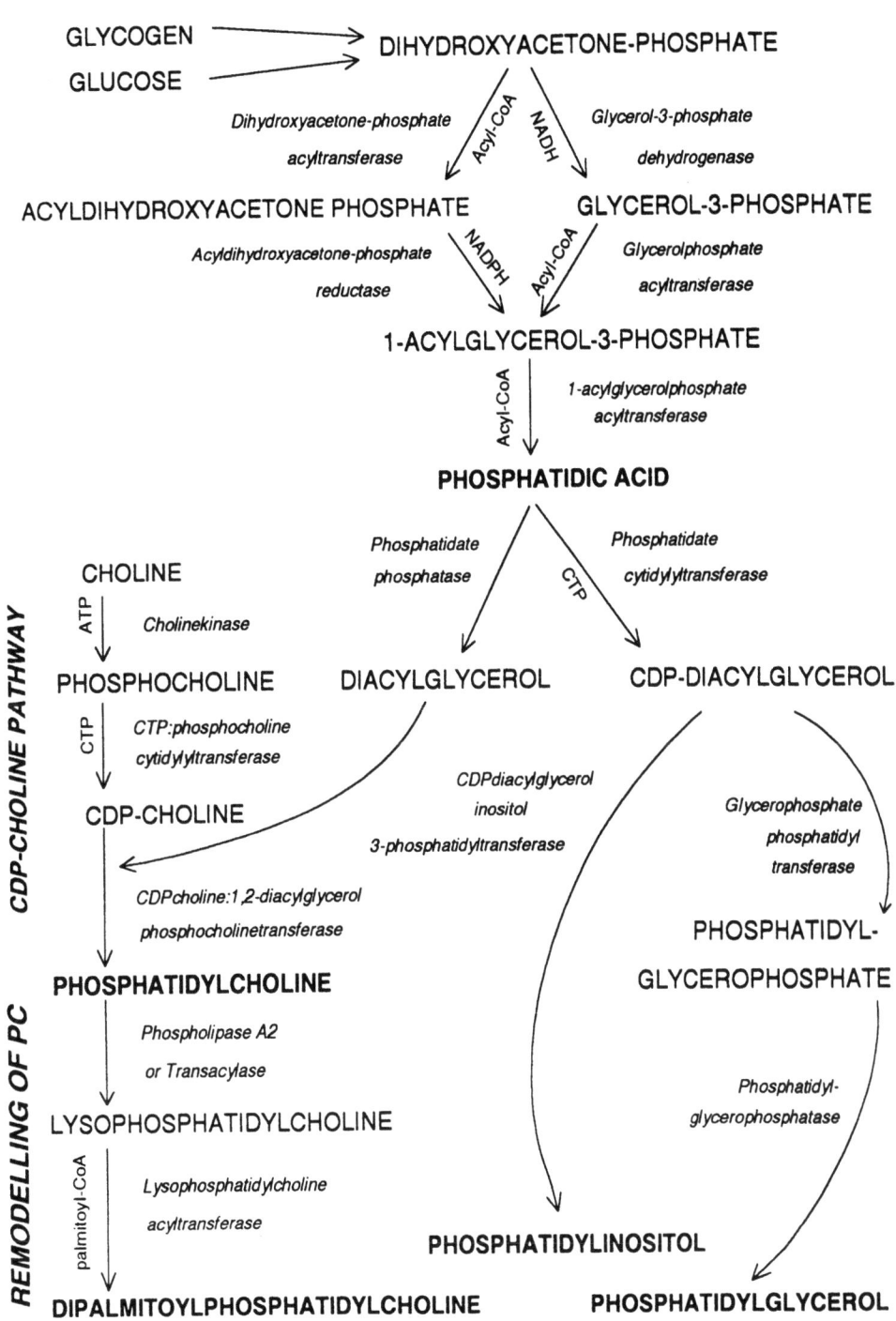

FIGURE 28.3. Pathways for the synthesis of the most important surfactant phospholipids. Note the key position of phosphatidic acid and that of CDP-diacylglycerol, which is the common precursor for the synthesis of phosphatidylglycerol and phosphatidylinositol. Phosphatidylcholine (PC) is produced via the CDP-choline pathway; a considerable part of the dipalmitoyl species of PC (DPPC) can also be formed by remodeling of de novo synthesized unsaturated PC.

dephosphorylated in intact cells[280–286] and that the phosphorylation state of the enzyme regulates its activity. The phosphorylation state of the enzyme is correlated with its location.[281,282,284–286] When the enzyme translocates from membranes to cytosol, it becomes subsequently phosphorylated. When it translocates from cytosol to membranes, it becomes dephosphorylated and active but the order of events and the precise significance is not yet clear. Protein phosphatases 1 and/or 2A have been shown to dephosphorylate the enzyme,[287,288] but which protein kinase is involved in the phosphorylation is still unclear. Protein kinase C and cAMP-dependent protein kinase are very unlikely candidates as is demonstrated by several investigations,[252,283,289–293] some of which involve fetal type II cells.[255,290] The number of investigations on the phosphorylation and dephosphorylation mechanism in developing lung are still very limited, and further investigations are required to elucidate the precise role of this mechanism in the regulation of CT activity.

In several cell types regulation of CT activity by diacylglycerols has been demonstrated,[293] but no convincing evidence exists for the fetal or adult lung.[239,256,272,294] The feedback inhibition of CT activity by increased PC in membranes[250,295-300] and the regulation of CT activity by altered membrane composition[300] may be very important mechanisms. Some evidence for them exists in type II cells.[301,302]

From recent experiments, it has become clear that the various mechanisms in the regulation of CT activity are closely interrelated. The precise role of these mechanisms and their interdependence has to be further investigated in the developing lung and isolated type II cells. Recent investigations show not only that the activity of CT is regulated, but also that CT protein expression is regulated at a pretranslational level in the type II cells of the developing lung.[254,279,303,304] The relative importance and the regulation of these mechanisms is not clear.

Other Regulatory Steps in Surfactant PC Synthesis

More controversy exists about a possible developmental regulation of the other two enzymes of the CDP-choline pathway—choline kinase and CDP-choline-1,2-diacylglycerol phosphocholinetransferase.[1,3,220] In most studies with whole lung of several species, including human lung, the choline kinase activity did not change, or even decrease, during the time of increased PC synthesis. In isolated rat fetal type II cells, no change in choline kinase activity was found during late gestation.[234] Most investigators found no developmental change in the activity of the phosphocholinetransferase, but some studies do report an increased activity, especially in the microsomal cell fraction, before term birth in several species.[1,3,220] In isolated rat fetal type II cells, no change of the activity of phosphocholinetransferase was found during late gestation when the activity was assayed with the use of endogenous diacylglycerols as substrate. However, a prenatal increase in activity was seen when the activity of phosphocholinetransferase was assayed in the presence of added exogenous diacylglycerols, suggesting a limitation in substrate for the enzyme.[234]

It has been reported that in type II cells only about half of the DSPC, the main surface tension lowering component of surfactant, is being synthesized directly by the de novo pathway using saturated diacylglycerols as precursors.[234,305] A considerable part of the disaturated species of PC is formed by remodeling of de novo synthesized unsaturated (in the 2-position) PC (Figure 28.3). The most important mechanism for this remodeling is a deacylation of PC at the 2-position by a phospholipase A$_2$ or by a transacylation with another phospholipid, followed by a reacylation step of the resulting lysophosphatidylcholine by the lysophosphatidylcholine acyltransferase (Figure 28.3).[1,2,20,220] The activity of the latter enzyme has been shown to be higher in type II cells than in whole lung, to increase during development, and to exhibit specificity toward palmitoyl–coenzyme A (CoA) as a substrate in fetal type II cells.[1,2,306]

As diacylglycerols are a necessary substrate for the enzyme phosphocholinetransferase during the process of PC synthesis (Figure 28.3), it is clear that the synthesis of these diacylglycerols needs to be regulated during the period of increased surfactant-associated PC synthesis. Zimmermann et al.[234] found an increased incorporation of radioactively labeled palmitate and glycerol into diacylglycerols in fetal rat type II cells before birth. Most likely there is a regulatory role for the enzyme phosphatidic acid phosphatase because of its key position in phospholipid synthesis (Figure 28.3). An increase in the activity of phosphatidic acid phosphatase in lung has been observed toward both aqueously dispersed phosphatidic acid and membrane-bound phosphatidic acid.[1,3,220] The membrane-bound substrate is probably more relevant during PC synthesis.

Role of Fatty Acid Synthesis in the Regulation of Perinatal PC Synthesis

Abundant evidence exists for an increase in fatty acid synthesis in fetal lung or isolated type II cells at the time of increased surfactant synthesis.[275] During normal lung development, fatty acids play at least two important roles in the de novo surfactant PC synthesis. Besides their role in regulating CT activity, fatty acids are a substrate for PC synthesis, and they are synthesized de novo by perinatal fetal type II cells at a high rate from a variety of substrates.[275]

The following observations point to the importance of de novo fatty acid synthesis for surfactant phospholipid formation in the perinatal period:[275,307] (1) In fetal rat lung the rate of fatty acid synthesis[308,309] and the specific activities of acetyl-CoA carboxylase[308,310] and fatty acid synthase[310,311] are increased in the period when surfactant production is accelerated. (2) Even in the presence of exogenous palmitate, inhibitors of fatty acid synthesis depress the rate of saturated PC formation in explants of fetal rat lung and isolated lung cells.[312,313] (3) In lungs of newborn rabbits, fatty acids synthesized from acetate are preferentially incorporated into saturated and total surfactant PC compared to exogenous palmitate.[314] All these findings support the importance of fatty acid synthesis in developing type II cells. These newly synthesized fatty acids play a role in the activation of cytosolic and microsomal CT, as described above. Weinhold et al.[276] found an increased amount of CT activity in lung microsomes shortly after birth in association with an increase in free fatty acid content in microsomes. Viscardi and McKenna[240] studied the fatty acid content of microsomal phospholipids in fetal and neonatal lung and showed an increase in these fatty acids together with increased microsomal CT activity. Free fatty acids were not measured. The increase of cytosolic H-form has been demonstrated in fetal lung following premature birth[238] and the role of free fatty acids has been shown in the transition of fetal to adult lung forms of cytosolic CT.[239,272] A progressive increase in cytosolic free fatty acids together with an increase in the H-form during lung development has not been demonstrated. Although free fatty acids can activate CT and possibly do so in the developing lung in vivo,[276] it is very possible that the activation of CT takes place after fatty acids have been incorporated into phospholipids or into diacylglycerols. The fact that free fatty acids can directly activate CT in different cells and do so in a reversible way, as shown by the addition of albumin,[276,281,315] within minutes,[281,316] would suggest a role for free fatty acids themselves. Furthermore, the role of free fatty acids in the activation of CT during hormonal stimulation, together with the importance of these hormones for lung development, would suggest a similar role for fatty acids during type II cell maturation.

Developmental Changes in Surfactant-Associated Proteins

From numerous investigations in the past decade it has become clear that the concentrations of all four surfactant-associated proteins increase during lung development. However, these changes seem to be regulated more or less independently for each protein[71,317-319] and to differ in several aspects from the changes in phospholipid content.[3] Concentrations of the surfactant-associated proteins during perinatal development have been measured by enzyme-linked immunosorbent assay (ELISA), especially for SP-A and SP-D, or estimated by immunohistochemistry. Their mRNAs have been quantified by Northern and dot blot analysis and by reverse-transcriptase polymerase chain reaction (PCR), estimated by in situ hybridization, or measured by solution hybridization analysis. In addition, information has been obtained from several animal species. From all these data, it is possible to extract the following general patterns:

SP-A can be detected in fetal rat lung on day 18[320] and in fetal rabbit lung on day 26 of gestation.[321] Thereafter, SP-A content increases rapidly until term, doubles in neonatal lung, then decreases somewhat and is subsequently increased severalfold in adult lung.[320-322] This pattern has been confirmed by immunohistochemistry analyses.[323-325] The developmental pattern of the levels of mRNA for SP-A correlates well with that of the SP-A protein content in rat[320,322,326-328] and rabbit lung.[137,329] With the use of sensitive techniques such as solution hybridization analysis, SP-A mRNA could be detected earlier, on day 22, during rabbit gestation but the pattern thereafter remained the same.[329] These findings suggest regulation of SP-A levels at the transcriptional level. In the baboon a similar pattern for SP-A mRNA was found, with the earliest detection at day 150.[330]

In the human lung the SP-A mRNA is low or almost undetectable by Northern or dot blot analysis until about 24 weeks' gestation.[331,332] However, with immunohistochemistry and in situ hybridization the SP-A and its mRNA were detected earlier in gestation.[153,333] In human amniotic fluid, small quantities of SP-A are detectable at around 20 weeks' gestation, with a gradual increase during the early third trimester.[334,335] From about 32 weeks SP-A is easily detected in amniotic fluid and the concentration increases rapidly from around 33 to 37 weeks toward term. This pattern very much resembles that of the surfactant-associated phospholipids.[336]

Messenger RNA for SP-C was detectable by Northern blot analysis on day 17 of gestation in the rat before the time when clearly recognizable type II cells with their lamellar bodies are present.[326] Low levels of SP-B mRNA were first found at day 18 of rat gestation. After day 18 the levels of SP-B and SP-C mRNAs increased dramatically toward day 21 and reached values similar to the adult levels at term.[326] Shimizu et al.[322] described a perinatal increase in SP-B with a peak occurring a few days after birth. In the rabbit similar patterns are observed compared to the rat, with the mRNA for SP-C first detected by Northern blot on day 22 of gestation and SP-B mRNA on day 26.[329,337] However, as for SP-A, SP-B mRNA could be detected in very low levels by more sensitive techniques on day 22 of rabbit gestation.[329] In baboons SP-B and SP-C mRNA were detected at 140 days' gestation and increased toward term.[330]

In the human lung, SP-B and SP-C mRNAs could be detected by Northern blot analysis as early as 13 weeks' gestation,[331] and the levels of these mRNAs increased between gestational weeks 16 and 20.[338] However, the mRNA levels for SP-B and SP-C were at these gestational ages much lower than in the adult lung.[338]

Only a few studies are available that describe the developmental pattern of SP-D. In the rat, the levels of SP-D mRNA and protein are low until late gestation, but as for SP-A a marked increase was found toward term and directly thereafter.[328,339] Then, SP-D concentrations remained fairly constant until adulthood.

In general, the content of all surfactant-associated proteins is high around term gestation, preparing the fetus for air breathing after birth. SP-A increased further into adulthood, but as is well established, SP-A appears to have a broader spectrum of functions such as an important role in lung defense (supra vide).

Hormonal Regulation of Surfactant Phospholipid and Protein Synthesis

Since the focus has been on the developmental aspects of the surfactant system, the role of hormonal regulation will be only briefly considered. For more detailed coverage of this topic the reader is referred to several excellent reviews.[1,220,241,318,336,340]

Corticosteroids: General Effects

Because of the important clinical consequences of the regulation of surfactant synthesis, and lung development in general, by corticosteroids, some experimental background is needed. Glucocorticoids have major effects on lung maturation and the maturation of several other organs in the immature fetus. The effects of exogenously administered corticosteroids on lung have been demonstrated in several animal species. They include improved pulmonary function or better surface tension properties, enhanced amounts of surfactant-associated phospholipids, accelerated morphologic maturity, and improved clinical parameters or survival of the animals.[241] The morphologic maturation of the lung is functionally probably even more important than the stimulation of surfactant synthesis. Not only exogenously administered corticosteroids but also endogenous fetal corticosteroids can stimulate lung maturation and surfactant synthesis and may play a very important role during normal lung maturation at the end of gestation (supra vide). This physiologic role of glucocorticosteroids during normal lung development is suggested by three types of evidence:[241] (1) temporal associations between fetal corticosteroid concentrations and lung maturation in several species, including humans, since the steroid concentration rises at the time of the increase in pulmonary surfactant;[341-346] (2) endocrine ablation studies in animals or the human anencephalic patient in which there is delayed lung maturation and a low cortisol concentration[347,348] and in decapitated fetal rats[349,350] or after chemical adrenalectomy;[351-353] and (3) the demonstration of specific receptors for corticosteroids in fetal lungs, including human fetal lungs, suggesting that fetal lung is a specific physiologic target tissue for corticosteroids.[354-359]

Corticosteroids: Effects on Surfactant PC Synthesis

In many studies corticosteroids have been shown to increase the amount of surfactant-associated phospholipids in fetal lung lavage and to enhance the incorporation of precursors into PC and PG in lung slices and lung explants.[1,220,241] The activities of many enzymes involved in the synthesis of PC (Figure 28.3) have been found to be increased by corticosteroids in animal experiments in vivo or in vitro.[1,220,241] Some of these findings are contradictory, which may be explained by the use of different animal species or experimental protocols. However, a definite role for CT, a rate regulatory enzyme in the synthesis of PC, seems to have been established. Studies with isolated type II cells[242,243] and mixed fetal lung cells[244] showed that the effect of corticosteroids on PC synthesis is most likely mediated through an activation of CT. Fatty acids may play a very important role in this activation of CT by corticosteroids as suggested from the following evidence:

First, fatty acid synthesis is regulated by corticosteroids. Dexamethasone has been shown to accelerate the normal developmental increase in fetal lung fatty acid synthesis in vivo and in vitro[309,360,361] and to enhance the activity of fatty acid synthase in fetal lung tissue.[311,360,362,363] Batenburg et al.[279,310] have demonstrated this in isolated fetal type II cells and have stressed that type II cell-fibroblast interactions are important in modulating the effect of hormones, not only on PC synthesis,[241-243,278] but also on fatty acid synthesis.[279,310] The effect of dexamethasone on fatty acid synthase activity in cultured fetal lung is due to enzyme induction[362] and is regulated at a pretranslational level.[279,303,364] Second, measurement of CT protein in fetal lung by immunotitration[251] and Western blotting[246] confirmed that CT enzyme mass is not increased by glucocorticoids. Earlier investigations suggested an activation of the enzyme instead of an increased enzyme mass, because the stimulatory effects of glucocorticoids could be severely diminished or abolished by assaying CT in the presence of lipid activators.[25,246,251,365,366] Third and most important, inhibitors of de novo fatty acid synthesis, which act at steps in the pathway prior to those catalyzed by fatty acid synthase, abolished the stimulatory effect of dexamethasone on CT activity in fetal rat lung explants.[365] The similar time course of fatty acid synthase and CT activity in these fetal rat lung explants cultured in the presence of dexamethasone further supports the importance of increased fatty acid synthesis through increased fatty acid synthase activity in the regulation of CT activity.[365] The role of a fatty acid–mediated activation of CT by corticosteroids has been further confirmed by the in vivo experiments performed by Mallampalli et al.[271] Maternal administration of betamethasone increased the total amount of free fatty acids associated with the cytosolic H-form (i.e., the high molecular weight form of CT, which is active) by 62%[271] in association with increased CT activity caused by a conversion of the L-form (i.e., low molecular weight form of CT, which has a low activity) to the H-form.[246,271] This finding supports a direct role for free fatty acids, but an effect of fatty acids after incorporation into (phospho) lipids or diacylglycerols cannot be excluded.

Taken together, the investigations support the following sequence for normal development: (1) exogenous or endogenous corticosteroids induce the production of fibroblast-pneumocyte factor (FPF) in lung fibroblasts adjacent to the alveolar epithelial cells[210] at a pretranslational level;[278] (2) FPF induces fatty acid synthase and other enzymes involved in fatty acid synthesis in fetal type II cells at a pretranslational level;[279] (3) this leads to an increase in fatty acid biosynthesis, and fatty acids, their metabolites, or lipids into which they become incorporated ultimately activate CT[25] by increasing the cytosolic H-form and possibly by translocation of CT from cytosol to microsomes. Studies by Zimmermann,[255] who used a rat model for congenital diaphragmatic hernia, demonstrated that this sequence can be disturbed by an abnormal lung development and reinforced the idea that it is at least as important to study mesenchyme and epithelial-mesenchymal interactions as it is to study epithelial cell functions. Several other hormones such as thyroid hormones, insulin and sex hormones, and several growth factors such as epidermal growth factor (EGF) and transforming growth factor-β (TGF-β) have been shown to influence this sequence of events either by influencing the production of FPF in lung fibroblasts or by modulating the effect of FPF on fetal type II cells.[241] That such regulatory mechanisms are important not only in cell culture or organ culture systems but also in clinical practice is illustrated by the success of the prenatal use of corticosteroids to prevent respiratory distress syndrome in premature neonates.[367,368] The recent suggestion to use antenatal corticosteroids and thyrotropin-releasing hormone for lung maturation in congenital diaphragmatic hernia[369] originates from laboratory data showing lung immaturity in different models of congenital diaphragmatic hernia.

It is clear that a better understanding of the mechanisms of regulation of surfactant PC synthesis can lead to more specific therapies. It has become commonplace to use antenatal corticosteroid therapy for women at risk of premature delivery. Recently, guidelines for the use of antenatal corticosteroids were prepared by the National Institutes of Health (NIH) Consensus Conference.[370] The benefits of antenatal administration of corticosteroids to fetuses at risk of preterm delivery vastly outweigh the potential risks. These benefits include not only a reduction in the risk of RDS but also a substantial reduction in mortality and intraventricular hemorrhage (IVH). All fetuses between 24 and 34 weeks' gestation at risk of preterm delivery should be considered candidates for antenatal treatment with corticosteroids.[370] These guidelines clearly take into account that corticosteroids not only stimulate surfactant synthesis but have a much wider spectrum of beneficial effects, such as the structural maturation of the lungs, brain, and other organs. New studies, many of them in progress, will further clarify the optimal dosing of corticosteroids, the possible benefit of repeating the dosing schedule after 1 or 2 weeks, the duration of the beneficial effect, and the possible benefit of direct fetal administration.

Effect of Corticosteroids on Surfactant-Associated Proteins

Maternal treatment with corticosteroids can increase the SP-A content of the fetal lungs. This effect is not straightforward and depends on several factors such as the dose, the length of treatment, and the duration of gestation, with the best effect being observed after day 18 of gestation in the rat.[371,372] Gross et al.[373] demonstrated that corticosteroids accelerate rather than initiate the formation of SP-A mRNA. Neonatal treatment with corticosteroids or treatment of the adult rat also increases SP-A or SP-A mRNA.[372–375] The effects of corticosteroids on SP-A seem to be both translational and pretranslational, as mRNA levels do not change in relation to the SP-A protein concentration.[327,374,376]

In human lung explants, corticosteroids have a biphasic dose response, with a low concentration being stimulatory on SP-A protein and its mRNA and high concentrations (i.e., 10^{-7} M or higher) being inhibitory.[377,378] Kari et al.[379] demonstrated that prenatal dexamethasone improved the surface activity of surfactant isolated from airway specimens of preterm neonates and tended to increase the ratio of SP-A to PC among recipients of exogenous surfactant. When dexamethasone was given postnatally to preterm neonates at risk for chronic lung disease, it transiently increased the concentration of SP-A in airway specimens.[380]

In fetal, neonatal, and adult rat lung, corticosteroids increase the mRNA levels for SP-B and SP-C,[322,327,374,381] and the effect is most pronounced on days 18 and 19 of gestation.[322,381] Also SP-B protein has been shown to increase after corticosteroids.[322,381] An increase in mRNAs for SP-B and SP-C after maternal administration of corticosteroids was also demonstrated in rabbits. SP-B and SP-C mRNAs were elevated in fetal human lung explants[331,338] and human lung adenocarcinoma cell lines[382,383] exposed to glucocorticosteroids.

Effects of Other Hormones

It is well known that several hormones and growth factors have an important role in lung maturation, and have effects on surfactant synthesis and/or turnover. β-Adrenergic agents have no important effects on surfactant PC synthesis, but stimulate surfactant secretion[384–388] from the type II cells into the alveolar space. They have important effects on fluid and ion transport across the alveolar barrier.[389] Many hormones that influence PC synthesis such as thyroid hormones, insulin and sex hormones, and several growth factors such as EGF and TGF-β have been shown to influence the sequence of events leading to increased PC synthesis by activation of

CT, either by influencing the production of FPF in lung fibroblasts or by modulating the effect of FPF on fetal type II cells.[241]

The increased incidence of RDS in neonates born to women with diabetes[223] can also be explained, at least in part, by the insulin inhibition of the glucocorticoid-induced production of FPF by fetal lung fibroblasts.[241] The antenatal administration of thyrotropin-releasing hormone (TRH) in combination with corticosteroids to accelerate lung maturity[390-392] originates from the insight gained from culture work and subsequent animal studies.[241]

Currently, hormones other than corticosteroids that increase lung maturation are being studied clinically. Thyroid hormones are known to accelerate fetal lung maturation in animal studies. However, the thyroid hormones T_3 and T_4 do not cross the placenta. This problem has been circumvented by maternal administration of TRH, which, via an increase in thyroid hormones, seems to have some theoretical disadvantages in that it inhibits maturation of antioxidant enzymes, at least in the rat, it does not stimulate or even inhibit surfactant protein production, and it inhibits fatty acid synthesis.[241] Clinical studies with maternal administration of a combination of TRH and corticosteroids suggested a slight advantage over corticosteroids alone in the prevention of bronchopulmonary dysplasia.[390,391] A recent multicenter trial found a worse outcome after prenatal corticosteroids and TRH compared to corticosteroids alone.[392] Further studies are required before this therapy can be generally recommended.

There appears to be a difference in the rate of lung maturation between the female and the male. In the human, the difference between the acceleration in lung maturation and surfactant synthesis is about 1 week. Male premature neonates have a higher incidence of respiratory distress syndrome[393] and a higher mortality with RDS[394] than female neonates. Sex differences in surfactant production have also been reported in several animal species.[1,220,241] This difference appears to be the result of a combination of the female advantage (i.e., estrogens stimulate PC synthesis and lung maturation) and the male disadvantage (i.e., androgens inhibit PC synthesis).[241]

The Importance of Surfactant Metabolism for Therapy of Surfactant Deficiency

The Pool Size of Surfactant Phosphatidylcholine at Birth and During Postnatal Development

As discussed above, surfactant synthesis increases with advancing gestation. From approximately 20 weeks' gestation in the human, surfactant accumulates within the primitive type II cells. Significant secretion from the type II cells into the alveolar space does not occur until approximately 34 to 35 weeks. Surfactant can be detected in the amniotic fluid and can be used as a measure of fetal pulmonary maturity. The alveolar pool size of surfactant is difficult to measure in the human. From animal studies in monkey,[395] it is known that the alveolar surfactant pool is about $100\,mg\cdot kg^{-1}$ at term. Adult animals, however, have an alveolar pool size of about 5 to $15\,mg\cdot kg^{-1}$. In several preterm animal models with RDS (rabbit, sheep and monkey) the amount of surfactant in alveolar washes was about $5\,mg\cdot kg^{-1}$. In the preterm monkey an increase in pool size was found from day 1 to days 3 to 4 when a concentration of more than $60\,mg\cdot kg^{-1}$ was measured. Thus, although secretory pathways are intact in the premature animal, the de novo synthesis is initially insufficient, but accelerates in the first few days after birth. This increase correlates with the well-known clinical improvement of RDS after 48 to 72 hours of life. In the human neonate with RDS similar but less reliable pool sizes of alveolar surfactant have been reported. Adams et al.[396] measured around $5\,mg\cdot kg^{-1}$ of surfactant in alveolar washes of neonates with RDS who had died. Hallman et al.[397] used PG as a marker to measure the surfactant phospholipid pool. As had been demonstrated earlier, the amount of PG was below the detection limit in tracheal aspirates of neonates with RDS. When such neonates were treated with a known amount of exogenous surfactant containing PG, the phospholipid pool size could be calculated from the dilution of PG, as measured in tracheal aspirates. A pool size of $<10\,mg\cdot kg^{-1}$ was reported. As phospholipids are taken up by type II cells and re-secreted (i.e., recycling), the pool size measured consists of the alveolar and cellular compartment together.

No reliable data exist relative to the change of the surfactant pool size after birth in the human. However, several recent investigations measured PC concentration in tracheal aspirates during the first few days of life in neonates with RDS. These PC concentrations can be expressed in different ways, depending on the denominator used. Commonly used are PC concentration per milliliter aspirate, which is dependent on the amount suctioned and the dilution with normal saline, or per milligram albumin or total protein, which is influenced by leakage of proteins into the alveoli in damaged immature lungs, or corrected for the sphingomyelin concentration (L/S ratio) or for total phospholipid concentration, reflecting composition more than amount of surfactant. The two most promising ways of expressing PC concentration seem to be the correction for dilution with the urea method and the use of the secretory component of immunoglobulin A (SC-IgA) as a reference protein. There is little experience so far with the use of SC-IgA as a correction for PC concentration in tracheal aspirates.[398] In the urea method there is the advantage that the urea concentrations in plasma and alveolar fluid are equal. Thus, PC concentration in tracheal aspirates is multiplied by $[urea]_{serum}/[urea]_{aspirate}$ to calculate the concentration of PC in epithelial lining fluid (ELF). Although this method has some flaws, it is simple and correlates quite well with data obtained from alveolar washes.[399] Hallman et al.[399] demonstrated a low $[PC]_{ELF}$ in tracheal aspirates of neonates with RDS on day 1 of a mean <1 mM compared to 6.1 mM in neonates without RDS, and an increase of $[PC]_{ELF}$ from day 1 to day 4 to concentrations comparable to those of neonates without RDS. These data are consistent with clinical improvement of RDS after 2 to 3 days and with animal data.

Bunt et al.[400] measured the fractional synthesis rate of palmitate in surfactant PC by infusing stable isotope labeled [U-^{13}C]glucose on the day of birth in six neonates with severe RDS treated with exogenous surfactant. Sequential tracheal aspirates were collected and analyzed. The label appeared in surfactant PC palmitate after about 20 hours and peaked at about 70 hours. The fractional synthesis rate from glucose was 5% of the palmitate PC pool per day, which was in absolute amounts estimated to be about $4 mg \cdot kg^{-1} \cdot d^{-1}$ of surfactant PC synthesis. These data are consistent with a low surfactant synthesis and an increase in surfactant pools after a few days.

The Initial Dose

Premature neonates with RDS have a relative surfactant deficiency ($5 mg \cdot dl^{-1}$) compared to term infants ($100 mg \cdot dl^{-1}$) and this deficiency temporarily lasts about 4 days. It seems logical to treat neonates with RDS once with exogenous surfactant at a dose of approximately $100 mg \cdot dl^{-1}$ to overcome the critical period when there is not yet enough surfactant synthesis. Indeed, in clinical trials with natural surfactants an initial surfactant dose of around $100 mg \cdot dl^{-1}$ body weight was optimal.[401] In a study with Alveofact, $100 mg \cdot dl^{-1}$ turned out to give better results than $50 mg \cdot dl^{-1}$. Similarly surfactant TA at a dose of $120 mg \cdot dl^{-1}$ did better than $60 mg \cdot dl^{-1}$.[402] Clinical trials with Curosurf, a porcine lung surfactant, suggest that $200 mg \cdot dl^{-1}$ is not better than $100 mg \cdot dl^{-1}$.

Prophylaxis or Rescue Treatment

From a theoretical point of view, prophylactic treatment before the first breath of neonates at risk for developing RDS is best. Surfactant deficiency exists immediately after birth and lung damage is initiated fast once alveolar collapse is allowed to occur. The distribution of surfactant in the lungs will be better if surfactant is administered soon after birth. However, surfactant treatment may interfere with initial delivery room resuscitation of the neonate. This may be a disadvantage, especially if the neonate was not surfactant deficient. Therefore, an argument can be made for the administration of surfactant after stabilization in the more controlled environment of the neonatal intensive care unit (NICU) and once early signs of RDS are present. This is known as rescue treatment. A few studies have directly compared prophylaxis with rescue treatment in a randomized way.[13] The results are somewhat contradictory, but overall no advantage of prophylaxis was found compared to rescue therapy. Using subgroup analysis, two investigations suggested that the smallest neonates (<26 weeks) who are at the highest risk of developing RDS may benefit from prophylactic surfactant treatment. Another interesting finding was revealed in the large OSIRIS trial,[403] which compared randomly 1344 neonates judged to be at high risk for RDS and treated before 2 hours of age with 1346 neonates who received surfactant treatment only when symptoms of RDS developed at a mean age of about 3 hours. A significant difference in death or oxygen dependency at term date was found favoring the early treatment. From these data together with animal data that show lung damage from RDS within a few hours, we conclude that prophylactic therapy does not seem to be necessary, except maybe for the smallest neonates. When rescue therapy is used, it should be used early, as soon as clinical signs of RDS appear, preferably before 2 hours of age.

Recycling of Surfactant Phosphatidylcholine After Surfactant Therapy

Studies with animals have suggested that in adults surfactant PC is recycled with an efficiency of about 50%.[395,404] In the term newborn animal, recycling efficiency is much higher (i.e., about 90–95%). De novo synthesis and catabolism of PC are very low compared to recycling. Surfactant PC remains in the lung. The metabolism of saturated PC was very similar in the lungs of preterm animals.[395,404] Studies with intravenously injected labeled precursors showed that there was a long time from synthesis to secretion of surfactant PC. When a tracer dose of radiolabeled surfactant PC was injected into the airways of preterm lambs, 40% became rapidly "lung associated" and could not be recovered from the alveolar wash. By 24 hours, about 80% was lung associated, probably because of uptake/recycling. However, almost 100% of the label could be recovered from a combined alveolar wash and lung tissue together. A turnover time of approximately 13 hours was calculated for alveolar PC in these preterm lambs. The turnover time for the total surfactant pool, including lamellar bodies, was several times longer. When radiolabeled treatment doses of surfactant ($100 mg \cdot dl^{-1}$) were used instead of tracer doses, the results were not different in these preterm lambs, despite a large increase in the surfactant pool.[395,404] Sixty percent of the label became quickly lung associated, and after 24 hours about 20% could be recovered from the alveolar wash. However, little of the label disappeared from the lung. That recycling takes place was demonstrated by the intratracheal injection of labeled lyso-PC, which was converted to PC and could be recovered from the alveolar wash. Again, adult animals may behave differently. In adult rabbits the clearance of surfactant was increased up to fivefold proportionally to the surfactant dose administered.[395,404]

Little information regarding surfactant PC metabolism in the human neonate is available. The few data that are available seem to be consistent with the animal data. The half-life of surfactant DPPC was studied by Hallman et al.[401] with the use of deuterium-labeled DPPC, which was mixed with the surfactant administered endotracheally. The half-life of DPPC was 39 to 59 hours. Bunt et al.[400] studied fatty acid composition of PC from tracheal aspirates of neonates with RDS who received surfactant. Fatty acids in PC consisted of 60% to 65% of palmitic acid before surfactant therapy. After treatment with Survanta, palmitic acid was 85%. The return to baseline composition occurred exponentially and allowed calculation of a half-life of 76 hours in four patients.[400] In the earlier mentioned studies with [U-^{13}C]glucose as a substrate for PC synthesis, Bunt et al.[400] estimated that the half-life of surfactant PC palmitate was 96 hours.

All these data are interpreted to suggest low synthesis and clearance rates for surfactant PC in the human neonate with RDS, a conclusion compatible with data from animal investigations.

Individual Response and the Transient Effect in Surfactant Therapy

If the exogenous surfactant remains in the lung and disappears with a half-life of more than 50 hours, then one dose of $100 mg \cdot dl^{-1}$ surfactant should be enough to cover the entire period from birth until the endogenous synthesis occurs. However, primary surfactant deficiency is not the only factor that plays a role in RDS. In the premature neonate with RDS, the lungs are structurally immature and will be damaged by asphyxia, infection, ventilation, and high oxygen concentrations, especially because the antioxidant systems are also immature. Surfactant function can be inhibited by several proteins that leak into the alveolar space, and surfactant can be inactivated by oxygen radicals and enzymes or by transformation into small vesicular surfactant forms. There is individual variability in the way neonates respond to surfactant treatment. Charon et al.[405] found that gross maldistribution of surfactant did not explain the variability in clinical response to surfactant therapy. We found a good to mild initial response in 86% of neonates, but about one third had a relapse with a worsening clinical condition. As was found by Charon et al.[405] a poor initial response to surfactant was associated with other factors such as asphyxia, infection, and patent ductus arteriosus. Before, but also after, surfactant therapy, there was a negative correlation between the concentration of PC in tracheal aspirates and the oxygen need. Hallman et al.[399] reported similar findings. Several studies have demonstrated a benefit of more than one dose of surfactant over a single dose.[406,407] It is not clear yet that more than two doses are beneficial. In the OSIRIS trial with Exosurf no difference in outcome was demonstrated between two and up to four doses.[403] We also did not find any difference in biochemical parameters (e.g., PC and surface tension lowering capacities in tracheal aspirates) or outcome in 49 infants with RDS randomized to either two or up to four doses of Survanta.[408]

In conclusion, the amount of surfactant that remains in the alveolar compartment in an active form after one dose of surfactant is not always enough to cope with such factors as surfactant inhibition and inactivation, but there is a limit to the additional effect of extra doses of surfactant. Further studies are required to understand the precise factors and their mechanisms that play a role in the response and effective duration of surfactant therapy.

Conclusions and Perspectives

In the past decade there has been spectacular development in both basic research on the pulmonary surfactant system and the clinical use of surfactant for treatment of neonatal RDS. In particular, knowledge of the molecular biology and physiologic roles of the four surfactant-associated proteins has expanded exponentially. It has been established that at least three of these proteins, the hydrophobic proteins SP-B and SP-C and the major hydrophilic protein SP-A, play crucial roles in the generation and maintenance of the surface film at the air-water interface. Several groups are currently modifying these proteins, either chemically or by site-directed mutagenesis, in order to study the consequences of such alterations for their functioning. Increasing evidence is becoming available that the hydrophilic surfactant proteins SP-A and SP-D may play an essential role in the innate defense system of the lungs. So far much of this evidence has been obtained in studies in vitro. Undoubtedly, knockout experiments with transgenic mice and studies with animal models for a variety of infectious diseases will be performed to further support a role of the hydrophilic surfactant proteins in lung defense.

Although the lung has no major functions before birth, its almost complete morphologic and biochemical development and maturation before birth is essential for survival immediately after birth. Adequate gas exchange is only possible from the beginning of the terminal saccular period of lung development, which is around 24 weeks in the human. From that time on, it is possible to recognize alveolar type II cells with their typical lamellar bodies. Maturation of the surfactant system takes place during this period of lung development with a rapid increase later in gestation, from 32 to 34 weeks until term and in the early neonatal period. The maturation occurs slightly earlier in females than in males. The content of glycogen increases in the type II cells and decreases again during the period of maximal surfactant synthesis. At the end of gestation there is a dramatic increase in the amount of surfactant phospholipids produced by the type II cells. The amount of PC increases up to 30-fold in lamellar bodies and lung lavage material. At the same time the percentage of saturated PC increases and an important change takes place in the composition of acidic phospholipids in the lung: the relative amount of PG increases, and PI decreases. The functional significance of this switch is not completely understood. The large changes in the concentration of surfactant-associated phospholipids are a reflection of increased biosynthesis and secretion of phospholipids by the alveolar type II cells.

Many investigations have demonstrated increased incorporation rates of radioactive precursors into phospholipids and especially into PC in fetal lung and isolated type II cells toward the end of gestation. The increased synthesis in surfactant phospholipids can be explained by an increase in the activities of the enzymes responsible for their synthesis. CTP-phosphocholine cytidylyltransferase (CT) has been shown to catalyze a rate-limiting step in the CDP-choline pathway, the primary pathway for de novo PC synthesis. The activity of this enzyme increases at the time of maximal surfactant PC synthesis. Recently, the purification of CT, the availability of antibodies against CT, and the cloning of cDNA for CT have made an important contribution to the progress in the understanding of the regulation of CT activity. Recent studies show not only that the activity of CT is regulated, but also that CT protein expression is regulated at a pretranslational level in the II cells of the developing lung.[254,279,303,304] The relative importance and the regulation of these mechanisms will be investigated in the future. It is expected that the gene sequence for CT will be determined, which will make it much easier to study the regulation of gene expression. Structure-function relationships will be further investigated with the help of site-directed mutagenesis and transgenic animals. New laboratory techniques will help to resolve the question of the recently suggested and intriguing possibility of the channeling of intermediates of the CDP-choline pathway from one enzyme to the next.[293,409,410] The role of the cytoskeleton in this channeling will be further examined.[293,410,411]

These new insights into the mechanisms of regulation of CT activity will lead to therapeutic implications.

Currently the use of prenatal corticosteroids is the treatment of choice for women at risk of premature delivery. Prenatal corticosteroids have been shown to increase fetal surfactant PC synthesis, and they do so via an intercellular interaction between lung fibroblasts and type II cells, which results in increased CT activity within the type II cells. The optimal schedule for prenatal treatment with corticosteroids and possibly other hormones or growth factors is a topic of investigation. All four surfactant-associated proteins increase during gestation and attain high concentrations at term gestation, but the exact timing and regulation of each of the proteins is variable. Corticosteroids, and other hormones, also influence the levels of the surfactant-associated proteins.

The increased synthesis at the end of gestation leads to an alveolar surfactant pool size of about $100\,\text{mg}\cdot\text{dl}^{-1}$ at term gestation. However, in preterm animals and in preterm neonates with RDS the surfactant pool size is only around $5\,\text{mg}\cdot\text{dl}^{-1}$. No reliable data exist for the changes in surfactant pool size after birth in the human. However, comparisons with animal data, measurements of surfactant PC concentrations in tracheal aspirates, and new studies of surfactant synthesis with stable isotopes all point to a significant increase in surfactant pool size over the first few days after birth. Because of the surfactant deficiency during these first few days in preterm neonates with RDS, surfactant replacement therapy with a dose of around $100\,\text{mg}\cdot\text{dl}^{-1}$ should be theoretically useful and has now been proven to be clinically successful. Delivery room prophylaxis with surfactant does not seem to be superior to early (i.e., preferably <2 hours after birth) rescue treatment of RDS, except maybe for the most premature neonates. Although the disappearance of endogenous and exogenous surfactant from the lungs is very slow with a half-life >2 days, it is frequently indicated to give more than one dose of exogenous surfactant to preterm neonates with RDS. Unfortunately, the response to surfactant is not always optimal. This can be explained by other factors such as structurally immature lungs and damage to the lungs by asphyxia, infection, ventilation, and oxygen-radicals. It is clear that more insight into the influence of such factors on surfactant function and metabolism should help the clinician to develop better therapeutic regimens and improve outcome of preterm neonates with RDS.

Acknowledgments. This work is supported by the Netherlands Foundation for Chemical Research, with financial aid from the Netherlands Organization for Scientific Research (NWO) and the Dutch Asthma Foundation (Nederlands Astma Fonds) (to L.M.G. van Golde) and by the Sophia Foundation for Medical Research (to L.J.I. Zimmermann).

References

1. Post M, Van Golde LMG. Metabolic and developmental aspects of pulmonary surfactant system. Biochim Biophys Acta 1988;947:249–286.
2. Batenburg JJ. Surfactant phospholipids: synthesis and storage. Am J Physiol 1992;262:L367–385.
3. Cockshutt AM, Possmayer F. Metabolism of surfactant lipids and proteins in the developing lung. In: Robertson B, van Golde LMG, Batenburg JJ, eds. Pulmonary surfactant: from molecular biology to clinical practice. Amsterdam: Elsevier, 1992:339–377.
4. Clements JA. Function of the alveolar lining. Am Rev Respir Dis 1979;115:67–71.
5. Van Golde LMG, Batenburg JJ, Robertson B. The pulmonary surfactant system: biochemical aspects and functional significance. Physiol Rev 1988;68:374–455.
6. Van Golde LMG, Batenburg JJ, Robertson B. The pulmonary surfactant system. News Physiol Sci 1994;9:13–20.
7. Enhorning G. Pulmonary surfactant function in alveoli and conducting airways. Can Respir J 1996;3:21–27.
8. Van Golde LMG. Potential role of surfactant proteins A and D in innate lung defense against pathogens. Biol Neonate 1995;67(suppl):2–17.
9. Pison U, Max M, Neuendank A, et al. Host defence capacities of pulmonary surfactant: evidence for "nonsurfactant" functions of the surfactant system. Eur J Clin Invest 1994;24:586–599.
10. Phelps DS. Pulmonary surfactant modulation of host-defense function. Appl Cardiopulmon Pathophysiol 1995;5:221–229.
11. Avery ME, Mead J. Surface properties in relation to atelectasis and hyaline membrane disease. Am J Dis Child 1959;97:517–523.
12. Walther FJ, Taeusch HW. Pathophysiology of neonatal surfactant insufficiency: clinical aspects. In: Robertson B, van Golde LMG, Batenburg JJ, eds. Pulmonary surfactant: from molecular biology to clinical practice. Amsterdam: Elsevier, 1992:485–523.
13. Jobe AH. Pulmonary surfactant therapy. N Engl J Med 1993;328:861–868.
14. Soll RF. Clinical trials of surfactant therapy in the newborn. In: Robertson B, Taeusch HW, eds. Surfactant therapy for lung diseases. New York: Marcel Dekker, 1995:407–442.
15. Possmayer F. A proposed nomenclature for pulmonary surfactant-associated proteins. Am Rev Respir Dis 1988;138:990–998.
16. Chevalier G, Collet AJ. In vivo incorporation of choline-3H, leucine-3H and galactose-3H in alveolar type II pneumocytes in relation to surfactant synthesis. A quantitative radioautographic study in mouse by electron microscopy. Anat Rec 1972;174:289–310.
17. Voorhout WF, Veenendaal T, Haagsman HP, et al. Intracellular processing of pulmonary surfactant protein B in an endosomal-lysosomal compartment. Am J Physiol 1992;263:L479–486.
18. Voorhout WF, Weaver TE, Haagsman HP, et al. Biosynthetic routing of pulmonary surfactant proteins in alveolar type II cells. Microsc Res Techn 1993;26:366–373.
19. Vorbroker DK, Voorhout WF, Weaver TE, et al. Post-translational processing of surfactant protein C in rat type II cells. Am J Physiol 1995;13:L727–733.
20. Van Golde LMG, Casals C. Metabolism of lipids. In: Crystal RG, West JB, Weibel E, Barnes PJ, eds. The lung. 2nd ed. Philadelphia: Lippincott-Raven, 1996:9–18.
21. Schlame M, Casals C, Rüstow B, et al. Molecular species of phosphatidylcholine and phosphatidylglycerol in rat lung surfactant and different pools of pneumocytes type II. Biochem J 1988;253:209–215.
22. Chander A, Fisher AB. Regulation of surfactant secretion. Am J Physiol 1990;258:L241–253.
23. Wright JR, Dobbs LG. Regulation of pulmonary surfactant secretion and clearance. Annu Rev Physiol 1991;53:395–414.
24. Mason RJ. Surfactant secretion. In: Robertson B, van Golde LMG, Batenburg JJ, eds. Pulmonary surfactant: from molecular biology to clinical practice. Amsterdam: Elsevier, 1992:295–312.
25. Rooney SA, Young SL, Mendelson CR. Molecular and cellular processing of lung surfactant. FASEB J 1994;8:957–967.
26. Oosterlaken-Dijksterhuis MA, van Eijk M, van Buel BLM, et al. Surfactant protein composition of lamellar bodies isolated from rat lung. Biochem J 1991;274:115–119.
27. Baritussio A, Alberti A, Quaglino D, et al. SP-A, SP-B, and SP-C in surfactant subtypes around birth: reexamination of alveolar life cycle of surfactant. Am J Physiol 1994;266:L436–447.
28. Voorhout WF, Veenendaal T, Haagsman HP, et al. Surfactant protein A is localized at the corners of the pulmonary tubular myelin lattice. J Histochem Cytochem 1991;39:1331–1336.
29. Doyle JR, Barr HA, Nicholas TE. Distribution of surfactant protein A in rat lung. Am J Respir Cell Mol Biol 1994;11:405–415.
30. Henry M, Ikegami M, Ueda T, et al. Surfactant protein B metabolism in newborn rabbits. Biochim Biophys Acta 1996;1300:97–102.
31. Ikegami M, Lewis JF, Tabor B, et al. Surfactant protein A metabolism in preterm ventilated lambs. Am J Physiol 1992;262:L765–772.
32. Ikegami M, Ueda T, Purtell J, et al. Surfactant protein A labeling kinetics in newborn and adult rabbits. Am J Respir Cell Mol Biol 1994;10:413–418.
33. Rice WR, Ross GF, Singleton FM, et al. Surfactant-associated protein inhibits phospholipid secretion from type II cells. J Appl Physiol 1987;63:692–698.
34. Dobbs LG, Wright JR, Hawgood S, et al. Pulmonary surfactant and its components inhibit secretion of phosphatidylcholine from cultured rat alveolar type II cells. Proc Natl Acad Sci USA 1987;84:1010–1014.
35. Bastacky J, Lee CYC, Goerke J, et al. Alveolar lining liquid layer is thin and continuous: low-temperature scanning electron microscopy of rat lung. J Appl Physiol 1995;79:1615–1628.
36. Wright JR, Clements JA. Metabolism and turnover of lung surfactant. Am Rev Respir Dis 1987;136:426–444.

37. Wright JR. Clearance and recycling of pulmonary surfactant. Am J Physiol 1990;259:L1–L12.
38. Notter RH, Penney DP, Finkelstein JN, et al. Adsorption of natural lung surfactant and phospholipid extracts related to tubular myelin formation. Pediatr Res 1986;20:97–101.
39. Breslin JS, Weaver TE. Binding, uptake, and localization of surfactant protein B in isolated rat alveolar type II cells. Am J Physiol 1992;262:L699–707.
40. Young SL, Fram EK, Larson E, et al. Recycling of surfactant lipid and apoprotein-A studied by electron microscopic autoradiography. Am J Physiol 1993;265:L19–26.
41. Pinto RA, Hawgood S, Clements JA, et al. Association of surfactant protein C with isolated alveolar type II cells. Biochim Biophys Acta 1995;1255:16–22.
42. Ueda T, Ikegami M, Jobe AH. Clearance of surfactant protein A from rabbit lungs. Am J Respir Cell Mol Biol 1995;12:89–94.
43. Ueda T, Ikegami M, Henry M, et al. Clearance of surfactant protein B from rabbit lungs. Am J Physiol 1995;268:L631–641.
44. Wright JR, Youmans DC. Degradation of surfactant lipids and surfactant protein A by alveolar macrophages. Am J Physiol 1995;268:L772–780.
45. Gross NJ, Narine KR. Surfactant subtypes in mice: characterization and quantitation. J Appl Physiol 1989;66:342–349.
46. Lewis JF, Ikegami M, Jobe AH. Altered surfactant function and metabolism in rabbits with acute lung injury. J Appl Physiol 1990;69:2303–2310.
47. Veldhuizen RA, Inchley K, Hearn SA, et al. Degradation of surfactant-associated protein B (SP-B) during in vitro conversion of large to small surfactant aggregates. Biochem J 1993;295:141–147.
48. Magoon MW, Wright JR, Baritussio A, et al. Subfractionation of lung surfactant: implications for metabolism and surface activity. Biochim Biophys Acta 1983;750:18–31.
49. Gross NJ. Extracellular metabolism of pulmonary surfactant. The role of a new serine protease. Annu Rev Physiol 1995;57:135–150.
50. Lewis JF, Veldhuizen R, Possmayer F, et al. Altered alveolar surfactant is an early marker of acute lung injury in septic adult sheep. Am J Respir Crit Care Med 1994;150:123–130.
51. Ueda T, Ikegami M, Jobe AH. Developmental changes of sheep surfactant: in vivo function and in vitro subtype conversion. J Appl Physiol 1994;76:2701–2706.
52. Kahn MC, Anderson GJ, Anyan WR, et al. Phosphatidylcholine molecular species of calf lung surfactant. Am J Physiol 1995;269:L567–573.
53. Montfoort A, van Golde LMG, van Deenen LLM. Molecular species of lecithins from various animal tissues. Biochim Biophys Acta 1971;231:335–341.
54. Schürch S, Possmayer F, Cheng S, et al. Pulmonary SP-A enhances adsorption and appears to induce surface sorting of lipid extract surfactant. Am J Physiol 1992;263:L210–218.
55. Pastrana-Rios B, Flach CR, Branner JW, et al. A direct test of the "squeeze-out" hypothesis of lung surfactant function. External reflection FT-IR at the air-water interface. Biochemistry 1994;33:5121–5127.
56. Bangham AD. Surface tensions in the lung. Biophys J 1995;68:1630–1631.
57. Keough KMW. Physical chemistry of pulmonary surfactant in the terminal air spaces. In: Robertson B, van Golde LMG, Batenburg JJ, eds. Pulmonary surfactant: from molecular biology to clinical practice. Amsterdam: Elsevier, 1992:109–164.
58. Rana FR, Harwood JS, Mautone AJ, et al. Identification of phosphocholine plasmalogen as a lipid component in mammalian pulmonary surfactant using high-resolution 31P-NMR spectroscopy. Biochemistry 1993;32:27–31.
59. Morand OH, Zoeller RA, Raetz CHR. Disappearance of plasmalogens from membranes of animal cells subjected to photosensitized oxidation. J Biol Chem 1988;263:11597–11606.
60. Haagsman HP. Toxicological aspects of the surfactant system. In: Robertson B, van Golde LMG, Batenburg JJ, eds. Pulmonary surfactant: from molecular biology to clinical practice. Amsterdam: Elsevier, 1992:705–734.
61. Rüstow B, Haupt R, Stevens PA, et al. Type II pneumocytes secrete vitamin E together with surfactant lipids. Am J Physiol 1993;265:L133–139.
62. Orgeig S, Barr HA, Nicholas TE. Effect of hyperpnea on the cholesterol to disaturated phospholipid ratio in alveolar surfactant of rats. Exp Lung Res 1995;21:157–174.
63. Baybutt RC, Smith JE, Yeh Y-Y. The effect of dietary fish oil on alveolar type II cell fatty acids and lung surfactant phospholipids. Lipids 1993;28:167–172.
64. Palombo JD, Lydon EE, Chen P-L, et al. Fatty acid composition of lung, macrophage and surfactant phospholipids after short-term enteral feeding with n-3 lipids. Lipids 1994;29:643–649.
65. Doyle IR, Jones ME, Barr HA, et al. Composition of human pulmonary surfactant varies with exercise and level of fitness. Am J Respir Crit Care Med 1994;149:1619–1627.
66. Jackson JC, Palmer S, Wilson CB, et al. Postnatal changes in lung phospholipids and alveolar macrophages in term newborn monkeys. Respir Physiol 1988;73:289–300.
67. Jobe AH, Ikegami M, Jacobs H. Changes in the amount of lung and airway phosphatidylcholine in 0.5–12 day old rabbits. Biochim Biophys Acta 1981;664:182–187.
68. Ohashi T, Pinkerton K, Ikegami M, et al. Changes in alveolar surface area, surfactant protein A, and saturated phosphatidylcholine with postnatal rat lung growth. Pediatr Res 1994;35:685–689.
69. Ratjen F, Rehn B, Costabel U, et al. Age-dependency of surfactant phospholipids and surfactant protein A in bronchoalveolar lavage fluid of children without bronchopulmonary disease. Eur Respir J 1996;9:328–333.
70. King RJ, Clements JA. Surface active materials from dog lung. II. Composition and physiological correlations. Am J Physiol 1972;223:715–726.
71. Weaver TE, Whitsett JA. Function and regulation of expression of pulmonary surfactant-associated proteins. Biochem J 1991;273:249–264.
72. Hawgood S. The hydrophilic surfactant protein SP-A: molecular biology, structure and function. In: Robertson B, van Golde LMG, Batenburg JJ, eds. Pulmonary sur-

factant: from molecular biology to clinical practice. Amsterdam: Elsevier, 1992:33–54.
73. Whitsett JA, Baatz JE. Hydrophobic surfactant proteins SP-B and SP-C: molecular biology, structure and function. In: Robertson B, van Golde LMG, Batenburg JJ, eds. Pulmonary surfactant: from molecular biology to clinical practice. Amsterdam: Elsevier, 1992:55–75.
74. Johansson J, Curstedt T, Robertson B. The proteins of the surfactant system. Eur Respir J 1994;7:372–391.
75. Kuroki Y, Voelker DR. Pulmonary surfactant proteins. J Biol Chem 1994;269:25943–25946.
76. Floros J, Karinch AM. Human SP-A: then and now. Am J Physiol 1995;268:L162–165.
77. Whitsett JA, Nogee LM, Weaver TE, et al. Human surfactant protein B: structure, function, regulation, and genetic disease. Physiol Rev 1995;75:749–757.
78. Phizackerley PJR, Town MH, Newman GE. Hydrophobic proteins of lamellated osmiophilic bodies isolated from pig lung. Biochem J 1979;183:731–736.
79. Curstedt T, Jörnvall H, Robertson B, et al. Two hydrophobic low-molecular-mass protein fractions of pulmonary surfactant. Characterization and biophysical activity. Eur J Biochem 1987;168:255–262.
80. Curstedt T, Johansson J, Barros-Söderling J, et al. Low-molecular-mass surfactant protein type 1. The primary structure of a hydrophobic 8 kDa polypeptide with eight half-cystine residues. Eur J Biochem 1988;172:521–525.
81. Johansson J, Jörnvall H, Curstedt T. Surfactant protein B: disulfide bridges, structural properties, and kringle similarities. Biochemistry 1991;30:6917–6921.
82. Johansson J, Jörnvall H, Curstedt T. Human surfactant polypeptide SP-B: disulfide bridges, C-terminal end, and peptide analysis of the airway form. FEBS Lett 1992; 301:165–167.
83. Vandenbussche G, Clercx A, Clercx M, et al. Secondary structure and orientation of the surfactant protein SP-B in a lipid environment. A Fourier transform infra-red spectroscopy study. Biochemistry 1992;31:9169–9176.
84. Vamvakopoulos NC, Modi WS, Floros J. Mapping the human pulmonary surfactant-associated protein B gene (SFTP3) to chromosome 2p12-p11.2. Cytogenet Cell Genet 1995;68:8–10.
85. Hawgood S, Benson BJ, Schilling J, et al. Nucleotide and amino acid sequences of pulmonary surfactant protein SP 18 and evidence for cooperation between SP 18 and SP 28–36 in surfactant lipid adsorption. Proc Natl Acad Sci USA 1987;84:66–70.
86. Glasser SW, Korfhagen TR, Weaver T, et al. cDNA and deduced amino acid sequence of human pulmonary surfactant-associated proteolipid SPL (Phe). Proc Natl Acad Sci USA 1987;84:4007–4011.
87. Jacobs KA, Phelps DS, Steinbrink R, et al. Isolation of a cDNA clone encoding a high molecular weight precursor to a 6-kDa pulmonary surfactant-associated protein. J Biol Chem 1987;262:9808–9811.
88. Emrie PA, Shannon JM, Mason RJ, et al. cDNA and deduced amino acid sequence for the rat hydrophobic pulmonary surfactant-associated protein, SP-B. Biochim Biophys Acta 1989;994:215–221.
89. Xu J, Richardson C, Ford C, et al. Isolation and characterization of the cDNA for pulmonary surfactant-associated protein-B (SP-B) in the rabbit. Biochem Biophys Res Commun 1989;160:325–332.
90. Weaver TE, Whitsett JA. Processing of hydrophobic pulmonary surfactant protein B in rat type II cells. Am J Physiol 1989;257:L100–108.
91. Weaver TE, Lin S, Bogucki B, et al. Processing of surfactant protein B proprotein by a cathepsin D-like protease. Am J Physiol 1992;263:L95–L103.
92. Suzuki Y, Fujita Y, Kogishi K. Reconstitution of tubular myelin from synthetic lipids and proteins associated with pig pulmonary surfactant. Am Rev Respir Dis 1989;140: 75–81.
93. Poulain FR, Allen L, Williams MC, et al. Effects of surfactant apolipoproteins on liposome structure: implications for tubular myelin formation. Am J Physiol 1992; 262:L730–739.
94. Williams MC, Hawgood S, Hamilton RL. Changes in lipid structure produced by surfactant proteins SP-A, SP-B, and SP-C. Am J Respir Cell Mol Biol 1991;5:41–50.
95. Oosterlaken-Dijksterhuis MA, van Eijk MA, van Golde LMG, et al. Lipid mixing is mediated by the hydrophobic protein SP-B but not by SP-C. Biochim Biophys Acta 1992;1110:45–50.
96. deMello DE, Nogee LM, Heyman S, et al. Molecular and phenotypic variability in the congenital alveolar proteinosis syndrome associated with inherited surfactant protein B deficiency. J Pediatr 1994;125:43–50.
97. Oosterlaken-Dijksterhuis MA, Haagsman HP, van Golde LMG, et al. Interaction of lipid vesicles with monomolecular layers containing lung surfactant proteins SP-B or SP-C. Biochemistry 1991;30:8276–8281.
98. Oosterlaken-Dijksterhuis MA, Haagsman HP, van Golde LMG, et al. Characterization of lipid insertion into monomolecular layers mediated by lung surfactant proteins SP-B and SP-C. Biochemistry 1991;30:10965–10971.
99. Revak SD, Merritt TA, Degryse E, et al. Use of human surfactant low molecular weight apoproteins in the reconstitution of surfactant biological activity. J Clin Invest 1988;81:826–833.
100. Cochrane CG, Revak SD. Pulmonary surfactant protein B (SP-B): structure-function relationships. Science 1991;254: 566–568.
101. Baatz JE, Elledge B, Whitsett JA. Surfactant protein SP-B induces ordering at the surface of model membrane layers. Biochemistry 1990;29:6714–6720.
102. Yu S-H, Possmayer F. Effect of pulmonary surfactant protein B (SP-B) and calcium on phospholipid adsorption and squeeze-out of phosphatidylglycerol from binary phospholipid monolayers containing dipalmitoylphosphatidylcholine. Biochim Biophys Acta 1992;1126:26–34.
103. Taneva SG, Keough KMW. Pulmonary surfactant proteins SP-B and SP-C in spread monolayers at the air-water interface: I. Monolayers of pulmonary surfactant protein SP-B and phospholipids. Biophys J 1994;66:1137–1148.
104. Taneva SG, Keough KMW. Dynamic surface properties of pulmonary surfactant proteins SP-B and SP-C and their

105. Günther A, Seeger W. Resistance to surfactant inactivation. In: Robertson B, Taeusch HW, eds. Surfactant therapy for lung disease. New York: Marcel Dekker, 1995:269–292.
106. Seeger W, Günther A, Thede C. Differential sensitivity to fibrinogen inhibition of SP-C vs. SP-B-based surfactants. Am J Physiol 1992;262:L286–291.
107. Robertson B, Kobayashi T, Ganzuka M, et al. Experimental neonatal respiratory failure induced by a monoclonal antibody to the hydrophobic surfactant-associated protein SP-B. Pediatr Res 1991;30:239–243.
108. Nogee LM, deMello DE, Dehner LP, et al. Brief report: deficiency of pulmonary surfactant protein B in congenital alveolar proteinosis. N Engl J Med 1993;328:406–410.
109. Hamvas A, Nogee LM, deMello DE, et al. Pathophysiology and treatment of surfactant protein-B deficiency. Biol Neonate 1995;67(suppl 1):18–31.
110. Nogee LM, Garnier G, Dietz HC, et al. A mutation in the surfactant protein B gene responsible for fatal neonatal respiratory disease in multiple kindreds. J Clin Invest 1994;93:1860–1863.
111. Clark JC, Wert SE, Bachurski CJ, et al. Targeted disruption of the surfactant protein B gene disrupts surfactant homeostasis, causing respiratory failure in newborn mice. Proc Natl Acad Sci USA 1995;92:7794–7798.
112. Pérez-Gil J, Cruz A, Casals C. Solubility of hydrophobic surfactant proteins in organic solvent/water mixtures. Structural studies on SP-B and SP-C in aqueous organic solvents and lipids. Biochim Biophys Acta 1993;1168:261–270.
113. Johansson J, Curstedt T, Robertson B, et al. Size and structure of the hydrophobic low molecular weight surfactant-associated polypeptide. Biochemistry 1988;27:3544–3547.
114. Johansson J, Jörnvall H, Eklund A, et al. Hydrophobic 3.7 kDa surfactant polypeptide: structural characterization of the human and bovine forms. FEBS Lett 1988;232:61–64.
115. Johansson J, Persson P, Löwenadler B, et al. Canine hydrophobic surfactant polypeptide SP-C: a lipopeptide with one thioester-linked palmitoyl group. FEBS Lett 1991;281:119–122.
116. Beers MF, Fisher AB. Surfactant protein C: a review of its unique properties and metabolism. Am J Physiol 1992;263:L151–160.
117. Curstedt T, Johansson J, Persson P, et al. Hydrophobic surfactant-associated polypeptides: SP-C is a lipopeptide with two palmitoylated cysteine residues, whereas SP-B lacks covalently linked fatty acyl groups. Proc Natl Acad Sci USA 1990;87:2985–2989.
118. Johansson J, Szyperski T, Curstedt T, et al. The NMR structure of the pulmonary surfactant-associated polypeptide SP-C in an apolar solvent contains a valyl-rich α-helix. Biochemistry 1994;33:6015–6023.
119. Pastrana B, Mautone AJ, Mendelsohn R. Fourier transform infra-red studies of secondary structure and orientation of pulmonary surfactant SP-C and its effect on the dynamic surface properties of phospholipids. Biochemistry 1991;30:10058–10064.
120. Vandenbussche G, Clercx A, Curstedt T, et al. Structure and orientation of the surfactant-associated protein C in a lipid bilayer. Eur J Biochem 1992;203:201–209.
121. Morrow MR, Taneva S, Simatos GA, et al. 2H NMR studies of the effect of pulmonary surfactant SP-C on the 1,2-dipalmitoyl-sn-glycerol-3-phosphocholine headgroup: a model for transbilayer peptides in surfactant and biological membranes. Biochemistry 1993;32:11338–11344.
122. Baatz JE, Smyth KL, Whitsett JA, et al. Structure and functions of a dimeric form of surfactant protein C: a Fourier transform infrared and surfactometry study. Chem Phys Lipids 1992;63:91–104.
123. Creuwels LAJM, Demel RA, van Golde LMG, et al. Characterization of a dimeric canine form of surfactant protein C (SP-C). Biochim Biophys Acta 1995;1254:326–332.
124. Glasser SW, Korfhagen TR, Weaver TE, et al. cDNA, deduced polypeptide structure and chromosomal assignment of human surfactant proteolipid SPL (pVal). J Biol Chem 1988;263:9–12.
125. Warr RG, Hawgood S, Buckley DI, et al. Low molecular weight human pulmonary surfactant protein (SP5): isolation, characterization and cDNA and amino acid sequences. Proc Natl Acad Sci USA 1987;84:7915–7919.
126. Fisher JH, Shannon JM, Hofmann T, et al. Nucleotide and deduced amino acid sequence of the hydrophobic surfactant protein SP-C from rat: expression in alveolar type II cells and homology with SP-C from other species. Biochim Biophys Acta 1989;995:225–230.
127. Beers MF, Lomax C. Synthesis and processing of hydrophobic surfactant protein C by isolated rat type II cells. Am J Physiol 1995;269:L744–753.
128. Yu S-H, Possmayer F. Role of bovine pulmonary surfactant-associated proteins in the surface-active property of phospholipid mixtures. Biochim Biophys Acta 1990;1046:233–241.
129. Takahashi A, Waring AJ, Amirkhanian J, et al. Structure-function relationships of bovine pulmonary surfactant proteins: SP-B and SP-C. Biochim Biophys Acta 1990;1044:43–49.
130. Creuwels LAJM, Boer EH, Demel RA, et al. Neutralization of the positive charges of surfactant protein C. Effects on structure and function. J Biol Chem 1995;270:16225–16229.
131. Taneva SG, Keough KMW. Pulmonary surfactant proteins SP-B and SP-C in spread monolayers at the air-water interface: II. Monolayers of pulmonary surfactant protein SP-C and phospholipids. Biophys J 1994;66:1149–1157.
132. Creuwels LAJM, Demel RA, van Golde LMG, et al. Effect of acylation on structure and function of surfactant protein C at the air-liquid interface. J Biol Chem 1993;268:26752–26758.
133. White RT, Damm D, Miller J, et al. Isolation and characterization of the human pulmonary surfactant apoprotein gene. Nature 1985;317:361–363.
134. Persson A, Chang D, Rust K, et al. Purification and biochemical characterization of CP4 (SP-D): a collagenous

surfactant associated protein. Biochemistry 1989;27:6361–6367.
135. Kuroki Y, Shiratori M, Ogasawara Y, et al. Characterization of pulmonary surfactant protein-D. Its copurification with lipids. Biochim Biophys Acta 1991;1086:185–190.
136. Benson B, Hawgood S, Schilling J, et al. Structure of canine pulmonary surfactant apoprotein: cDNA and complete amino acid sequence. Proc Natl Acad Sci USA 1985;82:6379–6383.
137. Boggaram V, Qing K, Mendelson CR. The major apoprotein of rabbit pulmonary surfactant. Elucidation of primary sequence and cyclic AMP and developmental regulation. J Biol Chem 1988;263:2939–2947.
138. Sano K, Fisher J, Mason RJ, et al. Isolation and sequence of a cDNA clone for the rat pulmonary surfactant-associated protein (PSP-A). Biochem Biophys Res Commun 1987;144:367–374.
139. Korfhagen TR, Bruno MD, Glasser SW, et al. Murine pulmonary surfactant SP-A gene: cloning, sequence, and transcriptional activity. Am J Physiol 1992;263:L546–554.
140. Voss T, Eistetter H, Schäfer K, et al. Macromolecular organization of natural and recombinant lung surfactant protein SP 28–36: structural homology with the complement factor C1q. J Mol Biol 1988;201:219–227.
141. Epstein J, Eichbaum Q, Sheriff S, et al. The collectins in innate immunity. Curr Opin Immunol 1996;8:29–35.
142. Hoppe H-J, Reid KBM. Collectins—soluble proteins containing collagenous regions and lectin domains—and their roles in innate immunity. Protein Sci 1994;3:1143–1158.
143. Haagsman HP, Hawgood S, Sargeant T, et al. The major lung surfactant protein, SP 28-36, is a calcium-dependent carbohydrate-binding protein. J Biol Chem 1987;262:13877–13880.
144. Haurum JS, Thiel S, Haagsman HP, et al. Studies on the carbohydrate-binding characteristics of human pulmonary surfactant-associated protein A and comparison with two other collectins: mannan-binding protein and conglutinin. Biochem J 1993;293:873–878.
145. Haagsman HP, White RT, Schilling J, et al. Studies on the structure of the lung surfactant protein, SP-A. Am J Physiol 1989;257:L421–429.
146. Drickamer K, Taylor ME. Biology of animal lectins. Annu Rev Cell Biol 1993;9:237–264.
147. Bruns G, Stroh H, Veldman GM, et al. The 35 kd pulmonary surfactant-associated protein is encoded on chromosome 10. Hum Genet 1987;76:58–62.
148. McCormick SM, Mendelson CR. Human SP-A1 and SP-A2 genes are differentially regulated during development and by cAMP and glucocorticoids. Am J Physiol 1994;266:L367–374.
149. Ogasawara Y, McCormack FX, Mason RJ, et al. Chimeras of surfactant proteins A and D identify the carbohydrate recognition domains as essential for phospholipid interaction. J Biol Chem 1994;269:29785–29792.
150. Kuroki Y, McCormack FX, Ogasawara Y, et al. Epitope mapping for monoclonal antibodies identifies functional domains of pulmonary surfactant protein A that interact with lipids. J Biol Chem 1994;269:29793–29800.
151. Hiraike N, Sohma H, Kuroki Y, et al. Epitope mapping for monoclonal antibody against human surfactant protein A (SP-A) that alters receptor binding of SP-A and the SP-A dependent regulation of phospholipid secretion by alveolar type II cells. Biochim Biophys Acta 1995;1257:214–222.
152. Voorhout WF, Veenendaal T, Kuroki Y, et al. Immunocytochemical localization of surfactant protein D (SP-D) in type II cells, Clara cells, and alveolar macrophages of rat lung. J Histochem Cytochem 1992;40:1589–1597.
153. Khoor A, Gray ME, Hull WM, et al. Developmental expression of SP-A and SP-A mRNA in the proximal and distal respiratory epithelium in the human fetus and newborn. J Histochem Cytochem 1993;41:1311–1319.
154. Rubio S, Lacazemas-Monteil T, Chailleyheu B, et al. Pulmonary surfactant protein A (SP-A) is expressed by epithelial cells of small and large intestine. J Biol Chem 1995;270:12162–12169.
155. deMello DE, Heyman S, Phelps DS, et al. Immunogold localization of SP-A in lungs of infants dying from respiratory distress syndrome. Am J Pathol 1993;142:1631–1640.
156. Veldhuizen RAW, Yao L-J, Hearn SA, et al. Surfactant-associated protein A is important for maintaining surfactant large-aggregate forms during surface-area cycling. Biochem J 1996;313:835–840.
157. Haagsman HP, Elfring RH, van Buel BLM, et al. The lung lectin surfactant protein A aggregates phospholipid vesicles via a novel mechanism. Biochem J 1991;275:273–276.
158. McCormack FX, Calvert HM, Watson PA, et al. The structure and function of surfactant protein A. Hydroxyproline- and carbohydrate-deficient mutant proteins. J Biol Chem 1994;269:5833–5841.
159. Ruano MLF, Miguel E, Perez-Gil J, et al. Comparison of lipid aggregation and self-aggregation activities of pulmonary surfactant-associated protein A. Biochem J 1996;313:683–689.
160. Pison U, Shiffer K, Hawgood S, et al. Effects of the surfactant-associated proteins, SP-A, SP-B, and SP-C, on phospholipid surface film formation. Progr Respir Res 1990;25:271–273.
161. Yamada T, Ikegami M, Tabor BL, et al. Effects of surfactant protein-A on surfactant function in preterm ventilated rabbits. Am Rev Respir Dis 1990;142:754–757.
162. Hallman M, Merritt TA, Akino T, et al. Surfactant protein A, phosphatidylcholine, and surfactant inhibitors in epithelial lining fluid. Correlation with surface activity, severity of respiratory distress syndrome, and outcome in small premature infants. Am Rev Respir Dis 1991;144:1376–1384.
163. Cockshutt AM, Weitz J, Possmayer F. Pulmonary surfactant-associated protein A enhances the surface activity of lipid extract surfactant and reverses inhibition by blood proteins in vitro. Biochemistry 1990;29:8424–8429.
164. Kuroki Y, Mason RJ, Voelker DR. Alveolar type II cells express a high-affinity receptor for pulmonary surfactant protein A. Proc Natl Acad Sci USA 1988;85:5566–5570.
165. Wright JR, Borchelt JD, Hawgood S. Lung surfactant apoprotein SP-A (26–36 kDa) binds with high affinity to isolated alveolar type II cells. Proc Natl Acad Sci USA 1989;86:5410–5414.
166. Wright JR, Wager RE, Hawgood S, et al. Surfactant apoprotein Mr = 26,000–36,000 enhances uptake of liposomes by type II cells. J Biol Chem 1987;262:2888–2894.

167. Tsuzuki A, Kuroki Y, Akino T. Pulmonary surfactant protein A-mediated uptake of phosphatidylcholine by alveolar type II cells. Am J Physiol 1993;265:L193–199.
168. Bates SR, Dodia C, Fisher AB. Surfactant protein A regulates uptake of pulmonary surfactant by lung type II cells on microporous membranes. Am J Physiol 1994;267:L753–760.
169. Horowitz AD, Moussavian B, Whitsett JA. Roles of SP-A, SP-B, and SP-C in modulation of lipid uptake by pulmonary epithelial cells in vitro. Am J Physiol 1996;270:L69–79.
170. Strayer DS, Yang SJ, Jerng HH. Surfactant protein-A-binding proteins. Characterization and structures. J Biol Chem 1993;268:18679–18684.
171. Stevens PA, Wissel H, Sieger D, et al. Identification of a new surfactant protein A binding protein at the cell membrane of rat type II cells. Biochem J 1995;308:77–81.
172. Wissel H, Looman AC, Fritzsche I, et al. The SP-A-binding protein BP55 is involved in surfactant endocytosis by type II pneumocytes. Am J Physiol 1996;15:432–440.
173. Yukitake K, Brown CL, Schlueter MA, et al. Surfactant apoprotein A modifies the inhibitory effect of plasma proteins on surfactant activity in vivo. Pediatr Res 1995;37:21–25.
174. Lu J, Willis AC, Reid KBM. Purification, characterization and cDNA cloning of human lung surfactant protein D. Biochem J 1992;284:795–802.
175. Crouch E, Rust K, Veile R, et al. Genomic organization of human surfactant protein D (SP-D). SP-D is encoded on chromosome 10q22.2-23.1. J Biol Chem 1993;268:2976–2983.
176. Shimizu H, Fisher JH, Papat P, et al. Primary structure of rat pulmonary surfactant protein D. cDNA and deduced amino acid sequence. J Biol Chem 1992;267:1853–1857.
177. Lim BL, Lu J, Reid KBM. Structural similarity between bovine conglutinin and bovine lung surfactant protein D and demonstration of liver as a site of synthesis of conglutinin. Immunology 1993;78:159–165.
178. Liou LS, Sastry R, Hartshorn KL, et al. Bovine conglutinin (BC) mRNA expressed in liver: cloning and characterization of the BC cDNA reveals strong homology to surfactant protein-D. Gene 1994;141:277–281.
179. Crouch E, Persson A, Chang D, et al. Molecular structure of pulmonary surfactant protein D (SP-D). J Biol Chem 1994;269:17311–17319.
180. Strang CJ, Slayter HS, Lachmann PJ, et al. Ultrastructure and composition of bovine conglutinin. Biochem J 1986;234:381–389.
181. Kölble K, Lu J, Mole SA, et al. Assignment of the human pulmonary surfactant protein D gene (SFTP4) to 10q22–q23 close to the surfactant protein A gene cluster. Genomics 1993;17:294–298.
182. Crouch E, Parghi D, Kuan SF, et al. Surfactant protein-D. Subcellular localization in nonciliated bronchiolar epithelial cells. Am J Physiol 1992;263:L60–66.
183. Fisher JH, Mason R. Expression of pulmonary surfactant protein D in gastric mucosa. Am J Respir Cell Mol Biol 1995;12:13–18.
184. Ogasawara Y, Kuroki Y, Akino T. Pulmonary surfactant protein D specifically binds to phosphatidylinositol. J Biol Chem 1992;267:21244–21249.
185. Persson AV, Gibbons BJ, Shoemaker JD, et al. The major glycolipid recognized by SP-D in surfactant is phosphatidylinositol. Biochemistry 1992;31:12183–12189.
186. Kuroki Y, Gasa S, Ogasawara Y, et al. Binding specificity of lung surfactant protein SP-D for glucosylceramide. Biochem Biophys Res Commun 1992;187:963–969.
187. Kuroki Y, Shiratori M, Murata Y, et al. Surfactant protein D (SP-D) counteracts the inhibitory effect of surfactant protein A (SP-A) on phospholipid secretion by alveolar type II cells. Biochem J 1991;279:115–119.
188. Sastry K, Ezekowitz RA. Collectins: pattern recognition molecules involved in first line host defense. Curr Opin Immunol 1993;5:59–66.
189. Holmskov U, Malhotra R, Sim RB, et al. Collectins: collagenous C-type lectins of the innate immune defense system. Immunol Today 1994;15:67–74.
190. Riddihough G. First-line defence. Nature 1994;372:114.
191. Hamm H, Kroegel C, Hohlfeld J. Surfactant: a review of its functions and relevance in adult respiratory disorders. Respir Med 1996;90:251–270.
192. Van Iwaarden F, Welmers B, Verhoef J, et al. Pulmonary surfactant protein A enhances the host-defense mechanism of rat alveolar macrophages. Am J Respir Cell Mol Biol 1990;2:91–98.
193. Weissbach S, Neuendank A, Petterson M, et al. Surfactant protein A modulates release of reactive oxygen species from alveolar macrophages. Am J Physiol 1994;267:L660–666.
194. Van Iwaarden JR, Shimizu H, van Golde PHM, et al. Rat surfactant protein D enhances the production of oxygen radicals by rat alveolar macrophages. Biochem J 1992;286:5–8.
195. Kremlev SG, Phelps DS. Surfactant protein A stimulation of inflammatory cytokine and immunoglobulin production. Am J Physiol 1994;267:L712–719.
196. Tenner AJ, Robinson SL, Borchelt J, et al. Human pulmonary surfactant protein (SP-A), a protein structurally homologous to C1q, can enhance FcR- and CR1-mediated phagocytosis. J Biol Chem 1989;264:13923–13928.
197. Manz-Keinke H, Plattner H, Schlepper-Schäfer J. Lung surfactant protein A (SP-A) enhances serum-independent phagocytosis of bacteria by alveolar macrophages. Eur J Cell Biol 1992;57:95–100.
198. Pikaar JC, Voorhout WF, van Golde LMG, et al. Opsonic activities of surfactant proteins A and D in phagocytosis of Gram-negative bacteria by alveolar macrophages. J Infect Dis 1995;172:481–489.
199. Ohmer-Schröck D, Schlatterer C, Plattner H, et al. Lung surfactant protein A (SP-A) enhances a phosphoinositide/calcium signaling pathway in alveolar macrophages. J Cell Sci 1995;108:3695–3702.
200. Kuan S-F, Rust K, Crouch E. Interactions of surfactant protein D with bacterial lipopolysaccharides. Surfactant protein D is an *Escherichia coli*–binding protein in bronchoalveolar lavage. J Clin Invest 1992;90:97–106.
201. Van Iwaarden JF, van Strijp JAG, Ebskamp MJM, et al. Surfactant protein A is an opsonin in the phagocytosis of herpes simplex virus type 1 by rat alveolar macrophages. Am J Physiol 1991;61;L204–209.

202. Van Iwaarden JF, Pikaar JC, Storm J, et al. Binding of surfactant protein A to the lipid A moiety of bacterial lipopolysaccharides. Biochem J 1994;303:407–411.
203. O'Riordan DM, Standing JE, Kwon K-Y, et al. Surfactant protein D interacts with *Pneumocystis carinii* and mediates organism adherence to alveolar macrophages. J Clin Invest 1995;95:2699–2710.
204. Benne CA, Kraaijeveld CA, van Strijp JAG, et al. Interactions of surfactant protein A with influenza A viruses: binding and neutralization. J Infect Dis 1995;171:335–341.
205. Hartshorn KL, Crouch EC, White MR, et al. Evidence for a protective role of pulmonary surfactant protein D (SP-D) against influenza A virus. J Clin Invest 1994;94:311–319.
206. Snyder JM, Mendelson CR, Johnston JM. The morphology of lung development in the human fetus. In: Nelson GH, ed. Pulmonary development. Transition from intrauterine to extrauterine life. (Lung biology in health and disease, vol. 27.). New York: Marcel Dekker, 1985:19–46.
207. Ten Have-Opbroek AAW. Immunological study of lung development in the mouse embryo. II. First appearance of the great alveolar cell, as shown by immunofluorescence microscopy. Dev Biol 1979;69:408–423.
208. Otto-Verberne CJM, Ten Have-Opbroek AAW. Development of the pulmonary acinus in fetal rat lung: a study based on an antiserum recognizing surfactant-associated proteins. Anat Embryol 1987;175:365–373.
209. Post M, Smith BT. Histochemical and immunocytochemical identification of alveolar type II epithelial cells isolated from fetal rat lung. Am Rev Respir Dis 1988;137:525–530.
210. Caniggia I, Tseu I, Han RNN, et al. Spatial and temporal differences in fibroblast behavior in fetal rat lung. Am J Physiol 1991;261:L424–433.
211. Carlson KS, Davies P, Smith BT, et al. Temporal linkage of glycogen and saturated phosphatidylcholine in fetal lung type II cells. Pediatr Res 1987;22:79–82.
212. Bourbon J, Jost A. Control of glycogen metabolism in the developing fetal lung. Pediatr Res 1982;16:50–56.
213. Maniscalco WM, Wilson CM, Gross I, et al. Development of glycogen and phospholipid metabolism in fetal and newborn rat lung. Biochim Biophys Acta 1978;530:333–346.
214. Kikkawa Y, Kaibara M, Motoyama EK, et al. Morphologic development of fetal rabbit lung and its acceleration with cortisol. Am J Pathol 1971;64:423–442.
215. Williams MC, Mason RJ. Development of the type II cell in the fetal rat lung. Am Rev Respir Dis 1977;115 (suppl):37–47.
216. Bourbon JR, Rieutort M, Engle MJ, et al. Utilization of glycogen for phospholipid synthesis in fetal rat lung. Biochim Biophys Acta 1982;712:382–389.
217. Farrell PM, Bourbon JR. Fetal lung surfactant lipid synthesis from glycogen during organ culture. Biochim Biophys Acta 1986;878:159–167.
218. Bhavnani BR. Ontogeny of some enzymes of glycogen metabolism in rabbit fetal heart, lungs, and liver. Can J Biochem Cell Biol 1983;61:191–197.
219. Bourbon JR, Doucet E, Rieutort M. Role of alpha-glucosidase in fetal lung maturation. Biochim Biophys Acta 1987;917:203–210.
220. Rooney SA. The surfactant system and lung phospholipid biochemistry. Am Rev Respir Dis 1985;131:439–460.
221. Hallman M. Antenatal diagnosis of lung maturity. In: Robertson B, van Golde LMG, Batenburg JJ, eds. Pulmonary surfactant: from molecular biology to clinical practice. Amsterdam: Elsevier, 1992:425–458.
222. Batenburg JJ, Hallman M. Developmental biochemistry of alveoli. In: Scarpelli EM, ed. Pulmonary physiology: fetus, newborn, child, and adolescent. 2nd ed. Philadelphia: Lea & Febiger, 1990:106–139.
223. Robert MF, Neff RK, Hubbell JP, et al. Association between maternal diabetes and respiratory distress syndrome in the newborn. N Engl J Med 1976;294:357–360.
224. Rooney S, Gobran LI, Wai-Lee TS. Stimulation of surfactant production by oxytocin-induced labor in the rabbit. J Clin Invest 1977;60:754–759.
225. Marino PA, Rooney SA. The effect of labor on surfactant secretion in newborn rabbit lung slices. Biochim Biophys Acta 1981;664:389–396.
226. Whittle MJ, Hill CM, Harkes A. Effect of labour on the lecithin/sphingomyelin ratio in serial samples of amniotic fluid. Br J Obstet Gynaecol 1977;84:500–503.
227. Egberts J, Noort WA. Gestational age-dependent changes in plasma inositol levels and surfactant composition in the fetal rat. Pediatr Res 1986;20:24–27.
228. Egberts J, Beintema-Dubbeldam A, de Boers A. Phosphatidylinositol and not phosphatidylglycerol is the important minor phospholipid in rhesus-monkey surfactant. Biochim Biophys Acta 1987;919:90–92.
229. Hallman M, Kulovich M, Kirkpatrick E, et al. Phosphatidylinositol and phosphatidylglycerol in amniotic fluid: indices of lung maturity. Am J Obstet Gynecol 1976;125:613–617.
230. Oulton M, Martin TR, Faulkner GT, et al. Developmental study of a lamellar body fraction isolated from human amniotic fluid. Pediatr Res 1980;14:722–728.
231. Hallman M, Epstein BL. Role of myo-inositol in the synthesis of phosphatidylglycerol and phosphatidylinositol in the lung. Biochem Biophys Res Commun 1980;92:1151–1159.
232. Hallman M, Slivka S, Wozniak P, et al. Perinatal development of myoinositol uptake into lung cells: surfactant phosphatidylglycerol and phosphatidylinositol synthesis in the rabbit. Pediatr Res 1986;20:179–185.
233. Quirk JG Jr, Bleasdale JE. Myo-inositol homeostasis in the human fetus. Obstet Gynecol 1983;62:41–44.
234. Zimmermann LJ, Hogan M, Carlson KS, et al. Regulation of phosphatidylcholine synthesis in fetal type II cells by CTP: phosphocholine cytidylyltransferase. Am J Physiol 1993;264:L575–580.
235. Gail DB, Farrell PM. Measurement of phosphatidylcholine precursors—choline, ethanolamine and methionine—in fetal and adult rat lung. Lung 1978;155:255–263.
236. Tokmakjian S, Possmayer F. Pool sizes of the precursors for phosphatidylcholine synthesis in developing rat lung. Biochim Biophys Acta 1981;666:176–180.
237. Post M, Batenburg JJ, van Golde LMG, et al. The rate limiting reaction in phosphatidylcholine synthesis by alveolar type II cells from fetal lung. Biochim Biophys Acta 1984;795:558–563.

238. Weinhold PA, Feldman DA, Quade MM, et al. Evidence for a regulatory role of CTP: cholinephosphate cytidylyltransferase in the synthesis of phosphatidylcholine in fetal lung following premature birth. Biochim Biophys Acta 1981;665:134–144.
239. Chu AJ, Rooney SA. Developmental differences in activation of cholinephosphate cytidylyltransferase by lipids in rabbit lung cytosol. Biochim Biophys Acta 1985;835:132–140.
240. Viscardi RM, McKenna MC. Developmental changes in cholinephosphate cytidylyltransferase activity and microsomal phospholipid fatty acid composition in alveolar type II cells. Life Sci 1994;54:1411–1421.
241. Post M, Smith BT. Hormonal control of surfactant metabolism. In: Robertson B, van Golde LMG, Batenburg JJ, eds. Pulmonary surfactant: from molecular biology to clinical practice. Amsterdam: Elsevier, 1992:379–424.
242. Post M, Barsoumian A, Smith BT. The cellular mechanism of glucocorticoid acceleration of fetal lung maturation. Fibroblast-pneumonocyte factor stimulates cholinephosphate cytidylyltransferase activity. J Biol Chem 1986;261:2179–2184.
243. Post M. Maternal administration of dexamethasone stimulates choline-phosphate cytidylyltransferase in fetal type II cells. Biochem J 1987;241:291–296.
244. Viscardi RM, Weinhold PA, Beals TM, et al. Cholinephosphate cytidylyltransferase in fetal rat lung cells: activity and subcellular distribution in response to dexamethasone, triiodothyronine, and fibroblast-conditioned medium. Exp Lung Res 1989;15:223–237.
245. Chu AJ, Rooney SA. Stimulation of cholinephosphate cytidylyltransferase activity by estrogen in fetal rabbit lung is mediated by phospholipids. Biochim Biophys Acta 1985;834:346–356.
246. Mallampalli RK, Walter ME, Peterson MW, et al. Betamethasone activation of CTP: cholinephosphate cytidylyltransferase in vivo is lipid dependent. Am J Respir Cell Mol Biol 1994;10:48–57.
247. Sharma A, Gonzales LW, Ballard PL. Hormonal regulation of cholinephosphate cytidylyltransferase in human fetal lung. Biochim Biophys Acta 1993;1170:237–244.
248. Weinhold PA, Rounsifer ME, Feldman DA. The purification and characterization of CTP: phosphorylcholine cytidylyltransferase from rat liver. J Biol Chem 1986;261:5104–5110.
249. Feldman DA, Weinhold PA. CTP: phosphorylcholine cytidylyltransferase from rat liver. Isolation and characterization of the catalytic subunit. J Biol Chem 1987;262:9075–9081.
250. Yao ZM, Jamil H, Vance DE. Choline deficiency causes translocation of CTP: phosphocholine cytidylyltransferase from cytosol to endoplasmic reticulum in rat liver. J Biol Chem 1990;265:4326–4331.
251. Rooney SA, Smart DA, Weinhold PA, et al. Dexamethasone increases the activity but not the amount of choline-phosphate cytidylyltransferase in fetal rat lung. Biochim Biophys Acta 1990;1044:385–389.
252. Jamil H, Utal AK, Vance DE. Evidence that cyclic AMP-induced inhibition of phosphatidylcholine biosynthesis is caused by a decrease in cellular diacylglycerol levels in cultured rat hepatocytes. J Biol Chem 1992;267:1752–1760.
253. Kalmar GB, Kay RJ, Lachance A, et al. Cloning and expression of rat liver CTP: phosphocholine cytidylyltransferase: an amphipathic protein that controls phosphatidylcholine synthesis. Proc Natl Acad Sci USA 1990;87:6029–6033.
254. Hogan M, Zimmermann LJ, Wang J, et al. Increased expression of CTP: phosphocholine cytidylyltransferase in maturing type II cells. Am J Physiol 1994;267:L25–32.
255. Zimmermann LJI. The regulation of CTP:phosphocholine cytidylyltransferase in fetal type II cells [PhD Thesis]. Erasmus University, Rotterdam, The Netherlands, 1995:277.
256. Zimmermann LJI, Lee W-S, Post M. Regulation of CTP:phosphocholine cytidylyltransferase by cytosolic lipids in rat type II pneumocytes during development. Pediatr Res 1995;38:864–869.
257. Wieder T, Geilen CC, Wieprecht M, et al. Identification of a putative membrane-interacting domain of CTP: phosphocholine cytidylyltransferase from rat liver. FEBS Lett 1994;345:207–210.
258. Craig L, Johnson JE, Cornell RB. Identification of the membrane-binding domain of rat liver CTP: phosphocholine cytidylyltransferase using chymotrypsin proteolysis. J Biol Chem 1994;269:3311–3317.
259. Johnson JE, Cornell RB. Membrane-binding amphipathic alpha-helical peptide derived from CTP: phosphocholine cytidylyltransferase. Biochemistry 1994;33:4327–4335.
260. Vance DE, Pelech SL. Enzyme translocation in the regulation of phosphatidylcholine biosynthesis. Trends Biochem Sci 1984;9:17–20.
261. Aeberhard EE, Barrett CT, Kaplan SA, et al. Stimulation of phosphatidylcholine synthesis by fatty acids in fetal rabbit type II pneumocytes. Biochim Biophys Acta 1986;875:6–11.
262. Burkhardt R, Von Wichert P, Batenburg JJ, et al. Fatty acids stimulate phosphatidylcholine synthesis and CTP: choline-phosphate cytidylyltransferase in type II pneumocytes isolated from adult rat lung. Biochem J 1988;254:495–500.
263. Chander A, Fisher AB. Choline-phosphate cytidyltransferase activity and phosphatidylcholine synthesis in rat granular pneumocytes are increased with exogenous fatty acids. Biochim Biophys Acta 1988;958:343–351.
264. Miller BE, Hook GE. Regulation of phosphatidylcholine biosynthesis in activated alveolar type II cells. Am J Respir Cell Mol Biol 1989;1:127–136.
265. Stern W, Kovac C, Weinhold PA. Activity and properties of CTP: cholinephosphate cytidylyltransferase in adult and fetal rat lung. Biochim Biophys Acta 1976;441:280–293.
266. Feldman DA, Dietrich JW, Weinhold PA. Comparison of the phospholipid requirements and molecular form of CTP:phosphocholine cytidylyltransferase from rat lung, kidney, brain and liver. Biochim Biophys Acta 1980;620:603–611.
267. Weinhold PA, Rounsifer ME, Charles L, et al. Characterization of cytosolic forms of CTP: choline-phosphate cytidylyltransferase in lung, isolated alveolar type II cells,

268. Mallampalli RK, Hunninghake GW. Expression of immunoreactive cytidine 5′-triphosphate: cholinephosphate cytidylyltransferase in developing rat lung. Pediatr Res 1993;34:502–511.
269. Weinhold PA, Charles L, Rounsifer ME, et al. Control of phosphatidylcholine synthesis in Hep G2 cells. Effect of fatty acids on the activity and immunoreactive content of choline phosphate cytidylyltransferase. J Biol Chem 1991;266:6093–6100.
270. Feldman DA, Rounsifer ME, Charles L, et al. CTP:phosphocholine cytidylyltransferase in rat lung: relationship between cytosolic and membrane forms. Biochim Biophys Acta 1990;1045:49–57.
271. Mallampalli RK, Salome RG, Li CH, et al. Betamethasone activation of CTP:cholinephosphate cytidylyltransferase is mediated by fatty acids. J Cell Physiol 1995;162:410–421.
272. Feldman DA, Brubaker PG, Weinhold PA. Activation of CTP:phosphocholine cytidylyltransferase in rat lung by fatty acids. Biochim Biophys Acta 1981;665:53–59.
273. Mallampalli RK, Salome RG, Hunninghake GW. Lung CTP:choline-phosphate cytidylyltransferase: activation of cytosolic species by unsaturated fatty acid. Am J Physiol 1993;265:L158–163.
274. Mallampalli RK, Salome RG, Spector AA. Regulation of CTP:choline-phosphate cytidylyltransferase by polyunsaturated n-3 fatty acids. Am J Physiol 1994;267:L641–648.
275. Rooney SA. Fatty acid biosynthesis in developing fetal lung. Am J Physiol 1989;257:L195–201.
276. Weinhold PA, Rounsifer ME, Williams SE, et al. CTP:phosphorylcholine cytidylyltransferase in rat lung. The effect of free fatty acids on the translocation of activity between microsomes and cytosol. J Biol Chem 1984;259:10315–10321.
277. Chan F, Harding PGR, Wong T, et al. Cellular distribution of enzymes involved in phosphatidylcholine synthesis in developing rat lung. Can J Biochem Cell Biol 1983;61:107–114.
278. Smith BT, Post M. Fibroblast-pneumocyte factor. Am J Physiol 1989;257:L174–178.
279. Batenburg JJ, Elfring RH. Pre-translational regulation by glucocorticoid of fatty acid and phosphatidylcholine synthesis in type II cells from fetal rat lung. FEBS Lett 1992;307:164–168.
280. MacDonald JI, Kent C. Identification of phosphorylation sites in rat liver CTP:phosphocholine cytidylyltransferase. J Biol Chem 1994;269:10529–10537.
281. Wang Y, MacDonald JI, Kent C. Regulation of CTP:phosphocholine cytidylyltransferase in HeLa cells. Effect of oleate on phosphorylation and intracellular localization. J Biol Chem 1993;268:5512–5518.
282. Hatch GM, Jamil H, Utal AK, et al. On the mechanism of the okadaic acid-induced inhibition of phosphatidylcholine biosynthesis in isolated rat hepatocytes. J Biol Chem 1992;267:15751–15758.
283. Watkins JD, Kent C. Phosphorylation of CTP:phosphocholine cytidylyltransferase in vivo. Lack of effect of phorbol ester treatment in HeLa cells. J Biol Chem 1990;265:2190–2197.
284. Watkins JD, Kent C. Regulation of CTP:phosphocholine cytidylyltransferase activity and subcellular location by phosphorylation in Chinese hamster ovary cells. The effect of phospholipase C treatment. J Biol Chem 1991;266:21113–21117.
285. Weinhold PA, Charles L, Feldman DA. Regulation of CTP:phosphocholine cytidylyltransferase in HepG2 cells: effect of choline depletion on phosphorylation, translocation and phosphatidylcholine levels. Biochim Biophys Acta 1994;1210:335–347.
286. Houweling M, Jamil H, Hatch GM, et al. Dephosphorylation of CTP-phosphocholine cytidylyltransferase is not required for binding to membranes. J Biol Chem 1994;269:7544–7551.
287. Radika K, Possmayer F. Inhibition of foetal pulmonary choline-phosphate cytidylyltransferase under conditions favouring protein phosphorylation. Biochem J 1985;232:833–840.
288. Zimmermann L, Post M. Regulation of CTP:phosphocholine cytidylyltransferase (CP-CYT) in fetal rat type II pneumocytes by phosphorylation and dephosphorylation. Pediatr Res 1991;29:56A.
289. Pelech SL, Pritchard PH, Vance DE. cAMP analogues inhibit phosphatidylcholine biosynthesis in cultured rat hepatocytes. J Biol Chem 1981;256:8283–8286.
290. Zimmermann LJ, Lee WS, Smith BT, et al. Cyclic AMP-dependent protein kinase does not regulate CTP:phosphocholine cytidylyltransferase activity in maturing type II cells. Biochim Biophys Acta 1994;1211:44–50.
291. Utal AK, Jamil H, Vance DE. Diacylglycerol signals the translocation of CTP:choline-phosphate cytidylyltransferase in HeLa cells treated with 12-O-tetradecanoylphorbol-13-acetate. J Biol Chem 1991;266:24084–24091.
292. Cook HW, Vance DE. Evaluation of possible mechanisms of phorbol ester stimulation of phosphatidylcholine synthesis in HeLa cells. Can J Biochem Cell Biol 1985;63:145–151.
293. Tronchere H, Record M, Terce F, et al. Phosphatidylcholine cycle and regulation of phosphatidylcholine biosynthesis by enzyme translocation. Biochim Biophys Acta 1994;1212:137–151.
294. Rosenberg IL, Smart DA, Gilfillan AM, et al. Effect of 1-oleoyl-2-acetylglycerol and other lipids on phosphatidylcholine synthesis and cholinephosphate cytidylyltransferase activity in cultured type II pneumocytes. Biochim Biophys Acta 1987;921:473–480.
295. Jamil H, Yao ZM, Vance DE. Feedback regulation of CTP:phosphocholine cytidylyltransferase translocation between cytosol and endoplasmic reticulum by phosphatidylcholine. J Biol Chem 1990;265:4332–4339.
296. Jamil H, Vance DE. Head-group specificity for feedback regulation of CTP:phosphocholine cytidylyltransferase. Biochem J 1990;270:749–754.
297. Geilen CC, Haase A, Wieder T, et al. Phospholipid analogues: side chain- and polar head group-dependent effects on phosphatidylcholine biosynthesis. J Lipid Res 1994;35:625–632.

298. Tijburg LBM, Houweling M, Geelen MJH, et al. Effects of dietary conditions on the pool sizes of precursors of phosphatidylcholine and phosphatidylethanolamine synthesis in rat liver. Biochim Biophys Acta 1988;959:1–8.
299. Sleight R, Kent C. Regulation of phosphatidylcholine biosynthesis in mammalian cells. II. Effects of phospholipase C treatment on the activity and subcellular distribution of CTP:phosphocholine cytidylyltransferase in Chinese hamster ovary and LM cell lines. J Biol Chem 1983;258:831–835.
300. Jamil H, Hatch GM, Vance DE. Evidence that binding of CTP:phosphocholine cytidylyltransferase to membranes in rat hepatocytes is modulated by the ratio of bilayer- to non-bilayer-forming lipids. Biochem J 1993;291:419–427.
301. Tesan M, Anceschi MM, Bleasdale JE. Regulation of CTP:phosphocholine cytidylyltransferase activity in type II pneumonocytes. Biochem J 1985;232:705–713.
302. Aeberhard EE, Barrett CT, Kaplan SA, et al. Regulation of phospholipid synthesis by intracellular phospholipases in fetal rabbit type II pneumocytes. Biochim Biophys Acta 1985;833:473–483.
303. Fraslon C, Batenburg JJ. Pre-translational regulation of lipid synthesizing enzymes and surfactant proteins in fetal rat lung in explant culture. FEBS Lett 1993;325:285–290.
304. Fraslon-Vanhulle C, Chailley-Heu B, Batenburg JJ, et al. Ontogeny of surfactant proteins and lipid-synthesizing enzymes in cultured fetal lung epithelial cells. Am J Physiol 1994;267:L375–383.
305. Post M, Schuurmans EAJM, Batenburg JJ, et al. Mechanisms involved in the synthesis of disaturated phosphatidylcholine by alveolar type II cells isolated from adult lung. Biochim Biophys Acta 1983;750:68–77.
306. de Vries ACJ, Batenburg JJ, van Golde LMG. Lysophosphatidylcholine acyltransferase and lysophosphatidylcholine:lysophosphatidylcholine acyltransferase in alveolar type II cells from fetal rat lung. Biochim Biophys Acta 1985;833:93–99.
307. Batenburg JJ. Biosynthesis of surfactant lipids. In: Robertson B, Van Golde LMG, Batenburg JJ, eds. Pulmonary surfactant: from molecular biology to clinical practice. Amsterdam: Elsevier, 1992:255–281.
308. Maniscalco WM, Finkelstein JN, Parkhurst AB. De novo fatty acid synthesis in developing rat lung. Biochim Biophys Acta 1982;711:49–58.
309. Rooney SA, Gobran LI, Chu AJ. Thyroid hormone opposes some glucocorticoid effects on glycogen content and lipid synthesis in developing fetal rat lung. Pediatr Res 1986;20:545–550.
310. Batenburg JJ, Den Breejen JN, Geelen MJH, et al. Phosphatidylcholine synthesis in type II cells and regulation of the fatty acid supply. Prog Respir Res 1990;25:96–103.
311. Pope TS, Rooney SA. Effects of glucocorticoid and thyroid hormones on regulatory enzymes of fatty acid synthesis and glycogen metabolism in developing fetal rat lung. Biochim Biophys Acta 1987;918:141–148.
312. Patterson CE, Davis KS, Rhoades RA. Regulation of fetal lung disaturated phosphatidylcholine synthesis by de novo palmitate supply. Biochim Biophys Acta 1988;958:60–69.
313. Maniscalco WM, Finkelstein JN, Parkhurst AB. Effects of exogenous fatty acids and inhibition of de novo fatty acid synthesis on disaturated phosphatidylcholine production by fetal lung cells and adult type II cells. Exp Lung Res 1989;15:473–489.
314. Jobe A, Ikegami M, Sarton-Miller I. The in vivo labeling with acetate and palmitate of lung phospholipids from developing and adult rabbits. Biochim Biophys Acta 1980;617:65–75.
315. Cornell R, Vance DE. Translocation of CTP:phosphocholine cytidylyltransferase from cytosol to membranes in HeLa cells: stimulation by fatty acid, fatty alcohol, mono- and diacylglycerol. Biochim Biophys Acta 1987;919:26–36.
316. Terce F, Record M, Tronchere H, et al. Reversible translocation of cytidylyltransferase between cytosol and endoplasmic reticulum occurs within minutes in whole cells. Biochem J 1992;282:333–338.
317. Stripp BR, Whitsett JA, Lattier DL. Strategies for analysis of gene expression: pulmonary surfactant proteins. Am J Physiol 1990;259:L185–197.
318. Ballard PL. Hormonal regulation of pulmonary surfactant. Endocr Rev 1989;10:165–181.
319. Mendelson CR, Boggaram V. Hormonal control of the surfactant system in fetal lung. Annu Rev Physiol 1991;53:415–440.
320. Katyal SL, Singh G. An enzyme-linked immunoassay of surfactant apoproteins. Its application to the study of fetal lung development in the rat. Pediatr Res 1983;17:439–443.
321. Snyder JM, Mendelson CR. Induction and characterization of the major surfactant apoprotein during rabbit fetal lung development. Biochim Biophys Acta 1987;920:226–236.
322. Shimizu H, Miyamura K, Kuroki Y. Appearance of surfactant proteins, SP-A and SP-B, in developing rat lung and the effects of in vivo dexamethasone treatment. Biochim Biophys Acta 1991;1081:53–60.
323. Katyal SL, Singh G. An immunologic study of the apoproteins of rat lung surfactant. Lab Invest 1979;40:562–567.
324. Williams MC, Benson BJ. Immunocytochemical localization and identification of the major surfactant protein in adult rat lung. J Histochem Cytochem 1981;29:291–305.
325. Sueishi K, Tanaka K, Oda T. Immunoultrastructural study of surfactant system. Distribution of specific protein of surface active material in rabbit lung. Lab Invest 1977;37:136–142.
326. Schellhase DE, Emrie PA, Fisher JH, et al. Ontogeny of surfactant apoproteins in the rat. Pediatr Res 1989;26:167–174.
327. Schellhase DE, Shannon JM. Effects of maternal dexamethasone on expression of SP-A, SP-B, and SP-C in the fetal rat lung. Am J Respir Cell Mol Biol 1991;4:304–312.
328. Ogasawara Y, Kuroki Y, Shiratori M, et al. Ontogeny of surfactant apoprotein D, SP-D, in the rat lung. Biochim Biophys Acta 1991;1083:252–256.
329. Connelly IH, Hammond GL, Harding PG, et al. Levels of surfactant-associated protein messenger ribonucleic acids in rabbit lung during perinatal development and after hormonal treatment. Endocrinology 1991;129:2583–2591.

330. Minoo P, Segura L, Coalson JJ, et al. Alterations in surfactant protein gene expression associated with premature birth and exposure to hyperoxia. Am J Physiol 1991; 261:L386–392.
331. Liley HG, White RT, Warr RG, et al. Regulation of messenger RNAs for the hydrophobic surfactant proteins in human lung. J Clin Invest 1989;83:1191–1197.
332. Ballard PL, Hawgood S, Liley H, et al. Regulation of pulmonary surfactant apoprotein SP 28–36 gene in fetal human lung. Proc Natl Acad Sci USA 1986;83:9527–9531.
333. Otto-Verberne CJM, Ten Have-Opbroek AAW, De Vries ECP. Expression of the major surfactant-associated protein, SP-A, in type II cells of human lung before 20 weeks of gestation. Eur J Cell Biol 1990;53:13–19.
334. King RJ, Ruch J, Gikas EG, et al. Appearance of apoproteins of pulmonary surfactant in human amniotic fluid. J Appl Physiol 1975;39:735–741.
335. Kuroki Y, Takahashi H, Fukada Y, et al. Two-site "simultaneous" immunoassay with monoclonal antibodies for the determination of surfactant apoproteins in human amniotic fluid. Pediatr Res 1985;19:1017–1020.
336. Snyder JM. The biology of surfactant-associated proteins. In: Bourbon JR, ed. Pulmonary surfactant: biochemical, functional, regulatory and clinical concepts. Boca Raton, FL: CRC Press, 1991:105–127.
337. Xu JJ, Richardson C, Ford C, et al. Isolation and characterization of the cDNA for pulmonary surfactant-associated protein-B (SP-B) in the rabbit. Biochem Biophys Res Commun 1989;160:325–332.
338. Whitsett JA, Weaver TE, Clark JC, et al. Glucocorticoid enhances surfactant proteolipid Phe and pVal synthesis and RNA in fetal lung. J Biol Chem 1987;262:15618–15623.
339. Crouch E, Rust K, Marienchek W, et al. Developmental expression of pulmonary surfactant protein D (SP-D). Am J Respir Cell Mol Biol 1991;5:13–18.
340. Gross I. Regulation of fetal lung maturation. Am J Physiol 1990;259:L337–344.
341. Smith BT. The role of pulmonary corticosteroid 11-reductase activity in lung maturation in the fetal rat. Pediatr Res 1978;12:12–14.
342. Mulay S, Giannopoulos G, Solomon S. Corticosteroid levels in the mother and fetus of the rabbit during gestation. Endocrinology 1973;93:1342–1348.
343. Kitterman JA, Liggins GC, Campos GA, et al. Prepartum maturation of the lung in fetal sheep: relation to cortisol. J Appl Physiol 1981;51:384–390.
344. de Fencl M, Tulchinsky D. Total cortisol in amniotic fluid and fetal lung maturation. N Engl J Med 1975;292:133–136.
345. Gewolb IH, Hobbins JC, Tan SY. Amniotic fluid cortisol as an index of fetal lung maturity. Obstet Gynecol 1977;49:462–465.
346. Sharp-Cageorge SM, Blicher BM, Gordon ER, et al. Amniotic-fluid cortisol and human fetal lung maturation. N Engl J Med 1977;296:89–92.
347. Weiss RR, Macri JN, Tejani N, et al. Antenatal diagnosis and lung maturation in anencephaly. Obstet Gynecol 1974;44:368–372.
348. Smith BT, Worthington D. Discordant lung maturation and corticosteroid levels in twins. Pediatr Res 1976;10:468A.
349. Blackburn WR, Travers H, Potter DM. The role of the pituitary-adrenal-thyroid axes in lung differentiation. I. Studies of the cytology and physical properties of anencephalic fetal rat lung. Lab Invest 1972;26:306–318.
350. Blackburn WR, Kelly JS, Dickman PS, et al. The role of the pituitary-adrenal-thyroid axes in lung differentiation. II. Biochemical studies of developing lung in anencephalic fetal rats. Lab Invest 1973;28:352–360.
351. Sosenko IR, Lewis PL, Frank L. Metyrapone delays surfactant and antioxidant enzyme maturation in developing rat lung. Pediatr Res 1986;20:672–675.
352. Vidyasagar D, Chernick V. Effect of metopirone on the synthesis of lung surfactant in does and fetal rabbits. Biol Neonate 1975;27:1–16.
353. Kling OR, Kotas RV. Endocrine influences on pulmonary maturation and the lecithin/sphingomyelin ratio in the fetal baboon. Am J Obstet Gynecol 1975;121:664–668.
354. Giannopoulos G, Mulay S, Solomon S. Cortisol receptors in rabbit fetal lung. Biochem Biophys Res Commun 1972;47:411–418.
355. Giannopoulos G. Glucocorticoid receptors in lung. I. Specific binding of glucocorticoids to cytoplasmic components of rabbit fetal lung. J Biol Chem 1973;248:3876–3883.
356. Giannopoulos G, Mulay S, Solomon S. Glucocorticoid receptors in lung. II. Specific binding of glucocorticoids to nuclear components of rabbit fetal lung. J Biol Chem 1973;248:5016–5023.
357. Ballard PL, Ballard RA, Gonzales LK, et al. Corticosteroid binding by fetal rat and rabbit lung in organ culture. J Steroid Biochem 1984;21:117–126.
358. Ballard PL, Ballard RA. Cytoplasmic receptor for glucocorticoids in lung of the human fetus and neonate. J Clin Invest 1974;53.
359. Sweezey N, Mawdsley C, Ghibu F, et al. Differential regulation of glucocorticoid receptor expression by ligand in fetal rat lung cells. Pediatr Res 1995;38:506–512.
360. Gonzales LW, Ertsey R, Ballard PL, et al. Glucocorticoid stimulation of fatty acid synthesis in explants of human fetal lung. Biochim Biophys Acta 1990;1042:1–12.
361. Maniscalco WM, Finkelstein JN, Parkhurst AB. Dexamethasone increases de novo fatty acid synthesis in fetal rabbit lung explants. Pediatr Res 1985;19:1272–1277.
362. Pope TS, Smart DA, Rooney SA. Hormonal effects on fatty-acid synthase in cultured fetal rat lung; induction by dexamethasone and inhibition of activity by triiodothyronine. Biochim Biophys Acta 1988;959:169–177.
363. Gonzales LW, Ballard PL, Ertsey R, et al. Effect of dexamethasone and cAMP on fatty acid synthethase in human fetal lung explants. FASEB J 1988;2:A492.
364. Xu ZX, Stenzel W, Sasic SM, et al. Glucocorticoid regulation of fatty acid synthase gene expression in fetal rat lung. Am J Physiol 1993;265:L140–147.
365. Xu ZX, Smart DA, Rooney SA. Glucocorticoid induction of fatty-acid synthase mediates the stimulatory effect of the hormone on choline-phosphate cytidylyltransferase

activity in fetal rat lung. Biochim Biophys Acta 1990; 1044:70–76.
366. Rooney SA, Dynia DW, Smart DA, et al. Glucocorticoid stimulation of choline-phosphate cytidylyltransferase activity in fetal rat lung: receptor-response relationships. Biochim Biophys Acta 1986;888:208–216.
367. Avery ME. Historical overview of antenatal steroid use. Pediatrics 1995;95:133–135.
368. Ryan CA, Finer NN. Antenatal corticosteroid therapy to prevent respiratory distress syndrome. J Pediatr 1995;126:317–319.
369. Suen HC, Bloch KD, Donahoe PK. Antenatal glucocorticoid corrects pulmonary immaturity in experimentally induced congenital diaphragmatic hernia in rats. Pediatr Res 1994;35:523–529.
370. NIH Consensus Conference. Effect of corticosteroids for fetal maturation on perinatal outcomes. JAMA 1995;273:413–418.
371. Hull WM, Breslin J, Weaver TE, et al. Distribution of surfactant proteins SP-A and SP-B in surfactant subfractions and lamellar bodies. Pediatr Res 1991;29:320A.
372. Phelps DS, Church S, Kourembanas S, et al. Increases in the 35 kDa surfactant-associated protein and its mRNA following in vivo dexamethasone treatment of fetal and neonatal rats. Electrophoresis 1987;8:235–238.
373. Gross I, Wilson CM, Floros J, et al. Initiation of fetal rat lung phospholipid and surfactant-associated protein A mRNA synthesis. Pediatr Res 1989;25:239–244.
374. Fisher JH, McCormack F, Park SS, et al. In vivo regulation of surfactant proteins by glucocorticoids. Am J Respir Cell Mol Biol 1991;5:63–70.
375. Young SL, Ho YS, Silbajoris RA. Surfactant apoprotein in adult rat lung compartments is increased by dexamethasone. Am J Physiol 1991;260:L161–167.
376. Boggaram V, Smith ME, Mendelson CR. Regulation of expression of the gene encoding the major surfactant protein (SP-A) in human fetal lung in vitro. Disparate effects of glucocorticoids on transcription and on mRNA stability. J Biol Chem 1989;264:11421–11427.
377. Odom MJ, Snyder JM, Boggaram V, et al. Glucocorticoid regulation of the major surfactant associated protein (SP-A) and its messenger ribonucleic acid and of morphological development of human fetal lung in vitro. Endocrinology 1988;123:1712–1720.
378. Liley HG, White RT, Benson BJ, et al. Glucocorticoids both stimulate and inhibit production of pulmonary surfactant protein A in fetal human lung. Proc Natl Acad Sci USA 1988;85:9096–9100.
379. Kari MA, Akino T, Hallman M. Prenatal dexamethasone and exogenous surfactant therapy: surface activity and surfactant components in airway specimens. Pediatr Res 1995;38:676–684.
380. Kari MA, Raivio KO, Venge P, et al. Dexamethasone treatment of infants at risk for chronic lung disease: surfactant components and inflammatory parameters in airway specimens. Pediatr Res 1994;36:387–393.
381. Phelps DS, Floros J. Dexamethasone in vivo raises surfactant protein B mRNA in alveolar and bronchiolar epithelium. Am J Physiol 1991;260:L146–152.

382. O'Reilly MA, Gazdar AF, Morris RE, et al. Differential effects of glucocorticoid on expression of surfactant proteins in a human lung adenocarcinoma cell line. Biochim Biophys Acta 1988;970:194–204.
383. O'Reilly MA, Gazdar AF, Clark JC, et al. Glucocorticoids regulate surfactant protein synthesis in a pulmonary adenocarcinoma cell line. Am J Physiol 1989;257:L385–392.
384. Dobbs LG, Mason RG. Pulmonary alveolar type II cells isolated from rats. Release of phosphatidylcholine in response to beta-adrenergic stimulation. J Clin Invest 1979;63:378–387.
385. Brown LA, Longmore WJ. Adrenergic and cholinergic regulation of lung surfactant secretion in the isolated perfused rat lung and in the alveolar type II cell in culture. J Biol Chem 1981;256:66–72.
386. Post M, Torday JS, Smith BT. Alveolar type II cells isolated from fetal rat lung organotypic cultures synthesize and secrete surfactant-associated phospholipids and respond to fibroblast-pneumonocyte factor. Exp Lung Res 1984;7:53–65.
387. Ballard PL, Ertsey R, Gonzales LK, et al. Isolation and characterization of differentiated alveolar type II cells from fetal human lung. Biochim Biophys Acta 1986;883:335–344.
388. Rasmusson MG, Scott JE, Oulton MR, et al. Characterization and comparison of the role of β-agonists on in vivo and in vitro surfactant-related phospholipid synthesis and secretion by fetal rabbit lung and isolated type II alveolar cells. Exp Lung Res 1988;14:811–822.
389. Walters DV. The role of pulmonary surfactant in transepithelial movement of liquid. In: Robertson B, van Golde LMG, Batenburg JJ, eds. Pulmonary surfactant: from molecular biology to clinical practice. Amsterdam: Elsevier, 1992:191–213.
390. Morales WJ, O'Brien WF, Angel JL, et al. Fetal lung maturation: the combined use of corticosteroids and thyrotropin-releasing hormone. Obstet Gynecol 1989;73:111–116.
391. Ballard RA, Ballard PL, Creasy RK, et al. Respiratory disease in very-low-birthweight infants after prenatal thyrotropin-releasing hormone and glucocorticoid. TRH Study Group. Lancet 1992;339:510–515.
392. ACTOBAT Study Group. Australian collaborative trial of antenatal thyrotropin-releasing hormone (ACTOBAT) for prevention of neonatal respiratory disease. Lancet 1995;345:877–882.
393. Miller HC, Futrakul P. Birth weight, gestational age, and sex as determining factors in the incidence of respiratory distress syndrome of prematurely born infants. J Pediatr 1968;72:628–635.
394. Farrell PM, Avery ME. Hyaline membrane disease. Am Rev Respir Dis 1975;111:657–688.
395. Jobe AH, Ikegami M. Surfactant metabolism. Clin Perinatol 1993;20:683–696.
396. Adams FH, Fujiwara T, Emmanouilides GC, et al. Lung phospholipid of the human fetus and infants with and without hyaline membrane disease. J Pediatr 1970;77:833.

397. Hallman M, Merritt TA, Pohjavuori M, et al. Effect of surfactant substitution on lung effluent phospholipids in respiratory distress syndrome: evaluation of surfactant phospholipid turnover, pool size, and the relationship to severity of respiratory failure. Pediatr Res 1986;20:1228–1235.
398. Dargaville PA, McDougall PN, South M. Comparison of tracheal aspirate and bronchoalveolar lavage for collection of surfactant specimens in ventilated infants. Appl Cardiopulmon Pathophysiol 1995;5:18–19 [abstr].
399. Hallman M, Merritt TA, Akino T, et al. Surfactant protein A, phosphatidylcholine, and surfactant inhibitors in epithelial lining fluid. Am Rev Respir Dis 1991;144:1376–1384.
400. Bunt JEH, Zimmermann LJI. Waltimena JLD, et al. Endogenous surfactant turnover in preterm infants measured with stable isotopes. Am J Resp Crit Care Med 1998; accepted for publication.
401. Hallman M, Merritt TA, Bry K. The fate of exogenous surfactant in neonates with respiratory distress syndrome. Clin Pharmacokinet 1994;26:215–232.
402. Konishi M, Fujiwara T, Nalto T, et al. Surfactant replacement therapy in neonatal respiratory distress syndrome. A multi-centre, randomized clinical trial: comparison of high- versus low-dose of Surfactant TA. Eur J Pediatr 1988;147:20–25.
403. The OSIRIS collaborative group. Early versus delayed neonatal administration of synthetic surfactant—the judgment of OSIRIS. Lancet 1992;340:1363–1369.
404. Jobe AH, Rider ED. Catabolism and recycling of surfactant. In: Robertson B, van Golde LMG, Batenburg JJ, eds. Pulmonary surfactant: from molecular biology to clinical practice. Amsterdam: Elsevier, 1992:313–337.
405. Charon A, Taeusch HW, Fitzgibbon C, et al. Factors associated with surfactant treatment response in infants with severe respiratory distress syndrome. Pediatrics 1989;83:348–354.
406. Dunn MS, Shennan AT, Possmayer F. Single- versus multiple-dose surfactant replacement therapy in neonates of 30 to 36 weeks' gestation with respiratory distress syndrome. Pediatrics 1990;86:564–571.
407. Speer CP, Robertson B, Curstedt T, et al. Randomized European Multicenter Trial of surfactant replacement therapy for severe neonatal respiratory distress syndrome: single versus multiple doses of Curosurf. Pediatrics 1992;89:13–20.
408. Zimmermann, LJI. Unpublished data.
409. Vance DE. Phosphatidylcholine metabolism: masochistic enzymology, metabolic regulation, and lipoprotein assembly. Biochem Cell Biol 1990;68:1151–1165.
410. Kent C, Carman GM, Spence MW, et al. Regulation of eukaryotic phospholipid metabolism. FASEB J 1991;5:2258–2266.
411. Hunt AN, Normand CS, Postle AD. CTP:cholinephosphate cytidylyltransferase in human and rat lung: association in vitro with cytoskeletal actin. Biochim Biophys Acta 1990;1043:19–26.

29
Liver Metabolism in the Fetus and Neonate

Jean-Paul Pégorier and Jean Girard

During the perinatal period important modifications occur in several physiologic functions and particularly dramatic changes in nutrition. In utero, the fetus receives a continuous intravenous supply of substrates for its growth and its oxidative metabolism and produces large quantities of CO_2 and urea.[1,2] Immediately after birth, the maternal supply of substrates ceases abruptly, and the neonate must withstand a brief period of starvation before being fed at intervals with milk, which is a high-fat and low-carbohydrate diet. The successful adaptation of the neonate to these changes of nutrition and environment require important modifications of glucose and fatty acid metabolism, which are orchestrated mainly by alterations in hormone secretion.

This chapter reviews the metabolic adaptations of glucose and fatty acid metabolism during the perinatal period. Most of the data on this subject come from experimental studies performed in various animal species and especially in the rat. The relevance of animal studies in the understanding of fuel homeostasis in the human neonate is considered (see Chapter 6).

Nutritional and Hormonal Changes During the Perinatal Period

Nutritional Changes

During pregnancy, the fetus is continuously supplied through the placenta with a diet rich in carbohydrate and amino acids and poor in fat (Figure 29.1).[1,2] In most species free fatty acids (FFAs) are poorly transferred across the placenta, and in the few species in which the placenta is permeable to FFA (e.g., the human, guinea pig, rabbit), FFAs are stored as triglycerides in liver and adipose tissue but are poorly oxidized by fetal tissues.[3,4] Immediately after birth, the neonate has to withstand a brief period of starvation before being fed at intervals with milk. From an energy point of view, milk is a high-fat low-carbohydrate diet (Figure 29.1).[3] In the rat, the lactose and fat content in milk represents respectively 3 and $10\,g \cdot 100\,g^{-1}$. In human milk, the lactose content is higher and the fat content is lower (i.e., respectively 7 and $4\,g \cdot 100\,g^{-1}$). Nevertheless, fat represents more than 50% of energy intake in the neonate of most species.[5] Lactose is the predominant carbohydrate in the milk, while 95% of milk fat is in the form of triglycerides. The nutrient content of milk depends on the stage of lactation. Colostrum is characterized by a lower lactose and a higher fat content than in mature milk.[5] The fatty acid composition of milk triglycerides shows marked species differences, depending on the chain length and the degree of saturation of fatty acid. For instance, milk from the human, guinea pig, or sow contains a very high proportion of long-chain fatty acids (i.e., respectively 85%, 98%, and 99% of triglycerides), whereas milk from the mare, rat, or rabbit contains a high proportion of medium-chain fatty acids (i.e., respectively 20%, 30%, and 70% of milk triglycerides).[6,7] Moreover, a significant amount of short-chain fatty acids is detectable in milk triglycerides of ruminants.[6,7]

Hormonal Changes

During the immediate postnatal period a large increase in plasma glucagon occurs in the neonate of different species—rat, rabbit, sheep, pig, and human (Figure 29.2).[8] In the rat, the increase in plasma glucagon concentration is observed both after vaginal delivery and cesarean section.[9,10] During the same period, plasma insulin concentration decreases rapidly or remains in a very low concentration (Figure 29.2).[8]

The transient hypoglycemia that supervenes in the neonatal rat and humans is not the factor triggering the changes in plasma glucagon and insulin concentrations because (1) they can occur in the absence of hypoglycemia,[11] and (2) the insensitivity of the A cells of the neonatal pancreas to acute changes (1–4 hours)

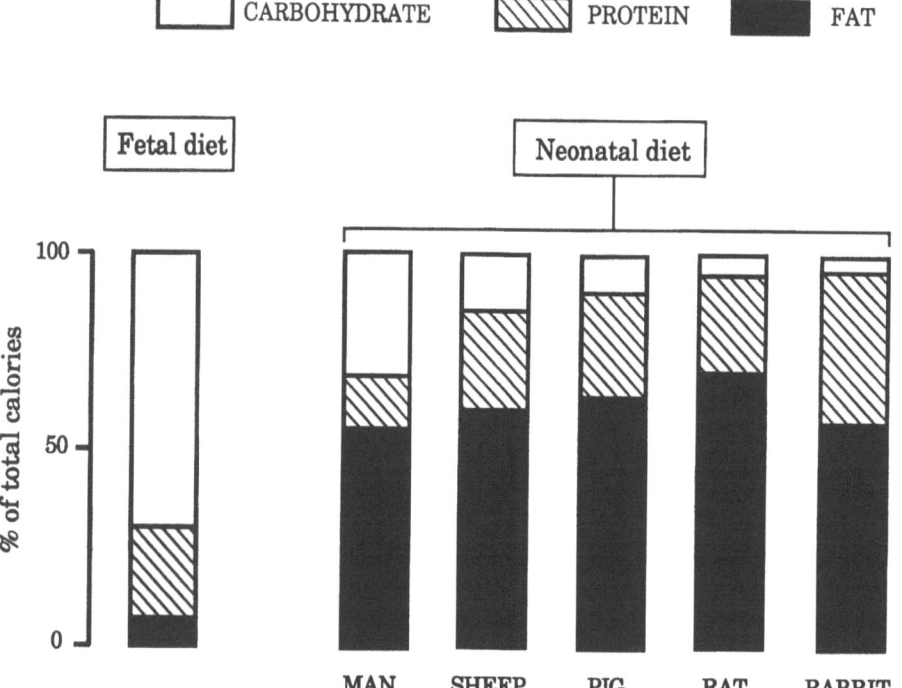

FIGURE 29.1 Composition of the diet in fetuses and neonates from different species. (Data from Battaglia and Meschia[1] and Girard and Ferré.[3])

in glycemia is well documented.[3,5] Although amino acids are potent stimulators of glucagon secretion by the fetal pancreas,[8] it is unlikely that they play a role in the surge of glucagon at birth since plasma amino acid concentration falls rapidly during this period.[12] A more likely mechanism to explain the acute neonatal increase in plasma glucagon concentration and the fall in plasma insulin concentration could be related to the stress of birth through an activation of the sympathetic nervous system.[3,5]

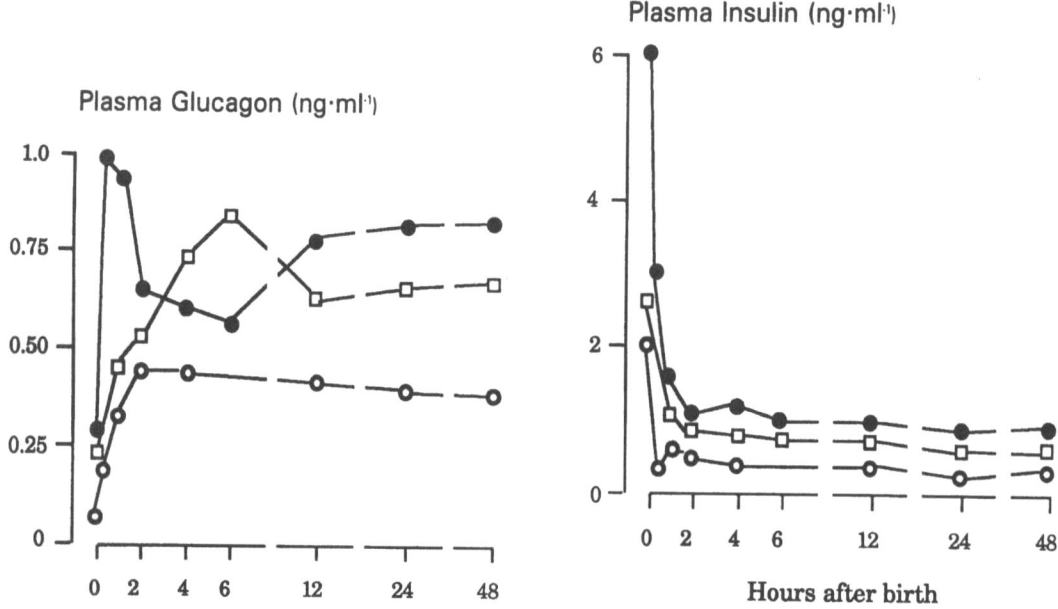

FIGURE 29.2. Plasma insulin and glucagon in fasting human (O—O), rabbit (□—□), and rat (●—●) neonates. (Data from Girard and Ferré,[3] Girard et al.,[9] and Callikan et al.,[63] with permission.)

Plasma cortisol or corticosterone concentrations are elevated in the plasma at delivery and rapidly decline during the first 24 hours following birth.[13,14] The concentration of growth hormone is very high at birth and remains elevated during the first 24 hours.[15,16]

In the sheep, pig, and human neonate, there is a marked rise in triiodothyronine (T_3) at 2 hours and a gradual increase in thyroxine (T_4) during the first 24 hours after birth.[17] In the rat, T_3 is undetectable in plasma at birth and T_4 is very low.

Regulation of Glucose Metabolism During the Perinatal Period

To meet the glucose needs of vital organs (e.g., brain, renal medulla) or cells (e.g., erythrocytes) that are partly or totally dependent on the oxidaton of this substrate for maintaining their functional activity,[3,18,19] the neonate must rapidly turn on the pathways for endogenous glucose production. The large glycogen stores accumulated in the liver during pregnancy are rapidly mobilized and are exhausted 12 hours after delivery.[20] After this period, the suckling neonate is entirely dependent on glucose supplied via the milk and on his capacity for an efficient gluconeogenesis to maintain his blood glucose concentration in the normal range. Thus, the liver has a crucial role in the adaptation of the neonate to extrauterine life (see Chapter 32).

These metabolic adaptations are tightly regulated by appropriate changes in hormone concentrations, such as insulin, glucagon, epinephrine, and sympathetic nervous system activity.

Mobilization of Liver Glycogen Stores

Liver glycogenolysis occurs at birth to maintain blood glucose concentration before other sources of energy become available from the milk. The importance of hepatic glycogen stores in maintaining normoglycemia in the postnatal period is illustrated by data from the intrauterine growth retarded human neonate. These neonates have reduced hepatic glycogen stores and rapidly become hypoglycemic during the early postnatal period.[21] In the human neonate, blood glucose concentration remains normal until liver glycogen concentration is reduced below $10 \, mg \cdot g^{-1}$.[22] However, as liver glycogen stores are exhausted 12 hours after birth whatever the nutritional environment,[5] exogenous glucose supply and an active gluconeogenesis are required thereafter for maintaining normoglycemia.

Changes in the Activities of Enzyme Controlling Glycogenolysis

Liver glycogenolysis results from the inactivation of glycogen synthase (GS) and the activation of glycogen phosphorylase (GP). The ratio of active forms of these enzymes is determined by their phosphorylation state, which is dependent on the activity of adenosine 3',5'-cyclic monophosphate (cAMP) protein kinase.[23] Prior to birth, GP and GS activities are present in fetal rat liver with a ratio of GS-a/GP-a that allows net glycogen synthesis.[24–27] Immediately after birth, GP messenger RNA (mRNA) levels and activity are slightly increased[27] and GS-a activity is decreased.[25,26,28] This suggests that the ratio of GP-a/GS-a(alpha) is a better indicator of neonatal liver glycogenolysis than the activity of GP-a itself.

It has been suggested that a part of liver glycogenolysis in the neonatal rat could involve the activation of acid α-glucosidase located in lysosomes,[29] which increases in neonatal rat liver.[30] The homozygous gsd (glycogen storage disease) rat has a genetic defect in liver GP kinase, which becomes rapidly hypoglycemic in the neonatal period.[31] This confirms the predominant role of GP-a in the regulation of glycogenolysis in the neonatal rat liver.

To participate in whole-body glucose homeostasis, glucose-6-phosphate derived from liver glycogenolysis must be hydrolyzed to glucose within the liver. The enzyme responsible for glucose-6-phosphate hydrolysis is glucose-6-phosphatase, which is located inside the microsome. Glucose-6-phosphatase is a key enzyme in glucose homeostasis since it catalyzes the final step of glycogenolysis and gluconeogenesis (vide infra). In the mouse having a deletion around the albinos locus on chromosome 7, the expression of glucose-6-phosphatase is reduced.[32] Homozygous deletion-mutant develops profound hypoglycemia immediately after birth,[33] showing the importance of that enzyme in the maintenance of glucose homeostasis in the immediate postnatal period. At the end of fetal life, liver glucose-6-phosphatase activity reaches 80% of adult levels and shows a postnatal increase.[34,35] These changes in glucose-6-phosphatase activity result from a stimulation of the transcription of its gene.[36] Then, the activity of glucose-6-phosphatase remains elevated, above the adult value, during all the suckling period.[36] This phenomenon can be regarded as a specific adaptation turned on by the change of environment at birth.

Hormonal Control of Glycogenolysis at Birth

The factors responsible for the stimulation of liver glycogenolysis at birth are not completely known. It has been suggested that the concomitant rise in plasma glucagon and catecholamine concentrations and the decline in plasma insulin concentration could be responsible for hepatic glycogen breakdown.[37] In vivo[38,39] and in vitro[18,40] studies have shown that glucagon stimulates glycogenolysis in fetal rat liver, whereas insulin prevents liver glycogenolysis.[41] Similarly, the infusion of somatostatin in the neonatal lamb lowers plasma insulin and glucagon concentrations and induces hypoglycemia. Reinfusion of glucagon during somatostatin infusion completely reverses hypoglycemia.[42] These experiments underline the primary role of glucagon in neonatal glucose production. The role of catecholamines depends on the species concerned. Adrenalectomy before parturition abolishes the postnatal increase of epinephrine and results in hypoglycemia in the neonatal sheep.[43] However, adrenalectomy of the rat at birth does not impair postnatal liver glycogen mobilization.[41]

The mechanisms by which glucagon or catecholamines stimulate liver glycogenolysis have not been completely elucidated. In the adult rat liver, catecholamines stimulate glycogenolysis via an increase in cytosolic Ca^{2+} concentration, secondarily to an activation of α_1-adrenergic receptors.[44] In the neonatal rat liver, catecholamine stimulates glycogenolysis via an increase in liver cAMP concentration, secondary to an activation of β_2-adrenergic receptors.[45,46] Since the increase in cytosolic Ca^{2+} in response to ionophore A23187 induces liver glycogenolysis in the fetal rat hepatocyte,[47] this suggests that the lack of response of perinatal liver to β-adrenergic agonists results from the low ratio of β/α adrenergic receptors.[48]

The administration of epinephrine, glucagon, or cAMP to the fetus near term induces liver glucose-6-phosphatase activity,[41,49] whereas insulin injection to the newborn rat prevents the rise in liver glucose-6-phosphatase activity.[41] Recent studies in the Fao rat hepatoma cell have shown that cAMP induces the accumulation of glucose-6-phosphatase mRNA, whereas insulin inhibits this effect.[50,51]

Exogenous Carbohydrate Supply

In most species, the initial milk (i.e., colostrum) is rich in fat and poor in carbohydrates.[5] Hydrolysis of lactose, the only carbohydrate present in milk, produces equal amounts of glucose and galactose which are taken up by the enterocyte via an active transport system[52,53] and after absorption are delivered to the liver via the portal vein. As liver glucose uptake is low during the neonatal period, glucose derived from lactose is delivered directly to peripheral tissue.[54]

The comparison of glucose supplied via the milk, with the rate of glucose utilization measured with stable or radioactive tracers, allows estimation of the contribution of exogenous glucose to neonatal glucose requirements. In all species in which these parameters have been measured, the glucose supplied by the milk accounts for less than 20% to 50% of glucose requirements of the neonate (Figure 29.3).[3,55,56] In contrast to glucose, galactose is almost exclusively taken up by the liver, where it is mainly converted to glucose since glycogen deposition is minimal during the neonatal period.[54] As the conversion of galactose to glucose requires an active glucose-6-phosphatase, it can be considered as a gluconeogenic precursor. The breast-fed suckling neonates are thus dependent on an active gluconeogenesis from galactose[54] and other substrates (e.g., lactate, amino acids, and glycerol) to sustain an efficient glucose production during the first week of life.

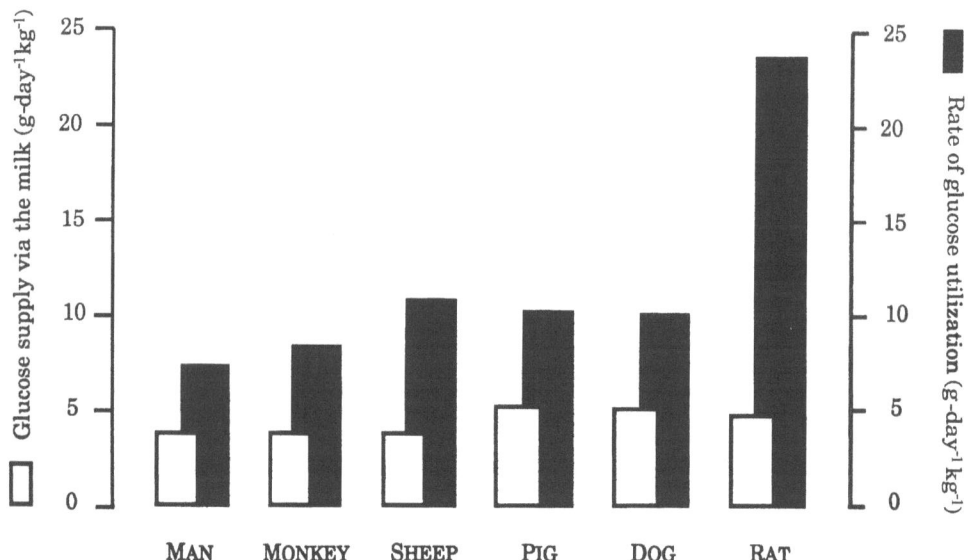

FIGURE 29.3. Comparison between glucose supplied via the milk and the rate of glucose utilization in newborns from various species. (Data from Girard and Ferré,[3] with permission.)

Development and Regulation of Gluconeogenesis

The Gluconeogenic Pathway

The pathway of gluconeogenesis involves specific enzymes located in different cell compartments. In the rat, phosphoenolpyruvate carboxykinase (PEPCK) and fructose-1,6-bisphosphatase are located in the cytosol, whereas pyruvate carboxylase is located in the mitochondrial matrix and glucose-6-phosphatase is located inside the microsomes. In most mammalian species (e.g., human, pig, guinea pig, sheep), PEPCK is also located both in cytosol and inside mitochondria. Mitochondrial PEPCK seems to be a constitutive enzyme whose activity does not vary in response to nutritional and/or hormonal changes, and it is considered to play a role only in basal gluconeogenesis. In contrast, it has been demonstrated that cytosolic PEPCK was an adaptative enzyme whose activity was directly correlated to the hepatic capacity for gluconeogenesis (Figure 29.4).[57] In the adult mammal, it has been shown that gluconeogenesis is regulated by short-term mechanisms involving phosphorylation/dephosphorylation or changes in allosteric effectors (fructose 2,6-bisphosphate). These short-term regulations occur at the level of pyruvate kinase, phosphofructokinase, and fructose-1,6-bisphosphatase.[58]

Increase in Gluconeogenic Enzyme Activities

The ability to synthesize glucose from lactate, pyruvate, and amino acids is very low in fetal liver and develops after birth in several species such as rat, rabbit, guinea pig, pig, and sheep.[5] Most of the enzymes involved in hepatic gluconeogenesis (i.e., pyruvate carboxylase, mitochondrial PEPCK, fructose-1-6-bisphosphatase, and glucose-6-phosphatase) have substantial activity (50–100% of adult value) in fetal liver. Although the cDNA coding for these enzymes has been cloned recently,[59–61] the developmental changes of their mRNA concentration is still unknown except for glucose-6-phosphatase (supra vide). In contrast, the activity of cytosolic PEPCK is low (0–25% of adult value) and increases markedly after birth.[62–65] Thus, cytosolic PEPCK is considered to be the rate-limiting enzyme in the gluconeogenic process.[57,64–66] Postnatal increase in cytosolic PEPCK activity is due to birth-associated factors rather than to nutritional and/or time-dependent factors.[41,67,68] The appearance of PEPCK at birth in the rat is due to de novo enzyme synthesis and to a low rate of degradation.[69,70] More recently, it has been reported that PEPCK mRNA levels are undetectable in fetal rat liver and accumulate within the first 2 hours after birth (Figure 29.4)[70–73] as the result of the stimulation of gene transcription.[73]

Recent studies have shown that the chromosomal deletion of the C^{3H} region in mouse chromosome 7 around the albinos locus[74] cause perinatal death from hypoglycemia.[33] This lethal albino deletion in the homozygous neonate is associated with a dramatic reduction in the activity of liver cytosol PEPCK.[75,76] The deficiency of PEPCK activity is not due to the possible inclusion of the PEPCK structural gene within the deleted sequences of chromosome 7, since it maps on chro-

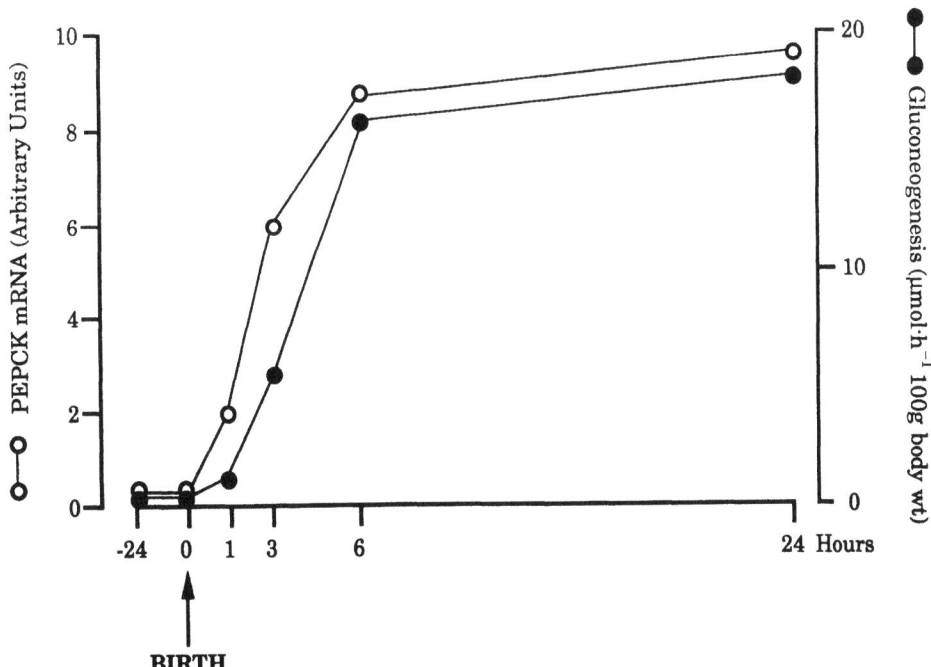

FIGURE 29.4. Postnatal changes in liver PEPCK mRNA concentration (data from Lyonnet et al.[73]) and gluconeogenic rate in vivo from [U-^{14}C] lactate. (Data from Girard et al.,[9] with permission.)

mosome 2. The mRNA levels of PEPCK are severely reduced and are not inducible by cAMP in the deletion homozygous neonate. Thus, the deletions are assumed to include a trans-acting regulatory gene specifically concerned with the developmental regulation of liver PEPCK and other liver-specific genes (supra vide). The trans-acting factor coded on chromosome 7 is postulated to render the structural gene of PEPCK competent to receive and respond to cAMP, perhaps by a change in chromatin conformation.[75,76] A trans-repressor factor (Tse-1) of PEPCK gene has been identified on chromosome 11 in the mouse using hybrids of the rat hepatoma cell and the mouse fibroblast.[77]

Indeed, transcribed genes reside in the domain of an altered chromatin structure in which the DNA is in an "open configuration" accessible to digestion by DNase I.[78] It has been suggested that hypomethylation of the PEPCK gene may be important for its activation. Indeed, the injection of the fetal rat with the methylase inhibitor 5-azacytidine results in the accumulation of PEPCK mRNA in the fetal liver.[79,80] This hypomethylation may be a prerequisite to liver PEPCK expression in the neonate. Two types of proteins that bind to DNA have been identified, and their sequential activation leads to PEPCK gene transcription: (1) differentiation factors, such as AF-1, which binds to the regulatory region of PEPCK gene early in development; (2) developmentally regulated factors, such as C/EBP, which bind to the regulatory region of PEPCK gene around the time of birth.[81]

Hormonal Regulation of Gluconeogenic Enzymes

Although little information is available on the hormonal regulation of pyruvate carboxylase, fructose-1-6-bisphosphatase, and glucose-6-phosphatase gene expression during the fetal-neonatal transition, the hormonal changes that occur at birth (Figure 30.2) (supra vide) could be involved. Indeed, it has been shown in the adult rat liver that glucagon via cAMP, insulin, and glucocorticoids regulated the gene expression coding for these enzymes.[50,58] In contrast, the hormonal control of PEPCK has been extensively studied during the fetal-neonatal transition.[5] Briefly, it was shown that injections of glucagon or cAMP in utero or insulin deficiency caused by streptozocin injections to the rat fetuses induced the premature appearance of PEPCK mRNA and activity.[41,71,82,83] In contrast, injections of insulin to the diabetic fetus or to the newborn rat at delivery impaired the induction of liver PEPCK.[41,82,84] The antagonistic effects of insulin and glucagon on liver PEPCK induction have been confirmed in the cultured hepatocyte from fetal rat in which glucagon and/or cAMP induce PEPCK mRNA accumulation,[85-88] whereas insulin[85] and epidermal growth factor (EGF)[88] oppose these effects. It has been demonstrated that prolonged maternal fasting during late gestation, prolongation of pregnancy, or phlorhizin administration to the pregnant rat induces changes in fetal plasma glucagon and insulin concentrations similar to those occurring at birth[9] and the premature appearance of liver PEPCK in the rat fetus.[89,90] Similarly, experimentally induced changes in the plasma insulin and glucagon concentrations are likewise associated with the premature appearance of hepatic cytosolic PEPCK in the fetal sheep.[91] Recent data suggest that glucagon is the dominant factor in the induction of liver PEPCK mRNA.[87] Indeed, glucagon alone is able to rapidly stimulate PEPCK mRNA accumulation in cultured fetal rat hepatocytes, whereas insulin is not able to antagonize the effects of maximal concentration of glucagon.[87]

Other Physiologic Factors Involved in the Initiation of Hepatic Gluconeogenesis

Three hypotheses have been proposed, in addition to the induction of cytosolic PEPCK, to explain the rapid increase in liver gluconeogenesis in the neonate: (1) an increase in liver oxygenation and a change in the liver redox state, (2) a maturation of mitochondrial oxidative capacity, and (3) a short-term control of fructose 6-phosphate/fructose 1,6-bisphosphate cycle.

Liver Oxygenation

In the term fetal sheep, despite the presence of gluconeogenic enzyme activities,[92,93] gluconeogenesis is inactive in utero and develops within few minutes after birth.[65] It has been suggested that gluconeogenesis could be inhibited in utero by the low adenosine triphosphate (ATP)/adenosine diphosphate (ADP) ratio and by the highly reduced cytosolic redox state [low nicotinamide adenine dinucleotide, oxidized (NAD^+)/nicotinamide adenine dinucleotide, reduced (NADH) ratio] prevailing in fetal liver.[62] It has been proposed that the appearance of gluconeogenesis in the neonatal liver would first involve a postnatal increase of blood PO_2,[65] which would result in an increase in the cytosolic cytosolic NAD^+/NADH ratio and in the degree of phosphorylation of adenine nucleotides, subsequently followed by an increase in liver cytosolic PEPCK. However, several data sets suggest that it is unlikely that acute postnatal liver oxygenation could account for the appearance of liver gluconeogenesis in the neonate. First, fetal liver O_2 consumption is high.[94] Second, it was shown that gluconeogenesis does not increase immediately after birth in the neonatal lamb, but progressively contributes to 30% of total hepatic glucose production 10 hours after birth.[95]

Mitochondrial Oxidative Capacity

The gluconeogenic pathway requires ATP or guanosine triphosphate (GTP) at several different steps (see Figure 29.10, supra vide). This suggests that mitochondrial oxidative capacity must be developed for liver gluconeogenesis to be fully active. It has been reported that pyruvate carboxylase activity increased severalfold soon after birth[96,97] as the result of a postnatal rise in the mitochondrial matrix adenine nucleotide content[98,99] or the ATP/ADP ratio.[100]

In mitochondria isolated from the term fetal rat liver, the respiratory control ratio (RCR), which estimates the degree of coupling between O_2 consumption and ATP synthesis, is lower than the corresponding ratio determined in the adult rat liver.[101–103] When mitochondria from the term fetal rat liver were incubated in the presence of 2,4-dinitrophenol, an uncoupler that allows the electron transport through the respiratory chain without the coupled process of ADP phosphorylation, the respiratory rate is markedly enhanced.[102,103] This suggests that the impaired energy transduction observed at birth arises from a decrease in ADP phosphorylation. The mitochondrial adenine nucleotide content [ATP + ADP + adenosine monophosphate (AMP)] is low at birth and rapidly increases within the first hours after birth in many mammalian species.[5] Then, the low RCR at birth may result from a limitation of intramitochondrial ADP, a precursor of ATP in the ATP synthetase system. The postnatal increase in mitochondrial respiratory capacity and oxidative phosphorylation is due to both a rapid increase in the rate of synthesis of succinate dehydrogenase and cytochrome c oxidase, and to the catalytic site of ATP synthetase (β-F1-ATPase).[104] The importance of the ATP synthetase system in the control of succinate oxidation rates in the neonatal liver mitochondria has been clearly demonstrated.[105] During development, the catalytic activity of ATP synthetase is regulated at both transcriptional and posttranscriptional levels. Indeed, it has been shown that the β-F1-ATPase mRNA accumulates in fetal rat liver[106] and translational efficiency increases immediately after birth.[106,107] The increase in mRNA coding for specific liver mitochondrial genes during the fetal life is considered as resulting from the proliferation of the organelles, whereas postnatal increase in translation of these specific proteins reflects organelle differentiation. Recently, it was shown that the stimulation of postnatal mitochondrial translation was due to the increase in adenine nucleotide content.[108,109]

The increased liver oxygenation as well as the decreased plasma insulin/glucagon molar ratio have been proposed as the stimulus for the increase in hepatic mitochondrial adenine nucleotide content in the neonatal rabbit.[99] If the neonate is exposed to hypoxia, the normal increase in mitochondrial adenine nucleotide content does not occur, and the related development of metabolic functions is suppressed.[99,110,111] In pups from diabetic mothers, characterized by high plasma insulin and low plasma glucagon concentrations, the postnatal increase in mitochondrial adenine nucleotide is suppressed, and the activation of pyruvate carboxylation is impaired.[110,112] Nevertheless, the two- to threefold increase of gluconeogenesis that could be due to enhanced pyruvate carboxylation is of minor importance when compared with the 50-fold increase that is due to the synthesis of cytosolic PEPCK.

Short-Term Control of Glycolysis/Gluconeogenesis

In the neonatal rabbit hepatocyte, the rate of gluconeogenesis from dihydroxyacetone (DHA), a substrate that enters the pathway upstream from the PEPCK is very low at birth, whereas the rate of glycolysis is high.[113] Within 6 hours after birth the partition of DHA between glycolysis and gluconeogenesis is completely reversed as the result of a decrease in fructose 2,6-bisphosphate concentration.[113] Fructose 2,6-bisphosphate, which is produced and hydrolyzed by the bifunctional 6-phosphofructo-2-kinase/fructose-2,6-bisphosphatase (PFK-2/FBPase-2) is a potent activator of 6-phosphofructo-1-kinase and an inhibitor of fructose-1,6-bisphosphatase.[114] In the fed adult rat, the high plasma insulin/glucagon ratio stimulates the dephosphorylation of the bifunctional enzyme and favors its kinase activity, leading to an increase in fructose 2,6-bisphosphate concentration and to an activation of 6-phosphofructo-1-kinase. Thus, the rapid fall in the plasma insulin/glucagon ratio immediately after birth might induce opposite changes in neonatal liver metabolism. For instance, the addition of glucagon to fetal pig hepatocytes immediately inhibits glycolysis and stimulates gluconeogenesis, supporting the role of glucagon in the short-term control of these pathways.[115] In contrast, the fructose 2,6-bisphosphate concentration is very low in the fetal rat liver[116] as the result of a decrease in PFK-2/FBPase-2 activity and gene expression during the last days of gestation.[117,118] Moreover, it has been reported that fetal rat liver contains an isoform of 6-phosphofructo-2-kinase that is not inhibited by glucagon or cAMP.[117,119] The total activity of liver 6-phosphofructo-2-kinase does not change during the perinatal period,[117] but the adult form of 6-phosphofructo-2-kinase appears after birth, and its activity and gene expression are induced by glucagon or cAMP.[119–121] Taken together, these data suggest that PFK-2/FBPase-2 bifunctional enzyme does not play a crucial role in setting the liver in the gluconeogenic mode in the newborn rat.

Regulation of Hepatic Fatty Acid Oxidation During the Perinatal Period

The concentration of plasma FFA increases markedly during the first hours following birth as the result of the mobilization of triglycerides stored in white adipose tissue and in the liver of the rabbit, guinea pig, and human, and from the hydrolysis of milk triglycerides.[5] To cover the energy needs of the neonate, fatty acid oxidation develops rapidly after birth in the liver and in many extrahepatic tissue such as heart, skeletal muscles, lung, kidney cortex, small intestine, and brown adipose tissue.[5] In the liver, the increased capacity for fatty acid oxidation results in a high rate of ketone body production, which is used as energetic substrates in many tissues and as lipogenic precursors in the brain.[5] Many in vitro studies have shown that the rates of fatty acid oxidation are very low in the fetal rat liver and markedly increase during the first 24 hours of extrauterine life[5] (see Chapters 36 and 38).

In mammalian liver, fatty acid oxidation can occur both in mitochondria and peroxisomes. During the past decade, the role and importance of peroxisomes have received considerable attention after the discovery that hypolipidemic drugs induce their proliferation and after the identification of peroxisomal diseases in humans.[122] During the fetal-neonatal transition, there is an increase in the number of peroxisomes and in the activities of specific enzymes.[123,124] However, the contribution of peroxisomal β-oxidation represents only 10% to 15% of total liver β-oxidation in the neonatal liver.[123,125]

Thus, this section is limited to a review of the mechanisms involved in the development and regulation of mitochondrial β-oxidation.

The Pathway of Fatty Acid Oxidation and Ketogenesis

Figure 29.5 summarizes the different steps of mitochondrial β-oxidation and ketogenesis. To be metabolized, long-chain fatty acids (LCFA) (i.e., more than 12 carbons) must be activated to their corresponding acyl–coenzyme A (CoA) by acyl-CoA synthetases located either on microsomal and peroxisomal membranes or on the outer mitochondrial membrane.[126] Long-chain

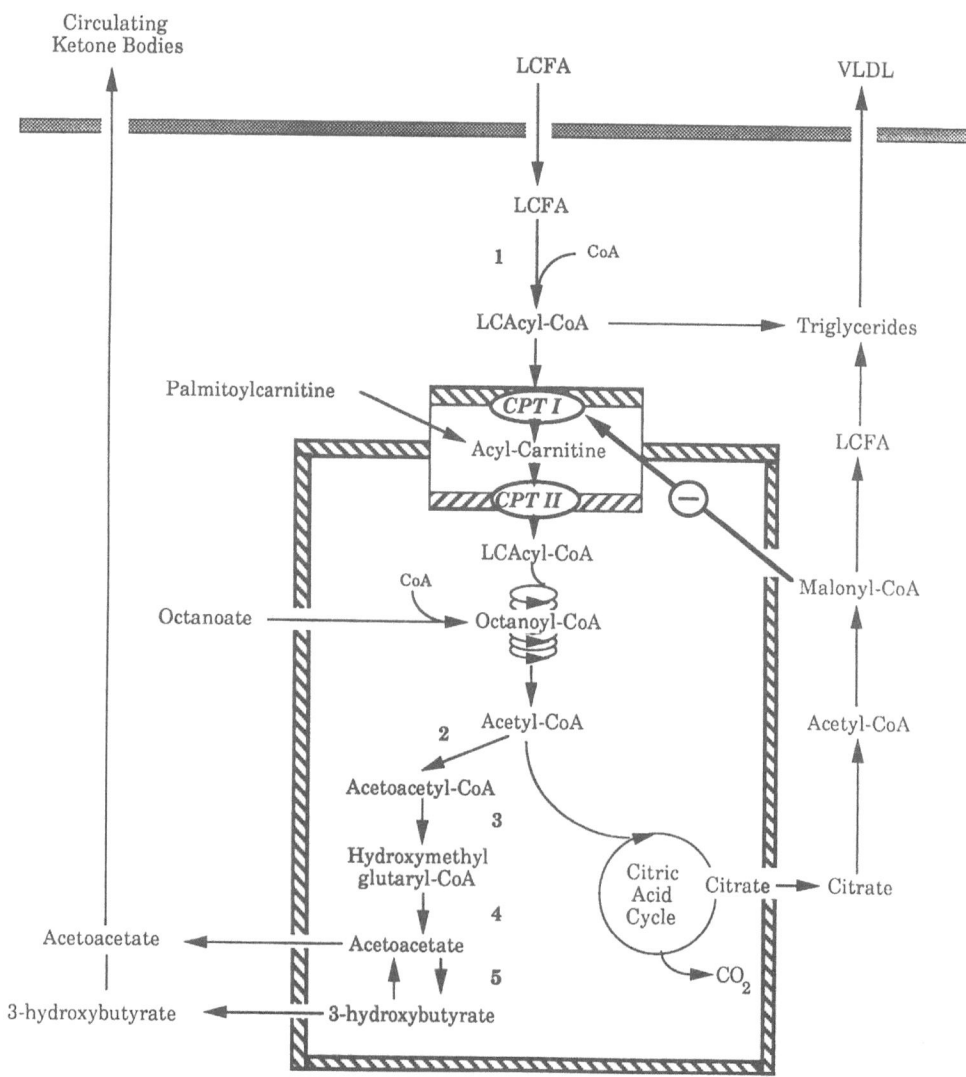

FIGURE 29.5. Intrahepatic metabolism of FFA. LCFA, long-chain fatty acid; LCAcyl-CoA, long-chain Acyl-CoA; VLDL, very low density lipoprotein; CPT I/II, carnitine palmitoyltransferase I and II; 1, long-chain acyl-CoA synthetase; 2, acetoacetyl-CoA thiolase; 3, hydroxymethylglutaryl-CoA synthase; 4, hydroxymethylglutaryl-CoA lyase; 5, hydroxybutyrate dehydrogenase.

(LC)Acyl-CoA can be either oxidized or reesterified depending on the physiologic state (Figure 29.5). The entry of LCAcyl-CoA into the mitochondrial matrix is ensured by the carnitine palmitoyltransferase (CPT) system, which consists of three distinct activities: the CPT I, located in the outer mitochondrial membrane; the carnitine-acylcarnitine translocase; and the CPT II, located in the inner membrane.[127] In contrast to LCFA, medium-chain fatty acid (MCFA) or short-chain fatty acid (SCFA) readily cross the mitochondrial membranes and are activated to their corresponding acyl-CoA by a short- or a medium-chain acyl-CoA synthetase located in the mitochondrial matrix.[126] Once inside the mitochondria, acyl-CoA, whatever its chain length, undergoes the successive steps of β-oxidation to yield molecules of acetyl-CoA and reduced equivalents [i.e., NADH and flavin adenine dinucleotide, reduced ($FADH_2$)]. In mitochondria of extrahepatic tissue, such as heart, skeletal muscles, kidney cortex, lung, and small intestine, acetyl-CoA undergoes oxidation into the Krebs cycle to yield CO_2, H_2O, GTP, and further reduced equivalents that may enter the electron transport chain to yield ATP. In liver mitochondria, acetyl-CoA produced by β-oxidation can undergo either the Krebs cycle or the hydroxymethylglutaryl (HMG)-CoA pathway for ketone body synthesis. Ketone bodies are then released into the circulation and transported to the peripheral tissues where they are used as respiratory fuels or as substrates for lipid biosynthesis.

Regulation of Fatty Acid Uptake and Acyl-CoA Formation

The transport of fatty acid across hepatocyte membrane is a matter of debate. For some it is a simple diffusion mechanism, whereas for others it represents a saturable process that involves various membrane proteins such as plasma membrane fatty acid binding protein ($FABP_{PM}$), fatty acid receptor (FAR), fatty acid translocase (FAT), fatty acid transport protein (FATP), or albumin binding protein.[128] Although the postnatal expression of these proteins is unknown, several lines of evidence suggest that neither the fatty acid concentration nor its cellular uptake represents the main regulatory steps for the development of hepatic fatty acid oxidation. For instance, when hepatocytes are incubated in the presence of similar concentration of FFA the rate of hepatic fatty acid oxidation is much lower in the term rat fetus than in the 24-hour-old neonate.[5,125,129,130] This suggests that transmembrane transport of fatty acid is not rate limiting for the onset of fatty acid oxidation.

Once inside the cell, FFA are bound to cytosolic fatty acid binding proteins (FABP).[128] The expression of the gene coding for FABPs is increased during the fetal-neonatal transition.[131,132] The function of FABPs is to increase the mobility of FFAs by decreasing their binding to membranes and enhancing the availability of FFAs for key metabolic pathways.[133] Prior to metabolization, FFAs are activated to their corresponding acyl-CoA ester by acyl-CoA synthetases specific to their chain length (Figure 29.5). Microsomal, peroxisomal, and mitochondrial LCAcyl-CoA synthetases share similar kinetic and immunologic properties.[134] Mitochondrial LCAcyl-CoA synthetase increases markedly after birth in the rat liver.[5] This probably results from an increase in its gene expression since LCAcyl-CoA synthetase mRNA concentration is very high during the suckling period.[135] LCAcyl-CoA binds with a very high affinity to acyl-CoA binding proteins (ACBP),[136] a step that seems required for utilization of LCAcyl-CoA either in β-oxidation or in triglyceride synthesis and to avoid degradation by acyl-CoA hydrolases.[137] The developmental changes in liver ACBP concentration is unknown.

During development, it seems that mitochondrial fatty acid oxidation is controlled by the partition of acyl-CoA derivatives between esterification and β-oxidation (Figure 29.5) rather than by the fatty acid activation process per se.[130,138,139]

Partition of LCAcyl-CoA into Triglyceride Synthesis or Acylcarnitine Formation

Little information is available concerning the partition of LCAcyl-CoA into acylglyceride and acylcarnitine synthesis during the neonatal period. However, it has been shown that the inhibition of mitochondrial fatty acid oxidation causes a marked accumulation of liver triglyceride concentration in the neonatal rat[140] as the result of an increased triglyceride synthesis.[130,138,139] This is consistent with the postnatal increase in the activity of microsomal enzymes of hepatic LCFA esterification[141] and in the rates of triglyceride synthesis.[142] This suggests that the development of mitochondrial LCFA oxidation at birth is controlled by acylcarnitine synthesis and/or oxidation rather than by a fall in the capacity for fatty acid esterification.

Changes in Activities of Enzymes Controlling Fatty Acid Oxidation and Ketogenesis

As the inner mitochondrial membrane is impermeable to acyl-CoA esters, their transfer inside the mitochondria is ensured by the carnitine palmitoyltransferase (CPT) system composed of three distinct entities (vide infra; Figure 29.5).[5] The activity of the overall CPT system rises markedly in the liver of the neonatal[5] as the result of an increase in CPT I activity, the activity of CPT II remaining unchanged (Figure 29.6).[143-145] The developmental changes in carnitine acylcarnitine translocase are unknown. The transcriptional and posttranscriptional fac-

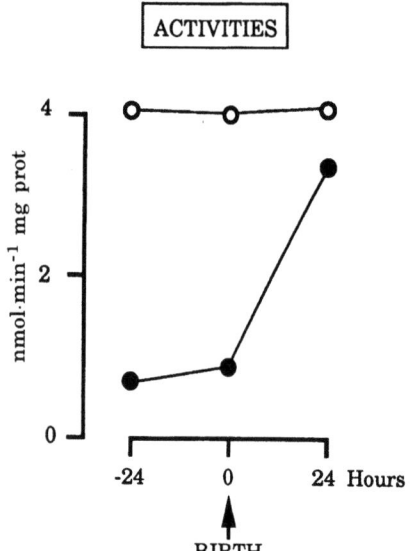
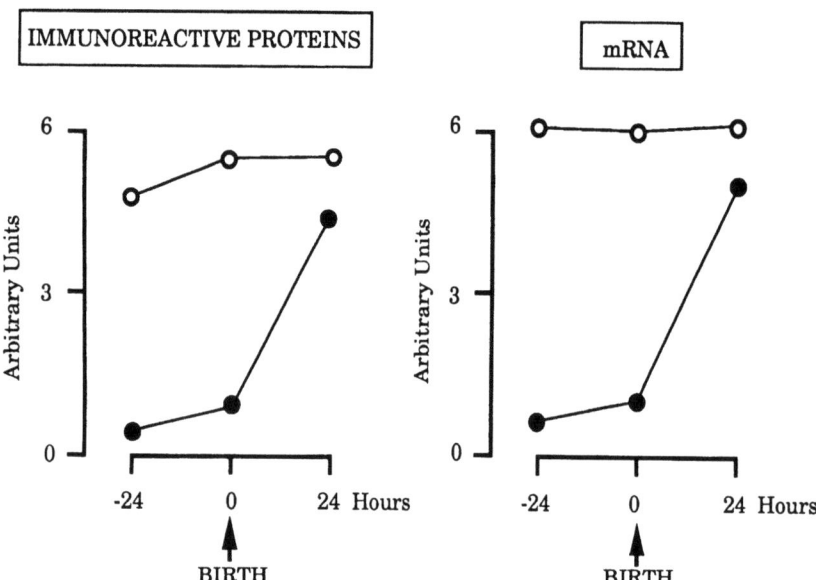

FIGURE 29.6. Postnatal changes in liver CPT I (●—● CPT I) and CPT II (○—○ CPT II) activities, immunoreactive protein, and mRNA concentrations in the rat. (Data from Thumelin et al.,[145] with permission.)

tors controlling CPT I activity at birth are discussed below. The first step of intramitochondrial β-oxidation is the catalyzation by acyl-CoA dehydrogenases of the specific fatty acid chain length. The activities of long-, medium-, and short-chain acyl-CoA dehydrogenases increase slightly after birth[144,146] as the result of stimulation of their gene expression.[147,148] The activities of the monofunctional short-chain enoyl-CoA hydratase, short chain 3-hydroxyacyl-CoA dehydrogenase, and 3-ketoacyl-CoA thiolase show an increase in activity but more slowly than does CPT I.[144,149] In contrast, the developmental changes in the long-chain enoyl-CoA hydratase/3-hydroxyacyl-CoA dehyrogenase/3-ketoacyl-CoA thiolase mitochondrial trifunctional protein[150,151] have not been studied.

This enzymatic cascade leads to the formation of a shortened acyl-CoA and a molecule of acetyl-CoA that may enter the Krebs cycle or be used for ketone body synthesis. The major pathway of acetoacetate formation is the 3-hydroxy-3-methylglucaryl-CoA pathway (HMG-CoA). First, acetyl-CoA is converted into acetoacetyl-CoA by acetoacetyl-CoA thiolase whose activity rises steadily after birth in rat liver mitochondria.[5] Then acetoacetyl-CoA is condensed with acetyl-CoA to form HMG-CoA owing to a mitochondrial HMG-CoA synthase activity, HMG-CoA being split into acetoacetate and acetyl-CoA by HMG-CoA lyase. The activities of these two mitochondrial enzymes exhibit very similar developmental patterns, with a marked increase within the first day after birth.[5] The activity of mitochondrial HMG-CoA synthase is lower than the activity of the other ketogenic enzymes at all stages of development.[152] Thus, it was considered as the rate-limiting step in the HMG-CoA pathway.[153,154] This is true if one considers ketogenesis as the metabolic pathway converting mitochondrial acetyl-CoA into ketones. However, if one considers ketogenesis as the metabolic pathway converting LCFA into ketone bodies, then CPT I is the rate-limiting enzyme since it controls the supply of acyl-CoA for β-oxidation and ketogenesis.[127,155] This has been clearly demonstrated in the adult rat hepatocyte using the flux control coefficient analysis.[156]

The transcriptional and posttranscriptional factors that control mitochondrial CPT I and HMG-CoA synthase are reviewed below.

Transcriptional and Posttranscriptional Regulation of CPT I and HMG-CoA Synthase Activities at Birth

The recent cloning of cDNAs of CPT I,[157] CPT II,[158] and mitochondrial HMG-CoA synthase,[159] and the availability of antibodies directed against these proteins,[154,160] has facilitated the study of the molecular mechanisms controlling the changes in mitochondrial CPT I, CPT II, and HMG-CoA synthase activities.

Transcriptional Regulation of Mitochondrial CPT I and HMG-CoA Synthase Genes

Changes in Hepatic CPT I Gene Expression

As mentioned above, the activity of CPT I is very low in the fetal rat liver and increases markedly after birth, whereas the activity of CPT II is already high in the fetal rat liver and does not change after birth (Figure 29.6).[143–145] This developmental pattern in CPT I and CPT II activities parallels that observed for immunoreactive protein concentrations.[145,161] The postnatal increase in the amount of CPT I protein results from a stimulation of its gene transcription,[162] which leads to a marked accumulation of hepatic CPT I mRNA concentration during the first 24 hours after birth.[145,163]

The liver CPT II mRNA and protein concentrations remain remarkably constant during development.[145,163] These data are consistent with previous observations showing that CPT II protein concentration[161] and activity[143] were not modified during the fetal-neonatal transition.

Changes in Hepatic Mitochondrial HMG-CoA Synthase Gene Expression

As reported above, the activity of mitochondrial HMG-CoA synthase increases during the immediate postnatal period. In the fetal rat liver, the mRNA coding for mitochondrial HMG-CoA synthase is not detectable before the 18th day of pregnancy and then increases slightly until the 21st day of pregnancy.[164] This increase could result from a progressive demethylation of the gene, since demethylation has been reported to be one of the factors responsible for the activation of mitochondrial HMG-CoA synthase gene transcription during the fetal-neonatal transition.[165] During the first 24 hours after birth, the concentration of mitochondrial HMG-CoA synthase mRNA increases markedly.[164,166]

Hormonal and Nutritional Regulation of Mitochondrial CPT I and HMG-CoA Synthase Genes

Modifications of fatty acid metabolism in the immediate postnatal period are attended by changes in plasma FFA, carnitine, and pancreatic hormone concentrations. The direct effect of pancreatic hormones on the induction of LCFA oxidation[139,167] and of CPT I[162] and mitochondrial HMG-CoA synthase[164] gene expression has been demonstrated using cultured fetal hepatocytes.

Interestingly, the postnatal increase in liver CPT I mRNA concentration is delayed in the 6-hour-old fasting rat when compared to a suckling one,[163] although their hormonal environment is similar.[9] This suggests that some factors contained in milk could affect CPT I gene transcription. Those factors could be FFAs since they have been shown to stimulate CPT I gene in the cultured fetal rat hepatocyte.[162] During the immediate postnatal period, plasma FFA levels increase in the suckling neonatal rat as the result of milk triglyceride hydrolysis, whereas they remain very low in the fasting neonatal rat since it is devoid of white adipose tissue.[5]

Mitochondrial CPT I. Addition of cAMP increases in a dose-dependent manner the accumulation of CPT I mRNA in cultured hepatocytes from the fetal rats, (Figure 29.7) whereas insulin antagonizes the effects of cAMP.[162] The cAMP-induced CPT I gene expression results from a stimulation of gene transcription that does not affect the CPT I mRNA half-life.[162] This suggests that the postnatal decrease in plasma insulin concentration potentiates the effects of increased plasma glucagon and liver cAMP concentrations. In terms of nutritional regulation of CPT I gene expression, it is noteworthy that carnitine, whose liver concentration increases markedly after birth,[168,169] has no effect on CPT I gene expression in the cultured fetal rat hepatocyte.[162] In contrast, saturated and polyunsaturated LCFAs induce CPT I mRNA accumulation in the cultured fetal hepatocytes as the result of both a stimulation of CPT I gene transcription and a stabilization of its mRNA.[162] MCFAs have no effect on CPT I gene expression.[162] The concentration of CPT II mRNA, which is already elevated in the cultured fetal hepatocyte, is unaffected by cAMP, insulin, or LCFA.[162] This is in agreement with the absence of the C/EBPα or CREB binding site in the promoter region of the CPT II gene.[170]

Several lines of evidence suggest that LCFAs must be transformed to their respective CoA esters to be active

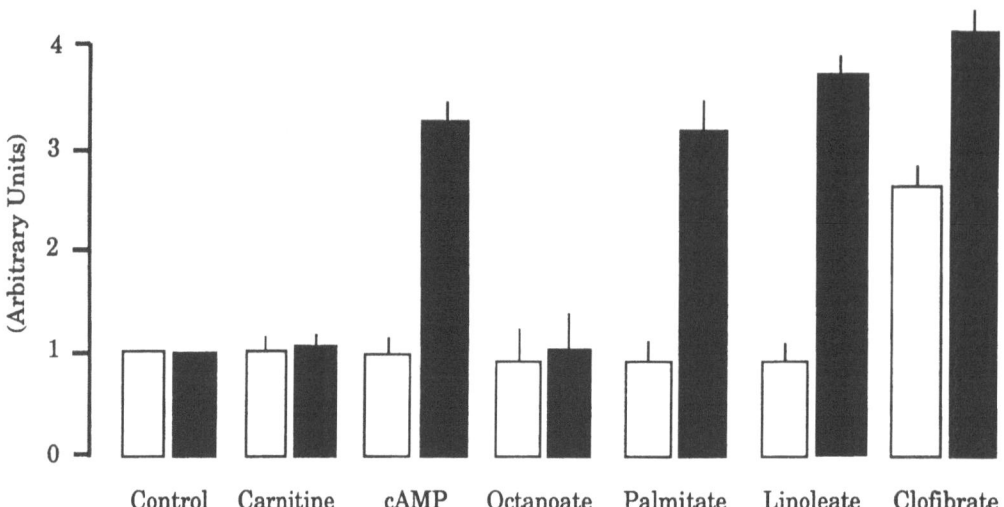

FIGURE 29.7. Effects of carnitine, dibutyryl cAMP, medium-chain fatty acid (octanoate), saturated (palmitate), or unsaturated (linoleate) long-chain fatty acids and of a peroxisome proliferator (clofibrate) on the accumulation of CPT I and CPT II mRNA in cultured hepatocytes from 20-day-old rat fetuses. (Data from Chatelain et al.,[162] with permission.)

in the induction of CPT I mRNA.[162] When the fetal rat hepatocyte is cultured in the presence of 2-bromopalmitate, which is a nonmetabolizable analogue of palmitate, the induction of CPT I mRNA is larger than in the presence of palmitate at the same concentration. Similarly, the inhibition of LCFA oxidation by tetradecylglycidic acid enhances the accumulation of CPT I mRNA in response to linoleate. Under these conditions, linolyl-CoA markedly accumulates in the cell since the fetal hepatocyte has a low capacity for esterification.[130] The mechanisms by which LCFAs stimulate gene transcription is unknown. Based on the comparison of the effects of LCFAs and peroxisome proliferators, it has been suggested that LCFAs could regulate gene transcription secondary to the activation of a nuclear receptor, the peroxisome proliferator activated receptor (PPAR).[171-173] The modulation of gene transcription is due to the binding of the heterodimer PPAR/RXR (retinoic acid receptor) to specific DNA sequences, such as the peroxisome proliferator responsive element (PPRE).[171-173] Whether this mechanism is involved in the control of CPT I gene transcription by LCFA remains to be determined. However, indirect evidence suggests that the regulation of CPT I gene transcription by LCFA and peroxisome proliferators is different. First, LCFA induces CPT I but not CPT II gene expression, whereas clofibrate, a potent peroxisome proliferator, enhances both CPT I and CPT II mRNA concentrations in the cultured fetal rat hepatocyte (Figure 29.7).[162] Second, when LCFA-induced CPT I mRNA accumulation is totally reversed by insulin, the clofibrate-induced CPT I and CPT II gene expression is not.[162]

Mitochondrial HMG-CoA Synthase. When the hepatocyte from the rat fetus was cultured in the presence of glucagon, mitochondrial HMG-CoA synthase mRNA accumulated in a dose-dependent manner,[164] with a half-maximal concentration of glucagon close to the concentration found in the plasma of the neonatal rat. These data are consistent with the finding of a cAMP responsive element in the promoter region of mitochondrial HMG-CoA synthase gene.[174]

The level of mitochondrial HMG-CoA synthase gene expression is also regulated by nutrients. As shown for CPT I, only LCFAs, whatever their degree of unsaturation, increase HMG-CoA synthase mRNA levels in the cultured fetal rat.[175] The absorption of large amounts of fats immediately after birth could promote the transcription of hepatic mitochondrial HMG-CoA synthase, since LCFAs have been shown to stimulate mitochondrial HMG-CoA synthase gene transcription through a PPAR-dependent mechanism.[176]

It is noteworthy that pancreatic hormones and/or LCFAs could also be involved in the transcriptional regulation of other enzymes of β-oxidation during the fetal neonatal transition. For instance, it has been shown that glucagon enhances the accumulation of liver mRNA coding for long-chain acyl-CoA dehydrogenase (LCAD), or medium-chain acyl-CoA dehydrogenase (MCAD),[148] whereas FFAs regulate the expression of

LCAcyl-CoA synthetase[135] and MCAD[177] genes in the adult rat liver.

Posttranscriptional Regulation of CPT I and HMG-CoA Synthase Activities by Metabolic Effectors

Following gene expression, protein translation, and protein import into the outer mitochondrial membrane (CPT I) or into the mitochondrial matrix (mitochondrial HMG-CoA synthase), the CPT I and HMG-CoA synthase activities are finely regulated by metabolic effectors whose concentrations can be modulated by pancreatic hormones.

Regulation of CPT I Activity

Carnitine is an essential factor for transferring LCAcyl-CoA inside the mitochondria. The hepatic concentration of carnitine increases rapidly after birth in the liver of the suckling rat.[168,169] This results from the transfer of carnitine from the mother to the pup via milk[168] since the neonatal rat has a reduced capacity to synthesize carnitine from butyrobetaine until 8 days after birth.[178] However, a postnatal increase in carnitine concentration does not appear to be the primary signal for the induction of LCFA oxidation and ketogenesis at birth. Indeed, the same degree of hyperketonemia is reached in the 16-hour-old starved rat fed with a triglyceride emulsion devoid of carnitine or supplemented with carnitine.[129]

Malonyl-CoA, the first committed intermediate in lipogenesis (Figure 29.5), is a potent inhibitor of CPT I.[179] The rate of hepatic lipogenesis decreases in the last 2 days of gestation in the fetal rat and is very low in the 1-day-old neonate.[5] This results from the inhibition of key lipogenic enzyme activities and gene expression due to the hormonal (i.e., high glucagon/low insulin plasma concentrations) and nutritional environment (i.e., high plasma FFA levels) of the newborn rats.[180] This allows the maintenance of a low intrahepatic malonyl-CoA concentration. The fall in malonyl-CoA concentration does not play a pivotal role in the development of fatty acid oxidation and ketogenesis.[5] Indeed, the decrease in hepatic malonyl-CoA concentration at birth[167] or induced by glucagon or cAMP in the cultured fetal rabbit hepatocyte[167] occurs 12 hours before any significant increase in LCFA oxidation. This suggests that additional mechanisms must be operating for an optimal initiation of fatty acid oxidation and ketogenesis at birth.

It has been shown in the adult rat liver that the inhibitory effect of malonyl-CoA on CPT I (i.e., the so-called sensitivity of CPT I to malonyl-CoA inhibition) was different depending on the physiologic and/or pathologic conditions.[127] The sensitivity of liver CPT I to malonyl-CoA inhibition is also markedly decreased in the first 24 hours following birth.[4,138,143,167] Glucagon and cAMP decrease the sensitivity of CPT I to malonyl-CoA inhibition in the cultured hepatocyte from the rabbit fetus, whereas insulin antagonizes their effects.[167] Although the molecular mechanisms responsible for these changes remain unknown, some hypotheses can be formulated. The delay required to change the sensitivity of CPT I to malonyl-CoA inhibition (8 to 12 hours) rules out a rapid regulation through a phosphorylation-dephosphorylation mechanism as suggested previously.[181] Moreover, it has been shown recently that changes in CPT I kinetic properties in the adult rat liver were not due to a phosphorylation of the enzyme.[182] Until recently, the location of the malonyl-CoA binding site was a matter of controversy. It was suggested that malonyl-CoA binding site could be located on a protein different from CPT I.[183,184] This hypothesis now can be excluded. Indeed, transfection of the CPT I cDNA into yeast cells, which are devoid of endogenous CPT I, leads to the expression of a membrane-associated CPT I that is active and has a sensitivity to malonyl-CoA inhibition close to that observed in mitochondria isolated from the starved adult rat liver.[185] Moreover, the expression of a truncated CPT I variant that lacks 82 N-terminal residues retains catalytic function but is less sensitive to malonyl-CoA inhibition.[185] This suggests that malonyl-CoA binds in the N-terminal region of the CPT I. The hormonal regulation of the sensitivity of CPT I to malonyl-CoA inhibition could include (1) an alteration in the spatial conformation of CPT I within the outer mitochondrial membrane,[186] and (2) a modification in the composition of the microenvironment of the CPT I[187-189] and/or in the fluidity of the mitochondrial membrane.[190]

Regulation of HMG-CoA Synthase Activity

As CPT I, the activity of HMG-CoA synthase is also regulated by metabolic effectors. Indeed, its activity is inhibited by succinyl-CoA through the succinylation of the enzyme. It has been reported that glucagon increases the ketogenesis flux in adult rat livers by lowering the intramitochondrial succinyl-CoA concentration leading to the desuccinylation and consequent activation of mitochondrial HMG-CoA synthase.[191-193] A similar mechanism exists also during induction of ketogenesis in the neonatal rat liver.[154]

Figure 29.8 summarizes all the known transcriptional and posttranscriptional mechanisms involved in the regulation of LCFA oxidation and ketogenesis.

Other Factors Involved in the Regulation of Hepatic Fatty Acid Oxidation

When the term rat fetal hepatocyte is incubated in the presence of octanoate whose oxidation is independent of CPT I (Figure 29.5), the rates of the ketone body are as

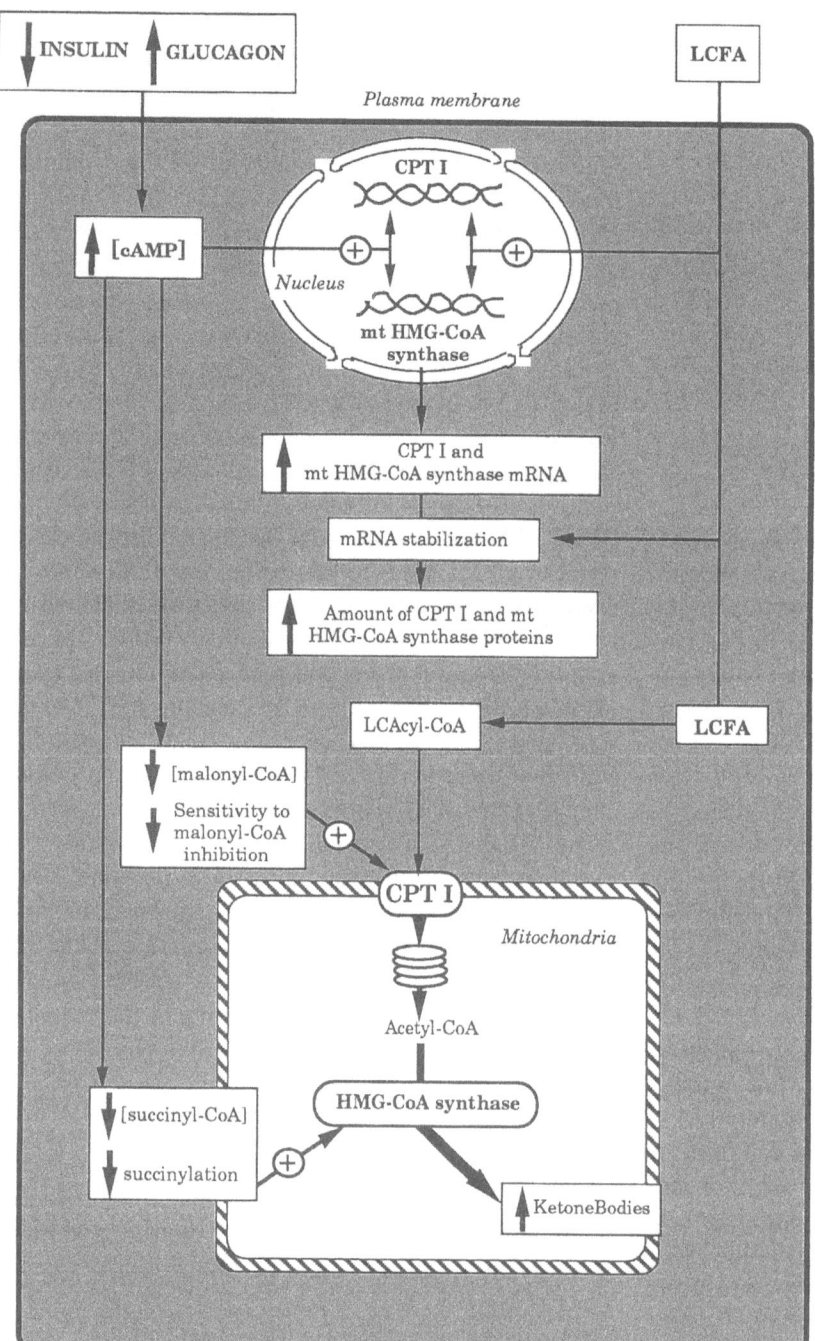

FIGURE 29.8. Schematic representation of the role of plasma insulin, glucagon, and long-chain fatty acids (LCFA) in the regulation of liver carnitine palmitoyltransferase (CPT) I and mitochondrial hydroxymethylglutaryl-CoA synthase (mt HMG-CoA synthase) at transcriptional and posttranscriptional levels.

low as from those measured from oleate.[130] Similarly, the oxidation of palmitoylcarnitine, which bypasses the CPT I step, is lower in liver mitochondria isolated from the rat fetus than in that isolated from the 24-hour-old neonate.[103] These data suggest that in the immediate postnatal period, fatty acid oxidation and ketogenesis are controlled at the level of CPT I or HMG-CoA synthase activities.

Maturation of Mitochondrial Oxidative Capacity

As discussed above, the emergence of fatty acid oxidation in the neonatal rat liver depends partly on an increase in the activity of enzyme of mitochondrial β-oxidation. This suggests that the enhanced capacity for fatty acid oxidation at birth could be related to an increase in the capacity of liver mitochondria for fatty acid oxidation. This successful postnatal adaptation results from both an increase in the number of mitochondria (i.e., proliferation) and an increase in functional capacity of preexisting mitochondria (i.e., differentiation).[194,195]

Within the first 24 hours after birth, the mitochondrial compartment relative to the volume of the hepatocyte increases.[194,195] However, it seems unlikely that changes in the mitochondrial mass could explain the increased capacity for fatty acid oxidation since it is decreased within the first hours after birth in the neonatal rat liver.[196] Similarly, it seems unlikely that the low rates of mitochondrial β-oxidation result from a defective coupling of the respiratory chain immediately after birth (supra vide), since the oxidation of palmitoylcarnitine, which bypasses the CPT I step, remains low at birth even in the presence of an uncoupler.[103]

In contrast, the low capacity for fatty acid oxidation may result from a reduced capacity for fatty acid activation inside the mitochondria. Indeed, the concentration of intramitochondrial CoA, which is required for the acyl moieties to enter β-oxidation, is very low at birth and increases markedly within 24 hours after birth in the neonatal rat liver. This could contribute to a low activation of fatty acid in fetal liver mitochondria, which in turn could limit their oxidation.[103]

Metabolic Fate of Mitochondrial Acetyl-CoA

Among the factors that could regulate ketogenesis in the neonatal liver, the large increase in gluconeogenesis (supra vide) is of prime importance for the channeling of acetyl-CoA between the tricarboxylic acid cycle and the ketogenic pathway (Figure 29.5). For instance, CO_2 production represents 45% of total oleate or octanoate oxidized by fetal hepatocytes, whereas it represents only 5% to 10% of total oleate or octanoate oxidized in neonatal hepatocytes.[125,139]

In the first 12 hours after birth, glycogenolysis provides large amounts of glucose-6-phosphate that are partly used in glycolysis. Oxaloacetate concentration is high and acetyl-CoA is condensed to citrate, which is used for lipogenesis. After this period, gluconeogenesis is well developed and the oxaloacetate concentration is low. Acetyl-CoA is then directed preferentially toward the formation of the ketone body. In keeping with this, it has been shown that inhibition of gluconeogenesis in the suckling neonate induces a rise in liver oxaloacetate concentration and a concomitant decrease in plasma ketone bodies.[197,198] Thus, it is clear that during the neonatal period, ketogenesis is controlled at the mitochondrial branch point of acetyl-CoA metabolism, but, from a quantitative point of view, this step is probably much less important than that controlled by CPT I.

Essential Role of Fatty Acid Oxidation in the Regulation of Hepatic Gluconeogenesis

In the suckling newborn rat, the inhibition of hepatic gluconeogenesis leads to a profound hypoglycemia.[197] Similarly, the 16-hour-old fasting newborn rat is severely hypoglycemic secondary to a deficiency of gluconeogenesis.[9,12] This suggests that an active liver gluconeogenesis is essential to maintain a normal blood glucose concentration in the neonate.

Because the activities of liver gluconeogenic enzymes and the hormonal environment of high plasma glucagon and low plasma insulin concentrations are appropriate for an active gluconeogenesis in the fasting neonate,[9,199] it has been suggested that the principal factors controlling the rate of gluconeogenesis at that time could be the supply of gluconeogenic precursors and the availability of FFA to the liver.[12] Indeed, the concentrations of gluconeogenic precursors and FFA are much lower in the plasma of the fasting than of the suckling neonate.[9,12,129] The very low concentration of plasma FFA in the fasting neonate results from the absence of adipose tissue at birth in the rat. In contrast, the suckling neonate receives FFA from the milk, which is a high-fat diet in the rat.

The reduced supply of gluconeogenic precursors cannot by itself explain the impairment of gluconeogenesis in the fasting neonate. First, the injection in vivo of a mixture of gluconeogenic substrates to the fasting neonate increases its glycemia, but the concentration achieved (36 mg·dl^{-1}; 2 mM) remains much lower than in the age-matched suckling newborn (90 mg·dl^{-1}; 5 mM), despite much higher concentrations of blood gluconeogenic substrates.[129] Second, the rate of gluconeogenesis from 10 mM lactate is five times lower in the isolated hepatocyte from the fasting neonate than from the suckling one.[200] In contrast, when the fasting neonate is fed a triglyceride emulsion containing long-chain (LCT) or medium-chain fatty acids (MCT), the glycemia is markedly increased (Figure 29.9).[129,201,202]

Several lines of evidence suggest that the increase in blood glucose concentration observed after LCT or MCT feeding results from a stimulation of gluconeogenesis. First, LCT or MCT feeding are associated with an increase in glucose turnover and in the conversion of labeled lactate to glucose.[129,201,202] Second, the rise in glycemia induced by LCT or MCT feeding is completely suppressed by simultaneous injection of an inhibitor of gluconeogenesis.[201,202] Third, the rate of gluconeogenesis from 10 mM lactate is markedly stimulated by addition of oleate or octanoate in isolated hepatocytes from fasting newborn rats.[200] The idea that an active fatty acid oxidation is essential to support a high rate of gluconeogenesis

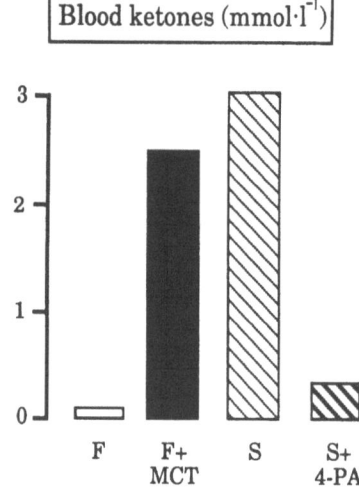

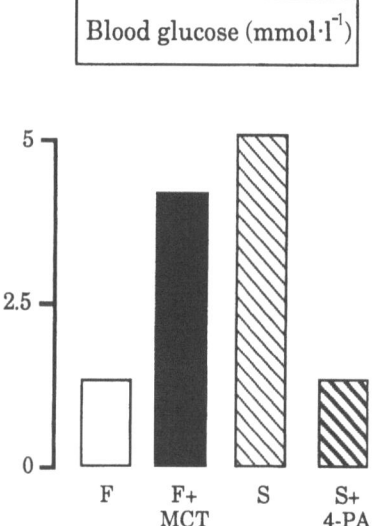

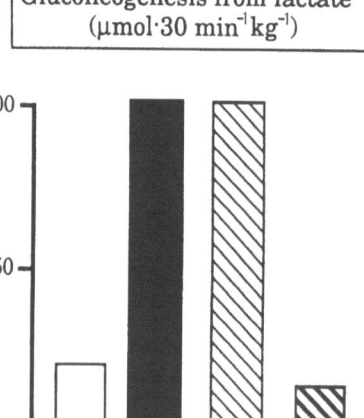

FIGURE 29.9 Effects of medium-chain triglyceride (MCT) feeding in 16-hour-old fasting rats (F) and of 4-pentenoic acid (4-PA) in 16-hour-old suckling rats (S) on blood ketones and glucose concentrations and on the rate of in vivo gluconeogenesis from [U-^{14}C] lactate. (Data from Pégorier et al.[202,203] and Turlan et al.[204].)

in the liver of the neonatal rat is also supported by the fact that the injection of 4-pentenoate or 2-tetradecylglycidate (TDGA) (i.e., inhibitors of long-chain fatty acid oxidation), to the suckling neonate causes an 80% decrease in gluconeogenesis and induces a dramatic fall in blood glucose concentration from 5 to less than 1 mM (Figure 29.9).[203,204] The administration of MCT to the neonate made hypoglycemic by TDGA restores a normal blood glucose concentration and gluconeogenic rate, since medium-chain fatty acids bypass the step inhibited by TDGA (i.e., CPT I).[204] The essential role of hepatic fatty acid oxidation for maintaining an active gluconeogenesis in the neonate has been confirmed in other species[66,115,198,205] including human neonates.

Using crossover plot analysis of gluconeogenic metabolites, it was shown that fatty acid oxidation supports hepatic gluconeogenesis by providing acetyl-CoA (an obligatory cofactor of pyruvate carboxylase), ATP, which enhances the reaction catalyzed by 3-phosphoglycerate kinase, and reducing equivalents (NADH) to displace the equilibrium reaction catalyzed by glyceraldehyde-3-phosphate dehydrogenase in the direction of gluconeogenesis.[206] Moreover, it has been shown in the adult rat hepatocyte that ketone bodies arising from fatty acid oxidation decrease the concentration of fructose

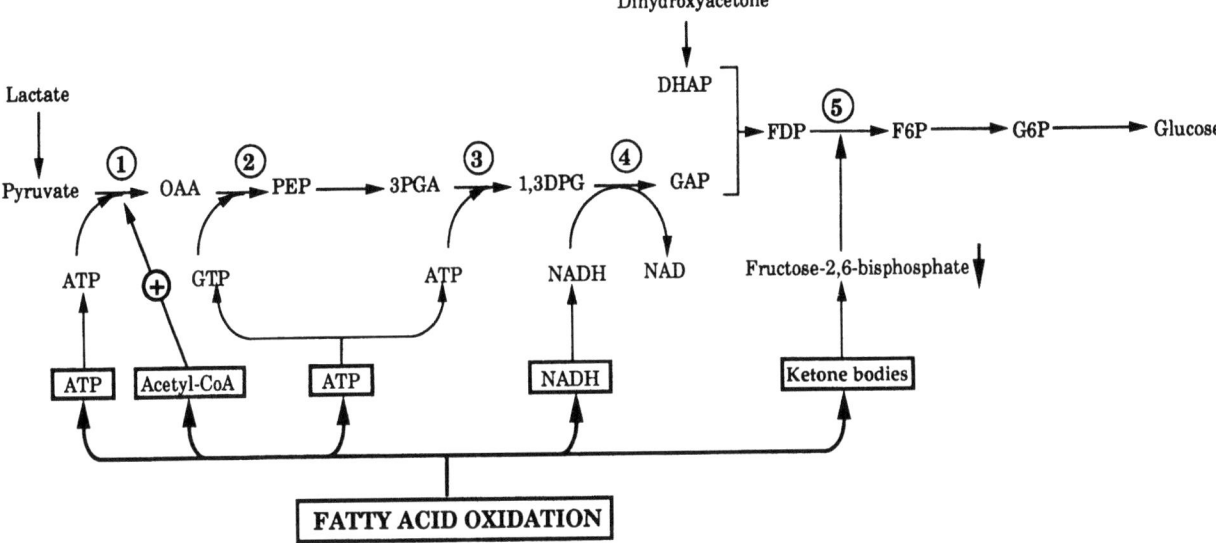

FIGURE 29.10. Schematic representation of the interrelationships between fatty acid oxidation and gluconeogenesis in the liver. 1, pyruvate carboxylase; 2, phosphoenolpyruvate carboxykinase; 3, phosphoglycerate kinase; 4, glyceraldehyde-3-phosphate dehydrogenase; 5, fructose-1,6-diphosphatase.

2,6-bisphosphate that in turn would also favor gluconeogenesis.[207]

Figure 29.10 summarizes the different steps of gluconeogenesis that are affected by products arising from fatty acid oxidation.

Glucose and Fatty Acid Metabolism in the Human Neonates

Animal studies have shown that changes in plasma pancreatic hormones and the development of active gluconeogenesis and fatty acid oxidation are crucial for glucose homeostasis in the neonatal period. To what extent these conclusions can be generalized to human neonates is considered in this section.

Hormonal Changes

Neonates from diabetic mothers have a marked hyperinsulinemia and a reduced hyperglucagonemia[208] in the immediate postnatal period, which results in a reduced hepatic glucose production[209] and hypoglycemia. When maternal diabetes is well controlled, the changes in insulin and glucagon secretion, the rate of hepatic glucose production, and the glycemia are similar to those occurring in the normal neonate.[210,211] In addition, the neonatals suffering from a congenital deficiency in pancreatic glucagon develops a severe neonatal hypoglycemia that can be corrected by administration of exogenous glucagon.[212,213] In one neonate presenting a marked hyperinsulinemia but a normal glucagonemia, hypoglycemia develops secondary to a reduced gluconeogenesis from alanine.[214] Taken together, these data suggest that appropriate changes in plasma insulin and glucagon are necessary to maintain a normal glucose homeostasis in human neonates (see Chapter 32).

Glucose and Fatty Acid Metabolism

Essential Role of Gluconeogenesis

Experiments using stable isotopes have clearly shown that carbon recycling and gluconeogenesis from alanine and glycerol are active in the immediate postnatal period in the human neonate,[215-218] thus confirming the importance of this metabolic pathway for glucose homeostasis in the human neonate. Moreover, the simple comparison of the amount of glucose supplied from milk and the rate of glucose utilization in the neonate shows that gluconeogenesis from galactose and other substrates is essential to support glucose homeostasis during the first week of life in the breast-fed neonate.

Development of Fatty Acid Oxidation and Ketogenesis

Within the first hours after delivery of the human neonate there is a fall in the respiratory quotient and a rise in the blood level of FFA, suggesting an increased fat oxidation.[5] In the term neonate, either fasted during the first 24 hours of life [219,220] or fed under current nursery practices,[217,221] the blood concentration of ketone bodies is maximal only 1 to 2 days after birth. It is noteworthy that the same degree of ketosis is achieved whether the human neonate is fed MCT formulas or breast-fed, i.e., with LCT suggesting that the regulation of hepatic fatty acid oxidation and ketogenesis seem not to be limited by the activity of the CPT system.[222] Indeed, it has been shown that total CPT activity in the fetal human liver is twice that found in the liver of the suckling rats[223] and that the liver of human fetuses is able to oxidize palmitate very actively.[224] Moreover, studies using stable isotopes have confirmed that ketogenesis is already mature in humans on the first day of life.[225,226] Hepatic ketogenesis is already active in infants born 10 weeks before normal term but for similar plasma FFA concentration the rate of daily ketone body synthesis is markedly lower than in normal term neonate.[226] This could be due to carnitine deficiency in the premature neonate.[227] Indeed, the development of ketogenesis in the human neonate is greatly dependent on the exogenous supply of carnitine because the liver has a limited capacity for de novo synthesis.[228] For instance, it has been shown that the degree of ketosis is higher in the breast-fed than in the formula-fed neonate; formula contains lower carnitine concentration than human milk[229] (see Chapters 36 and 38).

Interrelations Between Fatty Acid Oxidation and Gluconeogenesis

Unlike the rat, the normal term neonate has a high body fat content (i.e., 16% of body weight) and can survive prolonged starvation without hypoglycemia.[230] In contrast, the small-for-gestational-age (SGA) neonate has a low body fat content at birth and develops hypoglycemia after a short fast.[231] A defect in gluconeogenesis has been proposed to explain hypoglycemia in the SGA neonate,[14,232] and it has been shown that administration of triglycerides to the hypoglycemic SGA neonate increases its plasma glucose concentration,[233-236] secondary to a stimulation of hepatic glucose production.[237] Additional evidence for the role of hepatic fatty acid oxidation in the control of glucose homeostasis was provided by the studies of CPT I deficiency in the human neonate. Patients with CPT I deficiency present many metabolic disorders, especially recurrent episodes of hypoketotic hypoglycemia.[238] In keeping with this, an 8-month-old girl who developed marked hypoglycemia after a fast of 24 hours and had very low blood ketone body levels despite high plasma FFA concentrations was studied.[239] Further investigations have shown that the cultured fibroblasts of this girl had a reduced capacity to oxidize LCFA, but a normal capacity to oxidize medium- or short-chain fatty acids.[240] The defect in LCFA oxidation has been shown to result from a CPT I deficiency.[241,242] The administration of MCT to this hypoglycemic girl produced a rapid increase in her blood ketone body concentrations, since MCFAs enter the mitochondria by bypassing the CPT system. The restoration of normal β-oxidation was followed by a complete correction of her hypoglycemia.[239]

These data taken together thus confirm the essential relationship between fatty acid oxidation and gluconeogenesis in the liver of the human neonate.

Implications

The successful adaptation of the neonate to changes in nutrition and environment needs important modifications of glucose and fatty acid metabolism, which are orchestrated mainly by pancreatic hormone secretion.

The induction of hepatic glucose production (i.e., glycogenolysis and gluconeogenesis), fatty acid oxidation, and ketogenesis requires the activation of specific enzyme gene expression. For instance, hepatic glycogenolysis is partly dependent on the activation of glucose-6-phosphatase, whereas the development of gluconeogenesis is controlled mainly by the transcriptional induction of cytosolic PEPCK. Similarly, the appearance of liver fatty acid oxidation and ketogenesis requires the stimulation of mitochondrial CPT I and HMG-CoA synthase gene expression. The induction of these specific proteins is absolutely necessary but not sufficient. Except for PEPCK, whose regulation is only transcriptional, posttranscriptional modifications of these proteins also take place to allow the development of high rates of gluconeogenesis, fatty acid oxidation, and ketogenesis. Indeed, pyruvate kinase, phosphofructokinase, and fructose-1,6-bisphosphatase are finely controlled by phosphorylation/dephosphorylation or by allosteric (fructose 2,6-bisphosphate) mechanisms. Similarly, the decreased sensitivity of CPT I to malonyl-CoA inhibition and the desuccinylation of HMG-CoA synthase are crucial for the development of an active fatty acid oxidation and ketogenesis.

The postnatal increase in plasma glucagon and the decrease in plasma insulin, associated with the consequent rise in hepatic intracellular cAMP concentration, are directly involved in these transcriptional and posttranscriptional regulations. Moreover, fatty acids have been shown to participate, in concert with hormones, in the regulation of CPT I and HMG-CoA synthase gene expression during the immediate postnatal period.

This review also emphasizes that the development of an active gluconeogenesis in newborns is dependent on a high rate of fatty acid oxidation that provides obligatory cofactors (acetyl-CoA, ATP, NADH) for the gluconeogenic pathway.

Although species differences have been found in the regulation of postnatal metabolism, animal studies have been useful to understand the metabolic adaptations in the liver of human neonates.

Acknowledgment. The original work presented in this chapter has been supported by grants from Institut National de la Santé et de la Recherche Médicale, Ministère de l'Enseignement Supérieur et de la Recherche, and Fondation de la Recherche Médicale.

References

1. Battaglia FC, Meschia G. Principal substrates of fetal metabolism. Physiol Rev 1978;58:499–527.
2. Battaglia F, Meschia G. An introduction to fetal physiology. New York: Academic Press, 1986:257.
3. Girard J, Ferré P. Metabolic and hormonal changes around birth. In: Jones CT, ed. Biochemical development of the fetus and neonate. Amsterdam: Elsevier, 1982:517–551.
4. Girard J, Duée PH, Ferré P, et al. Fatty acid oxidation and ketogenesis during development. Reprod Nutr Dev 1985;25:309–319.
5. Girard J, Ferré P, Pégorier JP, Duée PH. Adaptations of glucose and fatty acid metabolism during the perinatal period and the suckling-weaning transition. Physiol Rev 1992;72:507–562.
6. Jenness R. Biosynthesis and composition of milk. J Invest Dermatol 1974;63:109–118.
7. Dils RR, Parker DS. Metabolic aspects of lactation and the supply of nutrients to the young. In: Jones CT, ed. Biochemical development of the fetus and neonate. Amsterdam: Elsevier, 1982:573–590.
8. Girard J, Sperling M. Glucagon in the fetus and the newborn. In: Lefebvre PJ, ed. Glucagon. Berlin: Springer-Verlag, 1983:251–274.
9. Girard JR, Cuendet GS, Marliss EB, et al. Fuels, hormones and liver metabolism at term and during the early postnatal period in the rat. J Clin Invest 1973;52:3190–3200.
10. Blazquez E, Sugase M, Blazquez M, Foa P. Neonatal changes in the concentration of liver cAMP and of serum glucose, FFA, insulin, pancreatic and total glucagon in man and in the rat. J Lab Clin Med 1974;83:957–967.
11. Kervran A, Gilbert M, Girard J, et al. Effect of environmental temperature on glucose-induced insulin response in the newborn rat. Diabetes 1976;25:1026–1030.
12. Girard J, Guillet I, Marty J, Marliss EB. Plasma amino acid levels and development of hepatic gluconeogenesis in the newborn rat. Am J Physiol 1975;229:466–473.
13. Malinowska KW, Hardy RN, Nathanielz PW. Plasma adrenocorticosteroid concentrations immediately after birth in infant rat, rabbit and guinea-pig. Experientia 1972;28:1366–1367.
14. Haymond MW, Karl I, Pagliara AS. Increased gluconeogenesis substrates in the small-for-gestational age infant. N Engl J Med 1974;291:322–328.
15. Cornblath M, Parker M, Reisner S, et al. Secretion and metabolism of growth hormone in premature and full term infants. J Clin Endocr Metab 1965;25:209–218.
16. Rieutort M. Pituitary content and plasma levels of growth hormone in foetal and weanling rats. J Endocrinol 1974;60:261–268.
17. Fisher D, Dussault J, Sack J, Chopra I. Ontogenesis of hypothalamic-pituitary-thyroid function and metabolism in man, sheep and rat. Recent Prog Horm Res 1977;33:59–107.
18. Jones C, Rolph T. Metabolic events associated with the preparation of the fetus for independent life. In: Ciba Foundation Symposium, Elliott K, Whelan J, eds. The fetus and independent life. London: Pitman 1981:241–258.
19. Jones CT, Rolph TP. Metabolism during fetal life: a functional assessment of metabolic development. Physiol Rev 1985;65:357–425.
20. Shelley HJ. Glycogen reserves and their changes at birth and in anoxia. Br Med Bull 1961;17:137–143.
21. Lubchenco L, Bard H. Incidence of hypoglycemia in newborn infants classified by birth weight and gestational age. Pediatrics 1971;47:831–838.
22. Shelley H, Neligan G. Neonatal hypoglycemia. Br Med Bull 1966;22:34–39.
23. Stalmans W. Glucagon and liver glycogen metabolism. In: Lefebvre PJ, ed. Glucagon. Berlin: Springer-Verlag, 1983:251–274.
24. Watts C, Gain KR. Glycogen metabolism in the liver of the developing rat. Biochem J 1973;160:263–270.
25. Khandelwal RL. Glycogen mobilizing enzyme activities in the developing rat liver. Int J Biochem 1982;14:1067–1073.
26. Margolis RN. Regulation of hepatic glycogen metabolism in pre- and postnatal rats. Endocrinology 1983;113:893–902.
27. Bloch CA, Ozbun MA, Khan SA. Glycogen phosphorylase: developmental expression in rat liver. Biol Neonate 1993;63:113–119.
28. Margolis RN, Tanner K. Glycogen metabolism in neonatal liver of the rat. Arch Biochem Biophys 1986;249:605–610.
29. Devos P, Hers HG. Random, presumably hydrolytic, and lysosomal glycogenolysis in livers of rats treated with phlorhizin and of newborn rats. Biochem J 1980;192:177–181.
30. Phillips MJ, Unakar G, Doorewaard G, Steiner JW. Glycogen depletion in the newborn rat liver. An electron microscopic and electron histochemical study. J Ultrastruct Res 1967;18:142–165.
31. Gain KR, Malthus R, Watts C. Glucose homeostasis during the perinatal period in normal rats with a glycogen storage disorder. J Clin Invest 1981;67:1569–1573.
32. Rupper S, Kelsey G, Schedl A, et al. Deficiency of an enzyme of tyrosine metabolism underlies altered gene expression in newborn liver lethal albino mice. Genes Dev 1992;6:1430–1443.
33. Glucksohn-Waelsch S. Genetic control of morphogenetic and biochemical differentiation: lethal albino deletions in the mouse. Cell 1979;15:227–237.
34. Dawkins MJR. Glycogen synthesis and breakdown in fetal and newborn rat liver. Ann NY Acad Sci 1963;111:203–211.

35. Burchell A, Leakey J. Development of the rat hepatic microsomal glucose-6-phosphatase system and its glucocorticoid inducibility. Biol Neonate 1988;54:107–115.
36. Haber BA, Chin S, Chuang E, et al. High levels of glucose-6-phosphate gene and protein expression reflect an adaptative response in proliferating liver and diabetes. J Clin Invest 1995;95:832–841.
37. Sperling MA. Glucose homeostasis after birth. In: Jones CT, ed. Fetal and neonatal development. Ithaca, NY: Perinatology Press, 1988:458–467.
38. Girard J, Bal D. Effets du glucagon-zinc sur la glycémie et la teneur en glycogène du foie fœtal du rat en fin de gestation. CR Acad Sci Paris 1970;267:777–779.
39. Greengard O, Dewey HK. The premature deposition or lysis of glycogen in livers of fetal rats injected with hydrocortisone or glucagon. Dev Biol 1970;21:452–461.
40. Plas C, Nunez J. Glycogenolytic response of cultured hepatocytes. Refractoriness following prior exposure to glucagon. J Biol Chem 1975;250:5304–5311.
41. Girard JR, Caquet D, Bal D, Guillet I. Control of rat liver phosphorylase, glucose-6-phosphatase and phosphoenolpyruvate carboxykinase activities by insulin and glucagon during the perinatal period. Enzyme 1973;15:272–285.
42. Sperling M, Grajwer L, Leake R, Fischer D. Effects of somatostatin infusion on glucose homeostasis in newborn lambs: evidence for a significant role of glucagon. Pediatr Res 1977;11:962–967.
43. Padbury J, Agata Y, Ludlow J, et al. Effect of fetal adrenalectomy on catecholamine release and physiologic adaptation at birth in sheep. J Clin Invest 1987;80:1096–1103.
44. Exton JH. Mechanisms of hormonal regulation of hepatic glucose metabolism. Diabetes Metab Rev 1987;3:163–183.
45. Sherline P, Eisen H, Glinsmann W. Acute hormonal regulation of cyclic AMP content and glycogen phosphorylase activity in fetal liver in organ culture. Endocrinology 1974;94:935–939.
46. Monancy MLJ, Plas C. Interactions of glucagon and epinephrine in the regulation of adenosine 3′,5′-monophosphate dependent glycogenolysis in the cultured fetal hepatocyte. Endocrinology 1980;107:1667–1675.
47. Freemark M, Handwerger S. Glycogenolytic effects of the calcium ionophore, but not vasopressin or angiotensin in foetal rat liver. Biochem J 1984;220:441–445.
48. Butlen D, Guillon G, Cantau B, Jard S. Comparison of the developmental patterns of vasopressin, glucagon and α-adrenergic receptors from rat liver membranes. Mol Cell Endrocrinol 1980;19:275–289.
49. Greengard O, Dewey HK. Initiation by glucagon of the premature development of tyrosine aminotransferase, serine dehydratase and glucose-6-phosphatase in fetal rat liver. J Biol Chem 1967;242:2986–2991.
50. Lange AJ, Argaud D, El-Maghrabi MR, et al. Isolation of a cDNA for the catalytic subunit of rat liver glucose-6-phosphatase: regulation of gene expression in FAO hepatoma cells by insulin, dexamethasone and cAMP. Biochem Biophys Res Commun 1994;201:302–309.
51. Argaud D, Zhang Q, Pan W, et al. Regulation of rat liver glucose-6-phosphatase gene expression in different nutritional and hormonal states. Gene structure and 5′-flanking sequence. Diabetes 1996;45:1563–1571.
52. Hamosh M. The development of the metabolic and transport function of the gastrointestinal system. In: Jones CT, ed. Biochemical development of the fetus and neonate. Amsterdam: Elsevier, 1982:591–619.
53. Buddington RK, Diamond JM. Ontogenetic development of intestinal nutrient transporters. Annu Rev Physiol 1989;51:601–619.
54. Kliegman RM, Sparks JW. Perinatal galactose metabolism. J Pediatr 1985;107:831–841.
55. Sparks JW. Augmentation of the glucose supply in the fetus and newborn. Semin Perinatol 1979;3:141–155.
56. Hay WJ. Fetal and neonatal glucose homeostasis and their relation to the small for gestational age infant. Semin Perinatol 1984;8:101–116.
57. Hanson R, Reshef L, Ballard F. Hormonal regulation of hepatic phosphoenolpyruvate carboxykinase (GTP) during development. Fed Proc 1975;34:166–171.
58. Pilkis SJ, Granner DK. Molecular physiology of the regulation of hepatic gluconeogenesis and glycolysis. Annu Rev Physiol 1992;54:885–909.
59. El-Maghrabi MR, Lange AJ, Kummel L, Pilkis SJ. The rat fructose-1-6-bisphosphatase gene. Structure and regulation of expression. J Biol Chem 1991;266:2115–2120.
60. Shelly LL, Lei KJ, Pan CJ, et al. Isolation of the gene for murine glucose-6-phosphatase, the enzyme deficient in glycogen storage disease type 1A. J Biol Chem 1993;268:21482–21485.
61. Jitrapakdee S, Booker GW, Cassady AI, Wallace JC. Cloning, sequencing and expression of rat liver pyruvate carboxylase. Biochemistry 1996;316:631–637.
62. Ballard FJ, Philippidis H. The development of gluconeogenic function in rat liver. In: Söling BW, ed. Regulation of gluconeogenesis. Stuttgart: Thieme-Verlag, 1971:66–81.
63. Callikan S, Ferré P, Pégorier JP, et al. Fuel metabolism in fasted newborn rabits. J Dev Physiol 1979;1:267–281.
64. Raghunatan R, Arinze IJ. Perinatal development of gluconeogenesis in guinea-pig liver. Int J Biochem 1977;8:737–743.
65. Warnes D, Seamark R, Ballard F. The appearance of gluconeogenesis at birth in sheep: activation of the pathway associated with blood oxygenation. Biochem J 1977;162:627–634.
66. El Manoubi L, Callikan S, Duée PH, et al. Development of gluconeogenesis in isolated hepatocytes from the rabbit. Am J Physiol 1983;244:E24–E30.
67. Yeung D, Oliver IT. Developement of gluconeogenesis in neonatal rat liver. Effect of premature delivery. Biochem J 1967;105:1229–1233.
68. Pearce PH, Buirchell BJ, Weaver PK, Oliver IT. The development of phosphoenolpyruvate carboxylase and gluconeogenesis in neonatal rats. Biol Neonate 1974;24:320–329.
69. Philippidis H, Hanson R, Reshef L, et al. The initial synthesis of proteins during development. Phosphoenolpyruvate carboxylase in rat liver at birth. Biochem J 1972;126:1127–1134.

70. Garcia-Ruiz JP, Ingram R, Hanson RW. Changes in hepatic mRNA for phosphoenolpyruvate carboxykinase (GTP) during development. Proc Natl Acad Sci USA 1978;75:4189–4193.
71. Cimbala MA, Lamers WH, Nelson K, et al. Rapid changes in the concentration of phosphoenolpyruvate carboxykinase mRNA in rat liver and kidney. Effects of insulin and cyclic AMP. J Biol Chem 1982;257:7629–7636.
72. Benvenisty N, Simchon EB, Cohen H, et al. Control of the activity of phosphoenolpyruvate carboxykinase and the level of its mRNA in livers of newborn rats. Effect of diabetes, glucose load and glucocorticoids. Eur J Biochem 1983;132:663–668.
73. Lyonnet S, Coupe C, Girard J, et al. In vivo regulation of glycolytic and gluconeogenic enzyme gene expression in newborn rat liver. J Clin Invest 1988;81:1682–1689.
74. Giometti CS, Gemmel MA, Taylor J, et al. Evidence for regulatory genes on mouse chromosome 7 that affect the quantitative expression of proteins in the fetal and newborn liver. Proc Natl Acad Sci USA 1992;89:2448–2452.
75. Gluecksohn-Waelsch S. Developmental genetics of hepatic gluconeogenic enzymes. Ann NY Acad Sci 1986;478:101–108.
76. Loose DS, Shaw PA, Krauter KS, et al. Transregulation of the PEPCK (GTP) gene, identified by deletions in chromosome 7 of the mouse. Proc Natl Acad Sci USA 1986;83:5184–5188.
77. Lem J, Chin AC, Thayer MJ, et al. Coordinate regulation of two genes encoding gluconeogenic enzymes by the trans-dominant locus Tse-1. Proc Natl Acad Sci USA 1988;85:7302–7306.
78. Benvenisty N, Reshef L. Developmental acquisition of DNase I sensitivity of the phosphoenolpyruvate carboxykinase (GTP) gene in rat liver. Proc Natl Acad Sci USA 1987;84:1132–1136.
79. Benvenisty N, Mencher D, Meyuhas O, et al. Sequential changes in DNA methylation patterns of the rat phosphoenolpyruvate carboxykinase gene during development. Proc Natl Acad Sci USA 1985;82:267–271.
80. Rothrock R, Lee K, Isham K, Kenney F. Changes in hepatic differentiation following treatment of rat fetuses with 5-azacytidine. Arch Biochem Biophys 1988;263:237–244.
81. Trus M, Benvenisty N, Cohen H, Reshef L. Developmentally regulated interactions of liver nuclear factors with the rat phosphoenolpyruvate carboxykinase promoter. Mol Cell Biol 1990;10:2418–2422.
82. Benvenisty N, Cohen N, Gidoni B, et al. Insulin-deficient diabetes in the perinatal period: ontogeny of gluconeogenesis and phosphoenolpyruvate carboxykinase. In: Shafrir E, Renold A, eds. Lessons from animal diabetes. London: J. Libbey, 1984:717–733.
83. Mencher D, Cohen H, Benvenisty N, et al. Primary activation of cytosolic phosphoenolpyruvate carboxykinase gene in fetal rat liver and the biogenesis of its mRNA. Eur J Biochem 1984;141:199–203.
84. Mencher DJ, Shouval D, Reshef L. Premature appearance of hepatic phosphoenolpyruvate carboxykinase in fetal rat, not mediated by cAMP. Eur J Biochem 1979;102:489–495.
85. Steele JG, McGrath M, Yeoh GCT, Oliver IT. Phosphoenolpyruvate carboxykinase in cultured foetal hepatocytes from the rat. Ontogeny of hormone inducibility and role of glucocorticoids and insulin in enzyme induction. Eur J Biochem 1980;104:91–99.
86. Van Roon MA, Zooneveld D, Charles R, Lamers WH. Accumulation of carbamoylphosphate synthase and phosphoenolpyruvate carboxykinase mRNA in embryonic rat hepatocytes: evidence for transcriptional control during the initial phase of specific gene expression in vitro. Eur J Biochem 1988;178:191–196.
87. Pégorier JP, Salvado J, Forestier M, Girard J. Dominant role of glucagon in the initial induction of phosphoenolpyruvate carboxykinase (PEPCK) mRNA in cultured hepatocytes from fetal rats. Eur J Biochem 1992;210:1053–1059.
88. Molero C, Valverde AM, Benito M, Lorenzo M. Phosphoenolpyruvate carboxykinase and glucose-6-phosphate dehydrogenase expression in fetal hepatocyte primary cultures under proliferative conditions. Exp Cell Res 1992;200:295–300.
89. Girard J, Ferré P, Gilbert M, et al. Fetal metabolic response to maternal fasting in the rat. Am J Physiol 1977;232:E456–E463.
90. Freund N, Kervran A, Assan R, et al. Fetal metabolic response to phlorhizin-induced hypoglycemia in pregnant rat. Biol Neonate 1980;38:321–327.
91. Narkewicz M, Carver T, Hay WJ. Induction of cytosolic phosphoenolpyruvate carboxykinase in the ovine fetal liver by chronic fetal hypoglycemia and hypoinsulinemia. Pediatr Res 1993;33:493–496.
92. Stevenson RE, Morris FH, Adock EW, Howell RR. Development of gluconeogenesis enzymes in fetal sheep liver and kidney. Dev Biol 1976;52:167–172.
93. Lemons J, Moorehead H, Hague G. Effects of fasting on gluconeogenic enzymes in the ovine fetus. Pediatr Res 1986;20:676–679.
94. Bristow J, Rudolph A, Itskovitz J, Barnes R. Hepatic oxygen and glucose metabolism in the fetal lamb. J Clin Invest 1983;71:1047–1061.
95. Townsend S, Rudolph C, Wood C, Rudolph A. Perinatal onset of hepatic gluconeogenesis in the lamb. J Dev Physiol 1989;12:329–335.
96. Ballard F, Hanson R. Changes in lipid synthesis in rat liver during development. Biochem J 1967;102:952–958.
97. Chang LO. The development of pyruvate carboxylase in rat liver mitochondria. Pediatr Res 1977;11:6–8.
98. Aprille JR, Yasmen P, Rulfs J. Acute postnatal regulation of pyruvate carboxylase activity by compartmentation of mitochondrial adenine nucleotide. Biochim Biophys Acta 1981;675:143–147.
99. Brennan WA Jr, Aprille JR. Regulation of hepatic gluconeogenesis in newborn rabbit: controlling factors in presuckling period. Am J Physiol 1985;249:E498–E505.
100. Cuezva JM, Fernandez E, Valcarce C, Medina JM. The role of ATP/ADP ratio in the control of hepatic gluconeogenesis in the early neonatal period. Biochim Biophys Acta 1983;759:292–295.

101. Pollak JK. The maturation of the inner membranes of fetal rat liver mitochondria. An example of positive-feedback mechanism. Biochem J 1975;150:477–488.
102. Aprille JR, Asimakis GK. Postnatal development of rat liver mitochondira: stage 3 respiration, adenine nucleotide translocase activity, and the net accumulation of adenine nucleotides. Arch Brochem Biophysl 1980;201:564–575.
103. Escriva F, Ferré P, Robin D, et al. Evidence that the development of hepatic fatty acid oxidation at birth in the rat is concomitant with an increased intramitochondrial CoA concentration. Eur J Biochem 1986;156:603–607.
104. Valcarce C, Navarette RM, Encabo P, et al. Postnatal development of rat liver mitochondrial functions. The role of protein synthesis and of adenine nucleotides. J Biol Chem 1988;263:7767–7775.
105. Baggetto L, Gautheron DC, Godinot C. Effects of ATP on various steps controlling the rate of oxidative phosphorylation in newborn rat liver mitochondria. Arch Biochem Biophys 1984;232:670–678.
106. Luis AM, Izquierdo JM, Ostronoff LK, et al. Translation regulation of mitochondrial differentiation in neonatal rat liver. Specific increase in the translational efficiency of the nuclear encoded mitochondrial β-F1-ATPase mRNA. J Biol Chem 1993;268:1868–1875.
107. Izquierdo JM, Ricart J, Ostronoff LK, et al. Changing patterns of transcriptional and post-transcriptional control of β-F1-ATPase gene expression during mitochondrial biogenesis in liver. J Biol Chem 1995;270:10342–10350.
108. Valcarce C, Izquierdo JM, Chamorro M, Cuezva JM. Mammalian adaptation to extrauterine environment: mitochondrial function impairment caused by prematurity. Biochem J 1994;303:855–862.
109. Joyal JL, Hagen T, Aprille JR. Intramitochondrial protein synthesis is regulated by matrix adenine nucleotide content requires calcium. Arch Biochem Biophys 1995;319:322–330.
110. Aprille JR, Nosek MT. Neonatal hypoxia or maternal diabetes delays postnatal development of liver mitochondria. Pediatr Res 1987;21:266–269.
111. Aprille JR. Regulation of the mitochondrial nucleotide pool size in liver: mechanism and metabolic role. FASEB J 1988;2:2547–2556.
112. Cuezva JM, Chitra CI, Patel MS. The newborn of diabetic rat. II. Impaired gluconeogenesis in the postnatal period. Pediatr Res 1982;16:638–643.
113. Duée PH, Pégorier JP, El Manoubi L, et al. Development of gluconeogenesis from different substrates in newborn rabbit hepatocytes. J Dev Physiol 1986;8:387–394.
114. Hers HG, Van Schaftingen E. Fructose 2,6-bisphosphate 2 years after its discovery. Biochem J 1982;206:1–12.
115. Duée PH, Pégorier JP, Peret P, Girard J. Separate effects of fatty acid oxidation and glucagon on gluconeogenesis in isolated hepatocytes from newborn pigs. Biol Neonate 1985;47:77–83.
116. Schubert C, Goltzsch W, Hofmann E. Perinatal changes of fructose 2,6 bisphosphate in the rat liver. Biochem Biophys Res Commun 1983;113:672–677.
117. Schubert C, Boehme HJ, Hofmann E. Hormonal control of fructose 2,6 bisphosphate concentration and phosphofructokinase 2 in rat liver during development. Biosci Rep 1986;6:513–518.
118. Casado M, Bosca L, Martin-Sanz P. Rat liver messenger ribonucleic acid and enzyme activity of 6-phosphofructo-2-kinase/fructose-2,6-bisphosphatase impairment during the late period of pregnancy. Endocrinology 1993;133:1044–1050.
119. Martin-Sanz P, Cascales M, Bosca L. Fructose 2,6 bisphosphate in isolated foetal hepatocytes. FEBS Lett 1987;225:37–42.
120. Martin-Sanz P, Cascales M, Bosca L. Glucagon-induced changes in fructose 2,6 bisphosphate and 6-phosphofructo-2-kinase in cultured rat foetal hepatocytes. Bichem J 1989;257:795–799.
121. Casado M, Bosca L, Martin-Sanz P. Differential regulation of the expression of 6-phosphofructo-2-kinase/fructose-2,6-bisphosphatase and pyruvate kinase by cyclic AMP in fetal and adult hepatocytes. J Cell Physiol 1995;165:630–638.
122. Reddy JK, Mannaerts GP. Peroxisomal lipid metabolism. Annu Rev Nutr 1994;14:343–370.
123. Krahling JB, Gee R, Gauger JA, Tolbert NE. Postnatal development of peroxisomal and mitochondrial enzymes in rat liver. J Cell Physiol 1979;101;375–390.
124. Cibelli A, Stefanini S, Ceru MP. Peroxisomal β-oxidation and catalase activities in fetal rat liver: effect of maternal treatment with clofibrate. Cell Mol Biol 1988;34:191–205.
125. Duée PH, Pégorier JP, El Manoubi L, et al. Hepatic triglyceride hydrolysis and development of ketogenesis in rabbits. Am J Physiol 1985;249:E478–E484.
126. Bremer J, Osmundsen H. Fatty acid oxidation and its regulation. In: Numa S, ed. Fatty acid metabolism and its regulation. Amsterdam: Elsevier Science, 1984:113–154.
127. McGarry JD, Woeltje KF, Kuwajima M, Foster DW. Regulation of ketogenesis and the renaissance of carnitine palmitoyltransferase. Diabetes/Metab Rev 1989;5:271–284.
128. Van Nieuwenhoven FA, Van der Vusse GJ, Glatz JFC. Membrane-associated and cytoplasmic fatty acid binding proteins. Lipids 1996;31:S223–S227.
129. Ferré P, Pégorier JP, Marliss EB, Girard J. Influence of exogenous fat and gluconeogenic substrates on glucose homeostasis in the newborn rat. Am J Physiol 1978;234:E129–E136.
130. Ferré P, Satabin P, Decaux JF, et al. Development and regulation of ketogenesis in hepatocytes isolated from newborn rats. Biochem J 1983;214;937–942.
131. Gordon JI, Elshourbagy N, Lowe JB, et al. Tissue specific expression and developmental regulation of two genes coding for the rat fatty acid binding proteins. J Biol Chem 1985;260:1995–1998.
132. Paulussen RJA, Jansen GPM, Veerkamp JH. Fatty-acid binding capacity of cytosolic proteins of various rat tissues: effect of postnatal development, starvation, sex, clofibrate feeding and light cycle. Biochim Biophys Acta 1986;877:342–349.
133. Luxon BA. Inhibition of binding to fatty acid binding protein reduces the intracellular transport of fatty acids. Am J Physiol 1996;271;G113–G120.

134. Miyazawa S, Hashimoto T, Yokota S. Identity of long-chain acyl coenzyme A synthethase of microsomes, mitochondria and peroxisomes in rat liver. J Biochem (Tokyo) 1985;98:723–733.
135. Schoonjans K, Staels B, Grimaldi P, Auwerx J. Acyl-CoA synthetase mRNA expression is controlled by fibric acid derivatives, feeding and liver proliferation. Eur J Biochem 1993;216:615–622.
136. Rosendal J, Ertbjerg P, Knudsen J. Characterization of ligand binding to acyl-CoA binding protein. Biochem J 1993;290:321–326.
137. Rasmussen JT, Rosendal J, Knudsen J. Interaction of acyl-CoA binding protein (ACBP) on process for which acyl-CoA is a substrate, product or inhibitor. Biochem J 1993;292:907–913.
138. Herbin C, Pégorier JP, Duée PH, et al. Regulation of fatty acid oxidation in isolated hepatocytes and liver mitochondria from newborn rabbits. Eur J Biochem 1987;165:201–207.
139. Pégorier JP, Garcia-Garcia MV, Prip-Buus C, et al. Induction of ketogenesis and fatty acid oxidation by glucagon and cyclic AMP in cultured hepatocytes from rabbit fetuses. Evidence for a decreased sensitivity of carnitine palmitoyltransferase I to malonyl-CoA inhibition after glucagon or cyclic AMP treatment. Biochem J 1989; 264:93–100.
140. Frost SC, Wells MA. A comparison of the utilization of medium and long-chain fatty acids for oxidation and ketogenesis in the suckling rat: in vivo and in vitro studies. Arch Biochem Biophys 1981;211:537–546.
141. Coleman A, Haynes EB. Hepatic monoacylglycerol acyltransferase. Characterization of an activity associated with the suckling period in rats. J Biol Chem 1984;259:8934–8938.
142. Jamdar SC. Glycerolipid biosynthesis in rat adipose tissue. Biochem J 1978;170;153–160.
143. Saggerson ED, Carpenter CA. Regulation of hepatic carnitine palmitoyltransferase activity during the foetal-neonatal transition. FEBS Lett 1982;150:177–180.
144. Chalk PA, Higham EC, Caswell AM, Bailey E. Hepatic mitochondrial fatty acid oxidation during the perinatal period in the rat. Int J Biochem 1983;15:531–538.
145. Thumelin S, Esser V, Charvy D, et al. Expression of liver carnitine palmitoyltransferase I and II genes during development of the rat. Biochem J 1994;300:583–587.
146. Carroll JE, McGuire BS, Chancey VF, Harrison KB. Acyl-CoA dehydrogenase enzymes during early postnatal development in the rat. Biol Neonate 1989;55:185–190.
147. Kelly DP, Gordon JI, Alpers R, Strauss AW. The tissue-specific expression and developmental regulation of two nuclear genes encoding rat mitochondrial proteins. Medium chain acyl-CoA dehydrogenase and mitochondrial malate dehydrogenase. J Biol Chem 1989;264:18921–18925.
148. Nagao M, Parimoo B, Tanaka K. Developmental, nutritional and hormonal regulation of tissue-specific expression of the genes encoding various acyl-CoA dehydrogenases and α-subunit of electron transfer flavoprotein in rat. J Biol Chem 1993;268:24114–24124.
149. Bailey E, Lockwood EA. Some aspects of fatty acid oxidation, and ketone body formation and utilization during development of the rat. Enzyme 1973;15:239–253.
150. Uchida Y, Izai K, Orii T, Hashimoto T. Novel fatty acid beta-oxidation enzymes in rat liver mitochondria. II. Purification and properties of enoyl-coenzyme A (CoA) hydratase/3-hydroxyacyl-CoA dehydrogenase/3-ketoacyl-CoA thiolase trifunctional protein. J Biol Chem 1992;267: 1034–1041.
151. Kamijo T, Aoyama T, Miyazaki JI, Hashimoto T. Molecular cloning of the cDNAs for the subunits of rat mitochondrial fatty acid β-oxidation multienzyme complex. Strutural and functional relationships to other mitochondrial and peroxisomal β-oxidation enzymes. J Biol Chem 1993;268:26452–26460.
152. Hipolito-Reis C, Bailey E, Bartley W. Factors involved in the control of the activity of enzymes of hepatic ketogenesis during development of the rat. Int J Biochem 1974;5:31–39.
153. Williamson DH, Bates MW, Krebs HA. Activity and intracellular distribution of enzymes of ketone-body metabolism in rat liver. Biochem J 1968;108:353–361.
154. Quant PA, Robin D, Robin P, et al. Control of hepatic mitochondrial 3-hydroxy-3-methylglutaryl-CoA synthase during the fœtal/neonatal transition, suckling and weaning in the rat. Eur J Biochem 1991;195;449–454.
155. McGarry JD, Foster DW. Regulation of hepatic fatty acid oxidation and ketone body production. Annu Rev Biochem 1980;49:395–420.
156. Drynan L, Quant PA, Zammit VA. Flux control exerted by mitochondrial outer membrane carnitine palmitoyltransferase over β-oxidation, ketogenesis and tricarboxylic acid cycle activity in hepatocytes isolated from rats in different metabolic states. Biochem J 1996;317:791–795.
157. Esser V, Britton CH, Weis BC, Foster DW, et al. Cloning, sequencing, and expression of a cDNA encoding rat liver carnitine palmitoyltransferase I. Direct evidence that a single polypeptide is involved in inhibitor interaction and catalytic function. J Biol Chem 1993;268:5817–5822.
158. Woeltje KF, Esser V, Weis BC, et al. Cloning, sequencing, and expression of a cDNA encoding rat liver mitochondrial carnitine palmitoyltransferase II. J Biol Chem 1990;265:10,720–10,725.
159. Ayté J, Gil-Gomez G, Haro D, et al. Rat mitochondrial and cytosolic 3-hydroxy-3-methylglutaryl-CoA synthases are encoded by two different genes. Proc Natl Acad Sci USA 1990;87:3874–3878.
160. Esser V, Kuwajima M, Britton CH, et al. Inhibitors of mitochondrial carnitine palmitoyltransferase I limit the action of proteases on the enzyme. Isolation and partial amino acid analysis of a truncated form of the rat liver isozyme. J Biol Chem 1993;268:5810–5816.
161. Kolodziej MP, Crilly PJ, Corstorphine CG, Zammit VA. Development and characterization of a polyclonal antibody against rat liver mitochondrial overt carnitine palmitoyltransferase (CPT I). Biochem J 1992;282:415–421.
162. Chatelain F, Kohl C, Esser V, et al. Cyclic AMP and fatty acids increase carnitine palmitoyltransferase I transcrip-

tion in cultured fetal rat hepatocytes. Eur J Biochem 1996;235:789–798.
163. Asins G, Serra D, Arias G, Hegardt FG. Developmental changes in carnitine palmitoyltransferases I and II gene expression in intestine and liver of suckling rats. Biochem J 1995;306:379–384.
164. Thumelin S, Forestier M, Girard J, Pégorier JP. Developmental changes in mitochondrial 3-hydroxy-3-methyl-glutaryl-CoA synthase gene expression in rat liver, intestine and kidney. Biochem J 1993;292:493–496.
165. Ayté J, Gil-Gomez G, Hegardt FG. Methylation of the regulatory region of the mitochondrial 3-hydroxy-3-methylglutaryl-CoA synthase gene leads to its transcriptional inactivation. Biochem J 1993;295:807–812.
166. Serra D, Asins G, Hegardt FG. Ketogenic mitochondrial 3-hydroxy-3-methylglutaryl-CoA synthase gene expression in intestine and liver of suckling rats. Arch Biochem Biophys 1993;301:445–448.
167. Prip-Buus C, Pégorier JP, Duée PH, et al. Evidence that the sensitivity of carnitine palmitoyltransferase I to inhibition by malonyl-CoA is an important site of regulation of hepatic fatty acid oxidation in the fetal and newborn rabbit. Perinatal development and effects of pancreatic hormones in cultured rabbit hepatocytes. Biochem J 1990;269:409–415.
168. Robles-Valdes C, McGarry JD, Foster DW. Maternal-fetal carnitine relationships and neonatal ketosis in the rat. J Biol Chem 1976;251:6007–6012.
169. Ferré P, Pégorier JP, Williamson DH, Girard J. The development of ketogenesis at birth in the rat. Biochem J 1978;176:759–765.
170. Gelb BD. Genomic structure of and a cardiac promoter for the mouse carnitine palmitoyltransferase II gene. Genomics 1993;18:651–655.
171. Keller H, Dreyer C, Medin J. et al. Fatty acids and retinoids control lipid metabolism through activation of peroxisome proliferator-activated receptor-retinoid X receptor heterodimers. Proc Natl Acad Sci USA 1993;90:2160–2164.
172. Clarke SD, Jump DB. Polyunsaturated fatty acid regulation of hepatic gene transcription. J Nutr 1996;126:1105S–1109S.
173. Schoonjans K, Staels B, Auwerx J. Role of the peroxisome proliferator-activated receptor (PPAR) in mediating the effects of fibrates and fatty acids on gene expression. J Lipid Res 1996;37:907–925.
174. Gil-Gomez G, Ayté J, Hegardt FG. The rat mitochondrial 3-hydroxy-3-methylglutaryl-CoA synthase gene contains elements that mediate its multihormonal regulation and tissue specificity. Eur J Biochem 1993;213;773–779.
175. Girard J, Chatelain F, Boileau J, et al. Nutrient regulation of gene expression. J Anim Sci 1997;75:46–57.
176. Rodriguez JC, Gil-Gomez G, Hegardt FC, Haro D. Peroxisome proliferator-activated receptor mediates induction of the mitochondrial 3-hydroxy-3-methylglutaryl-CoA synthase gene by fatty acids. J Biol Chem 1994;269:18,767–18,772.
177. Suzuki H, Kawarabayasi Y, Kondo J, et al. Structure and regulation of rat long-chain acyl-CoA synthethase. J Biol Chem 1990;265:8681–8685.
178. Hahn P. The development of carnitine synthesis from butyrobetaine in the rat. Life Sci 1981;29;1057–1060.
179. McGarry JD, Mannaerts GP, Foster DW. A possible role for malonyl-CoA in the regulation of hepatic fatty acid oxidation and ketogenesis. J Clin Invest 1977;60:265–270.
180. Girard J, Perdereau D, Foufelle F, et al. Regulation of lipogenic enzyme gene expression by nutrients and hormones. FASEB J 1994;8:36–42.
181. Harano Y, Kashiwagi A, Kojima H, et al. Phosphorylation of carnitine palmitoyltransferase and activation by glucagon in isolated rat hepatocytes. FEBS Lett 1985;188:267–272.
182. Guzman M, Kolodziej MP, Caldwell A, et al. Evidence against direct involvement of phosphorylation in the activation of carnitine palmitoyltransferase by okadaic acid in rat hepatocytes. Biochem J 1994;300:693–699.
183. Ghadiminejad I, Saggerson ED. The relationship of the rat liver overt carnitine palmitoyltransferase to the mitochondrial malonyl-CoA binding entity and to the latent palmitoyltransferase. Biochem J 1990;270:787–794.
184. Kerner J, Zaluzec E, Gage D, Bieber LL. Characterization of the malonyl-CoA-sensitive carnitine palmitoyltransferase (CPTo) of a rat heart mitochondrial particle. Evidence that the catalytic unit is CPTI. J Biol Chem 1994;269:8209–8219.
185. Brown NF, Esser V, Foster DW, McGarry JD. Expression of a cDNA for rat liver carnitine palmitoyltransferase I in yeast establishes that catalytic activity and malonyl-CoA sensitivity reside in a single polypeptide. J Biol Chem 1994;269:26,438–26,442.
186. Zammit VA, Corstorphine CG. Altered release of carnitine palmitoyltransferase activity by digitonin from liver mitochondria of rats in different physiological states. Biochem J 1985;230:389–394.
187. Brady LJ, Silverstein L, Hoppel C, Brady PS. Hepatic mitochondrial inner membrane properties and carnitine palmitoyltransferase A and B: effect of diabetes and starvation. Biochem J 1985;232:445–450.
188. Niot I, Pacot F, Bouchard P, et al. Involvement of microsomal vesicles in part of the sensitivity of carnitine palmitoyltransferase I to malonyl-CoA inhibition in mitochondrial fractions of rat liver. Biochem J 1994;304:577–584.
189. Mynatt RL, Greenhaw JJ, Cook GA. Cholate extracts of mitochondrial outer membranes increase inhibition by malonyl-CoA of carnitine palmitoyltransferase I by a mechanism involving phospholipids. Biochem J 1994;299:761–767.
190. Kolodziej MP, Zammit VA. Sensitivity of inhibition of rat liver mitochondrial outer-membrane carnitine palmitoyltransferase by malonyl-CoA to chemical and temperature-induced changes in membrane fluidity. Biochem J 1990;272:421–425.
191. Lowe DM, Tubbs PK. Succinylation and inactivation 3-hydroxy-3-methylglutaryl-CoA synthase by succinyl-CoA and its possible relevance to the control of ketogenesis. Biochem J 1985;232:37–42.
192. Quant PA, Tubbs PK, Brand MD. Treatment of rats with glucagon or mannoheptulose increases mitochondrial 3-hydroxy-3-methyl-CoA synthase activity and decreases

succinyl-CoA content in liver. Biochem J 1989;262:159–164.
193. Quant PA, Tubbs PK, Brand MD. Glucagon activates mitochondrial 3-hydroxy-3-methylglutaryl-CoA synthase in vivo by decreasing the extent of succinylation of the enzyme. Eur J Biochem 1990;187:169–174.
194. Aprille JR. Perinatal development of mitochondria in rat liver. In: Fiskum G, ed. Mitochondrial physiology and pathology. New York: Reinhold, 1986:66–99.
195. Cuezva JM, Valcarce C, Luis AM, et al. Postnatal mitochondrial differentiation in the newborn rat. In: Cuezva JM, Pascual-Leone AM, Patel MS, eds. Endocrine and biochemical development of fetus and neonate. New York: Plenum Press. 1990:113–135.
196. Escriva F, Decaux JF, Ferré P, Girard JR. Evidence that the hepatic mitochondrial mass decreases during the first sixteen hours following birth in starved newborn rats. Biol Neonate 1984;45:125–128.
197. Ferré P, Pégorier J-P, Girard J. The effects of inhibition of gluconeogenesis in suckling newborn rats. Biochem J 1977;162:209–212.
198. Pégorier JP, Duée PH, Girard J. Contribution of hepatic fatty acid oxidation and exogenous galactose supply to the regulation of glucose homeostasis in newborn rabbits. Biol Neonate 1987;51:31–39.
199. Girard J, Ferré P, Kervran A, et al. Role of insulin/glucagon molar ratio in the changes of hepatic metabolism during development in the rat. In: Foa PP, Bajaj JS, Foa NL, eds. Glucagon, its role in physiology and clinical medicine. New York: Springer-Verlag, 1977:563–581.
200. Ferré P, Satabin P, El Manoubi L, et al. Relationship between ketogenesis and gluconeogensis in isolated hepatocytes from newborn rats. Biochem J 1981;200:429–433.
201. Ferré P, Turlan P, Girard J. Effects of medium chain triglyceride feeding or glucose infusion on glucose kinetics in the newborn rat. J Dev Physiol 1985;7:37–46.
202. Pégorier JP, Leturque A, Ferré P, et al. Effects of medium-chain triglyceride feeding on glucose homeostasis in the newborn rat. Am J Physiol 1983;244:E329–E334.
203. Pégorier JP, Ferré P, Girard J. The effect of inhibition of fatty acid oxidation in suckling newborn rats. Biochem J 1977;166:631–634.
204. Turlan P, Ferré P, Girard J. Evidence that medium-chain fatty acid oxidation can support an active gluconeogenesis in the suckling newborn rat. Biol Neonate 1983;43:103–108.
205. Pégorier JP, Simoes-Nunes C, Duée PH, et al. Effects of intragastric triglyceride administration on glucose homeostasis in newborn pigs. Am J physiol 1985;249:E268-E275.
206. Ferré P, Pégorier JP, Williamson DH, Girard J. Interactions in vivo between oxidation of non-esterified fatty acids and gluconeogenesis in the newborn rat. Biochem J 1979;182:593–598.
207. Hue L, Maisin L, Rider MH. Palmitate inhibits liver glycolysis. Involvement of fructose-2,6-bisphosphate in the glucose/fatty acid cycle. Biochem J 1988;251:541–545.
208. Bloom S, Johnston D. Failure of glucagon release in infants of diabetic mothers. Br Med J 1972;4:453–454.
209. Kalhan SC, Savin SM, Adam PAJ, Attenuated glucose production rate in newborn infants of insulin-dependent diabetic mothers. N Engl J Med 1977;296:375–376.
210. Kuhl C, Andersen G, Hertel J, Molsted-Pedersen L. Metabolic events in infants of diabetic mothers during the first 24 hours after birth. I. Changes in plasma glucose, insulin and glucagon. Acta Paediatr Scand 1982;71:19–25.
211. Cowett RM, Susa IB, Giletti B, et al, Glucose kinetics in infants of diabetic mothers. Am J Obstet Gynecol 1983;146:781–786.
212. Kollee LA, Monnens LA, Cezka V, Wilms RH. Persistent neonatal hypoglycemia due to glucagon deficiency. Arch Dis Child 1978;53:422–424.
213. Vidnes J, Oyasaeter S. Glucagon deficiency causing severe neonatal hypoglycaemia in a patient with normal insulin secretion. Pediatr Res 1977;11:943–949.
214. Vidnes J, Oyasaeter S. Reduced gluconeogenesis due to hyperinsulinism: hormonal and metabolic studies in an infant with hypoglycemia. Pediatr Res 1978;12:619–624.
215. Kalhan SC, Bier DM, Savin SM, Adam PAJ. Estimation of glucose turnover and ^{13}C recycling in the human newborn by simultaneous [1-^{13}C] glucose and [6-6-$^2H_2$] glucose tracers. J Clin Endocrinol Metab 1980;50:456–460.
216. Frazer TE, Karl IE, Hillman LS, Bier DM. Direct measurement of gluconeogenesis from [$2,3$-$^{13}C_2$] alanine in the human neonate. Am J Physiol 1981;240:E615–E621.
217. Bougnères PF, Karl IE, Hillman LS, Bier DM. Lipid transport in the human newborn: palmitate and glycerol turnover and the contribution of glycerol to hepatic glucose output. J Clin Invest 1982;70;262–270.
218. Denne SC, Kalhan SC. Glucose carbon recycling and oxidation in human newborns. Am J Physiol 1986;251:E71–E77.
219. Melichar V, Drahota Z, Hahn P. Changes in the blood levels of acetoacetate and ketone bodies in newborn infants. Biol Neonate 1965;8:348–352.
220. Melichar V, Drahota Z, Hahn P. Ketone bodies in the blood of full term newborns, premature and dysmature infants and in infants of diabetic mothers. Biol Neonate 1967;11:23–28.
221. Anday EK, Stanley CA, Baker L, Delivoria-Papadopoulos M. Plasma ketones in newborn infants: absence of suckling ketosis. J Pediatr 1981;98:628–630.
222. Wu PYK, Edmeon J, Aeustad N, et al. Medium-chain triglycerides in infants formulas and their relation to plasma ketone body concentration. Pediatr Res 1986;20:338–341.
223. Hahn P, Skala J. Carnitine transferases in human fetal tissues. Biol Neonate 1973;22:9–15.
224. Roux JF, Yoshioka T, Myers RE. Conversion of palmitate to respiratory carbon dioxide by fetal tissues of man and monkey. Nature 1970;227:963–964.
225. Bougnères PF, Lemmel C, Ferré P, Bier DM. Ketone body transport in the human neonate and infant. J Clin Invest 1986;77:42–48.
226. deBoissieu D, Rocchiccioli F, Kalach N, Bougnères PF. Ketone body turnover at term and in premature newborns in the first 2 weeks after birth. Biol Neonate 1995;67:84–93.
227. Shenai JP, Borum PR. Tissue carnitine reserves of newborn infants. Pediatr Res 1984;18:679–687.

228. Rebouche CJ. Comparative aspects of carnitine biosynthesis in micro-organisms and mammals, with special attention to carnitine biosynthesis in man. In: Frenkel RA, McGarry JD, eds. Carnitine biosynthesis, metabolism and function. New York: Academic Press, 1980: 57–72.
229. Warshaw JB, Curry E. Comparison of serum carnitine and ketone body concentrations in breast and in formula-fed newborn infants. J Pediatr 1980;97:122–125.
230. Elphick M, Wilkinson A. The effects of starvation and surgical injury on the plasma levels of glucose, free fatty acids and neutral lipids in the newborn babies suffering from various congenital anomalies. Pediatr Res 1981;15:313–318.
231. Cornblath M, Schwartz R. Hypoglycemia in the neonate. J Pediatr Endocrinol 1993;6:113–129.
232. Mestyan J, Soltesz G, Schultz K, Horvath M. Hyperaminoacidemia due to accumulation of gluconeogenic amino acid precursors in hypoglycemic small for gestational age infants. J Pediatr 1975;87:409–414.
233. Mestyan J, Rubecz I, Soltesz G. Changes in blood glucose, free fatty acid and amino acids in low birth-weight infants receiving intravenous fat emulsion. Biol Neonate 1976;30:74–79.
234. Sabel KG, Olegard R, Mellander M, Hildingsson K. Interrelation between fatty acid oxidation and control of gluconeogenic substrates in small for gestational age (SGA) infants with hypoglycemia and with normoglycemia. Acta Paediatr Scand 1982;71:53–61.
235. Sann L, Divry P, Lasne Y, Ruitton A. Effect of oral lipid administration on glucose homeostasis in small-for-gestational age infants. Acta Paediatr Scand 1982;71:923–927.
236. Sann L, Mousson B, Rousson M, et al. Prevention of neonatal hypoglycemia by oral lipid supplementation in low birth-weight infants. Eur J Pediatr 1988;147:158–161.
237. Bougnères PF, Castano L, Rocchiccioli F, et al. Medium chain fatty acids increase glucose production in normal and low birth weight newborns. Am J Physiol 1989;256:E692–E697.
238. Bergman AJIW, Donckerwolcke RAMG, Duran M, et al. Rate-dependent distal renal tubular acidosis and carnitine palmitoyltransferase I deficiency. Pediatr Res 1994;36:582–588.
239. Bougnères PF, Saudubray JM, Marsac C, Fasting hypoglycemia resulting from carnitine palmitoyltransferase deficiency. J Pediatr 1981;98:742–746.
240. Saudubray JM, Coudé FX, Demaugre F, et al. Oxidation of fatty acids in cultured fibroblasts: a model system for the detection and study of defects in oxidation. Pediatr Res 1982;16:877–881.
241. Bougnères PF, Saudubray JM, Marsac C, et al. Decreased ketogenesis due to deficiency of hepatic carnitine acyltransferase. N Engl J Med 1980;302:123–124.
242. Demaugre F, Bonnefont JP, Mitchell G, et al. Hepatic and muscular presentations of carnitine palmitoyltransferase deficiency: two distinct entities. Pediatr Res 1988;24:308–312.

30
Gastrointestinal Tract Metabolism in the Fetus and Neonate

Robert E. Kimura

The transition from suckling to postweaned conditions in the developing rat provides a natural model for examining the effect of changes in energy requirements and oxidative substrates on intestinal metabolism. In the small intestine, oxidative substrates are not only delivered by the blood, but are immediately available from absorption of luminal substrates. Changes in the diet that occur during suckling and weaning have been shown to alter intracellular fatty acid concentrations in intestinal mucosal cells. The suckling rat pup diet consists of a high percentage of lipid (approximately 70% of total caloric content).[1] During suckling, the concentration of free fatty acids in serum is markedly elevated as compared with the adult concentration[2] and the intracellular concentrations of esterified fatty acids in jejunal mucosal cells are increased.[3] During weaning the rat pup's diet changes to one that is predominantly carbohydrate. Furthermore, the concentration of free fatty acids in the serum and the concentrations of esterified fatty acids in the mucosal cells decrease to those found in the adult. Finally, an increase in liver ketogenesis during the suckling period results in an increase in serum ketone concentrations. These abrupt changes in serum and intracellular concentrations of free and esterified fatty acids and ketone bodies provide a natural perturbation of substrates that can alter intestinal metabolism.

There are many studies of the changes in intestinal glucose,[4-6] fatty acid,[7] ketones,[8] and glutamine[9] metabolism during the transition between the suckling and the weaning period. This chapter reviews the data of these studies, which indicate possible dietary and functional control mechanisms of intestinal oxidative metabolism.

Intestinal Glucose Metabolism

Srivastav and Hubscher[10] reported that glycolysis is low in the intestine of the suckling pup relative to the postweaned pup. They correlated this increase in intestinal glycolysis in the postweaned rat with an increase in intestinal hexokinase activity. Similarly, Hahn and Skala[11] measured increases in intestinal activity of two glycolytic enzymes, glucose-6-phosphate dehydrogenase and pyruvate kinase activities at the time of weaning.

Developmental changes in the metabolism of glucose to CO_2, lactate, and pyruvate by the intestine during suckling and weaning periods have been evaluated. During the suckling period (i.e., 16 days of age), the rate of glucose oxidation to CO_2 is low compared with the rate in weaned rats[13] (Figure 30.1). During the weaning period (i.e., 18–21 days of age), and immediately after artificially induced weaning (i.e., 21 days of age), there is an abrupt increase in glucose oxidation, which peaks at 25 days of age. This increase in glucose oxidation subsequently decreases to adult levels following weaning yet remains higher than the activity seen during the suckling period.

CO_2 can be produced from glucose by glycolysis and pyruvate oxidation or by the hexosemonophosphate pathway. To differentiate the source of CO_2 production from glucose in developing rat intestine, [$^{14}CO_2$] production from [1-^{14}C]glucose and [6-^{14}C]glucose was examined (Table 30.1). [$^{14}CO_2$] production from the metabolism of [1-^{14}C]glucose can occur in both pathways, while glycolysis and pyruvate oxidation accounts for all of the [$^{14}CO_2$] produced from [6-^{14}C]glucose. [$^{14}CO_2$] produced from [1-^{14}C]glucose increased twofold after weaning. In contrast, [$^{14}CO_2$] produced from [6-^{14}C]glucose increased fivefold. Before weaning, the ratio of [$^{14}CO_2$] production from [1-^{14}C]glucose to [$^{14}CO_2$] from [6-^{14}C]glucose was 2.07 compared with 1.16 postweaning. This indicates a greater increase in CO_2 production from the glycolytic-pyruvate oxidation pathway compared with the hexosemonophosphate pathway at weaning.

Lactate production, which is an index of glycolytic activity,[10] in intestinal tissue slices of the developing rat increased from a prewean rate of 1.62 ± 0.08 nmol lactate produced·mg wet wt·min^{-1} to a postwean rate of 2.73 ± 0.10 (mean ± SEM).[6] The adult intestinal lactate

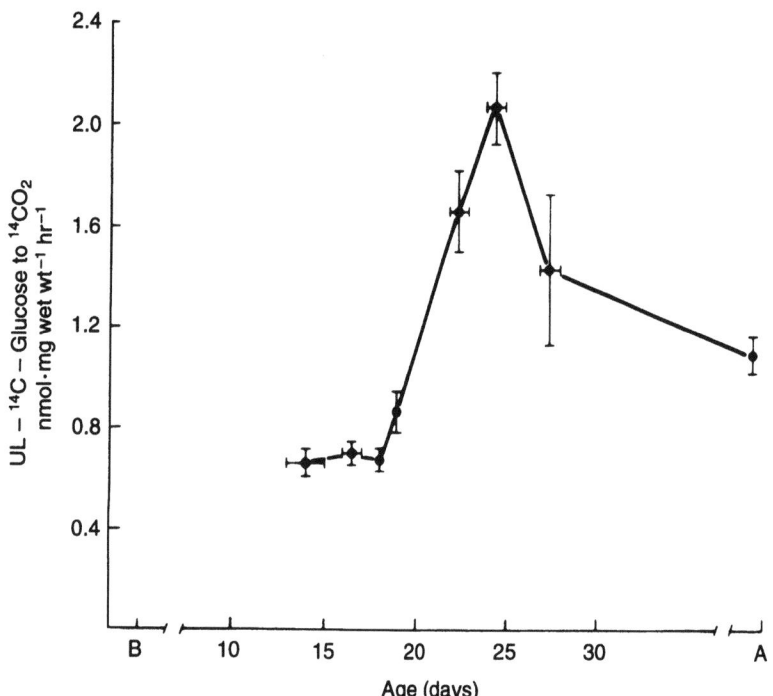

FIGURE 30.1. Developmental profile of [UL-^{14}C]glucose oxidation to [$^{14}CO_2$] by rat small intestinal tissue slices. Values are expressed as mean ± SEM (vertical symbols) of at least four observations (horizontal symbols define the range of age for the values). (From Kimura et al.,[6] with permission.)

production rate (1.93 ± 0.13) was comparable to suckling preweaned rats. In contrast to our studies, Srivastav and Hubscher,[10] reported that intestinal lactate production in homogenates prepared from intestinal mucosa was lower in the suckling rat compared to the adult. The disruption of mucosal cells and loss of endogenous controls in homogenate preparations used by Srivastav and Hubscher may account for the differences in these studies.

Under aerobic conditions, the rate of lactate production from glucose in adult intestine is greater than the rate of CO_2 production.[13,14] The studies of intestinal glucose metabolism in the developing rat are consistent with these adult studies. The ratios of [^{14}C]lactate to [^{14}C]CO_2 production from both [1-^{14}C]glucose and [6-^{14}C]glucose were greater than 18 for both pre- and postweaned rats (Table 30.1) The high rate of aerobic glycolysis in small intestine, measured in a tissue slice assay system, is similar to values obtained in adult rats using everted small intestine[13] and isolated mucosal cell.[13,14]

Control Mechanisms of Intestinal Glucose Metabolism in the Developing Rat

Pyruvate Dehydrogenase

The abrupt increase in intestinal glucose oxidation to CO_2 at weaning is mediated by pyruvate dehydrogenase activity. Pyruvate dehydrogenase in the active form, total

TABLE 30.1. Oxidation of [1-^{14}C]glucose and [6-^{14}C]glucose to CO_2 and lactate by developing rat intestine.

Age (days)	Product	[1-^{14}C]glucose oxidation		[6-^{14}C]glucose oxidation		[^{14}C] CO_2 [1-^{14}C]/[6-^{14}C]	[^{14}C]lactate
16	CO_2	0.87 ± 0.07	(18)	0.42 ± 0.04	(19)	2.07	
23	CO_2	2.24 ± 0.10	(6)*	1.93 ± 0.04	(6)*	1.16	
Adult	CO_2	1.19 ± 0.06	(5)*	0.79 ± 0.05	(5)*	1.51	
16	Lactate	25.7 ± 1.4	(17)	25.3 ± 1.4	(17)		1.01
23	Lactate	37.2 ± 0.7	(6)	35.8 ± 1.2	(6)*		1.04
Adult	Lactate	25.0 ± 0.7	(5)	26.7 ± 1.2	(5)		0.94

Data are expressed as nmol glucose oxidized · mg wet wt^{-1} h^{-1}.
Values expressed as mean ± SE (number of experiments).
*Value significantly different from 16 day old ($p < .01$).
From Kimura et al.,[6] with permission.

TABLE 30.2. Pyruvate dehydrogenase by developing rat intestine.

Age (days)	PDH active	PDH total	% Active
16	65 ± 15	274 ± 39	13
23	426 ± 31	559 ± 28	76

Data expressed as nmol [1-^{14}C]pyruvate decarboxylated to $^{14}CO_2$/g tissue/min.
Values expressed as mean ± SEM of five animals.
PDH active, the active form of pyruvate dehydrogenase; PDH total, total pyruvate dehydrogenase.
From Kimura et al.,[6] with permission.

pyruvate dehydrogenase activity, and the rate of pyruvate decarboxylation by intestinal tissue slices were measured (Table 30.2). There was a sixfold increase in the active form of pyruvate dehydrogenase activity at the time of weaning. The increased pyruvate dehydrogenase activity is the result of both an increase in the total amount of pyruvate dehydrogenase (i.e., twofold increase at the time of weaning) and an increase in the percentage of pyruvate dehydrogenase in the active form. The rate of decarboxylation of [1-^{14}C]pyruvate to [$^{14}CO_2$] also increased at the time of weaning from 3.02 ± 0.10^9 nmol·mg wet wt tissue^{-1} hr^{-1} in intestine of suckling rats to 4.80 ± 0.14^4 in intestine of the adult rat.

Citric Acid Cycle Activity

Another possible control mechanism of intestinal glucose oxidation in the developing rat during the suckling-weaning period is change in the citric acid cycle. The rate of acetate oxidation by mitochondria isolated from intestine (Table 30.3) of the suckling rat is 66% lower than the rate of the adult. This increase in intestinal mitochondrial acetate oxidation after weaning, which is reflective of citric acid cycle activity, is similar to the increase in intestinal oxidation of glucose.[6]

TABLE 30.3. The effect of acetoacetate on glucose oxidation in intestinal tissue slices of developing rat and acetate oxidation in intestinal mitochondria of developing rat.

Age (days)	Control	+1 mM Acetoacetate
Acetate oxidation to CO_2 in isolated mitochondria (nmol acetate oxidized·mg protein^{-1} hr^{-1})		
12–17	9.4 ± 2.7 (6)	24.5 ± 8.4 (6)
Adult	27.6 ± 4.9 (3)	14.0 ± 3.7 (3)
Glucose oxidation to CO_2 by intestinal tissue slices (nmol glucose oxidized·mg^{-1} wet wt tissue/h)		
15	0.49 ± 0.02 (6)	0.70 ± 0.09 (6)
Adult	2.49 ± 0.23 (3)	1.96 ± 0.25 (3)

Values are mean ± SEM (number rats).
Adapted from Kimura and Warshaw,[7] with permission.

Intramitochondrial [NADH]/[NAD$^+$]

In the heart,[15,16] it has been established that a decreased intramitochondrial nicotinamide adenine dinucleotide, reduced/nicotinamide adenine dinucleotide, oxidized [NADH]/[NAD$^+$] results in an increase in the active form of pyruvate dehydrogenase. Similarly, changes in the intramitochondrial [NADH]/[NAD$^+$] in the intestine of the developing rat correlate with changes in the active form of pyruvate dehydrogenase. We calculated the intramitochondrial [NADH]/[NAD$^+$] indirectly by determining tissue concentrations of 3-hydroxybutyrate and acetoacetate. The tissue concentration of 3-hydroxybutyrate during the suckling period was 10-fold greater than the concentration measured in the intestine of weaned rats (280 ± 34 nmol·g wet wt of tissue^{-1}). The concentration of acetoacetate was only 50% greater in the tissue from suckling animals (65 ± 7.3) compared with those from weaned rats (42.5 ± 2.5). Because the ratio of 3-hydroxybutyrate to acetoacetate decreases eightfold at the time of weaning, (4.47 to 0.54), the estimated intramitochondrial [NADH]/[NAD$^+$] decreased eightfold (the ratio of 3-hydroxybutyrate to acetoacetate was directly proportional to the intramitochondrial [NADH]/[NAD$^+$]). These studies suggest that, as in the heart, an increase in the intestinal pyruvate dehydrogenase activity is associated with a decrease in the intramitochondrial [NADH]/[NAD$^+$].

Citrate synthetase and isocitrate dehydrogenase, two enzyme systems that are controlled by intramitochondrial [NADH]/[NAD$^+$], have been shown to be the effective rate-limiting steps in other organ systems, such as the heart and muscle.[17] To determine if changes in intramitochondrial [NADH]/[NAD$^+$] of the intestine, in developing rat, control the increase in intestinal glucose oxidation to CO_2 during weaning, we investigated the effect of increasing the intramitochondrial [NADH]/[NAD$^+$] in intestine of postweaned rats on glucose oxidation.

The addition of exogenous 3-hydroxybutyrate causes a shift in the equilibrium of 3-hydroxybutyrate dehydrogenase to acetoacetate resulting in an increase in the intramitochondrial [NADH]/[NAD$^+$].[15] In the preweaned rat of 16 days of age in which the intramitochondrial [NADH]/[NAD$^+$] is already high, the addition of 3-hydroxybutyrate did not significantly inhibit intestinal glucose oxidation to CO_2 (Table 30.4). In the weaned rat, in which the intramitochondrial [NADH]/[NAD$^+$] is low, the addition of 3-hydroxybutyrate significantly inhibited glucose oxidation to CO_2 in intestine by 40% (Table 30.4). Similarly, addition of acetoacetate causes a decrease in the intramitochondrial [NADH]/[NAD$^+$]. Glucose oxidation by intestine of the suckling pup increased approximately 50% with the addition of acetoacetate, whereas in the intestine of the adult rat the addition of

TABLE 30.4. The effect of 3-hydroxybutyrate and glutamine on glucose oxidation by intestinal tissue slices of suckling and weaned rats.

	Control	+4 mM 3-Hydroxybutyrate	+2 mM Glutamine
16 d suckling	0.68 ± 0.03 (9)	0.63 ± 0.01 (4)	0.19 ± 0.01 (4)
Adult (weaned)	1.26 ± 0.08 (12)	0.69 ± 0.04 (8)	0.57 ± 0.02 (4)

Data expressed as nmol glucose oxidized to $CO_2 \cdot mg^{-1}$ wet wt·min^{-1}.
Values are mean ± SEM (number rats).
Adapted from Kimura et al.[5] and Kimura,[9] with permission.

acetoacetate decreased glucose oxidation by 25% (Table 30.3). These data suggest that in whole intestine the intramitochondrial [NADH]/[NAD⁺] regulates glucose oxidation in developing rat.

In the presence of 1 mM acetoacetate, the rate of acetate oxidation to CO_2, a measure of citric acid cycle activity, by mitochondria from suckling rat intestine increases threefold (Table 30.3). The addition of acetoacetate decreased acetate oxidation to CO_2 by isolated intestinal mitochondria from the adult animal. These studies suggest that citric acid cycle activity in isolated intestinal mitochondria is controlled by intramitochondrial [NADH]/[NAD⁺] and can account for the changes in glucose oxidation by intestine of developing rat.

Dietary Lipids

Hulsmann,[12] using perfused adult rat intestine, showed that when fatty acids are present in the perfusate, CO_2 production from glucose was markedly decreased and lactate production increased. Denton and Hughes[18] reported that the rat placed on high fat diet for 6 days showed a rapid decrease in adipose tissue pyruvate dehydrogenase activity, which is due primarily to a decrease in the active form of the enzyme. Adipose tissue from rats on a high-fat diet for 19 to 23 days had a significant decrease in total pyruvate dehydrogenase activity. These data are consistent with our own observation that the high-fat diet provided naturally during the suckling period causes a decrease in total pyruvate dehydrogenase activity and active pyruvate dehydrogenase in small intestine.

The Effect of Ketone on Intestinal Glucose Oxidation

Another possible influence on glucose metabolism during the suckling period is direct inhibition of the pyruvate dehydrogenase complex by serum ketones. During the suckling period, production of ketones by the liver is markedly elevated, resulting in an increased serum ketone concentration.[19] Windmueller and Spaeth[20] have reported that perfused adult rat jejunum oxidizes acetoacetate and 3-hydroxybutyrate and that the ketones are oxidized in preference to glucose and fatty acids. Other studies with perfused rat jejunum have shown that ketone bodies inhibit glucose oxidation to CO_2.[21] Lamers and Hulsmann[22] reported that pyruvate decarboxylation in adult rat intestine mucosal cells is inhibited by 5 mM DL-3-hydroxybutyrate.

It was determined that glucose oxidation in adult intestine was inhibited by 3-hydroxybutyrate while intestinal glucose oxidation of suckling pups was not altered by the presence of exogenous 3-hydroxybutyrate (Table 30.4). This suggests that during the suckling period the oxidation of glucose and pyruvate is already maximally inhibited by endogenous ketones, which are 10-fold greater in suckling than in postweaned rat intestine. Iemhoff et al.[13] reported that glucose oxidation to CO_2 in isolated mucosal cells from the fasted adult rat was one-third the rate seen in mucosal cells from the fed adult rat. One can speculate that increased endogenous pools of ketones, which are present in the starved state, cause the inhibition of CO_2 production. Hanson and Parson,[21] using perfused adult jejunum, reported that there is a significant decrease in the utilization of glucose by the intestines of the rat fasted for 48 hours compared with fed rat. They noted a decrease in the oxidation of glucose in the jejunum of fasted compared with fed rats. In addition, the presence of ketones in the perfusate decreased the oxidation of glucose in the fed rat jejunum, but completely inhibited the oxidation of glucose in the intestine of the fasted rat. The presence of physiologic ketosis, which is seen in the fasted state and during the suckling period, alters intestinal glucose metabolism. The increased sensitivity of glucose oxidation to the presence of exogenous ketones in the intestine of fasted rats may be secondary to alterations in the reduction-oxidation state of the intestine or the presence of endogenous ketones. Because lactate production from glucose was not affected by the presence of palmitate or 3-hydroxybutyrate in pre- or postweaned intestine, the concentration of palmitate and 3-hydroxybutyrate used in these experiments does not affect glycolytic activity or glucose uptake, which had been reported by Enser.[23]

Fatty Acid Oxidation

During the suckling period, rat pups absorb 75% of their caloric intake in the form of fatty acids.[1] This high fatty acid intake by the neonatal rat is associated with serum lipids that are twice that of the adult. Neonatal gut mucosa has a higher concentration of intracellular esterified fatty acids when compared to adult intestinal mucosal cells.[3,24] At the time of weaning there is a 4- to 10-fold decrease in the concentration of medium chain fatty acids in the triglycerides of small intestine. Iemhoff et al.[13] and Hulsmann[12] reported that mitochondria isolated from adult rat small intestinal epithelium oxidized sodium octanoate to CO_2 at high rates. These investigators reported that the rate of octanoate oxidation was approximately 15-fold that of palmitate. Hulsmann[12] further reported that palmitate was oxidized in preference to glucose in the adult rat small intestine. Windmueller and Spaeth,[20] using a jejunal segment preparation, reported that unesterified fatty acids contributed to less than 4% of all CO_2 production.

Medium- and long-chain fatty acid oxidation by isolated adult rat villus and crypt cells has been reported by Iemhoff et al.[13] Gangl and Ockner,[25] using a perfused intestinal rat model, reported that 42% of total radioactivity injected in the form of [^{14}C] palmitate can be recovered in a water-soluble metabolite pool that includes CO_2 and keto acids. Only 28% and 16% of the radioactivity was recovered as phospholipids and triglycerides, respectively.

The rate of oxidation of palmityl–coenzyme A (CoA) to CO_2 by isolated intestinal mitochondria of the developing rat pup increased 10-fold at the time of weaning (Figure 30.2). This was surprising in view of the high fat content of milk. A possible mechanism for the decrease in intestinal fatty acid oxidation in suckling rats is the inhibition of fatty acid β-oxidation by the high intramitochondrial [NADH]/[NAD$^+$] measured in intestine of suckling rats.[6] The rate of β-oxidation of fatty acids is regulated by the intramitochondrial [NADH]/[NAD$^+$].[26,27] Suppression of small intestinal fatty acid oxidation by an increase in intramitochondrial redox state has been previously reported by Gangl and Ockner.[25] To determine if oxidation in intestine is decreased during the suckling period, the presence of [^{14}C] in long-chain fatty acids in the assay medium after 1 hour of incubation was determined by saponifying and extracting long-chain fatty acids with pentane. There was no significant difference in the percent of [^{14}C] in the pentane extract between suckling and weaned rat intestine, suggesting similar rates of palmityl-CoA utilization. This suggests that fatty acid β-oxidation is not decreased in intestinal mitochondria of suckling rat pups.

A decrease in citric acid cycle activity in the intestine of suckling rats can account for the decrease in fatty acid

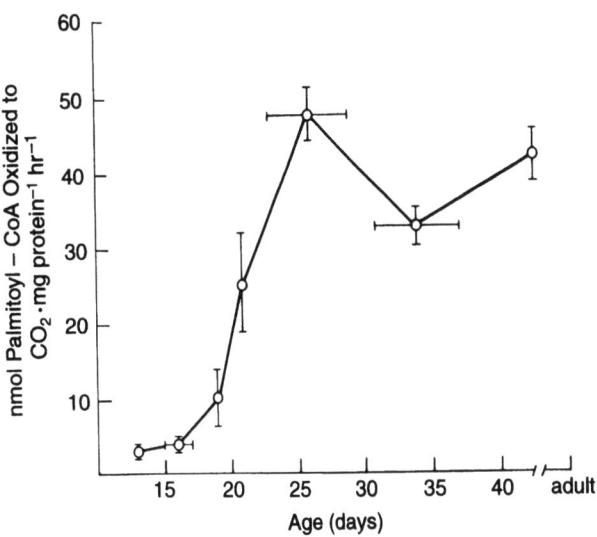

FIGURE 30.2. Developmental profile of oxidation of [1-^{14}C] palmityl-CoA to $^{14}CO_2$ by isolated mitochondria of rat small intestine. Values are expressed as mean ± SEM (vertical symbols) of at least four observations (horizontal symbols define the range of age for the values). (From Kimura and Warshaw,[7] with permission.)

oxidation to CO_2. The rate of acetate oxidation by mitochondria isolated from the intestine of suckling rats (Table 30.3) is one-third the rate in the adult. This increase in intestinal oxidation of acetate, which is reflective of citric acid cycle activity, is similar to that observed for intestinal oxidation of fatty acids and glucose.[6] When [^{14}C] was measured in the form of CO_2 and long-chain fatty acids, the total accountable [^{14}C] in adult intestinal mitochondria experiments was 53.8% and in suckling intestinal mitochondria experiments was 37%. The unaccountable [^{14}C] must be in a water-soluble fraction or short-chain fatty acids. This increase in the unaccountable [^{14}C] in suckling rat small intestinal mitochondria is consistent with a decrease in citric acid cycle activity. Acetate oxidation to CO_2 is suppressed in mitochondria of suckling rat intestine, supporting this conclusion.

Increases in intramitochondrial [NADH]/[NAD$^+$] have been reported to decrease citric acid cycle activity primarily at citrate synthetase (EC 4.1.3.7) and at isocitrate dehydrogenase (EC 1.1.1.41)[17] (Figure 30.3). Acetate and glucose oxidation by suckling rat intestine increased significantly when incubated with 1 mM acetoacetate. It previously has been reported that the addition of acetoacetate and 3-hydroxybutyrate can shift the intramitochondrial [NADH]/[NAD$^+$] through the activity of 3-hydroxybutyrate dehydrogenase. Hansford[28] has used changes in acetoacetate and 3-hydroxybutyrate concentrations in isolated heart mitochondria to determine the effect of changing the intramitochondrial redox state on pyruvate dehydrogenase activity. In these studies, rotenone was added to the assay mixture to prevent

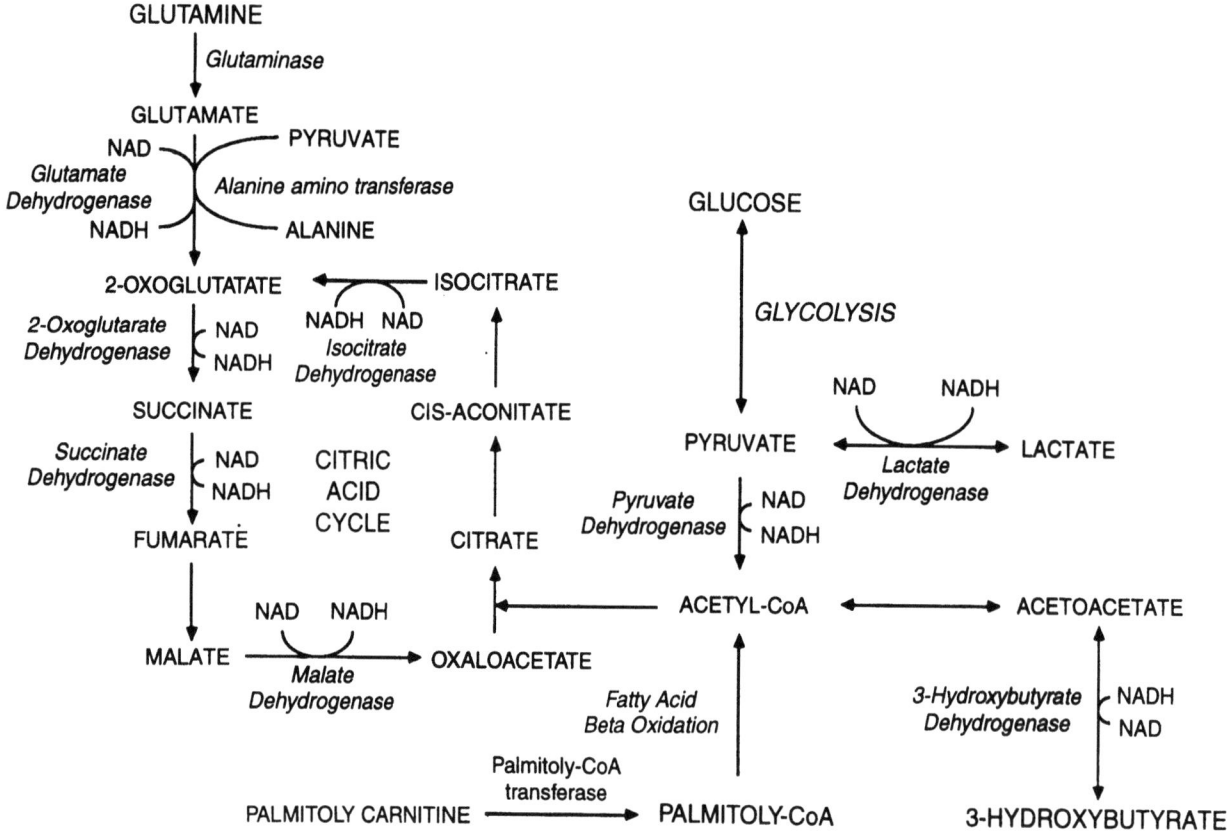

FIGURE 30.3. Biochemical pathways of substrate oxidation.

the oxidation of acetoacetate. A 100-fold increase in the 3-hydroxybutyrate to acetoacetate ratio resulted in an increase in the intramitochondrial [NADH]/[NAD$^+$] by 12-fold. Rotenone was not used because it would decrease oxidation. Short assay periods of 15 minutes in length were used and it was assumed that insignificant acetoacetate was oxidized. Under these conditions, the addition of acetoacetate would cause a decrease in the ratio of tissue concentrations of 3-hydroxybutyrate and acetoacetate, which would cause a decrease in intramitochondrial [NADH]/[NAD$^+$]. If acetoacetate is oxidized to acetyl-CoA, the resulting dilution of the acetate isotope at the intermediate acetyl-CoA would lower the calculated rate of oxidation. The stimulation of acetate oxidation may be greater than the calculated rate that was presented. The activation of acetate and glucose oxidation by the addition of acetoacetate in suckling rat intestine suggests a key regulatory role of intramitochondrial [NADH]/[NAD$^+$] during the suckling period.

In the postweaned animal, where the intestinal intramitochondrial [NADH]/[NAD$^+$] is low, the addition of acetoacetate decreased acetate oxidation (Table 30.3). The rate of oygen consumption by adult intestinal mitochondria is stimulated by the addition of acetate. This increase in oxygen consumption is inhibited by the addition of acetoacetate. This suggests that the decrease in [1-^{14}C] acetate oxidation to [^{14}CO$_2$] is secondary to inhibition of mitochondrial oxidation.

During the suckling period, oxidation of fatty acids by liver is elevated and appears to be regulated by an increase in carnitine palmitoyltransferase.[29] Aas and Daae[30] have shown an increase in carnitine palmitoyltransferase activity in the liver of rats provided a high-fat diet and an increase in fatty acid oxidation.[30] The activity of carnitine palmitoyltransferase of rat intestine mitochondria was determined to be elevated during the suckling period and it decreased after the time of weaning. The low rates of palmityl-CoA oxidation by intestinal mitochondria of suckling rats were seen despite high concentrations of carnitine palmitoyltransferase activity, which suggests that palmityl-CoA oxidation in mitochondria is not controlled by carnitine palmitoyltransferase. The data indicated that intestinal fatty acid oxidation to CO$_2$ is not controlled by carnitine palmitoyl transferase but by other factors such as intramitochondrial [NADH]/[NAD$^+$].

Glutamine Oxidation

In perfused adult rat intestinal models,[20,31–33] more than 25% of the total CO$_2$ production is produced from glutamine. Less than 20% comes from oxidation of the combination of fatty acids, glucose, and lactate, while

TABLE 30.5. Effect of increasing concentration of glutamine on glutamine oxidation by developing rat small intestine.

Age (days)	Glutamine concentration (mM)			
	0.5	1.0	2.0	4.0
15	1.27 ± 0.14 (7)	1.43 ± 0.13 (7)	1.54 ± 0.10 (19)	1.67 ± 0.20 (7)
Adult	0.48 ± 0.04 (3)	0.62 ± 0.08 (3)	0.88 ± 0.13 (10)	0.96 ± 0.11 (3)

Data expressed as nmol glutamine oxidized to $CO_2 \cdot mg^{-1}$ wet wt·min^{-1}.
Values are mean ± SEM (number rats).
Adapted from Kimura,[9] with permission.

50% to 60% comes from ketone bodies. Using tissue slices, the rate of glutamine oxidation to CO_2 by small intestine of suckling rat was approximately twice as great as that seen in the adult (Table 30.5). The rates of glutamine oxidation to CO_2 by isolated mitochondria from suckling and adult rat small intestine were 46.7 ± 4.8 and 57.6 ± 8.0 nmol glutamine oxidized·mg $protein^{-1}$ $hour^{-1}$, respectively. These data suggest that the rate of glutamine uptake by enterocytes is rate limiting in the small intestine of the developing rat. It has been reported that the uptake of a number of amino acids by developing rat small intestine is high postnatally and decreases after weaning.[34] These investigators have noted that the amino acid transport systems in the postnatal rat small intestine appear to be polyfunctional and become more specific after weaning. Although glutamine uptake was not measured by the present investigator, an increase in glutamine transport into enterocytes at weaning is consistent with the data.

An alternative explanation for the dependence of glutamine oxidation rate, on glutamine concentration in the intestine of adult rat, might be changes in the brush border of the intestine. The brush border of suckling rats is less developed than in the adult animal and diffusion of glutamine in the adult animal may be rate limiting.

It has been suggested that a cellular polarity exists among substrates absorbed from the vascular system and the intraluminal area.[25,31,35] Specifically, glutamine absorbed from the vascular space appears to be preferentially oxidized to CO_2 when compared to glutamine absorbed from the intraluminal space.[31] In the tissue studies, the sources of substrate from the vascular and intraluminal spaces were not delineated. These alterations in the rate of amino acid uptake from the intraluminal space may have profound effects on substrate availability to enterocytes.

Active glutamine oxidation in suckling rat small intestine may be similar to the sparing of glutamine oxidation in adult rats that are starved for 48 hours. Both the suckling pup and fasted adult rat have elevated blood ketone concentrations. Since glutamine oxidation is not affected by fasting and glucose oxidation is suppressed during the fasted state, Hanson and Parsons[31] reported that glutamine may play a larger role than glucose as an intestinal oxidative substrate. Similarly, studies of intestine of the suckling rat pup indicate that glucose oxidation is low (Figure 30.1) while glutamine oxidation is high (Table 30.6).

The intestinal oxidation of substrates that enter the citric acid cycle at the level of acetyl-CoA, glucose, and fatty acid is low in suckling rats as compared to adult rats. Intestinal glutamine oxidation, however, is active in the suckling rat, suggesting that the control of glutamine oxidation is different from glucose and fatty acid oxidation. It has been suggested that an alteration in intramitochondrial [NADH]/[NAD$^+$] may play a major role in controlling intestinal glucose oxidation in the developing rat.[6] An increase in intramitochondrial

TABLE 30.6. The effect of 3-hydroxybutyrate and glucose on glutamine oxidation in intestinal tissue slices of developing rat.

Age (d)	Control	+4 mM 3-Hydroxybutyrate	+5 mM Glucose
15–17	1.54 ± 0.1 (19)	1.53 ± 0.1 (10)	1.78 ± 0.12 (14)
20–25	0.98 ± 0.07 (10)	0.67 ± 0.03 (5)	0.91 ± 0.1 (10)
33–45	0.88 ± 0.13 (10)	0.57 ± 0.07 (10)	0.75 ± 0.09 (10)

In these studies 100 mM glutamine was used. The data are expressed as nmol glutamine oxidized to $CO_2 \cdot mg^{-1}$ wet wt·min^{-1}.
Values are mean ± SEM (4–5 rats).
Adapted from Kimura,[9] with permission.

[NADH]/[NAD⁺] was calculated by determining tissue concentration of 3-hydroxybutyrate and acetoacetate, and it was demonstrated that the addition of acetoacetate, which would decrease intramitochondrial [NADH]/[NAD⁺], enhances fatty acid oxidation to CO_2 in the suckling rat small intestine (Fig. 30.4).[7] Since the increased intramitochondrial [NADH]/[NAD⁺] in suckling rat small intestine does not affect glutamine oxidation, its effect on citric acid cycle activity must occur prior to the metabolic intermediate, 2-oxoglutarate. The sparing of glutamine oxidation in suckling rats suggests that citrate synthetase and/or isocitrate dehydrogenase are rate limiting, not 2-oxoglutarate dehydrogenase. These two enzyme systems, which are controlled by intramtiochondrial [NADH]/[NAD⁺], have been shown to be the effective rate-limiting steps in other organ systems, such as the heart and muscle.[17]

Glutamate, the metabolite of glutamine, is metabolized to 2-oxoglutarate by either alanine aminotransferase, aspartate aminotransferase, or glutamate dehydrogenase (Figure 30.3). It has been proposed that alanine aminotransferase is a major pathway of glutamate metabolism to 2-oxoglutarate in small intestine.[36] Alanine aminotransferase activity was determined using both whole tissue homogenates and subcellular fractions.[9] The majority of alanine aminotransferase activity was in the mitochondrial free supernatant in suckling and postweaned rat small intestine; less than 20% was in either the cell debris or the mitochondrial fractions.[9] In homogenates in which the cellular debris and nuclei were removed, alanine aminotransferase activity was 63% greater in the adult than in the suckling rat.[9] Bavere and Lund,[37] using isolated enterocytes and 1 mM amino-oxyacetate, a known inhibitor of both alanine and aspartate aminotransferase, reported that glutamine is still metabolized to CO_2 at approximately 40% of the uninhibited rate. Their data suggest that glutamate dehydrogenase is intact in the small intestine, but probably is not the preferred pathway from glutamate to oxoglutarate.

The effect of amino-oxyacetate, a known inhibitor of alanine aminotransferase, on glutamine and 3-hydroxybutyrate oxidation was determined.[9] With tissue slices, 10 mM amino-oxyacetate decreased suckling rat small intestinal glutamine oxidation to CO_2 by 95%, suggesting that glutamate dehydrogenase activity is low in developing rat intestine. In contrast, 10 mM amino-oxyacetate inhibited adult jejunal glutamine oxidation by 82%, a value significantly different from suckling rats ($p < .025$). One explanation for this variability in inhibition of glutamine oxidation is a difference in glutamate dehydrogenase activity. Greater inhibition in suckling jejunum suggests lower glutamate dehydrogenase activity as compared to the adult. One could speculate that during the suckling period, glutamate dehydroge-

TABLE 30.7. Substrate oxidation in intestinal tissue slices and isolated mitochondria of developing rat.

	Substrate oxidation in intestinal tissue slices		
Substrate	Glucose	Glutamine	3-Hydroxybutyrate
Suckling	0.68 ± 0.03 (9)	1.54 ± 0.12 (19)	0.15 ± 0.01 (8)
Weaned	1.26 ± 0.08 (12)	0.88 ± 0.13 (10)	0.58 ± 0.06 (8)

Data expressed as nmol substrate oxidized to $CO_2 \cdot mg^{-1}$ wet wt·min^{-1}. Values are mean ± SEM (number rats).

	Substrate oxidation in intestinal mitochondrial		
	Acetate	C16 CoA	3-Hydroxybutyrate
Suckling	9.4 ± 2.7 (6)	4 ± 1 (4)	8.6 ± 1.1 (9)
Weaned	27.6 ± 4.9 (3)	48 ± 3 (4)	16.2 ± 1.1 (7)

Data expressed as nmol substrate oxidized to $CO_2 \cdot protein^{-1} min^{-1}$. Values are mean ± SEM (number rats).
Adapted from Kimura,[9] Kimura and Ilich,[8] Kimura et al.,[6] and Kimura and Warshaw,[7] with permission.

nase is inhibited by high intramitochondrial [NADH]/[NAD⁺].

Ketone Oxidation

The suckling rat pup consumes a majority of its calories in the form of fatty acids and as a result of increased hepatic ketogenesis has high serum levels of 3-

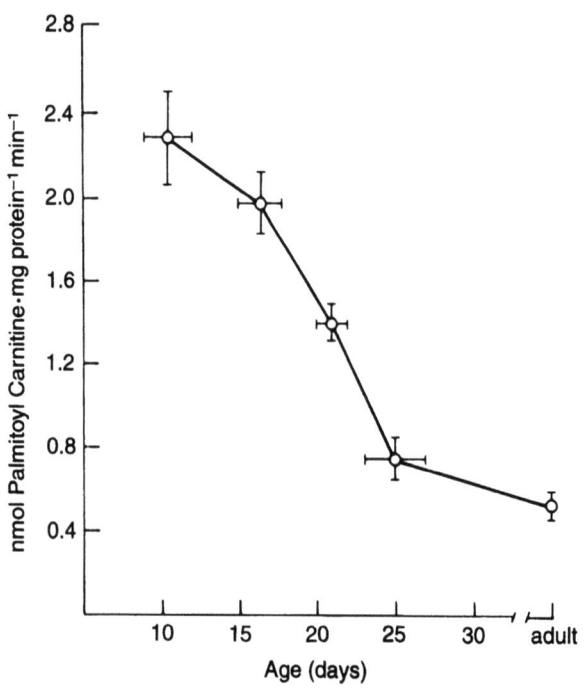

FIGURE 30.4. Developmental profile of carnitine palmitoyltransferase activity in isolated mitochondria of rat small intestine. Values are expressed as mean ± SEM (vertical symbols) of at least four observations (horizontal symbols define the range of age for the values). (From Kimura and Warshaw,[7] with permission.)

TABLE 30.8. Substrate oxidation in enterocytes of developing rat.

Age (days)	Glutamine	Glucose	3-Hydroxybutyrate
15–16 suckling	114 ± 12	8.4 ± 1.2	8.3 ± 1.3
23–24 weaned	87 ± 7	37.8 ± 3.6	15.0 ± 1.6

Data expressed as nmol substrate oxidized to $CO_2 \cdot protein^{-1} \cdot min^{-1}$.
Values are mean ± SEM (number rats).
Adapted from Kimura and Ilich,[8] with permission.

Carrington and Hanson[38] reported that in the adult rat the activity of intestinal 3-oxoacid CoA transferase was 8 to 10 µmol acetoacetate formation·min^{-1}g wet $weight^{-1}$. Williamson et al.[39] determined 3-oxoacid CoA-transferase activity both in the formation of acetoacetate and in the formation of acetoacetyl-CoA in different organs, and found that the ratio between acetoacetyl-CoA formation and acetoacetate formation was 1:6. 3-Oxoacid CoA-transferase activity was measured in the direction of acetoacetyl-CoA formation. The data, when hydroxybutyrate and acetoacetate. Page et al.[4] reported that serum 3-hydroxybutyrate concentration in the suckling rat was three times greater than in the weaned pup and six times greater than in the adult rat. This ketotic condition is similar to that seen in the fasting adult rat. The oxidation of ketone bodies accounts for 50% to 60% of CO_2 produced by autoperfused intestine of fasting adult rats, whereas glutamine oxidation accounts for 25% of CO_2 produced.[20] Like the intestines of the adult rat, the rate of oxidation of glutamine to CO_2 is high in the intestines of the suckling pup.[9] The oxidation of DL-3-hydroxybutyrate to CO_2 by intestines of suckling pups was less than the oxidation by intestines of weaned pups; 74.1% less using tissue slices (Table 30.7) and 44.6% less using enterocytes when expressed in terms of milligrams of protein (Table 30.8).

A possible control mechanism for the increase in intestinal ketone oxidation at weaning, would be a change in the activity of enzymes involved. Changes were measured in the activity of the enzymes involved with ketone oxidation, including 3-hydroxybutyrate dehydrogenase (EC 1.1.1.30), 3-oxoacid CoA-transferase (EC 2.8.3.5), and acetoacetyl-CoA thiolase (EC 2.3.1.9) in developing rat and adult rat intestines (Figure 30.5). Two of these enzymes, 3-hydroxybutyrate dehydrogenase and 3-oxoacid CoA-transferase, have been reported in significant amounts in adult jejunum.[38] The activity of 3-hydroxybutyrate dehydrogenase in the intestine of suckling rats was greater than the activity in the intestine of adults (Figure 30.5). Similarly, intestinal acetoacetyl-CoA thiolase activity in the suckling rat was twofold greater compared with the activity in the 24-day-old rat and the adult rat. In contrast, intestinal 3-oxoacid CoA-transferase activity was low in intestine of the suckling rat (0.28 ± 0.02 µmol·g wet weight $tissue^{-1} \cdot min^{-1}$) and increased two- to threefold in the weaned rat. Thus, of the three enzymes involved in ketone metabolism only changes in 3-oxoacid CoA-transferase activity follow the same developmental pattern as ketone oxidation. Similarly, Page et al.[4] have reported that in the brain of a developing rat, the activity of acetoacetyl-CoA thiolase decreased after weaning and 3-oxoacid CoA-transferase activity increased.

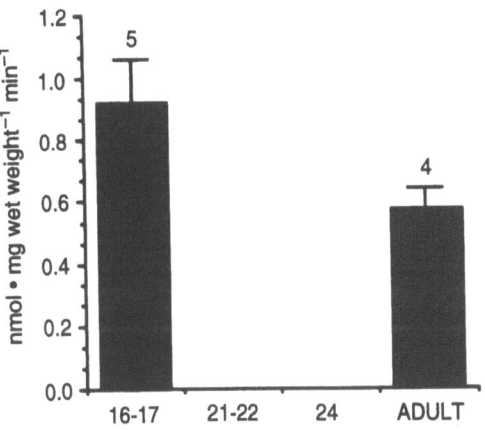
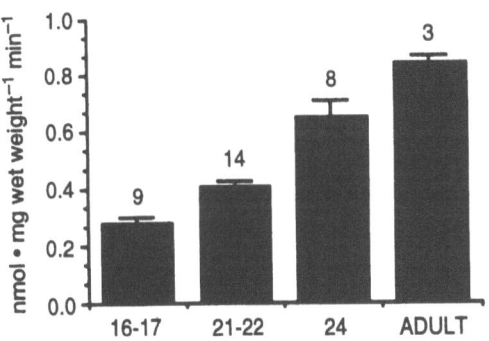
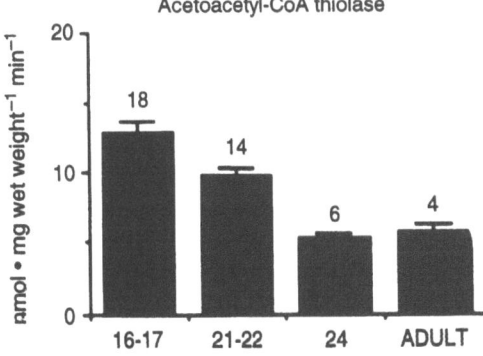

FIGURE 30.5. Changes in intestinal 3-hydroxybutyrate dehydrogenase, 3-oxoacid Co-A transferase, and acetoacetyl-CoA thiolase in developing rats. Values are expressed as means ± SEM (number of rats). (From Kimura and Ilich,[8] with permission.)

adjusted for the direction of acetoacetate formation, were comparable with Carrington's data.

Comparing the Oxidation of 3-Hydroxybutyrate, Glutamine, and Glucose by the Intestine of the Developing Rat

In studies of substrate oxidation by the intestine of adult rats, Windmueller and Spaeth[20,32,33] determined that glutamine is a significant oxidative substrate. To determine the effect of development on the significance of intestinal glutamine oxidation, the rates of oxidation of glutamine, glucose, and 3-hydroxybutyrate by the intestine of developing rat were compared. In tissue slices using a single oxidative substrate, glutamine oxidation in the intestine of suckling rat was 2- and 10-fold greater than glucose and 3-hydroxybutyrate oxidation, respectively (Table 30.7). In contrast, in postweaned rat, intestinal glucose oxidation was 30% and 54% greater than glutamine and 3-hydroxybutyrate oxidation, respectively. In the presence of glucose and glutamine, intestinal glutamine oxidation of suckling rats was 10 times greater than glucose oxidation (1.78 ± 0.12 vs 0.19 ± 0.01) (Tables 30.4 and 30.6), while in the postweaned rat, intestine glutamine oxidation was only 30% greater than glucose oxidation (0.75 ± 0.09 vs 0.57 ± 0.02).

The rate of L-glutamine oxidation to CO_2 by the enterocyte of the suckling and the weaned pups was comparable (Table 30.8). In contrast, the rate of glucose oxidation by enterocytes of suckling pups was 75% less than the rate of oxidation by enterocytes of weaned pups. The changes in glucose and glutamine enterocyte oxidation at the time of weaning is similar to changes in substrate oxidation measured using tissue slices. When evaluating absolute rates of substrate oxidation by enterocytes of developing rat, the rate of glutamine oxidation was 14-fold greater than glucose or ketone oxidation in enterocytes of suckling rat and 2- (glucose) and 6- (ketones) fold greater in enterocytes of postweaned rats.

The addition of 5mM D-glucose did not alter the CO_2 production from L-glutamine by enterocytes of suckling pups (Table 30.9). In contrast, CO_2 production from L-glutamine by enterocytes of weaned pups was increased by 32% with the addition of 5mM D-glucose, although this increase was not statistically significant. The addition of 4mM DL-3-hydroxybutyrate did not change production of CO_2 from L-glutamine by enterocytes of weaned pups. However, the addition of 4mM DL-3-hydroxybutyrate did result in a significant (27%) decrease in glutamine oxidation in the enterocytes of suckling pups. D-glucose oxidation to CO_2 by enterocytes of suckling and weaned pups decreased significantly (75% and 58%) in the presence of 5mM L-glutamine. However, the rate of CO_2 production from DL-3-hydroxybutyrate by enterocytes of suckling pups or weaned rats was not altered by the addition of 5mM L-glutamine.

The rate of CO_2 production from DL-3-hydroxybutyrate by enterocytes of suckling and weaned pups in the presence of 5mM L-glutamine was 12- and 6-fold less than the rate of CO_2 production from L-glutamine in the presence of 4mM DL-3-hydroxybutyrate (Table 30.9). The rate of CO_2 production from D-glucose by enterocytes of the suckling and weaned pups in the presence of 5mM L-glutamine was 54- and 7-fold less, respectively, than the rate of CO_2 production from L-glutamine in the presence of 5mM D-glucose.

The addition of glutamine caused a significant decrease in CO_2 production from D-glucose by enterocytes of both suckling and weaned pups. In contrast, the addition of glucose did not alter the rate of glutamine oxidation of enterocytes of developing rat intestine. This suggests that glutamine is the preferred oxidative substrate in enterocytes of developing rats when compared with glucose.

The intestinal oxidation of substrates that enter the citric acid cycle at the level of acetyl-CoA, glucose, and fatty acid, is low in suckling rats as compared to adult rats. Intestinal glutamine oxidation, however, is active in the suckling rat, suggesting that the control of glutamine oxidation is different from glucose and fatty acid oxidation. It has been suggested that an alteration in intramitochondrial [NADH]/[NAD$^+$] may play a major role in controlling intestinal glucose oxidation in the developing rat.[6] An increase in intramitochondrial

TABLE 30.9. Interaction of 3-hydroxybutyrate, glucose, and glutamine oxidation in enterocytes in developing rat.

Age (days)	Glutamine oxidation		
	Control	+Glucose	+3-Hydroxybutyrate
15–16 suckling	114 ± 12	114 ± 14	84 ± 12
23–adult weaned	87 ± 7	115 ± 13	88 ± 10

Age (days)	Glucose oxidation		
	Control	+Glutamine	+3-Hydroxybutyrate
15–16 suckling	8.4 ± 1.2	2.1 ± 0.3	4.5 ± 0.4
23–adult weaned	37.8 ± 3.6	16.0 ± 2.1	$27.5 + 3.7$

Age (days)	3-Hydroxybutyrate oxidation		
	Control	+Glutamine	+Glucose
15–16 suckling	8.3 ± 1.3	6.9 ± 1.3	11.1 ± 1.9
23–adult weaned	15.0 ± 1.6	14.4 ± 2.2	25.2 ± 4.3

Data expressed as rate of substrate oxidation to CO_2 (nmol·mg protein^{-1} hr^{-1}), mean ± SEM, $n = 4$–5.
Adapted from Kimura and Ilich,[8] with permission.

[NADH]/[NAD$^+$] was measured by determining tissue concentrations of 3-hydroxybutyrate and acetoacetate and it was demonstrated that the addition of acetoacetate, which would decrease intramitochondrial [NADH]/[NAD$^+$], enhances fatty acid oxidation to CO_2 in suckling rat small intestine. Since the increased intramitochondrial [NADH]/[NAD$^+$] in suckling rat small intestine does not affect glutamine oxidation, its affect on citric acid cycle activity must occur prior to the metabolic intermediate, 2-oxoglutarate. The sparing of glutamine oxidation in the suckling rat suggests that citrate synthetase and/or isocitrate dehydrogenase are rate limiting rather than 2-oxoglutarate deydrogenase. These two enzyme systems, which are controlled by intramitochondrial [NADH]/[NAD$^+$], have been shown to be the effective rate-limiting steps in other organ systems, such as the heart and muscle.[17]

It is difficult to interpret the experiments in which glucose and ketones are added to glutamine oxidation assays. A decrease in the calculated rate of oxidation may be related to an actual decrease in the rate of glutamine oxidation or may be secondary to dilution of the glutamine isotope. Since both glucose and 3-hydroxybutyrate oxidation increased at weaning, it is likely that some degree of dilution of the glutamine isotope did occur at the level of 2-oxoglutarate in the citric acid cycle (Figure 30.3). Utilizing [1-^{14}C] glutamine, suckling rat intestinal glutamine oxidation is not affected either by exogenous glucose or by 3-hydroxybutyrate in the suckling rat intestine, indicating that no significant dilution of the [1-^{14}C] glutamine occurs. Thus, glucose and 3-hydroxybutyrate oxidation in the suckling rat intestine must be insignificant compared to glutamine oxidation.

The Effect of Weaning and Steroids on Changes in Intestinal Metabolism

Fats provide 70% of the calories in a suckling rat diet. After rats are weaned to a solid diet, fats provide only 30% of the calories.[40] In addition to this abrupt change in diet, serum concentrations of corticosteroids and the number of intestinal glucocorticoid receptors increase 4 to 6 days before weaning.[41,42] During the last 4 days of the suckling period, changes occur in small intestinal function and structure. These changes include marked intestinal growth measured by length, weight, and protein content of the intestine,[43] development of brush border enzymes,[44] ileal pore closure to macromolecular absorption,[45] and morphologic differentiation of supranuclear vacuolar cells to mature appearing villous cells.[46]

Changes in enterocyte metabolism occur at the time of weaning. During the suckling period, serum free fatty acids are markedly elevated compared to adult concentrations.[3] The intracellular concentrations of esterified fatty acids in jejunal mucosal cells are increased.[47] After weaning, concentrations of serum free fatty acids[48] and esterified fatty acids in the mucosal cells fall to adult levels.[3] Both fatty acid and glucose oxidation by the small intestine increase at the time of weaning.[6] The estimated intramitochondrial [NADH]/[NAD$^+$] also decreases at this time.[6] Decreasing the intramitochondrial [NADH]/[NAD$^+$] stimulates fatty acid and glucose oxidation in mitochondria isolated from the small intestine of suckling rats. The in vitro addition of exogenous 3-hydroxybutyrate increases the intramitochondrial [NADH]/[NAD$^+$], and inhibits glucose oxidation in the weaned animal, but not in the suckling animal.[6] Since corticosteroids induce changes in intestinal structure and function in suckling animals, the relative contribution of glucocorticoids or diet on the increase in glucose oxidation after weaning was investigated.

Intestinal glycolysis, as measured by lactate production, did not change during suckling (Figures 30.6 and 30.7). When suckling is continued past the usual age of weaning, lactate production does not increase (Figure 30.7). Early glucocorticoid treatment also has no effect on lactate production in the suckling pup. After delayed weaning at 25 days, lactate production does increase. The lack of corticosteroid effect on lactate production in the suckling animal contrasts with the well-studied induction of brush border enzymes and other developmental changes.[43-46] Precocious weaning at 16 days of age is followed by a gradual increase in lactate production (Figure 30.8). Early steroid treatment does not change lactate production in suckling pups (Figures 30.6 and 30.7). After precocious weaning, however, lactate production increases sooner to postweaned levels in the treated pup (Figure 30.8). This change in lactate oxidation after precocious weaning indicates an effect by steroids on the glycolytic pathway in suckling animals. Glucose oxidation to CO_2 by the enterocyte, although much lower than oxidation to lactate, follows a similar developmental profile. Oxidation to CO_2 remains stable during suckling and increases only after weaning (Figures 30.6 and 30.7). Early cortisone treatment has no effect on CO_2 production during suckling. These studies clearly show that the increase in glucose metabolism to either lactate or CO_2 at weaning is not controlled by the endogenous glucocorticoid burst that occurs prior to weaning. Only after weaning does the increase in glucose metabolism occur. This suggests that changes associated with a modified diet at the time of weaning control intestinal glucose metabolism.

It has been shown that the decreased rate of glucose oxidation to CO_2 by intestine of suckling rats is associated with a lower rate of pyruvate decarboxylation and a decrease in active pyruvate dehydrogenase. Changes in the activity of pyruvate dehydrogenase during suckling and

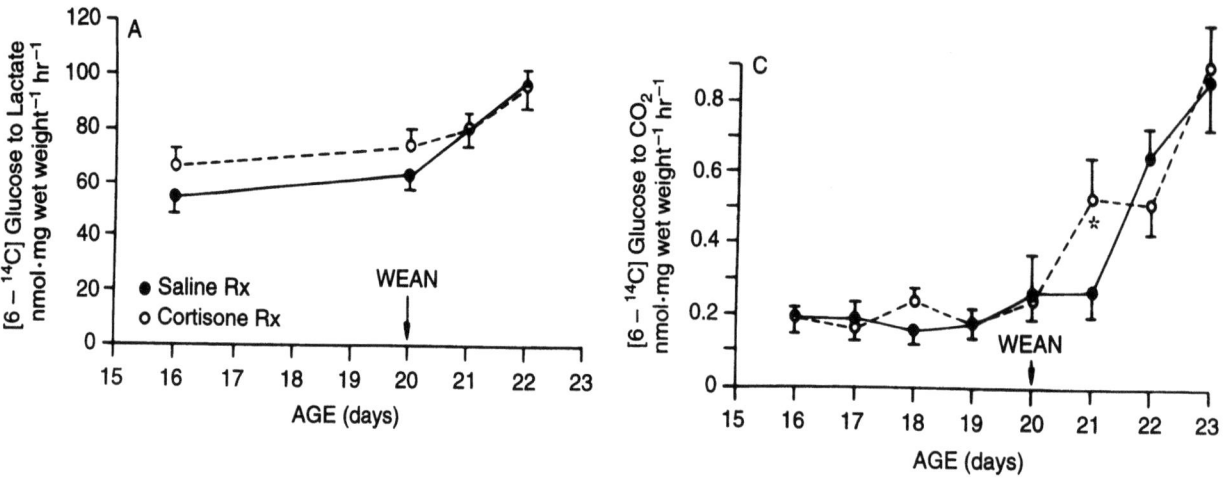

FIGURE 30.6. The effect of weaning at 20 days of age and cortisone treatment 10 to 13 days of age on glucose metabolism to lactate and CO_2. Points are mean ± SEM for 3 to 12 animals. (From Kimura and Reinersman,[5] with permission.)

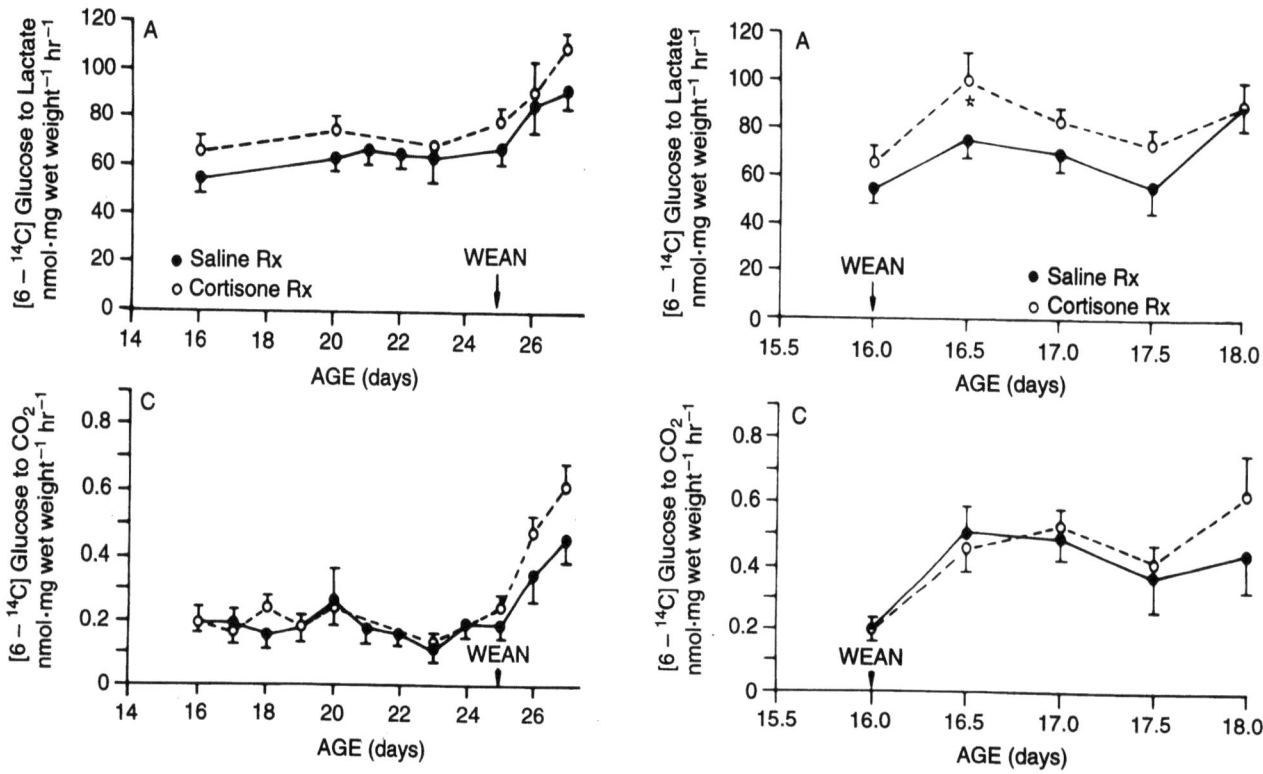

FIGURE 30.7. The effect of prolonged suckling to 25 days of age and cortisone treatment 10 to 13 days of age on glucose metabolism to lactate and CO_2. Points are mean ± SEM for 4 to 12 animals. (From Kimura and Reinersman,[5] with permission.)

FIGURE 30.8. The effect of precocious weaning at 16 days of age and cortisone treatment 10 to 13 days of age on glucose metabolism to lactate and CO_2. Points are mean ± SEM for 5 to 12 animals. (From Kimura and Reinersman,[5] with permission.)

weaning, periods of high and low fat intake, mediate changes in glucose oxidation to CO_2.

Clinical Implications

It is clear that glutamine is the preferred intestinal oxidative substrate in both the suckling and the weaned rat. In addition to providing energy by oxidative metabolism, a glutamine metabolite, ribose, is an important precursor for nucleotide synthesis. Because of these important intestinal functions, investigators have proposed supplementing total parenteral nutrition with glutamine. However, in the suckling rat, intestinal preference for glutamine oxidation is two- to three-fold greater than the weaned rat. This significant preference to glutamine oxidation in the suckling rat is controlled by intramitochondrial [NADH]/[NAD$^+$], which inhibits the oxidation of all substrates that enter into the citric acid cycle in the form of acetyl-CoA. The significance of glutamine as the preferred intestinal oxidative substrate in the suckling pup is that glutamine supplementation of total parenteral nutrition and in enteral feedings of the suckling neonates may have profound effects. Future studies regarding the effect of glutamine supplementation on neonatal intestinal function are needed.

Implications

In the presence of glutamine, glucose, and 3-hydroxybutyrate, glutamine is the preferred oxidative substrate in enterocytes of the suckling and the weaned rat. Studies of changes in intestinal metabolism in the developing rat clearly indicate that the oxidation of substrates that enter the citric acid cycle in the form of acetyl-CoA such as glucose, fatty acid, and lipids is low during the suckling period and increases after weaning. In contrast, glutamine that enters the citric acid cycle in the form of 2-oxoglutarate, is high during the suckling period and does not change during weaning. The control of the citric acid cycle appears to be the intramitochondrial [NADH]/[NAD$^+$], which is high during the suckling period and low in intestine of weaned rats. These studies demonstrate how evaluating changes in metabolism during a natural perturbation such as weaning can identify control mechanisms of metabolism. Finally, the changes in substrate oxidation during weaning are not controlled by the endogenous steroid burst that occurs at 16 days of age. Substrate oxidation changes only after weaning, suggesting that a change in diet is a significant factor in intestinal substrate oxidation.

References

1. Hahn P, Koldovsky O, Utilization of nutrients during postnatal development. Oxford: Pergamon Press, 1966:17.
2. Viktora J, Fodor J, Grafnetter D, et al. Studies of certain biochemical indices of fat metabolism during the ontogenesis of the rat. Cesk Fysiol 1960;9:63–64.
3. Dobiasova M, Hahn P, Koldovskv O. Fatty acid composition in developing rat. Biochem Biophys Acta 1964;84:538–549.
4. Page M, Krebs H, Williamson D. Activities of enzymes of ketone-body utilization in brain and other tissues of suckling rats. Biochem J 1971;121:49–53.
5. Kimura RE, Reinersman GT. Intestinal glucose metabolism during development: II. The role of glucocorticoids and weaning. Pediatr Res 1985;19:1313–1317.
6. Kimura RE, Thulin G, Warshaw JB, The effect of ketone bodies and fatty acid on intestinal glucose metabolism during development. Pediatr Res 1984;18:575–579.
7. Kimura RE, Warshaw JB. Control of fatty acid oxidation by intramitochondrial [NADH]/[NAD$^+$] in developing rat small intestine. Pediatr Res 1988;23:262–263.
8. Kimura RE, Ilich JZ. The oxidation of 3-hydroxybutyrate in developing rat jejunum. J Pediatr Gastroenterol Nutr 1991;13:347–353.
9. Kimura RE. Glutamine oxidation by developing rat small intestine. Pediatr Res 1987;21:214–217.
10. Srivastav L, Hubscher G. The effect of age on glycolytic and hexokinase activities in the mucosa of rat small intestine. Biochem J 1968;110:607–608.
11. Hahn P, Skala J. The development of some enzyme activities in the gut of the rat. Biol Neonate 1971;18:433–438.
12. Hulsmann WC. Preferential oxidation of fatty acids by rat small intestine. FEBS Lett 1971;17:35–37.
13. Iemhoff W, Van Den Berg J, DePijper A, Hulsmann WC. Metabolic aspects of isolated cells from rat small intestinal epithelium. Biochem Biophys Acta 1970;215:229–241.
14. Neptune E. Respirations and oxidation of various substrates by ileum in vitro. Am J Physiol 1965;209:329–332.
15. Hansford R, Cohen L. Relative importance of pyruvate dehydrogenase interconversion and feed-back inhibition in the effect of fatty acids on pyruvate oxidation by rat heart mitochondria. Arch Biochem Biophys 1978;191:65–81.
16. Kerby AL, Randle P, Cooper R, et al. Regulation of pyruvate dehydrogenase in rat heart. Biochem J 1976;154:327–348.
17. LaNoue KF, Bryla J, Williamson JR. Feedback interactions in the control of citric acid cycle activity in rat heart mitochondria. J Biol Chem 1972;247:667–679.
18. Denton RM, Hughes WA. Pyruvate dehydrogenase and the hormonal regulation of fat synthesis in mammalian tissues. Int J Biochem 1978;9:545–552.
19. Drahota Z, Hahn P, Klieninzeller A, Kostolanska A. Acetoacetate formation by liver slices from adult and infant rats. Biochem J 1964;93:61–65.
20. Windmueller H, Spaeth A. Identification of ketone bodies and glutamine as the major respiratory fuels in vivo for postabsorptive rat small intestine. J Biol Chem 1978;253:69–76.

21. Hanson P, Parsons D. Factors affecting the utilization of ketone bodies and other substrates by rat jejunum: effects of fasting and of diabetes. J Physiol 1978;278:55–67.
22. Lamers J, Hulsmann W. The effects of fatty acids on oxidation decarboxylation of pyruvate in rat small intestine. Biochem Biophys Acta 1974;343:215–225.
23. Enser M. Fatty acids and intestinal metabolism. Biochem J 1964;93:290–297.
24. Palkovic M, Skottova N, Hostacka A. Blood lipids during normal and early weaning in rats. Biol Neonate 1976;29:274–280.
25. Gangl A, Ockner R, Intestinal metabolism of plasma free fatty acids. Intracellular compartmentation and mechanisms of control. J Clin Invest 1975;55:803–813.
26. Pande S. On rate-controlling factors on long chain fatty acid oxidation. J Biol Chem 1971;246:5384–5390.
27. Bremer J, Wojtczak A. Factors controlling the rate of fatty acid oxidation in rat liver mitochondria. Biochim Biophys Acta 1971;280:515–530.
28. Hansford R. Studies on the effects of coenzyme A-SH: acetyl coenzyme A, nicotinamide adenine dinucleotide: reduced nicotinamide adenine dinucleotide and adenosine diphosphate: adenosine triphosphate ratios on the interconversion of active and inactive pyruvate dehydrogenase in isolated rat heart mitochondria. J Biol Chem 1976;251:5483–5489.
29. Augenfeld J, Fritz I. Carnitine palmitoyltransferase activity and fatty acid oxidation by livers from fetal and neonatal rats. Can J Biochem 1970;48:288–294.
30. Aas M, Daae L. Fatty acid activation and AGYL transfer in organs from rats in different nutritional states. Biochim Biophys Acta 1971;239:208–216.
31. Hanson P, Parsons D. Metabolism and transport of glutamine and glucose in vascularly perfused small intestine of rat. Biochem J 1977;166:509–519.
32. Windmueller H, Spaeth A. Uptake and metabolism of plasma glutamine by the small intestine. J Biol Chem 1974;249:5070–5079.
33. Windmueller H, Spaeth A. Respiratory fuels and nitrogen metabolism in vivo in small intestine of fed rats. Quantitative importance of glutamine, glutamate and aspartate. J Biol Chem 1980;255:107–112.
34. Younosza M, Smith C, Finch M. Comparison in vitro jejunal uptake of L-valine and L-lysine in the rat during maturation. J Pediatr Gastroenterol Nutr 1985;4:992–997.
35. Windmueller H, Spaeth A. Intestinal metabolism of glutamine and glutamate from the lumen as compared to glutamine from blood. Arch Biochem Biophys 1975;171:662–672.
36. Watford M, Lund P, Krebs H. Isolation and metabolic characteristics of rat and chicken enterocytes. Biochem J 1979;178:589–596.
37. Baveral IG, Lund P. A role for bicarbonate in the regulation of mammalian glutamine metabolism. Biochem J 1979;184:599–676.
38. Carrington JM, Hanson PJ. Distribution of activity of 3-oxoacid CoA-transferase and 3-hydroxybutyrate dehydrogenase in the gastrointestinal tract of fed and starved rats. Biochem Soc Trans 1981;9:55.
39. Williamson DH, Bates MW, Page MA, Krebs HA. Activities of enzymes involved in acetoacetate utilization in adult mammalian tissues. Biochem J 1971;121:41–47.
40. Cox WJ, Mueller A. Composition of milk from stock rats and apparatus for milking small laboratory animals. J Nutrition 1987;13:249–262.
41. Henning S, Ballard P, Kretchmer N. A study of the cytoplasmic receptors for glucocorticoids in intestine of pre- and post-weaning rats. J Biol Chem 1975;250:2073–2078.
42. Henning S. Plasma concentration of total and free corticosterone during development in the rat. Am J Physiol 1978;235:E451–E456.
43. Lee P, Lebenthal E. Early weaning and precocious development of small intestine in rats: genetic, dietary or hormonal control. Pediatr Res 1983;17:645–650.
44. Herbst J, Koldovsky O. Cell migration and cortisone induction of sucrase activity in jejunum and ileum. Biochem J 1972;126:471–476.
45. Daniels V, Hardy R, Malinowska K, Nathanielsz P. The influence of exogenous steroids on macromolecular uptake by the small intestine of the newborn rat. J Physiol 1973;299:681–695.
46. Carlile A, Beck F. Maturation of the ileal epithelium in the young rat. J Anat 1983;137:357–369.
47. Dobiasoa M, Hahn P, Koldovsky O. Fatty acid composition in developing rats. Fatty acid composition of triglycerides and phospholipids in some organs of the rat during postnatal development. Biochim Biophys Acta 1964;84:538–549.
48. Viktora J, Fodor J, Grafnetter D, et al. Studies of certain biochemical indices of fat metabolism during the ontogenesis of the rat. Cesk Fysiol 1964;9:63–64.

31
Muscle Metabolism in the Fetus and Neonate

Ulrich A. Walker and Armand F. Miranda

Skeletal muscle is derived from the mesoderm. Myogenesis involves a continuous and dynamic series of biosynthetic and restructuring events that result in the molding of fetal tissue, ultimately leading to adult muscle with its distinct metabolic, structural, and functional properties. During myogenesis many individual enzymes and structural proteins are replaced by other variants (i.e., isoforms), with modulated metabolic capabilities. The myogenic process is highly conserved in evolution. It involves the orderly expression of myogenic regulatory factors that act in concert with nonmyogenic tissue components, including the interaction with a competent nerve supply. The development of muscle is further complicated because it is a very heterogeneous tissue. Additional specific genetically regulated control elements are involved in the production and maintenance of functionally diverse muscle groups. During the past decade a wealth of new information has been gathered at the molecular level that sheds new light on the intricate genetic regulation of muscle cell commitment, development of muscle cell diversity, and muscle maturation. Most noteworthy is the discovery of several muscle regulatory genes, that can switch on the myogenic process in pluripotent cells.

Experimental studies in culture have demonstrated that the forced expression of any of these myogenic determination factors (MDFs) can induce the myogenic phenotype, even in cells that are otherwise destined to proceed into different lineages. Because sequential in vivo studies of human myogenesis are impossible to perform, some information presented in this chapter was derived from in vitro studies and corroborated from data obtained in a variety of other vertebrate systems. This chapter emphasizes those components of human myogenesis that appear to be most relevant to a basic understanding of normal skeletal muscle development and its metabolism. In addition, this information should provide a basis for understanding the etiology and developmental pathobiology of known genetic or acquired human myopathies. Moreover, a basic understanding of the mechanisms associated with muscle regeneration might help evaluate the use of myoblast transfer and gene therapy in genetic diseases of muscle.

The Myogenic Lineage

Skeletal muscle is derived from the embryonic mesodermal layer. Several types of muscle cells can be distinguished: Myogenic precursor cells (MPCs) are mononuclear cells that in their normal embryonic environment will become muscle, yet are not fully committed, because when they are experimentally transplanted to a different embryonic environment, these cells still display broad developmental capacity, behaving similarly to cells normally originating in the grafted environment.[1] Upon commitment the myogenic precursors become myoblasts. These mononuclear cells express at least one of the known myogenic determination factor genes: *MyoD*,[2] *myogenin*,[3] *myf-5*,[4] and *MRF-4*.[5] Following proliferation, myoblasts ultimately exit from the replicating cycle, nuclear DNA synthesis ceases, production of muscle-specific contractile and cytoskeletal proteins is initiated, and fusion to multinucleate syncytia ensues. Multinucleate muscle cells that are not fully differentiated are termed myotubes. It should be emphasized that myoblast fusion is not a prerequisite for differentiation, because in avian models in vivo, as well as in avian and mammalian muscle cultures, differentiated mononuclear cells can be observed.[6] Moreover, when myoblast fusion is experimentally inhibited, in vitro myodifferentiation can still occur.[7] In myotubes, the nuclei are centrally located as in myoblasts and muscle-specific proteins are rapidly synthesized. Myotubes then develop into myofibers, as the myonuclei, initially located centrally, migrate toward the periphery. Myofibrillar elements, such as actins and myosins, become organized and aligned to form well-organized contractile units (i.e., sarcomeres), and a well-developed acellular basal lamina becomes evident. Mitochondria, initially located centrally in the myotube, become wedged in the intermyofibrillar spaces of the developing myofiber and beneath the sarcolemma.[8] Transverse tubules appear.[9]

Myotube formation occurs in two waves, called primary and secondary. When myoblasts of early development birth dates synchronously fuse into myotubes, they give rise to primary myotubes, which form the initial basis for the embryonic muscle.[10] Primary myotube formation occurs synchronously. Initially, the primary myotubes are closely apposed. At later stages they separate and a basal lamina begins to ensheathe them. Secondary myotubes arise from subsequent asynchronous fusion of additional myoblasts emerging at later developmental time points.[10] Secondary myotube formation occurs between and along the scaffold of the primary myotubes.[10] Secondary myoblasts do not seem to fuse with primary myoblasts or myotubes[11] and differ from the latter not only in their temporal appearance, but also in morphology[12] and myosin chain expression.[13] Not all myoblasts fuse to form terminally differentiated muscle fibers. Some become quiescent cells, called satellite cells, that become wedged between the muscle cell surface membrane and the basal lamina of developing primary and secondary myotubes.[14] The satellite cells can be activated to proliferate and fuse during vigorous exercise, or following pathologic or mechanical muscle injury.[15] They can be considered a continuous source of muscle stem cells for muscle regeneration, even in mature muscle.[16] In cultures derived from adult muscle biopsies, satellite cells can proliferate, fuse, and differentiate, similar to myoblasts in vivo, thus representing an important source of muscle for experimental in vitro studies. Monoclonal antibodies that recognize the neural cell adhesion molecule (NCAM; CD56) bind specifically to activated, but not to resting, human satellite cells and can be used to distinguish the two populations.[17]

Satellite cells originate from the same somitically derived myogenic lineage as embryonic muscle cells;[18] however, they lack the pluripotency of the myogenic precursors in being unable to take part in muscle embryogenesis.[19] They are probably not lineal descendants of primary and secondary myoblasts.[20,21] In fact, three different myoblast populations can be distinguished based on their behavior in vitro and on the time when the cultures are started during embryonic development: embryonic, fetal, and adult. Embryonic and fetal myoblasts are cultured from embryonic or fetal muscle tissue, and are distinct from the above-discussed satellite cells (adult myoblasts).[13,20] Embryonic myoblasts are believed to be the in vitro correlate of primary myogenesis, whereas fetal myoblasts may represent the lineage responsible for secondary myotube formation. Support for the difference between adult myoblasts, e.g., mature muscle satellite cells and embryonic/fetal myoblasts come from differences in the expression of MDFs,[21] molecular forms of acetylcholine esterase,[22] myosins,[23,24] enolase,[25,26] desmin,[27] and from their response to growth factors.[28] Many other distinguishing features exist.[29] It is not known exactly at which stage satellite cells become a distinct class of myogenic cells. They seem to appear late during embryogenesis.[30,31] No counterparts of skeletal muscle satellite cells have been identified in cardiac muscle.

Embryonic Origin of Skeletal Muscle

Skeletal muscle can be divided into three classes (i.e., allotypes[32]) with respect to embryonic development, innervation, contractile properties, and involvement in myogenic or neurogenic disease. These allotypes encompass masticatory, extraocular,[33] and limb/trunk/diaphragm muscle. This discussion focuses on the musculature of limb and trunk, since this allotype represents the bulk of skeletal muscle. Contrary to skeletal muscle, heart and smooth muscle are derived from the splanchnic mesoderm. Smooth muscle does not fuse. Cardiac muscle does not have satellite cells and does not express any of the known MDFs characteristic for skeletal muscle differentiation.[34] Cardiomyocytes, although differentiated, are still able to undergo mitosis after partial disassembly of the contractile filaments.[34,35]

The myogenic lineage of limb and trunk muscle is presumed to be embryonically established during or after gastrulation with the formation of the mesoderm.[36] In contrast, striated head musculature and the striated sphincter pupillae arise differently, in that the former originates as a mixture of the four most anterior somites and the visceral arches[37] and the latter evolves from the neuroectoderm.[38] Somites arise from multiple embryonic cells that can be genetically heterogeneous, for example, because of X-chromosome inactivation and do not arise, as clones from a single cell.[39] In human embryos somites formation begins at day 20 in a rostrocaudal direction as mesodermal condensations of epithelial cells on either side of the neural tube (Figure 31.1A). Subsequently, these segmental structures segregate into the more dorsally located dermatomyotome and the more ventrally located sclerotome. During further development, at around the 5th week of gestation (Figure 31.1B), the cells of the sclerotome lose their epithelial morphology, condense around the notochord and the neural tube, and give rise to mesenchymal cells that are precursor cells of the axoskeleton (e.g., vertebrae, intervertebral disks, and ribs). The dermatomyotome diversifies into the dermatome, containing precursor cells for the dermis, and into the myotome. The mediodorsal part of the myotome constitutes postmitotic precursor cells for axial (i.e., back) muscles (i.e., epimere), its lateroventral part gives

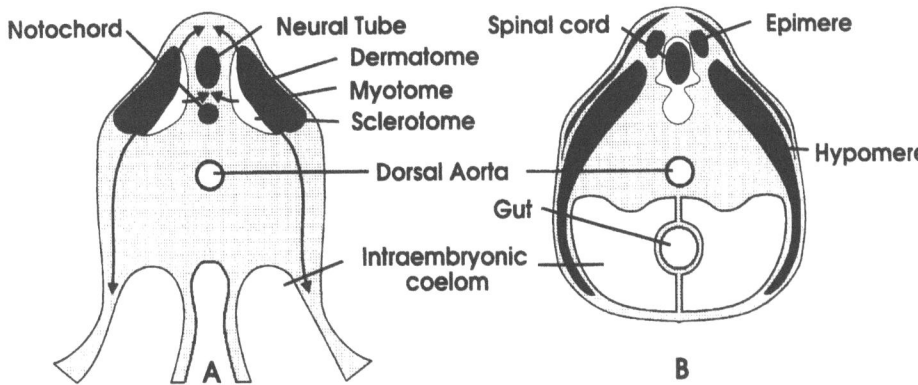

FIGURE 31.1. Transverse sections through the thoracic region of an early 4-week (A) and 5-week (B) human embryo. By the end of the 4th week of gestation, the dermatomes are starting to form the dermis. Myotome cells are migrating ventrolaterally and dorsomedially to form the hypo- and epimeres. Sclerotome cells condense to form the axoskeleton.

rise to muscle progenitors that migrate ventrally and generate intercostal, abdominal, and limb muscles (i.e., hypomere). The myotome compartment appears to be postmitotic, but the migrating cells that exit the myotome seem to become replenished, most likely by rapidly dividing cells from the overlying dermatome.[40]

The human limb buds form around the 28th embryonic day, the upper limb somewhat earlier than the lower one.[41] Furthermore limb muscle development is slightly more advanced proximally than distally. Limb myogenesis is distinctive to the myogenesis of the trunk. Whereas the cellular precursors of axial muscles express MDFs from the onset of myotome formation in the mesodermal somites,[20] limb muscles display a delay of myogenic determination gene expression until the limb muscle masses begin to coalesce (vide infra).[36] Furthermore the development of axial muscles seems to be strongly influenced by neural tube and notochord; in limb muscle differentiation, however, the limb mesoderm is the prime inducer of myogenesis.[42] The musculature of the axoskeleton is populated by myoblasts, migrating into their definitive location, whereas limb musculature is believed to be formed in situ. In day 35 in human embryos, the prospective limb muscle regions are histologically indistinguishable from the surrounding mesenchyme. But soon afterward, the now distinct, but still not compartmentalized, premuscle regions are likely to contain fibroblasts and myoblasts.[41]

The first multinucleated myotubes in limbs have been observed at day 45.[43] By day 50, all bone rudiments have formed and the major anatomical muscles are compartmentalized into their definite anatomical muscles by segregation from two premuscle masses that are located ventrally and dorsally from the prospective bone structures. At 9 to 10 weeks of gestation, primary myotubes have formed and between 13 and 18 weeks, they have become surrounded by secondary myotubes that are forming de novo during new waves of myoblast fusion along the scaffold of the primary myotubes. Elongation of the myotubes must occur very rapidly, because myotubes extend from the proximal to the distal region of the muscle almost immediately after muscle formation,[44] and because the limb grows very rapidly. Lengthening of myofibrils is accomplished by addition of new sarcomeres,[45] usually at the ends of the muscle fibers. By the end of the 3rd month cross-striations, typical for skeletal muscle, appear inside the myotubes. Rapid myoblast proliferation and accompanying fusion into myotubes continues until the 20th fetal week, when primary and secondary myotube formation is completed and only a few myoblasts persist. By then, cross-striated fibers predominate. Embryonic development of the striated extraocular muscles seems to be somewhat more advanced than that of limb muscle.[46]

Postnatally, human striated muscle fibers grow both in number, by addition of new myonuclei originating from the satellite cell compartment (i.e., hyperplasia), and in girth and length (i.e., hypertrophy), probably until at least the 4th postnatal month[47] and possibly into adult life[48] (Table 31.1). From 1 year until 5 years of age, the

TABLE 31.1. Mean muscle fiber diameters (μm) with standard deviations in infancy.

	4-lb Premature	Newborn	3 months	8 months	1 year	2 years
Diaphragm	13.2 (1.7)	11.5 (1.6)	15.2 (3.7)	20.7 (3.5)	18.2 (3.4)	17.9 (3.9)
Deltoid	6.2 (1.3)	6.8 (1.6)	9.8 (3.0)	8.2 (3.0)	10.3 (6.4)	10.3 (6.4)
Biceps	6.1 (1.3)	7.3 (1.9)	8.4 (1.9)	9.5 (2.2)	10.2 (2.9)	13.3 (3.7)
Gastrocnemius	7.1 (2.2)	6.2 (1.9)	9.1 (1.7)	8.0 (1.4)	16.0 (2.8)	18.8 (3.7)
Vastus lateralis	10.2 (1.8)	6.2 (1.9)	10.0 (1.6)	—	11.6 (1.6)	15.0 (4.5)

Modified from Bowden and Groyer,[539] with permission.

fiber diameter measured in paraffin-embedded muscle increases by 2 μm each year and in the subsequent 5 years by 3 μm each year.[49] Unlike in the adult, there are no sex differences in fiber girth.[50] The relative contribution of hyperplasia and hypertrophy to muscle enlargement is dependent on the individual species, as well as on the particular anatomical muscle.[51,52] In adult muscle, exercise generally seems to induce muscular hypertrophy, whereas continuous muscle stretching and overloading causes both hypertrophy and hyperplasia.[53,54] There seems to be a positive correlation between satellite cell population and muscle activity.[55,56]

Development of Fiber Specialization

Individual muscle fibers are not homogeneous within a single muscle; in fact, they are highly specialized in order to provide a wide range of forces, kinetics, and endurance. To accommodate this diversity, they must develop fine-tuned systems of energy delivery, which result in different metabolic profiles. In classic studies, the individual muscle fibers were morphologically divided into slowly contracting "red" fibers, and the faster contracting "white" fibers.[57] Myoglobin content contributes to the macroscopic differences in muscle color, since this oxygen-binding protein is more abundant in "slow" red muscle.[58]

Subsequently, the underlying biochemical features of fiber type specialization became evident, which has led to a more detailed classification of fiber types according to individual metabolic markers, such as their content of glycolytic and respiratory enzymes. Enzyme activity ratios could discriminate between fast- and slow-twitch fiber populations: examples are phosphofructokinase/citrate synthase, lactate dehydrogenase/malate dehydrogenase, glyceraldehydephosphate dehydrogenase/3-hydroxyacyl-CoA dehydrogenase.[58]

Three fiber types can now be demonstrated by histochemistry, using myofibrillar adenosine triphosphatase (ATPase) activity as a marker. This classification is based on the lability of myofibrillar ATPase following preincubation in either acidic, or alkaline buffers[59,60] (Table 31.2). Myofibrillar ATPase of type I (i.e., slow contracting) fibers is resistant to pH 4.3, but can be inhibited by incubation at pH 10.4. Type II (i.e., fast contracting) fibers have just the reverse properties. Type II fibers can be further subdivided according to their behavior at pH 4.6: whereas type IIA fibers show no ATPase activity, type IIB fibers do. In developing or regenerating fibers and under some circumstances in adult muscle, a continuum of staining patterns can be observed. Fibers that in addition to their stability at acidic pH are moderately stable at alkaline pH have been termed IC fibers, whereas alkaline stable fibers with moderate stability at acid pH have been termed IIC fibers. Although there is pronounced heterogeneity in enzyme ratios among the myosin-typed fibers, metabolic profiles are generally unable to reliably discriminate fibers beyond the major groups of fast- and slow-twitch fibers.[58]

With the discovery of individual isoforms of the myosin ATPase, distinguishable immunologically and the characterization of the contractile proteins at the gene level, understanding of fiber type specialization has entered a

TABLE 31.2. Myosin isoform profiles and histochemical fiber diversification in mammalian muscle.

		Fetus		Adult		
		Onset of fiber specialization	Activity compared to adult	Type I	Type IIA	Type IIB
Myosin ATPase	MHC	See Table 31.3		MHC_s	MHC_{fA}	MHC_{fB}
	MLC	See Table 31.3		$MLC1_s$, $MLC2_s$	$MLC1_f$, $MLC2_f$	$MLC1_f$, $MLC2_f$, $MLC3_f$
	ATPase pH 4.3	20 weeks		+++	+	+
	ATPase pH 4.6	20 weeks		+++	+	++
	ATPase pH 9.4	20 weeks		+	+++	+++
Oxidative phosphorylation	Mitochondria		↓	+++	++	+
	NADH dehydrogenase	20 weeks	↓	+++	++	+
	Succinate dehydrogenase		40% at birth	+++	++	+
	Cytochrome oxidase		↓	+++	++	+
	Myoglobin		↓	+++	++	+
Carbohydrate metabolism	Glycogen content	After birth	< 25 weeks:↓; afterward↔	+	+++	+++
	Phosphorylase		↓	+	++	+++
	Lactate dehydrogenase			+	++	+++
	Phosphofructokinase		50% at birth	++	+	+
Other	Myoadenylate deaminase		None	++	++	++

+/++/+++, low/intermediate/high enzymatic activity, respectively; MHC, myosin heavy chain; MLC, myosin light chain.

new era.[61,62] It became evident that fiber type diversity on the molecular level is actually much greater than can be observed biochemically or histochemically. Fiber type diversity is now linked to different molecular isoforms of the contractile protein components and their ratios in an individual fiber (vide infra). Indeed, fiber types are now often defined by the myosin heavy chain (MHC) isoform that they predominantly express. However, histochemical fiber type classification remains an important tool for the muscle pathologist and helps in understanding the metabolic adaptations accompanying diversification.

Histochemical differentiation of muscle fibers into the two main types becomes evident during the 5th gestational week (Table 31.2), at a time when a mature pattern of neuronal innervation has been established and is well established by the 26th week.[63–65] Type II fiber subtypes (type IIA and type IIB fibers) can be distinguished in the final 3 months of gestation, although even at term, some 15% to 20% remain undifferentiated (i.e., type IIC fibers).[63,66] Further fiber type differentiation continues throughout the first year of life and even throughout early childhood, although by 1 year of age the percentage of fiber types differs very little from the adult. As the demands on posture and weight bearing increase in the period between birth and 1 year of age, the total number of type I fibers increases, whereas the total number of type II fibers remains constant. However, the type II fiber subtype proportion changes, in that type IIB fibers increase and type IIA fibers decrease.[63] About 1% of undifferentiated fibers remain in the adult.[63]

The dichotomy of muscle fibers into slow- and fast-contracting elements is closely associated with qualitative differences of their contractile proteins. Virtually every contractile protein of muscle fibers exists in isoforms that occur in developmental succession and are distinct for fast- versus slow-twitch fibers. For some contractile proteins, isoforms arise by alternative splicing of a single gene, while in others they arise via differential expression of multigene families.[67,68] Species differences also exist. Commitment toward distinct expression of individual contractile protein isoforms can already be demonstrated in the early somites and during limb and trunk development.[20] The embryonic, fetal, and adult myoblasts are different committed cell populations that occur in sequential developmental succession. They are believed to participate primarily in the formation of primary myotubes, secondary myotubes, and satellite cells, respectively.[20] The term adult myoblasts is a misnomer, because muscle satellite cells are already present before birth. Whereas primary myotubes express fast, slow, or mixed fast/slow myosins, secondary myotubes express primarily fast myosins.[20]

The contractile proteins can be divided into thick and thin filaments (Figure 31.2). The thick filament of the sarcomere is composed primarily of myosin and small amounts (i.e., up to 15%) of additional proteins, such as the C protein, of largely unknown function.[69] The myosin molecule itself is a hexamer, consisting of two heavy chains (MHC), two alkali-dissociated, and two regulatory myosin light chains (MLC).[69,70] The myosin light chains

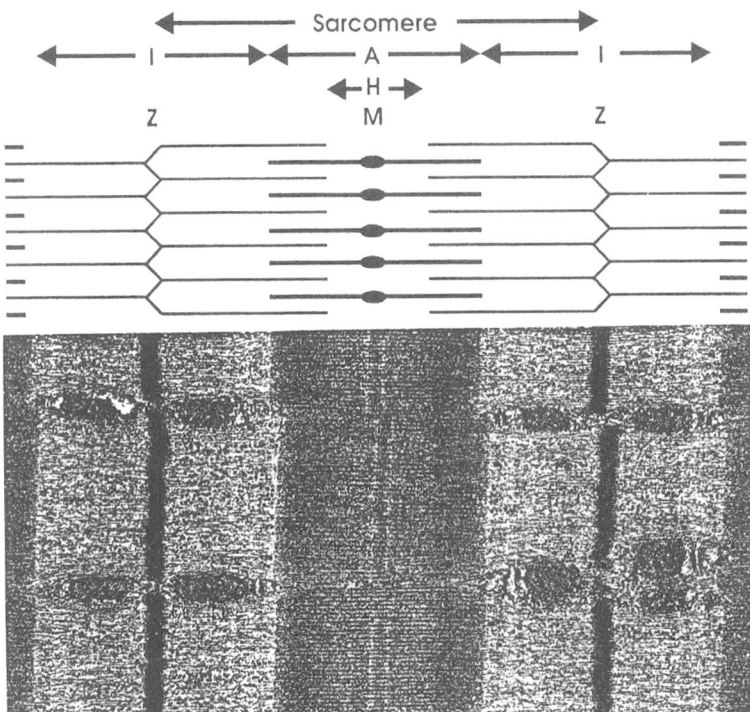

FIGURE 31.2. Electron micrograph of human striated skeletal muscle. The scheme shows the arrangement of the contractile myofibrillar lattice within the sarcomere. Thick myosin filaments (—●—) are bridged at the M line and interdigitate with thin actin filaments (——), attached to the Z line. I, I band (isotropic in polarized light); A, A band (anisotropic in polarized light); H, H zone. Note the intermyofibrillar mitochondria, located in the I band regions. (Photograph courtesy of Dr. Eduardo Bonilla.)

are associated with the globular head domains of the MHC molecule. The thin filament is composed of polymerized actin, associated with tropomyosin and the heterotrimer troponin.[71]

Until the final adult composition is reached, both MHC and MLC molecules undergo a series of isoform transitions that encompass a switch from embryonic via neonatal to adult isomyosins[20,58,67,70,72-76] (Table 31.3). Dividing myoblasts are believed to express little or no MHC.[77] Primary myotubes predominantly express embryonic (MHC_{emb}) and the slow myosin heavy chain (MHC_s). As primary myotubes mature, they discontinue the expression of MHC_{emb} and differentiate into slow fibers. Secondary myotubes express MHC_{emb} and neonatal MHC (MHC_{neo}), but no MHC_s and differentiate into adult fast (type IIA or IIB) fibers, each containing a different fast myosin isozyme (MHC_{fA} and MHC_{fB}, respectively).[58,67,76,78,79] Whereas adult slow muscle myosin contains two different slow MLC subunits ($MLC1_s$ and $MLC2_s$), three distinct light chains occur in mature fast muscle ($MLC1_f$, $MLC2_f$ and $MLC3_f$)[58,70] and a distinct embryonic light chain (MLC_{emb}) in developing fast fibers.[80] The light chains in the two adult fast-twitch subgroups are identical.[70]

Three actin isoforms have been identified. While α-actin is specific for mature muscle, the other isoforms (β- and γ- actin) are found in nonmuscle cells and in dividing myoblasts.[81,82] The tropomyosins, a family of actin binding proteins, have been extensively reviewed.[83,84] Four different genes have been identified in mammals and many more isoforms arise from alternative splicing and are expressed not only in muscle but also in nonmuscle cells. While the function of the different tropomyosin isoforms is still only poorly understood, it appears that mammalian type II muscle fibers express predominantly α and β forms, whereas type I fibers are characterized by β, γ and δ forms.[85] Other examples of isoforms in striated muscle are the C proteins, and the troponins T, I, and C.[58,67,68,86-88]

Fiber type differentiation is not irreversibly unidirectional. For example, in malignant transformation, such as in rhabdomyosarcoma, muscle tissue can lose its adult differentiation and fetal isoforms can reappear.[89]

Innervation

The fiber types are intermingled in a mosaic pattern in most muscle. Histochemical analysis on cross sections of muscle reveals a checkerboard pattern. The proportions of different fiber types vary in different muscles, depending on their functional requirements. Innervation follows the pattern of fiber type specialization in that each neuron innervates only fibers of a single fiber type (i.e., motor unit).[90,91]

The spinal motoneurons arise segmentally in the neural tube. They are among the first neurons that are formed.[92] Prospective motoneurons migrate to the ventral horn, axial motoneurons more medially, and limb motoneurons more laterally.[92] Motor innervation of embryonal limbs starts with pioneering nerve fibers between the 8th and the 10th week of gestation. Cholinergic axons, still unmyelinated but partly covered by Schwann cells derived from the neural crest, are guided by largely unknown mechanisms from the ventral horn through the plexus to the limb. They ultimately form knob-like structures with the central region of primary myotubes.[93]

The recognition process of the nerve terminal by the muscle fiber involves muscle activity[92] and several molecules synthesized by muscle and/or nerve, such as agrin[94] and NCAM. NCAM, a cell-cell adhesion molecule (vide infra), is initially present diffusely on the surface of both motoneurons and early myotubes, but becomes restricted to the neuromuscular junction after innervation has been established.[92,95] As the neuromuscular junction matures, synaptic vesicles begin to accumulate, the synaptic cleft widens, the postsynaptic membrane thickens, and there are alterations in the spatial and temporal behavior of acetylcholinesterase (AChE) and acetylcholine (ACh) expression.[93] AChE activity and ACh receptors (AChRs) are already detectable in myoblasts,[96-98] but it is only following myoblast fusion that they are increasingly expressed, although in a still spatially diffuse fashion rather than clearly membrane-bound.[99] With subsequent maturation, AChE activity and AChRs become segmentally confined to the junctional region and there is a switch in the use of the some 15 AChR genes.[99,100]

TABLE 31.3. Predominant myosin species in developing mammalian muscle fibers.

	Primary myogenesis (slow)	Secondary myogenesis (fast)
Embryonal period		
MHC	MHC_{emb}	MHC_{emb}
MLC (alkali)	$MLC\ 1_s$	$MLC\ 1_f$, $MLC\ 1_{emb}$
MLC (regulatory)	$MLC\ 2_s$	$MLC\ 2_f$
Fetal period		
MHC	$MHC_{emb} + MHC_s$	MHC_{neo}
MLC (alkali)	$MLC\ 1_s$	$MLC\ 1_f$, $MLC\ 3_f$, $MLC\ 1_{emb}$
MLC (regulatory)	$MLC\ 2_s$	$MLC\ 2_f$
Adult period		
MHC	MHC_s	MHC_{fA}, or MHC_{fB}
MLC (alkali)	$MLC\ 1_s$	$MLC\ 1_f$, $MLC\ 3_f$
MLC (regulatory)	$MLC\ 2_s$	$MLC\ 2_f$

Based on data from refs. 20 and 58. The scheme is an oversimplification, as, for example, developing primary and secondary fibers can synthesize both fast and slow MHCs.[20,132,540]

After the formation of the first synaptic contact of an individual muscle fiber, later arriving axons are restricted to making their contact at the site of the first-formed junction.[92] Initially, many different motoneurons might innervate the same muscle fiber at the same synaptic terminal (i.e., polyneuronal innervation), and an individual motoneuron might actually innervate most of the fibers of a muscle. As peripheral synapse formation continues, a large fraction of the motoneurons succumb to apoptotic cell death. The reason why this occurs and the mechanisms involved are not well understood.[101,102] After the period of motoneuron death, at around birth in mammals, there is a period where supernumerary synapses become eliminated, so that each synapse loses all but one of its innervating axons.[103,104] The eliminated terminals simply retract, but do not degenerate.[105] In that way, each motoneuron and each muscle fiber loses a large proportion of connections.[92] Consequently, motor units become more uniform in fiber type composition during the postnatal period.[106] The loss of polyneuronal innervation leads to a substantial decrease in the mean size of motor units, since the number of motor units per muscle does not decrease.[92,107] The maturation of the motor end plate requires several weeks and is completed within a few months of birth,[92] concomitant with the development of more pronounced metabolic differences between fast and slow muscle.[58]

Innervated primary myotubes are initially electrically connected by gap junctions.[108] However, as the primary myotubes move apart, they break down the gap junctions between them, but remain in contact with their original axons. The primary myotubes differentiate into slow motor units. Secondary myotubes, derived from lineally distinct secondary myoblasts and developing along the scaffold of the primary myotubes, also form an electrical syncytium by gap junctions, but there are no junctions between primary and secondary myotubes. Secondary myotubes are believed to become innervated in a second wave by trailing axons and develop mostly into larger and faster fibers that will make up the majority of adult muscle fibers. With secondary myogenesis, the primary myotubes are separated by the newly formed myogenic elements, their gap junctions are broken, and the different motor units become intermingled in the checkerboard pattern typical for most muscles. Although in the stage of polyneuronal innervation some motoneurons may rarely terminate on an inappropriate fiber,[92] the selectivity of early innervation of motoneurons with fast or slow characteristics to fast or slow fibers is the major factor in the generation of homogeneous motor units. However, exchange of wrongly connected fibers and selective elimination of supernumerary synapses may contribute to a lesser extent to the formation of a homogeneous motor unit in some muscles.[92] After the postnatal period, there appears to be very little metabolic variation between muscle fibers within a given motor unit.[58]

Initial studies on the influence of innervation on fiber type diversity supported the hypothesis that fast and slow motoneurons impose their own characteristics on developing muscle; cross-innervation experiments, inserting a fast nerve into a slow muscle or vice versa, showed that muscle fibers can change—at least to some extent—their properties upon foreign innervation.[80,109] Also muscle phenotypes can be altered by stimulating the nerve with the electrical pattern characteristic for a different fiber type.[70] However, commitment and heterogeneity toward the expression of specific MHC isoforms[20,110–112] has been observed in avian and mammalian myoblasts. It appears that genetic diversity of myoblasts specifies the diversity of fiber type in vertebrate muscles and that motoneurons might simply assist in muscle adaptation and maturation, rather than determining qualitative differences between fast and slow fibers. Whether this is also true for the human remains to be determined.[113] According to the current model, initial fiber type specialization results from the temporal, biphasic pattern of primary and secondary histogenesis that generates heterogeneous myoblast populations.[20,29,110,112,114] Subsequently, neural activity and other environmental stimuli can still modify fiber type properties, but only within certain limits.[80] Innervation also does not control muscle compartmentalization, since normal muscle pattern formation was observed in the absence of any innervation, as well as under the influence of the nervous system from another species and/or another segmental level.[115–118]

Afferent innervation of muscle can be observed after formation of primary myotubes. Sensory terminals form with a few primary myotubes and induce the formation of intrafusal fibers (i.e., muscle spindles).[119]

The Role of the Connective Tissue

Muscle is surrounded by three connective tissue layers derived from nonsomitic mesoderm: endomysium, surrounding individual muscle fibers; perimysium, surrounding groups of muscle fibers; and epimysium layers, surrounding the whole muscle. The connective tissue is composed of acellular (extracellular matrix; ECM[120]) and cellular elements. Cellular structures include fibroblasts, capillary endothelial cells, and fine motor and sympathetic nerve branches.

The endomysial ECM consists of a basal lamina (BL)[120,121] immediately adjacent to the muscle fiber plasma membrane (i.e., sarcolemma) and surrounding interstitial connective tissue. During the early stages of myotube formation, some primary and associated secondary muscle fibers can be seen to be surrounded by a single BL, but eventually each myotube acquires its own BL sheath.[120] Both, the cellular and acellular components of connective tissue as well as adhesion molecules on muscle cell membranes are important for myogenesis and the physical integration of muscle cells in their microenvironment and for muscle development.[121]

Cellular Components

As indicated above, muscle compartmentalization occurs during a very short time frame in limb embryogenesis. Homogeneous premuscle regions localized in posterior and anterior regions of the limb bud rapidly compartmentalize from proximal to distal into distinct longitudinal muscle bands and give rise to the individual extensor and flexor muscles. The exact mechanisms governing this muscle splitting are not known, but current evidence seems to point toward an important role for connective tissue.

The myogenic precursor itself does not possess intrinsic information guiding morphogenesis of anatomically correct muscles, since muscle compartmentalization is typically normal, even when the muscle progenitors are derived from other sources. This information is derived from reciprocal grafting experiments of embryonic tissues from quail to chick and vice versa.[122] Also, when myogenic cells are experimentally eliminated, morphologically appropriate tendons still form, even though they are not attached to true muscles.[123] Instead, fibroblasts become arranged to form a model of the muscle.[123] A major contribution of innervation in muscle compartmentalization is unlikely, since anatomically correct muscle formation occurs in denervated limb buds of the chick.[115] Other hypotheses, suggesting mechanical effects due to tendon and limb growth, are unlikely because normal muscle development occurs in the proximal limb after removal of the distal portion.[124]

The intermuscular cleavage zone was analyzed in the separation of limb muscles in the avian embryo.[125,126] The first indication of separation is an increase of the extracellular space between neighboring mesenchymal cells in the cleavage zone. The intermuscular cells subsequently acquire a more stellate morphology, characteristic of loose connective tissue cells. There is no indication of invasion of mesenchymal cells from outside the cleavage zone.

In summary, the differentiation of muscle cells and the morphogenesis (i.e., compartmentalization) of muscle, seem to be highly independent processes. Whereas myogenic cells, derived from somitic structures are necessary for the formation of skeletal muscle, they do not appear to contain information regulating muscle compartmentalization. Instead, pattern formation is controlled by interaction with the mesenchyme, into which the somitic cells migrate.

Acellular Components

Adhesion of the muscle cell to the extracellular matrix (ECM) is essential for the formation of skeletal muscle. ECM is not a homogeneous mesh of different structural proteins, because there are unique quantitative and qualitative differences in the distribution of the ECM materials between the three connective tissue layers surrounding muscle (e.g., epimysium, perimysium, and endomysium). Additionally, temporal changes in the ECM composition during limb development can be delineated.[127] ECM components are synthesized by both myogenic and connective tissue cells.[128,129]

The composition of ECM materials has important regulatory and structural consequences. Exactly which components of the ECM are important for myogenesis in vitro is still under investigation, but a variety of in vivo experiments have shown an important role of BL composition in the differentiation of myogenic precursors (MPCs). Many cellular adhesion molecules anchor on ECM components, and their distribution at the muscle surface might also be regulated by the ECM composition.[130,131] The most abundant glycoprotein of basement membranes is laminin.[132] It provides an anchor for muscle adhesion molecules of the integrin superfamily.[133,134] Muscle culture experiments have demonstrated that laminin can stimulate muscle proliferation and mediate morphologic alterations, such as elongation and motility.[135,136] Other muscle culture experiments have shown that basal membrane collagen (collagen type IV) can, unlike gelatin (collagen type I), enhance attachment and proliferation of chick embryonic MPCs whereas muscle differentiation and fusion is inhibited.[137] Other ECM components such as fibronectin[138] and hyaluronic acid[139] have similar effects.

Cell Adhesion Molecules

Cell adhesion molecules (Table 31.4) are anchor molecules located on the cell membrane. They mediate cell-cell or cell-matrix adhesion and are involved in transmembrane signaling. Adhesion molecules are essential for normal myogenesis.[140-142] Some of the best studied are the cell-cell adhesion molecules NCAM and N-cadherin. Both molecules are already expressed in somites.[143] NCAM, a member of the immunoglobulin superfamily, seems to promote myoblast fusion via Ca^{2+}-independent homophilic interaction. Its inhibition perturbs myotube formation[140] and its overexpression enhances myogenesis.[142] During myogenesis in vitro and in vivo, expression of NCAM undergoes isoform transition, mediated by differential RNA splicing of a single gene and various posttranslational modifications.[144-146] The isoform transition, encompassing the switch from a transmembrane to a membrane lipid anchored NCAM

TABLE 31.4. Developmental presence of selected adhesion molecules and of human histocompatibility antigens (HLAs) on muscle cells during myogenesis.

Surface antigen	Myoblast	Myotube	Satellite cell	Adult muscle fiber
HLA class I[167,541]	(+)	(+)		−
HLA class II[167,541]	−	−		
NCAM (CD56)[140,147,148]	+ Transmembrane isoform	+ Lipid anchored isoform	Activated + Dormant − Same as NCAM	Restricted to neuromuscular Junction/lower than perinatally Same as NCAM
N-cadherin[140,147,148]	+	(+)		
VLA-4[157]	+	+	−	−
VCAM-1[157]	+	+	(+)	−

VLA-4: very late activation antigen-4.
VCAM-1: vascular cell adhesion molecule-1.

isoform, precisely correlates with terminal myoblast differentiation and myotube formation, and is regulated by contractile activity.[146,147] In contrast to N-cadherin, myotubes continue to express NCAM at a high concentration until very late in development.[147] In embryonic myotubes and in myotubes derived from satellite cells that arise postnatally during muscle regeneration, NCAM is distributed along the entire muscle cell surface, but downregulated during subsequent maturation. In fully mature muscle it is restricted to the neuromuscular junction.[95,140] Down-regulation of NCAM was shown to be reversed following denervation and during aging.[148] NCAM was shown to promote neurite outgrowth,[149] probably by mediating muscle-nerve adhesion.[150]

Cadherins are a family of cell surface transmembrane glycoproteins that mediate Ca^{2+}-dependent cell-cell adhesion by interacting with identical cadherins on neighboring cells (i.e., homophilic adhesion). Their transmembrane domain interacts with the actin cytoskeleton inside the cell.[151] One member, N- (nerve-) cadherin, although neither tissue nor cell-type specific,[152] is expressed in the muscle cell throughout myogenesis both in vitro and in vivo. The receptor seems to be more abundant during primary than during secondary myogenesis.[140,141,147] N-cadherin expression is maximal in myoblasts just prior to fusion, high in young myotubes, and decreases as the myotubes mature.[147] Immunoinhibition of N-cadherin decreases the rate of myoblast fusion.[141] Like NCAM, N-cadherin is a marker for activated, but not dormant, satellite cells and expressed at a low concentration in mature muscle in vivo.[140] The molecule promotes neurite outgrowth, and is upregulated with denervation and downregulated with reinnervation.[153]

The integrins represent a third family of cell surface receptors and are composed of noncovalently associated α and β subunits that interact with ECM components, such as fibronectin and laminin,[154] thereby promoting mainly cell-matrix adhesion. Interaction with other receptors on adjacent cells can mediate cell-cell adhesion. On the internal cell surface the integrin molecule has a binding domain that interacts with microfilament components of the cytoskeleton, providing a link between the ECM and the muscle cytoskeleton.[155] The appearance of integrins on the cell surface is spatially and temporally regulated.[134] For example, expression of $\alpha_1\beta_1$-integrin, a laminin-collagen receptor, can be observed on the cell surface of somitic MPCs, on myoblasts migrating out of the somites, as well as on early myotubes, but it disappears as the differentiated myofibers begin to contract.[134] Another integrin, $\alpha_4\beta_1$ integrin or VLA-4, seems to be involved in cell-matrix interactions with fibronectin,[156] as well as in cell-cell interactions with its counterreceptor VCAM-1, a member of the immunoglobulin superfamily.[157] In myogenesis, the VLA-4/VCAM-1 interaction might contribute to the formation of secondary myotubes.[157] This set of adhesion molecules may play a role in the embryonic development of a variety of tissues other than muscle (Figure 31.3).[157-159] Disruption of β_1-integrin function can interfere with cell migration and reversibly block myotube formation by preventing myoblasts to withdraw from the cell cycle, potentially interfering with signal transduction,[133] thereby causing muscle abnormalities.[160]

Other cell surface molecules, which have important functions in the immune system, may have additional functions in developing muscle by promoting myoblast fusion.[161,162] For instance, histocompatibility leukocyte antigen (HLA) class I is constitutively expressed in aneurally cultured human myoblasts and myotubes.[163-165] The data are conflicting for HLA class II antigen expression in that it was found to be constitutively expressed on cultured human myoblasts and myotubes by some investigators,[163,166] whereas others failed to detect this surface marker.[164,165] HLA class II expression (HLA-DR) on both myoblasts and myotubes can be upregulated by interferon-γ (IFN-γ), but not by tumor necrosis factor-α (TNF-α).[164,165] Class II expression may enable the myoblast to act as antigen-presenting cell.[165] In normal muscle tissue in vivo, both HLA class I and class II are absent,[167] or limited,[168] but class II was found at the surface of satellite cells.[166] In inflammatory muscle disease, such as in polymyositis, dermatomyositis, and inclusion body myositis, upregulation of class II antigens (HLA-DR) in contrast to class I has not been detected.[167]

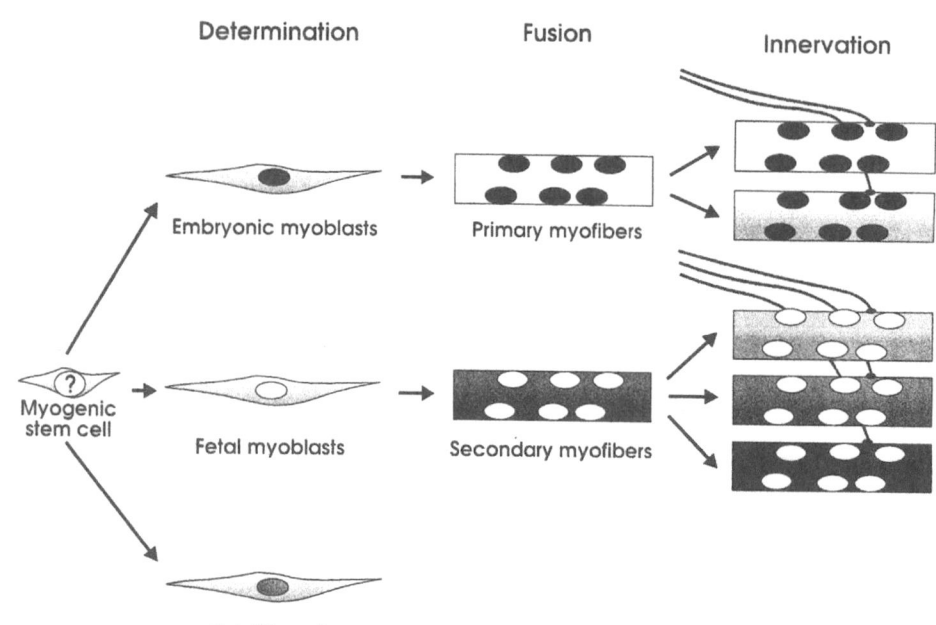

FIGURE 31.3. Hypothetical scheme of myogenesis and the origin of fiber diversity. The myogenic stem cell is not clearly defined. The color of the nucleus delineates commitment to a myoblast lineage. The sarcoplasmic shadings of the myofibers represent synthesis of particular myosin isoforms.

Qualitative Metabolic Markers of Muscle Differentiation: Isozymes

Most muscle-specific proteins appear as mononucleated myoblasts fuse to form multinucleated myotubes. Accompanying fusion, many muscle enzymes undergo not only quantitative changes but also qualitative alterations in the form of isoform switching. Isozyme transitions occur during ontogeny, regeneration, and in cultures derived from embryonic, neonatal, or adult muscle.[81,169-173] In many aspects, in vitro myogenesis can therefore provide an excellent model for in vivo myogenesis. However, although aneural muscle cultures fuse and differentiate remarkably well, they may not reach sufficient maturity to achieve full expression of the adult enzymatic phenotype.[174-176] Such advanced muscle maturation requires innervation, which in human cultures has been achieved by cocultivation with fetal rodent spinal cord complex.[177-179] In these nerve-muscle cultures functional innervation has been demonstrated electrophysiologically, ultrastructurally, and biochemically.[177] Tissue culture systems can be advantageous in the study of myogenesis, in that they facilitate the study of the appearance of muscle-specific isozymes sequentially during muscle development and maturation.[180] However, it should be emphasized that in vitro studies may not truly reflect the in vivo situation, because complex regulatory interactions imposed by other tissues in the intact organism may modulate the expression of muscle-specific enzymes quantitatively and qualitatively. In spite of this limitation, however, much useful information has been obtained from in vitro systems, data that are often difficult to derive from in vivo analysis. This section discusses some of the important enzymes of energy metabolism in muscle. Our selection includes those developmentally regulated enzymes that have been shown to cause human disease when deficient; hence, they have been studied genetically in more detail in human muscle in recent years.

Several of the enzymes discussed here occur in two or more tissue-specific isoforms that are developmentally regulated and are encoded by different genes. Other enzymes, that do not display muscle-specific isozymes and are expressed at all stages of development can be dysfunctional with severe pathologic consequences in brain, as well as other tissues. These enzymes include the lysosomal enzyme acid maltase,[181] the glycogen debrancher enzyme,[182] and phosphoglycerate kinase.[183,184] Since they are present in many tissues and at all stages of muscle development, the genetic defects of these proteins can often be diagnosed antenatally by performing biochemical assays in amniocytes or chorionic villus cells (Table 31.5). They can also be displayed in cultured muscle at the myoblast stage.[185,186] The glycogen brancher enzyme,[187] catalyzes the final step in glycogen synthesis and is somewhat exceptional, in that the human gene, located on chromosome 3,[188] has not yet been fully characterized. However, the existence of a developmentally regulated isozyme system has been suggested, based on a muscle-restricted expression and late onset of its defect.[189] The α subunit of another enzyme, phosphorylase b kinase, which is involved in the regulation of glycogen synthesis (glycogen synthase) and degradation (phosphorylase), occurs in at least two different isozymes, but the pathologic significance is still unclear.[190] The reader is referred to excellent reviews of the muscle enzymes that are involved in glycogen and glucose metabolism and their pathology.[191,192]

TABLE 31.5. Overview of enzymes in glycogen and glucose metabolism.

Enzyme	Isozymes	Disease	Onset of muscle symptoms	Prenatal diagnosis
1 Acid maltase	No	Glycogenosis II (Pompe)[181]	Infancy (childhood) adulthood	g, e[181,185]
2 Myophosphorylase	Yes	Glycogenosis V (McArdle)[542]	(Infancy) childhood (adulthood)	g
3 Debrancher	No	Glycogenosis III (Cori, Forbes)[182]	(Infancy, childhood) adulthood	g, e[185,543]
4 Phosphorylase b kinase	Yes	Glycogenosis VIII[190]	Infancy, childhood, adulthood	
5 Brancher	Likely	Glycogenosis IV (Andersen)[187]	Infancy	e[185]
6 Glucose-6-P dehydrogenase (G6PD)	No	Myoglobinuria (very rarely)[544]	Childhood, adulthood	
7 Phosphofructokinase (PFK)	Yes	Glycogenosis VII (Tarui)[221]	Infancy, childhood	g
8 Aldolase	Yes	Myoglobinuria[240]	Childhood (one case)	g
9 Phosphoglycerate kinase (PGK)	No	Glycogenosis IX[183,184]	Infancy, childhood, adulthood	g, e
10 Phosphoglycerate mutase (PGAM)	Yes	Glycogenosis X[247,250]	Childhood, adulthood	g
11 Enolase	Yes	Not described[25,259]		
12 Lactate dehydrogenase (LDH)	Yes	Glycogenosis XI[267]	Adolescence	g

There have been no reports on enolase deficiency.
Prenatal diagnosis: g, genetic (feasible if the mutation is known from an affected sibling); e, enzymatic.

It is not evident whether tissue-specific isoforms exist for the pyruvate dehydrogenase (PDH), a ubiquitous enzyme complex that catalyzes the decarboxylation of pyruvate to acetyl–coenzyme A (CoA) in a physiologically irreversible multistep reaction, connecting glycolysis with the Krebs cycle. Since the original description of PDH deficiency by Blass et al.,[193] more than 100 children have been identified, mostly with genetic defects in the subunit $E1_a$, encoded on the X chromosome. Although most cases appear to have a generalized defect with reduced enzymatic activity in brain, liver, kidney, muscle, heart, and circulating lymphocytes, as well as in cultured fibroblasts, one case was described in which the defect was restricted to the brain.[194] In others the defect was absent in cultured fibroblasts.[195–197] Furthermore, the extent of residual enzymatic activity may vary extensively between tissues from the same individual. These observations could on one hand be explained by tissue-specific isoforms of PDH subunits;[198] on the other hand, X-chromosome inactivation may result in mosaicism of various tissues and account for the observed pattern.[199] All affected PDH $E1_a$-deficient females analyzed so far have one normal and one mutant gene.[199] Therefore, X-chromosome inactivation prevents accurate prenatal prediction of the clinical phenotype of affected females.

Carbohydrate Metabolism—Glycolysis, Glycogen

Myophosphorylase

Glycogen phosphorylase (EC 2.4.1.1.) catalyzes the phosphorylytical cleavage of glucose-1-phosphate from 1-4-glycosyl residues at the outer branches of glycogen.[200] Three isozymes—M (muscle), L (liver) and B (brain)—have been identified and are dimers of identical subunits. The genes have been cloned and assigned to three different chromosomes.[201–203] The isozymes can be distinguished electrophoretically, by isoelectric focusing, or immunologically.[204–206] The human muscle isozyme gene is located on chromosome 11.

Glycogen phosphorylase activity is below the level of biochemical detection in human preimplantation embryos up to the blastocyst stage and is only about one fifth in fetal, as compared to adult, human muscle,[207] indicating that glycogen may not be an important substrate for muscle energy production during fetal life.[208] During development and differentiation of human skeletal muscle, the brain isozyme appears. The brain isozyme is the predominant isozyme of all fetal tissue. In normal mature human muscle, the brain dimer is subsequently almost completely replaced by the muscle isozyme[205,206] and in liver by the liver isozyme; however, the fetal brain isozyme prevails in adult brain and heart.[209,210]

Mutations in the gene encoding the muscle isozyme can lead to McArdle's disease (glycogenosis type V[199]). The condition is genetically heterogeneous, in that several point mutations, two deletions, and one insertion have been charted.[189,191] Whereas muscle glycogen phosphorylase deficiency is typically a disease of the young adult presenting with exercise-induced myalgia, cramps, and myoglobinuria, a few cases with onset during infancy have been described.[211,212]

Phosphorylase activity can be detected biochemically in aneural muscle cultures from McArdle's disease patients in contrast to muscle biopsy section.[205,213] This apparent paradox is explained by the reappearance of the fetal brain isozyme in muscle of these patients.[205,206] Whereas in aneural cultures the brain isozyme predominates and the muscle isozyme is only weakly expressed, a shift in the isozyme ratio toward the adult muscle pattern can be achieved in innervated cultures, along with an increase in total phosphorylase activity.[176,179,214,215]

Phosphofructokinase

Phosphofructokinase (PFK) (EC 2.7.1.11) catalyzes the physiologically irreversible phosphorylation of fructose-6-phosphate to fructose-1,6-diphosphate, a rate-limiting, highly regulated step in glycolysis (Figure 31.4). Human PFK was shown to be controlled by three different structural gene loci, located on chromosomes 1, 10, and 21, coding for the muscle (M), platelet (P), and liver (L) subunits, respectively.[216–219] Alternatively spliced gene transcripts exist.[220] The three subunits randomly assemble into 15 different homo- or heterotetrameric isozymes that are variably expressed in all fetal tissue.[173] Whereas in general there is a tendency toward uniformity in early fetal life, i.e., simultaneous expression of all three PFK loci, distinct tissue-specific isozyme patterns emerge with development.[173] Fetal skeletal muscle is composed mainly of hybrids between the M and P subunits, but also the L_4 tetramer and tetramers, consisting of the L subunit and M or P subunits, can be observed.[173] At about 20 weeks of gestation, first the L and then the P subunit containing isozymes disappear. Mature human skeletal muscle expresses exclusively the M_4 homotetramer.

Phosphofructokinase deficiency[189,191,221] (glycogenesis type VII, Tarui's disease) is a typically autosomally recessive inherited lack of functional M subunit, characterized by exercise intolerance of variable onset, myoglobinuria, and hemolytic anemia. A fatal infantile form has also been described.[222] There is no increase in venous lactate concentration in response to the ischemic exercise test. Several point mutations and deletions have been identified.[189,191,223]

In contrast to fetal skeletal muscle, normal cultured myogenic elements display predominantly the P and L subunits, regardless of the developmental stage.[224]

Aldolase

Fructosediphosphate aldolase (EC 4.1.2.13) converts fructose-1,6-diphosphate into glyceraldehyde phosphate and dihydroxyacetone phosphate. Like all glycolytic enzymes, the enzyme is ubiquitous in animal tissue. Animal aldolases are tetramers, usually composed of two of three different parental subunits: type A, the classic muscle form; type B, from the liver; and type C, from the brain.[225] Hybridization of two of these dissimilar subunits can give rise to five isozymes: two homotetramers and three heterotetramers (hybrids). Unlike lactate dehydrogenase (LDH) or creatine kinase (CK), aldolase tetramers are extremely stable, and subunit exchange does not seem to occur under physiologic conditions.[225]

Mature muscle in most animals and in the human contains only one isozyme (type A_4). However, during the period of embryonic development, muscle synthesizes the C subunit, which is combined with the A subunit into five isozyme forms. This five-membered isozyme pattern is observed in 6- to 8-week-old human embryos, whereas at 9 to 12 weeks of gestation, only four bands can be detected.[226] At 27 to 28 weeks only aldolase A_4 and a faint A_3C isozyme band are discernible.[226] In the perinatal and postnatal period from birth to 3 weeks, the A_4 isozyme is the only isozyme present and increases in specific activity.[227] The isozyme transition in muscle was studied in detail in the chick.[228,229] In "red" and "white" muscle, aldolase isozyme transitions coincided with a brisk increase of total enzyme activity, mainly due to aldolase A.[225,228]

What biologic advantage might these isozymes confer? With aldolase, both the A and C types are kinetically suited to glycolysis. The major established distinction between the forms appears to be their markedly different binding characteristics to actin-containing filaments.[230–233] Following tissue differentiation, aldolase C continues to maintain a strong presence in the brain and other organs where steady glycolysis is necessary. In contrast in muscle

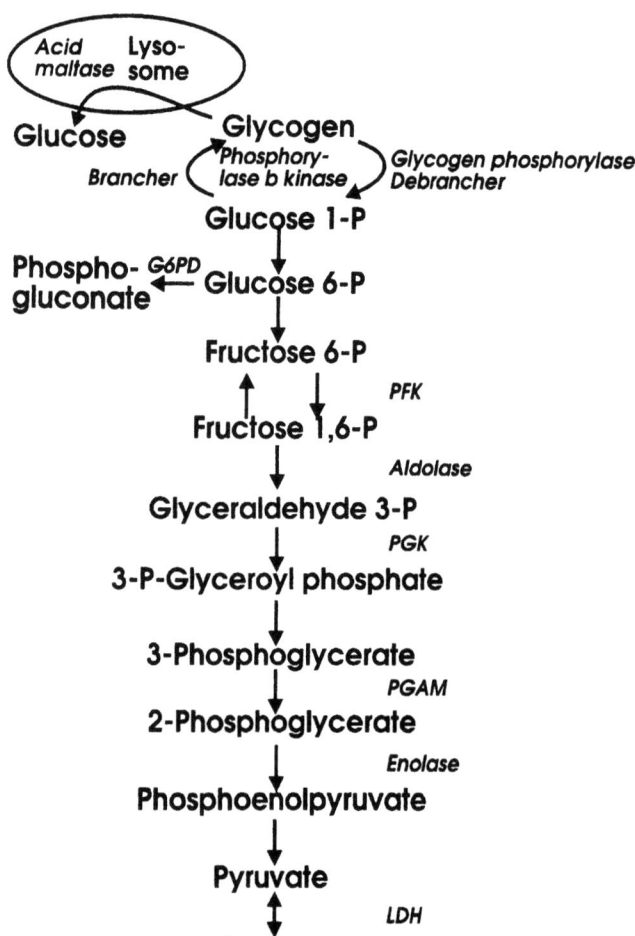

FIGURE 31.4. Overview of glycolysis and glycogen metabolism. G6PD, glucose-6-phosphate dehydrogenase; PFK, phosphofructokinase; PGK, phosphoglycerate kinase; PGAM, phosphoglycerate mutase; LDH, lactate dehydrogenase.

tissue, where at times acute and abrupt changes in energy demands might occur, aldolase A, which binds more tenaciously to actin, might be a more suitable catalyst, because it is positioned at subcellular sites, where energy is needed promptly.[234]

Regression toward the fetal isozyme patterns, (e.g., the appearance of A_3C, and sometimes even A_2C_2), was observed in muscle neoplasms[235] in patients with various genetic and acquired neuromuscular diseases[226] and experimentally in denervated rabbit muscle.[236]

In chick muscle cultures, the aldolase isozyme pattern changes rapidly after fusion from C_4 and AC_3 to all five A-C isozymes but the typical adult pattern (A_4) is not observed, not even 1 week after fusion.[237] If fusion is prevented by either calcium-deficient medium or medium-containing bromodeoxyuridine,[238] isozyme transition is not observed.[237]

Deficiency of functional aldolase A tetramers has been reported as a rare cause of hemolytic anemia in infancy and childhood[239] and of a myopathy with rhabdomyolysis.[240]

Phosphoglycerate Mutase

Phosphoglycerate mutase (PGAM) (EC 2.7.5.3) is an enzyme of the glycolytic pathway, that catalyzes the conversion of 3-phosphoglycerate to 2-phosphoglycerate. PGAM exists as three functional dimers[241]—PGAM-BB, MB, and MM. cDNAs of the M and the B subunits have been characterized and mapped to chromosomes 7 and 10.[242-244] The M subunit is specific for skeletal muscle and heart, but is also developmentally expressed in sperm from the spermatid stage onward.[245,246]

Developmental isozyme switching is quite similar to that with creatine kinase (CK). The isozyme pattern of fetal skeletal muscle includes all three dimers, but the MM isozyme becomes more prominent with increasing fetal age,[247,248] eventually replacing the MB and BB dimers almost completely.[204,247,249,250] During muscle differentiation in human cultures, transition from PGAM-BB to PGAM-MM, although incomplete, occurs somewhat later than that of the CK isoforms,[179,251] suggesting that the two enzymes might be under separate genetic control. As can be expected for a glycolytic enzyme, PGAM activity is much higher in fast-twitch type II fibers, as is CK activity, as compared to slow-twitch type I fibers.[252] In cardiac muscle, complete transition does not occur, and all the isozymes remain present even in the mature adult heart.

An autosomal-recessive deficiency of the M subunit of PGAM results in exercise intolerance, exercise-induced rhabdomyolysis, and an abnormally small increase of lactate on ischemic exercise (glycogenosis type X).[247,250] In some patients, point mutations of the PGAM-M gene on chromosome 7[244] have been identified.[189,253]

Enolase

Enolase (phosphopyruvate hydratase—EC 4.2.1.11) catalyzes the interconversion of 2-phosphoglycerate into phosphoenolpyruvate. Three isoforms exist as dimers of identical α, β, or γ subunits for which the genetic loci have been characterized.[254-256] Whereas the αα homodimer is exclusively expressed in liver and the predominant form in most other nonmuscle tissues, the γγ homodimer is found mainly in neuronal and neuroendocrine cells (i.e., neuron-specific enolase).

In early embryonic muscle, the αα isoform prevails.[26,257] Muscle-specific β-enolase, unlike most developmental protein markers of myogenesis, can already be demonstrated at the undifferentiated myoblast stage;[25,26] its appearance in fetal muscle seems to be linked to a distinct lineage of myoblasts evolving during secondary myogenesis.[25,26] The ββ homodimer is characteristic of mature muscle, where higher levels have been noted in type II fibers of fast-twitch muscle.[258,259]

Lactate Dehydrogenase

Lactate dehydrogenase (LDH) (EC 1.1.1.27) catalyzes the final step of glycolysis (i.e., the reduction of pyruvate to lactate). The five isozymes (M_4, M_3H_1, M_2M_2, M_1H_3, and H_4) of the tetrameric enzyme are generally permutations of two different subunits—LDH-M (LDH-A) and LDH-H (LDH-B). The isozymes are traditionally identified according to their different electrophoretic mobility; M_4 is the slowest migrating, H_4 the fastest, and the hybrids migrate to intermediate positions.[260] The third subunit, LDH-X (LDH-C) is expressed only in mature testis and sperm.[261] The genes encoding LDH-M and LDH-H have been localized to chromosomes 11[262] and 12,[263] respectively. There are marked differences between the M and H subunits in the inhibition of enzymatic activity by pyruvate. LDH-H is maximally active at low concentrations of pyruvate, but, unlike LDH-M, is strongly inhibited by high concentrations.[264] These characteristics guarantee the complete oxidation of pyruvate in the respiratory chain of the heart where LDH-H prevails and maintain an adequate energy supply in skeletal muscle where the M_4-tetramer is the predominant species, even in acute episodes of anaerobic exercise.[264] In mature skeletal muscle the LDH isozyme pattern varies in different fiber types. In "white" muscle, in which glycolysis is very active, M-tetramers predominate, whereas in metabolically aerobic "red" muscle, concerned mainly with postural duties, isozymes containing H subunits are found.

During ontogeny, transitions in the LDH isozyme pattern take place.[264-266] In early developmental stages of human skeletal muscle at 16 weeks gestation, the LDH pattern resembles more that of adult cardiac muscle, containing more H-subunit enzymes (M_2H_2 and M_3H_1).

Unlike other developmentally controlled isozymes of muscle, LDH-M$_4$ is abundant even in early, uninnervated myotubes in culture.[215,260] LDH deficiency (glycogenosis type XI) has been reported as an autosomal recessive trait.[267] Both, LDH-H[268] and LDH-M[189,267,269–272] subunit deficiencies have been described. The chief symptom of the M-subunit deficiency is exercise-induced rhabdomyolysis, but uterine stiffness in the early stage of delivery is not uncommon in females and often requires cesarean section.[272] A lack of LDH pattern maturation in muscle can be seen after birth in neurogenic atrophies, after experimental denervation, in muscle necrosis, and in situations of muscle regeneration, such as in muscular dystrophy.[264,273]

Mitochondrial Energy Metabolism

Oxidative Phosphorylation

When muscle cells contract, the myofibrillar myosin ATPase consumes chemical energy in the form of adenosine triphosphate (ATP). In muscle at rest, ATP is mainly supplied by mitochondria. The importance of these organelles in muscle energy metabolism might be inferred from the fact that mitochondrial protein in heart tissue is calculated to be 320 to 350 mg·g^{-1} of dry weight.[274,275] For their task mitochondria are equipped with an electron transport chain that is embedded in the extensively folded inner mitochondrial membrane. Electrons from substrate oxidation are shuttled through a series of enzymatic components (complexes I–V), each of which is assembled from numerous polypeptide subunits. Ultimately oxygen is reduced by oxidative phosphorylation (Figure 31.5; Table 31.6).

The mitochondrial respiratory chain (RC) is encoded by two separate genetic systems: mitochondrial DNA[276] (mtDNA) and nuclear DNA (nDNA). About 90% of the mitochondrial proteins and most of the subunits of the RC are not encoded by mtDNA but by nDNA. After synthesis as precursors, nuclear-encoded proteins are targeted from the cytoplasm to their correct mitochondrial

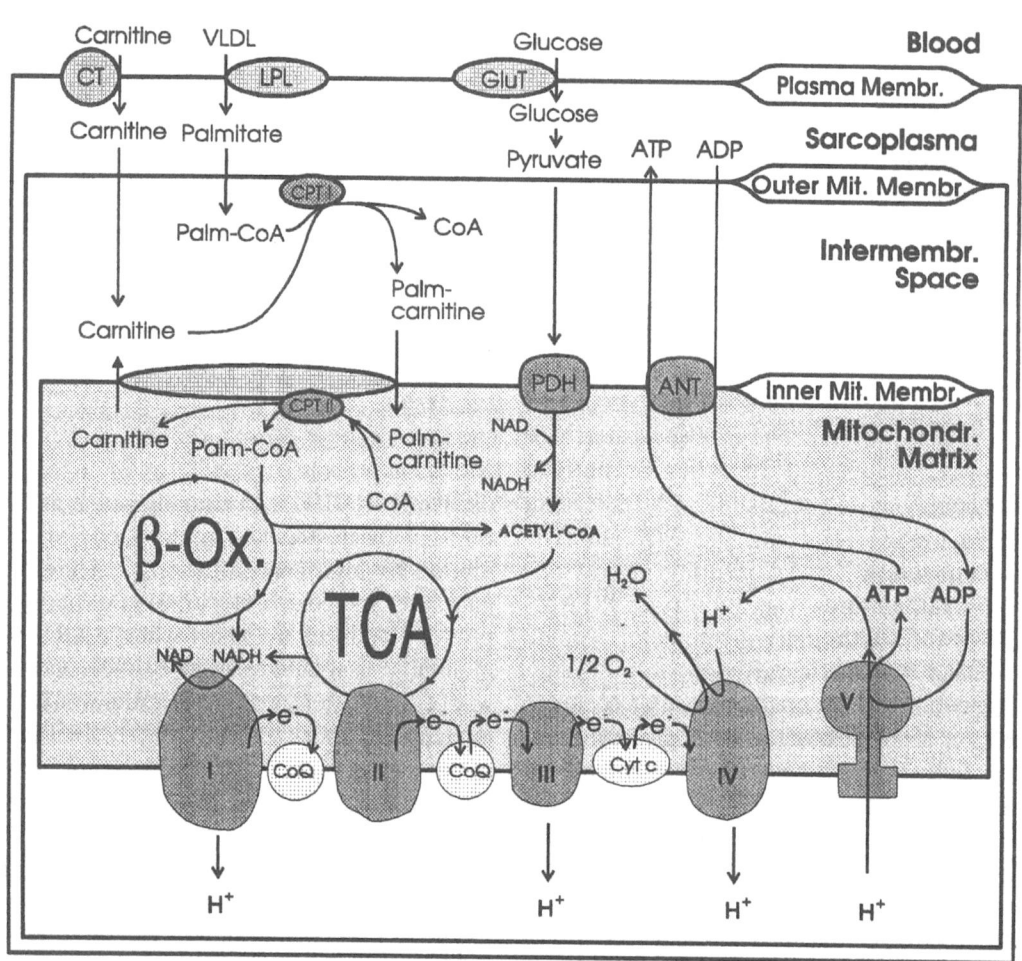

FIGURE 31.5. Oxidative metabolism of human skeletal muscle. ANT, adenine nucleotide translocase; CAT, carnitine acylcarnitine translocase; CoQ, coenzyme Q$_{10}$; CPT, carnitine palmitoyltransferase; Cyt c, cytochrome c; CT, carnitine transporter; GluT, glucose transporter; LPL, lipoprotein lipase; β-Ox., β-oxidation; PDH, pyruvate dehydrogenase complex; TCA, tricarboxylic acid (Krebs) cycle; VLDL, very low density lipoprotein; I, NADH-CoQ oxidoreductase; II, succinate-CoQ oxidoreductase; III, CoQ-Cyt c oxidoreductase; IV, cytochrome c oxidase; V, ATP-synthase.

TABLE 31.6. Defects of nuclear DNA (nDNA) leading to mitochondrial myopathies of infancy and childhood.

Mitochondrial substrate transport
    Fatal infantile form of CPT deficiency (CPTII)[545]
    Muscle form of CPT deficiency (CPTII)[546]
    Primary systemic carnitine deficiency[547,548]
    Primary muscle carnitine deficiency[549]
    Secondary carnitine deficiencies[417]
    Adenine nucleotide translocator (ANT) deficiency[295]
    Deficiency of the voltage-dependent anion channel (VDAC/porin)[550]
Defects of substrate utilization
    Pyruvate dehydrogenase complex deficiencies[551,552]
    Fumarase deficiency[553]
    Defects of fatty acid oxidation[417]
Respiratory chain defects
    Complex I deficiency[198]
    Complex II deficiency[198]
    Complex III deficiency[198]
    Complex IV deficiency[198]
    Coenzyme Q deficiency[554]
Defects of the energy transducing system
    Luft's disease[555]

location by means of positively charged amino-terminal leader sequences that bind to a specific membrane receptor. After translocation into the organelle, the leader sequences are cleaved by a mitochondrial peptidase to allow refolding of the protein.

Aside from the RC, mitochondria harbor other important biochemical pathways, such as the Krebs cycle, the urea cycle, and fatty acid β-oxidation. Human disease due to RC dysfunction can be biochemically classified according to the RC complex involved. A genetic classification traditionally distinguishes mendelian inherited mutations of nDNA from maternal inherited errors of mtDNA. New defects are being identified rapidly. Many mtDNA mutations have been linked to human disease, but now isozymes are known.[277,278] These conditions affect predominantly nondividing, postmitotic cells such as neurons and skeletal muscle fibers (Table 31.7).

One RC component that displays isozymes is complex IV, often referred to as cytochrome c oxidase (COX). The enzyme catalyzes the terminal transfer of electrons to oxygen, with the reduction of molecular oxygen to water. It contains 13 polypeptide subunits (I, II, III, IV, Va, Vb, VIa, VIb, VIc, VIIa, VIIb, VIIc, and VIII), two heme molecules, and two protein-bound copper atoms. The three largest subunits (I, II, and III) are encoded by mtDNA, and the rest by nDNA. In humans, there is evidence for tissue-specific isoforms of at least two COX subunits, both nuclear encoded: VIa and VIIa.[279–281] Both isoforms can be distinguished with immunologic[279,280] and molecular[281] techniques. Whereas the H (heart) isoforms of VIa and VIIa are found exclusively in human heart and skeletal muscle, the L (liver) isoforms can be detected in the kidney and the brain and in smooth muscle, as well as in striated muscle.[279,280] In an uninnervated human myoblast culture system, isoform switching of subunits VIa and VIIa was demonstrated at the transcriptional level, with reciprocal trends for heart- (upregulation) and liver-type subunits (downregulation).[282] In contrast to other species,[283] only a single isoform of subunit VIII seems to exist in the primate.[284,285]

Tissue-specific isoform switching from an unrecognized developmentally regulated muscle-specific isoform that is expressed in fetal muscle but downregulated during muscle maturation may be of clinical importance in a rare condition, known as benign infantile mitochondrial myopathy.[286–288] Soon after birth, affected neonates display a pure myopathy with generalized hypotonia, respiratory weakness, and severe lactic acidosis. The nuclear-encoded COX subunits VIIa and VIIb as well as the mtDNA-encoded subunit II are undetectable by immunohistochemistry in skeletal muscle, as is enzymatic COX activity.[288] Enzymatic COX activity is present in other tissues. By the age of 3, the enzymatic and immunohistochemical defect gradually vanishes, concomitant with spontaneous clinical recovery.

Adenine Nucleotide Translocase

Adenine nucleotide translocase (ANT) (EC 2.7.7) is the most abundant protein in the inner mitochondrial membrane and serves as an exchange carrier for adenosine diphosphate (ADP) and ATP, between mitochondrial matrix and cytosol (Figure 31.5). ANT seems to participate with mitochondrial creatine kinase (Mi-CK) (vide infra) in the functional maturation of the developing energy transduction system in sarcomeric tissues, since both enzymes are expressed in a 1:1 molar ratio in cardiac mitochondria and are functionally coupled.[289] Of the three isoforms that have been discovered so far, ANT2 and ANT3 are expressed in many tissues during the fetal stage and are downregulated in skeletal muscle during maturation, whereas ANT1, located on chromosome 4q,[290] is absent in myoblasts but is expressed strongly and specifically in mature sarcomeric tissues.[291–193] It is conceivable, that, as skeletal muscle matures and begins to express contractile elements, there is an increased need

TABLE 31.7. Disorders of early childhood caused by or affecting mitochondrial DNA (mtDNA) and disturbing respiratory chain activity.

Clinical presentation	Genetic defect
Subacute necrotizing encephalomyopathy— Leigh's syndrome[a,198]	Point mutations in ATPase gene and in tRNA genes, rearrangements (deletions/duplications)
Pearson's bone marrow/pancreas syndrome[556]	MtDNA rearrangements
Infantile non-Leigh encephalomyopathies[198]	As in Leigh's syndrome,[a] additionally mtDNA depletion[557,558]

[a] Leigh's syndrome also can be caused by several defects in nDNA encoded enzymes.

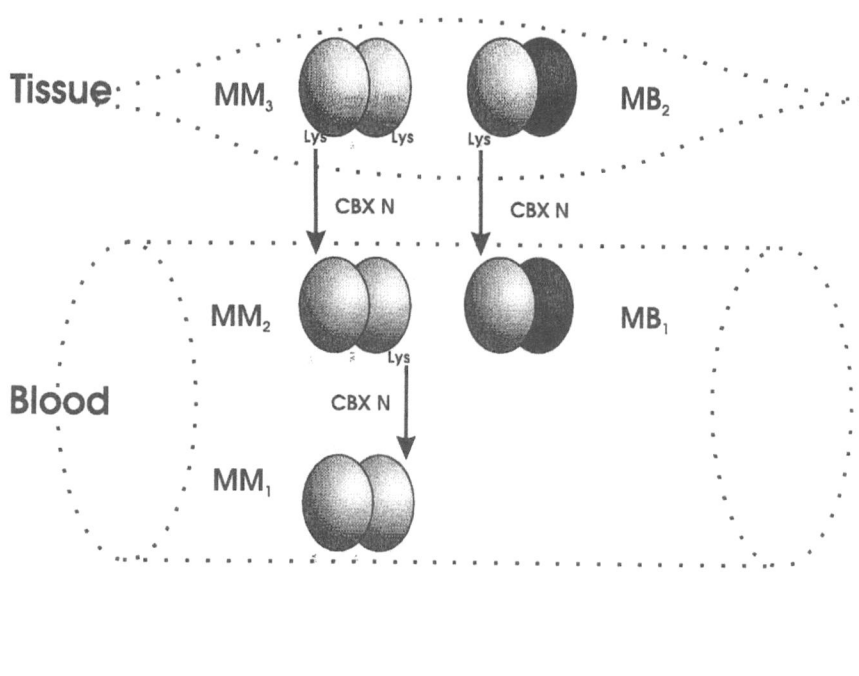

FIGURE 31.6. Creatine kinase (CK-) isoforms resulting from the postsynthetic conversion of cytosolic CK. Serum carboxykinase N (CBX N) cleaves the C-terminal lysine from the CK-M subunit.

for cytoplasmic ANT, requiring a more efficient ATP/ADP exchange system. Indeed, different kinetic properties of adenine nucleotide translocation have been reported for liver and heart mitochondria.[294]

A deficiency of the muscle specific ANT isozyme has recently been described in a 3.5-year-old boy with mitochondrial myopathy and lactic acidosis.[295]

Other Enzymes of Energy Metabolism

Creatine Kinase

Creatine kinase (CK) (EC 2.7.3.2.) catalyzes the reversible transphosphorylation between phosphocreatine and ATP and plays an important role in the regeneration of ATP levels and energy supply in muscle.[296] CK occurs as five different isozymes: one of three cytosolic isozymes is coexpressed with two mitochondrial species in a developmentally regulated and tissue-specific manner.[297]

Cytosolic CK is found mainly in skeletal muscle, heart, and brain.[298] The enzyme has a dimeric structure, with two subunits, M and B. The genes of the human M subunit and B subunits have been mapped to chromosomes 19 and 14, respectively.[299,300] The BB homodimer is the predominant form in brain, smooth muscle, and embryonic striated muscle and found in a variety of other tissues; CK-MM in contrast, is rather specific for differentiated sarcomeric muscle.[301] Mature skeletal muscle has almost exclusively MM isozyme (CK-MM); only 0% to 3% is composed of the third cytosolic isozyme, the CK-MB heterodimer.[302] Adult heart muscle in contrast has about 30% CK-MB activity, the rest being CK-MM. Subunit exchange among CK homodimers, as illustrated by the reaction CK-BB + CK-MM ↔ 2 CK-MB, is possible.[303] In mature heart or skeletal muscle, about 5% to 10% of CK-MM activity is associated with the myofibrillar fraction[304] and resides in protein, bound to the M-line of the sarcomere[305] (Figure 31.2). This location in the immediate vicinity of myosin-ATPase activity[304,305] is believed to guarantee the immediate energy supply of the sarcomere in resynthesizing ATP from ADP[305,306] and to provide a rapid feedback signal between contraction and mitochondrial respiration.[307]

The mitochondrial CK isozymes are composed of two subunit types with distinct structural and catalytic properties that have been purified from the outer surface of the inner mitochondrial membrane (Mi-CK).[308-313] The Mi-CKs are encoded by two separate genes[314] and the polypeptide products are believed to form mainly octameric aggregates.[296,313,315] Sarcomeric Mi-CK (sMi-CK) is restricted to skeletal muscle and heart; the other form is ubiquitous (uMi-CK), in that it also occurs in heart and skeletal muscle, but additionally in intestine, brain, kidney, placenta, and uterus.[296,313,314] Expression of Mi-CK messenger RNA (mRNA) in most tissues is 10- to 100-fold less than that of the cytosolic CK mRNAs[316] and Mi-CK protein activity amounts to 0.9% of total CK activity in adult human quadriceps muscle and to 9.0% in heart.[317] Both forms of Mi-CK are detectable in serum. Postsynthetic modifications to the cytoplasmic CK isozymes occur when the polypeptides are released from tissue into the blood, where serum carboxypeptidase N (CBX-N) cleaves the C-terminal lysine from the M subunit, leading to three isoforms of CK-MM and two isoforms of CK-MB[318] (Figure 31.6). Isoforms exhibit the same catalytic activity, but slightly different isoelectric points. The isoforms MM_3 and MB_2 are composed of unmodified tissue subunits. Conversion of one M subunit by serum carboxypeptidase N produces MM_2 and MB_1, respectively, whereas conversion of two M subunits produces MM_1. The isoforms can currently be distinguished electrophoretically or by immunoinhibition.[319-321] In normal serum, only trace amounts of tissue MM_3 are seen, but about equal amounts of tissue MB_2 and serum MB_1.[322] Measurement of the serum isoforms has special clinical relevance in the retrospective determination of the onset of acute myocardial ischemia,[318,323] or in the evaluation of success of myocardial reperfusion procedures.[321]

Development of total CK activity in human skeletal muscle is characterized by a sharp increase of predominantly CK-MM, during the fetal period and postpartum to adult levels between 40 days and 14 years of age.[324-326] These quantitative changes are accompanied by qualitative transitions of the cytosolic CK isozymes.[297,327-331] In the first 2 months of embryonic development, CK-BB is the principal isozyme. In fetal quadriceps, CK-MM rapidly increases between 6 and 16 weeks of gestation,[328] concomitant with fusion of myoblasts and accumulation and organization of the contractile machinery. The synthesis of CK-MM always precedes that of Mi-CK in both heart and skeletal muscle.[332,333] After 16 weeks of gestation, the predominant isozymes are MM and MB. BB may be present in low concentrations of less than 5% of total activity. Isozyme proportions in skeletal muscle and in heart have been analyzed.[328,334] CK-BB is the principal isozyme in fetal skeletal muscle during the first 2 months of gestation, followed by CK-MB, between the 8th and 11th week; at term, CK-MM was 78% to 92%, CK-MB 8% to 22%, and CK-BB 0% to 0.5%; in heart, the MB isozyme represents 16% to 20% of total cardiac CK activity at term. In normal adult skeletal muscle the MM isozyme prevails almost exclusively throughout life, although CK-MB may be detected with sensitive assays.[335] CK isozymes in the serum have been studied in healthy full-term neonates during the first 3 postnatal days.[336] Total CK serum activities and all CK isozyme activities increase and peak, generally between 5 hours and 33 hours after birth. Whereas CK-MM and CK-MB serum activities are low in neonates delivered by cesarean section compared to vaginal delivery, the CK-BB serum activity is not affected by the method of delivery.[336] The high CK-MB activity in the perinatal period is likely to originate in skeletal muscle rather than in heart. Although the reasons for the enzyme release are not completely understood, CK-MB leakage into the bloodstream might derive from immature muscle fibers that are damaged during muscle remodeling.

Unlike the cytosolic CK isozymes, there is no developmental isozyme switch between the Mi-CKs.[289] Total Mi-CK activity doubles in a linear fashion during the period from 29 weeks of gestation until term and subsequently increases by another factor of 2 to reach average adult levels.[331] In heart, there is virtually no expression of sMi-CK prior to birth,[289,307] but the activity of this sarcomere-specific mitochondrial isozyme rises sharply postnatally, concomitant with cardiac maturation and a postnatal shift from glycolytic to oxidative metabolism. The expression pattern of sMi-CK in skeletal muscle is similar to heart, although there is some prenatal enzyme activity.

There are developmental changes in the subcellular location of CK; for a review of the concept of metabolic compartmentalization in muscle cells see Wallimann et al.[296] and Hoerter et al.[333] Accompanying the progressive organization of the contractile proteins, some CK-MM, initially diffusely distributed in the cytosol, associates with the M line, which results in its functional coupling to myofibrillar ATPase. This was demonstrated to occur in the rat[337] and in the rabbit heart[332] during the first 2 postnatal weeks. Mi-CK is located close to the ATP/ADP translocase.[333] In this way, the cytosolic and the mitochondrial CK isoforms become critically located at sites of energy production and utilization.

During early stages of human innervated skeletal muscle cultures, as in aneural cultures, fetal patterns of CK-BB activity are characteristic,[251] but predominance of CK-MM, as is normally observed in mature muscle in vivo, appears only in spinal cord neuron-muscle coculture.[179,214,251] CK-MM expression precedes the appearance of enzymatically active muscle specific phosphoglycerate mutase (PGAM-MM), suggesting that these two systems might be under separate genetic control.[251] Mi-CK mRNA expression is sharply upregulated with the initiation of myoblast fusion, reaching greatest abundance 48 hours after myotube formation.[314]

The pattern of embryonal and in vitro isozyme development is recapitulated in situations of muscle regeneration, as in Duchenne's muscular dystrophy and other dystrophies.[338-340] A shift toward the fetal pattern can be detected with an increase in the MB isozyme fraction; occasionally BB isozyme is also seen. The changes in muscle isozymes are mirrored by serum CK,[341] since the amount of the MB isozyme in serum is so high, that the dystrophic heart alone cannot be its exclusive source.

Adenosine Monophosphate Deaminase

Adenosine Monophosphate Deaminase (AMPD) (EC 3.5.4.6.) catalyzes the irreversible hydrolytic deamination of adenosine monophosphate (AMP) to inosine monophosphate (IMP) and ammonia. The enzyme is ubiquitous among mammalian cell types and found in varying concentrations among different tissues. Exceptionally high concentrations are observed in skeletal muscle,[342] where AMPD preferentially occurs in type II fibers.[343] AMPD, together with the two AMP generating enzymes adenylosuccinate synthetase and adenylosuccinate lyase, forms the purine nucleotide cycle, the purpose of which in muscle contraction is not fully understood,[344] but it has a potentially important role for supplying ATP during intense exercise. In humans, three different isoforms of the tetrameric enzyme have been isolated from liver (L-AMPD), erythrocytes (E-AMPD), and muscle (M-AMPD—myoadenylate deaminase).[345,346] The isozymes have been assigned to three different genes: myoadenylate deaminase to the AMPD1 gene,[347] the L-form to AMPD2,[348] both located on chromosome 1, and the E-forms to AMPD3.[349] Each of the three genes produces multiple transcripts by alternative splicing.[350] During myogenesis, there is an early developmental transcript of the AMPD1 gene, which differs from the ultimate mature AMPD1 transcript in the removal of exon 2.[350-352] In cultures, at least some embryonic isozyme switches are recapitulated.[343,352,353] In human myoblasts, only the L and E isoforms prevail, with predominant perinuclear localization; the M isoform is undetectable.[343] With myotube formation, the M form appears and all three isoforms coexist,[343] but even in mature skeletal muscle in vivo, the L and E isoforms remain.[354]

Primary myoadenylate deaminase deficiency is an autosomal recessive trait, caused at least in part by a point mutation in exon 2 of the AMPD1 gene that leads to premature transcriptional termination.[344,355,356] The disease is characterized by muscular weakness, rapid fatigue, and cramps or myalgias following moderate exercise, accompanied by normal routine muscle histology.[344,355,357] Diagnostic procedures include ischemic forearm exercise[358] and histochemical or enzymatic assays of biopsied muscle. The AMPD carrier frequency in the general population is 20%, although only a minority of homozygous persons displays symptoms; in fact most of the affected individuals seem to be asymptomatic.[344,356] It is possible that in some of these cases the developmental alternative splicing event would remove the mutation, resulting in a functional polypeptide.[350,356] In cultures from AMPD-deficient patients, total enzyme activity was in the normal range, although the adult isozyme was not detectable in significant amounts. Nonmuscle isoforms can probably substitute AMPD activity in the incompletely developed muscle culture.[343,353,359,360] AMPD deficiency can be acquired secondary to many neuromuscular and rheumatologic diseases.[356]

Quantitative Metabolic Changes During Muscle Development

Not only are there significant alterations of the isozyme patterns in developing skeletal muscle, but there are substantial quantitative changes in the total enzymatic activity accompanying fetal muscle development during differentiation of myoblasts to myotubes and myofibers in vitro. These changes reflect the importance that several metabolic pathways acquire in a particular tissue as differentiation proceeds, in the integration of tissue-specific pathways to the needs of the organism as a whole, and in adaptation to the new extrauterine environment. In utero, fetal muscle is supplied with carbohydrates and amino acids at relatively constant and abundant rates by maternal metabolism. After birth, the neonate is subject to periods of starvation that demand special metabolic control. Furthermore, mother's milk is a diet relatively high in lipid and low in carbohydrate. Parturition calls for changes in skeletal muscle metabolism. A large body of data on the development of muscle metabolism has been accumulated from animal studies, but the maximal activity of enzymes in a particular pathway in vitro does not necessarily reflect its significance in vivo, because metabolic turnover is not only limited by enzyme concentration and type, but also by substrate availability and the presence of metabolic activators or inhibitors.

Carbohydrates

Enzymes involved in glycogen and glucose metabolism, such as glycogen phosphorylase, phosphoglucomutase, and PFK, experience an approximate 10-fold increase in activity after myotube formation,[361] which is attributable to upregulation in synthesis of muscle isozymes. Glycogen phosphorylase is assembled during myotube formation to yield the metabolically active enzyme.[362] Glycogen is deposited in the sarcoplasm mostly after fusion,[46] when muscle fibers acquire an insulin stimulated glucose transport system and respond to insulin by increased glucose uptake.[363]

Mammalian fetal muscle glycogen is of the normal branched structure.[207] Carbohydrates are generally reported to accumulate rapidly during late gestation, peak at birth, and rapidly decline postnatally.[364-366] The glycogen degrading enzyme phosphorylase is low during the fetal period and prenatally, but increases during the first 30 postnatal days.[207,367] Mammalian glycogenolysis is especially high in muscle near term.[364] At birth, plasma catecholamines increase acutely and may contribute to glycogenolysis in liver and skeletal muscle. The combustion of carbohydrate stores during the transition from the constant placental supply with glucose until the beginning of breast feeding ensures adequate substrate supply for the neonate.[364,366,368] Little is known about the endocrine control of fetal muscle glycogen content, but cortisol[369] and/or developmental changes in the expression of the receptors for insulin and the insulin-like growth factors[370] seem to be involved. During the first postpartum weeks, the disaccharide lactose, derived from milk, is the carbohydrate generally available to the neonate. Lactose is hydrolyzed by the intestinal mucosa into glucose and galactose, but only glucose is available as a glycolytic substrate to muscle.[371] Galactose, in contrast, can be utilized by the liver.[371]

An array of data indicates that in children the anaerobic energy metabolism pathway is immature. The maximal anaerobic power exerted by muscle on force-velocity testing is low.[372] Muscle enzymes involved in anaerobic glycolytic energy generation (e.g., aldolase, PFK,[373] and LDH[325]), their substrate (i.e., glycogen, vide supra), as well as their product (i.e., blood lactate[372]) are low between birth and puberty. On the other hand aerobic metabolism seems to be as developed in children as in adults, as indicated by measurements of maximal oxygen uptake (V_{O_2} max), adjusted for lean body mass.[372]

It has been reported, that the pentose phosphate shunt is negligible in normal adult muscle, but more active in fetal tissue.[374-376] The significance of this finding is discussed below.

Lipids and Oxidative Phosphorylation

Anabolic pathways of lipids in skeletal muscle have been studied in vivo[377-379] and in a variety of tissue culture systems, although human data are scarce.[380-385] When myoblasts fuse to form myotubes, there seems to be a decrease in lipid turnover[383,384] and a switch from predominant triacylglycerol synthesis to predominant phospholipid synthesis.[380,381,383,384]

A variety of enzymes involved in fatty acid synthesis were characterized in neonatal and adult skeletal muscle membranes, indicating a significantly higher de novo fatty acid biosynthesis in the neonate.[352,379] Changes in phospholipid composition have been observed in both sarcolemmar membranes[378,382] and in membranes of the sarcoplasmic reticulum.[377] Adult rabbit sarcolemma has a two- to threefold higher concentration of linoleic acid in the major phosphoglycerides and a 30% lower cholesterol content than neonatal membranes.[378] Whereas some phospholipid components were found to increase during muscle ontogeny, others were found to be unchanged or downregulated.[377,378,382,383]

Adult resting muscle produces energy by aerobic fatty acid oxidation almost exclusively, as indicated by a respiratory quotient close to 0.8,[386] and the same seems to be the case for developing fetal muscle at all stages,[387] although fetal muscle consumes less oxygen and produces more lactate per weight than adult muscle.[387] During breast-feeding, 70% of the caloric intake is in the form of lipid,[388] and muscle tissue seems to be well equipped for this increased lipid availability by increased lipid catabolism in the neonatal period. Lipoprotein lipase activity, is increased at birth.[162] The enzyme activities for fatty acid oxidation in skeletal muscle increase from early development until adulthood, irrespective of changes in mitochondrial mass, as indicated by studies of palmitate oxidation and enzymatic activities in porcine and rat muscle preparations.[389-391] Oxygen is delivered to the individual muscle cell by diffusion from blood capillaries. In the embryo, capillaries are formed from embryonic connective tissue and can be identified in fetal muscle as early as 9 weeks.[392] The extent of capillarization does not differ between children and adults,[392] but the oxygen tension of fetal blood is only 50% that of adult blood, and fetal muscle is deficient in myoglobin.[393,394] Skeletal muscle can adapt to low oxygen tension by upregulating glycolytic while reciprocally downregulating oxidative pathways.[395] On the other hand, reduced oxygen tension may impair oxidative phosphorylation.[396] Respiratory chain metabolism may be limited by diminished substrate delivery, such as in glycogen phosphorylase deficiency.[396]

The mitochondrial marker enzyme cytochrome c oxidase becomes detectable histochemically in a few muscle fibers at the 11th week of gestation and is present in about 90% of the fibers at the 28th week,[397] and other enzymes, such as citrate synthase in the Krebs cycle, behave similarly by steadily increasing to adult values.[391,398] The overall increase of mitochondrial oxidative capacity is attributed to a disproportional rise of mitochondrial enzyme activity, rather than an increase in mitochondrial number.[391] Neonatal muscle, as compared to adult skeletal muscle, displays relatively low activities of succinate dehydrogenase, citrate synthetase, and COX.[367,373,391] Human myotube formation from myoblasts in vitro is not accompanied by long-term changes in oxidative metabolism such as palmitate and pyruvate oxidation, COX, and citrate synthase,[399] but a transient three- to fivefold downregulation of mitochondrial enzymes and a reciprocal upregulation of glycolytic enzymes can be observed upon commitment.[291] Continuous motor excitement is a potent stimulus to mitochondrial biogenesis, enhancing expression of both nuclear and mitochondrial encoded respiratory chain components, as well as of regulators of mtDNA replication.[400-402] Fatty acid uptake seems to be similar in myoblasts and myotubes,[380] but modifications in carnitine uptake[385] and an increase in the number of mitochondria[403] have been described.

Carnitine, a quaternary amide, is an essential cofactor for two carnitine acyl-transferases—carnitine palmitoyltransferase (CPT) I and II—that catalyze the translocation of long-chain fatty acids from the cytosol into the mitochondria[404] and therefore play a pivotal role in β-oxidation. CPT I is located on the inner side of the outer mitochondrial membrane, whereas CPT II resides on the inner face of the inner mitochondrial membrane (Figure 31.5). In adults, carnitine is mainly synthesized in the liver. Dietary sources are red meat, poultry, fish, and dairy products.[366] In utero, the activity of an enzyme involved in carnitine biosynthesis is substantially reduced, and carnitine is acquired through transplacental transfer.[405–407] Because striated muscle cannot produce carnitine, it is dependent on the uptake from the blood via two specific transport systems of high and low affinity.[385,408] In infants, muscle has the highest carnitine concentration of all tissues and contains about 98% of the total body carnitine pool.[409–411] Unlike the liver and heart carnitine content, the muscle carnitine concentration correlates with gestational age, is still low at term, and reaches the adult concentration during the first 4 postnatal months.[410,412] Preterm neonates are born with very limited carnitine muscle reserves,[410] which further decline when carnitine is not exogenously supplied by human milk or some formulas, for example, during parenteral nutrition.[413,414] Although the carnitine concentration in blood is relatively high in the preterm neonate,[415] exogenous supplementation seems to increase the body stores of carnitine.[414] Primary and secondary carnitine deficiency syndromes can be distinguished. The former are rarely encountered and represent a decrease of intracellular carnitine without association to another condition; the latter can accompany a variety of other metabolic defects, systemic illnesses, or various drug regimens known to deplete carnitine stores.[416,417] Primary carnitine deficiency can occur in a systemic form, possibly due to a generalized defect in the high-affinity carnitine transporter, and in a form restricted to muscle.[408,417] An infantile form of primary myopathic carnitine deficiency has been described, although the disease most commonly presents in childhood or in young adults (see Chapter 38).[418]

Carnitine palmitoyltransferase deficiency is also a clinically, biochemically and genetically heterogeneous group of disorders.[419,420] Hepatic and multiorgan involvement is possible. CPT II deficiency typically presents in young adults, although an infantile form has been described.[421] It is the most common disorder of lipid muscle metabolism and the most frequent cause of hereditary myoglobinuria, and gene analysis is possible (see Chapter 38).[420]

Protein and Amino Acids

Adult skeletal muscle contains about 80% and fetal skeletal muscle about 40% of the total body protein.[422] Muscle is the body's principal site of degradation of branched amino acids and of synthesis of alanine and glutamine.[423] The amino acids that the fetus requires for its own muscle protein synthesis are actually supplied by maternal skeletal muscle.[424] During the first two trimesters of human pregnancy, when fetal demand is low, protein is stored in maternal muscle. The last trimester, when fetal demand is high, is characterized by increased maternal muscle catabolism, as evidenced by the increased urinary excretion of 3-methylhistidine, an amino acid mainly present in muscle contractile protein.[425] The overall negative protein balance of maternal muscle during this period may be initiated by an increased insulin resistance of maternal muscular tissue.[426,427] Insulin stimulates protein synthesis and inhibits protein degradation.[428]

Protein synthesis in fetal muscle must be faster than opposing protein degradation, to account for the positive protein balance in growing skeletal muscle. However, as fetal muscle develops, there is not only increased synthesis, but also faster degradation of protein.[429] The apparent paradox of increased protein degradation that leads to a faster protein turnover in growing, as opposed to nongrowing, muscle, may reflect remodeling processes. To accommodate the high demand in protein, the protein synthesis and remodeling apparatus of the muscle cell is well adjusted. For instance, avian muscle ribosomes are 90% polysomal,[430] amino acid reutilization is highly efficient, and molecules involved in protein folding, intracellular transport, and protein degradation, such as heat-shock protein 90 and ubiquitin, are developmentally upregulated.[431] However, the absolute rate of protein turnover in adult nongrowing skeletal muscle is relatively slow when compared with other organs. In mouse liver the turnover of stable proteins amounts to an average of 30%, approximately five to ten times faster than skeletal muscle.

Fusion of skeletal muscle is accompanied by important quantitative changes in muscle-specific protein, which encompasses about 60% of total muscle protein.[432] Genes encoding muscle-specific contractile proteins are activated, and other polypeptides, such as the acetylcholine receptor and enzymes, become significantly more abundant.[326,433–435] The immediate increase of total muscle protein after fusion is largely attributable to a sharp augmentation in the synthesis of muscle-specific contractile elements, whereas the sarcoplasmic protein fraction rises less sharply and to a minor extent.[326,436]

The developmentally increasing muscle mass can be estimated by measuring the urinary creatinine excretion. Creatine cooperates in the formation of creatine phosphate by CK and is synthesized in two steps in nonmuscle tissue,[437] since muscle itself lacks the enzymes necessary for creatine synthesis. The initial, rate-limiting step occurs in the kidney and is synthesized by the enzyme arginine-glycine amidinotransferase. The product guanidinoacetate is methylated in the liver to creatine, which is taken up by muscle by specific transporters.[438] The activity of arginine-glycine amidinotransferase in the rat kidney gradually increases during fetal development to reach adult levels at around 25 days after birth, the same time as CK.[435] Creatine phosphate is converted in muscle to creatinine, which is subsequently excreted by the kidney. In this fashion, about 2% of the total body pool of creatine in muscle is irreversibly lost in the urine each day.[439,440] Since creatinine formation occurs nonenzymatically, it is excreted at an essentially constant rate, at first-order kinetics. Therefore, creatinine urinary excretion is proportional to muscle creatinine and increases with development of the neonate, largely due to the expanding muscle mass.

Myoglobin is of relatively low abundance in fetal, as compared to adult, muscular tissue.[393,394] The muscle dipeptides carnosine and its methylated derivative anserine are found in large amounts only in skeletal muscle.[301] Their concentration is closely related to muscle activity and is higher in adult than in fetal tissue.[301,436] The dipeptide and free radical scavenger glutathione does not change dramatically around birth, but subsequently decreases to adult levels.[441] Tissue concentrations of amino acids are exceptionally high perinatally.[441]

Nucleic Acids

When myoblasts proliferate, synthesis of both nDNA and mtDNA is necessary. However, with myotube formation, replication of nDNA ceases[442] and 90% of the cytoplasmic DNA synthesis, mediated by a specific mitochondrial polymerase activity, is lost.[443] The remaining mtDNA polymerase activity seems to be important for normal muscle development, as can be deduced from the fact that a severe myopathy develops when the enzyme is iatrogenically inhibited by antiretroviral drugs, such as zidovudine (AZT).[444] With terminal differentiation and increasing protein synthesis, the DNA content per muscle wet weight decreases postnatally, whereas the RNA/DNA ratio increases.[326] A decrease of the RNA/protein ratio after fusion signifies rapid protein accumulation,[445] as well as reduced RNA synthesis.[171]

With myotube formation and terminating synthesis of nDNA, there is a decline in the demand for nucleic acid precursors. One essential component of nucleic acids is ribose, whose synthesis in turn requires an intact pentose phosphate cycle. The importance of this pathway for the provision of DNA precursors is illustrated by its enhanced activity in early fetal muscle tissue. Concomitant with decreasing nucleic acid turnover in terminally differentiating tissue, the pentose phosphate cycle loses its importance as demonstrated in vivo[446] and in vitro.[179] A parallel decline of key enzymes of the pentose phosphate shunt and mitotic index on one hand and RNA synthesis on the other hand have been demonstrated for the developing brain, another terminally differentiating tissue.[445] In non-postmitotic proliferating cells, such as in liver tissue, however, the pentose phosphate pathway activity seems to be unrelated to proliferative indices.[445]

Normal exercising muscle can release the purines inosine and hypoxanthine in substantial amounts from AMP deamination.[447] The release of these uric acid precursors may be accelerated under pathologic conditions such as in a variety of glycogeneses, where a block in glycolysis impairs ATP generation and promotes ADP and AMP formation.[448] The resulting increase in AMP deamination may lead to myogenic hyperuricemia.

Genetic Regulation of Myogenesis and Muscle Metabolism

Myogenic Determination Factors (MDFs)

Myogenesis begins with a restriction event that channels a population of mesenchymal somitic cells into a lineage committed to forming the muscle cell.[20] The molecular basis for this commitment involves the expression of a family of transcription factors that, acting as control switches, turn on muscle-specific gene expression in the premuscle cell. The muscle transcription factors are so powerful that they can experimentally convert numerous mesodermal and nonmesodermal cells into a myoblast phenotype.[2] The human family of MDFs, also called the MyoD gene family, is dispersed on different chromosomes and encoding four proteins (e.g., MyoD,[2] myogenin,[3] Myf-5,[4] and MRF4[5]). Their classification in a family is based on their secondary structure, which displays homologous basic and helix-loop-helix regions (bHLH).[449] Whereas the basic domain is required for DNA binding, the HLH domain is required for dimerization with other HLH proteins. Dimerization of two identical HLHs leads to MDF homodimers. Heterodimer formation of MDFs can efficiently result from the interaction with other MDFs, as well as another bHLH partner, E-protein.[449] Heterodimers are more efficient in promoting myogenesis than homodimers. The basic region of the MDF/E-protein homo- or heterodimer complexes mediates binding to specific target DNA sequences, called E-boxes.[450] Such E-boxes are located in the enhancer region of many muscle specific genes. For example, E-boxes were found in the enhancers of the gene for CK, the acetylcholine receptor α and δ subunits, desmin, myosin light chain, tropomyosin, troponin I, and vimentin. In addition to direct transcriptional activation of a large number of muscle-specific genes that contain E-boxes, the MDFs indirectly control the expression of muscle genes lacking the E-box. This is accomplished by the activation of myocyte enhancer factor-2 (MEF-2), an intermediate transcription factor, by MyoD. MEF-2 in turn binds and activates muscle-specific genes, lacking the E-box.[451,452] MEF-2 furthermore cooperatively amplifies the muscle specific gene activation signal provided by MyoD.[452] Like MyoD, MEF-2 expression is an early embryonic event in myogenesis.[453] In this way, the MDFs can coordinately regulate the gene expression of many muscle specific genes.

At least two proteins of the HLH family act as negative regulators of myogenic differentiation by competing with the promyogenic MyoD. So-called Id-protein (inhibitor of differentiation) can interact with E-proteins or MDFs via its HLH domain. The resulting heterodimer is unable to bind and activate E-box myogenic promoters, because Id lacks the basic region of the MDFs.[454] When Id is downregulated in myoblasts grown in high serum medium, containing high concentrations of mitogens, the E-proteins become available for binding with MDFs, which subsequently activates muscle-gene transcription.[455] The second bHLH-inhibitor of myogenesis is called twist. Twist was shown to inhibit myogenesis by blocking DNA binding by MyoD, by titrating E-proteins, and by inhibiting trans-activation by MEF2.[456]

The interaction of MDFs with members of another group of transcription factors, the leucine zipper family, the c-Fos, c-Jun, and JunB proteins, can lead to inhibition of both MDF and leucine zipper protein-dependent transcriptional activation.[457] Because Fos and Jun promote cell cycling, and MDFs have the opposite effect, the interaction between the two different classes of transcription factors might determine whether myoblasts proliferate or differentiate.[458] The permanent withdrawal of differentiating myoblasts from the cell cycle requires the interaction of the bHLH myogenic factors with yet another molecule, the tumor suppressor retinoblastoma protein (pRB).[459]

Almost immediately after somite generation, myogenic cells adjacent to the dorsal neural tube, destined to differentiate into medial myotome components, activate muscle-specific MyoD regulatory genes.[36,460-463] These cells differentiate into axial muscle. On the other hand, cells destined to migrate into dorsal and ventral muscle-forming region of the limb bud express MyoD genes later.[36,462,463] Smooth and cardiac muscle do not express MyoD, although they share some common muscle specific genes. Vertebrate twist protein, although expressed in the developing somite, is excluded from the myotome.[456]

The exact role of each individual MDF and its interaction in muscle development remains to be determined. The function of many more myogenic regulators is being characterized.[463] The existence of four MDFs probably represents some redundancy. For example, genetically engineered mice lacking functional MyoD have normal muscle.[464] On the other hand, mice lacking Myf-5 die of respiratory failure, due to rib cage abnormalities,[465] and mice lacking both MyoD and Myf-5 die because contractile proteins are absent in muscle.[466]

Regulation of Muscle-Specific Isozymes and Contractile Proteins

The mRNA levels of some muscle specific isozymes, such as those of glycogen phosphorylase, CK, and aldolase, increase simultaneously, suggesting coordinate transcriptional activation.[82,467] However, other muscle-specific gene products display temporal differences in their appearance after the activation of the myogenic program and are thought to be transcribed noncoordinately.[468,469] Coordination could be accomplished by common, muscle-specific trans-acting factors.[470,471] The regulatory regions of muscle genes contain enhancers and promoters targeted by their respective transcription factors. Muscle-specific enhancers have been found in many structural and nonstructural genes.[472-475] The same is true for promoters.[476,477] However, a muscle-specific gene is usually not controlled by a single element; rather, multiple regulators act in concert and often a combination of ubiquitous as well as muscle-specific factors assist to activate the genes.[82,478] For example, the human cardiac α-actin gene requires the interaction among three elements and their respective transcriptional activators,[477] whereas the troponin I gene was shown to require a different set of transcription proteins.[479] The control elements can be grouped into different families, and one is targeted by the transcription factors of the HLH family. The mechanisms by which fiber type specific gene regulation is initiated are unknown, but fiber-type specific transcriptional enhancers are likely to be involved.[480]

Epigenetic Regulators of Muscle Development and Metabolism: Hormones and Growth Factors

When a variety of metabolic characteristics of skeletal muscle were tested in twin and nontwin siblings, genetic effects were found to account for only 25% to 50% of the total phenotypic metabolic variation.[481] A variety of hormones and growth factors affect muscle proliferation and differentiation and assist in the adaptation of muscle metabolism to environmental changes. These mediators can be classified into those acting primarily on the cellular level, such as insulin-like and fibroblast growth factor, and others affecting the whole organism, such as growth hormone, thyroid hormones, glucocorticosteroids, and insulin.[482] The literature is often difficult to interpret, since the agent under investigation can have different effects, depending on the animal or dosage analyzed. In vivo alterations of the hormone under investigation are often correlated with changes in the level of other hormones. Insulin deficiency, for example, is accompanied by decreased plasma concentrations of thyroxine and increased concentrations of glucocorticoids and glucagon.[428] Studies in some noninnervated cell culture systems have yielded opposing results and innervated culture systems have not been investigated extensively. Negative results of an agent in a noninnervated system do not rule out possible action in innervated muscle cultures. Growth hormone receptors, for example, can be detected on muscle cells only in nerve-muscle cocultures.[482]

Growth hormone (GH) is one of the main anabolic regulators of muscle. It was shown to enhance many parameters of muscle metabolism,[482] such as amino acid transport and protein synthesis.[483] GH increases fatty acid oxidation[484] and reduces glucose utilization in muscle,[485] partly by causing insulin resistance.[486] Consequently, glycogen accumulates in the muscle of acromegalic patients.[487] Many, if not all, of the effects of GH on the cellular level are mediated by the insulin-like growth factors IGF-I and IGF-II, somatomedins. These peptides are produced in the liver in response to GH[482] and perhaps in muscle itself in an autocrine fashion.[488] The IGFs have mitogenic properties, but can stimulate myoblast differentiation.[40,482,489,490] There are two distinct IGF receptors, each displaying significant cross-reactivity for the other IGF type.[482] The type I receptor, unlike the type II receptor, additionally binds insulin.[482] The IGF receptors and the insulin receptor are developmentally regulated.[370,491]

Insulin has anabolic properties on muscle protein by increasing protein synthesis at the translational level and by decreasing protein degradation.[428] Unlike liver, hypoinsulinemic conditions, such as nutrient deprivation and diabetes, but also infections, can lead to proteolysis in muscle,[492] although it is not yet clear whether endotoxin itself or other cytokines are responsible for the protein catabolism during infections and septicemia.[428]

Thyroid hormone (T_4 and the more active T_3) promotes differentiation as well as satellite cell proliferation.[493] T_3 binding to a cytosolic receptor augments MyoD expression and directly targets the contractile protein genes[494] to induce fast MHC expression in slow fibers[494] and the synthesis of myosin ATPase.[495] In hypothyroidism the shortening time of muscle is prolonged.[496] In contrast, excessive amounts of T_3, as seen in thyrotoxicosis, act catabolically for proteins and carbohydrates.[496] The gene activation properties of the T_3 receptor complex are relatively inefficient, but are sharply enhanced by association with retinoid receptors.[494] Vitamin A deficiency or treatment with retinoid derivatives can therefore be teratogenic for muscle.[494,497] T_3 also regulates muscle capillarization and the expression of NCAM,[498] and augments protein synthesis, glycolytic activity, and amino acid[428] and carbohydrate transport. Furthermore, T_3 was shown to promote insulin resistance.[482,494,499–502] T_3 increases oxygen metabolism, since it is a major regulator of mitochondrial biogenesis and metabolism. Recently, an intramitochondrial factor with T_3-binding activity has been discovered.[503] It has been suggested that this protein might act as a T_3-dependent intramitochondrial transcription factor.[503]

Glucocorticosteroids are catabolic to muscle in vivo by increasing protein degradation at early stages after administration. At later stages and at higher doses they decrease amino acid transport and protein synthesis,[482,496] an effect that can be mitigated by physical activity.[504] Glucocorticoid action on carbohydrate metabolism, reducing glycogen phosphorylase and increasing glycogen synthetase activity, may largely be indirectly mediated by causing insulin resistance in muscle.[428,496] The glucocorticoid effects are more pronounced in type II as compared to type I fibers, since the former have a lesser ability to compensate for the loss in glycolytic energy metabolism by the relatively unimpaired oxidative phosphorylation.[428,496] Unlike their catabolic action in vivo, glucocorticoids have been reported to enhance proliferation and differentiation of cultured myoblasts, upregulate muscular IGF receptors,[482,505,506] and stimulate enzymatic activities, such as CK.[506] Adrenocorticotropin (ACTH) may have direct effects on muscle, regardless of its glucosteroid properties. For example, ACTH has mitogenic properties for satellite cells in tissue culture[29,507] and intramuscular ACTH application can lead to damaging fat deposition.[496] Therefore, an excess of ACTH may be myopathic by itself.[496] The steroid testosterone has its own cytoplasmic receptor in muscle,[508] but part of its anabolic action might be mediated by stimulating GH release from the pituitary gland.[509] The anabolic mechanism of estrogens has not been delineated.[482]

Various other peptide growth factors have been shown to influence myoblast differentiation at the cellular level. Members of the fibroblast growth factor (FGF) family,[489,510] platelet-derived growth factor (PDGF),[137,511] and transforming growth factor-β (TGF-β)[510] antagonize myoblast differentiation but stimulate satellite cell proliferation.[21,29] Both FGFs and TGF-β generally repress the transcription of MyoD;[512] the former may additionally regulate MDF function through a protein kinase C–dependent phosphorylation of its DNA binding domain[510] or by enhancing an MDF inhibitor, interacting stoichiometrically with the MDFs themselves, or with one of the MDF heterodimer partners[489,513] (see Chapter 20).

Muscle Regeneration and Gene Therapy

Muscle satellite cells are the only source of myogenic cells for adult muscle regeneration. Injured or lost muscle can be replaced only by proliferation and differentiation of this cellular compartment. After muscle damage has occurred, cellular debris is removed by macrophages; satellite cells leave their normal resting state (G_0) and enter the cell cycle. Satellite cells can be viewed as stem cells, fulfilling the three essential criteria of proliferation, production of specialized progeny, and self-maintenance.[514] Several experimental strategies have been employed to study muscle regeneration in vivo. The most selective method is to inject the muscle with bupivacaine hydrochloride (Marcaine), a local anesthetic that effectively kills myofibers without adversely affecting the proliferation of satellite cells.[515] The nerve and blood supply remain intact. Even after repeated injections of this agent, multiple cycles of regeneration can ensue, without depleting the satellite cell population.[516,517]

After injury, dormant myogenic cells become activated, start to express MDFs,[518] and initiate proliferation within 24 hours.[29] During divisions, the satellite cells appear to remain beneath the basal lamina. With fusion of the progeny, the original fiber is restored, MDF expression is downregulated,[518] and the satellite cells become quiescent. Likewise, when muscle tissue is trypsinized and placed in a culture dish, satellite cells begin to proliferate. The population doubling potential of satellite cells is, like all normal diploid cells, limited by senescence, although enormous. The adult muscle satellite cell can replicate 25 to 30 times, giving rise to >10^8 progeny (i.e., 27 divisions), whereas the fetal muscle cell can proliferate 60 to 70 times.[519,520] However, even this huge proliferative reservoir can become exhausted in cases of extensive muscle regeneration, such as in Duchenne's muscular dystrophy. Studies of cultured satellite cells from patients with muscular dystrophy clearly demonstrated a reduced number of doublings.[521]

Metabolic studies of skeletal muscle regeneration suggest an elimination of mitochondrial oxidative metabolism and, concomitant with DNA synthesis, an increase in pentose monophosphate shunt activity, as suggested by enhanced glucose-6-phosphate dehydrogenase (G6PD) and 6-phosphogluconate dehydrogenase.[522] Examining muscle homogenates, it has been suggested that glycolysis provides the necessary energy to support the subsequent regeneration processes, based on increased LDH activity.[523] On the other land, activities of glycogen synthetase, phosphorylase, PFK, and aldolase were found to be reduced.[524] Regenerating fibers are rich in RNA content, which is the basis of their basophilic reaction with the hematoxylin and eosin (H&E) stain. Muscle regeneration or atrophy, whether myogenic or neurogenic in origin,[525] is accompanied by a qualitative shift toward the fetal isozyme pattern, as detailed above for individual enzymes, such as LDH, CK, and aldolase, similar to that in cultures.

Understanding muscle differentiation has direct implications for the development of therapies to treat patients with a variety of genetic muscle diseases, such as inherited defects in muscle-specific isozymes or Duchenne's muscular dystrophy.[526,527] One treatment approach, myoblast transfer, involves the injection of normal allogenic or autologous myoblasts. Myoblasts can be expanded and genetically altered ex vivo, to replace a defective gene.[526,528,529] After injection the myoblasts disperse longitudinally and transversely within the muscle over considerable distances from the injection site and to add new functional nuclei to the defective muscle fiber,[29,528,530] but in practice still remain relatively localized (vide infra).[526] Myoblast transfer may require muscle regeneration following a mechanical lesion, especially with the use of adult, instead of neonatal, cells.[531] Other systems to deliver genetic material are viruses, liposomes,[532] and direct injection of naked DNA plasmids that are, for unknown reasons, preferentially taken up by heart and skeletal muscle.[529] Myoblasts are under investigation in the treatment of nonmuscle diseases. They can be designed to deliver a missing gene product, for example, growth hormone, clotting factors, or erythropoietin, into the circulatory system.[527,533] The genetically engineered myoblasts are expected to undergo terminal differentiation and become postmitotic at the site of administration, and this could prevent problems with tissue regeneration and transgene loss.

However, gene therapy still encounters a variety of technical difficulties. Retroviral vectors require DNA replication for insertion into genomic DNA and are unable to transduce terminally differentiated cells, such as myofibers. Adenoviral vectors lack sufficient numbers of receptors on differentiated muscle cells and may have the potential of infecting the germ line.[534,535] Furthermore, myoblasts and adenoviruses are immunogenic, which could lead to rejection or prevent repeated administration.[528,535] Retro- and adenoviral vectors can carry about 7 kb of genetic information,[535] but are not able to accommodate larger genes, like the dystrophin gene, whose product is absent in Duchenne's muscular dystrophy. In most diseases, the system of gene delivery must provide a mechanism of gene regulation, and strategies are being developed to achieve this requirement.[536,537] After myoblast fusion, the new gene product may remain in close spatial association with the newly transferred myonucleus where it is produced and may not migrate into other fiber areas. Such "territoriality" has been demonstrated for a variety of muscle proteins and organelles.[538] Despite all the difficulties, gene therapy is likely to belong to the therapeutic repertoire of the physician in the treatment of inherited muscle disorders in the future.

Acknowledgment. The authors thank Dr. M. Davidson and Dr. S. DiMauro for their critical review of the manuscript. This work was supported by the Deutscher Akademischer Austauschdienst (DAAD), the Muscular Dystrophy Association, and by National Institutes of Health grants HD 32062-02 and NS 11766-21.

References

1. Kato K, Gurdon JB. Single-cell transplantation determines the time when *Xenopus* muscle precursor cells acquire a capacity for autonomous differentiation. Proc Natl Acad Sci USA 1993;90:1310–1314.
2. Davis RL, Weintraub H, Lassar AB. Expression of a single transfected cDNA converts fibroblasts to myoblasts. Cell 1987;51:987–1000.
3. Wright WE, Sassoon DA, Lin VK. Myogenin, a factor regulating myogenesis has a domain homologous to MyoD. Cell 1989;56:607–617.
4. Braun T, Arnold HH. The four human muscle regulatory helix-loop-helix proteins Myf3-Myf6 exhibit similar hetero-dimerization and DNA binding properties. Nucleic Acids Res 1991;19:5645–5651.
5. Braun T, Bober E, Winter B, et al. Myf-6, a new member of the human gene family of myogenic determination factors: evidence for a gene cluster on chromosome 12. EMBO J 1990;9:821–831.
6. Przybylski RJ, Blumberg JM. Ultrastructural aspects of myogenesis in the chick. Lab Invest 1966;15:836–863.
7. Moss PS, Strohman RC. Myosin synthesis by fusion-arrested chick embryo myoblasts in cell culture. Dev Biol 1976;48:431–437.
8. Larson PF, Jenkison M, Hudgson P. The morphological development of chick embryo skeletal muscle grown in tissue culture as studied by electron microscopy. J Neurol Sci 1970;10:385–405.
9. Franzini-Armstrong C. The sarcoplasmic reticulum and the transverse tubules. In: Engel AG, Franzini-Armstrong C, eds. Myology. 2nd ed. New York: McGraw-Hill, 1994: 176–199.
10. Harris J, Duxson MJ, Fitzsimons RB, Rieger F. Myonuclear birthdate distinguish the origins of primary and secondary myotubes in embryonic mammalian skeletal muscles. Development 1989;107:771–789.
11. Miller JB, Crow MT, Stockdale FE. Slow and fast myosin heavy chain content defines three types of myotubes in early muscle cell cultures. J Cell Biol 1985;101:1643–1650.
12. Ross J, Duxson M, Harris A. Formation of primary and secondary myotubes in rat lumbrical muscles. Development 1987;100:383–394.
13. Pin CL, Merrifield PA. Embryonic and fetal rat myoblasts express different phenotypes following differentiation in vitro. Dev Genet 1993;14:356–368.
14. Bischoff R. The satellite cell and muscle regeneration. In: Engel AG, Franzini-Armstrong C, eds. Myology. 2nd ed. New York: McGraw-Hill, 1994:97–118.
15. Appell HJ, Forsberg S, Hollmann W. Satellite cell activation in human skeletal muscle after training: evidence for muscle fiber neoformation. Int J Sports Med 1988;9:297–299.
16. Schultz E. Satellite cell proliferative compartments in growing skeletal muscles. Dev Biol 1996;175:84–94.
17. Hurko O, Walsh FS. Human fetal muscle-specific antigen is restricted to regenerating myofibers of diseased adult muscle. Neurology 1983;33:737–743.
18. Armand O, Boutineau AM, Manger A, et al. Origin of satellite cells in avian skeletal muscles. Arch Anat Micr 1983;72:163–181.
19. Chevallier A, Pauto MP, Harris AJ, Kieny M. On the non-equivalence of skeletal muscle satellite cells and embryonic myoblasts. Arch Anat Micr 1987;75:161–166.
20. Stockdale FE. Myogenic cell lineages. Dev Biol 1992; 154:284–298.
21. Yablonka-Reuveni Z. Development and postnatal regulation of adult myoblast. Microsc Res Tech 1995;30:366–380.
22. Senni MI, Castrignano F, Poiana G, et al. Expression of adult fast pattern of acetylcholinesterase molecular forms by mouse satellite cells in culture. Differentiation 1987; 36:194–198.
23. Vivarelli E, Brown WE, Whalen RG, Cossu G. The experience of slow myosin during mammalian somitogenesis and limb bud differentiation. J Cell Biol 1988;107:2191–2197.
24. Hartley RS, Yablonka-Reuveni Z. Temporal differences in myosin heavy chain expression between descendents of satellite cells and embryonic myoblasts in vitro. J Cell Biol 1989;109:261a.
25. Peterson CA, Cho M, Rastinejad F, Blau HM. Beta-enolase is a marker of human myoblast heterogeneity prior to differentiation. Dev Biol 1992;151:626–629.
26. Barbieri G, De Angelis L, Feo S. et al. Differential expression of muscle-specific enolase in embryonic and fetal myogenic cells during mouse development. Differentiation 1990;45:179–184.
27. Yablonka-Reuveni Z, Nameroff M. Temporal differences in desmin expression between myoblasts from embryonic and adult chicken skeletal muscle. Differentiation 1990; 45:21–28.
28. Seed J, Hauschka SD. Clonal analysis of vertebrate myogenesis. VIII. Fibroblast growth factor (FGF)-dependent and FGF-independent muscle colony types during chick wing development. Dev Biol 1988;128:40–49.
29. Schultz E, McCormick KM. Skeletal muscle satellite cells. Rev Physiol Biochem Pharmacol 1994;123:213–257.
30. Hartley RS, Bandman E, Yablonka-Reuveni Z. Skeletal muscle satellite cells appear during late chicken embryogenesis. Dev Biol 1992;153:206–216.
31. Feldman JL, Stockdale FE. Temporal appearance of satellite cells during myogenesis. Dev Biol 1992;153:217–226.
32. Hoh JFY, Hughes S, Hugh G, Pozgaj I. Three hierarchies in skeletal muscle fiber classification: allotype, isotype and phenotype. In: Kedes LH, Stockdale FE, eds. Cellular and molecular biology of muscle development. New York: Alan R. Liss, 1989:15–26.

33. Porter JD, Baker RS. Muscles of a different "color": the unusual properties of the extraocular muscles may predispose or protect them in neurogenic and myogenic disease. Neurology 1996;46:30–37.
34. Tam SK, Gu W, Mahdavi V, Nadal-Ginard B. Cardiac myocyte terminal differentiation. Potential for cardiac regeneration. Ann N Y Acad Sci 1995;752:72–79.
35. Brodsky WY, Arefyeva AM, Uryvaeva IV. Mitotic polyploidization of mouse heart myocytes during the first postnatal week. Cell Tissue Res 1980;210:133–144.
36. Sassoon DA. Myogenic regulatory factors: dissecting their role and regulation during vertebrate embryogenesis. Dev Biol 1993;156:11–23.
37. Wachtler F, Christ B. The basic embryology of skeletal muscle formation in vertebrates: the avian model. Semin Dev Biol 1992;3:217–227.
38. Johnston MC, Noden DM, Hazelton RD, et al. Origins of avian ocular and periocular tissues. Exp Eye Res 1979;19:27–43.
39. Gearhart JD, Mintz B. Clonal origins of somites and their muscle derivatives: evidence from allophenic mice. Dev Biol 1972;29:27–37.
40. Allen RE, Boxhorn LA. Regulation of skeletal muscle satellite cell proliferation and differentiation by transforming growth factor-beta, insulin-like growth factor 1 and fibroblast growth factor. J Cell Physiol 1989;138:311–315.
41. Rutz R, Haney C, Hauschka SD. Spatial analysis of limb bud myogenesis: a proximodistal gradient of muscle colony-forming cells in chick embryo-leg buds. Dev Biol 1982;90:399–411.
42. Rong PM, Teillet MA, Ziller C, LeDouarin NM. The neural tube/notochord complex is necessary for vertebral, but not limb and body wall striated muscle differentiation. Development 1992;115:657–672.
43. Hauschka SD. Clonal analysis of vertebrate myogenesis: 3. Developmental changes in the muscle-colony-forming cells of the human fetal limb. Dev Biol 1974;37:345–368.
44. Bridge DT, Allbrook D. Growth of striated muscle in an Australian marsupial (*Setonix brachyurus*). J Anat 1970;106:285–295.
45. Williams PE, Goldspink G. Longitudinal growth of striated muscle fibers. J Cell Sci 1971;9:751–767.
46. Oguni M, Setogawa T, Matsui H, et al. Timing and sequence of the events in the development of extraocular muscles in staged human embryos: ultrastructural and histochemical study. Acta Anat 1992;143:195–198.
47. Montgomery RD. Growth of human striated muscle. Nature 1962;195:194–195.
48. Adams RD, de Reuck J. Metrics of muscle. In: Kakulas BA, ed. Basic research in myology. International Congress, Proc. second Intl. Congr. on Muscle Diseases. Amsterdam: Excerpta Medica, 1973:3–11.
49. Brooke MH, Engel WK. The histographic analysis of human muscle biopsies with regard to fiber types. 4. Children's biopsies. Neurology 1969;19:591–605.
50. Brooke MH, Engel WK. The histographic analysis of human muscle biopsies with regard to fiber types. 1. Adult male and female. Neurology 1969;19:221–233.
51. Ontell M, Dunn RF. Neonatal muscle growth. A quantitative study. Am J Anat 1978;152:539–555.
52. Ontell M, Kozeka K. Organogenesis of the mouse extensor digitorum longus muscle: a quantitative study. Am J Anat 1984;171:149–161.
53. McCormick KM, Schultz E. Mechanisms of nascent fiber formation during avian skeletal muscle hypertrophy. Dev Biol 1992;150:319–334.
54. Schiaffino S, Bormioli SP, Aloisi M. The fate of newly formed satellite cells during compensatory muscle hypertrophy. Virchows Arch 1976;21:113–118.
55. Schultz E, Darr KC, Macius A. Acute effects of hindlimb unweighting on satellite cells of growing skeletal muscle. J Appl Physiol 1994;76:266–270.
56. Darr KC, Schultz E. Exercise-induced satellite cell activation in growing and mature skeletal muscle. J Appl Physiol 1987;63:1816–1821.
57. Ranvier L. De quelques faits relatifs à l'histologie et à la physiologie des muscles striés. In: Brown-Séquard CE, Charcot JM, Vulpian AA, eds. Archives de physiologie normale et pathologique. 2nd ed. Paris: G. Masson, 1874:1–5.
58. Pette D, Staron RS. Cellular and molecular diversities of mammalian skeletal muscle fibers. Rev Physiol Biochem Pharmacol 1990;116:1–76.
59. Guth L, Samaha FJ. Qualitative differences between actomyosin ATPase of slow and fast mammalian muscle. Exp Neurol 1969;25:138–152.
60. Brooke MH, Kaiser KK. Three "myosin adenosine triphosphatase" systems. The nature of their pH lability and sulfhydryl dependence. J Histochem Cytochem 1970;18:670–672.
61. Nakamura A, Sreter F, Gergely J. Comparative studies of light meromyosin paracrystals derived from red, white, and cardiac muscle myosins. J Cell Biol 1971;49:883–898.
62. Arndt I, Pepe F. Antigenic specificity of red and white muscle myosins. J Histochem Cytochem 1975;23:159–168.
63. Colling-Saltin AS. Enzyme histochemistry on skeletal muscle of the human foetus. J Neurol Sci 1978;39:169–185.
64. Dubowitz V. Enzymatic maturation of skeletal muscle. Nature 1963;197:1215.
65. Dubowitz V. Enzyme histochemistry of developing human muscle. Nature 1966;211:884–885.
66. Farkas-Bargeton E, Diebler MF, Arsenio-Nunes ML, et al. Etude de la maturation histochimique, quantitative et ultrastructurale du muscle foetal humaine. J Neurol Sci 1977;31:245–260.
67. Kelly AM, Rubinstein NA. The diversity of muscle fiber types and its origin during development. In: Engel AG, Franzini-Armstrong C, eds. Myology. 2nd ed. New York: McGraw-Hill, 1994:119–133.
68. Bandman E. Contractile protein isoforms in muscle development. Dev Biol 1992;154:273–283.
69. Craig R. The structure of the contractile filaments. In: Engel AG, Franzini-Armstrong C, eds. Myology. 2nd ed. New York: McGraw-Hill, 1994:134–175.
70. Pette D, Vrbova G. Neural control of phenotypic expression in mammalian muscle fibers. Muscle Nerve 1985;8:676–689.

71. Potter JD. The content of troponin, tropomyosin, actin, and myosin in rabbit skeletal muscle myofibrils. Arch Biochem Biophys 1974;162:436–441.
72. Hoh JFY, Yeoh GPS. Rabbit skeletal myosin isoenzymes from fetal, fast-twitch and slow-twitch muscles. Nature 1979;280:321–322.
73. Lyons GE, Haselgrove J, Kelly AM, Rubinstein NA. Myosin transitions in developing fast and slow muscles of the rat hindlimb. Differentiation 1983;25:168–175.
74. Sreter FA, Balint M, Gergely J. Structural and functional changes of myosin during development. Comparison with adult fast, slow and cardiac myosin. Dev Biol 1975;46:317–325.
75. Whalen RG, Sell SM, Butler-Browne GS, et al. Three myosin heavy-chain isoenzymes appear sequentially in rat muscle development. Nature 1981;292:805–809.
76. Harris AJ, Fitzsimons RB, McEwan JC. Neural control of the sequence of expression of myosin heavy chain isoforms in foetal mammalian muscles. Development 1989;107:751–769.
77. Devlin RB, Emerson CP Jr. Coordinate regulation of contractile protein synthesis during myoblast differentiation. Cell 1978;13:599–611.
78. Gauthier GF, Lowey S. Distribution of myosin isoenzymes among skeletal muscle fibre types. J Cell Biol 1979;81:10–25.
79. Pierobon-Bormioli S, Sartore S, Dalla Libera L, et al. "Fast" isomyosins and fiber types in mammalian skeletal muscle. J Histochem Cytochem 1981;29:1179–1188.
80. Gauthier GF, Burke RE, Lowey S, Hobbs AW. Myosin isozymes in normal and cross-reinnervated cat skeletal muscle fibers. J Cell Biol 1982;92:471–484.
81. Whalen RG, Butler-Browne GS, Gros F. Protein synthesis and actin heterogeneity in calf muscle cells in culture. Proc Natl Acad Sci USA 1976;73:2018–2022.
82. Devlin RB, Emerson CP Jr. Coordinate accumulation of contractile protein mRNAs during myoblast differentiation. Dev Biol 1979;69:202–216.
83. Pittenger MF, Kazzaz JA, Helfman DM. Functional properties of non-muscle tropomyosin isoforms. Curr Opin Cell Biol 1994;6:96–104.
84. Nadal-Ginard B. Muscle cell differentiation and alternative splicing. Curr Opin Cell Biol 1990;2:1058–1064.
85. Perry SV. Activation of the contractile mechanism by calcium. In: Engel AG, Franzini-Armstrong C, eds. Myology. 2nd ed. New York: McGraw-Hill, 1994;529–552.
86. Reinach FC, Masaki T, Shafiq S, et al. Isoforms of C-protein in adult chicken skeletal muscle. Detection with monoclonal antibodies. J Cell Biol 1982;95:78–84.
87. Dhoot GD, Perry SV. Distribution of polymorphic forms of troponin components and tropomyosin in skeletal muscle. Nature 1979;278:714–718.
88. Zhu L, Lyons GE, Juhasz O, et al. Developmental regulation of troponin I isoform genes in striated muscles of transgenic mice. Dev Biol 1995;169:487–503.
89. Schiaffino S, Gorza L, Sartore S, et al. Embryonic myosin heavy chain as a differentiation marker of developing human skeletal muscle and rhabdomyosarcoma. Exp Cell Res 1986;163:211–220.
90. Kugelberg E. Histochemical composition, contraction speed and fatigability of rat soleus motor units. J Neurol Sci 1973;20:177–198.
91. Nemeth P, Pette D, Vrbova G. Comparison of enzyme activities among single muscle fibers within defined motor units. J Physio 1985;311:489–495.
92. Jansen JKS, Fladby T. The perinatal reorganization of the innervation of skeletal muscle in mammals. Progr Neurobiol 1990;34:39–90.
93. Fidzianska A. Human ontogenesis II. Development of the human neuromuscular junction. J Neuropathol Exp Neurol 1989;39:606–615.
94. Kleimann RJ, Reichardt LF. Testing the agrin hypothesis. Cell 1996;85:461–464.
95. Covault J, Sanes JR. Distribution of N-CAM in synaptic and extrasynaptic portions of developing and adult skeletal muscle. J Cell Biol 1986;102:716–730.
96. Larson PF, Park DC. Creatine kinase activity in the umbilical cord blood of aborted fetuses. J Neurol Sci 1974;23:33–36.
97. Mumenthaler M, Engel WK. Cytological localization of cholinesterase in developing chick embryo skeletal muscle. Acta Anat 1961;47:274–284.
98. Tennyson VM, Brzin M, Slotwiner P. The appearance of acetylcholine esterase in the myotome of the embryonic rabbit: an electron microscope cytochemical and biochemical study. J Cell Biol 1971;51:703–721.
99. Grubic Z, Komel R, Walker WF, Miranda A. Myoblast fusion and innervation with rat motor nerve alter distribution of acetylcholinesterase and its mRNA in cultures of human muscle. Neuron 1995;14:317–327.
100. Corriveau RA, Romano SJ, Conroy WG, et al. Expression of neuronal acetylcholine receptor genes in vertebrate skeletal muscle during development. J Neurosci 1995;15:1372–1383.
101. Houenou LJ, Li L, Lo AC, Yan Q, Oppenheim RW. Naturally occurring and axotomy-induced motoneuron death and its prevention by neurotrophic agents: a comparison between chick and mouse. Prog Brain Res 1994;102:217–226.
102. Oppenheim RW, Prevette D, Tytell M, Homma S. Naturally occurring and induced neuronal death in the chick embryo in vivo requires protein and RNA synthesis: evidence for the role of cell death genes. Dev Biol 1990;138:104–113.
103. Purves D, Lichtman JW, Elimination of synapses in the developing nervous system. Science 1980;210:153–157.
104. Jansen JKS, Van Essen DC, Brown MC. Formation and elimination of synapses in skeletal muscle of rat. Cold Spring Harbor Symp Quant Biol 1975;40:425–434.
105. Riley DA. Ultrastructural evidence for axon retraction during the spontaneous elimination of polyneuronal innervation of rat skeletal muscle. J Neurocytol 1981;10:425–440.
106. Fladby T, Jansen JK. Development of homogeneous fast and slow motor units in the neonatal mouse soleus muscle. Development 1990;109:723–732.
107. Korneliussen H, Jansen JKS. Morphological aspects of the elimination of polyneuronal innervation of skeletal

muscle fibers in new-born rats. J Neurocytol 1976;5:591–604.
108. Dennis MJ, Ziskind-Conhaim L, Harris AJ. Development of neuromuscular junctions in rat embryos. Dev Biol 1981;81:266–279.
109. Buller AJ, Eccles JC, Eccles RM. Differentiation of fast and slow muscles in the cat hindlimb. J Physiol 1960;150:399–416.
110. Stockdale FE, Miller JB. The cellular basis of myosin heavy chain isoform expression during development of avian skeletal muscles. Dev Biol 1987;123:1–9.
111. DiMario JX, Fernyak SE, Stockdale FE. Myoblasts transferred to limbs of embryos are committed to specific fiber fates. Nature 1993;362:165–167.
112. Miller JB, Stockdale FE. Developmental origins of skeletal muscle fibers: clonal analysis of myogenic cell lineages based on expression of fast and slow myosin heavy chains. Proc Natl Acad Sci USA 1986;83:3860–3864.
113. Cho M, Webster SG, Blau HM. Evidence for myoblast-extrinsic regulation of slow myosin heavy chain expression during muscle fiber formation in embryonic development. J Cell Biol 1993;121:795–810.
114. Kelly AM, Rubinstein NA. Development of neuromuscular specialization. Med Sci Sports Exerc 1986;18:292–298.
115. Shellswell GB. The formation of discrete muscles from the chick wing dorsal and ventral muscle masses in the absence of nerves. J Embryol Exp Morphol 1977;41:269–277.
116. Butler J, Cosmos E, Brierley J. Differentiation of muscle fiber types in aneurogenic brachial muscles of the chick embryo. J Exp Zool 1982;224:65–80.
117. Laing N, Lamb A. The distribution of muscle-fiber types in chick embryo wings transplanted to the pelvic region is normal. J Embryol Exp Morphol 1983;78:67–82.
118. Jacob HJ, Christ B, Grim M. Problems of muscle pattern formation and of neuromuscular relations in avian limb development. In: Kelley RO, Geotinck PF, MacCabe JA, eds. Limb development and regeneration. New York: Alan Liss, 1983:334–341.
119. Barker D, Banks RW. The muscle spindle. In: Engel AG, Franzini-Armstrong C, eds. Myology. 2nd ed. New York: McGraw-Hill, 1994:333–360.
120. Sanes JR. The extracellular matrix. In: Engel AG, Franzini-Armstrong C, eds. Myology. 2nd ed. New York: McGraw-Hill, 1994:242–260.
121. Paulsson M. Basement membrane proteins: structure, assembly, and cellular interactions. Crit Rev Biochem Mol Biol 1992;27:93–127.
122. Grim M. Control of muscle morphogenesis and endplate pattern in limb muscles of avian chimeras. In: Hinchliffe JR, Hurle JM, Summerbell D, eds. Developmental patterning of the vertebrate limb. New York: Plenum Press, 1992:293–297.
123. Grim M, Wachtler F. Muscle morphogenesis in the absence of myogenic cells. Anat Embryol 1991;183:67–70.
124. Pautou MP, Hedayat I, Kieny M. The pattern of muscle development in the chick leg. Arch Anat Microsc Morphol Exp 1982;71:193–206.
125. Schroeter S, Tosney KW. Ultrasound and morphometric analysis of the separation of two thigh muscles in the chick. Am J Anat 1991;191:351–368.
126. Schroeter S, Tosney KW. Spatial and temporal patterns of muscle cleavage in the chick thigh and their value as criteria for homology. Am J Anat 1991;191:325–350.
127. Fernandez MS, Dennis JE, Durshel RF, et al. The dynamics of compartmentalization of embryonic muscle by extracellular matrix molecules. Dev Biol 1991;147:46–61.
128. Kuhl U, Ocalan M, Timpl R, Van der Mark K. Synthesis of type IV collagen and laminin in cultures of skeletal muscle and their assembly on the surface of myotubes. Dev Biol 1982;93:344–354.
129. Nusgnes B, Delain D, Senechal H, et al. Metabolic changes in the extracellular matrix during differentiation of myoblasts of the L6 line and of a Myo- non-fusing mutant. Exp Cell Res 1986;162:51–62.
130. Dejana E, Colella S, Conforti G, et al. Fibronectin and vitronectin regulate the organization of their respective Arg-Gly-Asp receptors in cultured human epithelia cells. J Cell Biol 1988;107:1215–1223.
131. Roman J, LaChance RM, Broekelmann TJ, et al. The fibronectin receptor is organized by extracellular matrix fibronectin: implications for oncogenic transformation and for cell recognition of fibronectin matrices. J Cell Biol 1989:108:2529–2543.
132. Martin GR, Timpl R. Laminin and other basement membrane components. Annu Rev Cell Biol 1987;3:57–85.
133. Menko As, Boettiger D. Occupation of the cellular matrix receptor, integrin, is a control point for myogenic differentiation. Cell 1987;51:51–57.
134. Duband J-L, Belkin AM, Syfrig J, et al. Expression of alpha 1 integrin, a laminin-collagen receptor, during myogenesis and neurogenesis in the avian embryo. Development 1992;116:585–600.
135. Ocalan M, Goodman SL, Kuhl U, et al. Laminin alters cell shape and stimulates mobility and proliferation of murine skeletal myoblasts. Dev Biol 1988;125:158–167.
136. Foster RF, Thompson JM, Kaufmann SJ. A laminin substrate promotes myogenesis in rat skeletal muscle cultures: analysis of replication and development using antidesmin and anti-BrdUrd monoclonal antibodies. Dev Biol 1987;122;11–20.
137. Yablonka-Reuveni Z, Bowen-Pope DF, Harley RS. Proliferation and differentiation of myoblasts: the role of platelet derived growth factor and the basement membrane. In: Pette D, ed. The Dynamic state of muscle-fibres. Berlin: Walter de Gruyter, 1990:693–706.
138. Podleski TR, Greenberg I, Schlessinger J, Yamada KM. Fibronectin delays the fusion of L6 myoblasts. Exp Cell Res 1979;122:317–326.
139. Kujawa MJ, Pechak DG, Fiszman MY, Caplan AI. Hyaluronic acid bonded to cell culture surfaces inhibits the program of myogenesis. Dev Biol 1986;113:10–16.
140. Cifuentes-Diaz C, Nicolet M, Goudou D, et al. N-cadherin and N-CAM-mediated adhesion in development and regeneration of skeletal muscle. Neuromusc Disord 1993;3:361–365.
141. Knudsen K, Myers L, McElwee S. A role for the Ca^{2+}-dependent adhesion molecule, N-cadherin, in myoblast interaction during myogenesis. Exp Cell Res 1990;188:175–184.

142. Dickson G, Peck D, Moore SE, et al. Enhanced myogenesis in NCAM-transfected mouse myoblasts. Nature 1990;344:348–351.
143. Duband JL, Dufour S, Hatta K, et al. Adhesion molecules during somitogenesis in the avian embyro. J Cell Biol 1987;104:1361–1374.
144. Thompson J, Dickson G, Moore SE, et al. Alternative splicing of the neural cell adhesion molecule gene generates variant extracellular domain structure in skeletal muscle and brain. Genes Dev 1989;3:348–357.
145. Walsh FS, Dickson G. Generation of multiple N-CAM polypeptides from a single gene. Bioessays 1989;11:83–88.
146. Rafuse VE, Landmesser L. Contractile activity regulates isoform expression and polysialylation of NCAM in cultured myotubes: involvement of Ca^{2+} and protein kinase C. J Cell Biol 1996;132:969–983.
147. Fredette B, Rutishauser U, Landmesser L. Regulation and activity-dependence of N-cadherin, NCAM isoforms, and polysialic acid on chick myotubes during development. J Cell Biol 1993;123:1867–1888.
148. Andersson AM, Olsen M, Zhernosekov D, et al. Age-related changes in expression of the neural cell adhesion molecule in skeletal muscle: a comparative study of newborn, adult and aged rats. Biochem J 1993;290:641–648.
149. Doherty P, Fruns M, Seaton P, et al. A threshold effect of the major isoforms of NCAM on neurite outgrowth. Nature 1990;343:464–466.
150. Grumet M, Rutishauser U, Edelman GM. Neural cell adhesion molecule is on embryonic muscle cells and mediates adhesion to nerve cells in vitro. Nature 1982;295:693–695.
151. Hirano S, Nose A, Hatta K, et al. Calcium-dependent cell-cell adhesion molecules (cadherins): sub-class specificities and possible involvement of actin bundles. J Cell Biol 1987;105:2501–2510.
152. Knudsen KA. Cell adhesion molecules in myogenesis. Curr Opin Cell Biol 1990;2:902–906.
153. Doherty P, Rowett LH, Moore SE. Neurite outgrowth in response to transfected N-CAM and N-cadherin reveals fundamental differences in neuronal responsiveness to CAMs. Neuron 1991;6:247–258.
154. Horwitz A, Duggan K, Greggs R, et al. The cell substrate attachment (CSAT) antigen has properties of a receptor for laminin and fibronectin. J Cell Biol 1985;101:2134–2144.
155. Horwitz A, Duggan K, Buck C, et al. Interaction of plasma membrane fibronectin receptor with talin-a transmembrane linkage. Nature 1986;320:531–533.
156. Albeda SM, Buck CA. Integrins and other cell adhesion molecules. FASEB J 1990;4:2868–2880.
157. Rosen GD, Sanes JR, LaChance R, et al. Roles for the integrin VLA-4 and its counter receptor VCAM-1 in myogenesis. Cell 1992;69:1107–1119.
158. Sheppard AM, Onken MD, Rosen GD, et al. Expanding roles for alpha 4 integrin and its ligands in development. Cell Adhes Commun 1994;2:27–43.
159. Dean DC, Iademarco MF, Rosen GD, Sheppard AM. The integrin alpha 4 beta 1 and its counter receptor VCAM-1 in development and immune function. Am Rev Respir Dis 1993;148:S43–S46.
160. Jafredo T, Horwitz AF, Buck CA, et al. Myoblast migration specifically inhibited in the chick embryo by grafted CSAT hybridoma cells secreting anti-integrin antibody. Development 1988;103:431–446.
161. Honda H, Rostami A. Expression of major histocompatibility complex class I antigens in rat muscle cultures: the possible developmental role in myogenesis. Proc Natl Acad Sci USA 1989;86:7007–7011.
162. Cryer A, Jones HM. Developmental changes in the activity of lipoprotein lipase in rat lung, cardiac muscle, skeletal muscle and brown adipose tissue. Biochem J 1978;174:447–451.
163. Hardiman O, Faustman D, Li X, et al. Expression of major histocompatibility complex antigens in cultures of clonally derived human myoblasts. Neurology 1993;43:604–608.
164. Hohlfeld R, Engel AG. Induction of HLA-DR expression on human myoblasts with interferon-gamma. Am J Pathol 1990;136:503–508.
165. Goebels N, Michaelis D, Wekerle H, Hohlfeld R. Human myoblasts as antigen-presenting cells. J Immunol 1992;149:661–667.
166. Cifuentes-Diaz C, Delaporte C, Dautreaux B, et al. Class II MHC antigens in normal human skeletal muscle. Muscle Nerve 1992;15:295–302.
167. Karpati G, Pouliot Y, Carpenter S. Expression of immunoreactive major histocompatibility complex products in human skeletal muscles. Ann Neurol 1988;23:64–72.
168. McDouall RM, Dunn MJ, Dubovitz V. Expression of class I and class II MHC antigens in neuromuscular disease. J Neurol Sci 1989;89:213–226.
169. Fambrough D, Rash JE. Development of acetylcholine sensitivity during myogenesis. Dev Biol 1971;26:55–68.
170. Paterson BM, Stroman RC. Myosin synthesis in cultures of differentiating chicken embryo skeletal muscle. Dev Biol 1972;29:113–138.
171. Shainberg A, Yagil G, Yaffe D. Alterations of enzymatic activities during muscle differentiation in vitro. Dev Biol 1971;25:1–29.
172. Turner DC, Eppenberger HM. Developmental changes in creatine kinase and aldolase isoenzymes and their possible function in association with contractile elements. Enzyme 1973;15;224-238.
173. Davidson M, Collins M, Byrne J, Vora S. Alterations in phosphofructokinase isoenzymes during early human development. Establishment of adult organ-specific patterns. Biochem J 1983;214:703–710.
174. Miranda AF, Mongini T, DiMauro S. Hereditary metabolic myopathies. In: Strohman R, Wolf S, eds. Gene expression in muscle. New York: Plenum Press, 1985:25–42.
175. Iannaccone ST, Nagy B, Samaha FJ. Partial biochemical maturation of aneurally cultured human skeletal muscle. Neurology 1982;32:846–851.
176. Vita G, Askanas V, Martinuzzi A, Engel WK. Histoenzymatic profile of human muscle cultured in monolayer and innervated de novo by fetal rat spinal cord. Muscle Nerve 1988;11:1–9.
177. Peterson ER, Crain SM. Maturation of human muscle after innervation by fetal muscle spinal cord explants in

long-term cultures. In: Mauro A, ed. Muscle regeneration. New York: Raven Press, 1979:429–441.
178. Askanas V, Kwan H, Alvarez RB, et al. De novo neuromuscular junction formation on human muscle fibres cultured in monolayer and innervated by foetal rat spinal cord: ultrastructural and ultrastructural–cytochemical studies. J Neurocytol 1987;16:523–537.
179. Meola G, Sansone V, Radice S, et al. Enzymatic activity and morphological differentiation in de novo innervated human muscle cultures. Eur J Histochem 1994;38:125–136.
180. Turner DC, Gmür R, Siegrist M, et al. Differentiation in cultures derived from embryonic chicken muscle I. Muscle specific enzyme changes before fusion in EGTA-synchronized cultures. Dev Biol 1976;48:258–283.
181. Reuser AJ, Kroos MA, Hermans MM, et al. Glycogenosis type II (acid maltase deficiency). Muscle Nerve 1995;3:S61–S69.
182. Brunberg JA, McCormick WF, Schochet SS. Type 3 glycogenosis. An adult with diffuse weakness and muscle wasting. Arch Neurol 1971;25:171–178.
183. DiMauro S, Dalakas M, Miranda AF. Phosphoglycerate kinase deficiency: another cause of recurrent myoglobinuria. Ann Neurol 1983;13:11–19.
184. Bresolin N, Miranda A, Chang HW, et al. Phosphoglycerate kinase deficiency myopathy: biochemical and immunological studies of the mutant enzyme. Muscle Nerve 1984;7:542–551.
185. Shin YS. Diagnosis of glycogen storage disease. J Inherited Metab Dis 1990;13;419–434.
186. Miranda AF. Diseased muscle in tissue culture. In: Engel AG, Franzini-Armstrong C, eds. Myology. 2nd ed. New York: McGraw-Hill, 1994;1046–1071.
187. Fernandes J, Huijing F. Branching enzyme deficiency glycogenosis: studies in therapy. Arch Dis Child 1968; 43;347–352.
188. Thon VJ, Khalil M, Cannon JF. Isolation of human glycogen branching enzyme cDNAs by screening complementation in yeast. J Biol Chem 1993;268:7509–7513.
189. DiMauro S, Tsujino S, Shanske S, Rowland LP. Biochemistry and molecular genetics of human glycogenoses: an overview. Muscle Nerve 1995;3:S10–S17.
190. Van den Bergh IET, Berger R. Phosphorylase b kinase deficiency in man: a review. J Inherited Metab Dis 1990; 13:442–451.
191. DiMauro S, Tsujino S. Nonlysosomal glycogenoses. In: Engel AG, Franzini-Armstrong C, eds. Myology. 2nd ed. New York: McGraw-Hill, 1994;1554–1576.
192. Engel AG, Hirschhorn R. Metabolic disorders affecting muscle. In: Engel AG, Franzini-Armstrong C, eds. Myology. 2nd ed. New York: McGraw-Hill, 1994:1533–1553.
193. Blass JP, Avigan J, Uhlendorf BW. A defect in pyruvate decarboxylase in a child with intermittent movement disorder. J Clin Invest 1970;49:423–432.
194. Prick M, Gabreels F, Renier W, et al. Pyruvate dehydrogenase deficiency restricted to the brain. Neurology 1981; 31:398–404.
195. Kerr DS, Berry SA, Lusk MM, et al. A deficiency of both subunits of pyruvate dehydrogenase which is not expressed in fibroblasts. Pediatr Res 1988;24:95–100.
196. Willems JL, Monnens LAH, Trijbels JMF, et al. Pyruvate dehydrogenase deficiency in liver. N Engl J Med 1974;290: 406–407.
197. Miyabayashi S, Ito T, Narisawa K, et al. Biochemical study in 28 children with lactic acidosis in relation to Leigh's encephalomyopathy. Eur J Pediatr 1985;143:278–283.
198. Morgan-Hughes JA. Mitochondrial diseases. In: Engel AG, Franzini-Armstrong C, eds. Myology. 2nd ed. New York: McGraw-Hill, 1994:1610–1660.
199. Dahl H-H. Pyruvate dehydrogenase E1alpha deficiency: males and females differ yet again. Am J Hum Genet 1995;56:553–557.
200. Cori CF. Regulation of enzyme activity in muscle during work. In: Gaebler OH, ed. Units of biological structure and function. New York: Academic Press, 1956:573–583.
201. Lebo RV, Gorin F, Fletterick RJ, et al. High-resolution chromosome sorting and DNA spot-blot analysis assign McArdle's syndrome in chromosome 11. Science 1984; 225:57–59.
202. Newgard CB, Nakano K, Hwang PK, Fletterick RJ. Sequence analysis of the cDNA encoding human liver glycogen phosphorylase reveals tissue specific codon usage. Proc Natl Acad Sci USA 1986;83:8132–8136.
203. Newgard CB, Littman DR, van Genderen C, et al. Human brain glycogen phosphorylase. Cloning, sequence analysis, chromosomal mapping, tissue expression, and comparison with the human liver and muscle isozymes. J Biol Chem 1988;263:3850–3857.
204. Omenn GS, Cheung C-Y. Phosphoglycerate mutase isozyme marker for tissue differentiation in man. Am J Hum Genet 1974;26:393–399.
205. Sato K, Imai F, Hatayama I, Roelofs RI. Characterization of glycogen phosphorylase isoenzymes present in cultured skeletal muscle from patients with McArdle disease. Biochem Biophys Res Commun 1977;78:663–668.
206. DiMauro S, Arnold S, Miranda AF, Rowland LP. McArdle disease: the mystery of reappearing phosphorylase activity in muscle culture. A fetal isoenzyme. Ann Neurol 1978;3:60–66.
207. Ghosh S, Thakurta GG, Mukherjee KL. Glycogen content and structure and some enzymes of glycogen metabolism in human foetal organs. Indian J Med Res 1989;90:147–153.
208. Martin KL, Hardy K, Winston RM, Leese HJ. Activity of enzymes of energy metabolism in single human preimplantation embryos. J Reprod Fertil 1993;99:259–266.
209. Sato K, Morris HP, Weinhouse S. Phosphorylase: a new isozyme in rat hepatic tumors and fetal liver. Science 1972;178:879–881.
210. Sato K, Satoh K, Sato T, et al. Isoenzyme patterns of glycogen phosphorylase in rat tissues and transplantable hepatomas. Cancer Res 1976;36:487–495.
211. Milstein JM, Herron TM, Haas JE. Fatal infantile muscle phosphorylase deficiency. J Child Neurol 1989;4:186–188.
212. Cornelio F, Bresolin N, DiMauro S, et al. Congenital myopathy due to phosphorylase deficiency. Neurology 1983;33:1383–1385.
213. Roelofs RI, Engel WK, Chauvin PB. Histochemical phosphorylase activity in regenerating muscle fibers from

myophosphorylase-deficient patients. Science 1972;177: 795–797.
214. Martinuzzi A, Askanas V, Kobayashi T, et al. Expression of muscle-gene-specific isozymes of phosphorylase and creatine kinase in innervated cultured human muscle. J Cell Biol 1986;103:1423–1429.
215. Martinuzzi A, Askanas V, Kobayashi T, Engel WK. Asynchronous regulation of muscle specific isozymes of creatine kinase, glycogen phosphorylase, lactic dehydrogenase and phosphoglycerate mutase in innervated and non-innervated cultured human muscle. Neurosci Lett 1988; 89:216–222.
216. Vora S, Seaman C, Durham S, Piomelli S. Isozymes of human phosphofructokinase: identification and subunit structural characterization of a new system. Proc Natl Acad Sci USA 1980;77:62–66.
217. Weil D, Cottreau D, van Cong N, et al. Assignment of the gene for F-type phosphofructokinase to human chromosome 10 by somatic cell hybridization and specific immunoprecipitation. Ann Hum Genet 1980;44:11–16.
218. Vora S, Francke U. Assignment of the human gene for liver-type 6-phosphofructokinase isozyme (PFK) to chromosome 21 by using somatic cell hybrids and monoclonal anti-L antibody. Proc Natl Acad Sci USA 1981;78:3738–3742.
219. Vora S, Durham S, de Martinville B, et al. Assignment of the human gene for muscle-type phosphofructokinase (PFKM) to chromosome 1 (region cen-32) using somatic cell hybrids and monoclonal anti-M antibody. Somatic Cell Genet 1982;8:95–104.
220. Nakajima H, Kono N, Yamasaki T, et al. Tissue specificity in expression and alternative RNA splicing of human phosphofructokinase-M and L-genes. Biochem Biophys Res Commun 1990;173:1317–1321.
221. Tarui S, Okuno G, Ikua Y, et al. Phosphofructokinase deficiency in skeletal muscle: a new type of glycogenosis. Biochem Biophys Res Commun 1965;19:517–523.
222. Amit R, Bashan N, Abarbanel JM, et al. Fatal familial infantile glycogen storage disease: multisystem phosphofructokinase deficiency. Muscle Nerve 1992;15:455–458.
223. Nakajima H, Hamaguchi T, Yamasaki T, Tarui S. Phosphofructokinase deficiency: recent advances in molecular biology. Muscle Nerve 1995;3:S28–34.
224. Davidson M, Miranda AF, Bender AN, et al. Muscle phosphofructokinase deficiency. Biochemical and immunological studies of phosphofructokinase isozymes in muscle culture. J Clin Invest 1983;72:545–550.
225. Lebherz HG. On the regulation of fructose diphosphate aldolase isozyme concentrations in animal cells. In: Markert CL, ed. Isozymes, vol. 3. New York: Academic Press, 1975:253–279.
226. Tzvetanova E. Aldolase isoenzyes in serum and muscle from patients with progressive muscular dystrophy and from human foetus. J Neurol Sci 1971;14:483–489.
227. Reid S, Masters C. On the ontogeny of aldolase isozymes and their interactions with cellular structure. Mech Ageing Dev 1985;30:299–317.
228. Lebherz HG. Ontogeny and regulation of fructose diphosphate aldolase isoenzymes in "red" and "white" skeletal muscles of the chick. J Biol Chem 1975;250:5976–5981.
229. Lebherz HG, Rutter WJ. Distribution of fructose diphosphate aldolase variants in biological systems. Biochemistry 1969;8:109–121.
230. Murrell W, Crane D, Masters C. Ontogenic characteristics of cavian aldolase. Mech Ageing Dev 1992;65:35–50.
231. Parkhouse WS. Regulation of skeletal muscle metabolism by enzyme binding. Can J Physiol Pharmacol 1992;70:150–156.
232. Clarke FM, Masters CJ. On the reversible and selective absorption of aldolase isoenzymes in rat brain. Arch Biochem Biophys 1972;153:258–265.
233. Masters CJ. Interactions between glycolytic enzymes and components of the cytomatrix. J Cell Biol 1984;99:222s–225s.
234. Walsh TP, Clarke FM, Masters CJ. Modification of the kinetic parameters of aldolase on binding to the actin-containing filaments of skeletal muscle. Biochem J 1977; 165:165–167.
235. Schapira F. Aldolase isozymes in cancer. Eur J Cancer 1966;2:131–134.
236. Schapira F, Dreyfus J-C, Allard D. Les isozymes de la creatine kinase et de l'aldolase du muscle foetal et pathologique. Clin Chim Acta 1969;20:439–447.
237. Turner DC, Maier V, Eppenberger HM. Creatine kinase and aldolase isoenzyme transitions in cultures of chick skeletal muscle cells. Dev Biol 1974;37:63–89.
238. Tapscott SJ, Lassar AB, Davis RL, Weintraub H. 5-bromo-2'-deoxyuridine blocks myogenesis by extinguishing expression of MyoD1. Science 1989;245:532–536.
239. Miwa S, Fujji J, Tani K, et al. Two cases of red cell aldolase deficiency associated with hereditary hemolytic anemia in a Japanese family. Am J Hematol 1981;11:425–437.
240. Kreuder J, Borkhardt A, Repp R, et al. Brief report: inherited metabolic myopathy and hemolysis due to a mutation in aldolase A. N Engl J Med 1996;334:1100–1104.
241. Omenn GS, Hermodson MA. Human phosphoglycerate mutase: isozyme marker for differentiation and for neoplasia. In: Markert CL, ed. Isozymes, III. Developmental biology. New York: Academic Press, 1975:1005–1017.
242. Tsujino S, Sakoda S, Mizuno R, et al. Structure of the gene encoding the muscle-specific subunit of human phosphoglycerate mutase. J Biol Chem 1989;264:15334–15337.
243. Sakoda S, Shanske S, DiMauro S, Schon EA. Isolation of a cDNA encoding the B isozyme of human phosphoglycerate mutase (PGAM) and characterization of the PGAM gene family. J Biol Chem 1988;263:16899–16905.
244. Edwards YH, Sakoda S, Schon E, Povey S. The gene for human muscle-specific phosphoglycerate mutase, PGAM2, mapped to chromosome 7 by polymerase chain reaction. Genomics 1989;5:948–951.
245. Broceno C, Ruiz P, Reina M, et al. The muscle-specific phosphoglycerate mutase gene is specifically expressed in testis during spermatogenesis. Eur J Biochem 1995;227:629–635.
246. Fundele R, Winking H, Illmensee K, Jägerbauer EM. Developmental activation of phosphoglycerate mutase-2 in the testis of the mouse. Dev Biol 1996;124:562–566.

247. DiMauro S, Miranda AF, Khan S, et al. Human muscle phosphoglycerate mutase deficiency: a newly discovered metabolic myopathy. Science 1981;212:1277–1279.
248. DiMauro S, Miranda AF, Olarte M, et al. Muscle phosphoglycerate mutase deficiency. Neurology 1982;32:584–591.
249. Adamson ED. Isoenzyme transitions of creatine phosphokinase, aldolase and phosphoglycerate mutase in differentiating mouse cells. J Embryol Exp Morphol 1976; 35:355–367.
250. Bresolin N, Ro Y-I, Reyes M, et al. Muscle phosphoglycerate mutase (PGAM) deficiency: a second case. Neurology 1983;33:1049–1053.
251. Miranda AF, Peterson ER, Masurovsky EB. Differential expression of creatine kinase and phosphoglycerate mutase isozymes during development in aneural and innervated human muscle culture. Tissue Cell 1988;20:179–191.
252. Andres V, Cusso R, Carreras J. Distribution and developmental transition of phosphoglycerate mutase and creatine phosphokinase isozymes in rat muscles of different fiber-type composition. Differentiation 1989;41:72–77.
253. Tsujino S, Shanske S, Sakoda S, et al. The molecular genetic basis of muscle phosphoglycerate mutase (PGAM) deficiency. Am J Hum Genet 1993;52:472–477.
254. Giallongo A, Oliva D, Cali L, et al. Structure of the human gene for alpha-enolase. Eur J Biochem 1990;190:567–573.
255. Giallongo A, Venturella S, Oliva D, et al. Structural features of the human gene for muscle-specific enolase. Differential splicing in the 5′untranslated sequence generates two forms of mRNA. Eur J Biochem 1993;214:367–374.
256. Oliva D, Cali L, Feo S, Giallongo A. Complete structure of the human gene encoding neuron-specific enolase. Genomics 1991;10:157–165.
257. Rider CC, Taylor CB. Enolase isoenzymes in rat tissues. Electrophoretic, chromatographic, immunological and kinetic properties. Biochim Biophys Acta 1974;365:285–300.
258. Ibi T, Sahashi K, Kato K, Takahashi A, Sobue I. Immunohistochemical demonstration of beta-enolase in human skeletal muscle. Muscle Nerve 1983;6:661–663.
259. Matsushita H, Yamada S, Satoh T, et al. Muscle-specific beta-enolase concentrations after cross- and random innervation of soleus and extensor digitorum longus in rats. Exp Neurol 1986; 93:84–91.
260. Miranda AF, Somer H, DiMauro S. Isoenzymes as markers of differentiation. In: Mauro A, ed. Muscle regeneration. New York: Raven Press, 1979:453–473.
261. Markert CL, Shaklee JM, Whitt GS. Evolution of a gene: multiple genes for LDH isozymes provide a model of the evolution of gene structure, function, and regulation. Science 1975;189:102–114.
262. Boone CM, Chen TR, Ruddle FH. Assignment of three human genes to chromosomes (LDH-A to 11, TK to 17, and IDH to 20) and evidence for translocation between human and mouse chromosomes in somatic cell hybrids (thymidine kinase–lactate dehydrogenase A–isocitrate dehydrogenase–C-11, E-17, and F-20 chromosomes). Proc Natl Acad Sci USA 1972;69:510–514.
263. Chen TR, McMorris FA, Creagan R, et al. Assignment of the genes for malate oxidoreductase to chromosome 6 and peptidase B and lactate dehydrogenase B to chromosome 12 in man. Am J Hum Genet 1973;25:200–207.
264. Dawson DM, Goodfriend TL, Kaplan NO. Lactic dehydrogenases: functions of the two types. Science 1964;143: 929–933.
265. Cahn RD, Kaplan NO, Levine L, Zwilling E. Nature and development of lactic dehydrogenases. Science 1962;136: 962–969.
266. Philip J, Vesell ES. Sequential alterations of lactic dehydrogenase isoenzymes during embryonic development and in tissue culture. Proc Soc Exp Biol Med 1962;110: 582–585.
267. Kanno T, Sudo K, Takeuchi I, et al. Hereditary deficiency of lactate dehydrogenase M-subunit. Clin Chim Acta 1980; 108:267–276.
268. Kitamura M, Iijima N, Hashimoto F, Hiratsuka A. Hereditary deficiency of subunit H of lactate dehydrogenase. Clin Chim Acta 1971;34:419–423.
269. Maekawa M, Sudo K, Kanno T, Li SS-L. Molecular characterization of genetic mutation in human lactate dehydrogenase-A (M) deficiency. Biochem Biophys Res Commun 1990;168:677–682.
270. Maekawa M, Sudo K, Li SS-L, Kanno T. Analysis of genetic mutations in human lactate dehydrogenase deficiency using DNA conformation polymorphism in combination with polyacrilamide gel and silver staining. Biochem Biophys Res Commun 1991;180:1083–1090.
271. Tsujino S, Shanske S, Brownell AKU, et al. Molecular genetic studies of muscle lactate dehydrogenase deficiency in white patients. Ann Neurol 1994;36:661–665.
272. Kanno T, Maekawa M. Lactate dehydrogenase M-subunit deficiencies: clinical features, metabolic background, and genetic heterogeneities. Muscle Nerve 1995;3:S54–60.
273. Wiesmann U, Kaspar U, Mumenthaler M. Necrosis and regeneration of the tibialis anterior muscle in the rabbit. Arch Neurol 1969;21:373–380.
274. Idele-Wenger JA, Grotyohann LW, Neely JR. Regulation of fatty acid utilization in rat heart. J Mol Cell Cardiol 1982;14:413–417.
275. Carafoli E, Tiozzo R, Lugli G, et al. The release of calcium from heart mitochondria from sodium. J Mol Cell Cardiol 1974;6:361–371.
276. Anderson S, Bankier AT, Barell BG, et al. Sequence and organization of the human mitochondrial genome. Nature 1981;9:457–465.
277. Walker UA, Bernadette J-F, Byrne E. Impact of the 25th chromosome on mitochondrial dysfunction in human disease. J Clin Neurosci 1995;2:107–117.
278. DiMauro S, Moraes CT. Mitochondrial encephalomyopathies. Arch Neurol 1993;50:1197–1208.
279. Taanman JW, Hall RE, Tang C, et al. Tissue distribution of cytochrome c oxidase isoforms in mammals. Characterization with monoclonal and polyclonal antibodies. Biochim Biophys Acta 1993;1225:95–100.
280. Kennaway NG, Carrero-Valenzuela RD, Ewart G, et al. Isoforms of mammalian cytochrome c oxidase: correlation with human cytochrome c oxidase deficiency. Pediatr Res 1990;28:529–535.
281. Van Beeumen JJ, Van Kuilenburg ABP, Van Bun S, et al. Demonstration of two isoforms of subunit VIIa of cyto-

chrome c oxidase from human skeletal muscle. Implication for mitochondrial myopathies. FEBS Lett 1990; 263:213–216.
282. Taanman J-W, Herzberg NH, De Vries H, et al. Steady-state transcript levels of cytochrome c oxidase genes during human myogenesis indicate subunit switching of subunit VIa and co-expression of subunit VIIa isoforms. Biochim Biophys Acta 1992;1139:155–162.
283. Lightowlers R, Ewart G, Aggeler R, et al. Isolation and characterization of the cDNA's encoding two isoforms of subunit CIX of bovine cytochrome c oxidase. J Biol Chem 1990;265:2677–2681.
284. Van Kuilenburg ABP, Muijsers AO, Demol H, et al. Human heart cytochrome c oxidase subunit VIII. Purification and determination of the complete amino acid sequence. FEBS Lett 1988;240:127–132.
285. Rizutto R, Nakase H, Darras B, et al. A gene specifying subunit VIII of human cytochrome c oxidase is localized to chromosome 11 and is expressed in both muscle and nonmuscle tissues. J Biol Chem 1989;264:10595–10600.
286. DiMauro S, Nicholson JF, Hays AP, et al. Benign infantile mitochondrial myopathy due to reversible cytochrome c oxidase deficiency. Ann Neurol 1983;14:226–234.
287. Zeviani M, Peterson P, Servidei S, et al. Benign reversible muscle cytochrome c oxidase deficiency: a second case. Neurology 1987;37:64–67.
288. Tritschler H-J, Bonilla E, Lombes A, et al. Differential diagnosis of fatal and benign cytochrome c oxidase–deficient myopathies of infancy: an immunohistochemical approach. Neurology 1991;41:300–305.
289. Payne RM, Strauss AW. Expression of the mitochondrial creatine kinase genes. Mol Cell Biochem 1994;133–134:235–243.
290. Fan YS, Yang HM, Lin CC. Assignment of the human muscle adenine nucleotide translocator gene (ANT1) to 4q35 by fluorescence in situ hybridization. Cytogenet Cell Genet 1992;60:29–30.
291. Webster KA, Gunning P, Hardeman E, et al. Coordinate reciprocal trends in glycolytic and mitochondrial transcript accumulations during the in vitro differentiation of human myoblasts. J Cell Physiol 1990;142:566–573.
292. Lunardi J, Hurko O, Engel WK, Attardi G. The multiple ADP/ATP translocase genes are differentially expressed during human muscle development. J Biol Chem 1992; 267:15267–15270.
293. Stepien G, Torroni A, Chung AB, et al. Differential expression of adenine nucleotide translocator isoforms in mammalian tissues and during muscle cell differentiation. J Biol Chem 1992;267:14592–14597.
294. Klingenberg M, Martonosi AN, eds. The enzymes of biological membranes. New York: Plenum, 1985;4:511–553.
295. Bakker HD, Scholte HR, Van den Bogert C, et al. Deficiency of the adenine nucleotide translocator in muscle of a patient with myopathy and lactic acidosis: a new mitochondrial defect. Pediatr Res 1993;33:412–417.
296. Wallimann T, Wyss M, Brdiczka D, et al. Intracellular compartmentation, structure and function of creatine kinase isoenzymes in tissues with high and fluctuating energy demands: the 'phosphocreatine circuit' for cellular energy homeostasis. Biochem J 1992;281:21–40.
297. Trask RV, Billadello JJ. Tissue specific distribution and developmental regulation of M and B creatine kinase mRNAs. Biochim Biophys Acta 1990;1049:182–188.
298. Dawson DM, Fine IH. Creatine kinase in human tissues. Arch Neurol 1967;16:175–180.
299. Nigro JM, Schweinfest CW, Rajkovic A, et al. cDNA cloning and mapping of the creatine kinase M gene to 19q13. Am J Hum Genet 1987;40:115–125.
300. Stallings RL, Olson E, Strauss AW, et al. Human creatine kinase genes on chromosomes 15 and 19, and proximity of the gene for the muscle form to the genes for apolipoprotein C2 and excision repair. Am J Hum Genet 1988;43:144–151.
301. Boldrey AA, Severin S. The histidine-containing dipeptides, carnosine and anserine: distribution, properties and biological significance. In: Weber G, ed. Advances in enzyme regulation. New York: Pergamon Press, 1990:175–194.
302. Jockers-Wretou E, Pfleiderer G. Quantitation of creatine kinase isoenzymes in human tissue and sera by an immunological method. Clin Chim Acta 1975;58:223–232.
303. Lang H, Wuerzburg U. Creatine kinase, an enzyme of many forms. Clin Chem 1982;28:1439–1447.
304. Ventura-Clapier R, Saks VA, Vassort G, et al. Reversible MM-creatine kinase binding to cardiac myofibrils. Am J Physiol 1987;253:C444–C455.
305. Wallimann T, Eppenberger HM. Localization and function of M-line bound creatine kinase: M-band model and creatine phosphate shuttle. Cell Muscle Motil 1985;6:239–285.
306. Turner DC, Wallimann T, Eppenberger HM. A protein that binds specifically to the M-line of skeletal muscle is identified as the muscle form of creatine kinase. Proc Natl Acad Sci USA 1973;70:702–705.
307. Saks VA, Khuchua ZA, Vasilyeva EV, et al. Metabolic compartmentation and substrate channelling in muscle cells. Role of coupled creatine kinases in in vivo regulation of cellular respiration—a synthesis. Mol Cell Biochem 1994;133–134:155–192.
308. Jacobs H, Heldt WH, Klingenberg M. High activity of CK in mitochondria from muscle and brain. Evidence for a separate mitochondrial isoenzyme of CK. Biochem Biophys Res Commun 1964;16:516–521.
309. Jakobs H, Heldt HW, Klingenberg M. High activity of creatine kinase in mitochondria from muscle and brain and evidence for a separate mitochondrial isoenzyme of creatine kinase. Biochem Biophys Res Commun 1964;16:516–521.
310. Jacobus WE, Lehninger AL. Creatine kinase of rat heart mitochondria. Coupling of creatine phosphorylation to electron transport. J Biol Chem 1973;248:4803–4810.
311. Erickson-Viitanen S, Geiger PJ, Viitanen P, Bessman SP. Compartmentation of mitochondrial creatine phosphokinase II. The importance of the outer membrane for mitochondrial compartmentation. J Biol Chem 1982;252:14405–14411.

312. Blum HE, Deus B, Gerok W. Mitochondrial creatine kinase from human heart muscle: purification and characterization of the crystallized isoenzyme. J Biochem 1983;94:1247–1257.
313. Schlegel J, Wyss M, Schuerch U, et al. Mitochondrial creatine kinase from cardiac muscle and brain are two distinct isoenzymes but both form octameric molecules. J Biol Chem 1988;263:16963–16969.
314. Haas RC, Strauss AW. Separate nuclear genes encode sarcomere-specific and ubiquitous human mitochondrial creatine kinase isoenzymes. J Biol Chem 1990;265:6921–6927.
315. Fritz-Wolf K, Schnyder T, Wallimann T, Kabsch W. Structure of mitochondrial creatine kinase. Nature 1996;381:341–345.
316. Payne RM, Friedman DL, Grant JW, et al. Creatine kinase isoenzymes are highly regulated during pregnancy in rat uterus and placenta. Am J Physiol 1993;265:E624–E635.
317. Smeitink J, Wevers R, Hulshof J, et al. A method for quantitative measurement of mitochondrial creatine kinase in human skeletal muscle. Ann Clin Biochem 1992;29:196–201.
318. Wu AHB. Creatine kinase isoforms in ischemic heart disease. Clin Chem 1989;35:7–13.
319. Panteghini M. Serum isoforms of creatine kinase isoenzymes. Clin Biochem 1988;21:211–218.
320. Panteghini M, Bonora R, Pagani F. An immunoinhibition assay for determination of creatine kinase isoforms in serum. Eur J Clin Chem Clin Biochem 1994;32:383–389.
321. Yamashita T, Maruyama I, Toda H, et al. Detection of reperfusion 30 and 60 minutes after coronary recanalization by a rapid new assay of creatine kinase isoforms in acute myocardial infarction. Am Heart J 1993;125:649–656.
322. Puelo PR, Guadagno PA, Roberts R, Perryman MB. Sensitive, rapid assay of subforms of creatine kinase MB in plasma. Clin Chem 1989;35:7–13.
323. Puleo RR, Meyer D, Wathen C, et al. Use of a rapid assay of subforms of creatine kinase-MB to diagnose or rule out acute myocardial infarction. N Engl J Med 1994;331:561–566.
324. Ingwall JS, Kramer MF, Friedman WF. Developmental changes in heart creatine kinase. In: Jacobus WE, Ingwall JS, eds. Heart creatine kinase. Baltimore/London: Williams & Wilkins, 1980:9–17.
325. Hooft C, de Caey P, Lambert V. Etude comparative de l'activité enzymatique du tissu musculaire de l'enfant normal et des enfants atteints de dystrophie musculaire progressive aux stades differents de la maladie. Rev Fr Etud Clin Biol 1996;11:510.
326. Kloosterboer HJ, Stoker-DeVries SA, Hommes FA. The development of creatine kinase in rat skeletal muscle Changes in isoenzyme ratio, protein, RNA and DNA during development. Enzyme 1976;21:448–458.
327. Cao A, de Virgiliis S, Falorni A. The ontogeny of creatine kinase isoenzymes. Biol Neonate 1968;13:375–380.
328. Foxall DD, Emery AEH. Changes in creatine kinase and its isoenzymes in human fetal muscle during development. J Neurol Sci 1975;24:483–492.
329. Goto I, Nagamorie M, Katsuki S. Creatine phosphokinase isozymes in muscles. Human fetus and patients. Arch Neurol 1969;20:422–429.
330. Tzvetanova E. Creatine kinase isoenzymes in muscle tissue of patients with neuromuscular diseases and human fetuses. Enzyme 1971;12:279–288.
331. Smeitink J, Ruitenbeek W, van Lith T, et al. Maturation of mitochondrial and other isoenzymes of creatine kinase in skeletal muscle of preterm born infants. Ann Clin Biochem 1992;29:302–306.
332. Hoerter JA, Kuznetsov A, Ventura-Clapier R. Functional development of the creatine kinase system in perinatal rabbit heart. Circ Res 1991;69:665–676.
333. Hoerter JA, Ventura-Clapier R, Kuznetsov A. Compartmentation of creatine kinases during perinatal development of mammalian heart. Mol Cell Biochem 1994;133/134:277–286.
334. Schmidt EW, Bender W, Breinl H, et al. Creatinkinase und Creatinkinase-Isoenzymaktivitäten bei Neugeborenen. Entwicklung des organtypischen Isoenzymmusters während der Fetalperiode. Z Geburtsh Perinatol 1979;183:51–57.
335. Kar NC, Pearson CM. Creatine phosphokinase isoenzymes in muscle in human myopathies. Am J Clin Pathol 1965;43:207–209.
336. Jedeikin R, Makela SK, Shennan AT, et al. Creatine kinase isoenzymes in serum from cord blood and the blood of healthy full-term infants during the first three postnatal days. Clin Chem 1982;28:317–322.
337. Anversa P, Olivetti G, Bracchi PG, Loud AV. Postnatal development of the M-band in rat cardiac myofibrils. Circ Res 1981;48:561–568.
338. Kuby SA, Keutel HJ, Okabe K, et al. Isolation of the human ATP-creatine transphosphorylases (creatine phosphokinases) from tissues of patients with Duchenne muscular dystrophy. J Biol Chem 1977;252:8382–8390.
339. Somer H, Dubowitz V, Donner M. Creatine kinase isoenzymes in neuromuscular diseases. J Neurol Sci 1976;29:129–136.
340. Cavanagh NPC, Franklin GI, Hughes BP, et al. Creatine kinase isoenzymes in cultured human muscle cells. II. A study of carrier females for Duchenne muscular dystrophy by needle and open biopsy. Clin Chim Acta 1981;115:191–198.
341. Somer H, Donner M, Murros J, Konttinen A. A serum isozyme study in muscular dystrophy: particular reference to creatine kinase, aspartate aminotransferase, and lactic acid dehydrogenase isozymes. Arch Neurol 1973;29:343–345.
342. Conway EJ, Cooke R. The deaminases of adenosine and adenylic acid in blood and tissues. Biochem J 1939;33:479–492.
343. van Kuppevelt TH, Veerkamp JH, Fishbein WN, et al. Immunolocalization of AMP-deaminase isozymes in human skeletal muscle and cultured muscle cells: concentration of isoform M at the neuromuscular junction. J Histochem Cytochem 1994;42:861–868.
344. Van den Berghe G, Bontemps F, Vincent MF, Van den Bergh F. The purine nucleotide cycle and its molecular defects. Prog Neurobiol 1992;39:547–561.

345. Ogasawara N, Goto H, Yamada Y, et al. AMP deaminase isozyme in human tissues. Biochim Biophys Acta 1982; 714:298–306.
346. Ogasawara N, Goto H, Yamada Y, Watanabe T. Distribution of AMP deaminase isoenzymes in various human blood cells. Int J Biochem 1984;16:269–273.
347. Sabina RL, Morisaki T, Clarke P, et al. Characterization of the human and rat myoadenylate deaminase genes. J Biol Chem 1990;265:9423–9433.
348. Bausch-Jurken MT, Mahnke-Zizelman DK, Morisaki T, Sabina RL. Molecular cloning of AMP deaminase isoform L. Sequence and bacterial expression of human AMPD2 cDNA. J Biol Chem 1992;267:22407–22413.
349. Mahnke-Zizelman DK, Sabina RL. Cloning of human AMP deaminase isoform E cDNAs. Evidence for a third AMPG gene exhibiting alternative spliced 5′-exons. J Biol Chem 1992;267:20866–20877.
350. Morisaki H, Morisaki T, Newby LK, Holmes EW. Alternative splicing: a mechanism for phenotypic rescue of a common inherited defect. J Clin Invest 1993;92:2275–2280.
351. Kaletha K, Nowak G. Developmental forms of human skeletal-muscle AMP deaminase: the kinetic and regulatory properties of the enzyme. Biochem J 1988;249:255–261.
352. Sabina RL, Ogasawara N, Holmes EW. Expression of three stage-specific transcripts of AMP deaminase during myogenesis. Mol Cell Biol 1989;9:2244–2246.
353. Jacobs AE, Oosterhof A, Benders AA, Veerkamp JH. Expression of different isoenzymes of adenylate deaminase in cultured human muscle cells. Relation to myoadenylate deaminase deficiency. Biochim Biophys Acta 1992;1139:91–95.
354. Fishbein WN, Sabina R, Ogasawara N, Holmes EW. Immunologic evidence for the three isoforms of AMP deaminase (AMPD) in mature skeletal muscle. Biochim Biophys Acta 1993;1163:97–104.
355. Gross M. Molecular biology of AMP deaminase deficiency. Pharm World Sci 1994;16:55–61.
356. Sabina RL. Myoadenylate deaminase deficiency. In: Lane RJM, ed. Handbook of muscle disease. New York: Marcel Dekker, 1996:443–450.
357. Fishbein WN, Armbrustmacher VW, Griffin JL. Myoadenylate deaminase deficiency: a new disease of muscle. Science 1978;200:545–548.
358. Valen PA, Nakayama DA, Veum J, et al. Myoadenylate deaminase deficiency and forearm ischemic exercise testing. Arthritis Rheum 1987;30:661–668.
359. DiMauro S, Miranda AF, Hays AP, et al. Myoadenylate deaminase deficiency—muscle biopsy and muscle culture in a patient with gout. J Neurol Sci 1980;47:191–202.
360. Kaletha K, Nowak G. Myoadenylate deaminase deficiency studies on normal and deaminase-deficient skeletal muscle. Clin Chim Acta 1990;190:147–155.
361. Schudt C, Gaertner U, Dolken G, Pette D. Calcium-related changes of enzyme activities in energy metabolism of cultured embryonic chick myoblasts and myotubes. Eur J Biochem 1975;60:579–586.
362. Wahrmann JP, Recouvreur M, Favard-Sereno C. Development and regulation of the phosphorylase-glycogen complex in myogenic cells of the L6 line. J Cell Sci 1977;26:77–91.
363. Schudt C, Gaertner U, Pette D. Insulin action on glucose transport and calcium fluxes in developing muscle cells in vitro. Eur J Biochem 1976;68:103–111.
364. Bocek RM, Beatty CH. Glucogen metabolism in fetal, neonatal and infant muscle of the rhesus monkey. Pediatrics 1967;40:412–420.
365. Shelley HJ. Blood sugars and tissue carbohydrate in fetal and infant lambs and rhesus monkeys. J Physiol 1960;153:527–552.
366. Rebouche CJ. Carnitine function and requirements during life cycle. FASEB J 1992;6:3379–3386.
367. Novak M, Drummond GI, Skala J, Hahn P. Developmental changes in cyclic AMP, protein kinase, phosphorylase kinase, and phosphorylase in liver, heart, and skeletal muscle in the rat. Arch Biochem Biophys 1972;150:511.
368. Challiss RA, Ferré P. Integration of carbohydrate and lipid metabolism in skeletal muscle during postnatal development. Reprod Nutr Dev 1988;28:805–815.
369. Fowden AL, Comline RS, Silver M. The effects of cortisol on the concentration of glycogen in different tissues in the chronically catheterized fetal pig. Q J Exp Physiol 1985;85:23–35.
370. Alexandrides T, Moses AC, Smith RJ. Developmental expression of receptors for insulin, insulin-like growth factor I (IGF-I), and IGF-II in rat skeletal muscle. Endocrinology 1989;124:1064–1076.
371. Dombrowski GJ Jr, Swiatek KR. Lactate genesis by rat liver and muscle during development. Pediatr Res 1991;30:331–336.
372. Fellmann N, Coudert J. Physiologie de l'exercise musculaire chez l'enfant. Arch Pediatr 1994;1:827–840.
373. Colling-Saltin AS. Some quantitative biochemical evaluations of developing skeletal muscles in the human foetus. J Neurol Sci 1978;39:187–198.
374. Beatty CH, Basinger GM, Bocek RM. Pentose cycle activity in muscle from fetal, neonatal and infant rhesus monkeys. Arch Biochem Biophys 1965;117:275–281.
375. Beatty CH, Peterson RD, Basinger GM, Bocek RM. Major metabolic pathways for carbohydrate metabolism of voluntary skeletal muscle. Am J Physiol 1966;210:404–410.
376. Csapo A, Herrmann H. Quantitative changes in contractile proteins of chick skeletal muscle during and after development. Am J Physiol 1951;165:701–710.
377. Sarzale MG, Pilarska M. Phospholipid biosynthesis in sarcoplasmic reticulum membrane during development. Biochim Biophys Acta 1976;441:81–92.
378. Smith PB, Clark GF. Beta-adrenergic receptor-adenylate cyclase alterations during the postnatal development of skeletal muscle. Biochim Biophys Acta 1980;633;274–288.
379. Smith PB, Reitz RC, Kelley D. Acyl-CoA synthase and acyltransferase activity in developing skeletal muscle membranes. Biochim Biophys Acta 1982;713:128–135.
380. Sauro VS, Strickland KP. Changes in oleic acid oxidation and incorporation into lipids of differentiating L6 myoblasts cultured in normal or fatty acid-supplemented growth medium. Biochem J 1987;244:743–748.
381. Sauro VS, Strickland KP. Triacylglycerol synthesis and diacylglycerol acyltransferase activity during skeletal myogenesis. Biochem Cell Biol 1990;68:1393–1401.

382. Leskawa KC, Erwin RE, Hogan EL. Phospholipid biosynthesis during normal and dystrophic avian muscle cell differentiation in culture. Life Sci 1986;38:147–153.
353. Smith PB, Finch RA. Alterations in lipid metabolism of developing muscle cells in culture. Biochim Biophys Acta 1979;572:139–145.
384. Sandra A, Ionasescu VV. Alterations in lipid turnover in developing muscle. Biochem Biophys Res Commun 1980;93:898–905.
385. Martinuzzi A, Vergani L, Rosa M, Angelini C. L-Carnitine uptake in differentiating human cultured muscle. Biochim Biophys Acta 1992;1095:217–222.
386. Felig P, Wahren J. Fuel homeostasis during exercise. N Engl J Med 1975;293:1078–1084.
387. Beatty CH, Basinger GM, Bocek RM. Oxygen consumption and glycolysis in fetal, neonatal, and infant muscle of the rhesus monkey. Pediatrics 1968;42:5–16.
388. Ferré P, Decaux JF, Issad T, Girard JR. Changes in energy metabolism during the suckling and weaning period in the newborn. Reprod Nutr Dev 1986;26:619–631.
389. Carroll JE, McGuire BS, Chancey VF, Harrison KB. Acyl-CoA dehydrogenase enzymes during early postnatal development in the rat. Biol Neonate 1989;55:185–190.
390. Wolfe RG, Maxwell CV, Nelson EC. Effect of age and dietary fat level on fatty acid oxidation in the neonatal pig. J Nutr 1978;108:1621–1634.
391. Glatz JFC, Veerkamp JH. Postnatal development of palmitate oxidation and mitochondrial enzyme activities in rat cardiac and skeletal muscle. Biochim Biophys Acta 1982;711:327–335.
392. Jerusalem F. The microcirculation of muscle. In: Engel AG, Franzini-Armstrong C, eds. Myology. 2nd ed. New York: McGraw-Hill, 1994:361–374.
393. Kagen LJ, Christian CL. Immunologic measurement of myoglobin in human adult and fetal skeletal muscle. Am J Physiol 1966;211:656–660.
394. Weller PA, Prince M, Isenberg H, et al. Myoglobin expression: early induction and subsequent modulation of myoglobin and myoglobin mRNA during myogenesis. Mol Cell Biol 1986;6:4538–4547.
395. Webster KA. Regulation of glycolytic enzyme RNA transcriptional rates by oxygen availability in skeletal muscle cells. Mol Cell Biochem 1987;77:19–28.
396. De Stefano N, Argov Z, Matthews PM, et al. Impairment of muscle mitochondrial oxidative metabolism in McArdle's disease. Muscle Nerve 1996;19:764–769.
397. Moggio M, Bresolin N, Scarpini E, et al. Cytochrome c oxidase during human fetal development. Int J Dev Neurosci 1989;7:5–14.
398. Kloosterboer HJ, Stoker-DeVries SA, Hulstaert CE, Hommes FA. Quantitative analysis of morphological changes in skeletal muscle of the rat after hormone administration. Biol Neonate 1979;35:106–112.
399. Zuurveld JG, Oosterhof A, Veerkamp JH, van Moerkerk HT. Oxidative metabolism of cultured human skeletal muscle cells in comparison with biopsy material. Biochim Biophys Acta 1985;844:1–8.
400. Henriksson J, Chi MM-Y, Hintz CS, et al. Chronic stimulation of mammalian muscle: changes in enzymes of six metabolic pathways. Am J Physiol 1986;251:C614–C632.
401. Hood DA, Zak AR, Pette D. Chronic stimulation of rat skeletal muscle induces coordinate increases in mitochondrial and nuclear mRNAs of cytochrome-c-oxidase subunits. Eur J Biochem 1989;179:275–280.
402. Ordway GA, Li K, Hand GA, Williams RS. RNA subunit of mitochondrial RNA-processing enzyme is induced by contractile activity in striated muscle. Am J Physiol 1993;265:C1511–C1516.
403. Cooper WG, Konigsberg IR. Succinic dehydrogenase activity of muscle cells grown in vitro. Exp Cell Res 1961;23:576–581.
404. Bremer J. Carnitine metabolism and functions. Physiol Rev 1983;63:1420–1479.
405. Borum PR, Bennett SG. Carnitine as an essential nutrient. J Am Coll Nutr 1986;5:177–182.
406. Rebouche CJ. Comparative aspects of carnitine biosynthesis in microorganisms and mammals with attention to carnitine biosynthesis in man. In: Frenkel JD, ed. Carnitine biosynthesis, metabolism and functions. New York: Academic Press, 1980:57–72.
407. Girard J, Duee PH, Ferré P, et al. Fatty acid oxidation and ketogenesis during development. Reprod Nutr Dev 1985;25:303–319.
408. Treem WR, Stanley CA, Finegold DN, et al. Primary carnitine deficiency due to a failure of carnitine transport in kidney, muscle and fibroblasts. N Engl J Med 1988;319:1331–1336.
409. Borum PR. Variation in tissue carnitine concentrations with age and sex in the rat. Biochem J 1978;176:677–681.
410. Shenai JP, Borum PR. Tissue carnitine reserves of newborn infants. Pediatr Res 1984;18:679–682.
411. Engel AG, Rebouche CJ. Carnitine metabolism and inborn errors. J Inherited Metab Dis 1984;7(suppl 1):38–43.
412. Nakano C, Takashima S, Takeshita K. Carnitine concentration during the development of human tissues. Early Hum Dev 1989;19:21–27.
413. Penn D, Schmidt-Sommerfeld E, Pascu F. Decreased tissue carnitine concentrations in newborn infants receiving total parenteral nutrition. J Pediatr 1981;98:976–978.
414. Melegh B. Carnitine supplementation in the premature. Biol Neonate 1990;58(suppl 1):93–106.
415. Shenai JP, Borum PR, Mohan P, ConLevy SC. Carnitine status at birth of newborn infants of varying gestation. Pediatr Res 1983;17:579.
416. Pons R, DeVivo DC. Primary and secondary carnitine deficiency syndromes. J Child Neurol 1995;10(suppl):2S8–2S24.
417. DiDonato S. Disorders of lipid metabolism affecting skeletal muscle: carnitine deficiency syndromes, defects in the catabolic pathway, and chanarin disease. In: Engel AG, Franzini-Armstrong C, eds. Myology. 2nd ed. New York: McGraw-Hill, 1994:1587–1609.
418. Shapira Y, Glick B, Harel S, et al. Infantile idiopathic myopathic carnitine deficiency: treatment with L-carnitine. Pediatr Neurol 1993;9:35–38.
419. Zierz S. Carnitine palmitoyl transferase deficiency. In: Engel AG, Franzini-Armstrong C, eds. Myology. 2nd ed. New York: McGraw-Hill, 1994:1577–1586.
420. Verderio E, Cavadini P, Montermini L, et al. Carnitine palmitoyltransferase II deficiency: structure of the gene

421. Demaugre F, Bonnefont JP, Colonna M, et al. Infantile form of carnitine palmitoyltransferase II deficiency with hepatomuscular symptoms and sudden death. Physiopathological approach to carnitine palmitoyltransferase II deficiencies. J Clin Invest 1991;87:859–864.
422. Stave U. Perinatal changes of interorgan differences in cell metabolism. Biol Neonate 1975;26:318–332.
423. Tawa NE, Goldberg AL. Protein and amino acid metabolism in muscle. In: Engel AG, Franzini-Armstrong C, eds. Myology. 2nd ed. New York: McGraw-Hill, 1994:683–707.
424. Naismith DJ, Morgan BLG. The biphasic nature of protein metabolism during pregnancy in the rat. Br J Nutr 1976;36:563–566.
425. Naismith DJ, Emery PW. Excretion of 3-methyl-histidine by pregnant women: evidence for a biphasic system of protein metabolism in human pregnancy. Eur J Clin Nutr 1988;42:483–489.
426. Ryan EA, O'Sullivan MJ, Skyler JS. Insulin action during pregnancy. Studies with the euglycemic clamp technique. Diabetes 1985;34;380–389.
427. Leturque A, Ferré P, Burnol AF, et al. Glucose utilization rates and insulin sensitivity in vivo in tissues of virgin and pregnant rats. Diabetes 1986;35:172–177.
428. Sugden PH, Fuller SJ. Regulation of protein turnover in skeletal and cardiac muscle. Biochem J 1991;273:21–37.
429. Scornik OA. Protein synthesis and degradation during growth. In: Jones CT, ed. Biochemical development of the fetus and neonate. Amsterdam: Elsevier Biomedical Press, 1982:865–894.
430. Nwagwu M, Nana M. Quantitative measurement of active polysomes in developing muscle. Dev Biol 1974;41:1–13.
431. Bornman L, Polla BS, Gericke GS. Heat-shock protein 90 and ubiquitin: developmental regulation during myogenesis. Muscle Nerve 1996;19:574–580.
432. Ebashi S, Nonomura Y. Proteins of the myofibril. In: Bourne GH, ed. The structure and function of muscle. New York: Academic Press, 1973;3:286–352.
433. Schubert D, Tarikas H, Humpreys S, Heinemann S, Patrick J. Protein synthesis and secretion in a myogenic cell line. Dev Biol 1973;33:18–37.
434. Merlie JP, Buckingham ME, Whalen RG. Molecular aspects of myogenesis. Curr Top Dev Biol 1978;11:61–114.
435. Hommes FA, Oudman-Richters AR, Van der Zwaag P, et al. The development of enzymes of phosphocreatine biosynthesis in the rat. Dev Biol 1972;29:250–253.
436. Dreyfus JC, Schapira F. Biochemistry of muscle development. In: Stave U, Weech AA, eds. Perinatal physiology. 2nd ed. New York and London: Plenum, 1978; 715–725.
437. Walker JB. End-product repression in the creatine pathway of the developing chick embryo. Adv Enzyme Regul 1973;1:151–168.
438. Loike JD, Zalutsky DL, Kaback E, et al. Extracellular creatine regulates creatine transport in rat and human muscle cells. Proc Natl Acad Sci USA 1988;85:807–811.
439. Borsook H, Dubnoff JW. The hydrolysis of phosphocreatine and the origin of urinary creatine. J Biol Chem 1947;168:493–510.
440. Bloch K, Schoenheimer R, Rittenberg D. Rate of formation and disappearance of body creatine in normal animals. J Biol Chem 1941;138:155–166.
441. Stave U, Armstrong MD. Tissue free amino acid concentration in perinatal rabbits. Biol Neonate 1973;22;374–387.
442. Stockdale FE, O'Neill MC. Deoxyribonucleic acid synthesis, mitosis and skeletal muscle differentiation. In Vitro 1972;8:212–227.
443. Wicha M, Stockdale FE. DNA-dependent DNA polymerases in differentiating muscle cells. Biochem Biophys Res Commun 1972;48:1079–1087.
444. Arnaudo E, Dalakas M, Shanske S, et al. Depletion of muscle mitochondrial DNA in AIDS patients with zidovudine-induced myopathy. Lancet 1991;337:508–510.
445. Herrmann H, Tootle ML. Specific and general aspect of the development of enzymes and metabolic pathways. Physiol Rev 1964;44:289–371.
446. Lyles JM, Weill CL. Changes in glucose-6-phosphate dehydrogenase activity in developing embryonic chick skeletal muscle and spinal cord. Dev Neurosci 1986;8:44–52.
447. Sutton JR, Toews CJ, Ward GR, Fox IH. Purine metabolism during strenuous muscular exercise in man. Metabolism 1980;29:254–260.
448. Mineo I, Tarui S. Myogenic hyperuricemia: what can we learn from metabolic myopathies? Muscle Nerve 1995;3: S75–81.
449. Murre C, McCaw PS, Baltimore D. A new DNA binding motif in immunoglobulin enhancer binding, daughterless, MyoD, and myc proteins. Cell 1989;56:777–783.
450. Lassar AB, Buskin JN, Lockshon D, et al. MyoD is a sequence specific DNA binding protein requiring a region of myc homology to bind to the muscle creatine kinase enhancer. Cell 1989;58:823–831.
451. Gossett LA, Kelvin DJ, Sternberg EA, Olson EN. A new myocyte-specific enhancer-binding factor that recognizes a conserved element associated with multiple muscle-specific genes. Mol Cell Biol 1989;9:5022–5033.
452. Molkentin JD, Black BL, Martin JF, Olson EN. Cooperative activation of muscle gene expression by MEF2 and myogenic bHLH proteins. Cell 1995;83:1125–1136.
453. Edmondson D, Lyons GE, Martin JF, Olson EN. MEF2 gene expression marks the cardiac and skeletal muscle lineages during mouse embryogenesis. Mol Cell Biol 1994;120:1251–1263.
454. Benezra R, Davis RL, Lockshon D, et al. The protein Id: a negative regulator of helix-loop-helix DNA binding proteins. Cell 1990;61:49–59.
455. Dias P, Dilling M, Houghton P. The molecular basis of skeletal muscle differentiation. Semin Diagn Pathol 1994; 11:3–14.
456. Spicer DB, Rhee J, Cheung WL, Lassar AB. Inhibition of myogenic bHLH and MEF2 transcription factors by the bHLH protein twist. Science 1996;272:1477–1480.
457. Bengal E, Ransone L, Scharfmann R, et al. Functional antagonism between c-Jun and MyoD proteins: a direct physical association. Cell 1992;68:507–519.
458. Sorrentino V, Pepperkok R, Davis RL, et al. Cell proliferation inhibited by MyoDl independently of myogenic differentiation. Nature 1990;345:813–815.

459. Gu W, Schneider JW, Condorelli G, et al. Interaction of myogenic factors and the retinoblastoma protein mediates muscle cell commitment and differentiation. Cell 1993;72:309–324.
460. Pownall ME, Emerson CPJ. Sequential activation of three myogenic regulatory genes during somite morphogenesis in quail embryos. Dev Biol 1992;151:67–79.
461. Ott MO, Bober E, Lyons G, et al. Early expression of the myogenic regulatory gene, myf5, in precursor cells of skeletal muscle in the mouse embryo. Development 1991;111:1097–1107.
462. Emerson CP Jr. Embryonic signals for skeletal myogenesis: arriving at the beginning. Curr Opin Cell Biol 1993;5:1057–1064.
463. Cossu G, Tajbakhsh S, Buckingham M. How is myogenesis initiated in the embryo? Trends in Genetics 1996;12:218–223.
464. Rudnicki MA, Braun T, Hinuma S, Jaenisch R. Inactivation of MyoD in mice leads to upregulation of the myogenic HLH gene myf-5 and results in apparently normal muscle development. Cell 1992;71:383–390.
465. Braun T, Rudnicki MA, Arnold HH, Jaenisch R. Targeted inactivaton of the muscle regulatory gene myf-5 results in abnormal rib development and perinatal death. Cell 1992;71:369–382.
466. Rudnicki MA, Schnegelsberg PN, Stead RH, et al. MyoD or Myf-5 is required for the formation of skeletal muscle. Cell 1993;75:1351–1359.
467. Schweighoffer F, Maire P, Tuil D, et al. In vivo developmental modifications of the expression of genes encoding muscle-specific enzymes in rat. J Biol Chem 1986;261:10271–10276.
468. Sutherland CJ, Elsom VL, Gordon ML, et al. Coordination of skeletal muscle gene expression occurs late in mammalian development. Dev Biol 1991;146:167–178.
469. Gunning P, Hardeman E, Wade R, et al. Differential pattern of transcript accumulation during human myogenesis. Mol Cell Biol 1987;7100:4100–4114.
470. Melloul D, Aloni B, Calvo J, et al. Developmentally regulated expression of chimeric genes containing muscle actin DNA sequences in transfected myogenic cells. EMBO J 1984;3:983–990.
471. Nudel U, Greenberg D, Ordahl C, et al. Developmentally regulated expression of a chicken muscle specific gene in stably transfected rat myogenic cells. Proc Natl Acad Sci USA 1985;82:3106–3109.
472. Li K, Hodge JA, Wallace DC. OXBOX, a positive transcriptional element of the heart-skeletal muscle ADP/ATP translocator gene. J Biol Chem 1990;265:20585–20588.
473. Li Z, Paulin D. Different factors interact with myoblast specific and myotube-specific enhancer regions of the human desmin gene. J Biol Chem 1993;268:10403–10415.
474. Bassel-Duby R, Hernandez MD, Gonzalez MA, et al. A 40-kilodalton protein binds specifically to an upstream sequence element essential for muscle-specific transcription of the human myoglobin promoter. Mol Cell Biol 1992;12:5024.
475. Tapscott SJ, Lassar AB, Weintraub H. A novel myoblast enhancer element mediates MyoD transcription. Mol Cell Biol 1992;12:4994–5003.
476. Klamut HJ, Gangopadhyay SB, Worton RG, Ray PN. Molecular and functional analysis of the muscle-specific promoter region of the Duchenne muscular dystrophy gene. Mol Cell Biol 1990;10:193.
477. Sartorelli V, Webster KA, Kedes L. Muscle-specific expression of the cardiac alpha-actin gene requires MyoDl, CArG-box binding factor, and Sp1. Genes Dev 1990;4:1811–1822.
478. Cox RD, Buckingham ME. Actin and myosin genes are transcriptionally regulated during mouse skeletal muscle development. Dev Biol 1992;149:228–234.
479. Lin H. Yutzey K, Konieczny SF. Muscle-specific expression of the troponin I gene requires interactions between helix-loop-helix muscle regulatory factors and ubiquitous transcription factors. Mol Cell Biol 1991;11:267–280.
480. Corin SJ, Levitt LK, O'Mahoney JV, et al. Delineation of a slow-twitch-myofiber-specific transcriptional element by using in vivo somatic gene transfer. Proc Natl Acad Sci USA 1995;92:6185–6189.
481. Bouchard C, Simoneau JA, Lortie G, et al. Genetic effects in human skeletal muscle fiber type distribution and enzyme activities. Can J Physiol Pharmacol 1986;64:1245–1251.
482. Florini JR. Hormonal control of muscle growth. Muscle Nerve 1987;10:577–598.
483. Albertson-Wickland K, Edan S, Isaksson O. Analysis of early responses to growth hormone on amino acid transport and protein synthesis in diaphragms of young normal rats. Endocrinology 1980;106:298–305.
484. Winkler B, Steele R, Altszuler N, DeBodo RC. Effect of growth hormone on free fatty acid metabolism. Am J Physiol 1964;206:174–178.
485. Rabinowitz D, Zierler KL. Differentiation of active from inactive acromegaly by studies of forearm metabolism and response to intra-arterial insulin. Bull Johns Hopkins Hosp 1963;118:211–224.
486. Rosenfeld RG, Wilson DM, Dollar LA. Both human pituitary growth hormone and recombinant DNA-derived human growth hormone cause insulin resistance at postreceptor site. J Clin Endocrinol Metab 1982;54:1033–1038.
487. Pickett JBE, Layzer RB, Levin SR, et al. Neuromuscular complications of acromegaly. Neurology 1975;25:638–645.
488. Isgaard J, Nilsson A, Vikman K, Isakasson OGP. Growth hormone regulates the level of insulin-like growth factor-1 mRNA in rat skeletal muscles. J Endocr 1989;100:107–112.
489. Olwin BB, Hannon K, Kudla AJ. Are fibroblast growth factors regulators of myogenesis in vivo? Progr Growth Factor Res 1994;5:145–158.
490. Rosenthal SM, Cheng ZQ. Opposing early and late effects of insulin-like growth factor I on differentiation and the cell cycle regulatory retinoblastoma protein in skeletal myoblasts. Proc Natl Acad Sci USA 1995;92:10307–10311.
491. Moses AC, Nissley SP, Short PA, et al. Increased levels of multiplication-stimulating activity, an insulin-like growth factor, in fetal rat serum. Proc Natl Acad Sci USA 1980;77:3649–3653.

492. Garlick PJ, McNurlan MA. Isotopic methods for studying protein turnover. In: Raiha NCR, ed. Protein metabolism during infancy. Nestlé Nutrition Workshop Series, vol. 33. New York: Raven Press, 1994:29–47.
493. Beermann DH, Liboff M, Wilson DB, Hood LF. Effects of exogenous thyroxine and growth hormone on satellite cell and myonuclei populations in rapidly growing rat skeletal muscle. Growth 1983;47:179–184.
494. Muscat GE, Downes M, Dowhan DH. Regulation of vertebrate muscle differentiation by thyroid hormone: the role of the myoD gene family. Bioessays 1995;17:211–218.
495. Wiles CM, Young A, Jones DA, Edwards RHT. Muscular relaxation in rate, fibre-type composition and energy turnover in hyper- and hypothyroid patients. Clin Sci 1979;57:375–384.
496. Kaminski HJ, Ruff RL. Endocrine myopathies (hyper- and hypofunction of adrenal, thyroid, pituitary, and parathyroid glands and iatrogenic corticosteroid myopathy. In: Engel AG, Franzini-Armstrong C, eds. Myology. 2nd ed. New York: McGraw-Hill, 1994:1726–1753.
497. Hodak E, David M, Gadoth N, Sandbank M. Etretinate-induced skeletal muscle damage. Br J Dermatol 1987;116:623–626.
498. Thompson J, Moore SE, Walsh FS. Thyroid hormones regulate expresson of the neural cell adhesion molecule in adult skeletal muscle. FEBS Lett 1987;219:135–138.
499. Baldwin KM, Hooker AM, Campbell PJ, Lewis RE. Enzyme changes in neonatal skeletal muscle: effect of thyroid deficiency. Am J Physiol 1978;235:C97–C102.
500. Ianuzzo CD, Patel P, Oben V, et al. Thyroidal trophic influences on skeletal muscle myosin. Nature 1977;270:74–76.
501. Hausman GJ, Watson R. Regulation of fetal muscle development by thyroxine. Acta Anatomica 1994;149:21–30.
502. Celsing F, Blomstrand E, Melichna J, et al. Effect of hyperthyroidism of fibre-type composition, fibre area, glycogen content and enzyme activity in human skeletal muscle. Clin Physiol 1986;6:171–181.
503. Wrutniak C, Cassar-Malek I, Marchal S, et al. A 43-kDa protein related to c-Erb A α1 is located in the mitochondrial matrix of rat liver. J Biol Chem 1995;270:16347–16354.
504. Almon RR, Dubois DC. Fiber-type discrimination in disuse and glucocorticoid-induced atrophy. Med Sci Sports Exerc 1990;22:304–311.
505. Guerriero V, Florini JR. Dexamethasone effects on myoblast proliferation and differentiation. Endocrinology 1980;106:1198–1202.
506. Whitson PA, Stuart CA, Huls MH, et al. Dexamethasone effects on creatine kinase activity and insulin-like growth factor receptors in cultured muscle cells. J Cell Physiol 1989;140:8–17.
507. Cossu G, Cusella-De Angelis MG, Senni MI, et al. Adrenocorticotropin is a specific mitogen for mammalian myogenic cells. Dev Biol 1989;131:331–336.
508. Snochowski MF, Dahlberg E, Gustafsson JA. Characterization and quantification of the androgen and glucocorticoid receptors in cytosol from rat skeletal muscle. Eur J Biochem 1980;111:603–618.
509. Kawai K, Ogata E, Takano K, et al. Effects of testosterone and estradiol on serum somatomedin A and growth rate in rats. Endocrinol Jpn 1982;29:435–442.
510. Li L, Zhou J, James G, Heller-Harrison R, et al. FGF inactivates myogenic helix-loop-helix proteins through phosphorylation of a conserved protein kinase C site in their DNA-binding domains. Cell 1995;71:1181–1194.
511. Yablonka-Reuveni Z, Balestreri TM, Bowen-Pope DF. Regulation of proliferation and differentiation of myoblasts derived from adult mouse skeletal muscle by specific isoforms of PDGF. J Cell Biol 1990;111:1623–1629.
512. Vaidya TB, Rhodes SJ, Taparowsky EJ, Konieczny SF. Fibroblast growth factor and transforming growth factor beta repress transcription of the myogenic regulatory gene MyoD1. Mol Cell Biol 1989;9:3576–3579.
513. Weintraub H, Davis R, Tapscott S, et al. The myoD gene family: nodal point during specification of the muscle cell lineage. Science 1991;251:761–766.
514. Potten CS, Loeffler M. Stem cells: attributes, cycles, spirals, pitfalls and uncertainties. Development 1990;110:1001–1020.
515. Hall-Craggs EC. Rapid degeneration and regeneration of whole skeletal muscle following treatment with bupivacaine (marcaine). Exp Neurol 1974;43:349–358.
516. Morlet K, Grounds MD, McGeachie JK. Muscle precursor replication after repeated regeneration of skeletal muscle in mice. Anat Embryol 1989;180:471–478.
517. Mong FS. Satellite cells in the regenerated and regrafted skeletal muscles of rats. Experientia 1988;44:601–603.
518. Grounds MD, Garrett KL, Lai MC, et al. Identification of skeletal muscle precursor cells in vivo by use of MyoD1 and myogenin probes. Cell Tissue Res 1992;267:99–104.
519. Blau HM, Webster C. Isolation and characterization of human muscle cells. Proc Natl Acad Sci USA 1981;78:5623–5627.
520. Ham RG, St. Clair JA, Meyer SD. Improved media for rapid clonal growth of normal human skeletal muscle satellite cells. Adv Exp Med Biol 1990;280:193–199.
521. Wright WE. Myoblast senescence in muscular dystrophy. Exp Cell Res 1985;157:343–354.
522. Rifenberick DH, Koski Cl, Max SR. Metabolic studies of skeletal muscle regeneration. Exp Neurol 1974;45:527–540.
523. Snow MH. Metabolic activity during the degenerative and early regenerative stages of minced skeletal muscles. Anat Rec 1973;176:185–204.
524. Gallucci V, Novello F, Margreth A, Aloisi M. Biochemical correlates of discontinuous muscle regeneration in the rat. Br J Exp Pathol 1966;47:215–227.
525. Schapira F. Modification de specificité de l'aldolase musculaire au cours de l'atrophie. C R Acad Sci Ser D (Paris) 1966:2291.
526. Mendell JR, Kissel JT, Amato AA, et al. Myoblast transfer in the treatment of Duchenne's muscular dystrophy. N Engl J Med 1995;333:832–888.
527. Dhawan J, Pan LC, Pavlath GK, et al. Systemic delivery of human growth hormone by genetically engineered myoblasts. Science 1991;254:1509–1512.

528. Partridge TA, Invited review: myoblast transfer: a possible therapy for inherited myopathies? Muscle Nerve 1991;14:197–212.
529. Blau HM, Springer ML. Molecular medicine—muscle mediated gene therapy. N Engl J Med 1995;333:1554–1556.
530. Hughes SM, Blau HM. Migration of myoblasts across basal lamina during skeletal muscle development. Nature 1990;345:350–353.
531. Naffakh N, Pinset C, Montarras D, et al. Transplantation of adult-derived myoblasts in mice following gene transfer. Neuromuscul Disord 1993;3:413–417.
532. Trivedi RA, Dickson G. Liposome-mediated gene transfer into normal and dystrophin-deficient mouse myoblasts. J Neurochem 1995;64:2230–2238.
533. Hamamori Y, Samal B, Tian J, Kedes L. Myoblast transfer of human erythropoietin gene in a mouse model of renal failure. J Clin Invest 1995;95:1808–1813.
534. Acsadi G, Jani A, Massie B, Simoneau M, et al. A differential efficiency of adenovirus-mediated in vivo gene transfer into skeletal muscle cells of different maturity. Hum Mol Genet 1994;3:579–584.
535. Blau HM, Springer ML. Gene therapy—a novel form of drug delivery. N Engl J Med 1995;333:1204–1207.
536. Dahler A, Wade RP, Muscat GE, Waters MJ. Expression vectors encoding human growth hormone (hGH) controlled by human muscle-specific promoters: prospects for regulated production of hGH delivered by myoblast transfer or intravenous injection. Gene 1994;145:305–310.
537. Gossen M, Freundlieb S, Bender G, et al. Transcriptional activation by tetracyclines in mammalian cells. Science 1995;268:1766–1769.
538. Pavlath GK, Rich K, Webster SG, Blau H. Localization of muscle gene products in nuclear domains. Nature 1989;337:570–573.
539. Bowden DH, Groyer RA. The size of muscle fibers in infants and children. Arch Pathol 1960;69:188–189.
540. Stockdale FE, Raman N, Baden H. Myosin light chains and developmental origin of fast muscle. Proc Natl Acad Sci USA 1981;78:931–935.
541. Michaelis D, Goebels N, Hohlfeld R. Constitutive and cytokine-induced expression of human leukocyte antigens and cell adhesion molecules by human myotubes. Am J Pathol 1993;93:1142–1149.
542. Bartram C, Edwards RH, Beynon RJ. McArdle's disease: muscle glycogen phosphorylase deficiency. Biochim Biophys Acta 1995;1272:1–13.
543. Yang BZ, Ding JH, Brown BI, Chen YT. Definitive prenatal diagnosis for type III glycogen storage disease. Am J Hum Genet 1990;47(4):735–739.
544. Bresolin N, Bet L, Moggio M, et al. Muscle glucose-6-phosphate dehydrogenase deficiency. J Neurol 1989;236:193–198.
545. Hug G, Bove KE, Soukup S. Lethal neonatal multiorgan deficiency of carnitine palmitoyltransferase II. N Engl J Med 1991;91:1862–1864.
546. DiMauro S, DiMauro PM. Muscle carnitine palmityltransferase deficiency and myoglobinuria. Science 1973;73:929–931.
547. Morand P, Despert F, Carrier HN, et al. Myopathie lipidique avec cardiomyopathie sévère par déficit généralisé en carnitine. Arch Mal Coeur Vaiss 1979;79:536–544.
548. Tein I, De Vivo DC, Bierman F, et al. Impaired skin fibroblast carnitine uptake in primary systemic carnitine deficiency manifested by childhood carnitine-responsive cardiomyopathy. Pediatr Res 1990;90:247–255.
549. Rebouche CJ, Engel AG. Kinetic compartmental analysis of carnitine metabolism in the human carnitine deficiency syndromes. Evidence for alterations in tissue carnitine transport. J Clin Invest 1984;84:857–867.
550. Huizing M, Ruitenbeek W, Thinnes FP, et al. Deficiency of the voltage-dependent anion channel: a novel cause of mitochondriopathy. Pediatr Res 1996;39:760–765.
551. Robinson BH, MacMillan H, Petrova-Benedict R, Sherwood WG. Variable clinical presentation in patients with defective E1 component of pyruvate dehydrogenase complex. J Pediatr 1987;87:525–533.
552. Robinson BH, Chun K, Mackay N, et al. Isolated and combined deficiencies of the alpha-keto acid dehydrogenase complexes. Ann N Y Acad Sci 1989(Part VI);573:337–346.
553. Zinn AB, Kerr D, Hoppel CL. Fumarase deficiency: a new cause of mitochondrial encephalomyopathy. N Engl J Med 1986;315:469–475.
554. Ogasahara S, Engel A, Frens D, Mack D. Muscle coenzyme Q deficiency in familial mitochondrial encephalomyopathy. Proc Natl Acad Sci USA 1989;86:2379–2382.
555. Luft R, Ikkos D, Palmieri G, et al. A case of severe hypermetabolism of nonthyroid origin with a defect in the maintenance of mitochondrial respiratory control: a correlated clinical, biochemical, and morphological study. J Clin Invest 1962;41:1776–1804.
556. Rötig A, Cormier V, Blanche S, et al. Pearson's marrow-pancreas syndrome. A multisystem mitochondrial disorder in infancy. J Clin Invest 1990;86:1601–1608.
557. Tritschler HJ, Andreetta F, Moraes CT, et al. Mitochondrial myopathy of childhood associated with depletion of mitochondrial DNA. Neurology 1992;42:209–217.
558. Moraes CT, Shanske S, Tritschler H-J, et al. Mitochondrial DNA depletion with variable tissue expression: a novel genetic abnormality in mitochondrial diseases. Am J Hum Genet 1991;48:492–501.

Section V
Neonatal Metabolism

32
Neonatal Glucose Metabolism

Richard M. Cowett and Hussien M. Farrag

While the fetus is completely dependent on its mother for glucose and other nutrient transfer across the placenta, the adult is completely independent, especially one who is neither pregnant nor diabetic. The neonate is considered to be in a transition between the complete dependence of the fetus and the complete independence of the adult. The neonate must become independent after birth, balancing between glucose deficiency and excess to maintain euglycemia. The dependence of the conceptus on the mother for continuous substrate delivery in utero contrasts with the variable and intermittent exogenous oral intake that is the hallmark of the neonatal period and beyond. Development of carbohydrate homeostasis results from a balance between the specific morbidities to which the neonate is subject, developing hormonal, enzymatic, neural regulation, and substrate availability. Maturation of neonatal homeostasis is influenced by the integrity of the specific pathways of intermediary metabolism important in glucose metabolism (see Chapters 6 to 9, 29, and 31). The heterogeneity that is the hall-mark of neonatal glucose metabolism is illustrated by the multiplicity of conditions producing or associated with neonatal hypo- and hyperglycemia. The maintenance of euglycemia especially in the sick or low birth weight neonate is difficult, which reinforces the concept that the neonate is vulnerable to carbohydrate disequilibrium. This topic has been the subject of a number of recent evaluations.[1–10]

This chapter evaluates the definition of euglycemia by considering the range for hypo- and hyperglycemia and the various methodologies available to measure glucose concentration. We review the differential of hypo- and hyperglycemia, and consider the treatment of the altered states of glucose homeostasis. We evaluate those components influencing glucose homeostasis in the neonatal period, specifically glucose production and glucose utilization, and conclude by focusing on the relationship of glucose metabolism to the central nervous system.

Definition of Neonatal Euglycemia

A primary example of the heterogeneity that exists in our understanding of neonatal glucose metabolism is that there are no uniform standards accepted for specific limits of euglycemia. The definitions of what constitute hypo- and hyperglycemia are quite variable. It is well accepted that glucose is the major substrate of carbohydrate metabolism. At birth the maternal supply of glucose to the neonate, by definition, ceases abruptly. While the neonatal plasma glucose concentration is usually in the normoglycemic range at delivery, its actual concentration depends on such factors as the last maternal meal, the duration of labor, the route of delivery, and the type of intravenous fluid administered to the mother. As an example, Figure 32.1 depicts the mean plasma glucose and insulin concentrations of mothers and their neonates who received either no glucose (Ringer's lactate) ($N = 14$) or glucose (Ringer's lactate + 5% dextrose) ($N = 15$) as a bolus infusion during anesthesia for elective cesarean section.[11] Blood samples for plasma glucose and insulin concentrations were taken prior to intravenous fluid administration and at the time of delivery. Corresponding samples were taken from the neonate's umbilical vein and artery, subsequently at 30 minutes and hourly after birth for 4 hours. As noted in the figure, all mothers and neonates receiving glucose had hyperglycemia and hyperinsulinemia at delivery. The neonatal plasma glucose concentration declined rapidly during the first four hours of life. With one exception all neonates were euglycemic repeatedly and all were clinically asymptomatic. The changes in the neonate following glucose infusion to the mother reflect the differences that can occur in the neonate depending on the type of intravenous infusion administered at delivery.

After a normal delivery, the plasma glucose concentration declines to approximately $50\,mg \cdot dl^{-1}$ by 2 hours of age, but equilibrates at approximately $70\,mg \cdot dl^{-1}$ at 72 hours after birth.[10] Cornblath and Reisner[12] evaluated

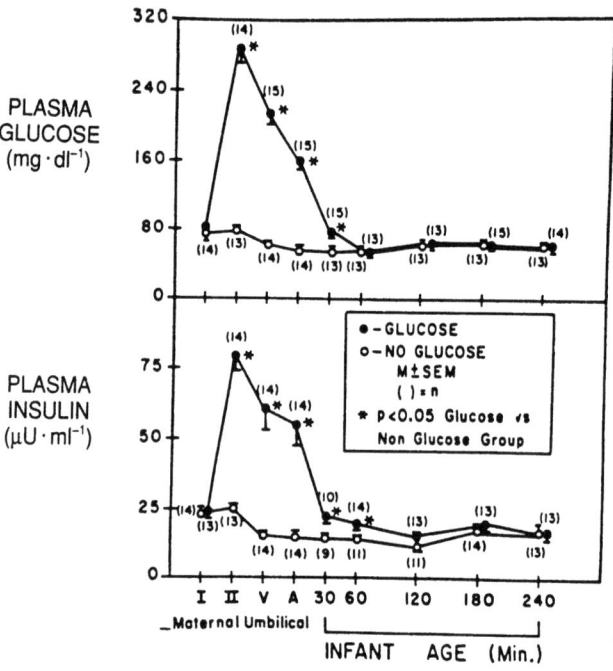

FIGURE 32.1. Plasma glucose and insulin concentration for the mothers and the neonates. Maternal I and II, samples obtained prior to fluid infusion and at delivery of infants, respectively, V, umbilical venous; A, umbilical arterial samples; (·), number of determinations. (From Cowett et al.,[11] with permission.)

the blood glucose concentration over time in a classic analysis of both the term and the low birth weight neonate. Their data suggested that a concentration below $40\,mg\cdot dl^{-1}$ or greater than $125\,mg\cdot dl^{-1}$ was abnormal after 3 days after birth. Critical adjustments are required by the neonate in the first 72 hours after birth to maintain glucose homeostasis.

Srinivasan et al.[13] evaluated the plasma glucose concentration in normal full-term neonates who weighed between 2500 and 4000g and were appropriate for age between 37 and 42 weeks of gestation. The predicted glucose concentrations during the first week of life are noted in Figure 32.2. All neonates were fed after 3 hours. The data indicated that the nadir in plasma glucose concentration is between 1 and 2 hours and that a significant rise occurs during the 3rd hour. The investigators suggested that a plasma glucose concentration $<35\,mg\cdot dl^{-1}$ should be of concern during the first 3 hours of postnatal life. They concluded that plasma glucose concentration $<40\,mg\cdot dl^{-1}$ between 3 and 24 hours and $<45\,mg\cdot dl^{-1}$ after 24 hours should be considered to be in the hypoglycemic range.

Another investigation of this topic was performed by Heck and Erenberg,[14] who evaluated the serum glucose concentration in the term neonate during the first 48 hours after birth. They concluded that a serum glucose concentration of $<30\,mg\cdot dl^{-1}$ on the first day of life and $<40\,mg\cdot dl^{-1}$ on the second day of life were the limits for the definition of hypoglycemia in the full-term neonate. Few similar evaluations of the limits of hypoglycemia have been reported for the preterm neonate.

The definition of hyperglycemia is equally unsettled.[15] However, a consensus exists that the range exceeds >125 to $150\,mg\cdot dl^{-1}$.[16-18]

Because the micropremie, i.e., the neonate born weighing ≤1000g birth weight (BW), represents a significant percentage of the neonates cared for in the neonatal intensive care setting, glucose homestasis was evaluated in a group of micropremies born over a period of 1 year in a large university-affiliated perinatal service.[19] Eighty-six neonates [(BW 770 ± 150g, range 460–1000g) (mean ± SD), gestational age (GA) 26 ± 2 weeks, range 23–32 weeks] had 1725 glucose determinations (20 ± 14 determinations for each neonate, range 0–90) performed over the course of the first month. Each neonate was evaluated relative to glucose concentration measured over that time period. The evaluation included how each neonate related to the demographics of the group as a whole, the intravenous and oral nutrition received (i.e., the volume, and rates of glucose, protein, and lipid administered), a clinical risk score, and the urine output measured relative to each glucose determination. There was a significant decline in mean plasma glucose concentration by incremental birth weight criterion over the range of weights of the neonates ($p < .0001$).

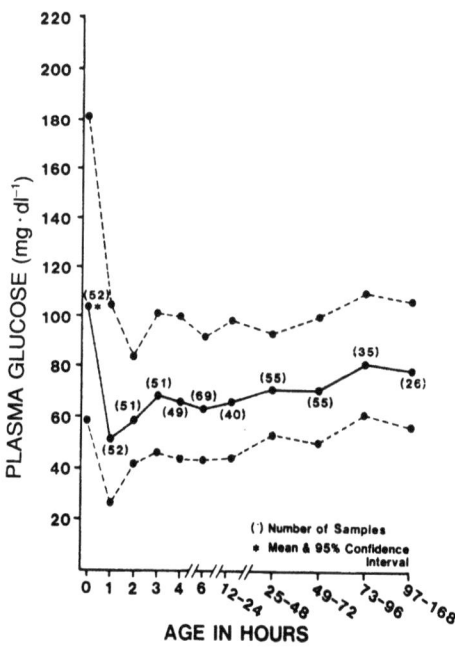

FIGURE 32.2. Plasma glucose concentrations in term neonates weighing 2.5 to 4.0 kg. (From Srinivasan et al.,[13] with permission.)

TABLE 32.1. Plasma glucose concentration by incremental birth weight criteria.

No. of neonates/no. of determinations*	2/9	19/225	16/542	14/365	23/306	10/248	2/23
Birth weight (g)	400–499	500–599	600–699	700–799	800–899	900–999	1000
Pl. glucose (mg·dl^{-1})	108 ± 88	218 ± 224	145 ± 86	158 ± 113	165 ± 126	123 ± 62	89 ± 26
Pl. glucose (mmol·L^{-1})	5.99 ± 4.88	12.10 ± 12.43	8.05 ± 4.77	8.77 ± 6.27	9.16 ± 6.99	6.83 ± 3.44	4.94 ± 1.44

Mean ± SD.
*Number of neonates in group/number of plasma glucose concentrations determined. To calculate mmol/L: mg/dl × 0.0555.
From Cowett et al.,[19] with permission.

Table 32.1 depicts the plasma glucose concentration subdivided into birth weight categories such that the evaluation represents the mean and standard error for all the plasma glucose determinations within each 100-g segment for the total period of the study. If one excludes the 400- to 499-g and 1000-g weight groups because of sample size, there appeared to be a general decline in concentration over weight. The investigators suggested that these data could be interpreted to indicate an improving physiologic adaptation, since there was a decline from a high of 218 ± 15 mg·dl^{-1} in the 500- to 599-g weight group to 124 ± 62 mg·dl^{-1} in the 900- to 999-g weight group. By SAS® mixed design analysis of administered substrate provided either by the intravenous or oral routes to each neonate, there was a significant relationship only between plasma glucose concentration and the amount of intravenous glucose administered ($p < .0002$). Significant relationships existed between plasma glucose concentration and the clinical risk score ($p < .0001$), but not urine output. The investigators concluded that hyperglycemia in the micropremie is related to an imbalance between physiologic immaturity, the rate of intravenous glucose administered, and the clinical condition of the neonate. Although this study could not be performed under conditions in which the neonates received only a saline infusion to determine basal glucose concentration, the data indicate the relative range that may be expected in this group of neonates receiving clinically standard rates of glucose infusion.

Parallel studies to the above are clearly necessary because of the general lack of consensus about the definition of both hypo- and hyperglycemia in the neonatal period. This lack of consensus was studied by Koh et al.,[20] who reported a range of hypoglycemia between 18 and 72 mg·dl^{-1} in the United Kingdom in a survey of health care professionals.

What should be apparent from this discussion is the variation not only in the definition of euglycemia but in the "normal" concentration of glucose at any point in time. An example is noted in Figure 32.3. In the four types of neonates commonly cared for in a neonatal unit—the term appropriate for gestational age (AGA), the term small for gestational age (SGA), the preterm AGA, and the preterm SGA—plasma glucose concentration changed constantly and in an apparently random fashion.[21] This chapter comprehensively catalogues the various etiologies of hypo- and hyperglycemia as well as the mechanisms controlling neonatal glucose homeostasis.

Measurement of Glucose Concentration in the Neonate

The difficulties involved in the definition of euglycemia are accentuated by the lack of attention to detail of measurement of neonatal glucose concentration. Failure to

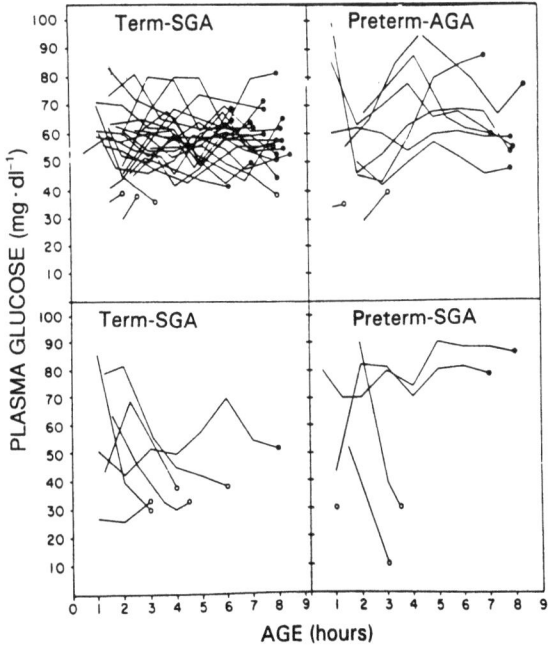

FIGURE 32.3. Plasma glucose concentration for the four groups of neonates studied during the first nine hours of life. (From Stanley et al.,[21] with permission.)

measure the glucose concentration rapidly enough accentuates red blood cell glycolysis, resulting in a falsely low concentration. A number of centers use the Dextrostix technique, which is thought to be reliable if directions are followed carefully. However, the manufacturer cautions that the reagent strips are not intended for use with a neonatal blood sample. An abnormal concentration, either in the hypoglycemic or hyperglycemic range, needs to be corroborated by laboratory determination of glucose concentration prior to correction of the suspected disequilibrium unless the patient is symptomatic.[7]

Some data allow one to question if the Dextrostix or like evaluation should be used at all. Several studies have evaluated various means of assessing blood glucose concentration. Frantz et al.[22] reported that the Dextrostix test strip is able to accurately identify a blood glucose concentration of $<50\,mg\cdot dl^{-1}$. However, they used fresh heparinized blood from the adult to evaluate reliability, which may not be applicable to the neonate. Perelman et al.[23] evaluated rapid glucose determination in the neonate, comparing the Dextrostix Ames Meter, Chemstrip bG test strip, and Stat Tek Meter methods with a glucose analyzer. The investigators concluded that there was modest accuracy in estimating whole blood glucose concentration. They suggested that confirmation by conventional laboratory techniques is necessary before therapeutic intervention. Wilkins and Kaira[24] compared blood glucose test strips for the detection of neonatal hypoglycemia. In 101 blood samples, results of three glucose test strip methods were compared with a laboratory determination of glucose concentration. Two test strips, the BM test glycemic 20–800 test strip and the Reflecto-Test hypoglycemia test strip, gave a rapid and reliable estimate, but the Dextrostix test strip tended to overestimate the blood glucose concentration.

In one report, Conrad et al.[25] suggested that the Glucostix, the Dextrostix, and the Chemstrip bG test strips were relatively unreliable, with r values of .73, .74, and .83, respectively, compared with the YSI analyzer in tests of 104 neonatal blood samples obtained by heelstick. They tested one glucose reflectance meter (i.e., the Glucometer M), which had an r value of .73 when correlated with the YSI analyzer. The investigators suggested that the YSI analyzer should be used preferentially to determine blood glucose concentration in the neonatal intensive care unit.

In an evaluation from an intensive care unit in an academic medical center, Lin et al.[26] evaluated four glucose reflectance meters. The manufacturers claimed that these meters could reliably measure whole blood glucose concentration as low as $20\,mg\cdot dl^{-1}$. To determine whether the accuracy of the determination would be affected by the technique of obtaining capillary blood by heelstick, cord arterial blood was evaluated from a separate group of neonates for comparison. All blood was sequentially analyzed five different times on each meter and the YSI analyzer. Evaluation of the data showed that accuracy was limited in heelstick blood whether one evaluated the percentage of difference between the means or the least squares regression for all the meters tested as noted in Table 32.2. The use of cord blood appeared to be associated with greater accuracy than the use of capillary blood obtained by heelstick in the analysis. The reason for the poor correlation with capillary samples and the high variability in the blood glucose concentration remains unclear. There was no relationship between accuracy and reliability of the various glucose reflectance meters as noted in Table 32.3. The Diascan S meter, which seemed to have accuracy closest to that of the YSI analyzer, was clearly not the most reliable in comparison with the YSI analyzer. On the other hand, the One Touch meter, which had the best reliability among the four glucose reflectance meters tested, was the least accurate. The

TABLE 32.3. Reliability of glucose analyzer and reflectance meters.

	Coefficient of variation %		
	Cord	Heel	p
YSI analyzer	3.2	3.3	NS
Glucometer M meter	5.6	5.8	NS
Diascan S meter	5.9	7.2	NS
Accu-Chek II meter	5.9	8.0	<0.01
One Touch meter	3.4	3.7	NS

From Lin et al.,[26] with permission.
NS, not significant.

TABLE 32.2. Accuracy of reflectance meters versus YSI glucose analyzer.

Reflectance meter	Cord	Heel	p
Difference between means (%)			
Glucometer M	−9.3	−23.2	
Diascan S	0.4	−0.4	
Accu-Chek II	1.2	16.4	
One Touch	35.2	25.6	
Correlation coefficient (r)			
Glucometer M	0.88	0.64	<0.05
Diascan S	0.96	0.71	<0.01
Accu-Chek II	0.91	0.71	<0.05
One Touch	0.92	0.86	NS

From Lin et al.,[26] with permission.
NS, not significant.

investigators concluded that, contrary to the manufacturers' claims, the glucose reflectance meter should probably not be used for evaluation of capillary blood glucose concentration in the high-risk neonate.

The conclusions of the study were reaffirmed when a parallel study was performed utilizing venous blood instead of heelstick blood.[27] There was no difference relative to reliability between venous blood and capillary heelstick blood for the various meters and the YSI analyzer.

Inanen et al.[28] evaluated the Ames Glucometer Elite glucose meter for use in the intensive care nursery in a study of point of service glucose testing. The glucose meter was compared with data obtained in the clinical laboratory on a Beckman CX 7 analyzer. Significant differences in data of the two methods were decreased when blood, sent to the laboratory for comparative testing, was delivered on ice to decrease the rate of glycolysis by the red blood cell. The investigators emphasized the importance of meticulous handling of the blood sample both for testing with the glucose meter as well as when blood is transported to the clinical laboratory. The use of ice to decrease the rate of glycolysis during transport is especially important if a significant length of time ensues between obtaining the sample and the actual laboratory determination. If further studies can corroborate this technique, it should become a standard methodology in the clinical determination of blood glucose concentration.

Holtrop et al.[29] evaluated the sensitivity and specificity of glucose oxidase peroxidase chromogen test strips by comparing values of 272 samples of serum glucose concentration with values obtained by Chemstrip bG. The diagnostic sensitivity of a test strip $\leq 40\,mg\cdot dl^{-1}$ to predict a serum glucose concentration $\leq 34\,mg\cdot dl^{-1}$ was 86%, with 78% specificity. The positive predictive value with a 21% prevalence of serum glucose concentration $\leq 34\,mg\cdot dl^{-1}$ was 52% with a negative predictive value of 95%. Fifty-eight of the serum glucose concentrations were $\leq 34\,mg\cdot dl^{-1}$ and the strips reported concentrations greater than $40\,mg\cdot dl^{-1}$ in eight. The investigators concluded that more sensitive and specific methods are required for the neonate.

It is important to remember that the blood glucose concentration is usually 10% to 15% lower than the corresponding plasma glucose concentration. Care must be taken when the test is performed because an erroneously high concentration can be caused by isopropyl alcohol mixing with the blood on the strip that is read by reflectance colorimetry.[30]

Jain et al.[31] reported the complexity inherent in the determination of glucose concentration when they found that measurement with the automated hexokinase method, rather than the oxidase method, may be interfered with by the combination of plasma free hemoglobin, bilirubin, and plasma triglycerides, which may be elevated in the plasma of the neonate. While a 1:1 dilution of plasma allowed for accurate determination of high plasma glucose concentration, this method was not acceptable at low plasma glucose concentration. The investigators concluded that glucose oxidase remains the method of choice for the determination of plasma glucose concentration.

Another factor of importance involves the concept that multiple sites can be utilized to obtain blood for the determination of glucose concentration in the neonate. Cowett and D'Amico[32] determined the variability in blood glucose concentration that may result from such sampling. Since pain and mechanical forces may be different because of the method used to obtain the capillary heelstick blood compared to a venous sample, the two sites were sampled simultaneously in 25 asymptomatic well neonates at 35.5 weeks gestational age. There was a significant ($p < .0001$) but weak correlation ($r^2 = .64$) between capillary blood and venous blood relative to blood glucose concentration. When the capillary heelstick-venous glucose concentration difference was compared to the mean of the capillary heelstick and venous glucose concentrations, a difference of $9\,mg\cdot dl^{-1}$ was noted in 3 of the 25 neonates. An appropriately obtained capillary heelstick blood sample provides measurement of blood glucose concentration, which is a variance compared to a venous sample, but which is probably not of significance physiologically.

Clinical Hypoglycemia in the Neonate

The close relationship between maternal and fetal glucose, the repetitive occurrence of wide swings of neonatal glucose concentration, and the retarded disappearance of an acute glucose load in both the term and preterm neonate indicate that the regulation of neonatal carbohydrate metabolism is poorly developed 72 hours after birth.[33] The birth process necessitates a period of readjustment to allow subsequent control. In the low birth weight neonate especially, this adjustment is delicate and may result in abnormal consequences such as hypo- or hyperglycemia. The difficulties relative to the definition of hypo- and hyperglycemia have already been discussed. One of the main clinical difficulties with these definitions is the nonspecific symptomatology, which includes the signs and symptoms listed in Table 32.4. These difficulties are compounded by the occurrence of symptoms at different blood glucose concentrations in different neonates and the lack of a universal threshold below or above which symptomatology may occur.[7,9] This is further considered at the end of the chapter when the relationship

TABLE 32.4. Signs and symptoms of neonatal hypoglycemia.

Abnormal cry	Hypothermia
Apathy	Hypotonia
Apnea	Jitteriness
Cardiac arrest	Lethargy
Convulsions	Tremors
Cyanosis	Tachypnea

between glucose homeostasis and the central nervous system is evaluated. These same conclusions were emphasized by a conference on hypoglycemia convened by the CIBA Foundation.[34]

A number of different classifications have been employed to categorize the various causes of hypoglycemia noted in the neonatal period. Cornblath and Schwartz[10] and others[35,36] have analyzed the various causes on the basis of clinical course, emphasizing time of presentation, duration, severity, and response to therapy. Another schema considers the biochemical and physiologic parameters and evaluates the relationship between hepatic production and/or uptake in contrast to peripheral utilization.[37,38] Differentiation of the various causes of hypoglycemia on the basis of physiologic and biochemical parameters would compare decreased hepatic glucose production due to substrate or enzymatic deficiencies to those secondary to increased insulin concentration. Inadequate glucose production includes those conditions involving decreased availability of substrate (e.g., glycogen, lactate, glycerol, and amino acids), altered sensitivity to neural or hormonal factors, and/or immature or altered enzymatic pathways (e.g., gluconeogenesis and/or increased peripheral utilization rates).

Pathophysiology of Hypoglycemia in the Neonate: Imprecise/Diminished Hepatic Glucose Production

Neonatal hypoglycemia not due to insulin excess is generally caused by diminished hepatic glucose production. The role of hepatic control of glucose homeostasis and its relationship to its disequilibrium in the neonate has received increasing attention in the literature. Conditions in the neonate that produce hypoglycemia relating to either imprecise control of glucose production or diminished substrate availability include the prematurely born neonate who is appropriate for gestational age, the small for gestational age neonate, the perinatally stressed and/or asphyxiated neonate, the cold-stressed neonate, and the neonate with either congenital heart disease or sepsis. The neonate may also be hypoglycemic because of glucagon deficiency or deficits in intermediary metabolic pathways such as glycogen storage disease type I or fructose-1,6-diphosphatase deficiency, reflecting a series of hereditary metabolic disorders in which hypoglycemia may be the initial or most obvious presenting feature.

The Preterm Appropriate for Gestational Age Neonate

The appropriate for gestation age neonate born before term may develop hypoglycemia. While the first report of this entity concerned the small for gestational age neonate,[39] subsequent studies documented hypoglycemia in the low birth weight neonate who was appropriate for gestational age. In 1968, Raivio and Hallman[40] reported a frequency of 1.4% of hypoglycemia in these neonates. Fluge[35] reported that as many as 14% of appropriate for gestational age neonates evidence neonatal hypoglycemia.

The diminished oral and parenteral intake in the low birth weight neonate in combination with the decreased concentration of substrates may explain the lower plasma glucose concentration seen in this neonate and his propensity for hypoglycemia. Functionally immature gluconeogenic and glycogenolytic enzyme systems present in the neonate potentiate these difficulties. The relatively increased size of the brain (i.e., 13% of the body mass in the neonate versus 2% in the adult) may be responsible for the greater proportion of glucose utilization during a period of fasting. This effect is magnified in the low birth weight neonate.

The Small for Gestational Age Neonate

Many centers have reported a relatively high frequency of hypoglycemia in the small for gestational age neonate ever since Cornblath et al.[39] in 1959 described its occurrence in eight infants born to mothers with toxemia. Lubchenco and Bard[41] and deLeeuw and deVries,[42] among others, have substantiated the occurrence of hypoglycemia in this neonate. Toxemia has been reported repeatedly to be associated with hypoglycemia, and its incidence has been shown to be highest (61%) in the neonate born to a mother with relatively low urinary estriols, compared to a frequency of 19% in the neonate born to a mother with a normal estriol concentration.[42,43] Reduction in energy reserves in the form of decreased glycogen deposition, combined with increased utilization of substrate, may account for the appearance of hypoglycemia (see Chapter 49).

Kliegman[44] studied the effect of maternal nutritional deprivation on fetal/neonatal metabolism in the dog. Besides reduced fetal weight at term (251 ± 7 vs 277 ± 7 g), the growth retarded pup evidenced lower glucose concentrations after 3, 6, and 9 hours of fasting, reduced plasma concentrations of free fatty acids at 9 and 24 hours, and a decreased ketone concentration at 24 hours compared to the control animal. While the systemic rates of palmitate and alanine turnover were not affected, systemic glucose production was reduced for 3 to 9 hours after birth, which resulted in the observed hypoglycemia. Kliegman speculated that reduced rates of gluconeogenesis from alanine and reduced oxidation of fuels such as free fatty acids contributed to the hypoglycemia. Free fatty acid recycling to triglyceride rather than oxidation contributed to the observed hypoglycemia.

Plasma insulin and blood glucose concentrations were measured in umbilical venous samples from 42 small for gestational age and 68 appropriate for gestational age fetuses by cordocentesis at 17 to 38 weeks' gestation.[45] In the appropriate for gestational age fetus plasma insulin concentration and the insulin-to-glucose ratio increased exponentially with gestation, suggesting maturation of the pancreas. The major determinant of fetal blood glucose concentration was maternal blood glucose concentration. The insulin-to-glucose ratio in the small for gestational age fetus was lower than in the appropriate for gestational age fetus, suggesting that hypoinsulinemia in the former was the result of hypoglycemia and pancreatic dysfunction. The degree of small for gestational age status did not correlate with plasma insulin concentration or the insulin-to-glucose ratio, which suggested to the investigators that insulin is not the primary determinant of fetal size.

Following bilateral maternal uterine artery ligation, Bussey et al.[46] studied the sequential changes in plasma glucose, insulin and glucagon concentrations, hepatic glycogen, and phosphoenolpyruvate carboxykinase during the first 4 hours in a growth-retarded rat pup model. Hypoglycemia was noted in the small for gestational age pup compared to control—an appropriate for gestational age pup—as well as reduced hepatic glycogen stores at birth. While plasma glucagon concentration increased, plasma insulin concentration declined. Phosphoenolpyruvate carboxykinase levels did not increase either. The investigators concluded that the small for gestational age pup develops hypoglycemia because of limited glycogen stores and retarded gluconeogenesis. The investigators speculated that delayed phosphoenolpyruvate carboxykinase induction in this animal may result from inadequate glycogen release at birth or decreased sensitivity to glucagon.

There have been a number of studies evaluating the intermediary metabolism of substrate available postnatally. A functional delay in the development of phosphoenolpyruvate carboxykinase, thought to be the rate-limiting enzyme of gluconogenesis, in the small for gestational age neonate was suggested by Haymond et al.[47] This was substantiated by Williams et al.,[48] who studied the effect of oral alanine feeding on glucose homeostasis in this neonate compared to the appropriate for gestational age neonate. Oral alanine feeding enhanced plasma glucagon concentration in both groups but stimulated hepatic glucose output only in the appropriate for gestational age neonate.

The effect of intravenously administered glucagon on plasma amino acid concentrations has been evaluated in various types of neonates including the small for gestational age neonate. This neonate in the first hours of life had significantly less total amino acids compared to a comparable group of appropriate for gestational age neonates, although the response to glucagon in the small for gestational age neonate mimicked the control group. It was speculated that the inability of the small for gestational age neonate to extract specific gluconeogenic amino acids could account for the susceptibility to hypoglycemia.[49]

Twenty-five neonates who were small for gestational age received $0.5\,mg\cdot day^{-1}$ glucagon to treat hypoglycemia.[50] Twenty of the 25 responded within 3 hours with an increase in blood glucose concentration to greater than $72\,mg\cdot dl^{-1}$. Five subsequently required hydrocortisone to maintain euglycemia. Rebound hypoglycemia occurred in nine following discontinuation of the glucagon. The response was poor after maternal beta blockade.

The role of glucagon was evaluated by Mestyan et al.[51] by measuring 17 amino acids before and during glucagon infusion in the normoglycemic and hypoglycemic small for gestational age neonates. In the normoglycemic group most amino acid concentrations declined significantly, but this did not occur in the neonate who was hypoglycemic. Although the effect was transient, these data reflect the ability of glucagon to produce acute changes in hepatic glucose homeostasis. This was demonstrated in the neonatal lamb between 1 and 3 days of age with infusions of somatostatin alone or in combination with insulin and glucagon during a 2-hour interval. Plasma glucose concentration declined when both insulin and glucagon were suppressed acutely, suggesting that the latter is of importance in maintaining glucose concentration during short-term fasting. It was suggested that the ratio between the two hormones acutely affected glucose homeostasis.[52]

The secretion of glucagon and insulin has been evaluated in the small for gestational age neonate. Both small and appropriate for gestational age neonates, after being fed oral glucose and protein at a rate of $1\,g\cdot kg^{-1}$ each after a 4-hour fast, had similar secretion of both pancreatic hormones. The investigators speculated that the instability of glucose metabolism in the small for gestational age neonate resulted from the rapid decline of glucose concentration and probably because of a transient deficiency of hepatic gluconeogenic enzymes, but not from an altered secretory pattern of the hormones.[53]

The adequacy of the hormonal response was reinforced in a study of the glucose infused small for gesttional age neonate who was evaluated by stable isotope kinetic analysis. Under stimulation of glucose infusion, this neonate and the appropriate for gestational age neonate had similar regulatory responses as well as functional integrity in handling glucose during the second day after birth.[54]

Using the newborn piglet model, Flecknell et al.[55] studied the effects of an intravenous glucose infusion on glucose homeostasis in the normal and growth-retarded neonatal piglet using a non–steady-state tracer technique. While suppression was noted in hepatic glucose output, hyperglycemia (i.e., pl glucose >150 mg·dl^{-1}) developed in the majority of study subjects. The mechanism of the hyperglycemia was thought to be failure to increase glucose utilization in response to the glucose infusion.

The possibility of hormonal excess producing growth retardation has been emphasized by Ogata et al.,[56] who adapted methodology to produce maternal hyperinsulinemia in a rat model. This resulted in decreased concentrations of glucose and amino acids in both the mother and fetus, which produced retarded fetal growth, limited hepatic glycogen deposition, and delayed neonatal phosphoenolpyruvate carboxykinase induction.

Sann et al.[57] evaluated the effect of hydrocortisone on intravenous glucose tolerance (i.e., 1 g·kg^{-1}) in eight term small for gestational age neonates compared to seven appropriate for gestational age neonates at a mean of 41 hours of age. The rate of glucose disappearance was decreased in the former neonate compared to the latter neonate. Plasma glucose concentration was similar in both groups while plasma insulin concentration did not change in the control group. After hydrocortisone administration, plasma insulin concentration increased. The investigators concluded that hydrocortisone induced a reduced peripheral uptake of glucose independent of insulin secretion.

In contrast, van Toledo-Eppinga et al.[58] evaluated leucine and glucose kinetics during growth hormone treatment in the intrauterine growth retarded preterm neonate. Seven neonates were studied and compared to eight appropriate for gestational age controls. The investigators concluded that postnatal treatment with recombinant human growth hormone supplementation was not effective in stimulating either protein gain or altering glucose kinetics in the intrauterine growth-retarded neonate.

The Neonate Experiencing Perinatal Stress/Hypoxia

The neonates that utilize glucose at an increased rate may be prone to hypoglycemia. Since the low birth weight neonate is subject to hypoxia, the combination of decreased substrate availability and increased rate of utilization may result in hypoglycemia. An increased rate of anaerobic glycolysis in combination with an increased rate of glycogenolysis is probably the underlying biochemical mechanism. Two moles of adenosine triphosphate (ATP) are generated by the Embden Meyerhof anaerobic pathway, whereas aerobic oxidation results in 36 mol of ATP. Eighteen times more glucose is required to generate the same amount of ATP. In addition, increased lactate production may result in an associated acidosis. Beard et al.[59,60] have emphasized the association between hypoxia and hypoglycemia in the low birth weight neonate and noted increased metabolic need out of proportion to substrate availability. The difficulties are accentuated in the neonate who is unable to replace substrate from the usual exogenous oral sources because of hypoxia or other clinical morbidity. Metabolic acidosis and lactic acidemia were noted during the first 24 hours of life in four term and 11 preterm neonates whose Apgar score had been 5 at 1 minute after birth and who were fed oral glucose loads.[61] Thus, not only may endogenous stores be depleted, but this neonate may be unable to tolerate an exogenous glucose load.

Another complication of perinatal stress is the presence of hyperinsulinism. In a report by Collins and Leonard[62] hyperinsulinism was noted unequivocally in three small for gestational age neonates and in three who were asphyxiated. The etiology of the hyperinsulinism was unclear.

A further evaluation of the metabolic effects of neonatal asphyxia was undertaken by Jansen et al.[63] Using a rat model, they showed that hypoxia drastically altered both metabolic fuel and glucoregulatory hormone availability. They suggested that persistence of the catecholamine surge, tissue hypoxia, and acidosis are responsible for the transient surge in glucose concentration and subsequent delay in the decline of insulin and increase of glucagon in the asphyxiated neonatal rat.

The Cold-Stressed Neonate

Hypoglycemia has been identified in the neonate who experiences cold injury. Mann and Elliott[64] described 14 neonates who suffered neonatal cold injury following prolonged exposure to environmental temperatures below 90°F. Marked hypoglycemia was documented in three of six neonates in whom it was measured. The hypoglycemia was presumed to be the result of free fatty acid elevation secondary to a cold-induced norepinephrine response.[65] Recognition of the potential association of hypoglycemia following cold stress should result in parenteral treatment, if necessary, in conjunction with the warming of the neonate. In addition, this relationship needs to be considered in the evaluation of blood glucose concentration in the neonate with temperature instability or in a suboptimal thermal environment.

Close et al.[66] evaluated the influence of environmental temperature on glucose tolerance and the insulin response in the neonatal piglet. Temperature was maintained at either 17°, 24°, or 33°C during which an intravenous infusion of 1 g glucose·kg^{-1} body weight was administered. Rectal temperature was maintained in all of the piglets subjected to the two higher temperatures, but not the lowest one in which 6 of 18 piglets became hypothermic. A higher glucose disappearance rate was noted; K_G: 200 and 2.32%/min was recorded for the animal maintaining homeothermic temperature during 17° and 24°C temperature conditions compared to those kept at thermal neutrality (1.66%/min). The insulin response was comparable. During hypothermia both K_G 0.76 ± 0.12% min and the insulin response were decreased. Glucose uptake by skeletal muscle was increased in the environmentally cold exposed homeothermic animal resulting in an increased metabolic rate (see Chapter 45).

The Neonate with Sepsis

Neonatal sepsis has been identified with increased frequency in association with hypoglycemia. Yeung[67] reported hypoglycemia in 20 of 56 neonates with signs of sepsis. He suggested that inadequate caloric intake in the infected neonate may predispose to its presence. The possibility of an increased metabolic rate was considered because the neonate in these studies was infused with 100 kcal·kg^{-1} day^{-1} intravenously. A decreased rate of gluconeogenesis has been documented in the laboratory animal following gram-negative bacterial infection.[68] The possibility of increased peripheral utilization because of enhanced insulin sensitivity in sepsis has been considered.[69] It is likely that one or more of these factors operate to produce the resultant hypoglycemia.

Fitzgerald et al.[70] further evaluated the effect of sepsis on carbohydrate metabolism by measuring plasma glucose, lactate, and insulin concentrations initially and then every 8 hours for 48 hours in a group of 29 neonates, six of whom had sepsis. Dextrose infusion, which was administered to maintain euglycemia, was elevated in the infected neonates, as was the plasma lactate concentration. The investigators concluded that these two parameters, plasma lactate concentration and the increased rate of dextrose infusion required, may be indicative of clinical sepsis in the early neonatal period.

The Neonate with Congenital Heart Disease/Congestive Heart Failure

An inverse relationship has been noted between the concentration of cardiac glycogen and the level of maturity of the neonate, exemplified by the decreased concentration in the offspring of mammalian species more mature at birth (e.g., humans, monkeys, sheep, etc.). These reserves are rapidly depleted during anoxia.[71] Benzing et al.[72] reported a series of 27 patients in whom the simultaneous occurrence of hypoglycemia and acute congestive heart failure was noted in association with congenital heart disease. Reduced dietary intake in association with diminished hepatic glycogen resulted in hypoglycemia. This has been further substantiated by Amatayakul et al.,[73] who noted the association of hypoglycemia with congestive heart failure in the neonate without a significant heart defect. The pathophysiology of hypoglycemia in cyanotic congenital heart disease was studied by Haymond et al.[74] Six subjects were evaluated between 13 and 67 months of age. Glucose and alanine turnover studies, utilizing stable isotope labeling in these neonates, were compared to control subjects. A subtle defect in hepatic extraction of gluconeogenic substrates was suspected, possibly secondary to decreased hepatic blood flow. It is apparent the presence of either hypoglycemia or congestive heart failure should be considered when either sign or symptom appears.

The interrelationship of hypoglycemia and pulmonary edema has been emphasized. Unfortunately, it was unclear whether the pulmonary edema was secondary to hypoglycemia or due to treatment of hypoglycemia since dextrose 20% in water ($D_{20}W$) was administered through an umbilical venous catheter into a branch of the left pulmonary vein.[75]

Nineteen neonates with symptomatic ventricular septal defect were examined by means of an intravenous glucose tolerance test and compared to 14 neonates who were healthy.[76] The neonate with ventricular septal defect was growth retarded with lower weight and length for age. Glucose tolerance was similar in both groups. Plasma insulin concentration was low in the neonate having a ventricular septal defect, but insulin secretion, as measured by C-peptide concentration, was elevated. The investigators speculated that increased insulin extraction occurs in the liver, but the mechanism is unknown.

The Neonate with Defective Gluconeogenesis/Glycogenolysis

Hypoglycemia has been noted in the neonate unable to sustain normal gluconeogenesis. Glucagon is important in hepatic glucose production since it enhances glycogenolysis and gluconeogenesis. There is a report of a neonate with isolated glucagon deficiency and neonatal hypoglycemia.[77] The diagnosis was based on a low basal glucagon concentration as well as a diminished response to hypoglycemia and alanine infusion, both potent stimulators of glucagon secretion, in a neonate with normal insulin secretion. Vidnes and Sovik[78,79] have reported three neonates with persistent neonatal hypoglycemia, one of whom evidenced an abnormal subcellular distribution of phosphoenolpyruvate carboxykinase in the extramitochondrial fraction.

A specific enzymatic deficiency that may affect gluconeogenesis in the neonate is type I glycogen storage disease with glucose-6-phosphatase deficiency. The deficiency is an autosomal recessive genetic defect that may occasionally present in the neonatal period with severe hypoglycemia and hepatomegaly. A second enzymatic defect, fructose-1,6-diphosphatase deficiency, has also been associated with hypoglycemia[80-82] (see Chapter 33).

Galactosemia may present after birth in the neonate who is septic and/or has hepatocellular jaundice. Later, at 1 month of age, the galactosemic infant may present with cataract formation. In some neonates, hypoglycemic symptoms have been reported and a positive reducing test noted in the urine to copper or iron. The usual biochemical defect is with galactose-1-phosphate uridyl transferase. The diagnosis involves the demonstration of a low true glucose concentration with the glucose oxidase technique in the presence of normal total hexoses, together with the determination of the enzymatic defect that can be analyzed in both the red and white blood cell. Exclusion of milk and milk products (i.e., lactose) is the treatment of choice. Because early intervention is preventative, routine neonatal screening has been recommended, since it is inherited as an autosomal recessive condition.[83]

Hereditary fructose intolerance may be diagnosed in the neonate who is old enough to ingest fruits or juices. The major intolerance is due to fructose-1-phosphate accumulation secondary to fructose-1-phosphate aldolase deficiency. The hypoglycemia is secondary to an inhibition of hepatic glucose release and absence of a hyperglycemic response to glucagon following ingestion or parenteral administration of fructose.

Pathophysiology of Hypoglycemia in the Neonate: Hyperinsulinism

Hypoglycemia secondary to increased plasma insulin concentration has now been associated with several discrete disorders of the pancreatic islet. It may be found in the infant of the diabetic mother (see Chapter 49), the neonate with hemolytic disease of the newborn, the neonate with nesidioblastosis or discrete or multiple islet cell adenomatosis, and the neonate requiring an exchange transfusion. The Beckwith-Wiedemann syndrome is another cause of hyperinsulinemic hypoglycemia, as is β-sympathomimetic treatment of the mother, following high umbilical artery catheter placement and following maternal ethanol consumption.

The Neonate with Rh Incompatibility

Hyperinsulinism has been implicated as the cause of the hypoglycemia seen in the neonate with severe Rh isoimmunization.[84-88] The neonate is invariably severely affected by his disease, with profound anemia and hepatosplenomegaly at birth. The shock and collapse seen on occasion may be caused primarily by profound hypoglycemia and, under such circumstances, glucose administration in addition to measures taken to correct the anemia may be necessary. The infant of the diabetic mother and severely Rh-affected neonate share several pathologic hallmarks. In addition to the hyperinsulinism and islet cell hyperplasia, both show almost identical edematous placental change. Both have excessive islands of extramedullary hematopoiesis in both liver and spleen. Although this latter finding may be the result of insulin stimulation, the precise cause of the hyperinsulinism itself in the Rh-affected neonate is uncertain. It has been suggested that an increase in reduced glutathione resulting from massive hemolysis of red blood cells may act as a stimulus to insulin release.

The Neonate Following Exchange Transfusion

Hypoglycemia, although not often considered, may be a significant problem following exchange transfusion. In this connection, the exchange blood and its preservatives are more critically important in the neonate in whom a double-volume washout is being undertaken than in an adult who is receiving 450 ml of the blood/preservative mixture to be diluted in the total 5 L or more, which is the blood volume.

Heparinized blood contains no added glucose. Moreover, the heparin, by raising the free fatty acid concentration, contributes to the hypoglycemic potential of the transfused blood, so that under some circumstances (e.g., severe Rh incompatibility with hyperinsulinism) its use would be contraindicated unless a concomitant intravenous glucose infusion is administered to prevent or treat hypoglycemia. With citrated blood, acid citrate dextrose (ACD), or citrate phosphate dextrose (CPD), the added dextrose yields a blood preservative mixture containing as much as 300 mg percent glucose. In this situation, although immediate hypoglycemia is usually not a problem, the high glucose load may result in a reactive insulin response. This response lags behind the glucose load being infused such that when the glucose "bolus" is suddenly terminated at the end of the exchange procedure, a state of hyperinsulinism ensues.[89] Studies documenting this occurrence have shown a precipitous 2-hour postexchange decline in blood glucose concentration to a value below that present prior to undertaking the exchange procedure.[90] Once again, the severely Rh-affected neonate is at greatest risk, but even the mildly affected and nonerythroblastotic neonate who undergoes an exchange transfusion may respond in such a manner. Recognition of this possibility should lead to its detection and treatment.

The Neonate with Beckwith-Wiedemann Syndrome

In 1964, Beckwith et al.[91] described a syndrome characterized by omphalocele, muscular macroglossia, and visceromegaly. Wiedemann[92] almost simultaneously described a similar clinical picture in three siblings. The etiology of the syndrome remains unclear. Pathologically, islet cell hyperplasia of the pancreas has been demonstrated in this neonate. It was subsequently shown that hypoglycemia may be an associated metabolic component of this syndrome, occurring in approximately 50% of the cases reported, with hyperinsulinism responsible for both the hypoglycemia and the somatic and visceral growth abnormalities. The hypoglycemia is ultimately self-limiting but may be protracted and difficult to control. In a patient with resistant hypoglycemia and hyperinsulinism, Schiff et al.[93] were ultimately able to achieve adequate control of glucose concentration with a combination of Sus-phrine and diazoxide therapy, which suppressed the release of basal and postprandial insulin secretion. The neonate presented at birth with an umbilical hernia, macroglossia, and hepatosplenomegaly as well as hyperinsulinism and severe, persistent hypoglycemia. Normal glucose control was achieved by 1 month of age. At 6 months, somatic growth was normal and hepatosplenomegaly had receded, but the macroglossia was still present. At 2 years of age growth was normal, and the tongue, although still large, could be kept within the oral cavity without any evidence of malocclusion.

The Neonate with Nesidioblastosis, Islet Cell Adenomas, or Adenomatosis

Although rare, nesidioblastosis,[94–97] discrete islet cell adenoma,[98,99] or adenomatosis[100,101] have been reported in the neonate and successfully treated. Hyperinsulinism without other apparent cause and resistant hypoglycemia should raise these rare but real possibilities. Preoperative confirmation may be sought either by means of ultrasound examination, regular GI radiographic studies, peritoneal air insufflation, or abdominal angiography, but surgical exploration may be necessary as a definitive diagnostic as well as therapeutic measure.

Solt'esz et al.[102] have reported 18 children with hyperinsulinemic hypoglycemia born to nondiabetic mothers. Thirteen presented within 3 days of birth, three by 20 months, and two by 9 years of age. The diagnosis was established by an altered insulin-to-glucose ratio with corresponding low ketone bodies, lactate, alanine, and glycerol concentrations. The subjects required increased rates of glucose administration of between 9 and 25 mg·kg^{-1}min^{-1} and had an increased glucose disappearance rate of K_G 7.6 ± 0.06%. The clinical course was quite variable: four subjects had transient hyperinsulinemia, two responded to diazoxide, two required both diazoxide and partial pancreatectomy, two responded to surgical excision of an isolated adenoma, five required total pancreatectomy for nesidioblastosis, and two were secondary to drug administration. In this series, heterogeneity existed in the clinical course of this condition.

Aynsley-Green et al.[103] evaluated plasma proinsulin and C-peptide concentrations in five children presenting with severe hyperinsulinemic hypoglycemia. Data were compared to those from 13 normal neonates. Three neonates and a 9-year-old required partial or total pancreatectomy. All evidenced an elevated proinsulin concentration and had an elevated C-peptide concentration as well, given the glucose concentration present. The investigators concluded that the insulin, proinsulin, and C-peptide concentration profile does not provide a reliable indicator for the underlying pathologic mechanism.

W'uthrich et al.[104] reported two siblings who had persistent neonatal hyperinsulinemic hypoglycemia who were successfully treated with diazoxide at a dose of 10 mg·kg^{-1}day^{-1} for 8 years and 1 year, respectively, without the necessity of surgery.

Bruining et al.[105] reported normalization of glucose homeostasis by utilization of a long-acting somatostatin analogue SMS 201-995 in a neonate with nesidioblastosis. Because a glucose infusion was unable to maintain euglycemia ≥36 mg·dl^{-1}, SMS 201-995 was administered. Coincident with its use, insulin concentration decreased and clinically apparent seizures disappeared. As in other cases, a subtotal pancreatectomy was performed as a primary treatment for the diagnosis of nesidioblastosis.

Glaser et al.[106] studied six neonates with persistent hypoglycemia secondary to hyperinsulinemia who were treated with somatostatin analogue SMS 201-995. Effective control by use of the drug alone was achieved in five of six neonates with administration of 10 to 40 μg·kg^{-1}day^{-1} given by subcutaneous injection. Most infants subsequently required subtotal pancreatectomy, but in one case long-term therapy with the drug alone achieved the therapeutic response necessary to maintain euglycemia.

However, nesidioblastosis may be noted in normal tissue and may not be the morphologic hallmark of hyperinsulinemic hypoglycemia.[107] The investigators suggested the term nesidiodysplasia, which includes increased, maldistributed, malregulated, or malprogrammed endocrine and amphocrine cells associated with cases of familial persistent hyperinsulinemic hypoglycemia of infancy.

The most likely inheritance is an autosomal recessive pattern.[108] The incidence of the condition has been estimated at 1/50,000 live births in a random mating population, but in Saudi Arabia the incidence is 1/2675 because 51% of births occur to parents who are first or second cousins. This epidemiologic situation provided the milieu to use a strategy known as homozygosity mapping to localize the gene responsible for the disease. The progeny of five families in whom this condition was present were studied by Thomas et al.[109] Glaser et al.[110] had reported linkage of this condition to chromosome 11p14-15.1, which was supported by the evaluation of these five families. Thomas et al.[109] localized this disorder to chromosome 11p between markers D11S1334 and D11S899 with a maximum logarithm base 10 of the odds ratio (LOD) score of 5.02 at marker D11S926. The investigators suggested that the gene responsible for familial persistent hyperinsulinemic hypoglycemia of infancy is likely to have an important role in the regulation of insulin release and normal pancreatic β-cell development.

The Neonate Whose Mother Received β-Sympathomimetics During Premature Labor

Investigations have described the potential for hypoglycemia after β-sympathomimetic tocolytic therapy, which is utilized increasingly to inhibit the premature onset of labor. A possible explanation of the relationship involves increased pancreatic secretion of insulin in response to a specific glucose concentration.[111,112] A prospective double-blind study of 35 patients in preterm labor with and without ruptured membranes was conducted by Leake et al.,[113] who evaluated the neonatal metabolic and cardiovascular effects of maternal Ritodine administration to the mother. Patients had received either intravenous and/or oral Ritodrine or a placebo. The shortest time from drug administration to delivery was 6 hours. No differences were noted in the Ritodrine group versus the control group relative to glucose concentration or cardiovascular evaluation. The investigators concluded that chronic oral administration did not significantly affect the neonate.

In an investigation of the etiology of the clinical situation, a neonatal lamb model was used to evaluate the drug.[114] Administration of Ritodrine produced both increased insulin secretion from the β cell and glucose production from the liver. Based on the mechanism(s) of action, it was concluded by the investigators that the presence of clinical hypoglycemia would depend on the time of administration prior to delivery.

The Neonate with an Umbilical Artery Catheter

Another cause of relative hyperinsulinism was reported to be secondary to malposition of an umbilical artery catheter. In a neonate requiring supplemental oxygen because of increasing respiratory distress, hypoglycemia was relieved only when a "high" catheter was repositioned from T11–12 to L-4. Following repositioning of the catheter, the child became euglycemic.[115] Malik and Wilson[116] reported two neonates who developed hyperinsulinism secondary to malposition of the umbilical arterial catheter. Repositioning resulted in cessation of the hyperinsulinemia. Puri et al.[117] reported the association of neonatal hypoglycemia associated with position of an umbilical catheter between the 8th and 9th thoracic vertebrae, which is the normal location. In this report, the catheter was moved and neonatal hypoglycemia resolved. Three neonates were reported whose catheter were placed between the 8th and 10th thoracic vertebrae. They were noted to have hypoglycemia that responded to catheter withdrawal to the 3rd to 4th lumbar region. The investigators speculated that the cause was significant streaming of glucose to the celiac axis. The mechanism of the hypoglycemia was postulated to be excessive insulin secretion following infusion into the celiac axis.[118]

This association was studied in a neonatal lamb model and the clinical suspicion was confirmed. The mechanism was felt to be decreased production of hepatic glucose secondary to the presumed increased portal insulin following "high" catheter placement.[119]

Jacob and Davis[120] studied differences in serum glucose concentration from different extremities in the neonate with an umbilical arterial catheter through which dextrose was infused. The neonate without a catheter evidenced no difference in simultaneous measurement of capillary glucose concentration, obtained from both lower extremities, while the neonate with a catheter did. Interestingly, the neonate with a high catheter did not. As expected, the highest concentration was confirmed from the extremity into which the catheter was placed. This is yet another study pointing out the heterogeneity possible in glucose determination depending on the location from which the blood is taken.

The Neonate Whose Mother Consumed Ethanol

The association of neonatal hypoglycemia and maternal ethanol ingestion has been reported. Singh et al.[121] evaluated glucose metabolism in a newborn rat model in which the mother was given ethanol. Blood glucose concentration, liver glycogen, and plasma insulin concentration were decreased in the ethanol-treated mother, as was liter size and average fetal body weight. The pup from an ethanol fed mother evidenced hypoglycemia and hypoinsulinemia. Within 1 hour after birth an elevation in blood glucose concentration was followed by a decrease to the hypoglycemic range. Liver glycogen stores, which were reduced, were quickly mobilized. The hypoglycemic tendency in the pup of an ethanol-treated mother disappeared after 4 days.

Witek-Janusek[122] examined the effect of maternal ethanol ingestion on the maternal and newborn glucose balance in a rat model. Controls were given an isocaloric liquid diet or ad libitum rat chow. Blood for glucose concentration and liver were sampled on days 21/22 and the pup was studied up to 24 hours after birth. Ethanol depressed not only maternal liver glycogen stores but also liver glycogen in the neonatal liver. Ethanol had no effect on plasma insulin concentration. Postnatal hypoglycemia could be observed following maternal ethanol ingestion. Singh et al.[123] evaluated the combined effect of chronic ethanol ingestion in the pregnant rat and the offspring. Fetal body weight and liver weight were reduced in the fetus of the alcohol fed mother. Blood glucose concentration was also lower, as was liver glycogen.

Other Causes of Hyperinsulinism

Isolated instances have been reported that mimic the problem of insulin excess and resultant hypoglycemia. Zucker and Simon[124] have reported symptomatic neonatal hypoglycemia in association with maternal administration of chlorpropamide. This resulted in stimulation of both the maternal as well as the fetal β cell. Because teratogenicity of the drug is a concern, its use is limited, especially since it provides poor control of glucose for the management of diabetes in pregnancy. Benzothiadiazide (i.e., thiazide) diuretics have been implicated in stimulating insulin secretion.[125] It has been suggested that these drugs produce an elevated maternal blood glucose concentration and stimulate the fetal islet with subsequent resultant neonatal hypoglycemia. There is a report of an neonate in whom hypoglycemia may have been due to an insulin-releasing substance, possibly from the gut.[126]

Hypoglycemia has been noted in individuals who are sensitive to leucine. This amino acid, among others, is known to be associated with increased insulin release and may be seen following ingestion of milk.[127] Recently, a fourth defect of leucine metabolism, 3-hydroxy-3-methyl glutaryl coenzyme A (CoA) lyase deficiency has been reported. Hypoglycemia was noted along with a characteristic excretory pattern of organic acids, but the exact mechanism resulting in the hypoglycemia was not apparent.[128]

Neonatal hypoglycemia has followed administration of salicylates, the suggested mechanism being an uncoupling of mitochondrial oxidative phosphorylation.[129] The association of congenital adrenal hyperplasia and hypoglycemia has been recorded.[130] Souto et al.[131] studied the effect of equivalent doses of insulin on the adrenal medulla of the neonatal and adult rat. Glycemia decreased to 33% of the control concentration in the adult while an equivalent dose of insulin to the neonate decreased glycemia to about 50%. Morphologic evaluation of the adrenal medulla supported the metabolic data. The investigators speculated that immaturity of the adrenal chromaffin tissue may be present in the neonate and is involved in hypoglycemic catecholamine counterregulation.

Artavia-Loria et al.[132] reported a survey of the frequency of hypoglycemia in 165 children who had primary adrenal insufficiency: 70% had congenital adrenal hyperplasia, 47% had Addison's disease, and 18% had hypoglycemia. One half of the episodes were in the neonatal period. The episodes of hypoglycemia were isolated in 13 children, four neonates with congenital adrenal hyperplasia and in one male with 11B-OH deficiency. Mechanistically, a significant correlation was noted between plasma glucose concentration and cortisol concentration during the episodes of hypoglycemia.

Hypoglycemia has been noted secondary to the treatment of indomethacin administered to the premature neonate with symptomatic patent ductus arteriosus. Unfortunately, the proposed mechanism of indomethacin (i.e., mediated lack of prostaglandin inhibition of insulin release) was not confirmed since there were no significant changes in plasma insulin concentration in one series.[133]

Evaluation of the Neonate with Hypoglycemia

As with any other diagnostic dilemma in neonatology, a detailed maternal history and thorough physical examination are required to determine the probable etiology of neonatal hypoglycemia. Maternal history including family history of diabetes or other glucose intolerance, drug ingestion (e.g., chlorpropamide, benzothiadiazide diuretics, salicylates, and ethanol), blood group incompatibility, preeclampsia, or pregnancy-induced hypertension, and the rate of dextrose administered to the mother during labor, should alert the physician to the potential etiology (i.e., the mechanism) of the observed hypoglycemia.

A thorough physical examination of the neonate indicates gestational age, and if the neonate is AGA, SGA, or large for gestational age (LGA). The appearance of the infant of the well-controlled diabetic of classes A, B, and C can usually be differentiated from that of the infant of classes D, E, and F who may be SGA. The neonate with Beckwith-Wiedemann syndrome is usually obvious with evidence of a protuberant tongue, umbilical hernia, and macrosomia. Prolonged jaundice and cataracts, which may not be apparent until 1 month of age, are indicative of galactosemia, as is the presence of reducing substances in the urine. Unexplained hepatomegaly may be indicative of glycogen storage disease (see Chapter 33). Abnormalities that may indicate central defects include abnormal genitalia, suggestive of pituitary abnormalities, and cleft lip and palate.

Appropriate laboratory evaluation should include evaluation of glucose, insulin, growth hormone, and cortisol concentrations, as well as thyroid function testing. Evaluation of pH, lactate, pyruvate, and ketone concentrations is indicated for glycogen storage disease. Studies are usually drawn when hypoglycemia is present or at a time following a fast of at least 3 to 4 hours. Tolerance tests are reserved for confirmation of a possible diagnosis such as a glucagon tolerance test if glycogen storage disease is suspected. A further clinical evaluation of the neonate, infant, and older child has been outlined by Sperling.[134] An evaluation of the neonate with a potential metabolic defect is comprehensively delineated in minute detail in Chapter 53.

Treatment of Hypoglycemia

Treatment of neonatal hypoglycemia begins with identification of its presence in the neonate at risk, documentation of its existence by appropriate laboratory measurement (vide supra), and corrective measures.

Oral administration of nutrients generally is advocated as either 5% dextrose or formula, but probably should be used only to maintain a glucose concentration already in the euglycemic range. With $6\,mg \cdot kg^{-1} min^{-1}$ used as the rate of glucose infusion required to maintain homeostasis, it is probably unreasonable to expect that oral feedings alone will provide for adequate glucose intake in the neonate who is diagnosed with hypoglycemia by laboratory analysis. Parenteral (i.e., intravenous) treatment of hypoglycemia with a constant infusion pump should avoid fluctuation in the rate of infusion that would result in variable insulin release. Oral feeding should be initiated as tolerated. Repeated documentation of blood or plasma glucose concentration should be an integral part of the treatment of any neonate. The glucose infusion rate should be gradually reduced rather than abruptly terminated so that sudden reactive hypoglycemia due to "uncovered" hyperinsulinism is avoided. Once oral feedings are initiated, evaluation of the glucose concentration just before a subsequent feeding provides documentation of the neonate's euglycemic status.

Parenteral therapy should begin with $6\,mg \cdot kg^{-1} min^{-1}$ followed by graded increases to achieve euglycemia with the minimal concentration of glucose required. A peripheral vein rather than an umbilical vessel is the preferred route of infusion. However, other than in an emergency, a concentration greater than 12.5% dextrose should be infused through a central venous route. A concentration greater than 20% dextrose is probably contraindicated by either route. Acute administration of 25% glucose by bolus infusion of up to $4\,ml \cdot kg^{-1}$, if required for relief of acute symptoms (e.g., seizures), must be followed by parenteral infusion until the effect of the bolus infusion on acute pancreatic insulin release subsides. However, more popular currently is an infusion of $2\,ml \cdot kg^{-1}$ of 10% dextrose in H$_2$O ($200\,mg \cdot kg^{-1}$) given over 1 minute, followed by a continuous dextrose infusion of $8\,mg \cdot kg^{-1} min^{-1}$ (Figure 32.4).[135]

Calculation of parenteral glucose therapy must include the actual concentration of glucose present in the administered fluid. A hydrated form of dextrose ($C_6H_{12}O_6 \cdot H_6O$) (molecular weight of 198) is used by most manufacturers to prepare the parenteral fluid so that the actual amount of glucose available is approximately 10% less.[136] This is of particular concern when the very low birth weight or severely hypoglycemic neonate is being treated.

There are increasing reports of the use of lipid infusion to assist in prevention of hypoglycemia. The mechanism of action is discussed later in this chapter. Sann et al.[137] evaluated the effect of oral lipid supplementation on the prevention of neonatal hypoglycemia in 28 low birth weight neonates whose mean gestational age was 36 ± 1 weeks and whose birth weight was $1778 \pm 230\,g$ compared to a control group of 23 neonates who had comparable demographic data. Hypoglycemia $\leq 31\,mg \cdot dl^{-1}$ occurred in 8 of 23 neonates in the control group versus 2 of 28 in the supplemented group receiving $2.9\,g \cdot day^{-1}$ of a solution containing 67% medium-chain triglycerides. This prospective study reported that lipid supplementation can

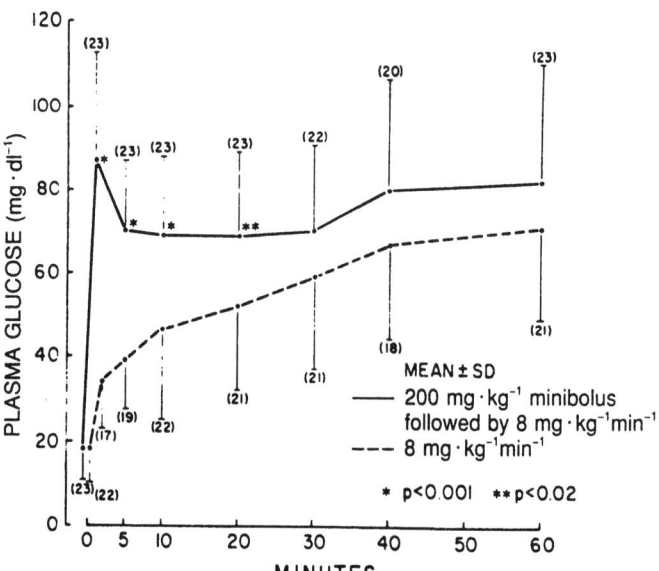

FIGURE 32.4. Plasma glucose concentrations in neonates treated with $200\,mg \cdot kg$ minibolus followed by $8\,mg \cdot kg^{-1} min^{-1}$ constant glucose infusion compared with plasma glucose concentration of neonates treated with constant infusion alone. (From Lilien et al.,[135] with permission.)

prevent the occurrence of hypoglycemia in the low birth weight neonate.

Treatment with a number of specific agents is indicated when parenteral therapy above 15 mg·kg^{-1}·min^{-1} is not effective in maintaining euglycemia. Corticosteroids have been shown to be effective in the therapy of hypoglycemia. Although several glucose-producing reactions are enhanced by the steroids, the major effect is probably that of gluconeogenesis from noncarbohydrate (i.e., protein) sources and decreased peripheral glucose utilization. Hydrocortisone is given in a dose of 5 mg·kg^{-1}·day^{-1} either intravenously or orally every 12 hours, or prednisone is used at a dose of 2 mg·kg^{-1}·day^{-1} orally. As with all forms of therapy, gradual diminution of the dosage administered, in concert with decreasing parenteral concentration of glucose and increasing oral intake of nutrients, should successfully wean the patient.

The use of glucagon provides a highly effective method of releasing glycogen from the liver and can indeed be a diagnostic therapeutic means of assessing whether or not the liver contains adequate stores. Its failure in some growth-retarded neonates is considered to be evidence for a lack of hepatic glycogen stores. In the infant of the diabetic mother, there is often a failure to respond to the usual doses (30 mg·kg^{-1}), despite the presence of more than adequate hepatic glycogen stores. The neonate frequently responds to a higher dose (300 mg·kg^{-1}) with prolonged and sustained hyperglycemia, so that the higher dose might well be used as initial therapy. Since glucagon may stimulate insulin release, its administration in all probability should be accompanied by an intravenous glucose infusion.

Like glucagon, epinephrine is capable of promoting glycogen to glucose conversion, but in far smaller quantities. For this effect glucagon is probably the drug of choice. The hyperglycemic potential of epinephrine in blocking glucose uptake by peripheral muscle presupposes an adequate blood concentration initially and is of little practical benefit in the hypoglycemic state. Epinephrine is a powerful anti-insulin hormone, a fact that explains its success as an effective antihypoglycemic agent in the infant of the diabetic mother as well as in other hyperinsulinemic neonates. The agent most commonly used is a 1:200 epinephrine in aqueous suspension (Sus-Phrine), which can be readily administered subcutaneously.[138]

Diazoxide, in a dose of 10 to 15 mg·kg^{-1}·day^{-1}, probably exerts its effect by suppressing pancreatic insulin secretion, although some investigators have suggested a direct effect on hepatic glucose production.[139,140] The drug should be used only when other modalities have failed.

Somatostatin, as described above, has been utilized to suppress insulin, as well as glucagon secretion and growth hormone, clinically as well as experimentally.[105,141]

Surgical intervention is indicated when an islet cell adenoma or adenomatosis has been confirmed.

Hyperglycemia in the Neonate

Hyperglycemia may be a problem for the neonate because of the theoretical potential for an osmotic diuresis and resultant dehydration.[142,143] Gentz and Cornblath[144] reviewed the problem of hyperglycemia in the SGA neonate with transient neonatal diabetes in the first 6 weeks of life. Symptoms included failure to thrive and dehydration despite adequate oral intake.

A major problem, in view of the widespread use of parenteral alimentation to nourish the low birth weight neonate, is the increasing number of reports of hyperglycemia that have been appearing in the literature over the past 30 years. The incidence will probably increase because of the growing prevalence of the very low birth weight neonates who are being cared for successfully in the intensive care setting.[19] Dweck and Cassady[16] originally reported on 43 of 50 neonates who weighed 1100 g or less who had a plasma glucose concentration of 125 mg·dl^{-1} or greater during parenteral glucose administration. Thirty-six of these infants had a plasma glucose concentration >300 mg·dl^{-1}, usually within 24 hours of birth. Diminished tolerance to glucose was inferred in the very low birth weight neonate who did not manifest the well-known adult Staub-Traugott effect (i.e., lower blood glucose concentration and increasingly rapid disappearance rates of glucose following its repeated administration).[145]

Zarif et al.[17] measured glucose, insulin, and growth hormone concentrations prospectively during the first 5 days of life in the low birth weight neonate receiving a parenteral or oral glucose load or a combination of both. Hyperglycemia was noted in 33 of 75 infants, and an association was noted between death and hyperglycemia. Insulin and growth hormone responses were not felt to be of etiologic significance. The investigators did report that most neonates had been stressed, suggesting the possibility of increased cortisol and/or catecholamine secretion.

A series of studies defined tolerance for glucose in 35 clinically healthy appropriate for gestational age neonates weighing 750 to 1500 g between 3 and 38 days of age.[18] Neonates were given graded doses of glucose at either 8, 11, or 14 mg·kg^{-1}·min^{-1} for 3 hours by continuous peripheral intravenous infusion. Plasma glucose and insulin concentrations and timed urine volume and glucose concentrations were measured. Nine neonates received 8 mg·kg^{-1}·min^{-1} and, in these neonates, plasma glucose and insulin concentrations were similar in the steady-state period. None of these neonates evidenced hyperglycemia. In contrast, 10 neonates receiving

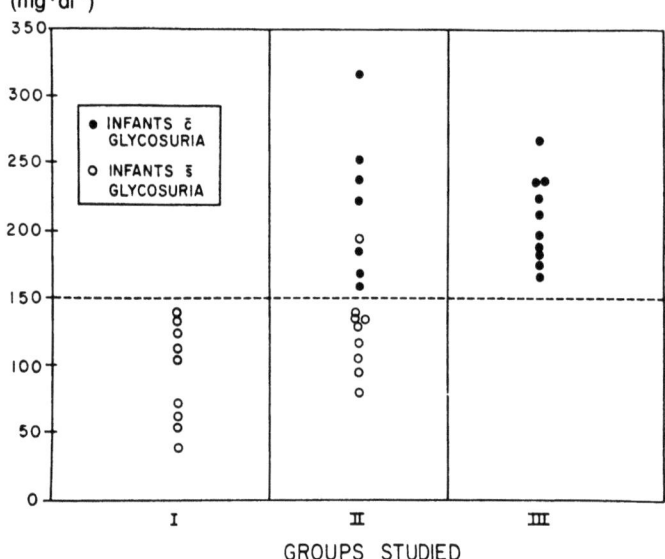

FIGURE 32.5. Maximum plasma glucose concentration in infants in the three groups. A plasma glucose concentration of 150 mg·kg^{-1}min^{-1} denoted hyperglycemia. (From Cowett et al.,[18] with permission.)

14 mg·kg^{-1}min^{-1} of exogenous glucose developed significantly higher plasma glucose and insulin concentrations in contrast to the neonates receiving 8 mg·kg^{-1}min^{-1} of infused glucose. Sixteen neonates received 11 mg·kg^{-1}min^{-1} and the plasma glucose concentration significantly increased to 140 to 160 mg·dl^{-1} in a comparable time period, but the plasma insulin concentration was not significantly different from baseline. Half of these neonates developed hyperglycemia (i.e., plasma glucose concentration >150 mg·dl^{-1}) with concomitant glycosuria as noted in Figure 32.5. At the time of study, all of these neonates had been clinically asymptomatic for at least 48 hours. These findings parallel the work of others who have also suggested that clinical morbidity may unfavorably affect neonatal glucose homeostasis.[146] Of importance, glycosuria did not exceed 6.4 mg·kg^{-1}min^{-1}, so that the glucose disposal rate (i.e., the retention rate) exceeded 90% of intake and an osmotic diuresis was not present in the glycosuric neonate. The presence of glycosuria was not related to neonatal postnatal age as depicted in Figure 32.6. The potential for an osmotic diuresis and dehydration may be more theoretic than real.

The interest in this clinical problem is noted by the increasing number of mechanisms that have been proposed to explain its presence clinically. Louik et al.[147] evaluated risk factors for neonatal hyperglycemia associated with 10% dextrose infusion as part of a drug surveillance program. A population of 1157 neonates was evaluated. Hyperglycemia, related to the 10% dextrose solution, was noted in 64 neonates, which was a frequency rate of 5.5%. This frequency is similar to that of the rate for hypoglycemia of 6.7%. There was an inverse correlation between frequency of hyperglycemia and decreasing birth weight. The risk of hyperglycemia was 18 times greater in the neonate of <1000 g birth weight than in the neonate of >2000 g birth weight. The risk also multiplied with increasing rate of glucose administration. These two risk factors were independent. Finally, specific stresses (e.g., increasing severity of respiratory distress and need to receive bicarbonate, used as an indirect measure of severity of illness), were associated with an increasing risk of hyperglycemia.

Wu et al.[148] have evaluated the occurrence of hyperglycemia in the neonate of ≤1000 g birth weight. The

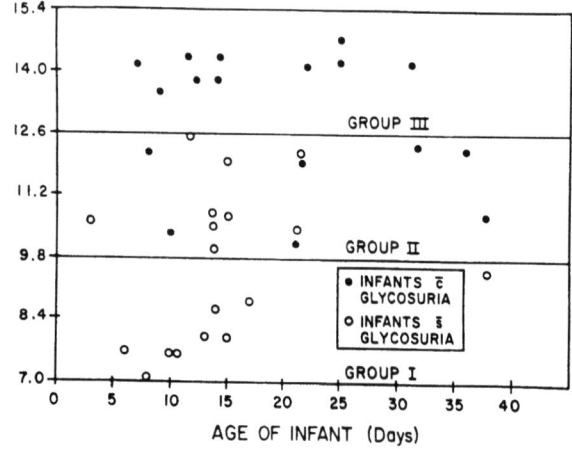

FIGURE 32.6. Rate of glucose infusion in the infants in the three groups plotted in relation to postnatal age at time of study. (From Cowett et al.,[18] with permission.)

mean birth weight was 802 ± 123 g and the gestational age was 27 ± 2 weeks. Correlation coefficients showed a correlation between the glucose infusion rate, caloric intake, and glucose concentration, but not between postnatal age and glucose concentration. Sixty-eight percent of the neonates had at least two values >150 mg·dl^{-1} associated with drugs, increased glucose infusion rate, or respiratory stress. These evaluations confirm the labile nature of neonatal glucose homeostasis in the micropremie.

The appearance of hyperglycemia in relation to neonatal surgery has been documented[149-154] (see Chapter 50). Srinivasan et al.[149] evaluated specific metabolic parameters of glucose homeostasis before, during, and following surgery in 16 term neonates. The rate of glucose infusion was maintained at 4.1 ± 1.2 mg·kg^{-1}min^{-1} and fluid losses during surgery were replaced without dextrose. The age of the patients was 1 day to 40 weeks and the surgical procedure lasted 83 ± 35 minutes. Both postinduction and postsurgical mean plasma glucose concentrations were elevated compared to the immediately preceding period. Both plasma insulin and plasma glucose concentrations were variable and inconsistent. The presence of hyperglycemia >150 mg·dl^{-1} was noted in 10 of 16 neonates and must be anticipated when a neonate requires surgery.

Steroids are being utilized commonly in the low birth weight neonate with bronchopulmonary dysplasia.[155-158] The untoward effect of hyperglycemia has been reported by Ferrara et al.[159] They evaluated a group of 77 very low birth weight neonates (mean birth weight 891 ± 209 g) who had a diagnosis of bronchopulmonary dysplasia. They were treated with dexamethasone to assist in weaning from mechanical ventilation. Besides other complications, glucose intolerance occurred in 40% (i.e., 29 of the 73 infants evaluated). Glucose intolerance resolved in all subjects following discontinuation of therapy. Increasing awareness is necessary to understand the prevalence of hyperglycemia with steroid use in the neonatal intensive care unit.

There is a case report of a neonate who had culture proven *Escherichia coli* sepsis in association with clinical evidence of hyperglycemia. Since the neonate's plasma insulin concentration was correspondingly low, the investigators postulated an inadequate insulin response as a mechanism of the observed hyperglycemia.[160] A recent report has documented the occurrence of hyperglycemia following administration of methylxanthines (e.g., theophylline) to the neonate. The mechanism of the hyperglycemia was postulated to be increased adenosine 3′,5′-cyclic monophosphate (cAMP) resulting in activation of hepatic glycogen phosphorylase and glycogen synthase. Both enzymes may increase the hepatic output of glucose.[161] The association of hyperglycemia and a chromosome deletion (46,xxDq-) on number 13 has been reported in an SGA neonate.[162]

Finally, the mechanisms involved in the clinical phenomenon of hyperglycemia in association with administration of parenteral alimentation and intravenous fat emulsion in the prematurely born neonate were studied by Yunis et al.[163] using stable isotopic glucose kinetic analysis. The investigators concluded that the increased plasma glucose concentration noted clinically was not due to enhanced glucose production, but rather probably the result of alterations in glucose utilization (vide infra).

Evaluation of the Neonate with Hyperglycemia

As noted previously in the discussion of the evaluation of neonatal hypoglycemia, a thorough evaluation of the maternal history and physical examination of the neonate is necessary to determine the diagnosis. This thorough review should provide clues to support one or more of the specific etiologies discussed above. It is necessary to calculate the rate of glucose/nutrient/fluid administered to confirm an appropriate rate of delivery. Measurement of plasma glucose concentration is necessary, as is measurement of urinary volume and glucose concentration to rule out the possibility of an osmotic diuresis, which, as discussed above may be unlikely except in specific circumstances.[19] Severity of the clinical course, the presence of infection or sepsis, and the need for surgery are major etiologic possibilities.

Treatment of Hyperglycemia

Treatment of hyperglycemia includes a decrease in the rate of glucose administration with ~6 mg·kg^{-1}min^{-1} equaling basal glucose production or administration of insulin. It would seem prudent to decrease the rate of carbohydrate administration first, rather than give insulin, as long as 60 kcal·kg^{-1}day^{-1} is provided to spare protein for subsequent somatic growth.[164] A number of investigators have documented the use of insulin in the treatment of hyperglycemia. Insulin has been administered to treat the extreme hyperglycemia that occurs without concomitant ketosis or acidosis. Subsequently, others have confirmed this treatment modality and suggested that deficient insulin secretion, production of a biologically inactive form of insulin, or altered conversion of proinsulin to insulin may be responsible for the clinical appearance of hyperglycemia.[165-167]

Exogenous insulin as a treatment for hyperglycemia to increase glucose disposal was reported in eight low birth weight neonates (1500 g) by Pollak et al.[168] A saline placebo was given during infusion of 14 mg·kg^{-1}min^{-1} of exogenous glucose on day 1 and was followed on day 2 by 10 mU·kg^{-1}min^{-1} of insulin infused over 50 minutes under similar conditions of glucose administration. Euglycemia resulted from the exogenous administration of the insulin. The investigators speculated that hyperglycemia during exogenous infusion of glucose was the result either of persistent endogenous hepatic glucose production or decreased peripheral utilization, but the two entities could not be differentiated. It appeared that an elevated plasma insulin concentration was required to achieve appropriate control of glucose homeostasis.

An extension of this concept was proposed by utilization of an "adult type" insulin pump to administer insulin to the very low birth weight neonate to improve glucose tolerance. Ostertag et al.,[169] a group that included an internist who has a great deal of experience in the use of the insulin pump, "borrowed" the pump from internal medicine and showed that it could be utilized successfully in the neonate for limited periods of time. Others have previously reported the administration of insulin to the neonate by more conventional intravenous therapy.[170,171] Until the report of Ostertag et al., the usual mode of administration was by retrograde infusion of 0.01 to 0.1 units·kg^{-1} for 2 to 4 hours in 0.25% salt-poor albumin concomitantly with a glucose infusion. In the small, sick, stressed neonate, insulin may be given safely as long as the glucose concentration is monitored appropriately, because of the relatively wide heterogeneous response that is possible following its administration. A great deal of experience needs to be gained, as well as miniaturization of the equipment, before the use of an insulin pump may be considered anything more than a research tool in the neonatal intensive care unit. It also needs to be shown that insulin delivery by use of the insulin pump is an improvement over the more conventional mechanical pumps presently in use.

An extension of the above, related to administration of insulin, was reported by Heron and Boucher.[172] They studied 15 preterm neonates whose mean gestation was 27 weeks and whose mean birth weight was 860g who were treated with insulin to counteract significant glucose intolerance. Energy intake increased from 61 ± 25 cal·kg^{-1}day^{-1} to 80 ± 25 cal·kg^{-1}day^{-1} and the dextrose infusion tolerated increased from 7.0 ± 2.7 mg·kg^{-1}min^{-1} to 9.2 ± 2.6 mg·kg^{-1}min^{-1} beginning at 5.3 days on the average and continuing for 1.5 to 17.5 days. The investigators cautioned about the need for repetitive monitoring of glucose concentration.

Binder et al.[173] treated the neonate whose birth weight was ≤1000g who had hyperglycemia and glycosuria with graded insulin infusion while energy intake was increased to 100 kcal·kg^{-1}day^{-1}. Of 76 neonates who survived, 34 received insulin and 42 did not. Those who required treatment were, as expected, smaller (767 ± 161g vs 872 ± 98g), and younger (26.8 ± 1.4 weeks vs 27.7 ± 2.0 weeks), and under more stress since they required ventilation longer (28 ± 19 days vs 17 ± 15 days). The treated neonates had a blood glucose concentration of 195 ± 60 mg·dl^{-1} during which time they received 7.9 ± 3.0 mg·kg^{-1}min^{-1}. Insulin improved glucose tolerance in the extremely low birth weight neonate.

In another study Collins et al.[174] conducted a prospective, randomized trial in 24 neonates whose birth weight mean was 772 + 128g to determine whether a continuous insulin infusion would improve glucose tolerance. Those neonates who received insulin for hyperglycemia tolerated higher glucose infusion rates, had greater nonprotein energy intake, and had better weight gain than the control neonates. The investigators appropriately cautioned that, before insulin is recommended for the routine care of the extremely low birth weight neonate, its effect on cellular metabolism and on the growth of specific tissue should be determined.

It is apparent that besides regulation of the rate of glucose administration and possible insulin delivery to treat hyperglycemia, there should be a concerted effort to identify the etiology that may be causing the problem. As noted, this may be secondary to the extreme prematurity of the neonate[19,147] or other significant stresses that are present clinically. Before lowering the concentration of parenteral glucose administered on the basis of hyperglycemia alone, one must measure urine concentration and volume to confirm the presence of an osmotic diuresis, which may be absent in the very low birth weight neonate. The concentration of hyperglycemia at which untoward central nervous system effects are first manifest has not been documented in the human. However, the presence of intracranial bleeding was documented in the newborn puppy in whom acute hyperglycemia was produced by "standard regimens" of glucose therapy.[175] Caution and further evaluation are necessary to define the effect of acute and chronic hyperglycemia on the central nervous system of the infant at risk (vide infra) (see Chapter 26).

Some investigators have suggested that early delivery of enteral feeding would assist in maintenance of glucose homeostasis in the prematurely born neonate who is hyperglycemic following intravenous glucose administration.[176] One mechanism may be enhanced gastrointestinal insulin release present in response to orogastric administration of a glucose load, which may occur when a threshold of glucose concentration has exceeded 105 mg·dl^{-1}.[177] Further investigation of this concept is necessary.

Control of Neonatal Glucose Homeostasis

There are a multiplicity of factors that influence neonatal glucose homeostasis. As noted in Table 32.5, specific clinical factors and maturational components influence glucose metabolism in the neonatal period. The gesta-

TABLE 32.5. Neonatal glucose homeostasis.

Clinical ⟷	Homeostasis ⟷	Maturation (control)
Gestational age		Hormonal
Term, preterm		Insulin
		Glucagon
		Sympathomimetics
Morbidity		Cortisol
IDM, SGA		Growth hormone
		Hormone receptors and
Substrate intake		glucose transporters
Exogenous		Enzymes
IV-Glucose		Glycogenolysis
IV-Lipid		Gluconeogenesis
		Substrate availability

IDM, infant of diabetic mother.

tional age of the neonate, whether term or preterm, and the degree of control that the neonate exhibits are important factors. Specific conditions such as whether the neonate is born to a diabetic mother or is small for gestational age affect the existing equilibrium (see Chapters 48 and 49). Another important consideration is the nutrients that are provided to the neonate. As has been discussed and will be further discussed subsequently in this chapter, the neonate may evidence hyperglycemia because of the administration of glucose and/or lipid intravenously. The influence of administration of glucose, amino acids, and lipids singly and in combination on glucose homeostasis is currently a topic of intense investigation in the field.

Relative to those factors that control glucose metabolism, the importance of hormonal factors has received a great deal of attention. Both insulin and the contrainsulin hormones are known to exert specific effects on glucose metabolism in the adult, and these factors are of current interest in neonatal metabolism. Hormone receptors and glucose transporters are also of interest from a mechanistic standpoint (see Chapter 7). Enzymatic components are of importance as well. Some work has been completed relative to maturation of intermediary metabolic pathways involving glycogenolyses and gluconeogenesis. As should be concluded from this discussion, the many etiologies of both hypo- and hyperglycemia reflect the transitional nature of neonatal glucose homeostasis that is under development in the perinatal-neonatal period.

Hormonal Regulation of Glucose Homeostasis

A number of investigations have focused on measurement of insulin and glucagon singly and in combination with each other relative to development of glucose homeostasis in the perinatal-neonatal period, as well as other counterregulatory hormones relative to insulin. Ktorza et al.[178] evaluated insulin and glucagon secretion during the perinatal period. They noted that insulin and glucagon are detected in most species early in gestation. The insulin to glucagon molar ratio is high in the fetus at term but then decreases dramatically after birth and remains low during the first hours after birth. This sets the stage in favor of glycogenolysis and gluconeogenesis after birth.

King et al.[179] studied postnatal development of insulin secretion in the premature neonate of 26 to 30 weeks' gestation for 110 days after birth and in the full-term neonate of 38 to 42 weeks' gestation for up to 47 days. Insulin concentration was measured before and after the beginning of a 30 minute glucose infusion given parenterally or enterally. The ratio of plasma insulin/plasma glucose at 30 minutes was used as the measurement. The premature neonate evidenced a small response to glucose on day 1, which gradually increased over the course of the study. The full-term neonate was more responsive. The investigators concluded that the premature neonate may take up to 18 weeks to fully respond to an increase in glucose concentration.

Immunoreactive glucagon (IRG) was analyzed between 12 hours and 60 days relative to four peaks—IRG >20,000, IRG 9000, IRG 3500 and IRG 2000—obtained by gel filtration.[180] Changes with age were confined to IRG 9000 and IRG 3500. IRG 9000 was nine times higher in the 12- to 36-hour-old dog compared to the adult (108 ± 24 pg·ml^{-1} vs 12 ± 3 pg·ml^{-1}) and declined to two times higher (27 ± 5 pg·ml^{-1}) at 31 to 60 hours. IRG 3500 was higher in the adult only during the first 36 hours after birth (36 ± 5 pg·ml^{-1} vs 15 ± 3 pg·ml^{-1}). Insulin infusion of 0.2 U·kg^{-1} IV produced hypoglycemia, but no change was noted in any immune-reactive glucagon component in the neonate. In response to an arginine infusion of 0.5 g·kg^{-1} over 15 minutes, there was an increase in plasma concentrations of IRG 9000 and 3500 in the neonate but an increase of only IRG 3500 in the adult. There appeared to be an impaired secretory response to hypoglycemia in the neonate.

Grasso et al.[181] infused either 1 g·kg^{-1} glucose or saline in 37 term and 35 preterm neonates and measured plasma glucagon, serum insulin, and blood glucose concentrations either before or after feeding during the first week after birth. Glucose infusion diminished plasma glucagon secretion by 61 ± 6% in the term neonate and 38 ± 4% in the preterm neonate. Serum insulin response to glucose infusion was variable, which attests to the heterogeneity of the neonatal period.

Mehta et al.[182] reported four neonates with severe hypoglycemia in whom the glucose production rate and the plasma concentrations of insulin and glucagon were measured. The hepatic glucose production rate was less than 20% of normal and plasma insulin concentration was never greater than $12\,\mu U\cdot ml^{-1}$. Two of the four neonates had low plasma glucagon concentration as well (i.e., $<60\,pg\cdot ml^{-1}$). A bolus infusion of glucagon restored the glucose production rate toward normal. In one neonate use of diazoxide further depressed an already low plasma insulin concentration from 4.2 to $1.6\,\mu U\cdot ml^{-1}$. The investigators speculated that the insulin-to-glucagon ratio may be more important than the absolute concentration of insulin in controlling glucose kinetics.

Others have focused on counterregulatory hormones besides glucagon in relation to insulin. Mayor and Cuezva[183] reviewed hormonal changes occurring in the perinatal period. Glucocorticoids and insulin mediate the rate of glycogen accumulation in fetal life. In the presuckling period, muscle glycogenolyses supplies lactate moieties, which are subsequently oxidized by neonatal tissue and act as an alternative substrate until glucose and ketones are available. The subsequent increase in plasma catecholamines and the decrease in the insulin-to-glucagon ratio resulted in liver glycogenolyses and gluconeogenesis to maintain euglycemia postnatally. During suckling, oxidation of free fatty acids, ketone body utilization, and gluconeogenesis supply energy for anabolism. Subsequently the increase in the insulin-to-glucagon ratio, occurring during feeding, resulted in the induction of lipogenesis.

Padbury et al.[184] evaluated the catecholamine surge at birth in the preterm lamb and term lamb in an exteriorized fetal lamb preparation in which the former was treated with surfactant before the first breath. There were similar baseline concentrations of catecholamines and a marked rise in circulating epinephrine and norepinephrine concentrations in both groups following cord cutting. However, the preterm lamb evidenced a delayed but exaggerated elevation of both catecholamine concentrations compared to the term group. Changes in heart rate were less profound and more gradual. Likewise, a blunted elevation in blood glucose concentration was noted. The catecholamine surge at birth appeared to be an adaptive physiologic component with specific variations in the preterm versus the term group.

Hagrevik et al.[185] evaluated the immediate postnatal adaption and sympathoadrenal activation in the neonate delivered vaginally compared with the neonate delivered by elective cesarean section. As might be expected, the vaginally delivered neonate evidenced higher catecholamine concentrations at birth compared to the neonate delivered by cesarean section under either epidural or general anesthesia. Likewise, umbilical arterial glucose concentration was higher in the former group compared to the two latter groups. The investigators speculated that, given the marked differences in catecholamine concentrations, the differences in metabolic adaptation were unexpectedly small, implying an attenuated metabolic response to sympathoadrenal stimulation in the neonate.

Gripois et al.[186] have evaluated the interrelationships between thyroid and adrenal medullary secretion in the neonatal rat. The adrenal medulla of the normal hypothyroid and hyperthyroid rat was stimulated by insulin-induced hypoglycemia. In the euthyroid animal, insulin-induced epinephrine secretion increased during the first 10 days of postnatal life. Hypothyroidism retarded the development of that response and hyperthyroidism accelerated that response. During adrenal medullary depletion following insulin-induced hypoglycemia, recovery was slower for the hyperthyroid animal than for the hypothyroid or euthyroid animals.

Kinetic analyses have been employed to evaluate hormonal control of neonatal glucose metabolism (see Chapter 1). Originally, an indirect technique of stepwise incremental glucose infusion was utilized to infer the rate of basal glucose output or glucose turnover in the neonate compared to the adult.[187] This inference was dependent on the assumption that the neonate was as sensitive to minimal changes in glucose concentration as the adult. Subsequently, studies in the puppy by Varma et al.[188] indicated that fine control is not developed. Kornhauser et al.[189] first utilized the Steele steady-state infusion technique to show that basal glucose production in the newborn puppy was two to three times the adult rate when expressed per unit body weight. Varma et al.'s data substantiated this.

Extending the investigation by Varma et al., Cowett et al.[190] hypothesized that insulin, specifically the insensitivity of the hepatocyte for insulin, appeared to have a dominant effect in controlling the turnover (i.e., production) rate of glucose. These studies began using the newborn lamb as a model. In this initial series it was hypothesized that the newborn lamb, unlike the adult sheep, would exhibit a developmentally blunted hepatic response with a persistent output of glucose in response to a glucose infusion. This hypothesis was evaluated in 26 unanesthetized mixed-breed term lambs and for comparison in eight 4- to 5-month-old mixed-breed sheep. After a 7-hour fast, basal plasma glucose, insulin, and glucagon concentrations were determined following which the term lambs received either 0, 5, 6, 11.7, or $21.7\,mg\,glucose\cdot kg^{-1}min^{-1}$ over a period of 6 hours. The older sheep received either 0 or $5.7\,mg\,glucose\cdot kg^{-1}min^{-1}$. Glucose turnover was determined by the prime constant infusion technique of Steele using D-[6-^{3}H] glucose during a 50-minute turnover period that followed the 6-hour infusion of 0.45% saline or varying doses of glucose. Both newborn and adult animals maintained a constant plasma glucose concentration and glucose-specific activity during the turnover period. Glucose production rates persisted in the term lamb until the infusion rate reached $21.7\,mg\cdot kg^{-1}min^{-1}$. In contrast, the adult lambs reduced the glucose production rate with a glucose infusion rate of $5.7\,mg\cdot kg^{-1}min^{-1}$. At the time the glucose production rate was significantly reduced, the plasma insulin concentration in the newborn lamb was fivefold greater than in the adult sheep (270 vs 56 μU·ml⁻¹). Blunted hepatic responsiveness to insulin appeared to be a major factor explaining the inefficiency in glucose homeostasis in the neonatal lamb.

In these studies, hyperglycemia and hyperinsulinemia were produced simultaneously. The effect of peripheral hyperinsulinemia could not be differentiated from that of hyperglycemia. Subsequently, varying concentrations of glucose and insulin were infused in six groups of newborn lambs for sufficient time to produce steady-state equilibrium conditions of euglycemia and hyperinsulinemia. Glucose production rates were measured as well as gluconeogenesis from lactate. This was accomplished by determining the ratio of [U-^{14}C]lactate/D-[6-^{3}H] glucose noted by "r" in Figure 32.7.

Increasing the rate of glucose infusion without administering insulin (groups II and III) produced a stepwise increase in plasma glucose and insulin concentrations when compared with controls (group I). Elevation of the plasma insulin concentration, induced by hyperglycemia, was associated with a significant ($p < .001$) reduction in the glucose production rate but was seen only when marked hyperglycemia and hyperinsulinemia were achieved (group III). With insulin administration, a significant ($p < .001$) and stepwise increase in plasma insulin concentration was observed depending on the dose of insulin administered. By simultaneous glucose infusion, a state of euglycemia or hyperglycemia was produced with concomitant hyperinsulinemia. With a slight increase in plasma insulin (61 μU·ml⁻¹) (group IV), a significant ($p < .001$) reduction in gluconeogenesis was noted together with a slight but not significant reduction in the rate of glucose production. When hyperinsulinemia was moderate to marked (236 and 481 μU·ml⁻¹) (groups V and VI), there was a significant ($p < .001$) reduction of both gluconeogenesis and the rate of glucose production. Insulin is known to inhibit glycogenolysis and gluconeogenesis while enhancing glycogenesis and results in the suppression of glucose production in the adult.[191-193] The data suggested that a moderate elevation of plasma insulin concentration effectively reduced gluconeogenesis (groups II and IV) but did not influence the endogenous glucose production. The latter was reduced only when a much higher insulin concentration was achieved (groups II, V, and VI). The conclusion was that insulin rather than glucose controls the rate of glucose production in newborn lambs.[194]

In neither previous study was the pancreatic β cell secretory activity evaluated. It was subsequently hypothesized that the pancreatic β cell response to glucose concentration was comparable in the term neonate and the older adult (i.e., there was no relatively decreased secretory activity of the neonatal β cell). To confirm this hypothesis of posthepatic insulin availability in the neonate, a steady-state insulin secretion study was performed using ^{131}I-insulin as the tracer.[195] Plasma glucose and insulin concentrations and insulin specific activity were determined. Endogenous posthepatic insulin secretion and the metabolic clearance rate were derived in the spontaneously delivered term lamb, betamethasone-

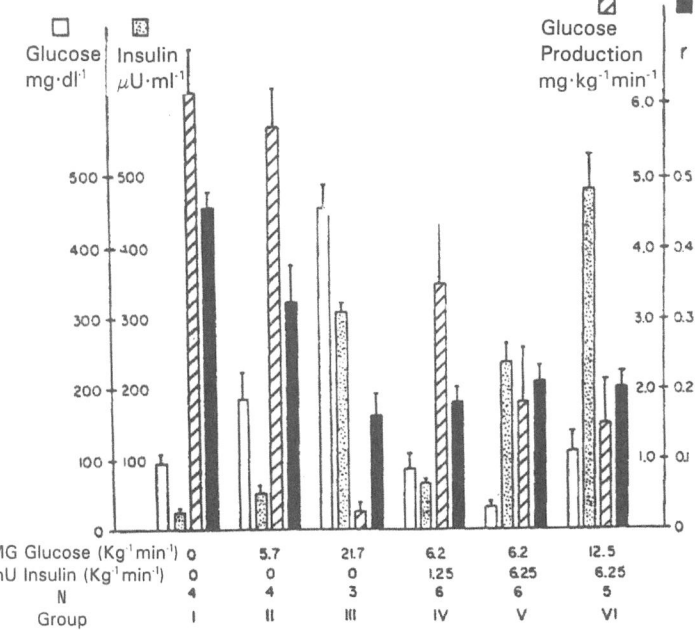

FIGURE 32.7. Plasma glucose and plasma insulin concentrations, glucose production rates and ratio of U[-^{14}C]lactate/D-[6-^{3}H] glucose for all groups. (From Susa et al.,[194] with permission.)

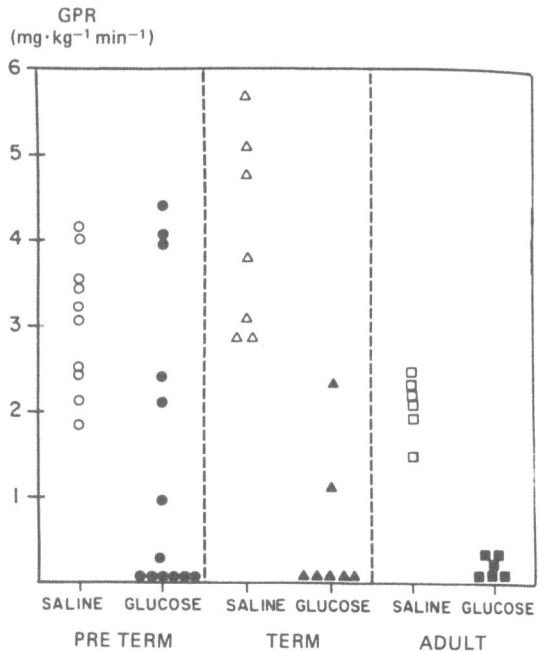

FIGURE 32.8. Glucose production rate for each neonate and adult during saline or glucose infusion. (From Cowett et al.,[196] with permission.)

treated preterm lamb, prematurely delivered, sheep, and the 4- to 5-month-old adult sheep. The posthepatic insulin secretion rate was not different in any of the three groups—term, premature, or adult—under influence of 45% saline infusion. Correspondingly, the similar posthepatic insulin secretion rate was noted when the three groups were infused with 5.7 mg·kg^{-1} min^{-1} of glucose. The metabolic clearance rate was not different in the groups. It was concluded that the posthepatic insulin secretion rate and the metabolic clearance rate were similar in term lamb and prematurely delivered lamb in comparison to 4- to 5-month-old adult sheep. Previously, it had been suggested that precise control of the rate of glucose production is characteristic of the mature (adult) animal, while the neonate evidence a decreased ability to suppress the rate of glucose production under glucose-infused conditions. The investigators concluded that this immaturity may be explained by neonatal hepatic unresponsiveness to insulin and is probably not related to secretory capacity of the pancreatic β cell.

As a nonruminant, the neonatal lamb is metabolically comparable to the human and it may be used to evaluate perinatal glucose homeostasis. However, kinetic studies in the human neonate would be of particular relevance physiologically. Following the development of stable isotope methodology in the laboratory, it was hypothesized that under conditions of glucose infusion, documentation of the degree of suppression of glucose production could be used to characterize the control of neonatal glucose homeostasis. Evaluation of the hormonal (e.g., insulin) factors associated with these observed changes in neonatal glucose homeostasis would also be possible. Figure 32.8 depicts the glucose production rate for the preterm and term neonates and adults who were studied. Five of 13 preterm and two of seven term neonates had persistent glucose production rates (GPR) (>1 mg·kg^{-1} min^{-1}) during glucose infusion. In contrast the glucose production rate in all adults was unmeasurable. There was no

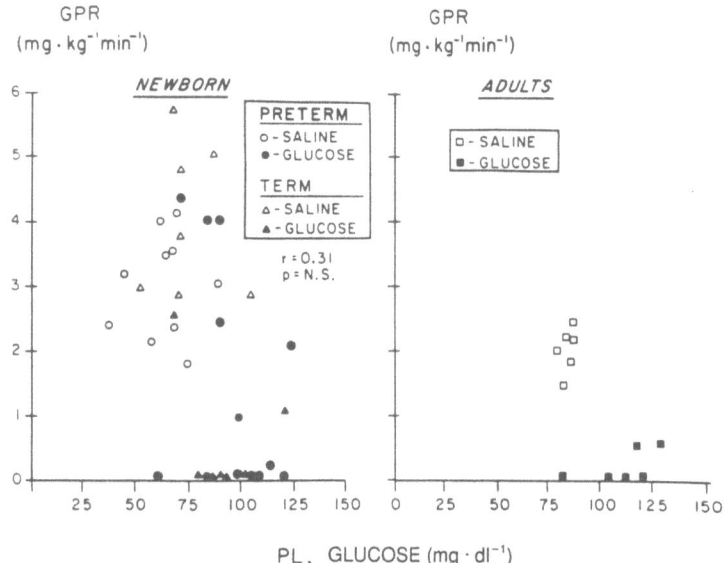

FIGURE 32.9. Correlation between the plasma glucose concentration during the turnover period and glucose production rate in the neonates and adults. (From Cowett et al.,[196] with permission.)

FIGURE 32.10. Correlation between the peripheral plasma insulin concentration during the turnover period and glucose production rate in the neonates and adults. (From Cowett et al.,[196] with permission.)

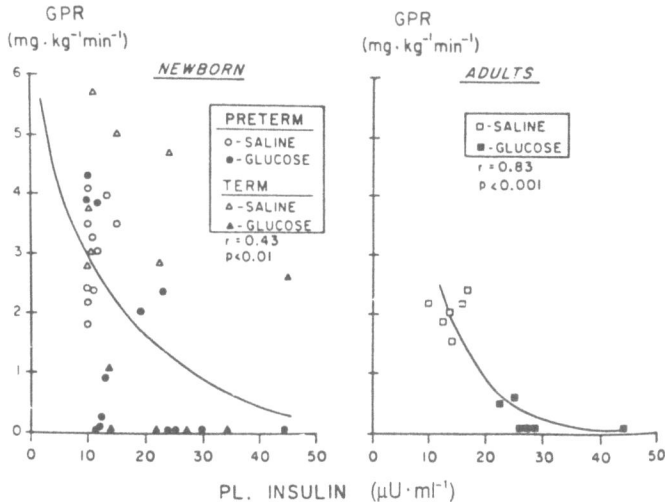

correlation between plasma glucose concentration and the glucose production rate in the neonate or in the adult as noted in Figure 32.9. Both the neonate and the adult did have a correlation between plasma insulin concentration and GPR. However, there was considerable variability in the neonate as noted in Figure 32.10. It was concluded that there are significant developmental differences in neonatal glucose homeostasis and that insulin is probably important in neonatal hormonal control of glucose production.[196]

A logical extension of the above discussion is the question of when does the neonate develop maturation (i.e., adult-like control) of glucose homeostasis. As noted above, suppression of the endogenous glucose production rate (i.e., GPR or Ra) is the adult response to glucose infusion. Persistent Ra (i.e., $\geq 1\,mg\cdot kg^{-1}\,min^{-1}$ and/or <80% decrease in Ra) in response to glucose infusion is evidence of a transitional homeostatic state in the neonate during the first days after birth. To determine if postnatal development produced an adult-like response, Ra was measured in 11 prematurely born neonates at 2 to 5 weeks after birth. In these paired studies, $4\,\mu g\cdot kg^{-1}\,min^{-1}$ D-[U-^{13}C] glucose tracer was infused by prime constant infusion to determine Ra, during either saline or glucose infusion, the latter at a rate of $5.3 \pm 0.2\,mg\cdot kg^{-1}\,min^{-1}$. When the data of the saline infusion turnover period were compared to those of the glucose infusion turnover period, plasma glucose concentration increased significantly from $88 \pm 3\,mg\cdot dl^{-1}$ to $101 \pm 4\,mg\cdot dl^{-1}$ ($p < .001$). Plasma insulin concentration remained unchanged ($12 \pm 5\,\mu U\cdot ml^{-1}$ vs $8 \pm 3\,\mu U\cdot ml^{-1}$). Ra was heterogeneous during glucose infusion and persistent Ra was present in 6 of 11 neonates as depicted in Figure 32.11. Of the five infants who showed decreased Ra during glucose infusion, three received glucose at a rate exceeding basal Ra.

Of the remaining six infants who evidenced persistent Ra during glucose infusion, three received glucose at a rate equal to or greater than of basal Ra. The conclusions were that glucose homeostasis in low birth weight infants is transitional throughout the neonatal period.[197]

A decreased response to epinephrine resulting in a decreased rate of production and decreased plasma

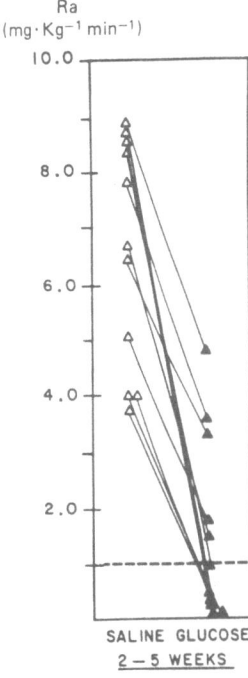

FIGURE 32.11. Endogenous glucose production rate (Ra) during saline and glucose infusion. (From Cowett et al.,[197] with permission.)

glucose concentration in the neonate in response to sympathomimetic stimulation of the neonatal lamb has been reported.[198,199] This lack of response to epinephrine correlated with the lack of response to insulin discussed above. It is possible, as noted by Hetenyi et al.,[200] that the decreased neonatal response to insulin and other hormones, for instance, glucagon and epinephrine, as discussed in these studies, may protect the neonate from rapid fluctuations in substrate such as glucose to allow its more ready availability for the developing brain. Diminished responsiveness to both insulin and counterregulatory insulin hormones should assist in maintaining glucose homeostasis in the neonate. Further investigations of insulin and the counterregulatory hormones are supplementing those studies that have been completed to date.[201–203]

Insulin Resistance and Sensitivity in the Neonate

Lack of the precise control of glucose homeostasis in the human neonate has been postulated as secondary to either a decreased sensitivity or resistance to insulin.[196,204] Although methods for assessing insulin resistance have varied considerably, many studies have evaluated only the insulin effect on plasma glucose concentration in the hyperglycemic, stressed neonate.[168–174] Fewer studies have evaluated the effects of insulin on glucose production in the healthy term or preterm neonate.[168,196,205] One methodology has been to study the effect of insulin in response to different glucose infusion rates.[196,205]

Hulman and Kliegman[206] and Kliegman et al.[207] are credited with the initial use of the euglycemic hyperinsulinemic clamp in the neonatal period in a beagle puppy model, after the model of DeFronzo et al.[208] Graded insulin infusions ranging from 3.75 to 100 mU·kg^{-1}min^{-1} were used in this animal model. The adult group had complete suppression of glucose production, while an 80% reduction was achieved in the newborn puppy group and the rate of glucose production persisted. The investigators attributed a lack of complete suppression of glucose production in the neonate to hepatic resistance to insulin and persistent gluconeogenesis.

Kahn[209] has defined insulin resistance and has provided a distinction between insulin insensitivity and insulin unresponsiveness. In the former, there is a shift to the right of the insulin dose-response curve such that a higher concentration of insulin is necessary to produce a half-maximal effect, with a maximal effect being achieved eventually. This is usually the result of decreased affinity or a decreased concentration of insulin receptors. During insulin unresponsiveness all responses to insulin are reduced including the maximal response, but the dose-response relationship that exists is normal, that is, the insulin concentration required to produce a half-maximal response is normal. This is usually the result of a postreceptor defect. Both forms of insulin resistance may combine such that a higher insulin concentration would be required to produce a half-maximal effect, and the maximal effect would be reduced compared to that of a normal response.

Farrag et al.[210] performed the euglycemic hyperinsulinemic clamp for the first time in the human neonate in a series of prematurely born neonates to evaluate insulin sensitivity in the neonatal period. As noted in Figure 32.12, one significant effect of insulin was to reduce hepatic glucose production in the preterm neonate at a relatively low insulin concentration during insulin infusion of 0.5 mU·kg^{-1}·min^{-1}. This effect did not significantly

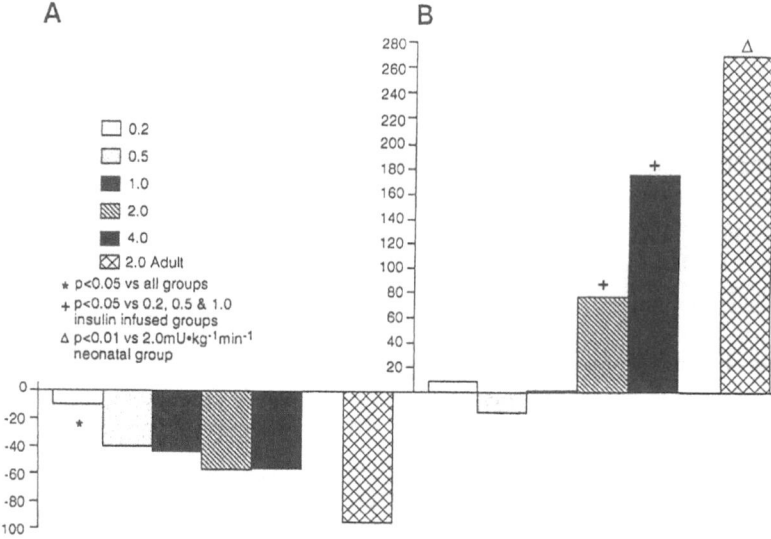

FIGURE 32.12. (A) The percent decrease in endogenous glucose production and (B) the percent increase in glucose utilization subdivided by the various insulin infusion rates that were administered to the neonate as well as the 2 mU·kg^{-1}min^{-1} insulin rate that was administered to the adult. (From Farrag et al.,[210] with permission.)

change despite the use of higher insulin infusion rates that resulted in as much as a 10-fold higher plasma insulin concentration. The percent reduction of endogenous glucose production ranged from 41% to 58% from that of basal rates, and persistent glucose production (i.e., $\geq 1 \text{ mg} \cdot \text{kg}^{-1} \cdot \text{min}^{-1}$) during steady-state insulin infusion was noted throughout. If one considers complete suppression of glucose production to be the maximal effect of insulin on the liver, the data demonstrate that this maximal effect could not be reached in the human preterm neonate. This pattern of response of glucose production to insulin is most consistent with the definition of nonresponsiveness to insulin and may be a postreceptor defect.[211] This mechanism may include factors at the membrane level aside from receptor concentration and affinity, such as the state of aggregation of the receptor or its ability to interact with other membrane proteins required for signal generation, as well as a variety of intracellular factors including all of the events that occur at steps distal to the membrane. This mechanism includes the stimulatory or inhibitory effect of insulin on glucose transporters and/or key enzymes in the glycolytic, glycogenolytic, or gluconeogenic pathways. Decreased receptor concentration and/or affinity is an unlikely explanation because, at least in the human adult, there are plenty of "spare" insulin receptors available after the number of receptor sites required to achieve a maximal response are occupied.[206,212] Also, there is an increase in both receptor concentration and affinity in the human neonate compared to that in the adult.[213] Finally, a reduction in receptor concentration below that required for a maximal response to take place will result not only in decreased responsiveness, but also in decreased sensitivity, which is not apparent in the present investigation.[209]

The indirect effect of insulin on endogenous glucose production has recently been evaluated.[214] Inhibition of lipolysis at the adipose tissue and reduction of free fatty acid concentrations were shown to act as signal to the liver to suppress endogenous glucose production. This particular issue is of current interest, but the limited amount of adipose tissue in the preterm neonate may potentially interfere with the indirect effect of insulin on endogenous glucose production.

Relative to peripheral glucose utilization, a significant increase from basal rates only at the 2 and $4 \text{ mU} \cdot \text{kg}^{-1} \cdot \text{min}^{-1}$ insulin infusion rates was demonstrated.[210] It was not possible to determine if a maximal effect on glucose utilization was achieved because a plateau was not reached. The data denote a significant increase in glucose utilization at a higher insulin concentration than what was required to significantly reduce the rate of glucose production. Despite the fact that the plateau was ultimately not reached at these insulin infusion rates, the neonatal glucose utilization response to insulin, even at a lower plasma insulin concentration, far exceeded that reported in the literature as the maximal response in the adult.[212]

Figure 32.13 depicts the respective correlations between endogenous glucose production and glucose utilization with plasma insulin concentration.

As noted previously, Goldman and Hirata[171] have suggested that an attenuated response to insulin in the very low birth weight neonate is the reason for the occurrence of hyperglycemia. They attributed this response to insulin resistance rather than to the lack of the β-cell response. They stated that absence of controls and the variable clinical status of the four neonates they studied were considerable limitations. Abrupt and sustained improve-

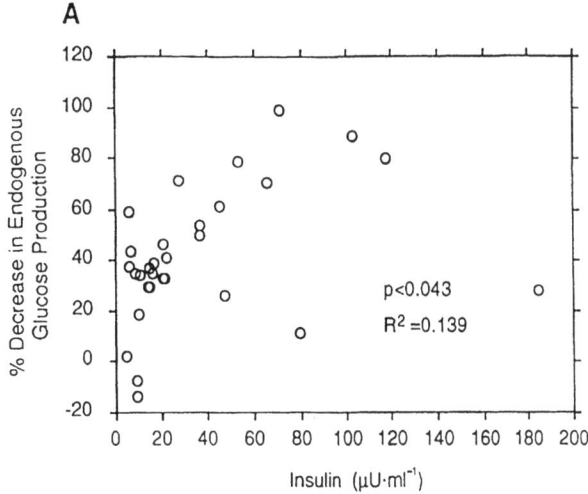

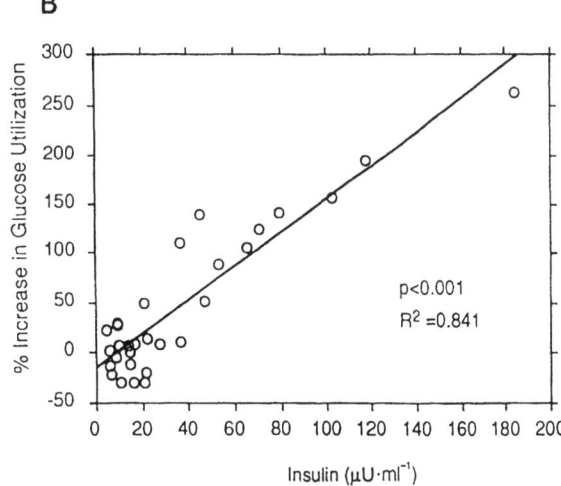

FIGURE 32.13. (A) A regression correlating the percent decrease in endogenous glucose production relative to plasma insulin concentration in the neonate. (B) A regression correlating the percent increase in glucose utilization relative to plasma insulin concentration in the neonate. (From Farrag et al.,[210] with permission.)

ment in glucose tolerance has been reported in response to short- and long-term insulin infusion.[168–174] Higher insulin infusion rates and plasma insulin concentrations were reported in these studies than in the present study, and no evaluation of glucose production or glucose utilization was documented.

An approximately 50% reduction in glucose production has been reported in response to an exogenous glucose infusion rate of ≈4–6 mg·kg^{-1}min^{-1} (i.e., similar to the basal glucose production rate in the neonate) that resulted in plasma insulin concentration ≈19 mU/ml.[196,205] There is a dichotomy in the literature in considering this reduction in glucose production to be primarily a response to either higher plasma insulin concentration or plasma glucose concentration.[196,205] At a similar plasma insulin concentration, as noted in Figure 33.12 (the 1.0 mU·kg^{-1}min^{-1} group), the reduction is in agreement with previous data, specifically that this reduction in glucose production can be explained as a result of an insulin response.[196] Kalhan et al.[205] suggested the glucose production rate was not in response to insulin, but to a higher plasma glucose concentration.

These data of Farrag et al.[210] are in agreement with those reported by Hertz et al.[215] relative to a strong positive correlation between plasma insulin concentration and glucose utilization. Hertz et al. also reported a complete suppression of glucose production when a high glucose infusion rate (i.e., 9.5 mg·kg^{-1}min^{-1}) was used, which resulted in a significant increase in both plasma glucose and insulin concentrations. At a similar plasma insulin concentration, a 41% reduction in glucose production was noted, so the combined effect of glucose and insulin seems necessary for complete suppression of glucose production. In contrast, a more recent investigation from that laboratory suggested that 5.5 mg·kg^{-1}min^{-1} glucose infusion rate resulted in a 90% suppression during intravenous infusion provided either alone or in combination with lipid.[216] Interestingly, suppression was achieved at a glucose concentration of approximately 90 mg·dl^{-1} and an extremely low insulin concentration of approximately 6 μU·ml^{-1}. The mechanisms that explain the dichotomy that exists in the two data sets are unclear.

Dose-response characteristics for effects of insulin on production and utilization of glucose in the adult have been described by Rizza et al.[212] The data of the adult group of Farrag et al.[210] are consistent with the data reported by Rizza et al. Farrag et al. chose a 2 mU·kg^{-1}min^{-1} infusion because at this rate Rizza et al. achieved maximal insulin effect on both the rates of glucose production and glucose utilization. The plasma insulin concentration was 200 to 300 mU·ml^{-1}. It had not been established what insulin concentration would result for a given insulin infusion rate in a neonate prior to Farrag et al.'s investigation.[210]

It is difficult to compare neonatal to adult data especially when both basal glucose production rates and glucose utilization rates are different, as are the plasma insulin concentrations. Similar to the adult, there is a strong positive linear correlation between plasma insulin concentration and the glucose utilization rate. The insulin effect on the glucose production rate started at a lower insulin concentration than that required for the glucose utilization rate. If one calculates insulin sensitivity at euglycemia, which is not confounded by non–insulin-mediated glucose utilization, as described by Bergman et al.,[217] it is apparent from the data that the neonate has a greater peripheral sensitivity to insulin compared to the adult. This may be due to a higher receptor concentration and affinity, provided that the postreceptor cascade is intact peripherally. On the other hand, contrary to the adult, complete suppression of glucose production could not be achieved in the human neonate. This is due to a nonresponsive component of glucose production response to the effect of insulin. The investigators concluded that, in contrast to the adult, the neonate has persistent glucose production and greater peripheral sensitivity to insulin.

Hormone Receptors in the Neonatal Period

Menon and Sperling[218] have summarized the changes in hepatic fetal receptors compared to corresponding adult receptors to emphasize their importance in maturation of homeostasis. They developed a hypothesis for the physiologic significance of insulin, glucagon, and epinephrine concentrations and receptor characteristics in the fetus and the neonate to explain the adaptation that occurs. As noted in Tables 32.6 and 32.7, the higher insulin receptor concentration facilitates anabolism and inhibits gluconeogenesis in the fetus. Decreased glucagon receptor number further limits the catabolic processes. Following delivery, the decreased insulin receptor number and insulin concentration in concert with a linkage of glucagon receptors and an increase in glucagon concentration results in mobilization of glucose and other nutrients. Likewise epinephrine enhances glucose production and lipolyses.

Development of Gluconeogenesis (Enzymatic Control) in the Neonatal Period

The maturation of enzymatic control has been summarized in detail by Girard[219] (see Chapter 29). As can be appreciated from what has been noted heretofore, the birth process requires major changes in glucose homeostasis. The ability of the fetus to synthesize glucose from gluconeogenic precursors such as lactate, pyruvate, and specific amino acids is quite depressed in the fetus. Enzymes involved in the gluconeogenic pathway include

TABLE 32.6. Hepatic fetal receptors compared to corresponding adult receptors.

Insulin	Glucagon	Epinephrine
Increased number (Ro)	Decreased number (Ro)	High β receptor (Ro)
Increased affinity (K)	Decreased or equal affinity (K)	Decreased α receptor number (Ro)
Downregulation absent	Downregulation—low Ro prevents assessment	
Autophosphorylation and tyrosine kinase activity—normal	Incomplete functional linkage to adenylate cyclase	Glycogenolysis-β mediated
Partial functional dissociation from some biologic actions	Functional linkage begins in late gestation	
Postnatally	Postnatally	Postnatally
Decrease in Ro amd K	Increase in Ro and perhaps K	Hepatic β receptors decrease in Ro
Functional linkage completed	Functional linkage completed	Hepatic α receptors increase in Ro
		Glycogenolysis gradually becomes α-mediated

From Manon and Sperling,[218] with permission.

TABLE 32.7. Hypothesis for the physiologic significance of insulin, glucagon, and epinephrine levels and receptor characteristics in the fetus and newborn.

Fetus	Newborn
Higher insulin receptor number (Ro) and affinity (K) should facilitate anabolic processes in some tissues leading to deposition of glycogen, protein, and fat despite low insulin levels	Following interruption of maternal nutrient supply, mobilization of glucose and other fuel stores is brought about by increase in epinephrine levels with functionally linked β receptors and increases in Ro of glucagon receptors, which are functionally linked to cAMP together with a surge in glucagon level
Low Ro and K and incomplete functional linkage of glucagon receptors and low glucagon levels limit glycogenolysis	Falling insulin levels and decreasing insulin receptor Ro and K facilitate glycogenolysis and gluconeogenesis
Fetus is dependent on maternal glucose supply, but in emergency (hypoxia), can initiate endogenous glucose production, via β-adrenergic–mediated glycogenolysis	

From Manon and Sperling,[218] with permission.

pyruvate carboxylase, mitochondrial phosphoenolpyruvate carboxykinase, fructose-6-diphosphatase and glucose-6-phosphatase. Girard and others have reported that the above activity in the near-term fetus is 50% to 100% while the activity of cytosolic phosphoenolpyruvate carboxykinase is low (i.e., 0–25%) and increases markedly after birth. Cytosolic phosphoenolpyruvate carboxykinase is induced by the process of birth rather than by temporal or nutritional factors. From a hormonal standpoint, it is the insulin-to-glucagon ratio rather than the absolute concentration of glucagon that stimulates induction of hepatic phosphoenolpyruvate carboxykinase. Furthermore, while it has been suggested that the rate of gluconeogenesis could be the limiting factor relative to gluconeogenic precursors and the availability of free fatty acids, Girard concluded that the evidence to date can be interpreted to suggest that the reduced supply of precursors cannot account for the impairment of gluconeogenesis in the fasted neonate.

In the human neonate, gluconeogenesis has been studied only to a limited degree. Although glycogen is stored by the fetus, its exclusive utilization represents only several hours of glucose precursor for production at a rate of 4 to 6 mg·kg^{-1} min^{-1}.[220] Frazer et al.[221] showed that the functional integrity of the gluconeogenic pathway existed by 6 hours after birth, the earliest sampling time in the study, by determining $^{13}C_2$ enrichment in blood glucose during the constant infusion of [2,3-^{13}C] alanine. Bougnères et al.[220] measured glycerol turnover and showed that 75% of transported glycerol was converted to glucose between 20 and 24 hours after birth, which represents 5% of hepatic glucose production. Gilfillan et al.[222] studied whether the fetus at term can produce alanine and showed that the fetus could, since there was a 42% decrease in ^{13}C enrichment of alanine between umbilical vein and artery. This would allow transfer of nitrogen from fetal muscle to the liver for utilization.

Gleason et al.[223] studied hepatic metabolism (i.e., oxygen consumption, lactate uptake, and glucose production) in the neonatal lamb using chronic catherization, microsphere techniques, and ^{14}C lactate to measure metabolism directly. The investigators reported that 38.4% of hepatic glucose production could be accounted for by lactate gluconeogenesis. Compared to a fetal liver preparation, the investigators concluded that blood flow and oxygen and substrate delivery to the liver was decreased in the neonate, but that the neonatal liver extracts more oxygen and substrate and that lactate gluconeogenesis occurs.

Data on glucose kinetics measuring total glucose production in infants and children utilizing either D-[6,6-^{2}H] glucose,[224,225] D-[1-^{13}C] glucose,[226,227] or both in combination,[228] and D-[U-^{13}C] glucose[196,229-231] originally appeared to evaluate control of neonatal glucose homeostasis. Parallel to our investigations,[231] Kalhan et al.[227] and King et al.[232] evaluated kinetics in the infant of the diabetic mother (see Chapter 49). Other investigators have studied leucine metabolism in the neonate[233] as well as neonatal glucose oxidation.[234-237]

In one series Denne and Kalhan[236] measured total carbohydrate oxidation, plasma glucose oxidation, and glucose carbon recycling in 11 fasted neonates. These investigators reported a rate of glucose production of 5.0 ± 0.4 mg·kg^{-1}·min^{-1}. Glucose was oxidized at a rate of 2.7 ± 0.3 mg·kg^{-1}·min^{-1}, representing 53% of glucose turnover. Recycling represented 36% of glucose production or 1.9 ± 0.7 mg·kg^{-1}·min^{-1}. The investigators concluded that recycling accounts for one third of glucose production, demonstrating active gluconeogenesis in the neonate. The remaining 20% represents local oxidation of tissue glycogen stores.

The actual measurement of gluconeogenesis has only recently been studied in detail because of the inability to measure the pathway. Kalhan et al.[238] have reported the utilization of an [^{2}H$_2$]O method to quantify gluconeogenesis and suggested that 20% of endogenous glucose produced in the preterm neonate of less than 32 weeks is via gluconeogenesis.

Likewise, Sunehag et al.[239] used mass isotopomer distribution analysis of circulating glucose to evaluate gluconeogenesis in the extremely premature neonate receiving parenteral alimentation. They concluded that glycogenolysis is a major source of glucose production for at least 10 hours after initiation of the study at 5 days after birth, although gluconeogenesis becomes an increasing contributor and may acount for at least 33% of glucose production at the same time.

Through a continuing series of investigations, Feng and Kliegman[240,241] and Feng et al.[242] have evaluated transcription of the genes for fructose-1,6-bisphosphatase, serine dehydrase, and hepatic cytosolic phosphoenolpyruvate carboxykinase. They concluded that persistent glucose production in the presence of hyperinsulinemia may be due to unsuppressed gluconeogenesis. They suggest that the stimulatory effect of epinephrine on gluconeogenesis, overriding insulin and glucose in the liver, may be one mechanism for the occurrence of neonatal hyperglycemia.

Substrate Availability in the Neonate

Significant investigations have focused on the differential of substrate availability versus physiologic hormonal control in the human, including the older child and the adult in evaluation of gluconeogenesis.[243-245] In the adult, Jahoor et al.[243] suggested that reduction in glucose turnover after an 86-hour fast was not secondary to a lack of gluconeogenic substrate. On the other hand, dependence of gluconeogenesis in those subjects on an adequate supply of precursors was demonstrated when reduction of lactate and alanine concentration with dichloroacetate caused a decrease in the rate of glucose production. Studies published of older children with diarrhea were interpreted by Bennish et al.[244] to suggest that defective gluconeogenesis was the etiology of the hypoglycemia. Haymond et al.[245] studied differences in circulating gluconeogenic substrates in men, women, and children subjected to short-term fasting and suggested that differences in glucose requirements among the three groups could be responsible for the differences noted in plasma substrate responses to fasting. The adult men and women evidenced nearly identical plasma lactate and pyruvate concentrations, while the initial venous lactate and pyruvate concentrations were highest in children and increased during the 6 hours of fasting. The investigators speculated that lactate production might be accelerated in the pediatric patient assuming normal hepatic substrate uptake. Neonates were not studied in that investigation. Others have evaluated the potential for lactate gluconeogenesis and found it to be accelerated in the preterm neonate compared to the adult. The speculation was that substrate acquisition may not be the primary problem in the development of glucose homeostasis neonatally.[246]

One of the issues of substrate availability related to glucose homeostasis involves the effect of glucose alone or in combination with other substrate on glucose production. In one series the endogenous glucose production rate was negligible under conditions in which glucose was infused as part of the hyperalimentation mixture prior to administration of an intravenous fat emulsion.[163] There is currently a clear dichotomy in studies evaluating the ability of the neonate to diminish endogenous glucose production, which occurs regularly in the adult.[204] In studies in the term neonate,[196,197,205] the infant of the diabetic mother,[231] and the premature neonate,[196] persistent endogenous glucose production >1.0 mg·kg^{-1}·min^{-1} was reported in response to administration of exogenous glucose infusion alone and in the newborn canine model using the euglycemic hyperinsulinemic clamp technique.[206] Others using different techniques such as the glucose clamp[235] or glucose and amino acid infusion[247] reported no persistent endogenous glucose production in the neonate. In the latter instance both an amino acid mixture and a relatively moderate rate of glucose was infused (~8mg·kg^{-1}min^{-1}). As pointed out by LaFeber et al.,[247] suppression may be incomplete under conditions in which less glucose is administered or it is the sole constituent of the infusate. The data reported in a recent study support this latter conclusion. No endogenous glucose production was noted when 6.8mg·kg^{-1}min^{-1} was being administered during the basal state with amino acids or following administration of glucose, amino acids, and the intravenous fat emulsion combined.[163] Further work is necessary to determine which component—the quantity of glucose administered, the addition of amino acids, and/or lipid emulsion—is the primary cause of the observed decline in endogenous glucose production in the neonate. Another question is the relative role of each of these substrates as a secretagogue for insulin. Such studies should assist in differentiating hormonal versus enzymatic control of neonatal glucose metabolism from the availability of substrate as a limiting factor in homeostasic maturation.

Glucose Utilization in the Neonate

The contribution of the oxidative and nonoxidative disposal of glucose to total glucose utilization in the neonate, especially the extremely low birth weight neonate, is important throughout the neonatal period. In one study, glucose production, glucose oxidation, and nonoxidative disposal were measured in 13 appropriate for gestational age preterm neonates (GA 25.5 ± 0.8 weeks, BW 757 ± 88g) by stable isotopic infusion of NaH^{13}CO$_3$, followed by [U-^{13}C]glucose.[248] To evaluate extrauterine maturation of these processes, the neonates were studied sequentially at two glucose infusion rates of 4 or 8mg·kg^{-1}min^{-1} early, at 53 ± 20 hours, and later, at 37 ± 8 days. Table 32.8 summarizes the data generated in this study. The mean blood glucose concentrations ranged from 58 to 102 mg·dl^{-1}. None of the neonates developed hyperglycemia, but in one (early) study of the 13 studies performed, one neonate was found to be hypoglycemic with blood glucose concentration of 28 mg·dl^{-1} while he was receiving an infusion of 8mg·kg^{-1}min^{-1} glucose. Although there was a trend toward a higher blood glucose concentration during the late versus the early study at the same glucose infusion, as well as a trend toward a higher blood glucose concentration in those who received 8mg·kg^{-1}min^{-1} compared to 4mg·kg^{-1}min^{-1} glucose infusion, none of these differences reached statistical significance. Mean plasma insulin concentrations were not significantly different among the groups. Although the group that received glucose infusion of 8mg·kg^{-1}min^{-1} early in the neonatal period had a higher mean plasma insulin concentration than the others, this difference did not reach statistical significance. Isotopic steady state was achieved in all study groups.

TABLE 32.8. Metabolic data.

Glucose infusion rate (mg·kg^{-1}min^{-1})	Early studies		Late studies	
	4	8	4	8
(n)	(6)	(7)	(6)	(7)
Bl. glucose (mg/dl)	58 ± 9	83 ± 14	85 ± 9	102 ± 11
Pl. insulin (μU/ml)	5.5 ± 0.6	18.3 ± 6.2	6.3 ± 1.6	8.1 ± 2.2
Total rate of appearance (mg·kg^{-1}min^{-1})	4.1 ± 0.1	7.8 ± 0.1	4.3 ± 0.3	8.2 ± 0.1
Glucose production rate (mg·kg^{-1}min^{-1})	0.2 ± 0.1	0.1 ± 0.1	0.4 ± 0.2	0.2 ± 0.1
Glucose oxidation rate (mg·kg^{-1}min^{-1})	2.8 ± 0.4	5.4 ± 0.7	2.1 ± 0.2	3.5 ± 0.5
Glucose oxidation rate (%)	67 ± 9.6	69 ± 9.1	49 ± 3.8	44 ± 6.7
Nonoxidative disposal (mg·kg^{-1}min^{-1})	1.4 ± 0.4	2.4 ± 0.7	2.2 ± 0.2	4.6 ± 0.6
Nonoxidative disposal (%)	34 ± 9.6	31 ± 9.1	51 ± 4.0	56 ± 6.7
Glucose clearance rate (ml·kg^{-1}min^{-1})	5.2 ± 0.6	9.1 ± 1.8	7.8 ± 1.0	12.0 ± 2.9

Note: See text for significant differences between groups. From Farrag et al.[248]

The mean rate of appearance (Ra) of glucose and the endogenous glucose production (EGP) rate during the steady-state glucose infusion for all groups are noted as well. In this study Ra reflects total glucose production rate, a combination of endogenously produced and exogenously administered glucose, during the steady-state glucose infusion. For each study group the mean Ra of glucose was not significantly different from that of the rate of glucose infused to the group. This indicated that in all study groups endogenous glucose production was completely suppressed (i.e., <1mg·kg^{-1}min^{-1}), probably because of the lack of substrate availability.

The mean rates of oxidative and nonoxidative disposal of glucose and the percentage of their contribution to total glucose utilization are listed as well. The glucose oxidation rate was significantly higher in those neonates who received 8mg·kg^{-1}min^{-1} glucose compared to 4mg·kg^{-1}min^{-1} glucose infusion during both the early ($p = .01$) and the late ($p = .03$) study. The contribution of glucose oxidation to total glucose utilization, as represented by the percent of glucose oxidation, was not significantly different in the group that received 4 mg·kg^{-1} min^{-1} versus 8 mg·kg^{-1} min^{-1} in either the early or late study. This contribution of glucose oxidation to total glucose utilization in the early studies was significantly higher than that calculated in the late studies ($p = .011$). The contribution of nonoxidative disposal (NOD) to total glucose utilization reflected the inverse of that of glucose oxidation; that is, its contribution (i.e., %NOD) was significantly higher in the late studies than in the early studies to the same degree ($p = .011$).

A significant linear and negative correlation was found between blood glucose concentration and the percent of glucose oxidized ($p < .001$, $r = -.61$), as depicted in Figure 32.14.

The higher rate of glucose oxidation in the neonate who received 8 mg·kg^{-1} min^{-1} versus 4 mg·kg^{-1} min^{-1} simply reflects the difference in glucose load. What is important to recognize in the current study is the ability of the extremely low birth weight neonates, soon after birth, to oxidize glucose at rates up to 5.4 mg·kg^{-1} min^{-1} (range 2.9–7.9 mg·kg^{-1} min^{-1}) when they received glucose infusion at a rate of 8 mg·kg^{-1} min^{-1}. This rate is almost twofold higher than what has been reported in the adult to be the maximum rate of glucose oxidation (~3 mg·kg^{-1} min^{-1}) during glucose infusion rates of up to 9 mg·kg^{-1} min^{-1}.[204,249,250] This is in agreement with the results of Sauer et al.,[237] who reported a mean glucose oxidation rate of 6.0 mg·kg^{-1} min^{-1} (range 3.8–9.7 mg·kg^{-1} min^{-1}) in the term and 5.8 mg·kg^{-1} min^{-1} (range 4.3–8.5 mg·kg^{-1} min^{-1}) in the larger preterm neonate. The fact that the extremely low birth weight neonate is able to oxidize such a rate of glucose should encourage the use of a relatively higher glucose infusion rate in these neonates. The current practice of using as low a glucose infusion rate as possible in these neonates to avoid hyperglycemia does not only limit energy intake from glucose, but also from fat and protein since the composition of the parenteral alimentation is usually administered proportionally.[7,8] Although hyperglycemia did not result from the rates of glucose infusion employed in these studies, the addition of fat and/or amino acids can increase the risk of this complication.[163,251] The risk of hyperglycemia should be weighed against the benefit of providing adequate energy especially when insulin infusion has been reported to significantly improve peripheral glucose utilization and enhance glucose tolerance in the preterm neonate, although as noted previously in this discussion the routine use of insulin awaits further investigation.[168,210]

In the early neonatal period the contribution of glucose oxidation to overall glucose utilization was significantly higher than that at the end of the neonatal period (67%/69% vs 49%/44%). It was also somewhat higher than that reported in the literature in larger preterm neonates who received total parenteral nutrition (63%), as well as those

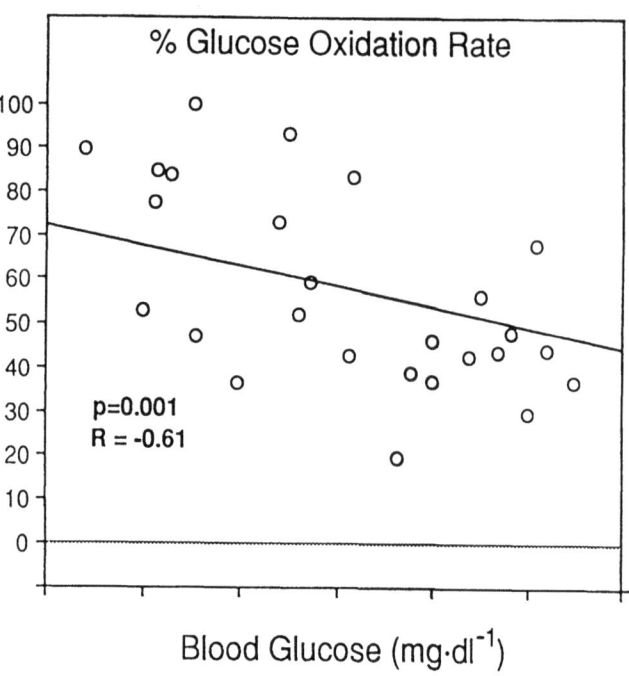

FIGURE 32.14. Negative correlation between blood glucose concentration and the percent glucose oxidized. (From Farrag et al.,[248] with permission.)

who utilized only glucose when they were studied at term (53%) or preterm (50%).[236,247,252] This probably reflects either a true difference in the contribution of glucose oxidation to total glucose utilization or the unavailability of other substrates for oxidation either from an endogenous source such as adipose tissue or from exogenous source such as parenteral nutrition.

The nonoxidative disposal of glucose represents its utilization by different metabolic pathways. In an anabolic state lipogenesis is a major route for nonoxidative disposal.[237] Other nonoxidative pathways for glucose may include glycogenesis, cycling in the pentose phosphate pathway, and/or formation of a carbon skeleton for amino acids.[253–255] The extrauterine developmental switch from a catabolic state (i.e., early studies) to an anabolic one (i.e., late studies) during the course of the current investigation can, at least in part, explain the significant increase in the contribution of the nonoxidative disposal of glucose to total energy metabolism in the late studies.

The data agree with those of van Goudoever et al.[252] in the preterm neonate. They reported that, at a glucose infusion rate of 4 mg·kg^{-1} min^{-1}, glucose oxidation rate on the first day of life was lower than the rate of glucose infusion. They also reported that the contribution of glucose oxidation, which averaged 2.9 mg·kg^{-1} min^{-1}, to the total energy expenditure was limited to about 30% of total energy expenditure. The above data further suggest that at a higher glucose infusion rate (i.e., 8 mg·kg^{-1}

min^{-1}), the average contribution of glucose oxidation to the total energy metabolism, based on arithmetic calculations, may increase to about 55% in the extremely low birth weight neonate in the first few days of life.

If glucose uptake by the neonatal brain saturates at low to moderate glycemic concentrations, as it does in the adult, the proportional contribution of the brain to total glucose utilization in the neonate would be greater at a lower than higher blood glucose concentration.[256] Because of the high brain to body weight ratio in the neonate, the contribution of the brain to total glucose utilization, primarily via glucose oxidation, is significant.[7,8] In this manner, at a higher blood glucose concentration, more glucose would be potentially available for utilization via nonoxidative pathways. In the present investigation this concept is supported by the negative correlation between blood glucose concentration and percent glucose oxidation as well as the positive one with percent nonoxidative disposal.

The investigators concluded that the extremely low birth weight neonate has the ability not only to oxidize a significant portion of the glucose load presented, but also to adjust the percent oxidized according to level of glycemia.[210] The changing pattern of the contribution of glucose oxidation and nonoxidative disposal to total glucose utilization was the main developmental change observed in the data. Other metabolic changes probably require maturation past the neonatal period.

Glucose Metabolism and the Central Nervous System

Glucose is the major substrate for brain metabolism.[257] Although ketones, glycerol, and lactate can support cerebral metabolism, the brain requires a constant supply of glucose, as discussed in Chapter 26. An initial problem related to glucose metabolism and the central nervous system is the definition of hypo- and hyperglycemia related to the nonspecific symptomatology that occurs at different concentrations of blood glucose in different neonates. There is a lack of a universal threshold below or above which symptomatology may occur. What has been accepted relatively universally is that it is in the brain that primary utilization of glucose occurs. This has been substantiated, at best indirectly, by a study of Bier et al.,[225] whose measurement of glucose production rate could be correlated with the estimated brain weight of the study subjects ranging from the premature neonate to the child weighing 25 kg compared to the adult. The neonate evidenced an increased rate of glucose production compared to the adults, as noted in Figure 32.15.

Recent investigations have emphasized the relationship between glucose production and central nervous system utilization. Huang et al.[258] evaluated the amount of systemic glucose production utilized by the cerebral cortex of a neonatal canine model. There was no correlation between systemic glucose production cerebral blood flow or cerebral glucose uptake with blood glucose concentration. Total cerebral glucose uptake was static across a wide range of glucose concentrations. The percent of glucose production utilized by the brain is an inverse of systemic glucose production. As one might expect, the cerebral extraction of glucose decreased as a function of increasing blood glucose concentration. The investigators concluded that canine glucose utilization was only 37% of systemic glucose production and that at a low rate a larger proportion of systemic glucose production is allotted to the brain.

Pryds et al.[259] measured cerebral blood flow, plasma epinephrine, and norepinephrine in 25 nonventilated preterm neonates (mean gestational age 30.4 weeks) 2 hours after birth during evaluation of hypoglycemia. When blood glucose concentration was low, cerebral blood flow increased and plasma epinephrine, but not

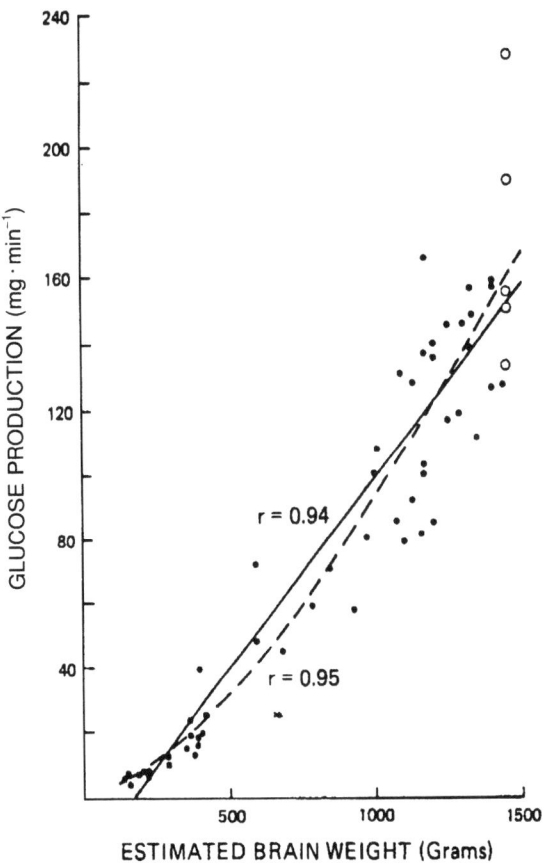

FIGURE 32.15. Relationship between glucose production rate and estimated brain weight in study subjects. (From Bier et al.,[225] with permission.)

norepinephrine concentration, was elevated. Following treatment with enteral and parenteral fluids, the blood glucose concentration increased and the cerebral blood flow declined by ~11.3%, but was still elevated (by 37.5%) in comparison to the control neonate. The investigators concluded that counterregulatory mechanisms result when blood glucose concentrations decrease to below 30 to 45 mg·dl^{-1}.

Anwar and Vannucci[260] studied cerebral blood flow responses to hypoglycemia in nine neonatal dogs treated with insulin to lower the blood glucose concentration to 1 to 35 mg·dl^{-1} with a mean 22 mg·dl^{-1}. Five animals served as controls. Increases in cerebral blood flow occurred in 17 of 20 structures of the brain in the hypoglycemic puppy ranging from 158% to 448% of the normoglycemic concentration. The percent increases in cerebral blood flow were greatest in the brain stem structures. A positive correlation existed between arterial blood pressure and cerebral cortical blood flow, suggesting a loss of autoregulation during the hypoglycemic episode. The mechanism of the increase in cerebral blood flow was hypothesized to be a stimulation of β-adrenergic receptors in the brain similar to what has been noted in the adult.

Cerebral blood flow was investigated in 24 preterm neonates of a mean 30.8 weeks of gestational age by intravenous 133-X_E clearance techniques during screening for hypoglycemia at a mean of 3 hours.[262] Cerebral blood flow was increased in 10 neonates with a blood glucose concentration of ≤30 mg·dl^{-1}, compared to the normoglycemic neonate, and decreased rapidly following treatment. Nine of the 10 were monitored by visual evoked cortical potentials, and EEGs were not less active during the hypoglycemic episodes. It was concluded that compensatory increases in cerebral blood flow may have supported cerebral metabolites during hypoglycemia.

Like Pryds et al.,[261] others have begun to evaluate neurophysiologic correlations. Koh et al.[20] have evaluated blood glucose concentration with changing patterns of auditory and somatosensory evoked potentials. Demonstration of abnormal neurophysiologic responses have been reported in the absence of symptoms. However, further correlation with plasma glucose concentration is necessary to understand the short- and long-term ramifications of specific glucose concentrations in the neonatal period.

Shen[262] has reported a prospective study of the neurosonographic findings in a series of 28 high-risk neonates who had been diagnosed with hypoglycemia. Most of the neonates were scanned initially on the first day and had a series of scans through 6 months of age. Findings included a diffuse increase in echogenicity, compressed ventricles, increased periventricular echogenicity, and hemorrhage early in the neonatal course. Later in the course, increased periventricular echogenicity, ventricular dilatation, and an increased gyral pattern were noted. In infants with neurologic sequelae, periventricular leukomalacia and brain atrophy were observed. While hypoglycemia probably did not account for all of the untoward findings, and could not be separated from the other insults such as asphyxia, the investigator suggested that early evaluation may provide critical information for vigorous treatment, while the later scans provide early prediction of potential poor neurologic outcome.

In another study of the relationship of glucose concentration to neurologic functioning, Cowett et al.[263] evaluated the effects of a wide range of glucose concentrations on brain stem conduction time I to V interpeak latency or prolonged wave V latency. Neonates were assessed by brain stem auditory-evoked response followed immediately by heelstick sampling to determine blood glucose concentration. Fifty neonates were studied who were between 33 and 40 weeks gestational age. No correlation was found between glucose concentration which ranged from 25 to 123 mg·dl^{-1} and the brain stem auditory-evoked response. The investigators concluded that alterations in glucose concentration within the generally accepted neonatal euglycemic range do not affect the functional status of the brain auditory pathway. This led to the interpretation that tighter clinical control of glucose homeostasis is probably not required in the neonatal period.

This need for research is even stronger relative to the problem of hyperglycemia. Relatively few data exist about the long-term neurophysiologic correlates at the high end of the spectrum as well. In one study, Pildes et al.[264] reported psychomotor developmental index aberrations in a neonate ≤1250 g at birth who was hyperglycemic in the neonatal period when he was subsequently evaluated at 1 to 2 years of age. By 3 to 4 years of age the differences disappeared.

An age-specific paradox exists relative to the effect of glucose on hypoxic-ischemic or ischemic brain damage. In the perinatal period research has been interpreted to suggest that pretreatment of perinatal animals with glucose infusion prolongs their survival under conditions of hypoxia, asphyxia, or cerebral ischemia, which is the exact opposite of what occirs in the adult. Vannucci et al.[265] studied this phenomenon in a rat model and concluded that the deleterious effects in the perinatal animal relate to preservation of tissue energy stores and less extensive tissue lactic acidosis than in the adult. This finding may relate to a more rapid clearance of lactic acid via either metabolism or transport.

One of the difficulties in this area of research is the quality of investigations of the relationship of hypoglycemia and hyperglycemia in the neonatal period with long-term neurodevelopmental outcome. A review of published studies by DiGiacomo and Hay[266] concluded that no definitive statements could be made relative to the interrelationship of hypoglycemia and long-term outcome. The necessity for prospective controlled studies is obvious.

Acknowledgments. Some of the work reported in this chapter was supported by National Institutes of Health grant HD27287 awarded to Dr. Cowett.

References

1. Cowett RM. Pathophysiology, diagnosis, and management of glucose homeostasis in the neonate. Curr Probl Pediatr 1985;15:1–47.
2. Cowett RM. Utilization of glucose during total parenteral nutrition. In: Lebenthal E, ed. Total parenteral nutrition in children: indications, complications and pathophysiological considerations. New York: Raven Press, 1986:17–27.
3. Ogata ES. Carbohydrate metabolism in the fetus and neonate and altered neonatal glucoregulation. Pediatr Clin North Am 1986;33:25–45.
4. Pildes RS, Pyati SP. Hypoglycemia and hyperglycemia in tiny infants. Clin Perinatol 1986;13:2351–2375.
5. Cowett RM, Stern L. Carbohydrate homeostasis in the fetus and newborn. In: Avery G, ed. Neonatology pathophysiology and management of the newborn. 3rd ed. Philadelphia: Lippincott, 1987:691–709.
6. Cowett RM, Schwartz R. Glucose homeostasis in the newborn. In: Stern L, Vert P, eds. Neonatal medicine. New York: Masson, 1987:809–831.
7. Cowett RM. Carbohydrate metabolism in the premature and compromised infant. In: Lebenthal E, ed. Textbook of gastroenterology and nutrition in early childhood. 2nd ed. New York: Raven Press, 1989:311–326.
8. Ogata ES. Problems of glucose metabolism in the extremely-low birth weight infant. In: Cowett RM, Hay WW, Jr, eds. The micropremie: the next frontier. Report of the ninety-ninth Ross Conference on Pediatric Research. Columbus, OH: Ross Laboratories, 1990:55–63.
9. Cowett RM. Hypo and hyperglycemia in the newborn. In: Polin RA, Fox WW, eds. Neonatal and fetal medicine; physiology and pathophysiology. Philadelphia: WB Saunders, 1992:406–418.
10. Cornblath M, Schwartz R. Disorders of carbohydrate metabolism in infancy. 3rd ed. Boston: Blackwell Scientific, 1991.
11. Cowett RM, Barcohana Y, Oh W. Human fetal and neonatal insulin response to maternal hyperglycemia at cesarean section (C/S). Pediatr Res 1981;15:506A.
12. Cornblath M, Reisner SH. Blood glucose in the neonate and its clinical significance. N Engl J Med 1965;273:378–381.
13. Srinivasan G, Pildes RS, Cattamanchi G, et al. Plasma glucose values in normal neonates: a new look. J Pediatr 1986;109:114–117.
14. Heck LJ, Erenberg A. Serum glucose levels in the term neonate during the first 48 hours of life. Pediatr Res 1987;110:119–122.
15. Pildes RS. Neonatal hyperglycemia. J Pediatr 1986;109:905–907.
16. Dweck HS, Cassady G. Glucose intolerance in infants of very low birth weight. I. Incidence of hyperglycemia in infants of birth weights 1100 grams or less. Pediatrics 1974;53:189–195.
17. Zarif M, Pildes RS, Vidyasagar D. Insulin and growth hormone responses in neonatal hyperglycemia. Diabetes 1976;25:428–433.
18. Cowett RW, Oh W, Pollak A, et al. Glucose disposal of low birth weight infants: steady state hyperglycemia produced by constant intravenous glucose infusion. Pediatrics 1979;63:389–396.
19. Cowett AA, Farrag HM, Gelardi NL, Cowett RM. Hyperglycemia in the micropremie: evaluation of the metabolic disequilibrium during the neonatal period. Prenatal and Neonatal Medicine (in press).
20. Koh TH, Aynsley-Green A, Tarbit M, et al. Neural dysfunction and hypoglycemia. Arch Dis Child 1988;63:1353–1358.
21. Stanley CA, Anday EX, Baker L, et al. Metabolic fuel and hormone response to fasting in newborn infants. Pediatrics 1979;64:613–619.
22. Frantz ID III, Medina G, Taeusch HW Jr. Correlation of Dextrostix values with true glucose in the range less than 50 mg/dl. J Pediatr 1975;87:417–420.
23. Perelman RH, Gutcher GR, Engle MJ, et al. Comparative analysis of four methods for rapid glucose determination in neonates. Am J Dis Child 1982;136:1051–1053.
24. Wilkins BH, Kaira D. Comparison of blood glucose test strips in the detection of neonatal hypoglycemia. Arch Dis Child 1982;57:948–960.
25. Conrad PD, Sparks JW, Osberg I, et al. Clinical application of a new glucose analyzer in the neonatal intensive care unit: comparison with other methods. J Pediatr 1989;114:281–287.
26. Lin HC, Maguire C, Oh W, et al. Accuracy and reliability of glucose reflectance meters in the high risk neonate. J Pediatr 1989;115:998–1000.
27. Cowett RM, D'Amico LB. Accuracy and reliability of glucose reflectance meters in the high risk neonate. Letter to the editor. J Pediatr 1992;120:1002.
28. Innanen VT, Deland ME, deCampos et al. Point-of care glucose testing in the neonatal intensive care unit is facilitated by the use of the Ames Glucometer Elite electrochemical glucose meter. J Pediatr 1997;130:151–155.
29. Holtrop PC, Madison KA, Kiechle FL, et al. A comparison of chromagen test strip (chemstrip bG) and serum glucose values in newborns. Am J Dis Child 1990;144:183–185.
30. Grazaitis DM, Sexton WR. Erroneously high dextostix values caused by isopropyl alcohol. Pediatrics 1980;66:221–223.
31. Jain R, Myers TF, Kahn SE, et al. How accurate is glucose analysis in the presence of multiple interfering substances in the neonate? (glucose analysis and interfering substances). J Clin Lab Anal 1995;10:13–16.
32. Cowett RM, D'Amico LB. Capillary (heelstick) versus venous blood sampling for the determination of glucose

concentration in the neonate. Biol Neonate 1992;62:32–36.
33. Shelley HJ, Bassett JM. Control of carbohydrate metabolism in the fetus and newborn. Br Med Bull 1975;31:37–43.
34. Cornblath M, Schwartz R, Aynsley-Green A, et al. Hypoglycemia in infancy: the need for a rationale definition. Pediatrics 1990;85:834–837.
35. Fluge G. Clinical aspects of neonatal hypoglycemia. Acta Paediatr Scand 1974;63:826–832.
36. Gutberlet RL, Cornblath M. Neonatal hypoglycemia revisited, 1975. Pediatrics 1976;58:10–17.
37. Milner RDG. Annotation—neonatal hypoglycemia. A critical appraisal. Arch Dis Child 1972;47:679–682.
38. Senior B. Current concepts. Neonatal hypoglycemia. N Engl J Med 1973;289:790–793.
39. Cornblath M, Odell GB, Levin EY. Symptomatic neonatal hypoglycemia associated with toxemia of pregnancy. J Pediatr 1959;55:545–562.
40. Raivio KO, Hallman N. Neonatal hypoglycemia. Occurrence of hypoglycemia in patients with various neonatal disorders. Acta Paediatr Scand 1968;57:517–521.
41. Lubchenco LO, Bard H. Incidence of hypoglycemia in newborn infants classified by birth weight and gestational age. Pediatrics 1971;47:831–838.
42. deLeeuw R, deVries IL. Hypoglycemia in small for dates newborn infants. Pediatrics 1976;58:18–22.
43. Koivisto M, Jouppila P. Neonatal hypoglycemia and maternal toxaemia. Acta Paediatr Scand 1974;63:743–749.
44. Kliegman R. Alterations of fasting glucose and fat metabolism in intrauterine growth retarded newborn dogs. Am J Physiol 1989;256:E380–E385.
45. Economides DL, Proudler A, Nicolardes KH. Plasma insulin in appropriate and small for gestational age fetuses. Am J Obstet Gynecol 1989;160:1091–1094.
46. Bussey ME, Finley S, LaBarbera A, et al. Hypoglycemia in the newborn growth retarded rat: delayed phosphoenol pyruvate carboxy kinase induction despite increased glucagon availability. Pediatr Res 1985;19:363–367.
47. Haymond MW, Karl IE, Pagliara AS. Increased gluconeogenic substrate in the small gestation age infant. N Engl J Med 1974;291:322–328.
48. Williams PR, Fiser RH Jr, Sperling MA, et al. Effects of oral alanine feeding of blood glucose, plasma glucagon, and insulin concentrations in small for gestational age infants. N Engl J Med 1975;292:612–614.
49. Reisner SH, Aranda JV, Colle E, et al. The effect of intravenous glucagon on plasma amino acids in the newborn. Pediatr Res 1973;7:184–191.
50. Carter PE, Lloyd DJ, Duffy P. Glucagon for hypoglycemia in infants small for gestational age. Arch Dis Child 1988;63:1264–1266.
51. Mestyan MJ, Schultz K, Soltesz G, et al. The metabolic effects of glucagon infusion in normoglycemic and hypoglycemic small for gestational age infants. Changes in plasma amino acids. Acta Paediatr Acad Sci Hung 1976;17:245–253.
52. Sperling MA, Grajwer L, Leake RD, et al. Effects of somatostatin (SRIF) infusion on glucose homeostasis in newborn lambs: evidence for a significant role of glucagon. Pediatr Res 1977;11:962–967.
53. Salle BL, Ruiton-Ugliengo A. Effects of oral glucose and protein load on plasma glucagon and insulin concentrations in small for gestational age infants. Pediatr Res 1977;11:108–112.
54. Cowett RM, Susa JB, Oh W, et al. Glucose kinetics in glucose infused small for gestational age infants. Pediatr Res 1984;18:74–79.
55. Flecknell PA, Wootton R, Royston JP, et al. Glucose homeostasis in the newborn: effects of an intravenous glucose infusion in normal and intrauterine growth retarded neonatal piglets. Biol Neonate 1987;52:205–215.
56. Ogata ES, Paul RI, Finley SL. Limited maternal field availability due to hyperinsulinemia retards fetal growth and development in the rat. Pediatr Res 1987;22:432–437.
57. Sann L, Morel Y, Lasne Y. Effect of hydrocortisone on intravenous glucose tolerance in small for gestational age infants. Helv Paediatr Acta 1983;38:475–482.
58. Van Toledo-Eppinga L, Houdijk MC, Delemarre-Van De Waal HA, et al. Leucine and glucose kinetics during growth hormone treatment in intrauterine growth retarded preterm infants. Am J Physiol 1996;270:E451–455.
59. Beard AG, Panos, TC, Marasigan, BV, et al. Perinatal stress and the premature neonate. Effect of fluid and caloric deprivation on blood glucose. J Pediatr 1966;68:329–343.
60. Beard AG. Neonatal hypoglycemia. J Perinatol Med 1975;3:219–225.
61. Tejani N, Lipshitz F, Harper RG. The responses to an oral glucose load during convalescence from hypoxia in newborn infants. J Pediatr 1979;94:792–796.
62. Collins JE, Leonard JV. Hyperinsulinism in asphyxiated and small for dates infants with hypoglycemia. Lancet 1984;1:311–313.
63. Jansen RD, Hayden MK, Ogata ES. Effects of asphyxia at birth on postnatal glucose regulation in the rat. J Dev Physiol 1984;6:473–483.
64. Mann TP, Elliott RIK. Neonatal cold injury due to accidental exposure to cold. Lancet 1957;1:229–234.
65. Schiff D, Stern L, Leduc J. Chemical thermogenesis in newborn infants: catecholamine excretion and the plasma nonesterified fatty acid response to cold exposure. Pediatrics 1966;37:577–582.
66. Close WH, LeDividish J, Dulee PH. Influence of environmental temperature on glucose tolerance and insulin response in the newborn piglet. Biol Neonate 1985;47:84–91.
67. Yeung CY. Hypoglycemia in neonatal sepsis. J Pediatr 1970;77:812–817.
68. LaNaoue KF, Mason AD Jr, Daniels JP. The impairment of glucogenesis by gram negative infection. Metabolism 1968;17:606–611.
69. Yeung CY, Lee VMY, Yeung CM. Glucose disappearance rate in neonatal infection. J Pediatr 1973;83:486–489.
70. Fitzgerald MJ, Goto M, Myers TF, et al. Early metabolic effects of sepsis in the preterm infant: lactic acidosis and

increased glucose requirement. J Pediatr 1992;121:951–955.
71. Shelley HJ. Glycogen reserves and their changes at birth and in anoxia. Br Med Bull 1972;17:137–143.
72. Benzing G, Schubert W, Hug G, et al. Simultaneous hypoglycemia and acute congestive heart failure. Circulation 1969;40:209–216.
73. Amatayakul O, Cumming GR, Haworth JC. Association of hypoglycemia with cardiac enlargement and heart failure in newborn infants. Arch Dis Child 1970;45:717–720.
74. Haymond MW, Strauss AW, Arnold KJ, et al. Glucose homeostasis in children with severe cyanotic congenital heart disease. J Pediatr 1979;95:220–227.
75. Kerkering KW, Robertson LW, Kodroff MB, et al. Grand rounds series: hypoglycemia and unilateral pulmonary edema in a newborn. Pediatrics 1980;65:326–330.
76. Lindell KH, Sabel KG, Eriksson BD, et al. Glucose metabolism and insulin secretion in infants with symptomatic ventricular septal defect. Acta Paediatr scand 1989;78:620–626.
77. Vidnes J, Oyasaeter S. Glucagon deficiency causing severe neonatal hypoglycemia in a patient with normal insulin secretion. Pediatr Res. 1977;11:943–949.
78. Vidnes J, Sovik O. Gluconeogenesis in infancy and childhood. Studies on the glucose production from alanine in three cases of persistent neonatal hypoglycaemia. Acta Paediatr Scand 1976;65:297–305.
79. Vidnes J, Sovik O. Gluconeogenesis in infancy and childhood. Deficiency of the extramitochondrial form of hepatic phosphoenolpyruvate carboxykinase in a case of persistent neonatal hypoglycemia. Acta Paediatr 1976;65:307–312.
80. Hers H-G, Van Hoof F, de Barsy T. Glycogen storage diseases. In: Scriver CR, Beaudet AI, Sly WS, et al., eds. The metabolic basis of inherited disease. 6th ed. New York: McGraw-Hill, 1989:425–452.
81. Pagliara AS, Karl IE, Keating JP, et al. Hepatic fructose-1,6-diphosphatase deficiency: a cause of lactate acidosis and hypoglycemia in infancy. J Clin Invest. 1972;51:2115–2123.
82. Ralleson ML, Mukle AW, Zigrang WD. Hypoglycemia and lactate acidosis associated with fructose-1,6-diphosphatase deficiency. J Pediatr 1979;94:933–936.
83. Levy HL, Hammersen G. Newborn screening for galactosemia and other galactose metabolic defects. J Pediatr 1978;92:871–887.
84. Barrett CT, Oliver TK Jr. Hypoglycemia and hyperinsulinism in infants with erythroblastosis fetalis. N Engl J Med 1968;278:1260–1263.
85. Molsted-Pedersen L, Trautner H, Jorgensen KR. Plasma insulin and k values during intravenous glucose tolerance test in newborn infants with erythroblastosis foetalis. Acta Paediatr Scand 1973;62:11–16.
86. Oh W, Yap LL, D'Amodio MD. Hypoglycemia in severely affected Rh erythroblastotic infants. J Pediatr 1969;74:813A.
87. Schiff D, Lowy C. Hypoglycemia and excretion of insulin in urine in hemolytic disease of the newborn. Pediatr Res 1970;4:280–285.
88. Katz CM, Taylor PM. Incidence of low birth weight in children with severe mental retardation. Am J Dis Child 1967;114:80–90.
89. Schiff D, Aranda JV, Chan G, et al. Metabolic effects of exchange transfusions. Effect of citrated and of heparinized blood on glucose, non-esterified fatty acids, 2-(4 hydroxybenzeneazo) benzoic acid binding and insulin. J Pediatr 1971;78:603–609.
90. Schiff D, Aranda JC, Colle E, et al. Metabolic effects of exchange transfusion. Delayed hypoglycemia following exchange transfusion with citriated blood. J Pediatr 1971;79:589–593.
91. Beckwith JB, Wang CI, Donel GN. Hyperplastic fetal visceromegaly with macroglossia, omphalocele, cytomegaly of adrenal fetal cortex, postnatal somatic gigantism, and other abnormalities. Newly recognized syndrome. Proceedings of the American Pediatrics Society, Seattle, 1964; June 16–18. (Abstract 41).
92. Wiedemann HR. Complexe malformatif familiale avec hernie ombilicale et macroglossie—un syndrome nouveau? J Genet Hum 1964;13:223.
93. Schiff D, Colle EC, Wells D, et al. Metabolic aspects of the Beckwith-Wiedemann syndrome. J Pediatr 1973;82:258–267.
94. Heitz PU, Kloppel G, Hacki WH, et al. Nesidioblastosis: the pathologic basis of persistent hyperinsulinemic hypoglycemia in infants. Diabetes 1977;26:637–642.
95. Schwartz SS, Rich BH, Lucky AW, et al. Familial nesidioblastosis: severe neonatal hypoglycemia in two families. Pediatrics 1979;95:44–53.
96. Woo D, Scopes JW, Polak JM. Idiopathic hypoglycemia in situ with morphological evidence of nesidioblastosis of the pancreas. Arch Dis Child 1976;51:528–531.
97. Hirsch HJ, Loo S, Evans N, et al. Hypoglycemia of infancy and nesidioblastosis studies with somatostatin. N Engl J Med 1977;296:1323–1326.
98. Baerentsen H. Case report: neonatal hypoglycemia due to an islet cell adenoma. Acta Paediatr Scand 1973;62:207–210.
99. Burst NRM, Campbell JR, Castro A. Congenital islet cell adenoma causing hypoglycemia in a newborn. Pediatrics 1971;47:605–610.
100. Habbick BJ, Cram RW, Miller KR. Neonatal hypoglycemia resulting from islet cell adenomatosis. Am J Dis Child 1977;131:210–212.
101. Gruppuso PA, DeLuca F, O'Shea PA, et al. Near total pancreatectomy for hyperinsulinism. Spontaneous remission of resultant diabetes. Acta Paediatr Scand 1985;74:311–315.
102. Solt'esz G, Jenkins PA, Aynsley-Green A. Hyperinsulinemic hypoglycemia in infancy and childhood: a practical approach to diagnosis and medical treatment based on experience of 18 cases. Acta Paediatr Hung 1984;25:319–332.
103. Aynsley-Green A, Jenkin P, Tronier B, et al. Plasma proinsulin and C peptide concentrations in children with hyperinsulinemic hypoglycemic. Acta Paediatr Scand 1984;73:359–363.
104. W'uthrich C, Schubiger G, Zuppinger K. Persistent neonatal hyperinsulinemia hypoglycemia in two siblings

successfully treated with diazoxide. Helv Paediatr Acta 1986;41:455–459.
105. Bruining GJ, Bosschaart AN, Aarsen RS, et al. Normalization of glucose homeostasis by a long acting somatostatin analog 201-995 in a newborn with nesidioblastosis. Acta Endocrinol Suppl (Copenh) 1986;279:275–278.
106. Glaser B, Landau H, Smilouici A, et al. Persistent hyperinsulinemic hypoglycemia of infancy: long term treatment with the somatostatin analogue sandostatin. Clin Endocrinol 1989;31:71–80.
107. Gould UE, Mamoli UA, Dardi LE, et al. Nesidiodysplasia and nesidioblastosis of infancy: structural and functional correlations with the syndrome of hyperinsulinemia hypoglycemia. Pediatr Pathol 1983;1:7–31.
108. Bruining GJ. Recent advances in hyperinsulinemism and the pathogenesis of diabetes mellitus. Curr Opin Pediatr 1990;2:758–765.
109. Thomas PM, Cote GJ, Hallman DM, et al. Homozygosity mapping to chromosome 11p, of the gene for familial hyperinsulinemic hypoglycemia of infancy. Am J Hum Genet 1995;56:416–421.
110. Glaser B, Chiu KC, Anker R, et al. Familial hyperinsulinemism maps to chromosome 11p14–15.1, 30cM centromeric to the insulin gene. Nat Genet 1994;7:185–188.
111. Epstein MF, Nicholls E, Stubblefield PG. Neonatal hypoglycemia after beta-sympathomimetic tocolytic therapy. J Pediatr 1979;94:449–453.
112. Procianoy RS, Pinheiro CEA. Neonatal hyperinsulinism after short term maternal beta sympathomimetic therapy. J Pediatr 1982;101:612–614.
113. Leake RD, Hobel CJ, Okada DM, et al. Neonatal metabolic effects of oral ritodrine hypochloride administration. Pediatr Pharmacol 1983;3:101–106.
114. Tenenbaum D, Cowett RM. The mechanisms of beta sympathomimetic action on neonatal glucose homeostasis in the lamb. J Pediatr 1985;107:588–592.
115. Nagel JW, Sims JS, Aplin CE, et al. Refractory hypoglycemia associated with a malpositioned umbilical artery catheter. Pediatrics 1979;64:315–317.
116. Malik M, Wilson DP. Umbilical artery catheterization. A potential cause of refractory hypoglycemia. Clin Pediatr 1987:26:181–182.
117. Puri AR, Alkalay AL, Pomerance JJ, et al. Neonatal hypoglycemia associated with umbilical artery catheter positioned at eighth to ninth thoracic vertebrae. Am J Perinatol 1987;4:195–197.
118. Carey BE, Zeilinger TC. Hypoglycemia due to high positioning of umbilical artery catheters. J Perinatol 1989;9:407–410.
119. Cowett RM, Tenenbaum D, Fatoba O, et al. The effects of glucose infusion above the celiac axis in the newborn lamb. Biol Neonate 1985;47:179–185.
120. Jacob J, Davis RF. Differences in serum glucose determinations in infants with umbilical artery catheters. J Perinatol 1988;8:40–42.
121. Singh SP, Sayder AK, Singh SF. Effects of ethanol ingestion on maternal and fetal glucose homeostasis. J Lab Clin Med 1984;104:176–184.
122. Witek-Janusek L. Maternal ethanol ingestion: effect on maternal and neonatal glucose balance. Am J Physiol 1986;251:E178–184.
123. Singh SP, Snyder AK, Pullen GL. Fetal alcohol syndrome—glucose and liver metabolism in term rat fetus and neonate. Alcoholism 1986;10:54–58.
124. Zucker P, Simon G. Prolonged symptomatic neonatal hypoglycemia associated with maternal chlorpropamide therapy. Pediatrics 1968;42:824–825.
125. Senior B, Slone D, Shapiro S, et al. Benzothiadiazides and neonatal hypoglycemia. Lancet 1976;2:377.
126. Stern C. Idiopathic hypoglycemia. Proc R Soc Med 1973;66:345–346.
127. Brown RE, Young RB. A possible role for the exocrine pancreas in the pathogenesis of neonatal leucine sensitive hypoglycemia. Am J Dig Dis 1970;15:65–72.
128. Schutgens RBH, Heymans H, Ketel A, et al. Lethal hypoglycemia in a child with a deficiency of 3-hydroxy-3-methyl glutaryl coenzyme A lyase. J Pediatr 1979;94:89–91.
129. Pickering D. Neonatal hypoglycemia due to salicylate poisoning. Proc R Soc Med 1968;61:1256.
130. Gemelli M, DeLuca R, Barberio G. Hypoglycemia and congenital adrenal hyperplasia. Acta Pediatr Scand 1979;68:285–286.
131. Souto M, Piezzi RS, Bianchi R. Effect of insulin on neonatal and adult adrenal medulla in the rat. Acta Anat (Base) 1985;122:216–219.
132. Artavia-Loria E, Chaussain JL, Bougneres PF, et al. Frequency of hypoglycemia in children with adrenal insufficiency. Acta Endocrinol Suppl (Copenh) 1986;279:275–278.
133. Lilien LD, Srinivasan G, Yeh TF, et al. Decreased plasma glucose following indomethacin therapy in premature infants with patent ductus arteriosus. Pediatr Pharmacol 1985;5:73–77.
134. Sperling MA. Hypoglycemia in the newborn infant, and child. In: Lifshitz F, ed. Pediatric endocrinology, a clinical guide. 2nd ed. New York: Marcel Dekker, 1990:803–838.
135. Lilien LD, Pildes RS, Srinivasan G, et al. Treatment of neonatal hypoglycemia with minibolus and intravenous glucose infusion. J Pediatr 1980;97:295–298.
136. Cowett RM, Susa JB, Schwartz R, et al. Concentration of parenteral glucose solution. Pediatrics 1977;59:791.
137. Sann L, Mousson B, Rousson M, et al. Prevention of neonatal hypoglycemia by oral lipid supplementation in low birth weight infants. Eur J Pediatr 1988;147:158–161.
138. McCann ML, Likly B. The role of epinephrine prophylactic therapy in infants of diabetic mothers. Proc Soc Pediatr Res 1967;3:5.
139. Victorin LH, Thorell JI. Plasma insulin and blood glucose during long-term treatment with diazoxide for infant hypoglycemia. Case report. Acta Paediatr Scand 1974;63:302–306.
140. Altszular N, Hampshire J, Moraru E. On the mechanism of diazoxide-induced hyperglycemia. Diabetes 1977;26:931–935.
141. Cowett RM, Tenenbaum D. Hepatic response to insulin in control of glucose homeostasis in the neonatal lamb. Metabolism 1987;36:1021–1026.

142. LeDune MA. Intravenous glucose tolerance and plasma insulin studies in small for date infants. Arch Dis Child 1972;47:111–114.
143. Fox HA, Krasna IN. Total intravenous nutrition by peripheral vein in neonatal surgical patients. Pediatrics 1973;52:14–20.
144. Gentz JCH, Cornblath M. Transient diabetes of the newborn. Adv Pediatr 1969;16:345–363.
145. Dweck HS, Brans YW, Sumners JE, et al. Glucose intolerance in infants of very low birth weight. Intravenous glucose tolerance tests in infants of birth weights 500–1380 grams. Biol Neonate 1976;30:261–267.
146. Lilien LO, Rosenfield RL, Baccaro MM, et al. Hyperglycemia in stressed small premature neonates. J Pediatr 1979;94:454–459.
147. Louik C, Mitchell AA, Epstein MF, et al. Risk factors for neonatal hyperglycemia associated with 10% dextrose infusion. Am J Dis Child 1985;139:783–786.
148. Wu S, Srinivasan G, Pildes RS, et al. Plasma glucose (G) values during the first month of life in infants <1000gm. Pediatr Res 1990;27:231A.
149. Srinivasan G, Jain R, Pildes RS, et al. Glucose homeostasis during anesthesia and surgery in infants. J Pediatr Surg 1986;21:718–721.
150. Arand KJS. Neonatal hyperglycemia during surgery. J Pediatr 1987;110:999.
151. Anand KJS, Brown MJ, Bloom SR, et al. Studies on the hormonal regulation of fuel metabolism in the human newborn infant undergoing anaesthesia and surgery. Horm Res 1985;22:115–128.
152. Anand KJS, Aynsley-Green A. Metabolic and endocrine effects of surgical ligation of patent ductus arteriosus in the human preterm neonate: Are there implications for further improvement of postoperative outcome? Mod Probl Pediatr 1985;23:143–157.
153. Anand KJS, Sippell WG, Aynsley-Green A. Randomised trial of fentanyl anaesthesia in preterm neonates undergoing surgery: effects on the stress response. Lancet 1987;1:243–248.
154. Anand KJS. The stress response to surgical trauma: from physiological basis to therapeutic implications. Prog Food Nutr Sci 1986;10:67–132.
155. Mammel MC, Green TP, Johnson DE, et al. Controlled trial of dexamethasone therapy in infants with bronchopulmonary dysplasia. Lancet 1983;1:1356–1358.
156. Avery GB, Fletcher AB, Kaplan M, et al. Controlled trial of dexamethasone in respirator-dependent infants with bronchopulmonary dysplasia. Pediatrics 1985;75:106–111.
157. Cummings JJ, Eugenio DB, Gross SJ. A controlled trial of dexamethasone in preterm infants at high risk for bronchopulmonary dysplasia. N Engl J Med 1989;320:1505–1510.
158. Harkavy KL, Scanlon JW, Chowdhry PK, et al. Dexamethasone therapy for chronic lung disease in ventilator- and oxygen-dependent infants: a controlled trial. J Pediatr 1989;115:979–983.
159. Ferrara TB, Coyser RJ, Haekstra RE. Side effects and long term follow up of corticosteroid therapy in very low birth weight infants with broncho-pulmonary dysplasia. J Perinatol 1990;10:137–142.
160. James T III, Blessa M, Boggs TR Jr, et al. Recurrent hyperglycemia associated with sepsis in a neonate. Am J Dis Child 1979;133:645–646.
161. Srinivasan G, Singh J, Gattamanchi G, et al. Plasma glucose changes in preterm infants during oral theophylline therapy. J Pediatr 1983;103:473–476.
162. Leisto J, Raivio K, Krohn K. Neonatal hyperglycemia and chromosome deletion (46,xx,Dq-). J Pediatr 1976;88:989–990.
163. Yunis KA, Oh W, Kalhan SC, Cowett RM. Glucose kinetics following administration of an intravenous fat emulsion to low birth weight neonates. Am J Physiol 1992;263:E844–849.
164. Anderson TL, Muttart CR, Bieher MA. A controlled trial of glucose versus glucose and amino acids in premature infants. J Pediatr 1978;94:949–951.
165. LeDune MA. Insulin studies in temporary neonatal hyperglycemia. Arch Dis Child 1971;16:392–394.
166. Sodoyez-Goffant F, Sodoyez JC. Transient diabetes mellitus in a neonate. J Pediatr 1977;91:395–399.
167. Gruppuso PA, Gorden P, Kahn CR, et al. Familial hyperproinsulinemia due to a proposed defect in conversion of proinsulin to insulin. N Engl J Med. 1984;331:629–635.
168. Pollak A, Cowett RM, Schwartz R, et al. Glucose disposal in low birth weight infants during steady state hyperglycemia: effects of exogenous insulin administration. Pediatrics 1978;61:546–549.
169. Ostertag SG, Jovanovic L, Lewis B, Auld PAM. Insulin pump therapy in the very low birth weight infant. Pediatrics 1986;78:625–630.
170. Vaucher YE, Walson PD, Morrow G III. Continuous insulin infusion in hyperglycemic very low birth weight infants. J Pediatr Gastroenterol Nutr 1982;2:211–217.
171. Goldman SL, Hirata T. Attenuated responses to insulin in very low birth weight infants. Pediatr Res 1980;14:50–53.
172. Heron P, Boucher D. Insulin infusion in infants of birthweight less than 1250g and with glucose tolerance. Aust Paediatr J 1988;24:362–365.
173. Binder ND, Raschzo PK, Benda GI, et al. Insulin infusion with parenteral nutrition in extremely low birth weight infants with hyperglycemia. J Pediatr 1989;114:273–280.
174. Collins JW, Hoppe M, Brown K, et al. A controlled trial of insulin infusion and parenteral nutrition in extremely low birth weight infants with glucose intolerance. J Pediatr 1991;118:921–927.
175. Arant BS Jr, Gooch WM III. Effects of acute hyperglycemia on brains of neonatal puppies. Pediatr Res 1979;13:488A.
176. Ekblad H, Kero P, Takala J. Stable glucose balance in premature infants with fluid restriction and early enteral feeding. Acta Paediatr Scand 1987;76:438–443.
177. Oliven A, King KC, Kalhan SC. Gastrointestinal enhanced insulin release in response to glucose in newborn infants. J Pediatr Gastroenterol Nutr 1986;5:220–225.
178. Ktorza A, Bihoreau MT, Nurjhan N, et al. Insulin and glucagon during the perinatal period secretion and metabolic effects on the liver. Biol Neonate 1985;48:204–220.

179. King RA, Smith RM, Dahlenberg GW. Long term postnatal development of insulin secretion in early premature neonates. Early Human Dev 1986;13:285–294.
180. Ghiglione M, Pascual JM, Rovira A, et al. Plasma glucagon-immunoreactive components in early life in dogs. Horm Metal Res 1985;17:387–390.
181. Grasso S, Fallucca F, Massone D. Inhibition of glucagon secretion in the human newborn by glucose infusion. Diabetes 1983;32:498–492.
182. Mehta A, Wootton R, Cheng KN, et al. Effect of diazoxide or glucagon on hepatic glucose production rate during extreme neonatal hypoglycemia. Arch Dis Child 1987;62:924–930.
183. Mayor F, Cuezva JM. Hormonal and metabolic changes in the perinatal period. Biol Neonate 1985;48:185–196.
184. Padbury JF, Polk DH, Newnham JP, et al. Neonatal adaptation greater sympathoadrenal response in preterm than full term fetal sheep at birth. Am J Physiol 1985;248:E443–449.
185. Hagrevik K, Faxelius G, Irestedt L, et al. Catecholamine surge and metabolic adaptation in the newborn after vaginal delivery and cesarean section. Acta Paediatr Scand 1984;73:602–609.
186. Gripois D, Valens M, Diarra A. Adrenal medullary responses to insulin induced hypoglycemia in the young rat. Influence of thyroid hormones. J Auton Nerv Syst 1986;15:165–178.
187. Adam PAJ, King KC, Schwartz R. Model for the investigation of intractable hypoglycemia: insulin-glucose interrelationship during steady state infusions. Pediatrics 1968;41:91–105.
188. Varma S, Nickerson H, Cowan JS, et al. Homeostasis response to glucose loading in newborn and young dogs. Metabolism 1973;22:1367–1375.
189. Kornhauser D, Adam PAJ, Schwartz R. Glucose production and utilization in the newborn puppy. Pediatr Res 1974;4:120–128.
190. Cowett RM, Susa JB, Oh W, et al. Endogenous glucose production during constant glucose infusion in the newborn lamb. Pediatr Res 1978;12:853–857.
191. Clark MG, Filsell OH, Jarrett IG. Gluconeogenesis in isolated intact lamb liver cells. Biochem J 1976;156:671.
192. Curnow RT, Rayfield EJ, George DT, et al. Control of hepatic glycogen metabolism in the rhesus monkey: effect of glucose, insulin, and glucagon administration. Am J Physiol 1975;228:E80–89.
193. Owen OE, Patel MS, Block BSB, et al. Gluconeogenesis in normal, cirrhotic and diabetic humans. In: Hanson RW, Mehlman MA, eds. Gluconeogenesis: its regulation in mammalian species. New York: Wiley Interscience, 1965:533.
194. Susa JB, Cowett RM, Oh W, et al. Suppression of gluconeogenesis and endogenous glucose production by exogenous insulin administration in the newborn lamb. Pediatr Res 1979;13:594–599.
195. Cowett RM, Susa JB, Warburton D, et al. Endogenous post-hepatic secretion and metabolic clearance rates in the neonatal lamb. Pediatr Res 1980;14:1391–1394.
196. Cowett RM, Oh W, Schwartz R. Persistent glucose production during glucose infusion in the human neonate. J Clin Invest 1983;71:467–475.
197. Cowett RM, Anderson GE, Maguire CA, et al. Ontogeny of glucose homeostasis in low birth weight infants. J Pediatr 1989;115:998–1000.
198. Cowett RM. Decreased response to catecholamines in the newborn: effect on glucose kinetics in the lamb. Metabolism 1988;37:736–740.
199. Cowett RM. Alpha adrenergic agonists stimulate neonatal glucose production less than beta adrenergic agonist in the lamb. Metabolism 1988;37:83–86.
200. Hetenyi C, Kovacevic N, Hall SEH, et al. Plasma glucagon in pups, decreased by fasting, unaffected by somatostatin or hyperglycemia. Am J Physiol 1976;231:1377–1382.
201. Cowett RM, Rapoza RE. Influence of glucagon as a contra insulin hormone in neonatal hyperinsulinemic hypoglycemia. Pediatr Res 1996;39:87A.
202. Cowett RM, Rapoza RE. Glucose does not autoregulate neonatal glucose homeostasis. Pediatr Res 1996;39:307A.
203. Cowett RM, Rapoza RE, Jawad G, et al. Sympathomimetics as contra-insulin hormones in neonatal hyperinsulinemic hypoglycemia. Pediatr Res 1997;41:230A.
204. Wolfe R, Allsop JR, Burke JF. Glucose metabolism in man: responses to intravenous glucose infusion. Metab Clin Exp 1979;28:210–220.
205. Kalhan SC, Oliver A, King KC, et al. Role of glucose in the regulation of endogenous glucose production in the human newborn. Pediatr Res 1986;20:49–52.
206. Hulman SE, Kliegman RM. Assessment of insulin resistance in newborn beagles with the euglycemic hyperinsulinemic clamp. Pediatr Res 1989;25:219–223.
207. Kliegman R, Trindade C, Hugan M, et al. Effects of euglycemic hyperinsulinemia on neonatal canine hepatic and muscle metabolism. Pediatr Res 1989;25:124–129.
208. DeFronzo RA, Tobin JD, Andres R. Glucose clamp technique: a method for quantifying insulin secretion and resistance. Am J Physiol 1979;237:E214–223.
209. Kahn CR. Insulin resistance, insulin insensitivity and insulin unresponsiveness: a necessary distinction. Metab Clin Exp 1978;27:1893–1902.
210. Farrag HM, Nawrath LM, Healey JE, et al. Persistent glucose production and greater peripheral sensitivity to insulin in the neonate vs. the adult. Am J Physiol 1997;272:E86–93.
211. Kono T, Barham FW. The relationship between the insulin-binding capacity of fat cells and the cellular response to insulin: studies with intact and trypsin-treated fat cells. J Biol Chem 1971;246:6210–6216.
212. Rizza RA, Mandarino LJ, Gerich JE. Dose response characteristics for effects of insulin on production and utilization of glucose in man. Am J Physiol 1981;240;E630–629.
213. Thorsson AV, Hintz RL. Insulin receptors in the newborn: increase in receptor affinity and number. N Engl J Med 1977;297:908–912.
214. Rebrin K, Steil GM, Getty L, et al. Free fatty acid as a link in the regulation of hepatic glucose output by peripheral insulin. Diabetes 1995;44:1038–1045.

215. Hertz DE, Karn CA, Liu YM, et al. Intravenous glucose suppresses glucose production but not proteolysis in extremely premature newborns. J Clin Invest 1993;92:1752–1758.
216. Denne SC, Karn CA, Wang J, et al. Effect of intravenous glucose and lipid on proteolysis and glucose production in normal newborns. Am J Physiol 1995;269:E361–E367.
217. Bergman RN, Hope ID, Yang YJ, et al. Assessment of insulin sensitivity in vivo; a critical review. Diabetes Metab Rev 1989;5:411–429.
218. Menon RK, Sperling MA. Carbohydrate metabolism. Semin Perinatol 1988;12:157–162.
219. Girard J. Gluconeogenesis in late fetal and early neonatal life. Biol Neonate 1986;50:237–258.
220. Bougnères PF, Karl IE, Hillman LS, et al. Lipid transport in the human newborn. Palmitate and glycerol turnover and the contribution of glycerol to neonatal hepatic glucose output. J Clin Invest. 1982;70:262–270.
221. Frazer TE, Karl IE, Hillman LS, et al. Direct measurement of gluconeogenesis from (2,3-^{13}C)alanine in the human neonate. Am J Physiol 1981;240:E615–621.
222. Gilfillan CA, Tserng KY, Kalhan SC. Alanine production by the human fetus at term gestation. Biol Neonate 1985;47:141–147.
223. Gleason CA, Roman C, Rudolph AM. Hepatic oxygen consumption, lactate uptake and glucose production in neonatal lambs. Pediatr Res 1985;19:1235–1239.
224. Bier DM, Arnold KF, Sherman WR, et al. In vivo measurement of glucose and alanine metabolism with stable isotopic tracers. Diabetes 1977;26:1005–1015.
225. Bier DM, Leake RD, Haymond MW, et al. Measurement of true glucose production rules in infancy and childhood with 6,6 dideutero glucose. Diabetes 1977;26:1016–1023.
226. Kalhan SC, Savin SM, Adam PAJ. Measurement of glucose turnover in the human newborn with glucose I-^{13}C. J Endocrinol Metab 1976;43:704–707.
227. Kalhan SC, Savin SM, Adam PAJ. Attenuated glucose production rate in newborn infants of insulin dependent diabetic mothers. N Engl J Med 1977;296:375–376.
228. Kalhan SC, Bier DM, Savin SM, et al. Estimation of glucose turnover and ^{13}C recycling in the human newborn by simultaneous [1-^{13}C]glucose and [6,6-^{2}H$_2$]glucose tracers. J Clin Endocrinol Metab 1980;50:456–460.
229. Kerr DS, Stevens MCG, Robinson HM. Fasting metabolism in infants. I. Effect of severe undernutrition on energy and protein utilization. Metabolism 1978;27:411–435.
230. Kerr DS, Stevens MCG, Picou DIM. Fasting metabolism in infants: II. The effect of severe undernutrition and infusion of alanine on glucose production estimated with 6-^{13}C-glucose. Metabolism 1978;27:831–848.
231. Cowett RM, Susa J, Gilleti B, et al. Glucose kinetics in infants of diabetic mothers. Am J Obstet Gynecol 1983;146:781–786.
232. King KC, Tserng KY, Kalhan SC. Regulation of glucose production in newborn infants of diabetic mothers. Pediatr Res 1982;16:608–612.
233. Denne SC, Kalhan SC. Leucine metabolism in human newborns. Am J Physiol 1987;253:E608–E615.
234. VanAerde JEE, Sauer PJJ, Pencharz PB, et al. The effect of energy intake and expenditure on the recovery of ^{13}CO$_2$ in the parenterally fed neonate during a 4 hour primed constant infusion of NAH^{13}CO$_3$. Pediatr Res 1985;19:806–810.
235. Zarlengo KM, Battaglia FC, Fennessey P, et al. Relationship between glucose utilization rate and glucose concentration in preterm infants. Biol Neonate 1986;49:181–189.
236. Denne SC, Kalhan SC. Glucose carbon recycling and oxidation in human newborns. Am J Physiol 1986;251:E71–77.
237. Sauer PJJ, VanAerde JEE, Pencharz PB, et al. Glucose oxidation rates in newborn infants measured with indirect calorimetry and [U-^{13}C]glucose. Clin Sci 1986;70:587–593.
238. Kalhan SC, Van Beek RHT, Sauer PJJ. Estimates of gluconeogenesis in the preterm infant. Pediatr Res 1997;41:233A.
239. Sunehag AL, Schanler RJ, Reeds PJ, et al. Gluconeogenesis in extremely premature infants receiving parenteral nutrition. Pediatr Res 1997;41:241A
240. Feng BC, Kliegman RM. Insulin resistance and neonatal canine gluconeogenesis: transcription of the fructose-1,6-bisphosphatase gene. Pediatr Res 1994;35:202A.
241. Feng BC, Li JX, Kliegman RM. Effects of insulin, epinephrine, and glucose on regulation of transcription of the serine dehydratase gene in newborn dogs. Biochem Mol Med 1996;57:91–96.
242. Feng BC, Li JX, Kliegman RM. Transcription of hepatic cytosolic phosphoenolpyruvate carboxykinase gene in newborn dogs. Biochem Mol Med 1996;59:13–19.
243. Jahoor F, Peters EJ, Wolfe RR. The relationship between gluconeogenic substrate supply and glucose production in humans. Am J Physiol 1990;258:E288–E296.
244. Bennish ML, Kalam AA, Rahman O, et al. Hypoglycemia during diarrhea in childhood: prevalance pathophysiology and outcome. N Engl J Med 1990;322:1357–1363.
245. Haymond MW, Karl IE, Clarke WL, et al. Differences in circulating gluconeogenic substances during short term fasting in men, women and children. Metabolism 1982;31:33–42.
246. Cowett RM, Wolfe RR. The potential for lactate gluconeogenesis is accelerated in the preterm neonate compared to the adult. J Dev Physiol 1991;16:341–347.
247. Lafeber HN, Sulkers EJ, Chapman T, et al. Glucose production and oxidation in preterm infants during total parenteral nutrition. Pediatr Res 1990;28:153–157.
248. Farrag HM, Nawrath LM, Dorcus EJ, et al. Ontogeny of glucose production and glucose oxidation in the extremely low birth weight [25–27 week] neonate. Submitted for publication.
249. Jacot E, Defronzo A, Jequier E, et al. The effect of hyperglycemia, hyperinsulinemia and route of glucose administration on glucose oxidation and glucose storage. Metabolism 1982;31:922–930.
250. Wolfe RR, O'Donell TF, Stone MD, et al. Investigation of factors determining the optimal glucose infusion rate in total parenteral nutrition. Metabolism 1980;29:892–900.
251. Savich RD, Finley SL, Ogata ES. Intravenous lipid and amino acids briskly increase plasma glucose concentra-

tions in small premature infants. Am J Perinatol 1988;5: 201–205.
252. van Goudoever JB, Sulkers EJ, Chapman TE, et al. Glucose kinetics and glucoregulatory hormone levels in ventilated preterm infants on the first day of life. Pediatr Res 1993;33:583–589.
253. Gleason VA, Hamm C, Jones MD Jr. Cerebral blood flow oxygenation and carbohydrate metabolism in immature fetal sheep in utero. Am J Physiol 1989;256:R1264–1268.
254. Altman DI, Perlman JM, Volpe JJ, et al. Cerebral oxygen metabolism in newborns. Pediatrics 1993;92:99–104.
255. Vannucci RC: Perinatal brain metabolism. In: Polin RA, WW Fox, eds. Fetal and neonatal physiology. Philadelphia: WB Saunders, 1992:1510–1519.
256. Best JD, Taborsky GJ Jr, Halter JB, et al. Glucose disposal is not proportional to plasma glucose in man. Diabetes 1981;30:847–850.
257. Volpe JJ. Hypoglycemia and brain injury. In: Neurology of the newborn. 2nd ed. Philadelphia: WB Saunders, 1987: 364–385.
258. Huang MM, Kliegman RM, Chau K. Partitioning and extraction of glucose regulates cerebral glucose utilization in newborn dogs. Biol Neonate 1989;55:290–297.
259. Pryds O, Christensen NJ, Friis-Hansen B. Increased cerebral blood flow and plasma epinephrine in hypoglycemic preterm neonates. Pediatrics 1990;85:172–176.
260. Anwar DU, Vannucci RC. Autoradiographic determination of regional cerebral blood flow during hypoglycemia on newborn dogs. Pediatr Res 1988;24:41–45.
261. Pryds O, Greisen G, Friis-Hansen B. Compensatory increase of CBF in preterm infants during hypoglycemia. Acta Paediatr Scand 1988;77:632–637.
262. Shen E-Y. Neurosonographic findings in high risk neonates with hypoglycemia. Acta Paediatr Sin 1996;37:248–252.
263. Cowett RM, Howard GM, Johnson J, et al. Brain auditory evoked response (BAER) in relation to neonatal glucose metabolism. Biol Neonate 1997;71:31–36.
264. Pildes RS, Wu SY, Henek T, et al. Early hyperglycemia: predictor of neonatal course and developmental outcome. Pediatr Res 1990;27:220A.
265. Vannucci RC, Brucklacher RM, Vannucci SJ. The effect of hyperglycemia on cerebral metabolism during hypoxia-ischemia in the immature rat. J Cereb Blood Flow Metab 1996;16:1026–1033.
266. DiGiacomo JE, Hay WW Jr. Abnormal glucose homeostasis. In: Sinclair JC, Bracken MB, eds. Effective care of the newborn infant. Oxford: Oxford University Press, 1992:590–601.

33
Inborn Errors of Carbohydrate Metabolism

Robert Schwartz

Many disorders of carbohydrate metabolism have an inherited, molecular basis,[1] but do not necessarily present in the perinatal period. This chapter discusses disorders that involve monosaccharide metabolism, intermediary metabolism, and glycogen metabolism, and is modified from a prior detailed evaluation.[1] Most disorders are clinically apparent by late infancy.[2]

Each section begins with a brief historical comment, followed by a clinical description. A subsequent section on pathogenesis, including molecular genetics, is followed by consideration of therapy and prognosis. The topics include:

- Galactosemia and variants
- Hereditary fructose intolerance and variants
- Disorders of gluconeogenesis:
    Pyruvate carboxylase
    Phosphoenolpyruvate carboxykinase deficiency
    Fructose-1,6-diphosphatase deficiency
- Glycogen storage diseases:
    Hepatic types I, III, VI, IX, XI
    Hepatic with cirrhosis IV
    Cardiac type II
    Muscular types V and VII

The initial metabolism of the three monosaccharides (e.g., glucose, fructose, galactose) important to the human depends on cellular membrane transport followed by phosphorylation by the specific kinases: glucokinase, fructokinase, and galactokinase. The less specific hexokinase contributes to this step depending on local conditions. Interestingly, only the consequences of galactokinase deficiency are of clinical significance (vide infra). None of these defects have a relationship to diabetes mellitus, type 1 or 2.

Disorders of Galactose Metabolism

Galactosemia is one of the better defined genetic, molecular diseases. The disease, as first described by Von Reuss[3] in 1908, was associated with failure to thrive, liver disease, and galactosuria. It was assumed that the latter was related to the ingestion of milk. Nine years later, Goppert[4] observed that the ingestion of galactose itself, as well as milk, resulted in galactosuria. The first patient described in the English-language literature was reported by Mason and Turner in 1935.[5] Subsequently, scattered cases and large series of cases have been reported through 1989,[6–13] including a report of the follow-up of Mason's original case by Townsend et al.[14] in 1951. Initially, attention was focused on (1) clinical description and course, (2) pathologic findings, and (3) physiologic disturbances of carbohydrate metabolism. These careful clinical investigations resulted in a plan of effective dietary therapy.

In 1933, Fanconi[15] described the first variant of a defect in galactose metabolism, which he called galactose diabetes, in a child, who presented only with cataracts. More recently, a number of modifications of the classic syndrome have been defined based on enzymatic,[16–18] metabolic,[17–19] and clinic[10,20] observations. These observations evolved from the classic basic investigations of Leloir,[21,22] who clarified the metabolic pathway for galactose and for galactose to glucose interconversion.

In the cell, galactose is phosphorylated from adenosine triphosphate (ATP) to galactose-1-phosphate by a specific galactokinase (Figure 33.1). The galactose-1-P reacts with uridine-diphosphoglucose (UDPG) in the presence of the specific enzyme P-gal uridyl transferase to form uridine-diphosphogalactose (UDPGal) and glucose-1-phosphate. UDPGal-4-epimerase with diphosphopyridine nucleotide (DPN) is necessary for the conversion of the UDPGal to UDPG. UDPG may be metabolized by several pathways.[13,23–26] It can react with pyrophosphate in the presence of UDPG pyrophosphorylase to form uridine triphosphate (UTP) and glucose-1-phosphate, or in the presence of glycogen synthase to form glycogen. Galactose may be reduced directly to galactitol by the enzyme aldose reductase

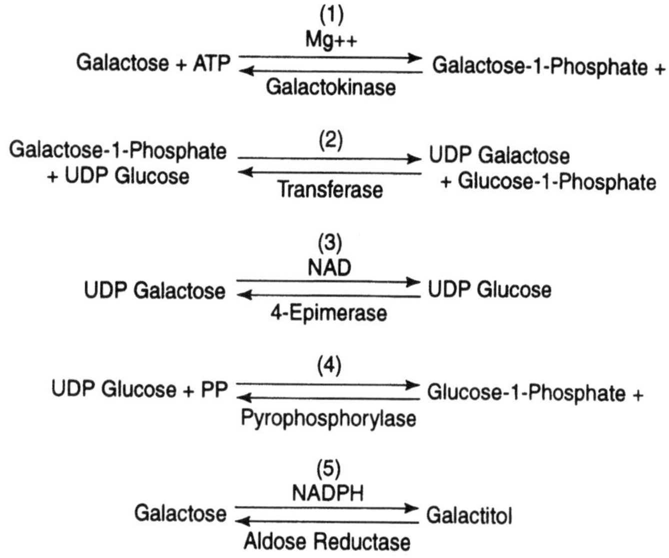

FIGURE 33.1. Galactose diabetes results from a deficiency of galactokinase (reaction 1), whereas classic galactosemia results from a deficiency of galactose-1-phosphate uridyl transferase (reaction 2). The transferase enzyme may occur in different molecular forms, thus accounting for some variants of enzyme activity. An absence of epimerase (reaction 3) has been reported to produce the classic syndrome.

$$\text{Galactose} + \text{ATP} \xrightleftharpoons[\text{Galactokinase}]{\overset{(1)}{\text{Mg}^{++}}} \text{Galactose-1-Phosphate}$$

$$\text{Galactose-1-Phosphate} + \text{UDP Glucose} \xrightleftharpoons[\text{Transferase}]{(2)} \text{UDP Galactose} + \text{Glucose-1-Phosphate}$$

$$\text{UDP Galactose} \xrightleftharpoons[\text{4-Epimerase}]{\overset{(3)}{\text{NAD}}} \text{UDP Glucose}$$

$$\text{UDP Glucose} + \text{PP} \xrightleftharpoons[\text{Pyrophosphorylase}]{(4)} \text{Glucose-1-Phosphate}$$

$$\text{Galactose} \xrightleftharpoons[\text{Aldose Reductase}]{\overset{(5)}{\text{NADPH}}} \text{Galactitol}$$

(Figure 33.1, reaction 5).[27] The explanation for the multiple clinical manifestations and syndromes that involve defects in galactose metabolism is beginning to be elucidated on a molecular basis. In 1995, Segal and Berry[13] reviewed the metabolism of galactose and its regulation at both the cellular and organ level. The specific enzymatic reactions and the alternate pathways for metabolism are detailed in their report. Gitzelman and Steinmann[28] have summarized the results of a recent workshop on galactosemia.

Galactosemia

Galactosemia is inherited as an autosomal recessive disorder and was reported by 1972 to occur worldwide in 1/10,000 to 1/187,000 births.[29] In the United States, routine newborn screening has detected from 1 in 14,500 (Maine) to as few as 1 in 119,000 (Ohio).[30] From screening 2,677,669 neonates in eight states, 35 affected infants were found for an average detection rate of 1 in 76,500.[30] The detection rate depends on sensitivity and specificity as well as precise confirmation. Improved methodology has been described.[31-35] In 1987, Ng et al.[36] reviewed worldwide frequencies of occurrence of galactosemia based on newborn screening data and reported rates of 1/26,000 in Ireland compared to 1/667,000 in Japan. The United States frequency was 1/62,000. Because of its rarity, newborn screening for galactosemia was stopped in Norway and not introduced in Great Britain, the Netherlands, and some states of the United States.[37] This decision has been made regarding screening despite the fact that the first symptoms may occur as early as 2 or 3 days of age.

Clinical Manifestations—Prenatal Effects

The newborn infant with galactosemia (P-gal uridyl transferase defect) is usually clinically normal at birth. In utero, the fetus may be exposed to variable amounts of lactose or galactose from the mother. The heterozygote mother may be unable to dispose of a galactose load as rapidly as a normal person can. This relative deficiency may result in increased levels of galactose reaching the fetus even under a normal dietary regimen. The presence of nuclear cataracts, which usually develop in the third fetal month and before lens development takes place, has been considered by Ritter and Cannon[38] to be a further indication of intrauterine fetal abnormalities related to galactose. Roe et al.[39] reported a Negro homozygous woman who was maintained on a lactose restricted diet since 1950 and gave birth in 1969 to a heterozygote male infant, who developed normally. Although lactose and galactitol were present in maternal urine, none was detected in maternal blood or amniotic fluid. In contrast, elevated galactitol has been found in amniotic fluid as early as 10 weeks of gestation with subsequent delivery of a neonate with classic galactosemia.[40]

The Problems of the Neonate

At birth the affected neonate appears normal, both physically and developmentally. But shortly after he begins to ingest milk, he develops a characteristic course that varies only in the severity and rapidity of the clinical manifestations.[9,40] Failure to gain weight in the first few days is common, as is jaundice, which increases and persists beyond the usual period of "physiologic jaundice." Subcutaneous bleeding may occur. Vomiting, diarrhea, and dehydration occur. The skin appears dry, rough, thick, and scaly. The liver enlarges and is smooth, firm, and nontender. If the disease is unrecognized, the course is one of progressive deterioration associated with liver disease (cirrhosis), cataracts, mental retardation, and even death. The characteristic abdominal distention is the combined result of ascites, hepatomegaly, and splenomegaly. Zonular or lamellar cataracts may be seen as early as 1 month of age. Mental retardation does not become manifest until later in the initial year of life. Malnutrition, extreme loss of subcutaneous fat tissue, and retarded growth become evident as the untreated disease progresses (Figure 33.2).

In contrast to these marked abnormalities, the onset in some infants may be subtle and the disease manifested only in a failure to feed well or to gain weight. The course progresses to a more characteristic clinical picture as they consume more lactose-containing foods. Mental retardation, which is the most serious consequence for untreated surviving children with this disorder, varies in severity.[41] Verbal dyspraxia, an unusual and characteristic speech disorder, appears with some regularity in children with classic galactosemia.[42] The heterozygote does not have clinical manifestations. Furthermore, the disease may be difficult to detect even in the homozygote. Hugh-Jones et al.[43] have reported a family with an affected homozygous grandfather of normal intelligence who had cataracts and hepatomegaly and was not diagnosed until the sixth decade of life.

Laboratory Data

Blood

The galactose concentration in the blood may not be diagnostic since it may be either normal or elevated postprandially after milk feedings in normal infants. Fasting blood glucose concentrations, as determined with specific glucose oxidase techniques, are normal, but may be low following the ingestion of galactose.[44,45] Morphologic studies may show no initial effects on the erythrocytes or leukocytes. No specific abnormalities in blood counts, acid base balance, or electrolyte concentrations occur unless extensive diarrhea or dehydration are present. Under these circumstances, azotemia and metabolic acidosis are found. A normocytic, hypoplastic anemia has been described later in the course of the disease. Liver function tests show variable results. Serum bilirubin and alkaline phosphatase, aspartate, and alanine amino transferases may be elevated. There is no characteristic pattern for other serum enzymes, including serum

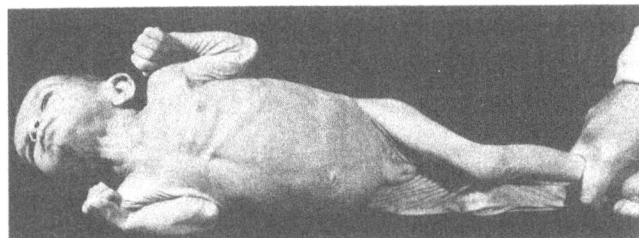
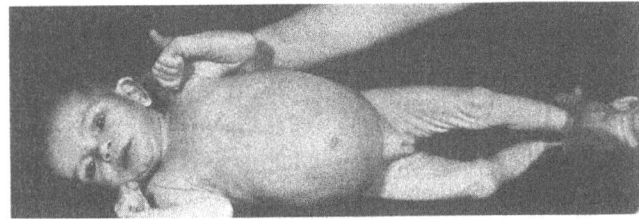
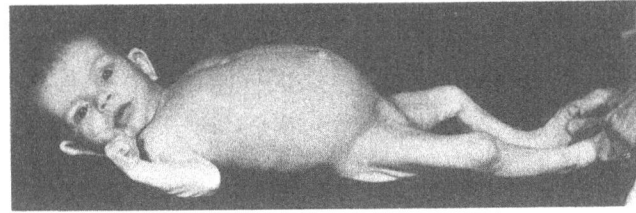

FIGURE 33.2. Infant with chronic diarrhea who was not discovered to have galactose intolerance until 5 months of age. Removal of lactose from the diet resulted in rapid improvement in nutrition.

glutamic–oxaloacetic transaminase (SGOT) and serum glutamic–pyruvic transaminase (SGPT).

Urine

Following milk feedings, abnormalities in the urine include generalized proteinuria, positive reducing substances, and a generalized aminoaciduria. The sediment is normal. The reducing substances are positive to Clinitest tablets in the absence of ketonuria. Specific analyses with glucose oxidase chemical reagent strips are negative or show a trace reaction, indicating that the reducing substance is not glucose. Further identification may be made by chromatography, including high performance liquid chromatography,[46] or by the specific enzymatic techniques that utilize galactose oxidase or galactose dehydrogenase.[47]

Ultrasound and/or Roentgen Findings

After a variable period of exposure to milk, ultrasonography and roentgen studies may show hepatomegaly, splenomegaly, and ascites. The kidneys are normal. Late roentgen changes may include generalized osteoporosis.

Diagnosis

A variety of diagnostic tests for this disorder have been devised and have been summarized by Kirkman,[48] Hsia,[49] Segal and Berry,[13] and Shin.[37] These include the identification of sugar in urine and specific enzyme tests on red or white blood cells. A variety of enzymatic techniques of variable specificity have been used for the erythrocytes and include a measurement of galactose-1-phosphate, UDPG consumption, and a methylene blue–coupled reaction with measurement of $^{14}CO_2$ from 1-^{14}C galactose.[13,49] The diagnostic enzymatic methods might not be available in all laboratories. Galactose tolerance tests are contraindicated and carry a risk of central nervous system toxicity.

Prenatal Diagnosis

When galactosemia is suspected from family history, prenatal diagnosis is indicated. The homozygous P-gal uridyl transferase deficiency has been diagnosed successfully in utero early in pregnancy in amnion cells by Nadler et al.[11] and confirmed by others.[50] The diagnosis has also been successfully made by enzyme analysis of chorionic villus biopsy.[51] Several groups have developed techniques, including a stable isotope dilution assay for galactitol in amniotic fluid.[52-54] The activities of galactose-1-phosphate uridyl transferase and of galactokinase have been studied in human fetal organs at various stages of gestation.[50,55]

Maximal specific activity for each enzyme was found at 28 weeks' gestation in the liver.

Postnatal Diagnosis

If not suspected prenatally, a urinalysis may be analyzed to determine whether reducing substances are present. This determination must be performed with Clinitest tablets and not with glucose oxidase reagents strips.[47,56] If a reducing substance other than glucose is found, the removal from the diet of lactose-containing foods (milk) should result in disappearance of the sugar (presumably galactose) from the urine within 24 to 72 hours. If galactosemia is suspected, the infant must be fed a galactose-free (milk-free) diet until enzyme studies in the red blood cells can be performed.[57] Galactose is not present in the urine of the neonate before onset of milk feedings. The specific diagnosis is established by the enzymatic methods that utilize red blood cells.

In the neonate suspected of having this disorder because of a positive family history or clinical manifestations, the diagnosis should be made by demonstrating the absence of galactose-1-P uridyl transferase in the red blood cells before the initiation of milk feedings, and not following the presence of reducing sugars in the urine.

Differential Diagnosis

Differential diagnosis in the neonate is concerned principally with melituria and with hyperbilirubinemia associated with hepatic disease. The latter includes consideration of sepsis, cytomegalic inclusion disease, toxoplasmosis, rubella, syphilis, biliary atresia, neonatal hepatitis, and congenital hypopituitarism with or without congenital optic nerve hypoplasia. A positive blood culture does not rule out galactosemia.

Reports have emphasized the occurrence of gram-negative (*Escherichia coli*) sepsis in infants with undiagnosed galactosemia and have suggested a relationship of substrate (lactose-galactose) requirement to the organism.[58,59] In the large U.S. survey noted above, of the 35 infants detected to be deficient in the transferase, 10 had significant neonatal infections. Of these, nine were fatal and four had *E. coli* infection.[30] A positive blood culture for *E. coli* in the neonate is an indication for a specific diagnostic test for galactosemia. However, the presence of minute amounts of galactose in the urine of the neonate, especially one who is low birth weight, may be a transient physiologic phenomenon related to a decreased tissue uptake of galactose.[60]

Later, the multiple causes for failure to thrive, diarrhea, cirrhosis, cataracts, albuminuria, and/or mental retardation must be considered in the differential diagnosis.

Therapy

In Utero

Once an in utero diagnosis is established, the mother should be given a galactose-lactose free diet. Some women who are known heterozygotes or homozygotes are advised to ingest the restricted diet before conception. Irons et al.[61] have observed a woman who maintained her blood concentration of galactose and galactose-1-phosphate at less than $1\,mg\cdot dl^{-1}$ throughout pregnancy. The affected fetus had a high level of galactose-1-phosphate ($4\,mg\cdot dl^{-1}$) in cord whole blood. There are over a dozen pregnancies reported with similar findings. Gitzelmann et al.[62] suggested that galactose-1-phosphate in the affected fetus of a mother on a restricted diet is endogenously produced from glucose-1-phosphate via the glucose-4-epimerase and the uridine diphosphogalactose pyrophosphorylase reactions (Figure 33.1).

Postnatal

The management of patients with this disorder requires meticulous attention to detail. The course changes dramatically when milk sugar (i.e., lactose) is removed from the diet. Even an infant with the full-blown disorder unrecognized for many months shows a remarkable response to the simple elimination of dietary lactose. His appetite increases, vomiting and diarrhea subside within a few days, weight gain ensues promptly, liver function improves, and jaundice subsides. Even the cataracts may disappear on a lactose-free diet. Holzel[40] has indicated that several of the low-galactose formulas are not devoid of oligosaccharides, which contain galactose. However, Gitzelmann and Auricchio[63] have examined critically the ability of a normal and a galactosemic child to metabolize soya α-galactosides. They detected no α-galactosidase activity in the human small intestine, no rise in erythrocyte galactose-1-phosphate after raffinose ingestion, and slow absorption of galactose from the colon of the galactosemic child. They concluded that soybean formulas are generally safe for galactosemic infants if they do not have diarrhea. Several satisfactory proprietary formulas are available.[64,65] In older children, avoidance of galactose is difficult because many foods contain unlabeled lactose. Candies and compounded foods, especially bread, sausage, and frankfurters, must be rigidly excluded unless their exact composition is known in detail.

Biochemical monitoring of erythrocyte galactose-1-phosphate is necessary to assure compliance with dietary recommendations.

Genetics

A careful family history is essential, as in all inherited disorders. Family counseling regarding further pregnancies can be more specific if enzymatic analysis of erythrocytes from all family members is performed to define heterozygotes. Family history has been inadequate in defining the individual heterozygote, but the enzymatic tests have made possible a more precise analysis of the genetic situation. Refinement of the assay system has resulted in the detection of a definite difference in transferase levels in normal adults and in parents of galactosemic children. Donnell et al.[66] studied 278 individuals, including 55 family members from 14 galactosemic families, and clearly identified the heterozygotes.

Molecular Genetics

The GALT (galactose-1-phosphate uridyltransferase) gene has been mapped to human chromosome 9 band p 13.[67] This is transmitted as an autosomal recessive trait with homozygotes estimated to occur in 1 in 50,000 newborns screened. There is no particular ethnic or geographic variation.[68]

Reichardt and Berg[69] have utilized a unique technique to clone and characterize the cDNA that encodes human galactose-1-phosphate uridyltransferase (GALT). The cDNA is 1400 bases in length and encodes a 43,000-M_r protein. The cloning strategy involved the identification of short peptide sequences conserved between the homologous enzymes from *E. coli* and yeast, and the construction of oligonucleotide pools corresponding to the conserved patches. These patches of conserved amino acids tend to be present in humans also.

Reichardt[70] has pursued these observations by studies of 15 galactosemic patients using molecular analysis of DNA, messenger RNA (mRNA), and protein by Southern, Northern, and Western blotting techniques. He concluded that galactosemia is caused by missense mutations. He found detectable enzyme activity in all 13 patients studied and speculated that this provided a threshold level of UDPGal, which is both the product of the GALT reaction and the substrate for the galactosylation of glycolipids and glycoproteins. He currently is analyzing glycolipids from patients to verify this hypothesis.

Reichardt[71] summarized in 1992 the genetic basis for galactosemia. He noted that nine missense mutations, three splicing mutations, three GALT protein polymorphisms, and one silent nucleotide substitution had been identified. The most common mutation is Q188R. He concluded that galactosemia is heterogeneous at the molecular level. In contrast to the Q188R defect, which is associated with a poor clinical course in white subjects, is another abnormality, S135L in blacks, with a good clinical outcome.[72] More recently, Elsas et al.[73] have presented a strategy to identify new biochemical phenotypes and molecular genotypes. Recent studies of DNA in galactose-1-phosphate uridyltransferase deficiency and the

Duarte variant (vide infra) in Germany found the Q188R in Caucasians in a frequency of 62% to 66%, while N314D was found in all Duarte alleles examined.[74]

Pathology

Pathologic studies indicate that the liver disease is a fatty infiltration with varying degrees of portal fibrosis resulting in a lobular pattern.[14] The hepatic cells may have a granular appearance. Infiltrates of leukocytes may be seen in the connective tissue. Medline and Medline[75] have described the early histologic changes in liver and this disease in twins. One died of aspiration at 9 days of age and the other shortly thereafter of sepsis. The liver was yellow and contained excessively large fatty droplets in virtually every hepatocyte. Extensive bile ductular proliferation was present in the periportal areas. There was no increase in fibrosis. Bell et al.[76] observed vacuolar changes in the epithelial cells of the proximal tubule of the kidney in one case. Crome[77] reported on the neuropathologic findings in a child with physical and mental retardation who survived to 8 years of age. He found microencephaly with pronounced fibrous gliosis of the white matter; the cerebellum showed marked loss of Purkinje's cells and less conspicuous loss of the granular layer. All the findings were considered nonspecific and could not be differentiated from those seen in other forms of mental retardation. Cataracts are usually lamellar or zonular, although a few nuclear or anterior cortical changes in the lens have been reported.[38] Levy et al.[78] have reported normal follicle development and abundant oocytes in the ovaries of a 5-day-old infant who died (vide infra).

Pathogenesis

Site of Defect

In classic galactosemia Schwarz et al.[79] found that galactose-1-phosphate accumulated in erythrocytes, suggesting that galactokinase was active normally and that the defect was beyond the first phosphorylation step. Kalckar et al.[80] demonstrated the defect to be an absence of the specific transferase, P-gal uridyltransferase, and with Isselbacher et al.[81] showed that the epimerase and UDPG pyrophosphorylase were normal. The latter investigations suggested that the reversibility of the epimerase reaction permitted synthesis of UDPGal under circumstances of dietary deprivation. This could account for normal galactolipid synthesis and central nervous system development in the absence of exogenous galactose.[81] Gitzelmann[82] has speculated that galactose-1-P is a pathogenic agent by inhibiting enzymes such as glucose-6-phosphatase, glucose-6-phosphate dehydrogenase, phosphoglucomutase, and glycogen phosphorylase.

In contrast, Reichardt[70] proposed that minimal transferase activity is required for survival to produce a threshold level of UDPGal for minimal galactosylation of glycoproteins and glycolipids. He suggested supplemental therapy with uridine in addition to galactose restriction. Kaufman et al.[83] have evaluated UDPGal in erythrocytes. Chronic administration of oral uridine resulted in normalization of erythrocyte UDPGal in two patients. This novel suggestion requires careful, critical evaluation and should be investigated further.

Mechanism of Toxicity

The mechanism of toxicity at the biochemical level is not entirely understood. The original suggestion of Mason and Turner that hypoglycemia was responsible for much of the symptomatology is untenable. The toxic effects appear to be more directly related to the accumulation of galactose-1-phosphate. Young rats fed diets high in galactose, up to 80% by weight, of total food, develop cataracts and renal disease.[84,85] The liver does not show histologic changes. Lerman[86] has shown that a 10-fold rise in the concentration of galactose-1-P is found in the lens in cataracts in experimental rats. Although little information is available about the metabolism of the human lens in this disease, transferase activity was apparently absent in the lens tissue from one galactosemic infant.[87] Several theories have been proposed to explain the cataracts that develop when there is galactose intolerance. One relates the changes to decreased oxidation of glucose and consequent interference with normal lens metabolism.[86] Another proposes conversion of galactose to its alcohol, galactitol, which accumulates with water to produce vacuoles in the lens.[88] The latter theory suggests that fiber rupture, secondary to the osmotic effects, precedes cataract formation. Another alcohol, mannitol has recently been identified in plasma of galactosemics by high-performance liquid chromatography (HPLC).[89]

The presence of galactose-1-P in erythrocytes impairs oxygen uptake. Tissue damage in liver, kidney, and brain is apparently related to this compound, although the mechanism of action is unknown. In vitro, galactose-1-P has been shown to inhibit phosphoglucomutase, glucose-6-phosphatase, or glucose-6-phosphate dehydrogenase, but how this might explain cellular damage is unknown.[89,90] From a clinical standpoint, both the rate of development and the rate of decline of toxicity suggest the slow accumulation of a toxic metabolite. This has been demonstrated with respect to aminoaciduria in the study of Cusworth et al.[91] They showed that a 3- to 5-day interval was necessary after initiation of a galactose diet before renal amino acid excretion increased. Similarly, removal of galactose from the diet resulted in a decrease in aminoaciduria only after a few days had passed. Although extensive liver disease might affect the plasma amino acid concentrations with overflow aminoaciduria, the studies of Hsia et al.[92] and of Cusworth et al. indicate that the primary effect is in the renal tubule, with minimal changes in plasma amino acids. The resultant aminoaciduria is the result of a reabsorptive alteration in the proximal tubule.

In addition to the well-described biochemical consequences of the transferase defect, there have been two studies indicating nonenzymatic galactosylation of proteins.[93-95] The significance of a more generalized galactosylation of proteins is unknown. Berry[96] has reviewed the evidence for toxicity of the polyols (e.g., galactitol and myoinositol).

Prognosis

The clinical manifestations are so highly variable that the ultimate course is unpredictable. In the undetected severe cases, death occurs in early infancy. In other untreated children, mental retardation and liver disease may be the major complications, with few surviving beyond childhood. Early diagnosis and careful dietary management can result in normal growth and development, both physically and mentally, without serious complications.[40,41] When the diagnosis has been delayed for several months, there may be some degree of permanent mental retardation, although other signs of galactose toxicity subside with diet therapy.

Reviews of experiences with dietary management in large numbers of patients have indicated a significant degree of psychosocial behavioral impairment. Komrower and Lee[97] investigated 60 galactosemic children whose physical health was good under therapy; however, intelligence scores were variable and tended to be low (i.e., I.Q. mean 80, range 30–118). They reported a recurrent pattern of learning difficulties and psychologic upset, which may, in part, have been environmental rather than inherent in the disorder. Similarly, Nadler et al.[11] reported on 55 patients whose mean IQ was lower than that of siblings; 80% of the children were one or more grades behind in school, and a specific learning disability was characterized by difficulty in mathematics and spatial relationships. Because of a short attention span, behavior problems were observed in school. Both investigators concluded that strict diet therapy beyond infancy (i.e., after 2 years of age) has not proved additionally beneficial relative to mental development.

Fishler et al.[98] described the intellectual and personality development of 23 girls and 22 boys treated from infancy and followed for up to 23 years. They noted the best developmental progress in the preschool age group. Schoolchildren aged 6 to 15 years had a mean IQ of 87, and nearly half had poor handwriting and difficulty in visual-perceptual function. Children who were diagnosed between birth and 1 month of age maintained more normal mental function as a group compared to those diagnosed between 4 and 11 months. The investigators also assessed the emotional-social aspects of behavior in their patients and concluded that poor self-image was related to their dietary restrictions, which set them apart from their peers. It should be noted that there was no significant difference among the mean IQs of the treated patients, their parents, and their unaffected siblings.

Subsequently, this group reported on the developmental follow-up status of 60 galactosemic infants.[99] The highest level of mental development was in the preschool age group. The lowest level, but still within normal limits, was in the school-age children. Mean IQ was 95 for the entire group with a range from 50 to 125. No correlation of IQ with diet compliance was found. One third of the patients studied by EEG were abnormal. It is unclear how much of the intellectual impairment may be avoided by prompt diagnosis and treatment.[100] Verbal dyspraxia is now recognized as a significant problem.[42]

Jan and Wilson[101] reported late, unusual neurologic findings in a 19-year-old who had been treated by rigid dietary restrictions since the age of 15 days. The patient showed progressive cerebellar and extrapyramidal disturbances. Although the investigators were uncertain as to the cause of the clinical finding, one can speculate that prolonged strict dietary control may not be indicated.

In addition to the long-term mental difficulties, reduced intelligence, and social maladjustment, Packman et al.[102] proposed that a subgroup of galactosemic children may develop a syndrome of mental retardation, tremor, and cerebellar dysfunction. Friedman et al.[103] have reported two adults, a 41-year-old man and a 46-year-old woman, one of whom developed complex partial seizures in the 4th decade and the other a severe cerebellar disorder in the 5th decade. They speculated that it seems likely that as galactosemic adults age, a spectrum of neurologic disorders occur, including seizures, cerebellar ataxia, extrapyramidal dysfunction, and apraxia. Whether this is due to the enzymatic defect alone, to other closely linked genetic abnormalities, or to therapy is unknown. Diagnosis at birth and early intervention with a galactose-free diet does not always assure an optimal outcome. Waisbren et al.[104] reported eight children diagnosed from 1 to 15 days of age, treated immediately and found to have no detectable galactose in the blood or urine and whole blood galactose-1-phosphate concentrations less than 2 mg/dl. At follow-up ages 3.6 and 11.6 years, variable deficits were identified in receptive language (i.e., comprehension), short-term memory, expressive language, and articulation. There is speculation that these long-term effects had originated in utero. Kaufman et al.[105] reported 45 subjects ages 4 to 39 years with classic galactosemia. Deficits of cognitive function were variable and not related to the age at diagnosis or to the severity of illness at presentation. A high incidence of abnormality was found on magnetic resonance imaging (MRI). Neurologic symptoms included ataxia, tremor, and dysmetria.

Tedesco et al.[106] have reported a normal pregnancy in a 17-year-old black galactosemic on dietary control, confirming the original report by Roe et al.[39] The newborn infant was normal and had heterozygote values of transferase and normal values of galactokinase activities in his erythrocytes. The placental tissue was deficient in transferase activity, which apparently had no deleterious effects on the fetus. Although these two pregnancies suggest that fertility and fetal development can be normal in galactosemic women under dietary control, infertility has emerged as a major problem in these patients.

Kaufman et al.[107] evaluated gonadal function in 18 female and 8 male subjects with galactosemia. The males were normal, but 12 females had hypergonadotropic hypogonadism. All the female patients had a 46xx karyotype, normal levels of thyroid hormone and prolactin, and no antiovarian antibodies. Urinary gonadotropins were biologically normal. Ovarian tissue was diminished or absent by ultrasonography. They speculated that the abnormality was acquired and related to galactose-1-phosphate toxicity. While there have been other reports substantiating these late findings, the etiology and time of onset have been questioned.[108–111] Subsequently, Q188R status was evaluated in patients with classic galactosemia.[112] No association was found for the mutation and primary amenorrhea. Timing of the onset of ovarian failure could not be explained by Q188R status alone.

Variants of Transferase Deficiency

Duarte Variant

In 1966, Beutler et al.[16,113] reported an extensive survey screening for the incidence of homozygous and heterozygous galactosemia in 1820 apparently normal individuals and in 352 subjects hospitalized in a mental institution utilizing a modification of the UDPG consumption technique. Thirty subjects had levels of transferase activity less than those of heterozygote parents of known galactosemic individuals. Nineteen subjects were Caucasian, 11 were unclassified, and none were black, Oriental, or American Indian. In family studies, abnormally low GALT activity suggested two general types of inheritance. In one, present in 15 of 34 subjects, enzyme activity was 50% of normal and indicated that a single gene was involved. In the second, enzyme activity was 75% of normal or greater than the level associated with the heterozygote carrier state in classic galactosemia. This abnormality has been termed the "Duarte variant." Individuals with red blood cell transferase activities that approximate 50% of normal levels could be either heterozygotes for classic galactosemia or homozygotes for the Duarte variant, an allelic gene. Heterozygotes for both the gene for galactosemia and the Duarte variant have approximately one-quarter normal enzyme activity. In this limited population survey, heterozygotes for galactosemia composed approximately 1.25% of the patients, while those for the Duarte variant, approximately 10% to 13%.

By electrophoretic mobility the transferases for the homozygous Duarte variant have a single band that differs from that of the normal.[114] Individuals who are heterozygous for the Duarte variant were found to have both distinct bands.

Gitzelmann et al.[115] reported two individuals in Switzerland (i.e., one infant and one parent of two known galactosemics) in whom family studies have suggested a pattern of enzyme activities similar to that of the Duarte variant. Starch-gel electrophoresis indicated a faster mobility of the patients' enzymes compared to that of normals.

While Levy et al.[116] reported no clinical manifestations for 10 individuals with either the homozygous or heterozygous form of the Duarte variant, Kelly[117] reported mild galactose intolerance in the Duarte/classic galactosemia variant. The heterozygous form of classic galactosemia has no clinical manifestations.

Negro Variant

Although relatively rare in African-Americans, classic galactosemia has been reported.[117,118] In studying whole-body metabolism of $1-^{14}C$-radiogalactose to $^{14}CO_2$ in vivo, Segal et al.[118] noted that 3 of 12 subjects with absent red cell transferase activity had normal net galactose metabolism. The three black individuals had had classic galactosemia in infancy, including cataract formation. The investigators suggested that certain individuals have a capacity to develop alternate pathways for galactose metabolism that circumvent the GALT reaction. This capacity has been designated as the "Negro variant."

Similar observations by other investigators have confirmed these differences among affected blacks. Studies of various tissues have not supported a global enzyme deficiency, thus white blood cell transferase may be present while erythrocytic activity is absent. Molecular techniques should clarify these differences.

Other Variants

In addition to the Duarte and Negro variants, there have been reports[119] of infants (i.e., homozygote variants) with symptoms of vomiting, failure to thrive, hepatomegaly, and cataracts who were found with transferase activity in erythrocytes that varied from 0% to 35% of normal. Electrophoretic mobility patterns were variable. These variants have been named for the place of origin: Indiana, Chicago, Rennes, Los Angeles, etc. These symptomatic infants are managed similarly to those with classic galactosemia.

Galactose-4-Epimerase

Gitzelmann[120] has reported on a deficiency of uridine diphosphate galactose-4-epimerase in erythrocytes from a normal infant. Several patients have been reported with the erythrocyte enzyme deficiency without clinical manifestation.

In contrast, in 1981, Holton et al.[121] reported an infant with classic galactosemia on day 5. The erythrocyte transferase activity was normal, as was galactokinase. There was a lack of activity of epimerase in both erythrocytes and skin fibroblasts. Concentrations of the proximal metabolites, uridine diphosphate galactose, and galactose-1-phosphate were increased in erythrocytes. The erythrocytes from the parents had decreased activity levels of epimerase.

In contrast to the classic transferase abnormality, management included an intake of small amounts of galactose at 1.5 g daily after 4 months of age. This small intake is essential for the biosynthesis of sphingolipids which are required for brain growth and development as well as for other galactosides. The classic transferase abnormality allows for some endogenous galactose synthesis from glucose via the intact epimerase reaction.

Studies of infants with this defect should permit an estimate of minimal galactose requirements for essential structural compounds.

Chromosomal Alterations and Galactose Metabolism

Transferase activities of either red or white blood cells have been reported to be increased in Down syndrome (trisomy 21), Cornelia de Lange's syndrome, and in other trisomy syndromes.[122,123] The significance of these observations remains obscure.

Galactokinase Deficiency

In 1933 in Zurich, a 9-year-old boy with von Recklinghausen's neurofibromatosis had an operation for bilaterally recurring cataracts. Fanconi[15] studied the melituria (2.2–5.8 g·100 ml^{-1}) in this patient and characterized the disorder as "galactose diabetes" because 50% to 87% of ingested galactose, 80% of galactose from ingested lactose, and 60% to 80% of milk lactose were excreted in the urine. The patient metabolized glucose, fructose, and other carbohydrates without melituria. Gitzelmann[18] restudied this patient at 43 years of age, at which time he appeared to have normal intelligence and no signs of cirrhosis, but was blind. His urine contained 2 g galactose and 0.04 g glucose per 100 ml. Studies of the patient's blood indicated that the hemolysate (1) metabolized galactose-1-phosphate normally, (2) had normal GALT activity, and (3) contained minimal concentrations of galactose-1-phosphate. Since these findings were not compatible with classic galactosemia, intact red blood cells were studied for both galactokinase and uridyltransferase activities utilizing ^{14}C-labeled galactose and its conversion to galactose-1-phosphate and uridine diphosphogalactose. In contrast to normal cells, red blood cells of the patient did not produce detectable amounts of either compound, indicating a deficiency of galactokinase. This patient was also studied for the possible relationship of polyol and galactitol to cataract formation.[27] He excreted excessive galactose in concentrations varying from 0.4 to 1.4 g and galactitol, from 0.03 to 0.77 g per 100 ml urine.

Subsequently, Gitzelmann[20] carried out extensive studies of the family members of the original propositus. An additional older sister had cataracts and galactokinase deficiency, while another sister with cataracts was suspected to have the defect. Gitzelmann postulated an absence of the enzyme in the liver as well because of the delayed clearance of galactose from the blood after the ingestion of milk. The net clearance of galactose was accomplished by its intact excretion and by its metabolism and excretion as galactitol. Of the approximately two thirds of dietary galactose accounted for, one fifth was excreted as galactitol and four fifths as galactose.

In a patient with hereditary galactokinase deficiency, Gitzelmann et al.[124] studied whole-body metabolism by measuring expired $^{14}CO_2$ after the administration of labeled ^{14}C-galactose, ^{14}C-galactitol, and ^{14}C-galactonate. The excretion of $^{14}CO_2$ was minimal, suggesting that the defect was extensive and involved all tissues. However, $^{14}CO_2$ was excreted more rapidly after the administration of ^{14}C-1-galactose than after ^{14}C-2-galactose, suggesting the possibility of an alternate oxidative pathway catalyzed by galactose dehydrogenase in this patient.

Galactokinase activity was measured in the red blood cells of 100 control subjects and 18 family members. In the latter, three groups were identified: (1) the two patients had virtually a complete deficiency of enzyme activity, (2) 10 relatives had intermediate values, and (3) six members had normal activities. All four of the children of the oldest patient had values in the intermediate group. Additional patients have been reported.[125-135]

Ng et al.[132] examined the developmental changes of galactokinase activity in human erythrocytes. Enzyme activities at 24 hours of age were approximately three times greater than those of the adult. Leukocyte buffy coats did not significantly affect the assay results. They speculated that a similar developmental pattern existed in the human liver. Dahlqvist et al.[127] noted higher galactokinase levels in erythrocytes from infants aged 2 to 4 months as compared to those of children and adults (i.e., aged 2 to 67 years). Vigneron et al.[133] reported similar control data, but found a transient galactokinase deficiency in a neonate. Repeated verification of the defect may be necessary during the first weeks of life.

Clinical Manifestations

The clinical manifestations are less severe than those of classic galactosemia. Mental retardation and liver disease do not appear to be significant. Cataract formation is a serious consequence with early onset. Thalhammer et al.'s[125] and Kerr et al.'s[129] infants had transient hepatosplenomegaly, although Cook et al.'s[128] and Kerr et al.'s infants were detected because of hyperbilirubinemia. Linneweh et al.'s[126] infant had a family history of cataracts as did the original patients of Gitzelmann.[20] All of the infants developed early changes of cataract formation while receiving milk feedings. These resolved promptly after the infants were given low-galactose feedings.

Monteleone et al.[130] reported a large kindred included two heterozygotes with cataracts and 6 of 10 siblings with cataracts in the third or fourth decade of life. The latter were not characterized by enzyme studies.

Laboratory Tests

Thalhammer et al.[125] noted a delay in the accumulation of blood galactose and galactosuria. They found low values for galactose on fasting blood samples early in the morning and suggested the optimal time to screen for excessive blood galactose was 1 hour after the second morning feed. Cook et al.[128] noted a low blood glucose value of $1.78\,mM$ ($32\,mg\cdot100\,ml^{-1}$) when his patient was 8 weeks of age, receiving a cow's milk formula. Blood galactose was $2.44\,mM$ ($44\,mg\cdot100\,ml^{-1}$) simultaneously. The mechanism of the hypoglycemia remains unclear.

Therapy

Therapy should be instituted promptly when either disorder is suspected. Proof of the specific enzymatic defect can then be obtained by analyzing the enzyme activities in red blood cells. A low galactose-lactose (i.e., milk) diet prevents the development of cataracts. Monteleone et al.[130] suggested that dietary control of the heterozygote may also be important in preventing cataracts.

Genetics and Prevalence

The disorder appears to be an autosomal recessive trait. Mayes[136] estimated the frequency of galactokinase deficiency, based on the incidence of heterozygotes, as 1 in 40,000 to 1 in 50,000. Cook et al.[128] suggested Mayes overestimated the carrier frequency and indicated a more realistic incidence of 1 in 100,000.

Pathogenesis

The common pathogenetic mechanisms in classic galactosemia and galactokinase deficiency suggest that the metabolism of galactose to galactitol in the lens is responsible for cataract formation. The absence of liver disease and mental retardation as well as of aminoaciduria in galactokinase deficiency is consistent with the consideration that galactose-1-phosphate is the major toxic metabolite in classic galactosemia. Galactokinase activity has been studied in several tissues of the human fetus. While most tissues showed maximal activity at 28 weeks' gestation, the brain is constant and high.[55,137]

The frequency of a deficiency of galactokinase as the etiologic factor in the cataracts of unknown origin is not well defined. In a survey of 210 persons who developed cataracts before the age of 40 years, Beutler et al.[138] assayed activities of galactokinase and of galactose-1-phosphate uridyltransferase in erythrocytes. Of 94 who developed cataracts before 1 year of age, two had a total deficiency of galactokinase and the remaining 92 a statistically significant reduction of enzyme activity. In contrast, those who developed cataracts in later life showed no abnormality in galactokinase activity. However, two had abnormalities of transferase activity with no activity in one and a reduction to 15% of normal in the other. The significance of partial enzyme deficiencies as demonstrated in red blood cells may be due to variants and will require further surveys of large populations and detailed genetic analyses.

All neonates should be screened for these readily detected enzyme defects.

Summary

Galactosemia is an autosomal recessive defect in the specific enzyme, galactose-1-phosphate uridyltransferase. Manifestations in early infancy may relate to liver disease, failure to thrive, cataracts, and mental retardation. Melituria and aminoaciduria are present. Avoidance of galactose (i.e., lactose) prevents progression of the symptoms and permits normal growth. Early recognition of this problem in the neonatal period and meticulous dietary control are essential to minimize the toxic effects of the accumulation of galactose-1-phosphate. Psychosocial, mental, and neurologic abnormalities may occur even with early rigid dietary management.

Several variants of the transferase deficiency are recognized: the Duarte variant with 50% of normal activity has no clinical manifestations, while the Negro variant may have classic galactosemia but an ability to metabolize galactose by alternate pathways.

A rare occurrence is the absence of uridine diphosphate galactose-4-epimerase, which is associated with classic symptoms of galactosemia. Treatment is a galactose-restricted diet that includes a small quantity of galactose intake to provide for synthesis of sphingolipids.

Galactokinase deficiency (i.e., galactose diabetes) is an autosomal recessive defect. The only clinical manifestation is cataracts. Galactokinase deficiency may be unrecognized for many years unless a urinalysis for reducing substances after lactose ingestion or routine enzyme screening in red blood cells in performed.

Hereditary Fructose Intolerance

Three distinct entities that result from abnormalities in the metabolism of fructose have been recognized: (1) essential or benign fructosuria,[139] (2) hereditary fructose intolerance (HFI),[140,141] and (3) fructose-1,6-diphosphatase deficiency.[142] Only HFI and those aspects of the other two defects necessary for a differential diagnosis are discussed. Detailed reviews have been presented by Perheentupa et al.,[143] Nikkila and Huttunen,[144] Froesch,[145] and, most recently, Gitzelmann et al.[146]

In 1956, Chambers and Pratt[140] described an adult with an "idiosyncrasy to fructose." The following year, Froesch et al.[141] were the first to describe fully the typical syndrome of HFI. They reported that the administration of fructose lowered the blood glucose concentration in affected patients and postulated that the primary defect was the absence of fructose-1-phosphate aldolase in the liver. Subsequently, over 150 patients with HFI have been reported from around the world,[143–159] except for Israel,[160] indicating a wide distribution of this genetic defect. The frequency of HFI is estimated by Gitzelmann and Baerlocher[161] to be 120,000 people in Switzerland.

Clinical manifestations occur only after the ingestion of fructose or fructose-containing food, e.g., sucrose (table sugar: a glucose/fructose disaccharide), fruits, honey, and similar foods. Another source of fructose may be sorbitol, a sugar alcohol quantitatively converted to fructose in the liver.[145,162] Sorbitol may be an ingredient of "diabetic" chocolate or a sugar substitute in intravenous infusion solutions. The severity and type of clinical presentation depend on the quantity of fructose in the diet and the age of the patient. The young infant is most vulnerable and may present with a serious chronic disease that begins with vomiting, failure to thrive, and hypoglycemia with the introduction of fructose in the diet, and progresses rapidly to liver damage[141,147–150,161] with hepatomegaly, jaundice, elevated serum levels of hepatic enzymes, hypoalbuminemia, ascites, and even death.[156,163–165] At least six deaths in infancy due to unrecognized HFI were reported between 1968 and 1972.[156,157,163–165]

Some infants at a relatively young age have been able "to convey their distaste for sweet-tasting foods" to a sensitive, alert mother and thus remain healthy.[143] A strong aversion for any sweet foods develops in all children and adults with HFI.

After infancy, abdominal pain, nausea, vomiting, malaise, excessive sweating, tremor, confusion, coma, and convulsions may follow the ingestion of foods containing fructose. In adults, the continual intake of fructose may result in renal tubular dysfunction and hypokalemia[166–168] leading to renal calculi,[169] polyuria, and periodic or progressive weakness or paralysis.[170]

It should be emphasized that fructosuria is not a constant finding and occurs only after the ingestion of fructose.

Although multiple forms of aldolase have been found in diverse tissues,[171,172] the primary enzyme defect has been shown to be an absence of activity of aldolase type B in liver,[172–177] in intestinal mucosa,[145,178] and in the renal cortex.[179] Cross et al.[180] identified the first mutation in the structural gene for B aldolase. The antibody to normal B aldolase cross-reacts with extracts of liver from some patients with HFI[177,181,182] and may even activate the mutant enzyme[183,184] (see Molecular Genetics, below).

In HFI, the secondary hypoglucosemia* that follows the ingestion or administration of parenteral fructose is due to an inhibition of hepatic glucose release and is accompanied by a fall in serum inorganic phosphorus[143,145,163,173] and by a rise in serum magnesium[162,163] and uric acid.[162,185] There is no hyperglycemic response to glucagon.[150,151,173] Infusing galactose either with[186] or after[151] fructose results in elevating the blood glucose, but glycerol and dihydroxyacetone do not.[164,186] In the majority of families studied, an autosomal recessive mode of inheritance has been suggested.

---

*Hypoglucosemia refers to a low plasma or blood glucose concentration irrespective of clinical symptoms. It is synonymous with asymptomatic hypoglycemia or chemical hypoglycemia. Hypoglycemia refers to the clinical syndrome associated with an abnormally low plasma or blood glucose concentration.

Clinical Manifestations

A variety of clinical signs and symptoms have been described in patients with HFI.[187,188] The manifestations depend on age, severity of the disease, the quantity and duration of the fructose ingestion or administration and other still-undetermined factors. If fructose-containing foods are avoided, the patients remain completely well and free of symptoms.

Young Infants

The most severe manifestations of this syndrome may occur in the young infant who is given either sucrose, glucose-fructose (e.g., as the carbohydrate supplement to his artificial formula), fruits, or fruit juices.[143,147,148,152,156–165,171,176,178,183,184,189–198] Breast-fed infants remain symptom-free. Generally, the firstborn infant with the disease may die or may suffer more than subsequently affected siblings who profit from the experience of the parents and the physician with the first child.

In the first few weeks to months of life, the infant may have anorexia, prolonged vomiting, failure to thrive, and hypochromic anemia. The vomitus may be projectile, blood-stained or just "spitting up." Periodic attacks of hypoglucosemia with apneic spells, occasional unconsciousness, and convulsions have been reported.[143,146–148,152,163,190] On examination, the infants are usually cachectic and stunted in growth. Jaundice, hepatomegaly, and, less often, splenomegaly may occur. If fructose-containing foods are continued, the disease progresses to more serious signs of liver failure, including hypoalbuminemia, abdominal distention with ascites, generalized edema, and deficiencies of hepatic coagulation factors.[141,147–150,161] Hemorrhagic manifestations have been prominent in some infants who have had prolonged prothrombin times, reductions in factors V, VII, X, and fibrinogen as well as elevations in factor VIII.[165,194] Some of these abnormalities in coagulation factors have been induced acutely following a diagnostic fructose tolerance test.[196] These infants may have elevated serum levels of bilirubin, of serum enzyme activities (SGOT, SGPT, etc.), and of the amino acids tyrosine and methionine.[191–193] On occasion, a severe metabolic acidosis may occur that is in part due to renal tubular dysfunction[163,166–168] and in part to the hyperlactic acidemia.[150,151] Albuminuria and aminoaciduria are usual. It must be reemphasized that a positive test for reducing sugars or fructosuria is not invariably present and may only appear after a significant exposure to fructose.

The liver at biopsy prior to dietary therapy or at autopsy shows extensive abnormal changes by both light and electron microscopy. These changes include focal areas of necrosis with or without storage material, widening and proliferation of biliary ducts, tubular formations extending through hepatic lobules, atypical pigments within the lumen of the pseudoacini, fatty degeneration of the peripheral lobules and portal fibrosis,[156,199] as well as biliary cirrhosis.[163]

The clinical syndrome of HFI in the infant may be highly variable. Some infants may have milder signs and symptoms if only minimal amounts of fructose are offered or if their disease is less marked.

Early diagnosis of this condition is necessary. If unrecognized or allowed to go untreated, death can ensue.[156,163–165] All the clinical and all the abnormal laboratory findings appear to be reversible once fructose has been removed from the diet. Striking improvement can occur dramatically within 24 to 48 hours— "*L'amelioration clinique est spectaculaire.*"[192] As in the infant suspected of having galactosemia, "any infant with an enlarged liver and proteinuria—or aminoaciduria" with vomiting, failure to thrive, and jaundice " ... is so suspect of having HFI that fructose should be excluded from the diet until the diagnosis has been ruled out." Similarly, parenteral fructose should be given only to patients "positively known to tolerate sugar."[143]

The more seriously ill infants have been reported from Europe.[147,148,150,156,163,165] One explanation might be that in Europe sucrose is used more commonly as the carbohydrate added to artificial feeding than in the United States, where corn syrups containing dextrins or maltose are used.

In instances in which the affected infants can reject or select foods, they develop a profound aversion to and distaste for anything sweet, to protect themselves from the toxic effects of fructose. This is particularly true in the adult in whom a chronic syndrome has never been reported, because he has learned what food to avoid. Some parents have recognized their infant's aversion to sweets as early as the first months of life, and one mother solved the problem for her daughter with HFI by breast-feeding her for 2.5 years.[163]

The Older Child and Adult

After the first year, vomiting may occur periodically and be attributed to ketosis,[200] which may simulate ketogenic hypoglycemia. In the older child and adult with HFI, fructose taken orally produces a varying response. Some patients may have severe epigastric pain, nausea, bloating, vomiting, and even diarrhea, with or without the symptoms specifically associated with hypoglycemia. Others, especially adults, may have little gastrointestinal discomfort and manifest only a delayed hypoglucosemic response. Phillips et al.[201] report proteinuria and striking changes by electron microscopy in a liver biopsy obtained 2 hours after the ingestion of 50 g of fructose by an adult man with HFI. They found that concentric and irregularly disposed membranous arrays occurred in the glycogen areas of most hepatocytes and were associated with marked rarefaction of hyaloplasm. Many of the membranous formations resemble cytolysomes. It is concluded that the lesions are a manifestation of focal cytoplasmic degeneration and a consequence of fructose toxicity in these patients. It is suggested that the formation of the lesions is related to the intracellular accumulation of substrates.

Renal calculi[169] may be found with polyuria. Periodic or progressive weakness and paralysis[170] have also been seen in some adults.

No severe gastrointestinal reactions, except for mild epigastric discomfort, have been observed following intravenous administration of fructose in patients with HFI. The onset of hypoglucosemia is essentially at the same time as that following oral fructose.[173] Epigastric pain of short duration has also been noted in 12 of 19 normal adults after 50 g of fructose were rapidly infused intravenously within a period of 20 minutes.[202]

Failure to thrive associated with recurrent vomiting, hepatomegaly, and frequently pronounced dysfunction of the liver and the renal tubule is characteristic of the chronic form of HFI in infancy. In contrast, older children have been reported to have subtle biochemical and clinical abnormalities. Hypoglycemia is not present, while hyperuricemia and hypermagnesemia are associated with increased urinary excretion rates for uric acid and magnesium. The most evident finding is severe growth retardation which may respond dramatically with catch-up growth to rigid restriction of dietary fructose at approximately 40 mg per kilogram per day.[203]

The patients with HFI usually have excellent teeth, with a minimal number of caries.[145,151,163,173] This is especially evident when patients are compared to nonaffected siblings.

Diagnosis

The diagnosis of HFI is dependent on a high index of suspicion and a careful nutritional history.[204] In contrast to the infant with galactosemia (Figure 33.2), the neonate with HFI remains perfectly well on breast-feedings. In the infant the onset of anorexia, vomiting, failure to thrive, drowsiness, and coma date from the introduction of fructose into the diet. With continued fructose feeding, hepatomegaly, jaundice, hemorrhagic manifestations, ascites, edema, and regression of neuromotor function can occur. Proteinuria and aminoaciduria are common. Reducing sugars are present in the urine only following the ingestion of fructose and must be distinguished from glucosuria. Infants with HFI have been considered to have pyloric stenosis, galactosemia, hereditary tyrosinemia or "acute tyrosinosis," hemorrhagic disease of the newborn, hepatitis, congenital cirrhosis, cytomegalic inclusion disease, or toxoplasmosis.

In the symptomatic young infant, a fructose-free diet must be instituted at once as a diagnostic-therapeutic test. A low blood glucose concentration, an elevated blood fructose concentration, and fructosuria following the ingestion of fructose establish the diagnosis. A complete reversal of symptoms occurs when fructose is eliminated from the diet.

In the older child and adult, there is a history of symptoms only following the ingestion of fructose-containing foods, as well as a marked avoidance of sweets.

Laboratory Diagnosis

Intravenous Fructose Tolerance Test

In the asymptomatic individual, an intravenous fructose tolerance test ($0.25 \text{g} \cdot \text{kg}^{-1} 5 \text{min}^{-1}$) produces a fall in plasma inorganic phosphorus[143,145,163,173] and prolonged hypoglucosemia; the latter may be overlooked unless a method specific for measuring glucose alone rather than all reducing sugars is used (Figure 33.3). A rise in plasma magnesium[162,163] and in uric acid[162,185] occurs as well. Because of the severe and often prolonged intestinal symptoms associated with the oral test, the intravenous test should be used in establishing the diagnosis, if at all possible. Fructosuria may be present after the tolerance test, but the amount detectable in the urine does not exceed 3% to 5% of administered load.[150]

Biopsy and Enzyme Activity Analysis

Characteristically, in liver,[172,173,175–177,183] kidney,[179] and intestine[178] the activity of aldolase B with fructose-1-P as substrate is markedly reduced to 0% to 12% of normal. In liver, the enzyme activity with fructose-1,6-diphosphate as substrate varies from 25% to 87% of normal. Thus, Schapira et al.[139,176,177] emphasized that the mean ratio of the activities, utilizing F-1-P and F-D-P as substrates, which in normal adult liver is 1.0 to 1.1, was 5.5 and always greater than 3 in patients with HFI, as originally reported by Hers and Joassin.[172] Since the responses to a fructose-free diet and to intravenous fructose are specific, biopsies are not necessary for clinical diagnosis but may be essential for basic biochemical investigations (vide infra).

Definitive diagnosis may be made utilizing leukocytes and identifying the gene abnormality on chromosome 9.[205]

Therapy

Therapy is simple and consists of the total elimination of fructose and all potential sources of fructose from the

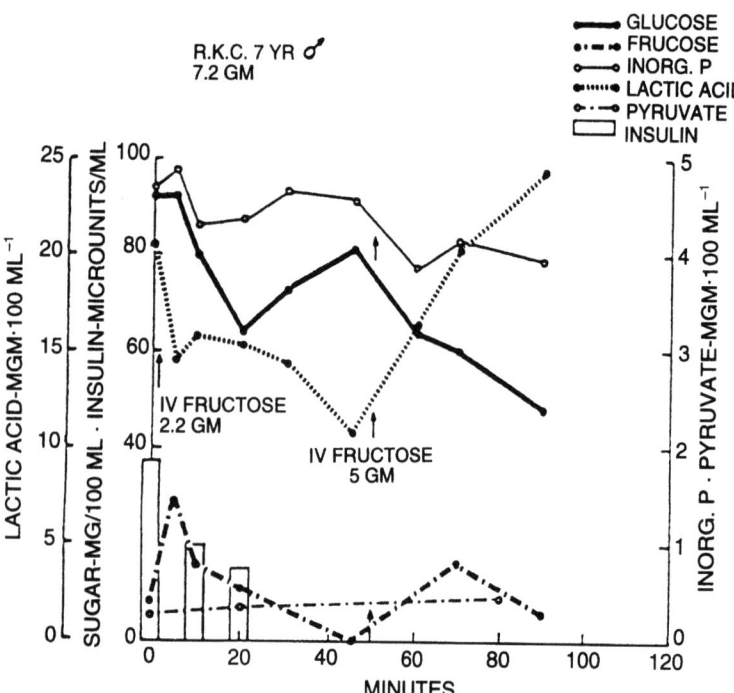

FIGURE 33.3. Intravenous fructose tolerance test in a patient (RKC) with HFI resulting in a fall in the levels of glucose, inorganic phosphorus, and insulin. Significant elevations of fructose and lactic acid levels occurred simultaneously. (From Cornblath et al.,[151] with permission)

diet.[57] Strict instruction with attention to detail and to the minor manifestations of HFI must be provided for the patient and his family. For example, potatoes may be a significant source of fructose, depending on the manner in which they are harvested, cooked, and stored.[260] If allowed to stand at room temperature for over 10 days, the fructose content diminishes significantly.[206] Certain vegetables, including broccoli, cucumber, gourds, and some brands of peas and rhubarb, contain a relatively small concentration of sucrose or fructose.[207] Obviously, each must be tested before being given to small infants. Among fruits that may contain a low concentration of fructose are avocados and some lemons. Another example of caution in therapy must be emphasized for the patient with HFI. Invert sugar, sorbitol, or levulose must never be administered as parenteral fluids to a patient with HFI since each can produce profound illness and even death.[157]

Intravenous glucose is given to treat the acute symptoms that are due to hypoglucosemia if the patient inadvertently eats or is given food containing fructose. There is no specific therapy for the intestinal manifestations. Some patients, as they become older, can tolerate small but increasing amounts of fructose.

Molecular Genetics

Hereditary fructose intolerance conforms to an autosomal recessive mode of inheritance[141] in almost all families reported. The exact genetic analysis of affected families is now possible with molecular genetic techniques applied to white cell DNA. Population studies with these new molecular probes are being carried out by Cross et al.[208]

Fructose 1,6-bisphosphate aldolase consists of four identical 40,000-dalton subunits in a tetrameric form. The three forms (A, B, and C) are distinguished by electrophoretic and catalytic properties. The isozymes are expressed in specific tissue patterns: aldolase A is found in developing embryo and increases greatly in adult muscle; aldolase B is dominant while aldolase A is repressed in adult liver, kidney, and intestine; and aldolase C is found equally with A in brain and nervous tissue.

In a remarkable series of observations, Cross et al.[180] identified a molecular lesion in the aldolase B gene from an affected person. They found a G → C transversion in exon 5 that creates a new recognition site for the restriction enzyme Ahall and results in an amino acid substitution (Ala → Pro) at position 149 of the protein within a region critical for substrate binding. These techniques were then used to specifically identify a genetic defect of HFI. Cross et al.[208] subsequently studied 50 subjects and found the Ala → Pro in 67% of alleles, while another mutation (Ala 174 Asp) was found in 16%. A third mutation (L288 delta C) carried a single base pair deletion causing a frame shift. Other mutations are likely.

One family was studied with polymerase chain reaction (PCR), which identified mutational heterogeneity of the proband. One allele was confirmed at A149P, the other was a 4-bp deletion found in exon 4, a deletion that causes a frame shift at codon 118, resulting in a truncated protein of 132 amino acids. The technique is rapid and efficient and should replace fructose tolerance tests or liver biopsy in diagnosis.[209]

In another study, the common allele A149P was again found; however, the other allele revealed the nucleotide sequence of exon 9 to have a 7-base deletion and 1-base insertion (7 + 1) at the 3' splice site of intron 8.[210]

Molecular analysis of common aldolase B alleles for HFI in North Americans indicated that 55% of the mutant alleles were A149P, similar to European populations. Two other alleles were A174D (11%) and N334K (2%). Significant differences between North American and European subjects were found.[211]

Cross et al.[208] extended their original studies to 41 European affected families. The mutation A149P was found in 67% of the alleles, more commonly in northern than southern Europe. Two other point mutations were A174D (16%). L288C carried a single base-pair deletion causing frame shift at codon 288 in Sicilian subjects. Despite regional differences, diagnosis is possible in over 95% of affected individuals.[208,212]

Ali et al.[213] established a diagnosis of HFI in a 16-year-old who died unexpectedly from hepatorenal failure following infusions of fructose and sorbitol. Two previously unknown mutations in aldolase B were identified in leukocytes from a brother. M-IT was inherited from the father; Y203X from the mother. A bit of archival necrotic liver was enhanced by PCR. Both mutations were found in the propositus.[213]

Pathogenesis

Before discussing the enzymatic deficiency and its secondary consequences in HFI, a description of the normal metabolism of fructose is required. As illustrated in Figure 33.4, fructose may be phosphorylated in the liver, kidney, and intestine by a specific fructokinase at the 1-position or by a nonspecific hexokinase at the 6-position. In other tissues of the body, phosphorylation of fructose occurs only at the 6-position. Glucose inhibits the phosphorylation of fructose in muscle, erythrocytes, leukocytes, and brain but not in adipose tissue.[214,215] The rapid uptake of fructose by adipose tissue is via a specific transport system that appears to operate independently of glucose or insulin.[214] Although fructose can be utilized in vitro by brain in the absence of glucose, fructose is unable to alleviate hypoglycemic manifestations in vivo because of its inability to cross the blood-brain barrier, according to Park et al.[216]

In the liver, kidney cortex, and mucosa of the small intestine, fructose-1-phosphate (F-1-P), in the presence of aldolase B, is split into the two trioses, glyceraldehyde and dihydroxyacetone phosphate, which may then enter the glycolytic cycle (Figure 33.5). Evidence has been obtained that liver aldolase in rabbit exists in a complex formation with fructose-1,6-bisphosphatase and acts in a coordinated manner in gluconeogenesis.[217]

Aldolase type B in liver both cleaves the phosphorylated hexoses F-1-P and F-1,6-diphosphate (FDP) equally and condenses the triosephosphates, glyceraldehyde phosphate and dihydroxyacetone phosphate, to FDP.[218,219] Normally, the cleaving activity ratio F-1-P/FDP is 1:2. Similar reactions occur in the mucosa of the small intestine and in the cortex of the kidney.[168] In contrast, aldolase type A or muscle type has a low affinity for F-1-P, while aldolase type C has an intermediate one.

Fructose-6-phosphate can be converted to glucose-6-phosphate by glucose phosphate isomerase or by being phosphorylated again by phosphofructokinase and ATP to FDP in the pathway common to the catabolism of glucose, galactose, and glycogen (Figure 33.5). The FDP is split to dihydroxyacetone phosphate and glyceraldehyde phosphate by aldolase B. FDP aldolase activity is diminished to a significantly lesser degree than that of F-1-P aldolase so that the activity ratio against the specific substrates exceeds 5.0.

The aldolases have been isolated from diverse tissues and characterized biochemically and immunologically. Enzyme activity has been studied as has genetic material. In studies in the rat, mRNA specific for aldolase B has

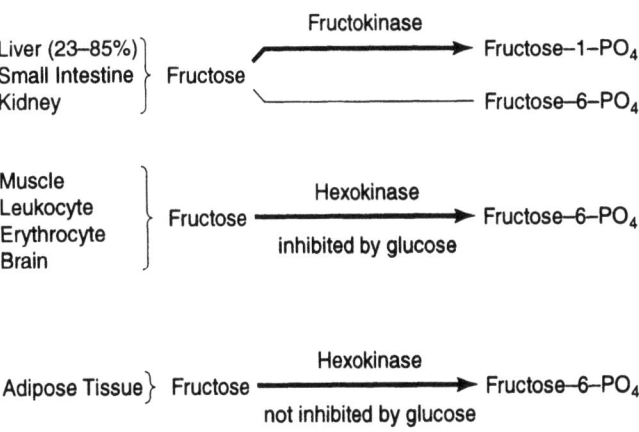

FIGURE 33.4. Normal fructose metabolism.

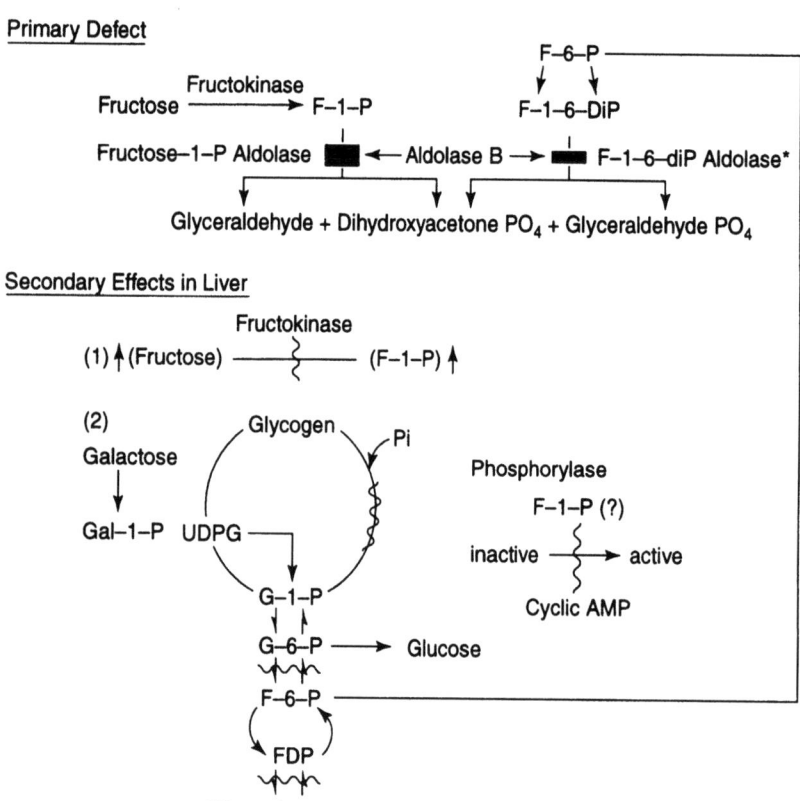

FIGURE 33.5. Hereditary fructose intolerance showing primary and secondary abnormalities.

been shown to vary with starvation and intake of carbohydrate. In vivo regulation of the aldolase B gene expression differs strongly in the liver, kidney, and small intestine.[220] In the liver, the synthesis of the mRNA requires the presence of dietary carbohydrates, the cessation of glucagon release, and the presence of permissive hormones, including insulin for glucose- and maltose-fed rats, but excludes them for fructose-fed animals. In the small intestine, the presence of both dietary carbohydrates and insulin (for maltose-fed rats) is required, but glucagon and adenosine 3′,5′-cyclic monophosphate (cAMP) are devoid of any effect. In the kidney, the synthesis of the mRNA is constitutive, poorly modulated by the diet, and unaffected by hormonal status.

The complete amino acid sequence for human aldolase B was derived from cDNA and genomic clones.[221] The amino acid and nucleotide sequences of aldolase were found to be strongly conserved even between different isozymes.

All the evidence supports the concept that the primary enzymatic deficiency in HFI is a marked reduction in the activity of aldolase B in hepatic parenchymal cells[139,172,173,175] and also in the cells of the intestinal villi[145,178] and renal cortex[168] (Figure 33.5). As a result of the enzyme deficiency, fructose-1-phosphate is not cleaved and accumulates in the liver, kidney, and intestine. The FDP is split by the aldolase A and aldolase C that have been shown to be present in livers from patients with HFI.[176,183] The abnormality involves the structural gene for aldolase B.

The genetically distinct cytosolic isoenzyme, aldolase B, expressed exclusively in liver, kidney, and intestine, was investigated in three affected individuals from a nonconsanguineous kindred by Cox et al.[222] The molecular basis of the enzymic defect was evaluated by diverse techniques, including affinity chromatography, immunodiffusion gels, immunoaffinity chromatography, radioimmunoassay, and electrofocusing. Cox et al. concluded that there is synthesis of an immunoreactive, but functionally and structurally modified, enzyme variant that results from a restricted genetic mutation. They further noted that the catalytic properties of the enzyme were profoundly modified in terms of both substrate affinity and absolute specific activity. Apparent specific activity for F-1-P cleavage was estimated to be reduced by almost one order of magnitude by radioimmunoassay and 100-fold by direct chemical assay. The enzyme determinations presented suggested that aldolase B in HFI has a very high FDP/F-1-P activity ratio and that the residual F-1-P aldolase activity in tissues is almost entirely accounted for by the presence of interfering amounts of isoenzymes A and C. In contrast, approximately one half of the liver FDP aldolase in HFI is due to the presence of modified aldolase B.

As a consequence of the basic enzymatic deficiency, a series of metabolic events occurs following the administration of fructose to a patient with HFI. Some are due to the accumulation of F-1-P with the sequestering of inorganic phosphate leading to intracellular deficiencies of both P_i and ATP. Others are the result of secondary inhibitions of critical steps in glycolysis, glycogenolysis, gluconeogenesis, and other homeostatic mechanisms within the cell that result in hypoglucosemia and acidosis.

Oberhaensli et al.[223] have observed an increase in sugar phosphates and decrease in inorganic phosphate in the liver of patients with hereditary fructose intolerance given small amounts of fructose before study by ^{31}P magnetic resonance spectroscopy.

An approach to a quantitative determination of the steps in the fructose to glucose conversion pathway in normal and HFI children, by analysis of [^{13}C]glucose isotopomers in plasma after [U-^{13}C]fructose administration, has also been developed.[224] The accepted pathway of fructose conversion to glucose, by F-1-P aldolase to triose phosphate, accounts for only 53% and 75% of the conversion in normal and HFI subjects, respectively. The significantly lower (by 67%) conversion of fructose to glucose in HFI as compared to control subjects after [U-^{13}C]fructose (~20 mg/kg) administration can serve as the basis of a safe diagnostic test for patients suspected of inborn errors of fructose metabolism.

As F-1-P accumulates in the cell, there is an inhibition of fructokinase,[141,173] accounting for the high blood levels of fructose. Ultimately, 80% to 90% of the fructose is utilized, probably in the adipose tissue.[173] The mechanisms of the gastrointestinal symptoms remain obscure, although the accumulation of fructose-1-phosphate in the brush border of the small intestine may be responsible.

With the rise in blood fructose concentration (Figure 33.3), there is a fall in P_i and an elevation of Mg^{2+} that suggest a significant depletion, even if temporary, of intracellular ATP and P_i. As a consequence, there is an increased degradation of adenosine monophosphate (AMP) to inosine 5′-phosphate and uric acid,[225] the latter of which increases in both plasma and urine.[143,162] Blood lactate concentration is also increased as a result of multiple interactions that include (1) competition for excretion with uric acid, (2) a secondary reaction to the renal tubular acidosis,[166–170,180,226] and (3) secretion of epinephrine.[143] The elevations noted in free fatty acids (FFA) appear to be secondary to the hypoglucosemia, insulinopenia, and hepatocellular dysfunction. It is noteworthy that although the elevation in lactate concentration was not blocked, that of FFA was by the simultaneous administration of glucose and fructose.[143]

The exact metabolic defects responsible for the low blood glucose concentration are being elucidated. The data indicate that the hypoglucosemia results from a block in hepatic glucose output due to the secondary inhibition of both glycogenolysis and gluconeogenesis and not from an increase in the peripheral utilization of glucose. Two studies support the concept of a block in hepatic glucose output. First, Dubois et al.[152] demonstrated a decreased rate of disappearance of intravenous glucose administered after fructose. In addition, the slope of the decline in specific activity of radioactive glucose given intravenously diminished significantly after fructose administration. This indicated that dilution of the glucose pool by nonlabeled hepatic glucose was markedly reduced. Second, whereas the patient with HFI responds to glucagon with a significant hyperglycemia when he is either fasting or at the end of a glucose tolerance test, he does not show a hyperglycemic response to glucagon after the ingestion of fructose.[150,151,173] Additional evidence against an increased utilization of glucose is lack of change or actual fall in the plasma insulin concentration as measured by immunoassay after fructose[151,173,227] (Figure 33.3).

The site of the secondary enzymatic blocks in the liver responsible for the hypoglucosemia has also been investigated. In studies in vitro F-1-P inhibited phosphoglucomutase.[228] However, the increase in the level of blood glucose after intravenous galactose indicates that the secondary block in glucose output is not due to the inhibition of phosphoglucomutase or glucose-6-phosphatase[151,186] or to the depletion of ATP. In addition, Hers[229] and others[163,193] have reported an increase in glucose-6-phosphatase activity in HFI livers. Therefore, it would appear that the increased fructose-1-phosphate and the deficiency in P_i inhibit glycogenolysis at the activation or action of phosphorylase. Fructose-1-phosphate, in the presence of low concentrations of inorganic phosphate (P_i), competitively inhibits phosphorylase A activity,[230–232] which explains the block in glycogenolysis. An infusion of sodium phosphates sufficient to maintain normal plasma levels of P_i given with fructose does not prevent the hypoglucosemia in patients with HFI.[143,190]

An inhibition of hepatic gluconeogenesis contributes to the hypoglucosemia as well. Neither dihydroxyacetone phosphate nor glycerol can correct the hypoglucosemia following fructose.[186] The block in gluconeogenesis could be present between the triose condensing activity of aldolase B and the formation of glucose-6-phosphate. Apparently, there is a secondary inhibition of both glucose phosphate isomerase[233] and the triosephosphate condensing activity of aldolase B[234] by F-1-P. In addition, the condensing activity is further affected by adenosine 5-phosphate.[234] Although the inhibition of the aldolase may be more complete, that of the glucose phosphate isomerase is not without clinical significance. Using trace quantities of fructose-6-^{14}C and lactate-1-^{14}C, Landau et al.[235] found that 12% to 20% of a fructose load is phosphorylated to fructose-6-phosphate in patients with HFI, whereas none was metabolized via this pathway in normal controls. Glucose phosphate isomerase would be critical in converting this intermediate to glucose. In conclusion, both the inhibition in glycogenolysis and gluconeogenesis effectively shut down hepatic glucose production after fructose administration in patients with HFI. The rate of onset of hypoglucosemia, which appears to be more rapid in younger patients, is the result of the degree of block in hepatic glucose production plus the rate of peripheral utilization.

Morris et al.[166,167,179] found extensive renal abnormalities following the administration of oral or intravenous fructose in subjects with HFI. These abnormalities included a variety of tubular defects, e.g., impaired reabsorption of phosphate, amino acids, glucose, and uric acid, indicating a complex dysfunction of the proximal renal tubule. In addition, they noted an acidification defect in which a decrease in proximal tubular reabsorption of bicarbonate exceeded 15% at a normal plasma bicarbonate concentration. During mild hyperchloremic acidosis associated with the administration of ammonium chloride and at a plasma bicarbonate concentration of 18 to $20 mEq \cdot L^{-1}$, urinary pH exceeded 6.0, and urinary excretion of net acid (titratable acid and ammonium ion minus bicarbonate) was inappropriately low for the degree of acidosis. Glomerular filtration rate was not affected. Titratable acid excretion was increased by infused phosphate, but urinary pH remained elevated. When plasma bicarbonate was decreased to less that $14 mEq \cdot L^{-1}$, urinary pH was reduced to less than 5, and excretion rates of titratable acid and ammonium were not reduced. These observations indicate that a hydrogen ion gradient can be normally developed in the distal tubule and that net acid excretion can be maintained provided that there is not an excess of bicarbonate in early distal tubular fluid. The primary acidification defect appears to be a limitation of proximal bicarbonate reabsorption so that excessive bicarbonate remains in the tubular fluid reaching the distal acidification site. The secretion of distal H^+ is insufficient to titrate this bicarbonate, so that there is a high urinary pH, bicarbonate wasting, and limited net hydrogen excretion unless severe acidosis occurs.

Summary

Hereditary fructose intolerance, a relatively new metabolic disorder, has been estimated to occur in 120,000 persons with a worldwide distribution. The defect in HFI appears to be a marked reduction in the activity of aldolase B in liver, kidney, and intestine, resulting in epigastric pain, bloating, nausea, and vomiting after the ingestion of fructose, and severe hypoglucosemia with its concomitant drowsiness, coma, and convulsions as a result of a secondary block in hepatic glucose production. A careful history makes the presence of this condition self-evident, and appropriate carbohydrate tolerance tests confirm the diagnosis.

If unrecognized in early infancy, hereditary fructose intolerance can be responsible for severe failure to thrive, protracted vomiting, hepatomegaly, stunted growth and development, liver failure, and, ultimately, death. Since all of these complications, except the last, are reversible with removal of fructose from the diet, it is critical that the diagnosis be made and therapy instituted promptly in early infancy. In reporting the death of a 3-year-old girl following intravenous fructose given postoperatively, Danks et al.[157] emphasized that "this case serves as a tragic reminder that the rarity of a disease is little consolation to those who suffer from it."

The patient with HFI manifests a wide variety of metabolic aberrations when given fructose. Additional investigations of these various parameters in patients with this congenital enzymatic defect may elucidate fundamental mechanisms in carbohydrate metabolism.

Benign or Essential Fructosuria

Essential fructosuria, a relatively rare disorder of metabolism, has been estimated to occur in 1:130,000 of the general population. This condition is considered to be inherited as an autosomal recessive trait.[236] Since the patient is asymptomatic and the condition is harmless, the actual incidence may be higher. The primary enzymatic disorder is a deficiency of the enzyme fructokinase (1) (Figure 33.4, reaction 1) that results in abnormally elevated levels of fructose in the blood, leading to fructosuria. In contrast to those with HFI, the patients with essential fructosuria are well and have no clinical disease.

Defects in Gluconeogenesis

Primary Defects

Defects in all four key enzymes in the pathway of gluconeogenesis have now been described (see Chapter 6). Deficiency of glucose-6-phosphatase activity is the most frequent (see Glycogen Storage Disease, below), followed by fructose-1,6-diphosphatase. Deficiencies of the other two enzymes, phosphoenolpyruvate carboxykinase and pyruvate carboxylase, are much less frequent. Lactic acidosis is common to all. Hypoglycemia is only present in the first two conditions in association with hepatomegaly.

Pyruvate Carboxylase Deficiency

Pyruvate carboxylase is one of a family of carboxylases that contains biotin.[237] It controls the first step in gluconeogenesis, i.e., pyruvate to oxaloacetate, and is allosterically inhibited by acetyl–coenzyme A (CoA). As a result of this defect, hypoglycemia would be expected to occur after a fast sufficient to deplete hepatic glycogen stores.[238,239] In fact, only half the cases reported have been hypoglycemic. One theoretical explanation is that the glycerol derived from lipolysis enters the gluconeogenic pathway beyond the enzymatic defect and provides substrate for glucose formation.

Two clinical entities have been described.[239,240] The original North American reports included infants with chronic or recurrent lactic acidosis, seizures, hypotonia, and delayed neurologic development. Hypoglycemia was not a constant finding. The acidosis was at times intractable to sodium bicarbonate therapy. In contrast, infants have been reported from France with a similar clinical presentation plus evidence of liver disease with elevated blood ammonia and plasma citrulline concentrations. The onset was early and progression to death rapid. In the former group lactate to pyruvate ratios were normal, whereas in the latter the L/P was elevated. This altered redox state was also seen in elevated acetoacetate to 3-hydroxybutyrate ratios. Plasma amino acids have not been remarkable; in particular, alanine concentrations have been high, normal, or low.

Molecular studies with cultured skin fibroblasts indicated that the patients with hyperammonemia did not synthesize a protein of the correct subunit molecular weight (M_r 125 K daltons) corresponding to pyruvate carboxylase.[241] In addition, they had no cross-reacting material (CRM) to antiserum against pyruvate carboxylase, whereas all the other patients did have CRM. They postulated two different mutations in the pyruvate carboxylase gene: one resulted in the synthesis of a relatively inactive pyruvate carboxylase protein CRM (+ve) and the other in the lack of expression of the gene in the form of a recognizable protein CRM (−ve).

Therapy is directed against the acidosis with sodium bicarbonate in which massive amounts may be required and the hypoglycemia with parenteral glucose infusion. Biotin has been effective in other carboxylase deficiencies, but has not been in this disorder.

Hepatic Phosphoenolpyruvate Carboxykinase (PEPCK) Deficiency

Fiser et al.[242] have reported a 9-month-old Mexican-American girl with episodic hypoglycemia first documented in the immediate neonatal period. Hormone concentrations were not remarkable; neither were the responses to fructose, galactose, or glycerol. Fasting alanine concentration was elevated, but alanine administration failed to increase the low plasma glucose concentration. A liver biopsy at 5.5 months of age indicated normal glycogenolytic and gluconeogenic enzyme activities, except for reduced pyruvate carboxylase and markedly low or undetectable PEPCK. Hommes et al.[243] have studied two unrelated infants who had an onset of hypoglycemia at 3 months and 19 months, respectively. The first infant had a large tongue and a grossly enlarged liver. Serum transaminase levels were elevated in both. The usual causes of hypoglycemia were ruled out and the course was one of rapid deterioration. Liver obtained at biopsy in the first case or immediately postmortem in both did not show abnormalities of the enzymes of glycogen metabolism; however, PEPCK activity was only detectable at low levels. The grossly fatty livers found at postmortem were considered to be due to increased fatty acid synthesis and related to decreased gluconeogenesis and modification of citrate-malate metabolism and the availability of acetyl-CoA. Whether this enzyme defect is primary or secondary is unknown. The relationship to acquired liver disease per se is unclear. These patients demonstrate the importance of hormone, substrate, and liver enzyme assays in defining the etiology of hypoglycemia.

Vidnes and Sovik[244] have studied three infants with persistent hypoglycemia but normoinsulinemia. In two there was reduced incorporation of ^{14}C-alanine to glucose. A defect in gluconeogenesis was postulated but not proven, possibly at phosphoenolpyruvate carboxykinase or pyruvate carboxylase. In one, they found an abnormal subcellular distribution of PEPCK with virtually no activity being detected in the extramitochondrial fraction of a liver homogenate.[245] PEPCK is a critical rate-limiting enzyme in the control of hepatic gluconeogenesis. It is coupled with pyruvate carboxylase to effect conversion of pyruvate to phosphoenolpyruvate via oxaloacetate. In its absence, glucose cannot be synthesized from precursor lactate or alanine. Because the enzyme is distributed both in the cytosol and mitochondria, biochemical analyses are difficult. As with other defects in gluconeogenesis, the metabolic lactic acidosis may be severe. There are insufficient numbers of reported cases to provide a genetic analysis.

Sudden infant death syndrome (SIDS) has been attributed to hypoglycemia secondary to a defect in gluconeogenesis by Lardy et al.[246] PEPCK has been studied in livers from infants dying unexpectedly due to SIDS. No abnormal activities have been noted. Sturner and Susa[247] have studied 52 infants ages 3 weeks to 7 months. Although the activity of phosphoenolpyruvate carboxykinase in liver was significantly reduced in SIDS ($p < .001$) and in SIDS with other findings ($p < .01$) compared to non-SIDS deaths, no differences were found in vitreous glucose concentration which is a reflection of plasma glucose concentration or liver glycogen. It is unlikely that hypoglycemia due to a defect in gluconeogenesis is of etiologic significance in SIDS.

Hepatic Fructose-1,6-Diphosphatase Deficiency

In 1970, an unusual form of hypoglycemia associated with ketosis was first reported by Baker and Winegrad.[248] Unlike other forms of "ketotic" hypoglycemia, lactic acidosis was noted as well. The triad could be induced by fasting, by feeding a high-fat diet, or by the administration of fructose, glycerol, or sorbitol.

Since the original report, other infants and children have been described with similar findings[249–259] and variable degrees of deficiencies in enzyme activity.[250,255,258,259] This disorder is unique to infancy. Sixty percent of affected subjects are female. At least half the cases reported had an onset in the newborn period with symptomatic hypoglycemia and/or acidosis. Since a nonfructose, high carbohydrate, intake may be protective, these infants do better on breast milk, which contains 6% to 8% lactose (i.e., glucose-galactose). Any event that limits intake and/or results in hypercatabolism, such as an intercurrent infection with fever, may produce hypoglycemia and metabolic acidosis. Hepatomegaly with a fatty liver may be present. Glucose administration is critical since these infants may rapidly succumb to hypoglycemia and severe lactic acidosis if the condition is not recognized. The firstborn affected infant is at greater risk for a fatal outcome because of failure to diagnose the initial serious event. In contrast, affected siblings are likely to have a benign course, including normal growth and development.

The aversion to sweets (i.e., sucrose) and the abdominal cramps so characteristic of hereditary fructose intolerance (vide supra) do not occur in these patients. In addition, patients with HFI do not develop hypoglycemia with fasting. These observations are important in the differential diagnosis.

The pathogenesis of this disorder has been defined by studies in individual patients by Baker and Winegrad[248] and Pagliara et al.[249] The major event is a total failure of gluconeogenesis as a result of the absence of the key enzyme, fructose-1,6-diphosphatase, in liver, although muscle is unaffected. As a result, functional studies by substrate loading with fructose, glycerol, alanine, sorbitol, or dihydroxyacetone fail to elevate blood glucose concentrations and may result in hypoglycemia and lactic acidosis (Figure 33.6). At this time, plasma insulin and magnesium concentrations are low while plasma FFA, ketones, phosphate, and uric acid concentrations are elevated. The latter is presumably due to renal tubular transport competition. In contrast, galactose is converted to glucose without difficulty. The subjects are variably sensitive to short overnight fasts and may not respond to glucagon since hepatic glycogen is depleted. Glucogenic amino acid concentrations, especially alanine, are elevated at the time of hypoglycemia. Increased urinary glycerol excretion during fasting has been observed.[260,262]

The diagnosis may be established by demonstrating the enzyme deficiency in liver[248,249] or jejunal mucosa.[250]

The use of leukocytes for assay of fructose-1,6-diphosphatase has been the subject of minor technical controversy.[254,261,263] It is apparent that meticulous attention to details of pH and instrumentation are essential to

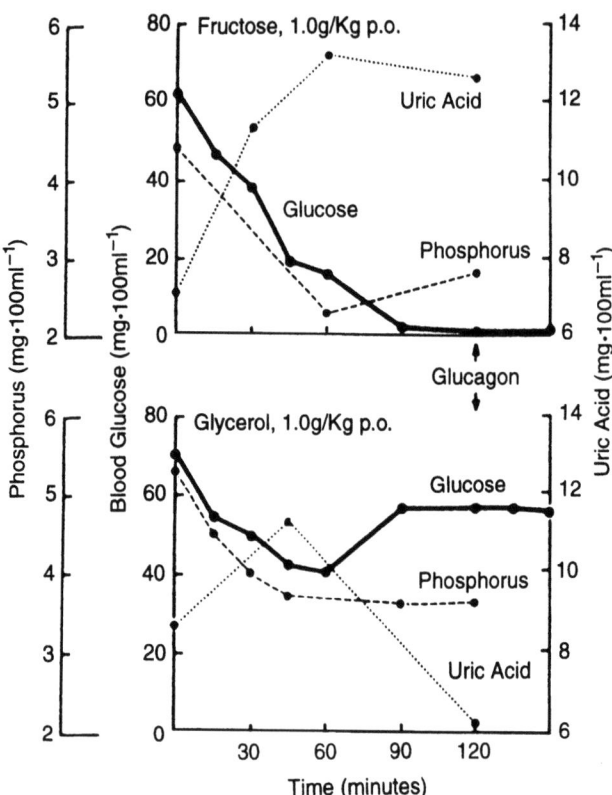

FIGURE 33.6. Fructose and glycerol tolerance tests in hepatic FDPase deficiency. (From Baker and Winegrad[248] with permission)

the development of a sensitive analysis. At least two techniques have been reported with relative similarities in the results.[264,265]

Variability of clinical responses to functional testing makes a definitive diagnosis dependent on tissue enzyme analysis. A presumptive diagnosis is possible utilizing fructose and glycerol tolerance tests[248] (Figure 33.6). The mechanisms responsible for the hypoglycemia that occurs in the postabsorptive state following the administration of fructose or glycerol are not well delineated. There is speculation concerning the role of phosphorylated intermediates that possibly inhibit glycogenolysis at the level of phosphorylase activity. Further specific in vitro studies are necessary to clarify this observation.

The enzyme is either absent in liver or markedly reduced. The normal enzyme contains four subunits of identical molecular weight 36,000. Its regulation is complex, but it is allosterically inhibited by AMP. Proteolytic degradation affects this property. Limited proteolysis may in part be responsible for residual activity in some subjects.

Management requires alertness on the part of the family and physician to any catabolic situation. Since hypoglycemia and lactic acidosis may occur rapidly with short periods of fasting or infection, intravenous glucose and sodium bicarbonate should be given prophylactically whenever an untoward event is anticipated.

Treatment consists of a diet free of sucrose, fructose, or sorbitol and low protein. A diet consisting of 56% calories as carbohydrate, 32% fat, and 12% protein has resulted in normal growth and development.[249]

The number of families studied suggests a simple autosomal recessive mode of inheritance. Preliminary studies suggest that intermediate levels of enzyme activity are present in liver and in white cells of parents. No molecular defect has been reported as yet.

Summary

Hypoglycemia, metabolic acidosis, and hepatomegaly can occur within hours after birth. Specific metabolic defects may be present in several disease pathways important to gluconeogenesis, including enzymes primarily concerned with gluconeogenesis, fatty acid metabolism, or specific amino acids (i.e., branched-chain AA).

Clinical signs and symptoms result in a high index of suspicion. Specific diagnosis requires quantification of metabolites in urine (e.g., gas chromatographic/mass spectroscopy for urinary organic acids) and/or plasma (e.g., amino acids). Enzyme analysis of leukocytes or skin fibroblasts may be necessary to establish a definitive diagnosis (see Chapter 53).

Management should be initiated concomitantly with diagnostic evaluation. Parenteral fluids with glucose and sodium bicarbonate therapy may be lifesaving. Ultimate management depends on understanding the pathogenetic mechanisms involved in specific metabolic defects.

Disorders of Glycogen Metabolism

A variety of types of disturbances of glycogen metabolism have been described over the past 60 years. The first patient was reported by Snapper and van Creveld[266] in 1928, who attributed the hepatomegaly, hypoglycemia, and ketonuria in a young boy to a defect in glycogen mobilization. This hepatic form of glycogen storage disease was further elucidated by pathologic studies (von Gierke[267]) and by biochemical studies (Schonheimer[268]). Von Gierke's patient had renal involvement, hence, the designation "hepatonephromegalia glycogenica." An apparently unrelated syndrome of glycogen accumulation in the heart of a young infant of 7 months was noted by Pompe[269] in 1932 and subsequently in skeletal muscle as well by van Creveld.[270,271] Van Creveld[270] reviewed the glycogen storage syndromes in detail in 1939 and emphasized the variations in the clinical and pathologic observations. Mason and Andersen[272] in 1941 reported a patient with hepatomegaly, hypoglycemia, and acidosis in the newborn period who died from infection at 2 months of age. The accumulation of excessive fat in the liver of these patients was emphasized by Debre.[273]

Initially, two categories of disease were apparent—hepatorenal and cardiomuscular. Two other distinct syndromes were described subsequently. Andersen[274] reported an increased concentration of an abnormal glycogen in the liver and a progressive course that terminated in cirrhosis with hepatic failure. McArdle[275] reported skeletal muscle involvement only and an onset in childhood but not usually diagnosed until adulthood. The classification based on clinical manifestations was then expanded to hepatorenal, cardiomuscular, hepatic cirrhotic, or muscular types of glycogen storage disease.

Biochemical classification was not possible until the details of the pathways of glycogen metabolism were elucidated by the Coris, Leloir, Kalckar, Colowick, the Stettens, Sutherland, Larner, Illingworth, and Hers.[276,277] Initially, the biochemical classification of the five glycogen storage diseases was presented by Cori[278] in 1954. Subsequently, this schema included six distinct biochemical and clinical types (Figure 33.7).[278] In addition, a number of specific enzymatic defects related to glycogen metabolism have been described and found to be associated with variable clinical manifestations. Various investigators have designated these types, ranging from type VII to type XI.[279,280]

Recent reviews have summarized the clinical findings as well as biochemical abnormalities in all of the glycogen storage diseases.[277,281,282]

Classification

Defects in glycogen metabolism could appear at any of the enzymatic steps described in Figure 33.8. The absence of glucose-6-phosphatase in liver was the first proven enzyme defect in the glycogen diseases.[283] The most intensely studied defects involve glucose-6-phosphatase, phosphorylase, and debrancher enzymes. Hers[284] has described a lysosomal system that hydrolyzes glycogen at an acid pH (i.e., acid α-glucosidase), which is important in regulating cytoplasmic glycogen accumulation. He first reported the absence of this enzyme in type II, the musculocardiac form of glycogen storage disease.

A classification based on the organs involved has been combined with that based on the biochemical defects to provide a useful clinical and physiologic approach to these inborn errors of metabolism (Table 33.1).

The hepatorenal glycogen diseases may result from deficiencies of four different enzymes: glucose-6-phosphatase (type Ia), glucose-6-phosphate translocase (type Ib), amylo-1,6-glucosidase (type III), and phosphorylase (type VI). Other rarer biochemical defects are absence of a stabilizing protein (IaSP), and defects in translocases for phosphate/pyrophosphate (type Ic) and for glucose (type Id). The other, rarer hepatic type (IV)

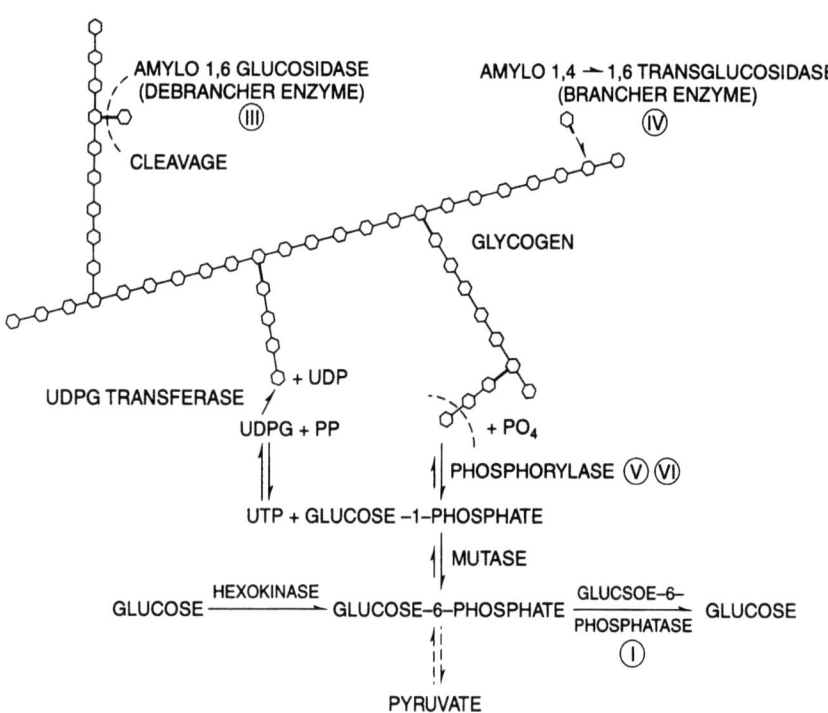

FIGURE 33.7. Schematic representation of glycogen synthesis. Numbers I to VI refer to sites of enzymatic defect in the various types of glycogen storage disease. Type II (alpha acid maltase) and type 0 (synthase or UDPG transferase) are not indicated specifically.

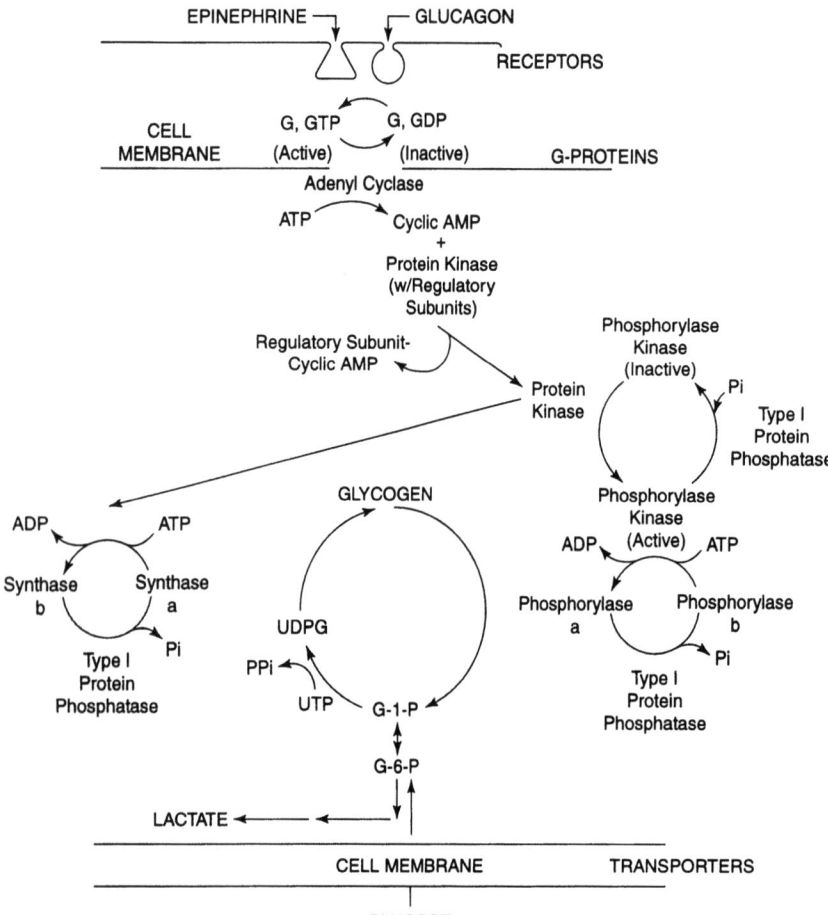

FIGURE 33.8. Hormonal regulation of glycogen metabolism via cyclic AMP. This schema omits release of glucose from the liver, as well as the mechanism(s) for branching and debranching of glycogen. The newly recognized phosphoinositide cascade also has been omitted.

33. Inborn Errors of Carbohydrate Metabolism

TABLE 33.1. Classification of major glycogen diseases.

Type	Organs involved	Glycogen content (g·100g^{-1})	Biochemical effects		Physiologic effects		
			Glycogen structure	Enzyme activity decreased	Blood glucose	Blood lactate	Others
Ia (von Gierke)	Liver Kidney Intestine	>8.0 Increased Increased	N N	Glucose-6-phosphatase Glucose-6-phosphatase Glucose-6-phosphatase	Very low	High	Pyruvate ↑ Urate ↑ FFA ↑ Lipids ↑
Ib	Liver			Glucose-6-phosphatase^a			
III* (Cori)	Generalized Esp. liver RBC WBC	Increased Increased N or H ?	Abnormal Abnormal Abnormal Abnormal	Amylo-1,6-glucosidase Amylo-1,6-glucosidase (±)	Very low or low	Normal	Lipids ↑ sl.
VI* (Hers)	Liver Kidney RBC WBC	Increased ? N or H ?	N? N N	Phosphorylase Phosphorylase	Low	Normal-high	Lipids ↑
V (McArdle)	Muscle RBC WBC Liver	Increased ?	N	Phosphorylase Normal Normal	Normal	Low	Myopathy
II (Pompe)	Generalized Liver Heart Muscle RBC WBC Amniotic cells	Increased Increased Increased Increased N ?	Normal	α 1,4-glucosidase α 1,4-glucosidase α 1,4-glucosidase α 1,4-glucosidase α 1,4-glucosidase α 1,4-glucosidase	Normal	Normal	Cardiomegaly Myopathy CNS
IV (Andersen)	Generalized Liver R-E system RBC WBC	Normal Normal	Abnormal Abnormal Abnormal	Amylo-1,4→ 1,6-transglucosidase Amylo-1,4→ 1,6-transglucosidase	Normal	Normal	Cirrhosis
0 (Lewis)	Liver Kidney RBC	Decreased	Normal	Glycogen synthase ? Normal	Very low	High^b	Fatty liver

* See text for variants.
N, normal; H, high.
^{a} Assayed on fresh liver; normal on frozen liver.
^{b} Postgalactose.

involves the deficiency or absence of amylo-1,4-1,6-transglucosidase. The muscular types include the cardiomuscular, with a general deficiency of acid maltase or α-glucosidase (type II); the skeletomuscular, with absence of phosphorylase (type V); or absence of phosphofructokinase (type VII) in muscle. A defect in hepatic glycogen synthase (type 0) has also been reported.[285] Abnormalities of the phosphorylase-activating (kinase) systems have been included as variants of type VI.[277]

Hepatic (Renal) Syndromes

Glucose-6-Phosphatase Defect (Type I)

The classic disease is manifested early in infancy by hepatomegaly without splenomegaly, with or without symptoms associated with hypoglycemia.[286] The liver is firm and smooth, and may extend to the iliac crest, filling a major portion of the protuberant abdomen. There are no signs of cirrhosis or portal hypertension. Although the kidneys are often enlarged, they may not be palpable because of the massive hepatomegaly. Cardiomegaly does not occur. The infant or child is short in stature but appears well nourished. The cheeks and extremities have excessive adipose tissue ("doll-like facies") (Figure 33.9), but the musculature is diminished and flabby. The face appears plethoric and may be moist with perspiration. If the patient is starved, agitated, or ill, respiration may be rapid and deep owing to acidosis. Easy bruising and a hemorrhagic tendency are common. Nose bleeds occur frequently. Some untreated patients have xanthomata, which appear as orange-colored papules over the upper

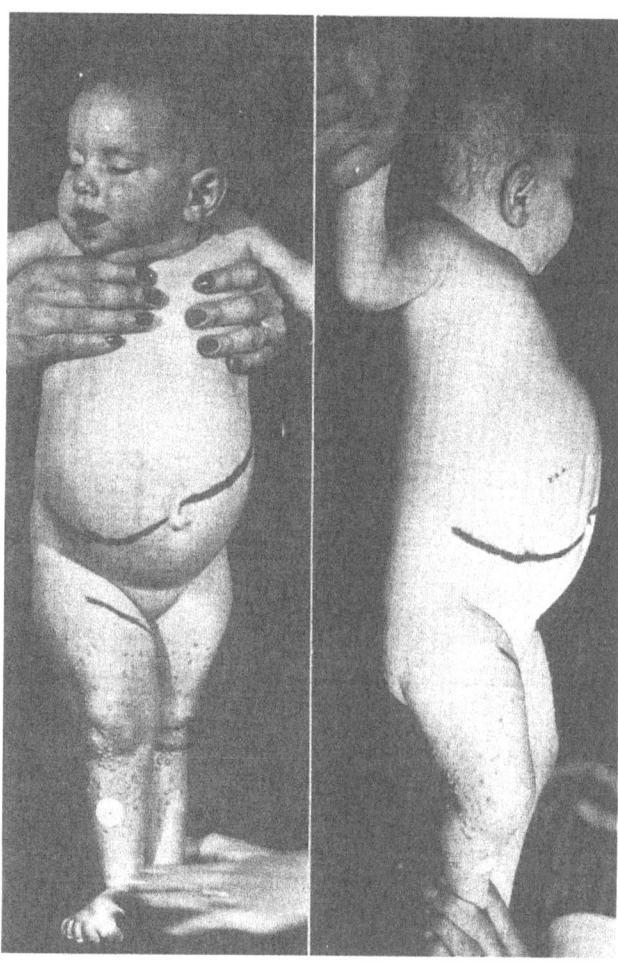

FIGURE 33.9. Infant with proven glycogen storage disease, glucose-6-phosphatase deficiency, showing the doll-like facies, hepatomegaly, and xanthomata on the lower extremities.

and lower extremities. Lipemia retinalis may also be noted. Ophthalmoscopic examination may reveal multiple bilateral, symmetrical, yellowish, nonelevated, discrete paramacular lesions.[287] The neurologic examination is unremarkable. Mental development varies: some children have been reported to be mentally retarded; others are normal. This appears to be unrelated to the hypoglycemia.

In the neonate, this syndrome may present as severe respiratory distress in the absence of pulmonary disease, which is due to profound metabolic lactic acidosis. The liver is markedly enlarged. Ketonuria[288] occurs in contrast to the older infant and child[289] and symptomatic hypoglycemia can be present as well. If undiagnosed, there may be rapid progression to death.[288]

Alternatively, the infant may be asymptomatic and only later in infancy or early childhood fail to thrive or grow and show a protuberant abdomen that is due to hepatomegaly.

Laboratory Tests

Lactic acidosis with a low pH is often present after a brief fast, although the routine urine and blood studies are usually within normal limits. Ketonuria has been observed transiently in very young infants[288] but not in older patients.[289] Thrombocytemia has been reported. The bleeding disorder includes prolonged bleeding time, low values for platelet adhesiveness, increased numbers of platelets, and high values for prothrombin and fibrinogen.[290] Routine chemical analyses usually reveal low or unmeasurable fasting blood glucose concentrations depending on the duration of the fast. Glycohemoglobin (HbA_{1c}) is normal, but HbA_{1a+b} is elevated.[291] The carbon dioxide content is low. Serum concentrations of Na, K, Cl, urea, and bilirubin are usually normal. Serum protein concentrations may be slightly elevated, with a normal electrophoretic pattern. The levels of glutamic oxaloacetic transaminase (SGOT), glutamic pyruvic transaminase (SGPT), fructose 1,6-diphosphate aldolase (ALD), and ornithine carbamoyl transferase (OCT) may be elevated, but lactic dehydrogenase (LDH) is normal.[292] Concentrations of lactate and pyruvate in blood are elevated, as may be those of urate and free fatty acids in plasma.[293] The plasma may be lactescent as a result of a generalized increase in lipids, including triglycerides, phospholipids, and cholesterol.[294] Plasma lipoprotein analyses have indicated the concentrations of very low density lipoprotein (VLDL) cholesterol and triglycerides are elevated, high-density lipoprotein (HDL) cholesterol is low, and low-density lipoprotein (LDL) cholesterol is within normal limits.

Ultrasound demonstrates the abdomen to be filled with a large liver mass and bilateral symmetrical enlargement of the kidneys.

Special Studies

Neither erythrocytes nor leukocyte analysis for glycogen content or structure[295] or enzyme activity[296,297] are diagnostic in type Ia glycogen storage disease (GSD) (see Genetics, below).

The diagnosis may be inferred from the results of tolerance tests that measure the breakdown of glycogen to glucose and lactate, and the conversion of hexoses (e.g., galactose or fructose) and other substrates (e.g., glycerol or dihydroxyacetone) to glucose. Glucagon, which acutely stimulates glycogenolysis and release of glucose from the liver,[298,299] is given following a short fast of 4 to 6 hours. It is given ($100 \mu g \cdot kg^{-1}$ to 1 mg maximum) intravenously or intramuscularly. Serial blood samples are obtained for 2 hours at 15-minute intervals for measuring both blood glucose and lactate concentrations. Blood glucose concentrations may decline to unmeasurable levels, remain unchanged, or increase slightly. Rarely, patients with undetectable hepatic glucose-6-phosphatase activity have responded to glucagon with a prompt, significant but subnormal hyperglycemia. The explanation for this unexpected reaction remains obscure. Blood lactate concentrations increase rapidly and markedly, occasionally to values over 150 mg·100 ml^{-1} within 30 to 60 minutes, in contrast to little or no rise in the normal individual.

In contrast to GSD I, failure of a rise in blood glucose concentration with a normal lactate response can be caused by a defect in amylo-1,6-glucosidase (III), phosphorylase (VI), phosphorylase kinase (VI), or deficient liver glycogen. The blood glucose response alone in the glucagon test is neither specific nor sufficient.

Another tolerance test to evaluate glucose-6-phosphatase activity indirectly and to bypass glycogenolysis is the intravenous galactose tolerance test described by Schwartz et al.[300] After a short fast of 4 to 6 hours, galactose (1 g·kg^{-1} body weight) is given rapidly intravenously as a 25% solution. Blood samples are taken to determine total hexose or galactose, glucose (i.e., glucose oxidase or hexokinase technique), and lactate concentrations at 10-minute intervals for 1 hour. Galactose disappears rapidly from the circulation. The absence of a rise in blood glucose (i.e., glucose oxidase) concentration with a significant increase in lactate concentration is presumptive evidence of a defect in glucose-6-phosphatase.

These tolerance tests can result in sufficient increases in lactic acid to produce reciprocal effects on buffer bicarbonate with decreased pH and CO_2 contents. If the patient is tachypneic and hyperpneic (i.e., acidotic) at the conclusion of the test, feedings should be supplemented with sodium bicarbonate in a dose of 2 mEq·kg^{-1} body weight^{-1}.

Biochemical Diagnosis

In the absence of genetic analyses (vide infra), the diagnosis is established by biochemical analysis of a liver biopsy. Prior to the biopsy, consultation and arrangements must be made with an experienced metabolic-biochemical laboratory to assure proper handling and analysis of the specimen. The laboratory will provide details for collecting and transporting the tissue.

Hers[279] has developed a technique for analysis of micro-quantities of tissue, which can be obtained safely from an infant by punch biopsy. Open biopsy at laparotomy carries the advantage of availability of larger tissue samples for multiple analyses as well as control of bleeding. The patient must be carefully evaluated for bleeding disorders and for the ability to withstand anesthesia. Lactic acidosis, hypoglycemia, and infection must be corrected prior to surgery (vide infra). The child is given a continuous infusion of glucose at 8 to 10 mg·kg^{-1}min^{-1} on the night before surgery and during exploration. An adequate biopsy sample must be immediately divided and one half analyzed fresh for the diagnosis of type Ib GSD. The other half is frozen on solid carbon dioxide (dry ice) or in liquid nitrogen (not in alcohol or acetone) for further biochemical and enzymatic analyses. Separate specimens should be placed in alcohol to allow for glycogen staining, as well as in Zenker's acetic acid and in formalin for routine histologic examination. At the time of laparotomy, muscle samples should also be obtained for biochemical and histologic examination, as described for the liver.

In every child who has an exploratory laparotomy for hepatomegaly of any cause, an adequate portion of the specimen should be frozen on solid carbon dioxide (i.e., dry ice) or in liquid nitrogen for possible future biochemical and enzymatic analyses.

The fresh and frozen biopsy material should be analyzed for glycogen content and structure and for activities of the enzymes of the glycogen cycle.[279,301] The liver specimen has a high glycogen content, greater than 5% of wet weight and a high fat content, greater than 4% to 8% of wet weight. The presence of excessive fat results in a falsely low glycogen content per unit total tissue.

A lack of glucose-6-phosphatase activity is evidence for the diagnosis of type Ia glycogen storage disease. Levels of 10% or less of normal glucose-6-phosphatase activity may represent nonspecific "alkaline" phosphatases or incomplete defects. Other enzyme activities, including those of glycogenolysis and glycolysis (phosphorylase, amylo-1,6-glucosidase, phosphoglucomutase, and phosphofructokinase) and glycogen synthesis (UDPG pyrophosphorylase and UDPG transglucosylase or synthase) have been found to be normal.

Glucose-6-phosphatase is bound inside the endoplasmic reticulum. A specific glucose-6-phosphate transporter is required to carry this substrate to the active site. At least two defects have been described. In type Ia, there is absence of the specific glucose-6-phosphatase. In type Ib, this enzyme is intact, but the transporter (i.e., glucose-6-phosphate translocase) is defective. This accounts for the differences observed between analyses performed on fresh versus frozen (i.e., disrupted) tissue.[302]

Pathology

At laparotomy, the liver is large and smooth with a gleaming capsule. It has a definite yellow, fatty appearance. There is no nodularity or irregularity in its surface. Microscopically, the hepatic cells are large and swollen with centrally placed nuclei. Staining with a standard hematoxylin and eosin preparation indicates normal preservation of lobular architecture without any inflammation, cirrhosis or tumor. There are many vacuolated areas, both within and apparently outside the hepatic cells. Examination of the alcohol-fixed specimens with Best's stain or with the Schiff's periodic acid (PAS) technique indicates numerous red- or purple-staining granules of carbohydrate in the hepatic cells. Vacuoles often persist, however, and are identified as fat by Sudan stain on Zenker's or formalin-fixed material. In some instances, the amount of fat exceeds that of glycogen. Examination of skeletal muscle in type I disease shows no particular abnormalities. The kidney is grossly enlarged and has normal architecture; microscopic examination indicates glycogen-laden proximal tubular cells.

Pathophysiology

The pathophysiology of this type I defect is best considered developmentally, beginning in utero. While the human fetus has been shown to have glucose-6-phosphatase activity as early as 10 weeks' gestation,[303] the primary energy source in utero is glucose derived transplacentally from the mother, relegating the fetal liver to a minor role in glucose homeostasis. Furthermore, the fetal circulation uniquely provides for a bypass of the liver via the ductus venosus so that only a fraction of the glucose supplied by the mother passes through the liver. The constant infusion of glucose from the mother maintains intact peripheral glucose metabolism, prevents hypoglycemia, and results in relatively normal intrauterine growth. The variable manifestations of type I disease in the newborn period may be related to differences in intrauterine hepatic blood flow.

Following delivery, the infant with complete absence of glucose-6-phosphatase is unable to sustain a normal blood glucose concentration, and hypoglycemia supervenes unless frequent glucose feedings are provided. Fortunately, feeding the infant by breast or formula every 3 to 4 hours may prevent hypoglycemia. Hepatic glycogen synthesis derives not only from excess glucose, but also from galactose and fructose. As the interval between feedings is extended, hypoglycemia occurs just prior to the next feeding.

During the period of starvation, the liver is unable to sustain a normal glucose concentration, resulting in a variety of secondary effects on hormone and substrate concentrations. The hormonal response to hypoglycemia includes an initial release of epinephrine, glucagon, and growth hormone, and later glucocorticoid. Phosphorylase is activated, hepatic glycogenolysis is increased, but glucose release from the liver only occurs by hydrolysis of branch points by amylo-1,6-glucosidase. This can result in approximately 8% free glucose release. Studies with stable isotopes, ^{13}C-glucose, have indicated a persistent hepatic glucose production of $2.0\,mg\cdot kg^{-1}min^{-1}$ with fasting.[304,305] This explains why hypoglycemia does not always accompany starvation and the minor rise in blood glucose concentration sometimes occurs with administration of glucagon.

Normally, lactate produced in the peripheral tissues, especially in erythrocytes and muscle, is removed from the circulation by the liver and either metabolized via the Krebs cycle or converted to glucose via the gluconeogenetic pathway. Mason and Sly[306] first reported the presence of excessive lactate in the blood of patients with glycogen storage disease. Several studies have confirmed this important observation and elucidated the origin of the lactate.[298,299] Intrahepatic changes of sugar phosphates and inorganic phosphate have been observed in patients with type Ia glycogen storage disease by P-31 magnetic resonance spectroscopy.[307]

The increased intrahepatic metabolism of glucose results in overactivity of all pathways from glucose-6-phosphate so that production of diphosphopyridine nucleotide, reduced (DPNH) and triphosphopyridine nucleotide, reduced (TPNH) is presumably increased.[293] These key cofactors are necessary for a variety of biochemical reactions, including the conversion of pyruvate to lactate and the synthesis of fatty acid, ketones, and cholesterol. The reason for hepatic fat accumulation and lactate formation may be secondary to the single defect, a failure to convert glucose-6-phosphate to glucose.[293] Decreased ketone formation may be due to increased malonyl-CoA, which inhibits carnitine acyl-transferase I.[293]

In addition to secondary effects, at least one tertiary effect has been noted—the rise in plasma urate concentration. This has been attributed to either an increase in purine metabolism or an increased tubular reabsorption. The latter appears most likely since it is related to the elevation in blood lactate concentration, which inhibits urate secretion in the renal tubule.[308] Roe and Kogut[309] inferred enhanced nucleotide catabolism from studies of responses to fructose or glucagon. Gout has been reported.[286]

Previously, growth retardation in inadequately treated patients, could not be satisfactorily explained on a biochemical or endocrinologic basis. However, the catch-up growth observed with intragastric continuous feedings or with administration of raw, uncooked cornstarch, make chronic hypoglycemia a major factor (vide infra).

Hypoglycemia

Previously, hypoglycemia without symptoms occurred frequently in this disease. Unmeasurable blood glucose concentrations (i.e., well under $10\,mg\cdot100\,ml^{-1}$) have been documented for several hours, without seizures or any symptoms of hypoglycemia. The implication is that, under these circumstances, the brain metabolizes a substrate or substrates other than glucose. Lactate is the likely substrate for brain in these children.[310]

Schulman and Saturen[288] reported electroencephalographic studies in two biochemically proven patients and could perceive no differences in electrical activity whether blood glucose concentrations were high or low. Both EEGs were interpreted as normal at very low blood sugar concentrations.

Now, with current management maintaining normoglycemia throughout the 24 hours, these patients manifest all of the clinical signs and symptoms of hypoglycemia when their blood glucose concentrations are low.[311] The full spectrum of neuroglycopenia, including death, has occurred in the treated patients.

Other problems can occur: (1) An intermittent diarrhea without intolerance to mono- or disaccharides or to fat remains unexplained.[312] (2) In older subjects, malignant changes may occur in the liver.[313] A 5-year-old boy with type Ia glycogen storage disease was reported to have multiple benign adenomata of the liver at postmortem.[314] Both radionuclide scintiscan and ultrasonography have been used to define these hepatic tumors.[315-317] Solitary and multiple lesions have been reported in adults. While most lesions are benign hepatomas, occasional transformation to carcinoma has been found. Cirrhosis does not precede this change. (3) Renal abnormalities have been reviewed by Moses[281] and include Fanconi's syndrome and uric acid nephropathy. Chen et al.[318] observed significant renal dysfunction in older patients. In some subjects initial microalbuminuria progressed to gross proteinuria and renal failure. Recently, hyperfiltration, hypercalcinuria, hypocitraturia, and nephrocalcinosis have also been reported.[319] Patients over 10 years of age should be assessed for renal dysfunction.

Therapy

The major objective of therapy, namely, maintenance of normoglycemia, anteceded the discovery of the specific enzyme defect. However, diet therapy was refined when hepatic glucose-6-phosphatase was found to be absent. A high protein diet was no longer recommended. Since neither gluconeogenesis nor the conversion of the monosaccharides (e.g., fructose and galactose) to glucose would support blood glucose concentrations, fruits and milk were to be avoided.

While diet therapy has improved over the past 40 years, the observations of Folkman et al.[294] placed renewed emphasis on maintenance of normoglycemia. In preparation for portocaval shunt surgery, they used continuous total parenteral nutrition with a central catheter for more than 30 days. They observed regression in size of the liver and correction of the lactic acidemia and hyperuricemia. In addition, hyperlipidemia (i.e., triglyceridemia and hypercholesterolemia) reverted to normal as did the platelet dysfunction. This was a remarkable demonstration of the effects of prolonged normoglycemia.

The next major advance occurred in the 1970s when Greene et al.[320] proposed continuous nighttime feedings. Several regimens evolved, including nasogastric administration of a high dextrose with or without amino acids, pump-controlled continuous feeding, or the installation of a permanent gastric button device for intermittent gastric insertion of the enteral feeding tube without reflux.[321] These regimens markedly increased growth in both height and weight and adolescent maturation but were not without risk. At least one fatality was reported from accidental malfunction of a pump during the night in a previously "hypoglycemic resistant" child.[311] The maintenance of normoglycemia appears to restore brain glucose sensitivity (i.e., primary dependence on glucose substrate) in contrast to the ability of the poorly controlled subject to utilize an alternate substrate, presumably lactate.

Another technique was intermittent nighttime feedings by the clock, every 3 hours. A 25-year-old man has grown normally, having reached adolescence with this regimen.

The next significant advance in diet therapy occurred in the 1980s when Chen et al.[322] described how raw, uncooked cornstarch maintained normal plasma glucose concentration for 4 to 6 hours. The underlying nutritional biochemistry has not yet been clarified. It is noteworthy that cooked starches (e.g., corn, potato, and rice) were rapidly hydrolyzed, absorbed, and have no prolonged effects on blood glucose concentration; these do not differ from dextrose (i.e., glucose monohydrate) or polycose (i.e., medium length polymers). Uncooked cornstarch is absorbed more slowly than raw potato or rice starch. The recommended dose is 1.75 to 2.5 g/kg per feeding in cool, chilled diet soda, Kool-Aid, or water. The exact dose and time interval should be evaluated by hourly monitoring of plasma glucose concentration and initiated in the hospital. Infants must be tested to determine their ability to digest and absorb the raw cornstarch before this therapy is instituted. After the initial evaluation, home blood glucose monitoring is used to evaluate dosage and effectiveness. In addition to safety, a major advantage of raw cornstarch therapy is in preventing and treating obesity induced by continuous or frequent night feeding. Consensus recommendations for treatment of the glycogen storage diseases were reported by representatives of the European communities[323] in 1988.

Diet therapy should include a caloric intake appropriate for age, ideal weight, and expected height, and an adequate protein intake according to National Research Council age-dependent standards. Carbohydrate sources should be only glucose or its polymers. Fructose and galactose and their disaccharides and polymers are to be avoided. Practically, this means no fruits, honey, or milk of any type. Appropriate sugar substitutes may be used. Stanley et al.[321] have suggested an average glucose rate of $10\,mg\cdot kg^{-1}min^{-1}$ to avoid lactic acidosis. This is equivalent to approximately $58\,kcal\cdot kg^{-1}day^{-1}$, an inordinately high carbohydrate intake for the older child. This recommendation has recently been questioned by Kalhan and Rossi[324] from stable isotope studies during nasogastric infusion. The recent European workshop suggested graded doses of glucose intake according to age.[323] These varied from 8 to 9 mg·kg^{-1}min^{-1} in infancy to 5 to 7 mg·kg^{-1}min^{-1} in the older child. The actual intake is best assessed with frequent blood glucose monitoring preprandially, day and night, for intake adjustment. Excessive caloric intake may contribute to abnormal weight gain and obesity.

Another important aspect of management is lactic acidosis, which can occur promptly with a decrease in blood glucose concentration or with infection. Under homeostatic conditions, normoglycemia prevents excessive lactic acid production. However, all children are vulnerable to this complication with intercurrent infections, especially those manifest by vomiting and diarrhea. The prophylactic administration of sodium bicarbonate (i.e., baking soda) at 2 mEq·kg^{-1}day^{-1} is remarkable. This is easily achieved by adding a single solution (1 tsp dry powder, i.e., 56 mEq/tsp, to 90 ml [3 oz] or 100 ml water) to a milk substitute or any liquid (e.g., Kool-Aid). All GSD patients are given a note with specific instructions to emergency room physicians to evaluate and treat with parenteral dextrose at 10 mg·kg^{-1}min^{-1} plus 75 mEq·L^{-1} of sodium bicarbonate, not sodium lactate or Ringer's lactate, until stable (i.e., no vomiting) and feeding is resumed.

Patients may have hyperuricemia and benefit from allopurinol therapy at 150 to 300 mg·day^{-1} depending on age.

Several surgical procedures to bypass the liver have been utilized in the past,[294,325] but none are recommended currently. Platelet dysfunction and abnormal bleeding, especially epistaxis, may occur. Even minor surgery, such as removal of a verruca, may result in uncontrolled bleeding. Elective surgery should be deferred until normoglycemia and reversal of the bleeding diathesis have been achieved.

Prognosis

Until the 1950s, infants with glycogen storage disease type I were usually diagnosed postmortem following minor illnesses that were fatal because of the associated metabolic lactic acidosis. Now, when the diagnosis is made and appropriate treatment instituted, early mortality associated with infections or hypoglycemia should be preventable.

Optimal management results in near normal growth and development. In particular, adolescent maturation is appropriate in well-controlled subjects. No significant adverse neurobehavioral effects of early-onset hypoglycemia have been reported.

Late complications associated with hyperuricemia have included pseudogout. Management with allopurinol has been effective. Maintenance of normoglycemia should minimize its occurrence.

A more significant late complication is the presence of hepatomata.[315–317] These tumors may be identified by ultrasound, CAT scan, or MRI. There are inadequate data to indicate that malignant transformation does occur. No specific therapy is known to prevent this complication.

Female patients have not only achieved successful physical and sexual maturation but have had successful normal pregnancies.[326] No untoward events have been reported for well-controlled pregnant individuals.

Genetics

Based on family history and the frequency of this disorder (type Ia) in siblings, it is considered a simple mendelian recessive that may affect either sex. There are fewer data to characterize the genetics of the type Ib defect. That frequency has not been estimated.

In 1993 investigators from the Human Genetics Branch of the National Institute of Child Health and Human Development reported the isolation of the cDNA and gene encoding human G6Pase, an enzyme associated with the endoplasmic reticulum (ER) and nuclear membranes. The human G6Pase transcription unit spans 12.5 kb and consists of five exons. The investigators identified mutations in the G6Pase gene of two patients diagnosed with GSD type 1a by PCR amplification of the coding region of each of the five exons and all exon/intron junctions.[327] Site-directed mutagenesis followed by transient expression assays confirmed that the mutations abolished G6Pase activity, establishing the molecular basis of GSD type 1a. Southern blot hybridization analysis using a panel of human-hamster hybrids showed that human G6Pase is a single-copy gene located on chromosome 17. To correlate specific defects with clinical manifestations of this disorder, the investigators identified mutations in the G6Pase gene of GSD type 1a patients.[328] In the G6Pase gene of a compound heterozygous patient (LLP), two mutations in exon 2 of one allele and exon 5 of the other allele were identified. The exon 2 mutation converts an arginine at codon 83 to a cysteine (R83C). This mutation, previously identified in another GSD type 1a patient, was shown to have no detectable phosphohydrolase activity. The exon 5 mutation in the G6Pase gene of LLP converted a glutamine codon at 347 to a stop (Q347SP). This Q347SP mutation was detected in all exon 5 subclones (i.e., five for each patient) of two homozygous patients, KB and CB, siblings of the same parents. The predicted Q347SP mutant G6Pase is a truncated protein of 346 amino acids, 11 amino acids shorter than the wild-type G6Pase of 357 residues. Site-directed mutagenesis and transient expression assays demonstrated that G6Pase-Q347SP was devoid of G6Pase activity. G6Pase is an ER membrane-associated protein containing an ER retention signal, two lysines (KK), located at residues 354 and 355. The investigators showed that the G6Pase-K355SP mutant containing a lysine-355 to stop codon mutation is enzymatically active. Their data demonstrate that the ER protein retention signal in human G6Pase is not essential for activity. However, residues 347 to 354 may be required for optimal G6Pase catalysis.

These molecular genetic studies have made possible exploration of the two models of glucose-6-P catalysis.[329] The translocase-catalytic unit model proposes that there are five GSD type 1 subgroups that correspond to defects in the G6Pase catalytic unit (1a), a stabilizing protein (1aSP), the glucose-6-P (1b), phosphate/pyrophosphate (1c), and glucose (1d) translocases. Conversely, the conformation-substrate-transport model suggests that G6Pase is a single multifunctional membrane channel protein possessing both catalytic and substrate, or product, transport activities. To elucidate whether mutations in the G6Pase gene are responsible for other GSD type 1 subgroups, the G6Pase gene of GSD types 1b, 1c, and 1aSP patients was characterized. The results showed that the G6Pase gene of GSD types 1b and 1c patients is normal, consistent with the translocase-catalytic unit model of G6Pase catalysis. However, a mutation in exon 2 that converts an Arg at codon 83 to a Cys (R83C) was identified in both G6Pase alleles of the type 1aSP patient. The R83C mutation was also demonstrated in one homozygous and five heterogeneous GSD type 1a patients, indicating that type 1aSP is a misclassification of GSD type 1a. These investigators also analyzed the G6Pase gene of seven additional type 1a patients and uncovered two new mutations that cause GSD type 1a.

Extension of these studies have included the six mutations of G6Pase gene in 12 unrelated type 1a patients.[330] There was one insertion (459 ins TA), one codon deletion (F327), and four missense. The structure-function relationships of amino acids 83, 222, and 295 and the role of carboxyl-terminal residues 348 to 354 in the catalytic activity of G6Pase were examined. Arg 83 was found to be essential, so no substitutions of other amino acids retained activity. His 119 was found to be essential, presumably as a phosphate acceptor. The carboxyl-terminal 8 residues are not essential.

With this background, 70 unrelated patients were studied utilizing SSPC analysis and DNA sequencing.[331] Sixteen mutations were found to abolish or greatly reduce G6Pase activity. R83 and Q347X are the most prevalent mutations found in Caucasians, 130X and R83C in Hispanics, and R83H in Chinese. The technology is noninvasive and can serve to establish a data base in screening and counseling patients clinically suspected of having the disease.

Japanese investigators[332] identified a novel mutation, a 91-nt deletion in exon 5. The 3' splicing occurred 91bp from the 5' site of exon 5 at position 732 in the coding region, causing a substitution of a single nucleotide (G to T) at position 727 in the coding region. Nine of ten patients have this mutation and 91% of patients and carriers in Japan are detectable by this splicing mutation.

Genetic studies of Israeli patients identified R83C in six Jews, but a novel V166G mutation in a Muslim Arab.[333] Diagnosis may now be made by pre- and postnatal analysis of DNA from blood, amniotic fluid or chorionic villus cells rather than from liver biopsy.

Variants of Type I

A subset (about 10%) of phenotypically similar patients have significant neutropenia and bacterial infections. Described in 1968, liver glucose-6-phosphatase activity was initially normal in frozen liver.[334,335] With the recognition of microsomal membrane transport systems for glucose-6-phosphate (T1) and for inorganic phosphate, pyrophosphate, and carbamyl phosphate (T2), subsequent studies on fresh liver demonstrated a deficiency of the glucose-6-phosphate translocase (type Ib).[336,337] Shin et al.[338] have developed a sensitive radioisotope method for glucose-6-phosphatase in polymorphonuclear leukocytes for the diagnosis of type Ib. Recent interest has focused on the impaired leukocyte function. Defects in glucose transport,[339,340] chemotaxis, and neutrophil function[341,342] have been reported. Except for the infections and impaired neutrophil function, these patients appear and are managed similarly to the classical von Gierke's, type Ia.

Summary

Hepatomegaly in a neonate, infant, or young child with a "doll-like" facies may be associated with epistaxis, hypoglycemia, lactic acidosis, and transient ketonuria. The basic problem is an inability to release glucose from the liver because of an absence of glucose-6-phosphatase activity. The diagnosis is dependent on an adequate biochemical analysis of liver tissue taken by biopsy or biochemical genetic analysis of leukocyte DNA. It may be inferred from glucagon and galactose tolerance tests. Complications associated with plasma lipid elevations, lactic acidemia, and hyperuricemia, may be minimized by maintaining normoglycemia by frequent feedings with raw cornstarch or by continuous nighttime nasogastric glucose administration.

Debrancher, Amylo-1,6-Glucosidase Deficiency (Type III)

Although the first documented case with an abnormal glycogen structure due to an absence of the enzyme amylo-1,6-glucosidase was studied by Illingworth and Cori[343] and reported by Forbes,[344] the original two cases described by van Creveld have been reevaluated and reclassified into this group.[286,345] The latter cases represent an experience extending over more than 30 years of careful clinical observation.

This disorder has clinical and physiologic abnormalities similar to those of type I disease. In the absence of biochemical analyses of liver tissue, distinction may be difficult. However, certain differences that are generally present enable the clinician to suspect this type of defect. The type III patients tend to have a milder disease and are not as seriously affected by minor infections. While hepatomegaly and hypoglycemia are present, the latter is usually not as severe as in type I disease. In addition, lactic acidosis, an important complication of type I disease, is less frequent and less severe. Ketonuria after fasting does occur,[289] but ketoacidosis is not a problem.

Diagnosis

The disease is often unsuspected until a protuberant abdomen and enlarged liver are found. Evaluation shows no evidence of liver dysfunction or splenomegaly. Laboratory studies may reveal nothing more than a low fasting blood glucose concentration. Mild elevation of plasma cholesterol concentration has been noted, but marked hyperlipemia is unusual. The blood glucose concentration is not well sustained during fasting. A glucagon stimulation test may give variable results. When performed after a brief period of starvation (i.e., 4 to 6 hours), a prompt, significant elevation of blood glucose concentration may be found. However, when performed after a 12- to 14- hour fast, there is usually no rise in blood glucose or lactic acid concentrations.[346] Both the galactose and fructose tolerance tests show normal disappearance of hexose, with prompt elevation of blood glucose (i.e., glucose oxidase). Types I, III, and VI have been differentiated by blood lactate response to oral hexoses or glucose.[347] The results of these tolerance tests may be used to make a presumptive diagnosis of type III disease.

The diagnosis may be further established by analysis of erythrocytes[295,348] or of leukocytes.[297,349] The erythrocytes may contain an excessive content of glycogen, which can be isolated and characterized to be a limited dextrin. The leukocytes have been shown to have a deficiency in debrancher enzyme activity. Definitive proof of the diagnosis is obtained by analysis of muscle and liver obtained at biopsy. The studies of Illingworth et al.[350] and Hers[279] have indicated the nature of the defect to be an absence of amylo-1,6-glucosidase, which results in a multi-branched glycogen with short outer chains. Recently, immunoblot analyses of glycogen debranching enzyme have been reported for different subtypes of glycogen storage disease type III.[351]

Histologically, the liver may be indistinguishable from that found in type I disease with accumulations of fat and glycogen in hepatic cells. Skeletal muscle from type III disease cannot be distinguished from type V, since glycogen accumulation is found beneath the sarcolemmal membrane in both.[352] Selective glycogenesis of Schwann cells in unmyelinated nerve fibers from intramuscular nerves has been reported.[353]

Course

The course of this disease appears to be milder than that of type I as evidenced by the survival to adulthood of van Creveld's patients[286] and many others.[277] With adolescence, the hepatomegaly becomes less prominent and ketonuria less severe. Growth is no longer impaired, and maturation, while delayed, does occur.[281] Although the underlying defect persists, no adverse consequences have been reported. The two patients of van Creveld had normal motor and intellectual development, were married, and had normal sons. Mental retardation does not appear to be a complication.

Recently, transient acute cortical blindness has been associated with hypoglycemia in a 7-year-old boy on two occasions.[354] High-voltage slowing on the electroencephalogram was observed over both occipital areas in both instances.

In a study of 16 patients with type III disease, Moses et al.[355] found widespread evidence of myopathy with heterogeneous expression. They also found a high incidence of cardiomyopathy by echocardiography and x-ray.[356]

Management

Management is directed toward maintenance of normoglycemia and prevention of progressive hepatic enlargement. Since blood glucose concentration cannot be sustained during prolonged starvation, the long overnight fast should be avoided and a feeding provided in the middle of the night. Excessive calories from any source should also be avoided. While galactose and fructose may be converted to glucose since glucose-6-phosphatase activity is intact, any excessive hexose would be converted to glycogen and stored in the liver. Protein and amino acids should be able to sustain blood glucose concentration through gluconeogenesis since glucose-6-phosphatase activity is normal; therefore, the suggestion of Bridge and Holt[357] for a night feeding high in protein is worthwhile. Hepatic fat accumulation can best be limited by maintenance of normoglycemia. A diet rich in proteins and containing starch as a major source of carbohydrate has been recommended.[358] As in type I disease, raw cornstarch is beneficial and prolongs the interval between feedings.

Prognosis

Prognosis in this disorder is good for attaining adulthood. Some patients may manifest a progressive myopathy in adult life, whereas others do not. All have elevated creatine phosphokinase activity. This myopathy is most evident in North African patients, in contrast to European and North American patients for reasons which are not evidently understood.[355]

Genetics

While the genetics of this disorder has not been clearly established, the occurrence in both sexes suggests simple autosomal recessive inheritance. In Israel, where there is a predominance of type III disease, a frequency of 1/5420 has been reported.[359]

It is interesting that eight of the nine patients reported by van Creveld and Huijing[360] were female. Huijing et al.[361] were unable to detect heterozygotes by leukocyte enzyme studies. Prenatal diagnosis may be made from analysis of cultured fibroblasts obtained by amniocentesis.[362] Ding et al.[363] reported marked molecular heterogeneity of mRNA. They had sequenced the cDNA of the debrancher enzyme.

Three major subtypes of debrancher enzyme phenotype have been identifed: the common form IIIa (78%) involves both liver and muscle; form IIIb (15%) lacks enzyme activity in liver, but muscle is intact; the rarest form, IIId (7%), lacks only transferase activity, but normal quantities of immunoreactive material are present in both liver and muscle.[364] The gene coding for the human debranching enzyme has been cloned and the nucleotide sequence determined.[365,366] The gene has been localized to chromosome 1 at band p21.[367,368] Recently, restriction fragment length polymorphisms (RFLPs) for linkage analysis were carried out in nine Middle East Jews. No major changes in gene structure were found.[369] Although the exact mutations causing GSD III in this population were not yet defined, the detection of intragenic EcoRI and TaqI RFLPs with a good informative value might enable linkage analysis for diagnostic purposes. Informative families may be amenable to heterozygote detection, as well as pre- and postnatal diagnosis.

Summary

Asymptomatic hepatomegaly in childhood may be associated with hypoglycemia and ketonuria, which are more apparent during a period of fasting. Absence of debrancher enzyme amylo-1,6-glucosidase may be noted in leukocytes and an excess quantity of an abnormal glycogen in erythrocytes. Normal growth and development, with diminution in hepatic size at adolescence, is usual. Prolonged fasting and excessive caloric intake should be avoided. Skeletal neuromyopathy and cardiomyopathy frequently are found later in the disease.

Liver Phosphorylase Defect (Type VI)

This disease, which is similar to types I and III clinically and therefore considered a form of hepatic glycogen storage disease, was identified biochemically in 1959 by Hers.[396] He has observed that one third of 1118 Europeans with GSD have this disorder.[277]

The disease has been described in siblings and usually has an early onset with hepatomegaly. Fasting blood glucose concentration and carbohydrate tolerance are variable; low or normal blood glucose concentrations are reported with fasting. The hyperglycemic responses to glucagon may be absent, subnormal or normal. The blood lactic acid concentration is not usually elevated, but ketonuria may be present. Galactose given intravenously produces a prompt elevation of blood glucose concentration.[85] Erythrocyte glycogen may be normal or elevated.

Biochemical Studies

Histologically, the liver is similar to that in type I, and has a high glycogen content with a normal structure. Enzyme analyses have shown normal activities of glucose-6-phosphatase and amylo-1,6-glucosidase, but depressed levels of phosphorylase as low as one-seventh normal activity.[371] Complete absence of the enzyme has not been reported.[301] Activators of the phosphorylase system appear intact, and inhibitors have not been found. Hers[370] emphasized the variability in this enzyme's activity in liver specimens obtained at biopsy and cautioned against overinterpretation of the biochemical data. Muscle phosphorylase activity in these patients is normal.

In normal individuals, phosphorylase activity is present in the leukocytes.[296,372,373] Low phosphorylase T but normal debrancher enzyme[301] activity levels have been reported in patients with type VI disease proved by biopsy of the liver.

The variability in responsiveness to tolerance tests (e.g., glucagon, galactose), in fasting hypoglycemia and in ketonuria may be due to the variations in the enzymatic defect. Even low levels of activity of this enzyme are apparently sufficient in some patients to produce adequate blood glucose elevations after administration of glucagon.

Course and Prognosis

The course and prognosis of the phosphorylase disease have not been adequately defined. Physiologically, greater similarity would be expected to type III, glycogen debrancher defect, than to type I, glucose-6-phosphatase deficiency. In contrast to type III disease, skeletal muscle is rarely involved. However, hepatic adenomata occur as in type I disease. In view of the site of the enzymatic defect, gluconeogenesis should be unimpaired and gluconeogenic substrates should be able to sustain the blood glucose concentration. A high protein diet with frequent feedings should be beneficial. In addition, glucocorticoids, which increased gluconeogenesis, may also be of value. It is not known to what extent the glucose formed will be released or synthesized to glycogen.

The natural history of X-linked form of phosphorylase kinase deficiency has been reported by Willems et al.[374] They had the unusual opportunity to observe two large kindreds with 41 affected males. Hepatomegaly was found in 92% on presentation; however, hypoglycemia and acidosis were rare in contrast to type I disease. Growth retardation was found in 68% of patients, while delay in motor development was observed in half (before 10 years of age). Laboratory observations included hypercholesterolemia (76%), hypertriglyceridemia (70%), elevation of glutamic pyruvic transaminase (GPT) (56%), and fasting hyperketosis (44%). During the initial years after onset, hypoglycemia (12%) and acidosis (2%) were infrequent findings. This remarkable disorder is associated with amelioration of both clinical and biochemical abnormalities, so that most adult subjects are asymptomatic.

Variants

The group considered to have a phosphorylase deficiency has been further characterized with reference to the adenylyl cyclase cascade. Christiansen et al.[375] reported a 2.5-month-old infant with hepatomegaly and normoglycemia. A hepatoma removed surgically had a defect in dephosphophosphorylase kinase. Hug et al.[376] first reported in 1966 a similar defect in a girl with increased hepatic glycogen. They subsequently reported five children with asymptomatic hepatomegaly without biochemical or clinical evidence of hypoglycemia who had less than 10% activation of liver phosphorylase in vitro.[377] The defect was overcome by addition of kinase in vitro, indicating the integrity of the phosphorylase enzyme. This deficiency in dephosphophosphorylase kinase was associated with glycogen accumulation both intercellularly and within the hepatocytes. Surprisingly, all five patients responded to glucagon acutely, but therapeutically its effectiveness was not clearly shown. Short stature occurred and mental development was normal. The long-term prognosis is unknown, and therapy is supportive only. Huijing and Fernandes[378] have observed different leukocyte responses in heterozygotes compared to Hug et al. They characterized phosphorylase kinase deficiency as an X-chromosomal defect. Hemolysate analysis has been used to distinguish two subgroups based on phosphorylase kinase activity, endogenous phosphorylase b and amylo-1,6-glucosidase activity.[379]

Shin et al.[380] have classified patients in four groups based on erythrocyte activities of phosphorylase kinase, phosphorylase, and amyloglucosidase. Tuchman et al.[381] studied a young child who did not have hypoglycemia, and who did not respond to a high-protein diet, but who did to a high-carbohydrate diet.

The phosphorylase system may be associated with defects[382] which result in (1) the X-linked phosphorylase b kinase deficiency, in which the muscle enzyme is unaffected; (2) the autosomal phosphorylase b kinase deficiency, which affects both liver and muscle; and (3) the deficiency of liver phsophorylase, which may be complete or partial. The gene coding for liver phosphorylase has been assigned to chromosome 14.[383] The α subunit of phosphorylase kinase has been assigned to the proximal long arm of the X chromosome, but the β subunit to chromosome 16.[384]

Summary

A decrease in hepatic and leukocytic phosphorylase activity has been found associated with hepatomegaly and hypoglycemia in early childhood. This entity is difficult to differentiate from the other two types of hepatic glycogen storage disease on clinical and physiologic observations alone. Multiple forms of this type of glycogen storage disease have been described, depending on the mechanism of the reduction in phosphorylase activity.

Glycogen Disease of Skeletal Muscle

Muscle Phosphorylase Deficiency (Type V), McArdle's Syndrome

This rare myopathy, first recognized in 1951, is of particular significance because it represents the first discovery of a genetic disease of muscle caused by the absence of a single, specific enzyme.[275]

Clinical Considerations

The disease is characterized by late onset. In early childhood the patient is relatively free of symptoms, except for muscle fatigue and thus an inability to keep up with one's playmates by the age of 7 years. Generally, symptoms are absent or minimal in the first decade. During the teens, muscle fatigue, particularly with strenuous exercise, may be more evident. Transient episodes of dark urine due to myoglobinuria may occur. Hepatomegaly is also absent, and the cardiopulmonary system is not remarkable.

Laboratory Studies

Laboratory studies, including blood and urine, are singularly unrewarding, except for the rare, postexercise episode of transient myoglobinuria. Serum enzyme and carbohydrate studies are particularly unremarkable. Electrolytes, including K and Ca, and concentrations of glucose, phosphate, lactate, and pyruvate are normal in the resting state.

Carbohydrate tests, including glucose tolerance, glucose and insulin tolerance, and epinephrine and glucagon tolerance, are all normal. The latter two tests indicate that liver phosphorylase is normal.

Physiologic Studies

McArdle[275] studied a 30-year-old male patient extensively and noted particularly a failure of ischemic exercise to produce an elevation in venous blood lactate concentration. Normally, prolonged exercise produces a significant elevation of the lactate concentration in venous blood, and ischemic exercise, depending on duration, similarly produces a characteristic elevation of from 25 to 30 mg·100 ml^{-1} above the basal concentrations.

Biochemical Studies

Biochemical studies of biopsied muscle have indicated an absence of phosphorylase a and b, but the presence of UDPG-glycogen synthase, phosphorylase kinase, and phosphoglucomutase.[385,386] Glycogen content in muscle in the three original cases was excessive at 2.4 to 4 g·100 g^{-1} (normal is less than 1% wet weight). The glycogen has been found to be structurally normal.

Pathology

Histologic examination of muscle has indicated variable tissue structure. In younger individuals, muscle appears normal, while in the older person with muscle atrophy hypertrophied fibers with blebs of raised sarcolemma are found.[387,388] The damaged fibers appear necrotic and may disappear altogether.

Pathogenesis

Resting muscle derives its energy mainly from oxidation of noncarbohydrate substances, although glucose uptake and degradation to lactate do occur.[389] Glycogen is not an important source of energy for resting muscle. In contrast, contracting muscle has an enormous demand for high-energy phosphates, which cannot be supplied adequately by substrates from the blood, even though blood flow increases with exercise. Under these conditions, glycogenolysis and the anaerobic metabolism of glucose with lactate production are important sources of energy to sustain muscle activity. The limitation of the individual with phosphorylase myopathy to sustain muscle during exercise is directly related to the inability to degrade glycogen.

Differential Diagnosis

Differential diagnosis is confined to other muscular disorders, including muscular dystrophy and congenital myotonia (i.e., Thomsen's disease). Defects in a variety of glycogenolytic and glycolytic enzymes of muscle must be considered, including phosphorylase b kinase, amylo-1,6-glucosidase, glucose phosphate isomerase, and type VII muscle phosphofructokinase.[390]

Course

The course of the disease is variably benign; longevity does not appear to be affected. Improvement in work and exercise tolerance has been reported following either glucagon injections and glucose or fructose ingestion (i.e., 30–45 g by mouth, three or four times daily).[391] Avoidence of strenuous activity is important.

Genetics

The genetics of this rare disease has been clarified in a detailed family study in which three cases (two proven) were found in a sibship of 13 individuals.[391] These findings suggest a single, completely recessive, rare, autosomal gene. Molecular genetic techniques have been used to assign this gene to chromosome 11.[392]

Summary

Myopathy due to the absence of muscle phosphorylase is a rare genetic disease manifest by intolerance to exercise. The abnormal response to ischemic exercise is characterized by a fall in venous lactate concentration. Muscle biopsy is necessary to demonstrate the biochemical defect. Other phosphorylases (e.g., liver, leukocyte, etc.) are not affected.

Muscle Phosphofructokinase Deficiency: Type VII

Glycogen storage in muscle from patients with a similar clinical picture to that of McArdle's disease has been reported by Tarui et al.[393] and Okuno et al.[394] In addition to the muscular disorder, the three young Japanese adult siblings had a nonspherocytic hemolytic anemia. Myoglobinuria was observed in one subject. As in phosphorylase deficiency, ischemic exercise failed to increase venous blood lactate. The low muscle phosphofructokinase activity was associated with increased concentrations of glucose-6-phosphate and fructose-6-phosphate in muscle, while fructose-1,6-diphosphate was low.

Muscle phosphofructokinase was found to be a different isozyme from that in liver, while erythrocytes normally have approximately half of each form. Tarui et al.[395] noted that total erythrocyte enzyme levels of phosphofructokinase were about 50% of normal, with absence of the muscle isozyme and persistence of the hepatic form. They related the reduced erythrocyte life span and hemolysis to the deficient red cell enzyme. Layzer et al.[396] have studied a similar patient from the United States.

They were unable to demonstrate any material in a muscle biopsy that would react with an antibody prepared against purified human muscle phosphofructokinase.

While only a few patients have been reported, the disorder is presumably inherited as an autosomal recessive, since it has been observed in both sexes and has been associated with reduced erythrocyte enzyme levels in parents.

Generalized Glycogen Storage Disease

Deficiency of α-Acid Glucosidase (Acid Maltase) (Type II) (Pompe's Disease)

Although this type of glycogen storage disease was one of the first to be described in terms of pathology,[269] the biochemical origin was unknown until the report of Hers in 1963.[284] This group of glycogen storage diseases represents a spectrum including idiopathic cardiomegaly of infancy, a neuromuscular disorder simulating amyotonia congenita and a diffuse cardioneuromuscular disease.[397,398] This disease is characterized by early onset, with a rapidly progressing deterioration to death, often within the first year of life and generally by the second year. The adult onset type may be benign in its course as noted in survivors.

In a review in 1950,[397] the criteria for a diagnosis of glycogen storage disease of the heart were as follows: (1) marked enlargement of the heart; (2) death within the first year of life; (3) typical "lacework" appearance of histologic sections of myocardium, resulting from the massive deposition of stored material in all cardiac fibers; and (4) chemical or histochemical demonstration of the material as glycogen.[397] These criteria were based on the original observations of Pompe[269] and van Creveld.[270,271]

However, these criteria are too rigid, since cases have been reported without cardiomegaly but with predominantly muscular involvement. The child may even live beyond the first year of life.[399]

Clinical Considerations

Onset can be at any time within the first year of life from the first day to a few months of age. In the generalized type, the clinical manifestations often include diffuse muscular weakness, respiratory difficulty, and progressive cardiac failure. Undernutrition due to difficult feeding, with failure to thrive and loss of subcutaneous fat, may be early manifestations. The muscles feel firm, although hypotonia may be present. Sometimes reflexes are totally absent. The heart is enlarged on percussion, but auscultation reveals no murmurs. The liver is normal or only minimally enlarged. The tongue may be large and protuberant, giving the infant the appearance of a cretin or of a baby with 21 trisomy. Progressive muscle weakness may involve the respiratory muscles, thus simulating amyotonia congenita. Cardiac enlargement progresses to failure, with dyspnea and cyanosis. Respiratory infection with fever is common and often is the precipitating terminal event.

In contrast to the fatal infantile form of this disease, there is an adult, milder form in which muscular weakness is most evident. Survival into middle decades is not unusual.

Laboratory Studies

Laboratory studies are remarkable in that they afford no clues pointing toward an abnormality of glycogen metabolism. Routine blood and urine analyses are merely consistent with the infant's nutritional and infection status. Low blood glucose concentration, when reported, has been due to inadequate nutrition since it is usually normal. Glucose, epinephrine, glucagon, and galactose tolerance tests have been normal. Blood lactic acid concentration is normal and rises normally after administration of epinephrine. Ketosis, ketonuria, and acidosis are not features of this disorder. Neostigmine responses and electromyography have not been diagnostic.

X-Ray Findings

Roentgen examination may reveal a large, globular heart that is diffusely involved and fills both sides of the thorax. Consolidation of the lungs may be present. The kidneys are not enlarged.

Cardiac Studies

The electrocardiogram is abnormal in those patients with involvement of the heart.[399] Supraventricular tachycardia has been reported as an initial presentation. The P-R interval is short, while the QRS complex may be high. Echocardiography indicates a diffusely symmetrically enlarged heart. Dincsoy et al.[400] observed endocardial fibroelastosis in two siblings.

Differential Diagnosis

The diagnosis, which can be suspected only from clinical evidence, depends on pathologic and biochemical studies. The patients with cardiac enlargement must be differentiated from the group of infants with primary endomyocardial disease, such as primary endocardial sclerosis, anomalous origin of a coronary artery, myocarditis, calcification of the coronary arteries, and idiopathic myocardial hypertrophy. Skeletal muscle involvement is a distinguishing feature. The latter must be differentiated from amyotonia congenita, a more common entity.[401] The general appearance of the infant with protuberant, large tongue and umbilical hernia may suggest Down syndrome or congenital hypothyroidism.

Diagnosis

The glycogen content of tissues, especially the heart and skeletal muscle, is high and can exceed 10% by wet weight. Glycogen structure is normal. The activity in liver of the enzymes phosphorylase, debrancher, and glucose-6-phosphatase have been normal. Erythrocyte glycogen is not elevated.[402] Acid maltase activity was low in the leukocytes of some patients with type II disease.[403,404]

Pathology

Tissues taken for histochemical analysis must be carefully handled, as the glycogen is highly soluble in water. The changes in cardiac, skeletal, and smooth muscle are similar—a honeycombed or lacework appearance due to extensive vacuolization is characteristic. Alcoholic PAS stains reveal heavy deposits of glycogen with intensively stained, closely packed granules of different sizes. Glycogen deposition granules may be found in a variety of tissues, including the central nervous system. This may occur diffusely and include brain, spinal cord, and peripheral nervous system, or be localized to specific areas such as the spinal cord and the autonomic nervous system.

Pathogenesis

Although an enzymic defect has been demonstrated, the pathogenesis is not entirely clear. Lejeune et al.[405] have localized α-acid glucosidase in the lysosomes in rat liver. These subcellular fractions contain a variety of hydrolases, which are capable of breakdown and digestion of localized areas within the cell. Apparently, there is a continual breakdown and synthesis of local cell constituents. Glycogen, which is synthesized normally and usually degraded by glycogenolytic enzymes (e.g., phosphorylase and debrancher), may also be degraded locally within the lysosome by α-acid glucosidase to maltose and glucose. In the absence of this enzyme, other lysosomal hydrolases might destroy the enzymes that usually break down glycogen, allowing normal glycogen to accumulate in the vacuoles. In other cellular sites, containing glycogen and the enzymes of synthesis and degradation, no physiologic defect in glucose metabolism is apparent. The accumulation of glycogen in localized vacuolated areas within the cell would be progressive, impair cellular function, and disrupt muscle fibers.

The enzyme α-acid glucosidase has been identified in a variety of tissues, including leukocytes, liver, and muscle. Skin fibroblasts and amniotic fluid cells have been cultured and assayed for α-glucosidase activity,[406,407] allowing in utero diagnosis.[408,409] Shin et al.[410] made a diagnosis in the first trimester by chorionic villus biopsy.

Genetics

The disease is familial, with as many as three affected siblings having been reported in a single family. Over 200 cases of this apparently genetically determined, autosomal recessive disorder have been cited.[411,412] Parents of affected children have decreased enzyme activity in cultured fibroblasts. Differences in enzyme activities between the infantile and late-onset form have been attributed to different allelic mutations.[413] The human gene for α-acid glucosidase has been cloned and assigned to chromosome 17.[413]

Prenatal diagnosis has progressed beyond enzymatic analysis to include mutation analysis.[414] Prenatal diagnosis of type II glycogen storage has been possible since the early 1970s with enzyme analysis of amniotic cells obtained in the 16th week.[415] Since 1984 chorionic villus biopsy at 10 to 12 weeks has assured earlier diagnosis.[416,417] The finding of two relatively common mutations in type II glycogen storage disease at ΔT525 and Δexon 18 makes carrier detection and prenatal diagnosis by mutation analysis in affected families feasible.[414] In most populations the incidence of infantile GSD II is estimated at 1 in 50,000, which implies a carrier frequency of 1 in 100 and a 0.25% risk that a proven carrier generates an affected child. The marked clinical differences between the infantile and adult forms of this disorder are associated with significant differences in α-glucosidase activity. Thus, α-glucosidase is virtually absent in the infantile form, whereas significant enzyme activity can be measured in the adult form.[418]

Therapy

As with other inherited molecular disorders, therapy has been unsuccessful and primarily supportive. Digitalization and surgical intervention have been notably without benefit. Exogenous enzyme administration has not been beneficial. Recombinant DNA biosynthesis or targeted gene therapy may be effective in the future.

Summary

Generalized glycogenosis is a progressive disorder of young infants in whom cardiac hypertrophy, skeletal muscle dysfunction, and central nervous system deterioration usually results in a fatal outcome in the first year of life. Abnormalities of carbohydrate physiology are not found, although excessive glycogen accumulation in a variety of tissues is characteristic. Diagnosis is established by muscle biopsy and the biochemical demonstration of an absence of α-acid glucosidase. The enzymatic defect may also be shown in the leukocyte and liver. There is no satisfactory therapy.

Storage of Abnormal Glycogen: Amylopectinosis Brancher Deficiency (Type IV) (α-1,4 Glucan: α-1,4 Glucan 6-Glycosyl Transferase)

This disorder was first described clinically by Andersen,[274] and the structure of the glycogen was characterized biochemically by Cori.[278] Absence of the enzyme in liver and leukocytes was reported by Brown and Brown.[419] The clinical course was uniform in the group in that the affected infant appeared normal at birth, grew well in the initial months, but failed to thrive early in infancy. By the sixth month of life, abdominal distention, hepatomegaly and splenomegaly appeared. Dilated superficial veins were present over the upper abdomen. Minimal icterus was present in Andersen's case.[274]

Laboratory Findings and Diagnosis

The hemogram indicats a mild anemia. Carbohydrate studies reveal a normal fasting blood glucose concentration, rarely as low as $30 \, mg \cdot 100 \, ml^{-1}$. Oral and intravenous glucose, galactose, and fructose tolerance tests are not remarkable. Response to administration of epinephrine and glucagon is variable, with a flat or delayed rise in blood glucose concentration. In contrast to other forms of glycogen storage disease, no abnormalities in blood concentrations of pyruvate, lactate, or urate have been observed either in the fasting state or during the tolerance tests.[420]

The major laboratory abnormalities are in liver function tests. SGOT rises as high as 240 units (normal <30), while SGPT reaches levels of 114 units (normal <30). In addition to transaminase, elevations of aldolase and lactate dehydrogenase, especially its isoenzyme, V form, occur.[421] Values for cholesterol and total lipids are not elevated. Serum electrolyte concentrations are not remarkable. A severe metabolic acidosis has been reported and thought to be of renal origin.[422]

Initial diagnosis, as determined by biopsy in early cases, was glycogen storage disease with diffuse early portal cirrhosis.

Course

The patients reported have had a similar course, with progressive liver or cardiac failure; most patients succumbed between 6 and 24 months, although survival until 4 years of age has been noted.[422] The complications of portal hypertension and cirrhosis predominate. Ascites, esophageal varices with hemorrhage, jaundice, and malnutrition are present. Hypoproteinemia occurs late in the course of the disease, while hypoprothrombinemia occurs early. Intercurrent infections are frequent.

Pathology

At postmortem the liver is large and firm with golden-yellow nodules. The spleen is large. The kidneys are enlarged but otherwise grossly normal on inspection. Histologically, the liver contains fibrous tissue and bile duct proliferation. Best's stain indicates the liver cells to be packed with red granules. On iodine stain, this material is a purplish-brown color instead of the usual reddish-brown characteristic of normal glycogen. Excess polysaccharide is identified histologically in many tissues, including liver, spleen, lymph nodes, intestinal mucosa, as well as kidneys, heart, muscle, reticuloendothelial system, and nervous system.

Andersen[274] noted difficulty in chemically isolating glycogen and submitted tissue to Cori for further biochemical analysis, who isolated the polysaccharide and characterized it as an amylopectin with abnormal inner and outer straight chains. On this basis, Andersen postulated a deficiency of brancher enzyme. Sidbury et al.[423] studied a variety of enzymes in liver and muscle and noted a general depression, without absence of a specific enzyme. They isolated and characterized the polysaccharide also as an amylopectin. It is of interest that the liver did not contain an excessive content of this glycogenlike material (0.18% to 2.86%) or of fat.

The diagnosis was suspected, in one case, from an analysis of red blood cell glycogen.[424] While the amount of material (i.e., polysaccharide) was not increased in content, the iodine spectrum was similar to that found with amylopectin and different from that of normal glycogen. Shin et al.[420] have measured the enzyme activity in erythrocytes in controls and in three affected children.

The diagnosis of type IV can be established by liver biopsy and accompanying histochemical and biochemical studies.[423,425] The liver glycogen content is usually below normal ($<5 \, g \cdot 100 \, g^{-1}$ liver) although a high value ($10.7 \, g \cdot 100 \, g^{-1}$) may occur.[422] One hypothesis suggested that the polysaccharide acts as a foreign body to produce a reaction in the reticuloendothelial system and in liver parenchymal cells.

Genetics

Although few cases have been reported, a familial incidence is evident. In one family, skin fibroblast studies from the propositus established the diagnosis, while those from the parents had enzyme values below those of controls. The disorder appears to be inherited as a simple autosomal recessive.

Therapy

Until recently, management has been nonspecific and supportive. Dietary therapy has been unsuccessful (high protein, low carbohydrate with corn oil). Portocaval transposition was attempted late in one patient without success.[425] Glucagon, both short and long acting, has not modified the course. Another patient survived with steroid therapy until 4 years of age.

A highly purified α-glucosidase from *Aspergillus niger* has been administered intravenously without success. No unfavorable reactions were observed. The liver did not diminish in size. This therapy did not modify the patient's course.

As noted earlier, the implications of substitution enzyme therapy in inherited molecular diseases may be great. Liver transplants have already begun to influence management in selected acquired (e.g., biliary atresia) and genetic diseases (e.g., hereditary tyrosinemia).[425,426] The possibility of intervention with liver transplant early in life may offer a mechanism for modifying this rapidly progressive disease.

Summary

The accumulation of an abnormal polysaccharide due to a deficiency of brancher enzyme results in pathologic changes in the reticuloendothelial system. In particular, cirrhosis occurs with progressive signs of hepatic dysfunction and, ultimately, death due to liver failure. The clinical and chemical picture cannot be distinguished from other causes of cirrhosis in infancy but is readily differentiated from hepatorenal forms of glycogen storage diseases. Identification of the abnormal glycogen in red blood cells, leukocytes, or in liver, or an analysis for the specific enzyme in fibroblasts or liver establishes the diagnosis. Liver transplant may be beneficial theoretically but has not been reported.

Glycogen Deficiency Disease

Glycogen Synthase Defect

The absence of glycogen synthase in the liver is the second clinical condition that may result from a defect in glycogen synthesis (vide supra). This is the first example of a defect in the synthetic pathway leading to inadequate glycogen formation.

First reported in 1963, a set of twins were found to be apneic at 46 and 40 hours of age prior to the initiation of feeding at 48 hours.[285] After 7 months of age, withdrawal of the night feeding was associated with pallor, transient strabismus, and then early morning convulsions prior to morning feeding. A 9-year-old girl had early morning hypoglycemia with onset after discontinuance of nighttime feeds as an infant.[427]

In another family[428] in which three prior siblings died in infancy with central nervous system signs, an infant did poorly with feedings during the first days of life, but thrived until $3\frac{1}{2}$ months of age. At 4 months she had an acute illness with 12 hours of marked lethargy and poor feeding followed by a "stiffening out spell" and unresponsiveness. She had "doll-like" facies and an enlarged liver. Her blood glucase concentration was $4\,\text{mg}\cdot100\,\text{ml}^{-1}$, although spinal fluid sugar was $40\,\text{mg}\cdot100\,\text{ml}^{-1}$. Glucagon, 3 hours after a meal, produced a prompt and significant elevation of the blood glucose concentration but had no effect after an overnight fast.

Diagnosis

Liver biopsy is necessary for enzyme analyses to establish the diagnosis. Although glycogen synthase activity has been demonstrated in the erythrocyte by Cornblath et al.[429] this tissue does not serve as a possible source for verification of the diagnosis. Erythrocytes from patients and other family members were found to contain normal glycogen synthase activity.[430] Thus, erythrocyte glycogen synthase appears to be unrelated to hepatic glycogen synthase.

A liver biopsy taken from one twin while the patient was maintained by intravenous glucose contained 0.45% glycogen and 9.8% total lipid. Histologically, there was glycogen depletion and pronounced fatty change of the liver. Enzyme studies revealed undetectable glycogen synthase activity, but normal activities of UDPG-pyrophosphorylase, phosphorylase, and glucose-6-phosphatase. Gitzelmann et al. found that the defect is not expressed in skin fibroblasts[431] or in erythrocytes.[432]

Genetics

The data are currently insufficient to establish the genetic aspects of this familial disease.

Pathogenesis

These three studies may represent a variant of the same basic defect, an absence of glycogen synthase. The pathophysiology and the precise biochemical defect remain to be defined. How glycogen synthesis occurs in the absence of this enzyme activity is unknown. Glycogen is apparently formed after meals, since there was a hyperglycemic response to glucagon at that time. This could result from the reversible phosphorylase action.[285] The failure of glycogen synthesis alone is inadequate to explain the hypoglycemia with fasting, since increased gluconeogenesis should compensate. It would appear that the inability to synthesize glycogen effectively may lead to secondary inhibition of gluconeogenesis.

Management

The management of these patients must be individualized. Dietary control with high-protein feedings appears to be effective in the mildly affected patient. When hypoglycemia is persistent and severe, raw cornstarch and/or glucocorticoid therapy may be indicated. Aynsley-Green et al.[433] were successful with frequent feedings of a high protein diet.

Prognosis

Dykes et al.[434] restudied the original family 7 years later. The twins had an improved ability to maintain a normal blood glucose concentration, but still had episodes of hypoglycemia. Glucagon responses at 3 and 20 hours after a meal were inadequate and interpreted to indicate diminished liver glycogen production. Galactose tolerance tests produced an elevation in both blood glucose and blood lactate concentrations.

Summary

A new familial disease characterized by hypoglycemia with starvation in early infancy has been associated with an absence of glycogen synthase in the liver and decreased glycogen stores. Signs of hypoglycemia may be severe, including convulsions before feeding. Diagnosis may be suspected from a failure of glucagon response after overnight fast, but requires enzyme studies of liver for its establishment.

References

1. Cornblath M, Schwartz R. Disorders of carbohydrate metabolism in infancy. Boston: Blackwell Scientific, 1991:7–10.
2. Scriver CR, Beaudet AL, Sly WS, Valle D, eds. The metabolic and molecular basis of inherited disease. 7th ed. New York: McGraw-Hill, 1995:Chapters 23–25.
3. Von Reuss A. Zuckerausscheidung im Saughlingsalter. Wien Med Wochenschr 1908;58:799–803.
4. Goppert F. Galacktosurie nach milchzuckergabe bei angelborenum, familiarem, chronischem leberleiden. Berl Klin Wochenschr 1917;54:473–477.
5. Mason HH, Turner ME. Chronic galactemia: report of case with studies on carbohydrates. Am J Dis Child 1935;50:359–374.
6. Goldbloom A, Brickman HF. Galactemia. J Pediatr 1946;28:674–691.
7. Donnell GN, Lann SH. Galactosemia. Pediatrics 1951;7:503–514.
8. Komrower GM, Schwarz V, Holzel A, Goldberg L. A clinical and biochemical study of galactosemia. Arch Dis Child 1956;31:254–264.
9. Hsia DY-Y, Walker FA. Variability in the clinical manifestations of galactosemia. J Pediatr 1961;59:872–883.
10. Hsia DY-Y. Clinical variants of galactosemia. Metabolism 1967;16:419–437.
11. Nadler HL, Inouye T, Hsia DY-Y. Classical galactosemia: a study of fifty-five cases. In: Hsia DY-Y, ed. Galactosemia. Springfield, IL: Charles C. Thomas, 1969:127–139.
12. Greenberg CR, Dilling LA, Thompson R, et al. Newborn screening for galactosemia: a new method used in Manitoba. Pediatrics 1989;84:331–335.
13. Segal S, Berry GT. Disorders of galactose metabolism. In: Scriver CR, Beaudet AL, Sly WS, Valle D, eds. The metabolic basis of inherited disease. 7th ed. New York: McGraw-Hill, 1995:967–1000.
14. Townsend EH Jr, Mason HH, Strong PS. Galactosemia and its relation to Laennec's cirrhosis; review of literature and presentation of 6 additional cases. Pediatrics 1951;7:760–773.
15. Fanconi G. Hochgradige galaktose intolerance (galaktose diabetes) bei einem kunde mit neurofibromatosis recklinghausen. Jahrbuch Kinderheilkunde 1933;138:1–8.
16. Beutler E, Blunda MC, Sturgeon P, Day RW. The genetics of galactose-1-phosphate uridyl transferase deficiency. J Lab Clin Med 1966;64:646–658.
17. Mellman WJ, Tedesco TA, Baker L. A new genetic abnormality. Lancet 1965;1:1395–1396.
18. Gitzelmann R. Deficiency of erythrocyte galactokinase in a patient with galactose diabetes. Lancet 1965;2:670–671.
19. Cuatrecasas P, Segal S. Galactose conversion to D-xylose: an alternate route of galactose metabolism. Science 1966;153:549–551.
20. Gitzelmann R. Hereditary galactokinase deficiency; a newly recognized cause of juvenile cataracts. Pediatr Res 1967;1:14–23.
21. Leloir LF. The metabolism of hexosephosphates. In: McElroy WD, Glass B, eds. Symposium on phosphorus metabolism, vol. 1. Baltimore: Johns Hopkins University Press, 1951:67–116.
22. Leloir LF. Enzymatic transformation of uridine diphosphate glucose into a galactose derivative. Arch Biochem Biophysics 1951;33:186–190.
23. Eisenberg FJR, Isselbacher KJ, Kalckar HM. Studies on metabolism of carbon-14-labelled galactose in a galactosemic individual. Science 1957;125:116–117.
24. Segal S, Blair A, Topper YJ. Oxidation of carbon-14-labelled galactose by subjects with congenital galactosemia. Science 1962;136:150–151.
25. Ng WG, Bergren WR, Donnell GN. Galactose-1-phosphate uridyl transferase activity in galactosemia. Nature 1964;203:845–847.
26. Isselbacher KJ. Evidence for an accessory pathway of galactose metabolism in mammalian liver. Science 1957;125:652–654.
27. Gitzelmann R, Curtis HC, Muller M. Galactitol excretion in the urine of a galactokinase-deficient man. Biochem Biophys Res Commun 1966;22:437–441.
28. Gitzelmann R, Steinman B, eds. Galactosemia symposium. Eur J Pediatr 1995;154(suppl):S1–S106.
29. Ellis C, Wilcox AR, Goldberg DM. Experience of routine live-birth screening for galactosemia in a British hospital

with emphasis on heterozygote detection. Arch Dis Child 1972;47:34–40.
30. Levy HL, Sepe SJ, Shih VE, et al. Sepsis due to *Escherichia coli* in neonates with galactosemia. N Engl J Med 1977;297:823–825.
31. Pesce MA, Bodourian SH. Clinical significance of plasma galactose and erythrocyte galactose-1-phosphate measurements in transferase-deficient galactosemia and in individuals with below-normal transferase activity. Clin Chem 1982;28(2):301–305.
32. Borden M. Screening for metabolic disease. In: Nyhan WL, ed. Abnormalities in amino acid metabolism in clinical medicine. Norwalk, CT: Appleton-Century, 1984:401–418.
33. Gitzelman R. Newborn screening for inherited disorders of galactose metabolism. In: Bickel H, Guthrie R, Hammersen G, eds. Neonatal screening for inborn errors of metabolism. Berlin: Springer-Verlag, 1980:67–79.
34. Paigen K, Pacholec F, Levy HL. A new method of screening for inherited disorders of galactose metabolism. J Lab Clin Med 1982;99:895–907.
35. Bowling FG, Brown ARD. Development of a protocol for newborn screening for disorders of the galactose metabolic pathway. J Inherited Metab Dis 1986;9:99–104.
36. Ng WG, Kawamura M, Donnell GN. Galactosemia screening: methodology and outcome from worldwide data collection. In: Therrell BL Jr, ed. Advances in neonatal screening. New York: Elsevier Science, 1987;243–249.
37. Schweitzer S. Newborn mass screening for galactosemia. Eur J Pediatr 1995;154(suppl 2):S37–S39.
38. Ritter JA, Cannon EJ. Galactosemia with cataracts; report of a case with notes on physiopathology. N Engl J Med 1955;252:747–752.
39. Roe TF, Hallatt JG, Donnell GN, Ng WG. Childbearing by a galactosemic woman. J Pediatr 1971;78:1026–1030.
40. Holzel A. Some aspects of galactosemia. Mod Probl Paediatr 1959;4:388 (Biblio-Paediatrica, fasc. 70).
41. Donnell GN, Collado M, Koch R. Growth and development of children with galactosemia. J Pediatr 1961;58:836–844.
42. Nelson D. Verbal dyspraxia in children with galactosemia. Eur J Pediatr 1995;154(suppl 2):S6–S7.
43. Hugh-Jones K, Newcomb AL, Hsia DY-Y. The genetic mechanism of galactosemia. Arch Dis Child 1960;35:521–528.
44. Mortensen O, Sondergaard G. Galactosemia (progress in pediatrics). Acta Paediatr 1954;43:467–477.
45. Isselbacher KJ. Galactosemia. In: Stanbury JB, Wyngaarden JB, Frederickson DS, eds. The metabolic basis of inherited diseases. New York: McGraw-Hill, 1960; 208–225.
46. Borden M. Screening for metabolic disease in abnormalities. In: Nyhan WL, ed. Amino acid metabolism in clinical medicine. Norwalk: Appleton-Century, 1984;401–418.
47. Dahlqvist A, Svenningsen NW. Galactose in the urine of newborn infants. J Pediatr 1969;75:454–462.
48. Kirkman HN. Galactosemia. Symposium on hereditary metabolic disease. Metabolism 1960;9:316–325.
49. Hsia DY-Y. Galactosemia: Biohemical methods. Charles C. Thomas, Publ. Springfield, IL. 1969:37–126.
50. Shin YS, Rieth WE, Schaub J. Prenatal diagnosis of galactosemia and properties of galactose-1-phosphate uridyl transferase in erythrocytes of galactosemic variants as well as in human fetal and adult organs. Clin Chim Acta 1983;128:271–281.
51. Rolland MO, Mandou G, Farriaux JP, Dorche C. Galactose-1-phosphate uridyl transferase activity in chorionic villus: a first trimester prenatal diagnosis of galactosemia. J Inherited Metab Dis 1986;9:284–286.
52. Holton B. Effects of galactosemia in utero. Eur J Pediatr 1995;154(suppl 2):S77–S81.
53. Allen JT, Gillett M, Holton JB, et al. Evidence of galactosemia in utero. Lancet 1980;1:603.
54. Jakobs C, Warner TG, Sweetman L, Nyhan WL. Stable isotope dilution analysis of galactitol in amniotic fluid: an accurate approach to the prenatal diagnosis of galactosemia. Pediatr Res 1984;18(4):714–718.
55. Shin-Buehring YS, Beier T, Tan A, et al. The activity of galactose-1-phosphate uridyl transferase and galactokinase in human fetal organs. Pediatr Res 1977;11:1045–1051.
56. Dahlqvist A. Test paper for galactose in urine. Scand J Clin Lab Invest 1966;18(suppl 92):101; 1968:22:87–93.
57. Cornblath M, Schwartz R. Disorders of carbohydrate metabolism in infancy. 3rd ed. Cambridge. MA: Blackwell Scientific, 1991:389–403.
58. Kelly S. Septicemia in galactosemia. JAMA 1971;216:330.
59. Shih VE, Levy HL, Karolkewicz BA, et al. Galactosemia screening of newborns in Massachusetts. N Engl J Med 1971;284:753–757.
60. Haworth JC, MacDonald MS. Reducing sugars in the urine and blood of premature babies. Arch Dis Child 1957; 32:417–421.
61. Irons M, Levy HL, Pueschel S, Castree K. Accumulation of galactose-1-phosphate in the galactosemic fetus despite maternal milk avoidance. J Pediatr 1985;107(2):261–263.
62. Gitzelmann R, Hansen RG. Galactose biogenesis and disposal in galactosemics. Biochim Biophys Acta 1974;372:374–378.
63. Gitzelmann R, Auricchio S. The handling of soya α-galactosides by a normal and a galactosemic child. Pediatrics 1965;36:231–235.
64. Holzel A, Komrower GM, Schwarz V. Low-lactose milk for congenital galactosaemia (letter to the editor). Lancet 1955;2:92.
65. Koch R, Acosta P, Ragsdale N, Donnell GN. Nutrition in the treatment of galactosemia. J Am Diet Assoc 1963; 43:216–222.
66. Donnell GN, Bergren WR, Bretthauer RK, Hansen RG. The enzymatic expression of heterozygosity in families of children with galactosemia. Pediatrics 1960;25:572–581.
67. Meera Khan P, Robson EB. Report of the committee on the genetic constitution of chromosome 9, Cytogen. Cell Genet 1978;22:106–110.
68. Levy HL, Hammersen G. Newborn screening for galactosemia and other galactose metabolism defects. J Pediatr 1978;92:871–877.
69. Reichardt JKV, Berg P. Cloning and characterization of a cDNA encoding human galactose-1-phosphate uridyl transferase. Mol Biol Med 1988;5:107–122.

70. Reichardt JKV. Galactosemia is caused by missense mutations: molecular studies and implications for therapy. Presented at the symposium "Galactosemia: New Frontiers in Research," sponsored by NICHHD and the Children's Hospital of Los Angeles, April 1989.
71. Reichardt JKV. Genetic basis of galactosemia. Human Mutat 1992;1:190–196.
72. Lai K, Langley SD, Singh RS, et al. A prevalent mutation for galactosemia among black Americans. J Pediatr 1996; 128:89–95.
73. Elsas LJ, Langley S, Steele E, et al. Galactosemia: a strategy to identify new biochemical phenotypes and molecular genotypes. Am J Hum Genet 1995;56:630–639.
74. Podskarbi T, Reichardt J, Shin YS. Studies of DNA in galactose-1-phosphate uridyl transferase deficiency and the Duarte variant in Germany. J Inherited Metab Dis 1994;17:179–150.
75. Medline A, Medline NM. Galactosemia: early structural changes in the liver. Can Med Assoc J 1972;107:877–878.
76. Bell LS, Blair WC, Lindsay S, Watson SJ. Lesions of galactose diabetes; pathological observations. Arch Pathol 1950;49:393–403.
77. Crome L. A case of galactosaemia with the pathological and neuropathological findings. Arch Dis Child 1962;37:415–421.
78. Levy HL, Driscoll SG, Porensky RS, Wender DF. Ovarian failure in galactosemia. N Engl J Med 1984;310:50.
79. Schwarz V, Goldberg L, Komrower GM, Holzel A. Some disturbances of erythrocyte metabolism in galactosemia. Biochem J 1956;62:34–40.
80. Kalckar HM, Anderson EP, Isselbacher KJ. Galactosemia, a congenital defect in a nucleotide transferase: a preliminary report. Proc Natl Acad Sci USA 1956;42:49–51.
81. Isselbacher KJ, Anderson EP, Kurahashi K, Kalckar HM. Congenital galactosemia, a single enzymatic block in galactose metabolism. Science 1956;123:635–636.
82. Gitzelmann R. Galactose-1-phosphate in the pathophysiology of galactosemia. Eur J Pediatr 1995;154(suppl 2):S45–S49.
83. Kaufman FR, Ng WG, Xu YK, et al. Treatment of patients (PTS) with classical galactosemia (G) with oral uridine. Pediatr Res 1989;25(4):142A.
84. Mitchell HS. Cataracts in rats fed on galactose. Proc Soc Exp Biol Med 1935;32:971–973.
85. Craig JM, Maddock CE. Observations on nature of galactose toxicity in rats. Arch Pathol 1953;55:118–130.
86. Lerman S. The lens in human and experimental galactosemia. NY J Med 1962;62:785–803.
87. Lerman S. The lens in congenital galactosemia. Arch Ophthalmol 1959;61:88–92.
88. Kinoshita JH. Selected topics in ophthalmic biochemistry. Arch Ophthalmol 1963;70:558–573.
89. Shin YS, Reiter K, Urban A, et al. Early manifestations of cataract in a child heterozygous for classical galactosemia and with diabetes mellitus type 1: increased plasma mannitol concentration in cataract patients. J Inherited Metab Dis 1994;17:151–153.
90. Sidbury JB Jr. The enzymatic lesions in galactosemia. J Clin Invest 1957;36:929(abstract).
91. Cusworth DC, Dent CE, Glynn FW. Amino-aciduria in galactosemia. Arch Dis Child 1955;30:150–154.
92. Hsia DY-Y, Hsia HH, Green S, et al. Amino-aciduria in galactosemia. Am J Dis Child 1954;88:458–465.
93. Urbanowski JC, Cohenford MA, Levy HL, et al. Nonenzymatically galactosylated serum albumin in a galactosemic infant. N Engl J Med 1982;306:84–86.
94. Coradello H, Pollak A, Scheibenveiter S, et al. Nichtenzymatische glykosylierung von hamoglobin und serumprotein bei kindern mit galaktosamie. Wien Klin Wochenschr 1983;95(22):804–809.
95. Segal S. Defective galactosylation in galactosemia: Is low cell UDP galactose an explanation? Eur J Pediatr 1995;154(suppl 2):S65–S71.
96. Berry GT. The role of polyols in the pathophysiology of hypergalactosemia. Eur J Pediatr 1995;154(suppl 2):S53–S64.
97. Komrower GM, Lee DH. Long-term follow-up of galactosemia. Arch Dis Child 1970;45:367–373.
98. Fishler K, Donnell GN, Bergren WR, Koch R. Intellectual and personality development in children with galactosemia. Pediatrics 1972;50:412–419.
99. Fishler K, Koch R, Donnell GN, Wenz E. Developmental aspects of galactosemia from infancy to childhood. Clin Pediatr 1980;19:38–44.
100. Gitzelmann R, Steinmann B. Galactosemia: How does long-term treatment change the outcome? Enzyme 1984; 32:37–46.
101. Jan JE, Wilson RA. Unusual late neurological sequelae in galactosemia. Dev Med Child Neurol 1973;15:72–74.
102. Packman S, Lo W, Schmidt K, et al. Neurologic sequelae in galactosemia. In: Therrell BL Jr, ed. Advances in neonatal screening. New York: Elsevier Science, 1987: 261.
103. Friedman JH, Levy HL, Boustany R-M. Late onset of distinct neurologic syndromes in galactosemic siblings. Neurology 1989;39:741–742.
104. Waisbren SE, Norman TR, Schnell RR, Levy HL. Speech and language deficits in early-treated children with galactosemia. J Pediatr 1983;102:75–77.
105. Kaufman FR, McBride-Chang C, Manis FR, et al. Cognitive functioning, neurologic status and brain imaging in classical galactosemia. Eur J Pediatr 1995;154(suppl 2):S2–S5.
106. Tedesco TA, Morrow G III, Mellman WJ. Normal pregnancy and childbirth in a galactosemic woman. J Pediatr 1972;81:1159–1161.
107. Kaufman FR, Kogut MD, Donnell GN, et al. Hypergonadotropic hypogonadism in female patients with galactosemia. N Engl J Med 1981;304:994–998.
108. Chen YT, Mattison DR, Schulman JD. Hypogonadism and galactosemia. N Engl J Med 1981;305:464–465.
109. Robinson ACR, Dockeray CJ, Cullen MJ, Sweeney EC. Hypergonadotrophic hypogonadism in classical galactosaemia: evidence for defective oogenesis. Case report. Br J Obstet Gynaecol 1984;91:199–200.

110. Kaufman FR, Donnell GN, Roe TF, Kogut MD. Gonadal function in patients with galactosaemia. J Inherited Metab Dis 1986;9:140–146.
111. Fraser IS, Shearman RP, Wilcken B, et al. Failure to identify heterozygotes for galactosaemia in women with premature ovarian failure. Lancet 1987;2(8558):566.
112. Kaufman FR, Reichardt JKV, Ng WG, et al. Correlation of cognitive, neurologic and ovarian outcome with the Q188R mutation of the galactose-1-phosphate uridyltransferase gene. J Pediatr 1994;125:225–227.
113. Beutler E, Baluda MC. An improved method for measuring galactose-1-phosphate uridyl transferase activity of erythrocytes. Clin Chim Acta 1966;13:369–379.
114. Mathai CK, Beutler E. Electrophoretic variation of galactose-1-phosphate uridyl transferase. Science 1966;154:1179–1180.
115. Gitzelmann R, Poley JR, Prader A. Partial galactose-1-phosphate uridyl transferase deficiency due to a variant enzyme. Helv Paediatr Acta 1967;22:252–257.
116. Levy HL, Sepe SJ, Walton DS, et al. Galactose-1-phosphate uridyl transferase deficiency due to Duarte/galactosemia variation: clinical and biochemical studies. J Pediatr 1978;92:390–393.
117. Kelly S. Significance of the Duarte/classical galactosemic genetic compound. J Pediatr 1979;92:937–940.
118. Segal S, Blair A, Roth H. The metabolism of galactose by patients with congenital galactosemia. Am J Med 1965;38:62–70.
119. Gitzelmann R, Hansen RG. Galactose metabolism, hereditary defects and their clinical significance. In: Burman D, Holton JB, Pennock CA, eds. Inherited disorders of carbohydrate metabolism. Lancaster: MTP Press, 1980:61–101.
120. Gitzelmann R. Deficiency of uridine diphosphate galactose 4-epimerase in blood cells of an apparently healthy infant. Helv Paediatr Acta 1972;27:125–130.
121. Holton JB, Gillett MG, MacFaul R, Young R. Galactosaemia: a new severe variant due to uridine diphosphate galactose-4-epimerase deficiency. Arch Dis Child 1981;56:885–887.
122. Brandt NJ, Forland A, Mikkelsen M, et al. Galactosemia locus and the Down's syndrome chromosome. Lancet 1963;2:700–703.
123. Dahlqvist A, Hall B, Kallen B. Blood galactose-1-phosphate uridyl transferase activity in dysplastic patients with and without chromosomal aberrations. Hum Hered 1969;19:628–640.
124. Gitzelmann R, Wells HJ, Segal S. Galactose metabolism in a patient with hereditary galactokinase deficiency. Eur J Clin Invest 1974;4:79–84.
125. Thalhammer O, Gitzelmann R, Pantlitschko MD. Hypergalactosemia and galactosuria due to galactokinase deficiency in a newborn. Pediatrics 1968;42:441–445.
126. Linneweh F, Schaumloffel E, Vetrella M. Galaktokinasedefekt bei einem neugeborenen. Klin Wochenschr 1970;48:31–33.
127. Dahlqvist A, Gamstorp I, Madsen H. A patient with hereditary galactokinase deficiency. Acta Paediatr Scand 1970;59:669–675.
128. Cook JGH, Don NA, Mann TP. Hereditary galactokinase deficiency. Arch Dis Child 1971;46:465–469.
129. Kerr MM. Logan RW, Cant JS, Hutchison JH. Galactokinase deficiency in a newborn infant. Arch Dis Child 1971;46:864–866.
130. Monteleone JA, Beutler E, Monteleone PL, et al. Cataracts, galactosuria, and hypergalactosemia due to galactokinase deficiency in a child. Am J Med 1971;50:403–407.
131. Olambiwonnu NO, McVie R, Ng WG, et al. Galactokinase deficiency in identical twins: clinical and biochemical studies. Pediatrics 1974;53:314–318.
132. Ng WG, Donnell GN, Bergren WR. Galactokinase activity in human erythrocytes of individuals at different ages. J Lab Clin Med 1965;66:115–121.
133. Vigneron C, Marchal C, Deifts C, et al. Deficit partiel et transitoire en galactokinase erythrocytaire chez un nouveau-ne. Arch Fr Pediatr 1970;27:523–531.
134. Gitzelmann R, Illig R. Inability of galactose to mobilize insulin in galactokinase-deficient individuals. Diabetologia 1969;5:143–145.
135. Gitzelmann R. Hereditary galactokinase deficiency. Citation Classics in Current Contents 1987;25:14.
136. Mayes JS. Screening for heterozygotes of the galactose enzyme deficiencies. In: Hsia DY-Y, ed. Galactosemia. Springfield, IL: Charles C. Thomas, 1969:291–296.
137. Shin-Buehring YS, Stuempfig L, Pouget E, et al. Characterization of galactose-1-phosphate uridyl-transferase and galactokinase in human organs from the fetus and adult. Clin Chim Acta 1981;112:257–265.
138. Beutler E, Matsumoto F, Kuhl W, et al. Galactokinase deficiency as a cause of cataracts. N Engl J Med 1973;288:1203–1206.
139. Schapira F, Schapira G, Dreyfus JC. La lesion enzymatique de la fructosurie benigne. Enzymol Biol Clin 1962;1:170–175.
140. Chambers RA, Pratt YTC. Idiosyncrasy to fructose. Lancet 1956;2:340.
141. Froesch ER, Prader A, Labhart R, et al. Die hereditare Fructoseintoleranz, eine bisher nicht bekannte kongenitale Stoffwechselstorung. Schweiz Med Wochenschr 1957;87:1168–1171.
142. Baker L, Winegrad AL. Fasting hypoglycemia and metabolic acidosis associated with deficiency of hepatic fructose-1,6-diphosphatase activity. Lancet 1970;2:13–16.
143. Perheentupa J, Raivio KO, Nikkila EA. Hereditary fructose intolerance. Acta Med Scand 1972;(suppl)542:65–75.
144. Nikkila EA, Huttunen JK, eds. Clinical and metabolic aspects of fructose (symposium). Acta Med Scand 1972 (suppl)542:1–244.
145. Froesch ER. Essential fructosuria and hereditary fructose intolerance. In: Stanbury JB, Wyngaarden JB, Fredricks DS, eds. The metabolic basis of inherited disease. 2nd ed. New York: McGraw-Hill, 1966:124–140.
146. Gitzelmann R, Steinmann B, Van Den Berghe G. Disorders of fructose metabolism. In: Scriver CR, Beaudet AL, Sly WS, Valle D, eds. Metabolic and molecular bases of inherited disease. 7th ed. New York: McGraw-Hill, 1995:905–934.

147. Jeune M, Planson E, Cotte J, et al. L'intolerance hereditaire au fructose. Pediatrie 1961;16:605–626.
148. Lelong M, Alagille D, Gentil J, et al. Cirrhose hepatique et tubulopathie par absence congenitale de l'aldolase hepatique. Bull Mem Soc Med Hop Paris 1962;113:58–70.
149. Lelong M, Alagille D, Gentil J, et al. L'intolerance hereditaire au fructose. Arch Fr Pediatr 1962;19:841–866.
150. Perheentupa J, Pitkanen E, Nikkila EA, et al. Hereditary fructose intolerance. A clinical study of four cases. Ann Paediatr Fenn 1962;8:221–235.
151. Cornblath M, Rosenthal IM, Reisner SH, et al. Hereditary fructose intolerance. N Engl J Med 1963;269:1271–1278.
152. Dubois R, Loeb H, Ooms HA, et al. Etude, d'un cas d'hypoglycemie fonctionelle par intolerance au fructose. Helvet Paediatr Acta 1961;16:90–96.
153. Wolfe H, Zschocke E, Wedemeyer FW, Hubner W. Angeborene hereditaire Fructose-intoleranze. Klin Wochenschr 1959;37:693–696.
154. Corsini F. L'intolleranza congenita al fruttosio. Clin Pediatr (Bologna) 1960;42:716–717.
155. Doherty RA, Williams HE, Field RA. Hereditary fructose intolerance. J Pediatr 1963;63:721(abstract).
156. Lindemann R, Gjessing LR, Merton B, Halvorsen S. Amino acid metabolism in hereditary fructosemia. Acta Paediatr Scand 1970;59:141–147.
157. Danks DM, Connellan JM, Solomon JR. Hereditary fructose intolerance: report of a case and comments on the hazards of fructose infusion. Aust Paediatr J 1972;8:282–286.
158. Kohlin P, Melin D. Hereditary fructose intolerance in four Swedish families. Acta Paediatr Scand 1968;57:24–32.
159. Baerlocher K, Gitzelmann R, Steinmann B. Clinical and genetic studies of disorders in fructose metabolism. In: Burman D, Holton JB, Pennock CA, eds. Inherited disorders of carbohydrate metabolism. Lancaster: MTP Press, 1980:163–190.
160. Steinitz H, Mizrahy O. Essential fructosuria and hereditary fructose intolerance (letter to the editor). N Engl J Med 1969;280:222.
161. Gitzelmann R, Baerlocher K. Vorteile und nachteile der fructose in der nahrung. Padiat Forbildiung Praxis 1973;37:40–55.
162. Steinman B, Baerlocher K, Gitzelmann R. Hereditare stoerungen des fruktosestoffwechsels: Belastungproben mit Fruktose, Sorbitol und Dihydroxyaceton. Nutr Metab 1975;18(suppl 1):115–132.
163. Levin B, Snodgrass GJAI, Oberholzer VG, et al. Fructosaemia. Am J Med 1968;45:826–838.
164. Rennert OM, Greer M. Hereditary fructosemia. Neurology 1970;20:421–425.
165. Cain AAR, Ryman BE. High liver glycogen in hereditary fructose intolerance. Gut 1971;12:929–932.
166. Morris RCM. An experimental renal acidification defect in patients with hereditary fructose intolerance. II. Its distinction from classic renal tubular acidosis, its resemblance to the renal acidification defect associated with the Fanconi syndrome of children with cystinosis. J Clin Invest 1968;47:1648–1663.
167. Morris RCJ. Renal tubular acidosis. N Engl J Med 1969;281:1405–1413.
168. Kranhold JF, Loh D, Morris RCJ. Renal fructose metabolizing enzymes: significance in hereditary fructose intolerance. Science 1969;165:402–403.
169. Higgins RB, Varney JK. Dissolution of renal calculi in a case of hereditary fructose intolerance and renal tubular acidosis. J Urol 1966;95:291–296.
170. Mass RE, Smith WR, Walsh JR. The association of hereditary fructose intolerance and renal tubular acidosis. Am J Med Sci 1966;251:516–523.
171. Penhoet E, Rajkumar R, Rutter WJ. Multiple forms of fructose diphosphate aldolase in mammalian tissue. Proc Natl Acad Sci USA 1966;56:1275–1282.
172. Hers HG, Joassin G. Anomalie de l'aldolase hepatique dans l'intolerance au fructose. Enzymol Biol Clin 1961;1:4–14.
173. Froesch ER, Wolfe HP, Baitsch H, et al. Hereditary fructose intolerance. An inborn defect of hepatic fructose-1-phosphate splitting aldolase. Am J Med 1963;34:151–167.
174. Metais P, Juif J, Sacrez R. Etude biochimique d'un cas d'intolerance hereditaire au fructose. Ann Biol Clin 1962;20:801–811.
175. Nikkila EA, Somersalo O, Pitkanen E, Perheentupa J. Hereditary fructose intolerance, an inborn deficiency of liver aldolase complex. Metabolism 1962;11:727–731.
176. Schapira F, Dreyfus JC. L'aldolase hepatique dans l'intolerance au fructose. Rev Fr Etud Clin Biol 1967;12:486–489.
177. Schapira F, Nordmann Y, Gregori C. Hereditary alterations of fructose metabolizing enzymes. Acta Med Scand 1972(suppl);542:77–83.
178. Nisell J, Linden L. Fructose-1-phosphate aldolase and fructose-1,6-diphosphate aldolase in the mucosa of the intestine in hereditary fructose intolerance. Scand J Gastroenterol 1968;3:80–82.
179. Morris RCJ, Euki I, Loh D, et al. Absence of renal fructose-1-phosphate aldolase activity in hereditary fructose intolerance. Nature (London) 1967:214:920–921.
180. Cross NCP, Tolan DR, Cox TM. Catalytic deficiency of human aldolase B in hereditary fructose intolerance caused by a common missense mutation. Cell 1988;53:881–885.
181. Schapira F, Nordmann Y, Dreyfus JC. La lesion biochimique de l'intolerance au fructose. Detection immunologique d'une aldolase modifiee. Rev Fr Etud Clin Biol 1968;13:267–269.
182. Schapira R, Hatzfeld A, Gregori C. Studies on liver aldolases in hereditary fructose intolerance. Enzyme 1974;18:73–83.
183. Gitzelmann R, Steinmann B, Bally C, Lebherz HC. Antibody activation of mutant human fructose diphosphate aldolase B in liver extracts of patients with hereditary fructose intolerance. Biochem Biophys Res Commun 1974;59:1270–1277.
184. Schapira F. Kinetic and immunological abnormalities of aldolase B in hereditary fructose intolerance. Proc Biochem Soc (Abstracts of Communications) 1975;3:232.
185. Perheentupa J, Raivio K. Fructose-induced hyperuricaemia. Lancet 1967;2:528–531.
186. Gentil C, Colin J, Valette AM, et al. Etude du metabolisme glucidique au cours de l'intolerance

187. Endres W, Sierck T, Shin YS. Clinical course of hereditary fructose intolerance in 56 patients. Acta Paediatr Jpn 1988;30:452–456.
188. Odievre M, Gentil C, Gautier M, Alagille D. Hereditary fructose intolerance in childhood. Am J Dis Child 1978; 132:605–608.
189. Levin B, Oberholzer VG, Snodgrass GJAI, et al. Fructosaemia, an inborn error of fructose metabolism. Arch Dis Child 1963;38:220–230.
190. Desbuquois B, Lardinois R, Gentil C, Odievre M. Effets d'une surcharge en phosphate de sodium sur l'hypoglucosemie. Arch Fr Pediatr 1969;26:21–35.
191. Grant DB, Allexander FW, Seakins JWT. Abnormal tyrosine metabolism in hereditary fructose intolerance. Acta Paediatr Scand 1970;59:432–434.
192. Willems C, Heusden A, Renson P, et al. Hypertyrosinemie avec hypermethioninemie neonatale dans un cas d'intolerance au fructose. Helv Paediatr Acta 1971;26:467–481.
193. Raju L, Chessells JM, Kemball M. Manifestation of hereditary fructose intolerance. Br Med J 1971;2:446–447.
194. Dominick H-Chr, Hosemann R, Diekmann L. Fructoseintoleranz bei 2 geschwistern. Biochemische und histologische untersuchungen. Monatsschr Kinderheilkd 1972;120:32–39.
195. Stampfler G, Heumann G, Schneegans E. Intolerance hereditaire au fructose et anomalies de la crase sanguine. Pediatrie 1972;27:169–179.
196. Bagnell P, Hug G, Walling L, Schubert WK. Biochemical and morphological observations in severe infantile fructose intolerance. Pediatr Res 1974;8:430(Abstract).
197. Baerlocher K, Gitzelmann R, Steinmann B, Gitzelmann-Cumarasamy N. Hereditary fructose intolerance in early childhood: a major diagnostic challenge. Helv Paediat Acta 1978;33:465–487.
198. Mercier JC, Bourrillon A, Beaufils F, Odievre M. Intolerance hereditaire au fructose a revelation precoce. Arch Franz Pediatr 1976;33:945–953.
199. Rossner JA, Feist D. Hereditare fructose intoleranz. Verh Dtsch Ges Pathol 1971;55:376–385.
200. Chaptal J, Jean R, Bonnet H, et al. Vomissement acetonemiques symptomatiques d'une intolerance congenitale qu fructose chez deux soeurs. Arch Fr Pediatr 1968;25:745–759.
201. Phillips JJ, Little JA, Ptak TW. Subcellular pathology of hereditary fructose intolerance. Am J Med 1968;44:910–921.
202. Saxon L, Papper S. Abdominal pain occurring during the rapid administration of fructose solutions. N Engl J Med 1957;256:132–133.
203. Mock DM, Perman JA, Thaler MM, Morris RC Jr. Chronic fructose intoxication after infancy in children with hereditary fructose intolerance. N Engl J Med 1983; 309:764–770.
204. Steinmann B, Gitzelmann R. The diagnosis of hereditary fructose intolerance. Helv Paediat Acta 1981;36:297–316.
205. Tolan DR, Penhoet EE. Characterization of the human aldolase B gene. Mol Biol Med 1986;3:245–264.
206. Klimmt G, Hubschmann K, Gmyrek D. Untersuchungen zur verminderung des fructosegehalts der Kartoffel. Ein beitrag zur diatetischen behandlung der hereditaren fructoseintoleranz. Monatsschr Kinderheilkd 1968;116:21.
207. Perheentupa J, Hallman N. Fructose intolerance. In: Gardner LI, ed. Endocrine and genetic diseases of childhood and adolescence. Philadelphia: WB Saunders, 1969:844–852.
208. Cross NC, deFranchis R, Sebastio G, et al. Molecular analysis of aldolase B genes in hereditary fructose intolerance. Lancet 1990;335:306–309.
209. Dazzo C, Tolan DR. Molecular evidence for compound heterozygosity in hereditary fructose intolerance. Am J Hum Genet 1990;46:1194–1199.
210. Brooks CC, Buist N, Tuerck J, Tolan DR. Identification of a splice-site mutation in the aldolase B gene from an individual with hereditary fructose intolerance. Am J Hum Genet 1991;49:1075–1081.
211. Tolan DR, Brooks CC. Molecular analysis of common aldolase B alleles for hereditary fructose intolerance in North Americans. Biochem Med Metab Biol 1992;48:19–25.
212. Cross NCP, Cox TM. Hereditary fructose intolerance. Int J Biochem 1990;22:685–689.
213. Ali M, Rosien U, Cox TM. DNA diagnosis of fatal fructose intolerance from archival tissue. Q J Med 1993;86:25–30.
214. Froesch ER, Ginsberg JL. Fructose metabolism of adipose tissue. I. Comparison of fructose and glucose metabolism in epididymal adipose tissue of normal rats. J Biol Chem 1962;237:3317–3324.
215. Froesch ER. Fructose metabolism in adipose tissue. Acta Med Scand 1972;(suppl)542:37–46.
216. Park CR, Johnson LH, Wright JH Jr, Batsel H. Effect of insulin on transport of several hexoses and pentoses into cells of muscle and brain. Am J Physiol 1957;191:13–18.
217. MacGregor S, Singh VN, Davoust S, et al. Evidence for formation of a rabbit liver aldolase-rabbit liver fructose-1,6-bisphosphatase complex. Proc Natl Acad Sci USA 1980;77:3889–3892.
218. Kaletta-Gmunder U, Wolf HP, Leuthardt F. Euber aldolasen. II. Chromatographische Trenning von 1-phosphofructaldolase und diphosphofructaldolase der Leber. Helv Chem Acta 1957;40:1027–1032.
219. Peanasky RJ, Lardy HA. Bovine liver aldolase. I. Isolation, crystallization and some general properties. J Biol Chem 1958;233:365–370.
220. Munnich A, Besmond C, Darquy S, et al. Dietary and hormonal regulation of aldolase B gene expression. J Clin Invest 1985;75:1045–1052.
221. Rottman WH, Tolan DR, Penhoet EE. Complete amino acid sequence for human aldolase B derived from cDNA and genomic clones. Proc Natl Acad Sci 1984;81:2738–2742.
222. Cox TM, O'Donnell MW, Camilleri M, Burghes AH. Isolation and characterization of a mutant liver aldolase in adult hereditary fructose intolerance. J Clin Invest 1983;72:201–213.

223. Oberhaensli RD, Taylor DJ, Rajagopalan B, et al. Study of hereditary fructose intolerance by use of ^{31}P magnetic resonance spectroscopy. Lancet 1987;2:931–934.
224. Gopher A, Vaisman N, Mandel H, Lapidot A. Determination of fructose metabolic pathways in normal and fructose intolerant children: A ^{13}C NMR study using [U-^{13}C]fructose. Proc Natl Acad Sci USA 1990;87:5449–5453.
225. Woods HF, Eggleston LV, Krebs HA. The cause of hepatic accumulation of fructose-1-phosphate on fructose loading. Biochem J 1970;119:501–510.
226. Morris RC Jr, McSherry E, Sebastian A. Modulation of experimental renal dysfunction of hereditary fructose intolerance by circulating parathyroid hormone. Proc Natl Acad Sci USA 1971;68:132–135.
227. Samols E, Dormandy TL. Insulin response to fructose and galactose. Lancet 1963;1:478–479.
228. Sidbury JB Jr. Zur Biochemie der hereditaren fructose-intoleranz (letter to the editor). Helvet Paediatr Acta 1959;14:317–318.
229. Hers H. Augmentation de l'activite de la glucose-6-phosphatase dans l'intolerance au fructose. Rev Int Hepatol 1962;12:777–782.
230. Thurston JH, Jonas EM, Hauhart RE. Decrease and inhibition of liver glycogen phosphorylase after fructose. Diabetes 1974;23:597–604.
231. Kaufmann U, Froesch ER. Inhibition of phosphorylase-a by fructose-1-phosphate, d-glycerophosphate and fructose-1,6-diphosphate: explanation for fructose-induced hypoglycemia in hereditary fructose intolerance and fructose-1,6-diphosphatase deficiency. Eur J Clin Invest 1973;3:407–413.
232. Van Den Berghe G, Hue L, Hers HG. Effect of the administration of fructose on the glycogenolytic action of glucagon. Biochem J 1973;134:637–645.
233. Zalitis J, Oliver IT. Inhibition of glucose-phosphate isomerase by metabolic intermediates of fructose. Biochem J 1967;102:753–759.
234. Bally C, Leuthardt F. Personal communication.
235. Landau BR, Marshall JS, Craig JW, et al. Quantitation of the pathways of fructose metabolism in normal and fructose-intolerant subjects. J Lab Clin Med 1971;78:608–618.
236. Lasker M. Essential fructosuria. Hum Biol 1941;13:51–63.
237. Nyhan WL. Inborn errors of biotin metabolism. Arch Dermatol 1987;123:1696–1698.
238. Saudubray J-M, Marsac C, Charpentier C, et al. Neonatal congenital lactic acidosis with pyruvate carboxylase deficiency in two siblings. Acta Paediatr Scand 1976;65:717–724.
239. Hommes FA, Schrijver J, Dias TL. Pyruvate carboxylase deficiency, studies on patients and on an animal model system. In: Burman D, Hallan JB, Pennook CA, eds. Inherited disorders of carbohydrate metabolism. Baltimore: University Park Press, 1979:269–286.
240. Haworth JC, Robinson BH, Perry TL. Lactic acidosis due to pyruvate carboxylase deficiency. J Inherited Metab Dis 1981;4:57–58.
241. Robinson BH, Oci J, Sherwood WG, et al. The molecular basis for the two different clinical presentations of classical pyruvate carboxylase deficiency. Am J Hum Genet 1984;36:283–294.
242. Fiser RH, Melsher HL, Fischer DA. Hepatic phosphoenolpyruvate carboxykinase deficiency: a new cause of hypoglycemia in childhood. Pediatr Res 1974;8:432 (Abstract).
243. Hommes KA, Bendien K, Elema JD, et al. Two cases of phosphoenolpyruvate carboxykinase deficiency. Acta Paediatr Scand 1976;65:233–240.
244. Vidnes J, Sovik O. Gluconeogenesis in infancy and childhood. II. Studies on the glucose production from alanine in three cases of persistent neonatal hypoglycaemia. Acta Paediatr Scand 1976;65:297–305.
245. Vidnes J, Sovik O. Gluconeogenesis in infancy and childhood. III. Deficiency of the extramitochondrial form of hepatic phosphoenolpyruvate carboxykinase in a case of persistent neonatal hypoglycaemia. Acta Paediatr Scand 1976;65:307–312.
246. Lardy HA, Bentle LA, Wagner MJ, et al. Defective phosphoenolpyruvate carboxykinase in victims of sudden infant death syndrome. National Institute of Child Health, Symposium on SIDS, July 1975.
247. Sturner WQ, Susa JB. Sudden infant death and liver phosphoenolpyruvate carboxykinase analysis. Forensic Sci Int 1980;16:19–28.
248. Baker L, Winegrad AI. Fasting hypoglycemia and metabolic acidosis associated with deficiency of hepatic fructose-1,6-dephosphatase activity. Lancet 1970;2:13–16.
249. Pagliara AS, Karl EI, Keating JP, et al. Hepatic fructose-1,6-diphosphatase deficiency. A cause of lactic acidosis and hypoglycemia in infancy. J Clin Invest 1972;51:2115–2123.
250. Baerlocher K, Gitzelmann R, Nussli R, Dumermuth G. Infantile lactic acidosis due to hereditary fructose-1,6-diphosphatase deficiency. Helv Paediatr Acta 1971;26:489–506.
251. Hulsmann WC, Fernandes J. A child with lactic-acidemia and fructose diphosphatase deficiency in the liver. Pediatr Res 1971;5:633–637.
252. Green HL, Stifel FB, Herman RH. Ketotic hypoglycemia due to hepatic fructose-1,6-diphosphatase deficiency. Treatment with folic acid. Am J Dis Child 1972;124:415–418.
253. Melancon SB, Khachadurian AK, Nadler HL, Brown BI. Metabolic and biochemical studies in fructose-1,6-diphosphatase deficiency. J Pediatr 1973;82:650–657.
254. Melancon SB, Nadler HL. Detection of fructose-1,6-diphosphatase with use of white blood cells. N Engl J Med 1972;286:731–732.
255. Saudubray JM, Dreyfus JC, Cepanec C, et al. Acidose lactique, hypoglycemie et hepatomegalie par deficit hereditaire en fructose-1,6-diphosphatase hepatique. Arch Fr Pediatr 1973;30:609–632.
256. Retbi JM. Acidose lactique et hypoglycemie par deficit congenital en fructose-1,6-diphosphatase hepatique. Thesis medicine. Paris: Rene Descartes, 1972.
257. Derosas FJ, Wapnir A, Lifshitz F, et al. Folic acid enhanced gluconeogenesis in glycerol-induced hypoglycemia and fructose-1,6-diphosphatase deficiency. The 56th An-

258. Odievre M, Brivet M, Moatti N, et al. Deficit en fructose-1,6-diphosphatase ches deux soeurs. Arch Fr Pediatr 1975;32:113–121.
259. Hopwood NJ, Holzman I, Drash AL. Fructose-1,6-diphosphatase deficiency. Am J Dis Child 1977;131:418–421.
260. Hommes FA, Campbell R, Steinhart C, et al. Biochemical observations on a case of hepatic fructose-1,6-diphosphatase deficiency. J Inherited Metab Dis 1985;8:169–173.
261. Shin YS. Diagnosis of fructose-1,6-disphosphatase deficiency using leukocytes: normal leukocyte enzyme activity in three female patients. Clin Invest 1993;71:115–118.
262. Dremsek PA, Sacher M, Stogmann W, et al. Fructose-1,6-diphosphatase deficiency: glycerol excretion during fasting test. Eur J Pediatr 1985;144:203–204.
263. Cahill J, Kirtley ME. FDPase activity in human leukocytes. N Engl J Med 1975;292:212–213.
264. Melancon SB, Nadler HL. Letter to the Editor. N Engl J Med 1975;292:212–213.
265. Schrijver J, Hommes FA. Activity of fructose-1,6-diphosphatase in human leukocytes. N Engl J Med 1975;292:1298–1299.
266. Snapper I, Van Creveld S. Un cas d'hypoglycemie avec acetonemie chez un enfant. Bull Mem Soc Med Hop (Paris) 1928;52:1315–1324.
267. Von Gierke E. Hepato-nephromegalia glycogenica (Glykogenspeicherkrankheit der leber und nieren). Beitr Pathol 1929;82:497–513.
268. Schonheimer R. Uber eine eigenartige storung des kohlehydrat-stoff-wechsels. Hoppe Seylers Z Physiol Chem 1929;182:148–150.
269. Pompe JC. Over idiopatische hypertrophie van het hart. Ned Tijdschr Geneeskd 1932;76:304–311.
270. Van Creveld S. Glycogen disease. Medicine 1939;18:1–128.
271. Van Creveld S. Investigations on glycogen disease. Arch Dis Child 1934;9:9–26.
272. Mason HH, Andersen DH. Glycogen disease. Am J Dis Child 1941;61:795–825.
273. Debre R. Les polyconles. Paris: Gaston Doin, 1947.
274. Andersen DH. Studies on glycogen disease with report of a case in which the glycogen was abnormal. In: Najjar VA, ed. Carbohydrate metabolism. Baltimore: Johns Hopkins University Press, 1952:28–42.
275. McArdle B. Myopathy due to a defect in muscle glycogen breakdown. Clin Sci 1951;10:13–35.
276. Stetten D Jr, Stetten MR. Glycogen metabolism. Physiol Rev 1960;40:505–537.
277. Hers H-G, Van Hoof F, de Barsy T. Glycogen storage diseases. In: Scriver CR, Beaudet AL, Sly WS, Valle D, eds. The metabolic basis of inherited disease. 6th ed. New York: McGraw-Hill, 1989:425–452.
278. Cori GT. Glycogen structure and enzyme deficiencies in glycogen storage disease. Harvey Lect (1952–53) 1954; 48:145–171.
279. Hers HG. Glycogen storage disease. In: Levine R, Luft R, eds. Advances in metabolic disorders. vol. 1. New York: Academic Press, 1964:1–44.
280. Spencer-Peet J, Norman ME, Lake BD, et al. Hepatic glycogen storage disease. Q J Med 1971;157:95–114.
281. Moses SW. Pathophysiology and dietary treatment of the glycogen storage diseases. J Pediatr Gastroenterol 1990;11:155–174.
282. Brown DH, Brown BI. Some inborn errors of carbohydrate metabolism. In: Whelan WJ, ed. MTP International review of science, vol. 5. Biochemistry of carbohydrates. London: Butterworth; Baltimore: University Park Press, 1975:391–426.
283. Cori GT, Cori CF. Glucose-6-phosphatase of the liver in glycogen storage disease. J Biol Chem 1952;199:661–667.
284. Hers HG. Glucosidase deficiency in generalized glycogen storage disease (Pompe's disease) Biochem J 1963;86:11.
285. Lewis GM, Spencer-Peet J, Stewart KM. Infantile hypoglycemia due to inherited deficiency of glycogen synthase in liver. Arch Dis Child 1963;38:40.
286. Van Creveld S. The Blackader lecture, 1962: the clinical course of glycogen disease. Can Med Assoc J 1963;88:1–15.
287. Fine RN, Wilson WA, Donnell GN. Retinal changes in glycogen storage disease type I. Am J Dis Child 1968;115:328–331.
288. Schulman JL, Saturen P. Glycogen storage disease of the liver. 1. Clinical studies during the early neonatal period. Pediatrics 1954;14:632–643.
289. Fernandes J, Pikaar NA. Ketosis in hepatic glycogenosis. Arch Dis Child 1972;47:41–46.
290. Nilsson IM, Ockerman PA. Bleeding disorder in hepatomegalic forms of glycogen storage disease. Acta Paediatr Scand 1970;59:127–133.
291. Zeller WP, Cornblath M, Schwartz HC, Schwartz R. Minor hemoglobins in disorders of carbohydrate metabolism. J Pediatr 1981;98:936–938.
292. Brante G, Kaijser K, Ockerman PA. Glycogenosis type I (lack of glucose-6-phosphatase) in four siblings. Acta Paediatr Scand 1964;(suppl)157:1–28.
293. Howell R, Ashton DM, Wyngaarden JB. Glucose-6-phosphatase deficiency glycogen storage disease. Studies on the interrelationships of carbohydrate, lipid and purine abnormalities. Pediatrics 1962;29:553–565.
294. Folkman J, Philippart A, Tze WJ, Crigler J JR. Portocaval shunt for glycogen storage disease: value of prolonged intravenous hyperalimentation before surgery. Surgery 1972;72:306–314.
295. Sidbury JB, Cornblath M, Fisher J, House E. Glycogen in erythrocytes of patient with glycogen storage disease. Pediatrics 1961;27:103–111.
296. Williams HE, Field JB. Further studies on leukocyte phosphorylase in glycogen storage disease. Metabolism 1963;12:464–466.
297. Williams HE, Kendig EM, Field JB. Leukocyte debranching enzyme in glycogen storage disease. J Clin Invest 1963;42:656–660.
298. Sokal JE, Lowe CU, Sarcione EJ, et al. Studies of glycogen metabolism in liver glycogen disease (von Gierke's

disease): six cases with similar metabolic abnormalities and responses to glucagon. J Clin Invest 1961;40:364–374.
299. Perkoff GT, Parker VJ, Hahn RF. The effects of glucagon in three forms of glycogen storage disease. J Clin Invest 1962;41:1099–1105.
300. Schwartz R, Ashmore J, Renold AE. Galactose tolerance in glycogen storage disease. Pediatrics 1957;19:585–595.
301. Illingworth B. Glycogen storage disease. Am J Clin Nutr 1961;9:683–690.
302. Tada K, Narisawa K, Igarashi Y, Kato S. Glycogen storage disease type IB: a new model of genetic disorders involving the transport system of intracellular membrane. Biochem Med 1985;33:215–222.
303. Villee CA. The intermediary metabolism of human fetal tissues. Cold Spring Harb Symp Quant Biol 1954;19:186–199.
304. Kalhan SC, Gilfillan C, Tserng K-Y, Savin SM. Glucose production in type I glycogen storage disease. J Pediatr 1982;101:159–160.
305. Tsalikian E, Simmons P, Gerich JE, et al. Glucose production and utilization in children with glycogen storage disease type I. Am J Physiol 1984;247:E513–E519.
306. Mason HH, Sly GE. Blood lactic acid in liver glycogen disease. Proc Soc Exp Biol 1943;53:145–147.
307. Oberhaensli RD, Rajagopalan B, Taylor DJ, et al. Study of liver metabolism in glucose-6-phosphatase deficiency (glycogen storage disease type 1A) by P-31 magnetic resonance spectroscopy. Pediatr Res 1988;23:375–380.
308. Fine RN, Strauss J, Donnell GN. Hyperuricemia in glycogen-storage disease type I. Am J Dis Child 1966;112:572–576.
309. Roe TF, Kogut MD. The pathogenesis of hyperuricemia in glycogen storage disease, type I. Pediatr Res 1977;11:664–669.
310. Fernandes J, Berger R, Smith GPA. Lactate as a cerebral metabolic fuel for glucose-6-phosphatase deficient children. Pediatr Res 1984;18:335–339.
311. Leonard JW, Dunger DB. Hypoglycaemia complicating feeding regimens for glycogen storage disease. Lancet 1978;2:1203–1204.
312. Fine RN, Kogut MD, Donnell GN. Intestinal absorption in type I glycogen storage disease. J Pediatr 1969;75:632–635.
313. Moses SW, Gutman A. Inborn errors of glycogen metabolism. Adv Pediatr 1972;19:95–169.
314. Resnick MB, Kozakewich HPW, Perez-Atayde AR. Hepatic adenoma in the pediatric age group. Am J Surg Pathol 1995;19(10):1181–1190.
315. Roe T, Kogut M, Buckingham B, et al. Hepatic tumors in glycogen storage disease type 1. Clin Res 1978;26:191A.
316. Grossman H, Ram PC, Coleman RA, et al. Hepatic ultrasonography in type I glycogen storage disease (von Gierke disease). Radiology 1981;141:753–756.
317. Brunelle F, Tammam S, Odierre M, Chaumont P. Liver adenomas in glycogen storage disease in children. Pediatr Radiol 1984;14:94–101.
318. Chen YT, Coleman RA, Scheinman JI, et al. Renal disease in type 1 glycogen storage disease. N Engl J Med 1988;381:7–11.
319. Restaino I, Stanley C, Baker L, et al. Renal tubular abnormalities and nephrocalcinosis in patients with type Ia glycogen storage disease. Pediatr Res 1990;27(4):337A.
320. Greene HL, Slonim AE, O'Neill JA Jr, Burr IM. Continuous nocturnal intragastric feeding for management of type 1 glycogen storage disease. N Engl J Med 1976;294:423–425.
321. Stanley CA, Mills JL, Baker L. Intragastric feeding in type I glycogen storage disease: factors affecting the control of lactic acidemia. Pediatr Res 1981;15:1504–1508.
322. Chen Y-T, Cornblath M, Sidbury JB. Cornstarch therapy in type I glycogen storage disease. N Engl J Med 1984;310:171–175.
323. Fernandes J, Leonard JV, Moses SW, et al. Glycogen storage disease: recommendations for treatment. Eur J Pediatr 1988;147:226–228.
324. Kalhan S, Rossi K. Glucose kinetics in type I and type III glycogen storage disease. In: Chapman TE, Berger R, Reijngoud DJ, eds. Stable isotopes in pediatrics nutritional and metabolic research. London: Intercept, 1990:237–247.
325. Starzl TE, Putnam CW, Porter KA, et al. Portal diversion for the treatment of glycogen storage disease in humans. Ann Surg 1973;178:525–539.
326. Johnson MP, Compton A, Drugan A, Evans MI. Metabolic control of von Gierke disease (glycogen storage disease type Ia) in pregnancy: maintenance of euglycemia with cornstarch. Obstet Gynecol 1990;75:507–510.
327. Lei K-J, Shelly LL, Pan C-J, et al. Mutations in the glucose-6-phosphatase genes that cause glycogen storage disease type 1a. Science 1993;262:580–583.
328. Lei K-J, Pan C-J, Shelly LL, et al. Identification of mutations in the gene for glucose-6-phosphatase, the enzyme deficient in glycogen storage disease type 1a. J Clin Invest 1994;93:1994–1999.
329. Lei K-J, Shelly LL, Lin B, et al. Mutations in the glucose-6-phosphatase gene are associated with glycogen storage disease type 1a and 1aSP, but not 1b and 1c. J Clin Invest 1995;95:234–240.
330. Lei K-J, Pan C-J, Liu J-L, et al. Structure-function analysis of human glucose-6-phosphatase, the enzyme deficient in glycogen storage disease type 1a. J Biol Chem 1995;270(20):11882–11886.
331. Lei K-J, Chen Y-T, Chen H, et al. Genetic basis of glycogen storage disease type 1a: prevalent mutations at the glucose-6-phosphatase locus. Am J Hum Genet 1995;57:766–771.
332. Kajihara S, Matsuhashi S, Yamamoto K, et al. Exon redefinition by a point mutation within exon 5 of the glucose-6-phosphatase gene is the major cause of glycogen storage disease type 1a in Japan. Am J Hum Genet 1995;57:549–555.
333. Parvari L, Moses S, Hershkovitz E, et al. Characterization of the mutations in the glucose-6-phosphatase gene in Israeli patients with glycogen storage disease type 1a: R83C in six Jews and a novel V166G mutation in a Muslim Arab. J Inherited Metab Dis 1995;18:21–27.
334. Field JB, Epstein S, Egan T. Studies in glycogen storage disease. I. Intestinal glucose-6-phosphatase activity in pa-

tients with von Gierke's disease and their parents. J Clin Invest 1965;44:1240–1247.
335. Senior B, Loridan L. Studies of liver glycogenoses, with particular reference to the metabolism of intravenously administered glycerol. N Engl J Med 1968;279:958–964.
336. Narisawa K, Igarashi Y, Otomo H, et al. A new variant of glycogen storage disease type 1 probably due to a defect in the glucose-6-phosphate transport system. Biochem Biophys Res Commun 1978;83:1360–1364.
337. Nordlie RC, Sukalski KA, Munoz JM, et al. Type 1c, a novel glycogenosis: underlying mechanisms. J Biol Chem 1983;258:9739–9744.
338. Shin YS, Rieth M, Tansendfreund J, Endres W. A sensitive radioisotopic method for glucose-6-phosphatase assay and diagnosis of glycogenosis type 1b using polymorphonuclear leukocytes. Personal communication.
339. Bashan N, Potashnik R, Hagai Y, Moses SW. Impaired glucose transport in polymorphonuclear leukocytes in glycogen storage disease Ib. J Inherited Metab Dis 1987;10:234–241.
340. Bashan N, Hagai Y, Potashnik R, Moses SW. Impaired carbohydrate metabolism of polymorphonuclear leukocytes in glycogen storage disease Ib. J Clin Invest 1988; 81:1317–1322.
341. Seger R, Steinmann B, Tiefenauer L, et al. Glycogenosis Ib: neutrophil microbicidal defects due to impaired hexose monophosphate shunt. Pediatr Res 1984;18:297–299.
342. Koven ML, Clark MM, Cody CS, et al. Impaired chemotaxis and neutrophil (polymorphonuclear leukocyte) function in glycogenosis type IB. Pediatr Res 1986;20:438–442.
343. Illingworth B, Cori GT. Structure of glycogens and amylopectins. III. Normal and abnormal human glycogen. J Biol Chem 1952;199:653–660.
344. Forbes GB. Glycogen storage disease. J Pediatr 1953;42: 645–653.
345. Van Creveld S, Huijing F. Differential diagnosis of the type of glycogen disease in two adult patients with long history of glycogenosis. Metabolism 1964;13:191–194.
346. Hug G, Krill CE Jr, Perrin EV, Guest GM. Cori's disease (amylo-1,6-glucosidase deficiency). N Engl J Med 1963; 268:113–120.
347. Fernandes J, Koster JF, Grose WF, Sorgedrager N. Hepatic phosphorylase deficiency. Its differentiation from other hepatic glycogenoses. Arch Dis Child 1974;49:186–191.
348. Moses SW, Chayoth R, Levin S, et al. Glucose and glycogen metabolism in erythrocytes from normal and glycogen storage disease type III subjects. J Clin Invest 1968;47: 1343–1348.
349. Huijing F. Enzymes of glycogen metabolism in leukocytes in relation to glycogen-storage disease. In: Whelan WJ, ed. Control of glycogen metabolism. Oslo: Oslo University Press (Universitetsforlaget), 1968:115–128.
350. Illingworth B, Cori GT, Cori CF. Amylo-1,6-glucosidase in muscle tissue in generalized glycogen storage disease. J Biol Chem 1956;218:123–129.
351. Ding SH, de Barsy T, Brown BI, et al. Immunoblot analyses of glycogen debranching enzyme in different subtypes of glycogen storage disease type III. J Pediatr 1990;116: 95–100.
352. Neustein HB. Fine structure of skeletal muscle in type III glycogenosis. Arch Pathol 1969;88:130–136.
353. Powell HC, Haas R, Hall CL, et al. Peripheral nerve in type III glycogenosis: selective involvement of unmyelinated fiber Schwann cells. Muscle Nerve 1985;8:667–671.
354. Garty BZ, Dinari G, Nitzan M. Transient acute cortical blindness associated with hypoglycemia. Pediatr Neurol 1987;3:169–170.
355. Moses SW, Gadoth N, Bashan N, et al. Neuromuscular involvement in glycogen storage disease type III. Acta Paediatr Scand 1986;75:289–296.
356. Moses SW, Wanderman KL, Myroz A, Frydman M. Cardiac involvement in glycogen storage disease type III. Eur J Pediatr 1989;148:764–766.
357. Bridge EM, Holt LE Jr. Glycogen storage disease; observations on the pathologic physiology of two cases of the hepatic form of the disease. J Pediatr 1945;27:299–315.
358. Fernandes J, Vande Kamer JH. Hexose and protein tolerance tests in children with liver glycogenosis caused by a deficiency of the debranching enzyme system. Pediatrics 1968;41:935–944.
359. Levin S, Moses SW, Chayoth R, et al. Glycogen storage disease in Israel. Isr J Med Sci 1967;3:397–410.
360. Van Creveld S, Huijing F. Glycogen storage disease. Biochemical and clinical data in sixteen cases. Am J Med 1965;38:554–561.
361. Huijing F, Obbink HJK, Van Creveld S. Activity of the debranching enzyme system in leukocytes. Acta Genet (Basel) 1968;18:128–136.
362. Milunsky A, Littlefield JW, Kanfer JN, et al. Prenatal genetic diagnosis. N Engl J Med 1970;283:1370–1381.
363. Ding JH, Harris DA, Bing-Zi Y, Chen YT. Cloning of cDNA for human muscle glycogen debrancher, the enzyme deficient in type III glycogen storage disease. Pediatr Res 1989;25:140A.
364. Hers HG, Van-Hoof F, DeBarsey T. The glycogen storage diseases. In: Scriver CR, Beaudet AL, Sly WS, Valle D, eds. The metabolism basis of inherited disease. 6th ed. New York: McGraw-Hill, 1989:425–452.
365. Yang BZ, Ding HG, Enghild JJ, et al. Molecular cloning and nucleotide sequence of cDNA encoding human muscle glycogen debranching enzyme. J Biol Chem 1992; 267:9294–9299.
366. Yang BZ, Ding HG, Bao Y, et al. Molecular basis of the enzymatic variability in type III glycogen storage disease (GSD III). Am J Hum Genet 1992;51(Suppl):A28.
367. Bao Y, Yang BZ, Chen YT. Structural organization of the multifunctional human glycogen debrancher gene. Am J Hum Genet 1993;53:662A.
368. Yang-Feng TL, Zheng K, Yu J, et al. Assignment of the human glycogen debrancher gene to chromosome 1p21. Genomics 1992;13:931–934.
369. Mishori-Dery A, Bashan N, Moses S, et al. RFLPs for linkage analysis in families with glycogen storage disease type III. J Inherited Metab Dis 1995;18:207–210.

370. Hers HG. Etudes enzymatiques sur fragments hépatiques; application a la classification des glycogenosés. Rev Int Hepatol 1959;9:35–55.
371. Lamy M, Dubois R, Rossier A, et al. La glycogenose par defici. Arch Fr Pediatr 1960;17:14–37.
372. Hulsmann WC, Oei TL, Van Creveld S. Phosphorylase activity in leukocytes from patients with glycogen storage disease. Lancet 1961;2:581–583.
373. Williams HE, Field JB. Low leukocyte phosphorylase in hepatic phosphorylase deficient glycogen storage disease. J Clin Invest 1961;40:1841–1845.
374. Willems PJ, Gerver WJ, Berger R, Fernandes J. The natural history of liver glycogenesis due to phosphorylase kinase deficiency: a longitudinal study of 41 patients. Eur J Pediatr 1990;149:268–271.
375. Christiansen RO, Page LA, Greenberg RE. Glycogen storage in a hepatoma: dephosphorylase kinase defect. Pediatrics 1968;42:694–696.
376. Hug G, Garancis JC, Schubert WK, Kaplan S. Glycogen storage disease, type II, III, VII and IX. Am J Dis Child 1966;111:457–474.
377. Hug G, Schubert WK, Chuck G. Deficient activity of dephosphorylase kinase and accumulation of glycogen in the liver. J Clin Invest 1969;48:704–715.
378. Huijing F, Fernandes J. X-Chromosomal inheritance of liver glycogenosis with phosphorylase kinase deficiency. Am J Hum Genet 1969;21:275–284.
379. Baussan C, Moatti N, Odievre M, Lemonnier A. Liver glycogenosis caused by a defective phosphorylase system. Hemolysate analysis. Pediatrics 1981;67:107–112.
380. Shin YS, Rieth M, Tausenfreund J, et al. Clinical and biochemical variability of phosphorylase B, kinase deficiency: its differentiation using erythrocyte parameters. Personal communication.
381. Tuchman M, Brown BI, Burke BA, Ulstrom RA. Clinical and laboratory observations in a child with hepatic phosphorylase kinase deficiency. Metabolism 1986;35:627–633.
382. Lederer B, Van Hoof F, Vanden Berghe G, Hers HG. Glycogen phosphorylase and its converter enzymes in haemolysates of normal human subjects and of patients with type VI glycogen storage disease. A study of phosphorylase kinase deficiency. Biochem J 1975;147:23–35.
383. Newgard CB, Fletterick RJ, Anderson LA, Lebo RV. The polymorphic locus for glycogen storage disease VI (liver glycogen phosphorylase) maps to chromosome 14. Am J Hum Genet 1987;40:351–364.
384. Francke U, Darras BT, Zander NF, Kiliman MW. Assignment of human genes for phosphorylase kinase subunits alpha (PHKA) to Xq12-q13 and beta (PHKB) to 16q12-q13. Am J Hum Genet 1989;45:276–282.
385. Larner J, Villar-Palasi C. Enzymes in glycogen storage myopathy. Proc Natl Acad Sci USA 1959;45:1234–1235.
386. Schmid R, Robbins PW, Traut RR. Glycogen synthesis in human muscle lacking phosphorylase. Proc Natl Acad Sci USA 1959;45:1236–1240.
387. Schmid R, Mahler R. Chronic progressive myopathy with myoglobinuria; demonstration of a glycogenolytic defect in the muscle. J Clin Invest 1959;38:2044–2058.
388. Pearson CM, Rimer DG, Mommaerts WFHM. A metabolic myopathy due to absence of muscle phosphorylase. Am J Med 1961;30:502–517.
389. Andres R, Cader G, Zierler KL. The quantitatively minor role of carbohydrate in oxidative metabolism by skeletal muscle in intact man in the basal state. Measurements of oxygen and glucose uptake and carbon dioxide and lactate production in the forearm. J Clin Invest 1956;35:671–682.
390. Mahler RF, McArdle B. Specific enzyme defect in glycogen breakdown causing a myopathy. Q J Med 1960;29:638 (Abstract).
391. Schmid R, Hammaker L. Hereditary absence of muscle phosphorylase (McArdle's syndrome). N Engl J Med 1961;264:223–225.
392. Lebo RV, Gorin F, Fletterick RJ, et al. High resolution chromosome sorting and DNA spot-blot analysis assign McArdle's syndrome to chromosome 11. Science 1984;225:57–59.
393. Tarui S, Okuno G, Ikara Y, et al. Phosphofructokinase deficiency in skeletal muscle. A new type of glycogenosis. Biochem Biophys Res Commun 1965;19:517–523.
394. Okuno G, Hizukuri S, Nishikawa M. Activities of glycogen synthetase and UDPGA-pyrophosphorylase in muscle of a patient with a new type of muscle glycogenosis caused by phosphofructokinase deficiency. Nature (Lond) 1966;212:1490–1491.
395. Tarui S, Koni N, Nasu T, Nishikawa M. Enzymatic basis for the co-existence of myopathy and hemolytic disease inherited muscle phosphofructokinase deficiency. Biochem Biophys Res Commun 1969;34:77–83.
396. Layzer RB, Rowland LP, Ranney HM. Muscle phosphofructokinase deficiency. Arch Neurol 1967;17:512–523.
397. DiSant'Agnese PA, Andersen DH, Mason HH, Bauman WA. Glycogen storage disease of the heart. I. Report of two cases in siblings with chemical and pathologic studies. Pediatrics 1950;6:402–424.
398. Brown BI, Zellweger H. α-1,4-glucosidase activity in leucocytes from the family of two brothers who lack this enzyme in muscle. Biochem J 1966;101:16C.
399. Nihill MR, Wilson DS, Hugh-Jones R. Generalized glycogenosis type II (Pompe's disease). Arch Dis Child 1070;45:122–129.
400. Dincsoy MY, Dincsoy HP, Kessler AD, et al. Generalized glycogenosis and associated endocardial fibroelastosis. J Pediatr 1965;67:728–740.
401. Clement DH, Godman GC. Glycogen disease resembling mongolism, cretinism and amyotonia congenita. J Pediatr 1950;36:11–30.
402. Kahana D, Telem C, Steinitz K, Solomon M. Generalized glycogenosis. J Pediatr 1964;65:243–251.
403. deBarsy T, Ferriere G, Fernandez-Alvarez E. Uncommon case of type II glycogenosis. Acta Neuropathol 1979;47:245–247.
404. Huijing F, Van Creveld S, Losekoot G. Diagnosis of generalized glycogen storage disease (Pompe's disease). J Pediatr 1963;63:984–987.
405. Lejeune N, Thines-Sempoux D, Hers HG. Tissue fractionation studies. 16. Intracellular distribution and properties of α-glucosidases in rat liver. Biochem J 1963;86:16–21.

406. Dancis J, Hutzler L, Lynfield L, Cox RP. Absence of acid maltase in glycogenosis type 2 (Pompe's disease) in tissue culture. Am J Dis Child 1969;117:108–111.
407. Nitowsky HM, Gounefeld A. Lysosomal α-glucosidases in type II glycogenosis. J Lab Clin Med 1967;69:472–484.
408. Nadler HG, Messina AM. In utero detection of type II glycogenosis (Pompe's disease). Lancet 1969;2:1277–1278.
409. Cox RP, Douglas G, Hutzler J, et al. In utero detection of Pompe's disease. Lancet 1970;1:893.
410. Shin YS, Rieth M, Tausenfreund J, Endres W. First trimester diagnosis of glycogenosis type II and type III. J Inherited Metab Dis 1989;12(suppl 2):289–291.
411. Bashan N, Potashnik R, Barash V, et al. Glycogen storage disease type II in Israel. Isr J Med Sci 1988;24:224–227.
412. Reuser AJJ, Koster JF, Hoogeveen A, et al. Biochemical, immunological and cell genetic studies in glycogenosis type II. Am J Hum Genet 1978;30:132–143.
413. D'Ancona GG, Wurm J, Croce CM. Genetics of type II glycogenosis: assignment of the human gene for acid alpha-glucosidase to chromosome 17. Proc Natl Acad Sci USA 1977;76:4526–4529.
414. Kleijer WJ, Vander Kraan M, Kroos MA, et al. Prenatal diagnosis of glycogen storage disease type II; enzyme assay or mutation analysis? Pediatr Res 1995;38:103–106.
415. Niermeijer MF, Kostar JF, Jahodova M, et al. Prenatal diagnosis of type II glycogenosis (Pompe's disease) using microchemical analyses. Pediatr Res 1975;9:498–503.
416. Besancon A-M, Gastelnau L, Nicolesco H, et al. Prenatal diagnosis of glycogenesis type II (Pompe's disease) using chorionic villi biopsy. Clin Genet 1985;27:479–482.
417. Grubisic A, Shin YS, Meyer W, et al. First trimester diagnoses of Pompe's disease (glycogenosis type II) with normal outcome: assay of acid α-glucosidase in chorionic villus biopsy using antibodies. Clin Genet 1986;30:298–301.
418. Reuser AJJ, Kroos MA, Hermans MMP, et al. Glycogenosis type II (acid maltase deficiency). Muscle Nerve 1995;18(suppl 3):S61–S69.
419. Brown BI, Brown DH. Lack of an α-1,4 glucan: α-1,4-glucan 6 glycosyl transferase in a case of type IV glycogenosis. Proc Natl Acad Sci USA 1966;56:725–729.
420. Shin YS, Steiguber H, Klemm P, et al. Branching enzyme in erythrocytes. Detection of type IV glycogenosis homozygotes and heterozygotes. J Inherited Metab Dis 1988;11(2):252–254.
421. Fernandes J, Huijing F. Branching enzyme-deficiency glycogenosis: studies in therapy. Arch Dis Child 1968;43:347–352.
422. Levin B, Burgess EA, Mortimer PE. Glycogen storage disease type IV, amylopectinosis. Arch Dis Child 1968;43:548–555.
423. Sidbury JB Jr, Mason J, Burns WB Jr, Reubner BH. Type IV glycogenosis. Report of a case proven by characterization of glycogen and studied at necropsy. Bull Johns Hopkins Hosp 1962;111:157–181.
424. Reed DB JR, Dixon LFP, Neustein HB, et al. Type IV glycogenosis. Lab Invest 1968;19:546–557.
425. Starzl TE, Zifelli BJ, Shaw BW, et al. Changing concepts of liver replacement for hereditary tyrosinemia and hepatoma. J Pediatr 1985;106:604–606.
426. Kleinman RE, Vacanti JP. Liver transplantation. In: Walker WA, Durie P, Hamilton JE, et al., eds. Pediatric gastrointestinal disease: pathophysiology, diagnosis and management. Ontario: BC Decker, 1991:1108–1124.
427. Aynsley-Green A, Williamson DH, Gitzelmann R. Hepatic glycogen synthetase deficiency. Definition of syndrome from metabolic and enzyme studies on a 9-year-old girl. Arch Dis Child 1977;52:573–579.
428. Parr J, Teree TM, Larner J. Symptomatic hypoglycemia, visceral fatty metamorphosis and aglycogenosis in an infant lacking glycogen synthetase and phosphorylase. Pediatrics 1965;35:770–777.
429. Cornblath M, Steiner DF, Bryan P, King J. Uridinediphosphoglucose glucosyl glucosyltransferase in human erythrocytes. Clin Chim Acta 1965;12:27–32.
430. Spencer-Peet J. Erythrocyte glycogen synthetase in glycogen storage deficiency resulting from the absence of this enzyme from liver. Clin Chim Acta 1964;10:481–483.
431. Gitzelmann R, Steinmann B, Aynsley-Green A. Hepatic glycogen synthetase deficiency not expressed in cultured skin fibroblasts. Clin Chim Acta 1983;130:111–115.
432. Gitzelmann R, Aynsley-Green A, Williamson DH. Blood cell glycogen synthetase activity in hepatic glycogen synthetase deficiency. Clin Chim Acta 1977;79:219–221.
433. Aynsley-Green A, Williamson DH, Gitzelmann R. The dietary treatment of hepatic glycogen synthetase deficiency. Helv Paediatr Acta 1977;32:71–75.
434. Dykes JRW, Spencer-Peet J. Hepatic glycogen synthetase deficiency. Further studies on a family. Arch Dis Child 1972;47:558–563.

34
Neonatal Protein Metabolism

Willi E. Heine

All living matter is based on the existence of protein. Protein plays an important role as the structural element of cells and extracellular matter, as the essential component of enzymes and hormones, as antibodies, and as many other endogenous compounds. Together with nucleic acids, protein forms inheritance factors that precisely reproduce the composition of numerous body proteins. Even minute changes in these factors can lead to severe disruption of protein metabolism.

Protein consists of only a few building blocks, including about 20 essential and nonessential amino acids and, as in the case of glycoproteins, various carbohydrates. The amino acids are assembled by intracellular enzymes to form proteins with different amino acid sequences, chain lengths, and three-dimensional structures. In this manner an enormous variety of proteins is constantly being synthesized.

All body proteins are in a state of continuous breakdown and renewal.[1] Birth and death of all living beings is permanently reflected in cells and tissues by protein synthesis and breakdown at the molecular level. Anabolism and catabolism rates differ among the various groups of organ proteins and are influenced by age, illness, and other conditions. Some 30% to 40% of the total body protein is involved in a steady flux.

In the fetus, total protein is 8.5% of the body weight. This percentage increases to about 11% at birth, approaches a maximum of about 17.5% in the adult, and declines with advancing age. Most of the protein of the adult is stored in striated muscle (46.8%), followed by the skeleton (18.6%), the skin (9.2%), and the adipose tissue (3.6%). The muscle mass constitutes about 43% of the total body mass in adults and about 21% in a 1.7 kg preterm neonate.[2] Hemoglobin accounts for 7.4% and albumin for 2.5% of the total body protein.[3] In the normal adult, the amount of metabolizable protein is estimated to be 6000 g. The amount of free tissue amino acids is 35 g, whereas the total masses of essential and nonessential plasma amino acids are only 0.2 g and 0.5 g, respectively.[4]

In the normal adult, body protein is in a state of dynamic equilibrium between protein synthesis and protein breakdown. Predominance of synthesis, as is the case in infancy and childhood, corresponds to net accumulation, whereas predominance of breakdown corresponds to net loss of body protein. Growth and aging, fasting, metabolic and hormonal disturbances, and infectious and traumatic diseases are known to affect this equilibrium. The steady state of protein metabolism is influenced by diurnal meal-related rhythms in the protein stores in different organs. Intake of protein-containing foods is accompanied by increased protein synthesis, leading to a net protein accumulation in the liver and other organs, followed by a corresponding net protein depletion between meals. Discontinuous secretion of human growth hormone and other anabolic hormones may change the equilibrium between protein synthesis and protein breakdown. For maintenance of the protein stores of the body, overall protein synthesis and protein breakdown are balanced over a period of 24 hours (see Chapter 6).

Molecular Biologic Aspects

Protein synthesis in mammalian cells is the result of a complicated interaction of various components. It takes place in the cell cytoplasm by interaction between ribosomes, messenger RNA (mRNA), transfer RNA (tRNA), amino acids, adenosine triphosphate (ATP), guanosine triphosphate (GTP), and numerous enzymes that catalyze the steps in protein synthesis. RNA is synthesized in the cell nucleus. RNA is the structural element in ribosomal RNA (rRNA), a carrier of amino acid sequence information (mRNA), and a chemical link between nucleic and amino acids (tRNA)[5] (see Chapters 3 and 4).

Access to the genetic code of DNA is gained by transcription of DNA into RNA. All single-stranded RNA molecules are inherently asymmetrical, having 5' and 3' ends. The primary RNA transcript is subsequently polyadenylized enzymatically at its 3' end. The 3' end of mRNA corresponds to the carboxy-terminal end of the protein, whereas the 5' end of the molecule corresponds to the amino-terminal end of the protein coded by the mRNA (Figure 34.1).

The transcribed RNA, a precursor of mRNA, is processed by removing RNA from the corresponding DNA sequences separating the coding regions. The originating mature mRNA is released from the cell nucleus into the cytoplasm, where it affixes to ribosomes. Its genetic information, which is read from the 5' to the 3' end, governs the order in which amino acids are linked by peptide bonds to form protein.

The amino acids are activated by 20 aminoacyl tRNA synthetases, each of which is specific for one particular amino acid. They are bonded to several tRNAs, carried to the ribosome, and linked to the peptide chain at its amino-terminal end. Translation takes place in three phases. Peptide chain initiation consists of establishment of the first peptide bond after the mRNA binds to the ribosome. The subsequent incorporation of amino acids into the growing peptide chain is called elongation; the completion of synthesis-release of the newly formed peptide chain and the mRNA from the ribosome is called termination. The mRNA molecule breaks down into its nucleotide building blocks, which can be used for the resynthesis of RNA.

In addition to adenine, guanine, cytosine, and uracil (i.e., the four main bases), the RNA species contain small quantities of modified components produced by various modifying enzymes during transcription. In contrast to the original nucleosides, the modified (i.e., methylated) nucleosides are not usually metabolized and reutilized, but are excreted renally.[6]

The turnover of rRNA is indicated by pseudouridine; 7-methylguanine and N^2,N^2-dimethylguanosine indicate the turnover of mRNA and tRNA, respectively. The ways that cells communicate with each other to stimulate protein synthesis have been unraveled more precisely in recent years. The signal transfer is brought about by numerous proteins, hormones, and growth factors that adhere to specialized receptors on the surface of the target cells. Insulin and growth factors such as epithelial growth factor and platelet-derived growth factor are known as the most important messengers that play a key role in initiating cellular protein synthesis. The pathway by which insulin initiates the process of translation after its binding to the receptor on the surface of protein synthesizing cells such as skeletal muscle fibers involves at least six intermediate proteins and enzymes before the signal activates an enzyme called mitogen activated protein (MAP) kinase. MAP kinase activates an intracellular

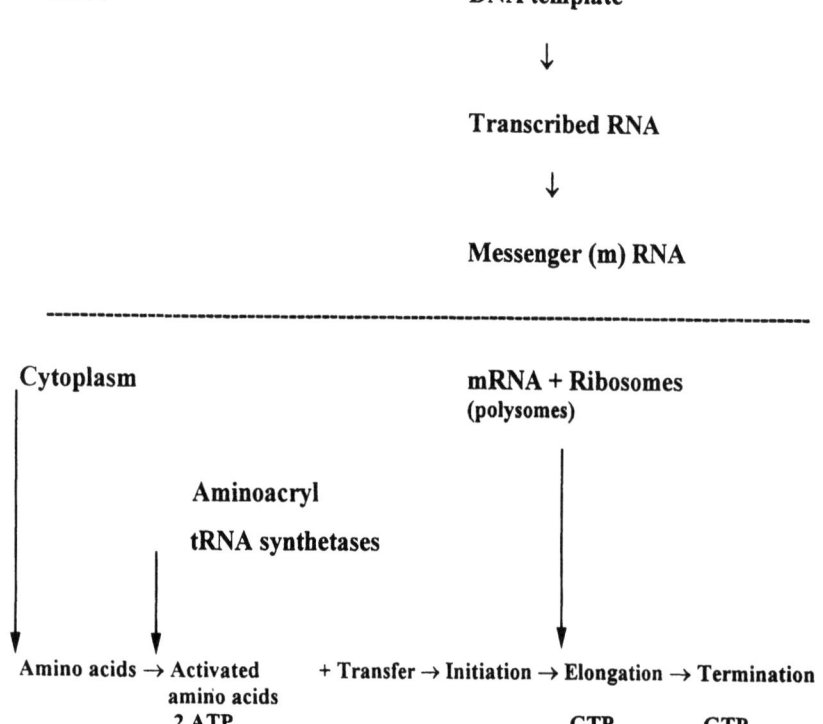

FIGURE 34.1. Formation of mRNA and its translation for protein synthesis.

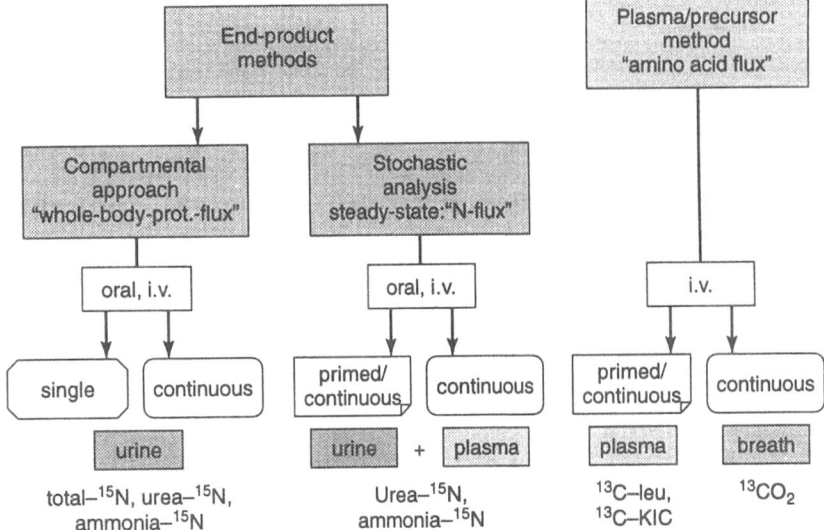

FIGURE 34.2. Methods for estimating whole-body protein parameters.

protein named PHASE-1 by phosphorylation, which together with other factors, initiates the mRNA-mediated translation process.[7]

Changes in the portion of tissue cells during the course of growth are accessible by DNA analysis. The DNA content of a diploid cell nucleus in humans is 6pg. The DNA concentration may serve for calculating the number of cells in an organ, whereas the protein-DNA relationship reflects the mean size of the cells.[8]

Protein synthesis is an energy-consuming process. The binding of amino acids to tRNA by aminoacyl tRNA synthetases requires two high-energy bonds from ATP for each amino acid. An additional high-energy bond from GTP is required for peptide chain elongation, and another is needed for the translation process. Four high-energy bonds are needed for each amino acid added to the peptide chain. The total mature cellular RNA consists of 70% to 80% rRNA, 15% to 20% tRNA, and 2% to 4% mRNA. The efficiency of the translational apparatus can be either enhanced or inhibited by changing the level or the activity of rate-limiting protein factors taking part in the process of translation. However, translation can be very specifically controlled by single mRNA or class of mRNA molecules acting on the initiation level. The specific knowledge of these mechanisms may become important in view of the development of new drugs and antisensitization technology directed to the expression of single proteins.[9]

Methods for Estimating Whole-Body Protein Parameters

The various approaches to measuring whole-body protein turnover have been compiled and critically reviewed by Waterlow et al. and Wolfe et al.[10–13] This chapter presents a comprehensive summary of the methods currently used to estimate whole-body protein parameters during the neonatal period. The sum of all protein synthesis and protein breakdown rates at any given time in the body is called the whole-body protein turnover. This parameter is closely related to energy metabolism and energy balance. The energy requirement for protein synthesis represents a significant fraction of the total metabolic rate in the neonate. In this connection, protein turnover is far more important for estimating protein metabolism than the classic nitrogen balance measurement. Current determinations for whole-body protein turnover are based on either compartmental or stochastic analysis and on amino acid kinetics plasma precursor methods (Figure 34.2).

Compartment Analysis

Compartment analysis uses the three-pool model originally proposed by Sprinson and Rittenberg[14] and its various modifications subsequently introduced by others. Winkler's modification is shown in Figure 34.3. With the three-pool model, cumulative ^{15}N excretion data can be used to calculate protein synthesis, protein breakdown, protein turnover, size of the nonprotein nitrogen pool, and endogenous urea excretion and nitrogen reutilization rates. The symbols used by Winkler and Faust[15,16] and the mathematical equations for calculating the above parameters, where K_{31} = protein excretion constant and K_{21} = protein synthesis constant, are as follows:

Metabolic (nonprotein) pool $\quad = Q_1 = \dfrac{R_{31}}{K_{31}}$

Protein synthesis $= R_{21} \quad = Q_1 \cdot K_{21}$

Protein degradation $\quad = R_{12} = R_{21} + R_{31} - R_{10}$

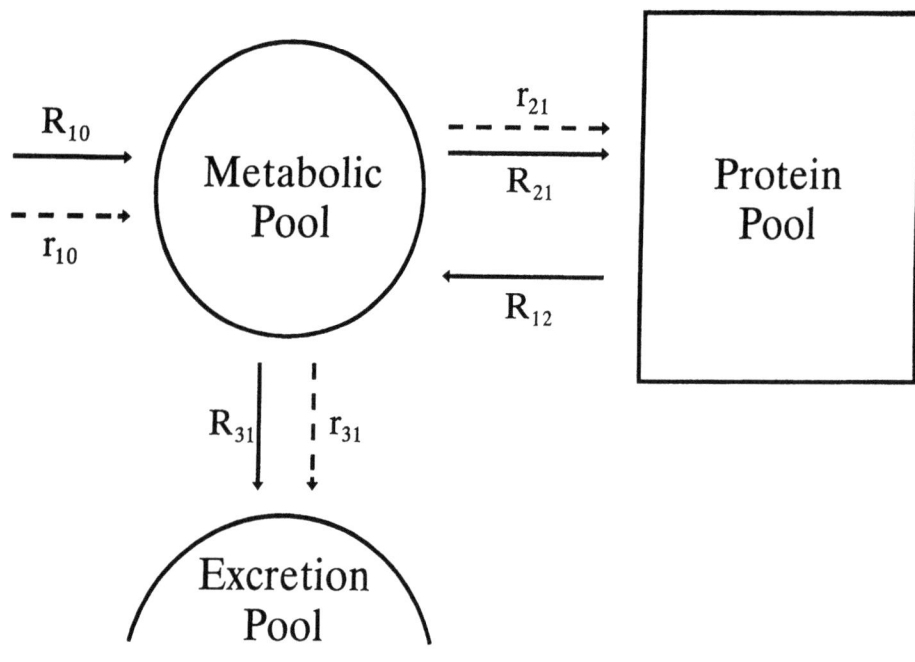

FIGURE 34.3. Three-pool model. Note the flux of nitrogen between the metabolic pool, protein pool, and excretion pool. R, flux of unlabeled nitrogen; r, flux of labeled nitrogen; R_{10}, intake of unlabeled nitrogen; r_{10}, intake of labeled nitrogen; R_{31}, excretion of unlabeled nitrogen; r_{31}, excretion of labeled nitrogen.

Rate of protein N gain $= R_{21} - R_{12}$

Protein turnover (flux) $= R_{21} + R_{31}$

Rate of endogenous urine N excretion (fraction of urinary) N derived from protein breakdown) $N = \dfrac{R_{31} \cdot R_{21}}{R_{21} + R_{31}}$

N reutilization rate = R_{12} – R of endogenous urine N $= \dfrac{R_{31} \cdot R_{12}}{R_{21} + R_{31}}$

Fractional reutilization rate $= \dfrac{R_{reut}}{R_{12}} \cdot 100$

Half-life of q_1 $= \dfrac{ln_2}{K_{21} + K_{31}}$

The calculation of flux rates and pool sizes has been described in detail by Plath et al.[17] and Wutzke et al.[18]

One of the indispensable assumptions for using the three-compartment model is the undisturbed renal excretion of nitrogen end products and water—a condition that is generally not fulfilled in the early neonatal period. For this reason and due to the rapid recycling of the tracer, the excretion plateau of ^{15}N in urinary nitrogen is frequently not reached in preterm infants. The order of magnitude of protein turnover rates, as determined by this method in the preterm infant, is decisively dependent on the amino acids used as tracer substances.

Stochastic Analysis

Stochastic analysis focuses on the overall metabolism of labeled substrates and ignores the various pools and components implicated in whole-body protein turnover. The tracers are administered either as a single bolus or by continuous infusion. If constant isotope infusion is used (i.e., if an isotope equilibrium is established), the existence of the various pools becomes irrelevant.

The constant-infusion technique was introduced by Picou and Taylor-Roberts[19] in 1969 using ^{15}N-glycine. The prerequisites for this model are a constant metabolic pool size during infusion, no recycling of the ^{15}N, no isotope discrimination, no difference in metabolism of amino acids from dietary intake and endogenous protein degradation, and the validity of ^{15}N-glycine as a tracer representing the total amino nitrogen.

The single-dose technique has the advantage of being suitable for clinical use, as it requires less effort. The rate of elevation to plateau level during constant infusion is equivalent to the inverse slope of the curve after single-pulse labeling.

Methods Relying on Amino Acid Kinetics

Parallel with the development of more sensitive mass spectrometers, methods for determining protein turnover rates relying on amino acid kinetics have been introduced (see Chapter 1). The tracer most commonly used with these methods is L-[1-^{13}C]leucine. Leucine is an essential amino acid and cannot be synthesized de novo.

The first step in tracer metabolism is deamination to [1-^{13}C]ketoisocaproic acid (KiCa). This metabolite is the precursor of all leucine oxidation. By its oxidative decarboxylation, $^{13}CO_2$ is released and exhaled by the lung. This pathway is used to measure the leucine oxidation rate by means of the [^{13}C]leucine breath test (see Chapter

2). Leucine oxidation varies inversely with the supply of carbohydrates.[20]

During constant infusion of [^{13}C]leucine, the tracer concentration in the plasma and expired air reaches a steady state within 1.5 to 2.0 hours after the infusion is begun.[21] Whole-body protein turnover can be estimated from the leucine oxidation rate measured via the $^{13}CO_2$ breath test and the [^{13}C]leucine level and [^{13}C]KiCa enrichment in the plasma (i.e., flux) as measured by gas chromatography-mass spectrometry. The estimation is based on the assumption that the whole-body protein consists of 7.8% leucine. This method has been validated for the human neonates in a comparison with [^{15}N]glycine techniques by Millward et al.[22]

There are objections to the use of labeled leucine as a tracer for measuring protein turnover rate.[23] Leucine kinetics are not representative of whole-body protein dynamics. The postabsorptive leucine flux of the plasma compartment may differ from that of other amino acids. Protein synthesis rates determined with L-[^{13}C]leucine are influenced by dietary leucine intake. Errors may result from the stimulation of insulin secretion by leucine and its degradation product, ketoisocaproic acid. This would simulate higher synthesis and accretion rates.

All these methods use intravenous tracer infusion and require repeated blood sampling. The necessity of developing noninvasive, economic, simple tracer kinetic methods that do not stress the patient and are ethically acceptable for metabolic studies has been repeatedly emphasized by Waterlow.[24] In pediatrics, these requirements are best satisfied by oral single-pulse labeling using reliable, stable isotope tracers. Protein turnover parameters can be calculated from the cumulative renal excretion of the nitrogen isotope by computer.

Protein Synthesis

Perinatal protein synthesis differs in many aspects from that in later life. The metabolic situation of the neonate is characterized by sudden interruption of the placental circulation. The availability of substrate for protein synthesis (e.g., amino acids, glucose, fatty acids, and glycerol) that was supplied throughout the fetal period by the parenteral route is abruptly interrupted by ligation of the umbilical cord. Substrate supply by the enteral route normally does not meet all requirements until the 7th day of postnatal life. The neonate is initially fasting and depends on glycogen, fat, and stored protein to maintain homeostasis. Although full-term neonates have sufficient energy stores for 28 days of survival without food intake, the survival of small premature neonates under such conditions is limited to approximately 4 days. This situation is due mainly to disruption of the protein metabolism owing to the severe reduction in protein supply. Further differences compared to later life are caused by the stress of delivery, expressed by fundamental changes in the hormonal patterns influencing protein, carbohydrate, and fat metabolism (Table 34.1).

In many respects the hormonal changes during the perinatal period resemble the hormonal disequilibrium caused by stress. Concentrations of hormones with counterregulatory effects (e.g., catecholamines, glucocorticosteroids, and growth hormone) are significantly elevated. These changes may be even more marked in stressed neonates after complicated deliveries. The postnatal hormonal situation can be considered an ingenious regulation mechanism to achieve adequate gluconeogenesis from gluconeogenic amino acids, lactate, and glycerol following the depletion of stored glycogen. It is comparable with the known stress-induced metabolic changes associated with a dangerous reduction in protein supply. This situation is enhanced because only half of the amino acids forming the protein are known to be suitable for gluconeogenesis. The elevation of (i.e., counterregulatory) hormone concentrations is accompanied by resistance of the peripheral tissues to insulin.

The role of prostaglandins, functioning as mediators in the hormonal control of protein metabolism in the neo-

TABLE 34.1. Hormonal changes influencing protein metabolism in the neonate.

Hormone	Concentration in plasma	Comments
Growth hormone	↑ to ↑↑	Diminishes to normal range after the 2nd week of life
Insulin-like growth factor	↓	Remains low until 3–5 years of age
ACTH	↑	↑↑ in cord blood
Cortisol	↑	↑↑ in mothers before delivery
17-Hydroxyprogesterone	↑	↑↑ in cord blood
Testosterone	(↑)	Higher values in male neonates
Epinephrine	↑	Higher values in preterm neonates
Norepinephrine	↑	
Insulin	(↑)	Increasing after stimulation (sucking and food intake)
Prostaglandins	↑	?

natal period, is not well known. Inhibition of prostaglandin synthesis by indomethacin and similar anti-inflammatory drugs can obviously improve muscle protein turnover.[25]

The increased renal nitrogen excretion, one of the most important components of the metabolic situation in the neonatal period, is due mainly to corticosteroids and glucagon. Renal nitrogen losses during the perinatal period are less serious than those associated with catabolism, possibly due to the concomitant increase in catecholamines, growth hormone, and androsterones.[26] Glucocorticosteroids and glucagon are known to have different effects on protein metabolism in the liver and muscle. Although they stimulate the synthesis of acute-phase protein in the liver, they also inhibit protein synthesis in the muscle. In this manner, amino acids that are released from the muscle can be used as a substrate for gluconeogenesis in the liver. However, the capacity for providing sufficient amounts of amino acids from protein breakdown in the muscle is restricted in the neonate, as the neonatal muscle mass per kilogram of body weight is only 50% of the corresponding value for the adult. The hormonal changes occurring during the neonatal period in response to stress and especially their influence on the link between protein metabolism and gestational age, adaptational difficulties, neonatal infection, and other complications are not completely understood. Special interest has been directed to the side effects of the therapeutical use of corticosteroids on neonatal protein metabolism.

Scott and Watterberg[27] described a reverse relationship between gestational age and plasma cortisol concentration in the postnatal preterm infants. The highest values were measured in the youngest infants. While healthy neonates of more than 27 weeks of gestational age showed a decrease of their cortisol concentrations from day 2 to day 6, ill infants were found to have increasing cortisol concentrations in this period of life. As corticosteroids are known to result in protein wasting, it is to be expected that these hormonal changes contribute to an excessive degradation of endogenous protein. Corresponding effects were reported due to corticosteroid treatment. Dexamethasone administered for bronchopulmonary dysplasia results in deterioration of nitrogen balance and increases the urinary 3-methylhistidine excretion, indicating loss of muscle tissue.[28] Protein breakdown and turnover rates were increased when measured on day 4 of dexamethasone treatment, whereas protein synthesis remained unchanged.[29]

Energy Requirements for Protein Synthesis

Among the fractional costs of energy expenditure, protein turnover rate is the highest energy demanding process in the neonatal period.[30] However, the exact effect of protein turnover on neonatal energy expenditure is not known. This is due to the diverging results obtained from the different methods for measurement of protein turnover currently in use.

The relationship between protein synthesis and energy requirements may be explained by some practical examples. The synthesis of one peptide bond requires four high-energy bonds from ATP and GTP.[10] Suppose a protein with a molecular weight of 48,000 daltons(d) has 400 peptide bonds. One mole of glucose is known to yield 38 mol of ATP under aerobic conditions, but only 2 mol of ATP under anaerobic conditions. For the synthesis of 48,000 g = 1 mol of protein, 1600 mol of ATP would be necessary, corresponding to 7578 g of glucose. The adult protein synthesis rate of $3 g \cdot kg^{-1} day^{-1}$ would require an energy equivalent of 0.57 g glucose, or 0.76 kcal/g protein synthesized.

The estimated protein synthesis rate of $12 g \cdot kg^{-1} day^{-1}$ for small preterm neonates would correspond to a demand of 2.27 g glucose. A protein synthesis rate of about $26 g \cdot kg^{-1} day^{-1}$ for neonates would require a glucose demand of around $5.0 g \cdot kg^{-1} day^{-1}$. This amount is probably half the amount of glucose that can be tolerated without inducing hyperglycemia in this age group and would exceed the volume and osmolality of fluids that can be administered clinically (see Chapter 32). These calculations do not include the additional energy requirement for protein degradation and the lower energy production from glucose under anaerobic conditions. From this point of view, the elevated protein synthesis rates reported for neonates in the past seem incredibly high and are probably a result of methodologic errors. The efficiency of protein gain in growing neonates (e.g., the relation between protein intake and protein gain) is affected by the biologic value of the food protein, the energy/protein ratio, perinatal growth-regulating factors, nutritional status, and intercurrent diseases. In very low birth weight neonates, 65% to 70% of the absorbed amino acids are used for protein accretion, and the remaining 30% to 35% are oxidized.[31]

Methods for establishing the metabolic cost of protein gain do not yield reliable results. The in vivo metabolic cost of protein gain was found to be $10 kcal \cdot g^{-1}$.[31] Based on an energy need of 6 mol ATP for the incorporation of 1 mol amino acid into the polypeptide chain, the cost of protein gain would be only $1 kcal \cdot g^{-1}$. This discrepancy may be explained by the high order of magnitude of protein synthesis and breakdown in the preterm and term neonate, provided the turnover is really 10 times higher than in later life, which is apparently not the case.

Protein Degradation

The importance of protein degradation is not as well known as that of protein synthesis. The high protein synthesis rates of the term and preterm neonate, as determined by tracer kinetic studies, are always accompanied by high protein breakdown rates. The energy supply for protein degradation appears to be necessary to maintain the acidic internal pH of the lysosomes, for protein transport into the lysosomes, and for the formation of organelles.[11] The exact energy requirement for protein degradation is not easily determined, as protein synthesis and breakdown are normally closely related. It seems certain that additional ATP consumption is needed for protein degradation and has to be considered when calculating the energy expenditure of the neonate.

Reutilization of Nitrogen from Protein Breakdown

The rate of reutilization of α-amino nitrogen from intracellular protein breakdown can be calculated from the protein synthesis rate and the rate of endogenous urinary nitrogen. The reutilization of nitrogen from amino acids reflects an adaptation to low protein intake and serves to maintain and increase the protein stores. Breast-feeding is generally accompanied by high reutilization rates of endogenous nitrogen, which provides for low urea synthesis rates and allows saving of energy.

Although the degradation of amino acids yields energy, a relatively large proportion is lost. This is due to the use of the degradation products for the synthesis of numerous body compounds and to energy-consuming processes such as urea and creatinine synthesis. Low-protein diets lead to a low serum urea concentration, which may reflect inadequate protein intake.[32] Diets high in protein may lead to elevated urea and α-amino nitrogen serum concentrations, indicating metabolic overloading. Large food protein intakes reduce the reutilization of amino acids derived from the cellular breakdown of protein. In preterm neonates (mean birth weight 2060 ± 4.5 g and 22.4 ± 6.8 days of age) receiving mother's milk, an endogenous nitrogen excretion rate of 2.13 ± 0.84 mg (0.152 ± 0.06 mmol)·kg^{-1}hr^{-1} was measured on day 16, whereas the corresponding value on a formula diet containing 1.8% protein was 4.12 ± 0.49 mg (0.294 ± 0.035 mmol)·kg^{-1}hr^{-1} on day 27 ($p < .005$). The corresponding reutilization rates were 94.63% and 89.67%, respectively. The endogenous nitrogen excretion rate and total renal nitrogen excretion were the only nitrogen metabolism parameters differing significantly between the human milk and protein-rich formula diets.[33]

In another group of five preterm neonates with a mean age of 30.4 ± 2.0 completed weeks of gestation and a mean body weight of 1592 ± 517 g fed on pooled human milk, the reutilization rate of endogenous nitrogen was 96% and 97%, at 31.6 ± 1.9 weeks' and 34.4 ± 1.9 weeks' gestation, respectively.[34] The reutilization of endogenous nitrogen on an oligopeptide diet used for dietary management of infants with diarrhea ranged between 74% and 91% (average 83%).[35] The lower reutilization rate on an oligopeptide diet and on a cow's milk–based formula than on a human milk diet correlates with the higher nitrogen intake, the chemical score of the peptides and proteins, and the additional losses of endogenous protein due to diarrhea. The reutilization of endogenous nitrogen does not involve only the α-amino nitrogen of amino acids from protein breakdown. There is evidence that urea nitrogen is at least partially reutilized. The urea content of mother's milk is approximately 300 mg·L^{-1}. Following administration of [^{15}N]urea-enriched human milk to six infants with a mean age of 1.4 months, nitrogen retention from the labeled urea was 16.7% to 61.4% (mean 40%) of the intake.[36] Fomon et al.,[37] feeding a formula diet with 1.5% protein, observed [^{15}N]urea nitrogen retention rates of only 13% for protein synthesis. This low rate may be due to the higher endogenous urea production rate on formula than on a human milk diet, differences in health status, or the greater age of the latter group. On a mother's milk diet, nitrogen retention from [^{15}N]urea was found to be only slightly higher than on a formula diet. The differences between the utilization rates of urea nitrogen reported by Heine et al.[36] and Fomon et al.[37,38] are probably due to differences in age and birth weight. In studies on preterm infants conducted by Donovan et al.,[39] the ^{15}N nitrogen retention from ^{15}N was 28% on average, whereas Wheeler et al.[40] reported on ^{15}N retention rates amounting to 90% of the recycled urea.

The results of these studies indicate that urea nitrogen from mother's milk is not fully available for protein synthesis, as hypothesized previously. The rate of nitrogen retention from dietary and endogenous urea is rather low in healthy neonates. It may increase if protein intake is low and protein needs are high during early infancy in premature neonates, and during catch-up growth.

After postnatal colonization of the intestinal tract, microbial nitrogen is available as an additional source for whole-body protein synthesis. Studies with oral and colonic administration of ^{15}N-labeled bifidobacteria revealed an absorption of 83% and retention of 73% of the microbial nitrogen within the protein pool.[41]

Nitrogen Balance

Nitrogen balance is defined as the difference between dietary nitrogen intake and nitrogen excretion. Definitions of the various nitrogen fractions used for nitrogen balance studies are given in Table 34.2.

The nitrogen content of biologic matter is conventionally determined by the Kjeldahl method. Another more rapid method based on the controlled combustion of the nitrogen-containing material in an oxygen stream and subsequent measurement of NO_2 by gas chromatography has been introduced.

TABLE 34.2. Nitrogen fractions used for nitrogen balance studies.

Fraction	Definition
Endogenous nitrogen (U_0)	Urinary nitrogen on nitrogen-free diet
Metabolic nitrogen (F_0)	Fecal nitrogen on nitrogen-free diet
Dietary nitrogen (D)	Nitrogen from food intake during test
Urinary nitrogen (U)	Urinary nitrogen under test conditions
Fecal nitrogen (F)	Fecal nitrogen during test
Nitrogen balance	$D - (U + F)$
Absorbed nitrogen	$D - (F - F_0)$
Digestibility (%)	$\dfrac{\text{Absorbed nitrogen} \times 100}{\text{Dietary nitrogen}}$
Retained nitrogen	$D - (F - F_0) - (U - U_0)$
Biologic value	$\dfrac{\text{Retained N}}{\text{Absorbed N}} \times 100$
Net protein value	Digestibility × biologic value

Modified from Beaton,[42] with permission.

Nitrogen is generally excreted renally as urea and ammonia. Fecal excretion of nitrogen may increase during the perinatal period as a result of diarrhea, maldigestion, malabsorption, and malexcretion. In such cases fecal nitrogen losses, which are normally neglected in nitrogen balance calculations, must be taken into account. Further nitrogen losses in sweat, skin cells, hair, and gaseous nitrogen are comparatively low and are generally ignored in nitrogen balance calculations. In very small premature neonates fecal losses amount to 10% of the gross nitrogen intake, and another 30% is excreted in the urine. The nitrogen retention is 60% of the intake.[31] During the first days of postnatal life the nitrogen balance of very small premature neonates is usually negative despite combined parenteral and enteral nutrition. Plath et al.[43] studied the nitrogen balance in 22 appropriate for gestational age (AGA) premature neonates on days 2, 4, 7, 14, 21, and 28 of postnatal life. Parenteral nutrition was initiated with a 10% glucose solution and was continued for 6 hours after birth with a mixture of 10% glucose and 4% amino acid solution in a 2:1 ratio. Pooled raw human milk feeding was introduced on days 2 to 4, with a gradual increase of milk amounts thereafter. The nitrogen balance became positive on day 7 of the feeding regimen (Table 34.3). At the beginning of the 2nd week of postnatal life, 60% of the nitrogen intake from human milk was retained. Fecal nitrogen losses amounted to 10% of the food nitrogen administered.

Positive nitrogen balance can be obtained earlier if fat emulsions are administered in addition.[44] As a source of energy, medium-chain triglycerides seem to improve the postnatal nitrogen balance of the preterm neonate better than long-chain triglycerides. Further improvement of the early postnatal nitrogen and energy balance can be considered to be both a crucial problem as well as a challenge in improving the care of the premature neonate. In full-term neonates receiving human milk, nitrogen retention is 200 to 240 mg·kg^{-1}day^{-1} at 2 weeks of age, 170 to 190 mg·kg^{-1}day^{-1} at 1 month, and 90 to 130 mg·kg^{-1} day at 3 months of age.[45] At higher protein intakes, nitrogen retention exceeds the calculated protein accretion even if "accelerated maturation" of the cells (e.g., a rapid increase in their nitrogen concentration) is assumed.[46,47]

There is a lack of information concerning the nitrogen balance of full-term neonates during the first days of life. Term neonates fed colostrum seem to achieve positive nitrogen balances 2 to 3 days after birth, although they continue to lose body weight during the first 7 days. This phenomenon is based on a dissociated balance between energy and protein metabolism, leading to a decrease in fat and fat-free body mass and a gain in protein.[30] Origi-

TABLE 34.3. Nitrogen intake, excretion, absorption, and retention in eight AGA preterm neonates.

Postnatal age (days)	Nitrogen intake (mg·kg^{-1}day^{-1})			Nitrogen excretion		Nitrogen absorption		Nitrogen retention	
	Oral	Parenteral	Total	Renal	Fecal	mg·kg^{-1}day^{-1}	%	mg·kg^{-1}day^{-1}	%
2	43.8 ± 88.4	202.6 ± 20.1	246.4 ± 78.8	379.8 ± 202.5	14.4 ± 9.1 (4%)	232.0 ± 73.4	94	−147.7 ± 231.0	−60
4	83.2 ± 130.5	205.7 ± 77.25	288.9 ± 62.4	396.3 ± 112.9	20.0 ± 17.7 (5%)	269.0 ± 61.3	93	−127.4 ± 125.6	−44
7	231.5 ± 108.1	97.4 ± 80.9	328.9 ± 39.0	223.1 ± 140.0	22.7 ± 9.3 (9%)	306.2 ± 37.0	91	83.2 ± 141.1	25
14	411.2 ± 47.7		411.2 ± 47.7	131.3 ± 44.8	45.1 ± 15.3 (10%)	366.1 ± 42.2	89	235.8 ± 68.8	57
21	430.5 ± 75.0		430.5 ± 75.0	116.4 ± 36.9	42.9 ± 13.1 (11%)	387.6 ± 73.6	90	271.2 ± 85.9	63
28 (29)	402.7 ± 95.4		402.7 ± 95.4	111.6 ± 40.4	34.6 ± 9.0 (10%)	368.1 ± 102.9	91	256.5 ± 116.2	64

Aged 2 to 29 days, mean gestational age 30.3 ± 1.5 completed weeks, mean body weight 1430 ± 270 g; fed on human milk, initially supported by administration of parenteral amino acid-glucose infusions.
From Plath et al.,[43] with permission.

nally it was assumed that the nitrogen balance of term and preterm neonates fed mature human milk remains negative for a longer period.[48] This conclusion needs to be reevaluated.

Nitrogen balance is mainly based on urinary excretion of urea, ammonia, and other nitrogen-containing degradation products. Urine excretion is known to be low, and urea clearance and renal concentration capacity are below normal during the early neonatal period.[26] This situation may cause retention of nitrogen-containing substances, which are usually excreted in the urine and simulate positive nitrogen balance. Irregularities in defecation frequency may contribute to methodologic errors in nitrogen balance studies during the early postnatal period. Because the minimum endogenous nitrogen loss amounts to approximately $0.9\,g$ protein $g\cdot kg^{-1}day^{-1}$, a positive nitrogen balance can hardly be expected in neonates fed on mother's milk before the 5th postnatal day. Higher nitrogen intake on formula diets may shorten this period. The limitations of the nitrogen balance method, especially during neonatal life, do not permit more accurate conclusions.

Net Protein Gain

Apart from late fetal life, there is no other period in life where growth and protein accretion are as intensive as immediately after birth. The postnatal period is characterized by further physiologic and metabolic maturation, which involves changes in the chemical composition of the body, such as increases in nitrogen content of cells and tissues. Protein accretion is usually measured by means of nitrogen balance. The total protein concentration of the human fetal body increases from the beginning of the perinatal period (e.g., the 20th week of gestation) from $22.5\,g$ (7.5% of body weight) to $388\,g$ (12.7%) at birth and approximately $469\,g$ (11.7%) at the end of the perinatal period (28 days after birth).[49,50] The relative contribution of isoleucine, lysine, methionine, phenylalanine, tryosine, and valine to the total amino acids in the body is similar to the concentration of these amino acids in plasma, but leucine is about twice as high and threonine 2.4 times lower in the fetal body. The levels of these two amino acids in the total fetal body are similar to those in mother's milk.

The differences between the nonessential amino acid concentrations in fetal plasma and those in the fetal body are more marked, especially for glycine. The glycine content has been found to be 3.5 times higher in the fetal body than in the fetal plasma and 5.6 times higher than in breast and cow's milk. These differences between extracellular and intracellular amino acid concentrations indicate the difficulty of comparing these concentrations in the two compartments. The increments of amino acids in fetal life calculated from amino acid analysis of the fetal body can be used to estimate daily postnatal requirements and may indicate the adequacy of human milk as a source of amino acids.

Widdowson et al.,[50] taking a 1000-g body as an example, stated that the amino acids in 200 ml of breast milk are just about sufficient for daily demands. Pohlandt and Kupferschmid[51] calculated the daily fetal protein accretion rate from the daily fetal weight gain and the protein content of the fetal body. Taking a net protein utilization of 80%, as proposed by Snyderman et al.,[52] they calculated the protein requirement of preterm neonates during the 32nd week of gestation to be not more than $2.7\,g\cdot kg^{-1}day^{-1}$. This applies to fetuses growing on the 50th weight percentile during the 30th to 31st postconceptional week. Most preterm and term neonates have lower requirements (Figure 34.4). A higher supply of human milk of approximately $250\,g\cdot kg^{-1}day^{-1}$ is necessary to meet the maximal protein requirement of $2.7\,g\cdot kg^{-1}day^{-1}$ during the 32nd week of gestation. Because of the limited tolerance to high volume loading in this age group, premature neonates must be fed either human milk enriched with protein or protein hydrolysates or formulas rich in protein. Commercial preterm infant formulas generally contain more than $2\,g$ protein$\cdot 100\,ml^{-1}$. Weight gain and protein accretion in preterm infants fed these formulas are significantly higher as compared with formulas containing lower protein concentrations.[53]

There is no convincing reason to assume that the intrauterine growth rate should be considered to be the optimal rate for the postnatal growth of preterm neonates.[54] The intrauterine growth rate is rarely achieved during postnatal life if taken as a goal for the nutritional management of preterm neonates. There is no evidence that a slower growth rate might be deleterious to the neonate. Rate and composition of postnatal weight gain are closely related to dietary protein and energy intakes. In preterm infants, high dietary protein/energy ratios were shown to be correlated with higher urinary nitrogen excretion, high blood urea nitrogen and amino acid concentrations, and a lower protein accretion rate as compared with higher energy intakes. The outcomes are predictable by a mathematical model.[55] There are deviations for individual neonates in the range of up to 30%, which make predictions between protein/energy intakes and the rate and composition of weight gain difficult. The high protein intakes necessary to achieve a normal level of intrauterine protein accretion may induce metabolic disturbances that are more likely to be harmful than a slightly delayed growth rate.

Casein-predominant formulas contain relatively high amounts of tyrosine and phenylalanine, which are poorly metabolized by the premature neonate and may reach toxic concentrations in the brain.[56] Whey protein-predominant mixtures of cow's milk proteins can have a greater similarity to the amino acid pattern of mother's

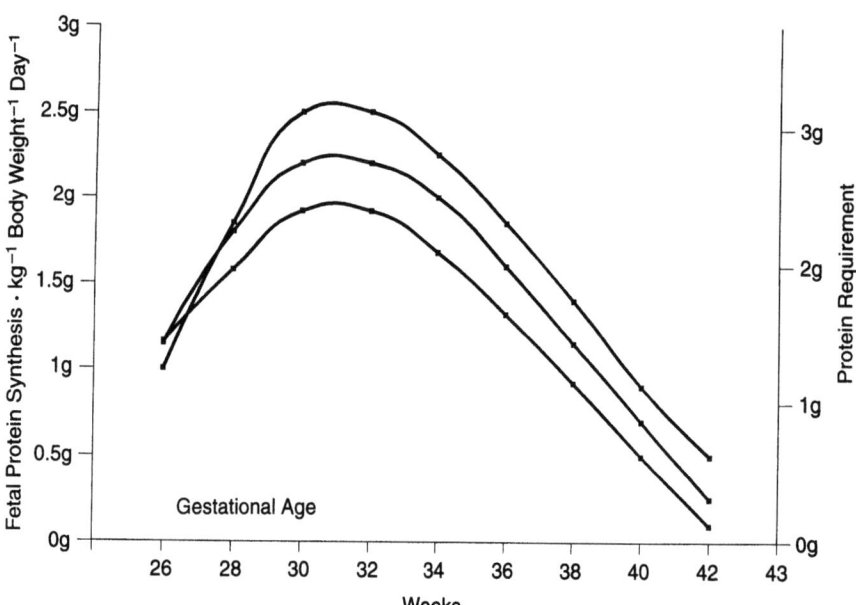

FIGURE 34.4. Fetal protein accretion (left axis) and the corresponding nutritional protein requirement (right axis) of preterm infants growing on the 90th, 50th, or 10th percentile according to Pohlandt and Kupferschmid.[51]

milk, although the threonine, methionine, and lysine concentrations are still distinctly higher than in human milk. Such mixtures represent the best adaptation that can be attained with mixtures based on commercially available whey protein and casein.

At present, the needs of premature neonates in terms of both quantity and quality of food protein are not completely understood. Numerous studies have compared the effects of various food protein intakes on the growth rates of preterm neonates and generally suggest that human milk feeding provides sufficient protein for the normal development of most preterm neonates. Moderately preterm neonates receiving their own mother's or donor's milk or protein-rich formula do not differ in body length, weight, or head circumference.[57,58]

In contrast, other pediatric nutritionists have recommended protein intakes of up to $5 g \cdot kg^{-1} day^{-1}$ for premature neonates. The originally recommended intakes reported by Gordon and Ganzor[59] ranged from 4 to $6 g \cdot kg^{-1} day^{-1}$. The recommendations of the Committee on Nutrition of the American Academy of Pediatrics[60] range between 2.25 and $5.0 g$ protein$\cdot g^{-1} day^{-1}$ and take into consideration a broad variation resulting from individual differences, gestational age, protein quality, digestibility, energy supply, and other factors. The corresponding recommendations of the Committee on Nutrition of the European Society for Pediatric Gastroenterology and Nutrition are 2.9 to $4.0 g \cdot kg^{-1} day^{-1}$.[61] On the basis of the fetal accretion rate of protein, the estimated requirements are 3.5 to $4.0 g \cdot kg^{-1} day^{-1}$.[60]

The protein requirements of very small premature neonates before the 30th postconceptional week may be difficult to meet from the calculated protein quantities, as the net protein utilization rates of these neonates may be lower than 80%. Even in full-term neonates the amount of protein available for nutrition in mother's milk, particularly secretory immunoglobulin A (IgA) and lactoferrin, is reduced during the early neonatal period.[62]

It is still unknown whether there is a delayed outcome on the health status induced by high protein intake in early infancy. There are tight correlations between the mode of early feeding and the body composition of infants. Butte et al.,[63] using the total electrical conductivity and ^{18}O-dilution method, found higher percentages of fat free body mass and total body water in formula-fed infants as compared with breast-fed infants, whereas the body fat proportion was lower. This is in accordance with the higher retention of nitrogen as observed in infants with high protein cow's milk formulas.[64] A further adaptation to the amino acid pattern of human milk protein, especially in view of the tryptophan and cystine supply,[65] can be obtained by α-lactalbumin supplementation of whey protein/casein mixtures.[66,67] Formulas produced in this way would allow decreasing the protein intake and avoid imbalances in amino acid metabolism, which may be deleterious for infants at risk.

Plasma Protein During the Perinatal Period

In human fetuses at midtrimester pregnancy, the total protein and albumin concentrations are lower and the α-fetoprotein concentrations are higher than in their mothers.[68] Premature neonates have significantly lower total protein, albumin, γ-globulin, and cholinesterase concentrations than term neonates. All proteins except $α_1$-globulin correlate positively with gestational age.[69] Serum albumin concentration rises from 1.9 g·dl^{-1} during the 26th week to 3.1 g·dl^{-1} during the 40th week of gestation and to 3.6 g·dl^{-1} within 3 weeks after birth.[70] The fractional and absolute synthesis rates for albumin is much higher in small premature neonates than in healthy young adults.[71]

Serum transferrin concentrations in preterm neonates are significantly lower than in term neonates. Transferrin concentration correlates positively with birth length, weight, gestational age, and albumin concentrations in all neonates.[72] Plasma pepsinogen concentrations are 1.0 to 1.5 times higher during the first week of life than in children and adults. In neonates the concentration of albumin and the following protein fraction in cord blood are lower than in later life: C-reactive protein, IgA, IgM, IgD, IgE, ceruloplasmin, haptoglobin, hemopexin, and transferrin. The concentrations of α-fetoprotein and α-amino nitrogen are higher.[26]

Serum concentrations of acute-phase proteins were found to be not different between term and preterm neonates with the exception of prealbumin apolipoprotein A, B, and C_4.[73] Prealbumin (i.e., trans-thyretin) concentration was found by Jain et al.[74] to be significantly lower in cord blood of neonates as compared with respective maternal concentrations (10.9 ± 0.5 vs 17.8 ± 0.8 mg·dl^{-1}). Concentration correlates with the birth weight of the neonate.

Acute-phase proteins such as C-reactive protein and granulocyte elastase have become important indicators for the diagnosis and differential diagnosis of infection. Even extremely low birth weight infants react with few exceptions promptly on inflammatory irritations, increasing their C-reactive protein and granulocyte elastase concentrations above the normal range of 10 mg·L^{-1} and 50 to 75 mg·L^{-1}, respectively. Deficiencies of coagulation-regulating protein C have been reported as a transient condition in neonates and especially in preterm infants with respiratory distress as well as in infants of diabetic mothers and in infants of twin gestations. Values of less than 0.1 unit·ml^{-1} reflect delayed maturation or increased turnover and are correlated with the subsequent onset of thrombosis.[75] Glycosylated plasma proteins exhibit distinctly lower concentrations in preterm born infants as compared with newborns born at term and adults (Table 34.4). Similar discrepancies between the reference concentrations of preterm infants, term-born neonates, and adults were recently described for histidine-rich glycoprotein.[76] Severely stressed neonates were found to have higher plasma concentrations of histidine-rich protein than normal control neonates.[77]

Serum insulin-like growth factors increase from 50 mg·ml^{-1} (IGF-I) and 350 ng·ml^{-1} (IGF-II) in the 33rd week of gestation to two to three times higher concentrations at term. IGF-I concentrations are significantly higher in fetuses with weights above the mean for gestational age. The binding proteins of IGF-I and IGF-II were found to be one third of the concentration of the adult.[78]

Fibronectin concentrations in plasma of newborns amounts to one third to one half of those found in the healthy adult. In respiratory distress syndrome, bacterial sepsis, intrauterine growth retardation, and postnatal malnutrition even lower fibronectin concentrations are registered. Low fibronectin concentrations in plasma are indicative for a functional insufficiency of the reticuloendothelial system and predispose to microbial infections.[79]

Regulation of Protein Turnover

Protein intake seems to stimulate both protein synthesis and protein degradation, apparently by stimulating insulin secretion and other hormonal changes.[80] Protein and nonprotein energy intakes appear to have additive effects on protein turnover and may stimulate protein accretion via different mechanisms.[81] The acute and adaptive responses to a high protein intake may consist of a decrease

TABLE 34.4. Plasma concentration of selected glycoproteins in preterm infants, neonates, and adults.

Glycoprotein	Proportion of carbohydrates (%)	A Preterm infants (mg·L^{-1})	B Term-born neonates (mg·L^{-1})	C Adults (mg·L^{-1})	A % of C	B % of C
Hemopexin	23	180 (65–250)	317 + 75	746 + 52	24	43
Haptoglobin	19.3	0	74 + 81	1470 (580–3730)	0	5
$α_1$-Antichymotrypsin	22.7	170 (41–821)	283 (132–493)	300–600	38	63
Ceruloplasmin	7.1	170 + 60	170 + 50	300 + 95	45	45
Orosomucoid	41.4	110 (27–539)	180 (83–412)	900 + 240	12	20
IgA	7.5	20 + 30	20 + 30	2000 + 610	1	1
IgM	12.0	73 + 38	110 + 50	990 + 27	7	11
IgD	11.3	0	0 (Traces)	44.8 (27.6–62.0)	0	0
Transferrin	5.9	1580 + 530	1620 + 540	2990 + 360	69	71
Albumin	0	25,800 + 4500	41,300 + 3200	38,000–4400	63	100

in the rate of protein degradation and an increase in the postabsorptive rates of both protein synthesis and breakdown, respectively.[82]

Protein synthesis and proteolysis inhibition in muscle preparation are greatly stimulated by branched-chain amino acids. Other amino acids do not have this effect. The in vivo effect of branched-chain amino acids is brought about by insulin release from the pancreatic islet cells caused by leucine and its degradation product ketoisocaproic acid.[83] Insulin is a powerful anabolic hormone stimulating the release of anabolic hormone that stimulates the synthesis of DNA, RNA, nucleic acids, and protein in target tissues. Lucas et al.[80] studied the hormonal and metabolic response to breast and cow's milk feeding in full-term neonates on the 6th postnatal day and found a significant postprandial rise in both groups. The plasma insulin concentration of the breast-fed group rose from $2.2 \pm 0.4\,\mu U \cdot ml^{-1}$ ($16 \pm 3\,mmol \cdot L^{-1}$) to a peak value of $14.0 \pm 2.5\,\mu U \cdot ml^{-1}$ ($102 \pm 18\,pmol \cdot L^{-1}$) after 55 minutes. The insulin response in the formula-fed group lasted significantly longer, the 90- and 150-minute concentrations exceeding those for the breast-fed neonates. The investigations observed no changes in plasma glucagon concentrations, whereas the lactate and pyruvate concentrations showed moderate phasic elevations after the formula feeding. These findings are consistent with the observation that insulin release is more strongly stimulated by amino acids than by glucose in the neonate and that the greatest release of insulin is caused by combined administration of amino acids and glucose.[84] This point is of practical importance relative to the development of maximally efficient infusion therapy during the early postnatal period.

Determination of Whole-Body Protein Turnover in the Term and Preterm Neonate: Order of Magnitude and Criticism of Methods

Despite the introduction of modern techniques based on the use of ^{15}N and ^{13}C amino acids as tracers for the study of neonatal protein turnover, there are few reliable data available concerning the order of magnitude of protein synthesis and breakdown in this age group. Protein synthesis and degradation are closely linked to the adequacy of energy supply, which is normally provided by the oxidation of glucose and triglycerides. If protein intake is high and energy intake low, the protein must be partially transformed to glucose to provide sufficient energy for protein accretion. Nitrogen balance, used for more than a hundred years to determine protein nitrogen accretion, does not provide insight into the dynamics of protein metabolism. The accretion of a certain amount of body protein may result from a high rate of protein synthesis concurrent with a high rate of protein degradation, but the same net protein gain can be obtained with low rates of synthesis and breakdown (Figure 34.5).

There are few reports on protein turnover during the early neonatal period. According to Young,[85] protein synthesis in the neonate amounts to $26\,g \cdot kg^{-1} day^{-1}$. This

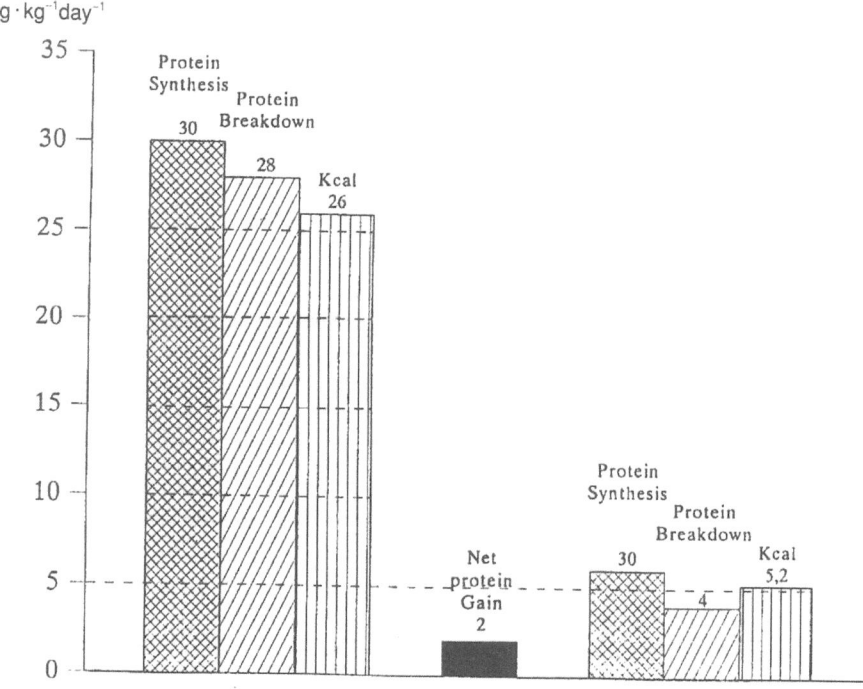

FIGURE 34.5. Net protein gain in relation to protein synthesis. Protein accretion may be achieved on the level of high or low synthesis and breakdown rates resulting in high or low energy needs.

figure appears to represent a waste of energy, as only 10% of the protein synthesized would serve for net protein gain.[86] Under such conditions the neonate would spend more than 20% of its energy expenditure on protein turnover, compared with only 6% in the adult.

The significance of this highly accelerated protein turnover during early life may be explainable by the need to provide sufficient amino acids for the synthesis of essential proteins. This theory has been confirmed only for prealbumin.[87]

Data obtained from experiments in newborn animals speak in favor of an amino acid shift from skeletal muscle to gastrointestinal tissue.[88] The existence of an analogous shift in the human neonate has not been proven.

Because renal nitrogen excretion during the neonatal period is comparatively low, almost complete reutilization of the endogenous nitrogen would be necessary to maintain nitrogen balance.[26] The high protein turnover during the neonatal period may be caused by the gluconeogenic pathway. The data of Frazer et al.[89] indicate that the human neonate has a high capacity for producing glucose from gluconeogenic amino acids and that this functional pathway is not impaired by growth retardation. The existence of these reported high turnover rates in neonates is questionable, as they may well be a result of methodologic shortcomings. During the past 5 years numerous studies have been directed to the improvement of the methods for determining protein turnover rates in preterm infants.[90–98] Tracer substances such as [^{15}N]glycine, [^{15}N]leucine, [^{13}C]leucine, and [^{15}N]-labeled yeast protein hydrolysate and different models were applied simultaneously for calculation of the turnover rates to clarify the causes of the deviating results of former studies. Van Goudoever et al.[98] compared the two most commonly used labeled amino acids [^{15}N]glycine and [1-^{13}C]leucine as tracer substances administered simultaneously for their suitability of determining whole-body protein turnover rates in appropriate for gestational age and small for gestational age preterm infants. Mean values of preterm turnover using [^{15}N]glycine and [1-^{13}C]leucine ranged from 10 to 14 g·kg^{-1}·d^{-1}.

Turnover rates were found to be higher when the end product method was used, pointing to the limited suitability of [^{15}N]glycine as a carrier for ^{15}N in protein turnover studies in preterm infants. The group of small for gestational age infants exhibited the lowest ^{15}N-urea enrichment, oxidized less leucine and retained significantly more nitrogen. Wutzke et al.[96] conducted a paired comparison study in preterm infants using [^{15}N]glycine, [^{15}N]leucine, and [^{15}N]yeast protein thermitase hydrolysate (YPTH) as tracers. Protein turnover rates were calculated by a three-pool model and the ammonia end product method (AEPM), respectively. The synthesis rates as calculated by the three-compartment model differed significantly among [^{15}N]leucine (9.1 g·kg^{-1}·d^{-1}) and [^{15}N]YPTH (5.9 g/kg·d^{-1}) (Figure 34.6). When the corresponding rates were determined from the excretion of label in ammonia, the results showed the opposite tendency (7.5 vs 14.4 vs 16.7 g·kg^{-1}·day^{-1}). The results of this study demonstrate the methodological errors connected with the AEPM and with the use of glycine and leucine as tracer substances for calculating whole-body protein parameters in preterm infants. They substantiate one of the main assumptions for tracer kinetic studies: the tracer nitrogen must be representative of the total amino nitrogen of the metabolic pool. Completely labeled mixtures of amino acids fulfill this requirement better than single amino acids. Considering this, protein synthesis rates of preterm infants are found to be much lower than originally claimed.

Compared with whole-body protein metabolism during the early neonatal period, that of full-term and

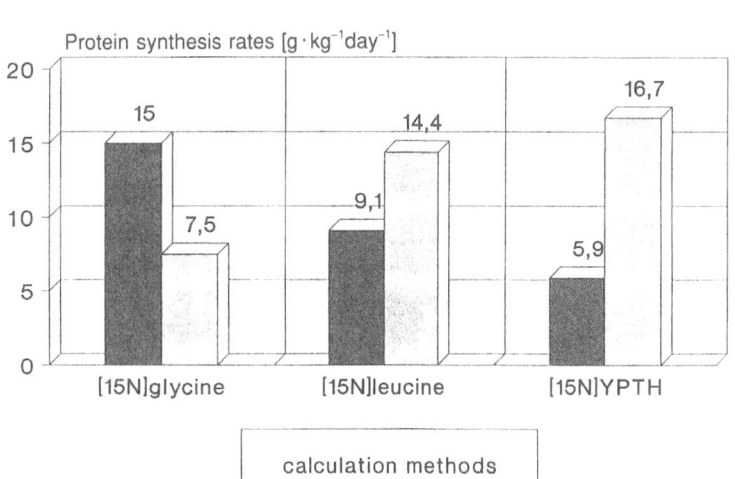

FIGURE 34.6. Protein synthesis rates in preterm infants as determined with three different tracer substances and two different models. [^{15}N]YPTH, [^{15}N]yeast protein thermitase hydrolysate; TCM, three compartment model; AEPM, ammonia end product method.

TABLE 34.5. Protein synthesis, protein breakdown, and protein N turnover in preterm neonates.

Gestational age (weeks)	Birth weight (g)	Postnatal age (days)	Protein synthesis (g·kg⁻¹day⁻¹)	Protein breakdown (g·kg⁻¹day⁻¹)	N turnover (g·kg⁻¹day⁻¹)	Ref.
—	2200–2380	29–68	12.7 (10.6–15.5)	—	—	64
30–36	1120–1758	1–45	26.3 ± 7.0	23.8 ± 7.4	4.35 ± 1.12	65
32 (31.5–33.0)	1055–1400	9–10	10.9 ± 3.4	9.3 ± 3.4	1.94 ± 0.54	69
26–37	800–1930	7–49	5.2–13.2	4.1–12.4	0.91–2.18	67
	1223 ± 166 (950–1420)		11.2	9.4		68
32.2 ± 0.8	1670 ± 181	26.3 ± 7.1	15.8 ± 2.6[a]	14.0 ± 2.7	2.6 ± 0.4	33
		23.3 ± 7.4	11.3 ± 3.1[b]	9.6 ± 3.0	1.9 ± 3.0	33

[a] [¹⁵N]Glycine.
[b] Amino acid mixtures as tracer substances. Data were compiled from the literature.

preterm neonates has been studied more intensively during the later postnatal phase. The values reported for protein synthesis and breakdown in premature neonates range from 5.2 to 26.3 g·kg⁻¹day⁻¹ and from 4.1 to 23.8 g·kg⁻¹day⁻¹, respectively[19,33,34,85,99-104] (Table 34.5). The changes in whole-body protein metabolism in very small preterm neonates in the course of postnatal life were determined by Plath et al.[34]

These studies were performed for different conceptional ages and were compared with data from preterm and term neonates fed human milk (Table 34.6). The data clearly show a decrease in protein synthesis and degradation as postconceptional age increases, although the values are probably overestimates due to the use of [¹⁵N]glycine as a tracer (vide supra).

Significant differences between the protein synthesis rates of preterm small for gestational age (SGA) neonates and preterm appropriate for gestational age (AGA) neonates were described by Cauderay et al.[105] Using repeated nasogastric [¹⁵N]glycine pulse labeling, these investigators found a higher rate of resting energy expenditure, a lower protein synthesis rate, and a 20% slower protein turnover in the SGA neonate, although the protein gain and the composition of the weight gain was similar in the two groups. Their conclusion that SGA neonates might tolerate slightly higher amounts of food protein is questionable. SGA neonates of very low birth weight tend to decompensate more easily on high protein intakes.[106,107]

The effects of different dietary regimens on the protein turnover in premature neonates were studied by Pencharz et al.[57] and Heine et al.[33] In preterm neonates weighing 1.5–2.0 kg who were given either mother's milk or casein- and whey-dominated formulas, respectively, no differences were found in nitrogen retention or growth in length and weight. Nitrogen absorption and net nitrogen utilization were higher in the human milk-fed group. Significantly higher rates of whole-body nitrogen flux, protein synthesis, and protein degradation were registered in the human milk-fed group.[57]

These findings are incompatible with the concept of evolutionary teleology: higher protein synthesis rates on a mother's milk diet would be equivalent to a higher energy expenditure. Further studies are needed to elucidate the mechanism causing these differences. Studies performed simultaneously by Heine et al.[33] on premature neonates fed either human milk or a formula diet revealed no differences between the two feeding regimens (Table 34.7).

All these data on protein turnover were obtained with [¹⁵N]glycine as a tracer. The mode of tracer administration differed from one study to another, which may explain why the rates sometimes diverge. Jackson et al.[99] used the continuous [¹⁵N]glycine infusion method of

TABLE 34.6. Daily protein turnover in preterm, moderately preterm, and term neonates.

	Preterm			
Measurement	Day 11	Day 31	Moderately preterm, day 16	Term, day 57 ± 20.5
Protein synthesis	14.3 ± 4.5	11.8 ± 2.9	7.9 ± 2.7	7.7 ± 1.4
Protein breakdown	12.1 ± 4.5	9.5 ± 3.0	6.0 ± 2.9	5.9 ± 1.5
Net protein gain	2.2 ± 0.2	2.3 ± 0.2	1.9 ± 3.0	1.8 ± 0.2
Nitrogen turnover	2.4 ± 0.7	2.0 ± 0.5	1.3 ± 0.5	1.3 ± 0.5

[a] Mean body weight of preterm neonates at birth was 1592 ± 517 g, that of moderately preterm neonates was 2064 ± 107 g, and that of term neonates was 3304 ± 801 g.
From Plath et al.[17] with permission.

TABLE 34.7. Daily protein turnover in preterm neonates fed mother's milk and formula diet.

Parameter	Mother's milk (x ± SEM)	Formula diet (n = 5) (x ± SEM)
Protein synthesis (g·kg^{-1}day^{-1})	7.87 ± 2.74	7.97 ± 2.09
Protein breakdown (g·kg^{-1}day^{-1})	5.95 ± 2.86	5.98 ± 1.87
Net protein gain (g·kg^{-1}day^{-1})	1.92 ± 0.26	1.98 ± 0.39
Protein turnover (g·kg^{-1}day^{-1})	8.33 ± 2.79	8.89 ± 1.98
Nonprotein N pool (g·kg^{-1})	0.634 ± 0.288	0.772 ± 0.130

From Heine et al.,[33] with permission.

Picou and Taylor-Roberts,[19] determining the rise of the isotope to plateau level in both urea and ammonia over a period of 72 hours. Under these conditions, urinary urea failed to become enriched at all in six of their eight studies. The same lack of ^{15}N enrichment of urinary urea was reported by Catzeflis et al.[104] in 5 of 16 preterm neonates to whom [^{15}N]glycine was administered for investigation of nitrogen turnover. The extremely high synthesis rates found by Pencharz et al.[102] were due to the short period of urine collection, which was not long enough for the cumulative urinary excretion of the tracer to reach a plateau. Single-pulse labeling according to the method of San Pietro and Rittenberg[108] performed by Nissim et al.,[103] Heine et al.,[33] and Plath et al.[34] or repeated oral administration of [^{15}N]glycine for 60 to 72 hours[104] led to comparable results.

There are further objections to the validity of using [^{15}N]glycine as a tracer for determining whole-body protein parameters in preterm and term neonates. Glycine fails to label the precursor pool adequately.[109,110] Adequate labeling of the precursor pool is one of the most important prerequisites for the tracer kinetic measurement of intermediary protein metabolism parameters.[111] Glycine accounts for 27% of all amino acids in the carcass proteins. In rapidly growing premature and term neonates it may become a semiessential amino acid.[99] Low dietary glycine intake (e.g., on a mother's milk diet) and low isotope dilution in [^{15}N]glycine pulse labeling may accelerate incorporation of tracer into rapidly growing collagen, simulating an increase in whole-body protein synthesis.

The link between the various organ systems in the context of whole-body protein turnover is illustrated in Figure 35.7. The intensity of isotope flux from the extracellular space and release of the label from the intracellular space of the organs may differ in many respects. The preferential incorporation of [^{15}N]glycine into rapidly growing carcass proteins and its involvement in other metabolic pathways may simulate high overall protein synthesis rates. Influences on whole-body protein metabolism may result from aberrations in the relative weights of the organ tissues and the metabolic activities of the organs during health and disease. It is assumed that mixtures of labeled amino acids or oligopeptides minimize the methodologic errors and more closely simulate the conditions needed for "true" whole-body protein turnover determination than single tracer amino acids.

The controversy surrounding the use of [^{15}N]glycine as a tracer for investigating protein metabolism, especially in patients with metabolic disturbances and in the preterm and term neonate, gave rise to comparative studies using different tracers. These studies were based on the assumption that mixtures of ^{15}N-labeled amino acids or a [^{15}N]yeast protein hydrolysate, which represent the α-amino nitrogen composition of the metabolic pool more closely, would be superior to [^{15}N] glycine.

Using the three-pool compartment model to determine nitrogen turnover, Plath et al.[17] found a 40% lower rate of protein synthesis and protein breakdown in very small preterm neonates after single-pulse labeling with a [^{15}N]amino acid mixture and [^{15}N]yeast protein hydrolysate, respectively, than after [^{15}N]glycine labeling. Because this model has not been fully validated by comparison with models with different assumptions, it is difficult to compare the corresponding results with those reported in the past.[112] The conditions provided by the paired study chosen for this experiment suggest that protein turnover rates in premature neonates could be determined more reliably with mixtures of ^{15}N-labeled amino acids. The drawbacks of the [^{15}N]yeast protein-pepsin-trypsin hydrolysate originally used by Plath et al.[17] as an alternative to the expensive [^{15}N]amino acid mixture have been overcome by the introduction of a [^{15}N]yeast protein thermitase hydrolysate, composed mainly of free amino acids, dipeptides, and tripeptides. In contrast to the [^{15}N]yeast protein pepsin-trypsin hydrolysate, this new tracer is rapidly absorbed and makes correction for fecal losses unnecessary (Table 34.8).

Comparative studies by Wutzke et al.[96] with [^{15}N]glycine, [^{15}N]leucine, and [^{15}N]yeast protein thermitase hydrolysate to determine protein turnover rates in preterm neonates revealed protein synthesis rates of 17, 11, and 6 g·kg^{-1}day^{-1}, respectively.

Low protein synthesis rates similar to those obtained with [^{15}N]yeast protein thermitase hydrolysate were determined by Beaufrere et al.,[113] in preterm neonates age

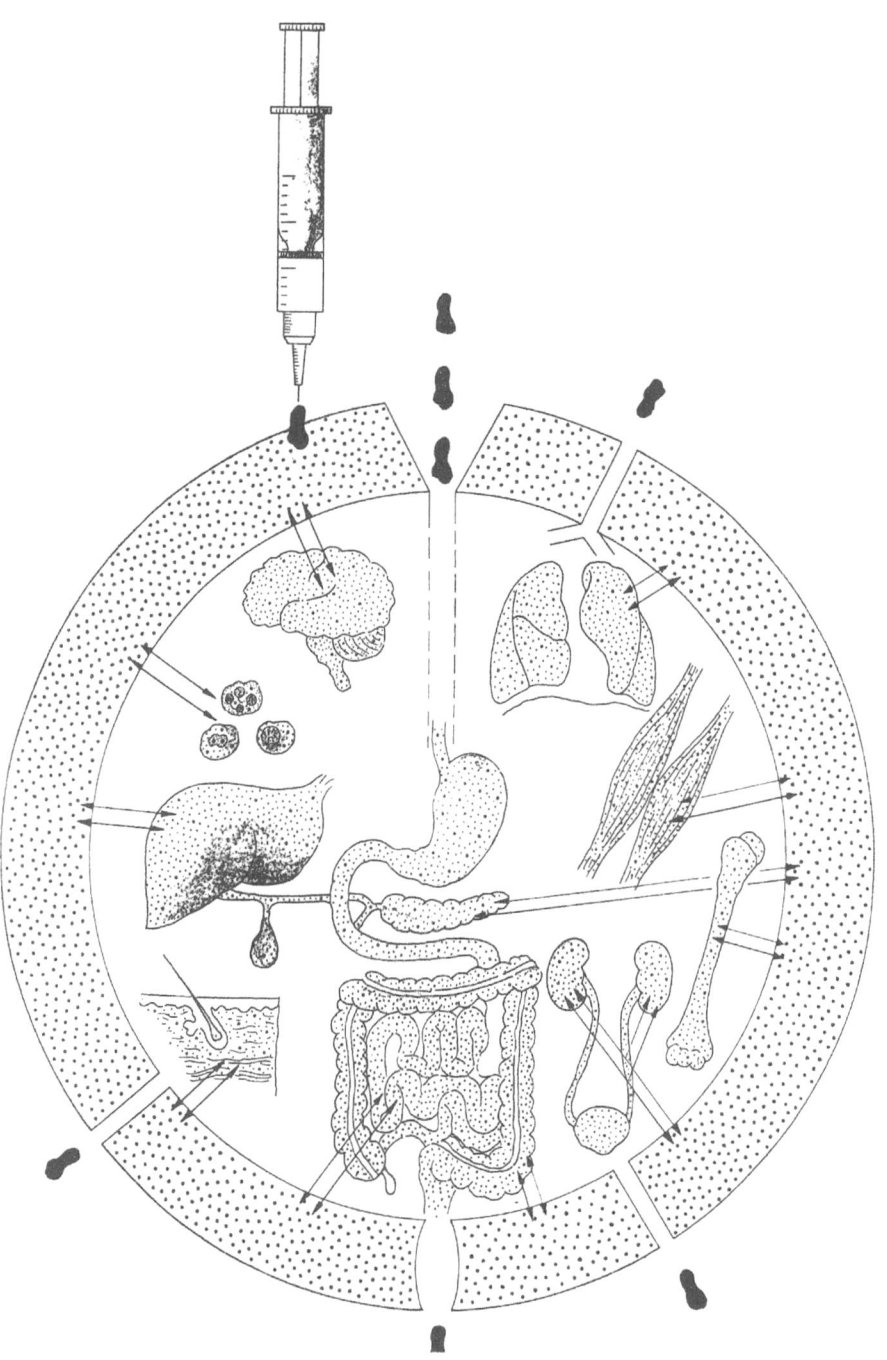

FIGURE 34.7. Tracer flux between the metabolic pool, protein pool of various organs, and excretion pool. Whole-body protein parameters result from the balanced interaction of all organ systems. Preferable incorporation of the tracer in various tissues, e.g., [^{15}N]glycine in fast-growing carcass protein may lead to an overestimation of protein synthesis rates.

TABLE 34.8. Fecal excretion of ^{15}N after oral administration of tracer substances in preterm neonates.

Tracer	No. of determination	% Excreted
[^{15}N]Glycine	4	0.7 ± 0.1
[^{15}N]Amino acid mixture	4	1.7 ± 0.1
[^{15}N]Yeast protein pepsin-trypsin hydrolysate	10	11.8 ± 5.0
[^{15}N]Yeast protein-thermitase hydrolysate	15	2.9 ± 1.0

[a] Feces collection period was 48 hours.

2.5 to 6.0 weeks and weighing 1650 to 1900 g. The neonates were fed on either human milk or enriched human milk. The investigators used a short, constant infusion of L-[1-^{13}C]leucine and calculated leucine turnover and leucine oxidation from [^{13}C]leucine in the plasma and ^{13}CO$_2$ abundance in breath. The resulting protein synthesis rates varied from 5 to 11 g·kg^{-1} day^{-1}.

Using ammonia as an end product, Stack et al.[93] studied the protein turnover in preterm neonates by means of a single oral bolus of [^{15}N]glycine and [^{15}N]yeast protein hydrolysate obtained by acidic hydrolysis. The investigators calculated considerably higher protein synthesis rates when [^{15}N]yeast protein hydrolysate was administered as a tracer substance in comparison to [^{15}N]glycine. An evaluation of this study without knowledge of the simultaneously excreted [^{15}N]urea is difficult. It is suspected that ammonia cannot serve as a reliable end product.

It can be concluded that the introduction of a uniformly labeled amino-oligopeptide mixture (e.g. [^{15}N]yeast protein thermitase hydrolysate) as a tracer for measuring protein nitrogen turnover rates will yield data that do not differ much from those measured in neonates and approximate more closely the true values for whole-body protein metabolism.

Schöch et al.[6] estimated the turnover rates of protein and RNA in preterm neonates and adults by measuring the renal excretion of 3-methylhistidine and modified one-way RNA catabolites. The turnover of actin and myosin, which serve as indicators of muscle and intestinal protein metabolism, are about three times higher in the preterm neonate than in the adult when the greater muscle weight of the latter is taken into account. The excretion rates for pseudouridine, 7-methylguanine, and N^2, N^2-dimethylguanosine are three to four times higher, reflecting the higher rRNA, tRNA, and mRNA turnover in the preterm neonates.[7] The calculated turnover rates in the group of premature neonates for rRNA, tRNA, and mRNA were, respectively, 0.10, 1.87, and 2.35 μmol·kg^{-1}·day^{-1}; the corresponding values for adults were 0.038, 0.66, and 0.64 μmol·kg^{-1}·day^{-1}. The relation of protein synthesis to plasma and cell amino acids in neonates was studied by Johnson and Metcoff[114] using neutrophils as a cell model and measuring the [^{3}H]leucine incorporation into the protein fraction of the granulocytes. The mean protein synthesis rate was 4067 ± 1763 pmol·hr^{-1}·mg^{-1} DNA. The protein synthesis rate was inversely related to birth weight and more closely related to a set of intracellular than to plasma amino acid concentrations. These and similar results cannot be applied to whole-body protein synthesis parameters.

In conclusion, the order of magnitude of protein turnover in term and preterm neonates is not as high as was originally determined. There is evidence that protein turnover rates in this age group are two to three times higher than during later life. The consequences in regard to optimal protein supply for preterm and term neonates remain controversial because energy and protein needs are known to vary among individuals and ethnic groups.[115]

Fasting and Protein Turnover

The relation between fasting and protein turnover has been studied in animals, children, and adults. The fetus is accustomed to a continuous supply of amino acids, glucose, fatty acids, and glycerol via the placental circulation throughout the fetal period, but must adapt after birth to an intermittent pattern of food intake, including an 8-hour nighttime fast. Little is known concerning the changes that occur in protein metabolism of neonates who are accentuated by the low food intake during the first days after birth. As measured by urea synthesis rate, neonates during fasting have an obligatory rate of protein oxidation of approximately 0.87 g·kg^{-1}·day^{-1}.[114] This corresponds to approximately 1% of the total protein of the body. In very small preterm infants, myofibrillar protein turnover, as measured by urinary excretion of N-t-methylhistidine, is higher than in larger neonates.[94]

Fasting seems to alter the rate of skeletal muscle protein growth to such an extent that the proportion of body protein partitioned into gastrointestinal tissue is preserved, while that of muscle protein is reduced. Intravenous feeding can decrease whole-body protein turnover and maintain visceral protein synthesis of approximately 4 g·kg^{-1}·day^{-1}.[94] Diurnal changes in nitrogen retention were measured in normal meal-fed children by Parsons et al.[117] using repeated oral [^{15}N]glycine tracer doses. Ingestion of food was followed by retention of nitrogen, although the excretion of urea increased. During the nightly fasting period, nitrogen losses increased. These requests are inconsistent with increased pulsatile human growth hormone excretion at night, which might protect the organism from the detrimental consequences of negative nitrogen balance related to the interruption of food intake. The diurnal changes in nitrogen retention are caused mainly by changes in body protein synthesis, whereas changes in the protein degradation rate in adults during experiments are more equivocal. This may be due to the unsatisfactory nature of the methods, which are based on the use of single tracer amino acids.[81,118] In experiments with healthy volunteers, Wernemann et al.[118] failed to show any meal-related diurnal variation in the capacity or the activity of protein synthesis in human skeletal muscle. They observed insulin peaks in response to food intake, whereas the cortisol concentration decreased continuously during the day.

The changes in protein synthesis that occur in skeletal muscle during fasting are greater than those in the body as a whole. Rennie et al.[119] showed that whole-body protein synthesis in fasting subjects fell by 35%, whereas the corresponding rate for skeletal muscle was 50%. Similar results had been reported earlier by Winterer et al.,[120] who used [^{15}N]glycine to study whole-body protein turnover in mildly obese subjects given a low-protein diet with a brief total fast. Garlick et al.[121] observed a 40% drop in whole-body protein synthesis in obese adults on a low-energy, protein-free diet. When the low-energy diet contained 50 g of protein, the protein synthesis rates were similar to those recorded with a normal diet.

Nutritional support prior to a preoperative 18-hour fast improved the whole-body protein synthesis rate by 42% and the muscle protein synthesis rate by 36% in adults.[122] Direct measurement of muscle protein metabolism across the forearm of normally fasting adults by means of L-[^{13}N]leucine and [^{15}N]leucine confirmed a significant, rapid decrease in muscle protein synthesis and a marked decrease in protein catabolism.[123]

Immobilization and Protein Turnover

Another aspect of protein metabolism of the neonate that has not been thoroughly investigated is the influence of motoric activity on protein synthesis and protein breakdown. Schönheyder et al.,[124] using [^{15}N]glycine as a tracer, observed that immobilization for several days caused a substantial negative nitrogen balance in adults. It was secondary to a fall in protein synthesis rather than an increase in protein breakdown. Correlations between bed rest and negative nitrogen balance were reported by Askanazi et al.[125]

These results were partly confirmed by immobilization experiments in rats.[126] The biochemical background of these observations is not well understood and requires further investigation. The human neonate, although practically immobilized for the first weeks of life, is known to have a positive nitrogen balance if adequately nourished.

Protein Metabolism During Metabolic Acidosis

The effects of metabolic acidosis on whole-body nitrogen turnover in healthy and sick neonates have not been studied. Metabolic acidosis is common during the early perinatal period in the presence of renal insufficiency and various congenital heart diseases, and leads to increased ammonia excretion. Experiments performed on dogs by Jeevanandam et al.,[127] using continuous hydrochloric acid infusions and pulse labeling with L-[^{15}N]alanine and [^{13}C]urea, revealed a 30% decrease in the total body protein synthesis rate. Protein breakdown fell by approximately the same degree. The urea pool size and excretion rate were reduced by 24% and 17%, respectively, confirming that the hepatic response during acidosis is decreased urea production. The results of this study point to the altered capacity of the organism to mobilize and utilize labile protein during acidosis. Other conditions of stress (e.g., sepsis, trauma, and burn injury) are known to have the opposite effect and may interfere with changes in protein turnover during acidosis. It has been suggested that the lower whole-body protein turnover caused by acidosis is related to changes in hepatic enzyme activity and has general effects on the cardiovascular system and sympathoadrenal regulation.

Digestion of Protein

The adaptation to intermittent enteral feeding following the interruption of intravenous nutrition via the placenta, although without complication in most individuals, is one of the most dramatic challenges for the neonate. Whereas all substrates needed for protein accretion are provided as building blocks during fetal life, enteral feeding involves the enzymatic breakdown of food protein into resorbable amino acids and oligopeptides. This protein degradation process depends on the perfect functioning of proteolytic enzymes in the stomach and pancreas as well as at the intestinal brush border. The digestive capacity for food proteins in term, and even preterm, neonates is surprisingly well developed, although proteolytic activity is subnormal in most neonates. This apparent contradiction between subnormal enzymatic activity and normal functioning of the biochemical processes during the neonatal period is a well-known but unexplained phenomenon.

Neonates are fed relatively small amounts of mother's milk during the first few days of life to permit gradual adaptation to the intraluminal digestion of food protein. The relatively high concentration of free amino acids and peptides in mother's milk probably enhances the release of hormones such as gastrin and cholecystokinin, which promote the release of proteolytic enzymes.[128]

At least two factors may interfere with the normal adaptation of the digestive tract during the perinatal period: (1) the initial "chaotic" colonization of the gastrointestinal tract after birth, and (2) the increased permeability of the mucosa enabling macromolecules to pass the mucosal barrier. It is not known to what extent microbial colonization of the upper intestinal tract and the lower proteolytic activity contribute potentially to the faster permeation of protein up to the 6th day after birth. The speculated closure of the mucosal barrier coincides with stabilization of the intestinal flora (i.e., the predominance of bifidobacteria in breast-fed neonates) improves antibacterial protection of the upper gastrointestinal tract by increasing hydrochloric acid concentration in the stomach, and protective components in mother's milk.

The permeation of heterologous food proteins through the mucosal wall during early postnatal life may induce hypersensitization to cow's milk and soy proteins if these substances are offered as human milk fortifier or as additional food because of the mother's hypogalactic state. This condition may be especially dangerous in atopic infants if mother's milk is replaced by a formula food during later infancy. By contrast, uninterrupted formula feeding from the beginning of the neonatal period seems to cause immunotolerance (e.g., controlled immunologic response to antigens). Partially hydrolyzed ("hypoallergenic") formulas were repeatedly shown to reduce the incidence of atopic dermatitis.[129-131] The immunologic background of this preventive effect is poorly understood and immunologists claim that only completely hydrolyzed proteins possess this preventive effect.[132]

Protein digestion starts in the stomach by pepsin and its isoenzymes. Peptic activity is maximal at pH 1.2 to 2.0. The pH of the gastric juice of neonates is rarely that low after the first hours after birth. Their peptic activity, the acidity of their gastric juice, and their basal and maximal acid output are distinctly lower during the perinatal period than in later infancy.[26] Pepsin is an endopeptidase. The main products of peptic digestion are large polypeptides, small amounts of oligopeptides, and amino acids (see Chapter 3). The peptic digestive function is still undergoing development during the perinatal period.

Peptic activity has been detected in the stomach as early as the 16th week of gestation, and increases three- to fourfold between the 28th and 40th week of gestation. Acid output and pepsin secretion have reached their maximum amounting to 50% of the corresponding adult values, by the 9th to 17th week of life.

In small premature neonates, basal acid output increases from $12 \pm 3 \mu mol \cdot kg^{-1} hr^{-1}$ to $26.5 \mu mol \cdot kg^{-1} hr^{-1}$ between the first week and second month after birth.[133] In term and preterm neonates fed on formulas, the intragastric pH rarely approaches the pH optimum for pepsin. This fact may affect the neonate's ability to destroy the antigenicity of food proteins and to break them into peptones by peptic digestion.[134]

Although the specific immunogenicity of cow's milk protein is rapidly reduced by peptic digestion at pH 2 to 3, tryptic digestion does not have a similar effect, probably because of high-molecular-weight residues, which can resist endopeptidase digestion despite a much higher α-amino nitrogen release from the protein in the case of tryptic digestion.[135] Tryptic activity in the duodenal juice is detectable at approximately 16 weeks of fetal life and increases markedly after the 28th week of gestation. Term and preterm neonates are known to secrete less tryptic enzyme in response to secretin-pancreozymin administration at birth.[136] Even in premature neonates intraluminal digestion of food proteins does not seem to be limited.[99] In contrast to the diminished secretion of tryptic enzymes, the absorption and intracellular digestion of peptides has been shown to be as efficient in the intestinal mucosa of the preterm neonate as in later life.[137]

Essential Amino Acids

The human cannot survive without a supply of eight essential amino acids: tryptophan, phenylalanine, leucine, isoleucine, threonine, methionine, lysine, and valine. This dependence is related to the carbon skeleton of most of these amino acids. The exceptions are lysine and threonine, which cannot be synthesized by transamination. The transient inability of preterm and term neonates to metabolize some essential and nonessential amino acids to a sufficient extent is well established. Increased plasma concentrations of phenylalanine, tyrosine, and methionine are common in premature neonates when food intake increases and indicate the limited metabolism of these amino acids. The capacity to synthesize glycine, proline, and other dispensable amino acids is probably below normal in the premature neonate. The rapidly growing, very small premature neonate has a high glycine requirement for carcass protein synthesis. The glycine supply from human milk is apparently too low for these neonates, who are unable to synthesize sufficient glycine from nonessential nitrogen sources. This fact may have consequences for the nutritional supply of glycine and for tracer kinetic studies of whole-body protein metabolism using [^{15}N]glycine as a tracer substance (vide supra). In view of the low activity of transsulfuration pathway enzymes in the fetal liver,[136] cystine[138] and taurine[139] are regarded as essential for neonates. Support for this notion comes from the high cystine and taurine concentrations in mother's milk. However, cystine is bound mainly in the secretory IgA, lactoferrin, and lysozyme fractions of human milk and is not fully available for protein synthesis during early neonatal life. Supplementation of formulas with taurine and cystine has not yielded convincing advantages.

It can be concluded from clinical experience that lower activities of enzymes for metabolizing amino acids do not generally coincide with changes in amino acid homeostasis. Preterm and term neonates are normally able to adapt to synthesizing most of the semiessential amino acids.[58] The significance of tyrosine, histidine, and arginine is not fully known. Experimental data obtained mainly by parenteral nutrition have suggested that amino acid solutions should be suitably supplemented with these amino acids.[140]

Estimation of Amino Acid Requirements in Preterm and Term Neonates

In the growing infant and child, essential and nonessential amino acids are required for the accretion of new tissue and for the replacement of basal or endogenous losses.[141] The essential amino acid requirements during early infancy were first determined between 1955 and 1964 by Snyderman et al., as cited by Jürgens.[140] The studies were performed on groups of six or seven young neonates who were fed mixtures of 18 free amino acids based on the pattern of the mother's milk protein. Following withdrawal of one special essential amino acid from the pattern, this amino acid was reintroduced until nitrogen balance approached the normal range obtained when feeding the complete amino acid mixture. The smallest amount of the amino acid that had to be added to the amino acid mixture to achieve this effect was considered to be equivalent to the minimal requirement. In this manner, the demands were determined for eight essential amino acids and histidine.

Jürgens[140] determined the amino acid requirements of 38 preterm neonates weighing 940 to 2400 g on total parenteral nutrition for 10-day periods. The nitrogen balance and serum amino acid pattern were used to determine optimal amino acid compositions for parenteral solutions.

The plasma transfer of amino acids after short-term infusions of amino acid solutions with different compositions was measured by Bürger and Wolf.[142] These investigators regarded the plasmatic transfer of the various amino acids to be identical to endogenous input requirement.

All of these methods have been shown to be lacking in various respects, although they have helped to improve the quality of amino acid solutions for the parenteral nutrition of preterm and term neonates.[140] Markedly elevated blood amino acid concentrations, indicating amino acid imbalance, were common side effects of the earlier generations of parenteral solutions. These effects have been avoided by the improved formulations, as have the toxic effects of amino acids due to excessive ammonia formation, azotemia, and acidosis. Immature human neonates have a relatively low tolerance to phenylalanine, tyrosine, and methionine.[143] Hyperphenylalaninemia is known to cause brain damage, and high tyrosine concentrations have been shown to correlate with learning difficulties in later life. If such conditions are produced by amino acid infusion therapy, similar disturbances are to be expected. High methionine plasma levels are commonly seen with parenteral nutrition during early infancy.[143]

Comparison of the amino acid inputs recommended by various investigators for human neonates receiving parenteral nutrition reveals broad method-related deviations for almost all essential and nonessential amino acids. The recommended concentrations sometimes differ by several hundred percent and can be used as reference only with caution.[144] For practical purposes, the amino acid pattern of human milk seems to be the most suitable reference, as even very small premature neonates are known to grow normally, retain nitrogen, and maintain an extracellular amino acid homeostasis comparable to those of term neonates, provided a sufficient quantity of mother's milk protein is offered. Such normality is limited by the volume of mother's milk necessary to meet this requirement. High volumes are suspected to cause cardiovascular and pulmonary disturbances. Additional elements of uncertainty may arise from differences in the results of amino acid analysis of mother's milk protein and the difficulty of manufacturing amino acid mixtures with a composition identical to that of mother's milk due to the low solubility and the instability of amino acids such as cystine, tyrosine, and glutamine. These difficulties may be overcome in the future by the use of dipeptides containing these amino acids.

Amino Acid Requirements for Parenteral Nutrition

The amounts of amino acids delivered by the placental bloodstream to the fetus far exceed those needed for fetal protein synthesis. The net umbilical uptake of the various amino acids by the human fetus is unknown. Animal experiments with fetal lambs revealed an uptake of 1 g nitrogen·kg^{-1}day^{-1} corresponding to 6.3 g protein·kg^{-1}day^{-1}.[145]

Because intrauterine growth rates and the corresponding protein accretion rates in fetal lambs are three times as high as in the human fetus, a distinctly lower umbilical amino acid uptake of approximately 2.1 g protein·kg^{-1}day^{-1} can be expected in the latter.

Moreover, a considerable fraction of the amino acids delivered from the placenta to fetal lambs is converted to urea, emphasizing the abundance of the amino acid supply.[146] Pohlandt[147] proposed that amino acid requirements for the parenteral nutrition of neonates should be estimated from the differences between the amino acid concentrations in the umbilical cord vein and those in the artery with an assumed blood flow of 108 L·kg^{-1}day^{-1}. In other studies by the same investigator, the amino acid consumption of neonates was established from neonates kept at the intrauterine steady-state amino acid blood concentration by constant infusion of amino acids on the basis of the data obtained from both models. The investigator recommended a total dose of 1.9 g amino acids·kg^{-1}day^{-1} for parenterally fed term neonates. This dose is distinctly lower than the current recommendations for the breast-fed neonate.

The effect of the stress of surgery on nitrogen metabolism of parenterally fed human neonates has been studied by Duffy and Pencharz.[148] They compared two amino acid intakes (2.3 and 3.9 g·kg^{-1}day^{-1}). The nonprotein energy intakes amounted to 81 kcal·kg^{-1}day^{-1} in both groups. There were no differences seen in flux, synthesis or breakdown, or urinary creatinine or 3-methylhistidine excretion between the two groups. The higher nitrogen intake correlated with the significantly higher net protein accretion because of the lower rate of endogenous protein breakdown (see Chapter 50).

Nitrogen intakes from amino acid solutions with a high biologic value of approximately 400 mg (2.5 g amino acids·kg^{-1}day^{-1}) and a nonprotein energy supply of about 80 kcal·kg^{-1}day^{-1} have been proposed to meet the needs of premature neonates during the immediate postoperative period.[149] The amino acid requirements of term neonates undergoing surgery were estimated by Zlotkin,[150] who recommended an amino acid intake of 2.3 to 2.7 g·kg^{-1}day^{-1}. Recommendations for intravenous amino acid intake of the term neonate vary from 2.5 to 5.0 g·kg^{-1}day^{-1},[150] as cited by Zlotkin.[111]

The higher figures were recommended when first-generation amino acid formulations were in use. Since adapted formulas have been available, the lower range has been recommended. Providing adequate amounts of energy, their use in lower dosage results in sufficiently high nitrogen retention and weight gain and reduces the risk of azotemia.[151]

Early postnatal amino acid administration was shown to improve whole-body protein turnover in preterm infants.[95,152] Protein breakdown and amino acid oxidation were higher when the nonprotein energy was administered as glucose in comparison with mixtures of glucose and fat emulsions.[153,154]

There were no differences in net protein gain, protein synthesis, and breakdown when amino acid solutions adapted to the amino acid pattern of human milk and egg protein, respectively, were compared.[155] However, this is not to be generalized, since commercial pediatric amino acid solutions differ broadly in the composition of their essential and nonessential amino acids.[144]

References

1. Schoenheimer R. The dynamic state of body constituents. Cambridge: Harvard University Press, 1942.
2. Sander G, Hülsemann I, Topp H, et al. Protein and RNA turnover. Ann Nutr Metab 1986;30:137–142.
3. Forbes RM, Cooper AR, Mitchel HH. The composition of the adult human body as determined by chemical analysis. J Biol Chem 1953;203:359–366.
4. Abumrad NN, Cerosimo E, Lacy WW. Physiologic role of branched chain amino and keto acids in vivo. In: Adibi SA, Fekl W, Langenbeck U, eds. Branched chain amino acids in health and disease. Basel: Karger, 1984;162–181.
5. Alberts B, Bray D, Lewis I, et al. Molecular biology of the cell. New York: Garland, 1983.
6. Schöch G, Topp H, Held A, et al. Interrelation between wholebody turnover rates of RNA and protein. Eur J Clin Natr 1990;44:647–658.
7. Tai-An X, Ming Kong X, Haystead TAJ, et al. PHAS-I AS a link between nitrogen activated protein kinase and translation initiation. Science 1994;266:653–656.
8. Cheek DB. Human growth. Philadelphia: Lea & Febiger, 1968.
9. Jansen M, De Moor CH, Sussenbach JS, Van den Brande JL. Translational control of gene expression. Pediatr Res 1995;37:681A.
10. Pain VM. Protein synthesis and its regulation. In: Waterlow JC, Garlick PJ, Millward DJ, eds. Protein turnover in mammalian tissues and in the whole body. Amsterdam: North Holland, 1978;15–54.
11. Waterlow JC, Garlick PJ, Millward DJ. Protein turnover in mammalian tissues and in the whole body. Amsterdam: North Holland, 1978.
12. Wolfe RR. Radioactive and stable isotope tracers in biomedicine. New York: Wiley-Liss, 1992.
13. Waterlow JC, Stephen JML. Protein metabolism in man. London, New York: Applied Science, 1981.
14. Sprinson DB, Rittenberg D. The rate of interaction of amino acids of the diet with the tissue proteins. J Biol Chem 1949;180:715–726.
15. Winkler E, Faust H. A mathematical model for the analysis of the turnover of protein mixtures. I. General mathematical formalism. Acta Biol Med Ger 1981;40:227–238.
16. Winkler E, Faust H. Theoretische Aspekte der Untersuchung des Stickstoffmetabolismus mit ^{15}N beim Menschen. I. Allgemeine Grundlagen. Isotopenpraxis 1978;14:349–352.
17. Plath C, Heine W, Wutzke KD, et al. ^{15}N Tracer kinetic studies of the validity of various ^{15}N-tracer substances for determining whole-body protein parameters in very small preterm infants. J Pediatr Gastroenterol Nutr 1987;6:400–408.
18. Wutzke KD, Heine W, Drescher U, et al. ^{15}N-labelled yeast protein—a valid tracer for calculating whole-body protein parameters in infants: a comparison between [^{15}N]-yeast protein and [^{15}N]-glycine. Hum Nutr Clin Nutr 1983;37C:317–327.
19. Picou D, Taylor-Roberts T. The measurement of total protein synthesis and catabolism and nitrogen turnover in infants in different nutritional states and receiving different amounts of dietary protein. Clin Sci 1969;36:283–296.
20. Park W, Faust H, Knoblach G, et al. Untersuchungen zur Dynamik des Proteinmetabolismus mit ^{13}C-markierten Aminosäuren. In: Eckardt I, Wolfram G, eds. Stabile Isotope in der Ernährungsforschung. Nicht-energetische Bedeutung von Fett. Reihe Klinische Ernährung. München: W. Zuckschwerdt, 1987;31:121–134.
21. Matthews DE, Motil KJ, Rohrbaugh DK, et al. Measurement of leucine metabolism in man from a primed continuous infusion of L [1-^{13}C]-leucine. Am J Physiol 1980;238:E473–E479.
22. Millward DJ, De Benoist B, Halliday D. The use of stable isotope in the measurement of whole body protein turnover in the human neonate. In: Dietze O, Kleinberger G, Wolfram G, eds. Clinical nutrition and metabolic research. Basel: Karger, 1986:178–191.
23. Bier DM, Young VR. Whole body protein turnover. Is leucine a representative tracer? In: Adibi SA, Fekl W, Langenbeck U, et al., eds. Branched chain amino acids in health and disease. Basel: Karger, 1984:147–161.
24. Waterlow JC. ^{15}N end-product methods for the study of whole body protein turnover. Proc Nutr Soc 1981;40:317–320.

25. Garlick PJ, Burns HJ, Palmer RM. Regulation of muscle protein turnover: possible implications for modifying the responses to trauma and nutrient intake. Baillieres Clin Gastroenterol 1988;2:915–940.
26. Plenert W, Heine W. Normalwerte. Berlin: Volk & Gesundheit, 1984.
27. Scott SM, Watterberg KL. Effect of gestational age, postnatal age, and illness on plasma cortisol concentrations in premature infants. Pediatr Res 1995;37:112A.
28. Brownlee KG, Ng PC, Henderson MJ, et al. Catabolic effect of dexamethasone in the preterm body. Arch Dis Child 1992;67:885 (7 Spec No).
29. Van Goudoever JB, Wattimena JD, Carnielli VP, et al. Effect of dexamethasone on protein metabolism in infants with bronchopulmonary dysplasia. J Pediatr 1994;124:112–118.
30. Micheli JL, Schisler K, Schutz Y, et al. Neonatal adaptation of energy and protein metabolism. J Perinatol Med 1991;19:87–106.
31. Micheli JL, Schutz Y, Pfister R, et al. Protein turnover and early postnatal growth in very low birth weight infants. In: Paust H, Park W, Helge H, eds. Use of stable isotopes in clinical research and practice. München: Zuckschwerdt, 1988;34:70–84.
32. Moro G, Minoli I, Fulconis F, et al. Low protein formula supports normal growth and protein metabolism in term infants. Pediatr Res 1987;21:433A.
33. Heine W, Plath C, Richter I, et al. ^{15}N-Tracer investigations into the nitrogen metabolism of preterm infants fed mother's milk and a formula diet. J Pediatr Gastroenterol Nutr 1983;2:606–612.
34. Plath C, Heine W, Krienke L, et al. ^{15}N Tracer-kinetic studies on the nitrogen metabolism of very small preterm infants on a diet of mother's milk. Hum Nutr Clin Nutr 1985;39C:399–409.
35. Heine W, Wutzke KD, Walther F, et al. Eiweißstoffwechsel und Fettbilanzen unter diätetischer Behandlung der akuten Säuglingsenteritis mit einer definierten, standardisierten Oligopeptidnahrung. Monatsschr Kinderheilkd 1987;135:99–102.
36. Heine W, Tiess M, Wutzke KD. ^{15}N Tracer investigations of the physiological availability of urea nitrogen in mother's milk. Acta Paediatr Scand 1986;75:439–443.
37. Fomon SJ, Matthews DE, Bier DM, et al. Bioavailability of dietary urea nitrogen in the infant. J Pediatr 1987;111:221–224.
38. Fomon SJ, Matthews DE, Bier DM, et al. Bioavailability of dietary urea nitrogen in the breast fed infant. Clin Lab Observ 1988;113:515–517.
39. Donovan SM, Lönnerdal B, Atkinson SA. Bioavailability of urea nitrogen for the low birthweight infant. Acta Paediatr Scand 1990;79:899–905.
40. Wheeler RA, Jackson AA, Griffith DM. Urea production and recycling in neonates. J Pediatr Surg 1991;26:1–3.
41. Heine W, Mohr C, Wutzke KD, Radke M. Symbiotic interactions between colonic microflora and protein metabolism in infants. Acta Paediatr Scand 1991;80:7–12.
42. Beaton GF. Nutrition. A comprehensive treatise. Orlando: Academic Press, 1964.
43. Plath C, Heine W, Massute G, et al. Stickstoffanalytische Untersuchungen zur Optimierung der Ernährung unreifer Frühgeborener durch Frauenmilchsupplementierung. Kinderarztl Prax 1987;55:19–30.
44. Hörnchen H, Neubrand W, Ioosten R, et al. Totale und partielle parenterale Ernährung bei Früh- und Neugeborenen. Stickstoffbilanzen und Aminosäurenchromatogramme. Infusionstherapie 1979;6:274–282.
45. Southgate DAT, Barrett M. The intake and excretion of caloric constituents of milk by babies. Br J Nutr 1966;20:363–372.
46. Fomon SJ. Nitrogen balance studies with normal fullterm infants receiving high intakes of protein. Pediatrics 1961;28:347–361.
47. Heine W, Gassmann B, Plenert W. Vergleichende Bilanzuntersuchungen an jungen Säuglingen unter Ernährung mit eiweißreichen und eiweißarmen Fertignahrungen. Padiatr Grenzgeb 1968;7:301–316.
48. Brock J. Biologische Daten für den Kinderarzt, vol. 2. Heidelberg: Springer, 1954:48–49.
49. Widdowson EM. The demands of the fetal and maternal tissues for nutrients and the bearing of these on the needs of the mother to "eat for two." In: Dobbing J, ed. Maternal nutrition in pregnancy. Eating for two? London: Academic Press, 1981:1–7.
50. Widdowson EM, Southgate DAT, Hey EN. Body composition of the fetus and infant. In: Visser HKA, ed. Nutrition and metabolism of the fetus and infant. Boston: Martinus Nijhoff, 1979:169–177.
51. Pohlandt F, Kupferschmid C. The protein requirement of preterm infants. Klin Pädiatr 1985;197:164–166.
52. Snyderman SE, Boyer A, Kogut D, et al. The protein requirement of the preterm infant. The effect of protein intake on the retention of nitrogen. J Pediatr 1969;74:872–880.
53. Wauben I, Westerterp K, Gerver WJ, et al. Effect of varying protein intake on energy balance, protein balance and estimated weight gain composition in premature infants. Eur J Clin Nutr 1995;49:11–16.
54. Heird WC. Feeding the premature infant: human milk or an artificial formula? Am J Dis Child 1977;131:468–469.
55. Kashyap S, Schulz K, Ramakrishnan R, et al. Evaluation of mathematical model for predicting the relationship between protein and energy intake of low birth weight infants and the rate and composition of weight gain. Pediatr Res 1994;35:704–712.
56. Guesry PR, Secretin MC, Goyens P. Neue Aspekte der Ernährung von Neugeborenen mit niedrigem Geburtsgewicht. Monatsschr Kinderheilkd 1985;134:508–515.
57. Pencharz PB, Farri L, Papageorgiou A. The effects of human milk and low protein-formulae on the rates of total body protein turnover and urinary 3-methyl histidine excretion of preterm infants. Clin Sci 1983;64:611–616.
58. Heine W. Zum Eiweißbedarf früh- und reifgeborener Säuglinge. Kinderaerztl Prax 1983;16:213–219.
59. Gordon HH, Ganzor AF. On the protein allowances for young infants. J Pediatr 1959;54:503–528.
60. Committee on Nutrition. American Academy of Pediatrics. Pediatric nutrition handbook. 2nd ed. Elk Grove Village, IL: 1985.

61. Committee on Nutrition of the Preterm Infant. European Society of Pediatric Gastroenterology and Nutrition. Nutrition and feeding of preterm infants. Acta Paediatr Scand Suppl 1987;336:1–14.
62. Prentice A, Ewing G, Roberts SB, et al. The nutritional role of breast milk IgA and lactoferrin. Acta Paediatr Scand 1987;76:592–598.
63. Butte NF, Wong WW, Fiorotto M, et al. Influence of early feeding mode on body composition of infants. Biol Neonate 1995;67:414–424.
64. Heine W, Gassmann B, Plenert W. Vergleichende Bilanzuntersuchungen an jungen Säuglingen unter Ernährung mit eiweißarmen und eiweißreichen Kuhmilchfertignahrungen. Pädiatr Grenzgeb 1968;7:301–316.
65. Heine W, Radke M, Wutzke KD. The significance of tryptophan in human milk. Amino Acids 1995;9:191–205.
66. Heine W. Qualitative aspects of protein in human milk and formula: amino acid pattern. In: Räihä N, ed. Protein metabolism during infancy. New York: Raven Press, 1994.
67. Heine W, Radke M, Wutzke KD, et al. α-Lactalbumin-enriched low-protein infant formulas: a comparison to breast milk feeding. Acta Paediatr 1996;85:1024–1028.
68. Forestier F, Daffos F, Rainaut M, et al. Blood chemistry of normal human fetuses at midtrimester of pregnancy. Pediatr Res 1987;21:579–583.
69. Ehrich JH, Rothganger S. Cholinesterase activity and protein concentration in the serum of premature and newborn infants. Klin Pädiatr 1987;199:98–102.
70. Cartlidge PHT, Rutter N. Serum albumin concentrations and oedema in the newborn. Arch Dis Child 1986;61:657–660.
71. Yudkoff M, Nissim I, McNellis W, et al. Albumin synthesis in premature infants: determination of turnover with ^{15}N-glycine. Pediatr Res 1987;21:49–53.
72. Misaki M, Kumazawa M, Sugita M, et al. A possible relationship between cord blood transferrin and birth length in infants. Horm Res 1987;25:228–231.
73. Colonna F, Calipa MT, Trappan A, et al. Proteine nutrizionali e della fase acuta nel neonato pretermine: standard di riferimento ed interrelazioni. Minerva Pediatr 1994;46:501–508.
74. Jain SK, Shah M, Ransonet L, et al. Maternal and neonatal plasma transthyretin concentrations and birth weight of newborn infants. Biol Neonate 1995;68:10–14.
75. Manco-Johnson MJ, Abshire TC, Jacobson LJ, et al. Severe neonatal protein C deficiency: prevalence and thrombolic risk. J Pediatr 1991;119:793–798.
76. Corrigan JJ Jr, Jeter MA. Histidine-rich glycoprotein and plasminogen plasma levels in term and preterm newborns. Am J Dis Child 1990;144:825–828.
77. Corrigan JJ Jr, Jeter MA. Tissue-type plasminogen activator inhibitor and histidine-rich glycoproteins in stressed human newborns. Pediatrics 1992;89:43–46.
78. Lassarre C, Hardouin S, Daffos F, et al. Serum insulin-like growth factors and insulin-like growth factor binding proteins in the human fetus. Relationship with growth in normal subjects and in subjects with intrauterine growth retardation. Pediatr Res 1991;29:219–225.
79. Polin RA. Role of fibronectin in diseases of newborn infants and children. Rev Infect Dis 1990;12(suppl 4):428–438.
80. Lucas A, Boyes S, Bloom SR, et al. Metabolic and endocrine responses to a milk feed in six day old term infants: differences between breast and cow's milk formula feeding. Acta Paediatr Scand 1981;70:195–200.
81. Reeds PJ, Fuller MF. Nutrient intake and protein turnover. Proc Nutr Soc 1983;42:463–471.
82. Garlick PJ, McNurlan MA, Ballmer PE. Influence of dietary protein intake on whole-body protein turnover in humans. Diabetes Care 1991;14:1189–1198.
83. Adibi SA, Fekl W, Langenbeck U, et al. Branched chain amino- and keto acids in health and disease. Basel: Karger, 1984.
84. Collu R, Ducharme JR, Guyda H. Pediatric endocrinology. New York: Raven Press, 1981.
85. Young VR. Protein energy interrelationship in the newborn: a brief consideration of some basis aspects. In: Lebenthal E, ed. Textbook of gastroenterology and nutrition in infancy. New York: Raven Press, 1981:257–263.
86. Roulet M. Der Proteinbedarf des reifen Neugeborenen und Frühgeborenen. Monatsschr Kinderheilkd 1983;131:480–482.
87. Giacoia GP, Watson S, West K. Rapid turnover transport proteins, plasma albumin and growth in low birth weight infants. J Parenter Enter Nutr 1984;8:367–370.
88. Ebner S, Schoknecht P, Reeds P, et al. Growth and metabolism of gastrointestinal and skeletal muscle tissues in protein-malnourished neonatal pigs. Am J Physiol 1994;266:1736–1743.
89. Frazer TE, Kare IE, Hillman LS, et al. Direct measurement of gluconeogenesis from 2.3-^{13}C2 alanine in the human neonate. Am J Physiol 1981;240:E615–E621.
90. Pencharz P, Beesley J, Sauer P, et al. A comparison of the estimates of whole-body protein turnover in parenterally fed neonates obtained using three different end products. Can J Physiol Pharmacol 1989;67:624–628.
91. Pencharz P, Beesley J, Sauer P, et al. Total-body protein turnover in parenterally fed neonates: effects of energy source studied by using [^{15}N]glycine and [1-^{13}C]leucine. Am J Clin Nutr 1989;50:1395–1400.
92. Stack T, Reeds P, Preston T, et al. A study of protein turnover in preterm neonates using ^{15}N enrichment of urinary ammonia. Eur J Clin Nutr 1990;44:231–234.
93. Stack T, Reeds P, Preston T, et al. ^{15}N tracer studies of protein metabolism in low birth weight preterm infants: a comparison of ^{15}N-glycine and ^{15}N-yeast protein hydrolysate and of human milk- and formula-fed babies. Pediatr Res 1989;25:167–172.
94. Pencharz PB. The 1987 Borden award lecture. Protein metabolism in premature infants. Can J Physiol Pharmacol 1988;66:1247–1252.
95. Van Lingen RA, van Goudoever JB, Luijendijk IH, et al. Effects of early amino acid administration during total parenteral nutrition on protein metabolism in preterm infants. Clin Sci 1992;82:199–203.
96. Wutzke KD, Heine W, Plath C, et al. Whole-body protein parameters in premature infants: a comparison on differ-

ent ^{15}N tracer substances and different methods. Pediatr Res 1992;31:95–101.
97. Beaufrère B. Protein turnover in low-birth-weight (LBW) infants. Acta Paediatr Suppl 1994;405:86–92.
98. Van Goudoever JB, Sulkers EJ, Halliday D, et al. Whole-body protein turnover in preterm appropriate for gestational age and small for gestational age infants: comparison of [^{15}N]glycine and [1-^{13}C]leucine administered simultaneously. Pediatr Res 1995;37:381–388.
99. Jackson AA, Shaw ICE, Barber A, et al. Nitrogen metabolism in preterm infants fed human donor breast milk: the possible essentiality of glycine. Pediatr Res 1981;15:1454–1461.
100. Nicholson JF. Rates of protein synthesis in premature infants. Pediatr Res 1970;4:389–404.
101. Pencharz PB, Steffee WP, Cochran W, et al. Protein metabolism in human neonates: nitrogen balance studies, estimated obligatory losses of nitrogen and whole-body turnover of nitrogen. Clin Sci Mol Med 1972;52:435–498.
102. Pencharz PB, Masson M, Desgranges F, et al. Total-body protein turnover in human premature neonates: effects of birth weight, intrauterine nutritional status and diet. Clin Sci 1981;61:207–215.
103. Nissim I, Yudkoff M, Pereira G, et al. Effects of conceptual age and dietary intake on protein metabolism in premature infants. J Pediatr Gastroenterol Nutr 1983;2:507–516.
104. Catzeflis C, Schutz Y, Micheli JL, et al. Whole body protein synthesis and energy expenditure in very low birth weight infants. Pediatr Res 1985;19:679–687.
105. Cauderay M, Schutz Y, Micheli JL, et al. Energy nitrogen balances and protein turnover in small and appropriate for gestational age low birth weight infants. Eur J Clin Nutr 1988;42:125–136.
106. Böhm G, Senger H, Braun W, et al. Metabolic differences between AGA and SGA infants of very low birth weight. I. Relationship to intrauterine growth retardation. Acta Paediatr Scand 1988;77:19–23.
107. Böhm G, Senger H, Müller DM, et al. Metabolic differences between AGA and SGA very low birth weight infants. II. Relationship to protein intake. Acta Paediatr Scand 1988;77:642–646.
108. San Pietro A, Rittenberg D. A study of the rate of protein synthesis in humans. II. Measurement of the metabolic pool and the rate of protein synthesis. J Biol Chem 1953;201:457–473.
109. Jackson AA, Golden MHN. Interrelationship of amino acid pools and protein turnover. In: Waterlow JC, Stephen JML, eds. Nitrogen metabolism in man. London, NJ: Applied Science, 1981:361–373.
110. Matthews DE, Conway JM, Young VR, et al. Glycine nitrogen metabolism in man. Metabolism 1981;30:886–893.
111. Fern EB, Garlick PJ, McNurlan MA, et al. The excretion of isotope in urea and ammonia for estimating protein turnover in man with [^{15}N]glycine. Clin Sci 1981;61:217–228.
112. Kien VL. ^{15}N-Tracers for studying whole body protein metabolism in premature infants. J Pediatr Gastroenterol Nutr 1987;6:321–323.
113. Beaufrere B, Putet G, Pachiaudi C, et al. Whole body protein turnover measured with ^{13}C-leucine and energy expenditure in preterm infants. Pediatr Res 1990;28:147–152.
114. Johnson C, Metcoff J. Relation of protein synthesis to plasma and cell amino acids in neonates. Pediatr Res 1986;20:140–146.
115. Schreier W. Einige quantitative und qualitative Aspekte der künstlichen Ernährung des neugeborenen Säuglings. In: Grüttner R, ed. Säuglings-ernährung heute. Berlin: Springer, 1982:27–49.
116. Kalhan SC. Rates of urea synthesis in the human newborn: effect of maternal diabetes and small size for gestational age. Pediatr Res 1993;34:801–804.
117. Parsons HG, Wood MM, Pencharz PB. Diurnal variation in urine [^{15}N]-urea content, estimates of whole body protein turnover, and isotope recycling in healthy meal-fed children with cystic fibrosis. Can J Physiol Pharmacol 1983;61:72–80.
118. Wernermann J, von der Decken A, Vinnars E. The diurnal pattern of protein synthesis in human skeletal muscle. Clin Nutr 1985;4:203–205.
119. Rennie MJ, Edwards RHT, Halliday D, et al. Muscle protein synthesis in man: effects of feeding and fasting. Clin Sci 1982;63:519–523.
120. Winterer J, Bistrian BR, Bilmazes C, et al. Whole body protein turnover, studied with ^{15}N-glycine, and muscle breakdown in mildly obese subjects during a protein-sparing diet and a brief total fast. Metabolism 1980;29:575–581.
121. Garlick PJ, Clugston GA, Waterlow JC. Influence of low-energy diets on whole-body protein turnover in obese subjects. Am J Physiol 1980;238:E235–E244.
122. Ward MWN, Halliday D, Matthews DE, et al. The effect of enteral nutritional support on skeletal muscle protein synthesis and whole body protein turnover in fasted surgical patients. Hum Nutr Clin Nutr 1983;37:453–458.
123. Cheng KN, Pacy PJ, Dworzak F, et al. Influence of fasting on leucine and muscle protein metabolism across human forearm determined using L-[1-^{13}C,^{15}N-]leucine as the tracer. Clin Sci 1987;73:241–246.
124. Schönheyder F, Heilskov NCS, Olesen K. Isotopic studies on the mechanism of negative nitrogen balance produced by immobilization. Scand J Clin Lab Invest 1954;6:178–188.
125. Askanazi I, Elwyn DH, Kinney IM, et al. Muscle and plasma amino acids after injury: the role of inactivity. Ann Surg 1978;188:797–803.
126. Goldspink DE. The influence of activity on muscle size and protein turnover. J Physiol 1977;264:283–296.
127. Jeevanandam M, Long CL, Birkhahn RH, et al. Evaluation of whole body nitrogen kinetics in acute metabolic acidosis. Am J Clin Nutr 1983;37:201–210.
128. Matthews DE. Protein digestion and absorption. In: Kretchmer N, Minkowski A, eds. Nutritional adaptation of the intestinal tract of the newborn. New York: Raven Press, 1983:73–91.
129. Chandra RK, Hamed A. Cumulative incidence of atopic disorders in high risk infants fed whey hydrolysate, soy,

129. and conventional cow's milk formulas. Ann Allergy 1991; 67:129–132.
130. Vandenplas Y, Hauser B, Van den Borre C, et al. Effect of a whey hydrolysate prophylaxis of atopic disease. Ann Allergy 1992;68:419–424.
131. Maroni A, Agosti M, Motta GA. Dietary prevention program including whey hydrolysed formula for high risk atopic babies: 0–24 month follow up. Dev Physiopathol Clin 1990;1:131–141.
132. Businco L, Dreborg S, Einarsson R, et al. Hydrolysed cow's milk formulae. Allergenicity and use in treatment and prevention. An ESPACI position paper. Pediatr Allergy Immunol 1993;4:101–111.
133. Clarke D, Hymon DE. Gastric secretory maturation of preterm infants. Pediatr Res 1984;18:193A.
134. Heine W, Fritzsch AK. Immunologische Veränderungen der Kuhmilchproteine bei der Magenverdauung. Kinderärztl Prax 1988;56:375–379.
135. Zoppi G, Andreotti G, Pajno-Ferrara F, et al. Exocrine pancreas function in premature and full term neonates. Pediatr Res 1973;6:880–886.
136. Hadorn B. Developmental aspects of intraluminal protein digestion. In: Lebenthal E, ed. Textbook of gastroenterology and nutrition in infancy. New York: Raven Press, 1981:365–373.
137. Auricchio S. Developmental aspects of brush border hydrolysis and absorption of peptides. In: Lebenthal E, ed. Textbook of gastroenterology and nutrition in infancy. New York: Raven Press, 1981:375–384.
138. Sturman IA, Gaull DE, Räihä NCR. Absence of cystathionase in human fetal liver: Is cystine essential? Science 1970;169:74–76.
139. Sturman IA, Rassin DK, Gaull DE. Taurine in development: Is it essential in the neonate? Pediatr Res 1976; 10:415A.
140. Jürgens P. Zum Aminosäurebedarf Früh- und Neugeborener sowie junger Säuglinge bei enteraler und parenteraler Ernährung. In: Bässler KH, Grünert A, Kleinberger G, eds. Contribution to infusion therapy and clinical nutrition. Basel, München: Karger, 1986;16:14–53.
141. Fomon SJ, De Maeyer EM, Owen GM. Urinary and fecal excretion of endogenous nitrogen by infants and children. J Nutr 1965;85:235–246.
142. Bürger U, Wolf H. Untersuchungen über die Verwertung parenteral zugeführter Aminosäuren bei Frühgeborenen und hypotrophen Neugeborenen. III. Zusammenstellung einer Aminosäurenlösung nach pharmakokinetischen Gesichtspunkten. Eur J Pediatr 1976;122:169–175.
143. Lindblad BS, Alfven G, Ginsburg EE. The intravenous and peroral requirements of amino acids in early infancy. In: Visser HKA, ed. Nutrition and metabolism of the fetus and infant. Boston: Martinus Nijhoff, 1979:325–339.
144. Heine W. Wieviel Eiweiß brauchen Frühgeborene. How much protein do preterm infants need? Ernährungsumschau 1995;42:51–56.
145. Lemons JA, Adcock EW, Jones UD Jr, et al. Umbilical uptake of amino acids in the unstressed fetal lamb. J Clin Invest 1976;58:1428–1434.
146. Gresham EL, James EJ, Raye IR, et al. Production and excretion of urea by the fetal lamb. Pediatrics 1972;50:372–379.
147. Pohlandt F. Studies on the requirement of amino acids in newborn infants receiving parenteral nutrition. In: Visser HKA, ed. Nutrition and metabolism of the fetus and infant. Boston: Martinus Nijhoff, 1979:341–364.
148. Duffy B, Pencharz PB. The effects of surgery on the nitrogen metabolism of parenterally fed human neonates. Pediatr Res 1986;20:32–35.
149. Duffy B, Gunn T, Colinge J, et al. The effect of varying protein quality and energy intake on the nitrogen metabolism of parenterally fed low birth weight (<1600 g) infants. Pediatr Res 1981;15:1040–1044.
150. Zlotkin SH. Intravenous nitrogen intake requirements in full term newborns undergoing surgery. Pediatrics 1984;73:493–496.
151. Heird WC, Winters RW. Total parenteral nutrition: the state of the art. J Pediatr 1975;86:2–16.
152. Rivera A Jr, Bell EF, Bier DM. Effect of intravenous amino acids on protein metabolism of preterm infants during the first three days of life. Pediatr Res 1993;33:106–111.
153. Salas-Salvado J, Molina J, Figueras J, et al. Effect of the quality of infused energy on substrate utilization in the newborn receiving total parenteral nutrition. Pediatr Res 1993;33:112–117.
154. Bresson JL, Bader B, Rocchiccioli F, et al. Proteinmetabolism kinetics and energy-substrate utilization in infants fed parenteral solutions with different glucose-fat ratios. Am J Clin Nutr 1992;55:481.
155. Mitton SG, Garlick PJ. Changes in protein turnover after the introduction of parenteral nutrition in premature infants: comparison of breast milk and egg protein-based amino acid solutions. Pediatr Res 1992;32(4):447–454.

de# 35
Inborn Errors of Amino Acid and Organic Acid Metabolism

Gerard T. Berry

Each of the 30 to 40 inborn errors of amino acid and or organic acid metabolism represent a rare occurrence in perinatal medicine. However, their combined incidence is about 1/4000 in the neonatal period. Their importance derives from what they tell us about intermediary metabolism and from the fact that these are generally treatable diseases if detected early. This chapter discusses the development of selected amino acid enzymes, pathways of amino acid and organic acid catabolism, and specific aminoacidopathies and organic acidurias that present in the neonatal period. These disorders include the organic acidemias such as propionic acidemia, methylmalonic acidemia, glutaric acidemia type II, multiple carboxylase deficiency, the urea cycle disorders, maple syrup urine disease, and nonketotic hyperglycinemia. The focus is on the biochemistry of these disorders, approaches to treatment and outcome (see Chapter 53).

Developmental Enzymology

The fetus requires nitrogen and amino acids for growth. As most of these compounds can cross the placental membrane by passive transport systems, there is less of a need for activity of fetal amino acid and organic acid metabolic pathways. Enzymatic activity appears to increase late in gestation, reaching adult levels in infancy.[1-3] Synthetic enzymes that follow this pattern include phenylalanine hydroxylase, glutamine synthetase, and ornithine aminotransferase.[4,5] Catabolic pathways, such as those in the urea cycle, evolve even more rapidly during this period.[6] The emergence of intramitochondrial enzymes, such as glutamate dehydrogenase and carbamyl phosphate synthetase I, increase in relation to the number of liver mitochondria.[7] Similar metabolic patterns to that in liver have been found in skeletal muscle,[8] kidney,[6] small intestine, stomach,[9] and brain.[10]

In human fetuses, Raiha and Suihkonen[11] found that urea synthetic activity was present by 22 weeks' gestation. However, very premature neonates of 29–31 weeks did not respond to increased protein intake with increased urea production, suggesting a limited ability to expand urea synthetic capacity. Urea synthetic activity could be induced by protein intake either after 31 weeks' gestation or beyond the postnatal age of 21 days in the more premature neonates.[12] A role for glucocorticoids and glucagon in hastening the maturation of urea cycle enzyme activity has been reported,[13] and suggests that small for gestational age neonates may have accentuated maturation of amino acid pathways.

The limited induction of urea synthetic activity with protein may account for the finding of an asymptomatic twofold elevation of plasma ammonium concentration during the first 4 to 6 weeks of life in most premature infants compared to that in term infants.[14] The etiology appears to involve arginine deficiency. Plasma concentrations of arginine and ornithine, intermediates in the urea cycle, are low, and arginine supplementation reduces ammonium concentration to normal.[15] This suggests that arginine may be an essential amino acid in the premature neonate.

The etiology of the more severe symptomatic transient hyperammonemia of prematurity,[16] is less clear. In this rare condition, premature neonates develop a plasma ammonium concentration in the range of 500 to 5000 μM associated with coma in the first 1 to 2 days of life. If the neonate survives this episode, he will recover without future episodes of hyperammonemia. However, many neonates will have suffered irreversible brain damage as a result of prolonged hyperammonemic coma. Hyperammonemia in this disorder does not respond to arginine supplementation and its etiology remains unclear.

Phenylalanine metabolism can also be transiently disturbed in the neonate, resulting in either neonatal tyrosinemia or hyperphenylalaninemia. Transient tyrosinemia is associated with increased excretion of tyrosine and its metabolites and is thought to be caused by a developmental immaturity of p-hybroxyphenylpyruvate oxidase.[17] It is exacerbated by increased protein and is less common in the breast-fed neonate. It appears that ascorbate (vitamin C) alleviates the tyrosinemia by protecting the enzyme from substrate inhibition. Although usually asymptomatic, transient tyrosinemia can be associated with lethargy and poor feeding.[18] This transient metabolic disturbance may be associated with future neurodevelopmental defects.[19,20]

Transient hyperphenylalaninemia is caused by delayed maturation of phenylalanine hydroxylase, the enzyme deficient in phenylketonuria (PKU).[18] Most neonates with this developmental aberration are detected by the PKU screening test, and a low phenylalanine formula is instituted on a short-term basis. The long-term consequences of transient hyperphenylalaninemia remain unknown.

Finally, the transsulfuration pathway involved in the synthesis of cysteine and taurine may be defective in the premature neonate. Fetal tissue and placenta lack cystathionase activity, which converts cystathionine to cysteine. As a result, cysteine, a nonessential amino acid in the adult, may be an essential amino acid in the premature neonate. Similarly taurine, being a product of the metabolism of methionine and cysteine, has been implicated as a semiessential amino acid in the premature neonate.[21] Supplementation with taurine has been shown to improve fat absorption and increase the maturation of auditory brain stem–evoked responses in the preterm neonate.[22] As a result cysteine and taurine are now added to many infant formulas.

In sum, amino acid metabolism appears to be deficient prior to full-term gestation. Yet, even the full-term neonate must adapt rapidly to the requirement of maintaining metabolic balance in the absence of the dialysis-like capabilities of the intact placenta. As a result the neonatal period is a time that inherited defects in amino acid and organic acid metabolism are most likely to surface at both the biochemical and clinical level. Because of the nature or severity of the enzymatic lesion, biochemical and/or clinical manifestations will be present even though the infant's diet is nutritionally replete. Examples include maple syrup urine disease, the organic acidemias, and the urea cycle disorders. In rare instances inborn errors have a prenatal origin; glutaric acidemia type II is an example of a lesion in mitochondrial energy metabolism that is associated with prenatal disease.[23]

Amino Acid Pathways Involved in Inborn Errors

In a broad sense, any biochemical disorder that affects the detoxification of ammonia or the catabolism of glucose or amino acids will be associated with manhandling of amino and/or organic acids. Defects in ureagenesis result in accumulation of waste nitrogen variably partitioned as ammonia itself, selective urea cycle enzyme substrates, certain nonessential amino acids, and pyrimidine metabolites. Inborn errors affecting disposal of the branched-chain amino acids of their organic acid breakdown products are responsible for most of the other disorders of amino or organic acid metabolism. The metabolism of amino acids, organic acids, and the urea cycle is part of the general scheme of intermediary metabolism involving anaerobic as well as aerobic metabolism of carbohydrates, fats, and amino acids. The interrelatedness of these generally catabolic pathways is shown in Figure 35.1.

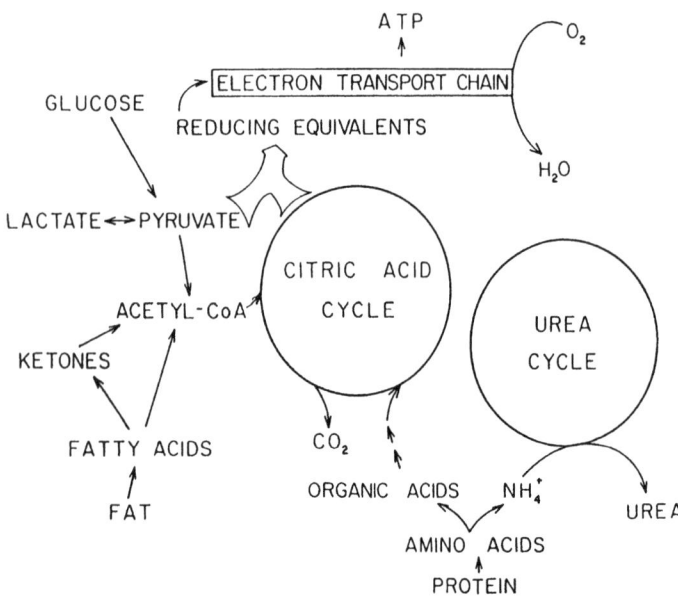

FIGURE 35.1. Intermediary metabolism: schematic representation of interactions between the glycolytic, citric acid, mitochondrial oxidation, amino acid, organic acid, and urea cycle pathways. Defects in these primarily catabolic pathways are the primary source of inborn errors of metabolism.

The Urea Cycle

While amino acids may be used for protein synthesis or conversion into special compounds such as neurotransmitters, their ultimate catabolic fate is to be broken down to CO_2, H_2O, and ammonia (NH_3). Flux through the catabolic pathway is accentuated by increased protein or amino acid intake and fasting-related muscle proteolysis. The urea cycle functions to maintain body NH_3 at a safe concentration by effecting conversion to excretable urea.

The urea cycle is depicted in Figure 35.2. Only liver contains all of the enzymes in amounts sufficient for effective urea cycle functioning. Activity of the cycle depends on hepatocyte ammonia concentration and on the supply of intramitochondrial ornithine to turn the cycle. The initial step is the condensation of NH_3, bicarbonate (HCO_3), and adenosine triphosphate (ATP) to generate carbamylphosphate. This is achieved in the mitochondrial matrix via carbamylphosphate synthetase I (CPS I). This enzyme requires N-acetylglutamate (NAG) for activation.[25] NAG is synthesized from acetyl–coenzyme A (CoA) and glutamate via mitochondrial N-acetylglutamate synthetase (NAGS). A positive effector for this enzyme is arginine, which is a urea cycle substrate.

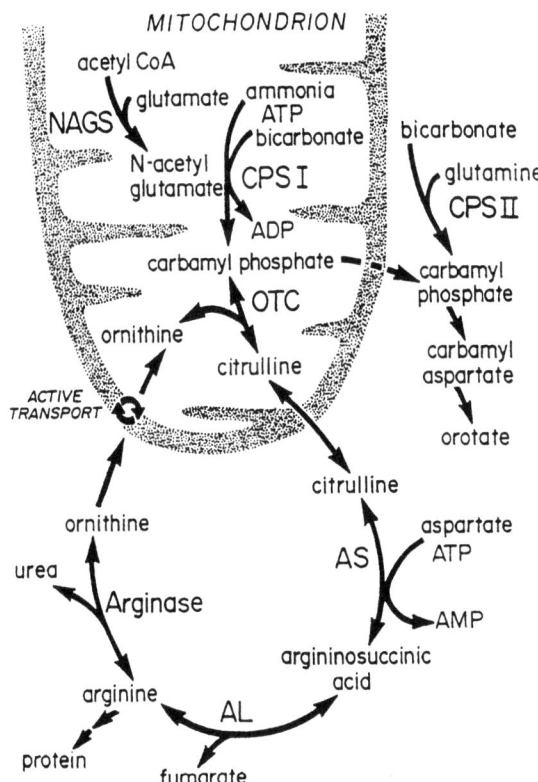

FIGURE 35.2. The urea cycle. NAGS, N-acetylglutamate synthetase; CPS, carbamyl phosphate synthetase; OTC, ornithine transcarbamylase; AS, argininosuccinate synthetase; AL, argininosuccinate lyase. (From Batshaw,[24] with permission.)

The second urea cycle enzyme, ornithine transcarbamylase (OTC), is located in the mitochondrial matrix, and allows carbamylphosphate to condense with ornithine to form citrulline. Both the mitochondrial uptake of ornithine and subsequent efflux of citrulline is carrier-mediated. Once in the cytosol, citrulline reacts with aspartate, which donates the second mole of waste nitrogen to form argininosuccinic acid (ASA). Argininosuccinate synthetase catalyzes this reaction, while argininosuccinase promotes the subsequent cleavage of argininosuccinic acid to arginine and fumaric acid. Another cytosolic enzyme, arginase, completes the cycle by promoting hydrolysis of arginine to ornithine and urea. It is important to note that the urea cycle is energy dependent, requiring an adequate supply of ATP for optimal activity.

Waste nitrogen enters the urea cycle either as NH_3 itself or as aspartate. Ammonia can be released from amino acids by a number of mechanisms. One is via mitochondrial glutamate dehydrogenase, which converts glutamate to the tricarboxylic acid cycle intermediate 2-ketoglutarate and ammonia. A second method is by the hydrolysis of glutamine, resulting in glutamate and ammonia via the enzyme glutaminase. Asparaginase similarly catalyzes the conversion of asparagine to aspartate and NH_3. Cystine may be directly desulfhydrated to ammonia, pyruvate, and hydrogen sulfide. Peroxisomal D-amino acid oxidases may affect direct production of ammonia from various D-amino acids.

Ammonia may be directly produced from adenosine, via adenosine deaminase or from the related nucleotide, adenosine monophosphate (AMP), during conversion to inosine monophosphate (IMP). Intermittently, the latter reaction may be an important source of free NH_3 in some cells or tissues such as skeletal muscle. However, most of the amine nitrogen in amino acids for disposal is ultimately shuttled to glutamate via transamination reactions, usually occurring in the cytosol and sometimes involving other nonessential amino acids such as aspartate and alanine.

Glycine Metabolism

Waste nitrogen can enter through the mitochondrial glycine cleavage enzyme complex, which results in the conversion of glycine and tetrahydrofolate (THF) to NH_3, CO_2, and methylenetetrahydrofolate. It is the major catabolic pathway for both glycine and serine. By a circuitous mechanism, this complex permits interconversion of glycine and serine. Four subunits, designated P, H, T, and L protein, compose this complex. Defects in this complex result in the inborn error nonketotic hyperglycinemia, which is described below. The reaction is initiated when glycine undergoes Schiff-base formation with the pyridoxal phosphate containing P protein.[26] Decarboxylation occurs as the aminomethyl moiety of glycine becomes covalently linked to the lipoamide-containing H protein. After release from the P protein, this one-carbon fragment of glycine is transferred from the lipoamide anchor on the H protein to tetrahydrofolate via the T protein. At this step, NH_3 is released. Lipoamide dehydrogenase, or nicotinamide adenine dinucleotide, oxidized (NAD^+)-dependent L protein, allows for subsequent reoxidation of the reduced sulphydryl group on the H protein. As most of these reactions are reversible, this complex may participate in the formation of serine via an oxidized form of tetrahydrofolate.

Branched-Chain Amino Acid Metabolism

Most of the hereditary defects in organic acid metabolism are the consequences of enzyme deficiencies of the branched-chain amino acids and are composed of the three essential aliphatic amino acids, leucine (Leu), isoleucine (Ile), and valine (Val). Their catabolism involves three steps: transamination, oxidative decarboxylation, and acyl-CoA dehydrogenation.

As shown in Figure 35.3, the initial step involves cytosolic conversion to corresponding branched-chain keto acids. These reactions are catalyzed by two transaminases, one of which utilizes leucine or isoleucene, while the other is specific for valine. Skeletal muscle is particularly enriched in branched-chain amino acid transaminase activities and accounts for the fact that branched-chain amino acids are primarily metabolized by muscle tissue and not liver. Liver is the prime location for catabolism of all other amino acids.

As opposed to the transaminases, there is only one branched-chain keto-acid decarboxylase enzyme (BCKAD) complex, and its activity is located principally in liver. A defect in this enzyme results in maple syrup urine disease (MSUD). The decarboxylase is under phosphorylation-dephosphorylation control and requires CoA, thiamine pyrophosphate, lipoic acid, NAD^+, and Mg^{2+} for activity. It is quite similar to the mitochondrial pyruvate dehydrogenase enzyme (PDH) complex in that there are three main subunits, E1, E2, and E3.[28,29] The E1 component has an $\alpha_2\beta_2$ structure and is associated with two regulatory enzymes, a kinase and a phosphatase.[28,30] A cDNA encoding the $E1_\alpha$, $E1_\beta$, E2, E3 and the kinase have been cloned.[31-42] The $E1_\alpha$ gene maps to 19q13.1-q13.2,[43] $E1_\beta$ to 6p21-p22,[44] E2 to 1p31,[44] and E3 to 7q31-q32.[45] One of the subunits, the E3 or lipoamide dehydrogenase, is in fact common to both BCKAD and PDH complexes. The BCKAD complex promotes the conversion of the leucine keto acid, 2-ketoisocaproic acid, into isovaleryl-CoA; the conversion of the isoleucine analogue 2-keto-3-methylvaleric acid to 2-methylbutyryl CoA; and the conversion of the valine analogue 2-ketoisovaleric acid to isobutyryl-CoA.

The product of the oxidative decarboxylation of the leucine kito acid, isovaleryl CoA, is subsequently metabolized via the flavin adenine dinucleotide (FAD)-dependent matrix enzyme, isovaleryl-CoA dehydrogenase, to 3-methylcrotonyl-CoA.[46] A defect in this dehydrogenase accounts for isovaleric acidemia. Separate dehydrogenases degrade the ester of isoleucine and valine. These flavin-containing soluble enzymes result in the formation of a double bond analogous to the dehydrogenation of fatty acyl-CoAs by chain length–specific acyl-CoA dehydrogenases during β-oxidation of fatty acids or dehydrogenation of the glutaric acid precursor, glutaryl-CoA. In the case of valine, the unsaturated product is methylacrylyl-CoA, while for isoleucine it is tiglyl-CoA. A generalized defect in acyl-CoA dehydrogenation has been implicated in glutaric acidemia, type II.

From this step, the oxidative mechanisms for the branched-chain organic acids deviate. Methacrylyl-CoA successively undergoes enolyl hydration, deacylation, oxidation, and thiol activation to form methylmalonyl-CoA. Analogous hydration of tiglyl-CoA results in the formation of 2-methyl-3-hydroxybutyryl CoA. The latter is oxidized to 2-methylacetoacetyl-CoA, which then undergoes thiolytic cleavage by the mitochondrial short-chain ketothiolase to propionyl-CoA and acetyl-CoA.

The further conversion of propionyl-CoA to D-methylmalonyl-CoA involves propionyl-CoA carboxylase, a biotin-containing enzyme.[47,48] A defect in this enzyme results in propionic acidemia. It is composed of α and β subunits.[47] Biotin is covalently linked to a lysine moiety on the α subunit.[48] The holocarboxylase appears to contain 6α and 6β subunits ($\alpha_6\beta_6$). A deficiency in holocarboxylase synthetase, the enzyme that attaches biotin to all the carboxylase apoenzymes,[49] leads to multiple carboxylase deficiency.

D-methylmalonyl-CoA is initially racemized to L-methylmalonyl-CoA,[50] which can then be converted to the tricarboxylic acid cycle intermediate, succinyl-CoA, via L-methylmalonyl-CoA mutase.[51] This enzyme utilizes the cofactor adenosylcobalamin to orchestrate this mechanistically complicated one-carbon movement.[52] Deficient enzyme or cofactor activity leads to methylmalonic acidemia. The enzyme is a dimer of identical subunits (α_2).[51] Unlike the isoleucine and valine pathways, leucine degradation does not result in the formation of methylmalonyl-CoA. Instead the biotin-containing enzyme, 3-methylcrotonyl-CoA carboxylase, helps to convert 3-methylcrotonyl-CoA to 3-methylglutaconyl-CoA. Enoyl hydration of the latter results in 3-hydroxy-3-methylglutaryl-CoA (HMG-CoA), which is the sole precursor for ketone body generation. During ketogenesis, it is primarily synthesized from the fatty acid metabolite, acetoacetyl-CoA, and acetyl-CoA via HMG-CoA synthetase. The final enzyme in the leucine pathway is HMG-CoA lyase, which catalyzes the

35. Inborn Errors of Amino Acid and Organic Acid Metabolism

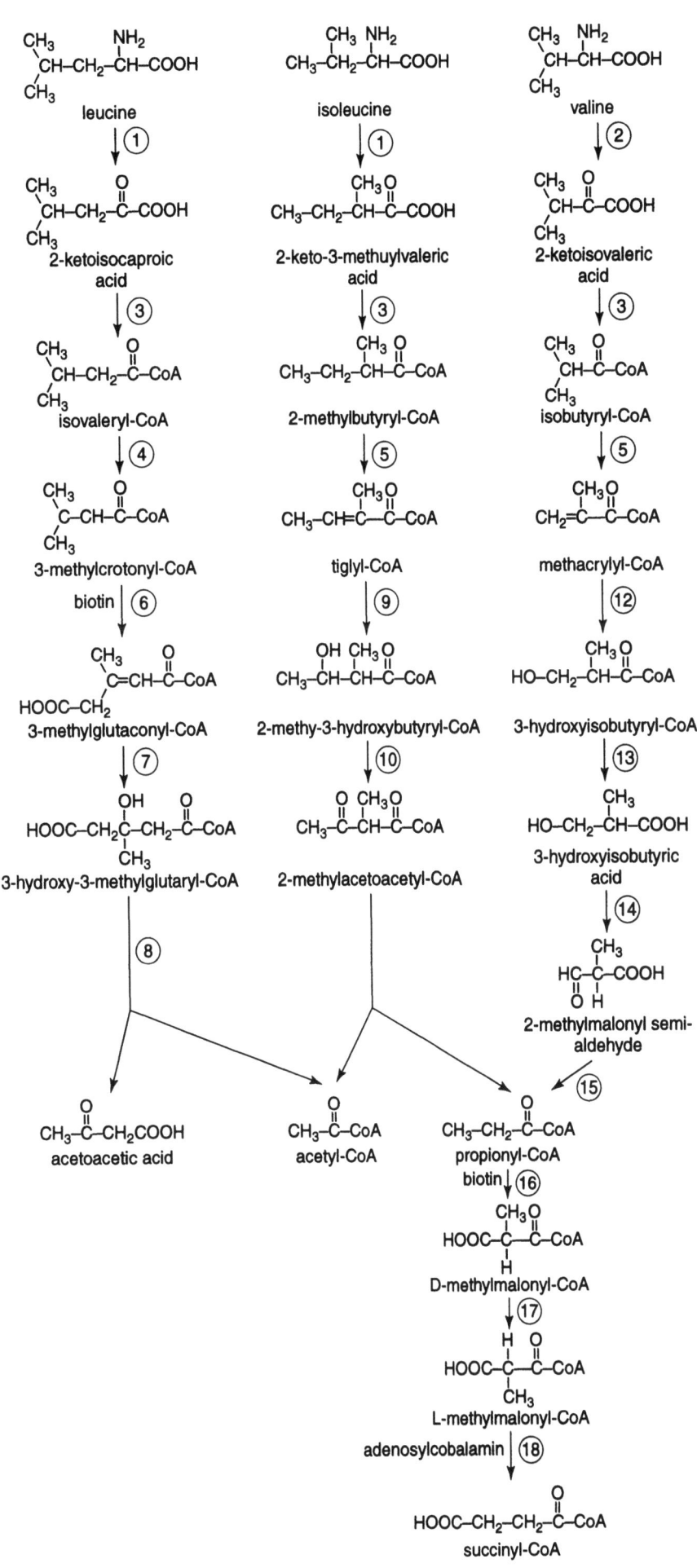

FIGURE 35.3. The three pathways for branched-chain amino acid catabolism. Enzymes are identified numerically: (1) leucine/isoleucine transaminase, (2) valine transaminase, (3) branched-chain 2-keto-acid dehydrogenase complex (the enzyme deficient in MSUD), (4) isovaleryl-CoA dehydrogenase (the enzyme defective in isovaleric acidemia), (5) isobutyryl-CoA/2-methylbutyryl-CoA dehydrogenase, (6) 3-methylcrotonyl-CoA carboxylase, (7) 3-methylglutaconyl-CoA hydratase, (8) 3-hydroxy-3-methylglutaryl-CoA lyase, (9) crotonase, (10) 2-methyl-3-hydroxybutyryl-CoA dehydrogenase, (11) 3-ketothiolase, (12) methylacryl-CoA hydratase, (13) 3-hydroxyisobutyryl-CoA deacylase, (14) 3-hydroxyisobutyrate dehydrogenase, (15) 2-methylmalonyl semialdehyde oxidase, (16) propionyl-CoA carboxylase (the enzyme deficient in propionic acidemia), (17) D-methylmalonyl-CoA racemase, and (18) L-methylmalonyl-CoA mutase (a cause of methylmalonic acidemia). (From Berry,[27] with permission.)

hydrolysis of HMG-CoA to acetyl-CoA and acetoacetate. A deficiency of this enzyme not only represents a defect in leucine oxidation but also results in an ultimate defect in ketogenesis.

Inborn Errors of Amino Acid Metabolism

This section is restricted to those inborn errors of amino acid metabolism that present clinical signs in the neonatal period. Most of these diseases have variants that present later in infancy or childhood and are associated with less severely deficient enzyme activity. The disorders discussed include organic acidemias (e.g., propionic acidemia, methylmalonic acidemia, glutaric acidemia types I and II, multiple carboxylase deficiency), inborn errors of urea synthesis, maple syrup urine disease, and nonketotic hyperglycinemia. All are autosomal recessively inherited disorders except for the urea cycle defect, ornithine transcarbamylase deficiency, which is transmitted as a sex-linked trait.[53]

Clinical Presentation of Inborn Errors in the Neonate

The neonate has relatively few ways of indicating severe illness. There is a commonality of symptoms between inborn errors of metabolism sepsis, gastrointestinal disorders, cardiopulmonary abnormalities, and intracranial hemorrhage. The neonate appears normal at birth and in the first 1 to 2 days of life. Thereafter, he manifests a progression of poor suck, hypotonia, vomiting, lethargy, grunting respirations, seizures, and coma.

Except for maple syrup urine disease, neonatal onset aminoacidopathies/organic acidemias all manifest varying degrees of hyperammonemia.[24] Each has a specific amino acid or organic acid profile. Most have effective treatment approaches. They inevitably lead to severe brain damage or death if not detected and treated within a few days of onset of clinical symptoms. It would seem reasonable to determine plasma ammonium and amino acid concentrations, and urinary organic acids as part of the workup of any neonate with the above symptom complex unless there is a clear explanation for the child's illness.

Treatment Approaches

Treatment approaches can be divided into rescuing the neonate from the acute crisis and the subsequent long-term management of the disease. In urea cycle disorders, at least, there is a significant correlation between the duration of metabolic coma and future intellectual outcome.[54] Therapy in the neonate should be started even before a definitive diagnosis is made. In fact, much of the therapy is the same irrespective of the diagnosis. Protein should be withheld and adequate calories provided. Vitamin cofactors, including biotin, cobalamin, and thiamine, are administered if an organic acidemia or maple syrup urine disease is suspected. Arginine, sodium benzoate, and sodium phenylacetate should be given if a urea cycle defect is probable.[24] Finally, peritoneal dialysis or preferably hemodialysis should be used in patients who have passed beyond stage II coma (i.e., unresponsive to painful stimuli).[55,56]

Chronic therapy of these disorders has been directed at (1) providing a deficient substrate, (2) restricting intake of substrates that directly or indirectly lead to accumulation of toxic intermediates, (3) using alternate pathways around the enzymatic block to deplete toxic intermediates, (4) amplifying residual enzyme activity using vitamin cofactors, (5) performing organ transplantation, and (6) using neuromodulators. In most cases combinations of these approaches are used and in the future the additional possibility of enzyme or gene replacement therapy may be envisioned.

In the discussion of specific enzyme deficiencies, each of these approaches is exemplified; for example, provision of arginine to the neonate with a urea cycle disorder is an example of replacing a deficient substrate.[57] Specific nitrogen-restricted diets are the mainstay of treatment for maple syrup urine disease[58] and propionic acidemia.[59] Sodium benzoate and sodium phenylacetate have been used to provide alternate pathways of waste nitrogen excretion in urea cycle disorders.[60] Vitamin cofactors have been used in treating multiple carboxylase deficiency and some cases of methylamalonic acidemia.[61] Liver transplantation has been utilized in certain urea cycle disorders.[62] Finally, neurotransmitter agents (e.g., L-dopa and 5-hydroxytryptophan) have been used to treat the dihydropteridine reductase form of phenylketonuria.[63]

Outcome

In general the neurologic outcome has been poor in children with neonatal-onset inborn errors of amino acid metabolism. This may be the result of delayed or ineffective treatment leading to prolonged coma. Besides coma, seizures, increased intracranial pressure, and intracranial hemorrhages have been common.[64] In the case of urea cycle disorders, there is evidence for a linear correlation between the duration of coma and both future IQ score and abnormalities seen on computed tomography of the brain.[54] That early treatment may improve prognosis in most of these disorders is suggested by studies of children with urea cycle disorders who were treated prospectively from birth as a result of a previously affected sibling.[65]

Their outcome was improved compared to that of their late-treated siblings. However, prospective treatment probably would not be helpful in glutaric acidemia type II or nonketotic hyperglycinemia, two inborn errors of amino acid metabolism that may have prenatal onset and for which effective therapy has yet to be developed.

Pathophysiology of Brain Damage

The neuropathology of children with inborn errors carries similarities across disease states. There are chronic abnormalities in myelin formation, alterations in the granular cell layer of the cerebellar cortex, and the presence of Alzheimer type II astrocytes. Acutely there can be cerebral edema and hemorrhage into various brain regions.[66]

These changes occur postnatally and the assumption has been that placental exchange protects the fetus in utero from the damaging effects of accumulating ammonia or amino acids. However, in some cases the protection may be incomplete and the neonate may suffer prenatal damage. In one child with ornithine transcarbamylase deficiency[67] there was evidence of brain cysts that had a prenatal origin. This may suggest incomplete protection by the heterozygous mother in this x-linked disorder. Certain children with glutaric acidemia type II have a dysmorphic appearance and organ malformations that clearly occurred early in embryogenesis.[68]

The mechanisms for both the prenatal and postnatal neuropathology are unclear. It is even uncertain what are the neurotoxic agents. For example, although it has been assumed that ammonia is directly neurotoxic, it is duration rather than peak height of ammonia during coma that correlates with subsequent brain damage.[54] This suggests the possibility of some secondary effect of ammonia on neurotransmitters. It has already been shown that some of the neurobehavioral alterations associated with hyperammonemia (e.g., anorexia, sleep disturbances, and hyperactivity) may be related to altered central serotonin metabolism. In one child, treatment with a diet low in tryptophan, the precursor of serotonin, resulted in improvement of these symptoms.[69]

It is unclear whether, in addition to ammonia, other intermediates in the urea cycle are neurotoxic. For example, there is some suggestion that children with citrullinemia and argininosuccinic aciduria have a worse intellectual outcome than those with carbamylphosphate synthetase and ornithine transcarbamylase deficiencies.[24] In the former two disorders citrulline and argininosuccinic acid accumulate in addition to ammonia, while in the latter conditions ammonia alone increases.

In another inborn error, nonketotic hyperglycinemia, severe seizures may not be a direct consequence of glycine accumulation. Instead they may be secondary to the effect of glycine on the epileptogenic glutamate receptors in the brain.[70] Improved knowledge of the neurotoxic elements in these disorders may lead to more effective means of protecting the brain during neonatal coma.

Inborn Errors of Urea Synthesis

Inherited deficiencies of each of the five enzymes of the urea cycle[64] and of N-acetylglutamate synthetase[71] have been described. Complete defects other than arginase deficiency present symptoms in the neonatal period, while partial defects present later in infancy or childhood. Arginase deficiency manifests in childhood as recurrent episodes of vomiting and lethargy and a progressive spastic diplegia.[72] The overall incidence of urea cycle disorders is about 1/30,000.[73]

The clinical presentation is similar in all the defects. The infant develops vomiting, lethargy, and coma in the first week of life and recurrent hyperammonemic episodes later in childhood, often associated with protein indiscretion or intercurrent illness. Untreated, these diseases are universally fatal.[74] Even with treatment there is only a 50% recovery from neonatal hyperammonemic coma.

In addition to hyperammonemic symptoms, infants with argininosuccinic aciduria develop a specific abnormality of the hair termed trichorrhexis nodosa.[75] Nodules appear on the hair shaft, and the hair is friable. A generalized erythematous maculopapular skin rash may appear in this disorder. Both the hair and skin conditions are associated with arginine deficiency and are corrected by arginine supplements.[76] Chronic hepatomegaly has been reported in patients with argininosuccinic aciduria, while in the other urea cycle disorders hepatomegaly is evident only during hyperammonemic episodes.[77,78] Pathologic examination of liver shows modest fatty infiltration and fibrosis. Although the etiology remains uncertain, carnitine concentration has been found to be decreased during hyperammonemic crises and may contribute to fatty infiltration.[79]

The differential diagnosis of the various urea cycle disorders usually can be made based on plasma amino acid concentration.[24] As citrulline is the product of carbamyl phosphate synthetase (CPS) and OTC and the substrate for argininosuccinate synthetase and argininosuccinase, its value is critical. In CPS and OTC deficiencies, plasma citrulline concentration is zero to a trace. With OTC deficiency there is increased urinary orotate excretion secondary to carbamyl phosphate accumulation and pyrimidine synthesis.[80] In CPS deficiency carbamylphosphate production is decreased or absent and orotate excretion is decreased. A defect in the production of the activator of CPS I, NAGS deficiency, resembles a partial CPS deficiency. In citrullinemia, plasma citrulline concentration is above 1000μM (normal 15–30μM). In argininosuccinic aciduria plasma citrulline concentration is moderately elevated, 100 to 300μM, and there are large peaks of argininosuccinic acid and its two anhydrides.

As children with these disorders have an impaired ability to excrete waste nitrogen as urea, long-term therapy was initially directed at reducing the intake of nitrogen, by decreasing protein intake and providing essential amino acids or their keto-acid analogues.[81] This approach theoretically permits adequate growth without an excessive nitrogen load. However, too great a restriction of protein leads to inadequate growth and excessive protein leads to hyperammonemia. The fine line of control was difficult to maintain. Furthermore, this approach fails when the infant is in a negative nitrogen balance, such as during an intercurrent infection. Fewer than 15% of children with neonatal onset urea cycle disorders survived the first year of life when only nitrogen restriction therapy was used.[74]

A more effective approach has involved combining nitrogen restriction with the replacement of a deficient substrate and the stimulation of alternative pathways of waste nitrogen excretion. Arginine plays a central role in this strategy. Plasma arginine concentration is deficient in all of the neonatal-onset urea cycle disorders.[57] In normal metabolism, arginine is required both to supply ornithine skeletons for OTC activity and to stimulate CPS I activity. Unless corrected, arginine deficiency will accentuate hyperammonemia by inhibiting residual urea synthetic activity. The second role of arginine is to stimulate alternate pathways of waste nitrogen excretion. It does so by promoting the synthesis and excretion of citrulline and argininosuccinic acid in citrullinemia and argininosuccinic aciduria, respectively.[82] Argininosuccinic acid contains both waste nitrogen atoms destined for excretion as urea. It has a renal clearance rate equal to the glomerular filtration rate. Provided it is continuously synthesized and excreted, argininosuccinic acid should serve as an effective substitute for urea as a waste nitrogen product. Like argininosuccinic acid, citrulline can be a means of waste nitrogen excretion. However, it contains only the one nitrogen atom derived from ammonium, lacking the second nitrogen derived from aspartic acid. Citrulline has a more limited urinary excretory capacity than argininosuccinic acid. Thus, therapy with arginine is less effective in citrullinemia.

In citrullinemia and other urea cycle disorders, arginine therapy is combined with sodium benzoate and/or sodium phenylacetate, which promote excretion of waste nitrogen.[83] Sodium benzoate is conjugated with glycine to form hippurate, which is cleared by the kidney at five times the glomerular filtration rate.

Theoretically, 1 mol of waste nitrogen is synthesized and excreted as hippurate for each mole of benzoate ingested. The hippurate synthetic mechanism rests primarily in hepatic mitochondria. The glycine consumed in this reaction can be replaced either by serine or by the reverse glycine cleavage pathway.

Sodium phenylacetate conjugates with glutamine to form phenylacetylglutamine, which is excreted by the kidney. Glutamine contains two nitrogen atoms, whereas glycine contains one. Two moles of waste nitrogen are removed for each mole of phenylacetate administered. Sodium phenylbutyrate may be used as on oral solution in lieu of sodium phenylacetate.[64] Phenylbutyrate is converted to phenylacetate in vivo.[64]

As a curative approach, liver transplantation[62] has been performed in children with CPS I and OTC deficiencies. The high cost as well as the mortality and morbidity associated with this procedure has limited its use.

Alternate pathway therapy has led to a 92% 1-year survival rate in neonates who recover from hyperammonemia coma.[60] Most of the survivors are mentally retarded.[54,84] There is a significant correlation between duration of neonatal hyperammonemic coma and IQ score at 12 months of age.[54] Four of the five children whose duration of coma was 2 days or less had normal IQ scores, while all seven children whose duration of coma was 5 days or more were severely mentally retarded. This illustrates the devastating effects of prolonged neonatal hyperammonemic coma and the importance of early diagnosis and treatment. Prenatal diagnosis is available by enzyme determination in amniocytes or chorionic villi for the cytosolic defects. Restriction fragment length polymorphism (RFLP) analysis was reported to be successful in providing prenatal diagnosis for approximately 70% of families with CPS or OTC deficiency.[85]

Propionic Acidemia

Propionic acidemia was the first described organic acidemia.[86] As noted above, the defect is in propionyl-CoA carboxylase, a biotin-requiring enzyme. Propionyl-CoA can be derived from oxidation of odd-numbered carbon-chain fatty acids, catabolism of isoleucine, valine, threonine, and methionine, and degradation of the three-carbon side chain of cholesterol. Increased dietary intake of the above precursors leads to increased blood concentration of propionic acid and increased urinary excretion of various propionate metabolites such as 3-hydroxypropionic acid, propionylglycine, tiglylglycine, and methylcitrate.

Patients with complete defects manifest clinical symptoms in the first week of life, while those with partial defects present later in infancy and childhood. In addition to the organic acidemia/aciduria, plasma ammonium concentration is in the range of 100 to 500μM, glycine concentration is in the range of 750 to 3000μM, and total serum carnitine concentration is significantly decreased.[59]

Leukopenia and thrombocytopenia are often evident during episodes of ketoacidosis. Unlike other organic acidemias, some patients with propionic acidemia do not manifest ketosis and/or metabolic acidosis during acute crises.[87,88]

As noted above, plasma ammonium concentration tends to be lower than that found in primary urea cycle defects. However, occasionally patients have had massive elevations in plasma ammonia. The mechanism of hyperammonemia appears to involve the partial inhibition of CPS I.[89] This is the result of both a direct inhibitory effect of the accumulated CoA esters on CPS I activity and an indirect effect on CPS I via impaired formation of its activator, N-acetylglutamate. There is a correlation between the plasma concentration of propionate and the degree of hyperammonemia.[90] An accumulation of CoA derivatives of organic acids accounts for the finding of hyperammonemia in other organic acidemias.

Carnitine deficiency is common in propionic acidemia as well as in other organic acidemias.[91] It results from decreased renal handling of filtered carnitine and from the conjugation of carnitine with the accumulating organic acid and the excretion of the formed acylcarnitine derivative. Secondary carnitine deficiency develops, and may contribute to muscle hypotonia and other clinical findings. Dietary supplementation will eradicate the carnitine deficiency and may provide a mechanism for detoxification (see Chapter 38).

Hyperglycinemia is another common finding in organic acidemia. In fact, the initial term for this group of inborn errors was ketotic hyperglycinemia.[86] It was to distinguish these disorders from nonketotic hyperglycinemia, in which there is a primary defect in the glycine cleavage enzyme complex.[92] In the organic acidopathies, glycine accumulates because of a secondary block in this enzyme complex, the mechanism of which is not understood.[93]

The accumulated organic acids result in bone marrow suppression. Studies of bone marrow in affected children reveal severely disturbed cellular morphology with trilineage dysmyelopoiesis, hemophagocytosis, and multinucleated histiocytes and megakaryocytes.[94] This defect may account for the predisposition of affected children for viral and bacterial infections.[95]

Therapy of propionic acidemia has primarily involved the use of a protein-restricted diet. Supplementation with carnitine is controversial. A special formula (e.g., Mead-Johnson or Ross Laboratories) that is deficient in the amino acid precursors of propionate has been used as adjunctive dietary therapy. This is supplemented with a proprietary formula and a non–protein-containing formula (e.g., 80056, Mead-Johnson, and Prophree, Ross Laboratories) to provide additional protein and calories. Although it was initially thought that a subgroup of children with propionic acidemia were responsive to large doses of biotin, more recent evidence indicates that these children actually had multiple carboxylase deficiency.[93] Although biotin supplementation has not led to a marked increase in enzyme activity in propionic acidemia, doses of 5 to 40 mg·d^{-1} may provide a nonspecific stimulation of residual enzyme activity.[96] Carnitine supplementation at a dose of 50 to 100 mg·kg^{-1}·d^{-1} can be given,[97] although the effectiveness has been questioned.

Neuropathologic studies show similarities to urea cycle disorders with cerebral edema, loss of subcortical myelinated fibers, Purkinje's cells, and the presence of Alzheimer type II astrocytes.[66] Discrete foci of status spongiosis have been noted in the thalamus. Survivors of neonatal onset propionic acidemia have a high incidence of developmental disabilities.

The α and the β subunits of propionyl-CoA carboxylase are encoded by genes on chromosomes 13 and 3, respectively.[98,99] A cDNA for both has been cloned and sequenced.[98,100,101] Two complementation groups, PccA and pccBC, have been identified and reflect mutations of the α and β subunit genes, respectively.[59] Single base and insertion/deletion mutation of the α gene have been described.[59,102,103] Prenatal diagnosis is possible by measuring propionyl-CoA carboxylase activity in amniocytes or chorionic villi.[59]

Multiple Carboxylase Deficiency

Multiple carboxylase deficiency was previously categorized as a biotin-responsive form of propionic acidemia.[104] Symptoms and biochemical abnormalities of the neonatal-onset form are similar to those described for propionic acidemia. In addition to propionate metabolites, there is increased urinary excretion of 3-methylcrotonylglycine and 3-hydroxyisovaleric acid.[105] This results from decreased functional activity of all four biotin-requiring carboxylases: propionyl-CoA carboxylase, pyruvate carboxylase, 3-methylcrotonyl-CoA carboxylase, and acetyl-CoA carboxylase.

There are two enzyme defects responsible for multiple carboxylase deficiency. Onset during the neonatal or early infantile period is usually due to the holocarboxylase synthetase deficiency[105,106] in which there is a variably elevated K_m of holocarboxylase synthetase for biotin. As discussed above, this enzyme covalently links biotin to the various inactive apoenzymes to form the active holocarboxylases. The more frequent form of multiple carboxylase deficiency usually presents in later infancy or childhood and is associated with a defect in biotinidase.[107] In this instance the holocarboxylase synthetase enzyme is normal, but cellular availability of biotin is reduced because there is a deficiency in biotinidase that regenerates biotin from the holocarboxylase degradation product, biocytin.[107]

Most children with the holocarboxylase synthetase deficiency have responded to biotin supplementation (i.e., 5–80 mg·d) with both an increase in activity of the carboxylases and the disappearance of organic aciduria. Despite effective therapy, neurologic outcome has not been good as there is often a delay in diagnosis leading to prolonged neonatal coma. Prenatal diagnosis is possible by measuring holocarboxylase synthetase activity in amniocytes or chorionic villi. This has permitted prenatal treatment with biotin in a few affected fetuses.[108] Although long-term follow-up has been lacking, one such prospectively treated infant appears to have had a good neurologic outcome.[109]

Methylmalonic Acidemia

There are several enzymatic defects that result in methylmalonic acidemia, including L-methylmalonyl-CoA mutase deficiency and several disorders of cobalamin metabolism. It is probably more common than the incidence of 1/48,000 noted in the 1981 Massachusetts screening survey of neonates.[110] While the exact incidence is unknown, methylmalonic acidemia, along with propionic acidemia, are the most common inborn errors of organic acid metabolism. Impaired breakdown of D- or L-methylmalonyl-CoA leads to its tissue accumulation and to increased concentration of its product of hydrolysis, methylmalonic acid (MMA). As noted above, the precursors of propionyl-CoA also affect MMA production because D-methylmalonyl-CoA is the product of the propionyl-CoA carboxylase reaction. Affected patients will have increased plasma and urine MMA concentration in addition to variably increased urinary excretion of the derivatives of propionic acid.

Phenotypic expression varies and seems dependent on the severity of the enzyme deficiency.[111] Major forms include (1) a life-threatening neonatal-onset disease, (2) a chronic infantile/childhood-onset type with failure to thrive and progressive psychomotor retardation associated with episodes of ketoacidosis, and (3) an intermittent childhood-onset form with acute episodes of metabolic decompensation but frequently normal development. Most of the patients with the neonatal-infantile–onset phenotype have severe deficiencies in L-methylmalonyl-CoA mutase activity. Cultured skin fibroblast cell studies have enabled patients to be categorized with one of seven genetically distinct groups, termed the complementation groups mut^0, mut$^-$, cbl A–D, and cblF.[59]

During episodes of ketoacidosis secondary abnormalities in intermediary metabolism including lactic acidosis, hyperammonemia, and occasional hypoglycemia occur. The patient with neonatal-onset methylmalonic acidemia may have very high plasma ammonium concentration.[112] As in other organic acidemias, plasma and urine glycine concentrations are increased and carnitine concentration is decreased. In infancy and childhood, there may be recurrent exacerbations precipitated by intercurrent infections or dietary indiscretions. These manifest as vomiting, ataxia, lethargy, and coma that simulate Reye's syndrome. Clinical sequelae in survivors include feeding difficulties, poor growth, hypotonia, mental retardation, and seizures.

Treatment using cobalamin derivatives has been attempted based on the knowledge that adenosylcobalamin is required for normal L-methylmalonyl-CoA mutase activity.[59] Unfortunately, neonatal onset patients usually are in the mut^0 or mut$^-$ categories and have either complete deficiencies of this enzyme or are unresponsive to cobalamin. Among the childhood-onset forms, some patients with adenosylcobalamin synthetase deficiency (i.e., cbl B group) have responded to pharmacologic therapy with hydroxocobalamin.[111]

Cobalamin responsiveness has been demonstrated in children with other defects in cobalamin metabolism (i.e., cbl C, D, F groups) that affect homocysteine metabolism.[59] cbl C and D involve defects in the conversion of oxidized cobalamin (Co^{+3}) to reduced cobalamin (Co^{+1}) that not only impair synthesis of adenosylcobalamin but also methylcobalamin, which is necessary for the conversion of homocysteine to methionine. This results in methylmalonic acidemia and homocystinuria and may be associated with hematologic abnormalities such as megaloblastic anemia as well as visual impairment and other neurologic abnormalities.[113] Finally, cobalamin responsivity has been reported in a single neonate with defective lysosomal release of transcobalamin II–bound cobalamin (designated cbl F).[114] Hypotonia, seizures, and stomatitis accompanied this form of methylmalonic acidemia.

The diagnosis of methylmalonic acidemia requires direct analysis of urine for organic acids by gas-liquid chromatography (GLC) or gas chromatography-mass spectrometry (GC-MS) to provide confirmatory evidence of the abnormal organic acid metabolites. Enzymatic analysis with MMA complementation group assignment can be performed on cultured skin fibroblasts. A cDNA-encoding human L-methylmalonyl-CoA mutase, as well as the gene, have been cloned and sequenced.[115-117] The gene has been mapped to 6p12–6p21.2.[118] Mutations producing mut^0 and mut$^-$ phenotypes have been identified.[119-121] Some patients were found to have no mutations involving the gene's open reading frame but decreased levels of messenger RNA (mRNA) on Northern blots.[122] Depending on the genotype, molecular diagnostic testing may be available. Prenatal diagnosis may be performed by measuring MMA in amniotic fluid, measuring enzyme activity in cultured amniocytes or in a chorionic villus biopsy sample, or, if feasible, by DNA mutational analyses on cells or tissues.[59]

The acute management of methylmalonic acidemia involves (1) protein elimination with the provision of adequate calories to suppress gluconeogenesis using intravenous fluids with glucose, (2) administration of intravenous bicarbonate to correct acidosis, and (3) pharmacologic doses of hydroxocobalamin (1 mg) in the new or undefined patient. Dialysis is usually not employed but may be necessary in some cases. As with propionic acidemia, the utility of L-carnitine in chronic management is controversial. However, it may play a useful role in promoting mitochondrial detoxification in the patient during acute metabolic decompensation.[97]

The mainstay of chronic therapy involves using a defined diet. Isoleucine, valine, methionine, and threonine catabolism may be reduced via the administration of a special formula that contains amino acids but is devoid of the above amino acids (e.g., OS1 or OS2, Mead Johnson, or Propinex, Ross Laboratories). Supplemental calories and fat are provided with a protein-free formula such as product 80056 (Mead-Johnson) or Prophree (Ross Laboratories). Patients with severe enzyme deficiencies may require daily alkali therapy. Carnitine supplementation has been tried. In patients with the cblC or cblD mutation, supplements of betaine and methionine have been used to treat the defect in methionine regeneration.[113]

The prognosis is good for patients with vitamin cofactor responsive forms of methylmalonic acidemia.[111] Unfortunately, the outlook is poor for patients with cobalamin-unresponsive neonatal-onset disease. Some neonates with onset in the first week of life will not survive despite aggressive treatment. Survivors who have had prolonged coma may have growth failure, mental retardation, cerebral palsy, and seizures. Prognosis for patients with chronic or intermediate forms in general depends on early diagnosis and the ability to effect good long-term metabolic control. However, some pathophysiologic aspects of methylmalonic acidemia remain undefined. Patients may develop chronic renal insufficiency, the natural history of which is unknown.[123–125] Acute episodes of metabolic decompensation with ketoacidosis can cause an extrapyramidal syndrome to develop secondary to acute necrosis of the globus pallidus.[126,127] Episodes of pancreatitis have been described.[128] This enigmatic complication has been reported in neonates with isovaleric acidemia and maple syrup urine disease.[128] Diverse cutaneous lesions that sometimes resemble acrodermatitis enteropathica have been reported in methylmalonic acidemia, and in propionic acidemia[129,130] (see Chapter 41).

General pathologic findings have included hepatic steatosis, and tubulointerstitial nephritis.[123–125,131–134] Neuropathology has involved dysmyelination of subcortical and other fibers, and bilateral status spongiosis of the globus pallidus.[112,135] Multiple neuropathologic lesions were detected in a 4-day-old preterm neonate, suggesting prenatal or early postnatal lesions.[136] In a recent review, the majority of patients with vitamin B_{12}–unresponsive early-onset disease were reported to have not survived beyond 2 years of age.[137]

Isovaleric Acidemia

A selective deficiency of the mitochondrial flavin-dependent enzyme isovaleryl-CoA dehydrogenase is responsible for this inborn error of leucine catabolism, isovaleric acidemia.[138] There are two clinical phenotypes: (1) an acute neonatal form characterized by overwhelming illness and resulting in death in over 60% of untreated infants; and (2) a chronic intermittent form with recurrent episodes of vomiting, lethargy, and ketoacidosis. The subsequent clinical course of patients who survive the newborn-onset disease is indistinguishable from that of patients with the chronic phenotype.

Biochemical alterations result from excessive leucine intake or muscle protein catabolism and include the accumulation of isovaleryl-CoA and isovaleric acid in blood and urine. As in the other organic acidemias, ketosis, lactic acidosis, hyperammonemia, hyperglycinemia, and hematocytopenia are evident during metabolic crises. However, there is an endogenous means of disposing of isovaleryl-CoA, by conjugation with glycine to form isovalerylglycine.[139] This is subsequently excreted in urine and forms the basis for treatment of isovaleric acidemia with glycine supplements.[140]

Newborns with the neonatal form are usually well for the first few days of life but then demonstrate poor intake, vomiting, hypotonia, and lethargy that progresses to coma. During this period, a characteristic odor, likened to that of "sweaty feet" or rancid butter, develops as isovaleric acid that accumulates in saliva, urine, and sweat. During infancy and childhood, affected patients have intercurrent episodes of decompensation similar to those found in other organic acidemias.

Whether well or acutely ill, the child excretes large amounts of isovalerylglycine. But during acute episodes, there is increased urinary excretion of 3-hydroxyisovaleric acid and increased amounts of free isovaleric acid in serum; plasma glycine concentration is variable. There is usually a metabolic acidosis with increased anion gap attributable to increased concentration of isovaleric acid, lactate, 3-hydroxybutyrate, and acetoacetate. Similar to other organic acidemias, plasma ammonia is usually increased and there is hematocytopenia.[139] The serum concentration of free carnitine is usually low, while the esterified carnitine content is increased, in the form of isovalerylcarnitine, which serves as another detoxification product.[141] The diagnosis of isovaleric acidemia may be confirmed by measuring enzyme activity in white blood cells or cultured skin fibroblasts. A cDNA has been cloned and sequenced.[142] The gene maps to chromosome 15q14–15.[143] Several mutations have been identified including a splice mutation that results in a loss of leader peptide.[144,145] Molecular diagnostic testing may yield useful results. Prenatal diagnosis has been accomplished by measuring isovaleryl-CoA dehydrogenase activity in amniocytes and isovalerylglycine in amniotic fluid.[146] Depending on the nature of the mutation, analysis of genomic DNA may be fruitful.

Therapy of isovaleric acidemia consists of protein restriction. Pharmacologic supplementation with both glycine (150–250 mg·kg^{-1}·d^{-1})[147] and L-carnitine (50–100 mg·kg^{-1}·d^{-1})[141] has been utilized. The restricted diet consists of natural protein, isoleucine and valines supplemented with a formula devoid of leucine (e.g., MSUD formula, Mead-Johnson). Occasionally platelet transfusions need to be given because of thrombocytopenia. Optimal maintenance therapy is associated with a reduction in the number of severe ketoacidotic attacks.[140] Most patients treated successfully from early infancy do not develop mental retardation, but are at increased risk for learning disabilities and attention deficit disorder.[138,140]

Glutaric Acidemia, Type I

Glutaric acidemia, type I (GAI) usually presents in infancy as an acute neurologic syndrome following an infection or as a slowly progressive neurodevelopmental disorder.[148] In the former, the sequelae of the acute encephalopathy resemble an extrapyramidal cerebral palsy syndrome with severe dystonia, dyskinesia, hypotonia, and motor delay or arrest. Dystonia and hypotonia may be found in the chronic phenotype. Episodes of vomiting and ketosis can occur in either form. Macrocephaly at birth is common. The brain computed tomography (CT) or magnetic resonance imaging (MRI) scans may reveal marked increases in the cerebrospinal fluid anterior to the temporal lobes and within the sylvian fissures. This may be found in apparently healthy neonates with GAI who are undergoing a workup for macrocephaly. Unlike glutaric acidemia, type II, the signs of overt disease in GAI do not appear in the neonate. Later on lesions of the caudate and putamen may be detected. However, some patients never manifest neurologic disease. The etiology of neither macrocrania nor the basal ganglia disease is known. This autosomal recessive disease is caused by a deficiency of glutaryl-CoA dehydrogenase activity and is associated with increased levels of glutaric and 3-hydroxyglutaric acid in urine.[149,150]

Glutaric Acidemia, Type II

Glutaric acidemia, type II (GAII) is different from the other inborn errors of amino acid metabolism in that signs are often evident from birth and there may be congenital abnormalities.[151] Neonates with glutaric acidemia, type II suffer intrauterine growth retardation and may have a dysmorphic appearance with dolichocephaly, high arched palate, rocker bottom feet, and hypospadias with chordee.[23] Cystic kidneys and cardiomyopathy have been reported so that the syndrome has similarities to Zellweger syndrome.[152] Biochemical alterations in GAII include hypo- or nonketotic hypoglycemia, metabolic acidosis, anemia, and hyperammonemia. Concentrations of lactic, glutaric, ethylmalonic, adipic, suberic, sebacic, 3-hydroxyisovalerate, 2-hydroxyglutaric, and 5-hydroxyhexanoic acids and isovalerylglycine, isobutyrylglycine, and 2-methyl-butyrylglycine are increased in urine.[149,151] Lactic acid is usually elevated in blood.[151]

Although initially called GAII because of the increased concentration of glutaric acid, it is a very different disease from GAI. GAII is more appropriately called multiple acyl-CoA dehydrogenase deficiency as it involves a defect in electron transfer from acyl-CoA dehydrogenases to coenzyme Q_{10} (CoQ_{10}) in the electron transfer chain.[153] This explains the increased excretion of the organic acid substrates of many flavoprotein dehydrogenases. Both electron transfer flavoprotein (ETF) and ETF dehydrogenase (the latter transfers electrons from ETF to the ubiquinone pool of the mitochondrial respiratory chain) function in this electron transfer. Deficiencies in either protein have been reported to cause GAII.[154]

Treatment attempts have involved supplements with riboflavin, a cofactor for the dehydrogenases.[155] Clinical improvement has been modest. Mortality is high and survivors are generally severely mentally retarded.[151] Pathologic abnormalities include subarachnoid hemorrhage and reactive gliosis with marked cerebral dysplasia and a wartlike surface.[156] Together with the anomalies noted above, this suggests abnormal tissue differentiation. The diagnosis can be made by measuring ETF and ETF dehydrogenase antigens by Western blot analysis or by direct assay of activities.[151] Prenatal diagnosis has been made by demonstrating large amounts of glutaric acid in amniotic fluid and/or impaired substrate oxidation in amniocytes.[157]

Maple Syrup Urine Disease

Maple syrup urine disease (MSUD) results from deficient activity of the branched-chain keto-acid dehydrogenase (BCKD) complex.[158] There are at least three phenotypes: The "classic" or neonatal-onset form is associated with a life-threatening disease. The less common chronic type usually presents in later infancy with poor growth, developmental delay, seizures, and acute episodes of ketoacidosis. There is a rare intermittent form occurring in older children and usually confined to acute episodic periods of metabolic decompensation.

The worldwide incidence of MSUD in the neonate is approximately 1/185,000.[158] Prevalence is highest in the Mennonite community, primarily centered in Pennsylvania, with a frequency of approximately 1/176 and is probably the consequence of a genetic founder effect.[158] Mutations involving single base changes, frame shifts, insertions, and deletions have been identified in the $E1_\alpha$, $E1_\beta$, E2, or E3 genes, with the majority of these types of mutations occurring in the E2 gene.[33,158] Most patients, which include Mennonite neonates, have classic early-onset disease. The biochemical lesion in Mennonites, however, involves deficiency of the $E1_\alpha$ subunit of the BCKAD complex[159,160] (vide supra). The majority of other patients with MSUD have had normal Western blot analyses of BCKAD proteins.[158] Rare patients have been reported with decreased affinity of the $E1_a$ subunit for the active vitamin B_1 cofactor, thiamine pyrophosphate.[161] These patients have responded to thiamine supplements. We expect most patients with E_2 deficiency[162] to manifest a classic phenotype.[158] Patients with the E_3 deficiency have deficiencies of the pyruvate and 2-ketoglutarate dehydrogenase complexes.[158] These patients demonstrate lactic acidosis and a progressive neurologic disorder.[163]

Untreated patients with MSUD have elevated concentrations of the branched-chain amino acids, leucine, isoleucine, and valine and the branched-chain keto acids 2-ketoisocaproic, 2-keto-3-methylvaleric, and 2-ketoisovaleric acids in blood and urine. Patients with the late-onset phenotype usually have elevated concentration only during acute episodes. High tissue concentrations of these compounds result in secondary biochemical disturbances such as ketosis, lactic acidosis, hypoalaninemia, and hypoglycemia.

Although neonates with classic MSUD are typically well for the first 3 to 4 days of life, it is possible to detect elevations in blood branched-chain amino acid concentrations as early as 6 to 12 hours after birth.[164] Elevated leucine is most related to clinical symptoms. As the blood leucine concentrations rises affected infants develop, in sequence, poor feeding, vomiting, the odor of maple syrup secondary to isoleucine metabolites, irritability, hypotonia/hypertonia, seizures, lethargy, periodic breathing/apnea, and coma. This progression of symptoms may take 1 to 2 weeks, by which time the neonates will require dialysis to remove the accumulated toxic metabolites.

The MSUD patients are at risk for recurrent episodes of metabolic decompensation throughout their lives, usually precipitated by infections. During these periods of stress and fasting, catabolism results in muscle protein breakdown and accumulation of branched-chain amino and keto acids. Symptoms range from vomiting, dehydration, lethargy, and ataxia to pyramidal tract dysfunction and coma. Mortality is likely attributable to increased intracranial pressure leading to herniation.[165–168]

Laboratory findings in untreated MSUD infants include increased plasma levels of isoleucine, valine, and leucine, the latter being markedly out of proportion to the other branched-chain amino acids.[169] Leucine concentration in the neonate may be more than 70 mg% (>5300 µM; normal <150 µM). There is the pathognomonic presence of alloisoleucine, an isomer of isoleucine. Plasma alanine concentration is inversely correlated to concentration of leucine, so that hypoalaninemia is most marked when leucine concentration is very high. There is increased urinary excretion of branched-chain keto acids and of the hydroxy derivatives of isoleucine and valine keto acids.

Although encephalopathy due to accumulation of branched-chain metabolites may present in the absence of ketoacidosis, a metabolic acidosis is a classic finding in MSUD. This may apply to ketosis, although in general ketonuria closely follows the degree of branched-chain amino acid and ketoacid excess. A raised anion gap may be largely attributable to accumulation of 3-hydroxybutyrate, acetoacetate, and lactate. Patients under chronic poor metabolic control usually have a hypochromic anemia.

The immediate diagnosis of MSUD requires amino acid chromatography. Gas-liquid chromatography of urine and/or plasma for branched-chain keto-acid measurements may be performed but is not essential. A useful, quick urine screening test is the 2,4-dinitrophenylhydrazine precipitation test, which is positive in the presence of large amounts of keto acids. The ferric chloride test (Phenistix) used in detecting phenylketonuria will also be positive in MSUD. The branched-chain keto-acid dehydrogenase enzyme activity can be measured in white blood cells and in cultured skin fibroblasts but is not necessary for diagnosis. Rapid prenatal diagnosis is feasible depending on which subunit is affected and the nature of the mutation[158] (see Chapter 53).

Pathologic findings in MSUD are confined to the central nervous system and consist of cortical atrophy, cerebellar degeneration, and white matter dysmyelination with spongiosis generally attributable to brain edema.[158,170]

The mainstay of therapy is dietary restriction of branched-chain amino acids. To allow for normal growth and development and to prevent metabolic decompensation, patients should receive the minimum required daily amounts of leucine, isoleucine, and valine, via proprietary infant formulas or table foods. This is supplemented with a branched-chain amino acid–free formula (e.g., Mead-Johnson or Ross Laboratories MSUD formula) to supply sufficient amounts of daily nitrogen. The ideal end points are normal growth and normal plasma concentrations of the branched-chain amino acids. If diets are too restrictive in these essential amino acids, deficiency states result in impaired growth and exfoliative skin rashes.[158,171] Conversely, excessive ingestion of protein causes branched-chain amino acid concentrations to rise and produces signs of illness.

The acute disease in the neonate requires peritoneal dialysis or preferably hemodialysis when the plasma leucine concentration is in excess of 30 to 40 mg%. Depending on the gastrointestinal tract status, neonates with more modest elevations in leucine can be treated with MSUD formula and isoleucine and valine supplementation, via continuous nasogastric tubal infusion. Special attention should be paid to the respiratory status and the occurrence of cerebral edema. Newly diagnosed patients should receive a course of thiamine on the rare chance that the neonate has the thiamine responsive variant of MSUD. Thiamine may help reduce branched-chain amino and keto acid concentrations in patients with residual enzyme activity but normal affinity for thiamine triphosphate (TPP) via TPP-induced stabilization of the mutant enzyme.[172]

In older infants episodes of decompensation, associated with acidosis and/or ketosis, should be treated by eliminating dietary protein, providing sufficient calories and "nontoxic" amino acids as MSUD formula and correcting the acid-base imbalance. Because of emesis, these infants often cannot tolerate enteral feedings. In these instances hyperalimentation using branched-chain amino acid–free solutions is beneficial.[173]

Nonketotic Hyperglycinemia

First described in 1962,[174] nonketotic hyperglycinemia (NKH) typically presents at 1 to 3 days of life with myoclonic seizures, lethargy, poor feeding, apneic spells, and hypotonia.[175] The comatose infant usually requires ventilatory support. The deep tendon reflexes and neonatal reflexes can disappear producing a clinical picture that resembles Werding-Hoffmann disease. A burst-suppressive pattern on EEG is very suggestive of NKH. Mortality is high and survivors are usually severely mentally retarded. Plasma glycine concentration is in the range of 700 to 2000 μM (normal <350 μM). Urinary excretion of glycine is increased. There is an increased cerebrospinal fluid (CSF)/plasma glycine ratio, 0.17 (0.01–0.03 in normals).[176] Urine organic acids fail to reveal significant organic aciduria, distinguishing this disorder from the organic acidemias that present with ketotic hyperglycinemia.

The defect in this disorder exists in the glycine cleavage enzyme complex, which degrades glycine via serine. The molecular nature of the defect in the glycine cleavage system has been studied in eight patients with neonatal-onset disease. Undetectable or extremely low levels of the complex were found in brain and liver.[177,178] There is evidence for some genetic heterogeneity in the enzyme defect, and atypical patients with late-onset disease have been described.[175] In a series of 30 patients, the majority with neonatal NKH had defects in the p protein.[179,180]

Treatment approaches have been directed at decreasing glycine concentrations or blocking glycine receptors in the brain. Results have been largely unsuccessful. Sodium benzoate has been used to decrease glycine concentration. At the commonly used dose, $250\,mg\cdot kg^{-1}\cdot d^{-1}$, there was little effect on plasma glycine concentration.[179] In one child, treatment with $500\,mg\cdot kg^{-1}\cdot d^{-1}$ was associated with a decrease in seizure activity.[181]

In nonketotic hyperglycinemia single carbon unit reactions generated from the pathways of the glycine cleavage system may be impaired. Methionine, choline, and folic acid have been used to provide single-carbon units.[182] Each has resulted in a decrease in plasma glycine concentration but with little clinical improvement.

Glycine primarily functions as an inhibitory neurotransmitter in the nervous system. A high concentration of glycine affects anterior horn cell function. Unlike the organic acidemias, nonketotic hyperglycinemia is associated with a preferential accumulation of glycine in the brain.[176] As a result, attempts have been directed at inhibiting the effect of glycine on brain function. Both strychnine and diazepam have been used as competitive inhibitors of glycine receptors.[183,184] Results have been equivocal in terms of clinical improvement.[185]

Glycine may act as a positive neuromodulator in other regions of the central nervous system. It is not clear whether glycine causes neuronal damage directly or indirectly stimulates the N-methyl-D-aspartate (NMDA) subgroup of glutamate receptors.[70] Glutamate has been implicated in seizures and in the brain damage caused by hypoxia, Huntington's disease, and Alzheimer's disease.[186] Theoretically, blocking access to these receptors might block brain damage. An approach might be to use noncompetitive inhibitors of NMDA receptors, such as dextromethorphan, phencyclidine, MK-801, indol-2-carboxylic acid, or ketamine.[187,188]

The pathology in nonketotic hyperglycinemia involves a dysmyelination and cellular differentiation with increased cellular density in cortex.[189] The neurons are slender and bipolar, and there is spongiosis of the white matter. Dysgenesis of the corpus callosum, including agenesis, has been reported.[190] These findings support a prenatal origin to the neuropathology that may limit the effectiveness of postnatal attempts at treatment. Prenatal diagnosis has been carried out successfully using enzymatic analysis of chorionic villus samples.[191,192]

Summary and Future Perspectives

In summary, forms of many inborn errors of amino acid metabolism are likely to present with acute symptoms in the first week of life. The underlying defects usually lie in the metabolic pathways of branched-chain amino acids, glycine, or the urea cycle. Clinical symptoms simulate sepsis and the diagnosis is likely to be missed if not specifically investigated by obtaining concentrations of ammonia and amino acids plasma and organic acids in urine. Early diagnosis is critical as untreated these disorders are usually fatal and late treatment generally leads to severe brain damage and mental retardation. Treatment approaches are available for all the conditions described, primarily involving restriction of nutrients, vitamin cofactor supplementation, and the stimulation of alternate metabolic pathways. The effectiveness of these approaches varies from excellent to borderline improvement. Once diagnosed, genetic counseling and prenatal diagnosis are also available as the disorders are inherited as mendelian traits.

Future knowledge about these disorders is likely to result from molecular biologic and neurochemical studies. Genetic heterogeneity of these disorders appears to be the rule rather than the exception. Further, curative treatment of inborn errors will probably rely on gene therapy involving the insertion of the cloned DNA sequence on a retroviral or an adenoviral-like carrier. This is already under active consideration for a number of disorders such as the ornithine transcarbamylase deficiency. In vitro, somatic gene therapy is already being realized. For example, lymphoblasts from patients with MSUD manifested normal decarboxylation activity following transduction with a retroviral vector bearing a full-length human El_α cDNA.[193]

As noted previously specific neuropathologic findings are rare or nonspecific. Yet, most of the late-treated children will suffer severe brain damage, manifest as mental retardation, seizure disorders, and cerebral palsy. It thus seems likely that inborn errors of metabolism may cause derangements in neurotransmitters or neuromodulators. Specific examples of this include dopamine deficiency in the dihydropteridine reductase deficient variant form of phenylketonuria[194] and serotonin excess in hyperammonemic disorders.[69] It is likely that additional neurochemical alterations will be identified in other inborn errors, shedding new light on the pathogenesis of these disorders.

It is of note that this is a "young" group of disorders with most diseases being described in the past 30 years and with new enzyme defects being identified yearly. Novel defects in mitochondrial fatty acid metabolism are described elsewhere (see Chapter 37). Additionally, new defects in peroxisomes, the posttranslational modification of proteins, oligosaccharides, and lysosomes have recently been described. One of the most recently identified group of inborn errors of metabolism involves defects in the previously little regarded peroxisome.[195] Peroxisomal oxidation defects have been implicated in pseudo-Zellweger syndrome,[196] as well as in the example par excellence of deficient biogenesis of peroxisomes, Zellweger syndrome.[195] A defect involving oligosaccharide metabolism, α-galactosidase B deficiency, has been described to explain one of the neuroaxonal dystrophies, Schindler disease.[197] A defect in lysosomal storage has been implicated in the newest form of methylmalonic acidemia (cbl F deficiency).[114] No longer are DNA mutations restricted to the nuclear genome. An ever-growing number of mutations involving mitochondrial DNA producing mitochondrial cytopathies or lactic acidosis syndromes are now being described.[198]

Finally, the previously drawn line between small molecular disorders and large molecular disorders has been eroded. It was previously taught that small molecular amino acid/organic acid disorders presented clinically as acute crises with vomiting, lethargy, and coma, while lysosomal storage disorders and other diseases with accumulation of large molecular weight compounds presented as subacute dementing diseases. However, it has been shown that Canavan leukodystrophy results from defects in aspartoacylase, which is involved in organic acid metabolism.[199] Obviously, intermediary metabolism still holds many secrets and its elucidation should aid in the care of the neonate.

References

1. Remesar X, Lopez-Tejero D, Pastor-Anglada M. Some aspects of amino acid metabolism in the rat fetus. Comp Biochem Physiol 1987;88B:719–725.
2. Miller AL, Chu P. The development of urea cycle enzyme activity in the liver of foetal and neonatal rats. Enzymol Biol Clin 1970;11:497–503.
3. Greengard O. Enzymic differentiation in mammalian tissues. Essays Biochem 1971;7:159–205.
4. Arola L, Palou A, Remesar X, et al. Changes in glutamine synthetase activity in the different organs of developing rats. Arch Int Physiol Biochim 1981;89:189–194.
5. Friedman PA, Kaufman S. A study of the development of phenylalanine hydroxylase in fetuses of several mammalian species. Arch Biochem Biophys 1971;146:321–326.
6. Arola L, Palou A, Remesar X, et al. Amino-acid enzyme activities in liver and kidney of developing rats. Arch Int Physiol Biochim 1982;90:163–171.
7. Jakovcic S, Haddock J, Getz GS, et al. Mitochondrial development in liver of foetal and newborn rats. Biochem J 1971;121:341–347.
8. Palou A, Remesar X, Arola L, et al. Ontogeny of amino-acid metabolism-enzymes in peripheral tissues of developing rats. Arch Int Physiol Biochim 1983;91:43–50.
9. Remesar X, Arola LI, Palou A, et al. Activities of amino acid metabolizing enzymes in the stomach and small intestine of developing rats. Reprod Nutr Dev 1985;25:861–866.
10. Arola LI, Palou A, Remesar X, et al. Amino acid enzyme activities in the brain of developing rats. IRCS Med Sci 1983;11:514–515.

11. Raiha NC, Suihkonen J. Development of urea synthesizing enzymes in human liver. Acta Paediatr Scand 1968; 57:121–124.
12. Boehm G, Muller DM, Beyreiss K, et al. Evidence for functional immaturity of the ornithine-urea cycle in very-low-birth-weight infants. Biol Neonate 1988;54:121–125.
13. Snell K. Protein, amino acid and urea metabolism in the neonate. In: Jones CT, ed. Biochemical development of the fetus and neonate. Amsterdam: Elsevier, 1982:651–695.
14. Batshaw ML, Brusilow SW. Asymptomatic hyperammonemia in low birthweight infants. Pediatr Res 1978;12:221–224.
15. Batshaw ML, Wachtel RC, Brusilow SW, et al. Arginine responsive asymptomatic hyperammonemia in the premature infant. J Pediatr 1984;105:86–91.
16. Hudak ML, Jones MD Jr, Brusilow SW. Differentiation of transient hyperammonemia of the newborn and urea cycle enzyme defects by clinical presentation. J Pediatr 1985; 107:712–719.
17. Rice DN, Houston IB, Lyon ICT, et al. Transient neonatal tyrosinaemia. J Inherited Metab Dis 1989;12:13–22.
18. Scriver CR, Kaufman S, Eisensmith RC, Woo SLC. The hyperphenylalaninemias. In: Scriver CR, Beaudet AL, Sly WS, Valle D, eds. The metabolic and molecular bases of inherited disease. 7th ed. New York: McGraw-Hill, 1995: 1015–1075.
19. Mamunes P, Prince PE, Thornton NH, et al. Intellectual deficits after transient tyrosinemia in the term neonate. Pediatrics 1976;57:675–680.
20. Menkes JH, Welcher DW, Levy HS, et al. Relationship of elevated blood tyrosine to the ultimate intellectual performance of premature infants. Pediatrics 1972;49:218–224.
21. Gaull G. Taurine in pediatric nutrition: review and update. Pediatrics 1989;83:433–442.
22. Tyson JE, Lasky R, Flood D, et al. Randomized trial of taurine supplementation for infants < 1300-gram weight: effect on auditory brainstem-evoked responses. Pediatrics 1989;83:406–415.
23. Goodman SI, Reale M, Berlow S. Glutaric acidemia type II: a form with deleterious intrauterine effects. J Pediatr 1983;102:411–413.
24. Batshaw ML. Hyperammonemia. Curr Probl Pediatr 1984;14(11):1–169.
25. Meijer AJ, Verhoeven AJ. N-acetylglutamate and urea synthesis. Biochem J 1984;223:559–560.
26. Kikuchi G. The glycine cleavage system: composition, reaction mechanism, and physiological significance. Mol Cell Biochem 1973;1:169–187.
27. Berry GT. Disorders of amino acid metabolism. In: Walker WA, Durie PR, Hamilton JR, et al., eds. Pediatric gastrointestinal disease. St. Louis: Mosby-Year Book, 1996:1137–1154.
28. Pettit FH, Yeaman SJ, Reed LJ. Purification and characterization of branched chain α-keto acid dehydrogenase complex of bovine kidney. Proc Natl Acad Sci USA 1978;75:4881–4885.
29. Danner DJ, Lemmon SK, Besharse JC, Elsas LJ. Purification and characterization of branched chain α-ketoacid dehydrogenase from bovine liver mitochondria. J Biol Chem 1979;254:5522–5526.
30. Reed LJ, Damuni Z, Merryfield ML. Regulation of mammalian pyruvate and branched-chain α-keto acid dehydrogenase complexes by phosphorylation-dephosphorylation. Curr Top Cell Regul 1985;27:41–49.
31. Zhang B, Kuntz MJ, Goodwin GW, et al. Molecular cloning of a cDNA for the elα subunit of rat liver branched chain α-ketoacid dehydrogenase. J Biol Chem 1987;262: 15220–15224.
32. Hu C-WC, Lau KS, Griffin TA, et al. Isolation and sequencing of a cDNA encoding the decarboxylase (El)α precursor of bovine branched-chain α-keto acid dehydrogenase complex. Expression of Elα mRNA and subunit in maple-syrup-urine-disease and 3T3-L1 cells. J Biol Chem 1988;263:9007–9014.
33. Fisher CW, Chuang JL, Griffin TA, et al. Molecular phenotypes in cultured maple syrup urine disease cells. Complete Elα cDNA sequence and mRNA and subunit contents of the human branched chain α-keto acid dehydrogenase complex. J Biol Chem 1989;264:3448–3453.
34. Zhang B, Crabb DW, Harris RA. Nucleotide and deduced amino acid sequence of the Elα subunit of human liver branched-chain α-ketoacid dehydrogenase. Gene 1988;69: 159–164.
35. Chuang JL, Cox RP, Chuang DT. Molecular cloning of the mature El-β subunit of human branched-chain α-keto acid dehydrogenase complex. FEBS Lett 1990;262:305–309.
36. Nobukuni Y, Mitsubuchi H, Endo F, et al. Maple syrup urine disease. Complete primary structure of the $E_1\beta$ subunit of human branched-chain α-ketoacid dehydrogenase complex deduced from the nucleotide sequence and a gene analysis of patients with this disease. J Clin Invest 1990;86:242–247.
37. Danner DJ, Litwer S, Herring WJ, Pruckler J. Construction and nucleotide sequence of a cDNA encoding the full-length preprotein for human branched chain acyltransferase. J Biol Chem 1989;264:7742–7746.
38. Nobukuni Y, Mitsubuchi H, Endo F, Matsuda I. Complete primary structure of the transacylase (E2b) subunit of the human branched chain α-keto acid dehydrogenase complex. Biochem Biophys Res Commun 1989;161:1035–1041.
39. Lau KS, Chuang JL, Herring WJ, et al. The complete cDNA sequence for dihydrolipoyl transacylase (E2) of human branched-chain α-ketoacid dehydrogenase complex. Biochem Biophys Acta 1992;1132:319–321.
40. Otulakowski G, Robinson BH. Isolation and sequence determination of cDNA clones for porcine and human lipoamide dehydrogenase. Homology to other disulfide oxidoreductases. J Biol Chem 1987;262:17313–17318.
41. Pons G, Raefsky-Estrin C, Carothers DJ, et al. Cloning and cDNIA sequence of the dihydrolipoamide dehydrogenase component of human a-ketoacid dehydrogenase complexes. Proc Natl Acad Sci USA 1988;85:1422–1426.
42. Popov KM, Zhao Y, Shimomura Y, et al. Branched-chain α-ketoacid dehydrogenase kinase. Molecular cloning, expression, and sequence similarity with histidine protein kinases. J Biol Chem 1992;267:13127–13130.
43. Fekete G, Plattner R, Crabb DW, et al. Localization of the human gene for the Elα subunit of branched chain keto

acid dehydrogenase (BCKDHA) to chromosome 19q13.1 → q13.2. Cytogenet Cell Genet 1989;50:236–237.
44. Zneimer SM, Lau KS, Eddy RL, et al. Regional assignment of two genes of the human branched-chain α-keto acid dehydrogenase complex: the E1β gene (BCKDHB) to chromosome 6p21–22 and the E2 gene (DBT) to chromosome 1p31. Genomics 1991;10:740–747.
45. Scherer SW, Otulakowski G, Robinson BH, Tsui LC. Localization of the human dihydrolipoamide dehydrogenase (DLD) to 7q31–q32. Ctyogenet Cell Genet 1991;56:176–177.
46. Rhead WJ, Tanaka K. Demonstration of a specific mitochondrial isovaleryl-CoA dehydrogenase deficiency in fibroblasts from patients with isovaleric acidemia. Proc Natl Acad Sci USA 1980;77:580–583.
47. Kalousek F, Darigo MD, Rosenberg LE. Isolation and characterization of propionyl-CoA carboxylase from normal human liver: evidence for a protomeric tetramer of nonidentical subunits. J Biol Chem 1980;255:60–65.
48. Gravel RA, Lam KF, Mahuran D, Kronis A. Purification of human liver propionyl-CoA carboxylase by carbon tetrachloride extraction and monomeric avidin affinity chromatography. Arch Biochem Biophys 1980;201:669–673.
49. Moss J, Lane MD. The biotin-dependent enzymes. Adv Enzymol 1971;35:321–442.
50. Mazumder R, Sasakawa T, Kaziro Y, Ochoa S. Metabolism of propionic acid in animal tissues. IX. Methylmalonyl coenzyme A racemase. J Biol Chem 1962;237:3065–3068.
51. Fenton WA, Hack AM, Willard HF, et al. Purification and properties of methylmalonyl CoA mutase from human liver. Arch Biochem Biophys 1982;214:815–823.
52. Babior BM. Cobamides as cofactors: adenosylcobamide dependent reactions. In: Babior BM, ed. Cobalamin biochemistry and pathophysiology. New York: John Wiley, 1975:141–212.
53. Ricciuti FC, Gelehrter TD, Rosenberg LE. X-chromosome inactivation in human liver: confirmation of X-linkage of ornithine transcarbamylase. Am J Hum Genet 1976;28:332–338.
54. Msall M, Batshaw ML, Suss R, et al. Neurologic outcome of children with inborn errors of urea synthesis. N Engl J Med 1984;310:1500–1505.
55. Donn SM, Swartz RD, Thoene JG. Comparison of exchange transfusion, peritoneal dialysis, and hemodialysis for the treatment of hyperammonemia in an anuric newborn infant. J Pediatr 1979;95:67–70.
56. Batshaw ML, Brusilow SW. Treatment of hyperammonemic coma caused by inborn errors of urea synthesis. J Pediatr 1980;97:893–900.
57. Brusilow SW. Arginine, an indispensable amino acid for patients with inborn errors of urea synthesis. J Clin Invest 1984;74:2144–2148.
58. Snyderman SE, Sansaricq C, Phansalkar SV, et al. The therapy of hyperammonemia due to ornithine transcarbamylase deficiency in a male neonate. Pediatrics 1975;56:65–73.
59. Fenton WA, Rosenberg LE. Disorders of propionate and methylmalonate metabolism. In: Scriver CR, Beaudet AL, Sly WS, Valle D, eds. The metabolic and molecular bases of inherited disease. 7th ed. New York: McGraw-Hill, 1995:1423–1449.
60. Batshaw ML, Brusilow SW, Waber L, et al. Treatment of inborn errors of urea synthesis: activation of alternative pathways of waste nitrogen synthesis and excretion. N Engl J Med 1982;306:1387–1392.
61. Wolf B, Hsia YE, Sweetman L, et al. Multiple carboxylase deficiency. Clinical and biochemical improvement following neonatal biotin treatment. Pediatrics 1981;68:113–118.
62. Tuchman M. Persistent acitrullinemia after liver transplantation for carbamylphosphate synthetase deficiency. N Engl J Med 1989;320:1498–1499.
63. Brewster TG, Moskowitz MA, Kaufman S, et al. Dihydropteridine reductase deficiency associated with severe neurologic disease and mild hyperphenylalaninemia. Pediatrics 1979;63:94–99.
64. Brusilow SW, Horwich AL. Urea cycle enzymes. In: Scriver CR, Beaudet AL, Sly WS, Valle D, eds. The metabolic and molecular bases of inherited disease. 7th ed. New York: McGraw-Hill, 1995;1221–1232.
65. Bartholomew D, Reichel R, Brusilow S. Prospective treatment of urea cycle disorders. J Pediatr 1991;119:923–928.
66. Steinman L, Clancy RR, Cann H, et al. The neuropathology of propionic acidemia. Dev Med Child Neurol 1983;25:87–94.
67. Filloux F, Townsend JJ, Leonard C. Ornithine transcarbamylase deficiency: neuropathologic changes acquired in utero. J Pediatr 1986;108:942–945.
68. Goodman SI, Stene DO, Mccabe ERB, et al. Glutaric acidemia type II: clinical, biochemical and morphologic considerations. J Pediatr 1982;100:946–950.
69. Hyman SL, Coyle JT, Parke JC, et al. Anorexia and altered serotonin metabolism in a patient with argininosuccinic aciduria. J Pediatr 1986;108:705–709.
70. Rothman SM, Olney JW. Excitotoxicity and the NMDA receptor. Trends in Neurosciences 1987;10:299–302.
71. Bachmann C, Colombo JP, Jaggi K. N-acetylglutamate synthetase deficiency: diagnosis, clinical observations and treatment. In: Lowenthal A, Mori A, Marescau B, eds. Urea cycle diseases. New York: Plenum Press, 1983;153:39–45.
72. Snyderman SE, Sansaricq C, Chem WJ, et al. Argininemia. J Pediatr 1977;90:563–568.
73. Holtzman NA, Batshaw ML, Valle DL. Genetic aspects of human nutrition. In: Goodhart RS, Shils ME, eds. Modern nutrition in health and disease. 6th ed. Philadelphia: Lea & Febiger, 1980:1193–1219.
74. Shih VE. Hereditary urea-cycle disorders. In: Grisolia S, Baguena R, Mayor F, eds. The urea cycle. New York: John Wiley, 1976:367–414.
75. Potter JL, Timmons GD, Silvida AA. Argininosuccinic aciduria—the hair abnormality revisited. Am J Dis Child 1980;134:1095–1096.
76. Kline JJ, Hug G, Schubert WK, et al. Arginine deficiency syndrome. Its occurrence in carbamyl phosphate synthetase deficiency. Am J Dis Child 1981;135:437–442.
77. Labrecque DR, Latham PS, Riely CA, et al. Heritable urea cycle enzyme deficiency-liver disease in 16 patients. J Pediatr 1979;94:580–587.

78. Farriaux JP, Dhondt JL, Formstecher P, et al. [Pathological and biochemical studies on a neonatal case of argininosuccinic aciduria]. Acta Neurol Belg 1976;76:26–34.
79. Ohtani Y, Ohyanagi K, Yamamoto S, et al. Secondary carnitine deficiency in hyperammonemic attacks of ornithine transcarbamylase deficiency. J Pediatr 1988;112:409–414.
80. Bachmann C, Colombo JP. Diagnostic value of orotic acid excretion in heritable disorders of the urea cycle and in hyperammonemia due to organic aciduria. Eur J Pediatr 1980;134:109–113.
81. Batshaw M, Brusilow S, Walser M. Treatment of carbamyl phosphate synthetase deficiency with ketoanalogues of essential amino acids. N Engl J Med 1975;292:1085–1090.
82. Brusilow SW, Batshaw ML. Arginine treatment of argininosuccinase deficiency. Lancet 1979;1:124–127.
83. Brusilow SW, Tinker J, Batshaw ML. Amino acid acylation: a mechanism of nitrogen excretion in inborn errors of urea synthesis. Science 1982;207:659–661.
84. Kendall BE, Kingsley DP, Leonard JV, et al. Neurological features and computed tomography of the brain in children with ornithine carbamoyl transferase deficiency. J Neurol Neurosurg Psychiatry 1983;46:28–34.
85. Rozen R, Fox JE, Hack AM, et al. DNA analysis for ornithine transcarbamylase deficiency. J Inherited Metab Dis 1986;9(suppl 1):49–57.
86. Childs B, Nyhan WL, Borden M, et al. Idiopathic hyperglycinemia and hyperglycinuria: a new disorder of amino acid metabolism. Pediatrics 1961;27:522–538.
87. Sweetman L, Nyhan WL, Cravens J, et al. Propionic acidaemia presenting with pancytopaenia in infancy. J Inherited Metab Dis 1980;56(2):65–69.
88. Harris DJ, Yang B, Wolf B, et al. Dysautonomia in an infant with secondary hyperammonemia due to propionyl CoA carboxylase deficiency. J Med Genet 1981;18:156–157.
89. Coude FX, Sweetman L, Nyhan WL. Inhibition by propionyl-coenzyme A of N-acetylglutamate synthetase in rat liver mitochondria: a possible explanation for hyperammonemia in propionic and methylmalonic acidemia. J Clin Invest 1979;64:1544–1551.
90. Wolf B, Hsia YE, Tanaka K, et al. Correlation between serum propionate and blood ammonia concentrations in propionic acidemia. J Pediatr 1978;93:471–473.
91. Chalmers RA, Roe CR, Stacey TE, et al. Urinary excretion of l-carnitine and acylcarnitines by patients with disorders of organic acid metabolism: evidence for secondary insufficiency of l-carnitine. Pediatr Res 1984;18:1325–1328.
92. Perry TL, Urquhart N, MacLean J, et al. Nonketotic hyperglycinemia. Glycine accumulation due to absence of glycine cleavage in brain. N Engl J Med 1975;292:1269–1273.
93. Wolf B, Hsia YE, Sweetman L, et al. Propionic acidemia: a clinical update. J Pediatr 1981;99:835–846.
94. Stork LC, Ambruso DR, Wallner SF, et al. Pancytopenia in propionic acidemia: hematologic evaluation and studies of hematopoiesis in vitro. Pediatr Res 1986;20:783–788.
95. Cowan WJ, Wara DW, Packman S, et al. Multiple biotin-dependent carboxylase deficiencies associated with defects in T-cell and B-cell immunity. Lancet 1979;2:115–118.
96. Wolf B. Reassessment of biotin-responsiveness in "unresponsive" propionyl CoA carboxylase deficiency. J Pediatr 1980;97:964–966.
97. Roe CR, Hoppel CL, Stacey TE, et al. Metabolic response to carnitine in methylmalonic aciduria. An effective strategy for elimination of propionyl groups. Arch Dis Child 1983;58:916–920.
98. Lamhonwah AM, Barankiewics TJ, Willard HF, et al. Isolation of cDNA clones coding for the α and β chains of human propionyl-CoA carboxylase: chromosomal assignments and DNA polymorphisms associated with PCCA and PCCB genes. Proc Natl Acad Sci USA 1986;83:4864–4868.
99. Kraus JP, Williamson CL, Firgaira FA, et al. Cloning and screening with nanogram amounts of immunopurified messenger RNAs: cDNA cloning and chromosomal mapping of cystathionine β-synthase and the β-subunit of propionyl CoA carboxylase. Proc Natl Acad Sci USA 1986;83:2047–2051.
100. Lamhonwah AM, Quan F, Gravel RA. Sequence homology around the biotin-binding site of human propionyl-CoA carboxylase and pyruvate carboxylase. Arch Biochem Biophys 1987;254:631–636.
101. Lamhonwah AM, Mahuran D, Gravel RA. Human mitochondrial propionyl-CoA carboxylase: localization of the N-terminus of the pro- and mature alpha chains in the deduced primary sequence of a full-length cDNA. Nucleic Acids Res 1989;17:4396.
102. Tahara T, Kraus JP, Rosenberg LE. An unusual insertion/deletion in the gene encoding the β-subunit of propionyl-CoA carboxylase is a frequent mutation in Caucasian propionic acidemia. Proc Natl Acad Sci USA 1990;87:1372–1376.
103. Tahara T, Kraus JP, Ohura T, Rosenberg LE, Fenton WA. Three independent mutations in the same exon of the PCCB gene. Differences between Caucasian and Japanese propionic acidemia. J Inherited Metab Dis 1993;16:353–360.
104. Saunders M, Sweetman L, Robinson B, et al. Biotin-responsive organic aciduria: multiple carboxylase defects and complementation studies with propionic acidemia in cultured fibroblasts. J Clin Invest 1979;64:1695–1702.
105. Sweetman L, Nyhan WL, Sakati NA, et al. Organic aciduria in neonatal multiple carboxylase deficiency. J Inherited Metab Dis 1982;5:49–53.
106. Roth KS, Yang W, Foremann JW, et al. Holocarboxylase synthetase deficiency: a biotin-responsive organic acidemia. J Pediatr 1980;96:845–849.
107. Wolf B, Grier RE, Allen RJ, et al. Biotinidase deficiency: the enzymatic defect in late-onset multiple carboxylase deficiency. Clin Chim Acta 1983;131:273–281.
108. Roth KS. Prenatal treatment of multiple carboxylase deficiency. Ann N Y Acad Sci 1985;447:263–271.
109. Michalski AJ, Berry GT, Segal S. Holocarboxylase synthetase deficiency: nine year follow-up of a patient on

chronic biotin therapy and a review of the literature. J Inherited Metab Dis 1989;12:312–316.
110. Coulombe JT, Shih VE, Levy HL. Massachusetts metabolic disorders screening program II. Methylmalonic aciduria. Pediatrics 1981;76:26–31.
111. Matsui SM, Mahoney MJ, Rosenberg LE. The natural history of the inherited methylmalonic acidemias. N Engl J Med 1983;308:857–861.
112. Shapiro LJ, Bocian ME, Raijman L, et al. Methylmalonyl-CoA mutase deficiency associated with severe neonatal hyperammonemia: activity of urea cycle enzymes. J Pediatr 1978;93:986–988.
113. Bartholomew DW, Batshaw ML, Allen RH, et al. Therapeutic approaches to cobalamin-C methylmalonic acidemia and homocystinuria. J Pediatr 1988;112:32–39.
114. Rosenblatt DS, Laframboise R, Pichette J, et al. New disorder of vitamin B_{12} metabolism (cobalamin F) presenting as methylmalonic aciduria. Pediatrics 1986;78:51–54.
115. Ledley FD, Lumetta M, Nguyen PN, et al. Molecular cloning of L-methylmalonyl-CoA mutase: gene transfer and analysis of mut cell lines. Proc Natl Acad Sci USA 1988;85:3518–3521.
116. Jansen R, Kalousek F, Fenton WA, et al. Cloning of full-length methylmalonyl-CoA mutase from a cDNA library using the polymerase chain reaction. Genomics 1989;4:198–205.
117. Nham S-U, Wilkemeyer MF, Ledley FD. Structure of the human methlmalonyl-CoA mutase (MUT) locus. Genomics 1990;8:710–716.
118. Ledley FD, Lumetta MR, Zoghbi HY, et al. Mapping of human methylmalonyl CoA mutase (MUT) locus on chromosome 6. Am J Hum Genet 1988;42:839–846.
119. Jansen R, Ledley FD. Heterozygous mutations at the mut locus in fibroblasts with mut^0 methylmalonic acidemia identified by polymerase-chain reaction cDNA cloning. Am J Hum Genet 1990;47:808–814.
120. Raff ML, Crane AM, Jansen R, et al. Genetic characterization of a MUT locus mutation discriminating heterogeneity in mut^0 and mut^- methylmalonic aciduria by interallelic complementation. J Clin Invest 1991;87:203–207.
121. Crane AM, Jansen R, Andrews ER, Ledley FD. Cloning and expression of a mutant methylmalonyl coenzyme A mutase with altered cobalamin affinity that causes mut^- methylmalonic aciduria. J Clin Invest 1992;89:385–391.
122. Ledley FD, Crane AM, Jumetta M. Heterogeneous alleles and expression of methylmalonyl CoA mutase in mut methylmalonic acidemia. Am J Hum Genet 1990;6:539–547.
123. Broyer M, Guesry P, Burgers EA, et al. Acidemic methyl malonique avec nephropathic hyperuricenique. Arch Fr Pediatr 1974;31:543–552.
124. Walter JH, Michalski A, Wilson WM, et al. Chronic renal failure in methylmalonic acidemia. Eur J Pediatr 1989;148:344–348.
125. Molteni KH, Oberly TD, Wolff JA, Friedman AL. Progressive renal insufficiency in methylmalonic acidemia. Pediatr Nephrol 1991;5:323–326.

126. Korf B, Wallman JK, Levy HL. Bilateral lucency of the globus pallidus complicating methylmalonic acidemia. Ann Neurol 1986;20:364–366.
127. Heidenreich R, Natowicz M, Hainline BE, et al. Acute extrapyramidal syndrome in methylmalonic acidemia: "metabolic stroke" involving the globus pallidus. J Pediatr 1988;113:1022–1027.
128. Kahler SG, Sherwood WG, Woolf D, et al. Pancreatitis in patients with organic acidemias. J Pediatr 1994;124:239–243.
129. Bodemer C, De Prost Y, Bachollet B, et al. Cutaneous manifestations of methylmalonic and propionic acidaemia: a description based on 38 cases. Br J Dermatol 1994;131:93–98.
130. De Raeve L, De Meirleir L, Ramet J, et al. Acrodermatitis enteropathica-like cutaneous lesions in organic aciduria. J Pediatr 1994;124:416–420.
131. Whelan DT, Ryan E, Spate M, et al. Methylmalonic acidemia: 6 years' clinical experience with two variants unresponsive to vitamin B12 therapy. Can Med Assoc J 1979;120:1230–1235.
132. Morita J, Ito Y, Yoshino M, et al. Persistent hyperkalemia in vitamin B_{12} unresponsive methylmalonic acidemia. J Inherited Metab Dis 1989;12:89–93.
133. Wolff JA, Strom C, Griswold W, et al. Renal tubular acidosis in methylmalonic acidemia. J Neurogenet 1991;2:31–39.
134. Rutledge SL, Geraghty M, Mroczek E, et al. Tubulointerstitial nephritis in methylmalonic acidemia. Pediatr Nephrol 1993;7:81–82.
135. Dayan AD, Ramsey RB. An inborn error of vitamin B12 metabolism associated with cellular deficiency of coenzyme forms of the vitamin. J Neurol Sci 1974;23:117–128.
136. Sum JM, Twiss JL, Horoupian DS. Selective death of immature neurons in methylmalonic acidemia of the neonate: a case report. Acta Neuropathol 1993;85:217–221.
137. van der Meer SB, Poggi F, Spada M, et al. Clinical outcome of long-term management of patients with vitamin B_{12}-unresponsive methylmalonic acidemia. J Pediatr 1994;125:903–908.
138. Sweetman L, Williams JC. Branched chain organic acidurias. In: Scriver CR, Beaudet AL, Sly WS, Valle D, eds. The metabolic and molecular bases of inherited disease. 7th ed. New York: McGraw-Hill, 1995:1387–1422.
139. Tanaka K, Isselbacher KJ. The isolation and identification of N-isovalerylglycine from urine of patients with isovaleric acidemia. J Biol Chem 1967;242:2966–2972.
140. Berry GT, Yudkoff M, Segal S. Isovaleric acidemia: medical and neurodevelopmental effects of long-term therapy. J Pediatr 1988;113:58–64.
141. Roe CR, Millington DS, Malthy DA, et al. L-carnitine therapy in isovaleric acidemia. J Clin Invest 1984;74:2290–2295.
142. Matsubara Y, Ito M, Glassberg R, et al. Nucleotide sequence of messenger RNA encoding human isovaleryl coenzyme A dehydrogenase and its expression in isovaleric acidemia fibroblasts. J Clin Invest 1990;85:1058–1064.

143. Kraus JP, Matsubara Y, Barton D, et al. Isolation of cDNA clones coding for rat isovaleryl-CoA dehydrogenase and assignment of the gene to human chromosome 15. Genomics 1987;1:264–269.
144. Vockley J, Parimoo B, Tanaka K. Molecular characterization of four different classes of mutations in the isovaleryl-CoA dehydrogenase gene responsible for isovaleric acidemia. Am J Hum Genet 1991;49:147–157.
145. Vockley J, Nagao M, Parimoo B, Tanaka K. The variant human isovaleryl-CoA dehydrogenase gene responsible for type II isovaleric acidemia determines an RNA splicing error, leading to the deletion of the entire second coding exon and the production of a truncated precursor protein that interacts poorly with mitochondrial import receptors. J Biol Chem 1992;267:2494–2501.
146. Hine DG, Hack AM, Goodman SI, et al. Stable isotope dilation analysis of isovalerylglycine in amniotic fluid and urine and its application for the prenatal diagnosis of isovaleric acidemia. Pediatr Res 1986;20:222–226.
147. Cohn RM, Yudkoff M, Rothman R, et al. Isovaleric acidemia: use of glycine therapy in neonates. N Engl J Med 1978;299:996–999.
148. Goodman SI, Frerman FE. Organic acidemias due to defects in lysine oxidation: 2-ketoadipic acidemia and glutaric acidemia. In: Scriver CR, Beaudet AL, Sly WS, Valle D, eds. The metabolic and molecular bases of inherited disease. 7th ed. New York: McGraw-Hill, 1995:1451–1460.
149. Goodman SI. Frerman FE, Loehr JP. Recent progress in understanding glutaric acidemias. Enzyme 1987;38:76–79.
150. Lipkin PH, Roe CR, Goodman SI, et al. A case of glutaric acidemia type I: effect of riboflavin and carnitine. J Pediatr 1988;112:62–65.
151. Frerman FE, Goodman SI. Nuclear-encoded defects of the mitochondrial respiratory chain including glutaric acidemia type II. In: Scriver CR, Beaudet AL, Sly WS, Valle D, eds. The metabolic and molecular bases of inherited disease. 7th ed. New York: McGraw-Hill, 1995:1611–1629.
152. Schutgens RBH, Wanders RJA, Nijenhuis A, et al. Genetic diseases caused by peroxisomal dysfunction. Enzyme 1987;38:161–176.
153. Amendt BA, Rhead WJ. The multiple acyl-coenzyme A dehydrogenation disorders, glutaric aciduria type II and ethylmalonic-adipic aciduria. Mitochondrial fatty acid oxidation, acyl-coenzyme A dehydrogenase, and electron transfer flavoprotein activities in fibroblasts. J Clin Invest 1986;78:205–213.
154. Hoganson G, Berlow S, Gilbert EF, et al. Glutaric acidemia type II and flavin-dependent enzymes in morphogenesis. Birth Defects 1987;23:65–74.
155. Gregersen N, Wintzensen H, Christensen SK, et al. C6-C10-dicarboxylic aciduria: investigations of a patient with riboflavin responsive multiple acyl-CoA dehydrogenation defects. Pediatr Res 1982;16:861–868.
156. Sweetman L, Nyhan WL, Trauner DA, et al. Glutaric aciduria type II. J Pediatr 1980;96:1020–1026.
157. Mitchell G, Saudubray JM, Benoit Y, et al. Antenatal diagnosis of glutaricaciduria type II. Lancet 1983;1:1099.
158. Chuang DT, Shih VE. Disorders of branched chain amino acid and keto acid metabolism. In: Scriver CR, Beaudet AL, Sly WS, Valle D, eds. The metabolic and molecular bases of inherited disease. 7th ed. New York: McGraw Hill, 1995:1239–1277.
159. Matsuda I, Nobukuni Y, Mitsubuchi H, et al. A T-to-A substitution in the E1α subunit gene of the branched-chain α-ketoacid dehydrogenase complex in two cell lines derived from Mennonite maple syrup urine disease patients. Biochem Biophys Res Commun 1990;172:646–651.
160. Fisher CR, Fisher CW, Chuang DT, Cox RP. Occurrence of a Tyr393 → Asn (Y393N) mutation in the E1α gene of the branched-chain α-keto acid dehydrogenase complex in maple syrup urine disease patients from a Mennonite population. Am J Hum Genet 1991;49:429–434.
161. Scriver CR, Mackenzie S, Clow CL, et al. Thiamine responsive maple syrup urine disease. Lancet 1971;1:310–312.
162. Danner DJ, Armstrong N, Heffelfinger SC, et al. Absence of branched chain acyl-transferase as a cause of maple syrup urine disease. J Clin Invest 1985;75:858–860.
163. Robinson BH, Taylor J, Sherwood WG. Deficiency of dihydrolipoyl dehydrogenase (a component of the pyruvate and alpha-ketoglutarate dehydrogenase complexes): a cause of congenital chronic lactic acidosis in infancy. Pediatr Res 1979;11:1198–1202.
164. DiGeorge AM, Rezvani I, Garibaldi LR, et al. Prospective study of maple-syrup-urine disease for the first four days of life. N Engl J Med 1982;307:1492–1495.
165. Mantovani JF, Naidich TP, Prensky AL, et al. MSUD: presentation with pseudotumor cerebri and CT abnormalities. J Pediatr 1980;96:279–281.
166. Mikati MA, Dudin GE, Der Kaloustian VM, et al. Maple syrup urine disease with increased intracranial pressure. Am J Dis Child 1982;136:642–643.
167. Lungarotti MS, Calabro A, Signorini E, et al. Cerebral edema in maple syrup urine disease. Am J Dis Child 1982;136:648.
168. Riviello JJ Jr, Rezvani I, Digeorge AM, Foley CM. Cerebral edema causing death in children with maple syrup urine disease. J Pediatr 1991;119:42–45.
169. Snyderman SE, Norton PM, Roitman E, et al. Maple syrup urine disease with particular reference to dietotherapy. Pediatrics 1964;34:454–472.
170. Silberman J, Dancis J, Feigin IH. Neuropathological observations in maple syrup urine disease: branched chain ketoaciduria. Arch Neurol 1961;5:351–363.
171. Kindt E, Halvorsen S. The need of essential amino acids in children: an evaluation based on the intake of phenylalanine tyrosine, leucine, isoleucine and valine in children with phenylketonuria, tyrosine amino transferase defect and maple syrup urine disease. Am J Clin Nutr 1980;33:279–286.
172. Fernhoff PM, Lubitz D, Danner DJ, et al. Thiamine response in maple syrup urine disease. Pediatr Res 1985;19:1011–1016.
173. Berry GT, Heidenreich RA, Kaplan P, et al. Branched-chain amino acid-free parenteral nutrition in the treatment of acute metabolic decompensation in patients with

173. maple syrup urine disease. N Engl J Med 1991;324(3):175–179.
174. Gerritsen T, Kaveggia E, Waisman HA. A new type of idiopathic hyperglycinemia with hypo-oxaluria. Pediatrics 1965;36:882–891.
175. Hamosh A, Johnston MV, Valle D. Nonketotic hyperglycinemia. In: Scriver CR, Beaudet AL, Sly WS, Valle D, eds. The metabolic and molecular bases of inherited disease. 7th ed. New York: McGraw-Hill, 1995:1337–1348.
176. Perry TL, Urquhart N, MacLean J, et al. Nonketotic hyperglycinemia. Glycine accumulation due to absence of glycine cleavage in brain. N Engl J Med 1975;292:1269–1273.
177. Perry TL, Urquhart N, Hansen S. Studies of the glycine cleavage enzyme system in brain from infants with glycine encephalopathy. Pediatr Res 1977;11:1192–1197.
178. Hayasaka K, Tada K, Fueki N, et al. Nonketotic hyperglycinemia: analyses of glycine cleavage system in typical and atypical cases. J Pediatr 1987;110:873–877.
179. Tada K. Nonketotic hyperglycinemia: clinical and metabolic aspects. Enzyme 1987;38:27–35.
180. Tada K, Hayasaka K. Non-ketotic hyperglycinaemia: clinical and biochemical aspects. Eur J Pediatr 1992;120:95.
181. Wolff JA, Kulovich S, Yu AL, et al. The effectiveness of benzoate in the management of seizures in nonketotic hyperglycinemia. Am J Dis Child 1986;140:596–602.
182. De Groot CJ, Troelstra JA, Hommes FA. Nonketotic hyperglycinemia: an in vitro study of the glycine-serine conversion in liver of three patients and the effect of dietary methionine. Pediatr Res 1970;4:238–243.
183. Gitzelmann R, Steinmann B, Otten A, et al. Nonketotic hyperglycinemia treated with strychnine, a glycine receptor antagonist. Helv Paediat Acta 1977;32:517–525.
184. Matalon R, Naidu S, Hughes JR, et al. Nonketotic hyperglycinemia: treatment with diazepam—a competitor for glycine receptors. Pediatrics 1983;71:581–584.
185. von Wendt L, Simila S. Saukkonen A-L, et al. Failure of strychnine treatment during the neonatal period in three Finnish children with nonketotic hyperglycinemia. Pediatrics 1980;65:1166–1169.
186. el-Defrawy SR, Boegman RJ, Jhamandas K, et al. The neurotoxic actions of quinolinic acid in the central nervous system. Can J Physiol Pharmacol 1986;64:369–375.
187. McDonald JW, Johnston MV. Non-ketotic hyperglycinemia: possible pathophysiological role of N-methyl-D-aspartate type excitatory amino acid receptors. Ann Neurol 1990;27:449–450.
188. Huettner JE. Indole-2-carboxylic acid: a competitive antagonist of potentiation by glycine at the NMDA receptor. Science 1989;243:1611–1613.
189. Brun A, Borjeson M, Hultberg B, et al. Neonatal nonketotic hyperglycinemia: a clinical, biochemical and neuropathological study including electron microscopic findings. Neuropadiatrie 1979;10:195–205.
190. Dobyns WB. Agenesis of the corpus callosum and gyral malformations are frequent manifestations of nonketotic hyperglycinemia. Neurology 1989;39:817–820.
191. Hayasaka K, Fueki N, Aikawa J. Prenatal diagnosis of non-ketotic hyperglycinemia: enzymatic analysis of the glycine cleavage system in chorionic villi. J Pediatr 1990;116:444–445.
192. Toone JR, Applegarth DA, Levy HL. Prenatal diagnosis of non-ketotic hyperglycinemia. J Inherited Metab Dis 1992;15:713–719.
193. Koyata H, Cox RP, Chuang DT. Stable correction of maple syrup urine disease in cells from a Mennonite patient by retroviral-mediated gene transfer. Biochem J 1993;295:635–639.
194. Butler IJ, Krumholz A, Holtzman A, et al. Dihydropteridine reductase deficiency variant of phenylketonuria: a disorder of neurotransmitters. Trans Am Neurol Assoc 1975;100:43–47.
195. Lazarow PB, Moser HW. Disorders of peroxisome biogenesis. In: Scriver CR, Beaudet AL, Sly WS, Valle D, eds. The metabolic and molecular bases of inherited disease. 7th ed. New York: McGraw-Hill, 1995:2287–2324.
196. Schram AW, Goldfischer S, van Roermund CWT, et al. Human peroxisomal 3-oxoacyl-coenzyme A thiolase deficiency. Proc Natl Acad Sci USA 1987;84:2494–2496.
197. Schindler D, Bishop DF, Wolfe DE, et al. Neuroaxonal dystrophy due to lysosomal alpha-N-acetylgalactosaminidase deficiency. N Engl J Med 1989;320:1735–1740.
198. Shoffner JM, Wallace DC. Oxidative phosphorylation diseases. In: Scriver CR, Beaudet AL, Sly WS, Valle D, eds. The metabolic and molecular bases of inherited disease. 7th ed. New York: McGraw-Hill, 1995:1535–1609.
199. Matalon R, Michals K, Sebesta D, et al. Aspartoacylase deficiency and N-acetylaspartic aciduria in patients with Canavan disease. Am J Med Genet 1988;29:463–471.

36
Neonatal Lipid Metabolism

Margit Hamosh

Fat is vital for normal growth and development, as it is the main energy source of the neonate. In addition to providing 40% to 50% of the total calories in human milk or formula, fat is essential to normal development because it provides the fatty acids necessary for brain development, it is an integral part of all cell membranes, and it is the sole vehicle for fat-soluble vitamins and hormones in milk.[1] These energy-rich lipids can be stored in the body in nearly unlimited amounts in contrast to the limited storage capacity for carbohydrate and protein. Before birth, glucose is the major energy source, whereas the fetal requirement for fatty acids is supplied mainly as free fatty acids from the maternal circulation. After birth, fat is supplied chiefly in the form of milk or formula triglycerides.[2]

Lipids are nonpolar or amphipathic substances that are insoluble in aqueous media (Figure 36.1). Absorption of fat permits efficient assimilation of a large number of hydrophobic (i.e., fat-soluble) chemicals, some beneficial (e.g., fat-soluble vitamins), and some detrimental (e.g., hydrophobic xenobiotics, drugs, and food additives).[3]

This chapter concentrates on lipid metabolism in general and on the specific aspects of fat metabolism that are different during the neonatal period. Topics discussed include the role of polyunsaturated fatty acids in infant nutrition and the possible late effects of early nutrition on obesity. In this overview the topics include fat structure; fat composition of human milk; fat digestion, absorption, and transport in the circulation; lipoproteins; the mechanisms of clearing circulating lipid; and the role of ketone bodies during the neonatal period. Finally, there is a brief discussion of inborn errors of lipid metabolism.

Fat Structure

The major lipid classes are glycerides, phospholipids, sterols (e.g., cholesterol), and free fatty acids (Figure 36.1).

Glycerides

Glycerides are non–phosphorus-containing lipids that are formed from the esterification of glycerol and fatty acids (Figure 36.1). Triglycerides (e.g., neutral fat) are the most abundant lipids in animal tissue and serve as an important energy source. In triglycerides all three of the carbon molecules of glycerol are esterified with fatty acids. Monoglycerides and diglycerides are compounds resulting from ester links between glycerol and one or two fatty acids, respectively.

Phospholipids

Phospholipids, phosphorus-containing lipid compounds, may be subdivided into three classes: derivatives of glycerol-3-phosphate (e.g., phosphatidyl choline, phosphatidyl ethanolamine, phosphatidyl serine, and phosphatidyl inositol), sphingosine, and the glycolipids. Phospholipids are found as structural components of all biologic membranes. They are important in oxidative phosphorylation, transport across cell membranes, and electron transport reactions. They are the main component of pulmonary surfactant.

Sterols

Sterols are alcohols with the cyclopentanoperhydrophenanthrene skeletal structure. The principal sterol is cholesterol, the parent compound of the steroids, including the adrenocortical, ovarian, and testicular hormones. The bile acids, degradative products of cholesterol, are important in gastrointestinal absorptive processes.

Fatty Acids

Fatty acids of animal origin are usually unbranched, monocarboxylic acids containing an even number of carbon atoms, varying from 2 to 24 in chain length. The fatty

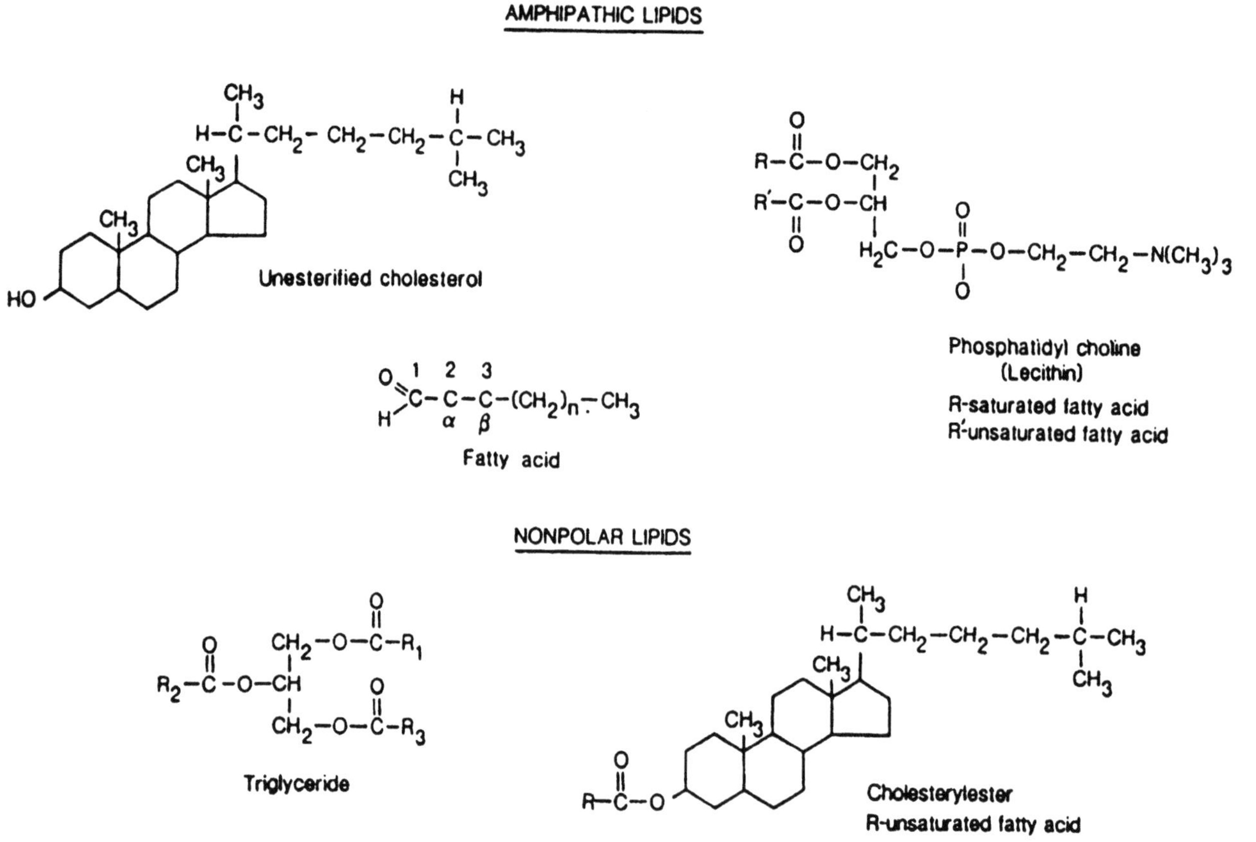

FIGURE 36.1. Principal dietary lipid components. (Adapted from Hamosh and Hamosh,[63] with permission.)

TABLE 36.1. Structure of fatty acids.

Descriptive name	Systemic name	Carbon atoms	Double bonds	Position of double bonds[a]	Unsaturated fatty acid class[b]
Acetic		2	0		
Butyric		4	0		
Caproic	Hexanoic	6	0		
Caprylic	Octanoic	8	0		
Capric	Decanoic	10	0		
Lauric	Dodecanoic	12	0		
Myristic	Tetradecanoic	14	0		
Palmitic	Hexadecanoic	16	0		
Palmitoleic	Hexadecanoic	16	1	9	n7
Stearic	Octadecanoic	18	0		
Oleic	Octadecanoic	18	1	9	n9
Linoleic	Octadecadienoic	18	2	9,12	n6
α-Linolenic	Octadecatrienoic	18	3	9,12,15	n3
γ-Linolenic	Octadecatrienoic	18	3	6,9,12	n6
Homolinolenic	Eicosatrienoic	20	3	8,11,14	n6
Arachidonic	Eicosatetraenoic	20	4	5,8,11,14	n6
	Eicosapentaenoic[c]	20	5	5,8,11,14,17	n3
	Docosahexaenoic[c]	22	6	4,7,10,12,15,19	n3

Fatty acids are classified according to structure as follows: medium-chain fatty acids, chain length ≤C12 carbon atoms; long-chain fatty acids, >C12 are divided into saturated (no double bonds) and unsaturated (6 double bonds). Saturated fats are considered atherogenic, whereas unsaturated fats have the opposite effect.
[a] Position of the one or more double bonds listed according to the number system. In this number system, only the first carbon of the pair is listed; i.e., 9 means position 9–10 starting from the carboxyl end.
[b] In the n number system, only the first double bond from the methyl end is listed and, as above, only the first carbon of the pair is written.
[c] No commonly used descriptive name.
Adapted from Montgomery et al.[241]

TABLE 36.2. Principal fat sources for infant formulas.

Milks and formula	Fat (%)	Source
Milks		
Human[a]	4.0[a]	
Cow	3.7	Buttermilk
Formulas		
Enfamil 20	3.7	Soy 80%, coconut oil 20%
Similac 20	3.6	Coconut and soy oils
Similac PM 60/40	3.8	Coconut and corn oils
SMA	3.6	Oleo, coconut, safflower, and soy oils
Lanolac	3.5	Coconut oil
ProSobee	3.6	Soy 80%, coconut oil 20%
Soyalac	4.0	Soybean oil
Isomil	3.6	Coconut and soy oils
Nutramigen	2.6	Corn oils
Portagen	3.2	MCT oil 88%, corn oil 12%
Pregestimil	2.7	Corn oil 60%, MCT oil 40%

[a] The composition of human milk fat is given in Tables 36.4 and 36.5.
MCT, medium-chain triglyceride.
From Hamosh,[1] with permission.

TABLE 36.3. Function of lipids in mammals.

Lipid class	Function
Glycerides	Fatty acid storage, metabolic intermediates
Phospholipids	Membrane structure, lung surfactant
Sterols	
Cholesterol	Membrane and lipoprotein structure; precursors of steroid hormones; degradation products are bile salts important in fat digestion and absorption
Cholesteryl ester	Storage and transport
Fatty acids	Major energy source, components of most lipids, precursors of prostaglandins

From Hamosh,[1] with permission.

acid chains may be either saturated or unsaturated (Table 36.1). Most biologically important fatty acids are esterified with glycerol, although a small portion are linked with other compounds or are free.

The fat composition of commercially available infant formulas is listed in Table 36.2. The composition of lipids in human milk is discussed in detail. The functions of the above-noted lipid classes are listed in Table 36.3. Storage lipid contains higher amounts of saturated fatty acids than do structural lipids.

Composition of Fat in Human Milk

Until this century human milk was the sole nourishment of the neonate. Indeed, although many milk substitutes are available commercially (Table 36.3), the aim of formula manufacturers is to duplicate as closely as possible the composition of human milk. Assuming that human milk is the "gold standard," a discussion of the fat composition of human milk is essential (see Chapter 52).

Mature human milk has a fat content of 3.5% to 4.5%. The fat in milk is contained within membrane enclosed milk fat globules.[4] The core of the globules consists of triglycerides (i.e., 98–99% of total milk fat), whereas the globule membrane is composed mainly of phospholipids, cholesterol, and proteins (Table 36.4). The packaging of triglyceride within the core of the globules permits the dispersion of these nonpolar lipids in the aqueous environment of milk and protects them from hydrolysis by milk lipases.[5,6]

Milk fat content and composition change during lactation. These changes are most pronounced during early lactation when colostrum is secreted 1 to 3 days postpartum, during the transition to mature milk within the following 2 to 3 days, and again during weaning. Mature milk maintains a constant fat composition.[7,8]

Total fat content increases gradually from colostrum (2.0%) through the transitional period (2.5–3.0%) to mature milk (3.5–4.5%).[9] Cholesterol content is highest in colostrum and decreases to a lower concentration in transitional and mature milks; it is distributed as 87% free cholesterol and 13% cholesteryl esters (Table 36.4). Phospholipids show a similar decrease from high concentrations in colostrum to lower concentrations in mature milk. The decline in phospholipid and cholesterol concentrations agrees well with an increase in the fat globule size and a decrease in the amount of membrane lipids containing about 60% of milk phospholipid and 85% of milk cholesterol.[10]

More than 98% of the fat in human milk is present in 11 major fatty acids from C_{10} to $C_{20:4}$ (Table 36.5). Medium-chain fatty acids amount to 10% of total fatty acids in mature milk of mothers of term neonates but contribute 17% of total fatty acids in milk produced by mothers of preterm neonates.[9]

TABLE 36.4. Composition of human milk fat.[a]

Component	%[b]	Comment
Glycerides (3.0–4.5 g·dl⁻¹)		
Triglycerides	98.7	Major component of the core of milk fat globules
Diglycerides	0.01	
Monoglycerides	0	
Free fatty acids	0.08	
Cholesterol (10–15 mg·dl⁻¹)		Major component of milk fat globule membrane
Phospholipids (15–20 mg·dl⁻¹)		
Sphingomyelin	37	
Phosphatidylcholine	28	
Phosphatidylserine	9	
Phosphatidylinositol	6	
Phosphatidylethanolamine	19	

[a] Mature milk from mothers of term neonates.
[b] Percent in lipid class.
Data from Hamosh et al.,[4] with permission.

TABLE 36.5. Fatty acid composition of human milk.[a]

Fatty acid	VPT (%) (26–30 weeks)	PT (%) (31–36 weeks)	T (%) (37–40 weeks)
10:0	1.37 ± 0.17	1.27 ± 0.18	0.97 ± 0.28
12:0	7.47 ± 0.72	6.55 ± 0.77	4.46 ± 1.17
14:0	8.41 ± 0.83	7.55 ± 0.89	5.68 ± 1.36
15:0	0.23 ± 0.04	0.27 ± 0.05	0.31 ± 0.07
16:0	20.13 ± 1.40	23.16 ± 1.49	22.20 ± 2.28
16:1	2.56 ± 1.40	2.92 ± 0.26	3.83 ± 0.39
17:0	0.34 ± 0.22	0.60 ± 0.24	0.49 ± 0.36
18:0	7.24 ± 1.13	7.25 ± 1.21	7.68 ± 1.85
18:1	33.41 ± 1.67	33.74 ± 1.79	35.51 ± 2.73
18:2	15.75 ± 1.22	13.74 ± 1.20	15.58 ± 1.99
18:3	0.76 ± 0.13	0.76 ± 0.14	1.03 ± 0.21
20:0	0.17 ± 0.13	0.09 ± 0.08	0.32 ± 0.11
20:2	0.35 ± 0.13	0.33 ± 0.13	0.18 ± 0.20
20:3	0.51 ± 0.09	0.43 ± 0.10	0.53 ± 0.15
20:4	0.55 ± 0.18	0.58 ± 0.19	0.60 ± 0.29
20:5	0.04 ± 0.05	0	0
21:0	0.05 ± 0.07	0.07 ± 0.08	0.17 ± 0.12
22:4	0.13 ± 0.10	0.24 ± 0.11	0.07 ± 0.16
22:5n6	0.11 ± 0.05	0.04 ± 0.05	0.03 ± 0.08
22:5n3	0.42 ± 0.09	0.12 ± 0.10	0.11 ± 0.15
22:6n3	0.24 ± 0.09	0.21 ± 0.09	0.23 ± 0.14

The data are means + SEM.
[a] Comparison of milk collected at 6 weeks of lactation from mothers who delivered at 26–30 weeks very preterm (VPT), 31–36 weeks preterm (PT), and 37–40 weeks term (T) of pregnancy.
Data are from Bitman et al.[9]

Saturated fatty acids constitute 42% and unsaturated fatty acids account for 57% of total lipid in human milk. Linoleic acid concentration is higher in more recent studies[9] than in earlier reports[11] and reflects the higher intake of polyunsaturated fats by the American population. Essential fatty acid concentrations are higher in colostrum and transitional milk than in mature milk.[9] Long-chain polyunsaturated fatty acids (LC-PUFA) derived from linoleic acid (18:2n6, 20:3, 20:4, 22:5n6) and from linolenic acid (18:3n3, 20:5, 22:5n3, 22:6) show a similar decrease throughout lactation. The concentration of these fatty acids is significantly higher in colostrum and milk of mothers of preterm neonates than mothers of term neonates.[9]

Table 36.6 lists the factors that affect milk fat content and composition. Length of gestation and length of lactation affect especially the content of the lipids that constitute the milk fat globule membrane phospholipid and cholesterol.[9] The latter are higher in the early stage of lactation (colostrum and transitional milk) because the milk fat globules are much smaller than in mature milk[10,11] and therefore the total "membrane" lipid level is higher in milk. Long-chain polyunsaturated fatty acids ($C_{20:4n6}$ and $C_{22:6n3}$) are essential for growth, brain development, and retinal function.[12] These fatty acids are stored in the fetus only in the last trimester of pregnancy; therefore, preterm infants depend exclusively on human milk for the provision of these essential nutrients. It has recently been shown that the concentration of n3 and n6 LC-PUFA are lower in pregnant and lactating women,[13] suggesting preferential transfer of these essential fatty acids from mother to fetus or to the neonate through milk, even at the cost of possible depletion of maternal reserves.[13] It has long been known that milk fat content changes drastically during each feed[14] and that milk fat composition is markedly affected by the maternal diet.[15] More recent data have shown that the mechanism for endogenous synthesis of fatty acids seems to be exhausted in women of very high parity,[16] that neonates who receive low fat-containing milk tend to nurse more frequently and for longer time periods, thereby causing an increase in milk volume,[17] and that there is a strong positive relationship between weight gain during pregnancy and milk fat content.[18] Low calorie intake leads to mobilization of fatty acids from maternal fat stores and their incorporation in milk triglycerides, leading to a more saturated milk fatty acid profile and higher concentrations of *trans* fatty acids.[19]

TABLE 36.6. Factors that affect milk fat content and composition.

Variable	Change
Gestation	LC-PUFA higher in preterm* and transitional milk
Lactation	Phospholipid, cholesterol higher in colostrum (preterm* > term*)
Parity	P10 +: lower endogenous synthesis of FA (C6–C16)
Volume	Low milk fat concentration associated with high volume
Feed	Fat: fore < mid < hind milk
Diet	
High CH	Increase in endogenous synthesis of FA (C6–C16)
Low calorie	Increase in palmitic acid (C16)
	Increase in *trans* fatty acids
Pregnancy weight gain	Positively associated with milk fat content

*Preterm and term refer to milk or colostrum of women who deliver prematurely or at term.
FA, fatty acids; CH, carbohydrate: LC-PUFA, long-chain polyunsaturated fatty acids.

Differences Between Human Milk and Formula Fat

The major differences between the fat in human milk and that in infant formulas are the absence of long-chain polyenoic fatty acids over C_{18} in formulas and the presence of only traces of cholesterol compared to an average cholesterol concentration of 10 to $15 mg \cdot dl^{-1}$ in human milk. Furthermore, whereas formulas deliver a constant amount of fat to the neonate during each feed, there are marked variations in the fat content of human milk, the fat concentration being lowest in fore-milk and gradually increasing to highest concentrations in hind-milk. In addition, fat content increases during the day, early morning milk having the lowest fat content.

Minerals, trace elements, and enzymes associated with the cream fraction of milk have similar diurnal variations. Nutrient content might vary in the milk secreted from the right or left breast at the same feeding.

In contrast to the changes in fat concentration, the fat composition of mature human milk is remarkably constant. Only drastic changes in the diet, such as consumption of excessively large amounts of polyunsaturated fats, carbohydrates, or severe limitations of total food intake, result in the increase of linoleic acid, palmitic acid, and medium-chain fatty acid concentrations, respectively. Studies show that the amount of eicosapentaenoic acid or *trans* fatty acids (i.e., geometric isomers of *cis* fatty acids, formed during partial hydrogenation of fat) increases markedly in milk of women who consume large amounts of fish oil[20] or hydrogenated fats,[19-21] respectively. The greatest increase in milk *trans* fatty acids occurs in women who are losing weight and consuming hydrogenated fat.[19] From these data it appears that *trans* fatty acids from the diet and from the mother's fat depots contribute to milk *trans* fatty acids.

Milk fat composition is markedly affected by maternal diseases such as cystic fibrosis,[22] diabetes,[23] and hyperlipemia.[24]

Effects of the Mode of Feeding on Later Life

In 1975, based on observations of the feeding habits of a single neonate, Hall[25] proposed that changes in the composition of human milk during each nursing might act as a cue for the duration of nursing. The marked increase in fat content during the feed might be associated with changes in the taste and texture of the milk, which might provide a signal to the neonate to stop feeding.[14,26] Hall's hypothesis suggested that in breast-fed neonates an appetite-control mechanism that protects from overfeeding develops early in life. Bottle-fed neonates would not develop such a control mechanism because of the uniform composition (i.e., fat content) of formula and because the amount consumed might be strongly affected by the mother's desire to "empty the bottle" at each feed. Although this attractive hypothesis has been widely quoted,[27] it has not been supported by a number of studies designed to test its validity.[28-30] Although milk fat content might not affect feeding patterns, there are distinct differences in the physiologic and metabolic responses to formula or milk feeding: (1) Differences exist in the pattern of milk intake in that breast-fed neonates have a lower rate of milk intake.[31,32] (2) Differences are seen in the pattern and rate of gastric emptying;[33,34] gastric emptying of human milk has a biphasic emptying pattern, with an initial fast phase, whereas gastric emptying of formula follows a linear pattern in both term and preterm neonates. Gastric emptying rates were earlier reported to be significantly slower ($p < .01$) in formula-fed than in milk-fed neonates, irrespective of gestational age. (3) Recent studies, however, show a similar gastric emptying pattern for formula or human milk.[35] Indeed there is no difference in gastric emptying rates of feeds identical in composition and calorie density given at volumes of about $20 ml \cdot kg^{-1}$.[36,37] Furthermore, the fatty acid composition of the feed of either formula or human milk does not seem to affect gastric emptying rate.[35,38]

Comparison of hormonal responses to feeding of human milk or formula have shown marked differences associated with these types of feeding and feeding-mode-dependent differences in gastrointestinal function as well as in pancreatic exocrine and endocrine function during the immediate neonatal period.[39,40]

The greater insulin secretion in bottle-fed neonates is of particular interest. As insulin stimulates fat deposition, it might affect the early development of adipose tissue and have a relation to cell number and cellular fat content of adipose tissue.[41,42]

Follow-up studies that compare the effect of breast-feeding and formula-feeding on growth, weight, fat content, and incidence of obesity have been carried out since the early 1970s. Whereas the early studies clearly show that breast-fed neonates have a tendency to be leaner than the bottle-fed group, more recent studies fail to show this effect. It seems that during the late 1960s and early 1970s bottle-fed neonates were often overfed, whereas more recently, with the greater awareness of good dietary habits, bottle-fed neonates receive volumes similar to those of neonates fed human milk; formula composition is also closer to that of human milk.

Follow-up studies on the effect of early nutrition on growth and obesity are more numerous for short-term than for long-term periods. In general, the young infant and toddler is protected to a certain extent from overweight by breast-feeding, but by 3 to 8 years of age the effect might be lost.[43] In long-term studies, some investigators reported a significant protective effect of breast-feeding against obesity in adolescents and young adults,[44] whereas others failed to find such protection.[45]

Other data suggest that energy requirements of neonates have been overestimated. Energy intakes have been shown to average about 70 kcal·kg^{-1} day^{-1} at 4 months of age in breast-fed infants compared to an intake of 110 kcal·kg^{-1} day^{-1} at 1 month after birth.[46–50] These studies indicate that the low energy intakes of breast-fed infants are not due to limitations in maternal milk production but represent physiologically regulated intakes.

In premature neonates there are differences in body composition between human milk-fed and formula-fed neonates, the former depositing less fat than the latter, despite the marked similarity in amount and energy provided by the two diets.[51,52]

Using the doubly labeled water method to quantitate simultaneously the energy expenditure, energy intake, milk volume intake, energy deposition, and energy content of breast milk, Lucas et al.[53] and Prentice et al.[54] found energy intake to be much lower than U.S. Department of Health and Human Services (DHHS) and Food and Agricultural Organization (FAO)/ World Health Organization (WHO) recommendations. An overestimation of human milk intake might have led to higher recommended daily allowance, which ultimately would lead to overfeeding of formula.

Careful analysis of milk intakes in the breast-fed neonates suggests a "characteristic volume for each mother-infant pair that is strongly related to infant weight at 1 month, suggesting that infant/or maternal factors coming into play during the first month of life are strong determinants of subsequent milk transfer to the infant."[55] This fine balance between a possible neonatal regulation of milk intake would be absent in the formula-fed neonate because of the possible maternal regulation of food intake.[56]

The different growth patterns of breast-fed and formula-fed infants indicate the need for separate growth curves of infants according to feeding mode. The WHO is now in the process of establishing such growth curves for exclusively breast-fed infants throughout the world.

White Adipose Tissue and Obesity

By definition obesity is an excess of adipose tissue relative to lean body mass. The reader is referred to the excellent reviews of these topics by Poissonnet et al.[57] and Bray.[58] It is necessary, to discuss certain aspects of development, especially because little is known from direct human studies and much is inferred from animal experiments.[58,59] Although in 1981 the Committee on Nutrition of the American Academy of Pediatrics emphasized "the need for studies on the pathogenesis of obesity in early life with an emphasis on the ontogeny of the fat organ," there is little new information on this topic.[60]

In the human, adipose tissue is present at 28 weeks' gestation.[57] Although preadipocytes might be present earlier, they can be located by standard techniques only after fat accumulation occurs within cells.[61] The earliest evidence of fat lobules is found in the buccal pad and gluteal areas of 14-week fetuses.[62] Because the third trimester is a period of rapid fat deposition in well-defined adipose tissue, the second trimester of pregnancy is considered a sensitive period for fat development.[57] Since detection of adipocytes is possible only after considerable fat accumulation, early markers for these cells have been sought. Lipid-accumulating enzymes (e.g., lipoprotein lipase), which hydrolyze circulating lipoprotein-triglyceride, promote the uptake of the released free fatty acids and monoglyceride by adipocytes.[63,64] This enzyme and lipolytic enzymes (e.g., the hormone-sensitive lipase that hydrolyzes triglycerides within the adipocytes, leading to release of free fatty acids from fat depots)[65] develop earlier than lipogenic enzymes, which synthesize fatty acids de novo within the tissue.[66–68] Animal and some human studies have shown that lipoprotein lipase is present in preadipocytes and has an important role in the lipid-filling process.[66–70] Lipoprotein lipase and hormone-stimulated lipase may play roles in initiating and maintaining the obese state in animals and humans.[71–75] Further studies are needed for a better understanding of these processes.

The number and size of adipocytes have received attention as early determinants of obesity. It was initially postulated that an increase in adipocyte number is limited to infancy,[41] ending in the human at about 2 years of age.[42,73] Later increases in adipose tissue mass were thought to occur chiefly by lipid filling of existing adipocytes. Studies by several investigators have identified two critical periods for proliferation of adipose tissue: One is before age 2 and the other during the adolescent growth spurt.[76,77] Infancy was assumed to be the period of adipocyte replication, suggesting that it may be directly related to nutrition, whereas during the adolescent growth spurt weight gain would result chiefly in adipocyte growth.[78] The excessive enlargement of adipocytes might also lead to adipocyte replication. The "fixed" cell theory (i.e., that by the age of 2 years each person has a well-defined number of adipocytes that ultimately determine adiposity throughout life) put excessive emphasis on early nutrition as a determinant of adult obesity. More recent studies show that adipocyte replication does not end during infancy,[79–84] that the excessive fat filling of adipocytes by overfeeding triggers cell division (i.e., when mean adipocyte size approaches 1.6 µg, new cells begin to appear)[81] and that there are site differences in the ability of adipose tissues to enlarge by hyperplasia, hypertrophy, or a combination of the two mechanisms.[82–87] Of special interest are the studies of Bjorntorp et al.[84] in the rat and of Lewis et al.[85–87] in the baboon. The studies of Bjorntorp et al. on the expansion of adipose tissue storage capacity at different ages in the rat concluded that expansion of adipocytes leads to recruitment of adipoblasts, which differentiate into preadipocytes when the increased demand for triglyceride storage can no longer be met by expansion of existing adipocytes.

The hypothesis that preweaning nutrition affects the fat cell number and adiposity in the adult was examined in carefully planned, longitudinal studies in the baboon by Lewis et al.[85–87] Neonatal baboons were fed similar formulas with caloric densities of 40.5 kcal (i.e., underfed), 67.5 kcal (i.e., fed normally), and 94.5 kcal (i.e., overfed) per 100 g formula. From weaning at 16 weeks until necropsy at 5 years of age, all baboons were fed the same diet. Fat cell size and number quantitated in 10 fat depots at sacrifice showed the following: Female baboons overfed as infants had markedly greater fat depot mass, primarily because of fat cell hypertrophy, than normally fed or underfed females. In overfed males, fat mass was greater in 4 of 10 depots compared with the other two feeding regimens. Underfeeding did not affect the body weight or adipose mass of either sex. These studies showed that, in the baboon, infant food intake does not have a major influence on fat cell number of the adult.

These studies show marked differences between the rat, a species on which most of our knowledge of adipose tissue development and physiology is based, and the baboon, a primate whose physiology should be closer to that of the human. A comparison between these two species raises questions that might be relevant to the premature neonate. Lewis et al. proposed that the degree of maturity at birth may determine the nature of preweaning fat mass increase by hyperplasia in the rat and hypertrophy in the baboon.[87] The less mature rat is similar at birth to the late gestational fetal primate with respect to the ontogeny of adipose tissue.[89] The size of fat depots is sensitive to intrauterine nutritional status.[90–93] The fat depots in which hyperplasia, in response to preweaning overfeeding, was seen in the baboon are either absent (e.g., groin, flank depots) or poorly developed (e.g., mesenteric) at birth.[87] Because the hyperplasia occurs in response to overfeeding at various ages in addition to infancy in the human, would premature neonates born early in the third trimester of pregnancy before the development of adipose tissue be even more vulnerable to obesity as infants as well as later in life?

Recent studies in the newborn seal, a species that secretes a very high fat content milk (35–55% fat) show very rapid fat deposition (1.9 ± 0.31 to 2.7 ± 0.17 kg·day^{-1} during early, days 1–5, and late, days 14–15, lactation, respectively) in the newborn.[94] This is a vital necessity for aquatic mammals, who have to deposit blubber immediately after birth for efficient insulation. Thus, the fat-storing function of white adipose tissue and lipoprotein lipase activity develop early and enable the rapid deposition of large amounts of dietary milk fat immediately after birth.[94]

The recent discovery of leptin, an important circulating signal for the regulation of body fat, its receptor, and the genes regulating their expression[95,96] and evidence for the presence of obesity-linked and region-specific regulation of the ob gene expression[97] suggest, however, that mode, quantity, and quality of early diet might be less important than previously assumed.

Brown Adipose Tissue

A detailed discussion of brown adipose tissue and its special role in thermogenesis is covered in Chapter 45. The tissue differs greatly from "white" adipose tissue (vide supra) in that the cells are multilocular (i.e., they contain several lipid droplets rather than the single large fat mass of "white" adipocytes) and are packed with many large mitochondria.[98] When the tissue is thermogenically inactive, the cells are filled with lipid and may resemble adipocytes. The cells are connected by gap junctions, which may provide electrical coupling between them, and they are innervated by sympathetic nerves.[99] Brown adipose tissue depots are located at specific sites (e.g., the interscapular, subscapular, axillary, and intercostal regions, as well as along the major blood vessels of the thorax and abdomen).[99]

The presence of this tissue differs among species. Nedergaard and Cannon[100] have divided these species into three groups: The first group comprises altricial species nest-dependent and underdeveloped at birth in which recruitment of brown adipose tissue starts at birth and reaches its peak several days postpartum. Rodents (e.g., rats and mice), belong to this group. Most of the knowledge of the development of brown adipose tissue is based on studies in the rat.[100] The second group of species are represented by immature neonates, where the recruitment of brown adipose tissue starts only when their central control systems have developed. The hamster and marsupials belong to this group. The third group has developed brown adipose tissue at birth that atrophies after birth. The guinea pig, calves, musk oxen, lambs, and goats belong to this group.

It is difficult to characterize the human neonate according to the above classification. It seems that there are marked similarities between human neonates and altricial species such as the rat.[99,100] The major function of brown adipose tissue in the neonate is to produce heat, which is accomplished by "nonshivering thermogenesis" and is dependent on the presence in brown adipose tissue of a specific mitochondrial protein (i.e., molecular weight 32,000) named thermogenin. This process is regulated by the hypothalamus, and the message is conveyed to the individual cells by the sympathetic nervous system.[100] The process of thermogenesis depends on the reversible uncoupling of mitochondria, enabling the oxidation of endogenous and exogenous substrates at high rates, independent of the need to phosphorylate adenosine diphosphate (ADP).[99] Thermogenin has been intensely studied by several groups and is known by different names: uncoupling protein, nucleotide binding protein, guanosine diphosphate (GDP)-binding protein, 32-kd protein, and the "proton conductance pathway." The reader is referred to several excellent reviews about the mechanism of thermogenesis, the chemistry of thermogenin, and the process that regulates its function.[100–102]

In the human, brown adipose tissue is present at birth but may continue to develop postnatally. Thermogenin concentration is high in children but has been reported even in adults.[103] The low thermogenic ability of preterm neonates is well known and is compensated for by the incubator.[100] Malnutrition in animals lowers the activity of brown adipose tissue. Hypothermia associated with malnutrition in the human neonate has been reported.[104] There are no reports of the effect of overfeeding on brown adipose tissue metabolism in the human, but in the rat postnatal overfeeding leads to increased metabolic activity of the tissue.[105] Inactivity of brown adipose tissue before the development of obesity in genetically obese animals is thought to be one of the causes of obesity.[106]

Nedergaard and Cannon[100] pointed out that a role for brown adipose tissue has been suggested in such rare diseases as Duchenne progressive muscular dystrophy, subcutaneous fat necrosis of the neonate, and brown fat necrosis with sudden infant death syndrome. They believe that in these unrelated diseases a sympathetic stimulation may lead to secondary effects on brown adipose tissue. There seems to be no evidence for a causative role of brown adipose tissue in these disorders.

Long-Chain Polyunsaturated Fatty Acids and Brain Development

In higher plants, animals, protozoa, and fungi, saturated fatty acids are acted on by desaturases to introduce double bonds, usually of the *cis* configuration. The introduction of the first double bond, a process that occurs in plants and animals, takes place in the cytosol. The resulting oleyl coenzyme A (CoA) can be converted to CoA derivatives of linoleic, linolenic, and other polyenoic acids by desaturation reactions that take place in the endoplasmic reticulum of plant cells and require nicotinamide adenine dinucleotide phosphate, reduced (NADPH) and

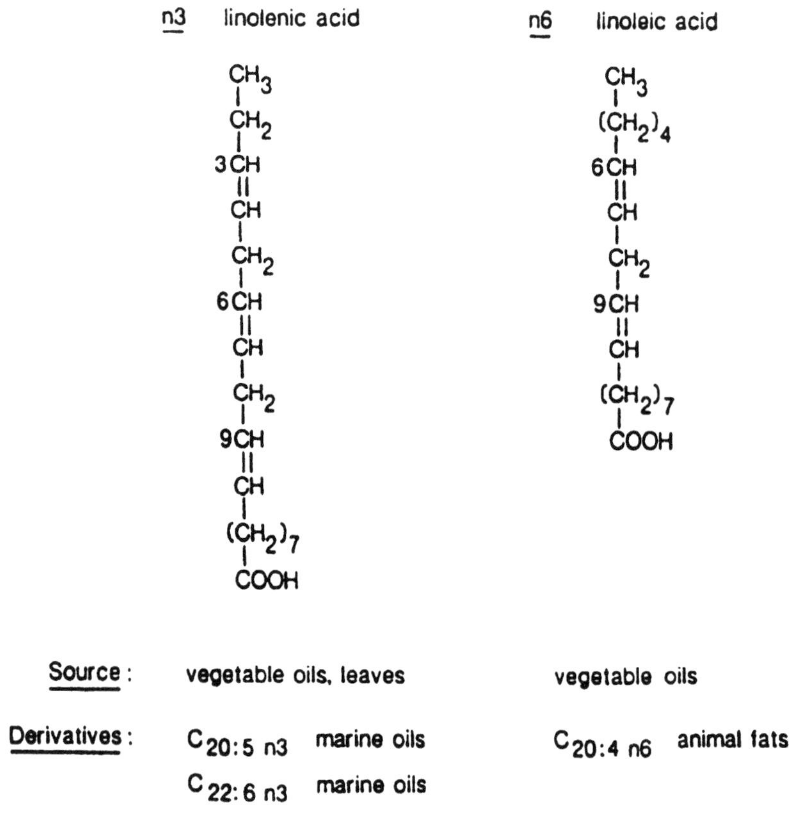

FIGURE 36.2. Families of fatty acids derived from the essential fatty acids.

TABLE 36.7. Characteristics of long-chain polyunsaturated fatty acids (LC-PUFA).

DHA (C_{22}:6n3)* essential for brain and retina development
AA (C_{20}:4n6)** essential for growth, precursor of prostaglandins, eicosanoids
Transferred to fetus mainly in last trimester
Transferred to newborn through mother's milk
Maternal plasma LC-PUFA decrease during pregnancy and lactation
Milk LC-PUFA decrease sharply after 3 months lactation
Multiple fetuses or successive pregnancy: lower LC-PUFA transfer to fetus
Elongation and desaturation of precursors inadequate in the newborn
Rates of conversion for n6 FA greater than n3 in the newborn

*Docosahexaenoic acid; **arachidonic acid.

light-generated ferredoxin as well as oxygen.[107] Because the conversion of oleyl CoA to linoleyl CoA does not occur in animals, polyenoic fatty acids such as linoleic and linolenic acids must be provided in the diet.

Essential fatty acids include two families distinguished by the position of the double bond closest to the methyl-terminal group of the fatty acid chain: n6 fatty acids, including linoleic acid (18:3 n6) and its longer-chain derivatives, and n3 fatty acids, comprising α-linolenic acid (18:3 n3) and its derivatives (Figure 36.2). These fatty acids are important to brain development, cell proliferation, myelination, and retinal function (Table 36.7).

Lipids are major constituents of the brain, where they are essential for the structure and function of neuronal and glial membranes, and are the main components of the myelin sheath. The biochemistry of brain development during the fetal and postnatal periods has been the subject of several reviews.[108,109] The specific subjects of lipid accretion in the fetus[110] and the very long chain fatty acids in the developing retina and brain[111] have been reviewed in depth. Lipids constitute about 60% of fetal brain solids—in myelin the weight of lipid amounts to 70% to 75% of dry weight.[112] The timing of growth and development of the human brain suggests that it might be more vulnerable to postnatal nutritional influence than previously assumed. The growth spurt is much more postnatal, ending only at 3 to 4 years after birth. The statement of Kuhn and Crawford,[113] "Human fetal development is a biological process in which both the blueprint (i.e., genetics) and building materials (i.e., nutrition) must be in good order for the construction of a healthy infant" is relevant not only to the fetal period but to infancy and childhood.[112] Because an increase in chain elongation-desaturation products does not occur for several weeks postpartum in preterm neonates, placental transfer of these fatty acids is of primary importance in accretion of these fatty acids in the fetus.[114] Based on quantitation of 22:6n3 and 22:5n3 in human milk,[9] our data show that preterm neonates fed their own mother's milk receive adequate amounts of long-chain polyunsaturated fatty acids that are sufficient to meet the estimated requirements for neural tissue synthesis.[114]

Brain growth is affected by nutrition at all steps of development but may be more vulnerable during critical periods of brain growth.[109] Whereas the mature brain is spared to a great extent the effects of malnutrition, during the early developmental period brain content and composition are affected by malnutrition, with myelin-associated lipids being particularly vulnerable, resulting in impaired myelination and synaptogenesis.[115] Although most of these studies have been carried out in animals, they might have great importance for human neonates, especially those born prematurely. The high content of 22:6n3 in brain lipids and the absence of this fatty acid from infant formulas, even those specially prepared for feeding the premature neonate, combined with good evidence for inadequate synthesis of this fatty acid from the precursor linolenic acid (18:3n3) have led to research aimed at adding long-chain polyunsaturated fatty acids to the diet of premature neonates (see Chapter 51).

Quantitation of 22:6n3 in individual red blood cell phospholipids in neonates born at less than 32 weeks' gestation has shown that this fatty acid decreased from a cord blood concentration while the neonates were receiving 60 kcal·kg^{-1}·day^{-1} from orogastric feedings. Similar 22:6n3 quantitation at 7 weeks of age has shown that this fatty acid increased in neonates fed preterm human milk, but continued to decline in neonates fed premature formula.[116] Studies to increase the level of 22:6n3 docosahexaenoic acid (DHA) by giving preterm neonates fish oil (MAX EPA) in the form of bolus or dispersed in the formula have shown an increased plasma phospholipid concentration of 22:6n3 with both modes of administration. The dispersed long-chain fatty acid was absorbed to a greater extent than when given as a bolus. These studies show that it is possible to prevent the postnatal decline in DHA and to maintain the serum concentrations of this fatty acid at a concentration seen in preterm neonates fed human milk by its careful addition to infant formulas.[117,118] It might be advisable to supplement infant formulas, not only with the long-chain polyunsaturated fatty acids of n3 series (e.g., DHA-22:6n3) but those of the n6 series[110] in order to maintain a concentration of fatty acids similar to that in human milk, and especially in the milk produced by women who deliver prematurely.[9]

A high concentrations of DHA (22:6n3) is present in the retina. Feeding of a diet low in 18:3n3 during pregnancy and after birth to the neonatal rhesus monkey results in a marked decrease of 22:6n3 content in retina and cerebral cortex to 50% of control values in the retina and 25% of control values in the cerebral cortex.[119] At 22 months of age the content of 22:6n3 in these tissues doubled in the control animals but failed to increase in the deficient group. Functionally, the deficient animal had subnormal visual acuity at 4 to 12 weeks of age and a prolonged recovery time of the dark-adapted electroretinogram after a saturating flash.[119] The disturbing effect of this early nutritional deficiency is the irreversible nature of the damage.[120] After 9 months of fish oil feeding, despite normalization of the DHA content of the retina, abnormal retinal function appears to be a persistent effect of n3 fatty acid deficiency during development. These studies indicate that primates, including the human, might not recover full brain function when early nutritional deficiencies are countered after the weaning period.[121] The avid uptake of polyunsaturated fatty acids by the developing brain, which increases steadily with increasing degrees of unsaturation,[122] indicates that these fatty acids have to be provided in optimal amounts for normal functional development.[123]

Recently LC-PUFA have been a major focus of research. Although considerable knowledge has been gathered, there is controversy over many basic questions relating to LC-PUFA and neonatal development. For instance, should the LC-PUFA concentration of human milk be the gold standard for the nutritional needs of the neonate? How important is antenatal deposition of LC-PUFA as compared to postnatal provision, i.e., maternal nutrition and stores as well as transfer to the fetus versus neonatal feeding mode—human milk or formula? While it is clear that the preterm neonate, who is born without LC-PUFA reserves formed primarily during the last trimester of gestation, needs an immediate postnatal supply, are the needs of the full-term neonate equally critical? Is a supply of DHA 22:6n3 essential for the development of visual acuity in the neonate? Is there a difference in DHA supply to the breast-fed as compared to the formula-fed neonate, resulting in higher brain DHA concentration, and is the latter related to better motor and cognitive function and higher IQ in the breast-fed child? Is the LC-PUFA composition of erythrocyte membranes representative of that in the developing brain? If infants, premature or full-term, are fed formula rather than mother's own milk, which provides an ample supply of arachidonic acid (AA) and DHA, how should these LC-PUFAs be supplemented?

Some of the questions can be answered now, while for others additional research will probably provide the information needed to reach meaningful conclusions. There is general consensus that the concentration of LC-PUFA (n3 and n6 series >20 carbons) in milk provides an ample supply of these essential fatty acids.[124] Furthermore, although the fatty acid profile of milk is affected by maternal diet, analysis of milk fat shows that the level of LC-PUFA in milk of women in Europe and Africa[125] is similar, and this similarity extends also to the United States,[9] indicating that LC-PUFA concentration in human milk is quite constant, with the exception of higher amounts of n3 LC-PUFA in the milk of women who consume large amounts of sea fish.[125,126]

Transfer of LC-PUFA to the fetus occurs even at the extent of relative deficiency in the maternal circulation, suggesting that dietary supplementation during pregnancy might be indicated.[127] Birth status of LC-PUFA can be assessed by analysis of plasma and erythrocyte phospholipid–fatty acids, but probably even better by analysis of the composition of umbilical cord arteries and veins of full-term and preterm neonates.[128] Birth concentration of LC-PUFA in plasma choline phosphoglycerides shows a strong correlation between AA (20:4n6) and fetal growth (e.g., weight and head circumference), while DHA (22:6n3) correlates strongly with length of gestation.[129] Indeed, a clinical trial to test the effect of fish oil supplementation on prolonging the duration of pregnancy was recently published.[130] Postnatal adequacy of LC-PUFA depends on the newborn's ability to convert the precursor linoleic and linolenic fatty acids to LC-PUFA through elongation and desaturation as well as on the exogenous supply of preformed LC-PUFA. There is currently controversy about whether these processes are well developed in the full-term neonate, while there is general consensus that LC-PUFAs have to be provided to the preterm neonate.[131]

The absence of LC-PUFA in infant formulas and the need for DHA for brain development and retinal function[132] have led to several studies that have examined whether the erythrocyte concentration is an indicator of brain and retina DHA. While earlier studies have shown such a relationship in the rat[133] recent studies fail to find one;[134] absence of such correlation has been reported in the piglet.[135] In the rhesus monkey[136] and the human,[137] however, there is a strong correlation between erythrocyte DHA and brain DHA, although no relationship was found between erythrocyte DHA and DHA concentration in the retina.[137] One may speculate on a possible relationship between higher brain content of DHA in breast-fed as compared to formula-fed infants[137,138] and improved neurodevelopment leading to higher IQ at school age of preterm infants fed human milk.[139] Delayed visual acuity development in animals and human has been attributed to low retinal DHA content.[140] In preterm infants retinal development is markedly affected by dietary DHA provided either as breast milk or as supplements to infant formula.[141-143]

The DHA-associated improvement in visual acuity might be a transient phenomenon lasting only for the first 4 months after premature birth.[140] A positive correlation between erythrocyte DHA concentration and visual acuity has also been reported in full-term neonates.[142,144] This further emphasizes the beneficial effect of feeding human milk rather than formula to the full-term as well as the preterm infant. Despite several recent studies that support the need for dietary supplementation of the full-term infant with DHA and AA,[145-147] one recent study failed to find a relationship between diet, blood lipid DHA, and visual acuity, and suggested that infant formula containing 1% linolenic acid "supports normal development of visual acuity of healthy term infants to 3 months of age."[148]

One drawback of supplementing infant formula with marine oil (rich in n3 LC-PUFA) is the gradual decrease in blood AA levels.[149] Because of the strong relationship between growth and AA levels, not only prenatally[129] but also during the first year after birth[149] and the AA lowering effect on n3 LC-PUFA in marine oil, it is advisable that the latter be added to infant formulas as purified DHA, which does not have this detrimental effect.

Maternal depletion of DHA and AA during pregnancy[150] and the relatively rapid decline of LC-PUFA in milk after the first 1 to 3 months of lactation[9,151,152] have raised the question of whether pregnant and nursing mothers should be supplemented with LC-PUFA. Very few such supplementation studies have been carried out, but from recent data it appears that supplementation with fish oil during pregnancy[153] or with DHA during lactation[154] results in markedly improved DHA status of the neonate and maintenance of a high milk DHA concentration during the first 3 months of lactation.

Although the highest concentration of DHA and AA have been reported in the milk of mothers of preterm infants during the first months of lactation,[9,151] it seems that they might not be sufficient to support postnatal LC-PUFA provision at intrauterine levels.[155] Given the recent stable isotope studies[156,157] that indicate that although the neonate is able to elongate and desaturate n3 and n6 precursor fatty acids, the amounts produced, especially for DHA, are inadequate to support the DHA concentration measured in the breast-fed infant,[156] while AA synthesis amounts to only 25% of neonatal plasma concentration.[154] The need for proper sources of LC-PUFA for maternal and/or infant supplementation could be met by DHA synthesized in algae and AA produced by fungi. These LC-PUFA have recently been found to be safe when given to healthy adults[158] or to lactating women.[154]

Although the debate over LC-PUFA supplementation will not be resolved in the near future, it might be necessary to arrive at a decision given the superior neurodevelopmental performance of term infants,[159] and the higher IQ at school age of preterm infants[160] given LC-PUFA supplements or mother's milk, respectively.

Medium-Chain Fatty Acids

Medium-chain fatty acids ($C_{8:0}$ to $C_{12:0}$) are present in low amounts in human milk and, as shown in Table 36.5, are present at higher concentrations in the milk of mothers of premature neonates.[9] They are mainly components of premature formulas, where they are added because of the poor absorption of cow's milk fat. The change in formula fat to vegetable fat blends, which contain high concentrations of unsaturated long-chain fatty acids, which are easier to solubilize and digest has resulted in similar absorption rates of formula fat containing either long-chain or medium-chain fatty acids. Medium-chain fatty acids are more easily released from triglycerides by lingual and gastric lipases. Earlier studies have shown that in experimental animals medium-chain fatty acids are absorbed directly from the stomach.[161,162] In other studies we have shown that in premature neonates fed formulas by gastric gavage, octanoic acid and, to a lesser extent, decanoic acid ($C_{8:0}$ to $C_{10:0}$, respectively) are rapidly absorbed through the gastric mucosa, providing a rapidly available energy source to the neonate.[163]

Medium-chain fatty acids are preferentially oxidized compared to long-chain fatty acids,[164] although storage of C_8, C_{10}, and C_{12} in adipose tissue has been reported.[165] Because medium-chain fatty acids can enter mitochondria without the need for carnitine-mediated transfer, they are a good source of ketone bodies. Care should be taken when adding medium-chain triglyceride (MCT) oil to fortify infant formula or human milk prior to feeding it to premature neonates. MCT oil tends to adhere to the feeding set when mixed with milk or formula prior to feeding.[166] To administer it efficiently, it should be fed directly through the gavage tube, followed by the infant's regular feed of either human milk or formula. The medium-chain fatty acids in premature formulas that contain high concentrations of this fat blend do not adhere to the gavage tube, probably because the fat is well blended into the formula.[167]

Fat Digestion, Absorption, and Transport

More than 95% of dietary fat, including that in human milk and infant formula, is triglyceride (Figure 36.1; Table 36.4). Digestion and absorption of dietary fat involve essentially the transport of water-insoluble molecules from one water phase—the lumen of the gastrointestinal tract—to another water phase—the lymph and plasma.[168-170] This process can be divided into three steps: (1) The luminal phase involves the solubilization and hydrolysis of triglycerides to free fatty acids, monoglycerides, and glycerol prior to their uptake by the intestinal mucosa; (2) The mucosal phase involves the reesterification of free fatty acids to form triglycerides, which are assimilated into chylomicrons and very low density lipoproteins (VLDL) prior to their release from the mucosal cell into the blood via the lymphatics; (3) During the transport and delivery phase, the fatty acids within chylomicrons and VLDL are taken up by the individual tissues for their metabolic needs.

Luminal Phase

Fat digestion requires adequate lipase activity and bile salt concentrations, the former for the breakdown of triglycerides and the latter for emulsification of fat prior to and during lipolysis. Fat digestion begins in the stomach with the action of lingual lipase, an enzyme secreted from lingual serous glands,[168] and of gastric lipase secreted from glands within the gastric mucosa.[169] Further digestion takes place in the small intestine through the action of pancreatic lipase (Figure 36.3).

Stomach

Initial hydrolysis of fat in the stomach leads to the formation of partial glycerides and free fatty acids.[170] This critical step is necessary for efficient fat absorption in the adult with adequate pancreatic function.[170-172] In the neonate and especially the preterm neonate, pancreatic lipase and intraduodenal bile acid concentrations, the major components of intestinal fat digestion, are low.[172] Efficient fat absorption in the neonate depends on alternate mechanisms for the digestion of dietary fat.

Of special importance is intragastric lipolysis in which lingual and gastric lipase compensate for low pancreatic lipase (Table 36.8).[168-173] In addition, the products of intragastric lipolysis, fatty acids and monoglycerides, compensate for low bile salt concentrations by emulsifying the lipid mixture.[174-176]

Rat lingual lipase and human gastric lipase have been cloned and expressed in *Escherichia coli* or yeast.[168,176]

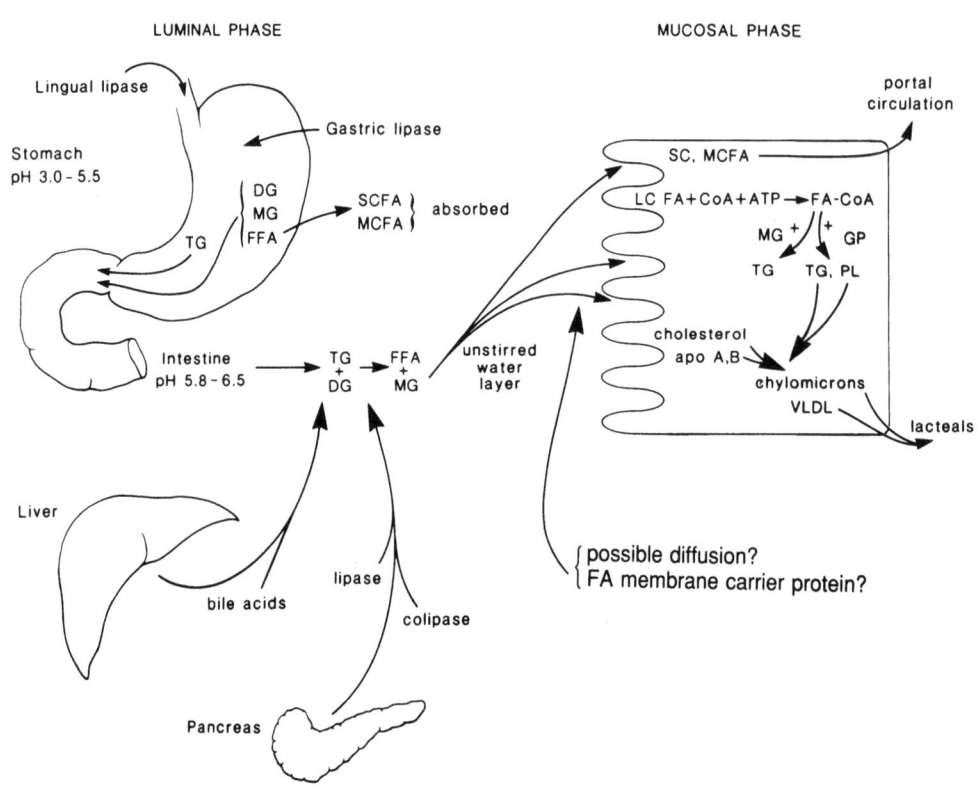

FIGURE 36.3. Fat digestion and absorption. Abbreviated scheme of major steps in fat hydrolysis in the lumen of stomach and intestine and reesterification in the intestinal mucosa. TG, triglyceride; DG, diglyceride; MG, monoglyceride; FFA, free fatty acids; GP, α-glycerophosphate; apoA, apoB, apoproteins A and B; PL, phospholipid. (From Hamosh,[1] with permission.)

TABLE 36.8. Compensatory digestive lipases in the neonate.

	Lipase in gastric aspirates	Milk bile salt stimulated lipase
Origin	Lingual serous glands; gastric mucosa	Mammary gland (human, gorilla, carnivores)
Ontogeny	Present from 24 weeks' gestation (in gastric tissue from 10 weeks' gestation)	Present after term and preterm (26–36 weeks) delivery and in prepartum mammary secretions
Site of action	Stomach (duodenum)	Intestine
Characteristics		
pH optimum	3.0–6.5	7.0–9.0
pH stability	>2.2	>3.5
Rate	MCT > LCT	MCT = LCT
	FA unsaturated > saturated	Water-soluble esters
Reaction products	FFA, DG, MG	FFA, glycerol, (MG?)
Bile salts	20–40% stimulation	Obligatory
Molecular weight	46,000–48,000	90,000–125,000
Function	Hydrolysis of 30–60% of ingested fat	Hydrolysis of 30–40% milk fat

MCT, medium-chain triglyceride; LCT, long-chain triglyceride; FA, fatty acids, FFA, free fatty acids; DG, diglycerides; MG, monoglycerides. Data from Hamosh et al.,[4] with permission.

They are glycoproteins of an approximate molecular weight of 52 kd and consist of 377 and 379 amino acid residues with an unglycosylated molecular weight of 42:56 kd and 43:16 kd for lingual and gastric lipase, respectively. The amino acid sequence of the two enzymes has an overall homology of 78%. Deglycosylation does not reduce catalytic activity; however, the terminal tetrapeptide, in particular lysine-4, is essential for enzymes binding to lipid-water interfaces. Rabbit and human gastric lipases have been crystallized recently.

Low pH optimum (2.5–6.5), absence of requirements for specific cofactors or bile salts, and stability to pepsin enable these enzymes to act in the stomach, and in certain diseases associated with pancreatic insufficiency such as cystic fibrosis and chronic alcoholism in the intestine.[177,178]

Substrate selectivity is relevant to specific aspects of neonatal digestion. Fatty acid and site selectivity (i.e., position of the fatty acid on the triglyceride molecule) of gastric lipase result in release of the fatty acids at the Sn3 position.[179] Long-chain polyunsaturated fatty acids of milk are located mainly at this position and are efficiently released by gastric lipase. Similar location of medium-chain fatty acids (MCFA) in milk fat leads to their preferential release in the stomach,[171] an observation that started the erroneous belief that gastric lipase is specific for MCFA. This site specificity indicates that fatty acids essential for infant development and growth, such as LC-PUFA as well as MCFA, an easily available energy source, are preferentially released.

The extent of gastric digestion of fat has been studied most extensively with mother's milk as the substrate. Depending on species, fat digestion in the stomach can account for 25% to 60% of total lipid digestion.[171] In the human, although gastric function and expression of gastric lipase are unaffected by diet, the extent of fat digestion is significantly greater in preterm infants fed mother's milk (25%) than formula (14%).[35] This difference is probably due to the structural differences in substrate presentation, that is, triglyceride within the milk fat globules or within formula fat particles.

The accessibility of triglyceride, the main energy source of the neonate to the other lipases that affect lipid digestion, has been examined. Earlier in vitro studies have shown that pancreatic colipase-dependent lipase cannot penetrate into milk fat globules and, therefore, is unable to hydrolyze the core triglyceride.[171,172] These studies have shown that gastric lipase and lingual lipase can hydrolyze the triglyceride within milk fat globules. Access to the core triglyceride is probably facilitated by the hydrophobic nature of lingual and gastric lipases, as well as by the fact that these enzymes do not hydrolyze the acyl bond of phospholipids,[168] or cholesteryl ester,[168] which are major components of the milk fat globule membrane.[168]

More recently, it became apparent that the milk bile salt-dependent lipase is unable to penetrate into milk fat globules, and that its activity in the hydrolysis of milk fat depends on initial partial hydrolysis by gastric lipase.[171,180] One can conclude that the phospholipid protein membrane of milk fat globules is not an obstacle to the action of preduodenal lipases. Phospholipids are a major barrier to triglyceride hydrolysis by milk bile salt-dependent lipase,[182] and a mixture of proteins and phospholipids prevents triglyceride hydrolysis by pancreatic colipase-dependent lipase.[182] Indeed, the hydrolysis of milk fat globule triglyceride by either of these enzymes depends on the initial predigestion by gastric lipase.[168,171]

Recent electron microscopy studies of milk fat globules at the end of 50 minutes of gastric digestion in infants show that the globules maintain their initial shape, and that the products of lipolysis are contained within the particles.[35] Similar milk fat globule–contained lipolysis products were previously reported during in vitro incubation of milk fat globules with lingual lipase and visualization by phase contrast or freeze etching techniques.[183] The free fatty acids and monoglycerides produced are more polar than the globule core trigylceride and migrate to the polar membrane. At this site, they might destabilize the membrane, which facilitates its breakdown in the intestine and facilitates subsequent action by pancreatic and milk lipases. Breaking of milk fat globule membranes is aided by bile salts, even at very low concentrations. Thus, contrary to the minimal contribution of the stomach to protein digestion, the stomach is essential to fat digestion not only because 30% to 60% of milk fat is digested at this site in the neonate, but also because partial hydrolysis in the stomach is a prerequisite for the subsequent intestinal digestion of fat. Furthermore, recent studies show that lipase activity and output in preterm infants are equal to that of healthy adults kept on a high-fat diet (23 ± 5 vs. 23 ± 3 U·kg^{-1} body weight, respectively) and is higher than in adults consuming a low-fat diet (5.2 ± 1.3 U·kg^{-1}).[184] The regulation of gastric lipase expression by dietary fat combined with the high fat consumption in infancy might explain the high gastric lipase activity even in very preterm infants.[184] Gastric lipolysis might also be of considerable importance during the transition from total parenteral nutrition (TPN) to gavage feeding because, contrary to intestinal and pancreatic digestive enzymes whose activity decreases during TPN,[185,186] gastric lipase activity is unaffected by mode of feeding.[187]

In gastric aspirates, lipase activity is high already at 25 weeks' gestation; activity remains constant up to 34 weeks, when it increases about 40% above the prior level and decreases again slightly before term delivery. In fetal gastric explants, lipase expression is evident at 10 to 13 weeks' gestation and the adult distribution,[188] that is, mainly in the body, with only traces of activity in the antrum, is established at 15 weeks' gestation. In contrast to pepsin, the secretion mechanism of lipase seems well developed at this time.[189]

Duodenum

Several lipases can participate in the intestinal digestion of dietary fat: pancreatic colipase-dependent lipase (CDL), carboxyl ester lipase (CEL), and in the breast-fed infant, milk bile salt-dependent lipase (BSDL). The latter two lipases are identical and are expressed in the pancreas (CEL) and in the mammary gland (BSDL).

Numerous investigators have reported the very slow development of CDL in the neonate[190,191] and have suggested that the efficient digestion of fat is probably accomplished by other lipases.[192,193] The "classic" CDL has a molecular weight of 48 kd, is glycosylated, has a serine at the catalytic site, and has a signal peptide that comprises the first 16 amino acids.[194] The preferred substrates of CDL are emulsions of triglycerides or insoluble micelles.[194] Water-soluble esters are hydrolyzed at much lower rates. CDL is inhibited by bile salts in concentrations found in the duodenum. This inhibition is reversed by pancreatic colipase, a 10-kd, 86 amino acid protein that is secreted as procolipase and is activated to colipase by trypsin through the cleavage of a pentapeptide activation peptide.[194,195] Pancreatic lipase, which has no activation peptide activity, might be regulated by the balance between colipase and procolipase.[194] The three-dimensional structure of pancreatic lipase has been determined and shows the presence of two domains: an amino terminal domain (residues 1–336) containing the active site, and a carboxyl terminal domain (residues 337–449).[196] Procolipase binds to the C-terminal domain of the lipase.[196] Recent studies show that lipase activity is regulated by a "lid," a surface helix covering the catalytic triad that moves, and thereby changes the hydrophobicity around the active site. This explains the interfacial activation of pancreatic lipase, that is, the increase in activity in the presence of a water-lipid interface. Pancreatic lipase is the major digestive lipase in the adult;[194] however, in the infant its contribution is limited. Lower lipase activity as compared with trypsin activity in small for gestational age (SGA) than in appropriate for gestational age (AGA) premature infants suggests that pancreatic lipase might be more susceptible to nutrient deprivation in utero than are proteolytic enzymes.[197]

Another lipase, the carboxylester lipase, a 100-kd glycoprotein, amounts to 4% of total protein in adult pancreatic juice.[198] As indicated above, this lipase is identical to the milk bile salt-dependent lipase. However, whereas the latter is assumed to contribute to fat digestion in the breast-fed infant, little is known about the contribution of pancreatic carboxylester lipase at this age in the human. The enzyme is, however, well represented among other species; it is the only pancreatic lipase in the shark[199] and it is the main pancreatic lipase in the suckling rat[200] before the development of CDL.

The pancreas also secretes a group of pancreatic lipase-related proteins (PLRP1 and PLRP2) whose characteristics differ from those of CDL by exhibiting high phospholipase activity, absence of interfacial activation, and absence of colipase effect in maintaining activity at high bile salt concentrations.[201] These pancreatic lipase-related proteins are under investigation in the human, as well as in several animal species. There is high homology between PLRP1 and PLRP2 and still remarkable but somewhat lower homology between these pancreatic proteins and CDL. Because of their high phospholipase activity and inhibition by bile salts that cannot be overcome by colipase, it has been recently suggested that they function mainly as phospholipases. The potential role of these additional members of the lipase gene family, especially PLRP1, which is present in high amounts only during the suckling period, in neonatal fat digestion is currently unknown.

The milk bile salt-dependent lipase (BSDL) is identical to the pancreatic carboxylester lipase. The characteristics of this milk lipase, as related to fat digestion in the neonate, have been reviewed recently.[173,202,203] There is indirect evidence that this lipase improves fat absorption in the neonate, and a greater body of evidence gathered from in vitro studies that the enzyme remains active in the infant's gastrointestinal tract and, therefore, might contribute significantly to fat digestion.[173] Because this lipase might have an important function in the neonate,[173,204,205] it remains the most extensively studied enzyme of human milk.

Milk bile salt-dependent lipase seems to be a constitutive enzyme of the mammary gland because it is independent of milk volume; that is, activity is similar before the onset of lactation and during weaning.[173] Furthermore, BSDL activity is high in the milk of women who deliver prematurely and is independent of duration of pregnancy. There is a high concentration of BSDL protein (i.e., 1% of total milk protein) in human and carnivore milk.[173,206] Activity varies among women, but it remains constant within each woman.[202]

The BSDL of human[207] and ferret[206] milk has been purified and characterized. The enzyme in human milk has recently been cloned.[208] Two variants of the cDNA for human BSDL[209] and two active forms of the enzyme with molecular masses of 97kd and 120kd have been reported. Some women produce two forms of this enzyme in approximately equal amounts.[209] The human milk lipase mRNA encodes a 748-residue protein, including a 23-residue signal peptide.[208] Recent studies suggest that the C-terminal part might not be necessary for some of the physiologic functions such as heat stability, stability to low pH, and resistance to proteolytic inactivation, and that physiologic and catalytic functions of BSDL reside in the conserved N-terminal domain.

The lack of positional or fatty acid specificity of the milk lipase indicates that it might be able to completely hydrolyze milk triglycerides. Recent studies in milk-fed full-term infants indicate, however, specificity for the Sn1 and Sn3 position and absorption of milk lipid as 2-monoglyceride and free fatty acids.[210] The combined action of gastric lipase and milk BSDL could, therefore, accomplish the process of milk fat digestion in the presence of very little pancreatic lipase. As discussed earlier, milk BSDL, similar to gastric lipase, is able to release LC-PUFA, whereas pancreatic lipase is unable to hydrolyze the carboxylic bond of LC-PUFA because of the proximity of the double bond to the carboxyl end of the fatty acid. Thus, LC-PUFA, especially DHA, which is essential for brain and retinal development, is efficiently taken up from milk fat, even in very premature infants.

Intragastric hydrolysis of milk fat produces relatively large amounts of monolauryl glyceride, a substance with antibacterial, antiviral, and antifungal activity, indicating that anti-infective agents are formed in the neonate's stomach during fat hydrolysis. Fat digestion in the stomach is probably quantitatively much more important for the neonate than for the healthy adult.

Even with a very low pancreatic lipase concentration, the neonate is able to absorb 90% to 95% of dietary fat through the combined action of gastric lipolysis and intestinal lipolysis by human milk lipase. Bile salt-stimulated lipase activity levels are similar in preterm and term milk and the enzyme is stable at low temperatures, indicating that preterm neonates fed their own mother's milk receive adequate digestive lipase even when fed previously stored milk.

Mucosal Phase

The products of luminal lipolysis pass into the enterocyte by passive diffusion.[211] Data suggest that fatty acid transport across the enterocyte could be facilitated by a specific membrane fatty acid binding protein.[212] Once inside the enterocyte the fatty acids are transported to the reesterification site, endoplasmic reticulum, by means of a soluble intracellular fatty acid binding protein.[213]

Fatty acid-binding proteins (FABPs) are a family of cytosolic proteins that bind hydrophobic ligands and are thought to be important in the uptake and intracellular transport of fatty acids in the enterocyte. Much progress has been achieved in our knowledge of these carrier proteins since their initial description.[213] The enterocyte expresses at least two such FABPs (I-FABP and L-FABP) identified by the organ in which they were first identified (i.e., the intestine and liver, respectively). These proteins are expressed at high levels (i.e., 1–2% of total cytosolic protein), their messenger RNAs (mRNAs) encoding up to 3% of total intestinal protein.[214] This topic was reviewed in 1994.[215,216] Briefly, there is evidence of extensive conservation of the primary structure of these genes with over 80% homology between rat and human liver and intestinal FABPs. These proteins increase at the time of birth in the rat[214] reaching highest concentrations in the adult. I-FABP and L-FABP are expressed only in villus cells with highest activity in the proximal small intestine. These binding proteins have been shown by histochemical techniques to be present also in the stomach. L-FABP, but not I-FABP, also binds cholesterol in a 1:1 molar ratio.[216]

After the fatty acids are activated to acyl-CoA, a step catalyzed by acyl-CoA ligase that occurs in the mitochondria, the reesterification to triglyceride occurs by two mechanisms: the monoglyceride and phosphatidic acid pathways.[217] In the first mechanism the acceptor of fatty acids is monoglyceride, whereas in the second pathway the acceptor is α-glycerophosphate produced from glucose metabolism. The monoglyceride pathway accounts for the reesterification of about 70% of absorbed fatty acids, whereas the phosphatidic acid pathway is the only mechanism for phospholipid synthesis in the intestinal mucosa (Figure 36.3).[217]

Studies in developing animals show that the mucosal phase of fat absorption is well developed and keeps pace with the higher fat intake of the neonatal period.[218–220]

The newly synthesized triglyceride, together with phospholipid, cholesterol, and protein, is assembled into lipoproteins (i.e., chylomicrons and VLDL). These large particles are released into the intercellular space by reverse pinocytosis, and they move across the basement membrane into the lymphatics.[221] Chylomicrons are released into the lacteals on the first day after birth, suggesting that this phase of fat assimilation is well developed in the neonate.

Transport of Lipid in the Circulation

Lipids are nonpolar or polar amphipathic substances (Figure 36.1) that are insoluble in aqueous media and can be transported in the circulation only in association with specific proteins. Polar lipids (e.g., free fatty acids and lysolecithin) bind to plasma albumin, whereas nonpolar lipids are transported within much larger particles, the lipoproteins. The nonpolar lipids (e.g., triglycerides and cholesteryl ester) form the hydrophobic core of the lipoproteins, whereas amphipathic lipids (e.g., phospholipids, cholesterol, small amounts of free fatty acids, and partial glycerides) combine with apoproteins to form the surface film.

The lipoproteins are generally divided into four categories: chylomicrons, VLDL, low-density lipoproteins (LDL), and high-density lipoproteins (HDL). The primary function of the lipoproteins is the transport of lipids, chiefly triglyceride (e.g., chylomicrons and VLDL) and cholesterol (e.g., LDL and HDL). In addition to their transport function—the solubilization of hydrophobic lipid in the aqueous environment of blood—the protein component of lipoproteins, the apolipoproteins, have important metabolic functions in the assembly and transport of fat from the intestine and in the transport and tissue uptake of the absorbed lipid, the lipoproteins. The apoprotein moieties of lipoproteins have been studied intensively in the past decade in various species, including the human. Apoproteins A-I, A-II, and B also have been studied during gut ontogeny. It is believed that they may be important in the fetus and neonate in preparing the intestinal mucosa for the high postnatal fat intake.[216] Apolipoprotein B is the major apoprotein of the triglyceride-rich chylomicrons and VLDL. This large hydrophobic protein, synthesized in liver and intestine, is the major structural protein of triglyceride-rich lipoproteins. It is present in two forms in the circulation: apo B-100 and apo B-48. The former is present in VLDL and LDL and the latter in chylomicrons.[215] Apo B-48 is colinear with the amino terminal of apo B-100 and does not contain the C-terminal region required for LDL receptor binding.[215,216] In the adult human, apo B-100 is synthesized in the liver and apo B-48 in the intestine. The rat liver produces both apo B-100 and apo B-48, whereas the rat intestine produces only apo B-48.

The functional significance of these two forms of apo B is related to specific lipid transport and delivery. Apo B-48 is expressed in the intestine and is the major lipid carrier for intestinally produced chylomicrons and VLDL, whereas production of apo B-100 in tissues other than intestine reflects their need for cholesterol. The early fetal development in the 9-week fetus of the editing mechanism (i.e., production of apo B-48) in the human prepares the fetus for the large influx of fat immediately after birth.[222]

Some apoproteins (e.g., apo B and apo AII) have a primary role in lipid transport, whereas others (e.g., apo CII and AI) are specific activators of enzymes involved in lipolysis (lipoprotein lipase) and interconversion of lipoproteins (e.g., lecithin: cholesterol acyltransferase; LCAT).

The catabolism of chylomicrons, VLDL, or Intralipid occurs by a stepwise reduction of the triglyceride core through the action of lipoprotein lipase, an enzyme that hydrolyzes lipoprotein triglyceride at the luminal surface of the capillary endothelium (Figure 36.4).[63,64] Concomitantly with triglyceride hydrolysis, surplus surface constituents (e.g., apoproteins and polar lipids, 60% of free cholesterol, 90% of phosphatidylcholine, and 100% of sphingomyelin) are removed from VLDL. These surface constituents are released in particulate form that associate into disk-shaped structures similar to nascent HDL precursors isolated from intestinal lymph or from rat liver perfusate.

The hydrolysis of chylomicrons and VLDL by lipoprotein lipase reduces the core of the lipoprotein particles, producing chylomicron remnants and LDL from chylomicrons and VLDL, respectively. The surplus surface constituents are the precursors of nascent HDL (Figure 36.4).[223]

A second lipase that hydrolyzes lipoprotein triglyceride is hepatic lipase, located in the endothelium of liver capillaries. The enzyme acts on VLDL triglyceride as well as on HDL phospholipids. Another enzyme with a key role in lipoprotein metabolism is LCAT, which is released from the liver into the circulation, where it acts specifically on plasma HDL by converting the lecithin and unesterified cholesterol of HDL to lysolecithin and

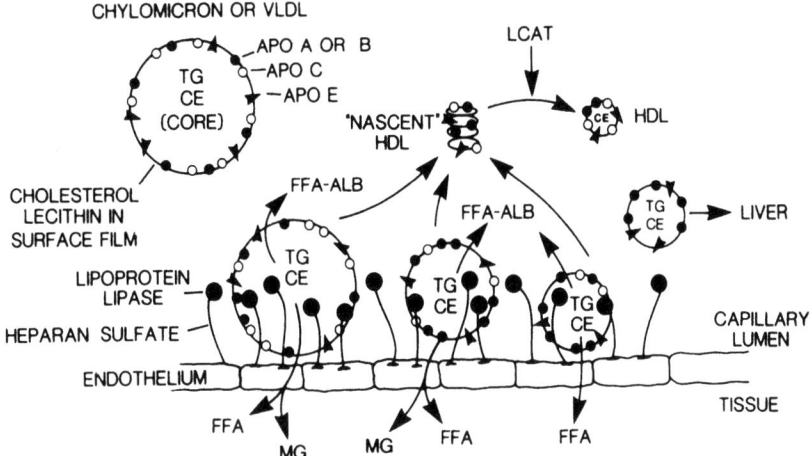

FIGURE 36.4. Hydrolysis of triglyceride in chylomicrons, VLDL, and Intralipid emulsion by endothelial lipoprotein lipase. Triglyceride-rich lipoproteins are represented as large particles containing a neutral lipid core of triglyceride (TG) and cholesteryl ester (CE) and a surface film composed of lecithin, cholesterol, and apoproteins. VLDLs are smaller than chylomicrons and contain different amounts of apoproteins. Lipoprotein lipase, bound to the endothelial surface through heparan sulfate, hydrolyzes lipoprotein TG to monoglyceride (MG) and free fatty acids (FFA). The latter are taken up by the tissues or are released into the circulation, where they bind to albumin (ALB). Shrinking of the particle core by lipolysis leaves an excess of surface components (broken line), which break off as disks similar to "nascent" high-density lipoprotein (HDL). These newly formed particles acquire cholesteryl ester via the lecithin: cholesteryl acyl transferase (LCAT) reaction, becoming spherical HDL particles. (From Hamosh and Hamosh,[63] with permission.)

cholesteryl ester.[224] Once esterified, the cholesteryl ester leaves the surface coat and moves into the nonpolar lipid core in the center of the particle, leading to transformation of the disk-shaped "nascent" HDL into spherical "mature" HDL.

Lipoprotein lipase, the key enzyme in removal of lipoprotein triglyceride, is important in the formation of both LDL and HDL lipoprotein (Figure 36.5). LCAT catalyzes the synthesis of almost the entire cholesterol ester of circulating lipoproteins. These two key enzymes differ in one important respect: lipoprotein lipase in active at the capillary wall and under normal conditions is found only in trace amounts in the circulation. This specific location probably facilitates the uptake of lipolytic products (e.g., free fatty acids and monoglycerides) into tissue. LCAT acts exclusively in plasma, where it accomplishes

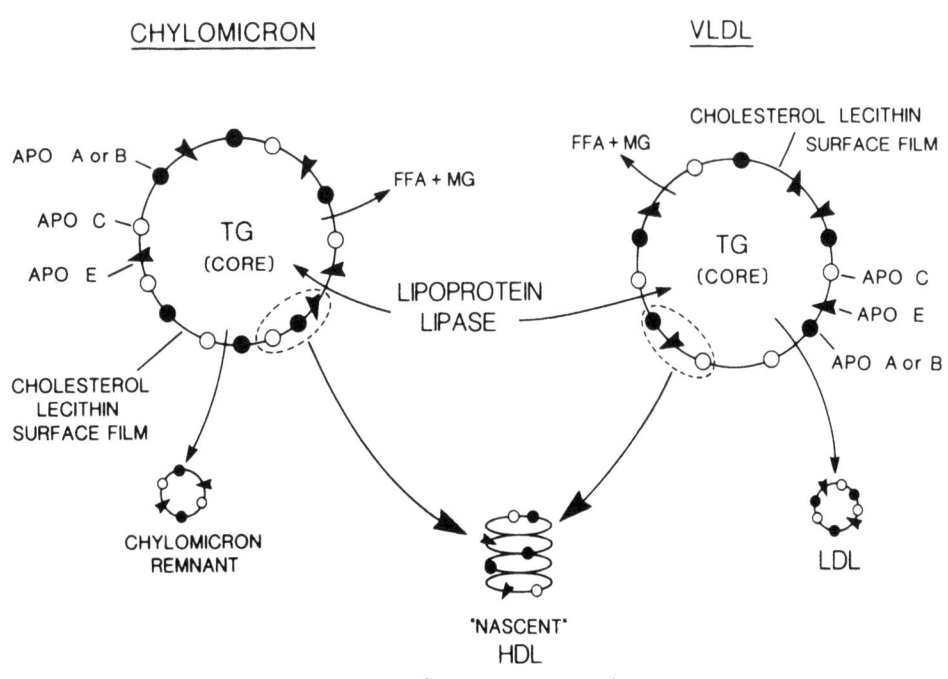

FIGURE 36.5. Central role of lipoprotein lipase in the formation of low-density and high-density lipoproteins. (From Hamosh,[1] with permission.)

TABLE 36.9. Lipid clearing enzymes: cofactors and mechanisms.

Enzyme cofactor	Characteristics	Substrate	Site of activity	Function	Deficiency
Lipoprotein lipase	Gene on Chr 8, 55-kd 475 AA	Chylomicron VLDL-TG IV lipid emulsion	Endothelium	Hydrolosis of TG to FFA and MG	Type I hyperlipidemia incidence 1:1,000,000 carrier Frequency 1:500
Apoprotein CII	Gene on Chr 19, 8.8-kd, 79 AA			Cofactor of LPL	Hyperlipidemia less severe than LPL deficiency 14 families, 8 mutations
Lecithin:cholesterol acyltransferase	Gene on Chr 16, 67-kD, 416 AA	HDL Lecithin, cholesterol	Plasma	Transesterification Synthesis of cholesteryl ester Transport of cholesterol from tissues	Familial LCAT deficiency; fish eye disease. 50 patients in 30 families
Apoprotein AI	Gene on Chr 11, 27-kd, 243 AA			Cofactor of LCAT	Less severe than LCAT deficiency

From Hamosh.[170] AA, amino acid; TC, triglyceride; FFA, free fatty acid; MG, monoglyceride; Chr, chromosome.

its function of continuous modulation of the cholesteryl ester content of circulating lipoproteins.

Lipoprotein lipase, localized exclusively in extraheptic tissues, is expressed in the liver during the immediate perinatal period,[222] where it has the same function as in other tissues, namely the hydrolysis of circulating triglyceride-rich lipoproteins.[225] Hormonal regulation of LPL is different in the neonatal liver from that in many peripheral tissues.[226] Message (mRNA) and expression (active LPL) become extinct within a few days after birth.[227] Lipoprotein lipase plays a special role in adipose tissue uptake of lipoprotein-triglyceride by the neonate. Indeed, in aquatic mammals, such as the gray seal, who transfer large amounts of fat through milk to their neonates in a relatively short time period of 1 to 2 weeks, milk fat content and pup body fat content are strongly correlated to LPL activity in mother and neonate, respectively.[94]

Studies in the neonatal piglet show that LCAT activity increases rapidly after birth and continues to rise throughout the first 3 weeks of life.[228] TPN depresses significantly the postnatal increase in LCAT activity.[228] Furthermore, at 3 weeks of TPN there is a marked decrease in LCAT activity[228] that coincides with TPN-induced cholestasis, characterized by markedly reduced bile salt–independent and –dependent bile flow and altered bile composition as compared to the mother suckled piglet.[229] Studies in the neonatal piglet might be relevant to the human neonate since recent studies indicate an 88% identity of cDNA and 93% identity at the protein level between human and porcine LCAT.[230]

The fatty acids taken up by peripheral tissues through the lipoprotein lipase-mediated hydrolysis of circulating lipoprotein triglyceride can be either deposited in adipose tissue, oxidized in most peripheral tissues, or reincorporated into lipoproteins (e.g., VLDL synthesis in the liver).

The first step in the catabolism of long-chain fatty acids is oxidation to H_2O and CO_2, which occurs in mitochondria and depends on the presence of carnitine. Long-chain fatty acids can cross the mitochondrial membrane only in the form of acylcarnitine. Carnitine is an essential cofactor for fatty acid oxidation, and acyl-CoA carnitine transferases are the key enzymes in fatty acid oxidation. The characteristics of the enzymes participating in lipid clearing and fatty acid oxidation are listed in Table 36.9 (see Chapter 38).

Ketone Bodies

Ketone bodies produced during fatty acid catabolism are important metabolites for the neonate. Ketone bodies give rise to acetoacetate. Acetoacetate is reduced by a specific inner-membrane mitochondrial β-hydroxybutyric acid dehydrogenase to yield β-hydroxybutyrate. The release of acetoacetate and β-hydroxybutyrate from the liver into the blood and their uptake by peripheral tissues is a constant, normal process.

Studies suggest that the capacity for ketone synthesis by the liver is low during the immediate neonatal period in the human and the guinea pig. Developmental changes in ketogenesis during the perinatal period have been reported in other species.

The activity of the enzymes of ketone body utilization (e.g., 3-oxoacid CoA transferase) in adult rat tissue is highest in kidney, heart, brown adipose tissue, and adrenal gland followed by submaxillary gland, lactating mammary gland, and brain. The liver has low activity of 3-oxoacid CoA transferase, which means that ketone bodies synthesized by the liver are not utilized by this organ but are directed to peripheral tissues. The enzymes of ketone body utilization show marked changes in activity during development of the rat, the pattern varying in different tissue. In the suckling rat, activity is high in brain and low in heart and kidney, resulting in channeling of ketone bodies to the developing brain in the suckling rat.

Although fatty acid oxidation does not occur in adult brain, it is present in fetal and neonatal brain, contributing as much as 25% of the metabolites entering the Krebs (i.e., tricarboxylic acid; TCA) cycle. Ketone bodies are a major source of energy for the developing brain in many species, including the human, in whom ketone bodies can be metabolized as early as 12 to 21 weeks' gestation. Such activity remains high during the remainder of gestation as well as postnatally.

In rat brain, permeability for β-hydroxybutyrate is sevenfold higher during suckling than at birth or in the adult. Milk fatty acids are the source of ketone bodies during this period. The brain is the major ketone body–using tissue in suckling mammals; activity of the enzymes that convert ketone bodies to acetyl-CoA increases rapidly after birth, reaches peak activity before weaning, and decreases thereafter. There is a direct relation between neurologic immaturity at birth and the extent of ketone body utilization.

Studies using stable isotopes show that ketone bodies can account for 25% of the neonate's basal energy requirements during the first few days of life.[231] Ketone body production and metabolism in the fetus and neonate have been reviewed elsewhere.[232–234]

Differences Between Preterm and Term Neonates

The differences between the premature and the term neonate in the various stages of fat metabolism have been discussed in this chapter. Because fat deposition and accretion of specific lipids occurs during the last trimester of intrauterine development, the very low birth weight neonate is deficient in specific metabolites (e.g., total adipose tissue mass, brain docosahexaenoic and eicosapentaenoic acids, and carnitine) as well as in the enzymes needed for fat digestion and metabolism (e.g., pancreatic lipase, fatty acid desaturation, and elongation). Furthermore, one of the most important differences in fat metabolism is that the very low birth weight neonate is often maintained on total parenteral nutrition for various periods after birth.

Lipids in Total Parenteral Nutrition

Improvement in the clinical nutritional management of the very low birth weight neonate has largely depended on methods of nutrient delivery. The addition of lipids to total parenteral nutrition has markedly advanced the growth of the very tiny neonate.

Lipid is administered to the neonate on an empirical basis; it is generally advised that it be given in amounts that do not cause lipemia (i.e., plasma triglycerides in excess of 100–150 mg·dl^{-1}).[235] The widespread use of lipid in parenteral nutrition is in marked contrast to the limited knowledge of the enzymes and cofactors active in the lipid-clearing process in low birth weight neonates.

Studies indicate that the infusion period and infusion rate affect the clearing of lipid in the low birth weight neonate maintained on total parenteral nutrition.[236] The presence of heparin in solutions prepared for intravenous use, even in the low concentrations of one unit per milliliter of intravenous fluid added to prevent clotting of catheters, might affect the lipid clearing process.[236] We reviewed elsewhere the enzymes and cofactors active in the mechanism of lipid clearing,[63] with special emphasis on the developmental period.[236,237]

The low birth weight neonate has lower levels of lipolytic enzymes (e.g., lipoprotein lipase and LCAT than the term neonate).[236–238] Studies in the weanling rat have shown that Intralipid infusion markedly lowers LCAT activity,[239] which is probably the reason for the hyperlipemia and hypercholesterolemia that develops in the very low birth weight neonate maintained on total parenteral nutrition with lipids in excess of 2 g·kg^{-1} day^{-1}.[236,237] The efficient clearing of 20% Intralipid might be related to the lower lecithin/triglyceride ratio, which is compatible with the low LCAT activity of the premature infant.[240]

Inborn Errors of Lipid Metabolism

Several inborn errors of metabolism have been described. They are rare and are usually described during the first year of life or later. Congenital absence of pancreatic lipase with normal activity of other exocrine pancreatic digestive enzymes and absence of colipase and normal lipase levels have been described.

Lipid clearing is impaired in type I hyperlipidemia, and it is most commonly due to absence of lipoprotein lipase activity; in rare cases, it is related to the specific absence of apoprotein CII, the cofactor of lipoprotein lipase. In the latter case lipoprotein lipase levels are normal, but the enzyme is unable to hydrolyze lipoprotein triglyceride because of the lack of apoprotein CII.

References

1. Hamosh M. Fat needs for term and preterm infants. In: Tsang RC, Nichols BL, eds. Nutrition during infancy. Philadelphia: Hanley & Belfus, 1988:133–159.
2. Hamosh M. Lipid metabolism in premature infants. Biol Neonate 1987;52(suppl):50–64.
3. Patton JS. Gastrointestinal lipid digestion. In: Johnson LR, ed. Physiology of the gastrointestinal tract. New York: Raven Press, 1981:1123–1146.

4. Hamosh M, Bitman J, Wood DL, et al. Lipids in milk and the first steps in their digestion. Pediatrics 1985;75(suppl):146–150.
5. Mehta NR, Jones JB, Hamosh M. Lipases in human milk: ontogeny and physiologic significance. J Pediatr Gastroenterol Nutr 1982;1:317–326.
6. Hamosh M. Physiological role of human milk lipases. In: Lebenthal E, ed. Gastrointestinal development and infant nutrition. New York: Raven Press, 1981:473–482.
7. Jensen RG. The lipids of human milk. Boca Raton, FL: CRC Press, 1989.
8. Hall B. Uniformity of human milk. Am J Clin Nutr 1979;32:304–310.
9. Bitman J, Wood DL, Hamosh M, et al. Comparison of the lipid composition of breast milk from mothers of term and preterm infants. Am J Clin Nutr 1983;38:300–312.
10. Reugg M, Blanc B. The fat globule size distribution in human milk. Biochim Biophys Acta 1981;666:7–13.
11. Simonin C, Ruegg M, Sidiropoulos D. Comparison of the fat content and fat globule size distribution of breast milk from mothers delivering term and preterm. Am J Clin Nutr 1984;40:820–826.
12. Innis SM. Essential fatty acids in growth and development. Prog Lipid Res 1991;30:39–103.
13. Holman RT, Johnson SB, Ogburn PL. Deficiency of essential fatty acids and membrane fluidity during pregnancy and lactation. Proc Natl Acad Sci USA 1991;88:4835–4839.
14. Hytten FE. Clinical and chemical studies in human lactation. II. Variation in major constituents during a feed. Br Med J 1977;1:176–179.
15. Insull W Jr, Hirsh J, James T, et al. The fatty acids of human milk. II. Alterations produced by manipulation of caloric balance and exchange of dietary fats. J Clin Invest 1959;38:443–450.
16. Prentice A, Jarjou LM, Drury PJ, et al. Breast-milk fatty acids of rural Gambian mothers: effects of diet and maternal parity. J Pediatr Gastroenterol Nutr 1989;8:486–490.
17. Tyson J, Burchfield J, Sentance F, et al. Adaptation of feeding to a low fat yield in breast milk. Pediatrics 1992;89:215–220.
18. Michaelsen KF, Larsen PS, Thomsen BL, et al. The Copenhagen cohort study on infant nutrition and growth: breast milk intake, human milk macronutrient content, and influencing factors. Am J Clin Nutr 1994;59:600–611.
19. Chappell JE, Clandinin MT, Kearney-Volpe C. Trace fatty acids in human milk lipids: influence of maternal diet and weight loss. Am J Clin Nutr 1985;42:49–56.
20. Harris WD, Connor WE, Lindsey S. Will dietary ω-3 fatty acids change the composition of human milk. Am J Clin Nutr 1984;40:780–785.
21. Craig-Schmidt MC, Weete JD, Faircloth SA, et al. The effect of hydrogenated fat in the diet of nursing mothers on lipid composition and prostaglandin content of human milk. Am J Clin Nutr 1984;39:778–786.
22. Bitman J, Hamosh M, Wood DL, et al. Lipid composition of milk from mothers with cystic fibrosis. Pediatrics 1987;80:927–932.
23. Bitman J, Hamosh M, Hamosh P, et al. Milk composition and volume during the onset of lactation in a diabetic mother. Am J Clin Nutr 1989;50:1364–1369.
24. Wang CS, Illingworth DR. Lipid composition and lipolytic activities in milk from a patient with homozygous familial hypobetalipoproteinemia. Am J Clin Nutr 1987;45:730–736.
25. Hall B. Changing composition of human milk and early development of an appetite control. Lancet 1975;1:779–781.
26. Lucas A, Lucas PJ, Baum JD. The nipple shield system: a device for measuring the dietary intake of breast fed infants. Early Hum Dev 1980;4:365–372.
27. Smart JL. Human milk fat and satiety: an appealing idea reappraised. Early Hum Dev 1978;2:395–397.
28. Woolridge MW, Baum JD, Drewett RF. Does a change in the composition of human milk affect sucking patterns and milk intake? Lancet 1980;2:192–194.
29. Drewett RF. Returning to the suckled breast: a further test of Hall's hypothesis. Early Hum Dev 1982;6:161–163.
30. Nysenbaum AN, Smart JL. Suckling behavior and milk intake of neonates in relation to milk fat content. Early Hum Dev 1982;6:205–213.
31. Lucas A, Lucas PJ, Baum JD. Pattern of milk flow in breast fed infants. Lancet 1979;2:57–58.
32. Lucas A, Lucas PJ, Baum JD. Differences in the pattern of milk intake between breast and bottle fed infants. Early Hum Dev 1981;5:195–199.
33. Cavell B. Gastric emptying in preterm infants. Acta Paediatr Scand 1979;68:725–730.
34. Cavell B. Gastric emptying in infants fed human milk or infant formula. Acta Paediatr Scand 1981;70:639–641.
35. Armand M, Hamosh M, Mehta NR, et al. Effect of human milk or infant formula on gastric function and fat digestion in the premature infant. Pediatr Res 1996;40:429–437.
36. Siegel M, Lebenthal E, Topper W, et al. Gastric emptying in prematures of isocaloric feedings with differing osmolalities. Pediatr Res 1982;16:141–147.
37. Siegel M, Lebenthal E, Krantz B. Effect of caloric density on gastric emptying in premature infants. J Pediatr 1984;104:118–122.
38. Sidebottom R, Curran JS, Williams PR, et al. Effects of long-chain vs. medium-chain triglycerides on gastric emptying time in premature infants. J Pediatr 1983;102:448–450.
39. Lucas A, Blackburn AM, Aynsley-Green A, et al. Breast vs bottle: endocrine responses are different with formula feeding. Lancet 1980;1:267–269.
40. Lucas A, Boyles S, Bloom SR, et al. Metabolic and endocrine responses to milk feed in six day old term infants: differences between breast and cow's milk formula feeding. Acta Paediatr Scand 1981;70:195–200.
41. Knittle JL, Hirsch J. Effect of early nutrition on the development of rat epididymal fat pads: cellularity and metabolism. J Clin Invest 1968;47:2091–2098.
42. Knittle JL. Obesity in childhood: a problem in adipose tissue cellular development. J Pediatr 1972;81:1048–1059.
43. Hamosh M, Hamosh P. Does nutrition in early life have long term metabolic effects: can animal models be used to predict these effects in the human? In: Goldman AS, Atkinson SA, Hanson LA, eds. Human lactation, vol. 3. The effects of human milk on the recipient infant. New York: Plenum Press, 1987:37–55.

44. Kramer MC. Do breast-feeding and delayed introduction of solid foods protect against subsequent obesity? J Pediatr 1981;98:883–887.
45. Marmot MG, Page CM, Atkins E, et al. Effect of breast feeding on plasma cholesterol and weight in young adults. J Epidemiol Commun Health 1980;34:164–167.
46. Dewey KG, Lonnerdal B. Milk and nutrient intake of breast fed infants from 1 to 6 months: relation to growth and fatness. J Pediatr Gastroenterol Nutr 1983;2:497–506.
47. Butte NF, Garza C, Smith EO, et al. Human milk intake and growth in exclusively breast fed infants. J Pediatr 1984;104:187–195.
48. Garza C, Stuff J, Butte NJ, et al. Complementation and weaning phases of lactation. In: Hamosh M, Goldman AS, eds. Human lactation, vol. 2. Maternal and environmental effects. New York: Plenum Press, 1986:155–163.
49. Dewey KG, Finley DA, Lonnerdal B. Breast milk volume and composition during late lactation (7–20 months). J Pediatr Gastroenterol Nutr 1984;3:713–720.
50. Neville MC, Oliva-Rasbach J. Is maternal milk production limiting for infant growth during the first year of life in breast fed infants? In: Goldman AS, Atkinson A, Hanson LA, eds. Human lactation, vol. 3. Effect of human milk upon the recipient infant. New York: Plenum Press, 1987:123–133.
51. Van Aerde J, Sauer P, Heim T, et al. Comparison of long-chain triglyceride formula vs own mother's milk feeding on growth, macronutrient and energy balance in very low birth weight infants. Pediatr Res 1987;21:439A.
52. Van Aerde J, Sauer P, Heim T, et al. Composition of weight gain and macronutrient storage in very low birth weight infants fed on mother's milk or medium chain triglyceride enriched formula. Pediatr Res 1987;21:281A.
53. Lucas A, Ewing G, Robert SB, et al. How much energy does the breast-fed consume and expend? Br Med J 1987;295:75–77.
54. Prentice AM, Lucas A, Vasquez-Valasquez L, et al. Are current dietary guidelines for young children a prescription for overfeeding? Lancet 1988;2:1066–1069.
55. Neville MC, Keller R, Seacat J, et al. Studies in human lactation: milk volumes in lactating women during the onset of lactation and full lactation. Am J Clin Nutr 1988;48:1375–1386.
56. Dewey KG, Lonnerdal B. Infant self-regulation of breast milk intake. Acta Paediatr Scand 1986;75:893–898.
57. Poissonnet CM, LaVelle M, Burdi AR. Growth and development of adipose tissue. Pediatrics 1988;113:1–9.
58. Bray GA. Obesity—a disease of nutrient or energy imbalance. Nutr Rev 1987;45:33–43.
59. Summary of workshop: fetal and infant nutrition and susceptibility to obesity. Nutr Rev 1978;36:122–126.
60. Committee on Nutrition, American Academy of Pediatrics. Nutritional aspects of obesity in infancy and childhood. Pediatrics 1981;68:880–883.
61. Stern J, Greenwood MRC. A review of development of adipose cellularity in man and animals. Fed Proc 1974;33:1952–1955.
62. Burdi AR, Poissonnet CM, Garn SM, et al. Adipose tissue growth pattern during human gestation: a histometric comparison of buccal and gluteal fat depots. Int J Obes 1985;9:247–256.
63. Hamosh M, Hamosh P. Lipoprotein lipase: its physiological and clinical significance. Mol Aspects Med 1983;6:199–289.
64. Borensztajn J. Lipoprotein lipase. Chicago: Evener, 1987.
65. Belfrage P, Fredrikson G, Stralfors P, et al. Adipose tissue lipases. In: Borgstrom B, Brockman HL, eds. Lipases. Amsterdam: Elsevier, 1984:365–416.
66. Bjorntorp P, Karlsson M, Petterson P, et al. Differentiation and function of rat adipocyte precursor cells in primary culture. J Lipid Res 1980;21:714–723.
67. Hietanen E, Greenwood MRC. A comparison of lipoprotein lipase activity and adipocyte differentiation in growing male rats. J Lipid Res 1977;18:480–490.
68. Johasson L, Hansson GK, Bondjers G, et al. Immunohistochemical localization of lipoprotein lipase in human adipose tissue. Atherosclerosis 1984;51:313–326.
69. Hausman GJ. Histochemically detectable lipoprotein lipase activity in adipose tissue of pigs of normal and decapitated pig fetuses. Acta Anat (Basel) 1982;114:281–290.
70. Vannier C, Jansen H, Negrel R, et al. Study of lipoprotein lipase content in Ob17 preadipocytes during adipose conversion. J Biol Chem 1982;257:1237–1239.
71. Eckel RH, Yost TJ. Weight reduction increases adipose tissue lipoprotein lipase responsiveness in obese women. J Clin Invest 1987;80:992–997.
72. Yost TJ, Eckel RH. Fat calories may be preferentially stored in reduced obese women: a permissive pathway for assumption of the obese state. J Clin Endocrinol Metab 1988;67:259–264.
73. Jacobson B, Smith U. Effect of cell size on lipolysis and antilipolytic action of insulin in human fat cells. J Lipid Res 1972;13:651–656.
74. Adebonjo OF, Coates PM, Cortner JA. Hormone sensitive lipase in human adipose tissue, isolated adipocytes and cultured adipocytes. Pediatr Res 1982;16:982–988.
75. Brook CGD, Lloyd JK, Wolf OH. Relation between age of onset of obesity and size and number of adipose cells. Br Med J 1972;2:25–27.
76. Hirsch J, Knittle JL. Cellularity of obese and non-obese human adipose tissue. Fed Proc 1970;29:1516–1521.
77. Brook CGD. Evidence for a sensitive period in adipose cell replication in man. Lancet 1972;2:624–627.
78. Hirsch J. Cell number and size as a determinant of subsequent obesity. Curr Concepts Nutr 1975;3:15–21.
79. Roche AF. The adipocyte-number hypothesis. Child Dev 1981;52:43–53.
80. Hager A, Sjostrom L, Arvidsson P, et al. Body fat and adipose tissue cellularity in infants: a longitudinal study. Metabolism 1977;26:607–614.
81. Knittle JL, Timmers K, Ginsberg-Fellner F, et al. The growth of adipose tissue in children and adolescents: cross sectional and longitudinal studies of adipose cell number and size. J Clin Invest 1979;63:239–246.
82. Faust IM, Johnson PR, Stern JS, et al. Diet-induced adipocyte number increase in adult rats: a new model of obesity. Am J Physiol 1978;235:E279–E286.

83. Faust IM, Johnson PR, Hirsch J. Long-term effects of early nutritional experience on the development of obesity in the rat. J Nutr 1980;110:2027–2034.
84. Bjorntorp P, Karlsson M, Petterson P. Expansion of adipose tissue storage capacity at different ages in rats. Metabolism 1982;31:366–373.
85. Lewis DS, Bertrand HA, Masoro EJ, et al. Preweaning nutrition and fat development in baboons. J Nutr 1983;113:2253–2259.
86. Lewis DS, Bertrand HA, Masoro EJ, et al. Effect of interaction of gender and energy intake on lean body mass and fat mass gain in infant baboons. J Nutr 1984;114:2021–2026.
87. Lewis DS, Bertrand HA, McMahan CA, et al. Preweaning food intake influences the adiposity of young adult baboons. J Clin Invest 1987;78:899–905.
88. Faust IM, Johnson PR, Hirsch J. Surgical removal of adipose tissue alters feeding behavior and the development of obesity in rats. Science 1977;197:393–396.
89. Dunlop M, Court JM, Hobbs JB, et al. Identification of small cells in fetal and infant adipose tissue. Pediatr Res 1978;12:905–907.
90. Enzi G, Zanardo V, Caretta F, et al. Intrauterine growth and adipose tissue development. Am J Clin Nutr 1981;34:1785–1790.
91. Ravelli GP, Stein ZA, Susser MW. Obesity in young men after famine exposure in utero and early infancy. N Engl J Med 1976;295:349–353.
92. Whitelaw AGL. Influence of maternal obesity on subcutaneous fat in the newborn. Br J Med 1976;1:985–986.
93. Whitelaw AGL. Subcutaneous fat in newborn infants of diabetic mothers: an indication of quality of diabetic control. Lancet 1977;1:15–18.
94. Iverson SJ, Hamosh M, Bowen WD. Lipoprotein lipase activity and its relationship to high milk fat transfer during lactation in grey seals. J Comp Physiol [B] 1995;165:384–395.
95. He Y, Chen H, Quon MJ, et al. The mouse obese gene. Genomic organization, promoter activity and activation by CCAAT/ enhancer-binding protein alpha. J Biol Chem 1995;270:28887–28891.
96. Tartaglia LA, Dembski M, Weng X, et al. Identification and expression cloning of a leptin receptor, OB-R. Cell 1995;83:1263–1271.
97. Masuzaki H, Hosoda K, Ogawa Y, et al. Augmented expression of obese (ob) gene during the process of obesity in genetically obese-hyperglycemic Wistar fatty (fa/fa) rats. FEBS Lett 1996;378:267–271.
98. Nedergaard J, Lindberg O. The brown fat cell. Int Rev Cytol 1982;74:187–286.
99. Himms-Hagen J. Brown adipose tissue metabolism and thermogenesis. Annu Rev Nutr 1985;5:69–94.
100. Nedergaard J, Cannon B. Brown adipose tissue: development and function. In: Polin RA, Fox WW, eds. Fetal and neonatal physiology. 2nd ed. Philadelphia: WB Saunders, 1998:478–488.
101. Nedergaard J, Conolly E, Cannon B, et al. Brown adipose tissue in the mammalian neonate. In: Trayhurn P, Nicholls DG, eds. Brown adipose tissue. London: Edward Arnold, 1986:152–213.
102. Trayhurn P, Nicholls DG, eds. Brown adipose tissue. London: Edward Arnold, 1986.
103. Lean MEJ, James WPT, Jennings G, et al. Brown adipose tissue uncoupling protein content in human infants, children and adults. Clin Sci 1986;71:291–297.
104. Brooke OG, Harris M, Salvosa CB. The response of malnourished babies to cold. J Physiol (Lond) 1973;233:75–91.
105. Moore BJ, Stern JS, Horwitz BA. Brown fat mediates energy expenditure of cold-exposed overfed neonatal rats. Am J Physiol 1986;251:R518–R524.
106. Goodbody AE, Trayhurn P. Studies on the activity of brown adipose tissue in suckling, pre-obese Ob/ob mice. Biochim Biophs Acta 1982;680:119–126.
107. Tinoco J. Dietary requirements and functions of α-linolenic acid in animals. Prog Lipid Res 1982;21:1–45.
108. Carey EM. The biochemistry of fetal brain development and myelination. In: Jones CT, ed. Biochemical development of the fetus and neonate. New York: Elsevier, 1982:287–336.
109. Meisami E, Timiras PS. Normal and abnormal biochemical development of the brain after birth. In: Jones CT, ed. The biochemical development of the fetus and neonate. New York: Elsevier, 1981:759–821.
110. Feldman M, Van Aerde JE, Clandinin MT. Lipid accretion in the fetus and newborn. In: Polin RA, Fox WW, eds. Neonatal and fetal medicine. Philadelphia: WB Saunders, 1991:299–314.
111. Carlson SE. Very long chain fatty acids in the developing retina and brain. In: Polin RA, Fox WW, eds. Fetal and neonatal physiology. 2nd ed. Philadelphia: WB Saunders, 1998:504–513.
112. Clandinin MT, Chappell JE, Heim T, et al. Fatty acid utilization in perinatal de novo synthesis of tissues. Early Hum Dev 1981;5:355–366.
113. Kuhn DC, Crawford M. Placental essential fatty acid transport and prostaglandin synthesis. Prog Lipid Res 1986;25:345–353.
114. Clandinin MT, Chappell JE, Heim T. Do low weight infants require nutrition with chain elongation desaturation products of essential fatty acids? Prog Lipid Res 1981;20:901–904.
115. Sastry PS. Lipids of nervous tissue: composition and metabolism. Prog Lipid Res 1985;24:69–176.
116. Carlson SE, Rhodes PG, Ferguson MG. Docosahexaenoic acid status of preterm infants at birth and following feeding with human milk or formula. Am J Clin Nutr 1985;44:798–804.
117. Liu CCF, Carlson SE, Rhodes PG, et al. Increase in plasma phospholipid docosahexaenoic and eicosapentaenoic acids as a reflection of their intake and mode of administration. Pediatr Res 1987;22:292–296.
118. Carlson SE, Rhodes PG, Roa VS, et al. Effect of fish oil supplementation on the n3 fatty acid content of red blood cell membranes in preterm infants. Pediatr Res 1987;21:507–510.
119. Neuringer M, Connor WE, Lin DS, et al. Biochemical and functional effects of prenatal and postnatal n3 deficiency on retina and brain of rhesus monkeys. Proc Natl Acad Sci USA 1986;83:4021–4025.

120. Neuringer M, Connor WE, Luck SL. Omega-3 fatty acid deficiency in rhesus monkeys: depletion of retinal docosahexaenoic acid and abnormal electroretinograms. Am J Clin Nutr 1985;43:706A.
121. Menon NK, Dhopeshwarkar GA. Essential fatty acid deficiency and brain development. Prog Lipid Res 1982;21:309–326.
122. Anderson GJ, Connor WE. Uptake of fatty acids by the developing rat brain. Lipids 1988;23:286–290.
123. Yamamoto N, Saito M. Moriuchi A, et al. Effect of dietary-linolenate/linoleate balance on brain lipid compositions and learning abilities of rats. J Lipid Res 1987;28:144–151.
124. Clandinin MT, Chappell JE, Van Aerde JEE. Requirements of newborns for long chain polyunsaturated fatty acids. Acta Paediatr Scand 1989;351:63–71.
125. Koletzko B, Thiel I, Obiodun PO. The fatty acid composition of human milk in Europe and Africa. J Pediatr 1992;120:S62–S70.
126. Innis SM, Kuhnlein HV. Long chain n-3 fatty acids in breast milk of Inuit women consuming traditional foods. Early Hum Dev 1988;18:185–189.
127. Holman RT, Johnson SB, Ogburn PL. Deficiency of essential fatty acids and membrane fluidity during pregnancy and lactation. Proc Natl Acad Sci USA 1991;88:4835–4839.
128. Hornstra G, Van Houwelingen AC, Simonis M, et al. Fatty acid composition of umbilical arteries and veins: possible implications for the fetal EFA-status. Lipids 1989;24:511–517.
129. Leaf AA, Leighfield MJ, Costeloe KL, et al. Long chain polyunsaturated fatty acids and fetal growth. Early Hum Dev 1992;30:183–191.
130. Olsen SF, Sorensen JD, Secher NJ, et al. Randomised controlled trial of effect of fish-oil supplementation on pregnancy duration. Lancet 1992;339:1002–1007.
131. Neuringer M, Anderson GJ, Connor WE. The essentiality of n-3 fatty acids for the development and function of the retina and brain. Annu Rev Nutr 1988;8:517–541.
132. Innis SM. Essential fatty acids in growth and development. Prog Lipid Res 1991;30:39–103.
133. Carlson SE, Carver JD, House SG. High fat diets varying in ratios of polyunsaturated to saturated fatty acids and linoleic to linolenic acid: a comparison of rat neural and red cell membrane phospholipids. J Nutr 1986;116:718–725.
134. Witchey K, Picciano MF, Yeh YY. Level of maternal dietary fat affects suckling pup plasma and erythrocyte but not brain phospholipid fatty acids. FASEB J 1994;8:174 (abstract).
135. Connor WE, Lin DS, Neuringer M. Is the docosahexaenoic acid (DHA, 22:6n-3) content of erythrocytes a marker for the DHA content of brain phospholipids? FASEB J 1993;7:152 (abstract).
136. Arbuckle LD, Innis SM. Docosahexaenoic acid is transferred through maternal diet to milk and to tissues of natural milk-fed piglets. J Nutr 1993;123:1668–1675.
137. Makrides M, Neumann MA, Byard RW, et al. Fatty acid composition of brain, retina and erythrocytes in breast-fed and formula infants. Am J Clin Nutr 1994;60:189–194.
138. Farquharson J, Cockburn F, Patrick WA, et al. Infant cerebral cortex phospholipid fatty-acid composition and diet. Lancet 1992;340:810–813.
139. Lucas A, Morley R, Cole TJ, et al. Breast milk and subsequent intelligence quotient in children born preterm. Lancet 1992;339:261–264.
140. Neuriger M, Connor WE, Van Petten C, et al. Dietary omega-3 fatty acid deficiency and visual loss in infant rhesus monkeys. J Clin Invest 1984;73:272–276.
141. Uauy R, Birch DG, Birch EE, et al. Effect of dietary omega-3 fatty acids on retinal function of very low birth weight neonates. Pediatr Res 1990;28:485–492.
142. Birch E, Birch D, Hoffman D, et al. Breast-feeding and optimal visual development. J Pediatr Opththalmol Strabismus 1993;30:33–38.
143. Carlson SE, Werkman SH, Rhodes PG, et al. Visual acuity development in healthy preterm infants: effect of marine oil supplementation. Am J Clin Nutr 1993;58:35–42.
144. Makrides M, Simmer K, Goggin M, et al. Erythrocyte docosahexaenoic acid correlates with the visual response of healthy, term infants. Pediatr Res 1993;33:425–427.
145. Decsi T, Thiel I, Koletzko B. Essential fatty acids in full term infants fed breast milk or formula. Arch Dis Child 1995;72:F23–F28.
146. Makrides M, Neumann MA, Byard RW, et al. Fatty acid composition of brain, retina and erythrocytes in breast- and formula fed infants. Am J Clin Nutr 1994;60:189–194.
147. Koletzko B, Decsi T, Demmelmair H. Arachidonic acid supply and metabolism in human infants born at full term. Lipids 1996;31:79–83.
148. Innis SM, Nelson CM, Rioux MF, et al. Development of visual acuity in relation to plasma and erythrocyte ω-6 and ω-3 fatty acids in healthy term gestation infants. Am J Clin Nutr 1994;60:347–352.
149. Carlson SE, Werkman SH, Peeples JM, et al. Arachidonic acid status correlates with first year growth in preterm infants. Proc Natl Acad Sci USA 1993;90:1073–1077.
150. Al MDM, Van Houwelingen AC, Kester ADM, et al. Maternal essential fatty acid patterns during normal pregnancy and their relationship to neonatal essential fatty acid status. Br J Nutr 1995;74:55–68.
151. Luukkainen P, Salo MK, Nikkari T. Changes in the fatty acid composition of preterm and term human milk from 1 week to 6 months of lactation. J Pediatr Gastroenterol Nutr 1994;18:355–360.
152. Hamosh M, Henderson TR, Hayman L. Long-chain polyunsaturated fatty acids in human milk during prolonged lactation. FASEB J 1996;10:A553.
153. Van Houwelingen AC, Sorensen JD, Hornstra G. Essential fatty acid status in neonates after fish-oil supplementation during late pregancy. Br J Nutr 1995;74:723–731.
154. Makrides M, Neumann MA, Gibson RA. Effect of maternal docosahexaenoic acid (DHA) supplementation on breast milk composition. Eur J Clin Nutr 1996;50:352–357.
155. Carnielli VP, Pederzini F, Vittorangeli R, et al. Plasma and red blood cell fatty acid of very low birth weight infants fed exclusively with expressed preterm human milk. Pediatr Res 1996;39:671–679.
156. Salem Jr N, Wegher B, Mena P, et al. Arachidonic and docosahexaenoic acids are biosynthesized from their 18-

carbon precursors in human infants. Proc Natl Acad Sci USA 1996;93:49–54.
157. Demmelmair H, Schenck U, Behrendt E, et al. Estimation of arachidonic acid synthesis in full term neonates using natural variation of ^{13}C content. J Pediatr Gastroenterol Nutr 1995;21:31–36.
158. Innis SM, Hansen JW. Plasma fatty acid responses, metabolic effects and safety of micro algal and fungal oils rich in arachidonic and docosahexaenoic acids in healthy adults. Am J Clin Nutr 1996;64:159–167.
159. Agostoni C, Trojan S, Belln R, et al. Neurodevelopmental quotient of healthy term infants at 4 months and feeding practice: the role of long chain polyunsaturated fatty acids. Pediatr Res 1995;38:262–266.
160. Lucas A, Morley R, et al. Breast milk and subsequent intelligence quotient in children born preterm. Lancet 1992;339:261–264.
161. Bitman J, Wood DL, Liao TH, et al. Gastric lipolysis of milk lipids in suckling rats. Biochim Biophys Acta 1985;834:58–64.
162. Aw TY, Grigor MR. Digestion and absorption of milk triacylglycerols in 14 day old suckling rats. J Nutr 1980;110:2133–2140.
163. Hamosh M, Bitman J, Liao TH, et al. Gastric lipolysis and fat absorption in preterm infants: effect of MCT or LCT containing formulas. Pediatrics 1989;83:86–92.
164. Putet G. Lipids as an energy source for the premature and full term neonate. In: Polin RA, Fox WW, eds. Neonatal and fetal medicine. Philadelphia: WB Saunders, 1997.
165. Sarda P, Lepage G, Roy CC, et al. Storage of medium-chain triglycerides in adipose tissue of orally fed infants. Am J Clin Nutr 1987;45:399–405.
166. Mehta NR, Hamosh M, Bitman J, et al. Adherence of medium-chain fatty acids to feeding tubes during gavage feeding of human milk fortified with medium-chain triglycerides. J Pediatr 1988;112:374–376.
167. Mehta NR, Hamosh M, Bitman J, et al. Adherence of medium chain fatty acids to feeding tubes of premature infants fed formula fortified with medium chain triglyceride. J Pediatr Gastroenterol Nutr 1991;13:267–269.
168. Hamosh M. Lingual and gastric lipases: their role in fat digestion. Boca Raton, FL: CRC Press, 1990.
169. Watkins JB. Mechanism of fat absorption and the development of gastrointestinal function. Pediatr Clin North Am 1975;22:721–730.
170. Hamosh M. Lipid metabolism in pediatric nutrition. Pediatr Clin North Am 1995;42:839–859.
171. Hamosh M, Iverson SJ, Kirk CL, et al. Milk lipids and neonatal fat digestion: relationship between fatty acids composition, endogenous and exogenous lipases and digestion of milk fat. World Rev Nutr Diet 1994;75:86–91.
172. Plucinski TM, Hamosh M, Hamosh P. Fat digestion in the rat: role of lingual lipase. Am J Physiol 1979;237:E541–E547.
173. Hamosh M. Digestion in the premature infant: the effects of human milk. Semin Perinatol 1994;18:485–494.
174. Hamosh M, Klaeveman HL, Wolf RO, et al. Pharyngeal lipase and digestion of dietary triglycerides in man. J Clin Invest 1975;55:908–913.
175. Roy CC, Roulet M, Lefebre D, et al. The role of gastric lipolysis in fat absorption and bile acid metabolism in the rat. Lipids 1979;14:811–814.
176. Bodmer MW, Angal S, Yanaton GT, et al. Molecular cloning of human gastric lipase and expression of the enzyme in yeast. Biochim Biophys Acta 1987;909:237–244.
177. Abrams CK, Hamosh M, Hubbard VS, et al. Lingual lipase in cystic fibrosis: quantitation of enzyme activity in the upper small intestine of patients with exocrine pancreatic insufficiency. J Clin Invest 1984;73:374–382.
178. Abrams CK, Hamosh M, Dutta SK, et al. Role of nonpancreatic lipolytic activity in exocrine pancreatic insufficiency. Gastroenterology 1987;92:125–129.
179. Hamosh M, Hamosh P. Selectivity of lipases: developmental physiology aspects. NATO ASI Series E: Applied Sciences 1996;317:31–49.
180. DiPalma J, Kirk C, Hamosh M, et al. Lipase and pepsin activity in the gastric mucosa of infants, children and adults. Gastroenterology 1991;101:116–121.
181. Bernback S, Blackberg L, Hernell O. The complete digestion of human milk triacylglycerol in vitro requires gastric lipase, pancreatic colipase-dependent lipase and bile salt stimulated lipase. J Clin Invest 1990;85:1221–1226.
182. Hamosh M. Digestion in the newborn. Clin Perinatol 1996;23:191–209.
183. Patton JS, Rigler MW, Liao TH, et al. Hydrolysis of triacylglycerol emulsions by lingual lipase—a microscopic study. Biochim Biophys Acta 1982;712:400–407.
184. Armand M, Hamosh M, DiPalma JS, et al. Dietary fat modulates gastric lipase activity in healthy humans. Am J Clin Nutr 1995;62:74–80.
185. Levine GM, Derren GG, Steiger E, et al. Role of oral intake in maintenance of gut mass and disaccharidase activity. Gastroenterology 1974;67:975–982.
186. Rossi TM. Effects of total parenteral nutrition on the digestive organs. In: Lebenthal E, ed. Total parenteral nutrition: indications, utilization, complications, and pathophysiological considerations. New York: Raven Press, 1986:173–184.
187. Mehta NR, Liao TH, Hamosh M, et al. Effect of total parenteral nutrition on lipase activity in the stomach of very low birth weight infants. Biol Neonate 1988;53:261–266.
188. Hamosh M, Scanlon JW, Ganot D, et al. Fat digestion in the newborn: characterization of lipase in gastric aspirates of premature and term infants. J Clin Invest 1981;67:838–846.
189. Menard D, Monfils E, Tremblay E. Ontogeny of human gastric lipase and pepsin activities. Gastroenterology 1995;108:1650–1656.
190. Boehm G, Bierbach U, Del Santo A, et al. Activities of trypsin and lipase in duodenal aspirates of healthy preterm infants: effects of gestational age and postnatal age. Biol Neonate 1995;67:248–253.
191. Lebenthal E, Lee PC. Development of functional response in human exocrine pancreas. Pediatrics 1980;66:556–560.
192. Hamosh M. Lingual and breast milk lipases. Adv Pediatr 1982;29:33–67.

193. Koldovsky O. Small and large intestine. In: Polin PA, Fox WW, eds. Fetal and neonatal physiology, vol. 2. Philadelphia: WB Saunders, 1992:1059–1077.
194. Lowe ME. The structure and function of pancreatic enzymes. In: Johnson LR, ed. Physiology of the gastrointestinal tract. 3rd ed. New York: Raven Press, 1994:1531–1542.
195. Erlanson-Albertsson C. Pancreatic colipase. Structural and physiological aspects. Biochim Biophys Acta 1992;1125:1–7.
196. Van Tilbeurgh H, Sarda L, Verger R, et al. Structure of the pancreatic lipase-procolipase complex. Nature 1992;359:159–162.
197. Boehm G, Bierback U, Senger H, et al. Activities of lipase and trypsin in duodenal juice of infants small for gestational age. J Pediatr Gastroenterol Nutr 1991;12:324–327.
198. Lombardo D, Guy O, Figarella C. Purification and characterization of carboxylester hydrolase from human pancreatic juice. Biochim Biophys Acta 1978;527:142–149.
199. Patton JS, Warner TG, Benson AA. Partial characterization of the bile salt-dependent triacylglycerol lipase from the leopard shard pancreas. Biochim Biophys Acta 1977;486:322–330.
200. Bradshaw WS, Rutter WJ. Multiple pancreatic lipases. Tissue distribution and pattern of accumulation during embryological development. Biochemistry 1972;11:1417–1528.
201. Giller T, Buchwald P, Koelin DB, et al. Two novel human pancreatic lipase related proteins hPLRP1 and hPLRP2. J Biol Chem 1992;267:16509–16513.
202. Hamosh M. Enzymes in human milk. In: Jensen RG, ed. Handbook of milk composition. San Diego: Academic Press, 1995:388–427.
203. Hui DY, Kissel JA. Sequence identity between human pancreatic cholesterol esterase and bile salt-stimulated milk lipase. FEBS Lett 1990;276:131–134.
204. Alemi B, Hamosh M, Scanlon JW, et al. Fat digestion in very low birth weight infants: effect of addition of human milk to low birth weight formula. Pediatrics 1981;68:484–489.
205. Williamson S, Finucane E, Ellis H, et al. Effect of heat treatment of human milk on absorption of nitrogen, fat, sodium, calcium and phosphorus by preterm infants. Arch Dis Child 1978;53:555–563.
206. Ellis LA, Hamosh M. Bile salt stimulated lipase: comparative studies in ferret milk and lactating mammary gland. Lipids 1992;27:917–922.
207. Wang C-S, Johnson D. Purification of human bile salt activated lipase. Anal Biochem 1983;133:457–461.
208. Nilsson J, Blackberg L, Carlsson P, et al. cDNA cloning of human milk bile salt-stimulated lipase and evidence for its identity to pancreatic carboxylic ester hydrolase. Eur J Biochem 1990;193:543–550.
209. Swan JS, Hoffman MM, Lord MK, et al. Two forms of human milk bile-salt stimulated lipase. Biochem J 1992;283:119–122.
210. Innis SM, Dyer R, Nelson CM. Evidence that palmitic acid is absorbed as Sn-2 monoacylglycerol from human milk by breast-fed infants. Lipids 1994;29:541–545.
211. Carey MC, Small DM, Bliss CM. Lipid digestion and absorption. Annu Rev Physiol 1983;45:651–677.
212. Stremmel W, Lotz G, Strohmeyer G, et al. Identification, isolation and partial characterization of a fatty acid binding protein from rat jejunal microvillus membranes. J Clin Invest 1985;75:1068–1076.
213. Ockner RK, Manning JM. Fatty acid binding protein in small intestine: identification, isolation and evidence for its role in cellular fatty acid transport. J Clin Invest 1974;54:326–338.
214. Gordon JI, Elshourbagy N, Lowe JB, et al. Tissue specific expression and developmental regulation of two genes coding for rat fatty acid binding proteins. J Biol Chem 1995;260:1985.
215. Davidson NO. Cellular and molecular mechanism of small intestinal lipid transport. In: Johnson LR, ed. Physiology of the gastrointestinal tract. 3rd. ed. New York: Raven Press, 1994:1909–1934.
216. Henning SJ, Rubin DC, Shulman RJ. Ontology of the intestinal mucosal. In: Johnson LR, ed. Physiology of the gastrointestinal tract. 3rd. ed. New York: Raven Press, 1994:571–611.
217. Johnston JM. Triglyceride biosynthesis in the intestinal mucosa. In: Rommell KH, Goebell H, Bohmer R, eds. Lipid absorption: biochemical and clinical aspects. Lancaster, UK: MTP, 1976:85–94.
218. Holzapple PG, Smith G, Kolodowsky O. Uptake, activation and esterification of fatty acids in the small intestine of the suckling rat. Pediatr Res 1975;9:786–791.
219. Flores CA, Hing SAO, Wells MA, et al. Rates of triolein absorption in suckling and adult rates. Am J Physiol 1989;257:G823–829.
220. Flores CA, Brannon PA, Wells MA, et al. Effect of diet on triolein absorption in weanling rats. Am J Physiol 1990;258:G38–G44.
221. Tso P, Balint JA. Formation and transport of chylomicrons by enterocytes to the lymphatics. Am J Physiol 1986;250:G715–G726.
222. Demmer LA, Levin MS, Elovson J, et al. Tissue-specific expression and developmental regulation of the rat apolipoprotein B gene. Proc Natl Acad Sci USA 1986;83:8102–8106.
223. Eisenberg S. Very low density lipoprotein metabolism. Prog Biochem Pharmacol 1979;15:139–165.
224. Glomset JA. Lecithin: cholesterol acyltransferase: an exercise in comparative biology. Prog Biochem Pharmacol 1976;15:41–46.
225. Gimenez-Llort L, Vilanove J, Skottova N. Lipoprotein lipase enable triacylglycerol hydrolysis by perfused newborn rat liver. Am J Physiol 1991;261:G641–647.
226. Peinado-Onsurbe J, Soler C, Soley M. Lipoprotein lipase activities are differentially regulated in isolated hepatocytes from neonatal rats. Biochim Biophys Acta 1992;1125:82–89.
227. Peinado-Onsurbe J, Staels B, Deeb S. Neonatal extinction of liver lipoprotein lipase expression. Biochem Biophys Acta 1992;1131:281–286.
228. Van Aerde JE, Hamosh M, Henderson TR, et al. Total parenteral nutrition delays the postnatal rise of lecithin: cholesterol acyltransferase. Pediatr Res 1995;37:321A.

229. Durksen DR, Van Aerdi JE, Chan G, et al. Total parenteral nutrition impairs bile flow and alters bile composition in newborn piglet. Dig Dis Sci 1996;41:1864–1870.
230. Hamosh A, Hamosh M, Henderson TR, et al. Unpublished observations.
231. Bougneres PF, Lemmel C, Ferre P, et al. Ketone body transport in the human neonate and infant. J Clin Invest 1986;77:42–48.
232. Edmond J, Anestad N, Robbins RA, Bergstrom JD. Ketone body metabolism in the neonate: development and effect of diet. Fed Proc 1985;44:2359–2364.
233. Yeh YY, Sheehan PM. Preferential utilization of ketone bodies in the brain and lung of newborn rats. Fed Proc 1985;44:2352–2358.
234. Williamson DH. Ketone body production and metabolism in the fetus and newborn. In: Polin RA, Fox WW, eds. Fetal and neonatal physiology. 2nd ed. Philadelphia: WB Saunders, 1998:493–503.
235. American Academy of Pediatrics, Committee on Nutrition. Nutritional needs of low-birth-weight infants. Pediatrics 1985;76:976–986.
236. Stahl GE, Spear ML, Hamosh M. Intravenous administration of lipid emulsion to premature infants. Clin Perinatol 1986;13:133–162.
237. Berkow SE, Spear LM, Stahl GE, et al. Total parenteral nutrition with Intralipid in premature infants receiving TPN with heparin: effect of plasma lipolytic enzymes, lipid and glucose. J Pediatr Gastroenterol Nutr 1987;366:598–604.
238. Papadopoulos A, Hamosh M, Chowdhry P, et al. Lecithin: cholesterol acyl transferase in the newborn: low activity level in preterm infants. J Pediatr 1988;113:896–898.
239. Amr S, Hamosh P, Hamosh M. Effect of Intralipid infusion on lecithin: cholesterol acyl transferase and lipoprotein lipase in young rats. Biochim Biophys Acta 1989;1001:145–149.
240. Goel R, Hamosh M, Stahol GE, et al. Plasma lecithin: cholesterol acyltransferase and plasma lipolytic activity in preterm infants given total parenteral nutrition with 10% or 20% Intralipid. Acta Paediatr 1995;84:1060–1064.
241. Montgomery R, Dryer RL, Conway TW, et al. Biochemistry: a case-oriented approach. 4th ed. St. Louis: Mosby, 1982.

37
Inborn Errors of Lipid Metabolism (Mitochondrial Fatty Acid Oxidation)

Charles A. Stanley

During fetal life, fatty acids and lipids are used almost exclusively for anabolism in cellular growth, synthesis, and differentiation. The fetal respiratory quotient of approximately 1.0 indicates that essentially no lipid is used as a fuel for energy production. After birth, there is an abrupt change in lipid metabolism with mitochondrial oxidation of stored fat and ketone synthesis suddenly becoming a critical pathway for survival during extrauterine life. Fatty acids are the preferred fuel for the heart and aerobically exercising skeletal muscle. Most importantly, as the constant supply of fuel via the placenta is replaced by cycles of intermittent feeding, fat becomes an essential store of fuel for energy production during long-term fasting. Developmental delay in maturation of fatty acid oxidation plays an important role in the susceptibility of the normal neonate to hypoglycemia in the immediate postnatal period. In addition, over a dozen genetic defects in mitochondrial fatty acid oxidation have been identified that may present in the newborn period with life-threatening illness.

Pathway of Mitochondrial Fatty Acid Oxidation

This topic has been the subject of detailed reviews.[1,2] In the fed state during extrauterine life, as in the fetus, fatty acids make little or no contribution to energy production. However, in prolonged fasting of 15 to 24 hours in infants or of 36 to 48 hours in adults, 90% of oxygen consumption is accounted for by oxidation of fatty acids. Tissues such as the heart utilize fatty acids efficiently and in direct proportion to their circulating concentrations. The brain is unable to use fatty acids, since these fuels cannot cross the blood-brain barrier. The liver oxidizes fatty acids incompletely to the level of acetyl-coenzyme A (CoA). The acetyl-CoA is condensed to form the ketones, acetoacetate and β-hydroxybutyrate, which are exported for use by peripheral tissues, particularly the brain. In this way, the brain is indirectly able to use fat stores as a fuel during fasting, thus sparing glucose consumption and the need for gluconeogenesis from essential body protein.

Mitochondrial fatty acid oxidation utilizes long-chain fatty acids of 16 to 18 carbons in length that are stored primarily as adipose tissue triglyceride. These fatty acids are released as the unesterified or free fatty acids and transported to liver and other organs bound to albumin. As shown in Figure 37.1, once taken up and activated in the cytosol to their coenzyme A esters, long-chain fatty acids may either be directed to resynthesis of triglyceride or to enter mitochondria for oxidation. Entry into mitochondria is regulated by the concentration of malonyl-CoA, the substrate for fatty acid synthesis and a noncompetitive inhibitor of carnitine palmitoyltransferase-1 (CPT-1), the first committed step in fatty acid oxidation. As shown in Figure 37.1, the carnitine cycle transports long-chain fatty acids across the barrier of the inner mitochondrial membrane (see Chapter 38). Repetitive cycles of β-oxidation sequentially shorten the fatty acid by two carbons until it is reduced to n/2 acetyl-CoA moieties. There are two to three different chain-length specific enzymes for each of the four steps of β-oxidation. The electrons produced in the first step, acyl-CoA dehydrogenase, are transferred to the electron transport chain via electron transfer flavoprotein (ETF) and ETF dehydrogenase (ETF-DH). In the liver, the majority of acetyl-CoA from fatty acid oxidation is converted to ketones via the β-hydroxy-β-methylglutaryl (HMG)-CoA cycle.

All of the enzymes of fatty acid oxidation (Table 37.1) are encoded by nuclear genes, synthesized in the cytosol, and transported across the mitochondrial membrane via specific signal peptide sequences recognized by membrane carrier proteins.[2] Most do not have tissue-specific isozymes. The exceptions include CPT-1 (i.e., liver-kidney-fibroblast isozymes different from muscle), HMG-CoA synthase (i.e., expressed only in liver and kidney, not in fibroblasts or muscle), and the plasma

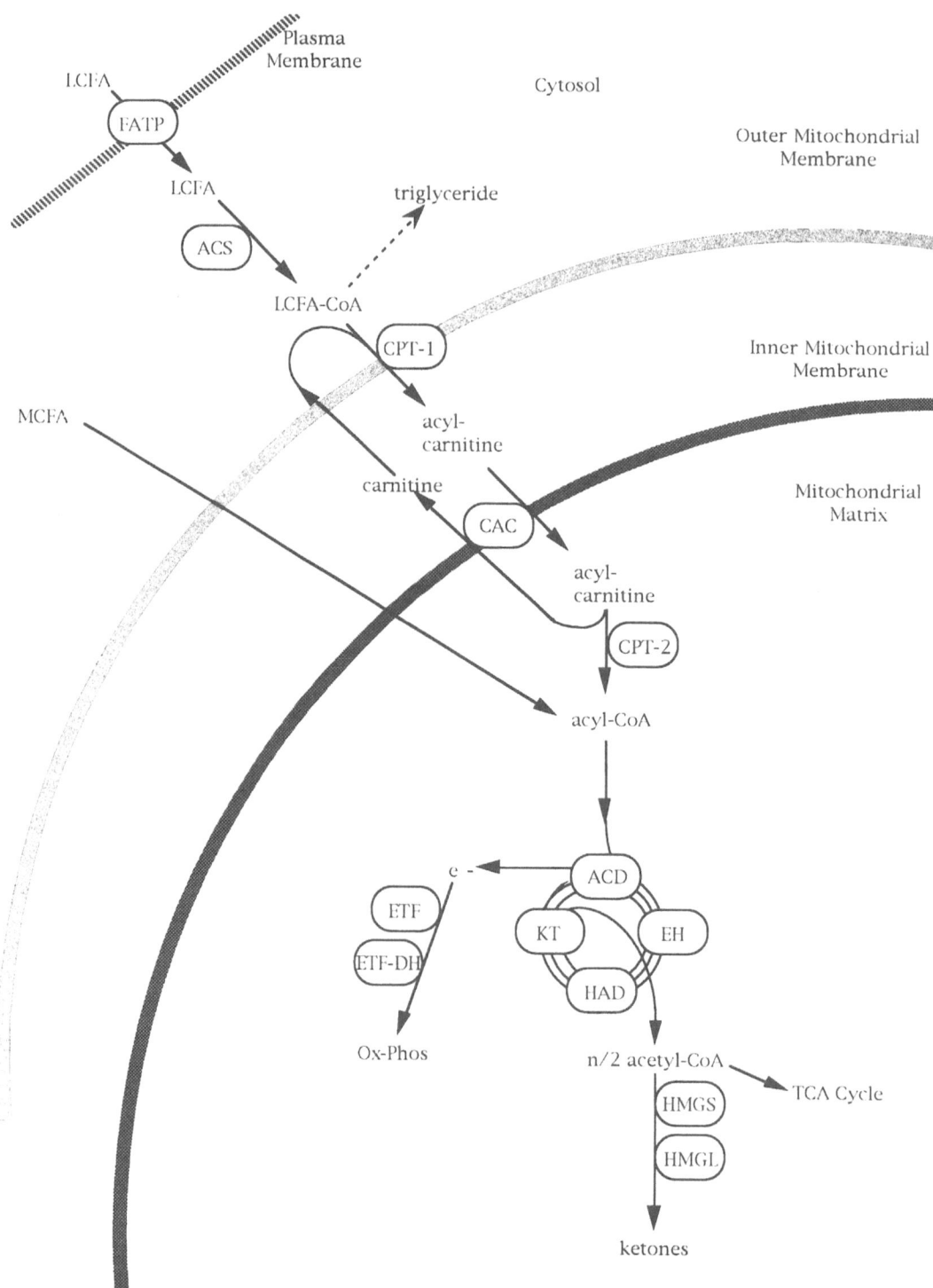

FIGURE 37.1. Pathway of fatty acid oxidation and ketone synthesis. Circulating long-chain fatty acids (LCFA) are transported into cells by a fatty acid transport protein (FATP) and activated to acyl-CoA by acyl-CoA synthetase (ACS). Fatty acids are transported into mitochondria by the combined action of carnitine palmitoyltransferase-1 (CPT-1), carnitine/acylcarnitine translocase (CAC), and CPT-2. Note that medium-chain fatty acids (MCFA) enter mitochondria directly. The β-oxidation cycle consists of acyl-CoA dehydrogenase (ACD), enoyl-CoA hydratase (EH), 3-hydroxyacyl-CoA dehydrogenase (HAD), and β-ketothiolase (KT) steps. Electrons are transferred from ACD by electron transfer flavoprotein (ETF) and electron transfer flavoprotein dehydrogenase (ETF-DH) to the electron transport chain (Ox-Phos). The n/2 moles of acetyl-CoA from each mole of LCFA oxidized are converted to ketones by β-hydroxy-β-methylglutaryl-CoA synthase and lyase (HMGS and HMGL).

37. Inborn Errors of Lipid Metabolism

TABLE 37.1. Enzymes of mitochondrial fatty acid oxidation.

Enzyme	Abbreviation
Fatty acid transport protein	FATP
Carnitine cycle	
Plasma membrane carnitine transporter	CT
Carnitine palmitoyltransferase-1	CPT-1
Carnitine/acylcarnitine carrier	CAC
Carnitine palmitoyltransferase-2	CPT-2
β-Oxidation cycle	
Acyl-CoA dehydrogenases	ACD
Very long-chain ACD (membrane)	VLCAD
Long-chain ACD (matrix)	LCAD
(? 2-methyl ACD)	
Medium-chain ACD	MCAD
Short-chain ACD	SCAD
Trifunctional protein	
Long-chain enoyl-CoA hydratase	EH
Long-chain 3-hydroxy ACD	LCHAD
Long-chain β-ketothiolase	LCKT
Crotonase (short chain EH)	
Short-chain β-ketothiolase	
Electron transfer	
Electron transfer flavoprotein	ETF
ETF dehydrogenase	ETF-DH
Ketone synthesis	
β-OH-β-methylglutaryl-CoA synthase	HMGS
β-OH-β-methylglutaryl-CoA lyase	HMG

membrane carnitine transporter (i.e., probably separate carriers in muscle-kidney-fibroblasts vs. liver).[3–5]

Development of Fatty Acid Oxidation in the Neonate

In both neonates and in laboratory animals there is evidence that the pathway of mitochondrial fatty acid oxidation is not developed at the time of delivery. Studies in normal neonates during the first 12 hours after birth show that, in contrast to older infants, children, and adults, fasting hypoglycemia is not accompanied by hyperketonemia.[6,7] Studies in animal models such as rats and guinea pigs have suggested that major developmental increases in the activity of CPT-1 occur in the second half of the first day after delivery.[8–10] Recent reports have confirmed that transcription of the CPT-1 gene is low until 12 hours after delivery.[9,10] Transcription of the mitochondrial HMG-CoA synthase gene required for hepatic ketone synthesis is also low during this time.[4,11–13] By 12 to 24 hours after delivery, the capacity for fatty acid oxidation and ketogenesis appears to be fully developed.[7] Exposure to dietary fat may serve as a signal for initiating transcription of CPT-1 and HMG-CoA synthase genes.[4]

This normal developmental delay in the capacity for fatty acid oxidation plays an important role in the well-documented high risk of hypoglycemia in normal neonates during the first day of life. In combination with the developmental delay in the enzymes of gluconeogenesis that occurs in the neonate, the delay in fatty acid oxidation means that the neonate is solely dependent on liver glycogen reserves as a source of fuel for the brain for up to 12 hours after delivery. In the absence of hepatic ketogenesis, the brain is not protected with any alternative substrates during neonatal transitional hypoglycemia. This provides an important rationale for not using a lower definition of hypoglycemia in neonates than in older children and adults.

Clinical Features of Genetic Defects in Fatty Acid Oxidation

The major roles of fatty acid oxidation are to provide energy for cardiac and skeletal muscle and to serve as a fuel during periods of prolonged fasting. The clinical features of the genetic defects in fatty acid oxidation reflect these three roles. Patients may present with primarily hepatic features of acute life-threatening coma triggered by excessive fasting, with cardiac features related to acute or chronic cardiomyopathy, or with acute or chronic muscle signs such as pain and rhabdomyolysis or weakness.[1,2,14–16]

Features of the hepatic mode of presentation may include nausea, vomiting, coma, or seizures associated with hypoglycemia, hypoketonemia and hypoketonuria, elevated transaminases and clotting times, hyperammonemia, and hyperuricemia. These features mimic Reye's syndrome, and defects in fatty acid oxidation should be considered as one of the causes of Reye's syndrome.[17] Patients are usually not acidemic or only mildly so, since ketones are inappropriately low for the degree of fasting stress. The liver may become moderately enlarged during acute attacks of illness due to accumulation of fat. Patients often appear normal between attacks and the illness may mimic Reye's syndrome or sudden infant death syndrome.[18,19] Attacks usually occur after more than 12 hours of fasting and are often triggered by intercurrent infections that cause either poor feeding or vomiting.

Cardiac features may include hypertrophic or dilated cardiomyopathy, which may appear only in association with fasting-induced acute illness or may be chronic. Muscle-like features may include episodes of rhabdomyolysis and myoglobinuria associated with prolonged exercise or fasting. In infants and children, weakness resembling muscular dystrophy is more common.

As shown in Table 37.2, the major clinical features of the known genetic defects in fatty acid oxidation are relatively similar and not specific to the site of defect. Since young neonates are usually not exposed to fasts of

TABLE 37.2. Clinical manifestations of genetic defects in mitochondrial fatty acid oxidation.

Defect	Liver	Heart	Muscle	Other
Carnitine cycle				
CT	+	+	+	
CPT-1	+[a]			
CAC[f]	+	+	+	
CPT-2[e,f]	+	+	+	+[b]
β-Oxidation cycle				
ACD				
VLCAD	+	+	+	
LCAD (no defects, yet)	?			
MCAD	+			
SCAD				g
Trifunctional protein				
EH				
LCHAD	+	+	+	+[c,d]
KT				
Crotonase (no defects, yet)				
SCHAD				g
SC-β-ketothiolase				g
Electron transfer				
ETF[e,f]	+	+	+	+[b]
ETF-DH[e,f]	+	+	+	+[b]
Ketone synthesis				
HMGS	+[a]			
HMGL	+			+

[a] Liver only.
[b] Fetal malformations.
[c] Retinopathy and neuropathy in some patients.
[d] Maternal acute fatty liver of pregnancy/HELLP syndrome.
[e] Mild and severe forms.
[f] No survivors.
[g] Atypical FAO defects.

12 hours or more, patients usually do not present until after 3 to 6 months of age. Exceptions to this rule include the most severe defects (e.g., translocase, severe CPT-2, and severe GA-2) and neonates with milder defects who are exposed to unusually prolonged fasting by attempted breast-feeding.[20] Not surprisingly, given the limited need for fatty acid oxidation in the fetus, most affected neonates have no clinical abnormalities either before or at delivery. However, brain and renal anomalies have been observed frequently in neonates with severe CPT-2 and severe GA-2 (ETF or ETF-DH deficiencies).[21] LCHAD is unusual in that some patients have evidence of progressive damage to tissues not considered to be dependent on fatty acid oxidation: progressive peripheral neuropathy and pigmented retinopathy.[22,23] LCHAD is distinctive for the apparently increased risk of HELLP syndrome, characterized by hemolyses elevated liver enzymes and low platelets, or acute fatty liver of pregnancy in heterozygote mothers, possibly independent of the disease status of the fetus.[24] The short-chain enzyme defects, short-chain acyl-CoA dehydrogenase (SCAD) and short-chain L-3-hydroxyacyl-CoA dehydrogenase (SCHAD), are un-

usual in the absence of acute fasting coma and a picture of chronic acidemia and delayed development.[25-27]

The following discussion highlights some of the noteworthy features of specific fatty acid oxidation disorders.

Carnitine Transport (CT) Deficiency

This disorder is distinguished by the presence of extremely low plasma and tissue carnitine concentrations ($\ll 5\%$ of normal). In contrast to most fatty acid oxidation defects, the initial presentation in the majority of these patients is progressive cardiomyopathy and weakness at 2 to 4 years of age.[5,14,28,29] Initial presentation with attacks of fasting coma and hypoglycemia is less common. It may be triggered at any time from birth through 1 to 2 years of age by prolonged fasting stress before evidence of chronic cardiomyopathy develops. Treatment with oral carnitine 50 to $100\,mg\cdot kg^{-1}$ does not fully normalize tissue concentrations, but appears to completely correct impaired fatty acid oxidation by liver and restore cardiac function to normal.[5,30] This is the only disorder that has been clearly demonstrated to respond to carnitine therapy.[14]

CPT-1 Deficiency

This disorder involves the liver isoform of CPT-1. Cardiac or muscle symptoms do not occur.[31,32]

Carnitine/Acylcarnitine Carrier (CAC) Deficiency

The few recognized patients with this disorder have been severely affected and only one has survived beyond the newborn period.[33,34]

CPT-2 Deficiency

There are two forms of this disorder: a severe, fatal neonatal form and a milder adult-onset form.[35-39] Fetal malformations, especially polycystic kidneys, have been observed in the former and in the severe neonatal form of ETF/ETF-DH deficiency.[21,40] The adult form of CPT-2 deficiency often presents with exercise-induced rhabdomyolysis and myoglobinuria.[41]

Very Long Chain Acyl-CoA Dehydrogenase (VLCAD) and Long-Chain Acyl-CoA Dehydrogenase (LCAD) Deficiency

Patients with either of these disorders were originally reported as LCAD deficiency.[42-44] This was based on in vitro assays showing impaired dehydrogenation of long-chain substrates prior to the time the separate membrane-bound VLCAD enzyme was recognized. It now appears that all previously diagnosed LCAD patients have VLCAD (or membrane associated LCAD) deficiency. No true matrix enzyme LCAD deficient patients have yet been identified; a recent report suggests that the real function of this protein may not involve the usual straight-chain fatty acids, but may be restricted to the minor role of 2-methyl branch-chain fatty acid oxidation.[45]

Medium-Chain Acyl-CoA Dehydrogenase (MCAD) Deficiency

This is the most commonly recognized fatty acid oxidation disorder.[1,46] Once diagnosed, with simple diet adjustments and appropriate care for acute illnesses, the disorder has an excellent prognosis with little impact on health in adult life. However, the disorder is life threatening, with 25% of patients dying prior to diagnosis and many suffering permanent brain damage from acute attacks of illness.[2,47]

LCHAD Deficiency

Unusual features of this disorder suggest chronic toxicity: retinopathy, peripheral neuropathy, as well as chronic and acute elevations of muscle creatine phosphokinase (CPK).[48] Several LCHAD heterozygote mothers have had severe illness late in pregnancy characterized as HELLP syndrome or acute fatty liver of pregnancy.[24] Whether this complication is related to the disease status of the fetus remains unclear.

SCAD and SCHAD Deficiencies

These short-chain fatty acid oxidation disorders do not present with features of hepatic, cardiac, or muscle involvement that are typical of other defects in the pathway. Rather than acute attacks of fasting hypoglycemic coma, these defects may not impair ketogenesis and patients have presented with more subtle, chronic problems of developmental delay, hypotonia, and metabolic acidosis.[25-27]

Short-Chain β-Ketothiolase Deficiency

This disorder presents primarily with attacks of hyperketonemia rather than hypoketosis, because peripheral ketone utilization is impaired.

ETF and ETF-DH Deficiencies (Glutaric Aciduria Type 2 or Ethylmalonic-Adipic Aciduria)

There are two forms of these defects: a severe, usually fatal neonatal form, and a milder form that resembles MCAD deficiency.[21] The severe form is associated with fetal malformations, especially of the kidney, similar to severe CPT-2 deficiency.

HMC Synthase (HMGS) Deficiency

Only one patient with this defect has been identified. Since the enzyme is present only in liver and kidney and is required only for ketone synthesis, the presentation was fasting hypoglycemia and hypoketotic coma.[49] Specific diagnosis represents a challenge, because no distinctive abnormalities were present in urinary organic acids, plasma total and free carnitine, or plasma acylcarnitine profile.

HMG Lyase (HMGL) Deficiency

Affected patients present with attacks of hypoketotic hypoglycemia. In contrast to other defects of ketone production, there is a marked metabolic acidosis due to accumulation of β-hydroxy-β-methylglutaric acid derived from leucine oxidation.

Epidemiology

The most frequently described fatty acid oxidation defects include MCAD, LCHAD, GA-2, and CPT-2. For the others, fewer than 50 patients have been identified to date. The incidence of MCAD, the most well recognized of the defects, occurs as high as 1 in 10,000 in individuals whose ethnic origin includes northwestern Europe and Britain.[2] LCHAD may be as common, but has not been as well studied. In combination, the incidence of the fatty acid oxidation disorders may approach 1 in 5,000, making them the most common of the inborn errors of intermediary metabolism.

Diagnosis (See Chapter 53)

Documentation of Impaired Fatty Acid Oxidation/Ketogenesis

Figure 37.2 is a study of fasting adaptation in a child with MCAD deficiency that demonstrates impaired hepatic fatty acid oxidation: inappropriately low plasma ketone concentrations despite high free fatty acids as hypoglycemia develops. This type of challenge can be used as a provocative test to diagnose patients with fatty acid oxidation disorders. The test may be dangerous and should be done only by experienced investigators. The same information can more easily be obtained at the time of presentation by using the critical samples of blood and urine that should be obtained prior to or immediately after treatment of acute illness is begun. In addition to

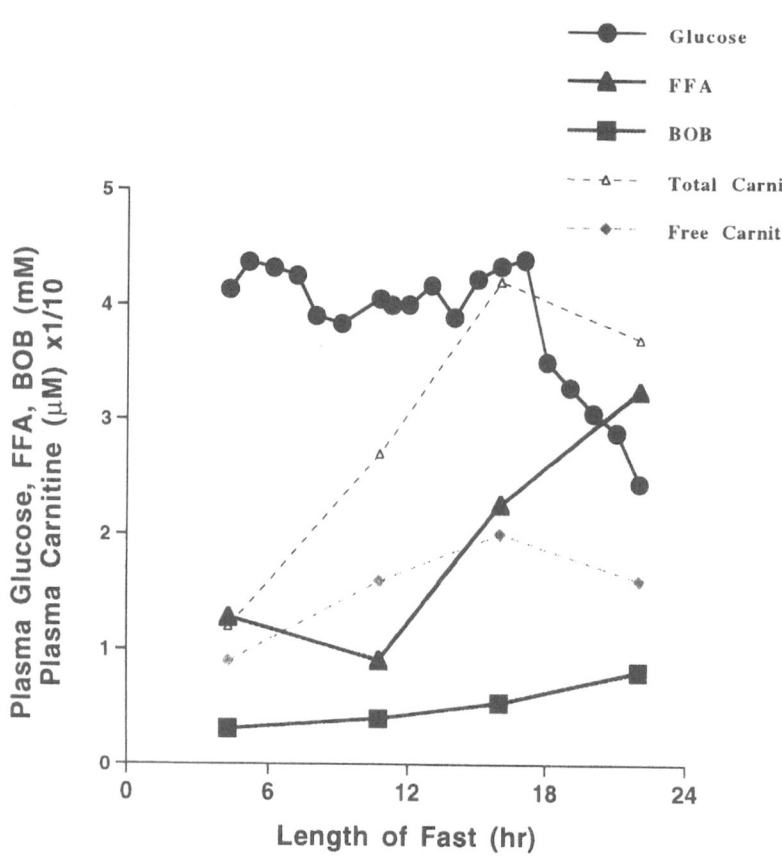

FIGURE 37.2. Fasting in a child with MCAD deficiency. Hypoglycemia occurs earlier than normal at 22 hours with inappropriately low β-hydroxybutyrate (BOB, normal 2–5 mM) and high free fatty acid (FFA, normal 1.5–2.5 mM) levels. Plasma total and free carnitine levels are low (normal 35–60, 30–55 μM) at the start and acylcarnitines rise markedly during the fast.

plasma ketones and free fatty acids, tests should include total and free plasma carnitine, plasma acylcarnitine profile by mass spectrometry, and urinary organic acid profile by gas chromatography-mass spectometry (Table 37.3). Plasma total carnitine concentrations obtained at times when patients are well are extremely low in CT deficiency, elevated in CPT-1 deficiency, normal in HMGS deficiency, and intermediately low in all other defects from CAC through HMGL deficiency.[14,33] The latter secondary carnitine deficiency disorders usually show abnormally high proportions of esterified carnitine. Studies of patients with several different secondary carnitine deficiency disorders indicate that carnitine concentrations are not lower because of excessive loss of acyl-carnitine metabolites. Rather, the mechanism of secondary carnitine deficiency appears to be an impairment of renal conservation of free carnitine. This may be due to competitive inhibition of carnitine transporter activity by accumulated acylcarnitines.[50] Tissue histology may reveal increased triglyceride deposits in liver, heart, or skeletal muscle.[51]

Diagnosis of Specific Fatty Acid Oxidation Disorders by Metabolite Analyses

This method is possible in less than half of the known defects (Table 37.3) (see Chapter 53). Recently, mass spectrometry methods have been developed for identifying specific acylcarnitines in newborn blood spot cards. This has made it possible to carry out newborn screening for MCAD deficiency, the most common of the known fatty acid oxidation disorders.[52]

Identification of the specific site of defect is often not straightforward in the fatty acid oxidation disorders. It

TABLE 37.3. Metabolites useful in diagnosis of fatty acid oxidation defects.

Urinary organic acid profile (GC-MS)	
MCAD	Hexanoyl-glycine
	Phenylpropionyl-glycine
	Suberyl-glycine
LCHAD	3-Hydroxy C8-C14 dicarboxylic acids
SCAD	Ethylmalonic acid
ETF/ETF-DH	Ethylmalonic
	Isovaleryl-glycine
	Glutaric acid
HMGL	β-Hydroxy-β-methylglutaric acid
Plasma acylcarnitine profile (MS-MS)	
VLCAD	C14:1 acylcarnitine
MCAD	C10:1 acylcarnitine
	Octanoyl-carnitine
SCAD	Butyryl-carnitine
ETF/ETF-DH	Isovaleryl-carnitine
	Glutaryl-carnitine
HMGL	β-Hydroxy-β-methylglutryl-carnitine

may be necessary to carry out detailed biochemical analyses using cultured fibroblasts or transformed lymphoblasts. Impairment of the overall fatty acid oxidation pathway can be demonstrated in vitro by measuring oxidation of radioactively labeled long-chain fatty acids in these cells.[53] Different chain-length substrates can be used to narrow down the probable location of the defect. Enzyme assays for specific steps are available in a small number of laboratories and can discriminate between affected individuals, carriers, and normals. Although experience is limited, cultured amniotic cells or chorionic villus biopsy may be useful for prenatal diagnosis.

Mutation Analysis

This method is useful in MCAD and, possibly, in LCHAD deficiencies for diagnosis and genetic studies, because single common point mutations account for the majority of mutant alleles in these two disorders. An A985G mutation, which yields an unstable enzyme protein, has been found in 90% to 95% of patients with MCAD deficiency, with over 80% of affected patients being homozygous.[54] Simple assays for the A985G mutation are available and may be useful in confirmation of the diagnosis of MCAD deficiency, in detection of affected but asymptomatic siblings, and in prenatal diagnosis. In LCHAD deficiency, a G1528C mutation that results in reduced enzyme activity has been detected in 24 of 26 unrelated patients.[55]

Therapy

The goal of both acute and long-term therapy for the disorders of fatty acid oxidation is to minimize the demand on the pathway by providing sufficient carbohydrate.[1,2] In milder disorders, such as MCAD deficiency, long-term therapy consists simply of avoiding fasts of more than 10 to 12 hours by ensuring a carbohydrate feeding at bedtime and not delaying breakfast. During intercurrent illness, extra carbohydrate snacks should be given since appetite may be poor. Early hospital care should be provided in case of gastroenteritis or other severe illness and intravenous dextrose given to maintain plasma glucose concentration above 4 to 5 mmol·L^{-1} (i.e., 10% dextrose at maintenance rates). It should be emphasized that blood glucose concentrations are not a reliable guide to illness in patients with fatty acid oxidation disorders, because symptoms develop in association with elevations of plasma free fatty acids before glucose reaches the hypoglycemic range. Ingestion of fat does not have an obvious effect on symptoms, especially in milder defects. It is reasonable to suggest lower than average intake of dietary fat. In more severe defects, additional efforts to minimize the need for fat oxidation may be useful, such as complete intravenous alimentation during recovery from acute illness and/or continuous intragastric tube feeding with a high-carbohdrate, low-fat formula such as Tolerex® for long-term management. In patients with defects specific to long-chain fatty acids, such as CPT-2 deficiency, medium-chain fatty acid oxidation is unimpaired. It has been suggested that medium-chain triglyceride (MCT) oil is a useful dietary supplement in these disorders. There is little reason to believe that this adds any benefit beyond simple high-carbohydrate feedings.

In specific disorders, additional therapies may be available. In the carnitine transporter defect (i.e., primary carnitine deficiency), carnitine therapy is essential and remarkably effective in correcting the disorder despite the fact that tissue concentrations are not raised beyond 5% to 10% of normal.[5,14,30] Although opinions on this point differ among investigators, there is no evidence that carnitine therapy has significant effects in any of the other fatty acid oxidation or organic acid oxidation disorders that are associated with secondary carnitine deficiency.[14] Some patients with mild forms of glutaric aciduria type 2 (ETF or ETF-DH deficiencies) or SCAD deficiency have been reported to benefit from treatment with high doses of riboflavin, the cofactor for these enzymes.[21,56]

Conclusion

The pathway of mitochondrial fatty acid oxidation and ketone synthesis becomes important to energy metabolism only after birth. The normal delay in development of this pathway is likely to play a major role in the high risk of hypoglycemia in neonates during the first day of life. Over a dozen different genetic defects in the pathway have been identified, mostly within the past decade. These disorders must be considered in neonates who present with acute, life-threatening illness, although most patients do not present until later in the first 1 to 2 years of life. Typical clinical features of genetic defects in fatty acid oxidation involve the following organs: liver, with attacks of fasting hypoketotic, hypoglycemic coma; heart, with acute or chronic cardiomyopthy; or skeletal muscle, with weakness or acute rhabdomyolysis. Specific diagnosis is aided by the recognition of the need for appropriate collection of the critical blood and urine samples at the time of initial illness. Long-term prognosis of these disorders ranges from uniformly fatal to excellent.

Acknowledgment. This work is supported in part by grants from the National Institutes of Health, RR-00240 and DK-43841.

References

1. Stanley CA. New genetic defects in mitochondrial fatty acid oxidation and carnitine deficiency. Adv Pediatr 1987;34:59–88.
2. Roe CR, Coates PM. Mitochondrial fatty acid oxidation disorders. In: Scriver CR, Beaudet AL, Sly WS, Valle D, eds. The metabolic and molecular bases of inherited disease. 6th ed. New York: McGraw-Hill, 1995:1501–1534.
3. Esser V, Britton CH, Weis BC, et al. Cloning, sequencing, and expression of a cDNA encoding rat liver carnitine palmitoyltransferase I. Direct evidence that a single polypeptide is involved in inhibitor interaction and catalytic function. J Biol Chem 1993;268:5817–5822.
4. Arias G, Matas R, Asins G, et al. The effect of fasting and insulin treatment on carnitine palmitoyl transferase I and mitochondrial 3-hydroxy-3-methylglutaryl coenzyme A synthase mRNA levels in liver from suckling rats. Biochem Soc Trans 1995;23A.
5. Stanley CA, DeLeeuw S, Coates PM, et al. Chronic cardiomyopathy and weakness or acute coma in children with a defect in carnitine uptake. Ann Neurol 1991;30:709–716.
6. Stanley CA, Anday EK, Baker L, Delivoria PM. Metabolic fuel and hormone responses to fasting in newborn infants. Pediatrics 1979;64:613–619.
7. Anday EK, Stanley CA, Baker L, Delivoria PM. Plasma ketones in newborn infants: absence of suckling ketosis. J Pediatr 1981;98:628–630.
8. Stanley CA, Gonzales E, Baker L. Development of hepatic fatty acid oxidation and ketogenesis in the newborn guinea pig. Pediatr Res 1983;17:224–229.
9. Thumelin S, Esser V, Charvy D, et al. Expression of liver carnitine palmitoyltransferase I and II genes during development in the rat. Biochem J 1994;300:583–587.
10. Asins G, Serra D, Arias G, Hegardt FG. Developmental changes in carnitine palmitoyltransferases I and II gene expression in intestine and liver of suckling rats. Biochem J 1995;306:379–384.
11. Prip BC, Thumelin S, Chatelain F, et al. Hormonal and nutritional control of liver fatty acid oxidation and ketogenesis during development. [Review]. Biochem Soc Trans 1995;23:500–506.
12. Thumelin S, Forestier M, Girard J, Developmental changes in mitochondrial 3-hydroxy-3-methylglutaryl-CoA synthase gene expression in rat liver, intestine and kidney. Biochem J 1993;292:493–496.
13. Duee PH, Pegorier JP, Quant PA, et al. Hepatic ketogenesis in newborn pigs is limited by low mitochondrial 3-hydroxy-3-methylglutaryl-CoA synthase activity. Biochem J 1994;298:207–212.
14. Stanley CA. Carnitine disorders. Adv Pediatr 1995;42:209–242.
15. Hale DE, Bennett MJ. Fatty acid oxidation disorders: a new class of metabolic diseases. J Pediatr 1992;121:1–11.
16. Bennett MJ, Hale DE, Coates PM, Stanley CA. Postmortem recognition of fatty acid oxidation disorders. Pediatr Pathol 1991;11:365–370.
17. Stanley CA, Coates PM. Inherited defects of fatty acid oxidation which resemble Reye's syndrome. In: Pollack JD, Redshaw PL, eds. Reye's syndrome IV. Bryan, OH: Natured Reye's Research Foundation, 1985:190–200.
18. Arens R, Gozal D, Jain K, et al. Prevalence of medium-chain acyl-coenzyme A dehydrogenase deficiency in sudden infant death syndrome. J Pediatr 1993;122:715–718.
19. Lundemose JB, Geregersen N, Kolvraa S, et al. The frequency of a disease-causing point mutation in the gene for medium-chain acyl-CoA dehydrogenase in sudden infant death syndrome. Acta Paediatr 1993;82:544–546.
20. Wilken B, Carpenter KH, Hammond J. Neonatal symptoms in medium chain acyl coenzyme A dehydrogenase deficiency. Arch Dis Child 1993;69:292–294.
21. Frerman FE, Goodman SI. Nuclear-encoded defect of the mitochondrial respiratory chain, including glutaric acidemia type II. In: Scriver CR, Beaudet AL, Sly WS, Valle D, eds. The metabolic basis of inherited disease. NY: McGraw-Hill, 1995:1611–1630.
22. Sewell AC, Bender SW, Wirth S, et al. Long-chain 3-hydroxyacyl-CoA dehydrogenase deficiency: a severe fatty acid oxidation disorder. Eur J Pediatr 1994;153:745–750.
23. Hale DE, Thorpe C, Braat K, et al. The L-3-hydroxyacyl-CoA dehydrogenase deficiency. Prog Clin Biol Res 1990;321:503–510.
24. Treem WR, Rinaldo P, Hale DE, et al. Acute fatty liver of pregnancy and long-chain 3-hydroxyacyl-coenzyme A dehydrogenase deficiency. Hepatology 1994;19:339–345.
25. Coates PM, Hale DE, Finocchiaro G, et al. Genetic deficiency of short-chain acyl-coenzyme A dehydrogenase in cultured fibroblasts from a patient with muscle carnitine deficiency and severe skeletal muscle weakness. J Clin Invest 1988;81:171–175.
26. Tein I, De VDC, Hale DE, et al. Short-chain L-3-hydroxyacyl-CoA dehydrogenase deficiency in muscle: a new cause for recurrent myoglobinuria and encephalopathy. Ann Neurol 1991;30:415–419.
27. Bennett MJ, Weinberger MJ, Kobori JA, et al. Mitochondrial short-chain L-3-hydroxyacyl-coenzyme A dehydrogenase deficiency: a new defect of fatty acid oxidation. Pediatr Res 1996;39:185–188.
28. Treem WR, Stanley CA, Finegold DN, et al. Primary carnitine deficiency due to a failure of carnitine transport in kidney, muscle, and fibroblasts. N Engl J Med 1988;319:1331–1336.
29. Stanley CA. Plasma and mitochondrial membrane carnitine transport defects. Prog Clin Biol Res 1992;375:289–300.
30. Tein I, DeVivo DC, Bierman F, et al. Impaired skin fibroblast carnitine uptake in primary systemic carnitine deficiency manifested by childhood carnitine-responsive cardiomyopathy. Pediatr Res 1990;28:247–255.
31. Stanley CA, Sunaryo F, Hale DE, et al. Elevated plasma carnitine in the hepatic form of carnitine palmitoyltransferase-1 deficiency. J Inherited Metab Dis 1992;15:785–789.
32. Tein I, Demaugre F, Bonnefont JP, Saudubray JM. Normal muscle CPT I and CPT II activities in hepatic presentation patients with CPT I deficiency in fibroblasts. Tissue specific isoforms of CPT I? J Neurol Sci 1989;92:229–245.

33. Stanley CA, Treem WR, Hale DE, Coates PM. A genetic defect in carnitine transport causing primary carnitine deficiency. Prog Clin Biol Res 1990;321:457–464.
34. Pande SV, Brivet B, Slama A, et al. Carnitine-acylcarnitine translocase deficiency with severe hypoglycemia and auriculoventricular block. Translocase assay in permeabilized fibroblasts. J Clin Invest 1993;91:1247–1252.
35. Bougneres PF, Saudubray JM, Marsac C, et al. Fasting hypoglycemia resulting from hepatic carnitine palmitoyl transferase deficiency. J Pediatr 1981;98:742–746.
36. Demaugre F, Bonnefont J, Mitchell G, et al. Hepatic and muscular presentations of carnitine palmitoyl transferase deficiency: two distinct entities. Pediatr Res 1988;24:308–311.
37. Bonnefont JP, Haas R, Wolff J, et al. Deficiency of carnitine palmitoyltransferase I. J Child Neurol 1989;4:198–203.
38. Demaugre F, Bonnefont JP, Colonna M, et al. Infantile form of carnitine palmitoyltransferase II deficiency with hepatomuscular symptoms and sudden death. Physiopathological approach to carnitine palmitoyltransferase II deficiencies. J Clin Invest 1991;87:859–864.
39. Saudubray J, Mitchell G, Bonnefont J, et al. Approach to the patient with a fatty acid oxidation disorder. Prog Clin Biol Res 1992;375:271–288.
40. Falik-Borenstein ZC, Jordan SC, Saudubray JM, et al. Brief report: renal tubular acidosis in carnitine palmitoyltransferase type 1 deficiency. N Engl J Med 1992;327:24–27.
41. DiMauro S, DiMauro PMM. Muscle carnitine palmityltransferase deficiency and myoglobinuria. Science 1973;182:929–931.
42. Hale DE, Batshaw ML, Coates PM, et al. Long-chain acyl coenzyme A dehydrogenase deficiency: an inherited cause of nonketotic hypoglycemia. Pediatr Res 1985;19:666–671.
43. Aoyama T, Uchida Y, Kelley RI, et al. A novel disease with deficiency of mitochondrial very-long-chain acyl-CoA dehydrogenase. Biochem Biophys Res Commun 1993;191:1369–1372.
44. Bertrand C, Largilliere C, Zabot MT, et al. Very long chain acyl-CoA dehydrogenase deficiency: identification of a new inborn error of mitochondrial fatty acid oxidation in fibroblasts. Biochim Biophys Acta 1993;1180:327–329.
45. Mao LF, Chu C, Luo MJ, et al. Mitochondrial beta-oxidation of 2-methyl fatty acids in rat liver. Arch Biochem Biophys 1995;321:221–228.
46. Stanley CA, Hale DE, Coates PM, et al. Medium-chain acyl-CoA dehydrogenase deficiency in children with nonketotic hypoglycemia and low carnitine levels. Pediatr Res 1983;17:877–884.
47. Iafolla AK, Thompson RJ, Roe CR. Medium-chain acyl-coenzyme A dehydrogenase deficiency: clinical course in 120 affected children. J Pediatr 1994;124:409–415.
48. Poll TBT, Billette DVT, Abitbol M, et al. Metabolic pigmentary retinopathies: diagnosis and therapeutic attempts. Eur J Pediatr 1992;151:2–11.
49. Thompson GN, Hsu YL, Pitt JJ, Treacy E, Stanley CA. Fasting hypoketotic: coma in a child with deficiency of mitochondrial 3-hydroxy-3-methylglutaryl-CoA synthase. New Eng J of Med 1997, in press.
50. Stanley CA, Berry GT, Bennett MJ, et al. Renal handling of carnitine in secondary carnitine deficiency disorders. Pediatr Res 1993;34:89–97.
51. Treem WR, Stanley CA. Massive hepatomegaly, steatosis, and secondary plasma carnitine deficiency in an infant with cystic fibrosis. Pediatrics 1989;83:993–997.
52. Hove JLKV, Zhang W, Kahler SG, et al. Medium chain acyl-CoA dehydrogenase deficiency: diagnosis by acylcarnitine analysis in blood. Am J Hum Genet 1993;52:958–966.
53. Saudubray J, Coude F, DeMaugre F, et al. Oxidation of fatty acids in cultured fibroblasts: a model system for the detection and study of defects in oxidation. Pediatr Res 1983;16:877–881.
54. Coates PM. Mutations causing medium-chain acyl-CoA dehydrogenase deficiency: a collaborative compilation of the data from 172 patients. Prog Clin Biol Res 1992;499–506.
55. Ijlst L, Wanders RJA, Ushikubo S, et al. Molecular basis of long-chain 3-hydroxyacyl-CoA dehydrogenase deficiency: identification of the major disease-causing mutation in the alpha-subunit of the mitochondrial trifunctional protein. Biochim Biophys Acta 1994;1215:347–350.
56. Bennett MJ, Pollitt RJ, Goodman SI, et al. Atypical riboflavin-responsive glutaric aciduria, and deficient peroxisomal glutaryl-CoA oxidase activity: a new peroxisomal disorder. J Inherited Metab Dis 1991;14:165–173.

38
Neonatal Carnitine Metabolism

Charles A. Stanley

Carnitine is a small, water-soluble molecule that plays a key role in transporting fatty acids across the barrier of the inner mitochondrial membrane for β-oxidation. Because of its central role in energy production from fatty acids, there has been considerable interest in the relation of carnitine to the development of fatty acid oxidation during the neonatal period. Information has become available on the role of carnitine in genetic and acquired disorders of fatty acid oxidation that provides some perspective on carnitine physiology in the neonate.[1-5] This topic has been the subject of multiple reviews.[1-5]

Physiology of Carnitine in the Adult Metabolic Role of Carnitine

As shown in Figure 38.1, carnitine participates in transporting long-chain fatty acids across the inner mitochondrial membrane in a three-step cycle involving a carnitine palmityl transferase enzyme associated with the outer aspect of the inner mitochondrial membrane (CPT-1), an inner membrane carnitine translocase, and a second carnitine palmityl transferase associated with the inner side of the inner mitochondrial membrane (CPT-2). Both CPT reactions catalyze the freely reversible exchange of the fatty acid between carnitine and coenzyme A (CoA).

In cells such as the hepatocyte, the entry of fatty acids into the mitochondrial oxidation path is regulated by the levels of malonyl-CoA, the substrate for fatty acid synthesis, which is a non-competitive inhibitor of CPT-1.[6] Fatty acid oxidation is suppressed when fatty acids are being synthesized and can proceed only when fatty acid synthesis is turned off.

Carnitine participates in similar exchange reactions with other CoA derivatives catalyzed by carnitine acetyl transferase in the case of acetyl-CoA or carnitine octanoyl transferase in the case of medium-chain and branched-chain fatty acyl-CoA substrates (Figure 38.2). These reactions may play a role in transporting acetyl and branched-chain acyl groups into and out of the mitochondrial matrix and probably serve the important function of buffering the esterified CoA pool and preventing the depletion of free CoA within the mitochondrial matrix. In peroxisomes, which oxidize very long-chain fatty acids only to the level of octanoic acid (C8), carnitine serves to transfer the octanoic acid into the mitochondria for final oxidation.

The three carnitine acyl-CoA transferase reactions are the only enzymatic reactions known to involve carnitine. In common with other trimethylated amino acid derivatives, it appears that carnitine is not subject to oxidation in the body but is excreted intact, primarily in the urine.

Maintenance of Tissue and Plasma Carnitine Concentrations

In most tissue carnitine concentration within the cell is 10 to 50 times higher than in plasma. In normal adults, plasma total carnitine concentration is 40 to 60 µmol·L^{-1}, whereas muscle total carnitine concentration ranges from 2500 to 3500 µmol·kg^{-1} (nmol·g^{-1}). This very high intracellular concentration of carnitine is achieved by a specific plasma membrane sodium-dependent transport system that couples the carnitine and sodium transmembrane gradients. There appear to be several carnitine transport systems: one for muscle, another for liver, and probably a separate intestinal/renal brush border system.[179] Within the cell, most of the carnitine is contained in the cytosol. Concentrations within the cytosol and mitochondria appear to be similar. Most (80–90%) of the intracellular and extracellular carnitine is in the free, unesterified form. The esterified fraction increases when fatty acid oxidation is activated (e.g., during fasting) and the intracellular acyl CoA/free CoA ratio is elevated.

Because carnitine is a metabolic end product, total body stores of carnitine are regulated by renal excretion.

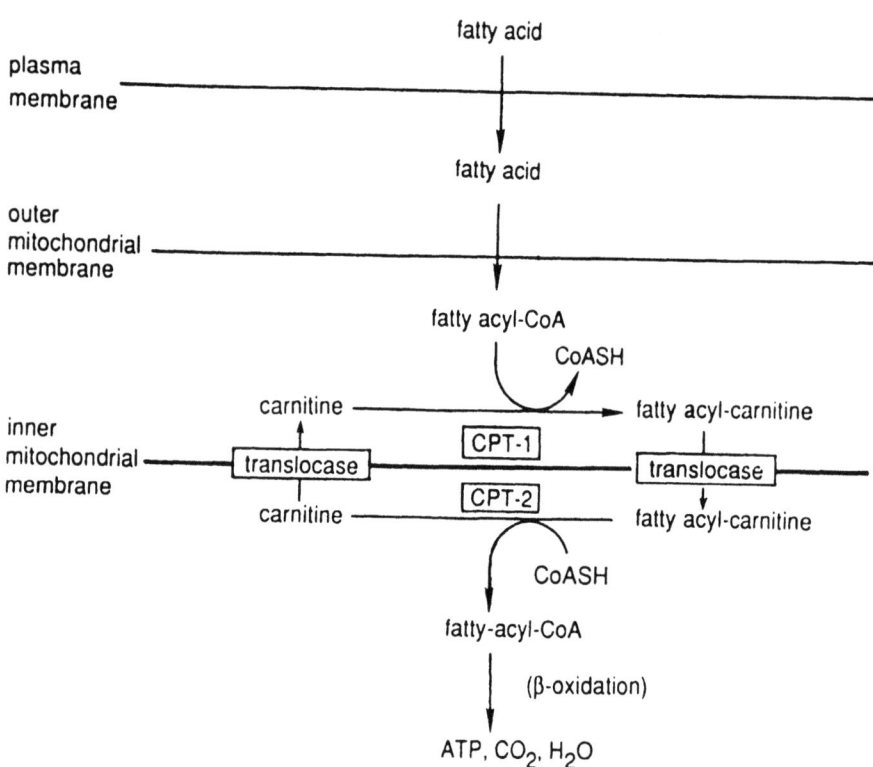

FIGURE 38.1. Role of carnitine in mitochondrial fatty acid oxidation. Carnitine shuttles fatty acids across the inner mitochondrial membrane in a cycle requiring carnitine palmityl transferases on the outer and inner aspect of the inner mitochondrial membrane (CPT-1 and CPT-2) and an inner membrane transport protein, carnitine translocase. Once inside the mitochondrial matrix, fatty acyl-CoA is β-oxidized to produce energy, CO_2, and H_2O.

The renal threshold for free carnitine excretion in adult humans is approximately $35\,\mu mol \cdot L^{-1}$, a value close to the normal plasma concentration.[10] At the normal plasma carnitine concentration, 95% to 98% of the filtered load of free carnitine is reabsorbed. Disorders that impair renal tubular function (e.g., renal Fanconi syndrome) result in lowering the plasma carnitine concentration.

During the 1970s, studies that showed an association between increased carnitine concentration and increased rates of fatty acid oxidation in rat liver during fasting initially suggested that tissue carnitine concentration might play a role in regulating fatty acid oxidation. Further work demonstrated that it was not the case, but that mitochondrial fatty acid oxidation is controlled by malonyl-CoA inhibition of CPT-I activity.[2,6] In addition, it was reported that hepatic fatty acid oxidation is not activated by the increase in carnitine concentration that occurs in the pregnant rat.[11] The significance of the increase in liver carnitine concentration during fasting in the rat remains unclear; it may be a species-specific phenomenon, as the concentration falls during fasting in the guinea pig.[12]

Although a high tissue concentration of carnitine does not increase fatty acid oxidation, there is no clear information as to how low the tissue carnitine concentration must be before fatty acid oxidation is limited. In vitro studies of human and rat tissue homogenates have been interpreted to suggest that fatty acid oxidation might become restricted at a carnitine concentration of about 10% of normal.[5,13] In children with the genetic disorder, primary carnitine deficiency, clinical manifestations of impaired muscle fatty acid oxidation appear to be completely corrected when the tissue carnitine concentration is raised from less than 1% of normal to as little

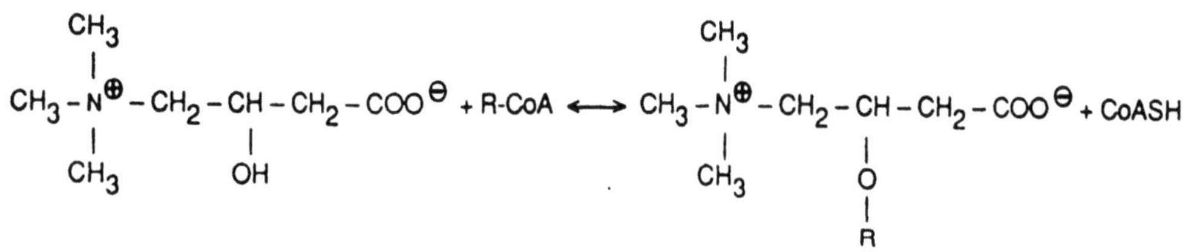

$$CH_3-\overset{CH_3}{\underset{CH_3}{\overset{|}{N^{\oplus}}}}-CH_2-CH(OH)-CH_2-COO^{\ominus} + R\text{-}CoA \longleftrightarrow CH_3-\overset{CH_3}{\underset{CH_3}{\overset{|}{N^{\oplus}}}}-CH_2-CH(O\text{-}R)-CH_2-COO^{\ominus} + CoASH$$

FIGURE 38.2. Reversible carnitine acyl transferase reaction. This reaction is carried out by separate chain-length specific enzymes: acetyl-carnitine transferase for short-chain fatty acids, octanoyl-carnitine transferase for medium-chain fatty acids, and two palmityl-carnitine transferases (CPT-1 and CPT-2) for long-chain fatty acids.

as 5% of normal.[14,15] These data indicate that the normal tissue carnitine concentration greatly exceeds what is required for metabolic pathways (e.g., fatty acid oxidation).

Sources of Carnitine

Diet

Carnitine is present in meats, from which the name carnitine derives, eggs, and milk products. Fruits and vegetables contain no carnitine. The normal adult diet contains 200 to 400 µmol·day^{-1}.[16] These small amounts of carnitine in the diet are efficiently absorbed in the small intestine via a high-affinity but low-capacity transport system. The daily urinary excretion of carnitine approximates the dietary intake, suggesting that exogenous sources account for most of the daily turnover of carnitine.[16] Large oral doses of carnitine are poorly absorbed and may cause mild diarrhea. Breast milk and milk-based infant formulas contain 50 to 100 µmol carnitine·liter^{-1}. Soy-protein formulas are usually supplemented with carnitine to this same level. Most elemental formulas and intravenous alimentation preparations contain no carnitine.

Endogenous Synthesis

Although the diet usually provides most of the daily carnitine turnover, carnitine is not a required nutrient, as it can be synthesized indirectly from lysine.[17] As shown in Figure 38.3, small amounts of lysine residues in protein are posttranslationally methylated to trimethyllysine. During protein degradation, the trimethyllysine residues are released and may be converted to carnitine by the enzyme steps shown in Figure 38.3. Most of this synthetic pathway occurs in muscle. The final step, catalyzed by γ-butyrobetaine hydroxylase, occurs predominantly in the kidney and, to a lesser extent, in the liver in man. The rate of trimethyllysine production appears to be the major determinant of the rate of carnitine biosynthesis.[18]

Human Disorders of Carnitine Deficiency

Discoveries of genetic disorders of fatty acid oxidation associated with carnitine deficiency provide important background for considering the possible role of carnitine in the metabolism of the neonate.[10,19] Primary carnitine deficiency is a recessively inherited defect in the plasma membrane carnitine transporter, which is associated with low (i.e., less than 1–2% of normal) concentrations of carnitine in plasma, heart, and skeletal muscle.[14,15] Patients with this disorder most commonly present after 18 to 24 months of age with gradually progressive cardiomyopathy and skeletal muscle weakness.[20] The separate liver transporter for carnitine appears to be unaffected, and hepatic ketogenesis may function normally in these patients. A few infants have presented at 3 to 12 months of age with fasting, hypoketotic hypoglycemia before manifesting myopathy. In these patients, plasma carnitine concentration was so low that liver carnitine concentration could not be maintained to permit fatty acid oxidation.

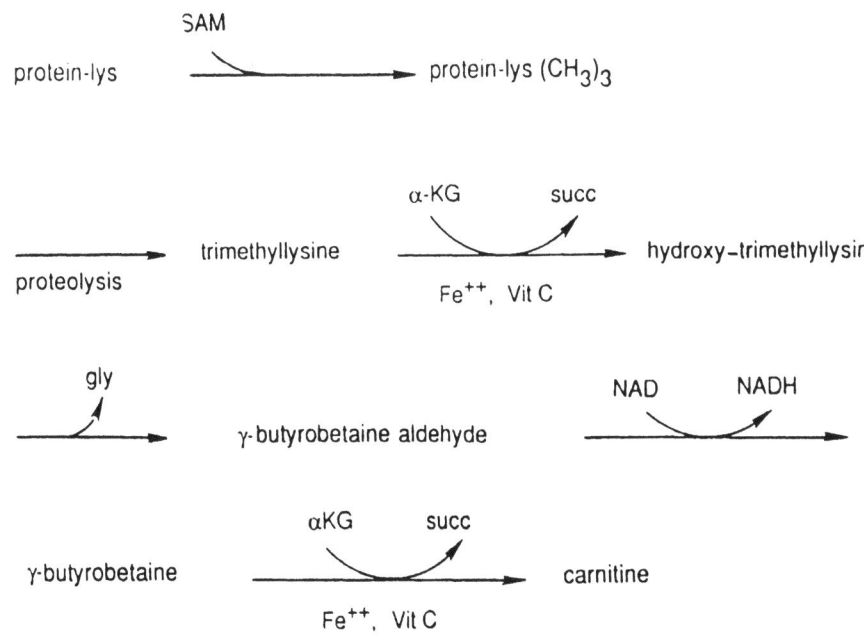

FIGURE 38.3. Pathway of carnitine biosynthesis from trimethyllysine residues in protein. The final step occurs only in kidney and liver. The other steps take place in all tissues, but predominantly in muscle.

Secondary carnitine deficiency is a feature of several genetic defects in which, although carnitine concentration is low, the primary cause of impaired fatty acid oxidation is a deficiency of one of the mitochondrial matrix enzymes required for fatty acid β-oxidation.[5,12] Carnitine concentrations in plasma and tissue are reduced to 25% to 50% of normal in these patients, and carnitine repletion does not correct the impairment in fatty acid oxidation. The mechanism of the secondary carnitine deficiency appears to be due to impaired transport of free carnitine.[21] Most commonly, these patients present at 3 to 24 months of age with episodes of fasting, hypoketotic hypoglycemia, and a marked dicarboxylic aciduria. In a few of these enzyme defects, there may be cardiomyopathy and skeletal muscle weakness. It should be emphasized that these genetic disorders of fatty acid oxidation, whether associated with primary or secondary carnitine deficiency, rarely present during the neonatal period because neonates are not usually exposed to fasts of such a length as to make fatty acid oxidation critical.

Neonatal Carnitine Metabolism

Carnitine and Developmental Changes in Fatty Acid Oxidation

Major developmental changes occur in fatty acid oxidation around the time of birth. The oxidation of fat makes little if any contribution to energy production before birth. After delivery, fat in milk provides 50% to 60% of calories in the human neonate and as much as 90% of calories in the neonatal rat. In the rat and guinea pig, there is a lag in maturation of hepatic fatty acid oxidation for several hours after delivery, primarily because CPT-1 activity is low in the fetus and does not increase to adult values until 12 hours or more after birth.[22-24] By 24 hours of age, hepatic fatty acid oxidation is well developed in the rat and the guinea pig. As a consequence of the high fat content of its diet, the neonatal rat displays a "suckling ketosis" with plasma total ketone concentrations peaking at 2.5 mmol·L^{-1} at 24 hours and remaining elevated to 1.5 mmol·L^{-1} through the first week of life.[11]

The human neonate seems to share some of these developmental changes in fatty acid oxidation, although it is much less dependent on fat as a fuel than the neonatal rat pup. The neonate appears to have a developmental delay in maturation of fatty acid oxidation similar to that in the rat and guinea pig, because neonates who develop fasting hypoglycemia during the first 8 hours of life do not have an appropriate elevation of ketones.[25] It seems likely that this reflects the same lag in the acquisition of CPT-1 activity in the human as in the rat or guinea pig. The ability to oxidize fatty acids seems to mature in the human neonate fairly rapidly after this initial postnatal lag period. Investigations of ketone concentration in neonates who do not receive full feedings until nearly the 5th day of life, show a low concentration during the first 24 hours and then a rise to above 1 mmol·L^{-1} by 24 to 36 hours after birth.[26,27] These data have sometimes been taken to mean that the human neonate manifests a "suckling ketosis" similar to that in the rat. However, studies in well-fed human neonates show plasma β-hydroxybutyrate concentration peaking at only 0.4 mmol·L^{-1} at 20 hours of age and remaining at about 0.2 to 0.3 mmol·L^{-1} through 72 hours of age.[28] The human neonate resembles the neonatal rat pup in terms of having a transient developmental deficit in fatty acid oxidation. Consistent with the differences in fat content of their respective milks, the human neonate differs from the rat by not showing the same extreme dependence on fat metabolism as postnatal feeding becomes established.

Plasma and tissue carnitine concentrations in human neonates and neonatal rats and guinea pigs are shown in Table 38.1. The most dramatic changes in tissue carnitine concentration occur in the rat.[11] In this species, liver carnitine concentration is slightly greater in the term fetus than in the fed adult, increases transiently by 24 hours to a concentration seen in the fasted adult rat, and then declines toward the fed adult concentration through the rest of the suckling period. Two factors may contribute to these changes in liver carnitine concentration. The first is that rat milk has a high concentration of carnitine during the first days of life (Table 38.2). Robles-Valdez et al.[11] have shown that carnitine is transferred from maternal liver through milk to the suckling pup. More important may be the high ketogenic activity of the liver in the rat pup at this time, as liver carnitine concentration is increased in the rat when hepatic fatty acid oxidation is stimulated. In contrast to liver, cardiac muscle carnitine

TABLE 38.1. Plasma and tissue total carnitine concentrations in the neonate.

Subject	Plasma (μmol·L^{-1})	Liver (nmol·g^{-1})	Muscle (nmol·g^{-1})	Heart (nmol·g^{-1})
Human				
Term	20–30	500	1500–2000	500–600
Preterm	20–30	400–500	500–1000	
Adult	40–60	900–1800	2500–3500	
Rat				
Term	40	225	–	175
Days 1–2	40	575	–	275
Days 10–14	40	275	–	625
Adult	50	160	–	650
Guinea pig				
Term	45	930	600	1300
Days 1–2	50	1000	700	1300
Day 10	50	470	850	1500
Adult	35	450	730	1500

Data are from Robles-Valdez et al.,[11] Stanley et al.,[23] Shenai et al.,[29] and Penn et al.,[31] with permission.

TABLE 38.2. Sources of carnitine in the neonate.

Subject	Total carnitine concentration ($\mu mol \cdot L^{-1}$)
Human maternal breast milk	
2–3 Days	73
2 Weeks	70
4 Weeks	65
Infant formulas	
Milk-based	50–150
Soy-based	
Pre-1988	nil
Post-1988	50–150
Special formulas	nil
Intravenous feedings	nil
Other species	
Rat milk	
Day 1	325
Day 3+	75
Cow milk	170
Sheep milk	940
Horse milk	75

Data are from Robles-Valdez,[11] Penn et al.,[32] Rubaltelli et al.,[33] with permission.

concentration is low in the term rat fetus and rises steadily to adult values by the end of the suckling period. The guinea pig, which is much more fully developed at birth than the rat, demonstrates changes in tissue carnitine concentration which roughly parallel those seen in the rat but are much less dramatic.[23] In this animal, heart and skeletal muscle carnitine concentrations are close to adult values at birth.

Limited data in the human, derived from neonates dying before 24 hours of age,[29,30] show slightly lower carnitine concentrations in liver and skeletal muscle compared to adult values. Premature neonates appear to have a slightly lower concentration in skeletal muscle, but similar concentrations in liver and cardiac muscle compared to term neonates. As discussed above, these concentrations of 25% to 50%, or more, of adult values are probably sufficient for fatty acid oxidation. There is no information on tissue concentration of carnitine beyond the first day in the human neonate to compare with the neonatal rat or guinea pig. Plasma total carnitine concentration in human neonates fed breast milk or carnitine-containing milk-based formulas is lower than in adults (25–35 versus 40–60 $\mu mol \cdot L^{-1}$). It most likely reflects a lower renal threshold for free carnitine. Melegh et al.[34] reported that the fractional excretion of free carnitine markedly increased from less than 5% to 30% of the filtered load in neonates whose plasma carnitine concentration was elevated into the normal adult range by feeding a formula supplemented with carnitine to 300 $\mu mol \cdot L^{-1}$.

Table 38.2 shows the sources of carnitine in the neonate. Human breast milk contains modest concentrations of carnitine, averaging 60 to 70 $\mu mol \cdot L^{-1}$. There is little change in breast milk carnitine with duration of nursing and no major difference in breast milk carnitine between mothers of term or premature neonates. In other species, there is a wide variation in milk carnitine content that appears to correlate with fat content, i.e., lowest in horse milk, which contains less than 2% fat, and highest in sheep milk, which contains more than 7% fat.[32] The basis for this relation is not known. Milk-based infant formulas provide greater amounts of carnitine than breast milk. Soy-protein formulas were devoid of carnitine before 1987 but are now supplemented to a concentration similar to that of breast milk. Elemental formulas and intravenous hyperalimentation solutions contain no carnitine.

The capacity to synthesize carnitine is thought to be intact in the human neonate. Although the activity of γ-butyrobetaine hydroxylase, the terminal step in carnitine synthesis, is low in the neonate, it does not appear to be a rate-limiting factor in carnitine biosynthesis.[35]

Carnitine Status of Neonates Fed Carnitine-Free Diets

Although the above data indicate that carnitine stores are probably adequate at birth, there have been several studies suggesting that a normal carnitine concentration cannot be maintained in neonates who are given carnitine-free diets.[36,37] This situation contrasts with that in older children and adults, who maintain a normal carnitine concentration over periods of months to years on carnitine-free diets.[4] Healthy infants fed a carnitine-free soy-protein formula for 3 months had a total plasma carnitine concentration of 20 $\mu mol \cdot L^{-1}$ compared to 50 $\mu mol \cdot L^{-1}$ in controls fed a formula containing carnitine at a concentration equal to that in breast milk.[37] Smith et al.[38] reported that the plasma carnitine concentration fell to a mean of 8 $\mu mol \cdot L^{-1}$ in a group of premature infants with birth weights less than 1000 g after an average of 30 days on carnitine-free oral and intravenous feedings. Less extreme lowering of carnitine concentration was observed in groups of neonates with birth weights greater than 1000 g who were on carnitine-free feedings for shorter lengths of time. In this study, it appeared that an oral carnitine intake of 40 to 60 $\mu mol \cdot day^{-1}$ was required to maintain a normal plasma carnitine concentration. Penn et al.[36] reported that postmortem tissue total carnitine concentration was as low as 20% of normal adult values in premature neonates who had received carnitine-free intravenous feedings for more than 2 weeks.

The clinical implications of low carnitine concentration in neonates fed carnitine-deficient diets have not been established. It is not known how low the tissue carnitine concentration must fall before deleterious effects might occur. As noted above, there are reasons to suspect that tissue carnitine concentration does not become a limiting factor in fatty acid oxidation until it drops to below 5% to 10% of normal.[5] This concentration is a more severe degree of carnitine deficiency than has been demonstrated in neonates. Second, there have been no reports of neonates developing clinical illness due to carnitine-free diets. Assuming that such illness has not been overlooked, it could mean either that neonates do not manifest signs of carnitine deficiency so long as they are otherwise being fed adequately or that, as in patients with primary carnitine deficiency, it takes months to years before clinical manifestations of carnitine deficiency become apparent. Finally, no investigations have been carried out in potentially carnitine-deficient neonates that are capable of demonstrating impairment of a carnitine-requiring process. Some data in neonates have examined ketone responses and the clearance of triglycerides following lipid infusions or the appearance of dicarboxylic acids in urine as an indicator of impaired fatty acid oxidation.[33,39-44] These investigations are difficult to interpret because, as previously emphasized, fatty acid oxidation is not active in the fed state. The discovery of the genetic primary carnitine deficiency disorder has made it clear that dicarboxylic aciduria is not a feature of impaired fatty acid oxidation due to carnitine deficiency.[14,20]

Clinical Correlations

It appears that neonates of all gestational ages have stores of carnitine at birth adequate to carry out fatty acid oxidation. There is a developmental lag in fatty acid oxidation during the first 8 to 24 hours after birth in the human neonate, similar to that in neonatal rats and guinea pigs. It most likely involves developmental changes in the activity of CPT-1, rather than in the tissue reserves of carnitine. After delivery, the neonate is much more dependent on exogenous sources of carnitine to maintain body stores of carnitine than are older children and adults. This fact may reflect a large demand for carnitine to meet the requirements of muscle tissue growth. A daily intake of 30 to 50 μmol carnitine seems sufficient to maintain normal plasma and normal tissue concentrations of carnitine. Breast milk and milk-based formulas contain sufficient carnitine to meet this demand, but intravenous alimentation solutions and some specialized infant formulas may provide no carnitine. Carnitine-free diets for periods of more than 1 to 2 weeks in neonates are likely to result in lower than normal plasma and tissue carnitine concentrations. It is particularly true for premature neonates because they are more likely to require such diets for extended periods. Whether the tissue concentration of carnitine falls low enough to have clinical consequences in the neonate remains speculative. The routine supplementation of soy-protein formulas with carnitine seems reasonable, and consideration should be given to providing carnitine supplements to neonates who require carnitine-free diets for more than a few weeks.

Acknowledgment. This work was supported by National Institutes of Health grants RR-00240 and DK-43841.

References

1. Bremer J. Carnitine—metabolism and functions. Physiol Rev 1983;63:1420–1480.
2. Frankel RA, McGarry JD, eds. Carnitine biosynthesis, metabolism and functions. Orlando: Academic Press, 1980.
3. Rebouche CJ, Paulson DJ. Carnitine metabolism and functions in humans. Annu Rev Nutr 1986;6:41–66.
4. Rebouche CJ. Is carnitine an essential nutrient for humans? J Nutr 1986;116:704–706.
5. Stanley CA. Carnitine disorders. Adv Pediatr 1995;42:209–242.
6. McGarry JD, Mannaerts GP, Foster DW. Characteristics of fatty acid oxidation in rat liver homogenates and the inhibitory effect of malonyl CoA. Biochim Biophys Acta 1978;530:305–313.
7. Vary TC, Neely JR. Characterization of carnitine transport in isolated perfused adult rat hearts. Am J Physiol 1982;242:H585–H592.
8. Christiansen RZ, Bremer J. Active transport of butyrobetaine and carnitine into isolated liver cells. Biochim Biophys Acta 1976;448:562–577.
9. Rebouche CJ, Mack DL. Sodium gradient-stimulated transport of L-carnitine into renal brush border membrane vesicles: kinetics, specificity, and regulation by dietary carnitine. Arch Biochem Biophys 1984;235:393–402.
10. Engel AG, Rebouche CJ, Wilson DM, et al. Primary systemic carnitine deficiency. II. Renal handling of carnitine. Neurology 1981;31:819–825.
11. Robles-Valdez C, McGarry JD, Foster DW. Maternal fetal carnitine relationships and neonatal ketosis in the rat. J Biol Chem 1976;251:6007–6012.
12. Stanley CA. New genetic defects in mitochondrial fatty acid oxidation and carnitine deficiency. Adv Pediatr 1987;34:59–88.
13. Long CS, Haller RG, Foster DW, et al. Kinetics of carnitine-dependent fatty acid oxidation: implications for human carnitine deficiency. Neurology 1982;32:663–666.
14. Treem WR, Stanley CA, Finegold DN, et al. Primary carnitine deficiency due to a failure of carnitine transport in kidney, muscle and fibroblasts. N Engl J Med 1988;319:331–336.
15. Stanley CA, DeLeeuw S, Coates PM, et al. Chronic cardiomyopathy and weakness or acute coma in children with a defect in carnitine uptake. Ann Neurol 1991;30:709–716.
16. Rudman D, Sewall CW, Ansley JD. Deficiency of carnitine in cachectic cirrhotic patients. J Clin Invest 1977;60:716–723.

17. Rebouche CJ. Comparative aspects of carnitine biosynthesis in man. In: Frenkel RA, McGarry JD, eds. Carnitine biosynthesis, metabolism and functions. Orlando: Academic Press, 1980:57–67.
18. Rebouche CJ, Lehman LJ, Olson AL. Epsilon-N-trimethyllsyine availability regulates the rate of carnitine biosynthesis in the growing rat. J Nutr 1986;116:751–759.
19. Roe CR, Coates PM. Acyl-CoA dehydrogenase deficiencies. In: Scriver CR, Beaudet AL, Sly WS, et al., eds. The metabolic basis of inherited disease. 6th ed. New York: McGraw-Hill, 1989.
20. Waber LJ, Valle D, Neill C, et al. Carnitine deficiency presenting a familial cardiomyopathy: a treatable defect in carnitine transport. J Pediatr 1982;101:700–705.
21. Stanley CA, Berry GT, Bennett MJ, et al. Renal handling of carnitine in secondary carnitine deficiency disorders. Pediatr Res 1993;34:89–97.
22. Foster PC, Bailey E. Changes in the activities of the enzymes of hepatic fatty acid oxidation during development of the rat. Biochem J 1976;154:49–56.
23. Stanley CA, Gonzales E, Baker L. Development of hepatic fatty acid oxidation and ketogenesis in the newborn guinea pig. Pediatr Res 1983;17:224–229.
24. Augenfeld J, Fritz IB. Carnitine palmitoyltransferase activity and fatty acid oxidation by livers from fetal and neonatal rats. Can J Biochem 1970;48:288–294.
25. Stanley CA, Anday EK, Baker L, et al. Metabolic fuel and hormone responses to fasting in newborn infants. Pediatrics 1979;64:613–619.
26. Melichor V, Drahota Z, Hahn P. Ketone bodies in the blood of full term newborn, premature and dysurature infants and infants of diabetic mothers. Biol Neonate 1967;11:23–28.
27. Persson B, Gentz J. The pattern of blood lipids and ketone bodies during the neonatal period, infancy and childhood. Acta Paediatr Scand 1966;55:353–362.
28. Anday EK, Stanley CA, Baker L, et al. Plasma ketones in newborn infants: absence of suckling ketosis. J Pediatr 1981;98:628–630.
29. Shenai JP, Borum PR, Mohan P, et al. Carnitine status at birth of newborn infants of varying gestation. Pediatr Res 1983;17:579–582.
30. Shenai JP, Borum PP. Tissue carnitine reserves of newborn infants. Pediatr Res 1984;18:678–681.
31. Penn D, Ludwigs B, Schmidt-Sommerfeld E, et al. Effect of nutrition on tissue carnitine concentrations in infants of different gestational ages. Biol Neonate 1985;471:130–135.
32. Penn D, Dolderer M, Schmidt-Sommerfeld E. Carnitine concentrations in the milk of different species and infant formulas. Biol Neonate 1987;52:70–79.
33. Rubaltelli FF, Orzali A, Rinaldo P, et al. Carnitine and the premature. Biol Neonate 1987;52(suppl):65–77.
34. Melegh B, Szucs L, Kerner J, et al. Changes of plasma free amino acids and renal clearance of carnitine in premature infants during L-carnitine supplemented human milk feeding. J Pediatr Gastroenterol Nutr 1988;7:424–429.
35. Olson AL, Rebouche CJ. γ-Butyrobetaine hydroxylase activity is not rate limiting for carnitine biosynthesis in the human infant. J Nutr 1987;117:1024–1031.
36. Penn D, Schmidt-Sommerfeld E, Pastcu F. Decreased tissue carnitine concentrations in newborn infants receiving total parenteral nutrition. J Pediatr 1981;98:976–978.
37. Novak M, Monkus EF, Buch M, et al. The effect of a L-carnitine supplemented soybean formula in the plasma lipids of infants. Acta Chir Scand Suppl 1983;517:149–155.
38. Smith RB, Sachan DS, Plattsmier J, et al. Plasma carnitine alterations in premature infants receiving various nutritional regimes. J Parenter Enteral Nutr 1988;12:37–42.
39. Sann L, Divry P, Cartier B, et al. Ketogenesis in hypoglycemic neonates: carnitine and dicarboxylic acids in neonatal hypoglycemia. Biol Neonate 1987;25:80–85.
40. Rubecz I, Sandor A, Hamar A, et al. Absence of responses in energy metabolism and respiratory quotient to carnitine infusion in premature infants. Acta Pediatr Hung 1985;26:227–231.
41. Coran AG, Drongowski RA, Baker PJ. The metabolic effects of oral L-carnitine administration in infants receiving total parenteral nutrition with fat. J Pediatr Surg 1985;20:758–764.
42. Yeh YY, Cooke RJ, Zee P. Impairment of lipid emulsion metabolism associated with carnitine insufficiency in premature infants. J Pediatr Gastroenterol Nutr 1985;4:795–798.
43. Rubecz I, Sandor A, Hamar A, et al. Blood levels of total carnitine and lipid utilization with and without carnitine supplementation in newborn infants. Acta Paediatr Hung 1984;25:165–171.
44. Orzali A, Maetzke G, Donzelli F, et al. Effect of carnitine on lipid metabolism in the neonate. II. Carnitine addition to lipid infusion during prolonged total parenteral nutrition. J Pediatr 1984;104:436–440.

39
Neonatal Bilirubin Metabolism

William J. Cashore

Jaundice is a common clinical finding in the neonate. During the first week after birth, visible jaundice may appear in as many as one third of them.[1] For most, clinical jaundice and transient elevation of serum bilirubin concentration are part of the physiologic maturation of bilirubin metabolism and excretion. In some neonates, however, severe or persistent hyperbilirubinemia results from underlying disorders of bilirubin production, conjugation, or excretion.

Bilirubin is the principal breakdown product of heme. Its main source is hemoglobin from senescent red cells, but small amounts of bilirubin are also derived from inefficient red cell production or from other heme-containing proteins.[2] The enzyme heme oxygenase responsible for the extraction of carbon monoxide from the heme ring is widespread in tissue, including brain, liver, spleen, and kidney.[2-4] As shown in Figure 39.1, heme oxygenase converts heme to biliverdin, with extraction of 1 mol of carbon monoxide per mole of biliverdin produced. Biliverdin reductase converts biliverdin to bilirubin, which in its predominant unconjugated form (bilirubin IX-α) is a weakly polar compound with several of its rings internally hydrogen bonded, partially soluble in lipid solvents but poorly soluble in water.[5] In the systemic circulation, unconjugated bilirubin is tightly bound to plasma albumin. In the hepatic microcirculation, albumin transports bilirubin to the space of Disse, where it is released from albumin and taken up at the hepatocyte cell membrane by a receptor protein known as ligandin.[6,7] Ligandin transports bilirubin within the cell to the smooth endoplasmic reticulum, where glucuronosyl transferase catalyzes the addition of glucuronide to the two carboxyl terminals of bilirubin in a stepwise fashion.[8,9] When partially mature, this enzyme system converts bilirubin IX-α to bilirubin monoglucuronide, a form of conjugated bilirubin commonly found in the bile secretions of the neonate and certain animal species. When fully mature, the conjugating system catalyzes the addition of a second glucuronide molecule to form bilirubin diglucuronide, the predominant form of conjugated bilirubin in the older child and human adult.

Most of the circulating bilirubin in the human fetus is unconjugated, because unconjugated bilirubin is sufficiently fat soluble to recross the placenta for maternal metabolism and excretion of bilirubin.[10,11] In the human fetus, this is a more favorable pathway, because the ultimate fate of bilirubin excreted in bile is further conversion in the large and small bowel, with the aid of acquired gastrointestinal flora, to water-soluble bile pigments that are excreted in the stool.[12] Because in fetal life the bowel is neither colonized nor functional, fetal hepatic conjugation of bilirubin would be a futile pathway, with no further opportunity for bilirubin excretion from the blood or bowel. Postnatally, the enzymatic system for conjugation and excretion of "direct" bilirubin matures in parallel with feeding, bowel colonization, and excretion of bile pigments in the stool. As shown in Figure 39.2, the first steps in the excretory process develop by monoglucuronide and diglucuronide formation and sinusoidal excretion into the bile, followed in the small bowel by deconjugation and further modification of the bilirubin to other bile pigments by bacterial and brush border enzymes, and in the large bowel by final conversion of bilirubin to its excretion products.[12] In most neonates, full maturation of this process takes 3 to 7 days. During the time required for this normal pathway to mature, some unconjugated bilirubin may accumulate in the circulation and tissues, resulting in visible jaundice.[1]

Is there a physiologic strategy or evolutionary advantage to this complex pathway for the metabolism and excretion of heme pigments? Alternate pathways for heme pigment excretion can be found in a number of species, and even exist as minor excretory pathways in the human. However, bilirubin and its immediate derivatives and precursors are moderately effective natural antioxidant compounds and may possibly function as antioxidants and free radical scavengers during the initial period of neonatal adaptation from a hypoxemic to a

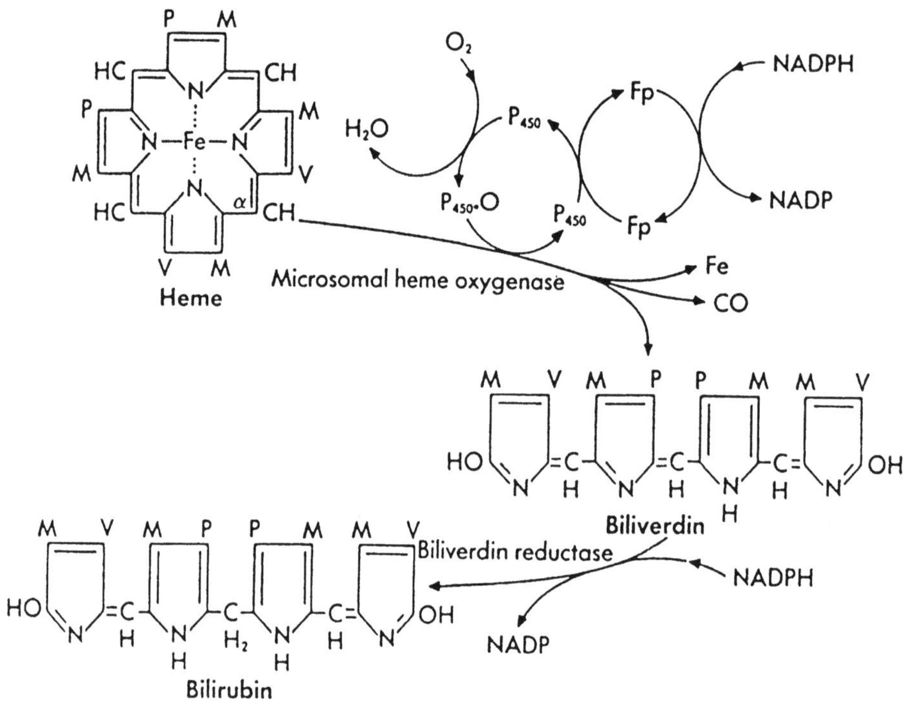

FIGURE 39.1 Formation of biliverdin and unconjugated bilirubin from heme, in a planar representation. (From Tenhunen et al.,[86] with permission.)

relatively hyperoxic environment.[13] The system by which heme binds oxygen and transports it to the tissue may have evolved as part of a defense system as well as a transport system to modulate both the distribution of oxygen to the tissues and the adverse effects of oxygen exposure. Bilirubin, a fat-soluble substance with multiple double bonds, derived from residual portions of the heme ring, may continue to serve an adaptive antioxidant function at "physiologic" concentrations during the immediate neonatal period.[14]

Definitions

Bilirubin: a primary degradation product of heme, via heme oxygenase and biliverdin reductase.

Unconjugated bilirubin: bilirubin IX-α prior to its conjugation as a mono- or diglucuronide, also known in laboratory testing as "indirect-reacting" bilirubin.

Conjugated bilirubin: Bilirubin mono- or diglucuronide. Often equated to "direct" bilirubin in laboratory

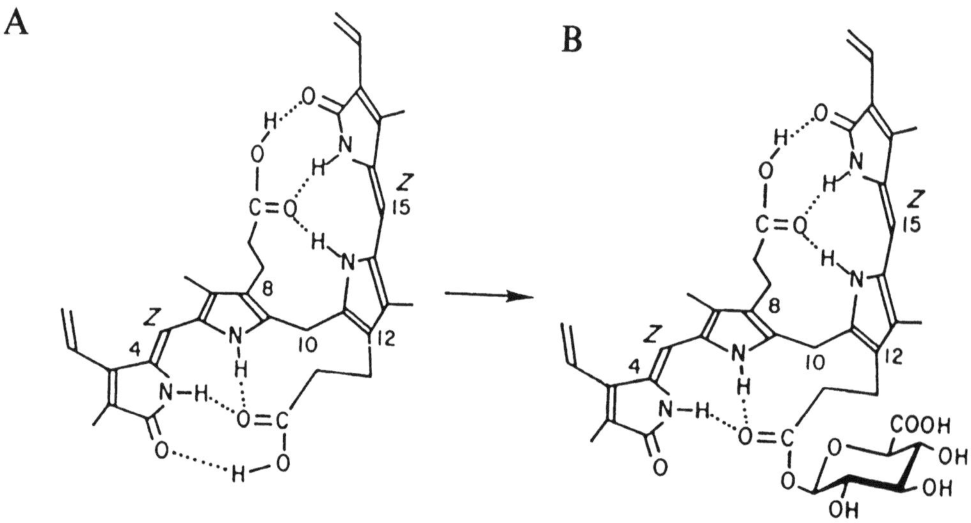

FIGURE 39.2 A: Characteristic structure of unconjugated bilirubin. At physiologic pH, hydrogen bonding between carboxyl and lactam groups maintains the molecule in a *cis* configuration (bilirubin IX-α, Z,Z) which is poorly soluble in water. B: Bilirubin monoglucuronide. Solubility and hepatic excretion of bilirubin are facilitated by conjugation of the carboxyl groups with glucuronic acid or light-induced excitation of the $C_{10}\alpha$-methene bridge, with realignment of the molecule in a more polar *trans* configuration (see text). (From McDonagh et al.,[87] with permission.)

terminology; however, direct bilirubin is not identical to its glucuronide conjugates, because the direct-reacting or water-soluble fraction of plasma bilirubin may contain small amounts of additional water-soluble derivatives.

Glucuronosyl transferase: An enzyme that catalyzes the stepwise addition of glucuronides to unconjugated bilirubin, to form bilirubin mono- and diglucuronides.

Photobilirubin: Isomers of bilirubin IX-α derived from exposure of double bonds in the α-methene bridge to incident light at 425 to 475 nanometers (i.e., "blue" light). These photo derivatives lack internal hydrogen bonds and are more soluble in water and bile than is bilirubin IX-α.

Disorders of Bilirubin Production

Conditions that decrease the red cell life span result in overproduction of bilirubin. The most frequent cause of bilirubin overproduction in the neonate is hemolysis.[2,3] Because the turnover of the fetal red cell is more rapid than that of adult red cell (i.e., 80–90 vs. 115–120 days), the normal physiologic rate of bilirubin production is somewhat higher in the fetus and neonate than in the older child or adult with predominance of hemoglobin A.[2] Nearly all genetically variant hemoglobins, as in the sickling or thalassemia syndromes, and most genetic variations in red cell formation and morphology (e.g., spherocytosis or elliptocytosis), have a decrease in red cell life expectancy and a concomitant increase in bilirubin production. Blood group incompatibility with maternal production of antibody, which attacks the fetal and neonatal red cell, is another source of bilirubin overproduction in the fetus and neonate. The most common scenario for red cell overproduction by antibody-mediated hemolysis is exposure of fetal A or B cells to preexisting anti-A or anti-B antibodies in the plasma of a group O mother. This condition, commonly called ABO incompatibility, is theoretically possible in 20% to 25% of normal pregnancies, but produces clinically detectable hemolysis in only 2% to 3% of neonates.[15] The induction of antibody against fetal red cells by maternal sensitization to the Rh group of antigens is less common, but generally more severe when it does occur. If the fetal red cell carries the predominant "RhD" antigen, but the mother is RhD negative, maternal exposure to fetal cells antenatally or at parturition may induce a maternal anti-D antibody response.

Bacterial sepsis appears to reduce the red cell life span in the neonate, and may impair the excretion of bilirubin from the liver.[16] The role of vertically transmitted viral infection in hemolysis is less certain, although maternal parvovirus infections can produce severe intrauterine hemolysis.[17] Extravascular collections of blood, such as cephalhematomata, bruises acquired during delivery, intraventricular cerebral hemorrhage in the premature, and other forms of enclosed hemorrhage (e.g., subdural, adrenal, peritoneal) may also be significant sources of extravascular red cell destruction and bilirubin production. Certain other pathophysiologic states, such as disseminated intravascular coagulation and acquired splenomegaly, may also decrease the red cell life span.

The rate of bilirubin production in neonates can be approximated by their rate of carbon monoxide production from heme.[2,3] Carbon monoxide production in expired breath increases with increased heme degradation. The rate of carbon monoxide excretion can be calibrated and bilirubin production estimated, since 1 mole of carbon monoxide is released per mole of heme converted to biliverdin. Breath analysis of carbon monoxide can be done noninvasively, but the assay must be calibrated for ambient carbon monoxide concentration. The assay may be less reliable in a setting with a high incidence of air pollution by external carbon monoxide production. Under carefully controlled conditions, carboxyhemoglobin content may also provide indirect estimates of the rate of biliverdin production from heme.[18] Clinical applications of these assays are not well established as indicators to predict jaundice or assist in the management of hyperbilirubinemia in the individual neonate. However, certain categories of neonates with an increased incidence of neonatal hyperbilirubinemia show evidence of increased bilirubin production. These include the premature neonate, the neonate with sepsis or congenital infections, the infant of the diabetic mother, the neonate with inherited disorders of red cell morphology or metabolism, and sometimes the neonate with large extravascular collections of blood.[3]

Neonatal Hyperbilirubinemia

The term hyperbilirubinemia is applied to conditions in which the neonate shows evidence of clinical jaundice that appears earlier than expected, increases above the expected limits of normal for age, or persists beyond the point at which spontaneous resolution of physiologic jaundice is expected.

Most neonatal hyperbilirubinemia appears to be an exaggeration of the normal physiologic accumulation of unconjugated bilirubin in the circulation, presenting a statistical departure from the expected normal pattern of neonatal jaundice, but not associated with a specific disease state. Furthermore, most cases represent only mild departures from the statistical limits of normal, and are not associated with major risk of an untoward outcome. However, the early or persistent appearance of jaundice in a neonate usually attracts the notice of parents and nurses and usually prompts some evaluation of jaundice by the physician caring for the neonate. In some cases, examination and observation are all that is needed. In other cases, however, more detailed clinical and laboratory evaluation are called for.[19] Often, the initial assessment is an attempt to distinguish hemolytic from nonhemolytic hyperbilirubinemia. The evaluation often begins with identification of the maternal blood type and past family history. If the mother is blood group O, the Rh type is negative, or maternal and neonatal blood groups are incompatible, antibody testing of maternal and neonatal specimens is indicated. Hemoglobin, hematocrit, estimation of red cell size, and hemoglobin content, reticulocyte, and peripheral blood smear for red cell morphology may be indicated, especially if anemia is present and hemolysis is suspected. An abnormal physical examination, abnormal morphology of the red cell, or a family history of a particular red cell disorder may prompt additional specific diagnostic tests.[20] In some populations, glucose-6-phosphate dehydrogenase deficiency is common and a potential source of neonatal hemolytic anemia.[17] In a few patients, underlying metabolic diseases, such as galactosemia or hypothyroidism, may present with persistent severe hyperbilirubinemia. There are also some congenital disorders of bilirubin conjugation and excretion, including Crigler-Najjar syndrome types I and II, Gilbert's disease, Dubin-Johnson syndrome, and Lucey-Driscoll syndrome.[9] These are disorders of bilirubin conjugation and transport that are variably inherited and characterized by various degrees of inability of the neonate to metabolize and excrete unconjugated bilirubin.[21-24]

Extensive laboratory evaluation is not justified in every case of neonatal jaundice.[19,20] Many cases that are merely "statistically abnormal" are self-limited and clinically benign. Other cases resulting from mild hemolytic conditions persist longer, but eventually resolve without specific treatment. Observation, reexamination, and reassurance are adequate in many cases. The clinician faced with early or persistent neonatal hyperbilirubinemia, however, should periodically monitor the patient by clinical or laboratory evaluation until the hyperbilirubinemia is resolved. Recent reported cases of bilirubin encephalopathy[25-27] have tended to occur in unobserved patients with somewhat obscure underlying conditions, whose hyperbilirubinemia was not followed after hospital discharge, or in some cases not noted by parents or physicians until a period of severe uncontrolled hyperbilirubinemia had passed.

Breast Milk Jaundice

Mild and persistent jaundice is more common in the breast-fed than in the formula-fed neonate.[1] Because the average serum bilirubin concentration is slightly higher, and the maximum serum bilirubin concentration is reached 1 or 2 days later than in the formula-fed neonate, hyperbilirubinemia is somewhat more often observed in the breast-fed neonate, and the statistical upper limits of "normal" serum bilirubin are somewhat more often exceeded than in the formula-fed neonate. Breast-feeding ought to represent the natural progression and resolution of neonatal jaundice; formula-feeding should be considered the experiment!

The origin of jaundice in the breast-fed neonate appears to be multifactorial.[12,28-30] Compared to the formula-fed neonate, during the first days volume intake may be slightly lower, extracellular and plasma water loss may be slightly higher, and colonization of the small and large bowel may be somewhat delayed. Concentration of the extracellular fluid during the postnatal period of adaptation and weight loss may slightly elevate the observed and measured concentration of plasma and tissue bilirubin. In addition, part of the elimination of bilirubin from the GI tract is achieved by peristalsis, and part by bacterial modification of bile pigments. Stasis of bile products in the underfed and uncolonized small bowel may promote reabsorption of bilirubin from the middle and distal small bowel, a condition known as the enterohepatic recirculation of bilirubin.[12,30] In addition, maternal factors in breast milk may either inhibit the transit of bilirubin through the liver by delaying its conjugation and excretion, or may actively promote the reuptake of bilirubin from the small bowel. These candidate substances in breast milk include multiply unsaturated fatty acids, β-glucuronidases, and hormonal inhibitors of bilirubin conjugation.[28,29] At one time, 3α, 20β-pregnane diol was thought to be a specific inhibitor of bilirubin conjugation ingested in maternal milk and then delaying hepatic metabolism of unconjugated bilirubin.[28] However, clinical confirmation of this and other candidate substances in maternal milk has been difficult to verify consistently. Further clinical evaluation is needed to clarify the symbiosis between maternal milk, bowel colonization, and occasional cases of severe persistent jaundice in the breast-fed neonate. Perhaps some of the antioxidant function of bilirubin noted earlier is preserved by persistence of jaundice in the breast-fed neonate.[13,14]

Bilirubin Toxicity

Unconjugated bilirubin is toxic to the central nervous system.[31-34] The exact mechanism of this toxicity is not known. Bilirubin is poorly soluble in water and somewhat soluble in fat, and has been shown to have affinity for phospholipids in cell membranes. Unconjugated bilirubin is the potentially toxic form, and acute and chronic bilirubin encephalopathy have been reported with severe or prolonged cases of unconjugated hyperbilirubinemia. Although clinically overt bilirubin encephalopathy is rare, it has serious long-term neurodevelopmental consequences when it does occur.[34]

Unconjugated bilirubin can bind to various types of cell membranes, including erythrocyte membranes, fat and skin cells, and neurons. Most of the bilirubin in the circulation and in the extravascular space is bound tightly to albumin.[4,35] In the circulation, albumin acts as a shuttle, transferring bilirubin from its sites of production and accumulation in the tissues to the liver for further metabolism.[5,7] In the extravascular extracellular space, albumin binds bilirubin to remove it from the tissue and carry it into the circulation for ultimate disposal. The binding of bilirubin to albumin is one of the important mechanisms by which it is kept out of the central nervous system.[31,35,36] Albumin extensively and tightly binds bilirubin and is the principal plasma protein for its binding and transport. One mole of albumin binds bilirubin very tightly, a second mole of bilirubin is bound somewhat less tightly, and then nonspecific binding and aggregation may account for the transport of additional bilirubin molecules on albumin.[4,35-38] In the plasma, the albumin concentration may be one of the determinants of maximum achievable serum bilirubin concentration in cases of extremely severe hyperbilirubinemia.

At physiologic and even most supraphysiologic concentrations of bilirubin, the albumin concentration is adequate to bind more than 99% of the bilirubin in the circulation. Small amounts of bilirubin are bound to the red cell membrane and possibly to other protein sites in the plasma, and the concentration of unbound or "free" bilirubin is very low.[31,39-41] "Free" bilirubin is important, however, as the probable medium by which bilirubin distributes between plasma proteins, tissues, and its sites of disposal. Free bilirubin can be displaced if albumin binding is inadequate, or if competing small molecules occupy the albumin binding sites for bilirubin in high concentrations. Examples of this displacement effect exist in clinical medicine as well as in experimental pharmacology.[42-44]

There are several hypotheses for the toxicity of bilirubin to neurons, none of them with enough experimental support at this time to be considered definitive.[34] One hypothesis is that single free bilirubin molecules attach to lipophilic sites on the external cell membrane.[39] As the lipophilic portion of bilirubin binds to the exterior of the cell, hydrophilic groups on the bilirubin molecule insert into the cytoplasm, where they can translocate protons inside the cell. This translocation of protons then causes alterations of charge and cation balance between the exterior and interior of the neuronal plasma membrane. The imbalance of cation concentration and charge would then trigger physiologic dysfunction in the neurons.[45]

The insolubility of bilirubin in water may promote aggregation of bilirubin at the cell surface, causing obstruction or impairment of receptors and ion channels.[4,33,35,41] The tendency of bilirubin to stain some lipid membranes, and the microscopic observation of bilirubin aggregates or crystals in the cell, would be consistent with this hypothesis. Specific biochemical mechanisms attributable to bilirubin precipitation or aggregation in neurons have not been described, but aggregation of bilirubin at receptor sites, transport mechanisms, and ion channels could be expected to produce severe nonspecific physiologic derangement of neurons.

Experimental evidence for the effects of bilirubin on neuronal membranes and metabolism does not yet yield a comprehensive pathophysiologic mechanism for bilirubin toxicity, but does allow for the tentative development of a theoretical framework for bilirubin toxicity, within which certain hypotheses can be tested:

1. Aggregation of bilirubin on membranes: A number of investigators, including Brodersen et al.[35,46] and Vasquez et al.,[47] have shown that bilirubin can bind to phospholipids and translocate to mitochondrial membranes.[48] Both morphologic observations and binding studies confirm the tendency of bilirubin to aggregate or bind to cell surfaces. In cultured neurons and synaptosomes, bilirubin can partition between outer cell and mitochondrial membranes.[48,49]

2. Cation transport: Synaptosomes or cultured cells exposed to external bilirubin showed decreased cation transport, with intracellular sodium and water retention.[50] This observation is consistent with the neuronal swelling seen in the early stages of bilirubin encephalopathy.[51]

3. Effects of bilirubin on membrane integrity. The neuroblastoma cell, exposed to bilirubin, shows a decreased ability for the cell and mitochondrial membranes to exclude trypan blue dye, another indicator of impaired membrane transport and defenses.[48,52]

4. Depolarization and repolarization: Exposure to bilirubin impairs drug or potassium induced depolarization in the synaptosome and hippocampal brain slices.[53-57] Resting potentials are decreased in synaptosomal membranes.[58] In intact synaptosomes and brain slices, action potentials are decreased in response to external depolarization.[56] The uptake of precursor, the synthesis of neurogenic amines, and possibly the reuptake of released neurotransmitters appear to be impaired.[53-57] A possible mechanism for the decrease in resting potential, stimulated depolarization, and neurotransmitter release is the translocation of protons by membrane bilirubin.[39] Both KCl- and veratridine-induced depolarization of synaptic membranes appears decreased, as shown by a decrease in dopamine release and synthesis, as well as by decreased action potentials.[54-56] These observations are consistent

with a decrease in membrane potential, or with a decrease in transport capabilities of the membrane. The exact effect of bilirubin on each part of the neurotransmitter pathway has not been elucidated.

5. Physiologic correlates. Clinical observations in the neonate as well as experimental observations in several species show decreased action potentials in brain slices[56] as well as decreased brain stem auditory evoked responses.[59] In several studies of the neonate, even moderate hyperbilirubinemia modifies the brain stem auditory evoked response,[60-62] and significant impairment of the brain stem auditory evoked response has been seen with severe hyperbilirubinemia.[62,63] Reversal with exchange transfusion or recovery from hyperbilirubinemia has also been seen. In naturally jaundiced Gunn rats, as well as in the experimentally jaundiced rat and piglet, the central components of brain stem auditory evoked response show decrease in amplitude, increase in latency, or both.[59,64,65] These observations are consistent with a deleterious effect of bilirubin on nerve transmission, and with the finding that central deafness is a not uncommon sequel of clinical bilirubin encephalopathy.[66]

Clinical Aspects of Bilirubin Toxicity

As noted above, clinical bilirubin encephalopathy is uncommon, even in the jaundiced neonate. The clinical findings show some overlap with other forms of basal ganglion and brain stem injury, and with dystonic cerebral palsy due to causes other than hyperbilirubinemia. Some biochemical aspects of bilirubin in CNS toxicity have been reviewed above.

The neonate with prolonged exposure to a very high bilirubin concentration has been reported to show decreased activity, tone, and sucking behavior.[67,68] As the clinical syndrome progresses, in a typical case the neonate first shows lethargy, decreased tone, and indifference to feeding or even difficulty with sucking and swallowing. The onset of these findings is usually subtle and gradual. As the clinical syndrome progresses, decreased tone changes to diffuse hypertonia, with rigid extension of the extremities, fisting, and posturing of the arms, crossed extension of the legs, and opisthotonos not relieved by comfort measures and difficult to relieve by flexion. Thrusting of the tongue and a high-pitched cry are observed, sometimes evolving into clinically overt seizures. Some neonates die during the acute stages of bilirubin encephalopathy. The survivors undergo a period of hypertonia and opisthotonos lasting several hours to several days, followed by hypotonia, lethargy, and poor responsiveness to handling and stimulation. The neonate so affected may be difficult to arouse and very difficult to feed. Hypotonia and developmental delay may persist for 3 to 6 months, usually then followed by the evolution of movement disorders and cranial nerve dysfunction toward the end of the first year.[69] The long-term outcome includes choreoathetosis, spasticity, and ataxic gait with overflow movements, and cranial nerve dysfunction including drooling and difficulty with swallowing, slurred speech, dyscoordination of eye movements, and central deafness.[69]

Careful study yields some clues of prodromal bilirubin effects on the central nervous system before overt bilirubin toxicity develops. Acoustic cry analysis shows subtle dyscoordination of the cry at a bilirubin concentration normally considered to have no long-term effect, and before a neurologically abnormal cry becomes obvious.[61,67] Recording of brain stem evoked responses shows decreased amplitude, prolonged central auditory brain stem conduction, or both in the moderately jaundiced neonate.[61-63] The moderately to severely jaundiced neonate also has subtle changes in auditory orientation responses. In the neonate, suppressed brain stem auditory evoked responses tend to normalize posttreatment for severe hyperbilirubinemia, and the neonate with a history of moderate to moderately severe neonatal hyperbilirubinemia seldom shows signs of permanent hearing loss.[19,62,63]

Some of the effects of acute bilirubin toxicity can be reproduced in the animal model, although no model completely reproduces the syndrome as seen in the human. Administration of exogenous bilirubin in high doses to the piglet results in suppression of brain stem auditory responses, extreme lethargy and hypotonia, and sometimes death with seizures, pulmonary edema, and pulmonary hemorrhage despite apparently normal pulmonary gas exchange before these events occur.[59] The artificially jaundiced laboratory rat and homozygous Gunn rat also show impaired auditory brain stem conduction, which in the case of the Gunn rat can be aggravated by the administration of small molecules that displace bilirubin (e.g., sulfonamides).[64] Some homozygous Gunn rats die with acute bilirubin encephalopathy at approximately 2 to 4 weeks of age. Others survive with persistent jaundice, ataxia, and impaired brain stem conduction.

Although most cases of bilirubin encephalopathy occur in the neonatal period, and most cases of bilirubin-related cerebral palsy are sequelae of severe neonatal hyperbilirubinemia, bilirubin encephalopathy can occasionally manifest as a chronic disorder or an acute disorder of later onset. Nearly all cases of type I Crigler-Najjar syndrome (i.e., congenital unconjugated hyperbilirubinemia) develop clinical signs of bilirubin encephalopathy later in life, even if overt encephalopathy was avoided by treatment during the neonatal period.[9] Occasional acquired cases of unconjugated hyperbilirubinemia produce acute bilirubin encephalopathy in the older child or young adult. Chronic or recurrent encephalopathy involving brain stem and cerebellum function has been reported in some patients with Crigler-Najjar syndrome, in a pattern different from the classic pattern of neonatal bilirubin encephalopathy.[70] Some of these patients develop sudden elevations of serum unconjugated bilirubin during unrelated illnesses (e.g., viral infections). With these sudden elevations of unconjugated bilirubin, they show deterioration of cerebellar and brain stem function. The resulting disabilities are sometimes transient rather than permanent, and tend to stabilize with resolution of the intercurrent illness and lowering of the serum bilirubin concentration. Eventually, nearly all individuals with a complete inability to conjugate bilirubin IX-α demonstrate some type of neurologic impairment unless they undergo liver transplantation.

From the range of abnormal findings just described, the clinician may inquire whether neonatal hyperbilirubinemia can result in subtle or minimal signs of chronic CNS dysfunction in later life. Most neurodevelopmental follow-up studies, however, do not show evidence for a dose-related syndrome of minimal brain damage related to a history of neonatal hyperbilirubinemia.[19,20,71] The clinical outcome for most cases of physiologic neonatal hyperbilirubinemia appears to be benign.

Low-Bilirubin Kernicterus

An unsolved problem in the evaluation of bilirubin toxicity is the unexpected appearance of basal ganglion staining and pathology in some minimally jaundiced high-risk neonates.[40,44,72,73] These findings were first reported in the high-risk premature neonate, who received standard therapy or sometimes no therapy at all for a serum bilirubin concentration generally considered physiologic and harmless. At autopsy, however, some neonates had bilirubin staining and histologic damage to the hippocampus and basal ganglia in the "classic" distribution and pattern seen in kernicterus.[74] For a time, multiple efforts were made to explain or prevent low-bilirubin kernicterus in high-risk and low birth weight neonates by the introduction of clinical tests for the binding of bilirubin to albumin, the early use of exchange transfusions, administration of albumin to increase bilirubin binding in the plasma, or the use of prophylactic phototherapy or medications to prevent hyperbilirubinemia or promote increased bilirubin excretion. However, the phenomenon of low-bilirubin kernicterus has never been satisfactorily explained. The condition was a frequent autopsy finding in some centers, but in others was seldom seen.

Efforts at classifying levels of risk according to birth weight, clinical condition, serum albumin concentrations, or experimental bilirubin binding tests proved impractical.[26,40,41] Some centers reported a high frequency of autopsy deaths diagnosed with low-bilirubin kernicterus, while other centers seldom encountered the problem. During the 1980s, the condition began to disappear from low birth weight autopsy series[75] without a suitable explanation for its occurrence or disappearance. In addition, few surviving low birth weight infants with bilirubin concentrations in the range sometimes considered hazardous, or with other conditions thought to increase the risk of low-bilirubin kernicterus, have shown any of the classic signs of postkernicteric bilirubin encephalopathy on neurodevelopmental follow-up. It is probable that the finding of low-bilirubin kernicterus in some autopsies represented agonal or postmortem staining of areas perhaps predisposed or previously damaged by hypoxic, ischemic, or toxic insults of another sort.[76] Although it is possible that low-bilirubin kernicterus was a uniformly fatal disorder when it occurred in the very high risk neonate, that conclusion seems unlikely in view of the general absence of postkernicteric abnormal neurologic findings in the low birthweight follow-up clinic.

The lack of a suitable explanation for low-bilirubin kernicterus and the virtual disappearance of this condition from autopsies of the high-risk infant also underscores the lack of a sound scientific basis for clinical management recommendations that stratify the neonate into risk groups by weight, clinical complications, or serum bilirubin and albumin concentrations.[26,77] Although various published recommendations to intervene earlier and at a lower serum bilirubin concentration in the high-risk neonate are still sometimes followed, many of the past and current algorithms for earlier treatment of the high-risk jaundiced neonate do not have adequate scientific or epidemiologic validation.

Evaluation and Management of Unconjugated Hyperbilirubinemia

Although bilirubin encephalopathy is now rare, it was common before treatment of severe hyperbilirubinemia secondary to Rh disease and other hemolytic states became possible. It is still important to identify, diagnose, and if possible, predict cases of severe neonatal hyperbilirubinemia to manage them preventively.

Inspection for the early onset or rapid progression of neonatal jaundice often leads to appropriate investigation in the immediate neonatal period. Jaundice that is readily apparent on the first hospital day, or resulting from known hemolytic states, should be followed with reexamination of the patient and appropriate laboratory studies. During prenatal care, the mother's blood type and Rh group should be determined. The Rh negative mother receives Rh immune antiglobulin at approximately 28 weeks' gestation, and again at term if her neonate is Rh positive. After birth, jaundice of early onset should prompt examination of the neonate for hepatosplenomegaly and review of the mother's and neonate's blood types. Routine blood typing of the neonate is not needed, but a cord or neonatal blood specimen should be reserved for determination of the neonate's blood type when requested.

The most common form of neonatal hemolytic jaundice, as noted above, is maternal versus fetal ABO incompatibility.[15] Although 20% to 25% of pregnancies are potentially at risk, only a minority of neonates are affected, most of them mildly. Hemolytic disease related to incompatibilities in the Rh antigen-antibody system tends to be more persistent and more severe. Unexpected, but sometimes severe, hyperbilirubinemia can also occur with red cell disorders such as glucose-6-phosphate dehydrogenase deficiency, heredity spherocytosis, and systemic metabolic disorders such as galactosemia.

Inspection of the neonate for jaundice on the first day or later for jaundice extending below the umbilicus will often lead the clinician to request measurements of total and direct bilirubin concentrations in the serum. If jaundice is present at birth, or if the serum bilirubin increases at a rate of more than 5 to $6\,mg\cdot dl^{-1}day^{-1}$, follow-up bilirubin determination and further studies for neonatal hemolysis are indicated. In some cases, serum bilirubin concentration reaches an early peak, and then sustains a plateau concentration that is still in a clinically acceptable range and requires no treatment. In others, hyperbilirubinemia increases persistently during the postnatal period. Serum bilirubin increasing more rapidly than 5 to $6\,mg\cdot dl^{-1}day^{-1}$, reaching a concentration of 12 to $15\,mg\cdot dl^{-1}$ during the first 48 hours, or exceeding $20\,mg\cdot dl^{-1}$ at any time, needs closer follow-up and often needs to be treated.

Neonatal hyperbilirubinemia is predominantly of the indirect reacting variety. Typical laboratory concentrations show an indirect fraction in the single numbers or teens, and a direct fraction $<1\,mg\cdot dl^{-1}$. In a few laboratory systems, the normal neonate may have a direct reacting fraction, slightly exceeding $1\,mg\cdot dl^{-1}$ but never greater than 15% of the total bilirubin. If the patient has indirect hyperbilirubinemia without obstructive liver disease, this slightly elevated direct fraction remains stable during the clinical course of the neonate's jaundice, and resolves as the indirect hyperbilirubinemia improves.

Antibody testing is indicated if blood group incompatibility is suspected. The direct antiglobulin test reacts the neonatal cell against an anti–human globulin to determine the presence of an antibody on the neonate's cells. The indirect antiglobulin test can be performed on neonatal or maternal serum, and reacts the serum against a panel of susceptible cells that agglutinate if a specific plasma antibody is present. In general, a positive direct antibody test is more diagnostic and predictive of hemolysis and hyperbilirubinemia than an indirect antiglobulin test, which documents the presence of an identifiable antibody in serum without proving that the antibody is an actual cause of neonatal hemolysis.

Treatment

Table 39.1 summarizes an incremental approach to the evaluation and management of neonatal jaundice in different birth weight categories. Although, as noted above, optimal bilirubin concentration for preventive or therapeutic intervention in the low birth weight neonate has never been reliably validated, it remains standard practice in most centers to evaluate and treat jaundice at a lower concentration in the premature than in the term neonate. This approach is maintained because of possible blood-brain barrier immaturity, lower mean plasma albumin concentration, and a longer clinical course of hyperbilirubinemia in the preterm neonate. In the low birth weight neonate, decisions to perform exchange transfusions should be individualized on the basis of available clinical and laboratory information, rather than constrained to specific formulas based on birth weight or bilirubin concentration.

For indirect hyperbilirubinemia from any cause, phototherapy is the initial treatment of choice.[78] Phototherapy in the blue part of the visible light spectrum excites the central double bonds of the bilirubin molecule, converting it to isomerized and more water-soluble forms that can be excreted from the liver without conjugation.[79,80] The production of photobilirubin depends on the intensity and wavelength distribution of light, the distance from the skin, and the amount of skin exposed. The initial isomerization phase is rapid, followed by a slower equilibration phase between the tissues and plasma and between the plasma and liver. The canalicular excretion phase may be rate limiting for the actual clinical effect of phototherapy in lowering serum bilirubin. Because the isomerization phase is rapid and persists for some time after the light source is re-

TABLE 39.1. Suggested guidelines of management of hyperbilirubinemia.

Weight	First BR	Phototherapy	Exchange Tx
≤750	Day 1	~5 mg%	>10 mg%
≤1000	Day 1	5–6 mg%	>10–12 mg%
≤1250	Day 1	6–7 mg%	12–15 mg%
≤1500	Day 1 or 2	8–10 mg%	>15 mg%
≤1750	Day 2 or when jaundiced	10–12 mg%	16–20 mg%
≤2000	When jaundiced	>12 mg%	~20 mg%
≤2500	When jaundiced	14–15 mg%	>20–25 mg%
≥2500	When jaundiced	16–20 mg%	≥22–25 mg%

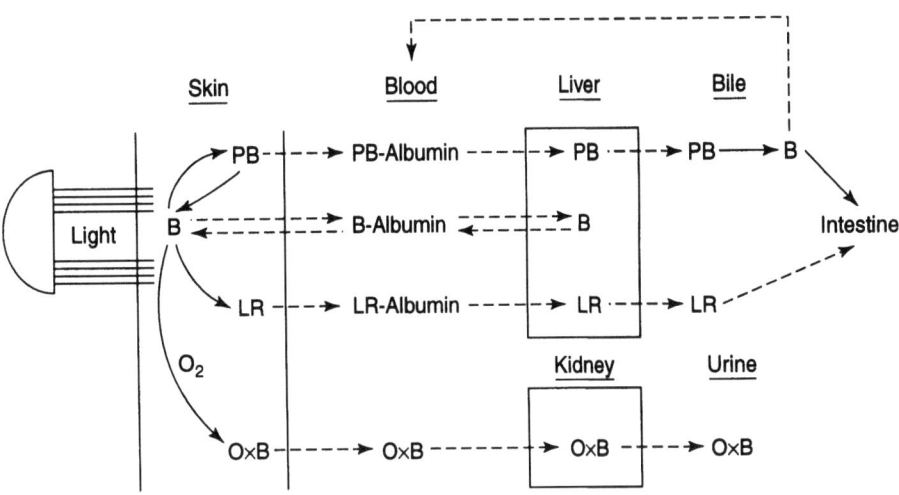

FIGURE 39.3 The cascade of phototherapy effects on the structure, distribution, and excretion of bilirubin. B, bilirubin IX-α (Z,Z configuration); PB, photobilirubin (E and Z isomer); LR, lumirubin (stable photo product); O_xB, bilirubin oxidation products. (From McDonagh et al.,[87] with permission.)

moved, intermittent phototherapy with high-intensity light is adequate and appropriate if the baby needs to be removed from the lights occasionally for feeding, diaper changes, etc. Figure 39.3 summarizes the effect of phototherapy on the structural rearrangement, distribution, and excretion of bilirubin and its photo-products.

Phototherapy does not alleviate or reverse the effects of hemolysis. In severe hemolytic states, phototherapy tends to be inadequate to control the serum bilirubin concentration completely within acceptable levels. Severe hemolytic states should also be treated with exchange transfusion, which more promptly lowers the high serum bilirubin concentration, replaces susceptible and damaged red cells with a red cell type not susceptible to the hemolytic influence, and partially lowers the antibody titer in the plasma. Even when exchange transfusion is planned, the neonate with severe jaundice should be treated with phototherapy to modify the course of his hyperbilirubinemia both before and after the exchange transfusion.

In hemolytic states, criteria for exchange transfusion include jaundice and anemia at birth, rapid postnatal increase in serum bilirubin, or indirect serum bilirubin concentrations exceeding $20\,mg\cdot dl^{-1}$ in the first few days after birth. The combination of exchange transfusion and phototherapy can be highly effective in maintaining serum bilirubin concentration below a "dangerous" range, and may be lifesaving in some instances. The two treatments, phototherapy and exchange transfusion, should be considered complementary rather than alternative treatments in severe hemolytic states. The occasional neonate with severe nonhemolytic hyperbilirubinemia (22–25 mg·dl^{-1} indirect bilirubin, or higher) should also be treated with exchange transfusion for prompt lowering of the excessive serum bilirubin levels, especially if the neonate has had unexpected onset of severe hyperbilirubinemia without close follow-up. In such cases, evaluation of the hyperbilirubinemia should proceed along with preparations for an exchange transfusion. Intensive phototherapy may be attempted, but exchange transfusion should be done within a few hours if the phototherapy by itself does not progressively lower serum bilirubin to a more acceptable concentration.[81]

Some breast-fed neonates with severe hyperbilirubinemia are nutritionally compromised, and a few are even dehydrated. The preferred route of rehydration is oral for most of these neonates, although initial IV hydration may be appropriate in a few with clinical dehydration. Prompt recognition of severe "breast milk jaundice" and treatment with phototherapy and adequate refeeding often reverse the trend in such neonates within a few hours, without the need for exchange transfusion. In a few neonates with jaundice related to breast-feeding, severe hyperbilirubinemia persists and requires an exchange transfusion.

Genetic Disorders of Bilirubin Metabolism

The hepatic conjugation of bilirubin is controlled by a gene complex on chromosome 2, at 2q37 (Figure 39.4). A family of glucuronosyl transferase isoforms with specific or related substrates is coded by exons 2 to 5 for a common carboxy terminal region, responsible for uridinediphosphoglucose (UDPG) binding to the enzyme, and by exons 1.1 to 1.7 for variable N-terminal regions, specific for bilirubin, phenols, and related anions and drugs that are bound to the N-terminal domain of the enzyme protein in the process of conjugation.[9,24] The isoform predominantly responsible for conjugation of bilirubin is termed UGT-1.[22] Activity of this enzyme matures gradually from mid-gestation until the adult level is reached several months after term. At birth, it is not yet fully mature. In the normal neonate and in the patient with certain mutations of UGT-1, increased enzyme activity is inducible by phenobarbital and some related small

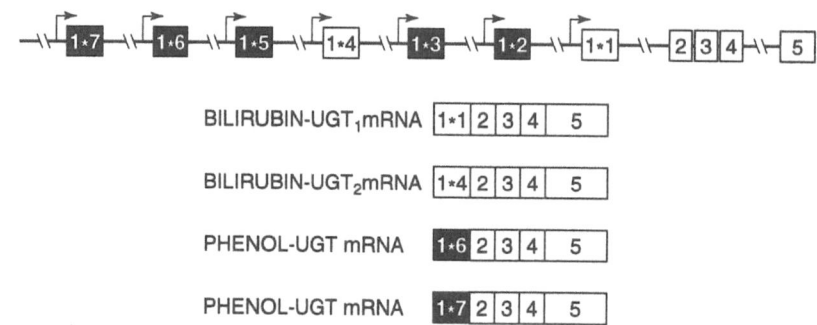

FIGURE 39.4 Diagram of the gene for glucuronide conjugation of bilirubin and related substrates. Exon 1.1, which codes specifically for the N-terminal peptide of bilirubin UDPGT-1, is one of at least seven identified exons (1.1–1.7) that code for N-terminal binding of bilirubin and other small molecules (e.g., phenols, drugs) in glucuronidation reactions. Exons 2–5 code for the carboxy terminal, which binds UDP glucuronic acid. (From Roy Chowdbury et al.,[9] with permission.)

molecules or perhaps by exposure to increased concentrations of unconjugated bilirubin. An isoform known as UGT-2 can be induced by phenobarbital to conjugate bilirubin in vitro, but generally appears to be physiologically inactive or ineffective in vivo, thus leaving its true physiologic role in bilirubin metabolism uncertain.[24]

Mutations can occur at several loci on the UGT-1 gene, and have been reported in exons 1, 2, and 4. Mutations of exon 1 alter the preference or affinity of the enzyme for bilirubin; mutations of exons 2 to 5 alter the enzyme's affinity for UDP glucuronide. In general, missense mutations or amino acid substitutions alter the enzyme's affinity or inducibility, while nonsense or stop mutations prevent synthesis or abolish activity of the enzyme.[9,21-24] Three phenotypes of congenital unconjugated hyperbilirubinemia correspond to several different reported mutations of the UGT-1 gene. These are summarized in Table 39.2.

Gilbert's disease presents with mild, recurrent unconjugated hyperbilirubinemia during both infancy and adult life. Patients with Gilbert's syndrome have been described with missense mutations in exons 1, 4, and 5, probably decreasing either synthesis of the enzyme or its affinity for bilirubin and UDP glucuronide. Patients heterozygous for these mutations should in theory have about 50% of normal activity and no clinical disease, but a number of recently reported heterozygous cases expressed only 14% to 30% of normal enzyme activity, inviting the conclusion that heterozygosity for the mutations of Gilbert's syndrome may downregulate bilirubin conjugation in a "dominant negative" fashion.[21]

Clinically, patients with Gilbert's syndrome have mild recurrent indirect hyperbilirubinemia that tends to be exaggerated by intercurrent illness (e.g., viral infections) and improved by administration in low doses of phenobarbital, which increases the activity of the conjugating

TABLE 39.2. Genetic errors in bilirubin conjugation.

Disorder	Gene defect(s)	Metabolic defect	Phenotype	Induction by phenobarbital	Inheritance
Crigler-Najjar syndrome, type I	Nonsense or "stop" mutations in the gene for UDPGT-1	No UDGPT-1 is synthesized, and no bilirubin glucuronides are produced	Permanent, severe unconjugated hyperbilirubinemia (25–45 mg·dl^{-1}); kernicterus in most cases	No	Autosomal recessive
Crigler-Najjar syndrome, type II	Missense mutations in UDPGT-1	Decreased enzyme synthesis and glucuronide formation (<10%)	Persistent, moderate hyperbilirubinemia (5–15 mg·dl^{-1}) kernicterus is uncommon	Yes (partial improvement)	Autosomal recessive
Gilbert's disease	Minor amino acid substitutions in UDPGT-1	Decreased enzyme activity (<50%) and possibly impaired binding of enzyme to substrates	Mild, recurrent hyperbilirubinemia (3–5 mg·dl^{-1})	Yes (substantial improvement)	Generally considered autosomal recessive, but a "negative dominant" effect is reported in some heterozygotes

enzymes. In all other respects, patients with this syndrome appear entirely normal and well. Gene mutations consistent with Gilbert's syndrome appear quite common, with 2% to 5% of the adult population estimated to be heterozygous for this trait.

Crigler-Najjar syndrome is a much rarer disorder of bilirubin conjugation, with two phenotypes, currently classified as Crigler-Najjar syndrome type I and type II (CN-I and CN-II). CN-I is a rare autosomal recessive disorder characterized by complete absence of bilirubin UDP-glucuronosyl transferase activity.[9,23] In some cases, UDPG-T isoforms for other substrates, such as phenols, are defective. Liver function is otherwise normal, except for the patient's inherited inability to conjugate bilirubin and sometimes other substrates. Severe hyperbilirubinemia appears in the neonatal period and persists throughout life. Most patients develop bilirubin encephalopathy, either as a neonate or later. Possible approaches to treatment include daily phototherapy and liver transplantation. Gene therapy is not yet possible, although the gene has been identified. Inheritance is autosomal recessive. CN-II is also rare and autosomal recessive.[9] Enzyme synthesis and activity are markedly decreased, but partly inducible by phenobarbital. The patient with CN-II develops persistent mild to moderate unconjugated hyperbilirubinemia beginning in the neonatal period, but kernicterus is uncommon.

The Lucey-Driscoll syndrome[9,78] appears to be an acquired but familial defect in bilirubin conjugation caused by a circulating inhibitor of glucuronyl transferase activity in maternal and neonatal plasma. Although the origin of the inhibitor is not known, familial recurrence is reported. The mother does not have signs of jaundice or liver disease. Neonatal jaundice may be severe and persistent, occasionally causing encephalopathy. After exchange transfusion, or with increasing postnatal age, the condition gradually resolves.

Conjugated (Direct) Hyperbilirubinemia

Some cases of neonatal conjugated hyperbilirubinemia are artifactual, since 15% of total bilirubin may show a direct reaction in jaundiced plasma. Among actual clinical cases of neonatal direct hyperbilirubinemia, approximately 50% are idiopathic and appear clinically benign.[82] In these cases, the direct-reacting bilirubin concentration in the serum remains elevated at 2 to 3 mg·dl^{-1} for several weeks after birth, but with no other signs of liver disease.

As shown in Table 39.3, neonatal conjugated hyperbilirubinemia has multiple causes. Some cases are secondary to intrahepatic inflammatory conditions or metabolic errors, and others are caused by primary or secondary obstruction of the biliary collecting system.

In the evaluation of neonatal direct hyperbilirubinemia, a useful distinction can be made between obstructive and hepatocellular cholestasis.[82] Obstruction may be anatomical or postinflammatory. Obstructive cholestasis generally progresses to a very high direct bilirubin concentration, with loss of stool pigment and minimal or no response to phenobarbital. Hepatocellular cholestasis may be postinflammatory, toxic, or metabolic. It is more likely to be mild to moderate, with a modest and more static increase in serum direct bilirubin, the appearance of some bile pigment in the stools, and often a partial or complete response to phenobarbital. Important to remember, however, is that chronic or recurrent inflammation of the liver from any cause may eventually lead to cirrhosis with scarring and obstruction to bile flow.

Ultrasonographic imaging of the liver is often useful to confirm the presence or absence, and location, of anatomical obstruction.[83] If the biliary tree is intact by ultrasound and the stools are pigmented, obstructive cholestasis is unlikely. If contrast imaging studies are indicated, the canalicular transport system is often primed with low-dose phenobarbital, and phenobarbital adminis-

TABLE 39.3. Neonatal hepatobiliary disorders.

Hepatocellular cholestasis
  Genetic and metabolic disorders
    α_1-antitrypsin deficiency
    Alagille's syndrome
    Cystic fibrosis
    Tyrosinemia
    Neonatal iron storage disease
    Fructose intolerance
    Galactosemia
    Storage diseases (Gaucher's, Niemann-Pick, Wilson's)
    Inborn errors of bile acid metabolism
    Posthemolytic "inspissated bile syndrome"
    Iatrogenic (TPN)
  Inflammatory (infectious) disorders
    Hepatitis (A,B,C,D, nonspecific)
    Herpesvirus hominis
    Cytomegalovirus
    Rubella
    HIV
    Toxoplasmosis
    Syphilis
    Bacteremia (usually gram-negative)
Noncholestatic syndromes
  Dubin-Johnson syndrome
  Rotor syndrome
Ductal cholestasis
  Biliary hypoplasia
  Biliary atresia[a]
  Choledochal cyst

[a] This may be postinflammatory, secondary to an intrauterine infection or other antenatal or perinatal inflammatory process.[85]

tration may begin to lower serum direct bilirubin, further supporting evidence for the presence of hepatocellular rather than ductal cholestasis. In a minority of cases of neonatal cholestasis, needle biopsy of the liver may be required for anatomical confirmation and prognostic staging of the cholestasis.

At present, the most common cause of neonatal hepatocellular cholestasis is iatrogenic, secondary to prolonged supplemental or total parenteral nutrition in the high-risk neonate. The mechanism for this manifestation of cholestasis is not known, but the condition appears both with and without the administration of intravenous fat emulsion. Fortunately, most cases resolve after discontinuation of the parenteral nutrients.

Ductal cholestasis is most often caused by anatomical obstruction or malformation of the intrahepatic or extrahepatic biliary collecting system. A choledochal duct cyst may obstruct bile flow at the level of the gallbladder. Biliary atresia is caused by malformation or destruction of the terminal collecting system, which fails to exit normally into the common bile duct. Chronic obstructive cholestasis leads to retention of biliary secretions, including retention of bile acids, which prolong and extend intrahepatic cellular and cirrhotic changes. A corrective operation or diversion procedure within 4 to 6 weeks of onset is often necessary to accomplish biliary drainage and ameliorate the chronic and progressive inflammatory changes caused by prolonged retention of bile acids. Liver transplantation may be the long-term therapy of choice for otherwise uncorrectable forms of congenital obstructive cholestasis.[84]

References

1. Maisels MJ, Gifford KL. Normal serum bilirubin levels in the newborn and the effect of breastfeeding. Pediatrics 1987;78:837–843.
2. Maisels MJ, Patlak A, Nelson NM, et al. Endogenous production of carbon monoxide in normal and erythroblastotic newborn infants. J Clin Invest 1971;50:1–13.
3. Bartoletti AL, Stevenson DK, Ostrander CR, et al. Pulmonary excretion of carbon monoxide in the human infant as an index of bilirubin production I. Effects of gestational age and postnatal age and some common neonatal abnormalities. J Pediatr 1979;94:952–955.
4. Rodgers PA, Stevenson DK. Developmental biology of heme oxygenase. Clin Perinatal. 1990;17:275–291.
5. Brodersen R. Aqueous solubility, albumin binding, and tissue distribution of bilirubin. In: Ostrow JD, ed. Bile pigments and jaundice. New York: Marcel Dekker, 1986:157–181.
6. Sorrentino D, Berk PD. Mechanistic aspects of hepatic bilirubin uptake. Semin Liver Dis 1988;8:119–136.
7. Levi AG, Gatmaitan Z, Arias IM. Two hepatic cytoplasmic protein fractions, Y and Z, and their possible role in the hepatic uptake of bilirubin, sulfobromophthalein, and other anions. J Clin Invest 1969;48:2156–2167.
8. Crawford JM, Hauser SC, Gollan JL. Formation, hepatic metabolism, and transport of bile pigments: a status report. Semin Liver Dis 1988;8:105–118.
9. Roy Chowdhury N, Attavar P, Roy Chowdhury J. Hereditary disorders of the liver and biliary system. In: Rimoin DL, Connor JM, Pyeritz RE, eds. Emery and Rimoin's principles and practice of medical genetics. 3rd ed. New York: Churchill Livingstone, 1977:1555–1578.
10. Lester R, Behrman RE, Lucey JF. Transfer of bilirubin ^{14}C across monkey placenta. Pediatrics 1963;32:416–419.
11. Schenker S, Mawber NH, Schmid R. Bilirubin metabolism in the fetus. J Clin Invest 1964;43:32–39.
12. Billing BH. Intestinal and renal metabolism of bilirubin including enterohepatic circulation. In: Ostrow JD, ed. Bile pigments and jaundice. New York: Marcel Dekker, 1986:255–269.
13. Stocker R, Yamamoto Y, McDonagh AF. Bilirubin is an anti-oxidant of possible physiological importance. Science 1987;235:1043–1046.
14. Stocker R, Glazer N, Ames BN. Antioxidant activity of albumin-bound bilirubin. Proc Natl Acad Sci USA 1987;84:5918–5922.
15. Zipursky A, Bowman JM. Isoimmune hemolytic diseases. In: Nathan DG, Oski FA, eds. Hematology of infancy and childhood. 4th ed. Philadelphia: WB Saunders, 1993:44–73.
16. Bernstein J, Brown AK. Sepsis and jaundice in early infancy. Pediatrics 1962;29:873–882.
17. Slusher TM, Vreman HJ, McLaren DW, et al. Glucose-6-phosphate dehydrogenase deficiency and carboxyhemoglobin concentrations associated with bilirubin-related morbidity and death in Nigerian infants. J Pediatr 1995;126:102–108.
18. Widness JA, Lowe LS, Stevenson DK, et al. Direct relationship of fetal carboxyhemoglobin with hemolysis in alloimmunized pregnancies. Pediatr Res 1994;35:713–719.
19. Newman TB, Maisels MJ. Evaluation and treatment of jaundice in the term newborn: a kinder, gentler approach. Pediatrics 1992;89:809–818.
20. Cashore WJ. Neonatal hyperbilirubinemia. In: Oski FA, DeAngelis CD, Feigin RD, et al., eds. Principles and practice of pediatrics. 2nd ed. Philadelphia: JB Lippincott, 1994:446–455.
21. Koiwai O, Nishizawa M, Hasada K, et al. Gilbert's syndrome is caused by a heterozygous missense mutation in the gene for bilirubin UDP-glucuronosyl transferase. Hum Mol Genet 1996;4:1183–1186.
22. Ritter JK, Chen F, Sheen YY, et al. A novel complex locus UGT1 encodes human bilirubin, phenol, and other UDP-glucuronyl transferase isozymes with identical carboxyl termini. J Biol Chem 1992;267:3257–3261.
23. Aono S, Yasakagu Y, Keino H, et al. A new type of defect in the gene for bilirubin uridine 5' diphosphate glucuronosyl-transferase in a patient with Crigler-Najjar syndrome type I. Pediatr Res 1994;35:629–632.
24. Burchell B, Nebert DW, Nelson DR, et al. The UDP glucuronosyltransferase gene superfamily: suggested nomenclature based on evolutionary divergence. DNA Cell Biol 1991;10:487–494.
25. Maisels MJ, Newman TB. Kernicterus in otherwise healthy, breast-fed term newborns. Pediatrics 1995;96:730–733.

26. Watchko JF, Claasen D. Kernicterus in premature infants: current prevalence and relationship to NICHD phototherapy study exchange criteria. Pediatrics 1994;93:996–999.
27. Penn AA, Enzmann DR, Hahn JS, Stevenson DK. Kernicterus in a full-term infant. Pediatrics 1994;93:1003–1006.
28. Foliot A, Ploussard JP, Housett E, et al. Breast milk jaundice: in vitro inhibition of rat liver bilirubin uridine diphosphate glucuronyl transferase activity and Z-protein bromosulfophthalein binding by human breast milk. Pediatr Res 1976;10:594–598.
29. Gourley GR, Anend RA. Beta-glucuronidase and hyperbilirubinemia in breast-fed and formula-fed babies. Lancet 1986;1:644–646.
30. Alonso EM, Whitington PF, Whitington SH, et al. Enterohepatic circulation of nonconjugated bilirubin in rats fed with human milk. J Pediatr 1991;118:425–430.
31. Karp WB. Biochemical alterations in neonatal hyperbilirubinemia and bilirubin encephalopathy. A review. Pediatrics 1979;64:361–368.
32. Diamond I, Schmid R. Oxidative phosphorylation in experimental bilirubin encephalopathy. Science 1967;155:1288–1289.
33. Brodersen R. Bilirubin transport in the newborn infant, reviewed with relation to kernicterus. J Pediatr 1980;96:349–356.
34. Cashore WJ. The neurotoxicity of bilirubin. Clin Perinatol 1990;17:437–447.
35. Brodersen R. Bilirubin: solubility and interaction with albumin and phospholipid. J Biol Chem 1979;254:2364–2369.
36. Diamond I, Schmid R. Experimental bilirubin encephalopathy. The mode of entry of bilirubin into the central nervous system. J Clin Invest 1966;45:678–689.
37. Lee C, Oh W, Stonestreet BS, et al. Permeability of the blood-brain barrier for ^{125}I-albumin bound bilirubin in newborn piglets. Pediatr Res 1989;25:452–456.
38. Wennberg RP, Hance AJ. Experimental bilirubin encephalopathy: importance of total protein, protein binding, and blood brain barrier. Pediatr Res 1986;20:789–792.
39. Wennberg RP. The importance of free bilirubin acid salt in bilirubin uptake by erythrocytes and mitochondria. Pediatr Res 1988;23:443–447.
40. Cashore WJ, Oh W. Ubound bilirubin and kernicterus in low-birth weight infants. Pediatrics 1982;69:481–485.
41. Cashore WJ, Oh W, Brodersen R. Reserve albumin and bilirubin toxicity index in infant serum. Acta Paediatr Scand 1983;72:415–419.
42. Øie S, Levy G. Effect of sulfisoxazole on pharmacokinetics of free and plasma protein bound bilirubin in experimental unconjugated hyperbilirubinemia. J Pharm Sci 1979;68:6–10.
43. Brodersen R. Competitive binding of bilirubin and drugs to human serum albumin, studied by enzymatic oxidation. J Clin Invest 1974;54:1353–1364.
44. Harris RC, Lucey JF, MacLean JR. Kernicterus in premature infants associated with low concentratios of bilirubin in the plasma. Pediatrics 1958;21:875–884.
45. Wennberg RP, Johanson BB, Folbergova J, Siesjo BK. Bilirubin-induced changes in brain energy metabolism after osmotic opening of the blood-brain barrier. Pediatr Res 1991;30:473–478.
46. Eriksen EF, Danielsen H, Brodersen R. Bilirubin-liposome interaction. J Biol Chem 1981;256:4269–4274.
47. Vasquez J, Garcia-Calvo M, Valdivieso F, et al. Interaction of bilirubin with the synaptosomal plasma membrane. J Biol Chem 1988;263:1255–1265.
48. Amit Y, Chan G, Fedunec S, et al. Bilirubin toxicity in a neuroblastoma cell line N-115: I. Effects on Na$^+$-K$^+$ ATPase, [^{3}H] thymidine uptake, L-[^{35}S] methionine incorporation, and mitochondrial function. Pediatr Res 1989;25:364–368.
49. Leonard M, Noy N, Zakim D. The interactions of bilirubin with model and biological membranes. J Biol Chem 1989;264:5648–5652.
50. Corchs JS, Serrani RE, Venri G, Palchik M. Inhibition of K$^+$ influx in Ehrlich ascites cells by bilirubin and ouabain. Experientia 1982;38:1069–1071.
51. Chen H-C, Wang C-H, Tsan K-W, Chen Y-C. An electron microscopic and radioautographic study of experimental kernicterus II. Bilirubin movement within neurons and release of waste products via astroglia. Am J Pathol 1971;64:45–66.
52. Amit Y, Poznansky MJ, Schiff D. Bilirubin toxicity in a neuroblastoma cell line N-115: II. Delayed effects and recovery. Pediatr Res 1989;25:364–368.
53. Cashore WJ, Kilguss NV. Inhibition of synaptosomal tyrosine uptake by bilirubin. Pediatr Res 1989;25:209A.
54. Cashore WJ, Kilguss NV, Chung CE. Effects of bilirubin and albumin on dopamine synthesis in striatal synaptosomes. Pediatr Res 1989;25:210A.
55. Amato MM, Kilguss NV, Gelardi NL, Cashore WJ. Dose-effect relationship of bilirubin on striatal synaptosomes in rats. Biol. Neonate 1994;66:288–293.
56. Hansen TWR, Paulsen O, Gjerstad L, Bratlid D. Short-term exposure to bilirubin reduces synaptic activation in rat transverse hippocampal slices. Pediatr Res 1988;23:453–456.
57. Ochoa ELM, Wennberg RP, An Y, et al. Interactions of bilirubin with isolated presynaptic nerve terminals: functional effects on the uptake and release of neurotransmitters. Cell Mol Neurobiol 1993;13:69–86.
58. Mayor F Jr, Diez-Guerra J, Valdivieso F, et al. Effects of bilirubin on the membrane potential of rat brain synaptosomes. J Neurochem 1986;47:363–369.
59. Hansen TWR, Cashore WJ, Oh W. Changes in piglet auditory brainstem response amplitudes without inreases in serum or cerebrospinal fluid neuron-specific enolase. Pediatr Res 1992;32:534–529.
60. Vohr BR, Lester B, Rapisardi G, et al. Abnormal brainstem function (brain-stem auditory evoked response) correlates with acoustic cry features in term infants with hyperbilirubinemia. J Pediatr 1989;115:303–308.
61. Vohr BR, Lester B, O'Shea C, et al. Behavioral changes correlated with brain term auditory evoked responses in term infants with moderate hyperbilirubinemia. J Pediatr 1990;117:288–291.

62. Nakamura H, Takada S, Shimabuku R, et al. Auditory nerve and brainstem responses in newborns with hyperbilirubinemia. Pediatrics 1985;75:703–708.
63. Nwaesei C, Van Aerde J, Boyden M, et al. Changes in auditory brainstem responses in hyperbilirubinemic infants before and after exchange transfusion. Pediatrics 1984;74:800–803.
64. Shapiro SM. Acute brainstem auditory evoked potential abnormalities in jaundiced Gunn rats given sulfonamide. Pediatr Res 1988;23:306–310.
65. Karplus M, Lee C, Cashore WJ, et al. The effects of brain bilirubin on brainstem auditory evoked response in rats. Early Hum Dev 1988;16:185–194.
66. Chisin R, Perlman M, Sohmer H. Cochlear and brainstem responses in hearing loss following neonatal hyperbilirubinemia. Ann Otol Rhinol Laryngol 1979;89:352–357.
67. Rapisardi G, Vohr B, Cashore WJ, et al. Assessment of infant cry variability in high-risk infants. Int J Pediatr Otorhinolaryngol 1989;27:19–29.
68. Connolly AM, Volpe JJ. Clinical features of bilirubin encephalopathy. Clin Perinatol 1990;17:371–379.
69. Byers RK, Paine RS, Crothers B. Extrapyramidal cerebral palsy with hearing loss following erythroblastosis. Pediatrics 1955;15:248–254.
70. Labrune PH, Myara A, Francoual J, et al. Cerebellar symptoms as the presenting manifestations of bilirubin encephalopathy in children with Crigler-Najjar type I disease. Pediatrics 1992;89:768–770.
71. Newman TB, Maisels MJ. Does hyperbilirubinemia damage the brain of healthy full-term infants? Clin Perinatol 1990;17:331–358.
72. Gartner LM, Synder RN, Chabon RS, et al. Kernicterus: high incidence in premature infants with low serum bilirubin concentrations. Pediatrics 1970;45:906–917.
73. Keenan WJ, Perlstein PH, Light IJ, et al. Kernicterus in small sick premature infants receiving phototherapy. Pediatrics 1972;49:652–655.
74. Ahdab-Barmada M, Moosy J. The neuropathology of kernicterus in the premature neonate. Diagnostic problems. J Neuropathol Exp Neurol 1984;43:45–55.
75. Jardine DS, Rogers I. Benzyl alcohol, kernicterus, intraventricular hemorrhage, and mortality in preterm infants. Pediatrics 1989;83:153–160.
76. Turkel SB, Miller CA, Guttenberg ME, et al. A clinical pathologic re-appraisal of kernicterus. Pediatrics 1982;69:267–272.
77. Lucey JF. Bilirubin and brain damage: A real mess! Pediatrics 1982;69:381–382.
78. Maisels MJ. Jaundice. In: Avery GB, Fletcher MA, MacDonald MG, eds. Neonatology, pathophysiology and management of the newborn. 4th ed. Philadelphia; JB Lippincott, 1994:630–725.
79. Ennever JF. Blue light, green light, white light, more light: treatment of neonatal jaundice. Clin Perinatol 1990;17:467–481.
80. MacDonagh AF, Plama LA, Trull FR, et al. Phototherapy for neonatal jaundice: configurational isomers of bilirubin. J Am chem Soc 1982;104:6865–6867.
81. AAP Subcommittee on Hyperbilirubinemia. Practice parameter: management of hyperbilirubinemia in the healthy term newborn. Pediatrics 1994;94:558–565.
82. Andres JM. Neonatal hepatobiliary disorders. Clin Perinatol 1996;23:321–352.
83. Ikeda S, Sera Y, Akagi M. Serial ultrasonic examination to differentiate biliary atresia from neonatal hepatitis: special reference to changes in size of the gall bladder. Eur J Pediatr 1989;148:396–400.
84. Kayaloghi M, D'Alessandro AM, Knechtle SJ, et al. Long-term results of liver transplantation for biliary atresia. Surgery 1993;114:711–718.
85. Yoon PW, Bresee JS, Olney RS, et al. Epidemiology of biliary atresia: a population-based study. Pediatrics 1997;99:376–382.
86. Tenhunen R, Marver HS, Schmid R. The enzymatic conversion of hemoglobin to bilirubin. Trans Assoc Am Physicians 1969;82:363–371.
87. McDonagh AF, Lightner DA. "Like a shrivelled blood orange"—Bilirubin, jaundice, and phototherapy. Pediatrics 1985;75:443–455.

40
Neonatal Calcium and Phosphorus Metabolism

Jeffrey L. Loughead and Reginald C. Tsang

The rapid advance of diagnostic and therapeutic technology has led to a shift in the emphases of research in prenatal mineral metabolism. Whereas the initial focus of investigation was aimed at the gross composition of the fetus and neonate,[1,2] more recently the focus has shifted to physiologic control and presently to subcellular control. Although the understanding is far from complete, there is a greater appreciation of the complex interrelations among the major mineral components of bone (e.g., calcium, phosphorus, and magnesium) and their recognized major hormonal regulators (e.g., parathyroid hormone, vitamin D, and calcitonin). This chapter reviews the physiologic basis of bone mineral metabolism in continuity from fetus to neonate. Each section begins with an overview of basic physiology, followed by a section on the impact of pregnancy including placental-fetal physiology, and ends with the dynamic period of the neonate.

Calcium

Calcium is the fifth most abundant inorganic element in the body; the adult human contains between 1100 and 1200g of calcium. Ninety-eight percent of total body calcium is complexed within the skeleton, and turnover of skeletal calcium is relatively slow. The remaining 2% of total body calcium is nearly equally divided between intracellular and extracellular spaces; the extracellular space contains the easily measured serum calcium. This calcium, as routinely measured, is total calcium representing three forms:

1. Protein-bound, primarily to albumin and making up approximately 45% of total calcium;
2. Complexed calcium, approximately 5% of the total, and complexed to bicarbonate, phosphate, citrate, or sulfate;
3. Ionized calcium, approximately 50% of total calcium and the metabolically active component.

In the well-nourished adult, serum total calcium concentration ranges from 9.0 to $10.5\,mg\cdot dl^{-1}$ (2.25 to $2.6\,mmol\cdot L^{-1}$) and is relatively stable. The ionized calcium concentration, although subject to changes directed by parathyroid hormone, calcitonin, vitamin D, and blood pH, is stable within an individual over prolonged periods and ranges from 4.8 to $5.2\,mg\cdot dl^{-1}$ (1.2 to $1.3\,mmol\cdot L^{-1}$).

These precisely regulated serum concentrations are the end result of the closely interlocking systems of dietary absorption, bone formation/resorption, and urinary and fecal excretion, all of which are regulated by at least three primary hormone systems. Calcium is readily available in the average diet, with the normal adult intake ranging between 500 and $2000\,mg\cdot day^{-1}$. This ingested calcium within the small intestine is absorbed 25% to 50%. Calcium absorption in the adult is a combination of two processes, one active and one passive. The active component is vitamin D dependent and is most pronounced in the proximal small intestine at less than $2\,g\cdot day^{-1}$ intake.[3] At greater intakes, the active component becomes saturated and absorption increases linearly, consistent with passive diffusion (Figure 40.1). There appears to be no practical upper limit of calcium absorption, although efficiency decreases with very high calcium intake.

Although calcium is important for muscle contraction, neurotransmission, enzyme function, and a variety of other important metabolic activities, most calcium is utilized in the formation and maintenance of bone. All ossified structures undergo slow, continual remodeling, and metabolism occurs primarily at the endosteal surface of the bone. Osteoprogenitor cells, when stimulated by parathyroid hormone and vitamin D, become osteoclasts, which resorb bone and release calcium, phosphorus, and magnesium into the circulation. Calcitonin, whose function is to decrease serum calcium concentrations, acts on osteoclasts, inhibits the action of parathyroid hormone, and promotes the conversion of osteoclasts to the

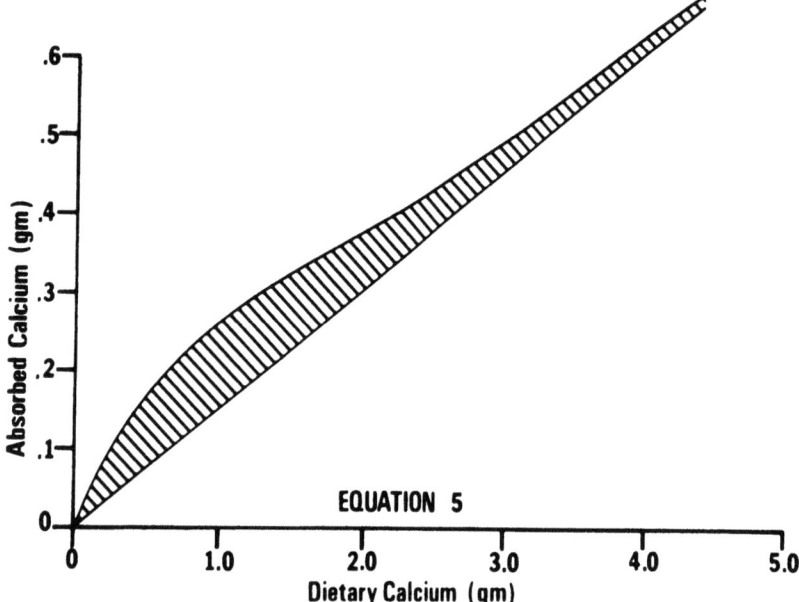

FIGURE 40.1. Mathematical relation of calcium absorption as a function of intake in adults. Upper line represents the active component of absorption and the lower line the passive component. At low intakes the active component is predominant. (From Heaney et al.,[3] with permission.)

bone-forming cells, the osteoblasts. The processes are ongoing and finitely coupled, allowing precise regulation of bone modeling and serum calcium concentration.

Calcium is primarily excreted from the body in either stool or urine. Most fecal calcium is unabsorbed dietary calcium. Calcium is present in all digestive secretions and represents apparently unregulated obligate calcium losses. This fecal endogenous calcium loss is stable and minimal in the healthy adult in comparison to urinary losses. Regulation of calcium excretion occurs at the kidney and calcium is filtered freely at the glomerulus. Although calcium is absorbed throughout the nephron, most of this filtered calcium is passively reabsorbed in the proximal tubule (50–55%) or actively reabsorbed within the distal tubule (10–15%). Control of the active calcium reabsorption component is not well defined, but appears to be controlled by parathyroid hormone (PTH) and vitamin D. Of these two hormones, PTH predominates, with increased PTH concentration leading to increased calcium reabsorption and phosphorus excretion. In the well-nourished adult, the net effect of the regulating influences results in mean urinary calcium losses of 185 mg·day^{-1} (4.6 mmol·d^{-1}).[4,5]

Calcium Metabolism in Pregnancy

Alterations in calcium homeostasis occur early in pregnancy (see Chapter 14). Changes in serum parathyroid hormone and vitamin D concentrations have been found within weeks of conception. Calcium balance studies performed early during the second trimester have shown increased net calcium retention.[6] These changes occur well in advance of when the developing fetus requires most of its calcium, suggesting an "anticipatory modification" of maternal calcium homeostasis. Such modification begins by increased intestinal absorption of calcium. This action is in part secondary to increased intake, but in the dietary range of 800 to 2000 mg calcium·day^{-1} it may be related to an elevation of 1,25-dihydroxyvitamin D [1,25(OH)$_2$D]. Serum concentrations of 1,25(OH)$_2$D rise early in pregnancy. This early rise may be artificial, as there is an associated rise in vitamin D–binding protein (VDBP) as well. Correction for the effect of increased VDBP concentration can be made mathematically by using the 1,25(OH)$_2$D/VDBP index. Using this correction, there is no significant early increase in "free" 1,25(OH)$_2$D. From the viewpoint that free 1,25(OH)$_2$D is probably the active component physiologically, an increase in 1,25(OH)$_2$D during pregnancy does not occur until 35 weeks' gestation. Whether changes in 1,25(OH)$_2$D concentration are responsible for the increase in calcium absorption noted early in pregnancy remain to be proved.

Urinary calcium excretion has been reported to be both increased and decreased during pregnancy. One cross-sectional study of more than 1000 pregnant women found a wide range of urinary calcium excretion of 30 to 620 mg·day^{-1} (0.75–15.5 mmol·d^{-1}).[7] The average urinary calcium was 136 mg·day^{-1} (3.4 mmol·d^{-1}); nearly one fifth of the women had urinary calcium excretion that exceeded the 95th percentile upper limit for nonpregnant women [350 mg·day^{-1} (8.75 mmol·d^{-1})]. The women had relatively similar diets, so the increased calcium excretion could not be explained by markedly variable dietary intakes. Pregnant women receiving low-calcium diets have increased urinary calcium.[8] Because urinary calcium excretion correlates with creatinine clearance,[7] the increased urinary calcium excretion is possibly the result of the increased glomerular filtration rate that occurs during pregnancy.

Serum total calcium concentration decreases progressively and significantly over the course of pregnancy. The decline reaches a nadir during the middle of the third trimester and rebounds slightly toward term.[9,10] This decline appears to follow that of serum albumin concentration, the major calcium-binding protein. Serum ionized calcium concentration in pregnancy has been found to increase,[10] decrease,[11] or remain steady.[9,12,13]

An important consideration in maternal calcium homeostasis is the mother's bone calcium stores. Studies in mice, using radioisotopes of calcium, have shown that as much as 30% of fetal calcium is derived from the maternal bone calcium.[14] Despite this finding, studies of human bone mineral content using photon absorptiometry have shown that in well-nourished women no measurable changes in maternal bone mineral content can be demonstrated related to current or past pregnancies.[15,16] Maternal bone stores appear to be protected through replenishment of bone losses, and an overall increase in bone turnover has been demonstrated during pregnancy.[6]

Calcium Metabolism in the Placenta

The placenta is the primary organ regulating transfer of calcium from mother to fetus and control of placental calcium transport appears to be largely on the fetal side at the syncytiotrophoblast. Calcium transfer is, at least in part, active, allowing fetal calcium concentration to exceed the maternal concentration during the last trimester. Because of this active transfer, the placenta "scavenges" calcium from the maternal circulation even in states of maternal calcium deficiency. Studies of neonates born to calcium-deficient mothers have shown that fetal calcium accretion is normal.[17]

Placental calcium transfer is likely by both paracellular diffusion and active transcellular movement with the paracellular component accounting for a minor portion of the total calcium transport. Three mechanisms are likely operative in the active transfer of calcium across the placenta: a carrier-mediated entry of calcium ions into the cell, an intracellular binding to maintain a low intracellular ionized calcium concentration, and extrusion of calcium to the fetal circulation.[18] Release of calcium to the fetal side is thought to be by two pathways. The first is a basic adenosine triphosphatase (ATPase)-independent, mediated transport in the placental basal plasma membrane. This is thought to be a facilitated diffusion that is saturable at high micromolar concentrations and inhibited by high magnesium concentrations.[18] The second is a high-affinity, magnesium and ATPase-dependent pump that extrudes calcium via vesicles to the fetal circulation.[19,20] This system is less saturable and is thought to play a major role in the supply of calcium to the human fetus.

Recently, a putative calcium sensor protein has been identified.[21] This protein is a 500-kd single-chain glycoprotein and has been found in human placental syncytiotrophoblast, parathyroid gland, and proximal kidney tubule brush border. It is likely that this protein occurs in a complex that requires other proteins and calcium in order to trigger the sensor. This sensor may be involved in mediating maternal-fetal calcium transport directly or indirectly though regulation of placental parathyroid–related peptide (pPTHrP) and placental production of 1,25(OH)$_2$D.

A protein similar to, if not identical to, intestinal calcium binding protein (iCaBP) has been found in the placenta.[22] Placental CaBP (pCaBP) increases with gestational age, paralleling the increase in placental calcium transfer.[23] Theoretically, pCaBP may augment the transfer of calcium within the placental cell as iCaBP augments transfer of calcium within the enterocyte while maintaining a stable intracellular ionized calcium concentration. Intestinal CaBP is 1,25(OH)$_2$D-dependent and pCaBP may be similarly regulated.[24,25] The finding of 25(OH)D-1α-hydroxylase in the placenta points to a possible local production and control of pCaBP and calcium transfer.[26,27] That calcium transfer may be under fetal control was suggested by Rodda et al.[28] in a report of fetal parathyroid function. Using thyroparathyroidectomized sheep, these investigators demonstrated that parathyroidectomy lead to an abrupt decline in the fetal serum calcium concentration and a reversal of the maternal-fetal calcium gradient. Infusion of immunoreactive PTH (iPTH) did not return the calcium gradient,[28,29] but infusion of crude parathyroid extract did (vide infra).[28] To what extent these factors contribute to total calcium transfer is the focus of further investigation.

Calcium Metabolism in the Fetus

The accumulation of calcium by the fetus is exponential with advancing gestation (Figure 40.2). Studies dating back to 1933 have shown marked increases in calcium accretion rates during the last trimester of gestation.[1,2,30] When comparison to body weight is made, calcium makes up an increasing percentage of fetal total body weight. An 800-g neonate has approximately 4.5 g of calcium, or 0.56% of total body weight; a 2000-g neonate has 15 g or 0.75% of total body weight; and a 3000-g term neonate has 25 to 30 g, or nearly 1% of total body weight as calcium.[2] The term fetus accumulates approximately 30 g of calcium, and approximately two thirds of it is accreted during the last trimester at a rate of up to 150 mg·kg^{-1}day^{-1}.[30] This transfer of calcium is against an increasingly positive maternal-fetal calcium gradient. Whereas the fetus during the mid–second trimester has a serum total calcium concentration of approximately 5.5 mg·dl^{-1} (1.37 mmol·L^{-1}), by term the total calcium con-

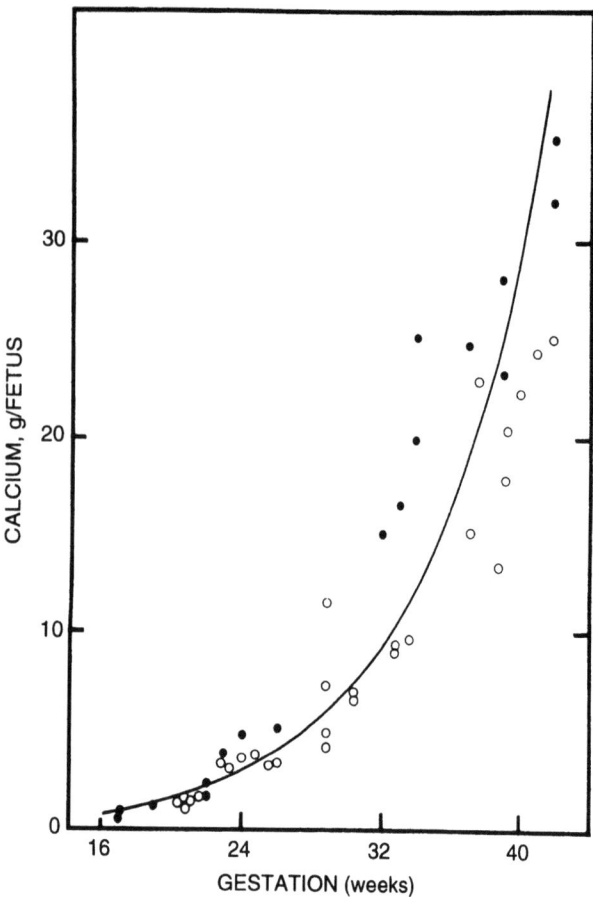

FIGURE 40.2. Calcium accretion in the human fetus from 16 to 40 weeks' gestation. (Data adapted from Widdowsen and Dickerson[265] (open circles) and Kelly et al.[266] (closed circles). (From Shaw,[30] with permission.)

centration has reached $11.0 \, mg \cdot dl^{-1}$ ($2.75 \, mmol \cdot L^{-1}$).[31,32] The role of these high fetal calcium concentrations is presumably to ensure an adequate supply of calcium for the fetus so it can continue its extraordinary growth rate with adequate bone mineralization. The fetus's hormonal response to this high calcium concentration appears to be unique and is discussed separately below.

Calcium Metabolism in the Neonate

With birth there is an instantaneous interruption of fetal calcium supply. Regardless of whether the neonate is fed or given intravenous fluids, calcium delivery over the first hours to days does not match the calcium delivery rate the fetus has been receiving. This fact sets the stage for a rapid and dramatic decline in serum total and ionized calcium concentration. Studies in the healthy term neonate have shown that at birth the neonate's cord blood total calcium concentration is nearly $11 \, mg \cdot dl^{-1}$ ($2.75 \, mmol \cdot L^{-1}$), and ionized calcium concentration is nearly $6 \, mg \cdot dl^{-1}$ ($1.5 \, mmol \cdot L^{-1}$).[32] By 2 hours of age the serum total calcium concentration declines by nearly 5%, and the full extent of this decline is in the ionized fraction. By 24 to 36 hours, the serum calcium concentration reaches its nadir of $9.0 \, mg \cdot dl$ ($2.25 \, mmol \cdot L$) for total calcium concentration [95% confidence range $7.8–10.2 \, mg \cdot dl^{-1}$ ($1.95–2.54 \, mmol \cdot L^{-1}$)] and $4.9 \, mg \cdot dl^{-1}$ ($1.22 \, mmol \cdot L^{-1}$) for ionized calcium [95% confidence range $4.4–5.4 \, mg \cdot dl^{-1}$ ($1.10–1.35 \, mmol \cdot L^{-1}$)] with the change in ionized calcium making up 75% of the change in total calcium.[32] After a period of stabilization, the serum calcium concentration slowly rises, reaching a concentration by 1 week of age similar to that found during childhood (Figure 40.3). Because of reduced oral intake and relatively low calcium concentrations in breast milk ($340 \, mg \cdot L$ or $8.5 \, mmol \cdot L$) and formula ($450 \, mg \cdot L^{-1}$ or $11 \, mmol \cdot L^{-1}$), diet has little role in the early stabilization of serum calcium concentration. As the neonate's intake increases over the first week of life, diet appears to have an increased role (see Chapters 51 and 52).

Parathyroid hormone and $1,25(OH)_2D$ concentrations in blood increase early in the postnatal period and remain elevated for several days postnatally. Studies of these

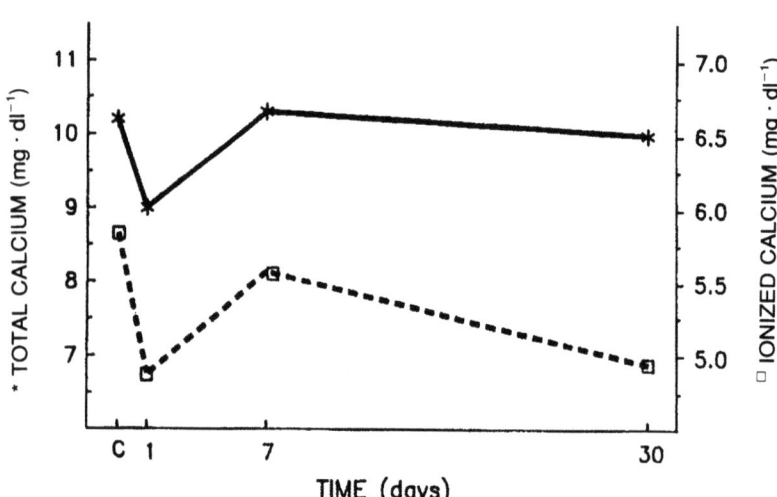

FIGURE 40.3. Serum total calcium and ionized calcium concentrations in term neonates over the first month of age. (Data were compiled from Loughead et al.[32] and Wandrup et al.[267])

hormones during the first day of life have found no consistent correlation between serum calcium concentration or changes in serum calcium concentration with either PTH or 1,25(OH)$_2$D concentrations. Over the course of the first week, the role of these hormones likely is enhanced.

Calcium absorption in the neonate depends on several factors: gestational and postnatal age, absolute calcium and phosphorus intake and the calcium/phosphorus ratio, the presence of lactose, fat, or magnesium in the diet, and possibly the vitamin D status of the neonate. Calcium absorption in the neonate appears to undergo a maturational process, with calcium absorption increasing with both gestational age[30,33] and postnatal age.[30,33–35] Intestinal absorption of calcium in the preterm neonate is thought to be slightly less than or equal to that in the term neonate.[35,36] During the early neonatal period, calcium absorption is intake-dependent,[35,37] consistent with passive absorption. As the neonate ages, preterm and term neonates have increased calcium absorption with a fractional absorption up to 80%,[30,36,38] consistent with an active transport adaptation.[35] Obtaining the true fractional absorption characteristic of neonates has been made difficult by the fact that, unlike adults, the excretion of endogenous calcium may be large.[30,38] Using stable isotope methodology, Barltrop et al.[37] reported endogenous calcium excretion ranging from 4 to 150 mg·dl^{-1} (1 to 37.5 mmol·L^{-1}). Such losses may markedly influence the measured fractional absorption by standard balance techniques.

Urinary calcium loss depends on gestation, serum calcium concentration, and glomerular filtration rate, but not intake.[39] Preterm neonates have lower glomerular filtration rates and lower tubular reabsorption of calcium than term neonates. The net result is that in the more preterm neonate there is higher urinary calcium loss. As the neonate ages, his glomerular filtration rate increases, but so does his tubular reabsorption, leading to improved calcium handling and a decrease in urine calcium.[39]

The usual dietary sources of calcium for the neonate are human milk and commercial formula. Human milk, both term and preterm, contains calcium at approximately 340 mg·dL^{-1} (8.5 mmol·L^{-1}),[40] and although there is significantly less calcium than most formulas [approximately 450 mg·L^{-1} (11 mmol·L^{-1})], human milk calcium appears to have higher bioavailability than that of formula.[38] Even with the greater bioavailability of human milk calcium and the higher concentration of calcium in formula, neither human milk nor standard formulas provide preterm neonates with sufficient calcium to meet their calculated mineral needs for bone growth. Rickets is common to the preterm neonate. Studies of bone mineral content of these neonates receiving either human milk or standard formulas have shown bone mineralization rates to be less than intrautrine rates; and even decreases in bone mineralization have been reported postnatally.[41–43] Emphasis has been placed on development of a formula that would meet the needs of the preterm neonate. Formulas high in calcium and phosphorus have resulted in bone mineralization rates comparable to intrauterine rates.[44] This approach necessitates high calcium and phosphorus concentrations in formula (1260 mg or 31 mmol Ca·L^{-1}, 780 mg or 25 mmol P·L^{-1}), which results in decreased mineral stability, and the potential for interference in absorption of lipids and other minerals such as magnesium and trace metals. In clinical practice these high-mineral formulas appear to be well tolerated by the preterm neonate.

Neonatal Hypocalcemia

An exaggeration of the "physiologic" fall in serum calcium concentration during the first days of life leads to neonatal hypocalcemia. The definition of neonatal hypocalcemia has been variously and arbitrarily defined in the past as a serum total calcium concentration of less than 8.0 (2 mmol·L^{-1}), less than 7.5 (1.87 mmol·L^{-1}), or less than 7.0 mg·dl^{-1} (1.75 mmol·L^{-1}). This variance in definition is, at least in part, due to the lack of clinical signs in many neonates, even at a very low serum total calcium concentration. Neonates at greatest risk for symptomatic or asymptomatic neonatal hypocalcemia, such as infants of diabetic mothers or preterm or asphyxiated neonates, frequently are sick for a multitude of reasons, and the contribution of neonatal hypocalcemia to signs related to their primary illness can be easily obscured. A better definition of neonatal hypocalcemia would be based on the metabolically active component of calcium, ionized calcium, as changes in ionized calcium concentration are more likely to have physiological significance.

Based on a study in carefully selected, healthy term neonates without maternal or perinatal conditions that could theoretically affect neonatal calcium concentration, a reasonable statistical definition of hypocalcemia for term neonates would be an ionized calcium concentration of less than 4.4 mg·dl^{-1} (1.1 mmol·L^{-1}).[32] This concentration represents two standard deviations below the mean at 24 hours, the "normal" physiologic nadir in term neonates. This definition is a statistical one and is based on assumptions of normal distributions of physiologic variables. Further investigation needs to define physiologically important limits for term and preterm neonates.

The pathogenesis of neonatal hypocalcemia is unclear, but in most cases is thought to be an exaggeration of the normal physiologic decline in serum calcium related to the abrupt interruption in calcium supply. Whether other factors add to this decline leading to neonatal hypocalcemia has been the source of much investigation.

Proposed factors include hypomagnesemia leading to impaired PTH response and action,[45] hypoparathyroidism leading to a blunted response to the falling serum calcium concentration,[46] hyperphosphatemia leading to decreased PTH response and possible enhancement of the action of calcitonin,[47] and hypercalcitoninemia leading to antagonism of PTH at the bone.[48] Each of these factors is discussed in more detail below.

The importance of developing a precise physiologic or practical definition of neonatal hypocalcemia is that therapy is not without risk. Oral therapy is frequently not possible in the sick neonate, and intravenous therapy carries the risk of cardiac dysrhythmia or subcutaneous extravasation and skin slough. However, when deemed appropriate for treatment, 10 to 20 mg·kg^{-1} of elemental calcium given as 1 to 2 ml·kg^{-1} of 10% calcium gluconate in a slow intravenous "bolus" infusion over a period of 10 to 20 minutes is suggested for symptomatic hypocalcemia. This is followed by an infusion of 60 to 75 mg·kg^{-1} day^{-1} of elemental calcium (i.e., as calcium gluconate) in intravenous fluids. The latter dosage of calcium may be used for asymptomatic hypocalcemia and frequently increases serum calcium concentrations to acceptable levels within 12 to 24 hours. The infusion rate may be halved in successive steps every 12 to 24 hours as the serum calcium concentration returns to within the normal range.

Late neonatal hypocalcemia, or hypocalcemia occurring after 3 to 5 days of age, has changed over the years. Historically, it was associated with the hyperphosphatemia as a result of feedings of cow milk or cow milk–based formulas high in phosphorus. With adjustment in the amount of phosphorus in formulas, hyperphosphatemic hypocalcemia is now a rarity, although anecdotal accounts of its occurrence are still reported.[48,49] Hyperphosphatemia results in hypocalcemia probably through a direct physiochemical effect of shifting calcium from blood to bone and soft tissues.

Apart from phosphate-induced conditions, hypocalcemia that begins late in the first week of life, or early neonatal hypocalcemia that requires continued therapy beyond the first week, is likely to be the result of a primary hormonal disturbance. Infants with late neonatal hypocalcemia should be investigated for hypoparathyroidism, vitamin D deficiency, primary malabsorption, or other mineral disturbance such as magnesium deficiency. DiGeorge syndrome (i.e., absence of parathyroid glands) and fetal parathyroid suppression secondary to maternal hyperparathyroidism and hypercalcemia, are examples of two hormonal disturbances causing late neonatal hypocalcemia.[50]

Neonatal Hypercalcemia

Hypercalcemia in the neonate is present when the serum total calcium concentration is more than 11.0 mg·dl (2.75 mmol·L);[32] it is rare except for iatrogenic causes. The obvious causes include excessive treatment for neonatal hypocalcemia, overzealous administration of calcium during cardiac arrest or blood volume exchange, the use of thiazide diuretics, prostaglandin excess, and excessive vitamin D supplements. More subtle is phosphorus deficiency in very low birth weight infants on parenteral nutrition or unfortified human milk. In phosphorus deficiency, there is an increase in serum 1,25(OH)$_2$D leading to a physiochemical shift of bone calcium to extracellular calcium and an increase in serum calcium. The calcium cannot be deposited in the bone due to the lack of available phosphorus. Diseases such as congenital hyperparathyroidism (e.g., either primary or secondary), idiopathic infantile hypercalcemia (i.e., Williams syndrome), familial hypocalciuric hypercalcemia, hypothyroidism, Bartter's syndrome (i.e., hyperprostaglandinemia), and fat necrosis have been associated with hypercalcemia that presents during the first month of life.

Clinical signs of hypercalcemia include lethargy, poor feeding, vomiting, constipation, polyuria, and hypertension. Persistence of hypercalcemia may result in seizures, metastatic calcifications, and nephrocalcinosis. Therapy includes removal of any iatrogenic cause, hydration with normal saline, and the use of calciuric diuretics such as furosemide or ethacrynic acid. In extreme cases, treatment with a glucocorticoid (e.g., cortisone 10 mg·kg^{-1} day^{-1}) or salmon calcitonin (4–8 IU·kg^{-1} dose^{-1} subcutaneously) has been advocated.[51] For long-term hypercalcemic conditions a low calcium, low iron, and low vitamin D formula (Calcilo, Ross Laboratories, Columbus, Ohio) is available. Most importantly, a thorough investigation for the underlying etiology of the hypercalcemia is necessary.

Phosphorus

Phosphorus constitutes nearly 1% of the total body mineral content of the adult and plays a critical role in the metabolism of both the adult and neonate. Of this phosphorus, 70% to 80% is complexed within bone, and most of the rest is intracellular. Of the intracellular phosphorus, nearly one half is in energy storage forms such as adenosine triphosphate (ATP), and the rest is involved in such vital structures as nucleic acids and cellular and organellar membranes. The total body phosphorus content is tightly regulated. Extracellular phosphorus concentration varies widely. Serum phosphorus concentration is high during childhood and declines into adulthood. Adult concentration varies by as much as 100%, with a normal range of 3.0 to 4.5 mg·dl^{-1} (1.0–1.45 mmol·L^{-1}), and has a circadian rhythm.

The wide variation in the serum phosphorus concentration may be secondary to few direct regulatory mechanisms. Parathyroid hormone (PTH), which has the greatest impact on the serum phosphorus concentration, primarily responds to changes in the ionized calcium concentration, not phosphorus. The kidney is the main organ regulating plasma phosphate concentration. Phosphorus is freely filtered at the glomerulus and presented to the renal tubule in a high concentration. The renal tubule reabsorbs phosphorus in the proximal and distal nephrons. In states of low PTH concentration, the renal tubular cells reabsorb up to 95% to 97% of filtered phosphorus. In states of high serum PTH concentration, reabsorption of phosphorus in proximal and distal tubules is inhibited, resulting in excretion of a high concentration of urinary phosphorus. Although markedly affected by PTH in the usual state, renal tubular cells appear to have a decreased responsiveness to PTH when there is severe phosphorus deficiency or overload. Phosphorus is reabsorbed in the face of high circulating PTH when there is severe phosphorus deficiency, and phosphorus is excreted despite low PTH concentration when serum phosphorus concentration is high.[52] These renal responses serve to protect phosphorus homeostasis at the extremes of phosphorus metabolism. Other hormones may have an effect on the excretion of phosphorus by the kidney. Growth hormone, 1,25(OH)$_2$D, insulin, and possibly somatomedins have been shown to increase renal tubular absorption of phosphorus.[53] The extent to which these hormones contribute to the normal regulation of serum phosphorus is unclear.

Phosphorus is prevalent in nearly all foods, and dietary deficiency is rare in adults. Phosphorus is absorbed in the small intestine, primarily in the jejunum, and the fractional absorption of dietary phosphorus is high. Fractional absorption declines slightly with age, but even in the adult the percent absorption of phosphorus has been measured at 60% to 75%.[53] The intestinal absorption of phosphorus by diffusion and vitamin D–dependent transfer appears to be independent of the active and passive calcium transport processes.[54] Studies in patients with undetectable serum 1,25(OH)$_2$D concentrations have shown phosphorus fractional absorption in the range of 30% to 40%,[53] and administration of 1,25(OH)$_2$D augments phosphorus absorption.[55]

Calcium and phosphorus are vital components of mineralized bone. In states of mineral sufficiency, calcium and phosphorus are deposited in an organized crystalline matrix in a calcium/phosphorus ratio of 2.1:1.0.[2] This mineralization is influenced by the hormones parathyroid hormone, calcitonin, and 1,25(OH)$_2$D. PTH stimulates the conversion of osteoprogenitor cells to osteoclasts, leading to the resorption of mineralized bone and release of both calcium and phosphorus into the extracellular space.[56] Calcitonin appears to inhibit bone resorption in a manner directly antagonistic to that of PTH. Calcitonin decreases the number and activity of osteoclasts, resulting in decreased bone resorptive release of calcium and phosphorus and in a lower serum phosphorus concentration.[57,58] 1,25(OH)$_2$D, whose production is regulated by PTH, facilitates the action of PTH at the bone surface, resulting in a release of calcium and phosphorus to the circulation. Serum phosphorus concentration appears to have a direct negative feedback effect on the hydroxylation of 25(OH)D: decreased serum phosphorus leads to increased production of 1,25(OH)$_2$D, and increased serum phosphorus leads to decreased 1,25(OH)$_2$D.[59]

Signs related to phosphorus deficiency include weakness, ataxia, irritability, seizures, paresthesias, metabolic acidosis, and cardiac and hepatic dysfunction. Clinical sequelae are rarely observed except in extreme hypophosphatemia ($<1-2$ mg·dl^{-1} or $<0.32-0.64$ mmol·L^{-1}). Signs of phosphorus excess largely relate to secondary hypocalcemia and include irritability, weakness, seizures, confusion, and tetany. High concentrations of phosphorus inhibit hydroxylation of 25(OH)D. Hence, long-term hyperphosphatemia may lead to signs of vitamin D deficiency.

Phosphorus Metabolism in Pregnancy

During pregnancy, serum phosphorus concentration falls progressively from conception to 29 to 32 weeks' gestation (see Chapter 14). At this point, phosphorus concentration reaches a nadir of approximately 13% below nonpregnant values and then rises slightly toward term.[9] The cause for this decline is not well understood. In that phosphorus is readily available in the diet and the percent intestinal absorption is high, dietary deficiency is not the cause for this decline. Parathyroid hormone, which may increase during pregnancy, would be expected to have a phosphaturic effect leading to hypophosphatemia. Excessive phosphorus losses have not been demonstrated during pregnancy. This progressive decline into the third trimester with the subsequent slight rebound toward term is the same pattern as for serum magnesium and total calcium concentrations. As for these other minerals, the change in extracellular volume during the third trimester of pregnancy may explain the change in the serum phosphorus concentration.

Phosphorus appears to be actively transferred across the placenta to the fetus. This action is inferred from the fact that during much of fetal life, the fetal serum phosphorus concentration markedly exceeds those of the pregnant female. Studies in the pregnant thyroparathyroidectomized rat on a low-phosphorus diet have shown that maternal serum phosphorus declines markedly. Fetal phosphorus accretion in these animals is normal, inferring that more than passive diffusion is responsible for the transfer.[60] Cord blood serum phosphorus concentration is inversely correlated with the gestational age of the fetus. In contrast to the serum calcium concentration which increases as the fetus reaches the third trimester, cord blood phosphorus concentration declines from nearly 14 mg·dl^{-1} (4.5 mmol·L^{-1}) during the second trimester to approximately 6 mg·dl^{-1} (1.9 mmol·L^{-1}) at term.[61] Despite this decline in the serum phosphorus concentration, the percent of total fetal body weight due to phosphorus increases with gestational age. Transfer of phosphorus and the amount accreted by the fetus increases exponentially over the duration of pregnancy.[62] This accretion reaches a maximum rate during the third trimester of approximately 60 to 74 mg·kg^{-1}·day^{-1} (1.94 to 2.39 mmol·kg^{-1}·day^{-1}) and is closely linked to the accretion of calcium with a calcium/phosphorus ratio of 1.7:1.0.[2]

Phosphorus Metabolism in the Neonate

At birth, the neonate's serum phosphorus concentration is relatively low in comparison to older neonatal or childhood values. In cord blood, the phosphorus concentration ranges from 3.7 to 8.1 mg·dl^{-1} (1.2 to 2.6 mmol·L^{-1}) with a mean value of 6.2 mg·dl^{-1} (2.0 mmol·L^{-1}); this figure compares to a mean phosphorus concentration of nearly 8.2 mg·dl^{-1} (2.6 mmol·L^{-1}) at 1 week of age for formula fed infants and 4.1 mg·dl^{-1} (1.3 mmol·L^{-1}) during childhood.[63] The relatively low initial concentration begins to rise shortly after birth reaching a peak by a week of age. The reason for this acute rise is not well understood. Diet theoretically has little effect owing to the relatively low enteral intake during this period. The lack of significant enteral intake may be associated with increased gluconeogenesis and endogenous phosphorus release. In that phosphorus homeostasis is largely under renal control, another explanation may be decreased glomerular filtration and decreased phosphorus filtration and excretion. A neonate has a relatively low glomerular filtration rate in the range of 25 to 35 ml·min^{-1} per 1.73 m^2, which in the adult has been shown to have a significant effect on reducing phosphorus excretion.[64] There might be decreased responsiveness of the renal tubules to the effects of PTH during this period. Parathyroid hormone is low at birth and rises over the first 24 to 48 hours of life. Urinary cyclic adenosine monophosphate (cAMP) is low during the first 24 hours of life, increasing and decreasing in parallel with the rise and fall in serum PTH. In a few neonates studied, the phosphaturic responsiveness of the kidney to exogenous PTH appears less during the first day of life compared to the same dose given on day 3 of life.[64,65] The early rise in the serum phosphorus concentration might be related to a combination of endogenous phosphorus release along with a decrease in phosphorus excretion. Because serum phosphorus concentration remains high even after PTH, cAMP, and urinary phosphorus excretion increases, other influences must play a role.

The intestinal absorption efficiency of phosphorus in the preterm and term neonate is high. Fractional absorption of phosphorus has been measured to be 86% to 97% regardless of phosphorus or calcium intake.[35] Phosphorus retention is influenced by calcium intake. With increased calcium intake there is increased phosphorus retention, probably secondary to the shared roles calcium and phosphorus play in bone mineralization. The pairing of retention is true for both enteral and parenteral administration of calcium and phosphorus. Studies using high concentrations of intravenous calcium alternating with phosphorus have shown poor retention rates compared to simultaneous infusion of these minerals.[66]

During the first month of life, serum phosphorus concentrations continue to rise in term and preterm neonates. These increased concentrations are maintained over the first several months of life and appear to be aimed at providing an adequate mineral supply for the extraordinary growth that occurs during the first several months of life. In states of phosphorus insufficiency, growth continues, albeit at a slower rate.[67] When supply is insufficient, phosphorus is preferentially used in the development of soft tissues and energy metabolism at the expense of bone mineralization, leading to the development of rickets. In states of phosphorus sufficiency, phosphorus itself appears to promote bone mineralization and development. In vitro studies have shown that increased phosphorus concentration leads to increased collagen synthesis and blunting of the resorptive effects of PTH in fetal bone.[68] The provision of sufficient dietary phosphorus appears to be vital for adequate growth and development of the neonate.

With the increasing tendency to use human milk as the primary source of nutrition, its mineral adequacy for term and preterm neonates has been studied. With respect to the term neonate, human milk generally appears to be adequate for delivery of phosphorus, although the forearm bone mineral content of these term neonates is lower or equal to those receiving cow milk derived formula. In that the human milk-fed neonate often is chosen, on a teleologic basis, as the "gold standard" for nutrition comparisons, one could argue that formula-fed neonates might be "overmineralized."[69] Supporting this concept is the lower serum ionized calcium concentration found in formula-fed infants compared to human milk-fed infants during the first 2 months.[70] This is likely due to the higher phosphorus content of the formulas, leading to an increased bone mineralization and a relatively low serum calcium concentration. Conversely, preterm neonates on human milk may demonstrate a "phosphorus deficiency syndrome" with increased urinary calcium, absence of urinary phosphorus, and decreased serum phosphorus concentration.[42,71-73] Relative to the needs of the preterm neonate, the low phosphorus content of human milk appears inadequate, with increases in bone mineral content significantly less than intrauterine rates and a high incidence of rickets.[43,74] The concentration of phosphorus in human milk declines with the duration of lactation, potentially accentuating its inadequacy as a source of phosphorus and limiting bone accretion. Various human milk fortifiers have been developed to more closely meet the needs of the preterm neonate. With mineral fortification, the absorption and retention of calcium and phosphorus may be increased relative to human milk alone. These absolute absorption and retention rates are still significantly less than that needed to match intrauterine accretion, and less than those found with available preterm infant formulas.[74,75] Further, liquid fortifiers have been shown to deliver greater amounts of calcium and phosphorus than powdered fortifiers.[76] The reason for these differences is thought to be the poorer solubility and bioavailability characteristics of the powders versus the liquids, and the chemical mixtures versus manufactured emulsions.

Preterm infant formulas have been developed for the specific needs of extrauterine preterm neonates. These formulas generally have calcium and phosphorus concentrations nearly four times those of human milk and are supplemented with relatively large quantities of vitamins and other minerals. Studies comparing these preterm infant formulas to human milk have shown improved calcium and phosphorus retention rates.[35,73,75,77] From these studies, a recommended calcium intake of 190 mg·kg^{-1}·day^{-1} (4.75 mmol·kg^{-1}·day^{-1}) and phosphorus intake of 100 mg·kg^{-1}·day^{-1} (3.2 mmol·kg^{-1}·day^{-1}) have been advocated.[78] Several studies using formulas that provide these high calcium and phosphorus intakes have demonstrated infant bone mineral content approximating the expected intrauterine bone mineral content and retention rates equal to, and even exceeding, intrauterine accretion rates.[41,42,44,79] At least one study using a preterm formula with a Ca/P ratio of 1.9:1.0 demonstrated a low serum phosphorus concentration with hypercalciuria and high tubular reabsorption of phosphate.[79] This pattern was thought to indicate too high a calcium/phosphorus ratio with relative phosphorus deficiency. Others have shown good calcium and phosphorus retention at variable ratios, concluding that the absolute quantities of the minerals are more important than their ratio.[35,80] With better understanding of the differing bioavailability of the various calcium and phosphorus salts, it may be that no single calcium and phosphorus intake or ratio will hold universally ideal. Specific recommendations may need to be developed for the various salts and for formulas versus human milk fortifiers.

Magnesium

Magnesium is the fourth most abundant cation and the second most abundant intracellular cation with a total body content in the adult of 20 to 28 g. Sixty-five percent of the total body magnesium is complexed within the skeleton, 34% in the intracellular space, and 1% in the extracellular space.[81] Of the magnesium within the extracellular space, only 25% is in the readily measurable intravascular plasma. Plasma magnesium is distributed in a fashion similar to calcium, with approximately 32% being protein-bound, 13% complexed to compounds such as citrate and lactate, and 55% in the free ionic form.[82] Changes in total body magnesium content are largely reflected in changes in skeletal magnesium and to a far lesser extent in the serum concentration. Recently, measurement of ionized magnesium has become clinically possible. Serum total magnesium concentration is very stable and there appears to be even less fluctuation in the serum ionized magnesium concentration.[83] Further, unlike total magnesium, the concentration of extracellular ionized magnesium is similar to that of intracellular magnesium.[84] As more knowledge is gained, a better understanding of serum ionized magnesium may reveal a closer relationship of serum ionized magnesium to total body magnesium.

The intracellular magnesium concentration is highly regulated and stable. This stability is a reflection of the many critical roles magnesium plays in cellular metabolism. Magnesium is important to the stabilization of DNA, RNA, and ribosomes.[85] It contributes to the synthesis and degradation of RNA and to the binding of messenger RNA to ribosomes necessary for protein synthesis, and it plays a role in carbohydrate metabolism. Magnesium is a cofactor in over 300 enzyme systems, including the ubiquitous adenyl cyclase system.[86,87] Magnesium increases the stimulus threshold in nerve fibers and high concentrations can have a curare-like effect.

Serum magnesium concentration is closely regulated in comparison to other serum components. Normal adult serum magnesium concentration ranges from 1.8 to 2.8 mg·dl^{-1} (0.75 to 1.2 mmol·L^{-1}) and varies little throughout the span of adult life. Although the relations are not as well defined as for calcium, many of the same hormones that regulate serum calcium concentration appear to affect serum magnesium concentration. Acute changes in serum magnesium concentration have effects on the PTH secretion similar to those produced by acute changes in calcium concentration.[88] An acute increase in serum magnesium concentration leads to a decline in serum PTH.[89] An acute decrease in the serum magnesium concentration results in an increase in PTH secretion similar to, but less than, that seen with comparable percentage changes in the serum calcium concentration. An increase in PTH secretion results in an increase in serum magnesium concentration probably via increased intestinal absorption, bone resorption, and, more importantly, decreased losses in the urine.[81,90]

Paradoxically, chronic magnesium deficiency results in decreased PTH secretion and a blunting of the action of PTH at target organs.[87,91-93] Decreased PTH secretion and action occur as a result of magnesium's role as a cofactor in the adenyl cyclase enzyme system. Adenyl cyclase converts ATP to cAMP, which is a primary messenger for secretion of PTH from parathyroid glands and for the action of PTH at its respective target organs.[94,95] Magnesium deficiency may lead to or exacerbate hypocalcemia by inhibiting the parathyroid response to declining serum calcium concentration.

The role of calcitonin in the regulation of serum magnesium concentration appears to be minimal. In vitro studies have shown that a 100% increase in the magnesium concentration of the extracellular bath leads to a discharge of calcitonin from the thyroid parafollicular cells.[96] This action compares to a similar calcitonin response with a 20% increase in the calcium concentration. A study of term and preterm infants who were infused with magnesium demonstrated no acute calcitonin response despite an increase of $1\,mg\cdot dl^{-1}$ ($0.4\,mmol\cdot L^{-1}$) to hypermagnesemic concentrations.[97] Likewise, a study in rats on a prolonged magnesium-deficient diet noted no calcitonin response despite significant decreases in serum magnesium.[98]

Vitamin D's influence on magnesium metabolism is not well defined. Although magnesium malabsorption has been reported in such vitamin D–deficient diseases as osteomalacia and rickets, magnesium deficiency may be related to malnutrition and decreased magnesium intake rather than vitamin D deficiency.[90] In one study, $1,25(OH)_2D$ given to vitamin D–replete adults showed no effect on the magnesium absorption.[53] In another study in which vitamin D was given to a population known to be at risk for vitamin D deficiency, the experimental group had a high serum calcium concentration but a low serum magnesium concentration relative to controls.[99] Animal studies have noted different findings. Both vitamin D–replete and –depleted animals responded to pharmacologic doses of $1,25(OH)_2D$ by increasing magnesium absorption.[100,101] Balancing this increased absorption, in both animals and humans, is an enhanced urinary loss with high doses of vitamin D resulting in no change or a decrease in net retention of magnesium.[102,103] Magnesium deficiency is associated with decreased $1,25(OH)_2D$ production in adults[104] and children.[105,106] Although the mechanism of this decreased production is unknown, it may be secondary to magnesium being a cofactor to $25(OH)D\text{-}1\alpha$-hydroxylase in renal tubular cells.[106] Magnesium supplementation to magnesium-deficient, hypocalcemic children results in an improved hormonal response to hypocalcemic diets with elevations in PTH and $1,25(OH)_2D$.[105]

Other hormones known to have a direct or indirect effect on the serum magnesium concentration are estrogen, thyroxin, and aldosterone, which lead to decreased serum magnesium concentrations, and epinephrine, glucocorticoids, and progesterone, which lead to an increased serum magnesium concentration. The overall effect of these hormones in the normal state appears to be minimal.

The average diet is plentiful in magnesium. Magnesium is absorbed in the distal small intestine, with colonic absorption occurring at low magnesium intakes. Unlike calcium, magnesium absorption is not predominantly active but a combination of facilitated diffusion and passive intercellular diffusion.[107] Facilitated diffusion, and a putative active colonic component, is most prominent at low intakes but is readily saturable at higher intakes.[108] Therefore, magnesium intake is nearly linear at all but the most restricted dietary intakes. Fractional absorption of magnesium appears to decrease with increasing age. The neonate has a fractional absorption of 55% to 75% depending on intake.[109,110] This figure compares with a fractional absorption of 35% to 49% in adults.[90,111] Absorption of magnesium depends on the composition of the intestinal content. Calcium, phosphorus, and long-chain triglycerides decrease the absorption of magnesium.[90] Calcium and magnesium appear to compete directly for absorptive sites in the intestine.[112]

The magnesium content of feces varies with intake, as the amount of endogenous magnesium excreted into the feces is small and stable despite the large quantities of magnesium in gastrointestinal secretions. The kidney is the primary site of magnesium regulation. Ionized magnesium is freely filtered at the glomerulus, and excretion is independent of glomerular filtration above a rate of $30\,ml\cdot min^{-1}$ per $1.73\,m^2$. The filtered ionized magnesium is primarily reabsorbed in the thick ascending loop of Henle.[113,114] This reabsorption is a function of the concentration of the magnesium presented to the tubule, effects of PTH, and, to a lesser extent, calcitonin.

Magnesium Metablism in Pregnancy

The Food and Nutrition Board of the National Academy of Sciences recommended dietary allowance for magnesium during pregnancy is $320\,mg\cdot day^{-1}$.[115] This figure compares with a typical adult diet of 300 to $360\,mg\cdot day^{-1}$.[111] Serum magnesium concentration in the pregnant woman falls slightly, reaching a nadir during the third trimester and rising during the last 4 to 6 weeks of pregnancy.[9,12] In that serum magnesium concentration makes up only a small fraction of the total body magnesium content, this fall may or may not reflect a biologically significant change in overall magnesium balance. This change in serum magnesium concentration resembles the change in serum total calcium concentration, which appears largely to reflect hemodilution due to an increased plasma volume.[116] Hemodilution does not fully explain this drop however. Handwerker et al.[83] noted that the percent decline in both serum ionized and total magnesium concentration was far less than the decrease in serum albumin during late pregnancy. Therefore, some regulatory mechanisms must be at work to maintain the serum magnesium concentration.

Transfer of magnesium from mother to fetus appears to be an active transport process. This is inferred from the fetal serum magnesium concentration being greater than the maternal serum concentration during much of intrauterine life. When magnesium radioisotopes were given to pregnant rabbits, the isotope was rapidly concentrated within the fetus.[117] As with most minerals, this transfer from pregnant female to fetus appears to increase exponentially over gestation. There is a sharp increase in the transfer of magnesium after the fifth month of gestation, reaching a peak of approximately 4.5 mg·day^{-1} (1.9 mmol·d^{-1}) by the eighth month. After the eighth month of gestation, there is a plateau in fetal total body magnesium content at approximately 1 g.[1] Serum total magnesium concentration in all but the markedly preterm neonate is similar to that of term neonate; however, serum ionized magnesium concentration may be higher in the less than 32-week gestation neonate than the term neonate.[118]

Although transfer of calcium and magnesium by the placenta are both active processes, they differ in at least one significant way. The placental transport system for calcium allows the fetus to be relatively independent of the calcium status of the pregnant female, whereas magnesium transport is more dependent. In maternal magnesium deficiency the pregnant female may maintain a normal intracellular magnesium concentration while her fetus has been shown, in at least one study, to be magnesium deficient.[119] Severe maternal magnesium deficiency has been associated with increased fetal loss in some species but no known human equivalent has yet been proved. A possible exception might be the infant of the diabetic mother. Pregnant insulin-dependent diabetic women have been shown to be at risk for true magnesium depletion due to high urinary magnesium losses and are at increased risk for fetal loss.[120] These women have impaired parathyroid function as well as blunted elevations in 1,25(OH)$_2$D in the third trimester.[121] These alterations may explain the increased risk for hypocalcemia and decreased bone mineral content seen in infants of diabetic mothers. Another study demonstrated that magnesium supplementation of pregnant women leads to fewer preterm births and a decrease in both maternal and neonatal days in the hospital.[122] Maternal hypermagnesemia results in fetal hypermagnesemia; the degree of the fetal hypermagnesemia corresponds to maternal hypermagnesemia much more than fetal hypercalcemia relates to maternal hypercalcemia.[123] With an acute increase in maternal serum magnesium concentration, there is a delay before an elevation is noted in the fetal concentration.[124,125] This delay is felt to be a protective effect of the placenta to acute mineral perturbations. However, over a period of days the fetal concentration will equilibrate and eventually exceed maternal concentration.[125]

Magnesium Metabolism in the Neonate

The preterm neonate at the eighth month of gestation has an average cord blood magnesium concentration similar to that of the term neonate, with a mean of 1.95 mg·dl^{-1} (0.8 mmol·L^{-1}) and ranging from 1.43 to 2.45 mg·dl^{-1} (0.6 to 1.0 mmol·L^{-1}).[126] Subsequently, there is an increase in serum magnesium concentration over the first week of life followed by a decline toward childhood values by the end of the first month.[127] A major cause of the change in serum magnesium concentration is the change in urinary magnesium excretion. Urinary magnesium excretion primarily depends on the glomerular filtration rate (GFR) and the effect of PTH. Term and preterm neonates have decreased GFRs over the first 48–72 hours of life, and urinary magnesium losses are markedly decreased to the range of 0.12 to 0.34 mg·kg^{-1}·day^{-1} over this period.[128] By 1 week of age, with an increase in dietary magnesium and an increase in GFR, there is an increase in magnesium excretion to the values more typical of the older child, 1.4 mg·kg^{-1}·day^{-1}. The preterm neonate whose GFR is decreased relative to the older infant has even lower magnesium excretion rate than the term neonate.[129] The very preterm are at risk for long-term magnesium deficiency due to renal immaturity. These infants have demonstrated high urinary magnesium losses even in a negative balance state and fail to achieve intrauterine retention rates despite intakes at the recommended 10 mg·kg^{-1}·day^{-1} (0.4 mmol·kg^{-1}·day^{-1}).[130]

The neonate's diet may vary widely in its content of magnesium, from human milk with 35 mg·L^{-1} (1.4 mmol·L^{-1}), to standard formulas with up to 81 mg·L^{-1} (3.4 mmol·L^{-1}). Human milk magnesium appears to be well absorbed by the term neonate, and there has been no documented report of magnesium deficiency in these neonates as a result of exclusive human milk feedings. However, in mothers who have delivered preterm neonates, magnesium concentration in milk decreases over time. One study noted an initial increase in the preterm neonate's serum magnesium concentration followed by a steady decline in serum magnesium concentration to 1 month of age.[127] The quantity of magnesium retained by these preterm neonates receiving their own mothers' milk did not meet the expected intrauterine accretion rates. This group of neonates was compared to a similar group fed a preterm formula with an increased magnesium concentration. In the latter group of neonates there was no decline in the serum magnesium concentration over the first month of life, and although these neonates had magnesium retention rates less than their intrauterine rates, they had greater retention that the human milk–fed neonates.

In another study of very low birth weight neonates, comparison was made between fortified preterm human milk and a preterm infant formula.[75] This study showed that supplementation could increase magnesium retention rates but that retention and intake were not correlated. A study using human milk fortified with minerals and components of powdered term human milk achieved magnesium retention rates greater than fetal accretion rates despite total magnesium concentrations in the milk less than that in many preterm infant formulas.[72]

It appears that bioavailability may be an important factor affecting magnesium status during the neonatal period. Formulas with high concentrations of calcium and phosphorus were shown in one study to decrease magnesium absorption such that magnesium retention rates are negative or fall below intrauterine rates.[130] As with calcium, magnesium is more efficiently absorbed from formulas containing short- or medium-chain triglycerides than long-chain triglycerides.[34] Although intrauterine accretion rates are being used as the "gold standard" for mineral requirements for preterm neonates, whether they are appropriate goals for the postnatal preterm neonate remains to be determined.

The relation between serum magnesium concentration and serum calcium concentration in the neonate is the focus of continued investigation. Theoretically, magnesium with its integral role in the secretion and function of PTH may have a permissive effect on the neonate's PTH response to a falling serum calcium concentration. A study of normal neonates demonstrated that the amplitude of the rise in serum PTH after birth correlated with neonatal serum magnesium concentration.[131] Further support for this permissive rule is found in the infant of the diabetic mother. These neonates have an increased incidence of hypomagnesemia and hypocalcemia and an apparently blunted PTH secretory response to hypocalcemia.[132,133] In infants of diabetic mothers, a decreased serum calcium concentration correlates well with the decreased serum magnesium concentration and decreased serum PTH secretory responsiveness.[132,134] Conversely, hypermagnesemic infants have increased serum calcium and often undetectable serum PTH concentrations.[135] This may indicate that magnesium influences the postnatal rise in serum calcium directly, in addition to acting on PTH secretion. Further study is necessary to better define the role of magnesium in neonatal calcium homeostasis.

Hypermagnesemia, defined as a magnesium concentration of more than $2.8 \text{ mg} \cdot \text{dl}^{-1}$ ($1.2 \text{ mmol} \cdot \text{L}^{-1}$), is a common iatrogenic result of therapy for maternal toxemia of pregnancy. When the pregnant woman is given magnesium sulfate the fetus's serum magnesium concentration rises in parallel. This fetal hypermagnesemia is a function of both the duration and degree of the maternal hypermagnesemia. A maternal serum concentration between 3 and $8 \text{ mg} \cdot \text{dl}^{-1}$ (1.24 and $3.3 \text{ mmol} \cdot \text{L}^{-1}$) is not uncommon.[135] High magnesium concentrations act as a natural calcium antagonist and have been shown to inhibit the release of acetylcholine at the neuromuscular junction. The signs of hypermagnesemia vary from individual to individual but generally increase with an increasing magnesium concentration. Signs such as lethargy, hypotonia, hypoventilation and apnea, hypotension, urinary retention, and prolonged atrioventricular conduction intervals are the result of magnesium's "calcium blocker" effect. Because of decreased urinary magnesium excretion of the first several days of life, the neonate may maintain an elevated serum magnesium concentration for the first 3 to 4 days of life. In many instances this hypermagnesemia is without sufficient symptomatology to warrant therapeutic intervention. For those neonates with severe or prolonged abnormal signs, hydration and a loop diuretic (e.g., furosemide or ethacrynic acid) may be helpful. For extreme cases with severe hypotension or cardiac dysrhythmias, double blood volume "exchange" transfusion may be used to rapidly reduce serum magnesium concentrations. Prolonged intrauterine hypermagnesemia may lead to the development of congenital rickets. Lamm et al.[136] reported five infants with long-term fetal exposure to hypermagnesemia that were born with osteopenia. The etiology is speculative but may involve heteroionic exchange of magnesium for calcium at the bone or inhibition of PTH production. With the increased use of magnesium as a tocolytic agent this warrants further investigation.

Neonatal hypomagnesemia is defined as a serum concentration of less than $1.6 \text{ mg} \cdot \text{dl}^{-1}$ ($0.66 \text{ mmol} \cdot \text{L}^{-1}$). Hypomagnesemia is common in asphyxiated neonates, intrauterine growth-retarded neonates, infants of diabetic mothers, and neonates born to magnesium-deficient mothers, such as those with malnutrition or malabsorptive conditions. Hypomagnesemia, hypocalcemia, and hypoparathyroidism are frequently encountered together, which is consistent with the theory that magnesium deficiency leads to a functional inhibition of parathyroid hormone secretion. The signs of hypomagnesemia are similar to those of hypocalcemia and occur most commonly with serum concentration less than $1.2 \text{ mg} \cdot \text{dl}^{-1}$ ($0.5 \text{ mmol} \cdot \text{L}^{-1}$).[129] Because hypomagnesemia and hypocalcemia are frequently found together, the exact contribution of each to clinical symptomatology is blurred. Signs commonly seen are irritability, tremor, hyperreflexia, and muscle weakness. Less common signs are hypertension, ST segment depression or T wave inversion, and seizures.

Therapy for hypomagnesemia is magnesium replacement enterally or parenterally. The minimum daily requirement of magnesium is estimated to be $6 \text{ mg} \cdot \text{kg}^{-1} \text{day}^{-1}$ ($0.25 \text{ mmol} \cdot \text{kg}^{-1} \text{day}^{-1}$) using elemental magnesium, and treatment for hypomagnesemia is two to three times the maintenance amount. It may be given enterally as magnesium sulfate, gluconate, lactate, or citrate. With an expected fractional absorption of only 55% to 75%, oral supplementation for hypomagnesemia should be in the range of 20 to 40 mg of element magnesium per kilogram per day. The daily dose of magnesium should be divided into at least four doses and diluted in feedings to minimize the diarrhea associated with enteral magnesium therapy.

For acutely symptomatic hypomagnesemia, parenteral therapy, intravenous or intramuscular, may be given. The preferred parenteral route is intramuscular using 50% magnesium sulfate (i.e., containing 50 mg elemental magnesium·ml^{-1}). A 50% magnesium sulfate dose of 0.1 to 0.2 mg·kg^{-1} (5–10 mg elemental magnesium per kilogram) may be given intramuscularly and may be repeated every 6 hours if hypomagnesemia persists. Intravenous infusion of magnesium sulfate must be given slowly and cautiously, with electrocardiographic and blood pressure monitoring to detect prolongation of the atrioventricular conduction time (i.e., long PR interval) or hypotension, which may occur with hypermagnesemia. A 0.12 ml·kg^{-1} dose of 50% magnesium sulfate diluted in a volume equal to 5 to 10 cc·kg^{-1}, given over 1 hour, has been shown to increase serum magnesium concentration by approximately 1 mg·dl^{-1} (0.4 mmol·L^{-1}). Intravenous therapy should be reserved for the symptomatic neonate.

Parathyroid Hormone

Parathyroid hormone (PTH) is a primary calcium-regulating hormone produced by the parathyroid glands. These glands are derived embryonically from the third and fourth endobranchial pouches. Because little hormone is stored within the parathyroid glands, polyribosomes of the rough endoplasmic reticulum of chief cells produce preproparathyroid hormone almost continually. Preproparathyroid hormone undergoes a series of two cleavage steps to produce the metabolically active 9500-dalton PTH. This protein is 84 amino acids long with the 1–34, N-terminal portion conferring bioactivity. Subtle decreases in serum calcium concentration induce the synthesis and release of PTH. The release of PTH from the gland is believed to be by exocytosis and is mediated by the magnesium-dependent adenyl cyclase enzyme system.[94] Although serum calcium is the primary regulator of PTH secretion, acute hypomagnesemia[137] decreases in 1,25(OH)$_2$D,[59,138] and increases in epinephrine[139] appear to stimulate the release of PTH. Receptors for 1,25(OH)$_2$D have been identified in the parathyroid gland and 1,25(OH)$_2$D may play a role in control of PTH secretion.[140,141]

Parathyroid hormone primarily affects three systems (e.g., the bone and kidney directly and the intestine indirectly to raise serum calcium concentration). At the bone, PTH in conjunction with 1,25(OH)$_2$D appears to induce a two-phase reaction. Initially, PTH inhibits bone-forming osteoblasts and induces conversion of osteoprogenitor cells to osteoclasts. The osteoclasts resorb bone and release calcium and phosphorus into the circulation. The second phase is a stimulatory effect on osteoblasts. The effect of PTH on bone is to initially increase resorption, then to increase both resorption and formation, or turnover of bone. PTH action at the kidney decreases reabsorption of calcium, phosphorus, sodium, and bicarbonate by the proximal tubule, which results in presentation of large concentrations of these minerals to the distal nephron.[142] PTH has its predominant effect by stimulating reabsorption of large quantities of calcium, with the net result of increased reabsorption of calcium and increased loss of phosphorus and bicarbonate.[143] PTH has an indirect effect on absorption of calcium from intestine through stimulation of the 25(OH)D-1α-hydroxylase system in the kidney. Under the influence of PTH, 25(OH)D is converted to 1,25(OH)$_2$D, which promotes increased calcium absorption from intestine, bone resorption, and urinary calcium reabsorption.

The actions of PTH at different target sites are likely mediated through a similar biochemical mechanism. In each of the target cells PTH is bound to a membrane receptor. Receptor binding induces production of a primary messenger termed an N or a G protein. The N protein stimulates a magnesium-dependent enzyme, adenyl cyclase, to convert ATP to cAMP. Cyclic-AMP increases both the efflux of calcium from the mitochondria and the influx of calcium from plasma to cytosal. It activates protein kinases, which promote phosphorylation of specific cytoplasmic proteins leading to cellular effects such as osteoclast activation, increased renal tubular cell calcium transport, and activation of 25(OH)-1α-hydroxylase in renal tubular cells.[144]

Parathyroid Hormone Metabolism in Pregnancy

Pregnancy has been described as a state of "physiologic hyperparathyroidism."[145] Although this concept has been recently challenged in several small studies,[13,146] the majority of studies have reported that by term the pregnant woman's serum PTH concentration may be elevated, even if not above the stated normal ranges, compared to the nonpregnant state.[9,10,12,145,147] Most studies have been cross-sectional and have shown a PTH increase during the third trimester with or without an earlier rise during the first trimester.[10,145] In two longitudinal studies, serum PTH concentration was found to increase progressively from early pregnancy to a peak at term;[9,12] at term the serum PTH concentration was 40% to 100% greater than that during early pregnancy. No correlation was found in any study between total calcium concentration and PTH. One study noted that serum PTH increased in parallel to the decline in calcium concentration.[10]

Parathyroid hormone does not appear to cross the placenta. Injection of radiolabeled PTH into the pregnant female of various animal species has not resulted in transfer to the fetus.[148,149] Human neonatal PTH concentration at delivery is significantly less than[10,150,151] or similar to maternal PTH concentration.[147,152,153] The fetus appears capable of secreting PTH early in the pregnancy. Histologic studies have noted PTH within the gland as early as the 10th to 12th week of gestation.[154] The role of the fetal parathyroid glands in calcium homeostasis is unclear. One study noted no detectable increase in parathyroid hormone secretion in fetal monkeys subjected to experimental hypocalcemia,[155] whereas another study reported a response.[156] Supporting a role for fetal parathyroid glands in calcium homeostasis are several animal studies. Thyroparathyroidectomized fetal rats demonstrated a decline in serum calcium concentration.[157] Injection of an anti-PTH antibody into fetal rats caused a decrease in the serum calcium concentration.[158] Parathyroidectomy of fetal lambs produced a decrease in serum calcium concentration of the fetus and a reversal of the maternal-fetal calcium gradient.[29] Infusion of bovine PTH (1–84) or rat PTH (1–34) did not reverse this change, but a crude parathyroid gland extract did.[28] This finding indicated that the parathyroid glands produce PTH-bioactive substances other than 1–34PTH, and that these other substances are, at least in part, responsible for the maternal-fetal calcium gradient. The molecule responsible for activation of the ovine placental calcium pump appears to be a parathyroid hormone–related protein (PTHrP) 1-86 amide, and the C-terminal portion is the active component.[159] However, this amide effect was not demonstrated in a perfused rat placental model and questions remain regarding the mechanism of human placental calcium transfer.[160]

Parathyroid Hormone Metabolism in the Neonate

Parathyroid hormone concentration in the cord blood of the neonate is low to undetectable[10,63,161] or is similar to the maternal value.[147,152,153,162] The differing results may be in part secondary to the numerous PTH assays used by various investigators to measure the whole molecule, midmolecule, C-terminal, or N-terminal components of PTH and its metabolites.[152] There is agreement that over the first 24 to 48 hours PTH concentration in the term neonate increases markedly.[63,132,161,163] After 48 hours, there appears to be a slight decline to a plateau in serum PTH concentration[132,161] (Figure 40.4). Preterm neonates have been shown to have a blunted rise in the serum PTH concentration over the first 24 to 48 hours by several investigators[43,63,152] and to have a PTH response similar to that of term neonates by another.[161] This blunted response is expressed as a delay in the onset of rise and as a lower peak value. These findings have led investigators to propose an initial relative hypoparathyroidism in the preterm neonate. This hypoparathyroidism is further demonstrated in the preterm neonate's response to hypocalcemic stress induced by exchange transfusion with citrated blood. Exchanges performed prior to 3 days of age were associated with little or no PTH response in both the preterm and term neonate. Preterm neonates more than 3 days of age demonstrated a PTH response greater than neonates less than age 72 hours, but it was

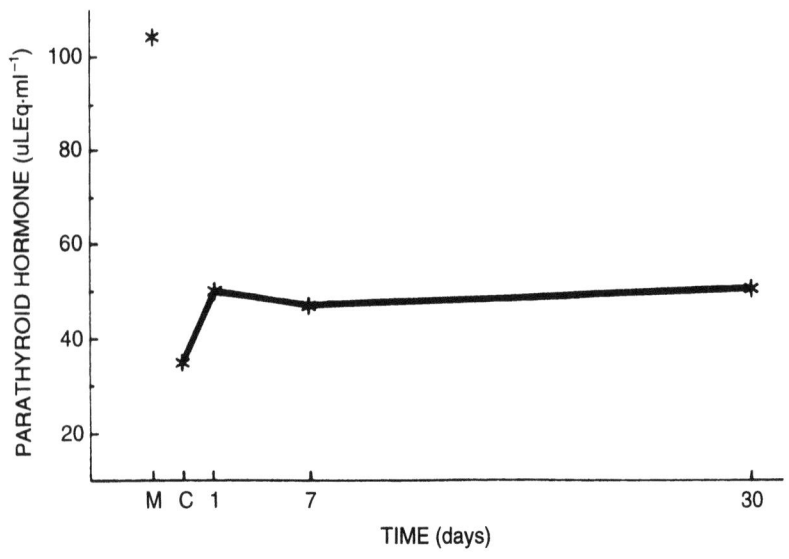

FIGURE 40.4. Cord, 1-, 7-, and 30-day serum parathyroid hormone concentration in the term neonate. Maternal (M) value at delivery. Normal adult range for this assay is 33 to 117 μlEq·ml^{-1}.

less than the PTH response of age-matched term neonates.[164] This finding indicates that there are both gestational and postnatal maturational changes in the PTH response, with the postnatal maturational changes being of more significance than the gestational changes.

Other factors affect the neonate's PTH response to hypocalcemia. Infants of diabetic mothers have an increased risk of hypocalcemia.[129,132,134] These neonates demonstrate a delayed and a decreased PTH response to hypocalcemia similar to that seen in the preterm neonate.[46,132] In that these neonates respond to exogenous PTH, there appears to be a functional hypoparathyroidism in the infant of the diabetic mother.[42] One hypothesis is that magnesium deficiency may contribute to this functional hypoparathyroidism.[97] It has been demonstrated that diabetic subjects are at risk for magnesium depletion and that infants of diabetic mothers have lower cord blood magnesium concentration than controls.[163] The PTH response to declining serum calcium concentrations is correlated to the infant's serum magnesium concentration, such that infants with lower cord serum magnesium concentrations have a blunted postnatal rise in PTH.

Asphyxia, as determined by Apgar score, is a risk factor for hypocalcemia. Studies of asphyxiated neonates have shown an increased PTH response over the first 72 hours of life.[46] The increase in PTH appeared to occur regardless of the extent of fall in serum calcium concentrations, which indicates that PTH secretion in these patients is not solely dependent on calcium concentration and that either an end-organ unresponsiveness to PTH (e.g., pseudohypoparathyroidism) or other factors associated with asphyxia override the calcemic effect of PTH.

Evidence for a pseudohypoparathyroid-like state in the term neonate has been proposed by studies evaluating urinary cAMP during the first 72 hours of life.[65,165] These studies demonstrated a decreased responsiveness to exogenous PTH on day 1 relative to day 3 of life, and an increase of nearly 30-fold in the levels of urinary cAMP with maturation. This pseudohypoparathyroid-like state is challenged by a study done in infants of diabetic mothers in which they were given PTH at 24 and 48 hours.[45] This study demonstrated a calcemic and phosphaturic response to exogenous PTH. Whether this response represents a physiologic or pharmacologic response has not been determined.

Neonatal Hyperparathyroidism

Primary neonatal hyperparathyroidism is a rare disease. It appears most commonly in the familial form and is assumed to be inherited as an autosomal recessive disorder.[166] More commonly, secondary hyperparathyroidism is found in the neonate. There have been 16 cases reported in the literature, often as a result of maternal hypoparathyroidism leading to maternal hypocalcemia.[167] The maternal hypocalcemia presumably leads to relative fetal hypocalcemia and hyperparathyroidism. The hyperparathyroid state may result in markedly demineralized bone and occasionally in neonatal hypercalcemia. Bone demineralization, if severe, may lead to intrauterine fractures and has been occasionally confused with such primary bone disorder as osteogenesis imperfecta.

Symptoms associated with neonatal hyperparathyroidism are related to the level of hypercalcemia and include vomiting, feeding intolerance, lethargy, and occasionally nephrolithiasis and hypertension. The radiologic findings include generalized bone demineralization with subperiosteal bone resorption and loss of the lamina dura surrounding the tooth buds.

A study of two neonates with secondary hyperparathyroidism showed that the biochemical changes associated with this type of hyperparathyroidism could resolve rapidly during the first 72 hours of life. Responsiveness of the parathyroid glands to ethylenediaminetetraacetic acid (EDTA)-induced hypocalcemia appeared to be normal by 12 days of age. Even with severe bone demineralization, routine care and feeding led to rapid remineralization by 1 month of age.[167]

Neonatal Hypoparathyroidism

Primary neonatal hypoparathyroidism may be present as an isolated defect or as part of a condition. It usually presents as persistent hypocalcemia of both total and ionized calcium with an undetectable serum PTH concentration. It has been suggested that a number of these patients may be part of the spectrum of the DiGeorge syndrome.[50] DiGeorge syndrome involves a series of anomalies involving the third and fourth endobranchial pouches resulting in abnormalities of the ear and mandible as well as the parathyroid, thymic, and cardiac systems. The pattern of inheritance has not been clearly established, but familial clusters have been reported.[168,169] It appears that many neonates with DiGeorge syndrome do not have complete absence of the thymus or parathyroid glands. If adequately supported throughout the neonatal period, the hypocalcemia and immunologic impairment may improve over the first year of life.

Transient neonatal hypoparathyroidism is another rare cause of neonatal hypocalcemia. The symptoms and signs are similar to those seen with other forms of neonatal hypoparathyroidism with an undetectable, or inappropriately low, PTH concentration during the neonatal period. The signs may be present within the first to several weeks of life and usually involve poor feeding, tremulousness, or tetany. Full recovery usually occurs within the first few months of life. One case report has shown that complete biochemical recovery may be prolonged and may not occur even as late as 22 months of age.[170]

Vitamin D

Vitamin D is available to the pregnant woman or neonate in one of two forms. Vitamin D_2, ergocalciferol, is produced naturally by plants and vitamin D_3, cholecalciferol, is produced in the skin and stored in the tissues of animals. Both are available in the diet, with vitamin D_3 being a readily supplied vitamin hormone for most sun exposed populations.

Vitamin D_3 is produced by animals in the epidermis by conversion of the cholesterol precursor 7-dehydrocholesterol to previtamin D. This conversion occurs when ultraviolet light splits the bonds between carbons 9 and 10, producing a conformation change in the second carbon ring. This change produces previtamin D_3, which is converted to vitamin D_3. Vitamin D_3 is carried by a specific carrier protein, vitamin D–binding protein (VDBP), to the liver (Figure 40.5).

Vitamin D, either as D_2 or D_3, when ingested in diet is absorbed pinocytotically in the small intestine, largely complexed with chylomicrons. These complexes are carried via the lymphatics or blood to the liver. In the liver, vitamin D_2 and vitamin D_3 undergo their first hydroxylation. This hydroxylation produces 25-hydroxyvitamin D_2 or 25-hydroxyvitamin D_3, [generally termed 25(OH)D] and may occur either in the endoplasmic reticulum, a high-affinity, low-capacity system, or in the mitochondria, a low-affinity, high-capacity system. Calcidiol, or 25(OH)D, is the most abundant form of circulating vitamin D and is the best indicator of vitamin D stores. There is feedback regulation at this hydroxylation step, but it appears to occur only at a very high serum concentration of 25(OH)D. With the ingestion of high doses of vitamin D or with greater sun exposure and increased production of vitamin D_3, there is only a transient elevation in circulating vitamin D concentration. However, concentrations of circulating 25(OH)D increase and remain high. Serum 25(OH)D is largely bound to VDBP and has a serum half-life of 2 to 3 weeks; 25(OH)D is bioactive but only at a high concentration, and the role of 25(OH)D appears to provide a readily available circulating pool of vitamin D.[171]

The second major hydroxylation of vitamin D occurs in the kidney. Under conditions of low serum phosphorous concentration, high parathyroid hormone concentration, and possibly low calcium concentration, 25(OH)D undergoes 1α-hydroxylation within the mitochondria of the proximal renal tubule cells. This conversation produces the most biologically active form of vitamin D, 1,25-dihydroxyvitamin D [1,25(OH)$_2$D], or calcitriol, which is carried in blood on VDBP. Measurements of serum 1,25(OH)$_2$D concentration increase with increasing VDBP concentrations. During periods of calcium and phosphorus deficiency or in the presence of a high concentration of circulating parathyroid hormone, serum

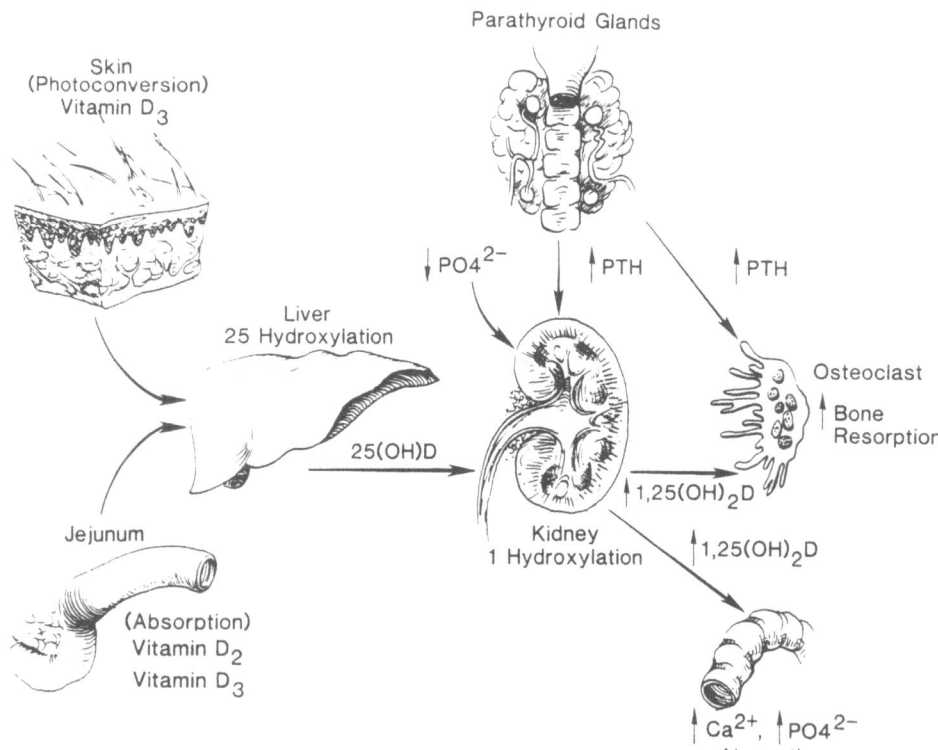

FIGURE 40.5. Vitamin D is derived from cholesterol in the skin or is absorbed in the diet. It is then transported to the liver to be converted to 25(OH)$_2$D. Under conditions of low serum calcium and phosphorus and increased PTH concentrations, 25(OH)D may then be further hydroxylated to 1,25(OH)$_2$D. 1,25(OH)$_2$D acts upon the bone, kidney, and intestine to increase serum calcium and phosphorus concentrations.

1,25(OH)$_2$D concentration is increased; 1,25(OH)$_2$D acts on intestine, bone, and kidney to increase the concentrations of circulating calcium and phosphorus. Also, 1,25(OH)$_2$D has a major effect at the enterocyte of the small intestine, stimulating production of calcium-binding protein within the enterocyte, facilitating transcellular calcium transport and markedly increasing active transport of calcium from intestine to blood.[172] Moreover, 1,25(OH)$_2$D acts in conjunction with PTH to release calcium and phosphorus from bone matrix. In the kidney, 1,25(OH)$_2$D acts on distal tubule cells to increase reabsorption of calcium, thereby decreasing urinary calcium losses.

With calcium and phosphorus sufficiency and a low concentration of circulating PTH, 25(OH)D undergoes an alternate hydroxylation in the kidney to 24,25-dihydroxyvitamin D [24,25(OH)$_2$D]. The precise role of this compound is not well defined. Increased concentration of 24,25(OH)$_2$D has been found during periods of rapid bone growth, such as in the fetus and early childhood, leading some to speculate that it plays a part in promoting fetal development and bone formation.[173-175]

Vitamin D Metabolism in Pregnancy

Alterations in calcium and vitamin D metabolism occur shortly after conception. These changes in vitamin D metabolism appear to be aimed at providing an optimal mineral environment for the fetus. A primary change in vitamin D metabolism is an increase in serum VDBP concentration. Serum VDBP has been shown to increase as early as the 10th week of pregnancy.[176] The concentration continues to rise during pregnancy, peaking between 34 and 36 weeks at approximately twice the nonpregnant concentration.[177,178] In that only a small portion of VDBP is complexed with a vitamin D sterol, the impact of this change on vitamin D metabolism is not entirely clear. But it appears to artificially elevate measured serum 1,25(OH)$_2$D concentrations.

The concentration of vitamin D itself does not change markedly during pregnancy from the nonpregnant serum concentration of 1 to 2 ng·ml^{-1}. The slight decrease to approximately 1 ng·ml^{-1} during pregnancy may be secondary to the increase in plasma volume that occurs during pregnancy.[179] Variations in dietary supplementation of vitamin D$_2$ and sunshine exposure influence the vitamin D$_2$/D$_3$ ratio in the circulation, with the sunshine exposure component being a major source of vitamin D.

Adequate vitamin D status during pregnancy is important for fetal bone ossification, postnatal calcium regulation, and odontogenesis. Infants born to mothers in northern climates and not supplemented with vitamin D have been found to have an increased incidence of delayed bone ossification, craniotabes, tooth enamel defects, and lack of postnatal rise in serum 1,25(OH)$_2$D.[180-185] Congenital rickets has been reported in neonates born to vitamin D–deficient mothers.[180,186] Maternal vitamin D supplementation reduced the incidence of delayed ossification and rickets in the population at risk for vitamin D deficiency.[185] Neonates born in summer have decreased bone mineral content compared with those born in winter.[187] These investigators speculated that maternal vitamin D status during early gestation (i.e., winter vitamin D status for infants born in summer) was important in ensuring optimal intrauterine bone mineralization. Concern remains on how to define adequate vitamin D stores and the issue of supplementation. Supplementation of 400 IU of vitamin D has been shown to be associated with vitamin D sufficiency but may be unnecessary in mothers receiving high sun exposure.

25(OH)D Metabolism During Pregnancy

Serum concentration of 25(OH)D during pregnancy, as in the nonpregnant state, is the best indicator of the mother's vitamin D status. In the unsupplemented pregnant woman, serum 25(OH)D concentration may[185,188] or may not[189,190] decrease over the term of her pregnancy. These differences in findings may be a consequence of the influence of seasonal changes in 25(OH)D concentration. Serum 25(OH)D concentration is increased by as much as threefold in August, compared to February.[189] Because of an individual's widely varying sun exposure and because of variances in climates, it might be desirable to supplement the pregnant woman with vitamin D during the term of her pregnancy. The standard vitamin D supplement in prenatal vitamins is 400 IU ergocalciferol (vitamin D$_2$) per day. Hollis and Pittard[179] showed that in a northern climate during the winter months this supplementation may lead 25(OH)D$_2$ to constitute as much as 50% of the mother's circulating 25(OH)D. These investigators showed that, despite supplementation, many patients had a 25(OH)D concentration in the low normal range, and one could suspect that without supplementation their 25(OH)D concentration would have been in the subnormal range. Alternate methods of supplementing the mother during pregnancy have been explored. Supplementing with 1000 units per day over the last trimester or with a single oral dose of 200,000 units of vitamin D during the seventh month of pregnancy significantly increases the maternal serum 25(OH)D concentration.[185,191] The safety of this regimen has not been adequately explored. Regardless of supplementation, sun exposure remains a major source of vitamin D and its metabolites for most women.[189]

The woman's 25(OH)D status is important in that 25(OH)D appears to be the major form of vitamin D transferred to the fetus. Such transfer appears to be passive in that the fetal concentration is approximately

70% to 80% of the maternal concentration.[192] Studies comparing cord blood serum 25(OH)D concentration to maternal concentration have noted a close correlation,[191,193-196] regardless of the gestational age of the fetus.[192,197] The discovery of a 25(OH)D sulfate ester has led to reevaluation of the maternal-fetal 25(OH)D relation.[198] The neonate's cord blood was found to contain a markedly greater concentration of 25(OH)D ester than was found in the mother. When 25(OH)D and 25(OH)D ester concentrations are combined, the fetal concentrations exceed the maternal combined total concentrations. Although there are sulfatases present in the placenta, they do not appear to deesterify the sulfated vitamin D ester, and it is unlikely that the ester crosses the placenta in either direction.[199] This ester theoretically may be produced by the placenta or fetus to inhibit the back-diffusion of 25(OH)D to the mother. It is suggested that esterification would trap or pool this vitamin D metabolite in the fetus. The role of 25(OH)D sulfates in fetal calcium metabolism has not been defined.

Maternal 25(OH)D may be hydroxylated within the placenta as well as simply passed to the fetus. Human placenta is capable of 1α-hydroxylation of 25(OH)D to 1,25(OH)$_2$D, and syncytiotrophoblasts contain specific 1,25(OH)$_2$D receptors.[200-202] Placental 24-hydroxylase activity has been demonstrated and appears to be the predominant 25(OH)D metabolic pathway regardless of the vitamin D status of the tissue.[203] The kidney contains both 1α- and 24-hydroxylases, but, in contrast, the hydroxylases act in a reciprocal fashion, with 1,25(OH)$_2$D generally suppressing the 1α-hydroxylase and stimulating the 24-hydroxylase. Thus, the 24-hydroxylase is active in the kidney only in states of vitamin D repletion. It is speculated that the predominant placental 24-hydroxylase activity may contribute to high fetal 24,25(OH)$_2$D concentrations and have important activity in fetoplacental function. The implications of these vitamin D–related hormones on fetal calcium supply and metabolism await further delineation.

In the fetus, 25(OH)D is stored primarily in blood, muscle, fat, kidney, and liver. The preterm neonate, with virtually no fat and decreased muscle mass, theoretically has decreased vitamin D stores compared to the larger term neonate, placing him at greater risk for postnatal vitamin D deficiency. One study found that preterm neonates, born with low serum 25(OH)D concentration, were unable to maintain or increase this concentration over the first several postnatal weeks.[197] Several investigations have demonstrated a steady increase in serum 25(OH)D concentration in preterm neonates given oral vitamin D supplements of 400 to 2100 IU·day^{-1}.[183,184,204,205] Although the preterm neonate may be born with diminished vitamin D stores, he appears able to increase or maintain his serum 25(OH)D concentration with relatively low amounts of vitamin D supplementation.

1,25-Vitamin D Metabolism in Pregnancy

Maternal 1,25(OH)$_2$D concentration increases soon after conception. A significant increase in plasma 1,25(OH)$_2$D concentration has been found by the 6th week of pregnancy, and there is progressive increase over the period of pregnancy.[206,207] The rapid early increase is surprising since, of the 30g of total calcium accreted by the fetus, two thirds is gained during the last trimester. Therefore, the maternal 1,25(OH)$_2$D concentration increases long before the mother is required to transfer any significant quantity of calcium to the fetus. At term, maternal 1,25(OH)$_2$D concentration is approximately double that of the nonpregnant woman.[207,208] In that maternal serum ionized calcium concentration is generally unchanged during pregnancy, the reason for the rapid and sustained increase in serum 1,25(OH)$_2$D concentration is not well understood. Parathyroid hormone is a primary stimulant to increased production of 1,25(OH)$_2$D in the nonpregnant person, but during pregnancy other hormonal influences have been implicated. In pregnant rats, 1,25(OH)$_2$D concentration increases equally in thyro-parathyroidectomized and control rats.[209] Estrogen, growth hormone, human placental lactogen (hPL), and human chorionic gonadotropin (hCG) increase during the first trimester.[207] Many of these hormones have been found to increase 1α-hydroxylase activity in animals.[210] Prolactin, which increases during early pregnancy, has been found pharmacologically to increase intestinal calcium absorption and the serum calcium concentration, without altering serum 1,25(OH)$_2$D concentration.[211] The hormones controlling calcium absorption and the extent of their interaction during pregnancy is an area for further research.

Transport of 1,25(OH)$_2$D from mother to fetus is controversial. In all studies, maternal serum 1,25(OH)$_2$D concentration is significantly higher than the fetal concentration. In some studies maternal-fetal concentrations do not correlate,[185,208,212] whereas in others there is good correlation.[176,213,214] When radiolabeled 1,25(OH)$_2$D has been given in therapeutic doses to the maternal rat, measurable quantities of labeled 1,25(OH)$_2$D have been found in the fetus.[215] Additionally, when radiolabeled 1,25(OH)$_2$D has been given to fetal sheep, measurable quantities have been found in the maternal circulation.[196] Maternal-fetal and fetal-maternal transfer of 1,25(OH)$_2$D appears possible, but more investigation is necessary.

The fetus is capable of producing 1,25(OH)$_2$D from 25(OH)D. Fetal kidney, in addition to the placenta, is capable of 1α-hydroxylation from very early in gestation.[26,27] The role of fetal 1,25(OH)$_2$D is not known. As the primary function of this hormone in the older individual is to increase absorption of calcium from the intestine, a function presumably not essential to the fetus, and since 1,25(OH)$_2$D acts on bone to mobilized calcium from bone, it is assumed that low concentrations of 1,25(OH)$_2$D may be beneficial in supporting fetal bone growth.[173,216]

Another possible role of fetal 1,25(OH)$_2$D is to stimulate production of calcium-binding protein (CaBP) in the placenta. A placental CaBP (pCaBP) has been identified similar to that found in the intestine.[22] The role of intestinal CaBP is to transport ionized calcium within the enterocyte, and it is speculated that the pCaBP plays a similar role in the placenta. It appears that pCaBP is 1,25(OH)$_2$D dependent.[24] The presence of 1α-hydroxylase in the placenta and the low but detectable fetal serum 1,25(OH)$_2$D concentration may signify a fetal role in the metabolic control of placental calcium transfer.

Vitamin D Metabolism in the Neonate

For most neonates access to direct sunlight and provision of vitamin D in the diet is low over the first several weeks to months after birth. The neonate theoretically is dependent on stores provided by the mother during intrauterine life. Vitamin D–deficient mothers have neonates with low serum 25(OH)D and calcium concentrations, and an increased incidence of late neonatal tetany.[217,218] These neonates have been shown to have decreased intestinal calcium absorption.[71] It has been speculated that this decreased serum 25(OH)D concentration would lead to a decreased ability to produce 1,25(OH)$_2$D and inhibit the neonate's intestinal absorption of calcium. A close relationship between serum 25(OH)D and 1,25(OH)$_2$D concentration of preterm neonates has been demonstrated.[183] Neonates born to mothers deficient in vitamin D have a low cord blood 25(OH)D concentration that remains low or falls, and they do not have a postnatal rise in 1,25(OH)$_2$D.[183,184] This low 25(OH)D concentration may persist for the first month of life before slowly rising to normal. Supplementation with as little as 500 IU vitamin D per day has been found to restore 25(OH)D and produce an increase in 1,25(OH)$_2$D concentration.[205] It appears that the 25(OH)D concentration may be the rate-limiting factor in the neonate's ability to increase 1,25(OH)$_2$D in the presence of low 25(OH)D concentration and decreased calcium absorption.

Preterm and term neonates born to vitamin D–sufficient mothers have similar cord blood 25(OH)D concentrations and appear to remain stable over the first week of life unless supplemented. Clements and Frasier,[219] using radiolabeled vitamin D$_3$, found that intrauterine transfer of vitamin D was the predominant source of vitamin D in the serum of the newborn rat pup over the first 1.5 to 2.0 weeks of life. There are analogous studies in humans; however, Specker et al.[220] found in exclusively breast-fed neonates that serum 25(OH)D concentration correlated well with maternal 25(OH)D concentration only up to 8 weeks of age. Another study confirmed this finding but showed correlation over only the first 2 weeks.[221] Breast milk 25(OH)D concentrations correlate well with maternal plasma values up to 5 to 8 weeks after delivery.[221,222] Maternally provided vitamin D, from either intrauterine or breast milk routes, appears to be the predominant source of 25(OH)D over the first several weeks to months in the unsupplemented neonate. The exclusively breast-fed infant may be at risk for vitamin D depletion after the first 1 to 2 months of age.

Enhancing the importance of maternally derived vitamin D, or 25(OH)D, is that diets available to the neonate may supply little vitamin D. Human milk's vitamin D content is apparently dependent on the mother's vitamin D status. Even in the vitamin D–supplemented mother, the content of vitamin D in human milk is low. The predominant forms of vitamin D in human milk are vitamin D and 25(OH)D. Taking into account all forms of vitamin D, human milk provides only 20 to 60 IU of vitamin D activity per liter. No difference between preterm or term human milk vitamin D activity has been demonstrated. Several studies have noted a steady decrease in serum 25(OH)D concentration in the unsupplemented, term, exclusively breast-fed neonate over the first 6 months of age.[220,223] One of these studies noted the marked influence of sunshine. Specker et al.[268] found that exclusively breast-fed neonates born during the summer had a steady decline in serum 25(OH)D concentrations during the winter months followed by an increase during the summer months (Figure 40.6). Neonates born during winter months show a steady increase with age during the summer, and then a decline toward winter. It appears that human milk alone in the non–sun-exposed neonate does not provide a significant source of vitamin D, and sun exposure is the predominant variable.

Infant formulas are supplemented with at least 400 IU vitamin D per liter, predominantly as ergocalciferol. These formulas would provide a 3.75-kg neonate, ingesting 200 ml·kg^{-1}·day^{-1}, the recommended dietary allowance (RDA) for neonates of 300 IU·day^{-1}. For the preterm neonate having a similar intake, a standard formula provides significantly less vitamin D than the USRDA for neonates. The concentration of vitamin D in some preterm infant formulas has been increased markedly to 1000 to 2000 IU·L^{-1} and would provide the 1-kg neonate ingesting 150 mg·kg^{-1}day^{-1} the equivalent of 150–300 IU of vitamin D activity per day. Whether this amount is optimal for these neonates is the focus of continued investigation.

In summary, there appears to be little change in serum vitamin D or 25(OH)D concentrations during pregnancy, with a progressive rise in 1,25(OH)$_2$D concentration;

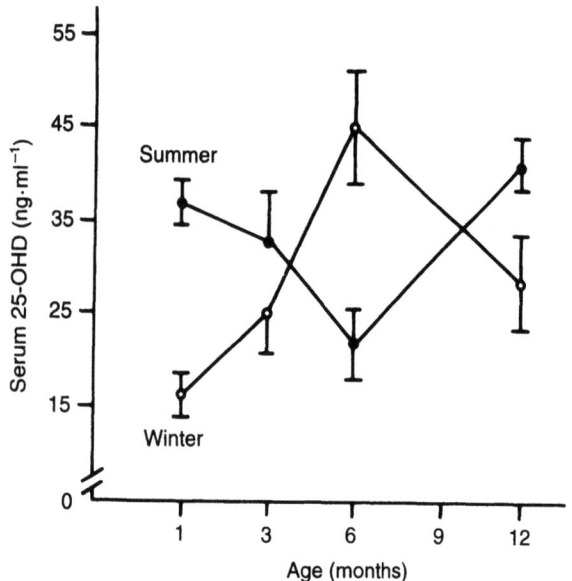

FIGURE 40.6. Changes in serum 25(OH)D concentration in relation to age and season. (From Specker and Tsang,[268] with permission.)

25(OH)D appears to be the predominantly transferred metabolite to the fetus. The fetus appears able to absorb 1α-hydroxylate 25(OH)D, yet the function of this metabolite during fetal life is unclear. Also 1,25(OH)$_2$D might be important in the placental transfer of calcium from mother to fetus for promotion of fetal bone mineralization. The initial stores of vitamin D for the young neonate appear to depend on the mother's vitamin D status and possibly the length of gestation. Serum 25(OH)D concentration remains stable in both preterm and term neonates for the first 1 to 2 months of age, if their initial concentration is normal. In vitamin D deficient preterm neonates, serum 25(OH)D concentration may remain low if unsupplemented. Serum 1,25(OH)$_2$D normally rises for the first week of life in the term and preterm neonates with adequate 25(OH)D stores. Because of the low quantity of vitamin D available in human milk, the neonate is dependent on prenatally acquired stores, sunshine exposure, or diet supplementation.

Calcitonin

Calcitonin is the predominant hormone known to decrease serum calcium concentration. Calcitonin is secreted from parafollicular (or "C") cells of the thyroid gland. These cells are of neural crest origin and are derived embryologically from the last endobranchial pouch. Calcitonin is a 32 amino acid polypeptide, and it appears that the entire chain is necessary to confer bioactivity. Adult serum calcitonin concentrations vary widely, ranging from undetectable to 50 pg·mL^{-1}.[224] The wide range of serum concentrations may be related to the technical difficulty of measuring picogram quantities, multiple factors affecting calcitonin secretion, and the circadian rhythm of secretion with a peak occurring at approximately noon.[225]

Secretion of calcitonin is influenced primarily by changes in serum ionized calcium concentration. An increase in serum calcium concentration leads to increase both the synthesis and secretion of calcitonin.[96] The role of calcitonin in calcium homeostasis appears to have a decreasing impact with increasing age.[57]

Magnesium, as the other major divalent cation of the body, affects calcitonin secretion. An increase in serum magnesium concentration has been shown in sheep to increase calcitonin secretion.[226] In the human, magnesium induces a rapid and striking decrease in circulating calcitonin concentrations in patients with hypercalcitoninemia secondary to medullary carcinoma of the thyroid.[227] These changes in serum magnesium concentration have been beyond the physiologic range, and the effect of magnesium on secretion of calcitonin in the normal state is not well defined.

Hormones such as gastrin, glucagon, cholecystokinin-pancreozymin, prostaglandin (PGE$_2$), and adrenergic agonists are calcitonin secretagogues.[228-230] With the exception of the adrenergic agonists, all of these hormones are involved in gastrointestinal digestion, which has led to speculation that calcitonin may play a role in the modulation of digestion as well as the serum calcium concentration.[231]

Calcitonin decreases the serum calcium concentration via an effect on bone and kidney. Calcitonin decreases bone resorption induced by vitamin D and PTH,[232] which is reflected by a decline in urinary hydroxyproline concentration.[233] Calcitonin decreases the number of osteoclasts, the cells responsible for bone resorption, and alters their ultrastructure.[58] Whereas it was initially thought that calcitonin inhibited the PTH effect on these cells, it now appears that calcitonin has a direct and independent effect.[234] Calcitonin, like PTH, stimulates adenyl cyclase, but instead of increasing the intracellular calcium concentration, there is a decrease.[235] In the kidney, calcitonin causes an increase in urinary calcium, phosphorus, magnesium, and cAMP.[236] Calcitonin does not appear to have a direct effect on intestinal absorption of calcium or phosphorus.[237,238] Calcitonin decreases secretion of gastrin and gastric acid, decreases gastric emptying and intestinal motility, impairs glucose tolerance, and decreases insulin secretion.[239] The impact of these effects on overall calcium homeostasis is not well defined.

Calcitonin has a half-life of approximately 10 to 15 minutes. Degradation of calcitonin occurs in the kidney primarily, but may occur in liver as well as placenta.[239,240]

Calcitonin Metabolism During Pregnancy

In cross-sectional studies, calcitonin concentration during pregnancy has been described as being elevated during all three trimesters of pregnancy.[190,241,242] In two longitudinal studies, a similar result was found when comparing the mean concentration of all patients.[9,12] Individual patients were highly variable, with no change, a decline, or an increase to the end of the second trimester followed by a decline to term. Calcitonin has been suggested to have a protective effect on the maternal skeleton during pregnancy. In rhesus monkeys there is increased calcitonin responsiveness to elevated serum calcium concentration during pregnancy.[243] In pregnant thyroidectomized rats there is a decrease in bone density relative to normal pregnant controls, leading to speculation that without calcitonin the maternal skeleton is at risk for demineralization.[242,244]

Calcitonin does not appear to cross the placenta.[245] However, there are calcitonin receptors on both the maternal side brush border (BBM) and the fetal side basal plasma membrane (BPM) of placental syncytiotrophoblasts.[246] There appear to be many more receptors on the BBM as compared to the fetal BPM.[246] Both membrane receptors activate that phosphoinositide pathway, but only the BPM receptors activate the adenyl cyclase system.[246,247] Thus, the role of calcitonin in modulating mineral transport across the placenta may be different at the maternal border versus the fetal side. Further, calcitonin may act to inhibit calcium transport from the mother and inhibit the back diffusion of calcium from the fetus during periods of high fetal serum calcium concentrations.

The fetus is capable of producing calcitonin as early as 14 weeks' gestation.[248] The human fetal thyroid contains a greater number of calcitonin-containing cells than does the adult thyroid.[249] Studies of cord blood have consistently noted a significantly greater calcitonin concentration than the corresponding maternal serum.[161,250,251] With high fetal serum calcitonin concentrations and no known placental calcitonin production, these findings favor a role for fetal calcitonin in the modulation of calcium, and possibly phosphate, transfer.[252] The nature of this interaction is still highly speculative.

Porcine, bovine, and ovine fetuses have greater calcitonin responsiveness to calcium infusions than do the adult.[253,254] Human amniotic fluid calcitonin concentration remains stable throughout pregnancy. It has been suggested that, although the fetal parafollicular cells are capable of responding to increased serum calcium concentration, there is no apparent increases in calcitonin secretion, as measured in amniotic fluid, despite marked fetal hypercalcemia.[255]

It is assumed that calcitonin assists in bone formation of the fetus. Based on vitro studies, calcitonin administered after bone formation has been initiated results in suppression of subsequent bone formation. When calcitonin is given during the initial phases of bone formation, there is an increase in bone formation due to stimulation of cartilage and bone precursor cells.[256] It is thought that calcitonin may have an enhanced role in the younger individual (e.g., the fetus, compared to that in the adult).

Calcitonin in the Neonate

Calcitonin concentration in cord blood of the neonate is elevated relative to maternal and nonpregnant concentrations. Cord blood calcitonin concentration decreases with increasing gestational age; neonates of less than 32 week's gestation have nearly three times the cord blood concentration of the term neonate.[48] In both the preterm and term neonate, calcitonin concentration increases after birth (Figure 40.7), with a peak at 24 to 48 hours of age followed by a decline to childhood values after 1 month of age.[48,250,257,258] Not only do neonates of less than 33 weeks' gestation have an increased cord blood calcitonin concentration, they appear to have a greater and more rapid response to a calcium infusion than gestationally older neonates.[164]

Elevated serum calcitonin concentration occurs in infants of diabetic mothers, neonates with low Apgar scores, and preterm neonates.[48,163] Because these three groups of neonates are at risk for early neonatal

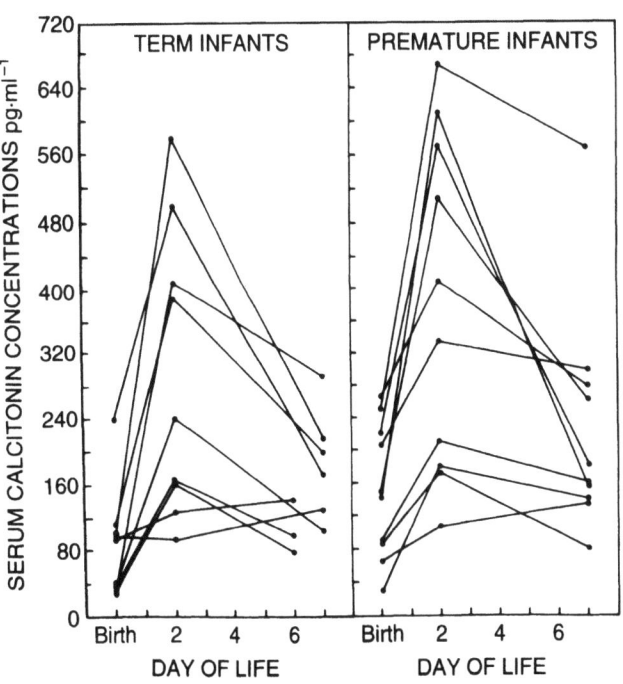

FIGURE 40.7. Cord, 48-hour, and 7-day serum calcitonin in term (left) and preterm (right) neonates. Adult (mean ± SEM) normal = 71.9 ± 6.6 pg·ml^{-1}. (From Hillman et al.,[161] with permission.)

hypocalcemia, it has been suggested that calcitonin may play a role in the etiology of this form of hypocalcemia.[161] One study has demonstrated a similar elevation in the postnatal calcitonin concentration over the first 24 hours of age in both the infant of the diabetic mother and in the normal term neonate.[163] No correlation between serum calcium concentration or the change in serum calcium concentration with serum calcitonin concentration was demonstrated in either group. The etiology for this rise in calcitonin is speculative. One hypothesis is that calcitonin may be increased as a result of the "stress" of birth with its resultant increase in adrenergic hormones. There is a postnatal rise in serum gastrin and glucagon concentrations, which are known calcitonin secretagogues.[257,259,260] These hormonal changes may explain the acute rise in calcitonin postnatally but do not explain the sustained increase over the first 28 days of life. Because of the effect of several gastrointestinal hormones on calcitonin secretion, there may be a role for calcitonin in the neonate's digestive adaptation. Suckling rats have an increased calcitonin concentration compared to weanling rates; and enteral calcium, lactose, and fat have been shown to increase the serum calcitonin concentration in the suckling rat.[261] Such increase in serum calcitonin concentration is associated with a decrease in gastric emptying and intestinal motility and a decrease in plasma triglyceride concentration.[262] It appears that, at least in the rat, calcitonin might have an effect on the absorption and clearance of several nutrients found in milk.

Serum calcitonin concentration in lactating women is elevated, and the concentration in milk may be 10 to 40 times greater than the serum concentration.[263] A study of lactating, totally thyroidectomized women noted that calcitonin concentrations in serum and milk were equal to those of lactating control women.[264] It was concluded that breast tissue might be capable of producing calcitonin independent of thyroidal influence. The high milk calcitonin concentration declined in both thyroidectomized and control women over the first 2 weeks of lactation.[264] As the milk volume is increasing markedly over the same period, it is unknown if there is an actual decrease in the production of calcitonin. The effect of lactational calcitonin on the suckling neonate is unknown.

Summary

Bone mineral homeostasis in the perinatal period is a complex interaction between mother, placenta, and fetus/infant. As our understanding of these relationships expands, the role of the placenta as an active contributor becomes more apparent. Calcium sensors have been located within the placenta that appear to modulate the active, and possibly passive, transfer of calcium to the fetus. The control of this sensor is unknown, but may receive instructions from the mother, fetus or placenta itself. In turn, the sensor may influence placental production of calcium regulatory hormones such as $1,25(OH)_2D$ and pPTHrP, as well as feedback to the maternal or fetal calcium regulatory hormones. The placenta is capable of hydroxylation of $25(OH)D$ to a variety of metabolites; the function and site of action are still speculative, but are

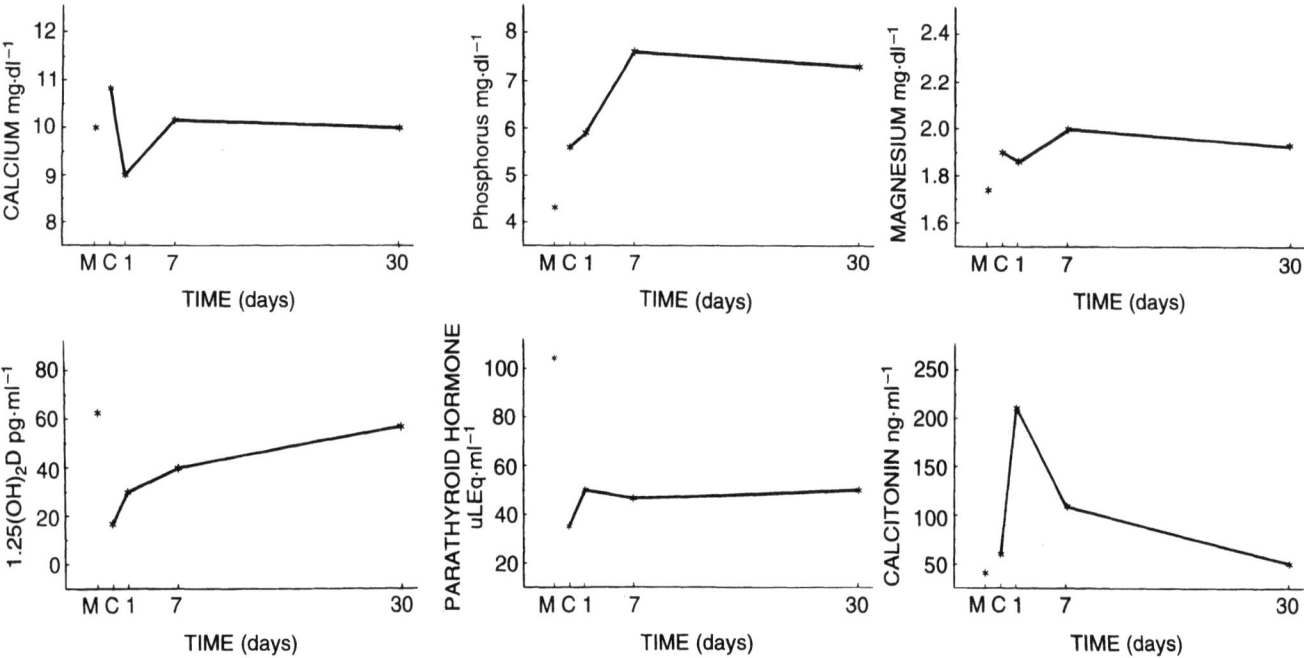

FIGURE 40.8. Relations over time of serum calcium, phosphorus, magnesium, vitamin D, parathyroid hormone, and calcitonin concentrations in the term neonate. Maternal (M) at delivery, cord blood (C), and 1-, 7-, and 30-day values are represented. Graphs demonstrate relations; actual values very depending on the measurement methodology.

likely to be at least locally active (e.g., as in stimulation of production of placental calcium binding protein). Clearly, the fetus demonstrates some control in calcium transfer as studies of thyroparathyroidectomized sheep have demonstrated. The sharply elevated fetal serum concentrations of calcitonin may influence early bone formation and mineralization, as well as a possible role in the transfer of calcium and phosphorus. After birth and removal of maternal and placental influences, the neonate must make rapid adjustments to new sources of minerals, provided intermittently and at lower concentrations. Preterm birth and its associated varied physiologic immaturities compound these challenges. As depicted in Figure 40.8 the first days of life of the term infant are marked by changes in all factors affecting bone mineralization, followed by a period of stabilization by 1 week of age. By the end of the first month, calcium and phosphorus and their regulatory hormones are at concentrations similar to those seen during childhood. Although much has been learned about the physiologic control of these changes, a greater understanding of the cellular and subcellular regulation of these changes is needed.

References

1. Givens MH, Macy IG. The chemical composition of the human fetus. J Biol Chem 1933;102:7–17.
2. Widdowsen EM, Spray CM. Chemical development. Arch Dis Child 1951;26:205–214.
3. Heaney RP, Saville PD, Recker RR. Calcium absorption as a function of calcium intake. J Lab Clin Med 1975;85:881–890.
4. Davis RH, Morgan DB, Rivlin RS. The excretion of calcium in the urine and its relation to calcium intake, sex and age. Clin Sci 1970;39:1–12.
5. Bulusu L, Hodgkinson A, Nordin BEC, et al. Urinary excretion of calcium and creatinine in relation to age and body weight in normal subjects and patients with renal calculus. Clin Sci 1970;38:601–612.
6. Heaney RP, Skillman TG. Calcium metabolism in normal human pregnancy. J Clin Endocrinol Metab 1971;33:881–890.
7. Howarth AT, Morgan DB, Payne RG. Urinary excretion of calcium in late pregnancy and its relation to creatinine clearance. Am J Obstet Gynecol 1977;129:499–502.
8. Duggin GG, Lyneham RC, Dale NE, et al. Calcium balance in pregnancy. Lancet 1974;2:926–927.
9. Pitkin RM, Reynolds WA, Williams GA, et al. Calcium metabolism in normal pregnancy: a longitudinal study. Am J Obstet Gynecol 1979;133:781–790.
10. Reitz RE, Daane TA, Woods JR, et al. Calcium, magnesium, phosphorus and parathyroid hormone interrelationships in pregnancy and newborn infant. Obstet Gynecol 1977;50:701–705.
11. Drake TS, Kaplan RA, Lewis TA. The physiologic hyperparathyroidism of pregnancy: Is it primary or secondary? Obstet Gynecol 1979;53:746–749.
12. Dahlman T, Sjoberg HE, Bucht. Calcium homeostasis in normal pregnancy and puerperium: a longitudinal study. Acta Obstet Gynecol Scand 1994;73:393–398.
13. Seki K, Makimura N, Mitsui C, et al. Calcium regulating hormones and osteocalcin levels during pregnancy: a longitudinal study. Am J Obstet Gynecol 1991;164:1248–1252.
14. Pecher CJ. Radio-calcium and radiostrontium metabolism in pregnant mice. Proc Soc Exp Biol Med 1941;46:91–94.
15. Christiansen C, Rodbro P, Heinild B. Unchanged total body calcium in normal human pregnancy. Acta Obstet Gynecol Scand 1976;55:141–143.
16. Walker ARP, Richardson B, Walker F. The influence of numerous pregnancies and lactations on bone dimensions in South African, Bantu and Caucasian mothers. Clin Sci 1972;42:189–195.
17. Booher LE, Hansmann GH. Studies in the clinical composition of the human skeleton. I. Calcification of the tibia of the normal newborn infant. J Biol Chem 1931;94:195–205.
18. Kamath SG, Haider N, Smith CH. ATP independent calcium transport and binding by basal plasma membrane of human placenta. Placenta 1994;14:147–155.
19. Whitsett JA, Tsang RC. Calcium uptake and binding by membrane fractions of human placenta. Pediatr Res 1980;14:769–775.
20. Fisher GJ, Kelley LK, Smith CH. ATP-dependent calcium transport across basal plasma membranes of human placental trophoblast. Am J Physiol 1987;252:C38–C46.
21. Lundgren S, Goran H, Hellman P, et al. A protein involved in calcium sensing of the human parathyroid and placental cytotrophoblast cells belongs to the LDL-receptor protein superfamily. Exp Cell Res 1994;212:344–350.
22. Umeki S, Nagao S, Nozawa Y. The purification and identification of calmodulin from human placenta. Biochem Biophys Acta 1981;674:319–326.
23. Bruns ME, Fausto A, Avioli LV. Placental calcium binding proteins in rats: apparent identity with vitamin D-dependent calcium binding protein from rat intestine. J Biol Chem 1978;253:3186–3190.
24. Bruns ME, Kellman E, Mills SE, et al. Immunochemical localization of vitamin D-dependent calcium binding protein in mouse placenta and yolk sac. Anat Rec 1985;213:514–517.
25. Lester GE. Cholecalciferol and placental calcium transport. Fed Proc 1986;45:2524–2527.
26. Tanaka Y, Halloran B, Schnoes HK, et al. In vitro production of 1,25-dihydroxyvitamin D_3 by rat placental tissue. Proc Natl Acad Sci USA 1979;76:5033–5035.
27. Weisman Y, Harell A, Edelstein S, et al. 1,25-Dihydroxyvitamin D_3 and 24,25-dihydroxyvitamin D in vitro synthesis by human decidua and placenta. Nature 1979;281:317–319.
28. Rodda CP, Kubota M, Heath JA, et al. Evidence for a novel parathyroid hormone-related protein in fetal lamb parathyroid glands and sheep placenta: comparisons with a similar protein implicated in humoral hypercalcemia of malignancy. J Endocrinol 1988;117:261–271.
29. Care AD, Caple IW, Abbas SK, et al. The roles of the parathyroid and thyroid glands on calcium homeostasis in the ovine fetus. In: Jones CT, Nathanielson PW, eds. The

physiological development of the fetus and newborn. London: Academic Press, 1985;135–145.
30. Shaw JCL. Evidence of defective skeletal mineralization in low birthweight infants: the absorption of calcium and fat. Pediatrics 1976;57:16–25.
31. Pitkin RM. Calcium metabolism in pregnancy: a review. Am J Obstet Gynecol 1975;121:724–737.
32. Loughead JL, Mimouni F, Tsang RC. Serum ionized calcium concentrations in normal neonates. Am J Dis Child 1988;142:516–518.
33. Okamoto E, Muttart C, Zucker C, et al. Use of medium chain triglycerides in feeding the low-birth-weight infant. Am J Dis Child 1982;136:428–431.
34. Tantibhedhyangkul P, Hashim S. Medium chain triglycerides feeding in premature infants: effects on calcium and magnesium absorption. Pediatrics 1987;61:537–545.
35. Giles MM, Fenton MH, Shaw B, et al. Sequential calcium and phosphorus balance studies in preterm infants. J Pediatr 1987;110:591–598.
36. Hillman LS, Tack E, Covell DG, et al. Measurement of true calcium absorption in premature infants using intravenous 46Ca and oral 44Ca. Pediatr Res 1988;23:589–594.
37. Barltrop D, Mole RH, Sutton A. Absorption and endogenous faecal excretion of calcium by low birth-weight infants on feeds with varying contents of calcium and phosphate. Arch Dis Child 1977;52:41–49.
38. Senterre J, Salle B. Calcium and phosphorus economy of the preterm infant and its interaction with vitamin D and its metabolites. Acta Pediatr Scand Suppl 1982;296:85–92.
39. Siegel SR, Hadeed A. Renal handling of calcium in the early newborn period. Kidney Int 1987;31:1181–1185.
40. Schanler RJ, Oh W. Composition of breast milk obtained from mothers of premature infants as compared to breast milk obtained from donors. J Pediatr 1980;96:679–681.
41. Greer FR, Steichen JJ, Tsang RC. Calcium and phosphate supplements in breast milk related rickets. Am J Dis Child 1982;136:581–583.
42. Chan GM, Mileur L, Hansen JW. Effects of increased calcium and phosphorous formulas and human milk on bone mineralization in preterm infants. J Pediatr Gastroenterol Nutr 1986;5:444–449.
43. Minton SD, Steichen JJ, Tsang RC. Bone mineral content in term and preterm appropriate for gestational age infants. J Pediatr 1979;95:1037–1042.
44. Steichen JJ, Grattan TL, Tsang RD. Osteopenia of prematurity: the cause and possible treatment. J Pediatr 1980;96:528–534.
45. Tsang RC, Kleinman LI, Sutherland JM, et al. Hypocalcemia in infants of diabetic mothers: studies in calcium, phosphorus and magnesium metabolism and parathormone responsiveness. J Pediatr 1972;80:384–395.
46. Schedewie HK, Odell WD, Fisher DA, et al. Parathormone and perinatal calcium homeostasis. Pediatr Res 1979;13:1–6.
47. Raisz LG. Physiologic-pharmacologic regulation of bone resorption. N Engl J Med 1970;282:909–916.
48. Venkataraman S, Tsang RC, Chem IW, et al. Pathogenesis of early neonatal hypocalcemia: studies of serum calcitonin, gastrin and plasma glucagon. J Pediatr 1987;110:599–603.
49. Bancroft JD. Late-onset hypocalcemic tetany. Am J Dis Child 1986;140:92.
50. Gidding SS, Minciotti AL, Langman CB. Unmasking of hypoparathyroidism in familial partial DiGeorge syndrome by challenging with disodium edatate. N Engl J Med 1988;319:1589–1591.
51. Anast CS, David LS. Human neonatal hypercalcemia. In: Holick MF, Gray TK, Anast CS, eds. Perinatal calcium and phosphorus metabolism. New York: Elsevier, 1983:363–385.
52. Gertner JM. Phosphorus metabolism and its disorders in childhood. Pediatr Ann 1987;16:957–965.
53. Wilz DR, Gray RW, Dominguez JH, et al. Plasma 1,25-$(OH)_2$-vitamin D concentrations and net intestinal calcium, phosphate and magnesium absorption in humans. Am J Clin Nutr 1979;32:2052–2060.
54. DeLuca HF. The vitamin D system in the regulation of calcium and phosphorus metabolism. Nutr Rev 1979;37:161–193.
55. Brickman AS, Hartenbower DL, Norman AW, et al. Actions of 1α-hydroxyvitamin D_3 and 1,25-dihydroxyvitamin D_3 on mineral metabolism in man. I. Effects on net absorption of phosphorus. Am J Clin Nutr 1977;30:1064–1069.
56. Rasmussan H, Bordier P, Kurokawa K, et al. Hormonal control of skeletal and mineral homeostasis. Am J Med 1974;56:751–758.
57. Foster GV, Byfield PGH, Gundmundson TV. Calcitonin. Clin Endocrinol (Oxf Metab) 1972;1:93–124.
58. Singer FR, Melvin KEW, Mills BG. Acute effects of calcitonin on osteoclasts in man. Clin Endocrinol (Oxf) 1976;5:333s–340s.
59. DeLuca HF. Some new concepts emanating from a study of the metabolism and function of vitamin D. Nutr Rev 1980;38:169–182.
60. Garel JM, Gilbert M. Dietary calcium and phosphorus manipulations in thyroparathyroidectomized pregnant rats and fetal liver glycogen stores. Reprod Nutr Rev 1981;21:969–972.
61. Pitkin RM. Calcium metabolism in pregnancy and the perinatal period: a review. Am J Obstet Gynecol 1985;151:99–109.
62. Ziegler EE, Biga RL, Forman SJ. Nutritional requirements of the premature infant. In: Suskind RM, ed. Textbook of pediatric nutrition. New York: Raven Press, 1981:29–40.
63. David L, Anast CS. Calcium metabolism in newborn infants. J Clin Invest 1974;54:287–296.
64. Parfitt AM, Kleerekoper M. Divalent ion homeostatic system physiology and metabolism of calcium, phosphorus, magnesium and bone. In: Maxel MH, Kleeman CR, eds. Clinical disorders of fluid and electrolyte metabolism. New York: McGraw-Hill, 1980:269–398.
65. Lineralli LG. Newborn urinary cAMP and developmental renal responsiveness to parathyroid hormone. Pediatrics 1972;50:14–23.
66. Hoehn GJ, Carey DE, Rowe JC, et al. Alternate day infusion of calcium and phosphate in very low birth weight infants: wasting of the infused mineral. J Pediatr Gastroenterol Nutr 1987;6:752–757.

67. Baylink D, Wergedal S, Stauffer M. Formation, mineralization and resorption of bone in hypophosphatemic rats. J Clin Invest 1971;50:2519–2530.
68. Raisz LG, Niemann I. Effect of phosphate, calcium and magnesium on bone resorption and hormonal responses in tissue culture. Endocrinology 1969;85:446–452.
69. Roberts CC, Chan GM, Folland D, et al. Adequate bone mineralization in breastfed infants. J Pediatr 1981;99:192–196.
70. Specker BL, Lichtenstein P, Mimouni F, et al. Calcium regulation hormones and minerals from birth to 18 months of age: a cross sectional study. II. Effects of sex, race, age, season and diet in serum minerals, parathyroid hormone and calcitonin. Pediatrics 1986;77:891–896.
71. Senterre J, Putet G, Salle B, et al. Effects of vitamin D and phosphorus supplementation of calcium retention in preterm infants fed banked human milk. J Pediatr 1983;103:305–307.
72. Schanler RJ, Garza C, Smith EO. Fortified mothers' milk for very low birth weight infants: results of macromineral balance studies. J Pediatr 1985;107:767–774.
73. Lyon AJ, McIntosh N. Calcium and phosphorus balance in extremely low birthweight infants in the first six weeks of life. Arch Dis Child 1984;59:1145–1150.
74. Greer F, McCromick A. Improved bone mineralization and growth in premature infants fed fortified own mother's milk. J Pediatr 1988;112:961–969.
75. Schanler RJ, Abrams SA, Garza C. Bioavailability of calcium and phosphorus in human milk fortifiers and formula for very low birth weight infants. J Pediatr 1988;113:95–100.
76. Bhatia J, Rassin DK, Human milk supplementation. Delivery of energy, calcium, phosphorus, magnesium, copper and iron. Am J Dis Child 1988;143:445–447.
77. Carey DE, Rowe JC, Goetz CA, et al. Growth and phosphorus metabolism in premature infants fed human milk, fortified human milk, or special premature formula. Am J Dis Child 1987;141:511–515.
78. Greer FR, Tsang RC. Calcium, phosphorus, magnesium and vitamin D requirements of the preterm infant. In: Tsang RC, ed. Vitamin and mineral requirements in preterm infants. New York: Marcell Dekker, 1985:99–136.
79. Rowe JC, Goetz CA, Carey DE, et al. Achievement of in utero retention of calcium and phosphorus accompanied by high calcium excretion in very low birth weight infants fed a fortified formula. J Pediatr 1987;110:581–585.
80. Steichen JH, Koo WWK. Mineral nutrition and bone mineralization in full-term infants. Monatsschr Kinderheilkd 1992;140(suppl):521–527.
81. Anast CS, Gardner DW. Magnesium metabolism. In: Bronner F, Coburn JW, eds. Disorders of mineral metabolism: pathophysiology of calcium, phosphorus and magnesium. Orlando: Academic Press, 1981:423–522.
82. Jukarainen E. Plasma magnesium levels during the first five days of life. Acta Pediatr Scand 1971;61:5–16.
83. Handwerker SM, Altura BT, Altura BM. Serum ionized magnesium and other electrolytes in the antenatal period of human pregnancy. J Am Coll Nutr 1996;15:26–43.
84. Altura BT, Burack JL, Caracco RQ, et al. Clinical studies with the NOVA ISE for iMg^{2+}. Scand J Clin Lab Invest 1994;54(suppl 217):53–67.
85. Wacker WEC, Parisi AF. Magnesium metabolism. N Engl J Med 1968;278:658–717.
86. Rall TW, Sutherland EW. Formation of a cyclic adenine ribonucleotide by tissue particles. J Biol Chem 1958;232:1065–1076.
87. Anast CS, Winnacker JL, Forte LR, et al. Impaired release of parathyroid hormone in magnesium deficiency. J Clin Endocrinol Metab 1976;42:707–717.
88. Buckle RM, Care AD, Cooper CW. The influence of plasma magnesium concentration of parathyroid hormone secretion. J Endocrinol 1968;42:529–534.
89. Cholst IN, Steinberg SF, Tropper PS, et al. The influence of hypermagnesemia on serum calcium and parathyroid hormone levels in human subjects. N Engl J Med 1984;310:1221–1225.
90. Wilkinson R. Absorption of calcium phosphorus and magnesium. In: Nordin BEC, ed. Calcium, phosphate and magnesium metabolism. Edinburgh: Churchill Livingstone, 1976:36–112.
91. Suh SM, Tashjian AH Jr, Matsuo N, et al. Pathogenesis of hypocalcemia in primary hypomagnesemia: normal end-organ responsiveness to parathyroid hormone, impaired parathyroid gland function. J Clin Invest 1973;52:153–160.
92. MacManus J, Heaton FW, Lucas PW. A decreased response to parathyroid hormone in magnesium deficiency. J Endocrinol 1971;49:253–258.
93. Freitag JJ, Martin KJ, Conrades MB, et al. Evidence for skeletal resistance to parathyroid hormone in magnesium deficiency. J Clin Invest 1979;64:1238–1244.
94. Abe M, Sherwood LM. Regulation of parathyroid hormone secretion by adenyl cyclase. Biochem Biophys Res Commun 1972;48:396–401.
95. Clemens TL, Holick MF. Recent advances in the hormonal regulation of calcium and phosphorus in adult animals and humans. In: Holick MF, Gray TK, Anast CS, eds. Perinatal calcium and phosphorus metabolism. New York: Elsevier, 1983:1–18.
96. Radde IC, Parkinson DK, Koo HSW. Magnesium and calcitonin; plasma magnesium levels in anemic children and in neonates. In: Proceedings of XIII International Congress Pediatrics, Metab Vorlag der Wiener Medizinishen Akademie, Wien, 1971;7:345.
97. Shaul PW, Mimouni F, Tsang RC, et al. The role of magnesium in neonatal calcium homeostasis: effects of magnesium infusion on calciotropic hormones and calcium. Pediatr Res 1987;22:319–323.
98. Planells E, Llopis J, Peran F, et al. Changes in tissue calcium and phosphorus content and plasma concentration of parathyroid hormone and calcitonin after long-term magnesium deficiency in rats. Am J Coll Nutr 1995;14:292–298.
99. Brown IRF, Brooke OG, Haswell DJ. Vitamin D and plasma magnesium in pregnancy. Clin Chim Acta 1981;111:109–111.
100. Karbach U, Ewe K. Calcium and magnesium transport and influence of 1,25(OH)$_2$D$_3$. Digestion 1987;37:35–42.
101. Levine BS, Brautbar N, Walling M, et al. Effects of vitamin D and diet magnesium on magnesium metabolism. Am J Physiol 1980;239:E515–E523.

102. Hodgkinson A, Marshall DH, Nordin BEC. Vitamin D and magnesium absorption in man. Clin Sci 1979;57:121–123.
103. Lifschitz F, Harrison HC, Harrison HE. Effects of vitamin D on magnesium metabolism in rats. Endocrinology 1967;81:849–853.
104. Rude RK, Adams JS, Ryzen E, et al. Low serum concentrations of 1,25-dihydroxyvitamin D in human magnesium deficiency. J Clin Endocrinol Metab 1985;61:933–940.
105. Saggese G, Federico G, Bertelloni S, et al. Hypomagnesemia and the parathyroid hormone-vitamin D endocrine system in children with insulin-dependent diabetes mellitus: effects of magnesium administration. J Pediatr 1991;118:220–225.
106. Ghazarian JG, DeLuca HF. 25-Hydroxycholecalciferol-1-hydroxylase: a specific requirement for NADPH and a hemoprotein component in chick kidney mitochondria. Arch Biochem Biophys 1974;160:63–72.
107. Brannan PG, Vergne-Marini D, Pat CYC, et al. Magnesium absorption in the human small intestine. J Clin Invest 1976;57:1412–1418.
108. Hardwick LL, Jones MR, Brautbar N, et al. Magnesium absorption: mechanisms and the influence of vitamin D, calcium, and phosphate. J Nutr 1991;121:13–23.
109. Skyberg D, Stromme JH, Nesbakken R, et al. Neonatal hypomagnesemia with selective malabsorption of magnesium—a clinical entity. Scand J Clin Lab Invest 1968;21:355–363.
110. Stromme JH, Nesbakken R, Normann T, et al. Familial hypomagnesemia. Acta Pediatr Scand 1969;58:433–444.
111. Levine BS, Coburn JW. Magnesium, the mimic/antagonist of calcium. N Engl J Med 1984;310:1253–1255.
112. Alcock N, MacIntyre I. Interrelationship of calcium and magnesium absorption. Clin Sci 1962;22:185–193.
113. Brunnette MG, Vignaoult N, Carriere S. Micropuncture study of Mg transport along the nephron in the young rat. Am J Physiol 1974;227:891–896.
114. Brunnette MG, Vignaoult N, Carriere S. Magnesium handling by the papilla of the young rat. Pfleugers Arch 1978;373:229–235.
115. Subcommittee on the RDAs. Minerals. In: Recommended Dietary Allowances. 10th ed. Washington DC: National Academy Press, 1989:174–194.
116. Pitkin RM. Maternal-fetal calcium homeostasis. In: Holick MF, Gray TK, Anast CS, eds. Perinatal calcium and phosphorus metabolism. New York: Elsevier, 1983:259–275.
117. Aikawa JK, Bruns PD. Placental transfer and fetal tissue uptake of Mg28 in the rabbit. Proc Soc Exp Biol Med 1960;105:95–98.
118. Marcus JC, Valencia BM, Altura BT, et al. Serum ionized magnesium (IMg) levels in premature and full-term infants. Neurology 1994;44:A145.
119. Dancis J, Springer D, Cohlan SA. Fetal homeostasis in maternal malnutrition. II. Magnesium deprivation. Pediatr Res 1971;55:131–136.
120. DeLeeuw I, Vertommen J, Abs R. The magnesium content of the trabecular bone in diabetic subjects. Biomedicine 1978;29:16–17.
121. Mimouni F, Tsang RC, Hertzberg VS, et al. Polycythemia, hypomagnesemia, and hypocalcemia in infants of diabetic mothers. Am J Dis Child 1986;140:798–800.
122. Spatling L, Spatling G. Magnesium supplementation in pregnancy. Br J Obstet Gynaecol 1988;95:120–125.
123. Green KW, Key TC, Coen R, et al. The effects of maternally administered magnesium sulfate on the neonate. Am J Obstet Gynecol 1983;146:29–33.
124. Hallak M, Cotton DB. Transfer of maternally administered magnesium sulfate into the fetal compartment of the rat: assessment of amniotic fluid, blood, and brain concentrations. Am J Obstet Gynecol 1993;169:427–431.
125. Hankins GD, Hammon TL, Yeomans ER. Amniotic cavity accumulation of magnesium with prolonged magnesium sulfate tocolysis. J Reprod Med 1991;36:446–449.
126. Anast CS. Serum magnesium levels in the newborn. Pediatrics 1964;33:969–974.
127. Atkinson SA, Radde IC, Anderson GH. Macromineral balances in premature infants fed their own mothers' milk or formula. J Pediatr 1983;102:99–106.
128. Tsang RC, Light IJ, Sutherland JM, et al. Possible pathogenic factors in neonatal hypocalcemia of prematurity. J Pediatr 1973;82:423–429.
129. Tsang RC, Oh W. Serum magnesium levels in low birth weight infants. Am J Dis Child 1970;120:44–48.
130. Giles MM, Laing IA, Elton RA, et al. Magnesium metabolism in preterm infants: effects of calcium, magnesium, phosphorus and of postnatal and gestational age. J Pediatr 1990;117:147–154.
131. Loughead JL, Mimouni F, Tsang RC, et al. A role for magnesium in neonatal parathyroid gland function? J Am Coll Nutr 1991;10:123–126.
132. Tsang RC, Chen IW, Friedman MA, et al. Parathyroid function in infants of diabetic mothers. J Pediatr 1975;86:399–404.
133. Mimouni F, Loughead JL, Miodovnik M, et al. Early neonatal predictors of neonatal hypocalcemia in infants of diabetic mothers: an epidemiologic study. Am J Perinatol 1990;7:203–206.
134. Noguchi A, Eren M, Tsang RC. Parathyroid hormone in hypocalcemic and normocalcemic infants of diabetic mothers. J Pediatr 1980;97:112–114.
135. Donovan EF, Tsang RC, Steichen JJ, et al. Neonatal hypermagnesemia: effect on parathyroid hormone and calcium homeostasis. Pediatrics 180;96:305–310.
136. Lamm CI, Norton KI, Murphy RJC, et al. Congenital rickets associated with magnesium sulfate infusion for tocolysis. J Pediatr 1988;113:1078–1082.
137. Habner JF, Potts JT. Relative effectiveness of magnesium and calcium on the secretion and biosynthesis of parathyroid hormone in vitro. Endocrinology 1976;98:197–202.
138. Rasmussen H, Feinblatt S. The relationship between the actions of vitamin D, parathyroid hormone and calcitonin. Calcif Tissue Res 1971;6:265–279.
139. Kukreja SC, Hargis GK, Browser EN, et al. Role of adrenergic stimuli in parathyroid hormone secretion in man. J Clin Endocrinol Metab 1975;40:478–481.
140. Care AD, Bates RF, Pickard DW, et al. The effects of vitamin D metabolites and their analogues on the secretion of parathyroid hormone. Calcif Tissue Res 1976;21:142–146.
141. Dietel M, Dorn G, Montz R, et al. Influence of vitamin D_3 and 24,25-dihydroxyvitamin D_3 parathyroid hormone

secretion, adenosine 3'5'-monophosphate release, and ultrastructure of parathyroid glands in organ culture. Endocrinology 1979;105:237–245.
142. Agus ZS, Puschett JB, Senesky D, et al. Mode of action of parathyroid hormone on cyclic adenosine 3'5'-monophosphate on renal tubular phosphate reabsorption in the dog. J Clin Invest 1971;50:517–626.
143. Norden BEC, Peacock M. Role of the kidney in regulation of plasma calcium. Lancet 1969;2:1280–1283.
144. Root AW, Harrison HE. Recent advances in calcium metabolism. II. Disorders of calcium homeostasis. J Pediatr 1976;88:177–199.
145. Cushard WG, Creditor MA, Canterbury, et al. Physiologic hyperparathyroidism in pregnancy. J Clin Endocrinol Metab 1976;34:767–771.
146. Gallacher SJ, Fraser WD, Owens OJ, et al. Changes in calciotrophic hormones and biochemical markers of bone turnover in normal human pregnancy. Eur J Endocrinol 1994;131:369–374.
147. Lequin RM, Hackeng WH, Schopman W. A radioimmunoassay for parathyroid hormone in man. II. Measurement of parathyroid hormone concentrations in human plasma by means of a radioimmunoassay for bovine hormone. Acta Endocrinol (Copenh) 1970;63:655–666.
148. Croley TE. The intracellular localization of calcium within the mature human placenta barrier. Am J Obstet Gynecol 1973;117:926–932.
149. Northrop G, Misenheimer HR, Becker FO. Failure of parathyroid hormone to cross the nonhuman primate placenta. Am J Obstet Gynecol 1977;129:449–453.
150. Samaan NA, Wigoda C, Castillo SG. Human serum calcitonin and parathyroid hormone levels in the maternal, umbilical cord blood and postpartum. In: Proceedings of the Fourth International Symposium of Endocrinology. London: Heineman, 1973:364–372.
151. Hillman LS, Slatopolsky E, Haddad JG. Perinatal vitamin D metabolism. IV. Maternal and cord serum 24,25-dihydroxyvitamin D concentrations. J Clin Endocrinol Metab 1978;47:1073–1077.
152. Tsang RC, Chen IW, Friedman M, et al. Neonatal parathyroid function: role of gestational and postnatal age. J Pediatr 1973;83:728–738.
153. Pitkin RM, Cruikshank DP, Schauberger CW, et al. Fetal calcitropic hormones and neonatal calcium homeostasis. Pediatrics 1980;66:77–82.
154. Leroyer-Alizon E, David L, Anast CS, et al. Immunocytologic evidence for parathyroid hormone in human parathyroid glands. J Clin Endocrinol Metab 1981;52:513–516.
155. Fleishman AR, Lerman S, Oakes GK, et al. Perinatal primate parathyroid hormone metabolism. Biol Neonate 1975;27:40–49.
156. Pitkin RM, Reynolds WA, Williams GA, et al. Maternal and fetal parathyroid hormone responsiveness in pregnant primates. J Clin Endocrinol Metab 1980;51:1044–1047.
157. Pic P, Maniey N, Jost A. Facteurs endocriniens reglant la calcemia foetale: indications sur le role des parathyroides. CR Soc Biol 1965;159:1274.
158. Garel JM. Effet de l'injection d'un serum "antiparathormone" chez le foetus de rat. CR Acad Sci 1970;271:349–350.
159. Care AD, Abbas SK, Pickard DW, et al. Stimulation of ovine placental transport of calcium and magnesium by mid-molecule fragments of human parathyroid hormone-related protein. Exp Phys 1990;75:605–608.
160. Shaw AJ, Moughal MZ, Maresh MJA, et al. Effects of two synthetic parathyroid hormone related protein fragments on maternal-fetal transfer of calcium and magnesium and release of cyclic AMP by the in-situ perfused rat placenta. J Endocrinol 1991;129:399–404.
161. Hillman LS, Rojanasathit S, Slatopolsky E, et al. Serial measurements of serum calcium, magnesium, parathyroid hormone, calcitonin, and 25-hydroxyvitamin D in premature and term infants during the first week of life. Pediatr Res 1977;11:739–744.
162. Delvin EE, Glorieux FH, Salle BL, et al. Control of vitamin D metabolism in preterm infants: feto-maternal relationships. Arch Dis Child 1982;57:754–757.
163. Mimouni F, Loughead JL, Tsang RC, et al. Postnatal surge in serum calcitonin concentrations: no contribution to neonatal hypocalcemia in infants of diabetic mothers. J Pediatr 1990;28:493–495.
164. Dincsoy MY, Tsang RC, Laskarzewski P, et al. The role of postnatal age and magnesium on parathyroid hormone responses during "exchange" blood transfusion in the newborn period. J Pediatr 1982;100:277–283.
165. Linerelli LG, Bobik C, Bobik J. Urinary cAMP and renal responsiveness to parathyroid hormone in premature hypocalcemic infants. Pediatr Res 1973;7:329A.
166. Hillman DA, Scriver CR, Pedvis S, et al. National familial primary hyperparathyroidism. N Engl J Med 1964;280:483–490.
167. Loughead JL, Mughal Z, Mimouni F, et al. The spectrum and natural history of congenital hyperparathyroidism secondary to maternal hypocalcemia. Am J Perinatol 1990;7:350–355.
168. Winter WE, Silverstein JH, Barrett DS, et al. Familial DiGeorge syndrome and tetralogy of Fallot and prolonged survival. Eur J Pediatr 1984;141:171–172.
169. Raatikka M, Rapola J, Tuuteri L, et al. Familial third and fourth pharyngeal pouch syndromes with truncus arteriosus: DiGeorge syndrome. Pediatrics 1981;67:172–175.
170. Bainbridge R, Mughal Z, Mimouni F, et al. Transient congenital hypoparathyroidism: How transient is it? J Pediatr 1987;111:866–868.
171. Bayard J, Bec P, Louvet D, et al. 25-Hydroxycholecalciferol dynamics in human plasma. In: IV International Congress of Endocrinology. Amsterdam: Excerpta Medica, 1972(abstract 597).
172. Bronner F, Pansu D, Stein WD. An analysis of intestinal calcium transport across the rat intestine. Am J Physiol 1986;250:6561–6569.
173. Bordier P, Rasmussen H, Marie P, et al. Vitamin D metabolites and bone mineralization in man. J Clin Endocrinol Metab 1978;46:284–294.
174. Kanis JA, Cundy T, Bartlett M, et al. Is 24,25-dihydroxycholecalciferol a calcium-regulating hormone in man? Br Med J 1978;1:1382–1386.
175. Henry HL, Norman AW. Vitamin D: two dihydroxylated metabolites are required for normal chicken egg hatchability. Science 1978;201:835–837.

176. Bouillon R, Van Assche FA, van Baelen H, et al. Influence of the vitamin D-binding protein in the serum concentration of 1,25-dihydroxyvitamin D_3. J Clin Invest 1981;67:589–596.
177. Bouillon R, Van Baelen H, DeMoor P. 25-Hydroxyvitamin D and its binding protein in maternal and cord blood serum. J Clin Endocrinol Metab 1977;45:679–684.
178. Haddad JG, Welgate J. Radioimmunoassay of the binding protein for vitamin D and its metabolites in human serum: concentration in normal subjects and patients with disorders of mineral homeostasis. J Clin Invest 1976;58:1217–1222.
179. Hollis BW, Pittard WB. Relative concentrations of 25-hydroxyvitamin D_2D_3 and 1,25-dihydroxyvitamin D_2D_3 in maternal plasma at delivery. Nutr Res 1984;4:27–32.
180. Specker BL, Ho M, Oestrich A, et al. Prospective study of vitamin D supplementation and rickets in China. J Pediatr 1992;120:733–739.
181. Brooke DG, Brown IRF, Bone CDM, et al. Vitamin D supplements in pregnant Asian women: effects on calcium states and fetal growth. Br Med J 1980;280:751–754.
182. Cockburn F, Belton NR, Purvis RJ, et al. Maternal vitamin D intake and mineral metabolism in mothers and their newborn infants. Br Med J 1980;231:1–10.
183. Glorieux FH, Salle B, Delvin EE, et al. Vitamin D metabolism in premature infants: serum calcitriol values during the first five days of life. J Pediatr 1981;99:640–643.
184. Salle B, Glorieux F, Delvin E, et al. Vitamin D metabolism in preterm infants. Acta Pediatr Scand 1983;72:203–206.
185. Delvin EE, Salle BL, Glorieux FH, et al. Vitamin D supplementation during pregnancy: effect on neonatal calcium homeostasis. J Pediatr 1986;109:328–334.
186. Moncrief M, Fadahunsi TO. Congenital rickets due to maternal vitamin D deficiency. Arch Dis Child 1974;48:810–811.
187. Namgung R, Tsang RC, Specker BL, et al. Low bone mineral content and high serum osteocalcin and $1,25(OH)_2D$ in summer- versus winter-born newborn infants: an early fetal effect. J Pediatr Gastroenterol Nutr 1994;19:220–227.
188. Reiter EO, Braunstein GD, Vargas A, et al. Changes in 25-hydroxyvitamin D and 24,25-dihydroxyvitamin D during pregnancy. Am J Obstet Gynecol 1979;135:227–229.
189. Hillman LS, Haddad JG. Perinatal vitamin D metabolism. III. Factors influencing late gestational human serum 25-hydroxyvitamin D. Am J Obstet Gynecol 1976;125:196–200.
190. Whitehead M, Lane G, Young O, et al. Interrelations of calcium-regulating hormones during normal pregnancy. Br Med J 1981;283:10–31.
191. Mallet E, Gugi B, Brunelle P, et al. Vitamin D supplementation in pregnancy: a controlled trial of two methods. Obstet Gynecol 1986;68:300–304.
192. Hillman LS, Haddad JG. Human perinatal vitamin D metabolism. I. 25-hydroxyvitamin D in maternal and cord blood. J Pediatr 1974;84:742–749.
193. Nehama H, Weintroub S, Eisenberg Z, et al. Seasonal variations in paired maternal-newborn serum. 25-hydroxyvitamin D and 24,25-dihydroxyvitamin D concentrations in Israel. J Med Sci 1987;23:274–277.
194. Bruns ME, Bruns DE. Vitamin D metabolism and function during pregnancy and the neonatal period. Anim Clin Lab Sci 1983;13:521–530.
195. Haddad JG, Boisseau V, Avioli LV. Placental transfer of vitamin D, and 25-hydroxycholecalciferol in the rat. J Lab Clin Med 1971;77:908–915.
196. Devaskar UP, Ho M, Devaskar S, et al. 25-Hydroxy- and 1,25-dihydroxyvitamin D; maternal-fetal relationship and the transfer of 1,25-dihydroxyvitamin D_3 across the placenta in an ovine model. Dev Pharmacol Ther 1984;7:213–220.
197. Hillman LS, Haddad JG. Perinatal vitamin D metabolism. II. Serial 25-hydroxyvitamin D concentrations in sera of term and premature infants. J Pediatr 1975;86:928–935.
198. Axelson M, Christensen NJ. Vitamin D metabolism in human pregnancy: concentrations of free and sulphated 25-hydroxyvitamin D_3 in maternal and fetal plasma at term. J Steroid Biochem 1988;31:35–39.
199. Epstein FH, Han A, Shackleton CH. Failure of steroid sulfatase to desulfate vitamin D_3 sulfate. J Invest Dermatol 1983;80:514–516.
200. Weisman Y, Harell A, Edelstein S, et al. 1,25-dihydroxyvitamin D_3 and 24,25-dihydroxyvitamin D_3 in vitro synthesis by human decidua and placenta. Nature 1979;281:317–319.
201. Whitsett JA, Ho M, Tsang RC, et al. Synthesis of 1,25-dihydroxyvitamin D_3 by human placenta in vitro. J Clin Endocrinol Metab 1981;53:484–488.
202. Pike JW, Grooze LL, Haussler MR. Biochemical evidence of $1,25(OH)_2D$ receptor macromolecules in parathyroid, pancreatic, pituitary and placental tissues. Life Sci 1980;26:407–414.
203. Rubin LP, Yeung B, Vouros P, et al. Evidence for human placental synthesis of 24,25-dihydroxyvitamin D_3 and 23,25-dihydroxyvitamin D_3. Pediatr Res 1993;34:98–104.
204. Robinson M, Merrett A, Teflow V, et al. Plasma 25-hydroxyvitamin D concentrations in preterm infants receiving oral vitamin D supplements. Arch Dis Child 1981;56:144–145.
205. Markestad T, Asknes L, Finne P, et al. Plasma concentrations of vitamin D metabolites in premature infants. Pediatr Res 1984;18:269–272.
206. Cross NA, Hillman LS, Allen SH, et al. Calcium homeostasis and bone metabolism during pregnancy, lactation, and postweaning: a longitudinal study. Am J Clin Nutr 1995;61:514–523.
207. Reddy GS, Norman AW, Willis DM, et al. Regulation of vitamin D metabolism in normal human pregnancy. J Clin Endocrinol Metab 1983;56:363–370.
208. Steichen JJ, Tsang RC, Grattan TL, et al. Vitamin D homeostasis in the perinatal period: 1,25-dihydroxyvitamin D in maternal, cord and neonatal blood. N Engl J Med 1980;302:315–319.
209. Nguyen TM, Halhale A, Guillozo H, et al. Thyroid and parathyroid-independent increase in plasma 1,25-dihydroxyvitamin D during late pregnancy in the rat. J Endocrinol 1988;116:381–385.

210. Spanos E, Brown DJ, Stevenson JC, et al. Stimulation of 1,25-dihydroxycholecalciferol production by prolactin and related peptides in intact renal cell preparation in vitro. Biochim Biophys Acta 1981;672:7–15.
211. Pahuja DW, DeLuca HF. Stimulation of intestinal calcium transport and bone calcium mobilization by prolactin in vitamin D deficient rats. Science 1981;214:1038–1039.
212. Fleischman AR, Rosen JF, Cole J, et al. Maternal and fetal serum 1,25-hydroxyvitamin D levels at term. J Pediatr 1980;97:640–642.
213. Hollis BW, Pittard WB. Evaluation of the total fetomaternal vitamin D relationship at term: evidence for racial differences. J Clin Endocrinol Metab 1984;59:652–657.
214. Weiland T, Fischer JA, Trechsel U, et al. Perinatal parathyroid, vitamin D metabolites, and calcitonin in man. Am J Physiol 1980;239:E385–E390.
215. Ross R, Care AD, Taylor CM, et al. The transplacental movement of metabolites of vitamin D in the sheep. In: Norman AW, Schaefer K. Coburn JW, et al., eds. Vitamin D basic research in its clinical application. Berlin: de Gruyter, 1979:341–344.
216. Somjen D, Binderman I, Weisman Y. The effects of 24R,25-dihydroxycholecalciferol and 1a,25-dihydroxycholecalciferol on ornithine decarboxylase activity and on DNA synthesis in the epiphysis and diaphysis of rat bone and in the duodenum. Biochem J 1983;214:293–298.
217. Paunier L, LaCourt G, Pilloud P, et al. 25-Hydroxyvitamin D and calcium levels in maternal, cord and infant serum in relation to maternal vitamin D intake. Helv Pediatr Acta 1978;33:95–103.
218. Heckmatt JZ, Peacock M, Davies AE, et al. Plasma 25-hydroxyvitamin D in pregnant Asian women and their babies. Lancet 1979;2:546–548.
219. Clements MR, Frasier DR. Vitamin D supply to the rate fetus and neonate. J Clin Invest 1988;81:1768–1773.
220. Specker BL, Tsang RC, Hollis BW. Effect of race and diet on human-milk vitamin D and 25 hydroxyvitamin D. Am J Dis Child 1985;139:1134–1137.
221. Hoogenboezem T, Degenhart HJ, DeMuinck PF, et al. Vitamin D metabolism in breast-fed infants and mothers. Pediatr Res 1989;25:623–628.
222. Hollis BW, Pittard WB, Reinhardt TA. Relationships among vitamin D, 25-hydroxyvitamin D, and vitamin D-binding protein concentrations in the plasma and milk of human subjects. J Clin Endocrinol Metab 1986;62:41–44.
223. Greer FR, Ho M, Dodson D, et al. Lack of 25-hydroxyvitamin D and 1,25-dihydroxyvitamin D in human milk. J Pediatr 1981;99:233–235.
224. Parthemore JG, Deftos LJ. Calcitonin secretion in normal human subjects. J Clin Endocrinol 1978;47:184–188.
225. Hillyard CJ, Cooke TJC, Coombes RC, et al. Normal plasma calcitonin: circadian variation and response to stimuli. Clin Endocrinol (Oxf) 1977;6:291–298.
226. Care AD, Bell NH, Bates RFL. The effect of hypermagnesemia on calcitonin secretion in vivo. J Endocrinol 1971;51:381–386.
227. Anast C, David L, Winnacker J, et al. Serum calcitonin-lowering effect of magnesium in patients with medullary carcinoma of the thyroid. J Clin Invest 1975;56:1615–1621.
228. Roos BA, Deftos LJ. Calcitonin secretion in vitro. II. Regulating effects on enteric mammalian polypeptide hormones on tract C-cell cultures. Endocrinology 1976;98:1284–1288.
229. Care AD. Effect of pancreozymin and secretion on calcitonin release. Fed Proc 1970;29:53A.
230. Cooper CW, Mahgoub AH. Stimulation of secretion of pig thyrocalcitonin by pentagastrin. Fed Proc 1971;30:417A.
231. Garel JM, Barlet JP, Kervran A. Metabolic effects of calcitonin in the newborn. Am J Physiol 1975;229:669–675.
232. Reynolds JJ. Inhibition by calcitonin of bone resorption induced in vitro by vitamin A. Proc R Soc Lond [Biol] 1968;170:61–69.
233. Krane SM, Harris ED Jr, Singer FR, et al. Acute effects of calcitonin on bone formation in man. Metabolism 1973;22:51–58.
234. Chambers TJ, McSheehy PMS, Thomson BM, et al. The effect of calcium-regulating hormones and prostaglandins on bone resorption by osteoclasts disaggregated from neonatal rabbit bones. Endocrinology 1985;60:234–239.
235. Marcus R, Heershe JNM, Aurbach GD. Effects of calcitonin on formation of 3'5'cyclic AMP in bone and kidney. In: Program of the Fifty-Third Annual Meeting US Endocrine Society 1971, abstract 57.
236. Potts JT Jr, Murray TM, Peacock M, et al. Parathyroid hormone: sequence synthesis, immunoassay studies. Am J Med 1971;50:639–649.
237. Cramer CF, Parkes CO, Copp D. The effect of chicken and hog calcitonin as some parameters of Ca, P and Mg metabolism in dogs. Can J Physiol Pharmacol 1969;47:181–184.
238. Robinson CJ, Matthews EW, MacIntyre I. The effect of parathyroid hormone and thyrocalcitonin on intestinal absorption of calcium and magnesium. In: Milhaud G, Owen M, Blackwood D, eds. Les Tissues Calcifies: Ve Symposium Europeen. Paris: Societe d'Edition d'Enseignement Superieur, 1968:279–282.
239. Garel JM, Milhaud G, Sizonenko PC. Inactivation de la calcitonine porcine par differents organes, foetaux et maternals du rat. CR Acad Sci 1970;270:2469.
240. Ardaillou R, Sizonenko P, Meyrier A, et al. Metabolic clearance rate of radioiodinated human calcitonin in man. J Clin Invest 1970;49:2345–2352.
241. Drake TS, Kaplan RA, Lewis TA. The physiologic hyperparathyroidism of pregnancy: Is it primary or secondary? Obstet Gynecol 1979;53:746–749.
242. Stevenson JC, Hillyard CS, MacIntyre I, et al. The physiological role for calcitonin: protection of the maternal skeleton. Lancet 1979;2:769–770.
243. Reynolds WA, Williams GA, Pitkin RM. Calcitropic hormone responsiveness during pregnancy. Am J Obstet Gynecol 1981;139:855–862.
244. Taylor TG, Lewis PE, Balderstone O. Role of calcitonin in protecting the skeleton during pregnancy and lactation. J Endocrinol 1975;66:297–308.
245. Milhaud G, Maukhtar MS, Perault-Straub AM, et al. Calcitonin. In: Taylor S, Foster GV, eds. Calcitonin,

Proceedings of the Second International Symposium. London: Heinemann, 1969:182–193.
246. Lafond J, Simouneau L, Savard R, et al. Calcitonin receptor in human placental syncytiotrophoblasts brush border and basal plasma membranes. Mol Cell Endocrinol 1994;99:285–292.
247. Lafond J, Auger D, Fortier J, et al. Hormone receptor in human placental syncytiotrophoblast brush border and basal plasma membranes. Endocrinology 1988;123:2834–2840.
248. Leroyer-Alizon E, David L, Dubois PM. Evidence for calcitonin in the thyroid gland of normal and anencephalic human fetuses: immunocytological localization, radioimmunoassay and gel filtration of thyroid extracts. J Clin Endocrinol 1980;50:316–321.
249. Pearse AGE. Calcitonin. In: Taylor S, Foster GV, eds. Calcitonin, Proceedings of the Second International Symposium. London: Heinemann, 1969:125.
250. Samaan NA, Anderson GD, Adam-Mayne ME. Immunoreactive calcitonin in the mother, neonate, child and adult. Am J Obstet Gynecol 1975;121:622–625.
251. David L, Salle BL, Putet G, et al. Serum immunoreactive calcitonin in low birth weight infants. Pediatr Res 1981;15:803–808.
252. Rebut-Bonneton C, Segond N, Demignon J, et al. Effects of calcitonin on human trophoblastic cells in culture: absence of autocrine control. Mol Cell Endocrinol 1992;85:65–71.
253. Littledike ET, Arnaud CD, Whipp SC. Calcitonin secretion in ovine, porcine and bovine fetuses. Proc Soc Exp Biol Med 1972;139:428–433.
254. Garel JM, Sajarol H, Barlet JP, et al. Dosage radioimmunoligique de la calcitone, chez le foetus de mouton. CR Acad Sci 1973;277:217–220.
255. Cruikshank DR, Pitkin RM, Reynolds WA, et al. Calcium regulating hormones and ions in amniotic fluid. Am J Obstet Gynecol 1980;136:621–625.
256. Weiss RE, Singer FR, Gorn AH, et al. Calcitonin stimulates bone formation when administered prior to initiation of osteogenesis. J Clin Invest 1981;68:815–818.
257. Bergman L, Kjellmer I, Selstam U. Calcitonin and parathyroid hormone: relation to early neonatal hypocalcemia in infants of diabetic mothers. Biol Neonate 1974;24:151–160.
258. Birge SJ, Avioli LV. Glucagon-induced hypocalcemia in man. J Clin Endocrinol 1969;29:213–218.
259. Johnston DI, Bloom SR. Plasma glucagon levels in the term human infant and the effect of hypoxia. Arch Dis Child 1973;48:451–454.
260. David L, Salle B, Chopard P, et al. Studies on circulating immunoreactive calcitonin in low birth weight infants during the first 48 hours of life. Helv Pediatr Acta 1977;32:39–44.
261. Garel JM, Besnard P. Milk factors controlling the plasma calcitonin level in the newborn rat. Endocrinology 1979;104:1617–1623.
262. Garel JM, Jullienne S. Plasma calcitonin levels in pregnant and newborn rats. J Endocrinol 1977;75:373–376.
263. Arver S, Bucht E, Sjoberg HE. Calcitonin-like immunoreactivity in human milk, longitudinal alterations and divalent cations. Acta Physiol Scand 1984;122:461–463.
264. Bucht E, Telenius-Berg M, Lundell G, et al. Immunoextracted calcitonin in milk and plasma from totally thyroidectomized women: evidence of monomeric calcitonin in plasma during pregnancy and lactation. Acta Endocrinol (Copenh) 1986;113:529–535.
265. Widdowsen EM, Dickerson JWT. Chemical composition of the body. In: Comar CL, Brunner F, eds. Mineral metabolism: an advanced treatise. vol 2, part A. Orlando: Academic Press, 1964:1–247.
266. Kelly HJ, Sloan RE, Hoffman W, et al. Accumulation of nitrogen and 6 minerals in the human foetus during gestation. Hum Biol 1951;23:61–74.
267. Wandrup J. Kancir C, Norgaard-Pedersen B. The concentration of free calcium ions in capillary blood from neonates on a routine basis using ICA2. Scand J Clin Lab Invest 1984;44:19–24.
268. Specker BL, Tsang RC. Cyclical serum 25-hydroxyvitamin D concentrations paralleling sunshine exposure in exclusively breast-fed infants. J Pediatr 1987;110:744–747.

41
Neonatal Trace Element Metabolism

Peter J. Aggett

A trace element is arbitrarily defined as an element that is present at a concentration of less than 100 parts per million (i.e., $100\,\mu g \cdot g^{-1}$ or $100\,mg \cdot kg^{-1}$).[1] At least nine elements (e.g., iron, zinc, copper, manganese, cobalt, chromium, selenium, molybdenum, and iodine) have proven to be essential. Additional studies in animal models have suggested that other elements (e.g., fluorine, nickel, tin, vanadium, silicon, arsenic, cadmium, lead, boron, and bromine), may be necessary for optimum health. This discussion focuses on the initial group of elements that have the highest potential relevance in the neonatal period.

To be considered essential the element must be ubiquitous in the body, although there may be specific tissue and intracellular concentrations that reflect its metabolism and function. Deprivation of the element induces reproducible features that are remedied by its reintroduction. The tissue concentration and body content of these elements are relatively constant throughout life, indicating the existence of systemic homeostatic control. In contrast, the tissue concentration for many nonessential elements may increase throughout life. Within a population such concentrations may have a skewed distribution, whereas those of essential elements have a normal distribution.

The disadvantage of the generic term trace element is that it obscures the important fact that each essential trace element has its own specific functions and systemic metabolic control. Each element should be considered independently. Trace elements function at such a fundamental level in cellular biochemistry that they interact extensively with other micronutrients and have considerable impact on the metabolism of the major nutrient substrate.

Systemic metabolic control of trace element distribution, utilization, and body burden is achieved by manipulation of their physicochemical properties, in particular, their oxidation states, and of their various affinities for organic ligands. This creates a chain of discrete physical and chemical compartments by which the elements are ultimately presented to their functional sites in appropriate forms and concentrations. Although these pathways have commonly come to be called metabolism, this term is inappropriate in that trace elements cannot be broken down or be extensively modified.

The trace elements can be regarded as forming three groups: (1) The cationic elements (e.g., zinc, iron, manganese, and copper) are transferred and utilized to a large extent as inorganic ions; they need specific carriers to effect their transfer across lipid membranes and to maintain their solubility at the physiological pH within extracellular and intracellular fluids. Their homeostasis is effected principally by the gastrointestinal tract and liver. (2) Elements that are used in an anionic form (e.g., molybdenum, selenium, iodine, chromium, and possibly fluorine) have a greater ability to cross lipid membranes spontaneously and are more soluble at physiological pH. They have efficient gastrointestinal uptake and transfer. Their systemic use and compartmentalization are achieved by exploiting their many oxidation states, and their homeostasis is achieved predominantly by renal excretion. (3) These elements are utilized as organic complexes, the most obvious example of which is the cobalt in vitamin B_{12}. Molybdenum is utilized as a molybdenum-pterin complex, and chromium may be metabolized as an organic chromium complex. The metabolism and roles of trace elements have been reviewed elsewhere.[1]

Iron

Function

The principal iron-dependent metalloproteins are shown in Table 41.1.[2-4] Additionally, iron may have a role in the function of ribonucleotide reductase and α-glycerophosphate dehydrogenase, but these compounds have not been characterized as iron metalloproteins.

TABLE 41.1. Some iron-dependent metalloproteins.

Metalloprotein	Function
Heme proteins	
Hemoglobin	Oxygen transport
Myoglobin	Oxygen storage
Cytochromes a,b,c	Electron transfer
Cytochrome c oxidase	Transfer of electrons to molecular oxygen at end of respiratory chain—requires copper also
Cytochrome P-450 + b_5	Microsomal mixed function oxidases
Catalase	Hydrogen peroxide breakdown
Peroxidases	Numerous electron donors
Sulfite oxidase metabolism	Mitochondrial membrane, sulfur
Tryptophan 2,3-dioxygenase	Pyridine metabolism
Iron-sulfur proteins	
Aldehyde oxidase	RCHO-RCOOH
Xanthine oxidase	Hypoxanthine—uric acid
Succinic dehydrogenase	At initial steps of oxidative phosphorylation
NADH dehydrogenase	
Phenylalanine hydroxylase	
Tyrosine hydroxylase	Pteridine-dependent
Tryptophan hydroxylase	
Prolyl hydroxylase	Collagen synthesis, need ascorbic acid and α-oxoglutarate
Lysyl hydroxylase	

Data from British Nutritional Foundation Task Force on Iron,[2] Hercberg et al.,[3] and Beard et al.,[4] with permission).
NADH, nicotinamide adenine dinucleotide, reduced.

In the adult hemoglobin and muscle myoglobin contains 60% to 70% and 10% of body iron, respectively. Most of the remaining iron is in storage pools, and only about 1% is incorporated in enzymes. An additional small pool is associated with the vascular transport glycoprotein transferrin.

The porphyrin-heme complex of hemoglobin and myoglobin contains iron that is maintained in the ferrous state, Fe(II), by an adjacent histidine residue of the globin, which provides electrons that protect this iron from being oxidized to the ferric state, Fe(III), facilitating a reversible association of iron with oxygen. In contrast, the heme proteins in the hemenzymes allow redox transitions; here the protein component appears to confer substrate specificity.

Metabolism

The intestinal uptake of iron occurs predominantly in the proximal small intestine.[4-6] Heme iron, released by intraluminal digestion, and inorganic iron and iron chelates are absorbed by separate carrier-mediated pathways, as well as by high-capacity nonspecific, probably diffusional, routes. Ferrous iron may be better absorbed than ferric iron, and ascorbic acid is probably important in facilitating absorption. Mucin and the mucosal glycoproteins might have an important role.[6] None of the processes involved are well characterized.

It has been proposed that transferrin and lactoferrin mediate the enterocytic uptake of iron, but this has not been confirmed. Enterocyte brush-border microvillus receptors for transferrin have not been identified, although they have been for lactoferrin. Homologous lactoferrin facilitates the intestinal uptake of iron in the animal model, but a similar role for this protein in the human has yet to be shown definitively. Some of this difficulty may arise from the variable species specificity of lactoferrin. Although bovine or monkey lactoferrin enhances enterocyte iron uptake in the anemic rat or mice pup, mouse lactoferrin does not do so in the monkey. Bovine lactoferrin is similarly ineffective regarding iron absorption by the human neonate.[7]

Transferrin receptors are present on the basolateral membrane of enterocytes. These receptors and their corresponding messenger RNA (mRNA) increase with iron deficiency, but because there is no defect in iron absorption with congenital atransferrinemia or in the hypotransferrinemic mice model, it is unclear if this receptor and the transferrin system participate directly in intestinal uptake and transfer of iron or in its regulation and in the sensing of systemic requirements for iron.[5] Both heme and nonheme iron are released by intraluminal digestion of food. At customary intakes the systemic iron burden is mainly regulated via altered uptake and transfer of iron by the intestinal mucosa such that there is an inverse relation between iron absorption and iron "status." However, the mucosal ligand and receptor involved and their regulation are unknown. The enterocytic basolateral membrane receptor for ferritin and transferrin enables them to sense and react to the systemic iron burden, as reflected by the plasma concentration of one or both of these proteins Through some unidentified process, apoferritin is induced within the enterocyte, which sequesters iron taken up by the mucosal cell and prevents its transfer to the body. The subsequent loss of ferritin with desquamated enterocytes is thought to provide the principal regulation of the transfer of iron to the body. Simultaneously, the ability of the enterocyte brush border to take up iron is down-regulated. The intraluminal iron concentration at which this mucosal control is overwhelmed is unknown.[4-6] Postabsorptive excretion of iron, if it occurs, is minimal.

With acute iron deficiency there is a delay before iron absorption increases. This delay may represent a need for the enterocytic pool of iron to be diminished before mucosal uptake increases or for the replacement on the mucosal villi of senescent enterocytes by ones that have been entrained with a higher capacity for the uptake and transfer of iron. After its mucosal uptake, heme is degraded by enterocytic heme oxygenase and the released iron forms a common transit pool with that of inorganic origin. The transit pool of iron has not been characterized. An iron-binding protein, mobilferrin, so named because it was discovered in Mobile, Alabama, which might enable the transcellular passage of iron, has been identified.[6] Mobilferrin is a homologue of calreticulin and it is able to bind zinc, copper, and calcium. It has been suggested that it might receive iron from membrane-bound integrin.

It is not clear how iron enters the portal circulation from the enterocyte. The characteristics of this process do not seem compatible with the known properties of transferrin, although transferrin is the protein with which the metal is subsequently associated in the circulation and extracellular fluid. This transferrin pool, albeit small, is the pivotal portal and systemic transport pool in iron metabolism, and about 35 mg of iron passes through it daily in the adult.

The binding of iron to apotransferrin requires its oxidation to Fe(III). This process is thought to be catalyzed by ceruloplasmin and possibly by another circulating cuproenzyme, ferroxidase II. This assumption is supported by gross disturbance of iron metabolism that occurs in aceruloplasminemia. Apotransferrin is a monomeric isoglycoprotein with a relative molecular mass approximately of 80,000 that contains two homologous C- and N-terminal binding sites, each with a different affinity for a molecule of Fe(III).[2] Transferrin is a member of a group of homologous proteins that includes ovotransferrin, lactoferrin, melanotransferrin, and hemiferrin.[2,4]

Within the plasma 39% of transferrin is iron-free apotransferrin: 11% is monoferric with the iron at the C-terminal binding site, and 23% has a single iron at the N-terminal. Only 20% of circulating transferrin is in the diferric form. The binding of iron to transferrin requires an associated anion, which is usually bicarbonate or carbonate. The protein can bind Cr(III), Mn(II), Cu(II), Co(III), Zn(II), and VO(II), but its role in the vascular transport of these ions is unknown. Transferrin is predominantly of hepatic origin, but it is synthesized in the brain, heart, spleen, kidney, testes, muscle, macrophages and T cells, and placenta. Transferrin is not synthesized by the intestinal mucosa, and that present in enterocytes is probably derived, via their basolateral membrane receptors, from the plasma.[4] The liver can produce up to 24 mg of the protein per kilogram body weight daily in the adult. The transferrin gene is on chromosome 3q and its expression is regulated by epidermal growth factor, insulin-like growth factor, platelet-derived growth factor, glucocoriticoid, metals, acute phase mediators, as well as by iron.[2]

The peripheral uptake of iron by tissue has been studied predominantly in hepatocytes and the reticulocytes.[2] In these cells it has been shown that transferrin binds to specific cell surface receptors that mediate the endocytic uptake of the intact molecule. A proton pump in the resultant vesicles reduces the intravesicular pH, releasing the iron, which is transported across the cell in vesicles and rapidly appears in mitochondrial enzymes and heme. Iron release from transferrin preferentially occurs from the C terminal and is more efficient at pH 5.6 rather than at pH 7.4, which would be consistent with the metal being liberated in intracellular endosomes. The residual apotransferrin and receptor complex is extruded and is recycled into the extracellular fluid. The expression of cell membrane transferrin receptors on cell surfaces is regulated by the iron requirement of the cells, the rate of hemoglobin synthesis in erythroid cells, and the proliferative state of the cell.

These transferrin receptors dimeric transmembrane glycoprotein gene, as for transferrin, is on chromosome 3, as is the gene for lactoferrin; however, apolactoferrin synthesis does not appear to be regulated by iron. It may reflect a concerted genetic control mechanism in iron metabolism, but clearly overall metabolic control is more complicated. Because the allele affected in the classic iron overload syndrome of hereditary hemochromatosis is on chromosome 6, and although lactoferrin has some 60% sequence homology with transferrin, there is no conclusive evidence that it is associated with the systemic metabolism of iron.[2]

In storage and systemic excess, cellular iron become associated with the proteins ferritin and hemosiderin.[2,4] In adults 100 to 500 mg iron is associated with ferritin and hemosiderin. Ferritin can bind up to 4500 atoms of iron per molecule. It is a hollow, porous 12 nm diameter spherical aggregate of 24 heavy (H) and light (L) isoferritins, each with a relative molecular mass of approximately 20,000, the proportions of which vary with their tissue of origin. The alleles for the H and L units are on chromosomes 11 and 19, respectively. It is envisaged that Fe(II) passes through the sphere's surface channels to the core, where it is oxidized and precipitated as a ferric hydroxide and possibly with phosphate, which might be involved in the subsequent release of the bound iron. The presence of iron is thought to derepress the synthesis of the ferritin subunit. Possibly tumor necrosis factor and cytokines can induce ferritin synthesis, which contributes to the hypoferrinemia associated with infection, inflammation, neoplasia, and similar stresses. The synthesis of the H and L monomers are differentially regulated; L subunits are regulated at both transcriptional and translational levels, whereas the H subunits are controlled only at the translational level. The relevance of this to intracellular iron metabolism is not known.

The release of iron from ferritin involves its reduction to Fe(II), which is possibly effected by dihydroflavin mononucleotides. In vitro studies have shown that ferritin can bind other metals including zinc, which it can release for the activation of zinc apoenzymes.[2,4] Ceruloplasmin may be necessary for the oxidation of the liberated iron.

Hemosiderin is produced by lysosomal denaturation of ferritin, which appears to be initiated at a threshold saturation of 4000 atoms of iron (i.e., about 85% saturation). Many intermediate compounds with differing degrees of protein degradation and proportionately increasing iron content exist between ferritin and hemosiderin, which can be detected especially in conditions of iron overload.

Deficiency Features

The classic accepted feature of iron deficiency is a microcytic hypochromic anemia, but the systemic effects of iron deficiency cannot be ascribed solely to a low hemoglobin concentration.[2,4,8] Tissue depletion of iron and biochemical defects arising from iron deprivation have been observed in skeletal and cardiac muscle, brain, intestine, and liver before anemia becomes obvious. Heme iron–dependent activities (e.g., skeletal and cardiac muscle cytochrome C and cytochrome oxidase activity) are less sensitive to iron deficiency than are respiratory enzymes, which are dependent on nonheme iron.

In the iron-deficient rat iron supplements induce rapid improvement of exercise endurance and muscle function associated with restored activity of α-glycerophosphate oxidase and reduced lactate production. Myoglobin concentration and cytochrome activities recover more slowly. Susceptibility to iron deprivation may vary among tissues. In the rat intestinal cytochrome and skeletal muscle succinate dehydrogenase activities are reduced before comparable phenomena are observed in the liver.

In the brain depressed aldehyde oxidase activity is thought to be responsible for increased production of serotonin and 5-hydroxyindole compounds, which may account for the depressed mental ability and shortened attention span that accompanies iron deficiency. Reduced activation of mitochondrial monoamine oxidase depresses liver and brain metabolism of phenylalanine and catecholamines with resultant increased urinary excretion of norepinephrine.

Altered metabolism of catecholamines and depressed mitochondrial succinate cytochrome C oxidase activity affecting the electron transport chain in the liver and other tissues may explain a variety of other metabolic defects in the iron-deficient model, such as impaired enterocytic function and an inability to maintain body temperature. The deiodination of thyroxine (T_4) to triiodothyronine (T_3) is disturbed in iron deficiency, and circulating T_4 concentration is elevated whereas that of T_3 is reduced.

Other biochemical defects arising from iron deficiency include reduced synthesis of DNA, abnormal collagen formation, and depressed neutrophil function with reduced activities of myeloperoxidase and impaired cell-mediated immunity.[3]

Pregnancy

Erythropoiesis and red cell mass are increased during pregnancy. Although the total pool increases, since the plasma volume expands to a greater degree there is a fall in the circulating concentrations of hemoglobin and iron. During pregnancy the intestinal uptake and transfer of iron are increased; in a longitudinal study in women the geometric mean of absorption of stable isotopically labeled iron added to a meal increased from 7% at 12 weeks' gestation to 36% and 64% at 26 and 36 weeks', respectively, and fell to 11% at 16 to 24 weeks postpartum.[9] The turnover of transferrin iron increases and the transferrin pool contains more penta and hexa sialylated forms during pregnancy. These forms have a higher and more specific affinity than the other forms of transferrin receptors on the placenta.[2] This maternal adaptation may well enable women to derive sufficient iron to meet their needs and those of their fetus from their customary dietary intakes. The recommendation that pregnant women should be given additional iron during pregnancy is not accepted universally.[10]

Placental Transfer of Iron

Placental iron transfer is established early in gestation, at which time the exocoelomic fluid is probably the main iron reservoir in early pregnancy, and the secondary yolk sac is probably the principal route of entry of iron to the embryo.[11]

The efficient acquisition of iron by the fetus is illustrated by fetal serum ferritin concentration, which steadily increases during gestation to reach a median concentration about 3.2 higher than that in the mother.[12] Similarly serum transferrin receptor concentration in fetus and neonate is higher than that in the adult.[13] These concentrations correlate not with iron status parameters but with gestational age and red cell mass, and are a good indicator of fetal erythropoiesis. Their independence of iron status probably reflects the predominant overall demand of proliferating tissues for iron.

The number of transferrin-binding sites on the placenta are regulated by other factors including endogenous growth factors (e.g., insulin and epidermal growth factor). The increased number of placental transferrin receptors in the diabetic pregnancy probably reflects this increase.[14]

Transferrin is taken up by transferrin receptor-mediated endocytosis into the syncytiotrophoblast. Intraplacental vesicles are formed, from which the iron is subsequently released and transferred by an uncharacterized mechanism into at least two probable pools: a ferritin pool and a mobile less avidly bound pool.[15]

Because the efficiency of iron uptake and transfer by the placenta is constantly increasing during gestation, it is difficult to determine precisely how this system responds to iron deficiency or overload, or to determine if there is any fetal control of placental uptake and transfer of iron.[15]

Severe iron deficiency impairs reproductive efficiency and is associated with intrauterine growth retardation. More marginal maternal iron deficiency does not appear to either reduce the fetal accumulation of iron or increase the subsequent risk of iron deficiency during infancy.[16,17] In one study the incidence of iron deficiency was compared in neonates born to two groups of mothers, one of which at delivery had a plasma ferritin concentration of 5 to $8\mu g \cdot L^{-1}$ (geometric mean $6.4\mu g \cdot L^{-1}$) and the other 10 to $32\mu g \cdot L^{-1}$ (geometric mean $18\mu g \cdot L^{-1}$). Cord blood plasma ferritin concentration of the two respective groups of neonates was 77 to $131\mu g \cdot L^{-1}$ (mean $100.5\mu g \cdot L^{-1}$) and 82 to $156\mu g \cdot L^{-1}$ (mean $117\mu g \cdot L^{-1}$). The plasma ferritin concentration of the two groups of neonates was similar at 6 weeks of age.[17]

Fetal and Neonatal Metabolism of Iron

The growing fetus contains approximately 58 and $94\mu g$ of iron per gram of fat-free tissue at 20 and 40 weeks' gestation, respectively.[18] The 1-kg fetus at 28 weeks' gestation contains about 64 mg of iron.[19] During the last trimester the fetus accumulates 1.7 to 2.0 mg of iron daily, and healthy term neonates contain 150 to 250 mg. During the last trimester, a major component of fetal weight gain is adipose tissue, so the amount of iron present on a body weight basis (70–80 $mg \cdot kg^{-1}$) remains relatively constant.[19]

Almost 80% of the body iron (i.e., 58 $mg \cdot kg^{-1}$ body weight) in the term neonate is in hemoglobin (1 g hemoglobin contains 3.4 mg of iron). Nine percent is in lean tissue, which contains 7 $mg \cdot kg^{-1}$ body weight and 14%; 10 $mg \cdot kg^{-1}$ body weight is in the reticuloendothelial and hepatic parenchymal iron depots.

The mean iron concentration in the fetal liver has been reported as 21.6 $\mu mol \cdot g^{-1}$ dry tissue with a range of 3.3 to 64.4 $\mu mol \cdot g^{-1}$; no correlation was noted between hepatic iron concentration and total storage iron or gestational age.[20]

The distribution of iron within the developing brain in the rat fetus is dependent on macrophages that convey iron from the choroid plexus to the cerebral hemisphere, the corpus callosum and internal capsule, and the tectum; after migration and donation of iron the macrophages transform to microglial cells. This observation might be of relevance to the impact of iron deprivation on neurological development.[21]

After delivery the neonate's increased Pao_2 depresses erythropoietin synthesis, which remains decreased for the next 8 weeks. The cessation of extramedullary erythropoiesis, increasing vascular volume, and hemolysis cause about a 30% fall in circulating hemoglobin concentration. The concentration stabilizes at 90 to 110 $g \cdot L^{-1}$ at 2 months, which is an overall decline of 1 g of hemoglobin weekly. The decline is more rapid postnatally than it is subsequently. The iron released from the degraded hemoglobin is retained in the reticuloendothelial system and is redistributed systemically. It is the major source of iron during the neonatal period and the ensuing 2 months. A fall in hemoglobin concentration of 60 $g \cdot L^{-1}$ would release 50 to 60 mg of iron, which would then be available to support lean tissue synthesis, which requires about 35 mg $Fe \cdot kg^{-1}$, and some accretion of iron stores. The latter would be reflected by the rapid increase in the circulating ferritin concentration that occurs during the neonatal period. At 1 month of age median serum ferritin concentration approximate 300 to 400 $\mu g \cdot L^{-1}$.[17,22]

This temporary increase in iron stores occurs irrespective of gestational age. Since hemoglobin declines with an attendant mobilization of iron in preterm neonates, their extrauterine requirements for iron are arguably less than they were in utero. Delayed clamping of the cord until it has stopped pulsing is associated with a 32% higher blood volume and a corresponding 30 to 50 mg increase in iron transferred to the neonate.[23]

The endogenous source of iron is finite. Eventually the demands of growth and resumed erythropoiesis result in a need for exogenous dietary iron. The time that this need occurs depends on the balance between the amount of body iron present initially, which is related to the neonate's initial hemoglobin concentration as well as to the rate at which iron is needed for anabolic processes or the rate at which it may be lost in blood or desquamated epithelial and intestinal cells.

Because erythropoiesis is not resumed until 2 to 3 months of life, the term neonate's requirement of exogenous iron is relatively small. Thereafter, iron stores become depleted rapidly, and if adequate iron is unavailable, the infant's circulating ferritin concentration, as evidence of iron depletion ($<10\,\mu g\cdot L^{-1}$), declines quickly.[17,22] As an approximation, the infant weight at which the iron reserves are potentially exhausted with a significant risk of iron deficiency can be calculated as a percentage of birth weight by multiplying the neonate's cord blood hemoglobin (grams per deciliter) by 11.5.[18]

The healthy term neonate has enough endogenous iron to meet his needs until about 4 months of age, irrespective of whether he is fed his own mother's milk or iron-supplemented or nonsupplemented formula. Owing to the more efficient absorption of iron from breast milk, some exclusively breast-fed infants show no evidence of iron depletion even at 9 months of age. Some of those fed unfortified formula show evidence of early iron depletion at 4 months of age, as do some breast-fed infants by 6 months. These ages should be considered the respective points at which to ensure that infants have an adequate supply of dietary iron.[24,25]

The preterm neonate needs, extra iron earlier than the term neonate does. Although the preterm neonate may have an iron content comparable to that of term neonate relative to body weight, the preterm neonate has a greater risk of iron deficiency. The initial hemoglobin concentration is lower (e.g., $90–110\cdot L^{-1}$ at 30–34 weeks' gestation), but a postnatal fall in hemoglobin still occurs. This decline would be exacerbated by blood loss from a venipuncture or other procedure. The faster growth rate of the preterm neonate depletes his iron stores rapidly, so that by 2 to 3 months of age the reserves are exhausted and he becomes dependent on exogenous iron. Similarly, the small for gestational age neonate has a greater need for iron. However, it seems that extra iron is not required during the neonatal period.

It is advised that the preterm infant needs 2 mg of elemental iron per kilogram body weight daily up to a maximum of 15 mg, which should be introduced by 8 weeks of age. The very low or extremely low birth weight neonate may need more than this amount. Regimens of daily iron supplements of 4, 3, and $2\,mg\cdot kg^{-1}$ for neonates weighing at birth less than 1 kg, 1.0 to 1.5 kg, and 1.5 to 2.5 kg, respectively, have been proposed.[26] Formula designed for the low birth weight neonate is fortified with sufficient iron, 12 mg ($215\,\mu mol\cdot L^{-1}$), to meet these estimates and to make supplemental iron unnecessary. On the other hand, the iron available from breast milk is inadequate for such neonates, and specific supplements are needed beginning at 6 to 8 weeks of age.

The iron content of human breast milk declines during lactation.[27,28] After 2 weeks lactation, human milk contains $0.56\,mg\cdot L^{-1}$ and after 5 months 0.3 mg of iron$\cdot L^{-1}$. In breast milk one third of iron is associated with lactoferrin, some with low molecular weight compounds and some with fat globules. Little is associated with casein.[29] The iron status of the mother has little effect on the iron content of breast milk and the provision of iron supplements for the lactating mother does not increase the milk iron content.

The need for fortification with iron of infant formula, particularly during the neonatal period, is uncertain. Studies of infants receiving formulas with 4 mg of iron$\cdot L^{-1}$ [30] or 3 mg of iron$\cdot L^{-1}$ [31] have found, on follow-up to about 6 months of age, no significant differences between breast-fed infants and those receiving formula with higher iron content with respect to hematologic features and conventional indicators of iron status. However, as an indication of relative cellular iron needs in the infant studies, one study found that these infants had higher circulating levels of transferrin receptors than infants on higher iron intakes from formulas.[30] Even so the highest transferrin receptor concentration were reported in a reference group of breast-fed infants.

Metabolic balance studies of the preterm and term neonate reveal net intestinal and whole-body loss of iron.[32,33] Other techniques using radioisotopes or stable isotopic labels have shown efficient intestinal uptake and transfer of iron by both groups of neonates. In animal models iron absorption is particularly efficient in the young animal, in whom it remains so even after parenteral loading with iron. Studies using whole-body counting and oral ^{59}Fe found retention of 5% to 35% in the term neonate and 8% to 37% in the preterm neonate. Retention of the label increases with postnatal age, and although it does not correlate with body weight, it is inversely proportional to the amount of histochemically demonstrable iron in the bone marrow.[34]

In another study of the preterm neonate in which the mean percent retention of ^{59}Fe was 18.9 and 40.9 at 2 to 3 and 5 to 6 weeks of age, respectively, the systemic utilization of the radiolabel was demonstrated by its incorporation into hemoglobin.[32] Although the retention of iron by the neonate does not correlate with body weight, the rate of incorporation of the radioisotope into hemoglobin is related directly to the rate of weight gain. These studies confirm efficient intestinal absorption of iron in the term and preterm infant.[35] The reason for this is uncertain. Studies in the developing guinea pig have shown enhanced ileal uptake of iron.[36] Newly absorbed iron in the gut mucosa is associated predominantly with a low molecular weight ligand rather than with ferritin, as would be the case in a mature animal.[37] These latter data could indicate that iron is in a transport rather than a sequestering pool.

The preterm neonate is in negative iron balance for the first month of life irrespective of intake, but the small for gestational age neonate is able to retain iron on intakes of 2.5 to 13.0 mg of iron.[32] In nontransfused neonates iron absorption is found to relate directly to daily intakes of 5 to 6 mg·kg^{-1}, and they achieve retention similar to that expected in utero. Evidence of systemic homeostasis is apparent in that this relation is lost in the neonate who has been transfused up to a hemoglobin concentration above 12 mg·dl^{-1}.

Iron losses via the gastrointestinal tract occur predominantly in desquamated enterocytes and by blood loss. Early introduction of unmodified cow's milk is associated with occult and occasionally gross gastrointestinal blood loss and hypoproteinemia.[38] It does not occur to the same extent with proprietary formula based on soy or cow's milk protein.

Inborn Errors of Iron Metabolism

Impaired Iron Absorption

Three siblings were reported who had a microcytic anemia and no evidence of systemic iron overload, but some evidence of impaired intestinal absorption of iron.[39]

Congenital Atransferrinemia

A rare autosomal defect, congenital atransferrinemia presents during early childhood with hypochromic microcytic anemia and a low-serum iron-binding capacity associated with low or absent transferrin.[40] The children reported had a systemic iron overload that did not involve the bone marrow. Intravenous infusions of transferrin were partially beneficial, but their prolonged care has not been described.

Defective Sialylation of Transferrin

Monozygous twin sisters with a syndrome of psychomotor retardation, raised cerebrospinal fluid (CSF) protein, reduced nerve conduction velocity, low serum iron, marginally reduced serum transferrin concentration, and normal hemoglobin concentration have been reported.[41] Because the transferrin had diminished sialic acid content, it was proposed that this disorder represented a basic defect affecting the sialylation and function of protein.

Impaired Uptake of Iron by Reticuloendothelial Cells

Iron-resistant hypochromic microcytic anemia was been reported in a brother and sister.[42] They had a high plasma iron concentration and a saturated transferrin. Their hepatocytes were laden with iron, but the reticuloendothelial cells in the liver and bone marrow had none. The underlying defect may have been impaired uptake of iron secondary to impaired binding of transferrin to the reticuloendothelial cells or in the subsequent translocation of iron.

Hereditary (Genetic or Idiopathic) Hemochromatosis

A syndrome of systemic iron overload without anemia, hereditary hemochromatosis (HH) is rarely symptomatic in children.[43] In this disease the intestinal mucosal uptake and transfer of iron is inappropriately high for the degree of iron overload. This defective homeostasis of iron appears to involve aberrant regulation of the mucosal transferrin receptor and ferritin with a resultant impaired inhibitory feedback by systemic iron on the mucosa. Duodenal enterocytes, but not other intestinal mucosal cells, from patients with HH have reduced contents of ferritin compared with those from normal individuals and from patients with other iron overload syndromes.[44]

Hereditary hemochromatosis is an autosomal recessive condition, and the responsible allele has been located on chromosome 6 as a gene that encodes a major histocompatibility complex protein called human leukocyte antigen (HLA)-H.[45,46] It has been suggested that HLA-H is located on the basolateral membrane of the enterocyte where it is involved with the regulation of iron uptake and transfer. The defect has a variable penetrance in homozygotes, and some heterozygotes have been reported to have altered iron metabolism.

Because in the Caucasian population as many as 11.0% and 0.5% may be heterozygous and homozygous, respectively, for HH, the elucidation of the basic defect may have undetermined implications for iron metabolism and requirements of the neonate. Studies of HLA linkages within pedigrees enables the detection of neonates at risk of developing HH, and criteria for its presymptomatic diagnosis in older children are being established.[43]

Perinatal (Neonatal) Hemochromatosis

This appears to be a heterogeneous condition and the possible involvement of an inborn error of iron metabolism is unclear. Neonatal hemochromatosis presents during early infancy.[47,48] Affected neonates have acute hepatic failure with hypoglycemia, hyperammonemia, hyperbilirubinemia, coagulation defects, and cardiac failure with hypotension. They invariably die at 1 to 4 months of age, although liver transplantation has been considered.

There is an increased hepatic content of iron, the periportal deposition of which is characteristic of hereditary hemochromatosis. Histologic examination shows a giant cell hepatitis with varying degrees of cellular necrosis. There is lobular disarray accompanied by diffuse fibrosis and regenerating nodules. Iron overload to a lesser extent affects the pancreas, heart, exocrine and endocrine glands, and thymus. The reticuloendothelial system is spared.

The inheritance of this defect is uncertain. The disorder affects both sexes equally. The excessive accumulation of iron is thought to start in utero, and for this reason some investigators prefer the term perinatal hemochromatosis for this syndrome.[49] The incidence is not increased in families with a known predisposition to hereditary hemochromatosis. There is no distinct linkage of the condition with HLA type, and no consistent abnormality of iron metabolism has been found in first-degree relatives.[50]

In a comparative study of hepatic morphology and siderosis, extrahepatic parenchymal siderosis, and iron burden of the infant with perinatal hemochromatosis (PH) and the infant with other forms of hepatic fibrosis or cirrhosis, hepatocellular siderosis varied widely in the latter group. It was suggested that iron does not have a primary etiologic in PH. The condition and its distinctive hepatic morphology is more related to the timing of liver disease or toxic damage during intrauterine life, when periportal hepatocytes normally contain hemosiderin. It was thought that environmental factors such as hypoxia, virus, and drugs might be responsible.[49] There has been a report of neonatal hepatitis and excessive hepatic iron deposition following intrauterine blood transfusion.[51]

Microcytic Anemia with Iron Malabsorption: An Inherited Disorder of Iron Metabolism

There is a report of two siblings with a hypoproliferative microcytic anemia and iron malabsorption, decreased serum iron, elevated serum total iron-binding capacity (TIBC), and decreased serum ferritin, despite prolonged treatment with oral iron and a poor response to systemic iron with only a partial correction of the hemoglobin, hematocrit, and microcytosis. The condition resembles a genetic anomaly: the microcytic mouse.[52]

Aceruloplasminemia

An inherited defect in ceruloplasmin synthesis has been reported to be associated with hemosiderosis. Loss of the ferroxidase activity of ceruloplasmin results in systemic iron deposition and hemosiderosis, and resultant tissue damage leads to diabetes mellitus and neurologic abnormalities. Iron is deposited in the basal ganglia and in the red and dentate nuclei. Eventually, in middle age, cerebellar ataxia, extrapyramidal signs, and dementia develop.[53]

Copper

Function

The transition between Cu(I) and Cu(II) enables copper to participate in a variety of catalytic electron transfer activities. The principal cuproenzymes are listed in Table 41.2, and the features of copper deficiency are largely attributable to impairment of these activities.[1,54,55]

Ceruloplasmin, a glycoprotein with a molecular weight of 135000, contains six copper atoms that are incorporated during its hepatocytic synthesis. Although it has a central role in copper metabolism, its precise function is unknown. In addition to systemic dissemination of copper, ceruloplasmin has numerous oxidase activities. Substrates for these activities include biogenic amines, adrenalin, serotonin, ascorbate, and sulfhydryl groups. Ceruloplasmin is the main oxidase activity necessary for the oxidation of Fe(II) and its incorporation of Fe(III) into transferrin, Similarly, ceruloplasmin may facilitate the incorporation of manganese into transferrin by oxidizing Mn(II) to Mn(III), and it may serve as a plasma free radical scavenger.

TABLE 41.2. Some mammalian cuproenzyme activities.

Enzyme	Comment
Cytochrome c oxidase	Mitochondrial; requires iron; oxidative phosphorylation
Superoxide dismutase	Cytosolic antioxidant: $2O_2^- + 2H^+ \rightarrow H_2O_2 + O_2$
Dopamine-13-monoxygenase	Synthesis of epinephrine and norepinephrine noradrenergic tissues
Tyrosinase	Tyrosine→dopa→dopaquinone in pigment production in choroid and epidermis
Uricase	Renal and hepatic metabolism of uric acid
Lysyl oxidase (and related enzymes)	Oxidative deamination peptidyl-lysine residues condensational cross-link formation in elastin and collagen[47]
Amine oxidases	Plasma and connective tissues
Thiol oxidase	Formation of disulfide linkages[46]
Ceruloplasmin	Multiple activities
Ferroxidase II	Fe(II) to Fe(III); ?vascular compartment

Data from Mertz,[1] Olivares and Uauy,[54] and Linder and Hazegh-Azam.[55]

Metabolism

In the adult the total body copper is 80 to 120 mg. Approximately 15%, 10%, and 40% of it is located in the liver, brain, and muscle, respectively. The copper content of various selected tissues is summarized in Table 41.3.[56,57] Highest concentrations are in the iris (105 µg·g dry weight^{-1}) and the choroid (88 µg·g dry weight^{-1}).

The daily intake of copper is 1 to 2 mg. From free solution, copper uptake and transfer occurs predominantly in the small intestine. Nonspecific binding sites and energy-dependent carrier-mediated specific mechanisms are probably involved.[54,55] As with other trace metals, copper is probably presented to the intestinal mucosa bound to low molecular weight ligands; glutathione, cysteine, lactose, starch, and glucose facilitate the intestinal absorption of copper. It is not known if copper is taken up by any specific cotransport pathway, but its intestinal uptake is improved when it is presented with L rather than with D amino acids. Additionally, the appearance of copper complexed with fatty acids and phosphatidic acid in the mesenteric lymph raises the possibility of another mechanism for intestinal absorption of the element.

Other cations such as zinc and iron impair the intestinal uptake and transfer of copper.[58] For example, excessive zinc supplements in infancy can cause copper deficiency,[59] and this interaction has long been exploited to reduce copper accumulation in patients with Wilson's disease.[60] These interactions may occur in the intestine at membrane-binding sites in transport mechanisms, or they may result from the induction of sequestering proteins (e.g., metallothionein) within the mucosa. Similar interactions may occur systemically.

Newly absorbed copper is transported on albumin and in binary complexes with low molecular weight ligands such as amino acids (e.g., histidine, threonine, and glutamine). Possibly it is also transported on other vascular proteins that are involved with the systemic transport of copper (e.g., an intermediate-sized relative molecular mass 280000 protein called transcuprein) and a histidine-rich glycoprotein (relative molecular mass 60000).[55] The affinity of albumin for copper varies among species. Because no abnormalities of copper metabolism have been seen in an animal with low-affinity albumin or in the adult with analbuminemia, its importance to copper metabolism must be questioned.

Sixty percent of an oral dose of copper appears in the liver 2 hours after ingestion. The hepatocytic uptake of this copper is carrier-mediated. It has been suggested that copper is removed from albumin in a binary complex with histidine, which then transfers the ionic metal, Cu(II), to a specific membrane-binding site. At this site competitive interaction with other metals (e.g., zinc) can occur. This mechanism is independent of that involved with ceruloplasmin.[61]

There are three major hepatic pools of the metal: (1) a pool involved in the production of ceruloplasmin, (2) a presumed storage depot; and (3) a pool destined for biliary excretion. Additionally, there is a small functional pool of cuproenzymes, and one in which copper is bound to metallothionein. Although there appears to be some communication between the minor pools and the former two major pools, there is none with the excretory pool of copper, which is a separate pathway.[55,62]

Although albumin binds copper in the vascular compartment, its hepatocytic precursor, proalbumin, does not, probably because the N-terminal copper binding site (histidine-alanine-asparagine-NH$_2$) is available to copper only after posttranslational modification of proalbumin. This sequence may avoid any interference by newly synthesized proalbumin with the hepatocytic metabolism of copper.

Metallothionein or, more precisely, the isometallothioneins are ubiquitous intracellular monomeric polypeptides with a relative molecular mass of 6500 comprising about 60 amino acids of which 30% are cysteine residues that are able to bind 6 to 10 atoms of metal per molecule.[62] The function of metallothionein is unknown. It binds copper, zinc, cadmium, and other metals, but only the first three are able to induce its synthesis. Cadmium is a more effective inducer than zinc, which is better than copper. Metallothionein is not inducible with zinc deficiency, which suggests that the primary role of the protein is in the metabolism of zinc. Other factors that induce its synthesis include endotoxemia, starvation, infection, glucocorticoids, hypothermia, exercise, and estrogen.

The proposed roles for metallothionein include (1) an intracellular zinc depot for the activation of apoenzymes; (2) a sequestering protein to protect against the potential damage of excessive intracellular accumulation of metals; (3) a regulator of zinc and copper metabolism, which because it binds copper more avidly than it does zinc, prevents copper from interfering with zinc binding sites;

TABLE 41.3. Approximate tissue copper content in adults, infants, and infants with Menkes syndrome.

Tissue	Copper content µg·g^{-1} (wet weight)		
	Adults	Infants	Menkes syndrome
Placenta	—	4.1–7.5	8.3–14.5
Liver	4.2–16.9	29.5–78.7	2.8–11.8
Brain	3.6–7.5	0.27–1.20	0.17–1.04
Intestine	1.2–3.4	4.1–7.5	6.4–12.4
Muscle	0.6–1.4	0.25–1.02	1.7–2.6
Spleen	0.90–1.68	0.6–1.9	6.4–15.4
Kidney	2.10–3.74	0.5–1.9	5.9–36.8
Lung	1.02–1.98	0.35–1.00	1.8–4.6

Data from Versieck[56] and Horn.[57]

(4) the homeostasis of zinc; and (5) an intracellular source of cysteine in the neonate and a source of reducing sulfhydryl antioxidant groups. It may well play a role in all of the above. However because its absence in zinc deficiency does not impair the metabolism of copper; metallothionein is probably not essential for copper metabolism.

The plasma compartment contains about 3 mg of copper. In the plasma some 60% to 70% of the element is in ceruloplasmin, 15% to 20% is bound to albumin, about 10% is present in transcuprein, and 10% or less is associated with low molecular weight ligands. The latter include glycyl-L-histidyl-lysine, a growth regulator that may facilitate cellular uptake of copper.[55]

Ceruloplasmin is more efficient than copper-albumin and copper–amino acid complexes in donating the metal to apoenzymes. This fact supports the postulated transport role for ceruloplasmin. Cellular mechanisms have been described for the endocytic uptake of ceruloplasmin, release of some of its copper, and recycling of the protein.

Homeostasis of copper is achieved by adjustment of biliary excretion; 0.5 to 1.5 mg of copper is lost by this route daily. In an animal model, administration of copper, either in free (i.e., ionic) solution or intact ceruloplasmin, results in the slow appearance of the metal in bile. Copper administered with desialylated ceruloplasmin appears more rapidly in bile. The copper complex is taken up probably by endocytosis following its association with a specific receptor on the hepatocytic brush border membrane. Afterward the intact copper complex may either enter the biliary canaliculi by means of vesicular transport or become associated with lysosomes in which it is degraded before excretion. It is conceivable that some copper enters the biliary canaliculi via parahepatocellular transepithelial pathways.[55,63]

The biliary content of copper responds rapidly to changes in the plasma concentration of nonceruloplasmin copper. A proportion of biliary copper is associated with protein fractions that are immunoprecipitable by antibodies to ceruloplasmin. Some of these proteins are further degraded during the secretion and storage of bile. Only 1% to 2% of biliary copper is associated with metallothionein. The metal is present in bile in association with micelles of phosphatidylcholine and bile acids and with conjugated bilirubin. Although biliary copper is apparently not effectively reabsorbed, the mechanism of this is not known.[54,55]

Copper Deficiency

Nearly all reports of symptomatic copper deficiency have occurred in infants as a result of either nutritional deprivation or an inborn error of metabolism known as Menkes' disease. The features of advanced copper deficiency are summarized in Table 41.4.[54,55,64–66] The differential diagnosis of the defective osteogenesis and skeletal changes include intrauterine infection, scurvy, rickets, and nonaccidental injury.[65]

Studies in a copper-derived animal model and adult human volunteers have shown a variety of other metabolic defects: inefficient cerebral and myocardial metabolism with cardiac dysrhythmias, conduction defects and bradycardia, degeneration of the exocrine pancreas,

TABLE 41.4. Clinical features of copper deficiency in infancy.

Failure to thrive
Pallor
Hypothermia, apneic attacks
Hypotonia, poor feeding
Skeletal changes (radiographic generalized and symmetrical)[64]
    Osteoporosis, fractures
    Metaphyseal irregularities, flaring and cupping, spurs, and chip fractures
    Epiphyseal porosis and separation
    Periosteal reaction and subperiosteal new bone formation
    Wormian bones, retarded bone age
Abnormal elastic and connective tissues, hernias, tortuous vasculature, varices, and aneurysms
Sideroblastic anemia
    Bone marrow: maturation arrest of erythroid and myeloid series
    Vacuolated cells, ringed sideroblasts
    Altered iron metabolism
    Hypochromic anemia, anisocytosis, microcytosis
    Neutropenia ($<1 \times 10^9 L^{-1}$)
Fish odor (?trimethylaminemia)[65]
Hypocupremia, hypoceruloplasminemia
Hypoproteinemia with edema

Data from Olivares and Uauy,[54] Linder and Hazegh-Azam,[55] Fell,[64] Grunebaum et al.,[65] and Blumenthal et al.[66]

defective thyroxine response to thyroid-stimulating hormone, altered metabolism of carbohydrates and lipids, impaired synthesis or release of enkephalins, increased turnover of norepinephrine, and altered synthesis of polypeptide hormones and coagulation factor V. In an animal model copper deficiency is accompanied by cardiac enlargement, with abnormal elastic laminae and connective tissue occasionally leading to cardiac rupture and aortic damage. Cytochrome C oxidase activity is reduced in all tissues, but impaired mitochondrial respiration occurs before any obvious effect on cytochrome C oxidase.[12] Although ceruloplasmin and ferroxidase facilitate the incorporation of iron into transferrin, it is noteworthy that iron and heme metabolism are not affected by hypoceruloplasminemia. Another mechanism such as the mitochondrial synthesis of heme may be pathogenic in the anemia of copper deficiency. Reduced activity of superoxide dismutase and possible increased susceptibility to oxidant damage is an early feature of copper deprivation, but the life span of active phagocytes is reduced before any fall in their superoxide dismutase activity.[12] A further compromise of antioxidant activity (e.g., reduced pulmonary and hepatic glutathione peroxidase activity) has been noted in the copper-deficient rat.

The susceptibility of immune mechanisms to copper deficiency is evident from studies in mice, cattle, and sheep.[12] Such models succumb to bacterial infection, and there are reduced numbers of antibody-producing cells and neutrophils. The reactivity of B and T cells to mitogens is reduced, as is neutrophilocidal activity. The copper-deficient neonate may still have a neutrophilic response to infection, but on the basis of experience in an animal model the life span and function of the neutrophils might be impaired.

Pregnancy

At term the total amount of copper in the fetus and placenta may be as much as 17% of that in the nonpregnant woman. This figure represents an accretion of about 45 mg of copper throughout pregnancy at an increased daily retention rate of 4%. It has been calculated that the overall daily accumulation of copper in the products of conception during the four quarters of pregnancy are 17, 61, 160, and 200 μg (0.27, 0.96, 2.50, and 3.20 μmol), respectively.[67]

The daily intake of copper (i.e., mean 1.4–2.8 mg) by pregnant women is similar to that of nonpregnant women.[67] It is likely that during pregnancy there is systemic adaptation of copper metabolism designed to meet the needs of the conceptus.

Metabolic balance studies suggest that midterm pregnant women need about 3 mg of copper daily to achieve reliable copper retention.[68] Similar studies of women eating animal- and plant-based diets supplying, respectively, 1.4 and 2.5 mg of copper daily find a marginally higher intestinal copper absorption in pregnant women than in nonpregnant women.[69]

Plasma and serum copper and ceruloplasmin concentrations rise steadily throughout pregnancy and after delivery return rapidly to nonpregnant concentrations. These concentrations at midpregnancy do not correlate with neonatal birth weight or with the outcome of pregnancy; reduced concentrations have been recorded in placental insufficiency, intrauterine death, and threatened abortion, and high concentrations accompany infection and toxemia.[70] The latter changes probably represent the hormonal influences of pregnancy and its complications. Anecdotal reports of reduced hepatic copper in pregnant women who have died in road traffic accidents or with late toxemia support the possibility that the increased circulating pool of copper arises from mobilization of the hepatic depot.[67]

The elevated total plasma copper concentration in maternal blood is due to an increase in the ceruloplasmin-bound metal, and the ultrafilterable amount bound to low molecular weight ligands is essentially unchanged. The concentration of copper in the fetus is higher than in the placenta. The concentration of copper in the maternal plasma exceeds that in the fetal circulation. Although this fact caused speculation that copper crosses the placenta by passive transfer along a concentration gradient, the uptake of copper by the isolated human trophoblast is temperature dependent and probably involves ceruloplasmin as the copper donor.[71]

The effects of antenatal copper deficiency in animal models are summarized in Table 41.5.[72] There have been no descriptions of maternal copper deficiency in human pregnancy. Abnormalities possibly secondary to the impaired supply of copper to tissues have been described in the offspring of women with cystinuria[73] or Wilson's disease[74] who had been treated with penicillamine. Both of the involved children had hernias and cutis laxa; one infant had hyperflexibility of joints, vascular anomalies, and hypertonia, and died with an overwhelming *Candida* septicemia; the other survived. Before attributing these

TABLE 41.5. Defects arising from prenatal deficiency of copper.

Fetal and early neonatal death
Neurologic abnormalities
   Fits, defective myelin synthesis
   Cerebral and/or cerebellar hypotrophy
Cardiovascular; aneurysms, varicosities, vascular fragility
Skeletal matrix defective (collagen and elastin)
Altered metabolism of energy and phospholipid
Impaired growth

Data from Hurley,[72] with permission.

phenomena entirely to copper deficiency, one should remember that penicillamine can chelate other trace elements and nutrients. The offspring of adequately treated women with Wilson's disease do not suffer any defects.[75]

Fetal and Neonatal Copper Metabolism

Body copper concentration is greater in the fetus and neonate than in the adult. The distribution of copper differs, and essentially the adult pattern of copper distribution is not achieved until late infancy (Table 41.3).

The calculated daily copper accumulation by a fetus is 51 µg (0.8 µmol)·kg body weight^{-1},[76] and the concentration of copper in the fetus increases from 3.5 mg·kg^{-1} of fat-free tissue at 20 weeks' gestation to about 4.6 mg·kg^{-1} at term when the total body copper is 20 mg.[19]

Between 20 weeks' gestation and term the hepatic copper concentration is approximately 5.3 mg·100 g wet weight^{-1} (200–400 µg·g dry weight^{-1}), which is at least ten times that of adult (15 µg·100 µg wet weight^{-1}). The fetal liver contains 3 mg at 26 weeks' gestation and 10 to 12 mg of copper at term (i.e., 50–60% of total body copper). There is considerable individual variation, with a reported range of 13 to 1218 µg·g dry weight^{-1}, and the distribution of copper in the liver may be uneven.[77] Assuming that the neonate requires about 25 µg·kg body weight^{-1} daily for lean tissue synthesis, the term neonate possibly has sufficient copper stores for 4 to 6 months and the preterm neonate enough for 2 to 3 months.

Much of the copper in the fetal liver is bound to metallothionein and is localized in the lysosomal fraction, in contrast to the nuclear and cytoplasmic distribution of zinc and metallothionein.[78] In further contrast to zinc, there is no correlation between the hepatic content of metallothionein and copper.[79] ^{64}Cu administered systemically to neonatal piglets is retained in the liver bound to metallothionein and high molecular weight proteins. It reappears slowly as ceruloplasmin in the circulation.[80]

In suckling rat pups intestinal uptake of radiocopper from aqueous solution, plasma, or of biliary origin is efficient (i.e., over 75%). This process may represent mucosal pinocytotic uptake of copper. After weaning, the uptake of biliary copper falls from 75% to 8% and that of plasma copper from 96% to 20%. This decline, which may represent gut closure, can be induced by steroid administration, although its relevance to the human neonate is unknown.[1]

Metabolic balance studies using stable isotopic labels of copper in the preterm and term neonate have shown that, despite having net intestinal secretion and net whole-body loss of the element, they have efficient intestinal uptake of the element.[81]

The copper content of human milk is highest in colostrum at 9.4 ± 1.9 µmol·L^{-1} (mean ± SD). It declines to 6.5 ± 0.63 µmol·L^{-1} at the end of 1 month lactation, subsequently declining to 3.46 ± 0.8 µmol·L^{-1}.[82] The latter value is still higher than that present in raw cow's milk (1.6–3.1 µmol·L^{-1}).

In human milk copper is associated with casein 7%, lipid 15%, whey protein 56%, and low molecular weight ligands 21%. By contrast, in cow's milk 44% of copper is associated with casein.[83] Dietary intake of copper has no influence on the copper concentration of breast milk.

Copper requirements of neonates are difficult to determine accurately because of the large endogenous stores in the term neonate and copper status is probably adequate in most populations. There is a risk, however, because milk is low in copper and adding copper in large amounts to formulas might cause oxidative damage to the organic constituents. Bioavailability of copper from cow milk and infant formula is low compared with that from human milk because of their different protein and mineral compositions. In a suckling rat model in which the hepatic uptake of radiolabeled copper is measured as a manifestation of copper absorption from intraintestinal milk, 25% and 23%, respectively, of the label is taken up from human milk and a cow's milk-based formula compared with only 10% of that in a soy protein-based formula.[84]

The normal range of plasma copper concentration in the adult is approximately 10 to 24 µmol·L^{-1}. Plasma concentrations of copper and ceruloplasmin gradually increase during infancy. They are lower in the preterm than in the term neonate and are related to postconceptional age (Tables 41.6 and 41.7).[85-88] This fact may represent developmental maturation of the hepatic synthesis of ceruloplasmin, since immunoreactive apoceruloplasmin concentration is lower in cord blood than in the adult circulation.[89] Despite these low plasma copper and ceruloplasmin concentrations, sufficient copper is transferred through this compartment to support peripheral requirements.

Neither the level of copper intake nor the timing of any supplementation have any influence on plasma or serum copper concentrations in the term or the preterm neonate.[90] In the term infant at 8 to 10 weeks postnatal age, plasma concentration was similar to that in the infants who had been fed their own mother's milk (copper content 5.8 µmol·L^{-1}) or formula containing either 0.47 or 6.3 µmol of copper·L^{-1}, respectively, providing 0.07 or 0.92 µmol copper·kg^{-1}daily^{-1}.[91]

The similarity of plasma copper concentration irrespective of the type of feed represents the maintenance of this concentration by the hepatic copper pool. It is likely that the infant on low copper intake may well have had more depleted stores than those on the higher intake.

Many infant formulas are supplemented with iron, and the iron/copper molar ratio in many formulas is higher

TABLE 41.6. Selected reference values for plasma or serum copper, by postconceptional age.[a]

Postconceptional age (weeks)	Barclay et al.[b] (plasma)	Sutton et al.[85] (plasma)	Halliday et al.[86] (serum)	Hillman[87] (serum)
25–28				4.5 (2.7)
29–30	3.7 (2.8–4.8)	5.5 (1.9–15.8)		4.3 (2.3)
31–32	4.8 (4.2–5.4)	5.6 (2.5–12.4)	5.9 (2.8–12.4)	4.9 (2.3)
33–34	5.1 (4.5–5.8)	5.5 (2.1–14.6)		5.7 (2.3)
35–36	5.8 (5.1–6.6)	6.1 (3.0–12.4)		6.1 (2.2)
			7.8 (3.8–16.0)	
37–38	6.3 (5.7–7.0)	7.3 (4.3–12.4)		7.4 (1.2)
39–40	7.6 (6.4–9.1)			8.2 (1.8)
41–42	8.9 (8.0–9.8)	9.8 (6.9–13.9)	11.1 (6.7–18.4)	9.4 (3.3)
43–44	9.4 (8.4–10.5)	10.2 (6.2–16.7)		11.0 (4.4)
45–46	11.4 (10.4–12.5)	11.5 (7.4–17.9)		10.2 (2.5)
			12.5 (8.1–19.3)	
47–48	11.0 (9.8–12.4)	13.9 (6.9–28.1)		12.8 (2.8)
49–50	11.5 (10.0–13.1)			
51–54	12.4 (11.2–13.6)		13.5 (9.9–18.4)	
55–59	12.9 (11.3–14.6)		16.0 (9.1–28.2)	

[a] Mean and 95% confidence level, except for Hillman's data, which are mean and SD.
[b] Unpublished data.

than that found in human breast milk which is about 1. A randomized crossover study has shown that the intestinal uptake and net whole-body retention of copper by infants fed formula containing either 38.6 or 9.5 times as much iron as copper (0.8 μmol·L^{-1}) produced net absorptions of 13.4% and 27.5%, respectively.[92] Similarly high intakes of zinc may impair copper absorption in humans, but in one study molar excess of 13:1 zinc to copper (i.e., at least four times that in breast milk) caused no obvious clinical or biochemical problems in preterm infants.[93] The occurrence of an iron-copper interaction is suggested by the reduced erythrocyte cupro-zinc superoxide dismutase activities (CuZnSOD) in low birth weight infants aged 5 months who had been receiving 13.7 mg of supplemental iron daily for 4 months.[94] Plasma copper concentration was similar in the latter group and CuZnSOD might be a more reliable indicator of any risk of copper deprivation. Plasma copper concentrations may be lower in the infant with rapid weight gain who might be at greater risk of copper depletion.[95] Similarly in a longitudinal study, infants from 0 to 6 months with the lowest CuZnSOD activity were those with the largest weight gains.[96]

In the growing infant copper deficiency has presented between 4 weeks and 8 months of age with a mean around 3 months postnatal age. The term infant presents around 6 months of age. None has presented during the first month of life, and there have been no reports of copper deficiency occurring in exclusively breast-fed or appropriately formula-fed term or preterm infants. The effectiveness of the hepatic copper store depends on its initial size, the relative rates of its depletion as it is redistributed to peripheral tissue, and repletion with absorbed dietary copper. It should be appreciated that imbalances causing copper deficiency arise from preterm delivery, total parenteral nutrition with inadequate copper supplements,[66,85] malnutrition and malabsorption syndromes, alkali therapy,[97] and the use of inappropriate diets such as unmodified cow's milk, some with added honey,[98] or a combination of these factors. The parenterally fed but not copper-supplemented preterm infant has been found to have higher plasma copper and ceruloplasmin concentrations than the enterally fed infant; however, the metabolic implications of this observation are not clear.[99]

Although reference ranges for the increasing plasma copper and ceruloplasmin concentrations of the term and the preterm neonate help interpret such concentrations in suspected deficiencies, the diagnosis ultimately depends on monitoring the clinical, hematologic, and

TABLE 41.7. Plasma ceruloplasmin and copper concentrations in healthy infants.

Postnatal age (months)	Plasma ceruloplasmin[a] (μmol·L^{-1})	Plasma copper (μmol·L^{-1})
Birth	0.90 (0.07–2.24)	4.57 (2.05–10.9)
2	1.64 (0.52–3.58)	11.2 (4.6–21.7)
4	2.09 (1.04–4.25)	13.1 (6.9–22.0)
6	2.54 (1.19–5.97)	15.28 (8.03–25.2)
12	3.21 (1.64–5.90)	19.7 (10.4–32.9)

Results are the means and ranges (in parentheses).
[a] SEM at each postnatal age was 0.07 μmol/L
Data from Salmenpera et al.,[88] with permission.

biochemical responses to a therapeutic trial of copper as copper acetate or sulfate (2.0–5.0 μmol·kg^{-1}daily^{-1}). Reticulocytosis is an early indication of a response to adequate treatment with copper that usually occurs within 4 to 7 days. The experience cited above demonstrates the potential usefulness of monitoring erythrocyte superoxide dismutase activity. Radiologic resolution of skeletal abnormalities appears after 3 weeks, and the retarded bone age is one of the last features to resolve.

The protective function of the hepatic reserves makes it difficult to assess the optimal copper intake for the neonate. For early infancy daily copper intakes of 1.26 μmol (80 μg)·kg^{-1} have been proposed, as has a "safe and adequate daily intake" of 6.3 to 9.5 μmol (400–600 μg).[100] An adequate parenteral intakes of 16 to 20 μg·kg^{-1} daily has been determined for the term neonate.[101] Similar amounts are probably adequate for the preterm neonate.[102]

Inborn Errors of Copper Metabolism

There are a number of inter- and intraspecies differences in the metabolism of copper (e.g., the tolerance of high copper intakes by sheep). In mice several mutants with manifestations of defective copper metabolism exist and present fascinating models for the study of copper metabolism.[103]

Menkes' Syndrome

An X-linked recessive disorder, Menkes' syndrome has a prevalence of about 1 in 35,000.[103] It is characterized by hypocupremia, hypoceruloplasminemia, and exaggerated features of gross copper deficiency. Whereas there are reduced concentrations of copper in the brain and liver, copper is increased in other tissue (Table 41.3). The incorporation of copper into its apoproteins is defective, creating a paradoxical condition of a functional copper deficiency when there is a systemic abundance of the element. As an example, the mitochondria from fibroblasts of patients have a reduced copper content, whereas the cells themselves are laden with the metal.[104] Much of the excess copper is associated with metallothionein. The basic defect is the production of an abnormal copper transport adenosine triphosphatase (ATPase), the gene for which (i.e., the Menkes gene) is located in a subregion of band Xq13.2–q13.3.[105,106] Various deletions and mutations of the gene have been found and this genotypic variation probably accounts for the increasingly appreciated heterogeneity of Menkes' disease.

Classically most affected boys present at about 3 months of age with developmental delay and regression, convulsions, apneic episodes, failure to thrive, and a propensity to infection. Their hair may be normal at birth, but by the time of presentation it has developed characteristic "kinky hair" defects. At birth the plasma copper and ceruloplasmin concentrations may be normal or even elevated compared with those normally seen in the term neonate. After 14 days they have declined to within normal neonatal limits but they do not subsequently rise to adult concentrations.[107] The diagnosis had been confirmed by demonstrating hypocupremia (<10 μmol·L^{-1} at 2 months), hypoceruloplasminemia, and low hepatic copper content on needle biopsy specimens, some of which still might be of some value as are the methods of prenatal diagnosis by measuring the elevated copper content and ^{64}Cu uptake in amniocytes, cultured chorionic villi, and fibroblast cultures.[108] However, genetic approaches and DNA analysis offer better opportunities for antenatal diagnosis[109] and early diagnosis, which might even enable the early institution of successful parenteral copper therapy in some genotypes.[110] Otherwise this treatment is disappointing. Although parenteral administration of copper may improve the circulating concentration of ceruloplasmin and the peripheral uptake of copper, and relieve some deficiency features such as the healing of fractures, it has a limited effect on psychomotor development and the overall prognosis for the condition. Features of Menkes' syndrome have been reported in heterozygotes.[111]

Familial Benign Copper Deficiency

An infant has been reported who developed seizures and hypotonic attacks, failure to thrive, frequent infections, mild hypochromic anemia, skeletal changes, persistent copper deficiency, and blond curly hair—but with normal psychomotor development and white blood cell count—who responded to oral copper supplements.[112] The child was hypocupremic (7–8 μmol·L^{-1}), but the serum ceruloplasmin concentration, measured by immunodiffusion, was said to be normal. The child's mother and paternal uncle had hypocupremia but normal immunoreactive ceruloplasmin. The interpretation of the latter data may well be limited because a copper-dependent functional assay of ceruloplasmin was not used.

Familial Hypoceruloplasminemia

Familial hypoceruloplasminemia has been noted as a autosomal recessive feature in an asymptomatic kindred who had low plasma copper and ceruloplasmin concentrations but normal urinary excretion of copper, normal hepatic histology, normal copper content, and normal hemoglobin concentration.[113]

Aceruloplasminemia

This is an autosomal recessive disorder of ceruloplasmin synthesis that is manifest as gross systemic disturbances of iron metabolism with increased tissue hemosiderosis leading in later life to a variety of endocrine and neurologic abnormalities.[53,114] Analysis of the cDNA of ceruloplasmin from one case showed the presence of a premature stop codon.[53] Increased lipid peroxidation occurs, not suprisingly, and the benefits of exogenous ceruloplasmin has been shown by the reduction of oxidation of plasma lipids.[114]

Wilson's Disease (Hepatolenticular Degeneration)

The affected allele for the recessive defect in copper metabolism known as Wilson's disease[103] is on chromosome 13.[115] The defective allele encodes a copper transporting P-type ATPase (ATP7B).[115] At least 25 mutations involving small insertions and deletions, and missense, nonsense, and splice site mutations, have been described and these probably account for the wide phenotypic presentation of the disease. The genotype can to a certain extent predict the age and probable presentation at onset. Mutations that completely disrupt the gene can produce liver disease in early childhood.

Even so the pathophysiology of the condition is still unclear. The hepatic incorporation of copper into ceruloplasmin is abnormal and there is defective biliary excretion of copper or ceruloplasmin or both.[116] There is a resultant characteristic hypocupremia, hypoceruloplasminemia, and hepatic retention of copper, leading eventually to a systemic overload with the element. Although the youngest reported age of presentation was 4 years, hepatocellular damage has been found at 1 year of age in an asymptomatic sibling of a known case. Diagnostic screening of patients and relatives can be facilitated by haplotype linkage data for the detection of mutations.[103] Those that are of most use are D13S314, D13S316, and D13S301.[117]

Chronic Dietary or Idiopathic Copper Toxicosis

Many cases of death during early childhood arising from excessive hepatic accumulation of copper with consequent hepatocellular failure have been described. The major example is Indian Childhood Cirrhosis in which the copper toxicity is thought to arise from copper contamination of milks stored and prepared in brass utensils.[118] Affected infants have greatly elevated hepatocytic and mesenchymal copper content, and the liver parenchyma shown ballooned and necrotic hepatocytes with increased Mallory bodies progressing to micronodular cirrhosis. Copper deposits have a panlobular distribution. Plasma copper and ceruloplasmin concentrations are initially normal. Similar cases have been encountered in the United States and Europe, and they may have a similar etiology. Cases in Bavaria have been associated with contamination of slightly acidic well water (pH 6.0) that was used to prepare infant formula with copper from copper piping. The water's copper content had increased from $0.4\,\mu mol \cdot L^{-1}$ to 35 to $53\,\mu mol \cdot L^{-1}$.[119] An endemic liver cirrhosis occurred in western Austria between 1900 and 1974. It resembled Indian Childhood Cirrhosis, and in the pedigrees of 138 cases followed an autosomal recessive inheritance.[120]

The importance of early feeding practices in the pathogenesis of this disorder is probably reflected in the reduced incidence of the disease in infants who have been breast-fed. In contrast to Wilson's disease, the lethal accumulations of copper in children with Idiopathic Copper Toxicoses (ICT) have been attributed primarily to an increased dietary intake of copper, but many infants without any adverse effect have similar intakes to reported cases. It has been argued that much of the epidemiologic evidence, such as that from Austria, is inconsistent with this being the sole cause, at least, of non-Indian Childhood Cirrhosis. Any such sensitivity to increased dietary copper intake probably occurs only in children with a genetic predisposition.[121]

Zinc

Zinc has a single oxidation state (Zn^{2+}). It does not undergo the electron transfer reactions characteristic of iron or copper. This relative stability enables it to participate in the structure of many organic molecules, to have a catalytic role in several enzymes, and to regulate some of the resultant activities.[122-124] More than 200 zinc-dependent enzyme activities have been identified in various species; some of those relevant to human metabolism are listed in Table 41.8.

Zinc has a structural and regulatory role in the activities of molecules such as thymulin,[125] the serum concentrations of which fall with zinc deprivation leading to quantitative and qualitative changes in lymphocyte function,[126] nerve growth factor, and in the presecretory hexamer of zinc. The presence of zinc in the insulin molecule protects it in vitro from free radical damage.[127]

The zinc finger configuration of protein was first identified in transcription factors but are now thought to be present in other proteins and to be involved in the association of peptide hormones with their receptors as well as those involving steroid molecules. The "zinc protein" metallothionein has been shown to donate zinc to the estrogen receptor.[128] Zinc is particularly abundant in the neocortex, pineal, and hippocampus. It is involved in excitatory neurotransmission and modification of other neurotransmitter activities and responses.

A number of proteins involved in the initiation and control of programmed cell death and apoptosis have an associated zinc molecule that might itself participate in the regulatory mechanisms. This observation might provide a basis for better understanding of the early phenomenon of zinc deficiency and, given the crucial role of programmed cell death in embryogenesis, for appreciating the teratogenic effects of even transient zinc deprivation.[129]

TABLE 41.8. Some mammalian zinc metalloproteins.

Activity	Role of zinc	Comment
Alcohol dehydrogenase	C,S	Also retinol dehydrogenase
Superoxide dismutase	S	Cytosolic activity
Alkaline phosphatase	C,S	? Intestinal mucosal phytase
Fructose-1,6-bisphosphatase	R,S	Gluconeogenesis
Aminopeptidases	C,(?R)	Hydrolysis of protein
Angiotensin-converting enzyme	C	Specific protease
Endopeptidase	C	Posttranslational protein modification; enkephalinase
Collagenase	C	
Carboxypeptidases	C	Probably including folate deconjugase for folate absorption
Carbonic anhydrase	C	Carbon dioxide transport
Aminolevulinic dehydratase	C	Heme synthesis
Glyceraldehyde-3-phosphate dehydrogenase		Pyridine nucleotide-dependent oxidoreductases
Lactate dehydrogenase	C	Glycolysis
Malate dehydrogenase		
Transcription factors	S	Retinoic acid, calcitriol, estrogen, nuclear receptors
Peptide hormone receptors	S	Zinc sandwiches, e.g., growth hormone

[a] C, catalytic; R, regulatory; S, structural.
From Vallee and Falchuk,[122] Coleman,[123] and Hooper,[124] with permission.

In contrast to iron and copper, the loss of specific enzyme activities is an inadequate basis for the features of zinc deficiency. Severe zinc deficiency occurs in animal models with no discernible changes in some zinc-dependent enzyme activities or in tissue composition of the element. Zinc is vital for optimal metabolism of protein, carbohydrate, and lipids. Tissues with high metabolic activity and turnover are most susceptible to zinc deficiency.

In an in vitro study of protein turnover in muscle and thymus in the rat, zinc deficiency was determined to reduce growth by impairing food intake, increasing tissue catabolism secondary to the reduced intake and hypercorticosteronism, and reducing protein synthesis.[130] The dependence of nitrogen metabolism and lean tissue synthesis, and insulin secretion and glucose tolerance on an adequate supply of zinc has been noted in the human adult on parenteral feeding and in convalescent malnourished children in whom marginal zinc supply is associated with an increased energy cost for new tissue deposition.[131] Zinc supplementation resulted in a greater net absorption of nitrogen and a higher rate of protein turnover, as estimated from urinary ammonia ^{15}N enrichment after oral [^{15}N]glycine.[132] This latter finding supports the important role of zinc in the synthesis of lean tissue. In such circumstances children with an adequate energy supply deposit adipose tissue instead and they have a higher energy cost of weight gain.

Zinc has a wide effect on lipid metabolism.[133] Its deficiency in the rat impairs apolipoproteins (apo) E and C synthesis, whereas circulating apo A-I levels are increased. These changes are associated with hypocholesterolemia. Although some of the changes in membrane, particularly microsomal membrane, phospholipids, and essential fatty acid metabolism that occur with zinc deprivation may be attributable to an attendant anorexia and malnutrition, some of the changes in prostaglandin synthesis may relate directly to zinc availability. Furthermore, zinc is essential for membrane integrity and resistance to oxidative damage.

Metabolism

The adult human contains approximately $30\,\mu g$ zinc·g fat free man^{-1}. The total body content is 1.4 to 2.0 g. It is not uniformly distributed, and the relative body pools are shown in Table 41.9.[134] These pools have different turnover rates, and the large amount of zinc deposited in hair, bone, and muscle has a relatively slow turnover. In contrast, that in the plasma, and by implication the extracellular pool, and the depot in the liver is relatively small but it has a rapid turnover and is the most labile.

TABLE 41.9. Relative sizes of tissue zinc pools in adults.

Tissue	Content (g)	Distribution (%)
Muscle	1.5	60
Bone	0.5–0.8	20–30
Skin and hair	0.21	8.0
Liver	0.10–0.15	4–6
Gastrointestinal tract and pancreas	0.03	2.0
Kidneys	0.02	0.8
Spleen	0.003	0.1
CNS	0.04	1.6
Blood	0.02	0.8
Plasma	0.003	0.1

Data from Jackson,[134] with permission.

Zinc is absorbed throughout the small intestine and possibly in the large bowel. Absorption is reported to be most efficient in the proximal gut.[135,136] Because there is large enteropancreatic circulation of zinc, perhaps two to three times the daily dietary intake, net intestinal absorption of the element in the human probably does not occur until the distal small intestine.[135] Zinc absorption is increased by protein, amino acids, and possibly lactose, and it is reduced by interactions with phytate, calcium, iron, and magnesium,[58,136] all of which need to be considered in the design of infant formula.

There are at least two classes of zinc binding involved in the uptake of the element across the enterocytic brush border: one is specific and carrier mediated, and the other is nonspecific. Passage of zinc across the apical membrane does not appear to be directly dependent on adenosine triphosphate (ATP), but that across the basolateral membrane probably is ATP-dependent, as is intestinal secretion of zinc.[136] There is no definitive evidence that these pathways involve cotransported ligands, but intestinal perfusion studies have shown that initial uptake of zinc is enhanced by oligopeptides such as diglycyl histidine and glycyl leucine. Zinc might also be absorbed by the paracellular route between the enterocytes.

Zinc in the portal circulation is taken up rapidly by the liver via hepatocytic saturable and nonsaturable mechanisms by which interactions with other minerals may occur. Hepatic uptake of zinc from plasma is stimulated by those factors that provoke the synthesis of metallothionein. It is mediated by interleukin-1 and possibly interleukin-6.[136] Subsequently the metal is redistributed systemically, although it is not known how this process is regulated. In the circulation, zinc is bound to albumin at sites different from those involved with copper: α_2-macroglobulin, low molecular weight protein, and possibly the histidine-rich protein (relative molecular mass 60000) that binds copper.[136] The general mechanisms for the uptake of zinc by peripheral tissues are unknown, but uptake by the exocrine pancreas has characteristics similar to those of hepatocytic uptake.

At adequate and marginally adequate dietary intake, homeostasis of zinc metabolism is effected primarily by the liver and intestine. When the body is at risk of zinc deprivation an upregulation of intestinal carrier sites and intestinal absorption of exogenous zinc increases and the intestinal loss of endogenous zinc is reduced and, to a lesser extent, renal conservation of the element is increased.[136,137] These mechanisms are important because with the exception of the possible hepatic pool there are no specific systemic stores of zinc and we are dependent on acquiring zinc from external sources.[134,136]

With high zinc intakes homeostasis is maintained by a reduced net intestinal uptake effected by downgrading of mucosal uptake. This results in a reduced absorption of dietary zinc with an increased loss of the endogenous element secreted into the intestinal lumen. Subsequently at high and unphysiologic intake the induction of metallothionein within enterocytes sequesters zinc within the mucosa and prevents its transfer to the body. Intestinal metallothionein mRNA and metallothionein protein are induced by both dietary and parenteral zinc. At high intakes of zinc the element accumulates in the skin and hair, and possibly bone.[136]

Deficiency Features

Because of the diverse role of zinc, it is possible to hypothesize a dependence of all the major cellular metabolic pathways on zinc. It is not surprising that the features of zinc deficiency are so protean (Table 41.10). They can resemble the features associated with deficiencies of essential amino acids, essential fatty acids, or vitamins A and E. Indeed, features of zinc deficiency in certain animal studies have been ameliorated by supplying these other nutrients. The onset of anorexia and growth retardation is rapid. There is a sensitivity to protein intake; blood ammonia and urea concentrations are elevated, and protein synthesis is decreased. Altered plasma and fatty acid profiles and altered prostaglandin metabolism develop in human zinc deficiency.[136]

Zinc deficiency has a profound adverse effect on immune function.[138] It causes thymic atrophy, reduced antibody [e.g., immunoglobulins G and M (IgG and IgM)] concentration, sheep red blood cell stimulated plaque-forming cells, natural killer cell activity, and cellular chemotaxis. Cell-mediated immunity is depressed with reduced cutaneous delayed hypersensitivity reactions. This condition manifests itself by the increased susceptibility to infection in patients with acrodermatitis enteropathica and by a variable inability to respond optimally to infestations with systemic and intestinal parasites in the animal model. The persistence of impaired antibody-mediated immunity in the subsequent two generations of zinc-deprived dams indicates a subtle effect of zinc deprivation on the entrainment of immunologic mechanisms.[139]

Neuropsychiatric features are prominent in human zinc deficiency. They indicate a role for the metal in functions such as appetite control, taste, olfactory func-

TABLE 41.10. Features of zinc deficiency during infancy.

Anorexia
Failure to thrive, weight loss
Tremor, jitteriness, hoarseness
Dermatitis (periorificial and extensor), vesiculobullous, pustular, hyperkeratotic, stomatitis, glossitis, paronychia, nail dystrophy
Fine brittle hair, tapered tips, alopecia
Loose frequent stools, malabsorption (disaccharide intolerance)
Increased susceptibility to infection

tion, vision and dark adaptation, abstract thought, and neuromuscular coordination.[140]

Pregnancy

Important examples of the effects of severe antenatal zinc deficiency on human pregnancy have been seen in women with acrodermatitis enteropathica.[67] Collectively this experience has shown that zinc deficiency may impair maternal growth. Physical factors may jeopardize prospective delivery and zinc deficiency may be teratogenic in human pregnancies. Achondroplasia and neural tube defects have affected the neonate, reflecting the teratogenic effect of the zinc deficiency model. Additionally, and as importantly, this experience has shown that pregnancy may exacerbate zinc deficiency. Pregnancy represents changes in the systemic metabolism of how zinc affects all women. It has been reported that women afflicted with several zinc deficiencies can still produce a normal neonate.

On the basis of studies in animal models, it is possible that the fetus is protected by zinc released adventitiously from maternal tissue that is being catabolized either as a result of the pregnancy or as a consequence of the zinc deficiency itself. Pregnant rats deprived of zinc can actually accumulate more zinc in their products of conception than they ingest during pregnancy. Additionally, even in the normal animal, some 30% of fetal zinc may come from maternal tissue. If in zinc-deprived models calcium and energy intakes are maintained to minimize tissue breakdown or skeletal turnover and the coincident released zinc is maintained, reproductive abnormalities characteristic of zinc deficiency can develop. Such phenomena have been observed in studies of zinc-deprived pregnant rhesus monkeys in which there is a negative correlation between food intake during the third trimester and their offspring's birth weight.[141,142] The zinc-deficient mothers become anorexic; they lose weight and have a smaller decline in plasma zinc concentration than those who eat normally. This may represent the release of zinc from catabolized maternal tissue increasing the availability of the element to the fetal-placental unit.

During pregnancy maternal intake of zinc differs little from that in nonpregnant women (range of the mean 7.9–14.4 mg daily). No problem can be attributed reliably to failure to achieve any of the published recommendations for zinc intake during pregnancy.

The calculated accumulation of zinc in increased tissue and body fluids arising from pregnancy shows daily extra maternal requirements of the order of 0.07, 0.24, 0.61, and 0.78 mg for each quartile of pregnancy, respectively. If these estimates are added to the possible basal daily requirement of approximately 2 mg, the respective physiologic requirements during pregnancy are 2.1, 2.2, 2.5 to 2.6, and 2.7 to 2.8 mg daily, respectively. At absorptive efficiencies between 20% and 50%, this requirement could be met by dietary zinc intakes of 14.0 to 5.6 mg daily. These figures match most observed intakes. If extra zinc is needed to sustain the products of conception, perhaps it is obtained by maternal systemic and intestinal adaptation and redistribution of the element.

Need for extra zinc during pregnancy depends on the population of women being considered. For example, a daily supplement of zinc of 25 mg given to healthy African-American mothers who had a low plasma zinc concentration below the median value from 19 weeks' gestation was associated with offspring with heavier mean birth weight and greater head circumference, particularly in the mothers whose body mass indices were below 26.[143] Analogous findings occurred in an adolescent population.[144] On the other hand, 44 mg of supplemental zinc daily given to healthy middle-class Danish mothers had no obvious effects.[145] In a United Kingdom study in which the daily zinc intake of a group of women was supplemented by 9 to 24 mg·day^{-1}, there was no beneficial effect on the progress of pregnancy and labor on fetal or neonatal welfare or growth compared to a group of unsupplemented women.[146]

Maternal smoking reduces the birth weight of the neonate and has been associated with reduced zinc content of maternal polymorphonuclear and mononuclear cells.[147] Smoking increases the body burden of cadmium, which is a potent antagonist of zinc metabolism. Placental zinc/cadmium ratios are related inversely to both maternal age and smoking. The mothers who smoke, compared to nonsmokers, have a higher placental concentration of bath cadmium and zinc, and their neonates have a lower plasma zinc concentration and lower birth weight.[148–150]

Recent studies in vitro show that cadmium-induced metallothionein binds zinc in the trophoblast, thereby restricting its availability to the fetus.[151] Cadmium inhibits by about 20% the uptake of zinc by microvillus border membranes prepared from the human trophoblast.[152]

Disturbed zinc metabolism may also contribute to the pathogenesis of fetal alcohol syndrome. In the rat even brief exposure to alcohol impairs the placental uptake and transfer of zinc as it does that of other nutrients. This defect is not overcome by zinc supplementation.[153]

Placental Transfer of Zinc

The placental transfer of zinc occurs against a gradient and is rate-limiting in the accumulation of zinc by the fetus.[154] The placenta binds zinc avidly and contains low molecular weight, cysteine-rich metal-binding proteins such as metallothionein, which may participate in zinc transfer.[155] Early investigations using the isolated dually perfused human placental lobule suggest that the placen-

TABLE 41.11. Defects arising from prenatal deficiency of zinc.

Impaired implantation
Embryonic and fetal death and resorption
Cleft lip and palate, micro- or anophthalmia
Anencephaly, hydrocephaly, neural tube defects
Spina bifida, syndactyly
Urogenital defects, cardiac malformations
Pulmonary malformations
Altered surfactant (low lecithin/sphingomyelin ratio)
Endocrine and exocrine pancreatic insufficiency
Immune defects
Delayed ossification, reduced bone density
Low birth weight (increased birth weight)
Inefficient labor, prolonged bleeding
Abnormal postnatal behavior in mother and neonate

From Golub et al.,[141,142,157] Leak et al.,[158] and Haynes.[159]

tal uptake of zinc at the maternal surface is carrier-mediated,[155] and this has been supported by studies using placental syncytiotrophoblast and microvillus brush border vesicles. An endocytic process might also be involved.[152,156]

The metal accumulates in the placenta where it diffuses across the fetal surface. There is no evidence to suggest that placental uptake and transfer of zinc is energy-dependent.

Both sustained and transient zinc deficiency in animal models cause a wide spectrum of reproductive abnormalities (Table 41.11).[141,142,157–159]

Fetal and Neonatal Metabolism

The overall concentration of zinc is $20\,mg\cdot kg^{-1}$ in fat free tissue or $38\,mg\cdot kg$ body weight^{-1} in the term neonate. At the 50th centile for weight, in utero zinc accumulates at a rate of $249\,\mu g\cdot kg^{-1}$ daily.[160] This accumulation amounts to $240\,\mu g$ and $675\,\mu g$ daily at 26 and 36 weeks' gestation, respectively. Although the zinc content of the heart, kidney, and brain is constant throughout gestation, the content in muscle increases from 110 to $160\,\mu g\cdot g^{-1}$ dry weight^{-1} at 20 and 40 weeks' gestational age, respectively.[161] In the neonate the liver contains 25% of the total body zinc, and the skeleton contains about 40% compared with 10% and 25%, respectively, in these tissues in the adult. Studies in piglets indicate that the pale unexercised muscles of the neonate contain less zinc than their mature counterparts. Mature red muscle contains three to four times as much zinc as white muscle. In the piglet this difference is not apparent at birth but develops during the first 8 weeks of life.[162] As with iron and copper, the metabolism of zinc in the neonate differs from that in the adult.

Changing concentration and intracellular distribution of zinc in the neonatal liver have been noted in a number of mammals including humans. Immunohistochemical localization of metallothionein in the liver of the rat pup shows that there is a diminution of intranuclear metallothionein between birth and 14 days postpartum, at which time the protein reaction is localized predominantly in the cytoplasmic pattern typical of adult animals. Although there is some interspecies variation in the time (i.e., late gestation or early infancy) at which hepatic metallothionein concentration is maximal, it declines to adult levels at around the age of weaning. This hepatic zinc-metallothionein may be a neonatal reserve of zinc, as is also suggested by observations that in the rat and the rhesus monkey, maternal deprivation of zinc during pregnancy reduces the content and stability of the hepatic zinc-metallothionein of the offspring.[163]

In human fetal liver, metallothionein concentration is high between 14 and 23 weeks' gestation.[164] Studies on human infant liver at postmortem from preterm or term neonates show that during the last trimester the concentration of metallothionein and zinc declines, although overall hepatic zinc content is relatively constant. Hepatic zinc and metallothionein concentrations correlate signficantly. During early life in term and preterm infants, hepatic metallothionein and zinc concentration decline rapidly to reach constant concentration at about the postnatal age of 4 months.[79] Zinc is homogeneously distributed in the liver with a mean zinc concentration in the term newborn liver of $639\,\mu g\cdot g$ dry weight^{-1} (range 300–$1400\,\mu g$). These concentrations are higher in neonates of 27 to 32 weeks' gestation.[165]

The intestinal absorption and secretion of zinc may change with maturation. Metabolic balance studies suggest that many preterm neonates have a net intestinal loss of zinc. Studies using stable isotopic markers have shown that they are able effectively to take up exogenous zinc and to adapt to reduced intake of the element by increasing uptake of dietary zinc and reducing the intestinal losses of endogenous zinc, both with formula and breast milk.[166,167] Similarly the preterm neonate can achieve true absorptions of dietary zinc in the order of 25% to 40%.[168,169]

Although systemic redistribution of zinc may meet the requirements of the neonate, breast milk is an important source of the element.

In human breast milk the zinc content ($\mu mol\cdot L^{-1}$) falls from 176 ± 72 in colostrum to 71.9 ± 18.3, 44.3 ± 10.7, and 7.6 ± 4.6 at 7 days, 1 month, and 7 months, respectively.[82] The zinc content of breast milk is not influenced by customary diet or by supplements. Zinc is absorbed less efficiently from soy isolate–based formulas than it is from cow's milk formula or human breast milk. The latter effect can be eradicated by removing phytate from the formula.[170]

Zinc deficiency has been described in preterm and term infants. The preterm neonates varied between 26 and 34 weeks' gestation and their birth weights varied between 710 and 2200g. Among reported cases, males predominated and most infants presented at about 3 months of age. One report suggested a similar occurrence in the infant fed a cow's milk–based formula.[171]

The pathogenesis of zinc deficiency in breast-fed infants may arise from a variety of factors including a preceding period of parenteral nutrition, impaired or immature intestinal absorption, homeostasis of zinc, and increased requirements imposed by rapid growth and inadequate intake from their mother's milk.[172,173] The likelihood of the last possibility is emphasized by the preceding unremarkable history of several such infants before presentation but who had low zinc intakes secondary to low contents of zinc in maternal milk.[174,175] Zimmerman et al.[175] studied one mother's milk when she was breast-feeding a subsequent neonate born at term. They reported the milk to have a low zinc content and surmised that the mother may have had defective mammary secretion of zinc. They and others have found that zinc supplements given to such mothers did not necessarily increase the zinc content of milk. In contrast, another case report described low zinc content in the milk of a woman whose breast-fed preterm neonate developed zinc deficiency. The mother subsequently had a normal zinc concentration in her milk during lactation after she had given birth at term. The low zinc content in some women may be a phenomenon of preterm milk.[176]

Severe zinc deficiency has been described in term breast-fed infants.[177-179] They had no antecedent predisposing factors, and like preterm infants, they presented at 3 to 5 months postnatally. The zinc content of the maternal breast milk was found to be low, and zinc supplementation failed to increase the zinc content of the milk.

The onset of symptoms for breast-fed infants argues against the diagnosis of acrodermatitis enteropathica in these children. They respond to smaller doses of zinc (i.e., 5–10 mg elemental zinc daily) than would be expected in a child with acrodermatitis enteropathica. These children continue to thrive after zinc supplements are withdrawn during later infancy.[174] Occasionally this challenge may need to be repeated. One preterm infant who developed zinc deficiency after prolonged intravenous feeding redeveloped features of zinc deficiency after the first attempt to withdraw zinc supplements.[172]

Symptomatic zinc deficiency, which has been reported in the term infant fed synthetic formula for metabolic disorders in the past, no longer appears to be a problem.[180,181]

Plasma zinc concentration in the healthy preterm neonate is close to that of the adult. A higher concentration has been noted in the breast-fed infant at 6 months than in those fed formula, which may reflect the efficiency of absorption of the metal.[182] In the preterm neonate there is a progressive decline in serum or plasma zinc concentration, with a nadir ($9-10 \pm 2.6$ prnol·L^{-1}) at about 6 to 12 weeks of age that increases subsequently. This depression correlates with the rate of weight gain, being greater in the infant who grows faster.[183] It is more marked in males, and it is noteworthy that the timing coincides with the peak incidence of symptomatic zinc deficiency. This finding is analogous to experience in convalescent malnourished children in whom attendant zinc deficiency impairs the energy efficiency of weight gain.[132,184]

If exogenous zinc availability is not sufficient to meet the amount needed for growth, zinc released adventitiously during skeletal remodeling would, with that from the liver, make up any deficit. Evidence of this possibility has been found in the zinc-deprived weanling rat in whom deposition and release of zinc from the skeleton could be induced by supplying high and low calcium intake, respectively.[185] A related phenomenon has been noted in the preterm infant with rickets and a presumed increased bone turnover who had the highest plasma zinc concentration.[186]

In the term infant at 2 weeks, and 3, 5, and 7 months of age zinc intakes from human milk were determined as 2.3 ± 0.68, 1.0 ± 0.43, 0.81 ± 0.42, and 0.52 ± 0.31 mg·day^{-1} respectively and were thought to be adequate. However, the concern was that growth limiting deficiencies might still be present.[187] Such concerns are best addressed by conducting supplementation studies. In one study an extra $4 mg·L^{-1}$ of zinc in formula was provided to healthy infants from birth to 12 months of age. At 6 months they had a higher serum zinc concentration ($13.0 \mu mol·L^{-1}$) than unsupplemented and breast-fed reference groups, which had a mean serum zinc concentration of $9.9 \mu mol/L$. However, after their diets had diversified this concentration fell to that of the other two groups. At no time was there any difference in the rate of weight gain or linear growth between the groups. A parallel study of zinc supplementation in the mothers found that 40 mg, but not 20 mg, of extra zinc daily reduced the decline in breast milk zinc content at 5 months' lactation. There was no discernible effect on the infants. The studies showed that low zinc concentrations in serum were not associated with impaired growth. Conversely, the infants with the highest rates of growth had the lowest zinc concentrations.[188,189] In a group of very low birth weight (VLBW) infants a zinc fortified formula (e.g., $11 mg·L^{-1}$ compared with $6.7 mg·L^{-1}$) is reported to have produced higher plasma zinc levels at 1 and 3 months, improved linear growth velocity, and maximum motor development scores.[190] For the parenterally fed preterm neonate daily intakes of $400 \mu g·kg^{-1}day^{-1}$ (about $6.0 \mu mol·kg^{-1}·d^{-1}$) has been proposed.[112]

Inborn Errors of Zinc Metabolism

Acrodermatitis Enteropathica

Acrodermatitis enteropathica is a rare autosomal recessive syndrome of zinc deficiency arising from a defect in intestinal absorption.[191,192] The infant fed formula presents sooner, but not usually during the neonatal period. The infant fed human breast milk has a delayed onset until an alternative formula and solids are introduced.

Familial Hyperzincemia

A kindred has been reported in which plasma zinc concentration was elevated up to five times normal.[193] This zinc was associated with plasma albumin. The affected individuals were asymptomatic and had no evidence indicative of other alterations in zinc metabolism.

Selenium

Function

The principal recognized role of selenium is as a component of the amino acid selenocysteine, which is present in a number of selenocysteine proteins. These include four glutathione peroxidases (e.g., two are cytosolic, one is a plasma form, and one is a phospholipid hydroperoxide glutathione peroxidase, which is the only form that reduces fatty acid hydroperoxides), and the iodothyronine deiodinases (e.g., types 1–3). Numerous other selenoproteins, the functions of which are still obscure, have been identified in mammalian tissue. These selenocysteine proteins, including possible xenobiotic oxidase activities and their genetic control, have not been completely characterized.[194–196] The antioxidant activities are synergistic with vitamin E, which is the major antioxidant in hydrophobic domains such as membrane lipids, and it is an important component of the intracellular defense against oxidant damage of membrane lipid, protein, and nucleic acids.

Metabolism

Selenium is absorbed efficiently at 60% to 80% of intake, irrespective of intake in the small intestine. Seleno amino acids such as selenocysteine and selenomethionine, in which selenium replaces the S component, are taken up by similar energy-dependent and sodium cotransport mechanisms to their sulfur analogues.[197] In healthy men on low dietary intakes of selenium, homeostatic retention of the element is achieved by increased intestinal absorption and reduced urinary excretion.[194,195]

It is probable that selenide is the pivotal compound in the metabolism of selenium. Seleno amino acids can be degraded to yield amino acid residues and selenite. Inorganic selenate and selenite are thought to be taken up by the red blood cells where they are reduced to selenide, which returns to the plasma where it binds readily to protein moieties, reducing its potential toxicity. Newly absorbed selenium appears to form a metabolic pool separate from the preexistent systemic element and is possibly the fraction preferentially excreted in the urine. Excess selenide becomes methylated by S-adenosylmethionine and is excreted as trimethylselenium and other derivatives in the urine. With grossly excessive intakes of selenium, a volatile dimethylated compound, $(CH_3)_2Se$, is formed that causes a characteristic garlic odor when lost via expired air.

Less than 2% of selenium in plasma exists as glutathione peroxidase. Most is associated with α_2- and β-globulins and with lipoproteins that are able in vitro to transfer the element to tissue.

Two selenium pools exist in tissue. One is selenomethionine in protein. This pool is subject to factors influencing methionine metabolism, and its constituent selenium is not readily available for selenium-dependent processes. At times of methionine deficiency selenomethionine is incorporated into S-methionine sites at the expense of repleting any possible concomitant selenium deficit. If methionine intake is adequate, selenium released from degraded selenomethionine is available to the active selenium pool.

Selenocysteine is the biologically active pool of selenium. In contrast to selenomethionine this amino acid can be synthesized systemically and it has a specific transfer RNA (tRNA). There is no evidence that it substitutes for its sulfur analogue. Selenocysteine is degraded by selenocysteine β-lyase.[194]

The total body content of selenium of 3 to 13 mg varies according to the geochemical environment and indigenous food intake. Customary adult daily intake of selenium varies between 20 and 300 ng. In some regions, such as the People's Republic of China, dietary intake ranges more extensively ($11–5000\,ng\cdot day^{-1}$), at which extremes of deficiency and toxicity syndromes occur.[198] The highest tissue concentrations are found in the liver ($1\,\mu g\cdot g$ wet weight^{-1}) and kidney ($0.1–0.4\,\mu g\cdot g$ wet weight^{-1}). This concentration may reflect the role of these organs in the metabolism of the element.

Reference ranges for whole blood and plasma selenium concentrations vary regionally according to the selenium intake for the population. In low selenium areas a whole blood selenium concentration of 45 to $60\,\mu g\cdot L^{-1}$ is encountered. In the United States concentration approximates $80\,\mu g\cdot L^{-1}$ or more. At a whole blood selenium concentration below $100\,\mu g\cdot L^{-1}$, a linear relation exists with glutathione peroxidase activity, at levels above this blood glutathione peroxidase activities become saturated and their activities plateau.[194,195] Clinical features of deficiency are not normally apparent until the whole blood selenium concentration is less than $10\,\mu g\cdot L^{-1}$, but increased red cell fragility can be detected when the level is below $40\,\mu g\cdot L^{-1}$.

Selenium Deficiency

In domestic livestock selenium deficiency causes extensive oxidative damage of the most exercised muscles, such as the heart, diaphragm, and those of the hind limb. Lesions may develop in the liver. In the rat selenium deficiency impairs the hepatic deiodination of thyroxine with resultant increased circulating levels of T_4, reduced T_3 concentrations, and thyroid enlargement.[196]

In humans the most striking selenium deficiency syndrome is seen with Keshan disease, which is a selenium-responsive cardiomyopathy that afflicts children, young adolescents, and pregnant women in the People's Republic of China.[194,195,199]

In patients on total parenteral nutrition. selenium-responsive cardiomyopathies have been described as having symptoms involving skeletal muscles with myofibrillar degeneration and increased plasma creatine kinase activities, macrocytosis, and lightening of skin and hair pigmentation.[200,201] With selenium supplementation changes in glutathione peroxidase activity appear successively at 7 to 14 days, 2 to 3 weeks, and 3 to 4 months in platelets, white blood cells, and red blood cells, respectively.[202]

Susceptibility to selenium deficiency and attendant oxidant damage is increased by other factors such as the availability of oxidizable substrate, the efficiency of other antioxidant mechanisms, and the relative amounts of oxidant generators. In an animal model parenteral supplementation with polyunsaturated fatty acids, iron, and copper can precipitate myopathies and other selenium-responsive defects. These observations could be pertinent to the pathogenesis of selenium-responsive features in the patient on intravenous alimentation.

Synthetic diets have a low selenium content (vide infra). Selenium repletion ($1\mu g$ Se·kg^{-1}day^{-1}) of a phenylalanine-restricted diet given to children improved their thyroid function indicators, presumably reflecting improved Se-dependent deiodinase activities in these patients.[203] Another important feature of selenium deprivation is its effect in the host on the virulence of benign coxsackie viruses. Amyocarditic strains on being passed through selenium-deficient mice acquire RNA genotypic changes, which confer myocarditic virulence. This effect might arise from oxidant damage since a similar phenomenon also occurs with vitamin E deficiency.[204]

Pregnancy

During pregnancy the products of conception require 3 to $5\mu g$ of selenium daily. Pregnant women consuming $150\mu g$ of selenium daily have been found to retain approximately $22\mu g \cdot day^{-1}$ more than nonpregnant women on a similar intake. This concentration is achieved by a reduction of the urinary excretion of selenium throughout pregnancy.[205]

During pregnancy, maternal plasma selenium concentration falls while that in the red blood cells remains unaltered. Maternal plasma concentration exceeds that in the fetal circulation, but it is not clear if this difference contributes to the transplacental passage of the element. Because selenate, but not selenite, inhibits the transfer of sulfate, it is possible that the fetus derives selenium via this sodium-dependent carrier-mediated pathway. Additionally, selenium as selenomethionine may reach the fetus via the placental pathways for transfer of methionine.[206]

Fetal and Neonatal Metabolism

The concentration of selenium in fetal tissue is similar to that in the adult. It has been calculated that the daily accumulation of selenium during the last trimester of gestation is $1\mu g \cdot kg^{-1}$. The intake of selenium by the breast-fed neonate is higher than that of formula-fed neonate. There is a geographical variability of breast milk selenium content that also varies with maternal intake.[207] It is highest in colostrum at 2 and 4 weeks' lactation with maternal foremilk containing 15.7 ± 4.9 and $14.4 \pm 1.6\mu g$ selenium·L^{-1}, respectively. Hind milk has a little more.[208] Infant formula based on cow's milk or soy protein contains approximately 5 to $8\mu g \cdot L^{-1}$. The efficiency of absorption of selenium is relatively efficient, being about 70% with a corresponding retention of about 55%.[209] However, these figures have a high variance of about 30%. It is difficult to assess the biologic significance of the reported difference of selenium absorption from cow's milk–based formula (64%) and that from soy-based products (49%).

Whole blood and serum selenium concentrations decline during the first months of life, reflecting the fall in red blood cell mass. In breast-fed neonates the plasma Se concentration remains stable, but their plasma glutathione peroxidase activities decrease. Formula-fed infants have a reduction in plasma Se concentration.[210] Selenium supplements given to the mother can to a certain extent ameliorate this occurrence.[211] Longitudinal studies in the infant show that by 3 months of age serum and whole blood concentrations of selenium increase and begin to correlate with selenium intake, possibly as a result of resumed erythropoiesis.[212] Infants on synthetic diets for the management of inborn errors of metabolism do not have low blood selenium concentrations until after the neonatal period.[212] Such infants have a whole blood selenium concentration similar to that of patients with Keshan disease, but they have no evidence of selenium deficiency. Because features of increased red blood cell fragility develop at whole blood selenium levels below

40 μg·L^{-1}, it has been recommended that one should try to maintain a concentration of 60 μg·L^{-1} for routine infant care. In New Zealand, which is a low-selenium area, this approach was followed, and infants given a formula containing 17 μg Se·L^{-1} had achieved plasma selenium and glutathione peroxidase activities of about 80% of adult levels at 3 months of age.[213] Similarly a study in Canada suggested that formula should probably contain 20 to 25 μg Se·L^{-1} (0.26–0.33 μmol·L^{-1}), particularly formula consumed by very low birth weight infants.[214] The fortification of a soy-based formula with selenate to a concentration of 0.17 μmol selenium·L^{-1} compared with a native content of 0.028 μmol·L^{-1} has also been found significantly to increase plasma and red cell selenium and glutathione peroxidase activities.[215] Selenium supplementation of parenteral nutrition with 3 μg·kg^{-1}day^{-1} of selenious acid has been found to improve similar parameters in the preterm infant.[216] Although the biologic significance of these changes is not clear for term infants, it has been reported that for preterm infants plasma selenium was significantly lower in infants at 28 days with chronic lung disease and bronchopulmonary dysplasia.[217]

Selenium toxicity has been described in China, where a blood selenium concentration of 3.2 mg·L^{-1} has been measured. Clinical features included hair loss, nail dystrophy, nausea, fatigue, dermatitis, and neuropathies. It has not been reported if human neonatal abnormalities occurred concurrently.[198]

The estimated safe and adequate intake of selenium during the first 6 months of life is 10 to 40 μg daily.[100] In the neonate an intake of 1.5 to 2.0 μg·kg^{-1} body weight is probably enough for parenteral nutrition.[102]

Iodine

Iodine maintains the effective conformation of thyroxine (T_4) and triiodothyronine (T_3). Adequate circulating concentrations of these thyroid hormones are necessary for optimum cellular metabolism and normal growth and development.[218,219]

Both organic and inorganic dietary iodide are absorbed efficiently up to 50% or more by the small intestine. Additionally, iodine or iodide can be acquired from topical disinfectants and diagnostic reagents. Extracellular fluid contains 10 to 15 μg iodine·L^{-1}. The total size of this pool is approximately 250 to 350 μg, but its precise mass varies with iodide intake. In the absence of specific dietary or exogenous supplementation, the total pool size corresponds closely to the amount of element entering the local food chain from the immediate geochemical environment. Plasma inorganic iodide is either loosely bound or free. It is cleared principally by the thyroid and kidney, but other tissue such as the gastrointestinal mucosa, mammary and salivary glands, and ovaries can actively concentrate the element. More than 75% of the 10 to 20 mg of iodide present in the normal adult is found in the thyroid gland. Iodide is taken up into the thyroid actively by a sodium-dependent carrier-mediated pathway that is stimulated by thyroid-stimulating hormone. This uptake mechanism is blocked by perchlorate and thiocyanate. The iodide is rapidly oxidized by the ferroheme enzyme thyroperoxidase (i.e., iodoperoxidase), and organified by iodination of tyrosyl residues in thyroglobulin. The resultant iodotyrosines are coupled to form iodothyronines. The major excretory route of iodide is via the urine, with the daily urinary excretion of the element being used as a convenient index of intake.

Thyroxine is deiodinated by hepatic deiodinase to T_3. Decreased circulatory levels of T_3 lead to a loss of the inhibitory feedback of T_4 on the release of hypothalamic thyrotropin-releasing hormone. Increased secretion of the latter increases the secretion of pituitary thyroid-stimulating hormone, which increases iodide uptake and causes thyroid hyperplasia and goiter.

The adult needs 40 to 100 μg of iodide daily to maintain iodide balance and optimum thyroid function. At intakes below this range, the incidence of goiter increases and a daily intake of 200 μg has been achieved by a current World Health Organization initiative designed to eradicate iodine deficiency disorders.[218,219]

Placental uptake of iodide is achieved by an active mechanism analogous to that in the thyroid gland. Similarly this process is inhibited by thiocyanate and perchlorate. In a model fetal plasma concentration of ^{131}I can be five times that in maternal plasma, but the transfer mechanism of iodide from the placenta to the fetus has not been characterized.[206]

It is now realized that a broad spectrum of iodine deficiency diseases exists of which goiter is just one extreme manifestation. Intrauterine iodine deficiency may arise from inadequate maternal intake or from the interference of goitrogens with iodine metabolism.[219]

Maternal iodine deficiency causes infertility, increased incidence of stillbirths, abortions, congenital abnormalities, and cretinism characterized by spastic diplegia, mental deficiency, and deaf mutism, usually in combination but occasionally as isolated defects. The latter is endemic in regions where the daily iodine intake is less than 25 μg, compared with the usual range of 80 to 150 μg. This deficiency can be ameliorated by maternal iodine supplementation, usually by intramuscular injection of iodized oil. This treatment is most effective if given preconceptionally or very early in pregnancy, which emphasizes the importance of maternal thyroid hormones in the neurodevelopment of the first trimester fetus. In Europe regional variations in biochemical thyroid function have been found in the neonate.[220] The preterm neonate has a higher risk of suboptimal thyroid function.[221]

The cord blood serum T_4 concentration in the term neonate ranges from 90 to 130 $\mu g \cdot L^{-1}$ compared to the adult value of 60 to 80 $\mu g \cdot L^{-1}$. The thyroid-stimulating hormone concentration in cord blood is 10 to 15 $mU \cdot L^{-1}$. This concentration increases transiently after birth but falls to the initial range by the third day of life. The circulating concentration of T_4 in the preterm neonate is low and increases slowly during the neonatal period. This might reflect the altered metabolism as well as the lower circulating concentration of thyroid binding globulin. Very low birth weight, especially small for gestational age, neonates exposed to topical iodine-containing products postnatally are at risk of transient hyperthyrotropinemia and transient hypothyroidism.[222] The small for gestational age infant has more labile thyroid function than normally grown iodine-exposed or control infants.

The recommended daily intake of 40 μg from 0 to 6 months of age is generous but probably corresponds with that achieved by breast-feeding. Intakes from breast milk vary with local geochemical availability of iodine; a range of breast milk iodine content of 29 to 490 $\mu g \cdot L^{-1}$ (mean 178 $\mu g \cdot L^{-1}$) has been reported. Infant formula contains at least 5 $\mu g \cdot 100 kcal^{-1}$.

Inherited defects affect iodide metabolism.[219] Defective active uptake of iodide by the thyroid is responsive to increased iodine intake, but inborn errors of iodide oxidation, iodination of tyrosyl residues, and coupling are not.

Manganese

Manganese is a component of arginase, pyruvate carboxylase, and mitochondrial superoxide dismutase. It participates in the activities of various hydrolases, kinases, decarboxylases, phosphotransferases, and glutamine synthetase. In the latter roles magnesium can replace manganese, but manganese seems to be particularly necessary for phosphoenol pyruvate carboxylase, prolidase, and glycosyl transferases.[223]

Daily intake of manganese is between 1 and 8 mg. The element is particularly abundant in plant foods and beverages such as tea. The intestinal absorption of manganese occurs throughout the length of the small intestine. Mucosal uptake appears to be mediated by two types of mucosal binding, one that is saturable with limited capacity and the other nonsaturable with an "infinite" capacity. The efficiency of manganese absorption in the adult is low, at a rate of approximately 10%. High concentrations of dietary calcium, phosphorus, and phytate impair the intestinal uptake of the element but are probably of limited significance because no well-documented case of human manganese deficiency has been reported.

Five hepatocellular pools associated with the element's metabolic roles and with its hepatobiliary excretion have been identified. The latter is the principal means of systemic homeostasis of the element. It is also lost into the intestinal lumen by pancreatic and mucosal secretion. There is no stable isotope of manganese available and as a result the metabolism of the element has not been well characterized particularly in the neonate. Difficulties also arise because it is hard to measure the element accurately.

Despite the difficulty characterizing the precise biochemical role of manganese, the manganese-deprived animal does display a variety of reproducible phenomena related to biochemical mechanisms involving manganese-dependent activities. Such features include growth retardation, impaired cartilage formation, and defective endochondrial osteogenesis leading to impaired development of the skeleton, and otoliths resulting in ataxia. Reduced glucose clearance and insulin secretion following a glucose load as well as reduced gluconeogenic response to glucagon and adrenaline have been reported. Hypocholesterolemia and altered lipid metabolism with accumulation of lipids in the liver and kidney with ultrastructural abnormalities in cellular and subcellular membranes have been described. In the rat manganese deficiency is associated with electroencephalographic abnormalities and increased susceptibility to convulsions.

Interest in possible manganese deprivation in humans has been stimulated by reports of manganese-responsive carbohydrate intolerance, reduced manganese concentration in the blood or hair or both of children on synthetic diets, and its association with Perthes disease, hip dislocation in Down syndrome, osteoporosis, Mseleni disease, and nontraumatic epilepsy. Manganese has been found in the hair of some mothers whose neonates had congenital abnormalities.[223]

During the last trimester of pregnancy, the human fetus accumulates 7 μg (0.13 μmol) manganese·g body weight^{-1} daily. Human breast milk contains 98 ± 29 and 67.4 ± 24 nmol manganese·L^{-1} at 2 days and 1 month, respectively. The intake of manganese from human milk by a neonate consuming 750 ml daily is about 1 to 3 μg irrespective of the infant's age.[82] The neonatal mouse and rat have delayed maturation of hepatobiliary excretion of manganese and increased intestinal uptake and transfer of the element. Metabolism of manganese has not been studied extensively in either term or preterm neonate.

In the animal model whole blood manganese concentration varies with extremes of manganese intake, but at more marginal intake than one would be clinically interested, there is no reliable index of manganese status.

During the first year of life a whole blood manganese concentration of 14 to 17 $\mu g \cdot L^{-1}$ has been reported, with the concentration in erythrocytes being 20 to 25 times higher than in serum. Erythrocytic manganese is high at birth at 376 ± 62.3 ng·g hemoglobin^{-1}, with a concentration of 435 ± 119 ng·g^{-1} at 1 month. Subsequently, it declines to a constant concentration of 151 ± 34 ng·g hemoglobin^{-1} at 4 months postnatal age.[224] In one study serum concentration of manganese in the formula-fed infant at 3 months of age (4.7 ± 1.6 µg·L^{-1}) was similar to that observed in breast-fed infants (4.4 ± 1.8 µg·L^{-1}), although the daily manganese intakes were 18.3 and 0.42 µg·kg^{-1}, respectively.[225] In the breast-fed infant a correlation exists between manganese intake and serum concentration. Overall these results suggest that the infant has some systemic regulation of manganese metabolism at 3 months of age. As manganese deficiency in the human has not been identified, it is not surprising that the dietary manganese requirement has not been assessed accurately. For the infant on parenteral feeding, a daily intake of 2 to 10 µg·kg^{-1} has been suggested.

Hypermanganesemia can occur in children with prolonged parenteral nutrition. Whole blood levels in the range of 615 to 1840 nmol·L^{-1} have occasioned concern about attendant risks of neurotoxicity. Some cases had clinical features of neurotoxicity, and others had basal ganglia changes evident on magnetic resonance imaging. The implications for the neonate and neonatal care have not yet been evaluated.[226]

A patient with prolidase deficiency (i.e., iminodipeptiduria) was found to have reduced arginase activity with accumulation of manganese in the erythrocytes. This case raised the suggestion that the disorder could represent an inherited abnormality in the incorporation of manganese into appropriate apoenzymes.[227]

Molybdenum

Molybdenum has several oxidation states, Mo(III) to Mo(VI). The pair that is exploited biochemically is that between Mo(V) and Mo(VI), which has a redox potential appropriate for electron exchange with flavin mononucleotide, enabling it to participate in enzyme activities (Table 41.12) involved in the metabolism of sulfur amino acids, xanthine, nucleotides, and uric acid. Although xanthine oxidase and aldehyde dehydrogenase have a similar broad range of substrates, they are nonetheless distinct enzymes. In these enzymes, which are dependent on iron, the molybdenum participates as a hepatically synthesized but incompletely characterized cofactor in which molybdate (MoO_4^{2-}) has a disulfide link with a pterin.[228,229]

Intestinal absorption of dietary molybdenum is highly efficient at a level of approximately 80%. The element is metabolized as an anion, and systemic homeostatic excretion is probably attained by renal excretion.

TABLE 41.12. Molybdenum-dependent enzyme activities in the human.

Activity	Cofactors	Comment
Xanthine oxidase	Flavin, "molybdenumpterin"	Many substrates including purines, pyrimidines, pteridines, pyridines
Aldehyde oxidase	Two iron-sulfur centers	N-heterocyclic compounds (e.g., quinolines)
Sulfite oxidase	Heme enzyme	Sulfite and bisulfite metabolism; mitochondrial

From Johnson and Wadman,[229] with permission.

Molybdenum deficiency in adult humans has occurred following a year of parenteral feeding.[230] An autosomal recessive syndrome that may result from defective synthesis of the molybdenum-pterin cofactor has been described in the infant.[229] In both circumstances the metabolism of sulfur amino acid and nucleotides is impaired. With prolonged intravenous feeding a patient develops irritability, night blindness, tachycardia, tachypnea, disorientation, and intolerance to intravenous sulfur amino acids, which induces encephalopathic features including coma. It is uncertain if the encephalopathy arises from sulfate deficiency, sulfite toxicity, or both. A patient had increased plasma concentrations of methionine, taurine, cysteine, hypouricemia, xanthinuria, and sulfituria, a 25-fold increase in urinary thiosulfite, and reduced urinary excretion of inorganic sulfate and uric acid. Unusually, S-sulfocysteine is present in the urine. A reduced intake of sulfur amino acids alleviates this feature, and all of the abnormalities respond rapidly to molybdenum (300 µg·day^{-1}) as ammonium molybdate.

The inborn error of metabolism involving molybdenum presents in neonates. They have dysmorphic features, feeding difficulties, bilateral dislocation of the lens, hypertonicity or less frequently hypotonicity, mental retardation, cerebral and cerebellar atrophy with encephalopathy, and generalized or partial epilepsy. The biochemical anomalies are those described above. The affected infant has undetectable activities of hepatic sulfite oxidase and xanthine dehydrogenase. No effective management of this disease has been developed, and death ensues during early childhood. The absence of sulfite oxidase activity in fibroblasts offers a means of antenatal diagnosis for this condition.

It is possible that molybdate, on the basis of an interaction with a sulfate pathway, crosses the placenta by a specific mechanism. In an animal model molybdenum deficiency reduces reproductive efficiency and neonatal survival.

Human breast milk molybdenum content falls from 15 ± 6.1 µg·L^{-1} on day 1 to an apparently constant concentration of 1 to 2 µg·L^{-1} at 1 month of age.[231] From the latter

TABLE 41.13. Other trace elements that may be essential.

Element	Model	Deficiency features
Arsenic	Chicks, mini-pig	Growth retardation, altered protein synthesis, elevated plasma uric acid
Boron	Chicks	Growth retardation, abnormal bones, interaction with cholecalciferol, metabolism of magnesium
Bromine	Chicks and mice	Can substitute for chloride and iodide
	Humans	Insomnia in renal dialysis patients
Fluorine	Rodents	Suboptimal iron utilization, anemia
	Humans	Dental health
Lithium	Goats, rats	Depressed growth and fertility
Nickel	Chick, cow, goat, mini-pig, rat, sheep	Depressed growth, hematopoieses, altered iron, zinc, and copper
Silicon	Chicks, rats	Impaired collagen formation and endochondrial ossification
Vanadium	Rats, chicks	Regulation of phosphoryl transfer enzyme Na + K + ATPase

From Neilsen,[235] with permission.

concentration it can be calculated that a breast-fed neonate would be receiving approximately 1.5 µg of molybdenum daily. It has been suggested that the neonate on parenteral nutrition needs between 1 and 2 µg·kg body weight^{-1} daily.

Chromium

The precise biologic role of chromium has not been established.[232,233] Studying chromium metabolism is difficult because of problems with analysis of the element. It may be necessary for the normalization of glucose tolerance, and it is reported to have been beneficial in the management of both hyperglycemic and hypoglycemic responses to glucose loads. It is thought that chromium facilitates the activity of insulin, possibly by optimizing the number of membrane insulin receptors. Its use in the management of patients with diabetes mellitus has produced inconsistent results. Such inconsistency has created skepticism about the essentiality of chromium. The element may have a role, direct or indirect, in the metabolism of lipids and nucleic acids.

The functions of chromium have been attributed to its involvement with nicotinic acid, cysteine, and glycine in a "glucose tolerance factor." This factor has not been fully characterized, and patients in whom chromium-responsive defects have been described have benefited from parenteral supplements of inorganic chromium. It has been suggested that some of the effects of chromium arise from a nonspecific effect on phosphoglucomutase.

Chromium deficiency has been described in adults and a child who were on prolonged parenteral nutrition. The features involved an insulin-resistant impaired glucose tolerance, elevated serum lipids, weight loss, ataxia, peripheral neuropathy, and encephalopathy. The adult patients responded to intravenous chromium chloride, but the response in the child was less conclusive.

Human breast milk contains 0.1 to 0.8 µg chromium· L^{-1} (mean 0.3 µg·L^{-1}).[234] A fully breast-fed infant at about 1 month of age would receive 0.2 to 0.5 µg·kg^{-1} daily. Most infant formula contains 10 to 20 pg·L^{-1}, and a safe and adequate daily dietary intake of 10 to 40 µg chromium has been suggested for the neonate.

The daily fetal accumulation of chromium during the last 12 weeks of gestation is approximately 0.1 to 0.2 µg·kg^{-1}. It has been calculated that 0.2 to 0.3 µg·kg^{-1} body weight intravenously would be adequate for neonates on parenteral nutrition.

Other Elements

The other trace elements that may prove to be essential and their functions are summarized in Table 41.13.[235] Little is known about their fetal and neonatal metabolism and consequently they are not analyzed in detail here.

The essentiality of fluoride is the most convincing because of its role in dental health. Because infant formulas, especially those reconstituted with fluoridated water, provide considerably more fluoride (300–1100 µg·day^{-1}) than that provided by breast milk (5–8 µg·day^{-1}), concern for the neonatal period has focused on the incipient risk of dental fluorosis. To avoid this problem it has been proposed that the upper limit of fluoride content in formula should be 0.4 mg·L^{-1} (i.e., 0.06–0.07 mg · 100 kcal^{-1}).[236]

References

1. Mertz W. Underwood's trace elements in human and animal nutrition. 4th ed. London: Academic Press, 1986.

2. British Nutrition Foundation Task Force on Iron. Iron: physiological and nutritional significance. London: Chapman and Hall, 1995.
3. Hercberg S, Galan P. Biochemical effects of iron deprivation. Acta Paediatr Scand Suppl 1989;361:63–70.
4. Beard JL, Dawson H, Pinero DJ. Iron metabolism: a comprehensive review. Nutr Rev 1996;54:295–317.
5. Flanagan PR. Mechanisms and regulation of intestinal uptake and transfer of iron. Acta Paediatr Scant Suppl 1989;361:21–30.
6. Conrad ME, Umbriet JN, Moore EG. Iron absorption and cellular uptake of iron. Adv Exp Med Biol 1994;356:69–79.
7. Fairweather-Tait SJ, Balmer SE, Scott PH, et al. Lactoferrin and iron absorption in newborn infants. Pediatr Res 1987;22:651–654.
8. Chesters JK, Arthur JR. Early biochemical defects caused by dietary trace element deficiencies. Nutr Res Rev 1988;1:39–56.
9. Barrett JFR, Whittaker PG, Williams JG, Lind T. Absorption of non-haem iron from food during normal pregnancy. Br Med J 1994;309:79–82.
10. US Preventive Services Task Force. Routine iron supplements during pregnancy. JAMA 1993;270:2846–2854.
11. Gulbis B, Jauniaux E, Decuyper J, et al. Distribution of iron and iron-binding proteins in first-trimester human pregnancies. Obstet Gynecol 1994;84:289–293.
12. Abbas A, Snijders RJ, Sadullah S, Nicolaides KH. Fetal blood ferritin and cobalamin in normal pregnancy. Fetal Diagn Ther 1994;9:14–18.
13. Carpani G, Buscaglia M, Ghisoni L, et al. Soluble transferrin receptor in the study of fetal erythropoietic activity. Am J Hematol 1996;52:192–196.
14. Petry CD, Wobken JD, McKay H, et al. Placental transferrin receptor in diabetic pregnancies with increased fetal iron demand. Am J Physiol 1994;267:E507–514.
15. Harris ED. New insights into placental iron transport. Nutr Rev 1992;50:329–331.
16. Sturgeon P. Studies of iron requirements in infants. III. Influence of supplemental iron during pregnancy on mother and infant. Br J Haematol 1959;5:45–55.
17. Rios E, Lipschitz DA, Cook JD, et al. Relationship of maternal and infant iron stores as assessed by determination of plasma ferritin. Pediatrics 1975;55:694–699.
18. Dallman PR. Nutritional anaemia of infancy, iron, folic acid and B_{12}. In: Tsang RC, Nichols BL, eds. Nutrition during infancy. Philadelphia: Hanely & Belfus, 1988:216–235.
19. Widdowson EM, Dickerson JWT. Chemical composition of the body. In: Comar CL, Bronner F, eds. Mineral metabolism: an advanced treatise vol. 2, part A. Orlando: Academic Press, 1964:1–247.
20. Faa G, Sciot R, Farci AM, et al. Iron concentration and distribution in the newborn liver. Liver 1994;14:193–199.
21. Moos T. Developmental profile of non-heme iron distribution in the rat brain during ontogenesis. Brain Res Dev Brain Res 1995;87:203–213.
22. Siimes MA, Addegio JE, Dallman PR. Ferritin in serum: diagnosis of iron deficiency and iron overload in infants and children. Blood 1974;43:581–590.
23. Pisacane A. Neonatal prevention of iron deficiency. Br Med J 1996;312:136–137.
24. Owen GM, Garry PJ, Hooper EM, et al. Iron nutriture of infants exclusively breast fed the first five months. J Pediatr 1981;99:237–240.
25. Siimes MA, Salmenpera L, Perheentupa J. Exclusive breast feeding for 9 months: risk of iron deficiency. J Pediatr 1984;104:196–199.
26. Siimes MA, Jarvenpaa A-L. Prevention of anaemia and iron deficiency in very low birth weight infants. J Pediatr 1982;101:277–280.
27. Vuori E. Intake of copper, iron, manganese and zinc by healthy, exclusively breast-fed infants during the first three months of life. Br J Nutr 1979;42:407–411.
28. Siimes MA, Vuori E, Kuitunen P. Breast milk iron—a declining concentration during the course of lactation. Acta Paediatr Scand 1979;68:29–31.
29. Franson G-B, Lonnerdal B. Iron in human milk. J Pediatr 1980;96:380–384.
30. Lonnerdal B, Hernell O. Iron, zinc, copper and selenium status of breast-fed infants and infants fed trace element fortified milk-based infant formula. Acta Paediatr 1994;83:367–373.
31. Haschke F, Vanura H, Male C, et al. Iron nutrition and growth of breast- and formula-fed infants during the first 9 months of life. J Pediatr Gastroenterol Nutr 1993;16:151–156.
32. Dauncey MJ, Davies CG, Shaw JCL, et al. Effect of iron supplements and blood transfusion on iron absorption by low birthweight infants fed pasteurised human breast milk. Pediatr Res 1978;12:899–904.
33. Widdowson EM, Cavell PA. Intakes and excretions of iron, copper and zinc in the neonatal period. Arch Dis Child 1964;39:496–501.
34. Bender-Ootze C, Schmerlinski E, Heinrich HC. Cytochemie des Nichthaemoglobineisens in Knochenmarkzellen und intestinale Eisenresorption bei verschiedenen Anamien des indesalters. Monatsschr Kinderheilkd 1971;119:13–19.
35. Gorten MK, Hepner R, Workman JB. Iron metabolism in premature infants. J Pediatr 963;63:1063–1071.
36. Chowrimootoo G, Gillett M, Debnam ES, et al. Iron-transferrin binding to isolated guinea pig enterocytes and the regional localisation of intestinal iron transfer during ontogeny. Biochim Biophys Acta 1992;1116:256–260.
37. Kozma MM, Chowrimootoo G, Debnam ES, et al. Developmental changes in mucosal iron binding proteins in the guinea pig. Expression of transferrin, H and L ferritin and binding of iron to a low molecular weight protein. Biochim Biophys Acta 1994;1201:229–234.
38. Fomon SJ, Ziegler EE, Nelson SE, et al. Cow's milk feeding in infancy: gastrointestinal blood loss and iron nutritional status. J Pediatr 1981;98:540–545.
39. Buchanan OR, Sheehan RG. Malabsorption and defective utilisation of iron in three siblings. J Pediatr 1981;98:725–728.
40. Goya N, Miyazaki S, Kodate S, Ushio B. A family of congenital transferrinemia. Blood 1972;40:239–245.
41. Jaeken J, van Eijk HO, van der Heul C, et al. Sialic acid-deficient serum and cerebrospinal fluid transferrin in a

41. newly recognised genetic syndrome. Clin Chim Acta 1984; 144:245–247.
42. Sahadi NT, Nathan DG, Diamond LK. Iron deficiency anaemia associated with an error of iron metabolism in two siblings. J Clin Invest 1964;43:510–521.
43. Bothwell TH, Charlton RW, Motulsky AG. Hemochromatosis. In: Scriver CR, Beaudet AL, Sly WS, Vallee D, eds. The metabolic and molecular bases of inherited disease. 7th ed. New York, London: McGraw-Hill, 1995: 2237–2269.
44. Fracanzani AL, Fargion S, Romano R, et al. Immunohistochemical evidence for a lack of ferritin in duodenal absorptive epithelial cells in idiopathic hemochromatosis. Gastroenterology 1989;96:1071–1078.
45. Feder JN, Gnirke A, Thomas W, et al. A novel MHC class 1-like gene is mutated in patients with heriditary hemochromatosis. Nat Genet 1996;13:399–408.
46. Fleet JC. Discovery of the hemochromatosis gene will require rethinking the regulation of iron metabolism. Nutr Rev 1996;54:285–292.
47. Knisley AS. Neonatal haemachromatosis. J Pediatr 1988; 113:871–874.
48. Barnard JA, Manci E. Idiopathic neonatal iron storage disease. Gastroenterology 1991;101:1420–1427.
49. Silver MM, Valberg LS, Cutz E, et al. Hepatic morphology and iron quantitation in perinatal hemochromatosis. Comparison with a large perinatal control population, including cases with chronic liver disease. Am J Pathol 1993;143: 1312–1325.
50. Dalhoj J, Kiaer H, Wiggers P, et al. Iron storage disease in parents and sibs of infants with neonatal hemochromatosis: 30-year follow-up. Am J Med Genet 1990;37:342–345.
51. Lasker MR, Eddleman K, Toor AH. Neonatal hepatitis and excessive hepatic iron deposition following intrauterine blood transfusion. Am J Perinatol 1995;12:14–17.
52. Hartman KR, Barker JA. Microcytic anemia with iron malabsorption: an inherited disorder of iron metabolism. Am J Hematol 1996;5:269–275.
53. Okamoto N, Wada S, Oga T, et al. Hereditary ceruloplasmin deficiency with hemosiderosis. Hum Genet 1996;97: 755–758.
54. Olivares M, Uauy R. Copper as an essential nutrient. Am J Clin Nutr 1996;63:791S–796S.
55. Linder MC, Hazegh-Azam M. Copper biochemistry and molecular biology. Am J Clin Nutr 1996;63:797S–811S.
56. Versieck J. Trace elements in human body fluids and tissues. CRC Crit Rev Clin Lab Sci 1985;22:97–184.
57. Horn N. Copper metabolism in Menkes' disease. In: Rennert OM, Chan W-Y, eds. Metabolism of trace metals in man, vol. 2. Boca Raton, FL: CRC Press, 1984:25–52.
58. Couzy F, Keen C, Gershwin ME, Mareschi JP. Nutritional implications of the interactions between minerals. Prog Food Nutr Res 1993;17:65–87.
59. Botash AS, Nasca J, Dubowy R, et al. Zinc-induced copper deficiency in an infant. Am J Dis Child 1992; 146:709–711.
60. Hoogenraad TU, Van Hattum J, Van den Hamer CJA. Management of Wilson's disease with zinc sulphate: experience in a series of 27 patients. J Neurol Sci 1987;77:137–146.
61. Ettinger MJ, Darwish HM, Schmitt RC. Mechanism of copper transport from plasma to hepatocytes. Fed Proc 1986;45:2800–2804.
62. Bremner I. Involvement of metallothionein to the hepatic metabolism of copper. J Nutr 1987;117:19–29.
63. Kressner MS, Stockert RJ, Morell AG, et al. Origins of biliary copper. Hepatology 1984;4:867–870.
64. Fell BF. Pathological consequences of copper deficiency and cobalt deficiency. Philos Trans R Soc Lond [Biol] 1981;294:153–169.
65. Grunebaum M, Horodinceanu C, Steinherz R. The radiographic manifestations of bone changes with copper deficiency. Pediatr Radiol 1980;9:101–104.
66. Blumenthal I, Lealman GT, Franklyn PP. Fracture of the femur, fish odour, and copper deficiency in a preterm infant. Arch Dis Child 1980;55:229–231.
67. Aggett PJ, Campbell DM, Page KR. The metabolism of trace elements in pregnancy. In: Chandra RK, ed. The metabolism of trace elements in children. New York: Raven Press, 1991:27–46.
68. Taper LJ, Olivia JT, Ritchey SI. Zinc and copper retention during pregnancy: the adequacy of prenatal diets with and without supplementation. Am J Clin Nutr 1985;41:1184–1192.
69. Turnlund JR, Swanson CA, King JC. Copper absorption and retention in pregnant women fed diets based on animal and plant proteins. J Nutr 1983;113:2346–2352.
70. Tuttle S, Aggett PJ, Campbell DM, et al. Zinc and copper nutrition in human pregnancy: a longitudinal study in normal primigravida and in primigravida at risk of delivering a growth retarded baby. Am J Clin Nutr 1985;41:1032–1041.
71. Mas A, Sarkar B. Uptake of ^{67}Cu by isolated human trophoblast cells. Biochim Biophys Acta 1992;1135:123–128.
72. Hurley LS. Teratogenic aspects of manganese, zinc and copper nutrition. Physiol Rev 1981;61:249–295.
73. Linares A, Zarranz Ji, Rodriguez-Alarcon J, et al. Reversible cutis laxa due to maternal penicillamine treatment. Lancet 1979;2:43.
74. Mjolnerod OK, Rasmussen K, Dommerud SA, et al. Congenital connective tissue defect due to D-penicillamine treatment in pregnancy. Lancet 1971;1:673–675.
75. Walshe JM. Pregnancy in Wilson's disease. Q J Med 1973; 46:73–83.
76. Shaw JCL. Trace elements in the fetus and young infant. II. Copper manganese, selenium, and chromium. Am J Dis Child 1980;134:74–81.
77. Faa G, Liguori C, Columbano A, et al. Uneven copper distribution in the human newborn liver. Hepatology 1987;7:838–842.
78. Ryden L, Deutsch HF. Preparation and properties of the major copper binding component of human fetal liver: its identification as metallothionein. J Biol Chem 1978; 253:519–524.
79. Zlotkin SH, Cherian MG. Hepatic metallothionein as a source of zinc and cysteine during the first year of life. Pediatr Res 1988;24:326–329.

80. Bingle CD, Srai SK, Whiteley OS, et al. Neonatal and adult Cu-64 metabolism in the pig and the possible relationship between the ontogeny of copper metabolism and Wilson's disease. Biol Neonate 1988;54:294–300.
81. Ehrenkranz RA, Gettner PA, Nelli CM, et al. Zinc and copper nutritional studies in very low birth weight infants: comparison of stable isotopic extrinsic tag and chemical balance methods. Pediatr Res 1989;26:298–307.
82. Casey CE, Neville MC, Hambidge KM. Studies in human lactation: secretion of zinc, copper, and manganese in human milk. Am J Clin Nutr 1989;49:773–785.
83. Fransson G, Lonnerdal B. Distribution of trace elements and minerals in human and cow's milk. Pediatr Res 1983;17:912–915.
84. Lonnerdal B. Bioavailability of copper. Am J Clin Nutr 1996;63:821S–829S.
85. Sutton AM, Harvie A, Cockburn F, et al. Copper deficiency in the preterm infant of very low birth-weight. Arch Dis Child 1985;60:644–651.
86. Halliday HL, Lappin TRJ, McMaster D, Patterson CC. Copper and the preterm infant. Arch Dis Child 1985;60:1105–1106.
87. Hillman LS. Serial serum copper concentrations in premature and SGA infants during the first 3 months of life. J Pediatr 1981;98:305–308.
88. Salmenpera L, Perheentupa I, Pakarinen P, et al. Cu nutrition in infants during prolonged exclusive breast feeding: low intake but rising serum concentrations of Cu and ceruloplasmin. Am J Clin Nutr 1986;43:251–257.
89. Matsuda I, Pearson T, Holtzman NA. Determination of apoceruloplasmin by radioimmunoassay in nutritional copper deficiency, Menkes' kinky hair syndrome, Wilson's disease and umbilical cord blood. Pediatr Res 1974;8:821–824.
90. Hillman LS, Martin L, Fiore B. Effect of oral copper supplementation on serum copper and caeruloplasmin concentrations in premature infants. J Pediatr 1981;98:311–313.
91. Salim S, Farquharson J, Arneil GC, et al. Dietary copper intake in artificially fed infants. Arch Dis Child 1986;61:1068–1075.
92. Haschke F, Ziegler EE, Edwards BB, et al. Effect of iron fortification of infant formula on trace mineral absorption. J Pediatr Gastroenterol Nutr 1986;5:768–773.
93. Haschke F, Singer P, Baumgartner D, et al. Growth, zinc and copper nutritional states of male premature infants with different zinc intake. Ann Nutr Metab 1985;29:95–102.
94. Barclay SM, Aggett PJ, Lloyd DJ, et al. Reduced erythrocyte superoxide dismutase activity in low birth weight infants given iron supplements. Pediatr Res 1991;29:297–301.
95. Burns J, Forsyth JS, Paterson CR. Factors associated with variation in plasma copper levels in preterm infants of very low birth weight. Eur J Pediatr 1993;152:240–243.
96. L'Abbe MR, Friel JK. Copper status of very low birth weight infants during the first 12 months of infancy. Pediatr Res 1992;32:183–188.
97. Nisai Y, Kittua E, Fikuda K, et al. Copper deficiency associated with alkali therapy in a patient with renal tubular acidosis. J Pediatr 1981;98:81–83.
98. Levy Y, Zeharia A, Grunebaum M, et al. Copper deficiency in infants fed cow milk. J Pediatr 1985;106:786–788.
99. Tyrala EE, Manser JI, Brodsky NL, et al. Distribution of copper in the serum of the parenterally fed premature infant. J Pediatr 1985;106:295–298.
100. Recommended Dietary Allowances. Food and Nutrition Board. National Research Council. 10th ed. Washington, DC: National Academy of Sciences, 1989.
101. Zlotkin SH, Buchanan BE. Meeting the zinc and copper intake requirements in the parenterally fed preterm and term infant. J Pediatr 1983;103:441–446.
102. Zlotkin SH, Atkinson S, Lockitch G. Trace elements in nutrition for premature infants. Clin Perinatol 1995;22:223–240.
103. Danks DM. Disorders of copper transport. In: Scriver CR, Beaudet AL, Sly WS, Vallee D, eds. The metabolic and molecular bases of inherited disease. ed. New York, London: McGraw-Hill, 1995:2211–2236.
104. Kodama H, Okabe I, Yanagisawa M, et al. Copper deficiency in the mitochondrial of cultured skin fibroblasts from patients with Menkes' syndrome. J Inherited Metab Dis 1989;12:386–389.
105. Davies K. Cloning the Menkes disease gene. Nature 1993;361:98.
106. Dierick HA, Ambrosini L, Spencer J, et al. Molecular structure of the Menkes disease gene. Genomics 1995;28:462–469.
107. Grover WD, Henkin RI. Trichopoliedystrophy (TPD): a fetal disorder of copper metabolism. Pediatr Res 1976;10:448A.
108. Tønnesen T, Horn N. Prenatal and postnatal diagnosis of Menkes' disease, an inherited disorder of copper metabolism. J Inherited Metab Dis 1989;12(suppl):207–214.
109. Tumer Z, Tonnesen T, Bohmann J, et al. First trimester prenatal diagnosis of Menkes disease by DNA analysis. J Med Genet 1994;31:615–617.
110. Kaler SG, Das S, Levinson B, et al. Successful early copper therapy in Menkes disease associated with a mutant transcript containing a small in-frame deletion. Biochem Mol Med 1996;57:37–46.
111. Iwakawa Y, Niwa T, Tomita M. Menkes kinky hair syndrome: a report on an autopsy case and his female sibling with similar clinical manifestations. Brain Dev 1979;11:260–266.
112. Mehes K, Petrovicz E. Familial benign copper deficiency. Arch Dis Child 1982;57:716–717.
113. Edwards CQ, Williams DM, Cartwright GE. Hereditary hypoceruloplasminemia. Clin Gen 1979;15:311–316.
114. Miyajima H, Takahashi Y, Serizawa M, et al. Increased plasma lipid peroxidation in patients with aceruloplasminemia. Free Radic Biol Med 1996;20:757–760.
115. Thomas GR, Forbes JR, Roberts EA, et al. The Wilson disease gene: spectrum of mutations and their consequences. Nat Genet 1995;9:210–217.
116. Chowrimootoo GF, Ahmed HA, Seymour CA. New insights into the pathogenesis of copper toxicosis in Wilson's disease: evidence for copper incorporation and defective

canalicular transport of caeruloplasmin. Biochem J 1996; 315:851–855.
117. Thomas GR, Roberts EA, Walshe JM, Cox DW. Haplotypes and mutations in Wilson disease. Am J Hum Genet 1995;56:1315–1319.
118. Bhave SA, Pandit AN, Tanner MS. Comparison of feeding history of children with Indian childhood cirrhosis and paired controls. J Pediatr Gastroenterol Nutr 1987;6:562–567.
119. Muller-Hocker J, Meyer U, Wiebecke B, et al. Copper storage disease of the liver and chronic dietary intoxication in two lurther German infants mimicking Indian childhood cirrhosis. Pathol Res Pract 1988;183:39–45.
120. Muller T, Feichtinger H, Berger H, Muller W. Endemic Tyrolean infantile cirrhosis: an ecogenetic disorder. Lancet 1996;347:877–880.
121. Scheinberg IH, Sternlieb I. Wilson disease and idiopathic copper toxicosis. Am J Clin Nutr 1996;63:842S–845S.
122. Vallee BL, Falchuk KH. The biochemical basis of zinc physiology. Physiol Rev 1993;73:79–118.
123. Coleman JE. Zinc proteins: enzymes, storage proteins, transcription factors, and replication proteins. Annu Rev Biochem 1992;61:897–946.
124. Hooper NM, ed. Zinc metalloproteases in health and disease. London; Bristol, PA: Taylor & Francis, 1996.
125. Cung MT, Marraud M, Lefrancier P, et al. NMR study of a lymphocyte differentiating thymic factor. J Biol Chem 1988;263:5574–5580.
126. Prasad AS, Meftah S, Abdallali J, et al. Serum thymulin in human zinc deficiency. J Clin Invest 1988;82:1202–1210.
127. Faure P, Lafond JL, Coudray C, et al. Zinc prevents the structural and functional properties of free radical treated-insulin. Biochim Biophys Acta 1994;1209:260–264.
128. Cano Gauci DF, Sarkar B. Reversible zinc exchange between metallothionein and the estrogen receptor zinc finger. FEBS Lett 1996;386(1):1–4.
129. Thompson CB. Apoptosis in the pathogenesis and treatment of disease. Science 1995;267:211–216.
130. Giugliana R, Millward DJ. The effects of severe zinc deficiency on protein turnover in muscle and thymus. Br J Nutr 1987;57:139–155.
131. Wolman SL, Anderson GH, Marliss EB, et al. Zinc in total parenteral nutrition: requirements and metabolic effects. Gastroenterology 1979;76:458–467.
132. Golden BE, Golden MH. Effect of zinc on lean tissue synthesis during recovery from malnutrition. Eur J Clin Nutr 1992;46:697–706.
133. Cunnane SC. Role of zinc in lipid and fatty acid metabolism and in membranes. Prog Food Nutr Sci 1988;12:151–188.
134. Jackson MJ. Physiology of zinc: General Aspects. In: Mills CF, ed. Zinc in human biology. New York: Springer-Verlag, 1989:1–14.
135. Matseshe JW, Philips SF, Malagelada JR, et al. Recovery of dietary iron and zinc from the proximal intestine of healthy man: studies of different meals and supplements. Am J Clin Nutr 1980;33:1946–1953.
136. Cousins RJ. Zinc. In: Zeigler EE, Filer LJ, eds. Present knowledge in Nutrition. 7th ed. Washington, DC: ILSI Press, 1996:293–306.
137. Taylor CM, Bacon JR, Aggett PJ, et al. The homeostatic regulation of zinc absorption and endogenous zinc losses in zinc deprived man. Am J Clin Nutr 1991;53:755–763.
138. Fraker PJ, Jardieu P, Cook J. Zinc deficiency and immune function. Arch Dermatol 1987;123:1699–1701.
139. Beach RS, Gershwin ME, Hurley LS. Gestational zinc deprivation in mice: persistence of immunodeficiency for three generations. Science 1982;218:469–471.
140. Wallwork JC. Zinc in the central nervous system. Prog Food Nutr Sci 1987;11:203–247.
141. Golub MS, Gershwin ME, Hurley LS, et al. Studies of marginal zinc deprivation in rhesus monkeys. 1. Influence on pregnant dams. Am J Clin Nutr 1984;39:265–280.
142. Golub MS, Gershwin ME, Hurley LS, et al. Studies of marginal zinc deprivation in rhesus monkeys: pregnancy outcome. Am J Clin Nutr 1984;39:879–887.
143. Goldenberg RL, Tamura T, Neggers Y, et al. The effect of zinc supplementation of pregnancy outcome. JAMA 1995;274:463–468.
144. Cherry FF, Sandstead HH, Rojas P, et al. Adolescent pregnancy: associations among body weight, zinc nutriture, and pregnancy outcome. Am J Clin Nutr 1989;50:945–954.
145. Jonsson B, Hauge B, Larsen MF, Hald F. Zinc supplementation during pregnancy: a double blind randomised controlled trial. Acta Obstet Gynecol Scand 1996;75:725–729.
146. Mahomed K, James DK, Golding I, et al. Zinc supplementation during pregnancy: a double blind randomised controlled trial. Br Med J 1989;299:826–830.
147. Simmer K, Thompson RPH. Maternal zinc and intrauterine growth retardation. Clin Sci 1985;68:359–399.
148. Kuhnert PM, Kuhnert BR, Erhard P, et al. The effect of smoking on placental and zinc status. Am J Obstet Gynecol 1987;157:1241–1246.
149. Kuhnert BR, Kuhnert PM, Debanne S, et al. The relationship between cadmium, zinc and birth weight in pregnant women who smoke. Am J Obstet Gynecol 1987;157:1247–1251.
150. Kuhnert BR, Kuhnert PM, Zarlingo TJ. Associations between placental cadmium and zinc and age and parity in pregnant women who smoke. Obstet Gynecol 1988;71:67–70.
151. Torreblanca A, Del Ramo J, Sarkar B. Cadmium effect on zinc metabolism in human trophoblast cells: involvement of cadmium-induced metallothionein. Toxicology 1992;72:167–174.
152. Page KR, Abramovich DR, Aggett PJ, et al. Uptake of zinc by human placental microvillus border membranes and characterisation of the effects of cadmium on this process. Placenta 1992;13:151–161.
153. Gishan FK, Green HC. Fetal alcohol syndrome: failure of zinc to reverse the effect of ethanol on placental transport of zinc. Pediatr Res 1983;17:529–531.
154. Nasrat H, Bloxam D, Nicolini et al. Midpregnancy plasma zinc in normal and growth retarded fetuses—a preliminary study. Br J Obstet Gynaecol 1992;99:646–650.
155. Page KR, Abramovich DR, Aggett PJ, et al. The transfer of zinc across the term dually perfused human placental lobule. Q J Exp Physiol 1988;73:585–593.

156. Bax CM, Bloxam DL. Two major pathways of zinc (II) acquisition by human placental syncytiotrophoblast. J Cell Physiol 1995;164(3):546–554.
157. Golub MS, Gershwin ME, Hurley LS, et al. Studies of marginal zinc deprivation: growth of infants in the first year. Am J Clin Nutr 1984;40:1192–1202.
158. Leek LC, Vogler lB, Gershwin ME, et al. Studies of marginal zinc deprivation in rhesus monkeys. V. Fetal and infant skeletal defects. Am J Clin Nutr 1984;40:1203–1212.
159. Haynes DC, Gershwin ME, Golub MS, et al. Studies of marginal zinc deprivation in rhesus monkeys. VI. Influence on the immunohaematology of infants in the first year. Am J Clin Nutr 1984;42:252–262.
160. Shaw JCL. Trace elements in the fetus and young infant. I. Zinc. Am J Dis Child 1979;133:1260–1268.
161. Casey CE, Robinson MF. Copper, manganese, zinc, nickel, cadmium and lead in human foetal tissues. Br J Nutr 1978;39:639–646.
162. Cassens RG, Hoekstra WG, Faltin EC, et al. Zinc content and subcellular distribution in red vs white porcine skeletal muscle. Am J Physiol 1967;212:688–692.
163. Keen CL, Lonnerdal B, Golub MS, et al. Influence of marginal maternal zinc deficiency on pregnancy outcome and zinc status in rhesus monkeys. Pediatr Res 1989;26:470–477.
164. Clough SR, Mitra RS, Kulkarni AP. Qualitative and quantitative aspects of human fetal liver metallothionein. Biol Neonate 1986;49:241–254.
165. Coni P, Ravarino A, Farci AM, et al. Zinc content and distribution in the newborn liver. J Pediatr Gastroextorol Nutr 1996;23:125–129.
166. Ziegler EE, Serfass RE, Nelson SE, et al. Effect of low zinc intake on absorption and excretion of zinc by infants studied with ^{70}Zn and extrinsic tag. J Nutr 1989;119:1647–1653.
167. Krebs NF, Reidinger CJ, Miller IV, Hambidge KM. Zinc homeostasis in breast-fed infants. Pediatr Res 1996;39:661–665.
168. Wastney ME, Angelus P, Barnes RM, Subramanian KN. Zinc kinetics in preterm infants: a compartmental model based on stable isotope data. Am J Physiol 1996;271:R1452–1459.
169. Friel JK, Andrews WL, Simmons BS, et al. Zinc absorption in premature infants: comparison of two isotopic methods. Am J Clin Nutr 1996;63:342–347.
170. Lonnerdal B, Bell I, Hendricks AG, et al. Effect of phytate removal on zinc absorption from soy formula. Am J Clin Nutr 1988;48:1301–1306.
171. Bonifazi E, Rigillo N, De Simone B, et al. Acquired dermatitis due to zinc deficiency in a premature infant. Acta Derm Venereol (Stockh) 1980;60:449–451.
172. Sivasubramanian KN, Henkin RI. Behavioural and dermatologic changes and a low serum zinc and copper concentration in two premature infants after parenteral alimentation. J Pediatr 1978;93:847–851.
173. Arakawa T, Tamura T, Igarashi Y, et al. Zinc deficiency in two infants during parenteral alimentation. Am J Clin Nutr 1976;29:197–204.
174. Aggett PJ, Atherton DJ, More, et al. Symptomatic zinc deficiency in a breast fed preterm infant. Arch Dis Child 1980;58:547–550.
175. Zimmerman AW, Hambidge KM, Leplow ML, et al. Acrodermatitis in breast-fed premature infants: evidence for a defect of mammary zinc secretion. Pediatrics 1982;69:176–183.
176. Murphy IF, Gray OP, Randall JR, et al. Zinc deficiency: a problem with preterm breast milk. Early Hum Dev 1985;10:303–307.
177. Roberts LJ, Shadwick CF, Bergstresser PR. Zinc deficiency in two full-term breast-fed infants. J Am Acad Dermatol 1987;16:301–304.
178. Kuramoto Y, Igarashi Y, Kato S, et al. Acquired zinc deficiency in two breast-fed mature infants. Acta Derm Venereol (Stockh) 1986;66:359–363.
179. Bye AME, Goodfellow A, Atherton DI. Transient zinc deficiency in a full-term breast-fed infant of normal birth weight. Pediatr Dermatol 1985;2:308–311.
180. Morishima Y, Tagi S, Kuwabara A, et al. An acquired form of acrodermatitis enteropathica due to long term lactose free milk alimentation. J Dermatol 1980;7:121–125.
181. Ermacora E, Benelli MG. Acrodermatite enteropatica in bambino fenilchetonurico. Minerva Dermatol 1968;41:523–524.
182. Tyrala EE, Manser JI, Brodsky NL, Tran N. Serum zinc concentrations in growing preterm infants. Acta Paediatr Scand 1983;72:695–698.
183. Altigani M, Murphy JF, Gray OP. Plasma zinc concentration and catchup growth in preterm infants. Acta Paediatr Scand Suppl 1989;357:20–33.
184. Golden BE, Golden MHN. Plasma zinc, rate of weight gain, and the energy cost of tissue deposition in children recovering from severe malnutrition on a cow's milk or soya protein based diet. Am J Clin Nutr 1981;34:892–899.
185. Murray EJ, Messer HH. Turnover of bone zinc during normal and accelerated bone loss in rats. J Nutr 1981;111:1641–1647.
186. Koo WWK, Succop P, Hambidge M. Serum alkaline phosphatase and serum zinc concentrations in preterm infants with rickets and fractures. Am J Dis Child 1989;143:1342–1345.
187. Krebs NF, Reidinger CJ, Robertson AD, Hambidge KM. Growth and intakes of energy and zinc in infants fed human milk. J Pediatr 1994;124:32–39.
188. Salmenpera L, Perheentupa J, Nanto V, Siimes MA. Low zinc intake during exclusive breast-feeding does not impair growth. J Pediatr Gastroenterol Nutr 1994;18:361–370.
189. Salmenpera L, Perheentupa J, Pakarinen P, Siimes MA. Zinc supplementation of infant formula. Am J Clin Nutr 1994;59:985–989.
190. Friel JK, Andrews WL, Matthew JD, et al. Zinc supplementation in very-low-birth-weight infants. J Pediatr Gastroenterol Nutr 1993;17:97–104.
191. Van Wouwe JP. Clinical and laboratory diagnosis of acrodermatis enteropathica. Eur J Paediatr 1989;49:2–8.
192. Aggett PJ. Acrodermatitis enteropathica. J Inherited Metab Dis 1983;6(suppl 1):22–30.

193. Failla ML, van de Verdonk M, Morgan WT, et al. Characterization of zinc binding proteins in plasma of patients with hyperzincaemia. J Lab Clin Med 1982;100:943–952.
194. Levander OA, Burk RF. Selenium. In: Zeigler EE, Filer LJ, eds. Present knowledge in nutrition. 7th ed. Washington, DC: ILSI Press, 1996:320–328.
195. Reilly C. Selenium in food and health. London: Chapman and Hall, 1996.
196. Arthur JR, Nicol F, Beckett GJ. Selenium deficiency, thyroid hormone metabolism, and thyroid hormone deiodinases. Am J Clin Nutr 1993;57:S236–S239.
197. Martin R, Janghorbani M, Young VR. Experimental selenium restriction in healthy adult humans: changes in selenium metabolism studied with stable isotope methodology. Am J Clin Nutr 1989;49:854–861.
198. Yang GX, Wang SX, Zhon RX, et al. Endemic selenium intoxication of humans in China. Am J Clin Nutr 1983;37:872–881.
199. Keshan Disease Research Group, Chinese Academy of Medical Sciences. Observations on the effect of sodium selenite in the prevention of Keshan disease. Chin Med J 1979;92:471–476.
200. Johnson RA, Baker SS, Fallon JT, et al. An occidental case of cardiomyopathy and selenium deficiency. N Engl J Med 1981;304:1210–1212.
201. Vinton NE, Dahlstrom KA, Strobel Ct, et al. Macrocytosis and pseudoalbinism: manifestations of selenium deficiency. J Pediatr 1987;111:711–717.
202. Cohen HJ, Brown MR, Hamilton D, et al. Glutathione peroxidase and selenium deficiency in patients receiving home parenteral nutrition: time course for development of deficiency and repletion of activity in plasma and blood cells. Am J Clin Nutr 1989;49:132–139.
203. Calomme MR, Vanderpas JB, Francois B, et al. Thyroid function parameters during a selenium repletion/depletion study in phenylketonuric subjects. Experientia 1995;51:1208–1215.
204. Beck MA, Shi Q, Morris VC, Levander OA. Rapid genomic evolution of a non-virulent coxsackievirus B3 in selenium-deficient mice results in identical virulent isolates. Nature Med 1995;1:433–436.
205. Swanson CA, Reamer DC, Veillon C, et al. Quantitative and qualitative aspects of selenium utilisation in pregnant and non-pregnant women: an application of stable isotope methodology. Am J Clin Nutr 1983;38:169–180.
206. Shennan DB, Boyd CAR. Review article: placental handling of trace elements. Placenta 1988;9:333–343.
207. Kumpulainen J, Salmenpera L, Siimes MA, et al. Selenium status of exclusively breast-fed infants as influenced by maternal organic or inorganic selenium supplementation. AM J Clin Nutr 1985;42:829–835.
208. Smith AM, Picciano MF, Milner JA. Selenium intakes and status of human milk and formula fed infants. Am J Clin Nutr 1982;35:521–526.
209. Ehrenkranz RA, Gettner PA, Nelli CM, et al. Selenium absorption and retention by very-low-birth-weight infants: studies with the extrinsic stable isotope tag 74Se. J Pediatr Gastroenterol Nutr 1991;13:125–133.
210. Jochum F, Fuchs A, Menzel H, Lombeck I. Selenium in German infants fed breast milk or different formulas. Acta Paediatr 1995;84:859–862.
211. McGuire MK, Burgert SL, Milner JA, et al. Selenium status of infants is influenced by supplementation of formula or maternal diets. AM J Clin Nutr 1993;58:643–648.
212. Lombeck I, Ebert KH, Kasperek K, et al. Selenium intake of infants and young children, healthy children and dietetically treated patients with phenylketonuria. Eur J Pediatr 1984;143:99–102.
213. Darlow BA, Inder TE, Sluis KB, et al. Selenium status of New Zealand infants fed either a selenium supplemented or a standard formula. J Paediatr Child Health 1995;31:339–344.
214. Friel JK, Andrews WL, Long DR, L'Abbe MR. Selenium status of very low birth weight infants. Pediatr Res 1993;34:293–296.
215. Smith AM, Chen LW, Thomas MR. Selenate fortification improves selenium status of term infants fed soy formula. Am J Clin Nutr 1995;61:44–47.
216. Daniels L, Gibson R, Simmer K. Randomised clinical trial of parenteral selenium supplementation in preterm infants. Arch Dis Child Fetal Neonatal 1996;74:F158–164.
217. Darlow BA, Inder TE, Graham PJ, et al. The relationship of selenium status to respiratory outcome in the very low birth weight infant. Pediatrics 1995;96:314–319.
218. Hetzel BS. Iodine deficiency disorders (IDD) and their eradication. Lancet 1982;2:1126–1129.
219. Stanbury JB. Iodine deficiency and the iodine deficiency disorders. In: Zeigler EE, Filer LJ, eds. Present knowledge in nutrition. 7th ed. Washington, DC: ILSI Press, 1996:378–383.
220. Delange F, Heidemann P, Bourdoux P, et al. Regional variations of iodine nutrition and thyroid function during the neonatal period in Europe. Biol Neonate 1986;49:322–330.
221. Delange F, Dalhem A, Bourdoux P, et al. Increased risk of primary hypothyroidism in preterm infants. J Pediatr 1984;105:462–469.
222. Parravicini E, Fontana C, Paterlini GL, et al. Iodine, thyroid function, and very low birth weight infants. Pediatrics 1996;98:730–734.
223. Keen CL, Zidenberg-Cherr S. Manganese. In: Zeigler EE, Filer LJ, eds. Present knowledge in nutrition. 7th ed. Washington, DC: ILSI Press, 1996:335–343.
224. Hatano S, Nishi Y, Usui T. Erythrocyte manganese concentration in healthy children, adults, and the elderly and in cord blood. Am J Clin Nutr 1983;37:457–460.
225. Stastny D, Vogel R, Picciano MF. Manganese intake and serum manganese concentrations of human milk-fed and formula-fed infants. Am J Clin Nutr 1984;39:872–878.
226. Fell JM, Reynolds AP, Meadows N, et al. Manganese toxicity in children receiving long-term parenteral nutrition. Lancet 1996;347:1992–1996.
227. Lombeck I, Wendel U, Versieck J, et al. Increased manganese content and reduced arginase activity in erythrocytes of a patient with prolidase deficiency (iminodipeptiduria). Eur J Pediatr 1986;144:571–573.
228. Rajagopalan KV. Molybdenum—an essential trace element. Nutr Rev 1987;45:321–328.
229. Johnson JL, Wadman SK. Molybdenum cofactor deficiency and isolated sulfite oxidase deficiency. In: Scriver CR, Beaudet AL, Sly WS, Vallee D, eds. The metabolic

and molecular bases of inherited disease. 7th ed. New York, London: McGraw-Hill, 1995:2271–2286.
230. Abumrad NN, Schneider AJ, Steel D, et al. Amino acid intolerance during prolonged total parenteral nutrition reversed by molybdate therapy. Am J Clin Nutr 1981;34:2551–2559.
231. Casey CE, Neville MC. Studies on human lactation. 3. Molybdenum and nickel in human milk during the first month of lactation. Am J Clin Nutr 1987;45:921–926.
232. Anonymous. Is chromium essential for humans? Nutr Rev 1988;46:17–20.
233. Stoecker BJ. Chromium. In: Zeigler EE, Filer LJ, eds. Present knowledge in nutrition. 7th ed. Washington, DC: ILSI Press, 1996:344–352.
234. Casey CE, Hambidge KM. Chromium in human milk from American mothers. Br J Nutr 1984;52:73–77.
235. Neilsen FH. Other trace elements. In: Zeigler EE, Filer LJ, eds. Present knowledge in nutrition. 7th ed. Washington, DC: ILSI Press, 1996:353–377.
236. Ekstrand J. Fluoride intake in early infancy. J Nutr 1989;119:1856–1860.

form# 42
Neonatal Vitamin Metabolism: Fat Soluble

Frank R. Greer and Richard D. Zachman

The fat-soluble vitamins are an exciting area of perinatal research. The nutrient-gene interaction of vitamin A is perhaps the best described of any nutrient and we are continually learning more about its important role in fetal development. Vitamin D, actually a prohormone, is not far behind in the description of its effects on DNA transcription and its impact on fetal development is one of growing importance. New vitamin K–dependent proteins, other than coagulation factors, are being described in many organ tissues and knowledge of vitamin K's role in perinatal metabolism is expanding. Of all the fat-soluble vitamins, vitamin E has the most proposed therapeutic benefits in the perinatal period. However, there are still no definite indications for its routine clinical use in pharmacologic quantities.

Vitamin A

The term vitamin A is used to describe the biologic activity of a group of compounds that includes both the naturally occurring and synthetically derived retinoids. The biologic activity of vitamin A is diverse. It is essential for vision, growth, reproduction, cell differentiation, and immunocompetency. By convention, the amount of vitamin A from all sources in the diet is converted into a single unit, a "retinol equivalent," which equals 1 µg of all-*trans* retinol.[1] Retinol is the naturally occurring alcohol form of the vitamin. Other metabolic forms include retinaldehyde (retinal), retinoic acid, and retinyl ester. A variety of naturally occurring metabolites of retinol have been identified, and advances in organic chemistry have led to the isolation of more than 1000 new synthetic retinoids, many of which have reached the marketplace.

Overview of Metabolism (Figure 42.1)

Ingested plant carotene or animal tissue retinyl esters are converted to free retinol in the proximal small intestine after the action of hydrolyses of the pancreas and intestinal brush border. Retinol is absorbed into the intestinal cells, esterified, and incorporated into chylomicrons that are transported via lymph into the circulation. The absorption process is facilitated by type II cellular retinol-binding protein (CRBP-II), which is found almost exclusively in the absorptive cells of the small intestine[2] and is distinctly different from the other cellular retinol-binding protein (CRBP) found in nearly all tissue.[3]

Chylomicron- and lipoprotein-bound retinyl esters are taken up by the liver for storage predominantly as retinyl palmitate. Retinyl ester, free retinol, and retinol-binding protein (RBP) are compartmentalized into various liver cell types.[1] A highly regulated hydrolysis process subsequently liberates free retinol for delivery to peripheral target tissues. Retinol is mobilized from the liver into the circulation as a specific complex with RBP and transthyretin.[4] After the circulating complex delivers retinol to the target tissue, the free RBP is rapidly excreted by the kidney and transthyretin is largely degraded by the liver. Target tissue may also take up retinyl esters directly from circulating chylomicron remnants.[5]

Target tissue cytosol contains CRBP-I and CRBP-II, the latter found only in intestinal cells, cellular retinoic acid-binding proteins (CRABP-I and -II), and other tissue-specific binding proteins.[3,6] Roles for these proteins are being identified and include the directing of retinoids to specific enzymes for esterification, hydrolysis, or oxidation, regulating free retinol and retinoic acid concentrations, and serving as a donor for catabolizing enzymes and enzymatic reactions in the visual cycle.[1,3,4,6,7]

The multiplicity of the effects of vitamin A was one of the considerations that led to the proposal that its mechanism of action was through gene regulation. The molecular biology of retinoids in regulating gene expression at specific body target sites has been one of the major thrusts of retinoid research in the past decade.[8–11] An action similar to that of steroid hormones has been found in which a specific retinoic acid–receptor protein complex

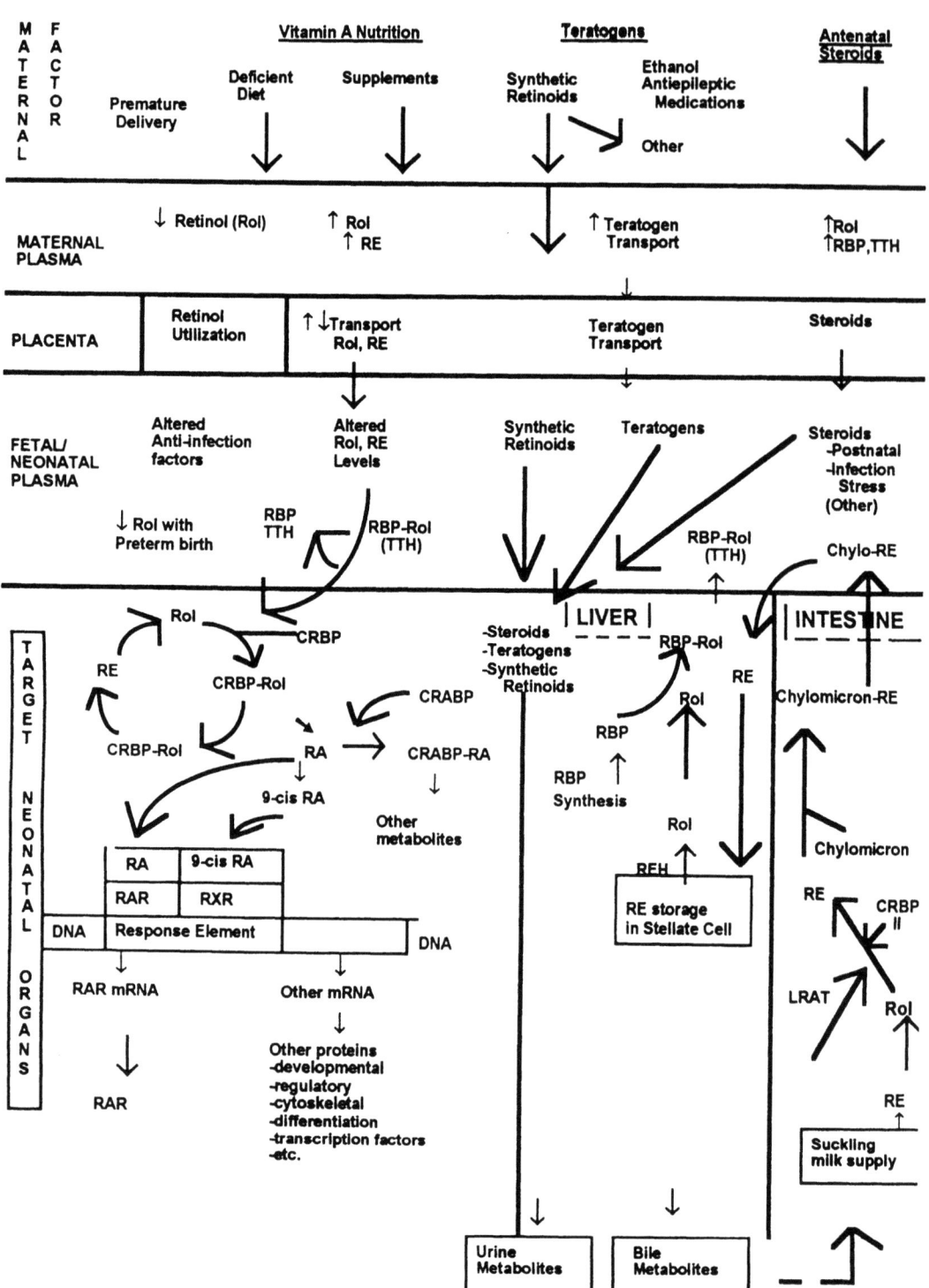

FIGURE 42.1. Aspects of vitamin A metabolism in the fetus and neonate. Several perinatal maternal factors can influence vitamin A metabolism resulting in changes in fetal development or neonatal vitamin A effects. Fetal vitamin A is less in maternal deficiency, higher if mother takes more than 10,000 IU daily supplements, with a possible increase in the occurrence of congenital anomalies. Certain synthetic retinoids, like isotretinoin can also be teratogenic. The mechanism of action of some other teratogens (e.g., ethanol, antiepileptic medication) may be through retinoids. Antenatal steroids affect fetal and maternal retinol and retinol-binding protein (RBP). The placenta utilizes some vitamin A and possibly makes RBP early in gestation, but more clarification of this organ's role is necessary. Preterm birth results in lower neonatal serum and liver storage levels of vitamin A. The transport of altered levels of retinoids and other factors passed to the neonatal plasma affect the storage of retinoids in liver and their function in other tissues. Both excess and low vitamin A intracellular levels can lead to altered gene products to the detriment of the developing embryo or neonatal function. Steroids, teratogens, and other factors can influence intracellular retinoid function. Rol, retinol; RE, retinyl ester; TTH, transthyretin; Chylo-RE, chylomicron containing retinyl ester; CRBP, cellular retinol binding protein; RA, retinoic acid; CRABP, cellular retinoic acid binding protein; 9-*cis*-RA, 9-*cis*-retinoic acid; RAR, retinoic acid receptor; RXR, 9-*cis*-retinoic acid receptor; DNA, deoxyribonucleic acid; mRNA, messenger ribonucleic acid; REH, retinyl ester hydrolase; LRAT, lecithin-retinol acyltransferase.

becomes bound to nuclear DNA, resulting in regulation of specific genes. Retinoic acid is a ligand for several nuclear retinoic acid receptors (RARs). In addition, 9-*cis* retinoic acid is a ligand for another set of retinoic acid nuclear receptors (RXRs). The identification of two distinct retinoid ligands and receptor systems has led to new versions of their signaling pathway. These RARs and RXRs bind as homodimers or heterodimers to specific DNA sequences known as nuclear response elements (Figure 42.1). They may even form heterodimers with other hormone receptors such as vitamin D or thyroid hormone.[10]

Many metabolites of retinol have been described. Retinol can be reversibly oxidized to retinaldehyde (retinal). Further nonreversible oxidation of retinal to retinoic acid accounts for the observation that retinoic acid can support growth but not the visual function of retinol. Retinoic acid cannot support reproductive activity. Epoxy derivative formation and β-glucuronidation of retinoic acid occur in the liver, and some metabolites are excreted into bile. A portion of the retinoic acid glucuronide undergoes enterohepatic circulation, but further oxidation, including chain shortening by decarboxylation, occurs in the intestine and other organs. Most of these biologic metabolites are excreted in the urine.[12]

Fetal-Maternal Metabolism

Placental Transfer

Pregnant mice and rats on a liberal supply of retinol transfer an adequate portion of the vitamin to the fetus. RBP appears coincident with retinol and increases with the growth of the fetus during midgestation in the rat (i.e., 11–14 days), suggesting transplacental transport of RBP-bound retinol.[13] A further increase in fetal liver retinol occurs later and another rise in RBP is attributed to the onset of fetal RBP synthesis. The fact that fetal rat liver microsomes can actively synthesize retinyl ester[14] suggests that retinol is delivered to fetal liver as the RBP-retinol complex, and is esterified and stored as retinyl ester, as it is in the mature animal.[12] Retinol is essential for normal rat placental growth. Placental uptake of radioactive retinol readily occurs, and both CRBP and CRABP have been demonstrated in the human placenta.[15,16]

Maternal transplacental transfer of retinol to the fetal rat is maintained until the mother is made deficient by low vitamin A.[17] The mechanism and regulation of retinol transport from the maternal circulation to the fetus through human placenta is not as established. Significant correlations between maternal and cord blood RBP concentrations have not been consistently found.[18-21] However, because cord blood and fetal liver concentrations of retinol are relatively constant over a wide range of maternal blood concentrations, it seems, based on the rat data cited above, that the fetus will be supplied with enough retinol unless the mother has obvious clinical signs of vitamin A deficiency.[17] Hence, the recommended daily allowance (RDA) during pregnancy is the same as in the nonpregnant state.[22]

Amniotic Fluid

Both retinol and RBP have been found in amniotic fluid,[23-26] but not retinyl esters. Although based on few data, it appears that the concentration of amniotic fluid retinol decreases close to term gestation (i.e., ≥36 weeks), and is approximately 10% to 20% of that found in the mother's serum or in cord blood. Amniotic fluid retinol concentration in pregnancies with fetal central nervous system defects (e.g., meningomyelocele, anencephaly) may be higher than normal (5.7 ± 1.6 vs $3.8 \pm 1.3 \mu g \cdot dl^{-1} \pm$ SD).[23,25] Cord blood retinol concentration in neonates has recently been reported to be lower in those with meningomyelocele than in neonates suffering from gastrointestinal abnormalities.[27] Perhaps loss of vitamin A via leaking cerebrospinal fluid (CSF) leads to the lower cord blood and higher amniotic fluid concentrations in the fetus with a neural tube defect.

In eight insulin-dependent diabetic and three toxemic pregnancies, amniotic fluid retinol was lower compared to the concentration of a normal population at a similar gestational age.[26] The investigators suggest that these maternal diseases alter the uteroplacental blood flow, affecting retinol transport across the placenta. The positive correlation between retinol and RBP amniotic fluid concentration in one study suggests retinol is transported from the maternal circulation into the amniotic fluid bound to RBP.[24] This reasoning is plausible, as it has been demonstrated that small proteins in amniotic fluid may originate from the maternal circulation.[28]

Teratology

It has been known for years that excess maternal vitamin A may cause congenital anomalies in the animal fetus,[29,30] and retinoic acid seems especially teratogenic.[31] A recent warning about the potential teratogenic effect of retinoids comes from the clinical study in which neonates born to women who took more that 10,000 IU (approximately 3000, retinal equivalents) of preformed vitamin A per day as a supplement had an increased frequency of birth defects. The highest rate of birth defects occurred with high vitamin A consumption prior to the 7th week of gestation.[32]

Data strongly implicate fetal embryopathy with isotretinoin (13-*cis*-retinoic acid) administration in humans.[33] The defects (e.g., most frequently craniofacial, cardiac, and thymic) result in a high mortality rate.[33-35] Retinol binding to CRBP, followed by esterification, thus protecting cells from potential toxicity, does not occur with the use of retinoic acid and its derivatives because the oxidation step between retinaldehyde and retinoic acid is irreversible. The use of such therapy in female patients of childbearing age must be undertaken with great caution. When retinoids are transported by plasma lipoproteins instead of RBP, as might be the case when RBP is saturated by excess retinol, or the plasma contains high concentrations of retinyl esters from excessive ingestion of these forms, the retinoids are delivered differently to biologic membranes, which may also lead to nonspecific toxic effects.[36]

The most recent insight into teratogenic mechanisms results from the data of the developmental roles of the RARs. First, null mutants in which a single RAR is knocked out results in few, if any, of the defects typically seen in vitamin A deficiency, so there is functional redundancy with the RARs. However, compound RAR null mutants die in utero or shortly after birth and histologically reveal most of the defects of vitamin A deficiency.[37] Second, there is an induction of the RAR-β gene expression in several systems that accompany retinoic acid induced fetal dysmorphogenesis.[38,39] On the other hand in RAR-γ gene–deleted mice, it took four times the usual retinoic acid teratogenic dose to produce the toxic effects seen in the wild-type mice.[40] Thus, some toxic effects of retinoids might act through specific RARs (Figure 42.1).

A third recent development is that some other teratogenic agents may act indirectly by altering the metabolism of retinoids, which would then be the final pathway for specified teratogenic effects. Prenatal ethanol ingestion known to cause fetal alcohol syndrome (FAS) might be such an example. Prenatal ethanol ingestion by the pregnant rat causes specific changes in concentrations of retinol, retinoic acid, and RAR messenger RNAs (mRNAs) in the whole embryo as well as target tissue such as fetal heart and brain.[41-43] The mechanism for such events has not been clarified. However, the information cited above about specific RARs being involved with teratogenesis fits with these observations. In addition, ethanol and retinoic acid might compete for the same retinoic acid nuclear response elements in the genes controlling the synthesis of oxidizing enzymes.[44] It has been found that children on anticonvulsant therapy have altered concentrations of retinoid metabolites in their serum.[45] The investigators suggested that because of the importance of retinoids for the signaling of crucial biologic events during embryonic development, altered retinoid metabolism might be highly significant in prenatally associated antiepileptic drug teratogenesis (Figure 42.1). Further work is needed in this area.

Fetal-Neonatal Vitamin A Metabolism

β-Carotene as a Precursor

There is little information on β-carotene uptake or its metabolism to vitamin A during the perinatal period. However, it has been known for years that β-carotene can meet the fetal and neonatal growth requirements for vitamin A. There is β-carotene in human cord blood, and there is a weakly positive correlation with gestational age and maternal serum β-carotene concentration.[46] In addition, human breast milk contains β-carotene, but the concentration on day 1 declines by 80% by day 5 of lactation.[46]

The perinatal role of carotenoids as antioxidants should be investigated further. There is obvious oxidant stress to lungs of the premature neonate during neonatal respiratory distress syndrome (RDS) with oxygen damage to the lung epithelial cell contributing to chronic lung disease. β-carotene can be metabolized to retinol, retinyl palmitate, and retinoic acid, which are all potential antioxidants, in isolated rat lung type II cells.[47] Data on the effect of carotene supplementation on developing or injured neonatal lung would be of interest.

Intestinal Absorption of Retinol

Dietary retinol originates mainly from the precursor β-carotene of plant origin or from the hydrolysis of long-chain retinyl esters from animal tissue consumption. In the neonate, the bile salt-stimulated lipase of human milk may contribute to enteral retinyl ester hydrolysis, but a nonspecific pancreatic carboxylic ester hydrolase is primarily responsible for intraluminal retinyl ester hydrolysis.[48] The retinol is incorporated into micelles for the microvillous membrane absorption. Intraluminal bile acid deficiency in the neonate may lead to inadequate micelle formation and affect retinol absorption.[48]

In the cells of the small intestine, CRBP-II is present at several times the concentration of CRBP-I, which is not specific to the small intestine. It is located in the microvilli and has the major role in the absorption of vitamin A.[4,48] This protein has the ability to bind both retinol and retinal from the cleavage of β-carotene, which would enhance its proposed function in intestinal absorption.[49] The developmental expression and regulation of these proteins have been described in the rat fetus.[50] Intestinal CRBP-II mRNA is first noted on the 19th day of gestation and increases 11-fold by day 21, then decreases after parturition. The increased CRBP-II mRNA during late fetal life corresponds to the proliferation of microvilli. On the other hand, CRBP, though present in the emerging small intestinal enterocyte early in the fetal rat, is no longer detected shortly before birth, suggesting that CRBP plays no role in retinol absorption during the perinatal period.[51,52] In the pregnant rat, both CRBP-II and its mRNA increase two- to fourfold in late pregnancy and remain elevated during at least 8 days of postpartum lactation, then decrease at the time of weaning. It has been suggested that this increase is to ensure increased availability of retinol for maternal absorption during the rapid development of the fetus and newborn pup.[53]

Early work suggested that nonspecific pancreatic and intestinal esterases were primarily responsible for reesterification of absorbed retinol in the intestine. However, more recent work identifies two other more specific retinol esterification mechanisms. One is the microsomal intestinal enzyme, acyl coenzyme A–retinol acyltransferase (ARAT). This enzyme may only have an important role in the absorption of retinol when retinol is in high concentrations, because when retinol is bound to CRBP-II it is not an effective substrate for ARAT. Instead, a lecithin-retinol acyltransferase (LRAT) is the primary retinol esterification enzyme.[48] The apparent K_m for LRAT is below that for retinol esterification by ARAT. LRAT accounts for the predominance of saturated fatty acid retinyl esters of retinyl palmitate and retinyl stearate, since LRAT uses only the fatty acid at position 1 of the donor, phosphatidylcholine. The relative contribution of ARAT and LRAT requires study. However, intestinal LRAT actively increases in the newborn intestine and remains high during the suckling period,[54] paralleling the concentration of CRBP II.

Storage of Retinol

The liver is the main storage organ for retinol, predominately as retinyl esters (Figure 42.1). Most of these esters are saturated to a level of 70% to 75%. The most abundant storage form is retinyl palmitate, the second most abundant being retinyl stearate. Although the retinyl esters are removed from the circulation almost entirely by parenchymal cells, over 90% of the storage occurs in the stellate cells under both normal and high vitamin intake environments.[4]

Vitamin A storage in stellate cells has been studied in mouse liver during late fetal and the neonatal periods.[55] This study showed that on the 15th day of gestation, radioactivity derived from [^{3}H] vitamin A administered to the mother was distributed in cells along the hepatic blood vessels that differ in ultrastructure from the vitamin A storing stellate cells of the adult liver. Storage later in gestation and in the adult mouse occurs in lipid droplet-containing stellate cells.

Both the stellate and parenchymal cells contain ARAT, LRAT, and the enzyme retinyl palmitate hydrolase, which hydrolyzes retinyl esters. In addition, stellate cells contain a high concentration of CRBP, which possibly directs retinol to esterification by LRAT, as was noted above for CRBP-II in the intestine. The perinatal developmental pattern of CRBP in the cell of the rat liver has been studied using immunohistochemical localization of the protein.[56] During the final prenatal week there is a progressive increase in CRBP in the parenchymal cells that continues until the second postnatal week, after which time it declines. After birth the most intense staining for CRBP is found in the stellate cells similar to the adult liver.[56]

The absolute amount and concentration of hepatic retinol storage increases during the perinatal period in the rat pup.[14,57,58] In the rat with low liver stores ($1.2 \mu g \cdot g^{-1}$), the distribution of vitamin A among parenchymal and stellate cells is altered, with 83% of the liver vitamin A present in the parenchymal cells.[59] With high liver stores, the stellate cell contains 82% of the vitamin. In addition, in the rat with low liver and plasma retinol concentrations there is a decreased turnover of retinol.[60] Although no similar data have been published for the human, many premature neonates are born with low or marginal liver vitamin A stores of less than $20 \mu g \cdot g^{-1}$ of liver tissue.[61-63] Therefore, altered liver distribution and changes in retinol turnover could also be present.

Fetal liver stores can be influenced somewhat by maternal retinol supplementation. Fetal and neonatal liver retinol stores are fourfold greater after a large dose of retinyl acetate to the pregnant mouse.[55] In the deficient maternal rat, subsequently supplemented with various intakes of retinol, the vitamin A content of lung, heart, liver, and brain increases dependent on the maternal retinol supplied.[64] Nutritional availability and intake of retinol may explain the exponential rise in liver vitamin A described in Swedish fetuses during the second and third trimester that did not occur in Ethiopian fetuses.[65]

There is a marked fall in lung retinyl ester stores in the fetus at the time of birth, even if the birth is premature.[58,66,67] This rapid decrease suggests a functional role for retinyl esters in the pulmonary cellular changes that occur during extrauterine adaptation. The amount of fetal lung retinol can be increased by supplementing the pregnant maternal rat with extra vitamin A.[68] However, it has not yet been determined that this is clinically important. Other tissues, even the lacrimal gland,[69] have small amounts of retinyl ester stores, but their status during the perinatal period has not been studied.

Mobilization of Retinol Stores

Retinyl ester stores must be hydrolyzed by the enzyme retinyl ester hydrolase (REH) as the first step in mobilization from the liver (Figure 42.1). REH has not been studied in the fetus or neonate.

A relation between REH and α-tocopherol (i.e., vitamin E) deficiency has been reported.[70] This study found that an α-tocopherol–deficient diet affects the steady-state concentration of retinol and retinyl esters in several organs of the rat.[70] In vitro studies on REH show that α-tocopherol inhibits this liver enzyme. Hence α-tocopherol deficiency could theoretically lead to increased hydrolysis resulting in lower total liver retinyl esters. In contrast, lung REH is stimulated by α-tocopherol in vitro. Premature neonates may have a lower tocopherol concentration.[71] Thus, it is conceivable that their retinol metabolism may be altered by some mechanism involving REH, but this question has not been studied.

Following retinol hydrolysis, the subsequent transport of retinol from the liver to other tissues for metabolism is dependent on liver RBP synthesis and secretion.[5] RBP is a single polypeptide chain of molecular weight 21,000 d that binds one molecule of retinol. Cloning and DNA sequencing of human RBP have been reported.[4,5] RBP is synthesized in both the liver parenchymal and stellate cells, and binding of retinol to RBP apparently results in the transport of the RBP-retinol complex from endoplasmic reticulum to the Golgi apparatus, from which secretion occurs. After secretion of the RBP-retinol complex, RBP binds in a 1:1 molar ratio with plasma transthyretin (Figure 42.1). The formation of this complex reduces the chance for glomerular filtration and renal catabolism of RBP.[5] The various factors that control the synthesis, release, and metabolism of RPB are reviewed in detail elsewhere.[5,72]

Plasma RBP concentration is lower in preterm neonates than term neonates and lower in the young child than in the adult.[73,74] In premature neonates the persistently low RBP concentration is consistent with lower protein and calorie intakes, as many sick premature neonates receive inadequate nutrition for a number of days because of other complicating medical problems. If RBP synthesis or release is altered by protein and calorie deprivation, delivery of retinol to target tissues in the premature neonate could be affected.

One investigation observed that RBP declined from day 0 to day 3 in the premature neonate with RDS and increased in a control group of premature neonates without RDS.[20] These is no explanation for this observation. However, premature neonates with RDS characteristically have a diuresis on days 3 to 5, which in conjunction with immature renal tubular function, may increase RBP turnover through renal losses in these premature neonates.

Adrenocortical hormones may accelerate retinol mobilization from the liver.[73] Dexamethasone stimulates the release of RBP from cultured rat liver cells.[75] Since antenatal steroids are used in mothers in premature labor to accelerate fetal lung surfactant maturation, an effect on RBP metabolism by antenatal steroids seems possible (Figure 42.1). In a study of the pregnant rhesus monkey receiving antenatal intramuscular dexamethasone to stimulate fetal lung maturation, both the maternal and fetal serum concentrations of RBP increased.[76] The increase in fetal serum RBP was dose-dependent. A similar effect of steroids on RBP was found in premature human neonates whose mothers were treated with antenatal steroids.[77] Cord blood transthyretin in premature neonates was elevated by maternal antenatal steroid administration.[78] It is unclear whether these changes of RBP and transthyretin are useful or detrimental to retinol metabolism and function in the human premature neonate.

Zinc deficiency may indirectly affect retinol stores. First, an enzyme that converts retinol into retinal is a zinc metalloenzyme. Second, retinal oxidase, which oxidizes retinol to retinoic acid, is a zinc-modulated enzyme. Finally, the synthesis of RBP and the retinol mobilization from the liver are decreased in severe zinc deficiency but return to normal when zinc is given. However, in two controlled studies with zinc supplementation in premature neonates, no differences in RBP concentrations were noted,[79,80] and premature neonates currently receiving zinc supplemented total intravenous nutrition do not have low zinc levels.

Further Tissue Metabolism of Retinol

The RBP-retinol-transthyretin complex in plasma delivers retinol to the target organ cell surface. It appears that the pigment-containing cells of the retina, liver parenchymal and stellate cells, and cells forming the blood-brain and blood-testes barriers, have specific RBP surface receptors. Other cells may utilize other mechanisms of uptake that are yet not fully defined.[4,5] Further utilization of retinol for function or metabolism occurs after binding with CRBP-I/II and CRABP-I/II. Though all the functions of the binding proteins are still not completely determined, their binding does facilitate esterification, regulates free retinol and retinoic acid levels, and aids in further catabolism of the vitamin.[4,5,12] Such binding may aid in the delivery of retinoic acid to the nucleus. Perinatal changes in concentrations of these cellular binding proteins do occur in some organs studied, including rat jejunum, ileum, liver, and lung.[56,81,82]

Nonoxidative metabolism of retinol to retinyl ester is the predominant metabolic reaction occurring in the intestine and liver.[83] Synthesis of retinyl esters can occur in the eye,[6] lung,[73] and most other tissue. A small amount of retinol appears in liver as glycosylated derivatives of retinyl phosphate, and their possible role in the function of retinol is being studied. Retinol is reversibly converted to retinal by oxidative metabolism. In the eye, all-*trans* retinal is further isomerized as part of the visual cycle, and the retinoids in photosensitive systems are being studied.[6] Irreversible oxidation of retinal to biologic active retinoic acid probably occurs in all tissue.[12,83]

Additional oxidized products of retinol metabolism appear in the urine and bile, most fecal metabolites probably arising from the latter (Figure 42.1). A portion of bile metabolites are reutilized because of enterohepatic circulation.[12,83] Numerous metabolites resulting from conjugation, decarboxylation, oxidation, epoxidation, and isomerization are formed and found in various tissue. A few of these metabolites have vitamin A activity, especially all-*trans*-retinol-β-glucuronide, but most do not.[12] There are few data on the activities of these other metabolites during the perinatal period.

Newer Areas of Potential Importance for Perinatal/Neonatal Vitamin A Metabolism

The newly defined roles of the nuclear retinoic acid receptors (e.g., RARs and RXRs) and of the metabolites retinoic acid and 9-*cis* retinoic acid on embryologic development have been noted. A few of the other areas specific to neonatal vitamin A metabolism and function are being actively studied.

Mild vitamin A deficiency is associated with an increased rate of infections in childhood, and in many studies supplemental vitamin A is accompanied by a decrease in mortality that accompanies infectious disease in infants and children.[84] It is observed in animal and in vitro studies that vitamin A has definite effects on lymphocytes, natural killer cells, phagocytic cells, and cytokines.[84-86] It is not surprising that vitamin A deficiency is one of the specific nutrient abnormalities associated with HIV-1 infection in the adult. Vitamin A deficiency is associated with an increased mortality rate with HIV-1 infection.[87] Furthermore, a recent study has shown the presence of maternal vitamin A deficiency increases the risk of maternal-infant transmission by a factor of four.[88] The exact reason for this increased transmission rate is not yet known, but the increased vertical transmission rate could occur in utero, during delivery, or through breast-feeding.

Vitamin A deficiency results in squamous cell metaplasia of columnar tracheal epithelium with the loss of cells that produce cilia and mucus. Necrotizing bronchiolitis and other histopathology similar to bronchopulmonary dysplasia (BPD) have been described.[89-94] Low liver retinyl ester stores have been documented after death in premature neonates (birth weight <1500g).[63] Conflicting and inconsistent data suggest that premature neonates developing BPD may have a lower initial plasma retinol concentration than do those who do not develop BPD.[20,95-101] Some clinical trials with supplemental vitamin A reported a decrease in the incidence of BPD and its associated morbidity in the premature neonates.[97,99,102-104] However, these observations remain controversial[105] and such supplements are not widely used. Even in neonates supplemented with vitamin A, 30% to 50% still develop BPD.[97,102,105]

It is becoming clear that vitamin A supplementation of the neonate by the enteral route is not as effective as that by intramuscular administration.[106,107] With the idea of increased supplements in preterm neonates at risk for BPD, there is an increased concern for vitamin A toxicity. One report states that vitamin A deficiency in preterm neonates can be safely corrected by supplementing feedings with 5000 IU (1500µg) daily for 32 days.[106] This is roughly twice the recommended RDA for the newborn and the infant. Another report states that one oral dose of 50,000 IU (15,000µg) given to neonates was associated with only rare and mild side effects.[108] However, clinical assessment of toxicity in a preterm neonate has not been studied, so guidelines in this area must be made carefully.

The question of the need for supplemental vitamin A in neonates with BPD is confounded by the prevalent use of glucocorticoids for treatment of BPD. Dexamethasone, the most commonly used steroid, affects the liver and lung vitamin A stores of neonatal rats,[109] and decreases the RAR-β expression in whole neonatal rat lung, explants, and pure lung epithelial cells.[110,111] In the human neonate, dexamethasone administration results in a transient rise followed by a decrease in serum retinol and RBP,[101,112] though it is not known what is happening to the liver stores of vitamin A.

Another confounding factor in evaluating the vitamin A status and determining the possible need for vitamin supplementation in the perinatal period is that previous investigations were based on a single plasma retinol concentration. Unfortunately, a single plasma retinol concentration does not correlate well with liver stores until they become very low [i.e., $<0.35\,\mu mol/L$ ($<10.0\,\mu g\cdot dl^{-1}$)][61,62,73,113-115] or extremely low [i.e., $<0.17\,\mu mol\cdot L^{-1}$ ($<5\,\mu g\cdot dl^{-1}$)].[116] Many investigators have noted this problem but the use of a single plasma retinol concentration continues in the evaluation of the premature neonate. A better method of confirming actual low vitamin A storage is through the determination of the relative dose response (RDR) following either the oral[117,118] or the intramuscular route of administration.[101] The obvious disadvantages of these methods are the need for a baseline plasma retinol concentration, an oral bolus or an injection of vitamin A, followed by a second plasma sample 5 hours later. A less invasive method of tissue retinoid assessment, such as the modified RDR,[119-121] may be more useful in the premature population if parenteral administration could be standardized. This remains an area that needs further study. While rat pups born to mothers on low vitamin A diets have liver concentrations about one-tenth the usual neonatal rat pup liver, the neonatal pups show no evidence of frank vitamin A deficiency until 1 month postpartum.[122] Therefore, a combination of low stores and other unknown factors may be necessary for a clinical diagnosis of vitamin A deficiency.

Vitamin D

Overview of Metabolism

Vitamin D, unlike the other fat-soluble vitamins, is essentially a prohormone. Although available from dietary sources, it is also synthesized in the skin from cholesterol, by a process that requires ultraviolet B light irradiation. The prohormone is transported from the skin by a spe-

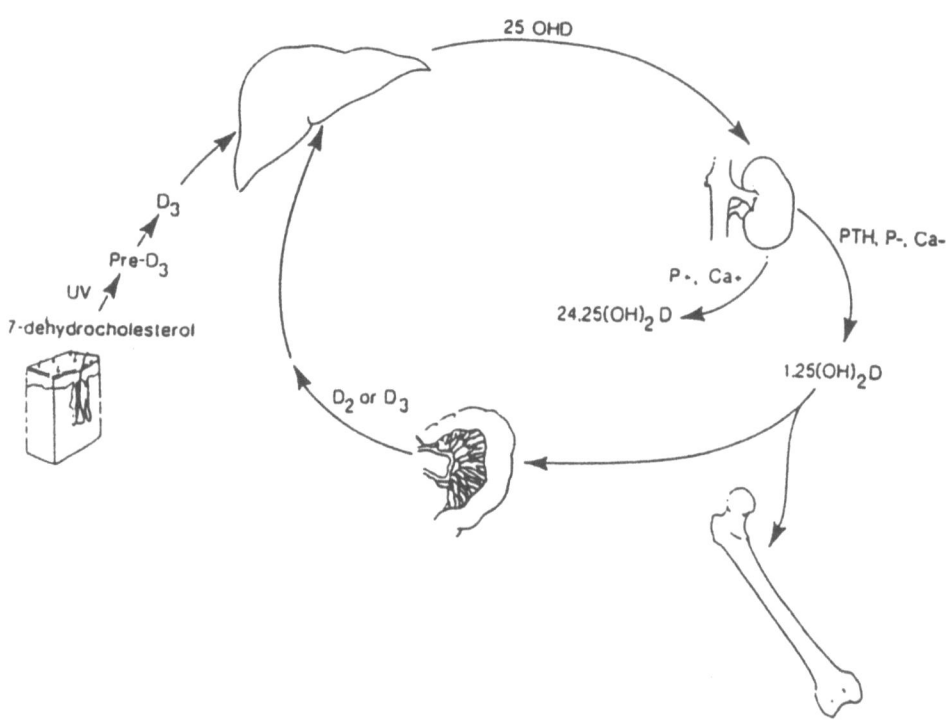

FIGURE 42.2. Vitamin D absorbed from the intestine or synthesized in the skin is hydroxylated in the liver to 25-hydroxyvitamin D, the major circulating vitamin D metabolite. 25-Hydroxyvitamin D is then converted to 1,25-dihydroxyvitamin D or 24,25-dihydroxyvitamin D in the kidney. 1,25-dihydroxyvitamin D stimulates intestinal calcium absorption and acts in concert with PTH to mobilize calcium from bone. (From Specker and Greer,[354] with permission.)

cific serum vitamin D–binding globulin to the liver, where it is converted by a cytochrome P-450–dependent enzyme, 25-hydroxylase, to 25-hydroxyvitamin D [25(OH)D], the major circulating form (Figure 42.2). 25(OH)D, largely bound to vitamin D–binding protein, is carried to the kidney where it is metabolized to either 1,25(OH)$_2$ vitamin D [1,25(OH)$_2$D] by the renal enzyme 1α-hydroxylase, or to 24,25(OH)$_2$ vitamin D [24,25(OH)$_2$D] by 24-hydroxlyase. It has been established that the proximal tubule is the renal site for the activity for 1α-hydroxylase, a cytochrome P-450–dependent monooxygenase enzyme.[123] Parathyroid hormone stimulates renal 1α-hydroxylase activity and enhances renal synthesis of 1,25(OH)$_2$D. The stimulating effect of parathyroid hormone (PTH) is mediated by cyclic adenosine monophosphate (cAMP), as exogenous cAMP restores the reduced 1α-hydroxylase activity in the proximal renal tubules of the parathyroidectomized, vitamin D–deficient rat.[123] It has been established that 1,25(OH)$_2$D induces renal production of 24-hydroxylase, which in turn produces 24,25(OH)$_2$D thereby reducing serum concentration of 1,25(OH)$_2$D[123] (see Chapter 40).

As described, 1,25(OH)$_2$D in concert with parathyroid hormone, maintains calcium and phosphorus homeostasis. This is accomplished by (1) increasing the intestinal absorption of these two elements, (2) affecting the renal handling of phosphate and to a lesser extent calcium, and (3) mobilizing these minerals from bone when necessary. 1,25(OH)$_2$D is the biologically active hormone whose synthesis is tightly regulated depending on the need for calcium and phosphorus. On the other hand, 24,25(OH)D, whose role in mineral metabolism is controversial, is predominantly produced during calcium and phosphorus sufficiency such that the serum concentrations of 1,25(OH)$_2$D and 24,25(OH)D are inversely proportional.

At the cellular level, 1,25(OH)$_2$D action is like that of steroidal hormones. In interacts with a specific receptor-binding protein in the cytosol. The hormone-protein complex becomes bound to nuclear chromatin. At a molecular level, similar to retinoic acid, radiolabeled ^{3}H-1,25(OH)$_2$D, when injected into cell preparations, localizes to the nucleus of many cell types, most of which have nothing to do with calcium homeostasis. Like thyroid hormone, steroidal hormones, and *trans*-retinoic acid, 1,25(OH)$_2$D has direct genomic effects via its binding to specific nuclear receptor proteins in the nucleus. This hormone-receptor protein complex then becomes a transcription factor, which binds to the nuclear response element on DNA. 1,25(OH)$_2$D, like retinoic acid, is involved in direct nuclear signaling. It is thought that binding of the hormone induces a conformational change within these DNA nuclear response elements that enables them to modulate the transcription activity of RNA polymerase II.[124] The nuclear response elements for 1,25(OH)$_2$D have been cloned and are likely the primary site of hormonal action regulating calcium homeostasis as well as other actions of 1,25(OH)$_2$D. These other actions include the regulation of the synthesis of bone proteins such as Ca-binding protein, osteocalcin, osteopontin, alkaline phosphatase, type I collagen, and integrin β$_3$, as well as many proteins involved in cell differentiation and proliferation, such as insulin-like and epidermal growth factors, transformin factor β, c-*myc*, c-*fos*, and c-*jun*.[125] Presumably, these vitamin D nuclear response elements are very important in development, and have been shown to be present by 13 days of gestation in the bone of the developing rat fetus.[125] How the vitamin D nuclear response elements may produce such a large number of different specific responses (e.g., protein synthesis) is unknown. The transcription factors for vitamin D may interact with those of retinoic acid and the thyroid/steroidal hormones on nuclear response elements to produce many specific proteins. This is an active area of research and speculation.[124]

Fetal-Maternal Metabolism

Calcitropic hormones are important in maintaining the serum concentrations of calcium in both mother and fetus. In the fetus and neonate, skin synthesis of vitamin D prohormone is not likely to be of major importance. It is apparent that vitamin D, the parent compound, and 25(OH)D readily cross the placenta from mother to fetus in humans, although the relatively low maternal serum concentration of the parent compound probably makes its placental transfer insignificant.[126] Its presence in relatively low concentrations in cord serum (i.e., 7% of maternal serum concentration) has been documented even in the neonate born to a woman with a daily intake of 100,000 IU of vitamin D.[127]

Most human studies have shown that cord 25(OH)D is generally lower than maternal 25(OH)D, with a range of 68% to 108% of maternal concentration being reported[128–139] (Table 42.1). In these studies there is a good correlation between maternal and cord serum concentrations. Additional evidence for 25(OH)D transport across the placenta is that the seasonal variation in serum 25(OH)D found in mothers is reflected in cord 25(OH)D concentration.[136–138,140]

The maternal-fetal relationship of 1,25(OH)$_2$D in the human is not as clear. This confusion is partially due to the various potential sources of fetal 1,25(OH)$_2$D, including fetal renal synthesis, maternal renal synthesis, as well as synthesis by the placenta. 1,25(OH)$_2$D synthesized by the maternal kidney from 25(OH)D does not appear to cross the placenta from mother to fetus in the rat[141,142] or the cow,[143] though it is likely to occur in sheep[144] and in the nonhuman primate.[145] In the human placental transfer of 1,25(OH)$_2$D has been demonstrated following large maternal oral doses,[146,147] as well as in the perfused placenta in vitro.[148] Cord blood concentration of 1,25(OH)$_2$D is generally lower than the maternal concentration and most research has found negative[149–151] rather than positive[128,135] correlations (Table 42.1) The importance of placental transfer of 1,25(OH)$_2$D from pregnant woman to the fetus remains unknown, particularly in the normal physiologic state.

Human placental tissue synthesizes 1,25(OH)$_2$D from 25(OH)D in vitro, and the data indicate that it is in the mitochondria of the fetal trophoblastic cell that this synthesis occurs.[152,153] Cytosolic receptors for 1,25(OH)$_2$D have been identified in the human and the rat placenta[154] where stimulation of calcium-binding protein would promote the role of this hormone in placental calcium transport. The placental 1,25(OH)$_2$D synthesized may even exceed the daily amount synthesized by the maternal kidney, accounting in part for the increased 1,25(OH)$_2$D seen in pregnancy in some investigations.[153] It has been speculated that placental 1,25(OH)$_2$D plays a role in the transport of calcium across the placenta from the pregnant woman to the fetus, though no regulator of the placental 25-hydroxylase has been identified.[153] Recent evidence now suggests that parathyroid hormone–related peptide (PTH-rp) may be even more important placental calcium transport (vide infra).

In the guinea pig, maternal administration of 1,25(OH)$_2$D has been demonstrated to increase the calcium content of the fetus.[155,156] In contrast, both maternal vitamin D deficiency and fetal nephrectomy in the rat do not affect fetal calcium content.[157,158] Transport of calcium across the placenta in the rat seems to be independent of vitamin D. These observations do not apply to the pregnant sheep. In this species, fetal nephrectomy results in fetal hypocalcemia,[159] though this may be due to the resulting fetal hyperphosphatemia.[160] Administration of 1,25(OH)$_2$D to the nephrectomized sheep fetus restores the fetal serum calcium concentration.

The issue of the role of PTH and PTH-rp in the transport of calcium across the placenta is even more complex.

TABLE 42.1. Relative calcium, phosphorus, vitamin D, and calciotropic hormone status in the mother, fetus (cord blood), and term infants at 24 hours of age.

Substance	Cord blood vs. maternal blood	Infant blood at 24 hr vs. cord blood
25-OH-vitamin D	↓	←→
1,25(OH)$_2$-vitamin D	↓	↑
24,25(OH)$_2$-vitamin D	↓	?
Calcium	↑	↓
Ionized calcium	↑	↓
Parathyroid hormone	↓	↑
Calcitonin	↑	↑
D-binding protein	↓	?

In the rat, fetal parathyroidectomy by decapitation results in a fall in ionized calcium concentration that can be restored by the infusion of PTH extract.[161] Obviously this PTH effect could be secondary to direct stimulation of 1,25(OH)$_2$D synthesis or due to the action of PTH on the placental calcium pump. In the fetal sheep, thyroid-parathyroidectomy with thyroxine replacement results in a rapid fall in serum ionized calcium. An infusion of a parathyroid gland extract restores the flux of calcium from mother to fetus.[162] However, infusion of bovine PTH(1-84) or rat PTH(1-34) does not restore the fetal-maternal calcium gradient in the sheep fetus.[162] This suggests that the sheep parathyroid gland contains a second peptide affecting calcium transport. Extract from the human lung tumor BEN cell line was subsequently shown to restore the calcium placental transport activity in the sheep placenta, again suggesting that PTH-rp is important to placental calcium transport in the sheep fetus.[162]

The PTH-rp is the humoral hypercalcemic factor of malignancy in humans and it has been speculated that it may be the molecule responsible for the activation of the placental calcium Na–adenosine triphosphatase (ATPase) pump. Its interaction with 1,25(OH)$_2$D is unknown, though it is thought that 1,25(OH)$_2$D can either up- or downregulate PTH-rp expression.[163] It is apparent that PTH-rp is produced throughout the maternal-fetal-placental unit during gestation. Human trophoblast tissue contains PTH-rp mRNA in both syncytio- and cytotrophoblasts. Amniotic fluid from humans has measurable PTH-rp by 16 weeks. PTH-rp is found in cord blood in both term and preterm infants, at concentrations within the normal adult range.[164] PTH-rp can stimulate placental calcium transfer in a placental perfusion model from the parathyroidectomized sheep fetus, and the detection of PTH-rp in fetal parathyroids suggests that PTH-rp is a candidate to regulate the placental calcium pump.[163]

The importance of the fetal kidney in 1,25(OH)$_2$D synthesis in vitro remains in question. In the nephrectomized fetal lamb the fall in fetal serum calcium concentration is evidence that the fetal kidney may be important.[165] In the pregnant rat, on the other hand, maternal nephrectomy does not prevent 1,25(OH)$_2$D synthesis from labeled (H^3) 25(OH)D, labeled 1,25(OH)$_2$D being found in both maternal and fetal circulation.[166]

In the human neonate there is preliminary evidence that 1,25(OH)$_2$D is decreased in infants with renal agenesis, without evidence of fetal hypocalcemia.[167] Simultaneous measurement of umbilical venous and arterial samples of neonate cord blood has shown mixed results. Two investigations found a significantly higher fetal umbilical arterial concentration of 1,25(OH)$_2$D compared to the umbilical venous concentration, suggesting fetal renal 1,25(OH)$_2$D production.[128,168] A third study failed to confirm these results.[169] All presently available evidence suggests that an extrarenal site of 1,25(OH)$_2$D synthesis exists (i.e., the placenta). This fact may be important in both fetal and maternal calcium metabolism, more so than fetal renal synthesis.

There is scant information on D-binding protein (DBP) in the fetus and neonate (Table 42.1). Although it is elevated during pregnancy, DBP concentration in the term neonate is equal to those in the nonpregnant adults.[170] DBP is apparently decreased in the premature neonate, the concentration being directly proportional to gestational age.[171,172]

Neonatal Vitamin D Metabolism

It is presumed that in the human neonate the major vitamin D source during the immediate postnatal period is placental transfer of maternal vitamin D or its metabolites during pregnancy. As discussed above, fetal 1,25(OH)$_2$D may be synthesized from 25(OH)D by the placenta or the fetal kidney. In the neonatal rat it has been shown that the primary neonatal source of vitamin D is of maternal origin by direct transfer across the placenta to the fetus.[173] In this study, the vitamin D–deficient female rat was given labeled vitamin D prior to mating. During pregnancy there was a linear increase in total fetal labeled 25(OH)D, 24,25(OH)D, and vitamin D itself (i.e., parent compound) between days 14 and 19 (full-term gestation is 21 days). The vitamin D present in the fetus was predominantly 25(OH)D (54%). During the 3-week suckling period, the stored labeled vitamin D accumulated in utero remained the primary determinant of vitamin D status in the pup, despite relatively high concentrations of vitamin D in rat milk (40–140 IU·L^{-1}) and a gradual decline in the total vitamin D content of the rat pup during the first 3 weeks of life. These data suggest that the vitamin D stores accumulated in the fetus in utero were readily available to the rat pups after birth. Although there are no similar data for the human, it is apparent from a number of clinical investigations in Asian immigrants to Great Britain[174] and in women in the People's Republic of China[139] that the neonatal vitamin D status is highly dependent on the maternal status. In the breast-fed human neonate without supplemental vitamin D, the vitamin D transferred across the placenta would remain the major source of vitamin D throughout the neonatal period, as the vitamin D content of human milk is low (<20 IU·L^{-1}).

For the formula-fed neonate, vitamin D intestinal absorption is probably significant as formulas in the United States generally contain a minimum of 400 IU·L^{-1}. Like the other fat-soluble vitamins, vitamin D is absorbed in the small intestine and transported in the intestinal lymph ducts associated with chylomicrons. In animals, the absorption rate of vitamin D is linearly related to doses of vitamin D, suggesting that absorption takes place by simple passive diffusion after solubilization by bile salts.[175] Vitamin D undergoes a certain amount of enterohepatic circulation, though 25-hydroxylation of the parent compound enhances the intestinal absorption and minimizes its loss during enterohepatic circulation.[176] In the term neonate with inoperable brain deformities, 13% to 23% of an oral dose of ^{14}C vitamin D was recovered from feces within 3 days.[177] There is no information on the absorptive capacity for vitamin D in the preterm neonate.

In the human term neonate within 24 hours of delivery, there is an increase in serum $1,25(OH)_2D$[150,178] (Table 42.1). This persists through the first 5 days of life.[178,179] In one report, serum $1,25(OH)_2D$ concentration was documented to decrease from day 5 to day 30 [100 ± 5 (SEM) vs 61 ± 4 pg·ml^{-1}]. In the premature neonate ≤32 weeks' gestation an increase in $1,25(OH)_2D$ occurred between birth and 24 hours and continued through day 5.[178] However, unlike the term neonate, $1,25(OH)_2D$ remained high for the first 7 to 9 weeks of life,[180,181] and by day 30 it was significantly higher than in the term neonate (i.e., 108 ± 3 vs 61 ± 4 pg·ml^{-1}). These figures may reflect the relative increased need for calcium in the premature neonate during this period of rapid postnatal growth.

Contrary to serum $1,25(OH)_2D$, serum $25(OH)D$ concentration shows no significant change during either the first 24 hours[150,178] (Table 42.1) or even during the first week of life in term and preterm neonates.[178] There is no significant correlation between serum $25(OH)D$ and $1,25(OH)_2D$ concentrations in these neonates during this early neonatal period.[180-182] In premature and term neonates, 1α-hydroxylation of $25(OH)D$ begins to occur shortly after birth, indicating the presence of renal 1α-hydroxylase during the immediate postnatal period (Table 42.1).[183] There is no information on $24,25(OH)_2D$ at 24 hours of age in term neonates. In one study, $24,25(OH)_2D$ was increased compared to cord blood by the fifth day of life.[129]

With termination of the placental calcium supply, the neonate must suddenly maintain its own calcium homeostasis. This rise in serum $1,25(OH)_2D$ concentration during the immediate postnatal period in term and preterm neonates parallels the decrease in serum calcium concentration that occurs after birth (Table 42.1). This period of relative hypocalcemia is exaggerated and prolonged in the premature neonate, perhaps again explaining the prolonged increase in serum $1,25(OH)_2D$ compared to the term neonate. This $1,25(OH)_2D$ increase is mediated by PTH, as the serum PTH concentration increases with decreasing serum calcium in preterm and term neonates[149,182,184,185] (Table 42.1). The rise in serum PTH can be blunted with an infusion of intravenous calcium, significantly increasing serum calcium in the premature neonate.[184,185]

It is of considerable interest that the hypocalcemia of prematurity persists in very low birth weight (VLBW) neonates despite the increase in serum PTH and $1,25(OH)_2D$. Even pharmacologic, intramuscular doses of $1,25(OH)_2D$ up to 3.0 μg·kg^{-1} do not affect the hypocalcemia in this group.[185] This may be explained in part by the fact that most of these neonates do not receive oral feedings during the immediate postnatal period so $1,25(OH)_2D$ cannot increase intestinal calcium absorption. It would not explain why adequate calcium is not mobilized effectively from bone in the face of falling serum calcium and rising PTH and $1,25(OH)_2D$ concentrations. Given the complexity and importance of $1,25(OH)_2D$ for fetal growth and development, this is difficult to explain.

Existing animal data support the hypothesis that the functional status of $1,25(OH)_2D$ intestinal receptors may account for the hypocalcemia of prematurity. As the rat gut is relatively immature at the time of birth, it may be somewhat comparable to the gut of the human premature neonate. In the neonatal suckling rat with a higher intake per kilogram of calcium than the human neonate it can be shown that the intestinal absorption of calcium after an injection of $1,25(OH)_2D$ does not increase until the time of weaning at 3 weeks of age,[186] and $1,25(OH)_2D$ acts at the intestinal level after being bound by specific receptors in the cytoplasm of the intestinal cell. Such receptors have been found to be present in low concentration in the intestine of the suckling rat at 7 and 14 days of life, but they increase at the time of weaning.[187] In the adult rat, the $1,25(OH)_2D$ receptor complex subsequently binds to nuclear chromatin and stimulates the synthesis of messenger RNA, which ultimately results in the synthesis of specific proteins responsible for the end-organ response to $1,25(OH)_2D$ (vide supra). The protein most commonly demonstrated to be the result of $1,25(OH)_2D$ action on intestinal epithelial cells is calcium-binding protein (CBP). The exact role of CBP in intestinal calcium transport is not clear, as it does not appear in the intestinal epithelial cells until calcium absorption is under way. With regard to human neonatal $1,25(OH)_2D$ receptors, it has been demonstrated in human cord blood lymphocytes from term and preterm neonates that, although these cells have the normal number of binding sites for $1,25(OH)_2D$, the $1,25(OH)_2D$ inhibition of mitogen-induced lymphocyte proliferation is considerably less than that of adult cells.[188] Before further observations on the inability of $1,25(OH)_2D$ to correct the hypocalcemia of prematurity can be made, additional information on the effect of $1,25(OH)_2D$ on the intestine, bone, and kidney in the premature neonate is necessary. Further data regarding the functioning of intestinal, bone, and renal cell nuclear receptors for 1,25(OH)$_2$D in the human neonate would be of great interest.

Little is known about the effects of vitamin D or its metabolites on the neonatal kidney. The older infant adapts well to retaining minerals such as calcium and phosphorus under conditions of increased needs, though almost all of the filtered calcium in the kidney is reabsorbed even in the absence of vitamin D. In the rat, 1,25(OH)$_2$D receptors have been identified in the proximal tubule of the nephron,[189] and a vitamin D–dependent calcium-binding protein has been found in the human kidney.[190] There is evidence that both phosphate and calcium reabsorption are stimulated by 1,25(OH)$_2$D in the mammalian kidney. Both of these actions apparently require protein synthesis, including renal CBP.[123]

One of the effects of 1,25(OH)$_2$D on bone is bone resorption, or remodeling, an essential function to maintain calcium homeostasis, as 98% of body calcium is located in bone. Bone resorption is carried out by osteoclasts, but vitamin D metabolites and PTH have no direct effect on osteoclasts, which lack receptors for 1,25(OH)$_2$D and PTH.[191] It is possible that osteoclast precursors have receptors, as 1,25(OH)$_2$D promotes osteoclast formation in bone organ cultures. Whereas PTH and 1,25(OH)$_2$D increase bone resorption and cAMP synthesis in bone organ cultures, in vitro PTH and 1,25(OH)$_2$D have no effect on bone resorption or motility of isolated osteoclasts.[191] The effects of 1,25(OH)$_2$D on osteoclasts must be mediated by other cells that have 1,25(OH)$_2$D receptors (i.e., osteoblasts).

Vitamin D and Vitamin K

In the important vitamin D function of bone resorption, there is a potential interrelationship with vitamin K. Osteocalcin or bone Gla protein (BGP) accounts for about 10% of the noncollagenous protein of bone. Its synthesis in bone cells requires the presence of vitamin K. This vitamin K–dependent gamma-carboxylation of the precursor of BGP accounts for the high affinity of BGP for calcium. In the vitamin K–deficient chick and rabbit with a low BGP concentration, bone mineralization is normal. Alternatively, as circulating BGP is involved in bone growth, bone turnover, or both, it has been hypothesized that BGP is involved in bone mineral mobilization.[192] In clinical studies of patients with diseases associated with increased rates of bone turnover (e.g., Paget's disease, hyperparathyroidism), blood BGP concentration is increased.

It has been shown that 1,25(OH)$_2$D stimulates BGP formation in rat osteosarcoma cell lines[193] and fetal rat calvariae.[194] BGP concentration is decreased in the vitamin D–deficient animal,[195] and in vivo administration of 1,25(OH)$_2$D to the human increases circulatory concentration of BGP in the adult,[196] the child,[197] and the premature neonate.[198] Whether 1,25(OH)$_2$D stimulation of BGP has anything to do with bone resorption can be questioned. In the rat calvaria model, PTH and epidermal growth factor, known to have the same effects as 1,25(OH)$_2$D on bone formation and resorption, do not stimulate BGP synthesis.[194]

It is likely that BGP does not cross the placenta, as there is not a significant positive correlation between maternal and cord blood concentrations.[178,199] In premature and term neonates at birth, BGP is markedly elevated to approximately three to four times the serum concentration of the normal adult.[178,199,200] BGP increases during the first 5 days of life in term and preterm neonates and along with serum 1,25(OH)$_2$D remains elevated through the first month of life compared to the concentration in the normal adult. However, there is no correlation between serum BGP and 1,25(OH)$_2$D in the neonate at any time during this period.[178]

Vitamin K

Vitamin K exists in three general forms (Figure 42.3). It was first isolated from alfalfa as a yellow oil, and this plant form of vitamin K is now known as vitamin K$_1$ or phylloquinone. A second form of this vitamin was isolated from putrefied fish meal and was originally called vitamin K$_2$ and is now a series of compounds with unsaturated side chains synthesized by bacteria, referred to as menaquinones. The basic structure of all vitamin K compounds is menadione, strictly a synthetic form (Figure 42.3).

Other than the standard initial injection of vitamin K, the neonate has several potential sources of vitamin K, including transplacental transfer, dietary sources from

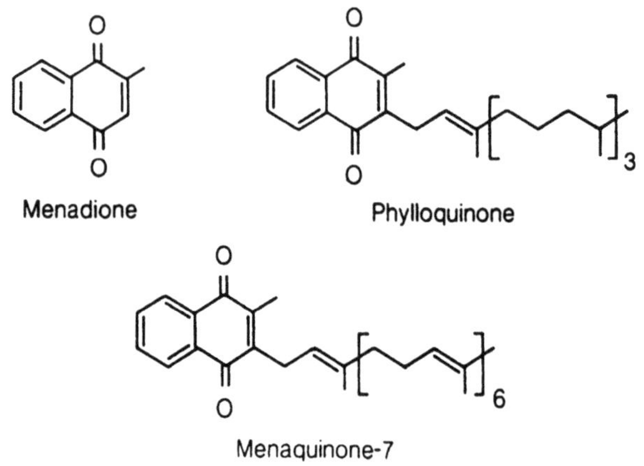

FIGURE 42.3. Biologically active forms of vitamin K. Vitamin K$_1$ (phylloquinone) is the major dietary from. Vitamin K$_2$ (menaquinones) is synthesized by bacteria. Menadione, a synthetic compound, is not important in human nutrition.

human milk or formula, and the possible absorption of menaquinones synthesized by the intestinal flora. Formulas available in the United States and Europe are fortified with phylloquinone (50–100 μg·ml^{-1}), whereas human milk generally contains less than 10 μg·ml^{-1}.[201–205] The notion that intestinal menaquinone, synthesized by intestinal bacteria, is absorbed and utilized as an important source of vitamin K in the human is one that has been overemphasized.[206]

Overview of Metabolism

Osteocalcin, or BGP, is just one of many vitamin K–dependent proteins, which include the plasma coagulation factors II (i.e., prothrombin), VII, IX, and X. Other vitamin K–dependent proteins are proteins C, S, and Z in plasma[207] and γ-carboxyglutamic acid–containing proteins in kidney, spleen, lung, uterus, placenta, pancreas, thyroid, thymus, testes, and bone.[208] Carboxylase activity has been detected in most of these tissues, including the human liver.[209] However, only osteocalcin (BGP) and matrix Gla protein (MGP) located in bone, of all the extrahepatic vitamin K–dependent proteins, have been completely characterized.[210]

All of the known vitamin K–dependent proteins have in common γ-carboxyglutamic acid (Gla), the unique amino acid formed by the postribosomal action of vitamin K–dependent carboxylase. These Gla residues, located in the homologous amino-terminal domain with a high degree of amino acid sequence identity[210] seen in all vitamin K–dependent proteins, are required for the calcium-mediated interaction of these proteins with a negatively charged phospholipid surface and are essential for the formation of the protein conformation that imparts this property.

The conversion of glutamyl residues to γ-carboxyglutamic acid residues on the vitamin K–dependent protein molecule creates effective calcium binding sites. Vitamin K is a necessary factor for the activity of this

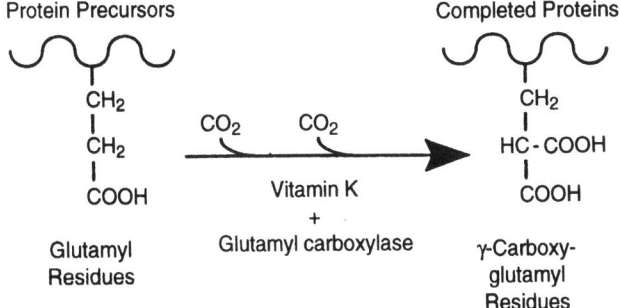

FIGURE 42.4. Vitamin K$_1$ functions as a cofactor with the microsomal enzyme glutamyl carboxylase to convert glutamyl residues to γ-carboxyglutamic acid residues on precursor proteins (i.e., prothrombin).

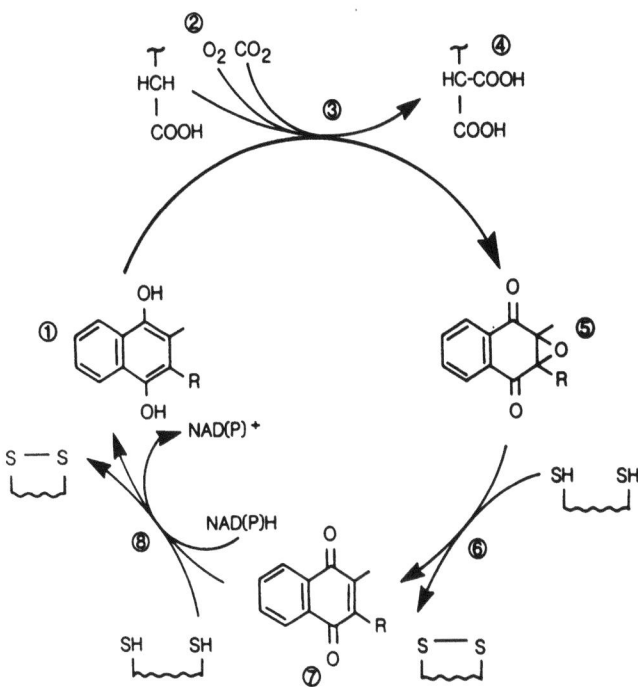

FIGURE 42.5. Metabolism of vitamin K$_1$ (1) in the liver. The conversion of a glutamyl residue on a vitamin K–dependent protein (2) to a γ-carboxyglutamyl (Gla) residue (4) by the enzyme glutamyl carboxylase (3) is dependent on the reduced vitamin K (1) and is coupled to the formation of vitamin K epoxide (5). The regeneration of vitamin K$_1$ from the epoxide form requires a dithiol (-SH)-dependent enzyme, epoxide reductase (6), to form the quinone form (7) of vitamin K and further reduction by a second dithiol-dependent enzyme (8), quinone reductase, to the hydroquinone vitamin K$_1$ (1). In this proposed vitamin K cycle, the two dithiol-dependent steps in vitamin K metabolism are blocked by the commonly used oral anticoagulants. (From Greer and Suttie,[355] with permission.)

microsomal glutamyl carboxylase (Figure 42.4). Studies of the microsomal vitamin K–dependent carboxylase have not elucidated the exact molecular role of vitamin K. Research has been hampered until very recently by the inability to purify the carboxylase.[210] It is apparent that during the posttranslational conversion of glutamyl to γ-carboxyglutamyl residues on the vitamin K–dependent peptides by carboxylase, vitamin K is converted to its 2,3-epoxide form (Figure 42.5).[207] Subsequently, the epoxide form of vitamin K is reduced to the quinone form by an epoxide reductase and to the active coenzyme form, the hydroquinone, by various microsomal quinone reductases. It is hypothesized that the role of vitamin K is to abstract the hydrogen of a glutamyl (Gla) residue as a proton from a vitamin K–dependent protein, leaving a carbon ion, which is attacked by free CO$_2$ to form a γ-carboxyglutamic acid (Figure 42.4).[207] The only source of energy needed to drive this unique carboxylation reaction comes from the reoxidation of the reduced vitamin.[210] Coumarin anticoagulants, such as warfarin apparently antagonize vitamin K action by inhibiting the epoxide and quinone reductase activities of liver. These actions increase the concentration of vitamin K epoxide and result in an insufficient amount of reduced vitamin K required for the action of carboxylase. The mechanism of action of vitamin K is reviewed elsewhere.[211]

Vitamin K is found in relatively high concentrations in liver, heart, and bone.[212,213] Other organs, such as brain, have low concentrations.

Menaquinones

Menaquinones can exhibit vitamin K activity in both in vitro and in vivo animal systems. They can participate in a vitamin K metabolic cycle such as that seen in Figure 42.5. We have very little information on menaquinones in the perinatal period in mothers or neonates. The significance of their role in perinatal, as well as in all human nutrition, is under study. As noted above, menaquinones are produced by colonic flora. Few of the bacteria composing the normal human intestinal flora produce menaquinones, including *Bifidobacterium*, *Lactobacillus*, and *Clostridium* species. Major producers include *Bacteroides fragilis* and *Escherichia coli*.

MK-6, MK-7, and MK-8 seem to be the most significant menaquinones and detectable concentrations have been found in human organs, plasma, and feces.[214-222] MK-7 and MK-8 are the predominant fecal forms in breast-feeding and formula-feeding infants,[223] though as might be expected, both phylloquinone and menaquinones are more prevalent in the stools of formula-fed neonates.[224] Menaquinones are the predominant form in human liver,[220,225-227] and even in the neonatal liver vitamin K_1 predominates over menaquinones (81 ± 73 vs 9 ± 2 pmol·g liver^{-1}).[228] However, evidence suggests that menaquinones are not readily available compared to phylloquinone from the hepatic pool.[229] Little is known about their absorption from the intestinal tract, plasma transport, or clearance from circulation. It should be pointed out, however, that most of the gut bacterial pool of menaquinone, located within bacterial membranes, is probably not available for absorption.

Menaquinone-4 (MK-4) should not be considered in the same context as other longer chained menaquinones, though it is of considerable research interest. It is not a major bacterial product. Most organs have detectable levels of MK-4, and with the exception of the liver in adults, MK-4 concentration is higher than that of phylloquinone. It seems likely that this MK-4 accumulation is due to synthesis rather than uptake. This would mean that individual organs contain an enzyme capable of converting phylloquinone to MK-4 via menadione (Figure 42.3). This is viewed by some to be very likely,[212,230,231] though a specific organ enzyme responsible for this conversion has not yet been demonstrated.

Fetal-Maternal Considerations

Vitamin K_1 or phylloquinone has been reported to be present in low (<2 µg·ml^{-1}) to undetectable concentrations in cord blood.[224,232-234] Our own recent data have shown that out of 156 cord blood in term neonates, none had measurable vitamin K.[235] There is no correlation between maternal and cord blood concentrations. All of the available evidence suggests that only very small quantities of vitamin K cross the placenta from mother to fetus. Indeed, even maternal pharmacologic doses of vitamin K have unpredictable effects on cord blood concentration.[224,232-234] In the rat, though physiologic concentrations are transported across the placenta, maternal pharmacologic doses do not increase placental transport proportionally.[236,237]

Neonatal Metabolism

Vitamin K, like all fat-soluble vitamins, is absorbed from the intestine into the lymphatic system, requiring the presence of both bile salts and pancreatic secretions.[238] Vitamin K deficiency has been observed in subjects with impaired fat absorption caused by obstructive jaundice, pancreatic insufficiency (e.g., cystic fibrosis), and adult celiac disease.[239,240] The lymphatic system is the major route of intestinal transport of absorbed phylloquinone in association with chylomicrons. Little is known of the existence of specific vitamin K carrier proteins, though cow's milk has been reported to contain a protein complex that is reversibly bound to vitamin K.[241]

In the rat, vitamin K_1 absorption occurs by an energy-dependent process in the proximal portion of the small intestine.[242] Absorption of menaquinones of bacterial origin has been found to be a passive, noncarrier-mediated process from the large and small intestines.[243,244] There is little specific information about the intestinal absorption of vitamin K in humans. In the neonate, 29% of an oral dose of vitamin K_1 is reported to be absorbed from the intestine.[245] The importance of the enterohepatic circulation of vitamin K in the human is unknown.

After the injection of vitamin K in the rat, vitamin K_1 is rapidly concentrated in liver but has a short half-life of 17 hours which is consistent with little long-term storage by this organ.[246] In the pig and the dog, vitamin K_1 and menaquinones are detected in the liver.[247] In the adult human it has been demonstrated with labeled vitamin K_1 that the total body pool of vitamin K is replaced approximately every 2.5 hours.[248] Compared to other fat-soluble vitamins, relatively small amounts of vitamin K have been reported in the liver of the neonate. Small amounts of menaquinones in the neonate could presumably be of bacterial origin, though as mentioned above we do not know about the liver's ability to convert phylloquinone to menaquinone-4 in the human.

In the neonate the concentrations of the vitamin K–dependent clotting factors (e.g., factors II, VII, IX, and X) are generally 25% to 70% of normal adult concentrations, and there is little difference at birth between 30 and 40 weeks' gestation.[249,250] Normal adult concentrations of these factors are not achieved until 6 months of age, and if anything, premature infants show an accelerated postnatal maturation toward adult levels compared to term infants. The prothrombin time shows a much wider range and variability in the neonate at birth (i.e., 11–16 seconds) compared to the adult (i.e., 11–14 seconds), and this persists through the first 6 months of life. The activated partial thromboplastin time shows a similar pattern compared to adults through the first 6 months of life.[249,250] Interestingly enough, in the neonate, injections of vitamin K_1 do not significantly alter these tests or the measurements of the individual clotting factors.[234,251] The differences in coagulation between the adult and the neonate cannot totally be ascribed to vitamin K "deficiency" and the carboxylase activity of the vitamin K cycle (Figure 42.5) may be limited by the number of precursor proteins, not the availability of vitamin K_1.

Human vitamin K deficiency results in the secretion of partially carboxylated prothrombin into the plasma, referred to as abnormal prothrombin or protein induced by vitamin K absence or antagonism (PIVKA).[252] PIVKA is a heterogeneous molecule. It consists of a pool of partially carboxylated prothrombin, as well as some completely acarboxylated prothrombin.[253] The number of acarboxylated sites (up to 10) per individual prothrombin molecule and the specific sites involved remain an area of investigation. Likewise, the degree of physiologic activity may vary with the number of carboxylated sites. A preparation lacking 20% of the γ-carboxylated sites, primarily at the more carboxy-terminal sites on the molecule, has been demonstrated to have near-normal physiologic activity.[253] Four methods have been described to measure PIVKA in the neonate, and recently these have been reviewed in detail.[252] However, only one of these methods is in widespread use at this time—specific antibody detection. The principle of this method is the preparation of a murine monoclonal antibody to PIVKA that is subsequently utilized in an enzyme-linked immunosorbent assay (ELISA). A number of such specific antibodies have now been described, which makes comparisons of clinical studies difficult.[254-257] This methodology has been used for measurements in cord blood and infants through 12 weeks of age. Detection rates of PIVKA in cord blood using this assay have ranged from 10% to 30%.[256-259] We have recently reported PIVKA values in a large series of full term neonates in the United States at the time of birth. Of 148 cord bloods, 49 (33%) were positive for PIVKA (≥ 0.2 Arbitrary units·ml^{-1}). A number of studies have shown that prophylactic vitamin K to the neonate results in near elimination of the positive PIVKA values that were present in cord blood.[260-263] The usefulness of this measurement for showing a subclinical vitamin K deficiency is a point of controversy. In a recent study of exclusively breast-feeding neonates who received vitamin K prophylaxis at birth by either oral or intramuscular route, there was no significant correlation between measurable PIVKA concentration and low plasma vitamin K concentration during the first 3 months of life.[235]

In essence, less is known about perinatal vitamin K metabolism than about other fat-soluble vitamins. Overt deficiency of vitamin K in the neonate is not a rare occurrence in parts of the world where vitamin K is not routinely administered at the time of birth. The associated hemorrhagic disease during the neonatal period remains a serious worldwide concern for infant morbidity and mortality. With the recent concerns over intramuscular newborn vitamin K_1 and associated childhood cancer in Europe, the incidence of hemorrhagic disease of the newborn has increased. These issues are reviewed in detail elsewhere.[264]

Vitamin E

The maternal-fetal and neonatal aspects of tocopherol nutrition have been a focus of vitamin E research ever since the discovery of this fat-soluble nutrient in 1922.[265] Lipids with vitamin E activity were isolated from wheat germ oil, and their chemical synthesis was achieved in 1938. The essentiality of vitamin E for humans was convincingly demonstrated only in 1967, when Oski and Barness[266] reported a hemolytic anemia state of the premature neonate that was responsive to α-tocopherol therapy. Despite growing interest since then, the vitamin remains somewhat of an enigma in regard to its precise subcellular role(s). It clearly can function in animals as a biologic antioxidant to prevent disease. The early years of research were characterized by descriptions of the disturbances in various vitamin E–deficient animals as the anatomical-clinical method of investigation was applied to this problem. Degeneration of the germinal epithelium in the male rat was found to be the underlying problem in testicular atrophy, whereas fetal resorption was clearly the major problem of the pregnant female. Paralysis associated with necrotic muscle and the occurrence of encephalomalacia was described in rodents and fowl.[267] In adult humans, much has been written in recent years on the role of vitamin E in ischemic heart disease, atherosclerosis, diabetes, cataracts, Parkinson's disease, and Alzheimer's disease. This recently has been reviewed elsewhere.[268]

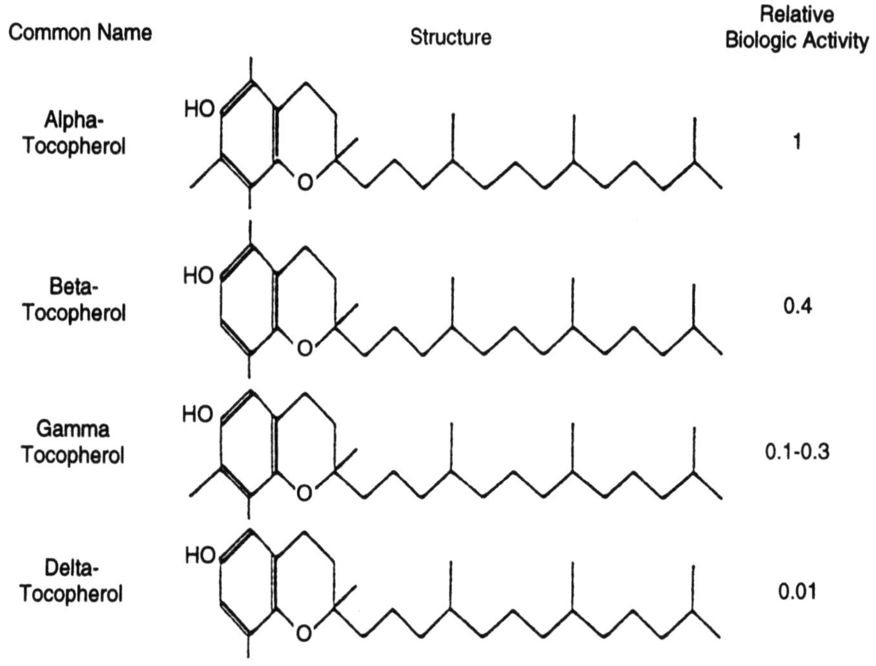

Common Name	Structure	Relative Biologic Activity
Alpha-Tocopherol		1
Beta-Tocopherol		0.4
Gamma-Tocopherol		0.1–0.3
Delta-Tocopherol		0.01

FIGURE 42.6. Chemical structure and relative biologic activities of tocopherols. The most active vitamer α-tocopherol, is referred to as 5,7,8-trimethyl tocol. The other three tocopherols differ only in the methyl substitutions on the benzene ring.

Studies during the 1940s and 1950s revealed that the premature neonate and the patient with malabsorption have a low concentration of blood tocopherol and abnormal hemolysis of erythrocytes incubated in the presence of hydrogen peroxide.[269,270] These studies indicated that cellular and subcellular membranes of lower animals and humans are susceptible to oxidative degeneration in the absence of vitamin E. Consequently, the vitamin was officially recognized in 1968 as an essential nutrient for the human by inclusion in the Recommended Dietary Allowances table of the National Academy of Sciences.[270] Other studies have clarified both biochemical and nutritional aspects of vitamin E.

Biochemistry

The biochemistry of vitamin E is complex, as there are eight naturally occurring compounds with characteristic biologic activities. Four are tocopherols (Figure 42.6) and four are tocotrienols. Detailed reviews on the nomenclature, stereochemistry, and biochemistry of vitamin E compounds have been published elsewhere.[271–273] The most abundant and active isomer is α-tocopherol (i.e., 5,7,8-trimethyl tocol). Vitamin E is found in foods as RRR–α-tocopherol, formerly known as d-α-tocopherol, whereas laboratory syntheses produces a mixture of eight epimers.

In addition to the α-vitamer, three other tocopherols with biologic activity are present in foods: β-, γ-, and δ-tocopherol. They differ from α-tocopherol only in regard to methyl substitutions on the benzene ring (Figure 42.6). The tocotrienols, which have not been as well studied, consist of four compounds similar to the corresponding tocopherols, but with unsaturated side chains. Only α-tocotrienol appears to have significant vitamin E activity.

The biologic activities of E vitamers vary considerably, but all show antioxidant capability (i.e., the ability to protect cellular and subcellular membranes from oxidative destruction initiated at the molecular level by lipid peroxidation).[272] Most of the data implicating the biologic antioxidant function have been generated by in vitro experiments. Evidence from in vivo studies confirm this role.[274] Some manifestations of vitamin E deficiency in the chick and the rat can be prevented by feeding synthetic antioxidants such as ethoxyquin. It is generally believed that all tocopherols function as free radical scavengers in membranes.[275] As illustrated in Figure 42.7, phospholipids in cellular and subcellular membranes contain polyunsaturated fatty acids (PUFA) that are susceptible to peroxidation. The fatty acid composition of membranes is influenced by diet.[276,277] To be effective, tocopherol must be localized in membrane sites exposed to free radicals. Vitamin E protects the esterified fatty acids by interrupting free radical reactions that otherwise can cause membrane damage in subcellular organelles. In this reaction, the phenolic hydroxyl group of tocopherol reacts with a peroxyl radical to form the corresponding organic hydroperoxide and the tocopherol radical (Vit E-O•):

$$ROO• + Vit\ E\text{-}OH \rightarrow ROOH + Vit\ E\text{-}O•$$

This effectively interrupts the chain of peroxidation reactions.[278]

Other cellular antioxidant systems such as glutathione peroxidase and superoxide dismutase may protect the cell from free radical attacks on peroxidizable fatty acids

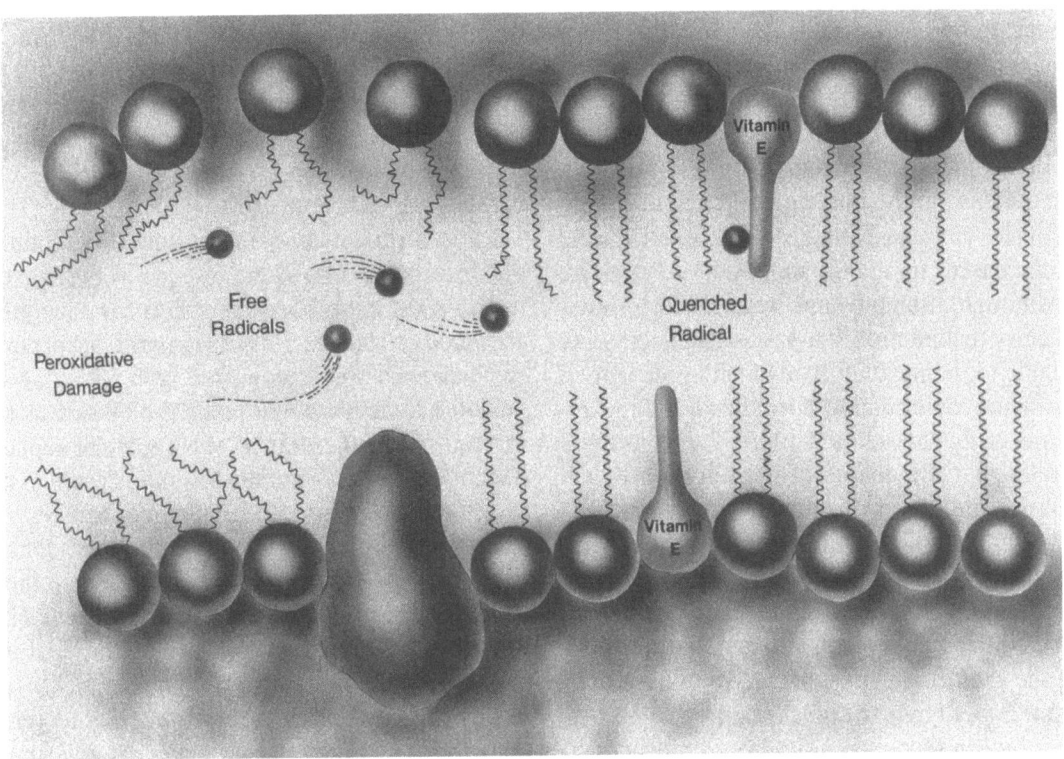

FIGURE 42.7. Biologic role of vitamin E as a membrane antioxidant, protecting polyunsaturated fatty acids that are esterified in the phospholipid bilayer by halting the chain reactions that can lead to peroxidative damage.

by "neutralizing" free radicals. Because of the relation between vitamin E and unsaturated fatty acids, the requirements for α-tocopherol are somewhat dependent on the amount and concentration of PUFA consumed and the resultant changes in membrane fatty acid composition.[276,277] The relation appears to be particularly important in the young growing animal in which formation of normal membrane structures and maintenance of their integrity are active biochemical processes. The susceptibility of developing tissues to pathologic changes in vitamin E deficiency is one of the characteristic features in the lower animal and the human.

The original international standard of vitamin E, synthesized from natural phytol and initially designated dl-α-tocopheryl acetate, is defined as having 1 IU·mg of activity. The corresponding value for naturally occurring RRR–α-tocopherol is 1.49 IU·mg. On the basis of in vivo bioassays, the approximate relative potencies of the other vitamers isomers compared to α-tocopherol are β 40% to 50%, γ 10% to 30%, and δ about 1%. The presence and location of methyl groups in the benzene ring is of great importance in determining biologic activity among the tocopherol isomers (Figure 42.6), perhaps because of an effect on membrane incorporation or turnover of a particular vitamer. The relative activity of a particular vitamin E isomer depends not only on the compound's structure but on its relative absorption, uptake by target tissues, and turnover rate. Consequently, results of in vitro assay systems do not yield the same results as in vivo bioassays. This point has led to disputes over the assignment of relative potencies, an important consideration with respect to dietary allowances.

Assessment of γ-tocopherol's relative activity is of importance because of the high content of this vitamer in the American diet, in infant formula preparations, and in some therapeutic lipid products marketed for intravenous use.[276,279] Although having only 10% of the activity of α-tocopherol traditionally,[273,276] more recent comparative assessment for lipid peroxidation in vivo in the iron-loaded rat suggests that γ-tocopherol may be 31% as effective as α-tocopherol.[280] In contrast to the in vivo bioassays, results obtained with in vitro tests indicate that γ-tocopherol shows more than 50% the activity of the α-vitamer.[276,281] The difference in γ-tocopherol's concentration of vitamin E activity in vitro has been attributed to a faster turnover rate than that for α-tocopherol.[276] Because of its uncertain bioavailability, dietary γ-tocopherol presently is assigned only 10% the activity of α-tocopherol.

Nutrient Interrelations

Several biochemical interactions have been identified between vitamin E and other nutrients. The interrelationship with vitamin A is described elsewhere (vide supra). As indicated previously, it is clear that the intake of PUFA markedly influences the vitamin E requirements of animals. There is good evidence that the tocopherol-PUFA relation is true in the human.[276,277,282-284] Varying the diets of adult men from beef fat to safflower oil causes an increase in the linoleic acid content of adipose tissue.[284] The vitamin E intake of these volunteers had to be increased to avoid abnormal erythrocyte hemolysis. Although attempts have been made to identify a fixed dietary tocopherol/PUFA ratio, sufficient data are not available to delineate this value with precision in the human. When determining tocopherol-PUFA requirements, not only the amount of PUFA consumed affects this ratio, but the degree of unsaturation of the fatty acids has an influence. In human diets where the primary fatty acid is linoleic, an α-tocopherol/PUFA ratio of $0.4\,\text{mg}\cdot\text{g}^{-1}$ seems nutritionally adequate. To provide a margin of safety, the American Academy of Pediatrics Committee on Nutrition has recommended that formulas designed for the preterm neonate provide a minimum of 1 IU of vitamin E per gram of linoleic acid.[285]

A relation between tocopherol and iron has been well established in animals and humans. Iron can catalyze peroxidation reactions and seems to be involved in the endogenous production of intracellular free radicals.[275] In the intestine the presence of iron consumed with vitamin E can lead to augmented destruction of tocopherol and a higher apparent vitamin E requirement. This point is pertinent to the premature neonate.[283,286] Interaction between tocopherol and selenium has been recognized for years. The basis of this interaction is the role of selenium as a cofactor in the function of the cytosolic antioxidant enzyme glutathione peroxidase.

Intestinal Absorption, Transport, and Metabolism of Tocopherols

Vitamin E must be absorbed, transported, delivered to cells, and integrated into lipid droplets, cellular membranes, and organelles of tissues to be effective. A variety of methods have been used to measure vitamin E absorption and transport.[270,276] Most of the quantitative information has been obtained by administering radioactive α-tocopherol and measuring fecal excretion of radioactivity, and it appears that transport processes are similar for the other tocopherol vitamers, although tissue storage and turnover are considerably different. The absorption of tocopherols is variable depending on total lipid absorption as with the other fat-soluble vitamins.[270] Bile salts and pancreatic enzymes are essential to the absorption process.[276,287] The efficiency of absorption decreases as larger amounts of tocopherol are consumed.[288] In the normal human, an average absorption of at least 50% and perhaps as high as 70% can be assumed for normal dietary intake of α-tocopherol (e.g., 0.4–1.0 mg in adults); however, the efficiency falls to less than 10% with pharmacologic intakes as high as 200 mg.[288] Decreased absorption of fat, as seen in the premature neonate and the patient with various forms of steatorrhea, results in a parallel loss of tocopherols.[270]

Little is known about the passage of vitamin E through the absorptive cells of the mucosa as no intestinal transfer proteins have been identified for tocopherol. Once absorbed, vitamin E isomers are incorporated into chylomicrons and transported with fat along with other fat-soluble vitamins via lymphatic vessels to the venous system. The concentration of tocopherol in plasma varies depending on the amount of lipid present. Tocopherols in plasma are associated with lipoproteins, no specific carrier protein having been conclusively identified. How they are liberated from chylomicrons and joined with the various lipoproteins is not exactly known. The enzyme lipoprotein lipase found on the endothelial surfaces of capillaries, are thought to be important. In any event, during the catabolism of chylomicrons to remnant particles, various forms of vitamin E are distributed to the circulating lipoproteins and ultimately to the tissue. It is thought that chylomicron remnant uptake directly by the liver may account for a major portion of absorbed tocopherols, just as it is important for retinol.

In the liver, newly absorbed lipids are incorporated into very low density lipoproteins (VLDL) and VLDL particles secreted by the liver are preferentially enriched with RRR–α-tocopherol. The liver is responsible for the control and release of RRR–α-tocopherol into human plasma.[289-295] It is now known that the function of the liver in maintaining plasma vitamin E concentration and the discrimination of the various forms of tocopherol are dependent on the cytosolic hepatic α-tocopherol transfer protein.[296] Originally identified,[297] purified, and characterized[298,299] in rat liver cytosol, it has now been isolated from human liver cytosol[300] and its complementary DNA sequence reported.[301] The human protein has a 94% homology with the rat protein and the gene has been localized to the 8q13.1–13.3 region of chromosome 8.[301,302] Furthermore, human deficiencies of this protein have now been reported that present as progressive peripheral neuropathy and ataxia.[303-306]

While being transported in the circulation, α-tocopherol is taken up by tissue other than the liver, including lung, heart, skeletal muscle, and adipose tissues. The concentration of tocopherol present in tissue is related to the amount of vitamin E consumed and the lipid content of the target organs. Fat accumulates α-tocopherol and can sequester it.[307] When the intake of vitamin E is high, the liver is a major repository, but the tocopherol pool in adipose tissue is much larger.

Although adipose tissue is sometimes considered a "store" of vitamin E, the tocopherol present in the adipocyte is not readily available to other tissue.[308] Intracellularly, vitamin E compounds are concentrated wherever there is abundant fatty acid, especially in phospholipid membrane–containing structures (e.g., mitochondria, microsomes, and plasma membranes).

The metabolism and turnover of α-tocopherol have been investigated only to a limited extent in the human and have not been adequately quantitated in any species. The major route of excretion of tocopherol metabolites appears to be fecal elimination, possibly in association with bile secretion and due to the fact that many forms of tocopherol in the diet are poorly absorbed. When a vitamin E–deficient diet is fed to animals, plasma and liver concentrations of α-tocopherol decrease rapidly. There seems to be two tocopherol pools present, at least in the rat: a rapidly metabolized pool (e.g., liver, plasma red cells) and a component that is retained for longer periods primarily present in adipose tissue, skeletal muscle, and neural tissue.[308]

Nutritional Assessment

In clinical studies, assessment for vitamin E status has depended on biochemical analysis of plasma or serum, erythrocytes, adipose tissue biopsies, and organs obtained at autopsy. In common practice, serum or plasma samples have been used most often to evaluate total tocopherol concentration. Most of the previous investigations utilizing colorimetric determination of total serum tocopherol have shown that a concentration about $0.5\,mg\cdot dl^{-1}$ indicates adequate nutritional status.[270] An improved assessment is obtained by measuring tocopherol isomers by high performance liquid chromatography, which provides precise determination of α-tocopherol concentrations as well as data on the other isomers.[309-311] Separation of the β and γ isomers is difficult. Consequently, these two vitamers are generally reported together as the β + γ fraction. Although 90% or more of the circulating vitamin E is normal α-tocopherol, large amounts of β + γ tocopherol and δ-tocopherol can be found in some circumstances. Unusually high proportions of β + γ tocopherol have been detected in adults on diets containing a predominance of γ-tocopherol (e.g., corn oil–supplemented diets).[312] Patients receiving the intravenous fat emulsion Intralipid have a high concentration of γ-tocopherol.[310]

In addition to measuring tocopherol concentration in blood, the peroxide hemolysis test is helpful in providing an index of antioxidant potential and vitamin E status. Although this test is not entirely specific, a normal result (<5% hemolysis during a 3-hour incubation in 2% H_2O_2) can be assumed to rule out vitamin E deficiency.[313]

Because of the marked influence of plasma lipids on circulating vitamin E concentration, tocopherol data have been expressed as a function of lipid concentration in many investigations.[313-315] These investigations have demonstrated that, although children have a significantly lower concentration of plasma vitamin E than the adult, a tocopherol/total lipid ratio of 0.6 to $0.8\,mg\cdot g^{-1}$ indicates adequate nutritional status.[313,314] Without the concurrent assessment of circulating lipids, it is possible that some individuals with low lipids are misclassified as vitamin E–deficient when they are actually normal.[313] Conversely, as demonstrated in studies of cholestatic children with marked hyperlipidemia, some hyperlipidemic subjects can have normal tocopherol concentrations per unit volume of plasma or serum but in reality may be significantly deficient in vitamin E.[315]

Maternal-Fetal Metabolism

A relatively low concentration of vitamin E is found in fetal tissues until body fat increases late in gestation. Although pregnancy is associated with a high maternal concentration of circulating vitamin E proportional to rising plasma lipids, transplacental delivery of tocopherols to the fetus is limited.[314] The ratio of maternal to fetal tocopherol concentration in blood is approximately 4:1, with the former concentration averaging $1.5\,mg\cdot dl^{-1}$ and the latter $0.38\,mg\cdot dl^{-1}$ in five series.[271] Similarly, neonatal tissue shows a relative paucity of vitamin E isomers. Not only is the neonatal tissue concentration generally low, but in the premature neonate the low proportion of adipose tissue further limits the total body vitamin E content.

There is a great interindividual variation in the human milk content of vitamin E. Colostrum contains relatively high concentrations of tocopherol isomers averaging $1.0 \pm 0.5\,mg\cdot dl^{-1}$.[316] After 2 weeks of lactation, the vitamin E concentration of human milk declines. Mature human milk contains all the expected isomers of tocopherol, but the vitamers other than α-tocopherol account for only about 2% of the vitamin E activity.[317] Generally, mature human milk contains 0.2 to $0.3\,mg\cdot dl^{-1}$ of α-tocopherol.[316] It is appropriate to examine milk vitamin E concentration in relation to PUFA. Although the lipid composition of human milk is influenced by maternal diet, it may be assumed that, on average, human milk provides approximately 6% of calories as linoleic acid. The amount of vitamin E concurrently ingested daily, approximately 2 mg of α-tocopherol equivalents in 750 ml of mature milk, appears to be adequate to prevent antioxidant deficiency in the term neonate. For the preterm infant, on the other hand, with lower initial stores and reduced intestinal absorption, human milk may not provide sufficient vitamin E.

Vitamin E Deficiency in Neonates

There have been three eras of investigation concerning vitamin E in neonates. From 1949 to 1967, generally stable neonates on enteral feedings were studied and their blood concentration of tocopherol were described along with some of the consequences of vitamin E deficiency (e.g., hemolysis).[266,269,270,318,319] When neonatal intensive care became routine during the 1970s, investigations were pursued on the vitamin E status of critically ill premature neonates leading to a better description of low vitamin E concentration and some of the associated clinical consequences and nutrient interactions.[283,320] During the 1980s more comprehensive investigations were performed on vitamin E status using sensitive microanalytical methods, and the interrelations between vitamin E and other nutrients have been more fully characterized.[310,311,321-323] The more recent reports have demonstrated that vitamin E deficiency is common among premature neonates receiving intensive care.[311,321-324] Some of these investigations have defined methods of correcting or preventing vitamin E deficiency in the critically ill, low birth weight neonate,[322,325-332] but they have identified toxicity associated with excessive doses of tocopherol preparations.[333]

The crisis in neonatal care associated with an alarming increase in retrolental fibroplasia during the late 1940s provided the occasion for the first demonstration that neonates are low in vitamin E. Owens and Owens[318] first called attention to this state of potential malnutrition in 1949 when they reported that a group of 46 premature infants, 2 to 8 weeks old, had serum total tocopherol concentrations averaging $0.2 \, mg \cdot dl^{-1}$, about one-half the mean value for adults. Shortly thereafter, this observation was confirmed.[319] In a series of 53 term and 32 premature neonates, all of whom had an uncomplicated hospital course, it was noted on the day of delivery that no significant differences were present in the serum tocopherol concentrations of the two groups.[319] However, whereas term neonates showed a significant increase in blood tocopherol concentration during the first week of life, the concentration in low birth weight infants did not increase until after 3 months of age.

The absorption of vitamin E in premature neonates has been studied primarily by the technique of administering large single dosages and measuring the blood concentration sequentially. From these results, it appears that neonates less than 32 weeks' gestation have significant malabsorption of tocopherol compared to term neonates and older children.[320] Prematurely delivered neonates may show evidence of vitamin E deficiency owing to several factors, including limited tissue storage at birth, intestinal malabsorption, and rapid growth rates that increase nutritional requirements in general. Many premature neonates may not be given enteral or even parenteral vitamin E for several days because of respiratory disorders requiring ventilator assistance. Even when they are given tocopherol supplements, premature neonates with respiratory distress syndrome may have a low blood tocopherol concentration.[311,320-322]

As reviewed elsewhere, the plasma tocopherol concentration in the premature neonate is far below the range found in the healthy adult ($0.5-1.5 \, mg \cdot dl^{-1}$).[270,323,324] Many studies have detected abnormally high rates of peroxide-induced erythrocyte hemolysis. Part of the explanation for low circulating tocopherol relates to decreased plasma lipids compared to the lipid concentration in adults. It is important to differentiate between tocopherol-sufficient and tocopherol-deficient premature neonates, particularly as parenteral vitamin E has been advocated in high doses for prophylaxis against neonatal disorders associated with oxygen toxicity.

To characterize further the apparent vitamin E deficiency of the premature neonate, a comprehensive analysis of vitamin E status was performed by analyzing tocopherol isomers, plasma lipids, and erythrocyte hemolysis in a group of 62 patients who received varied nutritional support over a 21-day study period.[311] The group of patients studied had a mean gestational age (±SD) of 31.2 ± 2.5 weeks (range 27–36 weeks) and a birth weight of 1475 ± 407 g (range 720–2240 g). There were no correlations between maternal and cord blood concentrations of β- and γ-tocopherol. However, for α-tocopherol there was a correlation ($r = 0.675, p < .01$) with neonates having about one-fourth the maternal concentration, as has been described by others. During the first 24 hours after delivery, in regard to total tocopherol and α-tocopherol concentrations, 95% and 98% of the neonates, respectively, were "abnormal" (i.e., below the lower limit of the adult normal range). The erythrocyte hemolysis test confirmed this vitamin E deficiency in 79% of those patients. Measures of vitamin E status rose during the 21-day study period. By using a well-established lower limit of normal peroxide hemolysis value to discriminate antioxidant status as a biologic index of vitamin E activity and mathematical or statistical modeling techniques, it was shown that the critical plasma tocopherol concentration is close to the $0.5 \, mg \cdot dl^{-1}$, conventionally accepted as the discriminator of vitamin E adequacy in the adult.[287,313]

Potential Consequences of Human Vitamin E Deficiency

As indicated in Table 42.2, several adverse consequences potentially attributable to vitamin E deficiency have been described in the medical literature in infants and children.[266,270,282,334-345] Unfortunately, controversy has surrounded almost all of the conditions attributed to human vitamin E deficiency or those claimed to be favorably

TABLE 42.2. Potential consequences of a low vitamin E concentration in children.

Hemolysis, which may lead to hemolytic anemia in premature infants[a]
Neuromuscular degeneration, characterized by axonal dystrophy in peripheral sensory nerves, posterior columns, and spinocerebellar tracts[b]
Increased risk of oxygen-toxicity conditions[c]
    Bronchopulmonary dysplasia
    Intraventricular hemorrhage
    Retinopathy of prematurity

---

[a] Susceptibility to anemia depends on other nutritional variables such as iron and polyunsaturated fatty acid intake.
[b] Neurologic dysfunction attributable to a low vitamin E concentration is especially common in chronic cholestatic hepatobiliary disorders such as biliary atresia but is not generally evident before 2 to 4 years of deficiency.
[c] As described in the text, controversy and dispute exist over the question of tocopherol's role and the relative risk of these three disorders in premature infants.

responsive to vitamin E therapy. Two lines of evidence have accumulated suggesting a role for tocopherol in human disease states: (1) signs and symptoms of a disorder potentially attributable to vitamin E deficiency have been documented and a corrective or preventative effect of vitamin E demonstrated (e.g., hemolytic anemia in premature infants); and (2) vitamin E supplementations, usually in pharmacologic amounts well above the recommended dietary allowance, have been utilized in clinical research protocols, and a lower incidence or severity of bronchopulmonary dysplasia and retinopathy of prematurity were initially reported. Despite numerous studies of this type, there have been relatively few clinical trials with adequate randomization and controlled conditions of study.

Hemolytic anemia of prematurity has been investigated repeatedly in relation to vitamin E therapy, ever since the first report by Oski and Barness[266] incriminating tocopherol deficiency as a responsible factor. As described in detail elsewhere, the conclusions from hematologic studies of vitamin E supplementation in the premature neonate differ depending on other variables that influence vitamin E status and requirements.[270,323] Nevertheless, the careful investigations of Gross and Melhorn[286] indicated the following: (1) an abnormal degree of hemolysis occurred in association with vitamin E deficiency; (2) supplementation of premature neonates with 25 IU of α-tocopherol acetate per day decreases the hemolysis and leads to a modest but significant increase in hemoglobin concentration; and (3) the hemolytic anemia associated with vitamin E deficiency is aggravated by ingestion of iron in iron-fortified formulas. It has been established that vitamin E deficiency under certain nutritional dietary conditions, contributes to accelerated hemolysis and causes prolonged anemia in the premature neonate.

A potential role of vitamin E supplementation in preventing or ameliorating retinopathy of prematurity was proposed in 1949 by Owens and Owens[318] and has remained controversial. It is difficult to interpret many clinical studies on this issue because of the predominant role of oxygen in injuring the immature retina and the fact that numerous variables have influenced every study. The assessment of retinopathy of prematurity has varied and often is subjective. The rationale for vitamin E therapy for this condition seems logical. The disease is characterized by a disorder of the control of retinal vascularization, leading to excessive proliferation of poorly organized fibrovascular tissue. In its severe form, retinopathy of prematurity causes retinal scarring, detachment, and blindness. Tocopherols are concentrated in the retinal tissue, where lipid concentrations are high and clearly can interrupt oxidation reactions that conceivably initiate the injury process. It has been proposed that vitamin E at a high concentration can suppress retinal neovascularization by inhibiting gap junction formation by spindle cells, the mesenchymal precursors of the inner retinal capillaries and putative inducers of neovascularization in this disease.[338,339]

Hittner et al.[337,338] were among the proponents of megasupplementation with vitamin E in premature neonates susceptible to retinopathy of prematurity. Their investigations, including a double-blind clinical trial, have shown an apparent beneficial effect when oral doses of tocopherol as high as $100 \text{ IU} \cdot \text{kg}^{-1} \text{day}^{-1}$ are given. The benefit is a reduced severity of the disease in susceptible neonates rather than its prevention. Another report has supported the use of vitamin E administration in high dosages.[336] In contrast, a negative controlled clinical trial was reported in which the investigators were unable to demonstrate prevention or amelioration of retinopathy of prematurity by vitamin E in large doses given intravenously.[344] It must be concluded that at present there is no conclusively demonstrated benefit to giving large doses of vitamin E for the intended purpose of preventing severe retinal disease.

Bronchopulmonary dysplasia is another condition of the premature neonate that was reported to be preventable by vitamin E therapy.[335] Further investigation of the role of vitamin E in bronchopulmonary dysplasia did not lead to confirmation of the original data, by either the same investigators[343] or others.[346,347] The rationale for this proposed effect is again logical, as tocopherols prevent oxidation-related injury of pulmonary membrane systems. In fact, the vitamin E–deficient animal showed an increased susceptibility to pulmonary oxygen toxicity. However, it cannot be claimed that vitamin E in large doses prevents bronchopulmonary dysplasia in the preterm infant.

Neurologic degeneration has been associated with chronic vitamin E deficiency. This topic has been reviewed in detail elsewhere.[340] Evidence suggests that between 1.5 and 4.0 years of age a low vitamin E concentration observed in children with cholestatic hepatobiliary disease and in other patients with malabsorption can cause neuromuscular degeneration. More specifically, axonal dystrophy has been observed in peripheral nerves and in spinal cord. Characteristic neurologic dysfunction may be prevented with appropriate vitamin E therapy.[340] This observation agrees well with studies of laboratory animals. There is now data suggesting vitamin E supplementation, if given in the first 12 hours of life, can reduce the incidence of intraventricular hemorrhage.[341,342,348,349] The hypothesis is that the effect is related to the vitamin's ability to scavenge free radicals, which then protects matrix capillary endothelial cells from hypoxic-ischemic injury. However, vitamin E in large doses cannot be recommended to prevent interventricular hemorrhage at this time. Further study is required.[350]

Vitamin E Requirements and Therapy

Because the neonate, especially the premature neonate, is born with low stores of α-tocopherol in addition to a decreased blood concentration, it is obvious that early provision of vitamin E is necessary to correct the deficiency state and prevent adverse consequences attributable to insufficient antioxidants. In the term neonate with normal intestinal absorption, it has been calculated from data obtained in studies of milk-fed neonates that $2\,mg \cdot day^{-1}$ is sufficient to raise blood and tissue concentrations. The amount is higher per kilogram than the 10 to 15 mg recommended for older children and adults. It is clear that normal blood and tissue concentrations of tocopherol can be achieved promptly in term neonates fed the usual volume of either breast milk or commercial formula.

The situation is different for the premature neonate. A variety of studies have been pursued to determine the vitamin E requirement of the premature neonate. Two kinds of investigation have been performed, the first dealing with neonates who received only parental nutrition support and the second investigating enterally fed neonates. The results in intravenously nourished neonates indicates that $1\,IU \cdot kg^{-1} day^{-1}$ eventually corrects the vitamin E deficiency state, but up to 7 to 10 days may be required.[350–352] Parenteral α-tocopherol acetate $3\,IU \cdot kg^{-1} day^{-1}$ rapidly corrects a low vitamin E concentration and abnormal peroxide hemolysis test within 24 hours.[322,325] Once a normal blood concentration of vitamin E is achieved, 1 to $2\,IU \cdot kg^{-1} day^{-1}$ can be given to maintain vitamin E sufficiency,[325] but without continued provision of tocopherol in the parenterally fed infant, insufficiency quickly develops.[322]

The pharmacokinetics of intravenously administered tocopherol preparations have been carefully studied.[332] Interestingly, it has been demonstrated that the acetate ester of α-tocopherol may not be adequately hydrolyzed when given intravenously. Accumulation of the acetate ester has been demonstrated in lung tissue. It is more likely that hydrolysis occurs in the intestine when preparations such as α-tocopherol acetate are provided by the enteral route.

In studies of enteral nutrition, it has been shown that a daily dose of 10 to 25 IU of water-miscible α-tocopherol acetate given to 0.6- to 1.5-kg neonates may be required to produce and maintain normal vitamin E status.[323–330] Six $IU \cdot kg^{-1} day^{-1}$ may be insufficient.[321] Even some neonates on this regimen may not maintain a plasma tocopherol concentration above $0.5\,mg \cdot dl^{-1}$, especially if they receive iron-fortified formula. Data from studies of enterally fed neonates are generally more difficult to interpret in relation to the dose and time required to correct a low blood E concentration. This point may be attributable to the variable intestinal absorption of tocopherol preparations in premature neonates, although some investigators dispute this.[353]

From studies of parenterally and enterally nourished premature neonates, it is reasonable to conclude that the immediate requirement of such neonates for absorbed vitamin E is 2 to $3\,IU \cdot kg^{-1} day^{-1}$ and that $1\,IU \cdot kg^{-1} day^{-1}$ suffices once the initial deficiency state is corrected and tissue stores are established. The decreased intestinal absorption that has been well demonstrated makes it necessary to give larger amounts (i.e., $10-25\,IU \cdot kg^{-1} day^{-1}$) when vitamin E supplements are provided enterally.

Megavitamin E supplementation of the premature neonate has been studied because of the interest of various groups to produce high tocopherol concentration in an effort to prevent or ameliorate severe retinopathy of prematurity.[336–339,344] These studies have been associated with oral doses as high as $100\,mg \cdot kg^{-1} day^{-1}$ and blood concentration of more than $3.5\,mg \cdot dl^{-1}$. It is difficult to recommend such doses, particularly because no protective effect on retinopathy was demonstrated in a randomized, controlled clinical trial.[344] Serious toxicity has been associated with megavitamin E supplement in premature neonates.[333] As reviewed elsewhere, the adverse effects may be attributable to the vehicle used for megavitamin E supplementation rather than the tocopherol preparation per se.[323] Doses of vitamin E of 1 to $3\,IU \cdot kg^{-1} day^{-1}$ by the parenteral route or $25\,IU \cdot kg^{-1} day^{-1}$ by the enteral route should be regarded as experimental and having potentially more risk than benefit for premature neonates at this time.

Summary

The four fat-soluble vitamins discussed in this chapter play important roles in perinatal metabolism and nutrition. They share many similarities with one another and there are relatively few major differences beyond their

TABLE 42.3. Comparison of fat-soluble vitamins (A, D, K, E).

Similarities

All are generic designations for a family of compounds; vitamins A and E are important antioxidants

Placental transfer—limited; maternal and fetal levels generally do not correlate, except for α-tocopherol

Absorbed from small intestine requiring bile salts and micellar formation; all are absorbed through the lymphatic system

All are stored in the liver; vitamin E stored in other tissues (fat and muscle) exceeds that in the liver

There are deficiency states unique to neonates; infant deficiency states of vitamins A and K are worldwide problems

Pharmacologic doses are used in neonates for prophylaxis and therapy

Pharmacologic doses have resulted in neonatal disasters

Plasma levels not sufficient to assess needs; vitamins A, E, and K have functional methods of assessment

Differences

Vitamin D is a prohormone

Vitamins A and D have specific cellular and circulating binding proteins; vitamins E and K are transported by nonspecific proteins, e.g., low-density and high-density lipoproteins

Vitamins A and D are involved in nuclear signaling and effect DNA transcription; vitamins E and K are not known to act at this level

Vitamin K is extremely low in human milk at all stages, compared to A, D, and E; deficiency states are described in breast-fed infants for vitamins K and D

Vitamin K can be synthesized by colonic bacteria

Vitamin K sufficiency may be assessed by a circulating abnormal protein

physiologic affect. These differences and similarities are summarized in Table 42.3.

References

1. Blomhoff R. Overview of vitamin A metabolism and function. In: Blomhoff R, ed. Vitamin A in health and disease. New York: Marcel Dekker, 1994:1–35.
2. Crow JA, Ong DE. Cell-specific immunohistochemical localization of cellular retinol-binding protein (type two) in the small intestine of rat. Proc Natl Acad Sci USA 1985;82:4707–4711.
3. Ong DE, Newcomer ME, Chytil F. Cellular retinol-binding proteins. In: Sporn MB, Roberts AB, Goodman DS, eds. The retinoids. 2nd ed. Orlando, FL: Academic Press, 1994:283–318.
4. Blomhoff R. Transport and metabolism of vitamin A. Nutr Rev 1994;52:513–523.
5. Soprano DR, Blaner WS. Plasma retinol-binding proteins. In: Sporn MB, Roberts AB, Goodman DS, eds. The retinoids. 2nd ed. Orlando, FL: Academic Press, 1994:257–282.
6. Saari JC. Retinoids in photosensitive systems. In: Sporn MB, Roberts AB, Goodman DS, eds. The retinoids. 2nd ed. Orlando, FL: Academic Press, 1994:351–386.
7. Napoli JL. Retinoic acid homeostasis: prospective roles of β carotene, retinol, CRBP and CRABP. In: Blomhoff R, ed. Vitamin A in health and disease. New York: Marcel Dekker, 1994:135–188.
8. Gudas LJ, Sporn MG, Roberts AB. Cellular biology and biochemistry of the retinoids. In: Sporn MG, Roberts AB, Goodman DS, eds. The retinoids. 2nd ed. Orlando, FL: Academic Press, 1994:443–520.
9. Chytil F. Vitamin A. Its role in differentiation and development in nutritional disease: research directions in comparative pathobiology. New York: Alan R. Liss 1986:21–31.
10. Mangelsdorf DJ, Umesono K, Evans RM. The retinoid receptors. In: Sporn MB, Roberts AB, Goodman DS, eds. The retinoids. 2nd ed. Orlando, FL: Academic Press, 1994:319–350.
11. Hofmann C, Eichele G. Retinoids in development. In: Sporn MB, Roberts AB, Goodman DS, eds. The retinoids. 2nd ed. Orlando, FL: Academic Press, 1994:387–441.
12. Blaner WS, Olson JA. Retinol and retinoic acid metabolism. In: Sporn MB, Roberts AB, Goodman DS, eds. The retinoids. 2nd ed. Orlando, FL: Academic Press, 1994:229–256.
13. Takahashi YI, Smith JE, Goodman DS. Vitamin A and retinol binding protein metabolism during fetal development in the rat. Am J Physiol 1977;233:E263–E272.
14. Rasmussen M, Petersen LB, Norum KR. Liver retinoids and retinol esterification in fetal and pregnant rats at term. Scand J Gastroenterol 1985;20:696–700.
15. Green T, Ford HC. Intracellular binding proteins for retinol and retinoic acid in early and term human placentas. Br J Obstet Gynaecol 1986;93:833–838.
16. Torma H, Vahlquist A. Uptake of vitamin A and retinol binding protein by human placenta in vitro. Placenta 1986;7:295–305.
17. Gardner EM, Ross AC. Dietary vitamin A restriction produces marginal vitamin A status in young rats. J Nutr 1993;123:1435–1443.
18. Dostalova L. Correlation of the vitamin status between mother and newborn at delivery. Dev Pharmacol Ther 1982;4:45–47.
19. Butte NF, Calloway DH. Proteins, vitamin A, carotene, folacin, ferritin and zinc in Navajo maternal and cord blood. Biol Neonate 1982;41:273–278.
20. Hustead VA, Gutcher GR, Anderson SA, et al. Relationship of vitamin A (retinol) status to lung disease in the preterm infant. J Pediatr 1984;105:610–615.
21. Vobecky JS, Vobecky J, Shapcott D, et al. Biochemical indices of nutritional status in maternal, cord, and early neonatal blood. Am J Clin Nutr 1982;36:630–642.
22. Underwood BA. Maternal vitamin A status and its importance in infancy and early childhood. Am J Clin Nutr 1994;59(suppl):517S–524S.
23. Sklan D, Shalit I, Lasebnik N, et al. Retinol transport proteins and concentrations in human amniotic fluid, placenta, and fetal and maternal sera. Br J Nutr 1985;54:577–583.
24. Wallingford JC, Milunsky A, Underwood BA. Vitamin A and retinol binding protein in amniotic fluid. Am J Clin Nutr 1983;38:377–381.
25. Parkinson CE, Tan JCY. Vitamin A concentration in amniotic fluid and maternal serum related to neural tube defects. Br J Obstet Gynaecol 1982;89:935–939.

26. Koskinin T, Valtonen P, Lehtovaara I, et al. Amniotic fluid retinol concentrations in late pregnancy. Biol Neonate 1986;49:81–84.
27. Drott P, Meurling S. Plasma concentrations of fat soluble vitamins A and E in neonates with myelomeningocele. Eur J Pediatr Surg 1992;2(5):265–268.
28. Burnett D, Bradwell AR. The origin of plasma proteins in human amniotic fluid: the significance of alpha-antichymotrypsin complexes. Biol Neonate 1980;37:302–307.
29. Robens JR. Teratogenic effects of hypervitaminosis A in the hamster and guinea pig. Toxicol Appl Pharmacol 1970;16:88–94.
30. Geelan JCA. Hypervitaminosis A-induced teratogenesis. CRC Crit Rev Toxicol 1979;6:351–375.
31. Shenefelt RE. Morphogenesis of malformations in hamsters caused by retinoic acid: relation to dose and stage at treatment. Teratology 1972;5:103–118.
32. Rothman KJ, Moore LL, Singer MR, et al. Teratogenicity of high vitamin A intake. N Engl J Med 1995;333:1369–1373.
33. Lammer EJ, Chen DT, Hoar RM, et al. Retinoic acid embryopathy. N Engl J Med 1985;313:837–841.
34. Benke PJ. The isotretinoin teratogen syndrome. JAMA 1984;251:3267–3269.
35. Lott IT, Bocian M, Pribram HW, et al. Fetal hydrocephalus and ear anomalies associated with maternal use of isotretinoin. J Pediatr 1984;105:597–602.
36. Goodman DS. Overview of current knowledge of metabolism of vitamin A and carotenoids. J Natl Cancer Inst 1984;73:1375–1379.
37. Lohnes D, Mark M, Mendelsohn C, et al. Developmental roles of the retinoic acid receptors. J Steroid Biochem Mol Biol 1995;53:475–486.
38. Soprano DR, Tairis N, Gyda M III, et al. Induction of RAR β2 gene expression in embryos and RAR β2 transactivation by the synthetic retinoid RO 13-6307 correlates with its high teratogenic potency. Toxicol Appl Pharmacol 1993;122:159–163.
39. Soprano DR, Gyda M III, Jiang H, et al. A sustained elevation in retinoic acid receptor β2 mRNA and protein occurs during retinoic acid-induced fetal dysmorphogenesis. Mech Dev 1994;45:243–253.
40. Look J, Landevehr J, Bauer F, et al. Marked resistance of RAR γ deficient mice to the toxic effects of retinoic acid. Am J Physiol 1995;269(Endocrinol Met 32):E91–E98.
41. Grummer MA, Zachman RD. The effect of ethanol ingestion on fetal vitamin A in the rat. Pediatr Res 1990;28:186–189.
42. DeJonge MH, Zachman RD. The effect of maternal ethanol ingestion on fetal rat vitamin A: a model for fetal alcohol syndrome. Pediatr Res 1995;37:418–423.
43. Grummer MA, Zachman RD. Prenatal ethanol consumption alters the expression of cellular retinol binding protein and retinoic acid receptor mRNA in fetal rat embryo and brain. Alcoholism Clin Exp Res 1995;19:1376–1381.
44. Duester G. Are ethanol-induced birth defects caused by functional retinoic acid deficiency? In: Blomhoff R, ed. Vitamin A in health and disease. New York: Marcel Dekker, 1994:343–363.
45. Nau H, Tzimas G, Mondry M, et al. Antiepileptic drugs alter endogenous retinoid concentrations: a possible mechanism of teratogenesis of anticonvulsant therapy. Life Sci 1995;57:53–60.
46. Ostrea EM Jr, Balum JE, Winkler R, et al. Influence of breastfeeding on the restoration of the low serum concentration of vitamin E and β-carotene in the newborn infant. Am J Obstet Gynecol 1986;154:1014–1017.
47. Zachman RD, Grummer MA. Uptake and metabolism of β-carotene in isolated rat lung type II cells. Pediatr Res 1989;25:333A.
48. Ong DE. Absorption of vitamin A. In: Blomhoff R, ed. Vitamin A in health and disease. New York: Marcel Dekker, 1994:37–72.
49. MacDonald PN, Ong DE. Binding specificities of cellular retinol-binding protein and cellular retinol-binding protein, type II. J Biol Chem 1987;262:10550–10556.
50. Li E, Demmer LA, Sweetser DA, et al. Rat cellular retinol-binding protein. II. Use of a cloned cDNA to define its primary structure, tissue specific expression and developmental regulation. Proc Natl Acad Sci USA 1986;83:5779–5783.
51. Ong DE, Lucas PC, Kakkad B, Quick TC. Ontogeny of two vitamin A-metabolizing enzymes and two retinol-binding proteins present in the small intestine of rat. J Lipid Res 1991;32:1521–1527.
52. Rubin DC, Ong DE, Gordon JI. Cellular differentiation in the emerging fetal rat small intestinal epithelium: mosaic patterns of gene expression. Proc Natl Acad Sci USA 1989;86:1278–1282.
53. Quick TC, Ong DE. Levels of cellular retinol binding proteins in the small intestine of rats during pregnancy and lactation. J Lipid Res 1989;30:1049–1054.
54. Herr F, MacDonald PN, Ong DE. Partial purification and characterization of lecithin-retinol acyltransferase from rat liver. J Nutr Biochem 1991;2:503–511.
55. Matsumoto E, Hirosawa K, Abe K, et al. Development of the vitamin A storing cell in mouse liver during late fetal and neonatal periods. Anat Embryol 1984;169:249–259.
56. Kato M, Kato K, Goodman DS. Immunochemical studies on the localization and on the concentration of cellular retinol-binding protein in rat liver during perinatal development. Lab Invest 1985;52:475–484.
57. Ismadi SD, Olson JA. Dynamics of the fetal distribution and transfer of vitamin A between rat fetuses and their mother. Int J Vitam Nutr Res 1982;52:111–118.
58. Zachman RD, Kakkad B, Chytil F. Perinatal rat lung retinol (vitamin A) and retinyl palmitate. Pediatr Res 1984;18:1297–1299.
59. Batres RO, Olson JA. A marginal vitamin A status alters the distribution of vitamin A among parenchymal and stellate cells in rat liver. J Nutr 1987;117:874–879.
60. Green MJ, Green JB, Lewis KC. Variation in retinol utilization rate with vitamin A status in rat. J Nutr 1987;117:694–703.
61. Olson JA. Recommended dietary intakes (RDI) of vitamin A in humans. Am J Clin Nutr 1987;45:704–716.
62. Olson JA, Gunning DB, Tilton RA. Liver concentrations of vitamin A and carotenoids, as a function of age and

other parameters of American children who died of various causes. Am J Clin Nutr 1984;39:903–910.
63. Shenai JP, Chytil F, Stahlman MT. Liver vitamin A reserves of very low birth weight neonates. Pediatr Res 1985;19:892–893.
64. Sharma HS, Misra UK. Postnatal distribution of vitamin A in liver, lung, heart and brain of the rat in relation to maternal vitamin A status. Biol Neonate 1986;50:345–350.
65. Gehre-Medhin M, Vahlquist A. Vitamin A nutrition in the human fetus. Acta Paediatr Scand 1984;73:333–340.
66. Zachman RD, Valceschini G. Effect of premature delivery on rat lung retinol (vitamin A) and retinyl ester stores. Biol Neonate 1988;54:285–288.
67. Shenai JP, Chytil F. Vitamin A storage in lungs during perinatal development in the rat. Biol Neonate 1990;57:126–132.
68. Shenai JP, Chytil F. Effect of maternal vitamin A administration on fetal lung vitamin A stores in the perinatal rat. Biol Neonate 1990;58:318–325.
69. Ubels JL, Osgood TB, Foley KM. Vitamin A is stored as fatty acyl esters of retinol in the lacrimal gland. Curr Eye Res 1988;7:1009–1016.
70. Napoli JL, McCormick AM, O'Meara B, et al. Vitamin A metabolism; alpha-tocopherol modulates tissue retinol levels in vivo, and retinyl palmitate hydrolase in vitro. Arch Biochem Biophys 1984;230:194–202.
71. Gutcher GR, Raynor WJ, Farrell PM. An evaluation of vitamin E status in premature infants. Am J Clin Nutr 1984;40:1078–1089.
72. Chen WYJ, James HO, Glover J. Retinol transport proteins. Biochem Soc Trans 1986;14:925–928.
73. Zachman RD. Retinol (vitamin A) and the neonates: special problem of the human premature infant. Am J Clin Nutr 1989;50:413–424.
74. Shenai JP, Chytil F, Jhaveri A, et al. Plasma vitamin A and retinol binding protein in premature and term neonates. J Pediatr 1981;99:302–305.
75. Borek C, Smith JE, Soprano DR, et al. Regulation of retinol-binding protein metabolism by glucocorticoid hormones in cultured H_4IIEC_3 liver cells. Endocrinology 1981;109:386–391.
76. Hustead VA, Zachman RD. The effect of antenatal dexamethasone on maternal and fetal retinol-binding protein. Am J Obstet Gynecol 1986;154:203–205.
77. Georgieff MK, Chockalingam UM, Sasanow SR, et al. The effect of antenatal betamethasone on cord blood concentrations of retinol-binding protein, transthyretin, transferrin, retinol and vitamin E. J Pediatr Gastroenterol Nutr 1988;7:713–718.
78. Georgieff MK, Susanow SR, Mammal MC, et al. Cord prealbumin values in newborn infants: effect of prenatal steroids, pulmonary maturity, and size for dates. J Pediatr 1986;108:972–976.
79. Hustead VA, Greger J, Gutcher GR. Zinc supplementation and plasma concentration of vitamin A in preterm infants. Am J Clin Nutr 1988;47:1017–1021.
80. Lockitch G, Godolphin W, Pendray MR, et al. Serum zinc, copper, retinol binding protein, pre-albumin, and ceruloplasmin concentrations in infants receiving intravenous zinc and copper supplementation. J Pediatr 1983;102:304–308.
81. Kylberg HK, Ong DE, Chytil F. Cellular retinol binding protein during postnatal development of the rat small intestine. Biol Neonate 1981;39:100–104.
82. Ong DE, Chytil F. Changes in levels of cellular retinol and retinol acid-binding proteins of liver and lung during perinatal development of rat. Proc Natl Acad Sci USA 1976;73:3976–3978.
83. Frolik CA. Metabolism of retinoids. In: Sporn MG, Roberts AB, Goodman DS, eds. The retinoids, vol. 2. Orlando, FL: Academic Press 1984:177–208.
84. West KP Jr. Vitamin A deficiency: its epidemiology and relation to child mortality and morbidity. In: Blomhoff R, ed. Vitamin A in health and disease. New York: Marcel Dekker, 1994:585–614.
85. Blomhoff HK, Smeland EB. Role of retinoids in normal hematopoiesis and the immune system. In: Blomhoff R, ed. Vitamin A in health and disease. New York: Marcel Dekker, 1994:451–484.
86. Ross AC. Vitamin A status: relationship to immunity and the antibody response. Proc Soc Exp Biol Med 1992;200:303–320.
87. Semba RD, Graham NMH, Caiaffa WT, et al. Increased mortality associated with vitamin A deficiency during human immunodeficiency virus type 1 infection. Arch Intern Med 1993;153:2149–2154.
88. Semba RD, Miotti PG, Chiphangivi JD, et al. Maternal vitamin A deficiency and mother to child transmission of HIV-1. Lancet 1994;343:1593–1597.
89. Rush MG, Hazinski TA. Current therapy of BPD. Clin Perinatol 1992;19:563–590.
90. Chytil F. The lungs and vitamin A. Am J Physiol 1992;262:L517–L527.
91. Blackfan KD, Wolach SB. Vitamin A deficiency in infants. A clinical and pathological study. J Pediatr 1933;3:679–706.
92. Harris CC, Sporn MB, Kaufman DG, et al. Histogenesis of squamous metaplasia in hamster tracheal epithelium caused by vitamin A deficiency or benzopyrene ferric oxide. J Natl Cancer Inst 1972;48:743–761.
93. Boren HG, Pauley J, Wright EG, et al. Cell population in the hamster tracheal epithelium in relation to vitamin A status. Int J Vitam Nutr Res 1974;44:382–390.
94. Northway WH, Rosan RC, Porter DY. Pulmonary disease following respirator therapy of hyaline-membrane disease. N Engl J Med 1967;276:357–368.
95. Mupanemunda RH, Lee DSC, Fraher LJ, et al. Postnatal changes in serum retinol status in very low birthweight infants. Early Hum Dev 1994;38:45–54.
96. Shenai JP, Chytil F, Stahlman MT. Vitamin A status of neonates with bronchopulmonary dysplasia. Pediatr Res 1985;19:185–188.
97. Shenai JP, Kennedy KA, Chytil F, et al. Clinical trial of vitamin A supplementation in infants susceptible to bronchopulmonary dysplasia. J Pediatr 1987;111:269–277.
98. Chan V, Greenough A, Cheeseman P, et al. Vitamin A levels at birth of high risk preterm infants. J Perinat Med 1993;21:147–151.
99. Papagaroufalis C, Caires M, Pantazataou E, et al. A trial of vitamin A supplementation for the prevention of

99. bronchopulmonary dysplasia (BPD) in very-low-birthweight (VLBW) infants. Pediatr Res 1988;23:518A(A).
100. Chabra S, Arnold JD, Leslie GI, et al. Vitamin A status in preterm neonates with and without chronic lung disease. J Paediatr Child Health 1994;30:432–435.
101. Zachman RD, Samuels DP, Brand JM, et al. Use of the intramuscular relative dose response test to predict bronchopulmonary dysplasia in premature infants. Am J Clin Nutr 1996;63:123–129.
102. Shenai JP, Rush MG, Stahlman MT, et al. Plasma retinol binding protein response to vitamin A administration in infants susceptible to bronchopulmonary dysplasia. J Pediatr 1990;116:607–614.
103. Shenai JP. Vitamin A in lung development and bronchopulmonary dysplasia. In: Blomhoff R, ed. Vitamin A in health and disease. New York: Marcel Dekker, 1994:323–342.
104. Robbins ST, Fletcher AB. Early vs. delayed vitamin A supplementation in very-low-birth-weight infants. J Parenter Enteral Nutr 1993;17:220–225.
105. Pearson E, Bose C, Snidow T, et al. Trial of vitamin A supplementation in very low birth weight infants at risk for bronchopulmonary dysplasia. J Pediatr 1992;121:420–427.
106. Landman J, Sive A, Heise HD, et al. Comparison of enteral and intramuscular vitamin A supplementation in preterm infants. Early Hum Dev 1992;30:163–170.
107. Rush MG, Shenai JP, Parker RA, et al. Intramuscular versus enteral vitamin A supplementation in very low birth weight neonates. J Pediatr 1994;125:458–462.
108. Agaoestina T, Humphrey JH, Taylor GA, et al. Safety of one 52-μmol (50,000 IU) oral dose of vitamin A administered to neonates. Bull World Health Org 1994;72:859–868.
109. McMenamy KR, Anderson MJ, Zachman RD. Effect of dexamethasone and oxygen exposure on neonatal rat lung retinoic acid receptor proteins. Pediatr Pulmonol 1994;18:232–238.
110. Grummer MA, Zachman RD. Postnatal rat lung retinoic acid receptor (RAR) mRNA expression and effects of dexamethasone of RAR β mRNA. Pediatr Pulmonol 1995;20:234–240.
111. Grummer MA, John ML, Zachman RD. The interaction of retinoic acid (RA) and dexamethasone (DEX) on retinoic acid receptors (RARs) and surfactant protein C (SP-C) in fetal rat lung explants (FLE) and the murine lung epithelial (MLE) cell line. Pediatr Res 1996;39:357A.
112. Georgieff MK, Mammel MC, Mills MM, et al. Effect of postnatal steroid administration on serum vitamin A concentration in newborn infants with respiratory compromise. J Pediatr 1989;114:301–304.
113. Underwood BA. Vitamin A in animal and human nutrition. In: Sporn MG, Goodman DS, eds. The retinoids, vol. 1. New York: Academic Press, 1984;281–392.
114. Meyer KA, Popper H, Steigmann F, et al. Comparison of vitamin A of liver biopsy specimens with plasma vitamin A in man. Proc Soc Exp Biol Med 1942;49:589–591.
115. Olson JA. Serum levels of vitamin A and carotenoids as reflectors of nutritional status. J Natl Cancer Inst 1984;73:1439–1444.
116. Montreewasuwat N, Olson JA. Serum and liver concentrations of vitamin A in Thai fetuses as a function of gestational age. Am J Clin Nutr 1979;32:601–606.
117. Loerch JD, Underwood AB, Lewis KC. Response of plasma levels of vitamin A to a dose of vitamin A as an indicator of hepatic vitamin A reserves in rats. J Nutr 1979;109:778–786.
118. Flores H, Campos F, Araujo C, et al. Assessment of marginal vitamin A deficiency in Brazilian children using the relative dose response procedure. Am J Clin Nutr 1984;40:1281–1289.
119. Tanumihardjo SA, Olson JA. A modified relative dose response assay employing 3,4-didehydroretinol (vitamin A2) in rats. J Nutr 1988;118:598–603.
120. Tanumihardjo SA, Koellner PG, Olson JA. The modified relative-dose-response assay as an indicator of vitamin A status in a population of well-nourished American children. Am J Clin Nutr 1990;52:1064–1067.
121. Tanumihardjo SA, Permaesih D, Dahro AM, et al. Comparison of vitamin A status assessment techniques in children from two Indonesian villages. Am J Clin Nutr 1994;60:136–141.
122. Garner EM, Ross AC. Dietary vitamin A restriction produces marginal vitamin A status in young rats. J Nutr 1993;123:1434–1443.
123. Kawashima H, Kurokawa K. Metabolism and sites of action of vitamin D in the kidney. Kidney Int 1986;29:98–107.
124. Carlberg C. Mechanisms of nuclear signaling by vitamin D_3 interplay with retinoid and thyroid hormone signaling. Eur J Biochem 1995;231:517–527.
125. Johnson JA, Grande JP, Roche PC, et al. Ontogeny of the 1,25-dihydroxyvitamin D_3 receptor in fetal rat bone. J Bone Miner Res 1996;11:56–61.
126. Hollis BW, Pittard WB. Evaluation of the total fetomaternal vitamin D relationships at term: evidence for social differences. J Clin Endocrinol Metab 1984;59:652–657.
127. Greer FR, Hollis BW, Napoli JL. High concentration of vitamin D_2 in human milk associated with pharmacologic doses of vitamin D_2. J Pediatr 1984;105:61–64.
128. Wieland P, Fischer JA, Trechsel IU, et al. Perinatal parathyroid hormone, vitamin D metabolites, and calcitonin in man. Am J Physiol 1980;239:E385–E390.
129. Seino Y, Ishida M, Yamaoka K. Serum calcium regulating hormones in the perinatal period. Calcif Tissue Int 1982;34:131–135.
130. Delvin EE, Glorieux FH, Salle BL, et al. Control of vitamin D metabolism in preterm infants: fetomaternal relationships. Arch Dis Child 1982;57:754–757.
131. Bouillon R, Van Baelen H, DeMoor P. 25-Hydroxyvitamin D and its binding protein in maternal and cord serum. J Clin Endocrinol Metab 1977;45:679–684.
132. Weisman Y, Occhipenti M, Knox G, et al. Concentration of 24,25-dihydroxyvitamin D and 25-hydroxyvitamin D in paired maternal-cord sera. Am J Obstet Gynecol 1978;130:704–707.
133. Paunier L, Lacoort G, Pelland P, et al. 25-Hydroxyvitamin D and calcium levels in maternal, cord and infant serum in relation to maternal vitamin D intake. Helv Paediat Acta 1978;33:95–103.

134. Shimotsuji T, Seino Y, Ishida M. Relations of plasma 25-hydroxyvitamin D levels in mothers, cord blood and newborn infants, and postnatal change in plasma 25-hydroxyvitamin D levels. J Nutr Sci Vitamin (Tokyo) 1979;25:79–86.
135. Gertner JM, Glassman MS, Coustan DR, et al. Feto-maternal vitamin D relationships at term. J Pediatr 1980;97:637–640.
136. Cockburn F, Belton NR, Purvis RJ, et al. Maternal vitamin D intake and mineral metabolism in mothers and their newborn infants. Br Med J 1980;281:11–14.
137. Kuroda E, Okano T, Mizuno N. Plasma levels of 25-hydroxyvitamin D_2 and 25-hydroxyvitamin D_3 in maternal cord and neonatal blood. J Nutr Sci Vitaminol 1981;27:55–65.
138. Verity CM, Burman D, Beadle PC, et al. Seasonal changes in perinatal vitamin D metabolism: maternal and cord blood biochemistry in normal pregnancies. Arch Dis Child 1981;56:943–948.
139. Zhao D, Xue Q, Xue, Y. Serum 25-OHD levels in maternal and cord blood in Beijing, China. Acta Paediatr Scand 1990;79:1240–1241.
140. Glasgow JFT, McBride J, Fairney A. The effect of local atmospheric temperature upon umbilical cord 25-hydroxyvitamin D. Br J Med Sci 1982;151:180–183.
141. Weisman Y, Sapir R, Harell A, et al. Maternal-perinatal interrelationships of vitamin D metabolism in rats. Biochim Biophy Acta 1976;428:388–395.
142. Rebut-Bonneton C, Demignon J, Cancela L, et al. Effect of 25-hydroxyvitamin D_3 and 1,25-dihydroxyvitamin D_3 maternal loads on maternal and fetal vitamin D metabolite level in the rat. Reprod Nutr Dev 1985;25:583–590.
143. Goff JP, Horst RI, Littledike ET. Effect of the maternal vitamin D status at parturition on the vitamin D status of the neonatal calf. J Nutr 1982;112:1387–1393.
144. Devaskar UP, Ho M, Devaskar SU, et al. 25-Hydroxy-and 1α,25-dihydroxyvitamin D. Maternal-fetal relationship and the transfer of 1,25-dihydroxyvitamin D_3 across the placenta in an ovine model. Dev Pharmacol Ther 1983;7:213–220.
145. Schedewie H, Slikker W, Hill D, et al. Transplacental transfer of 1,25(OH)$_2$ vitamin D in subhuman primates. Clin Res 1979;27:813A.
146. Marx SJ, Swart EG, Hamstra AJ, et al. Normal intrauterine development of the fetus of a woman receiving extraordinarily high doses of 1,25-dihydroxyvitamin D. J Clin Endocrinol Metab 1980;51:1138–1142.
147. Salle BL, Berthezene F, Glorieux FH, et al. Hypoparathyroidism during pregnancy: treatment with calcitriol. J Clin Endocrinol Metab 1981;52:810–813.
148. Ron M, Levitz J, Chuba J, et al. Transfer of 25-hydroxyvitamin D_3 and 1,25-dihydroxyvitamin D_3 across the perfused human placenta. Am J Obstet Gynecol 1984;148:370–374.
149. Fleischman AR, Rosen JF, Cole J, et al. Maternal and fetal serum 1,24-dihydroxyvitamin D levels at term. J Pediatr 1980;97:640–642.
150. Steichen JJ, Tsang RC, Gratton TL, et al. Vitamin D homeostasis in the perinatal period, 1,25-dihydroxyvitamin D in maternal, cord, and neonatal blood. N Engl J Med 1980;302:315–319.
151. Markestad T, Aksnes L, Alslein M, et al. 25-Hydroxyvitamin D and 1,25-dihydroxyvitamin D or D_2 and D_3 origin in maternal and umbilical cord serum after vitamin D_2 supplementation in human pregnancy. Am J Clin Nutr 1984;40:1057–1063.
152. Delvin EE, Arabian A, Glorieux FH, et al. In vitro metabolism of 25-hydroxycholecalciferol by isolated cells from human decidua. J Clin Endocrinol Metab 1985;60:880–885.
153. Zerwekh JE, Breslau NA. Human placental production of 1α,25-dihydroxyvitamin D_3: biochemical characterization and production in normal subjects and patients with pseudohypoparathyroidism. J Clin Endocrinol Metab 1986;62:192–196.
154. Pike JW, Gooze LL, Haussler MR. Biochemical evidence of 1,25-dihydroxyvitamin D receptor macromolecules in parathyroid, pancreatic, pituitary and placental tissues. Life Sci 1980;26:407–414.
155. Durand D, Barlet J-P, Braithwaite GD. The influence of 1,25-dihydroxycalciferol on the mineral content of foetal guinea-pigs. Reprod Nutr Dev 1983;23:235–244.
156. Durand D, Braithwaite GD, Barlet J-P. The effect of low hydroxycalciferol on the placental transfer of calcium and phosphate in sheep. Br J Nutr 1983;49:475–480.
157. Brommage R, DeLuca HF. Placental transport of calcium and phosphorus is not regulated by vitamin D. Am J Physiol 1984;246:F526–F529.
158. Care AD. The placental transfer of calcium. J Dev Physiol 1991;15:253–257.
159. Care AD. Calcium homeostasis in the foetus. J Dev Physiol 1980;2:85–99.
160. Moore ES, Langman CB, Favus MJ, et al. Role of fetal 1,25-dihydroxyvitamin D production in intrauterine phosphorus and calcium homeostasis. Pediatr Res 1985;19:566–569.
161. Garel J-M, Pic P, Jost A. Action de la parathormone chez le foetus de rat. Ann Endocrinol 1971;32:253–262.
162. Rodda CP, Kubota M, Heath JA, et al. Evidence for a novel parathyroid hormone-related protein in fetal lamb parathyroid glands and sheep placenta: comparisons with a similar protein implicated in humoral hypercalcaemia of malignancy. J Endocrinol 1988;117:261–271.
163. Moseley JM, Gillespi MT. Parathyroid hormone-related protein. Crit Rev Clin Lab Sci 1995;32:299–343.
164. Philbrick WM, Wysolmerski JJ, Galbraith S, et al. Defining the roles of parathyroid hormone-related protein in normal physiology. Physiol Rev 1996;76:127–173.
165. Ross R, Care AD, Robinson JS, et al. Perinatal 1,25(OH)$_2$D$_3$ in the sheep and its role in the maintenance of the transplacental calcium gradient. J Endocrinol 1980;87:17P–18P.
166. Lester GE, Gray TK, Lorenc RS. Evidence for maternal and fetal difference in vitamin D metabolism. Proc Soc Exp Biol Med 1978;159:303–307.
167. Salle BL, Glorieux FH, Delvin EE. Perinatal vitamin D metabolisms. Biol Neonate 1988;54:181–187.
168. Kuoppala T, Tuinrala R, Parvianinen M, et al. Can fetus regulate its calcium uptake? Br J Ob Gynaecol 1984;91:1912–1916.

169. Bouillon R, Van Assche FA, Van Baelen H. Influence of the vitamin D-binding protein on the serum concentration of 1,25-dihydroxyvitamin D_3: significance of the free 1,25-dihydroxyvitamin D_3 concentration. Clin Invest 1981;67:589–596.
170. Bouillon R, Van Baelen H, DeMoor P. 25-Hydroxyvitamin D and its binding protein in maternal and serum. J Clin Endocrinol Metab 1977;45:679–684.
171. Hillman LS, Haddad JG. Serial analyses of serum vitamin D binding protein in preterm infants from birth to postconceptual maturity. J Clin Endocrinol Metab 1983;56:189–191.
172. Auconi P, Biogini R, Colarizi P. Vitamin D-binding protein in the prenatal period. Eur J Pediatr 1985;144:228–229.
173. Clements MR, Fraser DR. Vitamin D supply to the fetus and neonate. J Clin Invest 1988;81:1768–1773.
174. Brooke OG, Brown IRF, Cleeve HJW. Observation on the vitamin D state of pregnant Asian women. Br J Obstet Gynaecol 1981;88:18–26.
175. Hollander D. Intestinal absorption of vitamins A and E. J Lab Clin Invest 1981;97:449–462.
176. Goldsmith R. Enterohepatic cycling of vitamin D and metabolites. Minerva Electrolyte Metab 1982;8:289–292.
177. Kodicek E. The fate of labeled vitamin D in rats and infants. In: Garattine S, Pauletti G, eds. Drugs affecting lipid metabolism. Amsterdam: Elsevier, 1961:515–519.
178. Delmas PO, Glorieux FH, Delvin EE, et al. Perinatal serum bone gla-protein and vitamin D metabolite preterm and full-term neonates. J Clin Endocrinol 1987;65:588–591.
179. Nishioka T, Yasuda T, Niimi H, et al. Evidence calcitonin plays a role in the postnatal increased serum $1\alpha,25$-dihydroxyvitamin D. Eur J Pediatr 1988;47:1148–1152.
180. Fetter WPF, Mettau JW, Degenhart HJ, et al. Plasma 1,25-dihydroxyvitamin D concentration in premature infants. Acta Paediatr Scand 1985;74:549–554.
181. Mawer EF, Stanbury SW, Robinson MJ, et al. Vitamin D nutrition and vitamin D metabolism in the premature human neonate. Clin Endocrinol (Oxf) 1986;25:641–649.
182. Hillman LS, Salmons S, Dokoh S. Serum 1,25-dihydroxyvitamin D concentration in premature infants: preliminary results. Calcif Tissue Int 1985;37:223–227.
183. Hillman LS, Hoff N, Salmans S, et al. Mineral homeostasis in very premature infants: serial evaluations of serum 25-hydroxyvitamin D, serum minerals, and bone mineralization. J Pediatr 1985;106:970–980.
184. Cooper TJ, Anast CS. Circulating immunoreactive parathyroid hormone levels in premature infants and the response to calcium therapy. Acta Paediatr Scand 1985;74:669–673.
185. Venkatarman PS, Blick KE, Fry HD, et al. Postnatal changes in calcium-regulation hormones in very-low birthweight infants. Am J Dis Child 1985;139:913–916.
186. Halloran BP, DeLuca HF. Calcium transport in small intestine during early development: role of vitamin D. Am J Physiol 1980;239:G473–G479.
187. Halloran BP, DeLuca HF. Appearance of the intestinal cytosolic receptor for 1,25-dihydroxyvitamin D during neonatal development in the rat. J Biol Chem 1981;256:7338–7342.
188. Ravid A, Koren R, Rotem C, et al. Mononuclear cells from human neonate are partially resistant to the action of 1,25-dihydroxyvitamin D. J Clin Endocrinol Metab 1988;67:755–759.
189. Chandler JS, Pike JW, Haussler MR. 1,25-Dihydroxyvitamin D_3 receptors in rat kidney cytosol. Biochem Biophys Res Commun 1979;90:1057–1063.
190. Morrissey RL, Rath DF. Purification of human renal calcium binding protein from necropsy specimen. Proc Soc Exp Biol Med 1974;145:699–703.
191. Huffer WE. Biology of disease: morphology and biochemistry of bone remodeling: possible control by vitamin D, parathyroid hormone, and other substances. Lab Invest 1988;59:418–442.
192. Anonymous. The function of the vitamin K-dependent protein, bone gla protein (BGP) and kidney gla protein (KGP). Nutr Rev 1984;42:230–233.
193. Price PA, Baukol SA. 1,25-Dihydroxyvitamin D_3 increases synthesis of the vitamin K-dependent bone protein by osteosarcoma cells. J Biol Chem 1980;255:11660–11663.
194. Lian JB, Coutts M, Canalis E. Studies of hormonal regulations of osteocalcin synthesis in cultured fetal rat calvariae. J Biol Chem 1985;260:8706–8710.
195. Lian JB, Glimcher MJ, Roufosse AH, et al. Alterations of the gamma-carboxyglutamic acid and osteocalcin concentrations in vitamin D-deficient chick bone. J Biol Chem 1982;257:4999–5003.
196. Markowitz ME, Gundberg CM, Rosen JF. The circadian rhythm of serum osteocalcin concentration: effects of 1,25-dihydroxyvitamin D administration. Calcif Tissue Int 1987;40:179–183.
197. Gundberg CM, Cole DEC, Lian JB, et al. Serum osteocalcin in the treatment of inherited rickets with 1,25-dihydroxyvitamin D_3. J Clin Endocrinol Metab 1983;56:1063–1067.
198. Koo WW, Tsang RC, Poser JW, et al. Elevated serum calcium and osteocalcin levels from calcitriol in preterm infants. Am J Dis Child 1986;140:1152–1158.
199. Shima M, Seino Y, Tanaka Y. Bone γ-carboxyglutamic acid containing protein in the perinatal period. Acta Paediatr Scand 1985;74:674–677.
200. Jie KG, Hamulyak K, Gijsbers BLMG, et al. Serum osteocalcin as a marker for vitamin K-status in pregnant women and their newborn babies. Thromb Haemost 1992;68:388–391.
201. Haroon Y, Shearer MJ, Rahim S, et al. The content of phylloquinone (vitamin K_1) in human milk, cow's milk and infant formula foods determined by high performance liquid chromatography. J Nutr 1982;112:1105–1117.
202. Motohara K, Matsukara M, Matsuda I, et al. Severe vitamin K deficiency in breast-fed infants. J Pediatr 1984;105:943–945.
203. Tamura T, Takasaki K, Hanaihara T, et al. Effect of vitamin K administration to the mother on prevention of vitamin K deficiency in the neonate. Acta Obst Gynaecol Jpn 1986;38:880–886.
204. Von Kries R, Shearer M, McCarthy PT, et al. Vitamin K_1 content of maternal milk: influence of the stage of lactation, lipid composition, and vitamin K_1 supplements given to the mother. Pediatr Res 1987;22:513–517.

205. Fournier B, Sann T, Guillaumont M, et al. Variations of phylloquinone concentration in human milk at various stages of lactation and in cow's milk at various seasons. Am J Clin Nutr 1987;45:551–558.
206. Lipsky JJ. Nutritional sources of vitamin K. Mayo Clin Proc 1994;69:462–466.
207. Suttie JW. Vitamin K-dependent carboxylase. Annu Rev Biochem 1985;54:459–477.
208. Dahlback B. Interaction between complement component C4b-binding protein and the vitamin K-dependent protein S. Scand J Clin Lab Invest 1985;45(suppl 177):33–41.
209. Soute BAM, DeMetz M, Vermeer C. Characteristics of vitamin K-dependent carboxylating systems from human liver and placenta. FEBS Lett 1982;146:365–368.
210. Suttie JW. Synthesis of vitamin K-dependent proteins. FASEB J 1993;7:445–452.
211. Dowd P, Ham SW, Naganathan S, et al. The mechanism of action of vitamin K. Annu Rev Nutr 1995;15:419–440.
212. Thijssen HH, Drittij-Reijnders MJ, Fischer MAJG. Phylloquinone and menaquinone-4 distribution in rats: synthesis rather than uptake determines menaquinone-4 organ concentrations. J Nutr 1996;126:537–543.
213. Hodges SJ, Bejui J, Leclercq M, et al. Detection and measurement of vitamins K_1 and K_2 in human cortical and trabecular bone. J Bone Miner Res 1993;8:1005–1008.
214. Hirauchi K, Sakano T, Morimoto A. Measurement of K vitamins in human and animal plasma by high-performance liquid chromatography with fluorometric detection. Chem Pharm Bull 1986;34:845–849.
215. Shino M. Determination of endogenous vitamin K (phylloquinone and menaquinone-n) in plasma by high-performance liquid chromatography using platinum oxide catalyst reduction and fluorescence detection. Analyst 1988;113:393–397.
216. Kindberg CG. Studies on vitamin K nutrition. PhD thesis. University of Wisconsin, Madison, 1987:219.
217. Hodges SJ, Akesson K, Vergnaud P, et al. Circulating levels of vitamin K_1 and K_2 decreased in elderly women with hip fractures. J Bone Miner Res 1993;8:1241–1245.
218. Hodges SJ, Pilkington MJ, Shearer MJ, et al. Age-related changes in the circulating levels of congeners of vitamin K_2, menaquinone-7 and menaquinone-8. Clin Sci 1990;787:63–66.
219. Hodges SJ, Pilkington MJ, Stamp TCB, et al. Depressed levels of circulating menaquinones in patients with osteoporotic fractures of the spine and femoral neck. Bone 1991;12:387–389.
220. McCarthy PT, Shearer MJ, Gau G, et al. Vitamin K content of human liver at different ages. Haemostasis 1986;16:84–85.
221. Kayata S, Kindberg C, Greer FR, et al. Vitamin K_1 and K_2 in infant human liver. J Pediatr Gastroenterol Nutr 1989;8:304–307.
222. Hodges SJ, Bejui J, Leclercq M, et al. Detection and measurement of vitamins K_1 and K_2 in human cortical and trabecular bone. J Bone Miner Res 1993;8:1005–1008.
223. Fujita K, Kakuya F, Ito S. Vitamin K_1 and K_2 status and fecal flora in breast fed and formula fed 1-month-old infants. Eur J Pediatr 1993;152:852–855.
224. Greer FR, Mummah-Schendel LL, Marshall S, et al. Vitamin K_1 (phylloquinone) and vitamin K_2 (menaquinone) status in newborn during the first week of life. Pediatrics 1988;81:137–140.
225. Uchida K, Komeno T. Relationships between dietary and intestinal vitamin K, clotting factor levels, plasma vitamin K and urinary Gla. In: Suttie JW, ed. Current advances in vitamin K research. New York: Elsevier Press, 1988:477–492.
226. Usui Y, Nishimura N, Kobayashi N, et al. Measurement of vitamin K in human liver by gradient elution high-performance liquid chromatography using platinum-black catalyst reduction and fluorometric detection. J Chromatogr 1989;489:291–301.
227. Usui Y, Tanimura H, Nishimura N, et al. Vitamin K concentrations in the plasma and liver of surgical patients. Am J Clin Nutr 1990;51:846–852.
228. Khayata S, Kindberg C, Greer FR, et al. Vitamin K_1 and K_2 in infant human liver. J Pediatr Gastroenterol Nutr 1989;8:304–307.
229. Suttie JW. The importance of menaquinones in human nutrition. Annu Rev Nutr 1995;15:399–417.
230. Will BH, Usui Y, Suttie JW. Comparative metabolism and requirement of vitamin K in chicks and rats. J Nutr 1992;122:2354–2360.
231. Guillaumont M, Weiser H, Sann L, et al. Hepatic concentration of vitamin K active compounds after application of phylloquinone to chickens on a vitamin K deficient or adequate diet. Int J Vitam Nutr Res 1992;62:15–20.
232. Shearer MJ, Barkhan P, Rahim S, et al. Plasma vitamin K_1 in mothers and their newborn babies. Lancet 1982;2:460–463.
233. Pietersma-deBruyn ALJM, Van Haard PMM. Vitamin K_1 in the newborn. Clin Chim Acta 1985;150:95–101.
234. Mandelbrot L, Guillaumont M, Leclercq M, et al. Placental transfer of vitamin K_1 and its implication in fetal haemostasis. Thromb Haemost 1988;60:39–43.
235. Greer FR, Smith DK, Marshall S, et al. Oral versus intramuscular vitamin K_1 prophylaxis: evaluation of a new oral mixed-micellar preparation in breastfeeding infants. In press.
236. Hamulyak K, DeBoer-van den Berg MAG, Thijssen HHW, et al. The placental transport of [^{3}H] vitamin K_1 in rats. Br J Haematol 1987;65:335–338.
237. Guillaumont MJ, Durr FM, Combet JM, et al. Vitamin K_1 diffusion across the placental barrier in the gravid female rat. Dev Pharmacol Ther 1988;11:57–64.
238. Blomstrand R, Forsgren L. Vitamin K_1 ^{3}H in man: its intestinal absorption and transport in the thoracic duct lymph. Int Z Vitam Forschung 1968;38:45–64.
239. Shearer MJ, McBurney A, Barkhan P. Studies on the absorption and metabolism of phylloquinone (vitamin K_1) in man. Vitam Horm 1974;32:513–542.
240. Corrigan JJ, Ulfers LL. Effect of vitamin E on prothrombin levels in warfarin-induced vitamin K deficiency. Am J Clin Nutr 1981;34:1701–1705.
241. Fournier B, Leclercq M, Andiger-Petit C, et al. Vitamin K_1 binding protein in milk. Int J Vitam Res 1987;57:145–150.

242. Hollander D, Rim E, Muralidhara KS. Vitamin K_1 intestinal absorption in vivo: influence of luminal contents on transport. Am J Physiol 1977;232:E69–E74.
243. Hollander D, Rim E. Vitamin K_2 absorption by rat everted small intestinal sacs. Am J Physiol 1976;231:415–419.
244. Hollander D, Muralidhara KS, Rim E. Colonic absorption of bacterially synthesized vitamin K_2 in the rat. Am J Physiol 1976;230;251–255.
245. Sann L, Leclercq M, Guillaumont M, et al. Serum vitamin K_1 concentrations after oral administration of vitamin K_1 in low birth weight infants. J Pediatr 1985;107:608–611.
246. Thierry MJ, Hermodson MA, Suttie JW. Vitamin K and warfarin distribution and metabolism in the warfarin-resistant rat. Am J Physiol 1970;219:854–859.
247. Duello TJ, Matschiner JT. Characterization of vitamin K from pig liver and dog liver. Arch Biochem Biophys 1971; 144:330–338.
248. Bjornsson TD, Meffin PG, Swezey SE, et al. Disposition and turnover of vitamin K_1 in man. In: Suttie JW, ed. Vitamin K metabolism and vitamin K-dependent proteins. Baltimore: University Park Press, 1980;328–332.
249. Andrew M, Paes B, Milner R, et al. Development of the human coagulation system in the full-term infant. Blood 1987;70:165–172.
250. Andrew M, Paes B, Milner R, et al. Development of the human coagulation system in the healthy premature infant. Blood 1988;72:1651–1657.
251. Göbel U, Sonnenschein-Kosenow S, Petrich C, et al. Vitamin K deficiency in the newborn. Lancet 1977;2:187–188.
252. Von Kries R, Greer FR, Suttie JW. Assessment of vitamin K status of the newborn infant. J Pediatr Gastroenterol Nutr 1993;16:231–238.
253. Liska DJ, Suttie JW. Location of gamma-carboxyglutamyl residues in partially carboxylated prothrombin preparations. Biochemistry 1988;27:8636–8641.
254. Amiral J, Grosley M, Plassart V, et al. Development of a monoclonal immunoassay for the direct measurement of decarboxyprothrombin on plasma (abstract). Thromb Haemost 1991;65:10.
255. Belle M, Brebank R, Guinet R, et al. Production of a new monoclonal antibody specific to human des-gamma-carboxyprothrombin in the presence of calcium ions. Application to the development of a sensitive ELISA-test. J Immunoassay 1995;16:213–229.
256. Bovill EG, Soll RF, Lynch M, et al. Vitamin K_1 metabolism and the production of descarboxyprothrombin and protein C in the term and premature neonate. Blood 1993; 81:77–83.
257. Motahara K, Endo F, Matsuda I. Effect of vitamin K administration on acarboxyprothrombin (PIVKA-II) levels in newborns. Lancet 1985;2:242–244.
258. Motohara K, Takayi S, Endo F, et al. Oral supplementation of vitamin K for pregnant women and effects on levels of plasma vitamin K and PIVKA-II in the neonate. J Pediatr Gastroenterol Nutr 1990;11:32–36.
259. Von Kries R, Shearer MJ, Widdershoven J, et al. Des-gamma-carboxyprothrombin (PIVKA-II) and plasma vitamin K_1 in newborns and their mothers. Thromb Haemost 1992;68:383–387.
260. Widdershoven J, Lambert W, Motohara K, et al. Plasma concentrations of vitamin K_1 and PIVKA-II in bottle-fed and breast-fed infants with and without vitamin K prophylaxis at birth. Eur J Pediatr 1988;148:139–142.
261. Cornelissen E, Kollée L, DeAbreu R, et al. Effects of oral and intramuscular vitamin K prophylaxis on vitamin K_1, PIVKA-II and clotting factors in breast-fed infants. Arch Dis Child 1992;67:1250–1254.
262. Cornelissen E, Kollée L, DeAbreu R, et al. Prevention of vitamin K deficiency in infancy by weekly administration of vitamin K. Acta Pediatr 1983;82:656–659.
263. Cornelissen E, Kollée L, van Lith T, et al. Evaluation of a daily dose of 25 mg vitamin K_1 to prevent vitamin K deficiency in breast-fed infants. J Pediatr Gastroenterol Nutr 1993;16:301–305.
264. Greer FR. Vitamin K deficiency and hemorrhage in infancy. Clin Perinatol 1995;22:759–777.
265. Evans HM, Bishop KS. On the existence of a hitherto unrecognized dietary factor essential for reproduction. Science 1922;56:650–651.
266. Oski FA, Barness LA. Vitamin E deficiency: a previously unrecognized cause of hemolytic anemia in the premature infant. J Pediatr 1967;70:211–220.
267. Nelson JA. Pathology of vitamin E deficiency. In: Machlin LJ, ed. Vitamin E. A comprehensive treatise. New York: Marcel Dekker, 1980:397–428.
268. Traber MG. Vitamin E in humans: demand and delivery. Annu Rev Nutr 1996;16:321–347.
269. Nitowsky HM, Cornblath M, Gordon HH. Studies of tocopherol deficiency in infants and children. II. Plasma tocopherol and erythrocyte hemolysis in hydrogen peroxide. Am J Dis Child 1956;92:164–174.
270. Farrell PM. Human health and disease. In: Machlin LJ, ed. Vitamin E. A comprehensive treatise. New York: Marcel Dekker, 1980:519–620.
271. Farrell PM. Vitamin E. In: Shils M, Young V, eds. Modern nutrition in health and disease. Philadelphia: Lea & Febeger, 1988:340–354.
272. Burton GW, Traber MG. Vitamin E: antioxidant activity, biokinetics and bioavailability. Annu Rev Nutr 1990;10: 357–382.
273. Bieri JG, McKenna MC. Expressing dietary values for fat-soluble vitamins: changes in concept and terminology. Am J Clin Nutr 1981;34:289–293.
274. McCay PB, King MM, Poyer JL, et al. An update on antioxidant theory: spin trapping of trichloromethyl radicals in vivo. Ann NY Acad Sci 1982;393–423.
275. McCay PB, King M. Biochemical function. In: Machlin LJ, ed. Vitamin E. A comprehensive treatise. New York: Marcel Dekker, 1980:289–317.
276. Bieri JG, Farrell PM. Vitamin E. Vitam Horm 1976;34: 31–75.
277. Farquahr JW, Ahrens EH. Effects of dietary fats on human erythrocyte fatty acid patterns. J Clin Invest 1963; 5:675–685.
278. Burton GW, Ingold KU. Vitamin E: application of the principles of physical organic chemistry to the exploration of its structure and function. Acc Chem Res 1986;19:194–201.

279. Bieri JG, Evarts RP. Gamma tocopherol: metabolism, biological activity, and significance in human vitamin E nutrition. Am J Clin Nutr 1974;27:980–986.
280. Dillard CJ, Gavino VC, Tappel AL. Relative antioxidant effectiveness of alpha-tocopherol and gamma-tocopherol in iron-loaded rats. J Nutr 1983;113:2226–2273.
281. Burton GW, Ingold KU. Antoxidation of biological molecules. I. The antioxidant activity of vitamin E and related chain-breaking phenolic antioxidants in vitro. J Am Chem Soc 1981;103:6472–6477.
282. Witting LA. The role of polyunsaturated fatty acids in determining vitamin E requirements. Ann NY Acad Sci 1972;203:192–198.
283. Williams ML, Shott RJ, O'Neal PL, et al. Role of dietary iron and fat on vitamin E deficiency anemia of infancy. N Engl J Med 1975;292:887–890.
284. Horwitt MK. Vitamin E and lipid metabolism in man. Am J Clin Nutr 1960;8:451–461.
285. Committe on Nutrition, American Academy of Pediatrics. Nutritional needs of low-birth-weight infants. Pediatrics 1985;75:976–986.
286. Gross S, Melhorn DK. Vitamin E, red cell lipids and red cell stability in prematurity. Ann NY Acad Sci 1972;203:141–162.
287. Farrell PM, Bieri JG, Fratantoni JF, et al. The occurrence and effects of human vitamin E deficiency: a study in patients with cystic fibrosis. J Clin Invest 1977;60:233–241.
288. Losowsky MS, Kelleher J, Walker BE. Intake and absorption of tocopherol. Ann NY Acad Sci 1972;203:212–222.
289. Traber MG, Burton GW, Hughes L, et al. Discrimination between forms of vitamin E by humans with and without genetic abnormalities of lipoprotein metabolism. J Lipid Res 1992;33:1171–1182.
290. Traber MG, Burton GW, Ingold KU, et al. *RRR*- and *SRR*-α-tocopherols are secreted without discrimination in human chylomicrons, but *RRR*-α-tocopherol is preferentially secreted in very low density lipoproteins. J Lipid Res 1990;31:675–685.
291. Traber MG, Ingold KU, Burton GW, et al. Absorption and transport of deuterium-substituted 2R,4′R,8′R-α-tocopherol in human lipoproteins. Lipids 1988;23:791–797.
292. Traber MG, Kayden HJ. Preferential incorporation of α-tocopherol vs. γ-tocopherol in human lipoproteins. Am J Clin Nutr 1989;49:517–526.
293. Traber MG, Kayden HJ. α-Tocopherol as compared with γ-tocopherol is preferentially secreted in human lipoproteins. Ann NY Acad Sci 1989;570:95–108.
294. Traber MG. Sokol RJH, Burton GW, et al. Impaired ability of patients with familial isolated vitamin E deficiency to incorporate α-tocopherol into lipoproteins secreted by the liver. J Clin Invest 1990;85:397–407.
295. Traber MG, Sokol RJ, Kohlschutter A, et al. Impaired discrimination between stereoisomers of α-tocopherol in patients with familial isolated vitamin E deficiency. J Lipid Res 1993;34:201–210.
296. Traber MG. Determinants of plasma vitamin E concentrations. Free Rad Biol Med 1994;16:229–239.
297. Catignani GL, Bieri, JG. Rat liver α-tocopherol binding protein. Biochim Biophys Acta 1977;497:349–357.
298. Sato Y, Hagiwara K, Arai H, et al. Purification and characterization of the α-tocopherol transfer protein from rat liver. FEBS Lett 1991;288:41–45.
299. Yoshida H, Yusin M, Ren I, et al. Identification, purification and immunochemical characterization of a tocopherol-binding protein in rat liver cytosol. J Lipid Res 1992;33:343–350.
300. Kuhlenkamp J, Ronk M, Yusin M, et al. Identification and purification of a human liver cytosolic tocopherol binding protein. Prot Exp Purif 1993;4:382–389.
301. Arita M, Sato Y, Miyata A, et al. Human alpha-tocopherol transfer protein: cDNA cloning, expression and chromosomal localization. Biochem J 1995;306:437–443.
302. Doerflinger N, Linder C, Puahchi K, et al. Ataxia with vitamin E deficiency: refinement of genetic localization and analysis of linkage disequilibrium by using new markers in 14 families. Am J Hum Genet 1995;56:1116–1124.
303. Sokol RJ, Kayden HJ, Bettis DB, et al. Isolated vitamin E deficiency in the absence of fat malabsorption—familial and sporadic cases: characterization and investigation of causes. J Lab Clin Med 1988;111:548–559.
304. Ben Hamida C, Doerflinger N, Belal S, et al. Localization of Friedrich's ataxia phenotype with selective vitamin E deficiency to chromosome 8q by homozygosity mapping. Nature Genet 1993;5:195–200.
305. Ben Hamida M, Belal S, Sirugo G, et al. Friedreich's ataxia phenotype not linked to chromosome 9 and associated with selective autosomal recessive vitamin E deficiency in two inbred Tunisian families. Neurology 1993;43:2179–2183.
306. Ouahchi K, Arita M, Kayden H, et al. Ataxia with isolated vitamin E deficiency is caused by mutations in the α-tocopherol transfer protein. Nature Genet 1995;9:141–145.
307. Bieri JG, Evarts RP. Effect of plasma lipid levels and obesity on tissue stores of α-tocopherol. Proc Soc Exp Biol Med 1975;149:500–502.
308. Bieri JG. Kinetics of tissue α-tocopherol depletion and repletion. Ann NY Acad Sci 1972;203:181–191.
309. Bieri JG, Tolliver LJ, Catignani GL. Simultaneous determination of α-tocopherol and retinol in plasma and red cells by high pressure liquid chromatography. Am J Clin Nutr 1979;32:2143–2149.
310. Gutcher GR, Lax AM, Farrell PM. Tocopherol isomers in intravenous lipid emulsions and resultant plasma concentrations. J Parenter Enteral Nutr 1984;8:269–273.
311. Gutcher GR, Raynor WJ, Farrell PM. An evaluation of vitamin E status in premature infants. Am J Clin Nutr 1984;40:1078–1089.
312. Horwitt MK, Harvey CC, Century B, et al. Polyunsaturated lipids and tocopherol requirements. J Am Diet Assoc 1961;38:231–235.
313. Farrell PM, Levine SL, Murphy MD, et al. Plasma tocopherol levels and tocopherol-lipid relationships in a normal population of children as compared to healthy adults. Am J Clin Nutr 1978;31:1720–1726.
314. Horwitt MK, Harvey CC, Dahm CH Jr, et al. Relationship between tocopherol and serum lipid levels for determination of nutritional adequacy. Ann NY Acad Sci 1972;203:223–226.

315. Sokol RJ, Heubi JE, Iannacone ST, et al. Vitamin E deficiency with normal serum vitamin E concentrations in children with chronic cholestasis. N Engl J Med 1984;310:1209–1212.
316. Lammi-Keefe CJ. Vitamin D and E in human milk. In: Jensen RG, ed. Handbook of milk composition. San Diego: Academic Press 1995:706–717.
317. Kobayaski H, Kanno C, Yamauchi K, et al. Identification of alpha-, beta-, gamma-, and delta-tocopherols and their contents in human milk. Biochim Biophys Acta 1975;380:282–290.
318. Owens WC, Owens EU. Retrolental fibroplasia in premature infants. Am J Ophthalmol 1949;32:1631–1637.
319. Moyer WT. Vitamin E levels in term and premature newborn infants. Pediatrics 1950;6:893–896.
320. Melhorn DK, Gross S. Vitamin E-dependent anemia in the premature infant. II. Relationships between gestational age and absorption of vitamin E. Pediatrics 1971;79:581–588.
321. Huijbers WAR, Schrijver J, Speek AJ, et al. Persistent low plasma vitamin E levels in premature infants surviving respiratory distress syndrome. Eur J Pediatr 1986;145:170–171.
322. Phillips B, Franck LS, Greene HL. Vitamin E levels in premature infants during and after intravenous multivitamin supplementation. Pediatrics 1987;80:680–683.
323. Slagle TA, Gross SJ. Vitamin E. In: Tsang RC, Nichols BL, eds. Nutrition during infancy. Philadelphia: Hanley & Belfus, 1988:277–288.
324. Farrell PM, Zachman RD, Gutcher GR. Fat soluble vitamins A, E, and K in the premature infants. In: Tsang RC, ed. Vitamin and mineral requirements in preterm infants. New York: Marcel Dekker, 1985:63–98.
325. Gutcher GR, Farrell PJM. Early intravenous correction of vitamin E deficiency in premature infants. J Pediatr Gastroenterol Nutr 1985;4:604–609.
326. Hittner HM, Speer ME, Rudolph AJ, et al. Retrolental fibroplasia and vitamin E in the preterm infant—comparison of oral versus intramuscular administration. Pediatrics 1984;73:238–249.
327. Gross SJ, Gabriel E. Vitamin E status in preterm infants fed human milk or infant formula. J Pediatr 1985;106:634–640.
328. Greene HL, Moore MEC, Phillips B, et al. Evaluation of a pediatric multiple vitamin preparation for total parenteral nutrition. II. Blood levels of vitamins A, D, and E. Pediatrics 1986;77:539–547.
329. Ronnholm KAR, Dostalova L, Simes MA. Vitamin E supplementation in very-low-birth-weight infants: long-term follow-up at two different levels of vitamin E supplementation. Am J Clin Nutr 1989;49:121–126.
330. Friedman CA, Wender DF, Temple DM, et al. Serum alpha-tocopherol concentrations in preterm infants receiving less than 25 mg/kg/day alpha-tocopherol acetate supplements. Dev Pharmacol Ther 1988;11:273–280.
331. Bougle D, Boutroy MJ, Heng J, et al. Plasma kinetics of parenteral tocopherol in premature infants. Dev Pharmacol Ther 1986;9:310–316.
332. Knight ME, Roberts RJ. Disposition of intravenously administered pharmacologic doses of vitamin E in newborn rabbits. J Pediatr 1986;108:145–150.
333. Balistreri WF, Farrell MK, Bove KE. Lessons from the E-ferol tragedy. Pediatrics 1986;78:503–506.
334. Horwitt MK, Bailey P. Cerebellar pathology in an infant resembling chick nutritional encephalomalacia. Arch Neurol Psychiatr 1959;95:869–872.
335. Ehrenkranz RA, Bonta BW, Ablow RC, et al. Amelioration of bronchopulmonary dysplasia after vitamin E administration: a preliminary report. N Engl J Med 1978;229:564–569.
336. Johnson L, Schaffer D, Quinn G, et al. Vitamin E supplementation and the retinopathy of prematurity. Ann NY Acad Sci 1982;393:473–484.
337. Hittner HM, Godio LB, Rudolph AJ, et al. Retrolental fibroplasia: efficacy of vitamin E in a double-blind clinical study of preterm infants. N Engl J Med 1981;305:1365–1371.
338. Hittner HM, Godio LB, Speer MI, et al. Retrolental fibroplasia: further clinical evidence and ultrastructural support for efficacy of vitamin E in the preterm infants. Pediatrics 1983;71:423–432.
339. Kretzer FL, Hittner JM, Johnson AT, et al. Vitamin E and retrolental fibroplasia: ultrastructural support of clinical efficacy. Ann NY Acad Sci 1982;393:145–164.
340. Sokol RJ. Vitamin E deficiency and neurologic disease. Annu Rev Nutr 1988;8:351–373.
341. Chiswick ML, Johnson M, Woodhall C, et al. Protective effect of vitamin E (dl-alpha-tocopherol) against intraventricular hemorrhage in premature babies. Br Med J 1983;287:81–84.
342. Speer ME, Blifeld C, Rudolph AJ, et al. Intraventricular hemorrhage and vitamin E in the very low-birth-weight infant: evidence of efficacy of early intramuscular vitamin E administration. Pediatrics 1984;74:1107–1112.
343. Ehrenkranz RA, Ablow RC, Warshaw JB. Effect of vitamin E on the development of oxygen-induced lung injury in neonates. Ann NY Acad Sci 1982;393:452–465.
344. Phelps DL, Rosenbaum AL, Isenberg SJ, et al. Tocopherol efficacy and safety for preventing retinopathy of prematurity: a randomized, controlled, double-masked trial. Pediatrics 1987;79:489–500.
345. Bell EF. Prevention of bronchopulmonary dysplasia: vitamin E and other antioxidants. In: Farrell PM, Tausing LM, eds. Bronchopulmonary dysplasia and related chronic respiratory disorders. Report of the Ninetieth Ross Conference on Pediatric Research, 1986:77–82.
346. Saldanha RL, Cepeda EE, Poland RL. The effect of vitamin E prophylaxis on the incidence and severity of bronchopulmonary dysplasia. J Pediatr 1982;101:89–93.
347. Watts JL, Milner R, Zipursky A, et al. Failure of supplementation with vitamin E to prevent bronchopulmonary dysplasia in infants <1500 g birthweight. Eur Respir J 1991;4:188–190.
348. Chiswick M, Gladman G, Sinba S, et al. Vitamin E supplementation and periventricular hemorrhage in the newborn. Am J Clin Nutr 1991;53:370S–372S.
349. Fish WH, Cohen M, Franzek E, et al. Effect of intramuscular vitamin E on mortality and intracranial hemorrhage in neonates of 1000 grams or less. Pediatrics 1990;85:578–584.

350. Laro MR, Wojewardine K, Wald NJ. Is routine vitamin E administration justified in very low-birthweight infants? Dev Med Child Neurol 1990;32:442–450.
351. Farrell PM. Vitamin E deficiency in premature infants. J Pediatr 1979;95:869–872.
352. Banagale RC, Bray JJ, Erenberg AP. Serum free tocopherol levels in premature infants (PI) receiving total parenteral nutrition (TPN). Pediatr Res 1981;15:492A.
353. Bell EF, Brown EJ, Milner R, et al. Vitamin E absorption in small premature infants. Pediatrics 1979;63:830–832.
354. Specker BL, Greer FR, Tsang RC, Vitamin D. In: Tsang RC, Nichols BL, eds. Nutrition during infancy. Philadelphia: Hanley & Belfus 1988:264–274.
355. Greer FR, Suttie VW, Vitamin K and the newborn. In: Tsang RC, Nichols BL, eds. Nutrition during infancy. Philadelphia: Hanley & Belfus 1988:289–297.

43
Neonatal Vitamin Metabolism: Water Soluble

Richard J. Schanler

Water-soluble vitamins play key roles in the developing human being. They function as cofactors for enzyme reactions of intermediary metabolism and therefore are dependent on the energy and protein contents of the diets as well as on the rates of growth and energy utilization of the individual. First elucidated as etiologic agents of diseases now known to be deficiency syndromes, their necessity was reiterated during the early development of artificial diets and parenteral feeding.

At birth, the concentration of water-soluble vitamins is greater in the neonate than in the mother. Active transport of water-soluble vitamins during pregnancy results in concentration gradients (1:1.5 to 1:6) favoring the fetus.[1] Significant correlations between maternal and full-term neonatal plasma water-soluble vitamin indices are reported.[2,3] Hypovitaminosis exists for many water-soluble vitamins in the absence of maternal supplementation during pregnancy.[4] Because of hemodilution and rapidly expanding body masses, problems arise in the interpretation of biochemical indices of vitamin sufficiency during pregnancy.[1,5]

With the exception of vitamin B_{12}, water-soluble vitamins are not stored in the body to any great extent and are rapidly depleted if intake is marginal. The status of the water-soluble vitamins, under usual circumstances in the United States, tends to be maintained throughout pregnancy and infancy in breast-fed, full-term infants, although maternal diet may affect vitamin sufficiency (Tables 43.1 and 43.2). Currently available commercial formulas also satisfy the vitamin needs of infancy (Tables 43.1 to 43.3). When deficiencies occur in developed countries, they generally are associated with chronic disease or substance abuse (e.g., alcohol, drugs). In contrast, deficiencies of water-soluble vitamins in developing countries are associated with protein-calorie malnutrition.[6]

The vitamin needs of the premature neonates are less clearly understood. Those fed human milk exclusively may not receive adequate amounts of certain vitamins. Commercial formulas designed for the premature infant tend to contain larger quantities of water-soluble vitamins than do standard infant formulas, perhaps in excess of needs.

Advisable intakes of water-soluble vitamins for full-term infants and children have been reported. Guidelines recommended by the Committee on Nutrition of the American Academy of Pediatrics (AAP) and those of the National Research Council, Recommended Dietary Allowances (RDA) generally are used (Table 43.4).[7,8] Additional recommendations have been published by the European Society of Pediatric Gastroenterology and Nutrition (ESPGAN) (Table 43.5).[9] Guidelines for premature infants generally follow the AAP but additional recommendations have been published by ESPGAN, the Nutrition Committee of the Canadian Paediatric Society (Table 43.5), and data from a variety of sources, including the European Community (EC), have been summarized (Table 43.5). For older children, the RDA often is used for reference intakes (Table 43.6). The RDA is one source used as a reference for pregnancy and lactation (Table 43.7).[5]

The gastrointestinal tract and liver modify orally ingested water-soluble vitamins. Parenteral administration of these vitamins, bypassing this barrier, may present the kidney with a large quantity of vitamins for excretion. The ability of the kidney to adapt to continuous parenteral administration of vitamins has not been determined. General guidelines for parenteral water-soluble vitamins for infants and children have been reported (Table 43.8).[10]

This chapter addresses the physiologic role and dietary adequacy pertinent to the pregnant woman and her developing infant for each of the water-soluble vitamins: thiamine, riboflavin, niacin, vitamin B_6, folate, vitamin B_{12}, pantothenic acid, biotin, and vitamin C.

TABLE 43.1. Milk concentrations of water-soluble vitamins (units·L^{-1}).

	Mature human milk[a]	Enfamil[b]	Similac[c]	Bovine milk[d]
Thiamine (µg)	220 (150–250)	520	676	375
Riboflavin (µg)	400 (300–600)	1000	1014	1650
Niacin (mg)	2.0 (1.8–2.3)	7.7	7.1	0.8
Vitamin B_6 (µg)	140 (90–200)	417	406	415
Folate (µg)	50 (40–85)	105	100	50
Vitamin B_{12} (µg)	0.7 (0.5–1.2)	1.6	1.7	3.6
Pantothenic acid (mg)	4.0 (2.5–6.7)	3.1	3.0	3.2
Biotin (µg)	5.0 (4–8)	15	30	50[e]
Vitamin C (mg)	50 (30–90)	54	60	12

[a] References—see text.
[b] 1993, Mead Johnson Nutritionals, Evansville, IN.
[c] 1994, Ross Laboratories, Columbus, OH.
[d] From Pennington,[27] with permission.
[e] From Bonjour,[145] with permission.

TABLE 43.2. Milk concentrations of water-soluble vitamins (units·100 kcal^{-1}).

	Human milk	Enfamil	Similac
Thiamine (µg)	31 (21–36)	78	100
Riboflavin (µg)	56 (42–85)	150	150
Niacin (mg)	0.29 (0.27–0.34)	1.1	1.1
Vitamin B_6 (µg)	20 (15–30)	62	60
Folate (µg)	7 (6–12)	15.6	15
Vitamin B_{12} (µg)	0.10 (0.07–0.16)	0.23	0.25
Pantothenic acid (mg)	0.6 (0.3–1.0)	0.5	0.4
Biotin (µg)	0.7 (0.6–1.1)	2.2	4.5
Vitamin C (mg)	8 (5–13)	8	9

TABLE 43.3. Milk content of water-soluble vitamins for premature infants (units·L^{-1}).

	Fortified Human milk[a]	Human milk and Similac Natural Care[b]	Similac Special Care[c]	Enfamil Premature Formula[d]
Thiamine (µg)	1730	1125	2030	1600
Riboflavin (µg)	2500	2717	5034	2400
Niacin (mg)	32.0	21.3	40.6	32.0
Vitamin B_6 (µg)	1280	1085	2030	1200
Folate (µg)	300	175	300	280
Vitamin B_{12} (µg)	2.5	2.6	4.5	2.0
Pantothenic acid (mg)	11.3	9.7	15.4	9.6
Biotin (µg)	32	152.5	300	32
Vitamin C (mg)	166	175	300	160

[a] Enfamil Human Milk Fortifier (1993, Mead Johnson Nutritionals, Evansville, IN), mixed as four packets per 100 ml mature human milk; data expressed per liter of milk.
[b] Mature human milk mixed 1:1 (vol:vol) with Similac Natural Care (1994, Ross Laboratories, Columbus, OH).
[c] Similac Special Care (1994, Ross Laboratories, Columbus, OH).
[d] Enfamil Premature Formula (1993, Mead Johnson Nutritionals, Evansville, IN).

Thiamine (Vitamin B_1)

General Metabolism

Thiamine is a thiazole moiety joined by a methylene bridge to a pyrimidine ring (Figure 43.1). The vitamin is absorbed in the proximal small intestine by both active and passive mechanisms and phosphorylated in the mucosal cells to yield the coenzyme thiamine pyrophosphate (TPP) and adenylic acid.[11,12] The absorption of thiamine is rate-limited and is slower in pregnancy and folate deficiency.[4] Thiamine is destroyed or inactivated by heat (cooking, pasteurization), alkaline solutions, and ionizing radiation.[13–15]

Thiamine pyrophosphate functions, with magnesium as a cofactor, in biochemical reactions related to carbohy-

TABLE 43.4. Advisable intakes of water-soluble vitamins for full-term infants.

	AAP[a] (units·100 kcal^{-1})	RDA[b] (units·day^{-1}) 0–6 mo	RDA[b] (units·day^{-1}) 6–12 mo	RDA (units·kg^{-1}·day^{-1}) 0–6 mo	RDA (units·kg^{-1}·day^{-1}) 6–12 mo
Thiamine (µg)	40	300	400	50	44
Riboflavin (µg)	60	400	500	67	56
Niacin (mg)	0.25 (0.8[c])	5[c]	6	0.8[c]	0.7
Vitamin B_6 (µg)[d]	35	300	600	50	67
Folate (µg)	4	25	35	4.2	3.9
Vitamin B_{12} (µg)	0.15	0.3	0.5	0.05	0.06
Pantothenic acid (mg)	0.3	2	3	0.3	0.3
Biotin (µg)	1.5	10	15	0.3	0.3
Vitamin C (mg)	8	30	35	5	3.9

[a] American Academy of Pediatrics.[7]
[b] Recommended Dietary Allowances.[8] Assume energy intake of 108 and 98 kcal·kg^{-1}·d^{-1} and body weight of 6 kg and 9 kg for 0–6 and 6–12 mo, respectively.
[c] As niacin equivalents.
[d] Assumes vitamin B_6/protein ratio of at least 15 µg·g^{-1}.

TABLE 43.5. Recommended enteral intakes of water-soluble vitamins for premature infants.

	ESPGAN[a]	Canadian	Other[33]
Thiamine (µg)	20 µg · 100 kcal^{-1}	40–50 µg · kg^{-1} · d^{-1}	240 µg · kg^{-1} · d^{-1}
Riboflavin (µg)	40–60 µg · 100 kcal^{-1}	360–460 µg · kg^{-1} · d^{-1}	360 µg · kg^{-1} · d^{-1}
Niacin (mg)	0.8 NE · 100 kcal^{-1}	0.86 NE · 100 kcal^{-1}	4.8 mg · kg^{-1} · d^{-1}
Vitamin B_6 (µg)	35–60 µg · 100 kcal^{-1}	15 µg · g protein^{-1}	180 µg · kg^{-1} · d^{-1}
Folate (µg)	60 µg · kg^{-1} · day^{-1}	50 µg · day^{-1}	50 µ · kg^{-1} · d^{-1}
Vitamin B_{12} (µg)	0.3 µg · day^{-1}	0.15 µg · day^{-1}	0.3 µg · kg^{-1} · d^{-1}
Pantothenic acid (mg)	0.33 mg · 100 kcal^{-1}	0.8–1.3 mg · kg^{-1} · d^{-1}	6.0 mg · kg^{-1} · d^{-1}
Biotin (µg)	1.2 µg · kg^{-1} · d^{-1}	1.5 µg · kg^{-1} · d^{-1}	17 µg · kg^{-1} · d^{-1}
Vitamin C (mg)	20–50 µg · day^{-1}	6–10 mg · kg^{-1} · d^{-1}	24 mg · kg^{-1} · d^{-1}

[a] ESPGAN, European Society of Pediatric Gastroenterology and Nutrition.[9]

TABLE 43.6. Advisable water-soluble vitamin intakes for children (units · day^{-1}).[8]

	1–3 years (13 kg)	4–6 years (20 kg)	7–10 years (28 kg)
Thiamine (µg)	700	900	1000
Riboflavin (µg)	800	1100	1200
Niacin (mg NE)	9	12	13
Vitamin B_6 (µg)	1000	1100	1400
Folate (µg)	50	75	100
Vitamin B_{12} (µg)	0.7	1.0	1.4
Pantothenic acid (mg)	3	3–4	4–5
Biotin (µg)	20	25	30
Vitamin C (mg)	40	45	45

TABLE 43.7. Advisable water-soluble vitamin intakes during pregnancy and lactation (units · day^{-1}).[8]

	Females (19–24 y)	Pregnancy	Lactation (0–6 mo)	Lactation (7–12 mo)
Thiamine (µg)	1100	1500	1600	1600
Riboflavin (µg)	1300	1600	1800	1700
Niacin (mg)	15	17	20	20
Vitamin B_6 (µg)	1600	2200	2100	2100
Folate (µg)	180	400	280	260
Vitamin B_{12} (µg)	2.0	2.2	2.6	2.6
Pantothenic acid (mg)	4–7	N/D	N/D	N/D
Biotin (µg)	30–100	N/D	N/D	N/D
Vitamin C (mg)	60	70	95	90

N/D, no available data.

TABLE 43.8. Parenteral intakes of water-soluble vitamins for infants and children.[10]

	Full-term infants and children (units · day^{-1})	Premature infants units · kg^{-1} day^{-1}[a]
Thiamine (µg)	1200	350
Riboflavin (µg)	1400	150
Niacin (mg)	17	6.8
Vitamin B_6 (µg)	1000	180
Folate (µg)	140	56
Vitamin B_{12} (µg)	1.0	0.30
Pantothenic acid (mg)	5	2.0
Biotin (µg)	20	6.0
Vitamin C (mg)	80	25

[a] Not to exceed full-term infant dose.

drate metabolism, i.e., active aldehyde transfer of two general types.[11,13,16] The first type is catalyzed by dehydrogenase complexes for the oxidative decarboxylation of α-keto acids: pyruvate to acetyl–coenzyme A (CoA), α-ketoglutarate to succinate, and the keto analogues of branched-chain amino acids. The dehydrogenase complexes are found in the mitochondria and are necessary for the initiation of the Krebs cycle. The second type of general reaction requiring TPP is the formation of α-ketols catalyzed by transketolase. This enzyme is located in the cytosol, especially in liver and blood cells. Transketolase supplies reduced nicotinamide adenine dinucleotide phosphate (NADPH) needed for biosynthetic reactions in the pentose phosphate pathway.

In addition to its coenzyme functions, thiamine is thought to play a specific role in neurophysiology. Thiamine and TPP are located in peripheral nerve membranes and may function to facilitate nerve conduction.[16,17]

Sources

The thiamine concentration in human milk increases from 20 µg · L^{-1} during the first 5 days of lactation to 220 µg · L^{-1} (31 µg · 100 kcal^{-1}, range 21–36 µg · 100 kcal^{-1}) in mature milk (Tables 43.1 and 43.2).[18–25] Milk thiamine can be increased by diet but only from the malnourished to the usual range of milk concentrations.[26] The thiamine contents of bovine milk and commercial formulas are provided in Tables 43.1 to 43.3.[20,27,28] Dietary sources of thiamine include meats, whole grains, enriched cereals, peas, potatoes, beans, nuts, and yeast.[20,27,29]

Perinatal Needs

The need for thiamine is directly related to the amount of metabolizable carbohydrate consumed. Practically, requirements are expressed in terms of energy content (µg · 100 kcal^{-1}). The minimum intake of the vitamin, 140

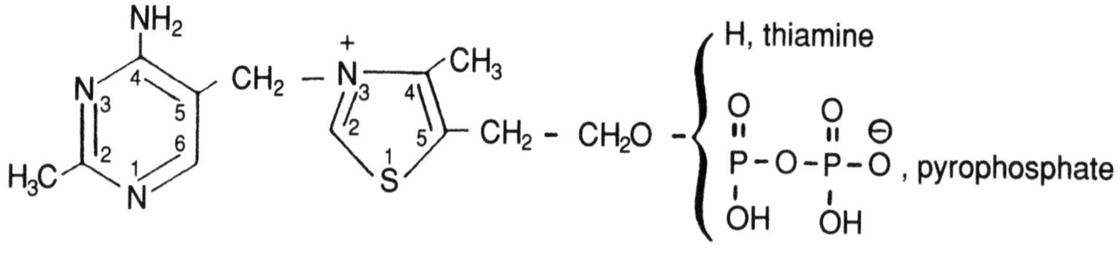

FIGURE 43.1. Thiamine and its pyrophosphate coenzyme.

to 200 μg·day^{-1}, was proposed because marked decreases in the urinary excretion of thiamine occurred in infants at intakes below this concentration.[30]

Although the thiamine concentration in human milk is slightly below the 40 μg thiamine·100 kcal^{-1} recommendation of the AAP (Table 43.4), the thiamine intake of full-term breast-fed neonates appears satisfactory, and thiamine deficiency in breast-fed neonates of well-nourished mothers has not been reported.[7] The AAP recommendation is similar to the RDA for infants.[7,8] The recommendations of ESPGAN are lower.[9] Because of variability in milk composition and the potential need for milk banking, which may include heat-treatment of the milk, the available thiamine in human milk may be inadequate for premature infants (Tables 43.1 and 43.5). Both full-term and premature formula-fed infants, however, receive sufficient thiamine to meet recommended vitamin needs (Tables 43.1 to 43.3 and 43.5).

The advisable intakes of thiamine for children, and for women during pregnancy and lactation are given in Tables 43.6 and 43.7. The vitamin requirements increase in pregnancy and lactation most likely because of the increased energy needs during that time.

Full-term neonates and children are thiamine sufficient during total parenteral nutrition (TPN) following parenteral thiamine hydrochloride intakes of 1.2 mg·day^{-1} (130 μg·100 kcal^{-1}).[31] Elevated whole blood thiamine concentrations after 50 and 115 days of TPN are reported in infants receiving 1.5 to 4.5 mg·day^{-1}.[32] Premature infants receiving 780 μg·day^{-1} thiamine hydrochloride (970 μg·100 kcal^{-1}, 720 μg·kg^{-1} day^{-1}) were thiamine-sufficient by transketolase assay.[31] That method of assessment did not distinguish excessive and potentially toxic concentrations from sufficient concentrations. Because the ratio of parenteral thiamine to energy intake probably was excessive, the dose used in premature neonates may be too high.[33]

The current recommendation for full-term infants, 1.2 mg·day^{-1}, based on guidelines of the American Medical Association Nutritional Advisory Group, probably is appropriate.[10,34] A consistent dose using 40% of a vial (MVI-Pediatric, Astra Pharmaceuticals, Westborough, MA) per kg·day^{-1} would supply 480 μg·kg^{-1} day^{-1}, but a more realistic dose for premature infants would be 350 μg·kg^{-1} day^{-1} (Table 43.8).[10]

To accommodate maternal and fetal growth and to account for the additional energy allowance, the thiamine allowance is increased in pregnancy (Table 43.7).[35]

Deficiency States

Thiamine deficiency occurs most frequently in areas of the world where the diet consists of unenriched white rice or flour. Consumption of large quantities of raw fish colonized with thiaminase-containing microorganisms, especially if dietary thiamine is decreased, may result in thiamine deficiency.[8] Because of its association with intermediary metabolism, thiamine deficiency usually manifests by abnormalities of carbohydrate metabolism, e.g., elevation of plasma pyruvate and lactate.[8] Marginal thiamine deficiency may be unmasked, therefore, by the administration of large carbohydrate loads.[36] Deficiency may be detected biochemically 1 week after removal of dietary thiamine. Chronic alcoholism, advanced age, malabsorption syndromes, prolonged antacid therapy, renal dialysis, folate deficiency, and chronic malnutrition, are additional causes of thiamine deficiency. Conditions resulting in large diuresis, such as that accompanying diuretic therapy, may increase the urinary excretion of thiamine.[13,14]

A deficiency of thiamine results in beriberi. The signs of this disease relate to the chronicity of the depletion, its severity, and associated stresses.[37] In adults, symptoms may include weakness, confusion, anorexia, peripheral neuropathy, and paresthesias. The illness has been described as "wet" or "dry" depending on the presence of edema or muscle wasting, respectively. In addition to neurologic manifestations, severe deficiency causes cardiovascular changes that may progress to fulminant cardiac failure ("cardiac beriberi").[14,38]

The Wernicke-Korsakoff syndrome results from severe, acute thiamine deficiency often observed in alcoholics and in pregnancies associated with severe vomiting. The high intake of calories solely derived from carbohydrate, coupled with decreased intake of nutritionally adequate foods, is associated with neuropsychiatric manifestations, including confusion, coma, ophthalmoplegia, nystagmus, ataxia, psychosis, and emotional disturbances.

Although thiamine deficiency in the infant may be either acute or chronic, the acute cardiac symptoms and signs generally predominate.[14] Anorexia, apathy, vomiting, restlessness, and pallor progress to dyspnea and cyanosis from cardiomegaly and congestive heart failure causing death in 24 to 48 hours. Acute cardiac failure at 4 days of age was the presenting sign in one neonate whose mother was thiamine deficient.[39] Cardiac beriberi has been reported in an adolescent girl who received an inadequate dose of thiamine (0.016 mg·100 kcal glucose^{-1}) while receiving TPN.[36]

"Infantile" beriberi may occur between 1 and 4 months of age in breast-fed infants whose mothers have a deficient thiamine intake.[38] Maternal signs of thiamine deficiency, however, may not be apparent. Infantile beriberi has been associated with maternal alcoholism and with improperly prepared or inadequately supplemented formula.[18,40,41] Symptoms generally include weak swallowing, nuchal rigidity, apnea, spasticity, ophthalmoplegia, hypothermia, and coma. The infant with beriberi may have a characteristically aphonic cry because of paralysis of the recurrent laryngeal nerve. A pseudomeningitic phase characterized by bulging fontanelle, seizures, and coma has been reported.[11,40,41]

Large doses of thiamine have been effective in the treatment of certain metabolic disorders, including a variant of maple syrup urine disease, Leigh's encephalopathy, thiamine-responsive megaloblastic anemia, and an abnormality in pyruvate decarboxylase characterized clinically by severe lactic acidosis.[11]

Although thiamine deficiency during pregnancy has been reported,[4,16] no correlation has been observed between maternal thiamine status and pregnancy outcome.[42] A 30% incidence of thiamine deficiency in pregnancy has been reported and has been explained on the basis of increasing metabolism, decreasing appetite, and persistent vomiting.[43] The fetomaternal gradient for thiamine favors the fetus and may protect it against maternal deficiency.[4,15,43]

Laboratory Assessment

The classic test for thiamine deficiency is the erythrocyte transketolase assay. In this assay, transketolase activity is measured before and after addition of thiamine pyrophosphate. The TPP effect entails enhancement of transketolase activity. Severe thiamine deficiency exists when this ratio is >25%, mild deficiency occurs when the ratio is 15% to 25%, and adequate status is suggested by a ratio of <15%.[13] The concentration of thiamine in whole blood or cerebrospinal fluid may be a better quantitative measure of vitamin status.[37,44] Urinary excretion of thiamine parallels dietary intake except at low concentrations of intake.[42] In excess of tissue needs, thiamine is excreted in the urine.[13] Plasma pyruvate and lactate are elevated in thiamine deficiency.

Simple thiamine deficiency can be treated orally with 5 mg of thiamine daily.[6] Severely ill children should be given 10 mg intravenously twice daily; those with fulminant congestive heart failure, 100 mg.[6]

Toxicity

Thiamine toxicity is rare. Large parenteral doses, however, may be associated with respiratory depression.[45] Anaphylaxis may occur with rapid intravenous administration.

Riboflavin (Vitamin B$_2$)

General Metabolism

Riboflavin and its coenzymes, flavin mononucleotide (FMN) and flavin adenine dinucleotide (FAD) are shown in Figure 43.2. The coenzymes function as electron donors and acceptors in biologic oxidation-reduction systems. They are intimately involved with a number of enzymatic reactions affecting the metabolism of glucose, fatty acids, and amino acids.

The vitamin is readily absorbed from the small intestine by a carrier-dependent pathway. In the intestinal mucosa, riboflavin is phosphorylated to riboflavin-5'-phosphate (also known as FMN) and further phosphorylated and adenylated to FAD. Absorption is reduced in biliary obstruction and in conditions that decrease intestinal transit time.[15] Urinary excretion of riboflavin depends on dietary intake and saturation of tissue stores.[46]

Riboflavin and its phosphates are decomposed by exposure to light and in strong alkaline solutions.[47,48] The concentration of riboflavin is reduced 50% after 8 hours of indirect sunlight.[49] Since parenteral MVI-Pediatric contains riboflavin-5'-phosphate, photodegradation should not be a problem. However, during parenteral administration, the compound is dephosphorylated to riboflavin and becomes susceptible to photodegradation.[50] Riboflavin is resistant to heat, acid, and oxidation. The processes of pasteurization, evaporation, and condensation of milk do not destroy the vitamin.[51]

Sources

The riboflavin concentration in human milk (Tables 43.1 and 43.2), 47 μg·100 kcal^{-1} (range 36–71 μg·100 kcal^{-1}),

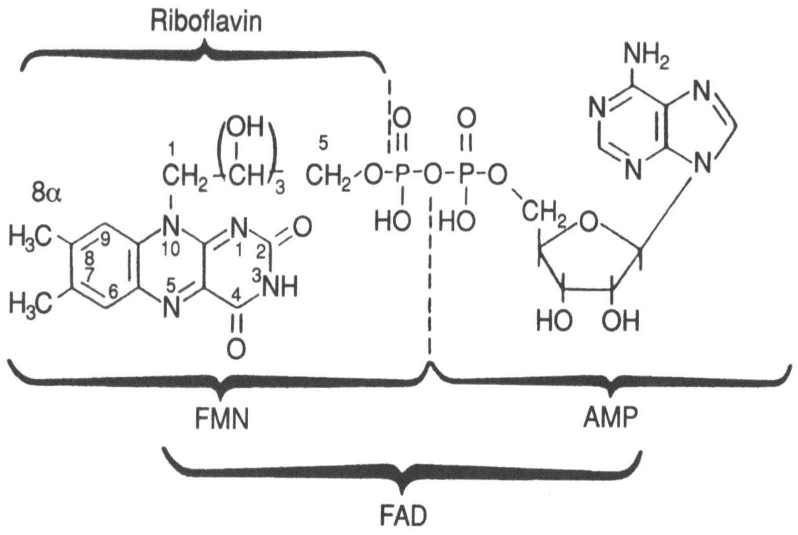

FIGURE 43.2. Riboflavin and its coenzyme forms, FMN and FAD.

remains uniform throughout lactation.[19–21,23,25,52,53] Vitamin supplementation is reflected in a greater milk riboflavin concentration only in extreme circumstances where maternal riboflavin intakes are below 1.7 mg·day^{-1} or greater than three times the RDA.[8,25,53,54] The riboflavin contents of standard formulas and bovine milk are given in Tables 43.1 to 43.3.[20,27,28] Riboflavin is present in a wide variety of foods: milk, cheese, eggs, leafy vegetables, meat, and whole-grain and enriched cereals.[29]

Perinatal Needs

Riboflavin is interrelated with protein metabolism, but riboflavin needs are based on caloric intake because of practical considerations, such as the close relationship between protein and calories and the similarity to the estimation of thiamine needs.[14]

Although the mean concentration of riboflavin in human milk differs both from the minimum recommendation specified by AAP (60 μg·100 kcal^{-1}) and from that calculated from the RDA (Table 43.4), breast-fed full-term neonates have satisfactory riboflavin status.[7,55] The discrepancy between recommendation and milk concentration relates to the more recent methods of determining the riboflavin concentration in human milk.

The premature neonate may have greater riboflavin needs due to the common, possibly prolonged, use of phototherapy. Exposure of stored milk to light also may reduce the amount of the vitamin available to the neonate. As a result, the riboflavin intake for the premature neonate fed human milk is inadequate.[56–58] The concentration of riboflavin in commercial formulas designed for premature neonates (Table 43.3), however, may lead to excessive intakes based on plasma and urine concentrations.[59]

Full-term neonates and children receiving TPN are riboflavin sufficient if they receive 1.4 mg·day^{-1} (150 μg·100 kcal^{-1}) of the vitamin.[31] Whole blood riboflavin concentrations after 50 and 115 days of TPN are adequate in children receiving 1.8 to 5.4 mg·day^{-1}.[32]

Premature infants who received 900 μg·day^{-1} (1180 μg·100 kcal^{-1}, 830 μg·kg^{-1} day^{-1}) have elevated riboflavin concentrations, especially if less than 1 kg birth weight.[31,33,60] The high plasma concentrations may result in renal accumulation and renal toxicity.[60] Despite potential photodegradation, the dose is excessive. The markedly elevated concentrations probably reflect excessive intake and poor renal clearance of riboflavin by the premature infant.[50]

The recommendation for the riboflavin content of TPN for the full-term neonate is 1.4 mg·day^{-1}.[58] The premature infant should receive significantly less than 40% of the vial (MVI-Pediatric) per kg·day^{-1}.[10] A dose of 150 μg·kg^{-1} day^{-1} probably is more realistic.[33,50]

Urinary riboflavin excretion declines during pregnancy and the erythrocyte glutathione reductase (EGR) activity ratio rises.[8] An additional 300 μg·day^{-1} is recommended to compensate for increased tissue needs during pregnancy (Table 43.7).[35]

Deficiency States

Generally, a deficiency of riboflavin occurs in conjunction with more generalized malnutrition and deficiencies of other vitamins. Ariboflavinosis is characterized by angular stomatitis, glossitis, cheilosis, seborrheic dermatitis around the nose and mouth, and eye changes that include reduced tearing, photophobia, corneal vascularization, and cataracts. Because these coenzymes are involved in the metabolism of vitamin B_6, the conversion of tryptophan to niacin is impaired in their absence. Riboflavin deficiency can occur within 7 days of a riboflavin-deficient diet.

Overt signs of deficiency are rare in inhabitants of developed countries. However, the 10-state nutrition survey revealed biochemical evidence of subclinical riboflavin deficiency in the following groups: women taking oral contraceptive agents, persons with diabetes, children from families of low socioeconomic status, children with chronic cardiac disease, the elderly, and infants undergoing phototherapy for hyperbilirubinemia.[51,55,56,61] Phototherapy treatment for hyperbilirubinemia may be associated with biochemical riboflavin deficiency especially in the breast-fed newborn neonate.[46–49,57,58]

Riboflavin deficiency in pregnancy has been reported in 25% patients during their first trimester to 40% patients at term.[43] In Gambia, riboflavin deficiency was present throughout pregnancy but peaked at parturition. That deficiency was unrelated to general malnutrition.[62] A response to maternal riboflavin supplementation ($5\,mg\cdot day^{-1}$) is observed.[63] Associations between decreased riboflavin intake and antenatal fetal mortality, prematurity, hyperemesis in pregnancy, and lactation failure have not consistently documented deleterious effects in infants.[43,64] For the infant born to the riboflavin-deficient mother, a dose of $400\,\mu g\cdot day^{-1}$ in the first year is suggested.[65]

Laboratory Assessment

The classic method for assessment of riboflavin deficiency is the activity of the enzyme EGR before and after FAD administration. An activation coefficient of 1.2 or greater (i.e., 20% increase) strongly suggests a deficient state.[9] The urinary excretion of riboflavin decreases in the early stages of deficiency. Plasma and red blood cell riboflavin, FMN, and FAD concentrations may be preferable to distinguish deficiency and toxicity states.[44,60]

Toxicity

There are no known toxic effects of riboflavin. Riboflavin does produce a yellow coloration of the urine.[45] Precipitation of riboflavin and obstructive uropathy were observed in a premature infant receiving parenteral nutrition who had plasma riboflavin concentrations 100-fold greater than cord blood concentrations.[60]

Niacin

General Metabolism

The word niacin refers to the compound nicotinic acid and its amide form, nicotinamide (niacinamide), shown in Figure 43.3. The vitamin is biologically active as a component of the coenzymes nicotinamide adenine dinucleotide (NAD) and nicotinamide adenine dinucleotide phosphate (NADP). The coenzymes are important in two-electron transfers and are involved in multiple metabolic processes, including fat synthesis, intracellular respiratory metabolism, and glycolysis.[66,67] The physiologic need for niacin is related to energy expenditure, because of the involvement of NAD and NADP in the respiratory chain.

Because excess dietary tryptophan is converted to niacin, the tryptophan content of the diet must be considered when describing the needs for niacin. Tryptophan pyrrolase converts tryptophan eventually to kynurenine and after multiple additional conversions to niacin. The conversion is catalyzed by riboflavin and vitamin B_6. In adults, approximately 3% of administered tryptophan is converted to niacin and 1 niacin equivalent (NE) equals 60 mg tryptophan or 1 mg niacin.[8,66] The conversion of tryptophan to niacin is more efficient during pregnancy, probably a result of estrogen.[8] There are no data available to determine the appropriate conversion factor for infants. Tryptophan accounts for 1.5% of the amino acids in proteins of animal origin.[66] Niacin is stable in foods and can withstand heating and prolonged storage.[67]

Sources

The concentration of niacin in human milk ($0.29\,mg\cdot 100\,kcal^{-1}$, range $0.27–0.34\,mg\cdot 100\,kcal^{-1}$) remains stable

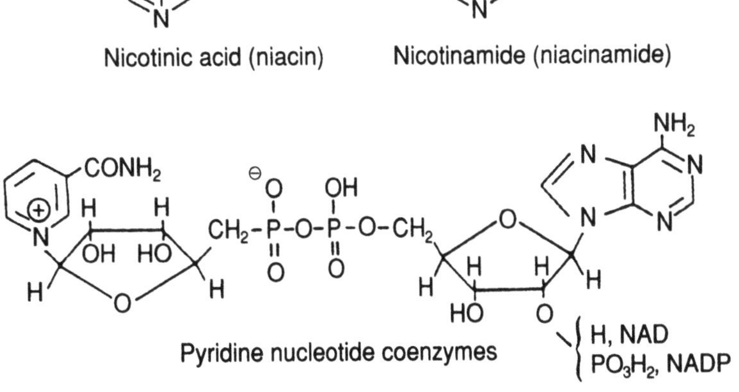

FIGURE 43.3. Niacin, niacinamide, and the pyridine nucleotide coenzymes.

throughout lactation (Tables 43.1 and 43.2).[19,25,34] If the mother is malnourished, niacin supplementation increases the concentration in the milk.[54] Approximately 70% of the total NEs in human milk are derived from tryptophan. The tryptophan content of human milk, 22 mg·dl^{-1} provides 3.8 NE·L^{-1}. The sum of preformed niacin and NEs derived from tryptophan in human milk is approximately 5.7 NE·L^{-1}.[8] In bovine milk, 90% of the NEs are derived from tryptophan.[66] Niacin is present in whole-grain cereals, meats, fish, eggs, and vegetables, including legumes.[29] Niacin in corn is present in a poorly absorbed form. Alkaline treatment of corn (e.g., the addition of lime water to corn in the preparation of corn tortillas as practiced in Mexico and Central America) makes the niacin more bioavailable.[68]

Perinatal Needs

In the infant, niacin status, as assessed by the urinary excretion of niacin metabolites, was normal when fed 6 NE·day^{-1} but not 4 NE·day^{-1}.[69] The recommended allowance for the full-term neonate is based on the NEs in human milk (Table 43.4). Neonates fed routine commercial formula receive adequate niacin (Tables 43.1 and 43.2). The distribution of preformed niacin versus tryptophan-derived niacin in milks has not been studied in relation to the estimated needs of this vitamin.

Full-term infants and children who receive 17 mg·day^{-1} of nicotinamide in TPN have adequate niacin status.[31] Children receiving 20 to 60 mg·day^{-1} for 15 to 90 days of TPN also have adequate vitamin status.[32] The whole blood niacin concentrations increased with the duration of TPN (from 0 to 90 days) and with increases in dosage of the vitamin (20 to 60 mg·day^{-1}).[32] Premature infants receiving 11 mg·day^{-1} were niacin-sufficient.[31] Although exogenous niacin needs may decrease if dietary tryptophan is excessive, the small amount of tryptophan available in pediatric parenteral nutrition formulations probably would not alter recommendations.

The recommendation for parenteral niacin intake in full-term infants and children is 17 mg·day^{-1}.[10] A recommendation for premature infants to use 40% of the vial (MVI-Pediatric) per kg/day or 6.8 mg·kg^{-1} day^{-1} would be consistent, but a dose of 5 mg·kg^{-1} day^{-1} may be more realistic.[10,33]

There is an increased urinary excretion of N^1-metabolites during pregnancy, which suggests an enhanced capacity for biosynthesis of niacin from tryptophan.[8] Because of increased energy needs, pregnant women should receive an additional 2 NE daily (Table 43.7).[35]

Deficiency States

A deficiency of niacin results in the clinical syndrome pellagra, a disease endemic to areas where corn is the primary staple.[66,67,70,71] Pellagra is observed in persons on a predominantly corn diet because corn is deficient in the amino acid tryptophan and the niacin is not well absorbed. The deficiency disease is characterized by weakness, lassitude, *dermatitis*, inflammation of mucous membranes, *diarrhea*, vomiting, dysphagia, and in severe cases, *dementia*, and *death* (i.e., the "4 D's"). Initially, cutaneous inflammation looks like a sunburn because only areas exposed to light are affected. A familial disorder of tryptophan-niacin metabolism, Hartnup disease, is an impaired absorption of monoamino/monocarboxylic acids, including tryptophan.[14,15,67,70-72]

The usual dose for the vitamin deficiency is 10 times the RDA.[6] In addition, a high-calorie, high-protein diet supplemented with all the B vitamins should be provided.[6]

Laboratory Assessment

In the liver, niacin is converted to multiple metabolites prior to its excretion in the urine. The measurement of the urinary excretion of niacin metabolites, N^1-methylniacinamide and N^1-methyl-6-pyridone-3-carboxamide ("pyridone"), is considered a good method for diagnosing niacin deficiency.[14,67,70] Although the excretion of the pyridone decreases earlier in niacin deficiency, it is the most difficult to assay. The ratio of N^1-methylniacinamide to creatinine in random urine samples is easy to use; values below 0.5 mg·g^{-1} creatinine suggest deficiency in adults.[14] Serum N^1-metabolites and nicotinamide can be assayed fluorimetrically.[67]

Toxicity

Excessive intakes of nicotinic acid in adults, which has been used as a pharmacologic agent to lower blood lipid concentrations, can cause cutaneous vasodilation, flushing, headache, pruritus, liver disease, skin rash, hyperuricemia, gastrointestinal ulcers, and impaired glucose tolerance.[6,34] However, nicotinamide (niacinamide) is not a cholesterol-lowering agent and does not have the same side effects. It is the latter form that is used in pediatric preparations.

Pyridoxine (Vitamin B$_6$)

General Metabolism

Pyridoxine, or vitamin B$_6$, shown in Figure 43.4, refers collectively to three naturally occurring pyridines—pyridoxine (PN, pyridoxol), pyridoxal (PL), and pyridoxamine (PM)—and their phosphorylated derivatives.[73] The vitamins are absorbed passively by intestinal mucosa cells, primarily in the proximal jejunum. There is rapid

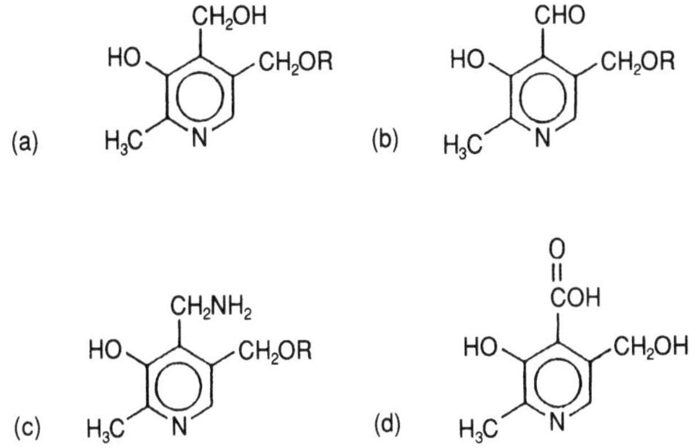

FIGURE 43.4. Forms of vitamin B_6. (a) R = H, pyridoxine; R = PO_3H_2, pyridoxine 5'-phosphate. (b) R = H, pyridoxal; R = PO_3H_2, pyridoxal 5'-phosphate. (c) R = H, pyridoxamine; R = PO_3H_2, pyridoxamine 5'-phosphate. (d) 4-pyridoxic acid.

transfer to the liver where phosphorylation occurs via a cytoplasmic pyridoxal kinase. The liver converts pyridoxine to pyridoxal and 4-pyridoxic acid (4-PA), the major excretory product. In the blood, the dominant forms of the vitamin are PL, PN, PLP (pyridoxal-5-phosphate), and 4-PA.

In the phosphorylated form (i.e., primarily PLP), vitamin B_6 plays a key role in metabolism by acting as a coenzyme.[73] The metabolic functions of vitamin B_6 include participation in interconversion reactions of amino acids, conversion of tryptophan to niacin and serotonin, neurotransmitter synthesis and metabolic reactions in the brain, carbohydrate metabolism, immune system development, and the biosynthesis of heme and prostaglandins. Because of the relationship between vitamin B_6 and protein metabolism, it is customary to consider the ratio of the factors when assessing needs. Ratios of vitamin B_6/protein of $15\,\mu g \cdot g^{-1}$ are appropriate and the two standard deviation lower limit is $11\,\mu g \cdot g^{-1}$.[74] In adults with vitamin B_6 deficient diets, abnormalities of tryptophan and methionine metabolism develop faster and vitamin B_6 concentrations decline more rapidly when protein intakes are high (80–160 vs 30–50 $g \cdot day^{-1}$).[74] During repletion studies, tryptophan and methionine metabolism and plasma vitamin concentrations normalize faster at low protein intakes. Similarly, studies in infants with B_6 deficiency and seizures had some relief of symptoms with high-carbohydrate diets and exacerbations of symptoms with high-protein diets.[74]

High-dietary protein intakes and the destruction of vitamin B_6 by light both increase vitamin B_6 needs. Heat destruction of the PL and PM vitamers probably was responsible for vitamin B_6 deficiency in infants fed improperly processed formulas.[75] The heat-stable vitamer, pyridoxine hydrochloride, is used for the fortification of commercial infant formulas.

Transport of vitamin B_6 becomes more active during the last trimester of pregnancy as assessed by the increased ratio of cord blood to maternal blood.[62,76] The vitamin concentrations are greater in cord blood when compared with those in maternal blood.[76,77] Cord blood contains PLP, pyridoxamine phosphate, and 4-PA in greatest quantities.[76] Indeed, of all water-soluble vitamins, vitamin B_6 has the greatest fetal/maternal ratio.[74,76] The intake of vitamin B_6 during the last trimester of pregnancy determines the nutritional state of the infant with respect to this vitamin.[76-78]

Sources

The vitamin B_6 content of human milk reflects the vitamin B_6 nutritional status of the mother.[54,79-84] A difference in vitamin B_6 content is observed between milks obtained from mothers who consumed the approximate RDA for vitamin B_6 (2.5 mg·day^{-1}) and mothers whose intake of vitamin B_6 differs from the RDA. The concentration of vitamin B_6 is $140\,\mu g \cdot L^{-1}$ ($20\,\mu g \cdot 100\,kcal^{-1}$, range 15–$30\,\mu g \cdot 100\,kcal^{-1}$) in milk obtained from mothers whose intake is below the RDA.[21,79,80,82,85] Milk concentrations of mothers who consumed between 2.5 and 5.9 mg·day^{-1} of vitamin B_6 average $30\,\mu g \cdot 100\,kcal^{-1}$ ($210\,\mu g \cdot L^{-1}$, range 150–$250\,\mu g \cdot L^{-1}$).[21,79,80,82,83,86] The milk vitamin concentration of those mothers consuming 10 to 20 mg·day^{-1} is $50\,\mu g \cdot 100\,kcal^{-1}$ ($340\,\mu g \cdot L^{-1}$, range 250–$530\,\mu g \cdot L^{-1}$).[79,86] The vitamin B_6 content of human milk may decline with prolonged lactation.[87] Milk vitamin B_6 content of women not receiving vitamin supplements is provided in Tables 43.1 and 43.2.

The vitamin B_6/protein ratio in milk, generally used to assess vitamin B_6 status, may decline to concentrations as low as $7\,\mu g \cdot g^{-1}$ in milk obtained from unsupplemented mothers.[79] However, a range of 8.5 to $30\,\mu g \cdot g^{-1}$ was reported depending on the maternal intake of vitamin B_6.[21,79,80,82,83,86] It seems prudent to recommend vitamin B_6 supplementation to lactating women (Table 43.7).

The range of vitamin B_6 concentrations in bovine milk and infant formulas is shown in Tables 43.1 to 43.3. Goat milk is deficient in vitamin B_6.[88] Vitamin B_6 is present in low concentrations in most plants and animals.[29]

Perinatal Needs

If the vitamin B_6 intake of a mother is adequate, the normal full-term neonate has sufficient stores of the vitamin to meet its needs during the first weeks of life. There is insufficient evidence to suggest that deficiency states exist in full-term breast-fed neonates, unless the vitamin B_6 content of their mothers' milk is low. The human milk–fed premature neonate would not receive adequate vitamin B_6.[88] For these reasons the ESPGAN[9] recommendations are greater than those specified by AAP.[7]

Clinical vitamin B_6 deficiency, manifested by seizures, has been reported in the formula-fed neonate who was given an improperly sterilized milk, which partially destroyed the vitamin.[85,89] The incidence of seizures was 0.3% when intakes of vitamin B_6 were 60 µg·day^{-1}.[74] A dose of vitamin B_6, 260 µg·day^{-1}, cured the seizure disorder, but 300 µg·day^{-1} normalized tryptophan metabolism.[74,85] Commercially available infant formulas contain sufficient vitamin B_6 to meet estimated needs of the full-term infant (Table 43.1). Formulas designed for premature infants, however, may contain excessive quantities of the vitamin.[59]

No deficiency of vitamin B_6 is observed in full-term infants and children receiving 1.0 mg or 3.0 mg·day^{-1} or 110 µg·100 kcal^{-1} of pyridoxine hydrochloride in TPN.[31,32] When premature infants received 650 µg·day^{-1} or 850 µg·100 kcal^{-1}, no deficiencies were observed.[31,32] However, as computed based on energy intakes, it is unclear whether the doses for premature infants are excessive.[33] Although there is a concern that premature infants of <30 weeks' gestation may be unable to convert parenterally administered pyridoxine to PLP, when given parenteral pyridoxine at doses of 300 to 700 µg·day^{-1} conversion of pyridoxine to other B_6 vitamers is observed.[33,90] PLP may not be the appropriate indicator for vitamin B_6 status in premature infants of <30 weeks' gestation.[91]

The recommended parenteral intake of vitamin B_6 in full-term infants is 1000 µg·day^{-1}.[10] A consistent parenteral vitamin B_6 intake of 300 µg·kg^{-1}day^{-1} provides adequate vitamin status for premature infants.[10]

Pregnancy is characterized by low dietary B_6 intake and by declining plasma PLP concentrations.[76,92,93] In one study, 60% of pregnant women were vitamin B_6 deficient, but no associated neonatal sequelae were observed.[43,74,92] Many studies report biochemical vitamin B_6 deficiency during pregnancy.[8,92,94] Although vitamin B_6 has been prescribed for morning sickness in pregnancy, no association between the status of that vitamin and the clinical signs has been found.[95]

Because of increased protein intakes in pregnancy, the needs for vitamin B_6 increase.[35,74] Urinary excretion of 4-PA is similar in pregnant and nonpregnant women, suggesting that vitamin absorption is adequate in pregnancy.[76] The lower plasma PLP concentrations during pregnancy may be attributed to fetal uptake and hemodilution.[8,76] Maternal plasma B_6 concentrations correlated with vitamin supplementation at 30 weeks and at term.[92] Intakes of 5.5 to 7.5 mg·day^{-1} were associated with stable plasma PLP concentrations throughout pregnancy. An intake of 1.4 mg·day^{-1} (only from dietary sources and no supplement) resulted in lower plasma PLP concentrations but no adverse outcomes in neonates at delivery were reported.[92] Gestational accumulation of vitamin B_6 affects the status of the full-term, breast-fed neonate.[78] Daily supplementation of the mother during pregnancy with >2 mg pyridoxine was associated with normal vitamin status in the infants through 4 months of lactation.[78] Therefore, an increment in vitamin B_6 intake during pregnancy appears appropriate (Table 43.7).

Deficiency States

In infants, dietary deprivation or malabsorption of vitamin B_6 results in hypochromic microcytic anemia, vomiting, diarrhea, failure to thrive, listlessness, hyperirritability, and seizures. In adults, vitamin B_6 deficiency may result in depression, confusion, peripheral neuritis, electroencephalograph abnormalities, and seizures.[75–77,79,86] As protein intake increases, the onset of vitamin deficiency becomes more rapid.

Vitamin B_6–dependent seizures in neonates respond to 5 to 10 mg pyridoxine given intravenously.[6] Affected neonates can be maintained on 10 to 25 mg·day^{-1}.[6]

Several conditions are associated with abnormalities in vitamin B_6 metabolism that require pharmacologic doses of the vitamin for adequate function. These vitamin B_6–dependency syndromes include the following conditions: pyridoxine-dependent seizures in the neonate, pyridoxine-responsive hypochromic microcytic anemia, xanthurenic aciduria, cystathioninuria, and homocystinuria. These conditions require massive doses of the vitamin, 200 to 600 mg·day^{-1}.[6] Routine vitamin B_6 supplementation is recommended for infants and children receiving isoniazid and for the breast-fed neonate whose mother receives isoniazid.[11]

Laboratory Assessment

Quantitative assays for total vitamin B_6 generally employ the microbiologic assay of *Saccharomyces uvarum*.[79–81,86] Methods for the assessment of vitamin B_6 nutritional status include the tryptophan load test, the measurement of 4-PA excretion, the plasma PLP concentration, and the measurement of erythrocyte activity of aspartate aminotransferase (glutamic-oxalacetic transaminase) and alanine aminotransferase (glutamic-pyruvic transaminase).[44,77] The erythrocyte glutamic-pyruvic transaminase (EGPT) index measures the enzyme activity before and after the addition of PLP. Normal individuals have an index of less than 1.25.[77,80]

Toxicity

Toxicity from large doses of the vitamin is rare. A sensory neuropathy occurs in adults taking large doses of the vitamin for a long period of time.[96]

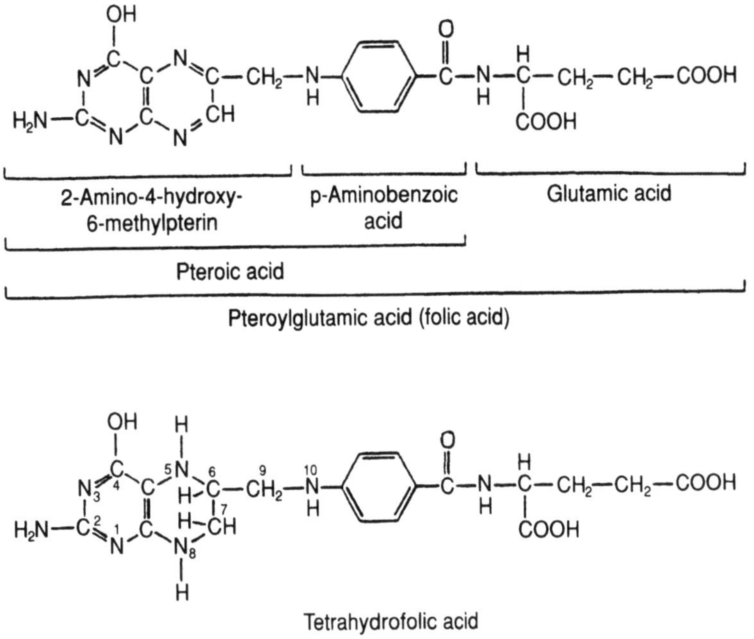

FIGURE 43.5. Folic acid and tetrahydrofolic acid.

Folate

General Metabolism

Folate is the general term that describes compounds having nutritional and chemical properties similar to folic acid (pteroylglutamic acid, PGA), shown in Figure 43.5. The parent compound is a pteridine moiety joined to para-aminobenzoic acid. Reduction of the pyrazine ring to yield tetrahydrofolate, addition of multiple glutamyl residues, and acquisition of one-carbon fragments result in activation of the vitamin. The coenzyme participates in the biosynthesis of purines and pyrimidines, in the metabolism of some amino acids, and in the catabolism of histidine.[97,98]

The vitamin is absorbed rapidly from the small intestine, primarily from the proximal third although the entire small bowel has absorptive capacity.[99] Dietary folate occurs predominantly as polyglutamate, usually as 5-methyl or 10-formyl pteroylpolyglutamate, which is hydrolyzed to the monoglutamate by the intestinal mucosa prior to absorption.[98] Zinc deficiency decreases the conjugase activity, resulting in decreased folate uptake.[100] Folate then enters the portal circulation as the free, monoglutamate derivative.[101] Absorption appears to be an active process that is enhanced by the presence of glucose.[102] The vitamin is inactivated by heat, canning, and light exposure.[9]

Folate homeostasis is regulated, at least in part, by the enterohepatic cycle.[103] Normally, bile folate is reabsorbed efficiently, which results in a total body folate turnover of only 1% per day in adults.[97] Because the biliary folate content is large, enterohepatic recirculation results in a long half-life of the vitamin.[97,101,104] The vitamin is synthesized by colonic bacteria.[8]

Sources

The folate content of human milk increases after the first postpartum week from 5 to $10\,\mu g \cdot L^{-1}$ to 20 to $40\,\mu g \cdot L^{-1}$ at 1 month and 50 to $100\,\mu g \cdot L^{-1}$ at 3 months.[9,75,82,98,101,105] The average folate contents of human and bovine milks, however, are similar, approximately $50\,\mu g \cdot L^{-1}$ ($7\,\mu g \cdot 100\,kcal^{-1}$) (Tables 43.1 and 43.2). Commercially prepared infant formulas contain a greater quantity of the vitamin (Tables 43.1 and 43.2). Folate supplementation increases the concentration of the vitamin in the milk of women who are malnourished.[54,82,106] Differences in folate concentrations between fore- and hindmilk have been reported.[107] Goat milk, containing $6\,\mu g \cdot L^{-1}$, is an inadequate source of folate.[98,101] Foods rich in folate include green leafy vegetables, organ meats, yeast, and fruit.[29] Folic acid supplements are absorbed better than polyglutamates found in food.

Perinatal Needs

The folate status of full-term neonates fed commercial formula appears adequate.[105,108,109] The U.S. RDA of $25\,\mu g \cdot day^{-1}$, which averages $4.2\,\mu g \cdot kg^{-1} day^{-1}$ during the first 6 months, provides a satisfactory intake of folate.[8] With respect to the content of folate in human milk, the AAP recommendation of $4\,\mu g \cdot 100\,kcal^{-1}$ appears appropriate and neither deficiency states nor low plasma folate concentrations have been reported in breast-fed full-term infants.[7,105,108–111] Indeed, a dose of 4 µg · 100 kcal^{-1} resulted in normal red cell morphology in a group of full-term infants.[112,113]

The recommendations for the premature neonate, however, are controversial.[9,112,114,115] No differences in rate of growth and hematologic indices have been reported in premature neonates given folate in doses of 100 µg·day^{-1} versus 3.5 µg·day^{-1}.[115] Ek et al.[116] evaluated formula-fed premature infants given folate in doses of either 65 µg·day^{-1} or 15 µg·day^{-1} for 1 year. Although differences in plasma and red cell folate concentrations were demonstrated at 2 to 6 months of age, no differences between groups were observed for growth and hematologic indices.[116] Current recommendations by ESPGAN differ from AAP and suggest that enterally fed premature infants should receive 60 to 65 µg·day^{-1}.[9] Because human milk may be inadequate for these infants, a supplement is recommended.[9]

Folate has been administered in TPN formulations to full-term neonates in doses of 140 µg·day^{-1} (15 µg · 100 kcal^{-1}).[31] At those intakes, cord red blood cell folate concentrations remained unchanged for 7 days, but increased at days 14 and 21. In children who received long-term TPN, red cell folate concentrations remained stable for 5 months. Adequate serum and red cell folate concentrations during 15 to 90 days of TPN were reported in children receiving 200 to 600 µg·day^{-1}.[32] An increase in plasma folate concentration was observed from 0 to 90 days and with increases in intakes from 200 to 600 µg·day^{-1}.[32] Red cell folate concentrations in premature neonates were slightly elevated when receiving parenteral doses of approximately 91 µg·day^{-1} (120 µg · 100 kcal^{-1} or 84 µg·kg^{-1} day^{-1}).[31]

The recommended TPN folate intake in full-term neonates and children is 140 µg·day^{-1}.[10] For premature neonates, a consistent daily dose of 40% of the vial (MVI-Pediatric) per kilogram body weight, 56 µg·kg^{-1} day^{-1}, would provide an adequate folate status. However, a more realistic dose for premature infants would be 40 µg·kg^{-1} day^{-1}.[10]

Low or marginally folate-deficient women may manifest folate deficiency during pregnancy.[8] In a study in Cambridge, pregnant women were receiving only 20% of the RDA for the vitamin. A decline in plasma folate concentrations during pregnancy is observed in most studies.[8,98,117] Supplementation to increase dietary folate to 400 µg·day^{-1} appears to provide sufficient vitamin to support fetal and maternal tissues (Table 43.5). The Centers for Disease Control and Prevention Advisory recommends 400 µg·day^{-1} for all women intending to conceive.[118–120] Higher doses, approximately 4 mg·day^{-1}, are suggested for women having a prior conception with a neural tube defect or suspected neural tube defect.[54,64,118]

Deficiency States

Nutritional folate deficiency is one of the most common hypovitaminoses in man.[98,101,102] Growth retardation, even in the absence of anemia, and abnormalities in bone marrow, neurologic status, and small intestinal morphology have been described in folate deficiency.[112] In a population of infants who consumed boiled and pasteurized bovine milk, which has a low folate concentration, supplementation of the vitamin was shown to improve growth at 4 to 6 months of age despite the absence of hematologic markers of deficiency.[121] Folate deficiency has been identified more commonly in small-for-gestational-age infants.[114] Correction of a folate-deficient maternal diet resulted in a 50% decrease in the incidence of small-for-gestational-age infants in India.[101] The fall in serum folate observed in the neonatal period reflects an increased need for folate for DNA and RNA synthesis.[122] Certain medications (e.g., phenobarbital, phenytoin, and sulfasalazine) may increase the need for the vitamin. Requirements for folate increase during pregnancy, periods of intense hematopoiesis, and growth.[9] Low folate concentrations are encountered in vitamin B_{12} deficiency. Treatment with folate may improve the hematologic manifestations of vitamin B_{12} deficiency, but does not affect the progressive neurologic degeneration associated with that deficiency state. Iron deficiency may lead to decreased utilization of folate.[123] Folic acid therapy may inhibit zinc absorption.[5]

The hematologic manifestations of folate deficiency include hypersegmentation of neutrophils (i.e., usually greater than 3.5 lobes), megaloblastosis, and anemia.[98,101,114] The sequential changes due to the ingestion of a folate-deficient diet have been described in adults.[101] The earliest finding, after 3 weeks of a deficient intake, is a low serum folate concentration. Continued deficient intake results in hypersegmentation of neutrophils by 5 weeks. At 13 weeks, there is an increased urinary formiminoglutamic acid (FIGLU) excretion. A diminished erythrocyte folate concentration is noted by 17 weeks, and megaloblastosis and anemia are evidenced by 20 weeks. Although megaloblastic anemia is reported in premature infants, anemia is a late sign of folate deficiency. Other more subtle changes in erythrocytes and neutrophils are more sensitive indicators of deficiency in the premature infant.

Folate doses as low as 5 µg·kg^{-1} day^{-1} produce a hematologic response in folate-deficient children, and daily doses of 1 to 5 mg are needed for maintenance.[6]

The incidence of congenital neural tube defects may be associated with preconceptional folate deficiency.[113,118] Significantly lower concentrations of red cell folate in mothers delivering infants with neural tube defects compared with control mothers have been reported.[124] Women who took multivitamin preparations during the periconceptional period appear to have a lower risk of delivering a neonate with a neural tube defect than women who did not take multivitamins.[125] Periconceptional use of multivitamins does not protect against neural tube deformities in all studies.[118,126] Although the data are conflicting, folate supplementation even before conception is advisable.[118]

Laboratory Assessment

Folate status is assessed by evaluating concentrations of the vitamin in sera and erythrocytes. Erythrocyte folate is less variable and is useful for assessing adequacy of long-term intake. Urinary excretion of FIGLU, an intermediate in the metabolism of histidine to glutamic acid, is an indicator of folate deficiency. Mean red blood cell volume (MCV) and the degree of granulocyte nuclear segmentation also are used to assess status.

Toxicity

Large doses of folate are infrequent because the vitamin has not been present in large quantities in over-the-counter preparations.[45] Folate may mask vitamin B_{12} deficiency and depress zinc absorption.[5]

Vitamin B_{12}

General Metabolism

The structure of vitamin B_{12} is shown in Figure 43.6. The corrin ring is a macrocyclic ring formed by the linkage of four reduced pyrrol rings. In the case of vitamin B_{12}, the center of the ring is cobalt. Perpendicular to the ring is a nucleotide (5,6-dimethylbenzimidazole) linked to the ring by D-1-amino-2-propanol. "Cobalamin" is used to describe vitamin B_{12} regardless of the moiety attached to the cobalt. Cyanocobalamin is the synthetic compound used in commercial preparations containing the vitamin. It is not found in significant amounts in food or in the human body and is not metabolically active until the cyanide moiety is removed. When the chemical was finally synthesized in 1947, it was called a B vitamin because of its water solubility and assigned the next available number, 12.[127]

Upon ingestion, vitamin B_{12} is released from food at gastric pH. It is then complexed with salivary R binder, which has greater affinity than intrinsic factor.[128] At the alkaline pH of the upper small bowel, pancreatic enzymes digest the R binder and release vitamin B_{12}. Intrinsic factor then binds vitamin B_{12} to facilitate Ca-dependent absorption, at alkaline pH, across ileal mucosa. Within the mucosa, intrinsic factor is replaced by a plasma transport protein.[129] One to three percent of

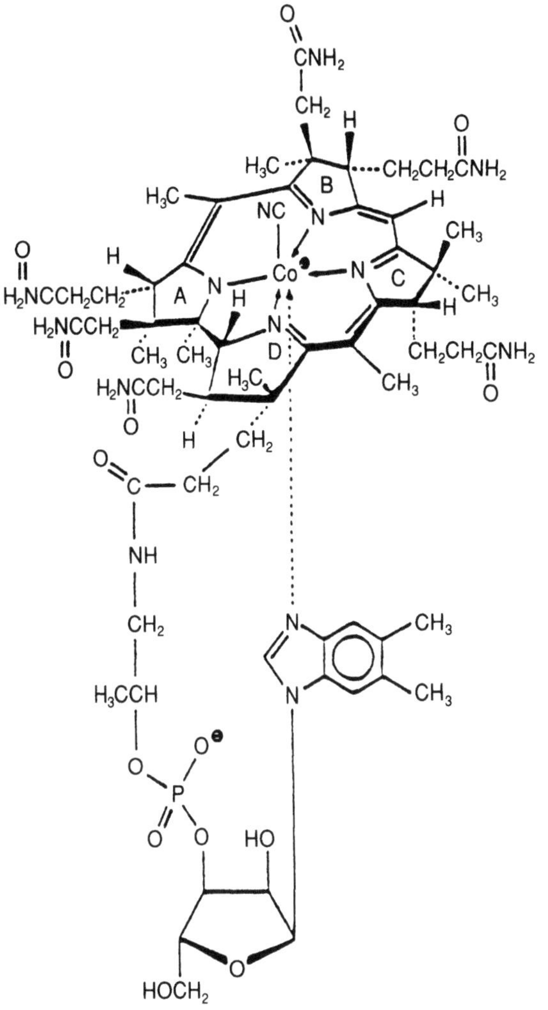

FIGURE 43.6. Vitamin B_{12} (cyanocobalamin).

vitamin B_{12} is absorbed passively. An effective enterohepatic circulation of vitamin B_{12} accounts for its long half-life.[129] Therefore, unlike other water-soluble vitamins, storage of vitamin B_{12} may last an adult 3 to 5 years.

Vitamin B_{12} is active in metabolism in two forms: methylcobalamin and 5-deoxyadenosylcobalamin (coenzyme B_{12}).[99] The methylated version is involved in one-carbon transfers. In particular, vitamin B_{12} transfers a methyl group from tetrahydrofolate to homocysteine for the synthesis of methionine. Vitamin B_{12} is necessary for the regeneration of tetrahydrofolate. In vitamin B_{12} deficiency, folate may be trapped in its demethylated form, and as such, it is unavailable for pyrimidine synthesis. This role of vitamin B_{12} in folate metabolism is responsible for the cellular folate deficiency.

Adenosylcobalamin participates in the reduction of purine and pyrimidine ribonucleotides to their corresponding deoxyribonucleotides necessary for DNA synthesis. The adenosyl form also is necessary for the conversion of methylmalonyl-CoA to succinyl-CoA. In this role, vitamin B_{12} is a key factor in the metabolism of fat, branched-chain amino acids, and carbohydrate.[99] A lack of vitamin B_{12} results in an accumulation of methylmalonic acid with subsequent excretion in the urine.

Sources

The vitamin B_{12} content of human milk ranges from $1.2\,\mu g \cdot L^{-1}$ at 1 week to $0.5\,\mu g \cdot L^{-1}$ at 6 months of lactation.[21,80,82] The average concentration is $0.7\,\mu g \cdot L^{-1}$ ($0.1\,\mu g \cdot 100\,kcal^{-1}$, range $0.07-0.18\,\mu g \cdot 100\,kcal^{-1}$) (Tables 43.1 and 43.2). Maternal supplementation with vitamin B_{12} tends to increase the vitamin content in the milk from the malnourished to the normal state.[54,80,82,130,131] The usual dietary sources are meat, fish, and eggs.[29] Meat products contain the adenosyl form of the vitamin and dairy products contain the methyl form.[6]

Perinatal Needs

Breast-fed neonates receive adequate amounts of vitamin B_{12} if maternal serum, and, therefore, milk, vitamin B_{12} concentrations are normal. Unless the maternal diet is deficient or conditions exist that impair maternal vitamin absorption, the breast-fed neonate has an adequate vitamin B_{12} status. Oral doses as little as $0.1\,\mu g \cdot day^{-1}$, however, correct or prevent a deficiency state in the breast-fed infant of a vegan.[129] The RDA of $0.3\,\mu g \cdot day^{-1}$ ($0.05\,\mu g \cdot kg^{-1} day^{-1}$) provides a substantial margin of sufficiency during infancy (Tables 43.4 and 43.6).

Vitamin B_{12} status during TPN has been reported for full-term neonates receiving $1\,\mu g \cdot day^{-1}$ ($0.1\,\mu g \cdot 100\,kcal^{-1}$).[31] Those neonates maintained vitamin B_{12} concentrations above reference controls, but these values tended to decline toward baseline cord blood values after 21 days of therapy. During the long-term administration of TPN in children, vitamin B_{12} concentrations remained above reference controls, especially while receiving doses of 2.5 to $7.5\,\mu g \cdot day^{-1}$.[31,32] The serum vitamin B_{12} concentration of premature neonates receiving $0.65\,\mu g \cdot day^{-1}$ ($0.85\,\mu g \cdot 100\,kcal^{-1}$, $0.6\,\mu g \cdot kg^{-1} day^{-1}$) remained elevated throughout the 28-day study.[31]

The recommended parenteral intake of vitamin B_{12} in full-term neonates and children of $1\,\mu g \cdot day^{-1}$ possibly is excessive, and a dose of $0.75\,\mu g \cdot day^{-1}$ may be more appropriate.[10] An estimate for the parenteral vitamin B_{12} intake of premature neonates based on 40% of a vial (MVI-Pediatric) per kg/day is $0.40\,\mu g \cdot kg^{-1} day^{-1}$. A more realistic dose for premature neonates is $0.30\,\mu g \cdot kg^{-1} day^{-1}$.[10]

Maternal vitamin B_{12} stores generally are satisfactory to meet the needs of pregnancy. The decline in plasma vitamin B_{12} concentrations during pregnancy are associated with increased macrocytic changes in erythrocytes.[117] A 10% increment in the vitamin intake in pregnancy appears appropriate (Table 43.5).

Deficiency States

The result of vitamin B_{12} deficiency is ineffective DNA synthesis, which is evident clinically as hypersegmentation of neutrophils and megaloblastic anemia. The sequential stages in the development of vitamin B_{12} deficiency have been described.[128]

Nerve damage is a consequence of vitamin B_{12} deficiency, because of inadequate myelin synthesis. An association between vitamin B_{12} and osteoblast-specific proteins has been reported.[132] Vitamin B_{12}–deficient adults had lower skeletal alkaline phosphatase activity and lower osteocalcin concentrations in plasma than did control subjects. Changes in the concentrations of those proteins were reported following vitamin B_{12} therapy.[132]

Because cobalamin stores greatly exceed daily needs, deficiency of this vitamin is encountered rarely. Clinical circumstances that produce vitamin B_{12} deficiency include lack of intrinsic factor (e.g., pernicious anemia, postgastrectomy, destruction of gastric mucosa), small bowel bacterial overgrowth, specific intestinal mucosal defects (e.g., celiac disease, ileal resection), inborn errors of metabolism, and drug interactions. Inadequate vitamin B_{12} status may result from a vegan diet.[129,133-135] In adults, the deficiency state is characterized by weakness, anemia, congestive heart failure, glossitis, lemon-colored skin, and neurologic conditions such as paresthesias, degeneration of posterior and lateral columns of the spinal cord, and peripheral neuritis.[133-135]

Vitamin B_{12} deficiency is reported in exclusively breast-fed infants whose mothers are strict vegans and take no vitamin supplements.[133] Delayed developmental milestones, coma, and hematologic findings (e.g., megaloblastic anemia, neutropenia, and thrombocytopenia) were the presenting findings. Urinary excretion of methylmalonic acid, glycine, methylcitric acid, and homocystine were elevated. A dramatic response to intramuscular vitamin B_{12} was noted.[133] Elevated urinary methylmalonic acid concentrations in lactating vegan women and in their infants decline following vitamin B_{12} therapy in infants and mothers.[135]

Resection of the terminal ileum, such as may occur as a result of necrotizing enterocolitis, may impair vitamin B_{12} absorption. Six of 14 children who had undergone ileal resection for necrotizing enterocolitis had evidence of malabsorption of the vitamin.[136] In these circumstances, therapy with parenteral vitamin B_{12} is needed every 1 to 3 months.[6]

Laboratory Assessment

The most commonly used test for the adequacy of vitamin B_{12} is serum concentration.[137] Red cell concentrations are less reliable because they overlap between normal and deficient subjects and because they are low in folate

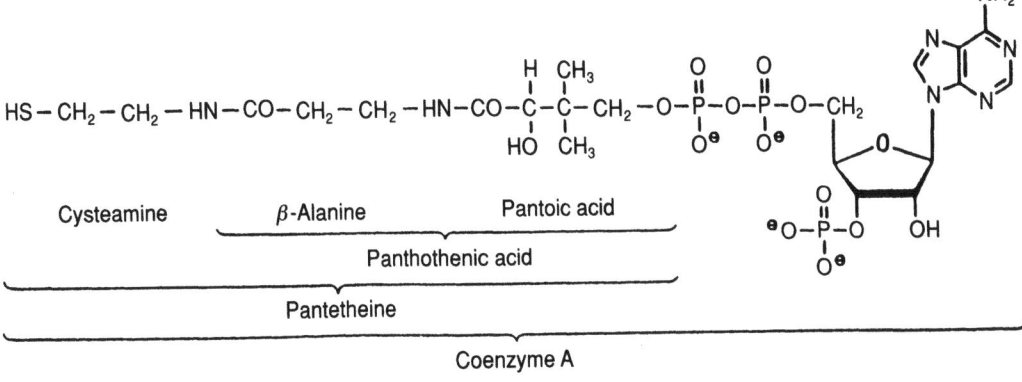

FIGURE 43.7. Pantothenic acid as part of coenzyme A.

and iron deficiency, despite adequate total body stores of vitamin B_{12}.[138] A functional test of vitamin B_{12} adequacy is the measurement of methylmalonic acid excretion with or without a loading dose of valine or isoleucine, but this test is less reliable and more complex.[137] The Schilling test also is used in the evaluation of vitamin B_{12} deficiency. Radiolabeled vitamin B_{12} is given orally and urinary excretion of labeled vitamin is measured both in the presence and absence of intrinsic factor. The test measures vitamin B_{12} absorption and the contribution of intrinsic factor to vitamin malabsorption.[139]

Toxicity

There are no reports of vitamin B_{12} toxicity.

Pantothenic Acid

General Metabolism

Pantothenic acid molecule (Figure 43.7) consists of β-alanine joined to pantoic acid (2,4-dihydroxy-3,3-dimethylbutyric acid) by an amide bond. It serves as an integral part of coenzyme A, which functions in acyl group transfers in the synthesis of fatty acids, cholesterol, steroids, the oxidation of fatty acids, pyruvate, and α-ketoglutarate, and in other acetylation reactions.[8,72,140,141]

Most pantothenic acid is ingested in the form of coenzyme A, which undergoes intestinal hydrolysis prior to absorption. The vitamin is transported in the blood as pantothenic acid, then resynthesized to coenzyme A locally. Endogenous synthesis of the vitamin from pantoic acid and β-alanine is reported. The plasma concentration of pantothenic acid in neonatal cord blood is severalfold greater than maternal blood.[140]

Sources

The concentration of pantothenic acid in mature human milk is approximately $4 mg \cdot L^{-1}$ ($0.6 mg \cdot 100 kcal^{-1}$, range $0.3-1.0 mg \cdot 100 kcal^{-1}$) (Tables 43.1 and 43.2).[23,142–144] Supplementation of malnourished women or consumption of extremely large quantities of the vitamin results in increases in the milk content of pantothenic acid.[54,142,143] In cow milk, 30% to 35% of the vitamin is lost in processing.[142,145]

Perinatal Needs

The safe and adequate intake of pantothenic acid is $2 mg \cdot day^{-1}$.[8] Infants receiving human milk or formula should ingest this amount during their first year.[8,142]

The vitamin needs during TPN have been evaluated in a small number of children.[31] Full-term neonates and children who received $5 mg \cdot day^{-1}$ maintained stable plasma concentrations for 21 days; premature neonates who received $3.2 mg \cdot day^{-1}$ ($2.9 mg \cdot kg^{-1} \cdot day^{-1}$) demonstrated slightly elevated plasma concentrations relative to their baseline and to controls.

The recommendation for parenteral pantothenic acid, $5 mg \cdot day^{-1}$, is appropriate for full-term neonates and children.[10] A consistent parenteral pantothenic acid intake of $1.5 mg \cdot kg^{-1} \cdot day^{-1}$ provides adequate vitamin status for the premature neonates.[10]

There are no data available to assess pantothenic acid needs in pregnancy.

Deficiency States

Because of the ubiquitous distribution of this vitamin, a clinical deficiency syndrome has not been reported.[141] The essential biologic role of pantothenic acid was defined in animal experiments, but extraordinary circumstances were required to produce the deficiency in man. For example, experimental deficiency has been produced in volunteers fed the antagonist ω-methylpantothenic acid as part of a pantothenic acid-deficient diet.[141] Subjects developed burning feet, gastrointestinal disturbances, headache, insomnia, fatigue, and muscle weakness. A deficiency of pantothenic acid also is observed in severe malnutrition. Pantothenic deficiency is considered to have caused the "burning feet syndrome" described in World War II prisoners in the Far East.[141]

Laboratory Assessment

Plasma concentration may be measured.[10]

Toxicity

Pantothenic acid toxicity has not been reported. High doses may be associated with water retention and diarrhea.[45] Anorexia, vomiting, hypotension, personality changes, and increased deep tendon reflexes have been associated with ingestion of high doses of the vitamin.[6]

Biotin

General Metabolism

Biotin (Figure 43.8) functions as a coenzyme for carboxylation, decarboxylation, and transcarboxylation reactions. As such, it plays an important role in the biosynthesis of amino and fatty acids and as a cofactor in gluconeogenesis. Biotin is absorbed by passive diffusion and transported bound to plasma proteins. Urinary excretion reflects dietary intake; fecal excretion, generally unaffected by intake, indicates enteric synthesis.[8,146]

Sources

The average biotin content of human milk during the first week of lactation is $0.7\,\mu g \cdot L^{-1}$.[8,23,147] The average biotin concentration in mature human milk is $5.0\,\mu g \cdot L^{-1}$ ($0.7\,\mu g \cdot 100\,kcal^{-1}$, range 0.6–$1.1\,\mu g \cdot 100\,kcal^{-1}$) (Tables 43.1 and 43.2).[23,144,146–148] Dietary supplementation of malnourished women results in a rise in the biotin content of the milk.[11] Cow's milk is a rich source of biotin (Table 43.1).[145]

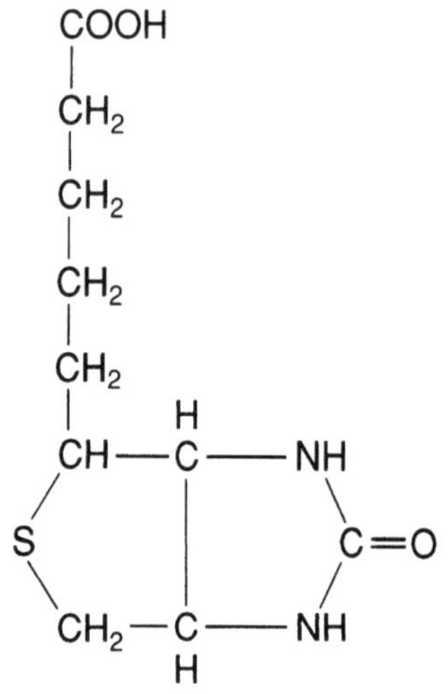

Small quantities of biotin are present in most plant and animal foods, including meats, yeast, egg yolks, dairy products, grains, fruits, and vegetables. A major source of biotin is intestinal bacteria.

Perinatal Needs

The bases for recommended intake for biotin have not been established. Urinary biotin excretion in the neonate increases in the first days of life and then declines until 6 months when, possibly related to diet, it rises gradually to adult concentration.[144] Biotin deficiency has not been reported in infants fed either human milk or formulas despite a wide range of intakes. The safe and adequate intake of biotin is $10\,\mu g \cdot day^{-1}$ for infants, which approximates the intake from human milk.[8]

The vitamin needs during TPN have been investigated.[31,32] Full-term infants and children receiving 20 to $90\,\mu g \cdot day^{-1}$ maintained stable, adequate plasma biotin concentrations for as long as 90 days. Premature neonates receiving $13\,\mu g \cdot day^{-1}$ ($12\,\mu g \cdot kg^{-1} \cdot day^{-1}$) had elevated plasma biotin concentrations, 10-fold greater than controls, during sampling intervals over a 28-day period.

The recommendation for TPN biotin intake for full-term neonates and children is $20\,\mu g \cdot day^{-1}$.[10] A consistent parenteral biotin intake of $6.0\,\mu g \cdot kg^{-1} \cdot day^{-1}$ would provide adequate vitamin status for premature neonates.[10]

Plasma biotin concentrations are lower in pregnancy and decline during gestation.[8] No data, however, are available to set specific allowances (Table 43.5).

Deficiency States

In individuals fed normal diets, a deficiency of biotin is unlikely to occur. A deficiency state is observed when gastrointestinal flora is suppressed or when biotin absorption is diminished, such as occurs in diets consisting of raw eggs.[146,148] Symptoms of biotin deficiency include anorexia, nausea, glossitis, pallor, mental changes, alopecia, and a fine maculosquamous dermatitis that becomes exfoliative.[72,149,150] Biotin deficiency has been reported in patients with short gut syndrome when the vitamin was omitted from TPN solutions.[147–150] A young girl receiving TPN for 6 months reportedly developed a scaly dermatitis, alopecia, pallor, irritability, lethargy, and markedly reduced urinary excretion and plasma concentration of biotin.[150] Administration of biotin corrected the abnormalities. Biotin-dependent carboxylase deficiency states have been described. The multiple carboxylase defect (e.g., pyruvate, propionyl-CoA, and methylcrotonyl-CoA carboxylase) has been shown to be

FIGURE 43.8. Biotin.

biotin responsive.[72] Antibiotics may affect biotin status by decreasing enteric synthesis of the vitamin.[148]

Laboratory Assessment

Plasma biotin concentration commonly is assayed by microbiologic methods and by competitive binding assays using avidin.[64,129]

Toxicity

There are no reports of biotin toxicity.

Vitamin C

General Metabolism

The two principal forms of vitamin C, shown in Figure 43.9, are L-ascorbic acid and the oxidized form, dehydroascorbic acid. L-ascorbic acid, the biologically more active form of the vitamin, is an antioxidant and accelerates hydroxylation reactions in many biosynthetic processes.[151] It may provide electrons to enzymes that require prosthetic metal ions in a reduced form to achieve full activity, such as the hydroxylation of proline and lysine in collagen synthesis.[151,152] Several functions of vitamin C–enhanced hydroxylase are known: the hydroxylation of lysine and methionine in carnitine biosynthesis, the catabolism of tyrosine, the synthesis of norepinephrine from dopamine, and the conversion of tryptophan to 5-hydroxytryptophan in the biosynthesis of serotonin. Vitamin C is of particular importance to the premature neonate because it enhances the activity of the immature hepatic enzyme, p-hydroxyphenylpyruvic acid oxidase, which increases the catabolism of tyrosine.[151–153] Transient tyrosinemia resulting from vitamin C deficiency or high tyrosine and/or protein intakes was a common problem for premature infants in the past.[72,153,154]

Vitamin C is involved in the synthesis of neurotransmitters. The human fetal brain contains 4 to 11 times the amount of vitamin C found in the adult brain.[155] The brain vitamin C content declines with increasing gestational age, but the content remains threefold greater than that in adults even after 4 weeks of age. The significance of the brain vitamin C concentration is unclear, but suggests that the provision of adequate vitamin C to the premature neonate may be important. The rise in serum vitamin C concentrations reported after intraventricular hemorrhage in premature neonates may be a marker of the disruption of the blood-brain barrier.[15,156] As an antioxidant, vitamin C may be important to the high-risk premature neonate exposed to hyperoxic environments and mechanical ventilation.[15,151,152]

Placental transfer results in a greater concentration of vitamin C in the fetus and in cord blood than in the mother.[153] With optimal nutrition, the maternal/cord vitamin C ratio is 0.5. If the mother is vitamin C deficient, however, the ratio declines to 0.25.[157] The fetus, therefore, appears to be protected from maternal vitamin C deficiency.[15] Scurvy has been reported, however, in the offspring of mothers who were clinically vitamin C deficient.[43] There is a decline in maternal concentrations of the vitamin during pregnancy that is independent of nutritional status.[155,156] Birth weight and gestational age are not correlated with concentrations of vitamin C in cord blood.[158]

Vitamin C is absorbed in the upper small intestine and excreted in the urine primarily as oxalic acid. At moderate intakes, urinary excretion is the main source of elimination. At high intakes the urinary excretion of the vitamin increases, and with intakes above $3 g \cdot day^{-1}$ the fecal excretion of the vitamin rises and protects against excessive intakes.[151,159]

The availability of vitamin C is influenced by its physical characteristics. The vitamin C content of human milk is reduced 90% by pasteurization.[151,160] Storage time, temperature, and oxidation affect vitamin C concentrations. The vitamin C content of pooled human milk is 50% lower than that of fresh milk.[160] Exposure of milk to copper, iron, and oxygen also reduces vitamin C concentrations. The plasma vitamin C concentration is reported to decline during febrile and gastrointestinal illnesses.

Sources

The vitamin C concentration of human milk generally is stable during lactation, averaging 50 mg/L (8 mg·100 kcal^{-1}, range 5–13 mg·100 kcal^{-1}) (Tables 43.1 and 43.2).[19–21,80,82,161–163] A 20% decline in milk concentration is reported after 6 to 25 months of lactation.[87,162] When the diet of a lactating mother is supplemented with vitamin C, an increase in milk concentration of the vitamin occurs only if her diet had been deficient in vitamin C.[54,161,164] No effect of routine supplementation on

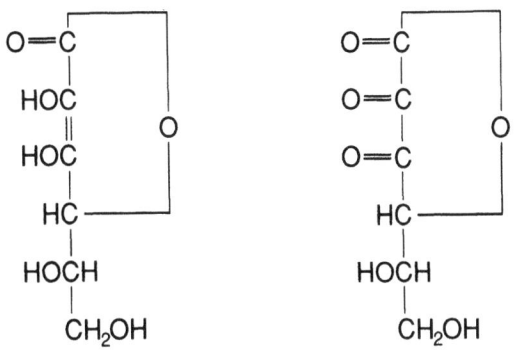

FIGURE 43.9. L-ascorbic acid and L-dehydroascorbic acid.

milk vitamin C concentration is reported for American women.[21,80,82,163]

Bovine milk contains a low concentration of vitamin C, probably because the cow is able to synthesize the vitamin (Table 43.1).[152,153,160] Commercially available infant formulas derived from bovine milk are fortified with the vitamin (Tables 43.1 and 43.2). Vitamin C is widely distributed in foods. The best sources are citrus fruits and green vegetables.[29]

Perinatal Needs

The vitamin C needs of the full-term neonate are obtained from estimates of the availability of the vitamin from human milk. Neonatal serum vitamin C concentrations decline during the first week and by 5 days are similar to maternal serum concentrations at delivery.[153] That low concentration is maintained in infants fed unsupplemented bovine milk. Based on studies of urinary excretion and body saturation, formula-fed full-term neonates require a minimum vitamin C supplement of $10\,mg \cdot day^{-1}$ to prevent scurvy.[151,153] If supplemented with $20\,mg \cdot day^{-1}$, formula-fed full-term neonates demonstrate serum concentrations similar to those of breast-fed infants.[153] Breast-fed full-term neonates appear to be saturated with respect to their vitamin C needs.[153,162]

When clinical conditions in premature neonates prevent early initiation of enteral nutrition, the delay of vitamin supplementation may lead to vitamin C deficiency. Vitamin C intakes in premature neonates of less than $5\,mg \cdot kg^{-1} \cdot day^{-1}$ result in a marked decline of plasma concentrations, from 1.56 to $0.48\,mg \cdot dl^{-1}$ during the first 14 days.[165] Normal plasma concentrations are maintained in premature neonates, however, when enteral feedings supplemented with vitamin C (5 to $10\,mg \cdot kg^{-1} \cdot day^{-1}$) are begun by 5 days of age.[165] The vitamin C needs of the premature neonate may be similar to the full-term neonate unless large quantities of tyrosine and/or protein ($>5\,g \cdot kg^{-1} \cdot day^{-1}$) are administered. To prevent hypertyrosinemia a daily intake of 75 to 100 mg of vitamin C has been suggested for premature neonates who receive high protein intakes.[153,154] Because protein intakes of 5 to $6\,g \cdot kg^{-1} \cdot day^{-1}$ are no longer recommended, this problem is of less significance today than in the past.[7] Furthermore, serum tyrosine concentrations in premature neonates fed human milk and whey-dominant formulas are lower when compared with those in similar neonates fed casein-dominant formulas.[166] It appears, therefore, that the vitamin C needs of premature neonates may not be significantly greater than those of full-term neonates, provided that human milk or whey-dominant formulas are used.

The AAP recommendations for the minimum vitamin C intake of premature neonate appear appropriate. The greater intakes recommended by ESPGAN would be appropriate in clinical circumstances of high protein and/or tyrosine consumption. Premature neonates fed pasteurized human milk, however, may receive inadequate vitamin C.[167]

Plasma vitamin C concentrations have been reported for full-term neonates and children to 11 years of age receiving TPN.[31] The infants and children who received 80 mg vitamin C daily maintained plasma concentrations of $1.1\,mg \cdot dl^{-1}$ for 21 days but by 2 to 5 months the plasma concentrations were marginal.[31] Plasma vitamin C concentrations in those children were similar to those reported in vitamin C–sufficient adults receiving long-term TPN.[168] Premature infants, however, who received 52 mg of vitamin C daily ($48\,mg \cdot kg^{-1} \cdot day^{-1}$) for 28 days had plasma concentrations two- to threefold greater (3.2 to $2.6\,mg \cdot dl^{-1}$) than their baseline and those of full-term infants.[31,156] Plasma concentrations were highest in the neonate with a birth weight <1 kg.

For full-term infants and children the TPN vitamin C intake is $80\,mg \cdot day^{-1}$ (Table 43.8).[10] When recommendations for premature infants are considered, a consistent dose of 40% of the vial (MVI-Pediatric) per $kg \cdot day^{-1}$ is $32\,mg \cdot kg^{-1} \cdot day^{-1}$. However, a more realistic recommendation for vitamin C intake from TPN is $25\,mg \cdot kg^{-1} \cdot day^{-1}$.[10,31]

The increment in fetal needs during pregnancy is 3 to $4\,mg \cdot kg^{-1} \cdot day^{-1}$. To offset losses from the mother's body pool, a $10\,mg \cdot day^{-1}$ increment in vitamin C is recommended (Table 43.7).[151] These recommendations closely approximate earlier studies evaluating plasma concentrations and tissue saturation studies.[153]

Deficiency States

A deficiency of vitamin C results in scurvy. Scurvy, the first dietary deficiency disease to be recognized, was not a matter of concern for infants until the end of the 19th century when the use of pasteurized milk and commercial formulas became prevalent. Infantile scurvy was observed in affluent families who purchased prepared infant formulas. The initial descriptions of scurvy in premature infants were associated with the exclusive feeding of pooled, pasteurized human milk.[160] The daily dose of vitamin C for premature infants, however, should approximate the amount contained in unpasteurized human milk. Today, infantile scurvy is reported occasionally in urban settings where children are fed unsupplemented bovine milk exclusively for their first 6 to 12 months.[72]

The earliest clinical manifestation of scurvy in adults is petechial hemorrhage, which indicates increased capillary fragility.[153] A classic manifestation of scurvy in adults is failure of wound healing. In that situation, collagen fibrils and intercellular cement are deposited improperly and bone growth ceases. Infantile scurvy is manifested by irritability and tenderness, swelling, and pseudoparalysis of the lower extremities. Enlargement of the costochondral junction (i.e., scorbutic rosary) is observed in scurvy and may be confused with rickets.[72] Characteristic radiologic abnormalities indicating a cessation of osteogenesis and marked bony changes, hyperkeratosis of hair follicles, and mental status changes characterize the progression of the illness.[72,169] Hemorrhagic manifestations in children include bleeding at the site of tooth eruption, bloody diarrhea, epistaxis, ocular bleeding, and petechiae at pressure points. Anemia, secondary to bleeding, decreased iron absorption, and abnormal folate metabolism, is a common finding.[152] Sepsis and failure to thrive are characteristics of premature infants reported with scurvy.

Infantile scurvy is treated with 25 mg vitamin C, four times per day for 4 to 5 days, followed by $25\,mg\cdot day^{-1}$ until healing occurs.[6]

Laboratory Assessment

Plasma and leukocyte vitamin C concentrations reflect recent intake of the vitamin and are reported most often in assessments of vitamin status. Acceptable plasma vitamin C concentration is $>0.6\,mg\cdot dl^{-1}$; values below $0.2\,mg\cdot dl^{-1}$ are observed in scurvy.[151,153] Subclinical vitamin C deficiency is likely when the concentration of vitamin C in leukocytes is below $100\,\mu g\cdot g^{-1}$.[9]

Toxicity

Prolonged intakes of vitamin C in adults, $>1.0\,g\cdot day^{-1}$, may cause oxaluria, uricosuria, and acidification of the urine.[34] Renal calculi may result from these changes. High doses may result in false-positive tests for urinary glucose, occult blood in feces, and exacerbations of glucose-6-phosphate deficiency. Excessive doses of vitamin C may alter bactericidal functions of white blood cells and also provoke "rebound scurvy." Rebound scurvy has been reported in adults who reduce their high vitamin intakes abruptly.[45,152,159] The rebound phenomenon has been reported also in neonates of mothers who took large doses of the vitamin during pregnancy.[34,72,151] Large doses of vitamin C may decrease the absorption of vitamin B_{12} and copper and increase the absorption of iron.

Conclusion

The best assessment of water-soluble vitamin needs in infancy is based on the human milk-fed full-term neonate in whom deficiencies of water-soluble vitamins are rare. The deficiencies that arise in human milk-fed neonates generally result from inadequacies in the maternal diet.

When we consider the variability in the concentrations of vitamins in human milk (Tables 43.1 and 43.2), it is curious that the human milk-fed neonate is protected from deficiencies of water-soluble vitamins.[170] Because we employ human milk as a model, the lack of consistency in vitamin concentrations makes precise recommendations difficult. For these reasons, ample allowances are given for infant formula guidelines.

The data suggest that periconceptional use of multivitamins may be beneficial in reducing neural tube and congenital heart defects in the neonate.[119,120,171] More data, however, are needed to assess the adequacy of water-soluble vitamins in pregnancy.

Acknowledgments. I appreciate the secretarial assistance of Idelle Tapper. This work is a publication of the USDA/ARS Children's Nutrition Research Center, Department of Pediatrics, Baylor College of Medicine and Texas Children's Hospital, Houston, Texas. This project has been funded in part with federal funds from the U.S. Department of Agriculture, Agricultural Research Service under Cooperative Agreement no. 58-6250-1-003. The contents of this publication do not necessarily reflect the views or policies of the U.S. Department of Agriculture, nor does mention of trade names, commercial products, or organizations imply endorsement by the U.S. Government.

References

1. King JC. Vitamin requirements during pregnancy. In: Campbell DM, Billmer MDG, eds. Nutrition in pregnancy. London: The Royal College of Obstetricians and Gynaecologists, 1983:33–45.
2. Dostalova L. Correlation of the vitamin status between mother and newborn during delivery. Dev Pharmacol Ther 1982;4:45–57.
3. Link G, Zempleni J. Intrauterine elimination of pyridoxal 5′-phosphate in full-term and preterm infants. Am J Clin Nutr 1996;64:184–189.
4. Baker H, Frank O, Thomson AD. Vitamin profiles of 174 mothers and newborns at parturition. Am J Clin Nutr 1975;28:56–65.
5. Newman V, Lyon RB, Anderson PO. Evaluation of prenatal vitamin-mineral supplements. Clin Pharm 1987;6:770–777.
6. Udall JN Jr, Greene HL. Vitamin update. Pediatr Rev 1992;13:185–194.
7. American Academy of Pediatrics, Committee on Nutrition. Nutritional needs of low-birth-weight infants. Pediatrics 1985;75:976–986.
8. National Research Council (U.S.), Subcommittee on the Tenth Edition of the RDAs. Recommended Dietary Allowances. Washington, DC: National Academy Press, 1989.
9. Wharton BA. Nutrition and feeding of preterm infants. Oxford: Blackwell Scientific, 1987.
10. Greene HL, Hambidge KM, Schanler R, Tsang RC. Guidelines for the use of vitamins, trace elements, calcium, magnesium, and phosphorus in infants and children receiving total parenteral nutrition: report of the Subcom-

mittee on Pediatric Parenteral Nutrient Requirements from the Committee on Clinical Practice Issues of the American Society for Clinical Nutrition. Am J Clin Nutr 1988;48:1324–1342.
11. Moran JR, Greene HL. The B vitamins and vitamin C in human nutrition I. General considerations and "obligatory" B vitamins. Am J Dis Child 1979;133:192–199.
12. Rindi G, Venura U. Thiamine intestinal transport. Physiol Rev 1972;52:821–827.
13. Gubler CJ. Thiamine. In: Machlin LJ, ed. Handbook of vitamins. New York: Marcel Dekker, 1991:233–282.
14. Goldsmith GA. Vitamin B complex. Thiamine, riboflavin, niacin, folic acid (folacin), vitamin B_{12}, biotin. Prog Food Nutr Sci 1975;1:559–609.
15. Schanler RJ, Nichols BL. The water soluble vitamins C, B_1, B_2, B_6, and niacin. In: Tsang RC, ed. Vitamin and mineral requirements in preterm infants. New York: Marcel Dekker, 1985:39–62.
16. Davis RE, Icke GC. Clinical chemistry of thiamine. Adv Clin Chem 1983;23:93–140.
17. Itokawa Y, Cooper JR. Ion movements and thiamine. II. Release of the vitamin from membrane fragments. Acta Biochim Biophys 1970;196:274–284.
18. Cochrane WA, Collins-Williams C, Donohue WL. Superior hemorrhagic polioencephalitis (Wernicke's disease) occurring in an infant—probably due to thiamine deficiency from use of a soya bean product. Pediatrics 1961;28:771–777.
19. Macy IG. Composition of human colostrum and milk. Am J Dis Child 1949;78:589–603.
20. Adams CF. Nutritive value of American foods. Washington, DC: Agricultural Research Service. 1975.
21. Thomas MR, Sneed SM, Wei C. The effects of vitamin C, vitamin B_6, vitamin B_{12}, folic acid, riboflavin, and thiamine on the breast milk and maternal status of well-nourished women at 6 months postpartum. Am J Clin Nutr 1980;33:2151–2156.
22. Knott EM, Kleiger SC, Torres-Bracamonte F. Factors affecting the thiamine content of breast milk. J Nutr 1943;25:49–58.
23. Ford JE, Zechalko A, Murphy J, Brooke OG. Comparison of the B vitamin composition of milk from mothers of preterm and term babies. Arch Dis Child 1983;58:367–372.
24. Roderuck CE, Williams HH, Macy IG. Human milk studies. XXIII. Free and total thiamine contents of colostrum and mature human milk. Am J Dis Child 1945;70:162–170.
25. Nail PA, Thomas MR, Eakin R. The effect of thiamine and riboflavin supplementation on the level of those vitamins in human breast milk and urine. Am J Clin Nutr 1980;33:198–204.
26. Pratt JP, Hamil BM, Moyer EZ, et al. Metabolism of women during the reproductive cycle. XVIII. The effect of multi-vitamin supplements on the secretion of B vitamins in human milk. J Nutr 1951;44:141–157.
27. Pennington JAT. Bowes & Church's food values of portions commonly used. Philadelphia: JB Lippincott, 1994.
28. Causeret J. La valeur vitaminique des laits animaux comparaison avec celle du lait de femme. Ann Nutr Alim 1971;25:A313–A334.
29. Zaloga GP, Bortenschlaer L. Vitamins. In: Gay SM, ed. Nutition in critical care. St. Louis: Mosby Year Book, 1994:217–242.
30. Holt LE Jr, Nemir RL, Snyderman SE, et al. The thiamine requirement of the normal infant. J Nutr 1949;37:53–66.
31. Moore MC, Greene HL, Phillips B, et al. Evaluation of a pediatrics multiple vitamin preparation for total parenteral nutrition in infants and children. I. Blood levels of water-soluble vitamins. Pediatrics 1986;77:530–538.
32. Marinier E, Gorski AM, Potier de Courcy G, et al. Blood levels of water soluble vitamins in pediatric patients on total parenteral nutrition using a multiple vitamin preparation. J Parenter Enteral Nutr 1989;13:176–184.
33. Greene HL, Porchelli P, Adcock E, Swift L. Vitamins for newborn infant formulas: a review of recommendations with emphasis on data from low birth-weight infants. Eur J Clin Nutr 1992;46:S1–S8.
34. American Medical Association, Council on Scientific Affairs. Vitamin preparations as dietary supplements and therapeutic agents. JAMA 1987;257:1929–1936.
35. Institute of Medicine, Subcommittee on Nutritional Status and Weight Gain During Pregnancy So. Nutrition during pregnancy. Washington, DC: National Academy Press, 1990.
36. La Selve P, Demolin P, Holzapfel L, et al. Shoshin beriberi: an unusual complication of prolonged parenteral nutrition. J Parenter Enteral Nutr 1986;10:102–103.
37. McCormick DB. Thiamin. In: Shils ME, Young VR, eds. Modern nutrition in health and disease. Philadelphia: Lea & Febiger, 1988:355–361.
38. Rascoff H. Beriberi heart in a 4 month old infant. JAMA 1942;120:1292–1293.
39. King EQ. Acute cardiac failure in the newborn due to thiamine deficiency. Exp Med Surg 1967;25:173–177.
40. Wyatt DT, Noetzel MJ, Hillman RE. Infantile beriberi presenting as subacute necrotizing encephalomyelopathy. J Pediatr 1987;110:888–891.
41. Van Gelder DW, Darby FU. Congenital and infantile beriberi. J Pediatr 1944;25:226–235.
42. Heller S, Salkeld RM, Korner WF. Vitamin B_1 status in pregnancy. Am J Clin Nutr 1974;27:1221–1224.
43. Malone JI. Vitamin passage across the placenta. Clin Perinatol 1975;2:295–307.
44. Powers JS, Zimmer J, Meurer K, et al. Direct assay of vitamins B_1, B_2, and B_6 in hospitalized patients: relationship to level of intake. JPEN 1993;17:315–316.
45. Alhadeff L, Gualtieri CT, Lipton M. Toxic effects of water soluble vitamins. Nutr Rev 1984;42:33–40.
46. Horwitt MK. Interpretations of requirements for thiamine, riboflavin, niacin-tryptophan, and vitamin E plus comments on balance studies and vitamin B_6. Am J Clin Nutr 1986;44:973–986.
47. Bates CJ, Liu DS, Fuller NJ, Lucas A. Susceptibility of riboflavin and vitamin A in breast milk to photodegradation and its implications for the use of banked breast milk in infant feeding. Acta Paediatr Scand 1985;74:40–44.
48. Fritz I, Said H, Harris C, et al. A new sensitive assay for plasma riboflavin using high performance liquid chromatography. J Am Coll Nutr 1987;6:449 (Abstract).

49. Chen MF, Boyce HW, Triplett L. Stability of the B vitamins in mixed parenteral nutrition solution. J Parenter Enteral Nutr 1983;7:462–464.
50. Porcelli PJ, Greene HL, Adcock EW. Retinol (vitamin A) and riboflavin (vitamin B_2) administration and metabolism in very low birth weight infants. Semin Perinatol 1992;16:170–180.
51. Cooperman JM, Lopez R. Riboflavin. In: Machlin LJ, ed. Handbook of vitamins. New York: Marcel Dekker, 1991:283–310.
52. Roderuck CE, Coryell MN, Williams HH. Human milk studies: XXIV. Free and total riboflavin contents of colostrum and mature milk. Am J Dis Child 1945;70:171–175.
53. Hughes J, Sanders TAB. Riboflavin levels in the diet and breast milk of vegans and omnivores. Proc Nutr Soc 1979;38:95A.
54. Deodhar AD, Rajalakshmi R, Ramakrishnan CV. Studies on human lactation—part III: effect of dietary vitamin supplementation on vitamin contents of breast milk. Acta Paediatr 1964;53:42–48.
55. Hovi L, Hekali R, Siimes MA. Evidence of riboflavin depletion in breast-fed newborns and its further acceleration during treatment of hyperbilirubinemia by phototherapy. Acta Paediatr Scand 1979;68:567–570.
56. Sisson TR. Photodegradation of riboflavin in neonates. Fed Proc 1987;46:1883–1885.
57. Ronnholm KAR. Need for riboflavin supplementation in small preterms fed with human milk. Am J Clin Nutr 1986;43:1–6.
58. Lucas A, Bates C. Transient riboflavin depletion in preterm infants. Arch Dis Child 1984;59:837–841.
59. Porcelli PJ, Adcock EW, DelPaggio D, et al. Plasma and urine riboflavin and pyridoxine concentrations in enterally fed very-low-birth-weight neonates. J Pediatr Gastroenterol Nutr 1996;23:141–146.
60. Baeckert PA, Greene HL, Fritz I, et al. Vitamin concentrations in very low birth weight infants given vitamins intravenously in a lipid emulsion: measurement of vitamins A, D, E, and riboflavin. J Pediatr 1988;113:1057–1065.
61. Lopez R, Cole HS, Montoya F, Cooperman JM. Riboflavin deficiency in a pediatric population of low socioeconomic status in New York City. J Pediatr 1975;105:420–422.
62. Reddy VAP, Bates CJ, Goh SGJ, et al. Riboflavin, folate and vitamin C status of Gambian women during pregnancy: a comparison between urban and rural communities. Trans R Soc Trop Med Hyg 1987;81:1033–1037.
63. Bates CJ, Prentice AM, Paul AA, et al. Riboflavin status in Gambian pregnant and lactating women and its implications for Recommended Dietary Allowances. Am J Clin Nutr 1981;34:928–935.
64. Brzezinski A, Bromberg YM, Braun K. Riboflavin deficiency in pregnancy. J Obstet Gynecol 1947;54:182–186.
65. Bates CJ, Prentice AM, Paul AA, et al. Riboflavin status in infants born in rural Gambia, and the effect of a weaning food supplement. Trans R Soc Trop Med Hyg 1982;76:253–258.
66. McCormick DB. Niacin. In: Shils ME, Young VR, eds. Modern nutrition in health and disease. Philadelphia: Lea & Febiger, 1988:370–375.
67. Hankes LV. Nicotinic acid and nicotinamide. In: Machlin LJ, ed. Handbook of vitamins. New York: Marcel Dekker, 1984:329–377.
68. Moran JR, Greene HL. Nutritional biochemistry of water-soluble vitamins. In: Grand RJ, Sutphen JL, Dietz WH Jr, eds. Pediatric nutrition theory and practice. Stoneham: Butterworth, 1987:51–67.
69. Holt LE Jr. The adolescence of nutrition. Arch Dis Child 1956;31:427–438.
70. Darby WJ, McNutt KW, Todhunter EN. Niacin. Nutr Rev 1975;33:289–297.
71. Spivak JL, Jackson DL. Pellagra: an analysis of 18 patients and a review of the literature. Johns Hopkins Med J 1977;140:295–309.
72. Moran JR, Greene HL. The B vitamins and vitamin C in human nutrition. II: "Conditional" B vitamins and vitamin C. Am J Dis Child 1979;133:308–314.
73. Lumeng L, Li TK, Lui A. The interorgan transport and metabolism of vitamin B_6. In: Reynolds RD, Leklem JE, eds. Vitamin B_6: its role in health and disease. New York: Alan R. Liss, 1985:35–54.
74. Bender DA. Vitamin B_6 requirements and recommendations. Eur J Clin Nutr 1989;43:289–309.
75. Fomon SJ. Nutrition of normal infants. St. Louis: Mosby-Year Book, 1993.
76. Contractor SF, Shane B. Blood and urine levels of vitamin B_6 in the mother and fetus before and after loading of the mother with vitamin B_6. Am J Obstet Gynecol 1970;107:635–640.
77. Driskell JA. Vitamin B_6. In: Machlin LJ, ed. Handbook of vitamins. New York: Marcel Dekker, 1984:379–401.
78. Heiskanen K, Siimes MA, Perheentupa J, Salmenpera L. Risk of low vitamin B_6 status in infants breast-fed exclusively beyond six months. J Pediatr Gastroenterol Nutr 1996;23:38–44.
79. Styslinger L, Kirksey A. Effects of different levels of vitamin B_6 supplementation on vitamin B_6 concentrations in human milk and vitamin B_6 intakes of breastfed infants. Am J Clin Nutr 1985;41:21–31.
80. Thomas MR, Kawamoto J, Sneed SM, Eakin R. The effects of vitamin C, vitamin B_6, and vitamin B_{12} supplementation on the breast milk and maternal status of well-nourished women. Am J Clin Nutr 1979;32:1679–1685.
81. Kirksey A, Udipi SA. Vitamin B_6 in human pregnancy and lactation. In: Reynolds RD, Leklem JE, eds. Vitamin B_6: its role in health and disease. New York: Alan R. Liss, 1985:57–77.
82. Sneed SM, Zane C, Thomas MR. The effects of ascorbic acid, vitamin B_6, vitamin B_{12}, and folic acid supplementation on the breast milk and maternal nutritional status of low socioeconomic lactating women. Am J Clin Nutr 1981;34:1338–1346.
83. West KD, Kirksey A. Influence of vitamin B_6 intake on the content of the vitamin in human milk. Am J Clin Nutr 1976;29:961–969.
84. Kirksey A, Roepke JLB. Vitamin B_6 nutriture of mothers of three breast-fed neonates with central nervous system disorders. Fed Proc 1981;40:864 (Abstract).
85. Bessey OA, Adam DJD, Hansen AE. Intake of vitamin B_6 and infantile convulsions: a first approximation of re-

quirements of pyridoxine in infants. Pediatrics 1957;20: 33–44.
86. Borschel MW, Kirksey A, Hannemann RE. Effects of vitamin B_6 intake on nutriture and growth of young infants. Am J Clin Nutr 1986;43:7–15.
87. Karra MV, Udipi SA, Kirksey A, Roepke JLB. Changes in specific nutrients in breast milk during extended lactation. Am J Clin Nutr 1986;43:495–503.
88. McCoy E, Strynadka K, Brunet K. Vitamin B_6 intake and whole blood levels of breast and formula fed infants: serial whole blood vitamin B_6 levels in premature infants. In: Reynolds RD, Leklem JE, eds. Vitamin B_6: its role in health and disease. New York: Alan R. Liss, 1985:79–96.
89. Molony CJ, Parmelee AH. Convulsions in young infants as a result of pyridoxine (vitamin B_6) deficiency. JAMA 1954;154:405–406.
90. Andon MB, Reynolds RD, Moser PB, et al. Impaired ability of premature infants 29 weeks gestational age to convert pyridoxine to pyridoxal phosphate. Fed Proc 1987;46:1016.
91. Raiten DJ, Reynolds RD, Andon MB, et al. Vitamin B-6 metabolism in premature infants. Am J Clin Nutr 1991; 53:78–83.
92. Schuster K, Bailey LB, Mahan CS. Effect of maternal pyridoxine-HCl supplementation on the vitamin B-6 status of mother and infant and on pregnancy outcome. J Nutr 1984;114:977–988.
93. Reynolds RD, Polansky M, Moser PB. Analyzed vitamin B-6 intakes of pregnant and postpartum lactating and nonlactating women. J Am Diet Assoc 1984;84:1339–1344.
94. Black AE, Wiles SJ, Paul AA. The nutrient intakes of pregnant and lactating mothers of good socio-economic status in Cambridge, UK: some implications for recommended daily allowances of minor nutrients. Br J Nutr 1986;56:59–72.
95. Schuster K, Bailey LB, Dimperio D, Mahan CS. Morning sickness and vitamin B_6 status of pregnant women. Hum Nutr Clin Nutr 1985;39C:75–79.
96. Schaumburg H, Kaplan J, Windebank A, et al. Sensory neuropathy from pyridoxine abuse—a new megavitamin syndrome. N Engl J Med 1983;309:445–448.
97. Brody T. Folic acid. In: Machlin LJ, ed. Handbook of vitamins. New York: Marcel Dekker, 1991:453–489.
98. Davis RE. Clinical chemistry of folic acid. Adv Clin Chem 1986;25:233–294.
99. Herbert VD, Colman N. Folic acid and vitamin B_{12}. In: Shils ME, Young VR, eds. Modern nutrition in health and disease. Philadelphia: Lea & Febiger, 1988:388–416.
100. Tamura T, Shane B, Baer MT, et al. Absorption of mono- and polyglutamyl folates in zinc-depleted man. Am J Clin Nutr 1978;31:1984–1987.
101. Herbert V. Recommended dietary intakes (RDI) of folate in humans. Am J Clin Nutr 1987;45:661–670.
102. Gerson CD, Cohen N, Hepner GW, et al. Folic acid absorption in man: enhancing effect of glucose. Gastroenterology 1971;61:224–227.
103. Hillman RS, McGuffin R, Campbell C. Alcohol interference with the folate enterohepatic cycle. Trans Assoc Am Phys 1977;90:145–156.
104. Herbert V, Das KC. The role of vitamin B-12 and folic acid in hemato- and other cell-poiesis. Vitam Horm 1976; 34:1–30.
105. Ek J, Magnus E. Plasma and red cell folate values and folate requirements in formula-fed term infants. J Pediatr 1982;100:738–744.
106. Metz J, Zalusky R, Herbert V. Folic acid binding by serum and milk. Am J Clin Nutr 1968;21:289–297.
107. Brown CM, Smith AM, Picciano MF. Forms of human milk folacin and variation patterns. J Pediatr Gastroenterol Nutr 1986;5:278–282.
108. Smith AM, Picciano MF, Deering RH. Folate intake and blood concentrations of term infants. Am J Clin Nutr 1985;41:590–598.
109. Salmenpera L, Perheentupa J, Siimes MA. Folate nutrition is optimal in exclusively breast-fed infants but inadequate in some of their mothers and formula-fed infants. J Pediatr Gastroenterol Nutr 1986;5:283–289.
110. Tamura T, Yoshimura Y, Arakawa T. Human milk folate and folate status in lactating mothers and their infants. Am J Clin Nutr 1980;33:193–197.
111. Ek J, Magnus EM. Plasma and red blood cell folate in breast-fed infants. Acta Paediatr Scand 1979;68:239–243.
112. Ek J. Folic acid and vitamin B_{12} requirements in premature infants. In: Tsang RC, ed. Vitamin and mineral requirements in preterm infants. New York: Marcel Dekker, 1985:23–38.
113. Edwards JH, Holmes-Siedle M, Lindenbaum RH. Vitamin supplementation and neural tube defects. Lancet 1982;1:275–276.
114. Strelling MK, Blackledge DG, Goodall HB. Diagnosis and management of folate deficiency in low birthweight infants. Arch Dis Child 1979;54:271–277.
115. Stevens D, Burman D, Strelling K, Morris A. Folic acid supplementation in low birth weight infants. Pediatrics 1979;64:333–335.
116. Ek J, Behneke L, Halvorsen KS, Magnus E. Plasma and red cell folate values and folate requirements in formula-fed premature infants. Eur J Pediatr 1984;142:78–82.
117. Bartels PC, Helleman PW, Soons JBJ. Investigation of red cell size-distribution histograms related to folate, vitamin B_{12} and iron state in the course of pregnancy. Scand J Clin Lab Invest 1989;49:763–771.
118. Rush D. Periconceptional folate and neural tube defect. Am J Clin Nutr 1994;59:511S–516S.
119. Daly LE, Kirke PN, Molloy A, et al. Folate levels and neural tube defects. Implications for prevention. JAMA 1996;274:1698–1702.
120. Rayburn WF, Stanley JR, Garrett ME. Periconceptional folate intake and neural tube defects. J Am Coll Nutr 1996;15:121–125.
121. Matoth Y, Zehavi E, Topper E, Klein T. Folate nutrition and growth in infancy. Arch Dis Child 1979;54:699–702.
122. Shojania AM, Hornady G. Folate metabolism in newborns and during early infancy. Pediatr Res 1970;4:422–426.
123. Rodriguez MS. A conspectus of research on folacin requirements of man. J Nutr 1978;108:1983–2075.
124. Smithells RW, Shepard S, Schorah CJ. Vitamin deficiencies and neural tube defects. Arch Dis Child 1976;51:944–950.

125. Mulinare J, Cordero JF, Erickson JD, Berry RJ. Periconceptional use of multivitamins and the occurrence of neural tube defects. JAMA 1988;260:3141–3145.
126. Mills JL, Rhoads GG, Simpson JL, et al. The absence of a relation between the periconceptional use of vitamins and neural-tube defects. N Engl J Med 1989;321:430–435.
127. Rickes EL, Brink NG, Koniuszy FR. Crystalline vitamin B_{12}. Science 1948;107:396–397.
128. Herbert V. The 1986 Herman Award Lecture. Nutrition science as a continually unfolding story: the folate and vitamin B-12 paradigm. Am J Clin Nutr 1987;46:387–402.
129. Herbert V. Recommended dietary intakes (RDI) of vitamin B-12 in humans. Am J Clin Nutr 1987;45:671–678.
130. Sandberg DP, Begley JA, Hall CA. The content, binding, and forms of vitamin B_{12} in milk. Am J Clin Nutr 1981;34:1717–1724.
131. Johnson PR Jr, Roloff JS. Vitamin B_{12} deficiency in an infant strictly breast-fed by a mother with latent pernicious anemia. J Pediatr 1982;100:917–919.
132. Carmel R, Lau KW, Baylink DJ, et al. Cobalamin and osteoblast-specific proteins. N Engl J Med 1988;319:70–75.
133. Higginbottom MC, Sweetman L, Nyhan WL. A syndrome of methylmalonic aciduria, homocystinuria, megaloblastic anemia and neurologic abnormalities in a vitamin B_{12}-deficient breast-fed infant of a strict vegetarian. N Engl J Med 1978;299:317–323.
134. Stollhoff K, Schulte FJ. Vitamin B_{12} and brain development. Eur J Pediatr 1987;146:201–205.
135. Specker BL, Miller D, Norman EJ, et al. Increased urinary methylmalonic acid excretion in breast-fed infants of vegetarian mothers and identification of an acceptable dietary source of vitamin B_{12}. Am J Clin Nutr 1988;47:89–92.
136. Collins JE, Rolles CJ, Sutton H, Ackery D. B_{12} absorption after necrotizing enterocolitis. Arch Dis Child 1984;59:731–734.
137. Herbert V. Vitamin B_{12}. In: Hegsted DM, Chichester CO, Darby WJ, et al., eds. Nutrition review's present knowledge in nutrition. New York: Nutrition Foundation, 1976:191–203.
138. Harrison RJ. Vitamin B-12 levels in erythrocytes in hypochromic anaemia. J Clin Pathol 1971;24:698–700.
139. Riedel BD, Greene HL, Vitamins. In: Hay WW Jr, ed. Neonatal nutrition and metabolism. St. Louis: Mosby Year Book, 1991:143–170.
140. Gross SJ. Choline, pantothenic acid, and biotin. In: Tsang RC, ed. Vitamin and mineral requirements in preterm infants. New York: Marcel Dekker, 1985:191–201.
141. Fox HM. Pantothenic acid. In: Machlin LJ, ed. Handbook of vitamins. New York: Marcel Dekker, 1984:437–458.
142. Song WO, Chan GM, Wyse BW, Hansen RG. Effect of pantothenic acid status on the content of the vitamin in human milk. Am J Clin Nutr 1984;40;317–324.
143. Johnston L, Vaughn L, Fox HM. Pantothenic acid content of human milk. Am J Clin Nutr 1981;34:2205–2209.
144. Coryell MN, Harris ME, Miller S. Human milk studies XXII. Nicotinic acid, pantothenic acid and biotin contents of colostrum and mature human milk. Am J Dis Child 1945;70:150–161.
145. Bonjour J. Biotin. In: Machlin LJ, ed. Handbook of vitamins. New York: Marcel Dekker, 1991:393–427.
146. Roth KS. Biotin in clinical medicine—a review. Am J Clin Nutr 1981;34:1967–1974.
147. Goldsmith SJ, Eitenmiller RR, Feeley RM, et al. Biotin content of human milk during early lactational stages. Nutr Res 1982;2:579–583.
148. Bonjour JP. Biotin in man's nutrition and therapy—a review. Int J Vitam Nutr Res 1977;47:107–118.
149. Hamil BM, Coryell M, Roderuck C, et al. Thiamine, riboflavin, nicotinic acid, pantothenic acid and biotin in the urine of newborn infants. Am J Dis Child 1947;74:434–446.
150. Mock DM, DeLorimer AA, Liebman WM, et al. Biotin deficiency: an unusual complication of parenteral alimentation. N Engl J Med 1981;304:820–823.
151. Olson JA, Hodges RE. Recommended dietary intakes (RDI) of vitamin C in humans. Am J Clin Nutr 1987;45:693–703.
152. Levine M. New concepts in the biology and biochemisty of ascorbic acid. N Engl J Med 1986;314:892–902.
153. Irwin MI, Hutchins BK. A conspectus of research on vitamin C requirements of man (2). J Nutr 1976;106:823–879.
154. Light IJ, Berry HK, Sutherland JM. Aminoacidemia of prematurity. Am J Dis Child 1966;112:229–236.
155. Adlard BPF, De Souza SW, Moon S. Ascorbic acid in the fetal human brain. Arch Dis Child 1974;49:278–282.
156. Arad ID, Eyal FG. High plasma ascorbic acid levels in preterm neonates with intraventricular hemorrhage. Am J Dis Child 1983;137:949–951.
157. Teel HM, Burke BS, Draper R. Vitamin C in human pregnancy and lactation. I. Studies during pregnancy. Am J Dis Child 1938;56:1004–1010.
158. Ibeziako PA, Ette SI. Plasma ascorbic acid levels in Nigerian mothers and newborns. Trop Pediatr 1981;27:263–266.
159. Jaffe GM. Vitamin C. In: Machlin LJ, ed. Handbook of vitamins. New York: Marcel Dekker, 1984:199–244.
160. Ingalls TH. Ascorbic acid requirements in early infancy. N Engl J Med 1938;218:872–875.
161. Selleg I, King CG. The vitamin C content of human milk and its variation with diet. J Nutr 1936;11:599–606.
162. Salmenpera L. Vitamin C nutrition during prolonged lactation: optimal in infants while marginal in some mothers. Am J Clin Nutr 1984;40:1050–1056.
163. Byerley LO, Kirksey A. Effects of different levels of vitamin C intake on the vitamin C concentration in human milk and the vitamin C intakes of breast-fed infants. Am J Clin Nutr 1985;41:665–671.
164. Bates CJ, Prentice AM, Prentice A, et al. The effect of vitamin C supplementation on lactating women in Keneba, a West African rural community. Int J Vitam Nutr Res 1983;53:68–76.
165. Arad ID, Sagi E, Eyal FG. Plasma ascorbic acid levels in preterm infants. Int J Vitam Nutr Res 1982;52:50–57.
166. Rassin DK, Gaull GE, Raiha NCR, Heinonen K. Milk protein quantity and quality in low-birth-weight infants. IV. Effects on tyrosine and phenylalanine in plasma and urine. J Pediatr 1977;90:356–360.
167. Heinonen K, Mononen I, Mononen T, et al. Plasma vitamin C levels are low in premature infants fed human milk. Am J Clin Nutr 1986;43:923–924.
168. Shils ME, Baker H, Frank O. Blood vitamin levels of long-term adult home total parenteral nutrition patients: the

efficacy of the AMA-FDA parenteral multivitamin formulation. J Parenter Enteral Nutr 1985;9:179–188.
169. Grewar D, Scurvy and its prevention by vitamin C fortified evaporated milk. Can Med Assoc J 1959;80:977–979.
170. Packard VS. Vitamins. In: Packard VS, ed. Human milk and infant formula. New York: Academic Press, 1982:29–49.
171. Botto LD, Khoury MJ, Mulinare J, Erickson JD. Periconceptional multivitamin use and the occurrence of conotruncal heart defects: results from a population-based, case-control study. Pediatrics 1996;98:911–917.

44
Neonatal Energy Metabolism

Pieter J.J. Sauer

It is a characteristic of all living individuals that they continuously consume energy and produce heat. Chemical energy is converted into a form of energy that can be used by the individual. Subsequently this energy is used for maintenance of the body: contraction of heart muscle, excretion of products by liver and kidney, etc. The energy used for these processes is finally given off as heat. Energy can also be used for activity and external work. All energy used for activity is given off as heat; during the process of external work, part of the energy consumed is given off as heat. When the neonate is nursed outside the thermoneutral environment (vide infra), energy is used especially for heat production. In the fetus and neonate energy is also needed for growth. This energy can be divided into that present in the components of new tissue (e.g., amino acids, fatty acids, single carbohydrates) and the energy needed to form the more complex molecules of the new tissue (e.g., DNA, lipoproteins). One of the most important laws of thermodynamics is the law of conservation of energy: energy can be transformed from one form into another, but can never be lost. The energy balance of a fetus or neonate can be written as:

$$Energy_{intake} = energy_{maintenance} + energy_{activity} + energy_{thermoregulation} + energy_{growth} + energy_{urine+feces}$$

where $Energy_{intake}$ = energy taken in with the food,
$Energy_{maintenance}$ = energy used for maintenance,
$Energy_{activity}$ = energy used for activity,
$Energy_{thermoregulation}$ = energy used for thermoregulation,
$Energy_{growth}$ = energy used for the synthesis and components of growth,
$Energy_{urine+feces}$ = energy lost in urine and feces.

Direct Calorimetry

All energy consumed within the body for maintenance, activity, and thermoregulation is finally converted into heat. This energy, the heat production of the body, is equal to heat loss plus heat stored within the body. The heat production can be measured by measuring total heat loss plus heat storage within the body. This method is called direct calorimetry and was performed for the first time in 1780 when Lavoisier and Laplace[1] measured the amount of ice melted by a guinea pig. Since that time many direct calorimeters have been built for use mainly for adults.[2-4] A few studies using direct calorimetry in neonates have been published.[5-9] Direct calorimeters are complicated to build, and because heat loss of the preterm and term neonate is rather low, it is difficult to quantify. The direct calorimeters used measure the heat flux by gradient layers, a series of thermocouples covering the wall of the calorimeter. The heat lost by radiation, convection, and conduction can be measured in this way. The difference in temperature between the air coming into and the air leaving the incubator must be added. The heat lost by evaporation is measured separately, usually by measuring the difference in humidity of the air entering and leaving the calorimeter. Another problem regarding direct calorimetry is the heat storage within the body, usually calculated by the following formula:[10]

$$Heat\ storage = body\ weight \times C_b \frac{0.6T_{int} + 0.4T_{skin}}{t}$$

where C_b = specific heat of body mass (0.84 kcal·kg·C°),
T_{int} = change in deep body temperature over time,
T_{skin} = change in skin temperature over time,
t = duration of study.

Calculation of heat storage is only an approximation and should be small compared with heat loss. The neonate should have almost no change in body temperature during a study, and a study should be conducted over at least a 4- to 6-hour period. Measurements of direct calorimetry completed over a period of less than 4 to 6 hours should be regarded with extreme caution.

An interesting direct calorimeter for adults has been designed by Webb et al.,[11,12] who designed a suit filled with water that covers the body completely. The heat production is calculated from the increase in water temperature, corrected for the change in body temperature. This technique has not been used in the neonate.

Indirect Calorimetry

Because of the problems related to direct calorimetry, other methods to measure heat production and heat loss have been developed. The most widely used method is indirect calorimetry. This method is based on the assumption that foodstuffs are oxidized in order to produce energy, using oxygen and producing carbon dioxide. By measuring the oxygen consumption and carbon dioxide production, with the nitrogen excretion as a product of protein oxidation, heat production can be calculated. This method has been reviewed extensively.[13–16]

Indirect calorimetry has been used to calculate the amount of the substrates (e.g., glucose and fat) that are oxidized. Lusk[17] published a table in 1924 from which the carbohydrate and fat oxidation could be calculated for a given oxygen consumption and the respiratory quotient (RQ) that is calculated as carbon dioxide production divided by oxygen consumption.[17] These tables were designed for the fasting adult. When glucose is the only source of energy the RQ is 1 compared with an RQ of 0.70 to 0.72 when all energy is derived from fat. This method has been used subsequently in the fed state. When these tables are used in the fed state, the possible conversion of one substrate into another is ignored, as only the end products, oxygen consumption, carbon dioxide production, and nitrogen excretion, are measured.[18] Energy is stored within the body in the fed state as fat, carbohydrate, and protein. During a high carbohydrate feeding, carbohydrates may be converted into fat for storage, and at the same time fat oxidation can take place. With indirect calorimetry this process cannot be differentiated from direct carbohydrate oxidation. Sauer's group compared glucose oxidation estimated from the data of indirect calorimetry with data obtained by infusing U-^{13}C glucose and collecting $^{13}CO_2$ in expired air, in the preterm and term infant and in the pregnant woman.[19–21] Glucose oxidation as measured with calorimetry gave significantly higher results compared to U-^{13}C glucose at high RQs but lower values at low RQs. These results can be explained from the conversion of glucose into lipids at a higher glucose intake, resulting in a high RQ. Intracellular glycogen oxidation at a low glucose intake resulted in a high fat oxidation and therefore low RQ, which can explain the underestimation at a low RQ. It seems more accurate to measure glucose oxidation with U-^{13}C glucose than with indirect calorimetry, especially at low and high RQs.

The carbohydrate utilization calculated from indirect calorimetry, at an RQ of less than 1, includes carbohydrate oxidation and the possible conversion of carbohydrate into fat when at the same time fat is being oxidized. An RQ of greater than 1 indicates that there is net accretion of fat from glucose; expressed differently, the lipogenesis from glucose is higher than any ongoing fat oxidation.

Another potentially complicating factor in the calculation of substrate utilization is the estimation of protein oxidation from urinary nitrogen excretion. Protein consists of various amino acids that have different RQs when oxidized. Usually an RQ of 0.81 is used as mean value for protein oxidation, but this figure is clearly an approximation. Errors in the measurement of urinary nitrogen hardly affect the estimation of energy expenditure but can have a significant influence on the calculation of substrate utilization.[18]

Another factor that must be taken into account in relation to the results of indirect calorimetry is the duration of the study. Oxygen consumption can fluctuate considerably with time even when all external factors are constant. Various investigators have studied the pattern of oxygen consumption over periods of hours to several days in the preterm neonate.[22–26] It can be concluded from these studies that a reliable estimate of the 24-hour energy expenditure needs continuous measurement over at least 4- to 6-hour periods. The variations found between short-term and long-term measurements are probably due to differences in activity and increased metabolic rate after a feeding.[22–26] In the adult the basal metabolic rate, defined as the lowest observed resting metabolic rate, measured in a healthy adult after an overnight fast of 12 hours at an environmental temperature of 22° to 27°C, has been introduced to decrease the variability in the estimate of oxygen consumption.[27] In the neonate it is impossible to use this definition, as it is unrealistic to starve a neonate for 12 hours. In the neonate the term resting metabolic rate has been considered to be the metabolic rate during sleep, or the lowest metabolic rate observed in each neonate. This rate may show quite some variation, depending on the period the oxygen consumption is measured. Not only can activity influence oxygen consumption, but oxygen consumption is different at different sleep states in the preterm neonate.[28–30]

As direct and indirect calorimetry have their limitations and are difficult to use in the ventilated neonate, other methods of measuring heat production have been sought. Chessex et al.[31] indicated a correlation between heart rate and oxygen consumption, suggesting that the heart rate might be used to estimate heat production. They showed that oxygen consumption increases when heart rate increases above 160 beats per minute (bpm). No correlation between heart rate and oxygen consumption was observed between 120 and 160 bpm, and almost 80% of the time the heart rate of the preterm neonate was within this range. The results of this study should be interpreted with caution: the method needs more validation before it can be used clinically.

Doubly Labeled Water

Another technique to estimate metabolic rate in the free-living individual is the use of doubly labeled water, $D_2^{18}O$. In 1955 Lifson et al.[32] described a method to calculate the CO_2 production from the difference in turnover rate between oxygen and hydrogen. This method is based on the principle that oxygen is lost via CO_2 and H_2O, whereas hydrogen is lost only via H_2O. The difference in turnover rate between oxygen and hydrogen is equal to CO_2 production (Figure 44.1). When a certain RQ is assumed, one can calculate the total energy expenditure. This method involves a number of assumptions as defined in the original report of Lifson et al. and discussed recently:[33-40]

1. The subject is in a steady state of body composition, so total body water, solids, and weight must remain constant.
2. All rates of intake and output remain constant.
3. Water is the only form in which the hydrogen of body water is lost from the body, and water plus CO_2 are the only forms in which the oxygen of body water is lost.
4. The enrichment of the hydrogen of water lost from the body is equal to that of the body water, and the enrichment of the oxygen of water and CO_2 lost from the body is equal to that of the body water.
5. The normal abundance of isotopic oxygen and hydrogen is the same in all substances involved in the material balance.
6. There is no isotopic reentry into the body or entry into the body of isotopic water vapor or CO_2.
7. The volume of distribution of labeled water is equal to the total body water (i.e., there is no incorporation of labeled hydrogen or oxygen of body water into other body constituents except in CO_2 in the case of O_2).

A number of these assumptions are not correct, and corrections must be made. First, the growing neonate is not in a steady state but increases body mass and body water with time. This problem can be overcome by measuring body composition at the beginning and the end of a 5-day period, over which time the turnover rate of oxygen and carbon dioxide is usually measured in the neonate. Second, the enrichment of all water lost by the body is not equal to the enrichment of body water. Specifically, the water lost by insensible water loss has an enrichment different from that of body water. For the different enrichments of water lost through the skin and via the lung, a correction factor has been introduced, as has a correction factor for the uptake of water through the skin and the lung.

The effects of fractionation are more important in the neonate compared with the adult owing to the high water turnover in the neonate relative to that in the adult. Finally, the precision by which the enrichment of body water can be measured is essential for this method. Fortunately, it has improved dramatically when using specially designed isotope ratio mass spectrometers with which enrichments as low as 0.0001% can be measured. Various studies have compared CO_2 production, calculated from the doubly labeled method with CO_2 production, and metabolic rate measured by indirect calorimetry. Studies in the adult showed a mean difference between the methods of 4% to 8%.[35,36]

A number of studies comparing indirect calorimetry with the $D_2^{18}O$ method were conducted in the preterm and term neonate. Roberts et al.[38] conducted a validation study in four preterm neonates. Indirect calorimetry was performed over almost 5 days with the decay curve of D_2O and $H_2^{18}O$ calculated from enrichment in urine. The mean difference between the methods of measuring CO_2 production was only 1.4% ± 4.8% (mean ± SD) and the difference in metabolic rate was 0.3% ± 2.6%. In this study a number of correction factors were used that have been debated by others. Jones et al.[39] showed that a change in the composition of the feeding during a study may cause a shift in baseline enrichment, resulting in a major error in the estimation of CO_2 production. The results of estimating CO_2 production using the doubly labeled water method with the results of indirect calorimetry are compared in Table 44.1. The doubly labeled water method can be regarded as a reliable method to measure total energy consumption in groups of individuals, including the preterm infant. The results in the individual patient, however, show rather large differences between indirect calorimetry and the doubly

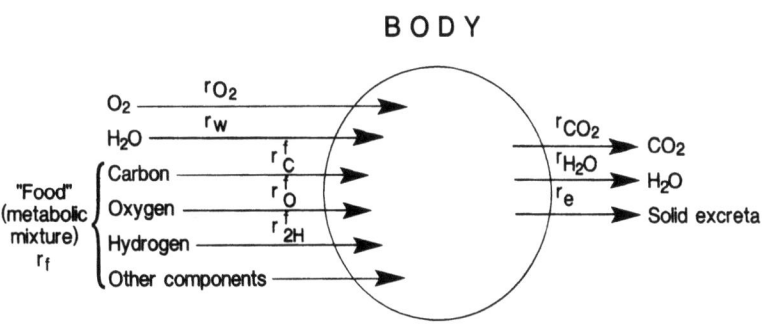

FIGURE 44.1. Material balance, assuming the body is in a steady state of composition.

TABLE 44.1. Carbon dioxide production rates and energy expenditure measured by indirect calorimetry and doubly labeled water method in neonates.

| Reference | Weight at study (g) | Postnatal age (days) | L·kg^{-1} day^{-1} | | % Difference | kcal·kg^{-1} day^{-1} | | |
			rCO$_2$ IDC	rCO$_2$ DLW		MR IDC	MR DLW RQ$_a$	MR DLW RQ$_b$
37	3100 ± 700	17 ± 19	10.5 ± 0.9	10.4 ± 1.1	−0.9 ± 6.2	57.4 ± 5.0	56.7 ± 5.0	58.6 ± 6.0
39	2670 ± 630	15 ± 18	10.4 ± 1.6	9.4 ± 1.1	−8.7 ± 12.9	NA	NA	NA
38	1635 ± 650	23 ± 10	10.9 ± 0.7	10.7 ± 0.3	−1.4 ± 4.8	58.4 ± 2.1	58.4 ± 1.4	NA
41	1556 ± 271	25 ± 6	10.5 ± 1.1	10.2 ± 1.0	−3.2 ± 8.8	58.8 ± 4.3	56.0 ± 5.5	57.6 ± 5.7

From Westerterp et al.,[41] with permission. RQ$_a$, RQ as used in original study (theoretical or measured); RQ$_b$, RQ of feeding; rCO$_2$, CO$_2$ production rate; MR, energy expenditure; IDC, indirect calorimetry; DLW, doubly labeled water method; NA, not available.

labeled method, making this last method rather unreliable. The method seems also not very accurate in the infant with changes in body water as, for instance, the bronchopulmonary dysplasia (BPD) patient. Finally, a stable baseline in $D_2^{18}O$ enrichments is critical.[39]

Comparison of Methods to Measure Heat Production

On theoretical grounds, direct calorimetry should be regarded as the gold standard against which the other methods of measuring heat production must be evaluated. Only a few studies in the neonate comparing direct and indirect calorimetry have been reported. Day and Hardy[5] were the first to conduct simultaneous measurements of direct and indirect calorimetry in the neonate. A reliable comparison between the results of direct and indirect calorimetry is not possible from their studies. The measurements of direct calorimetry cannot be regarded as accurate, as the duration of the studies was a relatively short period of approximately 1 hour, and the body temperature of the neonates changed considerably.

Sauer et al.[8] compared the results of direct and indirect calorimetry using 57 measurements in 14 preterm neonates. A higher metabolic rate calculated from indirect calorimetry was found in all neonates compared with the heat production measured by direct calorimetry; the mean difference was 4.9 kcal·kg^{-1} day^{-1}, or 7% of the indirect calorimetry value. The difference between indirect and direct calorimetry was considered equal to the energy needed for the synthesis of new tissue and stored within the body. These studies have not been confirmed.

Pittet et al.[42] reported the results of direct and indirect calorimetry in the adult. They showed no significant difference between the direct and indirect calorimetry during the period after a glucose, amino acid, or glucose plus amino acid meal. Webb et al.[11,12] compared direct and indirect calorimetry in the adult over a 24-hour period. Their results showed no difference between the methods when the subjects were at rest, but a higher result with indirect calorimetry during activity and semistarvation. No explanation for this difference was given. One can conclude, on the basis of the studies mentioned, that the results of direct calorimetry (i.e., heat production) and indirect calorimetry (i.e., metabolic rate) are comparable. In this chapter, as in the literature, the terms metabolic rate and heat production are used interchangeably.

Fetal Energy Requirements

The energy requirements of the fetus can be divided into energy for maintenance and energy for growth. These energy requirements can be calculated from either the energy supply to the fetus or the oxygen consumption of the fetus together with the energy stored with growth.

Most available data are from studies in the chronically instrumented pregnant sheep. The change in oxygen consumption of the fetal lamb with increasing gestational age is shown in Figure 44.2. It decreases with increasing gestational age when expressed per kilogram dry or wet weight.[43] The oxygen consumption of the fetal lamb at term is around 8 ml·kg^{-1} min^{-1}, equivalent to an energy consumption of approximately 40 kcal·kg^{-1} day^{-1}. The glucose consumption of the fetal lamb decreases with advancing gestational age from 9.4 to 4.9 mg·kg^{-1} min^{-1}.[44] It is questionable if the human fetal oxygen consumption can be estimated from data obtained in sheep. The brain of the fetal sheep is much smaller than that of the human fetus (1.2% vs 12% of body weight), while the brain is metabolically active. On the other hand, weight gain of the fetal lamb is higher than that of the human fetus. Despite differences in body composition and growth rate, the oxygen consumption of the human fetus is found to be almost equal to the values obtained in fetal lamb. Hay et al.[45,46] estimated the energy requirements of the fetal lamb from isotope studies. They calculated a total energy requirement of 86 kcal·kg^{-1} day^{-1}, of which 50 kcal·kg^{-1} day^{-1} is for maintenance and the remainder for growth. Most of the energy (45 kcal·kg^{-1} day^{-1}) was derived from amino acids; the remainder almost evenly split between glucose and lactate.

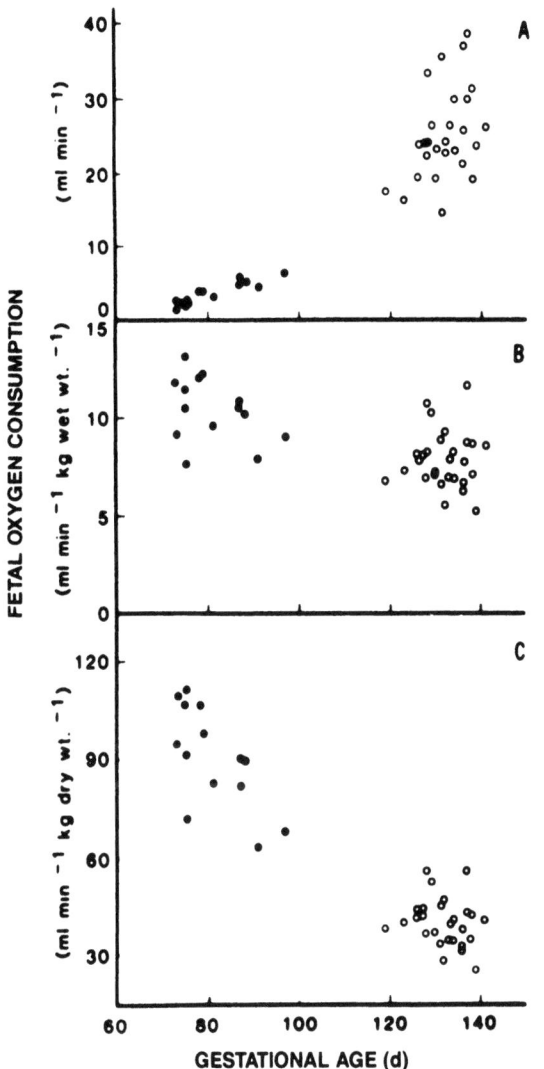

FIGURE 44.2. Relation between oxygen consumption of the fetal lamb and gestational age. (From Bell et al.[43] with permission.)

The oxygen consumption of the human fetus at term has been estimated as $5 \, ml \cdot kg^{-1} \, min^{-1}$ from the uterine blood flow and the oxygen content of blood from the uterine artery and vein.[47] A fetal oxygen consumption of $8 \, ml \cdot kg^{-1} \, min^{-1}$ was thought to be a more realistic value by Sparks et al.,[48] corresponding to an energy consumption of $40 \, kcal \cdot kg^{-1} \, day^{-1}$. Bonds et al.[49] calculated the oxygen consumption of the human fetus at term from the decrease in maternal oxygen consumption at delivery and found it to be $6.8 \, ml \cdot kg^{-1} \, min^{-1}$. Bozetti et al.[50] measured the oxygen content of fetal blood taken during fetoscopy at approximately 20 weeks. They found an oxygen saturation of 50% in presumed arterial versus 85% in venous fetal blood. Both values decreased with increasing gestation.[51] The fetal oxygen consumption can be calculated, using a mathematical model of fetal circulation as $8 \, ml \cdot kg^{-1} \, min^{-1}$.[52] The energy requirements of the fetus can be estimated from the increase in oxygen consumption of the mother (see Chapter 15). The increase in oxygen consumption in the mother results not only from oxygen consumption of the fetus but also from that of the mother herself owing to an increase in metabolically active tissue such as uterus and placenta and the resulting increase in cardiac output. Probably more than half the increase in oxygen consumption of the mother is due to the oxygen consumption of the placenta and uterus, the accretion of protein in placenta and uterus being higher than that of the fetus.[53] The increase in metabolic rate of the pregnant mother is around $400 \, kcal \cdot day^{-1}$. The energy consumption of a 3.5-kg neonate can thus be estimated to be $57 \, kcal \cdot kg^{-1} \, day^{-1}$ maximally.

The second part of the energy requirements of the fetus is the energy needed for growth. The energy for growth comprises the energy laid down in the components of new tissue and the energy needed to synthesize new tissue. The amount of energy laid down during life within the fetus can be calculated from the change in body composition of the fetus. It is usually calculated using the so-called reference fetus: data constructed from the body composition of those who died shortly before or after birth.[54,55] It should be emphasized that the body composition of the reference fetus is only an approximation of that of the growing fetus; strictly speaking, it is impossible to calculate changes in body composition (i.e., longitudinal data) from cross-sectional data. The published data on body composition are rather dated, from the time when the differentiation between appropriate for gestational age (AGA) and small for gestational age (SGA) was not appreciated. The disease that caused the death might have influenced the body composition. Taking these factors into consideration, one can still calculate the energy requirements for growth using these data, assuming the energy content of fat to be $9.2 \, kcal \cdot g^{-1}$, that of protein $5.6 \, kcal \cdot g^{-1}$, and that of glycogen $4 \, kcal \cdot g^{-1}$. The energy requirements for growth increase considerably during the last trimester of normal pregnancy (Figure 44.3) due to the large increase in body fat (Figure 44.4).[54–56]

The number of calories laid down at a gestational age of 26 weeks is around $12 \, kcal \cdot kg^{-1} \, day^{-1}$, of which 7 kcal is for nonfat tissue and 5 kcal for fat. At the end of a normal pregnancy the accumulation is $40 \, kcal \cdot kg^{-1} \, day^{-1}$ of which approximately $35 \, kcal \cdot kg^{-1} \, day^{-1}$ is for fat deposition.

The total caloric requirement of the growing fetus during the last trimester of the pregnancy can be estimated to be $96 \, kcal \cdot kg^{-1} \, day^{-1}$, consisting of $56 \, kcal \cdot kg^{-1} \, day^{-1}$ for maintenance and $40 \, kcal \cdot kg^{-1} \, day^{-1}$ for growth.[50] This energy requirement is almost equal to the energy requirement of the growing preterm neonate, as we shall discuss later. The energy requirement for individual patients can also be estimated from standard equations. For individual patients this is rather inaccurate, regarding the wide variability in energy metabolism among infants.[57]

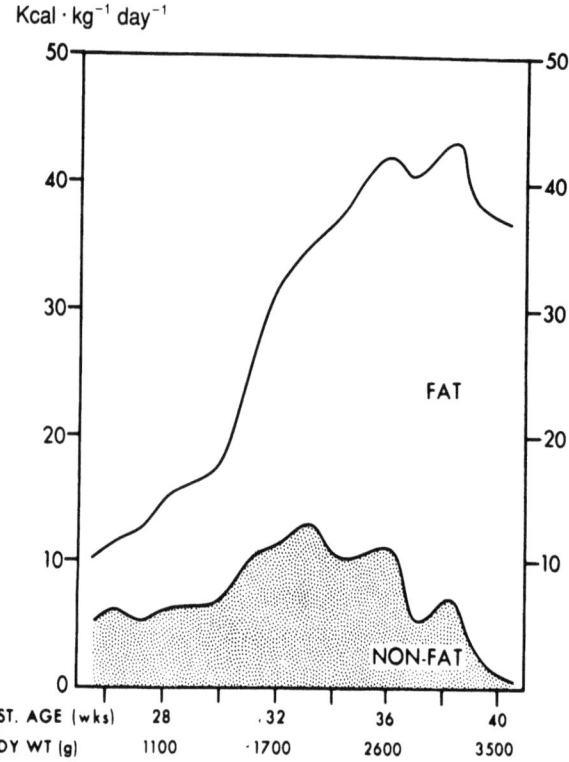

FIGURE 44.3. Relation between caloric accretion rates and gestational age of the human fetus. (From Heim,[56] with permission.)

Metabolic Rate After Birth

Oxygen consumption, as an indicator of total metabolic rate, increases rapidly after birth in animals and in the human neonate.[58,59] The total metabolic rate can be subdivided into resting metabolic rate and energy used for activity, for thermogenesis, and for growth. Different factors are found to affect metabolic rate, although no single factor regulating metabolic rate can be determined. Factors noted to influence metabolic rate in the neonate include postnatal age, energy intake, growth, composition of food, protein turnover, illness, specific dynamic action, activity, intrauterine growth retardation, and thermal environment. Each is discussed in detail.

Metabolic Rate and Postnatal Age

Resting and total metabolic rate increase rapidly during the first week of life.[58–63] Forsyth and Crighton[59] showed no significant increase in oxygen consumption of sick, ventilated neonate during the first days after birth, in contrast to an increase in the more healthy preterm neonate. Gudinchet et al.[63] found a small increase in total metabolic rate during the second week of life but no change thereafter. We demonstrated an increase in metabolic rate during the first week of life but no change in resting metabolic rate between the second and seventh postnatal weeks in the growing, preterm neonate.[8] The total metabolic rate expressed per kilogram body weight showed a slight increase owing to an increase in activity (Figure 44.5). Most studies on the relation between metabolic rate and postnatal age have been carried out in the preterm neonate. Only a few studies have been completed in the term neonate. There are no indications that the metabolic rate of the term neonate is significantly different from that of the preterm neonate.

Different explanations for the increase in metabolic rate after birth can be hypothesized. It is unlikely that postnatal age itself increases metabolic rate after birth. The correlation between postnatal age and metabolic rate is probably the result of other changes occurring at the same time.

The metabolic rate is usually expressed per kilogram body weight. After birth the body weight decreases, probably owing to a loss of water and solids.[64] The majority of the weight loss after birth is due to losses in body water, although there has to be a loss in solids as the energy intake is less than the energy expenditure at least during the first 3 to 4 days of life.[65,66] The loss of solids is mainly fat, which is metabolically inactive. When the percentage of metabolically active tissue per kilogram body weight is higher, there is an increase in the metabolic rate, expressed per kilogram body weight. How the metabolic rate should be expressed is an intriguing, unanswered question. Usually it is expressed per

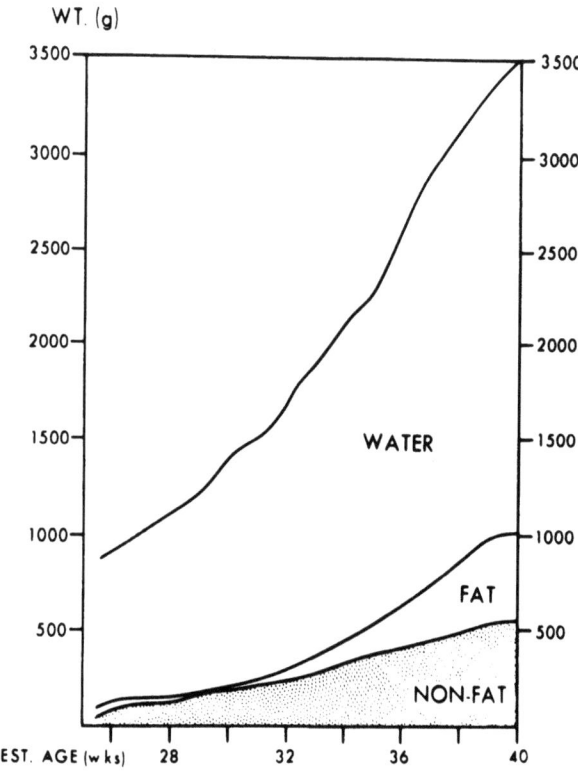

FIGURE 44.4. Relation between body composition and gestational age in the human fetus. (From Heim,[56] with permission.)

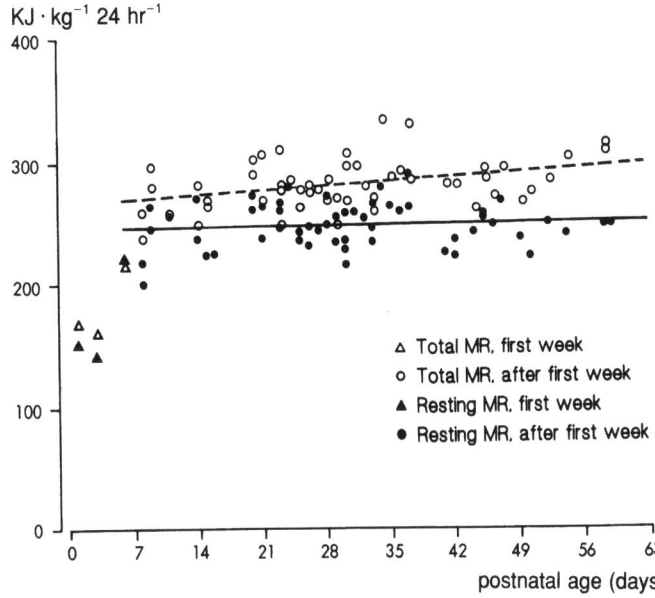

FIGURE 44.5. Relation between total and resting metabolic rate (MR) in preterm neonates versus postnatal age. The solid line represents the resting MR after the first week: y = 246 + 0.07x, showing no significant increase with increasing postnatal age. The dashed line represents the total MR after the first week: y = 269 + 0.40x, significantly increasing with postnatal age; $p < 0.05$. (From Sauer et al.,[8] with permission.)

kilogram body weight as the simplest measurement. It might be more appropriate to express metabolic rate per unit lean body mass or body cell mass. So long as it is impossible to measure lean body mass or body cell mass simple and accurately (see Chapter 47), the metabolic rate must be expressed per kilogram body weight. A second and more important factor that might explain the increase in metabolic rate after birth is the increase in energy intake that usually occurs during the first days after birth.

Effects of Energy Intake on Metabolic Rate

Bhakoo and Scopes[67] and Gentz et al.[61] found a difference in the increase in metabolic rate after birth according to the feeding regimen. A more rapid increase in energy intake is associated with a more rapid increase in oxygen consumption. Since that time, many studies have shown an influence of energy intake on metabolic rate. Increasing the intake of either carbohydrates, fat, or protein causes an increase in metabolic rate above the so-called basal metabolic rate. Long-term starvation results in a decreased metabolic rate, as shown in the adult.[68] Brooke[69] studied the effect of feeding solutions enriched with either peanut oil, medium-chain triglycerides (MCT), or sucrose on energy expenditure and growth in the preterm neonate. Although there was a clear trend of energy expenditure being higher with the enriched formula, it was significantly so only during the postprandial phase with two of the four enriched formulas. The increased energy expenditure was most likely due to the higher energy intake and not due to the addition of MCT, as two studies showed no change in energy expenditure when long-chain triglycerides (LCT) were replaced by MCT.[70,71]

Chessex et al.[62] reported a correlation between the increase in metabolic rate after birth and energy intake. Van Aerde studied the metabolic rate in the parenterally fed term neonate receiving either glucose only or a glucose-amino acid mixture.[72] Metabolic rate increased linearly when energy intake was above a level of approximately 40 kcal·kg^{-1}day^{-1}, at which point around 30% of the increase in energy intake was subsequently lost as heat (Figure 44.6). The addition of lipids to the glucose infusion, thereby increasing the energy intake, causes an increase in energy expenditure,[73] while the replacement of glucose by lipids has no effect on energy metabolism but causes a reduction in CO_2 production.[74-76] The latter can be explained by a reduction in lipogenesis.[21]

A different study evaluated the effect of increasing the energy intake, while keeping the composition of the feed

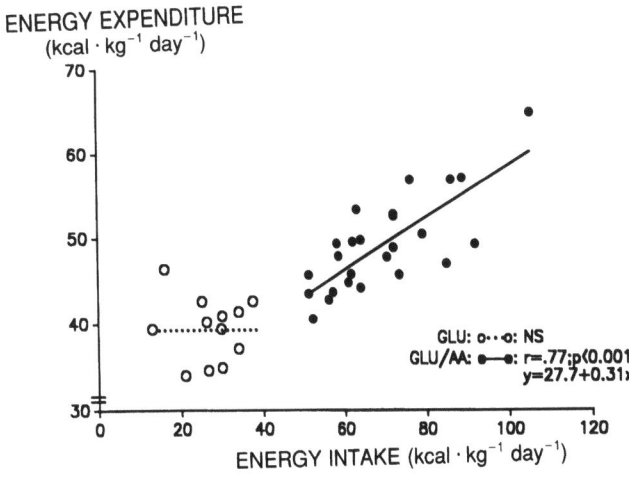

FIGURE 44.6. Relation between metabolic rate and energy intake in intravenously fed preterm neonates. (From Van Aerde,[72] with permission.)

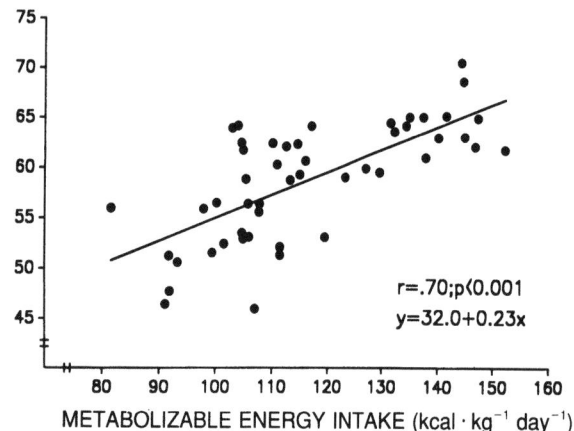

FIGURE 44.7. Relation between metabolic rate and metabolizable energy intake in orally fed preterm neonates. (From Van Aerde,[72] with permission.)

ing formula constant, on energy expenditure and growth in a group of orally fed preterm neonates.[77] The results show a linear relation between energy intake and metabolic rate when intake varied between 100 and 150 kcal·kg^{-1}·day^{-1} (Figure 44.7). In the Van Aerde study,[72] not only did energy intake increase, but protein intake increased at a corresponding rate. The increase in metabolic rate might have been due to an increase in protein intake. Kashyap et al.[78,79] and Schulze et al.[80] showed that energy expenditure was higher, though not statistically so, in a group of preterm neonates receiving 144 kcal·kg^{-1}·day^{-1} and protein at 3.9 g·kg^{-1}·day^{-1} compared with neonates receiving the same amount of protein and 120 kcal·kg^{-1}·day^{-1}. This finding confirms the importance of energy intake as a regulator of metabolic rate. The difference in energy expenditure was rather small: 64.3 ± 5.5 kcal·kg^{-1}·day^{-1} in the group receiving 120 kcal·kg^{-1}·day^{-1} versus 67.8 ± 3.0 kcal·kg^{-1}·day^{-1} in the group receiving 144 kcal·kg^{-1}·day^{-1}. The energy expenditure in a comparable group of neonates receiving 2.8 g·kg^{-1}·day^{-1} protein and 118 kcal·kg^{-1}·day^{-1} was lower than the energy expenditure in either group, 59.8 kcal·kg^{-1}·day^{-1}. This finding indicates an effect of both energy and protein intake on metabolic rate. Bell et al.[81,82] showed no difference in metabolic rate between neonates receiving either 120 or 100 kcal·kg^{-1}·day^{-1}. The protein intake in both groups of neonates was equal, 3.2 g·kg^{-1}·day^{-1}, raising the question of whether an increase in energy intake influences metabolic rate. The number of patients in this study was rather small, so no definitive conclusions could be drawn. Weinstein et al.[83] compared metabolic rate in three groups of preterm neonates receiving either dextrose only (38 or 64 kcal·kg^{-1}·day^{-1}) or dextrose plus amino acids (64 kcal·kg^{-1}·day^{-1}), providing 1 to 2 g of pro-

tein. Energy expenditure was higher when the energy intake increased. The addition of protein did not influence energy expenditure.

Several studies have investigated the relationship between energy and protein intake, metabolic rate, and gain in weight, length, and head circumference in the orally fed preterm neonate. A number of these studies are summarized in Table 44.2.

Figure 44.8 shows the relationship between metabolic rate and energy intake, calculated from the data in Table 44.2. If we perform multiple linear regression analysis (nonweighted) on these data, a model of protein intake and energy intake is more significant for metabolic rate ($p < .005$) than a model of energy intake alone:

$$MR = 17.6 + 5.3 * prot_{int} + 0.2 * energy_{int}$$
$$(r = 0.8;\ p < .00005)$$

It was concluded that metabolic rate is influenced by both energy and protein intake. The increase in metabolic rate after a feeding has been called specific dynamic action, "luxus consumption," thermic effect of feeding, or diet-induced thermogenesis. Two apparently distinct thermic responses to food ingestion have been described in the adult.[68,97-101] The first thermic response after a feeding is the increase in energy expenditure directly after a meal and is called the obligatory component. It is related to the digestion, absorption, and processing of nutrients. The second part of the thermic response after a feeding is an increase in basal metabolic rate, which occurs after chronic overfeeding and may be associated with diet-induced changes in thyroid hormones and the sympathetic nervous system. It is called the regulatory or facultative component. The exact biochemical regulation and clinical importance of the thermic effect of feeding in adults is currently uncertain.

Some of the factors known to influence the specific dynamic action in the adult are of potential importance to studies done in the neonate. Acheson et al.[99] showed that the thermic effect of a carbohydrate load in the adult is affected by the previously consumed diet. They administered 500 g carbohydrate to adults who had consumed either a high-fat, high-carbohydrate, or mixed diet several days before a study. The thermic effect was the highest in the subjects on a high carbohydrate diet. It was attributed to a higher conversion of carbohydrate to fat in this group. It was speculated that the only way carbohydrate could be stored in this group was as fat, as the glycogen stores were saturated after the high-carbohydrate feeding.

Using U-^{13}C glucose it has been shown that glucose is indeed converted by the preterm infant into lipids, also at the first day of life when the energy intake is less than expenditure.[102] Yunis et al.[103] found that the addition of lipids increased plasma glucose concentration. They found that this was not due to an increased glucose pro-

TABLE 44.2. Energy balance studies in the orally fed preterm neonate.

Ref.	Type of feeding	E_{in} (kcal·kg⁻¹·day⁻¹)	Losses: feces and urine (kcal·kg⁻¹·day⁻¹)	Metab energy (kcal·kg⁻¹·day⁻¹)	MR	Prot in (g·kg⁻¹·day⁻¹)	Prot ret (g·kg⁻¹·day⁻¹)	Protein (g·100 kcal⁻¹)	Weight gain (g·kg⁻¹·day⁻¹)	Length gain (cm·wk⁻¹)	Gain head circ. (cm·wk⁻¹)	% Prot·wt⁻¹	% Fat·wt⁻¹
84	LCT	149	18.2	131	62.6	3.2	1.9	2.1	16.8	1.0	0.9	11	21
85	EBM	136	31	105		3.5	1.6	2.6	15.6	0.8	0.9	10	
	LCT	151	29	122		3.8	2.0	2.5	21.5	1.4	1.1	9	
	MCT	145	32	113		2.5	1.2	1.7	15.3	0.9	0.9	8	
	MCT	143	38	105		3.7	1.8	2.6	13.7	0.8	0.7	13	
86	OMM	111	11	100	56	3.0	2.0	2.7	15.2	1.0	0.8	13	16.6
87	OMM	111	11	100	56	3.0	2.0	2.7	15.2	1	0.8	13.4	16.6
	LCT	149	18	141	63	3.2	2.6	2.1	18.8	1	0.9	12.5	33.8
88	LCT	126	11	115	58.4	2.7	1.7	2.1	16.9	0.9	0.9	10.1	27.7
	OMM	127	19	108	52.8	2.6	1.6	2.1	15.2	0.9	1.1	10.7	33.8
89	BM	106	11	95	48.6	2.5	1.6	2.3	14.2	1.0	1.0	11	15.5
	MCT	128	8	120	60.1	3.1	2.2	2.6	21.5	1.4	1.0	10.2	23.7
90	LCT	118	13	106	55.5	2.5	1.7	2.1	15.2	1.0	1.0	12	29
91	MCT	124	5.9	118	57	3.1	2.4	2.5	16.4	1.2	1.2	14	32
92	BM/MCT	114	14	99	58	3.0	1.8	3.0	15			12	23
73	BM	96	10	86		1.9	1.2	2.0	13.7	0.8		9	
	MCT	139	31	108		3.4	2.5	1.8	19.4	1.0		13	
26	MCT	123	13	100	68.4	3.3	2.0	2.6	16.6			12	20
70	MCT	134	10	123	62.7	3.0	2.1	2.2	21.2	1.3	1.1	10	25
	LCT	133	10	121	63.4	3.0	2.1	2.3	21.8	0.8	1.1	10	29
94	LCT	145	28	117		3.7	2.1	2.6	22.1	0.7	1.4	10	
	EBM	144	42	102		2.7	1.4	1.9	13.6	0.9	1.0	10	
95	BM	107	12	95	48.6	2.5	1.6	2.3	15.3	1.1	1.0	10	27
	BM + Prot	106	15	91	57.9	3.8	2.0	2.5	17.1	1.2	1.2	12	14
96	BM	125	19	106		2.9	1.9	2.3	16			12	
	MCT	125	23	102		2.8	1.9	2.2	14			14	
80	LCT	113	7	106	60	2.24	1.6	2.0	14.4			12	29
78	LCT	115	12	104	58	3.6	2.6	3.1	16.8			16	20
	LCT	149	11	137	69	3.5	2.6	2.3	21.7			12	28
79	LCT	119	9	110	59.8	2.8	2.2	2.3	16.0	1	1	13.7	24.6
	LCT	120	7	113	64.3	3.8	2.6	3.2	19.1	1.2	1.1	13.6	19
	LCT	144	6	138	67.8	3.9	2.9	2.7	21.5	1.3	1.2	13.5	26.2
71	MCT	120	10	110	59	3.3	2.4	2.8	16.6	0.9	1.2	15	25
	LCT	120	17	103	62	3.3	2.5	2.8	16.1	1.1	1.0	15	21

BM, breast milk; EBM, expressed breast milk; OMM, own mother's milk; LCT, preterm formula in which fat blend contains less than 5% medium-chain triglycerides; MCT, preterm formula in which 40–50% of fat blend is given as medium-chain triglycerides; E_{in}, energy intake; Metab energy, metabolizable energy intake; MR, metabolic rate; Prot in, protein intake; Prot ret, protein retention; % Prot/wtg, percentage of protein per gram weight gain; % Fat·wt⁻¹, percentage of fat per gram weight gain.

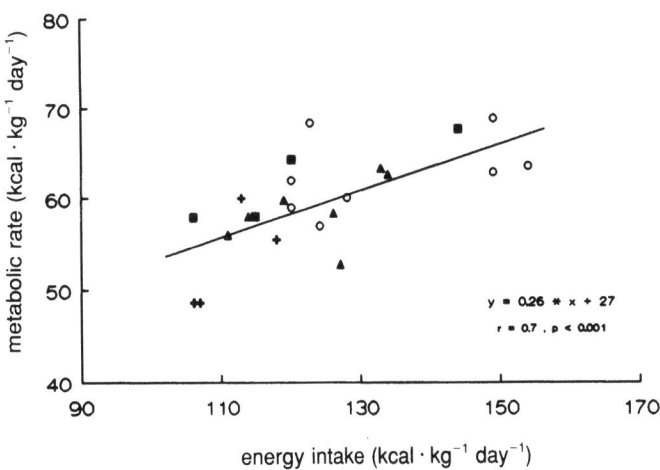

FIGURE 44.8. Relation between metabolic rate and energy intake in orally fed preterm neonates. Data are from Table 44.2.

duction but could be the result of alterations in glucose utilization. This study does have implications for studies in the neonate. When the effects of different feeding solutions (e.g., glucose only vs a glucose-fat mixture) are compared, one should take into consideration the body composition and glycogen stores prior to the study. Studies in which the prestudy feeding is not controlled or constant during at least 2 to 5 days should be regarded with caution.

The exact hormonal influences on metabolic rate are not yet known. Changes in thyroid hormones are related to slow changes in metabolic rate, but it has been argued that thyroid hormones do not influence metabolic rate but play a more permissive role.[104] Chikenji et al.[104] evaluated the effect of increasing glucose intake on nitrogen balance, energy expenditure, and fuel utilization in malnourished adults receiving parenteral nutrition with a constant nitrogen intake and a glucose intake below or slightly above energy expenditure. In this study the higher triiodothyronine (T_3)/thyroxine (T_4) ratio was found in the high glucose group, although the T_3 was not different between groups. The higher T_3/T_4 ratio might indicate a higher free T_3 concentration, which could result in an increase in metabolic rate. Yang et al.[105] could not detect any effect of a reduction in energy intake in rats on the levels of T_3 or T_4, or the free T_3 index. Energy reduction was correlated with a reduction in total insulin-like growth factors (IGF-I and -II). Various studies in adults have shown that changes in norepinephrine are responsible for more rapid changes in metabolic rate.[98-101] Acheson et al.[99] provided evidence that the rise in energy expenditure in excess of the obligatory requirements for processing and storing glucose after a high glucose load is completely mediated through sympathetic nervous activity. Schwartz et al.[100] could not detect any correlation between plasma epinephrine concentration and energy expenditure after a high-carbohydrate or a high-fat meal in the adult. The effect of thyroid hormones and sympathetic nervous activity in the neonate has hardly been studied. Weinstein et al.[83] measured T_4 and T_3 concentrations in the preterm neonate receiving either 38 or 64 kcal·kg^{-1}·day^{-1}. At the latter intake the calories were given either as glucose only or as a glucose-amino acid mixture. The oxygen consumption was higher at the higher energy intake, but amino acid intake had no influence. The T_4 and T_3 concentrations were not different between groups. These investigators measured the urinary epinephrine excretion as an indicator of sympathetic activity. It was significantly higher at the higher energy intake but was not influenced by amino acid intake. The role of different hormones, including insulin, glucagon, and somatomedins, in the regulation of the metabolic rate needs further study, specifically in the neonate.

Another mechanism that might contribute to the change in metabolic rate with a change in energy intake, and be part of the regulatory component of specific dynamic actions, is the futile metabolic cycles. These cycles are called futile because they have no obvious function. Substrates are recycled. These cycles consume energy and their function seems to be to produce heat. Alternatively, Crabtree and Newsholme[106] have demonstrated that substrate cycling can provide a mechanism of variable sensitivity for the control of substrate fluxes. They have shown theoretically that cycling amplifies the control of flux to a given change in regulator (e.g., hormone) concentration. An example of these cycles is the breakdown of glucose to three-carbon components as lactate and pyruvate and the resynthesis of these substrates to glucose in the liver. Another cycle is the continuous breakdown and reesterification of triglycerides. These cycles are at least partly controlled by hormones including insulin, glucagon, and norepinephrine.[107]

The exact importance of these cycles is unknown, but they are more active during septicemia and severe burns in the adult.[108-110] Other mechanisms considered to be related to the change in energy expenditure with altered energy intake are changes in oxidative phosphorylation and in the activity of the sodium-potassium pump. The role of these processes in the regulation of the energy expenditure in the neonate is unknown.

Some studies have found a difference in specific dynamic action between obese and nonobese individuals,[111,112] but these results have not been confirmed.[113] Whether an absence of specific dynamic action is important in the development of obesity in children remains unclear. Roberts et al.[114] studied total energy expenditure, using the doubly labeled water method and postprandial energy expenditure, measured by indirect calorimetry in neonates of mothers of normal weight and of mothers who were overweight. Fifty percent of the neonates of mothers who were overweight became overweight by the age of 1 year. The total energy expenditure of these neonates at 3 months was lower than that of the neonates with a normal weight at the age of 1 year. The postprandial energy expenditure measured at 0.1 and 3.0 months of age was not different between groups. Weight, length, skinfold thickness, and metabolizable energy intake did not differ at 3 months. It was suggested, but not supported by data, that the neonates who were overweight used less energy for activity than did their normal counterparts. Defective thermogenesis could not be ruled out in this study, as the measurements of postprandial energy expenditure were of short duration. More studies of the neonate at a very young age are needed to determine if a difference in the thermogenic metabolism of an obese child and adult is the cause or the result of obesity.

A different and, for the growing neonate, interesting explanation for the specific dynamic action (SDA) was given by Ashworth.[115] She showed a sharp increase in SDA in malnourished neonates during catch-up growth.

SDA was correlated with the rate of catch-up growth and declined after recovery. The energy cost of tissue synthesis was calculated from the increase in SDA as $0.3\,kcal\cdot g^{-1}$ weight gain. Mestyan et al.[116] and Brooke et al.[117] measured the increase in metabolic rate after feeding in the preterm neonate. In some neonates heat production was 40% to 50% above resting basal levels. Brooke and Ashworth[92] showed that the energy expenditure due to SDA was more than 10% of the daily intake. Freymond et al.[26] showed that this figure might be severely overestimated owing to interference with concomitant activity. In his study nine preterm neonates were observed for two consecutive days, during which time repeated measurements of energy expenditure were made using indirect calorimetry combined with a visual activity score. When the SDA was calculated from the increase in metabolic rate after a feeding, a thermogenic effect of the feeding of 9.5% ± 3.8% of the intake could be calculated. When this effect was corrected for the confounding effect of activity, the thermogenic effect amounted to only 3.1% ± 6.8% of the metabolizable energy intake.

TABLE 44.3. Energy cost of growth.

		kcal·g weight gain^{-1}		
Reference	Method	E_{comp}	E_{synth}	Total
117	Energy balance, preterm infants	4.0	1.7	5.7
62		3.6	0.4	4.0
8		2.8	0.3	3.1
63			0.5	
26		2.6		
78		2.6–3.3		
118	Energy balance, malnutrition	3.3	1.1	4.4
54	Carcass analysis	1.4	0.6	2.0
55		1.5	0.7	2.2
92	SDA			0.3
115			0.3	
62			0.4	
119	ATP equivalents	1.6	0.3	1.9

E_{comp} = energy present in the "building blocks" of new tissue; E_{synth} = energy needed for the synthesis of new tissue.

Effects of Growth on Metabolic Rate

The energy requirements for growth of the fetus or neonate include the fuels of energy transformation and the building materials for the production of new tissue. The energy present in the "building blocks" is equal to the difference between metabolizable energy intake (i.e., energy administered minus energy lost via feces and urine) and the metabolic rate. The second part of the energy cost of growth—the energy required for the synthesis of new tissue—is included in the metabolic rate. The faster the child is growing, the more energy is needed for this process. Several studies have shown a positive linear correlation between metabolic rate and weight gain in the preterm neonate,[62,63] as well as in the infant recovering from malnutrition.[92,118] The increase in metabolic rate due to growth represents the energy for tissue synthesis. Using the regression equation of weight gain versus energy expenditure, the energy cost of tissue synthesis has been calculated as 0.4 to $1.7\,kcal\cdot g^{-1}$ weight gain in the preterm neonate and 0.3 to $1.1\,kcal\cdot g^{-1}$ weight gain in the infant recovering from malnutrition.

Other methods to calculate the energy cost of tissue synthesis have produced data that are similar to these estimates (Table 44.3). Hommes[119] calculated the energy cost of growth on a theoretical basis from the adenosine triphosphate (ATP) equivalents required as $0.3\,kcal\cdot g^{-1}$ weight gain. Brooke and Ashworth[92] calculated the energy cost from the SDA in the malnourished infant as $0.3\,kcal\cdot g^{-1}$ weight gain. Sauer et al.[8] calculated the energy cost of tissue synthesis from the difference between the data of indirect and direct calorimetry. It was assumed that the energy needed for tissue synthesis is included in the measurement of indirect calorimetry, as food is oxidized to provide this energy. As the energy is stored within the body, this energy is not given off as heat and is not measured by direct calorimetry. The difference between the results of indirect and direct calorimetry represent the energy cost of tissue synthesis. The energy cost of synthesis calculated in this manner is $0.3\,kcal\cdot g^{-1}$ weight gain.

The energy cost of new tissue clearly depends on the composition of the weight gain. According to the recommendations of the Committee on Nutrition of the American Academy of Pediatrics, a preterm neonate should have a growth rate comparable to the intrauterine accretion rate,[120] while the optimal composition of weight gain can be calculated from the reference fetus constructed by Ziegler et al.[55] The protein content of new tissue is, irrespective of gestational age, approximately 12%, whereas the percentage of fat increases from 5% at 26 weeks to 20% at 40 weeks.

Effect of the Composition of Food Intake on Metabolic Rate

Studies in the intravenously fed adult have shown a higher metabolic rate and RQ when an infusate in which all, or almost all, energy is given as carbohydrate as compared to an infusate in which part of the energy is replaced by fat.[121,122] Heymsfield et al.[123] studied the metabolic rate, as measured by indirect calorimetry, and heat production, as measured by direct calorimetry, in the adult at different levels of oral energy intake. Metabolic rate remains virtually constant when the energy intake is increased from starving to a maintenance level. A further increase in energy intake causes a rise in both metabolic rate and heat production and no significant difference between the data is observed. A high carbohydrate formula, given continuously, results in an increase in both oxygen consumption and carbon dioxide production, but the increase in carbon dioxide production is higher than the increase in oxygen consumption. A high fat formula results in a smaller rise in metabolic rate and carbon dioxide production. These results are explained by a higher rate of lipogenesis during a high carbohydrate formula compared with a high fat formula.

Similar results have been obtained in the intravenously fed neonate, both preterm and term. Both oxygen consumption and carbon dioxide production decrease when part of the energy provided by glucose is isocalorically replaced by energy given as a fat emulsion.[74-76] The decrease in CO_2 production is more pronounced than the decrease in oxygen consumption, which results in a lower RQ in the mixed-fed group. In one study, Sauer et al.[19] measured carbohydrate oxidation simultaneously by indirect calorimetry and from the $^{13}CO_2$ excretion during a primed constant infusion of U-^{13}C-glucose. The difference between carbohydrate oxidation measured by indirect calorimetry and glucose oxidation measured by the $^{13}CO_2$ method was higher in the glucose-infused group compared with the glucose/fat-infused group. It was hypothesized that the differences in oxygen consumption and carbon dioxide production are due to a lower rate of lipogenesis in neonates receiving glucose plus fat, compared with those receiving glucose alone. Lipogenesis is a process in which 15% to 25% of the glucose calories are lost during the transformation into fat, while the RQ of this process is far above 1.

These results have clinical implications. Carbohydrates are often added to the diet of the neonate who shows insufficient weight gain in order to increase the energy intake. The beneficial effect of this addition is limited, as 25% of the energy is lost owing to the conversion of carbohydrates to fat in order to store the excess energy. Also, there is an increase in carbon dioxide production that may be harmful for the neonate with compromised lung function, causing or increasing respiratory failure.[124,125] Fat, which can be stored without almost any increase in metabolic rate or carbon dioxide production and loss of energy, has advantages over carbohydrate as an additional energy source.

The replacement of long-chain fatty acids by medium-chain fatty acids (MCT) has caused a reduction in weight gain in the adult, attributable to a higher metabolic rate in the MCT group.[126] Another study in the adult showed that excess energy given as MCT causes a higher metabolic rate compared with excess energy given as long-chain fatty acids (LCT).[127] This increased energy expenditure is attributable to less efficient storage of MCT as a result of lipogenesis in the liver.

Studies in the neonate have failed to show a difference in metabolic rate between the neonate fed either a formula in which all lipids are given as long-chain fatty acids or a formula in which 40% of the intake is MCT.[70,71] No effect of protein retention is observed either.[89,128] Sulkers et al.[129] found that almost 50% of the MCT is oxidized by the preterm neonate. In a study in which two groups of stable preterm neonates, both receiving 120 kcal·kg^{-1} day^{-1}, were fed a formula in which the lipids contained either 4% or 40% MCT, Sulkers et al.[71] found that the percentage of fat per gram weight gain is higher in the 40% MCT group than in the 4% MCT group. It is not due to a difference in metabolic rate but to slightly higher fat and energy resorption in the 40% MCT group. There were no differences in gain of length, weight, or head circumference. Using stable isotopes, Carnielli et al.[130] reported that at least part of the MCT was not oxidized, but was converted into long-chain fatty acids like palmitic acid. The effects of food components other than carbohydrates, fat, and protein on energy expenditure have not been studied in detail. Sulkers et al.[131] studied the effect of a high dose of carnitine on energy balance, nitrogen balance, and growth in the preterm neonate. Carnitine promotes the transport of long-chain fatty acids across the outer mitochondrial membrane, thereby promoting fat oxidation. This study reported evidence for a higher metabolic rate and a lower weight gain in the high carnitine group. More studies on the effects of substances such as carnitine on the energy balance are necessary (see Chapter 38).

Effects of Protein Turnover on Metabolic Rate

Protein is continuously synthesized from and broken down into amino acids (see Chapter 34). The protein turnover, calculated per body weight, is higher in the preterm neonate than at any other age. There is a fall in protein synthesis with age, with an increase during puberty, which might indicate that protein synthesis is related to growth[132] (Table 44.4).

The process of protein turnover consists of protein synthesis and protein breakdown. Protein synthesis is an energy-requiring process, and the energy liberated in the process of protein breakdown cannot be converted to energy-containing substances. Protein turnover is an energy-consuming process where almost all the energy consumed is given off as heat. Catzeflis et al.[133,134] estimated the energy cost of protein synthesis in the preterm neonate from the regression equation of protein synthesis versus energy expenditure. Based on this relation they found the energy required to synthesize 1 g of protein to be 2 kcal. Moore[135] calculated the energy requirement for protein synthesis on a theoretical basis to be 1 kcal/g protein. Assuming a protein synthesis rate in the preterm

TABLE 44.4. Total body protein synthesis and energy metabolism in children and young adults.

Age group	Protein synthesis (g·kg⁻¹ day⁻¹)	Basal metabolic rate (kcal·kg⁻¹ day⁻¹)	% of BMR used for protein synthesis[a]
Premature	14.4	55	26
Infants	6.1	52.8	12
Children	5.0	40.8	12
Adolescents	5.7	32.4	18
Adults	3.0	24	12

From Pencharz et al.,[132] with permission.
[a] Assuming an energy cost of protein synthesis of 1 kcal·g protein⁻¹.

neonate of 10 to 12 g·kg⁻¹day⁻¹, the energy requirement for protein synthesis accounts for 10 to 24 kcal·kg⁻¹ day⁻¹.[132,133] Energy intake, above a certain lower limit, seems not to affect protein synthesis or breakdown.[136,137] This might explain why increasing the energy intake by adding lipids in the intravenously fed infant did not improve protein balance.[138] The percentage of the resting metabolic rate that can be attributed to protein synthesis seems to be constant at all ages with the exception of a higher percentage at periods of rapid growth (Table 44.4). The difference in total metabolic rate between the hardly growing intravenously fed preterm neonate receiving approximately 75 kcal·kg⁻¹day⁻¹ and the metabolic rate of the rapidly growing orally fed preterm neonate receiving approximately 120 kcal·kg⁻¹day⁻¹ is around 20 kcal·kg⁻¹day⁻¹. Assuming a difference in weight gain of 10 g·kg⁻¹day⁻¹ (i.e., 5 vs 15 g·kg⁻¹day⁻¹) and a protein content of new tissue of 12%, the difference in protein gain is 1.2 g. When 6 g of protein have to be synthesized for the gain of 1 g of protein, it means a difference in protein synthesis of 6 g·kg⁻¹day⁻¹. The energy needed for this protein synthesis is approximately 6 to 12 kcal·kg⁻¹day⁻¹, or about half the difference in metabolic rate. Another contribution to the higher metabolic rate of the orally fed neonate is the energy needed for absorption of nutrients.

Protein intake is positively related to protein turnover; an increase in protein intake increases protein synthesis.[139] As protein synthesis is an energy-consuming process, part of the increase in energy expenditure found at a higher protein intake might be due to increased protein synthesis.[133,134] Young and Marchini[140] stressed the need for a generous intake of essential amino acids in humans, suggesting that an above minimal intake has advantages over the minimal intake, especially during a stressful stimulus. In the adult stressful stimuli cause an enhanced rate of protein breakdown and frequently a net loss of nitrogen from muscle. The reasons for the enhanced net rate of protein turnover have been summarized elsewhere.[106] They include (1) providing amino acids for protein synthesis required for repair processes and by cells of the immune system, (2) providing amino acids for gluconeogenesis in order to supply glucose as an obligatory energy substrate required for cells involved in repair and the immune system, and (3) providing branched-chain amino acids to serve as an additional energy source. Studies on protein turnover and gluconeogenesis in the ill term or preterm neonate have not been conducted. All studies done so far and referred to in this chapter have been conducted in relatively stable neonates.

Further studies on ill neonates are needed to observe if they might benefit from more liberal intake of protein or one or more essential amino acids than is regarded currently as necessary or even safe in the stable, healthy neonate.

Metabolic Rate and Illness

Various studies in the adult have investigated the effect of illness, injury, or burns on the metabolic rate. The response usually consists of a brief "ebb" phase, during which the metabolic rate is decreased, followed by a "flow" phase, during which the metabolic rate is increased.[141–143] A patient may go through different "ebb" and "flow" phases depending on the severity of the illness. During the flow phase there is increased protein breakdown, recycling of glucose, and recycling of fatty acids and triglycerides. Adequate nutritional support tends to reduce the increased substrate cycles but cannot normalize them.

Studies on the effect of illness on the metabolic rate of the neonate are incomplete. No studies have investigated the effect of infection (e.g., sepsis, pneumonia) on metabolic rate. A few studies have addressed the effect of respiratory distress on metabolic rate. Levison and Swyer[144] measured oxygen consumption in infants with respiratory distress syndrome (RDS). They found oxygen consumption below normal on the first day of life, gradually increasing to levels above normal on the fourth day of life, and returning to values found in the non–respiratory-stressed neonate around day 5 or 6. Richardson et al.[145] observed oxygen consumption in neonates with RDS to be above normal on the first day of life, gradually returning to normal in the days thereafter. Recent studies show conflicting results. Two studies found that the oxygen consumption during the first days of life was positively related to the severity of respiratory problems.[146,147] Forsyth and Crighton[59] observed a lower oxygen consumption during the first days of life in ventilated as compared to nonventilated infants. Hazan et al.[148] could not demonstrate an effect of decreasing the severity of respiratory problems through the administration of surfactant on oxygen consumptiom. Taking all studies together, there is a trend that the oxygen consumption is higher in the ventilated compared to the nonventilated neonate; however, this trend is not significant.[149]

The effect of chronic respiratory problems on metabolic rate has been studied. Weinstein and Oh[150] showed that neonates with bronchopulmonary dysplasia (BPD) have a 25% higher oxygen consumption than do control neonates of the same weight and age. Yeh et al.[151] found a higher metabolic rate in neonates with BPD compared to controls. The activity score of the BPD neonates tended to be higher than that of the controls.

Yunis and Oh[152] studied the effect of a glucose load 4 and 12 mg·g^{-1}min^{-1} on oxygen consumption and carbon dioxide production in the neonate with BPD after a 9-hour fast. This glucose load did not have an effect on either parameter in the control neonate. In neonates with BPD, oxygen consumption and carbon dioxide production increased significantly. In control neonates the RQ rose from 0.88 ± 0.15 to 0.92 ± 0.20 during the glucose infusion, probably owing to higher glucose oxidation. The RQ in the BPD neonate did not change—0.77 ± 0.15 at a glucose intake of 4 mg·kg^{-1}min^{-1} and 0.76 ± 0.15 at 12 g·kg^{-1}min^{-1}—surprisingly indicating that there was no increase in glucose oxidation during the glucose infusion in the BPD neonate. The large standard deviation in the RQ in both groups is also surprising, as it indicates that some neonates in the BPD group had an RQ of less than 0.7, which is physiologically impossible.

The results of these studies on the oxygen consumption of the neonate with BPD have been challenged.[153] All studies mentioned above were conducted using open circuit calorimeters, where the oxygen consumption was calculated from the difference in oxygen concentration between the incubator air and the ventilated hood. This difference in oxygen concentration is usually 0.2% to 0.4%. A very stable oxygen concentration in the incubator is needed, which is almost impossible to achieve when supplemental oxygen is added into the incubator. The higher oxygen consumption observed in the BPD neonate might be caused, at least partially, by measurement errors attributed to the instability of the enriched oxygen concentration in the incubator during calorimetry. The measurement of the carbon dioxide is not influenced by supplemental oxygen. Yunis and Oh[152] did not find a difference in carbon dioxide excretion between BPD and control neonates.

Another question that can be raised is whether the increased respiratory work, sometimes observed clinically in the BPD neonate, has a detectable effect on oxygen consumption. The energy cost of breathing is a small contribution to the total metabolic rate. Even a 100% increase in energy cost of breathing is difficult to detect by calorimetry. It is unlikely that the increase in metabolic rate found in the BPD neonate is due to an increased energy consumption of breathing. Two other explanations, in addition to the potential higher oxygen consumption, are given for the lower weight gain observed in infants with BPD. De Regnier et al.[154] attributed the lower growth to a lower energy and protein intake in the infant developing BPD during the initial phase of their illness. They observed that, once the infant received an energy and protein intake comparable to that of the non-BPD infant, growth rate was also comparable. Boehm et al.[155] found lower intraduodenal levels of lipase, trypsine, and bile acids in the infant who then went on to develop BPD. The resulting lower protein and fat intake might explain the growth failure, but a direct relationship between malabsorption and the development of BPD is unlikely.[155] Malnutrition can cause reduced production and release of surfactant as well as reduced capacity to repair damaged cellular and extracellular components. The respiratory drive can be reduced during protein and calorie malnutrition resulting in failure to wean from the ventilator and in muscle fatigue with apnea.[156] Almost all studies regarding the energy balance have been conducted in the relatively healthy neonate, although many neonates cared for in a neonatal intensive care nursery have significant problems. It is probably not justified to extrapolate results from the healthy to the sick neonate. To better care for the ill, immature neonate, more studies are necessary.

Effect of Activity on Metabolic Rate

Activity is a major contributor of energy expenditure in the adult. The preterm neonate hardly uses any energy for activity when he/she is lying quietly in the incubator or under a radiant warmer. The energy used for activity cannot be measured directly but is estimated from the difference between the total metabolic rate and the resting metabolic rate. This difference includes specific dynamic action, which might obscure the energy used for activity. Brooke et al.[117] estimated that activity increased the metabolic rate 23% to 34% above resting levels in the preterm neonate, comparable to the values derived by Rubecz and Mestyan,[157] who found 13 kcal·kg^{-1}day^{-1}, or approximately 18% of the energy intake.

A much lower energy expenditure for activity in the preterm neonate was found by others.[8,26,158,159] We calculated the energy for activity to be 7.4 kcal·kg^{-1}day^{-1}, or 6% of the energy intake.[8] Freymond et al.[26] found 3.6 kcal·kg^{-1}day^{-1}, or 5.3% of the metabolic rate. The preterm neonates can increase their metabolic rate during activity by 36% maximally, compared to 72% in the term neonates and 400% to 500% in adults.[159] An increase in energy used for activity with increasing postnatal age was observed according to clinical experience. In the studies performed in 1975 to 1980, neonates with more advanced postnatal and postconceptual age who were more active were studied.[117,157] The preterm neonates spend most of their time sleeping, 70% compared to 48% in the term neonates.[117] In adults, two distinct sleeping patterns can be defined: rapid eye movement (REM) and non-REM sleep. REM sleep is characterized as active sleep and non-REM as quiet sleep. Scoring the sleep states in the neonate may be based on clinical observations or on the combination of clinical observations and electroencephalographic (EEG) and electrooculographic (EOG) patterns. Stabell et al.[160] found no difference between quiet and active sleep. Schulze et al.[23] reported a higher oxygen consumption during REM sleep. Stothers and Warner[30] found significantly higher oxygen consumption during REM sleep when preceded by non-REM sleep but not in the reversed sequence. Dane et al.[28] observed a higher oxygen consumption during REM sleep with a threefold increase in variability.

It can be concluded that both activity and sleep state affect the metabolic rate in the preterm neonate; however, the effect is much lower than in the adult.

Intrauterine Growth Retardation and Metabolic Rate

Various studies have reported a higher metabolic rate in SGA neonates than in their AGA counterparts, when expressed per kilogram body weight.[71,129,161,162] Metabolic rate is also higher when it is expressed per lean body mass.[162] The higher metabolic rate in the SGA neonate cannot be explained only by differences in body composition (e.g., lower body fat and higher active-lean tissues). We did not find a difference between the protein turnover of AGA versus SGA neonates.[163] No definitive explanation for the higher energy metabolism in the SGA neonate can be given.

Abdulrazzaq and Brooke[164] explained the differences in metabolic rate by the increased head size in the SGA neonates. Although metabolic rate is significantly different between the SGA and AGA neonates when expressed per kilogram body weight, it is not different when expressed per head circumference or estimated brain weight. The higher metabolic rate in the SGA neonate has been used to estimate the oxygen consumption of the brain.[161]

Energy Losses in Stools and Urine

Part of the energy provided by the enteral route is subsequently lost via the feces. Another part of the energy intake is lost with nitrogen-containing substances in the urine. Factors affecting the intestinal absorption of dietary fats are the structure of the triacylglycerols, chain length and degree of saturation of the fatty acids, conditions at the site of lipolysis, availability of bile acids, lipolytic enzymes, maturity of the digestive system, and calcium and magnesium content of the feeding. The digestive tract is not fully developed in the preterm neonate, and the supply of bile acids may be inadequate. This point could be important, as the preterm formula contains up to 50% of its calories as fat. Early studies showed absorption of butterfat in the preterm neonate to be 45% to 60%.[165,166] Later, the absorption of unsaturated fatty acids was found to be approximately 80% and the absorption of MCT to be 95% to 100%.[167,168] Preterm formula was changed to have up to 50% of its fat as MCT in order to enhance fat absorption. Nitrogen retention was higher in one study when all fat was given as MCT.[169] Sulkers et al.[71] observed no difference in nitrogen absorption between infants receiving either 5% or 40% of fatty acids as MCT. Huston et al.[170] provided further evidence that the fat absorption of preterm neonates is dependent on chain length and degree of unsaturation. The absorption of unsaturated long-chain fatty acids (LCT) (C18-2) was 94.5%, whereas the absorption of C16-0 was only 74%. Chappell et al.[169] showed that the absorption might be dependent on other factors as well: fatty acids of equal length and saturation are better absorbed when given with the mother's own milk compared with preterm formula. An explanation for this finding is the stereoisomeric structure of triglycerides in human milk versus formula. Palmitic acid is mainly esterified to the Sn-2 position in human milk, while in formula it is bound to the outer positions of the glycerol molecule, the Sn-1 and Sn-3 positions. Pancreatic lipase mainly splits the fatty acid from the Sn-1 and Sn-3 positions. In human milk, the result is free unsaturated fatty acids from the Sn-1 and Sn-3 positions with a monoglyceride containing palmitic acid. The unsaturated fatty acids as well as the monoglyceride are well absorbed. In formulas the result of the splicing is free palmitic acid and a monoglyceride with an unsaturated fatty acid. The monoglyceride is well absorbed, the palmitic acid less well. A formula in which the palmitic acid is esterified on the Sn-2 position shows a higher fat absorption compared to a conventional formula.[171,172] Huston et al.[170] showed only a minor difference in fat absorption between neonates fed an MCT and those fed an LCT formula: 91% ± 6% versus 86% ± 4% resorption. They observed no effect of MCT on the absorption of calcium, phosphorus, or nitrogen. Hamosh et al.[173] were unable to show a difference between the absorption of MCT versus LCT in the preterm neonate. They found an absorption of 85% with MCT compared with 83% with an LCT formula. There is a clear relationship between fat and calcium excretion in the feces, in particular for palmitic acid. Palmitic acid forms soaps with calcium, causing less calcium and palmitic absorption.

Effects of Energy Intake on Nitrogen Balance

It has been known for years that the administration of energy positively influences nitrogen balance in the adult as well as in the neonate.[174] The protein-sparing effect of fat is thought to be secondary to the energy provided by fat, whereas the protein-sparing effect of carbohydrate is thought to be secondary to the reduction of gluconeogenesis. Baker et al.[175] showed in the adult that glucose and fat equally promote nitrogen retention. Pineault et al.[176] showed in the marginally preterm neonate of 34 to 36 weeks that an energy intake of 60 to 80 kcal·kg^{-1}day^{-1}, provided mainly as either glucose or fat, does not affect protein balance. Similar results were obtained by Heird et al.[177] Pencharz et al.[178] studied the effect of differences in the composition of energy intake on nitrogen balance and protein turnover. Administration of a high-carbohydrate or a high-fat solution intravenously at an energy intake of 80 to 90 kcal.kg^{-1}day^{-1} did not affect nitrogen balance or protein turnover. Neither is the protein balance affected when the energy intake is increased from 60 to 80 kcal.kg^{-1}d^{-1} by adding lipids.[138] That nitrogen retention increased when both protein and energy intake increased was shown also by De Curtis and Brooke.[179] They observed no effect of energy retention on the correlation between nitrogen intake and nitrogen retention in the preterm neonate fed banked human milk, probably because of a low nitrogen intake.

The protein-sparing effect of energy seems not to take place when the protein intake is low in relation to energy intake. From studies done in the orally fed preterm neonate with different energy and protein intakes (Table 44.2), it can be concluded that increasing the energy intake from 100 to 120 kcal·kg^{-1}day^{-1} does not influence protein retention at a constant level of protein intake. Protein retention, at that level of energy intake, is dependent only on protein intake. In one of the studies from the group from Columbia University, there was no effect on nitrogen retention when the energy intake was increased from 115 to 149 kcal·kg^{-1}day^{-1} and the protein intake was kept constant at 3.6 to 3.5 g·kg^{-1}day^{-1}.[78] This result is in contrast to results from a later study from the same group.[79] They concluded that weight gain is dependent on both energy and protein intake, as given by the following formula:[180]

$$\text{Weight gain} = 3.6\, protein_{in} + 0.095\, energy_{in} - 0.0047\, birth\ weight + 1.7\ (r = .8)$$

From the data in Table 44.2 the following multiple regression equation was constructed:

$$\text{Weight gain} = 0.12 * metabolizable\ energy_{in} + 1.9 * protein_{in} - 2.3\ (p < .00005;\ r = .75)$$

The studies summarized in Table 44.2 confirm that up to a protein intake of 3.6 g·kg^{-1}day^{-1} the nitrogen retention is dependent only on protein intake, provided the energy intake is more than 120 kcal·kg^{-1}day^{-1}.[180] When the protein/energy ratio is more than 3 g 100 kcal^{-1}, the energy might become the limiting factor in nitrogen retention and growth. There is a limit to the protein intake. A protein intake of more than 4 g·kg^{-1}day^{-1} is associated with high levels of amino acids and uremia. A protein intake of more than approximately 3.5 g·kg^{-1}day^{-1} does not seem advisable.

Nitrogen balance is influenced by protein intake not only at high levels of energy intake but at low levels of energy intake. Van Lingen et al.[139] have shown in the preterm neonate on the third or fourth day of life that the administration of an amino acid solution, 2.3 g·kg^{-1}day^{-1}, at an energy intake of 60 kcal·kg^{-1}day^{-1}, almost equal to the metabolic rate increases nitrogen retention and protein synthesis, but protein breakdown is not affected.

Effects of Protein and Energy Intake on Growth and Composition of Weight Gain in the Preterm Neonate

Various indicators are used to estimate growth in the neonate. The most widely used is weight gain, as it can be measured accurately and repeatedly. It is a rather poor estimate of growth, though, owing to the high water content of the preterm neonate. A small change in the percentage of water content of the body has a major effect on the measurement of weight gain. Weight gain should be measured over periods of at least 1 week, and the neonate should have a constant ratio of water versus solids. There can be a different composition of new tissue at equal weight gain. Measurement of weight gain should be combined with measurement of body composition. All studies conducted so far have used indirect measurements of the composition of weight gain. Length and head circumference are considered a reflection of increase in protein content of the body. Because the increase in the two parameters in small, it is difficult to detect any significant difference among small groups of neonates. Weight gain, as shown in the previous section, is dependent on both energy and protein retention (Figure 44.9). Some studies have suggested a correlation between gain in length and head circumference,[181] but no study showed a significant correlation. Taking all studies on orally fed, growing preterm neonates, as summarized in Table 44.2, a significant correlation between protein retention and gain in length can be found (Figure 44.10). No correlation between gain in head circumference and protein intake or retention is present. No correlation could be found between metabolizable energy intake and gain in length or head circumference.

The composition of weight gain of the preterm neonate and the fat content of new tissue can be manipulated by the amount of energy provided to the neonate. The percentage of protein per gram of new tissue is constant at different levels of protein intake and seems not to be

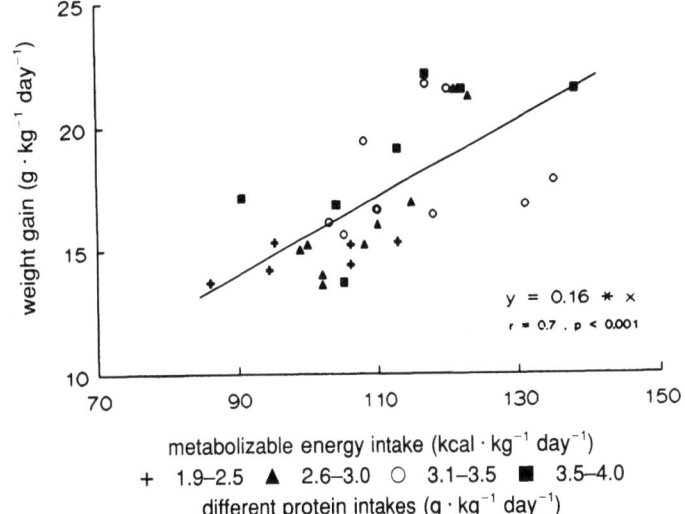

FIGURE 44.9. Relation between weight gain and metabolizable energy intake in orally fed preterm neonates. Data are from Table 44.2.

influenced by either protein or energy intake. The protein content per gram of new tissue of the fetus during the period of 26 to 36 weeks' gestation is 12% to 13%.[55] All studies in the orally fed preterm neonate show an almost equal percentage of protein, regardless of protein and energy intake (Table 44.2). The fat content of new tissue is influenced by the amount of energy given to the preterm neonate. The fat content per gram of new tissue of the fetus increases from approximately 0.05 g at 26 weeks to 0.2 g at 36 weeks. The fat content calculated from the studies shown in Table 44.2 ranges from 0.14 to 0.34 g/g weight gain, the higher fat content being correlated to the higher energy intake (Figure 44.11). The fat content per gram of new tissue is not equal to the intrauterine accretion. Decreasing the energy intake to around 100 kcal·kg⁻¹day⁻¹ might decrease the fat content per gram of weight gain. Weight gain is lower at a low energy intake. It is questionable if it is possible to obtain a weight gain equivalent to the intrauterine accretion (15–17 g·kg⁻¹day⁻¹) while keeping the fat content at intrauterine accretion rates.

No study has shown substantial evidence that a higher fat content per gram of new tissue is harmful to the preterm neonate either during the neonatal period or at follow-up. De Gamarra et al.[181] followed preterm infants until 6 months of age who were fed 118 ± 11 kcal·k⁻¹ day⁻¹ during the neonatal period and showed the percentage of fat per gram of weight gain to be 21% during that period. There was no indication of a higher fat content at 6 months compared to the normal term neonate, indicating that despite substantial fat accretion during the perinatal period it did not have lasting effects on body composition. It is doubtful if an increased fat content during the neonatal period found in the preterm neonate is harmful. It might even have advantages regarding the thermoregulation of the neonate (see Chapter 45). Another important aspect is that higher weight gain might reduce the hospital stay and costs.

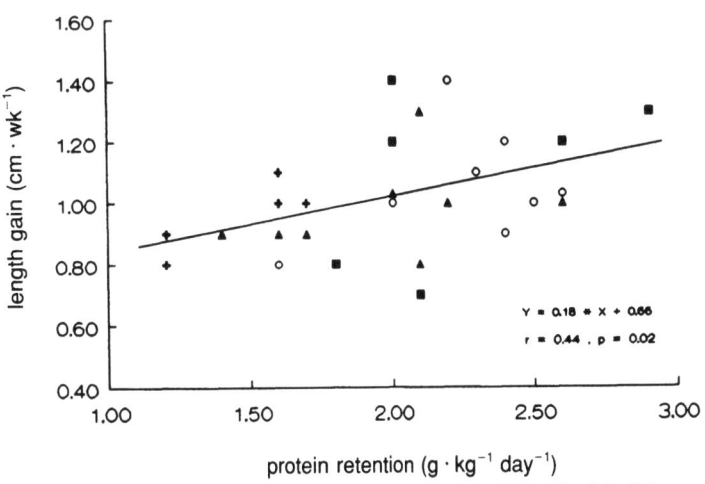

FIGURE 44.10. Relation between length gain and protein retention in orally fed preterm neonates. Data are from Table 44.2.

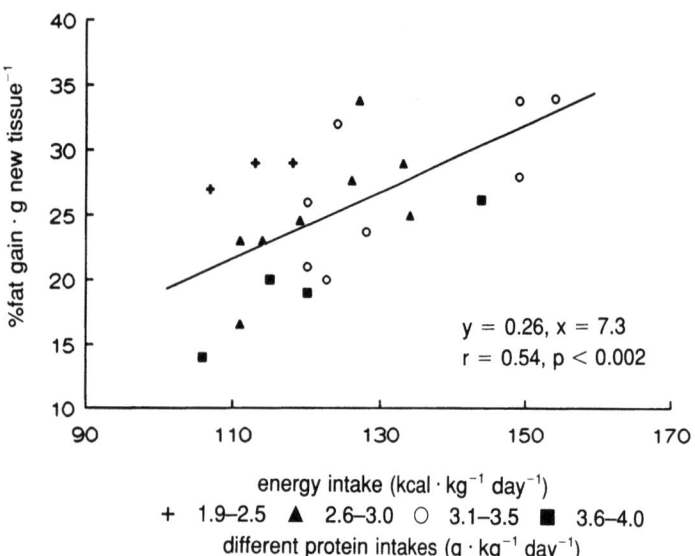

FIGURE 44.11. Relation between percent fat gain per gram of new tissue and energy intake in orally fed preterm neonates. Data are from Table 30.2.

Optimal Energy and Protein Intake of the Preterm Neonate

The energy and protein intake that can be advised for the preterm neonate is an important consideration. To address this point, one should first define the goal of the nutritional management. The Committee on Nutrition of the American Academy of Pediatrics issued the following statements in 1977 and in 1985 on the feeding of the low-birth weight neonate: "The goal of feeding regimens for low birth weight infant is to obtain a prompt postnatal resumption of growth to a rate approximating intrauterine growth because this is believed to provide the best possible conditions for subsequent normal development."[120,182] A few remarks can be made regarding this statement. Despite numerous studies, it has not been unequivocally shown that growth approximating the intrauterine growth provides the best condition for normal development. Most studies have evaluated growth only during the neonatal period. Only a few studies have evaluated the effect of nutrition during the neonatal period on subsequent neurodevelopmental outcome.

The optimal nutrition should be based not only on studies of growth and body composition during the neonatal period but perhaps mainly on the later outcome of these neonates. Neurodevelopmental outcome is one of the parameters that should be studied. Also, the tendency to be overweight and have higher cholesterol levels and more atherosclerosis that is found in adults who were born with low birth weight needs further follow-up.[183] Studies in animals have shown that nutrition during a critical period of development can have long-lasting effects. In baboons Lewis et al.[184] showed that the type of feeding during the first 4 months of life influences cholesterol turnover and the tendency to atherosclerosis in later life. A multicenter study in Finland showed that the cholesterol concentration of infants and children is correlated with the amount and quality of fat consumed during early life.[185] Some data on the effect of the type of nutrition on the developmental outcome of the preterm neonate are emerging from a prospective multicenter trial in England.[186-188] The first data of this study indicate that the neonate fed a preterm formula as the sole diet or as a supplement to mother's milk has a significant higher motor and developmental quotient at 9 and 18 months compared with the neonate fed a term formula or donor breast milk as a sole diet or supplement. These data are important, not only for defining the optimal energy and protein intake of the low birth weight neonate, but also because they show that nutrition of the preterm neonate can have lasting effects on the subsequent developmental outcome. The last trimester of the normal pregnancy can be regarded as a critical period for brain development that is influenced by the nutrition given during that period. So long as more studies on the long-term effect of the nutrition in the neonatal period on developmental outcome and other parameters as body composition are lacking, the definition of the optimal nutrition must be based on short-term studies in the preterm neonate.

A number of conclusions can be drawn from the data discussed:

1. A protein intake of less than $2.25\,g \cdot kg^{-1} day^{-1}$ is inadequate to promote normal growth. It has been shown to be insufficient to maintain plasma albumin and transthyretin concentrations.[78,177] Weight gain of up to $22\,g \cdot kg^{-1} day^{-1}$ is observed with a protein intake of 2.5 to $4.0\,g \cdot kg^{-1} day^{-1}$.

2. The combination of a high protein intake and high energy intake results in increased nitrogen retention.

3. Gain in length is influenced positively by protein retention.

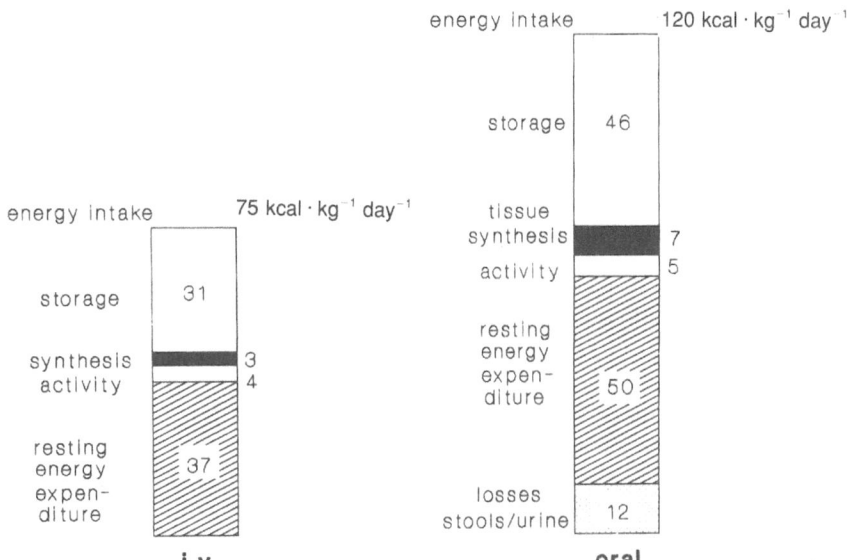

FIGURE 44.12. Estimated energy balance in intravenous and orally fed preterm neonates constructed from the data of various studies.[8,20,87,131]

4. The protein content per gram of weight gain is around $0.12 \, g \cdot g^{-1}$ weight gain^{-1} and is not influenced by protein intake.

5. Increasing the metabolizable energy intake above $120 \, kcal \cdot kg^{-1} day^{-1}$ results primarily in increased fat content per gram of weight gain without improving the weight gain.

6. A metabolizable energy intake of approximately $100 \, kcal \cdot kg^{-1} day^{-1}$ at a minimum is needed to achieve a weight gain comparable to the intrauterine accretion.

7. The fat content per gram of weight gain is higher than the intrauterine accretion at the energy intake needed to achieve the intrauterine weight gain. Achieving a weight gain comparable to the intrauterine accretion without a higher fat content per gram of new tissue might be impossible.

It is important to realize that all studies have been performed in the relatively healthy, stable, growing preterm neonate with a birth weight appropriate for gestational age and usually above 1000 g. It is impossible to extrapolate these conclusions to other groups of preterm neonates: unstable, ill, SGA, or tiny neonates with a birth weight of around 750 g or less. It is likely that the requirements of these neonates are higher compared to their stable, more mature counterparts (see Chapter 51).

Energy Balance

Combining the data from several studies, it is possible to construct an energy balance of the growing, stable preterm neonate fed 120 to $130 \, kcal \cdot kg^{-1} day^{-1}$ and protein at approximately $3 \, g \cdot kg^{-1} day^{-1}$. The preterm infant fed 120 to $135 \, kcal \cdot kg^{-1} day^{-1}$ uses $50 \, kcal \cdot kg^{-1} day^{-1}$ or 42% of the energy intake for maintenance, $5 \, kcal \cdot kg^{-1} day^{-1}$ or 4% for activity, $7 \, kcal \cdot kg^{-1} day^{-1}$ or 6% for tissue synthesis, and $46 \, kcal \cdot kg^{-1} day^{-1}$ or 38% for the components of new tissue (Figure 44.12). Approximately 10% of the energy intake is lost with feces and urine. The energy balance of the neonate fed intravenously an energy intake of $75 \, kcal \cdot kg^{-1} day^{-1}$ is shown in Figure 44.12. The metabolic rate and energy for growth is lower in these neonates, probably because of the lower energy intake. No energy is needed in this model for thermoregulation. When extra energy is needed for thermoregulation, it decreases the energy available for growth, as is discussed in Chapter 45.

References

1. Lavoisier AL, Laplace PS, Memoire sur la chaleur. Mem Math Phys Acad Sei 1780. Cited by Hull D, Smales ORC. In: Sinclair JC, ed. Temperature regulation and energy metabolism in the newborn. Orlando: Grune & Stratton, 1978:129–156.
2. Richet C. La chaleur animale. Bibliotheque Scientifique Internationale. Paris: Alcan, 1895.
3. Winslow CEA, Herrington LP, Gagge AP. Physiological reactions of the human body to varying environmental temperatures. Am J Physiol 1937;120:1–22.
4. Spinnler G, Jequier E, Favre R, et al. Human calorimeter with a new type of gradient layer. J Appl Physiol 1973;35:158–165.
5. Day R, Hardy JD. Respiratory metabolism in infancy and in childhood. XXVI. A calorimeter for measuring the heat loss of premature infants. Am J Dis Child 1942;63:1086–1095.
6. Ryser G, Jequier E. Study by direct calorimetry of thermal balance on the first day of life. Eur J Clin Invest 1972;2:176–187.
7. Dane HJ, Holland WPJ, Sauer PJJ, et al. A calorimetric system for metabolic studies of newborn infants. Clin Phys Physiol Meas 1985;6:36–46.

8. Sauer PJJ, Dane HJ, Visser HKA. Longitudinal studies on metabolic rate, heat loss, and energy cost of growth in low birth weight infants. Pediatr Res 1984;18:254–259.
9. Meis SJ, Dove EL, Bell EF, et al. A gradient-layer calorimeter for measurement of energy expenditure of infants. Am J Physiol 1994;266:1052–1060.
10. Silverman WA, Agate FJ Jr. Variation in cold resistance among small newborn infants. Biol Neonate 1964;6:113–127.
11. Webb P, Annis JF, Troutman SJ Jr. Human calorimetry with a water-cooled garment. J Appl Physiol 1972;32:412–418.
12. Webb P, Annis JF, Troutman SJ Jr. Energy balance in man measured by direct and indirect calorimetry. Am J Clin Nutr 1980;33:1287–1298.
13. Frayn KN. Calculation of substrate oxidation rates in vivo from gaseous exchange. J Appl Physiol 1983;55:628–634.
14. Ferrannini E. The theoretical bases of indirect calorimetry: a review. Metabolism 1988;37:287–301.
15. Ella M, Livesey G. Theory and validity of indirect calorimetry during net lipid synthesis. Am J Clin Nutr 1988;47:591–607.
16. Simonson DC, DeFronzo RA. Indirect calorimetry: methodological and interpretative problems. Am J Physiol 1990;258:E399–E412.
17. Lusk G. Analysis of the oxidation of carbohydrate and fat. J Biol Chem 1924;54:41–42.
18. Bursztein S, Saphar P, Singer P, et al. A mathematical analysis of indirect calorimetry measurements in acutely ill patients. Am J Clin Nutr 1989;50:227–230.
19. Sauer PJJ, Van Aerde J, Pencharz P, et al. Glucose oxidation rates in newborn infants measured with indirect calorimetry and U-^{13}C-glucose. Clin Sci 1986;70:587–593.
20. Van Aerde JEE, Sauer PJJ, Pencharz PB, et al. Effect of replacing glucose with lipid on the energy metabolism of newborn infants. Clin Sci 1989;76:581–588.
21. Glamour TS, McCullough AJ, Sauer PJJ, et al. Quantification of carbohydrate oxidation by respiratory gas exchange and isotopic tracers. Am J Physiol 1995;268:E789–E796.
22. Abdulrazzaq YM, Brooke OG. Respiratory metabolism in preterm infants; the measurement of oxygen consumption during prolonged periods. Pediatr Res 1984;18:928–931.
23. Schulze K, Kairam R, Stefanski M, et al. Spontaneous variability in minute ventilation oxygen consumption and heart rate of low birth weight infants. Pediatr Res 1981;15:1111–1116.
24. Marks KH, Nardis EE, Derr JA. Day-to-day energy expenditure variability in low birth weight neonates. Pediatr Res 1987;21:66–71.
25. Roberts SB, Murgatroyd PR, Crisp JA. Long-term variation in oxygen consumption rate in preterm infants. Biol Neonate 1987;52:1–8.
26. Freymond D, Schutz Y, Decombaz J, et al. Energy balance, physical activity, and thermogenic effect of feeding in premature infants. Pediatr Res 1986;20:638–645.
27. Bligh J, Johnson KG. Glossary of terms for thermal physiology. J Appl Physiol 1973;35:941–961.
28. Dane HJ, Sauer PJJ, Visser HKA. Oxygen consumption and CO_2 production of low-birth-weight infants in two sleep states. Biol Neonate 1985;47:205–210.
29. Hey EN. The relation between environmental temperature and oxygen consumption in the newborn baby. J Physiol (Lond) 1969;200:589–603.
30. Stothers JK, Warner RM. Oxygen consumption and neonatal sleep states. J Physiol (Lond) 1978;278:435–440.
31. Chessex P, Reichman BL, Verellen GJE, et al. Relation between heart rate and energy expenditure in the newborn. Pediatr Res 1981;15:1071–1082.
32. Lifson N, Gordon GB, McClintock R. Measurement of total carbon dioxide production by means of $D_2^{18}O$. J Appl Physiol 1955;7:704–710.
33. Lifson N, Little WS, Levitt DG, et al. $D_2^{18}O$ method for CO_2 output in small mammals and economic feasibility in man. J Appl Physiol 1975;39(4):657–664.
34. Schoeller DA. Energy expenditures from doubly labeled water: some fundamental considerations in humans. Am J Clin Nutr 1983;38:999–1005.
35. Schoeller DA, Webb P. Five-day comparison of the doubly labeled water method with respiratory gas exchange. Am J Clin Nutr 1984;40:153–158.
36. Klein PD, James WPT, Wong WW, et al. Calorimetric validation of the doubly-labelled water method for determination of energy expenditure in man. Hum Nutr Clin Nutr 1984;38C:95–106.
37. Jones PJH, Winthrop AL, Schoeller DA, et al. Validation of doubly labeled water for assessing energy expenditure in infants. Pediatr Res 1987;21:242–246.
38. Roberts SB, Coward WA, Schlingenseipen KH, et al. Comparison of the doubly labeled water ($^2H_2^{18}O$) method with indirect calorimetry and a nutrient-balance study for simultaneous determination of energy expenditure, water intake and metabolizable energy intake in preterm infants. Am J Clin Nutr 1986;44:315–322.
39. Jones PJH, Winthrop AL, Schoeller DA, et al. Evaluation of doubly labeled water for measuring energy expenditure during changing nutrition. Am J Clin Nutr 1988;47:799–804.
40. Pullicino E, Coward A, Elia M. Total energy expenditure in intravenously fed patients measured by the doubly labeled water technique. Metabolism 1993;42:58–64.
41. Westerterp KR, Lafeber HN, Sulkers EJ, et al. Comparison of short term indirect calorimetry and doubly labelled water method for the assessment of energy expenditure in preterm infants. Biol Neonate 1991;60:75–82.
42. Pittet PH, Gygax PH, Jequier E. Thermic effect of glucose and amino acids in man studied by direct and indirect calorimetry. Br J Nutr 1974;31:343–349.
43. Bell AW, Battaglia FC, Meschia G. Relation between metabolic rate and body size in the ovine fetus. J Nutr 1987;117:1181–1186.
44. Bell AW, Kennaugh JM, Battaglia FC, et al. Metabolic and circulatory studies of fetal lamb at midgestation. Am J Physiol 1986;250:E538–544.
45. Hay WW Jr. Fetal requirements and placental transfer of nitrogenous compounds. In: Polin RA, Fow WW, eds. Fetal and neontal physiology. Philadelphia: WB Saunders, 1992:441.
46. Hay WW Jr, DiGiacomo JE, Meznarich HK, et al. Effects of glucose and insulin on fetal glucose oxidation and oxygen consumption. Am J Physiol 1989;256:E704–713.

47. Romney SL, Reid DE, Metcalfe J, et al. Oxygen utilization by the human fetus in utero. Am J Obstet Gynecol 1955;70:791–799.
48. Sparks JW, Girard JR, Battaglia FC. An estimate of the caloric requirements of the human fetus. Biol Neonate 1980;38:113–119.
49. Bonds DR, Crosby LO, Cheek TG, et al. Estimation of human fetal-placental unit metabolic rate by application of the Bohr principle. J Dev Physiol 1986;8:49–54.
50. Bozetti P, Buscaglia M, Cetin I, et al. Respiratory gases, acid-base balance and lactate concentrations of the midterm human fetus. Biol Neonate 1987;51:188–197.
51. Economides DL, Nicolaides KH. Blood glucose and oxygen tension levels in small-for-gestational-age fetuses. Am J Obstet Gynecol 1989;160:385–389.
52. Huikeshoven FJ, Hope ID, Power GG, et al. Mathematical model of fetal circulation and oxygen delivery. Am J Physiol 1985;249:192–202.
53. Durnin JVGA, McKillop FM, Grant S, et al. Energy requirements of pregnancy in Scotland. Lancet 1987;2:897–900.
54. Widdowson EM. Changes in body proportions and composition during growth. In: Davis JA, Dobbing J, eds. Scientific foundation of paediatrics. London: Heineman, 1974:153–163.
55. Ziegler EE, O'Donnell A, Nelson SE, Fomon SJ. Body composition of the reference fetus. Growth 1976;40:329–341.
56. Heim T. Energy and lipid requirements of the fetus and the preterm infant. J Pediatr Gastroenterol Nutr 1983;2 (suppl 1):S16–S41.
57. Thomson MA, Bucolo S, Quirk P, et al. Measured versus predicted resting energy expenditure in infants: a need for reappraisal. J Pediatr 1995;126:21–27.
58. Scopes JW, Ahmed I. Minimal rates of oxygen consumption in sick and premature newborn infants. Arch Dis Child 1966;41:407–416.
59. Forsyth JS, Crighton A. Low birth weight infants and total parenteral nutrition immediately after birth. I. Energy expenditure and respiratory quotient of ventilated and non-ventilated infants. Arch Dis Child Fetal Neonatal Ed 1995;73:F4–7.
60. Hey EN. The relation between environmental temperature and oxygen consumption in the newborn baby. J Physiol (Lond) 1969;200:589–603.
61. Gentz J, Kellum M, Persson B. The effect of feeding on oxygen consumption, RQ and plasma levels of glucose, FFA and D-hydroxybutyrate in newborn infants of diabetic mothers and small-for-gestational age infants. Acta Paediatr Scand 1976;65:445–454.
62. Chessex P, Reichman BL, Verellen GJE, et al. Influence of postnatal age, energy intake, and weight gain on energy metabolism in the very low-birth-weight infant. J Pediatr 1981;99:761–766.
63. Gudinchet F, Schutz Y, Micheli JL, et al. Metabolic cost of growth in very low-birth-weight infants. Pediatr Res 1982;16:1025–1030.
64. van de Wagen A, Okken A, Zweens J, et al. Body composition at birth of growth-retarded newborn infants demonstrating catch-up growth in the first year of life. Biol Neonate 1986;49:121–125.
65. Bauer K, Cowett RM, Howard GM, et al. Effect of intrauterine growth retardation on postnatal weight change in preterm infants. J Pediatr 1993;123:301–306.
66. Micheli JL, Pfister R, Junod, et al. Water, energy and early postnatal growth in preterm infants. Acta Paediatr Suppl 1994;405:35–42.
67. Bhakoo ON, Scopes JW. Minimal rates of oxygen consumption in small-for-dates babies during the first week of life. Arch Dis Child 1974;49:583–585.
68. Horton ES. Introduction: an overview of the assessment and regulation of energy balance in humans. Am J Clin Nutr 1983;38:972–977.
69. Brooke OG. Energy balance and metabolic rate in preterm infants fed with standard and high-energy formulas. Br J Nutr 1980;44:13–23.
70. Whyte RK, Campbell D, Stanhope R, et al. Energy balance in low birth weight infants fed formula of high or low medium chain triglyceride content. J Pediatr 1986;108:964–971.
71. Sulkers EJ, Lafeber HN, Leunisse C, et al. Nitrogen and fat deposition in preterm infants fed a formula with 5 or 40% medium-chain triglycerides (MCT). J Pediatr Gastroenterol Nutr 1992;15:42–47.
72. Van Aerde J. Intravenous nutritional energy support and macronutrient utilization in the neonate. Acta Biomed Lovaniensia 1990;22:94–102.
73. Van Aerde J, Sauer PJJ, Pencharz PB, et al. Metabolic consequences of increasing energy intake by adding lipid to parenteral nutrition in full-term infants. Am J Clin Nutr 1994;59:659–662.
74. Chessex P, Belanger S, Piedboeuf B, et al. Influence of energy substrates on respiratory gas exchange during conventional mechanical ventilation of preterm infants. J Pediatr 1995;126:619–624.
75. Forsyth JS, Murdock N, Crighton A. Low birthweight infants and total parenteral nutrition immediately after birth. III. Randomised study of energy substrate utilisation, nitrogen balance, and carbon dioxide production. Arch Dis Child Fetal Neonatal Ed 1995;73:F13–16.
76. Salas-Salvado J, Molina J, Figueras J, et al. Effect of the quality of infused energy on substrate utilization in the newborn receiving total parenteral nutrition. Pediatr Res 1993;33:112–117.
77. Van Aerde J. Acute respiratory failure and bronchopulmonary dysplasia. In: Hay W, ed. Neonatal nutrition and metabolism. St. Louis: Mosby-Yearbook, 1991:476–506.
78. Kashyap S, Forsyth M, Zucker C, et al. Effects of varying protein and energy intakes on growth and metabolic response in low birth weight infants. J Pediatr 1986;108:955–963.
79. Kashyap S, Schulze KF, Forsyth M, et al. Growth nutrient retention, and metabolic response in low birth weight infants fed varying intakes of protein and energy. J Pediatr 1988;113:713–721.
80. Schulze K, Stefanski M, Masterson J, et al. Energy expenditure, energy balance, and composition of weight gain in

low birth weight infants fed diets of different protein and energy content. J Pediatr 1987;110:753–759.
81. Bell EF, Rios GR, Ungs CA, et al. Influence of energy and protein intake on energy utilization and body composition of small premature infants. Pediatr Res 1988;23:479A.
82. Bell EF. Diet and body composition of preterm infants. Acta Paediatr Suppl 1994;405:25–28.
83. Weinstein MR, Hanger K, Bauer JH, et al. Intravenous energy and amino acids in the preterm newborn infant: effects on metabolic rate and potential mechanism of action. J Pediatr 1987;111:119–123.
84. Reichman B, Chessex PH, Putet G, et al. Diet, fat accretion, and growth in premature infants. N Engl J Med 1981;305:1495–1500.
85. Brooke OG, Wood C, Barley J. Energy balance, nitrogen balance, and growth in preterm infants fed expressed breast milk, a premature infant formula, and two low-solute adapted formulae. Arch Dis Child 1982;57:898–904.
86. Chessex P, Reichman B, Verellen G, et al. Quality of growth in premature infants fed their own mothers' milk. J Pediatr 1983;102:107–112.
87. Reichman B, Chessex P, Verellen G, et al. Dietary composition and macronutrient storage in preterm infants. Pediatrics 1983;72:322–328.
88. Whyte RK, Haslam R, Vlainic C, et al. Energy balance and nitrogen balance in growing low birth weight infants fed human milk or formula. Pediatr Res 1983;17:891–898.
89. Putet G, Senterre J, Rigo J, et al. Nutrient balance, energy utilization, and composition of weight gain in very-low-birth-weight infants fed pooled human milk or a preterm formula. J Pediatr 1984;105:79–85.
90. Van Aerde J, Sauer P, Heim T, et al. Can intrauterine weight gain and body composition be simulated in the formula fed low birth weight infant? Pediatr Res 1985;19:164A.
91. Van Aerde J, Sauer P, Helm T, et al. Effect of medium chain triglyceride diet on energy and macronutrient utilization in the very low birth weight infant. Pediatr Res 1985;19:235A.
92. Brooke OG, Ashworth A. The influence of malnutrition on the postprandial metabolic rate and respiratory quotient. Br J Nutr 1972;27:407–415.
93. Roberts SB, Lucas A. The effects of two extremes of dietary intake on protein accretion in preterm infants. Early Hum Dev 1985;12:301–307.
94. Brooke OG, Onubogu O, Heath R, et al. Human milk and preterm formula compared for effects on growth and metabolism. Arch Dis Child 1987;62:917–923.
95. Putet G, Rigo J, Salle B, et al. Supplementation of pooled human milk with casein hydrolysate: energy and nitrogen balance and weight gain composition in very low birth weight infants. Pediatr Res 1987;21:458–461.
96. Schanler RJ, Garza C. Plasma amino acid differences in very low birth weight infants fed either human milk or whey-dominant cow milk formula. Pediatr Res 1987;21:301–305.
97. Danforth E. The role of thyroid hormones and insulin in the regulation of energy metabolism. Am J Clin Nutr 1983;38:1000–1017.
98. Landsberg L, Young JB. The role of the sympathetic nervous system and catecholamines in the regulation of energy metabolism. Am J Clin Nutr 1983;38:1018–1024.
99. Acheson KJ, Schutz Y, Bessard T, et al. Nutritional influences on lipogenesis and thermogenesis after a carbohydrate meal. Am J Physiol 1984;246:E62–E70.
100. Schwartz RS, Ravussin E, Massari M, et al. The thermic effect of carbohydrate versus fat feeding in man. Metabolism 1985;34:285–293.
101. King RFGJ, McMahon MJ, Almond DJ. Evidence for adaptive diet-induced thermogenesis in man during intravenous nutrition with hypertonic glucose. Clin Sci 1986;71:31–39.
102. Sauer PJJ, Carnielli VP, Sulkers EJ, et al. Substrate utilization during the first weeks of life. Acta Paediatr Suppl 1994;405:49–53.
103. Yunis KA, Oh W, Kalhan S, Cowett RM. Glucose kinetics following administration of an intravenous fat emulsion to low-birth-weight neonates. Am J Physiol 1992;263:E844–849.
104. Chikenji T, Elwyn DH, Gil KM, et al. Effects of increasing glucose intake on nitrogen balance and energy expenditure in malnourished adult patients receiving parenteral nutrition. Clin Sci 1987;72:489–501.
105. Yang H, Cree TC, Schalch DS. Effect of carbohydrate-restricted, calorie reduced diet on the growth of young rats and on serum growth hormone, somatomedins, total thyroxine and triiodothyronine, free T_4 index, and total corticosterone. Metabolism 1987;36:794–798.
106. Crabtree B, Newsholme EA. A systematic approach to describing and analyzing metabolic control systems. Trends Biochem Sci 1987;12:5–12.
107. Miyoshi H, Shulman GI, Peters EJ, et al. Hormonal control of substrate cycling in humans. J Clin Invest 1988;81:1545–1555.
108. Shaw JHF, Wolfe RR. Glucose, fatty acid, and urea kinetics in patients with severe pancreatitis. Ann Surg 1986;204:665–672.
109. Shaw JHF, Wolfe RR. An integrated analysis of glucose, fat, and protein metabolism in severely traumatized patients. Ann Surg 1989;209:63–72.
110. Jeevanandam M, Grote-Holman E, Chikenji T, et al. Effects of glucose on fuel utilization and glycerol turnover in normal and injured man. Crit Care Med 1990;18:125–135.
111. Pittet PH, Chappuis K, Acheson K, et al. Thermic effect of glucose in obese subjects studied by direct and indirect calorimetry. Br J Nutr 1976;35:281–292.
112. Schwartz RS, Halter JB, Bierman EL. Reduced thermic effect of feeding in obesity: role of norepinephrine. Metabolism 1983;32:114–117.
113. Felig P, Cunningham J, Levitt M, et al. Energy expenditure in obesity in fasting and postprandial state. Am J Physiol 1983;244:E45–51.
114. Roberts SB, Savage J, Coward WA, et al. Energy expenditure and intake in infants born to lean and overweight mothers. N Engl J Med 1988;318:461–466.
115. Ashworth A. Metabolic rates during recovery from protein-calorie malnutrition: the need for a new concept of specific dynamic action. Nature 1969;223:407–409.

116. Mestyan J, Jarai I, Fekete M, et al. Specific dynamic action in premature infants kept at and below the neutral temperature. Pediatr Res 1969;3:41–50.
117. Brooke OG, Alvear J, Arnold M. Energy retention, energy expenditure, and growth in healthy immature infants. Pediatr Res 1979;13:215–220.
118. Spady DW, Payne PR, Picou D, et al. Energy balance during recovery from malnutrition. Am J Clin Nutr 1976; 29:1073.
119. Hommes FA. The energy requirement for growth: a reevaluation. Nutr Metab 1980;24:110–113.
120. Committee on Nutrition, American Academy of Pediatrics. Nutritional needs of low-birth-weight infants. Pediatrics 1977;60:519–530.
121. Askanazi J, Rosenbaum H, Michelson C, et al. Increased body temperature secondary to total parenteral nutrition. Crit Care Med 1980;8:736–737.
122. Norderstrom J, Carpentier Y, Askanazi J, et al. Metabolic utilization of intravenous fat emulsion during total parenteral nutrition. Ann Surg 1982;196:221–231.
123. Heymsfield S, Head A, McManus C, et al. Respiratory, cardiovascular and metabolic effects of enteral hyperalimentation: influence of formula, dose and composition. Am J Clin Nutr 1984;40:116–130.
124. Billeaud C, Piedboeuf B, Chessex P. Respiratory gas exchange in response to fat-free parenteral nutrition: a comparison after thoracic or abdominal surgery in newborn infants. J Pediatr Surg 1993;28(1):11–13.
125. Chessex P, Gagne G, Pineault M, et al. Metabolic and clinical consequences of changing from high-glucose to high-fat regimens in parenterally fed newborn infants. J Pediatr 1989;115:992–997.
126. Geliebter A, Torbay N, Bracco EF, et al. Overfeeding with medium chain triglyceride diet results in diminished deposition of fat. Am J Clin Nutr 1983;37:1–4.
127. Hill JO, Peters JC, Yang D, et al. Thermogenesis in humans during overfeeding with medium-chain triglycerides. Metabolism 1989;38:641–648.
128. Sulkers EJ, Lafeber HN. Beaufrere B, et al. Glucose-metabolism in preterm infants fed a 40% MCT or a LCT formula. Pediatr Res 1990;27:292A.
129. Sulkers EJ, Lafeber HN, Sauer PJJ. Quantitation of oxidation of medium-chain triglycerides in preterm infants. Pediatr Res 1989;26:294–297.
130. Carnielli VP, Sulkers EJ, Moretti C, et al. Conversion of octanoic acid into long-chain saturated fatty acids in premature infants fed a formula containing medium-chain triglycerides. Metabolism 1994;43:1287–1292.
131. Sulkers EJ, Lafeber HN, Degenhart HJ, et al. Substrate utilization in low birth weight infants receiving total parenteral nutrition with high carnitine supplementation. Am J Clin Nutr 1990;52:889–894.
132. Pencharz PB, Parsons M, Motil K, et al. Total body protein turnover and growth in children, is it a futile cycle? Med Hypotheses 1981;7:115–160.
133. Catzeflis C, Schutz Y, Micheli JL, et al. Whole body protein synthesis and energy expenditure in very low birth weight infants. Pediatr Res 1985;19:679–687.
134. Beaufrere B. Protein turnover in low-birth-weight (LBW) infants. Acta Paediatr Suppl 1994;405:86–92.
135. Moore PB. Protein synthesis: elongation remodelled. Nature 1989;342:127–128.
136. Liechty EA, Boyle DW, Moorehead H, et al. Increased fetal glucose concentration decreases ovine fetal leucine oxidation independent of insulin. Am J Physiol 1993;265: E617–623.
137. Hertz DE, Karn CA, Liu YM, et al. Intravenous glucose suppresses glucose production but not proteolysis in extremely premature newborns. J Clin Invest 1993;92:1752–1758.
138. Van Aerde J, Sauer PJJ, Pencharz PB, et al. Metabolic consequences of increasing energy intake by adding lipid to parenteral nutrition in full-term infants. Am J Clin Nutr 1994;59:659–662.
139. van Lingen RA, van Goudoever JB, Luijendijk IL, et al. Effects of early amino acid administration during total parenteral nutrition on protein metabolism in pre-term infants. Clin Sci 1992;82:199–203.
140. Young VR, Marchini JS. Mechanisms and nutritional significance of metabolic responses to altered intakes of protein and amino acids, with reference to nutritional adaptation in humans. Am J Clin Nutr 1990;51:270–289.
141. Nelson KM, Long CL. Physiological basis for nutrition in sepsis. Nutr Clin Pract 1989;4:6–15.
142. Anonymous. Nutrition and the metabolic response to injury. Lancet 1989:995–997.
143. Jeevanandam M, Grote-Holman AE, Chikenji T, et al. Effects of glucose on fuel utilization and glycerol turnover in normal and injured man. Crit Care Med 1990;18: 125–135.
144. Levison H, Swyer PR. Oxygen consumption and the thermal environment in newly born infants. Biol Neonate 1964;7:305.
145. Richardson P, Bose CL, Bucciarelli RL, et al. Oxygen consumption of infants with respiratory distress syndrome. Biol Neonate 1984;46:53–56.
146. Wahlig TM, Gatto CW, Boros SJ, et al. Metabolic response of preterm infants to variable degrees of respiratory illness. J Pediatr 1994;124:283–288.
147. Billeaud C, Piedboeuf B, Chessex P. Energy expenditure and severity of respiratory disease in very low birth weight infants receiving long-term ventilatory support. J Pediatr 1992;120:461–464.
148. Hazan J, Chessex P, Piedboeuf B, et al. Energy expenditure during synthetic surfactant replacement therapy for neonatal respiratory distress syndrome. J Pediatr 1992; 120:S-29–33.
149. Wilson DC, McClure G, Dodge JA. The influence of nutrition on neonatal respiratory muscle function. Intensive Care Med 1992;18:105–108.
150. Weinstein MR, Oh W. Oxygen consumption in infants with bronchopulmonary dysplasia. J Pediatr 1981;99:958–961.
151. Yeh TF, McClenan DA, Ajayi OA, et al. Metabolic rate and energy balance in infants with bronchopulmonary dysplasia. J Pediatr 1989;114:448–451.
152. Yunis KA, Oh W. Effects of intravenous glucose, loading on oxygen consumption, carbon dioxide production and resting energy expenditure in infants with bronchopulmonary dysplasia. J Pediatr 1989;115:127–132.

153. Kalhan SC, Denne SC. Energy consumption in infants with bronchopulmonary dysplasia. J Pediatr 1990;116:662–664.
154. deRegnier RA, Guilbert TW, Mills MM, et al. Growth failure and altered body composition are established by one month of age in infants with bronchopulmonary dysplasia. J Nutr 1996;126:168–175.
155. Boehm G, Bierbach U, Moro G, et al. Limited fat digestion in infants with bronchopulmonary dysplasia. J Pediatr Gastroenterol Nutr 1996;22:161–166.
156. Frank L, Sosenko IRS. Undernutrition as a major contributing factor in the pathogenesis of bronchopulmonary dysplasia. Am Rev Respir Dis 1988;138:725–729.
157. Rubecz I, Mestyan J. The partition of maintenance energy expenditure and the pattern of substrate utilization in uterine malnourished newborn infants before and during recovery. Acta Paediatr Acad Sci Hung 1975;16:335–350.
158. Reichman BL, Chessex B, Putet G, et al. Partition of energy metabolism and energy cost of growth in the very low birth weight infant. Pediatrics 1982;69:446–451.
159. Billeaud C, Piedboeuf B, Jequier JC, et al. Relative contribution of physical activity to neonatal oxygen consumption. Early Hum Dev 1993;32:113–120.
160. Stabell U, Junge M, Fenner A. Metabolic rate and O_2 consumption in newborns during different states of vigilance. Biol Neonate 1977;31:27–31.
161. Chessex P, Reichman B, Verellen G, et al. Metabolic consequences of intrauterine growth retardation in very low birth weight infants. Pediatr Res 1984;18:709–713.
162. Davies PS, Clough H, Bishop NJ, et al. Total energy expenditure in small for gestational age infants. Arch Dis Child Fetal Neonatal Ed 1996;74:208–210.
163. Van Goudoever JB, Sulkers EJ, Halliday D, et al. Whole-body protein turnover in preterm appropriate for gestational age and small for gestational age infants: comparison of [15N]glycine and [1-(13)C]leucine administered simultaneously. Pediatr Res 1995;37:381–388.
164. Abdulrazzaq YM, Brooke OG. Is the raised metabolic rate of the small for gestation infant due to his relatively large brain size. Early Hum Dev 1988;16:253–261.
165. Davidson M, Bauer CH. Pattern of fat excretion in feces of premature infants fed various preparations of milk. Pediatrics 1960;25:375–384.
166. Zoula J, Melichar V, Novak M, et al. Nitrogen and fat retention in premature infants fed breast milk, "humanized" cows milk or half skimmed cows milk. Acta Pediatr Scand 1966;55:26–32.
167. Tantibhedhyangkul P, Hashim SA. Medium chain triglyceride feeding in premature infants: effects on fat and nitrogen absorption. Pediatrics 1975;55:359–369.
168. Roy CC, Ste-Marie M, Chartrand L, et al. Correction of the malabsorption of the preterm infant with a medium chain triglyceride formula. J Pediatr 1975;86:446–450.
169. Chappell JE, Clandinin MT, Kearney-Volpe C, et al. Fatty acid balance studies in premature infants fed human milk or formula: effect of calcium supplementation. J Pediatr 1986;108:439–447.
170. Huston RK, Reynolds JW, Jensen C, et al. Nutrient and mineral retention and vitamin D absorption in low birth weight infants: effect of medium-chain triglycerides. Pediatrics 1983;72:44–48.
171. Carnielli VP, Luijendijk IH, van Beek RH, et al. Effect of dietary triacylglycerol fatty acid positional distribution on plasma lipid classes and their fatty acid composition in preterm infants. Am J Clin Nutr 1995;62:776–781.
172. Carnielli VP, Luijendijk IH, van Goudoever JB, et al. Feeding premature newborn infants palmitic acid in amounts and stereoisomeric position similar to that of human milk: effects on fat and mineral balance. Am J Clin Nutr 1995;61:1037–1042.
173. Hamosh M, Bitman J, Liao TH. Gastric lipolysis and fat absorption in preterm infants: effect of medium-chain triglyceride or long-chain triglyceride-containing formulas. Pediatrics 1989;83:86–92.
174. Zlotkin CH, Bryan MH, Anderson GH. Intravenous nitrogen and energy intakes required to duplicate in utero nitrogen accretion in prematurely born human infants. J Pediatr 1981;99:115–120.
175. Baker JP, Detsky AS, Stewart S, et al. Randomized trial of total parenteral nutrition in critically ill patients: metabolic effects of varying glucose-lipid ratios as the energy source. Gastroenterology 1984;87:53–59.
176. Pineault M, Chessex P, Bisaillon S, et al. Total parenteral nutrition in the newborn: impact of the quality of infused energy on nitrogen metabolism. Am J Clin Nutr 1988;47:298–300.
177. Heird WC, Hay W, Helms RA, et al. Pediatric parenteral amino acid mixture in low birth weight infants. Pediatrics 1988;81:41–50.
178. Pencharz P, Beesley J, Sauer P, et al. Total-body protein turnover in parenterally fed neonates: effects of energy source studied by using [^{15}N]glycine and [I-^{13}C]leucine. Am J Clin Nutr 1989;50:1395–1400.
179. De Curtis M, Brooke OG. Energy and nitrogen balances in very low birth weight infants. Arch Dis Child 1987;62:830–832.
180. Heird WC, Kashyap S. Protein and energy requirement of low birth weight infants. Acta Pediatr Scand Suppl 1989;351:13–32.
181. De Gamarra ME, Schutz Y, Catzeflis C, et al. Composition of weight gain during the neonatal period and longitudinal growth follow-up in premature babies. Biol Neonate 1987;52:181–187.
182. Committee on Nutrition American Academy of Pediatrics. Nutritional needs of low birth weight infants. Pediatrics 1985;75:976–986.
183. Lucas A. Does early diet program future outcome? Acta Pediatr Scand Suppl 1990;365:58–67.
184. Lewis DS, Bertaut HA, McMahon A, et al. Preweaning food intake influences the adiposity of young adult baboons. J Clin Invest 1986;78:899–905.
185. Viikari J, Akerblom HK, Rasanen L, et al. Cardiovascular risk in young Finns. Acta Pediatr Scand Suppl 1990;365:13–19.
186. Lucas A, Morley R, Cole TJ, et al. Breast milk and subsequent intelligence quotient in children born preterm. Lancet 1992;339:261–264.

187. Lucas A, Morley R, Cole TJ, et al. A randomised multicentre study of human milk versus formula and later development in preterm infants. Arch Dis Child Fetal Neonatal Ed 1994;70:F141–146.

188. Lucas A, Fewtrell MS, Morley R, et al. Randomized outcome trial of human milk fortification and development outcome in preterm infants. Am J Clin Nutr 1996;64:142–151.

45
Neonatal Thermoregulation

Pieter J.J. Sauer

It has long been known that there is a direct relationship between body temperature and mortality of the low birth weight neonate. In 1900 Budin[1] showed that the mortality of the neonate with a birth weight of less than 2 kg was 98% when body temperature was less than 32°C compared to a mortality of 23% when body temperature was normal. Budin, together with Tarnier, introduced the use of the incubator to keep the neonate warm. Couney introduced the incubator to the general public by displaying it during the World Exhibitions between 1896 and 1939. The neonates cared for in the incubators during these exhibitions came from local hospitals. In 1958 Silverman et al.[2] noted a lower mortality of the low birth weight neonate nursed at 31° compared to 28°C. They also noted a lower mortality when the humidity of the air was increased,[3] as had been reported in 1933 by Blackfan and Yaglou.[4] Glass et al.,[5] from the same group, showed that environmental temperature and humidity influenced not only mortality but weight gain as well. They showed that the neonate nursed with an abdominal temperature of 36.5°C gained more weight compared to the neonate with a temperature of 35°C, but it could be overcome by increasing the energy intake.

The study of Silverman et al.[2] can be understood in relation to the studies reported by Mondhorst[6] in 1932. He had reported an increase in heat production in the low birth weight neonate as a reaction to a low environmental temperature. Day and Hardy[7] confirmed the results of Mondhorst, but these results were hardly noticed in the literature. The studies of Brück[8] and Brück et al.[9] attracted much attention. Brück et al. showed that the response of the low birth weight neonate to nursing in a relative cool environment is both an increase in heat production and, in order to reduce heat loss, a reduction in skin blood flow. They showed that the periods of quiet sleep increased at a higher environmental temperature.

Many studies were done during the period 1960 to 1980 regarding the response of the low birth weight infant to nursing in a cool environment. These studies have mainly investigated the change in oxygen consumption as a reaction to a change in environmental temperature of at least 3° to 4°C. Those studies are presently difficult to perform ethically, as the goal of treatment is to keep oxygen consumption as low as possible while keeping body temperature in the normal range. Important for understanding the thermoregulation of the neonate have been the studies of Hey et al.[10–12] They evaluated many aspects of the thermoregulatory response of the neonate and constructed guidelines for the optimal thermal environment. Hey[13] summarized all his studies in 1971.

Studies during the 1980s mainly dealt with methods to reduce heat loss and to improve incubators and radiant heaters and not with the question of how the term or very low birth weight neonate regulates body temperature. In recent years, a number of studies have been performed in animals regarding the onset of thermoregulation after birth. More is also known regarding the role and regulation of brown adipose tissue.

Principles of Thermoregulation

To effectively control body temperature, sensors are located in critical locations to respond to changes in the external and internal environment.[8,9,14] A central processing area receives, integrates, and responds to incoming signals. Heat production on one side and skin blood flow, sweating, respiration, and behavioral mechanisms on the other are balanced to keep body temperature constant using minimal amounts of energy. The questions that arise are about the localization of the temperature sensors and the number of sensors. Studies in the preterm neonate showing a relation between heat production and the difference between abdominal skin and incubator temperature,[15] as well as studies showing an increase in heat production as a reaction to cooling the skin in the absence of a change in core temperature, have indicated that the skin temperature plays a central role in the regulation of the heat production of the preterm neonate.[16] It is probably not only the skin temperature that regulates heat production; the central temperature may play a role as well.[17] The human body contains deep body thermosensors located in the preoptic area of the hypothalamus, the spinal cord, and the brain stem. The location of multiple thermosensors may indicate that body temperature is regulated by a multiple input mode; however, the exact regulation in the neonate is unknown. Body temperature is the result of a balance between heat production and heat loss. Heat is produced in all organs in the body. This heat can be stored in the body or transported from heat-producing organs to the surface area where it is lost. Heat loss can occur via four routes: convection, conduction, radiation, and evaporation.

Convection

Convection is the heat loss at the skin surface to the surrounding air. Convective heat loss is divided into natural convection and forced convection. Natural convection is the result of temperature differences in the air caused by heat loss from the body. Forced convection is due to air movements caused by a fan.

Convection can be defined as:

$$Q_{conv} = h_c \left(T_{sk} \times T_{air} \right)$$

where Q_{conv} = heat loss by convection,
T_{sk} = mean skin temperature,
T_{air} = mean air temperature.

The coefficient of heat transfer by convection (h_c) is defined as:

$$h_c = d^{0.67} \left(2.3 + 7.5 \, V^{0.67} \right)$$

where d = density of air,
V = velocity of the air (m·sec^{-1}).

The h_c in an incubator is estimated to be 4.0 to 5.4 $Wm^{-2}K^{-1}$.[18,19] The air velocity in most modern incubators is 0.05 to 0.20 m·sec^{-1}. The heat loss through convection, at this air velocity in an incubator, is almost equally divided between natural and forced convection, being approximately 20% to 30% of total heat loss. When radiant heaters are used, heat loss due to forced convection is the primary route.[20-22]

Conduction

Conduction is the transfer of heat directly through the body from the internal heat-producing organs to the skin surface and from the skin surface through material in contact with the skin. The general description of conduction is:

$$Q_{cond} = \frac{C_m \cdot S_{cond}}{d} \left(T_{sk} \cdot T_m \right)$$

where Q_{cond} = heat lost by conduction,
C_m = thermal conductivity of the material in contact with the skin,
S_{cond} = skin surface in contact with the material,
d = thickness of conducting material,
T_{sk} = mean skin temperature,
T_m = temperature of material.

Conduction is not important when a neonate is in an incubator but may be important when a radiant heater is used.[23]

Radiation

Radiation is the heat loss from a warmer surface to a cooler surface. It takes place irrespective of the temperature of the air. It is generally defined as:

$$Q_{rad} = h_r \cdot S \cdot \left(T_{sk} - T_w \right)$$

where Q_{rad} = heat loss of radiation,
h_r = heat transfer coefficient for radiation, 5 $Wm^{-2}K^{-1}$,
S = skin surface of the radiating skin surface,
T_{sk} = mean skin temperature,
T_w = temperature of the surrounding objects.

Heat loss through radiation is important for the very low birth weight neonate nursed in an incubator. Radiative heat loss can be reduced by placing a heat shield between the neonate and the incubator wall, by using a double-walled incubator, or by increasing the room temperature where the incubator is placed.

Evaporation

Evaporation of water from the skin or mucous membranes is an energy-consuming process that causes heat loss from the neonate. There are three distinct patterns of evaporative heat loss: (1) insensible evaporation from the skin surface, (2) evaporation of sweat, and (3) evaporation from the respiratory tract mucosa. The evaporation of 1 g of water causes a heat loss of approximately 0.58 kcal according to the formula:

$$Q_{evap} = evaporated \; water \; (g) \times 0.58 \; (kcal)$$

The evaporation is dependent on a number of factors associated with the neonate and the environment. The evaporative heat loss via the mucous membranes of the lung is given by the formula:

$$Q_{evap} = k \times E \times M \times \left(P_I - P_W \right)$$

where Q_{evap} = heat loss by evaporation on mucous membranes,
k = constant,
E = heat of evaporation,
M = metabolic rate,
P_1 = humidity of expired air,
P_w = humidity of environmental air.

The evaporative heat loss from the skin is given by the formula:

$$Q_{evap} = Lc \times E \times h_c \times f_w \times S \times (P_{sk} - P_W)$$

where Q_{evap} = evaporative heat loss on the skin,
L_c = constant,
E = heat of evaporation,
h_c = heat transfer coefficient,
f_w = fraction of the skin that is wet,
S = body surface area,
P_{sk} = humidity at skin temperature,
P_w = humidity of the environmental air.

The evaporative heat loss of the preterm neonate is dependent on gestational and postnatal age[24-27] (Figure 45.1). The evaporative heat loss can be even higher than total heat production.[26] Increasing the absolute humidity of the ambient air causes a reduction of evaporative heat loss.[24,27]

Evaporative heat loss is dependent on the absolute humidity of the environment and not on the relative humidity. Changing the environmental temperature without a change in the absolute humidity of the air results in a change in relative humidity but not in evaporative heat loss unless the neonate starts sweating.

Heat Balance

Heat balance of the individual can be reported as:

$$Q_{tot} = Q_{conv} + Q_{rad} + Q_{cond} + Q_{evap} + Q_{storage}$$

The different modes of heat loss are independent of each other. The amount of heat given off in different ways may vary, although total heat loss remains constant. When heat loss is greater than heat production, the neonate reduces skin perfusion resulting in a decreased skin temperature in order to reduce heat loss. The core temperature drops and results in a new equilibrium with the environment. The caregiver can change the environmental conditions in order to reduce heat loss, sometimes trying one or more methods. Under radiant heaters, as is discussed later, heat is gained by radiation and is lost through evaporation, convection, and conduction.

Fetal Thermoregulation

The fetus is continuously producing heat as a by-product of energy metabolism. This heat is subsequently lost to the mother, via either the amniotic fluid and uterine wall or the placenta. Abrams[28] and Abrams et al.[29] showed in their classic study in the sheep that the fetus has a 0.5°C higher body temperature than the mother but does follow changes in the temperature of the mother. The part of the heat that is lost via the placenta is indicated by a higher temperature of the umbilical artery compared with the umbilical vein. The fetal temperature represents a balance between the metabolic heat generated by the fetus and the loss of heat across the placenta (85%) and through the skin (15%).[30]

Adaptation After Birth

The neonate at birth moves from an environment of around 37°C to a cooler environment. This causes a drop in his temperature to the level normal after birth. Without adjustments, the temperature will drop further and the neonate will become hypothermic. The neonate has different ways of preventing this: vasoconstriction, pos-

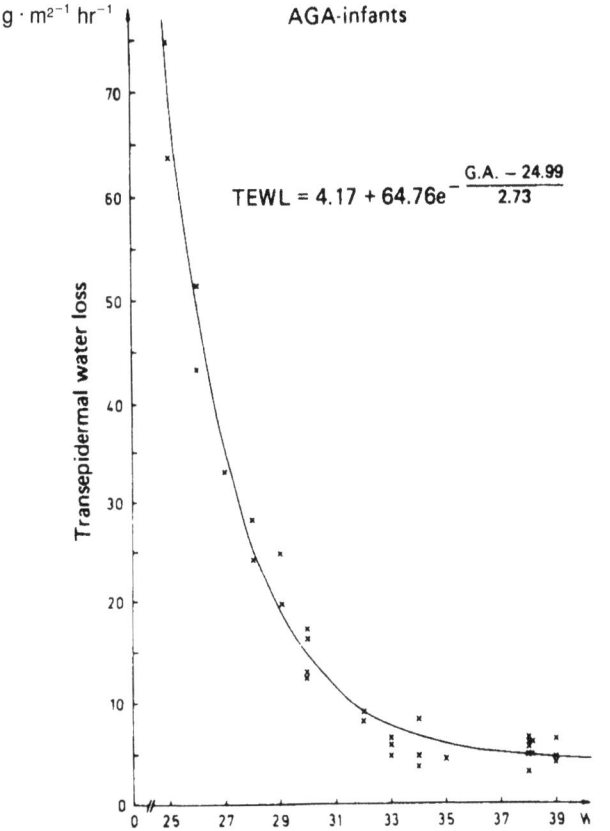

FIGURE 45.1. Transepidermal water loss (TEWL) in relation to gestational age on the first day of life. AGA, appropriate for gestational age; W, completed weeks of gestation. (From Hammarlund and Sedin,[24] with permission.)

tural changes, and an increase in heat production, either by shivering or nonshivering thermogenesis. Despite these adjustments, hypothermia is a frequent event in the neonate for the following reasons: (1) The body surface area/body weight ratio is much higher in the neonate than in the adult. The ratio in the preterm neonate is four times as high, and in term neonates it is 2.7 times as high. (2) The tissue insulation of the neonate is much less than that of the adult and remains rather low at maximal vasoconstriction. The tissue insulation is, at maximal vasoconstriction, one-third that of the adult value in the term neonate and one-fifth the adult value in the preterm neo-

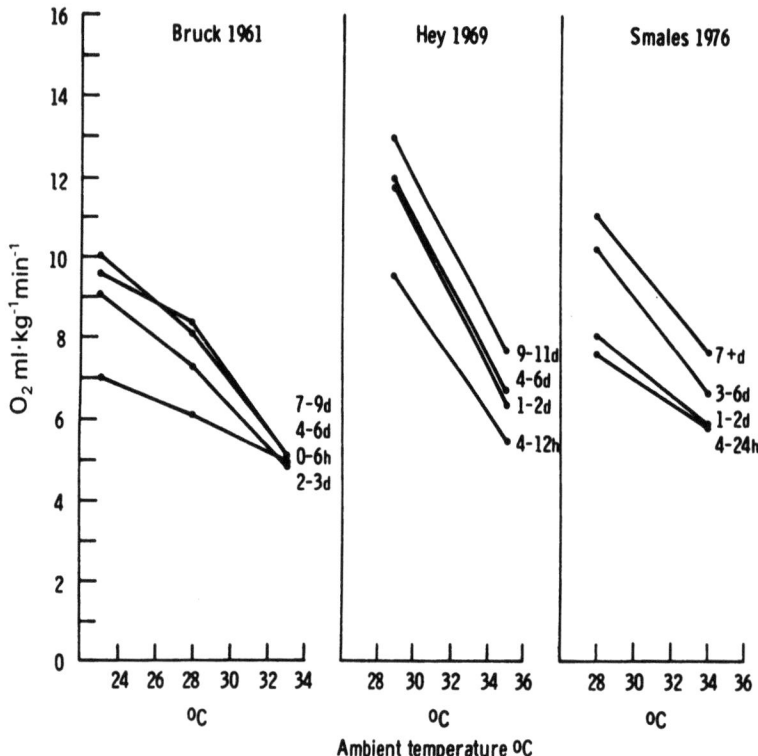

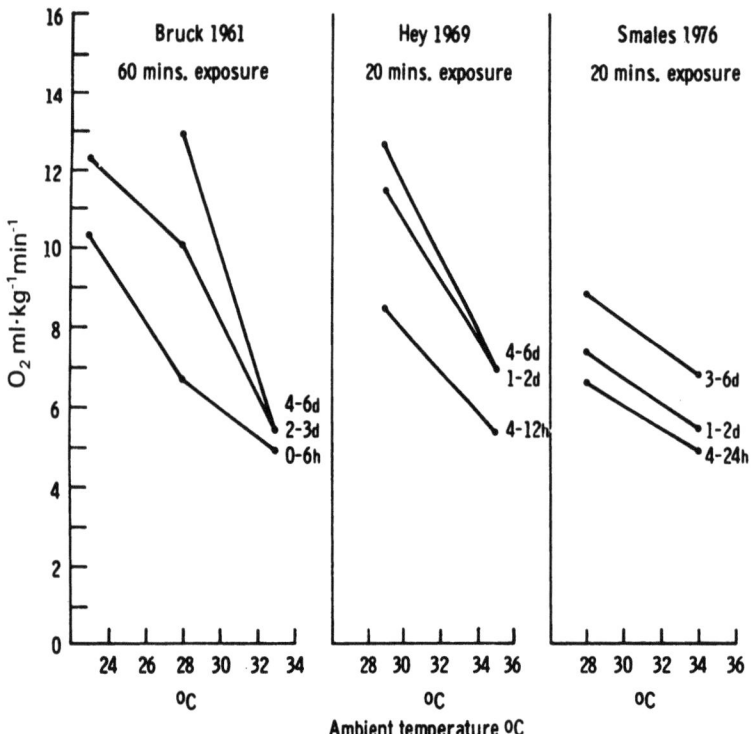

FIGURE 45.2. Average rates of oxygen consumption at term in the neonate. (From Sinclair.[127])

nate. (3) The flexion of the body of the neonate is higher than that of the adult, causing a higher convective heat loss in the neonate.[4] (4) The neonate has only a limited ability, especially the first days after birth, to increase its heat production. A fourfold higher heat production in the neonate compared to the adult would be needed to compensate for this higher heat loss. Effectively, the metabolic rate of both the term and preterm neonate at birth is only twice as high as that of the adult when expressed per kilogram of body weight.

The drop in body temperature is highly influenced by the temperature of the environment. Deep body temperature in the term neonate shows a decrease for 40 minutes at an environmental temperature of 24° to 26°C, whereas peripheral skin temperature continues to fall for 8 hours.[31] It is interesting to note that the environmental temperature at which the preterm and term neonate increase the metabolic rate is much higher than that of the adult.

The skin temperature of the preterm and term neonate at which an increase in oxygen consumption has been recorded is higher than that of the adult. This finding might indicate a setpoint for the thermoregulatory response in the neonate different from that in the adult.

The preterm neonate, especially one born before a gestational age of less than 30 weeks, is at far greater risk of a drop in body temperature compared to the more mature neonate. There is no difference in heat production when expressed per kilogram body weight. The heat production of the immature neonate is much less when expressed per body surface area. Also, the skin of the very immature neonate is very thin, only two to three cells thick, and since it contains little keratin, it leaks. Evaporation of the very preterm neonate is much higher compared with the more mature neonate (Figure 45.1), especially during the first 2 weeks after birth.[24-26] The effects of vasomotor changes and postural adjustments that can be seen in the very preterm neonate are much smaller compared with those of the term neonate. Finally, one has to realize that the ability to increase the metabolic rate in a cool environment is not maximal at birth; it increases with postnatal age and is more pronounced in the term than in the preterm neonate (Figure 45.2). How a neonate reacts to a cool environment might depend on the maturation of his or her thermoregulation center as well as on other factors.[34] In 1959 Hill[35] reported that the rise in metabolic rate as a result of a cold stress is reduced during hypoxia. Scopes and Ahmed[36] reported that asphyxia, infection, and birth injury adversely affect the defense of thermal stability. The mortality of the neonate, particularly of one with low birth weight, is markedly increased by hypothermia.[37,38] This fact might be related to a decreased function of neutrophils and reduced production of surfactant observed at a low body temperature.[39]

The human has two ways of increasing the heat production: shivering and nonshivering thermogenesis. Shivering is not observed in the neonate; the increased activity seen in a cool environment could be the equivalent. The most important thermogenesis is the heat production through the oxidation of substrates in the brown adipose tissue.

Brown Adipose Tissue

During the last trimester of the normal pregnancy brown adipose tissue (BAT) is formed in the human infant, expecially in the cervical and perirenal area (Figure 45.3). The structure of brown adipose tissue is specialized for heat production. This special function is demonstrated by the fact that, although brown fat accounts for only 1.5% of body fat, it accounts for 22% of cardiac output during cold stress[40] and about one-half the maximum thermogenic response.[41]

The presence of brown adipose tissue mediated thermogenesis was first suggested by Silverman et al., who found that the highest skin temperature after 1 hour of cold exposure is at the nape of the neck, above the brown fat. Other, probably larger stores of brown fat are found around the kidneys and adrenal glands. Further evidence for the existence of BAT was presented by Karlberg et al.[43] and Schiff et al.,[44] who showed increased oxygen consumption after norepinephrine infusion and increased urinary excretion of norepinephrine plus a rise in plasma nonesterfied free fatty acids in neonates exposed to cold. The blood glucose concentration was shown not to have an influence on the metabolic

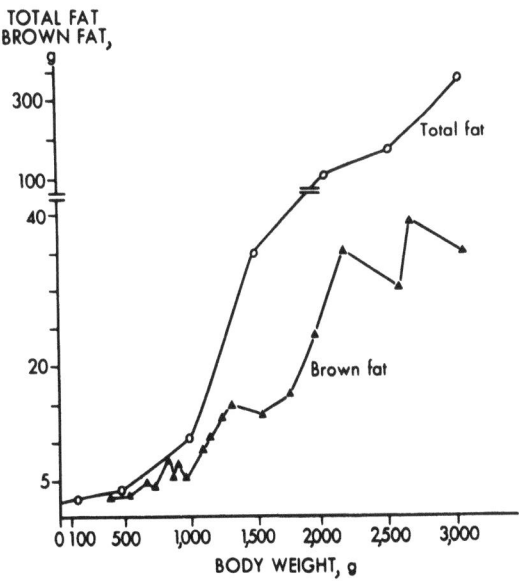

FIGURE 45.3. Total fat and brown fat plotted against body weight. (From Heim,[45] with permission.)

response to cold, in contrast to either endogenous or exogenous fat.[45] This can be explained by the fact that fatty acids and not glucose are the substrates for oxidation by BAT. Sufficient oxygen supply is a prerequisite for nonshivering thermogenesis. It is reported that brown adipose tissue metabolism is inhibited when the arterial Po_2 is below 30 mm Hg in the neonate and in the puppy.[31,46,47] The unique property of BAT that causes the remarkable thermogenic capacity is the presence of uncoupling protein. The uncoupling protein acts to short-circuit the proton electrochemical gradient generated during substrate oxidation and so promote dissipation of heat. Instead of converting energy into adenosine triphosphate (ATP) and other energy-rich compounds, as is the case in other tissues, all energy is converted into heat.

The presence of uncoupling protein in the mitochondria of BAT in human was first demonstrated by Lean et al.[48] The concentration of uncoupling protein is lower in the neonate than in the older infant; the lowest values are found in the preterm infant.[48]

Regulation of Brown Adipose Tissue

The capacity to increase heat production after birth is dependent on the thermogenesis in the BAT. It is important therefore to know what regulates the thermogenesis in BAT. According to many studies there are stimulators as well as inhibitors of BAT. Stimulators are the sympathetic nervous system, noradrenaline, adrenaline, and the thyroid hormones. Inhibitors are most likely prostaglandin E_2 and adenosine.

Development of the Sympathetic Nervous System

The sympathetic nervous system starts to appear halfway through gestation, but continues to develop after birth and in most species sympathetic innervation of autonomic end organs is absent or nonfunctioning at birth.[49] This may be the reason why the proportion of adrenergic receptor subtypes in many fetal tissues is very different from that found neonatally.[50] An explanation for these transitions in ontogenic development between fetal and neonatal life is to enable the newborn mammal to respond to specific stimuli associated with birth.[51] Consequently tissues such as BAT, which has a key role in thermoregulation after birth, contains several populations of sympathetic nerves[52] and innervation is completed close to term.[53] Following uterine contractions there is a 5- to 10-fold increase in fetal plasma noradrenaline concentration.[54] This enters the circulation as a result of spillover from postglanglionic sympathetic neurons rather than as adrenal medullary secretion.[52] The extent to which catecholamines are released in the circulation is dependent on fetal age and the type of delivery.[55] In the preterm neonate (i.e., less than 37 weeks of gestation) noradrenaline concentration in umbilical artery blood is 50% less than in the full-term neonate. The plasma noradrenaline concentration is much lower in the neonate delivered by cesarean section compared to vaginal delivery with this effect being magnified if general rather than epidural anesthesia is employed.[56,57]

There are several arguments that indicate that the sympathetic nervous system is involved in the regulation of the activity of BAT. In animals it is shown that the activity as well as the transcription of uncoupling protein is regulated by noradrenaline.[58,59] Noradrenaline is the natural neurotransmitter for BAT initiating thermogenesis, it has similar affinities for β_3- and α_1-adrenergic receptors. When brown adipocytes are stimulated in vitro with noradrenaline they increase their oxygen consumption to about 10 times the basal rate; about 80% of this increase is due to β_3- and 20% to α_1-adrenergic pathway.[60] There is a synergistic interaction between β_3- and α_1-adrenoreceptor stimulation.[61] Also, infusion of noradrenaline in the human neonate causes an increase in oxygen consumption, heat production, and plasma free fatty acids.[43,44] In addition, the neonate born after a cesarean section is more likely to develop hypothermia and have lower noradrenaline concentration compared to the neonate and the lamb born vaginally.[62,63] Finally, nonshivering thermogenesis can be blocked by chemical sympathectomy[53] and stimulated by the infusion of a β_3-adrenergic agonist in the newborn lamb.[64–66] Near-term newborn lamb, delivered by cesarean section showed a faster return to normal body temperature and an interruption of shivering thermogenesis after the infusion of a β_3-agonist.[65] Cesarean section delivery also caused a decrease in the level of noradrenaline content in BAT, consistent with what is observed in the vaginally delivered lamb.[66] Recent data have shown that both acute (i.e., 45-minute) and chronic (i.e., 8-day) treatment of normally delivered lamb with a β_3-agonist significantly enhances the thermogenic activity of BAT.[66]

Role of Thyroid Hormones

Thyroid hormones play an important role in regulating metabolism of both the mother and the fetus, which continues into neonatal life.[67–69] That thyroid hormones play an important role can be concluded from studies making the newborn animal hypothyroid. Sheep thyroidectomized in mid-gestation become profoundly hypothermic and die after delivery,[70] in contrast to the athyrotic human neonate. Thyroidectomy in fetal sheep 2 weeks before delivery leads to hypothermia and impaired nonshivering thermogenesis at birth.[67] Acute thyroidectomy at the time of delivery abolished the normal surge in T_3 concentration, but there was no decrease in oxygen consumption compared to the control newborn lamb probably because of the long half-life of T_4 in the neonate, which would allow the conversion of T_4 to T_3 to continue in the brown adipocyte.[67,71] The interaction of thyroid hormones and nonshivering thermogenesis has been clarified. Brown adipose tissue contains the enzyme type II iodothyroine 5′-monodeiodinase, which catalyzes the conversion of T_4 to T_3.[72] This enzyme is present in the BAT of the fetal sheep in the third trimester of gestation and increases with gestational age.[73] In response to cold exposure there is a remarkable increase in type II 5′-diiodinase in the BAT of the rat.[72] Intracellular T_3 concentration modulates the expression of the uncoupling protein in BAT. The thyroidectomized rat has a threefold reduction in the uncoupling protein concentration in BAT and becomes hypothermic. Replacement therapy with T_3 does not correct the hypothermia[74] or a low concentration of uncoupling protein, while replacement with T_4 corrects both very rapidly.[51] Thus, the optimal thermogenic function of BAT requires the intracellular conversion of T_4 to T_3 by 5′-diiodinase activation.[75–77] The euthyroid state is necessary for the perinatal increase in the uncoupling protein in RNA in BAT; in the hypothyroid rat pup the postnatal increase in uncoupling protein in RNA was very much reduced.[78,79] It can be concluded therefore that circulating T_4 and intracellular conversion to T_3 following birth are essential for neonatal thermogenesis rather than the surge in circulating T_3 and thyroid-stimulating hormone (TSH) following birth. The effect of intracellular T_3 is to increase the concentration of uncoupling protein by gene transcription and thereby to increase thermogenesis. Different factors regulating BAT are summarized in Figure 45.4.

Initiation of Thermoregulation after Birth

The temperature of the fetus, as stated before, parallels rather closely the temperature of the mother. The human neonate, like some animals, shows active thermoregulation soon after birth. The question arises, What regulates the switch to active thermoregulation after birth? Important data have been reported by the group of Gunn and Gluckman[80] in the fetal lamb. By placing a coil of tubing around the fetal trunk they were able to cool the fetus in utero. Cooling the fetus resulted in a rapid fall in temperature of the animal with rapidly developing acidosis. As a result the animal showed shivering that was markedly reduced during REM sleep, while shivering usually starts only when nonshivering thermogenesis or the activity of BAT is at a maximum.[81] Cooling the fetus did not result in the onset of respiration,[82] but there was a marked increase in the TSH concentration.[83] This did not, however, result in an increase in T_3 or T_4 concentrations. Cooling the fetus also resulted in an increase in cortisol and fetal plasma noradrenaline concentrations.[84] This was associated with a decrease in plasma insulin concentration and a marked increase in plasma glucose concentration. There was also an increase in heart rate and blood pressure, abolished by catecholamine antagonists.[84] Finally, cooling resulted in a reduction in skin blood flow and a marked increase in blood flow to brown fat.[82] The infusion of noradrenaline resulted only in a minor increase in lipolysis, which is a marker of activity

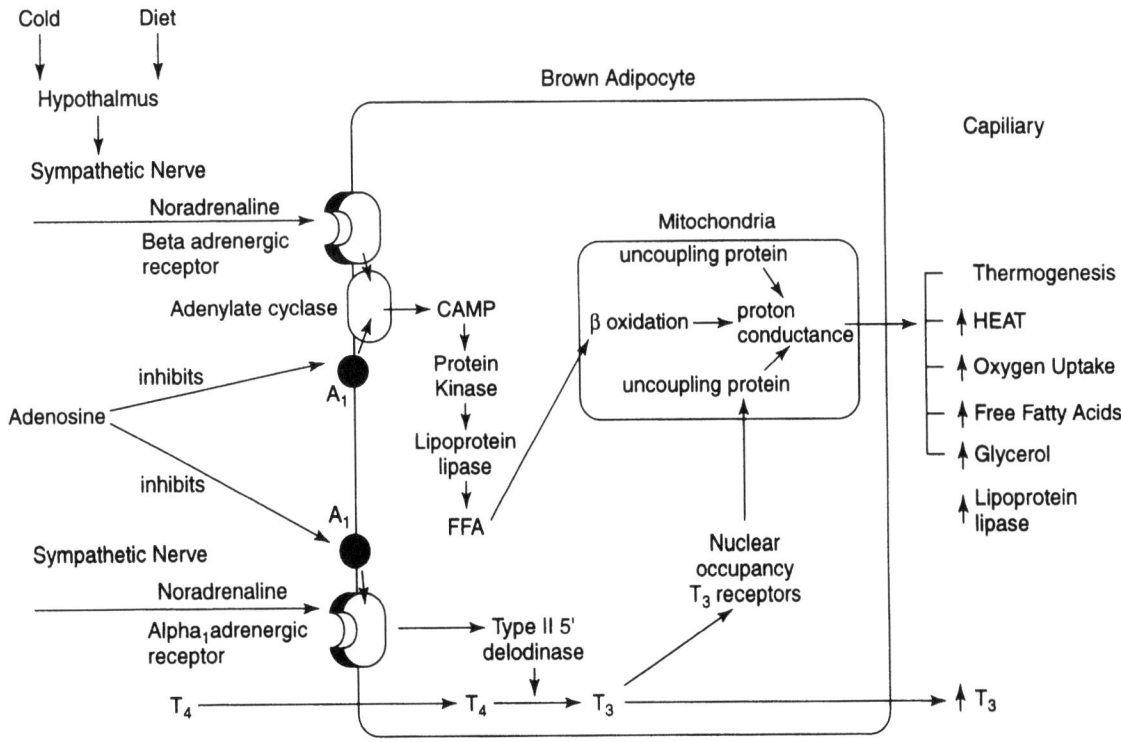

FIGURE 45.4. Some factors controlling nonshivering thermogenesis. (After Gunn and Gluckmann.[75])

of BAT[85] and oxygen consumption,[86] but no increase in body temperature.[87] The infusion of large doses of T_3 did not affect the level of nonshivering thermogenesis in the fetal lamb.[88] It can be concluded, therefore, that although all elements for thermoregulation are present in the fetal lamb, this process starts only after birth. In a next series of very elegant experiments Gunn et al.[89,90] were able to show that it must be inhibitors in the placental circulation that prevent thermoregulation. Cooling the fetus in utero resulted in a decline in fetal temperature that was only partly corrected by oxygenating the animal. The increases in glycerol and free fatty acid (FFA) concentrations were also rather limited (Figure 45.5). The occlusion of the umbilical cord resulted in rapid increases in body temperature, in the temperature of BAT, as well as an increase in glycerol and FFA concentrations.

Potential inhibitors of the fetal thermogenesis are prostaglandin E_2 and adenosin. Prostaglandin E_2 (PGE_2) has a potent antilipolytic effect. The infusion of indomethacin, a cyclooxygenase inhibitor that blocks the production of E_2, combined with cooling, resulted in a threefold increase in glycerol and FFA concentrations.[91] PGE_2 infusion resulted in a very rapid decrease in lipolysis, fetal temperature, and oxygen consumption during cord occlusion. Stopping the PGE_2 infusion resulted in a rapid increase of thermogenic indices.[91] Similar data were reported by Takeuchi et al.[92] recently.

Adenosine might also inhibit the thermogenic response before birth. It has antilipolytic properties,[93] is synthesized by the placenta,[94] and is rapidly metabolized.[95] Plasma adenosine concentration declined ≈50% after the occlusion of the umbilical cord, suggesting the placenta as a likely source of a significant fraction of circulating adenosine.[96] The infusion of an adenosine analogue resulted, in combination with cord occlusion, in a rapid fall in plasma FFA and glycerol concentration, core temperature, and oxygen consumption without a fall in blood pressure.[97]

It can be concluded from the studies summarized above that a combination of factors is required for the initiation of thermogenesis after birth. Important factors are the separation from the placenta, which will remove the inhibitors of thermogenesis, the stimulation of cutaneous cold receptors, the increase in oxygenation with breathing, and the increase in plasma noradrenaline and intracellular T_3 concentrations.

Effect of Mode of Delivery

The term neonate delivered by cesarean section evidences a more rapid decline in body temperature compared to the vaginally delivered neonate.[62] Similar observations are reported in the lamb.[63] A reduction in body temperature is seen especially in the neonate delivered after a cesarean section with general anesthesia as compared to epidural anesthesia. This might be related to lower noradrenaline concentration found in the neonate after birth following general anesthesia (3.2 nM), compared to epidural anesthesia (9.5 nM) and vaginal delivery (31.8 nM).[51] The ability to respond to a cool environment is influenced further by the environmental temperature after birth. Lambs were delivered by ce-

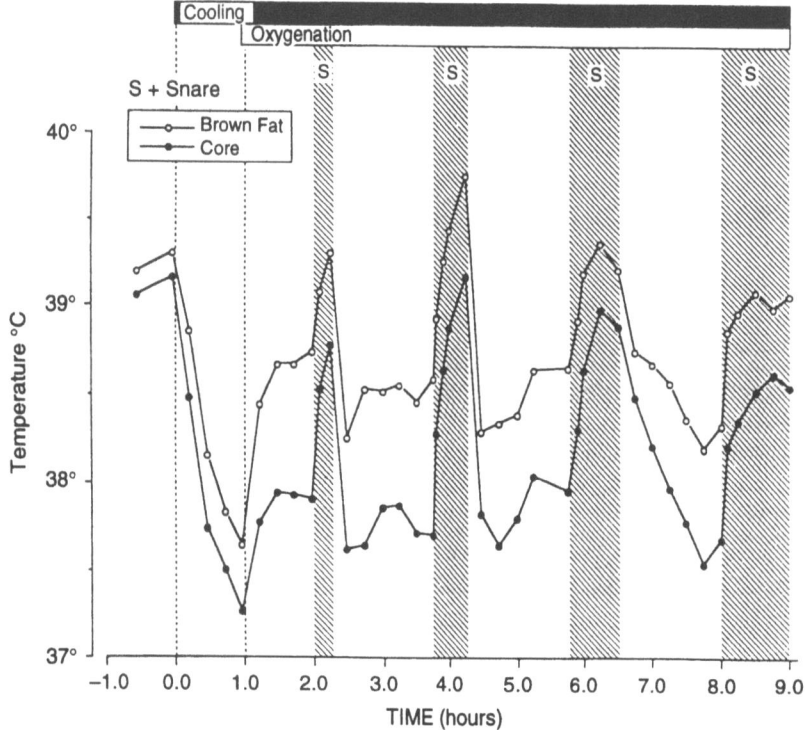

FIGURE 45.5. The time course of responses of fetal core (esophageal) and brown fat temperatures during cooling, oxygenation, and four episodes of umbilical cord occlusion (S) for one fetal sheep 141 days gestation over a 9-hour study. ●, core temperature, ○, brown fat temperature. (After Gunn and Gluckman.[90])

sarean section either in a warm (30°C) or a cool (15°C) environment.[63] There was no difference in heat production at an environmental temperature of 29°C, but the cool-delivered animals showed a 62% greater metabolic response at 14°C. Fifteen of the 18 studied lambs shivered during cold exposure, indicating a reduction in the ability to augment the heat production in BAT. Plasma T_3 and T_4 concentrations were increased in the cool- versus the warm-delivered animals. It seems therefore that delivering by cesarean section prevents the rise in BAT activity. Delivery into a cool environment increases the thyroid hormones, which benefits the newborn lamb by enabling a greater thermogenic response by shivering. Whether the same is true for the human neonate is unclear but not likely, since the human neonate cannot shiver.

Thermoregulation of the Very Low Birth Weight Neonate in the First Days After Birth

The neonate born after a short gestation (i.e., <30 weeks) or with a very low birth weight (i.e., <1 kg) is highly prone to develop hypothermia after birth. This can be explained by a number of factors, both physical and neuroendocrine. The heat loss of the neonate is increased due to the combination of low insulating capacity of the skin and a high skin temperature, high evaporative heat loss, and a limited capacity to reduce heat loss by vasoconstriction. Moreover, the body surface area is high in comparison to the weight of the neonate, making heat production per body surface area rather low. The capacity to increase heat production, especially in BAT is very limited. This can be explained by the limited presence of BAT, lower uncoupling protein concentration, the lower noradrenaline concentration of the neonate, and finally lower thyroid hormone concentrations.

Neutral Thermal Environment

The heat loss of the human body, according to the formulas described above, is dependent on factors in the environment (e.g., temperature of the air, walls, and surface contact area, air velocity, humidity), heat production, and the skin temperature of the individual. When the individual is capable of adjusting his or her heat loss to the extent that heat loss is equal to the heat produced as a result of the body's maintenance functions, the neonate is within the neutral thermal environment. No extra heat is produced to keep the body temperature constant. The thermoneutral environment is defined as the range of ambient temperature within which the metabolic rate is at a minimum and within which temperature regulation is achieved by nonevaporative physical processes alone.[98] A homeothermic individual, as a response to a cool environment, exhibits vasoconstriction, which results in a decline in skin temperature and a reduction in heat loss. The homeothermic individual starts to increase heat production when this reduction in heat loss is insufficient to prevent the core temperature from falling (Figure 45.6).

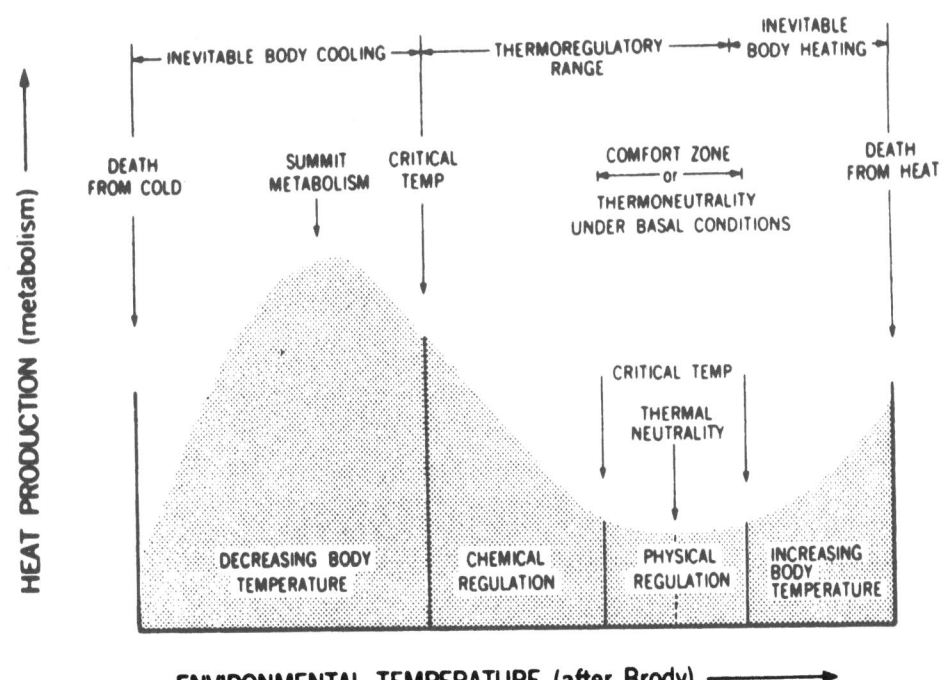

FIGURE 45.6. Homeothermic model (Brody). (From Sinclair,[128] with permission.)

Metabolic rate is supposed to increase at an environmental temperature above the so-called thermoneutral environment. This seems illogical, as heat production is already greater than heat loss under these conditions. Few data in the neonate have noted the effect of a higher than neutral temperature. One study, using direct calorimetry, showed a decrease in dry heat loss, an increase in wet heat loss, and an increase in body temperature.[99] Bell et al.[100] measured oxygen consumption, insensible water loss, and body temperature at different ambient temperatures in the low birth weight neonate.[100] Oxygen consumption was not significantly elevated at an ambient temperature above the presumed neutral temperature. Insensible water loss showed a significant increase. Wheldon and Harpin[101] found no increase in oxygen consumption in the term and preterm neonate when the incubator temperature was increased to increment body temperature so long as the neonate was quiet. Harpin et al.[102] showed that neonates, nursed at a high temperature, alter their posture from predominantly flexion to extension. The difference between core and skin temperature decreased while warming in order to increase heat loss. The term neonate is able to start sweating at birth, whereas the preterm neonate begins to sweat during the second week of life.[103] The temperature to induce sweating is higher in the preterm than in the term neonate, but the efficiency of sweating as a thermoregulatory process has been shown to be poor in both. The increased heat production at a temperature above the neutral temperature is probably due to increased activity as the result of discomfort and is not a true thermoregulatory response.

The adult does have, according to the definition, the lowest metabolic rate at the thermoneutral environment. There are clearly advantages to nursing the neonate in an environment where heat production is at a minimum, as an increase in heat production reduces energy available for growth. The definition of the neutral thermal environment given for the adult cannot be applied to define the optimal environment of the preterm neonate for the following reasons:

1. Studies showing an increase in metabolic rate at a lower environmental temperature have used temperatures several degrees below the suggested optimal temperature to provoke an increase in metabolic rate. Studies done in the small, very preterm neonate have failed to show an increase in metabolic rate as a result of a small change in environmental temperature.[104,105] Core and skin temperature and metabolic rate were increased continuously while changing the incubator temperature by 1°C and changes were detected in the trend of the core and skin temperature. Changes could not be distinguished in metabolic rate from spontaneous changes that occurred at a constant environmental temperature.[105] It was suggested that the small preterm neonate, on the first days of life, does not react as a true homeothermic individual but more as a poikilothermic individual by exerting little thermoregulatory control.[104–106]

2. Evaporative heat loss is an important part of heat loss in the preterm neonate.[24,26]

3. Oxygen consumption of the neonate shows a marked variation over the day. It is sometimes difficult, and it may take many hours, to define the minimal oxygen consumption.[107]

4. The definition of the neutral temperature cannot be used for each neonate individually, as it is impossible to measure oxygen consumption daily in each subject.

Based on the above data, new definitions and guidelines for the thermoneutral environment that can be used in clinical practice have been outlined.[105] These definitions are not based on the oxygen consumption of the neonate but on the trend in body temperature as a reaction to the environment. The optimal environment is so defined as the ambient temperature at which the core temperature of the neonate at rest is between 36.7° and 37.3°C and the core and mean skin temperature are changing less than 0.2° and 0.3°C·hour^{-1}, respectively. The absolute values of the body temperature, core, and skin and the trend in temperature that seems to be acceptable have been chosen arbitrarily. According to this definition, guidelines for the optimal thermal environment of the preterm neonate were devised based on measurements in a calorimeter (Figure 45.7). These data are in good agreement with the previously reported guidelines.[12,108] Only the temperatures of the very low birth neonate on the first few days of life are higher.

The Heat-Delivered Animal: Optimal Body Temperature After Birth

A severe drop in body temperature after birth is associated with an increased risk of death. It is therefore generally accepted that the neonate should be protected from cold stress after birth. Recent studies, however, have indicated that the neonate, born after severe asphyxia, might benefit from a drop in body temperature or rather a lower temperature of the brain. Data so far, however, are published only on the piglet. Thoresen et al.[109] and Edwards et al.[110] have shown that the delayed or secondary energy failure seen in the piglet made hypoxic after birth is highly reduced when the temperature of the piglet was reduced from the normal 38°C to 35°C. Comparable data were reported by Laptook et al.[111] Recently it was shown that cerebral injury after hypoxic/ischemia can be reduced in the rat by the infusion of adenosine.[112] Further data are needed to determine if this effect of adenosine is related to a reduced oxygen consumption in BAT.

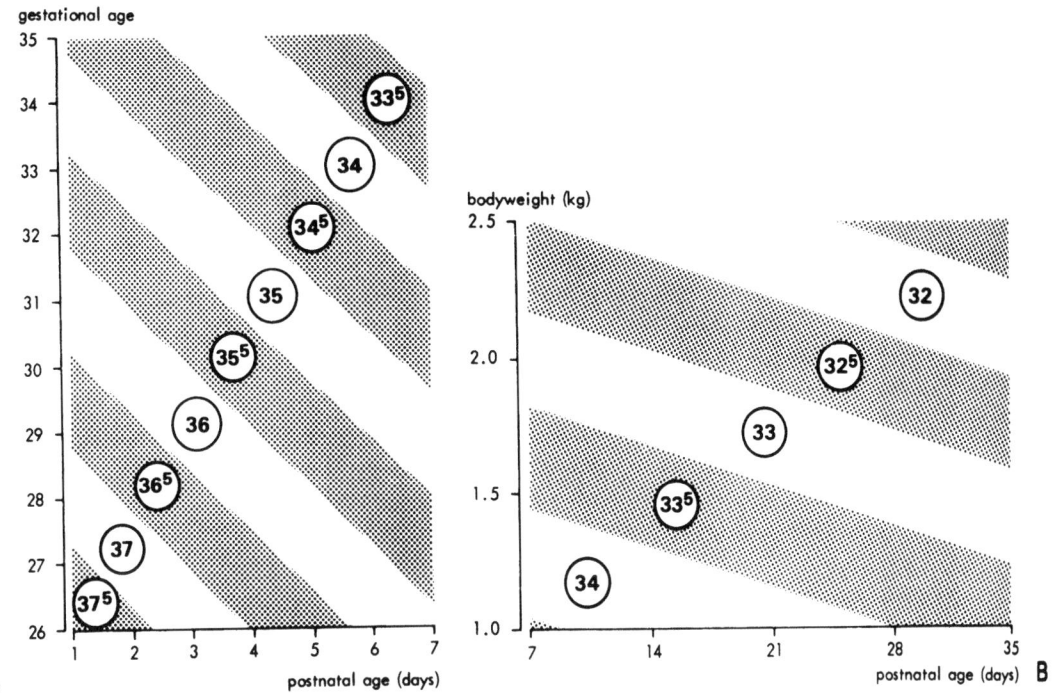

FIGURE 45.7. Guidelines for the optimal thermal environment at a humidity of the air defined as a dewpoint of 18°C and flow of 10 L/minute in relation to gestational age, weight, and postnatal age. Values below 29 weeks during the first week of life (A) and more than 2 kg after 7 days (B) are calculated by extrapolation. (From Sauer et al.,[105] with permission.)

Changes in Optimal Thermal Environment with Age

There is a decrease in optimal thermal environment with increasing gestational age, postnatal age, and weight. The first reason for the decrease in environmental temperature is the increase in metabolic rate after birth (see Chapter 44). The heat production not only increases when it is expressed per kilogram body weight, but increases more sharply and continues to increase after the first week of life when it is expressed per surface area (Figure 45.8).

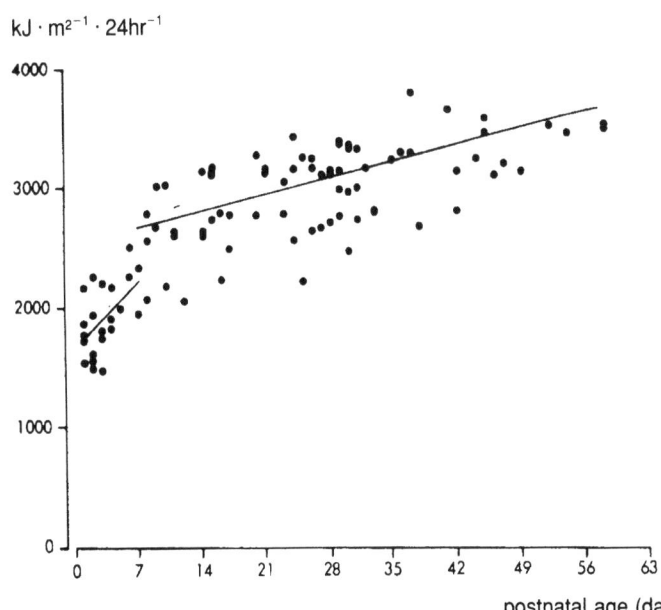

FIGURE 45.8. Resting metabolic rate at the thermoneutral environment. (From Sauer et al.,[105] with permission.)

Second, there is an increase in thermal insulation with increasing postnatal and gestational age. The skin of the preterm neonate evidences rapid maturation after birth.[113] The exact regulation of this skin maturation is not yet known, but the skin of a neonate born after 26 weeks matures rapidly after birth to be almost equal to the skin of a term neonate 2 weeks after birth. The increase in corneal layer thickness results in a decrease in heat loss. The skin not only matures histologically but functionally. Skin blood flow is inversely related to gestational age, being twice as high in the neonate born before 29 weeks as in the term neonate.[114] Term neonates show no change in skin blood flow during the first 7 days of life, whereas a significant drop is observed in the preterm neonate. The most pronounced reduction in skin blood flow is observed in the most premature neonate.

Probaly related to this skin maturation is the decline in evaporative heat loss after birth. The neonate born at less than 30 weeks' gestation has a high transepidermal fluid loss during the first days of life that decreases during the first weeks of life.[24,26] This evaporation is dependent on the humidity of the environment, being approximately 30% lower when the humidity is increased from an absolute humidity of 10 mm Hg to 25 mm Hg.[24,27] Evaporation is dependent more on gestational age than on birth weight.[27] A third explanation for a decrease in optimal thermal environment is the increase in subcutaneous fat observed during postnatal growth in the preterm neonate. It is interesting to observe the increase in subcutaneous fat when a neonate is transferred from an incubator to a cot.[116]

Regulation of Incubator Temperature

Because of the assumed central role of the abdominal skin temperature, incubators have been equipped to regulate air temperature as a feedback mechanism to the abdominal skin temperature. Even when it is accepted that the abdominal skin temperature has a major role in thermoregulatory heat production, there remains a question of which abdominal skin temperature is optimal.

There was no clear relationship between abdominal skin temperature and heat production in the preterm neonate when the abdominal skin temperature varied between 35.5° and 37.5°C.[17] It is unlikely, from a physiologic point of view, that the optimal abdominal skin temperature of all preterm neonates is 36.5°C. The skin after birth shows an increase in thickness and subcutaneous fat layer. The abdominal skin temperature, as a result, decreases. It is impossible to indicate one single optimal abdominal temperature for all neonates.

Studies have shown that the incubator air temperature is more stable when the air-mode control is used compared with the skin control.[34,117] It is true for modern incubators with proportional regulation instead of on-off regulation, even when the incubator temperature is not disturbed by, for instance, opening doors. The clinical significance of this point has not been proven. It was shown that fluctuations in incubator air temperature cause fluctuations in oxygen consumption, thereby putting a strain on energy metabolism and reducing potential growth.[34] Fluctuations in the incubator air temperature are associated with an increased incidence in apneic attacks.[118] One study showed no difference in global heat loss between air and skin servocontrol.[119] In another study an increased central-peripheral skin temperature gradient was observed during the first 2 days of life in the very preterm neonate in regard to skin control compared to servocontrol, indicating greater thermal stress during skin control.[106] It was concluded that skin control should not be used for the very preterm neonate during the first days of life.

There are a number of practical problems regarding the use of skin temperature probes. Potential pitfalls that lead to false skin temperature readings are a detached skin probe, the neonate or a cover lying on the probe, and phototherapy. Variations in body temperature due to infections of the neonate are more easily observed during air mode control than with skin control.

Chessex et al.[117] showed that the type of incubator might affect the optimal abdominal skin temperature. Neonates nursed in two different skin controlled incubators with the same abdominal skin temperature show differences in peripheral temperature and estimated heat loss. The high heat loss in one incubator can be overcome by increasing the abdominal temperature setting by 0.1°C.

It has been questioned whether strict stability of the ambient temperature is best for the preterm neonate. Variations in environmental temperature can help to establish a thermogenetic response (e.g., by the development of BAT). More studies in this area are needed. So long as it is unproven that some thermal stress might have advantages for the preterm neonate, it is advisable to pay attention to the negative effects of changes in environmental temperature and to keep the environmental temperature as stable as possible.

Different aspects of the incubator influence heat loss by the neonate (e.g., air temperature, wall temperature, air velocity, and humidity). Radiant heat loss by the neonate in the incubator depends on the temperature of the incubator wall. This temperature is dependent on the air temperature in a single-walled incubator and the temperature of the room, as discussed by Swyer.[120] In the double-walled incubator the temperature of the inner wall is almost independent of the temperature of the

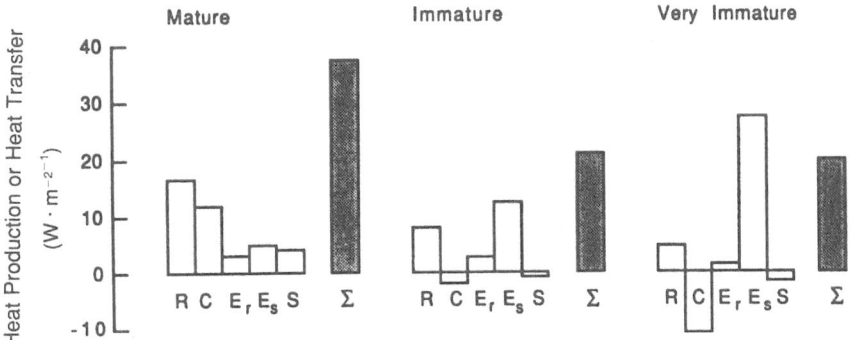

FIGURE 45.9. Heat exchanges in the term, 32-week, and under-28-week prematurely born neonate, nursed in an incubator. The neonates were nursed so their rectal temperatures were around 37°C. The very immature neonate gained heat by convection, and the surrounding air was warmer than the infant's surface temperature. R, radiation; C, convection; E, evaporation divided into that from the respiration tract (r) and that from the skin surface (s); S, heat storage. The shaded column on the right gives the net sum (Σ) of the heat exchanges. (From Hull,[115] with permission.)

room, and mainly influenced by the air temperature of the incubator. The inner wall of a double-walled incubator is usually warmer than the wall of a single-walled incubator, making this incubator especially suitable for the neonate of very low birth weight in whom a high environmental temperature more than 35°C is needed. The wall temperature of a single-walled incubator with an air temperature of 37°C placed in a room of 24°C is 33.6°C. The air temperature must be increased to 38.5° to 39.0°C to compensate for the radiant heat loss and to have an operative temperature of 37°C.[121] Another important aspect of the environmental conditions in the incubator is the humidity, especially for the neonate born at less than 30 weeks' gestation during the first days after birth. Increasing the humidity of the incubator air causes a marked reduction in evaporative heat loss in the neonate, allowing heat to be lost by convection and radiation.[122] Keeping the relative humidity at least 60% at all incubator air temperatures seems to be advisable, although these advantages must be balanced against potential risks of infection.[123] It might be impossible to achieve a thermoneutral environment for the very low birth weight neonate, even in double-walled incubators, unless the humidity is increased to the above-mentioned relative value of 60%. The mode of heat loss in an incubator for a term neonate, a preterm neonate born after 32 weeks, and a very preterm neonate born after 26 weeks—all kept at a core temperature of 37°C—are shown in Figure 45.9. The term neonate has heat loss due equally to radiation and convection and low heat loss due to evaporation, whereas the very premature neonate has a high heat loss due to evaporation, with heat gained by convection. The modes of heat loss depend on the type of incubator: In double-walled incubators radiant heat loss was found to be decreased but convective heat loss increased, causing an equal total heat loss.[124]

Heat Balance Using Radiant Heat

A completely different system for nursing the neonate is the use of radiant heat. This system consists of a powerful overhead radiant heat source that uniformly distributes radiant power over a mattress surface on an open bed. The mode of heat loss of this system is different from that seen with the incubator (Figure 45.10). Radiant heat loss is changed into heat gain by radiation, whereas heat losses by convection in the term neonate and by convection and evaporation in the preterm neonate are relatively high. A radiant temperature of 45°C may be needed to maintain core and skin temperatures within

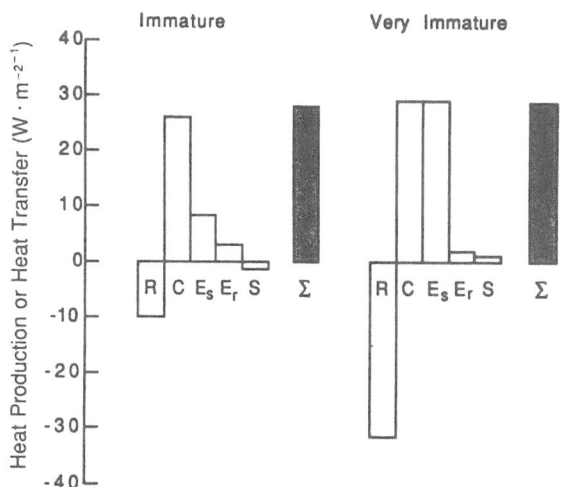

FIGURE 45.10. Heat exchanges of a 32-week neonate and an under 28-week neonate nursed under a radiant warmer. Large radiant heat gain is required by the very immature neonate to maintain body temperature. See Figure 45.9 for abbreviations. (From Hull,[115] with permission.)

the normal range. Radiant heaters are usually set using a servocontrol and a probe attached to the abdominal skin set between 36° and 37°C. The heat loss and heat gain are rather different at different sites of the body, resulting in marked differences in body temperature at different locations of the body[22] and a loss of the normal temperature difference between the core and the skin. It is not clear if this inhomogeneous body temperature and the heterogeneity of the environment cause a problem. Some studies have found a higher oxygen consumption in the neonate under a radiant heater,[21,125] but these data have not been confirmed by others.[115,126]

Implications

The body temperature of the preterm infant is the result of a balance between heat production within the body and heat loss. Heat loss in the neonate, and especially the very preterm neonate is high due to the properties of the skin: the low insulation, high evaporation, and limited capacity to vasoconstrict. The body surface area is high in relation to weight. Extra heat can be generated especially in brown adipose tissue; neonates do not show evidence of shivering. The heat production in brown adipose tissue is dependent on the uncoupling protein; its production and activity are regulated by noradenaline and the intracellular T_3 concentration.

Although the fetus has the capacity of active thermoregulation before birth, it passively follows the temperature of the mother. There is an inhibitor of thermoregulation, probably through prostaglandin E_2 amd adenosine.

After birth, the neonate shows a thermoregulatory response initiated by the clamping of the cord, cooling of the skin and initiation of breathing. The response found in the very preterm neonate, however, is rather limited, together with high heat loss causing a situation very prone for hypothermia. As a low body temperature is associated with an increased incidence in mortality and lower growth, the neonate should be protected from hypothermia and be nursed in a warm, humid environment. Whether this should also be advised for the term infant with severe asphyxia requires further study.

References

1. Budin P. "Le nourisson," alimentation et hygiene des enfants debiles—enfants nes a terme. Paris: Octave Dion, 1900.
2. Silverman WA, Fertig JW, Berger AP. The influence of the thermal environment upon the survival of newly born premature infants. Pediatrics 1958;22:876–886.
3. Silverman WA, Blanc WA. The effect of humidity on survival of newly born premature infants. Pediatrics 1957;20:477–487.
4. Blackfan KD, Yaglou CP. The premature infant: a study of the effects of atmospheric conditions on growth and on development. Am J Dis Child 1933;46:1175–1236.
5. Glass L, Silverman WA, Sinclair JC. Effect of the thermal environment on cold resistance and growth of small infants after the first week of life. Pediatrics 1968;41:1033–1046.
6. Mondhorst H. Uber die chemische Wärmeregulation frühgeborener Säuglinge. Monatsschr Kinderheilkd 1932;55:174–191.
7. Day R, Hardy JD. Respiratory metabolism in infancy and in childhood. XXVI. A calorimeter for measuring the heat loss of premature infants. Am J Dis Child 1942;63:1086–1095.
8. Brück K. Temperature regulation in the newborn infant. Blot Neonate 1961;3:65–119.
9. Brück K, Parmelee AH Jr, Brück M. Neutral temperature range of "thermal comfort" in premature infants. Biol Neonate 1962;4:31–51.
10. Hey EN, Mount LE. Heat losses from babies in incubators. Arch Dis Child 1967;42:75–84.
11. Hey EN, Maurice NP. Effect of humidity on production and loss of heat in the newborn baby. Arch Dis Child 1968;43:166–171.
12. Hey EN, Katz G. The optimum thermal environment of naked babies. Arch Dis Child 1970;45:328–334.
13. Hey EN. The care of babies in incubators. In: Gairdner D, Hull D, eds. Recent advances in paediatrics. London: Churchill Livingstone, 1971:171–215.
14. Darnall RA. The thermophysiology of the newborn infant. Med Instr 1987;21:16–22.
15. Adamsons K Jr, Gandy GM, James LS. The influence of thermal factors upon oxygen consumption of the newborn human infant. J Pediatr 1965;66:495–508.
16. Mestyan J, Jarai I, Fekete M. The significance of facial skin temperature in the chemical heat regulation of premature infants. Biol Neonate 1964;7:243–254.
17. Dane HJ. Temperature regulation in newborn infants. Thesis, Technical University, Delft, The Netherlands.
18. Wheldon AE. Energy balance in the newborn baby: use of a manikin to estimate radiant and convective heat loss. Phys Med Biol 1982;27:285–296.
19. LeBlanc MH, Edwards NK. Artifacts in the measurement of skin temperature under infant radiant warmers. Ann Biomed Eng 1985;13:443–450.
20. Baumgart S. Partitioning of heat losses and gains in premature newborn infants under radiant warmers. Pediatrics 1985;75:89–99.
21. Wheldon AE, Rutter N. The heat balance of small babies nursed in incubators and under radiant warmers. Early Hum Dev 1982;6:131–143.
22. Baumgart S. Radiant heat loss versus radiant heat gain in premature neonates under radiant warmers. Biol Neonate 1990;57:10–20.
23. Topper WH, Stewart TP. Thermal support for the very low birth weight infant: role of supplemental conductive heat. J Pediatr 1984;105:810–814.
24. Hammarlund K, Sedin G. Transepidermal water loss in newborn infants. III. Relation to gestational age. Acta Paediatr Scand 1979;68:795–801.

25. Hammarlund K, Sedin G, Strömberg B. Transepidermal water loss in newborn infants. VIII. Relation to gestational age and postnatal age in appropriate and small for gestational age infants. Acta Paediatr Scand 1983;72:721–727.
26. Rutter N, Hull D. Water loss from the skin of term and preterm babies. Arch Dis Child 1979;58:858–868.
27. Sauer PJJ, Dane HJ, Visser HKA. Influence of variations in the ambient humidity on insensible water loss and thermoneutral environment of low birth weight infants. Acta Paediatr Scand 1984;73:615–619.
28. Abrams RM. Energy exchange in utero. In: Moghissi KS, Hofez ESE, eds. The placenta: biological and clinical aspects. Springfield, IL: Charles C Thomas, 1974:28–53.
29. Abrams RM, Caton D, Clapp J, et al. Temperature differences in reproductive tract of nonpregnant ewe. Am J Obstet Gynecol 1971;110:370–375.
30. Gilbert RD, Schroder H. Kawamura T, et al. Heat transfer pathways between the fetal lamb and ewe. J Appl Physiol 1985;59:634–638.
31. Kubota S, Koyanagi T, Hori E, et al. Homeothermal adjustment in the immediate postdelivered infant monitored by continuous and simultaneous measurement of core and peripheral body temperatures. Biol Neonate 1988;54:79–85.
32. Hey EN. The relation between environmental temperature and oxygen consumption in the newborn baby. J Physiol (Lond) 1969;200:589–603.
33. Smales O. Simple method for measuring oxygen consumption in babies. Arch Dis Child 1978;53:53–57.
34. Heim T, Cser A, Jaszai V. Energy metabolism and thermal homeostasis in the newborn. In: Stern L, ed. Intensive care in the newborn II. New York: Masson, 1979:275–305.
35. Hill JR. The oxygen consumption of newborn and adult mammals. J Physiol (Lond) 1959;149:346–373.
36. Scopes JW, Ahmed J. Indirect assessment of oxygen requirements in newborn babies by monitoring deep body temperature. Arch Dis Child 1966;41:25–33.
37. Chance GW, O'Brien MJ, Swyer PR. Transportation of sick neonates 1972: an unsatisfactory aspect of medical care. Can Med Assoc J 1973;109:847–850.
38. Gunn TR, Outerbridge EW. Effectiveness of neonatal transport. Can Med Assoc J 1978;118:646–649.
39. Biggar WD, Bohn D, Kent G. Neutrophil circulation and release from bone marrow during hypothermia. Infect Immun 1983;40:708–712.
40. Alexander G, Bell AW. Hales JRS. Effects of cold exposure on tissue blood flow in the newborn lamb. J Physiol (Lond) 1973;23:65–77.
41. Alexander G, Williams D. Shivering and nonshivering thermogenesis during summit metabolism in young lambs. J Physiol (Lond) 1968;198:251–276.
42. Silverman WA, Zamelis A, Sinclair JC. Warm nape of the newborn. Pediatrics 1964;33:984–987.
43. Karlberg P, Moore RE, Oliver TK. Thermogenic and cardiovascular responses of the newborn baby to noradrenaline. Acta Paediatr Scand 1965;54:225–238.
44. Schiff D, Stern L, Leduc J. Chemical thermogenesis in newborn infants: catecholamine excretion and the plasma nonesterified fatty acid response to cold exposure. Pediatrics 1966;37:577–582.
45. Heim T. Energy requirements of thermoregulatory heat production in the newly born. In: Monset-Couchard M, Minnkowsky A, eds. Physiological and biochemical basis for perinatal medicine. Basel: Karger, 1981:158–174.
46. Heim T, Hull D. The blood flow and oxygen consumption of brown adipose tissue in the newborn rabbit to catecholamines, glucagon, corticotrophin and cold exposure. J Physiol (Lond) 1966;187:271–283.
47. Baum D, Anthony CL, Stowers C. Impairment of cold-stimulated lipolysis by acute hypoxia. Am J Dis Child 1971;121:115–119.
48. Lean ME, James WPT, Jennings G, et al. Brown adipose tissue uncoupling protein content in human infants, children and adults. Clin Sci 1986;71:291–297.
49. Slotkin TA, Seidler FJ. Adrenomedullary catecholamine release in the fetus and newborn: secretory mechanisms and their role in stress and survival. J Dev Physiol 1988;10:1–16.
50. Whitsett JA, Noguchi A, Moore JJ. Developmental aspects of α- and β-adrenergic receptors. Semin Perinatol 1982;6:125–141.
51. Symonds ME, Clarke L, Lomax MA. The regulation of neonatal metabolism and growth. In: Ward RHT, Smith SK, Donnai D, eds. Early fetal growth and development. London: RCOG Press, 1994:407–419.
52. Agata Y, Padbury JF, Ludlow JK, et al. The effect of chemical sympathectomy on catecholamine release at birth. Pediatr Res 1986;20:1338–1344.
53. Alexander G, Stevens G. Sympathetic innervation and the development of structure and function of brown adipose tissue: studies on lambs chemically sympathectomized in utero with 6-hydroxydopamine. J Dev Physiol 1980;2:119–137.
54. Eliot RJ, Klein AH, Glatz TH, et al. Plasma norepinephrine, epinephrine and dopamine concentrations in maternal and fetal sheep during spontaneous parturition and in premature sheep during cortisol-induced parturition. Endocrinology 1981;108:1678–1682.
55. Lagercrantz H, Bistoletti P. Catecholamine release in the newborn infant at birth. Pediatr Res 1973:11:889–893.
56. Falconer AD, Lake DM. Circumstances influencing umbilical-cord plasma catecholamines at delivery. Br J Obstet Gynaecol 1982;9:44–49.
57. Irestedt L, Lagercrantz H, Hjemdahl P, et al. Fetal and maternal plasma catecholamine levels at elective caesarean section under general or epidural anaesthesia versus vaginal delivery. Am J Obstet Gynaecol 1982;142:1004–1010.
58. Ricquier D, Bouillaud F. The brown adipose tissue mitochondrial uncoupling protein. In: Trayburn P, Nicholls BG, eds. Brown adipose tissue. London: Arnold.
59. Ricquier D, Bouillaud F, Toumelin P. Expression of uncoupling protein mRNA in thermogenic or weakly thermogenic brown adipose tissue. J Biochem Chem 1986;261:13905–13910.
60. Mohell N, Connolly E, Nedergaard J. Distinction between mechanisms underlying α and β adrenergic respiratory stimulation in brown fat cells. Am J Physiol 1987;253:C301–308.

61. Nicholls DG, Loche RM. Thermogenic mechanisms in brown fat. Physiol Rev 1984;64:1–64.
62. Christensson K, Siles C, Cabrera T, et al. Lower body temperatures in infants delivered by caesarean section than in vaginally delivered infants. Acta Pediatr 1993;82:128–131.
63. Clarke L, Darby CJ, Lomax MA, et al. Effect of ambient temperature during 1st day of life on thermoregulation in lambs delivered by caesarean section. J Appl Physiol 1994;76:1481–1488.
64. Champigny L, Holloway BR, Ricquier D. Regulation of UCP gene expression in brown adipocyte differentiated in primary culture. Effects of a new β-adrenoreceptor agonist. Mol Cell Endocrinol 1992;86:73–82.
65. Clarke L, Andrews DC, Crompton LA. Effects of B_3-adrenergic agonist administration on brown adipose tissue in the newborn lamb. J Physiol 1993;467;291P (abstr).
66. Symonds ME, Bird JA, Clarke L, et al. Manipulation of brown adipose tissue development in neonatal and postnatal lambs. In: Milton AS, ed. Temperature regulation. Switzerland: Birkhauser 1994:309–314.
67. Polk DH. Thyroid hormone effects on neonatal thermogenesis. Semin Perinatol 1988;12:151–156.
68. Symonds ME, Lomax MA. Maternal and environmental influences on thermoregulation in the neonate. Proc Nutr Soc 1992;51:165–172.
69. Fowden AL, Silver M. The effects of thyroxine deficiency on oxygen utilization by the sheep fetus. J Physiol 1993;459:328P (abstr).
70. Thorbum GD, Hopkins PS. Thyroid function in the foetal lamb. In: Comline KS, Cross KW, Dawes, et al., eds. Foetal and neonatal physiology. Cambridge: Cambridge University Press, 1973:488–507.
71. Breall JA, Rudolph AM, Heymann MA. Role of thyroid hormone in postnatal and metabolic adjustments. J Clin Invest 1984;73:1418–1424.
72. Silva JE, Larsen PR. Adrenergic activation of triiodothyronine production in brown adipose tissue. Nature 1983;305:712–713.
73. Wu SY, Polk DH, Fisher DA. Biochemical and ontogenic characterization of thyroxine 5'-monodeiodinase in brown adipose tissue from fetal and newborn lambs. Endocrinology 1986;118:1334–1339.
74. Whitaker EM, Hussain SH, Hervey GR, et al. Is increased metabolism in rats in the cold mediated by the thyroid? J Physiol 1990;431:543–556.
75. Gunn TR, Gluckmann PD. The endocrine control of the onset of thermogenesis at birth. In: Jones CT, ed. Baillière's clinical endocrinology and metabolism. London: Baillière Tindall, 1989:869–886.
76. Bianco AC, Silva JE. Optimal response of key enzymes and uncoupling protein to cold in BAT depends on local T_3 generation. Am J Physiol 1987;253:E255–263.
77. Bianco AC, Silva JE. Intracellular conversion of thyroxine to triiodothyronine is required for the optimal thermogenic function of brown adipose tissue. J Clin Invest 1987;79:295–300.
78. Obregon MJ, Pitamber J, Jacobsson A, et al. Euthyroid status is essential for the perinatal increase in thermogenin mRNA in brown adipose tissue of rat pups. Biochem Biophys Res Commun 1987;148:9–14.
79. Giralt M, Martin I, Iglesias R, et al. Ontogeny and perinatal modulation of gene expression in rat brown adipose tissue. Unaltered iodothyronine 5'-deiodinase activity is necessary for the response to environmental temperature at birth. Eur J Biochem 1990;193:297–302.
80. Gunn TR, Gluckman PD. The development of temperature regulation in the fetal sheep. J Dev Physiol Oxf 1983;5:167–179.
81. Gluckman PD, Gunn TR, Johnson BM. The effect of cooling on breathing and shivering in unanaesthetized fetal lambs in utero. J Physiol 1983;343:495–506.
82. Kawamura T, Gilbert RD, Power GG. Effect of cooling and heating on the regional distribution of blood flow in fetal sheep. J Dev Physiol Oxf 1986;8:11–22.
83. Fraser M, Gunn TR, Butler JH, et al. Circulating thyrotropin (TSH) in the ovine fetus: evidence for pulsatile release and the effect of hypothermia in utero. Pediatr Res 1985;19:208–212.
84. Gunn TR, Johnston BM, Iwamoto HS, et al. Haemodynamic and catecholamine responses to hypothermia in the fetal sheep in utero. J Dev Physiol 1985;7:241–249.
85. James E, Meschia G, Battaglia FC. A-V differences of free fatty acids and glycerol in the ovine umbilical circulation. Proc Soc Exp Biol Med 1971;138:823–826.
86. Lorijn RHW, Longo LD. Norepinephrine elevation in the fetal lamb: oxygen consumption and cardiac output. Am J Physiol 1980;239:R115–R122.
87. Hodgkin DD, Gilbert RD, Power GG. In vivo brown fat response to hypothermia and norepinephrine in the ovine fetus. J Dev Physiol Oxf 1988;10:383–391.
88. Power GG, Gunn TR, Johnstone BM. Umbilical cord occlusion but not increased plasma T_3 or norepinephrine stimulate brown adipose tissue thermogenesis in the fetal sheep. J Dev Physiol 1989;11:171–177.
89. Gunn TR, Ball KT, Gluckman PD. Reversible umbilical cord occlusion: effects on thermogenesis in utero. Pediatr Res 1991;30:513–517.
90. Gunn TR, Gluckman PD. Perinatal thermogeneses. Early Hum Dev 1995;42:169–183.
91. Gunn TR, Ball KT, Gluckman PD. Withdrawal of placental prostaglandins permits thermogenic responses in fetal sheep brown adipose tissue. J Appl Physiol 1993;73:998–1004.
92. Takeuchi M, Yoneyama Y, Power GG. Role of prostaglandin E2 and prostacyclin in nonshivering thermogenesis during simulated birth in utero. Prostaglandins Leukot Essent Fatty Acids 1994;51:373–380.
93. Woodward JA, Saggerson ED. Effect of adenosine deaminase. N^6-phenylisopropyladenosine and hypothyroidism on the responsiveness of rat brown adipocytes to noradrenaline. Biochem J 1986;238:395–403.
94. Slegel P, Kitagawa H, Maguire MH. Determination of adenosine in fetal perfusates of human placental cotyledons using fluorescence derivatization and reversed-phase high-performance liquid chromatography. Ann Biochem 1988;171:124–134.

95. Belle van H. Uptake and deamination of adenosine by blood. Species differences, effect of pH, ions, temperature and metabolic inhibitors. Biochem Biophys Acta 1969;192: 124–132.
96. Sawa R, Asakura H, Power GG. Changes in plasma adenosine during simulated birth of fetal sheep. J Appl Physiol 1991;70:1524–1528.
97. Ball KT, Gunn TR, Power GG, et al. A potential role for adenosine in the inhibition of nonshivering thermogenesis in the fetal sheep. Pediatr Res 1995;37:303–309.
98. Bligh J, Jonson KG. Glossary of terms for thermal physiology. J Appl Physiol 1973;35:941–961.
99. Sulyok E, Jequier E, Prod'hom LS. Thermal balance of the newborn infant in a heat gaining environment. Pediatr Res 1973;7:888–900.
100. Bell EF, Gray JC, Weinstein MR, et al. The effects of thermal environment on heat balance and insensible water loss in low-birth-weight infants. J Pediatr 1980;96:452–459.
101. Wheldon AE, Harpin VA. Metabolic rat in newborn babies in thermoneutral conditions and when overheated. Early Hum Dev 1982;6:249–252.
102. Harpin VA, Chellappah G, Rutter N. Responses of the newborn infant to overheating. Biol Neonate 1983;44:65–75.
103. Harpin VA, Rutter N. Sweating in preterm babies. J Pediatr 1982;100:614–619.
104. Wheldon AE, Hull D. Incubation of very immature infants. Arch Dis Child 1983;58:501–508.
105. Sauer PJJ, Dane HJ, Visser HKA. New standards for neutral thermal environment of healthy very low birth weight infants in week one of life. Arch Dis Child 1984; 59:18–22.
106. Ducker DA, Lyon AJ, Ross RR, et al. Incubator temperature control: effects on the very low birth weight infant. Arch Dis Child 1985;60:902–907.
107. Rutter N, Brown SM, Hull D. Variations in the resting oxygen consumption of small babies. Arch Dis Child 1978; 53:850–854.
108. American Academy of Pediatrics and American College of Obstetricians and Gynecologists. Guidelines for perinatal care. New York: March of Dimes Edition, 1988:274–281.
109. Thoresen M, Penrice J, Lorek A, et al. Mild hypothermia after severe transient hypoxia-ischemia ameliorates delayed cerebral energy failure in the newborn piglet. Pediatr Res 1995;37:667–670.
110. Edwards AD, Xue X, Squier MW, et al. Specific inhibition of apoptosis after cerebral hypoxia-ischaemia by moderate post-insult hypothermia. Biochem Biophys Res Commun 1995;217:1193–1199.
111. Laptook AR, Corbett RJ, Sterett R, et al. Modest hypothermia provides partial neuroprotection for ischemic neonatal brain. Pediatr Res 1994;35:436–442.
112. Gidday JM, Fitzgibbons JC, Shah AR, et al. Reduction in cerebral ischemic injury in the newborn rat by potentiation of endogenous adenosine. Pediatr Res 1995;38:306–311.
113. Evans NJ, Rutter N. Development of the epidermis in the newborn. Biol Neonate 1986;49:74–80.
114. Wu PYK, Wong WH, Guerra G, et al. Peripheral blood flow in the neonate. 1. Changes in total, skin, and muscle blood flow with gestational and postnatal age. Pediatr Res 1980;14:1374–1378.
115. Hull D. Thermal control in very immature infants. Br Med Bull 1988;44:971–983.
116. Heimler R, Sumners JE, Grausz JP, et al. Thermal environment change in growing premature infants: effect on general somatic growth and subcutaneous fat accumulation. Pediatrics 1981;68:82–86.
117. Chessex P, Blouet S, Voucher J. Environmental temperature control in very low birth weight infants (less than 1000 grams) cared for in double-walled incubators. J Pediatr 1988;113:373–380.
118. Perlstein PH, Edwards NK, Sutherland JM. Apnea in premature infants and incubator-air-temperature changes. N Engl J Med 1970;282:461–466.
119. Bell EF, Rios GR. Air versus skin temperature servo-control of infant incubators. J Pediatr 1983;103:954–958.
120. Swyer PR. Heat loss after birth. In: Sinclair JC, ed. Temperature regulation and energy metabolism in the newborn. Orlando: Grune & Stratton, 1978:91–128.
121. Sauer PJJ. Aspects of thermal regulation. In: Duc G, ed. Controversial issues in neonatal interventions. Stuttgart: Georg Thieme Verlag, 1989:94–108.
122. Sedin G, Hammarlund K, Riesenfeld T, et al. The influence of humidity. In: Duc G, ed. Controversial issues in neonatal interventions. Stuttgart: Georg Thieme Verlag, 1989:109–122.
123. Harpin VA, Rutter N. Humidification of incubators. Arch Dis Child 1985;60:219–224.
124. Bell EF, Rios GR. A double-walled incubator alters the partition of body heat loss of premature infants. Pediatr Res 1983;17:135–140.
125. LeBlanc MH. Relative efficacy of an incubator and an open warmer in producing thermoneutrality for the small premature infant. Pediatrics 1982;69:439.
126. Marks KH, Nardis EE, Momin MN. Energy metabolism and substrate utilization in low birth weight neonates under radiant warmers. Pediatrics 1986;78:465–472.
127. Sinclair JC, ed. Temperature regulation and preterm infants at different ages and different ambient and energy metabolism in the newborn. Orlando: Grune & Stratton, 1978:129–156.
128. Sinclair JC. Metabolic rate and temperature control in the newborn. In: Goodwin JW, Godden JO, Chance GW, eds. Perinatal medicine: the basic science underlying clinical practice. Baltimore: Williams & Wilkins, 1976:S58–S77.

46
Neonatal Water and Electrolyte Metabolism

Andrew T. Costarino and Stephen Baumgart

Water composes over 60% of all body matter in the adult, and close to 80% in the neonate.[1,2] Water serves as the vehicle to carry nutrients to the body's cells and remove its waste materials. The distribution of water determines the size of the body fluid compartments, and with water concentration, establishes the physiochemical milieu that allows cellular work to occur. Thus, water metabolism is integral to all life functions. This comprehensive review of water metabolism in the neonate, encompasses cellular regulation, cardiac and vascular physiology, as well as renal, neurologic, and hormonal functions.

Total body water volume (TBW) is usually expressed as a percent of total body weight. The plasma membranes of all of the body's cells establish two large divisions of the TBW: intracellular water (ICW), which is contained within the cells, and extracellular water (ECW), which surrounds the cells. This chapter begins with a presentation of the popular notion of the evolution of higher life forms[3,4] that provides the construct for understanding this distribution of TBW and the relationship of TBW to energy metabolism. Subsequent sections discuss cell volume regulation and the interface between the intracellular and the extracellular body fluid compartments, the control of the extracellular water through the interaction with the neonatal heart and kidney, and the hormonal modulation systems. Following sections emphasize the neonate's changes in water distribution during the transition from fetal to extrauterine life, and the premature neonatal adaptation to water loss upon exposure to a hostile environment (see Chapter 25).

Five common patient scenarios are presented in the final section to illustrate clinical manifestations of the basic principles developed in previous sections: the neonate with respiratory distress syndrome (RDS), the subsequent development of chronic pulmonary dysfunction (BPD), the critically ill premature neonate with shock and massive edema, the very low birth weight neonate of less than 26 weeks' gestation, and the growing premature neonate recovering from these conditions who manifests hyponatremia and edema.

Body Water Compartment Regulation

It is widely speculated that primitive, single-cell life forms first appeared in an ocean environment that was similar in composition to the ECW of modern mammals.[3,4] As these organisms evolved into more complicated multicellular, multitissue beings, they surrounded their cells with an internalized version of the primitive ocean allowing them to thrive in less constant external environments. The famous physiologist, Claude Bernard (1813–1878), called this the "milieu interior."[4] With such an organization, the internal cellular compartment is shielded from direct interface with the harsh modern environment, and can continue its primitive methods of regulating cell size and composition because it is buffered from sudden changes in solute and water content by the extracellular compartment. This arrangement, however, demands that the organism have a system to monitor the composition of the ECW, and have physiologic strategies to correct water and solute losses and gains resulting from its contact with the outside world.

Losses and gains of water and solute due to this interaction with the environment are coupled to the metabolic rate of an organism in a predictable way (Figure 46.1).[4,5] This interaction demands less than half the usual amount of energy a growing infant produces by metabolism.[5–7] The fuels oxidized to produce this metabolic energy are the carbon skeletons of carbohydrates, fats, and proteins. The by-products of energy production are carbon dioxide (CO_2), water, nitrogen waste, fixed acids, and heat. The fuels are carried into the organism with water, and the elimination of the waste products of metabolism results in water loss. Water is evaporated passively from the upper respiratory tract as CO_2 is exhaled during respiration. Excess heat is dissipated from the skin actively

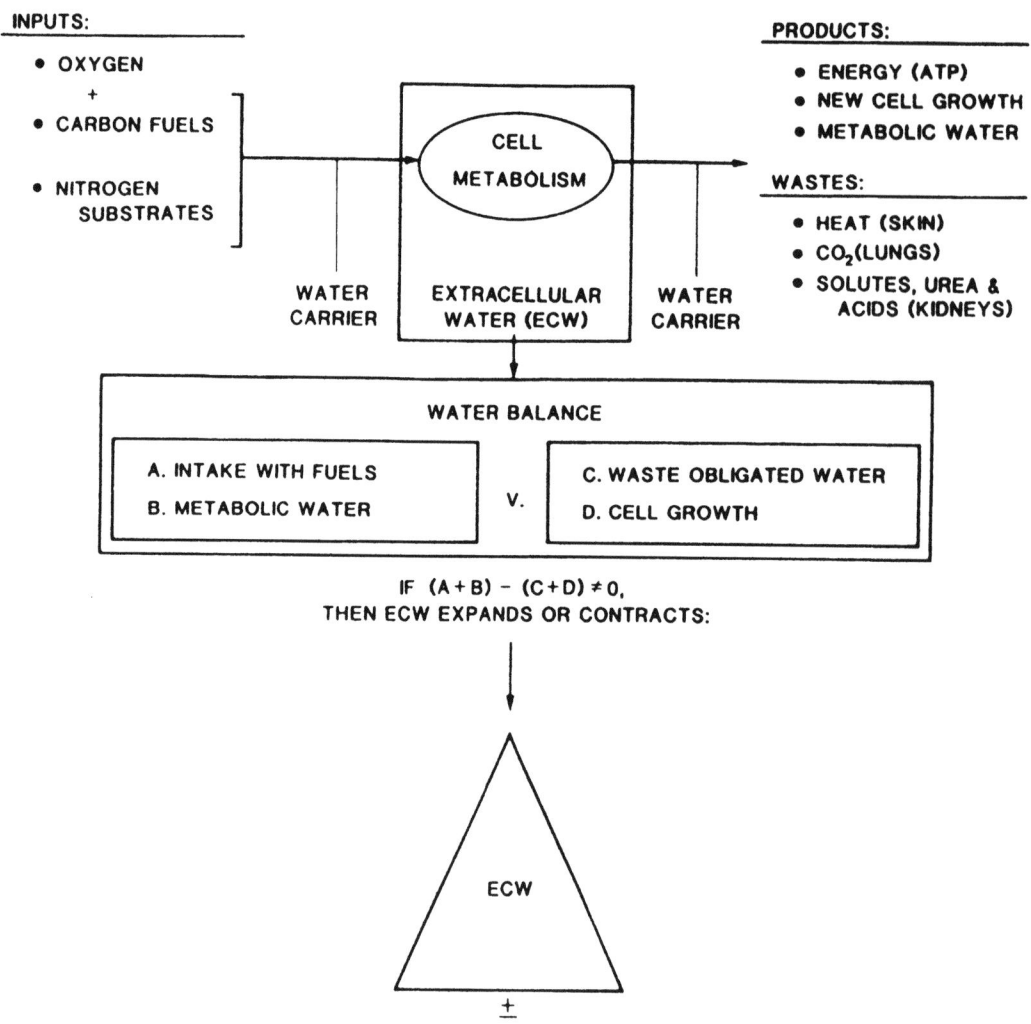

FIGURE 46.1. The relationship between the components of cellular metabolism and water balance in the extracellular compartment.

through sweating and passively through insensible evaporation of interstitial water. Nitrogen wastes and fixed acids are eliminated in the urine, necessitating renal water loss, while a small amount of water is lost from the gastrointestinal tract and a comparable small amount of water is gained from the oxidation of the carbon fuels. Finally, during growth, water is incorporated into new tissue in proportion to the quantity of intracellular solutes acquired. Regulation of all of these processes begins at the plasma membrane.

Osmolality and Osmotic Pressure

Like all chemicals, water spontaneously moves from a region of high concentration to one of low concentration. Such movement occurring through a semipermeable membrane, like the cell membrane, is called osmosis, from the Greek word for impulsation. The same Greek root provides the terms osmolality, quantity of water in solution, and osmotic pressure, the force that drives the movement of water between areas of different concentration.

Osmolality is the number of discrete particles of solute per kilogram of solvent.* The unit of measure of osmolality is the osmole. One osmole is the number of particles (Avogadro's number) in one gram molecular weight of a substance that does not dissociate in solution. If a solute dissociates into two ions when in solution, one gram mo-

---

*Solute concentration in body fluids is commonly measured by freezing point osmometry (one gram mole of solute per kilogram of water will lower its freezing point by 1.858°C).[8] The concentration of solute particles when expressed as the number of discrete particles per kilogram of solvent is properly termed osmolality. In physiologic studies, however, it is often more useful to know the number of discrete particles per liter of solution. The precise term for this quantity is osmolarity. Because the difference between the osmolality and osmolarity is small in physiologic solutions, the measured value for osmolality is commonly used as if it were the osmolarity and the term osmolality is used for either case.

lecular weight of that substance will contain two osmoles. In physiologic solutions the amount of solute is small so solute concentration is expressed in milliosmoles (mOsm) per kilogram.

Expressing the water concentration of a solution is confusing because water is the solvent in all body fluids. Although the same principle of osmolar concentration outlined above for the solutes applies to the solvent water particles, it is common to describe a solution by its concentration of solutes. For example, a solution of "pure" water contains 55.6 osmoles of water per kilogram (i.e., gram molecular weight of water = 18, therefore 1000 g/18 = 55.6 osmoles); but if sodium chloride or another solute were added to the solution, the water concentration would be diluted to less than this value. The second solution, however, is commonly described as having a higher osmolality due to its relatively higher concentration of sodium chloride. Thus, the concentration of water is expressed in the converse: solutions of low osmolality have a high concentration of water, and water is diluted in solutions with higher solute osmolality.

The water movement across semipermeable plasma membranes is important in regulating cell volume. The force driving water through a semipermeable membrane is called the osmotic pressure and its magnitude is proportional to the difference in the concentration of water on either side of the membrane. The van't Hoff equation expresses this force in terms of millimeters of mercury[9]:

$$P = cRT \qquad (1)$$

where P = osmotic pressure (mmHg),
c = solute concentration (osm/L),
R = the universal gas constant (62.3 mmHg) × L/(osm × °K),
T = the absolute temperature (°K).

Solving Equation 1 at body temperature demonstrates that $1\,mOsm \cdot L^{-1}$ of solution exerts 19.3 mmHg of osmotic pressure.[10] The osmolality of both the ECW and the ICW is normally between 270 and 300 mOsm, so on average the osmotic pressure in each compartment is 5500 mmHg. Since each compartment has the same or similar osmolality, there is no net movement of water. However, if a cell were suddenly placed into pure water, a force equal to 5500 mmHg would drive water into the cell. This is why hypotonic extracellular states may disrupt normal cell function, as when an intravenous infusion of sterile water causes hemolysis.

Regulation of the ICW

The principles of osmosis and osmotic pressure dictate that net movement of water between or within body fluids results only from differences in water concentration. The size of each compartment (e.g., the ICW and ECW), then, is determined by the volume of TBW and the quantity of diffusible and nondiffusible particles distributed within each.[11] In the mature mammal, approximately two thirds of all body solutes are found in the ICW and one third in the ECW. Therefore, the ICW is two times larger than the ECW. The percentage of TBW distributed to the each compartment, and by implication the distribution of body solutes, is dramatically different in the fetus, and large changes in both water and solutes occur during early neonatal life.[2,12,13]

The major solutes in the ICW are (1) the mass of intracellular proteins necessary for cell function, (2) organic phosphates associated with cellular energy production, and (3) the equivalent cations necessary to balance phosphate and protein anions.[1,11] The cell membrane is relatively impermeable to both the organic phosphates and the proteins, and it selectively pumps potassium into the cell in exchange for sodium. The result is that the major intracellular cation is potassium and the major extracellular cation is sodium.[1] Potential energy stored by creating a concentration difference for sodium and potassium between the ICW and the ECW allows cellular work.

Regulation of cellular production of the nondiffusible proteins and exchange of the diffusible sodium and potassium cations are the energy consuming, or active determinants of cellular size.[11] Because water movement is driven by osmotic pressure, any change in osmolality of the ECW is reflected in net movement of water into or out of the cell. The mechanisms that control the water concentration in ECW ultimately influence the volume of the ICW; however, cells have active methods for regulating their volume.[11,14,15] Cells respond to changes in volume by gaining or losing osmotically active solutes.[16] The most rapid response to cell volume change comes from control of the rate of potassium chloride uptake or loss. However, this system is not adequate to compensate for challenges to cell volume because large shifts in the concentration of intracellular potassium would have serious consequences on cell function. ICW volume is most likely regulated by organic osmolytes, small organic molecules that exist in the cytoplasm in high concentrations. Cells are able to alter the concentration of these compounds dramatically without harmful effects on cell structure or function. Three classes of organic osmolytes exist: the polyols (e.g., sorbitol and *myo*-inositol), amino acids (e.g., taurine, alanine, and proline), and the methylamines (e.g., betaine and glycerylphosphorylcholine).[11,15,16] Increased extracellular tonicity that tends to reduce cell volume will result in the accumulation of the organic osmolytes through their uptake from the extracellular space or changes in their production/degradation. These changes occur over hours. If an osmotic challenge occurs in the opposite direction, threatening cellular swelling, organic osmolytes decrease in concentration in two steps: first the osmolytes exit the cytoplasm through cell membrane channels that are activated by swelling, followed by reduction in the uptake or reduction in the production of these compounds.[16]

The effect of gestational development and of diseases of the fetus and neonate on the organic osmolyte system is incompletely understood, but recent study by Trachtman et al.[17] suggests that the cerebral ICW is greater in the developing mammal, and is associated with increased amounts of inorganic and organic osmolytes. The decrease in cell water content that occurs with maturation was most closely correlated with a decrease in the content of taurine. Taurine was the predominant organic osmolyte in the immature animal, as opposed to *myo-inositol* in the adult. These investigators concluded that the developing animal had a satisfactory ability to protect cerebral volume through the accumulation of organic and inorganic osmoles. They suggested that the developing animal responds as if it has a higher set point for intracellular osmolyte production in order to maintain a high brain water content.

Regulation of the ECW/ICW Interface: The Interstitial Compartment

The ECW compartment is subdivided into plasma water and nonplasma water (e.g., the intercellular or interstitial water) by the capillary endothelium.[1] The small but important differences between these two compartments allow the movement of water, with nutrients, from the circulating blood to the surrounding tissues. These differences are the result of a dynamic interaction of two forces: oncotic pressure (i.e., a result of the direct and indirect effects of the plasma proteins), and the hydrostatic pressure generated by the heart.[18] The principles of this interaction are important for understanding normal regulation of body water distribution and the pathophysiology of edema formation in the critically ill neonate.

Oncotic Pressure: A Special Case of Osmolality

Osmolality of body fluids is affected by the presence of large molecular weight plasma proteins, that is, molecules of larger than 40,000 daltons, sometimes called colloids.[19] These molecules do not pass freely through semipermeable membranes. Their particulate nature in solution exerts an osmotic force, and, because they are usually ionized at physiologic pH, there is an electromotive force associated with these molecules as well. These osmotic and electromotive forces cause an unequal distribution of the smaller diffusible ions (e.g., crystalloids) between body compartments known as the Gibbs-Donnan equilibrium (Figure 46.2).[9,20]

The high concentration of cations associated with the Gibbs-Donnan effect augments the osmotic pressure in the plasma compartment. The total increase in osmotic pressure of the plasma water, due to the protein plus cation content, is called the oncotic pressure, which is also termed colloid osmotic pressure. This force is approximately two thirds directly related to the nondiffus-

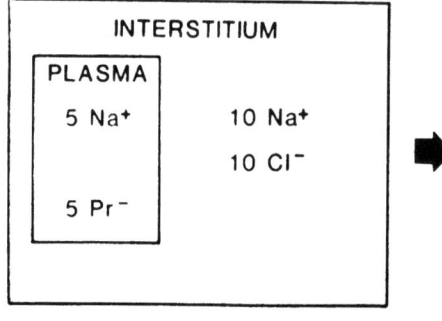 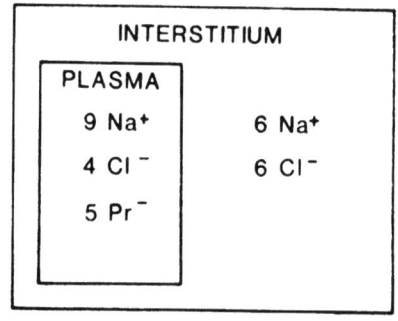

FIGURE 46.2. The Gibbs-Donnan equilibrium enhances the osmotic pressure in the protein rich plasma in the following way. The negatively charged plasma proteins allow a buildup of cations (e.g., mainly sodium) in plasma water against a concentration gradient. At equilibrium, both the plasma and the nonplasma water, separated by the capillary membrane, is electrically neutral (i.e., total cations equal total anions). Additionally, the product of the concentrations of the various diffusible ions on one side of the capillary membrane will equal the product of the concentrations of the same ions on the other; but there will be a higher concentration of diffusible ions in the plasma water. The presence of the nondiffusible plasma proteins by themselves results in increased osmotic pressure in the plasma water and this is enhanced by the the Gibbs-Donnan effect. The total increase in osmotic pressure of the plasma water due to the protein content is called the oncotic pressure. (From Valtin,[77] with permission.)

ible protein particles and one third a result of the difference in diffusible particles associated with the Gibbs-Donnan effect. Plasma oncotic pressure in the term neonate is in the range of 15 to 17 mm Hg compared to 25 to 28 mm Hg in the adult.[21,22] Although the Gibbs-Donnan equilibrium is especially important for the balance between the plasma and nonplasma water, it contributes to the osmolality of the ICW as well.

Hydrostatic/Osmotic Interaction: The Starling Relationship

Water movement across an idealized capillary wall is described by the relationship expressed in Equation 2 below. First described by Starling in 1896,[23] the formal mathematical treatment of the component forces leading to the equation was first presented only 45 years ago.[24,25]

$$J_V = K_F[(P_C - P_T) - \partial(\pi_P - \pi_T)] \quad (2)$$

where J_v = net flow across the capillary,
K_F = filtration coefficient,
P_C = capillary hydrostatic pressure,
P_T = interstitial hydrostatic pressure,
∂ = the Stavermann reflection coefficient,
π_P = plasma oncotic pressure,
π_T = interstitial oncotic pressure.

This relationship demonstrates that the movement of fluid out of the blood vessel is dependent on the product of the water permeability intrinsic to the capillaries (K_F), and the net driving pressure out of or into the capillary. That net driving pressure, $[(P_C - P_T) - \partial(\pi_P - \pi_T)]$, is a balance between the hydrostatic forces on either side of the capillary membrane ($P_C - P_T$), and the oncotic pressure on either side ($\pi_C - \pi_T$).[18,24,26]

Classically, the normal balance of these forces is thought to result in a small amount of water leaving the plasma at the arterial end of the capillary bed. Due to a fall in capillary hydrostatic pressure, much of it reenters the plasma at the venous end.[9] The small amount of fluid that remains in the interstitium is removed by lymphatic drainage.[27] In tissue in which the capillaries are not permeable to protein ($\partial > 0.8$), oncotic pressure differences across the vascular bed play an important role (e.g., brain, skin).[27] In tissue (or states) in which plasma proteins can pass easily through the capillary barrier (e.g., liver $\partial = 0.2 - 0.0$),[27,28] oncotic pressure forces do not counterbalance the tendency for hydrostatic forces to move water into the interstitium.

Disruption of the usual balance of forces within a tissue capillary bed may favor increased volume of fluid movement into the interstitium. For example, in conditions of high plasma hydrostatic pressure, increased vascular permeability, or low plasma oncotic pressure (Table 46.1), the lymphatic drainage must increase or tissue edema occurs.[9,29]

The ability to increase lymphatic drainage, like the other parameters related to capillary water exchange, varies among the different tissue beds. Thus, some organs are more or less prone to develop edema. Other factors affecting lymphatic drainage include (1) tissue movement, where lymphatic flow depends in part on tissue movement; (2) lymphatic obstruction due to tissue injury; and (3) mechanical factors (Table 46.1).[29]

K_F (Filtration Coefficient)

The filtration coefficient is proportional to two physical characteristics of the capillary bed: (1) permeability for water, or water conductance; and (2) the available capillary surface area.[9,24] Capillary permeability is largely

TABLE 46.1. Factors that promote water accumulation in the interstitial space.

Conditions of greater movement of water into the interstitium
I. High filtration coefficient
   Increased capillary permeability
     Tissues with large pores in the capillary endothelium
       Liver
       Spleen
     Conditions that injure the capillary membrane increasing permeability
       Sepsis
       Anaphylaxis
       Hypoxic tissue injury
   Increased capillary surface area
     Vasodilitation
II. Increased pressure gradient out of the capillary
   Increased hydrostatic pressure gradient
     Increased capillary hydrostatic pressure
       High cardiac output
       Venous obstruction
     Decreased tissue hydrostatic pressure
       Edematous states
   Decreased oncotic pressure gradient
     Decreased capillary oncotic pressure
       Prematurity
       Hyaline membrane disease
       Malnutrition
       Nephrotic syndrome
     Increased interstitial oncotic pressure
       Conditions associated with protein leak into the interstitium (prematurity, hyaline membrane disease, burns)

Conditions with decreased lymphatic drainage
I. Decreased muscle movement
   Therapeutic neuromuscular blockade or sedation
   Neurological injury
II. Lymphatic obstruction from scar
   Barotrauma/bronchopulmonary dysplasia
III. Mechanical factors
   Tight dressings around extremity
   High airway pressure obstructing lung lymphatics

determined by the number of pores (i.e., gaps) per square centimeter between endothelial cells that provide a channel for the water molecule. The number of these pores varies greatly among different tissue beds; for example, the capillaries of the liver are characterized by large numbers of very large openings, while those of the brain have almost none.[27,28]

Similarly, different tissues vary with regard to available capillary surface area. Thus, in experimental data, values for K_F are anywhere from 0.01 to 0.3 ml·min^{-1}mm Hg^{-1}100 g^{-1} tissue depending on the model.[26,27] Additionally, disease states, drugs, and mediators such as the leukotrienes (e.g., formerly, slow-reacting substance of anaphylaxis), histamine, and many of the prostaglandins alter K_F by affecting both the water conductance and the available surface area of the capillary bed.[30-32]

P_C (Capillary Hydrostatic Pressure)

The hydrostatic pressure in the capillary bed is dependent on the magnitude of the flow (i.e., the proportion of cardiac output) to that bed, and the resistance to flow at the venous end of the capillary bed.[9] P_C therefore will vary with the moment to moment changes in these determinants. Modulating influences on the determinants of P_C include systemic hormones, autonomic nervous system tone, and local tissue metabolic phenomenon.

P_T (Interstitial Hydrostatic Pressure)

The interstitium is filled with a hydrated gel composed of protein-bound substances called glycosaminoglycans.[32] Various forms of these compounds differ from tissue to tissue, but include hyaluronate, which is present in most tissue, heparin in liver, and keratin in bone.[33] These substances are produced by tissue fibroblasts and their function remains a matter of speculation; however, they do contribute to the shape of the various organs.[26,34] In relation to the transfer of water between the plasma and the nonplasma water, the interstitial gel is important because it determines the pressure-volume relationship (i.e., compliance) of the interstitial space (Figure 46.3).[34]

∂ (Stavermann Reflection Coefficient)

The reflection coefficient is the property of the capillary membrane that describes its permeability to plasma proteins. If the membrane is completely impermeable to protein, the value for ∂ will be 1.0.[18] Similar to the filtration coefficient (K_F), the value for ∂ differs greatly among capillary beds of different tissues and is influenced by vasoactive mediators of sepsis and inflammation.[9,26]

π_P (Plasma Oncotic Pressure)

Oncotic pressure was defined and its relationship to plasma proteins explained (vide supra). Clinical interest

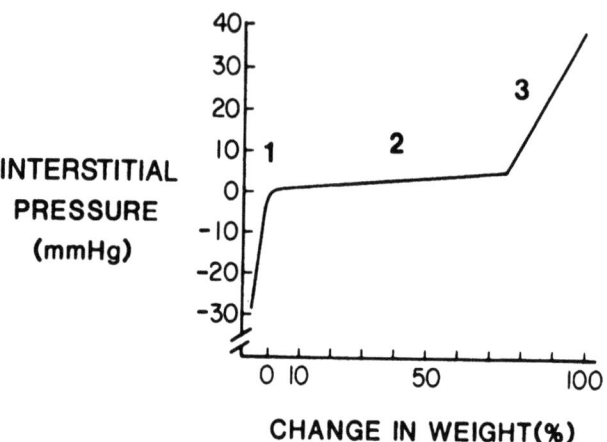

FIGURE 46.3. Guyton in the 1960s characterized tissue hydrostatic pressure and described a three-phase rise in tissue pressure with increasing volume. In health, interstitial pressure is negative to atmosphere and small increases in volume result in large increases in pressure (the compliance of the interstitium is low). This low compliance opposes fluid movement out of the capillary during normal conditions. The compliance increases once the interstitial pressure rises to atmospheric pressure. During this second phase, large amounts of fluid are accommodated in the interstitium without much change in the pressure until hard-pitting edema is manifest. Teleologically, this may occur so that during edema-producing disease states capillary perfusion may proceed even as large volumes of fluid leak out of the circulation. The second phase has been dubbed the edema safety factor. The third phase is one of low compliance. The volume of edema is large and increases further resulting in large increases in pressure due to limitation of tissue expansion from ridged structures such as skin, joint, or visceral capsules and muscle sheaths. (Modified from Civetta,[26] with permission.)

in plasma oncotic pressure has waxed and waned in recent years due to difficulty in its measurement and controversy surrounding the benefit of treating low oncotic pressure with colloid infusions.[19,26]

In the human neonate, measured values for plasma oncotic pressure are in the range of 15 to 17 mm Hg[21,22] for the neonate born at term, contrasting with values of 25 to 28 mm Hg in the normal adult. Values in the critically ill term neonate are not statistically different from the healthy neonate; however, the preterm neonates with respiratory distress syndrome have been noted to have lower plasma oncotic pressure (<12.0 mm Hg) when compared to their healthy counterparts (15.9 mm Hg).

During the 1950s, Guyton and Lindsey[36] demonstrated that pulmonary edema occurred at lower pulmonary vascular pressures when plasma oncotic pressure was lowered. Bland[37] has confirmed this experimental finding in the infant lamb. Despite these experimental findings, treating with colloid infusion to improve respiratory function in the premature neonate has not gained popularity for a number of reasons, including general success with other modalities, widespread clinical observation that colloid infusion does not dramatically improve pulmonary gas exchange, and fear that associated increases in hydrostatic pressure associated with such infusions will counterbalance any improvement in the oncotic forces and cause unwanted side effects (e.g., intraventricular hemorrhage).[20,38] Some investigators maintain that infused colloids may even promote pulmonary edema by leaking into the interstitium of a diseased lung (Figure 46.3).

π_T (Interstitial Oncotic Pressure)

Interstitial oncotic pressure is analogous to the plasma oncotic pressure. Although the gel matrix described above does contain negatively charged proteins, the osmotic pressure associated with these molecules is only one fourth to one half as great as that in the plasma.[9,27]

set point, which is usually between 275 and 290 mOsm·kg^{-1}.[40,41] The apparent monitored variables in the ECW control system are vascular pressure and osmolality, particularly sodium concentration, and the effectors are the heart itself, the kidney, and gastrointestinal intake relative to the thirst mechanism. In the critically ill neonate, whose intake is completely controlled by others, the latter effector is inactive. Modulators act at both the afferent and efferent limbs of the control system,[35,42] but this discussion focuses on the hormonal modulation of the kidney, including sympathetic catecholamines, the renin-angiotensin-aldosterone system, arginine vasopressin, and atrial natriuretic peptide.

The basic ECW control mechanism (Figure 46.4) functions as follows: An increase in ECW reflects an increase in plasma volume, which in turn increases blood

flow will then increase renal perfusion and urine formation. However, it is blood pressure rather than flow that is most directly correlated with increased urine production,[43,48] and it is pressure that serves as the prime stimulus to arterial mechanoreceptors that stimulate the hormonal response of the ECW control system modulators. Therefore, the systemic vascular resistance, as maintained by sympathetic nervous system tone and local metabolic needs, interacts with the direct effect of heart filling in the cardiovascular control of the ECW.[39,48]

The Kidney's Role in Regulation

The primitive single-cell organism alluded to above selectively transports solute from the surrounding ocean into the cell, and water passively follows.[2] By controlling solute, the organism can regulate volume. Similarly, volume of the extracellular space depends critically on the quantity of solute confined to this space. By modifying the balance of sodium and its anions, the kidney affects control of the ECW volume.[41]

The kidney's response to an increase in ECW volume comprises (1) increasing glomerular filtration rate (GFR), and (2) decreasing tubular resorption of filtered sodium and water. Both components include intrinsic renal mechanisms as well as renal function changes associated with the hormonal modulators of the ECW control system. The action of the kidney as an effector of ECW regulation is presented below in terms of the response to ECW expansion. In general, the response to ECW contraction is simply the converse.

The increase in GFR associated with ECW expansion is most probably a result of the increased hydrostatic pressure caused by the cardiovascular effects noted above. Additionally, if water expansion of the ECW dilutes plasma proteins, decreased oncotic pressure will favor filtration directly and indirectly through internal renal feedback mechanisms that alter the efferent arteriolar resistances.[49,50]

Minimal changes in GFR greatly increase the filtered load of sodium. For example, a 3500-g birth weight term neonate with a GFR of $17.0\,ml\cdot min^{-1}\,1.73\,m^{2-1}$ (2.2 ml· min^{-1})[51] and serum sodium concentration of $145\,mEq\cdot L^{-1}$ will filter approximately 460 mEq of sodium each day. A 5% increase in GFR will increase the filtered load to 485 mEq per day. To put these numbers into perspective, the total amount of sodium in such an infant's ECW is approximately 400 mEq, and maintenance sodium intake ($3.0\,mEq\cdot kg^{-1}\,day^{-1}$) is only $10.0\,mEq\cdot day^{-1}$. Each day, more than the entire ECW content of sodium is filtered and almost all is reabsorbed. Additionally, simply a 5% increase in GFR will increase sodium filtration by more than twice the standard daily sodium administration.

More important than the increase in GFR associated with an increased size of the ECW is the reduction in tubular reabsorption of filtered sodium. This change in tubular sodium reabsorption occurs by more than one mechanism.[49,50] In the proximal tubule, sodium reabsorption decreases because ECW volume expansion causes an increase in the peritubular hydrostatic pressure and a decrease in oncotic pressure that inhibits sodium transport.[50] Another intrarenal mechanism to increase sodium excretion may be the redistribution of renal plasma flow to the outer cortical nephrons.[52] These structures have shorter loops of Henle and, as a result, are less able to reabsorb solute. Commonly called the salt-losing nephrons, their perfusion is increased with expansion of the ECW.

Sodium excretion by the kidney, in response to ECW expansion, is further enhanced by the action of the hormone modulators on nephron function. In the distal tubule and collecting ducts a reduction in aldosterone effects increased sodium excretion. More importantly, release of atrial natriuretic peptides increase sodium excretion through their action at multiple nephron sites.[53] Lastly, expansion of ECW and concomitant decreases in compartment osmolality inhibit the secretion of arginine vasopressin, inhibiting thirst and promoting water diuresis.[54] The function of these modulators is presented in more detail (vide infra.)

The Role of the Modulators in ECW Regulation

Sympathetic and Renal Catecholamines

In animal studies both in vitro and in vivo, recent evidence has accumulated demonstrating sympathetic nervous system response to changes in extracellular volume that directly affect the kidney.[55-59] Norepinephrine not only produces changes in renal vascular tone limiting glomerular filtration, but also promotes a direct stimulatory effect on sodium-potassium (Na/K) adenosine triphosphatase (ATPase) in the tubular nephron, which restricts natriuresis. Volume expansion results in inhibition of sympathetic action on the kidney in sheep.[60,61] Sodium concentration may also affect sympathetic activity.[58] Although exact receptors and signaling have not been clearly defined, norepinephrine-induced sodium resorption in the tubules may be mediated by calcineurin (e.g., a norepinephrine-activated protein phosphatase) stimulating Na/K-ATPase activity in a rat model.[56]

Renal endogenous dopamine production has also been extensively investigated and reviewed.[55,56,58,59,62] Exogenously administered dopamine acts in the animal and adult kidney to produce vasodilatation, and in general an increase in glomerular filtration. This effect is mediated primarily by the dopamine receptor (DA_1). Dopamine produced endogenously by the proximal tubule of the kidney not only alters intrarenal hemodynamics, but also acts on renal tubular Na/K-ATPase via dopamine-specific protein phosphatase-1 inhibitor in a rat model to inhibit sodium resorption and to promote natriuresis and diuresis.[59] Further modulation of dopamine by interaction with other humoral regulators such as renin-angiotensin, kinins, and atrial natriuretic peptide has been reviewed.[55] Presumably, the counterregulatory roles of norepinephrine and dopamine on tubular Na/K-ATPase produce a balance homeostasis for sodium and water excretion by the kidney, and regulation of the extracellular space.

Renin-Angiotensin-Aldosterone System (RAAS)

Modulation by the RAAS of the heart and kidney's functions is another major component of the homeostatic mechanisms regulating the extracellular space. In health, RAAS output is more important for basal sodium and volume homeostasis and for response to ECW contraction than is lysis of the RAAS for response to ECW expansion. A decrease of the ECW volume results in lowering cardiac output and vascular perfusion pressure, which leads to a lower glomerular capillary pressure with reduced glomerular filtration.[53] The lower glomerular filtration reduces the delivery of sodium to the distal portion of the nephron. The juxtaglomerular cell responds to the change in capillary pressure and sodium delivery with an increase in the output of renin.[49,53,54]

Renin is an enzyme that has as its substrate a large glycoprotein of hepatic origin, the prohormone angiotensinogen. Renin cleaves from the N-terminal end of angiotensinogen a 10 amino acid structure with little physiologic action called angiotensin I (A-I). Another enzyme produced by the vascular endothelium, primarily in the lung, angiotensin-converting enzyme (ACE), removes two more amino acids from A-I to produce the potent vasoconstricting agent angiotensin II (A-II).[54]

The primary and secondary effects of A-II help stabilize the ECW. Recently, A-II has been demonstrated to be a potent stimulus for thirst, but the magnitude and role it plays in this response remain controversial and for practical purposes nonfunctional in the critically ill neonate whose intake is controlled.[46] A-II's effect on the circulation and the renal handling of solute and water have been more widely studied and are more important in ECW regulation in the critically ill neonate.

The vasoconstriction produced by A-II raises the perfusion pressure throughout the circulation, but at the same time it alters intrarenal fluid dynamics favoring sodium and water resorption by the proximal nephron.[63] Just as importantly, A-II is a potent stimulus on the zona glomerulosa cells of the adrenal gland to increase production and release of aldosterone. The action of aldosterone on the distal nephron epithelium augments the reabsorption of salt and water. Angiotensin II is not the only stimulus for aldosterone secretion. Hyperkalemia, hyponatremia, and adrenocorticotropic hormone (ACTH) secretion all stimulate its production directly or indirectly.[54] Angiotensin II has been described as a direct stimulant for renal tubular Na/K-ATPase activity, promoting resorption of water and salt in the proximal tubule in studies in the rat.[56]

Clinical assessment of the state of the RAAS is commonly performed through determination of plasma renin activity (PRA) and measurement of plasma or urinary aldosterone concentrations. Plasma renin activity is determined in vivo as the rate of A-I production when incubated with an endogenous concentration of angiotensinogen.[64]

Renal Kallikrein-Kinen System

Of recent interest in renal hemodynamic, and in salt and water handling is the kallikrein-kinen system.[55,65] Renal kallikrein comprises proteolytic enzyme activity produced locally in the renal cortex that hydrolyzes kininogens to produce bradykinins, which are potent vasodilators. Probably increasing intrarenal blood flow to the cortex, bradykinins may be modulated by kininase II, which is identical to ACE. Actions regarding vasodilatation in the renal papilla suggest a role in producing natriuresis as well. A direct effect on tubular sodium handling has been suggested.

Arginine Vasopressin (Antidiuretic Hormone, ADH)

Arginine vasopressin (AVP) is a nine amino acid peptide produced by neurons in the supraoptic and paraventricular nuclei of the hypothalamus. AVP is transferred down the axons of these cells that extend into the posterior pituitary gland. Depolarization of the axon cell membrane in response to stimulation from changes in blood osmolality, arterial blood pressure, and other stimuli, results in release of secretory granules containing AVP. These changes in osmolality and blood pressure and AVP release behave as a classic negative feedback control loop.

Increases in plasma osmolality are a much more potent stimulus for AVP secretion than are changes in arterial pressure, and not all osmotic agents provide a similar degree of stimulation.[66] Sodium chloride is the most potent osmotic substance and mannitol is very similar. An increase in blood osmolality from glucose, on the other hand, is a weak stimulus, and urea is intermediate between these extremes.[67] The primacy of osmolality over other stimuli for AVP release suggests that the AVP system is more important for maintaining the concentration of water in the ECW than it is for the total ECW volume. This role of AVP in control of water concentration rather than ECW volume is reflected in a state of excessive AVP release, i.e., the syndrome of inappropriate ADH (SIADH). In the patient with SIADH, increases in blood volume are small, usually not exceeding 5% to 10% above baseline, and urine output may be normal or increased depending on intake.[67]

Nonosmotic stimuli for AVP release include (1) hypovolemia, triggered by left atrial receptors and baroreceptors in the carotid sinus, along with elevated plasma angiotensin concentration; (2) nausea; and (3) pain or anxiety. These latter two are triggered centrally via brain stem and cortical output, respectively.

The action of AVP is to increase water reabsorption in the distal nephron. In the absence of this hormone, the tubule cell in this portion of the nephron is impermeable to water. AVP binds to the receptor on the surface of the cell membrane activating adenyl cyclase. The increased cellular concentration of adenosine 3′,5′-cyclic monophosphate (cAMP) then increases water permeability of the cell by mechanisms that have not been elucidate.[68] The osmolar gradient within the renal interstitium, to a large extent, determines the effect of AVP in increasing water reabsorption and urinary concentration.

Atrial Natriuretic Peptide

Regulation of water concentration (AVP), and salt and water volume (i.e., aldosterone modulation of the extracellular space) is complemented by a newly described and sensitive hormone system—the atrial natriuretic peptides (ANP).[69,70] Secretion sites for ANP are located diffusely in the left and right atria of the heart and are sensitive to increase in circulating blood volume with mechanical distortion of the atrial wall. Stretch results in prohormone release with a rise in circulating plasma concentrations. The prohormone is then cleaved by circulating enzymes to its active form. The principal action of ANP is to cause a fall in systemic blood pressure with the renal excretion of free water and sodium.[71,72] Although not all of the effects of the atrial natriuretic peptides are known, they appear to act by (1) increasing glomerular filtration, (2) decreasing renal renin production, (3) reducing both basal secretion of aldosterone and blocking the angiotensin II stimulation of adrenocortical aldosterone release, (4) inhibiting the action of aldosterone on the distal nephron, and (5) blocking angiotensin II vasoconstriction with a resultant reduction in blood pressure. The duration and action of ANP are probably very short-lived, a matter of minutes in one study on decreases in ANP concentration levels following ligation of a ductus arteiosus.[73]

Renal Prostaglandins

Prostaglandins are short-lived vasoactive hormones generated from the essential fatty acid, arachidonic acid, and have been reviewed with regard to local effects on the kidney.[55] Prostaglandin E_2 (PGE_2) is probably the predominant product in the renal tubule, promoting vasodilatation and natriuresis. PGE_2 moreover may act in concert with the kinins and modulate angiotensin II, yet increase renin secretion. Indomethacin inhibits prostaglandin production and results in a transient fall in glomerular filtration in the neonate. Development of prostaglandin synthesis in the fetal and neonatal kidney is described below.

Regulation of the ECW in the Neonate

Many of the abnormalities in the control of water metabolism in the critically ill or premature neonate result directly from developmental differences in the components of the ECW volume and concentration control system. Additionally, prematurity and other conditions associated with cardiorespiratory disease in the neonate and their associated therapies cause further dysfunction of the ECW control mechanism.

Neonatal Heart

This portion of the ECW control system appears to be limited in the neonate. Both term and preterm neonates exhibit a blunted Starling response to acute volume loading.[74] The limited reserve to increased cardiac preload is likely due to the morphology of the immature myocardium, which contains a high content of noncontractile tissue when compared to the adult heart. The result is a limited adaptive response to acute loading of the ECW.

Delivery of cardiac output to the neonatal kidney may nevertheless change with fetal development and neonatal transition. Blood pressure in the human neonate increases with gestational age at birth, and with postnatal age acutely during the first few weeks of life, and may parallel increases in renal blood flow as vascular resistance within the kidnay falls.[75-77] Seikaly and Arant[55] recently estimated that the human neonatal kidney receives 2% of cardiac output at term, 8.8% at 5 months, and 9.6% at 1 year of age. There are few reliable data to estimate the fraction of cardiac output received by the preterm kidney in the human. The adult fraction is estimated at approximately 15%.

The Neonatal Kidney

Numerous developmental differences occurring throughout gestation in renal physiologic function may compromise the efficiency of renal regulation of extracellular fluid balance as outlined above, particularly in the prematurely born human neonate. Prenatal urine formation has recently been reviewed by Aviles et al.[55] The amniotic fluid reflects fetal urine formation, derived largely from placental infusion of fluid and a lesser amount of swallowed amniotic fluid, which increases from $2\,ml\cdot hr^{-1}$ at 20 weeks' gestation to $>25\,ml\cdot hr^{-1}$ at term. Abnormalities of urine formation in utero may result in no bladder accumulation of urine on ultrasonography and oligohydramnios, as on renal dysgenesis, or increased bladder distention with oligohydramnios, as on obstructive uropathy with hydronephrosis.

Renal Blood and Plasma Flow, and Glomerular Filtration

The number of nephrons in the fetal kidney increases throughout pregnancy, until 34 to 36 weeks of gestational age when an almost full complement is realized.[78,79] Proliferation of glomeruli begins in the juxtamedullary parenchyma and continues outward with maturation. Only until well after birth is there a large cortical nephron population. Regional blood flow within the kidney's cortex is restricted by this anatomical progression prior to 34 weeks' gestation, with preferential perfusion of the cortical nephron in the outer kidney increasing only as nephrogenesis proceeds.[55] Moreover, early on, the glomerular capsule and mesangial capillaries are small, resulting in the surface area available for filtration being limited compared to that in the older infant and adult.[80,81] Fetal renal vascular resistance is high, restricting renal blood and contributing to a significantly lower glomerular filtration rate (vide infra).

Immediately after birth an abrupt change in renal physiology is superimposed on the gradual anatomic evolution of the fetal kidney when blood pressure increases in the first few hours to days of life and renal vascular resistance decreases.[75-77] These changes proceed over the first 1 to 3 weeks after birth even in the preterm neonate, probably resulting in increasing blood flow to the neonatal kidney as demonstrated in a recent color Doppler ultrasound study by Cleary et al.[77] (Figure 46.5). These investigators speculated that a decrease in renal vascular resistance occurred during the 0- to 3-week postnatal period, mitigating the increased renal artery blood flow velocities demonstrated even in the <34-week preterm neonate. Humoral mechanisms, which may affect these changes occurring upon and after birth, are described in more detail below, and include modulated sympathetic nervous system response with moderation of humoral catecholamine release, renal renin and angiotensin response, renal dopamine production, and prostaglandins.

Renal plasma flow, usually estimated from para-amino hippurate (PAH) infusions in the developing animal, and only occasionally in the human neonate, is difficult to evaluate since renal extraction of PAH occurs to a variable degree, resulting in underestimation of this parameter. As pointed out by Seikaly and Arant in a recent review, only one human neonatal study calculated PAH extraction, providing corrected estimates for renal plasma flow of about $140\,ml\cdot min^{-1}\,1.73\,m^{2-1}$ at 1 week of age, and $580\,ml\cdot min^{-1}\,m^{2-1}$ at 5 months, which equals 90% of adult values.[55,58] Based on these data, the investigators estimated renal blood flow values, adjusted for hematocrit, of approximately $250\,ml\cdot min^{-1}\,1.73\,m^{2-1}$ in the term neonate at a week of life.[55] Animal studies suggest that developmentally, values in the preterm are probably considerably lower than this for the anatomical and physiologic reasons cited above.

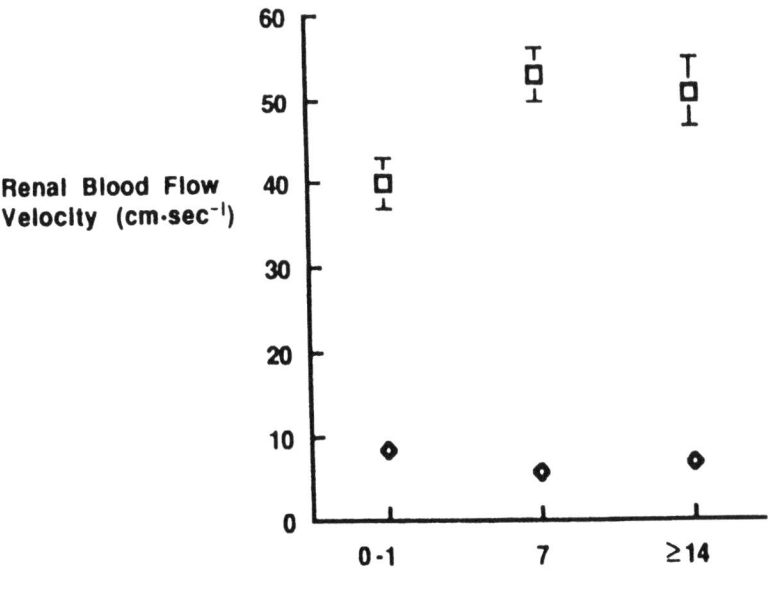

FIGURE 46.5. Mean (± SEM) systolic and diastolic renal artery blood flow velocities during weeks 1 to 3 of life in preterm infants. A significant increase occurs after the first week in systolic velocity. (From Cleary et al.,[77] with permission.)

Glomerular filtration rate increases concomitantly with changes in blood pressure, vascular resistance, and plasma flow, and continues to rise briskly throughout the first postnatal week following birth after 34 weeks' gestation when nephrogenesis is nearly complete.[51,83–85] Thereafter, glomerular maturation progresses more gradually, corresponding to differentiation of the cortical nephron into larger functional units postnatally. Such changes are commensurate with rapid growth during this early phase of postnatal development, and in general, the neonate at or near term is considered renal sufficient for high intakes of nutrition, fluid, and salt. In the premature neonate, however, at a gestational age of less than 34 weeks, the rapid increase in glomerular filtration may be blunted from the first weeks of life, despite increased renal perfusion suggested above. This would result in the observation of a lower glomerular filtration rate in the neonate.[51,78,83] The implication of these changes in glomerular function with regard to the regulation of the ECW is that the premature neonate, especially of very low birth weight, is less capable of excreting an excess water and salt load. Particular clinical scenarios for the consequences of developmentally low glomerular filtration in the preterm neonate with cardiopulmonary disease and severe prematurity in particular are discussed below.

Renal Tubular Transport Development

Probably the most important cellular transport process developing in several of the fetal organs, including the lung and kidney, is that of sodium/potassium (Na/K)-ATPase activity located within the cell wall. This process maintained by messenger RNA (mRNA) production, either stimulated by the concentrations of these ions in the intra- and extracellular fluids, or by numerous intrinsic and extrinsic hormone systems.[55,56,86–91] Many of the recognized active renal transport mechanisms are driven by the energy-dependent regulation of Na/K-ATPase activity in the proximal tubular cell's basolateral wall (Figure 46.6).[55,92] Natriuresis and concomitant water diuresis results from a combination of intrarenal hydrostatic forces with increased delivery of glomerular filtrate to the tubular lumen, and with modulation of Na/K-ATPase reclamation of tubular sodium to a level of 80% to 90% even in the developing kidney. Numerous humoral factors affecting proximal tubular balance are described below.

Recent evidence demonstrates in the maturing rat and dog animal model that production renal Na/K-ATPase increases simultaneously with gestation and with maturation of tubular regulatory function.[56,86] For example, glucocorticoids enhance Na/K-ATPase activity in both the lung and kidney in the neonatal rat at critical times around parturition, promoting natriuretic control.[87]

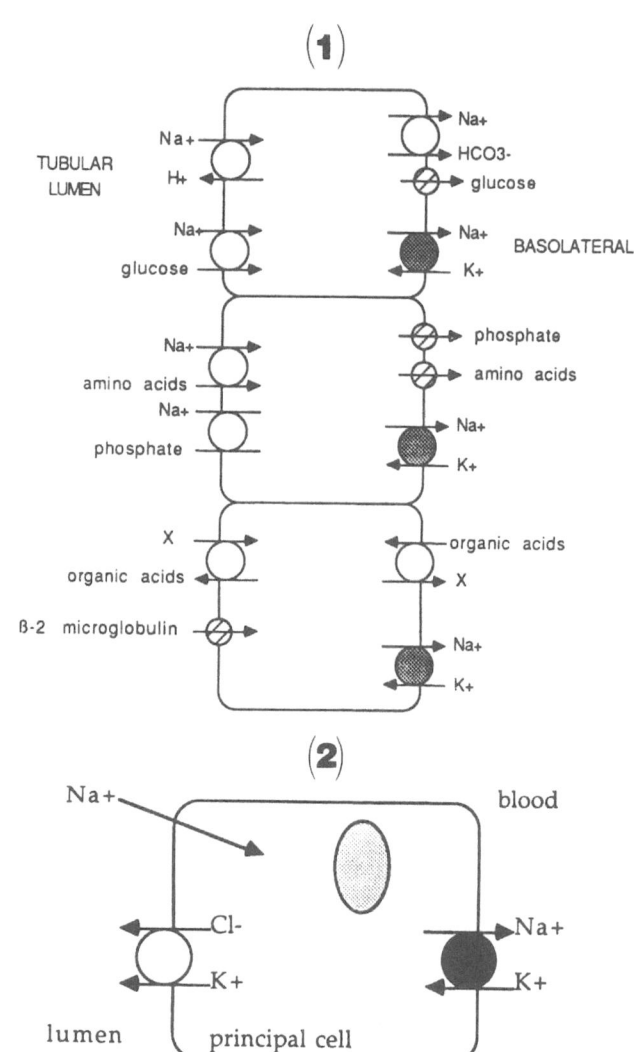

FIGURE 46.6. (1) Active transport of sodium across the proximal tubule cell in exchange for potassium is mediated by Na/K-ATPase located on the basolateral membrane (shaded circles). Countertransport of hydrogen ion (H⁺) and organic acids into the tubular lumen; and cotransport of sodium, glucose and amino acids, and phosphate may be powered by this enzyme activity. (2) In the collecting duct distally, passive reabsorption of sodium from the lumen favors an electrochemical gradient favorable for the secretion of potassium down its concentration gradient. (From Bailie,[55] with permission.)

Indomethacin seems to inhibit water excretion and natriuresis when administered prenatally, resulting in oliguria and diminishing amniotic fluid formation. This indomethacin effect may be ameliorated by glucocorticoids, suggesting a regulatory role for prostaglandins and glucocorticoids in the development of Na/K-ATPase activity.[88,89]

Finally, the development of the kidney's capacity for potassium secretion from the distal tubule and collecting system is dependent on maturation of the tubular basolateral membrane's Na/K-ATPase–dependent reclamation of sodium in an exchange ratio of 3:2 for potassium in the distal tubular cell. This uneven exchange results in an increased intracellular potassium concentration favoring potassium diffusion out to the tubular lumen and chloride exchange in, as well as for further resorption from, the lumen of filtered sodium.[55] Recently, immaturity in human Na/K-ATPase has been implicated in poor renal handling of potassium secretion from the very low birth weight preterm human kidney.[93] Also an endogenous source of potassium leakage from immature red cells results in an intrinsic hyperkalemia following birth with separation from placental control of body potassium concentration.[90,91]

Distal Tubular and Collecting Duct Diluting and Concentrating Capacity

In contrast to the renal cortex, medullary development of the distal tubule matures in early gestation.[78] The distal nephron of even the very premature neonate is able to produce a dilute urine when provided with adequate delivery of filtrate from the proximal tubule. The primary limitation of the fetal and early neonatal kidney in excreting excess water, therefore, occurs because of a limitation in glomerular function rather than in distal nephron function.[94]

Conversely, the premature neonate exhibits a reduced concentrating ability compared with the neonate at term and beyond. Urine concentration in excess of 600 mOsm·L^{-1} are seldom observed despite the frequent clinical observation at the bedside of high urine specific gravity.[76,95] Factors underlying diminished concentrating ability may include (1) a relatively low interstitial urea concentration,[96-99] (2) an anatomically shortened loop of Henle,[100] and (3) distal tubule and collecting system epithelium that is less responsive to AVP even with high circulating antidiuretic hormone concentrations present at birth.[97,98-100] Inability to concentrate urine output renders the preterm neonate vulnerable to ECW contraction and hypertonicity.

Sodium Balance

During fetal growth, urine flow is relatively low due to the decreased GFR associated with high renal vascular resistance.[80,81] Fractional reabsorption of filtered sodium increases with maturity so that urine is hypotonic relative to plasma by mid-gestation. Urine flow rate decreases toward term as the distal nephron becomes more responsive to fetal AVP.[52,99,101] This type of output coincides with the transport of large quantities of sodium chloride and obligate water into the fetus from the mother, ensuring a positive water and electrolyte balance for growth.[101,102] However, studies in chronic fetal lamb preparation suggest that by mid-gestation the fetus will respond to ECW volume expansion with a modulation of these high rates of proximal and distal tubular resorption.[103]

The term neonate continues to demonstrate positive sodium balance over a wide range of sodium intake.[52,102] This characteristic of the neonate's renal function is favorable during active growth and is maintained by a high circulating concentration of aldosterone.[52,99,101] The functional hyperaldosteronism is probably a result of a blunted negative feedback control on renin production.[52,104] Despite its functional advantages for the healthy neonate, the renal bias toward sodium reabsorption may limit the infant's ability to adjust excretion during acute ECW expansion.[105,106]

The premature neonate has a combination of difficulties with sodium homeostasis.[52,79,107] In contrast to the term neonate, the basal excretion of sodium in the premature neonate is high. With only a slight increase in GFR from the in utero rate, a relatively large percent of the filtered sodium chloride is excreted due to the less mature tubular response to aldosterone[79] and blunted adrenal production of aldosterone in response to renin-angiotensin stimulation.[108] Thus, the premature neonate is susceptible to both sodium wasting, resulting in ECW contraction, and an inability to accommodate ECW expansion due to the limited GFR.[52,105,109]

Potassium Balance

The glomerular filtrate of plasma potassium is almost entirely reclaimed by the proximal tubular cell, mediated by Na/K-ATPase activity described above. Potassium homeostasis by the neonatal kidney, then, is a result of the effect of filtrate flow, physical and chemical gradients, and hormonal influences on distal tubular secretion of potassium in exchange for sodium.[55,108,110] In the very immature kidney, the aldosterone signal may be sufficiently blunted to cause excessive suppression of baseline potassium secretion with sodium wastage.[52,93,111] Contributing to the problem of potassium regulation is leakage from the immature red cell, and perhaps other cell populations, resulting in an intrinsic hyperkalemia.[90,91] As a result, the very low birth weight neonate frequently exhibits hyperkalemia and an inability to tolerate intracellular and extracellular potassium overload.[93,112]

Function of the ECW Control Modulators in the Neonate

Sympathetic and Renal Catecholamines

Although the neonatal animal demonstrates a larger number of renal adrenergic receptors, there are species differences in the responses to α-adrenergic stimulation and inhibition. The neonatal lamb demonstrates greater natriuresis with adrenergic inhibition than the adult sheep, while the canine demonstrates less.[55,113] It is our speculation that a sympathetic surge following parturition in the neonatal subject contributes to an initial inhibition of natriuresis and water diuresis when compared to relatively higher rates of urine formation prenatally. Renal blood flow and sodium excretion are probably at least in part regulated by the sympathetic system in the neonatal period.

Renin-Angiotensin-Aldosterone System (RAAS)

A large number of investigations during the past 20 years have focused on the state of the RAAS in the neonatal period. Despite some contradictory findings, a clearer picture is beginning to emerge. These investigations demonstrate that PRA develops early in gestation and the neonate demonstrates very high values immediately after birth.[114,115] The premature neonate demonstrates levels even higher than the full-term neonate.[115,116] Some of the conflicting data regarding the pattern by which these values change in the weeks after birth are most probably related to differences in population and experimental technique. Furthermore, the neonatal animal and human demonstrate the expected response to the usual stimuli associated with increasing or decreasing production of PRA. For example, postural change (i.e., head up tilt) and hypoxia increase PRA, while volume loading and Lasix administration, causing increased distal solute delivery, decrease PRA.[117,118] A recurring observation is that the less mature neonate appears to have a more dramatic response to PRA stimuli, and a blunted response to inhibition.

Fewer data are available to describe the other components of the RAAS, but those that exist demonstrate a similar pattern for angiotensin and aldosterone production.[114,117-119] The few studies of ACE development suggest decreasing values with gestational age and higher levels in those premature neonates suffering from respiratory distress syndrome.[119,120]

A synthesis of the studies of RAAS and renal function in the term and preterm neonate provides a clearer picture. The RAAS matures early in gestation, and the combined effects of growth, immature feedback control on renin production, and poorly responsive renal tubules sustain the high levels characteristic of the premature neonate. As the neonate matures, the physiologic stimuli to the RAAS slowly decrease, reducing all the measures of RAAS.[52,117]

Superimposed on this pattern of development are the stimuli associated with cardiorespiratory disease and sodium administration in parenteral or enteral fluids. Respiratory disease, mechanical ventilation, and salt restriction are associated with increases in the RAAS indicators.[117,118,120]

Renal Kallikrein-Kinen System

El-Dahr[65] has recently demonstrated complete expression of the kallikrein-kinen system in the neonatal rat, with upregulation of mRNA related production increasing postnatally. In the human neonate, urinary kallikrein excretion is lower than later in life, and prematurity or illness may delay this development.[55] Functional studies seem less certain, since plasma renin activity is lower with increased urine kallikrein in the human neonate.

Arginine Vasopressin (Antidiuretic Hormone)

Studies of pathologic specimens demonstrate that fetal hypothalamic production and pituitary storage of arginine vasopressin (AVP) begin by 15 weeks' gestation. Although concentration increases throughout gestation, by the end of the second trimester tissue AVP concentration is near that of the term neonate.[121] Clinical studies demonstrate a high AVP concentration in umbilical cord blood samples obtained at parturition. AVP concentration in fetal samples is unrelated to AVP concentration in maternal blood, and studies of the anencephalic neonate demonstrate concentration.[122] Urinary AVP excretion during the immediate neonatal period does not vary with gestational age.[123] These studies indicate that AVP production is present at almost mature rates by midgestation.

During the neonatal period, high plasma AVP concentration associated with parturition declines rapidly during the first 24 hours, and continues to decrease during the first week of life. Again, prematurity appears to have little effect on this general pattern,[123] but other factors including vaginal delivery, birth asphyxia and meconium aspiration are associated with a higher concentrate.[122,124,125] Anesthetic administration to the parturient is associated with a lower concentration.[126] These data suggest that pain, hypoxia, and intracranial pressure are the cause of the high concentrate at birth. Not all data demonstrate an association between the Apgar score or need for delivery room resuscitation and postnatal AVP concentrate, indicating that other factors contribute to hypersecretion of AVP at birth.[124,127]

AVP release in response to hyperosmolality and hemorrhage in the fetal lamb and the human neonate indicates that, by mid-gestation, AVP response to both osmotic and baroreceptor stimulation is functional.[128-130] In addition to these responses, high urinary excretion of AVP is found in term and preterm neonates who are hypoxic or receiving positive pressure mechanical ventilation, those with pneumothorax, and those with intracranial hemorrhage.[123,129,131-133] These data are consistent with the nonosmotic release of AVP observed in the adult.[36] A high AVP concentration suggests that the syndrome of inappropriate antidiuretic hormone release (SIADH) contributes to the hyponatremia frequently seen in these neonates.[132,133] AVP release in response to pain in the neonate, which is another common cause of hypersecretion in adults, is less certain.[134-137]

During the latter half of gestation, fetal urine volume and free water clearance decrease while GFR and osmolar clearance increase.[130] Additionally, urinary concentration increases in the presence of exogenous administration of AVP.[138] Despite these findings, however, reabsorption of filtered water in the distal nephron, in response to AVP release, is blunted in the neonate compared to the adult. Both the term and preterm neonate exhibit increased urinary concentration with an increasing AVP concentration, but urine concentration plateaus at an osmolality of approximately 350 to 550 mOsm·kg^{-1}.[123,139] No further increase in urine osmolality occurs even as AVP concentration increases.

The etiology of the blunted response to AVP is multifactoral. Although tubular epithelial cell production of cAMP in response to AVP appears to be decreased in the less mature neonate,[98,140] this end-organ unresponsiveness probably plays a minor role in immature function. The major cause of an inability to concentrate urine is the limited solute concentration of the renal medullary interstitium.[141-143] The highly anabolic state of the neonate reduces the availability of both urea[141,143,144] and sodium[142,143,145] solutes. Increased postconceptional age, penetration of the loops of Henle from the outer cortical nephron into the renal medulla, and provision of a high-protein diet are associated with maturation of the urinary concentration in response to AVP.[141,143,144,146]

In summary, production and release of arginine vasopressin appears to be intact, even in the small premature neonate, but its effects on urinary water excretion is limited by the tubule's functional maturation and the renal medullary concentration gradient. Urine volume and concentration varies with postconceptional age, diet, and nephron maturity. The full characterization of the relationship of AVP to neonatal water balance is a topic of continuing research.

Atrial Natriuretic Peptide

Atrial natriuretic peptide in the neonate is infrequently studied; however, a few intriguing observations are available. Upon transition to extrauterine life, there occurs a surge in the extracellular water compartment's volume: (1) intracellular water shifts out of the cell into the interstitium,[13] (2) alveolar water in utero is forced by respiration into the pulmonary interstitium and lymphatics, and (3) there may be a placental transfusion of blood into the systemic venous circulation. There follows a brisk diuresis of free water and sodium excess into the urine over the next 2 to 3 days.[147] Measurements of ANP shortly after birth demonstrate significantly higher hormone concentration than in older children and adults.[148] If fed salt supplemented formula, the neonate persistently maintains elevated ANP and excretes salt.[149] In one report on the neonate, ANP was observed to initiate the diuresis of excess body edema fluid in the critically ill neonate with various lung disorders.[150] Ronconi et al.[151] have more recently reported that although urinary AVP concentration was consistently high in the preterm neonate with respiratory distress, who was receiving mechanical ventilation, human ANP increased significantly after birth by day 3, with the result that urine osmolar clearance and sodium excretion were enhanced with diuresis of 11% of body weight by day 5. Finally, another report suggests that although the ANP concentration may be very high at the inception of diuresis in the premature, mechanically ventilated neonate with RDS, there is no clear concordant renal response.[152] As in many other systems, prematurity may result in a blunted response to ANP not only in animal studies, but particularly in the neonate of less than 30 weeks' postconceptional age.[148,153]

Renal Prostaglandins

Prostaglandin synthesis can be demonstrated in the fetal animal, and receptor expression varies with postnatal age.[55] In the human neonate, urinary PGE$_2$ excretion is highest with premature birth, much lower in the term neonate, and it markedly decreases during childhood.[154] Since prostaglandins should increase renal blood flow and promote diuresis and natriuresis, indomethacin, which is often used to close a patent ductus arteriosus in the preterm neonate, should diminish urine flow, as observed clinically, and diminish sodium excretion, which is less often demonstrated. The role of prostaglandins in regulating the extracellular compartment in the neonate remains to be defined.

Transition to Extrauterine Life—The Redistribution of Body Water

During the fetus's transition from intrauterine homeostasis with growth to self-sufficient extrauterine life and continued growth, profound changes in extracellular and intracellular composition occur.[2] Almost immediately at birth, body water redistribution occurs with an efflux of volume and sodium into the extracellular space, followed by changes in cardiovascular and renal functions that flood the neonatal kidney, resulting in a diuresis.[13,155-157] Superimposed on these precipitous changes, slower escalation of nutritional intake of excess water, essential minerals, and nutrient substrates occurs, which results

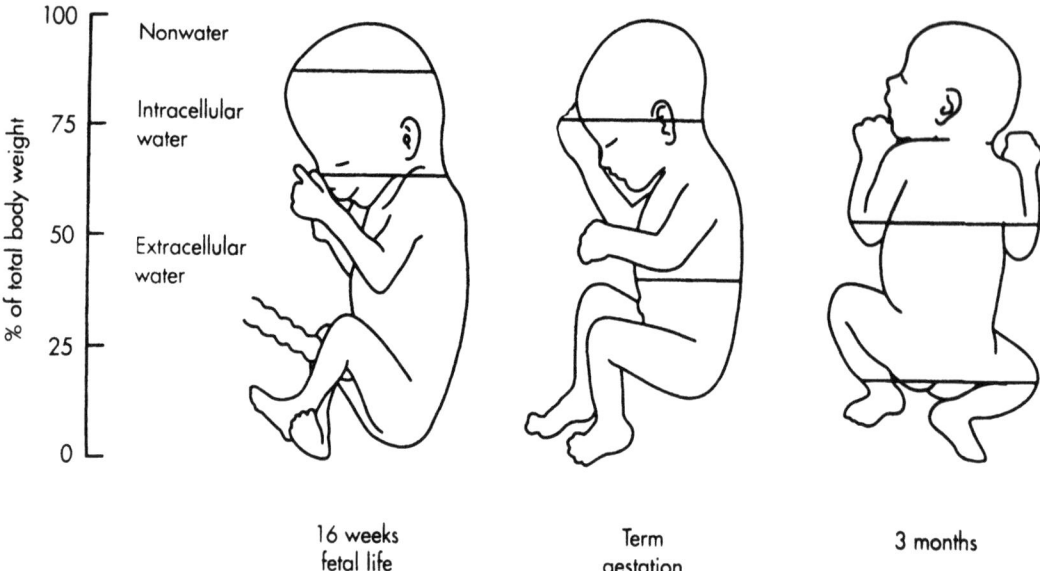

FIGURE 46.7. Changes in the composition of body fluids occurring during development. (From Costarino and Baumgart,[179] with permission.)

subsequently in a new homeostatic relationship between the entire organism and the extrauterine environment. This new relationship is characterized by growth.[2,12]

Third trimester fetal life is characterized by gradual increases in cell number, more rapid expansion of individual cell size, and differentiation into organized tissue and systems. During intrauterine growth, therefore, the relative proportion of water contained in the intracellular compartment expands more rapidly when compared to the extracellular fluid volume as total body water accrues. At 16 weeks' gestation, nearly 90% of body mass is water distributed in a roughly one-third ICW to two-thirds ECW proportion (Figure 46.7).[2,156] By term, this proportion is virtually reversed and is followed during postnatal growth by a gradual increase in proportional nonwater mass and an expanding intracellular water compartment.

Brans and Cassady[158] and Cheek and Talbert[159] have characterized the redistribution of body water following birth. The extracellular compartment expands acutely in the first hours to days of life as the result of placental transfusion, the resorption of lung fluid, and an efflux of intracellular water.[13] As the transitional circulation is "primed" by the increase in ECW, the pulmonary vascular bed opens and the lungs become fully perfused. A rebalancing of extracellular volume then occurs as kidney regulation and hormonal modulation of the ECW takes place. Initially, TBW contraction is proportionately greater from the ECW compared to the ICW, preserving cell volume, despite the initial efflux from the ICW that occurred in the first days after birth.[159]

For the neonates who are products of a difficult gestation or abnormal intrauterine growth, some investigators hold an additional view. Fluid excess at birth in these neonates is a result of cell injury. Initial efflux of intracellular water and ECW retention during the first week of life is a result of cell membrane dysfunction as manifested on physical examination as generalized edema. Recovery of cell membrane function is followed by a diuresis, which returns water distribution to normal. These proposed mechanisms help describe the alterations in body water distribution during the transition observed following pregnancies complicated by intrauterine asphyxia, growth retardation, maternal diabetes, and perhaps prematurity.[160]

Premature birth implies an early exposure of a large extracellular water and salt pool to the stresses of transition to extrauterine life. This surfeit volume is rapidly lost within the first days following birth as (1) a large insensible water loss is incurred,[161] and (2) a large volume of dilute urine is produced.[147,157] The result is an increased osmolality of the extracellular fluid compartment, which in turn drives a concurrent contraction in the intracellular water compartment. However, the contraction of the ICW is of a lesser magnitude because losses are "buffered" by the surrounding ECW.

In the critically ill premature neonate, diuresis may be delayed for days to weeks, resulting in fluid retention even if exogenous intake of water and salt is restricted.[162–165] Conversely, in the well neonate, excessive administration of fluid to artificially maintain body water weight is often futile, failing to keep pace with insensible water loss and brisk diuresis. Usually within 1 to 2 weeks the premature neonate recovers with a new relatively "dry" neonatal weight and composition. Tissue growth commences thereafter with expansion of cellular mass and the ICW.

Water Evaporation to the Environment

As outlined above, loss and gain of water through interaction with the environment demands about half of the energy produced by metabolism in order to maintain cellular integrity. The other 50% to 60% of the energy produced performs work (e.g., cerebral function, activity).[6] Oxidation of carbon fuels produces waste as well as energy. The wastes, including CO_2, water, nitrogen, fixed acids, and heat, are eliminated with obligate loss of water from the skin, respiratory system, and urinary and gastrointestinal tract. The evaporative water losses incurred by these elimination processes from the skin and lungs are not easily observed or measurable as liquid water. Together they are termed insensible water loss. The principles associated with such losses are especially important for understanding overall water metabolism in the premature neonate immediately upon exposure to the extrauterine environment.[159,164]

Respiration and Water Loss

Ventilation

Hydration is related to respiration by the physical evaporation of a small volume of water from the upper respiratory passages during spontaneous ventilation.[166] This volume is the respiratory contribution to net insensible water loss. At room temperature (25°C), atmospheric pressure (760 mm Hg), and 40% relative humidity, the average for a temperate climate at sea level, the healthy neonate in a thermally neutral metabolic steady state loses approximately 0.6 to $0.8\,ml\cdot kg^{-1}\,hr^{-1}$ to the environment through spontaneous ventilation of the tracheobronchial tree.[167] Consistently in infants, children, and adults, this volume makes up almost 30% of the total insensible water lost from the skin and respiratory passages combined.[168]

As seen in Table 46.2, however, a variety of conditions may alter the quantity of water the very low birth weight neonate exchanges with the ambient inspired environment. For example, the healthy 1.0-kg neonate comfortably breathing relatively dry nursery air (i.e., 25°C, humidity 40%) while managed on an open radiant warmer bed may theoretically exhale $0.83\,ml\cdot kg^{-1}\,hr^{-1}$ of water. Although extrapolation from adult data would suggest that a small amount of this water will be reclaimed immediately prior to exhalation in the slightly cooler nasopharynx,[167] empiric data in the premature neonate, nursed under these conditions, suggest this reclamation may not occur.[166]

Any disturbance of the resting, steady-state condition will result in an increase in ventilation and/or metabolic rate, requiring increased minute ventilation to meet tissue oxygen demands. Evaporation from the respiratory tract may then increase two to three times as noted in the second column of Table 46.2. Such increases in respiration frequently occur in the low birth weight neonate, particularly with cold distress during early stabilization and rewarming from delivery, or associated with infant agitation and activity, or as a manifestation of respiratory distress (e.g., RDS or pneumonia). The neonate, warmed in a nonhumidified incubator, supplemented with dry oxygen–enriched gasses, which is a common practice to avoid contamination with waterborne bacteria, will experience increased respiratory water loss, from a minimum of 1.0 to a maximum of over $2.0\,ml\cdot kg^{-1}\,hr^{-1}$. This will result in a water loss from respiration alone of more than $50\,ml\cdot kg^{-1}\,day^{-1}$. The tactic of incubator or head-hood humidification may reduce this "stressed" rate of evaporation; however, saturation of greater than 80% relative humidity may be required to achieve a rate of nonstressed exchange. Endotracheal incubation and mechanically supported infant ventilation with 100% saturated gas mixtures at body temperature may completely eliminate this component of water loss from the neonate in the intensive care setting regardless of stress or disease state.[161,169] However, care to eliminate particulate condensation in such a system is mandatory to avoid significant administration of liquid water to the patient.[170]

Respiration and Metabolic Water

Apart from physical evaporation during ventilation, another consideration of infant respiratory metabolism is the rate of water production as a by-product of carbohydrate, lipid, and protein oxidation. Traditionally, a healthy neonate's water of oxidation is considered to be less than 7% of net water exchange under resting steady-state conditions, and is balanced by an estimated 7% per day of fecal water loss.[167,168] However, in the critically ill or otherwise stressed preterm neonate who is at risk for higher metabolic rates of oxygen and carbon substrate consumption,[171,172] the production of water through oxidation may exceed $20\,ml\cdot kg^{-1}\,day^{-1}$ (Table 46.3). More-

TABLE 46.2. Estimated ventilatory water loss ($ml\cdot kg^{-1}\,hr^{-1}$) from a 1.0 kg infant breathing modified environments at theoretical resting and stressed (i.e., twice normal) minute ventilation.

Breathing environment (°C, % R.H., at 760 mm Hg)	Resting infant ventilation ($350\,ml\cdot kg^{-1}\,min^{-1}$)	Stressed infant ventilation ($700\,ml\cdot kg^{-1}\,min^{-1}$)
Room air (25°, 40%)	0.83	1.66
Saturated ventilator gas (37°, 100%)	0.0	0.0
Dry incubator air (34°, 0%)	1.05	2.10
Humid incubator air (34°, 80% max)	0.33	0.66

R.H., relative humidity.

TABLE 46.3. Variation in metabolic rate of water production with daily caloric expenditure (RQ assumed to be near 1.0).

Metabolic rate (kcal·kg^{-1} day^{-1})	Est'd metabolic water production (ml·kg^{-1} day^{-1})
50	7.5
100	15.0
150	22.5

over, evidence suggests that stool water losses in the premature neonate of less than 1.0 kg, prior to feeding, during the first week of life is negligible.[173]

The net water exchange for non–steady-state variations in an infant's respiration may be partially regulated by metabolic water production balanced by ventilatory water loss through evaporation from the respiratory passages. This net balance occurs only when the neonate is provided with a relatively temperate ambient breathing environment (i.e., not saturated), and usually does not equal zero (i.e., ventilatory water loss is generally twice the rate of metabolic water production). Nevertheless, the increase in water production that occurs with increases in metabolism is matched with proportional increases in ventilation and ventilatory evaporative loss. Therapeutic use of an artificially saturated environment in incubators to control excessive heat loss or in ventilator circuits to prevent airway desiccation may entirely obviate this balance and result in a bias toward free water retention.

Skin Water Loss

Most descriptions of water balance in the neonate combine ventilatory water loss and transepidermal water loss to consider net insensible water loss. The classic rule states that 23% of the normal infant's metabolically generated heat is dissipated through this insensible water loss, approximately 40 ml·kg^{-1} day^{-1}.[167,168] More recently, reported measurements of net insensible water loss in premature neonates (Table 46.4) are based, as in the past, on the observed neonatal weight change over time, and are sometimes corrected for the weights of metabolic gas exchange of oxygen and carbon dioxide.[174–179] The premature neonates in these studies, unlike previous work, however, constitute a heterogeneous group of different ages and sizes, receiving various modes of artificial incubation who may or may not be breathing humidity enriched gases.

Similar to the respiratory water exchange reviewed above, transepidermal water evaporation is subject to marked variations, independent of respiration and metabolism. In the premature neonate particularly, transcutaneous evaporation is a passive process wherein free water is lost from the exposed epithelium. It seems unlikely that sweat glands contribute much to the process of heat dissipation since (1) apocrine function is immature before 34 weeks' gestation, and (2) sympathetic innervation with an integrated sweat response to heat stimulation is blunted in the premature neonates.[180,181] Transcutaneous evaporation, therefore, remains predominantly insensible and cannot be viewed as a fixed proportion (i.e., 23%) of metabolic heat dissipation.

Indirect Assessment

Recent attempts to assess skin-only evaporation from the premature neonate utilize both direct and indirect methods. In the indirect techniques, respiratory water loss is isolated, then distinguished from the combined insensible water loss by subtraction from measured neonatal weight change. The difference is assumed to be the transcutaneous water loss. In the direct methods, transepidermal

TABLE 46.4. Measurements of insensible water loss in infants under radiant warmers and incubators.

Reference	Weight of infants (kilograms)	Incubator/radiant warmer	Insensible water loss (ml·kg^{-1} hr^{-1})
Fanaroff et al. 1972[174]	0.695–1.25	Incubator	3.45 ± 0.67
	1.250–1.80	Incubator	1.41 ± 0.71
Wu and Hodgman 1974[178]	<1.00	Incubator	2.68 ± 0.18
	1.00–1.25	Incubator	2.32 ± 0.31
	1.26–1.50	Incubator	1.60 ± 0.30
	1.51–1.75	Incubator	0.92 ± 0.25
	1.76–2.00	Incubator	0.71 ± 0.15
	<1.50	Radiant W.	2.45 ± 0.40
	>1.50	Radiant W.	1.49 ± 0.40
Williams and Oh 1974[175]	3.10 ± 0.13	Incubator	0.53 ± 0.05
	3.24 ± 0.97	Radiant W.	1.08 ± 0.12
Bell et al. 1979[177]	0.79–1.30	Incubator	1.58 ± 0.26
		Radiant W.	2.43 ± 0.24
Baumgart et al. 1981[176]	0.66–1.00	Radiant W.	5.27 ± 0.77
	1.01–1.50	Radiant W.	2.66 ± 0.20
	1.51–2.00	Radiant W.	0.52 ± 0.01

From Costarino and Baumgart,[179] with permission.

water evaporation is calculated from measurement of near-skin humidity gradients. Isolation of respiratory water loss, the indirect method, has been accomplished by means of a head hood,[181,182] and by use of an endotracheal breathing circuit.[169,176] In a steady-state thermal neutral environment, transcutaneous evaporation varies considerably in such studies. Infant size and gestation are important factors in each study influencing variation in evaporative rates, but variation in ambient vapor pressure and convective air currents in incubators and under radiant warmers may account for the differences between studies as well.[183,184]

Environment

Environmental impact on transepidermal water loss, independent of respiration has not been extensively evaluated using weight loss techniques. However, results describing the effects of infant incubation stagies on combined insensible water loss may be generalized to consider the largest contributing component, the skin. The most commonly employed strategy for the premature neonatal warming is the convectionally warmed incubator. Air temperatures suitable to maintain the low birth weight neonate in an isothermal condition at 36.5°C body temperature range in excess of 10.0°C above room air temperature. If not artificially humidified, which is a common practice to avoid bacterial contamination of the infant's skin and upper respiratory tract, ambient air relative humidity, and therefore vapor pressure, drops dramatically inside the incubator and facilitates evaporation. Compared to the diapered and bundled term neonate in a crib, the naked premature neonate in an incubator experiences an increased transepidermal evaporation much more than that necessary for heat dissipation (Table 46.4). Circulation of air inside the incubator by forced convection may further disturb evaporative gradients and increase water loss.[184]

Open exposure of the critically ill low birth weight neonate, nursed under a radiant warmer, results in a similar vapor pressure gradient that favors evaporation. The cool and dry room air passes over the neonate, is warmed and humidified at the skin surface, then increases by natural convection, carrying water gained from the infant's skin. Minor forced-convective air turbulence may facilitate evaporation under the radiant warmer by displacing the warm humid microenvironment layered within a few millimeters of the infant's surface.[182–185]

Infant epidermal water loss measured in the endotracheally intubated premature neonate receiving warmed, saturated breathing mixtures with no respiratory water loss was assessed under a radiant warmer as a function of body size in one study by Baumgart et al.[161,179] (Figure 46.8). These data suggest that very low birth weight in-

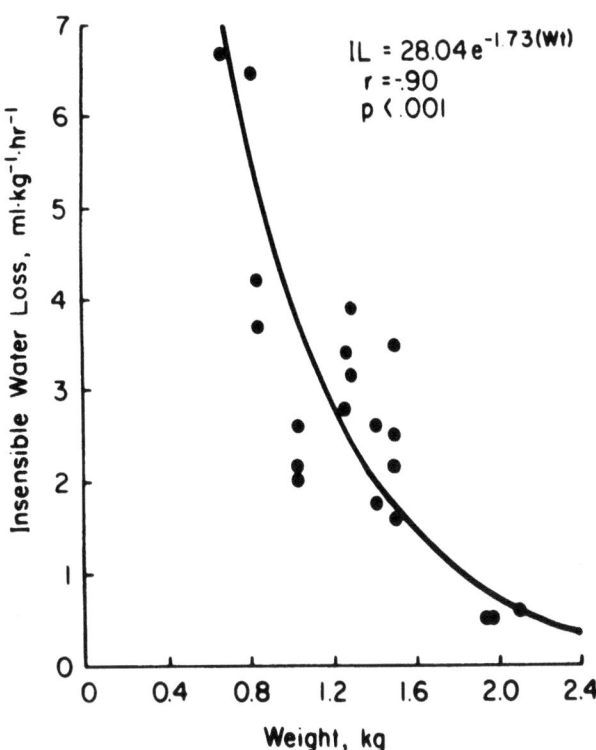

FIGURE 46.8. Insensible water loss increases with decreasing body weight (wt) in premature infants nursed under radiant warmers. (From Costarino and Baumgart,[179] with permission.)

fants (<1 kg) lose disproportionately more water from the skin alone than the more mature neonate. Two reasons are frequently cited for this phenomenon: (1) the immature neonate's epidermis is poorly cornified, presenting little barrier to passive evaporation from the underlying boundary epithelium, and (2) the tiny neonate's relative ratio of boundary surface exposure to body mass (i.e., water mass) increases geometrically with diminishing size (Table 46.5).[175–178,181,186,187] Both probably contribute to evaporative heat loss far in excess of the metabolic rate in the very low birth weight neonate.[182,184,188] Finally, a variety of clear plastic films and hoods have been advocated to preserve the microenvironment and reduce transepidermal evaporation.[183,189] Each application is unique in its net effect. Other neonatal environmental factors influencing insensible water loss have recently been reviewed and include skin blood

TABLE 46.5. Geometric increase in body surface area in proportion to diminishing body mass in low birthweight premature infants.

Weight (kg)	Calculated surface area (cm²)	Ratio (cm²·kg⁻¹)
2.0	1600	800
1.5	3000	870
1.0	1000	1000
0.5	650	1300

Calculated after Haycock et al.[187]

flow, phototherapy, clothing, and artificial skin-like membranes.[161,166,177,183,189-191]

Direct Assessment

In the direct method for assessing water loss from the skin, evaporation is calculated from the measured humidity and temperature gradients proximate to the skin's surface. The measurement probe is a small hollow cylinder, about 1.25 cm in diameter, held in place over the skin. Transepidermal water evaporation ($g \cdot m^{-1} hr^{-1}$) is calculated from temperature and humidity determinations sampled sequentially by a remote module. This technique is simple, noninvasive, and reproducible, and permits skin evaporation data to be obtained rapidly at the bedside. Investigations, utilizing this technique, have extended the previous observations on skin water loss performed under more artificial laboratory conditions to include the premature neonate nursed in a more relevant clinical environment. Much of the work summarized here has been reported by Hammerlund, Sedin, et al.[186,192] in an extensive series of studies.

As expected, larger transepidermal water loss was observed with early gestational neonates and postnatal infants compared to term infants (Figure 46.9).[186] Extremely high rates of water evaporation, as much as 13% body weight loss in the first day of life, correspond to the measurements previously presented (Figure 46.8).[161,179] Although environmental humidification as high as 60% relative humidity attenuated large water loss in the very low birth weight appropriate-for-gestational-age (AGA) neonate of <27 weeks' gestation, the transepidermal evaporation in these patients was never comparable to that in the more commonly encountered neonate of >28 weeks. These data further reinforce the contention that insensible water loss, particularly from the skin of the very immature neonate, does not represent a fixed proportion of metabolic heat dissipation.

Clinical Conditions Associated with Disordered Water Metabolism

Respiratory Distress Syndrome (RDS)

The premature neonate with surfactant deficiency has poor lung compliance, leading to alveolar atelectasis, elevated pulmonary vascular resistance, and abnormal pulmonary lymphatic drainage.[37,193] Additionally, this neonate has a low plasma oncotic pressure.[21,22] These abnormalities unbalance the Starling relationship in the pulmonary microvasculature and promote fluid movement out of the blood into the pulmonary interstium. Lung water content then increases, further hampering lung compliance and worsening gas exchange.[193,194] Oxygen and positive pressure ventilation may contribute to the endothelial injury and exacerbation of the fluid accumulation in the lung.

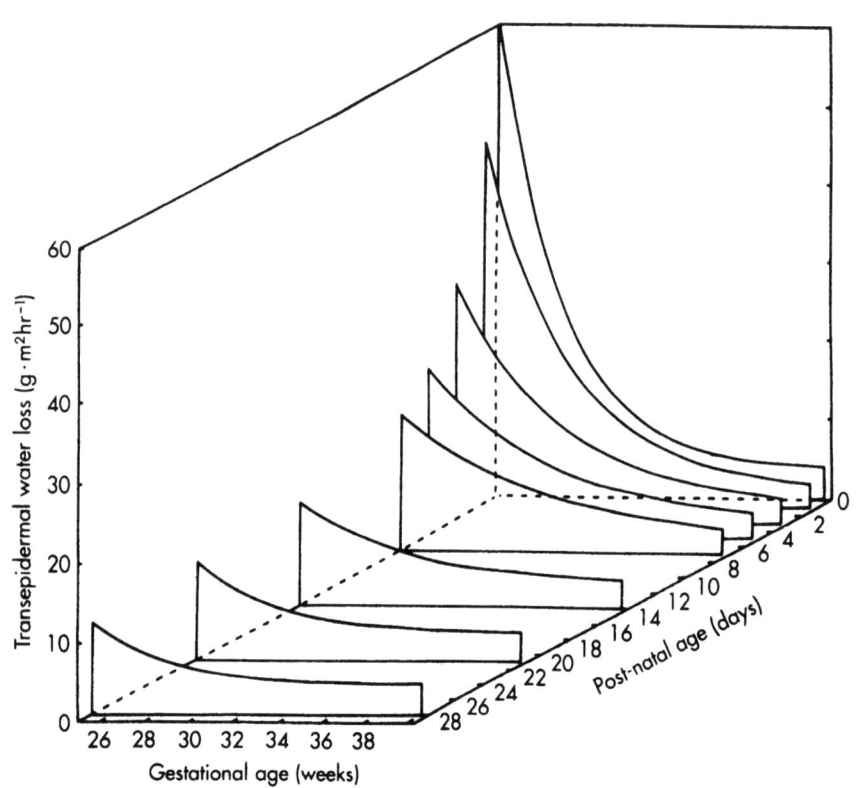

FIGURE 46.9. Transepidermal water loss in relation to gestational age at birth at different postnatal ages in appropriate-for-gestational age infants. (From Hammarlund and Sedin,[186] with permission.)

A diuresis usually occurs by the third day of the disease, perhaps a blunted expression of the physiologic diuresis occurring during the transition described above. Costarino et al.,[147] in a group of infants with RDS and >1.0 kg at birth, and others[195] have demonstrated that this diuresis is not a result of renal recovery from hypoxia, as previously suggested, because it precedes recovery. This change in urine flow is associated with a slight increase in GFR and a larger rise in free water clearance.[147,195] It is appealing to speculate that the origin of the diuretic fluid is the hypotonic edema from the lung. Indeed, some investigators have attempted to demonstrate improved pulmonary function following furosemide administration to enhance an earlier removal of excess salt and water. The improvements with this therapy are small and transient; hence, furosemide therapy has not achieved popular use. A report by Huet et al.[196] suggests that theophylline may also be used to augment glomerular filtration and salt and water diuresis.

More recently, Lorenz et al.[197] and Ramiro-Tolentino et al.[198] have investigated this diuresis in the very low birth weight neonatal population of <1.0 kg at birth. Analogous to the more mature population, prediuresis, diuresis, and postdiuretic phases of postnatal renal function were defined in 32 neonates over the first 5 days of life. Onset and cessation of diuresis occurred at greater than 24 hours and before 96 hours, respectively. During the prediuretic phase, glomerular filtration was relatively low and fractional excretion of sodium was on the order of 6% of the filtered sodium when adjusted for creatinine. During the diuretic phase, urine formation more than tripled, at twice the glomerular filtration rate, three times the sodium excretion, and double the fractional excretion of sodium (12%). Other investigators have reported a relatively high fractional excretion of sodium in this low birth weight population, and have attributed this state to acute renal failure[199] which seems unlikely. Urine osmolality remained constant, and bicarbonate was conserved in positive balance.[198] Weight indicated that a contraction alkalosis occurred during this diuresis. After the diuresis, glomerular filtration remained at the increased rate, while sodium excretion diminished. Shaffer and Meade[200] have recently demonstrated that bromide space, indicating the volume of the extracellular compartment, decreases in the premature neonate over the first 5 days of life, regardless of sodium intake. In general, the improvement in glomerular filtration and other renal function with postnatal age and the resolution of cardiorespiratory disease in the preterm neonate is consistent with other reports, although more often these studies demonstrated delayed diuresis with severe illness.[201-203]

In light of these findings, a modified approach to routine fluid and electrolyte maintenance in premature babies with RDS has been adopted (Figure 46.10).[179] The figure summarizes observed urine volume before, at the onset, during, and after diuresis in the premature neonate with RDS. Lung function (i.e., Aa-DO$_2$) may be seen to improve only after a large diuresis of free water occurs. In the fluid schedule, all predicted fluid losses are not replaced. TBW contracts in anticipation that the interstitial fluid volume well stabilize in a new, "dry" equilibrium between the pulmonary capillary and interstitium. Increasingly, the evidence suggests that fluid restriction during the acute phase of RDS prevents later development of pulmonary edema, patent ductus arteriosus with heart failure, and bronchopulmonary dysplasia.[164,204-207]

Bronchopulmonary Dysplasia (BPD)

Infants who develop chronic respiratory failure after acute RDS retain lung water persistently due to high pulmonary hydrostatic pressures, low capillary oncotic pressures, and a limitation of lymphatic drainage.[37,194] These abnormalities, in combination with scarring and distortion of lung anatomy, a large transpulmonary pressure, or high positive airway pressure, favor movement of water and albumin out of the plasma compartment, trapping it in the lung interstitium. Administration of excessive crystalloid- or colloid-enriched fluids often exacerbates the accumulation of pulmonary water, decreasing lung compliance and contributing to small airway obstruction.[208] Poor nutrition and increased metabolic demands in the infant with bronchopulmonary dysplasia result in hypoalbuminemia and poor capillary integrity in damaged tissue. Generalized body edema occurs as extracellular water accumulates outside the lung as well.

Whether high fluid intake, a patent ductus arteriosus, or the failure to generate a diuresis before 2 weeks of life contribute to the incidence of BPD is controversial. Further, the influence of treatment of these conditions with severe fluid restriction, indomethacin, and diuretics on the incidence or severity of BPD is speculative. Short of massive flooding, exogenous water administration is probably not the primary agent in the early pathogenesis of BPD, yet may contribute to this entity once established.

Pulmonary edema in BPD clearly impairs lung compliance, increases small airways resistance, and compromises gas exchange. One approach to therapy is modest water restriction with provision of substantial nutritional substrates to meet the increased metabolic energy demands.[172] In addition to parenteral nutrition, a variety of calorically dense premature formulations augmented with carbohydrate and/or lipids are advocated. Sparing use of diuretics with calcium and potassium supplementation has been demonstrated to be useful in the management of this disease; however, care must be exercised to avoid chronic wasting of sodium, potassium, and calcium salts to promote optimal growth recovery.

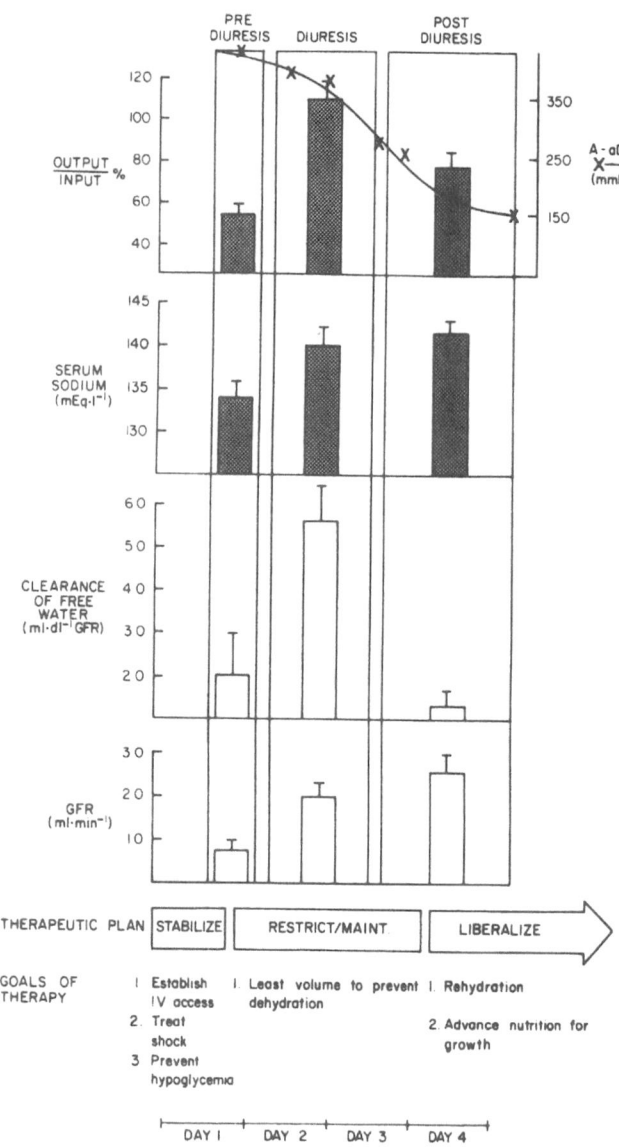

FIGURE 46.10. Diagram outlining the clinical course of infant respiratory distress syndrome in conjunction with the postnatal diuresis. A therapeutic schema is presented in three phases. (Adapted from Costarino et al.,[147,179] with permission.)

Shock and Edema

The neonate with severe perinatal asphyxiation or septic shock suffers diffuse tissue injury and cardiopulmonary dysfunction. Depending on the gestational age, vital organ function may be further compromised by immature development. Additionally, these patients manifest problems with the transition of circulation from the fetal to the extrauterine pattern. Oliguria and anasarca are commonly part of these patients' clinical presentation. Treatment of hypoxemia, acidemia, and hypotension in these neonates is difficult and may vary depending on the underlying cause. However, a few "intensive" therapies are typical of the most severe cases. Hypotension is treated initially with large volume intravenous infusions until compromise of pulmonary function by edema leads to the use of vasoactive inotropic agents. Hypocapnia is commonly a therapeutic target in order to minimize pulmonary vascular resistance and is often achieved only with high pressure, high-frequency mechanical ventilation, and neuromuscular blockade. Later in the patient's course, when the circulation is more stable, the clinician often administers diuretics to remove the obviously increased volume of body water in the hope that pulmonary function will improve.

Edema observed in these neonates is an abnormal accumulation of body water in the nonplasma ECW. The anasarca that complicates the course of the critically ill neonate commonly occurs in association with (1) conditions that unbalance the Starling forces such that water accumulates outside the plasma compartment; and (2) dysfunction of the underlying ECW control system (Figure 46.4), promoting abnormal ECW expansion through avid salt and water retention by the kidney. The kidney is discussed first.

The mechanism of the abnormal sodium and water retention in edema states has been a topic of active research since 1950. The observation that total ECW and plasma volumes are increased, yet salt and water excretion in the urine is diminished, suggests that there is either (1) a primary kidney abnormality (i.e., renal failure), or (2) some abnormal stimulus to the ECW control system's neurohumoral modulators.[141] The event underlying these abnormal functions has been postulated to be a loss of "effective circulating blood volume."[209]

The concept of effective blood volume has been criticized as undefinable, but recent studies by Schrier[39] and Shapiro et al.[48] indicate that an interaction between the cardiac output and vascular resistance on the arterial side of the circulation define it. In this schema (Figure 46.11), conditions of either low cardiac output, or high cardiac output with peripheral vasodilatation (e.g., sepsis), trigger the baroreceptors located in the central arteries. This signal then blocks tonic inhibition of the sympathetic nervous system, causing nonosmotic release of AVP and renin production, promoting salt and water retention by the kidney.

Elevated venous pressure augments edema formation both directly and indirectly (Figure 46.11).[39,209,210] Poor cardiac emptying with myocardial dysfunction distends the central veins and ultimately raises capillary pressure. The high capillary pressure promotes transudation of water out of the plasma compartment, reducing volume pumped into the arterial circulation. This indirect volume loss then triggers renal water retention.[211] Similarly, obstruction of central venous flow, from any cause, can initiate this vicious cycle. Indirect volume depletion associated with venous obstruction has long been postu-

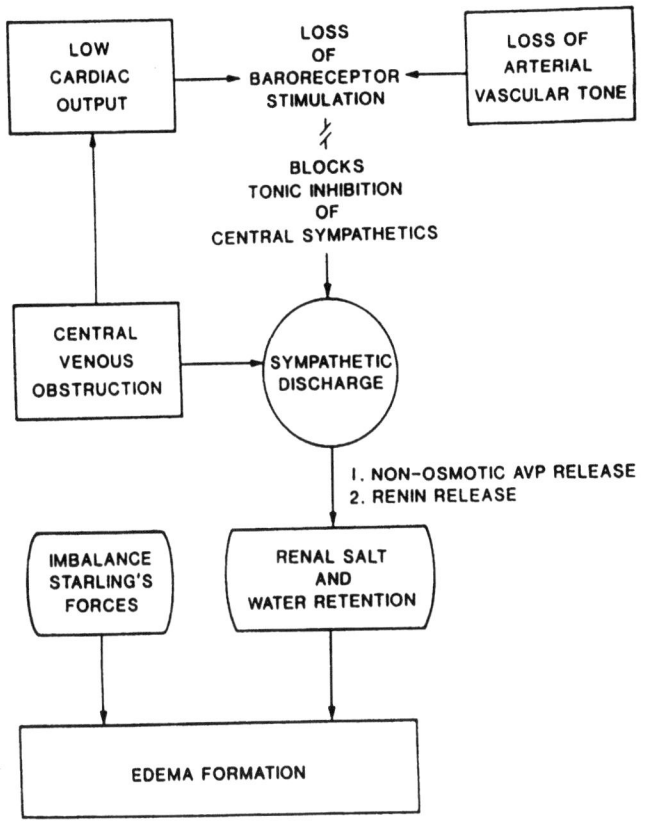

FIGURE 46.11. Mechanisms promoting edema formation in the critically ill neonate.

lated as the primary event in the ascites and edema of cirrhosis.

High venous pressure may directly contribute to renal water retention. In experimental models of cirrhosis, Levy and Wexler[212] established that renal retention of water and sodium precede any significant transudation of ascitic fluid or reduction in cardiac output. These findings suggest that intrahepatic venous hypertension directly stimulates renal sympathetic tone and results in increased renin release. A similar direct effect of renal venous hypertension has been demonstrated.[210]

Returning to the first component of edema formation, the disruption of the Starling forces, factors that interact to cause abnormal water accumulation in the nonplasma extracellular compartment are apparent. Disturbance of the normal Starling relationship (Equation 2) promotes transudation of water out of the capillary. Hydrostatic pressure is high secondary to circulatory failure and/or transmitted high airway pressure from mechanical ventilation.[132] Once edema is initiated, interstitial compliance increases (Figure 46.3).[26,33] Thus, the balance of the hydrostatic pressure component of Equation 2 favors water movement out of the vessel. Low plasma oncotic pressure, a characteristic of the neonate, is further impaired by nutritional deficiency in the critically ill patient. Vascular permeability to both water and solutes, and vasodilitation associated with release of the humoral mediators of shock, change the capillary filtration coefficient promoting edema formation. Accumulation of extravascular water is exacerbated in the neonate because lymphatic drainage may also be impaired. Lymphatic flow depends in part on tissue movement; therefore, the neonate who is paralyzed to aid respiratory care is more likely to form edema.[29]

The factors that contribute to formation of edema in the critically ill neonate are diagrammed in Figure 46.11. Myocardial dysfunction and vasodilation from sepsis, hypoxia, and associated metabolic derangements are sufficient to initiate these pathologic events. The mechanical effect of high airway pressure with assisted ventilation may contribute to edema by reducing cardiac chamber size (i.e., cardiac output), raising renal and splanchnic venous pressures and stimulating AVP release.[213,214] Birth asphyxia,[126,134] hypoxemia, pneumothora,[131] and intraventricular hemorrhage[125] directly stimulate the sympathetic nervous system with release of AVP, further complicating water balance.[123,132,213]

The Micropremie

The very low birth weight, extremely premature neonate, born weighing 500 to 1000 g, at less than 25 to 27 weeks' gestation, manifests a gelatinous-appearing skin so thin as to appear transparent, with little if any keratin content. As shown in Table 46.5, the ratio of this infant's body surface area to body water mass is six times greater than the adult's. Transepidermal water evaporation is geometrically higher than in larger premature neonates (Figures 46.8 and 46.9), resulting in loss of free water from the interstitial fluid acutely during the first 12 to 24 hours of life. The interstitial losses produce a hyperosmolar extracellular compartment characterized by hypernatremia often with hyperglycemia and hyperkalemia. The intracellular compartment ultimately shares the water loss secondary to high osmotic pressure in the extracellular space. This has been implicated as a contributor to the neurologic injuries sometimes seen.[179,215]

Most of the time, even as the serum sodium rises, urine flow with a high fractional excretion of sodium is maintained. Similarly, capillary perfusion, blood pressure, and peripheral tissue turgor survive the dehydration. However, persistent fluid and electrolyte aberrations beyond 24 to 72 hours of age are more commonly associated with shock and cardiac dysrhythmias. In particular, nonoliguric hyperkalemia, often associated with a hypernatremic, hyperosmolar state, has been described in the tiny neonate <800g at birth, with various mechanisms proposed for its development.[90,91,94,216,217] Gruskay et al.[93] originally demonstrated that the tiny premature neonate developing hyperkalemia in the absence of oliguric renal failure had similar glomerular filtration but higher fractional and absolute sodium excretion, with diminished potassium secretion in the urine. They proposed aldosterone insensitivity and functional immaturity of the distal collecting system's Na/K-ATPase activity.

In contrast, other investigators have suggested that glomerular immaturity with significantly higher serum creatinine and lower glomerular filtration results in a limited delivery of potassium into the distal tubule, resulting in hyperkalemia in the tiny infant.[216] Finally, recent calculations suggest that a shift of potassium occurs acutely after parturition, with separation from the placental exchange regulation of sodium and potassium, resulting in an endogenous shift of potassium from the intracellular to the extracellular compartment.[217] Stefano et al.[90] have recently provided experimental evidence in very low birth weight premature neonates demonstrating this latter effect. These investigators showed significantly lower Na/K-ATPase activity in carefully harvested erythrocytes in the infant developing hyperkalemia when contrasted with higher enzyme activity in those not developing hyperkalemia (Figure 46.12). They suggested that serum hypernatremia may disrupt this enzyme system, leaking sodium into cells unable to eject the ion in favor of potassium. Finally, they excluded tissue catabolism as a cause for hyperkalemia in these subjects.[91] Probably all of these proposed mechanisms contribute to the profound electrolyte disturbances reported.

Simply replacing the excess free water in the neonate prone to hypernatremia (100–200 or more ml·kg^{-1}·day^{-1}) may complicate the clinical situation. Inadvertent fluid and/or dextrose overloading may lead to a patent ductus arteriosus, pulmonary edema, and intraventricular hemorrhage.[215] Our approach to fluid therapy in these neonates is to apply the least amount of intravenous water volume replacement necessary to maintain serum sodium concentrations in the high-normal range (145–150 mEq·L^{-1}) during the first 24 to 72 hours of life.[179] Costarino et al.[218] have reported that sodium restriction during the first 5 days of life may be beneficial in reducing the occurrence of hypernatremia in the neonate who may already be receiving sodium in transfusions and a variety of medications. In this study, need for extra free water volume administration parenterally was reduced by this protocol. Sodium restriction, especially beyond the first week of life, may be controversial, however (vide infra).

To prevent the dehydration insult in the first place, application of a variety of plastic shields are advocated. These have been demonstrated to reliably reduce transcutaneous water loss.[189] Knauth et al.[191] have reported the use of a thin, semipermeable polyurethane membrane that is adherent to the skin. This technique can prevent excessive water loss, skin maceration, and dermal trauma, but further investigations are needed before this technique can be recommended generally. One preliminary report using this adherent membrane skin suggests effective restoration of fluid conservation with less hypernatremia, less fluid replacement volume, lower occurrence of patent ductus, and a reduced tendency for the development of BPD.[219] Some clinicians prefer to place the neonate into a warmed and humidified incubator to control free water loss by reducing the evaporation gradient near the skin. Care must be taken to avoid waterborne bacterial contamination with this practice.[220]

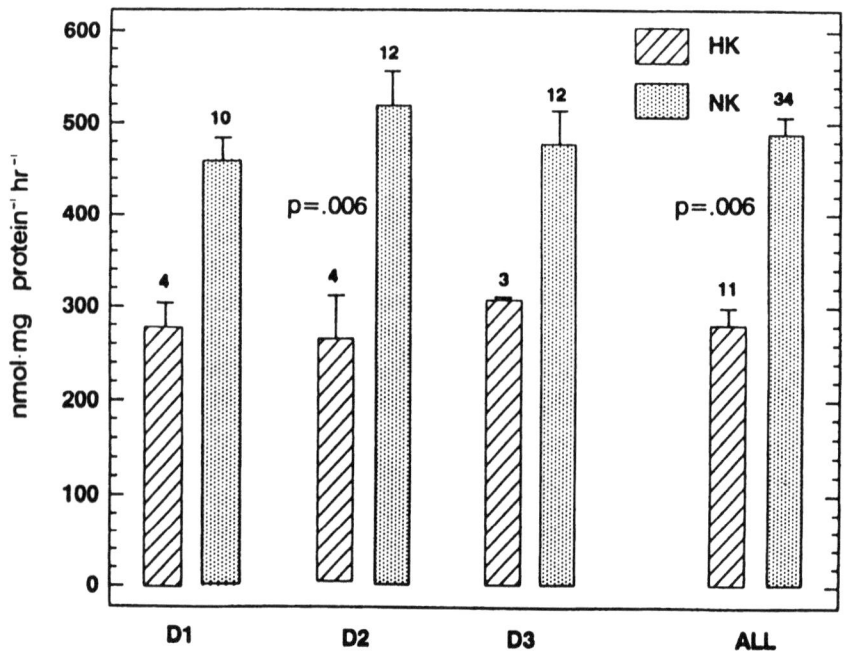

FIGURE 46.12. Na/K-ATPase activity in erythrocytes of very low birth weight infants with hyperkalemia (HK) versus normokalemia (NK) over 3 days. Lower activity is demonstrated in the HK group. (From Stefano et al.,[90] with permission.)

The Growing Premature Infant with Hyponatremia

A frequent finding in the nursery is that a clinically healthy infant, exhibiting adequate growth on enteral feedings, is mildly or moderately hyponatremic (serum sodium concentration 124–130 mEq·L^{-1}). This infant is usually 2 to 6 weeks old after birth at 26 to 30 weeks of gestation. Cardiorespiratory failure associated with prematurity has resolved or never existed and phototherapy treatment for hyperbilirubinemia is no longer necessary. The infant is not receiving parenteral fluids and is now beginning to accelerate on feedings. The clinical presentation often includes a hematocrit that is beginning to fall and the initiation of methylxanthine therapy for apnea of prematurity.

This characteristic hyponatremia in the healthy, growing very low birth weight infant was first noted by Sulyok[221] and Honour et al.[222] in the early 1970s and called to attention by Day et al.[107] and Roy et al.,[223] who coined the term late hyponatremia of prematurity. The pathogenesis of this syndrome is incompletely understood but much is known due to the continued work of Kovacs et al.[142] and Sulyok et al.[145,224]

In contrast to most hyponatremic states, the late hyponatremia of prematurity does not appear to be a result of a relative water excess, but rather is the result of a relative lack of sodium. Metabolic balance studies in these infants receiving recommended sodium intakes usually demonstrate that even with a high renal sodium excretion they are in a slightly positive sodium balance.[145,221,224] Glomerular filtration and urinary flow are increasing, as is expected with postconceptional age, and fractional excretion of sodium, although elevated, is similarly improving (i.e., decreasing) as expected. Distal tubular delivery of solute is increasing at a greater rate than the clearance of free water. Plasma renin activity, aldosterone, and arginine vasopressin are high in these infants.[139,145,221,222,224]

These experimental observations suggest that growth and immature renal function combine with limited sodium intake and other clinical factors to create the presentation described above. As glomerular filtration increases, delivery of solute to the distal nephron increases.[51,75] If proximal nephron resorption of sodium cannot keep pace with the rising GFR, distal solute delivery will increase even more.[101] Low hematocrit and plasma oncotic pressure as might exist will decrease proximal reabsorption of solute. Despite high plasma renin activity and aldosterone concentration, the insensitivity to aldosterone by the distal nephron results in relatively high excretion of sodium.[52] Sulyok et al.[225] have reported higher urinary AVP concentration in sodium supplemented preterm neonate (3–5 mEq·kg^{-1} day^{-1}) compared to the same neonate receiving a normal recommended salt intake (1.5–2.5 mEq·kg^{-1} day^{-1}) after the first week of life. Salt balance was more positive in the supplemented group but impact on water balance was not clearly demonstrated.

The patient described has recovered from the immediate stresses of prematurity—the skin has cornified, nursing on a radiant warmer bed is no longer necessary for emergency interventions, and phototherapy has been discontinued. Thus, the large insensible water loss that parallels or exceeds sodium loss during the first days of the very low birth weight neonate's life is greatly reduced. Enteral nutrition has been started in sufficient quantity to sustain an anabolic state, but frequently intolerance to feedings demands a relatively dilute formulation. The patient is often receiving theophylline, a drug that may promote diuresis and increase sodium loss.[223,224]

The typical patient with this disorder demonstrates a slightly positive sodium balance, but it is insufficient to meet demands for the growth of new tissue, particularly bone. The neonate incorporates sodium into tissues at a rate of 1.2 mEq·kg^{-1} day^{-1} during the third trimester, so a positive balance must meet this demand.[12] The renal tubular function of many of these neonates is inadequate to the task when provided with a dilute or nonsupplemented formula. Increased sodium losses that may occur with theophylline or diuretic therapy can compound the problem.

More recently, evidence has accumulated to suggest that during the first week of life, when the preterm neonate is usually most difficult to feed either parenterally, for reasons of fluid volume restriction elaborated above, or enterally, loss of sodium and water volume occurs despite variations in salt and water intake.[218,227,228] Heimler et al.[227] and Bauer et al.[228] used deuterium labeled heavy water (TBW), bromine or sucrose dilution (ECW), and Evan's blue dye (plasma volume) to demonstrate that while plasma and ICW volumes were maintained, ECW volume diminished during this period. Heimler et al.[227] suggested only the less stable neonate with inadequate nutritional energy intake experienced significant (>10%) weight loss than the adequately fed neonate (<5%). Bauer et al.,[228] in contrast, maintained that a positive nitrogen balance and minimal or no growth in total body solids mass characterized this period, and that weight loss comprised entirely the loss of salt and water from the ECW pool.

Costarino et al.,[218] Shaffer and Meade,[200] and Vanpee et al.[229] have proposed variously either short-term sodium restriction (<1 mEq·kg^{-1} day^{-1}) to prevent hypernatremia in the very low birth weight neonate (<800g), or excess sodium administration (3 vs 1 mEq·kg^{-1} day^{-1}) to avoid negative salt balance across an immature renal tubule and hyponatremia.[200,229] In a more recent set of data, the latter investigations have advocated 3 to 5 mEq·kg^{-1} day^{-1} sodium supplementation in the low birth weight preterm neonate by the first 2 weeks of life to prevent later onset of sodium deficiency and growth failure, which may be otherwise unrecoverable.[92,229] Of note, they suggest hypernatremia in the very low birth weight population is underevaluated in this regard, and that radiant warmers and insensible water loss may preclude such excess supplementation.[92] Early salt restriction should be considered for the shortest number of days based on serum electrolyte balance in the tiniest neonate, with liberalization of nutritional elements including sodium thereafter, even as water volume is restricted to avoid cardiopulmonary complications of water and salt overload.

References

1. Edelman IS, Liebman J. Anatomy of body electrolytes. Am J Med 1959;27:256–277.
2. Friis-Hansen B. Body water compartments in children. Pediatrics 1961;28:169–181.
3. Robertson JD. The habitat of the early vertebrates. Biol Rev 1957;32:156–187.
4. Dahlstrom H. Basal metabolism and extracellular fluid. Acta Physiol Scand 1950;21(suppl 71):5–80.
5. Wedgewood RJ, Bass DE, Klincis JA, et al. Relationship of body composition to basal metabolic rate in normal man. J Appl Physiol 1953;6:317–334.
6. Astrup J. Energy-requiring cell functions in the ischemic brain. J Neurol Surg 1982;56:282–497.
7. Valtin H. Renal function: mechanisms preserving fluid and solute balance in health. Boston: Little, Brown, 1973:22.
8. Weast RC, ed. Handbook of chemistry and physics. 69th ed. Boca Raton: CRC Press, 1988:D-269.
9. Michel CC. Fluid movements through capillary walls. In: Renkin EM, Michel CC, eds. Handbook of physiology, section II, Vol IV part (1). Bethesda, MD: American Physiologic Society, 1984:375–409.
10. Guyton AC. Textbook of medical physiology. 6th ed. Philadelphia: W.B. Saunders, 1981;339:41–54.
11. Macknight ADC, Leaf A. Regulation of cellular volume. Physiol Rev 1977;57:510–573.
12. Strauss J. Fluid and electrolyte composition of the fetus and newborn. Pediatr Clin North Am 1966;13:1077–1102.
13. MacLaurin JC. Changes in body water distribution during the first two weeks of life. Arch Dis Child 1966;41:286–291.
14. Trachtman H, Barbour R, Sturman JA, Finburg L. Taurine and osmoregulation: taurine is a cerebral osmoprotective molecule in chronic hypernatremic dehydration. Pediatr Res 1988;23:35–39.
15. Trachtman H. Cell volume regulation: a review of cerebral adaptive mechanisms and implications for clinical treatment of osmolal disturbances. Pediatr Nephrol 1991;5:743–750.
16. McManus MI, Churchwell KB, Strange K. Regulation of cell volume in health and disease. N Engl J Med 1995;333:1260–1266.
17. Trachtman H, Yancey PH, Gullans SR. Cerebral cell volume regulation during hypernatremia in developing rats. Brain Res 1995;693:155–162.
18. Landis EM, Pappenheimer JR. Exchange of substances through capillary walls. In: Hamilton WF, ed. Handbook of physiology. Circulation section II, Vol. II. Washington, D.C.: American Physiologic Society, 1963:961–1034.
19. Wiel MH, Henning RJ, Puri VK. Colloid oncotic pressure: clinical significance. Crit Care Med 1979:113–116.
20. Webster HL. Colloid osmotic pressure: Theoretical aspects and background. Clin Perinatol 1982;9:505–521.
21. Bhat R, Javed S, Malalis L, Vidyasagar D. Colloid osmotic pressure in healthy and sick neonates. Crit Care Med 1981;9:563–567.
22. Sola A, Gregory GA. Colloid osmotic pressure of normal newborns and premature infants. Crit Care Med 1981;9:568–572.
23. Starling EH. On the absorption of fluid from the connective tissue spaces. J Physiol (Lond) 1896;19:312–326.
24. Pappenheimer JR, Soto-Rivera. Effective osmotic pressure of the plasma proteins and other quantities associated with capillary circulation in the hind limb of cats and dogs. Am J Physiol 1948;152:471–491.
25. Landis EM. Capillary pressure and capillary permeability. Physiol Rev 1934;14:404–481.
26. Civetta JM. A new look at the Starling equation. Crit Care Med 1979;7:84–91.
27. Taylor AE. Capillary fluid filtration. Circ Res 1981;49:557–575.
28. Granger DN, Miller T, Allen R, et al. Permselectivity of cat liver blood-lymph barrier to endogenous macromolecules. Gastroenterology 1979;77:103–109.
29. Nicoll PA, Taylor AE. Lymph formation and flow. Annu Rev Physiol 1977;39:73–95.
30. Chien S, Sinclair DE, Dellenbeck RJ, et al. Effect of endotoxin on capillary permeability to macromolecules. Am J Physiol 1966;210:1401–1410.
31. Brigham KL, Bowers RE, Owen PS. Effects of antihistamines on lung vascular response to histamine in unanesthetized sheep. J Clin Invest 1976;58:391–398.
32. Comper WD, Laurent TC. Physiologic function of connective tissue polysaccharides. Physiol Rev 1978;58:255–315.
33. Guyton AC. Interstitial fluid pressure: II. Pressure volume curves of interstitial space. Circ Res 1965;16:452–460.
34. Guyton AC, Granger HJ, Taylor AE. Interstitial fluid. Physiol Rev 1971:527–563.
35. Guyton AC. Textbook of medical physiology. 6th ed. Philadelphia: WB Saunders, 1981:435–447.
36. Guyton AC, Lindsey AW. Effect of elevated left atrial pressure and decreased plasma protein concentration on the development of pulmonary edema. Circ Res 1959;7:649–657.
37. Bland RD. Edema formation in the newborn lung. Clin Perinatol 1982;9:593–611.
38. Barr PA, Bailey PE, Sumners J, Cassady G. Relation between arterial blood pressure and blood volume and effect of infused albumin in sick preterm infants. Pediatrics 1977;60:282–289.
39. Schrier RW. Pathogenesis of sodium and water retention in high output and low output cardiac failure, nephrotic syndrome, cirrhosis, and pregnancy. First of two parts. N Engl J Med 1988;319:1065–1071.

40. Robertson GL, Berl T. Water metabolism. In: Brenner BM, Rector FC, eds. The kidney. Philadelphia: WB Saunders, 1986:385–431.
41. Andersson B. Regulation of body fluids. Annu Rev Physiol 1977;39:185–200.
42. Gauer OH, Henry JP, Behn C. The regulation of extracellular fluid volume. Annu Rev Physiol 1970;32:547–595.
43. Guyton AC, Scanlon LJ, Armstrong GG. Effects of pressoreceptor reflex and cushing reflex on urinary output. Fed Proc 1952;11:61–62.
44. Hall JE, Guyton AC, Colemean TG, et al. Regulation of arterial pressure: role of pressure natriuresis and diuresis. Fed Proc 1986;45:2897–2903.
45. Mann JFE, Johnson AK, Gantten D, Eberhard R. Thirst and the renin-angiotensin system. Kidney Int 1987;32 (suppl 21):S27–S34.
46. Robertson GL, Shelton RL, Athar S. The osmoregulation of vasopressin. Kidney Int 1976;10:25–37.
47. DeTorrente A, Robertson GL, McDonald KM, Schrier RW. Mechanism of diuretic response to left atrial pressure in the anesthetized dog. Kidney Int 1975:355–361.
48. Shapiro MD, Nicholls KM, Groves BM, et al. Interrelationship between cardiac output and vascular resistance as determinants of effective arterial blood volume in cirrhotic patients. Kidney Int 1985;28:206–211.
49. Mills IH. Renal regulation of sodium excretion. Annu Rev Med 1970;21:75–98.
50. Brenner BM, Troy JL, Daugharty TM. On the mechanism of inhibition in fluid reabsorption by the renal proximal tubule of the volume expanded rat. J Clin Invest 1971;50:1596–1602.
51. Leake RD, Trygstad CW. Glomerular filtration rate during the period of adaptation to extrauterine life. Pediatr Res 1977;11:959–962.
52. Spitzer A. The role of the kidney in sodium homeostasis during maturation. Kidney Int 1982;21:539–545.
53. Laragh JH. Atrial natriuretic hormone: the renin aldosterone axis and blood pressure–electrolyte homeostasis. N Engl J Med 1985;313:1330–1340.
54. Laragh JH, Sealey JE. The renin-angiotensin-aldosterone hormonal system of sodium, potassium and blood pressure homeostasis. In: Orloff J, Berliner RN, eds. Handbook of physiology, section VIII, renal physiology. Washington, DC: American Physiologic Society, 1973:831–908.
55. Jones DP, Chesney RW. Development of tabular function. In: Bailie MD, ed. Renal function and disease. Clin Perinatol 1992;19:33–57.
56. Aperia A, Holtback U, Syren ML, et al. Activation/deactivation of renal Na+, K+ ATPase: a final common pathway for regulation of natriuresis. FASEB J 1994;8:436–439.
57. Ohtomo Y, Meister B, Hokfelt T, Aperia A. Coexisting NPY and NE synergistically regulate renal tubular Na+, K+ ATPase activity. Kidney Int 1994;45:1606–1613.
58. Ibarra F, Aperia A, Svensson LB, et al. Bidirectional regulation of Na+, K-ATPase activity by dopamine and an alpha-adrenergic agonist. Proc Natl Acad Sci USA 1993;90:21–24.
59. Meister B, Aperia A. Molecular mechanisms involved in catecholamine regulation of sodium transport. Semin Nephrol 1993;13:41–49.
60. Smith FG, Klindefus JM, Robillard JE. Effects of volume expansion on renal sympathetic nerve activity, cardiovascular and renal function in lambs. Am J Physiol 1992;262:R651–R658.
61. Smith FG, Sato T, McWeeny OJ, et al. Role of renal nerves in response to volume expansion in conscious, newborn lambs. Am J Physiol 1989;257:R1519–R1525.
62. Aperia A. Dopamine action and metabolism in the kidney. Curr Opinion Nephrol Hypertens 1994;3:39–45.
63. Johnson MD, Malvin RL. Stimulation of renal sodium reabsorption by angiotension II. Am J Physiol 1977;232:F298–F306.
64. Seifter JL, Skorecki KL, Stivelman JC, et al. Control of extracellular fluid volume and pathophysiology of edema formation. In: Brenner BM, Rector FC, eds. The kidney. Philadelphia: WB Saunders, 1986:343–384.
65. el-Dhar SS. Development biology of the renal kallikrein-kinin system. Pediatr Nephrol 1994;8:624–631.
66. Dunn FL, Brennon TJ, Nelson AE, Robertson GL. The role of blood osmolality and volume in regulating vasopressin secretion in the rat. J Clin Invest 1973;52:3212–3219.
67. Lasseter WE, Gottschalk CW. Regulation of water balance: urine concentration and dilution. In: Schrier RW, Gottschalk CW, eds. Diseases of the kidney, 4th ed. Boston: Little, Brown, 1988:119–142.
68. Grantham JJ, Burg MB. Effect of vasopressin and cyclic AMP on permeability of isolated collecting tubules. Am J Physiol 1966;211:255–259.
69. Sagnella GA, MacGregor GA. Cardiac peptides and the control of sodium excretion. Nature 1984;309:666–667.
70. Blaine EH. Emergence of a new cardiovascular control system: atrial natriuretic factor. Clin Exp Theor Pract 1985;A7(5&6):839–850.
71. Seymour AA. Renal and systemic effects of atrial natriuretic factor. Clin Exp Theor Pract 1985;A7(5&6):887–906.
72. Richards AM, Ikram H, Yanckle TG, et al. Renal, hemodynamic, and hormonal effects of human alpha atrial natriuretic peptide in healthy volunteers. Lancet 1985;1:545-548.
73. Andersson S, Tikkanen I, Pesonen E, et al. Atrial natriuretic peptide in patent ductus arteriosus. Pediatr Res 1987;21:396–398.
74. Baylen BG, Ogata H, Ikeganim M, et al. Left ventricular performance and contractility before and after volume infusion: a comparative study in preterm and full-term newborn. Circulation 1986;73:1042–1049.
75. Gruskin AB, Edelman CM Jr, Yuan S. Maturational changes in renal blood flow in piglets. Pediatr Res 1970;4:7-13.
76. Spitzer A. Renal physiology and function development. In: Edelman CM Jr, ed. The kidney and urinary tract, vol. 1. 1978:25–128.
77. Cleary GM, Higgins ST, Merton DA, et al. Developmental changes in renal artery blood flow velocity during the first three weeks of life in preterm neonates. J Pediatr 1996;129:251–257.
78. Robillard JE, Matson JR, Sessions C, et al. Maturational changes in the fetal glomerular filtration rate. Am J Obstet Gynecol 1975;122:601–606.

79. Robillard JE, Matson JR, Sessions C, et al. Developmental aspects of renal tubular reabsorption of water in the lamb fetus. Pediatr Res 1979;13:1172–1176.
80. Chung EE, Moore ES, Cevallos EE, et al. The effect of gestational age and arterial pressure on renal function in utero. Pediatr Res 1976;10:437A.
81. Rudolph AM, Heyman MA, Teramo KAW, et al. Studies on circulation of the previable human fetus. Pediatr Res 1971;5:452–465.
82. Calcagno PL, Rubin MI. Renal exaction of para-amino hippurate in infants and children. J Clin Invest 1963;42:1632–1639.
83. Aperia A, Broberger O, Elinder G, et al. Postnatal development of renal function in pre-term and full-term infants. Acta Pediatr Scand 1981;70:183–187.
84. Guignard JP, Torrado A, Mazouni SM, Gautier E. Renal function in respiratory distress syndrome. J Pediatr 1976;88:845–850.
85. Seitel H, Scopes J. Rates of creatinine clearance in babies less than one week of age. Arch Dis Child 1973;48:717–720.
86. Manuli MA, Lorenz JM. Extracellular pH modifies adaptive response to high K+ in cultured canine kidney cells. Am J Physiol 1992;262:F897–901.
87. Celsi G, Wang ZM, Akusjarvi G, Aperia A. Sensitive periods for glucocorticoids' regulation of Na+, K+ ATPase mRNA in the developing lung and kidney. Pediatr Res 1993;33:5–9.
88. Norton ME, Merrill J, Cooper BAB, et al. Neonatal complications after the administration of indomethacin for preterm labor. N Engl J Med 1993;329:1602–1607.
89. Van den Anker JN, Hop WCJ, de Groot R, et al. Effects of prenatal exposure to betamethasone and indomethacin on the glomerular filtration rate in the preterm infant. Pediatr Res 1994;36:578–581.
90. Stefano JL, Norman ME, Morales MC, et al. Decreased erythrocyte Na+, K+ ATPase activity associated with cellular potassium loss in extremely low birth weight infants with nonoliguric hyperkalemia. J Pediatr 1993;122:276–284.
91. Stefano JL, Norman ME. Nitrogen balance in extremely low birth weight infants with nonoliguric hyperkalemia. J Pediatr 1993;123:632–635.
92. Gaycock GB, Aperia A. Salt and the newborn kidney. Pediatr Nephrol 1991;5:65–70.
93. Gruskay JA, Costarino AT, Polin RA, Baumgart S. Nonoliguric hyperkalemia in the premature infant less than 1000 grams. J Pediatr 1988;113:381–386.
94. Leake RD, Zakandddin S, Trygstad CW, et al. The effects of large-volume intravenous fluid infusion on neonatal renal function. J Pediatr 1976;89:968–972.
95. Smith CA, Yudkin S, Young W, et al. Adjustment of electrolytes and water following premature births. Pediatrics 1949;3:34–48.
96. Edelman CM, Trompkon V, Barnett HL. Renal concentrating ability in newborn infants. Fed Proc 1959;18:40A.
97. Heller H. The renal function of newborn infants. J Physiol (Lond) 1944;102:429–440.
98. Imbert-Teboul M, Chabardes D, Cligue A, et al. Ontogenesis of hormone-dependent adenylate cyclase in isolated rat nephron segments. Am J Physiol 1984;247:F316–325.
99. Aperia A, Broberger O, Thodenius, et al. Development of renal control of salt and fluid homeostasis during the first year of life. Acta Pediatr Scand 1975;64:393–398.
100. Edelman CM, Barnett HL. Role of kidney in water metabolism in young infants. J Pediatr 1960;56:154–179.
101. Aperia A, Elinder G. Distal tubular sodium reabsorption in the developing rat kidney. Am J Physiol 1981;29:F487–491.
102. Aperia A, Broberger O, Thodenius K. Renal response to an oral sodium load in newborn full-term infants. Acta Pediatr Scand 1972;61:670–676.
103. Robillard JE, Sessions C, Kennedy RL, et al. Interrelationships between glomerular filtration rate and renal transport of sodium and chloride during fetal life. Am J Obstet Gynecol 1977;128:727–734.
104. Goldsmith DI, Drukker A, Blaufox MD, et al. Hemodynamic and excretory responses of the neonatal canine kidney to acute volume expansion. Am J Physiol 1979;237(5):F392–397.
105. Aperia A, Zetterstrom R. Renal control of fluid homeostasis in the newborn infant. Clin Perinatol 1982;9:523–533.
106. Drukker A, Goldsmith DI, Spitzer A, et al. The renin-angiotensin system in newborn dogs. Developmental patterns and response to acute saline loading. Pediatr Res 1980;14:304–307.
107. Day RL, Radde IC, Balfe JW, et al. Electrolyte abnormalities in very low birthweight infants. Pediatr Res 1976;10:522–526.
108. DeFronzo RA, Bia M, Smith D. Clinical disorders of hyperkalemia. Annu Rev Med 1982;33:521–554.
109. Aperia A, Broberger O, Thodenius K, et al. Developmental study of the renal response to an oral salt load in pre-term infants. Acta Pediatr Scand 1974;63:517–524.
110. Cox M. Potassium homeostasis. Med Clin North Am 1981;65:363–384.
111. Kaplan BS. Some thoughts on potassium and acetazolamide in developing kidneys. Dev Pharmacol Ther 1981;2:52–54.
112. Brion LP, Fleischman AR, Schwartz GJ. Hyperkalemia in very low birthweight infants with non-oliguric renal failure. Pediatr Res 1985;19:336A.
113. Fildes RD, Eisner GM, Calcagno PL, et al. Renal alpha-adrenoceptors and sodium excretion in the dog. Am J Physiol 1985;248:F128–F133.
114. Kotchen TA, Strickland AL, Rice MS, Walters DR. A study of the renin-angiotensin system in newborn infants. J Peds 1972;80:938–946.
115. Richer C, Hornych H, Amiel-Tison C. Plasma renin activity and its postnatal development in preterm infants. Biol Neonate 1977;31:301–304.
116. Csaba I, Ertyl T, Nemeth M, et al. Postnatal development of renin-angiotensin-aldosterone system, Raas, in relation to electrolyte balance in premature infants. Pediatr Res 1979;13:817–820.
117. Pipkin FB, Phil D, Smales ORC. A study of factors affecting blood pressure and angiotensin II in newborn infants. J Pediatr 1977;91:113–119.
118. Godard C, Geering JM, Geering K, Vallotton MB. Plasma renin activity related to sodium balance, renal function

and urinary vasopressin in the newborn infant. Pediatr Res 1979;13:742–745.
119. Bender JW, Davitt MK, Jose P. Angiotensin-I converting enzyme activity in term and premature infants. Biol Neonate 1978;34:19–23.
120. Mattioli L, Zakheim M, Mullis K, Molteni A. Angiotensin-I converting enzyme activity in idiopathic respiratory distress syndrome of the newborn infant and in experimental alveolar hypoxia in mice. J Pediatr 1975;87:97–101.
121. Schubert F, George JM, Rao MB. Vasopressin and oxytocin content of human fetal brain at different stages of gestation. Brain Res 1981;213:111–117.
122. Chard T, Hudson CN, Edwards CRW, Boyd NRH. Release of oxytocin and vasopressin by the human foetus during labour. Nature 1971;234:352–353.
123. Wiriyathian S, Rosenfeld CR, Arant BS, et al. Urinary arginine vasopressin: pattern of excretion in the neonatal period. Pediatr Res 1986;20:103–108.
124. Rees L, Forsling ML, Brook CGD, Vasopressin concentrations in the neonatal period. Clin Endocrinol 1980;12:357–362.
125. Hadeed AJ, Leake RD, Weitzman RE, Fisher DA. Possible mechanisms of high blood levels of vasopressin during the neonatal period. J Pediatr 1979;94:805–808.
126. Pohjavuouri M. Obstetric determinants of plasma vasopressin concentrations and renin activity at birth. J Pediatr 1983;103:966–968.
127. Polin RA, Hussain MK, James LS, Frantz AG. High vasopressin concentrations in human umbilical cord blood—lack of correlation with stress. J Perinatol Med 1977;5:114–119.
128. Weitzman RE, Fisher DE, Robillard JE, et al. Arginine vasopressin response to an osmotic stimulus in the fetal sheep. Pediatr Res 1978;12:35–38.
129. Robillard JE, Weitzman RE, Fisher DE, Smith FG. The dynamics of vasopressin release and blood volume regulation during fetal hemorrhage in the lamb fetus. Pediatr Res 1979;13:606–610.
130. Robillard JE, Matson JR, Sessions C, Smith FG. Developmental aspects of renal tubular reabsorption of water in the lamb fetus. Pediatr Res 1979;13:1172–1176.
131. Stern P, LaRochelle FT, Little GA. Vasopressin and pneumothorax in the neonate. Pediatrics 1981;68:499–503.
132. Leslie GI, Philips JB, Work J, et al. The effect of assisted ventilation on creatinine clearance and hormonal control of electrolyte balance in very low birth weight infants. Pediatr Res 1986;20:447–452.
133. Weinberg JA, Weitzman RE, Zakauddin S, Leake RD. Inappropriate secretion of antidiuretic hormone in a premature infant. Pediatrics 1977;90:111–114.
134. Hoppenstein JM, Miltenberger FW, Moran WH. The increase in blood levels of vasopressin in infants during birth and surgical procedures. Surg Gynecol Obstet 1968;127:966–974.
135. Waters CB, Weinberg JE, Leake RD, Fisher DA. Arginine vasopressin levels during painful stimulus in infancy. Pediatr Res 1982;16:569.
136. Kaplan SL, Feigin RD. Inappropriate secretion of antidiuretic hormone complicating neonatal hypoxic-ischemic encephalopathy. J Pediatr 1978;92:431–433.
137. Pohjavuori M. Obstetric determinants of plasma vasopressin concentrations and renin activity at birth. Pediatrics 1983;103:966–968.
138. Robillard JE, Weitzman RE. Developmental aspects of the fetal renal response to exogenous arginine vasopressin. Am J Physiol 1980;7:F407–414.
139. Rees L, Brook GD, Shaw JCL, Forsling ML. Hyponatremia in the first week of life in preterm infants. Part I arginine vasopressin secretion. Arch Dis Child 1984;59:414–422.
140. Schlondorff D, Weber H, Trizna W, Fine LG. Vasopressin responsiveness of renal adenylate cyclase in newborn rats and rabbits: Am J Physiol 1978;234:F16–F21.
141. Edelman CM, Wolfish NM. Dietary influence on renal maturation in preterm infants. Pediatr Res 1968;2:421.
142. Kovacs L, Sulyok E, Lichardus B, et al. Renal response to arginine vasopressin in premature infants with late hyponatraemia. Arch Dis Child 1986;61:1030–1032.
143. Svenningsen NW, Aronson AS. Postnatal development of renal concentration capacity as estimated by DDAVP-test in normal and asphyxiated neonates. Biol Neonate 1974;25:230–241.
144. Edelman CM, Barnett HL, Stark H. Effect of urea on concentration of urinary nonurea solute in premature infants. J Appl Physiol 1966;21:1021–1025.
145. Sulyok E, Kovacs L, Lichardus B, et al. Late hyponatremia in premature infants: role of aldosterone and arginine vasopressin. J Pediatr 1985;106:990–994.
146. Edelman CM. Developmental renal physiology. In: Gruskin AB, Norman ME, eds. Proceedings of the Fifth International Pediatric Nephrology Symposium. The Hague: Martinus Nijhoff, 1981:15–27.
147. Costarino AT, Baumgart S, Norman ME, Polin RA. Renal adaptation to extrauterine life in patients with respiratory distress syndrome. Am J Dis Child 1985;139:1060–1063.
148. Ekblad H, Kero P, Vuolteenaho O, et al. Atrial natriuretic peptide in the preterm infant: lack of correlation with natriuresis and diuresis. 1992;81:978–982.
149. Tulassay T, Rascher W, Seyberth HW, et al. The role of atrial natriuretic peptide in sodium homeostasis in premature infants. J Pediatr 1986;109:1023–1027.
150. Kojuma T, Hirata Y, Fukuda Y, et al. Plasma atrial natriuretic peptide and spontaneous diuresis in sick neonates. Arch Dis Child 1987;62:667–670.
151. Ronconi M, Fortunato A, Soffiati G, et al. Vasopressin, atrial natriuretic factor and renal water homeostasis in premature newborn infants with respiratory distress syndrome. J Perinatol Med 1995;23d:307–314.
152. Rozycki HJ, Baumgart S. Atrial natriuretic factor and renal function during diuresis in preterm infants. Clin Res 1987;35:556A.
153. Muchant DG, Thornhill BA, Belmonte DC, et al. Chronic sodium loading augments natriuretic response to acute volume expansion in the preweaned rat. Am J Physiol 1995;269:R15–R22.
154. Arant BS Jr. Functional immaturity of the newborn kidney: paradox or prostaglandin? In: Strauss J, ed. Homeostasis, nephrotoxicity and renal anomalies in the newborn. Boston: Martinus Nijhoff, 1984:271–278.

155. Cassady G. Effect of caesarian section on neonatal body water spaces. N Engl J Med 1971;285:887–891.
156. Costarino AT, Baumgart S. Controversies in fluid and electrolyte therapy for the premature infant. Clin Perinatol 1988;15:863–878.
157. Lorenz JM, Kleinman LI, Kotagal UR. Water balance in very low birthweight infants: relationship to water and sodium intake and effect on outcome. J Pediatr 1982;101:423–432.
158. Brans YW, Cassady G. Intrauterine growth and maturation in relation to fetal deprivation. In: Gruenwald P, ed. The placenta and its maternal supply line. London: Medical and Technical Publishing, 1975:307–334.
159. Cheek DB, Talbert JI. Extracellular volume (and sodium) and body water in infants. In: Cheek DB, ed. Human growth: body composition, cell growth, energy and intelligence. Philadelphia: Lea & Febiger, 1968:117–134.
160. Osler M, Pedersen J. The body composition of newborn infants of diabetic mothers. Pediatrics 1960;26:985–992.
161. Baumgart S, Langman CB, Sosulski R, et al. Fluid, electrolyte, and glucose maintenance in the very low birthweight infant. Clin Pediatr 1982;21:199–206.
162. Brown ER, Stark A, Sosenko I, et al. Bronchopulmonary dysplasia: possible relationships to pulmonary edema. J Pediatr 1978;92:982–984.
163. Bell EF, Warburton D, Stonestreet BS, et al. Effect of fluid administration on the development of symptomatic patient ductus arteriosus and congestive heart failure in premature infants. N Engl J Med 1980;302:598–604.
164. Spitzer AR, Fox WW, Delavoria-Papadopoulos M. Maximum diuresis: a factor in predicting recovery for respiratory distress sydrome and the development of bronchopulmonary dysplasia. J Pediatr 1981;98:476–479.
165. Arant BS. Adaptation of the infant to an external milieu. In: Gruskin AB, Norman ME, eds. Pediatric nephrology. Proceedings of the Fifth International Pediatric Nephrology Symposium 1980. The Hague: Martinus Nijhoff, 1981:265–272.
166. Sulyok E, Jequier E, Prod'hom LS. Respiratory contribution to the thermal balance of the newborn infant under various ambient conditions. Pediatrics 1973;51:641–650.
167. Sinclair JC. Metabolic rate and temperature control. In: Smith CA, Nelson NM, eds. The physiology of the newborn infant. 4th ed. Springfield, IL: Charles C. Thomas, 1976:354–415.
168. Winters RW. Maintenance fluid therapy. In: The body fluids in pediatrics. Boston: Little, Brown, 1973:113–133.
169. Sosulski R, Baumgart S. Respiratory water loss and heat balance in intubated premature infants receiving humidified air. J Pediatr 1983;103:307–310.
170. Rosenfield WN, Linshaw M, Fox HA. Water intoxication: a complication of nebulization with nasal CPAP. J Pediatr 1976;89:113–114.
171. Weinstein MR, Oh W. Oxygen consumption in infants with bronchopulmonary dysplasia. J Pediatr 1981;99:958–961.
172. Kurzner SI, Garg M, Bautista B, et al. Growth failure in bronchopulmonary dysplasia: elevated metabolic rates and pulmonary mechanics. J Pediatr 1988;112:73–80.
173. Jhaveri M, Kumar SP. Passage of the first stool in very low birthweight infants. Pediatrs 1987;79:1005–1007.
174. Fanaroff AA, Ward M, Gruber HS, et al. Insensible water loss in low birthweight infants. Pediatrics 1972;50:236–245.
175. Williams PR, Oh W. Effects of radiant warmer on insensible water loss in newborn infants. Am J Dis Child 1974;128:511–514.
176. Baumgart S, Engle WD, Fox WW, et al. Radiant warmer power and body size as determinants of insensible water loss in the critically ill neonate. Pediatr Res 1981;15:1495–1499.
177. Bell EF, Neidich GA, Cashore WJ, et al. Combined effect of radiant warmer and phototherapy on insensible water loss in low-birthweight infants. J Pediatr 1979;94:810–813.
178. Wu PYK, Hodgman JE. Insensible water loss in preterm infants: changes with postnatal development and non-ionizing radiant energy. Pediatrics 1974;54:704–712.
179. Costarino AT, Baumgart S. Modern fluid and electrolyte management of the critically ill premature infant. Pediatr Clin North Am 1986;33:153–178.
180. Bruck K. Heat production and temperature regulation. In: Stave U, ed. Perinatal physiology. New York: Plenum, 1978:455–498.
181. Hey EN, Katz G. Evaporative water loss in the newborn baby. J Physiol (Lond) 1969;200:605–619.
182. Wheldon AE, Rutter N. The heat balance of small babies nursed in incubators and under radiant warmers. Early Hum Dev 1982;6:131–143.
183. Baumgart S, Engle WD, Fox WW, et al. Effect of heat shielding on convection and evaporation, and radiant heat transfer in the premature infant. J Pediatr 1981;99:948–956.
184. Okken A, Blijhan C, Franz W, et al. Effects of forced convection of heated air on insensible water loss and heat loss in preterm infants in incubators. J Pediatr 1982;101:108–112.
185. Baumgart S. Radiant energy and insensible water loss in the premature newborn infant nursed under a radiant warmer. Clin Perinatol 1982;9:483–503.
186. Hammarlund K, Sedin G. Transepidermal water loss in newborn infants: VIII. Relation to gestational age and post-natal age in appropriate and small for gestational age infants. Acta Paediatr Scand 1983;72:721–728.
187. Haycock GB, Schwartz GJ, Wisotsky DH. Geometric method for measuring body surface areas: a height-weight formula validated in infants, children and adults. J Pediatr 1978;93:62–66.
188. Baumgart S. Partitioning of heat losses and gains in premature newborn infants under radiant warmers. Pediatrics 1985;75:89–99.
189. Baumgart S, Fox WW, Polin RA. Physiologic implications of two different heat shields for infants under radiant warmers. J Pediatr 1982;100:787–790.
190. Engle WD, Baumgart S, Schwartz JG, et al. Combined effect of radiant warmer power and phototherapy on insensible water loss in the critically ill neonate. Am J Dis Child 1981;135:516–520.
191. Knauth A, Gordin MS, McNelis W, Baumgart S. Semipermeable polyurethane membrane as an artificial skin for the premature neonate. Pediatrics 1989;83:945–950.
192. Sedin G, Hammarlund K, Nilsson GE, et al. Measurements of transepidermal water loss in newborn infants. Clin Perinatol 1985;12:79–96.

193. Lauweryns JM, Claessens S, Boussauw L. The pulmonary lymphatics in neonatal hyaline membrane disease. Pediatrics 1968;41:917–930.
194. Jefferies AL, Coates G, O'Brodovich H. Pulmonary epithelial permeability in hyaline membrane disease. N Engl J Med 1984;31:1075–1080.
195. Rees L, Shaw JCL, Brook GD, Forsling ML. Hyponatremia in the first week of life in preterm infants. Part II: sodium and water balance. Arch Dis Child 1984;59:423–429.
196. Huet F, Semama D, Grimaldi M, et al. Effects of theophylline on renal insufficiency in neonates with respiratory distress syndrome. Intensive Care Med 1995;21:511–514.
197. Lorenz JM, Kleinman LI, Ahmed G, Markarian K. Phases of fluid and electrolyte homeostasis in the extremely low birth weight infant. Pediatrics 1995;96:484–489.
198. Ramiro-Tolentino SB, Markarian K, Kleinman LI. Renal bicarbonate excretion in extremely low birth weight infants. Pediatrics 1996;98:256–261.
199. Ishizaki Y, Isozaki-Fukuda Y, Kojima T, et al. Evaluation of diagnositic criteria of acute renal failure in premature infants. Acta Paediatr Jpn 1993;35:311–315.
200. Shaffer SG, Meade VM. Sodium balance and extracellular volume regulation in very low birth weight infants. J Pediatr 1989;115:285–290.
201. Vanpee M, Ergander U, Herin P, Aperia A. Renal function in sick, very low-birth-weight infants. Acta Paediatr 1993;82:714–718.
202. Vanpee M, Blennow M, Linne T, et al. Renal function in very low birth weight infants: normal maturity reached during early childhood. J Pediatr 1992;121:784–788.
203. Bueva A, Guignard JP. Renal function in preterm neonates. Pediatr Res 1994;36:572–577.
204. Cornblath M, Forbes AE, Pildes RS, et al. A controlled study of early fluid administration on survival of low birthweight infants. Pediatrics 1966;38:547–554.
205. Spahr RC, Klein AM, Brown DR, et al. Fluid administration and bronchopulmonary dysplasia. Am J Dis Child 1980;134:958–960.
206. Gersony WM, Peckham GJ, Ellison RC, et al. Effects of indomethacin in premature infants with patent ductus arteriosus: results of a national collaborative study. J Pediatr 1983;102:895–906.
207. Van Marter LJ, Pagano M, Allred EN, et al. Rate of bronchopulmonary dysplasia as a function of neonatal intensive care practices. 1992;120:938–946.
208. Corbet A, Adams J. Current therapy in hyaline membrane disease. Clin Perinatol 1978;5:299–316.
209. Harris P. Role of arterial pressure in the oedema of heart disease. Lancet 1988;1:1036–1038.
210. Firth JD, Raine AEG, Ledingham JGG. Raised venous pressure: a direct cause of renal sodium retention in oedema? Lancet 1988;1:1033–1036.
211. Bichet DG, Vicki J, Van Putten BS, Schrier RW. Potential role of increased sympathetic activity in impaired sodium and water excretion in cirrhosis. N Engl J Med 1982;307:1552–1557.
212. Levy M, Wexler MJ. Sodium excretion in dogs with low-grade caval constriction: role of hepatic nerves. Am J Physiol 1987;253:F672–F678.
213. Kumar A, Pontoppidan H, Baratz RA, Laver MB. Inappropriate response to increased plasma ADH during mechanical ventilation in acute respiratory failure. Anesthesiology 1974;40:215–221.
214. Leslie G, Philips JB, Work J. The effect of assisted ventilation on creatinine clearance and hormonal control of electrolyte balance in very low birth weight infants. Pediatr Res 1986;20:447–452.
215. Finberg L. Dangers to infants caused by changes in osmolal concentration. Pediatrics 1967;40:1031–1034.
216. Shaffer SG, Kilbride HW, Hayen LK, et al. Hyperkalemia in very low birth weight infants. J Pediatr 1992;121:275–279.
217. Sato K, Kondo T, Iwao H, et al. Internal potassium shift in premature infants: cause of nonoliguric hyperkalemia. J Pediatr 1995;126:109–113.
218. Costarino T, Grusday JA, Corcoran L, et al. Sodium restriction versus daily maintenance replacement in very low birth weight premature neonates: a randomized, blind therapeutic trial. J Pediatr 1992;120:99–106.
219. Porot R, Brodsky N. Effect of Tegaderm use on outcome of extremely low birth weight (ELBW) infants. Pediatr Res 1993;33:231A.
220. Harpin A, Rutter N. Humidification of incubators. Arch Dis Child 1985;60:219–224.
221. Sulyok E. The relationship between electrolyte and acid base balance in premature infants during early postnatal life. Biol Neonate 1971;95:227–237.
222. Honour JW, Shackleton CHL, Valman HB. Sodium homeostasis in preterm infants. Lancet 1974;2:1147.
223. Roy RN, Chance CW, Radde IC, et al. Late hyponatremia in very low birthweight infants (1.3 kg). Pediatr Res 1976;10:526–531.
224. Sulyok E, Nemeth M, Teny IF, et al. Relationship between maturity, electrolyte balance, and the function of renin-angiotensin-aldosterone system in newborn infants. Biol Neonate 1979;35:60–65.
225. Sulyok E, Rascher W, Baranyai Z, et al. Influence of NaCL supplementation on vasopressin secretion and water excretion in premature infants. Biol Neonate 1993;64:201–208.
226. Harkavy KL, Scanlon JW, Jose P. The effects of theophylline on renal function in the premature newborn. Biol Neonate 1979;35:126–130.
227. Heimler R, Boumas BT, Jendrzejczak BM, et al. Relationship between nutrition, weight change, and fluid compartments in preterm infants during the first week of life. J Pediatr 1993;122:110–114.
228. Bauer K, Bovermann G, Roithmaier A, et al. Body composition, nutrition, and fluid balance during the first two weeks of life in preterm neonates weighing less than 1500 grams. J Pediatr 1991;118:615–620.
229. Vanpee M, Herin P, Broberger U, Aperia A. Sodium supplementation optimizes weight gain in preterm infants. Acta Paediatr 1995;84:1312–1314.

47
Body Composition of the Neonate

Kenneth J. Ellis

Linear growth during fetal development and neonatal life is accompanied by changes in the relative composition of the human body. During each phase of growth, changes occur in the general chemical composition of the major tissues in the body, their relative proportions of the total body weight, and in their physiologic and functional use. Although an individual's intrauterine growth may be under strong genetic controls, additional significant influences are attributable to the hormonal, nutritional, and health status of the mother.[1-6] Body composition data were initially derived from studies using whole-body chemical analyses of the human fetus and neonate. However, new in vivo methodologies are being developed that may provide more accurate standards. Estimates of fetal growth and changes in body composition during early infancy continue to provide reference standards for the nutritional assessment of neonates and may assist in their clinical care.

Historical Perspective on Body Composition Measurements

As analytical chemistry was being developed in the late 1800s, one of its many applications included analyses of the chemical content of human tissues and body fluids. Analyses of various tissues and fluids were performed for healthy subjects and for a number of clinical disorders. Chemical analyses of the whole body of human fetuses and infants, for example, can be traced to the early 20th century. These studies provided the first systematic scientific investigations of body composition during human development and its changes with neonatal growth. When these findings were compared with the information known about chemical composition of tissues obtained from adults, there were often differences. This, in part, led to the concept of "chemical maturity" for the adult body, especially for the lean tissues in the body.[7] This concept recognized that there are changes in the chemical makeup of various tissues after birth that are necessary before the composition of the body would reach the relatively constant proportions observed in adults. The age at which this chemical maturation would be attained may differ among tissues in the body and reach maturation at different times among the tissues.[8]

During the first three decades of this century, continued analyses of the human neonatal body, following abortion, stillbirth, or early death, were reported. At that time nutrition studies were undertaken to ascertain which foods might account for the growth increments occurring during fetal development and in early infancy. Metabolic balance studies were usually unsuccessful because of their lack of precision and difficulties in monitoring the infant's nutrient intake and energy expenditure. Starting in the late 1940s, there was a renewed interest in body composition of infants, especially that of the malnourished or preterm neonate, in terms of lowering the high neonatal mortality rate. More convenient methods were being developed to measure the nutrient content of foods. There was a parallel interest in having similar techniques to monitor the composition of growth in infants and children. Radioactive tracers developed to measure total body water and electrolytes were finding applications in studies of adults at about this time. The underwater weighing technique for the measurement of body density, as pioneered by Behnke et al.[9] during World War II, was starting to gain favor as a reference standard for body composition measurements in adults.

Over the past four decades these methods have been improved, and a number of new in vivo procedures have been developed or have expanded the older techniques to assess body composition, often with a focus on a specific subcompartment. Over the years many of these techniques have been discussed and evaluated in review articles.[10-18] This chapter provides a comprehensive summary of our current knowledge of human composition based on these in vivo methods, with an emphasis on estimating bone mass, lean tissue mass, the proportions of protein, muscle, and water content, and total body fat in the neonate and young infant.

Body Composition Models

Multicompartment Models

Most in vivo methods have been designed to measure the composition of the whole body. Many of these techniques provide only a single measure of some property of a subcomponent of the total body, usually for the nonfat or lean tissue mass. These techniques rely on the basic two-compartment model of body composition,

$$Wt = Fat + FFM$$

where Wt is body weight and FFM is the fat-free mass. The underwater weighing (UWW) technique is based on this two-compartment model concept. If the density of each compartment (e.g., fat and FFM) is known, and the weight of the body is obtained in air and totally submersed in water, one can calculate the relative proportions of each compartment needed to equal the weight of the body. Although this technique can be used with most healthy adults and older children, it is obviously not very applicable for use with neonates and infants. In addition to the technical difficulties of total submersion of the infant, there are the limitations of not knowing the true density of the nonfat tissues and having to correct for residual lung volume. Hence, the UWW technique has been long abandoned for use in infants and will not be discussed further in this chapter. However, the general principle is still used and is discussed later in this chapter with the air-displacement measurement technique.

Body composition modeling is not limited to the basic two-compartment model. At least five different levels of models can be easily constructed to describe body composition.[19] These are illustrated in Figure 47.1 along with the two-compartment model. To measure body composition as defined by the more elaborate models, an increasing number of independent measurements is needed, and each must have compartment specificity. To accurately monitor one of the subcompartments, a direct measure of some physical property unique to that compartment is required. As shown in Figure 47.1, the most basic framework or fundamental classification of body composition is based on the elemental content of the body. This model is considered by most investigators to be the "gold standard" for body composition.[19] The next higher model (level 2) is based on the combination of elements into chemical compounds that can be grouped into four major classifications: water, protein, minerals, and fat. The mathematical expression for this model is

$$Wt = Water + Protein + Minerals + Fat$$

and is often referred to as the four-compartment model of body composition. One can add a fifth compartment to account for the body's glycogen stores, but its mass is relatively small and it is assumed to be part (<0.5%) of the protein compartment. This four-compartment model is the one most often used when describing changes with growth, especially in terms of nutritional requirements. This model of body composition is the basis for most of the discussion in this chapter.

The level-3 model presents a physiologic view of body composition as it reflects the organization of the body

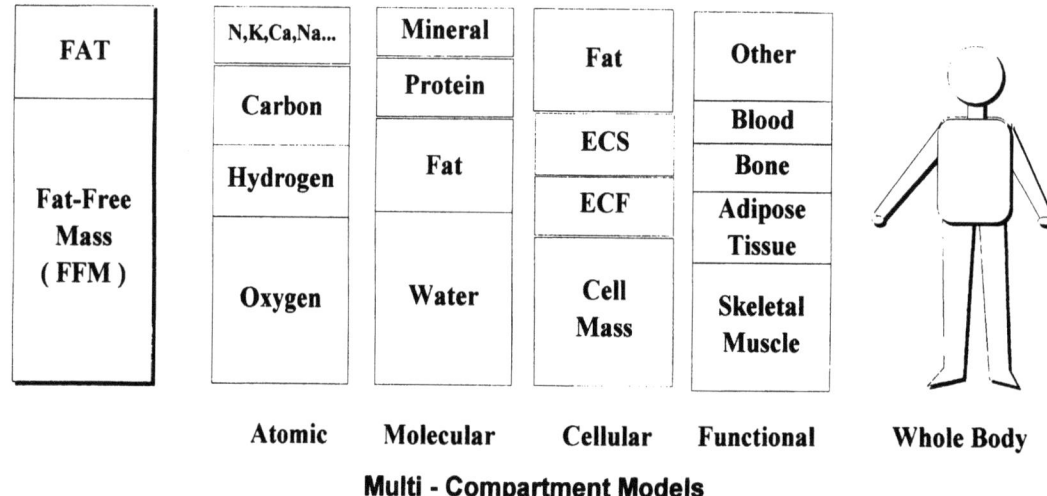

FIGURE 47.1. Models of body composition: basic two-compartment model, four multicompartment models, and the whole-body model.

into its intracellular and extracellular compartments. The intracellular compartment, called the body cell mass (BCM), combines its fluid and solids components. The extracellular compartment is subdivided into its extracellular water (ECW) and solids (ECS) subcomponents. This model is a three-compartment model of the fat-free mass, such that body weight is defined by the equation.

$$Wt = BCM + ECF + ECS + Fat.$$

The mineral content of the skeleton is the dominant component of the extracellular solids compartment. The BCM compartment was originally proposed by Moore et al.,[20] who questioned the usefulness of the FFM or lean body mass concept because it included the metabolically inactive extracellular compartment of the body's total nonfat mass. Moore et al. defined BCM as "that component of body composition containing the oxygen-exchanging, potassium-rich, glucose-oxidizing, work-performing tissue" of the body. The fact that these tissues are potassium-rich leads one to consider the measurement of total body potassium (TBK) or that of the intracellular water space as a measure of the BCM.[15,19]

The model at the fourth level of complexity considers the body's structural and functional components. Techniques such as magnetic resonance imaging (MRI), computed tomography (CT), and ultrasound imaging are providing information related to this model.[21] Dual-energy x-ray absorptiometry (DXA) provides information specific to the skeleton, although most investigators prefer to relate this technique to the level-2 model.

At the whole-body level of composition, one is measuring general properties of the body. The anthropometric measurements of body weight, stature or height, body circumferences, and weight-for-height ratio are the most common techniques. The bioelectrical methods would fit this classification, as they measure general properties of the body that must be related to a more direct assessment of body composition.[19]

Reference Models of Body Composition for the Fetus and Infant

Total body cadaver analyses have been reported by Fee and Weil,[3] Iob and Swanson,[22] Widdowson and Dickerson,[5,23] and Brozek et al.[24] These data are for the basic chemical model of body composition (level 1 of Figure 47.1). In addition, limited data for the water, protein, minerals, or fat content were provided in most of these studies. Fomon et al.[25,26] compiled these data to develop a "reference infant" model, while Ziegler et al.[2] used these data to construct a body composition model for the "reference fetus." These two models divide the body into four major compartments: water, protein, minerals, and fat (level 2 of Figure 47.1) and describe changes as a function of age. The mineral compartment was further subdivided into osseous (i.e., bone) and nonosseous (i.e., lean) components. It is interesting to note that Fomon and Ziegler and their colleagues chose not to use the cadaver data of Widdowson and Dickerson in these calculations on the basis that the gestational ages of the fetuses or preterm neonates were not adequately reported. Forbes[16] has shown that body weight is a more significant indicator of body composition than gestational age. Figure 47.2 presents the combined reference fetus and infant estimates with the data of Widdowson et al.[5,8,27] for the water, fat, mineral, and protein compartments as

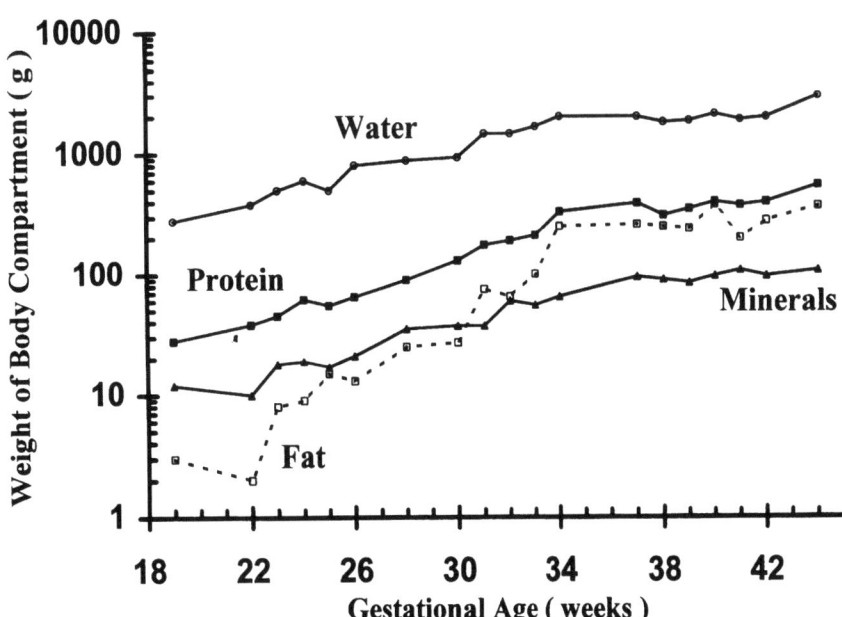

FIGURE 47.2. Body composition as a function of gestational age. (Values are the average of data reported by Ziegler et al.[2] and Widdowson et al.[5,27])

a function of body weight. It should be noted that these models are estimates of the average composition and do not consider the normal variations seen in individuals.

The scatter in individual values of elemental body composition for low birth weight infants as a function of body weight is illustrated in Figure 47.3. These data are those recently obtained from cadaver analyses using neutron activation analysis and whole-body counting.[28,29] Equations that describe these relationships for the neonate are given in Table 47.1. A significant observation reported in this study was that a minimum body potassium content, as an index of body cell mass, appeared critical for survival. The information presented in Figure 47.2 for body water, protein, mineral, and fat, and the elemental data presented in Figure 47.3 serve as the reference body composition curves during gestational growth.

Anthropometric Measurements

Basic anthropometric techniques consist of the physical measurements of body length, size, and circumferences of various body parts and regions, and body weight (level 5, Figure 47.1). These measurements have been per-

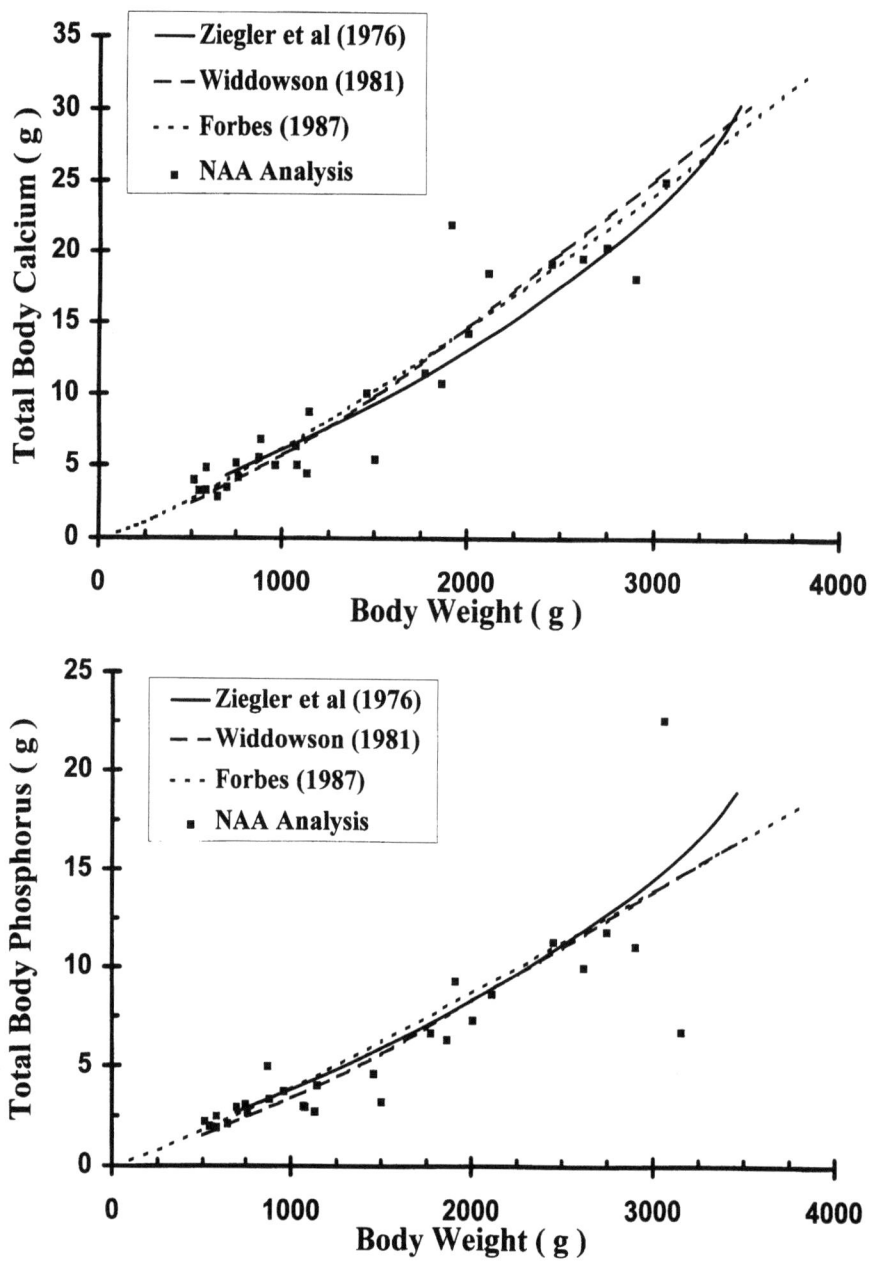

FIGURE 47.3. Elemental content for low birth weight infants. Individual data values obtained by cadaver neutron activation analysis. (The curves are based on the models of Ziegler et al.,[2] Widdowson et al.,[5,27] and Forbes.[16])

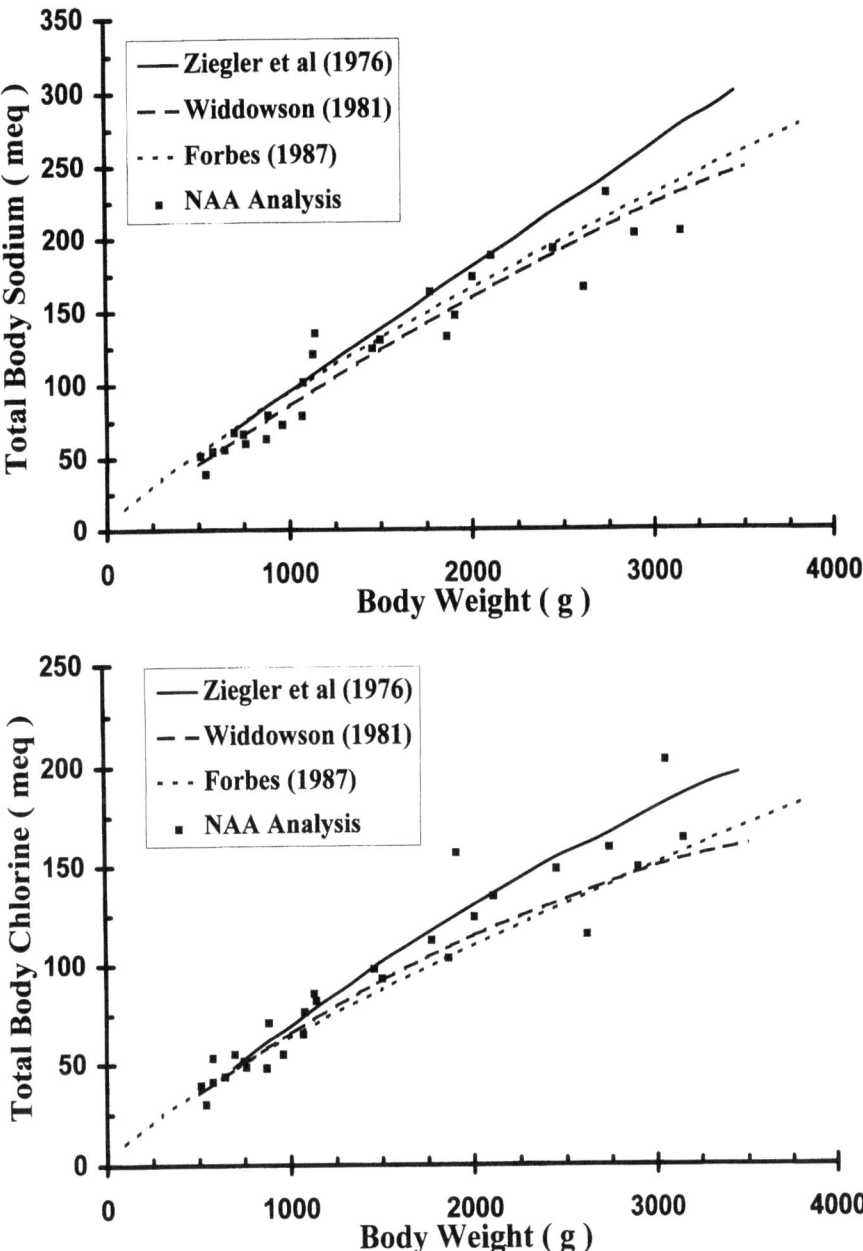

FIGURE 47.3. Continued.

TABLE 47.1. Exponential models of elemental body composition as a function of body weight.

Total body content	In vivo neutron activation analysis[a]	Chemical cadaver analysis[b]
Ca (g)	$0.00226 \, Wt^{1.148}$	$0.00117 \, Wt^{1.241}$
P (g)	$0.00412 \, Wt^{0.996}$	$0.00125 \, Wt^{1.164}$
Na (mEq)	$0.162 \, Wt^{0.902}$	$0.362 \, Wt^{0.806}$
Cl (mEq)	$0.183 \, Wt^{0.847}$	$0.284 \, Wt^{0.784}$
K (mEq)	$0.0716 \, Wt^{0.906}$	$0.0449 \, Wt^{0.989}$

[a] From Ellis et al.[28,29]
[b] From Forbes.[16]
Wt, body weight (g).

formed for many years and have been the basis for the estimation of body fat.[30] The relationships that have been developed appear adequate for describing a general population, but should be used with great caution when applied to the individual. Unfortunately, the anthropometric measurements lack sufficient precision for accurately estimating body composition in the individual, especially for the infant, and when the measurements are performed by untrained personnel. Nevertheless, reference tables of percentile distributions for body weight and stature for the infant are available.[31] To monitor growth, an infant's weight and stature are plotted on these charts to determine their relative percentile ranking at each age, malnutrition being defined mainly as an initial low weight percentile or a reduction in percentile with age.

The body mass index (BMI), defined as body weight divided by a power of height, has been used in an attempt to eliminate the variability in weight associated with differences in stature among individuals.[32] Using the "ideal" body weight values of the Metropolitan Life Insurance Company, the range of ideal BMIs (expressed as W/H^2) for normal men and women is 19 to $27\,kg \cdot m^{2-1}$.[16] Using this simple classification, individuals with a higher BMI value are classified as overweight, and those with a lower BMI value are called undernourished. This index range cannot be used with infants, as the normal range for healthy infants is about $13\,kg \cdot m^{2-1}$ at birth, increasing to about $18\,kg \cdot m^{2-1}$ at 1 year of age.[33]

Additionally, there is the measurement of skinfold thickness at various body sites. The basic assumption for this technique is that the mass of the subcutaneous adipose tissues is a constant fraction of the total body fat. Cadaver analyses of human fetuses have indicated that, although subcutaneous fat is a major portion of total body fat, its proportion of the total fat stores is not constant with gestational or postnatal age.[34,35] During growth in the third trimester, it has been estimated that subcutaneous fat is 70% to 80% of total body fat for the fetus, while reducing to approximately 42% for the full-term neonate. Even in the classic skinfold thickness studies of Lohman[36] and Durnin and Womersley,[37] the estimated mass of subcutaneous fat was only about one third of the total fat mass. The advantage of an inexpensive measurement, such as skinfold thickness obtained using calipers at specific sites of the body, must be weighed against the need for an accurate assessment of the individual. More recently, the inexpensive calipers have been replaced with instruments that use radiographic,[38] ultrasonographic,[39] or infrared interactance[40,41] measurements to determine the subcutaneous tissue thickness. These techniques remain as limited as the original mechanical measurements of skinfold thickness.

These limitations notwithstanding, numerous studies have correlated the subcutaneous fat thickness, measured at a number of sites on the body, with total body fat estimates and have provided prediction equations based solely on skinfold measurements. These equations tend to be population-specific, and are reported as inaccurate and misleading when used with other investigators' population norms. Going[42] has proposed that specific formulas for prediction of body density (i.e., body fatness) from skinfold thickness measurements are needed for specific populations. He calculated approximately a 3% to 9% error range for the estimation of body fat mass could be attributed to the inherent errors in the skinfold thickness measurements alone. Skinfold thickness measurements are for from ideal. After nearly four decades of use, there are still questions related to the selection of suitable body sites.

Body Water and Electrolyte Measurements

Total Body Water Measurements

Total body water (TBW) measurement of an individual can be obtained by direct dilution of an orally or intravenously administered tracer of labeled water or use of a chemical such as antipyrine that remains uniformly distributed in the water spaces.[43–45] For infants, this tracer is usually D_2O, although recent studies have used the more expensive tracer, $H_2^{18}O$, especially in conjunction with energy expenditure studies in infants.[46] If one can assume that the TBW is a constant fraction (k) of the nonfat mass, one can estimate body fat (Fat = Wt − TBW/k).

In 1945, Pace and Rathbun[47] summarized animal data and reported a mean water content of $732\,ml \cdot kg^{-1}$ (range: $69.9–76.3\,ml \cdot kg^{-1}$) for the fat-free mass. Although the use of this value as a constant has almost been enshrined as an absolute in body composition research in adults, its use has often been questioned, especially in children and older adults. Some 20 years earlier Moulton[7] had already indicated that the relative water content of the nonfat tissues at birth is substantially higher than that in adults with a subsequent gradual decline during growth. Consequently, the adult value of 73.2% water for the total lean mass is not appropriate for use in studies of neonates and young infants, since it leads to a significant underestimation of the body fat stores. Friis-Hansen[48] performed some of the earliest dilution studies for TBW measurements in children. The estimates were that approximately 80% of the FFM in the neonate is water, that it decreases through infancy, and does not reach a proportion similar to that in adults until about 3 years of age.[48] For this reason it is difficult, if not questionable, to estimate body fat mass or lean tissue mass in an infant on the basis of a body water measurement alone.

Sheng and Huggins[43] reviewed carcass analysis values for body water obtained for various species of animals with that obtained by the dilution techniques and reported that TBW could be overestimated by 5.7% to 23.1% of body weight. This overestimation seems to be most strongly associated with growth, pregnancy, weaning, and obesity.[43] In healthy adult humans this effect is estimated to be a 2% to 4% overestimation of the true TBW volume; however, during early life it may be substantially different.[49] The potential overestimation of TBW by the dilution technique, and the uncertainty in knowing the hydration level of the FFM of an individual neonate, should be considered when estimating the lean body mass or body fat stores as the difference between this compartment and body weight.

Total Body Electrical Conductivity Measurements

Total body electrical conductivity (TOBEC) continues to be evaluated as an in vivo technique for the assessment of body composition in infants.[50-53] This technique is based on the principle that the body's lean soft tissue, with its high water content and electrolytes, will conduct an electrical current better than fat or bone tissue. This technique would be a level-5 model, as it measures a general property of the whole body and not that of a specific tissue. The technique has been shown to be highly influenced by the geometry of the subject.[54] Separate instruments are needed for the neonate, infant, and adult. In each case, the TOBEC instruments have had to be calibrated with some other, more direct measure of the lean body mass or FFM. For adults, underwater weighing, TBW measurements from isotopic water, and ^{40}K measurements have served as the reference method to calibrate the TOBEC instrument. For the infant, only the water dilution technique has been used for this purpose, due in part to the difficulty of performing precise underwater weighing of the infant, and the lack of sensitivity with adult-sized whole-body counters. A prototype neonatal-sized TOBEC instrument, developed for testing (M. Fiorotto, Houston, TX, personal communication), was found to have inadequate precision and accuracy when assessing the body composition of very low birth weight neonates.

The infant TOBEC instrument has been calibrated for FFM and TBW using the data from direct carcass analyses of miniature piglets.[51,55] When the mean values obtained by TOBEC for FFM in neonates were compared to the mean values obtained by anthropometry and TBW, there were no differences.

The major pediatric application of TOBEC is the indirect measurement of body fat. TOBEC is used to first estimate FFM and then define fat as Wt-FFM. In the Netherlands, de Bruin et al.[56] performed TOBEC and anthropometric measurements in 435 healthy infants, ages 21 to 365 days. The equation to predict the fat-free mass is

$$FFM\,(kg) = 0.0264 \times (E\# \times Lc)^{0.5} - 0.0213$$

where $E\#$ is a raw number produced by the TOBEC instrument and Lc is the assumed conductive length of the body, defined as $Lc \times$ [crown-heel length − head circumference $\times \pi^{-1}$]. The standard error for FFM was 0.077 kg. The TOBEC-derived equation for total body fat, expressed as a function of age (days), is

$$Fat\,(g) = 384 + (1.19 \times Age) - (0.0164 \times Age^2)$$

with an r^2 value of 0.56 and a residual SD of 428 g. At each age, there was less variation in the body fat values obtained by TOBEC than those obtained using anthropometric equations.

Bioelectrical Impedance Measurements

Bioelectrical impedance analysis (BIA) has emerged as a popular in vivo technique for the assessment of body composition.[50-53,57,58] As with TOBEC, this technique is based on the principle that lean tissues conduct an electrical current better than fat tissues. The theoretical basis of the measurement has been questioned by a number of investigators.[59-61] Using the scheme presented in Figure 47.1, this method would be classified as a level-5 technique since it measures a general property of the whole body (i.e., body resistance). For single-frequency measurements, a 50-kHz frequency has been used. At this frequency, most of the current does not penetrate the cell membrane, but traverses through the extracellular fluid space. At higher frequencies, more of the current passes through cells, hence providing a measure of more than the extracellular compartment. Since the BIA measurement requires that electrodes be placed on one hand and foot, it can be used for all body sizes, from the neonate to an obese adult. This technique is sensitive to body geometry, especially that of the arms and legs. Use of an animal model to calibrate an instrument for use in humans is not feasible. To determine FFM a more direct measurement of this compartment (e.g., underwater weighing, TBW, and/or ^{40}K measurements) must be used as the calibration reference value.

Because each investigator has calibrated his/her own instrument on a reference population, many population-specific prediction equations have been produced regarding the BIA technique.[62] Most of these studies have been conducted in adults and children, while only a few have been performed in neonates and infants. The equations for infants are presented in Table 47.2. The BIA estimates of body composition, especially for body fat, have been equivocal. A National Institutes of Health technology assessment conference reached no consensus on an acceptable equation for BIA that would translate the body's resistance, impedance, or reactance value into a meaningful body composition value.[62] In the studies in infants, the addition of the BIA measurement did not substantially change or improve the estimates for body composition when compared with those derived from anthropometric measurements alone.[63-65] The basic height squared divided by resistance ($H^2 \cdot R^{-1}$) term was often found insufficient to accurately predict body water, and additional terms were added to the basic equation to

TABLE 47.2. Bioelectrical impedance prediction equations for infants and neonates.

Age Group	No. of subjects	Reference method	BIA equation $a(Ht^2 \cdot R^{-1}) + b$			Reference
			a	b	SEE	
<1 wk	5	TBW	0.62	0.04	—	Wilson et al.[78]
<1 wk	32	TBW	0.53	0.34	0.9	Mayfield et al.[77]
0.4–3 yr	30	TBW	0.67	0.48	0.36	Field et al.[79]

TBW, total body water (D_2O or $H_2^{18}O$ dilution method); SEE, standard error of the estimate of TBW; Ht, full height for age >1 month, otherwise it is the crown-heel length; R, BIA resistance value in ohms; a, slope; b, intercept.

reduce the prediction error. Clearly, the BIA technique needs to be studied systematically to establish its use in the neonate.

Body Water and Electrolytes

Marked changes in body water content occur during gestation and early neonatal life. There is a significant decrease in the body water compartment of the FFM, concurrent with a progressive rise in the proportion of solids (i.e., minerals) within the FFM. It is for this reason that measuring TBW without some knowledge of the hydration of the FFM can make it difficult to accurately estimate body fat mass, especially in an individual neonate.

Water content of the FFM decreases rapidly, from an estimated 90% at 20 weeks' gestation to approximately 83% at birth. Measurements of TBW using the dilution of stable isotopes of water such as D_2O or $H_2^{18}O$ clearly show that premature neonates have a higher water content than infants born at term.[66,67] The mean water content of preterm neonates is about 80% of body weight, compared with 72% for term neonates.[45,48] The relative volume of the extracellular and intracellular body water spaces changes during growth. Early gestation is characterized by an overexpanded extracellular compartment that normally decreases with increasing fetal age.[48,68] When expressed as a percentage of body weight, total body chloride, all of which is assumed to be in the extracellular compartment, decreases from about 62% of body weight at 20 weeks to 44% at 40 weeks.[27] During postnatal life, there is a continued decrease in the relative proportion of body weight that is the extracellular water space.[48] Bromide dilution studies in premature neonates have shown that the ECW is a greater percentage of weight than in healthy term neonates.[68–70] ICW, on the other hand, remains a relatively constant proportion of body weight, only increasing from 26% at 20 weeks to 28% at 40 weeks. After birth the relative proportion of ICW increases rapidly, reaching about 40% of body weight by 4 months.[48] The relative proportions of ECW and ICW in TBW shift markedly during fetal growth.

Using the D_2O and $H_2^{18}O$ dilution techniques, Butte and William[71] derived two prediction equations for total body water during early infancy. The D_2O equation, using body weight (kg) and body length (cm) as prediction variables, is

$$TBW(kg) = 0.389 \times Wt^{0.549} \times Ln^{0.306}$$

with an r^2 of 0.823 and standard error of the estimate for TBW of 0.060 kg. When compared with the TBW values based on the predictions of Friis-Hansen,[48,72] the Butte values averaged about 12% lower. Heimier et al.[73] investigated the relationship between weight change and redistribution of the fluid compartments during the first week of life of preterm neonates. D_2O and bromine (Br) dilution were used to monitor TBW and ECW, respectively. At 1 day of age, for mean body weight of 1.47 kg, the average TBW and ECW values were 1.24 L and 0.725 L, respectively. By day 7, ECW and TBW had decreased by about 16% in those neonates losing more than 10% body weight, while there was a change in ECW (−13%), but no change (−2%) in TBW for the weight-stable neonates. These investigators concluded that significant postnatal weight loss in less stable neonates was mainly reflective of contraction of the ECW when energy intake was inadequate. Singhi et al.[74,75] measured body water distribution in appropriate-for-gestational-age (AGA) neonates following normal births. The relative TBW content, normalized for body weight, were 777 ml·kg^{-1} and 737 ml·kg^{-1} for the preterm and term neonates, respectively. The corresponding ECW values were 349 ml·kg^{-1} for the preterm neonates, and 331 ml·kg^{-1} for the term group. The TBW ratio was comparable with that for white and black neonates, whereas the ECW ratio was lower. It should be noted that these investigators used sucrose dilution space to measure ECW and not the usual technique of Br dilution. The ECW/Wt ratio values were in agreement with those of other investigators who have used sucrose to estimate ECW in infants.[76]

Total body water measurements in conjunction with BIA have been reported in several neonatal studies.[77–79] Several equations to predict TBW in neonates using the

BIA technique are given in Table 47.2. Wilson et al.[78] reported the following BIA equation based on 17 observations in eight neonates with a mean birth weight of 760 g:

$$TBW = 0.55 \times (Ln^2/I) + 0.094$$

where I is body impedance (Ω) and Ln is body length (cm), and TBW is measured by $H_2^{18}O$ dilution.

Lean Body Mass Measurements

Body Density and Volume Measurements

Some investigators consider the densitometric method to be the "reference method" or "gold standard" for body composition measurements. This approach is based on the two-compartment model (i.e., fat and FFM) of body composition. Behnke et al.[9] showed that if the density of each component is known (assume d_{fat} = 0.9 g/cm^3 and d_{FFM} = 1.1 g/cm^3), the fat mass can be expressed as

$$Wt_{Fat} = 4.95(Wt/d) - 4.50 Wt$$

where Wt is body weight in air and d is total body density determined by underwater weighing. Accurate measurements of body weight and density are required in order to correctly predict body fat mass. Body weight can be measured easily and with an accuracy of ± 0.1 g. Body density is more difficult to measure, especially in infants and children, as the subject needs to be totally submerged. Adjustments are needed to correct for residual lung volume and possible gases in the gastrointesinal tract. The underwater method is not feasible for neonates, infants, or young children.

Alternative techniques have been developed for the measurement of body volume in neonates.[80–83] One approach is to measure the change in air pressure in a fixed-volume chamber when a neonate is placed in the chamber. The second method is an acoustical technique that makes use of the Helmholtz principle; the resonant frequency of a chamber is inversely proportional to the total volume of the chamber. The placement of the infant in the chamber reduces the volume and produces a new resonance frequency. A clear advantage of these two methods is that the infant is not submerged underwater; however, the corrections still apply for lung air and gastrointestinal gases.

Even with the assurance that body volume, and thus body density, can be measured with precision and accuracy for a given individual, limitations are imposed by the assumed density of the FFM. Changes in the chemical composition of FFM occur during normal growth.[5,26,28,29] A small change in the density of FFM substantially alters the estimate for body fat mass. If the density of the FFM of an infant is increased by 0.03 g·cm^{-1} above the assumed value of 1.064 g·cm^{-1}, the percentage fat content would double, from 11% to 23%. Brozek et al.[24] expressed reservations about the body density methods more than 30 years ago. These limitations remain today.

Recently, investigators have attempted to circumvent the restrictions imposed by a changing density value for FFM. The basic concepts used for the two-compartment model are expanded to the four-compartment model (water, fat, protein, minerals). If the density (g·cm^{-1}) values for water, fat, protein, and mineral are assumed to be 0.9937, 0.9007, 1.34, and 3.038, respectively, then the equation for estimating the mass of body fat becomes:

$$M_{fat} = 2.747 V_{total\,body} - 2.050 M_{total\,body} - 0.7145 M_{water} + 1.146 M_{mineral}$$

This approach attempts to correct the basic two-compartment model for individual variations in body water and mineral content. Three separate body composition measurements are required.

Total Body Potassium Measurements

The direct in vivo measurement of total body potassium (TBK) provides a unique chemical assay of the human body. The isotopic makeup of natural potassium includes the fractional content (0.0118%) of ^{40}K, a radioactive atom.[84] Although ^{40}K has a long half-life, 1 g of potassium emits approximately 209 photons of 1.46 MeV per minute. This energy is sufficient for most photons to exit the body, especially in the neonate. Therefore, if a photon detector has sufficient shielding, to reduce the natural background interferences, the natural ^{40}K signal from the body can be measured.[85] Figure 47.4 provides in vivo TBK data as a function of body weight for preterm neonates. TBK data on human neonatal cadavers are included for comparison. The values for the live neonates are in general agreement with the reference models developed by Ziegler et al.[2] and Fomon et al.[26] The TBK values for the cadavers, however, were generally below the reference model predictions. Low TBK values for ill neonates and low-weight neonates have been reported by Burmeister and Romahn.[86] Those ill neonates that survived for 10 days to return for a second TBK measurement had TBK/body weight^{-1} ratios that had returned to within the range observed for healthy neonates. Although Apte and Iyengar[1] did not report TBK values in their study of fetuses from malnourished mothers, the cadaver's total body nitrogen concentrations were lower than normal. Fee and Weil[3] attributed the death of several neonates in their study to a marked TBK deficiency. The difference in body weight between survival and nonsurvival was not associated with difference in body fat, but to the size and composition of the lean tissue mass. When coupled with these older studies, our own in

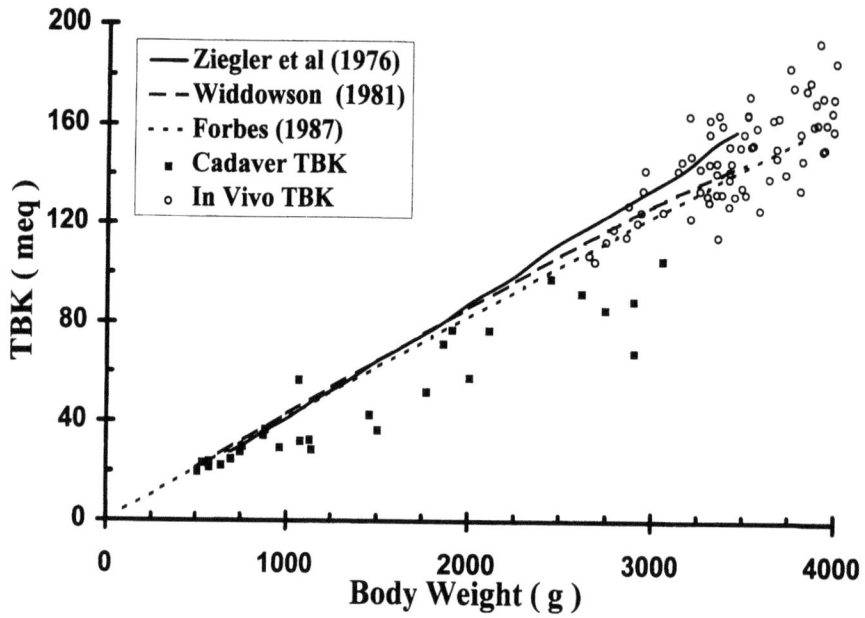

FIGURE 47.4. Total body potassium (TBK) vs body weight (Wt). Individual data are for preterm infant cadavers (■) and for live infants (○). (The curves are based on data from Ziegler et al.,[2] Widdowson et al.,[5,27] and Forbes.[16])

vivo observation clearly indicates that a critical or minimum body K content is essential to survival. Below this critical TBK content, life cannot be sustained.

Body Cell Mass and Intracellular Composition

The level-3 model of Figure 47.1 represents a physiologic approach to body composition. In this model, the FFM is divided into the functional components of (1) cellular mass, (2) extracellular fluid, and (3) extracellular solids (i.e., mainly that of the skeleton). As noted in the discussion on body water distribution, there is a progressive shift in the ratio of extracellular to intracellular water volume during normal fetal growth. Further evidence that the ICW/ECW ratio increases during fetal growth is indicated by the higher TBK/total body chlorine (TBCl) ratio observed in term neonates than in young fetuses.[5,28,29] The total body Na/K ratio decreases with increasing gestational age. During normal growth, there is an increase in body cell mass concurrent with a decrease in extracellular space during the second half of fetal development.

Intracellular water comprises a major portion of BCM. If the intracellular hydration of body tissues can be determined, one can estimate total BCM. If the average water content of the cells in the body is 70%, then BCM can be calculated as BCM = ICW/0.70. This approach requires knowledge of the ICW value. Unfortunately, no in vivo method has been developed for measuring ICW, and it can, at best, be approximated as the difference between TBW and ECW. In this case, the accuracy of the BCM estimate is dependent on the cumulative errors for both the TBW and ECW measurements, and the assumption of a fixed water content of the total cell mass.

The direct in vivo measurement of total body potassium by whole-body ^{40}K counting provides an alternate approach for estimating BCM. Moore et al.[20] developed the following equation for adults to calculate BCM from a body potassium measurement:

$$BCM(g) = 0.00833\, K\,(mEq)$$

where the constant is based on a cellular K/N ratio of $3\,mEq \cdot g^{-1}$ and a nitrogen content of $0.04\,g \cdot g$ wet tissue^{-1}. Using a similar approach, Burmeister and Romahn[86] obtained a value of $0.0111\,g$ BCM per mEq K for neonates.

The cellular K/N ratio used by Moore et al.[20] was based on chemical tissue data for adults. Spady et al.[87] used a lower K/N ratio value of $2.6\,mEq \cdot g^{-1}$ for their estimate of body composition in the premature neonate based, in part, on the reference fetus model of Ziegler et al.[2] The data of Widdowson and Dickerson[5] indicate that the whole body K/N ratio in the fetus decreases with age from about $3\,mEq \cdot g^{-1}$ at 20 weeks to $2.3\,mEq \cdot g^{-1}$ at 40 weeks. They reported a range of K/N ratios for various tissues, from $0.45\,mEq \cdot g^{-1}$ in skin to $5.0\,mEq \cdot g^{-1}$ in brain. Sheng and Huggins[88] have reported that the whole body K/N ratio changes significantly in the growing animal. Alternately, one can estimate the total body K/N ratio during human growth based on the ratio of the Forbes equations for these elements.[16] Combining these equations, one obtains the following expression for the K/N ratio for the human infant during growth;

$$K(mEq)/N(g) = 6.950\, Wt^{-0.147}$$

The K/N ratio decreases with increasing body weight and gestational age. At a body weight of 1000 g, the K/N ratio would be approximately 2.5 mEq·g^{-1}, decreasing to 2.1 mEq·g^{-1} at 3500 g body weight.

Bone Mineral Measurements

As noted in Figure 47.2, there is about a 10-fold increase in the total body mineral mass during the last 20 weeks of gestation. Rapid growth of the skeletal system is occurring during this time. This mineralization process is reflected by increases in both body calcium (Ca) and phosphorus (P). Body Ca increases slightly more than body P, so that the Ca/P ratio also increases with gestational age.[5] This change in the Ca/P ratio probably indicates a continued mineralization of the skeleton at bone sites that are initially cartilage-like tissues.[89] The skeletal mass approximately doubles during the second half of gestation, averaging an estimated 3.2% of body weight at full term.[90]

The development of the single-photon absorptiometry (SPA) instrument for measuring the bone status of neonates and infants has significantly increased our knowledge of the mineralization process during human growth. In particular, bone mineral content (BMC) of the low birth weight preterm neonate, as measured by SPA at the forearm, has been shown to be significantly lower than that of term neonates.[91-94] When fed exclusively human milk, many of these neonates continued to have low bone mineral status, which would place them at increased risk for fractures. Pittard et al.[93] reported that BMC values at 16 weeks of age are similar for term and preterm infants. When Rubinacci et al.[94] measured BMC at a common weight of 2 kg, they observed substantially lower BMC values for females compared with age- and weight-matched males. Venkataraman and Duke[95] reported BMC at the radius for 238 healthy term infants, and observed no gender difference or effect of maternal cigarette smoking. Sugimoto et al.[96] reported no gender differences in BMC at the radius for normal Japanese infants. On the other hand, Pohlandt and Mathers[97] reported lower BMC values at the mid-humerus for preterm neonates compared with term newborn neonates, yet the relative bone content of body weight was similar between the two groups. Horsman et al.[98] however, reported no differences in BMC of the mid-forearm between infants at 65 to 100 weeks postconception for preterm versus term births. Hillman et al.[99] followed longitudinal mineralization in term infants fed human milk, cow milk-based formula, or soy-based formula for 12 months. BMC at the radius significantly increased until about age 6 months, after which there was a plateau for the remaining 6 months of the study, independent of the food source. Nangung et al.[100] reported significant seasonal differences at birth in bone mineral content of infants, summer-born infants having lower BMC than those born in the winter months.

Until recently, it has been extremely difficult, if not impossible, to directly monitor in vivo changes in the total skeletal mass of the neonate or infant. For BMC the precision is reported at about 1.2% with an analytical sensitivity for infants estimated at 40 mg for bone calcium.[101] For the very small infant, Brunton et al.[102] obtained a less accurate estimate of the true BMC level when the DXA instrument was validated using chemical carcass analysis of piglets as the reference. More recently, Picaud et al.[103] reported on the reproducibility and accuracy of DXA using 13 piglets (1470-5510 g) and 30 term neonates (3.19 ± 0.22 kg). The ratio of BMC to carcass Ca content was 2.15, while the precision for BMC was about 2%. When applied to the infant measurements, the mean BMC during the first week of life was 54 ± 6 g or 26.4 ± 2.6 g calcium. Gotfredsen et al.[104] performed total body measurements in preterm neonates and found a fourfold increase in skeletal mass corresponding to the last 10 weeks of gestation. Those neonates that were small for gestational age (SGA) had less mineral mass than that observed for neonates of appropriate size for gestational age (AGA). Whether early dietary intervention can correct a deficiency in bone mineralization has not been adequately determined. Although dietary intervention may provide some improvement, the preterm neonate does not appear to attain bone mineralization comparable to that of age-matched term neonates. The preterm neonate does not attain the theoretical estimate for intrauterine mineralization. There must be a "catch-up" phase in postnatal growth, which may be lengthy, if the preterm infant is to achieve a bone mass similar to that of the term infant by 2 years of age.[105]

Recently, Koo et al.[106] reported the bone mineral status for 150 neonates (i.e., 85 preterm and 79 low birth weight) using DXA. The weight range at birth was 1002 to 3990 g, and gestational ages were 27 to 42 weeks. The predictive values of anthropometric measurements and race and gender were examined, body weight being the best single determinant of bone mineral status. The relationship between total body BMC (g) and neonatal body weight (kg), reported by Koo et al. is

$$BMC_{total\,body} = 24.2 \times Wt - 11.1$$

with an r^2 value of 0.95. The predicted mean values for total body BMC and the 95% confidence interval for the weight range 1 to 4 kg are illustrated in Figure 47.5. Included in this figure are the BMC values for 13 neonatal cadavers measured by DXA in our laboratory (Ellis, unpublished data).

Rupich et al.[107] have examined bone mass in older infants to determine whether there is a race or gender

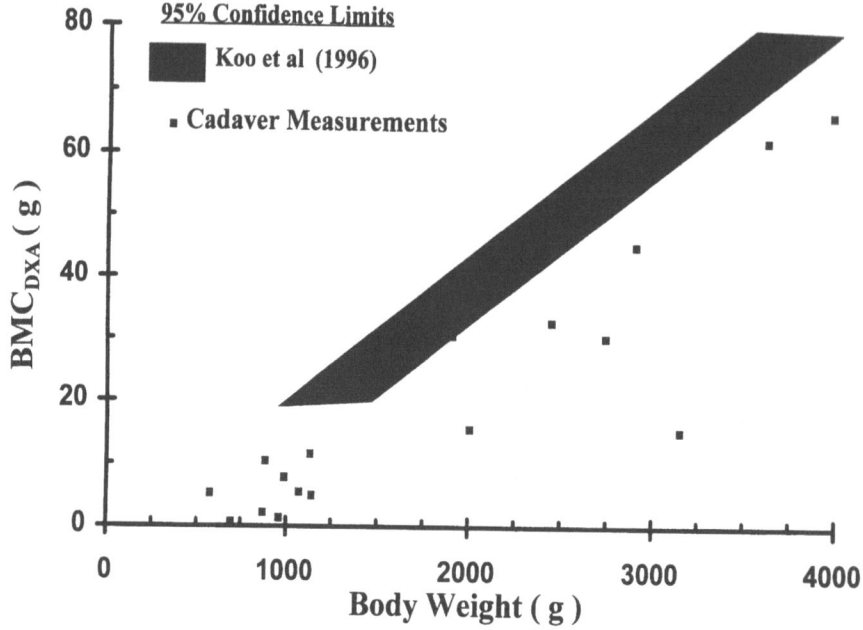

FIGURE 47.5. Bone mineral content (BMC) vs body weight (Wt) for preterm infant cadavers and live term infants. (The dashed region represents the 95% range for BMC reported by Koo et al.[106])

difference in BMC values. Total body measurements were performed in 64 healthy infants in the age range of 1 to 18 months, who were full term at birth. The prediction equation for BMC for this age range is

$$BMC\,[g] = 13.90 \times Wt\,[kg] + 5.72 \times Age\,[months] + 2.32 \times Race - 7.79 \times Gender + 30.46$$

where Race = 0 (white) or 1 (black), and Gender = 0 (male) or 1 (female). After accounting for the effects of age and body weight, the BMC values of males were greater than those of females. Differences in BMC between black and white children at these ages, were not evident.

Body Composition During Fetal and Neonatal Growth

Maternal Influence on Fetal Growth

Fetal growth can be influenced by the health and nutritional status of the mother during pregnancy. Maternal size appears to play an important role in defining the size of the neonate.[1-6,108] Although the exact nature of this influence is unknown, it may be partially the result of physical restraint, size of the placenta, physiologic limit in placental blood flow, and/or limited nutrient availability.[109] Physical restraint by the size of the uterus is clearly evident in multiple births.

Prerequisites for normal growth include adequate maternal nutrition and the general well-being of the mother. These requirements have been reviewed[110] and a number of studies have shown a positive association between maternal calorie reserves and neonatal body fat.[111,112] The neonate's birth weight and body fat content clearly can be influenced by the mother's health. Infants of diabetic mothers are often larger and fatter than average for their gestational age,[3] while excessive use of drugs[112] can result in growth retardation. There are no reported differences in the relative chemical composition of the FFM of fetuses of diabetic and nondiabetic mothers.

Irrespective of the cause, maternal malnutrition can play an important role in determining fetal growth and birth weight. Cigarette smoking and high alcohol consumption have been demonstrated to have negative effects on fetal growth.[113-115] In general, neonates born to mothers who smoke, compared to neonates of nonsmokers, are shorter, have lower weight, and have smaller head circumferences.[114] Since no differences in skinfold thickness measurements have been observed, it is assumed that the lower neonatal weight is due to reduced lean body mass and not less subcutaneous fat. This observation was confirmed by Spady et al.[116] who estimated the lean tissue content of the neonates by directly measuring body potassium using a whole-body counter. The severity of the effects of alcoholic consumption on fetal growth is directly related to the amount of alcohol ingested. Daily consumption of approximately 50 ml alcohol (i.e., two to three alcoholic drinks) significantly impairs fetal growth, resulting in low birth weight and an increased risk of premature birth.[113] A continued

TABLE 47.3. Effects of maternal malnutrition on body composition of the fetus.

Gestational age (weeks)	Normal weight[b] (g)	Malnourished weight (g)	Four-compartment model estimates[a]				
			Water (g)	Protein (g)	Minerals (g)	Fat (g)	%Fat
20	363	230	213	9	5	<3	<1%
28	1067	1065	870	128	29	38	3.5%
35	2393	1448	1180	170	37	61	4.2%
40	3311	2381	1871	231	55	224	9.4%

[a] Source: Apte and Iyengar.[1]
[b] Normal body weight for gestational age, derived from data used to construct Figure 47.2.

inadequacy in the nutrient supply to the fetus results in general growth retardation, including a slowing of the chemical maturity of all body tissues. The more severe the nutritional deprivation, the more marked is the growth retardation and the slower the development of critical body organs. The study of the chemical composition of fetuses of malnourished mothers in India clearly demonstrates the compositional consequences: higher body water, lower body protein and minerals, and lower body fat content (Table 47.3) than the average values for normal growth as illustrated in Figure 47.2.[1] As growth is impaired, there is a continued immaturity in the chemical composition of the fetus, resulting in an increasing percentage of body water. Garrow et al.[117] defined the infantile malnourished state as a significant reduction in body fat, and hyperhydration of the lean tissues accompanied by a depletion of body potassium and protein.

Unless there is specific evidence of drug, alcohol, or cigarette use, one can usually associate a low body weight at birth, independent of gestational age, with a lower-than-average body fat content. Whole-body chemical analyses of the malnourished Indian infants indicated an average body fat content of 4.5% at 35 to 37 weeks' and 9.3% at 40 weeks' gestation.[1] Mettau et al.,[118] using an in vivo xenon absorption technique, observed a similar range of body fat in nine preterm neonates. For neonates with appropriate body weights for gestational ages of 29 to 36 weeks, these investigators calculated the body fat content to average 7% of body weight. For the five full-term low birth weight neonates, with body weights more than 2 SD below normal, the average body fat content was about 7% of body weight, whereas in normal-weight full-term neonates, body fat content was about 14% of body weight.

Changes in Body Composition

The body composition of the human neonate changes significantly during gestation.[5,28,29,87] The impact of maternal nutrition has been discussed in the previous section. Based on the many chemical analyses of the whole body of human fetuses during the past 100 years,[1-5,35,28,29] we have been able to obtain reasonable estimates for the changes that occur during fetal growth and development. These studies have enabled the calculation of the elemental and body composition accretion of fat, protein, muscle, and bone minerals during the gestation period. These data can be used to develop estimates of the general nutrient needs of the fetus and neonate.[2,25,26] These models can be used to determine what fraction of total maternal nutritional needs is directly associated with the growth of the fetus. These models for fetal growth have served as the benchmark for assessing growth and the clinical efficacy of various approaches for the nutritional support of neonates born prematurely. The intrauterine nutrient accretion estimates provide a means to understanding the potential or natural growth patterns and the associated postnatal nutrient needs.

Fetal data reported by Widdowson and Dickerson[5] were from analyses made in their own laboratory, whereas Ziegler et al.[2] consolidated the literature on chemical analyses of fetuses and developed a composite model that they called the "reference fetus." The results of each of these two approaches, along with the individual cadaver data more recently reported by Ellis et al.[28,29] are shown for body Ca, K, Na, Cl, and P in Figure 47.3. These basic chemical data can be translated into the body composition compartments of water, fat, mineral, and protein as shown in Figure 47.2. Ziegler et al. excluded the fetal data of Widdowson and Dickerson because of their concern about the accuracy of the estimated gestational ages. Hytten and Leitch[109] have examined the lack of accuracy in obtaining an accurate gestational age and estimated the probable uncertainty of any quoted fetal age to be at least ±5 days. It seems reasonable to combine the Ziegler model and Widdowson's values to estimate average values of body composition at various ages. The changes in body composition at 6- to 8-week intervals are given in Table 47.4. As an alternate approach, Forbes[16] has calculated the accretion rate at various body weights by taking the first derivative of the exponential equations listed in Table 47.1. It is worthy of note that there is now a general consensus that body weight is a more important determinant of body composition of the fetus than is gestational

TABLE 47.4. Four-compartment model of body composition for normal fetal growth.

Gestational age (weeks)[a]	Normal Wt (g)	Water (g)	Protein (g)	Minerals (g)	Fat (g)	% Fat
20	363	322	27	10	<4	<1%
28	1067	898	106	35	28	2.6%
35	2393	1891	262	73	167	7.0%
40	3311	2381	407	116	407	12.3%
Average at birth[b]						
Male	3545	2484	459	116	486	13.7%
Female	3325	2284	424	108	509	15.3%

[a] Four-compartment model (From Ziegler et al.[2] and Widdowson and Dickerson.[5]
[b] Source: Ziegler et al.[2] and Fomon et al.[25,26]

age. These calculations represent only the average. It is evident that a wide range of fetal weights at a given gestational age can be expected even for normal healthy fetuses, as reflected by the range of normal weights at full-term births.

There is a ninefold increase in body weight, from about 363 g at 20 weeks to about 3300 g at birth, which gives an average gain of 21 g per day for this period. At the same time, the fetus doubles its body length, increasing from about 25 cm to approximately 50 cm. Forbes[16] has described the changes in elemental composition during this period using a single-component exponential model. These equations are provided in Table 47.1 along with those recently obtained by Ellis et al.,[28,29] who used nondestructive neutron activation analysis to examine the whole body of infant cadavers. Sheng and Nichols,[119] on the other hand, chose to present changes in weight and body composition as a logarithmic function of age. They calculated two periods of fetal growth: an initial phase that lasted to about 34 weeks of gestation, followed by a slower phase until birth. The relative weight increase was about 6.5-fold between 20 and 34 weeks and about 1.3-fold between 34 and 40 weeks. Physical constraints imposed by the uterus, the size of the placenta, and a relative decrease in uterine blood flow have been suggested as factors contributing to this decrease.[109]

Changes in the body composition compartments of fat, water, protein, and minerals as a function of age are shown in Figure 47.2. Alternatively, one can calculate the accretion rate using the equations provided in Table 47.1. Based on the model presented in Figure 47.2, there is the rapid accumulation of body mass up to about 34 weeks' gestation, followed by a slower rate of increase until birth. These changes are similar to that derived on the basis of body weight as calculated by Forbes[16] and Ellis et al.[28,29] It is important to note that although there is a slowing of the rates of increase in mass during the last 6 weeks of gestation, physiologic maturation continues in order to prepare the fetus for postnatal life.

One of the most prominent features during the last half of human gestation is that there is more than a 200-fold increase in body fat. At full-term birth, it is estimated that 12% to 15% of body weight is fat. The percentage is higher for infants of diabetic mothers, while lower when there is maternal malnutrition.[1,3] The changes in the other body composition compartments of water, protein, and minerals are less dramatic (Figure 47.2 and Table 47.4). Body protein increases about 14-fold, while total body water increased about sevenfold. As the body grows, the relative proportion of water is reduced. The mass of the mineral content has about a 10-fold increase, but remains about 3% of body weight. When the cumulative increases for the last half of the gestation period are used to calculate daily accretions, the averages are: fat, $2.9\,\text{g}\cdot\text{day}^{-1}$; water, $14.8\,\text{g}\cdot\text{day}^{-1}$; protein, $2.7\,\text{g}\cdot\text{day}^{-1}$; and mineral, $0.7\,\text{g}\cdot\text{day}^{-1}$; combining for an average weight gain of $21\,\text{g}\cdot\text{day}^{-1}$. These values provide only average estimates of the nutrient retention during this period of growth. A number of genetic and maternal factors could be expected to cause individual variations in these rates.

Measurements of an increase in the subcutaneous fat layers in neonates provided evidence that total body fat content increases as body weight and gestational age increase. The sum of average skinfold thickness measurements of the subscapular, triceps, rib, abdomen, and anterior thigh for a series of neonates with birth weights in the range 1.2 to 5.2 kg were positively correlated ($r = 0.6$) with birth weight.[120] On average, a 1.2-mm increase in skinfold thickness occurred for each kilogram increase in birth weight. In a separate study, this observation was confirmed for neonates born at a gestational age of 26 to 42 weeks.[121] Skinfold thicknesses were obtained at eight sites, with an average summed increase of 1.4 mm per week for the 26 to 42 weeks. Similar studies performed by McGowan et al.[122] on neonates born at a gestational age of 36 to 42 weeks demonstrated correlations between birth weight and individual skinfold thickness at the biceps, triceps, quadriceps, and subscapular and thigh sites ($r = 0.47$–0.7). Oakley et al.[123] reported that triceps and subscapular skinfold thickness increase to a maximum at about 37 to 39 weeks gestational age and that a positive relation exists between skinfold thickness at each of the sites and birth weight (2.0–4.5 kg) of the neonates.

In each of these studies, variability in skinfold thickness increases progressively with body weight. This may support the concept that variability in body fat content is already established by late fetal life and may be reflective of the range seen in children and adults. The physiologic or biochemical factors that produce variability in fat deposition may already be operative during fetal growth. As with adults, the variations in body weight, irrespective of birth age and sex of the fetus, are primarily the result of variations in body fat content. Lean tissue mass is relatively constant among healthy term neonates and contributes only slightly to variations in body weight. Maternal nutrition and health are important factors influencing the variability of fetal body fat content.

During fetal growth, skinfold thickness and body fat increase. Skinfold thickness measurements give, at best, only an indirect estimate of total body fat because the relative distribution of total body fat in neonates during growth shifts between the external and internal fat depots. During the last 10 weeks of gestation, there is an 18-fold increase in subcutaneous fat deposits while deep visceral fat is increased only eightfold.[35] Subcutaneous fat is estimated to be 60% to 80% of total body fat, a range significantly higher than the 42% value reported by Forbes[34] for one full-term neonate. Some investigators have reported total body fat values for neonates using DXA, although the lack of accurate calibration at these body weights and for this low range of %fat values,[124] suggest that DXA estimates should be viewed with caution.

Implications

Although discrepancies in the estimates of body composition in neonates and infants may be attributed to the relatively small number of neonates examined in some studies, and to the individual variations among neonates, a major factor appears to be related to the in vivo measurement technique and its method of calibration or verification. Before one can expect compatibility among the various techniques, there must be good agreement among different manufacturers using the same basic technique (e.g., BIA, TOBEC, DXA, etc). All BIA measurements of an infant should obtain the same value for body resistance, independent of the instrument. Likewise, all DXA instruments should give the same BMC and body fat values within the instruments' precision for individual. Standardization is needed if body composition measurements are to be accepted as accurate, reliable indices of the neonate's nutritional status.

Further research is needed to better understand the effects of diet and its relative nutrient composition on the growth pattern of neonates, especially that of the low birth weight neonate. Although weight gain, stature, and skinfold thicknesses will continue to be used in most studies, one can expect that direct in vivo measurements of body composition will begin to better establish these requirements. Weight gain alone is insufficient to accurately assess the nutritional status of an infant, as there are substantial differences among infants in the rate of lean, fat, and bone deposition, concurrent with the relative loss of body water. The reference fetus model appears adequate for estimating the average intrauterine changes, but one should be careful when using this model to estimate growth in postnatal life, especially in individual cases.

With continued interest in precise techniques to estimate body composition in neonates, one can expect the adaptation of some of the more sophisticated techniques being developed for adults. Each of these techniques shows great potential for the estimation of the anatomical distribution and composition of lean, fat, and bone tissues. The instrumentation is often expensive and will remain relatively unavailable for routine clinical measurements, with placement largely confined to pediatric research centers. A chemical profile of the body remains the preferred assay, but with the exception of TBK, its application to infants is prohibited by the dose of ionizing radiation required. A similar dose consideration eliminates the use of computed tomography for body composition studies. Images depicting fat and muscle components of various body regions can be obtained with nuclear magnetic resonance (NMR) imaging.[125] It may become feasible to measure in vivo, the body's content of phosphorus, fluoride, and sodium, and TBW[125-129] using magnetic resonance spectroscopy. Continued improvements in DXA technology are already providing useful morphologic information on bone structural changes in aging. This type of application can be expected to be extended into the study of bone growth in infants, and children especially if there is a defect in mineral metabolism. A resonant gamma absorption technique (David Vartsky, Soreq, Israel, personal communication, 1996) has the potential for the measurement of body nitrogen at a dose comparable with that of DXA. The bioelectrical techniques continue to hold promise but need further refinement and verification of their applicability, especially in cases of abnormal hydration.[62]

References

1. Apte SV, Iyengar L. Composition of the human foetus. Brit J Nutr 1972;27:305–312.
2. Ziegler EE, O'Donnell AM, Nelson SE, et al. Body composition of the reference fetus. Growth 1976;40;329–341.
3. Fee BA, Weil WB Jr. Body composition of infants of diabetic mothers by direct analysis. Ann NY Acad Sci 1963;110:869–897.
4. Silliman K, Kretchmer N. Maternal obesity and body composition of the neonate. Biol Neonate 1995;68:384–393.
5. Widdowson EM, Dickerson JWT. Chemical composition of the body. In: Comar CL, Bronner F, eds. Mineral metabolism, vol. 2. Orlando: Academic Press, 1972:1–247.
6. Gormican A, Valentine J, Satter E. Relationships of maternal weight gain, prepregnancy weight and infant birth weight. J Am Diet Assoc 1980;77:662–667.
7. Moulton CR. Age and chemical development in mammals. J Biol Chem 1923;57:79–97.

8. Spray CM, Widdowson EM. The effect of growth and development on the composition of mammals. Br J Nutr 1950;4:332–353.
9. Behnke AR, Feen BG, Welham WC. The specific gravity of healthy men: body weight and volume as an index to obesity. JAMA 1942;118:495–498.
10. Brozek J, Henschel A, eds. Techniques for measuring body composition. Washington, DC: National Academy Press, 1961.
11. Brozek J, ed. Body composition. Ann NY Acad Sci 1963; 110:1–1018.
12. Brozek J, ed. Human body composition: approaches and applications. New York: Pergamon, 1965.
13. National Academy of Sciences. Body composition in animals and man. Washington, DC: National Academy Press, 1968.
14. Garrow JS. New approaches to body composition. Am J Clin Nutr 1982;35:1152–1158.
15. Lohman TG. Research in progress validation of laboratory methods of assessing body composition. Med Sci Sports Exerc 1984;16:596–603.
16. Forbes GB. Human Body Composition: Growth, Aging, Nutrition, and Activity. New York: Springer-Verlag, 1987.
17. Lukaski HC. Methods for the assessment of human body composition: traditional and new. Am J Clin Nutr 1987;46: 537–556.
18. Sheng H-P. Methodologies for measuring body composition in humans. In: Designing foods. Animal product options in the marketplace. Washington, DC: National Academy Press, 1988:242–250.
19. Wang ZM, Pierson RN Jr, Heymsfield SB. The five-level model: a new approach to organizing body composition research. Am J Clin Nutr 1992;56:19–28.
20. Moore FD, Olesen KH, McMurrey JD, et al. The body cell mass and its supporting environment. Philadelphia: Saunders, 1963.
21. Fuller MF, Fowler PA, McNeill G, Foster MA. Imaging techniques for the assessment of body composition. J Nutr 1994;124:1545s–1550s.
22. Iob V, Swanson WW. Mineral growth of the human fetus. Am J Dis Child 1934;47:302–306.
23. Widdowson EM. Importance of nutrition in development, with special reference to feeding low-birth-weight infants. In: Nutritional goals for low-birth-weight infants. Columbus, OH: Ross Laboratories, 1982:4–11.
24. Brozek J, Grande F, Anderson JT, et al. Densitometric analysis of body composition: revision of some quantitative assumptions. Ann NY Acad Sci 1963;110:113–140.
25. Fomon SJ. Body composition of the male reference infant during the first year of life. Pediatrics 1967;40:863–870.
26. Fomon SJ, Haschke F, Ziegler EE, et al. Body composition of reference children from birth to age 10 years. Am J Clin Nutr 1982;35:1169–1175.
27. Widdowson EM, Spray CM. Chemical development in utero. Arch Dis Child 1951;26:205–214.
28. Ellis KJ, Shypailo RJ, Schanler R, Langston C. Body elemental composition for the neonate: new reference data. Am J Hum Biol 1993;5:232–330.
29. Ellis KJ, Shypailo RJ, Schanler RJ. Body composition of the pre-term infant. Ann Hum Biol 1994;21:533–545.
30. Dauncey MJ, Gandy G, Gairdner D. Assessment of total body fat in infancy from skinfold thickness measurements. Arch Dis Child 1977;52:223–227.
31. Tanner JM. Standards for birth weight or intra-uterine growth. Pediatrics 1970;46:1–6.
32. Keys A, Fidanza F, Karvonen MJ, et al. Indices of relative weight and obesity. J Chronic Dis 1972;25:329–343.
33. Rolland-Cachera MF, Sempe M, Guill-Bataille M, et al. Adiposity indices in children. Am J Clin Nutr 1982;36:178–184.
34. Forbes GB. Methods for determining composition of the human body. Pediatrics 1962;29:477–494.
35. Southgate DAT, Hey En. Chemical and biochemical development of the human fetus. In: Roberts DF, Thomson AM, eds. Biology of human fetal growth. New York: Halsted Press, 1976:195–209.
36. Lohman TG. Skinfolds and body density and their relation to body fatness: a review. Hum Biol 1981;53:181–225.
37. Durnin JVGA, Womersley J. Body fat assessed from total body density and its estimation from skinfold thickness: measurements on 481 men and women aged from 16 to 72 years. Br J Nutr 1974;32:77–97.
38. Garn SM. Roentgenogrammetric determinations of body composition. Hum Biol 1957;29:337–353.
39. Borkan GA, Hults DE, Cardarelli J, et al. Comparison of ultrasound and skinfold measurements in assessment of subcutaneous and total fatness. Am J Phys Anthropol 1982;58:307–313.
40. Cassady SL, Nielsen DH, Janz KF, et al. Validity of near infrared body composition analysis in children and adolescents. Med Sci Sports Exerc 1993;25:1185–1191.
41. Conway JM, Norris KH, Bodwell CE. A new approach for the estimation of body composition: infrared interactance. Am J Clin Nutr 1984;40:1123–1130.
42. Going SB. Densitometry. In: Roche AF, Heymsfield SB, Lohman TG, eds. Human body composition. Champaign, IL: Human Kinetics, 1996:3–24.
43. Sheng H-P, Huggins RA. A review of body composition studies with emphasis on total body water and fat. Am J Clin Nutr 1979;32:630–647.
44. Schoeller DA, van Santen E, Peterson DW, et al. Total body water measurement in humans with ^{18}O and ^{2}H labeled water. Am J Clin Nutr 1980;33:2686–2693.
45. Trowbridge FL, Graham GG, Wong WW, et al. Body water measurements in premature and older infants using H_2 ^{18}O isotopic determinations. Pediatr Res 1984;18:524–527.
46. Micheli JL, Pfister R, Junod S, et al. Water, energy and early postnatal growth in preterm infants. Acta Paediatr Suppl 1994;405:35–42.
47. Pace N, Rathbun EN. Studies on body composition. III. The body water and chemically combined nitrogen content in relation to fat content. J Biol Chem 1945;158:685–691.
48. Friis-Hansen B. Body water compartments in children: changes during growth and related changes in body composition. Pediatrics 1961;28:169–181.

49. Sheng H-P, Huggins RA. Tritiated water as a measure of body water in immature rats growing at different rates. J Appl Physiol 1989;66:476–480.
50. Harrison GG, Van Itallie TB. Estimation of body composition: a new approach based on electromagnetic principles. Am J Clin Nutr 1982;35:1176–1179.
51. Cochran WJ, Klish WJ, Wong WW, et al. Total body electrical conductivity used to determine body composition in infants. Pediatr Res 1986;20:561–564.
52. Segal KR, Gutin B, Presta E, et al. Estimation of human body composition by electrical impedance methods: a comparative study. J Appl Physiol 1985;58:1565–1571.
53. Lukaski HC, Johnson PE, Bolonchunk WW, et al. Assessment of fat-free mass using bioelectrical impedance measurements of the human body. Am J Clin Nutr 1985;41:810–817.
54. Sutcliffe JF, Smye SW, Smith MA. A further assessment of an electromagnetic method to measure body composition. Phys Med Biol 1995;40:659–670.
55. Fiorotto ML, Cochran WJ, Funk RC, et al. Total body electrical conductivity measurements: effects of body composition and geometry. Am J Physiol 1987;252:R794–R800.
56. De Bruin NC, Luijendijk IHT, Visser HKA, Degenhart HJ. The effect of alterations in physical and chemical characteristics on TOBEC-derived body composition estimates: validation with non-human models. Phys Med Biol 1994;39:1143–1156.
57. Kushner RF. Bioelectrical impedance analysis: a review of principles and applications. J Am Coll Nutr 1992;11:199–209.
58. Deurenberg P, Schutz Y. Body composition: overview of methods and future directions of research. Ann Nutr Metab 1995;39:325–333.
59. Forbes GB, Simon W, Amatruda JM. Is bioimpedance a good predictor of body-composition change? Am J Clin Nutr 1992;56:4–6.
60. Lichtenbelt WDV, Westerterp KR, Wouters L. How solid is the theoretical basis for bioelectrical impedance analysis? Am J Clin Nutr 1995;61:1307–1308.
61. Deurenberg P, Weststrate JA, Hautvast JG, van der Kooy K. Is the bioelectrical-impedance method valid? Am J Clin Nutr 1991;53:179.
62. National Institutes of Health. Technology Assessment Conference Statement: Biological impedance analysis in body composition measurement. Washington, DC: NIH, 1994.
63. Gartner A, Maire B, Delpeuch F, et al. The use of bioelectrical impedance analysis in newborns, the need for standardization. In: Ellis KJ, Eastman JD, eds. Human body composition: methods, models, and assessment. New York: Plenum Press, 1993:165–168.
64. Kabir I, Malek MA, Rahman MM, et al. Changes in body composition of malnourished children after dietary supplementation as measured by bioelectrical impedance. Am J Clin Nutr 1994;59:5–9.
65. Sidhu JS, Charles BG, Triggs EJ, et al. Assessment of bioelectrical impedance for individualising gentamicin therapy in neonates. Eur J Clin Pharmacol 1993;44:253–258.
66. Singhi SC, Ganguli NK, Bhakoo ON, et al. Body water distribution in newborn infants appropriate for gestational age. Indian J Med Res 1995;101:193–200.
67. Brans YW, Andrew DS, Dutton EB, et al. Dilution kinetics of chemicals used for estimation of water content of body compartments in perinatal medicine. Pediatr Res 1989;25:377–382.
68. Cassady G, Milstead RR. Antipyrine space studies and cell water estimates in infants of low birth weight. Pediatr Res 1971;5:673–682.
69. Shaffer SG, Meade VM. Sodium balance and extracellular volume regulation in very low birth weight infants. J Pediatr 1989;115:285–290.
70. Morkeger JC, Sheng HP, Huggins RA. A comparison of chloride, bromide, and sucrose dilution volumes in neonatal pigs. Proc Soc Exp Biol Med 1991;196:344–350.
71. Butte NF, Wong WW, Garza C. Prediction equations for total body water during early infancy. Acta Paediatrica 1992;80:264–265.
72. Friis-Hansen B. The body density of newborn infants. Acta Paediar 1963;52:513–521.
73. Heimier R, Doumas BT, Jendrzejczak BM, et al. Relationship between nutrition, weight change, and fluid compartments in preterm infants during the first week of life. J Pediatr 1993;122:110–114.
74. Singhi S, Sood V, Bhakoo ON, Ganguly NK. Effect of intrauterine growth retardation on postnatal changes in body composition of preterm infants. Indian J Med Res 1995;102:275–280.
75. Singhi S, Sood V, Bhakoo ON, et al. Composition of postnatal weight loss and subsequent weight gain in preterm infants. Indian J Med Res 1995;101:157–162.
76. Van der Wagen A, Okken A, Zweens J, et al. Composition of postnatal weight loss and subsequent weight gain in small for dates newborn infants. Acta Paediatr (Stockh) 1985;74:57–61.
77. Mayfield SR, Uauy R, Waidelich D. Body composition of low-birth weight infants determined by using bioelectrical resistance and reactance. Am J Clin Nutr 1991;54:296–303.
78. Wilson DC, Baird T, Scrimgeour CM, et al. Total body water measurements in very low birth weight infants using bioelectrical impedance (abstract). Proc Nutr Soc 1991;54:296–303.
79. Fjeld CR, Freundt-Thume J, Schoeller DA. Total body water measured by ^{18}O dilution and bioelectrical impedance in well and malnourished children. Pediatr Res 1990;27:98–102.
80. Faulkner F. An air displacement method of measuring body volume in babies: a preliminary communication. Ann NY Acad Sci 1963;110:75–79.
81. Taylor A, Aksoy Y, Scopes JW, et al. Development of an air displacement method for whole body volume measurement of infants. J Biomed Eng 1985;7:9–17.
82. Dell RB, Aksoy Y, Kashyap S, et al. Relationship between density and body weight in prematurely born infants receiving different diets. In: Ellis KJ, Yasumura S, Morgan WD, eds. In vivo body composition studies. London: Institute of Physical Medicine, 1987:91–97.
83. Sheng H-P, Dang T, Adolph AL, et al. Infant body volume measurements by acoustic plethysmography. In: Ellis KJ,

Yasumura S, Morgan WD, eds. In vivo body composition studies. London: Institute of Physical Medicine, 1987:415–420.
84. Forbes GB. Potassium: the story of an element. Perspect Biol Med 1995;38:554–566.
85. Ellis KJ. Whole-body counting and neutron activation analysis. In: Roche AF, Heymsfield SB, Lohman TG, eds. Human body composition. Champaign, IL: Human Kinetics, 1996:45–61.
86. Burmeister W, Romahn A. Potassium content in full term and premature babies: energies for the synthesis of body cell mass. In: Linneweh F, ed. Current aspects of perinatology and physiology of chidren. New York: Springer-Verlag, 1973:139–156.
87. Spady DW, Schiff D, Szymanski WA. A description of the changing body composition of the growing premature infant. J Pediatr Gastroenterol Nutr 1987;6:730–738.
88. Sheng HP, Huggins RA. Body cell mass and lean body mass in the growing beagle. Proc Soc Exp Biol Med 1973;142:175–180.
89. Dickerson JWT. Changes in the composition of the human femur during growth. Biochem J 1962;82:56–61.
90. Trotter M, Peterson RR. Weight of bone during the fetal period. Growth 1969;33:169–184.
91. Gotfredsen A, Jensen J, Borg J, et al. Measurement of lean body mass and total body fat using dual photon absorptiometry. Metabolism 1986;35:88–93.
92. Minton SD, Steichen JJ, Tsang RC. Bone mineral content in term and preterm appropriate-for-gestational age infants. J Pediatr 1979;95:1037–1042.
93. Pittard WB III, Geddes KM, Hulsey TC, Hollis BW. Osteocalcin, skeletal alkaline phosphatase, and bone mineral content in very low birth weight infants: a longitudinal assessment. Pediatr Res 1992;31:181–185.
94. Rubinacci A, Sirtori P, Moro G, et al. Is there an impact of birth weight and early life nutrition on bone mineral content in preterm born infants and children? Acta Paediatr 1993;82:711–713.
95. Venkataraman PS, Duke JC. Bone mineral content of healthy, full-term neonates. Am J Dis Child 1991;145:1310–1312.
96. Sugimoto T, Nishino M, Tsunenari T, et al. Radial bone mineral content of normal Japanese infants and prepubertal children: influence of age, sex, and body size. Bone Miner 1994;24:189–200.
97. Pohlandt F, Mathers N. Bone mineral content of appropriate and light for gestational age preterm and term newborn infants. Acta Paediatr Scand 1989;78:835–839.
98. Horsman A, Ryan SW, Congdon RJ, et al. Bone mineral content and body size 65 to 100 weeks' postconception in preterm and full term infants. Arch Dis Child 1989;64:1579–1586.
99. Hillman LS, Chow W, Salmons SS, et al. Vitamin D metabolism, mineral homeostasis, and bone mineralization in term infants fed human milk, cow milk-based formula, or soy-based formula. J Pediatr 1988;112:864–874.
100. Nangung R, Tsang RC, Specker BL, et al. Low bone mineral content and high serum osteocalcin and 1,25-dihydroxyvitamin D in summer- versus winter-born newborn infants: an early fetal effect. J Pediatr Gastroenterol Nutr 1994;19:220–227.
101. Going SB, Massett MP, Hall MC, et al. Detection of small changes in body composition by dual-energy x-ray absorptiometry. Am J Clin Nutr 1993;57:845–850.
102. Brunton JA, Bayley HS, Atkinson SA. Validation and application of dual-energy x-ray absorptiometry to measure bone mass and body composition in small infants. Am J Clin Nutr 1993;58:839.
103. Picaud J-C, Rigo J, Nyamugabo k, et al. Evaluation of dual-energy x-ray absorptiometry for body-composition assessment in piglets and term human neonates. Am J Clin Nutr 1996;63:157–163.
104. Gotfredsen A, Petersen A, Hassager C, et al. Body composition in infants by dual-photon 153-Gd absorptiometry (DPA). In: Ellis KJ, Yasumura S, Morgan WD, eds. In vivo body composition studies. London: Institute of Physical Medicine, 1987:83–86.
105. Steichen JJ, Asch PAS, Tsang RC. Bone mineral content measurement in small infants by single-photon absorptiometry: current methodologic issues. J Pediatr 1988;113:181–187.
106. Koo WWK, Walters J, Bush AJ, et al. Dual-energy x-ray absorptiometry studies of bone mineral status in newborn infants. J Bone Miner Res 1996;11:997–1002.
107. Rupich RC, Specker BL, Lieuw-A-Fa M, Ho M. Gender and race differences in bone mass during infancy. Cal Tissue Int 1996;58:395–397.
108. Garn SM, Pesick SD. Relationship between various maternal body mass measures and size of the newborn. Am J Clin Nutr 1982;36:664–668.
109. Hytten FE, Leitch I. The physiology of human pregnancy. London: Blackwell Scientific Publications, 1971.
110. Metcoff J. Association of fetal growth with maternal nutrition. In: Faulkner F, Tanner JM, eds. Human growth: principles and prenatal growth, vol. 1. New York: Plenum, 1978:417–425.
111. Frisancho AR, Klayman JE, Matos J. Influence of maternal nutritional status on prenatal growth in a Peruvian urban population. Am J Phys Anthropol 1977;46:265–274.
112. Frank DA, Bresnahan K, Zuckerman BS. Maternal cocaine use: impact on child health and development. In: Barnes LA, ed. Advances in pediatrics, vol. 40. Chicago: Mosby, 1993:65–99.
113. Hingson R, Alpert JJ, Day N, et al. Effects of maternal drinking and marijuana use on fetal growth and development. Pediatrics 1982;70:539–546.
114. Harrison GG, Branson RS, Vaucher YE. Association of maternal smoking with body composition of the newborn. Am J Clin Nutr 1983;38:757–762.
115. Zaren B, Lindmark G, Grebre-Medhin M. Maternal smoking and body composition of the newborn. Acta Paediatr 1996;85:213–219.
116. Spady DW, Atrens MA, Szymanski WA. Effects of mother's smoking on their infants' body composition as determined by total body potassium. Pediatr Res 1986;20:716–719.
117. Garrow JS, Flecher K, Halliday D. Body composition in severe infantile malnutrition. J Clin Invest 1965;44:417–425.
118. Mettau JW, Degenhart HJ, Visser HKA. Measurement of total body fat in newborns and infants by absorption and

desorption of nonradioactive xenon. Pediatr Res 1977;11: 1097–1101.
119. Sheng HP, Nichols BL Jr. Body composition of the neonate. In: Cowett RM, ed. Principles of perinatal-neonatal metabolism. New York: Springer-Verlag, 1991: 650–670.
120. Farr V. Skinfold thickness as an indication of maturity of the newborn. Arch Dis Child 1966;41:301–308.
121. Whitelaw A. Subcutaneous fat measurement as an indication of nutrition of the fetus and newborn. In: Visser HKA, ed. Nutrition and metabolism of the fetus and infant. Boston: Martinus Nijhoff, 1979:131–143.
122. McGowan A, Jordan M, MacGregor J. Skinfold thickness in neonates. Biol Neonate 1975;25:66–84.
123. Oakley Jr, Parsons RJ, Whitelaw AGL. Standards for skinfold thickness in British newborn infants. Arch Dis Child 1977;52:287–290.
124. Brunton JA, Bayley HS, Atkinson SA. Body composition analysis by dual energy x-ray absorptiometry compared to chemical analysis of fat, lean, and bone mass in small piglets. In: Ellis KJ, Eastman JD, eds. Human body composition: methods, models, and assessment. New York: Plenum Press, 1993:157–160.
125. Fuller MF, Foster MA, Hutchinson JMS. Estimation of body fat by nuclear magnetic resonance imaging. Proc Nutr Soc 1985;44:108A.
126. Lewis DS, Rollowitz WL, Bertrand HA, et al. Use of NMR for measurement of total body water and estimation of body fat. J Appl Physiol 1986;60:836–840.
127. Li L. A new technique for solid NMR imaging and application to phosphorus imaging in solid bone. Phys Med Biol 1991;36:199–206.
128. Ebifegha ME, Code RF, Harrison JE, et al. In vivo analysis of bone fluoride content via NMR. Phys Med Biol 1987;32:439–451.
129. Ra JB, Hilal Sk, Oh CH, Mun IK. In vivo magnetic resonance imaging of sodium in the human body. Magn Reson Med 1988;7:11–22.

48
The Small-for-Gestational-Age Neonate

Edward S. Ogata

Until 1961 all neonates with birth weights of 2500g or less were considered to have been born prematurely. It then became recognized that birth weight could be discordant with gestational age. Neonates were subsequently classified as appropriate (AGA), small (SGA), or large for gestational age (LGA)[1] (Figure 48.1). This chapter reviews some of the mechanisms responsible for intrauterine growth retardation and focuses on the metabolic morbidities to which the SGA neonate is prone.

Intrauterine growth retardation is a frequently occurring complication of pregnancy and is associated with numerous perinatal morbidities. This problem is of increased relevance to perinatologists and neonatologists, as many of the tiniest premature neonates receiving neonatal intensive care are probably SGA. The incidence of intrauterine growth retardation has been estimated to range from 38% to 80% of all low birth weight neonates.[2,3] This discrepancy underscores the fact that no uniform definition of intrauterine growth retardation exists. Even when a normal intrauterine growth pattern in established for a population, somewhat arbitrary criteria must be used to define growth retardation. Birth weight less than 2 standard deviations (SD) from the mean or below the third percentile are often used to define SGA. Numerous mathematical relations attempting to quantitate ponderance have been formulated to define abnormal growth. Neonates may not fulfill any of these criteria for SGA but still appear wasted or undernourished. Such neonates generally have limited subcutaneous tissue and are often referred to as being "dysmature."

Intrauterine growth retardation alters a number of physiologic and metabolic functions in the fetus and neonate that result in a number of morbidities. Not only are these altered functions potentially life-threatening to the fetus, they also pose questions concerning the relationship between delayed fetal growth and altered metabolic and fetal development. Delineation of the factors that limit growth and those that alter development would add to our understanding of the linkage between mechanisms responsible for normal and abnormal intrauterine growth and development.

Patterns of Altered Growth

Neonates with intrauterine growth retardation are classified as demonstrating either symmetrical or asymmetrical growth. Symmetrical growth retardation implies that both brain and body growth are limited; asymmetrical growth indicates that although body growth is retarded, gross brain growth is "spared." Factors intrinsic to the fetus in general cause symmetrical growth retardation, whereas external factors cause asymmetrical growth. Patterns of symmetrical growth retardation develop early during fetal life, reflecting their intrinsic nature. Asymmetrical patterns generally develop during the third trimester, a period normally of rapid fetal growth. Improvements in fetal surveillance methodology have challenged this concept, as asymmetrical growth retardation has been identified during the second trimester.[4] In addition, many extremely premature neonates (<600g) are probably SGA. These observations support the concept that the extrinsic factors that can retard fetal growth can exert and manifest their effects during the second trimester.

Etiologies

Fetal growth normally varies greatly. Mean birth weight for neonates born in New Guinea is 2400g;[5] normal weights in other populations can exceed 4000g.[6] These variations of normal must be considered when the criteria for diagnosis of SGA are developed. Similarly, normal data for the growth of the head, femur, and other variables of growth must be considered.

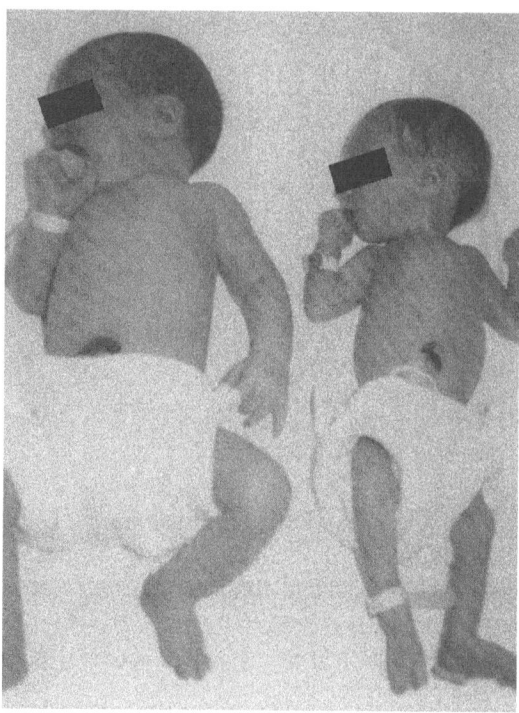

FIGURE 48.1. Discordant twins. The mechanisms for the development of this phenomenon are not well understood but probably include altered blood flow, limited metabolic fuel availability, and diminished uterine volume.

Symmetrical Growth Retardation

Factors that are well recognized to limit the growth of both the fetal brain and body include chromosomal anomalies (e.g., particularly trisomy conditions), congenital infection [toxoplasmosis, rubella, cytomegalovirus, and herpes simplex (TORCH)], dwarf syndromes, and some inborn errors of metabolism. These conditions retard growth by altering multiple factors.

Intrauterine infection should be considered whenever symmetrical growth retardation is noted. TORCH and syphilis retard fetal growth. Toxoplasmosis is associated with microcephaly, chorioretinitis, and intracranial calcifications. Congenital rubella infections often cause heart defects, glaucoma, cataracts, and deafness. Syphilis may cause intrauterine growth retardation by interfering with placental blood flow as a result of placentitis, which directly affects fetal growth.

Numerous drugs are teratogenic to the fetus and can cause malformation syndromes. In addition, maternal alcohol, cigarette, and addictive drug usage retard fetal growth.[2,7] The mechanisms by which it occurs are multifactorial.

Asymmetrical Growth Retardation

The late second and third trimesters are the first periods during gestation that some of the transplacentally derived metabolic fuels provided to the fetus can be channeled from ongoing growth to energy storage in the form of fat and glycogen.[8] This process is critical preparation for normal adaptation to extrauterine life. When it is interrupted, asymmetrical growth retardation results. Although not quantitated, it is likely that a slight reduction of fuel provision might first limit fat and glycogen storage but would allow continued carcass and brain growth. More extreme limitation would affect both growth and energy storage. The timing is of importance; perhaps with an early decrease of fuel provision, growth might be more profoundly affected. A later diminution might result in the "dysmature" neonate. Although general clinical teaching suggests that brain growth is spared under these circumstances, the mechanisms for this phenomenon are unclear. It should be remembered that although gross brain growth might be preserved, functional capability could be affected by the factors causing growth retardation.

Factors Responsible for Retarding Growth

Hormones and Growth Factors

Metabolic fuel availability alone is an important factor but not the only one responsible for affecting fetal growth. A number of hormones and growth factors interact to modulate normal growth. Alterations in their availability are probably important in retarding fetal growth. Insulin is a critical growth-stimulating hormone for the fetus (see Chapter 8). Numerous in vivo and in vitro observations indicate that insulin stimulates the growth of specific insulin-sensitive tissues: muscle, connective, hepatic, and adipose.[9] Insulin does not stimulate the growth of neural tissues, which explains why although hyperinsulinemic infants of diabetic mothers are fat and have organomegaly they have a normal-sized brain (see Chapter 49). The role of insulin in growth is further emphasized by those rare infants with neonatal diabetes mellitus. These insulinopenic infants are always growth-retarded.[10] Insulin has been found to be decreased in SGA fetuses.[11] Other growth-stimulating hormones, including growth hormone, thyroxine and steroids, that do not have a major role in stimulating fetal growth have been found to be normal.[12]

The role of growth hormone in stimulating fetal growth is not known. Both insulin and growth hormone are present in the human fetal circulation by 9 to 11 weeks' gestation.[13] It is generally believed that the role of growth hormone is minimal. Anencephalic fetuses, which often have an interrupted or absent hypothalamic-pituitary axis and have no measurable growth hormone, grow appropriately to term. On the other hand, growth hormone has been demonstrated to have slight but significant growth-stimulating effects on certain growth hormone–sensitive tissues in the rat.[14]

Insulin is the dominant growth-stimulating hormone for the fetus and its effect extends beyond the neonatal period. It is unclear when insulin ceases to be the primary modulator of growth and when growth hormone assumes this role. Data from congenital growth hormone–deficient dwarfs suggest that this might occur at 6 to 12 months of life because it is at this point that these infants first demonstrate diminished growth.[15]

Insulin-like growth factors (IGF) probably contribute to the regulation of fetal growth. Alterations in their availability may contribute to the development of growth retardation. Cord plasma IGF concentrations correlate directly with birth weight.[12] Studies of human fetal tissue suggest that the IGFs may exert their effects in an autocrine-paracrine manner, i.e., mesenchymal cells may synthesize and release IGF to stimulate the growth of adjacent tissues.[16,17] The six IGF binding proteins may modulate IGF's effects through direct binding; certain binding proteins may also inhibit cell growth directly.[18] Plasma concentrations of both IGF-I and IGF-II directly correlate with body mass in growth-retarded rat fetuses; IGF binding protein correlates indirectly with body mass (see Chapter 20).[19]

Metabolic Fuels and Placental Function

Altered placental handling and transport of metabolic fuels contribute to the development of fetal growth retardation. The physiologic factors that influence placental transport of metabolic fuels, acid-base status, and exchange of O_2 and CO_2 are maternal (i.e., uterine) blood flow and the availability of maternally derived metabolic fuels. Of note, changes in these variables are often ascribed to "uteroplacental insufficiency," a poorly defined clinical term.

Alterations in placental handling as well as transport of a metabolic substance cause growth retardation. With respect to glucose, three glucose pools—maternal, placental, and fetal—must be considered (see Chapter 17). Under normal circumstances, there is considerable bidirectional flux between the fetal and maternal pools. The placenta not only transfers glucose in both directions but also rapidly metabolizes glucose.[20,21] Indeed, in the sheep, the fetal glucose pool contributes approximately 40% of the glucose metabolized by the placenta. In various animal models of fetal growth retardation, either or both glucose flux and placental metabolism of glucose are altered.

Little information is available concerning placental glucose transport under conditions of growth retardation. Umbilical venous arterial differences (UVAD) of glucose have been reported to be similar in cord blood of normal and growth-retarded fetuses.[22] On the other hand, growth-retarded fetuses appear to have lower UVAD of amino acid concentrations. These observations suggest that alterations of amino acid may be more important than glucose in the development of growth retardation in the human.

Glucose transporters (Glut) are structurally similar proteins encoded by a family of genes and expressed in a tissue-specific manner[23,24] (see Chapter 7). They have been identified on the syncytiotrophoblast, cytotrophoblast, and endothelial cells of the human placenta and of several animals. Glut 1 appears to be the dominant isoform in human placenta. Its expression may not be altered in the placenta of human growth-retarded fetuses.[25] On the other hand, the placenta of the growth-retarded rat expresses Glut 1 messenger RNA (mRNA) and protein to a greater extent than normal.[26] The upregulation of Glut 1 may be an attempt to compensate for diminished glucose provision to the intrauterine growth-retarded (IUGR) rat fetus. Despite the upregulation of Glut 1, fetal plasma glucose is diminished in the IUGR rat fetus. This suggests that Glut 1 expression is probably not rate limiting in the transfer of glucose under IUGR conditions in the rat.

The transplacental provision of amino acids is critically important for fetal growth and development (see Chapter 18). Amino acids are substrates for synthesis and oxidative metabolism. Understanding of the placental transport of amino acids under conditions of growth retardation is rudimentary. This is due to the complexity of amino acid transporters.[27] While amino acid transporters are highly stereospecific, transporting L- more effectively than D-amino acids, they have low substrate specificity, i.e., one transporter may carry a number of different amino acids and different transporters may have overlapping specificities. As with glucose transporters, amino acid transporter density and populations may differ between the microvillous and basal membranes.

In several animal models of intrauterine growth retardation, placental Na-dependent amino acid transport is diminished.[27,28] The expression and function of a transporter with system A characteristics are significantly decreased in placentas from growth-retarded human fetuses.[29-31] The V_{max} of the system A transporter has been found to be decreased in the placenta of human growth-retarded infants.[32]

Quantification in the human of amino acid flux and fetal plasma concentrations under IUGR and normal

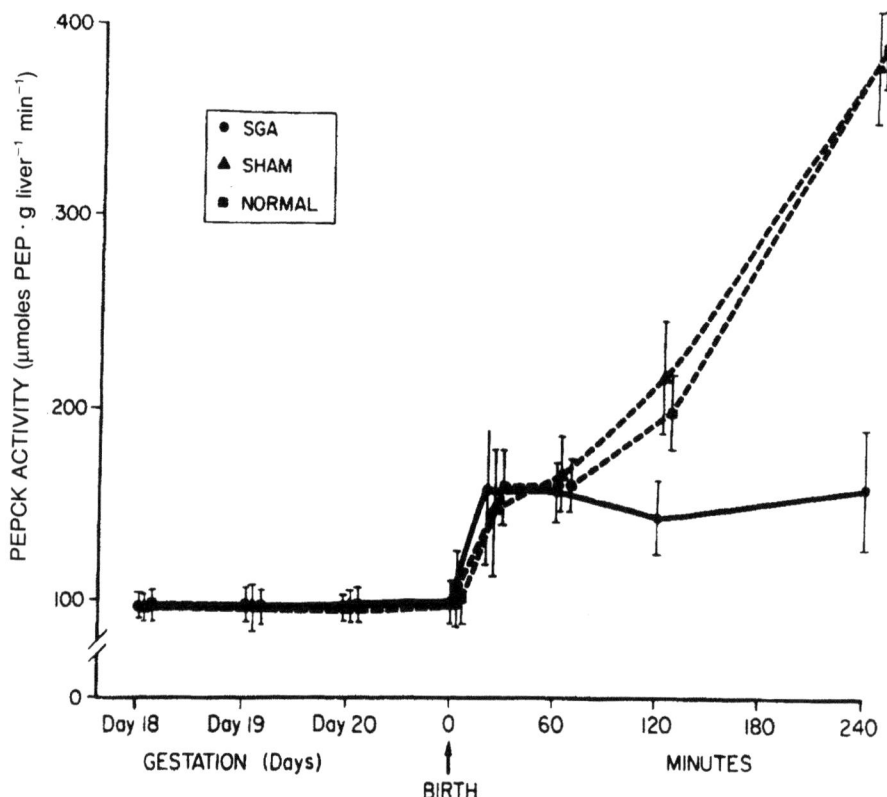

FIGURE 48.2. Fetal plasma concentrations of amino acids in growth-retarded (triangle) and normal (circle) fetuses. The concentration of valine, leucine, and isoleucine are significantly diminished in the growth-retarded fetus.

conditions are limited. The cordocentesis method has allowed measurement of human fetal plasma amino acid concentrations during mid- and late gestation in the human. Total alpha amino nitrogen and branched-chain amino acids are diminished in the umbilical venous circulation of growth-retarded fetuses. The maternal/fetal ratio of amino acids confirm that transport is reduced under conditions of growth retardation[33,34] (Figure 48.2). Similar reductions in plasma branched-chain amino acid concentrations have been reported in the growth-retarded fetal rat.[35]

The fact that the branched-chain amino acids, particularly leucine, are diminished in the circulations of both the growth-retarded human and rat fetus is intriguing and emphasizes the important role of these essential amino acids in fetal growth. The branched-chain amino acids are central for protein synthesis and oxidative metabolism. Indeed, under conditions of maternal fuel deprivation, fetal leucine oxidation increases greatly. Further support of the importance of the branched-chain amino acids comes from studies of normal pregnancy, which indicate that these amino acids are preferentially transported to the fetal circulation. Maternal heat stress in the ewe retards fetal growth.[36] Placental leucine transport, oxidation, and fetal disposal are all significantly reduced.[37] The precise manner in which the transport of branched-chain amino acids is altered to contribute to the development of growth retardation is unclear.

Clinical Conditions

Multiple gestation often results in growth retardation. Although the mechanisms in the human have not been identified, it has long been recognized in polytocous animals that fetal growth is inversely related to litter number.[38] In ablation studies of the fetal rat, blood flow to the surviving fetuses of a litter is enhanced, resulting in increased metabolic fuel availability. This situation stimulates insulin secretion and accelerates the growth of surviving fetuses.[39] It may be that with increased litter number the converse situation exists and fetal growth is limited.

A variety of maternal conditions appear to cause "uteroplacental insufficiency" and retard fetal growth. Chronic maternal hypertension caused by renal disease or of an "essential" nature without a specific identified etiology increases the risk of intrauterine growth retardation. Pregnancy-induced hypertension may reduce uteroplacental perfusion long before the clinical signs of edema, proteinuria, and hypertension develop.[40] Vascular insufficiency caused by long-standing maternal diabetes mellitus can cause growth retardation despite the development of hyperglycemia. It may be due to altered metabolic fuel availability early in gestation.[41] Women with severe lupus erythematosus and the lupus anticoagulant are at risk of hypertension and growth retardation. Maternal cyanotic heart disease and pregnancy at high altitude can increase the incidence of growth retardation.

All of these conditions primarily retard fetal growth by altering gaseous exchange and pH. Limitation of maternally derived metabolic fuels, if extreme, can retard fetal growth even if gaseous exchange remains normal. Severe maternal caloric restriction due to famine or impoverishment have been associated with a high incidence of growth retardation.[42] A condition has been described in which pregnant women do not develop the normally expected "diabetogenic" state of normal pregnancy. Rather than demonstrating a blunted clearance of glucose, such women clear glucose from their circulations as if they were not pregnant.[43,44] Twenty to thirty percent of these women deliver SGA neonates. The mechanisms are not understood. It is possible that such women do not effectively secrete the normally expected anti-insulin factors as placental lactogen and progesterone during gestation.

Neonatal Problems

Numerous morbidities are frequent in the SGA neonate (Table 48.1).

Birth Stress

The fetus that is already stressed by "uteroplacental insufficiency" is at great risk of suffering perinatal asphyxia, as the additional burden of uterine contractions compromises an already insufficient blood supply. In the human SGA fetus, it is unclear to what extent the stress of labor causes hypoxia, acidosis, or hypercarbia. These alterations not only directly cause organ damage but may alter metabolic functions; for example, such stresses stimulate catecholamine secretion, which can deplete hepatic and mitochondrial glyogen stores.

Hypocalcemia

Birth stress may result in hypocalcemia. The mechanisms are not well understood but are related to calcium compartment shifts due to acidosis and possibly to enhanced calcitonin release. Nothing intrinsically predisposes an SGA neonate to develop hypocalcemia. If birth stress is avoided, hypocalcemia does not develop. Another consequence of the stress of labor on the SGA fetus is meconium passage during the antepartum and intrapartum period. This problem can result in the meconium aspiration syndrome. Persistent pulmonary hypertension of the neonate may develop as a consequence of birth stress or with meconium aspiration syndrome. These conditions threaten the survival of the SGA neonate.

Hypoglycemia

Neonates who are SGA develop hypoglycemia as a consequence of limited hepatic glycogen stores and, in some neonates, a delay in the ability to sustain gluconeogenesis (see Chapter 32). Glycogenolysis is a major means by which the neonate maintains glucose homeostasis following birth. The limitation in glycogen stores is a primary cause of the early transient hypoglycemia that many SGA neonates develop.[45] A subgroup of SGA neonates develop hypoglycemia that can last for days. Limited studies in human SGA neonates suggest that this may be due to impaired gluconeogenic capability. Such hypoglycemic SGA neonates have increased plasma concentrations of gluconeogenic precursors.[46] Administration of alanine to SGA neonates does not increase plasma glucose concentrations as it does in AGA neonates.[47] These observations suggest that impaired gluconeogenic capability, rather than limitation of gluconeogenic substrate, is responsible for the prolonged hypoglycemia that develops in some SGA infants.

Studies of several animal models of intrauterine growth retardation indicate that the induction of one, if not several, of the critical gluconeogenic enzymes is delayed.[48] The mechanisms responsible are unknown. In the SGA neonatal rat in which hepatic phosphoenolpyruvate carboxykinase activity is reduced, the mechanism responsible for this delayed induction is unknown. Fetal and neonatal SGA rats have significantly increased plasma glucagon and decreased insulin concentrations, a relationship that should enhance gluconeogenic enzyme induction (Figure 48.3).[49] Whether this results from a deficiency in receptor number, binding capacity, or postreceptor signals is unclear. These animal studies explain why corticosteroid therapy is often useful for treating prolonged hypoglycemia in SGA neonates, as steroids are potent inducers of hepatic gluconeogenic enzymes. These hormonal relations demonstrate a link between growth and metabolic development, as the limitation of insulin contributes to limited growth.

Limited body fat stores and an inability to metabolize lipids are other factors that contribute to the development of hypoglycemia in SGA neonates. Plasma glucose concentration correlates directly with plasma free fatty

TABLE 48.1. Morbidities in the SGA neonate.

Morbidity	Mechanism
Birth stress, meconium aspiration syndrome	Compromised uteroplacental blood flow
Hypocalcemia	Birth asphyxia
Hypoglycemia	Diminished glycogen stores
	Delayed induction of gluconeogenic capability
Polycythemia	Enhanced placental transfusion
	Chronic intrauterine hypoxia

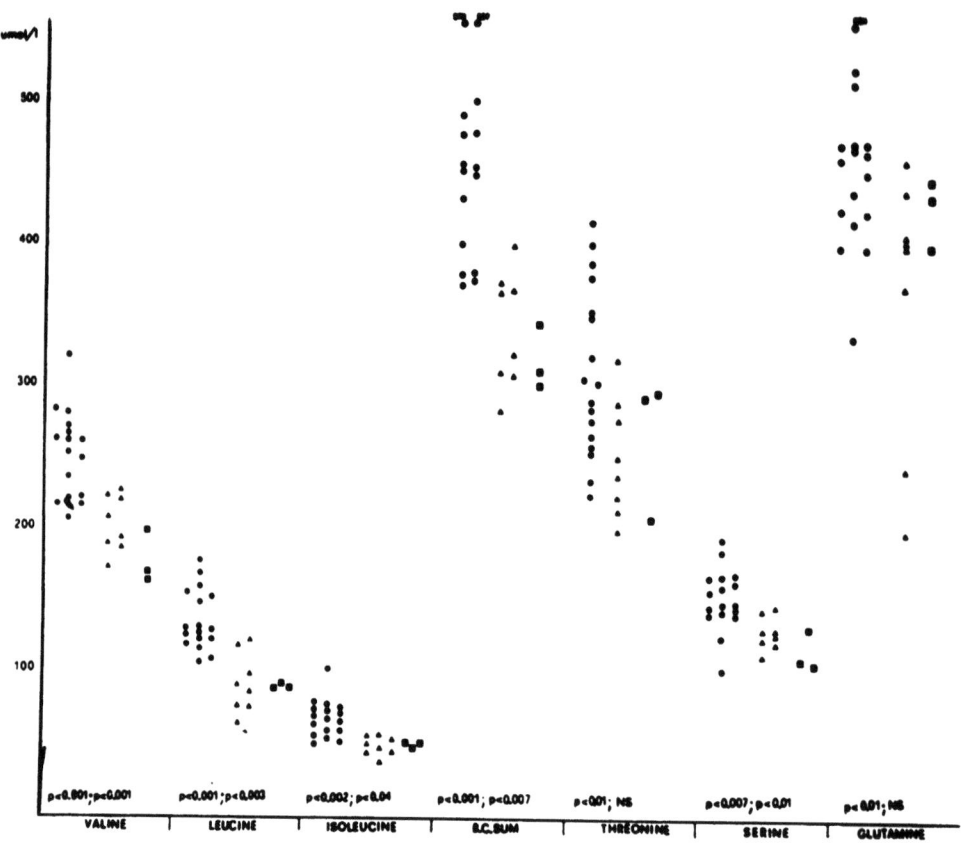

FIGURE 48.3. Phosphoenolpyruvate carboxykinase (PEPCK) activity in fetal and neonatal rats. Rats growth-retarded by maternal uterine artery ligation (i.e., SGA) did not increase hepatic PEPCK activity during the neonatal period, whereas the fetuses of sham-operated and normal mothers did. These direct measurements of gluconeogenic capability are consistent with the inferential observation in the human SGA infant that gluconeogenic capability is transiently impaired during the neonatal period.

acid concentrations in fasted SGA neonates. SGA neonates receiving exogenous lipids develop elevated plasma free fatty acid and triglyceride concentrations, but do not form ketone bodies.[50] These observations suggest that not only does the SGA neonate have limited fat stores but its ability to utilize and oxidize lipids is impaired. Because fatty acid oxidation is linked to gluconeogenesis, these limitations may contribute to the development of hypoglycemia.

Measurements of oxygen consumption and related metabolic variables suggest that SGA neonates have elevated metabolic rates.[51] The mechanisms are unclear. Teleologically, it may represent an attempt to compensate for the chronic intrauterine caloric deprivation. In this regard, the SGA fetal rat significantly increases glucose utilization in a number or organs as gestation progresses. These increased compensatory glucose requirements may contribute to the development of hypoglycemia.

Ketotic hypoglycemia of infancy may be a potential long-term consequence of intrauterine growth retardation. This disorder, which is the most common cause of hypoglycemia during infancy, often develops in children who were SGA.[52] Whether the alterations of intrauterine life are directly responsible for the development of ketotic hypoglycemia of infancy is unclear. It is known that the SGA rat pup, when fasted at 3 weeks of life, develops hypoglycemia and ketosis as a result of limited substrate availability.[53]

Polycythemia/Hyperviscosity

The SGA neonate is more likely than the AGA neonate to have an increased red blood cell mass. The mechanisms responsible are not completely understood. It is likely that chronic intrauterine hypoxia may stimulate fetal erythropoietin synthesis causing polycythemia. Placental transfusion may be exaggerated in SGA fetuses. The development of polycythemia-hyperviscosity with its associated complications increases the risk of morbidity in SGA neonates.[54]

Outcome

The long-term physical growth and neurodevelopmental outcome of the SGA neonate has not been completely defined. It is well established that neonates whose intrauterine growth was retarded as a result of chromosomal anomalies, syndrome anomalads, or congenital infections generally remain microcephalic and small throughout life. Their cognitive and psychomotor development is impaired in relation to the etiology of their growth retardation.

The outcome for asymmetrical SGA neonates is less clear. Most studies indicate that many term SGA neonates never meet their full growth potential and remain smaller than expected.[55] Exogenous growth hormone has not been clearly demonstrated to correct postnatal growth. Early studies indicated that such neonates are at increased risk of cognitive and psychomotor delay.[56] Other data indicate that term SGA neonates, if they do not suffer birth asphyxia, demonstrate normal cognitive and psychomotor development.[57]

Outcome data for prematurely born SGA neonates are less clear. Early studies indicated that premature SGA neonates were at greater risk of cognitive and psychomotor delay than were premature AGA neonates.[58] More recent results, perhaps reflecting improved neonatal care, suggest that premature SGA neonates, although at risk for long-term developmental problems, are at no greater risk than premature AGA neonates.[59,60]

References

1. Public health aspects of low birth weight. WHO Techn Rep Ser 1961;217:245–251.
2. Stein ZA, Susser M. Intrauterine growth retardation: epidemiological issues and public health significance. Semin Perinatol 1984;8:5–14.
3. Gruenwald P. Infants of low birth weight among 5000 deliveries. Pediatrics 1964;34:157–168.
4. Sabbagha RE. Intrauterine growth retardation. In: Sabbagha RE, ed. Ultrasound applied to obstetrics and gynecology. Philadelphia: Lippincott, 1987:112–131.
5. Wark L, Malcolm LA. Growth and development of the Lumi child in the Sepik district of New Guinea. Med J Aust 1969;2:129–138.
6. Ashcroft MT, Buchanan IC, Lovell HG, et al. Growth of infants and preschool children in St. Christopher-Nevis-Anguilla West Indies. Am J Clin Nutr 1966;19:37–59.
7. Ouellette EM, Rosett HC, Rosman NP, et al. Adverse effects on offspring of maternal alcohol abuse during pregnancy. N Engl J Med 1977;297:528–530.
8. Hill RDG. Insulin as a growth factor. Pediatr Res 1985;19:879–886.
9. Freinkel N. Of pregnancy and progeny. Diabetes 1980;29:1023–1035.
10. Schiff P, Colle E, Stern L. Metabolic and growth patterns in transient neonatal diabetes. N Engl J Med 1972;287:119–124.
11. Gewolb IH, Warshaw JB. Influences on fetal growth. In: Warshaw JB, ed. The biological basis of reproductive and developmental medicine. New York: Elsevier, 1983:364–389.
12. Ashton IK, Vesey J. Somatomedin activity in human cord plasma and relationship to birth size, insulin, growth hormone, and prolactin. Early Hum Dev 1978;2:115–122.
13. Ashworth MA, Leach FW, Milner RDG. Development of insulin secretion in the human fetus. Arch Dis Child 1973;48:151–156.
14. Glasscock GF, Gelber SE, Lamson G, et al. Pituitary control of growth in the neonatal rat: effects of neonatal hypophysectomy on somatic and organ growth, serum insulin-like growth factors, (IGF-1 and IGF-2 levels), and expression of IGF binding proteins. Endocrinology 1990;127:1792–1803.
15. Kaplan SL, Underwood LE. Clinical studies with recombinant DNA derived methionyl human growth hormone in growth hormone deficient children. Lancet 1986;1:679–701.
16. Hall K, Sara VR. Growth and somatomedins. Vitam Horm 1983;40:175–253.
17. D'Ercole AJ, Stiles A, Underwood L. Tissue concentrations of somatomedin C: further evidence of multiple sites of synthesis and paracrine or autocrine mechanisms of action. Proc Natl Acad Sci USA 1989;81:935–939.
18. Romanus J, Terrel J, Yang Y. Insulin-like growth factor carrier proteins in neonatal and adult rat serum are immunologically different: demonstration using a new radioimmunoassay for the carrier protein from BRL-3A rat liver cells. Endocrinology 1986;118:1743–1758.
19. Unterman TG, Simmons RA, Glick RP, Ogata ES. Circulating levels of insulin, insulin-like growth factor I (IGF-I), IGF-II, and IGF-binding proteins in the small for gestational age fetal rat. Endocrinology 1993;132:327–336.
20. Hay W, Sparks J, Battaglia F, Meschia G. Maternal fetal glucose exchange: necessity of a three pool model. Am J Physiol 1984;246:E528–E534.
21. Hay W, Molina R, DeGiacomma J, Meschia G. Model of placental glucose consumption and glucose transfer. Am J Physiol 1990;258:R569–R570.
22. Cetin I, Marconi A, Bozetti P, et al. Umbilical amino acid concentrations in appropriate and small for gestational age infants: a biochemical difference present in utero. Am J Obstet Gynecol 1988;158:120–126.
23. Bell GI, Kayano T, Buse JB, et al. Molecular biology of mammalian glucose transporters. Diabetes Care 1990;13:198–208.
24. Devaskar S, Mueckler M. The mammalian glucose transporter. Pediatr Res 1992;31:1–13.
25. Jansson T, Wennergren M, Illsley N. Glucose transporter protein expression in human placenta throughout gestation and in intrauterine growth retardation. J Clin Endocrinol Metab 1993;77:1554–1562.
26. Reid GJ, Lane RH, Flozak AS, Simmons RA. Placenta expression of glucose transporter protein (Glut 1) in fetal overgrowth. Pediatr Res 1996;39:318A.
27. McGiven J, Pastor Angladi A. Regulatory and molecular aspects of mammalian amino acids transport. Biohem J 1993;299:321–334.

28. Nitzan M, Orloff S, Shulman J. Placental transfer of analogs of glucose and amino acids in experimental intrauterine growth retardation. Pediatr Res 1979;13:100–103.
29. Jansson T, Persson E. Placental transfer of glucose and amino acids in intrauterine growth retardation: studies with substrate analogs in the awake guinea pig. Pediatr Res 1990; 28:203–208.
30. Mahendran D, Donnai P, Glazier JD, et al. Amino acid (system A) transporter activity in microvillous membrane vesicles from the placentas of appropriate and small for gestational age babies. Pediatr Res 1993;34:661–666.
31. Glazier J, Sibley CP, Carter M. Effect of fetal growth restriction on system A amino acid transporter activity in the maternal facing plasma membrane of rat syncytiotrophoblast. Pediatr Res, in press.
32. Dicke J, Henderson G. Placental amino acid uptake in normal and complicated pregnancies. Am J Med Sci 1988; 295:223–227.
33. Cetin I, Marconi A, Buzzetti P, et al. Umbilical amino acid concentrations in appropriate and small for gestational age infants: a biochemical difference present in utero. Am J Obstet Gynecol 1988;158:120–126.
34. Cetin I, Marconi A, Corbetta C, et al. Fetal amino acids in normal pregnancies and in pregnancies complicated by intrauterine growth retardation. Early Hum Dev 1992;29: 183–186.
35. Ogata ES, Bussey M, Finley S. Altered gas exchange, limited glucose, branched chain amino acids and hyperinsulinism retard fetal growth in the rat. Metabolism 1986; 35:950–977.
36. Thureen P, Tremble K, Meschia G, et al. Placental glucose transport in heat induced fetal growth retardation. Am J Physiol 1992;263:R578–R585.
37. Ross J, Fennessey R, Wilkening R, et al. Placental transport and fetal utilization of leucine in a model of fetal growth retardation. Am J Physiol 1996;270:E491–E503.
38. Barr M, Jensch R, Brent R. Prenatal growth in the albino rat: effects of number, intrauterine position, and resorption. Am J Anat 1970;128:413–428.
39. Ogata ES, Finley S. Selective ligation of uterine artery branches accelerates fetal growth in the rat. Pediatr Res 1988;24:384–390.
40. Sibai B, Andersen G. Pregnancy outcome of intensive therapy in severe hypertension in first trimester. Obstet Gynecol 1986;67:517–523.
41. Pedersen JF, Molsted Pedersen L, Mortensen HB. Fetal growth delay and maternal hemoglobin A_{ic} in early diabetic pregnancy. Obstet Gynecol 1984;64:351–352.
42. Ravelli GP, Stein ZA, Susser MA. Obesity in young men after famine exposure in utero and early infancy. N Engl J Med 1976;295:349–353.
43. Khouzami V, Ginshang DS, Daikoku NH, et al. The glucose tolerance test as a means of identifying intrauterine growth retardation. Am J Obstet Gynecol 1981;139:423–430.
44. Sokol RD, Kazzi GH, Kalhan S. Identifying the pregnancy at risk for intrauterine growth retardation: possible usefulness of the intravenous glucose tolerance test. Am J Obstet Gynecol 1982;143:220–223.
45. Shelley NJ, Neligan GA. Neonatal hypoglycemia. Br Med Biol 1966;22:34–39.
46. Mestiyan J, Soltesz G, Schultz K, et al. Hyperaminoacidemia due to the accumulation of gluconeogenic precursors in the small for gestational age infant. N Engl J Med 1974;291:322–328.
47. Williams PR, Fiser R, Sperling MA, et al. Effects of oral alanine feeding on blood glucose, plasma glucagon and insulin concentrations in small for gestational age infants. N Engl J Med 1975;292:612–614.
48. Kollee LAA, Monneus LAH, Tribels IMF, et al. Experimental intrauterine growth retardation in the rat: evaluation of the Wigglesworth model. Early Hum Dev 1979;3: 295–300.
49. Bussey M, Finley S, Ogata ES. Hypoglycemia in the newborn growth retarded rat: delayed phosphoenolpyruvate carboxykinase induction despite increased glucagon availability. Pediatr Res 1985;19:363–367.
50. Sabel K, Olegard R, Victorn I. Interrelation between fatty acid oxidation and control of gluconeogenic substrates in small-for-gestational age (SGA) infants with hypoglycemia and with normoglycemia. Acta Paediatr Scand 1982;71:53–62.
51. Sinclair JC, Silverman WA. Intrauterine growth in active tissue mass of the human fetus with particular reference to the undergrown baby. Pediatrics 1966;38:48–57.
52. Haymond WM, Karl IE, Pagliari AS. Ketotic hypoglycemia: an amino acid substrate limited disorder. J Clin Endocrinol Metab 1975;42:846–853.
53. Ogata ES, Bussey M, Finley S, et al. Altered growth, hypoglycemia, hypoalaninemia, and ketonemia in the young rat: postnatal consequences of intrauterine growth retardation. Pediatr Res 1985;19:32–37.
54. Yao A, Lind J. Placental transfusion. Am J Dis Child 1974; 27:128–136.
55. Fitzhardinge P, Stevens E. The small for date infant. I. Later growth patterns. Pediatrics 1972;49:671–678.
56. Fitzhardinge P, Stevens E. The small for date infant. II. Neurological and intellectual sequelae. Pediatr Res 1972; 50:50–56.
57. Westwood M, Kramer M, Munoz D, et al. Growth and development of full-term non-asphyxiated small for gestational age newborns: follow-up through adolescence. Pediatrics 1983;71:376–382.
58. Commey MB, Fitzhardinge PM. Handicap in the preterm small for gestational age infant. J Pediatr 1979;5:779–786.
59. Vohr BR, Oh W, Rosenfield AG, et al. The preterm small for gestational age infant: a two-year follow-up study. Am J Obstet Gynecol 1979;133:425–431.
60. Pena IC, Teberg AJ, Finello KM. The premature small-for-gestational age infant during the first year of life: comparison by birth weight and gestational age. J Pediatr 1988;113: 1066–1073.

49
The Infant of the Diabetic Mother

Richard M. Cowett

The infant of the diabetic mother (IDM) is the premier metabolic example of the morbidity that may exist in the neonate secondary to maternal disease (i.e., diabetes) (Figure 49.1) (see Chapter 10). From a development standpoint the normal neonate is in a transitional state of glucose homeostasis. The fetus is completely dependent on its mother for glucose delivery, and the adult is considered to have control of glucose homeostasis since plasma glucose concentration is regulated to a precise degree.[1] In contrast, maintenance of glucose homeostasis may be a major problem even for the normal neonate[2] (see Chapter 32). The precarious nature of this equilibrium is emphasized by the numerous morbidities producing or associated with neonatal hypo- and hyperglycemia during this period of development. Analysis of the IDM documents not only how far we have come in understanding the pathophysiology of the dysequilibrium that may exist, but also how much more research is necessary to fully understand the operative mechanisms. From the discussion to follow it will be apparent that more data are needed to fully understand the metabolic derangements that exist. The topic of the IDM has been evaluated previously in extensive reviews.[3-5]

Although many IDMs have an uneventful perinatal course, there is still an increased risk of complications. Many of these can be minimized with appropriate obstetric and pediatric intervention; consequently, the obstetrician and pediatrician must be knowledgeable about these potential problems. This chapter enumerates many of the difficulties that the IDM may encounter and evaluates the pathophysiologic basis of their occurrence.

Perinatal Mortality and Morbidity

While the IDM may have greater morbidity than the neonate of the nondiabetic woman, many infants of insulin-dependent diabetic women experience an uneventful clinical course, and even more infants of gestational diabetic women do well.[3-5] Theoretically, the more closely metabolically controlled the diabetic pregnant patient is, the greater the potential for producing a normal neonate. Over the past decade or so, perinatal mortality, except for congenital anomalies, has approached that for the neonate born to a nondiabetic mother.[6,7]

The physician responsible for the care and delivery of the mother must inform the physician responsible for the care of the neonate of the mother's status well in advance of delivery. Certainly the pregnancy of the diabetic mother should be considered to be of high risk. Knowledge of the character of the maternal diabetes, prior pregnancy history, and complications occurring during pregnancy allows the physician caring for the neonate to anticipate many of the potential fetal and neonatal complications and to be present at delivery (Table 49.1). One review has considered the question of whether centralized hospital care made a difference in the management of insulin-dependent pregnant diabetics in Northern Ireland.[8] After evaluating perinatal loss rates and the incidence of congenital anomalies, the investigators concluded that peripheral hospitals away from a centralized facility should offer to manage the pregnant diabetic only if they have an antenatal/endocrine unit and a neonatal intensive care unit.

Studies of perinatal morbidity and mortality from diverse centers attest to the improving success of the above principle. In 1974, Pedersen et al.[9] published a review of their experiences over a 26-year period with an analysis of 1332 diabetic pregnancies. Perinatal mortality varied directly with maternal severity of diabetes as judged by two commonly used maternal classification schema: White's original classification of diabetes in pregnancy and Pedersen's Prognostically Bad Signs in Pregnancy (PBSP) classification. White's revised classification (Table 49.2) is based on duration of diabetes and the presence of late vascular complications,[10] while the PBSP classification (Table 49.3) includes abnormalities of the current pregnancy.

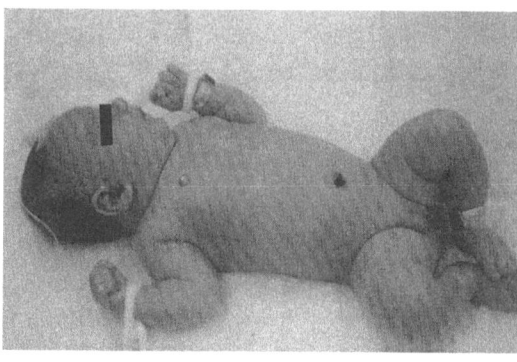

FIGURE 49.1. The infant of a diabetic mother. This infant weighed more than 4000 g at birth.

A report from the Joslin Clinic service supports the importance of these factors, especially preeclampsia (pretoxemia) as a significant morbidity in the pregnant diabetic. Of 420 patients in the series with insulin-dependent type I diabetes, 110 or 26.2% delivered before 37 weeks compared to an incidence of 9.7% in the nondiabetic population. One third of the premature deliveries related to preeclampsia. The investigators concluded that a major problem of the diabetic pregnancy relates to the problem of preeclampsia producing prematurity.[11] The risk to the fetus was increased when the PBSP classification was "added" to the White classification.

The relationship between the two was emphasized by Diamond et al.,[12] who studied 199 pregnancies from 1977 to 1983. They noted that the presence of PBSP increased the perinatal mortality rate from 7.3 to 17.1% and was predictive of pulmonary morbidity in general (31.6% vs 16.3%). The investigators concluded that the combination of the two are still as predictive as had been noted by Pedersen. While these investigators noted an improvement in nondiabetic pregnancy outcome during this same period, they emphasized that the improved classification schema and increased experience were the major reasons for the improved results in the diabetic pregnancy. This improved perinatal mortality has been confirmed at many centers in the United States and in Europe. While the frequency of macrosomia has decreased, the rate is still higher than that in the neonate born to the nondiabetic woman. In a survey of macrosomic neonates (i.e., large for gestational age, >95 percentile weight for gestational age), most of these neonates have been born to obese mothers, not all of whom have glucose intolerance as judged by postpartum glycohemoglobin studies.[13,14] Nevertheless, the gestational diabetic with glucose intolerance during late pregnancy often remains undiagnosed and may have a neonate with a greater risk for perinatal complications.

Hemoglobin (Hb)A_1C has been widely touted as a measure of long-term control of the diabetic. However, published data reflect increasing disenchantment relative to its reliability. While a higher HbA_1 was noted in the woman diagnosed as having gestational diabetes, a relatively low sensitivity in detecting gestational diabetes was confirmed. HbA_1 and oral glucose tolerance test parameters did not correlate, and delivery of the large-for-gestational-age (LGA) neonate was not associated with higher HbA_1.[15]

TABLE 49.1. Morbidities in the IDM.

Asphyxia
Birth injury
Caudal regression
Congenital anomalies
Double outlet right ventricle
Heart failure
Hyperbilirubinemia
Hypocalcemia
Hypoglycemia
Hypomagnesemia
Increased blood volume
Macrosomia
Neurologic instability
Organomegaly
Polycythemia and hyperviscosity
Respiratory distress
Respiratory distress syndrome
Septal hypertrophy
Small left colon syndrome
Transient hematuria
Truncus arteriosus

TABLE 49.2 White's classification of diabetes in pregnancy (modified).

Gestational diabetes	Abnormal glucose tolerance test, but euglycemia maintained by diet alone or diet alone insufficient, insulin required
Class A	Diet alone, any duration or onset age
Class B	Onset age 20 years or older and duration less than 10 years
Class C	Onset age 10 to 19 years or duration 10 to 19 years
Class D	Onset age under 10 years, duration over 20 years, background retinopathy, or hypertension (not preeclampsia)
Class R	Proliferative retinopathy or vitreous hemorrhage
Class F	Nephropathy with over 500 mg/day proteinuria
Class RF	Criteria for both R and F coexist
Class H	Arteriosclerotic heart disease clinically evident
Class T	Prior renal transplantation

TABLE 49.3. Prognostically bad signs of pregnancy (PBSP).

Chemical pyelonephritis
Precoma or severe acidosis
Toxemia
"Neglecters"

Cano et al.[16] studied the relationship between maternal glycosylated hemoglobin and fetal β cell activity in relation to birth weight. A population of 40 maternal-neonatal pairs was studied of whom 17 were diabetic pregnancies. Insulin and C-peptide concentrations were measured in cord blood and compared to that of maternal HbA_1. The latter did not relate to the birth weight ratio, while insulin and C-peptide concentrations did. The investigators suggested that in populations in good control, blood glucose concentration, as monitored by HbA_1, is not the major determinant of fetal growth.

In contrast, Pollak et al.[17] studied the estimation of glucitollysine content of umbilical cord extracts as a spin-off of the measurement of glycation processes in biologic samples. The data of 12 samples from the IDM were compared to 14 samples from the non-IDM. Using ion exchange chromatography followed by reverse-phase high-pressure liquid chromatography, they noted a higher glucitollysine concentration in the IDM compared to controls. The concentration was even higher in the IDM with congenital malformations. The investigators suggested that nonenzymatic glycation of fetal tissue does occur as a result of in utero exposure to cumulative glycemia.

Relative to perinatal mortality, Teramo et al.[18] published data from Helsinki, Finland. Their study focused on two time periods: 1970–1971 and 1975–1977. In 1974, the principles of obstetric monitoring and the treatment of the pregnant diabetic and her neonate were updated. Their review focused on the differences resulting from those changes in management. Specifically this involved increased monitoring and more frequent hospitalization for metabolic control, especially in the third trimester. In 1975–1977 all diabetic patients were hospitalized from the 32nd week of pregnancy until delivery. Strict maintenance of normoglycemia (i.e., blood glucose $<120\,mg\cdot dl^{-1}$) was the goal of management and, in the latter years, a permanent interdisciplinary team was in charge of the treatment of the patient. Gestational age of the neonate was increased significantly; however, mean birth weight was unchanged. The perinatal mortality rate fell markedly as did neonatal morbidity. The investigators concluded that while advances were apparent, the final answers were far from settled because of the significant percentage of neonatal morbidities still present.

Similar conclusions about strict metabolic control were reported by Jerwell et al.,[19] who evaluated their experience in Norway between 1967 and 1976. A total of 1035 births to diabetic mothers were registered during the 10-year period. Not only did perinatal mortality fall by 30%, but the duration of gestation increased from 35.5 to 37 weeks over the same period. The number of neonates who were appropriate for gestational age (AGA) increased from 53.3% to 70.0%. The care of these pregnant diabetics occurred more commonly in university clinics and regional hospitals, from 38.7% in 1967–1968 to 77.1% in 1975–1976. The impact of these interventions did not affect the malformation rate, which was still more common by a factor of 50% in the infant born to the diabetic woman compared with the general population.

Maternal glucose variability has been studied in 154 pregnant diabetic patients who were hospitalized for a month prior to delivery.[20] An evaluation of the correlation for within day plasma glucose variability showed that there was a significant association between maternal glucose variability and enhanced neonatal outcome (i.e., decreased incidence of complications) and that there was no correlation between maternal glucose variability and the birth weight of the neonate. The investigators acknowledged that absence of glucose variability would not ensure prevention of neonatal complications.

Roberts and Pattison[21] reported on a 20-year experience involving 1528 pregnancies of diabetic women: 571 had type I diabetes and 957 had gestational diabetes. The perinatal mortality rate decreased from 15.2% to 2% for those with type I diabetes and from 6.7% to 0.5% for those with gestational diabetes. The investigators related the improvement in mortality to improved management of glucose control. They reported, as noted by others, the major outstanding problem is the persistent high incidence of congenital malformations.

Another evaluation was performed in which euglycemia was maintained in the diabetic woman who evidenced vascular compromise.[22] While improvement was noted in many of the side effects of vascular compromise such as proteinuria and retinopathy, there was a wide range noted in the neonatal birth weight in spite of a normal hemoglobin A_1 determination.

Coustan and Imarah[23] attempted to use prophylactic insulin treatment of the gestational diabetic to reduce the incidence of macrosomia, operative delivery, and birth trauma. The data showed a partial decline of complications with tightened maternal metabolic control. Subsequently the same investigators evaluated a randomized clinical trial of insulin pump or intensive conventional therapy. Twenty-two pregnant diabetic women were randomized to conventional therapy or insulin pump therapy. No significant differences were found with either regimen. Excellent therapy was achieved with both.[24]

The use of insulin therapy was reported by Thompson et al.[25] One hundred and eight gestational diabetics were randomized to receive diet plus insulin or diet alone to maintain glycemic control. The investigators reported that if the patient was treated for at least 6 weeks with diet plus insulin, the mean birth weight, the incidence of macrosomia, and the ponderal index were reduced. No patient who weighed less than 200 lb and maintained euglycemic control delivered a neonate who weighed more than 4000 g. The investigators concluded that maternal obesity or failure to achieve glycemic control should alert the clinician to an increased risk of macrosomia.

This same conclusion was reached by Larsen et al.,[26] who concluded that maternal obesity (i.e., >95%) was associated with a 2.2 odds ratio of macrosomia (i.e., BW > 4000 g) compared to 1.0 for women who weighed between the 25th and the 75th percentile.

An extension of the above was reported by Nordlander et al.,[27] who evaluated factors that influence neonatal morbidity in gestational diabetes. Perinatal morbidity was significantly more frequent in the gestational diabetic (i.e., 23%) than in the control group (i.e., 13%). The occurrence of a large-for-gestational-age neonate was not different between groups. Of those born to the gestational diabetic, the neonate who presented with morbidities was of an earlier gestational age at delivery, was delivered more frequently by cesarean section, and had a mother who had higher prepregnancy weight and greater area under the glucose tolerance curve. Gestational age at delivery and maternal prepregnancy weight were the most significant factors. The investigators concluded that factors besides blood glucose control during pregnancy were critical relative to neonatal outcome in the gestational diabetic pregnancy.

A population-based study of 68 diabetics requiring insulin treatment and 403 treated with diet alone were compared to a random sample of 1 in 12 of 893 nondiabetic women who delivered in one regional hospital.[28] No relationship was noted between maternal glycosylated hemoglobin at delivery and the neonatal birth weight. At each week of gestation the infant born to the diabetic was heavier than the infant born to the nondiabetic ($p < .05$). No differences were noted in maternal glycosylated hemoglobin between the two groups throughout pregnancy. Factors affecting birth weight included diabetes, ethnic origin, and parity. The investigators concluded that substrates other than glucose, which induce hyperinsulinemia, may be related to the higher birth weight of the neonate.

Hanson et al.[29] evaluated factors influencing neonatal morbidity in the diabetic pregnancy. They evaluated maternal duration of diabetes, third trimester blood glucose control, gestational age at delivery, mode of delivery, and hypertension in 92 consecutive pregnancies of White's classes B through F. Morbidities were classified as none, minor, or severe. No differences were noted in the former two groups. Those with severe morbidity had longer duration of maternal diabetes, shorter gestational age at birth, higher rates of cesarean section, and higher frequency of toxemia. The most significant single factor was the gestational age of the pregnancy. Glucose control between 70 and 153 mg·dl^{-1} did not influence morbidity.

Finally, Hod et al.[30] reported data evaluating the effect of patient compliance, fasting plasma glucose on the oral glucose tolerance test, maternal body constitution, and method of treatment on perinatal outcome of the patient with gestational diabetes mellitus; 470 patients were compared to 250 control nondiabetics. Patient compliance reduced the rate of macrosomia (14.4%) and neonatal hypoglycemia (3.4%) but not to the level of the control population (5.2% and 1.2%, respectively). Intensified insulin treatment was beneficial in terms of reducing the rate of perinatal complications in the obese parturient but, again, not to the level of the control group.

While most investigators have agreed on the importance of maintenance of euglycemia, the most optimal method clinically has not been established. DeVeciana et al.[31] compared the efficacy of postprandial and preprandial monitoring to achieve glycemic control in the gestational diabetic woman. Sixty-six women who were 30 weeks or earlier were studied; they were treated with insulin therapy following either preprandial monitoring or postprandial monitoring 1 hour after a meal. The change in glycosylated hemoglobin was greater in the postprandial group and the birth weight of the neonate was lower as well. Similarly, there was a lower rate of neonatal hypoglycemia in the large-for-gestational-age neonate, and a lower delivery rate by cesarean section.

The maintenance of a normal metabolic state, including euglycemia, should diminish, but not completely eradicate, the increased perinatal and neonatal mortalities and morbidities noted in the diabetic pregnancy. The mechanisms for this clinical observation are discussed below.

Pathogenesis of the Effects of Maternal Diabetes on the Fetus

As yet, no single pathogenic mechanism has been clearly defined to explain the diverse problems observed in the IDM. Nevertheless, many of the effects can be attributed to maternal metabolic (i.e., glucose) control. Pedersen[32] originally emphasized the relationship between maternal glucose concentration and neonatal hypoglycemia (Table 49.4). His simplified hypothesis recognized that maternal hyperglycemia resulted in fetal hyperglycemia, which stimulated the fetal pancreas, resulting in islet cell hyper-

TABLE 49.4. Components for the hypothesis of "hyperinsulinism" in the IDM.

Islet hyperplasia and β-cell hypertrophy
Obesity and macrosomia
Hypoglycemia with low FFA concentration
Rapid glucose disappearance rate
    Higher plasma insulin-like activity after glucose
    Umbilical vein reactive immunoinsulin increase
C-peptide and proinsulin concentrations elevated

trophy and β cell hyperplasia with increased insulin availability. Following delivery, the neonate was no longer supported by placental glucose transfer and neonatal hypoglycemia occurred.

Hyperinsulinemia in utero affects diverse organ systems, including the placenta. Insulin acts as the primary anabolic hormone of fetal growth and development, resulting in visceromegaly, especially of heart and liver, and macrosomia. In the presence of excess substrate such as glucose, increased fat synthesis and deposition occur during the third trimester. Fetal macrosomia is reflected by increased body fat, muscle mass, and organomegaly but not an increased size of the brain or kidney.[33,34] After delivery there is a rapid fall in plasma glucose concentration with persistently low concentrations of plasma free fatty acids (FFA), glycerol, and beta-hydroxybutyrate. In response to an intravenous glucose stimulus, plasma insulin-like activity is increased as is plasma immunoreactive insulin, determined in the absence of maternal insulin antibodies and plasma C-peptide concentration.[35] The insulin response to intravenous arginine is also exaggerated in the infant of a gestationally diabetic mother.[36]

In a follow-up study using the chronic hyperinsulinemic fetal rhesus monkey, Susa et al.[37] investigated neonatal insulin secretion following delivery. They gave glucagon at a dose of $300\,\mu g \cdot kg^{-1}$ to stimulate insulin secretion. Compared to controls, the experimental group evidenced a blunted insulin and C-peptide response to the glucagon infusion. The investigators suggested that fetal hyperinsulinemia inhibited its own synthesis and secretion in utero and that these alterations persisted after birth.

MacFarlane and Tsakalakos[38] suggested that the initial increase in fetal size due to fetal hyperinsulinemia produced developing hypoxemia. The limitation in fetal oxygen availability altered differential utilization of glucose and increased α-glycerophosphate synthesis in the fetal adipocyte, which resulted in fetal adiposity.

Schwartz et al.[39] evaluated whether macrosomia in the fetus of the diabetic mother is related to fetal hyperinsulinemia and whether hyperinsulinemia and macrosomia are related to maternal metabolic control. Ninety-five nondiabetic pregnant women were compared to 155 insulin-treated pregnant women who were subdivided according to the White classification, the presence of hypertension, the birth weight, and the mode of delivery. Optimal care was provided and the neonate was evaluated. Macrosomia (≥97.5%) was noted in 10% to 27% of the diabetic groups and was correlated with umbilical total insulin, free insulin, and C-peptide concentrations. Glycosylated hemoglobin was only a weak predictor of birth weight and fetal hyperinsulinemia. The investigators concluded that the etiology of macrosomia essentially remains unexplained, but that hyperinsulinemia remains the major stimulus for excessive fetal growth.

On the other hand, Gloria-Bottini et al.[40] studied 230 diabetic mothers and showed that macrosomia is associated with two specific genomic sites: phosphoglucomutase locus-1 (PMG-1)-Rh blood group linkage group (chromosome 1), and Hind III restriction fragment length polymorphism (RFLP) linked to insulin-like growth factor-I (IGF-I) (chromosome 12). In the PMG-1 mother carrying the E allele, there was a proportion of 8.7% of macrosomic neonates compared with 39.6% in mothers with other genotypes. The proportion of macrosomic neonates was much lower among neonates carrying the IGF-IHS allele of the Hind III RFLP linked to IGF-I (20%) than among IGF-IF/IGF-IHF neonates (55%).

The response to an oral glucose load results in an earlier plasma insulin concentration increase compared with the normal neonate, although the area under the insulin curve is similar.[41] During the initial hours after birth, the response to an acute intravenous bolus of glucose is a rapid rate of glucose disappearance from the plasma in the IDM compared with the normal.[42] In contrast, the increase in plasma glucose concentration following stepwise hourly increases in the rate of continuously infused glucose results in an elevation even at normal rates, that is, 4 to $6\,mg \cdot kg^{-1} min^{-1}$.[43,44] The latter may be attributed to a persistence of hepatic glucose output that is similar to that noted in the normal neonate.

Alterations of plasma glucocorticoids and growth hormone have not been significant in IDMs in all published data. Definitive studies of the somatomedins (IGF-I, IGF-II) have been reported. As an example, Hill et al.[45] studied IGFs in fetal macrosomia in the neonate whose mother did or did not have diabetes. Cord concentrations of IGF-I, total IGF, and IGF binding protein were determined in 15 term IDMs and 29 term neonates of nondiabetic mothers. While there was a relationship between cord IGF and total IGF concentration in the LGA versus AGA neonate of the nondiabetic, there was no such relationship in the IDM. IGF binding proteins were not different in any group. The investigators concluded that the absence of increased IGF in the IDM was interpreted to suggest that these growth factors are not involved in the development of macrosomia in the IDM.

On the other hand, Roth et al.[46] hypothesized that macrosomia in the IDM may be due to either a perturbation of a putative placental-fetal growth axis involving, among other factors, IGF-I and -II, the ubiquitous peptides that share structural homology with insulin. Placental IGF-I and -II messenger RNA concentrations in placenta and IGF-I and -II peptide concentrations in cord serum were measured in the nonmacrosomic neonate of the nondiabetic (i.e., controls), in the macrosomic IDM, and in the nonmacrosomic IDM. IGF-I in cord serum in the macrosomic diabetic group was significantly higher compared to the other two groups. The concentration was directly correlated with neonatal birth weight irrespective of the diabetic state. The IGF-II concentration in the mother who was diabetic was elevated but was not correlated with neonatal birth weight, nor was there a concomitant increase in placental IGF-II concentration.

In contrast, urinary excretion of catecholamines was diminished, especially in the neonate with a low plasma glucose concentration.[47] In addition, plasma glucagon concentration was less elevated after delivery in comparison to the normal neonate.[48]

Studies of the insulin receptor in the fetal monocyte, isolated from placental blood of the infant of gestationally diabetic mother (IGDM) at delivery, indicate that the IGDM has more receptor sites per monocyte than the normal adult or normal neonate.[49] Monocytes from both the normal neonate and IGDM show greater affinity for insulin than do those from the adult. Furthermore, in the presence of an increased ambient concentration of plasma insulin, monocytes of the IGDM seem to develop an increased, not decreased, concentration of insulin receptors as well as increased affinity for the hormone. The significance of these observations for the physiologic effects of insulin are unclear. However, there are implications for competition of insulin and its antibody for receptor sites and metabolically insulin-sensitive tissue.

The role of the insulin receptor in macrosomia and the tendency to hypoglycemia was studied in the IDM and the neonate, born to the nondiabetic mother, of between 3 and 14 days of age. The IDMs were macrosomic. Plasma free insulin concentration in cord blood was 15-fold higher in the IDM compared to the control, and threefold higher in peripheral venous blood. Hypoglycemia was noted in 12 of 17 IDMs but in none of the control neonates. In umbilical blood, insulin binding to erythrocytes was not different between groups, but decreased during the first weeks at a more rapid rate in the IDM. This was due to decreased receptor affinity and receptor concentration. Thus, insulin binding was similar in spite of gross hyperinsulinemia in the IDM, the latter resulting in macrosomia and hypoglycemia that decreased early on in the neonatal period.[50]

To evaluate the effect of diabetes on umbilical cord blood erythrocyte insulin receptor characteristics, 13 normal and 14 diabetic pregnancies were studied relative to fetal insulin binding.[51] Specific binding of insulin to erythrocytes was comparable. The IDM evidenced a fourfold decrease in receptor affinity and fourfold increase in receptor sites in spite of significant hyperinsulinemia. The investigators concluded that the fetus of the diabetic mother exhibits a low-affinity/high-capacity insulin binding system that allows it to maintain normal insulin sensitivity in the presence of hyperinsulinemia.

Krew et al.[52] compared fetal insulin production, as estimated by amniotic fluid C peptide, and neonatal body fat as estimated by anthropometrics and total body electrical conductivity. They concluded that fetal insulin production, as estimated by amniotic fluid C-peptide concentration, influences fetal growth primarily through increasing fetal fat deposition rather than lean body mass.

Relative to specific material factors, adiposity in the neonate born to the gestational diabetic mother, in comparison to a control group of neonates, was studied by Vohr et al.,[53] 119 term neonates born to gestational diabetic women, 57 of whom were LGA and 62 of whom were AGA, were compared to 143 term control neonates, 74 of whom were LGA and 69 of whom were AGA. Multiple regression analyses to determine effects of significant maternal factors on neonatal body mass index suggested that pregnancy weight and weight gain were significant predictors for both groups. Second and third trimester glucose concentrations were significant predictors for the body mass index of the gestational diabetic, while a significant glucose screen predicted body mass index in the control group. Increased adiposity in the IGDM was related to increased neonatal blood pressure.

Lipase activities were measured in the placenta of rats made diabetic by streptozocin treatment and in the placenta of women identified as having type II diabetes (i.e., impaired glucose tolerance) and/or type I with or without vascular complications.[54] Normals were evaluated for comparison. At pH 4 lipase activity increased in the placenta both in the rat and the human in comparison to controls. In the women a correlation was present between placental lipase activity at pH 4 and birth weight in impaired glucose tolerance patients, suggesting that increased activity may contribute to increased fetal weight by contributing to increase fat transfer across the placenta.

An interesting variation on the theme of the effects on maternal diabetes on the fetus was addressed by Homko et al.,[55] who evaluated the relationship between ethnicity and gestational diabetes relative to macrosomia in an urban diabetes program in an academic setting. Between 1991 and 1994 gestational diabetes mellitus was diagnosed in 103 African-American women and 36 Latino women. All factors being equal, macrosomia developed in 50% of the neonates of the Latino women versus 19% of the neonates of the African-American women. The investigators suggested that, at least in this series, an ethnic variation in fetal growth may be present.

Finally, the cause of macrosomia in the infant of the diabetic woman was further evaluated by the National Institute of Child Health and Human Development's Diabetes in Early Pregnancy Study, which recruited insulin-dependent diabetic and control women before conception, and provided an opportunity to evaluate the relationship between maternal glycemia and percentile birth weight.[56] Data were analyzed from 323 diabetic and

361 control women. Fasting and nonfasting venous plasma glucose concentrations were measured on alternate weeks in the first trimester and monthly thereafter. Glycosylated hemoglobin was measured weekly in the first trimester and monthly thereafter. More infants of the diabetic women were at or above the 90th percentile for birth weight than infants of control women (28.5% vs 13.1%, $p < .001$). The third-trimester nonfasting glucose concentration, adjusted for data in prior trimesters, was the stronger predictor of percentile birth weight ($p = .001$). After adjusting for maternal hypertension, smoking, and ponderal index, the investigators concluded that monitoring of nonfasting glucose concentration rather than the fasting concentration, which is the more commonly monitored in clinical practice, is necessary to prevent macrosomia.

Kinetic Analysis of the IDM

Application of in vivo kinetic analysis has been utilized by numerous investigators to evaluate the IDMA metabolically. An early study using stable nonradioactive isotopes was reported by Kalhan et al.[57] using [1-^{13}C] glucose and the prime constant infusion technique. The investigators measured systemic glucose production rates in five normal nondiabetic neonates and five infants of insulin-dependent diabetics at 2 hours of age. As expected, the infant of the diabetic mother had a lower glucose concentration during the study time compared to the infant of the nondiabetic mother. For the first time, the investigators reported that the IDM had a lower systemic glucose production rate. They suggested that decreased glucose output was related to inhibited glycogenolysis. They speculated that increased insulin and decreased glucagon concentrations and catecholamine responses resulted in decreased systemic output. What was fascinating about their data was that, for the late 1970s, the diabetic women were considered to be in excellent control. They had been hospitalized during the last 4 weeks of the pregnancy to achieve strict metabolic control with maternal blood glucose between 50 and 150 mg·dl^{-1}. Yet the systemic glucose production rate of these neonates was lower than that of the control neonates.

A further evaluation of the IDM was reported by the same group 5 years later.[58] Again focusing on the neonate of the mother in "strict control," the investigators evaluated systemic glucose production in five infants of insulin-dependent mothers, one neonate of a gestational diabetic and five neonates born to nondiabetic women. The blood glucose data were in a more restrictive range of 36 to 104 mg·dl^{-1} compared to that of the previous series and the mothers were controlled in a hospital setting for 3 to 4 weeks prior to delivery. In this series the systemic glucose production rate was similar in the infant of the diabetic compared to the control neonate. However, the investigators, like other groups,[59] carried their analysis a significant step further. They infused exogenous glucose, which can diminish endogenous glucose production because of the precise control known to be the hallmark of the adult. The IDM did not evidence as great a suppression of endogenous glucose production as the adult. The investigators concluded that altered regulation of glucose production may be secondary to intermittent maternal hyperglycemia even in the strictly controlled woman.

These studies parallel the work of the Brown University group that has studied glucose kinetics in the neonate using 78% enriched D[U-^{13}C] glucose. Sixteen infants of diabetic women, of whom 10 were insulin dependent and six were chemical dependent, were compared to five infants of nondiabetic women. Four infants of insulin-dependent mothers and five infants of chemical-dependent diabetic mothers received 0.45% saline as the stable isotopic tracer diluent to determine basal endogenous glucose production (Figure 49.2). All of the mothers were evaluated relative to control mothers by utilization of hemoglobin A$_1$C and maternal plasma glucose and/or cord vein glucose at delivery. None of the women were maintained in the hospital prior to study. There was a similarity between the basal glucose produc-

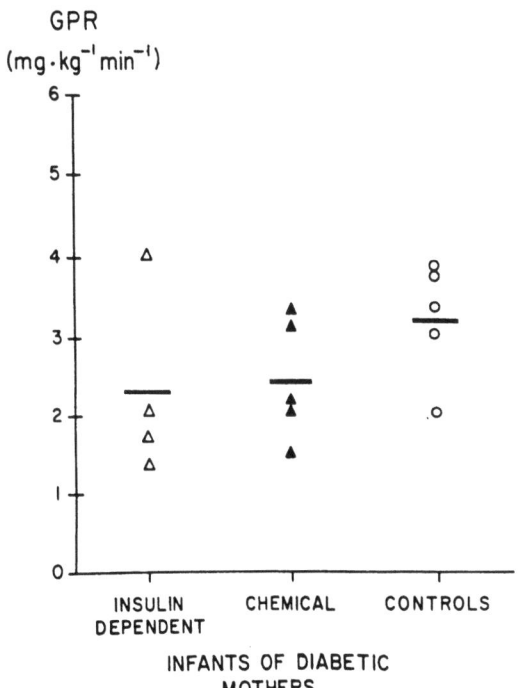

FIGURE 49.2. Glucose production rate (GPR) for the study neonates. The solid bar indicates the mean rate of production within each group. The solid figures denote neonates who received exogenous glucose as the isotopic tracer diluent and the open figures denote neonates who received 0.45% saline as the isotopic tracer diluent. (From Cowett et al.,[59,60] with permission.)

tion rate in the neonate studied with no exogenous glucose infused. The investigators concluded that good metabolic control of the maternal diabetic state would help maintain euglycemia.[60] However, in a subsequent analysis where neonates of nondiabetic mothers received glucose exogenously to maintain euglycemia, a heterogeneity continued to exist in the ability of the neonate to depress endogenous glucose production.[61] These latter data parallel other work from the same group that reflects the transitional nature of glucose metabolism in the term and preterm neonate, both born to the diabetic and the nondiabetic parturient[59,62] (see Chapter 32).

Baarsma et al.[63] followed 15 mother-infant pairs from the beginning of pregnancy until birth. Glucose kinetics were measured on the first day of life with stable isotopic dilution. In association with the above, free fatty acids, and ketones were also measured. The neonates received $3.4 \pm 0.7 \, mg \cdot kg^{-1} min^{-1}$ glucose during the study. No relationship existed between maternal control and glucose kinetics in the neonate. Total production was $5.2 \pm 1.1 \, mg \cdot kg^{-1} min^{-1}$ and endogenous glucose production was $1.8 \pm 1.1 \, mg \cdot kg^{-1} min^{-1}$ following subtraction of the glucose infusion. Endogenous glucose production was significantly lower in the neonates studied at the end of the first day of life (Figure 49.3). The lower production rate was associated with an increased concentration of ketone bodies, which suggested increased production (Figure 49.4). The investigators concluded that glucose kinetics in the infant of the tightly controlled diabetic mother are probably normal.

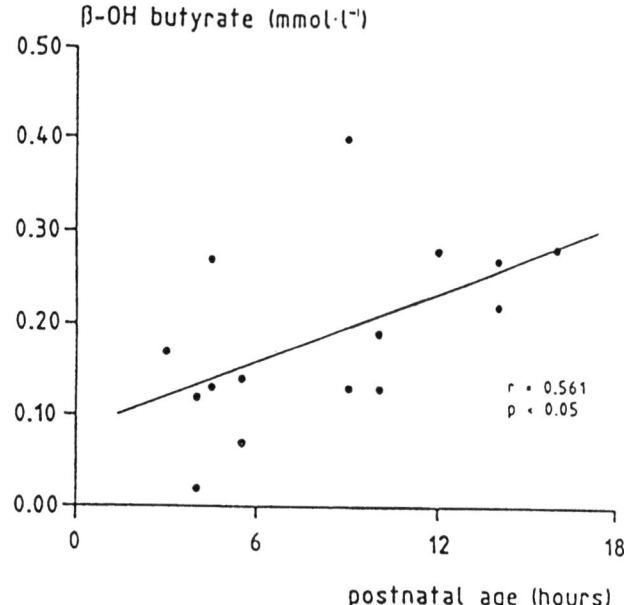

FIGURE 49.4. In the infants of mothers with tightly controlled diabetes, the 3OHB (β hydroxybutyrate) concentration is significantly correlated with postnatal age. (From Baarsma et al.,[63] with permission.)

The realization that neonatal glucose homeostasis is in a transitional state and is not the only factor affecting neonatal birth weight is further supported by studies in which maternal control was evaluated in a group of gestationally diabetic women relative to the birth weight of the neonate.[64] If the Pedersen hypothesis was correct, birth weight of the neonate should correlate with the degree of control of the mother during the pregnancy. There was a lack of correlation between birth weight and mean maternal plasma glucose concentration during the third trimester of pregnancy in this group of gestational diabetics (Figure 49.5). This lack of correlation further supports the heterogeneity of the diabetic state and suggests that while control of glucose homeostasis is multifactorial, control of fetal growth is likewise. Similar conclusions led Freinkel and others to conclude that mixed nutrients (e.g., amino acids, free fatty acids, etc.) other than glucose are important in fetal-neonatal metabolic control as noted in the schematic[65,66] (Figure 49.6). This concept is an important one for ongoing research.

Support for this concept has been provided by Kalkhoff et al.,[67] who studied the relationship between neonatal birth weight and maternal plasma amino acid profiles in lean and obese nondiabetic woman and in type I diabetic pregnant woman. HbA_1, plasma glucose concentration, and total amino acid profiles were elevated in the diabetic patient compared with controls. No differences were present between obese and lean control groups. Plasma glucose concentrations and profiles of HbA_1 did not correlate with relative weight of the neonate while average total plasma amino acids concentra-

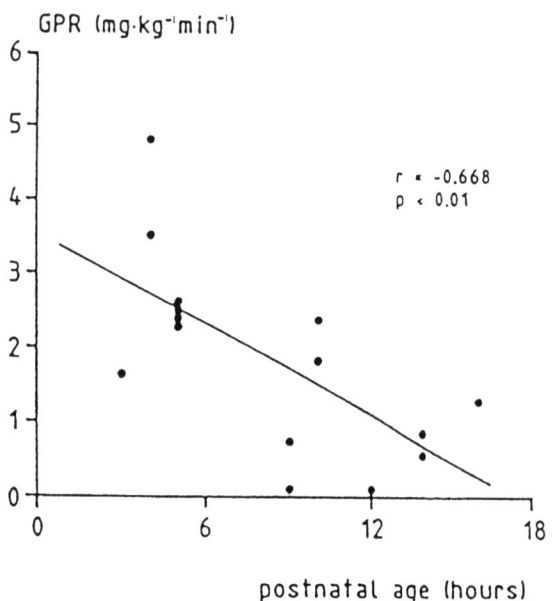

FIGURE 49.3. Correlation between endogenous glucose production and postnatal age, determined cross sectionally in 15 infants of diabetic mothers. (From Baarsma et al.,[63] with permission.)

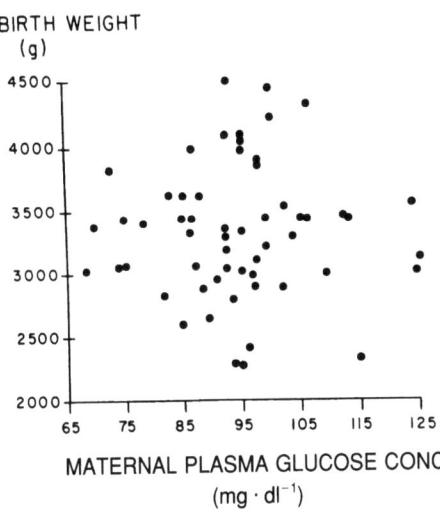

FIGURE 49.5. Lack of correlation between birth weight of the neonate and mean maternal plasma glucose concentration (mg/dl) during the last trimester of pregnancy in the glucose-intolerant group. (From Widness et al.,[64] with permission.)

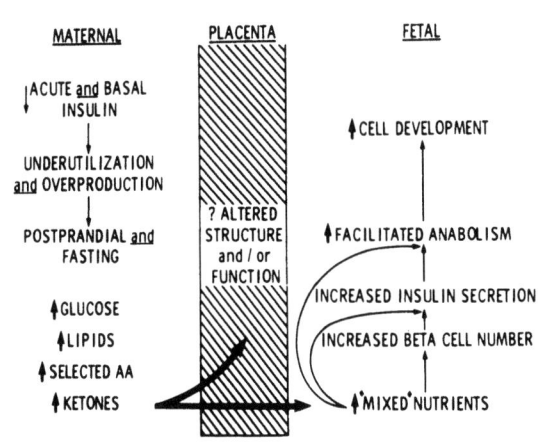

FIGURE 49.6. Fetal development in insulinogenic diabetic pregnancy utilizing maternal mixed nutrients as controlling factors. (From Freinkel,[65] with permission.)

tions did. The investigators concluded that maternal plasma amino acid profiles may influence fetal weight generally and affect the development of neonatal macrosomia.

Another data set, focusing on the relationship between neonatal birth weight and substrate, was a study by Knopp et al.,[68] who evaluated that relationship relative to plasma triglyceride concentration. They drew plasma samples for a number of metabolic parameters 1 hour after a 50-g glucose load in 521 randomly selected negatively screened individuals, 264 positively screened individuals with a negative glucose tolerance test, and 96 positively screened individuals with a positive glucose tolerance test at 24 to 28 weeks of gestation. Plasma triglyceride concentration was the only test elevated in the gestational diabetic subject, but not in the negative glucose tolerance test group. Plasma triglyceride concentration was the only test besides glucose that was significantly related to birth weight ratio, that is, birth weight corrected for gestational age, and to glucose intolerance. The investigators concluded that plasma triglyceride may be a physiologic contributor to neonatal birth weight (Figure 49.7) (see Chapters 12 and 13).

Patel and Kalhan[69] have evaluated glycerol kinetics in the IDM. They noted the possibility of intermittent hyperglycemia and hyperinsulinemia in utero in the IDM and suggested that lower concentration of plasma FFAs, concomitant with lower plasma glucose concentration, was secondary to decreased mobilization of fatty acid from adipose tissue. Since glycerol is released in a 1:3 molar ratio with fatty acids, they measured glycerol turnover using [2-^{13}C]glycerol. Unexpectedly in the macrosomic IDMs that were studied, a normal adaptive response to fasting was noted, which could assist in maintaining euglycemia.

There is increasing recognition that further work is necessary to understand the relationship between glucose and other substrates relative to neonatal birth weight especially in the IDM born to the well controlled as well as the poorly controlled diabetic (vide supra).

Congenital Anomalies

While most of the morbidity and mortality data for the IDM have shown definite improvement with time, congenital anomalies remain a significant unresolved problem. The three- to fourfold increase in the incidence of congenital anomalies in the offspring of diabetic women has been noted in most centers for a long time and remains the most frequent contributor to perinatal mortality.[6,7,70,71]

In a population-based study of 7958 infants over a 12-year span from 1968 to 1980, Becerra et al.[72] documented differences between the IDM and the non-IDM relative to congenital malformations. The relative rate for major malformations in the neonate born to the mother with insulin-dependent diabetes mellitus was 7.9 compared to the neonate of the nondiabetic mother. Likewise, the relative risk for central nervous system and cardiovascular system defects was 15.5 and 18.0, respectively. Interestingly, the neonate of the mother who had gestational diabetes and required insulin therapy was 20.6 times as likely to have a cardiovascular malformation as the neonate of the nondiabetic mother. This finding came at a time when centers were reporting perinatal mortalities in

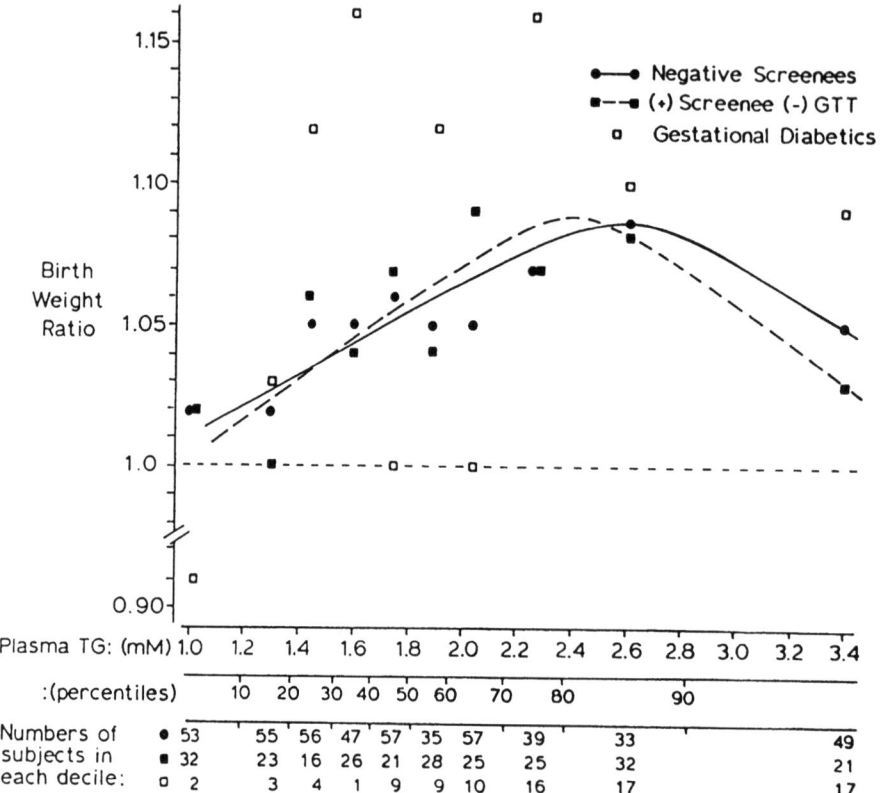

FIGURE 49.7. Relationship between birth weight ratio (neonatal birth weight adjusted for gestational age) and plasma triglyceride concentration. (From Knopp et al.,[68] with permission.)

offspring of insulin-dependent diabetic women that were no different from nondiabetics after correction for death due to congenital anomalies.[6,7,73]

The pathogenesis of the increase in congenital anomalies among IDMs has remained obscure, although several etiologies have been proposed to account for these, including (1) hyperglycemia, either preconceptional or postconceptional; (2) hypoglycemia; (3) fetal hyperinsulinemia; (4) uteroplacental vascular disease; and/or (5) genetic predisposition. A review has cogently summarized the relevant data obtained from investigations during the 1980s.[74] While there are data to support each of these proposed mechanisms, currently the best evidence supports the postconceptional hyperglycemia etiology.

If a preconceptional influence of hyperglycemia, or hypoglycemia, or a genetic predisposition for congenital anomalies were operative, then one might anticipate that the offspring of the diabetic father as well as the diabetic mother would have an increased incidence of anomalies. This assumes that the sperm and egg would be equally affected by the physiologic and biochemical permutations of maternal diabetes. In a careful hospital chart review by Neave[75] of 1262 offspring of diabetic fathers, only a slight increase in anomalies of questionable significance was found when compared with matched controls. In this same study, a marked increase in anomalies was found in the offspring of the diabetic mother compared with both the offspring of the diabetic father and an independent control group.

Studies of normalization of blood glucose concentration before conception in the diabetic woman have been reported. One large European diabetic population from Karlsburg, Germany, including nonpregnant women who were cared for in an ongoing diabetic outpatient program to normalize blood glucose concentration, had a markedly lower incidence of congenital anomalies compared with a simultaneously studied group of women who had no such therapeutic diabetic regimen applied prenatally.[76]

These conclusions were also confirmed by Goldman et al.[77] in a group of 75 insulin-dependent diabetic women of whom 44 were followed preconceptionally. Glycemic control was obtained by intensified insulin therapy. Compared to a control group that was not seen preconceptionally, there were no congenital malformations in the intensively followed group compared with a frequency of 9.6% congenital anomalies in the control group.

In a series of gestational diabetes, 136 women underwent preconceptional counseling at least 2 months before conception. Evaluation included oral glucose tolerance testing, mean blood glucose, glycosylated hemoglobin, and management by self-monitoring as well as nutritional counseling compared to a group of 154 women who did not undergo this program. Those who participated delivered their neonate without congenital malformations.[78]

There are scant human data on the association of hyperglycemia and anomalies. This may be due in part to the fact that organogenesis is taking place at a time during pregnancy when many diabetic women are not usually carefully evaluated for hyperglycemia. HbA$_1$C, which reflects ambient plasma glucose concentration over the previous 4 to 6 weeks, has the potential advantage of offering one indicator of integrated "chronic" blood glucose control. A report of initial visit first trimester maternal HbA$_1$C values in a group of insulin-dependent subjects found higher values in those diabetic women giving birth to a neonate with an anomaly.[79]

In recent years, a multiplicity of studies have reported the strong association of preconceptional testing and control with a marked diminution in the incidence of congenital anomalies. These data parallel other reports suggesting that later control after the first trimester did not result in a fall in the incidence of congenital malformations, although other morbidity did decrease. In fact, the neonatal malformation rate rose and was not influenced by maternal age or diabetic class.[80]

Hypoglycemia may play a teratogenic role in the diabetic pregnancy. Symptomatic hypoglycemia during the first trimester is a frequently observed morbidity in the insulin-dependent diabetic, although quantification has been difficult. Although the injection of insulin into the chick embryo has induced rumplessness,[81] current data indicate that the primate placenta probably acts as a complete barrier to maternal insulin from mid-gestation onward.[82] The failure of insulin to cross the placenta in the rat during the critical period of organogenesis has been considered by Widness et al.[83] using iodinated insulin.

An epidemiologic study was conducted evaluating a series of 2587 IDMs between 1926 and 1983. An overall malformation rate of 6.6% was reported. The series was divided into five consecutive periods of 500 infants each. During the final period of study, between 1979 and 1983, a decrease in severity and frequency of congenital malformations was noted. Interestingly, the investigators suggested that the fetus that was statistically smaller than normal in early pregnancy carried a higher risk of being malformed. They concluded that preconceptional metabolic control was necessary for optimal fetal outcome.[84]

The growth in anomalies with increasing duration and severity by White's classification of diabetes has been interpreted to indicate the degree to which maternal vascular disease may play a role.[32] Although anomalies in the offspring of the diabetic mother tend to encompass a spectrum of organ systems rather than a specific, discrete syndrome, some individual patterns tend to occur more frequently. Major congenital heart disease, musculoskeletal deformities, including the caudal regression syndrome, central nervous system deformities such as anencephaly spina bifida, and hydrocephalus have been reported. Based on these findings, the critical period of teratogenesis for the pregnant diabetic has been inferred to take place before the seventh week following conception. A study has highlighted the use of ultrasound for the early diagnosis of congenital anomalies, specifically, the caudal regression syndrome at 18 to 20 weeks of gestation.[85]

One rare congenital defect that increased in frequency in the IDM is the small left colon syndrome.[86] The etiology of this deformity is obscure. With conservative medical management, the condition usually resolves spontaneously within the neonatal period.

While the IDM is known to have signs of congestive heart failure, the spectrum of cardiomyopathy ranges from congestive failure to hypertrophic cardiomyopathy. A number of studies have evaluated the presence of hypertrophic cardiomyopathy in the infant of the poorly controlled diabetic woman. In one study, 11 IDMs were followed for 30 to 40 months after presenting with signs of respiratory distress; they all had septal hypertrophy on echocardiogram.[87] The natural history appeared to be resolution of symptoms within 2 to 4 weeks and of hypertrophy within 2 to 12 months. In another study, 34 infants of diabetic mothers were found to have hypertrophy of the interventricular septum and of the walls of the right and left ventricles.[88] The presence of hypertrophy was seen predominantly in the neonate whose mother was under poor diabetic control. Similar conclusions were reached in a third series, in which septal hypertrophy was noted in 6 of 18 IDMs, all of whom had profound hypoglycemia after birth, in contrast to the neonate without hypertrophy.[89] These findings are consistent with the metabolic effects of neonatal hyperinsulinism present in the fetus. It was suggested that fetal hyperinsulinism contributes directly to the septal hypertrophy. Primary fetal hyperinsulinemia in the rhesus fetus has been found by Susa et al.[34] to be associated with significant muscular hypertrophy and cardiomegaly.

Although cardiac hypertrophy apart from congenital heart disease has been recognized in the autopsy of the IDM for the past three decades, it has been only in the past 15 years that attention has been directed to a peculiar form of subaortic stenosis similar to the idiopathic hypertrophic subaortic stenosis found in the adult.[90] This particular entity may be associated with symptomatic congestive heart failure. As with the adult variant, in the neonate therapy with digoxin is contraindicated since the resultant increased myocardial contractility has been reported to be deleterious. Propranolol appears to be the therapeutic drug of choice. Clinically, this disorder resolves spontaneously over a period of weeks to months with correction of the echocardiographic features as well.

A further evaluation of the association of maternal diabetes and cardiovascular malformations was reported by Ferencz et al.[91] from the Baltimore-Washington Infant Study, a population-based case control study of cardiovascular malformations. The strongest associations with overt type I diabetes were with double-outlet right ventricle and truncus arteriosus. No associations were noted with gestational diabetes.

In a reevaluation of a previous study of the neonate with gestational diabetes who had altered left ventricular filling, Mehta et al.[92] reported that cardiac alterations in this neonate were not secondary to a preponderance of macrosomia, but were rather a consequence of an altered metabolic in utero environment.

Weber et al.[93] suggest that hypertrophic cardiomyopathy and abnormal ventricular diastolic filling in the IDM is related to poor maternal glycemic control. These investigators evaluated the fetuses of the well-controlled mother and of the nondiabetic mother. Evaluation of cardiac growth and ventricular diastolic filling took place 20 to 26, 27 to 33, 34 to 40, and 48 to 72 hours after birth. No differences were noted between groups during any period; however, progression of diastolic filling is abnormally delayed in the fetus of the diabetic woman and is presumably more likely in the poorly controlled diabetic.

Two reports have described the association of maternal insulin-dependent diabetes and the DiGeorge anomaly with the presence of renal agenesis, which may be either unilateral or bilateral. Clearly, the presence of maternal diabetes should prompt at least a consideration of these two possibilities.[94,95] Another report by Lupski et al.[96] noted an infant of a diabetic mother who presented with hypocalcemia and congenital heart disease; a truncus arteriosus type I cytogenetic analysis showed $45_1X,-Y,-22,+der-(Y)+(Y;22)$ with a del (22) (q11.1). The autopsy showed a truncus arteriosus type II and thymic aplasia consistent with the DiGeorge anomaly.

Three infants with left right asymmetry have also been reported: one with left isomerism and asplenia, one with polysplenia, and one with situs inversus and a neural tube defect. Two of the three had increased Hg A_1C, indicative of poor glycemic control.[97]

Finally, a number of studies have raised the possibility that vitamin E may provide a protective effect against the diabetic embryopathy through its well-known antioxidant effect.[98–100] Further research is required to determine the clinical applicability of these data.

Macrosomia, Birth Injury, and Asphyxia

At birth, the infant of the poorly controlled diabetic often appears macrosomic in contrast to the infant born to either the well-controlled diabetic or the nondiabetic, nonobese mother. At birth, a consequence of undetected fetal macrosomia may be a difficult vaginal delivery due to shoulder dystocia with resultant birth injury and/or asphyxia. These potential birth injuries include cephalhematoma, subdural hemorrhage, facial palsy, ocular hemorrhage, brachial plexus injuries, and clavicular fracture. Injury to the brachial plexus may appear with a variety of presentations because the nerves of the brachial plexus may be variably damaged. In addition to the obvious injury to the nerves of the arm, diaphragmatic paralysis occurs when the phrenic nerve is injured. Because of the associated organomegaly in the IDM, hemorrhage in the abdominal organs is possible, specifically the liver and the adrenal gland. Hemorrhage into the external genitalia of the large neonate has been reported.

In a study of the incidence and predisposing factors for clavicular fracture in the neonate, a group of 46 of 3030 neonates (1.5%) were diagnosed with clavicular fracture. When compared to a control group of 52 neonates without a fracture, the neonate with a fracture had a higher birth weight, an older mother, a longer second stage of labor, a higher rate of instrumented delivery, and shoulder dystocia. Eighty percent of the neonates weighed less than 4000 g. Through multivariate analysis two predisposing variables—birth weight over 3500 g and maternal age >29 years—were significant.[101]

Because the subjects are at high risk, intrapartum monitoring is essential to minimize potential complications. Clearly, early identification of macrosomia is critical. Mintz et al.[102] suggested that shoulder soft tissue measurements and abdominal circumference may be the best individual predictors of the potential for macrosomia. The combination of abdominal circumference >90th percentile and shoulder soft tissue width >12 mm was the best predictor with a sensitivity of 96%, specificity of 89%, and accuracy of 93%. At delivery, the physician evaluating the neonate should assign Apgar scores at 1 and 5 minutes to document the presence or absence of asphyxia. While the specific etiology of asphyxia is unclear, it may be due to difficulty in the intrapartum period because of relative macrosomia.

Asphyxia may have diverse consequences for the neonate. Acutely, asphyxia may affect respiratory, renal, and central nervous system function. Decreased fluid intake is usually recommended until the degree of injury to the renal and central nervous systems can be ascertained. An important complication of asphyxia in the neonate may be later respiratory difficulty. Mimouni et al.[103] studied the problem of asphyxia in the infant of insulin-dependent diabetic. They suggested that poor glycemic control in the third trimester, diabetic vascular disease, preeclampsia, and smoking are significant risk factors for perinatal asphyxia. They prospectively studied 162 infants born to 149 diabetic mothers of White class B-R-T. Forty-four neonates (27.2%) had evidence of asphyxia.

Its presence did not correlate with third trimester control or with the other factors listed, but did correlate with nephropathy occurring in pregnancy, maternal hyperglycemia before delivery, and prematurity. The investigators concluded that in the pregnant diabetic, maternal and subsequently fetal hyperglycemia before delivery leads to fetal hypoxemia.

Using a fetal lamb preparation, Philipps et al.[104,105] attempted to evaluate the mechanism of perturbations of fetal fuel and showed that fetal hyperglycemia stimulated fetal oxidative metabolism. This resulted in fetal glucose and lactate entry and stimulation of fetal oxygen consumption. If the stimulus was great enough, fetal hypoxia with metabolic acidosis and demise resulted.

Current management of the pregnant diabetic includes determining the degree of pulmonary maturity by the lecithin/sphingomyelin (L/S) ratio, the presence of phosphatidyl glycerol, and/or foam stability test (FST) prior to elective delivery. A false-positive L/S ratio may be associated with asphyxia. In one study in 150 women who had an amniocentesis within 72 hours of delivery with an L/S ratio ≥2.1, the incidence of respiratory distress syndrome (RDS) was significantly increased in the neonate who had a low Apgar score at 1 and 5 minutes. This was independent of whether or not the mother had diabetes mellitus.[106]

Others have reported success with the regular use of the biophysical profile in the pregnancy complicated by insulin-dependent diabetes. Dicker et al.[107] reported on 98 insulin-dependent diabetic pregnant mothers who underwent monitoring by use of the biophysical profile from 28 weeks until parturition. Only 2.9% had scores <7, suggesting an abnormality. If the prolife was recorded within 2 days before birth, a normal profile predicted a normal 1-minute Apgar score in 92% and normal 5-minute Apgar score in 99%. While the specificity was good in 80% to 90% of cases, the predictive value of an abnormal test result and sensitivity was poor.

One study reported a rare occurrence of gangrene in an IDM.[108] Gangrene was noted in an upper extremity with massive muscle necrosis of the forearm requiring debridement. It was postulated that gangrene developed from a propensity for thrombosis in the IDM. Another case was reported of an IDM who in utero was diagnosed as having a brachial artery thrombosis. Of 32 neonates reported in the literature, the seven who had peripartum limb gangrene were IDMs. The investigators speculated that the IDM may be at increased risk for thrombosis if an umbilical artery catheter was placed.[109]

Identification of maternal diabetes and maintenance of good metabolic control in the pregnant diabetic should diminish the frequency and magnitude of macrosomia and its attendant complications; careful obstetric management should prevent birth injury and asphyxia. Ogata et al.[110] reported data that seem to confirm this concept. Serial studies to estimate fetal biparietal diameter and abdominal circumference were used as differential inducers of intrauterine growth in fetuses of mothers who were White class A to C. Biparietal diameter was similar in fetuses of both groups. However, abdominal circumference was noted to be normal or enhanced. The latter group had an increased insulin concentration, weighed more at birth, and had more subcutaneous fat. The investigators concluded that ultrasound was shown to be useful in the preliminary detection of macrosomia.

A recent study evaluated whether macrosomia is associated with increased perinatal morbidity and mortality. The question was whether the birth of a previous macrosomic neonate heralded the risk for a subsequent macrosomic neonate. A population-based cohort study utilizing birth data from Washington State between 1984 and 1990 identified a 7.0 times risk in this clinical situation. The overall prevalence was 22% and was interpreted to suggest that a mother with one macrosomic neonate is at markedly increased risk for a subsequent one.[111]

Respiratory Distress Syndrome

Respiratory distress, including respiratory distress syndrome (RDS), may be a relatively frequent and potentially severe complication in the IDM. While the clinical association has been long recognized, published data have increased our understanding of the pathophysiologic interrelationships. Neonatal RDS, the pathologic correlate of which is hyaline membrane disease, develops because of lung immaturity in the neonate and may be a major cause of morbidity. RDS has a typical course that is manifest by an increasing oxygen requirement due to progressive respiratory compromise. Tachypnea, intercostal and subcostal retractions, nasal flaring, and expiratory grunting appearing in the first few minutes to hours of life are the cardinal signs of the disease. In uncomplicated cases, the disease may peak by 72 hours of age. Complications commonly associated with the disease include the presence of a persistent patent ductus arteriosus (PDA) in the very small (<1250g) neonate and bronchopulmonary dysplasia in the neonate requiring prolonged ventilatory support and high ambient oxygen concentration. Both of these conditions may significantly lengthen the clinical course of an otherwise self-limited disease.

Surfactant is produced in the type II pneumocyte and is composed of protein and phospholipid. It normally functions to diminish surface tension at the air-alveolar interface. Absence of this material results in pulmonary atelectasis and the characteristic clinical picture described above. On roentgen examination of the chest, a diffuse reticulogranular pattern and air bronchograms are observed. The phospholipid components of surfactant progressively increase with advancing gestational age and are the basis for utilization of specific laboratory tests of pulmonary maturity including phosphatidyl glycerol determination, L/S ratio, and/or the foam stability test.

While the increased susceptibility to RDS has been suspected in the IDM, a definitive retrospective analysis by Robert et al.[112] evaluated the relative risk of RDS in the IDM in a large series of diabetic pregnancies from the Joslin Clinic and the Boston Hospital for Women. The relative risk of RDS in the IDM was higher in comparison to the infant of the nondiabetic mother. If specific confounding variables are excluded, including gestational age, delivery by cesarean section, presence of labor, birth weight, sex, Apgar score at 5 minutes, hemorrhage, presence of hydramnios, maternal anemia, and maternal age, the relative risk is 5.6 times higher in the IDM. This effect is primarily confined to the neonate whose gestational age is ≤38 weeks. Present obstetric management has been noted to markedly reduce the frequency of RDS.

Warburton et al.[113] provided biochemical correlation of the association between RDS and diabetes in a fetal lamb model. Glucose infusion of $14\,mg\cdot kg^{-1}\,min^{-1}$ before 113 days' gestation resulted in pulmonary desaturated phosphatidylcholine being 1.5-fold higher compared to controls. After this point in gestation, it increased in the control but not in the glucose-infused fetus. Lung stability to air inflation was 2.0-fold greater in the control as well. The investigators concluded that following chronic glucose infusion in fetal lamb lung, desaturated phosphatidylcholine and lung stability were comparable with a predisposition of the fetus to develop RDS.

Recognition that RDS occurs in the IDM led to evaluation of alternative tests of amniotic fluid that might better predict the potential of an infant having RDS. In 1973, two years after initially reporting on the value of the L/S ratio in normal pregnancies, Gluck and Kulovich[114] noted that diabetes mellitus was associated with a delay in maturation of the ratio for White classes A, B, and C, while an acceleration was found for classes D, E, and F diabetic pregnancies evaluated at specific gestational ages. When an L/S ratio equals 2.0, there may be an increased frequency of false positives in all diabetic classes.

Further refinements in the L/S ratio include quantitative chromatographic assays of surfactant phosphatides to define the presence of phosphatidyl glycerol (PG), the absence of which has been correlated with increased incidence of RDS even with an L/S ratio of ≥2.0.[114] It has been shown that the presence of PG in amniotic fluid may increase the probability that a neonate can be delivered without signs of respiratory distress due to surfactant deficiency. Hallman and Teramo[115] measured phospholipids in amniotic fluid from diabetic pregnancies and compared the results with data from normal pregnancies. While there was little difference in the L/S ratio, the PG remained low and phosphatidylinositol (PI) remained high even when the L/S ratio was ≥2.0.

Surfactant production increases near term and probably results from the activation of the pathway for dipalmitoyl lecithin, which in turn may be mediated through increases in fetal plasma cortisol concentration. While plasma cortisol production rates are normal in the IDM, it has been shown that insulin can interfere with incorporation of choline into lecithin even when cortisol is present.[116] Neufeld et al.[117] have reported that incorporation of labeled glucose and fatty acid residues into saturated phosphatidylcholine was reduced in fetal rabbit lung slices in the presence of insulin. Endogenous insulin, known to be increased in the fetus of the poorly controlled pregnant diabetic, may play a significant role in delaying pulmonary maturation. While the specific biochemical mechanisms are not completely understood, these data correlate with the clinical situation in which not only is pulmonary maturation delayed in the IDM, but also RDS may be noted with L/S ratios ≥2.0.

An extension of the above concepts was reported by Curet et al.[118] Samples of amniotic fluid were analyzed for phospholipid content and correlated with the incidence of RDS. The incidence of RDS was 4.5% in the infant of the diabetic and 5.3% in the infant of the nondiabetic. If phosphatidyl glycerol was present, no neonate developed RDS; if PG was absent, RDS occurred in 16.7% and 14.4% of infants of diabetics and nondiabetics, respectively. After 37 weeks RDS did not occur in infants of diabetic mothers and only in 0.6% of the infants of nondiabetic mothers. The investigators suggested that dating of the pregnancy decreases the need for phospholipid analysis.

One possible biochemical component of importance is SAP-35,[119] a surfactant-associated protein of M 28,000 to 35,000 present as a glycoprotein in the alveolus of the lung. This protein has impact on the structural organization of surfactant phospholipid and provides regulatory information controlling surfactant phospholipid secretion and metabolism. While its expression is enhanced by adenosine 3',5'-cyclic monophosphate (cAMP) and epidermal growth factor, it is inhibited by transforming growth factor and insulin. Decreased SAP-35 has been noted in amniotic fluid of the diabetic pregnant patient. An increase to a normal concentration in SAP-35 with tight metabolic control has been noted in association with a decrease in the incidence of RDS.

In a clinical correlation analysis, Ylinen[120] related high maternal HbA_1, generally >8.0, and delayed fetal lung maturation in the insulin-dependent diabetic pregnancy.

The trend to deliver the diabetic patient later in gestation rather than earlier is increasing markedly. Previously, early delivery was advised to diminish the risk of intrauterine fetal death, but increasing assessment of fetal well-being by biophysical profiling and specific evaluation of pulmonary maturation for elective delivery affords the obstetrician the opportunity of delivering the patient at the optimal time.

Hypoglycemia

A decline in plasma glucose concentration following delivery is characteristic of the IDM. Values less than 35 mg·dl^{-1} in the term neonate and less than 25 mg·dl^{-1} in preterm neonate are abnormal and may occur within 30 minutes after clamping the umbilical cord. Factors that are known to influence the degree of hypoglycemia include prior maternal glucose homeostasis and maternal glycemia during delivery. An inadequately controlled pregnant diabetic will have stimulated the fetal pancreas to synthesize excessive insulin, which may be readily released. Administration of intravenous dextrose during the intrapartum period, which results in maternal hyperglycemia (>125 mg·dl^{-1}) will be reflected in the fetus and will exaggerate the normal postdelivery fall in plasma glucose concentration. In addition, hypoglycemia may persist for 48 hours or may develop after 24 hours.

As noted previously, fetal hyperinsulinemia is associated with a suppressed concentration of plasma free fatty acids and/or variably diminished hepatic glucose production in the neonate (Figure 49.2). Other factors that may contribute to the development of hypoglycemia include defective counterregulation by catecholamines and glucagon.

The neonate exhibits transitional control of glucose metabolism, which suggests that a multiplicity of factors affect homeostasis. Many of the factors are similar to those that influence homeostasis in the adult. What is different in the neonate are the various stages of maturation that exist. Prior work in conjunction with glucose infusion studies can be summarized to suggest that there is blunted splanchnic (hepatic) responsiveness to insulin in the neonate both in the IDM as well as in the preterm and term neonate of the nondiabetic mother, compared to the adult.[61] What has not been studied, but what is of particular interest, are the many contrainsulin hormones that influence metabolism. If insulin is the primary glucoregulatory hormone, then contrainsulin hormones assist in balancing the effect of insulin and other factors.

One should probably evaluate all of the contrainsulin hormones but those that have been of particular interest in the IDM have been those of the sympathoadrenal neural axis. Many studies have evaluated epinephrine and norepinephrine concentrations in the IDM. The results are quite variable. An early study involved 11 infants of diabetic mothers, only two of whom were gestational diabetics. Urinary excretion of catecholamines was measured and compared to that in 10 infants of normal mothers. Urinary norepinephrine and epinephrine concentrations did not increase in the infant of the diabetic woman who was severely hypoglycemic, but did increase in the neonate whose mother was mildly hypoglycemia.[47]

These results parallel investigations of Stern et al.,[121] who suggested that hypoglycemia may be secondary to an adrenal medullary exhaustion phenomenon. This would be secondary to long-standing hypoglycemia in the IDM, which would presumably be secondary to poor control of the maternal diabetic. In further studies, Keenan et al.[122] noted that when normal plasma glucose concentration increases, plasma insulin concentration declines, and plasma free fatty acid concentration increases in response to exogenous administration of epinephrine. This confirmed the exhaustion theory. A parallel explanation was given by Young et al.[123] to explain the high plasma norepinephrine concentration in the IDM whose degree of euglycemic control was not reported, except that some of the neonates were borderline large for gestational age. The investigators speculated that the IDM, exposed to excessive quantities of glucose, may be subject to chronic sympathoadrenal stimulation.

In another series, Artel et al.[124] measured plasma epinephrine and norepinephrine concentrations in the IDM. Elevated concentrations of both hormones were reported, although variation was markedly increased in the IDM. The investigators speculated that hypoglycemia after birth may be secondary to adrenal exhaustion, producing temporary depletion later in the neonatal period. This might account for the appearance of hypoglycemia noted clinically by others. In a follow-up of this concept, to evaluate whether the neonatal changes were related to maternal metabolic control, plasma glucose, catecholamines, and glucagon concentrations were measured in the neonatal period in 10 neonates of class B diabetics who were well controlled. Good control resulted in appropriate counterregulatory hormone responses comparable to the neonate of the nondiabetic mother. The investigators concluded that epinephrine and glucagon concentrations were significant in perinatal glucose homeostasis.[125]

A series by Broberger et al.[126] evaluated sympathoadrenal activity in the first 12 hours after birth in the IDM of whom nine were of type I diabetes and 13 were of insulin-treated gestational diabetes. Failure to observe differences in plasma epinephrine and norepinephrine concentrations between the IDM and the control neonate was felt to be secondary to good metabolic control of the diabetic mother.

Other factors related to sympathoadrenal activity in the neonate may be of importance. In a continuing evaluation of the transitional nature of neonatal glucose metabolism, both of insulin and contrainsulin factors, epinephrine was infused in two doses (50mg or 500mg·kg^{-1} min^{-1}) in a newborn lamb model and glucose kinetics (turnover) were measured with [6-^{3}H]glucose. The newborn lamb showed a blunted response to the lower dose of epinephrine infused. The investigators speculated that the newborn lamb evidenced blunted responsiveness to this important contrainsulin stimulus.[127,128] This tendency was reaffirmed by recent data from the same laboratory.[129] It is possible that, if this occurs in the diabetic state, it would partially account for the presence of hypoglycemia noted clinically.

Thus, the IDM is a prime example of the potential of glucose dysequilibrium in the neonate. Because of the transitional nature of glucose homeostasis in the neonatal period in general, accentuation of the dysequilibrium may be enhanced in the IDM secondary to metabolic alterations present in the maternal diabetic. A great deal of work is necessary to fully appreciate the operative mechanisms.

The infant of the diabetic mother is generally asymptomatic with a relatively low plasma glucose concentration. This may be due to the initial brain stores of glycogen, although the exact biochemistry is undefined. Signs and symptoms that may be observed in the asymptomatic neonate are nonspecific and include tachypnea, apnea, tremulousness, sweating, irritability, and seizures. The asymptomatic neonate generally does not require parenteral treatment for maintenance of carbohydrate homeostasis. Early oral feeding at 3 to 4 hours of age may be beneficial to maintain plasma glucose concentration that is not severely depressed.

Therapy is preventive, including rigid maternal control of blood glucose concentration during pregnancy and delivery. Plasma glucose concentration should be obtained at delivery from the umbilical vein. Subsequently, the neonate should be screened at 1, 2, and 4 hours and then prior to each feeding until the plasma glucose concentration is consistently in the euglycemic range. Glucose concentration requires measurement by laboratory chemical analysis.[130,131]

The symptomatic infant should be treated with parenteral fluid. Lilien et al.[132] have reported successful treatment with a "minibolus" infusion of 2ml·kg^{-1} of 10% dextrose in water (200mg·kg^{-1}) given over 1 minute followed by a continuous infusion of dextrose at a rate of 8mg·kg^{-1} min^{-1}. Bolus injections alone without subsequent infusion only exaggerate hypoglycemia by a rebound mechanism and are contraindicated. Once the plasma glucose stabilizes above 45mg·kg^{-1}, the infusion may be slowly decreased while oral feeds are initiated and advanced. If symptomatic hypoglycemia persists, higher glucose rates of 8 to 12mg·kg^{-1} min^{-1} or more may be necessary.

Glucagon has been administered within 15 minutes after delivery to prevent hypoglycemia. Since the majority of neonates are asymptomatic, this is probably not warranted in most patients. Furthermore, glucagon may stimulate insulin release, which may exaggerate the tendency to hypoglycemia.

Prompt recognition and treatment of symptomatic neonates has minimized sequelae. To date, there is no uniformity of opinion about the potential of long-term sequelae secondary to hypoglycemia in the neonate.[133]

Hypocalcemia and Hypomagnesemia

Besides hypoglycemia, hypocalcemia ranks as one of the important metabolic derangements observed in the IDM.[134] Serum calcium concentration is elevated following an increase in parathyroid hormone (PTH) concentration by three mechanisms: mobilization of bone calcium, reabsorption of calcium in the kidney, and increased absorption of calcium in the intestine through action of vitamin D. In contrast, serum calcium concentration is decreased following an increase in calcitonin, which antagonizes the action of PTH. Serum calcium concentration may be increased by vitamin D (1,25-dihydroxyvitamin D), which improves both absorption of calcium in the intestine after feeding as well as reabsorption from bone (see Chapter 40).

During pregnancy, calcium is transferred from mother to fetus, concomitant with an increasing hyperparathyroid state in the mother. Calcium concentration is higher in the fetus than in the mother. This hyperparathyroid state functions as a homeostatic compensation to restore the maternal calcium that is diverted to the fetus. Neither calcitonin nor parathyroid hormone cross the placenta.

At birth, because of the concentration of calcitonin, and 1,25-dihydroxyvitamin D, serum calcium concentration declines following interruption of maternal-fetal calcium transfer. Increases in PTH and 1,25-dihydroxyvitamin D as early as 24 hours of age ensure correction of the low serum calcium concentration.

Tsang et al.[135–137] have shown that the neonate is prone to hypocalcemia, particularly the prematurely born neonate, the one who is asphyxiated, and the IDM. Approximately 50% of the neonates born to insulin-dependent diabetic women develop hypocalcemia (≤7 mg·dl^{-1}) during the first 3 days of life.[134] This increased incidence of hypocalcemia is not seen in the infant of the gestational diabetic woman when compared with controls. Evaluation of the operative mechanisms has failed to establish prematurity or asphyxia per se, which may be present in the IDMs as contributing factors. However, the frequency and severity of serum hypocalcemia is directly related to the severity of diabetes and potentiated if birth asphyxia is superimposed on the clinical state. It has been postulated that the mechanism at least partially responsible for hypocalcemia is hyperphosphatemia, which is present during the initial 48 hours after birth (see Chapter 40).

In the infant of the insulin-dependent diabetic, a failure of an appropriate increase in PTH concentration in response to hypocalcemia has been reported in contrast to both the infant of the gestational diabetic and the nondiabetic. The PTH response in the normal neonate, which occurs on the second to third day, does not occur in the infant of the insulin-dependent diabetic patient until 48 hours or later on the third or fourth day.

In an extension of the above studies, Noguchi et al.[138] evaluated parathyroid function in the hypocalcemic versus the normocalcemic IDM. In the hypocalcemic IDM serum PTH concentration did not increase in response to low serum calcium concentration, while in the normocalcemic IDM the PTH concentration did increase in response to a slight decline in serum calcium concentration. These data in the IDM are interpreted to suggest that maternal diabetes may be an independent factor related to suppressed neonatal parathyroid function.

Martinez et al.[139] measured osteocalcin and PTH serum concentrations in 41 insulin-dependent diabetic pregnant women throughout pregnancy and in the umbilical cord and during the first days after birth. The data were interpreted to suggest that diabetes decreases bone turnover during pregnancy in the mother and during the perinatal period in the offspring.

Hypomagnesemia ($<1.5\,\text{mg}\cdot\text{dl}^{-1}$) has been found in as many as 33% of IDMs. As with hypocalcemia, the frequency and severity of clinical symptoms are correlated with the maternal status. Noguchi et al.[138] have correlated the neonatal magnesium concentration with that of the mother, as well as with the maternal insulin requirement and concentration of intravenous glucose administered to the neonate. They speculated that hypocalcemia in the IDM may be secondary to decreased hypoparathyroid function as a result of the hypomagnesemia. In a subsequent evaluation, these investigators correlated decreased maternal serum magnesium concentration with adverse fetal outcome in the insulin-dependent diabetic woman. They speculated that decreased magnesium concentration may contribute to the high spontaneous abortion and malformation rate in the insulin-dependent diabetic pregnancy.[140]

Hypocalcemia and hypomagnesemia, which have clinical manifestations similar to those of hypoglycemia, must be evaluated and treated appropriately. The long-term potential deleterious effects of either hypocalcemia or hypomagnesemia are unknown.

Hyperbilirubinemia and Polycythemia

Hyperbilirubinemia is observed more frequently in the IDM than in the normal neonate. Although a number of hypotheses have been suggested, the pathogenesis remains uncertain. Prematurity, that is biochemical immaturity, which is present in many of these neonates, was one explanation that was rejected after gestational age–matched comparisons with non-IDMs showed the IDMs to be more jaundiced.[141] The increased incidence of Coombs positive ABO incompatibility reported in some IDMs in one study has not been confirmed.[142] Other etiologies of the hyperbilirubinemia have been related to hemolysis with decreased red cell survival. Red cell life span, osmotic fragility, and deformability have not been found to be appreciably different in the IDM; neither an increased umbilical cord bilirubin concentration nor an increased postnatal rate of hemoglobin decline has been demonstrated. In an evaluation, Peevy et al.[143] suggested that only the macrosomic IDM was at risk for hyperbilirubinemia and that increased hemoglobin turnover was a significant factor in its pathogenesis. However, Stevenson et al.[144,145] suggested that delayed clearance of the bilirubin load was a factor, as measured by pulmonary excretion of carbon monoxide, as an index of bilirubin production.

The polycythemia frequently observed in the IDM may well be the most important factor associated with hyperbilirubinemia. A venous hematocrit ≥65% has been observed in 20% to 40% of IDMs during the first days after birth and has infrequently been associated with such signs and symptoms of neonatal polycythemia, as jitteriness, seizures, tachypnea, priapism, and oliguria. Therapy with a partial exchange transfusion of 10% to 15% of the total blood volume through the umbilical vein using plasmanate or 5% albumin has been associated with rapid resolution of symptoms. Careful studies examining the relationship of neonatal polycythemia to maternal blood glucose control and/or other perinatal factors associated with the diabetic pregnancy have not been completed.

Indirect evidence for fetal hypoxia in the IDM may explain the neonatal preponderance for polycythemia and hyperbilirubinemia. Umbilical cord erythropoietin concentration, measured at birth using a highly sensitive and specific radioimmunoassay, which is stimulated by hypoxia, has been found to be above the narrow range for the control neonate in one third of a group of 61 IDMs.[146] There was an association with relative hyperinsulinemia at birth. The fetal monkey, hyperinsulinemic in the last third of gestation in the absence of maternal diabetes, has been shown to have markedly elevated plasma erythropoietin concentration as well as other evidence of increased fetal erythropoiesis, such as an elevated reticulocyte count.[147] In addition, chronically catheterized fetal sheep that have been made hyperglycemic have been found to have increased oxygen consumption and decreased distal aortic arterial oxygen content.[148] Similar speculation was suggested by Mimouni et al.[149] following their finding of a 29.4% incidence of polycythemia in the IDM versus 5.9% in the control neonate.

Another consideration is the concept of ineffective erythropoiesis in the IDM. Further support for this concept comes from a study of gestational age–matched controls and IDMs in whom increased carbon monoxide excretion, derived from heme metabolism, was observed.[144,145] Hemoglobin concentration was not significantly higher in the IDM. Hemolysis was not evident by evaluation of the possibility of Coombs positive blood group incompatibility. Increased ineffective erythropoiesis, defined as erythroid precursors harbored in body organs such as the liver and spleen and not released into the peripheral circulation, was postulated as an etiology for the observed increased bilirubin concentration in the IDM. In related data, Perrine et al.[150] reported delay in the fetal globin switch in the IDM. The mechanism of this delay is unknown.

In an attempt to correlate glucose control early in pregnancy with subsequent development of neonatal outcome, Morris et al.[151] studied whether glycosylated hemoglobin early in pregnancy could be correlated with the bilirubin concentration noted in the neonate. There was an association in which lower glycosylated hemoglobin concentration before 17 weeks was subsequently associated with fewer neonates with hyperbilirubinemia. The investigators concluded that a glycosylated hemoglobin increase, even in the second trimester, is associated with perinatal morbidity.

In a study of 32 mother-infant pairs, Green et al.[152] published data indicating a correlation between maternal total glycolsylated hemoglobin at delivery and neonatal hematocrit. The investigators concluded that improved maternal glycemic control during late gestation may decrease the incidence of neonatal polycythemia.

In a study of the mechanisms involving neonatal polycythemia in the IDM, a complete blood count, serum iron, transferrin, and ferritin concentrations were evaluated in samples from the umbilical cord of neonates born to nine gestational diabetic mothers, 21 non–insulin-dependent diabetic mothers, and eight insulin-dependent diabetic mothers. While there were no differences in serum iron concentration, transferrin concentration was higher and ferritin concentration was significantly lower in the IDM compared to a control population. The investigators concluded that iron storage is reduced in the fetus of the diabetic mother.[153]

Renal Vein Thrombosis

Renal vein thrombosis is a severe, life-threatening, but rare occurrence in the perinatal period.[154] Its occurrence is more frequently associated with maternal diabetes mellitus compared to the normal nondiabetic population. Although Pedersen[32] failed to mention this condition in his monograph, in one postmortem survey of 16 cases of neonatal renal vein thrombosis, five were found in the IDM.[155] Seven other neonates were born to mothers without known diabetes but with fetal macrosomia and pancreatic β-cell hypertrophy and hyperplasia. Another center reported a case of an IDM who had nearly a totally occlusive thrombosis in the umbilical vein.[156]

The pathogenesis of this lesion remains obscure, although most of the speculation has centered on the possible etiologic role of polycythemia. Sludging of the red cell, combined with a further reduction in cardiac output as a result of diabetic cardiomyopathy, may be a contributing factor. Stuart et al.[157] have suggested that because platelet endoperoxides are increased in the IDM, the normal balance between proaggregatory platelets and antiaggregatory vascular prostaglandins is disrupted in the IDM, favoring the development of thrombosis. In a subsequent study, Stuart et al.[158] evaluated abnormalities in vascular arachidonic acid metabolism in the IDM. They noted that decreased prostacyclin formation has been suggested as a cause of an atherothrombotic tendency in the adult. The investigators studied 6-ketoprostaglandin F_1 in the IDM in whom it was normal in an umbilical cord sample, if the mother was in good control. Inhibition of 6-keto $F_{1\alpha}$ was noted if the mother's HbA_1C was elevated, indicating poor diabetic control. The investigators suggested that the correlation observed between plasma 6-keto $F_{1\alpha}$ prostaglandin formation and endogenous vascular prostaglandin formation in the IDM indicated that an in vitro deficiency of prostacyclin formation reflected a concomitant in vivo abnormality. Why this lesion shows selectivity for the kidney is obscure. Birth trauma is an unlikely initiating factor, since this lesion has been observed in both the stillborn and the IDM delivered by cesarean section. Another case has been reported in a stillborn IDM whose mother received oxytocin induction.[159]

In the neonate the diagnosis is usually made in the first hours or days after birth, with the findings of hematuria and flank masses as the most salient features. Therapy is aimed at careful fluid and electrolyte management and correction of polycythemia. A pediatric surgical consultation is indicated for evaluation of a possible nephrectomy. The role of heparinization in the therapy of this entity remains controversial.

Long-Term Prognosis and Follow-Up

The previous discussion has focused on problems primarily encountered during the neonatal period. Of equal concern and perhaps of greater ultimate importance are the long-term effects on growth and development, on psychosocial intellectual capabilities, and finally on the risk to the neonate of subsequently developing diabetes. One of the most important factors influencing long-term prognosis is the improvement in management of the pregnant diabetic and her neonate. Assuming that many of the deleterious effects of the diabetic pregnancy are being modified by normalization of metabolic status in both the pregnant woman and her conceptus, the poor prognoses that have been reported in previous retrospective studies should be ameliorated in future prospective evaluations.

In spite of the frequency of the clinical presentation of the infant of the diabetic mother, there are relatively few prospective studies of the infant's growth and development. Farquhar's[160] analysis of 231 of a group of 320 neonates is significant in that more children up to 15 years of age declined to below the third percentile for height than exceeded the 97th percentile (i.e., 21 vs 5). Weight, in contrast, seemed to be equally divided both above and below the normal range. This was confirmed by evaluating the weight-to-height index of each child, expressed as a percentage of the 50th percentile for age and sex. Evaluation of these criteria suggested that excessive weight is almost 10 times more common than unusually low weight. Farquhar suggests that this may represent a potential "return to obesity" noted at birth in this group.

In another study, Bibergeil et al.[161] noted that height was elevated in 16.7% but below normal in 9.3%. Neonates greater than 4 kg had significant elevations of height or weight at time of entrance to school. Somatic growth of children of diabetic mothers was studied by Vohr et al.[162] They suggested that macrosomia in the IDM may be a predisposing factor for later obesity, since at 7 years of age 8 of 19 offspring of diabetics who had been large for gestational age at birth were obese, whereas only 1 of 14 who had been appropriate for gestational age was obese.

Gerlini et al.[163] evaluated body weight, length, and head circumference from birth through 48 months of age. In the IDM no specific differences related to the White classification. Children of mothers exhibiting poor control during pregnancy showed higher values for weight and the weight/height ratio in infancy compared to the neonate of the well-controlled diabetic. Female offspring contributed most to the observed differences.

Silverman et al.[164] tested the hypothesis that long-term postnatal development may be modified by the in utero metabolic experience. They enrolled offspring of women with insulin-dependent diabetes mellitus, non–insulin-dependent diabetes mellitus, and gestational diabetes in a prospective study from 1977 through 1983. Fetal β cell function was assessed by measurement of amniotic fluid insulin at 32 to 38 weeks' gestation. Postnatally, plasma glucose and insulin concentrations were measured yearly from 1.5 years of age after fasting and 2 hours after 1.75 g·kg^{-1} oral glucose tolerance test. Control subjects had a single oral glucose challenge at 10 to 16 years of age. In the offspring of the diabetic mother, the prevalence of impaired glucose tolerance was 1.2% at <5 years, 5.4% at 5 to 9 years, and 19.3% at 10 to 16 years. The 88 offspring of diabetic mothers (12.3 ± 1.7 years), when compared with 80 control subjects of the same age and pubertal stage, had higher 2-hour glucose and insulin concentrations. Impaired glucose tolerance was not associated with the etiology of the mother's diabetes or macrosomia at birth. Impaired glucose tolerance was recorded in only 3.7% of adolescents whose amniotic fluid insulin as normal and 33.3% of those with elevated concentrations. The investigators concluded that impaired glucose tolerance in the offspring is a long-term complication of maternal diabetes. Excessive insulin secretion in utero, as assessed by amniotic fluid insulin concentration, is a strong predictor of impaired glucose tolerance in childhood.

In consideration of neuropsychological development, the high frequency of congenital malformations may be directly or indirectly associated with neuropsychological handicaps. In a large series, Yssing[165] found that 36% of 265 children had evidence of cerebral dysfunction or related conditions. Cerebral palsy and epilepsy were found to be three to five times higher in comparison with the normal population, but mental retardation was not noted to be different. When present, the difficulties seemed to be related to extremes of maternal age, severity of diabetes, low birth weight for gestational age, or complications during pregnancy.

The outcome of children at 1, 3, and 5 years of age was evaluated by Stehbens et al.[166] Psychological evaluations suggested that at 3 and 5 years of age, the IDM was more vulnerable to intellectual impairment, especially if the neonate was born small for gestational age or if the pregnancy was complicated by acetonuria. This concept was reinforced by the work of Petersen et al.[167] They studied early growth delay in diabetic pregnancy in relation to psychomotor development at age 4. Their studies of 99 consecutive insulin-dependent and 101 nondiabetic pregnant women led them to conclude that the children with a history of growth delay in early diabetic pregnancy should be examined at 4 to 5 years of age by Denver developmental screening for possible impairment.

The presence of hypoglycemia per se has not been related to later neuropsychological defects. Persson and Gentz[168] found no evidence that asymptomatic hypoglycemia leads to intellectual impairment by 5 years of age. No obvious relationship was found between maternal acetonuria during pregnancy, infant birth weight, blood glucose during the first hours after birth, or neonatal complications and the IQ of the children. A correlation did exist between maternal and child IQ. Hadden et al.[169] studied 123 children of type I insulin-dependent diabetic mothers and 124 children of nondiabetic mothers. No differences were found following pediatric assessment or by a psychologically based maternal and teacher questionnaire of the emotional state or academic achievement of the child.

Questioning to what extent maternal metabolism during pregnancy affects cognitive and behavioral function of the offspring by altering brain development, Rizzo et al.[170] correlated measures of metabolism in pregnant diabetic and nondiabetic women with intellectual development of their offspring. Of 223 pregnant women, 89 had pregestational diabetes mellitus, 99 had gestational diabetes, and 35 had normal carbohydrate metabolism. Carbohydrate and lipid metabolism were evaluated with respect to two measures of infant development: the Bayley scale at age 2 years and the Stanford-Binet at ages 3, 4, and 5 years. The Bayley scale at 2 years of age correlated inversely with the mother's third trimester plasma beta-hydroxylbutyrate concentration, and the Stanford-Binet correlated inversely with third trimester plasma beta-hydroxybutyrate and free fatty acid concentrations. The investigators concluded that ketoacidosis and accelerated starvation should be avoided in pregnancy because of its potential long-term adverse consequences.

Finally, the question of whether the IDM has an increased likelihood of becoming diabetic is important and has been the subject of a number of analyses. If a parent has insulin-dependent mellitus, the empirical risk of his or her offspring developing insulin-dependent diabetes mellitus is in the range of 1% to 5%.[171] While family aggregates do exist, transmitted both through and within generations, a simple mode of inheritance is inconsistent with the reported data. Some have suggested that a polygenic multifactorial model best explains the reported observations.[172] It appears that the neonate born to a mother with diabetes is at increased risk for developing the disease in comparison to the normal population. There is one case report of a unique infant whose an insulin-dependent diabetic mother, was diagnosed by 4 months of age. The neonate was reported to have developed glucosuria by 2 weeks after birth at a gestational age 36 weeks at birth and to have required insulin by 5 months of age.[173]

After documenting the decline in perinatal mortality from 23% prior to 1961 to 14% from 1961 to 1975, and then to around 4% subsequently, Warram et al.[174] evaluated the number of neonates who subsequently developed diabetes in a cohort of 1319 neonates. Insulin-dependent diabetes had developed in 21, a risk of 2.1 ± 0.5% by 20 years of age. The risk of diabetes in the offspring of the diabetic mother was increased in the young mother and is independent of the risk factors for perinatal mortality. This is one third of the risk previously reported for the offspring of fathers with insulin-dependent diabetes. The investigators speculated that exposure in utero to an affected mother may protect the fetus from developing insulin-dependent diabetes later in life.

Acknowledgment. Some of the work reported in this chapter was supported by National Institutes of Health grant HD 27287 awarded to Dr. Cowett. We wish to express our appreciation to Ms. Patricia Knight for her expert secretarial assistance.

References

1. Wolfe RR, Allsop J, Burke JF. Glucose metabolism in man: responses to intravenous glucose. Metab Clin Exp 1979;28:210–220.
2. Cowett RM. Neonatal glucose metabolism. In: Cowett RM, ed. Principles of perinatal neonatal metabolism. New York: Springer Verlag, 1991:356–371.
3. Cowett RM. The metabolic sequelae in the infant of the diabetic mother. In: Jovanovic L, ed. Controversies in diabetes and pregnancy. New York: Springer-Verlag, 1988:149–171.
4. Cowett RM. The infant of the diabetic mother. In: Hay WW Jr, ed. Neonatal nutrition and metabolism. Chicago: Yearbook, 1991:419–431.
5. Cowett RM. The infant of the diabetic mother. In: Sweet AY, Brown E, eds. Medical and surgical complications of pregnancy: effects on the fetus and newborn. Chicago: Yearbook, 1991:302–319.
6. Jovanovic L, Druzin M, Peterson CM. Effects of euglycemia on the outcome of pregnancy in insulin-dependent diabetic women as compared with normal control subjects. Am J Med 1980;68:105–112.
7. Kitzmiller JL, Cloherty JP, Younger MD, et al. Diabetic pregnancy and perinatal morbidity. Am J Obstet Gynecol 1978;131:560–568.
8. Traub AI, Harley JM, Cooper TK, et al. Is centralized hospital care necessary for all insulin-dependent pregnant diabetics? Br J Obstet Gynaecol 1987;94:957–962.
9. Pedersen J, Molsted-Pedersen L, Andersen B. Assessors of fetal perinatal mortality in diabetic pregnancy. Analyses of 1332 pregnancies in the Copenhagen series 1946–1972. Diabetes 1974;23:302–305.
10. Hare JW, White P. Gestational diabetes and the White classification. Diabetes Care 1980;3:394.
11. Greene MF, Hare JW, Krache M, et al. Prematurity among insulin requiring diabetic gravid women. Am J Obstet Gynecol 1989;161:106–111.
12. Diamond MD, Salyer SL, Vaughn WK, et al. Reassessment of White's clarification and Pedersen's prognostically bad signs of diabetic pregnancies in insulin dependent diabetic pregnancies. Am J Obstet Gynecol 1987;156:599–604.
13. Pollak A, Brehm R, Havelec L, et al. Total glycosylated hemoglobin in mothers of large for gestational age infants: a postpartum test for undetected maternal diabetes? Biol Neonate 1983;40:129–135.

14. Widness JA, Schwartz HC, Zeller WP, et al. Glycohemoglobin in postpartum women. Obstet Gynecol 1983;57:414–421.
15. Cocilovo G, Guerra S, Colla F, et al. Glycosylated hemoglobin (HbA₁) assay as a test for detection and surveillance of gestational diabetes. A reappraisal. Diabetes Metab 1987;13:426–430.
16. Cano A, Barcelo F, Fuentet T, et al. Relationship of maternal glycosylated hemoglobin and fetal beta cell activity with birthweight. Gynecol Obstet Invest 1986;22:91–96.
17. Pollak A, Salzer HR, Lischka A, Hayde M. Nonenzymatic glycation of fetal tissue in diabetic pregnancy. Estimation of the glucitollysine content of umbilical cord extracts. Acta Paediatr Scand 1988;77:481–484.
18. Teramo K, Kuusisto AN, Raivio KO. Perinatal outcome of insulin-dependent diabetic pregnancies. Ann Clin Res 1979;11:146–155.
19. Jerwell J, Bjerkedal T, Moe N. Outcome of pregnancies in diabetic mothers in Norway 1967–1976. Diabetologia 1980;18:131–134.
20. Artal R, Golde SH, Dorey F, et al. The effect of plasma glucose variability on neonatal outcome in the pregnant diabetic patient. Am J Obstet Gynecol 1983;147:537–541.
21. Roberts AB, Pattison NS. Pregnancy in women with diabetes mellitus, twenty-years experience: 1968–1987. N Z Med J 1990;103:211–213.
22. Jovanovic R, Jovanovic L. Obstetric management when normoglycemia is maintained in diabetic women with vascular compromise. Am J Obstet Gynecol 1984;149:617–623.
23. Coustan DR, Imarah J. Prophylactic insulin treatment of gestational diabetes reduces the incidence of macrosomia, operative delivery, and birth trauma. Am J Obstet Gynecol 1984;150:836–842.
24. Coustan DR, Reece EA, Sherwin RS, et al. A randomized clinical trial of the insulin pump vs intensive conventional therapy in diabetic pregnancies. JAMA 1986;108:329–330.
25. Thompson DJ, Porter KB, Gunnells DJ, et al. Prophylactic insulin in the management of gestational diabetes. Obstet Gynecol 1990;75:960–964.
26. Larsen CE, Serdula MK, Sullivan KM. Macrosomia: influence of maternal overweight among a low income population. Am J Obstet Gynecol 1990;162:490–494.
27. Nordlander E, Hanson U, Persson B. Factors influencing neonatal morbidity in gestational diabetic pregnancy. Br J Obstet Gynecol 1989;96:671–678.
28. Fraser D, Weitzman S, Leiberman JR, et al. Factors influencing birth weight in newborns of diabetic and non-diabetic women. A population based study. Eur J Epidemiol 1990;6:427–431.
29. Hanson U, Persson B, Stangenberg M. Factors influencing neonatal morbidity in diabetic pregnancy. Diabetes Res 1986;3:71–76.
30. Hod M, Rabinerson D, Kaplan B, et al. Perinatal complications following gestational diabetes mellitus: how sweet is ill? Acta Obstet Gynecol Scand 1996;75:809–815.
31. DeVeciana M, Major CA, Morgan MA, et al. Postprandial versus preprandial blood glucose monitoring in women with gestational diabetes mellitus requiring insulin therapy. N Eng J Med 1995;333:1237–1241.
32. Pedersen J. The pregnant diabetic and her newborn. 2nd ed. Baltimore: Williams & Wilkins, 1977.
33. Naeye RL. Infants of diabetic mothers: a quantitative morphologic study. Pediatric 1964;35:980–988.
34. Susa JB, McCormick KL, Widness JA, et al. Chronic hyperinsulinemia in the fetal rhesus monkey. Effects on fetal growth and composition. Diabetes 1979;28:1058–1063.
35. Block MD, Pildes RS, Mossabhou NA, et al. C-peptide immunoreactivity (CRP): a new method for studying infants of insulin-treated diabetic mothers. Pediatrics 1974;53:923–928.
36. King KC, Adam PAJ, Yamaguchi K, et al. Insulin response to arginine in normal newborn infants and infants of diabetic mothers. Diabetes 1974;23:816–820.
37. Susa JB, Boylan JM, Sehgal P, et al. Impaired insulin secretion in the neonatal rhesus monkey after chronic hyperinsulinemia in utero. Proc Soc Exp Biol Med 1990;194:209–215.
38. MacFarlane CM, Tsakalakos N. The extended Pedersen hypothesis. Clin Physiol Biochem 1988;6:68–73.
39. Schwartz R, Gruppuso PA, Pelzold K, et al. Hyperinsulinemia and macrosomia in the fetus of the diabetic mother. Diabetes Care 1994;17:640–648.
40. Gloria-Bottini F, Gerlini G, Lucarini N. Both maternal and foetal genetic factors contribute to macrosomia of diabetic pregnancy. Hum Hered 1994;44:24–30.
41. Pildes RS, Hart RJ, Warrner R, et al. Plasma insulin response during oral glucose tolerance tests in newborns of normal and gestational diabetic mothers. Pediatrics 1969;44:76–82.
42. Isles PE, Dickson M, Farquhar JW. Glucose intolerance and plasma insulin in newborn infants of normal and diabetic mothers. Pediatr Res 1966;2:198–208.
43. Adam PAJ, King KC, Schwartz R. Model for investigation of intractable hypoglycemia. Insulin glucose interrelationships during steady state infusion. Pediatrics 1968;41:91–105.
44. King KC, Adam PAJ, Clements GA, et al. Infants of diabetic mothers: attenuated glucose uptake without hyperinsulinemia during continuous glucose infusions. Pediatrics 1969;44:381–392.
45. Hill WC, Pelle-Day G, Kitzmiller JL, et al. Insulin like growth factors in fetal macrosomia with and without maternal diabetes. Hormone Res 1989;32:178–182.
46. Roth S, Abernathy MP, Lee WH, et al. Insulin-like growth factors I and II peptide and messenger RNA levels in macrosomic infants of diabetic pregnancies. J Soc Gynecol Invest 1996;3:78–84.
47. Light IJ, Sutherland JM, Loggie JM, et al. Impaired epinephrine release in hypoglycemic infants of diabetic mothers. N Engl J Med 1967;277:394–398.
48. Bloom SR, Johnston DT. Failure of glucagon release in infants of diabetic mothers. Br Med J 1972;4:453–454.
49. Kaplan SA, Neufeld ND, Lippe BM, et al. Maternal diabetes and the development of the insulin receptor. In: Merkatz IR, Adam PAJ, eds. The diabetic pregnancy. A perinatal perspective. New York: Grune & Stratton, 1979:169–173.

50. Lautala P, Puukka R, Knip M, et al. Postnatal decrease in insulin binding to erythrocytes in infants of diabetic mothers. J Clin Endocrinol Metab 1988;66:696–701.
51. Rigg LA, Becher SG. ^{125}I insulin receptor binding characteristics on umbilical cord blood erythrocytes from normal and diabetic pregnancies. Am J Perinatol 1991;8:209–213.
52. Krew MA, Kehl RJ, Thomas A, et al. Relation of amniotic fluid C peptide levels to neonatal body composition. Obstet Gynecol 1994;84:96–100.
53. Vohr BR, McGarvey ST, Coll CG. Effects of maternal gestational diabetes and adiposity on neonatal adiposity and blood pressure. Diabetes Care 1995;18:467–475.
54. Kaminsky S, Silbley CP, Maresh M. The effects of diabetes on placental lipase activity in the rat and human. Pediatr Res 1991;30:541–543.
55. Homko CJ, Sivan E, Nyirjesy P, et al. The interrelationship between ethnicity and gestational diabetes in fetal macrosomia. Diabetes Care 1995;18:1442–1445.
56. Jovanovic-Peterson, Peterson CM, Reed GF, et al. Maternal postprandial glucose levels and infant birth weight: the Diabetes in Early Pregnancy Study. Am J Obstet Gynecol 1991;164:103–111.
57. Kalhan SC, Savin SM, Adam PAJ. Attenuated glucose production rate in newborn infants of insulin-dependent diabetic mothers. N Engl J Med 1977;296:375–376.
58. King KC, Tserng KY, Kalhan SC. Regulation of glucose production in newborn infants of diabetic mothers. Pediatr Res 1982;16:608–612.
59. Cowett RM, Susa JB, Giletti B, et al. Variability of endogenous glucose production in infants of insulin dependent diabetic mothers. Pediatr Res 1980;14:570A.
60. Cowett RM, Susa JB, Giletti B, et al. Glucose kinetics in infants of diabetic mothers. Am J Obstet Gynecol 1983;146:781–786.
61. Cowett RM, Oh W, Schwartz R, et al. Persistent glucose production during glucose infusion in the neonate. J Clin Invest 1983;71:467–473.
62. Cowett RM, Andersen GE, Maguire CA, et al. Ontogeny of glucose kinetics in low birth weight infants. J Pediatr 1988;112:462–465.
63. Baarsma R, Reijngoud DJ, van Asselt WA, et al. Postnatal glucose kinetics in newborns of lightly controlled insulin dependent diabetic mothers. Pediatr Res 1993;34:443–447.
64. Widness JA, Cowett RM, Coustan DR, et al. Neonatal morbidities in infants of mothers with glucose intolerance in pregnancy. Diabetes 1985;34(suppl 2):61–65.
65. Freinkel N. Of pregnancy and progeny: Banting Lecture. Diabetes 1980;29:1023–1035.
66. Milner RDG. Amino acids and beta cell growth in structure & function. In: Merkatz IR, Adam PAJ, eds. The diabetic pregnancy. A perinatal perspective. New York: Grune & Stratton 1979;37:145–153.
67. Kalkhoff RK, Kandaraki E, Morrow PG, et al. Relationship between neonatal birth weight and maternal plasma amino acid profiles in lean and obese nondiabetic women and in type I diabetic pregnant women. Metabolism 1988;37:234–239.
68. Knopp RH, Magee MS, Walden CE, et al. Prediction of infant birth weight by GDM screening tests: importance of plasma triglyceride. Diabetes Care 1992;15:1605–1613.
69. Patel D, Kalhan S. Glycerol metabolism and triglyceride-fatty acid cycling in the human newborn: effect of maternal diabetes and intrauterine growth retardation. Pediatr Res 1992;31:52–58.
70. Kucera J. Rate and type of congenital anomalies among offspring of diabetic women. J Reprod Med 1971;7:61–70.
71. Pedersen LM, Tygstrup I, Pedersen J. Congenital malformations in newborn infants of diabetic women. Correlation with maternal diabetic vascular complication. Lancet 1964;1:1124–1126.
72. Becerra JE, Koury MJ, Cordero JF, et al. Diabetes mellitus during pregnancy and the risks for specific birth defects: a population based case control study. Pediatrics 1990;85:1–9.
73. Roversi GD, Gugiulo M, Nicolini U, et al. A new approach to the treatment of diabetic pregnant women. Am J Obstet Gynecol 1979;135:567–576.
74. Metzger BE, Buchanan TA, eds. Diabetes and birth defects: insights from the 1980's, prevention in the 1990's. Diabetes Spectrum 1990;3:149–189.
75. Neave C. Congenital malformation in offspring of diabetics. Perspect Pediatr Pathol 1984;8:213–222.
76. Fuhrmann K, Reiher H, Semmler K, et al. Prevention of congenital malformations in infants of insulin dependent diabetic mothers. Diabetes Care 1983;6:219–223.
77. Goldman JA, Dicker D, Feldberg D, et al. Pregnancy outcome in patients with insulin-dependent diabetes mellitus with preconceptional diabetic control: a comparative study. Am J Obstet Gynecol 1986;155:293–297.
78. Dicker D, Feldberg D, Yeshaya A, et al. Pregnancy outcome in gestational diabetes with preconceptional diabetes counseling. Aust N Z J Obstet Gynaecol 1987;27:184–187.
79. Miller E, Hare JW, Cloherty JP, et al. Elevated maternal hemoglobin A_{1c} in early pregnancy and major congenital anomalies in infants of diabetic mothers. N Engl J Med 1981;304:1331–1334.
80. Ballard JL, Holroyde J, Tsang RC, et al. High malformation rates and decreased mortality in infants of diabetic mothers managed after the first trimester (1956–1978). Am J Obstet Gynecol 1984;148:111–118.
81. Landauer W. Rumplessness in chicken embryos produced by the injection of insulin and other chemicals. J Exp Zool 1945;98:65–77.
82. Adam PAJ, Teramo K, Raiha N, et al. Human fetal insulin metabolism early in gestation. Diabetes 1969;18:409–416.
83. Widness JA, Goldman AS, Susa JB, et al. Impermeability of the rat placenta to insulin during organogenesis. Teratology 1983;28:327–332.
84. Molsted-Pedersen L, Pedersen JF. Congenital malformations in diabetic pregnancies. Acta Paediatr Scand Suppl 1985;32:79–84.
85. Perrot LJ, Williamson S, Jimenex JF. The caudal regression syndrome in infants of diabetic mothers. Ann Clin Lab Sci 1987;17:211–220.
86. Davis WS, Allen RP, Favara BE, et al. Neonatal small left colon syndrome. Am J Roent Rad Ther Nucl Med 1974;120:327–329.

87. Way GL, Wolfe RR, Eshughpour E, et al. The natural history of hypertrophic cardiomyopathy in infants of diabetic mothers. J Pediatr 1979;95:1020–1025.
88. Mace S, Hirschfeld SS, Riggs T, et al. Echocardiographic abnormalities in infants of diabetic mothers. J Pediatr 1979;95:1013–1019.
89. Breitweser JA, Mayer RA, Sperling MA, et al. Cardiac septal hypertrophy in hyperinsulinemic infants. J Pediatr 1980;96:535–539.
90. Halliday HL. Hypertrophic cardiomyopathy in infants of poorly controlled diabetic mothers. Arch Dis Child 1981;56:258–263.
91. Ferencz C, Rubin JD, McCarter RJ, et al. Maternal diabetes and cardiovascular malformations: predominance of double outlet right ventricle and truncus arteriosus. Teratology 1990;41:319–326.
92. Mehta S, Nuamah I, Kalhan S. Altered diastolic function in infants of mothers with gestational diabetes: no relation to macrosomia. Pediatr Cardiol 1995;16:24–27.
93. Weber HS, Botti JJ, Baylen BG. Sequential longitudinal evaluation of cardiac growth and ventricular diastolic telling in fetuses of well controlled diabetic mothers. Pediatr Cardiol 1994;15:184–189.
94. Novak RW, Robinson HB. Coincident DiGeorge anomaly and renal agenesis and its relation to maternal diabetes. Am J Med Genet 1994;50:311–312.
95. Wilson TA, Bletlen SL, Vallone A, et al. DiGeorge anomaly with renal agenesis in infants of mothers with diabetes. Am J Med Genet 1993;47:1078–1082.
96. Lupski JR, Langston C, Friedman R, et al. DiGeorge anomaly associated with a de novo Y.22 translocation resulting in monosomy del (22) (q11.2). Am J Med Genet 1991;40:196–198.
97. Slavotinek A, Hellen E, Gould S, et al. Three infants of diabetic mothers with malformations of left right asymmetry—further evidence of the aetiological role of diabetes in the malformation spectrum. Clin Dysmorphol 1996;5:241–247.
98. Viana M, Herrera E, Bonet B. Teratogenic effects of diabetes mellitus in the rat. Prevention by vitamin E. Diabetologia 1996;39:1041–1046.
99. Sivan E, Reece EA, Wu YK. Dietary vitamin E prophylaxis and diabetic embryopathy. Morphologic and biochemical analyses. Am J Obstet Gynecol 1996;175:793–799.
100. Fosberg H, Borg LA, Cagliero E, et al. Altered levels of scavenging enzymes in embryos subjected to a diabetic environment. Free Radical Res 1996;24:451–459.
101. Many A, Brenner SH, Yaron Y. Prospective study of incidence and predisposing factors for clavicular fracture in the newborn. Acta Obstet Gynecol Scand 1996;75:378–381.
102. Mintz MC, Landon MB, Gabbe SG, et al. Shoulder soft tissue width as a predictor of macrosomia in diabetic pregnancies. Am J Perinatol 1989;6:240–243.
103. Mimouni F, Miodounik M, Siddigi TA, et al. Perinatal asphyxia in infants of insulin dependent diabetic mothers. J Pediatr 1988;113:345–353.
104. Philipps AF, Porte PJ, Stablinsky S, et al. Effects of chronic fetal hyperglycemia upon oxygen consumption in the ovine uterus and conceptus. J Clin Invest 1984;74:279–286.
105. Philipps AF, Rosenkranz TS, Raye J. Consequences of perturbations of fetal fuels in ovine pregnancy. Diabetes 1985;34(suppl 2):32–35.
106. Cruz AC, Buhi WC, Birk SA, et al. Respiratory distress syndrome with mature lecithin/sphingomyelin ratios, diabetes mellitus and low Apgar scores. Am Obstet Gynecol 1976;126:78–82.
107. Dicker D, Feldberg D, Yeshaya A, et al. Fetal surveillance in insulin dependent diabetic pregnancy: predictive value of the biophysical profile. Am J Obstet Gynecol 1988;159:800–804.
108. Hsi AC, Davis DJ, Sherman FC. Neonatal gangrene in the newborn infants of diabetic mothers. J Pediatr Orthop 1985;5:358–360.
109. VanAllen MI, Jackson JC, Knopp RH, et al. In utero thrombosis and neonatal gangrene in an infant of a diabetic mother. Am J Med Genet 1989;33:323–327.
110. Ogata ES, Sabbagha R, Metzger BE, et al. Serial ultrasonography to assess evolving fetal macrosomia. Studies in 23 pregnant women. JAMA 1980;243:2405–2408.
111. Davis R, Woelk G, Mueller BA, et al. The role of previous birthweight on risk for macrosomia on a subsequent birth. Epidemiology 1995;6:607–611.
112. Robert MD, Nel RK, Hubbell JP, et al. Association between maternal diabetes and the respiratory distress syndrome in the newborn. N Engl J Med 1976;294:357–360.
113. Warburton D, Parton L, Buckley S, et al. Effects of glucose infusion on surfactant and glycogen regulation in fetal lamb lung. J Appl Physiol 1987;63:1750–1756.
114. Gluck L, Kulovich MV. Lecithin/sphingomyelin ratios in amniotic fluid in normal and abnormal pregnancies. Am J Obstet Gynecol 1973;115:539–546.
115. Hallman M, Teramo K. Amniotic fluid phospholipid profile as a predictor of fetal maturity in diabetic pregnancies. Obstet Gynecol 1979;54:703–707.
116. Smith BT, Giroud CJP, Robert M, et al. Insulin antagonism of cortisol action on lecithin synthesis by cultured fetal lung cells. J Pediatr 1975;87:953–955.
117. Neufeld ND, Sevanian A, Barrett CT, et al. Inhibition of surfactant production by insulin in fetal rabbit lung slices. Pediatr Res 1979;13:752–754.
118. Curet LB, Tsao FH, Zachman RD, et al. Phosphalidyl glycerol, lecithin/sphingomyelin ratio and respiratory distress syndrome in diabetic and nondiabetic pregnancies. Int J Obstet Gynecol 1989;30:105–108.
119. Nogee L, McMahon M, Whitsett JA. Hyaline membrane disease and surfactant protein SAP 35 in diabetes in pregnancy. Am J Perinatol 1988;5:374–377.
120. Ylinen K. High maternal levels of hemoglobin A_{lc} associated with delayed lung maturation in insulin-dependent diabetic pregnancies. Acta Obstet Gynecol Scand 1987;66:263–266.
121. Stern L, Ramos A, Leduc J. Urinary catecholamine excretion in infants of diabetic mothers. Pediatrics 1968;42:598–605.
122. Keenan WJ, Light IJ, Sutherland JM. Effects of exogenous epinephrine on glucose and insulin levels in infants of diabetic mothers. Biol Neonate 1972;21:44–53.

123. Young BJ, Cohen WR, Rappaport EB, et al. High plasma norepinephrine concentrations at birth in infants of diabetic mothers. Diabetes 1979;28:697–699.
124. Artel R, Platt LD, Kummula RK, et al. Sympatho-adrenal activity in infants of diabetic mothers. Am J Obstet Gynecol 1982;42:436–439.
125. Artal R, Doug N, Wu P, et al. Circulating catecholamesus and glucagon in infants of strictly controlled diabetic mothers. Biol Neonate 1988;53:121–125.
126. Broberger U, Hansson U, Lagercrantz H, et al. Sympatho-adrenal activity and metabolic adjustment during the first 12 hours after birth in infants of diabetic mothers. Acta Pediatr Scand 1984;73:620–625.
127. Cowett RM. Decreased response to catecholamines in the newborn: effect on glucose kinetics in the lamb. Metabolism 1988;37:736–740.
128. Cowett RM. Alpha adrenergic agonists stimulate neonatal glucose production less than beta adrenergic agonists in the lamb. Metabolism 1988;37:831–836.
129. Cowett RM, Rapoza RE, Jawed G, Gelardi NL. Sympathomimetic responses as contra-insulin hormones in neonatal hyperinsulinemic hypoglycemia. Pediatr Res 1997;41:230A.
130. Lin HC, Maguire CA, Oh W, et al. Accuracy and reliability of glucose reflectance meters in the neonatal intensive care unit (NICU). J Pediatr 1989;115:998–1000.
131. Conrad PD, Sparks JW, Osberg I, et al. Clinical application of a new glucose analyzer in the neonatal intensive care unit: comparison with other methods. J Pediatr 1989;114:281–287.
132. Lilien LD, Pildes RS, Srainivasan G, et al. Treatment of neonatal hypoglycemia with minibolus and intravenous glucose infusion. J Pediatr 1980;97:295–298.
133. Cornblath M, Schwartz R, Aynsley-Green A, et al. Hypoglycemia in infancy: the need for a rational definition. Pediatrics 1990;85:834–837.
134. Tsang RC, Brown DR, Steichen JJ. Diabetes and calcium disturbances in infants of diabetic mothers. In: Merkatz IR, Adam PAJ, eds. The diabetic pregnancy. A perinatal perspective. New York: Grune & Stratton, 1979:207–225.
135. Tsang RC, Kleinman L, Sutherland JM. Hypocalcemia in infants of diabetic mothers: studies in Ca, P and Mg metabolism and in parathyroid hormone responsiveness. J Pediatr 1973;80:384–395.
136. Tsang RC, Light IJ, Sutherland JM, et al. Possible pathogenetic factors in neonatal hypocalcemia of prematurity. J Pediatr 1973;82:423–429.
137. Tsang RC, Chen I, Atkinson W, et al. Neonatal hypocalcemia in birth asphyxia. J Pediatr 1974;84:428–433.
138. Noguchi A, Erin M, Tsang RC. Parathyroid hormone in hypocalcemia and normocalcemic infants of diabetic mothers. J Pediatr 1980;97:112–114.
139. Martinez ME, Catalan P, Lisbona A, et al. Serum osteocalcin concentrations in diabetic pregnant women and their newborns. Horm Metab Res 1994;26:338–342.
140. Mimouni F, Miodovnik M, Tsang RC, et al. Decreased maternal serum magnesium concentration and adverse fetal outcome in insulin-dependent diabetic women. Obstet Gynecol 1987;80:85–88.
141. Taylor PM, Wolfson J, Bright NH, et al. Hyperbilirubinemia in infants of diabetic mothers. Biol Neonate 1963;5:289–298.
142. Zetterstrom R, Strindberg B, Arnold RG. Hyperbilirubinemia in ABO hemolytic disease in newborn infants of diabetic mothers. Acta Paediatr 1958;47:238–250.
143. Peevy KJ, Landaw SA, Gross SA. Hyperbilirubinemia in infants of diabetic mothers. Pediatrics 1980;66:417–419.
144. Stevenson DF, Ostrander CR, Cohen RS, et al. Pulmonary excretion of carbon monoxide in the human infant as an index of bilirubin production. Eur J Pediatr 1981;137:255–259.
145. Stevenson DR, Ostrander CR, Hopper AO, et al. Pulmonary excretion of carbon monoxide as an index of bilirubin production. IIa. Evidence for possible delayed clearance of bilirubin in infants of diabetic mothers. J Pediatr 1981;98:822–824.
146. Widness JA, Susa J, Garcia JF, et al. Increased erythropoiesis and elevated erythropoietin in infants born to diabetic mothers and in hyprinsulinemic rhesus fetuses. J Clin Invest 1981;67:637–642.
147. Carson BS, Philipps AF, Simmons MA, et al. Effects of a sustained insulin infusion upon glucose uptake and oxygenation of the ovine fetus. Pediatr Res 1980;14:147–152.
148. Philipps AF, Widness JA, Garcia JF, et al. Erythropoietin elevation in the chronically hyperglycemia fetal lamb. Proc Soc Exp Biol Med 1982;170:42–47.
149. Mimouni F, Miodovnik M, Siddiqi TA, et al. Neonatal polycythemia in infants of insulin-dependent diabetic mothers. Obstet Gynecol 1986;68:370–372.
150. Perrine SP, Greene MF, Faller DV. Delay in the fetal globin switch in infants of diabetic mothers. N Engl J Med 1985;312:334–338.
151. Morris MA, Grandis AS, Litton JC. Glycosylated hemoglobin concentration in early gestation associated with neonatal outcome. Am J Obstet Gynecol 1985;153:651–654.
152. Green DW, Khoury J, Mimouni F. Neonatal hematocrit and maternal glycemic control in insulin dependent diabetes. J Pediatr 1992;120:302–305.
153. Murata K, Toyoda N, Ichio T, et al. Cord transferrin and ferritin values for erythropoiesis in newborn infants of diabetic mothers. Endocrinol Jpn 1989;36:827–832.
154. Avery ME, Oppenheimer EH, Gordon HH. Renal vein thrombosis in newborn infants of diabetic mothers. N Engl J Med 1957;265:1134–1138.
155. Takeuchi A, Benirschke K. Renal vein thrombosis of the newborn and its relation to maternal diabetes. Biol Neonate 1961;3:237–256.
156. Fritz MA, Christopher CR. Umbilical vein thrombosis and maternal diabetes mellitus. J Reprod Med 1981;26:320–323.
157. Stuart MJ, Sunderji-Shirazali G, Allen JB. Decreased prostacyclin production in the infant of the diabetic mother. J Lab Clin Med 1981;98:412–416.
158. Stuart M, Sunderje SC, Walenga RW, et al. Abnormalities in vascular arachidonic acid metabolism in the infant of the diabetic mother. Br Med J 1985;290:1700–1702.

159. Al-Samarrai SF, Kato A, Urano Y. Renal vein thrombosis in stillborn infants of diabetic mothers. Acta Pathol Jpn 1983;34:1411–1447.
160. Farquhar JW. Prognosis for babies born to diabetic mothers in Edinburgh. Arch Dis Child 1960;44:36–47.
161. Bibergeil H, Bodel E, Amendt P. Diabetes and pregnancy: early and late prognoses of children of diabetic mothers. In: Camerini-Davalos RA, Cole HS, eds. Early diabetes in early life. New York: Academic Press, 1975:427–434.
162. Vohr BR, Lipsitt LP, Oh W. Somatic growth of children of diabetic mothers with reference to birth size. J Pediatr 1980;97:196–199.
163. Gerlini G, Arachi S, Gori MG, et al. Developmental aspects of the offspring of diabetic mothers. Acta Endocrinol Suppl 1986;277:150–155.
164. Silverman BL, Metzger BE, Chon H, et al. Impaired glucose tolerance in adolescent offspring of diabetic mothers. Relationship to fetal hyperinsulinemia. Diabetes Care 1995;18:611–617.
165. Yssing M. Long-term prognosis of children born to mothers diabetic when pregnant. In: Camerini-Davalos RA, Cole HS, eds. Early diabetes in early life. New York: Academic Press, 1975:575–586.
166. Stehbens JA, Baker GL, Kitchell M. Outcome at ages 1, 3, and 5 years of children born to diabetic women. Am J Obstet Gynecol 1977;127:408–413.
167. Petersen MB, Pedersen SA, Greisen G, et al. Early growth delay in diabetic pregnancy: relation to psychomotor development at age 4. Br Med J 1988;296:598–600.
168. Persson B, Gentz J. Follow up of children of insulin dependent and gestational diabetic mothers. Neuropsychological outcome. Acta Paediatr Scand 1983;73:349–358.
169. Hadden DR, Bryne E, Trotter I, et al. Physical and psychological health of children of type 1 (insulin dependent) diabetic mothers. Diabetologia 1983;26:250–254.
170. Rizzo T, Metzger RE, Burns WJ, et al. Correlations between antepartum maternal metabolism and child intelligence. N Engl J Med 1991;325:911–916.
171. Anderson CE, Rotter JI, Rimoin DL. Genetics of diabetes mellitus. In: Rifkin H, Raskin P, eds. Diabetes mellitus, vol 5. New York: Prentice Hall, 1981:79–85.
172. Simpson JL. Genetics of diabetes mellitus and anomalies in offspring of diabetic mothers. In: Merkatz IR, Adam PAJ, eds. The diabetic pregnancy. A perinatal perspective. New York: Grune & Stratton 1979:249–260.
173. Widness JA, Cowett RM, Zeller WP, et al. Permanent neonatal diabetes in an infant of an insulin-dependent mother. J Pediatr 1982;100:926–929.
174. Warram JH, Krolewski AS, Kahn CR. Determinants of IDM and perinatal mortality in children of diabetic mothers. Diabetes 1988;37:1328–1334.

50
Metabolism of the Neonate Requiring Surgery

Arnold G. Coran, Agostino Pierro, and David J. Schmeling

Postoperative or posttraumatic morbidity and mortality in the high-risk adult have been correlated with, and may be precipitated by, the magnitude and duration of the metabolic response to the stressful event. Complications such as severe weight loss, cardiopulmonary insufficiency, thromboembolic disorders, gastric stress ulcers, impaired immunologic function, prolonged convalescence, and death have been related to aspects of the metabolic response to surgical or traumatic stress.[1,2]

These metabolic responses to operative stress in the adult (Table 50.1) have been the subject of laboratory and clinical investigation for the past century; similar responses in the neonate are not as well documented. Metabolic complications or aberrations induced by operative stress may upset the delicate metabolic balance of a neonate already involved in the process of adaptation to its postnatal environment. The normal neonatal reserves of nutrients (e.g., carbohydrate, protein, and fat) are limited, and the energy-consuming processes of rapid growth and maturation are occurring simultaneously with the additional demands produced by surgery. This concept is supported by experimental data, which demonstrate higher morbidity and mortality in the neonate than in the older child or adult subjected to similar procedures.[3,4] It is evident that knowledge of specific aspects of the neonatal stress response is of more importance in comparison to similar responses in the adult. Knowledge of this response is imperative for those providing care to the neonate.

Metabolic studies, even in the normal neonate, are few owing to limitations caused by insensitive assays, the difficulties inherent in conducting prolonged observations, and the limited amount of blood that can be withdrawn ethically. It is apparent that postoperative treatment would be greatly improved if a thorough understanding of the metabolic consequences of operative stress were achieved. The evidence suggests that the neonate frequently responds to trauma and stress in a manner different from that of the older child or adult.

The metabolic response to a surgical operation may be a considerable challenge to the homeostasis of the high-risk patient. This is particularly true of the neonate, whose metabolism is readily disturbed by environmental and other factors, which is reflected in the higher morbidity and mortality reported.[3] Anand and Hickey[5] have suggested that reducing the metabolic response to operative stress may lead to an improvement in the survival of these infants. In a randomized trial, these investigators have shown that the neonate who received deep anesthesia with sufentanil had a significantly decreased incidence of sepsis, metabolic acidosis, and disseminated intravascular coagulation and fewer postoperative deaths in comparison with the neonate who received lighter anesthesia with halothane plus morphine. Interestingly, in the neonate who received sufentanil anesthesia, the hormonal response to operative stress was significantly reduced.

Historical Background

Justus von Liebig, a German organic chemist, is credited with being the first to recognize the process of metabolism, which in 1848, he aptly defined as "the sum of chemical changes of materials under the influence of living cells."[6] This definition remains accurate today.

The interest in metabolic changes following surgical trauma began in 1872, when Joseph Bauer[7] documented increased nitrogen elimination from the body following hemorrhages. Subsequently, J.D. Malcolm,[8] in 1893, postulated an increased metabolic rate after abdominal surgery as the explanation for his observation of increased urea excretion following surgery. Experimental support for these observations was provided by Aub and Wu,[9] who developed a feline laboratory model for traumatic shock and demonstrated a marked postshock decline in basal metabolic rate as well as a rise in the nonprotein nitrogen, urea, creatinine, and glucose concentrations in blood.[9]

TABLE 50.1. Metabolic response to operative stress in the adult and neonate.

Metabolite	Adult response	Neonatal response
Metabolic rate and oxygen consumption	↓ Briefly, then ↑	↓ Comparable to that in adults (minimal change compared to age-matched controls)
Carbohydrate	↑ Hyperglycemia response ↑ Gluconeogenesis and ↓ glucose utilization	↑ Glucose 2× normal immediately postoperatively (less persistent ↑ than in adults); probably secondary to glycogenolysis rather than ↑ gluconeogenesis; neonates may be unable to carry out hepatic gluconeogenesis secondary to lack of key enzyme
Protein	Negative nitrogen balance Slight ↑ protein breakdown, dependent on severity of stress; ↑ with increased severity; ↓ protein synthesis in extrahepatic tissues ↑ Amino acid utilization for gluconeogenesis, acute phase reactant synthesis, and synthesis of components of healing process ↑ Nitrogen excretion sustained up to 5 days	Negative nitrogen balance during the first 2–3 days Oxidation of fat stores to spare protein
Fat	Adipose tissue lipolysis → mobilization of nonesterified fatty acids and ↑ ketone body formation About 75–90% of postoperative requirements supplied by fat metabolism (10–25% by protein)	↑ Lipolysis + ketogenesis (? catecholamine stimulated) → ↑ total ketone bodies, ↑ glycerol, ↑ nonesterified fatty acids Postoperative fat utilization exceeds rate of mobilization of free fatty acids

Claude Bernard[10] was centrally involved in early studies of mammalian metabolism with particular interest in the role of the central nervous system (CNS) in metabolic regulations. He was able to produce glycosuria and a diabetic condition in dogs through CNS manipulation, and in 1855 he postulated a central role for an adrenal gland-derived substance in the control of blood glucose.[11] Subsequently, Bernard[12] published his classic treatise on stress-induced physiologic changes, in which he demonstrated an increase in blood glucose concentration associated with simultaneous depletion of hepatic glycogen stores as a result of hemorrhage and trauma. Brown-Séquard[13,14] confirmed Bernard's hypothesis by successfully demonstrating the presence of adrenaline in the secretion of the adrenal gland. Further early observations on postoperative changes include Harold Pringle et al.'s[15] observation in 1905 that surgical operations were frequently followed by oliguria. G.H. Evans[16] in 1911 demonstrated that salt retention was common during the postoperative period.

W.B. Cannon[17] further focused attention on the endocrine response to injury in his Shattuck Lecture of 1917. He described a condition of wound shock that produced a marked increase in sympathetic nervous system activity. He described stimulation of the output of an adrenaline-like substance and a significant increase in blood glucose concentration as a result of these changes. Cannon[18,19] later introduced the idea of "homeostasis" to represent the constancy of the cellular environment, and proposed that operative or traumatic injury poses a threat to the body's "homeostatic" mechanism.[18,19]

Cuthbertson,[20] in 1929, characterized a catabolic postoperative response to injury consisting of increased losses of nitrogen, sulfur, and phosphorus in urine. He was the first to propose that skeletal muscle was being catabolized after injury and coined the term catabolic response to injury, which he thought accounted for the changes he observed in urine.[21] He subsequently demonstrated that diets high in protein and energy content are capable of diminishing the posttraumatic nitrogen losses but are unable to completely abolish this response.[22] In 1946, Hans Selye[23] described a "general adaptation syndrome" in response to stress. He demonstrated that this adaptive process is associated with hypercalcemia, acidosis, and a negative nitrogen balance.

Moore and Ball[24] are well known for their important contributions to the field of postsurgical metabolism in the adult. Their textbook remains a classic resource. Among their most important contributions is the demonstration that surgical stress causes decreased carbohydrate utilization, a marked increase in fat oxidation, and a net nitrogen loss. They characterized response to surgery as occurring in four phases: (1) adrenergic-corticoid phase; (2) corticoid withdrawal phase; (3) spontaneous anabolic phase; and (4) fat gain phase.

Hayes and Coller[25] demonstrated that cation excretion is determined primarily by the magnitude of the adrenocortical response, and that postoperative water excretion is controlled by vasopressin secretion. They demonstrated that the postoperative use of intravenous fluids is associated with maintenance of normal water exchange. As more sophisticated physiologic and biochemical assays were developed, advances in hormonal metabolism and physiology were greatly facilitated. In 1954, Sandberg et al.[26] demonstrated a marked increase in 17-hydroxycorticosteroids intraoperatively, with a smaller rise noted immediately upon induction of anesthesia. These early investigations into the hormonal response to operative stress culminated with the 1959 observations of Hume and Egdahl,[27] which established the hypothalamus as the center of control for initiation of the hormonal response to surgical and nonsurgical stress.

Investigations of normal neonatal metabolism originated with Albert von Bezold's[28,29] studies of a stillborn fetus in 1857-1858. In 1916, Ylppo[30] documented the presence of an "acidotic condition" in the neonate. His data were substantiated in studies by Marples and Lippard[31,32] in 1932-1933, who demonstrated that all normal premature and term neonates are prone to develop acidosis. W.M. Marriott,[33] in the 1919 Harvey Lecture, described the many disastrous effects of dehydration in the neonate.

Early investigations suggested that the physiologic disturbances associated with operative stress in the neonate are the same as in the adult and differ only in the degree of change.[34,35] To facilitate the acquisition data and to optimize perioperative care of the surgical neonate, Peter Rickham[36] carried out extensive investigations in the neonate modeled after the investigations reported in the adult by Moore and Ball.[24] His 1957 monograph on the metabolic response to neonatal surgery remains a classic work.[36] As a result of his data and alterations in perioperative care based on those data, Rickham[36] noted that the mortality for major surgical procedures performed on the neonate decreased from 76% in 1949 to about 25% in 1952.

Since the publications of Moore and Ball and Rickham, a great number of investigators have been involved in the study of postoperative metabolic changes in the neonate and the adult. This chapter summarizes the current knowledge of these responses in the neonate.

Energy Metabolism and Thermogenesis

Cuthbertson[37,38] demonstrated that trauma or surgery significantly affects energy metabolism in the adult. There is a brief "ebb" period of a depressed metabolic rate immediately following the trauma, which is followed by a "flow phase" characterized by an increase in oxygen consumption.[37,38] Subsequent studies in the adult have demonstrated that resting energy expenditure (REE) increases after an operation, although to a lesser degree than after multiple trauma and burns.[39-42] This increase has been attributed to the energy requirements of the injured tissue, heat losses from the wound, and an increased futile cycling of metabolic substrates,[43-46] and is believed to be mediated by catecholamines, glucagon, and cortisol, which are released in response to stress.[47-51]

Several studies in the infant and child have not been able to demonstrate any increase in REE following operation.[52-56] In a study of oxygen consumption (V_{O_2}) in the postoperative neonate, Ito et al.[52] demonstrated that the V_{O_2} of a term, normally fed neonate increases with advancing age until approximately the second or third week of life. Ito et al.'s study demonstrated no postoperative increase in V_{O_2} in the neonate other than that expected for a normal neonate of that age. On the contrary, they observed that some neonates, predominantly those undergoing major abdominal operations, demonstrate lower postoperative oxygen consumption than would be expected in a normal neonate of the same age. They concluded that postoperative V_{O_2} in the neonate is better correlated with caloric intake than with the intensity of the operative stress. It has been postulated that the infant and child are able to convert energy expended on growth to energy spent on wound repair and healing, avoiding the overall increase in energy expenditure seen in the adult.[53] However, these studies are at odds with the findings of other investigators,[57-60] who have demonstrated changes in hormones, and metabolic substrates following stress, similar to those observed in the adult. A possible explanation for this discrepancy centers on the different timing of the various investigations. The maximum endocrine and biochemical changes were observed immediately after operation and gradually returned to normal over the next 24 hours. By contrast, several studies of resting energy expenditure[53-56] have been performed at least 24 hours after the end of the operation, by which time any changes may have already occurred.

In a recent study on 19 neonates Jones et al.[61] demonstrated that oxygen consumption (V_{O_2}) and resting energy expenditure increase after the operation by approximately 15%, peaking 4 hours after the start of the operation, and then return to baseline levels by 12 to 24 hours. The timing of these changes corresponds with the postoperative increase in catecholamine levels described by Anand et al.[57,58] Moreover, Jones et al.[62] demonstrated in the neonate that interleukin-6 increases maximally by 12 hours after surgery. A linear correlation exists between the increase in interleukin-6 and the operative stress score, indicating that this cytokine is a marker of the stress response.

The increase in resting energy expenditure observed by Jones et al.[61] was significantly greater in the neonate having a major operation than in the neonate having a minor operation. Among the former, the increase in resting energy expenditure was significantly greater in those neonates more than 48 hours old than in those less than 48 hours old. A possible explanation for this may be related to the secretion of endogenous opioids by the neonate. It has been suggested that nociceptive stimuli during the operation are responsible for the endocrine and metabolic stress responses, and that these stimuli may be inhibited by opioids.[58,63] This is supported by data showing that moderate doses of opioids blunt the endocrine and metabolic responses to operative stress in infancy.[5,58] The concentration of endogenous opioids in the cord blood of the neonate is five times higher than plasma concentration in the resting adult.[63,64] It is possible that the reduced metabolic stress response observed in the neonate less than 48 hours old is related to a higher circulating concentration of endogenous opioids. This might constitute a protective mechanism blunting the response to stress in the perinatal period.

Chwals et al.[65] demonstrated that the postoperative increase in REE can result from severe underlying acute illness, such as sepsis or intense inflammation, that frequently necessitates surgery. REE is directly proportional to growth rate in the healthy neonate, and growth is retarded during acute metabolic stress. These investigators suggested that increased energy is utilized for growth recovery following the earlier resolution of the acute injury response in the surgical neonate with no sepsis or major inflammation. The investigators indicated that serial postoperative REE can be used to stratify injury severity and may be an effective parameter to monitor the return of normal growth metabolism.

Infants and children undergoing operations under general anesthesia are exposed to a variety of stress factors, such as cold, anesthetic agents, the operation itself, and starvation, that may have detrimental effects on heat production (i.e., energy expenditure) and core temperature.[61] Studies on thermogenic response to surgery have been performed almost exclusively in the experimental animal.[66-68] Indirect calorimetry provides a noninvasive method of calculating the whole-body heat production by measuring the oxygen consumption (Vo_2) and the carbon dioxide production and converting these values to an equivalent quantity of heat. In a recent study using indirect calorimetry before, during, and after major abdominal operations, Fasoli et al.[69] demonstrated that oxidative metabolism and body temperature in infants and children vary before, during, and after major abdominal operations. The metabolic and thermogenic response to operative stress is age-related: during the operation infants decrease metabolic rate and tend to maintain stable body core temperature, whereas children increase both metabolic rate and body core temperature.

Oxidative breakdown of nutrients releases energy that is converted to usable chemical fuel [i.e., adenosine triphosphate (ATP)] in the mithocondria of cells by oxidative phosphorylation. This is used to drive energy consuming processes in the body. During oxidative phosphorylation protons are pumped from the mitochondrial matrix to the intermembrane space. Proton-pumping is directly proportional to the rate of Vo_2 and generates and maintains a difference in electrochemical potential of protons across the inner membrane. Protons turn back into the matrix by one of two routes: the "phosphorylating pathway," which generates ATP, or the "leak pathway," which is nonproductive and releases energy as heat. A significant proportion (i.e., 20–30%) of oxygen consumed by resting hepatocytes from adult rats is used to drive the heat-producing proton leak.[70] This leak pathway in the liver and other organs is a significant contributor to the reactions that make up the standard resting energy expenditure and, therefore, results in significant resting heat production.[71,72] The proton permeability of the inner mitochondrial membrane in the rat liver mitochondria is high in the fetus, significantly reduced during early neonatal life, and reaches the lowest maintained level in the adult.[73] These investigators suggested that this could provide a physiologic protective mechanism for thermal adaptation of newborn rats during the perinatal period before the establishment of brown adipose tissue thermogenesis.[73]

It is conceivable that the neonate is "preprogrammed" with similar protective mechanisms for surviving the stresses of birth (i.e., cold adaptation), surgery (i.e., cord division), and starvation (i.e., transient hypoglycemia). Such mechanisms include a reduction in energy expenditure to spare nutrient energy reserves and an ability to increase the proton leak to generate heat before nonshivering brown adipose tissue thermogenesis is established. These survival mechanisms may persist during the neonatal period. As intraoperative stress and birth trauma are similar in nature, it is possible that the intraoperative reduction in energy expenditure described by Fasoli et al.[69] in early infancy represents a "protective survival mechanism" and that the core temperature may be maintained by a relative increase in the proton leak. During an operation and cold exposure, infants seem to utilize a lower proportion of available energy (i.e., proton gradient) to drive ATP synthesis and dissipate a greater proportion as heat (i.e., proton leak) to maintain body temperature.

The neonate is not able to respond to cold exposure by shivering, but has a highly specialized tissue, brown fat, capable of generating heat without shivering (i.e., nonshivering thermogenesis). As environmental temperature decreases, an increased blood flow to brown fat stores is observed and heat is produced in brown fat mitochondria. Nonshivering thermogenesis is inhibited by anesthetic agents in the experimental animal.[66,67] Albanese et al.[66] have shown that in rabbits termination of general anesthesia during cold exposure causes a rapid and profound increase in nonshivering thermogenesis.

This may explain the sudden and rapid increase in energy expenditure observed in the young infant at the end of an operation (see Chapters 44 and 45).[61,69]

Carbohydrate Metabolism

Adult postoperative change in carbohydrate metabolism can be summarized as a significant hyperglycemic response during and after surgery. This effect may be the result of an increase in glucose production as well as diminution in peripheral glucose utilization, with a relative decrease in insulin concentration.[74–82]

Pioneering work early in this century by Benedict and Talbot,[83] who monitored the respiratory quotient (RQ) of the normal neonate, demonstrated that as much as 80% of the energy requirements are fulfilled by calories derived from fat. This point is interesting because carbohydrates provide the main source of energy in the fetus. Soon after birth and even before feeding is started, a rapid fall in glycogen reserves has been demonstrated.[84] The blood glucose concentration is known to fall during the early postnatal period.[85] An increase of plasma free fatty acids (FFAs) and ketone bodies has been documented to occur concurrent with these changes in glucose and glycogen, adding support to the importance of fat-derived calories in the neonate.[86,87] Unfortunately, an operation on the neonate is frequently accompanied by a period of starvation that may be prolonged, especially if the gastrointestinal tract is involved. The advent of hyperalimentation has aided somewhat in altering this pattern. It is known that depot fat accounts for 10% to 15% of the body weight of the normal human neonate, and it may provide the main source of energy during the period of starvation soon after birth.[88,89]

In 1968 an intravenous glucose tolerance test was performed on 14 neonates undergoing surgery for abnormalities of the alimentary tract.[90] The investigators observed that 6 of the 14 neonates had a greatly reduced tolerance to glucose administered by intravenous infusion. They noted a constant rate of glucose disappearance that was unrelated to the absolute glucose concentration, in contrast to data in older children and adults. They postulated, as an explanation for these observations, that (1) the neonate may be less able than the adult to form glycogen from glucose, (2) there may be a temporary increased insulin dependency in the neonate, and (3) the uptake of glucose by the tissues may be reduced by high circulating hormonal concentrations of adrenaline and growth hormone. These investigators noted depression of the concentration of FFAs after the injection of glucose, which suggests that the administered glucose may have a fat-sparing action even when the K_t values (percent clearance of administered glucose from blood per minute) are low. They concluded that the prolonged use of a parenteral glucose solution might lead to severe hyperglycemia, and the capacity of the neonate to handle infused glucose is variable among individuals (see Chapter 32).

Elphick and Wilkinson[91] demonstrated a postoperative increase in the blood glucose concentration to approximately two times preoperative levels in neonates but noted that the glucose concentration returns to normal within 12 hours. This finding is in contrast to data from the adult surgical patient, showing that the blood glucose concentration may remain high for several days. These investigators noted the similarity of their findings to those of Pinter[92] and proposed that the elevation in blood glucose concentration noted in the postoperative period may be due to either increased production or decreased utilization of glucose, or a combination of the two. In an earlier study of glucose tolerance testing in postoperative neonates, diminished glucose utilization had been demonstrated by these investigators.[90] In attempting to explain this relative intolerance, they cited the type of anesthesia as one important contributory factor. The mechanism postulated is a direct effect by endogenous catecholamines resulting in altered glucose metabolism, with variations in anesthesia methods causing alterations in the catecholamine response. This concept has been confirmed in experimental studies with the neonatal rabbit and puppy.[93,94] The conclusion from these data was that endogenous sources of energy are supplying a sufficient number of calories to satisfy the requirements of the normal neonate during starvation secondary to congenital anomalies and after the surgical correction of these anomalies, but at significant metabolic cost.

When evaluating starvation, a condition frequently linked with operative stress in neonates, Elphick and Wilkinson[91] were unable to document hypoglycemia in normal birth weight neonates starved for up to a week. They postulated that the glucose-sparing action of FFAs was responsible and suggested a relation between maintenance of a normal blood glucose concentration during starvation and body fat stores.

In contrast to what is reported above, studies of substrate utilization that involve indirect calorimetry in the neonate receiving a constant intravenous infusion of dextrose have shown that the respiratory quotient did not change significantly in the immediate postoperative period.[61] This indicates that substrate utilization is unaltered by the operative stress in the neonate. Energy needs may even be decreased after surgery because of growth inhibition (resulting from catabolic stress metabolism), decreased insensible losses, and inactivity. Recently Letton et al.[95] have shown that during the early postoperative period, lipogenesis with increased CO_2 production is substantial. Lipogenesis seems to occur even at a reduced caloric delivery rate that exceeds REE by only 50%. These data suggest that caloric requirements after operative stress are likely to be equal to or only minimally in excess of the normal requirement.

In a study utilizing stable isotopes, Kalhan et al.[96] examined glucose turnover, systemic glucose production rate, and recycling of glucose carbon as an indicator of gluconeogenesis. They studied six normal neonates ranging in age from 2 hours to 3 days. The human fetus is known to be dependent on the mother for its glucose needs, and no fetal glucose production has been demonstrated during intrauterine life.[97] There is, however, the potential for fetal gluconeogenesis. The presence of key gluconeogenic enzymes in fetal liver specimens has been documented.[98] Kalhan et al. concluded that gluconeogenesis is not expressed in utero. During the perinatal period when the placental or maternal supply of substrate including glucose to the fetus or neonate is abruptly interrupted, the neonate demonstrates a normal capacity for systemic glucose production in order to meet its metabolic needs. Their studies suggested that the source of the available glucose is chiefly from the process of glycogenolysis rather than gluconeogenesis. These investigators did demonstrate that gluconeogenesis via the Cori cycle may be possible at as early as 2 hours of life. They noted that the contribution of recycled carbon to systemic glucose production does not increase during the neonatal period and that glycogenolysis continues to play the key role in maintaining adequate glucose availability for metabolic needs. They postulated that this predominant role of glycogenolysis over gluconeogenesis may be the result of the ready availability of sufficient glycogen stores due to the frequent feeding of the neonate. It is not difficult to imagine that this system may be interfered with by the stresses placed on a neonate by surgery and interruption of dietary intake as well as alteration in gastrointestinal function.

Similar stable isotope studies to elucidate stress-induced changes in postoperative glucose homeostatic mechanisms in neonates have not been reported. It has been documented through elaborate arteriovenous catheterization study in the adult patient with major injury and sepsis that there is increased splanchnic production of glucose in this state.[99] Concomitant increased uptake of gluconeogenic amino acids, primarily alanine, and increased production of glucose and urea implicate increased gluconeogenesis rather than glycogenolysis as the source of the glucose generated. Exogenous glucose sources were found by these investigators to diminish the observed gluconeogenic response in the normal control subject but not in the septic or postoperative patient.

The available evidence in the adult suggests that increased glucose production from the splanchnic tissues may contribute substantially to the hyperglycemic response to surgical stress. Elphick and Wilkinson's[90,91] studies showing altered glucose tolerance suggest a role for decreased glucose utilization in this state. The hyperglycemic response is complex and multifactorial. Not only is the ability to utilize glucose in peripheral tissue in an impaired state but the mechanism of utilization may be altered. In an experimental model of skin healing utilizing ^{14}C-labeled glucose to assess the various pathways of glucose metabolism in wounded tissue resulting in ATP production, Im and Hoopes[100] demonstrated a marked increase in glycolytic capacity (i.e., Embden-Meyerhof pathway), as well as increased activity of the pentose shunt and decreased activity of the Krebs cycle. Their wounded skin model is characterized by increased glucose utilization and lactate production. Seventy percent of the ATP produced is through the Embden-Meyerhof pathway in wounded tissue, rather than through the Krebs cycle as in normal skin.

Another postulated mechanism for the observed postsurgical hyperglycemia and increase in blood lactate and pyruvate concentrations is the elevated adrenaline concentration in response to the operative stress, resulting in activation of the Cori cycle. Although the precise mechanism for the hyperglycemic response is not clear, the clinical implications of significant hyperglycemia in a neonate are important. Significant changes in plasma osmolality can result from alterations in glucose concentration. It has been documented in the neonate that an increase in plasma osmolality of more than 25 mOsm·kg^{-1} over a period of 4 hours can have profound detrimental effects on the renal cortex and cerebral cortex and may even precipitate intracranial hemorrhage in the neonate.[101,102]

In addition to the marked postoperative hyperglycemia, a number of investigators have demonstrated increases in blood lactate and pyruvate concentrations in the postoperative adult patient.[103,104] Arteriovenous catheterization studies in the adult have demonstrated that adrenaline release during surgery increases lactate and pyruvate production due to glycogen breakdown in peripheral tissues.[75] In addition, it is well known that injured tissue around the surgical wound derive their energy mainly from glycolysis, which may contribute to the increased lactate production after surgery.[78,100] Other factors involved in the increased lactate concentration noted include tissue hypoperfusion and hypoxia during surgery.[100] These changes may be related to the anesthesia or be secondary to hypotension as a result of excessive blood loss or altered circulatory patterns during surgery.[105] As shown by double isotope turnover studies in the normal neonate, many of these metabolites are removed from the circulation by the liver and are used as substrate for hepatic gluconeogenesis, although it may not be the case in the stressed neonate.[96]

The significance of elevated blood alanine concentration in the neonate is much less clear. Although alanine is known to be the key gluconeogenic amino acid in the adult, some data have documented hypoalaninemia in neonates receiving glucagon.[106,107] This effect was postulated to be secondary to increased splanchnic utilization of alanine for glucagon-stimulated gluconeogenesis. In a subsequent study of the relationship between neonatal plasma alanine, glucagon, and insulin concentration, no correlation was observed between changes in alanine and glucose concentration.[108] These data further cloud the role of gluconeogenic substrates and the process of gluconeogenesis in the hyperglycemic response.

In their 1987 study of the effect of fentanyl on postoperative metabolic changes in neonates, Anand et al.[58] demonstrated increases in blood lactate and pyruvate concentrations during surgery in the nonfentanyl group but noted no similar changes in the fentanyl-treated patient. Twenty-four hours postoperatively the blood lactate and pyruvate concentrations had fallen below preoperative levels in the nonfentanyl group. Quantitative blood concentrations of total gluconeogenic substrates, measured as the sum of the blood concentrations of lactate, pyruvate, alanine, and glycerol, in the nonfentanyl group of neonates, increased substantially during surgery, but fell by 24% postoperatively. These changes in the postoperative period were attributed to the utilization of these substrates for gluconeogenesis with excess glucose production in the nonfentanyl-treated neonate. The differences between the fentanyl and nonfentanyl groups were postulated to be due to blunting of the stress-induced catecholamine response in the fentanyl group with resultant diminution of catecholamine-induced postoperative changes.

An earlier study from Anand's groups provides support for this concept.[57] Significant increases in blood concentrations of lactate, pyruvate, total ketone bodies (e.g., acetoacetate and hydroxybutyrate), and glycerol were noted during surgery in their experimental group, which consisted of preterm and the term neonate. In this study, the blood lactate concentration remained elevated until 12 hours after surgery, whereas all other metabolites measured returned to preoperative concentrations by 6 hours postoperatively. No significant changes were seen in the blood concentration of the gluconeogenic amino acid alanine during or after surgery. Blood lactate concentration showed a high degree of correlation with the plasma adrenaline concentration at the end of surgery and 6 hours after surgery. There was a significant correlation between blood glycerol concentration and plasma adrenaline and noradrenaline concentrations at the end of surgery.

When examining the response of a subgroup of six term and preterm neonates matched for degree of surgical stress and anesthetic technique, some interesting findings are noted in the above study. No significant differences in blood glucose, pyruvate, total ketone bodies, or glycerol concentrations were noted between these two groups of neonates either before or after surgery. Preterm neonates demonstrated a significant rise in blood lactate concentration during surgery, whereas no similar change was noted in the subgroup of the term neonate.

In summarizing their observations, these investigators suggested that the importance of the changes noted in their study may be in the provision of substrate for hepatic gluconeogenesis during the postoperative period. The significant hyperlactacidemia noted during surgery in the premature neonate is postulated to be due to deficiency of the key hepatic gluconeogenic enzymes, although separate studies by Kalhan et al.[97] and Marsac et al.[98] do not support this hypothesis.

It is conceivable that the greater degree of hyperlactacidemia in the preterm neonate is related to less rich glycogen stores in their skeletal muscle in comparison with the term neonate, with resultant increased dependence on gluconeogenesis for substrate provision in the face of an immature gluconeogenic mechanism. The rise in blood lactate concentration may be due to tissue hypoxia caused by changes in peripheral circulation during anesthesia and surgery.

From the above discussion, it is apparent that the hyperglycemic response to surgery may result from a combination of increased production and decreased utilization of glucose. Many of the hormonal changes affecting the hyperglycemic response have been described. These hormonal changes are capable of inducing glycogenolysis as well as gluconeogenesis following surgery. These responses are accompanied by a decreased rate of glucose utilization, particularly during the surgical procedure. The relative contributions of each of these mechanisms may depend on a variety of factors including the degree of surgical trauma, the gestational age of the patient, the body composition, as well as particulars of the anesthetic management. In addition, nutritional supplementation seems to play a modulating role (see Chapter 32).

Protein Metabolism

Acute malnutrition as a result of insufficient nutrient intake or of the increased metabolic demands of illness or trauma leads to increased catabolism of muscle protein and a negative nitrogen balance. These changes along with rapid utilization of energy substrate stores at a time when nutritional intake is often reduced drastically affects the ability to heal wounds, combat infection, and have sufficient muscular strength to breathe adequately, all resulting in increased morbidity and mortality.[109] Even the well-nourished may experience periods of debility after the injury of major surgery, which may relate to the reduction of protein reserves and energy stores.[110]

Major operative stress in adult patients results in a negative nitrogen balance. A compilation of factors accounts for this result. Among those well-documented factors are increased protein breakdown and decreased protein synthesis in extrahepatic tissues. There is increased utilization of amino acids for alternate purposes such as gluconeogenesis, synthesis of acute phase reactants by the liver, and synthesis of components of the healing process in injured tissues. The patient experiencing trauma or sepsis has been demonstrated to have rapid onset of muscle wasting, protein depletion, and elevated urea excretion.[111,112] An increased supply of amino acids is made available during sepsis or trauma for energy production by gluconeogenesis and oxidation. These additional amino acids satisfy the requirements of the liver and other visceral tissue for greatly accelerated synthesis of the proteins essential to immunologic defense, healing of wounds, and maintenance of functions in the vital organs. The adult response to starvation is characterized by sacrifice of visceral protein to furnish amino acids for gluconeogenesis and other purposes, whereas in stressful situations (e.g., trauma or sepsis) muscle protein is degraded and the liver increases its protein content.[113]

Important as this metabolic response may be to survival, prolonged mobilization of amino acids leads to devastating muscle weakness. In some patients muscle weakness is so great that ventilation is insufficient to overcome the respiratory insufficiency associated with trauma. Depletion of protein is accompanied by deterioration of cellular structure, insufficient production of acute-phase reactants, and reduced synthesis of other necessary proteins. Under such conditions, the patient is prone to perish from overwhelming infection, culminating in multisystem failure.[114]

The ill neonate is particularly susceptible to the adverse metabolic effects a major illness or surgical operation imposes. Perioperative protein metabolic and nutritional status must be given special consideration in this population because of smaller body size, rapid growth, highly variable fluid requirements, and the immaturity of certain organ systems. These factors, as well as low caloric reserves in the premature neonate and ill child, make an adequate caloric and amino acid intake particularly important. Consequently, the neonate whose nutritional needs are not met as a result of functional or organic disorder of the gastrointestinal tract can rapidly develop protein-calorie malnutrition and associated complications.[115]

The most important clinical consequence of a catabolic stress reaction is thought to be increased protein breakdown after surgery.[116] The consequences could be particularly deleterious in a postoperative neonate whose nutritional status is already tenuous.

Adult urinary nitrogen excretion is increased after major surgery and may remain elevated for as long as 5 days postoperatively.[117] Johnston's[118] study suggests that an adult patient's nitrogen losses are equivalent to 500 g of lean muscle tissue per day. An important determinant of the magnitude and duration of the postoperative nitrogen loss appears to be the severity of surgical stress.[117] There is some evidence in the adult patient that the availability of ketone bodies as a metabolic fuel for peripheral tissues may result in a decreased need for amino acid oxidation in extrahepatic tissue, specifically skeletal muscle, and may ultimately result in decreased nitrogen loss and sparing of muscle protein sources.[119]

In an elaborate study of muscle protein degradation in the nonoperated premature neonates, Ballard et al.[116] examined correlations between energy input, nitrogen retention, weight gained, and subsequent survival. They demonstrated that approximately 5% of total muscle protein is degraded daily. The total and fractional rates of protein breakdown demonstrate significant reverse correlations with nitrogen retention but have no relation to total energy input. Not surprisingly, protein degradation is higher than average in neonates who are losing weight at the time of the balance study, and lower in neonates who demonstrate weight gain. Protein degradation was higher in neonates who died within 2 weeks of the study. It is unclear whether this increased degradation in preterminal neonates is related to events that stimulated muscle proteolysis (e.g., sepsis), or is due to the underlying nitrogen status of the patient.[120] Significantly, myofibrillar protein breakdown is not different between neonates fed orally and those receiving parenteral nutrition. These investigators commented that the effects of nitrogen and energy status on muscle protein degradation in the premature neonate are different from changes reported in the adult human or the adult rat. To explain these findings they postulated that the limited energy reserves of the premature neonate may be responsible for the differences observed. They were unable to demonstrate any correlation between energy input in the premature neonate and rate of muscle protein breakdown. This finding is in contrast to large increases in total muscle protein breakdown seen in the rat subjected to total energy restriction and a slight decrease in muscle protein breakdown in long-term fasting in the obese adult human.[121,122] They attempted to explain the differences between their data and those of other studies mentioned above on the basis of the size of the fat reserves, as there is evidence that ketonemia produced by fat mobilization is accompanied by a lower rate of muscle protein breakdown, and because the premature neonate clearly has little adipose tissue, it would explain the difference.[119]

Ballard et al.[116] reported an increase in muscle protein degradation in premature neonates by demonstrating a negative nitrogen balance or minimal retention of nitrogen daily. They postulated that it may be due to increased protein breakdown as a result of a demand for amino acids, which cannot be met simply by a decrease in protein synthesis. They stated that the response observed "is surely catastrophic if prolonged for any length of time," thus arguing forcefully that a substantial nitrogen supply to the premature infant should be maintained. They noted that the muscle/total body protein degradation ratio is 7%, in contrast to a value of 30% found in the adult. They attribute this difference to the small pool of muscle protein in the premature neonate.[123] They speculated on the tissue sites of the remaining 93% of protein degradation in the premature neonate and postulated that organs that account for greater relative ratios of neonatal body weight (e.g., brain, liver, or skin) may contribute significantly to total body protein degradation. The result of this visceral protein breakdown could be disastrous.

Colle and Paulsen[124] in a 1959 study of postoperative neonates, demonstrated urinary nitrogen losses of 200 to 300 mg·kg^{-1} 24 hours^{-1} in contrast to 80 mg·kg^{-1} 24 hours^{-1} in normal neonates. These losses were transient and not sustained. Rickham during the late 1950s demonstrated a postoperative increase in nitrogen excretion in the neonate, but added that, as in the adult, this increase is no greater than that found when the patient is starved.[36] Rickham noted that a crude protein infusion in the form of plasma results in rapid utilization of the infused protein. He thought that a postoperative plasma infusion serves the double purpose of maintaining a normal plasma volume and restoring the plasma protein concentration. Winthrop et al.[56] demonstrated, in a prospective evaluation of the pediatric trauma patient, significant increases in basal metabolic rate (BMR), whole-body protein turnover, protein synthesis, and urinary nitrogen excretion. These patients were found to have a negative nitrogen balance since protein breakdown increased relatively more than protein synthesis. The increase in protein breakdown/turnover, synthesis, and nitrogen excretion was found to have greatly exceeded the increase noted in BMR (i.e., 93%, 82%, and 56%, respectively, vs 14% increase in BMR) in the young (i.e., <10 years old) posttrauma patient. The investigators were unable to demonstrate a correlation between BMR and whole-body protein turnover, suggesting that changes in energy expenditure and protein metabolism following injury may be mediated by different mechanisms. They concluded that the metabolic response of the pediatric patient to multiple trauma differs from that of the adult and noted that the pediatric trauma patient requires not only increased caloric intake but, more importantly, a significant increase in protein intake in an attempt to optimize the balance between protein synthesis and breakdown. The differences from the adult include a much smaller change in total energy expenditure in the child and the lack of correlation between an increased metabolic rate and whole-body protein turnover.

Minor or moderate surgical stress is capable of significantly decreasing plasma concentrations of total amino acids.[125,126] Primarily responsible for this decrease is the reduction in the plasma concentrations of gluconeogenic amino acids, especially alanine. As mentioned earlier, Stjernstrom et al.[75] demonstrated, through catheterization studies of muscle vascular beds, that peripheral release of gluconeogenic amino acids accompanies abdominal operations. Postoperative production of gluconeogenic amino acids may be a result of skeletal muscle catabolism.[128,129] Gluconeogenesis can occur as these amino acids are selectively taken up in the splanchnic, hepatic, and renal tissues.[99,130] In contrast to the decreased systemic concentrations of gluconeogenic amino acids noted above, there is evidence for elevation of branched-chained amino acid (BCAA) concentrations in blood and within skeletal muscle.[125,126,131,132] This finding is in contrast to the decreased concentrations documented in the patient with liver disease.[133,134]

Stress-induced muscle protein catabolism results in the release of gluconeogenic amino acids, which are rapidly cleared from the blood to be metabolized by the liver and splanchnic tissue, as well as release of BCAAs into the circulation. These BCAAs are not normally metabolized in the liver but, initially, in muscle and other peripheral tissue. Anabolism is diminished in the stressed state, resulting in minimal utilization of these BCAAs.[131,135,136]

In addition to being indicators of increased proteolytic activity or altered protein metabolism, there may be a functional role for the alteration in amino acid patterns. It has been suggested that arginine may have an immunoregulatory effect as well as an effect of promoting nitrogen retention and wound healing.[137] Arginine may be important because of its effects in augmenting immune responsiveness and in diminishing protein catabolism.[138,139] Arginine is known to stimulate secretion of pituitary and pancreatic hormones.[137,140] Any of these roles may be important in the postoperative stressed state.

Studies by Clowes et al.[141] have demonstrated a nearly identical relationship between the amino acid composition of hydrolyzed muscle protein and the molar proportion of amino acids released into the bloodstream during sepsis or after trauma, implicating the breakdown of muscle protein as the source of these amino acids. A significant breakthrough in the understanding of this proteolytic response was made when Clowes et al.[142] demonstrated a circulatory peptide capable of inducing muscle proteolysis in sepsis and trauma. They suggested that the proteolysis-inducing factor they isolated from plasma is not one of the hormones usually secreted in stressful situations. They postulated that it may be a product released from leukocytes or macrophages in association with the activation of complement in the presence of infection or the tissue damage associated with trauma or surgery. This theory was substantiated by the observation that septic patients' plasma could induce proteolytic changes when incubated with normal skeletal muscle. They reiterated that the increased supply of amino acids is made available in sepsis or trauma not only for energy production or oxidation but, more importantly, to satisfy the requirements of the liver and other visceral tissue for a greatly accelerated synthesis of the protein essential for immunologic defense, healing of wounds, and maintenance of function in vital organs.

Finley et al.[143] examined the effect of major operative trauma on skeletal muscle metabolism in the adult patient receiving a constant preoperative infusion of nutrients. They noted a significant postoperative decrease in the plasma concentrations of the following amino acids: taurine, threonine, serine, glycine, alanine, citralline, amino-N-butyrate, methionine, histidine, arginine, glutamine, glutamate, and BCAAs including valine and isoleucine. There is a postoperative increase in amino acid release from a forearm muscle bed, which is made up in large part of an increase in the glycogenic amino acids serine, threonine, glycine, and alanine; by a marked increase in the release of BCAAs; and by an efflux of taurine, methionine, phenylalanine, lysine, and arginine. They suggested that the visceral production of glucose is quantitatively matched by the net uptake of glucose precursors across the splanchnic bed.[144] They noted that infused nutrients suppress visceral gluconeogenesis in these patients. Their results showed that new glucose production is lower than what is observed in the fasting human suffering from trauma.[145] Finley et al.[143] speculated that the increased release of proline, methionine, arginine, and phenylalanine from muscle may be related to higher requirements by healing wounds and an increased demand for the precursors of catecholamines.

In 1985, Hulton et al.[146] demonstrated in an animal model that hormonal blockade of the catabolic responses to surgery by phentolamine and propranolol inhibits net skeletal muscle protein catabolism without altering whole-body nitrogen loss. This fact may prove clinically useful in that hormonal blockade may attenuate the posttraumatic catabolic response, preventing accelerated skeletal muscle breakdown and body protein loss. Total-body nitrogen loss in this study was unaffected, indicating that skeletal muscle is spared at the expense of other sources of amino nitrogen. The investigators speculated that these other amino acids are derived from the viscera. It is possible that hormonal blockade could prevent the obligatory loss of skeletal muscle protein in critically ill patients. Simultaneous nutritional support might provide the amino acids necessary for acute-phase protein synthesis, gluconeogenesis, and wound repair.

Warner et al.,[147] in an experimental animal model, demonstrated that infusion of a catabolic hormone (e.g., glucagon, epinephrine, cortisol) results in increased amino acid uptake in the liver. These catabolic hormones have no effect on amino acid uptake in skeletal muscle. Total plasma amino acids are reduced in the hormone-infused animal. These investigators concluded that stress-induced elevations of catabolic hormones are, at least in part, responsible for the augmented liver amino acid uptake but that they are not responsible for the reduced muscle amino acid uptake characteristic of sepsis or severe trauma.[148]

Moyer et al.,[2] studying the critically ill adult patient who was septic or posttraumatic, examined concentrations of various plasma substances in an effort to identify plasma profiles reflective of the patient's progress. They were able to identify numerous amino acid fractional concentrations and patterns that had specific predictive value.

Studies of postoperative nitrogen balance in the term neonate originated with Rickham in 1957.[36] Since that time, several investigators have substantiated a strongly negative nitrogen balance in response to surgical stress and have demonstrated that it may persist for 72 to 96 hours.[124,149-151] These data demonstrate that the severity of the surgical stress is correlated with the degree of nitrogen loss. It has been noted that nitrogen loss postoperatively is greater in the neonatal age group than in the older infant subjected to similar degrees of surgical stress.[152,153] In a study of the neonate undergoing major or minor operative procedures, a direct relation was noted between the degree of stress and the quantity of nitrogen loss.[154]

In 1984, Zlotkin[155] published a study assessing postoperative nitrogen balance in the term neonate who had received parenteral nutrition containing nitrogen at 300 to $600 \text{mg} \cdot \text{kg}^{-1}$ 24 hours^{-1}. He demonstrated nitrogen retention in the neonate and correlated it with increasing nitrogen intake. He calculated that a nitrogen intake of $280 \text{mg} \cdot \text{kg}^{-1}$ 24 hours^{-1} would be required to duplicate the nitrogen accretion rate of a breast-fed neonate. These neonates had undergone variable degrees of surgical stress and represented a heterogeneous group. The studies were carried out at least 72 hours after surgery, a time when the major hormonal and metabolic alterations induced by operative stress have returned to baseline.

A subsequent study of 18 preterm neonates undergoing a variety of surgical procedures examined early (i.e., 0–72 hours postoperatively) changes in nitrogen retention, protein synthesis, and protein turnover.[156] One group of neonates received $2.3 \pm 0.4 \text{g}$ of amino acid·kg^{-1} day^{-1} and the other $3.9 \pm 0.5 \text{g} \cdot \text{kg}^{-1}$ day^{-1}. The investigators showed a strong correlation between nitrogen intake and net nitrogen retention. The group receiving the higher amino acid intake had significantly greater net protein synthesis rates (i.e., synthesis-breakdown). The improved nitrogen utilization in this group was achieved principally by a reduction in endogenous protein breakdown. There were no differences between the two groups in urinary creatinine or 3-methylhistidine excretion. Because these two parameters reflect skeletal muscle protein turnover, the differences between the groups in terms of nitrogen retention and protein turnover appear to be mediated through visceral protein sparing.

Another marker of endogenous protein breakdown that has received widespread attention is the molar 3-methylhistidine/creatinine ratio (3-MH/Cr).[157] The rationale for use of the 3-MH/Cr ratio is the belief that 3-methylhistidine originates from the breakdown of skeletal muscle actin and myosin. A significant series of assumptions accompany use of this ratio. First, this molecule is excreted quantitatively in the urine following its liberation from myofibrils. Second, the contribution of nonskeletal muscle (i.e., skin and gastrointestinal muscle) to the total 3-methylhistidine pool is negligible. Additionally, this amino acid is not metabolized further and is not used for de novo protein synthesis following its liberation into the circulation. Numerous studies have demonstrated that the urinary 3-MH/Cr ratio correlates closely with the net nitrogen balance in preterm and term neonates.[116,158,159] The preterm neonate, stressed by severe clinical illness and manifesting a negative nitrogen balance and weight loss at the time of study, has demonstrated a markedly elevated 3-MH/Cr ratio.[160] Additional data in the postoperative term neonate have demonstrated a significant increase in the 3-MH/Cr ratio and in nitrogen loss during the first 72 hours after surgery.[159] This finding was later confirmed by the same investigators in the preterm neonate undergoing surgery.[58] Reduction of the surgical stress responses in preterm and term neonates by using different anesthesia techniques such as halothane supplementation or fentanyl was found to inhibit these changes in the urinary 3-MH/Cr ratio.[58,59]

The most important clinical consequence of the catabolic stress reaction has been said to be the increased protein breakdown after surgery.[160] During the first few days after birth, neonates lose weight before resuming the rapid weight gain associated with intrauterine development.[116] Although much of the weight loss is water, some of it reflects the breakdown of carbohydrate and lipid stores and the relatively high rate of total body and muscle protein degradation, which may further contribute to the catabolic state.[123,161] The previous study failed to demonstrate any correlation between energy input in the premature neonate and the rate of muscle protein breakdown,[116] in contrast to the findings of Zlotkin[155] and Duffy and Pencharz.[156] Ballard et al.[116] thought it may be due in part to the size of the fat reserve, as there is evidence that ketonemia produced by fat mobilization is accompanied by a lower rate of muscle protein breakdown. They pointed out that the preterm neonate has relatively little adipose tissue and may be expected to demonstrate increased muscle protein catabolism when energy intake is minimal. They concluded by stating, "Nevertheless we consider it is not possible at the present time to reconcile all of the findings on energy restriction in such a way that an expected response on muscle protein breakdown can be stated."

Pinter[92] in 1973 examined the nonessential/essential amino acid ratio in 17 neonates undergoing surgery. He demonstrated a fall in the ratio during surgery with a gradual postoperative rise. α-Amino nitrogen demonstrated a slight, insignificant increase during surgery and remained at a constant concentration. Postoperatively, a pronounced decrease in α-amino nitrogen was observed. Due to the rise in the combined concentrations of the essential amino acids leucine, isoleucine, valine, and methionine, the nonessential/essential amino acid plasma ratio decreased. The changes in the α-amino nitrogen concentration indicate a marked redistribution of the circulating free amino acids. The rise in blood urea nitrogen observed during the early postoperative period is probably due to several factors (e.g., enhanced protein breakdown, hemoconcentration, and oliguria) which are well-known consequences of surgery.

In a later study of 29 neonates undergoing a moderate degree of surgical stress for correction of various congenital anomalies, Pinter[162] was unable to demonstrate a statistically significant change in the nonessential/essential amino acid ratio. No significant change in the α-amino nitrogen concentration was noted. They did suggest that the plasma free amino acid pool changes dramatically both during and after surgery.

From the adult studies outlined, it can be concluded that the negative nitrogen balance seen after moderate surgical stress is due mainly to a decrease in the rate of protein synthesis, whereas the rate of protein breakdown is unaltered or slightly increased. Protein metabolism in the patient exposed to severe degrees of surgery, trauma, or sepsis is characterized by a massive breakdown of tissue protein, with the protein synthesis rate being unaltered, decreased, or in some cases slightly increased.

The infant has a far greater avidity for nitrogen than the adult, and positive nitrogen balance can be readily restored by increasing nitrogen and caloric intake. The neonatal surgical data indicate that the negative nitrogen balance observed in adults is limited to the early postoperative period. Duffy and Pencharz[156] documented both an improved nitrogen balance in association with an increased nitrogen intake and postoperative nitrogen accretion, even during the 3 days immediately after surgery, but they noted that nitrogen utilization may be partially impaired postoperatively. Metabolic studies in the stable neonate in the anabolic phase after surgery (i.e., after 5 days following surgery) demonstrate that protein balance is maintained, even during a hypocaloric nutritional regimen.[56,163] Nitrogen balance can be obtained with as little as 20 kcal·kg^{-1} day^{-1} of metabolizable energy intake at the expense of continuous depletion of fat stores.[56] Protein retention correlates significantly with protein intake, total energy intake, and energy storage. Therefore, greater protein retention can be obtained by increasing either the protein or the energy intake. However, to achieve increased protein retention, it is preferable to add more energy than more protein because of the likelihood of azotemia, hyperammonemia, and metabolic acidosis in the patient receiving a high quantity of intravenous amino acids. Pierro et al.[163] have demonstrated that protein retention is almost 90% when $2\,g \cdot kg^{-1} day^{-1}$ and 75 nonprotein calories·$kg^{-1} day^{-1}$ are administered to the stable infant after at least 2 days following surgery. The influence of different energy substrates on nitrogen balance is controversial. Nitrogen retention can be enhanced by giving carbohydrate or fat, which are said to be protein sparing. Although some studies have suggested that the protein-sparing effect of carbohydrate is greater than that of fat,[164] other studies have suggested that the protein-sparing effect of fat may be either equivalent to or greater than that of carbohydrate.[163,165,166] Recent protein turnover studies utilizing stable isotope tracer techniques have shown that carbohydrate and fat have an equivalent effect on whole-body protein flux, protein synthesis, and protein breakdown[166,167] (see Chapter 34).

Fat Metabolism

The postoperative state in the adult patient produces a catabolic response that, in addition to the already-mentioned changes in carbohydrate and protein metabolism, results in the mobilization of nonesterified fatty acids (NEFAs) from adipose tissue as well as increased formation of ketone bodies. These changes may be of prime importance in providing an endogenous energy source in the posttraumatic state.

Three decades ago Allison et al.[168] documented increased plasma concentrations of NEFAs associated with decreased glucose tolerance in a group of patients suffering burn injuries. Subsequent studies by this same group in postoperative patients demonstrated an increase in plasma NEFAs.[169] This increase was noted both pre- and intraoperatively. The preoperative increase was attributed to the catabolic stimulus provided by the emotional stress of anticipating surgery. An increase of NEFAs following trauma was confirmed in 1974; the extent of the response was correlated with the severity of trauma.[170]

The importance of the contribution of fat to energy supply in a stressed state was illustrated by Kinney et al.[171] in a 1970 study in which they demonstrated, by indirect calorimetry, that as much as 75% to 90% of postoperative energy requirements are supplied by fat metabolism and the remainder is provided by protein. It may be necessary for these NEFAs to undergo conversion by the liver to ketone bodies prior to their utilization as an energy source.[172]

Lipolysis of stored triglycerides and the control of adipocyte lipolysis are important for mobilizing lipid in the injured patient. Lipolysis in the adipocyte is carried out by the hormone-sensitive lipase (HSL) enzyme.[173] This enzyme complex is affected by a number of other circulating hormones, including the catecholamines.

Forse et al.,[174] in an in vitro study, noted that with trauma the β-adrenergic responsiveness of the adipocyte and the catecholamine receptor on these cells are significantly decreased. It may be interpreted as desensitization of the β-receptors with downregulation and indicates increased in vivo lipolysis early after injury. After 4 days these changes had returned to normal.

Wolfe et al.,[175] in a study of patients suffering from severe burn injury, utilized stable isotope tracers to demonstrate changes in the substrate cycle involving the simultaneous breakdown and synthesis of stored triglycerides (i.e., triglyceride–fatty acid cycle).[175] The rates of triglyceride–fatty acid and glycolytic-gluconeogenic cycling are elevated in these patients by 450% and 250%, respectively. These investigators concluded that increased substrate cycling contributes to the increased thermogenesis and energy expenditure seen with a severe burn and that increased triglyceride–fatty acid cycling is due to β-adrenergic stimulation. The increased metabolic rate observed may be secondary to increased substrate cycling and not secondary to increased rates of protein synthesis.[176]

Because the stress response associated with surgery causes an elevation of plasma nonesterified fatty acids and decreased insulin secretion, one would expect an increased production of ketone bodies in response to operative stress. Several studies have shown that the concentration ranges from no change to a mild elevation to a substantial increase.[177-180] It has been demonstrated that the patient who remains normoketonemic after major surgery is likely to manifest an increased nitrogen loss in comparison with the patient who is hyperketonemic postoperatively.[119] Studies in the trauma patient suggest that the lack of ketogenesis is due to postinjury vasopressin release, the degree of which is directly proportional to the severity of injury.[162,172] Vasopressin may exacerbate protein catabolism and muscle wasting by suppressing ketogenesis in the patients subjected to severe trauma, major surgical stress, or sepsis.

In the human neonate, depot fat accounts for 10% to 15% of body weight. From metabolic balance data, Hughes et al.[89] calculated that only about 8% of body protein is catabolized when a 3-kg neonate is starved for 12 days, yet 39% of the neonate's fat is consumed. Because of this low metabolic conversion of protein, the ability to reduce peripheral glucose utilization would be of advantage to the starving neonate. Whether high FFA turnover can result in reduced peripheral glucose uptake remains to be confirmed. Glycerol released from adipose tissue during lipolysis could be a source for supplementation or maintenance of blood glucose concentration.

In their experimental study in perinatal rats, Mayor and Cuezva[181] noted that during the suckling period the oxidation of fatty acids, ketone body utilization, and active gluconeogenesis supply the bulk of energy and carbon components required to support the rapid growth rate during this period. This metabolic process begins with an increase in the insulin/glucagon ratio that occurs with the change to a carbohydrate-rich diet, which initiates the induction of lipogenesis at weaning.

Anand et al.[57] demonstrated an increase in blood concentrations of total ketone bodies and glycerol during neonatal surgery. They believed this increase is a reflection of catecholamine-stimulated lipolysis and ketogenesis. They noted a strong correlation between serum concentrations of glycerol and adrenaline and noradrenaline at the end of surgery. In addition to their use as an energy source, they postulated that the ketone bodies in peripheral tissues, through the formation of citrate and the inhibition of phosphofructokinase, may further inhibit the peripheral utilization of glucose and contribute to the postoperative hyperglycemia seen in the neonate.[182,183] In a study of the effectiveness of improved anesthetic management through the use of halothane, they demonstrated that concentrations of ketone bodies increase during surgery in the group not receiving halothane, but are unchanged in the group receiving halothane, with a significant difference at the end of surgery.[58] Plasma concentrations of NEFAs are significantly higher in the group not receiving halothane than in the halothane group at the end of the operation and 6 hours later. These responses indicate a greater degree of lipolysis, probably mediated by the release of catecholamines in the nonhalothane group and facilitated by the decrease in the insulin/glucagon ratio during surgery in that group. Halothane suppresses the catecholamine response, which results in decreased lipolysis and formation of NEFAs.

Further data from this study have shown that, although there is marked hyperglycemia and mobilization of gluconeogenic substrates during and after surgery, it is likely that these substrates are utilized during the perioperative period.[184] They postulated that the primary sources of energy in the surgical neonate are provided by the mobilization of NEFAs from adipose tissue and their conversion to ketone bodies in the liver. Despite this potential physiologic importance, fat metabolism in the surgical neonate and infant has undergone little study. Pinter[92] reported a substantial increase in plasma NEFA concentration during surgery with a further significant increase postoperatively, whereas Elphick and Wilkinson[91] found no significant changes in NEFAs during the preoperative period. In the later study, a decrease in plasma triglyceride concentration was documented postoperatively, whereas the plasma concentrations of lipoproteins, phospholipids, and cholesterol were unchanged during and after surgery. These responses could be altered, at least partially, by starvation, as the neonates in both the above studies received no nutritional support for variable periods before and during the study.

Studies in the term neonate have shown that circulating concentrations of NEFAs, glycerol, and total ketone bodies increase significantly during surgery, but revert to preoperative values by 6 hours postoperatively.[185] The significant increase in free fatty acids, glycerol, and total ketone bodies during surgery is indicative of lypolysis and ketogenesis, mediated by intraoperative catecholamine release, as evidenced by the strong correlation between blood glycerol and plasma adrenaline and noradrenaline concentrations at the end of surgery. An earlier study in the older infant, undergoing inguinal herniorrhaphy, documented a significant increase in plasma NEFA concentration during surgery and concluded that it is indicative of lipolysis in response to the surgical stress.[186] In contrast, in studies of the neonate undergoing various operative procedures, including cardiac surgery, blood concentrations of total ketone bodies were found to be decreased significantly at the end of surgery and remained below preoperative concentrations at 6 hours postoperatively.[57] These changes have been attributed to the effects of cardiopulmonary bypass (CPB). Two mechanisms have been postulated to account for them: (1) the substantial increase in blood glycerol concentration noted may be caused by the heparinization of blood just prior to CPB, resulting in activation of lipoprotein lipase and subsequent breakdown of plasma triglycerides; and (2) the markedly decreased hepatic circulation and decreased metabolic rate during CPB with deep hypothermia and circulatory arrest. This would prevent the utilization of glycerol for gluconeogenesis and the conversion of circulating NEFAs into ketone bodies.

In addition to serving as an energy source, studies of glycerol turnover in neonates have shown that 75% of glycerol formed from lipolysis enters the gluconeogenic pathway in the neonatal liver and contributes to 5% of hepatic glucose production.[187] The oxidation of FFAs by the neonatal liver may further stimulate postoperative gluconeogenesis through the generation of ATP to support gluconeogenesis, the production of acetyl–coenzyme A, which activates pyruvate carboxylase, and the provision of reducing equivalents for glyceraldehyde-3-phosphate dehydrogenase.[188]

In a study on patent ductus arteriosus ligation in the term and preterm neonate, there was a significant rise in blood concentrations of lactate, pyruvate, total ketone bodies, and glycerol by the end of the operative procedure. By 6 hours postoperatively the concentrations of all these metabolites had reverted to their preoperative levels.[189]

In the nonoperated neonate who has not yet been fed, the respiratory quotient, the blood glucose concentration, and the serum FFA concentration increase, indicating a rapid change from carbohydrate to fat metabolism soon after birth.[90] In addition, liver and muscle glycogen reserves are reduced, and the rate of disappearance of glucose administered by intravenous infusion is decreased.[85,189,190–192] It appears that protein is less easily utilized for energy purposes during starvation.[193,194] These findings indicate that fat, rather than protein or carbohydrate, is being used for energy production in the neonate.

In a recent study, various surgical procedures led to variable changes in the plasma concentration of FFAs.[91] In addition, 4 to 24 hours after surgery the plasma triglyceride concentration fell by an average of 25% but later rose. In this study, during starvation, plasma FFA concentration rose during the first 2 days of life and was very high between days 3 and 5. Plasma triglycerides, cholesterol, phospholipids, and total esterified fatty acids increased after birth. These data suggest that during starvation in the neonate there is rapid mobilization of fat from adipose tissue stores and a reduction in the peripheral utilization of glucose. There is no evidence to suggest any impairment of fat mobilization or metabolism even after 7 days of starvation. After surgery, even though there is more rapid mobilization of fat, the rate of utilization is greater than the rate of mobilization, resulting in variable and even reduced concentrations of the various lipids. These data led these investigators to speculate that the neonate who is of normal birth weight may be more able to cope with starvation and surgical injury than is generally realized through this rapid mobilization of stored fat.

Pinter[92] demonstrated that the average plasma FFA concentration shows a slight but significant increase at the end of surgery. At the 6th and 12th postoperative hours this increase is already more pronounced. The plasma FFA concentration shows great individual variation. Although in most cases a marked increase in plasma FFA concentration occurs, the average increase, because of the significantly different initial concentration, did not achieve statistical significance. At 24 hours postoperatively, the increase persisted. As an explanation for the occasional absence of an increase in FFA postoperatively, Pinter postulated that pronounced hyperglycemia directly or indirectly inhibits the mobilization of FFA. The fact that after surgery a rapid fall in blood glucagon concentration is accompanied by a rise in plasma FFA concentration lends support to this explanation.

Pinter,[162] in a study of 29 neonates being operated on for congenital anomalies, described their metabolic characteristics between the first and seventh postoperative day. In these investigations, a decreased FFA concentration was observed between the second and seventh days, whereas during surgery, as well as on the first postoperative day, a well-defined increase in the FFA concentration occurred, which might have been caused by the response to the anesthesia and surgery (i.e., an increased release of catecholamines and steroids, metabolic effects of anesthetics, hypoxia, hypothermia, acidosis). Although the FFA concentration showed a tendency to decrease postoperatively, it remained higher than the preoperative concentration. This pattern of fat metabolism can be explained by two factors: (1) during the postoperative period the complex hormonal and metabolic changes evoked by surgery are returning to their preoperative concentration; and (2) the state of hypoalimentation. These combined hormonal and metabolic processes, which are typical of the adaptation to extrauterine life, explain why it is difficult to find a reciprocal relation between glucose and FFA metabolism.[195,196] Elphick[197] failed to demonstrate a relation between glucose and FFA concentrations in neonates after surgery.

Studies in the adult have indicated that the concentration of circulating FFAs varies in response to surgical stress.[198] Talbert et al.'s[186] study examined neonates undergoing bilateral inguinal hernia repair. Eleven of 13 patients demonstrated a significant elevation in FFA concentration following surgery. The plasma FFAs have been identified as the major metabolite from the mobilization of body adipose tissue/depot fat to be used as an energy source.[195,199] The hydrolysis of triglycerides is the major biochemical reaction in fat stores for the production of energy precursors. Mobilization of fatty acids is mediated by three central mechanisms: metabolic, hormonal, and neural.[200] Under conditions of starvation a net release of FFAs from the peripheral fat depots is observed.

Various hormones have been demonstrated to be active in the regulation of fatty acid mobilization.[201] Among the most important of these hormonal regulators are the catecholamines. These compounds have been recognized as potent stimulants of FFA mobilization.[202] A concomitant increase in the rate of glycerol production verifies that an elevation in plasma FFAs is due to an absolute increase in the rate of hydrolysis of triglycerides. Animal experiments have emphasized the importance of this mechanism in producing postoperative elevations in plasma FFAs.[203] The importance of the innervation of fat stores in facilitating FFA mobilization has been verified by experiments with innervated and denervated tissues.[201] The sympathetic nervous system is a critical component of this process. Because norepinephrine is the chemical mediator at the postganglionic sympathetic nerve ending, the final mechanism of action may be similar to that observed following parenteral administration of this compound. The importance of this system as a mechanism for mobilizing FFAs has been documented in the adult during emotional stress.[204] It is evident that circulating concentration of FFAs are regulated by a variety of factors, many of which participate in the neonate's response to stress. The importance of this composite action is suggested in Talbert et al.'s[186] experiments, in which they demonstrated an increase in plasma FFA in the absence of a discernible increase in circulating catecholamines. Previous investigators have demonstrated an elevation of FFAs in the adult following cholecystectomy and inguinal herniorrhaphy.[198] These data substantiate the sensitivity of FFA mobilization to the stimulus of surgical trauma and suggest the usefulness of the plasma FFA concentration as an index of the neonate's stress response.

In addition to the mobilization of body fat stores, renewal of these stores has been suggested as a response to surgery. Winthrop et al.[56] showed that body fat increased postoperatively from day 0 to day 7 from 12.9% ± 0.6% to 14% ± 0.6% ($p < .05$) in 13 term neonates undergoing surgery at approximately 10 days of life. Although it is a small but statistically significant increase in body fat, the magnitude of the change falls within the range of experimental error for anthropometry. In this study, fat accounted for almost 60% of the new solid tissue synthesized, which is in agreement with Fomon et al.'s[205] figure of 56.6%[205] (see Chapter 36).

Implications

It is apparent that the adult patient demonstrates a catabolic response to the stresses induced by operative or accidental trauma. The degree of this catabolic response may be quantitatively related to the extent of the trauma or the magnitude of associated complications such as infection. The host response to infection, traumatic injury, or major operative stress is characterized by such events as fever, pituitary and stress hormone elaboration, mineral redistribution, and increased acute-phase protein synthesis.[206]

The beneficial effects of this stress response lie in providing alternate energy sources to meet metabolic demands as well as providing essential building blocks for synthetic activities that occur during the postoperative period. It has been suggested that the hyperglycemia response is essential in supplying the increased glucose requirements of injured tissue.[100] The proteolytic component of the stress response provides the necessary amino acid components for reparative protein synthesis and production of acute-phase reactants by the liver. The changes in metabolic patterns induced by the stress response are satisfied in part by increased lipolysis and ketogenesis to provide an alternate source of metabolic fuel for tissues such as the brain and skeletal muscle. Additionally, the observed gluconeogenesis may aid in maintaining the glucose supply for vital organs principally dependent on glucose.[78,207] This metabolic response has been shown to potentiate many adverse conditions during the postoperative period and to further exacerbate the stress response. Examples include a hypermetabolic state with attendant increased oxygen consumption, increased energy requirements, increased temperature, elevated cardiac output, and altered or impaired inflammatory or immune responsiveness. Numerous investigators have demonstrated that the adult patient exposed to severe degrees of traumatic stress is subjected to greatly increased complications, such as cardiac or pulmonary insufficiency, myocardial infarction, impaired hepatic or renal function, gastric stress ulcers, and sepsis. Evidence exists to suggest that this response may be life-threatening if the induced catabolic activity remains excessive or unchecked for a prolonged period. Moyer et al.[2] were able to identify with a great degree of certainty the patients who were likely to succumb based on a single analysis of a variety of plasma-borne substrates obtained up to 9 days prior to death.

It is apparent that modulating or blunting the catabolic response induced by the stress state may have beneficial effects. In studies of postoperative pain management, improved pain control resulted in reduction of postoperative nitrogen loss and shortened periods of convalescence following operation.[208,209] However, few attempts have been made to modify the response of the neonate to postoperative pain and stress. The techniques of neonatal anesthesia have been based in the past on the assumption that responses to pain and surgical stress is not clinically important in the neonate and that the use of lighter anesthesia may prevent respiratory and circulatory complications in the postoperative period.[5]

It is evident from the preceding review that the human neonate, even the one born prematurely, is capable of mounting a metabolic response to operative stress. Unfortunately, many of the areas for which a relatively well-characterized response exists in the adult are poorly documented in the neonate. As is the case in the adult, the response seems to be primarily catabolic in nature because the combined hormonal changes include increased release of catabolic hormones such as catecholamines, glucagon, and cortisol coupled with suppression of and peripheral resistance to the effects of the primary anabolic hormone insulin.

The catecholamines may be the agents of primary importance in this response and may modulate the remaining components of the hormonal response to stress as well as the metabolic changes, including inhibition of insulin release, marked hyperglycemia, and a breakdown of the neonate's stores of nutrients. These reactions result in the release of glucose, NEFAs, ketone bodies, and amino acids. Although these metabolic by-products are necessary to meet the body's altered energy needs in a time of increased metabolic demands, it is possible that a severe or prolonged response would be detrimental to a previously ill neonate with limited reserves of nutrients and already high metabolic demands imposed by rapid growth, organ maturation, and adaptation to the postnatal environment. Anand and Hickey[5] have shown that alterations in anesthesia technique with the addition of agents such as sufentanil and postoperative analgesia with high doses of opioids are able to significantly blunt this catabolic response. These investigators have shown that the neonate who received deeper anesthesia had a decreased incidence of sepsis, metabolic acidosis, disseminated intravascular coagulation, and fewer postoperative deaths in comparison with the neonate who received lighter anesthesia. It appears that modulation of the postoperative catabolic response may greatly affect the immune response.

It is hoped that future developments and the acquisition of more detailed knowledge of the response will allow modification of the stress response in postoperative neonates in order to further decrease their mortality and morbidity.

References

1. Kehlet H. Stress-free anaesthesia and surgery. Acta Anaesthesiol Scand 1979;23:503-504.
2. Moyer E, Cerra F, Chenier R, et al. Multiple systems organ failure. VI. Death predictors in the traumaseptic state—the most critical determinants. J Trauma 1981;21:862-869.
3. Rackow H, Salanitre E, Green LT. Frequency of cardiac arrest associated with anesthesia in infants and children. Pediatrics 1961;28:697-704.
4. Schweiss JF, Pennington DG. Anesthetic management of neonates undergoing palliative operations for congenital heart defects. Cleve Clin Q 1981;48:153-165.
5. Anand KJS, Hickey PR. Halothane-morphine compared with high-dose sufentanil for anesthesia and postoperative analgesia in neonatal cardiac surgery. N Engl J Med 1992;326:1-9.
6. Liebig J. Die Organische Chemie in ihrer Anwendung auf Physiologie und Pathologic. New York: Braunschweig, Wiley and Putnam, 1848.
7. Bauer J. Ilbur Zerretzungsvorgange in Thierkirper unter dem Kinflusse von Blutentziehunger. Z Biol 1872;8:567-603.
8. Malcolm JD. The physiology of death from traumatic fever; a study in abdominal surgery. Lancet 1893;1:408-410,460-462,519-521.
9. Aub JC, Wu H. Studies in experimental traumatic shock. II. Chemical changes in the blood. Am J Physiol 1920;54:416-424.
10. Bernard C. Chiens rendus diabetiques. C R Soc Biol 1849;1:60-63.
11. Bernard C. Lecons de physiologie experimentelle au College de France, Paris, 1855.
12. Bernard C. Lecons de physiologie operatoire. Paris: Baillière, 1879.
13. Brown-Séquard C.-E. Des effets produits chez l'homme par des injections souscutanées d'un liquide retire des testicules frais de cobae et de chien. C R Soc Biol 1889;9:415-454.
14. Brown-Séquard C.-E. The effects produced on man by subcutaneous injections of a liquid obtained from the testicles of animals. Lancet 1889;2:105-107.
15. Pringle H, Maunsell RCB, Pringle S. Clinical effects of ether anaesthesia on renal activity. Br Med J 1905;2:542-543.
16. Evans GH. The abuse of normal salt solutions. JAMA 1911;57:2126-2127.
17. Cannon WB. The Shattuck Lecture: the physiological factors concerned in surgical shock. Boston Med Surg J 1917;176:859-867.
18. Cannon WB. A consideration of the nature of wound shock. JAMA 1918;70:611-617.
19. Cannon WB. The wisdom of the body. New York: Norton, 1932.
20. Cuthbertson DP. The influence of prolonged muscular rest on metabolism. Biochem J 1929;23:13281-13345.
21. Cuthbertson DP. Observations on the disturbance of metabolism produced by injury to the limbs. Q J Med 1932;1:233-246.
22. Cuthbertson DP, Munro AN. A study of the effect of overfeeding on the protein metabolism of man. Biochem J 1937;31:694-705.
23. Selye H. The general adaptation syndrome and the diseases of adaptation. J Clin Endocrinol 1946;6:117-230.
24. Moore FD, Ball MR. The metabolic response to surgery. Springfield, IL: Charles C Thomas, 1952.
25. Hayes MH, Coller FA. The neuroendocrine control of water and electrolyte excretion during surgical anesthesia. Surg Gynecol Obstet 1952;95:142-149.
26. Sandberg AA, Elk-Nes K, Sammels LT, et al. The effects of surgery on the blood levels and metabolism of 17-hydroxy-corticosteroids in man. J Clin Invest 1954;33:1509-1516.
27. Hume DM, Egdahl RH. The importance of the brain in the endocrine response to injury. Ann Surg 1959;150:697-712.
28. Von Bezold A. Untersuchungen über die Vertheilung von Wasser, organischer Materie und anorganischen Verbindugen in Thierreiche. Z Wissensch Zool 1857;8:487-524.
29. Von Bezold A. Das Chemische Shebett der Wirkelthiere. Z Wissensch Zool 1858;9:240-269.
30. Ylppo A. Neugehofenen-, Hunger- und Intoxikatations Acidosis in ihren Bezichungen Zueinander. Z Kinderheilkd 1916;14:268-448.
31. Marples F, Lippard VW. Acid-base balance of newborn infants. II. Consideration of the low alkaline reserve of normal newborn infants. Am J Dis Child 1932;44:31-39.
32. Marples E, Lippard VW. Acid-base balance of newborn infants. III. Influence of cow's milk on the acid base balance of the blood of newborn infants. Am J Dis Child 1933;45:294-306.

33. Marriott WM. Some phases of the pathology of nutrition in infancy. Harvey Lect 1919;15:121–151.
34. Moore RM. Acute intestinal obstruction in infants and children: physiological and pathological considerations. Miss Doctor 1946;23:554–556.
35. Santulli TV. Intestinal obstruction in the newborn infant. J Pediatr 1954;44:317–337.
36. Rickham PP. The metabolic response to neonatal surgery. Cambridge: Harvard University Press, 1957.
37. Cuthbertson DP. Post-shock metabolic response. Lancet 1942;1:433–437.
38. Cuthbertson DP. Protein metabolism in relation to energy needs. Metabolism 1959;8:787–808.
39. Carli F, Aber VR. Thermogenesis after major elective surgical procedures. Br J Surg 1987;74:1041–1045.
40. Elwyn DH, Kinney JM, Askanazy J. Energy expenditure in surgical patients. Surg Clin North Am 1981;61:545–556.
41. Kinney JM. Assessment of energy metabolism in health and disease. Columbus, OH: Ross Laboratories, 1980.
42. Long CL, Schaffel N, Geiger JW, et al. Metabolic response to injury and illness: estimation of energy and protein needs from indirect calorimetry and nitrogen balance. J Parenteral Enteral Nutr 1979;3:452–456.
43. Caldwell FT, Hammell HT, Dolan F. Determination of energy balance following thermal burns by using gradient calorimetry. Surg Forum 1965;16:486–488.
44. Wilmore DW, Long JM, Mason AD, et al. Catecholamines: mediator of the hypermetabolic response to thermal injury. Ann Surg 1974;180:653–668.
45. Wilmore DW, Aulick LH, Mason AD, Pruitt BA. Influence of the burn wound on local and systemic responses to injury. Ann Surg 1977;186:444–458.
46. Wilmore DW. The wound as an organ. In: Little RA, Frayn KN, eds. The scientific basis for the care of the critically ill. Manchester, UK: Manchester University Press, 1986:45–49.
47. Fellows IW, Bennett T, MacDonald IA. The effect of adrenaline upon cardiovascular and metabolic functions in man. Clin Sci 1985;69:215–222.
48. Frayn KN, Little RA, Maycock PF, Stonor HB. The relationship of plasma catecholamines to acute metabolic and hormonal responses to injury in man. Circ Shock 1985;16:229–240.
49. Jaattela A, Alho A, Avikainen V, et al. Personal communication.
50. Marchuk JB, Finley RJ, Groves AC, et al. Catabolic hormones and substrate patterns in septic patients. J Surg Res 1977;23:177–182.
51. Sjostrom L, Schutz Y, Gudinchet F, et al. Epinephrine sensitivity with respect to metabolic rate and other variables in women. Am J Physiol 1983;245:E431–E442.
52. Ito T, Iyomasa Y, Inoue T. Changes of the postoperative minimal oxygen consumption of the newborn. J Pediatr Surg 1976;11:495–503.
53. Groner JI, Brown MF, Stallings VA, et al. Resting energy expenditure in children following major operative procedures. J Pediatr Surg 1989;24(8):825–828.
54. Shanbhogue RLK, Jackson M, Lloyd DA. Operation does not increase resting energy expenditure in the neonate. J Pediatr Surg 1991;26:578–580.
55. Shanbhogue RLK, Lloyd DA. Absence of hypermetabolism after operation in the newborn infant. J Parenter Enteral Nutr 1992;16:333–336.
56. Winthrop AL, Jones PJH, Schoeller DA, et al. Changes in the body composition of the surgical infant in the early postoperative period. J Pediatr Surg 1987;22:546–549.
57. Anand KJS, Brown MI, Causon RC, et al. Can the human neonate mount an endocrine and metabolic response to surgery? J Pediatr Surg 1985;20:41–48.
58. Anand KJS, Sippell MA, Aynsley-Green A. Randomised trial of fentanyl anaesthesia in preterm babies undergoing surgery: effects on the stress response. Lancet 1987;1:243–248.
59. Anand KJS, Sippell WG, Schofield NM, et al. Does halothane anaesthesia decrease the metabolic and endocrine stress response of newborn infants undergoing operation? Br Med J 1988;296:668–672.
60. Ward-Platt MP, Tarbit MJ, Aynsley-Green A. The effects of anesthesia and surgery on metabolic homeostasis in infancy and childhood. J Pediatr Surg 1990;25:472–478.
61. Jones MO, Pierro A, Hammond P, Lloyd DA. The metabolic response to operative stress in infants. J Pediatr Surg 1993;28:1258–1263.
62. Jones MO, Pierro A, Hashim IA, et al. Postoperative changes in resting energy expenditure and interleukin-6 in infants. Br J Surg 1994;81:536–538.
63. Csontos K, Rust M, Hollt V, et al. Elevated plasma β-endorphin levels in pregnant women and their neonates. Life Sci 1979;25:835–844.
64. Facchinetti F, Bagnoli F, Bracci R, Genazzani AR. Plasma opioids in the first hours of life. Pediatr Res 1982;16:95–98.
65. Chwals WJ, Letton RW, Jamie A, Charles B. Stratification of injury severity using energy expenditure response in surgical infants. J Pediatr Surg 1995;30:1161–1164.
66. Albanese CT, Nour BM, Rowe MI. Anesthesia blocks nonshivering thermogenesis in the neonatal rabbit. J Pediatr Surg 1994;29:983–986.
67. Ohlson KBE, Mohell N, Cannon B, et al. Thermogenesis in brown adipocytes is inhibited by volatile anesthetic agents. A factor contributing to hypothermia in infants? Anesthesiology 1994;81:176–183.
68. Nour BM, Boudreauz JP, Rowe MI. An experimental model to study thermogenesis in the neonatal surgical patient. J Pediatr Surg 1984;19:764–770.
69. Fasoli L, Okada Y, Quant PA, Pierro A. Intraoperative stress causes a different thermogenic and metabolic response in infants compared to children. Personal communication.
70. Brand MD. The proton leak across the mitochondrial inner membrane. Biochim Biophys Acta 1990;1018:128–133.
71. Rolfe DFS, Hulbert AJ, Brand MD. Characteristics of mitochondrial proton leak and control of oxidative phosphorylation in the major oxygen-consuming tissues of the rat. Biochim Biophys Acta 1994;1188:405–416.
72. Brand MD, Chien LF, Ainscow EK, et al. The causes and functions of mitochondrial proton leak. Biochim Biophys Acta 1994;1187:132–139.
73. Valcarce C, Vitorica J, Satrústegui J, et al. Rapid postnatal developmental changes in the passive proton permeability

of the inner membrane in rat liver mitochondria. J Biochem 1990;108:642–645.
74. Watters JM, Bessey PQ, Dinarello CA, et al. Both inflammatory and endocrine mediators stimulate host response to sepsis. Arch Surg 1986;121:179–190.
75. Stjernstrom H, Jorfeldt L, Wiklund L. The influence of abdominal surgical trauma upon the turnover of some blood borne metabolites in the human leg. J Parenter Enteral Nutr 1981;5:207–214.
76. Ross H, Johnston IDA, Welborn TA, et al. Effect of abdominal operation on glucose tolerance and serum levels of insulin, growth hormone and hydrocortisone. Lancet 1966;2:563–566.
77. Wright PD, Henderson K, Johnston IDA. Glucose utilization and insulin secretion during surgery in man. Br J Surg 1974;61:5–8.
78. Wilmore DW. Glucose metabolism following severe injury. J Trauma 1981;21:705–707.
79. Alberti KGMM, Batstone GF, Foster KJ, et al. Relative role of various hormones mediating the metabolic response to injury. J Parenter Enteral Nutr 1980;4:141–146.
80. Bromage PR, Shibata HR, Willoughby HW. Influence of prolonged epidural blockade on blood sugar and cortisol response to operations upon the upper part of the abdomen and thorax. Surg Gynecol Obstet 1971;132:1051–1056.
81. Kusaka M, Ui M. Activation of the Cori cycle by epinephrine. Am J Physiol 1977;232:E145–E155.
82. Mills NL, Beaudet RL, lsom OW, et al. Hyperglycaemia during cardiopulmonary bypass. Ann Surg 1973;177:203–205.
83. Benedict FG, Talbot FB. The physiology of the newborn infant: character and amount of the catabolism. Carnegie Institute Publ. No. 233, Washington, DC, 1915.
84. Shelley HJ. Glycogen reserves and their changes at birth and in anoxia. Br Med Bull 1961;17:137–143.
85. Cornblath M, Ganzon AF, Nicolopoulos D, et al. Studies of carbohydrate metabolism in the newborn infant. III. Some factors influencing the capillary blood sugar and the response to glucagon during the first hours of life. Pediatrics 1961;27:378–389.
86. Novak M, Metichar V, Hahn P, et al. Levels of lipids in the blood of newborn infants and the effect of glucose administration. Physiol Bohemoslov 1961;10:488–492.
87. Persson B, Gentz J. The pattern of blood lipids, glycerol and ketone bodies during the neonatal period, infancy and childhood. Acta Paediatr Scand 1966;55:353–362.
88. Widdowson EM, Spray CM. Chemical development in-utero. Arch Dis Child 1951;26:205–214.
89. Hughes EA, Stevens LH, Wilkinson AW. Some aspects of starvation in the newborn baby. Arch Dis Child 1964;39:598–604.
90. Elphick MC, Wilkinson AW. Glucose intolerance in newborn infants undergoing surgery for alimentary tract anomalies. Lancet 1968;2:539–554.
91. Elphick MC, Wilkinson AW. The effects of starvation and surgical injury on the plasma levels of glucose, free fatty acids, and neutral lipids in newborn babies suffering from various congenital anomalies. Pediatr Res 1981;15:313–318.
92. Pinter A. The metabolic effects of anesthesia and surgery in the newborn infant. Z Kinderchir 1973;12:149–162.
93. Elphick MC. The effect of starvation and injury on the utilization of glucose in newborn rabbits. Biot Neonate 1971;17:399–409.
94. Pinter A, Schafer J. Metabolic effects of anesthesia and surgery newborn: blood glucose, plasma free fatty acids, free amino acid and blood lactate level in newborn puppies. Acta Paediatr Acad Sci Hung 1973;14:85–90.
95. Letton RW, Chwals WJ, Jamie A, Charles B. Early postoperative alterations in infant energy use increase the risk of overfeeding. J Pediatr Surg 1995;30:988–992.
96. Kalhan SC, Bier DM, Savin SM, et al. Estimation of glucose turnover and ^{13}C recycling in the human newborn by simultaneous [1-^{13}C]glucose and [6.6-$^{2}H_2$]glucose tracers. J Clin Endocrinol Metab 1980;50:456–460.
97. Kalhan SC, D'Angelo LJ, Savin S, et al. Glucose production in pregnant women at term gestation: sources of glucose for human fetus. J Clin Invest 1979;63:388–394.
98. Marsac C, Saudubray JM, Moncion A, et al. Development of gluconeogenic enzymes in the liver of human newborns. Biol Neonate 1976;28:317–325.
99. Gump FE, Long CL, Geiger JW, et al. The significance of altered gluconeogenesis in surgical catabolism. J Trauma 1975;15:704–712.
100. Im MJC, Hoopes JE. Energy metabolism in healing skin wounds. J Surg Res 1970;10:459–466.
101. Finberg L. Dangers to infants caused by changes in osmolal concentration. Pediatrics 1967;40:1031–1034.
102. Arant BS, Gooch WM. Effects of acute hyperglycemia on the central nervous system of neonatal puppies. Pediatr Res 1978;12:549A.
103. Bent IM, Paterson JL, Mashiter K, et al. Effects of high-dose fentanyl anesthesia on the established metabolic and endocrine response to surgery. Anesthesia 1984;39:19–23.
104. Walsh ES, Traynor C, Paterson JL, et al. Effect of different intraoperative fluid regimens on circulating metabolites and insulin during abdominal surgery. Br J Anaesth 1983;55:135–140.
105. Bunker JP. Metabolic acidosis during anesthesia and surgery. Anesthesiology 1962;23:107–123.
106. Felig P, Pozefsky T, Marliss E, et al. Alanine: key role in gluconeogenesis. Science 1970;167:1003–1004.
107. Reisner SH, Aranda JV, Colle E, et al. The effect of intravenous glucagon on plasma amino acids in the newborn. Pediatr Res 1973;7:184–191.
108. DeLamater PV, Sperling MA, Fiser RH, et al. Plasma alanine: relation to plasma glucose, glucagon and insulin in the neonate. J Pediatr 1974;85:702–706.
109. Studley HO. Percentage of weight loss: a basic indicator of surgical risk in patients with chronic peptide ulcer. JAMA 1936;106:458–460.
110. Christensen J, Kehlet H. Postoperative fatigue and changes and nutritional status. Br J Surg 1985;71:473–476.
111. Cuthbertson DP. The disturbance of metabolism produced by bony and nonbony injury, with notes on certain abnormal conditions of bone. Biochem J 1930;24:1244–1263.

112. Duke JH, Jorgensen SB, Broell JR, et al. Contribution of protein to caloric expenditure following injury. Surgery 1970;68:168–174.
113. Ryan NT. Metabolic adaptations for energy production during trauma and sepsis. Surg Clin North Am 1976;56:1073–1090.
114. McMenamy RH, Birkhahn R, Oswald G, et al. Multiple systems organ failure. I. The basal state. J Trauma 1981;21:99–114.
115. Coran AG. Nutrition of the surgical patient. In: Welch KJ, ed. Pediatric surgery. 4th ed. Chicago: Year Book, 1986:96–108.
116. Ballard EJ, Tomas FM, Pope LM, et al. Muscle protein degradation in premature human infants. Clin Sci 1979;57:535–544.
117. Fleck A. Protein metabolism after surgery. Proc Nutr Soc 1980;39:125–132.
118. Johnston IDA. Endocrine aspects of the metabolic response to surgical operation. Ann R Coll Surg Engl 1964;35:270–286.
119. Rich AJ, Wright PD. Ketosis and nitrogen excretion in undernourished surgical patients. J Parenter Enteral Nutr 1979;3:350–354.
120. Wannemacher RW, Dinterman RE. Total body protein catabolism in starved and infected rats. Am J Clin Nutr 1977;30:1510–1511.
121. Ogata ES, Foung SKH, Holliday MA. The effects of starvation and refeeding on muscle protein synthesis and catabolism in the young rat. J Nutr 1978;108:759–765.
122. Marliss EB, Murray FT, Nakhooda AF. The metabolic response to hypocaloric protein diets in obese man. J Clin Invest 1978;62:468–479.
123. Tomas FM, Ballard FJ, Pope LM. Age dependent changes in the rate of myofibrillar protein degradation in humans as assessed by 3-methylhistidine and urinative excretion. Clin Sci 1979;56:341–346.
124. Colle E, Paulsen EP. Response of the newborn infant to major surgery. I. Effects on water, electrolyte, and nitrogen balance. Pediatrics 1959;23:1063–1084.
125. Johnston IDA, Dale G, Craig RP, et al. Plasma amino acid concentrations in surgical patients. J Parenter Enteral Nutr 1980;4:161–164.
126. Vinnars E, Bergstrom J, Furst P. Influence of postoperative state on the intracellular free amino acids in human muscle tissue. Ann Surg 1975;182:665–671.
127. Elia M, Ilic V, Bacon S, et al. Relationship between the basal blood alanine concentration and the removal of an alanine load in various clinical states in man. Clin Sci 1980;58:301–304.
128. Karl IE, Garber AI, Kipnis DM. Alanine and glutamine synthesis and release from skeletal muscle. J Biol Chem 1976;251:844–860.
129. Muhlbacher F, Kapadia CF, Colpoys MF, et al. Effects of glucocorticoids on glutamine metabolism in skeletal muscle. Am J Physiol 1984;10:E75–E83.
130. Lund P, Williamson DH. Inter-tissue nitrogen fluxes. Br Med Bull 1985;41:251–256.
131. Dale G, Young G, Latner AL, et al. The effect of surgical operation on venous plasma amino acids. Surgery 1977;81:295–301.
132. Wedge JH, DeCampos R, Kerr A. Branched-chain amino acids: nitrogen excretion and injury in man. Clin Sci Mol Med 1976;50:393–399.
133. Fischer JE, Yoshimura N, Aguire A, et al. Plasma amino acids in patients with hepatic encephalopathy. Am J Surg 1974;127:40–47.
134. Ansley JD, Issacs JW, Rikkers LF, et al. Quantitative tests on nitrogen metabolism in cirrhosis in relation to other manifestations of liver disease. Gastroenterology 1978;75:570–579.
135. McMenamy RM, Shoemaker WC, Richmond JE, et al. Uptake and metabolism of amino acids by the dog liver perfused in situ. Am J Physiol 1962;202:407–414.
136. Elia M, Farrell R, Ilic V, et al. The removal of infused leucine after injury, starvation and other conditions in man. Clin Sci 1980;59:275–283.
137. Barbul A. Arginine: biochemistry, physiology and therapeutic implications. J Parenter Enteral Nutr 1986;10:227–238.
138. Saito H, Trockic O, Wang S, et al. Metabolic and immune effects of dietary arginine supplementation after burn. Arch Surg 1987;122:784–789.
139. Sitren HS, Fisher H. Nitrogen retention in rats fed on diets enriched with arginine and glycine. I. Improved N retention after trauma. Br J Nutr 1977;37:195–208.
140. Mulloy AL, Kari FW, Visek WJ. Dietary arginine, insulin secretion, glucose tolerance and liver lipids during repletion of protein depleted rats. Horm Metab Res 1982;14:471–475.
141. Clowes JHA Jr, Randall HT, Cha CJ. Amino acid and energy metabolism in septic and traumatized patients. J Parenter Enteral Nutr 1980;4:195–205.
142. Clowes JHA, George BC, Villee CA, et al. Muscle proteolysis induced by a circulating peptide in patients with sepsis or trauma. N Engl J Med 1983;308:545–552.
143. Finley RJ, Inculet RI, Pace R, et al. Major operative trauma increases peripheral amino acid release during the steady-state infusion of total parenteral nutrition in man. Surgery 1986;99:491–499.
144. Garber AJ, Menzel PH, Boden G, et al. Hepatic ketogenesis and gluconeogenesis in humans. J Clin Invest 1971;54:981–989.
145. Wilmore DW, Goodwin CW, Aulick LH, et al. Effect of injury and infection on visceral metabolism and circulation. Ann Surg 1980;192:491–504.
146. Hulton N, Johnson DJ, Smith RJ, et al. Hormonal blockade modifies post-traumatic protein catabolism. J Surg Res 1985;39:310–315.
147. Warner BW, James JH, Hasselgren PO, et al. Effect of catabolic hormone infusion on organ amino acid uptake. J Surg Res 1987;42:418–424.
148. Hasselgren PO, James JH, Fischer JE. Inhibited muscle amino acid uptake in sepsis. Ann Surg 1986;203:360–365.
149. Knutrud O. The water and electrolyte metabolism in the newborn child after major surgery. Oslo: Universitetsforiaget, 1965.
150. Hughes EA, Stevens LH, Toms DA, et al. Esophageal atresia: metabolic effects of operation. Br J Surg 1965;52:403–410.

151. Wilkinson AW, Hughes EA, Stevens LH. Neonatal duodenal obstruction: the influence of treatment on the metabolic effects of operation. Br J Surg 1965;52:410–424.
152. Sukarochano K, Motai Y, Slim M, et al. Postoperative protein metabolism in pediatric surgery. Surg Gynecol Obstet 1965;121:79–90.
153. Grewal RS, Mampilly J, Misra TR. Postoperative protein metabolism and electrolyte changes in pediatric surgery. Int Surg 1969;51:142–148.
154. Greenall MJ, Kettlewell MGW, Gouch MH. Nitrogen requirements for postoperative parenteral nutrition in neonates. Acta Ther 1983;9:5–10.
155. Zlotkin SH. Intravenous nitrogen intake requirements in full-term newborns undergoing surgery. Pediatrics 1984;73:493–496.
156. Duffy B, Pencharz P. The effects of surgery on the nitrogen metabolism of parenterally fed human neonates. Pediatr Res 1986;20:32–35.
157. Young VR, Munro HN. N T-methylhistidine (3-methylhistidine) and muscle protein turnover; an overview. Fed Proc 1978;37:2291–2300.
158. Burgoyne JL, Ballard FJ, Tomas FM, et al. Measurements of myofibrillar protein breakdown in newborn human infants. Clin Sci 1982;63:421–427.
159. Anand KJS. Metabolic and endocrine effects of surgery and anesthesia in the human newborn infant. Doctoral thesis, University of Oxford, 1985.
160. Seashore JH, Huszar G, Davis EM. Urinary 3-methylhistidine/creatinine ratio as a clinical tool: correlation between 3-methylhistidine excretion and metabolic and clinical states in healthy and stressed premature infants. Metabolism 1981;30:959–969.
161. Pencharz PB, Steffee WP, Cochran W, et al. Protein metabolism in human neonates: nitrogen balance studies, estimated obligatory losses of nitrogen and whole-body turnover of nitrogen. Clin Sci Mol Med 1977;52:485–498.
162. Pinter A. Metabolic changes in newborn infants following surgical operations. Acta Pediatr Acad Sci Hung 1975;16:171–180.
163. Pierro A, Carnielli V, Filler RM, et al. Characteristics of protein sparing effect of total parenteral nutrition in the surgical infant. J Pediatr Surg 1988;23:538–542.
164. Chessex P, Gagne G, Pineault M, et al. Metabolic consequences of changing from high glucose to high fat regimens in parenterally fed newborn infants. J Pediatr 1989;115:992–997.
165. Pineault M, Chessex P, Bisaillon S, Brisson G. Total parenteral nutrition in the newborn: impact of the quality of infused energy on nitrogen metabolism. Am J Clin Nutr 1988;47:298–304.
166. Pencharz P, Beesley J, Sauer P, et al. Total body protein turnover in parenterally fed neonates: effects of energy source studied by using 15 N glycine and 13 C leucine. Am J Clin Nutr 1989;50:1395–1400.
167. Pierro, 1995. Unpublished observations.
168. Allison SP, Hinton P, Chamberlain MJ. Intravenous glucose tolerance, insulin and free fatty acid levels in burned patients. Lancet 1968;1:1113–1116.
169. Allison SP, Tomlin PJ, Chamberlain MJ. Some effects of anaesthesia and surgery on carbohydrate and fat metabolism. Br J Anaesth 1969;41:588–593.
170. Meguid MM, Brennan MF, Aoki TT, et al. Hormone substrate interrelationships following trauma. Arch Surg 1974;109:776–783.
171. Kinney JM, Duke JH, Long CL, et al. Tissue fuel and weight loss after injury. J Clin Pathol 1970;23:65–72.
172. Williamson DH. Regulation of ketone body metabolism and the effects of injury. Acta Chir Scand Suppl 1981;52:22–29.
173. Steinberg D, Khoo JC. Hormone sensitive lipase of adipose tissue. Fed Proc 1977;36:1986–1990.
174. Forse RA, Leibel R, Askanazi J, et al. Adrenergic control of adipocyte lipolysis in trauma and sepsis. Ann Surg 1987;206:744–751.
175. Wolfe RR, Herndon DN, Jahoor F, et al. Effect of severe burn injury on substrate cycling by glucose and fatty acids. N Engl J Med 1987;317:403–408.
176. Wolfe RR, Herndon DN, Peters EJ, et al. Regulation of lipolysis in severely burned children. Ann Surg 1987;206:214–221.
177. Cooper GM, Holdcroft A, Hall GM, et al. Epidural analgesia and the metabolic response to surgery. Can Anaesth Soc J 1979;26:381–385.
178. Foster KJ, Alberti KGMM, Binder C, et al. Lipid metabolites and nitrogen balance after abdominal surgery in man. Br J Surg 1979;66:242–245.
179. Oppenheim WL, Williamson DH, Smigh R. Early biochemical changes and severity of injury in man. J Trauma 1980;20(2):135–140.
180. Kehlet HI, Brandt MR, Hansen AP, et al. Effect of epidural analgesia on metabolic profiles during and after surgery. Br J Surg 1979;66:543–546.
181. Mayor F, Cuezva JM. Hormonal and metabolic changes in the perinatal period. Biol Neonate 1985;48:185–196.
182. Anand KJS, Aynsley-Green A. Metabolic and endocrine effects of surgical ligation of patent ductus arteriosus in the human preterm neonate: Are there implications for further improvement of postoperative outcome? Mod Probl Pediatr 1985;23:143–157.
183. Williamson DH. The production and utilization of ketone bodies in the neonate: In: Jones CT, ed. Biochemical development of the fetus and neonate. Amsterdam: Elsevier, 1982:621–650.
184. Anand KJS. Hormonal and metabolic functions of neonates and infants undergoing surgery. Curr Opin Cardiol 1986;1:681–689.
185. Anand KJS, Brown MJ, Bloom SR, et al. Studies on the hormonal regulation of fuel metabolism in the human newborn infant undergoing anesthesia and surgery. Horm Res 1985;22:115–128.
186. Talbert JL, Karmen A, Graystone JE, et al. Assessment of the infants response to stress. Surgery 1967;61:626–633.
187. Bougneres PF, Karl IE, Hillman LS, et al. Lipid transport in the human newborn: palmitate and glycerol turnover and the contribution of glycerol to neonatal hepatic glucose output. J Clin Invest 1982;70:262–270.

188. Williamson JR. Role of anion transport in the regulation of metabolism. In: Hanson RW, Mehlman MA, eds. Gluconeogenesis, its regulation in mammalian species. New York: Wiley, 1976:165–220.
189. Shelley HJ. Carbohydrate reserves in the newborn infant. Br Med J 1964;1:273–275.
190. Heard CRC, Stewart RJC. Protein malnutrition and disorders of the endocrine glands: biochemical changes. Acta Endocrinol Suppl (Copenh) 1960;51:1277–1278.
191. Baird JD, Farquhar JW. Insulin-secreting capacity in newborn infants of normal and diabetic women. Lancet 1962;1:71–74.
192. Bowie MD, Mulligan PB, Schwartz R. Intravenous glucose tolerance in the normal newborn infant: the effects of a double dose of glucose and insulin. Pediatrics 1963;31:590–598.
193. Hahn P, Koldovsky O. Utilization of nutrients during postnatal development. New York: Pergamon Press, 1966.
194. McCance PA, Strangeways WMB. Protein catabolism and oxygen consumption during starvation in infants, young adults and old men. Br J Nutr 1954;8:21–32.
195. Dole VP. A relation between non-esterified fatty acids in plasma and the metabolism of glucose. J Clin Invest 1956;35:150–154.
196. Randle PJ, Garland PB, Hales CN, et al. The glucose fatty-acid cycle: its role in insulin sensitivity and the metabolic disturbances of diabetes mellitus. Lancet 1963;1:785–789.
197. Elphick MC. Some aspects of fat and carbohydrate metabolism in the newborn. PhD thesis, London, 1972.
198. Wadstrom LB. Plasma lipids and surgical trauma: a methodological, experimental and clinical study. Acta Chir Scand Suppl 1959;238:1–19.
199. Gordon RS, Cherkes A. Unesterified fatty acid in human blood plasma. J Clin Invest 1956;35:206–212.
200. Steinberg D. Catecholamine stimulation of fat mobilization and its metabolic consequences. Pharmacol Rev 1966;18:217–235.
201. Vaughan M, Steinberg D. Effect of hormones on lipolysis and esterification of free fatty acids during incubation of adipose tissue in vitro. J Lipid Res 1963;4:193–199.
202. Steinberg D. Fatty acid mobilization—mechanisms of regulation and metabolic consequences. In: Grant JK, ed. The control of lipid metabolism. Orlando, FL: Academic Press, 1963:111–143.
203. Carlson LA, Liljedahl SO. Lipid metabolism and trauma. Acta Med Scand 1963;173:25–34.
204. Bogdonoff MD, Estes EH, Trout D. Acute effect of physiologic stimuli upon plasma nonesterified fatty acid level. Proc Soc Exp Biol Med 1959;100:503–504.
205. Fomon SJ, Haschke F, Zeigler EE, et at. Body composition of reference children from birth to age 10 years. Am J Clin Nutr 1982;35:1169–1175.
206. Bessey PQ, Watters JM, Aoki TT, et al. Combined hormonal infusion stimulates the metabolic response to injury. Ann Surg 1984;200:264–288.
207. Elliott M, Albert KGMM. The hormonal and metabolic response to surgery and trauma. In: Kleinberger G. Deutsch E, eds. New aspects of clinical nutrition. Basel: Karger, 1983:247–270.
208. Kerri-Szanto M. Demand analgesia. Br J Anesth 1983;55:919–920.
209. Brandt MR, Fernandez A, Mordhurst R, et al. Epidural analgesia improves postoperative nitrogen balance. Br Med J 1978;1:1106–1108.

51
Nutritional Support of the Neonate I: Alternate Fuels and Routes of Administration

Jane P. Balint and Robert M. Kliegman

Since the advent of modern neonatal intensive care we have witnessed the survival of many critically ill very low birth weight (VLBW) neonates. Many of the technical advances that have contributed to the improved survival of these neonates have been focused on the treatment of cardiopulmonary disease. These important intensive care technologies include state of the art ventilators, medical or surgical therapy for patent ductus arteriosus, and surfactant therapy of respiratory distress syndrome.[1-3]

The approach to the nutritional support of these technology dependent VLBW neonates has been partially impeded by the very nature of the technological advances (e.g., endotracheal intubation, general anesthesia/surgery, extracorporeal membrane oxygenation, drugs used to support the infant with multisystem organ failure), by the immaturity of the premature neonate's gastrointestinal system, by the developmentally related intolerance to various nutrients, and by poorly evaluated feeding regimens. These problems have resulted in a group of nutritional disorders due to specific nutrient deficiencies or excesses (Table 51.1). (See chapters in Section V for evaluation of specific deficiencies.) Among the most critically ill technology-dependent chronic patients in neonatal intensive care units (NICU), the incidence of malnutrition approaches 25%.

Considering the recognized importance of nutritional support for these critically ill neonates, it is interesting to note the many controversies and unresolved issues related to the nutritional approach to the VLBW neonate (Table 51.2). Some of these controversies may be due to an uncertainty of the appropriate reference standard for postnatal growth. The nutritional requirements and the actual tissue composition that constitutes normal extrauterine growth of the VLBW neonate have not been determined.

The marked differences between the in utero and extrauterine environments, the immaturity of metabolic homeostasis, the excretory systems, and the digestion processes, and the stresses of being critically ill explain many of the nutritional disorders in the VLBW neonate. Extrauterine growth is not always able to parallel the intrauterine growth characteristics of the fetus had it remained in utero. One reasonable goal for the alimentation of the VLBW neonate is to provide sufficient, safe quantities of nutrients to support extrauterine growth without producing adverse effects related to the function and growth of individual organ systems. During the acute stressful illness (usually birth through 3–5 days of life), the goal is to prevent excessive catabolism and nutritional deficiencies. Thereafter, the goal is to support nutrient retention and growth.[4]

Historical Perspective of Neonatal Feeding

At the turn of the 20th century, nutrition and the provision of a warm environment were the principal methods of care for the premature neonate. During the period 1910–1930 wet nurses provided human milk for those premature neonates who survived long enough to receive enteral alimentation.[2] During 1940–1950 pediatricians who cared for sick premature neonates became concerned about the potential risks of oral alimentation with milk. These physicians worried that milk feedings could cause aspiration pneumonia, abdominal distention, cyanosis, or diarrhea. The practice at this time kept the sickest and smallest neonates without nutrition or water for longer periods than the healthier, larger neonates. It was during the decade beginning in 1960 that physicians conducted carefully controlled clinical investigations that documented the safety of early alimentation and reported the complications of fasting and thirsting.[3,5-8] The immediate adverse effects of these practices included dehydration (hyperbilirubinemia, azotemia, oliguria, hypernatremia, and fever in term neonates) and the metabolic effects of substrate deficiency (hypoglycemia, hypothermia, decreased oxygen consumption, gas-

TABLE 51.1. Potential nutritional disorders of very low birth weight neonates.

Nutritional factor	Disorder
Deficiencies	
Fluids	Hypernatremia, hyperbilirubinemia, azotemia, oliguria, hypothermia, weight loss
Glucose	Hypoglycemia, hypothermia, weight loss
Protein	Hypoalbuminemia
Sodium	Hyponatremia
Calcium	Osteopenia
Phosphorus	Osteopenia
Vitamin D	Osteopenia
Linoleic acid	Essential fatty acid deficiency
Linolenic acid	Abnormal neuroretinal development
Vitamin E	Anemia, edema, neuronal damage
Zinc	Dermatitis, diarrhea, poor growth, immune dysfunction
Vitamin K	Hemorrhage
Carnitine	Decreased ketogenesis
Excesses	
Fluids	PDA, BPD
Glucose	Hyperglycemia, potential osmotic diuresis, sepsis, increased CO_2 production
Calories	Increased resting metabolic rate, increased adipose tissue deposition
Protein	Increased BUN, abnormal plasma aminogram, hyperammonemia, acidosis
Calcium	Milk-bolus intestinal obstruction
MCT oil	Bezoars, diarrhea, emesis, distention
Intralipid	High prostaglandin levels, hypertriglyceridemia, impaired host defense (sepsis?)
Vitamin E	Infection (NEC?)
Iron	Hemolysis
Carnitine	Enhanced lipolysis, increased oxygen consumption

TABLE 51.2. Issues in neonatal feeding.

How—Enteral (nasojejunal, nasogastric, nipple) vs IV
When—Early vs late enteral feeds
Frequency—Continuous vs bolus (q1,2,3h) enteral feeds
Which food—Human milk vs special formula
To supplement—Protein, calories, minerals, vitamins
Growth standard—In utero vs postnatal growth curves
Avoiding adverse effects—Iatrogenesis; well meaning but untested therapies vs randomized controlled clinical trials

trointestinal mucosal atrophy). The long-term consequences of poor nutrition include reduced tissue growth (e.g., lung), respiratory muscle weakness, immunodeficiency with increased risk of infection, and compromised neurodevelopmental potential.[9]

Developmental Aspects of Fasting Energy Metabolism

The metabolic alterations during fasting have been determined in adult humans, who serve as an important comparison to the fasted term and VLBW neonate.[10,11] The neonate often demonstrates more severe abnormalities of fasting metabolism than the adult. The abnormal metabolic control of the neonate may be due to deficient nutrient precursors, attenuated storage pool availability (e.g., glycogen), reduced regulatory enzyme activity (e.g., phosphoenolpyruvate carboxykinase), and diminished counterregulatory hormone responses (e.g., epinephrine, glucagon) due to reduced hormone secretion or reduced receptor activity and increased substrate utilization compared with that of the adult. Fasting in the adult is characterized by hormonal and metabolic changes that eventually result in the mobilization of stored nutrients (e.g., glycogen, triglycerides) and the provision of alternate fuels (e.g., free fatty acids, ketones) that spare tissue glucose utilization. During a short period of starvation in adults, glycogenolysis contributes to basal hepatic glucose production of approximately $2 mg \cdot kg^{-1} min^{-1}$. This is in contrast to the much higher rate of glucose utilization of premature neonates ($4-6 mg \cdot kg^{-1} min^{-1}$).[12] Glycogenolysis is activated by a reduction in blood glucose and insulin concentrations and by an increased concentration of circulating glucagon, which raises the tissue levels of cyclic adenosine monophosphate (cAMP). The net result is conversion of glycogen phosphorylase to its more active state with the reciprocal conversion of glycogen synthase to its less active glucose-6-phosphate dependent state. Hepatic glycogen stores become depleted after approximately 24 hours of fasting in adults. Hepatic and later renal gluconeogenesis become activated as the mobilization of gluconeogenic amino acids from muscle (e.g., alanine, glutamine) provide precursors for ongoing glucose production. In addition to the mobilization of gluconeogenic precursors, induction of the synthesis of rate-limiting gluconeogenic enzymes (e.g., phosphenolpyruvate carboxykinase) is required for new glucose production. At the same time glycerol (gluconeogenic) and free fatty acids (FFAs) become mobilized from tissue triglyceride stores. This mobilization may be due to the reduced availability of circulating glucose, a lower serum insulin concentration, or increased catecholamine and glucagon concentrations.[10,11] FFAs serve many important metabolic roles during fasting. They are excellent alternate sources of acetylcoenzyme A (CoA), which is both a regulator of glycolytic flux and a carbon source for the Krebs cycle. FFAs spare some glucose utilization in liver, muscle, and heart by inhibiting glycolysis and by the provision of acetyl CoA for the Krebs cycle. Under these conditions pyruvate is directed away from oxidation to the gluconeogenic pathway following conversion to oxaloacetate by the enzyme pyruvate carboxylase. The partial oxidation of FFAs produces ketones. Ketone production provides an alternate fuel that can partially spare glucose utilization by the brain. Ketones reduce muscle proteolysis and maintain the muscle mass. Ketones alter renal acid-base status and facilitate renal gluconeogenesis. Hepatic FFA oxidation enhances gluconeogenesis by the production of adenosine triphosphate (ATP) and nicotinamide adenine dinucleotide, reduced (NADH), which are both needed in the energy-requiring process of gluconeogenesis. Fasting-induced lipolysis increases the availability of glycerol, which serves as another precursor for gluconeogenesis.[10,11]

Current practice does not allow a term or premature neonate to be fasted for more than a few hours after birth. Compared to the adult, the term neonate has reduced tissue fuel stores, as depicted by triglycerides (i.e., 100,000 vs 4800 kcal), glycogen (i.e., 600 vs 136 kcal), and protein (i.e., 25,000 vs 1600 kcal). The premature neonate born at 28 weeks' gestation has even less lipid (e.g., 90 kcal), glycogen (e.g., 18 kcal), and protein (e.g., 340 kcal) stores.[10] Based on these data it is estimated that the adult may survive total starvation for as long as 90 days, whereas the term (e.g., 33 days) and premature neonate (e.g., 4 days) would survive such fasting for a much shorter time.[13] In addition to quantitative differences of stored fuels, the rate and duration of mobilization of alternate fuels are modified by prematurity. Compared with 1- to 4-year-old children, term and premature neonates develop hypoglycemia and demonstrate much lower serum levels of FFAs and ketones during a comparable fast.[10] Oxygen consumption are significantly reduced in fasted low birth weight neonates.[14] Oxygen consumption increases with the provision of exogenous substrates to these neonates.

Fasting energy metabolism has been extensively examined in the neonatal rat. Because of the absence of subcutaneous fat stores and relatively immature neurologic status, the term rat may be analogous to the premature human.[10,15] Compared with the adult (i.e., 10–20% fat) the 28-week human neonate has only 2% to 5% adipose tissue. During a 16-hour fast, neonatal rat pups demonstrate hypoglycemia and reduced serum concentrations of lactate, FFAs, glycerol, and ketones.[15] Before 16 hours of age, lipolysis is noted by a transient increase of serum FFAs, glycerol, and ketone bodies. With more prolonged starvation, substrate deficiency develops as noted by attenuated concentrations of these oxidizable substrates.[15,16] By providing an exogenous source of nutrients (e.g., triglycerides), after 16 hours of fasting the neonatal rat demonstrates an approximately sixfold rise in blood glucose, plasma FFA, and ketone body concentrations.[15] The increment of blood glucose concentration is due to enhanced gluconeogenesis by the various mechanisms discussed above. Similar observations have been noted in other fasted neonatal mammals.[16–18] Indeed, in preterm neonates exogenous lipids reduce glucose oxidation and utilization and increase blood glucose concentrations.[19–22] These observations emphasize the precarious nature of substrate availability in the fasted newborn mammal. The data highlight the importance of alternate substrate utilization to maintain glucose homeostasis and the avoidance of neonatal hypoglycemia. Because endogenous fuels become depleted more rapidly in VLBW neonates, there is an urgent need to provide exogenous nutrients by the enteral or parenteral route.

Problem of Neonatal Hypoglycemia

Hypoglycemia is a common metabolic problem among fasted neonates in general and in particular among high-risk VLBW neonates. In addition to premature neonates, others at increased risk for neonatal hypoglycemia include those subjected to fetal distress, cold stress, asphyxia, sepsis, intrauterine growth retardation, maternal diabetes mellitus, polycythemia, and congenital heart disease, as well as those exposed to excessive glucose loads during labor following dextrose administration to the mother.[1,10,11,23] (For complete discussion of this problem see Chapter 32.)

Neonatal hypoglycemia may be due to one of two common mechanisms. First, hyperinsulinemia may be present as in the infant of the diabetic mother, or with the Beckwith-Wiedemann syndrome, nesidioblastosis, or erythroblastosis fetalis; or it may occur following excessive dextrose administration to the mother during labor. The pathophysiology related to hyperinsulinemia, in some cases, is due to transfer of glucose by facilitative diffusion across the placenta to the fetus. Blood glucose concentration in the fetus increases rapidly after intravenous glucose administration to the mother during labor or during maternal diabetes, with fetal levels approaching 75% to 80% of maternal blood glucose concentrations. Fetal hyperglycemia causes subsequent pancreatic insulin secretion and a hyperinsulinemic state. After birth the hyperinsulinemia persists, and if no exogenous glucose is provided, hypoglycemia may develop. Hyperinsulinemia may be associated with an attenuated counterregulatory hormone response, as the serum concentrations of glucagon or epinephrine may be lower than expected for the degree of neonatal hypoglycemia in some patients.

The second common mechanism for neonatal hypoglycemia is related to substrate deficiency due to depletion of substrate storage pools such as glycogen or triglycerides. This mechanism is noted in the stressed, fasted, premature neonate or the one with intrauterine growth retardation. Compared with term neonates, these low birth weight neonates have low stores of tissue glycogen and lipid. In addition, with episodes of fetal or neonatal distress, these stores may be rapidly depleted (e.g., glycogen due to anoxia-ischemia) following catecholamine release or the increased glycolytic flux during anaerobic glycolysis.[10,11,17] Rare causes of neonatal hypoglycemia are hepatic failure or inborn errors of metabolism such as galactosemia, tyrosinemia, glycogen storage disease, and disorders of oxidative metabolism of fats or carbohydrates (mitochondrial defects)[10] (see Chapter 35).

The signs and symptoms of neonatal hypoglycemia are due to cerebral glucopenia (e.g., apnea, coma, seizures, irritability, hypotonia) or catecholamine release (e.g., pallor, tachycardia). Nonspecific signs may include heart failure, cyanosis, persistent fetal circulation, or hypothermia. Many patients with neonatal hypoglycemia do not demonstrate detectable manifestations and are considered to have asymptomatic hypoglycemia. The signs of neonatal hypoglycemia may be subtle.[24,25] Animal models of neonatal hypoglycemia have demonstrated reduced cerebral ATP in asymptomatic mammals, and studies in asymptomatic hypoglycemic human neonates have demonstrated unexpected neurologic dysfunction.[24,26,27] The latter investigation among human infants demonstrates abnormal sensory-evoked responses as determined by brain stem auditory-evoked potentials or somatosensory-evoked potentials. In some asymptomatic patients the abnormal evoked potentials return to normal with glucose administration.[24] The follow-up of patients with asymptomatic neonatal hypoglycemia has yielded contradictory results regarding the effect of hypoglycemia on subsequent neurodevelopmental outcome. Evidence suggests that hypoglycemic patients are at increased risk for developmental delay, independent of covariable or confounding neonatal risk factors.[28] In this study if hypoglycemia was present for longer than 5 days, severe neurologic dysfunction was present on follow-up at 18 months of age.[28]

In studies of hypoglycemia in the NICU, the risks for hypoglycemia have been associated with birth weight less than 1000 g, intrauterine growth retardation, birth asphyxia, and a low ponderal index.[28] In this study the incidence of acute hypoglycemia was inversely related to the severity of the depression of the plasma glucose concentrations, as concentrations less than $11 \text{mg} \cdot \text{dl}^{-1}$ were noted in 10%, concentrations less than $29 \text{mg} \cdot \text{dl}^{-1}$ were noted in 28%, and concentrations less than $47 \text{mg} \cdot \text{dl}^{-1}$ were seen in 66% of the patients. The incidence of prolonged hypoglycemia (>3 days) increased as the severity of hypoglycemia decreased and was 1.4%, 4%, and 16% in the severe ($11 \text{mg} \cdot \text{dl}^{-1}$), moderate ($29 \text{mg} \cdot \text{dl}^{-1}$), and mild ($47 \text{mg} \cdot \text{dl}^{-1}$) categories, respectively. Using a cutoff value of $40 \text{mg} \cdot \text{dl}^{-1}$, others have demonstrated an incidence of hypoglycemia of 30% among low- or high-risk infants.[29,30] The incidence of hypoglycemia is always greatest during the first 6 hours after birth.[31]

The definition of hypoglycemia was challenged with the publication of a series of papers between 1984 and 1988. The original definition of hypoglycemia was based on a statistical analysis of patients subjected to routine fasting while admitted to the NICU during the 1960s.[1] Premature neonates were considered hypoglycemic with two plasma glucose concentrations less than $25 \text{mg} \cdot \text{dl}^{-1}$, whereas the defined plasma glucose concentration in the term neonate was less than $35 \text{mg} \cdot \text{dl}^{-1}$, both occurring during the 72 hours after birth. Thereafter, a plasma glucose concentration of less than $45 \text{mg} \cdot \text{dl}^{-1}$ was considered hypoglycemic.[1,10] With the evidence that abnormal sensory-evoked potentials are present at plasma glucose levels of $47 \text{mg} \cdot \text{dl}^{-1}$ in low birth weight infants, and that premature neonates with a blood glucose concentration less than $47 \text{mg} \cdot \text{dl}^{-1}$ for more than 5 days have abnormal developmental follow-up at 18 months, we must reconsider our definition of neonatal hypoglycemia.[24,25,28]

It would be prudent to treat all neonates with plasma glucose concentration less than $45 \text{mg} \cdot \text{dl}^{-1}$ at any time of their hospitalization. In asymptomatic, otherwise healthy neonates, the nutrients provided by milk feeding may be all that is needed, whereas in the sick premature neonate an intravenous infusion of glucose at a rate of 6 to $8 \text{mg} \cdot \text{kg}^{-1} \text{min}^{-1}$ may correct the hypoglycemia. Symptomatic hypoglycemia requires a bolus of intravenous glucose of approximately $200 \text{mg} \cdot \text{kg}^{-1}$, followed by a continuous intravenous infusion of glucose given by a pump at a rate of $8 \text{mg} \cdot \text{kg}^{-1} \text{min}^{-1}$.[32] Careful evaluation of the plasma glucose concentration is required to titrate the glucose infusion rate to maintain plasma glucose concentrations above $45 \text{mg} \cdot \text{dl}^{-1}$. Patients with protracted or refractory hypoglycemia require detailed investigations to determine the etiology, which may include hyperinsulinemic states or inborn errors of metabolism.

Caloric Requirements of the VLBW Neonate

The energy requirements of the VLBW neonate can be divided into two important components: that needed for maintenance of body functions and that needed for growth. Maintenance energy requirements include the turnover of body macromolecules, maintenance of electrochemical gradients, and other internal processes that make up the basal metabolic rate. Because the VLBW neonate always receives some nutrient intake, the resting metabolic rate (10% or so higher than the basal rate) is usually the closest approximation of the basal rate. The resting metabolic rate expends approximately 45 to $60 \text{kcal} \cdot \text{kg}^{-1} \text{day}^{-1}$.[33-36] Muscle activity ($5-10 \text{kcal} \cdot \text{kg}^{-1} \text{day}^{-1}$) and heat generation ($5-10 \text{kcal} \cdot \text{kg}^{-1} \text{day}^{-1}$) needed for temperature regulation, if exposed to an environment below the neutral thermal environment (NTE), are additional energy-requiring processes that should be considered independent of the caloric requirements needed for maintenance or growth. The wide range of caloric needs for the above energy-requiring processes and the caloric requirements noted below for growth reflect (1) the difficulty of measuring energy consumption in sick VLBW infants; (2) different feeding protocols or environment conditions; and (3) differences inherent in patient populations, e.g., age, duration of feeding, activity, NTE, growth status: small (SGA), appropriate (AGA), or large (LGA) for gestational age. (For a further discussion see Chapters 44 and 45.)

Whenever feeding is initiated there are two additional energy-losing processes: diet-induced thermogenesis and malabsorption of nutrients lost in feces. The thermic effect of food results in a postprandial elevation of oxygen consumption of 10% to 15%. In 24 hours postprandial oxygen consumption may amount to $5 kcal \cdot kg^{-1}$. As the caloric intake of milk increases, the heat expended as the postprandial elevation of oxygen consumption increases. The metabolic rate rises proportionately to increases in the caloric intake of the neonate.[33,37,38] This diet-induced thermogenesis represents many processes, such as the transfer and conversion of nutrient precursors to their storage forms, and the metabolic costs of tissue synthesis (vide infra). The energy lost in feces owing to malabsorption varies greatly depending on the milk composition, the neonate's birth weight, and postnatal age. Overall, fecal nutrient losses in enterally fed infants represent 5 to $20 kcal \cdot kg^{-1} day^{-1}$.

In general, energy (i.e., calories) metabolism is balanced, as energy intake is equal to energy stored plus energy expended plus energy excreted. *Metabolizable energy* is the energy intake minus that excreted in stool. Energy stored varies with the composition of the newly synthesized tissue and corresponds to fat, protein, and glycogen deposited (vide infra). Energy expended represents the basal metabolism, temperature regulation, activity, and the calories required for the synthesis of new tissues. The net caloric requirement for all of these processes ranges from 90 to $165 kcal \cdot kg^{-1} day^{-1}$, with most neonates attaining satisfactory growth on 105 to $130 kcal \cdot kg^{-1} day^{-1}$.[4,39,40]

The energy requirement for growth relates to the energy content (i.e., storage) of the actual tissue and is dependent on the composition (i.e., percent fat) of the tissue. In addition, the energy cost of growth is dependent on the energy used to synthesize the new tissue. Overall tissue growth (i.e., synthesis and storage) requires 40 to $55 kcal \cdot kg^{-1} day^{-1}$ and is a large component of the total caloric requirement of the VLBW neonate. The *synthetic caloric* needs are 10 to $35 kcal \cdot kg^{-1} day^{-1}$, or an average of 0.5 to $1.7 kcal \cdot g^{-1}$ of tissue (e.g., the proportion of fat, protein, or water). The energy requirements for tissue nutrient *storage* (i.e., $20–30 kcal \cdot kg^{-1} day^{-1}$), or an average of 3.0 to $5.7 kcal \cdot g^{-1}$ of tissue, are dependent on the fat, protein, and water composition of new tissue.[35,37–39] The energy stored as protein is $11 kcal \cdot kg^{-1} day^{-1}$, and that in fat is much greater at $30 kcal \cdot kg^{-1} day^{-1}$.[36]

The content of the synthesized tissue determines the energy requirement as fat requires more caloric input than protein. Growth of the SGA neonate is characterized by more protein and water deposition and that of the AGA neonate by high rates of fat storage. The cost of tissue growth in SGA neonates is less than that for the AGA neonate. SGA neonates may demonstrate growth at a lower caloric intake than the AGA neonate. On average, the energy cost of tissue growth (i.e., synthesis and storage) is 3 to $4.5 kcal \cdot g^{-1}$.

Although the macromolecular composition of the synthesized tissue requires varying energy intakes, changes in energy intake may have profound effects on the composition of new tissue, resting energy expenditure, diet-induced thermogenesis, and gastrointestinal nutrient losses. In VLBW neonates the percent of calories lost in the stool increases as the enteral energy intake increases.[37] In one study there was a poor relation between energy intake or retention and the weight gained. Interestingly, substitution of medium-chain triglycerides for the milk's long-chain fat does not improve energy retention or weight gain.[37,41] With increases of energy intake there are corresponding increases of basal and postprandial oxygen consumption and the energy cost of tissue growth.[33] These data suggest that with high energy intake the composition of the new tissue has a higher fat content than the tissue synthesized and nutrients stored at lower caloric intakes. Compared with the fetus of 28 to 34 weeks' gestation, the extrauterine nourished premature neonate fed formula demonstrates a much higher tissue fat content.[42,43] Despite rates of weight gain that are similar to the in utero weight gain of the fetus, the VLBW neonate fed after birth experiences a fat retention rate approximately threefold that of the fetus. In the VLBW neonate, protein ($1.9 g \cdot kg^{-1} day^{-1}$), carbohydrate ($1.8 g \cdot kg^{-1} day^{-1}$), and fat ($5.4 g \cdot kg^{-1} day^{-1}$) synthesis determines the energy costs of growth. In contrast the fetal fat accretion rate is only 1 to $2 g \cdot kg^{-1} day^{-1}$ during the similar period of gestation.[43]

Current recommendations for energy and nutrient intake are based on the assumption that the extrauterine premature neonate requires the same nutrient retention as the fetus and that the VLBW neonate should achieve the comparable intrauterine growth rate for the respective gestational age.[39] This assumption may be inappropriate for many reasons related to the marked differences between the intrauterine and extrauterine environment (thermal, activity), the routes of administration (placenta, vein, or intestine), the abnormal composition of the postnatal tissue growth with present feeding practices, the technical problems of delivering nutrients by vein (calcium, phosphorus, glucose) or by enteral (calcium, fat, lactose) routes, and the metabolic intolerances of

TABLE 51.3. Nutritional assessment of premature neonates.

Nutrient history
    Alimentation fluid
    Lipids
    Formula (type, volume, calories per kilogram)
    Supplements
    Time of first enteral feeding
    Episodes when enteral feedings stopped, reason

Medical history
    Birth history
    Gestational age
    In utero growth (e.g., AGA vs SGA vs LGA)
    Short bowel syndrome
    BPD
    Cholestatic jaundice
    Osteopenia
    Infection
    Congenital anomalies

Growth history
    Current weight, length, head circumference
    Growth curves related to initial birth weight
    Daily weight gain
    Weekly head circumference and length
    Skinfold thickness
    Mid-arm circumference
    Ponderal index

Gastrointestinal history
    Gastroesophageal reflux
    Emesis (aspirates)
    Diarrhea (acute, chronic)
    Distended abdomen
    Ileus
    Constipation
    Necrotizing enterocolitis

Laboratory studies
    Hemoglobin
    White blood cell count
    Lymphocyte count
    Glucose
    Calcium, phosphorus
    Alkaline phosphatase
    Prothrombin time
    Albumin
    Prealbumin
    Retinol binding protein
    Triglycerides
    Bicarbonate
    Electrolytes
    Urine pH
    BUN
    Hand radiograph (bone mineralization)
    Bone densitometry

Physical examination
    Dermatitis (zinc, biotin, vitamins, essential fatty acids)
    Fractures (calcium, vitamin D, phosphorus, copper)
    Pallor
    Edema
    Jaundice
    Muscle mass
    Hair growth, texture

AGA, appropriate for gestational age; SGA, small for gestational age; LGA, large for gestational age.

parenteral (e.g., glucose, protein, fat) or enteral (e.g., lactose, fat) feedings (vide infra). Because it may be difficult to reproduce the rate and composition of fetal growth after the birth of the premature neonate, we must strive to provide safe quantities of nutrients to support continued growth, without producing adverse metabolic effects or nutritional deficiency syndromes. We have learned to appreciate the immaturity of the metabolic pathways, hepatic clearance, renal excretion, and gastrointestinal absorption of the VLBW neonate. We must balance these intolerances with judicious quantities of high-quality utilizable nutrients. The continuous nutritional assessment of the VLBW neonate requires particular attention to the multiple variables noted in Table 51.3.

Nutrient Requirements of the VLBW Neonate

The specific macronutrient and micronutrient requirements depend on the route of administration (Table 51.4).[4,39,44–47] As discussed above, the caloric needs of the VLBW neonate vary between 90 and 165 kcal·kg^{-1}·day^{-1}. The Committee on Nutrition of the American Academy of Pediatrics recommends 105 to 130 kcal·kg^{-1}·day^{-1} for the neonate who is fed enterally.[39] The caloric needs vary depending on the neonate's activity, maintenance of the neutral thermal environment, fecal losses, and the composition of new tissue deposition.

The protein needs of the VLBW neonate vary depending on the route of administration. Enteral protein intake of 2.5 to 4.0 g·kg^{-1}·day^{-1} has supported growth among VLBW neonates. At lower protein intakes there is the risk of poor growth and hypoalbuminemia, and at higher rates of protein intake there is the risk of hyperaminoacidemia, metabolic acidosis, azotemia, and hyperammonemia. The Nutrition Committee of the Canadian Paediatric Society recommends 1 to 3 g·kg^{-1}·day^{-1} during days 0 to 7 and 3.5 to 4 g·kg^{-1}·day^{-1} for infants <1 kg or 3 to 3.6 g·kg^{-1}·day^{-1} for infants >1 kg after the first week of life.[4]

Fats are an excellent source of calories and are required at least for the provision of essential fatty acids, which include linoleic acid (18:2 ω-6) a precursor to arachidonic acid and linolenic acid (18:3 ω-3) a precursor to docosahexaenoic acid (DHA) (Figure 51.1). DHA is a precursor to phospholipids, which are integral structural macromolecules in the cell membrane.[9,48–51] Human milk contains linoleic acid as 5% to 7% of its calories; linolenic acid represents approximately 10% of the essential fatty acids in human milk. Soy oils and marine oils are other sources for linolenic acid. Safflower oil is a poor source for linolenic acid. At least 3% of the total calories should be provided as these essential fatty acids. Without the ω-6 and ω-3 fatty acids a deficiency state develops

TABLE 51.4. Nutritional needs of low-birth-weight neonates.

	Enteral units·kg^{-1} day^{-1}	Parenteral units·kg^{-1} day^{-1}	Comment
Calories (kcal)	105–130	90–100	Additional calories needed in certain disease states
Protein (g)	3.0–4.0 whey predominant	2.5–3.5 crystalline amino acids	In enteral feeding, 2.5–3.5 g·kg^{-1} day^{-1} high quality protein can support growth without metabolic stress
Fat (g)	5.0–7.0 40–50% of calories	2.0–3.5 up to 45% of calories	At least 3% of calories as linoleic acid and a small amount as linolenic acid
Carbohydrate (g)	10–14	10–16	Lactose enhances enteral calcium absorption
Sodium (meq)	2.5–4.0	2.0–4.0	May need 4–8 meq·kg^{-1}day^{-1} to prevent hyponatremia in VLBW due to high FeNa
Potassium (meq)	2.0–3.0	2.0–3.0	
Calcium (mg)	170–230	80–100	
Phosphorus (mg)	100–140	60–80	
Magnesium (mg)	7–10	5–7	
Zinc (mcg)	1000	400	
Copper (mcg)	80–150	20	Omit from TPN with cholestasis
Selenium (mcg)	1.0–3.0	1.5–2.0	Omit from TPN in renal dysfunction
Manganese (mcg)	2.0–7.5	1	Omit from TPN with cholestasis
Chromium (mcg)	0.1–0.5	0.2	Omit from TPN in renal dysfunction
Molybdenum (mcg)	0.2–0.5	0.25	Not needed in TPN except for long-term use
Iron (mg)	2–4	0.1–0.2	Not necessary for first 6–8 weeks
Vitamin D (IU)	400 IU·day^{-1}	160 IU·kg^{-1} day^{-1}	For infant on TPN 2 ml·kg^{-1} day^{-1} of pediatric MVI provides vitamin needs
Method	Tube feeding if sick or until adequate suck and swallow. Advance over 10–14 days if <1500 g; and over 6–8 days if >1500 g	Start at 6 mg·kg^{-1} min^{-1} glucose 0.5–1 g·kg^{-1} day^{-1} fat 0.5–1 g·kg^{-1} day^{-1} protein	Hyperglycemia common with parenteral glucose in <1000 g neonate; advance to 12 mg·kg^{-1} min^{-1} maximum Monitor serum triglycerides as parenteral lipids increased

Source: Data from Nutrition Committee, Canadian Paediatric Society[4]; Committee on Nutrition, American Academy of Pediatrics[39]; Clark[44]; Greene, Hambridge, Schanler, et al.[45]; Pereira[46]; Zlotkin, Atkinson, Lockitch.[47]

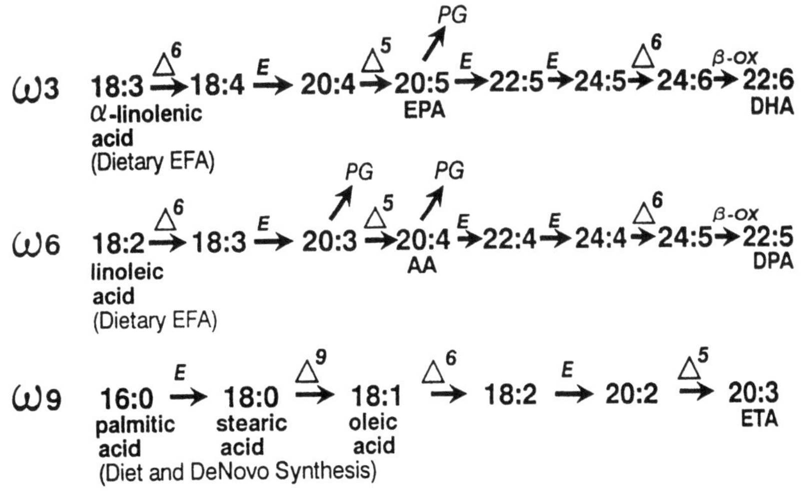

FIGURE 51.1. Metabolism of long chain polyunsaturated fatty acids (PUFA). Parent essential fatty acids (EFA) are derived from dietary sources for both ω-3 (18:3, α-linolenic acid) and ω-6 (18:2, linoleic acid) series. Elongation occurs two carbons at a time and delta desaturases (Δ9, Δ6, Δ5) introduce double bonds at 9, 6 and 5 carbons from the carbonyl moiety. The final step in the formation of ω-3 and ω-6 end-products is catalyzed by a peroxisomal beta-oxidation. Long chain PUFA of significance include: 20:4ω-6(AA), 22:5ω-6 (DPA), 20:3ω-9 (ETA), 20:5ω-3 (EPA) and 22:6ω-3 (DHA). EPA, AA and 20:3ω-6 are immediate precursors of prostaglandins (PG) and other eicosanoids. AA = arachidonic acid; DPA = docosapentaenoic acid; ETA = eicosatrienoic acid; EPA = eicosapentaenoic acid; DHA = docosahexaenoic acid. From: Uauy-Dagach R, Mena P, Hoffman DR[50] with permission.

that is characterized by poor growth, weeping scaling dermatitis, hypotonia, electroencephalographic and electrocardiographic changes, poor wound healing, and immunodeficiency.[51] The diagnosis of essential fatty acid deficiency is confirmed by measuring low serum concentrations of linoleic and arachidonic acids and increased concentrations of 5,8,11-eicosatrienoic acid. The serum triene/tetraene ratio is greater than 0.4.[52]

There is increasing evidence that a deficiency of ω-3 fatty acids (linolenic acid) alone produces symptoms in humans.[9,48–51] Manifestations may include peripheral neuropathy, dermatitis, and abnormal visual function.[49–51] Indeed, neurodevelopmental outcome in neonates may be adversely affected by ω-3 fatty acid deficiency.[9,48] There are also potential risks associated with excessive administration of polyunsaturated essential fatty acids including oxidant stress, hemolysis, bronchopulmonary dysplasia, retinopathy of prematurity, and platelet dysfunction with subsequent hemorrhage. These risks have not been proven to date in neonates. Uauy-Dagach and colleagues[50] recommend that VLBW infants receive 0.5 to 0.7 $g \cdot kg^{-1} day^{-1}$ of linoleic acid and 70 to 150 $mg \cdot kg^{-1} day^{-1}$ of linolenic acid.

Carbohydrates are given as lactose or glucose polymers enterally or glucose parenterally and are an important source of calories (i.e., 40% enterally, variable parenterally) for the VLBW neonate. The specific formulation, routes, intolerances, and complications related to these nutrients are discussed individually in the following sections, which concentrate on parenteral or enteral nutrition.

Parenteral Nutrition of the VLBW Neonate

The initial parenteral fluid given to VLBW neonates is either D_5W or $D_{10}W$ at rates sufficient to deliver glucose at 6 to 8 $mg \cdot kg^{-1} min^{-1}$. The fluid infusion rates vary between 70 and 150 $ml \cdot kg^{-1} day^{-1}$ and depend on the state of hydration, insensible water losses, electrolyte disorders, and any unusual fluid losses.

Carbohydrate

When provided at the above rates by parenteral routes, glucose solutions reduce negative nitrogen balance and lipolysis, prevent hypoglycemia, and replace fluid lost through insensible water losses and through the obligate water needed to excrete the renal solute load. Glucose is an obligate fuel for the brain, peripheral nerves, retina, bone marrow, erythrocytes, and renal medulla. In addition to its role as an oxidative fuel, glucose serves as an important precursor for lipogenesis.[20]

Nonetheless, excessive glucose administration may result in hyperglycemia. The usual glucose intolerance of the VLBW neonate may be exacerbated by sepsis, catecholamine or steroid administration, birth weight less than 1000 g, age less than 1 week, cardiopulmonary instability, and pancreatic endocrine insufficiency (e.g., anatomic or relative).[53] Hyperglycemia may theoretically result in a hypertonic plasma, hyperosmolar coma, glycosuria, osmotic diuresis, and dehydration, although it is unlikely in the neonate.[54] In addition, hyperglycemic VLBW neonates frequently have increased morbidity and mortality when compared with the weight-matched euglycemic neonate.[53] The incidence of hyperglycemia may be as high as 30% among neonates weighing less than 1000 g.[55] It should be noted that all glycosuric infants are not always hyperglycemic. Hyperglycemia is defined as a plasma glucose level greater than 150 $mg \cdot dl^{-1}$.[53]

The pathophysiology of neonatal hyperglycemia relates to two basic mechanisms of glucose homeostasis.[10,53,56–58] First, the premature neonate demonstrates an attenuated pancreatic insulin secretion response to hyperglycemia.[12,59] This relative insulinopenia is probably not the primary defect, because exogenous administration of insulin does not always improve the hyperglycemia.[57] The most probable mechanism is a failure of tissue to respond to insulin. In the presence of hyperglycemia and hyperinsulinemia, neonates do not completely suppress their own endogenous hepatic glucose production.[10,12,56,57,60] The adult responds to exogenous glucose and endogenous insulin with complete suppression of endogenous hepatic glucose production.[56,60] If the neonate does not suppress endogenous systemic glucose output, hyperglycemia develops. In addition to an attenuated hepatic response to insulin and glucose in neonates, insulin-dependent peripheral tissue (e.g., muscle) demonstrates a reduced capacity to utilize glucose in the presence of insulin.[56] Both insulin-stimulated tissue glucose utilization and the suppression of ongoing hepatic glucose production are attenuated in the newborn compared with the adult. (For a complete discussion of this entity see Chapter 32.)

This defect could be due to excessively high levels of counterregulatory factors such as catecholamines, corticosteroids, or FFAs. A defect at the level of the insulin receptor may be present. Because neonatal tissue has increased numbers of insulin receptors compared with adults and because the response to glucose at maximum insulin stimulation is reduced, the defect is thought to be a postreceptor defect.[56] The site of this postbinding insulin resistance may be the autophosphorylation by the receptor tyrosine kinase of the receptor's β-subunit, translocation of the glucose carrier from the cytoplasm to the cell membrane, or other transmembrane signaling mechanisms involved in insulin action.

Incomplete suppression of hepatic gluconeogenesis is responsible, in part, for the persistent systemic glucose production in newborn mammals.[61] This is one manifestation of neonatal insulin resistance at the level of a postreceptor defect. The regulation of hepatic gluconeogenesis is related to the activation and synthesis of key regulatory enzymes. The genetic expression of these regulatory gluconeogenic enzymes is controlled by the interaction of various hormone ligands with the respective hormone responsive (e.g., binding) elements in the upstream regulatory region of that enzyme's gene. In adult mammals insulin has a dominant effect over other hormonal regulators (e.g., epinephrine, glucagon) and usually suppresses the transcription of the gluconeogenic gene. In the neonate, insulin has an attenuated response resulting in continued transcription of the gluconeogenic enzyme's gene.[61] In addition, insulin's action is not dominant as gluconeogenic gene transcription is stimulated by epinephrine and hyperglycemia despite the presence of significant hyperinsulinemia.[61]

The treatment of hyperglycemia includes reduction of the glucose infusion rate and the concentration from $D_{10}W$ to D_5W or even $D_{2.5}W$.[53] Alternately, exogenous intravenous insulin can be given by pump to enhance tissue glucose uptake and attempt to inhibit endogenous glucose production.[58,62,63] With careful monitoring of blood glucose and serum potassium concentrations, insulin rates of 0.02 to 0.4 U·hour^{-1} can reduce blood glucose concentration and enhance the provision of additional calories.[64-66] With intravenous insulin, glucose infusion rates have increased by 60%, and total caloric intake from glucose has increased from 49 to 70 kcal·kg^{-1}·day^{-1}.[62] Hypoglycemia, hypokalemia, and excessive lipogenesis are added risks associated with insulin therapy.

Galactose is another carbohydrate source that can reduce hyperglycemia and can potentially be utilized without the need for insulin.[67-73] Galactose, an epimer of glucose, represents 50% of carbohydrate calories when lactose is the disaccharide in milk. Galactose can stabilize glucose homeostasis by its more rapid uptake by the liver, by producing a reduced rate of systemic carbohydrate appearance, and by producing a lower rate of glucose clearance relative to administered glucose. Galactose and glucose demonstrate equal rates of enteral absorption. Plasma galactose concentration is much lower than glucose concentration. This difference may be due to rapid clearance by the liver and storage of galactose in hepatic glycogen or hepatic metabolism of galactose to glucose. In experimental conditions substitution of some galactose for part of the intravenous glucose load has been demonstrated to improve glucose intolerance to enhance net carbohydrate administration in hyperglycemic glycosuric VLBW neonates.[71] During one study serum galactose levels increased to 15 mg·dl^{-1}, a concentration usually not encountered in VLBW neonates.[53] Because intravenous galactose is currently not available, nor is it approved for parenteral alimentation for VLBW neonates, enteral feeding with lactose-containing milks remains the only source of galactose.

The approach to neonatal hyperglycemia must take into consideration the infant's clinical condition and the observation that hyperglycemia is usually transient and often present only during the first few days after birth. Initial treatment should include a reduction of the glucose infusion rate. This solution is only temporary, as more calories will be needed to prevent proteolysis and weight loss. If hyperglycemia persists at low rates of glucose infusion, intravenous human recombinant insulin may be cautiously initiated. Alternatively, small enteral feedings with lactose-containing milk may help improve the glucose intolerance. Throughout this evaluation, causes for hyperglycemia other than metabolic-endocrine immaturity should be considered (e.g., sepsis).

Excessive intravenous glucose loads have been associated with fatty liver, cholestatic jaundice, lactic acid production, increased serum cortisol and catecholamine levels, and hypercarbia.[33] Hypercarbia results from the excessive carbon dioxide production relative to simultaneous oxygen consumption associated with the oxidation of glucose (e.g., respiratory quotient, RQ = 1) or during the synthesis of lipids from glucose carbon precursors (e.g., RQ > 1).[74] Hypercarbia has been noted to occur in cycles during "window" periods of parenteral alimentation when glucose was the only fuel provided.[74] This observation has relevance to specific groups of VLBW neonates with chronic lung disease (vide infra).

Protein

The protein requirements of the parenterally alimented neonate are provided by crystalline amino acids.[10,33,39,75-78] Because of immature metabolic pathways, the premature neonate's requirement for essential amino acids includes those traditional essential amino acids of older infants and adults plus cysteine, histidine, tyrosine, and possibly taurine.[79] In utero the fetus, at 28 weeks' gestation, retains nitrogen at approximately 350 mg·kg^{-1}·day^{-1}, whereas the term fetus retains approximately 150 mg·kg^{-1}·day^{-1}.[79] This figure corresponds to a protein intake of 2.2 g·kg^{-1}·day^{-1} for the premature neonate. This amount of protein assumes no catabolism of amino acids, the provision of an ideal mixture of essential amino acids, sufficient nonprotein calories to meet energy costs of growth and maintenance, and other potential variables effecting nitrogen utilization. The Committee on Nutrition of the Academy of Pediatrics currently recommends the provision of essential crystalline amino acids at a rate of 2.5 to 3.5 g·kg^{-1}·day^{-1} for the VLBW neonate (Table 51.4).[39] Excessive amounts of intravenous amino acids (e.g., casein hydrolysate, crystalline amino acids) have resulted in hyperammonemia, high blood urea nitrogen (BUN) concentration, hyperaminoacidemia, abnormal serum amino acid profiles (e.g., high phenylalanine, glycine, methionine concentrations; low branched-chain amino acids or tyrosine concentrations), metabolic acidosis, increased renal solute loads, and cholestatic jaundice (Table 51.5) (see Chapter 34).

Crystalline amino acids must be given with nonprotein calories, which usually constitute varying ratios of carbohydrate and lipid.[80] Nitrogen retention may be optimal when 8% of calories are provided as amino acids, 60% as glucose, and 32% as fat. Under these conditions, the resting metabolic rate and respiratory quotient decline and nitrogen retention increases relative to a high carbohydrate (i.e., 87%) and low fat (i.e., 5%) mixture.[80] Growth among premature neonates has been demonstrated with as little as 80 to 90 kcal·kg^{-1}·day^{-1} while receiving crystalline amino acids at 2.5 g·kg^{-1}·day^{-1}.[81] Below 80 kcal·kg^{-1}·day^{-1} the weight status is stabilized at constant weight without net gain. When total caloric intake is below this level, the amino acids are not always incorporated into new protein but serve as replacement for tissue turnover or as oxidative fuels to support energy production.

Because various amino acid solutions result in abnormal serum amino acid profiles among parenterally alimented compared with enterally fed VLBW neonates, new preparations of intravenous amino acids have been developed.[75,76] The newer preparations (e.g., Trophamine and Aminosyn PF) have been reported to normalize the serum amino acid profiles of parenterally alimented neonates. In addition to the usual amino acids, newer neonatal products may contain *N*-acetyl-L-tyrosine, *N*-acetyl-L-cysteine, and cysteine HCl.[82–84] Additional hopes for the newer amino acid solutions are that they will enhance growth and reduce the incidence of liver injury manifested as cholestatic jaundice.

Lipid

Intravenous lipids have greatly enhanced our ability to provide essential fatty acids and serve as well as an efficient, relatively safe isotonic, high-density parenteral caloric source.[33,52,85,86] The nitrogen-sparing capacity of intravenous lipids is probably equivalent to an isocaloric amount of glucose.[52] Intravenous lipids result in a lowered RQ, less carbon dioxide production, and equivalent nitrogen retention as high glucose solutions[80,85] (see Chapter 36).

Intravenous lipids come as an emulsion of soy (e.g., Intralipid, Travamulsion) or safflower (e.g., Liposyn) oils. The latter preparation has a lower concentration of linolenic acid and may result in a linolenic acid deficiency state.[85] Most solutions come prepared as a 10% (1.1 cal/ml) or 20% solution. The 20% solution is preferred as it

TABLE 51.5. Potential complications of total parenteral alimentation.

Catheter related
  Superior vena cava syndrome
  Pulmonary thromboembolism
  Pulmonary hypertension
  Pneumothorax
  Pleural or pericardial effusions (extravasated solution)
  Cardiac arrhythmias
  Mural thrombosis (cardiac)
  Intramyocardial infusion
  Cutaneous slough
  Hemorrhage
  Plasticizer release?
  Flocculation, precipitation of nutrients by mixing incompatibilities

Infections
  Staphylococcal sepsis (*S. aureus*, *S. epidermidis*)
  Candida sepsis
  Malassezia furfur
  Diphtheroids
  Gram-negative sepsis (with short gut syndrome)
  Local phlebitis (exit wound, tract)
  Contaminated solutions (rare organisms)
  Endocarditis

Electrolyte (minerals)
  Hyponatremia
  Hypernatremia
  Hypokalemia
  Hyperkalemia
  Hypophosphatemia
  Trace mineral deficiency (Zn, Cu, Mg, Fe)

Metabolic complications
  Hypoglycemia (infusion stopped)
  Hyperglycemia (hyperosmolar state)
  Hyperaminoacidemia
  Hyperammonemia
  Azotemia
  Essential fatty acid deficiency
  Metabolic acidosis
  Phototherapy alterations of hyperalimentation fluid components
  Hypertriglyceridemia
  Hyperphospholipidemia

Systemic complications
  Cholestasis (hepatic dysfunction)
  Fatty infiltration (liver, monocytes, lung, Intralipid)
  Altered myocardial function (decreased PO_4)
  Intestinal mucosal atrophy
  Gastrointestinal hyposecretion
  Altered intestinal motility
  Platelet dysfunction (Intralipid)
  ? Hemolysis (Intralipid)
  Osmotic diuresis (glucose)
  Bone disease (rickets)
  Isosmolar coma (protein)
  Hypoxia (Intralipid)
  Aluminum toxicity

is associated with a lower risk of hypertriglyceridemia and hyperphospholipidemia.[87] Older preparations of intravenous lipids had large lipid molecules (1 μm), which produced a fat overload syndrome, bleeding, and liver damage.[88,89] Newer preparations are 0.4 to 0.5 μm in size and are composed of triglycerides, egg phospholipid as an emulsifier, and glycerin to produce an isotonic solution (280 mOsm·L^{-1}). Intravenous lipids undergo metabolism at the endothelial cell membrane of muscle and adipose tissues.[52,89] At the capillary endothelium the fixed lipoprotein lipase causes hydrolysis of the triglyceride moiety to FFAs, which can then be oxidized or reesterified to triglycerides. The latter triglycerides can be stored or incorporated into very low density lipoproteins (VLDLs) and transported in the circulation. In addition to metabolism by the endothelial lipoprotein lipase, a postheparin circulating lipase contributes to the metabolism of intravenous lipids.[52] Postheparin lipolytic activity may be derived from hepatic and extrahepatic sources. Together, endothelial cell and postheparin lipases contribute to the clearance and subsequent utilization of intravenous lipids. Clearance (or tolerance) of lipids may be reduced in premature neonates (i.e., <27 weeks) during the first week of life, following intrauterine growth retardation, during hypoxia or sepsis, and following surgery or trauma. The initial intolerance to intravenous lipids improves in the premature neonate with time after the first week of life. This intolerance may be due to decreased adipose tissue mass, diminished lipoprotein lipase, or reduced postheparin plasma lipase activity.

Intravenous lipids are usually infused during a 24-hour period and at initial rates of 0.5 to 1.0 g·kg^{-1}·day^{-1}. Maximum rates as high as 3.5 g·kg^{-1}·day^{-1} given throughout the 24-hour period are usually safe, well tolerated, and without significant adverse metabolic or idiosyncratic effects (Tables 51.4 and 51.5).[52,85,86,90–99] Two important effects theoretically associated with intravenous lipids are its potential effect on bilirubin binding to albumin and its effect on pulmonary function.[52,85,86,90–93]

Following hydrolysis triglycerides may result in increased levels of FFAs. FFAs may bind to albumin and displace unconjugated bilirubin resulting in an increased free (i.e., unbound) bilirubin concentration. The latter is significant because the free component of unconjugated bilirubin has been associated with bilirubin encephalopathy (kernicterus). If the FFA/albumin ratio is less than 4:1, bilirubin should not be displaced by FFAs.[91] At usual rates of intravenous lipid infusion, the plasma FFA levels rarely exceed 1 to 2 mEq·L^{-1}, which does not usually cause displacement of bilirubin.[91,100] The safety of intravenous lipids can be maximized by avoiding infusion rates of lipids greater than 3.5 g·kg^{-1}·day^{-1} and by using a continuous infusion throughout the 24-hour period.[91] If the VLBW neonate has a serum unconjugated (i.e., indirect) bilirubin concentration above 10 mg·dl^{-1}, intravenous lipids may need to be infused at the lower rates (e.g., 0.5–1.0 g·kg^{-1}·day^{-1}).[85]

Intravenous fat has been associated with the development of hypoxia in some humans and experimental animals.[84,101] This hypoxia has been thought to be due to various proposed mechanisms that may affect oxygenation (e.g., lipid coating the erythrocyte, fat emboli in pulmonary arteries, fatty lesions in pulmonary endothelial cells, fat incorporation into pulmonary macrophages, and venous admixture with increased pulmonary artery pressure). A direct embolic effect of Intralipid has been proposed. However, these observations have been shown to be due to a postmortem artifact resulting in insoluble fat globules.[86,88,90,94,95] High doses of intrapulmonary (i.e., tracheal) or intravenous fat can produce an adult respiratory distress-like syndrome. In these models, intravenous fat produces hypoxia, abnormal ventilation/perfusion ratios, and increased pulmonary vascular resistance.[92,93] In these investigations local vasoactive prostaglandin concentrations increase markedly, and indomethacin (a prostaglandin synthesis inhibitor) prevents the abnormal pulmonary vascular responses. Although these effects have been demonstrated in laboratory models, they are probably not operable in VLBW neonates who receive the recommended amounts of intravenous lipids at the suggested 24-hour infusion rate.

Intravenous fat emulsions containing medium-chain triglycerides in addition to long-chain triglycerides have been studied in Europe. The theoretical benefits of these solutions include increased nitrogen retention, decreased dependence on carnitine for lipid metabolism, less displacement of bilirubin, more rapid hydrolysis, and less effect on the pulmonary system.[102,103] Further data are needed to determine the clinical benefit of these newer products.

Carnitine is essential for the oxidative metabolism of fatty acids. Carnitine is endogenously synthesized from lysine and methionine but is also available from dietary sources.[66,104] Supplementation of intravenously alimented infants with (50 μg·kg^{-1}·day^{-1}) carnitine results in an increase in serum ketone levels, the ability to tolerate more intravenous lipid and greater weight gain during the first 2 weeks of life.[104] If this study is confirmed, carnitine may be an additional nutrient that should be provided to support fatty acid utilization in VLBW infants. Nonetheless, unwise use of carnitine may produce lipolysis, increased nitrogen excretion, and an elevation of the oxygen consumption[66] (see Chapter 38).

Methods and Complications

The availability of safe, efficient sources of essential amino acids, glucose, and lipids in addition to vitamins, trace minerals, and electrolytes has enhanced the ability to offer total parenteral nutrition to specific populations of high-risk neonates. All VLBW neonates do not need total parenteral alimentation because many can receive partial or total enteral nutritional support. Early in life VLBW neonates usually receive parenteral nutrients to supplement enteral milk feedings. As the amount of milk tolerated by the VLBW neonate increases, parenteral nutrients can be weaned. VLBW neonates often require 2 to 3 weeks to achieve all caloric intake by the enteral route. During this time important calories, nitrogen, vitamins, and trace minerals can be given by peripheral vein to supplement the enteral feedings. The content of nitrogen, fat, and glucose is gradually increased as needed according to both the tolerance of the neonate and the expected period of time the neonate requires intravenous supplementation of enteral feedings.

If the infant requires enhanced amounts of parenteral calories a percutaneously placed small central venous line is needed to provide hypertonic glucose. Central venous lines are not required for many neonates because enteral feedings can be initiated successfully in most VLBW neonates during the first 1 to 2 weeks of life. Nonetheless, there are neonates (usually <1000g), who require total parenteral nutrition because they have severe feeding intolerance and cannot be successfully fed by the enteral route. Additional indications for total parenteral nutrition include severe necrotizing enterocolitis (NEC), short bowel syndrome, serious gastrointestinal malformations, chylothorax unresponsive to medium-chain triglycerides (MCT) oil-based formula, and the unusual child with intractable diarrhea who cannot tolerate any enteral feedings.

Total parenteral alimentation can adequately support growth in VLBW neonates.[77,78,105] The hormone and circulating fuels during parenteral alimentation vary depending on the fat content of the solution. Elevated plasma FFA and ketone concentrations and decreased plasma glucose, lactate, and insulin concentrations are noted when lipids constitute a high proportion of infused nutrients compared with glucose-predominant solutions.[10] Nonetheless, nitrogen balance should not be different between glucose- or fat-predominant intravenous solutions. Compared with enterally fed neonates, parenterally alimented VLBW neonates can maintain normal profiles of amino acids and hormones.[75,76] The mixture of nutrients should be given continuously and extended throughout the 24-hour period to avoid cyclic fluctuations of glucose, insulin, lactate, ketones, and carbon dioxide.[74,106,107] Complications of total parenteral nutrition are common and include those related to the catheter (mechanical), infections, electrolyte and metabolic imbalances, and systemic effects such as osteopenia and cholestatic jaundice (Table 51.5). The latter two complications are disturbingly common among VLBW neonates who require prolonged periods of parenteral alimentation.

Osteopenia of prematurity, also known as rickets of prematurity, is a possible complication of total parenteral alimentation among VLBW neonates.[108] Decreased bone mineralization is noted among adult patients receiving total parenteral alimentation.[109] Osteopenia of prematurity may occur among formula-fed VLBW neonates, so it is not exclusively related to parenteral feedings.[110] Osteopenia of prematurity is associated with reduced intake of calcium, phosphorus, and vitamin D but may be exacerbated by acidosis, diuretic-induced calciuria, aluminum toxicity, and hepatic dysfunction. In adult patients receiving parenteral alimentation, osteopenia has improved when excessive intravenous doses of vitamin D are reduced. Presently there is no one clear etiology of the osteopenia of prematurity. When enterally alimented VLBW neonates receive additional supplementation with calcium, phosphorus, and vitamin D, bone mineralization improves and bone fractures heal, suggesting that a combined approach to this disease is beneficial. If the VLBW neonate who receives all nutrition by the parenteral route develops osteopenia, the calcium and phosphorus content of the solution should be increased. Judicious care is taken to avoid precipitation of calcium salts in the solution.[110-112] High doses of intravenous or intramuscular vitamin D have been successful in improving the bone mineralization status of these neonates (see Chapters 40 and 42).

Cholestatic jaundice is a common problem among parenterally fed VLBW neonates. The incidence increases with decreasing gestational age and may be present in as many as 33% of VLBW neonates.[113-115] Cholestatic liver disease is unusual among enterally fed neonates. Various components of the intravenous formulary including excessive carbohydrates and amino acids have been implicated with the development of neonatal hepatic injury and cholestasis. In vitro studies and animal models have suggested that certain cholestatic amino acids can cause cholestatic liver disease in neonates. New intravenous amino acid preparations have tried to balance the amino acid mixture in an attempt to lower the incidence of cholestasis.[76] Overall the incidence of cholestatic liver disease increases with the duration of intravenous alimentation, the period of time the neonate receives nothing by mouth (NPO), the presence of gastrointestinal disturbances such as NEC, the presence of sepsis, hypotension, and endotoxemia, the use of diuretics, and the lower the neonate's birth weight.[113,114,116] These factors may contribute to reduced bile flow, bile sludging, and obstruction of intrahepatic bile ducts.

Gallbladder stones may develop in this environment, as the concentration of bilirubin or bile salts exceeds their solubility—and stones form. Most neonates with cholelithiasis have calcium bilirubinate stones visible on plain radiographs or with ultrasonography.[116] Cholestatic jaundice is usually reversible once enteral feedings are

TABLE 51.6. Potential adverse effects of intravenous lipids.

Problem	Comments
Allergic-type signs	Chills, fever, eosinophilia; rare in VLBW
Pulmonary fat embolization	May be postmortem artifact
Hypoxia	Lipids increase prostaglandins; increases mean pulmonary artery pressure, lung lymph flow, and V/Q mismatch
Leukocyte dysfunction	Controversial; probably not significant
Infection	*Malassezia furfur*; lipid required as growth factor; *Staphylococcus epidermidis* sepsis; lipid accumulation in macrophages
Hyperglycemia	Rare; insulin resistance, increased gluconeogensis, glucose-sparing effect
Fat agglutination	Mixing with other parenteral nutrients or certain serums
Hyperbilirubinemia/kernicterus	Not a problem at recommended doses and with continuous 24-hour infusion
Platelet dysfunction	Rare; hypercoagulopathy, bleeding
Spurious hyponatremia	Laboratory test artifact as triglycerides displace plasma water
Hypertriglyceridemia	Most common in SGA; sepsis or hypoxia
Fatty liver	May be nonspecific
Linolenic acid deficiency	Low level of the essential fatty acid in safflower oil-based preparations
Erythrocyte membrane	Coating with lipids; unknown effect; bizarre cells (Burr cells, acanthocytes) seen with liver disease and elevated triglycerides
Triglyceride hydroperoxide formation	Cover intravenous tubing during phototherapy; add ascorbic acid to intravenous solution
Increased work of breathing	Related to increased Pco_2 or CO_2 production with or without decreased Po_2; increased minute ventilation

initiated. Unfortunately, some VLBW neonates cannot be fed by the enteral route and require prolonged periods of time on parenteral nutrition. These neonates are at risk for cirrhosis, end-stage liver failure, and rarely hepatocellular carcinoma[117,118] (Table 51.5). The most common causes of death among infants with short bowel syndrome who require total parenteral alimentation for prolonged periods are hepatic failure and complications of cirrhosis. Cholestatic liver disease in VLBW neonates is also associated with increased serum copper levels and the development of Kayser-Fleischer corneal rings.[113] These two observations are reversible with the institution of enteral feedings. Unfortunately, end-stage liver disease is not a reversible disorder and requires liver transplantation if a donor is available.

Although the association between prolonged periods of total parenteral alimentation seems to be an obvious contributing factor for cholestatic jaundice of neonates, there is another hypothesis. Prolonged periods of being NPO significantly alters gastrointestinal growth and function[114,119-124] (see Hypocaloric Enteral Feeding, below). An animal receiving all nutrients by vein and none by the enteral route develops mucosal atrophy of the small intestine.[123,124] In addition, there are marked abnormalities of local intestinal hormones among these patients. Without these local gut hormones (e.g., secretin, gastrin, cholecystokinin), there is no signal to increase bile or pancreatic flow or to increase mucosal cell growth. When enteral feedings are initiated in VLBW neonates, plasma concentrations of gastrin, enteroglucagon, insulin, gastric inhibitory peptide, pancreatic polypeptide, neurotensin, secretin, and motilin increase.[121,122] These hormones may have endocrine (i.e., systemic) effects, but they have local paracrine effects on gastrointestinal growth and function. Local availability of nutrients in the intestine may have similar trophic effects independent of gut hormones. Local nutrients may directly stimulate intestinal growth and function, Rather than hepatotoxic substances being present in parenteral nutrition solutions, the cause of the cholestatic jaundice of the VLBW neonate may be related to being NPO, with the infant not experiencing the beneficial trophic and secretory influences of the various gut hormones.[114,119] The incidence of cholestatic jaundice can be reduced among VLBW neonates who receive a small proportion of their total nutrients by the enteral route.[114] The potential adverse effects associated with intravenous lipids are outlined in Table 51.6.

Enteral Alimentation of the VLBW Neonate

Many neonatologists avoid enteral alimentation of the ill VLBW neonate until the patient's serious cardiopulmonary diseases have resolved. There are concerns that enteral alimentation during the first few weeks of life may not be possible owing to relative hypomotility of the intestine and limited gastric capacity in these VLBW neonates.[33] Some believe that these physiologic limitations preclude the use of enteral feedings among the smallest, sickest VLBW neonates or even among healthier VLBW neonates during the first week of life. Because the coordination of sucking and swallowing may not be present until 32 to 34 weeks, and the gag reflex may be delayed until this time, neonatologists have been concerned that these neonates are at risk for regurgitation, aspiration pneumonia, hypoxia, and gastric distention (Table 51.7).

TABLE 51.7. Potential problems in enterally fed preterm neonates.

General problems
　Abdominal distention, gastric retention, constipation
　Gastroesophageal reflux, regurgitation
　Aspiration pneumonia, laryngospasm
　Apnea, bradycardia, decreased Pao$_2$, decreased FRC
　Necrotizing enterocolitis
　Endotoxemia
Methodology[a-d]
　Gastrointestinal perforation[a]
　Nasopharyngeal irritation[a]
　Esophagitis/reflux[a]
　Otitis/sinusitis[a]
　Occult blood in stool[a]
　Plasticizer toxicity?[a]
　Reflux[b]
　Tracheal catheterization[a]
　Abnormal upper gastrointestinal tract colonization[c]
　Jejunojejunal intussusception[c]
　Fat malabsorption[c]
　Pyloric stenosis[c]
　Poor motor development[d]
Formula
　Milk protein allergy (cow, soy)
　Lactobezoars (MCT oil, calcium supplements, casein)
　Systemic metabolic intolerances (e.g., late metabolic acidosis, protein, galactosemia)
　Deficiency states (rickets: soy formula)
　Necrotizing enterocolitis (hyperosmotic formula)
　Toxins (aluminum)
　Abdominal distention, diarrhea (MCT, lactose)
　Lactose intolerance
　Contaminated formula (bacteria)

[a] Feeding tube.
[b] Intragastric feeds.
[c] Transpyloric feeds.
[d] Gastrostomy feeds.
FRC, functional residual capacity.

Other concerns include the purported risk of NEC if fed with an umbilical catheter in place (vide infra). In addition to these general concerns, there are specific complications related to the methods of feeding and to the formula fed to these high-risk VLBW neonates (Table 51.7).[10] Although the risks of fasting and thirsting have been demonstrated by randomized controlled trials, the advent of parenteral nutrition solutions have provided VLBW patients with a source of nutrition without the risks of enteral feedings. Parenteral alimentation is not without risks and is associated with specific and potentially serious adverse effects (Table 51.5). The neonatologist must balance both methods of alimentation against their potential risks.

Current enteral feeding practices of the VLBW neonate reflect many of the concerns related to the risks associated with enteral alimentation. Added to these concerns are the ever present risks of developing NEC, which is relatively rare among parenterally fed neonates (vide infra).[10,106,125] Many neonatologists avoid enteral alimentation among neonates less than 1000 g for at least 1 week after birth.[126] Larger VLBW neonates may receive some enteral alimentation between 3 and 5 days of life. Usually the VLBW neonate continues to receive a combination of parenteral and enteral feedings after beginning recovery from the common cardiopulmonary diseases of the neonatal period. In many neonatal centers full enteral feedings, with reciprocal reduction of intravenous alimentation, is not achieved until 2 to 4 weeks of life.[114,127] During the critical stages of acute neonatal diseases [respiratory distress syndrome (RDS), persistent fetal circulation (PFC), patent ductus arteriosus (PDA)] most VLBW neonates receive all calories by vein and are kept NPO.

There are studies suggesting that early enteral alimentation, even during episodes of RDS, are safe and beneficial to the VLBW neonate.[3,114,128-130] Indeed, in 1974 Brans et al.[128] demonstrated that fed patients with RDS who were enterally fed did as well as those enterally alimented with additional intravenous nutrient supplementation. The latter supplemented group nonetheless had a higher incidence of hyperglycemia, hyperosmolality, and acidosis. In another randomized investigation comparing parenteral and enteral alimentation, the intravenously fed group exhibited more sepsis, azotemia, and cholestatic jaundice but demonstrated a lower incidence of NEC during the 2-week study period.[105] More recent investigations have not demonstrated an increased overall incidence of NEC in VLBW neonates fed on day 1 versus day 7.[131] Delaying enteral alimentation for 2 weeks failed to prevent the development of NEC during the patients' hospitalization.[132] Withholding enteral feedings did not reduce the incidence but may delay the day of onset of NEC.

Enteral alimentation has potential beneficial effects. Early enteral alimentation may provide greater quantities of nutrients than parenteral alimentation. Those neonates who were given early (day 1) enteral feedings received more protein and calories during the first week of life.[131] A similar study demonstrated greater calcium, phosphorus, and vitamin D intake among VLBW neonates fed with umbilical catheters in place during the first week of life than among those who were parenterally alimented.[114] There appears to be no added risk if an umbilical catheter is in place.[133] In addition to these potential benefits of enteral alimentation, there are significant effects on intestinal mucosal growth and function (vide supra).

Digestion

The physiology of nutrient digestion and absorption is modified by the milk or formula fed to the neonate and by developmental differences of intestinal function.

Although the intestinal structure is present at the time of birth, the functions (e.g., motility, digestion, absorption) of the immature intestine are relatively underdeveloped. Digestion of carbohydrate and fats may be reduced and potentially contribute to malabsorption in VLBW neonates. If significant fecal nutrient loss occurs, there may be poor postnatal growth among enterally alimented VLBW neonates.[33,134,135]

Carbohydrates

The predominant carbohydrate fed by the enteral route to the VLBW neonate is lactose. This disaccharide of glucose and galactose is often supplemented with glucose polymers of varying carbon lengths in the formulas made for the VLBW neonate. The concentration of lactose in breast milk is approximately $7 g \cdot L^{-1}$. Lactose is converted to glucose and galactose by the brush border disaccharidase lactase.[33,134,135] Lactase mucosal enzyme activity is lower in the preterm neonate than in the term neonate. At 28 to 32 weeks the mucosal activity of lactase is 30% of the activity at term gestation.

Lactose malabsorption in the small intestine may cause lactose to enter the colon where the colonic flora ferment lactose to hydrogen gas and short-chain organic acids. Hydrogen gas diffuses to the portal vein and is eventually excreted by the lungs. As a reflection of this malabsorption, breath hydrogen concentration is increased among normal premature neonates compared with the low levels of hydrogen excreted by term neonates.[134,135] The organic acids produced by colonic bacterial fermentation may be metabolized by the colonic mucosa or absorbed into the portal circulation. This colonic salvage of organic acid products of malabsorption may avoid excessive nutrient losses in the stool and support enterocyte growth.

With excessive lactose administration there may be more lactose malabsorption than can be salvaged by the colon. This degree of malabsorption would result in an osmotic watery, acidic diarrhea (i.e., positive stool-reducing substances), feeding intolerance, flatulence, abdominal distention, borborygmi, and organic acidosis.[134–136] One benefit of lactose is that it enhances enteric calcium absorption.[134,135]

It is recommended that 40% to 45% of the calories in formula for VLBW neonates be in the form of carbohydrates.[33,134,135] Because lactose intolerance is a problem in some VLBW neonates, specialized formulas for premature neonates contain 50% to 60% of their carbohydrate as glucose polymers. Glucose polymers enhance the caloric density of a formula, but because of their long chain length they do not increase the osmolality of the formula.[134] Nonetheless, the preterm neonate has low pancreatic amylase activity (i.e., 10% of adult values), which could limit glucose polymer digestion to absorbable single glucose molecules. Other digestive enzymes improve glucose polymer hydrolysis. In addition to salivary amylase and breast milk amylase, the preterm neonate has high concentrations (i.e., 50–100 times adult values) of the small intestinal mucosal glucoamylase (previously called maltase).[33,134,135] Because of these digestive enzymes glucose polymers are considered to be as good a source of carbohydrate for VLBW neonates as lactose is for term neonates.

Lipid

Fat digestion is dependent on the chain lengths (e.g., medium vs long-chain fatty acids) and the presence of various lipases (e.g., lingual, breast milk, gastric, pancreatic) and bile salts. Fat in the form of triglycerides represents 40% to 50% of the calories of formula. Fat is a high-energy fuel that provides the essential fatty acids (e.g., linoleic and linolenic acids). Some degree of fat malabsorption is present during the neonatal period. Preterm neonates demonstrate more steatorrhea than term infants.[33] Vegetable fats are absorbed better than animal fats, and unsaturated fatty acids and human milk fat are absorbed better than saturated fats and the fat source of formula, respectively. The enhanced absorption of human milk may relate to complete hydrolysis of triglycerides at the 1 and 3 positions, with palmitate monoglyceride being readily absorbed. Alternatively, human milk fats may have a digestive advantage compared with formula due to the presence of a human milk lipase. Human milk lipase combines with lingual and gastric lipases to aid triglyceride hydrolysis by pancreatic lipase. Heating of human milk denatures human milk lipase, resulting in a greater amount of malabsorbed fat.[137] Calcium salt supplementation may exacerbate fat malabsorption.[11,33,135] Bile salt concentrations are low in the preterm neonate but not always below the critical micellar concentration required to enhance fat absorption. Bile salts stimulate human milk lipase activity. Overall, 10% to 20% of ingested fat may be malabsorbed by VLBW neonates.

Because long-chain fatty acids require lipases and bile salts, whereas MCTs can be absorbed directly into the portal venous system without digestion, it is thought that MCTs offer a nutritional advantage to the VLBW neonate.[33,135] Unfortunately, despite the popularity of MCT oil in premature formulas, there is no evidence to suggest that MCTs improve energy balance when compared to formula containing long-chain triglycerides.[41,138,139] Indeed MCT oil may produce adverse effects (e.g., feeding intolerance, diarrhea, abdominal distention, emesis, gastric bezoars).

Protein

Protein digestion is efficient in the VLBW neonate.[135] The levels of pancreatic proteases and brush border peptidases are sufficient to absorb the usual protein loads given these neonates. Although protein digestion and absorption are efficient, there are specific problems related to the systemic metabolic effects of protein deficiency or excess. In addition to the quantity of protein, the quality of the protein as measured by the whey/casein ratio affects the metabolic tolerance to the protein load. Although its role is not yet determined, taurine is now added to most infant formulas.[140]

Too little protein may result in poor weight gain, hypoalbuminemia, and edema. Too much protein can result in hyperaminoacidemia (e.g., methionine, tyrosine, cystine, phenylalanine), hyperammonemia, azotemia, metabolic acidosis, mental retardation, and an increased renal solute load.[33] Whey proteins (e.g., α-lactalbumin, lactoferrin, and immunoglobulin G in human milk; β-lactoglobulin in formula) are associated with fewer metabolic intolerances (e.g., azotemia, acidosis) than casein proteins. A safe range of good quality protein intake varies between 2.5 and $4.0 g \cdot kg^{-1} day^{-1}$ (Table 51.4).[34] Studies have demonstrated that growth of the VLBW neonate is augmented if fed $115 kcal \cdot kg^{-1} day^{-1}$ with the protein content at 3.6 rather than $2.2 g \cdot kg^{-1} day^{-1}$.[141] Increasing the energy content of the diet beyond $115 kcal \cdot kg^{-1} day^{-1}$ resulted in even greater weight gain. This weight gain followed active lipogenesis and greater adipose tissue deposition. In another study weight gain and nitrogen retention were enhanced in VLBW neonates fed isocaloric formulas with 3.8 versus 2.8 $g \cdot kg^{-1} day^{-1}$ of protein.[142] The lower rate of protein intake was associated with nitrogen accretion rates similar to the in utero fetal nitrogen retention. This group demonstrated a normal serum albumin concentration. In contrast, the group given protein at $3.8 g \cdot kg^{-1} day^{-1}$ demonstrated higher serum amino acids and BUN.[142] In these neonates the protein intake may have exceeded that needed for tissue synthesis, resulting in amino acid catabolism and ureagenesis. The higher plasma amino acid concentrations may reflect amino acid provision in excess of the tissue's ability to use these precursors of protein. Increased protein intake in excess of tissue synthetic needs increases energy expenditure as diet-induced thermogenesis. In this study and others discussed previously excessive caloric intake results in fat storage and not necessarily more protein synthesis.[142]

Human Milk Feeding of the VLBW Neonate

The beneficial immunologic and nutritional effects of human milk have been known for years (Table 51.8) (see Chapter 52). Some human milk nutrients are digested and absorbed more efficiently than those of commercial formula. These effects may be due to the macromolecular structure and composition of human milk or to digestive enzymes secreted by the mammary gland into human milk (lipases, amylases). Nonetheless, human milk, especially pooled mature milk, has certain limitations as a nutrient source for VLBW neonates (Table 51.9). Pooled mature human milk may be deficient in protein, calcium, and sodium if fed to VLBW neonates. Poor growth, hypoalbuminemia, edema, osteopenia, poor bone mineralization, fractures, and hyponatremia may develop in VLBW neonates fed pooled mature human milk.[3,143,144]

Human milk expressed from mothers who deliver premature neonates contains higher concentrations of protein, sodium, and occasionally calories when compared with pooled mature term milk.[144-147] Studies have demonstrated greater weight gain, normal serum albumin con-

TABLE 51.8. Beneficial effects of human milk for VLBW neonates.

Immunologic effects (cellular, immunoglobulin A, antibacterial enzymes)

Nutritional effects
  Enhanced absorption of fat, iron, calcium
  Whey protein of higher quality
  Fewer metabolic intolerances
  Presence of trophic factors for intestinal development and growth (epidermal growth factor, gastrin, prostaglandin, thyroid hormone)
  Preterm human milk: higher levels of protein and sodium
  Low renal solute load
  Provision of linoleic and linolenic acids

Other effects
  Reduced risk of NEC
  Increased IQ
  Prevents cow-soy-milk protein allergy
  Enhances gut closure to potential allergens
  Psychological interaction and bonding

TABLE 51.9. Potential limitations of human milk for VLBW neonates.

Infections/immunological limitations
  Viral agents (HIV, CMV, hepatitis B)
  Other infections (syphilis, tuberculosis, *Listeria*)
  Contamination with skin flora during manual expression
  Heat treatment destroys enzymes and immunocompetent cells

Nutritional limitations
  Relatively deficient in calcium, phosphorus, sodium, vitamin D, vitamin K
  Possibly deficient in protein (especially if pooled mature milk)
  Occasionally deficient in zinc
  Heat treatment destroys lipase and amylase

Other limitations
  Drugs enter milk and may produce toxicity to VLBW neonate (pharmaceuticals, toxins)
  VLBW neonates require gavage feeding, not direct breast-feeding
  Psychological stresses—lactation failure

CMV, cytomegalovirus.

centration, and lower serum alkaline phosphatase levels in VLBW neonates fed preterm human milk from their own mothers than in VLBW mature neonates fed pooled, term milk.[144,147] Pasteurization of preterm milk may reduce some of the beneficial effects of preterm human milk.[148] Energy expenditure is lower in VLBW neonates fed preterm human milk compared with formula, despite equivalent weight gain.[149] Neonates fed preterm human milk demonstrate a lower metabolic rate, higher fat oxidation, lower fat accretion (i.e., 16% vs 33%) and similar rates of protein accretion. Growth, assessed by weight, length, and head circumference, is the same in VLBW neonates fed human preterm milk or formula. Because of the reduced percentage of body fat and equal retention of nitrogen, human preterm milk-fed neonates produce tissue with greater water content. Although substrate utilization is different in human milk–fed neonates, net weight gain is unaffected.[42] Nonetheless, with high rates of human milk feeding, the caloric intake becomes directly related to the percent body fat deposited.[42]

Protein supplementation of human milk results in higher serum albumin concentration in the supplemented group and elevated serum amino acid and BUN concentrations.[150] Supplementation with energy, protein, calcium, phosphorus, sodium, and vitamin D, as available from commercial milk fortifiers, enhances weight gain and shortens the hospital stay of VLBW infants.[4] Another study compared the effect of supplementing banked human milk with protein and MCT oil.[138] MCT does not influence growth, whereas protein supplementation improves weight gain and serum albumin concentration. This study used pooled human milk, and the VLBW neonates had an initial protein intake of only $1.8 \text{g} \cdot \text{kg}^{-1} \text{day}^{-1}$. It is currently unknown if lower serum albumin concentration in the unsupplemented yet growing VLBW neonates (i.e., receiving human milk) has the same (i.e., assumed) significance as the hypoalbuminemia associated with protein-calorie malnutrition.

Because the calcium intake of human milk may be too low to support bone mineralization of the VLBW neonate, calcium supplementation has been recommended by some.[111,151-154] The in utero calcium accretion rate of the 28- to 32-week fetus approaches 100 to $150 \text{mg} \cdot \text{kg}^{-1} \text{day}^{-1}$. Human milk cannot supply this amount of calcium to the VLBW neonate. Human milk feedings may predispose the VLBW neonate to decreased bone mineralization compared with the reference fetus or formula-fed VLBW neonate after birth.[112] Fortification of human milk with calcium and phosphorus may improve bone mineral content and reduce serum alkaline phosphatase levels.[153] Similar improvements in bone metabolism may be noted with phosphorus and vitamin D supplementation.[151] It is not certain if the moderate elevation of serum alkaline phosphatase with decreased bone mineralization, in the absence of fractures, in the growing human-milk-fed VLBW neonate is a significant problem. With continued human milk feedings over time, these infants demonstrate improvement of bone mineral content and lower serum alkaline phosphatase levels. They usually maintain normal serum calcium and phosphorus concentrations. Excessive calcium salt supplementation may result in nephrocalcinosis, intestinal intolerance, or calcium-induced intestinal obstruction, perforation, and subsequent peritonitis.[155]

Methods of Enteral Feeding of VLBW Neonates

Because the VLBW neonate of less than 32–34 weeks' gestation cannot coordinate sucking, swallowing, uvula and epiglottic closure, esophageal propulsion and peristalsis, and gastric motility, they are usually fed by nasogastric or orogastric tube. Gravity drip or intermittent gavage and intragastric feedings are common choices among neonatologists. VLBW neonates initially are fed every hour, and the frequency extends to every 2 to 3 hours with increasing postnatal age and greater tolerance of the feedings.[125]

Continuous enteral feedings have been successful but may be associated with a higher risk of tube complications and reduced nutrient availability. The latter results from the separation of fat from the milk in the tubing during continuous infusions. In most infants, there is no demonstrable benefit of continuous versus intermittent feedings. In some patients, intermittent gavage feedings may cause a reduction of the tidal volume and of minute ventilation with an increase in pulmonary resistance.[156] The clinical significance of these findings has yet to be determined.

Intragastric feedings permit gastric digestion of various nutrients, provide some antimicrobial properties from gastric acidity, are not associated with dumping syndrome, and may improve the tolerance of high osmotic loads.[135] Nasojejunal or transpyloric feeding avoids reflux or regurgitation and the risk of aspiration pneumonia. This type of feeding may be beneficial for neonates with a poor gag reflex, gastroesophageal reflux, and emesis with depressed levels of consciousness. Transpyloric feedings may overcome delayed gastric emptying times noted in some VLBW neonates. Transpyloric feedings have been associated with fat malabsorption, dumping of hypertonic formula, diarrhea, and abnormal colonization of the upper small intestine.[10,157-159] Additional problems associated with tube feedings are listed in Table 51.7.

The rate of advancing enteral nutrition among VLBW neonates may have a significant effect on the incidence of gastrointestinal intolerance, diarrhea, or NEC.[125] Among VLBW neonates, caloric density usually is initiated at half-strength formula (10 calories per ounce) and advanced slowly to full-strength formula over 24 to 48 hours. Thereafter the volume of formula is increased so that full enteral nutrition (i.e., 150 ml·kg^{-1}day^{-1}) is achieved 7 to 14 days after the initiation of milk feeding.[125] Signs of emesis, abdominal distention, diarrhea, or elevated gastric residuals should require that the rate of the increment of milk volume be reduced to allow for individual patient differences. Significant clinical manifestations such as abdominal tenderness, hematochezia, hematemesis, hypothermia, apnea/bradycardia, abdominal wall erythema, an abdominal mass, and persistent bloody stools suggest the diagnosis of NEC.[125] Laboratory evidence of NEC includes acidosis, neutropenia, and thrombocytopenia; radiographic signs includes pneumatosis intestinalis, portal venous gas, and pneumoperitoneum.[125]

Necrotizing enterocolitis is a disease of unknown etiology. It is almost universally noted among enterally fed neonates, as 95% have been fed formula or, less often, human milk. NEC can occur on any day of life after the initiation of enteral feedings but usually is noted within 7 to 10 days of milk feeding. Delaying enteral alimentation does not reduce the incidence of NEC.[131] Rapid increases in milk volume and hyperosmotic formula have been associated with the development of NEC.[125] In some studies the incidence of rapid volume changes during enteral alimentation is noted more frequently in patients with NEC than among age-matched controls.[125] Patients who later developed NEC had daily enteral volume increments of 57 ml·kg^{-1}day^{-1} versus 22 ml·kg^{-1}day^{-1} among patients who did not develop NEC. Although slower feeding protocols have not yet been proved to reduce the incidence of NEC in a prospective clinical trial, it would be prudent to avoid daily formula volume increments of more than 20 ml·kg^{-1}day^{-1}.

Hypocaloric Enteral Feeding of the VLBW Neonate

There are significant advantages for the VLBW neonate given enteral feedings (Table 51.10). Although there have been various risks associated with enteral alimentation, they can be minimized by judicious use of appropriate formula or preterm maternal milk, slow increments of milk volume, and careful monitoring of the neonate's status. Currently, infants with RDS, umbilical artery catheters, PDA, and bronchopulmonary dysplasia can benefit from enteral nutrients as early as the first week of life. This route of alimentation is physiologic and can provide a greater density of macronutrients, trace elements, and minerals than the parenteral route. Trophic intraluminal nutrients may stimulate mucosal growth; these nutrients may include glucose, amino acids, glutamine, nucleotides, and the short-chain fatty acids.[160]

TABLE 51.10. Beneficial effects of hypocaloric enteral feedings.

Direct (nutrient) or indirect (paracrine, endocrine) trophic effects on mucosal growth
Stimulation of biliary-pancreatic secretion
Improved glucose tolerance
Reduced indirect hyperbilirubinemia
Reduced cholestatic jaundice
Reduced osteopenia of prematurity
Reduced risk of central catheter complications including sepsis
Faster achievement of full enteral feeds
Faster maturation of gastrointestinal motility
Reduced feeding intolerance
Improved weight gain
No increased risk for necrotizing enterocolitis

Intravenous nutrition should supplement enteral alimentation during the period when the intragastric feeding volume is advanced.

Dunn et al.[114] have demonstrated the safety and beneficial effects of early hypocaloric feedings in VLBW neonates. Twenty neonates were kept NPO for 10 days and received parenteral alimentation, and 19 VLBW (mean gestational age 26.8 weeks and birth weight 989 g) received parenteral alimentation in addition to hypocaloric enteral feedings beginning on the second day of life. Most of these neonates had RDS, umbilical artery catheters, and PDA; all required endotracheal intubation and mechanical ventilation. Hypocaloric feedings, named "gut stimulation" by the nursery staff, were initiated with half-strength premature formula at 48 hours of age. Neonates were fed every hour or every 2 hours and received 0.5 to 2.0 ml per feeding depending on their weight. The total daily volume was 15 to 20 ml·kg^{-1}day^{-1} and the formula was advanced to full strength as tolerated. Neonates received enteral feedings for 10 days of the study, after which time the clinician could decide to initiate or advance enteral feedings in either the NPO group or the hypocaloric group, respectively.

Because of the trophic effects of enteral nutrition on the intestinal mucosa and its beneficial effect on bile flow, it was hypothesized that the hypocaloric-fed neonates would demonstrate improved feeding tolerance and less cholestatic jaundice. Compared with the group kept NPO for 10 days, the hypocaloric-fed group demonstrated a faster time to full enteral alimentation, fewer days with physiologic jaundice, fewer days on phototherapy, a lower incidence of cholestatic jaundice, lower serum alkaline phosphatase levels, and improved oral glucose tolerance.[114] Ill VLBW neonates who were intubated and had umbilical arterial catheters in place benefited from early hypocaloric feedings as demonstrated by a lower incidence of cholestatic jaundice and osteopenia of prematurity. There were no episodes of aspiration pneumonia, nor were there more cases of NEC in this group than in the control NPO group. Improved feeding tolerance and no untoward effects were noted also in other studies that gave small enteral feedings to VLBW neonates.[129,161,162]

An appropriate approach to the alimentation of the ill VLBW neonate includes both parenteral and enteral nutritional support. The results of randomized controlled trials of hypocaloric feeding have demonstrated significant beneficial effects related to the many common nutritional problems of the VLBW neonate. Hypocaloric enteral feeding helps to reduce the incidence of metabolic bone disease, cholestatic jaundice, and glucose intolerance. These beneficial responses are not associated with added risks, as the incidence of NEC and aspiration pneumonia is not greater in the enterally fed patients than in those kept NPO. Feeding tolerance appears to be improved by prior hypocaloric alimentation. The presence of an endotracheal tube or an umbilical artery catheter does not influence the success or increase the risks associated with enteral alimentation (e.g., NEC). Early enteral alimentation may be initiated during the first week of life and be maintained at a fixed level during this time. Once the patient demonstrates tolerance to enteral feedings the volume can be increased slowly (not more than $20\,\text{ml}\cdot\text{kg}^{-1}\,\text{day}^{-1}$) to achieve full enteral feeding ($150\,\text{ml}\cdot\text{kg}^{-1}\,\text{day}^{-1}$) within 7 to 14 days of the onset of enteral nutrition.

Parenteral alimentation can supplement the enteral feedings. Total parenteral nutrition should be reserved for the unusual patient populations discussed previously.

Special Nutritional Problems of the VLBW Neonate

Short Bowel Syndrome

Short bowel syndrome is a significant problem in the NICU. Congenital anomalies of the bowel (e.g., volvulus, gastroschisis), cystic fibrosis (e.g., meconium ileus, atresia, peritonitis), and NEC are common gastrointestinal diseases that result in short bowel syndrome. The nutritional support of patients with short bowel syndrome requires a combination of parenteral and enteral alimentation.[136,163] Malabsorption is a common problem for these neonates. The severity of malabsorption does not always correspond to the length of the remaining bowel. Nevertheless, the shorter the remaining intestine, the greater the incidence of malabsorption and diarrhea. The absence of an ileocecal valve further increases this incidence. Although neonates have survived with as little as 10 to 15 cm of small bowel with or without an ileocecal valve, most neonates with this limited length of intestine do not survive without prolonged parenteral nutrition and possibly transplantation.[164-166]

The diarrhea associated with short bowel syndrome has multiple etiologies, including reduced absorptive area, intestinal bacterial overgrowth, malabsorption of fat, osmotic diarrhea due to lactose malabsorption, bile salt deconjugation, viral agents (e.g., enteric adenovirus), and hypergastrinemia with excessive gastric acid secretion. Nutritional disorders include malabsorption of fat or carbohydrates, calcium, fat-soluble vitamins, and in the long term, vitamin B_{12} (Table 51.11).

Total parenteral nutrition has improved the immediate outcome of these infants. The chronic debilitating problems of osteopenia, cholestatic jaundice, central venous catheter-related sepsis, and end-stage hepatic failure significantly contribute to the morbidity and mortality of patients with short bowel syndrome. Whenever possible, parenteral nutrition support should be supplemented with low-volume enteral feedings. Elemental formula, carbohydrate free (replaced with fructose or glucose), or formula with casein hydrolysates and polymerized glucose with or without MCT oil, have been successfully employed to improve the nutritional care. Hydrolyzed casein is more trophic to the intestinal mucosa than whole protein, while long-chain fatty acids are more trophic than medium-chain triglycerides.[167] Enteral alimentation is often frustrating, with exacerbations of diarrhea associated with increases of the volume of oral feedings.

Care must be given to the fluid and electrolyte balance of these infants during the immediate postoperative and convalescent stages. A simple episode of gastroenteritis can cause severe ileostomy fluid losses resulting in dehydration, hyponatremia, and metabolic acidosis. If possible, the ileostomy should be closed and the small and large bowel reconnected to take advantage of the colon's

TABLE 51.11. Complications of short gut syndrome.

Acute
   Hyponatremia—hypokalemia (end jejunostomy syndrome)
   Diarrhea induced hypovolemia
   Adenoviral (other viral) superimposed diarrhea
   Malabsorption (osmotic diarrhea)
   Hypergastrinemia (secretory diarrhea)
   Bile salt malabsorption (cholerrheic-secretory diarrhea)
   Acidosis (bicarbonate losses)

Chronic
   Failure to thrive
   TPN-hepatic disease (cholestasis)
   Cholelithiasis
   Catheter complications (sepsis, thrombosis, dislodgement)
   Bacterial overgrowth
   D-lactic acidemia (coma, mental status changes)
   Colitis-ileitis-like lesions
   Vitamin A, D, E, K, and B_{12} deficiency
   Trace mineral deficiency (zinc, etc.)
   Anastomotic strictures
   Bile salt deficiency (steatorrhea)
   Oxalate nephrolithiasis
   Malabsorption of oral drugs (antibiotics, etc.)
   Metabolic (TPN-induced) bone disease

great ability to reabsorb water and electrolytes.[125] Added care should be given to avoid the development of various nutritional deficiencies, such as those due to fat-soluble vitamin (e.g., D, E, A, K), trace minerals (e.g., copper, zinc), and essential fatty acids. If these deficiency syndromes are not treated, they contribute to somatic growth failure and impede intestinal recovery.

Therapy must be carefully balanced and titrated. Cholestyramine is of value in the therapy of bile salt associated diarrhea but may result in bile salt malabsorption and bile salt depletion. Loperamide may be helpful in reducing a rapid transit time, but if transit becomes too slow, intestinal bacterial overgrowth may develop. Somatostatin may improve a secretory diarrhea but inhibit the growth of the villus. Surgical placement of valves may slow intestinal transport but increases the risk of intestinal bacterial overgrowth.

Bronchopulmonary Dysplasia

Bronchopulmonary dysplasia (BPD) is another significant sequela of VLBW neonates following prolonged periods of oxygen therapy and mechanical ventilation.[136] Patients with BPD often remain oxygen and mechanical ventilator dependent for many months after birth. The pulmonary pathology of BPD includes fibrosis, atelectasis, and focal emphysema, which creates serious ventilation-perfusion inequalities and chronic hypoxia and hypercarbia. Chronic respiratory acidosis and hypoxia may produce pulmonary hypertension and cor pulmonale. Episodes of fluid retention produce left-sided heart failure with pulmonary edema, which further exacerbates the chronic underlying pulmonary parenchymal disease.

Because of the risk of cor pulmonale, left-sided heart failure, and pulmonary edema, the fluid status of infants with BPD is often tenuous. Heart failure may be precipitated by receiving too much fluid, whereas, alternatively, BPD may produce renal sodium retention with resultant fluid overload and pulmonary edema. The medical management of patients with BPD includes diuretics and moderate fluid restriction to reduce the risk of heart failure and pulmonary edema. Diuretic therapy is unfortunately associated with adverse effects, such as the development of a hypokalemic hypochloremic metabolic alkalosis, hypercalciuria with nephrocalcinosis and nephrolithiasis, diminished bone mineralization, and gallbladder sludge or stones. Hypokalemic alkalosis may be treated with potassium chloride, and diminished bone mineralization may require supplementation with calcium and vitamin D.

Fluid restriction has been accomplished by feeding BPD patients hypercaloric formula concentrated to 24, 27, or even 30 calories per ounce. Enhanced caloric provisions are necessary to balance the increased oxygen consumption (i.e., energy expenditures) and the negative effects on growth of steroid therapy.[168,169] Increasing the caloric density decreases the fluid intake but also adds new potential nutritional problems. High caloric density formula enriched with added carbohydrates may exacerbate carbohydrate malabsorption and produce watery diarrhea, emesis, flatulence, borborygmi, abdominal distention, and feeding intolerance. High MCT oil formula enrichment is associated with emesis, diarrhea, and abdominal distention. Excessive concentration of the formula may increase the renal solute load. As discussed above, there is currently no proved biologic advantage as determined by energy balance studies for preferring MCT when compared with long-chain triglycerides. The signs and symptoms associated with feeding intolerances due to MCT or carbohydrate enrichment can be confused with more serious neonatal gastrointestinal conditions, such as infectious diarrhea, NEC, or intestinal obstruction. Repeated episodes of feeding intolerance may result in multiple lengthy periods of patients being placed NPO with further dependence on parenteral alimentation and the added risks associated with intravenous nutrition. Hypercaloric enteral alimentation, as discussed in previous sections, may have other detrimental effects. The added calories may produce an increase in basal and postprandial oxygen consumption, and hence carbon dioxide production. The net effect in patients with BPD may be an added stress to an already compromised respiratory system.[101,170] Growth may not be enhanced as well as one would expect from these additional calories. The added calories may result in an increase in expended energy or fat deposition or both, which may not benefit new lean tissue growth, especially that needed the most for the healing lung. Oxygen consumption is reported to be higher in patients with BPD than in age-matched controls. This fact may be related to a presumed increased work of breathing due to increased elastic recoil of the lung and increased size of the physiologic dead space. Alternatively, the increased oxygen consumption in BPD patients may be related to their high caloric intake. Energy is required for lung and somatic growth. Nonetheless, there must be a balance between energy intake to meet these patients' needs with energy expenditure in the basal and postprandial states.

Another theoretical nutritional aspect of caring for patients with BPD relates to the composition of the nutrient intake. Alimentation with a high carbohydrate load (enteral or parenteral) results in a high carbon dioxide production with a respiratory quotient (RQ) near 1. The RQ may actually exceed 1 if the carbohydrates serve as precursors for lipogenesis. Fat-based alimentation results in a lower carbon dioxide production rate and may decrease the carbon dioxide needed to be excreted by the sick lung.[101,170] Cyclic hypercapnea has been reported in adults during periods of carbohydrate-based alimentation. Modified liquid diets with increased fat content have been used with some success to improve lung function among adult patients with chronic obstructive lung disease.[171-174] In one study of infants receiving an intravenous glucose load of 4 and 12 mg·kg^{-1}·min^{-1} on two consecutive days, basal oxygen consumption, basal carbon dioxide production, and resting energy expenditure were increased in infants with BPD compared to control infants.[175]

The prudent nutritional approach to infants with BPD is to provide sufficient formula to permit growth of 10 to 20 g·kg^{-1}·day^{-1} without excessive fluid intake, which might exacerbate heart failure. Use of MCT supplementation is theoretically preferable to supplementation with glucose polymers in an attempt to lower carbon dioxide production. Excessive caloric intake should be monitored carefully, as it may increase energy expenditure. Diuretics should be added if fluid balance results in heart failure. Potassium chloride supplement should be given to prevent hypokalemia alkalosis. Nevertheless, the principal treatment of BPD is oxygen in sufficient amounts to prevent arterial desaturation. Repeated or persistent episodes of hypoxia exacerbate pulmonary hypertension and cause deterioration of the right side of the heart. Appropriate nutritional management cannot reverse the harmful effects of arterial hypoxemia. All attempts should be made to maintain the arterial saturation above 90%. If this level can be achieved, nutritional support will result in successful weight gain and linear growth.

The Critically Ill Neonate: Systemic Inflammatory Response Syndrome (SIRS)

Critical illness, especially that associated with the SIRS is associated with specific metabolic and nutritional perturbations due to accelerated catabolism and attenuated nutrient utilization (Table 51.12). SIRS in an acute, though often subacute, inflammatory response to infection, necrotizing enterocolitis, asphyxia, burns, trauma, or surgery and is frequently associated with the multiple organ dysfunction syndrome (MODS), such as respiratory or renal insufficiency, hepatic failure, central nervous system depression, or cardiac pump failure.[102,176]

Infammatory mediators such as tumor necrosis factor (TNF) (previously called cachexin) result in many of the manifestations of SIRS and MODS. Indeed, prior treatment with antibody to TNF in animal models may attenuate these symptoms. Gastrointestinal and nutritional manifestations of SIRS and MODS often include ileus, gastric atony, splanchnic hypoperfusion, hepatic synthetic and detoxification failure, poor growth, and poor wound healing.

TABLE 51.12. Potential metabolic perturbations during systemic inflammatory response syndrome.

Oxygen consumption-energy metabolism
  Hypermetabolism—excessive oxygen consumption (increased resting energy expenditure)
  Poor distribution of microcirculation—regional ischemia including mesenteric circulation
  Oxygen delivery—consumption regional mismatch
  Hypo-hyperthermia
Carbohydrate metabolism
  Hyperglycemia
  Enhanced gluconeogenesis and glycogenolysis
  Insulin resistance
  Enhanced counterregulatory hormone secretion (epinephrine, norepinephrine, glucagon, cortisol, prolactin, growth hormone)
  Hypoglycemia
  Lactic acidosis
  Elevated CO_2 production
Protein-amino acids
  Enhanced proteolysis
  Enhanced negative nitrogen balance
  Synthesis of acute phase reactants, cytokines, etc.
  Hyperaminoacidemia (tyrosine, phenylalanine)
  Hypoaminoacidemia (valine, leucine, isoleucine)
  Hypoalbuminemia
Lipids
  Enhanced lipolysis
  Hypertriglyceridemia
  Hyper or hypoketonemia
  Altered oxidation of free fatty acids
  Reduced lipogenesis

In addition to the effects of SIRS on metabolism (see Table 51.12), nutrients may adversely contribute to morbidity. Therefore, in SIRS, poor utilization of infused or ingested nutrients may produce an added metabolic stress for the patient. Excessive provision of glucose may produce hyperglycemia or lactic acidosis, while excessive protein or amino acid intake may contribute to hyperammonemia.[176] Intralipids may exacerbate a ventilation-perfusion mismatch, while excessive glucose loading will increase carbon dioxide production and add to the work of breathing. Attempts to overcome the negative nitrogen balance noted during SIRS may not enhance growth or tissue healing but may produce significant metabolic disturbances.

Nonetheless, poor nutrient intake may contribute to muscle weakness (e.g., hypophosphatemia, protein losses), pulmonary surfactant synthetic defects, immunodeficiency, hypoalbuminemia, specific nutrient deficiencies, or osteopenia. Thus, optimal nutritional support may improve outcome if used judiciously. If the stress of SIRS can be predicted (e.g., date of surgical repair of congenital heart disease), then preoperative nutritional support (e.g., continuous 24 hour nasogastric tube feedings) may improve the nutritional status of the patient at the time of surgery.

Considerable discussion has centered on the route of nutrient support during or after SIRS. The enteral route is preferred by some authorities as it is simple, less costly, associated with fewer risks and because it enhances intestinal mucosal growth and integrity.[177] The latter consideration is important because excessive mucosal permeability during SIRS may contribute to sepsis following translocation of bacteria or endotoxin from the intestinal lumen, through the mucosa to the systemic circulation. Others believe total parenteral nutrition is equally beneficial.[178] To date there is little evidence of the value of either method of nutrition in the VLBW infant with SIRS. Considering the developmental immaturity, together with the added nutrient intolerance associated with SIRS, it is prudent to provide sufficient calories in the form of glucose in the first 1 to 2 days of a SIRS-like illness to support oxidative metabolism and to avoid hypoglycemia and excessive rates of negative nitrogen balance. Thereafter, intravenous amino acids may be added at 48 to 72 hours. The authors do not recommend early use of intravenous lipid in neonates with SIRS. In addition, enteral feedings, although theoretically beneficial, must be balanced with the gastric atony and small bowel dysmotility problems associated with SIRS and with prematurity.

Acknowledgment. The authors wish to express their gratitude for the expert assistance in the preparation of this manuscript to Ms. Sandy Ingram.

References

1. Kliegman R. The fetus and the neonatal infant. In: Behrman R, Kliegman R, Arvin A, eds. Nelson textbook of pediatrics. 15th ed. Philadelphia: Saunders, 1996:431–513.
2. Davies DP. The first feed of low birthweight infants. Arch Dis Child 1978;53:187–192.
3. Brooke OG. Nutrition in the preterm infant. Lancet 1983; 2:514–516.
4. Nutrition Committee, Canadian Paediatric Society. Nutrient needs and feeding of premature infants. Can Med Assoc J 1995;152:1765–1785.
5. Auld PAM, Bhangananda P, Mehta S. The influence of an early caloric intake with I-V glucose on catabolism of premature infants. Pediatrics 1966;37:592–596.
6. Cornblath M, Forbes AE, Pildes RS, et al. A controlled study of early fluid administration on survival of low birth weight infants. Pediatrics 1960;38:547–554.
7. Wu PYK, Teilmann P, Gabler M, et al. "Early" versus "late" feeding of low birth weight neonates: effect on serum bilirubin, blood sugar, and responses to glucagon and epinephrine tolerance tests. Pediatrics 1967;39:733–739.
8. Rabor IF, Oh W, Wu PYK, et al. The effects of early and late feeding of intrauterine fetally malnourished (IUM) infants. Pediatrics 1968;42:261–269.
9. Wilson DC. Nutrition of the preterm baby. Br J Obstet Gynaecol 1995;102:854–860.
10. Kliegman R, Fanaroff A. Developmental metabolism and nutrition. In: Gregory G, ed. Pediatric anesthesia. 2nd ed. New York: Churchill Livingstone, 1989:201–286.
11. Kliegman R, Hulman S. Intrauterine growth retardation: determinants of aberrant fetal growth. In: Fanaroff A, Martin R, eds. Neonatal perinatal medicine: diseases of the fetus and newborn. 4th ed. St. Louis: Mosby, 1987:69–114.
12. Sunehag A, Gustafsson J, Ewald U. Very immature infants (≤30 wk) respond to glucose infusion with incomplete suppression of glucose production. Pediatr Res 1994;36:550–555.
13. Heird WC, Driscoll JM, Schullinger N, et al. Intravenous alimentation in pediatric patients. J Pediatr 1972;80:351–372.
14. Bhakoo ON, Scopes JW. Minimal rates of oxygen consumption in small-for-dates babies during the first week of life. Arch Dis Child 1974;49:583–584.
15. Ferre P, Pegorier J-P, Marliss EB, et al. Influence of exogenous fat and gluconeogenic substrates on glucose homeostasis in the newborn rat. Am J Physiol 1978;234: E129–E136.
16. Kliegman RM, Morton S. The metabolic response of the canine neonate to twenty-four hours of fasting. Metabolism 1987;36:521–526.
17. Kliegman RM, Miettinen EL, Adam PAJ. Fetal and neonatal responses to maternal canine starvation: circulating fuels and neonatal glucose production. Pediatr Res 1981;15:945–951.
18. Miettinen E-L, Kliegman RM, Tserng K-Y. Fetal neonatal responses to extended maternal canine starvation. I. Circulating fuels and glucose and lactate turnover. Pediatr Res 1983;17:634–638.
19. Hawdon JM, Aynsley-Green A, Ward Platt MP. Neonatal blood glucose concentrations: metabolic effects of intravenous glucagon and intragastric medium chain triglyceride. Arch Dis Child 1993;68:255–261.
20. Sauer PJJ, Carnielli VP, Sulkers EJ, et al. Substrate utilization during the first weeks of life. Acta Paediatr Suppl 1994;405:49–53.
21. Sulkers EJ, Lafeber HN, van Goudoever JB, et al. Decreased glucose oxidation in preterm infants fed a formula containing medium-chain triglycerides. Pediatr Res 1993; 33:101–105.
22. Yunis KA, Oh W, Kalhan S, et al. Glucose kinetics following administration of an intravenous fat emulsion to low-birth-weight neonates. Am J Physiol 1992;263:E844–E849.
23. Grylack LJ, Chu SS, Scanlon JW. Use of intravenous fluids before cesarean section: effects on perinatal glucose, insulin, and sodium homeostasis. Obstet Gynecol 1984;63:654–658.
24. Koh THHG, Aynsley-Green A, Tarbit M, et al. Neural dysfunction during hypoglycaemia. Arch Dis Child 1988; 63:1353–1358.
25. Koh THHG, Eyre JA, Aynsley-Green A. Neonatal hypoglycaemia—the controversy regarding definition. Arch Dis Child 1988;63:1386–1398.

26. Kliegman RM. Cerebral metabolic intermediate response following severe canine intrauterine growth retardation. Pediatr Res 1986;20:662–667.
27. Kliegman RM. Cerebral metabolic response to neonatal hypoglycemia in growth-retarded dogs. Pediatr Res 1988;24:649–652.
28. Lucas A, Morley R, Cole TJ. Adverse neurodevelopmental outcome of moderate neonatal hypoglycaemia. Br Med J 1988;297:1304–1308.
29. Sexson WR. Incidence of neonatal hypoglycemia: a matter of definition. J Pediatr 1984;105:149–150.
30. Heck LJ, Erenberg A. Serum glucose levels in term neonates during the first 48 hours of life. J Pediatr 1987;110:119–122.
31. Srinivasan G, Pildes RS, Cattamanchi G, et al. Plasma glucose values in normal neonates: a new look. J Pediatr 1986;109:114–117.
32. Lilien LD, Pildes RS, Srinivasan G, et al. Treatment of neonatal hypoglycemia with minibolus and intravenous glucose infusion. J Pediatr 1980;97:295–298.
33. Tsang R, Nichols B. Eds. Nutrition during infancy. St. Louis: Mosby, 1988.
34. Wharton B. Nutrition and feeding of preterm infants. Oxford: Blackwell, 1987.
35. Fomon S, Heird W. Energy and protein needs during infancy. Orlando: Academic Press, 1986.
36. Freymond D, Schutz Y, Decombaz J, et al. Energy balance, physical activity, and thermogenic effect of feeding in premature infants. Pediatr Res 1986;20:638–645.
37. Brooke OG. Energy balance and metabolic rate in preterm infants fed with standard and high-energy formulas. Br J Nutr 1980;44:13–23.
38. Brooke OG, Alvear J, Arnold M. Energy retention, energy expenditure, and growth in healthy immature infants. Pediatr Res 1979;13:215–220.
39. Committee on Nutrition, American Academy of Pediatrics. Nutritional needs of preterm infants. Pediatric nutrition handbook. Elk Grove Village, IL: American Academy of Pediatrics, 1993:64–89.
40. Committee on Nutrition of the Preterm Infant, European Society of Paediatric Gastroenterology and Nutrition. Nutrition and feeding of preterm infants. Acta Paediatr Scand 1987;suppl 336:1–14.
41. Whyte RK, Campbell D, Stanhope R, et al. Energy balance in low birth weight infants fed formula of high or low medium-chain triglyceride content. J Pediatr 1986;108:964–971.
42. Reichman B, Chessex P, Verellen G, et al. Dietary composition and macronutrient storage in preterm infants. Pediatrics 1983;72:322–328.
43. Reichman B, Chessex P, Putet G, et al. Diet, fat accretion, and growth in premature infants. N Engl J Med 1981;305:1495–1500.
44. Clark DA. Nutritional requirements of the premature and small for gestational age infant. In: Suskind RM, Lewinter-Suskind L, eds. Textbook of pediatric nutrition. 2nd ed. New York: Raven Press, 1993:23–31.
45. Greene HL, Hambridge M, Schanler R, et al. Guidelines for the use of vitamins, trace elements, calcium, magnesium, and phosphorus in infants and children receiving total parenteral nutrition: report of the Subcommittee on Pediatric Parenteral Nutrient Requirements from the Committee on Clinical Practice Issues of the American Society for Clinical Nutrition. Am J Clin Nutr 1988;48:1324–1342.
46. Pereira GR. Nutritional care of the extremely premature infant. Clin Perinatol 1995;22:61–75.
47. Zlotkin SH, Atkinson S, Lockitch G. Trace elements in nutrition for premature infants. Clin Perinatol 1995;22:223–240.
48. Innis SM, Lupton BA, Nelson CM. Biochemical and functional approaches to study of fatty acid requirements for very premature infants. Nutrition 1994;10:72–76.
49. Uauy R, Hoffman DR, Birch EE, et al. Safety and efficacy of omega-3 fatty acids in the nutrition of very low birth weight infants: soy oil and marine oil supplementation of formula. J Pediatr 1994;124:612–620.
50. Uauy-Dagach R, Mena P, Hoffman DR. Essential fatty acid metabolism and requirements for LBW infants. Acta Paediatr Suppl 1994;405:78–85.
51. Uauy-Dagach R, Mena P. Nutritional role of omega-3 fatty acids during the perinatal period. Clin Perinatol 1995;22:157–175.
52. Stahl G, Spear ML, Hamosh M. Intravenous administration of lipid emulsions to premature infants. Clin Perinatol 1986;13:133–162.
53. Pildes P. Neonatal hyperglycemia. J Pediatr 1986;109:905–907.
54. Cowett RM, Oh W, Pollak A, et al. Glucose disposal of low birth weight infants: steady state hyperglycemia produced by constant intravenous glucose infusion. Pediatrics 1979;63:389–396.
55. Louik C, Mitchell AA, Epstein MF, et al. Risk factors for neonatal hyperglycemia associated with 10% dextrose infusion. Am J Dis Child 1985;139:783–786.
56. Hulman S, Kliegman R, Heng J, et al. Relationship of substrate level to turnover rate in fasted adult and newborn dogs. Am J Physiol 1988;254:E137–E143.
57. Pollak A, Cowett RM, Schwartz R, et al. Glucose disposal in low-birth-weight infants during steady-state hyperglycemia: effects of exogenous insulin administration. Pediatrics 1978;61:546–549.
58. Goldman SL, Hirata T. Attenuated response to insulin in very low birthweight infants. Pediatr Res 1980;14:50–53.
59. Hertz DE, Karn CA, Liu YM, et al. Intravenous glucose suppresses glucose production but not proteolysis in extremely premature newborns. J Clin Invest 1993;92:1752–1758.
60. Cowett RM, Oh W, Schwartz R. Persistent glucose production during glucose infusion in the human neonate. J Clin Invest 1983;71:467–475.
61. Feng B-C, Li J, Kliegman RM. Effects of insulin, epinephrine and glucose on regulation of transcription of the serine dehydratase gene in newborn dogs. Biochem Mol Med 1996;57:91–96.
62. Sparks J, Lynch A, Chez R, et al. Glycogen regulation in isolated perfused near term monkey liver. Pediatr Res 1976;10:51–58.

63. Ostertag SG, Jovanovic L, Lewis B, et al. Insulin pump therapy in the very low birth weight infant. Pediatrics 1986;78:625–630.
64. Binder ND, Raschko PK, Benda GI, et al. Insulin infusion with parenteral nutrition in extremely low birth weight infants with hyperglycemia. J Pediatr 1989;114:273–280.
65. Collins JW, Hoppe M, Brown K, et al. A controlled trial of insulin infusion and parenteral nutrition in extremely low birth weight infants with glucose intolerance. J Pediatr 1991;118:921–927.
66. Lipsky CL, Spear ML. Recent advances in parenteral nutrition. Clin Perinatol 1995;22:141–155.
67. Kliegman RM, Sparks JW. Perinatal galactose metabolism. J Pediatr 1985;107:831–841.
68. Kliegman RM, Morton S. Galactose assimilation in pups of diabetic canine mothers. Diabetes 1987;36:1280–1285.
69. Kliegman RM, Miettinen EL, Kalhan SC, et al. The effect of enteric galactose on neonatal canine carbohydrate metabolism. Metabolism 1981;30:1109–1118.
70. Pribylova J, Kozlova J. Glucose and galactose infusions in newborns of diabetic and healthy mothers. Biol Neonate 1979;36:193–199.
71. Sparks J, Avery G, Fletcher A, et al. Parenteral galactose therapy in the glucose intolerant premature infant. J Pediatr 1982;100:255–261.
72. Kliegman RM, Morton S. Sequential intrahepatic metabolic effects of enteric galactose alimentation in newborn rats. Pediatr Res 1988;24:302–307.
73. Kaempf JW, Li H-Q, Groothius JR, et al. Galactose, glucose, and lactate concentrations in the portal venous and arterial circulations of newborn lambs after nursing. Pediatr Res 1988;23:598–602.
74. Jannace PW, Lerman RH, Dennis RG, et al. Total parenteral nutrition-induced cyclic hypercapnia. Crit Care Med 1988;16:727–728.
75. Heird WC, Hay W, Helms RA, et al. Pediatric parenteral amino acid mixture in low birth weight infants. Pediatrics 1988;81:41–50.
76. Heird WC, Dell RB, Helms RA, et al. Amino acid mixture designed to maintain normal plasma amino acid patterns in infants and children requiring parenteral nutrition. Pediatrics 1987;80:401–408.
77. Kerner JA. Parenteral nutrition in the premature infant. Part I. Perinatol Neonatal 1988;12:18–22.
78. Kerner JA. Parenteral nutrition in the premature infant. Part II. New information on specific nutrient requirements. Perinatol Neonatol 1988;12:8–33.
79. Lemons JA, Neal P, Ernst J. Nitrogen sources for parenteral nutrition in the newborn infant. Clin Perinatol 1986;13:91–109.
80. Nose O, Tipton JR, Ament ME, et al. Effect of the energy source on changes in energy expenditure, respiratory quotient, and nitrogen balance during total parenteral nutrition in children. Pediatr Res 1987;21:538–541.
81. Zlotkin SH. Trophamine. Pediatrics 1988;82:388–389.
82. Adamkin D, Radmacher P, Rosen P. Comparison of a neonatal versus general-purpose amino acid formulation in preterm neonates. J Perinatal 1995;15:108–113.
83. Heird WC. Amino acid and energy needs of pediatric patients receiving parenteral nutrition. Pediatr Clin North Am 1995;42:765–789.
84. Mitton SG. Amino acids and lipid in total parenteral nutrition for the newborn. J Pediatr Gastroenterol Nutr 1994;18:25–31.
85. Committee on Nutrition. Use of intravenous fat emulsions in pediatric patients. Pediatrics 1981;68:738–793.
86. Dainow II. Safety of Intralipid. Lancet 1980;2:1020–1021.
87. Helbock HJ, Ames BN. Use of intravenous lipids in neonates. J Pediatr 1995;126:747–748.
88. Hertel J, Tygstrup I, Andersen GE. Intravascular fat accumulation after Intralipid infusion in the very low-birth-weight infant. J Pediatr 1982;100:975–976.
89. Kretchmer N, Minkowski A. Nutritional adaptation of the gastrointestinal tract of the newborn. New York: Raven Press, 1983.
90. Levene MI, Wigglesworth JS, Desai R. Pulmonary fat accumulation after Intralipid infusion in the preterm infant. Lancet 1980;2:815–818.
91. Brans YW, Ritter DA, Kenny JD, et al. Influence of intravenous fat emulsion on serum bilirubin in very low birth-weight neonates. Arch Dis Child 1987;62:156–160.
92. Skeie B, Askanazi J, Rothkopf MM, et al. Intravenous fat emulsions and lung function: a review. Crit Care Med 1988;16:183–194.
93. Venus B, Prager R, Patel CB, et al. Cardiopulmonary effects of Intralipid infusion in critically ill patients. Crit Care Med 1988;16:587–590.
94. Schroder H, Paust H, Schmidt R. Pulmonary fat embolism after Intralipid therapy—a post-mortem artefact? Light and electron microscopic investigations in low-birth-weight infants. Acta Paediatr Scand 1984;73:461–464.
95. Schroder H, Paust H, Schmidt R. Pulmonary fat embolism after Intralipid therapy—a post-mortem artefact? Light and electron microscopic investigations in low-birth-weight infants. Acta Paediatr Scand 1984;73:461–464.
96. Greer FR, McCormick A, Locker J. Changes in fat concentration of human milk during delivery by intermittent bolus and continuous mechanical pump infusion. J Pediatr 1984;105:745–749.
97. Etzioni A, Meshulam T, Zeltzer M, et al. Intralipid effects on preterm neonate serum: chemoattractant and opsonizing capacities. J Pediatr Gastroenterol Nutr 1987; 6:105–108.
98. Usmani SA, Harper RG, Usmani SF. Effect of a lipid emulsion (Intralipid) on polymorphonuclear leukocyte functions in the neonate. J Pediatr 1988;113:132–136.
99. Fischer GW, Hunter KW, Wilson SR, et al. Diminished bacterial defenses with Intralipid. Lancet 1980;2:819–820.
100. Adamkin D, Radmacher PG, Klingbeil RL. Use of intravenous lipid and hyperbilirubinemia in the first week. J Pediatr Gastroenterol Nutr 1992;14:135–139.
101. Chessex P, Belanger S, Piedboeuf B, et al. Influence of energy substrates on respiratory gas exchange during conventional mechanical ventilation of preterm infants. J Pediatr 1995;126:619–624.
102. Adan D, LaGamma EF, Browne LE. Nutritional management and the multisystem organ failure/systemic inflam-

103. Ulrich H, Pastores SM, Katz DP, et al. Parenteral use of medium-chain triglycerides: a reappraisal. Nutr 1996;12:231–238.
104. Bonner CM, DeBrie KL, Hug G, et al. Effects of parenteral L-carnitine supplementation on fat metabolism and nutrition in premature neonates. J Pediatr 1995;126:287–292.
105. Yu VYH, James B, Hendry P, et al. Total parenteral nutrition in very low birthweight infants: a controlled trial. Arch Dis Child 1979;54:653–661.
106. Kanarek KS, Villavecess C, Duckett G, et al. Serum concentrations of growth hormone, insulin, free thyroxine, thyrotropin, and cortisol in very-low-birth-weight infants receiving total parenteral nutrition. Am J Dis Child 1988;142:993–995.
107. Whitfield MF, Spitz L, Milner RDG. Clinical and metabolic consequences of two regimens of total parenteral nutrition in the newborn. Arch Dis Child 1983;58:168–175.
108. Brooke OG, Lucas A. Metabolic bone disease in preterm infants. Arch Dis Child 1985;60:682–685.
109. Klein GL, Ament ME, Bluestone R, et al. Bone disease associated with total parenteral nutrition. Lancet 1980;2:1041–1044.
110. Steichen JJ, Gratton TL, Tsang RC. Osteopenia of prematurity: the cause and possible treatment. J Pediatr 1980;96:528–534.
111. Chan GM, Mileur L, Hansen JW. Effects of increased calcium and phosphorus formulas and human milk on bone mineralization in preterm infants. J Pediatr Gastroenterol Nutr 1986;5:444–449.
112. Chan GM, Mileur L, Hansen JW. Calcium and phosphorus requirements in bone mineralization of preterm infants. J Pediatr 1988;113:225–229.
113. Dunn LL, Annable WL, Kliegman RM. Pigmented corneal rings in neonates with liver disease. J Pediatr 1987;110:771–776.
114. Dunn L, Hulman S, Weiner J, et al. Beneficial effects of early hypocaloric enteral feeding on neonatal gastrointestinal function: preliminary report of a randomized trial. J Pediatr 1988;112:622–629.
115. Beal EF, Nelson RM, Pucciarelli RL, et al. Intrahepatic cholestasis associated with parenteral nutrition in premature infants. Pediatrics 1979;64:342–347.
116. Farrell MK, Balistreri WF. Parenteral nutrition and hepatobiliary dysfunction. Clin Perinatol 1986;13:197–226.
117. Hodes JE, Grosfeld JL, Weber TR, et al. Hepatic failure in infants on total parenteral nutrition (TPN): clinical histopathologic observations. J Pediatr Surg 1982;17:463–468.
118. Patterson K, Kapur SP, Chandra RS. Hepatocellular carcinoma in a noncirrhotic infant after prolonged parenteral nutrition. J Pediatr 1985;106:797–800.
119. Rager R, Finegold MJ. Cholestasis in immature newborn infants: is parenteral alimentation responsible? J Pediatr 1975;826:264–269.
120. Balistreri W, Farrell M, eds. Enteral feeding: scientific basis and clinical applications. Report of Ninety-Fourth Ross Conference on Pediatric Research, Columbus, Ohio, Ross Laboratories 1988:1–161.
121. Aynsley-Green A. Hormones and postnatal adaptation to enteral nutrition. J Pediatr Gastroenterol Nutr 1983;2:2418–2427.
122. Aynsley-Green A. The adaptation of the human neonate to extrauterine nutrition: a pre-requisite for postnatal growth. In: Cockburn F, ed. Fetal and neonatal growth. New York: Wiley, 1988:153–193.
123. Dworkin LD, Levin GM, Farber NJ, Spector MH. Small intestinal mass of the rat is partially determined by indirect effects of intraluminal nutrition. Gastroenterology 1976;71:626–630.
124. Feldman E, Dowling R, McNaughton J, Peters T. Effects of oral versus intravenous nutrition on intestinal adaptation after small bowel resection in the dog. Gastroenterology 1974;70:712–719.
125. Kliegman R, Walsh M. Neonatal necrotizing enterocolitis: pathogenesis, classification and spectrum of illness. Curr Probl Pediatr 1987;17:215–288.
126. Churella HR, Bachhuber WL, MacLean WC. Survey: methods of feeding low-birth-weight infants. Pediatrics 1985;76:243–249.
127. Moyer-Mileur L, Chan GM. Nutritional support of very-low-birth-weight infants requiring prolonged assisted ventilation. Am J Dis Child 1986;140:929–932.
128. Brans YW, Sumners JE, Dweck HS, et al. Feeding the low birth weight infant: orally or parenterally? Preliminary results of a comparative study. Pediatrics 1974;54:15–22.
129. Slagle TA, Gross SJ. Effect of early low-volume enteral substrate on subsequent feeding tolerance in very low birth weight infants. J Pediatr 1988;113:526–531.
130. Unger A, Goetzman BW, Chan C, et al. Nutritional practices and outcome of extremely premature infants. Am J Dis Child 1986;140:1027–1033.
131. Ostertag SG, LaGamma EF, Reisen CE, Ferrentino FL. Early enteral feeding does not affect the incidence of necrotizing enterocolitis. Pediatrics 1986;77:275–280.
132. LaGamma EF, Ostertag MNS, Birenbaum H. Failure of delayed oral feedings to prevent necrotizing enterocolitis: results of study in very-low-birth-weight neonates. Am J Dis Child 1985;139:385–389.
133. Davey AM, Wagner CL, Cox C, et al. Feeding premature infants while low umbilical artery catheters are in place: a prospective, randomized trial. J Pediatr 1994;124:795–799.
134. Lebenthal E, Tucker N. Carbohydrate digestion: development in early infancy. Clin Perinatol 1986;13:37–57.
135. Lebenthal E, Leung Y. Feeding the premature and compromised infant: gastrointestinal considerations. Pediatr Clin North Am 1988;35:215–238.
136. Ballard R. Pediatric care of the ICN graduate. Philadelphia: Saunders, 1988.
137. Williamson S, Finucane E, Ellis H, et al. Effect of heat treatment of human milk on absorption of nitrogen, fat, sodium, calcium, and phosphorus by preterm infants. Arch Dis Child 1978;53:555–563.
138. Ronnholm KAR, Perheentupa J, Siimes MA. Supplementation with human milk protein improves growth of

138. small premature infants fed human milk. Pediatrics 1986; 77:649–653.
139. Bustamante SA, Fiello A, Pollack PF. Growth of premature infants fed formulas with 10%, 30% or 50% medium-chain triglycerides. Am J Dis Child 1987;141:516–519.
140. Greer FR. Formulas for the healthy term infant. Pediatr Rev 1995;16:107–112.
141. Schulze KF, Stefanski M, Masterson J, et al. Energy expenditure, energy balance, and composition of weight gain in low birth weight infants fed diets of different protein and energy content. J Pediatr 1987;110:753–759.
142. Kashyap S, Schulze KF, Forsyth M, et al. Growth, nutrient retention, and metabolic response in low birth weight infants fed varying intakes of protein and energy. J Pediatr 1988;113:713–721.
143. Davies DP. Adequacy of expressed breast milk for early growth of preterm infants. Arch Dis Child 1977;52:296–301.
144. Gross SJ. Growth and biochemical response of preterm infants fed human milk or modified infant formula. N Engl J Med 1983;308:237–241.
145. Lemons P, Stuart M, Lemons MA. Breast-feeding the premature infant. Clin Perinatol 1986;13:111–122.
146. Anonymous. Breast not necessarily best. Lancet 1988;1:624–625.
147. Atkinson SA, Bryan MH, Anderson GH. Human milk feeding in premature infants: protein, fat, and carbohydrate balances in the first two weeks of life. J Pediatr 1981;99:617–624.
148. Stein H, Cohen D, Herman AAB, et al. Pooled pasteurized breast milk and untreated own mother's milk in the feeding of very low birth weight babies: a randomized controlled trial. J Pediatr Gastroenterol Nutr 1986;5:242–247.
149. Whyte RK, Haslam R, Vlainic C, et al. Energy balance and nitrogen balance in growing low birthweight infants fed human milk or formula. Pediatr Res 1983;17:891–898.
150. Ronnholm KAR, Sipila I, Siimes MA. Human milk protein supplementation for the prevention of hypoproteinemia without metabolic imbalance in breast milk-fed, very low-birth-weight infants. J Pediatr 1982;101:243–247.
151. Senterre J, Putet G, Salle B, et al. Effects of vitamin D and phosphorus supplementation on calcium retention in preterm infants fed banked human milk. J Pediatr 1983;103:305–307.
152. Modanlou HD, Lim MO, Hansen JW, et al. Growth, biochemical status, and mineral metabolism in very-low-birth-weight infants receiving fortified preterm human milk. J Pediatr Gastroenterol Nutr 1986;5:762–767.
153. Venkataraman PS, Blick KE. Effect of mineral supplementation of human milk on bone mineral content and trace element metabolism. J Pediatr 1988;113:220–224.
154. Ehrenkranz RA, Gettner PA, Nelli CM. Nutrient balance studies in premature infants fed premature formula or fortified preterm human milk. J Pediatr Gastroenterol Nutr 1989;8:58–67.
155. Koketzko B, Tangermann R, von Kries R, et al. Intestinal milk-bolus obstruction in formula-fed premature infants given high doses of calcium. J Pediatr Gastroenterol Nutr 1988;7:548–553.
156. Blondheim O, Abbasi S, Fox WW, et al. Effect of enteral gavage feeding rate on pulmonary functions of very low birth weight infants. J Pediatr 1993;122:751–755.
157. Pereira GR, Zucker A. Nutritional deficiencies in the neonate. Clin Perinatol 1986;13:175–189.
158. Pereira GR, Lemons JA. Controlled study of transpyloric and intermittent gavage feeding in the small preterm infant. Pediatrics 1981;67:68–72.
159. Whitfield MF. Poor weight gain of the low birthweight infant fed nasojejunally. Arch Dis Child 1982;57:597–601.
160. LeLeiko NS, Walsh MJ. The role of glutamine, short-chain fatty acids, and nucleotides in intestinal adaptation to gastrointestinal disease. Pediatr Clin North Am 1996;43:451–469.
161. Berseth CL. Effect of early feeding on maturation of the preterm infant's small intestine. J Pediatr 1992;120:947–953.
162. Troche B, Harvey-Wilkes K, Engle WD, et al. Early minimal feedings promote growth in critically ill premature infants. Biol Neonate 1995;67:172–181.
163. Ziegler MM. Short bowel syndrome in infancy: etiology and management. Clin Perinatol 1986;13:163–173.
164. Collins JB, Georgeson KE, Vicente Y, et al. Short bowel syndrome. Semin Pediatr Surg 1995;4:60–73.
165. Shanbhogue LKR, Molenaar JC. Short bowel syndrome: metabolic and surgical management. Br J Surg 1994;81:P486–499.
166. Vanderhoof JA. Short bowel syndrome in children and small intestinal transplantation. Pediatr Clin North Am 1996;43:533–550.
167. Vanderhoof JA. Short bowel syndrome in children. Curr Opin Pediatr 1995;7:560–568.
168. Van Goudoever JB, Wattimena JDL, Carnielli VP, et al. Effect of dexamethasone on protein metabolism in infants with bronchopulmonary dysplasia. J Pediatr 1994;124:112–118.
169. Wu PYK, Edmond J, Morrow JW, et al. Gastrointestinal tolerance, fat absorption, plasma ketone and urinary dicarboxylic acid levels in low-birth-weight infants fed different amounts of medium-chain triglycerides in formula. J Pediatr Gastroenterol Nutr 1993;17:145–152.
170. Pereira GR, Baumgart S, Bennett MJ, et al. Use of high-fat formula for premature infants with bronchopulmonary dysplasia: metabolic, pulmonary, and nutritional studies. J Pediatr 1994;124:605–611.
171. Tirlapur VG, Mir MA. Effect of low calorie intake on abnormal pulmonary physiology in patients with chronic hypercapneic respiratory failure. Am J Med 1984;77:987–994.
172. Herve P, Simonnearu G, Girard P, et al. Hypercapnic acidosis induced by nutrition in mechanically ventilated patients: glucose versus fat. Crit Care Med 1985;13:537–540.
173. Kwan R, Mir MA. Beneficial effects of dietary carbohydrate restriction in chronic cor pulmonale. Am J Med 1987;82:751–758.
174. Pingleton SK. Harmon GS. Nutritional management in acute respiratory failure. JAMA 1987;257:3094–3099.

175. Yunis KA, Oh W. Effects of intravenous glucose loading on oxygen consumption, carbon dioxide production, and resting energy expenditure in infants with bronchopulmonary dysplasia. J Pediatr 1989;115:127–132.
176. Wahlig TM, Georgieff MK. The effects of illness on neonatal metabolism and nutritional management. Clin Perinatol 1995;22:77–96.
177. Sax HC. Early nutritional support in critical illness is important. Crit Care Clin 1996;12:661–666.
178. Marino PL, Finnegan MJ. Nutrition support is not beneficial and can be harmful in critically ill patients. Crit Care Clin 1996;12:667–676.

52
Nutritional Support of the Neonate II: The Rationale for Human Milk Feeding

Richard J. Schanler

Human milk is recommended as the exclusive nutrient source for feeding full-term infants during the first 6 months after birth and should be continued, with the addition of solid foods, at least through the first 12 months.[1,2] The recommendation for human milk feeding arises because of its acknowledged benefits with respect to infant nutrition, gastrointestinal function, host defense, and psychological well-being. The recognition of beneficial effects in premature infants is emerging to support the feeding of human milk.[3] Favorable outcomes of breast-feeding are reported for both infants and mothers.

This chapter focuses on the rationale for breast-feeding by describing the unique milk composition and the functional outcomes of breast-feeding for infants and mothers, as well as the management of lactation for full-term and premature infants (see also Chapter 51).

Milk Composition

Nutritional Aspects

It is important to understand the unique specificity of the components in human milk.[2] Many factors have dual roles, one as a nutrient source or to facilitate nutrient absorption and the other to promote host defense or gastrointestinal function. The composition of human milk is remarkable for its variability. This variability may serve to improve nutrient composition in a way that is specifically adapted to the needs of the full-term infant.[4]

Protein (Nitrogen)

In the first few weeks after birth, the total nitrogen content of milk from mothers who deliver premature infants (i.e., preterm milk) is greater than milk obtained from women delivering full-term infants (i.e., term milk).[5-8] Usually beyond the first few weeks of lactation, the total nitrogen content in both milks declines similarly to approach what we call mature milk.[7,8] Approximately 20% of the total nitrogen is in the form of nonprotein nitrogen-containing compounds, such as free amino acids and urea, in contrast to bovine milk in which the nonprotein nitrogen is 5% of total nitrogen.[9,10] There is a debate as to how much of these nonprotein nitrogen-containing compounds contribute to nitrogen utilization.[11,12] The rate of absorption of nonprotein nitrogen, determined by stable isotope methods, has been estimated at 13% to 43%.[11,12]

The protein quality (i.e., proportion of whey and casein proteins) of human milk (e.g., 30% casein and 70% whey) differs from that in bovine milk (e.g., 82% casein and 18% whey).[10] The caseins are a group of proteins with low solubility in acid media. Whey proteins remain in solution after acid precipitation. Generally, the soluble proteins in the whey fraction are more easily digested and are associated with more rapid gastric emptying.[13] The whey protein fraction provides lower concentrations of phenylalanine, tyrosine, and methionine, and higher concentrations of taurine, than the casein fraction of milk.[14-17] The resulting plasma amino acid patterns are particularly distinct in premature infants. Since potentially toxic imbalances in the levels of various amino acids are avoided, the plasma amino acid pattern found in full-term breast-fed infants is used as a reference in infant nutrition.[18,19]

The type of proteins contained in the whey fraction differs between human and bovine milks. The major human whey protein is α-lactalbumin, a protein involved in the mammary gland synthesis of lactose and a nutritional protein for the infant. Lactoferrin, lysozyme, and secretory immunoglobulin A (sIgA) are specific human whey proteins involved in host defense.[20-22] Because these host defense proteins resist proteolytic digestion, they are capable of a first line of defense by lining the gastrointestinal tract. The three host defense proteins essentially are absent in bovine milk. The major whey protein in bovine milk is β-lactoglobulin.[10]

Lipid

The lipid system in human milk, responsible for providing approximately 50% of the calories in the milk, is structured to facilitate superior fat digestion and absorption.[4,23] The lipid system is comprised of an organized milk fat globule, a pattern of fatty acids (e.g., high in palmitic 16:0, oleic 18:1, and the essential fatty acids, linoleic 18:2ω-6, and linolenic 18:3ω-3) characteristically distributed on the triglyceride molecule (i.e., 16:0 at the 2 position of the molecule), and bile salt-stimulated lipase.[24,25] As the lipase is heat-labile, it is important to recognize that the superior fat absorption from human milk is reported only when unprocessed milk is fed.[24] Fat absorption is increased when human milk is added to formula, suggesting that the milk lipase is active on exogenous lipid.[26] The mixture of fatty acids in commercial formulas differs from that in human milk. Generally, to meet the fat absorption from human milk, commercial formulas have a greater quantity of medium-chain fatty acids than human milk.

Of the macronutrients in human milk, fat is the most variable in content.[25,27,28] The fat content rises slightly throughout lactation, changes over the course of one day, increases within the feeding, and varies from mother to mother.[27,29,30] The interindividual variation tracks through lactation and is not affected by diet but may be affected by maternal body composition.[31,32] As the fat is not homogenized, it may separate from the milk upon standing in a container.[33,34] The separated fat may adhere to collection containers and feeding tubes and syringes. In that case, the infant is robbed of the needed calories. For premature infants, the variability in composition and homogeneity may affect fat intake from expressed human milk.

The pattern of fatty acids in human milk is unique in its content of very long chain fatty acids. Arachidonic acid (20:4ω-6) and docosahexaenoic acid (22:6ω-3), derivatives of linoleic and linolenic acids, respectively, are found in human, but not bovine milk. Arachidonic and docosahexaenoic acids functionally have been associated with cognition, growth, and vision.[35-37]

Carbohydrate

The carbohydrate composition of human milk is important as a nutritional source of lactose and for the presence of oligosaccharides. Although studies in full-term infants demonstrate a small proportion of unabsorbed lactose in the feces, the presence of lactose is assumed to be a normal physiologic effect of feeding human milk.[38,39] A softer stool consistency, more nonpathogenic bacterial fecal flora, and improved absorption of minerals have been attributed to the presence of small quantities of unabsorbed lactose from human milk feeding.[40,41]

Mineral and Trace Elements

The concentration of calcium and phosphorus in human milk is significantly lower than bovine milk and infant formula. The content of these macrominerals is relatively constant through lactation. The macrominerals in human milk are more bioavailable than those in infant formula because of the manner in which they are packaged. In human milk, the minerals are bound to digestible proteins and are also present in complexed and ionized states, which are readily bioavailable.[42]

The concentrations of iron, zinc, and copper decline through lactation.[43,44] The concentrations of copper and zinc, despite their decline through lactation, appear adequate to meet the infant's nutritional needs. The concentration of iron, however, may not meet the infant's needs beyond 6 months of breast-feeding,[44-46] at which time, most authorities agree, an iron supplement is indicated to prevent subsequent iron deficiency anemia.

Vitamins

Maternal vitamin status may affect the content of vitamins in the milk.[47] Generally, maternal deficiency may result in low concentrations in milk that increase in response to dietary supplementation. This is more common for water-soluble than fat-soluble vitamins.[47]

Vitamin K deficiency may be a concern in the breast-fed infant.[48] Bacterial flora are responsible for providing adequate vitamin K. The intestinal flora of the breast-fed infant make less menaquinone and the content of vitamin K in human milk is low. This necessitates that a single dose of vitamin K be given at birth.[48]

The vitamin D needs of breast-fed infants are controversial and have been reviewed.[49] Maternal diet and sunshine exposure are the major factors affecting vitamin D status of the breast-fed infant. Insofar as only a little exposure to sunshine is necessary for vitamin D synthesis, there is no need for a vitamin D supplement. Should the exposure be questioned or the climate forbidding, a daily dose of 400 IU vitamin D is recommended for infants.[49]

Nonnutritional Factors

Nucleotides

Although they can be synthesized endogenously, it appears that exogenous nucleotides may have a role in a variety of metabolic functions in infants.[50] Nucleotides consist of either a purine (e.g., uracil, cytosine, thymine) or pyrimidine (e.g, adenine, guanine, hypoxanthine, xanthine) base and a pentose sugar (e.g, ribose or deoxyribose) joined by mono-, di-, or triphosphate esters. As such, they serve as immediate precursors for RNA and

DNA synthesis. Functions generally attributed to dietary nucleotides include effects on lymphoid, intestinal, and hepatic tissues and in lipid metabolism.[50,51] The growth of *Bifidobacterium* in stool flora is affected positively by exogenous nucleotides.[51]

Gastrointestinal Factors

Many hormones (e.g., cortisol, somatomedin-C, insulin-like growth factors, insulin, thyroid hormone), growth factors (e.g., epidermal growth factor, nerve growth factor), and gastrointestinal mediators (e.g., neurotensin, motilin) are present in human milk that may affect gastrointestinal function and/or body composition.[52-54] Epidermal growth factor (EGF) is a polypeptide that stimulates DNA synthesis, protein synthesis, and cellular proliferation in intestinal cells.[55] EGF resists proteolytic digestion and is found in the intestinal lumen in suckling animals. Nerve growth factor may play a role in the innervation of the intestinal tract. The hormonal components in milk may affect intestinal growth and mucosal function. Free amino acids may exert dual roles in infants. Taurine may be trophic for intestinal growth and glutamine may be a fuel for the small intestine.[55]

Host Defense Factors

A variety of heterogeneous agents that possess antimicrobial activity are found in human milk.[20,22,56,57] Many of these agents persist through lactation and are resistant to the gastrointestinal digestive enzymes in the infant. The antimicrobial activities generally are found at mucosal surfaces.

Specific factors such as lactoferrin, lysozyme, and sIgA compose the whey fraction of human milk protein, generally resist proteolytic degradation, and line mucosal surfaces preventing microbial attachment and inhibiting microbial activity.[20-22,58] Lactoferrin has antimicrobial activity when not conjugated to iron (apolactoferrin).[59] It may function with other host defense proteins to effect microbial killing. Lysozyme is active against bacteria by cleaving cell walls. sIgA is synthesized by plasma cells against specific antigens.[60] The enteromammary and bronchomammary immune systems summarize the important part of the protective nature of human milk.[60-62] In these systems the mother produces sIgA antibody when exposed to foreign antigens either via her respiratory or gastrointestinal tracts. The plasma cells traverse the lymphatic system and are secreted at mucosal surfaces, including the mammary gland. Ingestion of milk provides the infant with passive sIgA antibody against the offending antigen. The systems are active in infants against a variety of antigens.[20,61,62]

The products of lipid hydrolysis, free fatty acids and monoglycerides, may exhibit antimicrobial activity against a variety of pathogens, e.g., by preventing attachment and infection with viruses and protozoa, such as *Giardia*.[63]

Oligosaccharides and glucoconjugates of protein affect intestinal bacterial flora to facilitate the growth of *Lactobacillus* species. These agents mimic bacterial epithelial receptors in the respiratory tract and in doing so, prevent attachment of pathogenic agents to epithelial lining of mucosal surfaces. There are a variety of oligosaccharides and glycoproteins that act as receptor analogues for multiple antimicrobial agents.[56,64]

There are white cells 90% of which are neutrophils and macrophages in human milk that contribute to the antimicrobial activity through phagocytosis and intracellular killing.[21] The lymphocytes in human milk may contribute to cytokine production (e.g., T cells) or IgA production (e.g., B cells).[21,57,65]

In summary, the composition of human milk is a complex mixture of compounds with several roles in nutrition, gastrointestinal function, and host defense. The components are in a dynamic state, occasionally affected by maternal diet and well-being, and appear to be uniquely suited to the human infant. A representation of the composition of human milk is difficult because of the dynamic nature of the nutrients, but for comparative purposes the tabulation of mature human milk and bovine milk compositions is given in Table 52.1.

Milk Volume

Milk transfer from mother to infant generally is measured by the test-weighing technique, weighing the infant before and after each feeding for at least 24 hours. Mean milk volumes reported for healthy, exclusively breast-fed infants range from about 750 to $800 \text{ g} \cdot \text{day}^{-1}$, but milk intakes for an individual infant may be as low as $450 \text{ g} \cdot \text{day}^{-1}$ or as high as $1200 \text{ g} \cdot \text{day}^{-1}$.[66] The low milk intakes on the first 2 days increase markedly on days 3 and 4, and then gradually increase to levels seen in full lactation.[67] Infant demand rather than maternal lactation capacity determines milk intake.[68,69] A decline in human milk volume is associated with the addition of milk substitutes or solid foods. Instead of being supplementary, milk substitutes and solid foods have been shown to displace human milk.[70,71]

Maternal factors that influence milk volumes have been investigated in a number of studies. In well-nourished women, age, parity, current weight, body mass index, body fat, and weight gain during pregnancy have not been shown to influence milk production.[32,72,73] Maternal stress, anxiety, fatigue, and/or illness may affect milk production.[74] Incomplete breast emptying and infrequent milk expression reduce milk production.[75] Smoking has been shown to have a deleterious effect on milk production.[76-78] Combined estrogen/progesterone oral contra-

TABLE 52.1. Composition of mature human milk and bovine milk.

Component, units·L^{-1}	Human milk	Bovine milk
Energy, kcal	680	680
Protein, g	10	33
% Whey/casein	72/28	18/82
Fat, g	39	38
% MCT/LCT	2/98	8/92
Carbohydrate, g	72	47
% Lactose	100	100
Calcium, mg	280	1200
Phosphorus, mg	140	920
Magnesium, mg	35	120
Sodium, mg	180	480
Potassium, mg	525	1570
Chloride, mg	420	1020
Zinc, μg	1200	3500
Copper, μg	250	100
Iron, μg	300	460
Vitamin A, IU	2230	1000
Vitamin D, IU	22	24
Vitamin E, IU	2.3	0.9
Vitamin K, μg	2.1	4.9
Thiamin (vitamin B$_1$), μg	210	300
Riboflavin (vitamin B$_2$), μg	350	1750
Pyridoxine (vitamin B$_6$), μg	93	470
Niacin, mg	1.5	0.8
Biotin, μg	4	35
Pantothenic acid, mg	1.8	3.5
Folic acid, μg	85	50
Vitamin B$_{12}$, μg	1	4
Ascorbic acid, mg	40	17

From Greer et al.,[48] Institute of Medicine,[66] American Academy of Pediatrics,[264] Blanc,[265] Dallman[266] and Schanler.[267]

ceptives have a moderate inhibitory effect on milk yield, whereas progesterone-only preparations have no effect on milk yield or breast-feeding duration.[79] Skin-to-skin contact practiced in neonatal nurseries may increase milk production.[80]

Effect of Maternal Nutrition on Milk Composition

The evidence derived from a variety of populations suggests that the capacity to produce milk of sufficient quantity and quality to support the growth of infants is satisfactory, even when the mother's dietary supply of nutrients is limited.[66] Lactation does require additional nutrients for the mother, but diet does not have to be changed drastically. However, a chronically deficient diet resulting in depletion of maternal nutrient stores may adversely affect milk composition.

With the exception of extreme dietary deprivation, maternal energy intake seems to have only a weak or indirect effect on milk volume.[32,81] Short-term diet restriction to 1500 kcal·day^{-1} for 1 week did not compromise milk production rates, but diets with less than 1500 kcal·day^{-1} may do so.[82] A 20-hour fast did not alter milk production.[83] A 10-week weight reduction program that achieved a 538-kcal deficit did not affect milk volume or composition.[84]

There is no consistent evidence that diet affects the concentration of milk protein, even in malnourished populations.[85-87] The effects of protein supplementation on milk protein concentration are less consistent. Increasing the protein intake from 46 to 134 g·day^{-1} increased milk total nitrogen and nonprotein nitrogen concentration.[88]

The types of fatty acids in human milk, but not the quantity, are affected by the type and proportion of fat in the diet.[89,90] The fraction of milk lipids derived from endogenous fat synthesis within the mammary gland is increased on low fat diets. A shift in dietary fat from 40% to 10% of total calories caused an increase in the milk content of short-chain saturated fatty acids.[91] Vegetarians have a higher concentration of linoleic acid in their milk.[92]

In general, the concentration of fat-soluble vitamins in milk are somewhat susceptible to the vitamin status of the mother, but the water-soluble vitamins in milk are more responsive to maternal diet. Maternal vitamin A deficiency is associated with decreased levels of vitamin A in milk.[93,94] Milk vitamin D is directly affected by maternal vitamin D status.[95] The vitamin K concentration in human milk is responsive to maternal dietary supplementation.[96]

Although influenced by diet, water-soluble vitamin concentrations in milk generally are regulated so as not to exceed a reasonable upper limit.[97-99] Vitamin-deficient diets will lower the vitamin content in the milk. Milk B$_6$ depends largely on maternal intake and responds to supplementation.[100] Although folate is preferentially secreted into milk at the expense of the mother's folate stores, milk concentrations can decline with severe folate deficiency. Milk vitamin B$_{12}$ content is lower in vegans, malnourished women, and those with latent pernicious anemia.[101] The vegan mother who eats no meat products or takes no vitamin supplements is at risk of vitamin B$_{12}$ deficiency. Her infant may be at risk for vitamin B$_{12}$ deficiency and may show signs of deficiency before the mother.[102] Maternal vitamin B$_{12}$ supplementation will provide vitamin sufficiency to mother and infant.[103]

Milk concentrations of calcium, phosphorus, and magnesium, which are tightly regulated in the plasma, may be affected by malnutrition and length of lactation.[66,104,105] Iron and copper in human milk are independent of nutrient status.[106-108] Zinc supplementation (i.e., 15 mg·day^{-1} for 7 months) did not affect milk zinc concentration in well-nourished women.[109] Selenium concentration in milk is related to plasma concentrations.[110]

Infection Control Issues

It is unwarranted to consider breast-feeding a means of transmitting disease to the infant. It is appropriate to recommend breast-feeding to the mother who has mastitis and is undergoing treatment for the condition. Maternal herpes infections localized to the perineal area or the oral mucosa do not pose a risk to the breast-fed infant.[111] Maternal herpetic lesions localized to the mammary areola, however, do pose a risk and the infant should not be breast-fed while these lesions remain. Cytomegalovirus excretion is common in human milk, the mothers being seropositive for the virus.[112] In the full-term infant, this is not a concern with respect to breast-feeding. Maternal rubella or maternal rubella immunization does not increase the risk of disease in the breast-fed infant.[111,113] To date, most authorities recommend breast-feeding for mothers exposed to and infected with the hepatitis viruses.[114] Although mothers with active miliary tuberculosis should not breast-feed, mothers who are seroconverters or receiving antituberculosis therapy may do so.

The data for human immunodeficiency virus are a concern.[111,115–117] Although transplacental transmission may occur in 30% of cases when the mother is seropositive during pregnancy, the data for lactation are less clear. The virus has been isolated from human milk and there are suggestions of transmission of HIV from breast-feeding. There are reports, however, that human milk protects the recipient infant from HIV. Until more data are accumulated, the guidelines from the U.S. Centers for Disease Control and Prevention suggest that mothers who are seropositive for HIV should not breast-feed. The World Health Organization advises that because the transmission of HIV in milk is uncertain, breast-feeding should be encouraged, especially in developing countries. In that recommendation, the risk/benefit ratio of not breast-feeding was greater in developing countries than the risk of transmission of HIV.

The data regarding potential transmission of disease via breast-feeding have been summarized in the Red Book, Report of the Committee on Infectious Diseases of the American Academy of Pediatrics.[118]

Xenobiotics in Lactation

A number of drugs may be secreted into human milk, but only a few are thought to be contraindications to breast-feeding.[119] These include chemotherapeutic agents, radioactive isotopes, drugs of abuse, lithium, ergotamine, and drugs that suppress lactation. In addition, anticonvulsants, antihistamines, sulfa drugs, and salicylates may have effects on some breast-feeding infants. Potential exposures from environmental agents should be considered. Caffeine may enter milk, but maternal consumption of one or two caffeine-containing beverages per day may not be associated with significant manifestations in the infant.[120] The use of alcohol is controversial. Some studies have indicated that alcohol may affect the infant's behavior adversely.[121,122] Some changes in developmental outcomes at one year have been attributed to the maternal ingestion of alcohol.[122] Cigarette smoking may affect milk volume.[76,77]

Secretion of medications into milk is affected by dose schedule and duration, feeding pattern of the infant, and the infant's total diet and age. The timing of breast-feeding should avoid peak blood concentrations of selected medications. For some medications, the stage of lactation (i.e., age of the infant) determines the safety of the agent. Sulfa drugs would not be indicated in the first month of lactation, but may pose no concern to the infant who is several months of age. The mother should be encouraged to discuss any medication with her physician.

Benefits of Breast Feeding

Benefits for the Neonate

Body Composition

Although lower concentrations of calcium and phosphorus are observed in human milk compared with formula, measures of bone mineralization are similar between human milk– or formula-fed full-term infants during the first year of life.[123–126]

Gastrointestinal Function

Gastric emptying is faster following the feeding of human milk than with commercial milk-based formula.[13] The clinical impression is that large gastric residual volumes are reported less frequently in premature infants fed human milk. Many factors in human milk may stimulate gastrointestinal growth and motility, and enhance maturity of the gastrointestinal tract.

Morbidity

There are numerous studies from developing countries that delineate the protective effects of breast-feeding. In developing areas, the incidence of gastroenteritis and respiratory disease and overall morbidity and mortality are lower in breast-fed infants than infants fed milk substitutes.[127,128] In the United States, breast-fed infants have lower rates of diarrhea, lower respiratory tract illness, acute and recurrent otitis media, and urinary tract infection.[129–131] Not only is the attack rate lower, but the duration and severity of illness appear to be shortened in the breast-fed infant.[132]

In developed countries, even in affluent groups, a reduction is found in the incidence of gastroenteritis.[127,133] The incidence of diarrheal disease in infants breast-fed for 12 months was one-half that of formula-fed infants.[132] Infants who were breast-fed for at least 13 weeks were found to have significantly lower incidence of gastroenteritis (e.g., vomiting or diarrhea as a discrete illness lasting 48 hours or more) to 1 year of age than infants fed formula from birth.[134] These observations were significant even when controlled for confounding variables such as sibling number, day care attendance, social class, maternal age, and maternal smoking.

Respiratory illnesses are reduced in frequency and/or in duration in breast-fed infants.[133-136] The incidence of wheezing is less and overall lower respiratory tract infection is decreased.[136,137] The incidence of otitis media and recurrent otitis media were reduced in infants breast-fed for 4 or more months.[138,139] Not only was the incidence of otitis media reduced in infants breast-fed for 1 year, but the duration of each episode was reduced significantly compared with formula-fed infants.[132]

The incidence of urinary tract infection is reduced in breast-fed infants.[140] This observation may be a result of the excretion of bioactive substances in the urine (e.g., oligosaccharides, lactoferrin, sIgA).[141,142]

Premature infants fed human milk have a lower incidence of necrotizing enterocolitis (NEC) if they receive human milk compared with receiving commercial formula.[143,144] The lower incidence of NEC is observed even if the supply of mother's milk is low and formula is used as a supplement. Thus, partial and exclusive use of mother's milk appears to protect the premature infant from this devastating condition. Although, the mechanism for the protection from NEC is unclear, the feeding of IgA-IgG preparations appears to reduce its incidence.[145] These data suggest that by lining the gastrointestinal tract with host defense proteins, the infant is protected from this inflammatory condition. The incidence of sepsis and a variety of neonatal infections is also reduced in premature infants receiving human milk.[144,146-152]

Chronic Disease

Perhaps the most intriguing data are those suggesting that specific chronic disorders have a lower incidence in children who were breast-fed as infants. There may be protective effects of breast-feeding against Crohn's disease, lymphoma, specific genotypes of type I juvenile diabetes mellitus, and certain allergic conditions.[153-155] There are conflicting data regarding the protection against allergy afforded by breast-feeding, possibly because maternal diet did not exclude the potentially offending antigens.[156] Breast-feeding appears to be protective against food allergies.[22,56] Atopic dermatitis may be lessened in infants whose mothers follow a restricted diet. A lower incidence of atopic conditions is reported in breast-fed infants with a family history of atopy.[157]

There appears to be a relationship between breast-feeding and the development of type I insulin-dependent diabetes mellitus (IDDM).[155] IDDM was more likely when breast-feeding lasted less than 3 months and bovine milk proteins were introduced before 4 months of age.[155] Elevated concentrations of specific IgG antibody to bovine serum albumin that cross-reacts with β cell–specific surface protein have been identified in children with IDDM.[158] It is estimated that up to 30% of type I IDDM could be prevented by removing bovine milk from the diet for the first 3 months.[155]

In summary, a large quantity of data demonstrates the marked protective effects of breast-feeding, in the developed world as in the developing world.

Neurobehavioral Aspects

Maternal-infant bonding is enhanced during breast-feeding. In addition, improved long-term cognitive and motor abilities in full-term infants have been directly correlated with the duration of breast-feeding. Even when adjusted for socioeconomic status and parent education, at 3, 4, and 5 years there were significant increments in cognitive test scores that correlated positively with the duration of breast-feeding.[159] Improved long-term cognitive development in premature infants also has been correlated with the receipt of human milk during their hospitalization.[160,161] A series of studies has indicated that human milk–fed full-term and premature infants have improved visual function compared with formula-fed infants.[35,37,162,163] The relationship between diet and visual function becomes even more profound when we relate these effects to beneficial long-term cognitive outcomes.

Benefits for the Mother

Recovery from childbirth is accelerated by the oxytocin's action on uterine involution.[164] Although breast-feeding should not be considered a reliable means of contraception, breast-feeding prolongs the period of postpartum amenorrhea.[165] Menstruation resumes between 34 and 65 weeks postpartum and ovulation between 30 and 40 weeks postpartum. Frequency, intensity, and timing of feedings affect the endocrinologic responses that modulate ovulatory status.[166]

Studies examining whether breast-feeding promotes postpartum weight loss are conflicting.[167-173] Prolonged breast-feeding may confer some advantage in terms of weight loss. Compared with nonlactating women, weight loss of lactating women was greater from 1 to 12 months postpartum, but not from 12 to 24 months postpartum.[167]

Bone mineralization declines during lactation, with a compensatory remineralization after weaning.[174-177] Lactation has been shown to confer a protective effect against osteoporosis and bone fracture in later life,[178-181] but this has not been confirmed in all studies.[182-184]

A protective effect of breast-feeding against breast cancer has been found in a number of studies,[185-195] but not in other studies.[190-195] Breast-feeding and the duration of breast-feeding were associated with a reduction in cancer risk in premenopausal women.[190] The effects were even greater in premenopausal women who had a cumulative total of 24 months of breast-feeding or who were 20 years or younger when they first lactated.

Management of the Full-Term Neonate

General Management

Breast-feeding can begin as soon after delivery as both mother and baby are stable. Correct positioning and proper breast-feeding technique are necessary to ensure effective nipple stimulation and optimal breast emptying with minimal discomfort. Maternal anxiety may impair the letdown response and lead to a poor lactation experience.

Rigid time restrictions should not be imposed. Some clinicians suggest that nursing be conducted for 5 minutes per breast at each feeding the first day, 10 minutes on each side the second day, and 15 minutes or more thereafter. It must be noted that the time for complete milk transfer is variable and may take as long as 20 minutes. To maximize milk intake and optimally stimulate and empty both breasts, it is preferable to nurse at both breasts during each feeding. In the presence of well-conditioned letdown, or milk ejection reflex, a vigorous infant can obtain most of the available milk in 5 to 7 minutes. Additional sucking, however, ensures complete breast emptying and facilitates milk production as well as satisfying the infant's sucking urge. The mother should alternate the side on which she begins feedings so that the breast last suckled is the first one used at the next feeding. To prevent nipple trauma, the mother should break suction gently after nursing by inserting her finger between the breast and the baby's gums.

In the first few weeks after birth, an infant is adequately nourished if at least 8 to 12 feedings are received each day and the infant sleeps contentedly between feedings. Some infants may feed 12 or more times a day. Infants should not refuse to latch on or be too sleepy to feed. Long nighttime intervals (i.e., greater than 5 hours) without feeding should be avoided in the first few weeks. By the third postpartum day, breast-fed infants should have stopped losing weight and be able to latch on to the breast appropriately. In the first few days after delivery, it is important to monitor the adequacy of milk intake each day by counting the number of wet diapers, the number and quantity of stools, and, if necessary, weight gain (i.e., avoid body weight loss >7%).[196] In the first day, the infant should go no longer than 24 hours without a wet diaper and stool. On day 3, infants should have six wet diapers and at least three stools; meconium should be absent from stools, stools should appear yellow, and "milk" stools should be noted. Later in the first week after birth, there should be six pale yellow diapers per day and a yellow stool with each feeding. Later in the month, the stool frequency may diminish to three per day.[196,197]

The mother also should be assessed.[196,197] By day 3, she should have some breast engorgement and notice milk dripping from the opposite breast during feeding. She should be breast-feeding every 3 hours, at least eight times in 24 hours. She should know how to find knowledgeable help with respect to breast-feeding.

Early hospital discharge programs pose a concern for monitoring the breast-fed infant. An early home or office visit 24 to 48 hours after discharge is important to assess breast-feeding and clinical status. This early visit should assess the adequacy of hydration, milk intake, and weight gain; the presence of jaundice; and the state of the mother (anxiety, concerns). One breast-feeding episode should be observed during this first visit. The next visit should be within 2 weeks of hospital discharge. Telephone contact should be encouraged if questions arise. The availability of community, office, and/or hospital lactation resources should be reinforced.

Breast Care

Lactogenesis, or the onset of milk secretion, usually occurs on the second to fourth postpartum day and is associated with engorgement or swelling of the breasts. Breast engorgement is an uncomfortable and sometimes painful swelling. It is due to increased blood and lymph flow to the breast at the onset of lactogenesis. Poor or infrequent emptying of the breast exacerbates this condition. Engorgement can cause the nipple-areola junction to be tense and convex, making it difficult for the infant to grasp correctly. Manual or mechanical (i.e., breast pump) expression of milk prior to nursing will soften the areola area and facilitate the infant's latch-on.

Cracked or fissured nipples are usually the result of improper latch-on, improper disengagement, or the use of abrasive soaps or alcohol on the breast. Treatment of this condition involves keeping the nipples dry. Because the glands of Montgomery provide the best of lubrication for the areola and nipple throughout pregnancy, no additional lubricants are needed.

Localized areas of breast discomfort may be due to plugged ducts. These are focal areas of breast engorgement caused by milk stasis. The condition results from irregular nursing, skipped feedings, and inadequate breast emptying. This condition of localized tenderness and mass in an area of the breast should be differentiated from mastitis. The plugged duct may be a precursor of mastitis. Treatment of a plugged duct involves starting consecutive feedings on the affected side and changing nursing position to facilitate emptying different lobes of the breast. Additional relief is provided by gently massaging the affected area during nursing or pumping while applying moist heat. Frequent nursing is recommended.

Hospital Routines

Because the initial hospital experience may affect ultimate breast-feeding outcome, programs have been designed to facilitate breast-feeding in a normal physiologic manner.[198] In 1991, UNICEF and the World Health Organization (WHO) began an international campaign to promote breast-feeding following a ten-step program. The U.S. Baby Friendly Hospital Initiative modified the steps for use in the U.S. (Table 52.2).[199–201] To accomplish successful breast-feeding, postpartum units must maintain a written policy on breast-feeding that is communicated to the entire staff. All health care staff must be trained in the implementation of this policy. Pregnant women should be informed of the benefits for breast-feeding. Breast-feeding should commence within 1 hour of birth unless medically not indicated. Health care staff must be able to demonstrate appropriate breast-feeding skills to mothers. Infants should be given nothing but breast milk unless medically indicated. There is no reason to supply glucose water or formula to the exclusively breast-fed infant who is otherwise healthy. Rooming-in for 24 hours per day should be practiced to allow unrestricted breast-feeding. No pacifiers should be given to the infants, as any need for sucking should be met with breast-feeding. Each hospital should establish breast-feeding support groups or work with organized community support groups so that families have a resource upon leaving the hospital. The success of this program in the U.S. has been reviewed.[202]

Supplements

Under normal conditions, an infant should not be bottle fed for the first 2 weeks, after which time lactation usually is well established. Infants may be confused by a rubber nipple or pacifier, which require different tongue and jaw motions. Furthermore, if the appetite or the sucking response is partially satiated by water or formula, the infant will take less from the breast, causing diminished milk production, which may lead to lactation failure. Sterile water and glucose water supplements may exacerbate hyperbilirubinemia because they prevent adequate milk (i.e., calorie) intake.[48,203]

The healthy, breast-fed, full-term infant requires little in the way of vitamin and mineral supplements. The breast-fed infant must rely on a vitamin K supplement given at birth.[48] The vitamin D concentration in human milk may be insufficient to prevent rickets, especially in dark-skinned infants.[204] Such infants may need a vitamin D supplement if not exposed to adequate amounts of sunlight.[125,126,205] Iron absorption from human milk is excellent, but because the concentration of iron declines during lactation, the breast-fed infant requires an iron supplement after 6 months of age.[44,46]

Growth Patterns

There is substantial evidence that the growth patterns of healthy breast-fed infants are distinct from formula-fed infants who conform more closely to the National Center for Health Statistics (NCHS) growth reference.[206–211] Breast-fed infants weight gain is faster in the first 2 months, and slower thereafter when compared with the NCHS reference. Deviation from the NCHS curves is explained in part by the fact that the curves were based on predominantly formula-fed infants. Relative to the NCHS growth reference, it might be inferred that the growth of breast-fed infants is unsatisfactory resulting in early food supplementation and cessation of breast-feeding. Further investigations have shown that the growth of the breast-fed infant is appropriate.[212] Slower growth velocity in breast-fed infants is not associated with obvious deleterious functional consequences. A U.S. study showed no association between energy intake and morbidity or achievement of developmental milestones in breast-fed infants through their first year.[71] Awareness of these distinct growth patterns should factor into the clinician's evaluation of infant growth and minimize the risk of introducing unnecessary complementary foods to breast-fed infants.

TABLE 52.2. Baby Friendly Hospital Initiative: 10 steps to successful breast-feeding.

1.	Written breast-feeding policy should be available.
2.	Health care staff should be trained to implement the policy.
3.	Educate pregnant women in prenatal classes and visits.
4.	Initiate breast-feeding within one hour of birth.
5.	Demonstrate how to breast-feed and maintain lactation.
6.	Use only breast milk, unless medically not indicated.
7.	Practice rooming-in 24 hours/day.
8.	Encourage breast-feeding on demand.
9.	Give no artificial nipples or pacifiers.
10.	Facilitate the development of breast-feeding support groups.

From World Health Organization[199] and UNICEF.[201]

Management of the Premature Neonate

Nutritional Concerns

Despite the profound benefits of human milk, the premature infant may be at risk for nutritional deficits. Human milk–fed premature infants manifest slower growth rates and inadequate intakes of specific nutrients to meet their greater needs.[213-219] Nutrient inadequacies may result from the compositional variability of human milk; losses associated with collection, storage, and feeding procedures; or inherently lower concentrations than those needed by growing premature infants.[7,8,27,29] The decline in the milk content of protein and sodium through lactation has been associated with reduced nutrient delivery to the premature infant.[7] Fat and vitamin losses have been associated with feeding procedures.[33,220] The content of calcium and phosphorus in human milk is never sufficient to meet the premature infant's demands for growth and skeletal mineralization.[219,221,222]

As noted earlier, the most variable nutrient component in human milk is fat.[25,28] Such variability presents a problem in determining the adequacy of energy intake for premature infants. After the initial few weeks of feeding, the lower protein intakes in human milk–fed premature infants may become a concern.[7] Lower serum albumin, total protein, and blood urea nitrogen (BUN) concentrations have been observed in human milk–fed premature infants compared with infants fed either whey- or casein-dominant commercial formulas.[215,223-225] These data suggest that protein inadequacy may manifest in premature infants fed human milk. Similarly, hyponatremia has been observed in premature infants fed human milk.[226,227]

The deficient intake of calcium and phosphorus from human milk, throughout lactation, is a problem because they are far below the mineral intakes needed by premature infants to achieve intrauterine accretion rates for Ca and P.[217,219,222,228-230] Balance studies indicate the magnitude of the deficit in Ca and P that accumulates during the 2- to 3-month hospitalization of the premature infant.[219] The approximate Ca intake from unfortified human milk is $44 mg \cdot kg^{-1} day^{-1}$ and excretory losses (urine plus feces) average $24 mg \cdot kg^{-1} day^{-1}$, resulting in a net Ca retention of $20 mg \cdot kg^{-1} day^{-1}$. This value is significantly below the intrauterine Ca accretion rate of 100 to $120 mg \cdot kg^{-1} day^{-1}$.[229] A cumulative deficit in bone mineral mass, therefore, might be expected with the continued feeding of unfortified human milk throughout the hospitalization. This mineral deficit has been noted on skeletal radiographs, which reveal poor bone mineralization, rickets, and fractures.[231,232]

Biochemical markers of deficient Ca and P intakes include low serum and urine phosphorus concentrations, elevated serum alkaline phosphatase activity, and elevated serum and urine calcium concentrations.[221,222,228,232-234] Serum phosphorus concentration is the best indicator of Ca and P status in human milk–fed premature infants. Prolonged deficiency of Ca and P tends to stimulate bone resorption to attempt a normalization of serum calcium concentration. This bone activity often is correlated with elevated serum alkaline phosphatase activity. In a comparison of human milk versus formula, the majority of premature infants having an elevated serum alkaline phosphatase activity were those fed human milk.[233] Moreover, at 9 and 18 months follow-up, linear growth was significantly lower in the group of premature infants having the highest serum activity of alkaline phosphatase in the neonatal period.[234]

Vitamin A and riboflavin concentrations decline with tube-feeding; vitamin C activity may be reduced secondary to oxidative effects.[235]

Thus, the potential of human milk for nutritional inadequacies in the premature infant versus its positive effects on host defense and infant development poses a dilemma: How can clinicians use human milk to the best advantage for the premature infant?

General Nutritional Support

The emerging host defense data warrant extraordinary efforts to provide nutritionally adequate milk to the high-risk population of premature infants. The data emphasize that even partial human milk feeding should be encouraged because of the protection afforded. We could accomplish some nutritional benefit by avoiding the use of restricted volumes of milk. The use of mother's own milk is associated with greater rates of growth than pasteurized donor human milk.[236] There are additional concerns with the use of donor human milk that include the potential transmission of infectious agents and other contaminants.[237]

The manner in which human milk is used in the nursery may result in nutrient losses. The use of continuous milk infusion systems may result in a great loss of available fat.[34] Milk infusion systems employing a syringe and pump, with the syringe oriented upright, ensure optimal delivery of fat.[34] Procedures also should be adopted during the collection and preparation phases that avoid losses of fat. The separation of nutrients in milk is a concern when using any additives to human milk.[238]

Hindmilk has been used in selected cases to provide the premature infant with additional energy.[30] Fractionation of each milk expression into two portions, foremilk and hindmilk, is practical if the mothers have sufficient milk production. The fat content of hindmilk may be 1.5- to threefold greater than that of foremilk.[29,30,239] The additional fat, and therefore, energy intake from hindmilk has been shown to improve the body weight gain in premature infants.[30]

Despite such precautionary measures, without the addition of supplemental nutrients, human milk–fed premature infants may not receive adequate intakes of protein, calcium, and phosphorus, and possibly zinc and copper. Multivitamin and iron supplements are necessary for premature infants.

Human Milk Fortification

Growth rates and serum protein and BUN concentrations in premature infants are increased when human milk feedings are fortified with protein.[215,224,240-243] Multicomponent fortifiers are needed to increase rates of growth and normalize biochemical indices of nutritional status in premature infants.[234,244-246] Calcium and phosphorus fortification using a powdered multicomponent fortifier meets the needs for achieving intrauterine nutrient accretion rates.[247] Fat absorption, however, may be affected by multicomponent fortification of human milk.[247] Further modifications, therefore, may be needed to achieve optimal growth rates.

Nutritional recommendations for the breast-fed premature infant are needed to cover the period after hospital discharge. Growth and biochemical indices should be monitored serially after discharge to ensure optimum nutritional status. The bone mineral content of premature infants fed fortified human milk during hospitalization took 2 years to catch up to similar infants fed formula after discharge.[248]

The preferred diet for the premature infant is fortified mother's milk.[3] Currently, commercial formulations in the United States are available in a powder form (i.e., Enfamil Human Milk Fortifier, Mead Johnson Nutritional Division, Evansville, IN) and in a liquid form (i.e., Similac Natural Care 24, Ross Laboratories, Columbus, OH). The preparations differ in their composition (Table 52.3).

Mothers of premature infants may not have sufficient milk for complete enteral feeding. Because the benefits to host defense accrue from partial human milk feeding, alternating fortified human milk with preterm formula may be appropriate.[249] Using that alternate feeding approach, net nutrient retention and growth were equivalent to intrauterine accretion rates and lower milk intakes were needed than when feeding fortified human milk alone.

Mother's own, unfortified milk is used in the initial feedings; the freshest milk is used if a long interval elapses from birth to initial feeding. Generally, commercial fortifiers are used in all human milk–fed premature infants who require tube-feeding. This target population includes infants less than 2 kg body weight and 35 weeks'

TABLE 52.3. Comparison of the nutrient composition of human milk from early lactation (1 week), later lactation (1 month), fortified human milks, and preterm formulas.

	Human milk, 1 week	Mature human milk (MM), 1 month	EHMF[a] + MM	SNC[b] + MM	EPF[c] 24	SSC[d] 24
Volume, ml	100	100	100	100	100	100
Energy, kcal	67	70	84	76	81	81
Protein, g	2.4	1.8	2.5	2.0	2.4	2.2
% Whey/casein	70/30	70/30	70/30	65/35	60/40	60/40
Fat, g	3.8	4.0	4.0	4.2	4.1	4.4
% MCT/LCT	2/98	2/98	2/98	25/75	40/60	40/60
Carbohydrate, g	6.1	7.0	9.7	7.8	9.0	8.6
% Lactose	100	100	72	72	50	50
Calcium, mg	25	22	112	116	134	146
Phosphorus, mg	14	14	59	60	67	73
Magnesium, mg	3.1	2.5	3.5	6.1	5.5	9.7
Sodium, mg	50	30	37	33	32	35
Potassium, mg	70	60	75	82	83	104
Chloride, mg	90	60	78	63	69	66
Zinc, µg	500	320	1030	770	1215	1215
Copper, µg	80	60	120	130	100	200
Vitamin A, IU	560	400	1350	475	1013	550
Vitamin D, IU	4	4	214	63	219	122
Vitamin C, mg	5.4	5.6	17.2	17.8	16	30
Vitamin E, IU	1.0	0.3	4.9	1.8	5.1	3.2

From Butte et al.,[6] Gross et al.,[8] Telemo et al.,[60] and Newman et al.[268]
[a] Enfamil Human Milk Fortifier (1993, Mead Johnson Nutritionals, Evansville, IN), four packets + 100 ml mature human milk.
[b] Similac Natural Care 24 (1994, Ross Laboratories, Columbus, OH) diluted 1:1 with mature human milk.
[c] Enfamil Premature Formula 24 (1993, Mead Johnson Nutritionals, Evansville, IN).
[d] Similac Special Care 24 (1994, Ross Laboratories, Columbus, OH).

52. Nutritional Support of the Neonate II

gestation. Milk volumes, if indicated clinically, are allowed to increase from 150 ml·kg^{-1} day^{-1} to a maximum of 200 ml·kg^{-1} day^{-1}. The fortifier is added when the infants demonstrate clinical tolerance to human milk feeding at volumes of 100 ml·kg^{-1} day^{-1}. To provide optimal mineral intakes, if unfortified human milk is used for more than 1 week, a fortifier should be added despite the volume consumed. Hindmilk is used if an infant's weight gain is less than 15 g·kg^{-1} day^{-1} and the mother's milk production exceeds her infant's needs by approximately 30%. Iron is supplemented when complete enteral tube-feeding is achieved.

Thus, it appears that commercial formulations designed to fortify human milk provide nutrients to approach the needs of premature infants, but newer formulations may be required to meet all the nutritional needs of premature infants.

Monitoring Nutritional Status

The nutritional status of premature infants fed human milk is monitored serially. Optimal rates of growth generally should exceed a weight gain of 15 g·kg^{-1} day^{-1} and a length increment of approximately 1.0 cm/week. Biochemical monitoring of nutritional status includes serum phosphorus, alkaline phosphatase activity, sodium, albumin, and BUN concentrations. Urinary biochemical indices may be helpful in gauging calcium and phosphorus supplementation. Approximations for the urinary excretion of calcium should be less than 6 mg·kg^{-1} day^{-1} and phosphorus greater than 4 mg·kg^{-1} day^{-1}.

Hospital-Based Lactation Support

Mother's Own Milk Bank

All mothers who desire to provide milk for their infants should meet with an experienced lactation specialist soon after delivery to learn how to initiate lactation and plan home-based collection of milk for the hospitalized neonate.

Mothers should be encouraged to initiate milk expression soon after delivery. Milk production in mothers of premature infants is negatively correlated with the day milk expression is initiated.[75] Manual and mechanical methods for milk expression should be offered. The use of mechanical methods generally is associated with greater milk production.[74,250] The double pumping method of milk expression, which allows for simultaneous pumping of both breasts, is available with most electric breast pumps. The double pumping system reportedly results in greater serum prolactin concentration, milk production, milk fat concentration, and maternal preference when compared with other artificial methods of milk expression.[251,252] It is helpful to have a pump rental service at or near the hospital.

The establishment at the hospital of a mother's own milk bank provides quality control over such practices as the initiation of milk expression, use and maintenance of breast pumps, methods for milk collection, and transport and storage; it serves as a liaison between mother and nursery to identify when and how much milk is needed for the infant; and it helps clinicians in determining the acceptability of milk if the mother is ill or using medications. Guidelines for the establishment of a hospital-based mother's own milk bank have been published.[74,250] The bank also provides the appropriate clean environment for milk handling, for the addition of fortifiers, and for aliquoting appropriate volumes for the infants' daily needs. In addition, it provides a quiet place for mothers to express milk when visiting their infants and for breastfeeding.

Milk should be collected in either glass or hard plastic containers. Plastic bags are not advisable because of the loss of immune components and the potential for contamination.[74] One milk expression should be collected separately in each milk container. Milk to be fed within 24 hours can be refrigerated after collection. Milk to be fed after that time should be frozen immediately at −15° to −20°C. All milk must be transported to the hospital on ice in an enclosed, thermally protected chest. Maternal compliance with milk collection can be monitored by bacteriologic screening of a milk sample.

Of great concern to the mother of a premature infant is the maintenance of a milk supply sufficient to meet the infant's needs, both currently and in the future. Mothers of premature infants should be informed that their potential for lactation is good.[253] Early emphasis should be placed on frequency and duration of milk expression. Milk expression should occur at least six times per day, with the longest nonpumping period no greater than 5 hours.[254] Strategies to minimize maternal stress before and during pumping (e.g., muscle relaxation techniques, audio relaxation tape, picture of infant on pump) may facilitate milk ejection.[255,256]

Skin-to-Skin Contact

Skin-to-skin contact between infant and mother has been a useful method to assist milk production. Skin-to-skin contact should be commenced as soon as the infant is physiologically stable. The technique involves placing the diaper-clad infant upright between the maternal breasts. While in skin-to-skin contact, premature infants have normal body temperature, diminished apnea and bradycardia, and higher oxygen saturation.[257–260] This intervention tends to enhance maternal self-confidence, facilitates earlier hospital discharge, increases milk production, and lengthens lactation.[257,259,261,262]

Progression to Breast-Feeding

Once the premature infant achieves full enteral feeding via the oro- or nasogastric route, early breast-feeding should be considered. Usually, the lactation specialist meets with the mother and infant to instruct the mother, and to gauge the infant's success at latch-on and the coordination of sucking and swallowing with respiration. Generally, nonnutritive breast-feedings increase in duration as the infant matures. Once the infant demonstrates the ability, one breast-feeding is substituted for a single bolus tube-feeding. As the infant is observed to feed satisfactorily and daily weight gain ensues, a second breast-feeding is added. Milk intake during breast-feeding can be measured by the test-weighing technique.[67,263] Successful breast-feeding often can be achieved without bottle-feeding if the mother is available. When the infant demonstrates success at two breast-feedings in a day, the mother usually can breast-feed exclusively each day for a given interval (e.g., 6 hours of ad libitum breast-feeding). After the breast-feeding interval concludes, the bolus tube-feeding protocol is reinstituted. The exclusive breast-feeding sessions can be lengthened as the mother's schedule allows.

Near the time of hospital discharge, a decision is made about the adequacy of the mother's milk volume for ad libitum breast-feeding at home. The lactation specialist should be available for home follow-up to ensure a successful breast-feeding outcome.

Acknowledgments. I thank Idelle Tapper for secretarial assistance. This work is a publication of the USDA/ARS Children's Nutrition Research Center, Department of Pediatrics, Baylor College of Medicine, Houston, TX, and has been funded in part with federal funds from the U.S. Department of Agriculture, Agricultural Research Service, under cooperative agreement 58-6250-1-003, and from the National Institutes of Health, Clinical Research Centers Branch, grant M01 RR-00188-30. The contents of this publication do not necessarily reflect the views or policies of the U.S. Department of Agriculture, nor does mention of trade names, commercial products, or organizations imply endorsement by the U.S. government.

References

1. American Academy of Pediatrics, Committee on Nutrition. Encouraging breast-feeding. Pediatrics 1980;65:657–658.
2. Nutrition Committee of the Canadian Paediatric Society, Committee on Nutrition of the American Academy of Pediatrics. Breast-feeding. Pediatrics 1978;62:591–601.
3. Nutrition Committee, Canadian Paediatric Society. Nutrient needs and feeding of premature infants. Can Med Assoc J 1995;152:1765–1785.
4. American Academy of Pediatrics, Committee on Nutrition. Nutrition and lactation. Pediatrics 1981;68:435–433.
5. Atkinson SA, Bryan MH, Anderson GH. Human milk: difference in nitrogen concentration in milk from mothers of term and premature infants. J Pediatr 1978;93:67–69.
6. Butte NF, Garza C, Johnson CA, et al. Longitudinal changes in milk composition of mothers delivering preterm and term infants. Early Hum Dev 1984;9:153–162.
7. Schanler RJ, Oh W. Composition of breast milk obtained from mothers of premature infants as compared to breast milk obtained from donors. J Pediatr 1980;96:679–681.
8. Gross SJ, David RJ, Bauman L, et al. Nutritional composition of milk produced by mothers delivering preterm. J Pediatr 1980;96:641–644.
9. Carlson SE. Human milk nonprotein nitrogen: occurrence and possible functions. In: Barness LA, ed. Advances in pediatrics. Chicago: Year Book Medical 1985:43–70.
10. Hambraeus L. Proprietary milk versus human breast milk in infant feeding, a critical appraisal from the nutritional point of view. Pediatr Clin North Am 1977;24:17–35.
11. Heine W, Tiess M, Wutzke KD. 15N tracer investigations of the physiological availability of urea nitrogen in mother's milk. Acta Paediatr Scand 1986;75:439–443.
12. Fomon SJ, Bier DM, Matthews DE, et al. Bioavailability of dietary urea nitrogen in the breast-fed infant. J Pediatr 1988; 113:515–517.
13. Billeaud C, Guillet J, Sandler B. Gastric emptying in infants with or without gastro-oesophageal reflux according to the type of milk. Eur J Clin Nutr 1990;44:577–583.
14. Rassin DK, Gaull GE, Raiha NCR, et al. Milk protein quantity and quality in low-birth-weight infants. IV. Effects on tyrosine and phenylalanine in plasma and urine. J Pediatr 1977;90:356–360.
15. Gaull GE, Rassin DK, Raiha NCR, et al. Milk protein quantity and quality in low-birthweight infants. III. Effects on sulfur amino acids in plasma and urine. J Pediatr 1977;90:348–355.
16. Jarvenpaa AL, Raiha NC, Rassin DK. Feeding the low-birth-weight infant: I. Taurine and cholesterol supplementation of formula does not affect growth and metabolism. Pediatrics 1983;71:171–178.
17. Jarvenpaa AL, Rassin DK, Raiha NCR, et al. Milk protein quantity and quality in the term infant. II. Effects on acidic and neutral amino acids. Pediatrics 1982;70:221–230.
18. Rassin DK. Amino acid responses in neonatal nutrition and their implications for the central nervous system. In: Barness L, ed. Protein requirements in the term infant. Princeton: Excerpta Medica, 1988:3–9.
19. Lindblad BS, Alfven G, Zetterstrom R. Plasma free amino acid concentrations of breast-fed infants. Acta Paediatr Scand 1978;67:659–663.
20. Goldman AS, Chheda S, Keeney SE, et al. Immunologic protection of the premature newborn by human milk. Semin Perinatol 1994;18:495–501.
21. Lonnerdal B. Biochemistry and physiological function of human milk proteins. Am J Clin Nutr 1985;42:1299–1317.
22. Hanson LA, Ahlstedt S, Andersson B, et al. Protective factors in milk and the development of the immune system. Pediatrics 1985;75(suppl):172–176.

23. Hernell O, Blackberg L. Human milk bile salt-stimulated lipase: functional and molecular aspects. J Pediatr 1994; 125:S56–61.
24. Jensen RG, Hagerty MM, McMahon KE. Lipids of human milk and infant formulas: a review. Am J Clin Nutr 1978; 31:990–1016.
25. Jensen RG, Jensen GL. Specialty lipids for infant nutrition. I. Milks and formulas. J Pediatr Gastroenterol Nutr 1992;15:232–245.
26. Alemi B, Hamosh M, Scanlon JW, et al. Fat digestion in very low-birthweight infants: effect of addition of human milk to low birthweight formula. Pediatrics 1981;68:484–489.
27. Butte NF, Garza C, Smith EO. Variability of macronutrient concentrations in human milk. Eur J Clin Nutr 1988;42:345–349.
28. Hamosh M. Lipid metabolism in premature infants. Biol Neonate 1987;52(suppl 1):50–64.
29. Neville MC, Keller RP, Seacat J, et al. Studies on human lactation. I. Within-feed and between-breast variation in selected components of human milk. Am J Clin Nutr 1984; 40:635–646.
30. Valentine CJ, Hurst NM, Schanler RJ. Hindmilk improves weight gain in low-birth-weight infants fed human milk. J Pediatr Gastroenterol Nutr 1994;18:474–477.
31. Nommsen LA, Lovelady CA, Heinig MJ, et al. Determinants of energy, protein, lipid, and lactose concentrations in human milk during the first 12 months of lactation: the DARLING study. Am J Clin Nutr 1991;53:457–465.
32. Butte NF, Garza C, Stuff JE, et al. Effect of maternal diet and body composition on lactational performance. Am J Clin Nutr 1984;39:296–306.
33. Greer FR, McCormick A, Loker J. Changes in fat concentration of human milk during delivery by intermittent bolus and continuous mechanical pump infusion. J Pediatr 1984;105:745–749.
34. Schanler RJ. Special methods in feeding the preterm infant. In: Tsang RC, Nichols BL, eds. Nutrition during infancy. Philadelphia: Hanley & Belfus, 1988:314–325.
35. Uauy R, Hoffman DR. Essential fatty acid requirements for normal eye and brain development. Semin Perinatol 1991;15:449–455.
36. Innis SM. Human milk and formula fatty acids. J Pediatr 1992;120:S56–S61.
37. Carlson SE, Werkman SH, Rhodes PG, et al. Visual-acuity development in healthy preterm infants: effect of marine-oil supplementation. Am J Clin Nutr 1993;58:35–42.
38. Whyte RK, Homer R, Pennock CA. Faecal excretion of oligosaccharides and other carbohydrates in normal neonates. Arch Dis Child 1978;53:913–915.
39. MacLean WC, Fink BB. Lactose malabsorption by premature infants: magnitude and clinical significance. J Pediatr 1980;97:383–388.
40. Ziegler EE, Fomon SJ. Lactose enhances mineral absorption in infancy. J Pediatr Gastroenterol Nutr 1983;2:288–294.
41. Schanler RJ. Suitability of human milk for the low birth-weight infant. Clin Perinatol 1995;22:207–222.
42. Neville MC, Watters CD. Secretion of calcium into milk: a review. J Dairy Sci 1983;66:371–380.
43. Casey CE, Hambidge KM, Neville MC. Studies in human lactation: zinc, copper, manganese, and chromium in human milk in the first month of lactation. Am J Clin Nutr 1985;41:1193–1200.
44. Dallman PR, Siimes MA, Stekel A. Iron deficiency in infancy and childhood. Am J Clin Nutr 1980;33:86–118.
45. Saarinen UM. Need for iron supplementation in infants on prolonged breast-feeding. J Pediatr 1978;93:177–180.
46. Lonnerdal B, Hernell O. Iron, zinc, copper and selenium status of breast-fed infants and infants fed trace element fortified milk-based infant formula. Acta Pediatr 1994;83:367–373.
47. Schanler RJ, Prestridge LL. Neonatal vitamin metabolism—water soluble. In: Cowett RM, ed. Principles of perinatal-neonatal metabolsim. New York: Springer-Verlag, 1991:559–582.
48. Greer FR, Suttie JW. Vitamin K and the newborn. In: Tsang RC, Nichols BL, eds. Nutrition during infancy. Philadelphia: Hanley & Belfus, 1988:289–297.
49. Specker BL, Greer F, Tsang RC. Vitamin D. In: Tsang RC, Nichols BL, eds. Nutrition during infancy. Philadelphia: Hanley & Belfus, 1988:264–276.
50. Carver JD, Walker WA. The role of nucleotides in human nutrition. Nutr Biochem 1995;6:58–72.
51. Uauy R, Quan R, Gil A. Role of nucleotides in intestinal development and repair: implications for infant nutrition. J Nutr 1994;124:1436S–1441S.
52. Koldovsky O. The potential physiological significance of milk-borne hormonally active substances for the neonate. J Mammary Gland Biol Neoplasia 1996;1:317–323.
53. Prosser CG. Insulin-like growth factors in milk and mammary gland. J Mammary Gland Biol Neoplasia 1996; 1:297–306.
54. Ellis LA, Mastro AM, Picciano MF. Milk-borne prolactin and neonatal development. J Mammary Gland Biol Neoplasia 1996;1:259–269.
55. Sheard NF, Walker WA. The role of breast milk in the development of the gastrointestinal tract. Nutr Rev 1988;46:1–8.
56. Hanson LA, Adlerberth I, Carlsson B, et al. Host defense of the neonate and the intestinal flora. Acta Paediatr Scand Suppl 1989;351:122–125.
57. Goldman AS, Sharpe LW, Goldblum RM. Anti-inflammatory properties of human milk. Acta Paediatr Scand 1986;75:689–695.
58. Goldman AS, Smith CW. Host resistance factors in human milk. J Pediatr 1973;82:1082–1090.
59. Nuijens JH, van Berkel PHC, Schanbacher FL. Structure and biological actions of lactoferrin. J Mammary Gland Biol Neoplasia 1996;1:285–295.
60. Telemo E, Hanson LA. Antibodies in milk. J Mammary Gland Biol Neoplasia 1996;1:243–249.
61. Kleinman RE, Walker WA. The enteromammary immune system. Dig Dis Sci 1979;24:876–882.
62. Fishaut M, Murphy D, Neifert M, et al. Bronchomammary axis in the immune response to respiratory syncytial virus. J Pediatr 1981;99:186–191.

63. Isaacs CE, Kashyap S, Heird WC, et al. Antiviral and antibacterial lipids in human milk and infant formula feeds. Arch Dis Child 1990;65:861–864.
64. Newburg DS. Oligosaccharides and glycoconjugates in human milk: their role in host defense. J Mammary Gland Biol Neoplasia 1996;1:271–283.
65. Goldman AS, Chheda S, Garofalo R, et al. Cytokines in human milk: properties and potential effects upon the mammary gland and the neonate. J Mammary Gland Biol Neoplasia 1996;1:351–358.
66. Institute of Medicine, Subcommittee on Nutrition During Lactation. Nutrition during lactation. Washington, DC: National Academy Press, 1991.
67. Neville MC, Keller R, Seacat J, et al. Studies in human lactation: milk volumes in lactating women during the onset of lactation and full lactation. Am J Clin Nutr 1988;48:1375–1386.
68. Macy IG, Hunscher HA, Donelson E, et al. Human milk flow. J Dis Child 1930;39:1186–1204.
69. Saint L, Maggiore P, Hartmann PE. Yield and nutrient content of milk in eight women breast-feeding twins and one woman breast-feeding triplets. Br J Nutr 1986;56:87–95.
70. Stuff JE, Nichols BL. Nutrient intake and growth performance of older infants fed human milk. J Pediatr 1989;116:959–968.
71. Dewey KG, Heinig MJ, Nommsen LA, et al. Adequacy of energy intake among breast-fed infants in the DARLING study: relationships to growth velocity, morbidity, and activity levels. J Pediatr 1991;119:538–547.
72. Dewey KG, Heinig MJ, Nommsen LA, et al. Maternal vs infant factors related to breast milk intake and residual milk volume: the DARLING study. Pediatrics 1991;87:829–837.
73. Michaelsen KF, Larsen PS, Thomsen BL, et al. Weight, length, head circumference, and growth velocity in a longitudinal study of Danish infants. Dan Med Bull 1994;41:577–585.
74. Schanler RJ, Hurst NM. Human milk for the hospitalized preterm infant. Semin Perinatol 1994;18:476–484.
75. Hopkinson JM, Schanler RJ, Garza C. Milk production by mothers of premature infants. Pediatrics 1988;81:815–820.
76. Hopkinson JM, Schanler RJ, Fraley JK, et al. Milk production by mothers of premature infants: influence of cigarette smoking. Pediatrics 1992;90:934–938.
77. Vio F, Salazar G, Infante C. Smoking during pregnancy and lactation and its effect on breast-milk volume. Am J Clin Nutr 1991;54:1011–1016.
78. Andersen AN, Lund-Andersen C, Larsen JF, et al. Suppressed prolactin but normal neurophysin levels in cigarette smoking breast-feeding women. Clin Endocrinol 1982;17:363–368.
79. Winikoff B, Semeraro P, Zimmerman M. Contraception during breast-feeding: a clinician's handbook. New York: Population Council, 1988.
80. Hurst N, Valentine C, Renfro L, et al. Skin-to-skin holding in the neonatal intensive care influences maternal milk volume. J Perinatol 1997;36:551–559.
81. Prentice A, Paul A, Black A, et al. Cross-cultural differences in lactational performance. In: Hamosh M, Goldman AS, eds. Human lactation 2: maternal and environmental factors. New York: Plenum Press, 1986:13–44.
82. Strode MA, Dewey KG, Lonnerdal B. Effects of short-term caloric restriction on lactational performance of well-nourished women. Acta Paediatr Scand 1986;75:222–229.
83. Neville M, Oliva-Rasbach J. Is maternal milk production limiting for infant growth during the first year of life in breast-fed infants? In: Goldman AS, Atkinson SA, Hanson LA, eds. Human lactation 3: the effects of human milk on the recipient infant. New York: Plenum Press, 1987:123–133.
84. Dusdieker LB, Hemingway DL, Stumbo PJ. Is milk production impaired by dieting during lactation? Am J Clin Nutr 1994;59:833–840.
85. Lonnerdal B, Forsum E, Gebre-Medhin M, et al. Breast milk composition in Ethiopian and Swedish mothers. II. Lactose, nitrogen, and protein contents. Am J Clin Nutr 1976;29:1134–1141.
86. Villalpando SF, Butte NF, Wong WW, et al. Lactation performance of rural Mesoamerindians. Eur J Clin Nutr 1992;46:337–348.
87. Sanchez-Pozo A, Lopez-Morles J, Izquierdo A, et al. Protein composition of human milk in relation to mother's weight and socioeconomic status. Hum Nutr Clin Nutr 1987;41C:115–125.
88. Forsum E, Lonnerdal B. Effect of protein intake on protein and nitrogen composition of breast milk. Am J Clin Nutr 1980;33:1809–1813.
89. Jensen RG. The lipids of human milk. Boca Raton, FL: CRC Press, 1989.
90. Chappell JE, Francis T, Clandinin MT. Vitamin A and E content of human milk at early stages of lactation. Early Hum Dev 1985;11:157–167.
91. Hachey DL, Silber GH, Wong WW, et al. Human lactation II: endogenous fatty acid synthesis by the mammary gland. Pediatrics 1989;25:63–68.
92. Sanders THB, Ellis TR, Dickerson JWT. Studies of vegans: the fatty acid composition of plasma cholinephosphoglycerides, erythrocytes, adipose tissue, breast milk and some indicators of susceptibility to ischemic heart disease in vegans and omnivore controls. Am J Clin Nutr 1978;31:805–813.
93. Butte NF, Calloway DH. Evaluation of lactational performance of Navajo women. Am J Clin Nutr 1981;34:2210–2215.
94. Gebre-Medhin M, Vahlquist A, Hofvander Y, et al. Breast milk composition in Ethiopian and Swedish mothers. I. Vitamin A and β-carotene. Am J Clin Nutr 1976;29:441–451.
95. Hollis BW, Lambert PW, Horst RL. Factors affecting the antirachitic sterol content of native milk. In: Holick MF, Gray TK, Anast CS, eds. Perinatal calcium and phosphorous metabolism. Amsterdam: Elsevier, 1983:157–182.
96. von Kries R, Shearer M, McCarthy PT, et al. Vitamin K_1 content of maternal milk: influence of the stage of lactation, lipid composition, and vitamin K_1 supplements given to the mother. Pediatr Res 1987;22:513–517.
97. Bates CJ, Prentice AM, Prentice A, et al. The effect of vitamin C supplementation on lactating women in

Keneba, a West African rural community. Int J Vitam Nutr Res 1983;53:68–76.
98. Byerley LO, Kirksey A. Effects of different levels of vitamin C intake on the vitamin C concentration in human milk and the vitamin C intakes of breast-fed infants. Am J Clin Nutr 1985;41:665–671.
99. Pratt JP, Hamil BM, Moyer EZ, et al. Metabolism of women during the reproductive cycle. XVIII. The effect of multi-vitamin supplements on the secretion of B vitamins in human milk. J Nutr 1951;44:141–157.
100. Kirksey A, Roepke JLB. Vitamin B_6 nutriture of mothers of three breast-fed neonates with central nervous system disorders. Fed Proc 1981;40:864.
101. Johnson PR Jr, Roloff JS. Vitamin B_{12} deficiency in an infant strictly breast-fed by a mother with latent pernicious anemia. J Pediatr 1982;100:917–919.
102. Higginbottom MC, Sweetman L, Nyhan WL. A syndrome of methylmalonic aciduria, homocystinuria, megaloblastic anemia and neurologic abnormalities in a vitamin B_{12}-deficient breast-fed infant of a strict vegetarian. N Engl J Med 1978;299:317–323.
103. Specker BL, Miller D, Norman EJ, et al. Increased urinary methylmalonic acid excretion in breast-fed infants of vegetarian mothers and identification of an acceptable dietary source of vitamin B_{12}. Am J Clin Nutr 1988;47:89–92.
104. Laskey MA, Prentice A, Shaw J, et al. Breast-milk calcium concentrations during prolonged lactation in British and rural Gambian mothers. Acta Paediatr Scand 1990;79:507–512.
105. Prentice A, Barclay DV. Breast-milk calcium and phosphorus concentrations of mothers in rural Zaïre. Eur J Clin Nutr 1991;45:611–617.
106. Dallman PR. Iron deficiency in the weaning: a nutritional problem on the way to resolution. Acta Paediatr Scand 1986;S323:59–67.
107. Siimes MA, Salmenpera L, Perheentupa J. Exclusive breast-feeding for 9 months: risk of iron deficiency. J Pediatr 1984;104:196–199.
108. Lonnerdal B, Keen CL, Hurley LS. Iron, copper, zinc, and manganese in milk. Annu Rev Nutr 1981;1:149–174.
109. Krebs NF, Reidinger CJ, Hartley S, et al. Zinc supplementation during lactation: effects on maternal status and milk zinc concentrations. Am J Clin Nutr 1995;61:1030–1036.
110. Mannan S, Picciano MF, Influence of maternal selenium status on human milk selenium concentration and glutathione peroxidase activity. Am J Clin Nutr 1987;46:95–100.
111. Ruff AJ. Breastmilk, breastfeeding, and transmission of viruses to the neonate. Semin Perinatol 1994;18:510–516.
112. Dworsky M, Yow M, Stagno S, et al. Cytomegalovirus infection of breast milk and transmission in infancy. Pediatrics 1983;72:295–299.
113. Krogh V, Duffy C, Wong D, et al. Postpartum immunization with rubella virus vaccine and antibody response in breast-feeding infants. J Lab Clin Med 1989;113:695–699.
114. Martino MD, Appendino C, Resti M, et al. Should hepatitis B surface antigen positive mothers breast-feed? Arch Dis Child 1985;60:972–974.
115. Dunn DT, Newell ML, Ades AE, et al. Risk of human immunodeficiency virus type 1 transmission through breast-feeding. Lancet 1992;340:585–588.
116. Palasanthiran P, Ziegler JB, Stewart GJ, et al. Breast-feeding during primary maternal human immunodeficiency virus infection and risk of transmission from mother to infant. J Infect Dis 1993;167:441–444.
117. Oxtoby MJ. Human immunodeficiency virus and other viruses in human milk: placing the issues in broader perspective. Pediatr Infect Dis J 1988;7:825–835.
118. American Academy of Pediatrics, Peter G, ed. 1997 Red Book: Report of the Committee on Infectious Diseases. 24nd ed. Elk Grove Village, IL: AAP, 1994.
119. American Academy of Pediatrics, Committee on Drugs. The transfer of drugs and other chemicals into human milk. Pediatrics 1994;93:137–150.
120. Berlin CM, Denson M, Daniel CH, et al. Disposition of dietary caffeine in milk, saliva, and plasma of lactating women. Pediatrics 1984;73:59–63.
121. Menella JA, Beauchamp GK. The transfer of alcohol to human milk. Effects on flavor and the infant's behavior. N Engl J Med 1991;325:981–985.
122. Little RE, Anderson KW, Ervin CH, et al. Maternal alcohol use during breast-feeding and infant mental and motor development at one year. N Engl J Med 1989;321:425–430.
123. Hillman LS, Chow W, Salmons SS, et al. Vitamin D metabolism, mineral homeostasis, and bone mineralization in term infants fed human milk, cow milk-based formula, or soy-based formula. J Pediatr 1988;112:864–874.
124. Venkataraman PS, Luhar H, Neylan MJ. Bone mineral metabolism in full-term infants fed human milk, cow milk-based, and soy-based formulas. Am J Dis Child 1992;146:1302–1305.
125. Greer FR, Searcy JE, Levin RS, et al. Bone mineral content and serum 25-hydroxyvitamin D concentration in breast-fed infants with and without supplemental vitamin D. J Pediatr 1981;98:696–701.
126. Greer FR, Searcy JE, Levin RS, et al. Bone mineral content and serum 25-OH D concentrations in breast-fed infants with and without supplemental vitamin D: one year follow-up. J Pediatr 1982;100:919–922.
127. Popkin BM, Adair L, Akin JS, et al. Breast-feeding and diarrheal morbidity. Pediatrics 1990;86:874–882.
128. Glass RI, Stoll BJ. The protective effect of human milk against diarrhea. Acta Paediatr Scand 1989;351:131–136.
129. Cunningham AS. Morbidity in breast-fed and artificially fed infants. J Pediatr 1977;90:726–769.
130. Cunningham AS. Morbidity in breast-fed and artificially fed infants. II. J Pediatr 1979;95:685–689.
131. Cunningham AS, Jelliffe DB, Jelliffe EFP. Breast-feeding and health in the 1980s: a global epidemiologic review. J Pediatr 1991;118:659–666.
132. Dewey KG, Heinig MJ, Nommsen-Rivers LA. Differences in morbidity between breastfed and formula-fed infants. J Pediatr 1995;126:696–702.
133. Kovar MG, Serdula MD, Marks JS, et al. Review of the epidemiologic evidence for an association between infant feeding and infant health. Pediatrics 1984;74:S615–638.

134. Howie PW, Forsyth JS, Ogston SA, et al. Protective effect of breast-feeding against infection. Br Med J 1990;300:11–16.
135. Frank AL, Taber LH, Glezen WP, et al. Breast-feeding and respiratory virus infection. Pediatrics 1982;70:239–245.
136. Wright AL, Holberg CJ, Martinez FD, et al. Breast feeding and lower respiratory tract illness in the first year of life. Br Med J 1989;299:945–948.
137. World Health Organization, United Nations Children's Fund. Protecting, promoting and supporting breast-feeding: the special role of maternity services. Geneva, Switzerland: WHO, 1989.
138. Rubin DH, Leventhal JM, Krasilnikoff PA, et al. Relationship between infant feeding and infectious illness: a prospective study of infants during the first year of life. Pediatrics 1990;85:464–471.
139. Duncan B, Ey J, Holberg CJ, et al. Exclusive breast-feeding for at least 4 months protects against otitis media. Pediatrics 1993;91:867–872.
140. Pisacane A, Graziano L, Mazzarella G, et al. Breast-feeding and urinary tract infection. J Pediatr 1992;120:87–89.
141. Coppa GV, Gabrielli O, Giorgi P, et al. Preliminary study of breast-feeding and bacterial adhesion to uroepithelial cells. Lancet 1990;335:569–571.
142. Goldblum RM, Schanler RJ, Garza C, et al. Human milk feeding enhances the urinary excretion of immunologic factors in low birth weight infants. Pediatr Res 1989;25:184–188.
143. Lucas A, Cole TJ. Breast milk and neonatal necrotizing enterocolitis. Lancet 1990;336:1519–1523.
144. Schanler RJ, Shulman RJ, Lau C. Fortified human milk improves the health of the premature infant. Pediatr Res 1996;40:548A.
145. Eibl MM, Wolf HM, Furnkranz H, et al. Prevention of necrotizing enterocolitis in low-birth-weight infants by IgA-IgG feeding. N Engl J Med 1988;319:1–7.
146. Narayanan I, Prakash K, Bala S, et al. Partial supplementation with expressed breast-milk for prevention of infection in low-birth-weight infants. Lancet 1980;2:561–563.
147. Narayanan I, Prakash K, Gujral VV. The value of human milk in the prevention of infection in the high-risk low-birth-weight infant. J Pediatr 1981;99:496–498.
148. Narayanan I, Prakash K, Murthy NS, et al. Randomised controlled trial of effect of raw and holder pasteurised human milk and of formula supplements on incidence of neonatal infection. Lancet 1984;2:1111–1113.
149. El-Mohandes AAE, Picard M, Simmens SJ. Human milk utilization in the ICN decreases the incidence of bacterial sepsis. Pediatr Res 1995;37:306A.
150. Covert RF, Barman N, Domanico RS, et al. Prior enteral nutrition with human milk protects against intestinal perforation in infants who develop necrotizing enterocolitis. Pediatr Res 1995;37:305A.
151. Narayanan I, Prakash K, Verma RK, et al. Administration of colostrum for the prevention of infection in the low birth weight infant in a developing country. J Trop Pediatr 1983;29:197–200.
152. Contreras-Lemus J, Flores-Huerta S, Cisneros-Silva I, et al. Disminucion de la morbilidad en neonatos pretermino alimentados con leche de su propia madre. Biol Med Hosp Infant Mex 1992;49:671–677.
153. Davis MK, Savitz DA, Graubard BI. Infant feeding and childhood cancer. Lancet 1988;1:365–368.
154. Koletzko S, Sherman P, Corey M, et al. Role of infant feeding practices in development of Crohn's disease in childhood. Br Med J 1989;298:1617–1618.
155. Gerstein HC. Cow's milk exposure and type I diabetes mellitus. Diabetes Care 1994;17:13–19.
156. Kramer MS. Does breast feeding help protect against atopic disease? Biology, methodology, and a golden jubilee of controversy. J Pediatr 1988;112:181–190.
157. Saarinen UM, Backman A, Kajosaari M, et al. Prolonged breast-feeding as prophylaxis for atopic disease. Lancet 1979;2:163–166.
158. Karjalainen J, Martin JM, Knip M, et al. A bovine albumin peptide as a possible trigger of insulin-dependent diabetes mellitus. N Engl J Med 1992;327:302–307.
159. Rogan WJ, Gladen BC. Breast-feeding and cognitive development. Early Hum Dev 1993;31:181–193.
160. Lucas A, Morley R, Cole TJ, et al. A randomised multicentre study of human milk versus formula and later development in preterm infants. Arch Dis Child 1994;70:F141–146.
161. Lucas A, Morley R, Cole TJ, et al. Breast milk and subsequent intelligence quotient in children born preterm. Lancet 1992;339:261–264.
162. Crawford MA. The role of essential fatty acids in neural development: implications for perinatal nutrition. Am J Clin Nutr 1993;57:703S–710S.
163. Anderson GJ, Connor WE, Corliss JD. Docosahexaenoic acid is the preferred dietary n-3 fatty acid for the development of the brain and retina. Pediatr Res 1990;27:89–97.
164. Riordan J. Anatomy and psychophysiology of lactation. In: Riordan J, Auerbach KG, eds. Breast-feeding and human lactation. Boston: Jones and Bartlett, 1993:81–104.
165. Wang IY, Fraser IS. Reproductive function and contraception in the postpartum period. Obster Gynecol Surv 1994;49:56–63.
166. Campbell OM, Gray RH. Characteristics and determinants of postpartum ovarian function in women in the United States. Am J Obstet Gynecol 1993;169:55–60.
167. Dewey KG, Heinig MJ, Nommsen LA. Maternal weight-loss patterns during prolonged lactation. Am J Clin Nutr 1993;58:162–166.
168. Ohlin A, Rossner S. Maternal body weight development after pregnancy. Int J Obes 1990;15:159–173.
169. Greene GW, Smiciklas-Weight H, School TO, et al. Postpartum weight change: How much of the weight gained in pregnancy will be lost after delivery? Obstet Gynecol 1988;71:701–717.
170. Rookus MA, Rokebrand P, Burema J, et al. The effect of pregnancy on the body mass index 9 months postpartum in 49 women. Int J Obes 1987;11:609–618.
171. Potter S, Hannum S, McFarlin B, et al. Does infant feeding method influence maternal weight loss? J Am Diet Assoc 1991;91:441–446.

172. Dugdale AE, Eaton-Evans J. The effect of lactation and other factors on post-partum changes in body-weight and triceps skinfold thickness. Br J Nutr 1989;61:149–153.
173. Manning-Dalton C, Allen LH. The effects of lactation on energy and protein consumption, postpartum weight change and body composition of well nourished North American women. Nutr Res 1983;3:293–308.
174. Kent GN, Price RI, Gutteridge DH, et al. Human lactation: forearm trabecular bone loss, increased bone turnover, and renal conservation of calcium and inorganic phosphate with recovery of bone mass following weaning. J Bone Min Res 1990;5:361–369.
175. Lamke B, Brundin J, Moberg P. Changes in bone mineral content during pregnancy and lactation. Acta Obstet Gynecol Scand 1977;56:217–219.
176. Specker BL, Tsang RC, Ho ML. Changes in calcium homeostasis over the first year postpartum: effect of lactation and weaning. Obstet Gynecol 1991;78:56–62.
177. Sowers MF, Corton G, Shapiro B, et al. Changes in bone density with lactation. JAMA 1993;269:3130–3135.
178. Aloia JF, Cohn SH, Vaswani A, et al. Risk factors for postmenopausal osteoporosis. Am J Med 1985;78:95–100.
179. Feldblum PJ, Zhang J, Rich LE, et al. Lactation history and bone mineral density among perimenopausal women. Epidemiology 1992;3:527–531.
180. Kreiger N, Kelsey JL, Holford TR, et al. An epidemiologic study of hip fracture in postmenopausal women. Epidemiology 1982;116:141–148.
181. Cumming RG, Klineberg RJ. Breast-feeding and other reproductive factors and the risk of hip fracture in elderly women. Int J Epidemiol 1993;2:684–691.
182. Bauer DC, Browner WS, Cauley JA, et al. Factors associated with appendicular bone mass in older women. Ann Intern Med 1993;118:657–665.
183. Fox KM, Magaziner J, Sherwin R, et al. Reproductive correlates of bone mass in elderly women. J Bone Miner Res 1993;8:901–908.
184. Kritz-Silverstein D, Barett-Connor E, Hollenbach KA. Pregnancy and lactation as determinants of bone mineral density in postmenopausal women. Am J Epidemiol 1992;136:1052–1059.
185. Byers TS, Graham S, Rzepka T, et al. Lactation and breast cancer: evidence for a negative association in premenopausal women. Am J Epidemiol 1985;121:664–674.
186. Layde PM, Webster LA, Baughman AL, et al. The independent associations of parity, age at first full term pregnancy, and duration of breast-feeding with the risk of breast cancer. Cancer and Steroid Hormone Study Group. J Clin Epidemiol 1989;42:963–973.
187. McTiernan A, Thomas DB. Evidence for a protective effect of lactation on risk of breast cancer in young women: results from a case control study. Am J Epidemiol 1986; 124:353–358.
188. Yoo K, Tajima K, Kuroishi T, et al. Independent protective effect of lactation against breast cancer: a case control study in Japan. Am J Epidemiol 1992;135:726–733.
189. Newcomb PA, Storer BE, Longnecker MP, et al. Lactation and a reduced risk of premenopausal breast cancer. N Engl J Med 1994;330:81–87.
190. Kvale G, Heuch I. Lactation and cancer risk: Is there a relation specific to breast cancer? J Epidemiol Community Health 1987;42:30–37.
191. Wynder EL, MacCornack FA, Stellman SD. The epidemiology of breast cancer in 785 United States Caucasian women. Cancer 1978;41:2341–2354.
192. Brinton LA, Hoover R, Fraumeni JF. Reproductive factors in the aetiology of breast cancer. Br J Cancer 1983;47:757–762.
193. London SJ, Colditz GA, Stampfer MJ, et al. Lactation and risk of breast cancer in a cohort of US women. Am J Epidemiol 1990;132:17–26.
194. Siskind V, Schofield F, Rice D, et al. Breast cancer and breast-feeding: results from an Australian case-control study. Am J Epidemiol 1989;130:229–236.
195. Thomas DB, Noonan EA. Breast cancer and prolonged lactation. The WHO Collaborative Study of Neoplasia and Steroid Contraceptives. Int J Epidemiol 1993;22:619–626.
196. Lawrence RA. Early discharge alert. Pediatrics 1995;96:966–967.
197. Neifert M. Early assessment of the breast-feeding infant. Contemp Pediatr 1996;13(10):142–166.
198. Powers NG, Naylor AJ, Wester RA. Hospital policies: crucial to breast-feeding success. Semin Perinatol 1994;18:517–524.
199. World Health Organization, UNICEF, Protecting, promoting, and supporting breastfeeding: the special role of maternity services. Geneva, Switzerland: World Health Organization, 1989.
200. UNICEF. Innocenti declaration on the protection, promotion, and support of breast-feeding. New York: UNICEF, Nutrition Cluster (H-8F), 1990.
201. UNICEF. Take the Baby-Friendly Hospital Initiative! A global effort with hospitals, health services, and parents to breast-feed babies for the best start in life. New York: UNICEF, 1991.
202. Wright A, Rice S, Wells S. Changing hospital practices to increase the duration of breast-feeding. Pediatr 1996;97:669–675.
203. DeCarvalho M, Hall M, Harvey D. Effects of water supplementation on physiological jaundice in breast-fed babies. Arch Dis Child 1981;56:568–569.
204. Bachrach S, Fisher J, Parks JS. An outbreak of vitamin D deficiency rickets in a susceptible population. Pediatrics 1979;64:871–877.
205. Roberts CC, Chan GM, Folland D, et al. Adequate bone mineralization in breast-fed infants. J Pediatr 1981;99:192–196.
206. U.S. Department of Health Education and Welfare. National Center For Health Statistics (NCHS) growth curves for children, birth–18 years. Publication No. (PHS) 78-1650. Washington, DC: DHEW, 1977.
207. Ahn CH, MacLean WC. Growth of the exclusively breast-fed infant. Am J Clin Nutr 1980;33:183–192.
208. Dewey KG, Heinig MJ, Nommsen LA, et al. Growth of breast-fed and formula-fed infants from 0 to 18 months: the DARLING study. Pediatrics 1992;89:1035–1041.
209. Nelson SE, Rogers RR, Ziegler EE, et al. Gain in weight and length during early infancy. Early Hum Dev 1989; 19:223–239.

210. Salmenpera L, Perheentupa J, Siimes MA. Exclusively breast-fed healthy infants grow slower than reference infants. Pediatr Res 1985;19:307–312.
211. Whitehead RG, Paul AA, Cole TJ. Diet and the growth of healthy infants. J Hum Nutr Diet 1989;2:73–84.
212. Heinig MJ, Nommsen LA, Peerson JM, et al. Intake and growth of breast-fed and formula-fed infants in relation to the timing of introduction of complementary foods: the DARLING study. Acta Paediatr 1993;82:999–1006.
213. De Curtis M, Brooke OG. Energy and nitrogen balances in very low birthweight infants. Arch Dis Child 1987;62:830–832.
214. Brooke OG, Onubogu O, Heath R, et al. Human milk and preterm formula compared for effects on growth and metabolism. Arch Dis Child 1987;62:917–923.
215. Kashyap S, Schulze KF, Forsyth M, et al. Growth, nutrient retention, and metabolic response of low-birth-weight infants fed supplemented and unsupplemented preterm human milk. Am J Clin Nutr 1990;52:254–262.
216. Cooper PA, Rothberg AD, Pettifor JM, et al. Growth and biochemical response of premature infants fed pooled preterm milk or special formula. J Pediatr Gastroenterol Nutr 1984;3:749–754.
217. Gross SJ. Growth and biochemical response of preterm infants fed human milk or modified infant formula. N Engl J Med 1983;308:237–241.
218. Atkinson SA, Bryan MH, Anderson GH. Human milk feeding in premature infants: protein, fat and carbohydrate balances in the first two weeks of life. J Pediatr 1981;99:617–624.
219. Schanler RJ, Oh W. Nitrogen and mineral balance in preterm infants fed human milks or formula. J Pediatr Gastroenterol Nutr 1985;4:214–219.
220. Bates CJ, Liu DS, Fuller NJ, et al. Susceptibility of riboflavin and vitamin A in breast milk to photodegradation and its implications for the use of banked breast milk in infant feeding. Acta Paediatr Scand 1985;74:40–44.
221. Rowe JC, Wood DH, Rowe DW, et al. Nutritional hypophosphatemic rickets in a premature infant fed breast milk. N Engl J Med 1979;300:293–296.
222. Atkinson SA, Radde IC, Anderson GH. Macromineral balances in premature infants fed their own mothers' milk or formula. J Pediatr 1983;102:99–106.
223. Raiha NCR, Heinonen K, Rassin DK, et al. Milk protein quantity and quality in low-birth-weight infants. I. Metabolic responses and effects on growth. Pediatrics 1976;57:659–674.
224. Ronnholm KAR, Sipila I, Siimes MA. Human milk protein supplementation for the prevention of hypoproteinemia without metabolic imbalance in breast milk-fed, very low birth weight infants. J Pediatr 1982;101:243–247.
225. Polberger SKT, Axelsson IE, Räihä NCR. Urinary and serum urea as indicators of protein metabolism in very low birthweight infants fed varying human milk protein intakes. Acta Paediatr Scand 1990;79:737–742.
226. Roy RN, Chance GW, Radde IC, et al. Late hyponatremia in very low birthweight infants. Pediatr Res 1976:526–531.
227. Kumar SP, Sacks LM. Hyponatremia in very low-birthweight infants and human milk feedings. J Pediatr 1978;93:1026–1027.
228. Schanler RJ. Calcium and phosphorus absorption and retention in preterm infants. Exp Med 1991;2:24–36.
229. Ziegler EE, O'Donnell AM, Nelson SE, et al. Body composition of the reference fetus. Growth 1976;40:329–341.
230. American Academy of Pediatrics, Committee on Nutrition. Nutritional needs of low-birth-weight infants. Pediatrics 1985;75:976–986.
231. Koo WWK, Sherman R, Succop P, et al. Sequential bone mineral content in small preterm infants with and without fractures and rickets. J Bone Miner Res 1988;3:193–197.
232. Pettifor JM, Stein H, Herman A. Mineral homeostasis in very low birth weight infants fed either own mother's milk or pooled pasteurized preterm milk. J Pediatr Gastroenterol Nutr 1986;5:248–253.
233. Lucas A, Brooke OG, Baker BA, et al. High alkaline phosphatase activity and growth in preterm neonates. Arch Dis Child 1989;64:902–909.
234. Senterre J, Putet G, Salle B, et al. Effects of vitamin D and phosphorus supplementation on calcium retention in preterm infants fed banked human milk. J Pediatr 1983;103:305–307.
235. Heinonen K, Mononen I, Mononen T, et al. Plasma vitamin C levels are low in premature infants fed human milk. Am J Clin Nutr 1986;43:923–924.
236. Stein H, Cohen D, Herman AAB. Pooled pasteurized breast milk and untreated own mother's milk in the feeding of very low birth weight babies: a randomized controlled trial. J Pediatr Gastroenterol Nutr 1986;5:242–247.
237. Garza C. Banked human milk for very low birth weight infants. In: Atkinson SA, Hanson LA, Chandra RK, eds. Breast-feeding, nutrition, infection and infant growth in developed and emerging countries. St. John's, Newfoundland, Canada: ARTS Biomedical, 1990:25–34.
238. Bhatia J, Rassin DK. Human milk supplementation: delivery of energy, calcium, phosphorus, magnesium, copper and zinc. Am J Dis Child 1988;142:445–447.
239. Hall B. Uniformity of human milk. Am J Clin Nutr 1979;32:304–312.
240. Moro GE, Fulconis F, Minoli I, et al. Growth and plasma amino acid concentrations in very low birthweight infants fed either human milk, protein fortified human milk or whey-predominant formula. Acta Paediatr Scand 1989;78:18–22.
241. Polberger SKT, Axelsson IA, Raiha NCR. Growth of very low birth weight infants on varying amounts of human milk protein. Pediatr Res 1989;25:414–419.
242. Ronnholm KAR, Perheentupa J, Siimes MA. Supplementation with human milk protein improves growth of small premature infants fed human milk. Pediatrics 1986;77:649–653.
243. Putet G, Rigo J, Salle B, et al. Supplementation of pooled human milk with casein hydrolysate: energy and nitrogen balance and weight gain composition in very low birth weight infants. Pediatr Res 1987;21:458–461.
244. Schanler RJ, Garza C. Improved mineral balance in very low birth weight infants fed fortified human milk. J Pediatr 1987;112:452–456.
245. Greer FR, McCormick A. Improved bone mineralization and growth in premature infants fed fortified own mother's milk. J Pediatr 1988;112:961–969.

246. Ehrenkranz RA, Gettner PA, Nelli CM. Nutrient balance studies in premature infants fed premature formula or fortified preterm human milk. J Pediatr Gastroenterol Nutr 1989;8:58–67.
247. Schanler RJ, Abrams SA. Postnatal attainment of intrauterine macromineral accretion rates in low birth weight infants fed fortified human milk. J Pediatr 1995;126:441–447.
248. Schanler RJ, Burns PA, Abrams SA, et al. Bone mineralization outcomes in human milk-fed preterm infants. Pediatr Res 1992;31:583–586.
249. Rifka MG, Schanler RJ. Can we meet intrauterine calcium (Ca) and phosphorus (P) accretion rates by feeding very low birth weight infants (VLBWI) fortified human milk? Pediatr Res 1994;35:319A.
250. Arnold LDW. Recommendations for collection, storage, and handling of a mother's milk for her own infant in the hospital setting. West Hartford, CT: Human Milk Banking Association of North America, 1993.
251. Zinaman MJ, Hughes V, Queenan JT, et al. Acute prolactin and oxytocin responses and milk yield to infant suckling and artificial methods of expression in lactating women. Pediatrics 1992;89:437–440.
252. Auerbach KG. Sequential and simultaneous breast pumping: a comparison. Int J Nurs Stud 1990;27:257–265.
253. Lefebvre F, Ducharme M. Incidence and duration of lactation and lactational performance among mothers of low-birth-weight and term infants. Can Med Assoc J 1989;140:1159–1164.
254. DeCarvalho M, Robertson S, Friedman A, et al. Effect of frequent breast-feeding on early milk production and infant weight gain. Pediatrics 1983;72:307–311.
255. Miles MS. Parents of critically ill premature infants: sources of stress. Crit Care Nurs Q 1989:69–74.
256. Cross BA. Neurohormonal mechanisms in emotional inhibition of milk ejection. J Endocrinol 1977;41:193–210.
257. Whitelaw A, Sleath K. Myth of the marsupial mother: home care of very low birthweight babies in Bogota, Colombia. Lancet 1985;2:1206–1209.
258. DeLeeuw R, Colin EM, Dunnebier EA, et al. Physiological effects of kangaroo care in very small preterm infants. Biol Neonate 1991;59:149–155.
259. Wahlberg V. Alternative care for premature infants. The "kangaroo method." Advantages, risks, and ethical questions. Neonatologica 1987;4:362–367.
260. Acolet D, Sleath K, Whitelaw A. Oxygenation, heart rate and temperature in very low birth infants during skin-to-skin contact with their mothers. Acta Paediatr Scand 1989;78:189–193.
261. Hurst NM, Valentine CJ, Renfro L, et al. The effect of skin-to-skin holding of low birth weight infants (<1500 gm) on maternal milk volume. Pediatr Res 1995;37:309A.
262. McCormick DB. Water-soluble vitamins: bases for suggested upper limits for infant formulas. J Nutr 1989;119:1818–1819.
263. Coward WA. Measuring milk intake in breast-fed babies. J Pediatr Gastroenterol Nutr 1984;3:275–279.
264. American Academy of Pediatrics, Committee on Nutrition. Zinc. Pediatrics 1978;62:408–412.
265. Blanc B. Biochemical aspects of human milk—comparison with bovine milk. World Rev Nutr Diet 1981;36:1–89.
266. Dallman PR. Nutritional anemia in infancy: iron, folic acid, and vitamin B_{12}. In: Tsang RC, Nichols BL, eds. Nutrition during infancy. Philadelphia: Hanley & Belfus, 1988:216–235.
267. Schanler RJ. Water soluble vitamins: C, B_1, B_2, B_6, niacin, biotin, and pantothenic acid. In: Tsang RC, Nichols BL, eds. Nutrition during infancy. Philadelphia: Hanley & Belfus, 1988:236–252.
268. Newman V. Vitamin A and breast-feeding: a comparison of data from developed and developing countries. Food Nutr Bull 1994;15:161–176.

53
Evaluation of the Neonate with a Potential Metabolic Defect

Pinar T. Ozand

The significant metabolic transition that the neonate experiences in the first few days after birth, makes him particularly vulnerable to the manifestation of a disease of intermediary metabolism. Such disorders as propionic acidemia,[1] methylmalonic acidemia,[2] the urea cycle diseases,[3] fructose-1,6-diphosphatase deficiency,[4] and galactosemia (PGal transferase deficiency)[5] may lead to severe symptomatology within 2 to 3 days of the neonatal period. Severe forms of fatty acid oxidation[6] and respiratory chain diseases disorders[7] appear immediately after birth and may cause morbidity while the neonatologist is attempting to make a diagnosis. To make matters worse, cell-mediated immunodeficiency associated with some of these disorders may cause early neonatal bronchopneumonia or sepsis, confusing the clinician who, while treating the infection, misses the underlying metabolic disease, resulting in a neurologically crippled infant. Many of these diseases cause enough alterations in the acid-base balance, glucose, and ammonia homeostasis that a rapid metabolic workup is necessary to diagnose and appropriately treat the neonate before irreversible damage occurs.

The mode of inheritance of most of these diseases is autosomal recessive. In many instances, a careful family history reveals the death of a previous neonate or a young infant due to a similar disease. When there is consanguinity, the history of the extended family reveals the presence of relatives with infants with the same disease. At times the disease is confined to certain communities or tribes, such as the high incidence of maple syrup urine disease (MSUD; or branched-chain amino acidemia) among the Mennonite population of North America[8] and 3-hydroxy-3-methylglutaryl coenzyme A (CoA) lyase deficiency in a certain tribe of Saudi Arabia,[9] both of which are due to a founder effect. If a diagnosis has already been confirmed in the previous sibling, it is usually safe to conclude the neonate has the same disorder. This concept greatly expedites the necessary studies and treatment. Detailed diagnostic studies must be conducted in any neonate with a suspected metabolic disease, even if it is a postmortem examination. This is of paramount importance not only for treatment of a subsequent sibling, but also for genetic counseling. Many of these diseases can be accurately diagnosed antenatally, either by biochemical or molecular genetic techniques. The parents should be aware that there is a 25% chance in every subsequent pregnancy of having a neonate with the same disease. They may request prenatal diagnosis and elect abortion of an affected fetus.

At times there may be a readily observable clinical symptom, such as an intrauterine growth defect that indicates an energy-deprived fetus such as the one with pyruvate dehydrogenase deficiency.[10] At other times there may be no clinical biochemical warning signs, and the neonate will remain a puzzle, until a diagnosis is reached by chance. A good example is the extreme neonatal hypotonia that may cause severe ventilation problems requiring respiratory support, as may be the case in a severe phenotype of 4-hydroxybutyric aciduria.[11]

In other neonates, an encephalopathic picture evolves after the initial metabolic transition is achieved. Such an infant is unable to maintain his or her own metabolism. A good example is MSUD, which usually manifests at 5 to 7 days of neonatal life,[12] since it takes about 4 to 5 days for the branched-chain amino acids to increase to a concentration that will cause acute brain edema,[13] brain stem lesions, and the unmistakable signs of a neurologic catastrophe.[14] Another good example is methylenetetrahydrofolate (Me-H_4-folate) reductase deficiency, where it takes approximately 1 week to deplete the methionine supply received from the mother, and apneic symptoms of the disease usually appear after 1 to 2 weeks.[15]

The fetus may be so compromised by the teratogenic effect of a disturbed biochemical function that he or she will be born with multisystemic developmental abnormalities, including dysmorphic features. Good examples of this are multiple acyl-CoA dehydrogenase deficiency (glutaric aciduria type 2; GAT-2),[16] and severe forms of peroxisomal diseases such as Zellweger syndrome.[17]

The fetus may be damaged due to the accumulation of a storage substance, causing nonimmune hydrops fetalis. If there is no hematologic or chromosomal abnormality underlying the hydrops, it is always wise to rule out a storage disease. A large number of lysosomal storage diseases are known to produce a neonate with anasarca, causing diagnostic confusion. Such diseases include Gaucher disease type 2,[18] G_{M1} gangliosidosis,[19] β-glucuronidase deficiency,[20] sialidosis,[21] galactosialidosis,[22] and severe forms of a lysosomal enzyme processing defect, "I cell" disease.[23]

This brief introduction confirms that the neonatologist must be thoroughly aware of the potential presence of an inborn error of metabolism in any neonate with unusual symptoms, and must initiate a reasonable workup to rule out such a condition. This is important for patients of any ethnic group, but particularly for those with heavy consanguinity or, if there is a positive family history, when the presence of an inborn error of metabolism in the neonate is to be anticipated.

Given these considerations, it is prudent to screen all neonates for potentially treatable inborn errors of metabolism (see Neonatal Screening, below). This is now feasible through tandem mass spectrometric (MS)-based techniques.[24,25] Medically it is of a higher priority to screen immediately for diseases that manifest within the first days of life, in preference to those diseases that cause damage some time later such as hyperphenylalaninemia [phenylketonuria (PKU)]. When such a screening program is not available, the responsibility is on the neonatologist who must be alert to the possibility of an early manifesting inborn error of metabolism. This chapter provides "decision trees" based on the clinical and biochemical presentation of this latter group of diseases.

Presentation of Neonatal Metabolic Diseases

A metabolic workup starts with the initial clinical observations. Although it is not always possible to provide clear demarcation lines, a convenient classification, which may be used at the bedside, is as follows:

1. A neonate with acute metabolic decompensation; devastating metabolic disease of the neonate. This group can be further subdivided:
   a. Neonates with manageable/treatable diseases.
   b. Neonates with primary lactic acidosis, which is not always treatable.
2. A neonate with primarily an encephalopathic presentation and stupor.
3. Teratogenic disorder in a neonate.
4. A neonate with features of a lysosomal storage disease.

Acute Metabolic Decompensation in a Neonate

Neonates with Manageable/Treatable Diseases

It is not unusual to encounter a neonate who is normal during the first few hours to few days of life, but rapidly evolves to a disease state with coma. Usually a prodrome of lethargy, refusal to feed, and vomiting progresses into full coma with symptoms suggesting severe global central nervous system (CNS) involvement. A neonate that cannot be aroused presents with altered muscle tone of central origin and seizures. The vomiting may be so severe that it may be mistaken for pyloric stenosis.[26,27] This symptom complex, known as devastating metabolic disease of the neonate, is a true pediatric emergency, and unless diagnosed and treated immediately, will cause death or severe neurologic crippling.[28] Diseases known to cause such an acute metabolic decompensation are listed in Table 53.1. They can be classified into organic acid disorders, primary lactic acidosis, amino acid disorders, and those carbohydrate diseases that may manifest neonatally. Certain fatty acid oxidation disorders as short-chain acyl-CoA dehydrogenase deficiency[29] and some amino acid disorders such as tyrosinemia type 1[30] rarely cause symptoms in early neonatal age. Some milder phenotypes of the listed organic acid and amino acid carbohydrate disorders and primary lactic acidosis may manifest first, during later infancy.[31] In the same family, one infant with isovaleric acidemia (IVA) may be symptomatic at 2 to 3 days, while the other sibling may not show an acute decompensation until 2 years of age. Hormonal diseases, such as congenital adrenal hyperplasia and hyperinsulinism, may lead to a picture that may be confused with the devastating metabolic disease of the neonate.

In some of these diseases, there are useful clinical clues that may help the neonatologist (as noted in Table 53.2). Most patients with propionic acidemia and methylmalonic acidemia have a depressed nasal bridge and abnormalities of the philtrum, indicating prenatal onset of these diseases (Figures 53.1 and 53.2).

In addition, the time of the appearance of symptoms provides another valuable clinical clue. The severe phenotypes of fatty acid oxidation disorders,[6] multiple carboxylase deficiency,[32] 3-hydroxy-3-methylglutaryl-CoA lyase deficiency,[9] and severe forms of primary lactic acidosis,[33] including 3-methylglutaconic aciduria,[34] usually produce severe symptoms before the first 24 hours of life. While the hyperammonemic symptoms of ornithine transcarbamylase[35] and carbamylphosphate synthetase

TABLE 53.1. Diseases that are known to cause acute metabolic decompensation during the first 2 weeks of life.

Various organic acidemias	Primary lactic acidosis	Amino acid disorders	Carbohydrate disorders
Propionic acidemia	Pyruvate dehydrogenase deficiency	Maple syrup urine disease (MSUD)	Fructose-1-6-diphosphatase deficiency
Methylmalonic acidemia	Pyruvate carboxylase deficiency	Carbamylphosphate synthetase deficiency	Fructose-1-phosphate aldolase deficiency
Isovaleric acidemia	Complex I deficiency	Ornithine transcarbamylase deficiency	Galactosemia (P Gal transferase deficiency)
3-hydroxy-3-methylglutaryl-CoA lyase deficiency	Complex IV deficiency	Citrullinemia (argininosuccinate synthetase deficiency)	
Multiple carboxylase deficiency due to deficiency of holocarboxylase synthetase	3-Methylglutaconic aciduria	Argininosuccinic aciduria (argininosuccinate lyase deficiency)	
3-Methylcrotonyl-CoA carboxylase deficiency		Tyrosinemia type 1 (rare in neonate)	
Short-chain acyl-CoA dehydrogenase deficiency (rare in neonate)			
Medium-chain acyl-CoA dehydrogenase deficiency			
Long-chain acyl-CoA dehydrogenase deficiency			
3-Hydroxy-long-chain acyl-CoA dehydrogenase deficiency			
Carnitine/acyl carnitine translocase deficiency			
Multiple acyl-CoA dehydrogenase deficiency (type 2 glutaric aciduria)			
Pyroglutamic aciduria (5-oxoprolinuria)			

deficiencies[36] usually appear at 24 to 48 hours, citrullinemia (argininosuccinic acid synthetase [ASA-S] deficiency)[37] and argininosuccinic aciduria (ASAuria; ASA-lyase [ASA-L] deficiency)[38] present at 48 to 72 hours, and MSUD usually at 5 to 7 days. Severe phenotypes of propionic acidemia, methylmalonic acidemia, and isovaleric acidemia may first cause acute acidosis at 2 to 3 days of age. Galactosemia may first appear with *Escherichia coli* sepsis before hypoglycemia is suspected.[39] The hypoglycemia of fructose-1,6-diphosphatase deficiency rarely manifests in a neonate, unless the baby is kept fasting.[40]

Routine Laboratory Tests

Unfortunately, the clinical symptoms and their time of appearance are not specific, and unless laboratory tests are used, a correct diagnosis may not be reached.

A rapid laboratory investigation of the cause of the acute metabolic decompensation must be immediately initiated. These tests include clinical biochemical studies, followed by more specialized biochemical tests. The routine tests that must be secured in a neonate with acute decompensation are listed in Table 53.3.

Pathophysiology

The severe CNS symptoms (e.g., seizures, stupor, coma, tone changes, etc.) accompanying the acute event indicates severe involvement of the cerebral gray matter and in certain disorders, such as MSUD, of the brain globally.[41] This may be due primarily to the inhibition of pathways involved in energy production by the accumulating toxic metabolites or brain edema caused by excessive glutamine accumulation in the brain due to hyperammonemia.[42] It may be due secondarily to severe systemic acidosis or hypoglycemia, decreasing energy production in the CNS.

Neonates with Primary Lactic Acidosis

A significant percentage of patients with acute metabolic decompensation have a primary or congenital lactic acidosis due to the defects of pyruvate metabolism or of

TABLE 53.2. Some alerting physical signs in a neonate with devastating metabolic disease of the newborn.

Disease	Clinical sign
Propionic acidemia	"Organic acid face"; nipple anomalies, usually severe central hypotonia; sepsis with *Candida* or gram-negative organisms
Methylmalonic acidemia	"Organic acid face"; increased or unchanged muscle tone
Isovaleric acidemia	Increased or unchanged muscle tone; "sweaty feet" smell
3-Hydroxy-3-methylglutaryl-CoA lyase deficiency	No distinguishing features; except almost invariably the acute metabolic decompensation occurs a few hours after the first feeding
Holocarboxylase synthetase and pyruvate carboxylase deficiencies	Central hypotonia is very severe; more severe than that seen in other diseases of the newborn period
MCAD (medium-chain acyl-CoA dehydrogenase deficiency)	Hydrops fetalis, congenital anomalies of the muscle, such as diaphragmatic abnormalities
Long-chain, 3-hydroxy-long-chain acyl-CoA dehydrogenase and translocase deficiencies	Severe and early cardiac failure with cardiomyopathy, hepatomegaly in a neonate who may have also myopathy, but otherwise looks normal
Glutaric aciduria type 2	In some patients facial dysmorphia with high forehead, low-set ears, hypoplastic mid-face, hypertelorism with rings under the eyes, as well as rocker-bottom feet, muscular defects of abdominal wall, anomalies of external genitalia including hypospadias and chordee
Pyruvate dehydrogenase deficiency	Intrauterine growth retarded neonate (always; even if the neonate is only a symptomatic heterozygote) with epicanthic folds, hepatomegaly, and severe hypotonia; features of an infant with fetal alcohol syndrome
3-Methylglutaconic aciduria	Various dysmorphic features, undescended testicle, mild hepatomegaly, and stupor
MSUD	Alternating changes in muscle tone; severe early myoclonic eye movements; sweet burnt sugar or maple syrup smell in diaper, hair, under armpits, or ear wax; sepsis with gram-negative or positive organisms
Urea cycle diseases	Coma is earlier and deeper than others
Fructose-1,6-diphosphatase deficiency	Delayed feeding triggers the initial acute decompensation
Galactosemia	Cataracts, severe hepatomegaly, early sepsis
Nesidioblastosis	Growth parameters >90%

the respiratory chain.[43] Although no reliable frequency can be stated,[28,44,45] this syndrome accounts for 10% to 25% of all instances of acute metabolic decompensation in the neonate. As the term primary lactic acidosis implies, there are few, if any, clinical or rapid biochemical tests available to identify its etiology without resorting to specific tests. There are five important diseases that cause severe primary lactic acidosis in the neonate: two are related to the metabolism of pyruvate—deficiency of pyruvate dehydrogenase complex[46] and deficiency of pyruvate carboxylase;[47] two others are respiratory chain diseases; deficiency of complex I[48] and IV (cytochrome oxidase).[49] Although it is not proven, the neonatal form of 3-methylglutaconic the fifth one is another aciduria, one is another less important cause of primary lactic acidosis. It is probably caused by a yet unknown defect in mitochondrial oxidation.[34,50] This group of diseases is invariably lethal, causing death by 4 to 5 months of age. Diseases with primary lactic acidosis have only experimental therapies. Their diagnosis is usually made for purposes of genetic counseling or for academic interest, with the hope that a novel treatment procedure may become available in the future, for application at the time of delivery.

Primary lactic acidosis manifests with severe encephalopathy and its symptoms are not specific. These symptoms occur early, and they are severe and difficult to correct: metabolic acidosis with stupor or coma, grunting respirations, and seizures in a severely hypotonic newborn.[51] Systemic manifestations in association with encephalopathy, such as acute liver derangement, renal involvement, and cardiomyopathy, are encountered in complex IV deficiency,[52] and less commonly in complex I deficiency,[53] and 3-methylglutaconic aciduria.[50]

A neonate with the deficiency of pyruvate dehydrogenase (PDH) may show dysmorphic features, signifying

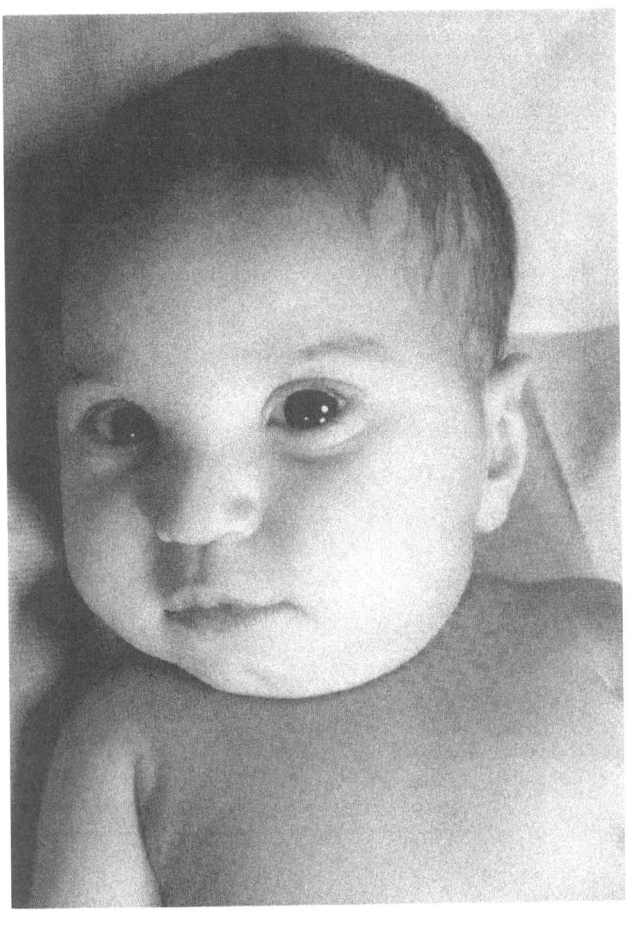

FIGURE 53.1. Facial photo of a young infant with propionic acidemia.

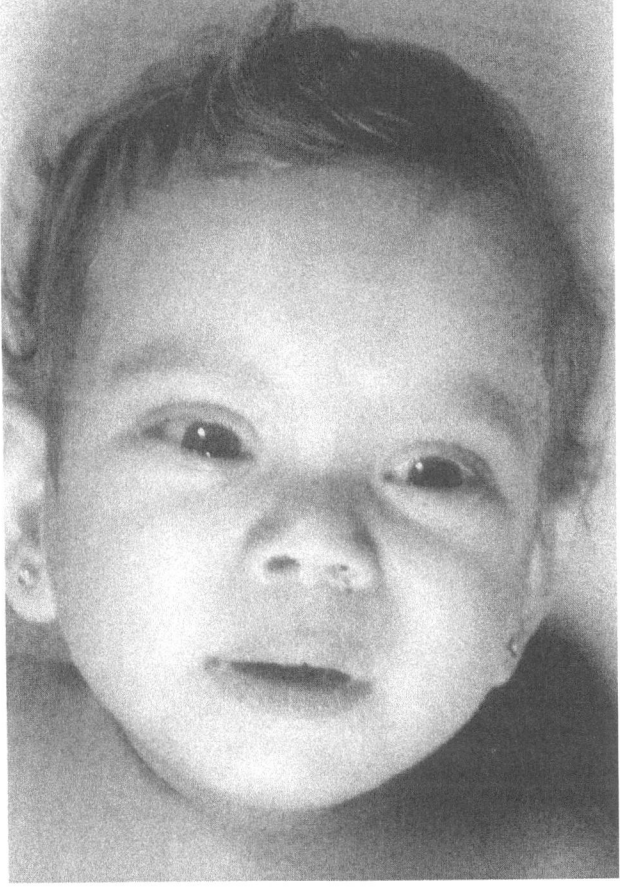

FIGURE 53.2. Facial photo of a young infant with methylmalonic acidemia.

the prenatal onset of the effects of this deficiency (Figure 53.3).[54] The facial features resemble those seen in fetal alcohol syndrome.[10] In fact both disorders may share a common etiology, and fetal alcohol syndrome is probably caused by the inhibition of PDH by the acetaldehyde produced from ethanol. Less subtle dysmorphic changes are seen in the patient with complex IV deficiency and 3-methylglutaconic aciduria.[50] No dysmorphic features have been described in the patient with complex I and pyruvate carboxylase deficiencies.

Routine Laboratory Tests

The recommended tests are listed in Table 53.3; in this instance the ratio of lactate/pyruvate, and 3-hydroxybutyrate/acetoacetate in blood are most helpful.[55-59]

Pathophysiology

The brain depends on a high rate of aerobic glycolysis. It is estimated that the brain in a normal neonate oxidizes 125 g glucose a day.[60,61] The rate-limiting step in aerobic glycolysis in the brain is the PDH reaction, which is subject to many diverse metabolic controls. Fully active PDH in brain can oxidize a maximum of 180 g of glucose a day, which does not leave much room for a compensatory mechanism when there is a deficiency of PDH.[60,61] Since PDH activity is a rate-limiting step in the aerobic oxidation of glucose in brain, when PDH or respiratory chain enzymes are deficient, the level of lactate in CSF increases over that in the blood, resulting in so-called cerebral lactic acidosis.[62] It is interesting to note that the symptoms of severe Menkes' disease in a neonate is an encephalopathy similar to that seen in complex IV deficiency, except there is no lactic acidosis. In this instance the deficiency of cerebral copper leads to the deficient activities of copper-heme proteins and of cytochrome c oxidase, which are copper-dependent activities.[63]

Since the majority of mitochondrial proteins are encoded in the nuclear genome, most cases of primary lactic acidosis are caused by abnormalities in nuclear genes. The mutational events leading to deficiencies of PDH[64-66] and pyruvate carboxylase have been detailed.[67] Those mutations in mitochondrial (mt)-DNA, are usually asso-

TABLE 53.3. Routine laboratory tests for a neonate suspected of having a metabolic disease.

Routine blood tests	Blood tests for primary lactic acidosis		Indicates
	Lactate/pyruvate (normal 10–25)	3-Hydroxybutyrate/ acetoacetate ratio (normal 2–5)	
pH, base excess, p_{CO_2}*			
Ammonia*			
Glucose*			
Lactate and pyruvate*			
3-Hydroxybutyrate and acetoacetate*	Normal or low	No or minimal postprandial ketosis	Pyruvate dehydrogenase deficiency
Red blood cell, leukocyte and platelet counts*			
Liver enzymes	Elevated (>30)	Normal or low postprandial value	Pyruvate carboxylase deficiency
Creatine kinase			
Lactic dehydrogenase (muscle and liver types)	Elevated (>30)	Elevated (>5)	Respiratory chain diseases
Prothrombin time and PTT			
Red blood cell and plasma folate			
Uric acid			
Cholesterol	Tests for lysosomal storage disorders:		
	Blood tests:		
	Peripheral blood film for vacuolated lymphocytes and metachromatic granules		
Routine urine tests	Bone marrow biopsy for storage cells		
Reducing substance			
Ferricyanide test	Urine tests:		
Sulfite screening test	urine screen for mucopolysacchariduria		
2,4-dinitrophenylhydrazine (DNPH) screening test			

*Changes in these parameters are presented in detail in Table 53.7.

ciated clinically with later-onset diseases of infancy. The molecular genetics of PDH deficiency have been studied extensively. The enzyme contains three subunits: E_1, which in turn contains two subunits $E_{1\alpha}$ and $E_{1\beta}$, E_2, and E_3. The PDH complex is activated by a specific PDH phosphatase and inactivated by a PDH phosphokinase.[68] The gene of the $E_{1\alpha}$ subunit is on chromosome X, and the chromosomal locations of other subunits have also been established.[69,70] The E_2 requires protein X for its catalytic function. Although mutations for almost all of these subunits have been described,[71,72] most patients with PDH deficiency have mutations in $E_{1\alpha}$.[73,74]

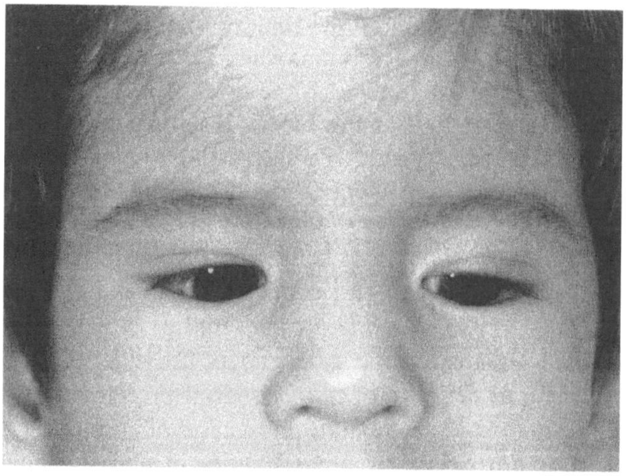

Significance of Initial Chemical Measurements

In many instances, the routine laboratory tests secured initially will help the pediatrician reach a preliminary diagnosis.

Measurement of Acid-Base Balance

The measurement of changes in blood pH is the most essential initial step in the workup. It is a universally recommended procedure to document the blood pH and base excess. The diseases that cause acute metabolic decompensation can be classified into two groups: those that cause acidosis, and those that lead to respiratory alkalosis (Table 53.4). Most of the organic acidemias are associated with a decrease in blood pH. The three major organic acidemias of the neonate—propionic acidemia,[75] methylmalonic acidemia,[76] and isovaleric acidemia[77]—all cause significant ketosis. They may show some lactic acidosis, but the drop in blood pH is due to the mobilization

FIGURE 53.3. Facial features of an infant with pyruvate dehydrogenase deficiency.

TABLE 53.4. Differential diagnosis of changes in blood acid-base balance in a neonate with acute metabolic decompensation.

Metabolic acidosis[a] (organic acidemia)			Respiratory alkalosis (urea cycle disorders)		
Mainly ketosis	Mainly lactic acidosis	Mixed keto-lactic acidosis	Blood lactic acid normal	Blood lactic acid; mildly to moderately high	Mild or no changes
Methylmalonic acidemia	3-Hydroxy-3-methylglutaryl-CoA lyase deficiency	Multiple carboxylase deficiency due to holocarboxylase synthetase deficiency	Carbamylphosphate synthetase deficiency	Citrullinemia (argininosuccinate synthetase deficiency)	Maple syrup urine disease
Propionic acidemia	Pyruvate dehydrogenase deficiency	3-Methylcrotonyl-CoA carboxylase deficiency	Ornithine transcarbamylase deficiency	Argininosuccinic aciduria (argininosuccinate lyase deficiency)	
Isovaleric acidemia	Pyruvate carboxylase deficiency	Fructose-1,6-diphosphatase deficiency			
	3-Methylglutaconic aciduria				
	Respiratory chain diseases				
	Fatty acid oxidation disorders[b]				

[a] Pyroglutamic aciduria causes periodic acidosis without lactic acidosis or ketosis but with hemolytic anemia.
[b] During severe acute metabolic decompensation and shock.

of ketone bodies. The neonatal form of multiple carboxylase deficiency,[78–80] and at times 3-methylglutaconic aciduria,[34,50] respiratory chain diseases,[81] and fructose-1,6-diphosphatase[82] deficiencies, may show mixed keto-lactic acidosis. Others like fatty acid oxidation disorders, 3-hydroxy-3-methylglutaryl-CoA lyase,[9] pyruvate dehydrogenase,[61] multiple acyl-CoA dehydrogenase,[6] and pyruvate carboxylase[83] deficiencies, cause mainly lactic acidosis with only mild to absent ketosis. The only organic acidemia of the neonate that causes acidosis with no associated lactic acidemia or ketosis is 5-oxoprolinuria (pyroglutamic aciduria).[84]

The diseases of the urea cycle are almost always associated with respiratory alkalosis.[85] Hypoventilation is a common finding in pyruvate dehydrogenase deficiency.[86] In patients with citrullinemia and argininosuccinic aciduria the moderately large negative base excess (BE) is due to the associated lactic acidemia and may confuse the clinician.[87] The crisis of MSUD in the neonate is almost never associated with hypoglycemia or with a disturbed acid-base balance;[88] when a mild acidosis is present in such a neonate, it is due to mild ketonemia.

Pathopysiology

The acute encephalopathy caused by the organic acidemias has been explained by the relative deficiency of CoA, trapped intracellularly as the organic acid-CoA ester, leading to the deficiency of free reduced coenzyme A (CoASH).[88,89] Free carnitine is rapidly depleted by the excessively generated acyl-CoA esters that are transacetylated into acylcarnitines.[90] The rationale for the therapeutic use of L-carnitine, as well as the diagnosis of an organic acidemia through either low blood free carnitine or elevated acylcarnitines by tandem MS, depend on these observations.[90,91]

Both methylmalonyl-CoA and propionyl-CoA inhibit transmitochondrial shuttle of malate and pyruvate carboxylase, leading to decreased gluconeogenesis, hypoglycemia, and lactic acidosis, and indirectly to ketosis.[88–92] Both compounds, particularly propionyl-CoA, inhibit glycine cleaving enzyme, leading to hyperglycinemia.[94,95] The acute CNS symptoms of these organic acidemias probably represent a combined effect of acidosis, hypoglycemia, and hyperammonemia, leading to depressed brain utilization of glucose and to the toxic effect of intracerebrally accumulating glycine. In the patient with respiratory chain diseases such as complex IV deficiency, the brain and other organ systems are deprived of energy, which is the cause of encephalopathy and derangement of the liver.[49,52,60,62]

The following case histories for two patients illustrate the sequence of presenting symptoms and laboratory workup used for diagnosis.

Case History: Methylmalonic Acidemia

This male neonate was the product of normal pregnancy and delivery with normal 1- and 5-minute Apgar scores. He developed lethargy at 48 hours of life, with tachypnea.

He had a grade 2/6 systolic murmur at the left upper sternal border. His liver edge was firm and was 3 cm below the right costal margin. The parents were first cousins, and this was the first child of the family. The neonate's primitive reflexes were diminished, with poor sucking, and the muscle tone was increased. The initial laboratory workup indicated pH of 7.19 with a BE of −16; lactate 6 mM, ammonia 333 μM, normoglycemia, and urine ketones 2+. A preliminary diagnosis of an organic acidemia was made. A blood sample sent for tandem MS revealed within hours elevated propionylcarnitine with a ratio of C_3-/C_2-carnitine of 1.7 (normal is 0.4), and low free carnitine 6 μM (normal >20 μM). Blood glycine by tandem MS was only borderline elevated. A subsequent urine sample sent for gas chromatography GC/MS studies revealed increased 3-hydroxypropionic, methylmalonic, and methylcitric acids. These findings confirmed that the neonate had methylmalonic acidemia (MMA). Echocardiographic studies indicated a cribriform ventricular septal defect (VSD), and patent ductus arteriosus (PDA). The computed tomography (CT) of the brain indicated decreased attenuation of central white matter. The electroencephalogram (EEG), visual evoked potentials (VEP), and brain stem auditory evoked potentials (BAEP) were not remarkable. The patient was transferred to our service at 72 hours of age, and was given IV carnitine 50 mg·kg^{-1} 6 hourly^{-1} IM, 1 mg hydroxycobalamin daily, and the appropriate amount of bicarbonate, glucose, and fluids 1500 ml·m^{-1}, for 3 days. His ammonia and acid-base balance were normal within 18 hours. He could be started on MMA formula at 6 days of age, and was discharged at 10 days as a healthy baby on MMA formula, oral carnitine (200 mg·kg^{-1} day^{-1}), polycitra 5 ml·kg^{-1} day^{-1}, digoxin 15 μg bid, and Lasix 2 mg bid. His PDA closed spontaneously while in the hospital, and the VSD closed at 4 months of age, with cardiac medications soon discontinued after discharge. He did not have a second metabolic decompensation during the next 2 years. His growth was parallel to normal growth lines. The complementation studies by geneticist Dr. W. Fenton of Yale University showed the patient had cobalamin A (cbl A) mutation. Two years later, a brother was born; he was found to have MMA by selective screening through tandem MS and by urine studies through GC/MS. He was immediately placed on treatment with IV glucose and IV carnitine, and did not have acute metabolic decompensation neonatally or later in life.

Case History: Propionic Acidemia

This female neonate was one of twins born to a first cousin marriage. Her twin brother was and remained normal. She developed lethargy, poor sucking, and vomiting at the age of 7 days, and was admitted to the hospital. She was found to be extremely floppy, with absent neonatal reflexes, and to have normoglycemia, mild acidosis, pH 7.27, BE −11, with lactic acid 4 mM, ammonia 230 μM, and urine ketones 2+. A blood sample revealed elevated propionylcarnitine C_3-/C_2-carnitine of 2.5 (normal <0.4), glycine 520 μM (normal <400 μM), and free carnitine of 12 μM (normal >20 μM) by tandem MS. A presumptive diagnosis of PA was made, and the baby was transferred to the service at the age of 10 days. On admission her platelets were 50,000/mm^3, and WBC 3100/mm^3. The platelets further decreased to 30,000/mm^3 within 24 hours and she had to be given a platelet transfusion. She received appropriate amount of glucose and bicarbonate with IV carnitine (50 mg·kg^{-1} 6 hourly^{-1}) for the next 3 days. The GC/MS studies indicated highly elevated 3-hydroxypropionic acid, propionylglycine, and 3-methylcitric acid, and the putative clinical diagnosis of propionic acidemia (PA) was confirmed. She was started on PA formula and oral medications at 12 days of age. However, her sucking was not adequate and she had to receive nasogastric (NG) tube feeding for the next 2 weeks. Her CT brain revealed diffuse central white matter disease, interpreted as cerebral edema. Her video-EEG was markedly abnormal due to continuous electrical and clinical seizure activity. Her clinical myoclonic seizures were controlled by phenobarbital. She was discharged on oral carnitine (200 mg·kg^{-1} d^{-1}), polycitra 5 ml·kg^{-1} d^{-1}, and PA formula. She started to develop, albeit slowly, but her tone and deep tendon reflexes remained diminished. A repeat magnetic resonance imaging (MRI) of the brain at 4 months of age indicated better myelination and resolution of the brain edema. A positron emission tomography (PET) scan of the brain with ^{19}fluoro-2-deoxyglucose (F-2-DG) at 5 months of age, indicated mildly decreased glucose uptake diffusely, particularly marked at the frontal lobes, and an intense small area of uptake in the right frontal cortex interpreted as a focus for her seizures. Putaminal glucose uptake was mildly reduced, with asymmetric uptake of glucose at the heads of the caudate, the right less than the left. Further clinical course was complicated by chronic vomiting and frequent bronchopneumonia due to aspiration, which required repeated hospitalizations. At 18 months she was still severely hypotonic, spoke little, and could sit independently but could not walk.

Case History: Maple Syrup Urine Disease

The acute encephalopathy caused by MSUD is due to the toxic effect of elevated concentrations of branched-chain amino acids (BCAA), particularly of leucine, leading to acute generalized brain edema,[14,96] including brain stem involvement, and subsequent clinical symptoms of apnea, opisthotonus, seizures, and tone changes. The MRI of the brain of a neonate with MSUD shows severe edema in the central white matter, cerebellum, and brain stem

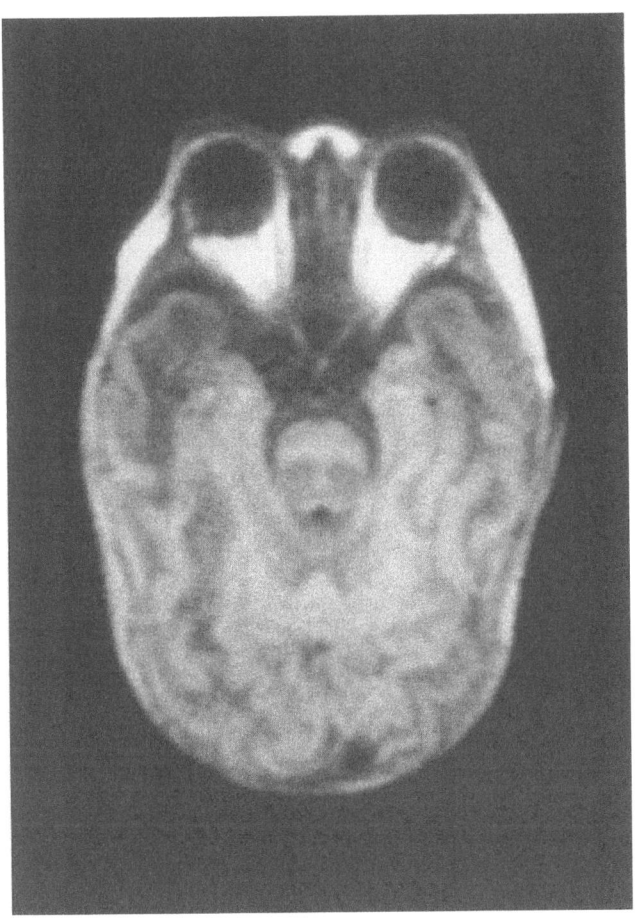

FIGURE 53.4. MRI of the brain of a neonate with maple syrup urine disease, showing severe edema of central white matter, and cerebral peduncle.

(Figure 53.4). This neuroradiologic appearance is so characteristic that an experienced radiologist will immediately diagnose MSUD. An illustrative case history follows:

This female neonate was referred at 38 days of age with an already-diagnosed MSUD. The mother was 16 years old, she was gravida 4, para 3, living 2. The parents, who were first cousins, had already lost a male infant to the same disease at 1 month of age. The female infant had normal Apgar scores but was small for gestational age. At home she developed refusal to feed, irritability, and lethargy at 10 days. She was suspected to have sepsis, query metabolic disease, and was admitted to the neonatal ICU (NICU) of the referral hospital. Her blood gases, pH, glucose, lactic acid, and ammonia were normal. She was placed on IV fluids with dextrose, and a blood and urine sample revealed leucine 2.3 mM (normal <0.12 mM), isoleucine 0.6 mM (normal <0.1 mM), and valine 0.8 mM (normal <0.33 mM). Urine GC/MS showed greatly elevated branched-chain α-keto acids (BCKA). The diagnosis of MSUD was made. Instructions for the management and MSUD formula were sent to the referring hospital, and she was transferred 3 weeks later, at the age of 38 days, for a comprehensive workup. At the time of admission she was lethargic, with severe midline hypotonia and bilateral ankle clonus. She were found to have bilateral optic atrophy. The EEG revealed bilateral independent spikes; VEP (visual evoked potentials) indicated prolonged latency of the first wave; although amplitudes were considered to be normal, the shape of the potentials was abnormal, containing several components. The BAEP (brain auditory evoked potentials) indicated normal latency for peaks 1 and 5, but pronounced latency of peak 3. The MRI of the brain indicated severe edema in the cerebral and cerebellar hemispheres, with involvement of cerebral peduncles and pons. She was kept on treatment with MSUD formula and was discharged 10 days later with blood leucine of 0.61, isoleucine 0.29, and valine 0.2 mM. Valine was supplemented to the formula at $30\,mg \cdot kg^{-1} \cdot day^{-1}$ since she showed perineal dermatitis.

She was next admitted at 9 months of age for severe, perineal rash, failure to thrive (4.1 kg), and some spasticity. She had good visual pursuit, she could roll from side to side, and spoke a few words. The background of her EEG was well developed but she had photic activated right occipital focus of discharge. She was given valine and isoleucine supplements, and antibiotic plus steroid ointment for her dermatitis. She improved within a week and was discharged. She had no major complaint for the next 2 years.

At the age of 3 years she was admitted for the workup of seizures and bronchopneumonia. She had hypotonia, increased deep tendon reflexes, and bilateral ankle clonus. The cerebrospinal fluid (CSF) and blood workup were not remarkable, and no organism grew from these sources. The blood leucine on admission was 0.9, isoleucine 0.3, and valine 0.4 mM. Despite a history of grandmal seizures, the EEG was found to be nearly normal; it had improved as compared to the previous study at 2 years of age. The psychometric evaluation revealed borderline global developmental delay. Since then she has had several seizures, despite treatment with phenobarbital and adequate blood levels of the drug. She was admitted once for mild ataxia that the father had noted, and the MRI of the brain revealed moderate cerebellar involvement. At present she is 7 years old, and her last psychometric assessment indicated normal cognitive function, with mildly delayed language skills; however, she has marked motor clumsiness and attention deficit disorder. She has very mild ataxia. Her blood branched-chain amino acids (BCAA) have remained within normal limits for the past 3 years. She is a lovely girl attending regular school.

Measurement of Blood Ammonia

Another valuable laboratory analysis is the determination of blood ammonia. Blood ammonia is elevated both in organic acidemias and urea cycle disorders.[26,97] The accumulating organic acids and their coenzyme A esters inhibit the intramitochondrial carbamylphosphate synthetase (CPS-1) and the synthesis of its activator N-acetylglutamate (NAG).[98] Therefore, hyperammonemia is also a feature observed in organic acid disorders, including severe phenotypes of PDH deficiency.

Three major organic acidemias of the neonate—propionic acidemia, methylmalonic acidemia, and isovaleric acidemia—cause significant hyperammonemia, usually >300μM, during the initial acute metabolic crisis,[99–101] while during repeated episodes later in infancy, the hyperammonemia caused by these disorders is usually mild.[102] The hyperammonemia caused by urea cycle disorders is usually precipitous and rapidly exceeds 1000μM if not treated. Differential diagnosis in a hyperammonemic infant is listed in Table 53.5.

Pathophysiology

Hyperammonemia in urea cycle disorders (UCD), and in conjunction with acidosis and hypoglycemia in organic acidemias, is the main cause of the acute encephalopathy in a neonate.[103–107] Hyperammonemia is associated with increased intracranial pressure,[105–107] brain edema, and in severe cases, such as a UCD, respiratory alkalosis. The brain edema is a consequence of astrocyte swelling probably secondary to the osmotic effect of increased glutamine synthesis due to hyperammonemia and its accumulation in these cells.[42,108] The severe brain edema in a patient with missed diagnosis of citrullinemia is shown in Figure 53.5. In experimental animals, brain edema

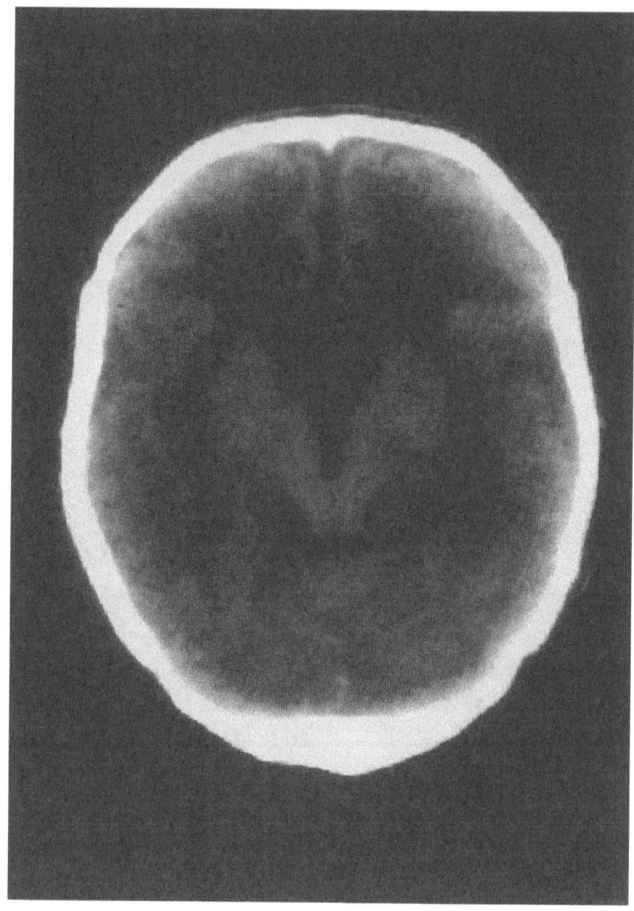

FIGURE 53.5. Severe brain edema in CT brain of a patient with citrullinemia whose diagnosis was missed for 1 week.

TABLE 53.5. Differential diagnosis of hyperammonemia in a newborn with acute metabolic decompensation.

Hyperammonemia with acidosis	Hyperammonemia with respiratory alkalosis or normal gases
Propionic acidemia	Carbamylphosphate synthetase deficiency
Methylmalonic acidemia	Ornithine transcarbamylase deficiency
Isovaleric acidemia	Citrullinemia (argininosuccinate synthetase deficiency)
3-Hydroxy-3-methylglutaryl-CoA lyase deficiency	Argininosuccinic aciduria (argininosuccinate lyase deficiency)
Holocarboxylase synthetase deficiency	
3-Methylcrotonyl-CoA carboxylase deficiency	
Pyruvate dehydrogenase deficiency (severe phenotype)	

caused by hyperammonemia can be prevented when glutamine synthetase is inhibited with methionine sulfoximine.[109–111] During the hyperammonemic coma, the CSF concentration of glutamine, e.g., in ornithine transcarbamylase deficiency[112] or in argininosuccinic aciduria,[113] is extraordinarily high, usually to 10- to 15-fold higher than normal. The MRI spectroscopy of the brain in patients with ornithine transcarbamylase deficiency has confirmed the increased glutamine accumulation in CNS.[114]

The case histories of two patients with two different types of urea cycle disorder follow.

Case History: Citrullinemia

This female neonate was discharged from the referral hospital at 3 days of age with the diagnosis of pulmonary stenosis. She developed lethargy, progressing to coma on day 4, and developed hypoxia. These symptoms were attributed to the cardiac disease and she remained in the coma until 7 days, at which time she was transferred. On admission she was in deep coma, with absent neonatal reflexes, and with an oxygen saturation of 50%. A metabolic workup revealed blood pH 7.513 with a BE of −1.5, and blood ammonia value of 1080 μM (normal for age <95 μM). An emergency tandem MS revealed blood citrulline to be >2 mM (normal is 50 μM). She was immediately placed on peritoneal dialysis, since no hemodialysis was available; she was given a bolus of IV L-arginine 600 mg·kg^{-1}, and was placed on IV L-arginine 600 mg·kg^{-1}day^{-1} and ucephan 500 mg·kg^{-1}day^{-1} (a mixture of sodium benzoate and phenylacetate 250 mg·kg^{-1}day^{-1} each) given in four equal doses. Her blood ammonia decreased to 207 μM in less than 24 hours. During the next 2 days the blood pyruvate and lactate levels varied between 128 and 216 μM (normal <80 μM) and 5.9 to 7.4 mM (normal <2 mM), respectively. A urine GC/MS study indicated massive excretion of orotic acid. An EEG on admission revealed severe intermittent background discontinuity, and multifocal EEG seizures. A CT of the brain indicated massive brain edema. At 2 weeks of age she was stabilized and a balloon dilatation with valvulostomy was achieved successfully, reducing the ventriculopulmonary arterial gradient. She developed coagulase positive *Staphylococcus aureus* sepsis at the third week, with disseminated intravascular coagulopathy (DIC). She required ventilatory support for 2 weeks, with adequate antibiotic coverage and fresh frozen plasma. She developed seizures, which were controlled by clonazepam and phenobarbital. During this period she received total parenteral nutrition (TPN) with only 0.7 to 0.9 g·kg^{-1}day^{-1} amino acid mixture and lipids. The daily ammonia concentration, after the initial episode, never exceeded 60 μM. She gradually could be taken off the respirator, and her clinical condition could be stabilized. She could not suck and had to be fed the UCD formula, L-arginine, and ucephan through an NG tube. A repeat CT brain revealed lessening of the cerebral edema with dilated ventricles. At 2 months of age she was showing fluctuating consciousness, occasionally opening her eyes and blinking, with some spontaneous movement of her extremities; however, she could not fix her gaze. Her condition has improved slowly. At 3 months she started to vocalize and smile. At 1 year of age she has severe spastic quadriplegia, and can say one or two words. She has a difficult to control seizure disorder.

Case History: Argininosuccinic Aciduria or ASA-lyase Deficiency

This female neonate was born in our nursery and was the product of normal pregnancy and delivery with Apgar scores of 8 and 9 at 1 and 5 minutes, respectively. Her birth weight, height, head circumference, physical examination, and neonatal reflexes were all within normal limits. The family history was interesting: The parents were first cousins. The mother, a Bedouin, was 35 years old, gravida 13, term 11, para 1, abortion 0, and living 7. She described the disease and the death of her four previous neonates succinctly as: "They would get sick with refusal to feed, sleeping, and unresponsive on the third sun rise, and they would be dead on the third sundown." The neonate's blood tandem MS at 24 hours revealed trace, and at 48 hours significant ASA. The blood citrulline value was five times normal and urine contained moderate orotic aciduria. At this point a blood ammonia was found to be 287 μM. Her blood pH and gases remained normal. She was immediately given a bolus of L-arginine, 600 mg·kg^{-1}, and placed on IV L-arginine at 600 mg·kg^{-1}day^{-1} for 48 hours. She was also placed on ucephan and UCD formula. Her blood ammonia became <60 μM in 12 hours. She never got sick, and was discharged home in 2 days, on oral L-arginine, ucephan, and UCD formula (1 g·kg^{-1}day^{-1}), and milk (1 g·kg^{-1}day^{-1} milk protein). At outpatient visits at 2, 3, and 4 months of age, she was normal except for mild spasticity, and some difficulty in fixing her gaze, but with normal neonatal reflexes. Ucephan therapy was discontinued. At 1 year of age she was normal, and started to walk and speak. At present she is 2 years old and totally normal.

Measurement of Blood Glucose

Blood glucose may be normal or mildly decreased in a number of organic acidemias and in amino acid disorders.[88] However, in a large group of organic acidemias it may be significantly low. The pediatrician must first be sure that the low concentration of blood glucose is correct. If the blood sample is left at room temperature for a long while without separating the red blood cells from serum or plasma, before it is sent to the laboratory, or if it is collected on trichloroacetic acid, which inhibits the glucose oxidase reaction even when neutralized, falsely low blood glucose results will be obtained.

Severe hypoglycemia is the presenting symptom in fatty acid oxidation disorders,[115] such as medium-chain acyl-CoA dehydrogenase,[116] long-chain acyl-CoA dehydrogenase,[117] 3-hydroxy-long-chain acyl-CoA dehydrogenase,[118] carnitine/acylcarnitine translocase,[119] and multiple acyl-CoA dehydrogenase[120] deficiencies. In 3-hydroxy-3-methylglutaryl-CoA lyase deficiency, during acute metabolic decompensation the hypoglycemia will be severe (glycemia usually <9 mg·dl^{-1}) with lactic acidosis often exceeding 15 mM.[9] Holocarboxylase synthetase deficiency may be associated with normal or mild hypoglycemia.[121] The hypoglycemia of fatty acid oxidation disorders is usually associated with absent or trace ketones in the urine.[115-117] Unfortunately, hypoketotic hypoglycemia is encountered in the hyperinsulinism states of the newborn, such as nesidioblastosis. Frequently, the height and weight of neonates with

TABLE 53.6. Differential diagnosis of hypoglycemia in a neonate with acute metabolic decompensation.

Hypoglycemia with ketoacidosis	Hypoglycemia with lactic acidosis	Hypoglycemia with keto-lactic acidosis	Hypoglycemia and absent ketosis[a]	Hypoglycemia with liver failure/ hepatomegaly
Propionic acidemia	3-Hydroxy-3-methylglutaryl-CoA lyase deficiency	Holocarboxylase synthetase deficiency	Medium-chain fatty acyl-CoA dehydrogenase deficiency	Galactosemia
Methylmalonic acidemia	Pyruvate carboxylase deficiency (mild and late)	3-Methylcrotonyl-CoA carboxylase deficiency	Long-chain and very long-chain fatty acyl-CoA dehydrogenase deficiency	Tyrosinemia type 1
Isovaleric acidemia		Short-chain fatty acyl-CoA dehydrogenase deficiency	3-Hydroxy-fatty acyl-CoA dehydrogenase deficiency	Fructose-1-phosphate aldolase deficiency
		Fructose-1,6-diphosphatase deficiency	Carnitine/acylcarnitine translocase deficiency	
			Multiple acyl-CoA dehydrogenase deficiency (glutaric aciduria type 2)	
			Nesidioblastosis Adrenal insufficiency	

[a] Fatty acid oxidation disorders may be associated with mild to moderate lactic acidosis, particularly if the patient is in shock.

nesidioblastosis is above 90%; the occurrence of hypoglycemia is unpredictable, often occurring in the fed state, and responding rapidly to glucagon injection.[122] The clinical features may nevertheless be confusing, and in all neonates with hypoketotic hypoglycemia a specialized workup to rule out a fatty acid oxidation disorder must be ordered. In such neonates, a urine GC/MS and blood tandem MS studies must be routinely secured. Serial measurements of blood insulin, particularly while the infant is hypoglycemic, or pancreatic venous sampling for insulin concentration,[123] must be obtained to rule out hyperinsulinism. Adrenal insufficiencies of all types should be considered in the neonate with hypoglycemia, particularly if there is severe dehydration, shock, and hyponatremia. A differential diagnosis of hypoglycemia is listed in Table 53.6.

It must be emphasized that MSUD in a neonate does not cause hypoglycemia or acidosis. The MSUD crisis in a neonate is not accompanied by significant changes in routine clinical biochemical tests, while acute metabolic decompensation of MSUD that occurs at 6 months or later is almost always associated with mild to moderate hypoglycemia and ketosis.[12,88]

Summary

In Table 53.7 a decision tree for various clinical laboratory tests is summarized. These tests are available at most health care centers; the neonatologist can reach a preliminary diagnosis using these guidelines promptly initiating treatment while waiting for the final correct diagnosis.

Specialized Biochemical Studies

More specialized biochemical tests must be immediately ordered to confirm the preliminary diagnosis. Such special tests include organic acid studies by GC/MS in the

TABLE 53.7. Clinical and laboratory findings in a neonate with acute decompensating metabolic disease.

Disease	Blood pH	Lactic acidemia	Blood ammonia	Blood glucose	Keto-nuria	Hematologic findings	Blood culture	Miscellaneous findings
Propionic acidemia	Acidosis	Mild to moderate	Moderate elevation	Normal to mild hypoglycemia	2–3+	Mild neutropenia; severe thrombocytopenia	Usually +; Candida or unusual Gram (−) or (+) organisms	
Methylmalonic acidemia	Acidosis	Mild to moderate	Moderate elevation	Normal to mild hypoglycemia	2–3+	Mild neutropenia, thrombocytopenia	Rare, when present usually Gram (+)	
Isovaleric acidemia	Acidosis	Usually normal	Moderate elevation	Normal to mild hypoglycemia	2–3+	Moderate to severe thrombocytopenia	Usually Gram (−) or (+) organisms	"Sweaty feet" smell of urine and diaper
3-Hydroxy-3-methyl-glutaryl-CoA lyase deficiency	Acidosis	Severe, usually >15 mM	Mild elevation	Hypoglycemia usually < 1 mM during crisis	Absent	Normal	Usually sterile	Mildly elevated liver enzymes as ALT and AST

53. Evaluation of the Neonate with a Potential Metabolic Defect

TABLE 53.7. Continued.

Disease	Blood pH	Lactic acidemia	Blood ammonia	Blood glucose	Keto-nuria	Hematologic findings	Blood culture	Miscellaneous findings
Holocarboxylase synthetase and 3-methylcrotonyl-CoA carboxylase deficiency	Acidosis	Moderate to severe	Mild to moderate elevation	Moderate hypoglycemia	1–2+	Normal	Usually positive	
Medium-, long-chain acyl-CoA, 3-hydroxy-acyl-CoA dehydrogenase and carnitine / acylcarnitine translocase case deficiencies	Moderate acidosis (severe if there is peripheral shock)	Mild to moderate (severe if there is peripheral shock)	Usually normal	Severe hypoglycemia during crisis, mild to moderate hypoglycemia otherwise	Absent	Normal	Usually sterile	Elevated heart and muscle enzymes such as creatine kinase and heart and muscle-type lactic dehydrogenase
Multiple acyl-CoA dehydrogenase deficiency (glutaric aciduria 2)	Normal to mild acidosis	Mild to moderate	Usually normal	Severe hypoglycemia	Absent	Normal	Usually sterile	Mildly disturbed liver enzymes despite hepatomegaly
Pyruvate dehydrogenase deficiency	Acidosis	Severe (high in CSF)	May be elevated	Normal	Normal to trace	Normal	Usually sterile	Normal to low lactic acid/pyruvate ratio
Pyruvate carboxylase deficiency	Acidosis	Severe (high in CSF)	Normal	Normal or mild hypoglycemia	Mild+	Normal	Usually sterile	Elevated lactate/pyruvate ratio
Respiratory chain diseases	Acidosis	Severe (high in CSF)	Normal	Normal	2–3+	Normal	Usually sterile	Elevated lactate/pyruvate and 3-hydroxybutyrate/acetoacetate ratios
3-Methylglutaconic aciduria	Acidosis	Moderate when present	Normal	Severe hypoglycemia when present	Trace	Normal	Usually sterile	
Pyroglutamic aciduria (5-oxoprolinuria)	Acidosis	Absent	Normal	Normal	Absent	Hemolytic anemia reticulocytosis, low haptoglobins	Occasionally positive	Hemoglobinuria
Fructose-1, 6-diphosphatase deficiency	Acidosis	Severe	Normal	Severe hypoglycemia	2–3+	Normal	Usually sterile	Elevated ALT and AST during crisis
Maple syrup urine disease	Normal	Normal	Normal	Usually normal, at times mild hypoglycemia	Normal to trace	Normal	Usually positive with unusual Gram (+) and (–) organisms	"Maple syrup" smell in urine, diaper, armpits, hair, and cerumen
Carbamylphosphate synthetase and ornithine transcarbamylase deficiencies	Normal or respiratory alkalosis	Normal	Very high, exceeding 1000 μM by day 2–3	Normal	Normal	Normal	Occasionally positive	
Citrullinemia and argininosuccinic aciduria	Normal or respiratory alkalosis	During crisis: 4–6 mM	High and reaching 1000 μM by 4–5 days	Normal	Normal	Normal	Occasionally positive	
Galactosemia	Normal	Normal	Normal	Moderate to severe hypoglycemia	Normal	Normal	Almost always (+) usually E. Coli sepsis	Elevated ALT and AST; findings of renal Fanconi syndrome
Fructose-1-phosphate aldolase deficiency	Normal	Normal	Normal	Severe hypoglycemia	Normal	Normal	Usually sterile	Elevated ALT and AST; findings of renal Fanconi syndrome
Tyrosinemia-1 (when present in a neonate)	Normal	Normal	Normal	Mild hypoglycemia	Normal	Prolonged PT and PTT, thrombocytopenia	Usually sterile	Elevated bilirubin, mildly elevated ALT, AST, renal Fanconi syndrome

urine,[124] and amino acid measurements in the blood by chromatographic techniques.[125] Conventionally GC/MS studies are always performed in freshly collected urine,[124] which can be frozen until it reaches the diagnostic laboratory. High-pressure liquid chromatography (HPLC) is usually employed for amino acids.[125] It is always advisable to measure amino acids in the blood, unless a renal proximal tubular derangement is suspected.

Among disorders of carbohydrate metabolism, galactosemia may be diagnosed through measurement of the defective enzyme PGal transferase[126] in freshly collected red blood cells, or alternatively by measuring galactose in blood or urine by using specific enzymes for galactose such as galactose oxidase or galactose dehydrogenase.[127] Unless stored with correct preservatives such as dithiothreitol plus ethylenediaminetetraacetic acid (EDTA), blood samples show low PGal transferase activity even if they are stored frozen at $-70°C$. The disorders of fructose metabolism are best diagnosed by the measurement of specific enzymes in a liver biopsy,[128-132] as their measurement in lymphocytes[129] is not always reliable. An alternative approach is to give IV fructose,[133] 100 to $200 mg \cdot kg^{-1}$, and to follow the ensuing mild hypoglycemia and lactic acidosis over a period of 4 hours. In a patient with fructose-1,6-diphosphatase deficiency, mild hypoglycemia and mild lactic acidosis will appear by 90 to 120 minutes. Oral fructose loading is not advisable.

In patients with primary lactic acidosis, measurement of pyruvate dehydrogenase[134-137] and pyruvate carboxylase[138,139] are best performed in cultured fibroblasts or in a biopsy material. The complex I and IV are measured through direct determination of oxidation in mitochondria isolated from the biopsy material (e.g., liver or muscle).[140-143] The diagnosis of 3-methylglutaconic aciduria depends on the measurement of the compound in urine by GC/MS.[34,50]

In a busy laboratory the results of a routine GC/MS and HPLC amino acids are usually not available for 48 hours or more. Other special tests such as enzyme studies are even more time-consuming, and the results may not become available for 1 to 8 weeks.

The selection of blood or urine for analysis, or any of the aforementioned tests, depends on the easy access to the test within the center, as well as the type of disease suspected. Almost all disorders of amino acid metabolism require measurement of individual amino acids. The exceptions are deficiencies of carbamylphosphate synthetase (CPS) and ornithine transcarbamylase (OTC). In OTC deficiency, detection of orotic aciduria in the urine through GC/MS[144,145] is required to differentiate the disease from CPS deficiency in a male infant who has hyperammonemia.

As a rule, organic acid disorders are best diagnosed by the GC/MS studies in the urine. Some laboratories use urine GC/MS to identify MSUD through the increased excretion of branched-chain α-keto acids. This is advisable when E_3 deficiency, a variant of pyruvate dehydrogenase deficiency, is suspected because of a mildly elevated blood level of branched-chain amino acids. In addition to the branched-chain α-ketoaciduria, pathognomonic elevations of α-ketoglutaric aciduria and lactic aciduria indicate E_3 deficiency.[146,147]

The recent availability of tandem MS has facilitated the management of these diseases, since it provides a correct diagnosis within hours.[148] Most of the disorders listed in Table 53.1 require immediate intervention and management; therefore, tandem MS is a must for centers that encounter these disorders.

A summary of the results of these specialized tests is shown in Table 53.8. The urine GC/MS findings in certain fatty acid oxidation disorders, such as defects involving the oxidation of long-chain species, may be nonspecific and misleading, because long-chain fatty acid esters are preferentially excreted in the bile.[149] Tandem MS is the gold standard for the diagnosis of fatty acid oxidation diseases.[150]

Some problems occur with organic acid analyses. It is not possible to differentiate between ethylmalonic aciduria and short-chain acyl-CoA dehydrogenase deficiency, since both yield similar data in the urine GC/MS and tandem MS studies;[25] however, the clinical presentation of the diseases differ. Since no structural analysis is inherent in tandem MS, elevation of hydroxy-C5 carnitine can be seen not only in isovaleric acidemia, but also in β-ketothiolase and 3-hydroxy-3-methylglutaryl-CoA lyase deficiencies.[25] False elevations of C5 carnitine may be observed, albeit mild, if antibiotics that contain, or catabolize to yield, pivalic acid have been given to the mother. Krebs cycle intermediates in the urine,[151] particularly 2-ketoglutarate, are mainly encountered in diseases of respiratory chain,[152] glycogen storage disease type 1,[153] and fructose-1,6-diphosphatase[152] deficiency. In the United States and Europe, the common mutation of the medium-chain fatty acyl-CoA dehydrogenase deficiency may be used easily for molecular genetic study–based diagnosis since a single type of mutation accounts for approximately 90% of the cases.[154-158]

Tandem MS does not discriminate propionic acidemia (PA) from methylmalonic acidemia (MMA), which can be achieved only by urine GC/MS.[25] The clinical symptoms of these two disorders are somewhat different, and appropriate treatment is common to both diseases (i.e., IV carnitine, alkalinizing solutions, and the special PA diet). It may be given to the infant while waiting for the result of urine GC/MS studies.[25,26] In patients with MMA, complementation studies[159,160] or studies of urinary excretion of methylmalonic acid should be done before and after vitamin B_{12} therapy is undertaken,[161] since the management and prognosis of various complementation groups of MMA (e.g., vitamin B_{12}–responsive or –unresponsive

TABLE 53.8. Specialized biochemical tests required to confirm the diagnosis.

Disease	Urine organic acids by GC/MS studies	Blood amino acid studies	Blood tandem MS studies	Enzyme studies; special tests
Propionic acidemia	3-Hydroxypropionic acid, methylcitric acid, and propionylglycine	Glycine	Propionylcarnitine and glycine are high; free carnitine is low	Propionyl-CoA carboxylase in L and F
Methylmalonic acidemia	Same organic acids seen in propionic acidemia are high; methylmalonic aciduria is also present	Glycine may be borderline elevated	Same changes in carnitine and carnitine esters as in propionic acidemia	Complementation studies are required in F to find the Mut^0, Mut^-, cobalamin A and B types
Isovaleric acidemia	Isovaleric, 3- and 4- hydroxy isovaleric acids, isovalerylglycine	Glycine may be borderline elevated	C5-carnitine and hydroxy-C5 carnitine	Radioactive label release based enzyme assay in L and F
3-Hydroxy-3-methylglutaryl-CoA lyase deficiency	3-Hydroxy-3-methylglutaric, 3-methylglutaric, 3-methylglutaconic, 3-hydroxyisovaleric and lactic acids	N.H.	3-Methylglutarylcarnitine and hydroxy-C5 carnitine	3-hydroxy-3-methylglutaryl-CoA lyase assay in L and F
Holocarboxylase synthetase and 3-methylcrotonyl-CoA carboxylase deficiencies	3-Hydroxypropionic acid, 3-methylcrotonyl- and propionyl-glycine, methylcitric acid	N.H.	Propionylcarnitine, 3-methylcrotonylcarnitine, hydroxy-C5 carnitine	Assays for propionyl-CoA carboxylase, pyruvate and 3-methylcrotonyl-CoA carboxylase, holocarboxylase synthetase in L and F
Short-chain acyl-CoA dehydrogenase deficiency	Ethylmalonic, methylsuccinic acids	N.H.	C4- and C-5 carnitine esters	Enzyme assay in F
Medium-chain acyl-CoA dehydrogenase deficiency	Adipic, sebacic, suberic, 5-hydroxyhexanoic acid and hexanoylglycine	N.H.	C6:0, C8:0, C8-1, C10:0, and C10:1 carnitines	Enzyme assay in F; molecular genetic studies for $A_{985} \to G$ transition*
Long- and very long-chain acyl-CoA dehydrogenase deficiencies	C_6 to C_8 dicarboxylic acids	N.H.	5-cis C14:1 carnitine is pathognomonic, C16:0, C16:1, C18:1, C18:2 carnitine (blood and bile)	ETF-based or label release based activity are measured in F
3-Hydroxylong-chain acyl-CoA dehydrogenase assay	3-hydroxy-carboxylic aciduria of C_{14} to C_{16} chain length	N.H.	Hydroxy C14:0, C16:0 C18:1, C18:2 carnitines	Enzyme measurement with 3-ketoacyl substrates in F
Carnitine/acylcarnitine translocase deficiency	Not reported	N.H.	Very low free carnitine is pathognomonic; high C16:0, C18:0, C18:1 carnitine esters	Enzyme assay in F
Multiple acyl-CoA dehydrogenase deficiency (glutaric aciduria type 2)	Lactic, ethylmalonic, glutaric, 2-hydroxyglutaric, adipic, sebacic, suberic, C_{12}-dioic acids	N.H.	Carnitine esters observed in short-, medium-, and long-chain acyl-CoA dehydrogenase deficiencies and glutarylcarnitine	ETF and ETF-QO measurement, and label release assays in F
Pyruvate dehydrogenase deficiency	Lactic, pyruvic acids	Alanine	N.H.	Enzyme assay in F
Pyruvate carboxylase deficiency	Lactic, pyruvic acids	Alanine	N.H.	Enzyme assay in L and F
Respiratory chain diseases	Lactic, pyruvic and 2-oxoglutaric acids	Alanine	N.H.	Measurement of oxygen uptake in liver or muscle mitochondria
3-Methylglutaconic aciduria	3-methylglutaconic, 3 methylglutaric, 3-hydroxy-C5	N.H.	N.H.	Hydratase assay in F for hydratase deficiency
Pyroglutamic aciduria	Pyroglutamic acid	Glutathione absent in RBC	Pyroglutamic acid (blood and urine)	

TABLE 53.8. Continued.

Disease	Urine organic acids by GC/MS studies	Blood amino acid studies	Blood tandem MS studies	Enzyme studies; special tests
Maple syrup urine disease	2-keto branched chain acids	Leucine, isoleucine, valine	Leucine, isoleucine, valine	Enzyme assay in L and F
Carbamylphosphate synthetase deficiency	N.H., absent orotic acid	High glutamine and alanine; low citrulline	High glutamine and alanine	Enzyme measurement in liver biopsy
Ornithine transcarbamylase deficiency	Orotic acid	High glutamine and alanine; low citrulline	High glutamine and alanine	Increased orotic acid excretion following allopurinol load (for late onset forms and hemizygote females)
Citrullinemia	Lactic, orotic acids	Very high citrulline	Citrulline	
Argininosuccinic aciduria	Lactic, orotic	Argininosuccinic acid (urine)	Argininosuccinic acid in blood and urine	
Galactosemia	N.H.	Generalized aminoaciduria	N.H.	Enzyme assay in RBC
Fructose-1,6-diphosphatase deficiency	Lactic, 2-oxoglutaric acids	N.H.	N.H.	Cautious IV fructose loading (100–200 mg/kg/dose), enzyme assay in liver biopsy
Fructose-1-phosphate aldolase deficiency	N.H.	Generalized aminoaciduria	N.H.	Enzyme assay in liver biopsy
Tyrosinemia type 1	Succinylacetone and δ-aminolevulinic acid	Tyrosine and methionine	Tyrosine and methionine	Very high plasma α-fetoprotein

The indicated organic, amino acids, and carnitine esters are elevated. N.H., not helpful; F, cultured skin fibroblasts; L, leukocytes or lymphoblastic cell lines; C_N; the number indicates the length of the acyl group; $C_{N:0}$ or $C_{N:1}$ the number of double bonds in the fatty acyl-moiety; ETF and ETF-QO: electron transport flavoprotein and ETF-ubiquinone oxido-reductase.
* The indicated transition is the common mutation in U.S. and Europe.

phenotypes), or phenotypes in association with homocystinuria, are different.[162,163] The detection of methylcitric acid by GC/MS in urine[164] almost always indicates PA or MMA, even when other compounds characteristic of these diseases are low or absent. Tandem MS also does not differentiate between pipecolic[165] and pyroglutamic aciduria; when it is detected, the clinician has to use his/her judgment for diagnosis, which is not difficult, since the clinical symptoms of pyroglutamic aciduria is different from those of Zellweger syndrome.

Tandem MS does not differentiate between leucine and isoleucine, and once MSUD is detected, an HPLC amino acid determination technique must then be used to monitor the therapy. The concentrations of isoleucine and valine usually are reduced rapidly following the use of special MSUD formula, leading to a disturbed ratio of branched-chain amino acids, which is the cause of severe dermatitis, the so-called scalded skin syndrome (Figure 53.6).[166]

Orotic aciduria occurs not only in OTC deficiency but also, to a lesser degree, in citrullinemia (ASA-S deficiency) and argininosuccinic aciduria (ASA-L deficiency).[144,145] The degree of citrullinemia in ASA-S deficiency is much higher than that seen in ASA-L deficiency.[167] ASA has a high clearance rate[168,169] and it may be missed in HPLC-based amino acid analysis in blood. Tandem MS is the gold standard for the detection of ASD-L deficiency, since it can detect trace amounts of ASA in the blood specifically.[170] If the diagnosis of ASA-L deficiency is based on HPLC amino acid analysis, urine measurements for argininosuccinic acid is preferable.

Transient tyrosinemia is common in the neonate,[171] particularly among the premature.[172,173] Elevated tyrosine and methionine are common findings in a neonate with hepatitis,[174] and unless urine succinylacetone and δ-aminolevulinate are determined, tyrosinemia type 1 diagnosis must not be made.[175,176] Renal Fanconi syndrome may be seen not only in tyrosinemia type 1,[177] but also in galactosemia[178] and fructose-1-phosphate (F-1-P) aldolase deficiency.[179]

Finally, it is important to emphasize that the neonate may expire despite all attempts. It is imperative that se-

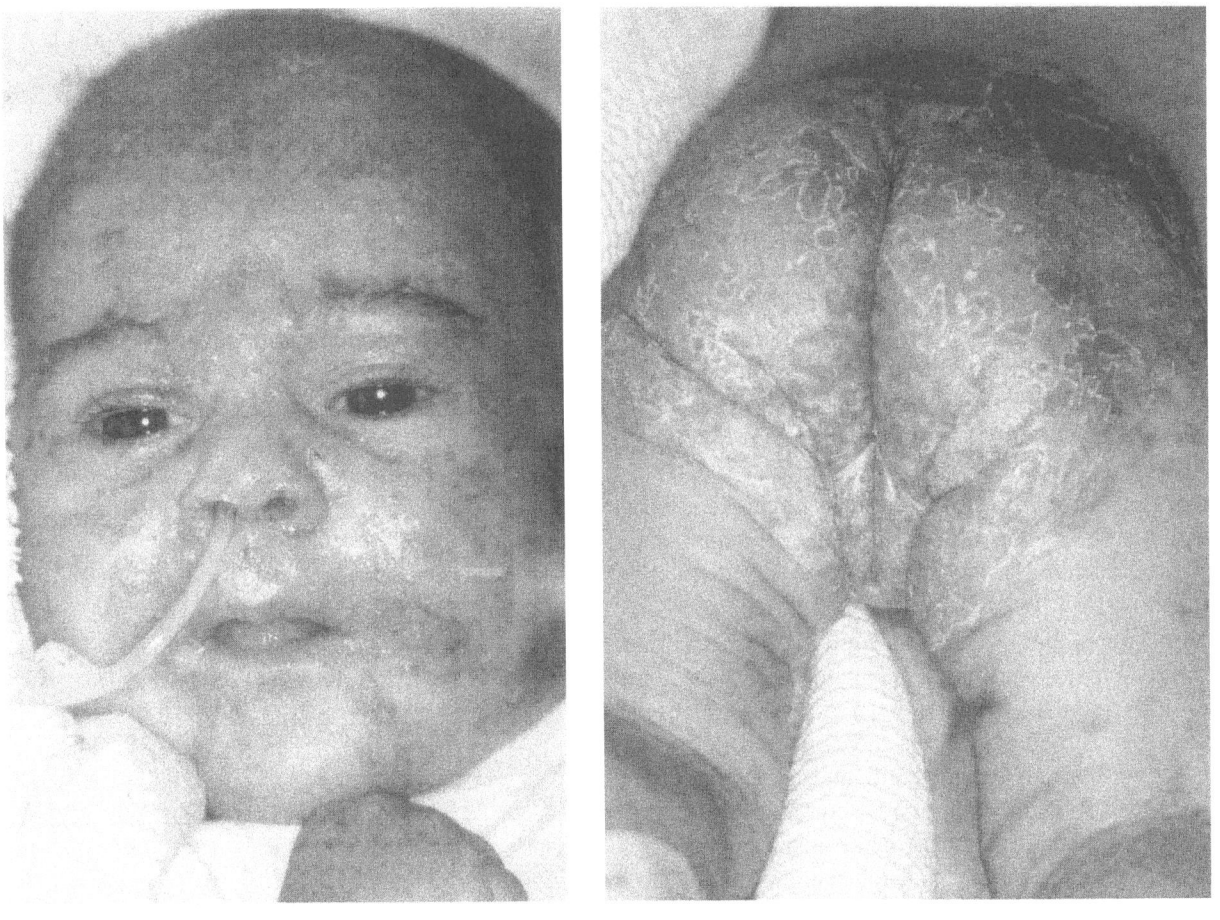

FIGURE 53.6. Scalded skin of a patient with maple syrup urine disease, whose valine and isoleucine values were reduced far below normal by diet given: (A) facial erythroderma; (B) appearance of buttocks.

rum, urine, and when possible CSF samples from such a neonate be kept frozen in a repository. Since a dried blood spot is the preferred matrix for tandem MS studies, several drops of blood should be dried on Guthrie paper and stored for future use. Diagnostic considerations may evolve after the demise of the neonate; it is also imperative that a living specimen, such as a fibroblast or lymphoblast culture, is secured and kept in a cell culture repository. Such material is indispensable for biochemical and molecular genetic studies at a later date. In our experience, successful fibroblast cultures can be established even 1 day after death if the body is kept cold.

Neonatal Screening

The idea of neonatal screening for potentially treatable diseases stemmed from the successful treatment of hyperphenylalaninemia (PKU) when diagnosed early in infancy. Worldwide, a large number of screening procedures and programs have been employed[180–186] to detect PKU,[187–189] galactosemia,[190,191] biotinidase deficiency,[192] MSUD,[193] cystic fibrosis,[194] hypothyroidism,[195] congenital adrenal hyperplasia,[196] glucose-6-phosphate dehydrogenase deficiency,[197] Duchenne muscular dystrophy,[198] peroxisomal disorders,[199] hemoglobin variants,[200] familial hypercholesterolemia,[201] and neuroblastoma.[202] An early diagnosis of some of these disorders prevents the disease and its complications, such as galactosemia, MSUD, biotinidase deficiency, hypothyroidism, and congenital adrenal hyperplasia. In some, a diagnosis within the first days of life is not very important, and can be delayed for a week or two with impunity, such as PKU and cystic fibrosis. In some others diagnosis does not require intervention, since the disease is not treatable but may have future potential treatments, such as Duchenne muscular dystrophy and peroxisomal diseases. Considering the cost factor involved in any screening program, it is best to concentrate efforts on the detection of diseases with significant cost/benefit ratio and with potential cure or benefit to the neonate.

The incidence of some organic and amino acid disorders has been studied in large populations of neonates in New England[186,203] and Quebec.[182] Such screening programs have been ongoing in the United Kingdom,[195] Denmark,[180] Australia,[194] France,[187-189] Germany,[184] and Sweden.[185] Fortunately, these disorders are not very common in North America and Europe. Worldwide figures for the incidence of some these disorders, e.g., biotinidase, is available.[192] In consanguineous communities, such as those in the Middle East, they are common diseases, and their frequency is at least two magnitudes higher.

While a large number of organic and amino acid disorders cause early neonatal disease requiring immediate diagnosis and management, a convenient comprehensive neonatal screening method for them has not been available until recently. The identification of these ever-increasing numbers of disorders that cause significant morbidity and mortality in the neonate required a novel technology. The introduction of tandem mass spectrometry for this purpose has been fortunate. This is a technique first developed by Millington et al.[204] It depends on separation, estimation, and identification based on molecular weight.[25] It bypasses a chromatographic preparative procedure that is time-consuming. The machine contains two mass spectrometers in tandem, separated by a collision chamber where molecules are fragmented. The first spectrometer separates and estimates molecules according to their molecular weight, and the second spectrometer identifies the compounds separated in the first mass spectrometer through fragments of specific molecular weights generated in the collision chamber. Each class of compound generates specific fragments with a specific molecular weight. Therefore, identification and measurement of different compounds within a given biochemical group can be achieved rapidly, within seconds. Tandem MS can also be programmed to measure components of different classes of compounds, for example, individual carnitine esters and amino acids, sequentially during the same analytic run.[148]

This technique has already been applied to the detection of a large number of metabolic diseases in two different screening programs, one in the United States[205] and another one in Saudi Arabia,[206,207] with rewarding results. It requires a minimal amount of blood or urine sample; a drop on the Guthrie paper usually is sufficient.[208] The sample can be sent to the central laboratory by mail. Except for the initial cost of purchasing the equipment, the operating cost is negligible; the chemicals required are inexpensive and technical support required is minimal. Tandem MS detects many diseases simultaneously. The analytical time is rapid, usually less than 2 minutes per sample, permitting the analysis of 600 to 800 samples per day, and the results become available in less than 24 hours. False-positive and false-negative results are rare.[148]

Although tandem MS detects 34 or more inborn errors of metabolism all at once, those diseases that are pertinent to the acute metabolic decompensation in a neonate are listed in Table 53.9. Comparative frequencies of these disorders as detected through tandem MS based within a selective and neonatal screening program in the United States[205] and Saudi Arabia[206,207] are presented in the same table. The gratifying results in the management of an early detected disease and the wide spectrum of treatable diseases that can be diagnosed rapidly make tandem MS technique a most valuable tool for neonatal medicine. An unexpected result of the tandem MS and molecular genetic investigation-based neonatal screening in the Pittsburgh area has been the detection of significant numbers of neonates and carriers with medium-chain acyl-CoA dehydrogenase deficiency.[209] The tandem MS from a patient with MSUD and from patients with medium-chain, long-chain, and 3-hydroxy-fatty acyl-CoA dehydrogenase deficiencies are shown together with normal tandem MS amino acid and carnitine profiles in Figures 53.7 and 53.8.

TABLE 53.9. Diseases that present in neonatal period that can be screened by the tandem MS technique.

Organic acidemias	Pittsburgh program ($n = 255,063$)	Saudi program ($n = 26,063$)
Propionic acidemia	2	42
Methylmalonic acidemia	1	46
Isovaleric acidemia	0	21
3-Hydroxy-3-methylglutaryl-CoA lyase deficiency	1	16
Multiple carboxylase deficiency (severe neonatal form)	0	15
Short-chain acyl-CoA dehydrogenase deficiency	0	10
Medium-chain acyl-CoA dehydrogenase deficiency	18	15
Long- or very long-chain acyl-CoA dehydrogenase deficiency	0	12
Carnitine/acylcarnitine translocase deficiency	0	4
Multiple acyl-CoA dehydrogenase deficiency (glutaric aciduria 2)	0	14
Pyroglutamic aciduria	0	4
Pipecolic aciduria	0	3
Amino acid disorders		
Maple syrup urine disease	2	30
Hypomethioninemia	0	1
Citrullinemia	0	7
Argininosuccinic aciduria	0	13
Nonketotic hyperglycinemia	0	12
Carbohydrate diseases		
Galactosemia*	No information	2*
Adrenal hyperplasia*	No information	No information

The numbers observed in the Pittsburgh[205] and Saudi[206] programs, combined for neonatal and selective screening, are compared. Both programs use tandem MS. The number of patients screened in each program is indicated (n); those diseases that don't have a tandem MS procedure but is detected by other techniques are indicated (*).

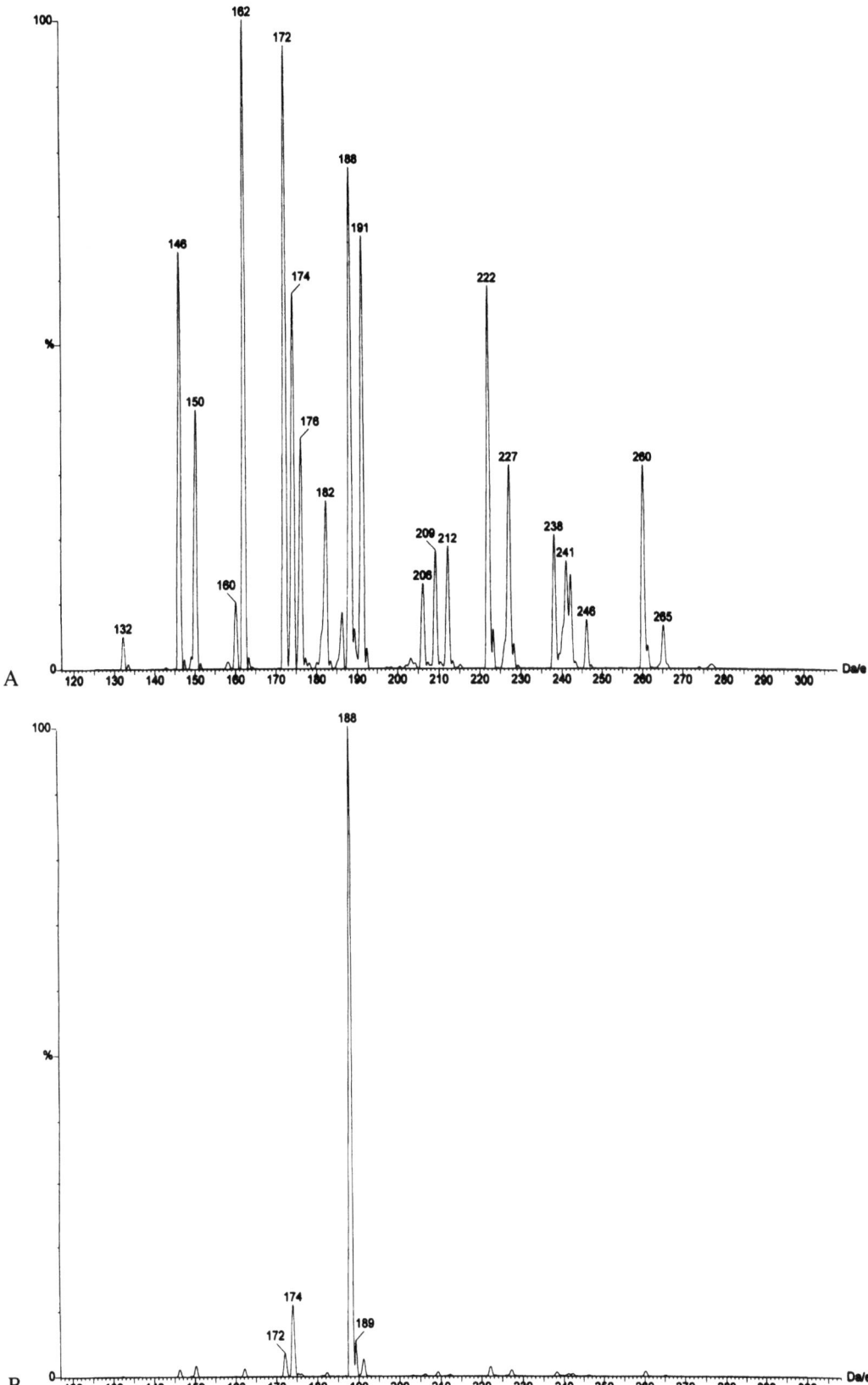

FIGURE 53.7. Tandem MS profile of amino acids in a normal neonate (A), as compared to a patient with maple syrup urine disease (B). The leucine (188) and valine (174) peaks predominate.

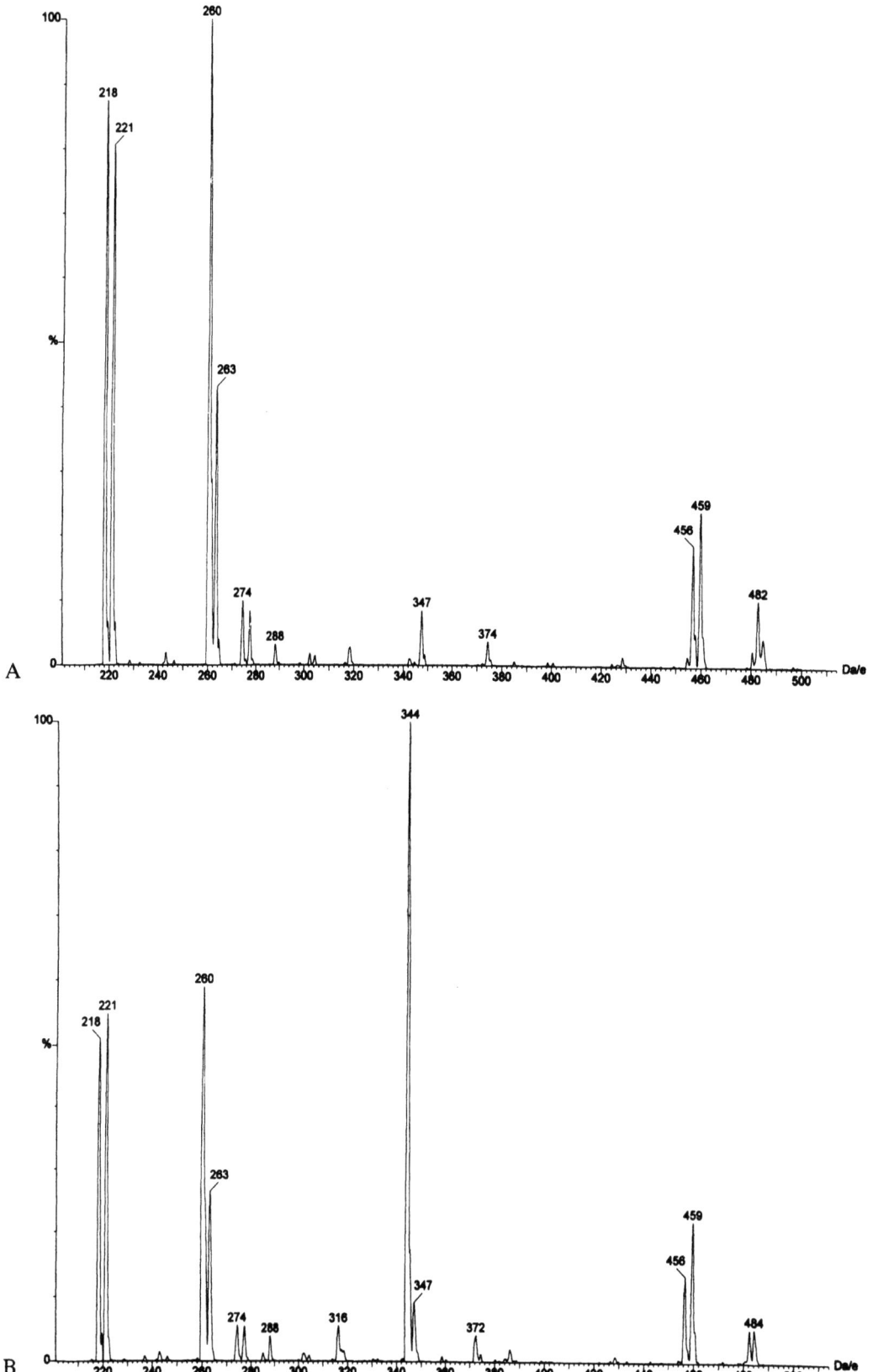

FIGURE 53.8. Tandem MS profiles in a normal infant (A), as compared to the profiles seen in medium-chain, long-chain, and 3-hydroxy-long-chain acyl-CoA dehydrogenase deficiencies (B, C, and D respectively). A: In a normal infant the predominant species is 260 (acetyl carnitine). B: In medium-chain acyl-CoA dehydrogenase deficiency the main peak is C8:0 (octanoyl carnitine) (344) with lesser peaks of C6:0 (316) and C10:0 (372), all of which are medium-chain acylcarnitines. C: In long-chain acyl-CoA dehydrogenase deficiency, long-chain acylcarnitines C12:0 (400); C14:1 (426); C14:0 (428); C16:0 (456); C16:2 (454); and C16:1 (452) are the predominant peaks. D: In 3-hydroxy-long-chain acyl-CoA dehydrogenase deficiency, in addition to long-chain acylcarnitines, carnitine esters of hydroxylated species of C12 (416), C14 (440), C16 (472), and C18 (490) are also present. The internal standards are deuterated (D_3) acetyl carnitine (263), octanoyl carnitine (347), and palmitoyl carnitine (459).

53. Evaluation of the Neonate with a Potential Metabolic Defect

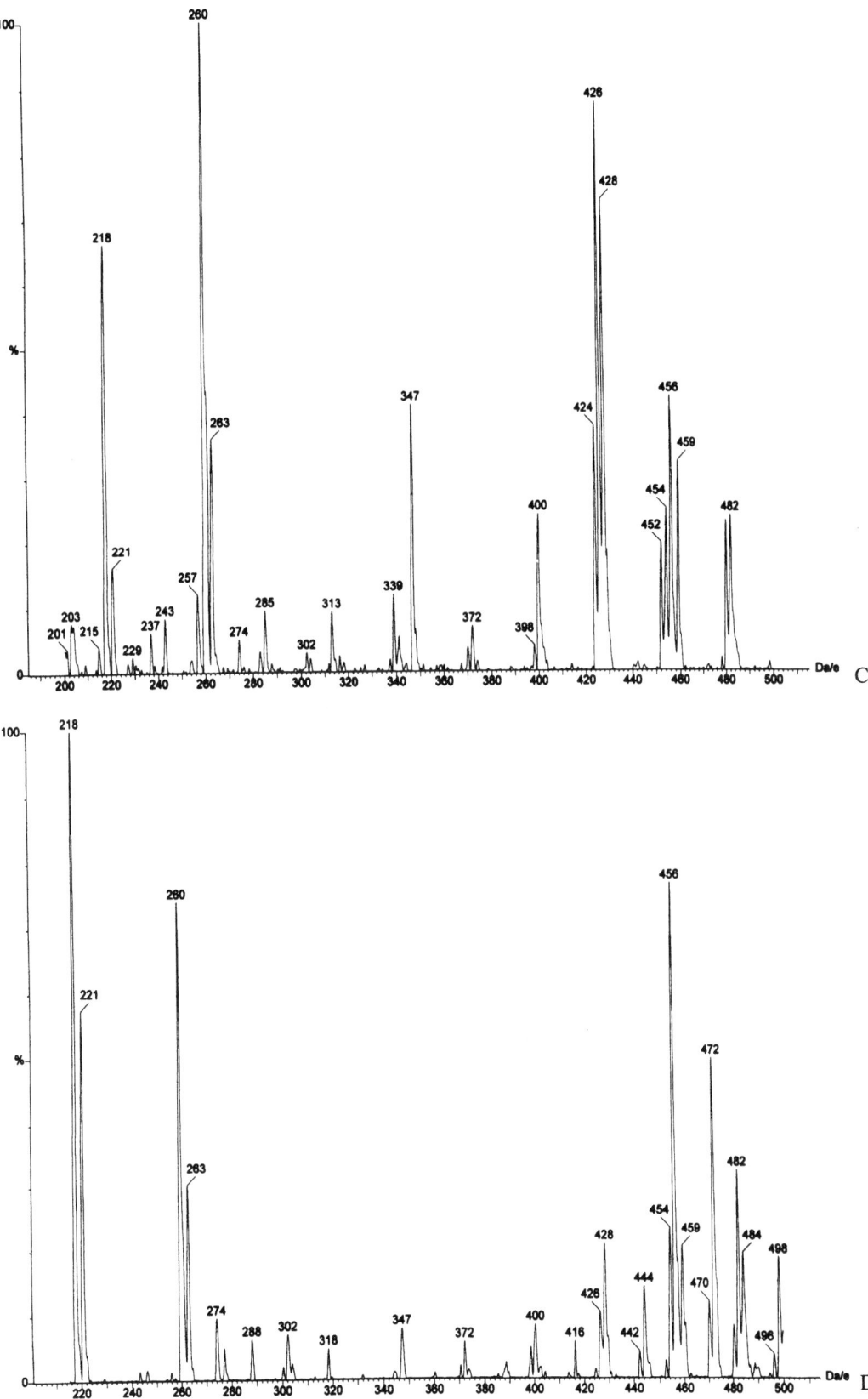

FIGURE 53.8. *Continued.*

Most countries do not have a well-organized network of health services, hindering an efficient neonatal screening program. In such instances, selective screening of neonates suspected of having a metabolic disease,[210–213] or of high-risk newborns from families that have an older child with an organic or amino-acidemia, is performed. This is a second-best choice. The safety window of neonatal onset organic acidemias and MSUD are only a few days. Unless an efficient neonatal screening program is in place, the neonate will develop the symptoms of the disease by the time the sample is received in the screening laboratory. Therefore, a neonatal screening effort becomes a selective screening procedure. Given the fact that most of these disorders can be treated with success, if diagnosed early during a metabolic decompensation, tandem MS–based screening should be the method of choice in countries that do not have an efficient neonatal screening program in place. In our experience, selective screening of the high-risk neonate, or testing all other presymptomatic children in the extended family has resulted in the most rewarding results, saving many of them from neurologic crippling and death.

Management of Acute Metabolic Decompensation

A most vigorous and urgent intervention is needed to correct dehydration by giving appropriate amounts of fluid and saline, and acidosis by administering alkaline solutions such as bicarbonate and by giving glucose to manage the hypoglycemia (Table 53.10). The only exception to this is patients with primary lactic acidosis, in whom sodium bicarbonate administration should be done cautiously, using isotonic solutions in moderate amounts. It has been shown that the use of massive doses of bicarbonate in such patients produces a large amount of CO_2 in the blood, which diffuses across the blood-brain barrier, lowering the pH in CSF, which indicates the aggravated acidosis in the brain.[214]

Once a preliminary diagnosis is reached, the patient should be placed on appropriate specific treatment without delay. If the diagnosis is established before the acute metabolic decompensation, or even if within 24 to 36 hours of the crisis, these specific therapies will provide rewarding results. The chance of residual neurologic damage increases substantially in patients with delayed diagnosis and delayed treatment. There are good management protocols for approximately two thirds of the diseases listed in Table 53.1.

The neonatologist should always keep in mind that the phenotypic presentation of these diseases is always variable, even in the same family. A good example is primary lactic acidosis caused by pyruvate carboxylase (PC) deficiency.[47,57,67,139,215–219] This disease, as well as holocarboxylase synthetase deficiency in a neonate, is usually not treatable, but biotin-responsive forms have been reported. Experience in our hospital shows that 10% of either PC or multiple carboxylase deficiencies are responsive to biotin. In these families, while the index neonate died within 1 week, the next sibling with the disease is alive with minimal or no neurologic sequelae. A patient with the severe form of long-chain acyl-CoA dehydrogenase deficiency rapidly expires due to cardiac arrhythmia and cardiomyopathy[220–222] within a few days, unless vigorous IV carnitine treatment is given to clear the heart muscle of the accumulated long-chain fatty acyl-CoA esters. A guideline for the management of acute crisis is shown in Table 53.10. Our hospital has had many success stories in the neonatal period when the disease was diagnosed and treated satisfactorily either before or early in the acute metabolic decompensation.

A universally accepted rule is that the acute crisis of PA is treated with a great number of calories,[223,224] and that of MMA with a large amount of fluids.[224] These therapies are given until 48 hours after the disappearance of ketones from the urine. The initial crisis of both PA and MSUD may be so severe that an insulin drip has to be added to rapidly reach the anabolic state.[225] Recently, special amino acid mixtures that do not contain branched-chain amino acids have become available and should be used in the TPN (Pharma Thera Inc., Memphis, TN). Metronidazole has been used in patients with PA and MMA with satisfactory results; this drug decreases propionic acid production by anaerobic gut flora.[226] A patient with acute crisis of PA always develops severe thrombocytopenia 3 to 4 days after the onset of crisis,[26] and if unrecognized it will cause intracerebral hemorrhage and death.

Use of carnitine,[227–230] particularly of IV carnitine, has been a lifesaving method in most instances. During an acute metabolic decompensation, the parenteral route should always be preferred to the oral administration of this drug, since only a fraction of the L-carnitine, 5% to 10%, is absorbed orally. In most instances, IV carnitine will correct the hyperammonemia of an organic acidemia within 12 to 18 hours.

In all neonates with primary lactic acidosis, carnitine, biotin, and thiamine must be given for at least a week to see if they have a beneficial effect. The protocols for the treatment of primary lactic acidosis are largely experimental.[231,232] Some centers use coenzyme Q, phytanedione (vitamin K_1),[231,232] and ascorbic acid on a blind basis when a neonate is found to have primary lactic acidosis. The lactic acidosis of patients with $E_{1\alpha}$ deficiency of PDH usually can be controlled by administering an activator of PDH phosphatase, dichloroacetate.[233,234] However, little or no improvement of encephalopathy accompanies the normalization of lactic acidemia. Patients with E_2 deficiency have been

TABLE 53.10. Medications used for the management of the acute metabolic decompensation in the neonate.

Disease	Compound to be restricted	Specific management during the acute metabolic decompensation
Propionic acidemia	Isoleucine, valine, threonine and methionine; in TPN 1–1.2 g/kg amino acid mixture, or specific mixture of amino acids for the disease	Carnitine 100 mg/kg bolus followed by 50 mg·kg^{-1} 6 hourly^{-1}; 12.5% dextrose in TPN, after 6 hours, insulin drip is added starting from 0.05 U/kg/hour, the amount of glucose is increased gradually up to 15–17.5%, and insulin drip is adjusted according to glycemia; metronidazole may be used at 30 mg·kg^{-1} day^{-1}; hemodialysis is recommended in severe metabolic crisis
Methylmalonic acidemia	Same as for propionic acidemia	Carnitine dose and frequency as in propionic acidemia; generous amounts of fluid are given; daily hydroxycobalamin 1 mg IM; insulin drip is usually not needed
Isovaleric acidemia	Restricted leucine, in TPN; if specific amino acid mixture is available, use the one recommended for MSUD	Carnitine dose and frequency is as in propionic acidemia; glycine 500 mg·kg^{-1} day^{-1} in three or four divided doses is given through a nasogastric tube
3-Hydroxy-3-methylglutaryl-CoA lyase deficiency	Restrict leucine	Carnitine may be used as doses as indicated above; however, infusion of glucose and bicarbonate are usually sufficient
Multiple carboxylase deficiency (severe neonatal forms of the disease)	Same restrictions as in propionic acidemia	Same therapy as used for propionic acidemia; add biotin 5–10 mg·kg^{-1} day^{-1} to be given through a nasogastric (NG) tube
Fatty acid oxidation disorders as short-, medium-, long-acyl-CoA, 3-hydroxyacyl long-chain CoA dehydrogenase, translocase deficiencies	Restrict lipids in the TPN mixture	Carnitine IV, 100 mg·kg^{-1} bolus, followed by 50 mg·kg^{-1} every 6 hours
Multiple acyl-CoA dehydrogenase deficiency	Restrict lipids in TPN	Riboflavin 100 mg·kg^{-1} d^{-1}, glycine 500 mg·kg^{-1} d^{-1} through an NG tube
Primary lactic acidosis (pyruvate dehydrogenase, pyruvate carboxylase deficiencies, respiratory chain diseases and 3-methylglutaconic aciduria)	Use isotonic bicarbonate solutions cautiously	Pyruvate dehydrogenase deficiency: thiamine 20–50 mg·kg^{-1} day^{-1} carnitine 200 mg·kg^{-1} day^{-1} through NG tube; sodium dichloroacetate 100 mg·kg IV twice daily may be tried Pyruvate carboxylase deficiency: biotin 10 mg·kg^{-1} day^{-1} through NG tube Other disorders: coenzyme Q 25 mg day, phytanedione 5 mg day, and ascorbic acid 100 mg day may be tried
Pyroglutamic aciduria	Same restrictions as for glucose-6-phosphate dehydrogenase deficiency	
Maple syrup urine disease	Leucine, isoleucine, valine; use the specific amino acid mixture when available; otherwise 1–1.2 g·kg^{-1} amino acid mixture in TPN	12.5% dextrose in TPN; after 6 hours, insulin drip is added starting from 0.05 U/kg/hour, the amount of glucose is increased gradually up to 15–17.5%, and insulin drip is adjusted according to glycemia; hemodialysis is recommended in severe metabolic crisis; trial of thiamine 10–20 mg·kg^{-1} day^{-1} through NG tube
Carbamylphosphate synthetase and ornithine transcarbamylase deficiencies, citrullinemia and argininosuccinic aciduria	Special mixture of amino acids, or 1–1.2 g·kg^{-1} amino acids in TPN	Mixture of 100 mg/ml each of sodium benzoate and sodium phenylacetate (Ucephan) IV 2.5 ml/kg diluted 1/10 in 5% dextrose given as bolus over 90 minutes; same dose is divided into four and given over next 24 hours with the same precautions; IV L-arginine 600 mg·kg (6 ml of 10% solution) diluted 1/10 in 5% dextrose as bolus; same dose divided into four given next 24 hours
Tyrosinemia type 1	Avoid barbiturates and other medications that can aggravate porphyria	10–15% glucose is given through a central line to combat its neurologic crisis; hypokalemia, hyponatremia and hypophosphatemia must be treated appropriately
Fructose-1,6-diphosphatase deficiency		IV glucose and sodium bicarbonate are sufficient

Fluid, electrolyte, glucose and bicarbonate treatment are standard therapies, provided as required by the laboratory findings. The L-arginine used should be the solution for IV therapy. When TPN is provided the amounts of compounds to be restricted are indicated. For the acute management of most of these disorders, it is preferable to use the special amino acid mixtures available for the disease as discussed in the text.

reported to benefit from the administration of lipoic acid, its cofactor.

The hyperammonemia of a urea cycle disorder (UCD) is a serious medical emergency, and must be immediately managed by hemodialysis.[235,236] This is particularly true for CPS and OTC deficiencies. When the ammonia concentration exceeds 400 μM, significant sequelae of the encephalopathy will remain; after 1,000 μM, even for a brief period, the infant will remain quadriplegic despite vigorous therapy. The evolution of hyperammonemia in citrullinemia and argininosuccinic aciduria are somewhat more indolent; the blood ammonia in these latter disorders can be restored to normal within 12 to 18 hours with vigorous use of IV L-arginine. In all UCD patients, while waiting for hemodialysis and diagnosis, the treatment with IV sodium benzoate, phenylacetate, and arginine should be initiated immediately.[237–239]

Chronic Management

Once the acute decompensation is treated, these diseases must then be managed with special diets (Table 53.11) and medications. These patients should never be permitted to fast, and even minor infections should be treated by hospitalization, with IV therapy to prevent the catabolic state created by a metabolic stress. Usually the diseases listed in Table 53.1 will cause recurrent crises later during infancy and early childhood that should be managed as vigorously as the initial metabolic decompensation. This is usually easier since the diagnosis has already been established, and the treatment can be initiated rapidly. It must always be remembered that patients with PA, MMA, and MSUD are immune compromised and they must receive antibiotics with potential effect on unusual gram(−) and (+) bacteria.

The medications for chronic management are listed in Table 56.10, except now the oral route, e.g., carnitine syrup, arginine, and sodium benzoate[237] powder, may be used. Most centers prefer not to use sodium benzoate and to use only sodium phenylacetate, since it is more effective. Sodium phenylbutyrate is preferred to sodium phenylacetate[238,239] since it has a better taste. This compound is broken down to phenylacetate normally in liver and is an effective medication for urea cycle disorders. In a patient with fructose-1, 6-diphosphatase deficiency, the clinician should always remember that most pediatric medications contain sucrose and their use will only aggravate the hypoglycemia and lactic acidosis due to fasting or to metabolic stress caused by an infection. When possible, capsules, tablets, and suppositories should be prescribed for these infants.

TABLE 53.11. Chronic management of diseases that cause acute metabolic decompensation.

Disease	Commercial formulas available	Compounds restricted in the formulas or special diets
Propionic acidemia, methylmalonic acidemia, multiple carboxylase deficiency	PROPINEX-2 (Ross)	L-isoleucine, L-valine, L-threonine, L-methionine
3-Hydroxy-3-methylglutaryl-CoA lyase and 3-Methylcrotonyl-CoA carboxylase deficiencies and isovaleric acidemia	MSUD diet powder. MSUD 1, or MSUD 2 (Mead Johnson); KETONEX-1 (Ross) with addition of glycine, isoleucine and valine	L-leucine; also a low-fat diet
Medium-chain acyl-CoA dehydrogenase deficiency		Strict avoidance of fasting with frequent feeding of a high-carbohydrate diet
Long chain, and long-chain 3-hydroxyacyl-CoA dehydrogenase deficiencies		Medium-chain triglycerides $1 \text{g} \cdot \text{kg}^{-1} \text{ day}^{-1}$; fats with long-chain fatty acids, are restricted; high-carbohydrate diet
Multiple acyl-CoA dehydrogenase deficiency		A low-fat, high-carbohydrate diet
Maple syrup urine disease	MSUD diet powder. MSUD 1, or MSUD 2 (Mead Johnson); KETONEX-1 (Ross)	Branched-chain amino acids
Tyrosinemia type 1	Low phenylalanine/tyrosine diet powder; TYR 1, TYR 2 (Mead Johnson); XPHEN, TYR; TYROMEX-1 (Ross)	Phenylalanine and tyrosine
Urea cycle disorders	UCD 1, UCD 2 (Mead Johnson); CYCLINEX-1 (Ross)	Contains only essential amino acids in an optimum ratio
FDPase deficiency		Strict restriction of sucrose and fructose intake; avoid fasting
Galactosemia	Pregestemil	Strict restriction of galactose and lactose intake
Any disorder that requires restricted nitrogen intake	Protein-free diet powder; MODUCAL (Mead Johnson): PORPHREE (Ross)	
Any disorder of leucine metabolism	XLEU (Ross)	
Protein-base supplementation	PROVIMIN (Ross); for fatty acid oxidation disorders	

FDPase, fructose diphosphatase.

53. Evaluation of the Neonate with a Potential Metabolic Defect

These management procedures require a team effort. A dietitian specialized in the management of these diseases, a social worker, a home health care nurse, and physician are the essential components of such a team.

Diagnosis and Management of a Neonate with Stupor

An encephalopathy may be present at birth, characterized by central hypotonia, seizures, and stupor. More common disorders are listed in Table 53.12. Despite their dramatic clinical presentations, these are difficult diseases to diagnose since most of them are not accompanied by disturbances in the common clinical laboratory tests.

It must be remembered that in the neonatal age group a seizure, as a rule, is either tonic or myoclonic, not grand mal. Primitive neurologic reflexes may be greatly diminished or absent, even cry may be absent. Such a neonate shows severe hypotonia. This symptomatology may be confused with perinatal anoxia, chromosomal aberrations, Werdnig-Hoffmann disease, congenital myasthenia, congenital myopathies, congenital muscular dystrophy, congenital myotonia, or congenital polyneuropathy. The important clinical and laboratory presentations of neonatal encephalopathies with stupor are listed in Table 53.12.

Among organic acid disorders, 3-methylglutaconic aciduria is a disease with unknown etiology and in at least one third of patients there would be no neonatal hypoglycemia or lactic acidosis.[34,50] There may be no associated dysmorphic features, and the diagnosis is first

TABLE 53.12. Main clinical and laboratory findings, and experimental treatment of neonatal diseases with stupor.

Disease	Main clinical findings	Main laboratory findings	Experimental therapeutic modalities
3-Methylglutaconic aciduria	Severe central hypotonia, stupor, blindness, deafness, usually myoclonic seizures and minor dysmorphic features	Urine GC/MS shows two isomers of 3-methylglutaconic acid; mild/moderate lactic acidemia; MRI of brain reveals cerebral and cerebellar dysgenesis with central white matter disease; absent VEP and BAEP	Same experimental therapy as outlined in Table 53.10
Severe phenotype of 4-hydroxybutyric aciduria	Severe hypotonia, apnea due to poor respiratory efforts and diaphragmatic paresis; stupor, severe atonic/myoclonic seizures; occasional lens cataracts and retinitis pigmentosa	Urine GC/MS studies show 4-hydroxy-butyric acid, and intermediates suggestive of impaired beta-oxidation as well as those encountered in type 2 glutaric aciduria; mild/severe subcortical white matter disease in MRI of brain	γ-vinyl GABA (Vigabatrin) 35–50 mg·kg^{-1}·day^{-1} alone or in combination with dextromethorphan 25 mg·kg^{-1}·day^{-1}
Nonketotic hyperglycinemia	Severe early hypotonia often requiring ventilatory support, hiccups that can be observed even in fetus; myoclonic jerks	Increased blood and CSF glycine (usually 5- to 10-fold); CSF/blood glycine >0.08. MRI of brain frequently shows dysgenesis of corpus callosum; EEG shows burst suppression pattern	Dextromethorphan starting from 20 increasing to 35 mg·kg^{-1}·day^{-1} together with sodium benzoate 500 mg·kg^{-1}·day^{-1}
Methylene-tetrahydro (Me-H$_4$)-reductase deficiency	Central apnea, hypotonia, myoclonic seizures, microophthalmia	Positive ferricyanide test in fresh urine; blood methionine is <5 μM, homocystinuria, cystathioninuria, increased blood homocysteine and low RBC folate	Folinic acid 1–2 mg·kg^{-1}·day^{-1}; methionine up to 100 mg·kg^{-1}·day^{-1}; betaine 100 mg·kg^{-1}·day^{-1}; hydroxycobalamin 1 mg IM, once every 1–2 weeks
Menkes' disease, early severe neonatal form	X-linked inheritance; stupor, hypothermia, hypopigmentation, myoclonic seizures, unusual face with sagging cheeks, hair abnormalities (observed later)	Low plasma copper and ceruloplasmin; by 3–4 months of age subdural hematoma may occur; cerebral arteriograms show early tortuosity	Intramuscular injections of chelated copper-histidinate 1 mg·day^{-1}
Sulfite oxidase and molybdenum cofactor deficiencies	Severe, early myoclonic seizures not responsive to anticonvulsive treatment, opisthotonus, blindness, nystagmus	Urine sulfite oxide test is positive; low plasma and urinary uric acid, in urine S-sulfocysteine is present	Restricted intake of sulfur amino acids to minimum permissible; ammonium molybdate in patients with molybdenum cofactor deficiency

reached from a urine GC/MS study ordered as a routine workup of a hypotonic neonate.

The clinical presentation of severe phenotypes of 4-hydroxybutyric aciduria may be stupor and severe hypotonia.[11,240] This is a disease of γ-aminobutyric acid (GABA) metabolism,[241-243] in which the dehydrogenase that oxidizes the transamination product of GABA, succinic-semialdehyde, is missing. The succinic-semialdehyde that accumulates is reduced by a reductase to 4-hydroxybutyric acid, which has potent pharmacologic actions in CNS.[244]

Among amino acid disorders, nonketotic hyperglycinemia (NKH) is a common disorder[245-248] with seizures, severe central hypotonia, and various types of brain dysgenesis. It is important to establish a diagnosis of NKH, since it is a potentially treatable disease.[245,249-251] Blood glycine concentration in this disorder may vary greatly, and NKH is best diagnosed by the simultaneous measurement of blood and CSF glycine.[252] A high CSF/blood glycine ratio (>0.08) always indicates the presence of NKH. One form of NKH is associated with D-glyceric aciduria.[253] An illustrative case history follows.

Case History: Nonketotic Hyperglycinemia

This male neonate was 1 month old, a product of a normal pregnancy and delivery with normal 1-, 5-, and 10-minute Apgar scores. The parents were first cousins and they had lost two infants previously to a neonatal disease with coma within 1 month. Soon after birth he developed lethargy progressing to coma requiring ventilatory support. He had no primitive neonatal reflexes and was severely hypotonic. Blood chemistries, liver function, pH, lactate, pyruvate, and ammonia were normal. A tandem MS study revealed blood glycine 900 μM (normal <400 μM) and CSF glycine 280 μM (normal <4 μM), with a CSF/blood glycine ratio of 0.31 (normal <0.08). The EEG revealed diffuse disorganization of the background with interhemispheric asymmetry. The MRI of the brain revealed a thin corpus callosum with delayed myelination in centrum ovale. He was placed on $25\,mg\cdot kg^{-1}\,day^{-1}$ dextromethorphan and $500\,mg\cdot kg^{-1}\,day^{-1}$ sodium benzoate. He came out of coma within 3 days and was discharged after 1 week. He did remarkably well, achieving normal milestones of infancy. At 11 months of age he started to sit independently despite moderate hypotonia, had appropriate vocalization and good social skills.

Another cause of hypotonia, seizures, stupor, and central apnea is hypomethioninemia due to methylenetetrahydro (Me-H$_4$)-folate reductase deficiency.[15,254] This folate metabolic abnormality must be considered in any neonate with central apnea with no readily explainable cause. A simple nitroprusside test in a freshly collected urine sample rapidly reveals the disease since it is associated with homocystinuria.[254] The treatment with folinic acid, methionine,[255] and betaine[256] should be initiated immediately, while waiting for specialized biochemical tests to confirm the diagnosis. In such a patient methylmalonic aciduria is absent. If methylmalonic aciduria occurs within this myriad of biochemical findings, the disease is due to an abnormality of vitamin B$_{12}$ metabolism (cbl E and G mutations).[257] However, this latter group of disorders usually manifests later during infancy or early childhood. An illustrative case history follows.

Case History: Putative Me-H$_4$-Folate Reductase Deficiency

This female neonate was 1 month old, a product of a normal pregnancy and delivery. The parents were first cousins and had lost their first baby to a disease with apnea, requiring ventilatory support progressing to *Candida* sepsis, DIC, and death at 2 months of age. The patient was normal until 10 days of age, at which time the parents noted her to have depressed respiratory activity and cyanosis. A congenital heart disease was suspected and was admitted to a peripheral hospital for workup. The cardiac studies and CT brain were normal. She was discharged, and the parents decided to take her to a tertiary care center. She suffered apnea en route and had to be resuscitated in the emergency room of the referring hospital. She was worked up for a CNS, pulmonary, or cardiac disease while receiving ventilatory support. She had microophthalmia and pronounced hypotonia with diminished reflexes. She had macrocytosis, and red blood cell (RBC) volume was 100 μl; a blood folate concentiation was not obtained. No cause was found for her central apnea; a blood sample was sent for analysis by tandem MS. It revealed hypomethioninemia, 2.1 μM (normal >7 μM), and no propionylcarnitine. A urine sample was found to contain no methylmalonic acid but, by tandem MS, large amounts of homocystine and cystathionine. This symptom complex suggested a folate metabolic abnormality, possibly Me-H$_4$-folate reductase or methionine synthetase deficiency. She was immediately given 15 mg folinic acid. Next day she was taken off the ventilator, breathing on her own, with great general improvement particularly in the muscle tone. Methionine $100\,mg\cdot kg^{-1}\,day^{-1}$ and betaine $100\,mg\cdot kg^{-1}\,day^{-1}$ were added to her medications and she was discharged 1 week later. She suffered an intraventricular hemorrhage at home at 2 months of age and had to be hospitalized. The reason for this hemorrhage could not be found. A ventriculoperitoneal shunt was placed for the acquired hydrocephalus. The further clinical course was not remarkable. She required methionine supplementation, and when methionine was discontinued blood levels decreased to <5 μM within a week, with apnea reappearing. Betaine supplementation did not restore blood methionine to normal levels. Although no enzyme measurements are available, the clinical symptomatology including apnea, and the biochemical findings support a diagnosis of Me-H_4-folate reductase deficiency. A follow-up MRI study indicates that she has severe brain atrophy. At the age of 1 year she has not achieved any developmental milestones. Whether the clinical course would have been this unsatisfactory if she were diagnosed at birth is unknown.

The severe type of Menkes' disease appears at birth with hypotonia, seizures and stupor.[258] Its inheritance is X-linked. The copper and ceruloplasmin concentrations are low, and these two biochemical parameters should be measured in all hypotonic male neonates. The neonatal manifestation of either molybdenum cofactor[259] or sulfite oxidase[260] deficiency is severe, intractable seizures and hypotonia. The characteristic feature of these diseases, dislocated lens and cataract, may not appear until late infancy. The disease usually, but not always, is detected in freshly collected urine by using a sulfite detecting paper (Merck Sharpe & Dohme, NJ). Decreased functions of sulfite oxidase and molybdenum cofactor lead to a decreased blood concentration of uric acid, which should be determined in any neonate with intractable seizures.[261]

Procedures of Management

The treatments available are mostly experimental. However, because these are such serious diseases, such therapies are justifiable (Table 53.12).

The neonatal forms of 3-methylglutaconic aciduria in some instances[50] may benefit from the use of medications used in the management of mitochondriopathies, such as coenzyme Q, phytonadione, and ascorbic acid.[231,232]

In some patients with 4-hydroxybutyric aciduria (4-OHB), the use of vigabatrin (γ-vinyl GABA), a GABA-transaminase noncompetitive inhibitor, has been beneficial. The neonate can form such a large amount of succinic-semialdehyde, the precursor of 4-OHB, that it is almost impossible to reduce the formation of 4-OHB, through vigabatrin, to a low concentration.[242,243] In some instances, dextromethorphan, an N-methyl-D-aspartate (NMDA) receptor antagonist, has been beneficial.[250]

The therapeutic results with dextromethorphan and sodium benzoate in nonketotic hyperglycinemia,[249–251] have also been mixed, with no beneficial effect in some and improvement in others. In our experience seizures and hypotonia respond to the outlined treatment if it is administered early. With such therapy, at least in one of the neonates diagnosed and treated at birth, the subsequent motor and mental development have been normal.

Mixed results have been obtained in the therapy of methylenetetrahydro (Me-H_4)-folate reductase deficiency. In this disorder folinic acid should be used,[255] since it can enter into the CNS. Frequent monitoring of blood methionine must be performed to assure an adequate concentration of blood methionine. The rationale for the use of betaine is to reduce homocysteinemia.[256]

Mixed results have been reported with chelated copper therapy in Menkes' disease.[262] Early therapy, which can be given even in utero, before the blood-brain barrier matures, may be beneficial. For this reason, labor may be induced early (i.e., 32 weeks of gestation), in order to start the injections of the copper-histidinate.

No beneficial therapy has so far been proposed for sulfite oxidase deficiency, and severe malnutrition may evolve by prolonged restriction of sulfur amino acids, the source of sulfite, in the diet. In patients with molybdenum cofactor deficiency, the use of ammonium molybdate has been recommended.

Teratogenic Disorders in the Neonate

It is not unusual to encounter a neonate with dysmorphic features. Some of these are due to chromosome abnormalities such as Downs syndrome and can be confused with pyruvate dehydrogenase deficiency or fetal alcohol syndrome. Some are due to metabolic disturbances in the mother such as maternal PKU, alcoholism, drug use (e.g., Dilantin, warfarin, methotrexate), uncontrolled diabetes mellitus, maternal riboflavin avitaminosis, or abnormal sensitivity to vitamin D (e.g., Williams-Beuren syndrome). Others are due to inborn errors of metabolism, and the more commonly encountered disorders are listed in Table 53.13.

Peroxisomal Disorders of the Neonate

The most important disorders that disturb morphogenesis are peroxisomal disease. Among these are Zellweger syndrome (ZS),[263] neonatal adrenoleukodystrophy (NALD),[264] and rhizomelic chondrodysplasia punctata (RCDP).[265] The mode of inheritance of these disorders is autosomal recessive.

The features of ZS (Table 53.13) include a characteristic craniofacial appearance with high forehead, flat occiput, large fontanel, low nasal bridge, external ear deformity, particularly with a crease in the ear lobe, micrognathia, and redundant skin folds in the neck. Cataract of lens, abnormal retinal pigmentation, enlarged liver, and such abnormal neurologic findings as diminished/absent neonatal reflexes, severe central hypotonia, and myoclonic seizures are almost always encountered. The typical face of a patient with ZS is shown in Figure 53.9.

The clinical appearance of a neonate with NALD is that of a milder form of ZS. The seizures in NALD are severe and intractable; the NALD patient is often de-

TABLE 53.13. Clinical and laboratory features of teratogenic disorders of the neonate.

Disease	Clinical features	Laboratory features
Zellweger syndrome	Characteristic craniofacial dysmorphia, ear lobe abnormalities, cataract, retinitis pigmentosa, hepatomegaly, myoclonic seizures, severe central hypotonia, diminished neonatal reflexes	Stippled epiphyses, central white matter disease, gyral abnormalities and heterotopias in MRI of brain, cysts in liver and kidney, accumulation of C26:0 fatty acid in blood, tissues and organs, low docosahexaenoic acid, abnormal bile acids in plasma, pipecolic aciduria, decreased plasmalogens in red blood cells, empty peroxisomes in brain and liver biopsy by EM, impaired phytanic acid oxidation, decreased plasmalogen in tissues, medium-chain dicarboxylic aciduria
Neonatal adrenoleukodystrophy	Similar features to Zellweger syndrome, except milder, and dysmorphic features may be absent; severe myoclonic seizures	More pronounced white matter disease and less pronounced brain dysmorphia as compared to Zellweger syndrome; same biochemical findings
Rhizomelic chondrodysplasia punctata	Rhizomelic dwarfism, joint contractures	Pronounced punctate chondrodysplasia, coronal clefts of vertebral bodies, normal blood C26:0; decreased plasmalogen in tissues and red blood cells
Multiple acyl-CoA dehydrogenase deficiency (glutaric aciduria type 2)	Refer to Table 53.2	Refer to Table 53.8
Mevalonic aciduria	Characteristic craniofacial abnormalities, with a "button" nose and wide forehead, hypotonia, early failure to thrive, diarrhea, rash	Increased mevalonic acid and its lactone in urine by GC/MS
Carbohydrate-deficient glycoprotein syndrome	Characteristic face, inverted nipples, hypotonia	Poorly glycosylated transferrin

scribed as a continuously shivering neonate. In this disorder, as compared to ZS, cerebral demyelination is more impressive; chondrodysplasia and renal cysts are absent.

The RCDP patient is easily diagnosed because of the rhizomelic dwarfism (e.g., shortened proximal limbs), joint contractures (Figure 53.10), coronal clefts of vertebral bodies on lateral x-ray of the spine, and more severe and widespread chondrodysplasia punctata than seen in ZS (Figure 53.11). However, RCDP must be differentiated from Conradi-Hünermann syndrome,[266] and X-linked dominant[267] and X-linked recessive[268] forms of chondrodysplasia. In Conradi-Hünermann syndrome, the limb length is normal; the syndrome is inherited as an autosomal dominant trait. Infants with these latter disorders live longer, while RCDP is a lethal disease of infancy.

Pathogenesis

Peroxisomal proteins are synthesized by genes coded in the nucleus.[269] They are synthesized at their final sizes and are imported into the peroxisomes that are on a network of peroxisomal reticulum. This leads to enlargement of the peroxisomes, which then bud or divide into new peroxisomes.[269,270] Complementation studies indicate that ZS and NALD belong to the same complementation group, and there are 10 different groups in ZS and 6 in NALD.[271] ZS is usually due to a defect in peroxisomal assembly factor (PAF1), a 35-kd membrane protein,[272] or due to mutations in yet another peroxisomal membrane protein, PMP 70.[273] These lead to absent formation of peroxisomes. In NALD as well, there is a failure to import peroxisomal proteins. Therefore, in ZS and NALD virtually all peroxisomal functions, notably peroxisomal β-oxidation, are absent. The peroxisomal enzymes remain in cytosol, and are degraded. Under electron microscopy (EM), peroxisomes are either absent or empty.[274] In both disorders hexacosanoic acid (C26:0) accumulates and accounts for 25% of fatty acids in CNS and retina.[275] Oxidation of a long-chain fatty acid, lignoceric acid (C24:0), is impaired in both disorders.[276] Absent peroxisomal functions lead to various abnormalities in morphogenesis, particularly abnormal neuronal migration leading to microgyria and pachygyria.[277] In both disorders the accumulating C26:0 is probably the cause of impaired morphogenesis, since similar clinical features are not seen in RCDP, where C26:0 is normal.

In patients with disorders of peroxisomal biogenesis, levels of docosahexaenoic acid (DHA; C22-cis 4, 7, 10, 13, 16, 19 hexaenoic acid) in the brain, retina, liver, and blood are low.[278,279] DHA is important for the integrity of both the brain and retina, so its deficiency may play a role in the pathogenesis of some of the clinical manifestations. Pipecolic aciduria observed in ZS and NALD is due to failure of its breakdown, which normally takes place in peroxisomes.[280] Bile acids are metabolized to deoxycholic

53. Evaluation of the Neonate with a Potential Metabolic Defect

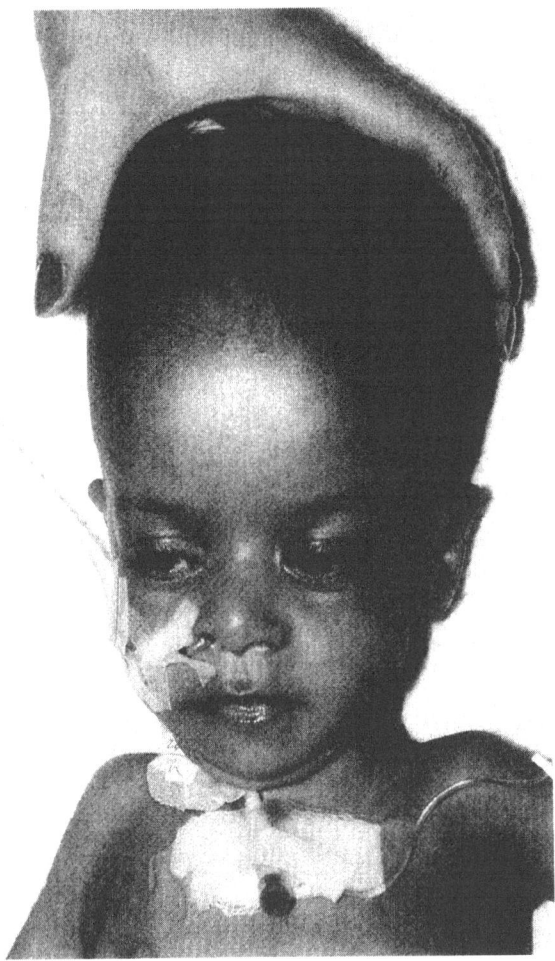

FIGURE 53.9. The typical facial appearance of a neonate with Zellweger syndrome.

Other Teratogenic Disorders in the Neonate

The neonatal-onset forms of glutaric aciduria type 2 (GAT-2) may, or may not, exist with dysmorphic features.[284] The dysmorphic features are summarized in Table 53.2. There is prominent hepatomegaly, seizures, and severe central hypotonia. The neonatal forms of this disorder present with severe hypoglycemia, and often with lactic acidosis within 24 hours. Most neonates expire within the first week of life; others may die of cardiomyopathy later during early infancy. A few have been described to be responsive to therapy with riboflavin.

Pathogenesis

Either electron-transport flavoprotein (ETF) of ETF-ubiquinone oxidoreductase (ETF-QO) are defective. This leads to functional deficiencies of multiple riboflavin-linked dehydrogenases such as short-, medium-, long-

acid in peroxisomes, and their precursors are increased in ZS and NALD, since bile acid oxidation is impaired. This could relate to the pathogenesis of hepatic abnormality, elevated liver enzymes, and hepatic fibrosis.[281] The medium-chain dicarboxylic aciduria (e.g., adipic, sebacic, suberic acids) observed in ZS is due to the impaired peroxisomal β-oxidation, leading to increased ω-oxidation of fatty acids by the P_{450}-mediated oxidation in ribosomes.[282] Dicarboxylic aciduria is more severe in fatty acid oxidation disorders.

In RCDP, a single peroxisomal enzyme responsible for the synthesis of plasmalogens, dihydroxyacetonephosphate (DHAP)-acyl transferase, is absent.[265,283] There may be defective oxidation of phytanic acid, another peroxisomal function. In RCDP the blood level of C26:0 is normal. The skeletal defects are probably linked to defective plasmalogen formation.[283]

The special biochemical tests used in the diagnosis of this group of disorders are listed in Table 53.13. There is no known treatment for neonatal peroxisomal diseases; DHA 250 g·day^{-1} has been recommended in view of its important role for the integrity of brain and retina.

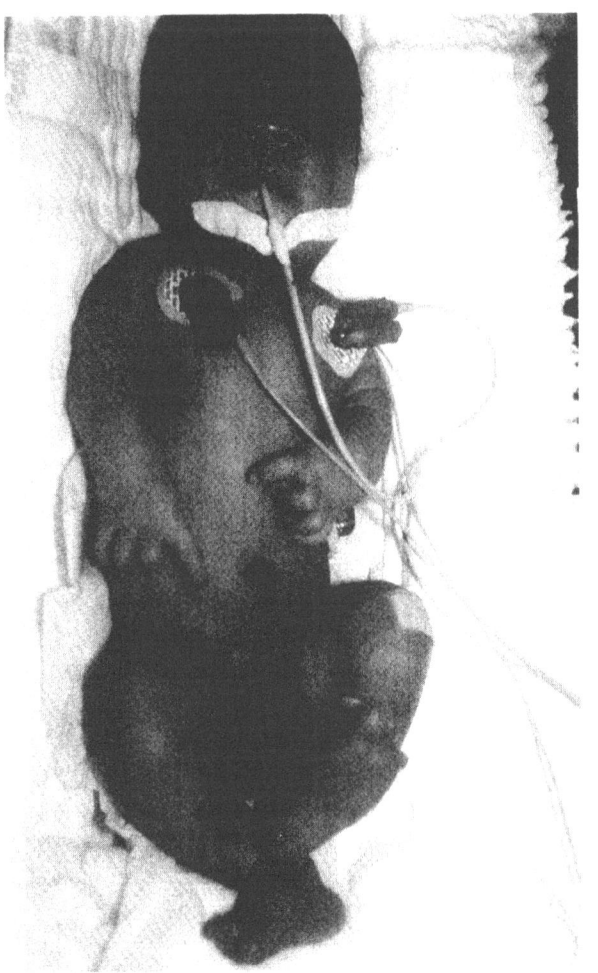

FIGURE 53.10. The appearance of a neonate with rhizomelic chondrodysplasia punctata.

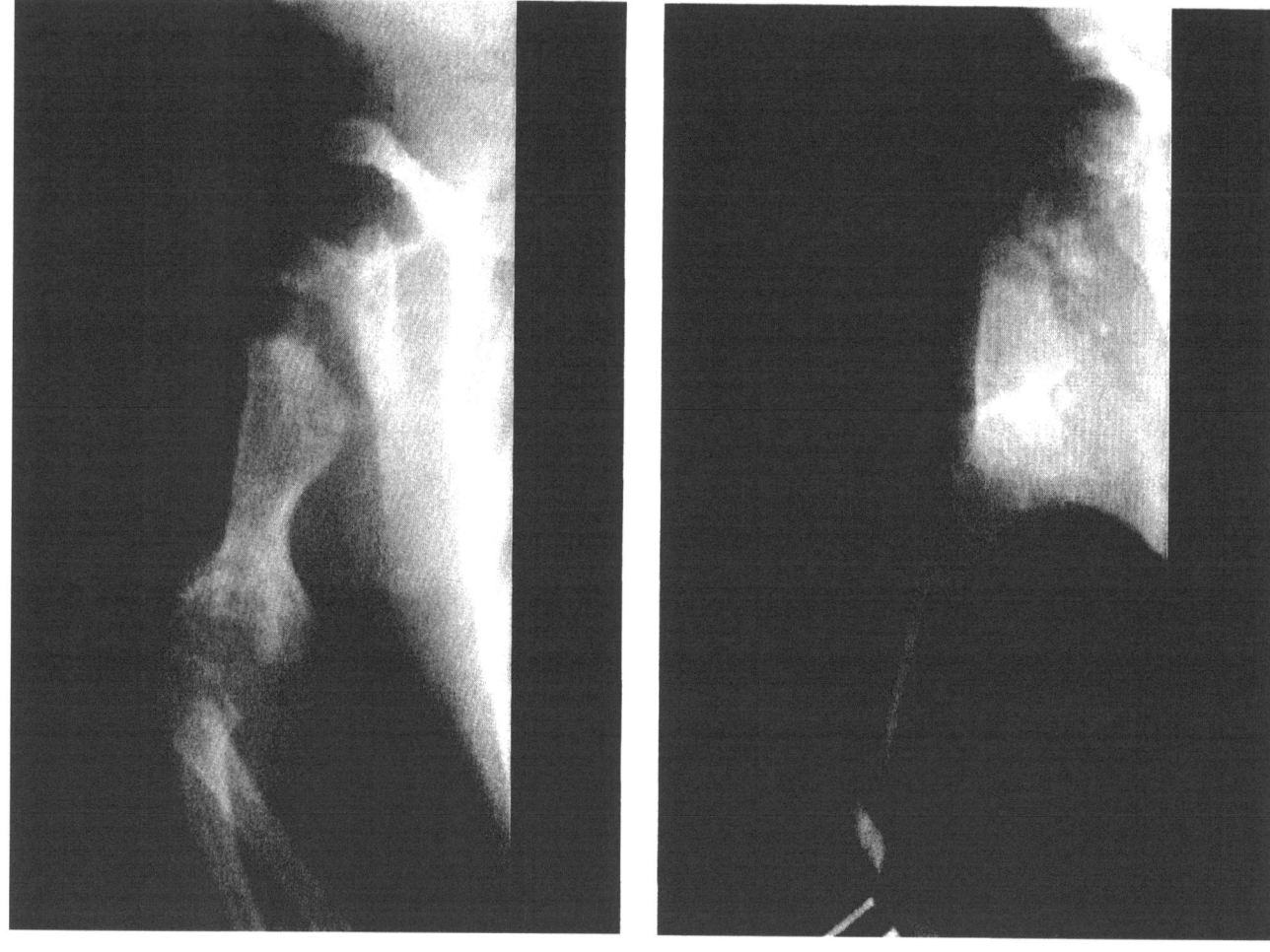

FIGURE 53.11. The x-ray of right humerus, frontal (A) and lateral (B) views in a patient with rhizomelic chondrodysplasia punctata indicating very short humerus, chondrodysplasia, and severe calcified, punctate stippling.

and very long chain acyl-CoA, glutaryl-CoA, isovaleryl-CoA, and 2-methylbutyryl-CoA dehydrogenases, dimethylglycine, and sarcosine oxidases, which must function through ETF and ETF-QO.[284,285] The blood acylcarnitine profile and the urine dicarboxylic acids reflect these multiple dehydrogenase deficiencies. In Figure 53.12, the blood tandem MS of a neonate with GAT-2 is shown, indicating the deficient activities of multiple acyl-CoA dehydrogenases. The teratogenic effect is due to absent riboflavin function, and can also be seen in the neonate from a mother who has an abnormality in the metabolism of riboflavin.[286] All patients show severe microvesicular fatty changes in the liver, in the proximal renal tubule, and in the myocardium. In some, renal abnormalities may be present as cysts that occupy renal cortex and medulla. In the brain, abnormal neuronal migration, neuronal loss, and gliosis may be observed. The experimental treatment for GAT-2 is listed in Table 53.10.

Mevalonic aciduria is caused by the deficiency of mevalonate kinase, which initiates the synthetic pathways of dolichol, cholesterol, and ubiquinone.[287] It is an autosomal recessive disease with such dysmorphic features as dolicocephaly, triangular face, downward slanted eyes, underdeveloped nasal bridge, and large posteriorly rotated and low set ears (Table 53.13). Most patients show early and severe failure to thrive, hypotonia, and recurrent crisis with fever, rash, vomiting, diarrhea, and central hypotonia. Since mevalonic acid is readily cleared through the kidney, metabolic acidosis is not observed. Although cholesterol synthesis is blocked, exogenous sources supply enough cholesterol, and hypocholesterolemia is not usually present. The disease is readily diagnosed since in urine GC/MS large amounts of mevalonic acid and mevalonolactone are found. There is no known treatment for mevalonic aciduria; a diet high in cholesterol and ubiquinone supplementation may be tried.

Carbohydrate-deficient glycoprotein syndrome (CDGS) is a disease of later infancy and childhood (Table 53.13). However, its dysmorphic features such as high nasal bridge, prominent jaw, large ears, and, particularly, inverted nipples may be observed at birth.[288] The neonate may be hypotonic from birth on. Inverted

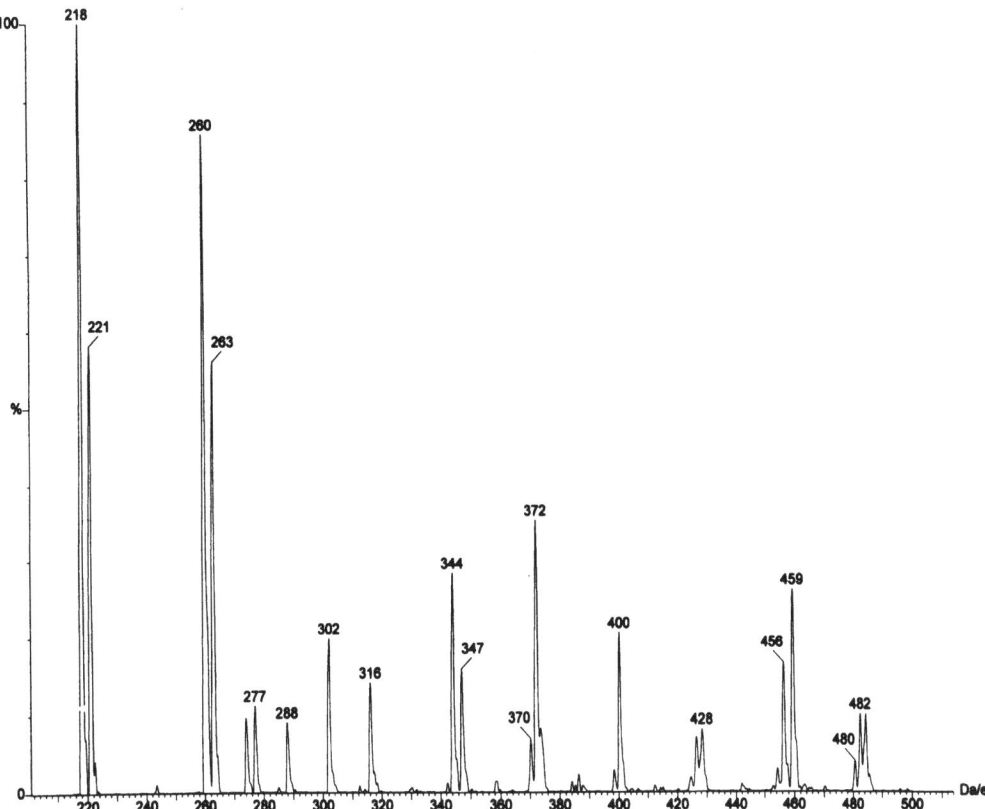

FIGURE 53.12. Tandem MS of blood, in a patient with glutaric aciduria type 2; showing almost all the peaks of fatty acyl carnitines between C4 and C18, in addition to glutarylcarnitine (388).

nipples may be observed in a variety of dysmorphic syndromes, such as Weaver syndrome.[289] The neonate with the latter disease is usually large at birth and shows early advanced skeletal maturation during infancy. CDGS is an autosomal recessive disease in which some aspect of N-linked oligosaccharide synthesis or transfer is defective. When inverted nipples are present in a neonate with hypotonia, the state of glycosylation of transferrin must be determined; it is poor in CDGS.[290]

Lysosomal Storage Diseases Encountered in the Neonate

The severe phenotypes of lysosomal storage diseases manifest in the neonate. Hydrops fetalis, in addition to either cardiomyopathy, hepatosplenomegaly, or dysmorphic and storage features of a mucopolysaccharidosis (MPS), including dysostosis multiplex, are present. Vacuolated lymphocytes and macrophages with storage substance are found in light microscopy and EM. These diseases are listed in Table 53.14. Their mode of inheritance is autosomal recessive and can be diagnosed prenatally by chorionic villus biopsy or by analysis of cultured amniocytes.

Most of the diseases listed in Table 53.14 usually manifest in early infancy; however, the severe phenotypes will affect the fetus, causing hydrops fetalis. Besides evidence of fetal edema and anasarca, the clinical symptoms and laboratory findings of these diseases in a neonate are summarized in Table 53.14.

In the severe phenotype of Gaucher disease type 2, besides hydrops fetalis, there may be associated ichthyosis.[18] Early hepatosplenomegaly is a rule, and even bone erosion can be seen in x-ray studies. Oculomotor abnormalities such as apraxia and bilateral fixed strabismus, bulbar signs such as stridor and opisthotonus, and global CNS involvement such as seizures and choreoathetoid movements may be observed. This variant of Gaucher disease is lethal and the infant expires within a few months. The enzyme measurement in leukocytes and fibroblasts, as well as the presence of Gaucher cells in a bone marrow biopsy, indicates the disease. There is no treatment available for this phenotype of Gaucher disease.

Infants with the severe form of G_{M1} gangliosidosis show macrosomia; early hepatosplenomegaly; and dysmorphic features similar to those in patients with MPS, such as coarse face, thick skin, hirsutism of forehead, gingival hyperplasia, and macroglossia.[19] Evidence of dysostosis multiplex, central hypotonia, and poor sucking is seen

TABLE 53.14. Clinical and laboratory features of lysosomal diseases that cause hydrops fetalis.

Disease	Clinical features	Laboratory features
Neonatal Gaucher disease	Hepatosplenomegaly, bone erosion, oculomotor apraxia, stridor, bulbar signs, and at times ichthyosis	Deficient acidic β-glucosidase activity in leukocytes and fibroblasts; Gaucher cells in bone marrow biopsy
G_{M1} gangliosidosis	Features of MPS at birth, such as coarse face visceromegaly, hernia, dysostosis multiplex, and cherry-red macula	Deficient β-galactosidase activity in leukocytes and fibroblasts
Galactosialidosis	Recurrent abortions in the family; features of mucopolysaccharidosis at birth, such as coarse face visceromegaly, hernias, dysostosis multiplex, and cherry-red macula	Deficient neuraminidase, β-galactosidase, and carboxypeptidase Y activities in lymphocytes, or fibroblasts
Sialidosis	Features of mucopolysaccharidosis at birth, such as coarse face visceromegaly, hernias, dysostosis multiplex, cherry-red macula, stippled epiphyses, and periosteal cloaking	Deficient neuraminidase with preserved activity of β-galactosidase in fibroblasts and leukocytes
β-Glucuronidase deficiency	Recurrent abortions in the family; features of mucopolysaccharidosis at birth, such as coarse face, visceromegaly, hernias, and dysostosis multiplex	Deficient β-glucuronidase activity in leukocytes or fibroblasts
Mucolipidosis II or "I-cell" disease	Features of mucopolysaccharidosis at birth, such as coarse face visceromegaly, hernias, dysostosis multiplex, cardiac valvular defects, and striking gingival hyperplasia	Increased lysosomal enzymes in plasma and urine, decreased lysosomal enzymes in leukocytes or fibroblasts; deficient phosphotransferase activity in cells
Niemann-Pick disease type C	Early, prolonged neonatal jaundice, death due to hepatic or pulmonary failure	Intense perinuclear fluorescence staining by filipin in fibroblasts

frequently. An arrest in growth and rapid progression of encephalopathy appear early following the neonatal period. The "cherry-red macula" (Figure 53.13), and optic atrophy are seen later in infancy. This variant of G_{M1} gangliosidosis is lethal and the infant expires within a few months. A simple analysis of β-galactosidase in leukocytes or fibroblasts establishes the diagnosis. There is no treatment available.

Galactosialidosis is a variant form of G_{M1} gangliosidosis, except the fundamental defect is different. A protein, carboxypeptidase Y, or the protective protein is absent. This protein is responsible for binding and protecting both β-galactosidase and sialidase against proteolytic degradation during their passage through the cytosol. Therefore, there is a combined deficiency of both β-galactosidase and sialidase with the accumulation of sialyloligosaccharides in lysosomes. The disease may manifest at any age between birth and adolescence. The neonatal form is associated with hydrops fetalis; in fact, it has been reported to cause recurrent fetal loss due to hydrops fetalis.[22] The picture of an infant with anasarca due to galactosialidosis is shown in Figure 53.14. The neonate shows a coarse face, inguinal hernias, visceromegaly, and mild dysostosis multiplex. Cardiomegaly, and thickened septum may be present. Proteinuria indicates renal involvement. Corneal clouding and cherry-red macula are observed later in infancy.

In severe phenotypes of sialidase deficiency, a similar clinical picture with hydrops fetalis may also be observed.[21] The differential diagnosis of these latter disorders is through the determination of β-galactosidase, sialidase or carboxypeptidase Y in leukocytes and fibroblasts. There is no treatment.

The neonatal presentation of severe phenotype of β-glucuronidase deficiency is similar to galactosialidosis. A family with recurrent abortions due to hydrops fetalis caused by β-glucuronidase deficiency has been reported.[20] The disease is diagnosed by the absence of β-glucuronidase in leukocytes and fibroblasts.

Mucolipidosis II or "I-cell" disease manifests with features characteristic of MPS at birth.[23] Neonates with I-cell

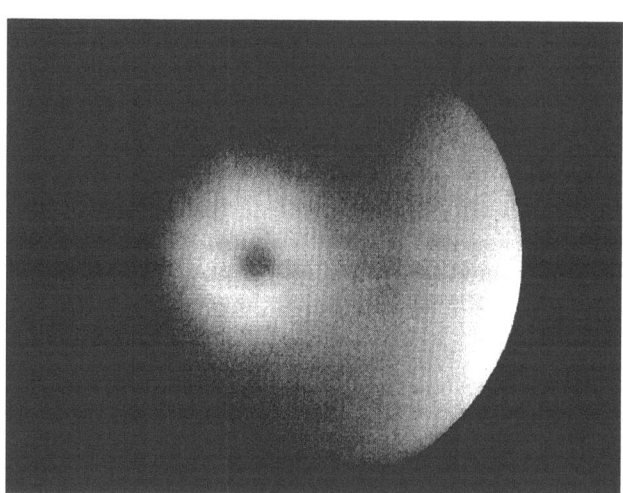

FIGURE 53.13. Cherry red macula in an infant with G_{M1} gangliosidosis.

53. Evaluation of the Neonate with a Potential Metabolic Defect

increased levels of lysosomal enzymes in plasma and urine, while they are deficient in leukocytes and fibroblasts. The phosphotransferase assay is also a sensitive and reliable way to establish the diagnosis. There is no treatment.

The phenotypic presentation of Niemann-Pick disease type C is a prolonged neonatal cholestatic jaundice. In contrast to other types of Niemann-Pick, the defect in type C is not in sphingomyelinase but in the cellular trafficking of exogenous cholesterol accumulating as unesterified cholesterol in lysosomes.[291] Although the disease becomes first symptomatic in early childhood, it may present in a neonate with ascites and early hepatosplenomegaly.[292] In the severe neonatal form, terminal hepatic failure without neurologic signs ensues rapidly during early infancy.[293] The neonate may also show early pulmonary infiltration by foam cells and will die in early infancy due to either hepatic or pulmonary failure.[294] The diagnosis is made by demonstrating the accumulation of unesterified cholesterol in the lysosomes of fibroblasts by intense perinuclear fluorescence observed on filipin staining. The disease has no treatment.

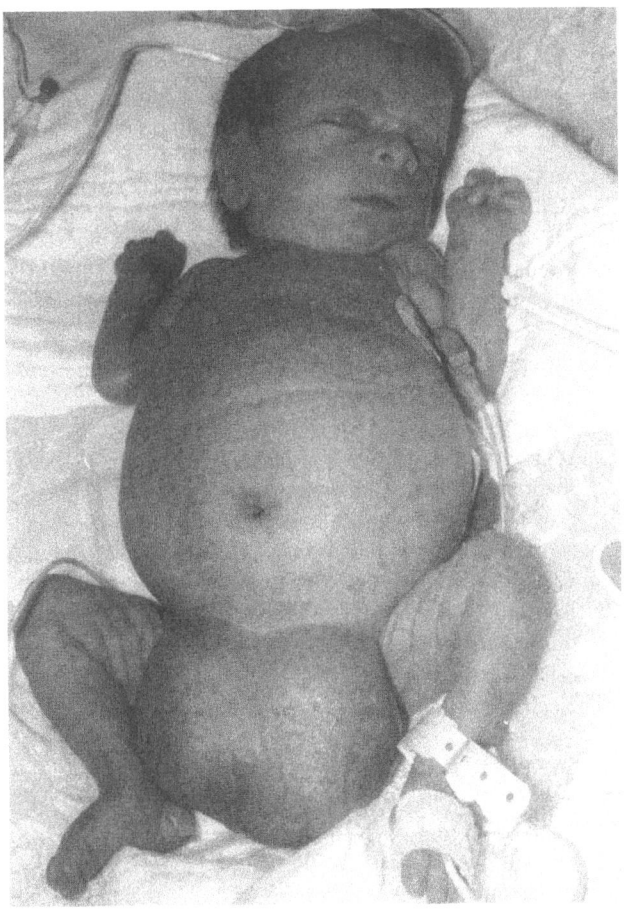

FIGURE 53.14. A neonate with galactosialidosis; severe anasarca gives her labia majora the appearance of a scrotum.

disease usually show coarse face, restricted joint movement, cardiac valvular abnormalities, generalized hypotonia, congenital hip dislocation, and bilateral talipes equinovarus. Gingival hyperplasia is striking. The picture of an infant with I-cell disease is shown in Figure 53.15. Fibroblasts of I-cell disease show characteristic membrane-bound vacuoles containing electron-lucent or fibrillogranular material from which the disease is named. The defect is in the processing of lysosomal enzymes at the endoplasmic reticulum where mannose oligosaccharides are attached, trimmed, and transferred to the Golgi apparatus. In the Golgi apparatus an α-N-acetylglucosamine-l-phosphate is attached to the mannose, with subsequent removal of the N-acetylglucosamine, leaving the phosphate on mannose as mannose-6-phosphate. Lysosomal enzymes tagged with mannose-6-phosphate can then be recognized by specific receptors on lysosomes and can be transferred into the intralysosomal compartment. In I-cell disease, the attachment of N-acetylglucosamine-l-phosphate step is defective, leading to the simultaneous deficiency of several lysosomal enzymes. The disease is readily diagnosed by

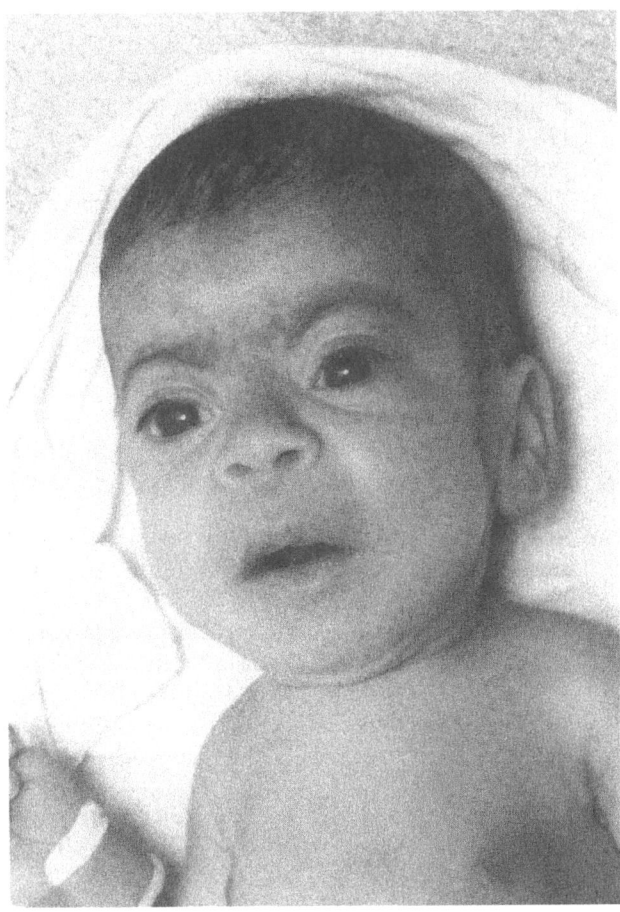

FIGURE 53.15. A neonate with "I-cell" disease showing the dysmorphic features of mucopolysaccharidosis.

References

1. Wolf B, Hsia YE, Sweetman L, et al. Propionic acidemia: a clinical update. J Pediatr 1981;99:335–346.
2. Stokke O, Eldjarn L, Norum KR, et al. Methylmalonic acidemia: a new inborn error of metabolism which may cause fatal acidosis in the neonatal period. Scand J Lab Clin Invest 1967;20:313–328.
3. Brusilow SW, Batshaw ML, Waber L. Neonatal hyperammonemic coma. Adv Pediatr 1982;29:69–103.
4. Buhrdel P, Bohme H-J, Didt L. Biochemical and clinical observations in four patients with fructose-1,6-diphospatase deficiency. Eur J Pediatr 1990;149:574–576.
5. Gitzelmann R, Hansen RG. Galactose metabolism, hereditary defects and their clinical significance. In: Burman D, Holton JB, Pennock CA, eds. Inherited disorders of carbohydrate metabolism. Baltimore: University Park Press, 1980:61–101.
6. Stanley CA. New genetic defects in mitochondrial fatty acid oxidation and carnitine deficiency. Adv Pediatr 1987;34:59–88.
7. Kuroda Y, Naito E, Takeda E, et al. Congenital lactic acidosis. Enzyme 1987;38:108–114.
8. Fisher CR, Chuang JL, Cox RP, et al. Maple syrup urine disease in Mennonites. Evidence that the Y393N mutation in E1 alpha impedes assembly of the E1 component of branched-chain alpha-keto acid dehydrogenase complex. J Clin Invest 1991;88:1034–1037.
9. Ozand PT, Al Aqeel A, Gascon G, et al. 3-Hydroxy-3-methylglutaryl-coenzyme A (HMG-CoA) lyase deficiency in Saudi Arabia. J Inherited Metab Dis 1991;14:174–188.
10. Robinson BH, MacMillan H, Petrova-Benedict R, et al. Variable clinical presentation in patients with defiective E_1 component of pyruvate dehydrogenase complex. A review of 30 cases with a defect in the E_1 component of the complex. J Pediatr 1987;111:525–533.
11. Rahbeeni Z, Ozand PT, Rashed M, et al. 4-Hydroxybutyric aciduria. Brain Dev 1994;16(suppl):64–71.
12. Peinemann F, Danner DJ. Maple syrup urine disease: 1954 to 1993. J Inherited Metab Dis 1994;17:3–15.
13. Mantovani JF, Naidich TP, Prensky AL, et al. MSUD presentation with pseudotumor cerebri and CT abnormalities. J Pediatr 1980;96:279–281.
14. Brismar J, Aqeel A, Brismar G, et al. Maple syrup urine disease: findings on CT and MR scans of the brain in 10 infants. AJNR 1990;11:1219–1228.
15. Narisawa K, Wada Y, Saito T, et al. Infantile type of homocystinuria with N5, 10-methylenetetrahydrofolate reductase defect. Tohoku J Exp Med 1977;121:185–194.
16. Mitchell G, Saudubray JM, Gubler MC, et al. Congenital anomalies in glutaric aciduria type 2. J Pediatr 1984;104:961–962.
17. Schutgens RB, Heymans HA, Wanders RJ, et al. Peroxisomal disorders: a newly recognized group of genetic diseases. Eur J Pediatr 1986;144:430–440.
18. Lui K, Commens C, Choong R, et al. Collodion babies with Gaucher's disease. Arch Dis Child 1988;63:854–856.
19. O'Brien JS. Ganglioside storage diseases. Adv Hum Genet 1972;3:39–98.
20. Stangenberg M, Lingman G, Roberts G, et al. Brief clinical report: mucopolysaccharidosis VII as a cause of fetal hydrops in early pregnancy. Am J Med Genet 1992;44:142–144.
21. Beck M, Bender SW, Reiter HL, et al. Neuraminidase deficiency presenting as non-immune hydrops fetalis. Eur J Pediatr 1984;143:135–139.
22. Kleijer WJ, Hoogeveen A, Verheijen FW, et al. Prenatal diagnosis of sialidosis with combined neuraminidase and β-galactosidase deficiency. Clin Genet 1979;16:60–61.
23. Sprigz RA, Doughty RA, Spackman TJ, et al. Neonatal presentation of I-cell disease. J Pediatr 1978;93:954–958.
24. Millington DS, Terada N, Chace DH, et al. New developments in fatty acid oxidation. In: Coates PM, Tanaka K, eds. The role of tandem mass spectrometry in the diagnosis of fatty acid oxidation disorders. New York: Wiley-Liss 1992;339–354.
25. Rashed MS, Ozand PT, Bucknall MP, et al. Diagnosis of inborn errors of metabolism from blood spots by acylcarnitines and amino acids profiling using automated electrospray tandem mass spectrometry. Pediatr Res 1995;38:324–331.
26. Ozand PT, Rashed M, Gascon GG, et al. Unusual presentations of propionic acidemia. Brain Dev 1994;16(suppl):46–57.
27. Lehnert W, Junker A, Wehinger H, et al. Propionic Ä cidamie mit Hypertrophischer Pylorusstenose und Entgleisungen im Glukosstoffwechsel. Monatsschr Kinderheilkd 1980;128:720–723.
28. Saudubray JM, Ogier H, Bonnefont JP, et al. Clinical approach to inherited metabolic diseases in the neonatal period. A 20 year survey. J Inherited Metab Dis 1989;12(suppl 1):25–41.
29. Amendt BA, Greene C, Sweetman L, et al. Short chain acyl CoA dehydrogenase deficiency. Clinical and biochemical studies in two patients. J Clin Invest 1987;79:1303–1309.
30. Gray RG, Patrick AD, Preston FE, et al. Acute hereditary tyrosinemia type 1: clinical, biochemical and haematological studies in twins. J Inherited Metab Dis 1981;4:37–40.
31. Robinson BH, Taylor J, Sherwood WG. The genetic heterogeneity of lactic acidosis: occurrence of recognizable inborn errors of metabolism in a pediatric population with lactic acidosis. Pediatr Res 1980;14:956–962.
32. Packman S, Sweetman L, Baker H, et al. The neonatal form of biotin responsive multiple carboxylase deficiency. J Pediatr 1981;99:418–420.
33. Lombes A, Romero NB, Touati G, et al. Clinical and molecular heterogeneity of cytochrome c oxidase deficiency in the newborn. J Inherited Metab Dis 1996;19:286–295.
34. Gibson KM, Nyhan WL, Sweetman L, et al. 3-Methylglutaconic aciduria: a phenotype in which the activity of 3-methylglutaconyl-coenzyme A hydratase is normal. Eur J Pediatr 1988;148:76–82.

35. Kang ES, Snodgrass PJ, Gerald PS. Ornithine transcarbamylase deficiency in the newborn infant. J Pediatr 1973;82:642–649.
36. Hommes FA, DeGroot CJ, Wilmink CW, et al. Carbamylphosphate synthetase deficiency in an infant with severe cerebral damage. Arch Dis Child 1969;44:688–693.
37. Danks DM, Tippett P, Zentner G. Severe neonatal citrullinemia. Arch Dis Child 1974;49:579–581.
38. Carton D, De Shrijver F, Kint J, et al. Argininosuccinic aciduria. Neonatal variant with rapid fatal course. Acta Paediatr Scand 1969;58:528–534.
39. Levy HL, Sepe SJ, Shih VE, et al. Sepsis due to *Escherichia coli* in neonates with galactosemia. N Engl J Med 1977;297:823–825.
40. Retbi JM, Gabilan JC, Marsac C. Acidose lactique et hypoglycémie à début néonatal par déficit congénital en fructose-1-6-diphosphatase hépatique. Arch Fr Pediatr 1975;32:367–380.
41. Romero FJ, Ibarra B, Rovira M, et al. Cerebral computed tomography in maple syrup urine disease. J Comput Assist Tomogr 1984;8:410–411.
42. Hawkins RA, Mans AM. Brain metabolism in encephalopathy caused by hyperammonemia. Adv Exp Med Biol 1994;368:11–21.
43. Miyabashi S, Ito T, Narisawa K, et al. Biochemical studies in 28 children with lactic acidosis in relation to Leigh's encephalomyelopathy. Eur J Pediatr 1985;143:278–283.
44. Rashed M, Ozand PT, Al Aqeel A, et al. Experience of King Faisal Specialist Hospital and Research Center with Saudi organic acid disorders. Brain Dev 1994;16(suppl):1–6.
45. Chavez-Carballo E. Detection of inherited neurometabolic disorders. Pediatr Neurol 1992;39:801–819.
46. Brown GK, Brown RM, Scholem RD, et al. The clinical and biochemical spectrum of human pyruvate dehydrogenase complex deficiency. Ann NY Acad Sci 1989;573:360–368.
47. Robinson BH, Oei J, Sherwood WG, et al. The molecular basis for the two different clinical presentations of classical pyruvate carboxylase deficiency. Am J Hum Genet 1984;36:283–294.
48. Hoppel CL, Kerr DS, Dahms B, et al. Deficiency of the reduced adenine dinucleotide dehydrogenase component of complex I mitochondrial electron transport. Fatal infantile lactic acidosis and hypermetabolism with skeletal-cardiac myopathy and encephalopathy. J Clin Invest 1987;80:71–77.
49. Zeviani M, Van Dyke DH, Servidei S, et al. Myopathy and fatal cardiopathy due to cytochrome c oxidase deficiency. Arch Neurol 1986;43:1198–1202.
50. Al Aqeel Rashed M, Ozand PT, et al. 3-Methylglutaconic aciduria: ten cases with a possible new phenotype. Brain Dev 1994;16(suppl):23–32.
51. Matsuo M, Ookita K, Takemine H, et al. Fatal case of pyruvate dehydrogenase deficiency. Acta Paediatr Scand 1985;74:140–142.
52. Zeviani M, Nonaka I, Bonilla E, et al. Fatal infantile mitochondrial myopathy and renal dysfunction caused by cytochrome c oxidase deficiency: immunological studies in a new patient. Ann Neurol 1985;17:414–417.
53. Bentlage HA, Wendel U, Schagger H, et al. Lethal infantile mitochondrial disease with isolated complex I deficiency in fibroblasts but with combined complex I and IV deficiencies in muscle. Neurology 1986;47:243–248.
54. Sherwood WG, Robinson BH. Dysmorphism in congenital lactic acidosis syndrome. Pediatr Res 1984;18:300A.
55. Morris AA, Leonard JV, Brown GK, et al. Deficiency of respiratory chain complex I is a common cause of Leigh disease. Ann Neurol 1996;40:25–30.
56. Stansbie D, Sherriff RJ. Fructose load test—an in vivo screening test designed to assess pyruvate dehydrogenase activity and interconversion. J Inherited Metab Dis 1978;1:163–165.
57. Saudubray JM, Marsac C, Cathelineau CL, et al. Neonatal congenital lactic acidosis with pyruvate carboxylase deficiency in two siblings. Acta Paediatr Scand 1976;65:717–724.
58. Rotig A, Cormier V, Blanche S, et al. Pearson's marrow-pancreas syndrome. A multisystem mitochondrial disorder in infancy. J Clin Invest 1990;86:1601–1608.
59. Moreadith RW, Batshaw ML, Ohnishi T, et al. Deficiency of the iron-sulfur clusters of mitochondrial reduced nicotinamide-adenine dinucleotide-ubiquinone oxidoreductase (complex I) in an infant with congenital lactic acidosis. J Clin Invest 1984;74:685–697.
60. Robinson BH, Sherwood WG. Lactic acidemia, the prevalence of pyruvate decarboxylase deficiency. J Inherited Metab Dis 1986;7(suppl 1):69–73.
61. Robinson BH: Lactic acidemia (disorders of pyruvate carboxylase, pyruvate dehydrogenase). In: Scriver CR, Beaudet AL, Sly WS, Valle D, eds. The metabolic and molecular basis of inherited disease. New York: McGraw-Hill, 1995:1479–1500.
62. Brown GK, Haan EA, Kirby DM, et al. "Cerebral" lactic acidosis: defects in pyruvate metabolism with profound brain damage and minimal systemic acidosis. Eur J Pediatr 1988;147:10–4.
63. Kodama H, Okabe I, Yanagisawa M, et al. Copper deficiency in the mitochondria of cultured skin fibroblasts from patients with Menkes syndrome. J Inherited Metab Dis 1989;12:386–389.
64. Dahl H-HM, Brown GK, Brown RM, et al. Mutations and polymorphisms in the pyruvate dehydrogenase $E_{1\alpha}$ gene. (Review). Hum Mutat 1992;1:97–102.
65. Endo H, Hasegawa K, Narisawa K. Defective gene in lactic acidosis: abnormal pyruvate dehydrogenase $E_{1\alpha}$-subunit caused by a frameshift. Am J Hum Genet 1989;44:358–364.
66. Robinson BH, MacKay N, Petrova-Benedict R, et al. Defects in the E_2 lipoyl transacetylase and X-lipoyl containing component of the pyruvate dehydrogenase complex in patients with lactic acidemia. J Clin Invest 1990;85:1821–1824.
67. Robinson BH, Oei J, Saudubray JM, et al. The French and North American phenotypes of pyruvate carboxylase deficiency, correlation with biotin containing protein by ^{3}H-biotin incorporation, ^{35}S-streptavidin labeling, and

Northern blotting with a cloned cDNA probe. Am J Hum Genet 1987;40:50–59.
68. Reed LJ. Regulation of mammalian pyruvate dehydrogenase complex by a phosphorylation-dephosphorylation cycle. Curr Top Cell Reg 1981;18:95–106.
69. Szabo P, Sheu KF, Robinson RM, et al. The gene for alpha polypeptide of pyruvate dehydrogenase is X-linked in humans. Am J Hum Genet 1990;46:874–878.
70. Olson S, Song BJ, Huh TL, et al. Three genes for enzymes of pyruvate dehydrogenase complex map to human chromosomes 3, 7 and X. Am J Hum Genet 1990;46:340–349.
71. Robinson BH, Sherwood WG. Pyruvate dehydrogenase phosphatase deficiency: a cause of chronic congenital lactic acidosis in infancy. Pediatr Res 1975;9:935–939.
72. Geoffroy V, Fouque F, Benelli C, et al. Defect in the X-lipoyl containing component of the pyruvate dehydrogenase complex in a patient with a neonatal lactic acidemia. Pediatrics 1996;97:267–272.
73. Hansen LL, Brown GK, Kirby DM. Characterization of the mutations in three patients with pyruvate dehydrogenase $E_{1\alpha}$ deficiency. J Inherited Metab Dis 1991;14:140–151.
74. DeMeirleir L, Lissens W, Benelli C, et al. Aberrant splicing of exon 6 in the pyruvate dehydrogenase-$E_{1\alpha}$ mRNA linked to a silent mutation in a large family with Leigh's encephalomyelopathy. Pediatr Res 1994;36:707–712.
75. Ando T, Rasmussen K, Nyhan WL, et al. Propionic acidemia in patients with ketotic hyperglycinemia. J Pediatr 1971;78:827–832.
76. Lindblad B, Lindblad BS, Olin P, et al. Methylmalonic acidemia: a disorder associated with acidosis, hyperglycinemia and hyperlactatemia. Acta Paediatr Scand 1968;57:417–424.
77. Spirer Z, Swirsky-Fein S, Zakut V, et al. Acute neonatal isovaleric acidemia. A report of two cases. Israel J Med Sci 1975;11:1005–1010.
78. Koboru JA, Johnston K, Sweetman L. Isolated 3-methylcrotonyl CoA carboxylase deficiency presenting as Reye-like syndrome. Pediatr Res 1989;25:142A.
79. Roth K, Cohn R, Yandrasitz J, et al. Beta-methylcrotonic aciduria associated with lactic acidosis. J Pediatr 1976;88:229–235.
80. Sherwood WG, Saunders M, Robinson BH, et al. Lactic acidosis in biotin-responsive multiple carboxylase deficiency caused by holocarboxylase synthetase deficiency of early and late onset. J Pediatr 1982;101:546–550.
81. Edery P, Gerard B, Chretien D, et al. Liver cytochrome c oxidase deficiency in a case of neonatal-onset hepatic failure. Eur J Pediatr 1994;153:190–194.
82. Baerlocher K, Gitzelmann R, Nussli R, et al. Infantile lactic acidosis due to hereditary fructose-1,6-diphosphatase deficiency. Helv Paediatr Acta 1971;26:489–506.
83. Maeska H, Komiya K, Misugi K, et al. Hyperalaninemia, hyperpyruvicemia and lactic acidosis due to pyruvate carboxylase deficiency of the liver; treatment with thiamine and lipoic acid. Eur J Pediatr 1976;122:159–168.
84. Hagenfeldt L, Larsson A, Zetterstrom R. Pyroglutamic aciduria. Studies in an infant with chronic metabolic acidosis. Acta Paediatr Scand 1974;63:1–8.
85. Wichser J, Kazemi H. Ammonia and ventilation: site and mechanism of action. Resp Physiol 1974;20:393–406.
86. Johnston K, Newth CJL, Sheu K-FR, et al. Central hypoventilation syndrome in pyruvate complex deficiency. Pediatrics 1984;74:1034–1040.
87. van der Heiden C, Gerards LJ, van Biervliét JPGM, et al. Lethal neonatal argininosuccinate lyase deficiency in four children from same sibship. Helv Paediatr Acta 1976;31:407–417.
88. Worthen HG, Al Ashwal A, Ozand PT, et al. Comparative frequency and severity of hypoglycemia in selected organic acidemias, branched-chain amino acidemia, and disorders of fructose metabolism. Brain Dev 1994;16:(suppl):81–85.
89. Halperin ML, Schiller CM, Fritz IB. The inhibition of methylmalonic acid of malate transport by the dicarboxylate carrier in rat liver mitochondria: a possible explanation for hypoglycemia in methylmalonic acidemia. J Clin Invest 1971;50:2276–2281.
90. Stumpf DA, Parker WD, Angelini C. Carnitine deficiency, organic acidemias and Reye syndrome. Neurology 1985;35:1041–1045.
91. Millington DS, Roe CR, Maltby DA. Application of high resolution fast atom bombardment and constant B/E ratio linked scanning to the identification and analysis of acylcarnitines in metabolic disease. Biomed Mass Spectr 1984;11:236–241.
92. Evangeliou A, Stumpf DA, Parks JC. Citrate synthase inhibition by acyl CoA esters. Ann Neurol 1985;18:383–384.
93. Cheema-Dhadli S, Leznoff CC, Halperin M. Effect of 2-methylcitrate on citrate metabolism: implications for the management of patients with propionic acidemia and methylmalonic aciduria. Pediatr Res 1975;9:905–908.
94. Hillman RE, Sowers LH, Cohen JL. Inhibition of glycine oxidation in cultured fibroblasts by isoleucine. Pediatr Res 1973;7:945–947.
95. Hillman RE, Otto EF. Inhibition of glycine-serine interconversion in cultured human fibroblasts by products of isoleucine catabolism. Pediatr Res 1974;8:941–945.
96. Brismar J, Ozand PT. CT and MR of the brain in the diagnosis of organic acidemias. Experiences with 107 patients. Brain Dev 1994;16(suppl):104–124.
97. Stewart PM, Walser M. Failure of normal ureagenic response to amino acids in organic acid loaded rats: A proposed mechanism for the hyperammonemia of propionic and methylmalonic acidemia. J Clin Invest 1980;66:484–492.
98. Coude FX, Sweetman L, Nyhan WL. Inhibition by propionyl CoA of N-acetylglutamate synthetase in rat liver mitochondria. A possible explanation for hyperammonemia in propionic and methylmalonic acidemia. J Clin Invest 1979;64:1544–1551.
99. Packman S, Mahoney MJ, Tanaka K, et al. Severe hyperammonemia in a newborn infant with methylmalonyl CoA mutase deficiency. J Pediatr 1978;92:769–771.
100. Wilson WG, Audenaert SM, Squillaro EJ. Hyperammonemia in a preterm infant with isovaleric acidemia. J Inherited Metab Dis 1984;7:71.

101. Mendiola J Jr, Robotham JL, Liehr JG, et al. Neonatal lethargy due to isovaleric acidemia and hyperammonemia. Tex Med 1984;80:52–54.
102. Cathelineau L, Briand P, Ogier H, et al. Occurrence of hyperammonemia in the course of 17 cases of methylmalonic acidemia. J Pediatr 1981;99:279–280.
103. Treem WR. Inherited and acquired syndromes of hyperammonemia and encephalopathy in children. (Review). Semin Liver Dis 1994;14:236–258.
104. Gjedde A, Lockwood AH, Duffy TE, et al. Cerebral blood flow and metabolism in chronically hyperammonemic rats: effect of an acute ammonia challenge. Ann Neurol 1978;3:325–330.
105. Barzilay Z, Britten AG, Koehler RC, et al. Interaction of CO_2 and ammonia on cerebral blood flow and O_2 consumption in dogs. Am J Physiol 1985;248:H500–H507.
106. Chodobski A, Szmydynger-Chodobska J, Urbanska A, et al. Intracranial pressure, cerebral blood flow and cerebrospinal fluid formation during hyperammonemia in cat. J Neurosurg 1986;65:86–91.
107. Voorhies TM, Ehrlich ME, Duffy TE, et al. Acute hyperammonemia in the young primate: physiologic and neuropathologic correlates. Pediatr Res 1983;17:970–975.
108. Takahashi H, Koehler RC, Brusilow SW, et al. Inhibition of brain glutamine accumulation prevents cerebral edema in hyperammonemic rats. Am J Physiol 1991;261:H825–H829.
109. Takahashi H, Koehler RC, Hirata T, et al. Restoration of cerebrovascular CO_2 responsitivity by glutamine synthesis inhibition in hyperammonemic rats. Circ Res 1992;71:1220–1230.
110. Jessy J, DeJoseph MR, Hawkins RA. Hyperammonemia depresses glucose consumption throughout the brain. Biochem J 1991;227:693–696.
111. Hawkins RA, Jessy J. Hyperammonemia does not impair brain function in the absence of net glutamine synthesis. Biochem J 1991;277:697–703.
112. Levin B, Abraham JM, Oberholzer VG, et al. Hyperammonemia: a deficiency of liver ornithine transcarbamylase. Occurrence in mother and child. Arch Dis Child 1969;44:152–161.
113. van der Zee SP, Trijbels JM, Monnens LA, et al. Citrullinemia with rapidly fatal neonatal course. Arch Dis Child 1971;46:847–851.
114. Connelly A, Cross JH, Gadian DG, et al. Magnetic resonance spectroscopy shows increased brain glutamine in ornithine carbamoyl transferase deficiency. Pediatr Res 1993;33:77–81.
115. Divry P, David M, Gregersen N, et al. Dicarboxylic aciduria due to medium chain acyl CoA dehydrogenase defect. A cause of hypoglycemia in childhood. Acta Paediatr Scand 1983;72:943–949.
116. Stanley CA, Hale DE, Coates PM, et al. Medium-chain acyl-CoA dehydrogenase deficiency in children with nonketotic hypoglycemia and low carnitine levels. Pediatr Res 1983;17:877–884.
117. Treem WR, Stanley CA, Hale DE, et al. Hypoglycemia, hypotonia, and cardiomyopathy: the evolving picture of long-chain acyl-CoA dehydrogenase deficiency. Pediatrics 1991;87:328–333.
118. Poll-The BT, Bonnefont JP, Ogier H, et al. Familial hypoketotic hypoglycemia associated with peripheral neuropathy, pigmented retinopathy and C_6-C_{14} hydroxydicarboxylic aciduria. A new defect in fatty acid oxidation? J Inherited Metab Dis 1988;11(suppl 2):183–185.
119. Stanley CA, Hale DE, Berry GT, et al. Brief report: a deficiency of carnitine-acylcarnitine translocase in the inner mitochondrial membrane. N Engl J Med 1992;327:19–23.
120. Niederwieser A, Steinmann B, Exner U, et al. Multiple acyl-CoA dehydrogenation deficiency (MADD) in a boy with nonketotic hypoglycemia, hepatomegaly, muscle hypotonia and cardiomyopathy: Detection of N-isovalerylglutamic acid and its monoamide. Helv Paediatr Acta 1983;38:9–26.
121. Leonard JV, Seakins JW, Bartlett K, et al. Inherited disorders of 3-methyl-crotonyl CoA carboxylation. Arch Dis Child 1981;56:53–59.
122. Labrune P, Bonnefont JP, Nihoul-Fekete CN, et al. Evaluation des méthodes diagnostiques et thérapeutiques de l'hyperinsulinisme du nouvauné et du nourisson. Arch Fr Pediatr 1989;46:167–173.
123. Brunelle F, Negre V, Barth MO, et al. Pancreatic venous sampling in infants and children with primary hyperinsulinism. Pediatr Radiol 1989;19:100–103.
124. Sweetman L. Organic acid analysis. In: Hommes FA, ed. Techniques in diagnostic human biochemical genetics. New York: Wiley-Liss, 1991:143–176.
125. Hill DW, Walther FH, Wilson TD, et al. High performance liquid chromatographic determination of amino acids in the picomole range. Anal Chem 1979;51:1338–1341.
126. Nelson K, Hsia DY. Screening for galactosemia and glucose-6-phosphate dehydrogenase deficiency in newborn infants. J Pediatr 1967;71:582–585.
127. Dahlqvist A. Test paper for galactose in urine. Scand J Clin Lab Invest 1968;22:87–93.
128. Pagliara AS, Karl IE, Keating JP, et al. Hepatic fructose-1,6-diphosphatase deficiency. A cause of lactic acidosis and hypoglycemia in infancy. J Clin Invest 1972;51:2115–2123.
129. Alexander D, Assaf M, Khudr A, et al. Fructose-1,6-diphosphatase deficiency: diagnosis using leukocytes and detection of heterozygotes with radiochemical and spectrophotometric method. J Inherited Metab Dis 1985;8:174–177.
130. Corbeel L, Eggermont E, Eeckles R, et al. Recurrent ketotic acidosis associated with fructose-1,6-diphosphatase deficiency. Acta Paediatr Belg 1976;29:29–34.
131. Steinmann B, Gitzelmann R. The diagnosis of hereditary fructose intolerance. Helv Paediatr Acta 1981;36:297–316.
132. Baker L, Winegrad AI. Fasting hypoglycaemia and metabolic acidosis associated with deficiency of hepatic fructose-1,6-diphosphatase activity. Lancet 1970;2:13–16.
133. Steinmann B, Gitzelmann R. Fruktose und sorbitol in infusionsflüssigkeiten sind nicht immer harmlos. Int Zeit Vit Ernahrungforsc 1976;15(suppl):289–294.
134. Farrell DF, Clark AF, Scott CR, et al. Absence of pyruvate decarboxylase activity in man: a cause of congenital lactic acidosis. Science 1975;187:1082–1084.

135. Haas RH, Thompson J, Morris B, et al. Pyruvate dehydrogenase activity in osmotically-shocked rat brain mitochondria: stimulation by oxaloacetate. J Neurochem 1988;50:673–680.
136. Sheu KF, Hu CC, Utter MF. Pyruvate dehydrogenase complex activity in normal and deficient fibroblasts. J Clin Invest 1981;67:1463–1471.
137. Reed LJ, Willms CR. Purification and resolution of the pyruvate dehydrogenase complex (*Escherichia coli*). Methods Enzymol 1966;9:247–265.
138. DeVivo DC, Haymond MW, Leckie MP, et al. The clinical and biochemical implications of pyruvate carboxylase deficiency. J Clin Endocrinol Metab 1977;45:1281–1296.
139. Tsuchiyama A, Oyanagi K, Hirano S, et al. A case of pyruvate carboxylase deficiency with late prenatal diagnosis of an unaffected sibling. J Inherited Metab Dis 1983;6:85–88.
140. Zheng XX, Shoffner JM, Voljavec AS, et al. Evaluation of procedures for assaying oxidative phosphorylation enzyme activities in mitochondrial myopathy muscle biopsies (review). Biochim Biophys Acta 1990;1019:1–10.
141. Benecke R, Strumper P, Weiss H. Electron transfer complex I defect in idiopathic dystonia. Ann Neurol 1992;32:683–686.
142. Land JM, Morgan-Hughes JA, Clark JB. Mitochondrial myopathy. Biochemical studies revealing a deficiency of NADH-cytochrome b reductase activity. J Neurol Sci 1981;50:1–13.
143. Shoffner JM, Wallace DC. Oxidative phosphorylation diseases. In: Scriver CR, Beaudet AL, Sly WS, Valle D, eds. The metabolic and molecular basis of inherited disease. New York: McGraw-Hill, 1995:1535–1609.
144. Webster DR, Simmons HA, Berry DMJ, et al. Pyrimidine and purine metabolites in ornithine transcarbamylase deficiency. J Inherited Metab Dis 1981;4:27–31.
145. van Gennip AH, van Bree-Blom EJ, Grift J, et al. Urinary purines and pyrimidines in patients with hyperammonemia of various origins. Clin Chim Acta 1980;104:227–239.
146. Munnich A, Saudubray JM, Taylor J, et al. Congenital lactic acidosis, alpha-ketoglutaric aciduria and variant form maple syrup urine disease due to a single enzyme defect: dihydrolipoyl dehydrogenase deficiency. Acta Paediatr Scand 1982;71:167–171.
147. Liu TC, Kim H, Arizmendi C, et al. Identification of two missense mutations in a dihydrolipoamide dehydrogenase-deficient patient. Proc Natl Acad Sci USA 1993;90:5186–5190.
148. Rashed MS, Bucknall MP, Little D, et al. Screening for inborn errors of metabolism by electrospray tandem mass spectrometry and a computer-assisted metabolic profiling algorithm for automated flagging of abnormal profiles. Clin Chem 1997;43:1129–1141.
149. Rashed MS, Ozand PT, Bennett MJ, et al. Inborn errors of metabolism diagnosed in sudden infant death cases by acylcarnitine analysis of postmortem bile. Clin Chem 1995;41:1109–1114.
150. Rashed MS, Ozand PT, Harrison ME, et al. Electrospray mass spectrometry in the diagnosis of organic acidemias. Rapid Commun Mass Spectrom 1994;8:129–133.
151. Israels S, Haworth JC, Dunn HG, et al. Lactic acidosis in childhood. Adv Pediatr 1976;22:267–303.
152. Chalmers RA. Organic acids in urine of patients with congenital lactic acidoses: an aid to differential diagnosis. J Inherited Metab Dis 1984;7(suppl):79–89.
153. Fernandes J, Berger R. Urinary excretion of lactate, 2-oxoglutarate, citrate and glycerol in patients with glycogenosis type 1. Pediatr Res 1987;21:279–282.
154. Yokota I, Indo Y, Coates PM, et al. Molecular basis of medium chain acyl-coenzyme A dehydrogenase deficiency. An A to G transition at position 985 that causes a lysine-304 to glutamate substitution in the mature protein is the single prevalent mutation. J Clin Invest 1990;86:1000–1003.
155. Tanaka K, Yokota I, Coates PM, et al. Mutations in the medium-chain acyl-CoA dehydrogenase (MCAD) gene. Hum Mutat 1992;1:271–279.
156. Matsubara Y, Narisawa K, Miyabayashi S, et al. Identification of a common mutation in patients with medium-chain acyl-CoA dehydrogenase deficiency. Biochem Biophys Res Commun 1990;171:498–505.
157. Yokota I, Coates PM, Hale DE, et al. Molecular survey of a prevalent mutation, ^{985}A-to-G transition, and identification of five infrequent mutations in the medium-chain acyl-CoA dehydrogenase (MCAD) gene in 55 patients with MCAD deficiency. Am J Hum Genet 1991;49:1280–1291.
158. Matsubara Y, Narisawa K, Tada K. Medium-chain acyl-CoA dehydrogenase deficiency: molecular aspects (review). Eur J Pediatr 1992;151:154–159.
159. Gravel RA, Mahoney MJ, Ruddle FH, et al. Genetic complementation in heterokaryons of human fibroblasts defective in cobalamin metabolism. Proc Natl Acad Sci USA 1975;72:3181–3185.
160. Willard HF, Mellman IS, Rosenberg LE. Genetic complementation among inherited deficiencies of methylmalonyl CoA mutase activity: evidence for a new class of human cobalamin mutant. Am J Hum Genet 1978;30:1–13.
161. Lindblad B, Lindstrand K, Svanberg B, et al. The effect of cobamide coenzyme in methylmalonic acidemia. Acta Paediatr Scand 1969;58:178–180.
162. Matsui SM, Mahoney MJ, Rosenberg LE. The natural history of the inherited methylmalonic acidemias. N Engl J Med 1983;308:857–861.
163. Shevell MA, Matiaszuk N, Ledley FD, et al. Varying neurological phenotypes among mut^0 and mut$^-$ patients with methylmalonyl CoA mutase deficiency. Am J Med Genet 1993;45:619–624.
164. Ando T, Rasmussen K, Wright JM, et al. Isolation and identification of methylcitrate, a major metabolic product of propionate in patients with propionic acidemia. J Biol Chem 1972;247:2200–2204.
165. Danks DM, Tipett P, Adams C, et al. Cerebro-hepatorenal syndrome of. Zellweger: a report of eight cases with comments on the incidence, the liver lesion, and a fault in pipecolic acid metabolism. J Pediatr 1975;86:382–387.
166. Northrup H, Sigman ES, Herbert AA. Exfoliative erythroderma resulting from inadequate intake of branched-chain amino acids in infants with maple syrup urine disease. Arch Dermatol 1993;129:384–385.

167. Batshaw ML, Thomas GH, Brusilow SW. New approaches to the diagnosis and treatment of inborn errors of urea synthesis. Pediatrics 1981;68:290–297.
168. Brusilow SW, Batshaw ML. Arginine therapy of argininosuccinase deficiency. Lancet 1979;1:124–127.
169. Brusilow SW, Valle DL, Batshaw ML. New pathways of nitrogen excretion in inborn errors of urea synthesis. Lancet 1979;2:452–454.
170. Millington DS, Maltby DA, Roe CR. Rapid detection of argininosuccinic aciduria and citrullinuria by fast atom bombardment and tandem mass spectrometry. Clin Chim Acta 1986;155:173–188.
171. Levy HL, Shih VE, Madigan PM, et al. Transient tyrosinemia in full-term infants. JAMA 1969;209:249–250.
172. Fernbach SA, Summons RE, Pereira WE, et al. Metabolic studies of transient tyrosinemia in premature infants. Pediatr Res 1975;9:172–176.
173. Partington MW, Mathews J. The relation of plasma tyrosine level to weight gain of premature infants. J Pediatr 1966;68:749–753.
174. Sharp HL, Lindahl JA, Freese DK, et al. A new hepato-pancreato-renal disorder resembling tyrosinemia involving neuropathy and abnormal metabolism of polyunsaturated acids. J Pediatr Gastroenterol Nutr 1988;7:167–176.
175. Sassa S, Fujita H, Kappas A. Succinylacetone and delta-aminolevulinic acid dehydratase in hereditary tyrosinemia; immunochemical study of the enzyme. Pediatrics 1990;86:84–86.
176. Strife CF, Zuroweste EL, Emmett EA, et al. Tyrosinemia with acute intermittent porphyria: aminolevulinic acid dehydratase deficiency related to elevated urinary aminolevulinic acid levels. J Pediatr 1977;90:400–404.
177. Roth KS, Carter BE, Higgins ES. Succinylacetone effects on renal tubular phosphate metabolism: a model for experimental renal Fanconi syndrome. Proc Soc Exp Biol Med 1991;196:428–431.
178. Gitzelmann R, Hansen RG. Galactose metabolism, hereditary defects and their clinical significance. In: Burman D, Holton JB, Pennock CA, eds. Baltimore: University Park Press, 1980:61–101.
179. Richardson RM, Little JA, Patten RL, et al. Pathogenesis of acidosis in hereditary fructose intolerance. Metabolism 1979;28:1133–1138.
180. Norgaard-Pedersen B. Towards acceptable practices for antenatal and neonatal screening for disease or disease risk. Clin Genet 1994;46:152–159.
181. Seashore MR. Neonatal screening for inborn errors of metabolism: update (review). Semin Perinatol 1990;14:431–438.
182. Lemieux B, Auray-Blais C, Giguere R, et al. Newborn urine screening experience with over one million infants in the Quebec network of genetic medicine. J Inherited Metab Dis 1988;11:45–55.
183. Grenier A, Morisette J, Dussault JH, et al. Hereditary metabolic diseases in Quebec: blood screening. Union Med Canada 1980;109:591–595.
184. Mathias D, Bickel H. Follow-up study of 16 years neonatal screening for inborn errors of metabolism in West Germany. Eur J Pediatr 1986;145:310–312.
185. Alm J, Larsson A. Evaluation of nation-wide neonatal metabolic screening programme in Sweden 1965–1979. Acta Paediatr Scand 1981;70:601–607.
186. Bennett AJ. New England regional newborn screening program. N Engl J Med 1977;197:1178–1179.
187. Farriaux JP. Results of screening for phenylketonuria in France. Presse Med 1987;16:1072–1074.
188. Dhondt JL, Farriaux JP, Sailly JC. Economic evaluation of cost-benefit ratio of neonatal screening procedure for phenylketonuria and hypothyroidism. J Inherited Metab Dis 1991;14:633–639.
189. Briard ML. Neonatal screening for phenylketonuria and hypothyroidism in France. A 12 year experience. Ann Biol Clin 1988;46:387–392.
190. Misuma H, Wada H, Kawakami M, et al. Galactose and galactose-1-phosphate spot test for galactosemia screening. Clin Chim Acta 1981;111:27–32.
191. Bowing FG, Brown AR. Development of a protocol for newborn screening for disorders of the galactose metabolic pathway. J Inherited Metab Dis 1986;9:99–104.
192. Wolf B. Worldwide survey of neonatal screening for biotinidase deficiency. J Inherited Metab Dis 1991;14:923–927.
193. Naylor EW. Newborn screening for maple syrup urine disease. In: Therell BL, ed. Laboratory methods for neonatal screening. Washington DC: American Public Health Association, 1993:115–124.
194. Wilcken B, Wiley V, Sherry G, et al. Neonatal screening for cystic fibrosis: a comparison of two strategies for case detection in 1.2 million babies. J Pediatr 1995;127:965–970.
195. Gruters A, Delange F, Giovanelli G, et al. Guidelines for neonatal screening programs for congenital hypothyroidism. European Society for Pediatric Endocrinology Working Group on Congenital Hypothyroidism. Horm Res 1994;41:1–2.
196. Kelnar CJ. Congenital adrenal hyperplasia (CAH)—the place for prenatal treatment and neonatal screening. Early Hum Dev 1993;35:81–90.
197. Kaplan M, Hammerman C, Kvit R, et al. Neonatal screening for glucose-6-phosphate dehydrogenase deficiency: sex distribution. Arch Dis Child 1994;71:F59–60.
198. Rosenberg T, Jacobs HK, Thompson R, et al. Cost-effectiveness of neonatal screening for Duchenne muscular dystrophy—how does this compare to existing neonatal screening for metabolic disorders. Soc Sci Med 1993;37:541–547.
199. Jakobs C, van den Heuvel CM, Stellaard F, et al. Diagnosis of Zellweger syndrome by analysis of very long-chain fatty acids in stored blood spots collected at neonatal screening. J Inherited Metab Dis 1993;16:63–66.
200. Henderson SJ, Fishlock K, Horn ME, et al. Neonatal screening for hemoglobin variants using filter-paper dried blood specimens. Clin Lab Hematol 1991;13:327–334.
201. Wilcken DE, Blades BL, Dudman NP. A neonatal screening approach to the detection of familial hypercholesterolaemia and family-based coronary prevention (review). J Inherited Metab Dis 1988;11(suppl):87–90.
202. Woods WG, Lemieux B, Leclerc JM, et al. Screening for neuroblastoma (NB) in North America: the Quebec project. Prog Clin Biol Res 1994;385:377–382.

203. Coulombe JT, Shih VE, Levy HL. Massachusetts metabolic disorders screening program. II. Methylmalonic aciduria. Pediatrics 1981;67:26–31.
204. Millington DS, Kodo N, Norwood DL, et al. Tandem mass spectrometry: a new method for acylcarnitine profiling with potential for neonatal screening for inborn errors of metabolism. J Inherited Metab Dis 1990;13:321–324.
205. Naylor E. Disorders detected by the expanded supplemental newborn screening program at Neo Gen Screening Inc. Third International Meeting of the Society for Neonatal Screening, Boston, MA, October 21–24, 1996.
206. Ozand PT, Rashed MS. Tandem mass spectrometry with computer-assisted metabolic profiling in screening for inborn errors of metabolism. Fourth Asian-European Workshop on Inborn Errors of Metabolism, Munich, Germany, August 25–September 1, 1996.
207. Ozand PT, Rashed MS. Results of neonatal and selective screening in Saudi Arabia during a period of nine months; new experience gained. Fourth Asian-European Workshop on Inborn Errors of Metabolism, Munich, Germany, August 25–September 1, 1996.
208. Barns RJ, Bowling FG, Brown G, et al. Carnitine in dried blood spots: a method suitable for neonatal screening. Clin Chim Acta 1991;197:27–33.
209. Ziadeh R, Hoffman EP, Finegold DN, et al. Medium-chain acyl-CoA dehydrogenase deficiency in Pennsylvania: neonatal screening shows high incidence and unexpected mutation frequencies. Pediatr Res 1995;37:675–678.
210. Lehnert W. Long-term results of selective screening for inborn errors of metabolism. Eur J Pediatr 1994;153(suppl 1):S9–13.
211. Duran M, Dorland L, De Bree PK, et al. Selective screening for amino acid disorders. Eur J Pediatr 1994;153(suppl 1):S33–37.
212. Duran M, Dorland L, Wadman SK, et al. Group tests for selective screening of inborn errors of metabolism. Eur J Pediatr 1994;153(suppl 1):S27–32.
213. Hoffman GF. Selective screening for inborn errors of metabolism—past, present, and future (review). Eur J Pediatr 1994;153(suppl 1):S2–8.
214. Stacpoole PW. Lactic acidosis: the case against bicarbonate therapy. Ann Intern Med 1986;105:276–279.
215. Bartlett K, Ghneim HK, Stirk JH, et al. Pyruvate carboxylase deficiency. J Inherited Metab Dis 1984;7(suppl 1):74–78.
216. Oizumi J, Shaw KN, Giudici TA, et al. Neonatal pyruvate carboxylase deficiency with renal tubular acidosis and cystinuria. J Inherited Metab Dis 1983;6:89–94.
217. Sagy M, Barzilay Z, Barash V, et al. Congenital lactic acidosis associated with pyruvate carboxylase deficiency. Isr J Med Sci 1981;17:1159–1163.
218. Haworth JC, Robinson BH, Perry TL. Lactic acidosis due to pyruvate carboxylase deficiency. J Inherited Metab Dis 1981;4:57–58.
219. Murphy JV, Isohashi F, Weinberg MB, et al. Pyruvate carboxylase deficiency: an alleged biochemical cause of Leigh's disease. Pediatrics 1981;68:401–404.
220. Corr PB, Creer MH, Yamada KA, et al. Prophylaxis of early ventricular fibrillation by inhibition of acylcarnitine accumulation. J Clin Invest 1989;83:927–936.
221. Hug G, Bove KE, Soukup S. Lethal multiorgan deficiency of carnitine palmitoyl-transferase II. N Engl J Med 1991;325:1862–1864.
222. Tein I, DeVivo DC, Bierman F, et al. Impaired skin fibroblast carnitine uptake in primary systemic carnitine deficiency manifested by childhood carnitine-responsive cardiomyopathy (review). Pediatr Res 1990;28:247–255.
223. Thompson GN, Chalmers RA. Increased urinary metabolite excretion during fasting in disorders of propionate metabolism. Pediatr Res 1990;27:413–416.
224. Saudubray JM, Ogier H, Charpentier C, et al. Neonatal management of organic acidurias. Clinical update. J Inherited Metab Dis 1984;7(suppl 1):2–9.
225. Kalloghlian A, Gleispach H, Ozand PT. A patient with propionic acidemia managed with continuous insulin infusion and total parenteral nutrition. J Child Neurol 1992;7(suppl):S88–91.
226. Thompson GN, Chalmers RA, Walter JH, et al. The use of metronidazole in the management of methylmalonic and propionic acidemias. Eur J Pediatr 1990;149:792–796.
227. Roe CR, Bohan TP. L-carnitine therapy in propionic acidemia. Lancet 1982;1:1411–1412.
228. Roe CR, Hoppel CL, Stacey TE, et al. Metabolic response to carnitine in methylmalonic aciduria. An effective strategy for elimination of propionyl groups. Arch Dis Child 1983;58:916–920.
229. Wolff JA, Carroll JE, Le Phuc Thuy, et al. Carnitine reduces fasting ketogenesis in patients with disorders of propionate metabolism. Lancet 1986;1:289–291.
230. van der Meer SB, Poggi F, Spada M, et al. Clinical outcome of long-term management of patients with vitamin B_{12}-unresponsive methylmalonic acidemia. J Pediatr 1994;125:903–908.
231. Goda S, Hamada T, Ishimoto S, et al. Clinical improvement after administration of coenzyme Q10 in a patient with mitochondrial encephalomyopathy. J Neurol 1987;234:62–63.
232. Bresolin N, Bet L, Binda A, et al. Clinical and biochemical correlations in mitochondrial myopathies treated with coenzyme Q10. Neurology 1988;38:892–899.
233. Stacpoole PW, Harman EM, Curry SH, et al. Treatment of lactic acidosis with dichloroacetate. N Engl J Med 1983;309:390–396.
234. Stacpoole PW, Lorenz AC, Thomas RG, et al. Dichloroacetate in the treatment of lactic acidosis. Ann Intern Med 1988;108:58–63.
235. Donn SM, Swartz RD, Thoene JG. Comparison of exchange transfusion, peritoneal dialysis and hemodialysis for the treatment of hyperammonemia in an anuric newborn infant. J Pediatr 1979;95:67–70.
236. Wiegand C, Thompson T, Bock GH, et al. The management of life-threatening hyperammonemia: a comparison of several therapeutic modalities. J Pediatr 1980;96:142–144.
237. Brusilow W, Tinker J, Batshaw ML. Amino acid acylation: a mechanism of nitrogen excretion in inborn errors of urea synthesis. Science 1980;207:659–661.
238. James MO, Smith RL, Williams RT, et al. The conjugation of phenylacetic acid in man, sub-human primates and some non-primate species. Proc R Soc Lond [B] 1972;182:25–35.

239. Brusilow SW. Phenylacetylglutamine may replace urea as a vehicle for waste nitrogen excretion. Pediatr Res 1991; 29:147–150.
240. Rating D, Hanefeld F, Siemes H, et al. 4-Hydroxybutyric aciduria: a new inborn error of metabolism. I. Clinical review. J Inherited Metab Dis 1984;7(suppl 1):90–92.
241. Brown GK, Cromby CH, Manning NJ, et al. Urinary organic acids in succinic semialdehyde dehydrogenase deficiency: evidence of alpha-oxidation of 4-hydroxy-butyric acid, interaction of succinic semialdehyde with pyruvate dehydrogenase and possible secondary inhibition of mitochondrial beta-oxidation. J Inherited Metab Dis 1987;10:367–375.
242. Jakobs C, Michael T, Jaeger E, et al. Further evaluation of vigabatrin therapy in 4-hydroxybutyric aciduria. Eur J Pediatr 1992;151:466.
243. Gibson KM, DeVivo DC, Jakobs C. Vigabatrin therapy in patient with succinic semialdehyde dehydrogenase deficiency. Lancet 1989;2:1105–1106.
244. Snead OC. Gamma hydroxybutyrate. Life Sci 1977;20:1935–1944.
245. Langan TJ, Pueschel SM. Nonketotic hyperglycinemia: clinical, biochemical, and therapeutic considerations (review). Cur Probl Pediatr 1983;13:1–30.
246. Dobyns WB. Agenesis of corpus callosum and gyral malformations are frequent manifestations of nonketotic hyperglycinemia. Neurology 1989;39:817–820.
247. Von Wendt L, Similä S, Saukkonen A-L, et al. Prenatal brain damage in nonketotic hyperglycinemia. Am J Dis Child 1981;135:1072.
248. Perry TL, Urquhart N, Maclean J, et al. Nonketotic hyperglycinemia. Glycine accumulation due to absence of glycine cleavage in brain. N Engl J Med 1975;292:1269–1273.
249. Wolff JA, Kulovich S, Yu AL, et al. The effectiveness of benzoate in the management of seizures in nonketotic hyperglycinemia. Am J Dis Child 1986;140:596–602.
250. Schmitt B, Steinmann B, Gitzelmann R, et al. Nonketotic hyperglycinemia: clinical and electrophysiologic effects of dextromethorphan, an antagonist of the NMDA receptor. Neurology 1993;43:421–424.
251. Hamosh A, McDonald JW, Valle D, et al. Dextromethorphan and high-dose benzoate therapy for nonketotic hyperglycinemia in an infant. J Pediatr 1992;121:131–135.
252. Scriver CR, White A, Sprague W, et al. Plasma-CSF glycine ratios in normal and nonketotic hyperglycinemia subjects. N Engl J Med 1975;293:778.
253. Brandt NJ, Rasmussen K, Brandt S, et al. D-glyceric acidemia, and non-ketotic hyperglycinaemia. Clinical and biochemical findings in a new syndrome. Acta Paediatr Scand 1976;65:17–22.
254. Nishimura M, Yoshino K, Tomita Y, et al. Central and peripheral nervous system pathology of homocystinuria due to 5,10-methylenetetrahydrofolate reductase deficiency. Ped Neurol 1985;1:375–378.
255. Harpey JP, Rosenblatt DS, Cooper BA, et al. Homocystinuria caused by 5,10-methylenetetrahydrofolate reductase deficiency. A case in an infant responding to methionine, folinic acid, and pyridoxine and vitamin B_{12} therapy. J Pediatr 1981;98:275–278.
256. Wendel U, Bremer HJ. Betaine in the treatment of homocystinuria due to 5,10-methylene THF reductase deficiency. Eur J Pediatr 1984;142:147–150.
257. Watkins D, Rosenblatt DS. Functional methionine synthase deficiency (cblE and cblG): clinical and biochemical heterogeneity (review). J Med Genet 1989;34:427–434.
258. Danks DM, Campbell PE, Stevens BJ, et al. Menkes' kinky hair syndrome: an inherited defect in copper absorption with widespread effects. Pediatrics 1972;50:188–201.
259. Aukett A, Bennett MJ, Hosking GP. Molybdenum cofactor deficiency: an easily missed inborn error of metabolism. Dev Med Child Neurol 1988;30:531–535.
260. Brown GK, Scholem RD, Croll HB, et al. Sulfite oxidase deficiency: clinical, neuroradiologic, and biochemical features in two new patients. Neurology 1989;39:252–257.
261. Shih VE, Abroms IF, Johnson JL, et al. Sulfite oxidase deficiency. Biochemical and clinical investigations of a hereditary metabolic disorder in sulfur metabolism. N Engl J Med 1977;297:1022–1028.
262. Sherwood G, Sarkar B, Sass Kortsak A. Copper histidinate therapy in Menkes' disease. Prevention of progressive neurodegeneration. J Inherited Metab Dis 1989;12(suppl 2):393–396.
263. Wilson GN, Holmes RG, Custer J, et al. Zellweger syndrome: diagnostic assays, syndrome delineation, and potential therapy. Am J Med Genet 1986;24:69–82.
264. Aubourg P, Scotto J, Rocchiccioli F, et al. Neonatal adrenoleukodystrophy. J Neurol Neurosurg Psychiatry 1986;49:77–86.
265. Heymans HS, Oorthuys JW, Nelck G, et al. Rhizomelic chondrodysplasia punctata: another peroxisomal disorder. N Engl J Med 1985;313:187–188.
266. Spranger JW, Opitz JM, Bidder U. Heterogeneity of chondrodysplasia punctata. Humangenetik 1971;11:190–212.
267. Happle R. X-linked dominant chondrodysplasia punctata. Review of literature and report of a case. Hum Genet 1979;53:65–73.
268. Curry CJ, Magenis RE, Brown M, et al. Inherited chondrodysplasia punctata due to a deletion of the terminal short arm of an X-chromosome. N Engl J Med 1984;311:1010–1015.
269. Lazarow PH, Fujiki Y. Biogenesis of peroxisomes. Annu Rev Cell Biol 1985;1:489–530.
270. Lazarow PB, Robbi M, Fujiki Y, et al. Biogenesis of peroxisomal proteins in vivo and in vitro. Ann NY Acad Sci 1982;386:285–300.
271. Yajima S, Suzuki T, Shimozawa N, et al. Complementation study of peroxisome-deficient disorders by immunofluorescence staining and characterization of fused cells. Hum Genet 1992;88:491–499.
272. Shimozawa N, Tsukamoto T, Suzuki Y, et al. A human gene responsible for Zellweger syndrome that affects peroxisomal assembly. Science 1992;255:1132–1134.
273. Gartner J, Moser H, Valle D. Mutations in the 70 K peroxisomal membrane protein gene in Zellweger syndrome. Nature Genet 1992;1:16–23.
274. Santos MJ, Imanaka T, Shio H, et al. Peroxisomal membrane ghosts in Zellweger syndrome—aberrant organelle assembly. Science 1988;239:1536–1538.

275. Goldfischer S, Collins J, Rapin I, et al. Peroxisomal defects in the neonatal onset and X-linked adrenoleukodystrophy. Science 1985;227:67–70.
276. Suzuki Y, Orii T, Mori M, et al. Deficient activities and proteins of peroxisomal β-oxidation enzymes in infants with Zellweger syndrome. Clin Chim Acta 1986;156:191–196.
277. Evrard P, Caviness VS Jr., Prats-Vinas J, et al. The mechanism of arrest of neuronal migration in the Zellweger malformation: an hypothesis bases upon cytoarchitectonic analysis. Acta Neuropathol (Berl) 1978;41:109–117.
278. Martinez M. Abnormal profiles of polyunsaturated fatty acids in the brain, liver, kidney, and retina of patients with peroxisomal disorders. Brain Res 1992;583:171–182.
279. Martinez M. Severe deficiency of docosahexaenoic acid in peroxisomal disorders. A defect of delta-4 desaturations? Neurology 1990;40:1292–1298.
280. Wanders RJ, Romeyn GJ, van Roermund CWT, et al. Identification of L-pipecolate oxidase in human liver and its deficiency in the Zellweger syndrome. Biochem Biophys Res Commun 1988;154:33–38.
281. Hanson RF, Szczepanick-vanLeeuwen P, Williams GC, et al. Defects of bile acid synthesis in Zellweger's syndrome. Science 1979;203:1107–1108.
282. Rocchiccioli F, Aubourg P, Bougneres PF. Medium- and long-chain dicarboxylic aciduria in patients with Zellweger syndrome and neonatal adrenoleukodystrophy. Pediatr Res 1986;20:62–66.
283. Hoefler G, Hoefler S, Watkins PA, et al. Biochemical abnormalities in rhizomelic chondrodysplasia punctata. J Pediatr 1988;112:726–733.
284. Goodman SI, Frerman FE. Glutaric acidemia type II (multiple acyl-CoA dehydrogenation deficiency). J Inherited Metab Dis 1984;7(suppl 1):33–37.
285. Loehr JP, Goodman SI, Frerman FE. Glutaric acidemia type II: heterogeneity of clinical and biochemical phenotypes. Pediatr Res 1990;27:311–315.
286. Harpey JP, Charpentier C, Goodman SI, et al. Multiple acyl-CoA dehydrogenase deficiency occurring in pregnancy and caused by a defect in riboflavin metabolism in the mother. Study of a kindred with seven deaths in infancy. Value of riboflavin therapy in preventing this syndrome. J Pediatr 1983;103:394–398.
287. Hoffman G, Gibson KM, Brandt IK, et al. Mevalonic aciduria—an inborn error of cholesterol and nonsterol isoprene biosynthesis. N Engl J Med 1986;314:1610–1614.
288. Jaeken J, Stibler H, Hagberg B. The carbohydrate-deficient glycoprotein syndrome: a new inherited multisystemic disease with severe nervous system involvement. Acta Paediatr Scand 1991;suppl 375:1–71.
289. Weaver DD, Graham CB, Thomas IT, et al. A new overgrowth syndrome with accelerated skeletal maturation, unusual face and camptodactyly. J Pediatr 1974;84:547–552.
290. Jaeken J, van Eijk HG, van der Heul C, et al. Sialic acid-deficient serum and cerebrospinal fluid transferrin in a newly recognized genetic syndrome. Clin Clim Acta 1984;144:245–247.
291. Vanier MT, Rodriguez-Lafrasse C, Rousson R, et al. Type C Niemann-Pick disease: spectrum of phenotypic variation in disruption of intracellular LDL-derived cholesterol processing. Biochim Biophys Acta 1991;1096:328–337.
292. Manning DJ, Price WI, Pearse RG. Fetal ascites: an unusual presentation of Niemann-Pick disease type C. Arch Dis Child 1990;65:335–336.
293. Rutledge JC. Progressive neonatal liver failure due to type C Niemann-Pick disease. Pediatr Pathol 1989;9:779–784.
294. Pin I, Pradines S, Pincemaille O, et al. Forme respiratoire mortelle de maladie de Niemann-Pick Type C. Arch Fr Pediatr 1990;47:373–375.

Index

A

ABCA. *See* Automated Breath Carbon Analyzer
ABO incompatibility, 867
  and hyperbilirubinemia, 872
Absorption
  cholesterol during pregnancy, 228–229
  copper, and zinc impairment of absorption, 917, 921
  fat, 221–222, 228–229, 835–836
  glucose, renal absorption of, 122–123
  intestinal fat, 98
  magnesium, 285–287, 887–891, 890
  medium-chain fatty acids, 1015
  phosphorus, 885
  retinol, 946–947
  vitamin A, 946–947
  vitamin E, 960
ACE. *See* Angiotensin-converting enzyme
A-cell function
  and diabetes mellitus, 161
  hormonal influences, 158
Aceruloplasminemia
  copper metabolism defect, 922–923
  iron metabolism defect, 916
Acetyl-CoA, fatty acid oxidation in neonate, 610, 615, 847
Acid-base regulation, maternal/fetal placental, 466–470
  and bicarbonate, 467–468
  and buffers, 469
  and carbon dioxide, 467–471
  imbalance, causes of, 470, 471
Acidemia, and maternal/fetal acid-base balance, 470
α-acid glucoside deficiency (Type II), 756–758
  cardiac studies, 756
  diagnosis of, 757
  differential diagnosis, 756–757
  genetic factors, 757
  laboratory studies, 756
  pathogenesis, 757
  pathology, 757
  signs of, 756
  treatment of, 757
  X-ray findings, 756
Acidosis, and maternal/fetal acid-base balance, 470
Acoustical method, body composition measure, 1085
Acrodermatitis enteropathica, 928–929
  and zinc deficiency, 288, 928–929
ACTH
  and cortisol formation, 169
  and cortisol secretion, 170
  and skeletal muscle, 663
Activin, 415
Activity
  and energy metabolism in neonate, 1014–1015
  reduced activity effects, 316–317
  See also Exercise
Acute care, for metabolic disease, 1222–1224
Acute metabolic decompensation, management of, 1222–1225
  and carnitine therapy, 1222
  and infant formulas, 1224
  treatment of, 1224–1225
Acyl-CoA
  in fatty acid oxidation in neonate, 609
  in lipid metabolism, 556–557
Adenine nucleotide translocase (ANT)
  deficiency, signs of, 656
  skeletal muscle, 655–656
Adenohypophysial hormones, ontogeny of, 430
Adenohypophysis, 429–430
Adenomatosis, 693–694
Adenosine
  and ductus arteriosus after birth, 504
  and lipid metabolism, 99–100
  thermoregulation inhibition, 1034
Adenosine diphosphate (ADP)
  conversion from ATP, 537
  Krebs cycle regulation, 558
Adenosine monophosphate deaminase (AMPD)
  deficiency, signs of, 658
  skeletal muscle, 657–658
Adenosine triphosphate (ATP)
  brain, fetus/neonate, 537–539, 541
  conversion to ADP, 537
  and exercise, 325, 326
  and galactose metabolism, 723–724
  heart, production/utilization of, 551, 558–559, 561
  and lipid metabolism, 557
  and liver gluconeogenesis in neonate, 606–607
  oxidative phosphorylation, 537–538
  and phosphorous, 884
  and protein metabolism in neonate, 778
  skeletal muscle metabolism, 644, 654–655
  stability of concentration, 537
Adenylate cyclase, measurement of, 62
Adenylate kinase reaction, ADP to ATP conversion, 537
Adipocytes, and fatty acids, 147
Adipose tissue
  brown, 827–828, 1031–1032
  and triglycerides, 99
  white, 826–827
Adolase, skeletal muscle, 652–653
Adrenal gland
  congenital defect of, 426
  development of, 425–426
  steroid hormone synthesis/secretion, 426
Adrenal hyperplasia, 426, 695

Adrenaline. *See* Epinephrine
α-adrenergic receptors, 440
   and catecholamines, 162, 164, 440
   and growth hormone, 166
   subtypes of, 162, 440
β-adrenergic receptor kinases, 444, 445
β-adrenergic receptors, 440–445
   and catecholamines, 162, 164
   desensitization of, 444–445
   hormonal regulation of, 441–444
   subtypes of, 441
Adrenocorticotropin. *See* ACTH
Adult, cardiac output in, 493–496
AF. *See* Amniotic fluid
Afterload changes, and cardiac output, 495–496
Agarose gels, protein separation, 48
Age
   and lung surfactant, 570
   and protein synthesis, 106
   and thermoregulation, 1037–1038
AIB. *See* Aminoisobutyric acid
Alanine
   and glucose metabolism, 92
   metabolism in pregnancy, 210–211
Albumin
   and fatty acid transfer to fetus, 391
   fatty acid transfer to heart, 552
Alcohol consumption, and fetal growth, 1088–1089
Aldolase
   deficiency, signs of, 653
   skeletal muscle, 652–653
Aldosterone, and sodium metabolism in pregnancy, 282
Allantoic fluid (ALLF), 522
ALLF. *See* Allantoic fluid
Altitude
   and fetal growth retardation, 1101
   and fetal respiration, 473
Alveofact, 585
Alveolar type II cells
   fetal lung development, 576
   surfactant reentry to, 569
   surfactant secretion, 568
   surfactant synthesis, 567–568
Ames Glucometer Elite, glucose measure, 687
Amino acid metabolism
   branched-chain amino acids, 802–804
   in heart, 557, 560
   in neonate, 791
   and skeletal muscle, 660–661
Amino acid/organic acid metabolism disorders
   and ammonia, 804
   brain damage, mechanisms for, 805
   and branched-chain amino acid metabolism, 802–804
   developmental factors, 799–800
   diagnostic approach, 1214–1215, 1218–1221
   glutaric acidemia, Type I, 810
   glutaric acidemia, Type II, 810
   and glycine metabolism, 801–802
   isovaleric acidemia, 809–810
   maple syrup urine disease, 810–812
   methylmalonic acidemia, 808–809
   multiple carboxylase deficiency, 807–808
   nonketotic hyperglycinemia, 812
   prognosis, 804–805
   propionic acidemia, 806–807
   screening programs, 1217–1218
   signs in neonate, 804
   treatment approaches, 804
   and urea cycle, 801
   urea synthesis disorders, 805–806
Amino acids
   branched-chain, 108–109
   and codons, 42
   in enteral feeding, 1167–1168
   essential amino acids, 791, 1013
   as fatty acid synthesis precursor, 394
   fetal nitrogen accretion, 373–375
   and glucagon secretion, 158
   kinetic experiments in fetus, 371–373
   neonatal requirements, 791–792
   in parenteral feeding, 1161–1162
   and parenteral nutrition, 792
   placental transport, 1099–1100
   and protein synthesis in pregnancy, 207–209
   protein turnover as recycling of, 112
   tracer studies, 776–777
   uptake and liver, 93
Amino acid kinetics, 383–384
Amino acid transporters, 384
Aminoisobutyric acid (AIB), 384
Amino-oxyacetate, effect on glutamine, 634
Aminosyn PF, 1162
Ammonia
   in amino acid metabolism disorders, 804
   and urea cycle, 801
   See also Hyperammonemia
Amniotic fluid (AF), 522–524
   and brain natriuretic peptide, 524
   functions of, 522
   hormones/peptides in, 523–525
   reserve function, 523
   retinol in, 945
   volume changes, 523
AMPD. *See* Adenosine monophosphate deaminase
Amylin, 171
   and insulin-resistance, 171
Amylopectinosis brancher deficiency (Type IV), 758–759
   course of disease, 758
   diagnosis of, 758
   genetic factors, 758
   laboratory findings, 758
   pathology of, 758
   treatment of, 759
Anaerobic threshold, definition of, 326
Androgens, fetal protection from maternal, 427
Androstenedione, 427
Anemia
   and hydrops fetalis, 525
   iron deficiency, 290, 291
   maternal, placental effects, 459
Angiotensin-converting enzyme (ACE), 521–522
Angiotensin-converting enzyme inhibitors, effects on fetus, 521–522
Angiotensin-II
   maternal/fetal placental blood flow mediation, 463
   and renal function, 522, 1053
Animal models
   bioengineered rodents, use of, 82–83
   cardiac output, 493–494
   fetal cardiac output, 491, 492, 493–494
   fetal growth studies, farm animals, 83–86
   and fetal macrosomia study, 81–82
   glucose metabolism in pregnancy, 199–200
   human versus nonhuman differences, 80
   ideal model, features of, 80–81, 87
   intrauterine growth retardation (IUGR), 382–383
   organ systems study, 80
   placental studies, 80–81
   usefulness of, 79
   variation of metabolic factors among mammals, 86–87
ANT. *See* Adenine nucleotide translocase
Anthropometric measurements, 1080–1082
Antibodies, in immunoassays, 28–29
Anticoagulants, 955–956
Antidiuretic hormone
   and neonate, 1058–1059
   and water/electrolyte balance, 1053–1054
Apo A-I, 230–231
Apo A-II, 230–231
Apoptosis, 406
Aquaporins, 513–516
   sites of expression, 514
Arachidonic acid, 259, 263
   cascade, 261, 262

Index

and fetal growth, 265–267
during labor, 265, 266
ARAT, 947
A-retinol acyltransferase. *See* ARAT
Arginine therapy, for urea synthesis disorders, 806
Arginine vasopressin
and neonate, 1058–1059
stimulators for release, 1054
and water channels, 513
and water/electrolyte metabolism, 1053–1054
Argininosuccinic aciduria, 1211
case example, 1211
laboratory findings, 1211
treatment of, 1211
Ariboflavinosis, signs of, 982
Arsenic, deficiency features, 934
Artificial placenta, 476
Asphyxia
and hypocalcemia, 893
infant of diabetic mother, 1116–1117
Aspirin therapy, and preeclampsia prevention, 269
Asymmetrical growth retardation, 1097, 1098
ATP. *See* Adenosine triphosphate
Atrial natriuretic peptide, 511–512
actions of, 512, 1054
maternal/fetal placental blood flow mediation, 464
in neonate, 1059
during pregnancy, 512
sites of secretion, 1054
and sodium balance, 281
and water/electrolyte metabolism, 1054
Autocrine secretion, growth factor stimulation, 403–404
Automated Breath Carbon Analyzer (ABCA), 18
Autoradiogram, 66–67
Avogadro's number, 1046

B

Baroflex regulation, fetal circulation, 497
Bartter's syndrome, 884
Basal metabolic rate (BMR), in pregnancy, 312
Basic fibroblast growth factors (bFGF), and morphogenesis, 407
Baylor College of Medicine Human Genome Center, Web site, 45
Beckwith-Wiedemann syndrome, 379
and hypoglycemia in neonate, 693
physical signs, 695
Behavioral problems, and galactosemia, 729
Bekman CX 7 analyzer, glucose measure, 687
Bergman minimal model technique, 187
Beriberi, thiamine deficiency, 980, 981
Bicarbonate, and acid-base regulation, maternal/fetal placental, 467–468
Bilirubin
and carbon monoxide production from heme, 867
conjugated, 866–867
metabolism and excretion, 865–866
photobilirubin, 867
source of, 865, 866
unconjugated, 865, 866, 868, 869
Bilirubin metabolism, 865–876
bilirubin toxicity, 868–871
breast milk jaundice, 868
conjugated hyperbilirubinemia, 875–876
Crigler-Najjar syndrome, 875
definitions, 866–867
genetic factors, 873–875
Gilbert's disease, 874–875
hyperbilirubinemia, 867–867
low-bilirubin kernicterus, 871
Lucey-Driscoll syndrome, 875
treatment of, 871–872
Bilirubin toxicity, 868–871
animal studies, 870
in Crigler-Najjar syndrome, 870–871
in older child, 870–871
rationale for, 869–870
signs of, 870
and unconjugated bilirubin, 868–869
Bioelectrical impedance measurement, 1083–1084
Bioengineered rodents, experimental use of, 82–83
BioInformation on the World Wide Web, 41–42
Biosynthesis
and catecholamines, 162
of cortisol, 169
of epinephrine, 162
of glucagon, 155
of growth hormone, 166
of insulin, 135–138
of norepinephrine, 162
of prostaglandins, 259–263
Biotin, 992–993
deficiency features, 992–993
laboratory assessment of, 993
metabolism of, 992
neonatal needs, 992
sources of, 992
Biotin therapy, for multiple carboxylase deficiency, 808
Birth
and cardiac output, 505
cardiac output after, 504–505
and ductus arteriosus, 502–503
ductus arteriosus after, 502–503
and fetal circulation, 501
fetal circulation after, 501
glucose concentration at, 683–684
hypoglycemia after birth, 547
and kidney function, 1055–1056
lungs at, 584–585
metabolic rate after, 1006–1007
and myocardial contractility, 505
myocardial contractility after, 505
neonatal circulatory changes, 501
norepinephrine release at, 439–440
thermoregulation at, 1033–1034, 1037
and water/electrolyte balance in neonate, 1059–1066
Birth injury, infant of diabetic mother, 1116
Birth stress, and small-for-gestational-age (SGA) infant, 1101
Birth weight
and hypoglycemia, 685, 688, 697, 699, 1156
and iron deficiency, 291
and lead exposure, 293–294
neonatal classifications, 1097
and zinc deficiency, 289
See also Fetal growth; Intrauterine growth retardation (IUGR); Small-for-gestational-age (SGA) infants
Blood flow
changes in pregnancy, 320
and exercise, 321
and exercise in pregnancy, 323
and water/electrolyte metabolism, 1051–1052
Blood flow, maternal/fetal placental, 460–466
chemical mediation of, 462–465
increase and gestation, 461
and preeclampsia, 465–466
regulation of, 461–462
regulation of placental blood flow, 518–519
uterine blood flow, 461
See also Fetal circulation
Blood pressure
and ductus arteriosus, 490, 497
fetal, 490
and heart rate, 498–499
Blood transfusion, hyperbilirubinemia, 873
BMR. *See* Basal metabolic rate
Body composition
fetal growth, 1088–1091
maternal influences, 1088–1089
Body composition measures
acoustical method, 1085

anthropometric measurements, 1080–1082
bioelectrical impedance measurement, 1083–1084
body cell mass measure, 1079, 1086
body mass index, 1082
bone mineral measurement, 1087–1088
densitometric method, 1085
historical view, 1077
imaging methods, 1079
multicompartment models, 1078–1079
reference models, 1079–1080, 1089
skinfold measures, 1082
total body electrical conductivity measurement, 1083
total body potassium measurement, 1085–1086
total body water measurement, 1082, 1084
underwater weighing method, 1078
Body mass index, 1082
Body water compartment regulation, 1045–1046
Bohr effect, 459, 470
Bone mineral measurement, 1087–1088
Boron, deficiency features, 934
Bound ligands, 55
Bradycardia, and hypoxemia, 498–499
Bradykinin
 ductus closure after birth, 503
 production of, 1053
 pulmonary vasodilator, 502
Brain
 and adenosine triphosphate, 537–539, 541
 cerebral glucose metabolism, 543–547
 development and breast feeding, 830–831
 development and fatty acids, 828–831
 and essential fatty acids, 259
 and facilitative glucose transporters, 127–128
 glucose transporter proteins, 544–547
 and ketone bodies, 98, 105
 See also Cerebral metabolism in fetus/neonate
Brain damage, mechanisms for, 805
Brain natriuretic peptide, in amniotic fluid, 524
Branched-chain amino acids
 and growth-retarded fetus, 1100
 metabolism of, 802–804
 and protein metabolism, 108–109
 and protein metabolism in fetal-placental unit, 377–379
Breast care, 1187–1188

Breastfeeding
 benefits for mother, 1186–1187
 benefits for neonate, 1185–1186
 and brain development, 830–831
 breast care, 1187–1188
 and cognitive development, 1186
 and disease transmission to neonate, 1185
 compared to formula feeding, 825–826
 guidelines for, 1187
 hospital programs for, 1188
 and infant formulas, compared to, 825–826
 and infant growth, 1188
 and later life, 825–826
 milk expression/collection, 1191
 physiologic/metabolic responses to, 825
 and preterm infant, 1189–1192
 and skin-to-skin contact, 1191
 stop feeding mechanism, 825
 and supplements, 1188
 vegans and vitamin B^{12} deficiency, 990
 and zinc deficiency, 928, 929
 See also Human milk
Breast milk jaundice, 868
 causes of, 868
 treatment of, 873
Breath testing, ^{13}C
 advantages to use, 22
 analysis of samples, 21
 application to neonatology, 21–22
 categories of, 18
 commercial use, 18–19
 and health care delivery costs, 20–21
 medical efficacy of, 19–20
 origins of, 17–18
 possible outcomes of, 19–20
 regulatory approval of, 20
 time of administration, 22
Bromine, deficiency features, 934
Bronchopulmonary dysplasia, 323, 1172–1173
 complications of, 1172
 effect on metabolic rate, 1014
 nutritional intervention, 1172–1173
 pulmonary edema in, 1065, 1172
 and water/electrolyte balance defect, 1065
Brown adipose tissue
 disorders related to, 828
 regulation of, 1032
 and thermoregulation, 827–828, 1031–1032
Buffers, and maternal/fetal acid-base regulation, 469
Bunsen solubility coefficient, 455
Burning feet syndrome, 992

C
Cadherins, 649
Calcitonin, 898–900
 and diabetic mothers, 899–900
 fetal production of, 899
 functions of, 879–880, 885, 898
 and magnesium regulation, 888
 metabolism in neonate, 899–900
 metabolism in pregnancy, 899
 secretion, regulation of, 898, 900
Calcium, 283–284, 879–884
 bioavailability of, 283
 calcitonin effects, 898
 calcium/phosphorous ratio in feeding, 887
 excretion of, 880, 883
 food sources for neonate, 883
 functions of, 879–880
 hypercalcemia, 884
 hypocalcemia, 883–884
 metabolism in fetus, 881–882
 metabolism in neonate, 882–883
 metabolism of, 283
 metabolism in placenta, 881, 889
 metabolism in pregnancy, 283–284, 880–881
 and pregnancy-induced hypertension (PIH), 284
 for prevention of preeclampsia, 284
 requirements in pregnancy, 283
 and vitamin D, 284, 953–954
Calcium-binding protein, 897
Calcium ions, and hormonal secretion, 62–63
Calcium/phosphorous ratio in feeding, 887
Calories
 fetal requirements, 1005
 very low birthweight infant requirements, 1156–1158
Calorimetry
 direct, 1001–1002
 indirect, 1002
cAMP
 and actions of glucagon, 160
 and β-adrenergic receptors, 162
 control of levels in liver, 146
 cyclic, formation of, 62
 gene expression regulation, 444
 hormonal regulation role, 427
 measurement of, 62
 response element binding protein, 147
Capillary hydrostatic pressure, and water/electrolyte metabolism, 1050
Caracass analysis methods, protein metabolism in fetal-placental unit, 369–370
Carbohydrate-deficient glycoprotein syndrome, 1230–1231

Index

signs of, 1230–1231
Carbohydrate homeostasis, and glucagon, 158–159
Carbohydrate metabolism disorders, 723–760
  α-acid glucoside deficiency (Type II), 756–758
  amylopectinosis brancher deficiency (Type IV), 758–759
  Debrancher, amylo-1,6-glucosidase deficiency (Type III), 751–753
  fructose intolerance, 733–740
  galactokinase deficiency, 731–733
  galactose-4-epimerase, 731
  galactosemia, 723–730
  glucose-6-phosphatase defect (Type I), 745–751
  glycogen synthase defect, 759–760
  hepatic fructose-1,6-diphosphatase deficiency, 741–743
  hepatic phosphoenolpyruvate carboxykinase (PEPCK) deficiency, 741
  liver phosphorylase defect (Type VI), 753–754
  muscle phosphofructokinase deficiency (Type VII), 755–756
  muscle phosphorylase deficiency (Type V), 754–755
  pyruvate carboxylase deficiency, 740–741
  and surgery, 1135–1137
Carbohydrates
  and energy metabolism in neonate, 1012
  in enteral feeding, 1167
  and exercise, 326
  as fatty acid synthesis precursor, 394
  in human milk, 1182
  in parenteral feeding, 1160–1161
  for very low birth weight infant, 1160–1161, 1167
Carbon dioxide
  and acid-base regulation, maternal/fetal placental, 467–471
  and fetal glucose oxidation, 343
  fetal imbalances, causes of, 470
  forms carried in blood, 468
  and glutamine oxidation, 633, 636
  and ketone bodies, 630
  placental efficiency, 472
  placental exchange compared to lung, 470, 472
  production in neonatal intestine, 627
Carbon magnetic resonance, 6
Carbon monoxide, and bilirubin production, 867
Carcass analysis, 369–340
Cardiac failure, thiamine deficiency, 981

Cardiac metabolism, 551–563
  amino acid metabolism, 557
  ATP concentration, 551
  ATP production, 551, 558, 561
  ATP utilization, 551, 559
  carbohydrate metabolism, 552–556
  catabolic pathways, 552
  cellular compartmentation, 559–560
  enzymatic regulation, 552
  and free fatty acids, 552, 556–557
  glucose transport, 551–552
  and ketone bodies, 557
  lipid metabolism, 556–557
  oxidative phosphorylation, 558–559
  and phosphocreatine, 559
  protein synthesis, 560–561
  pyruvate metabolism, 555
  substrate entry in heart, 551–552
  tricarboxylic cycle, 558
Cardiac metabolism in fetus/neonate, 561–563
  and changing organism, 561
  glucose metabolism, 562–563
  and long-chain fatty acids, 561–562
  mitochondrial volume increase, 561
  oxygen consumption/metabolism, 561
Cardiac output, 493–496
  in adult, 493
  animal studies, 493–494
  birth events, effects of, 504–505
  changes in pregnancy, 319, 322
  and exercise, 320–321
  and heart rate, 494–495
  and oxygen consumption, 504
  and preload/afterload, 495–496
  preload/afterload effects, 495–496
  regulation in fetus, 494–496
  sheep compared to humans, 494
  and thyroid hormone, 504–505
  use of term in context of fetus, 493
Cardiovascular defects, infant of diabetic mother, 1114, 1115–1116
Cardiovascular system
  exercise (nonpregnant state), 320–321
  and exercise in pregnancy, 322–323
  during pregnancy, 319–320
Caries protection, fluoride, 295, 296
Carnitine, 857–862
  carnitine-free diets, 861–862
  concentrations in neonate, 860–861
  and developmental changes, 860–861
  dietary sources, 859
  dietary sources for neonate, 861
  endogenous synthesis, 859
  functions of, 857
  lipid metabolism in neonate, 613
  lipid metabolism in skeletal muscle, 659–660

maintenance of concentrations of, 857–859
metabolic role of, 857
in parenteral nutrition, 1163
and preterm infants, 660
recommended daily intake, 862
synthesis in neonate, 861
Carnitine/acylcarnitine carrier deficiency, 850
  signs of, 850
  treatment of, 850
Carnitine acyltransferase (CAT), 100, 398
  and lipid metabolism, 556
Carnitine deficiency, 660, 852, 859–860
  age of presentation, 860
  carnitine palmitoyltransferase-1 deficiency (CPT-1), 850
  carnitine palmitoyltransferase-2 (CPT-2) deficiency, 850
  carnitine transport deficiency, 850
  genetic factors, 859, 860
  signs of, 859, 860
Carnitine metabolism, 857–862
  carnitine-free diets, and neonates, 861–862
  clinical conditions, 862
  concentrations, maintenance of, 857–859
  deficiency, disorders of, 859–860
  and fatty acid oxidation, 860–861
  physiology of, 857
  sources of, 859
Carnitine palmitoyltransferase-1, 398, 847, 848, 849
Carnitine palmitoyltransferase (CPT) system
  deficiency, 660
  fatty acid oxidation in neonate, 609–613
  intestinal tract of neonate, 632
  metabolic effectors and regulation of, 613
  transcriptional/posttransscriptional regulation at birth, 611–613
Carnitine therapy
  for acute metabolic decompensation, 1222
  for carnitine/acylcarnitine carrier deficiency, 850 for propionic acidemia, 807
β-carotene, as vitamin A precursor, 946
CAT. See Carnitine acyltransferase
Catabolic pathways, 552
Catabolism of glucagon, 157–158
Cataracts
  and galactokinase deficiency, 732
  and galactosemia, 725, 728
Catecholamines
  and α-adrenergic receptors, 162, 440

and β-adrenergic receptors, 162, 440–445
biosynthesis, 162
chemical structure, 161
degradation of, 162
elimination of, 162
epinephrine, 161–165
and exercise, 327
and free fatty acid mobilization, 1144
and glucose metabolism in neonate, 702
inactivation of, 162
and liver glycogenolysis in neonate, 604
mechanisms of action, 162
metabolic actions, 163
and metabolic regulation, 164
and myocardial contractility, 505
perinatal metabolism of, 437–438
perinatal secretion, 438–440
release at birth, 439–440
release of, 162
renal, 1052–1053, 1057–1058
secretion, regulation of, 163
types of, 161
and water/electrolyte metabolism, 1052–1053
Catechol-O-methyl transferase (COMT), and catecholamine degradation, 162
CDKs. See Cell-cycle dependent protein kinases
CDNA, rapid amplification of, 53
Cell adhesion molecules, 648–649
cadherins, 649
integrins, 649
Cell-cycle dependent protein kinases (CDKs), and cell proliferation, 404–405
Cells
apoptosis, 406
differentiation of, 406
migration and motility, 406–407
morphogenesis, 407
negative cell cycle, 405
organogenesis, 407
proliferation of, 404–406
water channels, 513–516
Cell signaling, 53–54
and receptor binding, 53–54
Cellular compartmentation, 559–560
Cellular ritincol-binding protein. See CRBP I and II
Cellular techniques, 41–42
Central nervous system
and glucose metabolism in neonate, 713–715
and glycose metabolism, 91
Cerebral energy
metabolism of, 537

utilization of, 541–542
Cerebral glucose metabolism, 543–547
Cerebral metabolism in fetus/neonate
adenosine triphosphate (ATP), 537–539, 541
cerebral blood flow measurement, 542–543
cerebral metabolic rate for oxygen, 539–540
energy utilization, 541–542
flow-metabolism couple, 542–543
glucose transporters, 544–547
glucose utilization, 543–544
glycolysis, 540–541
mitochondria, 541
oxidative metabolism, 539–540
substitute fuels for metabolism, 547–548
Cesarean section, and thermoregulation, 1034
CGP. See Chorionic growth hormone-prolactin
CHEF. See Contour-clamp homogeneous electric field electrophoresis
Chemoreflex regulation, fetal circulation, 497–498
Chemstrip bG test strip, glucose measure, 686, 687
Chloramphenicol acetyltransferase (CAT), uses of, 67
Cholestasis
and conjugated hyperbilirubinemia, 875–876
and parenteral nutrition, 1164–1165
Cholesterol, 221–222
absorption and synthesis in pregnancy, 228–229
conversion to triglycerides, 223
derivation of, 821
excretion of, 224
high density lipoproteins (HDL), 223–224
low density lipoproteins (LDL), 223–224
in lung surfactant, 570
placental transport, 238
recycling of, 223
source of, 426–427
storage and metabolism of, 221–222, 223
very low density lipoproteins (VLDL), 223
Cholesterol acyltransferase (ACAT), 427
Chorionic growth hormone-prolactin (CGP), 427
Chromatin, arrangement of, 42
Chromium, 934
deficiency, signs of, 934

functions of, 934
neonate requirements, 934
Chronic care for metabolic disease, 1224–1225
Chylomicrons, synthesis in neonate, 836, 837
Cigarette smoking
and fetal growth, 1088
and placental respiratory gas exchange, 474–475
and zinc deficiency, 926
Citric acid cycle. See Krebs cycle
Citrullinemia, 805–806, 1210–1211
case example, 1210–1211
laboratory findings, 1211
treatment of, 1211
Class II receptors, 60
Class I receptors, 60
Clinical Laboratories Improvement Act, 21
Clinitest tablets, 726
Cloning
insulin gene, 138–139
See also Recombinant DNA
Cobalamin therapy, for methylmalonic acidemia, 808
Cocaine abuse, and fetal respiration, 474
Codons, and amino acids, 42
Cognitive functioning
and breastfeeding, 1186
and galactosemia, 729
infant of diabetic mother, 1123–1124
See also Mental retardation
Cold-stressed neonate, hypoglycemia in, 690–691
Colostrum
carbohydrate content of, 604
lactose and fat content of, 601
Combined ventricular output, 491
Compartmenalization, skeletal muscle, 648
Compartment analysis, protein metabolism study, 775–776
Compartmentation, cardiac metabolism, 559–560
Competitive immunoassay, 30–31
Concurrent model, placental exchange, 451
Conduction principle, thermoregulation, 1028
Congenital adrenal hyperplasia, and neonatal hypoglycemia, 695
Congenital atransferrinemia, 915
Congenital defects
adrenal gland, 426
infants of diabetic mothers, 1114–1116
left-to-right shunt, 490
and neonatal hypoglycemia, 691, 695

Congenital lipoid adrenal hyperplasia, cause of, 426
Conjugated hyperbilirubinemia, 875–876
   causes of, 875
   evaluation for, 875–876
   treatment approaches, 876
Connective tissue, composition of, 647–648
Constant-infusion method, protein metabolism study, 776
Contour-clamp homogeneous electric field electrophoresis (CHEF), 45
Contrainsulin hormones
   amylin, 171
   cortisol, 168–171
   epinephrine, 161–165
   glucagon, 155–161
   growth hormone, 165–168
   leptin, 172
   tumor necrosis factor-α, 172
Convection principle, thermoregulation, 1028
Copper, 294–295, 916–923
   bioavailability of, 294
   deficiency features, 918–919, 921
   fetal/neonatal metabolism of, 920–922
   functions of, 916
   metabolism of, 294, 916–918
   metabolism in pregnancy, 294–295, 919–920
   and pregnancy outcome, 295
   regulation of, 918
   zinc impairment of absorption, 917, 921
Copper intoxication, 923
   causes of, 923
   signs of, 923
Copper metabolism defects
   aceruloplasminemia, 922–923
   copper intoxication, 923
   familial benign copper deficiency, 922
   familial hypoceruloplsminemia, 922
   genetic factors, 922–923
   Menkes' syndrome, 922
   Wilson's disease, 923
Cori cycle, and glucose metabolism, 92
Corticosteroids
   and β-adrenergic receptor regulation, 441–442
   fetal lungs, effects on, 582–582
   hypoglycemia treatment, 697
   and lactate production, 637
   and protein metabolism in neonate, 778
Corticotropin-releasing factor (CRF), placental production/release of, 428
Cortisol, 168–171
   biosynthesis of, 169
   degradation of, 169
   and diabetes mellitus, 171
   and ductus arteriosis after birth, 503
   elimination of, 169
   exercise effects, 329
   and glucose metabolism in fetal-placental unit, 355
   and glucose metabolism in pregnancy, 191, 192
   mechanism of action, 169–170
   metabolic functions of, 170
   and metabolic regulation, 170–171
   and protein metabolism in neonate, 778
   release of, 169
   secretion, regulation of, 170
   transport of, 169
Cosmids, recombinant DNA, 50
Countercurrent exchange model, placental exchange, 451–453
Counterregulatory hormones. *See* Contrainsulin hormones
C peptide, and insulin biosynthesis, 136–138
CPT-1. *See* Carnitine deficiency
CPT-2. *See* Carnitine deficiency
CRBP I and II, 943–947
Creatine kinase
   and developmental changes, 657
   skeletal muscle, 656–657, 660–661
Creatine phosphokinase, and ATP to ADP conversion, 537
Cretinism, and iodine deficiency, 297
CRF. *See* Corticotropin-releasing factor
Crigler-Najjar syndrome, 868, 870, 875
   features of, 875
   treatment approaches, 875
Cross-reactivity in immunoassay, 30
Cultural differences, weight gain, 310–311, 312–313
Culture, and energy metabolism in pregnancy, 310–317
Curosurf, 585
Current Opinion in Cell Biology, 42
Cyclic adenosine monophosphate. *See* cAMP
Cyclic nucleotides, immunoassay measurement, 36
Cyclooxygenase metabolites, maternal/fetal placental blood flow mediation, 462–463
Cytidylytransferase
   phosphorylation sites, 578–579
   regulation of, 578–579
Cytochrome c oxidase, 659

D

Dawn phenomenon, and growth hormone, 168
Debrancher, amylo-1,6-glucosidase deficiency (Type III), 751–753
   course of, 752
   diagnosis of, 752
   genetic factors, 753
   management of, 752
   prognosis of, 752–753
Degradation
   of cortisol, 168–171
   of growth hormone, 166
Dehydroepiandrosterone, 427
Dehydroepiandrosterone sulfate, 427
Deiodination, thyroid hormones, 432–434
Densitometric method, body composition measure, 1085
Dental caries, fluoride supplementation, 934
Deoxyribonucleic acid. *See* entries under DNA
Desensitization of target cells, 59–60
   causes of, 59
   process of, 59
   versus supersensitivity, 59
Developmental endocrinology, 425–434
   adrenal gland, development of, 425–426
   estrogen, 425–426
   follicle-stimulating hormone (FSH), 430–431
   growth hormone, 430
   human chorionic gonadotropin (hCG), 427
   hypothalamic peptides, 428
   hypothalamus, development of, 428–429
   inhibin, 428
   luteinizing hormone (LH), 430–431
   maternal androgens, fetal protection from, 427
   pituitary gland, development of, 429–430
   placental lactogen, 427–428
   progesterone, 426–427
   steroids, 425–427
   thyroid gland, development of, 432
   thyroid hormone, 432–434
   thyroid-releasing hormone (TRH), 431–432
Developmental enzymology, 799–800
Dexamethasone, and vitamin A mobilization, 948
Dextromethorphan, 1227
Dextrostix method, glucose measure, 686
Diabetes mellitus
   A-cell dysfunction in, 161
   animal models of maternal diabetes, 81–82
   and cortisol, 171

dawn phenomenon, 168
and epinephrine, 164–165
and glucagon, 160–161
and glucose metabolism in pregnancy, 194–196
and GLUT 4, 125–126
and lipid metabolism in pregnancy, 243–244
salicylates, effects on insulin response, 270
Somogyi phenomenon, 168
See also Gestational diabetes mellitus; Infant of diabetic mother; Insulin-dependent diabetes mellitus; Non-insulin dependent diabetes mellitus
Diabetic mother, infant of. *See* Infant of diabetic mother
Diagnosis of metabolic disease. *See* Metabolic disease evaluation
Diagnostic methods
immunoassay, 27–37
mass spectometry, 4
modeling, 9–10
nuclear magnetic resonance (MRI), 4–6
positron emission tomography, 6–7
stable isotope tracers, 7–9
Diascan S meter, glucose measure, 686
Diazoxide, hypoglycemia treatment, 697
DiGeorge syndrome, 893
and maternal diabetes, 1116
Digestion
fat in neonate, 831–835
of human milk, 1185
and prostaglandins, 264
of protein in neonate, 790–791
and very low birth weight infant nutrition, 1166–1167
See also Gastrointestinal tract of fetus/neonate
Digestive lipases, 832–834
Diglycerides, 821
Dipalmitoylphosphatidylcholine (DCCP), in lung surfactant, 568–570
Direct calorimetry, 1001–1002
Disease transmission, and breastfeeding, 1185
DNase footprinting, 66
DNA sequencing
characterizing DNA sequences, 44
coding regions, 42–43
hybridization methods, 44–45
preparation from nucleated cells, 43–44
restriction enzymes and sequencing, 44
sequencing cloned fragments, 45

Southern blot hybridization, 44–45
structure of, 42–43
DNA synthesis, and skeletal muscle, 661
DOPA, 162
Dopamine, 161
biosynthesis of, 162
effects on kidney, 1052–1053
Dot blot/slot blot apparatus, RNA sequencing, 46
Double layer method, protein separation, 49
Doubly labeled water
energy metabolism measurement, 1003–1004
compared to indirect calorimetry, 1003–1004
Drugs, and fetal morbidity, 521
Duarte variant, galactosemia, 730
Dubin-Johnson syndrome, 868
Duchenne's muscular dystrophy, 657
and brown adipose tissue, 828
Ductus arteriosus
after birth, 502–503
fetal circulation, 502
and vascular pressure, 490, 497
Duodenum, fat digestion, 834–835

E
Eadie-Hofstee equation, 58
Echocardiography, fetal cardiac output study, 492
Eclampsia, and lipid peroxides, 241
Edema
brain, and hyperammonemia, 1210
mechanisms related to, 1066–1067
pulmonary, 1065
water/electrolyte metabolism defect, 1066–1067
EDRF. *See* Endothelium-derived relaxing factor
EGF. *See* Epidermal growth factor
Eicosanoids, 259
Electroblotting apparatus, 48
Electrolytes. *See* entries under Water/electrolyte metabolism
Electromagnetic flowmeters, fetal cardiac output study, 492
Electron transfer flavoprotein, 847, 848
Electron transfer flavoprotein deficiency, 851, 1229–1230
forms of, 851
Electron transfer flavoprotein dehydrogenase, 847, 848
Electron transfer flavoprotein dehydrogenase deficiency, 851
Electron transport chain, and heart, 558–559
Electrophoresis, protein separation, 47–48

Electrophoresis mobility shift assay (EMSA), 66
ELISA immunoassay, steps in use, 37
Embryo, and facilitative glucose transporters, 126–127
EMSA. *See* Electrophoresis mobility shift assay
Endogenous growth hormone, 167–168
Endogenous fat, 99–100
Endogenous synthesis, 859
Endometriosis, and prostaglandins, 265
Endothelial relaxing factor (EDRF), pulmonary vasodilation, 502
Endothelins
in amniotic fluid, 523–524
regulation of placental blood flow, 519
Endothelium-derived relaxing factor (EDRF), and fetal/placental blood flow, 464, 465
Energy balance computations, 1019
Energy balance equation, 1001
Energy metabolism
and exercise, 325–326
skeletal muscle, 654–658
Energy metabolism in fetal-placental unit
caloric requirements, 1005
energy requirements, 1005
and oxygen consumption, 1005
and protein metabolism, 376–377
Energy metabolism measurement
comparison of methods, 1004
direct calorimetry, 1001–1002
doubly labeled water, 1003–1004
heat storage equation, 1001
indirect calorimetry, 1002
Energy metabolism in neonate
and activity, 1014–1015
energy balance computations, 1019
energy balance equation, 1001
energy intake effects, 1007–1011
enriched formulas and metabolic rate, 1007–1010
food composition effects, 1011–1012
futile metabolic cycles, 1010
growth effects, 1011
and illness, 1013–1014
and intrauterine growth retardation, 1015
metabolic rate after birth, 1006–1007
and nitrogen balance, 1015–1016
optimal energy/protein intake, 1018–1019
preterm infants, 1014–1015
protein turnover effects, 1012–1013
resting metabolic rate, 1002
and sleep states, 1015
and specific dynamic action, 1010–1011

Index

stools/urine and energy loss, 1015
and surgery, 1133–1134
and thyroid hormones, 1010
and weight gain, 1016–1017
Energy metabolism in pregnancy
basal metabolic rate (BMR), 312
baseline data, 313–314
cross-cultural view, 310–317
energy costs, 309
energy intake measurement, 314–316
energy requirements, 313–314
energy savings, 314
and exercise, 326–327
fat increase, 309–311
reduced activity effects, 316–317
running costs, 312
total energy cost, 312–313
Enolase, skeletal muscle, 653
Enteral feeding
advantages of, 1166
and amino acids, 1167–1168
complications of, 1166, 1170
hypocaloric feeding, 1170–1171
methods of, 1169–1170
very low birth weight infant, 1165–1171
Enzymatic regulation, 552
Enzymes
isozymes, 650–654
restriction enzymes, listing of, 44
signaling enzymes, fetal-placental unit, 408–411
Epidermal growth factor (EGF), 411–412
functions of, 412
in human milk, 1183
and lipid metabolism in fetal-placental unit, 395
receptor for, 407
synthesis of, 411
types of, 412
Epidermal growth factor precursor (preproEGF) gene, 43
Epinephrine, 161–165
biosynthesis of, 162
degradation of, 162
and diabetes mellitus, 164–165
elimination of, 162
and exercise, 327
and glucose metabolism in neonate, 705–706
as hormone, 161
hypoglycemia treatment, 697
inactivation of, 162
lipolytic effect of, 99
mechanisms of action, 162
metabolic functions of, 163–164
and metabolic regulation, 164
release of, 162
secretion, regulation of, 163

Essential amino acids
importance of intake, 1013
types of, 791
Essential fatty acids
deficiency, measurement of, 1160
functions of, 259
and lipid metabolism, 221
omega-3 series, 221
omega-6 series, 259
and prostaglandin production, 259–263
in very low birth weight infant feeding, 1158–1160
Estrogen, 425–426
and glucose metabolism in pregnancy, 191
and lipid metabolism in pregnancy, 224–225
maternal/fetal placental blood flow mediation, 464
synthesis in fetal-placental unit, 425–426, 427
Ethanol ingestion
effects on retinol, 946
maternal, and hypoglycemia in neonate, 694–695
Euglycemic-hyperinsulinemic clamp
in adults, 187
in newborns, 706–707
Eukaryotic gene activity, 65
European Molecular Biology Laboratory, Web site, 45
Evaporation, and thermoregulation, 1028–1029
Exercise
anaerobic threshold, meaning of, 326
and carbohydrate intake, 326
cardiovascular effect, 319–321
duration effects, 326
and energy metabolism, 325–326
and glucose metabolism, 102
intensity effects, 325
and lactate concentration, 325–326
and lactate threshold, 325–326
respiratory effect, 322
Exercise in pregnancy
cardiovascular effects, 322–323
and cortisol, 329
energy metabolism, 326–327
and fat stores, 325
fetal effects, 324–325
glucose concentration, 327–329
and growth hormone, 329
and norepinephrine, 327
recovery phase, 324
respiratory effects, 322–323
Exogenous carbohydrate supply, 604
Exons, 43
Exosurf, 586

Experimental treatments for metabolic disease, 1225
Extracellular matrix, skeletal muscle, 648
Extracellular signaling factors, 403
Extracellular water compartment, 1048
Extracellular water regulation, 1051–1054

F
Facilitated anabolism, 384
Facilitative glucose transporters, 123–129
and brain, 127–128
and embryo, 126–127
functions of, 123
GLUT 1, 123–124
GLUT 2, 124–125
GLUT 3, 125
GLUT 4, 125–126
GLUT 5, 126
GLUT 7, 126
and kidney, 129
and liver, 128
and lungs, 128
and muscle, 128–129
and placenta, 127
topology of transporters, 123
Familial benign copper deficiency, 922
Familial hypoceruloplsminemia, 922
Family history, metabolic disease evaluation, 1201
Farm animals, maternal diabetes study, 83–86
Fasting
and glucagon secretion, 158
and glucose metabolism, 93, 94, 104
and lipolysis, 104
maternal, and fetal protein metabolism, 377–379
metabolic changes in adult, 1154
metabolic changes in preterm infant, 1154–1155
and protein metabolism, 106–107, 108
and protein metabolism in neonate, 789–790
and protein metabolism in pregnancy, 208–209
Fasting/feeding response, 208–209
Fat absorption, 228–229, 835–836
Fat deposition measurement, 310
Fat digestion, 831–835
Fat-free mass, 309
Fat metabolism, and surgery, 1142–1145
Fat storage, 241–243
Fat stores in pregnancy, 309–311
cultural patterns and weight gain, 310–311, 312–313

energy cost of, 309–310
and energy during exercise, 325
fat deposition measurement, 310
fat-free mass, 309
importance of, 310
and lactation, 310
and postpartum period, 310
weight and fat gain, 310–311
Fatty acid-binding proteins, 609
role in fatty acid transport, 835–836
Fatty acid chain length, 391
Fatty acid oxidation defects
carnitine/acylcarnitine carrier deficiency, 850
carnitine palmitoyltransferase-1 deficiency, 850
carnitine palmitoyltransferase-2 deficiency, 850
carnitine transport deficiency, 850
diagnosis of, 851–853
electron transfer flavoprotein deficiency, 851
electron transfer flavoprotein dehydrogenase deficiency, 851
epidemiology, 851
features of, 849–850
genetic factors, 849–850
ketone synthesis deficiencies, 851
long-chain acyl-CoA dehydrogenase deficiency, 850–851
long-chain 3-hydroxyacyl-CoA dehydrogenase deficiency, 851
medium-chain acyl-CoA dehydrogenase deficiency, 851
metabolite analyses, 852–853
mutation analysis, 853
short-chain acyl-CoA dehydrogenase deficiency, 851
short-chain β-ketothiolase deficiency, 851
short-chain fatty acid oxidation deficiency, 851
treatment of, 853
very long chain acyl-CoA dehydrogenase deficiency, 850–851
Fatty acid oxidation in neonate, 607–617
acylcarnitine formation, 609
acyl-CoA formation, 609
carnitine palmitoyltransferase (CPT) system, 609–613
enzyme activities, 609–610
gastrointestinal system, 631–632
glucose, role of, 617–618
and hepatic gluconeogenesis, 615–617
hormonal factors, 611–612
and mitochondrial oxidative capacity, 611–612, 614–615
pathway for, 608–609
relationship to hepatic gluconeogenesis, 615–617
tissue related to, 608
triglyceride synthesis, 609
Fatty acid receptor, 609
Fatty acids, 821–823
adipocyte metabolism, 147
fetal lungs, 580–581
fetus, transfer to, 391
heart, transfer to, 552
insulin effects, 147
medium-chain fatty acids, 831, 1012
names of, 822
oxidation in fetus, 397–399
oxidation pathways, 396–397
placental transfer, 390–391
structure of, 821–822
synthesis, pathways of, 392–393
See also Essential fatty acids; Free fatty acids; Long-chain fatty acids; Medium-chain fatty acids
Fatty acid translocase, 609
Fatty acid transport protein, 609
Federated 2-D PAGE Database, 49
Feeding. See Breastfeeding; Human milk; Infant formulas; Nutritional support; Very low birth weight infant nutrition
Fertilization, and prostaglandins, 264–265
Fetal albumin concentration, 391
Fetal blood gases, 490
Fetal circulation
baroflex regulation, 497
cardiac output, 493–496, 504–506
changes after birth, 501
chemoreflex regulation, 497–498
ductus arteriosus, 502–504
fetal blood gases, 490
fetal heart and blood flow, 488
fetal liver and blood flow, 487–488
methods of study of, 491–492
mixing of oxygenated/systemic venous blood, 488, 490
myocardial contractility, 496–497
oxygen saturation, 490
postnatal circulation, 487
and prostaglandins, 269–270
pulmonary circulation, 501–502
reduced oxygen delivery, effects of, 498–501
vascular pressures, 490
Fetal effects
from copper deficiency, 295
from diabetic mother, 200, 271, 272–273, 358
from lead exposure, 292–293
from magnesium overload, 286
maternal exercise, 324–325
from zinc deficiency, 289
Fetal glucose oxidation, 343
Fetal growth
altitude, effects of, 1101
and arachidonic acid, 265–266
farm animal models, 83–86
lipids, effect of, 241–243
and maternal alcohol consumption, 1088–1089
and maternal cigarette smoking, 1089
and maternal diabetes, 200, 1110, 1111
and maternal fatty acid concentrations, 241–243
and maternal malnutrition, 1089
and maternal metabolism, 384
and trimesters of pregnancy, 266
See also Birth weight; Intrauterine growth retardation (IUGR); Small-for-gestational-age (SGA) infants
Fetal heart rate, and maternal exercise, 324–325
Fetal lipid accumulation, and placental transfer, 390, 392
Fetal lipid metabolism. See Lipid metabolism in the fetal-placental unit
Fetal neurotoxicity, and lead, 292–293
Fetal nitrogen accretion, and amino acids, 373–375
Fetal placental respiration, 451–476
acid-base regulation, 466–470
and altitude, 473
artificial placenta, 476
Bohr effect, 459
and cigarette smoking, 474–475
and cocaine abuse, 474
factors affecting oxygen transfer, 453–454
and fetal surgery, 475–476
and Fick's first law, 454
gas exchange and placenta, 451, 470–473
Haldane effect, 459
hemoglobin and oxygen delivery, 457–459
and maternal exercise, 325
maternal/fetal oxygen partial pressures, 456–457
maternal/fetal placental blood flow, 460–466
placental diffusing capacity, 454–456
placental insufficiency, compensatory factors, 457–458
placental oxygen transfer, 453–454
placenta compared to lung, 470–473
Fetal-placental unit
circulation in, 487–506
developmental endocrinology, 425–434

Index

glucose metabolism, 337–361
lipid metabolism, 389–399
protein metabolism, 369–384
respiration in, 451–476
sympathoadrenal system, 437–445
water and electrolyte metabolism, 511–526
Fetal respiration, effects of altitude on, 473
Fetal secretion, 427, 430
Fetuin, and fatty acid transfer to fetus, 391
Fetus
  calcitonin production, 899
  calcium metabolism, 881–882
  caloric requirements, 1005
  growth/body composition of, 1089–1091
  growth retarded, 1100
  iron concentration, 913
  iron metabolism, 913–914
  and kinetic experiments, 371–373
  and protein metabolism in pregnancy, 217–128
  thermoregulation of, 1029, 1033–1034
  vitamin D stores, 896
  See also Fetus/neonate
Fetus/neonate
  cardiac metabolism, 561–563
  cerebral metabolism, 540–547
  gastrointestinal tract metabolism, 627–639
  liver metabolism, 601–619
  lung development, 575–587
  skeletal muscle metabolism, 641–655
FFAs. See Free fatty acids
FGF. See Fibroblast growth factor
Fibroblast growth factor (FGF), 416–417
  functions of, 417
  receptors for, 416–417
  and skeletal muscle, 663
  types of, 416
Fibroblast-pneumocyte factor (FPF), 578, 583
Fick principle
  amino acids in, 370
  Fick's first law, equation for, 454
  glucose metabolism in fetal-placental unit, 337–339
  villous surface area of placenta, 454, 455
Field inversion gels (FIG), 45
FIG. See Field inversion gels
First messengers, activity from, 60
Flow-metabolism couple, cerebral metabolism in fetus/neonate, 542–543
Flowmeters, fetal cardiac output study, 492

Fluid balance, in lungs, 516–517
Fluoride, 295–296
  bioavailability of, 295
  caries protection, 295, 296
  in infant formula, 934
  metabolism in pregnancy, 295–296
  prenatal fluoride, 296
Fluorine, deficiency features, 934
Folate, 987–989
  deficiency features, 988–989
  laboratory assessment, 989
  metabolism of, 987
  needs during pregnancy, 988
  neonatal needs, 987–988
  sources of, 987
  toxicity, 989
Folate metabolism defect, 1226–1227
  case example, 1226–1227
  laboratory findings, 1226
Folinic acid, 1227
Follicle-stimulating hormone (FSH), 430–431
  fetal production of, 430–431
Food composition, and metabolic rate, 1011–1012
Formulas. See Infant formulas
FPF. See Fibroblast-pneumocyte factor
Fractional synthetic rate, of protein, 371
Frank-Starling mechanism, 494
  and exercise, 321
Free fatty acids (FFAs)
  and cardiac metabolism, 552, 556–557
  and cardiac metabolism of fetus/neonate, 561–562
  for energy in exercise state, 325, 326
  energy source and heart, 552
  and fasting, 1154–1155
  in fetal circulation, 562
  and fetal growth, 242
  and glucagon secretion, 158
  and glucose utilization, 97, 184
  and lipid metabolism in pregnancy, 228
  β-oxidation, 556–557
  oxidation, regulation of, 100–103
  placenta and transport, 236–237
  and preeclampsia, 268–269
  and prostaglandins, 266
  release of, 99–100
  and surgery, 1144–1145
Free radical damage, and selenium deficiency, 298
Fructose, placental production, 351
Fructose diphosphate, conversion to fructose-6-phosphate, 94
Fructose intolerance, 692, 733–740
  biopsy and enzyme activity analysis, 735

enzyme defect in, 733, 738–739
genetic factors, 736–737
intravenous fructose tolerance test, 735
pathogenesis, 737–740
signs in older children/adults, 734–735
signs in young infants, 733, 734
treatment of, 736–737
Fructose-phosphate, and fructose intolerance, 737–740
FSH. See Follicle-stimulating hormone
Futile metabolic cycles, events of, 1010
  in glucose metabolism, 94

G

Galactokinase deficiency, 731–733
  clinical signs, 732
  genetic factors, 732
  laboratory tests, 732
  pathogenesis, 732
  treatment of, 732
Galactose
  phosphorylation of, 723–724
  treatment for hyperglycemia, 1161
  uptake in neonatal liver, 604
Galactose-4-epimerase and galactosemia, 731
Galactosemia, 692, 723–730
  and behavioral problems, 729
  blood work up, 725–726, 1214
  differential diagnosis, 726
  Duarte variant, 730
  galactose-4-epimerase, 731
  genetic factors, 724, 727–728
  Negro variant, 730
  neonatal abnormalities, 724–725
  pathologic studies, 728
  postnatal diagnosis, 726
  postnatal treatment, 727
  prenatal diagnosis, 726
  prognosis, 729–730
  signs of, 724
  site of defect, 728
  toxicity, mechanism of, 728–729
  ultrasound findings, 726
  urine work up, 726
  in utero treatment, 727
Galactose-phosphate uridyltransferase (GALT), cloning of, 727
Galactose uptake, 604
Galactosialidosis, 1232
  pathogenesis, 1232
  signs of, 1323
Gallbladder stones, and parenteral nutrition, 1164–1165
GALT. See Galactose-phosphate uridyltransferase
Gangrene, infant of diabetic mother, 1117

Gastrointesintal tract of fetus/neonate
  fatty acid oxidation, 631–632
  glutamine oxidation, 632–634, 636–637
  intestinal glucose metabolism, 627–630
  ketone oxidation, 634–635
  and weaning, 637
Gating, meaning of, 60
Gaucher disease, 1231
  severe type, 1231
Gene ablation, 68–69
  knockout method, goal of, 68
Gene mutations, 139
Gene regulation, 64–68
  DNA regulatory region, 64
  levels related to, 64
  molecular analysis of, 66–68
  response elements, 65
  TATA box, 64–65
Gene therapy
  difficulties related to, 664
  skeletal muscle, 663
Genetic disease, recombinant DNA diagnosis, 51–52
Genetic factors
  α-acid glucoside deficiency (Type II), 757
  amylopectinosis brancher deficiency (Type IV), 758
  bilirubin metabolism defects, 873–875
  carnitine deficiency, 859–860
  copper metabolism defects, 922–923
  Debrancher, amylo-1,6-glucosidase deficiency (Type III), 753
  fatty acid oxidation defects, 849–850
  fructose intolerance, 736–737
  galactokinase deficiency, 732
  galactosemia, 724, 727–728
  and gestational diabetes mellitus, 198–199
  Gilbert's disease, 868, 874–875
  glucose-6-phosphatase defect (Type I), 750–751
  insulin-dependent diabetes mellitus, 194
  iron metabolism defects, 915
  liver phosphorylase defect (Type VI), 754
  maple syrup urine disease, 811
  metabolic disease, 1201
  metabolism, 41
  muscle phosphorylase deficiency (Type V), 755
Genomic DNA, analysis of, 43–45
Gestational diabetes mellitus
  associated features, 127
  β-cell response changes, 198
  and fetal growth, 200
  genetic factors, 198–199
  insulin receptor defects, 197–198
  insulin studies, importance of, 199
  insulin therapy, 1107–1108
  long-term effects of, 199–200
  and non-insulin dependent women, 195–196
  tumor necrosis factor-α, 198
  tyrosine phosphatase activity alteration, 198
GHF. *See* Growth hormone factor
Gibbs-Donnan equilibrium, 1048, 1049
Gilbert's disease, 868, 874–875
  genetic factors, 874, 875
Glomerular filtration rate (GFR)
  and angiotensin-converting enzyme inhibitors, 522
  in neonate, 1056
  and sodium metabolism in pregnancy, 282
  water/electrolyte balance, 1052
Glucagon, 155–161
  biosynthesis, 155
  and cAMP, 160
  and carbohydrate homeostasis, 158–159, 183–184
  catabolism of, 157–158
  and diabetes mellitus, 160–161
  and exercise in pregnancy, 329
  and fatty acid oxidation, 398
  and glucose metabolism in neonate, 701–702
  hypoglycemia treatment, 697, 1120
  and ketone body homeostasis, 159–160
  and liver glycogenolysis in neonate, 604
  mechanism of action, 160
  plasma glucagon, 155–157
  in postnatal period, 601–602
  protein metabolism, 111
  and protein metabolism in fetal-placental unit, 382
  secretion, regulation of, 158
  secretion of, 156–158
  storage of, 156
Glucocorticoid response element (GRE), 65–66
Glucocorticosteroids, and skeletal muscle, 663
Glucometer M, glucose measure, 686
Gluconeogenesis
  fetal production, 359–360
  liver, in fetus/neonate, 605–607, 617, 618
  in neonate, 709–710
  process of, 91–93
Gluconeogenesis disorders
  hepatic fructose-1,6-diphosphatase deficiency, 741–743
  hepatic phosphoenolpyruvate carboxykinase (PEPCK) deficiency, 741
  and hypoglycemia, 691–692
  pyruvate carboxylase deficiency, 740–741
Glucose
  availability and metabolism, 104–105
  concentration at birth, 683–684
  epinephrine effects, 163–162
  and fatty acid oxidation, 103–104
  and fatty acid oxidation in neonate, 617–618
  feeding for hypoglycemia, 156, 1156
  feeding for very low birth weight infant, 1160–1161
  functions of, 121
  heart and transport of, 551–552
  infused, physiologic response to, 97–98
  and insulin secretion, 139–140
  measurement in neonate, 685–687
  organs of production of, 91
  plasma glucose concentration at birth, 683–684
  production of, 91
  and protein metabolism, 109
  regulation of utilization, 96
Glucose-fatty acid cycle, 103–108
  endogenous fat as energy source, 99–100
  free-fatty acid oxidation, regulation of, 100–103
  glucose availability and metabolism, 104–105
  glucose effects on fatty acid oxidation, 103–104
  glucose effects on lipolysis, 103
  glycerol, 105
  hepatic triglyceride synthesis, 98–99
  hormones in, 99
  inhibition of glucose uptake, 101–102
  intestinal fat absorption, 98
  ketones, 105
  lipid clearance from blood, 99
  support for theory, 101
Glucose metabolism, 91–103
  and alanine, 92
  cerebral glucose metabolism, 543–547
  control mechanisms, 93
  fructose diphosphate, conversion to fructose-6-phosphate, 94
  futile cycles, 94
  and glucagon, 158–159
  gluconeogenesis, 91–93
  glucose uptake, 95
  glucose utilization, regulation of, 96
  glycogen deposition, 96
  glycogenolysis, 91

Index

glycolysis, 95–96
in heart, 552–556
in heart of fetus/neonate, 562–563
and hepatic triglyceride synthesis, 98–99
hexose monophosphate shunt, 96
infused glucose, physiologic response to, 97–98
and insulin, 95, 97, 125, 144–146, 184–186
and intestinal fat absorption, 98
intestinal tract of neonate, 627–630
and lipids. See Glucose-fatty acid cycle
and liver, 91, 93–94, 95, 96, 145–146
muscle uptake of glucose, 97
in perinatal period. See Liver glyconeogenesis in neonate
physiologic control of, 95
postabsorptive state, 183–184
postprandial state, 184
pyruvate, conversion to phosphoenolpyruvate (PEP), 93–94
pyruvate oxidation, 96
renal gluconeogenesis, 93
in skeletal muscle, 651–654, 658–659
substrate regulation, 93
Glucose metabolism in fetal-placental unit
and cortisol, 355
and fat synthesis, 358–359
Fick principle, 337–339
and gestational changes, 350
gluconeogenesis, 359–360
glucose oxidation, 356–357
glucose oxidation rate, 343–344
glucose production, 344–345, 360
glucose transporters, 123–129, 345–346, 356
glucose uptake, 352
glucose utilization, 352–354, 360
glycogen formation, 351, 357–358
insulin effects on, 353–354
insulin receptors, 346
insulin secretion, 140, 352–353
and intrauterine growth factors (IGF), 355–356
and maternal glucose concentration, 347–348
net flux measurements, 337–339
net utilization versus turnover, 338–339
placental glucose metabolism, 351–352
placental glucose transport, 346–351, 1099
placental surface area effects, 349
and protein metabolism, 360–361
three-pool glucose utilization model, 341–343
and thyroid hormone, 354–355
tracer methods for measurement, 338–341
two-pool glucose utilization model, 341
Glucose metabolism in neonate
and catecholamines, 702
and central nervous system, 713–715
clinical hypoglycemia, 687–697
disorders of. See Carbohydrate metabolism disorders
and epinephrine, 705–706
euglycemia, definition of, 683–684
and glucagon, 701–702
gluconeogenesis, 709–710
glucose measurement, 685–687
glucose utilization, 711–713
hormone receptors, 709
hyperglycemia in neonate, 697–700
hypoglycemia, definition of, 684–685
and insulin, 701–705
insulin resistance/sensitivity, 706–708
plasma glucose concentration at birth, 683–684
substrate availability, 710–711
and surgery, 1135–1137
Glucose metabolism in pregnancy
animal models, 199–200
and cortisol, 191, 192
early gestation, 186–188
and estrogen, 191
during exercise, 327–329
and gestational diabetes. See Gestational diabetes mellitus
hepatic glucose output, control of, 192
and human placental lactogen, 191–192
and insulin-dependent diabetes mellitus, 194
insulin secretion, 192–193
late gestation, 188–191
compared to nongravid persons, 183–186
and non-insulin dependent diabetes mellitus, 194–196
postabsorptive state, 186–187, 189
postprandial state, 187–188, 189–191
and progesterone, 191
and prolactin, 192
and prostaglandins, 270–273
proximal post-insulin receptor defects, 197–198
skeletal muscle metabolism, 193–194
and tyrosine phosphatase, 198
and weight gain, 188
Glucose oxidation, 356–357
Glucose oxidation rate, 343–344
Glucose-6-phosphatase
genetic factors, 750–751
liver glycogenolysis in neonate, 603
measurement of, 747
Glucose-6-phosphatase defect (Type I), 692, 745–751
biochemical diagnosis, 747
genetic factors, 750–751
and hypoglycemia, 748–749
and jaundice, 868
laboratory tests, 746
pathology, 747–748
pathophysiology, 748
prognosis of, 750
signs of, 745–746
tolerance tests, 746–747
treatment of, 749–750
variants of, 751
Glucose production, 344–345, 360
Glucose therapy
and hyperglycemia in neonate, 156, 696
for very low birth weight infant, 1160–1161
Glucose transporter proteins, 544–547
Glucose transporters
and brain, 544–547
facilitative. See Facilitative glucose transporters
in fetal-placental unit, 123–129, 345–346, 356
insulin regulation of, 144–145
sites of expression, 122
sodium-dependent transporters, 121–123
Glucose turnover
net utilization versus turnover, 338–339
use of term, 338
Glucose uptake, 352
Glucose utilization, 352–354, 360
β-glucuronidase deficiency, 1232
Glucuronosyl transferase, 867
GLUT 1, 123–124, 145
and brain, 127, 545–547
and embryo, 126–127
and liver, 128
and lung, 128
and placenta, 127, 345–346
GLUT 2, 124–125, 192
and embryo, 127
and kidney, 129
and liver, 128
GLUT 3, 125
and brain, 127–128, 546, 547
and embryo, 127
and placenta, 127, 345
GLUT 4, 125–126, 145, 186
and gestational diabetes mellitus, 197
and liver, 128

GLUT 5, 126
and brain, 546
GLUT 7, 126
Glutamate, production of, 634
Glutamic-oxaloacetic transaminase (GOT), and amino acid metabolism, 557
Glutamic-pyruvic transaminase (GPT), and amino acid metabolism, 557
Glutamine
inhibition of oxidation, 634
oxidation, gastrointesinal tract of fetus/neonate, 632–634, 636–637
uptake from placenta, 358
Glutaric acidemia, Type I, 810
prognosis, 810
signs of, 810
Glutaric acidemia, Type II, 810
prognosis, 810
signs of, 810
treatment approach, 810
Glycerides, nature of, 821
Glycerol
production of, 105
release of, 93
Glyceryl trinitrate (GTN), modulation of nitric oxide (NO), 466
Glycine
metabolism of, 801–802
and nonketotic hyperglycinemia, 812
Glycogen formation, 351, 357–358
Glycogenesis type VII, 652
Glycogen metabolism
deposition and glucose metabolism, 96
fetal heart, 562
fetal-placental unit, 351, 357–358
in heart, 553–554
and insulin, 145–146
in lungs of fetus/neonate, 576–577
skeletal muscle, 658–659
Glycogen metabolism disorders
α-acid glucoside deficiency (Type II), 756–757
amylopectinosis brancher deficiency (Type IV), 758–759
classification of, 743–745
Debrancher, amylo-1,6-glucosidase deficiency (Type III), 751–753
glucose-6-phosphatase defect (Type I), 745–751
glycogen synthase defect, 759–760
liver phosphorylase defect (Type VI), 753–754
muscle phosphofructokinase deficiency (Type VII), 755–756
Glycogenolysis
in fetus/neonate, 603–604
in heart, 553–554
process of, 91

Glycogen phosphorylase, liver glycogenolysis in neonate, 603
Glycogen synthase defect, 759–760
diagnosis of, 759
management of, 760
pathogenesis, 759
prognosis, 760
Glycogen synthetase
liver glycogenolysis in neonate, 603
regulation of, 553
Glycolysis
aerobic glycolysis, 540
in brain, fetus/neonate, 540–541
in heart, 554–555
hypoxia, effects on, 556
inhibition of, 555
intestinal tract of fetus/neonate, 627–628
process of, 95–96
Glyconeogenesis, renal, process of, 93
G_{M1}, gangliosidosis, 1231–1232
signs of, 1231–1232
Gonadotropin-releasing hormone (GnRH), placental production/release of, 428, 431
G proteins, receptor binding with, 61–62
GRE. See Glucocorticoid-response element
Great vessels, fetal blood flow, 488
Growth
effects on metabolic rate, 1011
See also Fetal growth
Growth factors, 61, 403
insulin, 148
use of term, 403
Growth factors in fetal-placental unit
apoptosis from, 406
and cell migration/motility, 406–407
and cell morphogenesis, 407
cellular differentiation from, 406
cellular proliferation from, 404–406
epidermal growth factor (EGF), 411–412
fibroblast growth factor (FGF), 416–417
hepatocyte growth factor (HGF), 417
insulin-like growth factors (IGFs), 412–414
nerve growth factor (NGF), 417
platelet-derived growth factor (PDGF), 414–415
receptors for, 407–408
signaling enzymes, 408–411
site of secretion and action, 403–404
transforming growth factor-α, 411–412
transforming growth factor-β, 415–416

Growth hormone, 165–168
and α-adrenergic receptors, 166
biosynthesis of, 166
degradation of, 166
endogenous growth hormone, role of, 167–168
exercise effects, 329
fetal secretion, 430
and intrauterine growth retardation (IUGR), 1098–1099
mechanism of action, 167
metabolic functions of, 166–167
and protein metabolism, 111
releasing factors, 166
secretion, regulation of, 166
and skeletal muscle, 663
structure of, 165–166
Growth hormone factor, 429–430
Growth-hormone releasing hormone (GRH), 166
Growth retardation, 1097, 1098
Growth retarded fetus, 1100

H
Haldane effect, 459, 470
Hales-Randle effect, 184
Hartnup disease, niacin deficiency, 984
Harvard University, Web site, 45
hCG. See Human chorionic gonadotropin
HCS. See Human chorionic somatomammotropin
HDL. See High density lipoproteins
Heart
adenosine triphosphate, production/utilization of, 551, 558–559, 561
blood flow in fetal heart, 488
changes in pregnancy, 319
and water/electrolyte metabolism, 1051–1052
and water/electrolyte metabolism in neonate, 1054
See also Cardiac metabolism
Heart defects
cardiac hypertrophy, 115
infant of diabetic mother, 1115–1116
left-to-right shunt, 490
and neonatal hypoglycemia, 691
Heart rate
and blood pressure, 498–499
and cardiac output, 494–495
Heat balance equation, 1029
Heat storage equation, 1001
Heme and non-heme sources of iron, 289
Hemoglobin
diabetes control, 1106–1107
and placental oxygen delivery, 457–459
in pregnancy, 290

Index

Hemosiderin, 912
Henderson-Hasselbach equation, 467
Hepatic fructose-1,6-diphosphatase deficiency, 741–743
 diagnosis of, 742
 management of, 742–743
 pathogenesis of, 742
 signs of, 742
Hepatic glucose output, control of, 192
Hepatic phosphoenolpyruvate carboxykinase (PEPCK) deficiency, 741
 molecular defect, 741
 signs of, 741
 and sudden infant death syndrome (SIDS), 741
Hepatic triglyceride lipase (HTGL), 234
Hepatocyte growth factor (HGF), 417
 in amniotic fluid, 524
 chemical structure, 417
 functions of, 417
 receptors for, 417
Hepatolenticular degeneration. See Wilson's disease
Hereditary fructose intolerance. See Fructose intolerance
Hereditary hemochromatosis, 915
Hexose monophosphate shunt, glucose metabolism, 96
HGF. See Heptocyte growth factor
High density lipoproteins (HDL)
 androgen effects, 225
 estrogen effects, 224–225
 and fetal growth, 243
 and lactating women, 248
 metabolism of, 223–224
 placental transport, 237, 238–239
 in pregnancy, 229–230, 232–236, 238–239
High-resolution 2-D PAGE, protein separation, 48
Hill-Langmuir equation, 57
Histocompatiblity leukocyte antigen (HLA), and skeletal muscle development, 649
HIV. See Human immunodeficiency virus
HLA. See Histocompatibility leukocyte antigen; Human leukocyte antigen
Horizontal protein blotting, protein separation, 48
Hormones
 in amniotic fluid, 523, 524
 and calcitonin secretion, 898
 contrainsulin hormones, 155–172
 and diabetes mellitus, 161
 and energy metabolism in neonate, 1010
 and glucose metabolism in normal adult, 91, 94
 and glucose metabolism in neonate, 701–706
 and glucose metabolism in pregnancy, 191, 191–192
 in human milk, 1183
 and intrauterine growth retardation (IUGR), 1098–1099
 and lipid metabolism in pregnancy, 224–225
 and lipid synthesis, 99
 and lungs of fetus/neonate, 582–584
 and magnesium metabolism, 888
 and phosphorous concentration, 885
 and protein metabolism, 109–112
 and protein metabolism in neonate, 777–778
 and regulation of β-adrenergic receptors, 441–444
 and skeletal muscle, 662–663
 See also Developmental endocrinology; specific hormones
HTGL. See Hepatic triglyceride lipase
Human chorionic gonadotropin (hCG), 427
 chromosomal location of gene coding, 427
 fetal secretion, 427
 hormone regulators of, 427
 physiological functions of, 427
 and sexual differentiation, 427
Human chorionic somatomammotropin (HCS), 165–166, 427
Human Genome Project, 42, 52
Human immunodeficiency virus (HIV), transmission from breastfeeding, 1185
Human leukocyte antigen (HLA), 915
Human milk
 biotin content, 992
 calcium content, 883
 carbohydrates in, 1182
 carnitine in, 861
 chromium in, 934
 content and course of lactation, 823, 824, 825
 digestion of, 1185
 drugs secreted into, 1185
 factors affecting composition of, 824, 825
 fat content in, 823–824
 fatty acid composition of, 824
 folate content, 987
 compared to formula, 825
 fortification of, 887, 1169, 1190–1191
 growth factors in, 1183
 hormones in, 1183
 host defense factors, 1183
 iron content, 914
 magnesium content, 889
 manganese content, 932
 maternal influences, 1183–1184
 and maternal nutrition, 1184
 minerals/trace elements in, 1182
 molybdenum in, 933–934
 niacin content, 983–984
 nucleotides in, 1182–1183
 pantothenic acid content, 991
 and phosphorous deficiency, 886–887
 protein quality of, 1181–1182
 pyridoxine content, 985
 riboflavin content, 981–982
 thiamine content, 980
 trans fatty acids in, 825
 and vegan mothers, 1184
 for very low birth weight infant, 1168–1169
 vitamin B_{12} content, 990
 vitamin C content, 993
 vitamin D content, 897, 952, 1182, 1184
 vitamin E content, 961
 vitamin K deficiency, 1182, 1184
 volumes, 1183
 zinc content, 927–928
 See also Breastfeeding
Human placental lactogen, 427–428
 daily production of, 428
 fetal secretion, 428
 genetic location of, 427
 and glucose metabolism in pregnancy, 191–192
 terms related to, 427
Hybridization methods, DNA, 44–45
Hybridoma, 28–29
Hydatiform mole, 519
Hydrallantois, 523
Hydrops fetalis
 causes of, 525
 immune type, 525
 nonimmune type, 525
Hydrostatic/osmotic interaction, 1049–1051
16α-hydroxydehydroepiandrosterone sulfate, 425
Hyperammonemia
 differential diagnosis, 1201
 laboratory findings, 1210
 pathophysiology for, 1210
Hyperbilirubinemia, 867–867
 and ABO incompatibility, 872
 conjugated hyperbilirubinemia, 875–876
 evaluation for, 868, 872
 infant of diabetic mother, 1121
 management of, 872–873
 and Rh incompatibility, 871–872
 underlying causes, 868
Hypercalcemia, 884
 causes of, 884

signs of, 884
Hypercarbia, causes of, 1161
Hypercholesterolemia, management of, 249
Hyperglucagonemia, 158
Hyperglycemia in fetus, 352–353
Hyperglycemia in neonate, 697–700
 evaluation of, 699
 and infant death, 697
 infant of diabetic mother, 1108–1109
 and parenteral nutrition, 697–698
 pathophysiology of, 1160
 and sepsis, 699
 and steroid therapy, 699
 and surgery, 699, 1135, 1136, 1137
 treatment of, 699–700, 1161
 and very low birth weight infant, 697, 1160–1161
Hyperglycinemia, in propionic acidemia, 807
Hyperinsulinemia
 and Beckwith-Wiedemann syndrome, 693, 1155
 disorders related to, 138
 and exercise, 328
 familial, 138
 gene mutations, 139
 and hypoglycemia in neonate, 690, 692–695, 1155
 infant of diabetic mother, 273, 1109, 1155
 and leucine sensitivity, 695
 and maternal β-sympathomimetic therapy, 694
 and nesidioblastosis, 693–694
 pathophysiology of, 1155
 and Rh incompatibility, 692–693
Hyperkalemia, very low birth weight infant, 1057
Hyperlipidemia, Type I, 839
Hypermagnesemia, 889, 890
 definition of, 890
 fetus, 890
 management of, 890
 neonate, 890
 signs of, 890
Hypermanganesemia, 933
Hyperparathyroidism, 893
 and pregnancy, 891
 signs of, 893
Hypertension. See Pregnancy-induced hypertension (PIH)
Hypertriglyceridemia, management of, 249
Hyperventilation, and maternal/fetal acid-base balance, 470
Hyperzincemia, 929
Hypoaminoacidemia, 110
Hypocalcemia, 883–884
 and asphyxia, 893
 and hypoparathyroidism, 893–894
 infant of diabetic mother, 1120–1121
 pathogenesis, 883–884
 risk factors for neonates, 883, 893
 small-for-gestational-age (SGA) infant, 1101
 treatment of, 884
 underlying conditions, 884
 and vitamin D, 953
Hypocaloric feedings, very low birth weight infant, 1170–1171
Hypoglycemia
 after birth, 547
 control and growth hormone, 167–168
 and cortisol, 170–171
 and fructose intolerance, 734–735
 and glucagon secretion, 158, 617
 glucose-6–phosphatase defect (Type I), 748–749
 Somogyi phenomenon, 168
Hypoglycemia in neonate, 687–697, 1155–1156
 and Beckwith-Wiedemann syndrome, 693
 and birth weight, 685, 688, 697, 699, 1156
 causes of, 1155–1156, 1211
 cold-stressed neonate, 690–691
 and congenital adrenal hyperplasia, 695
 and congenital heart disease, 691
 definition of, 684, 1156
 differential diagnosis, 1212
 evaluation of, 695–696, 1211–1212
 glucagon treatment, 697, 1120
 gluconeogesis defects, 691–692
 and hyperinsulinemia, 690, 1155
 and hypoxia, 690
 immediate newborn period, 547
 infant of diabetic mother, 200, 271, 617, 1115, 1119–1120
 intrauterine growth retardation (IUGR), 127, 690
 and leucine sensitivity, 695
 and maternal β-sympathomimetics therapy, 694
 and maternal ethanol ingestion, 694–695
 and nesidioblastosis, 693–694
 in postnatal period, 601–602, 617
 preterm infant, 688
 and Rh incompatibility, 692
 and sepsis, 691
 signs/symptoms of, 688, 1156
 small-for-gestational-age (SGA) infant, 618, 688–690, 1101–1102, 1156
 and toxemia, 688
 treatment of, 696–697, 1120, 1156
 and umbilical artery catheter, 694
Hypomagnesemia, 890–891
 causes in neonate, 890
 definition of, 890
 infant of diabetic mother, 1121
 management of, 890–891
Hyponatremia, of prematurity, 1069–1070
Hypoparathyroidism, 893–895
 DiGeorge syndrome, 893
 and hypocalcemia, 893–894
 in preterm infant, 892–893
Hypotension, treatment of, 1066
Hypothalamic peptides, 428
 corticotropin-releasing factor (CRF), 428
 gonadotropin-releasing hormone (GnRH), 428
 placental production/release of, 428
Hypothalamus
 development of, 428–429
 and glycose metabolism, 91
 hypothalamic peptides, 428–429
Hypoxemia
 and bradycardia, 498–499
 and fetal circulation, 498–499
Hypoxia
 as glycolysis trigger, 556
 and hypoglycemia in neonate, 690
 and parenteral nutrition, 1163

I

Ichthyosis, hormonal factors, 425
Illness, and metabolism rate in neonate, 1013–1014
Imaging methods, body composition measures, 1079
Immobilization, and protein turnover, 790
Immune system
 and human milk, 1183
 and prostaglandins, 264
 and vitamin A deficiency, 949
 and zinc deficiency, 925
Immunoassay
 antibodies used, 28–29
 antibody characterization, 29–30
 competitive immunoassay, 30–31
 cross-reactivity, 30
 cyclic nucleotides measurement, 36
 development/design of, 28
 ELISA format, 37
 goals of, 28
 immunometric assay, 31–33
 kit directories, 36
 kit versus in-house assay, 36–37
 liquid-phase, 33
 nonisotopic method, 34
 ordering information, 37
 peptides in, 35
 precision of, 28

Index

prostaglandin measurement, 36
proteins used, 34–35
separation methods, 33
signaling methods, 33–34
solid-phase, 33
specificity of, 28
steroid measurement, 35
thyroid hormones measurement, 35–36
Immunohistochemistry, 58–59
Immunometric assay, 31–33
Inborn errors
  amino acid/organic acid metabolism disorders, 804–813
  branched-chain amino acid metabolism, 802–803
  carbohydrate metabolism disorders, 723–760
  diagnosis of. See Metabolic disease evaluation
  fatty acid oxidation defects, 839, 847–853
  gylcine metabolism, 801–802
  urea cycle, 801
Incubator, 1027, 1038–1039
  and preterm infant, 1038
  single versus double walled, 1038–1039
  temperature regulation, 1038
  and water loss, 1062, 1063
Indirect calorimetry, 1002
  compared to doubly labeled water, 1003–1004
Infant of diabetic mother
  asphyxia, 1116–1117
  birth injury, 1116
  calcitonin elevations in neonate, 899–900
  cardiovascular defects, 1114, 1115–1116
  early/late delivery issue, 1118–1119
  ethnic factors, 1110
  and fetal body composition, 1110
  fetal growth, 200, 1110, 1111
  fetal problems resulting from, 271, 272–273, 358
  gangrene, 1117
  hyperbilirubinemia, 1121
  hyperglycemia, 1108–1109
  hyperinsulinemia of, 273, 1109
  hypocalcemia, 893, 1120–1121
  hypoglycemia, 1119–1120
  hypomagnesemia, 1121
  infant mortality and diabetes control, 1107–1108
  insulin-dependent mother, fetal effects, 271
  insulin therapy for mother and outcome, 1107–1108
  kinetic analysis of, 1111–1113

macrosomia, 81–82, 200, 271, 379, 1109–1110, 1116, 1117
maternal classification (White's scheme), 1106
perinatal mortality, 1106
polycythemia, 1121–1122
pre-birth monitoring studies, 1117
preeclampsia, 1106
prenatal care and outcome, 1105, 1107–1108, 1111–1112, 1114–1115
prognosis for, 1122–1124
Prognostically Bad Signs of Pregnancy, 1105, 1106
renal vein thrombosis, 1122
and respiratory distress syndrome, 577, 1117–1119
small left colon syndrome, 1115
vitamin E as protectant, 1116
Infant formulas
  for acute metabolic decompensation, 1224
  and brain development, 830–831
  and breastfeeding, compared to, 825–826
  calcium content, 883
  carnitine in, 861
  composition and metabolic rate, 1007–1010
  enriched, and metabolic rate, 1007–1010
  fluoride in, 934
  compared to human milk, 825
  human milk fortifiers, 1190
  iron fortification, 914
  lipids in, 823
  and magnesium absorption, 890
  phosphorous content, 886
  for preterm infants, 887, 897, 1015
  product names, 823
  vitamin D content, 897, 952–953
  water-soluble vitamin contents, 978
Infantile beriberi, thiamine deficiency, 981
Infection, and protein synthesis, 108
Infertility, and prostaglandins, 264, 265
Infused glucose, 97–98
Inhibin, 428
  functions of, 428
  organs for production of, 428
Innervation, of skeletal muscle, 646–647
In situ hybridization, RNA, 46–47
Insulin
  and adipocyte fatty acid synthesis, 147
  and amylin, 171
  anabolic effect of, 109
  biosynthesis of, 135–138
  counterregulatory hormones. See Contrainsulin hormones

dawn phenomenon, 168
epinephrine effects, 164
and exercise in pregnancy, 328–329
fetal secretion, 352–354
gene, cloning of, 138–139
and gluconeogenesis in liver, 146
glucose effects, 139–140
glucose-FFA-cycle issue, 97
and glucose metabolism in neonate, 701–705
and glucose production, 95
and glucose transport, 144–145, 184–185
and glucose utilization, 97, 125
and glycogen metabolism, 145–146
and glycolysis in liver, 146
as growth factor, 148
insulin gene, 138–139
insulin receptor, 140–142
and intrauterine growth retardation (IUGR), 1099
and lipid metabolism, 99, 147
and lipid metabolism in fetal-placental unit, 394–395
and myocardial protein balance, 561
postreceptor events, 142–144
and pregnancy. See Glucose metabolism in pregnancy
and protein metabolism, 109–112, 147–149
and protein metabolism in fetal-placental unit, 379–381
regulation of release, 139–140
resistance to, 171
second messenger, 144
sex-differences in concentrations of, 226
and skeletal muscle, 663
structure of, 135
Insulin-dependent diabetes mellitus
  and breast fed infants, 1186
  genetic factors, 194
  glucose metabolism in pregnancy, 194
  and magnesium depletion, 889
  Somogyi effect, 168
Insulin-like growth factors (IGF), 412–414
  animal models, 83–86
  and cell differentiation, 406
  chromosomal location of, 412
  EGF receptor knockout mice studies, 412
  and energy metabolism, 85
  and glucose metabolism in fetal-placental unit, 355–356
  IGF binding proteins, 413–414
  IGF-I, 412, 413
  IGF-II, 412–413

and intrauterine growth retardation
(IUGR), 1099
modulation of, 83
physiological actions of, 413
promoter region for, 413
and protein metabolism in fetal-
placental unit, 381–382
synthesis of, 414
Insulin receptors, 140–142
fetal-placental unit, 346
Insulin receptor substrate (IRS-1),
functions of, 142–143
Insulin resistance
compared to insulin
unresponsiveness, 706
in neonate, 706–708
Insulin secretion, 140, 192–193, 352–353
Insulin signaling, 184–186
Insulin therapy
in gestational diabetes, 1107–1108
hyperglycemia treatment in neonate,
699–700
Integrins, 649
Intellectual impairment, infant of
diabetic mother, 1123
Interorgan metabolism, 377
Interstitial hydrostatic pressure, and
water/electrolyte metabolism, 1050
Interstitial oncotic pressure, and water/
electrolyte metabolism, 1051
Intestinal tract of neonate, 632
Intestines, breath tests, 18
Intracellular water regulation,
1047–1048
Intralipid, 1162, 1163
Intrauterine growth retardation
(IUGR)
amino acid kinetics studies, 383–384
and amino acid transport system, 384
animal studies, 382–383
areas of investigation, 383
asymmetrical growth retardation,
1097, 1098
and energy metabolism in neonate,
1015
and growth hormone, 1098–1099
and hypoglycemia, 127, 690
and increased placental blood flow,
465
and insulin, 1099
and insulin-like growth factors
(IGF), 1099
and iron deficiency, 913
maternal conditions related to,
1100–1111
and multiple gestation, 1100
and nutritional regulation, 381–382
and placental transport of metabolic
fuels, 1099–1100

and protein metabolism in fetal-
placental unit, 382–384
symmetrical growth retardation,
1097, 1098
Intravenous fructose tolerance test, 735
In utero surgery, and placental
respiratory gas exchange, 475–476
Iodide, placental permeability to, 432
Iodine, 296–297, 931–932
bioavailability of, 296
defective uptake, 932
deficiency features, 931–932
deficiency and fetal effects, 297
functions of, 931
metabolism defects, 932
metabolism of, 296, 931
metabolism in pregnancy, 296–297
placental transfer, 931
and thyroid hormones, 931–932
Iron, 289–292, 909–916
bioavailability, 289
deficiency features, 912
deficiency in pregnancy, 290–292
fetal/neonatal metabolism of,
913–915
function of, 909–910
heme and non-heme sources, 289
iron deficiency anemia, 290, 291
iron-dependent metalloproteins, 909,
910
metabolism of, 289–290, 910–912
metabolism in pregnancy, 290, 912
neonatal deficiency, 913
placental transfer of, 912–913
and preterm infants, 914–915
recommended daily intake, 290
supplementation in pregnancy,
291–292
uptake by tissue, 911
and vitamin E, 960
Iron deficiency anemia, 290, 291
Iron-dependent metalloproteins, 909,
910
Iron fortification in infant formulas,
914
Iron metabolism defects, 915–916
aceruloplasminemia, 916
and birth weight, 291
congenital atransferrinemia, 915
defective sialylation of transferrin,
915
hereditary hemochromatosis, 915
impaired absorption, 915
impaired iron uptake, 915
microcytic anemia, 916
perinatal hemochromatosis, 915–916
Ischemia, and glycolysis inhibition, 555
Islet cell adenoma, 693–694
Isotopic tracer measures of turnover,
211–212

Isovaleric acidemia, 809–810
biochemical alterations in, 809–810
forms of, 809
signs of, 809
treatment of, 810
Isozymes
genetic defects related to, 650, 651
regulation of, 662
skeletal muscle, 650–654
See also Skeletal muscle metabolism
IUGR. See Intrauterine growth
retardation

J

Jackson mice, 430
JAKS (Janus kinases), 408
Jaundice, 865
and glucose-6-phosphatase defect,
868
and parenteral feeding, 1164
See also Bilirubin metabolism
defects
Jun N-terminal kinase (JNK) system,
growth factor signal transduction,
410–411

K

KAL gene, 429
Kallikrein-kinen system
in neonate, 1058
and water/electrolyte metabolism,
1053
Kallman's syndrome, hormonal factors,
429
Keratinocyte growth factor (KGF), 416
and skin development, 407
Keshan disease, 930
Ketogenesis
and insulin, 147
in neonate, 608–609, 617–618
Ketone bodies
and cardiac metabolism, 557
as fatty acid synthesis precursor, 394
fuel for perinatal brain, 547
glucagon and homeostasis of,
159–160
and glucagon secretion, 158
importance for neonate, 838
and intestinal glucose oxidation in
neonate, 630
oxidation and fetal development, 399
oxidation and gastrointestinal tract
of fetus/neonate, 634–635
oxidation and neonatal intestinal
tract, 634–635
production of, 105, 159
and protein metabolism, 109
suckling ketosis, 860
and surgery, 1142–1143
utilization by brain, 98, 105

Index

utilization in neonate, 838–839
Ketone body homeostasis, 159–160
Ketone synthesis deficiencies, 851
Kidney
  catacholamine effects, 1052–1053
  and facilitative glucose transporters, 129
  function after birth, 1055–1056
  gluconeogenesis, 93
  and glycagon catabolism, 157–158
  of neonate, 1054–1059
  of preterm infant, 1069–1070
  and prostaglandins, 264
  sodium excretion, 1052
  and water/electrolyte metabolism, 1052
  and water/electrolyte metabolism in neonate, 1054–1059
Kinetic analysis, infant of diabetic mother, 1111–1113
Kinetic experiments, 371–373
Kinetic techniques, 1–10
Kit directories, 36
Kit versus in-house assay, 36–37
Kjeldahl method, nitrogen balance, 779
Knockout method of gene ablation, 68
Krebs cycle, 538, 539
  and ADP regulation, 558
  of heart, 554, 558
  intestinal tract of neonate, 629, 631

L

Labor
  and arachidonic acid, 265
  prostaglandins during, 265
Lactate
  and cardiac metabolism, 555–556, 557
  and cardiac metabolism of fetus/neonate, 562
  conversion and pyruvate, 394, 555
  elevation in fetus, causes of, 470
  and exercise, 325–326
  as fatty acid synthesis precursor, 394
  and fetal fatty acid oxidation, 399
  and glucose metabolism, 92
  Pasteur effect, 555
  production and neonatal intestine, 627–628
Lactate acidosis, primary, 1203–1206
Lactate dehydrogenase
  deficiency, signs of, 654
  skeletal muscle, 653–654
Lactation
  and fat stores in pregnancy, 310
  and maternal lipid metabolism, 244, 247–249
Lactic acid, fuel for perinatal brain, 547–548
Lactogen, placental, 427–428
Lactose, in enteral nutrition, 1167
Lactose intolerance, 1167
LDL. *See* Low density lipoproteins
Lead, 292–294
  bioavailability of, 292
  and birth weight, 293–294
  fetal neurotoxicity, 292–293
  high exposure effects, 292
  metabolism in pregnancy, 292
  and pregnancy outcome, 293–294
  treatment of exposure, 292
  and VACTERL syndrome, 293
Lecithin-retinol acyltransferase. *See* LRAT
Left-to-right shunt, 490
Leptin, 172
  concentrations, affecting factors, 172
  functions of, 172
  and obesity, 827
Leucine
  and growth-retarded fetus, 1100
  and protein metabolism, 108
  turnover in pregnancy, 212–124
  utilization in fetal-placental unit, 376, 383
Leucine sensitivity, and hypoglycemia in neonate, 695
Leukotrines, 263
  pulmonary vasodilation, 502
LH. *See* Luteinizing hormone
LHRH. *See* Leuteinizing hormone-releasing hormone
Ligand-gated ion channels, types of, 60
Ligand recognition, 54–58
Ligands
  bound and unbound, 55
  receptor activation and binding, 53–58
  tagging procedure, 55
  types of, 53
Limb myogenesis, 643
Limbs, limb bud formation, 643
Lineweaver-Burk equation, 57
Linoleic acid, 259, 1158
Linolenic acid, 259, 1158
Lipid clearing enzymes, 838
Lipid dosorders, management of, 249–250
Lipid metabolism
  and adenosine, 99–100
  and cholesterol ingestion, 221–222
  and epinephrine, 164
  and essential fatty acids, 221
  fat absorption, 221–222
  fatty acid oxidation pathway, 847–849
  in heart, 556–557
  in heart of fetus/neonate, 561–562
  and insulin, 99, 147
  lipoprotein cascade, 222–224
  and liver, 100, 104, 147
  sex differences in, 225–226
  in skeletal muscle, 659–660
Lipid metabolism in fetal-placental unit
  and body composition changes, 390
  control factors in lipid transfer, 390
  and epidermal growth factor (EGF), 395
  fatty acid chain length, 391
  fatty acid oxidation, 396–399
  fatty acid synthesis pathways, 392–393
  fetal albumin concentration, 391
  fetal lipid accumulation and placental transfer, 390, 392
  fetuin concentration, 391
  future studies, 395–396
  and gestational age, 392, 393–394
  glucose carbon effects, 358–359
  and insulin, 394–395
  ketone oxidation, 399
  lipogenesis precursors, 394
  neural factors, 395
  placental metabolism of lipids, 391
  processes in, 389
  transplacental fatty acid gradient, 390–391
Lipid metabolism in neonate
  and brain development, 828–831
  digestive lipases, 832–834
  disorders of. *See* Fatty acid oxidation defects
  and duodenum, 834–835
  fat absorption, 835–836
  fat digestion, 831–835
  inborn errors of, 839
  ketone bodies, 838–839
  lipid clearing enzymes, 838
  medium-chain fatty acids, 831
  mitochondrial fatty acid oxidation, 849
  and parenteral nutrition, 839
  and preterm infants, 839
  and stomach, 832–834
  and surgery, 1142–1145
  transport of lipids, 836–838
Lipid metabolism in pregnancy
  and appetite regulation, 226–228
  and diabetes mellitus, 243–244
  and estrogen, 224–225
  fat absorption, 228–229
  fat storage, 226–227
  and fetal growth, 241–243
  and free fatty acids, 228
  lactation, 244, 247–249
  lipid disorders, management of, 249–250
  lipoprotein lipid metabolism, 227–236

placenta and lipid transport, 236–239
placenta and modified lipoproteins, 239–241
and progestins, 225
and prostaglandins, 265–266
and toxemic pregnancy, 241
Lipids
in enteral feeding, 1167
fatty acids, 821–823
functions in mammals, 823
and glucose metabolism. See Glucose-fatty acid cycle
glycerides, 821
in human milk, 823–824
in infant formulas, 823
lung surfactant lipids, 569–570, 577–578
in parenteral feeding, 1162–1163
phospholipids, 821
sterols, 821
for very low birth weight infant, 839, 1162–1163, 1167
Lipid supplementation, for hypoglycemia in neonate, 696–697
Lipogenesis, 392–395
Lipoprotein cascade, 222–224
Lipoprotein lipase (LPL), 99, 222, 838
function of, 222
regulation of, 222
Lipoprotein lipid metabolism, 227–236
Lipoproteins
chylomicrons, 836, 837
function of, 836
high density lipoproteins (HDL), 223–224
lipid transport in neonate, 836–838
low density lipoproteins, 223–224
very low density lipoproteins (VLDL), 223
Lipoproteins and pregnancy
causes of lipid level change, 231–235
changes in lipid levels, 229–231
diabetes, effects of, 243–244
and fetal growth, 241–243
high density lipoproteins (HDL), 229–230, 232–236, 238–239
hormonal effects, 235–236
and lactation, 244, 247–249
lipid transfer across placenta, 236–239
low density lipoproteins (LDL), 229–230, 232–236, 238–241
placenta and modified lipoproteins, 239–241
very low density lipoproteins (VLDL), 229–230, 232–235, 237, 238
Liposyn, 1162
Lipoxygenase products, 263
Liquid-phase immunoassay, 33

Lithium, deficiency features, 934
Liver
blood flow in fetal liver, 487–488
breath tests, 18
and facilitative glucose transporters, 128
and glucose metabolism, 91, 93–94, 95, 96
glucose output in pregnancy, 192
and glycagon catabolism, 157
glycogen metabolism, 145–146
ketogenesis, 147
lipid metabolism, 100, 104, 147
protein breakdown, 110
protein metabolism in pregnancy, 217
triglyceride synthesis, 98–99
vitamin A storage/mobilization, 947–948
Liver glycogenolysis in neonate, 603–607
carbohydrates supplied via milk, 604
enzyme activities, 603, 605–606
and galactose uptake, 604
glycogenolysis, 603–604
glyconeogenesis, 605–607, 617, 618
glyconeogenic pathway, 605
hormonal factors, 603, 606
and liver glycogen stores, 603
liver oxygenation, 606
mitochondrial oxidative capacity, 606–607
relationship to fatty acid oxidation, 615–617
short term control of, 607
Liver metabolism in fetus/neonate
fatty acid oxidation. See Fatty acid oxidation in neonate
glucose metabolism. See Liver glyconeogeneis in neonate
and hormonal changes, 601–603, 617
and nutritional changes, 601
Liver phosphorylase defect (Type VI), 753–754
biochemical studies, 753
course of, 753–754
genetic factors, 754
prognosis of, 754
variants of, 754
Long-chain acyl-CoA dehydrogenase deficiency, 850–851
Long-chain fatty acids
and brain development, 828–831
and cardiac metabolism in fetus/neonate, 561–562
characteristics of, 828
liver glyconeogenesis in neonate, 608–609
and mitochondrial fatty acid oxidation, 847

Long-chain 3-hydroxy acyl-CoA dehydrogenase deficiency, 851
signs of, 851
Low-bilirubin kernicterus, 871
preventive measures, 871
Low density lipoprotein receptor (LDL-R), exons and encoding of functional domains, 43
Low density lipoproteins (LDL)
in eclaptic and preeclamptic women, 241
metabolism of, 223–224
placental transport, 239–241
in pregnancy, 227, 229–230, 232–236, 238–241
as source of cholesterol, 426–427
as steroid hormones precursor, 425, 426
synthesis in neonate, 836–837
Lowry decapitation technique, 541, 542
Low-salt diet, 519–520, 521
LPL. See Lipoprotein lipase
LRAT, 947
Lucey-Driscoll syndrome, 868, 875
Lund gefense mechanisms, 575
Lungs, 567–575
age and surfactant, 570
alveolar type II cells, 567–568
dipalmitoylphosphatidylcholine (DCCP), 568–570
and facilitative glucose transporters, 128
fetal/neonatal pulmonary circulation, 501–502
fluid balance of, 516–517
gas exchange compared to placenta, 470–473
lung defense mechanisms, 575
phosphatidylcholine (PC), 569–560
phosphatidylglycerol (PG), 570
pulmonary vasodilation, 502
SP-A protein, 573–574
SP-B protein, 571–572
SP-C protein, 572–573
SP-D protein, 574–575
surfactant lipids, 569–570, 1118
surfactant metabolism, extracellular, 568–569
surfactant secretion, 568
surfactant synthesis, 567–568
Lungs of fetus/neonate, 575–587
alveolar type II cells, 576
and corticosteriods, 582–582
cytidylytransferase, regulation of, 578–579
fatty acid synthesis, 580–581
glycogen metabolism, 576–577
phosphatidylcholine (PC) accumulation, 577, 578

phosphatidylcholine (PC) at birth, 584–585
phosphatidylcholine (PC) synthesis, 579, 580–581
and respiratory distress syndrome, 584–587
sex differences, 584
stages of development, 575–576
surfactant lipids and development, 577–578
surfactant pool size at birth, 584–585
surfactant proteins and development, 581
and thyroid hormones, 583–584
Luteinizing hormone (LH), 430–431
fetal production of, 430–431
Luteinizing hormone-releasing hormone
(LHRH), fetal production of, 427
Lysine, utilization in fetal-placental unit, 376
Lysomal storage diseases, in the neonate, 1231–1233

M
Macrosomia
and animal models, 81–82
early identification, 1116
infant of diabetic mother, 200, 271, 379, 1109–1110, 1116, 1117
and maternal obesity, 1108
Magnesium, 285–287, 887–891, 890
absorption of, 888
bioavailability of, 285
and calcitonin regulation, 888
and calcitonin secretion, 898
concentrations in body, 887
high doses, fetal effects, 286
hypermagnesemia, 889
hypomagnesemia, 890–891
maternal deficiency, effects of, 889
metabolism in neonate, 889–891
metabolism of, 285
metabolism in pregnancy, 285, 888–889
and parathyroid hormone secretion, 887–888
placental transport of, 285–286
preterm labor prevention, 286
regulation of, 887–888
status and pregnancy outcome, 286–287
transfer to fetus, 889
Magnesium sulfate, for preeclampsia, 267, 268
Major intrinsic protein (MIP), 514
Male, sex differentiation, hormonal factors, 427
Malnutrition, maternal, and fetal growth, 1089, 1101

Malonyl-CoA, and lipid metabolism in neonate, 613, 847
Mammalian genomic structure, 42–43
Manganese, 932–933
deprivation, effects of, 932
functions of, 932
hypermanganesemia, 933
MAO. *See* Monozmine oxidase
Maple syrup urine disease, 810–812, 1209
case example, 1209
enzyme defect, 802
genetic factors, 811
laboratory findings, 811, 1209
treatment of, 811–812, 1209
types of, 810
Maracaine, 664
Mass spectometry
basic principles of, 4
diagnosis with, 4
Maternal alcohol consumption, 1088–1089
Maternal androgens, fetal protection from, 427
Maternal anemia, 459
Maternal cigarette smoking, 1089
Maternal diabetes, 200, 1110, 1111
animal models of, 81–82
Maternal ethanol ingestion, 694–605
Maternal fatty acid concentrations, 241–243
Maternal/fetal acid-base balance, 470
Maternal/fetal placental blood flow mediation, 463, 464
Maternal glucose concentration, 347–348
Maternal lipid metabolism, 244, 247–249
changes in, 390
Maternal malnutrition, 1089, 1101
Maternal metabolism, 384
Maternal β-sympathomimetics therapy, 694
Mathematical modeling, 9–10
McArdle's disease, 5
muscle isozyme defect, 651
See also Muscle phosphorylase deficiency (Type V)
MDI. *See* Monodeiodinase enzyme
Medications for metabolic disease, 1223, 1225, 1227
Medium-chain acyl-CoA dehydrogenase deficiency, 851
prognosis, 851
treatment of, 851
Medium-chain fatty acids
consumption and metabolic rate, 1012
in enteral nutrition, 1167
feeding complications from, 1172

and infant absorption, 1015
synthesis in neonate, 831
Menaquinones
bacterial producers of, 956
and vitamin K metabolism, 956
Menkes' syndrome, 922, 1226
and copper metabolism, 294, 922
management of, 922, 1227
severe form, 1226
signs of, 922
Menstruation, and prostaglandins, 265
Mental retardation
and galactosemia, 725, 729
and nonketotic hyperglycinemia, 812
and urea synthesis disorders, 806
Mercurial-insensitive water channel, 516
Messenger molecules
interaction with receptors, 53
types of, 53
Metabolic acidosis
and protein metabolism in neonate, 790
and starvation, 93
Metabolic defects, 916, 922–923
Metabolic disease evaluation
acute metabolic decompensation, management of, 1222–1225
for argininosuccinic aciduria, 1211
for carbohydrate-deficient glycoprotein syndrome, 1230–1231
for citrullinemia, 1210–1211
classification of disorders, 1202
clinical/laboratory findings, 1212–1213, 1225
family history, 1201
for galactosialidosis, 1232
for Gaucher disease, 1231
for β-glucuronidase deficiency, 1232
for glutaric aciduria, Type, 2, 12290
for G_{M1}, gangliosidosis, 1231–1232
for hyperammonemia, 1210
for hypoglycemia, 1211–1212
for manageable/treatable disease, 1202–1203
for maple syrup urine disease, 1209
for Menkes disease, 1226–1227
for methylmalonic acidemia, 1207–1208
for mevalonic aciduria, 1230
for mucolipidosis II, 1232–1233
for Neimann-Pick disease, 1233
for neonatal adrenoleukodystrophy, 1227–1229
neonatal screening, 1217–1222
for nonketotic hyperglycemia, 1226
for primary lactic acidosis, 1203–1206
for propionic acidemia, 1208–1209

for rhizomelic chondrodysplasia punctata, 1227–1229
routine laboratory tests, 1206
for sialidosis, 1232
specialized tests, 1214–1217
tandem MS, 1214–1215, 1218–1221
time of appearance of symptoms, 1202–1203
for Zellweger syndrome, 1227–1229
Metabolic disease management
acute care, 1222–1224
for amino acid disorders, 1227
chronic care, 1224–1225
experimental treatments, 1225
medications used, 1223, 1225, 1227
nutritional support, 1222–1224
Metabolic effectors, and regulation of carnitine palmitroyltransferase, 613
Metabolic factors, variations among mammals, 86–87
Metabolic research, limitations of, 3
Metabolism
and bronchopulmonary dysplasia, 1014
cellular events in, 41
genetic influences, 41
glucose-fatty acid cycle, 103–108
glucose metabolism, 91–103
protein metabolism, 105–112
response to surgery. *See* Surgery, neonate
variations among mammals, 86–87
See also entries under Energy metabolism
Metabolism, methodology for study of, 27. *See* Immunoassay
3-methylhistidine (3-MH), excretion in pregnancy, 216
Methylmalonic acidemia, 808–809, 1207–1208
case example, 1207–1208
and cobalamin therapy, 808
diagnosis of, 808, 1208
dietary control, 809
enzyme defect in, 808
forms of, 808
pathologic findings, 809
prognosis, 809
treatment approach, 808, 809, 1208
Mevalonic aciduria, 1230
signs of, 1230
Mice, EGF receptor studies, 412
Mice, transgenic, 68
Michaelis-Menten equation, 57
Microcytic anemia, 916
Milk
avoiding in glucose-6-phosphatase defect (Type I), 749

avoiding in galactokinase deficiency, 732
avoiding in galactosemia, 692, 727
and gluconeogenesis in neonate, 604
and glucose requirements of neonate, 604
lactose and fat content of, 601
water-soluble vitamins in, 978
See also Human milk
Milk bile salt-dependent lipase, 835
Milk expression/collection, 1191
Mineral metabolism in pregnancy
calcium, 283–284
copper, 294–295
fluoride, 295–296
iodine, 296–297
iron, 289–292
lead, 292–294
magnesium, 285–287
selenium, 297–298
sodium, 281–283
zinc, 287–289
Minerals
fetal acquisition of, 518
in human milk, 1182
Mineral transport, and placenta, 518
MIP. *See* Major intrinsic protein
Mitochondria
and cardia metabolism, 561
in fatty acid oxidation in neonate, 611–612, 614–615
fatty acid oxidation pathway, 847–849
of fetal/neonatal brain, 541
muscle metabolism, 654–655
respiratory chain, 654–655
Mitochondrial development, 541
Mitochondrial fatty acid oxidation, 847–849. *See also* Fatty acid oxidation defects
Mitochondrial oxidative capacity, 606–607
Mitogen-activated protein (MAP) kinase, growth factor signal transduction, 409–411
M-mode echocardiography, 319
Modeling
diagnosis with, 9–10
model-independent approach, 9
system models, 9
Modified lipoproteins, 239–241
MODS. *See* Multiple organ dysfunction syndrome
Molecular techniques
cell signaling, 53–54
desensitization of target cells, 59–60
DNA sequencing, 42–45
future view, 69
gene ablation, 68–69
gene regulation, 64–68

ligand recognition, 54–58
polymerase chain reaction, 52–53
protein separation, 47–49
receptor purification and analysis, 58–59
receptor types, 60
recombinant DNA, 49–52
RNA sequencing, 45–47
second messengers, role of, 62–64
signal transduction pathways, 61–62
transgenic techniques, 68
Molybdenum, 933–934
deficiency features, 933
metabolism defects, signs of, 933
metabolism of, 933
Monoamine oxidase (MAO), and catecholamine degradation, 162
Monoclonal antibodies, in immunoassay, 28
Monoclonal antibody probes, 48
Monodeiodinase (MDI) enzyme, 432–433
Monoglycerides, 821
Morphogenesis, 407
Morphologic techniques, 58–59
Motoric activity, and protein metabolism, 790
Mucolipidosis II, 1232–1233
pathogenesis, 1233
signs of, 1233
Multiple adenergic receptors, 440–441
Multiple carboxylase deficiency, 807–808
enzyme defects in, 807
prenatal diagnosis, 808
treatment approach, 808
Multiple gestation, 1100
Multiple organ dysfunction syndrome (MODS), 1173
Multivillous stream system, 451–452
Muscle isozyme defect, 651
Muscle metabolism, and mitochondria, 654–655
Muscle phosphofructokinase deficiency (Type VII), 755–756
signs of, 755
Muscle phosphorylase deficiency (Type V), 754–755
biochemical studies, 755
course of disease, 755
differential diagnosis, 755
genetic factors, 755
laboratory studies, 754–755
pathogenesis, 755
pathology, 755
physiologic studies, 755
signs of, 754
Muscle. *See* Skeletal muscle; Skeletal muscle metabolism

Mutation analysis, fatty acid oxidation defects, 853
Myoblasts, 641, 642, 646
  gene therapy, 664
Myocardial contractility
  affecting factors, 496–497
  after birth, 505
  and catecholamines, 505
  fetal circulation, 496–497
Myofibers, 641–642
Myogenic determination factors (MDFs), 641, 642, 643, 661–662
  genetic regulation, 661–662
Myogenic precursor cells, 641, 648
Myophosphorylase, skeletal muscle, 651
Myotubes, 641–643, 647

N

NAD. *See* Nicotinamide adenine dinucleotide
NADP. *See* Nicotinamide adenine dinucleotide phosphate
Natriuretic peptides, 511–512
  actions of, 512
  atrial natriuretic peptide, 511–512
  gene coding for prohormones of, 511–512
  sites of production, 511–512
Necrotizing enterocolitis
  and enteral feeding, 1170
  and human milk, 1186
Negative cell cycle, 405
Negro variant, galactosemia, 730
Neimann-Pick disease, 1233
  signs of, 1233
Neonatal adrenoleukodystrophy, 1227–1229
  pathogenesis, 1228–1229
  signs of, 1227–1228
Neonatal bilirubin metabolism. *See* Neonatal bilirubin metabolism
Neonatal carnitine metabolism. *See* Carnitine metabolism
Neonatal euglycemia, 683–685
Neonatal glucose homeostasis, control of, 700–713
Neonatal screening, 1217–1222
Neonate
  amino acid/organic acid metabolism disorders, 804–813
  amino acids, requirements for, 791–792
  bilirubin metabolism defects, 867–876
  body composition, 1088–1091
  breastfeeding of, 1181–1192
  calcitonin metabolism, 899–900
  calcium metabolism, 882–883
  carbohydrate metabolism disorders, 723–760
  carnitine metabolism, 860–862
  energy metabolism, 1001–1019
  fatty acid oxidation defects, 847–853
  glucose metabolism, 683–715
  hypoglycemia, 694
  infant of diabetic mother, 1105–1124
  lipid metabolism, 831–839
  magnesium metabolism, 888–889
  metabolic disease evaluation, 1201–1233
  parathyroid hormone metabolism, 892–893
  phosphorous metabolism, 886–887
  protein metabolism, 773–793
  surgery of, 1131–1146
  thermoregulation, 1027–1040
  trace element metabolism, 909–934
  vitamin D metabolism, 897–898
  vitamin metabolism, fat soluble vitamins, 943–964
  water/electrolyte metabolism, 1054–1070
  See also Fetus/neonate
Nerve damage, and Vitamin B^{12} deficiency, 990
Nerve growth factor (NGF), 417
  and cell differentiation, 406
  chemical structure, 417
  functions of, 417
Nesidioblastosis, 379
  and hypoglycemia in neonate, 693–694
Net flux measurements of glucose, 337–339
Net protein gain, 781–782
Neural tube defects
  and folate deficiency, 988–989
  and zinc, 289
Neurological disorders
  and amino acid metabolism disorders, 805
  and galactosemia, 729–730
  and glutaric acidemia, 810
NGF. *See* Nerve growth factor
Niacin, 983–984
  deficiency features, 984
  laboratory assessment of, 984
  metabolism of, 983
  neonatal needs, 984
  sources of, 983–984
  toxicity, 984
Niacinamide, 983, 984
Nickel, deficiency features, 934
Nicotinamide adenine dinucleotide (NAD), 394, 537, 983
  and glycolysis, 95
  intestinal tract of neonate, 629–630, 631–632, 636–637
Nicotinamide adenine dinucleotide phosphate (NADP), 983
Nicotinic acid, 983, 984
Nitric oxide (NO)
  maternal/fetal placental blood flow mediation, 464–465
  modulation of release of, 466
  and preeclampsia, 466
Nitric oxide synthase (NOS), 464, 465
Nitrogen accretion, fetus, 373–375
Nitrogen balance, 779–781
  definition of, 779
  and energy intake, 1015–1016
  fractions used in nitrogen balance studies, 780
  measurement methods, 779
  of neonates, 780–781
  positive balance, 780
  and protein intake, 1016
  and surgical stress, 1138, 1140, 1141
  and urinary excretion, 780, 781
Nitrogen kinetics, 209–210, 212, 214
Nitrogen metabolism
  fetal-placental unit, 379–382
  during pregnancy, 209–210
Nitrogen, reutilization of, 779
NMR. *See* Nuclear magnetic resonance
Non-insulin dependent diabetes mellitus
  and gestational diabetes mellitus, 195
  glucose metabolism in pregnancy, 194–198
  pathophysiology of, 194–195
Nonisotopic method of immunoassay, 34
Nonketotic hyperglycinemia, 812, 1226
  case example, 1226
  enzyme defect in, 812
  prenatal diagnosis, 812
  signs of, 812, 1226
  treatment approaches, 812, 1226
Nonoxidative glucose disposal, 193
Nonpregnant glucose metabolism, 183–186
Norepinephrine, 161
  biosynthesis of, 162
  effects on kidney, 1052
  and exercise, 321–322
  and exercise in pregnancy, 327
  and myocardial contractility, 496
  norepinephrine transporter (NET) messenger RNA, 438
  perinatal metabolism of, 437–438
  perinatal secretion of, 438–440
  release at birth, 439–440
Northern blotting, RNA sequencing, 46–47
NOS. *See* Nitric oxide synthase
Nuclear magnetic resonance (NMR)
  basic principles of, 5

carbon magnetic resonance, 6
diagnosis with, 4–6
proton magnetic resonance, 6
Nucleated cells, 43–44
Nucleic acid synthesis, and skeletal muscle, 661
Nucleotides, in human milk, 1182–1183
Nutritional support
for acute metabolic decompensation, 1222–1224
and bronchopulmonary dysplasis, 1172–1173
enteral feeding, 1165–1171
historical view, 1153–1154
and hypoglycemia, 1155–1156
parenteral nutrition, 1160–1165
and short bowel syndrome, 1171–1172
and systemic inflammatory response syndrome (SIRS), 1173–1174
and very low birth weight infant, 1156–1173
See also Breastfeeding; Human milk; Infant formulas; Very low birth weight infant nutrition

O

Obesity
and breastfeeding versus formula feeding, 825–826
definition of, 826
energy expenditure and age, 1010
and leptin, 827
and white adipose tissue, 826–827
Oct-1, 429
Oct-2, 429
Oleate oxidation, 398
Oleic acid, in diabetic pregnancy, 271–272
Oligohydramnios, and fetal urine output, 523
Omega-3 fatty acids, 221
benefits during pregnancy, 268
Omega-6 fatty acids, 259
Oncotic pressure, 1048–1049
One Touch meter, glucose measure, 686
Online Mendelian Inheritance in Man database, 51–52
Optimal energy/protein intake, 1018–1019
Organic acid disorders. See Amino acid/organic acid metabolism disorders
Organogenesis, and growth factors, 407
Organ systems, animal models for study of, 80–81
Orotic aciduria, 1215
Osmolality, 1046–1047
measurement of, 1046–1047

oncotic pressure, 1048–1049
of solution, 1047
Osmotic pressure, van Hoff equation, 1047
Osteocalcin, 955
Osteopenia of prematurity, 1164
Ovulation, and prostaglandins, 265
Oxaloacetate, 93
Oxidation
and fetal development, 399
and gastrointestinal tract, 634–635
and neonatal intestinal tract, 624–635
Oxidative metabolism, cerebral metabolism in fetus/neonate, 539–540
Oxidative phosphorylation
ATP and brain, 537–538
ATP and heart, 558–559
skeletal muscle, 654–655
Oxygen
consumption and respiratory problems, 1013–1014
fetal oxygen consumption, 1005
placental exchange compared to lung, 470, 472
reduced delivery and fetal circulation, 498–499
saturation in fetal blood, 490
Oxygen consumption metabolism, 561
Oxygen delivered, fetal effects of reduction in, 498–501
Oxygen saturation, 490
Oxygen transfer
factors affecting, 453–454
and fetal placental respiration, 452, 453–461, 466
Oxygen uptake
and exercise, 320
and exercise in pregnancy, 322, 323
in pregnancy, 320
Oxytocin, 266

P

Pancreas
breath tests, 18
glycagon, 155–161
Pantothenic acid, 991–992
deficiency features, 991–992
metabolism of, 991
neonatal needs, 991
sources of, 991
toxicity, 992
Paracrine, 403
Parathyroid hormone (PTH), 43, 891–895
actions of, 891
and calcium metabolism, 283, 882–883, 884, 891
hyperparathyroidism, 891, 893

hypoparathyroidism, 892, 893–895
and magnesium concentration, 887–888, 890
and magnesium metabolism, 285
metabolism in neonate, 892–893
metabolism in pregnancy, 891–892
and phosphorous concentration, 884–885, 886
Parathyroid hormone-relate peptide (PTHrP), 43, 286
in amniotic fluid, 523, 524
Parenteral nutrition
and amino acids, 792
amino acids in, 1161–1162
carbohydrates in, 1160–1161
complications of, 1161, 1163, 1164–1165
and hyperglycemia in neonate, 696–698
lipids in, 839, 1162–1163, 1165
methods for, 1164
and short bowel syndrome, 1171–1172
very low birth weight infant, 1160–1165
vitamin E in, 964
Pasteur effect, 555
Pathogenesis, galactokinase deficiency, 732
PC. See Phosphatidylcholine
PCR. See Polymerase chain reaction
PDGF. See Platelet-derived growth factor
Pellagra, niacin deficiency, 984
Pentose phosphate pathway, 96
PEP. See Phosphoenolpyruvate
PEPCK. See Phosphoenolpyruvate carboxykinase
Peptide bonds, and protein metabolism, 377
Peptide growth factors, and skeletal muscle, 663
Peptides
and amniotic fluid, 523–525
immunoassay measurement, 35
Perinatal hemochromatosis, 915–916
causation, 916
signs of, 915
Perinatal metabolism of catecholamines, 437–438
Perinatal secretion, and catecholamines, 438–440
Peroxisomal disorders, in the neonate, 1227–1229
PFGE. See Pulsed-field gel electrophoresis
PG. See Phosphatidylglycerol
Phenistix, 811
Phenylalanine, metabolic disturbance in neonate, 799–800

Phenylketonuria (PKU), 1217
  enzyme deficiency, 800
Phosphatidylcholine (PC)
  and fatty acid synthesis, 580–581
  fetal lung accumulation, 578, 579
  in lung surfactant, 569–570
  pool size at birth, 584–585
  synthesis of, 579, 580–581
Phosphatidylglycerol (PG), of lung surfactant, 570
Phosphocreatine, and ATP utilization in heart, 559
Phosphoenolpyruvate carboxykinase (PEPCK), 146
  and gluconeogenesis in neonate, 605–607
Phosphoenolpyruvate (PEP)
  conversion from pyruvate, 93–94
  and glycolysis, 95–96
Phosphofructokinase
  deficiency, signs of, 652
  and glycolysis, 555
  skeletal muscle, 652
  stimulation of, 555
Phosphoglycerate mutase
  deficiency, sign of, 653
  skeletal muscle, 653
Phospholipids
  classes of, 821
  nature of, 821
Phosphorus, 884–887
  and adenosine triphosphate, 884
  absorption of, 885
  calcium/phosphorous ratio in feeding, 887
  deficiency, signs of, 885
  excess, signs of, 885
  functions of, 884, 885
  metabolism in neonate, 886–887
  metabolism in pregnancy, 885–886
  regulatory mechanisms, 884–885
Phosphorylase, and glycogen synthesis, 553–554
Phosphorylaion sites, 578–579
Photobilirubin, 867
Phototherapy, for hyperbilirubinemia, 872–873
Phylloquinone, 956
PIH. See Pregnancy-induced hypertension
Pit-1. See Growth hormone factor
Pituitary gland
  cell types of, 429
  development of, 429–430
  follicle-stimulating hormone (FSH), 430–431
  growth hormone (GH), 430
  luteinizing hormone (LH), 430–431
  transcription factors, 429–430
PKU. See Phenylketonuria

Placenta
  animal models for study of, 80–81, 86
  architecture of, 452
  artificial placenta, 476
  blood exchange, 451
  blood flow activity, 460–466
  blood flow regulation, 518–519
  calcium metabolism in, 881
  components of, 451
  concurrent exchange model, 451
  countercurrent exchange model, 451–453
  defective transport and intrauterine growth retardation (IUGR), 1099–1100
  diffusing capacity of, 454–456
  doubling over gestational course, 456
  and fetal respiration. See Fetal placental respiration
  glucose metabolism, 351–352
  iodine transfer, 931
  iron transfer, 912–913
  maternal anemia, effects of, 459
  metabolism of maternal lipids, 391
  mineral transport, 518
  multivillous stream system, 451–452
  physiological classification of types, 451–453
  variability in venous drainage, 453
  villous surface area (VSA), 454–455
  vitamin A transfer, 945
  vitamin D synthesis, 951
  zinc transfer, 926–927
  See also Fetal-placental unit
Placental amino acid transport, 1099–1011
Placental blood flow, regulation of, 518–519
Placental diffusing capacity, 454–456
Placental fatty acid transfer, 390–391
Placental glucose metabolism, 351–352
Placental glucose transport, 346–351, 1099
Placental lactogen, 427–428
Placental oxygen transfer, 453–454
Placental repiratory gas exchange
  and cigarette smoking, 474–475
  and in utero surgery, 475–476
Placental sulfatase, deficiency and ichthyosis, 425
Placental surface area effects, 349
Placental transport
  and amino acids, 1099–1100
  glucose transport, 127, 346–351
  lipid transport, 236–239
  magnesium, 285–286
  modified lipoproteins, 239–241
Plasma, increase in volume during pregnancy, 512–513

Plasma amino acids, 207–209
Plasma glucagon, 155–157
Plasma oncotic pressure, and water/electrolyte metabolism, 1050–1051
Platelet-derived growth factor (PDGF), 414–415
  chemical structure, 414
  functions of, 415
  receptors for, 414–415
  and skeletal muscle, 663
Polyacrylamide gel electrophoresis, protein separation, 48
Polyclonal antibodies, in immunoassay, 28
Polycythemia
  infant of diabetic mother, 1121–1122
  small-for-gestational-age (SGA) infant, 1102
Polyhydramnios, and excess urine production, 523
Polymerase chain reaction (PCR), 52–53
  benefits of, 52
  cDNA, rapid amplification of, 53
  DNA ligase, use of, 52
  RNA sequencing, 47
  transcription mapping, 52
Pompe's disease. See α-acid glucoside deficiency (Type II)
Positron emission tomography
  basic principles of, 6
  and cerebral protein synthesis studies, 7
  diagnosis with, 6–7
Postabsorptive glucose metabolism, 183–184, 186–187, 189
Postnatal circulation, fetal, 487
Postprandial glucose metabolism, 184, 187–188, 189–191
Potassium balance, neonate, 1056–1057
Potassium measurement, body composition measures, 1085–1086
Pre-birth monitoring studies, 1117
Preeclampsia, 519–521
  abnormalities in pregnancy, 519–521
  aspirin therapy for, 269
  and blood flow, 465–466
  calcium and prevention, 284
  characteristics of, 266–267
  and diabetic mother, 1106
  and free fatty acids, 268–269
  hormonal changes, theory of, 284
  and lipid peroxides, 241
  low-dose aspirin therapy, 269
  and low-salt diet, 519–520, 521
  magnesium sulfate therapy, 267, 268, 286
  and nitric oxide (NO), 466
  and placental blood flow, 465–466
  and selenium deficiency, 298

and sodium metabolism, 282–283, 520
and thromboxane, 267–268
time of development, 519
volume abnormality, 519–520
Pregnancy
and alanine, 210–211
and atrial natriuretic peptide, 512
blood flow, changes in 320
energy metabolism in, 309–329
essential fatty acids in, 221, 259–263
exercise in, 322–329
facilitated anabolism in, 384
fat stores in, 309–311
gestational diabetes mellitus, 195–200
glucose metabolism in, 183–200
lipid metabolism in, 221–250
mineral metabolism in, 281–298
prostaglandins in, 260, 263–266, 270–274
protein metabolism in, 207–218
trimesters of, 266
and water/electrolyte balance, 511–518
Pregnancy-induced hypertension (PIH)
and calcium, 284
drugs and fetal morbidity, 521
and fetal growth retardation, 1100
Preload changes, and cardiac output, 495–496
Premature rupture of membranes (PROM), and lead exposure, 293
Prenatal care, 1105, 1107–1108, 1111–1112, 1114–1115
Prenatal diagnosis, galactosemia, 726
Prenatal fluoride, 296
Preterm infants
breastfeeding of, 1189–1192
carnitine deficiency, 660
energy expenditure of, 1014–1015
human milk fortifiers for, 886–887
hypocalcemia of, 953
hypoglycemia in, 688
hyponatremia in, 1069–1070
hypoparathyroidism in, 892–893
and incubator temperature, 1038
infant formulas for, 887, 897, 1015
iron requirements, 914–915
lipid metabolism in, 839, 1015
magnesium intake/retention, 889–890
protein intake recommendations, 1018–1019
protein metabolism, 786–789
and protein metabolism, 783
respiration problems. See Respiratory distress syndrome
riboflavin needs, 982
sodium homeostasis, 1057
and thermoregulation, 1036

thiamin requirements, 980
vitamin C needs, 994
and vitamin E, 962, 964
water/electrolyte balance, 1060
water soluble vitamin requirements, 979
zinc deficiency, 927–928
See also entries under Very low birth weigh infant
Preterm labor
and lead exposure, 293
magnesium and prevention, 286
and prostaglandins, 273–274
zinc and prevention, 288
Primary lactic acidosis, 1203–1206
laboratory tests, 1205, 1214
pathophysiology, 1205–1206
signs of, 1204–1205
Probe hybridization, recombinant DNA, 50
Progesterone
and glucose metabolism in pregnancy, 191
maternal/fetal placental blood flow mediation, 464
placental secretion of, 426
Progestins, and lipid metabolism in pregnancy, 225
Prognostically Bad Signs of Pregnancy, 1105, 1106
Proinsulin, conversion to insulin, 135–138. See also Insulin
Prolactin
in amniotic fluid, 523
and fetal adrenal gland development, 426
and glucose metabolism in pregnancy, 192
Prolidase deficiency, 933
PROM. See Premature rupture of membranes
Propionic acidemia, 806–807, 1208–1209
and carnitine deficiency, 807
case example, 1208
diagnosis of, 1208
enzyme defect in, 806
signs of, 806–807
treatment approach, 807, 1208
Prostacyclin, 267
maternal/fetal placental blood flow mediation, 463
pulmonary vasodilator, 502
Prostaglandins
A series, 273
biosynthesis of, 259–263
chemical inhibitors of, 262–263
and digestion, 264
and ductus arteriosus after birth, 503–504

E series, 263, 265, 273, 503
and fetal circulation, 269–270
F series, 263, 265, 273
and glucose metabolism in pregnancy, 270–273
and immune system, 264
immunoassay measurement, 36
and kidney, 264, 1054, 1059
and labor, 265
and lipid metabolism in pregnancy, 265–266
lipoxygenase products, 263
and male fertility, 264
measurement methods, 260
and neonate, 1059
and preterm labor, 273–274
and protein metabolism in neonate, 777–778
reproduction, roles in, 264–265
and respiratory system, 264
structure of, 260–261
therapeutic uses in pregnancy, 273
thermoregulation inhibition, 1034
and vascular system, 263–264
and water/electrolyte metabolism, 1054, 1059
Prostanoids, maternal/fetal placental blood flow mediation, 463
Protein 21 (p21), and negative cell cycle, 405
Protein
in enteral feeding, 1167–1168
in human milk, 1181–1182
immunoassay measurement, 34–35
intake for preterm infant, 1018–1019
and neonatal growth, 1016–1017
and nitrogen balance, 1016
in parenteral feeding, 1161–1162
for very low birth weight infant, 1161–1162, 1167–1168
Protein hormones
human chorionic gonadotropin (hCG), 427
inhibin, 428
placental lactogen, 427–428
Protein metabolism, 105–112
age effects on, 106
and adenosine triphosphate, 778
and branched-chain amino acids, 108–109
and exercise, 325
feeding and fasting effects, 106–107
glucagon, 111
and glucose, 109
and growth hormone, 111
in heart, 560–561
and insulin, 109–112, 147–149
and ketone bodies, 109
liver protein breakdown, 110
and preterm infants, 786–789

Index

protein intake effects, 107–108
rate of turnover, significance of, 112
regulation of, 105–106
and skeletal muscle, 660–661
and surgery, 1137–1142
and testosterone, 111–112
and thyroid metabolism, 111
Protein metabolism in fetal-placental unit
 branched-chain amino acids, 377–379
 caracass analysis methods, 369–370
 and energy metabolism, 376–377
 in gastrointestinal tissue, 375–376
 and glucagon, 382
 and glucose production, 360–361
 and insulin, 379–381
 interorgan metabolism, 377
 and intrauterine growth retardation (IUGR), 382–384
 kinetics of amino acids in fetal arterial free amino acid pool, 371–373
 leucine uptake and utilization, 376
 maternal fasting effects, 377–379
 net arteriovenous balance determinations, 370
 nitrogen accretion, 373–375
 nitrogen metabolism, 379–382
 and peptide bonds, 377
 placental amino acid transport, 1099–1011
 rate of incorporation of tracer amino acid into fetal protein measure, 370–371
Protein metabolism in neonate
 amino acid kinetics studies, 776–777
 compartment analysis, 775–776
 and corticosteroids, 778
 and cortisol, 778
 digestion of protein, 790–791
 energy requirements, 778
 essential amino acids, 791
 and fasting, 789–790
 compared to later age, 777
 during metabolic acidosis, 790
 molecular aspects, 773–774
 and motoric activity, 790
 net protein gain, 781–782
 nitrogen balance, 779–781
 nitrogen reutilization, 779
 plasma protein of newborn, 782–783
 and preterm infants, 783
 and prostaglandins, 777–778
 protein degradation, 778–779
 protein turnover, 784–790
 protein turnover regulation, 783–784
 stochastic analysis, 776
 and surgery, 1137–1142
Protein metabolism in pregnancy
 alanine metabolism, 210–211

fasting/feeding response, 208–209
and fetus, 217–128
isotopic tracer measures of turnover, 211–212
leucine turnover, 212–124
liver, 217
and nitrogen kinetics, 209–210, 212, 214
plasma amino acids, 207–209
protein costs in pregnancy, 207
protein turnover, 211–215
skeletal muscle protein, 216
tyrosine turnover, 213–214
urea synthesis, 209–210
and uterus, 217
Protein separation, 47–49
 double layer method, 49
 high-resolution 2-D PAGE, 48, 49
 horizontal protein blotting, 48
 polyacrylamide gel electrophoresis, 48
 reverse-phase high-performance liquid chromatography (RP-HPLC), 47
 sodium dodecyl sulfate-PAGE (SDA-PAGE), 48
 vertical protein electroblotting apparatus, 48
 Western blot, 48, 49
 zonal electrophoresis, 47–48
Protein turnover
 and amino acid recycling, 112
 effects on metabolic rate, 1012–1013
 and immobilization, 790
 neonate, 211–215, 783–784
 in pregnancy, 211–215
 process of, 1012
 and protein intake, 1013
Protein synthesis, 207–209
Proton magnetic resonance, 6
Proximal post-insulin receptor defects, 197–198
PTH. See Parathyroid hormone
Pulmonary circulation, fetal, 501–502
Pulmonary edema
 and bronchopulmonary dysplasia, 1065, 1072
 and hypoglycemia, 691
Pulmonary vasodilators, 502
Pulmonary surfactant, life cycle of, 567–569
Pulsed-field gel electrophoresis (PFGE), 45
Pyridoxine (Vitamin B^6), 984–986
 deficiency features, 986
 laboratory assessment of, 986
 metabolism of, 984–985
 needs in pregnancy, 986
 neonatal needs, 985–986
 sources of, 985

toxicity, 986
Pyruvate
 and cardiac metabolism, 555
 conversion and lactate, 394, 555
 conversion to phosphoenolpyruvate (PEP), 93–94
 and Krebs cycle, 554–555
 oxidation, 96
Pyruvate carboxylase, 93
Pyruvate carboxylase deficiency, 740–741
 molecular studies of, 741
 signs of, 741
 treatment of, 741
Pyruvate dehydrogenase, 555
 intestinal tract of neonate, 628–629

R
Radiant heaters, 1039–1040
 temperature settings, 1039–1040
 and water loss, 1062, 1063
Radiation principle, thermoregulation, 1028
Radiolabeled antigens, in immunoassay, 33–34
Radionuclide-labeled microsphere method, fetal cardiac output study, 491–492
Radioreceptor assay, 56
Rapid temperature cycling, uses of, 53
rasGAP, 409–410
Rathke's pouch, 429
Receiver operational characterization (ROC) curve, 20
Receptor autoradiography, 58–59
Receptor binding
 and cell signaling, 53–54
 ligand-receptor interactions, 56–58
 receptor binding assays, criteria for, 55
 receptor binding parameters, 55
Receptor purification and analysis, 58–59
 applications for, 59
 purification strategy, 59
 removing receptors from cell membrane, 59
Receptors
 activation, 54
 categories of, 60
 Class I/II receptors, 60
 and desensitization of target cells, 59–60
 growth factor receptors, 407–408
 hormone receptors and neonate, 709
 insulin receptor, 140–142
 reaction with several proteins, 61–62
 receptor antibodies, 54
 and signal transduction pathways, 60–62

target cell desensitization, 59–60
Recombinant DNA, 49–52
  cloning vectors, criteria for, 49
  cosmids, 50
  diagnosis of metabolic disease with, 51–52
  genomic libraries, use of, 50–51
  isolating DNA sequences, 50
  molecular cloning process, 49
  plasmid design features, 49–50
  probe hybridization, 50
  size of DNA fragments, 49
  sources of DNA for, 50
REH, 947
Relaxin, and water/electrolyte metabolism in pregnancy, 517–518
Renal function, and angiotensin-II, 522, 1053
Renal gluconeogenesis, 93
Renal glycosuria, and sodium-dependent glucose transport, 122–123
Renal vein thrombosis, infant of diabetic mother, 1122
Renin
  in amniotic fluid, 524–525
  production of, 1053
Renin-angiotensin-aldosterone system
  components of system, 521–522
  maternal/fetal placental blood flow mediation, 463–464
  in neonate, 1058
  and preeclampsia, 520
  and sodium balance, 281
  and water/electrolyte metabolism, 1053
Reporter genes, introduced in mammalian cells, 66–67
Reproduction, roles of prostaglandins in, 264–265
Respiration
  and exercise (nonpregnant state), 322
  and exercise in pregnancy, 322–323
  fetal-placental unit. See Fetal placental respiration
  during pregnancy, 320
  and water loss, 1061–1062
Respiratory distress syndrome, 584–587
  complications of, 1117
  exogenous surfactant treatment, 585
  individual response to treatment, 586
  and infant of diabetic mother, 577, 1117–1119
  and metabolic rate, 1014
  and oxygen consumption, 1013
  and phosphatidylcholine (PC) pool size, 584–585
  phosphatidylcholine (PC) after treatment, 585–586

prophylaxis, 585
rescue treatment, 585
surfactant deficiency, 585, 1117–1118
and water/electrolyte balance problems, 1064–1065
Respiratory gas exchange, and placenta, 451
Respiratory problems, See also Bronchopulmonary dysplasia; Respiratory distress syndrome
Respiratory system
  and prostaglandins, 264
  See also Lungs
Response elements, 65
  functions of, 65
  glucocorticoid-response element (GRE), 65–66
Restriction enzymes
  common enzymes, listing of, 44
  and DNA sequencing, 44
Restriction fragment length polymorphisms (RFLPs)
  and diagnosis of disease, 51
  functions of, 51
  informative types, 51
Retinoic acid, 945
Retinol, 943
  and amniotic fluid, 945
  intestinal absorption, 946–947
  metabolites of, 945
  storage of, 947
  See also Vitamin A
Retinyl ester hydrolase. See REH
Reverse-phase high-performance liquid chromatography (RP-HPLC), protein separation, 47
Reverse transcription, RNA sequencing, 47
RFLPs. See Restruction fragment length polymorphisms
Rhesus monkey, 82
Rh incompatibility
  and hyperbilirubinemia prevention, 871–872
  and hypoglycemia in neonate, 692
Rhizomelic chondrodysplasia punctata, 1227–1229
  pathogenesis, 1229
  signs of, 1228
Riboflavin (Vitamin B_2), 981–983
  deficiency features, 982–983
  laboratory assessment of, 983
  metabolism of, 981
  neonatal needs, 982
  sources of, 981–982
  toxicity, 983
Ribonucleic acid. See entries under RNA
Riboprobe, 47

Rickets of prematurity, 1164
RNase protection assay (RPA), RNA sequencing, 47
RNA sequencing
  dot blot/slot blot apparatus, 46
  instability of molecule, 46
  multiple sequences from single gene, 46
  northern blotting, 46–47
  percent in mammalian cell, 46
  polymerase chain reaction, 47
  reverse transcription, 47
  RNase protection assay (RPA), 47
  sequencing methods, 46–47
  in situ hybridization, 46–47
  structure of, 45–46
  synthesis from DNA, 45
RNA synthesis
  protein metabolism in neonate, 773–775
  and skeletal muscle, 661
ROC. See Receiver operational characterization curve
Rodents, bioengineered, 82–83
Rosenthal-Scatchard equation, 57, 58
RPA. See RNase protection assay

S

Salicylates, effects on insulin response, 270
Satellite cells, 642
Scatchard analysis, 29
Screening programs, for amino acid/organic acid metabolism disorders, 1217–1218
Scurvy, vitamin C deficiency, 994–995
Second messengers, 62–64
  activity from, 60
  cAMP, 62
  insulin, 144
  properties of, 62–64
  types of, 62–63
Seizure prophylaxis, and magnesium, 286
Seizures, and vitamin B_6 deficiency, 986
Selenium, 297–298, 929–931
  bioavailability, 297
  deficiency, effects of, 298
  deficiency features, 930
  fetal/neonatal metabolism, 930–931
  function of, 929
  metabolism of, 929
  metabolism in pregnancy, 298, 930
  and pregnancy outcome, 298
Separation methods, immunoassay, 33
Sepsis
  and bilirubin problems, 867
  and galactosemia, 726
  and hyperglycemia in neonate, 699

Index

and hypoglycemia in neonate, 691
Sequence-tagged site markers, 52
Seven-transmembrane (7-TM) segment receptors, 60
Sex differences
  insulin concentrations, 226
  lipid metabolism, 225–226
  lungs of fetus/neonate, 584
Sex differentiation, 431
  and human chorionic gonadotropin (hCG), 427
SGA. See Small-for-gestational-age infant
Sheep, cardiac output of, 494
Shock, and water/electrolye balance defect, 1066
Short bowel syndrome, 1171–1172
  complications of, 1171
  nutritional intervention, 1171–1172
Short-chain acyl-CoA dehydrogenase deficiency, 851
Short-chain fatty acid oxidation deficiency, 851
Short-chain β-ketothiolase deficiency, 851
Short gut syndrome, biotin deficiency, 992
Sialidosis, 1232
Sickle cell anemia, polymerase chain reaction detection, 53
SIDS. See Sudden infant death syndrome
Signaling enzymes, growth factors in fetal-placental unit, 408–411
Signaling methods, immunoassay, 33–34
Signal transduction pathways, 61–62
  initiation of signal transduction, 61
  ligand-gated ion channel receptors, 60
Silicon, deficiency features, 934
Single-channel recording methods, 60
Single-photon absorptiometry, bone status measure, 1087
Single-transmembrane segment receptors, 60
  types of, 60–61
SIRS. See Systemic inflammatory response syndrome
Skeletal muscle
  and ACTH, 663
  and aldolase, 652–653
  cell adhesion molecules, 648–649
  compartmenalization, 648
  and connective tissue, 647–648
  embryonic development of, 642–644
  extracellular matrix, 648
  and facilitative glucose transporters, 128–129
  fiber specialization, 644–646

gene therapy, 663
and glucocorticosteroids, 663
glucose metabolism in pregnancy, 193–194
and glucose uptake, 97
and glucose utilization, 96, 97, 184
and growth hormone, 663
innervation, 646–647
and insulin, 663
isozymes, 650–654
limb myogenesis, 643
muscle cells, 641–642
myogenic determination factors (MDFs), 641, 642, 643, 661–662
and peptide growth factors, 663
protein metabolism in pregnancy, 216
regeneration of, 663
and thyroid hormone, 663
Skeletal muscle metabolism
  adenine nucleotide translocase (ANT), 655–656
  adenosine monophosphate deaminase (AMPD), 657–658
  adolase, 652–653
  carbohydrate metabolism, 651–654, 658–659
  changes and development, 658–661
  creatine kinase, 656–657
  enolase, 653
  lactate dehydrogenase, 653–654
  lipid metabolism, 659–660
  mitochondrial energy metabolism, 654–658
  myophosphorylase, 651
  nucleic acid synthesis, 661
  oxidative phosphorylation, 654–655
  phosphofructokinase, 652
  phosphoglycerate mutase, 653
  protein synthesis, 660–661
  and surgery, 1140
Skin, and water loss, 1062–1064
Skin development, and KGF, 416
Skinfold
  measures, 1082
  thicknesses, 188
Sleep, metabolic rate during, 1015
Small-for-gestational-age (SGA) infant
  birth stress to, 1101
  and folate deficiency, 988
  hypocalcemia, 1101
  hypoglycemia, 1101–1102
  hypoglycemia in, 618, 688–690
  outcome for, 1103
  polycythemia-hyperviscosity, 1102
  See also Intrauterine growth retardation (IUGR)
Small intestine, sodium-dependent glucose transporters, 121–122

Small left colon syndrome, infant of diabetic mother, 1115
Snell mice, 430
Sodium, 281–283
  balance, maintenance of, 281
  balance and neonate, 1057
  bioavailability of, 281
  kidney and excretion of, 1052
  metabolism in pregnancy, 281–282
  placental transport, 518
  and preeclampsia, 282–283, 519–520, 521
Sodium benzoate, 1227
Sodium-dependent glucose transporters, 121–123
  and renal absorption of glucose, 122–123
  SGLT1, 121, 122, 123
  SGLT2, 121, 122
Sodium dodecyl sulfate-PAGE (SDA-PAGE), protein separation, 48
Sodium metabolism, and aldosterone, 282
Somatostatin, 166, 428
  hypoglycemia treatment, 697
Somites, skeletal muscle, 642, 662
Somogyi phenomenon, and growth hormone, 168
Son of sevenless (SOS), 143
Southern blot, DNA hybridization, 44–45
SP-A, 573–574, 581
SP-B, 571–572, 581
SP-C, 572–573, 581
SP-D, 574–575, 581
Specific dynamic action, 1010–1011
Stable isotope tracers
  basic principles of, 7–8
  diagnosis with, 7–9
  several tracers, benefits of, 8
  types of studies with, 8–9
StAR. See Steroidogenic acute regulatory protein
Starling relationship, water/electrolyte balance, 1049–1051
Starvation, and metabolic acidosis, 93
STAT proteins, growth factor signal transduction, 408
Stat Tek Meter, glucose measure, 686
Stavermann relection coefficient, and water/electrolyte metabolism, 1050
Steroid hormones, 425–427
  and adrenal gland, 425–425
  estrogen, 425–426
  immunoassay measurement, 35
  precursor for, 425, 426
  progesterone, 426
Steroidogenic acute regulatory protein (StAR), 426

Steroid therapy, and hyperglycemia in neonate, 699
Sterols, nature of, 821
Stimulus-secretion coupling, 62–63
Stochastic analysis, protein metabolism study, 776
Stomach
 breath tests, 18
 fat digestion, 832–834
Stuck twin syndrome, 523
Stupor, in neonate, 1225–1226
Substrate availability, glucose metabolism in neonate, 710–711
Substrates. *See* Branched-chain amino acids; Glucose; Ketone bodies; Hormones
Suckling ketosis, 860
Sudden infant death syndrome (SIDS)
 and brown adipose tissue, 828
 hepatic phosphoenolpyruvate carboxykinase (PEPCK) deficiency, 741
Surfactant deficiency. *See* Respiratory distress syndrome
Surfactant proteins, 581
 biogenesis of, 571, 572, 573
 corticosteroids, effects on, 582–583
 developmental changes in, 581
 functions of, 571–573, 574, 575
 SP-A, 573–574, 581
 SP-B, 571–572, 581
 SP-C, 572–573, 581
 SP-D, 574–575, 581
 structure of, 571, 572, 573, 574
 See also Lungs; Lungs of fetus/neonate
Surgery, neonatal
 and carbohydrate metabolism, 1135–1137
 and energy metabolism, 1133–1134
 and fat metabolism, 1142–1145
 historical view, 1131–1133
 and hyperglycemia, 699, 1135, 1136, 1137
 and protein metabolism, 1137–1142
 and thermoregulation, 1134
Surgery, in utero, and placental respiratory gas exchange, 475
Survanta, 586
Symmetrical growth retardation, 1097, 1098
Sympathetic nervous system, and thermoregulation, 1032
Sympathoadrenal system, 437–445
 α-adrenergic receptors, 440
 β-adrenergic receptors, 440–445
 importance of, 437
 multiple adenergic receptors, 440–441

 perinatal catecholamine metabolism, 437–438
 perinatal catecholamine secretion, 438–440
 β-sympathomimetic therapy, and neonatal hypoglycemia, 694
Systemic inflammatory response syndrome (SIRS), 1173–1174
 metabolic effects, 1173
 nutritional complications of, 1173
 nutritional intervention, 1173–1174

T
Tachyphylaxis, meaning of, 59
Tandem MS studies, 1214–1215, 1218–1221
 diseases screened by, 1218
 examples of profiles, 1219–1221
Target cells, desensitization of, 59–60
Tarui's disease, 652
TATA box, 64–65
TBASE. *See* Transgenic/Targeted Mutation Database
Temperature, and glucose tolerance, 690–691
Teratogenic disorders, in the neonate, 12271229–1231
Teratogens
 and intrauterine growth retardation (IUGR), 1098
 vitamin A, 945–946
Testosterone
 in fetal-placental unit, 427
 and protein metabolism, 111–112
Thermogenesis, 1133–1135
Thermoregulation, 1027–1040
 and age, 1037–1038
 and brown adipose tissue, 827–828, 1031–1032
 conduction principle, 1028
 convection principle, 1028
 environmental factors, 1035–1036
 evaporation, 1028–1029
 of fetus, 1029, 1033–1034
 heat balance equation, 1029
 incubator, 1027, 1038–1039
 inhibitors of, 1034
 and mode of delivery, 1034–1035
 of neonate, 1029–1031
 of neonate during surgery, 1134
 post-birth, 1033–1034, 1037
 and preterm infant, 1036
 radiant heat source, 1039–1040
 radiation principle, 1028
 and surgery, 1134
 and sympathetic nervous system, 1032
 and thyroid hormones, 1032–1033
 and very low birth weight infant, 1035

Thiamine (Vitamin B_1), 978–981
 deficiency features, 980–981
 laboratory assessment of, 981
 megasupplementation, disorders for, 981
 metabolism of, 978–980
 neonatal needs, 980
 sources of, 980
 toxicity, 981
Three-pool model, maternal-fetal glucose exchange, 341–343
Thromboxane, and preeclampsia, 267–268
Thyroid gland, development of, 432
Thyroid hormones, 432–434
 and β-adrenergic receptor regulation, 441–442
 deiodination, 432–434
 and energy metabolism in neonate, 1010
 and fetal cardiac output, 504–505
 fetal lungs, effects on, 583–584
 and glucose metabolism in fetal-placental unit, 354–355
 immunoassay measurement, 35–36
 and iodine, 931–932
 and skeletal muscle, 663
 synthesis of, 432
 and thermoregulation, 1032–1033
 thyroid-releasing hormone (TRH), 431–432
Thyroid metabolism, and protein metabolism, 111
Thyroid-releasing hormone (TRH), 431–432
 secretion in fetus, 433
Thyroid response elements (TRE), 442
Tissue synthesis, and metabolic rate, 1011
Tocolysis, and magnesium, 286
Tocopherols. *See* Vitamin E
Tolerex, 853
Topology of facilitative glucose transporters, 123
TORCH, and intrauterine growth retardation (IUGR), 1098
Total body electrical conductivity measurement, 1083
Total body potassium measurement, 1085–1086
Total body water measurement, 1082, 1084
Total body water volume, components of, 1045
Toxemia, and hypoglycemia, 688
Toxemic pregnancy, 241
Trace elements
 categories of, 909
 chromium, 934
 copper, 916–923

Index

essential, functions of, 909
fluoride, 934
in human milk, 1182
iodine, 931–932
iron, 909–916
manganese, 932–933
miscellaneous elements, 934
molybdenum, 933–934
selenium, 929–931
zinc, 923–929
Tracer methods
    amino acid kinetics studies, 776–777
    fetal amino acid kinetics, 371–373, 376
    measurement of fetal-placental glucose, 338–341
Transcription Factors Database, 442
Transcription mapping, master catalog of genes, 52
Trans fatty acids, in human milk, 825
Transferrin, defective sialylation of transferrin, 915
Transforming growth factor-α, 411–412
Transforming growth factor-β, 404, 415–416
    functions of, 415, 416
    multiple signaling pathways for, 415–416
    receptors for, 415
    and skeletal muscle, 663
Transgenic/Targeted Mutation Database (TBASE), 69
Transgenic techniques, 68–69
    transgenic mice, creation of, 68
Transient hyperphenylalaninemia, cause of, 800
Transplacental fatty acid gradient, 390–391
Travamulsion, 1162
Tricarboxylic cycle, of heart, 558
Triglycerides
    and cardiac metabolism, 557
    clearance from adipose tissue, 99
    and glucose metabolism, 98–99
    and lipid metabolism, 223
    liver and synthesis of, 98–99
    nature of, 821
    in pregnancy, 232–238
Trophamine, 1162
Tumor necrosis factor-α, 172
    functions of, 172
    and gestational diabetes mellitus, 198
    mechanisms of action, 172
    and systemic inflammatory response syndrome, 1173
2-D PAGE
    databases on, 49
    protein separation, 48, 49

Two-pool model, maternal-fetal glucose exchange, 341
Two-to-four transmembrane (2-TM, 3-TM, 4-TM), 60
Tyrosine, turnover in pregnancy, 213–214
Tyrosine hydroxylase, and catecholamine biosynthesis, 162
Tyrosine kinases, growth factor signal transduction, 408–409
Tyrosinemia, 1215
Tyrosine phosphatase, and gestational diabetes mellitus, 198
Tyrosine phosphorylation, and insulin receptor, 141

U

Ultrasonic flowmeters, fetal cardiac output study, 492
Umbilical artery catheter, hypoglycemia in neonate, 694
Umbilical cord compression, fetal circulatory response, 500–501
Unbound ligands, 55
Unconjugated bilirubin, 865, 866, 868, 869
Underwater weighing method, body composition measure, 1078
University of Aix-Marseille, Web site, 45
Urea, synthesis in pregnancy, 209–210
Urea cycle, 801
    ammonia production/release, 801
    events in, 801
Urea synthesis disorders, 805–806
    arginine therapy for, 806
    differential diagnosis, 805
    plasma profile, 805–806
    prenatal testing, 806
    signs of, 805
    treatment approach, 806
Uremia, hyperglucagonemia, 158
Uridine triphosphate (UTP)
    galactose synthesis, 723–724
    glycogen synthesis, 553
Urine
    and energy loss in neonate, 1015
    manifestations in galactosemia, 726
Urine flow
    abnormal, consequences of, 523
    fetal, 523
Uterine blood flow, 461
Uterus, and protein metabolism in pregnancy, 217
UTP. *See* Uridine triphosphate

V

VACTERL syndrome, 293
Vanadium, deficiency features, 934

Van Hoff equation, osmotic pressure, 1047
Vanillylmandelic acid (VMA), formation of, 162
Vascular volume, altering sense of, 513
Vascular system, and prostaglandins, 263–264
Vasodilation, bradykinin, 502, 503, 1053
Vegans, and vitamin B_{12} deficiency, 990, 1184
Venous drainage, variability in, 453
Venous plasma glucose, 163
Ventilatory threshold, and exercise, 322
Verbal dyspraxia, and galactosemia, 725
Vertical protein electroblotting apparatus, protein separation, 48
Very long chain acyl-CoA dehydrogenase deficiency, 850–851
Very low birth weight infant
    and hyperglycemia, 697
    potassium imbalance, 1057
    and thermoregulation, 1035
    and water/electrolyte metabolism, 1067–1068
Very low birth weight infant nutrition, 1156–1173
    and bronchopulmonary dysplasia, 1172–1173
    caloric requirements of infant, 1156–1158
    carbohydrate sources, 1160–1161, 1167
    complications of feeding, 1161, 1163, 1164–1165, 1170
    and digestion, 1166–1167
    enteral feeding, 1165–1171
    human milk, 1168–1169
    for hyperglycemia, 1160–1161
    hypocaloric feedings, 1170–1171
    lipids, 839, 1162–1163, 1167
    nutrient requirements, 1158–1160
    nutritional assessment, 1158
    nutritional disorders, 839, 1154
    parenteral nutrition, 1160–1165
    protein sources, 1161–1162, 1167–1168
    for short bowel syndrome, 1171–1172
    and systemic inflammatory response syndrome, (SIRS), 1173–1174
Very low density lipoproteins (VLDL)
    estrogen effects, 224
    and lactating women, 248
    and lipolysis, 98, 99, 103
    metabolism of, 223
    placental transport, 237
    in pregnancy, 229–230, 232–235, 237, 238

progestin effects, 225
synthesis in neonate, 836–837
Vigabatrin, 1227
Villous surface area (VSA), of placenta, 454–455
Vitamin A, 943–949
  in amniotic fluid, 945
  β-carotene precursor, 946
  deficiency features, 949
  fetal/neonatal metabolism, 946–949
  functions of, 943
  intestinal absorption, 946–947
  metabolism of, 943–945
  mobilization from liver, 947–948
  placental transfer, 945
  storage of retinol, 947
  supplementation in neonate, 949
  as teratogen, 945–946
  and zinc deficiency, 948
Vitamin B_1. See Thiamine (Vitamin B^1)
Vitamin B_2. See Riboflavin (Vitamin B_2)
Vitamin B_6. See Pyridoxine (Vitamin B_6)
Vitamin B_{12}, 989–991
  deficiency features, 990
  forms of, 989
  laboratory assessment of, 990–991
  metabolism of, 989–990
  neonatal needs, 990
  sources of, 990
  and vegans, 990, 1184
Vitamin C, 993–995
  deficiency features, 994–995
  laboratory assessment, 995
  metabolism of, 993
  neonatal needs, 994
  preterm infant needs, 994
  sources of, 993–994
  toxicity, 995
Vitamin D, 894–898, 949–954, 950–953
  and breastfed infants, 1182, 1184
  and calcium, 284, 953–954
  in fetus, 896
  hydroxylation of, 894–895, 896
  and magnesium metabolism, 888
  maternal-fetal metabolism, 951–952
  metabolism in neonate, 897–898, 952–954
  metabolism of, 949–951
  metabolism in pregnancy, 895–897
  1,25(OH)D, 896–897, 950–954
  placental synthesis, 951
  skin and production of, 894
  sources of, 894
  supplementation dose, 895
  transport to fetus, 896, 898
  25(OH)D, 895–896
  and vitamin K, 954
Vitamin E, 957–964
  absorption of, 960
  assessment of status, 961
  biochemistry of, 958–959
  deficiency effects, 962–964
  deficiency features, 962
  diabetic mothers, fetal protection, 1116
  functions of, 957–958
  iron effects, 960
  maternal-fetal metabolism, 961
  megavitamin supplementation, 964
  metabolism of, 961
  nutrient interactions, 959–960
  in parenteral nutrition, 964
  and preterm infant, 964
  transport of, 960–961
Vitamin K, 954–957
  deficiency, 957
  forms of, 954
  low level in human milk, 1182, 1184
  maternal-fetal metabolism, 956
  measurement of, 957
  and menaquinones, 956
  metabolism in neonate, 956–957
  metabolism of, 955–956
  sources for neonate, 954–955
  transport of, 956
  and vitamin D, 954
Vitamin metabolism, fat soluble vitamins, 943–964
  vitamin A, 943–949
  vitamin D, 949–954
  vitamin E, 957–964
  vitamin K, 954–957
Vitamin metabolism, water soluble vitamins
  biotin, 992–993
  folate, 987–989
  niacin, 983–984
  pantothenic acid, 991–992
  pyridoxine (Vitamin B_6), 984–986
  riboflavin (Vitamin B_2), 981–983
  thiamine (Vitamin B_1), 978–981
  vitamin B_{12}, 989–991
  vitamin C, 993–995
Vivonex, 853
VLDL. See Very low density lipoproteins
VSA. See Villous surface area

W

Water channels, 513–516
  aquaporins, 513–516, 517
  characteristics of, 513
  types of tissue containing, 513, 514
Water/electrolyte measurement, body composition measures, 1082–1085
Water/electrolyte metabolism, 1045–1054
  and arginine vasopressin, 1053–1054
  and atrial natriuretic peptide, 1054
  and blood flow, 1051–1052
  body water compartment regulation, 1045–1046
  and capillary hydrostatic pressure, 1050
  and catecholamines, 1052–1053
  extracellular water compartment, 1048
  extracellular water regulation, 1051–1054
  and heart, 1051–1052
  hydrostatic/osmotic interaction, 1049–1051
  intersititial compartment, 1048–1051
  intracellular water regulation, 1047–1048
  and kallikrein-kinen system, 1053
  and kidney, 1052
  oncotic pressure, 1048–1049
  osmolality, 1046–1047
  osmotic pressure, 1047
  and prostaglandins, 1054
  and renin-angiotensin-aldosterone system, 1053
  Starling relationship, 1049–1051
  total body water volume, 1045
Water/electrolyte metabolism defects
  and bronchopulmonary dysplasia, 1065
  and edema, 1066–1067
  and preterm infant, 1069–1070
  and respiratory distress syndrome, 1064–1065
  and shock, 1066
  and very low birth weight infant, 1067–1068
Water/electrolyte metabolism, fetal-placental unit
  amniotic fluid, role of, 522–523
  angiotensin-converting enzyme, 521–522
  and brain natriuretic peptide, 524
  and endothelins, 523–524
  and hepatocyte growth factor, 524
  hydrops fetalis, 525
  lungs and fluid balance, 516–517
  mineral acquisition by fetus, 518
  placental blood flow maintenance, 518–519
  preeclampsia, 519–521
  and prolactin, 523
  and renin, 524–525
Water/electrolyte metabolism in neonate
  and birth, 1059–1066
  and heart, 1054
  and kidney, 1054–1059
  and preterm infants, 1060

Water loss and respiration, 1061–1062
water loss and skin, 1062–1064
Water/electrolyte metabolism in pregnancy, 511–518
and natriuretic peptides, 511–512
plasma volume increase, 512–513
and relaxin, 517–518
water channels, 513–516
Water loss
direct assessment of, 1064
and incubator, 1062, 1063
indirect assessment of, 1062–1063
and radiant heating, 1062, 1063
and respiration, 1061–0162
and skin, 1062–1064
Water soluble vitamins
in milk/infant formulas, 978
recommended intake for children, 979
recommended intake during pregnancy/lactation, 979
recommended intake for preterm infants, 979
See also Vitamin metabolism, water-soluble vitamins
Weaning, and intestinal metabolism, 637
Weight gain
fat increase and metabolism, 309–311
and glucose metabolism in pregnancy, 188
Wernicke-Korsakoff syndrome, thiamine deficiency, 980–981
Western blot, protein separation, 48, 49
White adipose tissue, and obesity, 826–827
Whole-body protein, 775–776, 784–791
Williams-Beuren syndrome, 1227
Williams syndrome, 884
Wilson's disease, 923
and copper metabolism, 294, 923
diagnosis of, 923
signs of, 923
World Wide Web
bioinformation on, 41–42
databases for nucleotide searches/analysis, 45
Online Mendelian Inheritance in Man database, 51–52
Transgenic/Targeted Mutation Database (TBASE), 69
2-D PAGE databases, 49

Y
YSI analyzer, glucose measure, 686

Z
Zellweger syndrome, 1227–1229
pathogenesis, 1228–1229
signs of, 1227
Zinc, 287–289, 923–929
bioavailability of, 287
and birth weight, 289
breastfeeding and deficiency, 928, 929
cigarette smoking effects, 926
deficiency features, 924, 925–926
deficiency and vitamin A, 948
fetal/neonatal metabolism, 927–928
functions of, 923, 924
and lipid metabolism, 924
metabolism of, 287, 924–925
metabolism in pregnancy, 287–288, 926
and neural tube defects, 289
placental transfer, 926–927
and pregnancy outcome, 288–289
recommended dose in pregnancy, 287
regulation of, 925
uptake of, 925
zinc metalloproteins, 924
Zinc fingers, 287
Zinc metabolism defects
acrodermatitis enteropathica, 928–929
and birth weight, 289
hyperzincemia, 929
Zonal electrophoresis, protein separation, 47–48

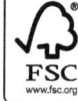

If you have any concerns about our products,
you can contact us on
ProductSafety@springernature.com

In case Publisher is established outside the EU,
the EU authorized representative is:
**Springer Nature Customer Service Center GmbH
Europaplatz 3, 69115 Heidelberg, Germany**

Printed by Libri Plureos GmbH
in Hamburg, Germany